Textbook of Pain

For Churchill Livingstone

Commissioning Editor: Geoff Nuttall
Co-ordinating Editor: Isobel Black
Production Controller: Mark Sanderson
Sales Promotion Executive: Caroline Boyd

Textbook of Pain

Edited by

Patrick D. Wall FRS DM FRCP
Professor Emeritus of Physiology
St Thomas' Hospital
London, UK

Ronald Melzack FRSC PhD
E. P. Taylor Professor of Psychology
McGill University
Montreal, Quebec, Canada

THIRD EDITION

Clinical consultants
John J. Bonica MD DSc DMedSc (Hon) FRCAnaes (Hon)
Harold Merskey DM FRCP FRCPsych FRCP(C) FAPA
Michael J. Cousins MB BS MD FFARACS FFARCS
Howard L. Fields MD PhD
Issy Pilowsky MB ChB MD DPM FRANZCP FRCPsych FRACP FASSA AM

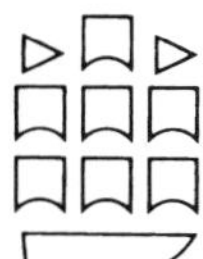

CHURCHILL LIVINGSTONE
EDINBURGH LONDON MADRID MELBOURNE NEW YORK AND TOKYO 1994

CHURCHILL LIVINGSTONE
Medical Division of Longman Group UK Limited

Distributed in the United States of America by Churchill Livingstone Inc., 650 Avenue of the Americas, New York, N.Y. 10011, and by associated companies, branches and representatives throughout the world.

First edition 1984
Second edition 1989
Third edition 1994
Reprinted 1994 (three times)

ISBN 0-443-04757-X

British Library Cataloguing in Publication Data
A catalogue record for this book is available from the British Library.

Library of Congress Cataloging in Publication Data
Textbook of pain/edited by Patrick D. Wall, Ronald Melzack; clinical consultants, John J. Bonica . . . [et al.]. -- 3rd ed.
p. cm.
Includes bibliographical references and index.
ISBN 0-443-04757-X
1. Pain. I. Wall, Patrick D. II. Melzack, Ronald. III. Bonica, John J., 1917-.
[DNLM: 1. Pain. WL 704 T355 1994]
RB127.T45 1994
616'. 0472--dc20
DNLM/DLC
for Library of Congress 93-29873

Printed and bound in Great Britain by
Butler & Tanner Ltd, Frome and London

The publisher's policy is to use **paper manufactured from sustainable forests**

Contributors

Ronald G. Barr MA MDCM FRCP(C)
Professor of Pediatrics and Psychiatry, McGill University-Montreal Children's Hospital Research Institute; Head, Child Development Programme, Montreal Children's Hospital, Montreal, Quebec, Canada

Allan I. Basbaum PhD
Associate Professor, Departments of Anatomy and Physiology and Keck Center for Integrative Neuroscience, University of California, San Francisco, USA

R. W. Beard MD FRCOG
Chairman, Department of Obstetrics and Gynaecology, St Mary's Hospital Medical School, London, UK

Gary J. Bennett PhD
Chief, Neuropathic Pain and Pain Measurement Section, Neurobiology and Anesthesiology Branch, National Institute of Dental Research, National Institutes of Health, Bethesda, Maryland, USA

Charles B. Berde MD PhD
Director, Pain Treatment Service, Children's Hospital, Boston; Associate Professor of Anaesthesia (Pediatrics), Harvard Medical School, Boston, Massachusetts, USA

Jean-François Bernard MD PhD
Chargé de Recherche, Institut National de la Santé et de la Recherche Medicale, Paris, France

Jean-Marie Besson DSc
Director, Unité de Recherches de Physiopharmacologie du Système Nerveux, INSERM, Paris, France

Stuart Bevan PhD
Head, Section of Biology, Sandoz Institute for Medical Research, London, UK

Laurence M. Blendis MD FRCP(C) FRCP
Professor of Medicine, University of Toronto, Toronto General Hospital, Ontario, Canada

Helmut Blumberg PD Dr.med.
Head of Outpatient Unit, Department of Neurosurgery, University of Freiburg, Freiburg, Germany

Jörgen Boivie MD PhD
Senior Consultant, Department of Neurology, Unviersity Hospital, Linköping, Sweden

John J. Bonica MD DSc DMedSc(Hon) FRCAnaes(Hon)
Professor and Chairman Emeritus, Department of Anesthesiology, University of Washington School of Medicine; Director Emeritus, Multidisciplinary Pain Center, University of Washington Medical Center, Seattle, Washington, USA

Anthony J. Bouckoms MB ChB
Associate Professor of Psychiatry, University of Connecticut; Director, Consultation-Liaison Psychiatry, Hartford Hospital, Hartford, Connecticut, USA

William Breitbart MD FAPM
Assistant Attending Psychiatrist, Memorial Sloan-Kettering Cancer Center, New York, New York, USA

Francis M. Bush DMD PhD MS
Professor and Director, TMJ-Orofacial Pain Center, Virginia Commonwealth University School of Dentistry, Richmond, Virginia, USA

Stephen H. Butler MD
Associate Professor, Department of Anesthesiology, University of Washington School of Medicine, Seattle, Washington, USA

James N. Campbell MD
Professor of Neurosurgery, Johns Hopkins University School of Medicine, Baltimore, Maryland, USA

Sharon J. Carmanico MA
Graduate Teaching Fellow, Department of Psychology, Virginia Commonwealth University, Richmond, Virginia, USA

John M. Cavanaugh MD
Research Scientist, Wayne State University, Bioengineering Center, Detroit, Michigan, USA

Nathan I. Cherny MBBS FRACP
Pain Service, Department of Neurology, Memorial Sloan-Kettering Cancer Center, New York, New York, USA; Lecturer in Palliative Medicine, Department of Medicine, Monash University, Melbourne, Australia

Manon Choinière PhD
Research Scholar, Burn Centre, Hôtel-Dieu Hospital of Montreal; Research Assistant Professor, Department of Surgery, Faculty of Medicine, University of Montreal; Research Associate, Department of Anaesthesia, Faculty of Medicine, University of Montreal, Montreal, Quebec, Canada

Michael J. Cousins MB BS MD(Syd) FANZCA FRCA
Head, Department of Anaesthesia and Pain Management, Royal North Shore Hospital, Sydney; Chair of Pain Management, Sydney University, Sydney, Australia

Kenneth D. Craig PhD
Professor of Psychology, University of British Columbia, Vancouver, British Columbia, Canada

Janet Cushnaghan MSc MCSP
Clinical Research Assistant, Rheumatology Unit, University Department of Medicine, Bristol, UK

Marshall Devor PhD
Professor and Chairman, Department of Cell and Animal Biology, Life Sciences Institute, Hebrew University of Jerusalem, Israel

Paul Dieppe BSc MD FRCP
ARC Professor of Rheumatology, University of Bristol, Bristol, UK

Andy Dray PhD
Head, Section of Pharmacology, Sandoz Institute for Medical Research, London, UK

Ronald Dubner DDS PhD
Chief, Neurobiology and Anesthesiology Branch, National Institute of Dental Research, National Institutes of Health, Bethesda, Maryland, USA

David Dubuisson MD PhD
Assistant Professor of Surgery, Harvard Medical School, Boston, Massachusetts, USA

Richard H. T. Edwards PhD FRCP
Head, Department of Medicine, University of Liverpool, Liverpool, UK

Mostafa M. Elhilali MD PhD FRCS(C)
Professor and Chairman, Division of Urology, McGill University; Urologist-in-Chief, Royal Victoria Hospital and Montreal General Hospital, Montreal, Quebec, Canada

Jacqueline A. Ellis
Department of Psychology, Carleton University, Ottawa, Ontario, Canada

Howard L. Fields MD PhD
Professor of Neurology and Physiology, University of California, San Francisco, California, USA

Maria Fitzgerald BA PhD
Reader in Neurobiology, Department of Anatomy and Developmental Biology, University College London, London, UK

Xochitl Gallegos MA PhD RegPsych
Psychologist, Workers' Compensation Board, Richmond, British Columbia, Canada

Kevin F. Gangar MA FRCS MRCOG
Lecturer in Obstetrics and Gynaecology, St Mary's Hospital, London, UK

Richard H. Gracely PhD
Neuropathic Pain and Pain Measurement Section' Neurobiology and Anesthesiology Branch, National Institute of Dental Research, National Institutes of Health, Bethesda, Maryland, USA

D. M. Grennan MD PhD FRCP
Department of Rheumatology, Royal North Shore Hospital, St Leonards, New South Wales, Australia

Gisèle Guilbaud MD DSc
Directeur de Recherches, INSERM, Paris, France

Jan M. Gybels MD PhD
Professor of Neurology and Neurosurgery; Chief of Clinic of the Department of Neurosurgery; Director, Laboratory of Experimental Neurology, KUL University of Leuven, Leuven, Belgium

Scott Haldeman DC MD PhD FRCP(C)
Associate Clinical Professor, Department of Neurology, University of California, Irvine, California, USA

John G. Hannington-Kiff BSc(Hons) MBBS MRCS LRCP FRCA
Director, Pain Relief Centre, Frimley Park Hospital, Surrey, UK

Stephen W. Harkins PhD
Professor, Department of Gerontology, Psychiatry and Psychology, Virginia Commonwealth University, Richmond, Virginia, USA

R. A. Hitchings FRCS FCOphth
Consultant Ophthalmic Surgeon, Moorfields Eye Hospital, London, UK

Constance S. Houck MD
Instructor of Anaesthesia (Pediatrics), Harvard Medical School; Assistant in Anesthesia (Pediatrics), Children's Hospital, Boston; Associate Director, Pain Treatment Service, Boston, Massachusetts, USA

Andrew M. Hoy BSc MBBS MRCP DMRT FRCR
Medical Director, The Princess Alice Hospice, Esher, Surrey; Honorary Consultant in Radiotherapy and Oncology, St Thomas' Hospital, London, UK

Wilfrid Jänig MD
Professor, Physiologisches Institut, Christian-Albrechts Universität, Kiel, Germany

Malcolm I. V. Jayson MD FRCP
Professor of Rheumatology, Rheumatic Diseases Centre, University of Manchester, UK

Mary Ellen Jeans RN PhD
Professor, School of Nursing, McGill University, Montreal, Quebec, Canada

Troels Staehelin Jensen MD PhD
Associate Professor, Department of Neurology, Aarhus University Hospital, Aarhus, Denmark

Barton A. Jessup PhD
Director, Leslie R. Peterson Rehabilitation Centre, Workers' Compensation Board of British Columbia, Richmond, British Columbia; Adjunct Professor, Psychology Department, Simon Fraser University, Burnaby, British Columbia, Canada

Joel Katz PhD CPsych
Research Psychologist, Department of Psychology, and Acute Pain Research Unit, Department of Anaesthesia, The Toronto Hospital; Assistant Professor, Department of Behavioural Science and Department of Anaesthesia, University of Toronto, Toronto, Ontario, Canada

Francis J. Keefe PhD
Associate Professor of Medical Psychology and Psychology-Social and Health Sciences; Director, Pain Management Program, Duke Medical Center, Durham, North Carolina, USA

Jörg-Ulrich Krainick DrMed
Professor of Neurosurgery, St Elisabeth Krankenhaus, Kiel, Germany

Barbara J. de Lateur MD MS
Professor, Department of Rehabilitation Medicine, School of Medicine, University of Washington; Physiatrist-in-Chief, Harborview Medical Center, Seattle, Washington, USA

John C. Lefebvre BA
Department of Psychology, Social and Health Sciences, Duke University, Durham, North Carolina, USA

Sandra M. LeFort PhD(Cand) MN RN
School of Nursing, McGill University, Montreal, Quebec, Canada

Justus F. Lehmann MD
Professor, Department of Rehabilitation Medicine, School of Medicine, University of Washington, Seattle, Washington, USA

Eva Lessard BPT BA BScPT
Assistant Academic Coordinator of Clinical Education-Physiotherapy and Faculty Lecturer, School of Physical and Occupational Therapy, McGill University, Montreal, Quebec, Canada

Jon D. Levine MD PhD
Professor, Departments of Medicine, Anatomy, Neuroscience and Oral Surgery, University of California, San Francisco, California, USA

John D. Loeser MD
Professor, Neurological Surgery and Anesthesiology; Director, Multidisciplinary Pain Center, University of Washington, Seattle, Washington, USA

Caroline F. Lucas BSc BMBCh DCH MRCP DMRT
Consultant in Palliative Medicine, North West Surrey; Deputy Medical Director, The Princess Alice Hospice, Esher, Surrey, UK

Glenn Alan McCain MD FRCP FACP
Associate Director, Pain Therapy Center of Charlotte, Presbyterian Hospital, Charlotte, North Carolina, USA

Conor J. McCarthy MB MRCPI
Research Fellow, Rheumatology Unit, Bristol Royal Infirmary, Bristol, UK

Patricia A. McGrath PhD
Director, Child Health Research Institute; Associate Professor of Paediatrics, University of Western Ontario, London, Ontario, Canada

Patrick J. McGrath PhD
Professor of Psychology, Pediatrics, Psychiatry and Occupational Therapy, Dalhousie University, Halifax, Nova Scotia, Canada

Robert F. McLain MD
Assistant Professor of Orthopaedic Surgery, University of California, Davis, School of Medicine, Sacramento, California, USA

Stephen B. McMahon BSc PhD
Senior Lecturer, Department of Physiology, St Thomas' Hospital Medical School (UMDS), London, UK

H. J. McQuay DM FRCA
Clinical Reader in Pain Relief, University of Oxford, Churchill Hospital, Oxford, UK

Alain Maertens de Noordhout MD PhD
University Department of Neurology, Hopital de la Citadelle, Liège, Belgium

Annika B. Malmberg MScPharm
Doctoral Student, Department of Clinical Pharmacology, Salgrenska University Hospital, Göteborg, Sweden; Department of Anesthesiology, University of California, San Diego, California, USA

Marco Maresca MD
Researcher, Pain Centre, University of Florence, Florence, Italy

Donald Meichenbaum PhD
Professor of Psychology, University of Waterloo, Waterloo, Ontario, Canada

Ronald Melzack FRSC PhD
E. P. Taylor Professor of Psychology, McGill University, Montreal, Quebec, Canada

George Mendelson MB BS MD FRANZCP
Honorary Senior Lecturer, Department of Psychological Medicine, Monash University, Melbourne; Consultant Psychiatrist, Pain Management Centre, Caulfield General Medical Centre, Melbourne, Victoria, Australia

Harold Merskey DM FRCP FRCPsych FRCP(C) FAPA
Professor of Psychiatry, University of Western Ontario; Director of Research, London Psychiatric Hospital, London, Ontario, Canada

Richard A. Meyer MS
Associate Professor of Neurological Surgery and of Biomedical Engineering, School of Medicine; Principal Staff, Applied Physics Laboratory, Johns Hopkins University, Baltimore, Maryland, USA

John Miles MB BCh FRCS
Senior Consultant Neurosurgeon, Walton Centre for Neurology and Neurosurgery, Liverpool; Director, Pain Relief Foundation, UK

K. R. Mills PhD MRCP
University Lecturer in Clinical Neurophysiology, The Radcliffe Infirmary, Oxford; Fellow of Green College, Oxford, UK

Richard C. Monks MDCM FRCP(C)
Associate Professor of Psychiatry, McGill University, Montreal, Quebec, Canada

D. J. Newham MCSP PhD
Professor and Head of Physiotherapy, Biomedical Sciences Division, Kings College, London, UK

Nancy Z. Olson BA MPS
Research Director, Analgesic Development Ltd, New York, New York, USA

Steven D. Passik PhD
Clinical Assistant Attending Psychologist, Memorial Sloan-Kettering Cancer Center; Instructor of Psychology in Psychiatry, Cornell University Medical Center, New York, New York, USA

Shirley Pearce BA(Oxon) MPhil PhD
Senior Lecturer in Psychology, University College London, London, UK

Issy Pilowsky MB ChB MD DPM FRANZCP FRCPsych FRACP FASSA AM
Professor and Head, Department of Psychiatry, University of Adelaide; Head of Psychiatric Service and Consultant to Pain Clinic, Royal Adelaide Hospital, Adelaide, Australia

Charles E. Poletti MD
Associate Visiting Neurosurgeon, Massachusetts General Hospital, Boston, Massachusetts, USA

Russell K. Portenoy MD
Associate Professor of Neurology, Cornell University Medical College, New York; Associate Attending Neurologist, Memorial Sloan-Kettering Cancer Center, New York, New York, USA

Donald D. Price PhD
Professor and Director of Research, Department of Anesthesiology, Medical College of Virginia, Richmond, Virginia, USA

Paolo Procacci MD
Professor of Internal Medicine, Director of the Pain Centre, University of Florence, Florence, Italy

Srinivasa N. Raja MD
Associate Professor and Director, Pain Management Services, Department of Anesthesiology and Critical Care Medicine, Johns Hopkins University School of Medicine, Baltimore, Maryland, USA

H. P. Rang MB BS MA DPhil FRS
Director, Sandoz Institute for Medical Research, London, UK

Peter Rasmussen MD PhD
Professor Emeritus of Neurosurgery, Aarhus University Hospital, Aarhus, Denmark

Patricia C. Rinaldi PhD
Associate Professor, Department of Neurosurgery, University of California, Irvine, California, USA

Barry D. Rosenfeld PhD
Clinical/Ethics Fellow, Memorial Sloan-Kettering Cancer Center, New York, New York, USA

Kathleen M. Rowat BScN MSc PhD
Associate Professor, School of Nursing, McGill University, Montreal, Quebec, Canada

Dame Cicely Saunders OM DBE FRCP
Founder and Chairman, St Christopher's Hospice, London, UK

John W. Scadding BSc MD FRCP
Consultant Neurologist, National Hospital for Neurology and Neurosurgery; Senior Lecturer, Institute of Neurology, London, UK

Jean Schoenen MD Agrégé
Research Director, NFSR, University of Liège, Belgium

Yair Sharav DMD MS
Professor of Oral Medicine, Hebrew University; Chairman, Department of Oral Diagnosis, Oral Medicine and Oral Radiology, School of Dental Medicine, Hebrew University-Hadassah, Jerusalem, Israel

Ralph E. Small PharmD
Professor of Pharmacy and Pharmaceutics; Professor of Medicine, Medical College of Virginia, Virginia Commonwealth University, Richmond, Virginia, USA

M. A. Smith FRCS
Consultant Surgeon, Department of Orthopaedics, St Thomas' Hospital, London, UK

Anders E. Sola MD MS
Clinical Assistant Professor, Department of Anaesthesiology and Pain Service, University of Washington School of Medicine, Seattle, Washington, USA

Erik Spangfort MD PhD
Associate Professor of Orthopaedic Surgery, Karolinska Institute, Stockholm, Sweden

Nicholas P. Spanos PhD
Professor of Psychology and Director of the Laboratory for Experimental Hypnosis, Carleton University, Ottawa, Ontario, Canada

Abraham Sunshine BA MA MD
Professor of Clinical Medicine, NYU Medical Center, New York; Attending Physician, Tisch Hospital, New York; Attending Physician, Bellevue Hospital, New York; President and Medical Director, Analgesic Development Ltd, New York, New York, USA

William H. Sweet MD DSc
Emeritus Professor of Surgery, Harvard Medical School; Senior Neurosurgeon, Massachusetts General Hospital, Boston, Massachusetts, USA

Yetunde Taiwo
Rheumatology Division, University of California, San Francisco, USA

Ronald R. Tasker MD FRCS(C)
Professor, Department of Surgery, University of Toronto; Division of Neurosurgery, The Toronto Hospital, Toronto, Ontario, Canada

U. Thoden MD
Professor and Director, Neurological Department, Klinikum Landshut, Landshut, Germany

John W. Thompson MBBS PhD FRCP
Director of Studies and Honorary Physician, St Oswald's Hospice, Newcastle upon Tyne; Emeritus Consultant Clinical Pharmacologist, Newcastle Health Authority; formerly Director, Pain Relief Clinic, Royal Victoria Infirmary; Emeritus Professor of Pharmacology, University of Newcastle upon Tyne, UK

Todd Troshynski
Department of Anaesthesia, Harvard Medical School and Children's Hospital, Boston, Massachusetts, USA

Dennis C. Turk PhD
Profesor of Psychiatry, Anesthesiology and Behavior Science; Director, Pain Evaluation and Treatment Institute, University of Pittsburgh Medical Center, Pittsburgh, Pennsylvania, USA

Robert G. Twycross MA DM FRCP
Macmillan Clinical Reader in Palliative Medicine, University of Oxford; Consultant Physician, Sir Michael Sobell House, Churchill Hospital, Oxford, UK

Anita M. Unruh BSc(OT) MSW
Assistant Professor of Occupational Therapy, Dalhousie University, Halifax, Nova Scotia, Canada

Patrick D. Wall FRS DM FRCP
Professor Emeritus of Physiology, St Thomas' Hospital, London, UK

James N. Weinstein DO
Endowed Professor, University of Iowa Department of Orthopaedic Surgery; Director, Spine Diagnostic and Treatment Center, Iowa City, Iowa, USA

Matisyohu Weisenberg PhD
Professor, Department of Psychology, Bar-Ilan University, Ramat-Gan, Israel

Patricia A. Wells MSc
Associate Professor, School of Physical and Occupational Therapy, McGill University. Montreal, Quebec, Canada

Howard N. Winfield MD FRCS(C)
Department of Urology, Royal Victoria Hospital, Montreal, Quebec, Canada

Clifford J. Woolf MB BCh PhD MRCP
Professor of Neurobiology, Department of Anatomy and Developmental Biology, University College London, London, UK

C. B. Wynn Parry MBE MA DM FRCP FRCS DPhysMed
Director of Rehabilitation, Royal National Orthopaedic Hospital, London; King Edward VII Hospital, Midhurst, UK

Tony L. Yaksh PhD
Professor and Vice-Chairman for Research, Department of Anesthesiology, University of California, San Diego La Jolla, California, USA

Anthony Yates MD FRCP
Emeritus Consultant Rheumatologist, St Thomas' Hospital, London, UK

Ronald F. Young MD
Clinical Professor of Neurosurgery, University of California, Irvine, California; Director, Neuroscience Center, Northwest Hospital, Seattle, Washington, USA

Massimo Zoppi MD
Associate Professor of Rheumatology, University of Florence, Florence, Italy

Contents

Quick reference index to chapter titles and key words

The comprehensive index is at the back of the book.

Introduction to the edition after this one

Patrick D. Wall

Introductions tend to dullness: lightweight hors d'oeuvres skipped by the hungry reader who goes straight for the meat in the chapters which follow. The authors and editors in this book have done their best to summarise where we stand in an extraordinarily rapidly moving field. What more is there to say? The speed of change surprised the authors of chapters in previous editions who all found radical revision a necessity. New emphasis points have appeared which required new sections and authors. Rather than covert boasting as an introduction, it may be better to point to the remaining overt failures which will hopefully be acceptable topics by the next edition. No one, except dedicated masochists, enjoys self-criticism. Instead we place a taboo on failures and cover them with nonchalant scrapings like cats in the garden, looking innocently around as though nothing was happening. I propose to use this space to list some of those unmentionable topics which, nonetheless, show signs of future solution.

INTRACTABLE PAIN

There are those who have led the hugely successful fight against tractable pains with the remarkably effective use of narcotics in the control of the majority of cancer pains. Their success not only over the pains but also over the resistance of their colleagues naturally encourages them to continue the same logical strategy. For them, there are no intractable pains, only intractable doctors. Good luck to them. In a sense they are correct since it is certainly possible to hold a patient in a continuous state which approaches general anaesthesia. However there is also a group of highly skilled physicians and surgeons who are deeply distressed by their inability to control some types of pain in certain patients, short of demolition.

By far the commonest group of these patients have suffered peripheral or central nerve damage. Amputees, nerve injury cases and the various neuropathies make up the largest numbers. Talking to such chronic cases tells one a lot about their disease and about their doctors. They move on like draught horses, uncomplaining, heads down in continuous driving snow. Not only have their multiple treatments failed but they have suffered the indignity of being told that their pain will go away and/or that it is all in their head. They have learnt that to continue to complain is to alienate and to isolate. These stoical characters plod on, often counted as cured because they no longer go to the doctors or take their ineffective medicine.

Fortunately there is a real future hope for these unfortunates. The basis of that hope can be seen in a number of the basic chapters in this book. Now that most scientists have abandoned the idea of a line labelled pain dedicated hard wired nervous system, we are moving into a period of acceptance of plasticity and control. Mechanisms are being discovered by which nerve impulses drive the nervous system into a continuous state of pain production. More relevant to these deafferentation states is a quite different mechanism. The nervous system is the master of homeostasis. When central nerve cells discover that they are isolated from their normal source of afferent input, they react by increasing their excitability in an attempt to compensate for the decreased input.The mechanisms by which these cells achieve their exalted states of excitability are being unravelled and clearly offer the possibility of new radical therapy. A quite different approach centres around the question of how deafferented cells 'know' that they have lost their input. The answers appear to relate to substances which are transported or fail to be transported. This has led to intense studies on growth factors produced by tissue and distributed by the transport mechanism within nerve fibres. These studies offer considerable hope for the future elimination of intractable pains but single 'magic bullets' are highly unlikely since there are multiple mechanisms by which nerve cells maintain their stable state even when that state is pathological.

CHRONIC PAIN

I have always been puzzled by the meaning of this phrase as distinct from intractable pain. Does it mean that there is a group of patients with tractable pains who never had access to a competent doctor? Does it mean that some patients progress through a treatable stage which is neglected and then later evolve into a perpetual intractable state? Or does it mean that the prolonged experience of pain can itself induce a separate and independent irreversible psychopathological state? As an outsider I read allusions to these questions but find mixed confusing answers.

One aspect of the phrase is clear. There are many conditions which are treatable but only up to a point. Arthritis is the commonest example. Even where hip replacement is followed by pain relief in two-thirds of the patients, the rationale is a complete mystery as described in the chapter here on osteoarthritis (Ch. 20). Medicinal treatments ameliorate the pain in most patients but there are few who can tolerate the long-term side-effects of the full doses which completely relieve the minority. For this reason one particularly welcomes the intense revival of interest in the nature of inflammation as described here. The subject lay fallow for almost a century after Virchow. The discovery of the prostaglandins opened the door to the full power of modern molecular biology. It now becomes apparent that a huge orchestrated cascade of changes form up under the single umbrella word, inflammation. Each offers a future of therapeutic interest but it is highly unlikely that silencing one member of the orchestra will silence the entire cacophonous symphony.

EUTHANASIA

In early 1993, the Dutch parliament was the first in the world to free doctors from prosecution if they deliberately ended a patient's life under precicely defined conditions. These conditions include the formal request of the alert patient, the agreement of two independent doctors and the presence of intolerable pain. I include this matter here not because of the vast philosophical, practical, ethical and religious issues but because it forewarns doctors concerned with pain that they will find themselves in a position where they are required to make legal public pronouncements on the existence of intractable pain in particular cases. In 1992, a British rheumatologist was found guilty and given a suspended sentence for injecting a patient with a lethal dose of potassium chloride. The 71-year-old patient had been in the rheumatologist's care for many years with rheumatic heart disease, widespread progressive rheumatoid arthritis and, eventually, collapsed vertebrae and infection. She legally requested a withdrawal of all therapy except for pain control. Within a few days, she was rapidly deteriorating and was clearly soon to die but intravenous narcotics were failing to control her pain. On the urging of the patient and her two sons, the doctor terminated this shambles. After his conviction, the doctor's case was naturally referred to the General Medical Council who are responsible for the licences permitting medical practice. It was decided that the doctor should not be suspended but a condition was attached that the doctor must take a training course in established pain management clinics. I describe this case because it is clear that doctors concerned with pain will have to become quite clear about their responsibility to individual patients and also their responsibility in training their fellow physicians.

EPIDEMIOLOGY AND WOMEN

The aim of most general surveys is to establish the prevalence of pain. They stress the huge economic loss and the lack of available medical care for social financial reasons. They should also discuss the social reputation of doctors and their treatments and the reasons for the growing popularity of alternative medicine. In a recent anonymous survey of an entire class of clinical medical students, the same array and frequency of painful conditions (headaches, backaches, dysmenorrhea, old injuries, etc.) were reported as in a class of law students. What was surprising was that many of the medical students who obviously were familiar with many pains and with the physicians in their hospital and had access to a free medical service had never consulted a physician. One can only surmise that they must have suffered fear or shame or guilt or disillusionment with medicine along with their pain. Here is pain as a taboo subject operating on the informed individual. It raises the question of the reliability of the sample which haunts every aspect of epidemiology.

The other aim of epidemiology is to establish cause. Tropical medicine contains many spectacular examples where careful study of geographical distribution and particular habits and habitats led directly to the identification of the causative organism. We do not have enough examples of such studies in painful conditions. For example, we still do not know if low back pain is related to the way in which muscles were used before the pain. A recent large study of low back pain among factory workers found it related only to job satisfaction. This conclusion was welcomed by those who suspected workers with back pain as being just general complainers. Others found the conclusion less satisfactory when it was noted that the sample did not include all workers but only those who complained to the company doctor, who might well be a target of the work dissatisfied.

The most obvious unequal distribution of pain occurs between men and women. Apart from the special case of pain from uterus, ovaries, breasts and vulva, there is a marked preponderance of women over men in a surprising number of specific conditions. These include migraine, atypical facial neuralgia, temporomandibular joint syndrome, fibromyalgia, post encephalitic myalgia, irritable bowel syndrome, rheumatoid arthritis and multiple sclerosis. This evident liability of women to a series of very different painful conditions contrasts with the universal longer life expectancy of women. Surely these facts must contain a series of clues worth serious analysis. Instead there is a subculture of flippant and sexist pseudo explanations which permits the imbalance to be ignored. The commonest myth is that women have lower pain thresholds and a high tendency to complain. The experimental literature on this confirms and denies the differences in a horrible confusion. The commonest sources of the confusion are failures to take into account the meaning of the stimulus to the subject, the situation, the familiarity of the stimulus, the sex and social status of the observers, and the presence of peers who set approved standards of response. In a recent example, two male experimenters found no difference between men and women subjected to painful hot and cold stimuli. However, women were significantly more sensitive and less tolerant to electric shocks than men. My reaction is that men are usually familiar with electric shocks in the course of car maintenance and in fixing electrical gadgets while the most liberated of women still tend to show a sensible respect for bare wires. I await a resolution of the question but my reading of the literature is that no difference has been shown between men and women subjected to brief harmless stimuli. I also doubt the other common myth that the difference is explained by hormones. The striking female preponderance of rheumatoid arthritis and multiple sclerosis is hard to attribute to a major endocrine difference. Perhaps the best case can be made for migraine. When this disease is diagnosed by accepted criteria in children, the sex ratio is equal and only diverges in favour of women after the age of 12. It is frequently relieved in pregnancy and after menopause the ratio declines. For the individual with migraine, the nature of an attack is identical in men and women. Rather than considering hormones as the cause of migraine, it would seem that men and women equally may possess a design defect which explodes as migraine but that hormones secondarily may exaggerate the defect. An alternative hypothesis would be that migraine is a partially sex linked genetic disease since migraine appears to run in families. There is more than hormones in the difference of men and women. For example hypermotility which is evident in children is more common in women and is present in a high percentage of chronic low back pain patients.

Where a condition is unevenly spread in the population, hard work on critical classical epidemiology can unravel genetic and environmental factors.

PREVENTION

A surprising number of pain complaints are predictable. The most obvious example is pain after elective surgery. In nerve damage, there is usually a prolonged time course of evolution. In the case of some neuropathies, such as diabetic neuropathy, the condition is usually diagnosed long before it becomes painful. Postherpetic neuralgia slowly emerges from the florid acute state. Even when pain occurs immediately after damage to a single nerve, the pain is at first limited to part of the territory of the damaged nerve and only slowly enlarges over months to incorporate neighbouring tissue. This means that the physician has time to consider preemptive therapies which might influence the subsequent misery.

The possibility of ameliorating postoperative pain is at present under intense investigation. Since my 1988 proposal, there have been 20 clinical investigations, the majority positive but with some clear negative results. The background for these efforts is explained in the chapter by Woolf (Ch. 63), himself a major contributor. Briefly, it has become apparent that the arrival of impulses in unmyelinated afferents in the spinal cord sets off very prolonged increases of excitability of nerve cells involved in provoking pain. The nature and chemistry of the long acting neurotransmitters and of the changes in the cells are becoming defined. These prolonged hyperexcitabilities can be prevented in animals either by preventing the input volley with local anaesthetics or by preventing the cell reaction with narcotics or more recent compounds. The hypothesis for test in man is that the patient in postoperative pain is complaining partly of impulses arriving over his afferents at the time of his complaint and partly of the long lasting increased excitability induced during the surgery. The clinical trials in progress are testing the relative effectiveness of local anaesthesia in the various tissues damaged during surgery and of local or systemic narcotics given before surgery and of various anti-inflammatory agents. These prior therapies are being combined with various regimes of continuous postoperative analgesia. It seems likely that no one approach will eliminate pain but that combinations may lead to marked improvement not only of pain but of lung malfunction and other sequelae.

In cases of nerve damage, the time available for intervention is much longer but the problems are more complex and quite new therapies may be necessary. We do not yet understand the relative role of nerve impulses and of transported substances, both of which may play a part in the subsequent changes in central nerve cells. Furthermore there may be combined multiple sites of pain provoking pathology from the site of axon damage to the dorsal root ganglia and on to the central cells. These are covered in a number of the basic chapters. If the source of prolonged pain is caused by the nerve impulses generated during surgery for elective amputation or during the acute stages of neuropathic damage, they should be controllable by variations of conventional therapy. If however transported chemicals are the major source of the problem, a lot of fundamental research and ingenuity will be required. Promising agents are the growth factors such as NGF and BDNF, some of which can be made in therapeutic quantities by genetic engineering. The situation is exciting and hopeful but since combined therapies are the likely outcome, hard and difficult clinical trials will be necessary. For example, acute herpes zoster, even in the elderly, normally resolves without pain. If it is decided that vigorous therapy of the acute phase will prevent the development of post herpetic neuralgia, as many believe, it will be necessary to treat very large numbers of acute patients in order to prove a significant decrease of the minority who go on to develop post herpetic neuralgia.

PAIN WITHOUT PERIPHERAL PATHOLOGY

Modern medical diagnosis is firmly based on a 200-year development of pathology: initially on morphological pathology and, since the turn of the century, on chemical pathology. Furthermore classical neurology taught that pain was initiated by impulses in nociceptive peripheral afferents activated by a pathological state in peripheral tissue. However, we are faced with a crisis epidemic of painful states where no peripheral pathology has been discovered or, if apparent, is clearly secondary to some primary change. These conditions now include tension headaches, migraine, temporomandibular joint syndrome, trigeminal neuralgia, the majority of neck and back pains, fibromyalgia, interstitial cystitis, etc. To add to this problem, it is emerging that, even where overt pathology is clearly present, the extent of the peripheral pathology is poorly related to the amount of pain. These conditions include myocardial ischaemia, arthritis, amputation, neuropathies, etc. The extent of this paradox is emphasised in the same individual where successive episodes of cardiac ischaemia fail to indicate the amount of ischaemic muscle in terms of pain and even worse where a patient, with two unequally osteoarthritic hips at the same time, complains only of the less damaged hip.

The standard response to this problem is given by the great majority of doctors in two stages. First, the normal sensory nervous system is a reliable accurate witness to currently observable peripheral pathology. Second, any deviation from this first rule is a mental aberration. These two rigid rules are simple restatements of Cartesian dualism. I firmly believe that there are three alternative possibilities. First, I find it unwise arrogance to believe that our present techniques of diagnosis are capable of detecting all relevant forms of peripheral pathology. Second, we are now beginning to realise, as described in the first ten chapters of this book, that a peripheral event may trigger long lasting changes in the spinal cord and brain by way of nerve impulses and transported substances. This means that overt peripheral pathology is capable of initiating a cascade of changes which may persist in the central nervous system long after peripheral pathology has disappeared. Third, we are now beginning to discover that sensory systems are not dedicated and hard wired but are normally held in a stable state by elaborate dynamic control mechanisms. The rules of the physiology of these control mechanisms allows them to be pushed outside their normal working range in which state they will oscillate or fire continuously. As with all known mechanical and biological control systems, it is also possible for them to drift idiopathically into an unstable state as described elsewhere (Wall 1988) as pain control system diseases.

The contemporary custom of assigning the cause of pain either to peripheral pathology or to mental pathology is too simple because it ignores the subtle dynamic properties of peripheral tissue and of the nervous system of which three examples have been given, which could explain many of the diseases listed and which have previously been attributed to mental disorders.

THE SILENCE OF PSYCHIATRISTS AND THE BURDEN ON PSYCHOLOGISTS

The small cohort of distinguished psychiatrists who have contributed to this book would be the first to admit that they are in a minority of psychiatrists. The problem of pain has failed to penetrate mainstream psychiatry. This is particularly unfortunate when the classical psychiatric subject of hysteria has been shifted to the apparently meaningful phrase 'somatisation' and applied to a very large number of pain patients.

The consequence of the progress I have been describing is that a huge burden has been placed on clinical psychologists. The full power of the classical medical profession which is pathologically based has concluded that there is 'nothing wrong' in pathological terms with the great majority of chronic pain patients. Since this conclusion is unquestioned and since the only generally accepted alternative is that there must be a design fault in human mental processing which permits the generation or gross exaggeration of pain states, then the psychologist is presented with compulsory questions. It becomes the duty of the profession of psychologists to find an answer to the questions: 'What is the nature of the personality liable to create pain?' or 'What is the personality liable to exaggerate subclinical disorders into crippling states?' Most would agree that there has been a failure to answer these questions. Is that because psychology is inadequate or because they were asked the wrong questions? Their problem was exaggerated by the obvious necessity to start with people in pain and to look backwards in an attempt to define the personal nature of pain patients. This inevitably required them to attempt to unravel the consequences of pain from the causes of pain. In the course of this exploration, they took on responsibility for effective therapies such as cognitive and behaviour therapies. The rationale for these beneficial treatments is taken either as affecting the premorbid personality or as a pragmatic learning to cope with existing pain. This profession needs and deserves our intellectual support in answering the conundrum we and the patients have set.

Descartes to Eccles and Popper

STIMULUS⟶TRANSMISSION⟶SENSATION⟶PERCEPTION

Fig. I.1 Dualism.

A SCHEME FOR PAIN MECHANISMS

We live in an age where ideas have taken a minor and tertiary role. James Watson proclaims that science progresses from technique to data to ideas, and most agree. I disagree and believe that old accepted ideas form an 'eminence grise' which covertly drives the nature of the questions and the techniques they are meant to solve and therefore the data represent self-fulfilling answers to doubtful questions. For that reason, I believe we need to generate new ideas as possible testable solutions to the hugely puzzling questions about pain. My chapter on the placebo (Ch. 71) responds to such a challenge. The artificial intelligence modellers of the brain produce marvellous new electronics but fail to influence biology. The contemporary philosophers still trudge in the funeral procession of Aristotle (Searle 1992) and fail to incorporate the neurosciences.

Any one thinking inevitably produces a scheme that incorporates cause and effect. Experimentalists also require a plan on which to organize their questions and, usually implicitly, without statement, adopt one of the philosophical schemata. With almost vanishing rarity, the experimental findings have affected philosophical thought. There are four classical plans upon which experiments to discover the nature of sensory processing have been based and I wish to propose a fifth for the future. The four plans are complementary and each has generated undoubted facts that have to be incorporated in any plan.

DUALISM

This scheme remains the main basis on which most neurophysiology is based. It predicts that identifiable components of the brain will reliably detect, transmit and deliver specific fractions of sensation. My own and many others' inability to detect any such system which could be reasonably labelled a pain system led me to reject the plans as a plausible generator of the sensation of pain (Wall & Jones 1992). Light pressure on the skin usually provokes a sensation of touch but in other circumstances, i.e. tenderness, the same stimulus to the same skin is very painful. The plasticity of the relation of the stimulus to response and the changeable properties of the neurons made it impossible to view this sensory system as line-labelled, modality-dedicated and hard-wired as required by the Cartesian system. From Descartes on to Eccles and Popper, an absolute separation is made between the reliable body machinery which produces sensation and the subsequent mental process of perception (Fig. I.1)

HIERARCHIES

250 years after Descartes and contemporary with Darwin, a scheme for subdivision of the nervous system into higher and lower levels was introduced (Fig. I.2) but it has been interpreted incorrectly in three ways. First, it has been taken to mean that 'higher' is the same as 'more recently evolved'. This, in turn, is taken to justify the dogma that the mind is in the cerebral cortex. What a leap (in the dark)! Second, while evolution is much discussed in Hughlings Jackson's writing and while his guru Spencer originated the phrase of 'survival of the fittest', they used evolution to mean something quite different from Darwin. Spencerian evolution relates to thermodynamics and to entropy and is therefore reversible, while Darwinian evolution is not reversible. The third incorrect interpretation was a trivialisation that has dominated the use of the scheme in the 20th century. Three crucial discoveries had been made by Jackson's time: there are anatomically separate inputs and outputs to the central nervous system (Bell and Magendie); there are anatomically separate input and output pathways within the central nervous system (Brown-Séquard); there are reflex pathways within the spinal cord which link inputs and outputs (Sechenow). Even the simplest neurologist and the most sophisticated textbook writer could cope with these three ideas. Therefore they took Jackson and his subtle followers to mean that there was a short reflex pathway which runs through the spinal cord, a longer one through the brain stem and the longest one which looped through the cortex. In fact, Jackson and Sherrington were very specific that there were internal loops connecting the various levels, which makes the pathways far more complex than a simple set of reflex loops. Jackson's greatest neurological discoveries came from epileptics. In the commonest form of grand mal epilepsy, the convulsive phase of the attack is preceded by a sensory aura in which the patient has a sensory experience. This can vary among patients from a simple tingling on one finger to an elaborate scene with people, music and a landscape. These are not hallucinations in the sense that the patient believes they are actually happening. On the contrary, the patient is angry and terrified because he knows he is about to have a fit. Auras are brilliantly described by Dostoyevsky, himself an epileptic, in *The Idiot*. The importance for our present

Hughlings Jackson and Herbert Spencer to Sherrington

STIMULUS ⇆ SPECIFICS ⇆ INTEGRATION ⇆ HIGHER CENTRES

Fig. I.2 Hierarchies.

discussion is that the brain is capable of creating virtual reality without reference to or stimulation from the sensory nervous system. This depends on long-range feedback mechanisms within the central nervous system, which do not reach out into the periphery.

CYBERNETICS

Claude Bernard was concerned with the maintenance of a stable internal environment. As he and those who followed studied how stability was achieved, they began to realize that a series of components must exist. This was formalized by Norbert Wiener as cybernetics (Fig. I.3). First there had to be an internal standard which was compared with the actual situation. A comparator measured the mismatch between a sensory input which signalled the actual situation and an internal standard which signalled the ideal situation. This mismatch signal was amplified and triggered a series of graded output patterns which, in turn, fed back onto the actual input to reverse its trend and thereby to reduce the mismatch signal. Physiologists have identified many of the components. In cooling, for example, the dropping temperature is the stimulus which deviates from the standard. The mismatch difference signal triggers an orchestrated series of output patterns as the difference grows – vasoconstriction, piloerection, release of thyroid hormone, insulin and adrenaline to increase metabolism, shivering, rigors.

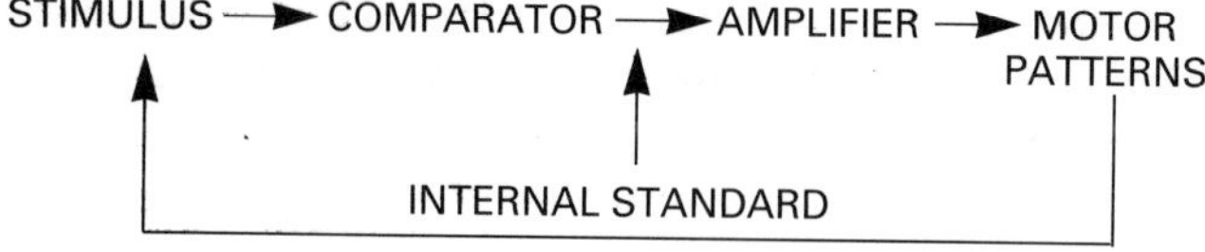

Fig. I.3 Cybernetics.

ETHOLOGY

This spectacular development of old-fashioned nature study defined a series of stages between stimulus and response (Fig. I.4). The sensory input is used twice, to decide first what to do and then how to do it. In the initial stage, a combination of sensory signals from outside and from inside assigns a priority to one feature in the behavioural repertoire. This releases the motor pattern which is most relevant to the biological situation. The successful achievement of this motor pattern requires a second consultation with the sensory system. Where is the enemy, mate, nest or chick and is it being approached on the optimal course? Experimental studies have been very successful in identifying the sensory patterns and the motor pattern generators but less so the priority-assignment mechanism.

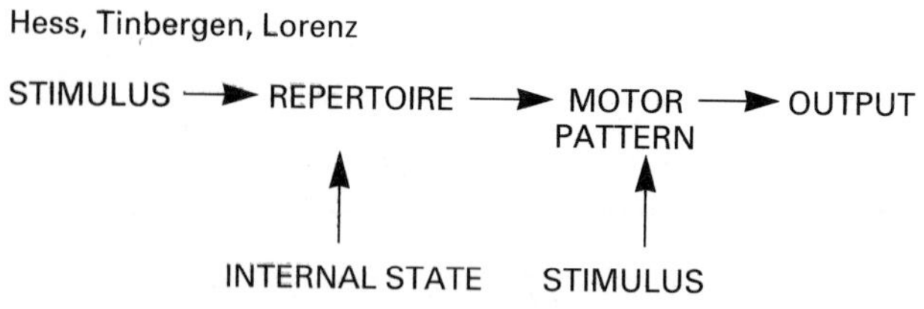

Hess, Tinbergen, Lorenz

STIMULUS → REPERTOIRE → MOTOR PATTERN → OUTPUT

INTERNAL STATE (→ REPERTOIRE) STIMULUS (→ MOTOR PATTERN)

Fig. I.4 Ethology.

REALITY–VIRTUAL REALITY

I wish to propose here that advanced brains contain both the Jackson version of a hierarchical system and the Tinbergen-Lorenz version of an ethological system. The ethological component sequence of repertoire-priority-motor pattern contains an inherent fraction of species-specific components heavily modified by experience and learning. This machinery is entirely responsible for the domestic and skilled actions of everyday life and does not involve consciousness. However, on occasions, a combination of internal and external stimuli occur for which there is no biologically appropriate response available in the repertoire-priority-motor pattern system. When this mismatch occurs, an attentional switch diverts the input into a quite different system. Before going further I wish to give two illustrative examples.

The phantom limb has been a challenging paradox for philosophers and neurologists. Descartes was aware that he had set a trap for himself in the very rigidity of his proposed sensory mechanism. He writes in *Meditations on first philosophy* (1641):

> It is manifest that notwithstanding the sovereign goodness of God, the nature of man, in so far as it is a composite of mind and body, must sometimes be at fault and deceptive. For should some cause, not in the foot but in another part of the nerves that extend from the foot to the brain, or even in the brain itself, give rise to the motion ordinarily excited when the foot is injuriously affected, pain will be felt just as though it were in the foot and thus naturally the sense will be deceived: for since the same motion in the brain cannot but give rise in the mind always to the same sensation and since this sensation is much more frequently due to a cause that is injurious to the foot than by one acting in another quarter, it is reasonable that it should convey to the mind pain as in the foot.

The brilliance of Descartes here introduces the idea of the false signal but at the same time has to define the mind as a passive slave of the sensory apparatus. Three centuries later, Bromage & Melzack (1974) considered the results of adding local anaesthetic to nerves supplying a body part. Far from producing signals, these agents block the normal trickle of signals which reaches the brain. A startling phantom phenomenon appears in the area of anaesthesia. This phantom is not an imitation of the real limb, it is more real, swollen and attention grabbing. In the scheme under discussion, the repertoire-priority component of the brain is presented with a sensory input which is simply not in the repertoire. In that situation, the attention switch operates to bring into action the sensation perception mechanism, which, in the absence of a sensory input, creates a virtual limb. Seeking a confirmatory sensory input, the patient visually explores the limb and palpates it and the phantom disappears.

The second example comes from the work of Dubner et al (1981), Bushnell et al (1984) and Duncan et al (1987), which is so startling and novel that it has yet to intrude on theory. They recorded in monkeys from first-order central cells which receive information from nerve fibres from the skin. By all classical criteria, these cells fulfil perfectly the requirements of Cartesian sensory transmission cells i.e their discharge rigidly and reliably reflects a particular stimulus applied to a unique area of skin. The cells signal in a lawful fashion the location, intensity and nature of the stimulus with such reliability that the signal was the same in awake or anaesthetized monkeys. These workers then trained the animals to use a stimulus in a discrimination task in which the correct response was rewarded. The form of the trial was that the animal was first given a warning signal that the trial was about to begin, then the stimulus was applied and then the animal was rewarded with a drink of orange juice if it reached out and pushed a button if, and only if, the stimulus was of a particular intensity. When the training began, of course, the cell responded only to the skin stimulus and not to the warning signal or any of the other events. However, when the animal had successfully solved the problem and was fully trained, many cells produced a brief burst of activity after the warning signal. This novel period of cell discharge mimicked the discharge of the cell which always occurred after the stimulus to be discriminated was presented. This means that the trained brain had created a virtual input which ran over the same pathway as the input provoked by the real stimulus. A precise model of the expected input precedes the input actually provoked by the expected stimulus. The literature contains several examples of this creation of inputs without stimuli in classical and operant conditioning.

Returning to the scheme, it proposes that the brain is capable of generating a virtual reality (Fig. I.5). It is further proposed that this experimental theatre is brought into action only when the repertoire–priority system fails to provide a biologically appropriate motor pattern. The Jacksonian reality–virtual reality experimental theatre is simultaneously author, director, stage, actors and audience. In the situation of a fully mastered discriminant task, the expectations of the stage play precisely mimic reality. That is pantomime. In chronic pain, no amount of rewriting or changing of cast and scenery provides a resolution to match and cancel reality. That is tragedy.

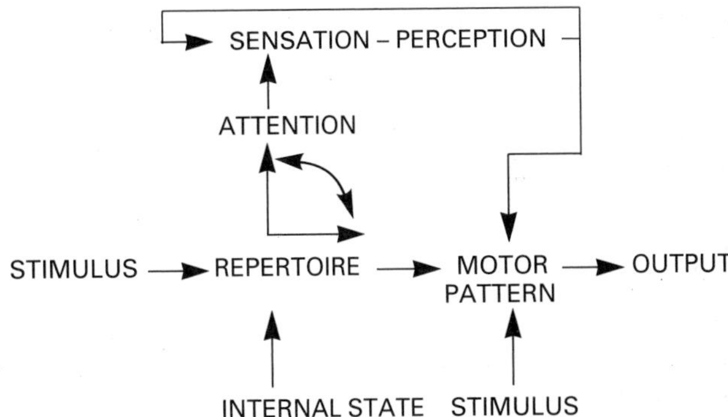

Fig. I.5 Reality–virtual reality.

In summary, it is proposed that there are two alternate brain mechanisms superimposed on each other and which can use some of the same neural elements. They do not operate simultaneously. The 'reality' circuit which does not involve conscious perception operates when one form of behaviour has been assigned a high priority. This is the situation during emergency analgesia when a reaction such as escape has been assigned a higher biological priority than attending to pain. This circuit is also in action during the placebo reaction when expectation has assigned pain a low priority because it is inappropriate. The other circuit, the 'virtual reality' circuit operates and continuously re-examines the input as modified by the possible repertoire of alternate behaviours when the normal circuitry can assign no evident priority to the repertoire of behaviours which would remove the stimulus. I proposed that the operation of this circuit which is consciousness is in action during perceived pain.

REFERENCES

Bromage P R, Melzack R 1974 Phantom limbs and the body schema. Canadian Anaesthetists Society Journal 21: 267–274

Bushnell M C, Duncan G H, Dubner R, He L F 1984 Activity of trigeminothalamic neurons in monkey trained in a thermal discrimination task. Journal of Neurophysiology 52: 170–187

Descartes R 1641 Meditation on a first philosophy. Paris

Dubner R, Hoffman D S, Hayes R L 1981 Task related responses and their functional role. Journal of Neurophysiology 46: 444–464

Duncan G H, Bushnell M C, Bates R, Dubner R 1987 Task related responses of monkey medullary dorsal horn neurones. Journal of Neurophysiology 57: 289–310

Searle J 1992 The rediscovery of the mind. MIT Press, Cambridge, Mass.

Wall P D 1988 Stability and instability of central pain mechanisms. The John J. Bonica Distinguished Lecture. In: Dubner R, Gebhart G F, Bond M R (eds) Pain research and clinical management, vol. 3. Proceedings of the Vth World Congress on Pain, Hamburg 2–7 August 1987. Elsevier, Amsterdam

Wall P D, Jones M 1992 Defeating pain. Plenum Press, New York

Wall P D, Safran J W 1986 Artefactual intelligence. In: Rose S, Appignanesi L (eds) Science and beyond. Blackwell, Oxford, p 115–130

SECTION 1

Basic aspects

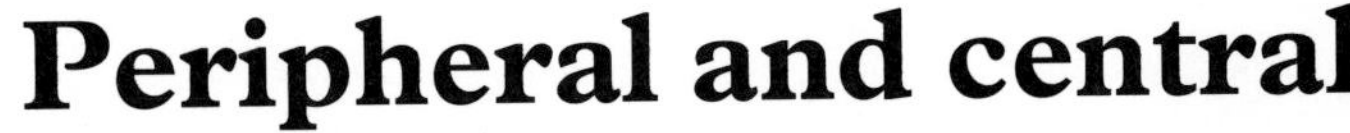

Peripheral and central

1. Peripheral neural mechanisms of nociception

Richard A. Meyer, James N. Campbell and Srinivasa N. Raja

One of the vital functions of the nervous system is to provide information about the occurrence or threat of injury. The sensation of pain, by its inherent aversive nature, contributes to this function. In this chapter, we shall consider the peripheral neural apparatus that responds to noxious (injurious or potentially injurious) stimuli and thus provides a signal to alert the organism of potential injury. This apparatus must respond to the multiple energy forms that produce injury (such as heat, mechanical and chemical stimuli) and provide information to the central nervous system regarding the location and intensity of noxious stimuli.

We consider first the nociceptive apparatus associated with skin, since skin has been the most extensively studied tissue. Investigators have studied cutaneous sensibility by recording from single nerve fibres in different species, including man. Stimuli are applied to the receptive field (i.e., area of the tissue responsive to the applied stimulus) of single fibres, and the characteristics of the neural response are noted. This analysis is particularly powerful when combined with correlative psychophysical studies, in which identical stimuli are rated by human subjects.

Highly specialized sensory fibres, alone or in concert with other specialized fibres, provide information to the central nervous system not only about the environment, but also about the state of the organism itself. In the case of the sensory capacity of the skin, cutaneous stimuli may evoke a sense of cooling, warmth, or touch. Accordingly, there are sensory fibres that are selectively sensitive to these stimuli. Warm fibres, which are predominantly unmyelinated fibres, are exquisitely sensitive to gentle warming of their punctate receptive fields. These fibres have been shown to signal exclusively the quality and intensity of warmth sensation (Konietzny & Hensel 1975; Darian-Smith et al 1979a, 1979b; Johnson et al 1979). Similar types of studies have shown that a subpopulation of the thinly myelinated, Aδ-fibres responds selectively to gentle cooling stimuli and encodes the sense of cooling (Darian-Smith et al 1973). For the sense of touch there are different classes of mechanoreceptive afferent fibres that are exquisitely sensitive to deformations of the skin. These low-threshold mechanoreceptors encode such features as texture and shape.

The remaining class of cutaneous receptors are distinguished by a relatively high threshold to the adequate stimulus, be it heat, mechanical, or cooling stimuli. Because these receptors respond preferentially to noxious stimuli, they are termed nociceptors (Sherrington 1906). Nociceptors are sub-classified with respect to three criteria:

1. unmyelinated (C-fibre) versus myelinated (A-fibre) parent nerve fibre
2. modalities of stimulation that evoke a response
3. response characteristics.

We will consider the properties of cutaneous nociceptors, and then review how their function is thought to relate to the sensation of pain.

Once tissue is damaged, a cascade of events results in enhanced pain to natural stimuli, termed hyperalgesia. A corresponding increase in the responsiveness of nociceptors, called sensitization, occurs. The characteristics of hyperalgesia and its neurophysiological counterpart, sensitization, will be discussed in a later section.

PROPERTIES OF NOCICEPTORS IN UNINJURED SKIN

The receptive field of a nociceptor is often first localized by use of mechanical stimuli. Various other stimulus modalities are then applied to this receptive field. Unlike other types of cutaneous receptors, many nociceptors respond to multiple stimulus modalities, including mechanical, heat, cold, and chemical stimuli (Bessou & Perl 1969; Szolcsányi 1980; Van Hees & Gybels 1981; Beck & Handwerker 1974). Hence, the term polymodal nociceptor is often appropriate. However, in most systematic studies of nociceptors, only heat and mechanical stimuli have been used. Therefore the nomenclature of CMH and AMH has been adopted to refer to C-fibre mechano-heat sensitive nociceptors and A-fibre mechano-heat sensitive nociceptors, respectively.

C-FIBRE MECHANO-HEAT NOCICEPTORS (CMHs)

The heat threshold of CMHs in primates is typically greater than 38°C, but less than 50°C. The response of a typical CMH to a random sequence of heat stimuli ranging from 41–49°C is shown in Figure 1.1. It can be seen that the response increases monotonically with stimulus intensity over this temperature range which encompasses the pain threshold in humans.

The response of CMHs is strongly influenced by the stimulus history. Both suppression and sensitization are observed. One example of suppression is the observation that the response to the second of two identical heat stimuli is less than the response to the first stimulus (Fig. 1.2). This suppression is dependent on the time between stimuli, with full recovery taking more than 10 minutes (Tillman 1992). A similar reduction in the pain intensity of repeated heat stimuli is observed in human subjects (LaMotte & Campbell 1978). Suppression is also apparent in Figure 1.1B where the response to a given stimulus varied inversely with the intensity of the preceding stimulus. The enhanced response, or sensitization, that may occur in CMHs after tissue injury will be described below in the section on hyperalgesia.

Low-threshold C-fibre mechanoreceptors which do not respond to heat have been described in cat (Bessou & Perl 1969), rabbit (Shea & Perl 1985a), primate (Kumazawa & Perl 1977) and man (Nordin 1990). The role of these fibres in sensation is unclear.

A-FIBRE MECHANO-HEAT NOCICEPTORS (AMHs)

Two types of AMHs have been identified (Dubner et al 1977; Campbell & Meyer 1986). Type I AMHs have very high heat thresholds under normal circumstances and, because of this, are referred to as high threshold mechanoreceptors (HTMs) by many investigators (Burgess & Perl 1967; Burgess et al 1968; Perl 1968). Some have thresholds below 50°C, though the majority have thresholds of 53°C or greater. However, most can be shown to respond to heat if the heat stimulus is of sufficient intensity and duration. Type I AMHs are particularly prevalent on the glabrous skin of the hand in monkey (Campbell et al 1979) and have also been described in cat and rabbit (Fitzgerald & Lynn 1977; Roberts & Elardo 1985a). The mean conduction velocity for Type I AMHs in monkey is 30 m/s and extends as high as 55 m/s. Thus, by conduction velocity criteria, Type I AMHs fall into a category between that of Aδ- and Aβ-fibres.

Type II AMHs have been most extensively studied on the monkey face (Dubner et al 1977) but are known to exist in other hairy skin areas. Notably they have *not* been found on the glabrous skin of the hand. The major distinguishing feature of Type II AMHs is that their threshold to

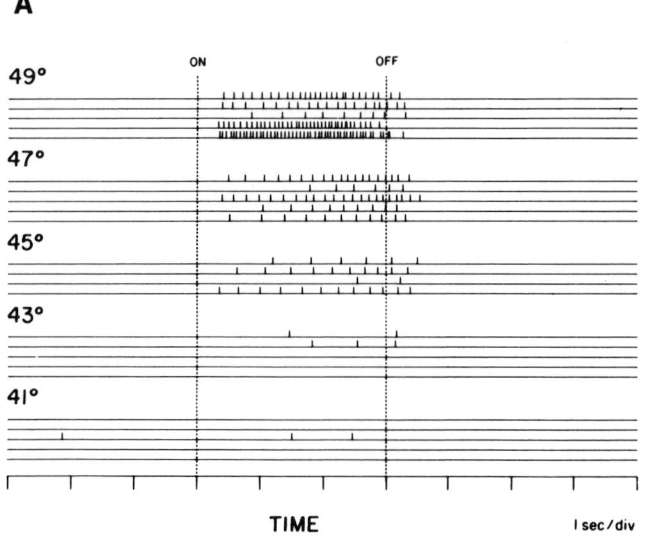

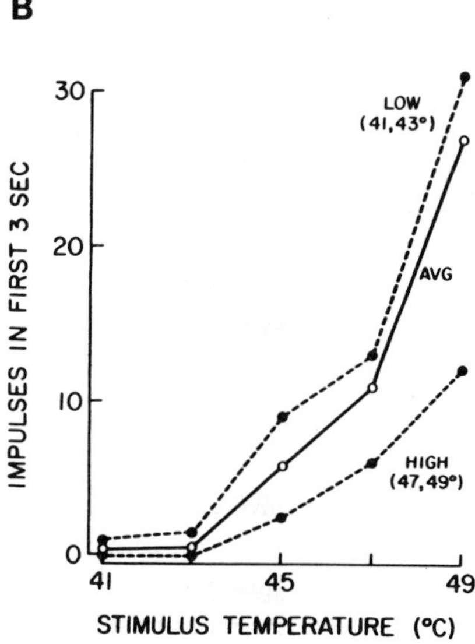

Fig. 1.1 Response of a typical C-fibre nociceptor to heat stimuli. 3 s duration heat stimuli, ranging from 41–49°C, were presented at 25 s interstimulus intervals to the glabrous skin of the monkey hand. Each stimulus occurred with equal frequency and was preceded by every other stimulus an equal number of times. Within these constraints, the order of stimulus presentation was randomized. Base temperature was 38°C. **A** Replicas of the response. Each horizontal line corresponds to one trial, and the trials are grouped by stimulus temperature. Each vertical tick corresponds to an action potential. **B** Stimulus-response function for this nociceptor. The solid line represents the total response to a given temperature averaged across all presentations. The dotted lines represent the stimulus-response functions obtained when the preceding temperature was of low (41 and 43°C) or high (47 and 49°C) intensity. (From LaMotte & Campbell 1978 with permission.)

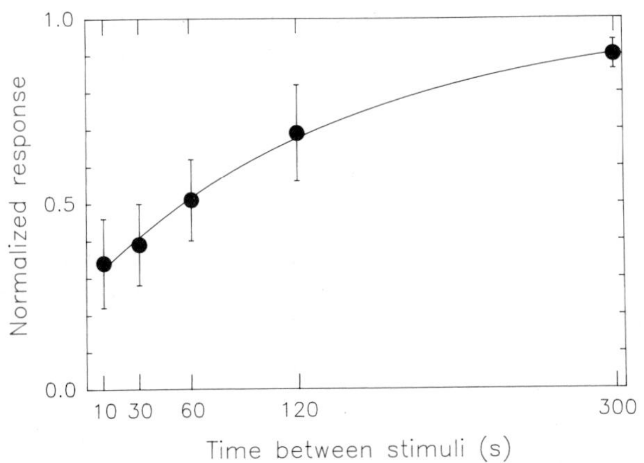

Fig. 1.2 Suppression of response of C-fibre nociceptors to repeated heat stimuli depends on time interval between stimuli. The response to the second stimulus is expressed as a fraction of the response to the first stimulus. Suppression was greatest at the short interstimulus intervals. (n = 13, mean ± S.D., adapted from Tillman 1992 with permission.)

heat is substantially lower than that of Type I AMHs. The mean conduction velocity, 15 m/s, is also lower than that of Type I AMHs. As will be noted later, Type II AMHs are thought to signal first pain sensation.

Examples of the differing responses of the two types of AMHs to a heat stimulus are shown in Figure 1.3. The receptor utilization time (time between stimulus onset and activation of the receptor) for Type II AMHs is much shorter than for Type I AMHs. In addition, Type II AMHs exhibit a burst of activity at the onset of a stepped heat stimulus, whereas the response of Type I AMHs does not adapt quickly (Treede et al 1991).

MECHANICALLY INSENSITIVE AFFERENTS

Not all cutaneous nociceptors respond to mechanical stimuli. Recent evidence suggests that about half of the Aδ-fibre nociceptors and 30% of the C-fibre nociceptors either have very high mechanical thresholds (> 6 bar = 600 kPa = 60 g/mm²) or are unresponsive to mechanical stimuli (Meyer et al 1991; Handwerker et al 1991b; Kress et al 1992). These nociceptors are referred to as mechanically insensitive afferents (MIAs). Similar afferent fibres have been reported in knee joint (Schaible & Schmidt 1985), viscera (Häbler et al 1988) and cornea (Tanelian 1991).

As shown in Figure 1.4, some cutaneous MIAs may be chemospecific receptors (LaMotte et al 1987; Meyer et al 1988; Meyer et al 1991; Kress et al 1992; Davis et al 1993). Others respond to intense cold or heat stimuli (LaMotte & Thalhammer 1982; Meyer et al 1991; Kress et al 1992). In the knee joint, MIAs become responsive to mechanical stimuli after inflammation (Grigg et al 1986). Similar sensitization to mechanical stimuli after administration of inflammatory agents or after cutaneous injury

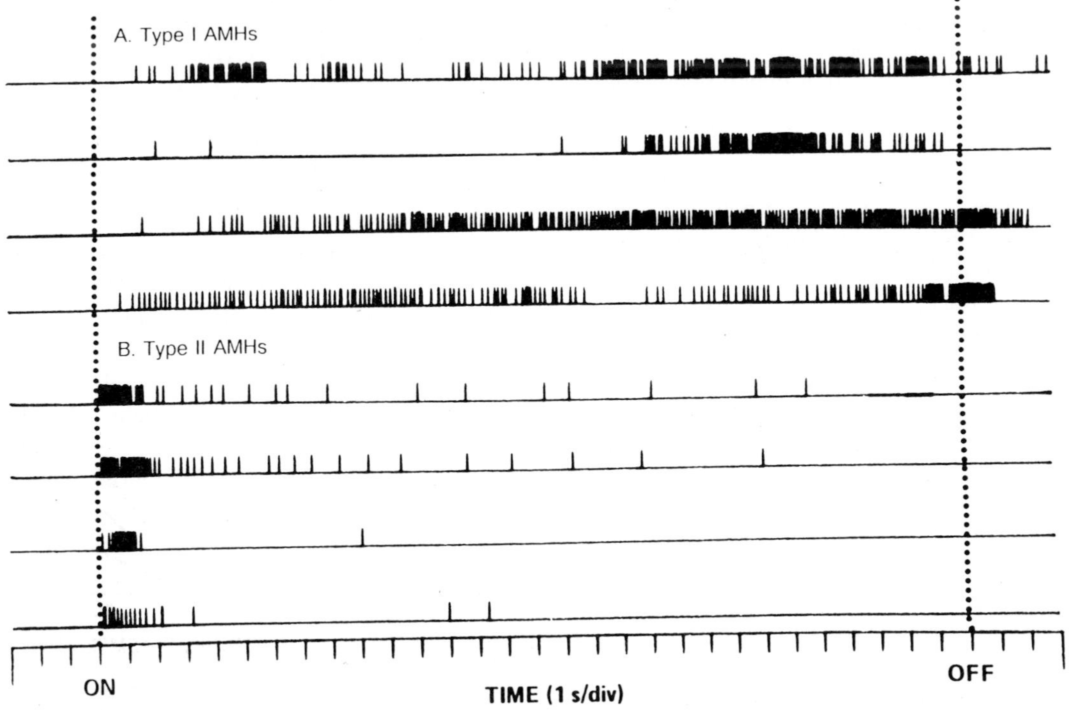

Fig. 1.3 Responses of four Type I and four Type II AMHs to a stepped heat stimulus (53°C, 30 s). **A** The Type I AMHs have a longer receptor utilization time with a peak discharge frequency near the end of the stimulus. **B** The Type II AMHs have a short receptor utilization time and show a quickly adapting response to stepped heat stimuli. The Type I AMHs play an important role in hyperalgesia to heat, while the Type II AMHs are likely candidates for signalling first pain sensation.

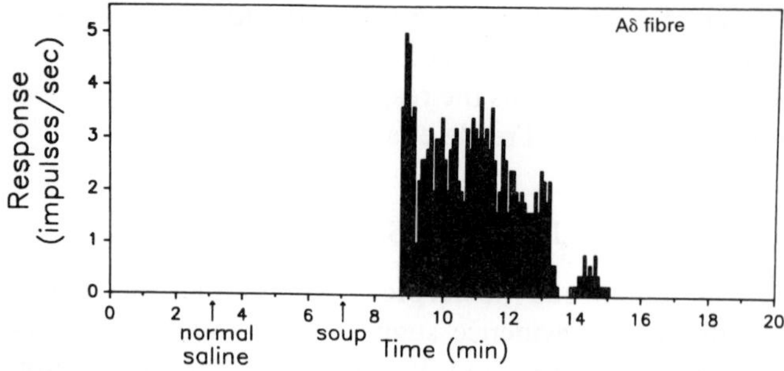

Fig. 1.4 Response of an Aδ-fibre nociceptor to injection of a mixture of inflammatory mediators. The nociceptor was a mechanically-insensitive afferent (MIA) that did not respond to heat or mechanical stimuli or to injections of saline. This MIA responded vigorously to a 10 μl intradermal injection of a chemical soup containing 10 nmol bradykinin, 0.3 nmol prostaglandin E_1, 30 nmol serotonin, and 30 nmol histamine (bin size = 5 s). (From Meyer et al 1991 with permission.)

has been observed in cutaneous MIAs (Meyer et al 1991; Handwerker et al 1991b; Davis et al 1993).

COUPLING BETWEEN C-FIBRE NOCICEPTORS

Coupling of action potential activity occurs between C-fibres in the normal peripheral nerve of monkey (Meyer et al 1985b). Coupling frequently involves conventional CMHs. The coupling is eliminated by injection of small amounts of local anaesthetic at the receptive field of the CMH, indicating that the site of coupling is near the receptor. Collision studies indicate that the coupling is bidirectional. Sympathetic fibres appear not to be involved in this coupling as demonstrated by experiments where the sympathetic chain is stimulated or ablated (Meyer & Campbell 1987). The role of coupling is unknown, but may relate to the flare response or other efferent functions of nociceptors (see below). Coupling between peripheral nerve fibres is also one of the pathological changes associated with nerve injury (Wall & Gutnick 1974; Seltzer & Devor 1979; Blumberg & Jänig 1982; Meyer et al 1985c). In this case, coupling occurs at the site of axotomy.

ANATOMICAL STUDIES OF CUTANEOUS NOCICEPTORS

The terminals of Type I AMHs have been traced anatomically into the skin of cat (Kruger et al 1981). Thinly myelinated axons are found in regions identified as having punctate sensitivity to mechanical stimuli. At the papillary layer, the myelin sheath is lost. Within the epidermal basal lamina, the axons lose association with Schwann cell processes and are surrounded by keratinocytes. Both clear round and large dense core vesicles are noted at the epidermal penetration site. The vesicles are similar morphologically to vesicles present in other cells involved in hormone and neurotransmitter secretion. C-fibre nociceptors are also thought to contain vesicles in their terminals. It is presumed that these vesicles secrete their contents into the tissues upon activation (see efferent role of nociceptors below).

DEVELOPMENT OF NOCICEPTORS

Sensory neurons in the dorsal root ganglia of rat in utero and shortly after birth depend on nerve growth factor (NGF) for survival. In adults, this dependence on NGF disappears. Recent data support the contention that Aδ-nociceptors (Ritter et al 1991; Lewin et al 1992) and C-fibre nociceptors (Mendell & Lewin 1992) in the postnatal period depend on the presence of NGF for development. NGF is abundant in the epidermis and may provide an important neurotrophic factor for nociceptors. During a critical postnatal period, treatment with anti-NGF leads Aδ-fibres to develop into low-threshold mechanoreceptors instead of nociceptors. This suggests that NGF is necessary for development of nociceptors and that, in the absence of NGF, what would be nociceptors develop instead into mechanoreceptors. Cell death as a result of anti-NGF treatment in this critical period was not evident. Intracellular recordings from the dorsal root ganglia in anti-NGF treatment animals reveal reduced numbers of cells with action potential characteristics of Aδ-nociceptors. The influence of neurotrophic factors on nociceptors in tissues other than skin is not yet known.

THE RELATIONSHIP OF NOCICEPTOR ACTIVITY TO PAIN SENSATIONS

CMHs SIGNAL PAIN FROM HEAT STIMULI TO GLABROUS SKIN

We now examine the evidence that CMHs signal pain. In normal glabrous skin of the hand, two types of fibres, the CMH nociceptors (not AMHs) and the warm fibres, respond to heat stimuli at temperatures near the pain threshold in humans (i.e. around 45°C). It is of interest, therefore, to compare how warm fibres and CMHs encode information about noxious heat stimuli. Warm fibres respond vigorously to gentle warming of the skin (Konietzny & Hensel 1975; Darian-Smith et al 1979b). An example of the response of a warm fibre to stimuli in the noxious heat range is shown in Figure 1.5. The response of warm fibres is not monotonic over this temperature range. In the example shown in Figure 1.5, the total evoked response at 49°C was less than that at 45°C. Psychophysical studies done in man demonstrate that pain increases monotonically with stimulus intensities between 40 and 50°C (LaMotte & Campbell 1978). Because the responses of CMHs increase monotonically over this temperature range (Fig. 1.1) and the responses of warm fibres do not (Fig. 1.5), it follows that CMHs signal the

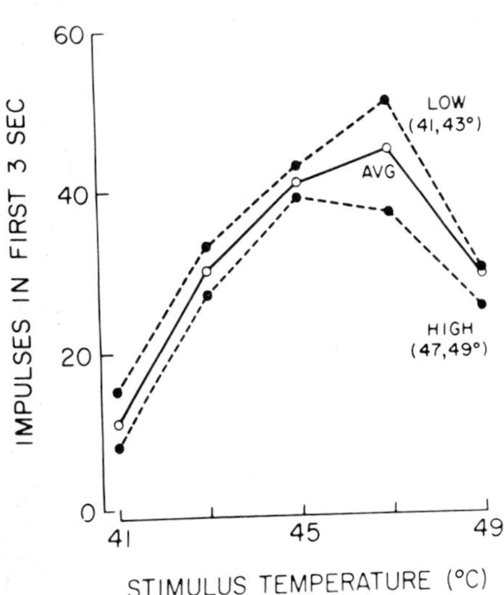

Fig. 1.5 Non-monotonic response of a warm fibre to heat stimuli in the noxious range. Stimulus presentation paradigm same as for Figure 1.1. The total response during the 3 s stimulus interval is plotted as a function of stimulus temperature. (From LaMotte & Campbell 1978 with permission.)

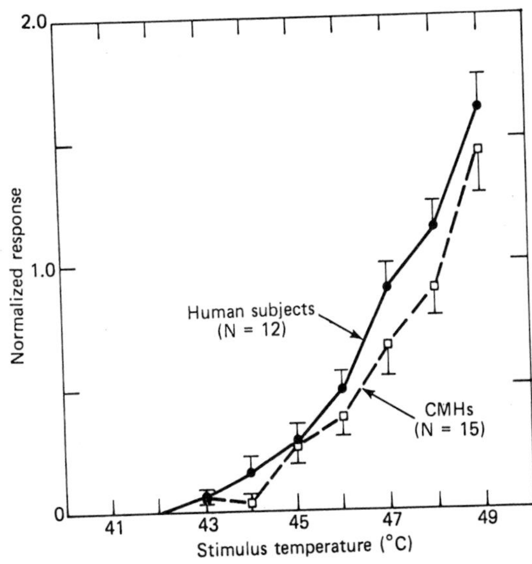

Fig. 1.6 Correlation of response of C-fibre nociceptors in monkey with pain ratings of human subjects. The close match between the curves supports a role of C-fibre nociceptors in heat pain sensation from the glabrous skin. The first stimulus of the heat sequence was always 45°C. The remaining nine stimuli ranged from 41–49°C in 1°C increments and were presented in random order. Human judgments of pain were measured with a magnitude-estimation technique: subjects assigned an arbitrary number (the modulus) to the magnitude of pain evoked by the first 45°C stimulus and judged the painfulness of all subsequent stimuli as a ratio of this modulus. The response to a given stimulus was normalized by dividing by the modulus for each human subject or by the average response to the first 45°C stimulus for the CMHs. (From Meyer & Campbell 1981b with permission.)

sensation of heat pain to the glabrous skin of the hand (LaMotte & Campbell 1978).

Other evidence in support of a role of CMHs in pain sensation includes:

1. Human judgments of pain to stimuli over the range of 41–49°C correlate well with the activity of CMH nociceptors over this range (Fig. 1.6, Meyer & Campbell 1981b).
2. Selective A-fibre ischaemic blocks or C-fibre (local anaesthetic) blocks indicate that C-fibre function is necessary for thermal pain perception near the pain threshold (Sinclair & Hinshaw 1950; Torebjörk & Hallin 1973).
3. Stimulus interaction effects observed in psychophysical experiments (LaMotte & Campbell 1978) are also observed in recordings from CMHs (Figs 1.1 and 1.2).
4. The latency to pain sensation on glabrous skin following stepped temperature changes is long and consistent with input from CMHs (Campbell & LaMotte 1983).
5. In patients with congenital insensitivity to pain, microscopic examination of the peripheral nerves indicates absence of C-fibres (Bischoff 1979).

HUMAN MICRONEUROGRAPHIC RECORDINGS

Microneurography has been used to record from nociceptive afferents in awake humans. The technique involves percutaneous insertion of a microelectrode into fascicles of nerves such as the superficial radial nerve at the wrist. These studies have demonstrated that the properties of nociceptors in man and monkey are similar (Hagbarth & Vallbo 1967; Ochoa & Torebjörk 1983). Microneurographic studies allow direct correlations between the discharges of CMHs and the reported sensations of the subject. In some experiments, the microelectrode is also used to stimulate the identified, single nerve fibre in awake human subjects, evoking specific sensations. With stimulation of CMHs, subjects report pain (or sometimes itch, see below). Some argue that the size of the stimulating electrode is too large to stimulate individual units (Wall & McMahon 1985). Given this reservation the following evidence from microneurographic studies in humans points to the capacity of activity in CMHs to evoke pain:

1. Intraneural electrical stimulation of presumed single identified CMHs in humans elicits pain (Torebjörk & Ochoa 1980).
2. The heat threshold for activation of CMHs recorded in awake humans is just below the pain threshold (Gybels et al 1979; Van Hees & Gybels 1981).
3. A linear relationship exists between responses of CMHs recorded in awake humans and ratings of pain over the temperature range 39–51°C (Torebjörk et al 1984).

AMHs AND PAIN

As shown in Figure 1.7, a long duration heat stimulus applied to the glabrous skin of the hand in human subjects evokes substantial pain for the duration of the stimulus.

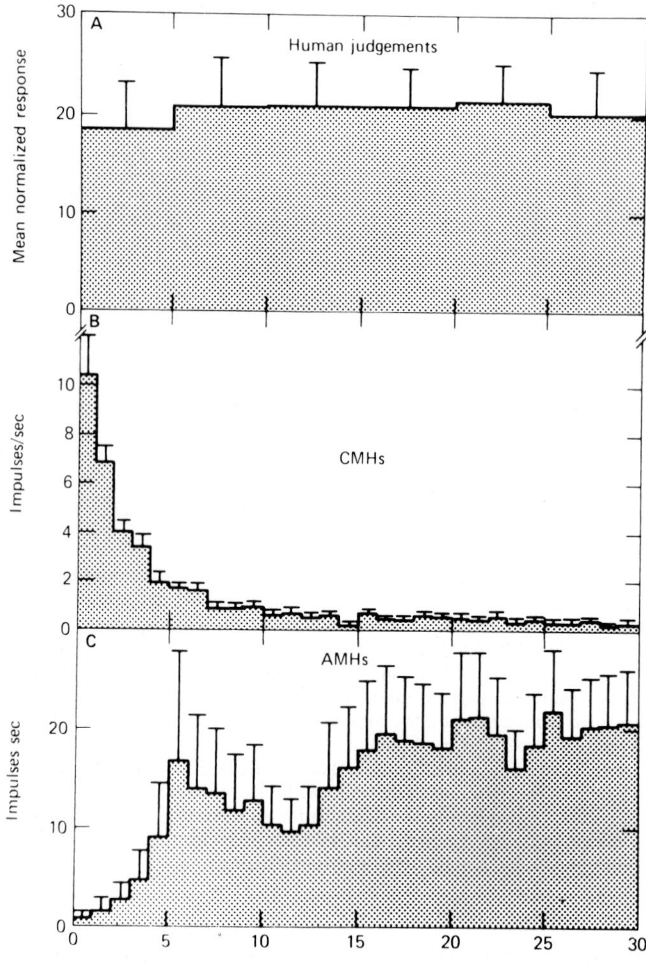

Fig. 1.7 Ratings of pain by human subjects during a long-duration, intense heat stimulus (53°C, 30 s) applied to the glabrous hand are compared with responses of CMHs and Type I AMHs. **A** Pain was intense throughout the stimulus (n = 8). **B** The brisk response of the CMHs at the beginning of the stimulus changed to a low rate of discharge after 5 s (n =15). **C** The response of the Type I AMHs increased during the first 5 s and remained high throughout the stimulus (n = 14). (From Meyer & Campbell 1981a with permission.)

CMHs have a prominent discharge during the early phase of the stimulus, but this response adapts within seconds to a low level. In contrast, Type I AMHs are initially unresponsive, but then discharge vigorously. Therefore, it is likely that Type I AMHs contribute to the pain during a sustained high intensity heat stimulus (Meyer & Campbell 1981a).

In the hairy skin, stepped heat stimuli evoke a double pain sensation (Lewis & Pochin 1937; Campbell & LaMotte 1983). The first perception is a sharp pricking sensation, and the second sensation is a burning feeling that occurs after a momentary lull during which little if anything is felt. Myelinated afferent fibres must signal the first pain, since the latency of response to first pain is too quick to be carried by slowly conducting C-fibres (Campbell & LaMotte 1983). Type II AMHs (Fig. 1.3) are ideally suited to signal this first pain sensation:

1. The thermal threshold is near the threshold temperature for first pain (Dubner et al 1977)
2. The receptor utilization time (time between stimulus onset and receptor activation) is short (Meyer et al 1985a)
3. The burst of activity at the onset of the heat stimulus is consistent with the percept of a momentary pricking sensation.

The absence of a first pain sensation to heat stimuli applied to the glabrous skin of the human hand (Campbell & LaMotte 1983) correlates with the failure to find Type II AMHs on the glabrous skin of the hand in monkey.

A dual pain sensation is also perceived in response to sharp mechanical stimuli presented to both hairy and glabrous skin. The first pain is likely signalled by activity in a subset of A-fibre nociceptors.

The preceding discussion indicates that nociceptors may signal pain. However, two caveats are in order:

1. This does not mean that activity in CMHs always signals pain. It is clear that low level discharge rates in nociceptors do not always lead to sensation (e.g. Van Hees & Gybels 1981; Adriaensen et al 1984a). Central mechanisms for attention quite obviously play a crucial role in whether and how much nociceptor activity leads to the perception of pain.

2. It is probable that receptors other than nociceptors signal pain in certain circumstances. For example, the pain to light touch that occurs after certain nerve injuries or with tissue injury appears to be signalled by activity in low-threshold mechanoreceptors (see discussion below).

NOCICEPTOR RESPONSES TO CONTROLLED MECHANICAL STIMULI

The most commonly studied nociceptors respond to both heat and mechanical stimuli. The area of the receptive field that responds to mechanical stimuli has also been found to respond to heat stimuli (Treede et al 1990a). However, the transducer elements that account for mechanosensitivity are likely to be different from those responsible for heat. Analgesia to heat but not mechanical stimuli was observed following application of capsaicin to the skin of humans (Simone & Ochoa 1991; Davis et al 1992). Similarly, when capsaicin was administered to C-fibre polymodal nociceptors in the cornea, their response to heat and chemical stimuli was eliminated, but they still responded to mechanical stimuli (Belmonte et al 1991). This suggests that the mechanical and heat transducer mechanisms are different.

A paradox with regard to mechanically induced pain is that a mechanical stimulus that evokes the same level of activity in a C-fibre nociceptor as a heat stimulus, evokes less pain than the heat stimulus (e.g. Van Hees & Gybels 1981). In addition, the mechanical threshold for activating nociceptors is well below the pain threshold. This apparent discrepancy could be due to the spatial summation (i.e. recruitment of more nociceptors) associated with the larger area heat stimulus. Alternatively, the coactivation of low-threshold mechanoreceptors with the mechanical, but not the heat, stimulus could result in suppression of pain.

Nociceptive afferents are often vigorously activated by mechanical stimuli that are reported to be non-painful (Gybels et al 1979; Van Hees & Gybels 1981). As shown in Figure 1.8, C-fibre nociceptors in humans display a monotonically increasing response for short-duration mechanical stimuli increasing into the noxious range. In this study, the mechanical stimulus was a light metal cylinder (0.3 g) that was shot at the skin at different velocities. All of the C-fibres studied responded to stimuli that were not rated as painful by human subjects. At the mean pain threshold (11 m/s), the mean evoked response was nine action potentials (Koltzenburg & Handwerker 1993).

For long-duration mechanical stimuli, the response of nociceptors to suprathreshold stimuli adapts with time. In contrast, when similar long-duration mechanical stimuli are applied to human subjects, pain increases throughout the stimulus (Adriaensen et al 1984b). Reeh et al (1987) postulated that recruitment of activity in nociceptors that innervate nearby skin might explain the increased pain with time. When a stimulus was applied outside the receptive field of A-fibre nociceptors, the evoked response began several seconds after the stimulus onset and did not adapt. A similar delayed response of C-fibre nociceptors has been demonstrated for long-duration mechanical stimuli that are initially below threshold (White et al 1991).

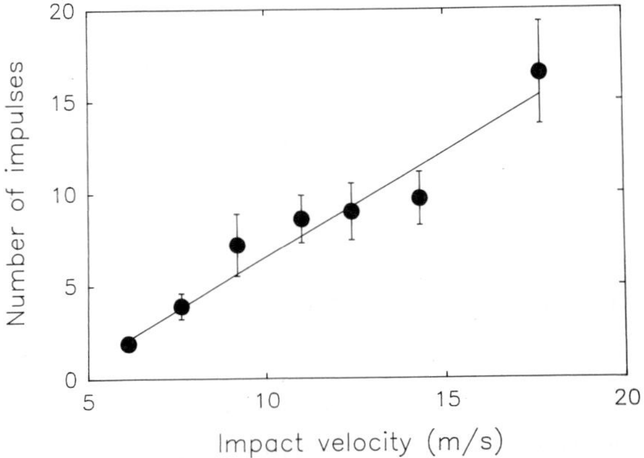

Fig. 1.8 Monotonically increasing response of C-fibre nociceptors in humans to noxious mechanical stimuli. A light metal cylinder (0.3 g) was shot perpendicular to the skin at different velocities. The mean response of 9 fibres is plotted. In psychophysical studies, the mean pain threshold was 11 m/s. (Adapted from Koltzenburg & Handwerker 1993 with permission.)

NOCICEPTORS AND COLD PAIN SENSATION

CMHs and AMHs in general respond meagrely to cooling stimuli. What then is the peripheral neural basis for cold induced pain? Klement & Arndt (1992) demonstrated that cold pain could be evoked by cold stimuli applied within the veins of human subjects. A local anaesthetic applied within the vein, but not in the overlying skin, abolished cold pain sensibility. It is therefore possible that cold pain is served by vascular receptors.

HYPERALGESIA: ROLE OF NOCICEPTORS AND OTHER AFFERENT FIBRES

To understand the peripheral neural mechanisms of pain to noxious stimuli is to understand only one aspect of pain sensibility. There is, in fact, a dynamic plasticity that relates stimulus intensity and sensation. Of great biological importance in this regard is the phenomenon of *hyperalgesia*. Hyperalgesia is defined as a *leftward shift of the stimulus-response function that relates magnitude of pain to stimulus intensity*. An example of this is seen in Figure 1.9, which shows human judgments of pain to heat stimuli before and after a burn. It is evident that threshold for pain is lowered and pain to suprathreshold stimuli is enhanced.

Hyperalgesia is a consistent feature of tissue injury and inflammation. Pharyngitis is associated with hyperalgesia in the pharyngeal tissues, such that merely swallowing induces pain. Micturition in the presence of a urinary tract infection is painful, again reflecting the presence of hyperalgesia. In inflammatory arthritis, slight motion of the joint leads to pain. Ironically, with most diseases we think in terms of loss of function, whereas neuropathic conditions sometimes lead to enhanced function, i.e. hyperalgesia. Hyperalgesia may be prominent in neuropathic conditions such as post-herpetic neuralgia, certain cases of diabetic neuropathy, and certain cases of traumatic nerve injury.

The peripheral neural mechanisms of hyperalgesia have been studied in the joint, cornea, testicle, bladder and other tissues. Much of the theoretical work on hyperalgesia, however, has evolved from studies of the skin, and it is this work that will receive attention here. Neural mechanisms in other tissues will be discussed in later sections.

Hyperalgesia occurs not only at the site of injury but also in the surrounding uninjured area. Hyperalgesia at the site of injury is termed *primary hyperalgesia*, while hyperalgesia in the uninjured skin surrounding the injury is termed *secondary hyperalgesia* (Lewis 1935, 1942). As we will see, the neural mechanisms for primary and secondary hyperalgesia differ.

In discussing hyperalgesia, it is useful to consider the following variables:

1. energy form of the *injury*
2. type of *tissue* involved

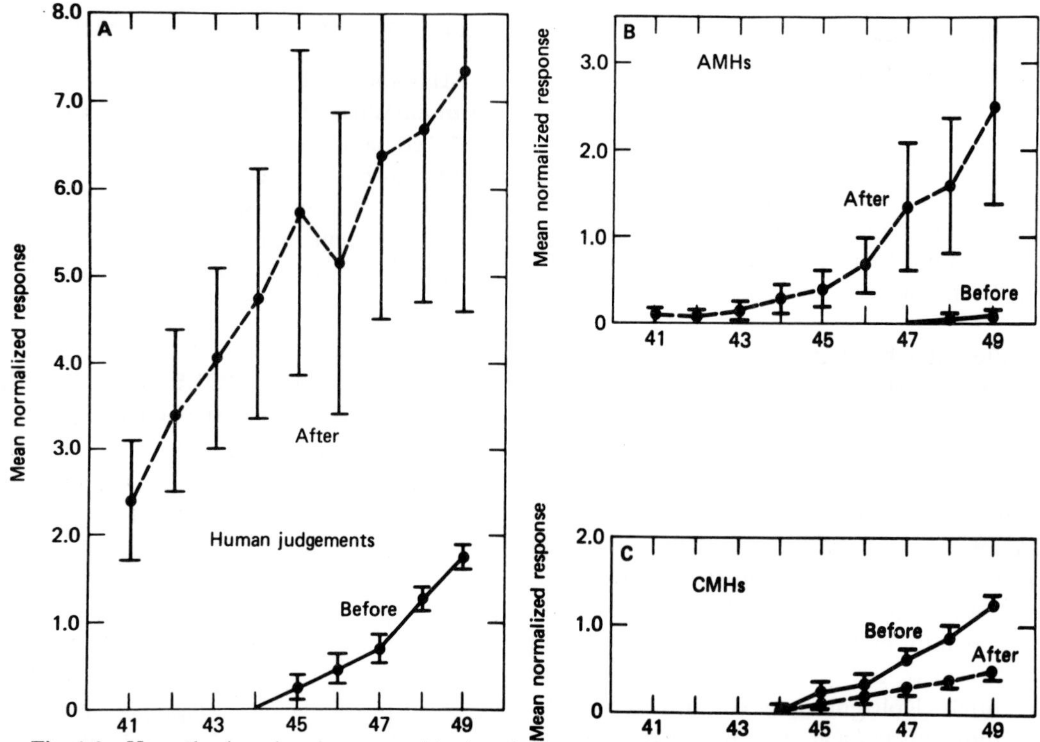

Fig. 1.9 Hyperalgesia and nociceptor sensitization after a cutaneous burn injury. Responses to heat stimuli were obtained 5 min before and 10 min after a 53°C, 30 s burn to the glabrous skin of the hand. The burn resulted in increases in the magnitude of pain (hyperalgesia) in human subjects that were matched by enhanced responses (sensitization) in Type I AMHs in monkey. In contrast, CMHs exhibited decreased sensitivity after the burn. **A** Human judgments of pain (n = 8). **B** Responses of A-fibre nociceptive afferents (Type I AMHs) in monkeys (n = 14). **C** Responses of C-fibre nociceptive afferents (CMHs) in monkeys (n = 15). The same type of random heat sequence and normalization described in Figure 1.6 was used. Because the AMHs did not respond to the 45°C stimulus before the burn, the AMH data were normalized by dividing by the response to the first 45°C after the burn. (From Meyer & Campbell 1981a with permission.)

3. energy form of the *test stimulus*
4. *location of the testing* relative to the area injured.

These variables interact in complex ways. For example, it will be shown that nociceptors will sensitize to mechanical stimuli (the energy form of the test stimulus), but only after certain forms of injury (viz. injection of inflammatory mediators).

An experimental design frequently used for the study of the neural mechanisms of hyperalgesia is to characterize the response properties of a given cell, then apply a manipulation which under usual circumstances would produce hyperalgesia, and finally assess whether this manipulation has altered the response properties of the cell in question. As shown in Figure 1.10, the relative locations of the injury site, the test site, and the receptive field of the sensory neuron being studied dictate whether the experiment provides information regarding the mechanisms of primary or secondary hyperalgesia (Treede et al 1992). These three variables may interact in any of six ways. As shown in Figure 1.10, when the injury and the test site coincide (Fig. 1.10A,B), the study has provided a basis by which to consider the mechanism for primary hyperalgesia, whereas when the test site and the injury site diverge (Fig. 1.10C–F), the study has provided a basis by which to account for secondary hyperalgesia.

When the paradigms shown in Figure 1.10A and B are used, it is found that, under certain circumstances, nociceptors have an increased response to the test stimulus. Thus peripheral neural mechanisms are likely to account for at least some aspects of primary hyperalgesia. In contrast, nociceptors do not develop an enhanced response to the test stimulus when the paradigms shown in Figure 1.10C–F are investigated. By default, therefore, the mechanism for secondary hyperalgesia must reside within the central nervous system (CNS).

PRIMARY HYPERALGESIA

Hyperalgesia to heat stimuli

We consider first the situation where a burn injury is applied to the skin, where the test stimulus is heat applied to the location of the burn injury. When a burn is applied to the glabrous skin of the hand, marked hyperalgesia to heat develops as shown in Figure 1.9A (Meyer & Campbell 1981a). The hyperalgesia is manifest as a leftward shift of the stimulus-response function that

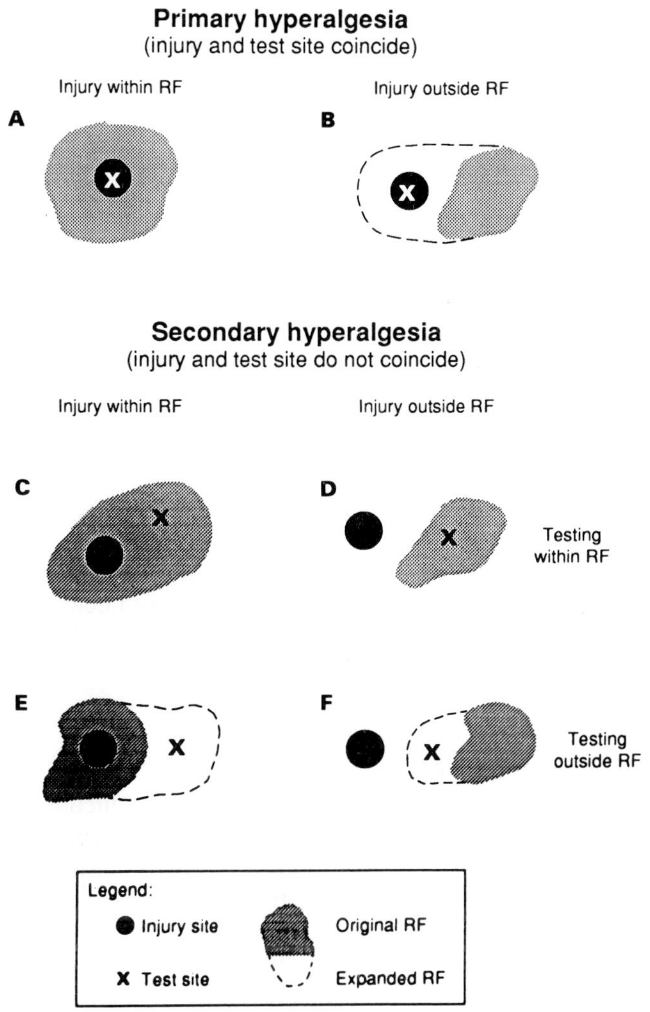

Primary hyperalgesia
(injury and test site coincide)

Injury within RF — A
Injury outside RF — B

Secondary hyperalgesia
(injury and test site do not coincide)

Injury within RF — C, E
Injury outside RF — D, F

Testing within RF
Testing outside RF

Legend:
Injury site
Original RF
X Test site
Expanded RF

Fig. 1.10 Experimental configurations for testing the neural mechanisms of primary and secondary hyperalgesia. To study primary hyperalgesia, the site of injury (indicated by filled circle) and the site of testing (indicated by the X) must coincide. Alterations of the stimulus-response functions from stimuli applied to the original receptive field (A) or expansion of the receptive field towards the injury site (B) are substrates for primary hyperalgesia. To study secondary hyperalgesia, the site of injury and the site of testing must not coincide (C–F). A sensitization of the stimulus-response function revealed by testing within the original receptive field may occur following injuries within (C) or outside the receptive field (D). An expansion of the receptive field to include a test site outside the original receptive field may occur for injuries within (E) or outside (F) the receptive field. (From Treede et al 1992 with permission.)

relates magnitude of pain to stimulus intensity. For example, the 41°C stimulus after injury was as painful as the 49°C stimulus prior to injury.

Peripheral sensitization as a mechanism for primary hyperalgesia to heat stimuli

Substantial evidence favours the concept that the primary hyperalgesia to heat stimuli that develops at the site of a burn injury is mediated by sensitization of nociceptors

Table 1.1 Comparison of characteristics of hyperalgesia and sensitization

Hyperalgesia (subject response)	Sensitization (fibre response)
Decreased pain threshold	Decreased threshold for response
Increased pain to suprathreshold stimuli	Increased response to suprathreshold stimuli
Spontaneous pain	Spontaneous activity

(Meyer & Campbell 1981a; LaMotte et al 1982). *Sensitization* is defined as a *leftward shift of the stimulus-response function that relates magnitude of the neural response to stimulus intensity.* Sensitization is characterized by a decrease in threshold, an augmented response to suprathreshold stimuli, and ongoing spontaneous activity (Bessou & Perl 1969; Beck et al 1974; Beitel & Dubner 1976). These properties correspond to the properties of hyperalgesia (Table 1.1).

To explain the hyperalgesia that occurs with a burn to the glabrous skin of the hand, a correlative analysis of subjective ratings of pain in humans with responses of nociceptors (CMHs and Type I AMHs) in anaesthetized monkeys was performed (Meyer & Campbell 1981a). Test heat stimuli were applied to the glabrous skin of the hand before and after a 53°C, 30-second burn. The burn led to prominent hyperalgesia in the human subjects (Fig. 1.9A). The CMHs showed a decreased response following the burn (Fig. 1.9C), whereas the Type I AMHs were markedly sensitized (Fig. 1.9B). Thus, it is likely that, for thermal injuries to the glabrous skin of the hand, AMHs, not CMHs, code for the heat hyperalgesia.

Sensitization is not a uniform property of nociceptors. Tissue type and the nature of the injury are important variables. For example, CMHs that innervate the glabrous skin of the hand do not sensitize to a burn injury, whereas CMHs that innervate hairy skin do (Campbell & Meyer 1983). Thus, CMHs appear to play a role in accounting for hyperalgesia to heat stimuli on hairy skin (LaMotte et al 1983; Torebjörk et al 1984). These data support the conclusion that the hyperalgesia to heat stimuli that occurs at the site of an injury is due to sensitization of primary afferent nociceptors.

Hyperalgesia to mechanical stimuli

In some respects distinguishing hyperalgesia to mechanical stimuli in the primary and secondary zone may be incorrect. There is evidence that the mechanism for hyperalgesia in the two zones may be the same. The mechanisms discussed in this section, however, will be limited to those which may be applicable to the primary zone.

There are at least two different forms of mechanical hyperalgesia. One form of mechanical hyperalgesia is evident when the skin is gently stroked with a cotton swab and may be called *stroking hyperalgesia*, dynamic hyperalgesia, or allodynia. The second form of hyperalgesia is evident when punctate stimuli, such as von Frey probes, are applied and accordingly has been termed *punctate hyperalgesia*. As will be discussed in the section on secondary hyperalgesia, the mechanisms for these two forms of mechanical hyperalgesia are likely different.

Nociceptor sensitization as a mechanism for mechanical hyperalgesia in the primary zone

It was initially presumed that sensitization of nociceptors accounts for mechanical hyperalgesia, particularly in the area of primary hyperalgesia. However, within the original receptive field, thresholds to mechanical stimulation of either CMHs or AMHs, as measured with von Frey hairs (a punctate stimulus), are not changed by heat or mechanical injury (Campbell et al 1979; Thalhammer & LaMotte 1982; Campbell et al 1988).

Expansion of the receptive field of a nociceptor into an adjacent area of injury (Fig.1.11) is an alternate peripheral mechanism that may account for primary hyperalgesia to mechanical, as well as heat, stimuli. The receptive fields of AMH fibres as well as some CMH fibres expand modestly into the area of an adjacent heat (Thalhammer & LaMotte 1982) or mechanical (Reeh et al 1987) injury. As a result of this expansion, heat or mechanical stimuli delivered after the injury will activate a greater number of fibres. This spatial summation would be expected to induce more pain. The physiological basis of this expansion is unknown. Since the mechanical thresholds within the expansion areas are similar to those in the original receptive fields (Thalhammer & LaMotte 1982), this form of sensitization is not likely to account for the significant decrease in threshold associated with stroking hyperalgesia.

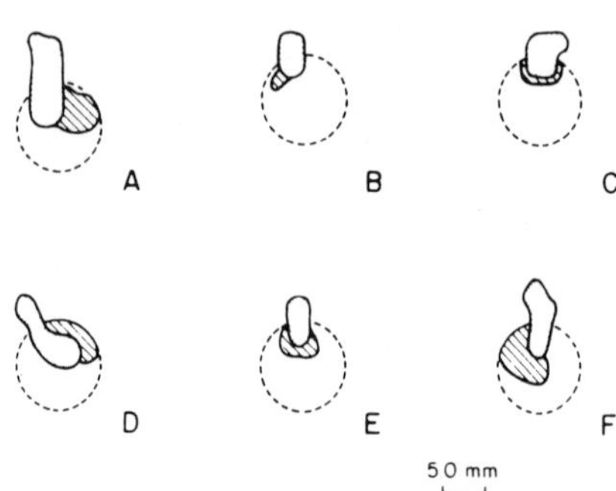

Fig. 1.11 Receptive field expansion in primary nociceptive afferents following a cutaneous injury. The shape of the receptive fields of six nociceptors was determined with the same von Frey hair before and after a conditioning stimulus of 56°C for 7 s that was delivered to the location indicated by the dashed circle. The solid line indicates the receptive field before the conditioning stimulus; the hatched area indicates the enlargement that was evident 22 min after the conditioning stimulus. **A–E** AMHs, **F** CMH. (From Thalhammer & LaMotte 1982 with permission.)

Loss of central inhibition as a mechanism of mechanical hyperalgesia in the primary zone

Under usual circumstances, the production of pain from activation of nociceptors with mechanical stimuli is inhibited in the CNS by the concurrent activation of low-threshold mechanoreceptors (Noordenbos 1959; Van Hees & Gybels 1981; Bini et al 1984). There is evidence that injury decreases the responsiveness of low-threshold mechanoreceptors. A decrease in responsiveness of low-threshold mechanoreceptors in the cat footpad was observed when the receptive field was heated to noxious temperatures (Beck et al 1974). In addition, slowly-adapting, low-threshold mechanoreceptors in the primate have a reduced response to mechanical stimuli after a burn to their receptive field (Khan, Meyer, Campbell, unpublished observations). Hyperalgesia to mechanical stimuli in the primary zone could therefore be due to injury to low-threshold mechanoreceptors, which would lead to a central disinhibition of nociceptor input and thus result in enhanced pain (viz. hyperalgesia).

Nociceptor sensitization after exposure to chemicals

Although a burn injury does not lead to a reduction in mechanical threshold for nociceptors, exposure of nociceptors to the mediators thought to be responsible for inflammatory pain nevertheless may cause nociceptors to become sensitized to mechanical as well as heat stimuli (Martin et al 1987; Davis et al 1993). Figure 1.12 shows the response of an Aδ-fibre nociceptor to mechanical stimuli before and after exposure to a mixture of algesic inflammatory mediators (bradykinin, histamine, serotonin, and prostaglandin E_1).

SECONDARY HYPERALGESIA

An understanding of secondary hyperalgesia is important not only with regard to understanding the neural mechanisms of inflammatory pain, but also with regard to understanding many aspects of chronic pain. We will consider in this section the nature of secondary hyperalgesia and its possible peripheral and central mechanisms.

Primary hyperalgesia is characterized by the presence of enhanced pain to heat *and* mechanical stimuli, whereas secondary hyperalgesia is characterized by enhanced pain to *only* mechanical stimuli. To compare the sensory changes that occur in the zones of primary and secondary hyperalgesia, burn injuries were applied to two locations on the glabrous skin of the hand in human subjects (Fig. 1.13). Within minutes of the injury, lightly touching the skin caused pain both at the site of the two burns as well as in a large area surrounding the burns. The decrease in the pain threshold to von Frey hairs in the

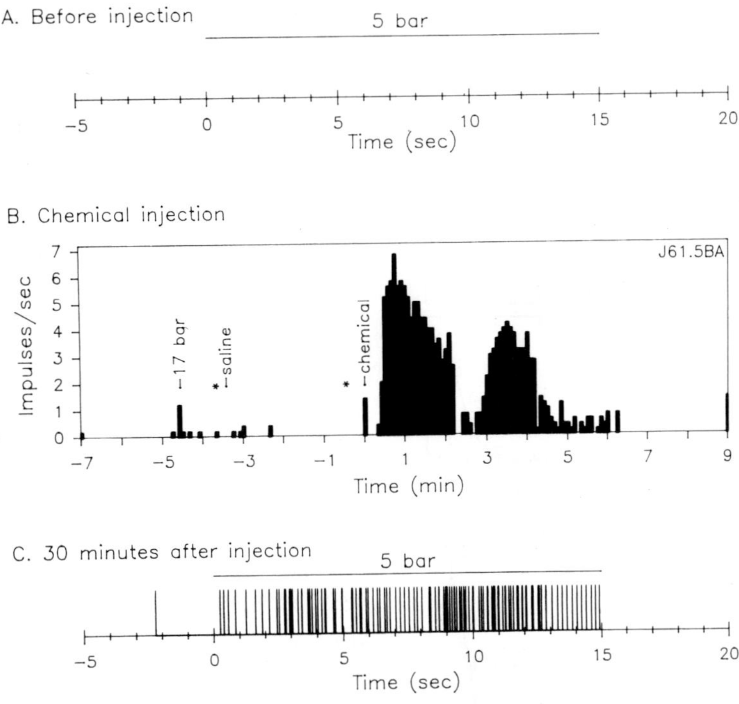

Fig. 1.12 Example of sensitization to mechanical stimuli following a chemical injection for an Aδ-fibre nociceptor. The inflammatory mixture described in Figure 1.4 was used. **A** The fibre did not respond to application of a 5-bar stimulus for 15 s to the most sensitive area within its receptive field. The initial mechanical threshold for this fibre was 10 bar, and therefore it was a mechanically-insensitive afferent (MIA). **B** This fibre had a strong response following injection of the chemical mixture into its RF. (Each asterisk indicates time of needle insertion; bin size = 5 s.) **C** Sensitization to mechanical stimuli was demonstrated in this fibre 30 min after the chemical injection. The fibre now responded to application of the 5-bar stimulus. Each vertical tick corresponds to time of occurrence of an action potential. The von Frey threshold decreased (from 10 bar to 4 bar) and the receptive field area increased (from 9 mm^2 to 88 mm^2). No response to heat was observed either before or after the injection. (From Davis et al 1993 with permission.)

primary (injured) zone was similar to that in the area of secondary hyperalgesia (Fig. 1.13B). Marked hyperalgesia to heat was observed in the area of primary hyperalgesia (site A, the injury site; Fig. 1.13C). In the uninjured region between the two burns, however, the painfulness of the heat stimuli actually decreased (Fig. 1.13D). Notably, the area between the burns was *hyp*algesic to heat, while being *hyper*algesic to mechanical stimuli.

In the discussion of primary hyperalgesia, it was necessary to account for hyperalgesia to both heat and mechanical stimuli. In the case of secondary hyperalgesia, it is necessary to account only for mechanical hyperalgesia. Hyperalgesia to cooling and heating stimuli does not occur. As noted above and as will be clarified further in this section, the distinction between primary and secondary hyperalgesia is to some extent artificial. The mechanisms that account for hyperalgesia to mechanical stimuli in the secondary zone may very well account for mechanical hyperalgesia in the primary zone.

Spreading sensitization of nociceptors does not occur

Activation of nociceptors leads to a flare response. This response is neurogenic in the sense that it depends on intact innervation of the skin by nociceptors. The flare response extends well outside the area of initial injury. One explanation of the flare response is that it involves a spreading activation of nociceptors. Activation of one nociceptor leads to release of chemicals, such as substance P, which activate neighbouring nociceptors, leading to further release of chemicals and activation of additional nociceptors. Lewis (1942) believed that a similar mechanism, which he termed *spreading sensitization*, accounted for secondary hyperalgesia. Activation and sensitization of one nociceptor lead to spread of this sensitization to another nociceptor, due possibly to the effects of a sensitizing substance released from the nociceptor initially activated.

One way to test this hypothesis is to stimulate electri-

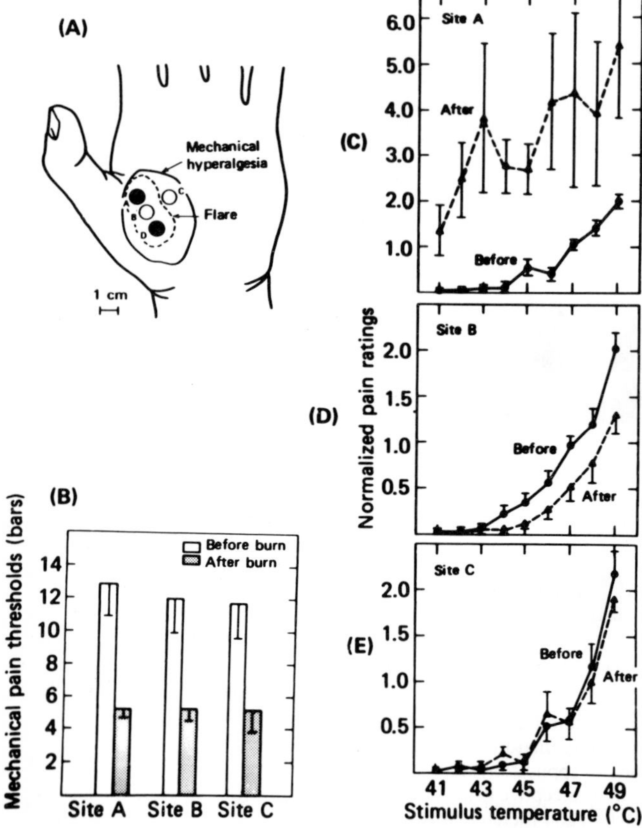

Fig. 1.13 Hyperalgesia to mechanical and heat stimuli develops at the site of injury (zone of primary hyperalgesia), whereas hyperalgesia to mechanical, but not heat, stimuli develops in the uninjured area surrounding an injury (zone of secondary hyperalgesia). **A** Two burns (53°C, 30 s) were applied to the glabrous skin of the hand (sites A and D). Mechanical thresholds for pain and ratings of pain to heat stimuli were recorded before and after the burns at one of the injury sites (site A), in the uninjured skin between the two burns (site B), and at an adjacent site (site C). The areas of flare and mechanical hyperalgesia following the burns in one subject are also shown. In all subjects, the area of mechanical hyperalgesia was larger than the area of flare. Mechanical hyperalgesia was present even after the flare disappeared. **B** Mean mechanical thresholds for pain before and after burns are shown for seven subjects. The mechanical threshold for pain was significantly decreased following the burns. The mechanical hyperalgesia was of similar magnitude at each of the three test spots (A, B, C). **C–E** Mean normalized ratings of painfulness of heat stimuli (same as described in Fig. 1.6) before and after burns are shown. **C** At burn site A, all the characteristics of heat hyperalgesia (i.e. decrease in pain threshold, increased pain to suprathreshold stimuli, and spontaneous pain) were observed after the burns (n = 8). **D** In the uninjured area between the two burns (site B), pain ratings decreased after the burns. Thus, heat *hyp*algesia was observed (n = 9). **E** At site C, pain ratings before and after the burns were not significantly different (n = 8). (From Raja et al 1984 with permission.)

cally nociceptive fibres along the nerve trunk to determine if this induces sensitization of the nociceptors. Antidromic stimulation of nociceptive fibres in monkey (Meyer et al 1988) and rat (Reeh et al 1986) was found not to cause sensitization.

Pursuant to the paradigm shown in Figure 1.10C, heat injury to one half of the receptive field of nociceptors does not alter sensitivity of the other half to heat stimuli (Thalhammer & LaMotte 1983). Pursuant to the paradigm shown in Figure 1.10D, an injury adjacent to the receptive field of nociceptors fails to alter the responses of CMHs in monkey (Campbell et al 1988) and rat (Reeh et al 1986).

Other differences exist between flare and secondary hyperalgesia:

1. The zone of secondary hyperalgesia is generally larger than the zone of flare (Raja et al 1984; LaMotte et al 1991; Koltzenburg et al 1992b).
2. Flare can be induced without inducing secondary hyperalgesia (for example with histamine), and secondary hyperalgesia can be induced without a flare response (LaMotte et al 1991).
3. Secondary hyperalgesia does not spread beyond the body's midline, whereas the flare response does (LaMotte et al 1991).

Spreading sensitization, an exception

Although antidromic stimulation and certain injuries (e.g. cuts, burns, and certain chemical injuries) applied adjacent to receptive fields do not sensitize nociceptors, one type of injury does appear to lead to spreading sensitization. A prolonged, intense, pressure stimulus applied immediately adjacent to mechanically sensitive A-fibre, but not C-fibre, nociceptors leads to a lowered mechanical threshold within the receptive field (Reeh et al 1987).

Central mechanisms of secondary hyperalgesia

If peripheral sensitization does not account for secondary hyperalgesia, the mechanisms noted in Figure 1.10C–F should be examined in the CNS. Indeed, it has been relatively easy to demonstrate enhanced responsiveness of the CNS neurons to mechanical stimuli after cutaneous injury (e.g. Simone et al 1991b). Substantial evidence favours this important tenet: *the peripheral signal for pain does not reside exclusively with nociceptors. Under pathological circumstances, other receptor types, which are normally associated with the sensation of touch, acquire the capacity to evoke pain.* This principle applies not only to secondary hyperalgesia, but also to neuropathic pain states in general. This condition arises through augmentation of responsiveness of central pain-signalling neurons to input from low-threshold mechanoreceptors, a phenomenon often termed *central sensitization*. One possible mechanism for central sensitization is that central pain-signalling neurons develop strengthened synaptic links with normally ineffectual inputs of low-threshold mechanoreceptors.

Studies with capsaicin

Many of the insights acquired about secondary hyperalgesia have been gained from studies with capsaicin, the active ingredient in hot peppers. Investigators have been drawn to the use of capsaicin as the 'injury' stimulus for several reasons:

1. Capsaicin selectively activates nociceptors (Szolcsányi 1990).
2. Capsaicin causes intense pain and a large zone of secondary hyperalgesia when applied topically or intradermally to the skin (Simone et al 1989).
3. Injection of capsaicin into the skin does not produce any apparent tissue injury.
4. The characteristics of hyperalgesia resemble those for heat or cut injuries.

Immediately around the injection site, heat and mechanical hyperalgesia are present. Outside this area of primary hyperalgesia is a large zone of secondary hyperalgesia that is characterized by mechanical hyperalgesia but *not* heat hyperalgesia.

LaMotte and colleagues recently performed a number of experiments to determine the relative importance of peripheral and central sensitization in secondary hyperalgesia (LaMotte et al 1991). To test whether peripheral nerve fibres are sensitized, capsaicin was administered under conditions of a proximal nerve block, and the magnitude of hyperalgesia was determined after the effects of the anaesthetic dissipated. When the relevant nerve is blocked proximal to the capsaicin injection site, the CNS is spared the nociceptive input generated at the time of injection. The peripheral nervous system effects of the capsaicin are not affected, since the nerve block is proximal to the area of capsaicin application. Figure 1.14 shows the results of this experiment in one subject. No hyperalgesia was present after the block had worn off. Thus, when the CNS is spared the input of nociceptors at the time of the acute insult, the hyperalgesia is sharply curtailed. Central sensitization, therefore, plays a major role in secondary hyperalgesia.

Another experiment indicates that this central sensitization is dependent on events in the peripheral nervous system. When the capsaicin injection site is cooled or anaesthetized after the injection, signs of secondary hyperalgesia are either eliminated or substantially reduced (LaMotte et al 1991). Thus, input from the sensitized nociceptive neurons in the zone of primary hyperalgesia is required to maintain the secondary hyperalgesia. This theme of central sensitization requiring an ongoing peripheral nociceptive input will reemerge in the discussion below of sympathetically maintained pain.

As noted earlier, there are two forms of mechanical hyperalgesia, stroking and punctate. We will consider first stroking hyperalgesia (allodynia). Stroking hyperalgesia appears to be mediated by activity in low-threshold mechanoreceptors. When a pressure cuff was used to selectively block myelinated fibres, the pain to stroking disappeared at a time when touch sensation was lost, but

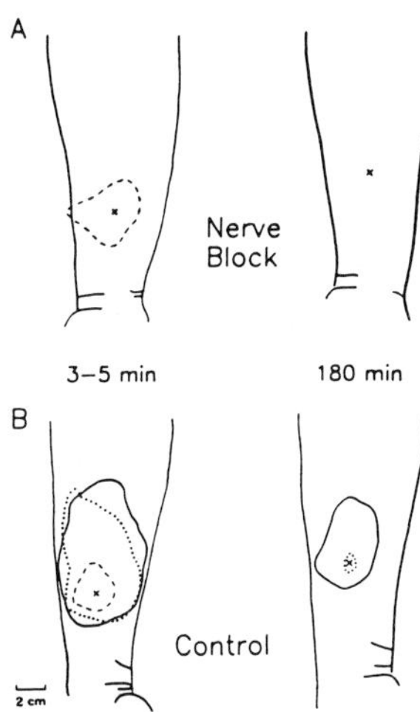

Fig. 1.14 A proximal nerve block prevents the development of secondary hyperalgesia. **A** After blockade of the lateral antebrachial nerve with 1% xylocaine, capsaicin (100 µg in 10 µl) was injected into the anaesthetic skin. A flare (dashed line) developed within 5 min. No hyperalgesia was present 180 min after the capsaicin injection when the local anaesthetic block had recovered. **B** On the control arm, normal flare and hyperalgesia to stroking (dotted line) and punctate (solid line) stimuli developed within 5 min, and hyperalgesia to punctate stimuli was still present 180 min after the capsaicin injection. (From LaMotte et al 1991 with permission.)

when heat and cold sensation were still present (LaMotte et al 1991; Koltzenburg et al 1992b). In another series of experiments, Torebjörk and colleagues performed intraneural microstimulation in awake human subjects (Torebjörk et al 1992). A microelectrode was placed within the nerve so that electrical stimulation evoked tactile paraesthesias referable to a particular area. Then capsaicin was injected adjacent to this area so that secondary hyperalgesia was created in the area of referred paraesthesias. When the same electrical stimulus was repeated, it now evoked pain (Fig. 1.15). Thus, stimulation of primary afferent fibres normally concerned with tactile sensibility evoked pain when (but not before) secondary hyperalgesia was produced.

A model for secondary hyperalgesia to stroking stimuli is shown in Figure 1.16. In normal tissue, a noxious stimulus activates primary afferent nociceptors. The resulting action potentials propagate to second order neurons in the dorsal horn. In this functional block diagram, we refer to these second order neurons as central pain-signalling neurons. Signals from the central pain-signalling neurons ascend to higher neural centres and eventually result in the perception of pain. Normally, activity in low-threshold mechanoreceptors is not painful. A large afferent barrage in nociceptors leads to a selective modulation of the central pain-signalling neurons such that the input from low-threshold receptors is augmented. This selective sensitization may be due to an enhancement of the synaptic efficacy of low-threshold mechanoreceptors onto the central pain-signalling neurons. Light tactile

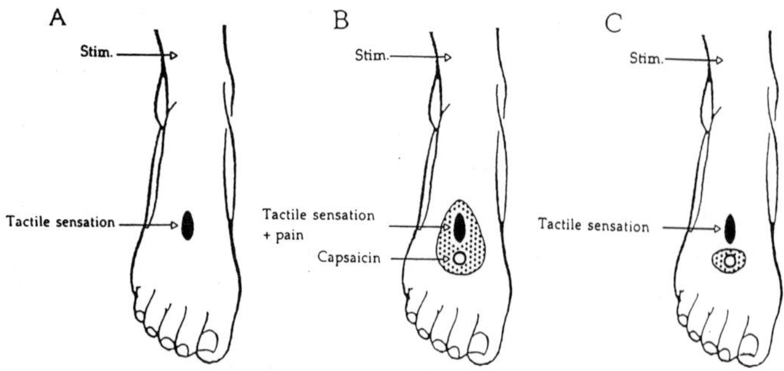

Fig. 1.15 Microneurographic evidence that large-diameter myelinated fibres are involved in the pain observed in the zone of secondary hyperalgesia. **A** Intraneural electrical stimulation of the superficial peroneal nerve at a fixed intensity and frequency evoked a purely tactile (non-painful) sensation projected to a small skin area on the dorsum of the foot (black area). **B** After intradermal injection of capsaicin (100 μg in 10 μl) adjacent to the projected zone (at the site indicated by the open circle), a zone of secondary hyperalgesia developed that overlapped the sensory projection field. Now, intraneural stimulation at the same intensity and frequency as in **A** was perceived as a tactile sensation accompanied by pain. **C** When the zone of secondary hyperalgesia no longer overlapped the sensory projection field, the intraneural stimulation was again perceived as purely tactile, without any pain component. (From Torebjörk et al 1992 with permission.)

stimuli that activate low-threshold mechanoreceptors result in action potentials that now gain enhanced access to central pain-signalling neurons, leading to the perception of pain to gentle mechanical stimuli. This central sensitization is maintained by spontaneous activity in nociceptors at the injury site; when this nociceptor activity is reduced or eliminated, the central sensitized state diminishes.

If capsaicin is injected beside a thin strip of local anaesthesia (Fig. 1.17), the secondary hyperalgesia does not spread beyond the area of the anaesthetic strip (LaMotte et al 1991). Upon initial evaluation, this finding might be taken as evidence for spreading sensitization. However, the proximal nerve block experiment described above argues against spreading sensitization of primary afferent fibres. To account for the findings of the anaesthetic strip experiment, LaMotte hypothesized that chemospecific nociceptors responsive to capsaicin exist which have very large receptive fields (LaMotte et al 1991; LaMotte 1992). CNS input from these fibres is needed to produce widespread central sensitization. The anaesthetic strip blocks conduction of the action potentials from the branches of the fibres to the CNS. This blockade of nociceptor input to the CNS prevents the development of hyperalgesia in the region beyond the anaesthetic strip. This mechanism requires a close somatotopic relationship between the area rendered allodynic and the area served by the nociceptor input.

Different mechanisms for stroking and punctate hyperalgesia

Whereas stroking hyperalgesia appears to be mediated by activity in low-threshold mechanoreceptors, several lines of evidence indicate that punctate hyperalgesia has a different neural mechanism and is mediated by activity in nociceptors:

1. In the zone of secondary hyperalgesia, the area of punctate hyperalgesia is consistently larger than that of stroking hyperalgesia (e.g. Figs 1.14 and 1.17).

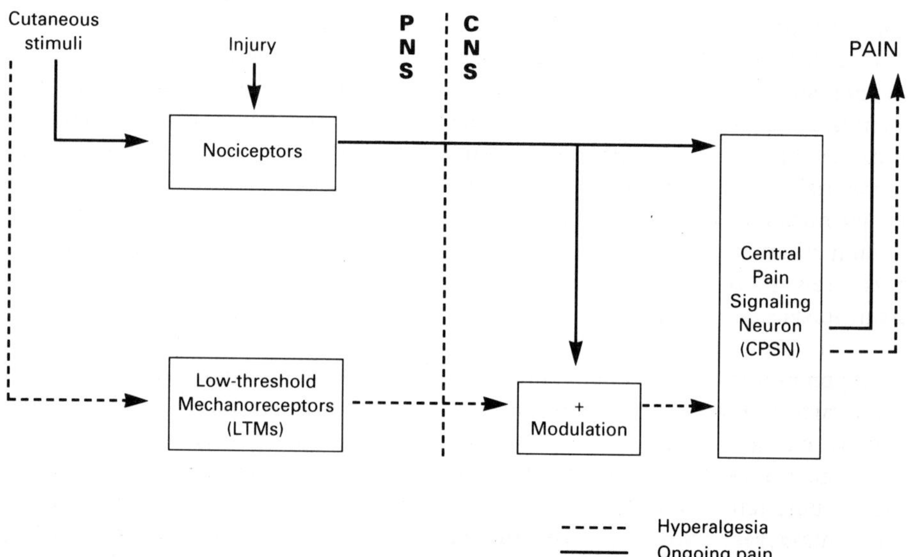

Fig. 1.16 Model of secondary hyperalgesia to stroking stimuli. The afferent barrage in nociceptors at the time of injury results in a sensitization of the central pain-signalling neurons (CPSNs). Now, input from low-threshold mechanoreceptors produces an augmented response in these CPSNs. This central sensitization is maintained by low-grade activity in the nociceptors.

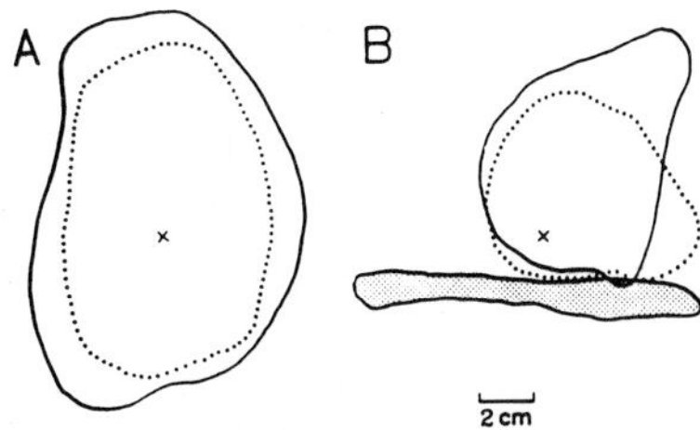

Fig. 1.17 A local anaesthetic strip blocks the spread of secondary hyperalgesia. **A** Normal areas of hyperalgesia to stroking (dotted line) and punctate (solid line) stimuli after intradermal injection of capsaicin (100 μg in 10 μl) at the site marked by an X on the volar forearm. **B** When the capsaicin was injected beside a strip of skin that was made anaesthetic by intradermal injections of xylocaine, the hyperalgesia did not cross to the other side of the anaesthetic strip. (From LaMotte et al 1991 with permission.)

2. Stroking hyperalgesia after capsaicin injection lasts 1–2 hours, whereas punctate hyperalgesia lasts 13–24 hours (LaMotte et al 1991).

3. Punctate hyperalgesia, not stroking hyperalgesia, developed after intradermal capsaicin injection into the arm of a patient with a severe large fibre neuropathy (Treede & Cole 1993). This evidence suggests that punctate hyperalgesia is mediated by small-diameter (presumably nociceptive) fibres.

4. The pain produced by touching the skin with different wool fabrics was greatly increased in the region of secondary hyperalgesia (Cervero et al 1993). The pain was proportional to the prickliness of the fabrics. Since nociceptors, and not low-threshold mechanoreceptors, exhibit a differential response to different wool fabrics (Garnsworthy et al 1988), activity in nociceptors likely contributes to this form of secondary hyperalgesia to wool fabrics.

Other observations support the concept that punctate hyperalgesia is due to central sensitization to input from nociceptive fibres. Like stroking hyperalgesia, punctate hyperalgesia is abolished or markedly reduced when capsaicin is injected into an area rendered temporarily anaesthetic by a proximal nerve block (LaMotte et al 1991). Thus the initial nociceptive input is important in the induction of stroking and punctate hyperalgesia. When the area of primary hyperalgesia is anaesthetized, however, punctate hyperalgesia persists, whereas stroking hyperalgesia is eliminated. Therefore, stroking hyperalgesia has an ongoing dependence on inputs from the sensitized area, whereas punctate hyperalgesia is more enduring and less dependent on ongoing discharge from the sensitized area.

Since hyperalgesia to heat does not occur in the zone of secondary hyperalgesia, punctate hyperalgesia cannot be due to generalized central sensitization to polymodal nociceptive inputs. The data appear to require that the central sensitization applies only to the inputs from nociceptors sensitive to mechanical stimuli and not to inputs from nociceptors sensitive to heat stimuli.

NOCICEPTORS AND THE SYMPATHETIC NERVOUS SYSTEM

Activity in nociceptors induces an increase in sympathetic discharge. Under usual circumstances, the converse is not true: sympathetic activity has no impact on the discharge of nociceptive neurons. In certain patients, however, nociceptors appear to be under the influence of the sympathetic nervous system. Under these circumstances, patients are said to have *sympathetically maintained pain* (SMP).

Sometimes referred to as reflex sympathetic dystrophy or causalgia, SMP can be manifest in a variety of situations. For example, pain that arises from acute herpes zoster, soft tissue trauma, metabolic neuropathies, nerve injury, as well as other conditions *may* be based on activity in the sympathetic nervous system. Certain nerve lesions in animals produce a state that resembles neuropathic pain in man and which can be eliminated by a sympathectomy (Shir & Seltzer 1991; Kim & Chung 1991; Neil et al 1991).

In SMP, anaesthetic blockade of the sympathetic nervous system relieves pain. If norepinephrine is then injected into the previously painful skin, pain can be again induced (Wallin et al 1976; Davis et al 1991). Norepinephrine injected into normal subjects evokes no pain. Therefore, in SMP, norepinephrine that normally is released from the sympathetic terminals acquires the capacity to evoke pain.

This production of pain is mediated through activation of alpha receptors. Phentolamine, an alpha-adrenergic antagonist, relieves pain when given to patients with SMP (Raja et al 1991). Clonidine, an alpha$_2$-adrenergic agonist, also relieves pain when applied topically in patients with SMP (Davis et al 1991). Activation of alpha$_2$-adrenergic receptors, located on sympathetic terminals, blocks norepinephrine release. Thus, clonidine appears to relieve pain by blocking norepinephrine release. When phenylephrine, a selective alpha$_1$-adrenergic agonist, was applied to the clonidine-treated area, pain was rekindled in patients with SMP (Davis et al 1991). Thus, clinical data suggest that the alpha$_1$-adrenergic receptor plays a pivotal role in SMP. This leads to the hypothesis that nociceptors develop sensitivity to norepinephrine through expression of alpha$_1$ receptors. This may involve a phenotypic change in nociceptors such that nociceptors acquire an abnormal sensitivity to norepinephrine. An alternate hypothesis is that alpha$_2$-inhibitory receptors develop on nociceptors.

One model that explains SMP is shown in Figure 1.18. This model is similar to that shown in Figure 1.16 for secondary hyperalgesia. In SMP, nociceptors are thought to develop an alpha-adrenergic sensitivity, probably as the result of the expression of alpha$_1$-adrenergic receptors on their terminals. In this pathological situation, sympathetic efferent activity leads to low-grade ongoing activity in the nociceptors. This ongoing activity in the nociceptors

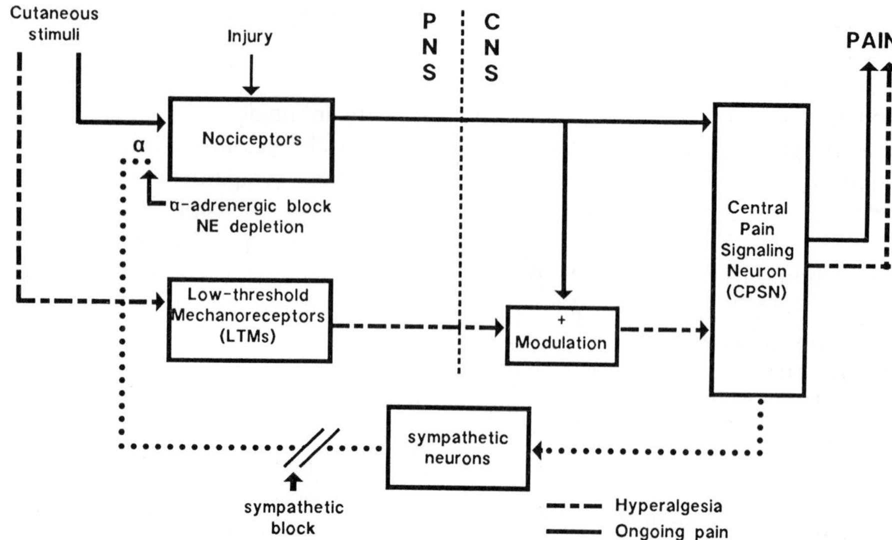

Fig. 1.18 Model to explain the hyperalgesia that develops in sympathetically-maintained pain. Like secondary hyperalgesia (Fig. 1.16), pain to light touch is signalled by activity in low-threshold mechanoreceptors that have an enhanced connectivity to the central pain-signalling neurons. In SMP, nociceptors develop adrenergic sensitivity such that the release of norepinephrine by the sympathetic nervous system produces spontaneous activity in the nociceptors. This spontaneous activity maintains the CNS in a sensitized state. An anaesthetic block of the sympathetic neurons or a peripheral adrenergic block will eliminate this ongoing activity in the nociceptors and thus lead to reversal of the central sensitized state.

maintains the central pain-signalling neurons in a sensitized state such that input from low-threshold mechanoreceptors produces pain. The ongoing nociceptor activity probably also contributes to the ongoing pain perceived by the patients.

Therapeutic measures that are aimed at eliminating the ongoing activity in the nociceptors should lead to relief of the ongoing pain and the pain to light touch (Fig. 1.18). For SMP, procedures that reduce or eliminate the excitation of the alpha$_1$-receptor will be successful. An anaesthetic block of the sympathetic ganglia is effective because it eliminates the efferent drive. Topical application of clonidine is effective because it activates the alpha$_2$-autoreceptor which reduces the release of norepinephrine from the sympathetic terminals. Systemic phentolamine, phenoxybenzamine, and prazocin are alpha-adrenergic receptor antagonists and therefore block the activation of the nociceptors. Intravenous regional guanethidine eliminates the norepinephrine stores in the sympathetic terminals.

Nociceptors normally do not respond to sympathetic stimulation (Shea & Perl 1985b; Roberts & Elardo 1985a, 1985b; Barasi & Lynn 1986). After axotomy however, some fibres that innervate the resulting neuroma respond to local catechol application and to sympathetic stimulation (Wall & Gutnick 1974; Devor & Jänig 1981; Scadding 1981; Häbler et al 1987). Some investigators have noted that intact nociceptors may have or acquire catechol sensitivity (Kieschke et al 1988). Inflammation may also lead to catechol sensitization (Sanjue & Jun 1989: Sato et al 1992).

After partial nerve section, many of the remaining intact nociceptive fibres develop sensitivity to sympathetic stimulation (Sato & Perl 1991). Notably, these effects are antagonized by the alpha$_2$-antagonists, yohimbine and rauwolscine. These observations, though in agreement with the above observations that the sympathetic-adrenergic interactions are mediated via an alpha receptor, are at odds with clinical observations that the alpha$_1$-receptor is the culprit in SMP. Further work will be necessary to determine the mechanism for catechol sensitization and to determine the receptor subtype responsible for this interaction.

CHEMICAL SENSITIVITY OF NOCICEPTORS

Injury results in the local release of numerous chemicals which mediate or facilitate the inflammatory process. These include bradykinin, prostaglandins, leukotrienes, serotonin, histamine, substance P, thromboxanes, platelet activating factor, protons, and free radicals. Some of these chemicals activate nociceptors and therefore are directly involved in producing pain, while others lead to a sensitization of the nociceptor response to natural stimuli and therefore play a role in primary hyperalgesia.

BRADYKININ

Bradykinin is released upon tissue injury and is present in inflammatory exudates (Melmon et al 1967; Rocha e Silva

& Rosenthal 1961; DiRosa et al 1971). Bradykinin has been shown to produce pain in man when given intradermally, intraarterially or intraperitoneally (Cormia & Dougherty 1960; Guzman et al 1962; Coffman 1966; Lim et al 1967; Ferreira et al 1971; Ferreira 1983; Manning et al 1991). As illustrated in Figure 1.19A, intradermal injection of bradykinin produces hyperalgesia to heat stimuli (Manning et al 1991).

Administration of bradykinin in the region of the receptive field of unmyelinated and myelinated nociceptors results in an evoked response in the fibres (Beck & Handwerker 1974; Handwerker 1976a, 1976b; Lang et al 1990; Mizumura et al 1990; Khan et al 1992). A pronounced tachyphylaxis of the evoked response is observed following repeated presentations of bradykinin. As illustrated in Figure 1.19B, bradykinin administration leads to a transient sensitization of the response of nociceptors to heat stimuli (Kumazawa et al 1991; Khan et al 1992; Koltzenburg et al 1992a) that correlates with the transient hyperalgesia to heat observed in humans.

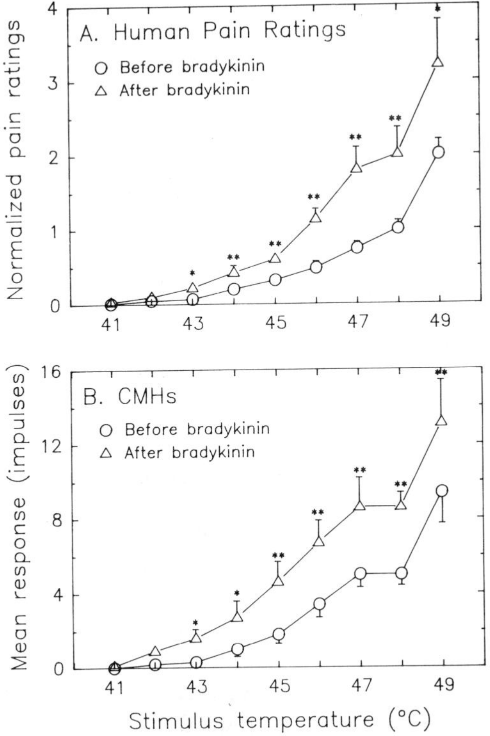

Fig. 1.19 Intradermal injection of bradykinin leads to hyperalgesia to heat in human subjects and sensitization to heat in CMH receptors of monkey. Heat testing was done before and after intradermal injection of bradykinin (10 nmol in 10 μl). The heat sequence described in Figure 1.6 was used. **A** Bradykinin produces hyperalgesia to heat stimuli in human subjects. Pain ratings to heat stimuli presented to the volar forearm were obtained before and after injections of bradykinin (n = 22, adapted from Manning et al 1991 with permission). **B** Bradykinin produces sensitization to heat of CMHs in monkey (n = 10, adapted from Khan et al 1992 with permission).

PROTONS

The low pH levels found in inflamed tissues have led to the hypothesis that local acidosis may contribute to the pain and hyperalgesia associated with inflammation. Continuous administration of low pH solutions causes pain and hyperalgesia to mechanical stimuli (Steen & Reeh 1992). This correlates with the recent observation that protons selectively activate nociceptors and produce a sensitization of nociceptors to mechanical stimuli (Steen et al 1992).

SEROTONIN

Mast cells, upon degranulation, release platelet activating factor which in turn leads to serotonin release from platelets. Serotonin causes pain when applied to a human blister base (Richardson & Engel 1986) and can activate nociceptors (Fock & Mense 1976; Lang et al 1990). Serotonin can also potentiate the pain induced by bradykinin (Sicuteri et al 1965; Fock & Mense 1976; Richardson & Engel 1986) and enhance the response of nociceptors to bradykinin (Fjallbrant & Iggo 1961; Hiss & Mense 1976; Nakano & Taira 1976; Mense 1981; Lang et al 1990).

HISTAMINE

Substance P released from nociceptor terminals can cause the release of histamine from mast cells. Histamine can lead to a variety of responses, including vasodilation and oedema. The role of histamine in pain sensation is unclear, since application of exogenous histamine to the skin produces itch and not pain sensations (Simone et al 1991a).

ARACHIDONIC ACID METABOLITES

The prostaglandins, thromboxanes and leukotrienes are a large family of arachidonic acid metabolites collectively known as eicosanoids. The eicosanoids are generally considered not to activate nociceptors directly, but rather to sensitize the nociceptors to natural stimuli and other endogenous chemicals (Ferreira et al 1974). This sensitizing effect of eicosanoids may play an important role in hyperalgesia associated with inflammation.

Inhibition of prostaglandin production by administration of cyclooxygenase inhibitors decreases pain associated with inflammation. Of the different prostaglandins, PGI_2, PGE_1, PGE_2, and PGD_2 are most likely to have a role in inflammatory pain. Of the leukotrienes (metabolites of the lipoxygenase pathway), LTD_4 and LTB_4 have been suggested to play a role in hyperalgesia (Levine et al 1984b; Denzlinger et al 1985; Bisgaard & Kristensen 1985).

MOLECULAR MECHANISMS OF CHEMICAL EXCITATION

Chemicals act on endings of nociceptive afferents by altering the conductance of membrane channels (Rang et al 1991). Some chemicals act on membrane receptors that are directly linked to ion channels to cause membrane depolarization. For example, serotonin, ATP, and capsaicin are thought to act through receptor-gated ion channels. Other chemicals act indirectly through membrane receptors that are linked to intracellular, second-messenger systems. For example, activation of the bradykinin receptor results in activation of phospholipase C which stimulates production of diacylglycerol. This leads to the activation of protein kinase C which opens a membrane cation channel leading to membrane depolarization.

EFFERENT FUNCTIONS OF NOCICEPTORS

Cutaneous nerves have more than a fourfold higher number of small diameter Aδ- and C-fibres than the larger, myelinated Aβ-fibres (Ochoa & Mair 1969). Why does the rarely activated nociceptive system require many more signal lines than the mechanoreceptor system that provides information for the more commonly utilized and complex tactile detection system? A possible explanation is that nociceptors, apart from signalling pain, serve other regulatory and trophic functions (Kruger 1988; McMahon & Koltzenburg 1990). An efferent role for nociceptors was suggested years ago by Lewis (1937) to account for the flare that surrounds an acute injury. Experimental evidence suggests that small-diameter afferent fibres may have several effector functions such as regulation of blood flow and vascular permeability in somatic and visceral tissues; trophic functions, such as maintenance and repair of skin integrity; and immunological processes, such as emigration of leucocytes at sites of tissue injury (Nilsson et al 1985; Kjartansson et al 1987). Afferent fibres are also considered to play a role in the regulation of activity of autonomic ganglia and visceral smooth muscles (for reviews see Szolcsányi 1984; Holzer 1988; Maggi & Meli 1988).

Antidromic stimulation of dorsal roots induces plasma extravasation, not only in cutaneous tissues, but also in a wide variety of internal organs (Szolcsányi 1988). The principal lines of evidence indicating that afferent neurons are involved in antidromic vasodilation, neurogenic inflammation and axon reflex flare are:

1. The responses are abolished by surgical or chemical ablation (e.g. with capsaicin) of the sensory innervation of the involved tissues (Jansco et al 1977; Lembeck & Holzer 1979; Gamse et al 1980; Carpenter & Lynn 1981; Szolcsányi 1988).
2. The responses occur independently of the autonomic nervous system (Couture et al 1985; Blumberg & Wallin 1987).

The fibres involved in the reflex vasodilation are polymodal nociceptive C-fibres that are capsaicin-sensitive (Jansco et al 1967, 1968). Low-firing frequencies (<1 Hz) in C-fibres can generate significant vasodilation (Lynn & Shakhanbeh 1988). Recent reports indicate that stimulation of Aδ-fibres may also result in a flare response (Jänig & Lisney 1989).

Several lines of evidence indicate that the mechanism for flare is different from the mechanisms for pain. First the size of the flare does not correlate with the intensity of pain induced by the stimulus. For example, the area of flare is much greater around an injection of histamine in comparison to the flare induced by an equally painful heat stimulus (Treede 1992). In man, observations that low firing frequencies of nociceptors may not be associated with any conscious sensation (Gybels et al 1979) may offer an explanation for flare not always being associated with pain. Secondly, strong mechanical stimulation adequate to excite most polymodal C-fibres does not cause neurogenic vasodilation (Lynn & Cotsell 1992). Thus, flare and pain may represent two different aspects of cutaneous small fibre function.

Flare is thought to be due to a peripheral axon reflex. Activation of one branch of a nociceptive receptor by a noxious stimulus results in the antidromic invasion of action potentials into adjacent branches of the nociceptor which, in turn, causes the release of vasoactive substances from the terminals of the nociceptor. However, the extent of the flare far exceeds the receptive field size of conventional nociceptors (Beitel & Dubner 1976; Kumazawa & Perl 1977; Campbell & Meyer 1983; Raja et al 1984; Treede et al 1990b). Possible explanations for this discrepancy might include the following (Fig. 1.20):

1. Flare is mediated by a subpopulation of chemosensitive nociceptive fibres with large receptive fields (Fig. 1.20A, Lewis 1937). Some C-fibres with large, complex receptive fields have been reported (Meyer et al 1991). Recent observations on the time course of spread of flare from the stimulus site, however, suggest that the spread is too slow to be accounted for by conduction within terminal arborizations of single afferent neurons (Lynn & Cotsell 1992).
2. Axo-axonal coupling between small fibres may be responsible for the spread of the flare reaction (Fig. 1.20B, Mathews 1976; Meyer et al 1985b).
3. Flare results from spreading depolarization along adjacent nociceptive terminals via a daisy-chain cascade mechanism (Fig. 1.20C, Lembeck & Gamse 1982).

Anatomical, immunological and histochemical studies have revealed the presence of several peptides in sensory neurons and their peripheral and central projections.

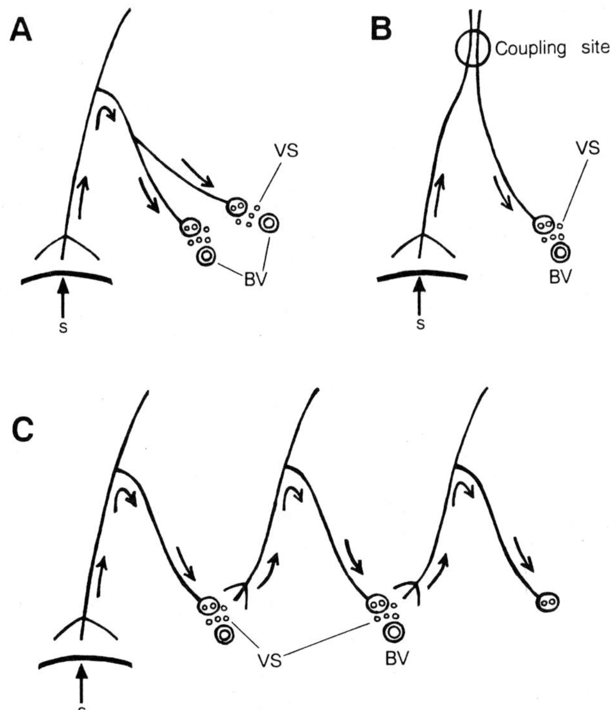

Fig. 1.20 Schematic models for possible mechanisms of flare mediated by primary afferent fibres. **A** Activation of one branch of a nociceptor leads to antidromic invasion of action potentials into adjacent branches that leads to release of vasoactive substances (VS). **B** Nociceptors are coupled to other fibres which release vasoactive substances. **C** A chemical cascade exists whereby substances released by one nociceptor cause vasodilation as well as activation of adjacent nociceptors which leads in turn to a spread of the flare. (BV = blood vessel, S = stimulus that evokes a flare response.)

These peptides include substance P and other tachykinins, such as neurokinins A and K, calcitonin-gene-related peptide (CGRP), somatostatin and vasoactive intestinal polypeptide (Lembeck & Gamse 1982; Holzer 1988; Micevych & Kruger 1992). The presence and release of tachykinins such as substance P from capsaicin-sensitive sensory nerve endings and their ability to induce many of the signs of acute inflammation, including vasodilation and plasma extravasation, indicate that tachykinins are the principal mediators of neurogenic inflammation and axon reflex flare (Saria 1984; Helme et al 1986). The vasodilation induced by substance P may be, at least in part, an indirect effect related to histamine release from mast cells (Hagermark et al 1978; Barnes et al 1986; Ebertz et al 1987). CGRP also has potent and prolonged vasodilator properties in humans and may be one of the mediators of neurogenic vasodilation, possibly playing a role in long-term vascular responses to injury (Levine et al 1984a; Brain et al 1985, 1986; Piotrowski & Foreman 1986; Pedersen-Bjergaard et al 1991).

Substance P, neurokinin A, and CGRP are also released from trigeminovascular axons in the pial and dural circulations, resulting in vasodilation and plasma extravasation (Moskowitz et al 1983, 1989). This release of vasoactive neuropeptides from perivascular sensory nerves via axon reflex-like mechanisms may play an important role in the pathophysiology of vascular headache and cerebral hyperperfusion syndromes (Macfarlane et al 1991; Moskowitz 1991).

Szolcsányi and coworkers (Szolcsányi 1988) propose that single nociceptor terminals may possess a dual sensory and efferent function. The mediator release mechanism is resistant to blockade by local anaesthetics and tetrodotoxin, suggesting that propagating action potentials are not essential.

NEURAL MECHANISMS OF ITCH

Itch is the common sensory phenomenon associated with the desire to scratch. Like pain, itch can be produced by chemical, mechanical, thermal or electrical stimuli. However, itch differs from pain in that itch can be evoked only from the superficial layers of skin, mucosa, and conjunctiva, and not from deep tissues. In addition, itch and pain usually do not occur simultaneously from the same skin region and, in fact, mild painful stimuli (e.g. scratching) are effective in abolishing itch.

Itch appears to be signalled in the periphery by activity in unmyelinated and perhaps thinly myelinated fibres:

1. Itch persists during a selective block of A-fibre function (Bickford 1938; Handwerker et al 1987).
2. Electrical stimulation of itch spots produces itch at a long latency consistent with conduction in C-fibres (Arthur & Shelley 1959).
3. Intraneural microstimulation of identified C-fiber receptors leads to the perception of itch (Torebjörk & Ochoa 1981).
4. Topical application of capsaicin, which desensitizes receptors of unmyelinated fibres, leads to a decrease in itch sensitivity (Toth-Kasa et al 1986; Handwerker et al 1987; Simone & Ochoa 1991).

The neural basis for itch sensation is not well understood. A number of different theories have been proposed including the three summarized below (McMahon & Koltzenburg 1992):

1. *Specificity theory.* According to the specificity theory, a group of afferents exists that responds specifically to pruritic substances. Activation of this labelled line then leads to itch sensation. A small percentage of C-fibre receptors responds to pruritic substances such as histamine (Khan et al 1987; Handwerker 1992). However, these histamine-sensitive receptors also respond to algesic substances (e.g. mustard oil) and other noxious stimuli (Tuckett & Wei 1987; Handwerker et al 1991a) and, thus, are polymodal receptors similar to typical nociceptors decribed above. Whether some mechanically insensitive

afferents (see section on MIAs above) respond specifically to pruritic substances has not been determined yet. Since itch can be produced by mechanical and heat stimuli, it is reasonable to expect that 'itch receptors' are polymodal in nature.

2. *Pattern theory.* According to the pattern theory, the temporal pattern of neural activity in nociceptors is used to distinguish between itch and pain. One possibility is that itch is perceived at low levels of nociceptor activity and pain is perceived at higher levels of nociceptor activity. However, this possibility seems unlikely since electrical stimulation of itch spots produces itch at a low stimulation frequency which becomes intense itch, but not pain, at higher frequencies of stimulation (Tuckett 1982). Similarly, intrafascicular electrical stimulation of presumed single C-fibre afferents in humans could produce pure itch sensation which did not become pain at higher stimulus frequencies (Torebjörk & Ochoa 1981).

3. *Central processing theory.* According to this theory, pruritic and noxious stimuli excite a largely overlapping population of primary afferent nociceptors, and the perception of itch or pain depends on central processing. One possibility is that pruritic stimuli result in activation of one subpopulation of central neurons whereas noxious stimuli activate another (Fig. 1.21). Another possibility is that noxious stimuli result in an inhibition of activity in the subpopulation that is activated by pruritic stimuli.

Pruritic stimuli may also lead to 'itchy skin' in the region surrounding the stimulus site where mechanical stimuli elicit the sensation of itch (Bickford 1938). This is analogous to the region of secondary hyperalgesia to mechanical stimuli that surrounds a noxious stimulus. This area of itchy skin appears to be due to an alteration in

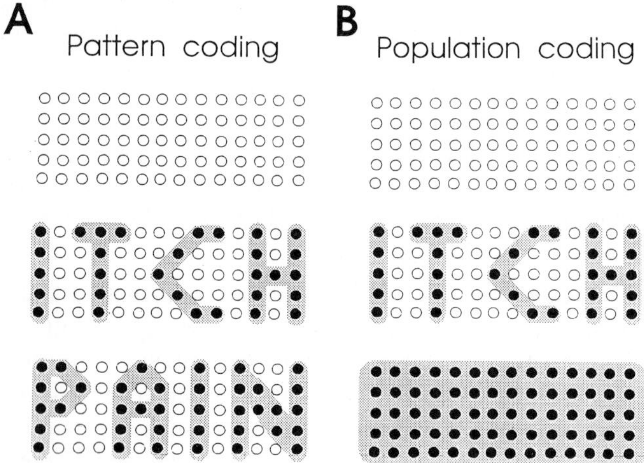

Fig. 1.21 Schematic illustrations of how a differential response of different populations of central neurons could explain itch and pain sensation. Open circles represent inactive cells and filled circles represent excited neurons. Top panels: no pain or itch sensation. Middle panels: itch sensation. Bottom panels: pain sensation. (From McMahon & Koltzenburg 1993 with permission.)

central processing such that tactile stimuli are able to activate central neurons responsible for itch (Simone et al 1991a; LaMotte 1992).

The sense of prickle is often confused with itch. Prickle also appears to be signalled by activity in nociceptors. When wool fabrics that were rated by human subjects as slightly prickly to very prickly were applied to the receptive fields of primary afferents, the response of nociceptors increased with the prickliness of the fabric whereas the response of low-threshold mechanoreceptors was independent of the prickliness of the fabric (Garnsworthy et al 1988).

NOCICEPTORS IN TISSUES OTHER THAN SKIN

As understanding of nociception has advanced in studies of the skin, increased attention has turned to other organs. Psychophysical correlations with physiological studies of nociceptor function in organs other than the skin, however, have proved difficult. In deeper tissues, the demonstration that a receptor has a high threshold does not necessarily mean that it signals pain. Receptive properties of afferents are dependent on the properties of the tissues in which they are embedded. Differences in receptor sensitivity reflect, in part, variations in the position of the transducing element within the tissue with respect to the experimental stimulus.

For many tissues (e.g. tooth pulp and cornea), only pain sensations can be evoked. Thus, the afferent fibres probably signal pain. For other deep tissues, such as muscle, fascia, joints, bone, vascular structures and viscera, multifarious perceptual possibilities complicate analysis. Some afferent fibres may be important in normal organ function without being involved in conscious sensation. Others may be involved in sensations other than pain.

While studies on somatic afferents have provided considerable support for the specificity theory of pain, the mode of encoding noxious events by visceral afferents has remained controversial (Cervero & Jänig 1992). Behavioural and clinical studies indicate that there are important differences between cutaneous and deep pain. For example, unlike cutaneous pain, deep pain is diffuse and poorly localized. Deep pain may be associated with strong autonomic responses such as sweating and changes in heart rate, blood pressure and respiration. In addition, deep pain may be produced by stimuli that are not tissue damaging, e.g. distension of bowel and bladder (Dubner 1991; Ness & Gebhart 1990). Finally, visceral pains may be associated with referred pain as well as cutaneous and deep tissue hyperalgesia. Recently, there has been a renewed interest in understanding the neurobiological basis of pain associated with deep tissues. A detailed discussion of the physiological mechanisms of pain originating from visceral tissues is beyond the scope of this chapter, and the reader is referred to comprehensive reviews (Ness & Gebhart 1990; Meller & Gebhart 1992).

CORNEA

Though threshold for activation serves as a reasonable criterion to distinguish nociceptors from other afferent fibre types in the skin, the cornea illustrates the problem with use of this criterion alone for other tissue types. The mean threshold for activation of primary afferent fibres that innervate the cornea is comparable to the threshold for activation of low-threshold mechanoreceptors in the skin (Belmonte & Giraldez 1981; Tanelian & Beuerman 1984). It is likely, however, that mild stimuli may injure the cornea, and it is certainly clear that low intensity stimuli to the cornea induce pain. Thus, it is reasonable to label the afferent fibres that innervate the cornea nociceptors, since, in the spirit of Sherrington's original usage, these receptors are concerned with the detection of injury. The lesson for study of other tissues, where psychophysical data are sparse, is clear. Threshold for activation is a precarious parameter by which to judge a receptor or a nociceptor.

Although pain is generally thought to be the only sensation that can be elicited from stimulation of the cornea, some studies have suggested that thermal and mechanical stimuli can be differentiated (Lele & Weddell 1959; Kenshalo 1960; Beuerman & Tanelian 1979). There are no obvious specialized sense organs. Sensory terminals end in the intraepithelial tissue as unmyelinated fibres. The innervation density is 300–600 times that of the skin (Rozsa & Beuerman 1982). The mechanical receptive fields of the nociceptors are uniformly sensitive and broad, covering as much as 20% of the corneal surface.

TOOTH PULP AND PERIODONTAL LIGAMENT

Though it is disputed whether pain is the only sensation evoked by stimulation of the tooth pulp, certainly pain is the predominant sensation. The tooth pulp and dentin are innervated by Aδ- and C-fibres (Harris & Griffin 1968; Byers 1984) that form an interlacing network, the subodontoblastic plexus. From this plexus, nerve fibres extend to the odontoblastic layer, predentin, and dentin and terminate as free nerve endings. The sensory receptors respond to chemical, thermal and mechanical stimuli and thus are polymodal (Funakoshi & Zotterman 1963; Haegerstam et al 1975; Mathews 1977; Dubner 1978). Single fibre recordings suggest that Aδ-fibres, but not C-fibres, respond to stimuli associated with cavity preparation, such as drilling, desiccation or scraping of dentin (Narhi et al 1982). Pulpal C-fibres respond to gradual warming of the tooth to noxious temperatures. Thus, it appears that Aδ-fibres are responsible for dentinal pain, whereas C-fibres may respond to pain originating from the pulp (Narhi 1985a, 1985b; Trowbridge 1985). Recent studies indicate that periodontal C-fibres are predominantly nociceptive, and the polymodal response characteristics of most of these fibres are similar to the response characteristics of pulpal C-fibres (Jyväsjärvi & Kniffki 1989; Mengel et al 1992).

MUSCLE

Muscle pain is a frequently experienced sensation that occurs after strenuous exercise, direct trauma, inflammation and during sustained muscular contractions (for recent reviews, see Mense 1990, 1991). Torebjörk et al (1984) demonstrated with electrical stimulation of nerve fascicles in awake humans that deep muscle pain is dependent on activation of small-diameter afferent fibres. It has been observed that pain can be produced by noxious stimulation of muscle, fascia and tendons. The many free nerve endings found in the connective tissue of the muscle, between muscle fibres, in blood vessel walls and in tendons are thought to be the receptors for the muscle's nociceptive afferent fibres.

The small myelinated afferent fibres found in muscle are labelled group III fibres and have conduction velocities from 2.5–20 m/s (Paintal 1960). The unmyelinated fibres are termed group IV fibres and have conduction velocities less than 2.5 m/s (Mense & Schmidt 1974; Fock & Mense 1976; Hiss & Mense 1976). Of all the group III and IV fibres, 40% are thought to be nociceptors. Another 20% are contraction-sensitive and are thought to be involved in the cardiopulmonary adjustments that occur during exercise (Hnik et al 1969; McCloskey & Mitchell 1972). Approximately 30% are low-threshold mechanoreceptors and may signal deep pressure sensations. The final 10% are thermally responsive and may be involved in thermoregulation (Mense & Meyer 1985).

In several species, the group III and IV muscle afferent fibres have been characterized by their vigorous response to endogenous substances such as bradykinin, serotonin, histamine and potassium. In contrast, muscle spindles and tendon organs do not exhibit comparable responses (Paintal 1960; Kumazawa & Mizumura 1976; Mense 1977). Fibres responsive to bradykinin have also been observed to be selectively sensitive to high intensity mechanical stimuli (Paintal 1961). In addition, muscle nociceptors may be sensitized by catecholamines (Kieschke et al 1988) and by changes in the biochemical environment resulting from hypoxia and impaired metabolism. Sensitization of muscle nociceptors by the release of endogenous chemicals may explain the local tenderness often associated with muscle trauma or unaccustomed exercise.

JOINT

Much of what is known about joint afferent fibres is based on studies in cat (for reviews see Guilbaud 1988; Schaible et al 1989; Sessle & Hu 1991). Nerve fibre counts in the articular nerves of the knee reveal that the afferent fibres are predominantly group III (thinly myelinated) and group IV (unmyelinated) (Skoglund 1956; Freeman & Wyke 1967; Langford & Schmidt 1983). Nociceptors in the joint are located in the joint capsule and ligaments, bone, periosteum, articular fat pads and perivascular sites, but probably not in the joint cartilage. The sensory endings of the group III and IV nerve fibres lack a myelin sheath and are not surrounded by perineurium. The branched, terminal trees of these fibres have a string-of-beads appearance that may represent multiple receptive sites in the nerve endings (Heppelman et al 1990). At the sites of the axonal beads, a large proportion of the axolemma is devoid of a Schwann cell covering, and the axon fibre has a number of vesicles (Fig. 1.22).

Based on their sensitivities to pressure and joint movements, afferent fibres of the knee joint have been classified under five categories:

1. & 2. Low-threshold units that are excited strongly or weakly, respectively, by innocuous pressure and movements of the knee joint.
3. High-threshold units that are activated only by noxious pressure or movements exceeding the working range of the joint.
4. Units that respond to strong pressure to the knee, but not to movement.
5. Units that do not react to any mechanical stimulus to the normal joint, referred to as 'silent nociceptors' (Schaible & Schmidt 1988a).

It is suggested that, in the normal joint, the high-threshold units signal pain evoked by extreme joint movement (Schaible & Schmidt 1983a, 1983b; Grigg et al 1986).

Experimentally-induced arthritis is associated with dramatic changes in the response properties of joint afferents (Heppelman et al 1985; Schaible & Schmidt 1985; Heppelman et al 1987). Sensitization is observed in all types of afferent fibres. This sensitization may take the form of afferent activation by movements in the working range, activation by pressure, or an induction or increase in resting discharges. Of particular interest is the sensitization of fibres in categories 4 and 5 that were initially insensitive to joint movements. Sensitization in these fibres occurs in the second to third hour after injection of the inflammatory compounds, a time course that matches the behavioural changes in test animals (Schaible & Schmidt 1988a; Neugebauer & Schaible 1988). Chemical mediators of inflammation, such as bradykinin, prostaglandins, leukotrienes, potassium ions, serotonin and possibly interleukins, are considered to play an important role in the sensitization of joint afferent fibres (Heppelman et al 1985; Schaible & Schmidt 1988b; Herbert & Schmidt 1992). This inflammation-induced sensitization of articular afferents is likely to contribute to the enhanced pain that accompanies arthritis. Studies by Levine and coworkers have suggested that substances such as substance P released from the peripheral terminals of small diameter afferent fibres (see section on efferent functions of nociceptors) may contribute to the severity of joint injury (Levine et al 1984a, 1985). Articular tissues are also innervated by sympathetic efferents, and a modulatory role for these fibres via a prostaglandin-mediated mechanism has been suggested in arthritis (see Basbaum & Levine 1991 for review).

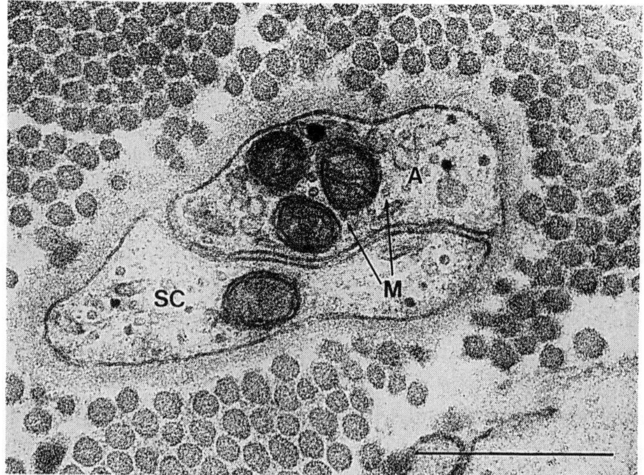

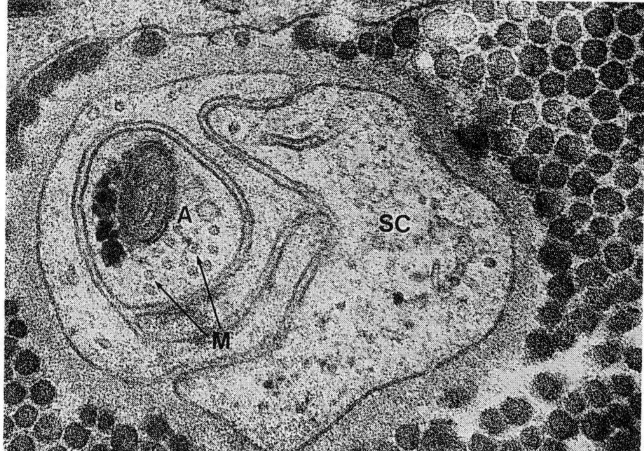

Fig. 1.22 Electron micrographs of sensory endings of group IV nerve endings in the knee joint capsule. Top: cross section of the nerve fibre at the site of an axonal bead showing mitochondria, glycogen particles and vesicles. The major part of the axolemma is devoid of Schwann cell covering and directly abuts the basal lamina. Bottom: section close to a waist-like region of the nerve fibre about 47 μm distant from top section. At this level the axon is completely wrapped by Schwann cell lamellae. (A = sensory axon; SC = Schwann cell; M = microtubules; × 93 000; Bar = 0.5 μm.) (From Heppelman et al 1990 with permission.)

THE RESPIRATORY SYSTEM

A large percentage of mucosal sensory C-fibres have the characteristic attributes of cutaneous polymodal nociceptors, except that they also respond to air-borne stimuli. A large percentage of the myelinated laryngeal afferent fibres are pressure sensitive and respond to irritant gases. Their role in sensation is not known. Unmyelinated afferent fibres that innervate the larynx have not been well studied (for reviews, see Coleridge & Coleridge 1984; Paintal 1986; Widdicombe 1986; Martling 1987).

Three main groups of receptors have been characterized which innervate the tracheobronchial tree and lungs:

1. Slowly-adapting stretch receptors are localized in airway smooth muscle and are involved in reflexes. Their activity does not appear to reach consciousness.
2. The rapidly-adapting 'irritant' stretch receptors respond to inflation and deflation of the airways and lungs. They are also sensitive to inhaled dusts and irritant chemicals. Like cutaneous polymodal receptors these receptors are also stimulated by a number of chemical mediators such as histamine, serotonin, and acetylcholine. Prostaglandin $F_2\alpha$ and E_2 potentiate mechanical responsiveness. The discharge and sensitivity of these receptors are increased in a number of pathological conditions.
3. The C-fibre receptors first studied by Paintal (1955) and termed J receptors have many properties in common with the rapidly adapting mechanoreceptors. They have little tonic discharge normally and are stimulated or sensitized in a variety of lung conditions such as congestion, lung oedema and pneumonia. These receptors are activated by endogenous chemical mediators and are also activated by some inhaled gases. The evidence that unpleasant sensations are derived from these lung receptors is circumspect. The burning sensation produced by an endotracheal/bronchial catheter can be abolished by vagal block (Klassen et al 1951). Certain conditions, such as pulmonary congestion, intravascular injection of lobeline (nicotinic ganglionic agonist), and rigorous physical exercise, strongly excite lung C-fibre receptors in animals. A subpopulation of afferent fibres in the lung that are activated by capsaicin contain neuropeptides of the tachykinin family (substance P, neurokinin A and neuropeptide K) as well as CGRP (Lundberg & Saria 1987). The release of the neuropeptides induces protein extravasation, increases local blood flow and causes bronchoconstriction (Martling 1987).

THE CARDIOVASCULAR SYSTEM

Puncture of the arterial wall in humans induces pain. The neural apparatus for this effect probably resides in the nervi-vasorum, but to date these receptors have been little studied. Psychophysical studies (Arndt & Klement 1991) have been performed by applying noxious stimuli to isolated vein segments in human subjects. Osmotic, stretching, cold and heat stimuli evoke similar sensations. This suggests that the venous wall is invested with polymodal nociceptive fibres.

Pain from endogenous or exogenous stimulation of the heart usually occurs only under certain pathological conditions. It is unclear whether pain from the heart is signalled by sympathetic afferent fibres or the parasympathetic afferent fibres in the vagus nerve (Coleridge & Coleridge 1980, 1981; Baker et al 1980; Kaufman et al 1980; Malliani et al 1986). Traditionally, the sympathetic afferents are considered to be solely responsible for signalling pain arising from the heart. Based on an extensive review of the literature, Meller & Gebhart (1992) propose that vagal afferents may also contribute to pain associated with myocardial ischemia. Many sympathetic afferent nerve fibres innervating the heart respond to bradykinin (Baker et al 1980; Lombardi et al 1981). However, there is conflicting evidence as to whether bradykinin causes pain when injected into coronary arteries (Malliani et al 1984; Pagani et al 1985). Other chemical mediators of cardiac pain may include serotonin (Takahashi 1985; James et al 1988), adenosine (Sylvén et al 1986a, 1986b; Crea et al 1990), histamine (Guzman et al 1962), prostaglandins, lactate, and potassium (for reviews see Sylvén 1989; Meller & Gebhart 1992).

THE DIGESTIVE SYSTEM

Progress in understanding visceral pain from the gastrointestinal tract has been limited by the lack of an agreement on an adequate noxious, visceral stimulus. Recent studies have demonstrated that colorectal distension is a reliable noxious visceral stimulus that induces pain in humans (Ness & Gebhart 1988; Ness et al 1990).

Clinically, visceral pain of reflux oesophagitis may mimic angina pectoris, as the pain is often referred to the same somatic regions (Lee et al 1985; Richter et al 1989). A likely explanation for the above clinical phenomenon is the recent observations that the somatic input from the upper thoracic dermatomes and the visceral inputs from the distal oesophagus and the heart converge on the same spinal neurons (Garrison et al 1992).

Afferent fibres that serve the digestive system are, as with the heart, found in conjunction with the motor fibres of both the sympathetic and parasympathetic systems. Afferent fibres that course with the vagus nerve are known to be responsible for nociceptive reactions to stimuli applied to the upper oesophagus and for certain forms of gastrointestinal discomfort associated with ulcers (Mei 1983). Pain of lower oesophageal and intestinal origin is usually signalled by afferent fibres in the thoracic sympathetic chain or the splanchnic nerves (Sengupta et al 1990). Visceral afferents from the lower oesophagus are either rapidly adapting, slowly adapting or have a slow adaptation with an after discharge to a sustained distension (Sengupta et al 1990). Studies on the distal oesophagus indicate that the inflamed gut is more sensitive to distension than a noninflamed viscera (Garrison et al 1992).

The majority of the visceral afferent fibres from the colon and rectum are Aδ- and C-fibres that course with the parasympathetic nerves (Vera & Nadelhaft 1990b). Many of these afferent fibres respond to non-noxious stimulation and also have a monotonically increasing response to stimuli in the noxious range (Blumberg et al 1983; Cervero & Sharkey 1988; Jänig & Koltzenburg 1991a).

Functionally different subpopulations of primary afferents that innervate the colon and anal canal have been described (Blumberg et al 1983; Jänig & Koltzenburg 1991a). Afferent fibres in the digestive system can be subdivided into those with specific properties, such as digestive chemoreceptors, thermoreceptors, and low-threshold mechanoreceptors, and those with polymodal sensitivity. Except for the mesenteric Pacinian corpuscles, the remainder of the Aδ- and C-fibre mechanoreceptors have slowly adapting properties (Morrison 1977; Bahns et al 1986). Haupt et al (1983) demonstrated that ischaemia of the colon excites afferent fibres that also respond to distention and to bradykinin. Cervero (1982, 1983) identified a group of units in the ferret that innervate the bile duct and respond preferentially to high luminal pressure. More recent studies have identified a large number of unmyelinated afferent fibres from the colon that are not activated by innocuous and noxious mechanical stimulation. It has been speculated that these fibres are the visceral counterparts of the 'silent nociceptors' described in somatic structures (Jänig & Koltzenburg 1991a).

Detailed anatomical studies have demonstrated important differences in the distribution of central terminals of visceral and somatic primary afferent fibres (Sugiura et al 1989). For example, in the guinea pig the terminal branches of somatic C-fibre afferents are circumscribed extending about 400 μm rostrocaudally and 100 μm mediolaterally. However, visceral C-fibres have many terminal regions extending over several spinal segments. The extensive rostrocaudal distribution of the visceral C-fibre afferents may provide the basis for the diffuse nature of visceral pain from the gut.

THE UROGENITAL SYSTEM

The differences between mechanisms of nociception in the skin and viscera are emphasized by studies on the response properties of visceral afferents from the urinary tract. There is ongoing controversy as to whether visceral pain is mediated by a specific subgroup of nociceptive fibres (specificity theory) or by the spatial and temporal patterns of discharges in non-specific afferent fibres (pattern theory) (Jänig & Morrison 1986; Cervero 1988; Cervero & Jänig 1992). Two distinct groups of afferent fibres capable of signalling noxious stimuli have been identified in the urinary bladder. Most visceral afferents from the urinary bladder are unmyelinated fibres, although a population of myelinated Aδ- fibres is also present (Vera & Nadelhaft 1990a). The majority of visceral primary afferents from the bladder, urethra, and reproductive and other pelvic organs encode for both noxious and non-noxious stimuli (Bahns et al 1986, 1987; Berkley et al 1990; Häbler et al 1990). As shown in Figure 1.23, a subset of the unmyelinated fibres accurately encode intravesical pressure changes in the noxious range (Häbler et al 1990). In addition, a subpopulation of C-fibre visceral afferents has been identified that is not mechanically sensitive, but is excited by chemical irritants (Koltzenburg & McMahon 1986; Häbler et al 1988, 1990). Reflexes evoked by urinary bladder distention in rats are increased by mucosal inflammation. Thus, pain originating from the bladder may be intensified by the presence of inflammation (McMahon & Abel 1987; McMahon 1988; Häbler et al 1988, 1990).

Recent studies indicate that uterine afferent fibres are present both in the hypogastric and pelvic nerves. These fibres are capable of signalling information about temporal and spatial aspects of mechanical and chemical stimulation of the uterus (Floyd et al 1977; Berkley et al 1988, 1990). The afferents are mostly C-fibres, although Aδ-fibres are also present.

Free nerve endings derived from Aδ- or C-fibres are abundant throughout the glans penis (Johnson & Halata 1991). The two fibre types associated with these endings appear to be slowly adapting low-threshold stretch receptors and high-threshold mechanoreceptors (Kitchell et al 1982; Johnson & Kitchell 1987).

Kumazawa and colleagues (1986) studied the sensory innervation of the testes of the dog. More than 95% of the fibres of the superior spermatic nerve are unmyelinated with the great majority having polymodal properties (i.e. responding to mechanical, chemical and thermal stimuli). Responses of the polymodal receptor are augmented by application of prostaglandins E_2 and I_2 (Mizumura et al 1991) and of bradykinin acting via a B_2 receptor (Mizumura et al 1990). The prostaglandins are less potent in their ability to excite nociceptors as compared to their efficacy as potentiators of the response to bradykinin (Mizumura et al 1991). The effects of algesic substances on the testicular polymodal nociceptors may result from Ca^{2+} dependent membrane surface potential changes (Sato et al 1989).

BRAIN AND MENINGES

Clinically, headache and visceral pain have several common features; both are diffuse, poorly localized, and are often associated with intense autonomic responses. Considerable experimental evidence indicates that nociceptive information from cranial blood vessels, in particular the vessels within the dura mater and the

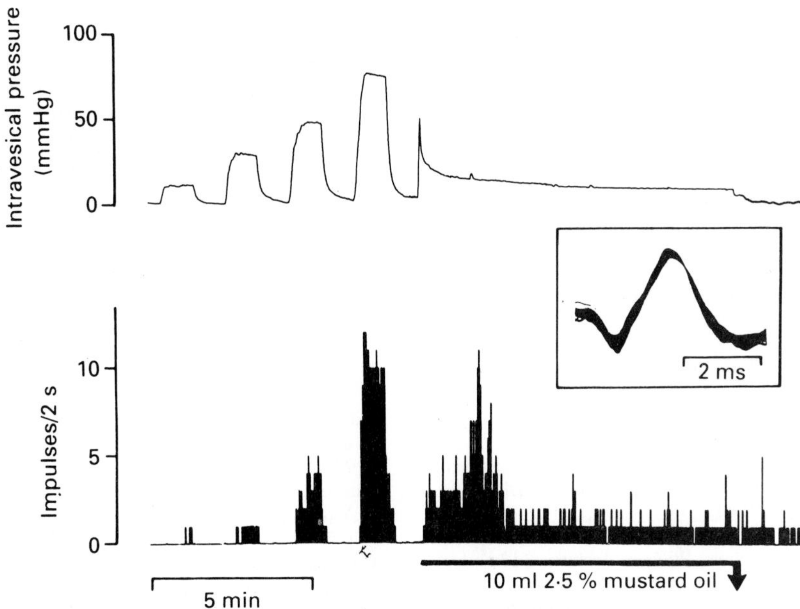

Fig. 1.23 Recordings from an unmyelinated afferent fibre from the urinary bladder. Top: pressure recordings from the lumen of the bladder in response to distension of the bladder with saline. Bottom: response of afferent fibre to increasing intravesicular pressures and to application of mustard oil. (From Häbler et al 1990 with permission.)

leptomeninges, play an important role in headache (for reviews, see Moskowitz et al 1989; Moskowitz 1991). The meningeal blood vessels are surrounded by a dense plexus of sensory axons emanating from the cells in the trigeminal ganglia and from the upper cervical dorsal root ganglia (Mayberg et al 1981; Arbab et al 1986). Each ganglion cell has divergent axon collaterals that innervate multiple large vessels supplying both brain parenchyma and the overlying dura mater (Arbab et al 1986; O'Connor & Van der Kooy 1986). The trigeminovascular nerves are predominantly C-fibres that have free nerve endings with vesicles. The vesicles contain several polypeptides, including substance P, neurokinin A, CGRP and galanin. Electrical stimulation of the trigeminal ganglia or infusion of tachykinins results in vasodilation and plasma protein leakage in rat dura mater (Markowitz et al 1987). Ergot alkaloids that are therapeutically useful in the management of vascular headaches may act by blockade of the small fibre mediated neurogenic inflammation in the dura mater (Saito et al 1988). Recent physiological studies also indicate that the trigeminovascular axons within the dura have $5HT_{1B/D}$-like receptors. Agonists of this receptor (e.g. sumatriptan) block neurogenic plasma extravasation and are clinically useful in the management of vascular headaches (Buzzi & Moskowitz 1990).

Anatomical studies have demonstrated that the pia mater covering the spinal cord and its roots has considerable unmyelinated fibre innervation. Little is known about the physiology of these primary afferent fibres innervating the spinal meninges. A recent report indicates that a subpopulation of unmyelinated fibres in the ventral root serves as primary afferent fibres innervating the root proper or its sheath (Jänig & Koltzenburg 1991b). These pial afferents have no resting discharges and appear to be maximally activated by noxious stimuli.

Acknowledgements

We appreciate the assistance of J. L. Turnquist and T. V. Hartke. This research was supported by NIH grants NS-14447 and NS-26363. R. A. Meyer was supported in part by the US Navy (N00039–92–C–0001).

REFERENCES

Adriaensen H, Gybels J, Handwerker H O, Van Hees J 1984a Suppression of C-fiber discharges upon repeated heat stimulation may explain characteristics of concomitant pain sensations. Brain Research 302: 203–211

Adriaensen H, Gybels J, Handwerker H O, Van Hees J 1984b Nociceptor discharges and sensations due to prolonged noxious mechanical stimulation—a paradox. Human Neurobiology 3: 53–58

Arbab M A R, Wiklund L, Svengaard N D 1986 The distribution of cerebral vascular innervation from superior cervical, trigeminal, and spinal ganglia investigated with retrograde and anterograde WGA-HRP tracing in the rat. Neuroscience 19: 695–708

Arndt J O, Klement W 1991 Pain evoked by polymodal stimulation of the hand veins in humans. Journal of Physiology (London) 440: 467–778

Arthur R P, Shelley W B 1959 The peripheral mechanisms of itch in man. In: Wolstenholme G E W, O'Connor M (eds) Pain and itch: nervous mechanisms. Little, Brown & Co., Boston

Bahns E, Ernsberger U, Jänig W, Nelke A 1986 Functional characteristics of lumbar visceral afferent fibres from the urinary bladder and the urethra in the cat. Pflügers Archives 407: 510–518

Bahns E, Halsband U, Jänig W 1987 Functional characteristics of sacral afferent fibres from the urinary bladder, urethra, colon, and anus. Pflügers Archives 410: 296–303

Baker D G, Coleridge H M, Coleridge J C G, Nerdrum T 1980 Search for a cardiac nociceptor: Stimulation by bradykinin of sympathetic afferent nerve endings in the heart of the cat. Journal of Physiology (London) 306: 519–536

Barasi S, Lynn B 1986 Effects of sympathetic stimulation on mechanoreceptive and nociceptive afferent units from the rabbit pinna. Brain Research 378: 21–27

Barnes P J, Brown M J, Dollery C T, Fuller R W, Heavey D J, Ind P W 1986 Histamine is released from skin by substance P but does not act as the final vasodilator in the axon reflex. British Journal of Pharmacology 88: 741–774

Basbaum A I, Levine J D 1991 The contribution of the nervous system to inflammation and inflammatory disease. Canadian Journal of Physiology and Pharmacology 69: 647–651

Beck P W, Handwerker H O 1974 Bradykinin and serotonin effects on various types of cutaneous nerve fibers. Pflügers Archives 347: 209–222

Beck P W, Handwerker H O, Zimmermann M 1974 Nervous outflow from the cat's foot during noxious radiant heat stimulation. Brain Research 67: 373–386

Beitel R E, Dubner R 1976 Response of unmyelinated (C) polymodal nociceptors to thermal stimuli applied to monkey's face. Journal of Neurophysiology 39: 1160–1175

Belmonte C, Giraldez F 1981 Responses of cat corneal sensory receptors to mechanical and thermal stimulation. Journal of Physiology (London) 321: 355–368

Belmonte C, Gallar J, Pozo M A, Rebollo I 1991 Excitation by irritant chemical substances of sensory afferent units in the cat's cornea. Journal of Physiology (London) 437: 709–725

Berkley K J, Robbins A, Sato Y 1988 Afferent fibers supplying the uterus in the rat. Journal of Neurophysiology 59: 142–163

Berkley K J, Hotta H, Robbins A, Sato Y 1990 Functional properties of afferent fibers supplying reproductive and other pelvic organs in pelvic nerve of female rat. Journal of Neurophysiology 63: 256–272

Bessou P, Perl E R 1969 Response of cutaneous sensory units with unmyelinated fibers to noxious stimuli. Journal of Neurophysiology 32: 1025–1043

Beuerman R W, Tanelian D L 1979 Corneal pain evoked by thermal stimulation. Pain 7: 1–14

Bickford R G 1938 Experiments relating to the itch sensation, its peripheral mechanism and central pathways. Clinical Science 3: 377–386

Bini G, Crucci G, Hagbarth K E, Schady W, Torebjörk E 1984 Analgesic effect of vibration and cooling on pain induced by intraneural electrical stimulation. Pain 18: 239–248

Bischoff A 1979 Congenital insensitivity to pain with anhidrosis. A morphometric study of sural nerve and cutaneous receptors in the human prepuce. In: Bonica J J, Liebeskind J C, Albe-Fessard D G (eds) Advances in pain research and therapy. Raven Press, New York, p 53–65

Bisgaard H, Kristensen J K 1985 Leukotriene B produces hyperalgesia in humans. Prostaglandins 30: 791–797

Blumberg H, Jänig W 1982 Activation of fibers via experimentally produced stump neuromas of skin nerves: Ephaptic transmission or retrograde sprouting. Experimental Neurology 76: 468–482

Blumberg H, Wallin B G 1987 Direct evidence of neurally mediated vasodilatation in hairy skin of the human foot. Journal of Physiology (London) 382: 105–121

Blumberg H, Haupt P, Jänig W, Kohler W 1983 Encoding of visceral noxious stimuli in the discharge patterns of visceral afferent fibres from the colon. Pflügers Archives 398: 33–40

Brain S D, Williams T J, Tippins J R, Morris H R, MacIntyre I 1985 Calcitonin gene related peptide is a potent vasodilator. Nature 313: 54–56

Brain S D, Tippins J R, Morris H R, MacIntyre I, Williams T 1986 Potent vasodilator activity of calcitonin gene-related peptide in human skin. Journal of Investigative Dermatology 87: 533–536

Burgess P R, Perl E R 1967 Myelinated afferent fibres responding specifically to noxious stimulation of the skin. Journal of Physiology (London) 190: 541–562

Burgess P R, Petit D, Warren R M 1968 Receptor types in cat hairy skin supplied by myelinated fibers. Journal of Neurophysiology 31: 833–848

Buzzi M G, Moskowitz M A 1990 The antimigraine drug, sumatriptan (GR43175), selectively blocks neurogenic plasma extravasation from blood vessels in dura mater. British Journal of Pharmacology 99: 202–206

Byers M R 1984 Dental sensory receptors. International Review of Neurobiology 25: 39–94

Campbell J N, Lamotte R H 1983 Latency to detection of first pain. Brain Research 266: 203–208

Campbell J N, Meyer R A 1983 Sensitization of unmyelinated nociceptive afferents in the monkey varies with skin type. Journal of Neurophysiology 49: 98–110

Campbell J N, Meyer R A 1986 Primary afferents and hyperalgesia. In: Yaksh T L (ed) Spinal afferent processing. Plenum Press, New York, p 59–81

Campbell J N, Meyer R A, LaMotte R H 1979 Sensitization of myelinated nociceptive afferents that innervate monkey hand. Journal of Neurophysiology 42: 1669–1679

Campbell J N, Khan A A, Meyer R A, Raja S N 1988 Responses to heat of C-fiber nociceptors in monkey are altered by injury in the receptive field but not by adjacent injury. Pain 32: 327–332

Carpenter S E, Lynn B 1981 Vascular and sensory responses of human skin to mild injury after topical treatment with capsaicin. British Journal of Pharmacology 73: 755–758

Cervero F 1982 Afferent activity evoked by natural stimulation of the biliary system in the ferret. Pain 13: 137–151

Cervero F 1983 Mechanisms of visceral pain. In: Lipton S, Miles J (eds) Persistent pain. Academic Press, London, p 1–19

Cervero F 1988 Visceral pain. In: Dubner R, Gebhart G F, Bond M R (eds) Proceedings of the Vth World Congress on Pain. Elsevier, Amsterdam, p 216–226

Cervero F, Jänig W 1992 Visceral nociceptors: A new world order. Trends in Neuroscience 15: 374–378

Cervero F, Sharkey K A 1988 An electrophysiological and anatomical study of intestinal afferent fibres in the rat. Journal of Physiology (London) 410: 381–397

Cervero F, Meyer R A, Campbell J N 1993 Does secondary hyperalgesia involve central sensitization to nociceptive input. Pain (in press)

Coffman J D 1966 The effect of aspirin on pain and hand flow responses to intra-arterial injection of bradykinin in man. Clinical Pharmacology and Therapeutics 7: 26–37

Coleridge H M, Coleridge J C G 1980 Cardiovascular afferents involved in regulation of peripheral vessels. Annual Review of Physiology 42: 413–427

Coleridge H M, Coleridge J C G 1981 Afferent fibres involved in defence reflexes from the respiratory tract. In: Hutas I, Debreczeni L A (eds) Advances in physiological sciences. Pergamon Press, Budapest, p 467–477

Coleridge J C G, Coleridge H M 1984 Afferent vagal C-fibre innervation of the lungs and airways and its functional significance. Review of Physiology Biochemistry and Pharmacology 99: 1–110

Cormia F E, Dougherty J W 1960 Proteolytic activity in development of pain and itching: Cutaneous reactions to bradykinin and kallikrein. Journal of Investigative Dermatology 35: 21–26

Couture R, Cuello A C, Henry J L 1985 Trigeminal antidromic vasodilation and plasma extravasation in the rat: effects of sensory, autonomic, and motor denervation. Brain Research 346: 108–114

Crea F M, Giuseppe P, Galassi A R, Hassan E T, Kaski J C, Davies G, Maseri A 1990 A role of adenosine in pathogenesis of anginal pain. Circulation 81: 164–172

Darian-Smith I, Johnson K O, Dykes R 1973 'Cold' fiber population innervating palmar and digital skin of the monkey: Responses to cooling pulses. Journal of Neurophysiology 36: 325–346

Darian-Smith I, Johnson K O, LaMotte C, Kenins P, Shigenaga P, Ming V C 1979a Coding of incremental changes in skin temperature

by single warm fibers in the monkey. Journal of Neurophysiology 5: 1316–1331
Darian-Smith I, Johnson K O, LaMotte C, Shigenaga Y, Kenins P, Champness P 1979b Warm fibers innervating palmar and digital skin of the monkey: Responses to thermal stimuli. Journal of Neurophysiology 42: 1297–1315
Davis K D, Treede R D, Raja S N, Meyer R A, Campbell J N 1991 Topical application of clonidine relieves hyperalgesia in patients with sympathetically-maintained pain. Pain 47: 309–317
Davis K D, Meyer R A, Turnquist J L, Pappagallo M, Filloon T G, Campbell J N 1992 Cutaneous injection of the capsaicin analog, NE-21610, produces analgesia to heat but not to mechanical stimuli. Society for Neuroscience Abstracts 18: 285
Davis K D, Meyer R A, Campbell J N 1993 Chemosensitivity and sensitization of nociceptive afferents that innervate the hairy skin of monkey. Journal of Neurophysiology 69: 1071–1081
Denzlinger C, Rapp S, Hagmann W, Keppler D 1985 Leukotrienes as mediators in tissue trauma. Science 230: 330–332
Devor M, Jänig W 1981 Activation of myelinated afferents ending in a neuroma by stimulation of the sympathetic supply in the rat. Neuroscience Letters 24: 43–47
DiRosa M, Giroud J P, Willoughby D A 1971 Studies of the mediators of the acute inflammatory response induced in rats in different sites by carrageenan and turpentine. Journal of Pathology 104: 15–29
Dubner R 1978 Neurophysiology of pain. Dental Clinics of North America 22: 11–30
Dubner R 1991 I. Introductory remarks: Basic mechanisms of pain associated with deep tissues. Canadian Journal of Physiology and Pharmacology 69: 607–609
Dubner R, Price D D, Beitel R E, Hu J W 1977 Peripheral neural correlates of behavior in monkey and human related to sensory-discriminative aspects of pain. In: Anderson D J, Mathews B (eds) Pain in the trigeminal region. Elsevier, Amsterdam, p 57–66
Ebertz J M, Hirshman C A, Kettelkamp N S, Uno H, Hanifin J M 1987 Substance P-induced histamine release in human cutaneous mast cells. Journal of Investigative Dermatology 88: 682–685
Ferreira S H 1983 Peripheral and central analgesia. In: Bonica J J, Lindblom U, Iggo A (eds) Advances in pain research and therapy, vol 5. Raven Press, New York, p 627–634
Ferreira S H, Moncada S, Vane J R 1971 Indomethacin and aspirin abolish prostaglandin release from the spleen. Nature 231: 237–239
Ferreira S H, Moncada S, Vane J R 1974 Proceedings: Potentiation by prostaglandins of the nociceptive activity of bradykinin in the dog knee joint. British Journal of Pharmacology 50: 461P
Fitzgerald M, Lynn B 1977 The sensitization of high threshold mechanoreceptors with myelinated axons by repeated heating. Journal of Physiology (London) 265: 549–563
Fjallbrant N, Iggo A 1961 The effect of histamine, 5-hydroxytryptamine and acetycholine on cutaneous afferent fibres. Journal of Physiology (London) 156: 578–590
Floyd K, Hick V E, Morrison J F B 1977 Mechanosensitive afferent units in the hypogastric nerve of the cat. Journal of Physiology (London) 259: 457–471
Fock S, Mense S 1976 Excitatory effects of 5-hydroxytryptamine, histamine and potassium ions on muscular group IV afferent units: A comparison with bradykinin. Brain Research 105: 459–469
Freeman M A R, Wyke B 1967 The innervation of the knee joint. An anatomical and histological study in the cat. Journal of Anatomy 101: 505–532
Funakoshi M, Zotterman Y 1963 A study in the excitation of dental nerve fibers. In: Anderson D J (ed) Sensory mechanism in dentine. Pergamon, Oxford, p 60–72
Gamse R, Holzer P, Lembeck F 1980 Decrease of substance P in primary afferent neurones and impairment of neurogenic plasma extravasation by capsaicin. British Journal of Pharmacology 68: 207–213
Garnsworthy R K, Gully R L, Kenins P, Mayfield R J, Westerman R A 1988 Identification of the physical stimulus and the neural basis of fabric-evoked prickle. Journal of Neurophysiology 59: 1083–1097
Garrison D W, Chandler M J, Foreman R D 1992 Viscerosomatic convergence onto feline spinal neurons from esophagus, heart and somatic fields: Effects of inflammation. Pain 49: 373–382
Grigg P, Schaible H G, Schmidt R I 1986 Mechanical sensitivity of group III and IV afferents from posterior articular nerve in normal and inflamed cat knee. Journal of Neurophysiology 55: 635–643
Guilbaud G 1988 Peripheral and central electrophysiological mechanisms of joint and muscle pain. In: Dubner R, Gebhart G F, Bond M R (eds) Proceedings of the Vth World Congress on Pain. Elsevier, Amsterdam, p 201–215
Guzman F, Braun C, Lim R K S 1962 Visceral pain and the pseudaffective response to intra-arterial injection of bradykinin and other algesic agents. Archives of International Pharmacodynamics 136: 353–384
Gybels J, Handwerker H O, Van Hees J 1979 A comparison between the discharges of human nociceptive nerve fibers and the subjects ratings of his sensations. Journal of Physiology (London) 292: 193–206
Häbler H-J, Jänig W, Koltzenburg M 1987 Activation of unmyelinated afferents in chronically lesioned nerves by adrenaline and excitation of sympathetic efferents in the cat. Neuroscience Letters 82: 35–40
Häbler H-J, Jänig W, Koltzenburg M 1988 A novel type of unmyelinated chemosensitive nociceptor in the acutely inflamed urinary bladder. Agents and Actions 25: 219–221
Häbler H-J, Jänig W, Koltzenburg M 1990 Activation of unmyelinated afferent fibres by mechanical stimuli and inflammation of the urinary bladder in the cat. Journal of Physiology (London) 425: 545–562
Haegerstam G, Olgart L, Edwall L 1975 The excitatory action of acetylcholine on intradental sensory units. Acta Physiologica Scandinavica 93: 113–118
Hagbarth K E, Vallbo A B 1967 Mechanoreceptor activity recorded percutaneously with semimicroelectrodes in human peripheral nerves. Acta Physiologica Scandinavica 69: 121–122
Hagermark O, Hökfelt T, Pernow B 1978 Flare and itch induced by substance P in human skin. Journal of Investigative Dermatology 71: 233–235
Handwerker H O 1976a Pharmacological modulation of the discharge of nociceptive C fibers. In: Zotterman Y (ed) Sensory functions of the skin in primates. Pergamon Press, Oxford, p 427–439
Handwerker H O 1976b Influences of algogenic substances and prostaglandins on the discharges of unmyelinated cutaneous nerve fibers identified as nociceptors. In: Bonica J J, Albe-Fessard D (eds) Advances in pain research and therapy, vol 1. Raven Press, New York, p 41–45
Handwerker H O 1992 Pain and allodynia, itch and alloknesis: An alternative hypothesis. American Pain Society Journal 1: 135–138
Handwerker H O, Magerl W, Klemm F, Lang E, Westerman R A 1987 Quantitative evaluation of itch sensation. In: Schmidt R F, Schaible H G, Vahle-Hinz C (eds) Fine afferent nerve fibers and pain. Weinheim, New York, p 461–473
Handwerker H O, Forster C, Kirchhoff C 1991a Discharge partterns of human C-fibers induced by itching and burning stimuli. Journal of Neurophysiology 66: 307–315
Handwerker H O, Kilo S, Reeh P W 1991b Unresponsive afferent nerve fibres in the sural nerve of the rat. Journal of Physiology (London) 435: 229–242
Harris R, Griffin C J 1968 Fine structure of nerve endings in the human dental pulp. Archives of Oral Biology 13: 773–778
Haupt P, Jänig W, Kohler W 1983 Response pattern of visceral afferent fibres, supplying the colon, upon chemical and mechanical stimuli. Pflügers Archives 398: 41–47
Helme R D, Koschorke G M, Zimmermann M 1986 Immunoreactive substance P release from skin nerves in the rat by noxious thermal stimulation. Neuroscience Letters 63: 295–299
Heppelman B, Schaible H G, Schmidt R F 1985 Effects of prostaglandins E_1 and E_2 on the mechanosensitivity of group III afferents from normal and inflamed cat knee joints. In: Fields H L, Dubner R, Cervero F (eds) Advances in pain research and therapy, vol 9. Raven Press, New York, p 91–102
Heppelman B, Hebert M K, Schaible H G, Schmidt R F 1987 Morphological and physiological characteristics of the innervation of cats normal and arthritic knee joint. In: Pubols L S, Sessle B J, Liss A R (eds) Effects of injury in trigeminal and spinal somatosensory system. Alan R. Liss, New York, p 19–27
Heppelman B, Messlinger K, Neiss W F, Schmidt R F 1990 Ultrastructural three-dimensional reconstruction of group III and group IV sensory nerve endings ('free nerve endings') in the knee joint capsule of the cat: Evidence for multiple receptive sites. Journal of Comparative Neurology 292: 103–166

Herbert M D, Schmidt R F 1992 Activation of normal and inflamed fine articular afferent units by serotonin. Pain 50: 79–80

Hiss E, Mense S 1976 Evidence for the existence of different receptor sites for algesic agents at the endings of muscular group IV afferent units. Pflügers Archives 362: 141–146

Hnik P, Hudlicka O, Kuchera J, Payne R 1969 Activation of muscle afferents by nonproprioceptive stimuli. American Journal of Physiology 217: 1451–1458

Holzer P 1988 Local effector functions of capsaicin-sensitive sensory nerve endings: Involvement of tachykinins, calcitonin gene-related peptide and other neuropeptides. Neuroscience 24: 739–768

James T N, Rossi L, Hagerman G R 1988 On the pathogenesis of angina pectoris. Annals of Thoracic Surgery 41: 572–578

Jansco N, Jansco-Gabor A, Szolcsányi J 1967 Direct evidence for neurogenic inflammation and its prevention by denervation and by pretreatment with capsaicin. British Journal of Pharmacology and Chemotherapy 31: 138–151

Jansco N, Jansco-Gabor A, Szolcsányi J 1968 The role of sensory nerve endings in neurogenic inflammation induced in human skin and in the eye and paw of the rat. Journal of Pharmacology and Chemotherapy 32: 32–41

Jansco G, Kiraly E, Jansco-Gabor A 1977 Pharmacologically induced selective degeneration of chemosensitive primary sensory neurones. Nature 270: 741–743

Jänig W, Koltzenburg M 1991a Receptive properties of sacral primary afferent neurons supplying the colon. Journal of Neurophysiology 65: 1067–1077

Jänig W, Koltzenburg M 1991b Receptive properties of pial afferents. Pain 45: 77–85

Jänig W, Lisney J W 1989 Small diameter myelinated afferents produce vasodilation but not plasma extravasation in rat skin. Journal of Physiology 415: 477–486

Jänig W, Morrison J F B 1986 Functional properties of spinal visceral afferents supplying abdominal and pelvic organs, with special emphasis on visceral nociception. In: Cervero F, Morrison J F B (eds) Progress in brain research: visceral sensation. Elsevier, Amsterdam, p 87–114

Johnson K O, Darian-Smith I, LaMotte C, Johnson B, Oldfield S 1979 Coding of incremental changes in skin temperature by a monkey: Correlation with intensity discrimination in man. Journal of Neurophysiology 42(5): 1332–1353

Johnson R D, Halata Z 1991 Topography and ultrastructure of sensory nerve endings in the glans penis of the rat. Journal of Comparative Neurology 312: 299–310

Johnson R D, Kitchell R L 1987 Mechanoreceptor response to mechanical and thermal stimuli in the glans penis of the dog. Journal of Neurophysiology 57: 1813–1836

Jyväsjärvi E, Kniffki K-D 1989 Afferent C fibre innervation of cat tooth pulp: Confirmation by electrophysiological methods. Journal of Physiology 411: 663–675

Kaufman M P, Baker D G, Coleridge H M, Coleridge J C 1980 Stimulation by bradykinin of afferent vagal C-fibers with chemosensitive endings in the heart and aorta of the dog. Circulation Research 46: 476–484

Kenshalo D R 1960 Comparison of thermal sensitivity of the forehead, lip, conjunctiva, and cornea. Journal of Applied Physiology 15: 987–991

Khan A A, Meyer R A, Campbell J N 1987 Responses of unmyelinated nociceptive afferents to histamine. Society for Neuroscience Abstracts 13: 779

Khan A A, Raja S N, Manning D C, Campbell J N, Meyer R A 1992 The effects of bradykinin and sequence-related analogs on the response properties of cutaneous nociceptors in monkeys. Somatosensory and Motor Research 9: 97–106

Kieschke J, Mense S, Prabhakar N R 1988 Influence of adrenaline and hypoxia on rat muscle receptors in vitro. In: Hamann W, Iggo A (eds) Progress in brain research. Elsevier, Amsterdam, p 91–97

Kim S H, Chung J M 1991 Sympathectomy alleviates mechanical allodynia in an experimental animal model for neuropathy in the rat. Neuroscience Letters 134: 131–134

Kitchell R L, Gilanpour H, Johnson R D 1982 Electrophysiologic studies of penile mechanoreceptors in the rat. Experimental Neurology 75: 229–244

Kjartansson J, Dalsgaard C J, Jonsson C E 1987 Decreased survival of experimental critical flaps in rats after sensory denervation with capsaicin. Plastic and Reconstructive Surgery 79: 218–221

Klassen K P, Morton D R, Curtis G M 1951 The clinical physiology of the human bronchi. III. The effect of the vagus section on the cough reflex, bronchial caliber and clearance of bronchial secretions. Surgery 29: 483–490

Klement W, Arndt J O 1992 The role of nociceptors of cutaneous veins in the mediation of cold pain in man. Journal of Physiology (London) 449: 73–83

Koltzenburg M, Handwerker H O 1993 Differential ability of human cutaneous nociceptors to signal mechanical pain and to produce vasodilation. Journal of Neuroscience (in press)

Koltzenburg M, McMahon S B 1986 Plasma extravasation in the rat urinary bladder following mechanical, electrical and chemical stimuli: evidence for a new population of chemosensitive primary sensory afferents. Neuroscience Letters 72: 352–356

Koltzenburg M, Kress M, Reeh P W 1992a The nociceptor sensitization by bradykinin does not depend on sympathetic neurons. Neuroscience 46: 465–473

Koltzenburg M, Lundberg L E R, Torebjörk H E 1992b Dynamic and static components of mechanical hyperalgesia in human hairy skin . Pain 51: 207–219

Konietzny F, Hensel H 1975 Warm fiber activity in human skin nerves. European Journal of Physiology 359: 265–267

Kress M, Koltzenburg M, Reeh P W, Handwerker H O 1992 Responsiveness and functional attributes of electrically localized terminals of cutaneous C-fibres in vivo and in vitro. Journal of Neurology 68: 581–595

Kruger L 1988 Morphological features of thin sensory afferent fibers: a new interpretation of 'nociceptor' function. In: Hamann W, Iggo A (eds) Progress in brain research. Elsevier, Amsterdam, p 253–257

Kruger L, Perl E R, Sedivec M J 1981 Fine structure of myelinated mechanical nociceptor endings in cat hairy skin. Journal of Comparative Neurology 198: 137–154

Kumazawa T 1986 Sensory innervation of reproductive organs. In: Cervero F, Morrison J F B (eds) Progress in brain research: visceral sensation. Elsevier, Amsterdam, p 115–132

Kumazawa T, Mizumura K 1976 The polymodal C-fiber receptor in the muscle of the dog. Brain Research 101: 589–593

Kumazawa T, Perl E R 1977 Primate cutaneous sensory units with unmyelinated (C) afferent fibers. Journal of Neurophysiology 40: 1325–1338

Kumazawa T, Mizumura K, Minagawa M, Tsujii Y 1991 Sensitizing effects of bradykinin on the heat responses of the visceral nociceptor. Journal of Neurophysiology 66: 1819–1824

LaMotte R H 1992 Subpopulations of 'nocifensor neurons' contributing to pain and allodynia, itch and alloknesis. American Pain Society Journal 2: 115–126

LaMotte R H Campbell J N 1978 Comparison of responses of warm and nociceptive C-fiber afferents in monkey with human judgements of thermal pain. Journal of Neurophysiology 41: 509–528

LaMotte R H, Thalhammer J G 1982 Response properties of high-threshold cutaneous cold receptors in the primate. Brain Research 244: 279–287

LaMotte R H, Thalhammer J G, Torebjörk H E, Robinson C J 1982 Peripheral neural mechanisms of cutaneous hyperalgesia following mild injury by heat. Journal of Neuroscience 2: 765–781

LaMotte R H, Thalhammer J G, Robinson C J 1983 Peripheral neural correlates of magnitude of cutaneous pain and hyperalgesia: a comparison of neural events in monkey with sensory judgements in human. Journal of Neurophysiology 50: 1–26

LaMotte R H, Simone D A, Baumann T K, Shain C N, Alreja M 1987 Hypothesis for novel classes of chemoreceptors mediating chemogenic pain and itch. Pain (Suppl. 4): S15

LaMotte R H, Shain C N, Simone D A, Tsai E-F P 1991 Neurogenic hyperalgesia: Psychophysical studies of underlying mechanisms. Journal of Neurophysiology 66: 190–211

Lang E, Novak A, Reeh P W, Handwerker H O 1990 Chemosensitivity of fine afferents from rat skin in vitro. Journal of Neurophysiology 63: 887–901

Langford L A, Schmidt R F 1983 Afferent and efferent axons in the

medial and posterior articular nerves of the cat. Anatomical Record 206: 71–78
Lee M G, Sullivan S N, Watson W C, Melendez L 1985 Chest pain-esophageal disease. Gastroenterology 29: 719–743
Lele P P, Weddell G 1959 Sensory nerves of the cornea and cutaneous sensibility. Experimental Neurology 1: 334–359
Lembeck F, Gamse R 1982 Substance P in peripheral sensory processes. Ciba Foundation Symposium 91: 35–54
Lembeck F, Holzer P 1979 Substance P as neurogenic mediator of antidromic vasodilation and neurogenic plasma extravasation. Naunyn-Schmiedeberg's Archives of Pharmacology 310: 175–183
Levine J D, Clark R, Devor M, Helms C, Moskowitz M A, Basbaum A I 1984a Intraneuronal substance P contributes to the severity of experimental arthritis. Science 226: 547–549
Levine J D, Lau W, Kwiat G, Goetzl E J 1984b Leukotriene B4 produces hyperalgesia that is dependent on polymorphonuclear leukocytes. Science 225: 743–745
Levine J D, Dardick S J, Basbaum A I, Scipio E 1985 Reflex neurogenic inflammation. I. Contribution of the peripheral nervous system to spatially remote inflammatory responses that follow injury. Journal of Neuroscience 5: 1380–1386
Lewin G R, Ritter A M, Mendell L M 1992 On the role of nerve growth factor in the development of myelinated nociceptors. Journal of Neuroscience 12: 1896–1905
Lewis T 1935 Experiments relating to cutaneous hyperalgesia and its spread through somatic fibres. Clinical Science 2: 373–423
Lewis T 1937 The nocifensor system of nerves and its reactions. British Medical Journal 431–435
Lewis T 1942 Pain. Macmillan, New York
Lewis T, Pochin E E 1937 The double pain response of the human skin to a single stimulus. Clinical Science 3: 67–76
Lim R K S, Miller D G, Guzman F et al 1967 Pain and analgesia evaluated by intraperitoneal bradykinin-evoked pain method in man. Clinical Pharmacology and Therapeutics 8: 521–542
Lombardi F, Della Bella P, Casati R, Malliani A 1981 Effects of intracoronary administration of bradykinin on the impulse activity of afferent sympathetic unmyelinated fibres with left ventricular endings in the cat. Circulation Research 48: 69–75
Lundberg J M, Saria A 1987 Polypeptide-containing neurons in airway smooth muscle. Annual Review of Physiology 49: 557–572
Lynn B, Cotsell B 1992 Blood flow increases in the skin of the anaesthetized rat that follow antidromic sensory nerve stimulation and strong mechanical stimulation. Neuroscience Letters 137: 249–252
Lynn B, Shakhanbeh J 1988 Neurogenic inflammation in the skin of the rabbit. Agents and Actions 25: 228–230
McCloskey D I, Mitchell J H 1972 Reflex cardiovascular and respiratory responses originating in exercising muscle. Journal of Physiology (London) 224: 173–186
Macfarlane R, Moskowitz M A, Sakas D E, Tasdemiroglu E, Wei E P, Kontos H A 1991 The role of neuroeffector mechanisms in cerebral hyperfusion syndromes. Journal of Neurosurgery 75: 845–855
McMahon S B 1988 Neuronal and behavioural consequences of chemical inflammation of rat urinary bladder. Agents and Actions 25: 231–233
McMahon S B, Abel C 1987 A model for the study of visceral pain states: Chronic inflammation of the chronic decerebrate rat urinary bladder by irritant chemicals. Pain 28: 109–127
McMahon S B, Koltzenburg M 1990 Novel classes of nociceptors: Beyond Sherrington. Trends in Neuroscience 13: 199–201
McMahon S B, Koltzenburg M 1992 Itching for an explanation. Trends in Neuroscience 15: 497–501
Maggi C A, Meli A 1988 The sensory-efferent function of capsaicin-sensitive sensory neurons. General Pharmacology 19: 1–43
Malliani A, Pagani M, Lombardi F 1984 Visceral versus somatic mechanisms. In: Wall P D, Melzack R (eds) Textbook of pain. Churchill Livingstone, Edinburgh, p 100–109
Malliani A, Lombardi F, Pagani M 1986 Sensory innervation of the heart. In: Cervero F, Morrison J F B (eds) Progress in brain research: visceral sensation. Elsevier, Amsterdam, p 39–48
Manning D C, Raja S N, Meyer R A, Campbell J N 1991 Pain and hyperalgesia after intradermal injection of bradykinin in humans. Clinical Pharmacology and Therapeutics 50: 721–729
Markowitz S, Saito K, Moskowitz M A 1987 Neurogenically mediated leakage of plasma proteins occurs from blood vessels of dura mater in the rat brain. Journal of Neuroscience 7: 4129–4136
Martin H A, Basbaum A I, Kwiat G C, Goetzl E J, Levine J D 1987 Leukotriene and prostaglandin sensitization of cutaneous high-threshold C- and A-delta mechanonociceptors in the hairy skin of rat hindlimbs. Neuroscience 22: 651–659
Martling C R 1987 Sensory nerves containing tachykinins and CGRP in the lower airways. Functional implications for bronchoconstriction, vasodilatation and protein extravasation. Acta Physiologica Scandinavica (Suppl) 563: 1–57
Mathews B 1976 Coupling between cutaneous nerves. Journal of Physiology 254: 37P–38P
Mathews B 1977 Responses of intradental nerves to electrical and thermal stimulation of teeth in dogs. Journal of Physiology (London) 264: 641–664
Mayberg M, Langer R S, Zervas N T, Moskowitz M A 1981 Perivascular meningeal projections from cat trigeminal ganglia: Possible pathway for vascular headaches in man. Science 213: 228–230
Mei N 1983 Sensory structures in the viscera. In: Ottoson D (ed) Sensory physiology 4. Springer-Verlag, New York, p 2–42
Meller S T, Gebhart G F 1992 A critical review of the afferent pathways and the potential chemical mediators involved in cardiac pain. Neuroscience 48: 501–524
Melmon K L, Webster M E, Goldfinger S E, Seegmiller J E 1967 The presence of a kinin in inflammatory synovial effusion from arthritides of varying etiologies. Arthritis and Rheumatism 10: 13–20
Mendell L M, Lewin G R 1992 Regulation of cutaneous C-fiber heat nociceptors by NGF in the developing rat. Society for Neuroscience Abstracts 18: 130
Mengel M K C, Jyväsjärvi E, Kniffki K-D 1992 Identification and characterization of afferent periodontal C-fibres in the cat. Pain 48: 413–420
Mense S 1977 Muscular nociceptors. Journal of Physiology 73: 233–240
Mense S 1981 Sensitization of group IV muscle receptors to bradykinin by 5-hydroxytryptamine and prostaglandin E_2. Brain Research 225: 95–105
Mense S 1990 Physiology of nociception in muscles. In: Fricton J R, Awad E A (eds) Advances in pain research and therapy, vol 17. Raven Press, New York, p 67–85
Mense S 1991 Considerations concerning the neurobiological basis of muscle pain. Canadian Journal of Physiology and Pharmacology 69: 610–616
Mense S, Meyer H 1985 Different types of slowly conducting afferent units in cat skeletal muscle and tendon. Journal of Physiology (London) 363: 403–417
Mense S, Schmidt R F 1974 Activation of group IV afferent units from muscle by algesic agents. Brain Research 72: 305–310
Meyer R A, Campbell J N 1981a Myelinated nociceptive afferents account for the hyperalgesia that follows a burn to the hand. Science 213: 1527–1529
Meyer R A, Campbell J N 1981b Peripheral neural coding of pain sensation. Johns Hopkins Applied Physics Laboratory Technical Digest 2: 164–171
Meyer R A, Campbell J N 1987 Coupling between unmyelinated peripheral nerve fibers does not involve sympathetic efferent fibers. Brain Research 437: 181–182
Meyer R A, Campbell J N, Raja S N 1985a Peripheral neural mechanisms of cutaneous hyperalgesia. In: Fields H L, Dubner R, Cervero F (eds) Advances in pain research and therapy, vol 9. Raven Press, New York, p 53–71
Meyer R A, Raja S N, Campbell J N 1985b Coupling of action potential activity between unmyelinated fibers in the peripheral nerve of monkey. Science 227: 184–187
Meyer R A, Raja S N, Campbell J N, MacKinnon S E, Dellon A L 1985c Neural activity originating from a neuroma in the baboon. Brain Research 325: 255–260
Meyer R A, Campbell J N, Raja S N 1988 Antidromic nerve stimulation in monkey does not sensitize unmyelinated nociceptors to heat. Brain Research 441: 168–172
Meyer R A, Davis K D, Cohen R H, Treede R-D, Campbell J N 1991

Mechanically insensitive afferents (MIAs) in cutaneous nerves of monkey. Brain Research 561: 252–261

Micevych P E, Kruger L 1992 The status of calcitonin gene-related peptide as an effector peptide. Annals of the New York Academy of Sciences 657: 379–396

Mizumura K, Minagawa M, Tsujii Y, Kumazawa T 1990 The effects of bradykinin agonists and antagonists on visceral polymodal receptor activities. Pain 40: 221–227

Mizumura K, Sato J, Kumazawa T 1991 Comparison of the effects of prostaglandins E_2 and I_2 on testicular nociceptor activities studied in vitro. Naunyn Schmiedebergs Archives of Pharmacology 344: 368–376

Morrison J F B 1977 The sensory innervation of the gastro-intestinal tract. In: Brooks F P, Evers P (eds) Nerves and the gut. Charles Slack, Thorofare, p 297–326

Moskowitz M A 1991 The visceral organ brain: implications for the pathophysiology of vascular head pain. Neurology 41: 182–186

Moskowitz M A, Brody M, Liu-Chen L-Y 1983 In vitro release of immuno-reactive substance P from putative afferent nerve endings in bovine pia-arachnoid. Neuroscience 9: 809–814

Moskowitz M A, Buzzi M G, Sakas D E, Linnik M D 1989 Pain mechanisms underlying vascular headaches. Review of Neurology (Paris) 145: 181–193

Nakano T, Taira N 1976 5-Hydroxytryptamine as a sensitizer of somatic nociceptors for pain-producing substances. European Journal of Pharmacology 38: 23–29

Narhi M V O 1985a Dentin sensitivity: a review. Journal of Biology Buccale 13: 75–96

Narhi M V O 1985b The characteristics of intradental sensory units and their responses to stimulation. Journal of Dental Research 64: 546–571

Narhi M V O, Jyväsjärvi E, Hirvonen T, Huopaniemi T 1982 Activation of heat-sensitive nerve fibers in the dental pulp of the cat. Pain 14: 317–326

Neil A, Attal N, Guilbaud G 1991 Effects of guanethidine on sensitization to natural stimuli and self-mutilating behaviour in rats with a peripheral neuropathy. Brain Research 565: 237–246

Ness T J, Gebhart G F 1988 Colorectal distension as a noxious visceral stimulus: Physiologic and pharmacologic characterization of pseudaffective reflexes in the rat. Brain Research 450: 153–169

Ness T J, Gebhart G F 1990 Visceral pain: A review of experimental studies. Pain 41: 167–234

Ness T J, Metcalf A M, Gebhart G F 1990 A psychophysiological study in humans using phasic colonic distension as a noxious visceral stimulus. Pain 43: 377–386

Neugebauer V, Schaible H-G 1988 Peripheral and spinal components of the sensitization of spinal neurons during an acute experimental arthritis. Agents and Actions 25: 234–236

Nilsson J, von Euler A M, Dalsgaard C-J 1985 Stimulation of connective tissue cell growth by substance P and substance K. Nature 315: 61–63

Noordenbos W 1959 Pain. Elsevier, Amsterdam, p 1–182

Nordin M 1990 Low-threshold mechanoreceptive and nociceptive units with unmyelinated (C) fibers in the human supraorbital nerve. Journal of Physiology (London) 426: 229–240

Ochoa J, Mair W G P 1969 The normal sural nerve in man. I. Ultrastructure and numbers of fibres and cells. Acta Neuropathologica (Berlin) 13: 197–216

Ochoa J L, Torebjörk H E 1983 Sensations evoked by intraneural microstimulation of single mechanoreceptor units innervating the human hand. Journal of Physiology (London) 342: 633–654

O'Connor T P, Van der Kooy D 1986 Pattern of intracranial and extracranial projections of trigeminal ganglion cells. Journal of Neuroscience 6: 2200–2207

Pagani M, Pizzinelli P, Furlan R et al 1985 Analysis of the pressor sympathetic reflex produced by intracoronary injections of bradykinin in conscious dogs. Circulation Research 56: 175–183

Paintal A S 1955 Impulses in vagal afferent fibres from specific pulmonary deflation receptors. The response of these receptors to phenyl diguanide, potato starch, 5-hydroxytryptamine and nicotine, and their role in respiratory and cardiovascular reflexes. Quarterly Journal of Experimental Physiology 40: 89–111

Paintal A S 1960 Functional analysis of group III afferent fibers of mammalian muscle. Journal of Physiology (London) 152: 250–270

Paintal A S 1961 Participation by pressure-pain receptors of mammalian muscles in the flexion reflex. Journal of Physiology (London) 156: 498–514

Paintal A S 1986 The visceral sensations—some basic mechanisms. Progress in Brain Research 67: 3–19

Pedersen-Bjergaard U, Neilsen L B, Jensen K, Edvinsson L, Jansen I, Olesen J 1991 Calcitonin gene-related peptide, neurokinin A and substance P: Effects on nociception and neurogenic inflammation in human skin and temporal muscle. Peptides 12: 333–337

Perl E R 1968 Myelinated afferent fibres innervating the primate skin and their response to noxious stimuli. Journal of Physiology (London) 197: 593–615

Piotrowski W, Foreman J C 1986 Some effects of calcitonin gene-related peptide in human skin and on histamine release. British Journal of Dermatology 114: 37–46

Raja S N, Campbell J N, Meyer R A 1984 Evidence for different mechanisms of primary and secondary hyperalgesia following heat injury to the glabrous skin. Brain 107: 1179–1188

Raja S N, Treede R-D, Davis K D, Campbell J N 1991 Systemic alpha-adrenergic blockade with phentolamine: A diagnostic test for sympathetically maintained pain. Anesthesiology 74: 691–698

Rang H P, Bevan S, Dray A 1991 Chemical activation of nociceptive peripheral neurones. British Medical Bulletin 47: 534–548

Reeh P W, Kocher L, Jung S 1986 Does neurogenic inflammation alter the sensitivity of unmyelinated nociceptors in the rat? Brain Research 384: 42–50

Reeh P W, Bayer J, Kocher L, Handwerker H O 1987 Sensitization of nociceptive cutaneous nerve fibers from the rat tail by noxious mechanical stimulation. Experimental Brain Research 65: 505–512

Richardson B P, Engel G 1986 The pharmacology and function of 5-HT3 receptors. Trends in Neuroscience 9: 424–427

Richter J E, Bradley L A, Castell D O 1989 Esophageal chest pain: current controversies in pathogenesis, diagnosis, and therapy. Annals of Internal Medicine 110: 66–78

Ritter A M, Lewin G R, Kremer N E, Mendell L M 1991 Requirement for nerve growth factor in the development of myelinated nociceptors *in vivo*. Nature 350: 500–502

Roberts W J, Elardo S M 1985a Sympathetic activation of A-delta nociceptors. Somatosensory Research 3: 33–44

Roberts W J, Elardo S M 1985b Sympathetic activation of unmyelinated mechanoreceptors in cat skin. Brain Research 339: 123–125

Rocha e Silva M, Rosenthal S R 1961 Release of pharmacologically active substances from the rat skin in vivo following thermal injury. Journal of Pharmacology and Experimental Therapeutics 132: 110–116

Rozsa A J, Beuerman R W 1982 Density and organization of free nerve endings in the corneal epithelium of the rabbit. Pain 14: 105–120

Saito K, Markowitz S, Moskowitz M A 1988 Ergot alkaloids block neurogenic extravasation in dura mater: Proposed action in vascular headaches. Annals of Neurology 24: 732–737

Sanjue H, Jun Z 1989 Sympathetic facilitation of sustained discharges of polymodal nociceptors. Pain 38: 85–90

Saria A 1984 Substance P in sensory nerve fibres contributes to the development of oedema in the rat hind paw after thermal injury. British Journal of Pharmacology 82: 217–222

Sato J, Perl E R 1991 Adrenergic excitation of cutaneous pain receptors induced by peripheral nerve injury. Science 251: 1608–1610

Sato J, Mizumura K, Kumazawa T 1989 Effects of ionic calcium on the responses of canine testicular polymodal receptors to algesic substances. Journal of Neurophysiology 62: 119–125

Sato J, Suzuki S, Iseki T, Kumazawa T 1992 Adrenergic excitation of cutaneous nociceptors in adjuvant-induced arthritic rats. Society for Neuroscience Abstracts 18: 134

Scadding J W 1981 Development of ongoing activity, mechanosensitivity and adrenaline sensitivity in severed peripheral nerve axons. Experimental Neurology 73: 345–364

Schaible H G, Schmidt R F 1983a Activation of groups III and IV sensory units in medial articular nerve by local mechanical stimulation of knee joint. Journal of Neurophysiology 49: 35–44

Schaible H G, Schmidt R F 1983b Responses of fine medial articular nerve afferents to passive movements of knee joint. Journal of Neurophysiology 49: 1118–1126

Schaible H G, Schmidt R F 1985 Effects of an experimental arthritis on the sensory properties of fine articular afferent units. Journal of Neurophysiology 54: 1109–1122
Schaible H-G, Schmidt R F 1988a Time course of mechanosensitivity changes in articular afferents during a developing experimental arthritis. Journal of Neurophysiology 60: 2180–2195
Schaible H G, Schmidt R F 1988b Excitation and sensitization of fine articular afferents from cat's knee joint by prostaglandin E_2. Journal of Physiology (London) 403: 91–104
Schaible H G, Neugebauer V, Schmidt R F 1989 Osteoarthritis and pain. Seminars in Arthritis and Rheumatology 18: 30–34
Seltzer Z, Devor M 1979 Ephaptic transmission in chronically damaged peripheral nerves. Neurology 29: 1061–1064
Sengupta J N, Saha J K, Goyal R K 1990 Stimulus-response function studies of esophageal mechanosensitive nociceptors in sympathetic afferents of opossum. Journal of Neurophysiology 64: 796–812
Sessle B J, Hu J W 1991 Mechanisms of pain arising from articular tissues. Canadian Journal of Physiology and Pharmacology 69: 617–626
Shea V K, Perl E R 1985a Sensory receptors with unmyelinated (C) fibers innervating the skin of the rabbit's ear. Journal of Neurophysiology 54: 491–501
Shea V K, Perl E R 1985b Failure of sympathetic stimulation to affect responsiveness of rabbit polymodal nociceptors. Journal of Neurophysiology 54: 513–519
Sherrington C S 1906 The integrative action of the nervous system. Scribner, New York
Shir Y, Seltzer Z 1991 Effects of sympathectomy in a model of causalgiform pain produced by partial sciatic nerve injury in rats. Pain 45: 309–320
Sicuteri F, Fanciullacci M, Franchi G, Del Bianco P L 1965 Serotonin-bradykinin potentiation on the pain receptors in man. Life Sciences 4: 309–316
Simone D A, Ochoa J 1991 Early and late effects of prolonged topical capsaicin on cutaneous sensibility and neurogenic vasodilatation in humans. Pain 47: 285–294
Simone D A, Baumann T K, LaMotte R H 1989 Dose-dependent pain and mechanical hyperalgesia in humans after intradermal injection of capsaicin. Pain 380: 99–107
Simone D A, Alreja M, LaMotte R H 1991a Psychophysical studies of the itch sensation and itchy skin ('alloknesis') produced by intracutaneous injection of histamine. Somatosensory and Motor Research 8: 271–279
Simone D A, Sorkin L S, Oh U et al 1991b Neurogenic hyperalgesia: central neural correlates in responses of spinothalamic tract neurons. Journal of Neurophysiology 66: 228–246
Sinclair D C, Hinshaw J R 1950 A comparison of the sensory dissociation produced by procaine and by limb compression. Brain 73: 480–498
Skoglund S 1956 Anatomical and physiological studies of knee joint innervation in the cat. Acta Physiologica Scandinavica 36 (Suppl 124): 1–101
Steen K H, Reeh P W1992 Sustained graded pain and hyperalgesia from experimental tissue acidosis in human subjects. Society for Neuroscience Abstracts 18: 384
Steen K H, Reeh P W, Anton F, Handwerker H O 1992 Protons selectively induce long lasting excitation and sensitization to mechanical stimulation of nociceptors in rat skin, in vitro. Journal of Neuroscience 12: 86–95
Sugiura Y, Terui N, Hosoya Y 1989 Difference in distribution of central terminals between visceral and somatic unmyelinated (C) primary afferent fibers. Journal of Neurophysiology 62(4): 834–840
Sylvén C 1989 Angina pectoris. Clinical characteristics, neurophysiological and molecular mechanisms. Pain 36: 145–167
Sylvén C, Beermann B, Jonzon B, Brandt R 1986a Angina pectoris-like pain provoked by intravenous adenosine in healthy volunteers. British Medical Journal 293: 227–230
Sylvén C, Edlund A, Brandt R, Beermann B, Jonzon B 1986b Angina pectoris-like pain provoked by intravenous adenosine. British Medical Journal 293: 1027–1028
Szolcsányi J 1980 Effect of pain-producing chemical agents on the activity of slowly conducting afferent fibres. Acta Physiologica Academiae Scientiarum Hungaricae 56: 86
Szolcsányi J 1984 Capsaicin and neurogenic inflammation: history and early findings. In: Chahl L A, Szolcsányi J, Lembeck F (eds) Antidromic vasodilatation and neurogenic inflammation. Akademiai Kiado, Budapest, p 7–25
Szolcsányi J 1988 Antidromic vasodilation and neurogenic inflammation. Agents and Actions 23: 4–11
Szolcsányi J 1990 Capsaicin, irritation, and desensitization: neurophysiological basis and future perspectives. In: Green B G, Mason J R, Kare M R (eds) Chemical senses, vol 2–Irritation. Marcel Dekker, New York, p 141–169
Takahashi H 1985 Cardiovascular and sympathetic responses to intracarotid and intravenous injections of serotonin in rats. Naunyn-Schmiedebergs Archives of Pharmacology 329: 222–226
Tanelian D L 1991 Cholinergic activation of a population of corneal afferent nerves. Experimental Brain Research 86: 414–420
Tanelian D L, Beuerman R W 1984 Responses of rabbit corneal nociceptors to mechanical and thermal stimulation. Experimental Neurology 84: 165–178
Thalhammer J G, LaMotte R H 1982 Spatial properties of nociceptor sensitization following heat injury of the skin. Brain Research 231: 257–265
Thalhammer J G, LaMotte R H 1983 Heat sensitization of one-half of a cutaneous nociceptor's receptive field does not alter the sensitivity of the other half. In: Bonica J J, Lindblom U, Iggo A (eds) Advances in pain research and therapy, vol 5. Raven Press, New York, p 71–75
Tillman D B 1992 Heat response properties of unmyelinated nociceptors. Doctoral dissertation. Johns Hopkins University. Baltimore, MD
Torebjörk H E, Hallin R G 1973 Perceptual changes accompanying controlled preferential blocking of A and C fibre responses in intact human skin nerves. Experimental Brain Research 16: 321–332
Torebjörk H E, Ochoa J 1980 Specific sensations evoked by activity in single identified sensory units in man. Acta Physiologica Scandinavica 110: 445–447
Torebjörk H E, Ochoa J L 1981 Pain and itch from C-fiber stimulation. Society for Neuroscience Abstracts 7: 228
Torebjörk H E, LaMotte R H, Robinson C J 1984 Peripheral neural correlates of magnitude of cutaneous pain and hyperalgesia: simultaneous recordings in humans of sensory judgments of pain and evoked responses in nociceptors with C-fibers. Journal of Neurophysiology 51: 325–339
Torebjörk H E, Lundberg L E R, LaMotte R H 1992 Central changes in processing of mechanoreceptive input in capsaicin-induced secondary hyperalgesia in humans. Journal of Physiology (London) 448: 765–780
Toth-Kasa I, Jansco G, Bognar A, Husz S, Obal F Jr 1986 Capsaicin prevents histamine-induced itching. International Journal of Clinical Pharmacological Research 6: 163–169
Treede R-D 1992 Vasodilator flare due to activation of superficial cutaneous afferents in humans: heat-sensitive versus histamine-sensitive fibers. Neuroscience Letters 141: 169–172
Treede R-D, Cole J D 1993 Dissociated secondary hyperalgesia in subject with large fibre sensory neuropathy. Pain 53: 169–174
Treede R-D, Meyer R A, Campbell J N 1990a Comparison of heat and mechanical receptive fields of cutaneous C-fibre nociceptors in monkey. Journal of Neurophysiology 64: 1502–1513
Treede R-D, Meyer R A, Davis K D, Campbell J N 1990b Intradermal injections of bradykinin or histamine cause a flare-like vasodilatation in monkey. Evidence from laser Doppler studies. Neuroscience Letters 115: 201–206
Treede R-D, Meyer R A, Campbell J N 1991 Classification of primate A-fiber nociceptors according to their heat response properties. Pflügers Archives (Suppl 1) 418: R42
Treede R-D, Meyer R A, Raja S N, Campbell J N 1992 Peripheral and central mechanisms of cutaneous hyperalgesia. Progress in Neurobiology 38: 397–421
Trowbridge H O 1985 Intradental sensory units: Physiological and clinical considerations. Journal of Endodontics 11: 489–498
Tuckett R P 1982 Itch evoked by electrical stimulation of the skin. Journal of Investigative Dermatology 79: 368–373
Tuckett R P, Wei J Y 1987 Response to an itch-producing substance in cat. II. Cutaneous receptor populations with unmyelinated axons. Brain Research 413: 95–103

Van Hees J, Gybels J C 1981 Nociceptor activity in human nerve during painful and nonpainful skin stimulation. Journal of Neurology, Neurosurgery and Psychiatry 44: 600–607

Vera P L, Nadelhaft I 1990a Conduction velocity distribution of afferent fibers innervating the rat urinary bladder. Brain Research 520: 83–89

Vera P L, Nadelhaft I 1990b The conduction velocity and segmental distribution of afferent fibers in the rectal nerves of the female rat. Brain Research 526: 342–354

Wall P D, Gutnick M 1974 Ongoing activity in peripheral nerves: The physiology and pharmacology of impulses originating from a neuroma. Experimental Neurology 43: 580–593

Wall P D, McMahon S B 1985 Microneurography and its relation to perceived sensation. A critical review. Pain 21: 209–229

Wallin B G, Torebjörk E, Hallin R G 1976 Preliminary observations on the pathophysiology of hyperalgesia in the causalgic pain syndrome. In: Zotterman Y (ed) Sensory functions of the skin of primates with special reference to man. Pergamon, Oxford, p 489–499

White D M, Taiwo Y O, Coderre T J, Levine J D 1991 Delayed activation of nociceptors: correlation with delayed pain sensations induced by sustained stimuli. Journal of Neurophysiology 66: 729–734

Widdicombe J 1986 The neural reflexes in the airways. European Journal of Respiratory Disease (Suppl) 144:1–33

2. Inflammatory pain

Jon Levine and Yetunde Taiwo

INTRODUCTION

The inflammatory process, a complex series of biochemical and cellular events, is activated in response to tissue injury or to the presence of foreign substances. Inflammation not only removes the injured tissue or foreign material, but also contributes to the process of tissue repair and healing. The cardinal signs of inflammation: rubor (redness), calor (heat), tumor (swelling), dolor (pain) and functio lasea (loss of function) are presently, at least partly, understood in terms of the action of specific inflammatory mediators. This chapter describes mechanisms by which these inflammatory mediators have been shown to produce pain and enhance pain.

THE STUDY OF ENHANCED PAIN SENSATION

Studies mapping functional neural pathways have demonstrated that sensory neurons responding to stimuli capable of producing tissue damage have either myelinated small-diameter (Aδ) or unmyelinated (C) fibre axons (Torebjörk & Hallin 1974; Handwerker 1976). In primates, unmyelinated C-fibres account for most identified nociceptive afferents (Kumazawa & Perl 1977a, 1977b). These nociceptive neurons are activated by noxious heat (>44°C), intense mechanical pressure, or chemical mediators of inflammation, such as bradykinin, serotonin and elevated hydrogen ion concentration (Gilfort & Klanni 1965; Beck & Handwerker 1974; Richardson & Engel 1986; Dray & Perkins 1988; Bevan & Yeats 1991; Kumazawa et al 1991). A subset of C-fibres called 'silent' fibres have been described which are apparently non-responsive to mechanical and thermal stimuli, although some have been described to be chemosensitive (see Chs 1 and 7 for more discussion).

Interestingly, even though pain is a major complaint of patients with ongoing inflammation, the majority of these patients do not experience pain continually. Rather, patients experience pain predominantly when the inflamed site is moved or touched, i.e. there is tenderness rather than overt pain. This lowered threshold to produce a pain sensation is referred to as hyperalgesia. It has been shown that in the presence of inflammation, individual nociceptors become sensitized so that activation is now produced by stimuli usually not intense enough to cause activation; at the same time a usually noxious stimulus produces an even greater sensation of pain. The electrophysiological correlates of this altered pain response include a lowered threshold for nociceptor activation, increased spontaneous activity and an increased frequency of firing after a suprathreshold stimulus (Fig. 2.1). The different classes of nociceptors have been shown to develop a lowered threshold at inflammatory sites and after injection of inflammatory mediators by various routes (intradermal, intraarterial and intraarticular). There is also a phenomenon of secondary hyperalgesia by which input by small-diameter afferents in the spinal cord results in pain

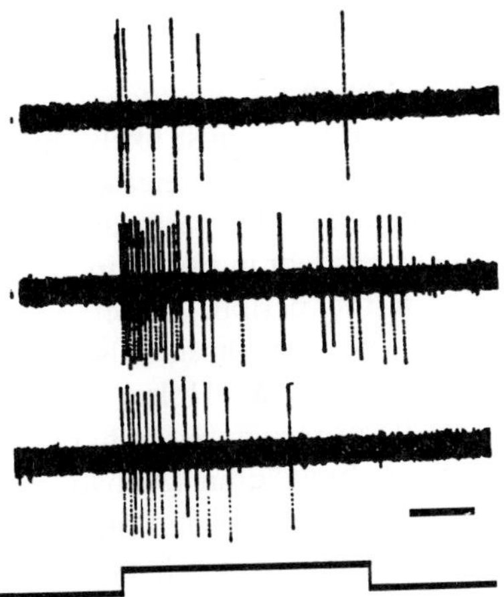

Fig. 2.1 An example of sensitization of a C-fibre nociceptor in the presence of the inflammatory mediator bradykinin. The top trace shows the response of an isolated C fibre to a threshold von Frey hair stimulus (3.6 g). After the injection of bradykinin this C fibre shows an enhanced response to the 3.6 g stimulus (middle trace). The bottom trace shows that the fibre now responds to a previously subthreshold stimulus (1.48 g). The onset and duration of the stimulus is indicated below the bottom trace. The horizontal bar represents 1 second.

experienced by stimulation of large-diameter fibres in the area providing the site of sensitization (see Chs 1 and 7 for more details).

Because some inflammatory mediators like bradykinin both activate and sensitize nociceptors, it has been assumed that activation and sensitization have a common mechanism. In fact, recent evidence from investigations of second messenger systems has revealed a protein kinase C (PKC)-mediated increase in sodium conductance involved in activation (Dray & Perkins 1988; Burgess et al 1989; however see Dunn & Rang 1990) and involvement of the cAMP second messenger system in sensitization (Ferreira & Nakamura 1979a; Taiwo et al 1989).

Various techniques have been useful in studying mechanisms by which inflammatory mediators lower nociceptive threshold and cause inflammatory pain. The technique of obtaining recordings from nerve fibres in awake humans has allowed direct correlation between discharges from these nociceptors and the report of pain but is limited by practical considerations. Instead, both behavioural techniques employing nociceptive reflex tests in animals and electrophysiological recordings from single fibres have been employed extensively to study the mechanisms underlying inflammatory pain (Bessou & Perl 1969; Beck & Handwerker 1974; Mense & Schmidt, 1976; Meyer & Campbell 1981; LaMotte et al 1982; 1983; Reeh et al 1987; Schaible & Schmidt 1988; Mense & Meyer 1988; Neugabauer et al 1989; Habler et al 1990; Cohen & Perl, 1990; Kirchoff et al 1990; White et al 1990; Kumazawa et al 1991; Cooper et al 1991; Koltzenburg et al 1992).

THE ROLE OF INFLAMMATORY MEDIATORS IN ALTERING PAIN SENSATION

Altered pain sensation in the presence of the inflammation is thought to be produced, most likely, by cytokines and other inflammatory mediators released from circulating leucocytes and platelets, by vascular endothelial cells, from immune cells resident in tissue (including mast cells) and from cells in the peripheral nervous system. The primary afferent neuron itself also contributes to inflammation (Lembeck & Holzer 1979). The first inflammatory mediator recognized to have potent hyperalgesic properties was bradykinin (Armstrong et al 1953). Since then, a host of cytokines and other mediators have been identified that might be hyperalgesic, including prostaglandins, leukotrienes, serotonin, adenosine, histamine, interleukin-1, interleukin-8, nerve growth factor octapeptide (NGF-OP) and substance P, which is released by the primary afferent itself. Some of these inflammatory mediators are believed to act directly on the nociceptor to lower thresholds (prostaglandins, serotonin, adenosine, 8(R), 15(S)-diHETE) while others are believed to produce hyperalgesia indirectly by acting first on other cells, such as the sympathetic postganglionic neuron or neutrophils (Fig. 2.2).

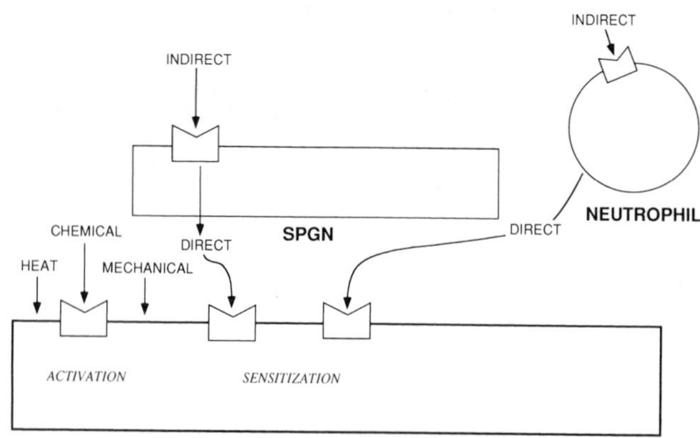

Fig. 2.2 Sensitization of the primary afferent nociceptor by indirect and direct mechanisms. Some inflammatory mediators are believed to act directly on the primary afferent to sensitize them to heat, mechanical, or chemical stimulation. The primary afferent can also be sensitized indirectly by other inflammatory mediators which first act on neutrophils or the sympathetic postganglionic neuron (SPGN) terminal. Direct action is characterized by a very short latency to hyperalgesia, persistence after elimination of the known indirect targets and confirmation by action on nociceptors in tissue culture.

PRIMARY AFFERENT SENSITIZATION BY DIRECT ACTION

Prostaglandins are considered prototypic sensitizing agents. Their administration does not elicit overt pain (Crunkhorn & Willis 1971) yet they decrease nociceptive threshold in behavioural tests in animals (Ferreira & Nakamura 1979a; Taiwo et al 1987; Taiwo & Levine 1989a) and produce tenderness in humans (Ferreira 1972). In electrophysiological studies in animals, prostaglandin E_2 sensitizes high-threshold somatic and visceral afferents when administered systemically (Handwerker 1976; Juan & Lembeck 1974; Fowler et al 1985) or when injected directly into the receptive field of a nociceptive afferent (Pateromichelakis & Rood 1981; Martin et al 1986).

Prostaglandins are not stored; rather, in response to an inflammatory mediator or to trauma, their de novo synthesis (from arachidonic acid released from membrane phospholipids) is stimulated (Kunze & Vogt 1971; Irvine 1982; O'Flaherty 1987). Free arachidonic acid is metabolized to prostanoids by the cyclooxygenase pathway (Samuelsson 1972, 1983) or to leukotrienes, by the lipoxygenase pathway (Roth & Siok 1978; Mizuno et al 1982) (Fig. 2.3). Prostaglandin E_2 and prostaglandin I_2 have been found to mediate directly bradykinin and norepinephrine hyperalgesia, respectively. 8(R),15(S)-diHETE has been found to mediate the neutrophil-

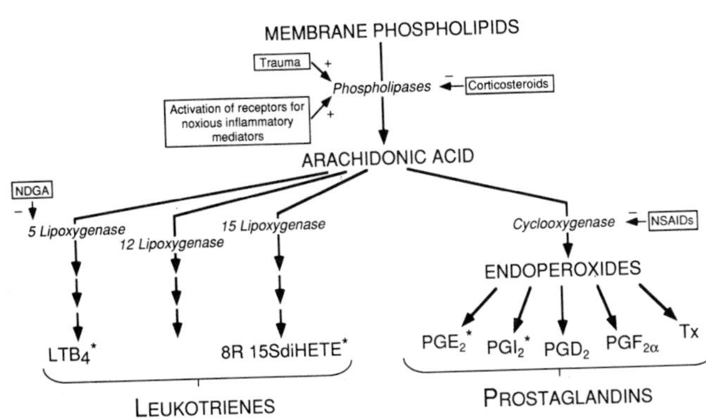

Fig. 2.3 Cascade for the production of hyperalgesic leukotrienes and prostaglandins after activation of membrane phospholipases by trauma or inflammatory mediators. The cascade can be modulated at several points by corticosteroids, nonsteroidal antiinflammatory drugs (NSAIDs) and nordihydroguaiaretic acid (NDGA). Metabolites that have been shown to be hyperalgesic are marked by an asterisk. LTB_4= leukotriene B_4; 8(R),15(S) -diHETE = 8(R),15(S) -dihydroxyicosatetraenoic acid; PGE_2 = prostaglandin E_2; PGI_2 = prostaglandin I_2; PGD_2 = prostaglandin D_2; $PGF_{2\alpha}$ = prostaglandin $F_{2\alpha}$; Tx = thromboxane.

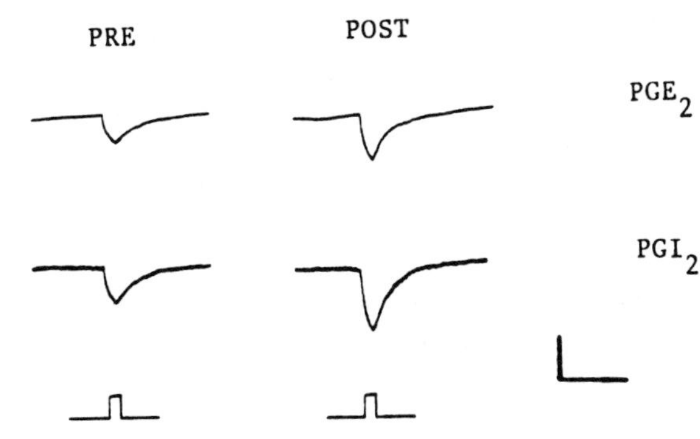

Fig. 2.4 Enhancement of capsaicin-induced inward current in whole cell patch clamp studies of presumed nociceptors in culture after hyperalgesic prostaglandins. Under PRE are responses to a 2 s capsaicin stimulus (represented by square wave pulse), which results in a maximum current of approximately 110 picoamps. The POST responses demonstrate enhanced current induced by capsaicin in the presence of prostaglandin E_2 (PGE_2) or prostaglandin I_2 (PGI_2). The demonstration of enhancement of capsaicin current in neuron tissue culture has been used as a criterion for direct sensitization by hyperalgesic mediators. The horizontal bar represents 10 s and the vertical bar 100 picoamps.

dependent hyperalgesia of leukotriene B_4. Prostaglandin $F_{2\alpha}$, prostaglandin D_2, 12(S) hydroxyheptadecatrienoic acid and thromboxane B_2 appear not to be hyperalgesic, although there is one report of prostaglandin D_2-induced hyperalgesia (Okhubo et al 1983). The analgesic properties of aspirin, indomethacin and other nonsteroidal antiinflammatory analgesics (NSAIDs), which inhibit the cyclooxygenase pathway (Smith & Willis 1971; Vane 1971; Ferreira et al 1973) emphasize the clinical importance of prostaglandin hyperalgesia. The sensitization of nociceptors by prostaglandins is particularly important since they enhance the response of nociceptors to other inflammatory mediators, such as vasoactive amines and kinins (Fock & Mense 1976).

The extremely rapid onset of hyperalgesia following intradermal injection of the arachidonic acid metabolites (Taiwo et al 1987) and the persistence of this hyperalgesia following the elimination of inflammatory cells (Taiwo & Levine 1989a) or the sympathetic postganglionic neuron suggest a direct action on the primary afferent (Taiwo et al 1987; Taiwo & Levine 1989a). The most convincing evidence that prostanoids act on the primary afferent neuron and do not require intermediary cells, has come from studies on cultured neurons (Baccaglini & Hogan 1983; Pitchford & Levine 1991). Whole cell patch clamp electrophysiology recordings performed on cells identified as nociceptors (Pitchford & Levine 1991, Petersen & LaMotte 1992) have demonstrated that direct micropipette application of either prostaglandin E_2 or prostaglandin I_2 significantly enhances the magnitude of the inward current produced by capsaicin (Fig. 2.4).

8(R),15(S) -diHETE, the mediator of leukotriene B_4 neutrophil-dependent hyperalgesia, also appears to act directly at a receptor on the primary afferent (Levine et al 1986b; Taiwo et al 1987), and on a different receptor than those for the prostaglandins as demonstrated by selective antagonism by the stereoisomer 8(S),15(S) -diHETE (Levine et al 1986b; White et al 1990).

Adenosine, which is generated in large amounts during inflammatory tissue hypoxia (Edlund et al 1983; Fredholm & Sandberg 1983) has been shown to activate unmyelinated afferents (Katholi et al 1985; Cherniack et al 1987; Moteiro & Ribeiro 1987; Runold et al 1987), to produce pain in humans (Bleehen & Keele 1977; Sylven et al 1988) and to elicit nociceptive behaviour in animals (Collier et al 1966). Adenosine was also found to produce hyperalgesia, probably by a direct action on the primary afferent neuron (Taiwo & Levine 1990). Based on studies using selective antagonists and agonists, adenosine hyperalgesia appears to be mediated by action on the adenosine A_2 type receptor.

Serotonin, released from activated platelets, is also significantly elevated in inflammatory exudates and has been reported to cause pain in humans, probably by action at the $5HT_3$ receptor (Richardson et al 1985; Richardson & Engle 1986; Giordano & Dyche 1989; Giordano & LaVerne 1989) present on primary afferents (Fozard 1984). Serotonin may also potentiate the pain induced by other inflammatory mediators such as bradykinin (Douglas & Ritchie 1957; Fjallbrant & Iggo 1961; Sicuteri et al 1965; Beck & Handwerker 1974; Fock & Mense 1976; Hiss & Mense 1976; Neto 1978; Nakano & Taira 1976; Mense 1981; Richardson et al 1985). Recent behavioural studies suggest that serotonin can also produce hyperalgesia, by action at a different receptor, most likely the $5HT_{1a}$ receptor (Taiwo & Levine 1992a). Direct action is suggested by the extremely short latency and independence from the sympathetic postganglionic neuron, neutrophil, and prostaglandin synthesis (Taiwo & Levine 1992b).

SECOND MESSENGERS FOR PRIMARY AFFERENT HYPERALGESIA

The identification of a diverse group of hyperalgesic agents producing hyperalgesia by action at different receptors on the primary afferent nociceptor prompted a search for a common second messenger. Prostaglandins (Hamprecht & Schultz 1973; Collier & Roy 1974) and adenosine (Saltin & Rall 1970; Daly 1977; Daly et al 1984; Snyder 1985) had been shown to elevate intracellular cAMP in numerous tissues. In studies designed to evaluate cAMP as the common second messenger, a membrane permeable analogue of cAMP (8-bromo cAMP) and forskolin, an agent which directly activates adenylyl cyclase to increase cAMP (Seamon et al 1981; DeSouza et al 1983; Schimmel 1984; Schmidt & Kukovetz 1989), were both found to produce hyperalgesia (Taiwo et al 1989). In addition, inhibitors of the enzyme that degrades cAMP, phosphodiesterase, significantly prolongs 8-bromo cAMP hyperalgesia and that produced by other directly-acting agents (Taiwo et al 1989; Taiwo & Levine 1990, 1992a). Hyperalgesia is also inhibited by blocking the phosphorylation of cAMP-dependent protein kinase (protein kinase A, PKA) (Botelho et al 1988; Braumann & Jastroff 1985, Taiwo & Levine 1991a). These results are all consistent with a critical role of the cAMP second messenger system in the mediation of sensitization of the primary afferent nociceptor. The hypothesis was further strengthened by patch clamp electrophysiology studies employing presumed nociceptors from cultured dorsal root ganglion neurons (Pitchford & Levine 1991) in which 8-bromo cAMP mimicked the effect of prostaglandin E_2 (Pitchford & Levine 1991).

Coupling of receptors located on the primary afferent nociceptor to adenylyl cyclase activity appears to be via a stimulatory guanine nucleotide regulatory protein (G_s) (Taiwo & Levine 1989b). Agents which activate inhibitory guanine nucleotide regulatory protein (G_i), such as opioids and, interestingly, adenosine acting at the A_1-receptor (Levine & Taiwo 1989; Taiwo & Levine 1990, 1991b), inhibit hyperalgesia. A schematic representation of the role of the cAMP second messenger system in inflammatory hyperalgesia and its modulation is shown in Figure 2.5.

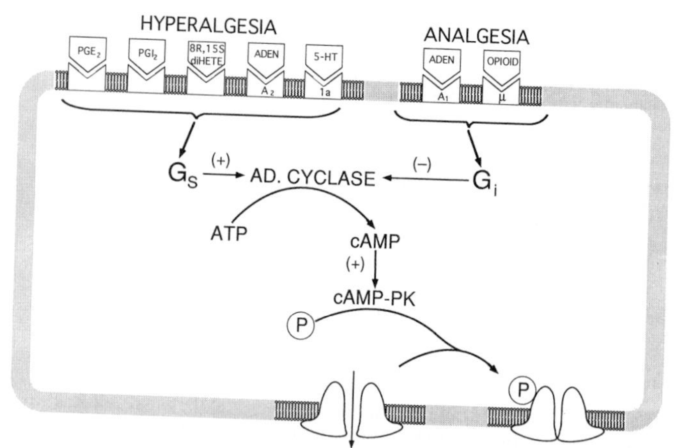

Fig. 2.5 The cyclic AMP second messenger system mediates primary afferent hyperalgesia via a stimulatory G-protein. Phosphorylation by activated cAMP-dependent protein kinase is necessary; its specific substrate is unknown. It may be that a membrane channel protein is phosphorylated to decrease membrane conductance, as shown. Analgesia (or more correctly inhibition of hyperalgesia) can be mediated by activation of an inhibitory G-protein. PGE_2 = prostaglandin E_2; PGI_2 = prostaglandin I_2; 8R,15S-diHETE = 8(R),15(S) -dihydroxyicosatetraenoic acid; Aden = Adenosine; 5-HT = serotonin; A_2 = A_2-type adenosine receptor; 1a = 1a-type serotonin receptor; A_1 = A_1-type adenosine receptor; G_s = stimulatory G-protein; AD = adenylyl cyclase; G_i = inhibitory G-protein; ATP = adenosine triphosphate; cAMP = cyclic adenosine monophosphate; cAMP-PK = cAMP-dependent protein kinase; P = phosphorus.

INDIRECT HYPERALGESIA

SYMPATHETIC NEURON-DEPENDENT HYPERALGESIA

While activity in the sympathetic nervous system rarely if ever causes pain, following tissue or nerve injury, the activity of nociceptors can be modulated by catecholamines, and this phenomenon may play an important role in the development of certain pain syndromes, including reflex sympathetic dystrophies, causalgia and some types of headache (White & Sweet 1969; Appenzeller 1976). Interestingly, several inflammatory mediators (e.g. bradykinin, interleukin-8 and norepinephrine) have been demonstrated to require the postganglionic sympathetic neuron for expression of hyperalgesia.

One such inflammatory mediator is bradykinin, a nonapeptide cleaved from α_2-globulins by kallikreins circulating in the plasma and activated at sites of tissue injury (Edery & Lewis 1963; Garrison 1990) (Fig. 2.6). Bradykinin has been found to be present in large amounts in inflammatory exudates (Rocha et al 1961; Melmon et al 1967; DiRosa et al 1971). Its injection in humans produces pain (Cormia & Dougherty 1960; Guzman et al 1962; Coffman 1966; Lim et al 1967; Ferreira et al 1971; Ferreira 1983) and single fibre recordings from peripheral nerves have shown that bradykinin activates primary afferent neurons (Dray & Perkins 1988; Haley et al 1989; Whalley et al 1989; Kumazawa et al 1991). Bradykinin has also been shown to excite dorsal root ganglion and trigeminal ganglion cells in culture (Baccaglini & Hogan 1983). Activation by bradykinin has been proposed to involve the generation of diacyl glycerol and activation of protein kinase C, leading to an increase in sodium

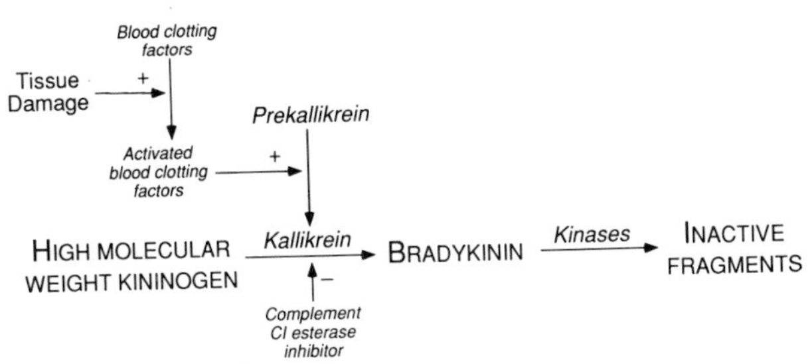

Fig. 2.6 Liberation of bradykinin after tissue damage. A series of steps occurring after tissue injury leads to the liberation of the inflammatory mediator bradykinin, which is both a primary afferent activator and sensitizer. Circulating clotting factors, an α_2-globulin (high molecular kininogen), and activated enzymes (kallikreins) are involved. Bradykinin is rapidly inactivated by kinases present at the sites of inflammation. Production of bradykinin can also be inhibited by endogenous substances (e.g. by complement C1 esterase inhibitor).

conductance (Dray & Perkins 1988; Burgess et al 1989; however, see Dunn & Rang 1990).

In addition to the overt production of pain, bradykinin also sensitizes nociceptors to produce hyperalgesia (Beck & Handwerker 1974; Handwerker 1976; Khan et al 1986; Mense & Meyer 1988; Neugabauer et al 1989) and has been shown to lower nociceptive thresholds in animal behavioural studies (Levine et al 1986c; Taiwo & Levine 1988b). Bradykinin-induced sensitization of primary afferent neurons and mechanical hyperalgesia have been shown to depend on sympathetic postganglionic neuron production of prostaglandins (Lembeck et al 1976; Levine et al 1986c; Taiwo & Levine 1988a; Kumazawa et al 1991). Thermal sensitization by bradykinin (albeit brief) (Raja et al 1990; Kumazawa et al 1991; Koltzenburg et al 1992), which also depends on prostaglandin synthesis (Kumazawa et al 1991), is reported to be unaffected by surgical sympathectomy, but that technique is less complete than chemical sympathectomy (Fischer et al 1964; Thoenen 1972).

The catecholamine, norepinephrine, has also been reported to produce hyperalgesia, but interestingly, only in the presence of tissue injury, such as exists during inflammation, and increased intracellular calcium may play a role (Taiwo et al 1990). Early studies of experimentally-induced neuromas had suggested that norepinephrine produced hyperalgesia via upregulation of α-adrenergic receptors on injured primary afferent nociceptors (Wall & Gutnick 1974; Devor & Janig 1981; Devor 1983; Blumberg & Janig 1984), but such upregulation of α-adrenergic receptors on primary afferents and coupling to nociceptive mechanisms has not been demonstrated.

Alternatively, norepinephrine may act on the sympathetic postganglionic neuron, stimulating production of hyperalgesic prostaglandins (Gonzales et al 1989), a hypothesis supported by the observation that sympathectomy attenuates norepinephrine hyperalgesia (Levine et al 1986c). The clinical observation that iontophoresis of norepinephrine into the skin of patients with causalgia or reflex sympathetic dystrophy reactivates quiescent pain and hyperalgesia, suggests that these mechanisms have clinical relevance in sympathetically-maintained pain syndromes; the latency of approximately 10 minutes (Wallin et al 1976) is also consistent with an indirect action of norepinephrine. Mechanical hyperalgesia produced by both bradykinin or by norepinephrine appear to be dependent on the production of hyperalgesic prostaglandins by sympathetic postganglionic neurons. But these two mediators appear to stimulate production of different prostaglandins (Taiwo & Levine 1988a, Taiwo et al 1990). Bradykinin activates phospholipase A_2 to yield prostaglandin E_2 while norepinephrine activates phospholipase C to yield prostaglandin I_2 (Taiwo et al 1990) (Fig. 2.7). Bradykinin has also been demonstrated to release norepinephrine from sympathetic postganglionic neuron terminals and is, therefore, able to activate both pathways.

Interleukin-1 is a cytokine, produced by leucocytes in response to exposure to bacterial toxins or to inflammatory mediators (Dinarello 1989). Both interleukin-1β and interleukin-1α polypeptides produce hyperalgesia, although interleukin-1β is a thousand times more potent (Ferreira et al 1988). Like bradykinin and norepinephrine, interleukin-1 induces E-type prostaglandin production in non-neuronal cells (Dayer et al 1986) and interleukin-1 hyperalgesia is probably also mediated by prostaglandins

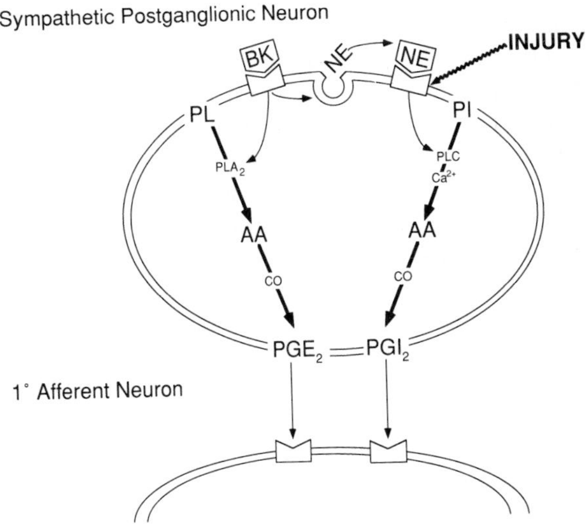

Fig. 2.7 Bradykinin (BK) and norepinephrine (NE) act on the sympathetic postganglionic neuron to produce hyperalgesia. The hyperalgesia is indirect, being mediated by prostaglandin E_2 (PGE_2) and prostaglandin I_2 (PGI_2), respectively and involves different metabolic pathways. While bradykinin hyperalgesia occurs in normal tissue, norepinephrine hyperalgesia only occurs in the presence of tissue injury. The sympathetic postganglionic neuron terminal itself is a source of NE. PL = phospholipid; PI = phosphatidyl inositol; PLA_2 = phospholipase A_2; PLC = phospholipase C; Ca^{2+} = calcium; AA = arachidonic acid; CO = cyclooxygenase.

(Ferreira et al 1988). Another cytokine, interleukin-8, has been demonstrated to produce a sympathetic-dependent hyperalgesia that does not appear to be mediated by prostaglandins (Cunha et al 1991).

Nerve growth factor (NGF) production is markedly increased following nerve injury (Heumann et al 1987) and by interleukin-1 (Heumann et al 1987; Lindholm et al 1987). The amino terminal octapeptide fragment of NGF, which is readily cleaved from NGF (Burton et al 1978), is structurally similar to bradykinin (Bothwell et al 1979) and has been demonstrated to induce a hyperalgesia attenuated by sympathectomy and by indomethacin (Taiwo et al 1991). Like norepinephrine-hyperalgesia, NGF-octapeptide hyperalgesia is present only after injury.

In summary, there are numerous inflammatory mediators that are likely to play a role in the production of inflammatory pain and employ the common mechanism of sympathetic postganglionic neuron stimulation and prostaglandin production.

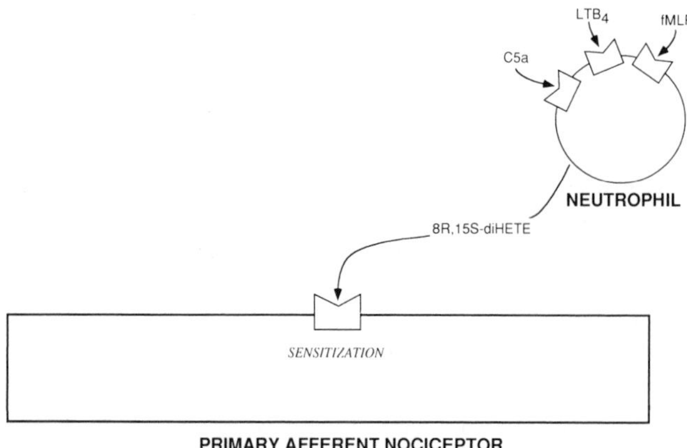

Fig. 2.8 The neutrophil is an intermediary in the hyperalgesia produced by C5a, a fragment of the fifth component of the complement cascade, the leukotriene, leukotriene B_4 and the bacterial cell wall peptide, fMLP (formyl methionyl-leucylphenylalanine). Sensitization of the primary afferent is produced by direct action of the hyperalgesic leukotriene, 8(R),15(S) -diHETE, released from the neutrophil.

NEUTROPHIL-DEPENDENT HYPERALGESIA

The polymorphonuclear leucocyte (neutrophil) is a principal effector cell in inflammatory reactions. It accumulates at sites of inflammation primarily to destroy and evacuate antigenic material. The accumulation of neutrophils is commonly associated with a marked hyperalgesia as, for example, in gout. A specific inflammatory mediator, leukotriene B_4 (LTB_4), which is a potent neutrophil attractant (Goetzl & Pickett 1980; Goldman & Goetzl 1982) has been shown to produce hyperalgesia both in humans (Lewis et al 1981; Bisgaard & Kristensen 1985) and in animals (Rackham & Ford-Hutchinson 1983; Levine et al 1984, 1985, 1986b) and that produced by intradermal injection of leukotriene B_4 in rats is dependent on the presence of circulating leucocytes (Levine et al 1984). Leukotriene B_4 hyperalgesia appears to be explained by the attraction and activation of neutrophils and release of a hyperalgesic substance, 8(R),15(S) -diHETE, which directly sensitizes primary afferent nociceptors (Levine et al 1984, 1986b).

The identification of the neutrophil as an important element in leukotriene B_4-mediated hyperalgesia suggested that other substances that attract and activate neutrophils might, by a similar indirect action, cause hyperalgesia. Indeed, two additional substances – C_{5a}, the anaphylactoid fragment of the fifth component of the complement cascade, and formyl methionyl-leucylphenylalanine (fMLP), a tripeptide bacterial cell wall fragment – have also been shown to produce neutrophil-dependent hyperalgesia, by eliciting the production of the same leukotriene, 8(R),15(S) -diHETE (Levine et al 1985). Mechanisms of neutrophil-dependent hyperalgesia are diagrammed in Figure 2.8.

OTHER POSSIBLE TYPES OF HYPERALGESIA

Substance P, an undecapeptide located in one tenth to one third of dorsal root ganglion neurons and transported to the peripheral primary afferent terminals (Brimjoin et al 1980; Harmar & Keen 1982) is released peripherally after afferent activation (Bill et al 1979; Brodin et al 1981; Moskowitz et al 1983; White & Helme 1985). Substance P contributes to the inflammatory response by causing vasodilation, increased vascular permeability (Lembeck & Holzer 1979; Saria 1984), increased production and release of lysosomal enzymes (Johnson & Erdos 1973), release of prostaglandin E_2, e.g. from synoviocytes (Lotz et al 1987), and release of interleukin-1 and the neutrophil chemoattractant interleukin-6 (Lotz et al 1988). In addition, it has been reported to attract and activate leucocytes (Helme & Andrews 1985; Saito et al 1986; Payan et al 1984; Bar-Shavit et al 1980; Hartung et al 1988), although such an action does not appear to cause the release of 8(R),15(S) -diHETE from neutrophils. While recent electrophysiological experiments (Cohen & Perl 1990) suggest that substance P has no direct effect on cutaneous nociceptors, the possibility of a contribution to hyperalgesia secondary to its numerous proinflammatory effects remains a possibility. Histamine, which is one of the first of the sequentially released mast cell inflammatory – mediators (Di Rosa et al 1971) appears to produce itch but not hyperalgesia or pain (Lewis 1933; LaMotte et al 1988). Finally, it should be noted that hyperalgesia mediated by large-diameter fibres which are not nociceptors can also occur in areas surrounding inflammation (secondary hyperalgesia) (Lewis 1935, 1942) and there is also evidence for a contribution of the central nervous system (CNS) to hyperalgesia (Cook et al 1987; Laird & Cervero 1989; Simone et al 1989).

Table 2.1 Mediators of inflammatory pain and hyperalgesia

Agents	Action on primary afferent	Mediator/ second messenger
Prostaglandin E_2 (PGE_2)	Direct	cAMP
Prostaglandin I_2 (Prostacyclin, PGI_2)	Direct	cAMP
8(R),15(S) -diHETE	Direct	cAMP
Adenosine	Direct	cAMP
Serotonin		
a) activation	Direct	(?)
b) sensitization	Direct	cAMP
Bradykinin		
a) activation	Direct	Protein kinase C
b) sensitization	Indirect (SPGN)	Prostaglandin E_2
Norepinephrine	Indirect (SPGN)	Prostaglandin I_2
Interleukin 1	Indirect (SPGN)	Prostaglandin
Interleukin 8	Indirect (SPGN)	(?)
NGF octapeptide	Indirect (SPGN)	Prostaglandin
Leukotriene B_4 (LTB_4)	Indirect (neutrophil)	8(R),15(S) -diHETE
fMLP	Indirect (neutrophil)	8(R),15(S) -diHETE
C_{5a}	Indirect (neutrophil)	8(R),15(S) -diHETE
Substance P (?)	(?)	(?)

A summary of the direct and indirect mediators of hyperalgesia is shown in Table 2.1.

PHARMACOTHERAPY FOR INFLAMMATORY PAIN

NSAIDS

Nonsteroidal antiinflammatory drugs (NSAIDs) are the most commonly used analgesics for the treatment of inflammatory pain. Their primary action appears to be the inhibition of prostaglandin synthesis at peripheral sites of inflammation (Lim et al 1964; Ferreira et al 1971; Ferreira 1972), although there is mounting evidence that they may also alter nociception by acting within the CNS (Ferreira et al 1978; Yaksh 1982; Devoghel 1983; Taiwo & Levine 1988). At sites of inflammation, inhibition of prostaglandin synthesis not only eliminates the direct hyperalgesic action of these mediators but also results in a decrease in the sensitizing effects of other inflammatory mediators (Fock & Mense 1976). NSAIDs are useful for a variety of mild to moderate inflammatory pains and also for severe pains, such as ureteral and biliary colic and severe dysmenorrhoea, subsequent to the introduction of injectable and rectal suppository NSAIDs that allow higher doses to be well tolerated (Thornell et al 1979; Marsala 1980). NSAIDs have been remarkably successful in preventing postoperative pain, when administered prophylactically (Dionne & Cooper 1978). Nevertheless, despite these successes, a variety of inflammatory pain states remain poorly managed by NSAIDs, probably due to the multiplicity of mediators that are capable of directly sensitizing the primary afferent.

CORTICOSTEROIDS

Corticosteroids have been used to control pain, particularly in clinical syndromes that are recalcitrant to NSAIDs. The success of corticosteroids can be understood in view of their potent action to inhibit phospholipase A_2 and, therefore, to prevent the release of arachidonic acid, thereby attenuating synthesis of both hyperalgesic prostaglandins and leukotrienes (Levine et al 1984, 1985, 1986b). The use of corticosteroids is quite limited, however, by their significant systemic side-effects, especially with chronic use.

SYMPATHOLYTIC THERAPY

Although the mechanism by which sympathetic postganglionic neuron terminals contribute to pain is incompletely understood (Koltzenburg & McMahon 1991) a number of diverse painful clinical conditions can be effectively relieved by sympathetic ablation (Glynn et al 1971; Loh & Nathan 1978; Levine et al 1986a), especially those characterized by an altered autonomic control in effector organs. The necessary contribution of the sympathetic nervous system to the action of various hyperalgesic inflammatory mediators such as bradykinin, norepinephrine, interleukin-1β and NGF-octapeptide, may explain the efficacy of sympatholysis.

MEDIATOR ANTAGONISTS

The identification of inflammatory mediators, present in inflammatory and neuropathic pain states, that alter pain sensation has also led to interest in the possible development of specific mediator receptor antagonists. To this end, antagonists to prostaglandins (Sanner 1969; Rakovska & Milenov 1984), bradykinin (particularly B_2 receptors; Whalley et al 1989), interleukin-1β (Ferreira et al 1988) and neurokinins, including substance P (Ganet et al 1991), are in various stages of development as analgesic agents. The enhanced selectivity of action of these agents may also reduce side-effects.

Another approach to selective inhibition of inflammatory mediator action is the development of inhibitors of the specific enzymes involved in mediator synthesis. Enzyme targets under investigation include phospholipases, lipoxygenases and kallikreins.

The elucidation of the cAMP second messenger system as a common mediator of primary afferent hyperalgesia allows the possibility of another novel approach to the treatment of inflammatory pain, namely antagonism of the cAMP second messenger system. Agents inhibiting stimulatory G-protein activity or activating inhibitory G-proteins would be potential analgesics and might allow single agent analgesia. Mu-opioids, which are known to activate inhibitory G-proteins and decrease intracellular cAMP (Law et al 1981; Childers & LaRiviere 1984; Sharma et al 1975; Makman et al 1988) have recently been shown to produce naloxone antagonizable analgesia when injected into sites of inflammation (hyperalgesic tissue) (Ferreira & Nakamura 1979b; Hargreaves et al 1987; Stein et al 1988a, 1988b, 1989, 1991; Levine & Taiwo 1989).

Interestingly, delta and kappa receptor specific opioid agonists have also been shown to produce antinociception in inflamed tissue (Stein et al 1988b, 1989). They do not inhibit direct hyperalgesia, such as that of prostaglandin E_2 (Levine & Taiwo 1989), but inhibit sympathetic postganglionic neuron-dependent hyperalgesia (Taiwo & Levine 1991b), probably by acting on kappa and delta opioid receptors known to be present on sympathetic postganglionic neuron terminals (Hughes et al 1981; Illes et al 1985; Berzetei et al 1988).

Finally, other specific antagonists, e.g. those directed at inhibiting receptor action of substance P, interleukin and bradykinin are all potential agents for the treatment of inflammatory pain and hyperalgesia. Advances in the understanding of inflammatory pain, including the discovery of as yet unknown mediator actions as well as better understanding of the mechanism in the primary afferent to produce sensitization and activation, will undoubtedly suggest even more approaches to the treatment of inflammatory pain.

REFERENCES

Appenzeller O 1976 The autonomic nervous system: an introduction to Basic and Clinical Concepts, 2nd edn. Elsevier, Amsterdam

Armstrong D, Dry R M L, Keele C A, Markham J W 1953 Observations on chemical excitant of cutaneous pain in man. Journal of Physiology (London) 120: 326–351

Baccaglini P L, Hogan P G 1983 Some sensory neurons in culture express characteristics of differentiated pain sensory neurons. Proceedings of the National Academy of Sciences (USA) 80: 594–598

Bar-Shavit Z, Goldman R, Stabinsky Y et al 1980 Enhancement of phagocytosis—a newly found activity of substance P residing in its N-terminal tetrapeptide. Biochemical and Biophysical Research Communications 94: 1445–1451

Beck P W, Handwerker H O 1974 Bradykinin and serotonin effects on various types of cutaneous nerve fibers. Pflügers Archives 347: 209–222

Berzetei I P, Fong A, Yamamura H I, Duckles S P 1988 Characterization of kappa opioid receptors in the rabbit ear artery. European Journal of Pharmacology 151: 449–455

Bessou P, Perl E R 1969 Response of cutaneous sensory units with unmyelinated fibers to noxious stimuli. Journal of Neurophysiology 32: 1025–1043

Bevan S, Yeats J 1991 Protons activate a cation conductance in a sub-population of rat dorsal root ganglion neurones. Journal of Physiology (London) 433: 145–161

Bill A, Stjernschatz J, Mandahl A, Brodin E, Nilsson G 1979 Substance P release on trigeminal nerve stimulation effects in the eye. Acta Physiologica Scandinavica 106: 371–373

Bisgaard H, Kristensen J K 1985 Leukotriene B produces hyperalgesia in humans. Prostaglandins 30: 791–797

Bleehen T, Keele C A 1977 Observation on the algogenic actions of adenosine compounds on the human blister base preparation. Pain 3: 367–377

Blumberg H, Janig W 1984 Discharge pattern of afferent fibers from a neuroma. Pain 20: 335–344

Botelho L H P, Rothermel J D, Coombs R V, Jastorff B 1988 cAMP analog antagonist of cAMP action. Methods in Enzymology 159: 159–172

Bothwell M A, Wilson W H, Shooter E M 1979 The relationship between glandular kallikrein and growth factor-processing proteases of the mouse submaxillary gland. Journal of Biological Chemistry 254: 7287–7294

Braumann T, Jastroff B 1985 Physicochemical characterization of cyclic nucleotides by reversed phase high performance liquid chromatography. II. Quantitative determination of hydrophobicity. Journal of Chromatography 350: 105–118

Brimjoin S, Lundberg J M, Brodin E, Hokfelt T, Nilsson G 1980 Axonal transport of substance P in the vagus and sciatic nerves of the guinea-pig. Brain Research 191: 443–457

Brodin E, Gazelius B, Olgart L, Nilsson G 1981 Tissue concentration and release of substance P in the vagus and sciatic nerves of the guinea-pig. Brain Research 191: 443–457

Burgess G M, Mullaney I, McNeill M, Dunn P M, Rang H P 1989 Second messengers involved in the mechanism of action of bradykinin in sensory neurones in culture. Journal of Neuroscience 9: 3314–3325

Burton L E, Wilson W H, Shooter E M 1978 Nerve growth factor in mouse saliva. Rapid isolation procedures for and characterization of 7S nerve growth factor. Journal of Biological Chemistry 253: 7807–7812

Cherniack N S, Runold M, Prabhakar N R, Mitra J 1987 Effect of adenosine on vagal sensory pulmonary afferents. Federation Proceedings, American Societies for Experimental Biology 46: 825

Childers S R, LaRiviere G 1984 Modification of guanine nucleotide-regulatory components in brain membranes. I. Relationship of guanosine 5'-triphosphate effects on opiate receptor binding and coupling receptors with adenylate cyclase. Journal of Neuroscience 4: 2764–2771

Coffman J D 1966 The effect of aspirin on pain and blood flow responses to intra-arterial injection of bradykinin in man. Clinical Pharmacology and Therapeutics 7: 26–37

Cohen R E, Perl, E R 1990 Contribution of arachidonic and derivatives and substance P to the sensitization of cutaneous nociceptors. Journal of Neurophysiology 64: 457–464

Collier H O J, James G W L, Schneider C 1966 Antagonism by aspirin and fenamates of bronchoconstriction and nociception induced by adenosine-5' triphosphate. Nature 212: 411–412

Collier H O J, Roy A O 1974 Morphine-like drugs inhibit the stimulation by E prostaglandins of cyclic AMP formation by rat brain homogenate. Nature 248: 24–25

Cook A J, Woolf C J, Wall P D, McMahon S B 1987 Dynamic receptive field plasticity in rat spinal cord dorsal horn following C-primary afferent input. Nature (London) 325: 151–153

Cooper B, Alquist M, Friedman R M, Lebanc J 1991 Properties of high-threshold mechanoreceptors in the goat oral mucosa. II. Dynamic and static reactivity in carrageenan-inflamed mucosa. Journal of Neurophysiology 66: 1280–1290

Cormia F E, Dougherty J W 1960 Proteolytic activity in development of pain and itching: cutaneous reactions to bradykinin and kallikrein. Journal of Investigative Dermatology 35: 21–26

Crunkhorn P, Willis A L 1971 Cutaneous reactions to intradermal prostaglandins. British Journal of Pharmacology 41: 49–56

Cunha F Q, Lorenzetti B B, Poole S, Ferreira S H 1991 Interleukin-8 as a mediator of sympathetic pain. British Journal of Pharmacology 104: 765p–767p
Daly J W 1977 Cyclic nucleotides in the nervous system. Plenum Press, New York
Daly J W, Butts-Lamb P, Padgett W 1984 Subclasses of adenosine receptors in the central nervous system: interaction with caffeine and related methyl xanthines. Cellular and Molecular Neurobiology 3: 69–80
Dayer J M, de Rochenouteix B, Burrus B, Demczut S, Dinarello J-M 1986 Human recombinant interleukin-1 stimulates collagenase and prostaglandin E-2 production by human synovial cells. Journal of Clinical Investigation 77: 645–648
De Souza N J, Dohadwalla A N, Reden J 1983 Forskolin: a labdane diterpenoid with antihypertensive positive and adenylate cyclase activating properties. Medicinal Research Reviews 3: 201–219
Devoghel J C 1983 Small intrathecal doses of lysine-acetylsalicylate relieve intractable pain in man. Journal of International Medical Research 11: 90–91
Devor M 1983 Nerve pathophysiology and mechanisms of pain and analgesia. Journal of the Autonomic Nervous System 7: 371–384
Devor M, Janig W 1981 Activation of myelinated afferents ending in a neuroma by stimulation of the sympathetic supply in the rat. Neuroscience Letters 24: 43–47
Dinarello C A 1989 Interleukin-1 and other growth factors. In: Kelley W N, Harris E D Jr, Ruddy S, Sledge C B (eds) Textbook of rheumatology. W B Saunders, New York, p 285–299
Dionne R A, Cooper S A 1978 Evaluation of preoperative ibuprofen for postoperative pain after removal of third molars. Oral Surgery, Oral Medicine, Oral Pathology 45: 851–856
Di Rosa M, Giroud J P, Willoughby D A 1971 Studies of the mediators of the acute inflammatory response induced in rats in different sites by carrageenan and turpentine. Journal of Pathology 104: 15–29
Douglas W W, Ritchie J M 1957 On excitation of non-medullated afferent fibers in the vagus and aortic nerves by pharmacological agents. Journal of Physiology (London) 138: 31–43
Dray A, Perkins M N 1988 Bradykinin activates peripheral capsaicin-sensitive fibers via a second messenger system. Agents and Actions 25: 214–215
Dunn P M, Rang H P 1990 Bradykinin-induced depolarization of primary afferent terminals in the neonatal rat spinal cord in vitro. British Journal of Pharmacology 100: 656–660
Edery H, Lewis G P 1963 Kinin forming activity and histamine in lymph after tissue injury. Journal of Physiology (London) 169: 568–583
Edlund A, Fredholm B B, Patiguani P, Patroro C, Wennmalm A, Wennmalm M 1983 Release of two vasodilators – adenosine and prostacycline from isolated rabbit hearts during controlled hypoxia. Journal of Physiology (London) 340: 487–501
Ferreira S H 1972 Prostaglandins, aspirin-like drugs and analgesia. Nature 240: 200–203
Ferreira S H 1983 Peripheral and central analgesia. In: Bonica J J, Lindblom U, Iggo A, (eds) Advances in pain research and therapy, vol 5. Raven Press, New York, p 627–634
Ferreira S H, Nakamura M 1979a I. Prostaglandin hyperalgesia, cAMP/Ca^{2+} dependent process. Prostaglandins 18: 179–190
Ferreira S H, Nakamura M 1979b Prostaglandin hyperalgesia: the peripheral analgesic activity of morphine, enkephalin and opioid antagonist. Prostaglandins 18: 191–200
Ferreira S H, Moncada S, Vane J R 1971 Indomethacin and aspirin abolish prostaglandin release from the spleen. Nature 231: 237–239
Ferreira S H, Moncada S, Vane J R 1973 Prostaglandins and the mechanisms of analgesia produced by aspirin-like drugs. British Journal of Pharmacology 49: 86–97
Ferreira S H, Lorenzetti B B, Correa F M A 1978 Central and peripheral antialgesic actions of aspirin-like drugs. European Journal of Pharmacology 53: 39–48
Ferreira S H, Lorenzetti B B, Bristow A F, Poole S 1988 Interleukin-1 beta as a potent hyperalgesic agent antagonized by a tripeptide analogue. Nature 334: 698–700
Fischer J E, Kopin I J, Wurtman R J 1964 Effects of lumbar sympathectomy on the uterine uptake of catecholamine. Nature 203: 939–949
Fjallbrant N, Iggo A 1961 The effect of histamine, 5-hydroxytryptamine and acetylcholine on cutaneous afferent fibers. Journal of Physiology (London) 156: 578–590
Fock S, Mense S 1976 Excitatory effects of 5-hyroxytryptamine, histamine and potassium ions on muscular group IV afferent units: a comparison with bradykinin. Brain Research 105: 459–469
Fowler J C, Greene R, Weinreich D 1985 Two calcium-sensitive spike after hyperpolarization in visceral sensory neurons of the rabbit. Journal of Physiology (London) 365: 59–75
Fozard J R 1984 Neuronal 5-HT receptors in the periphery. Neuropharmacology 23: 1473–1486
Fredholm B B, Sandberg G 1983 Inhibition by xanthine derivatives of adenosine receptor-stimulated cyclic adenosine 3',5'monophosphate accumulation in rat and guinea-pig thymocytes. British Journal of Pharmacology 80: 639–644
Ganet C, Carruette A, Fardin V et al 1991 Pharmacological properties of a potent and selective non peptide substance P antagonist. Proceedings of the National Academy of Sciences (USA) 88: 10208–10212
Garrison J C 1990 Histamine, bradykinin, 5-hydroxytryptamine and their antagonists. In Goodman A G, Rall T W, Nies A S, Taylor P (eds) The pharmacological basis of therapeutics, 8th edn. Macmillan, New York, p 575–599
Gilfort T M, Klanni I 1965 5-Hydroxytryptamine, bradykinin and histamine as mediators of inflammatory hyperesthesia. Journal of Physiology (London) 208: 867–876
Giordano J, Dyche J 1989 Differential analgesic actions of serotonin 5-HT_3 receptor antagonists in the mouse. Neuropharmacology 28: 423–427
Giordano J, LaVerne R 1989 Peripherally administered serotonin 5-HT_3 receptor antagonists reduce inflammation pain in rats. European Journal of Pharmacology 170: 83–86
Glynn C J, Basedow R W, Walsh H A 1971 Pain relief following postganglionic sympathetic blockade with IV guanethidine. British Journal of Anaesthesia 53: 559–562
Goetzl E J, Pickett W C 1980 The human PMN leukocyte chemotactic activity of complex hydroxyeicosatraenoic acids (HETEs) Journal of Immunology 125: 1789–1791
Goldman D W, Goetzl E J 1982 Specific binding of leukotriene B_4 to receptors on human polymorphonuclear leukocytes. Journal of Immunology 129: 1600–1604
Gonzales R, Goldyne M E, Taiwo Y O, Levine J D 1989 Production of hyperalgesic prostaglandins by sympathetic postganglionic neurons. Journal of Neurochemistry 53: 1595–1598
Guzman F, Braun C, Lim R K S 1962 Visceral pain and the pseudoaffective response to intra-arterial injection of bradykinin and other algesic agents. Archives Internationales de Pharmacodynamie et de Therapie 136: 353–384
Habler H J, Janig W, Koltzenburg M 1990 Activation of unmyelinated afferent fibers by mechanical stimuli and inflammation of the urinary bladder in the cat. Journal of Physiology (London) 425: 545–562
Haley J E, Dickenson A H, Schachter M 1989 Electrophysiological evidence for a role of bradykinin in chemical nociception in the rat. Neuroscience Letters 97: 198–202
Hamprecht D, Schultz J 1973 Stimulation by prostaglandin E_1 of adenosine 3',5'-cyclic monophosphate formation in neuroblastoma cells in the presence of phosphodiesterase inhibitors. Federation of European Biochemical Societies Letters 34: 85–89
Handwerker H O 1976 Influence of algogenic substances and prostaglandin on the discharge of unmyelinated cutaneous nerve fibers identified as nociceptors. In: Bonica J J et al (eds) Advances in pain research and therapy, vol 1. Raven Press, New York, p 41–45
Hargreaves K, Joris J, Dubner R 1987 Peripheral actions of opiates in the blockade of carrageenan-induced cutaneous hyperalgesia. Pain 4 (Suppl): s17
Harmar A, Keen P 1982 Synthesis and central and peripheral axonal transport of substance P in a dorsal root ganglion-nerve preparation in vitro. Brain Research 231: 379–385
Hartung H-P, Wolters K, Tokya K V 1988 Substance P binding properties and studies on cellular response in guinea-pig macrophages. Journal of Immunology 136: 3856–3863
Helme R D, Andrews P V 1985 The effect of nerve lesions on the inflammatory response to injury. Journal of Neuroscience Research 13: 453–459

Heumann R, Korsching S, Bandtlow C, Thoenen H 1987 Changes of nerve growth factor synthesis in non neuronal cells in response to sciatic nerve transection. Journal of Cell Biology 104: 1623–1631

Hiss E, Mense S 1976 Evidence for the existence of different receptor sites for algesic agents at the endings of muscular group IV afferent units. Pflügers Archives 362: 141–146

Hughes J, Kosterlitz H W, Leslie F M 1981 Effect of morphine on adrenergic transmission in the mouse vas deferens. Assessment of agonist and antagonist potencies of narcotic analgesics. British Journal of Pharmacology 53: 371–381

Illes P N, Pfeiffer I, Von Kugelgen I, Starke K 1985 Presynaptic receptor subtypes in the rabbit ear artery. Journal of Pharmacology and Experimental Therapeutics 232: 526–533

Irvine R F 1982 How is the level of free arachidonic acid controlled in mammalian cells? Biochemistry Journal 204: 3–16

Johnson A R, Erdos G G 1973 Release of histamine from mast cells by vasoactive peptides. Proceedings of the Society for Experimental Biology and Medicine 142: 1252–1256

Juan H, Lembeck F 1974 Action of peptides and other algesic agents on paravascular pain receptors of the isolated perfused rabbit ear. Naunyn-Schmiedebergs Archives of Pharmacology 283: 151–166

Katholi R E, McCann W P, Woods W T 1985 Intrarenal adenosine produces hypertension via renal nerves in the one-kidney, one clip rat. Hypertension 7 (Suppl. 1): 188–193

Khan A A, Raja S N, Campbell J N, Hartke T V, Meyer R A 1986 Bradykinin sensitizes nociceptors to heat stimuli. Society for Neuroscience Abstract 12 (part 1): 219

Kirchoff C, Jung S, Reeh P W, Handwerker H O 1990 Carrageenan inflammation increases bradykinin sensitivity of rat cutaneous nociceptors. Neuroscience Letters 111: 206–210

Koltzenburg M, McMahon S 1991 The enigmatic role of the sympathetic nervous system in chronic pain. Trends in Pharmacological Sciences 12: 399–402

Koltzenburg M, Kress M, Reeh P W 1992 The nociceptor sensitization by bradykinin does not depend on sympathetic neurones. Neuroscience 46: 465–474

Kumazawa T, Perl E R 1977a Primate cutaneous receptors with unmyelinated (C) fibers and their projection to the substantia gelatinosa. Journal of Physiology (Paris) 73: 287–304

Kumazawa T, Perl E R 1977b Primate cutaneous sensory units with unmyelinated (C) afferent fibers. Journal of Neurophysiology 40: 1325–1338

Kumazawa T, Mizumura T, Minigawa M, Tsuji Y 1991 Sensitizing effects of bradykinin on the heat response of the visceral nociceptor. Journal of Neurophysiology 66: 1819–1824

Kunze H, Vogt W 1971 Significance of phospholipase A for formation of prostaglandins. Annals of the New York Academy of Sciences 180: 123–125

Laird J M A, Cervero F 1989 A comparative study of the changes in receptive-field properties of multireceptive and nocireceptive rat dorsal horn neurons following noxious mechanical stimulation. Journal of Neurophysiology 62: 854–863

LaMotte R H, Thalhammer J G, Torebjörk H E, Robinson C J 1982 Peripheral neural mechanisms of cutaneous hyperalgesia following mild injury to heat. Journal of Neuroscience 2: 765–781

LaMotte R H, Thalhammer J G, Robinson C J 1983 Peripheral neural correlates of magnitude of cutaneous pain and hyperalgesia: comparison of neural events in monkey with sensory judgements in humans. Journal of Neurophysiology 50: 1–26

LaMotte R H, Simone D A, Baumann T K, Shain C N, Alreja M 1988 Hypothesis for novel classes of chemoreceptors mediating chemogenic pain and itch. In: Dubner R, Gebhart G F, Bond M R (eds) Proceedings of the Vth World Congress of Pain. Elsevier, Amsterdam, p 529–535

Law P Y,Wu J, Koehler J E, Loh H H 1981 Demonstration and characterization of opiate inhibition of the striatal adenylate cyclase activity. Journal of Neurochemistry 36: 1834–1846

Lembeck F, Holzer P 1979 Substance P as neurogenic mediator of antidromic vasodilatation and neurogenic plasma extravasation. Naunyn-Schmiedebergs Archives of Pharmacology 310: 175–183

Lembeck F, Popper H, Juan H 1976 Release of prostaglandins and the mechanisms of analgesia produced by aspirin-like drugs. British Journal of Pharmacology 49: 86–97

Levine J D, Taiwo Y O 1989 Involvement of the mu-opiate receptor in peripheral analgesia. Neuroscience 32: 571–575

Levine J D, Lau W, Kwiat G, Goetzl E J 1984 Leukotriene B_4 produces hyperalgesia that is dependent on polymorphonuclear leukocytes. Science 225: 743–745

Levine J D, Gooding J, Donatoni P, Borden L, Goetzl E J 1985 The role of the polymorphonuclear leukocyte in hyperalgesia. Journal of Neuroscience 5: 3025–3029

Levine J D, Fye K, Heller P, Basbaum A I, Whiting-O'Keefe Q 1986a Clinical response to regional intravenous guanethidine in patients with rheumatoid arthritis. Journal of Rheumatology 13: 1040–1043

Levine J D, Lam D, Taiwo Y O, Donatoni P, Goetzl E J 1986b Hyperalgesic properties of 15-lipoxygenase products of arachidonic acid. Proceedings of the National Academy of Sciences (USA) 83: 5331–5334

Levine J D, Taiwo Y O, Collins S D, Tam J K 1986c Noradrenaline hyperalgesia is mediated through interaction with sympathetic post ganglionic neurone terminals rather than activation of primary afferent nociceptors. Nature 323: 158–160

Lewis R A, Soter N A, Corey E J, Austen K F 1981 Local effects of synthetic leukotrienes (LTs) on monkey (M) and human (H) skin. Clinical Research 29: 492A

Lewis T 1933 Clinical observations and experiments reacting to burning pain in extremeties, and to so-called erythromelalgia in particular. Clinical Science 1: 175–211

Lewis T 1935 Experiments relating to cutaneous hyperalgesia and its spread through somatic fibers. Clinical Science 2: 373–423

Lewis T 1942 Pain. MacMillan, New York

Lim R K S, Guzman F, Roders D W et al 1964 Site of action of narcotic and non-narcotic analgesics determined by blocking bradykinin evoked visceral pain. Archives Internationales de Pharmacodynamie et de Therapie 152: 25–58

Lim R K S, Miller D G, Guzman F et al 1967 Pain and analgesia evaluated by intraperitoneal bradykinin-evoked pain method in man. Clinical Pharmacology and Therapeutics 8: 521–542

Lindholm D, Heumann R, Meyer M, Thoenen H 1987 Interleukin-1 regulates synthesis of nerve growth factors in non-neuronal cells in sciatic nerve. Nature 330: 658–659

Loh L, Nathan P 1978 Painful peripheral states and sympathetic blocks. Journal of Neurology, Neurosurgery and Psychiatry 41: 664–671

Lotz M, Carson D A, Vaughan J H 1987 Substance P activation of rheumatoid synoviocytes: neural pathway in the pathogenesis of arthritis. Science 235: 893–895

Lotz M, Vaughan J H, Carson D A 1988 Effect of neuropeptides on production of inflammatory cytokines by human monocytes. Science 241: 1218–1221

Makman M H, Dvorkin B, Crain S M 1988 Modulation of adenylate cyclase activity of mouse spinal cord-ganglion explants by opioids, serotonin and pertussis toxin. Brain Research 445: 303–313

Marsala F 1980 Treatment of ureteral and biliary pain with an injectable salt of indomethacin. Pharmacotherapeutica 2: 237–362

Martin H A, Basbaum A I, Kwiat G C, Goetzl E J, Levine J D 1986 Leukotriene and prostaglandin sensitization of cutaneous high-threshold C-mechanonociceptors in the rat. Neuroscience 22: 651–659

Melmon K L, Webster M E, Goldfinger S E, Seegmiller J E 1967 The presence of a kinin in inflammatory synovial effusion from arthritides of varying etiologies. Arthritis and Rheumatism 10: 13–20

Mense S 1981 Sensitization of group IV muscle receptors to bradykinin by 5-Hydroxytryptamine and prostaglandin E_2. Brain Research 225: 95–105

Mense S, Meyer H 1988 Bradykinin-induced modulation of the response behaviour of different types of feline group II and IV muscle receptors. Journal of Physiology (London) 398: 49–63

Mense S, Schmidt R F 1976 Activation of group IV afferent units from muscle by algesic agents. Brain Research 72: 305–310

Meyer R A, Campbell J N 1981 Myelinated nociceptive afferents account for the hyperalgesia that follows a burn to the hand. Science 213: 1527–1529

Mizuno K, Yamamoto S, Lands W 1982 Effects of non-steroidal anti-inflammatory drugs on fatty acid cyclooxygenase and prostaglandin hydroperoxidase activities. Prostaglandins 23: 743–757

Moskowitz M A, Brody M, Liu-Chen L-Y 1983 In vitro release of immunoreactive substance P from putative afferent nerve endings in bovine pia arachnoid. Neuroscience 9: 809–814

Moteiro E C, Ribeiro J A 1987 Ventilatory effects of adenosine mediated by carotid body chemoreceptors in the rat. Naunyn-Schmiedebergs Archives of Pharmacology 335: 143–148

Nakano T, Taira N 1976 5-Hydroxytryptamine as a sensitizer of somatic nociceptors for pain producing substances. European Journal of Pharmacology 38: 23–29

Neto F R 1978 The depolarizing action of 5-HT on mammalian non-myelinated nerve fibers. European Journal of Pharmacology 49: 351–356

Neugabauer V, Schaible H G, Schmidt F 1989 Sensitization of articular afferents to mechanical stimuli by bradykinin. Pflügers Archives 415: 330–335

O'Flaherty J T 1987 Phospholipid metabolism and stimulus response coupling. Biochemical Pharmacology 36: 407–412

Okhubo T, Shibata M, Takahashi H, Inoki R 1983 Effect of prostaglandin D_2 on pain and inflammation. Japanese Journal of Pharmacology 33: 264–266

Pateromichelakis S, Rood J P 1981 Prostaglandin induced sensitization of A-delta moderate pressure mechanoreceptors. Brain Research 232: 89–96

Payan D G, Levine J D, Goetzl E J 1984 Modulation of immunity and hypersensitivity by sensory neuropeptides. Journal of Immunology 132: 1601–1604

Petersen M, LaMotte R H 1992 Sensitization of the capsaicin evoked inward current by protons. European Journal of Physiology 420(Supp. 1): R45

Pitchford S, Levine J D 1991 Prostaglandins sensitize nociceptors in cell culture. Neuroscience Letters 132: 105–108

Rackham A, Ford-Hutchinson A W 1983 Inflammation and pain sensitivity effects of leukotrienes D_4, B_4 and prostaglandin E_1 in the rat paw. Prostaglandins 25: 588–616

Raja S N, Kozak S L, Manning D C, Meyer R A, Campbell J N 1990 Intradermal bradykinin induces hyperalgesia to heat stimuli in man. Pain (Suppl) 5: s130

Rakovska A, Milenov K 1984 Antagonist effect of SC19220 on the response of guinea-pig gastric muscle to prostaglandins E_1, E_2 and F_2 alpha. Archives Internationales de Pharmacodynamie et de Therapie 268: 59–69

Reeh P W, Bayer J, Kocher L, Handwerker H O 1987 Sensitization of nociceptive cutaneous nerve fibers from the rat's tail by noxious stimulation. Experimental Brain Research 65: 505–512

Richardson B P, Engel G 1986 The pharmacology and function of $5\text{-}HT_3$ receptors. Trends in Neurosciences 9: 424–428

Richardson B P, Engel G, Donatsch P, Stadler P A 1985 Identification of serotonin-M receptor subtypes and their specific blockade by a new class of drugs. Nature 316: 126–131

Rocha E, Silver M, Rosenthal S R 1961 Release of pharmacologically active substances from the rat skin in vivo following thermal injury. Journal of Pharmacology and Experimental Therapeutics 132: 110–116

Roth G R, Siok C J 1978 Acetylation of the NH_2-terminal serine of prostaglandin synthetase by aspirin. Journal of Biological Chemistry 253: 3782–3784

Runold M, Prabhakar N R, Mitra J, Cherniack N S 1987 Adenosine stimulates respiration by acting on vagal receptors. Federation Proceedings, American Societies for Experimental Biology 46: 825, C Thomas, Springfield, Illinois

Saito A, Kimura S, Goto K 1986 Calcitonin gene-related peptide as potential neurotransmitter in guinea-pig right atrium. American Journal of Physiology 256: H693–H698

Saltin A, Rall T W 1970 The effect of adenosine and adenine nucleotides on the cyclic adenosine 3',5' phosphate content of the guinea-pig cerebral cortex slices. Molecular Pharmacology 6: 13–23

Samuelsson B 1972 Biosynthesis of prostaglandins. Federation Proceedings 31: 1442–1460

Samuelsson B 1983 Leukotriene mediators of immediate hypersensitivity reactions and inflammation. Science 220: 568–575

Sanner J H 1969 Antagonism of prostaglandin E_2 by 1-acetyl-2-(8-chloro-10,11,-dihydrodibenz (b.f.) oxazepine-10-carbonyl hydrazine (SC19220). Archives Internationales de Pharmacodynamie et de Therapie 180: 46–56

Saria A 1984 Substance P in sensory nerve fibers contributes to the development of oedema in the rat hindpaw after thermal injury. British Journal of Pharmacology 323: 341–342

Schaible H G, Schmidt R F 1988 Excitation and sensitization of fine articular afferents from cat's knee joint by prostaglandin E_2. Journal of Physiology (London) 403: 91–104

Schimmel R J 1984 Stimulation of cAMP accumulation and lipolysis in hamster adipocytes with forskolin. American Journal of Physiology 246: C63–C68

Schmidt K, Kukovetz W R 1989 Mediation of the cardiac effects of forskolin by specific binding sites. American Journal of Physiology 246: C63–C68; Journal of Physiology (London) 403: 91–104

Seamon K B, Padgett W, Daly J W 1981 Forskolin: unique diterpene activator of adenylate cyclase in membranes and in intact cells. Proceedings of the National Academy of Sciences (USA) 78: 3363–3367

Sharma S K, Nirenberg M, Klee W A 1975 Morphine receptors as regulators of adenylate cyclase activity. Proceedings of the National Academy of Sciences (USA) 72: 590–594

Sicuteri F, Franciullacci M, Franchi G, Del Bianco P L 1965 Serotonin-bradykinin potentiation on the pain receptors in man. Life Sciences 4: 309–316

Simone D A, Baumann T K, Collins J G, LaMotte R H 1989 Sensitization of cat dorsal horn neurons to innocuous mechanical stimulation after intradermal injection of capsaicin. Brain Research 486: 185–189

Smith J B, Willis A L 1971 Aspirin selectively inhibits prostaglandin production in human platelets. Nature (London) New Biology 231: 235–237

Snyder S H 1985 Adenosine as a neuromodulator. Annual Review of Neuroscience 8: 103–124

Stein C, Millan M J, Shippenberg T S, Herz A 1988a Peripheral effect of fentanyl upon nociception in inflamed tissue of the rat. Neuroscience Letters 84: 225–228

Stein C, Millan M J, Yassouridis A, Herz A 1988b Antinociceptive effects of mu and kappa-agonists in inflammation are enhanced due to a peripheral opioid receptor-specific mechanism. European Journal of Pharmacology 155: 255–264

Stein C, Millan M J, Shippenberg T S, Peter K, Herz A 1989 Peripheral opioid receptors mediating antinociception in inflammation. Evidence for involvement of mu, delta and kappa receptors. Journal of Pharmacology and Experimental Therapeutics 248: 1269–1275

Stein C, Hassan A H S, Prezewlocki R, Gramsch C, Peter K, Herz A 1991 Opioids from immunocytes interact with receptors on sensory nerves to inhibit nociception in inflammation. Proceedings of the National Academy of Sciences (USA) 87: 5935–5939

Sylven C, Jonzon B, Fredholm B B, Kaijser L 1988 Adenosine injection into the brachial artery produces ischemia like pain or discomfort in the forearm. Cardiovascular Research 22: 664–678

Taiwo Y O, Levine J D 1988a Prostaglandins inhibit endogenous pain control mechanisms by blocking transmission at spinal noradrenergic synapses. Journal of Neuroscience 8: 1346–1349

Taiwo Y O, Levine J D 1988b Characterization of the arachidonic metabolites mediating bradykinin and noradrenaline hyperalgesia. Brain Research 458: 402–406

Taiwo Y O, Levine J D 1989a Prostaglandin effects after elimination of indirect hyperalgesic mechanisms in the skin of the rat. Brain Research 492: 397–399

Taiwo Y O, Levine J D 1989b Contribution of guanine nucleotide regulatory proteins to prostaglandin hyperalgesia in the rat. Brain Research 492: 397–399

Taiwo Y O, Levine J D 1990 Direct cutaneous hyperalgesia induced by adenosine. Neuroscience 38: 757–762

Taiwo Y O, Levine J D 1991a Further confirmation of the role of adenyl cyclase and of cAMP-dependent protein kinase in primary afferent hyperalgesia. Neuroscience 44: 131–135

Taiwo Y O, Levine J D 1991b Kappa and delta opioids block sympathetically dependent hyperalgesia. Journal of Neurosciences 11: 928–932

Taiwo Y O, Levine J D 1992a Mediation of serotonin hyperalgesia by the cAMP second messenger system. Neuroscience 48: 479–483

Taiwo Y O, Levine J D 1992b Serotonin is a directly acting hyperalgesic agent in the rat. Neuroscience 48: 485–490

Taiwo Y O, Goetzl E J, Levine J D 1987 Hyperalgesia onset latency suggests a hierarchy of action. Brain Research 423: 333–337

Taiwo Y O, Bjerknes L, Goetzl E J, Levine J D 1989 Mediation of primary afferent hyperalgesia by the cAMP second messenger system. Neuroscience 32: 577–580

Taiwo Y O, Heller P H, Levine J D 1990 Characterization of distinct phospholipases mediating bradykinin and adrenaline hyperalgesia. Neuroscience 39: 523–531

Taiwo Y O, Levine J D, Burch R M, Woo J E, Mobley W C 1991 Hyperalgesia induced in the rat by the amino-terminal octapeptide of nerve growth factor. Proceedings of the National Academy of Sciences (USA) 88: 5144–5148

Thoenen H 1972 Surgical immunological and chemical sympathectomy, their application in the investigation of the physiology and pharmacology of the sympathetic nervous system. In: Blaschko H, Muscholl E (eds) Catecholamine. Springer-Verlag, Berlin, p 813–844

Thornell E, Jansson R, Kral J G, Svanvik J 1979 Inhibition of prostaglandin synthesis as a treatment for biliary pain. Lancet i(8116): 584

Torebjörk H E, Hallin R G 1974 Identification of afferent C units in intact human skin nerves. Brain Research 67: 387–403

Vane J R 1971 Inhibition of prostaglandin synthesis as a mechanism of action for aspirin-like drugs. Nature (London) New Biology 231: 232–235

Wall P D, Gutnick M 1974 Ongoing activity in peripheral nerves: the physiology and pharmacology of impulses originating from a neuroma. Experimental Neurology 43: 580–593

Wallin G, Torebjörk E, Hallin R 1976 In: Zotterman Y (ed) Sensory functions of the primate skin with special reference to man. Pergamon, Oxford, p 489–502

Whalley E T, Clegg S, Steward J M, Vavrek R J 1989 Antagonism of the algesic action of bradykinin on the human blister base. Advances in Experimental Medicine and Biology 247A: 261–268

White D M, Helme R D 1985 Release of substance P from peripheral nerve terminals following electrical stimulation of the sciatic nerve. Brain Research 336: 27–31

White D M, Basbaum A I, Goetzl E J, Levine J D 1990 The 15-lipoxygenase product, 8R,15S-diHETE, stereospecifically sensitizes C-fiber mechano-heat nociceptors in the hairy skin of the rat. Journal of Neurophysiology 63: 966–970

White J C, Sweet W H 1969 Pain and the neurosurgeon: a forty year experience. C C Thomas, Springfield

Yaksh T L 1982 Central and peripheral mechanisms for the analgesic action of acetylsalicyclic acid. In: Barnett H J M, Mustard J F (eds) Acetylsalicyclic acid: new uses for an old drug. Raven Press, New York, p 137–151

3. Nociceptive peripheral neurons: cellular properties

H. P. Rang, S. Bevan and A. Dray

INTRODUCTION

The process of nociception involves the generation of nerve impulses by the peripheral terminals of small-diameter sensory neurons, the propagation of these impulses to the spinal cord, and the release of mediators in the dorsal horn. As well as serving as a vehicle for this type of afferent signalling, nociceptive neurons may also subserve other types of communication. For example, they have a peripheral effector role causing responses associated with neurogenic inflammation (vasodilation, vascular leakage) and neuroimmune regulation. In addition they can also control smooth muscle contraction and glandular secretion in various organs, such as the airways, gastrointestinal and urinary tracts (Maggi & Meli 1988; Holzer 1988).

At the cellular level, there are several characteristic features of nociceptive afferent neurons:

1. They are sensitive to a variety of different kinds of noxious stimulus (thermal, mechanical, chemical), their chemosensitivity being particularly pronounced
2. They contain and release a wide variety of neuropeptides
3. They are sensitive to particular growth factors, most notably nerve growth factor (NGF).

Their role in inflammatory states is particularly important, partly because many inflammatory mediators cause excitation or enhanced responsiveness of nociceptive afferent terminals, and partly because the neuropeptides released from the terminals themselves accentuate the inflammatory response. Longer term modulation of the properties of nociceptive neurons by cytokines and growth factors may also be important in the functional changes that are associated with various chronic pain states. In inflammatory pain, the interactions are mainly between the local inflammatory cells and the nociceptive nerve terminals, though it is also likely that cytokines may access distant sites via the circulation. In other types of chronic pain, it has long been recognized that sympathetic nerve terminals also play an important role (McMahon 1991). However the nature of the interaction between sympathetic and nociceptive nerve terminals is still rather poorly understood. The interplay of these cellular components – inflammatory cells, sympathetic neurons and nociceptive neurons – is summarized in Figure 3.1, in which some of the key chemical mediators are also identified.

In this chapter, we focus on the cellular characteristics of nociceptive afferent neurons, and discuss the ways in which they contribute to the function of these cells under normal and pathological circumstances. The main themes covered are:

1. The membrane properties of sensory neurons
2. Chemical excitation and sensitization of nociceptive afferent terminals by inflammatory mediators and other agents
3. The synthesis and release of mediators (neuropeptides and fast transmitters) by nociceptive afferent neurons
4. The effects of cytokines and growth factors on nociceptive afferent neurons.

MEMBRANE PROPERTIES OF SENSORY NEURONS

As with all other excitable cells, excitation of nociceptive neurons involves the interplay of voltage-sensitive ion channels, particularly sodium, potassium and calcium channels. Sensory neurons possess special membrane mechanisms rendering them sensitive to external stimuli. Many of the effective stimuli are chemicals which operate through a variety of receptors coupled to various transduction mechanisms through which the functional effects of the ligand-receptor interaction are produced. Mechanosensitive ion channels are well known in various cell types, and it is likely that similar mechanisms confer mechanosensitivity on sensory neurons. The way in which neurons respond to thermal stimuli is very poorly understood. It is not known whether temperature changes affect excitability

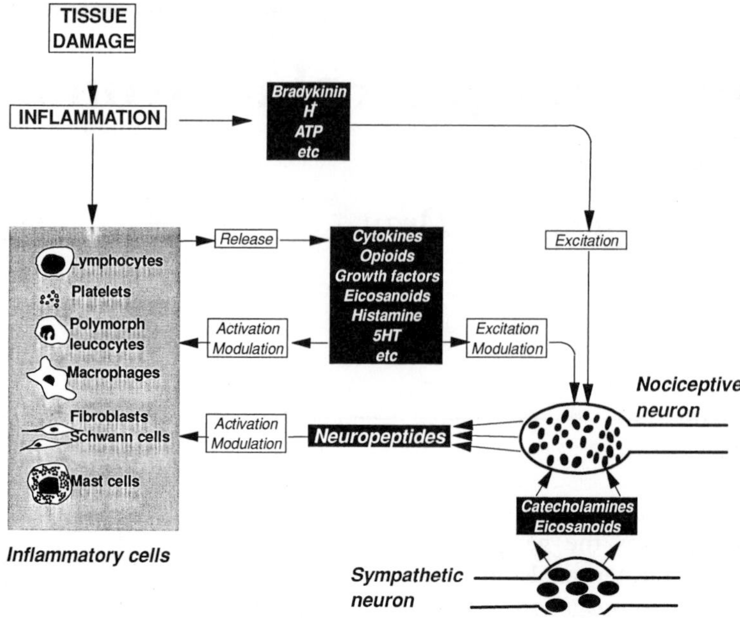

Fig. 3.1 Scheme illustrating various mediators produced by injury and inflammation. A number of factors are released from damaged tissue, from immune cells and other blood cells. These can act directly on nociceptors or can stimulate the production and release of other mediators from immune cells and sympathetic neurons.

indirectly by altering the concentration of one or more chemical mediator, or more directly through specific thermosensitive ion channels.

ION CHANNELS OF SENSORY NEURONS

Studies on the cell soma membrane of dorsal root ganglion neurons, either in situ, in freshly isolated cells or cells maintained in tissue culture, show that the same types of ion channel occur in sensory neurons as in other excitable cells (Scott 1992). However, we cannot be sure how exactly the properties of the nerve terminal membrane, where the processes of transduction and encoding take place, resemble those of the soma. Furthermore, cultured sensory neurons are normally exposed to high concentrations of nerve growth factor, which is known to alter ion channel expression and affect membrane properties (see below).

In general activation of inward (depolarizing) membrane currents, or inactivation of outward currents, will lead to increased excitability of the membrane, whereas the opposite changes will inhibit the cell from firing. It is convenient to divide membrane ion channels into those that are gated by changes in membrane potential, and those that are gated by chemical ligands. In making this distinction, it must be borne in mind that many voltage-gated channels are modulated (usually on a longer time-scale), by chemical mediators, and that many ligand-gated ion channels also show some voltage-sensitivity. The physiological responses of nociceptive neurons that need to be better understood in terms of ion channel behaviour are:

1. Normal excitation by noxious stimuli (chemical, thermal, mechanical)
2. Pathological sensitization (increased response to low-intensity stimuli)
3. Spontaneous activity associated with neuronal damage.

VOLTAGE-GATED ION CHANNELS

The main channels responsible for inward membrane currents are the voltage-activated sodium and calcium channels, since these are the main ions for which a large inward electrochemical gradient is maintained (Nowycky 1992). Increased chloride permeability also depolarizes sensory neurons, though less strongly, since the equilibrium potential for chloride is much less positive (~−20 mV) than that for sodium (~ +40 mV) or calcium (>+60 mV). Outward current is carried mainly by potassium ions. For each of these principal ions, there are several distinct types of voltage-gated channel (see below). Many modulatory factors that control the excitability of neurons do so by activating or inhibiting one or more types of potassium conductance.

Sodium channels

Sodium channels, which open rapidly and transiently when the membrane is depolarized beyond about −40mV, are essential in most neurons for action potential generation and conduction. Studies on sensory neurons in vitro show that the C-cells, which have unmyelinated axons, and correspond mainly to the physiologically-defined polymodal nociceptive neurons, usually have slow action potentials, with a clearly defined inflection on the falling phase. They can be distinguished from A-cells, which have myelinated axons and much faster action potentials, though there is some overlap between the thinly myelinated Aδ- and C-cell populations (Koerber & Mendell 1992). The electrophysiological properties of A- and C-cells are summarized in Table 3.1. One difference is that the action potentials of C-cells are largely resistant to block by tetrodotoxin (TTX), because they possess a distinct population of TTX-insensitive sodium channels, which activate more slowly than the TTX-sensitive channels which predominate in A-cells (Koerber & Mendell 1992). These TTX-insensitive channels differ from the TTX-sensitive channels also in requiring a greater depolarization for activation and inactivation (Kostyuk et al 1981a; McLean et al 1988). These differences mean that C-cells have a higher depolarization threshold for action potential generation, and are also less liable than A-cells to become refractory. TTX-insensitive sodium channels occur also in skeletal and cardiac muscle (Stephan & Agnew 1991) but it is not known whether they are identical to those of sensory neurons.

Table 3.1 Comparison of electrophysiological properties of A and C cell membranes

Characteristic	A-cells	C-cells
Action potential properties†		
Amplitude (mV)	73	82
Overshoot (mV)	20	32
Rate of rise (V/S)	458	227
Duration (ms)	1.0	5.0
Inflection on falling phase	No	Yes
Blocked by TTX	Yes	Partly
After-potential ampl (mV)	−5.9	−8.2*
After-potential duration (ms)	3.8	12.9*
Voltage-dependent channels		
Na currents		
TTX-sensitive	+	+
TTX-insensitive	−	+
K currents		
Delayed rectifier	++	+
Transient (A-current)	−	+ (some cells)
Ca currents		
Low threshold (T)	−	+
High threshold (L)	+	++
High threshold (N)	+	+

*Some C-cells of nodose ganglion have slow, long-lasting (>10 s) AHP in addition to fast AHP (Fowler et al 1985)

† Data from Harper & Lawson (1985)

Sodium channels as therapeutic targets

Spontaneous action potential discharge is known to occur in sensory nerve neuromas and may account for the pain associated with such lesions (see Ch. 4; it is possible that the accumulation of additional sodium channels in the axonal membrane proximal to the site of nerve transection (Devor et al 1989) is a factor in this altered membrane behaviour. Addition of extra sodium channels is, however, unlikely to be sufficient by itself to elicit spontaneous activity, since sodium channels do not open until the membrane is considerably depolarized. Most probably, as in the heart and in other types of spontaneously active neurons (Hille 1991), other types of voltage-dependent 'pacemaker' channels with relatively slow opening and closing kinetics are involved in the patterning and frequency-coding of sensory neuron activity, but more work is needed to characterize such channels in sensory neurons. However, the possibility that the sodium channels underlying the excitability of nociceptive neurons are pharmacologically distinct from those of most other neurons offers the prospect of new therapeutic approaches to neuropathic pain. This mechanism may underlie the clinical observation that some sodium channel blocking agents, such as phenytoin, carbamazepine and tocainide, may be efficaceous analgesics in neuropathic pain (Lindstrom & Lindblom 1987; Tanelian & Brose 1991), though it is not known whether this is due to an action on sensory neuron excitability.

Potassium channels

Regulation of cell excitability through the opening and closing of potassium channels is important in many physiological contexts, and the variety of different mechanisms is reflected in a great heterogeneity of potassium channel subtypes. In addition to the two main types of voltage-gated channels in sensory neurons, summarized in Table 3.2 (Nowycky 1992), many other types have been described (Cook 1990; Hille 1991).

K-channels (I_K; delayed rectifier) that open in response to depolarization occur in most neurons, and are largely responsible for the rapid repolarization of the membrane that terminates the action potential; I_K determines the action potential configuration, but has little effect on the excitability of the membrane or the firing pattern. A second type of K-channel (I_A), also found in many neurons (Rogawski 1985), opens more rapidly in response to depolarization, but also inactivates if the membrane remains even slightly depolarized. This current effectively opposes the rapidly-activating Na-current needed to generate an action potential. Thus when I_A is inactivated by a small resting depolarization of the membrane, the Na-current is effectively unopposed, and membrane excitability is increased. The rapid switch-on of I_A during

Table 3.2 Properties of voltage-gated ion channels of sensory neurons

Ion	Channel type	Act^n range (mv)	Act^n time course (msec)	Inact^n	Blockers	Modulated by	Function	Notes
Na	TTX-sensitive	–37	~1	Yes fast	TTX local anaesthetics	Not known	Fast AP upstroke	Main Na current of A-cells; less pronounced in C-cells
	TTX-insensitive	–25	~5	Yes slow	local anaesthetics	NGF	Slow TTX-resistant AP	Expressed in most C-cells
K	Delayed rectifier (I_K)	~–30	10–30	No	TEA dendrotoxin	Not known	AP repolarization	Less marked in C- than A-cells. Fast and slow-activating subtypes identified
	Transient (I_A)	–20 (fast) 0 (slow)	~1 (fast) ~5 (slow)	Yes fast ~20 ms slow 1–2 s	4-amino-pyridine	Not known	Control of repetitive firing frequency, and excitability of membrane at resting potential	
Na /K	Delayed inward rectifier (I_h)	–90	~200	No	Cs	Not known	Not known. Requires membrane hyperpolarization for activation	Mainly A-cells
Ca	Low threshold (T)	~–50	1–5	Yes 10–40 ms	Ni Amiloride Relatively insensitive to Cd	Few examples (opiates)	Can cause delayed depolarization and repetitive firing (inward Ca current) Contributes to AP repolarization and after-hyperpolarization (Ca-activated K-channels)	Absent in A-cells Abundant in medium and small DRG neurons; absent in capsaicin-sensitive neurons
	High threshold, non-inactivating (L)	~–10	slow ~50 ms	Very slow or absent	Cd Dihydropyridines	Many drugs and mediators (e.g. opiates, noradrenaline, dopamine, somatostatin, eicosanoids, GABA)	Causes 'hump' on action potential Spike after hyperpolarization Transmitter release (partly)	More in C- than in A-cells
	High threshold, inactivating (N)	~–20	~50 ms	Fast ~50 ms	Cd ω-conotoxin	As L channels	As L channels. Mainly responsible for transmitter release	Similar in all sensory neurons

an action potential means that the K-conductance of the membrane is high immediately afterwards, so the neuron cannot fire again until I_A has subsided. I_A is therefore regarded as one of the main factors regulating the maximum firing frequency of neurons (Connor & Stevens 1971). Many studies have reported A-channels in sensory neurons (e.g. Kostyuk et al 1981b; Kasai et al 1986; McFarlane & Cooper 1991) but it is not known whether there are differences between A- and C-cells. Suppression of the A-current could, in principle, give rise to the type of spontaneous activity associated with damage to sensory neurons.

Calcium-activated potassium channels

Calcium-activated K-channels ($I_{K(Ca)}$) occur in many types of cell. In neurons there are two main types (Cook 1990) and they are responsible for the later phases of the after-hyperpolarization (AHP) that follows an action potential. Calcium-activated K-channels impose a period of reduced excitability after each action potential, and are thus important in regulating the firing pattern of the neuron (Hille 1991). The channels are opened by the influx of calcium through voltage-activated calcium channels, which open during the action potential (see below). Sensory neurons, like various brain neurons, show two distinct types of spike after-hyperpolarization (Fig. 3.2), with different time-courses (Higashi et al 1984; Fowler et al 1985), which appear to be associated with the two types of Ca-activated channel. The fast AHP, which decays within a few milliseconds, is mainly due to the rapid opening of the 'big' conductance (BK) channels, and occurs in all sensory neurons. More interesting is the very prolonged AHP, lasting for several

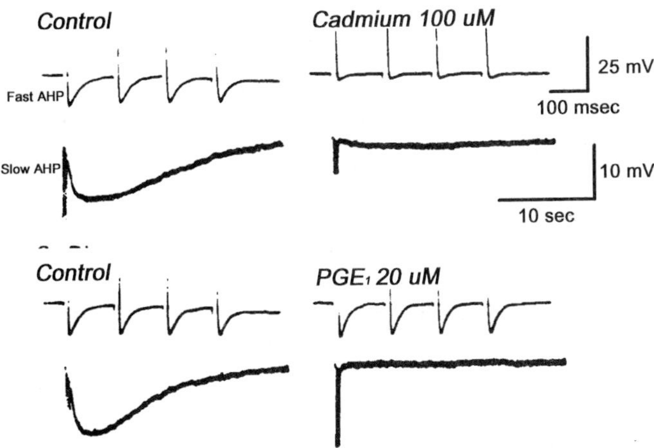

Fig. 3.2 Evidence that PGE_1 inhibits the slow calcium activated after-hyperpolarization in a visceral sensory neuron. Top two traces show that addition of cadmium, which blocks I_{Ca}, abolishes both fast and slow AHPs. Bottom two traces show that PGE_1 selectively blocks the slow AHP. (From Fowler et al 1985 with permission.)

seconds, which is seen only in a subpopulation of C-neurons, but not in A-neurons. This is associated with the opening of 'small' conductance (SK) channels, and has a major influence on the ability of the neuron to fire repetitively in response to a maintained depolarization (Weinreich & Wonderlin 1987); it is also susceptible to inhibition by inflammatory mediators such as prostaglandins (Fig. 3.3; Weinreich & Wonderlin 1987), bradykinin (Weinreich 1986) and 5-hydroxytryptamine (Christian et al 1989). It is one of the few examples so far where it has been possible to account for the physiological modulation of sensory neuron properties in terms of a defined effect on the cell membrane. The slow AHP has been recorded in visceral afferent (nodose ganglion) neurons of the rabbit, but it is not known whether it is a general property of C-neurons.

Slow inward rectifier channels

Sensory neurons also express another kind of voltage-dependent cation channel, the inward rectifier channel which is unusual among ion channels in being activated by membrane hyperpolarization. In sensory neurons, these channels are permeable to both sodium and potassium ions, and they are activated only when the membrane is hyperpolarized beyond its normal resting potential of about -70 mV (Mayer & Westbrook 1983). Among sensory neurons, inward rectification is largely confined to A-cells (Nowycky 1992), but its physiological role is unknown. One of the effects of infection of sensory neurons with herpes simplex virus is to block this inward rectifier current; however, the loss of excitability that the virus produces is most probably due to loss of functional sodium channels (Mayer et al 1986).

A. Direct ligand-gated channel type

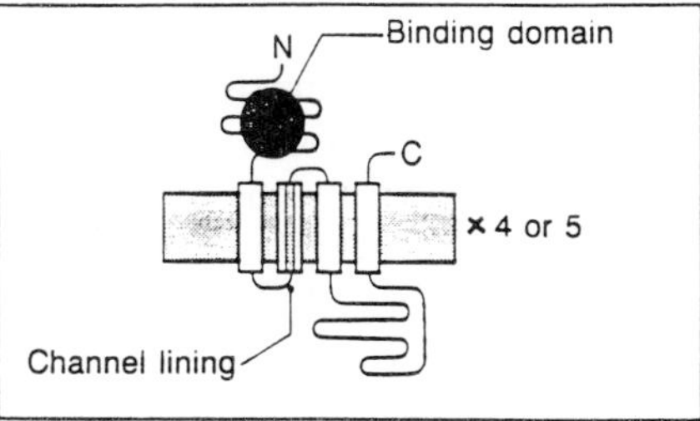

B. G-protein-coupled type

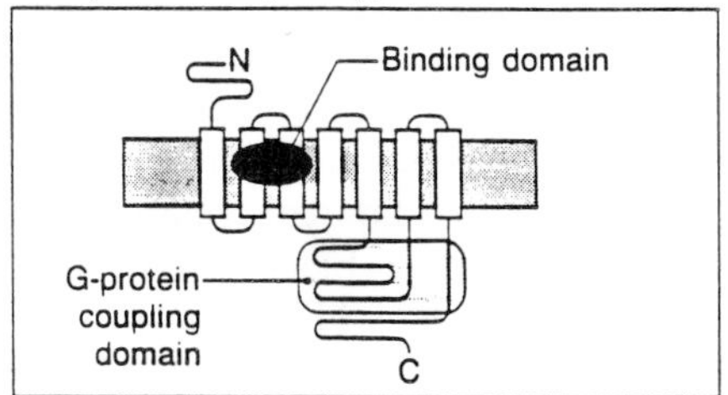

C. Tyrosine-kinase-linked type

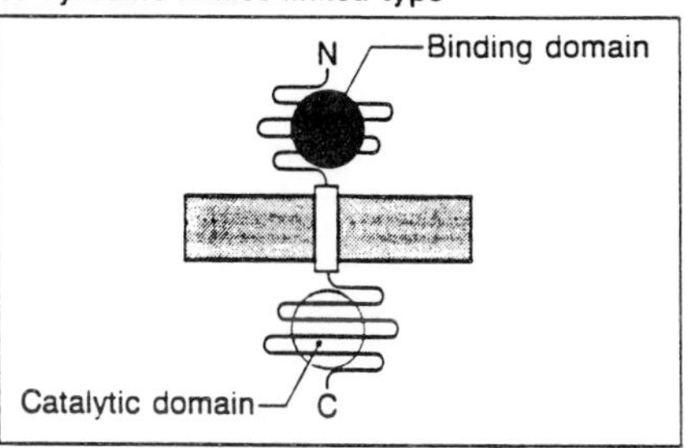

D. Intracellular steroid/thyroid type

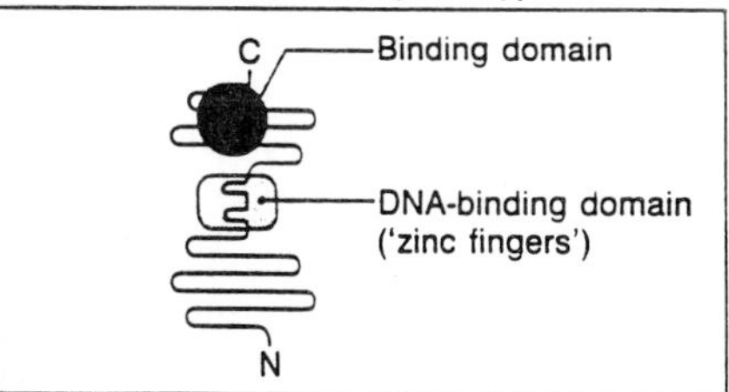

Fig. 3.3 General structure of four receptor families. The hydrophobic transmembrane domains are shown as rectangles. **A** Type I – fast ligand-gated ion channels: involved mainly in fast neuronal activity and composed of 4–5 sub-units of the type shown. The channel and the ligand binding site form part of the same protein molecule, and are coupled allosterically, with no intervening biochemical processes. **B** Type II – G-protein coupled receptors: possess a distinct intracellular domain through which they couple to G-proteins, this association occurring only when the receptor is occupied by a ligand molecule. The activated G-proteins associate with an effector molecule, which is usually an enzyme such as adenylate cyclase. The enzyme may be activated or inhibited, thus changing the concentration of one or more intracellular second messengers (e.g. cyclic nucleotides, inositol phosphates, calcium ions). **C** Type III – Tyrosine-kinase-linked receptors: involved mainly in the actions of growth factors such as NGF. The extracellular ligand-binding domain of the receptor is coupled directly to an intracellular catalytic domain, which is activated when the ligand is bound, causing phosphorylation of tyrosine residues of particular substrate proteins. **D** Type IV – Steroid/thyroid hormone receptors: bind to and regulate specific DNA sequences in the cell nucleus, thereby controlling transcription of particular genes, and the expression of particular proteins by the cell. Little is known about their role in sensory neurons. (From Rang & Dale 1991 with permission.)

Calcium channels

Voltage-activated calcium channels are expressed in many types of cell (Hess 1990; Scott et al 1991). Sensory neurons have been shown to possess three main kinds, termed L-, N- and T-channels respectively. They are distinguished on the basis of the degree of membrane depolarization needed to activate the currents (activation threshold), their inactivation characteristics and their pharmacological properties (Table 3.2). T-channels, sometimes referred to as LVA (low voltage-activated) channels, form a well-defined class, characterized by a low threshold for activation. The distinction between N- and L-channels is based on their different inactivation characteristics and on their different pharmacological properties (L-channels being blocked by dihydropyridine calcium antagonists, while N-channels are blocked by ω-conotoxin). Recent studies on the distribution of these channel subtypes in sensory neurons (Scroggs & Fox 1992; Table 3.1) show that T-channels are absent in large-diameter neurons (presumably A-cells), very abundant in medium-diameter neurons, and present at lower abundance in small-diameter, capsaicin-sensitive, neurons (presumably C-cells). N-channel currents appear to be similar in all cells, but dihydropyridine-sensitive (L) channel currents were predominant in small-diameter cells. In medium- and large-diameter cells, Scroggs & Fox (1992) found that a large proportion of the calcium current was carried by channels that were neither low-threshold (T) nor blocked by dihydropyridine (L) or ω-conotoxin (N), implying the presence of another kind of channel.

With regard to cell function, calcium entry through voltage-gated Ca-channels can affect many cellular processes, including activation of other membrane channels, release of transmitters, and regulation of many enzymes (especially kinases and phosphatases) which initiate a variety of other short- and long-term cellular effects. The inward current contributes directly to membrane depolarization, and the characteristic 'hump' on the falling phase of the C-cell action potential is due to a Ca-current. It is known to be sensitive to many agents (e.g. baclofen, noradrenaline, dopamine, somatostatin, opiates) which are known to inhibit high-threshold (L and/or N) channels in sensory neurons (Scott et al 1991; Cox & Dunlap 1992). T-currents can also carry a substantial depolarizing current, and may be responsible for repetitive firing of sensory neurons following a single stimulus (White et al 1989). T-channels appear to be unaffected by most of the inhibitory modulators that act on L- and/or N-channels, although Schroeder et al (1991) found that opiates inhibited T-currents as well as high-threshold currents. In contrast, the entry of calcium through high-threshold (L or N) channels, which depends greatly on the amplitude and duration of the action potential, is modulated by chemical agents (see below). In general, calcium entry through T-channels appears to be involved mainly in the control of neuronal firing patterns, partly on account of the inward current itself, and partly through the opening of various calcium-activated ion channels, whereas calcium entry through high-threshold channels controls transmitter release. In sensory neurons, neuropeptide release is blocked by ω-conotoxin, but relatively insensitive to dihydropyridines (Perney et al 1986; Santicolli et al 1992), suggesting that N-channels are the main portal of entry for the calcium involved in peptide release.

CHEMICAL EXCITATION AND SENSITIZATION OF SENSORY NEURONS

To respond to chemical signals, sensory neurons are provided with specific recognition proteins (receptors). There are four distinct types of receptor (Fig. 3.3) involved in chemical signalling, whose architecture reflects their different transduction mechanisms (Rang & Dale 1991).

In general, Type I receptors are involved in fast neuronal excitation or inhibition, working on the millisecond time scale; Type II receptors are associated mainly with modulatory processes, acting over a timescale of seconds to minutes; Type III and IV receptors generally produce their effects through changes in gene transcription, and act in hours or days. This is an over-simplification, however, since the biochemical processes controlled by each type of receptor may interact strongly. For example, the opening of membrane calcium channels by capsaicin (Type I mechanism) may disrupt axonal transport, and thus prevent access of nerve growth factor (Type III mechanism) to the cell body, thereby inhibiting neuropeptide synthesis (Otten et al 1983). For general accounts of the role of chemical ligands and their receptors in the control of neuronal function, see Kandel et al 1991; Levitan & Kaczmarek 1991.

AGENTS ACTING ON SENSORY NEURONS

Table 3.3 summarizes the various types of receptor which are found on sensory neurons and indicates the way in which membrane properties are affected. Figure 3.4 shows some of the molecular events which can occur at the nociceptor terminal.

Protons and capsaicin

The pH of the extracellular environment is known to fall in a number of pathophysiological conditions such as hypoxia/anoxia as well as in inflammation (Jacobus et al 1977; Corbe & Poole-Wilson 1980). For example, recent studies have reported that the pH of synovial fluid from

Table 3.3 Different receptor types on sensory neurons and their cellular effects

Receptor type	Link to ion channel	Example (receptor subtype)	Cellular effect
Type I	Direct	Capsaicin/RTX H^+ 5-HT (5-HT_3) ATP (P_2) Glutamate (kainate) GABA ($GABA_a$)	Excitation
Type II	G-protein linked	GABA ($GABA_b$) Somatostatin Opiates Adenosine Adrenoreceptors Neuropeptide Y 5-HT (5-$HT_{1 \text{ or } 2}$)	Inhibition of transmitter and peptide release: presynaptic inhibition
		Bradykinin (B_2) 5-HT (5-$HT_{1\text{-like and } 2}$) Histamine ($H_1$) Eicosanoids Adrenoreceptors (α_2) PGE_2	Excitation and/or sensitization
Type III	None	NGF (trk a)	Modifies gene expression

inflamed joints is significantly more acid than that from normal joints with the pH of 'bulk fluid' as low as pH 6.6-6.8 (Ward & Steigbigel 1978). Indeed the local, pericellular pH around sensory terminals may be even more acidic than the bulk fluid.

Low pH solutions evoke a prolonged activation of sensory nerves (Steen et al 1992) and produce a sharp stinging pain (Lindahl 1962). Protons evoke two types of depolarizing ionic current in sensory neurons. One current is evoked by rapid changes in pH in the normal physiological range, 7.4–7.0 (Krishtal & Pidoplichko 1980; Konnerth et al 1987). As this current and the resultant depolarization lasts only a few seconds, it is unlikely to contribute to any prolonged nociceptive response. The second current has a different ionic basis to the initial current and is evoked by a greater lowering of extracellular pH. These low pH levels are required to produce the sustained nerve activation seen in intact preparations. This current shows a much slower rate of inactivation and can be sustained for several minutes (Bevan & Yeats 1991). The membrane depolarization evoked by this current is the probable basis for the prolonged sensory neuron activation seen with low pH solutions (Steen et al 1992).

Capsaicin, the pungent principle in *Capsicum* peppers, has a highly specific action on a subpopulation of sensory neurons. Capsaicin activates nociceptive neurons, notably the polymodal nociceptors, to evoke the sensation of burning pain (LaMotte et al 1992). Visceral afferents can also be activated by capsaicin (Maggi 1992) and this activation results in autonomic effects either through reflex actions or by the direct release of sensory neuropeptides from the peripheral terminals of these sensory axons. Several pieces of evidence indicate that capsaicin interacts with a specific membrane receptor: the effects are cell specific, small modifications to the structure of capsaicin can have large effects on activity with a clear structure-

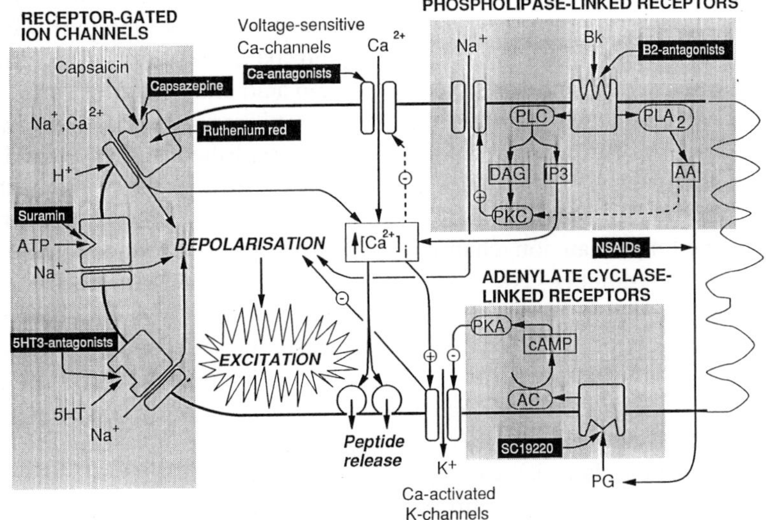

Fig. 3.4 Simplified scheme illustrating some of the molecular events that control the excitability of nociceptive peripheral neurons.
Abbreviations: PLC = phospholipase C; PLA_2 = phospholipase A_2; DAG = diacylglycerol; IP3 = inositol-1,4,5-trisphosphate; PKC = protein kinase C; AA = arachidonic acid; PG = prostaglandin; AC = adenylate cylcase; cAMP = cyclic adenosine monophosphate; PKA = cAMP-dependent protein kinase; Bk = bradykinin; 5HT = 5-hydroxytryptamine; NSAIDs = nonsteroidal antiinflammatory drugs. (From Rang et al 1991 with permission.)

activity relationship demonstrated (Szolcsanyi & Jansco-Gabor 1975), and the effects of capsaicin can be inhibited by a newly discovered competitive antagonist, capsazepine (Dickenson & Dray 1991; Bevan et al 1992). The interaction between capsaicin and its receptor opens an ion channel that is permeable to both monovalent and divalent cations (Bevan & Szolcsanyi 1990). The resultant ion flow produces an inward membrane current that depolarizes and activates the neuron.

The normal physiological role for the unique capsaicin-sensitive ion channel is not known. So far no endogenous capsaicin-like molecule has been identified, but the sustained membrane current evoked by protons shows a striking similarity to that evoked by capsaicin (Bevan et al 1993). The two responses have a common ionic basis and both capsaicin and protons activate neuronal channels with similar characteristics. Furthermore responsiveness to both agents is controlled by nerve growth factor (Winter et al 1988). Although protons can activate the capsaicin-operated ion channels the binding site for protons and capsaicin appears to differ as capsazepine, a competitive capsaicin antagonist, has no effect on the sensory nerve activation by protons (Bevan et al 1993). Another structurally related toxin, resiniferatoxin (RTX) is some 100-1000 times more potent than capsaicin (Szallasi & Blumberg 1989) and activates the same ion channel (Winter et al 1990). The binding of RTX to sensory neuronal membranes can be displaced by capsaicin (Szallasi & Blumberg 1990) and the effects of RTX are inhibited competitively by capsazepine, indicating that the binding sites for RTX and capsaicin are in close proximity or overlap.

Adenosine triphosphate (ATP) and adenosine

ATP is present at millimolar levels in cells and is released by tissue damage where it can act on the surrounding cells including the sensory neurons. Intradermal injection of micromolar concentrations of ATP produces a sharp, transient pain. In rat sensory neurons, this activation by ATP is due to the opening of an ion channel permeable to both monovalent (notably Na^+) and divalent (Ca^{2+}) ions (Krishtal et al 1988; Bean et al 1990) and can be blocked by a purinergic P_2-receptor antagonist, suramin.

ATP receptors are also found on inflammatory cells, notably macrophages. Macrophage activation by ATP liberates various cytokines and prostanoids which can act, either directly or indirectly, to sensitize sensory neurons (see below). In addition adenosine formed by the breakdown of ATP also provokes pain when administered to a human blister base (Bleehen & Keele 1977). Adenosine can induce hyperalgesia in animals when administered intradermally (Taiwo & Levine 1990) and produces pain in human volunteers when administered intravenously (Sylven 1989). The observation that cat myelinated and unmyelinated vagal afferents are sensitized by intravenous adenosine (Cherniak et al 1987) is consistent with the human data. The mechanisms of action of adenosine are not well understood but its actions are thought to be due to a direct effect on sensory neurons rather than by activation of other cell types. Activation of an A_2-receptor producing a rise in cAMP levels has been implicated in the hyperalgesia induced in animals (Taiwo & Levine 1990). Other studies have failed, however, to find evidence that activation of either A_1 or A_2-receptors influences the discharge of mechanoreceptive neurons in normal and arthritic ankle joints in the rat (Ashgar et al 1992).

Excitatory amino acids

Glutamate depolarizes sensory neurons by directly opening ion channels (Huettner 1990). Studies on both isolated sensory neurons and dorsal root preparations from neonatal rats have shown that the receptor has a unique pharmacology. There are three major classes of glutamate receptors directly linked to ion channels. These have been categorized on the basis of their preferential activation by certain agonists and sensitivity to antagonists. NMDA receptors are activated by N-methyl-D-aspartate, AMPA receptors by (±) 2-amino-3-hydroxy-5-methyl-4-isoxazole-proprionic acid and kainate receptors by kainic acid. The general pharmacological profile of the sensory neuron receptor places it in the kainate preferring class; AMPA is far less active than kainate and NMDA is inactive. However, the sensory neuron receptor differs from the kainate receptors in other neurons (e.g. motoneurons) as it displays a much higher affinity for agonists such as domoate (Huettner 1990; Ishida & Shinozaki 1991) and has a different selectivity for some amino acid antagonists (Evans et al 1987). The physiological significance of the sensitivity to glutamate has not been established and it is unclear whether glutamate is released from tissues to activate sensory neurons. Nevertheless in animal experiments, local injection of glutamate can produce inflammation and hyperalgesia (Follenfant & Nakamura-Craig 1992), although in the latter case the available data with specific antagonists suggest that NMDA-type receptors rather than kainate receptors are involved.

Bradykinin

Bradykinin, a 9-residue peptide formed by proteolytic cleavage of a circulating precursor protein, is an important inflammatory mediator. Its effects include contraction or relaxation of visceral and vascular smooth muscle, secretion from epithelial cells, and stimulation of nociceptive neurons (Marceau et al 1983; Proud & Kaplan 1988; Dray & Perkins 1993).

Algogenic effects

Bradykinin stimulates nociceptive nerve terminals and causes pain (Kumazawa & Mizumura 1980; Manning et al 1991). It is the most potent endogenous algogenic agent known. In addition to activating nociceptive nerve terminals directly, bradykinin sensitizes them to other stimuli, including mechanical and thermal stimulation (Mense & Meyer 1988; Manning et al 1991). There is also a strong synergism between the excitatory action of bradykinin and that of other algogenic substances, such as prostaglandins and 5-hydroxytryptamine (Lembeck & Juan 1974), and bradykinin itself evokes the release of prostaglandins (see below). In the skin, bradykinin excites mainly the C-polymodal nociceptors (Beck & Handwerker 1974; Lang et al 1990) but some other classes of C- and Aδ-units may also be activated. In joint and muscle afferents (Kanaka et al 1985) nonmyelinated Group IV, and thinly-myelinated Group III afferents seem to be equally sensitive to bradykinin. In general bradykinin-sensitive fibres form a subpopulation of the capsaicin-sensitive group (Lang et al 1990); there is a broad, but incomplete, overlap between the populations of fibres that respond to bradykinin and to other algogenic agents, such as histamine and 5-hydroxytryptamine.

Bradykinin receptors on sensory neurons

Two main classes of bradykinin receptor (B_1 and B_2) have been defined pharmacologically (Farmer & Burch 1992). The B_1 receptor is selectively activated by des-Arg^9-bradykinin, which can be formed from bradykinin by the action of a tissue peptidase. Another analogue, des-Arg^9-Leu^8-bradykinin, acts as a selective antagonist for the B1 receptor. The B1 receptor is constitutively expressed in certain vascular tissues, but in other tissues it appears only to be expressed (or unmasked) under conditions of inflammation or other kinds of tissue insult. The physiological significance of this unusual behaviour of the B_1 receptor is not yet clear. The B_2 receptor is much better characterized, and accounts for the majority of the pharmacological effects of bradykinin. Recently discovered peptide antagonists of bradykinin (e.g. NPC 567, Steranka et al 1988, HOE140, Hock et al 1991), selective for the B2 receptor, have helped to establish that bradykinin makes a significant contribution to inflammatory pain and hyperalgesia and that the direct effects of bradykinin on sensory neurons are mediated by B_2 receptors (Whalley et al 1987; Steranka et al 1988). Normally B_1-receptor agonists do not mimic, nor do B_1-receptor antagonists block, the excitatory effects of bradykinin (Whalley et al 1987). However under conditions where inflammatory hyperalgesia persists for a few days or longer, there may be a significant contribution of B_1 receptors to the hyperalgesia (Perkins et al 1993; Dray & Perkins 1993). Clearly, therefore, kinins are important mediators in both acute pain and in the subsequent hyperalgesia produced by injury and inflammation. Prevention of their effects with receptor antagonists will most certainly provide new therapies for pain and inflammation.

Mechanism of action of bradykinin

Both molecular cloning (McEachern et al 1991; Hess et al 1992) and biochemical studies (Farmer & Burch 1992) indicate that B_2. receptors belong to Type II (see above), and couple to effector molecules via G-proteins. Studies on sensory neurons in culture (Burgess et al 1989a; McGehee et al 1992) show that the excitatory effect of bradykinin is associated with an inward (depolarizing) current and an increase in membrane conductance, mainly to sodium ions. Compared with the response to agents such as capsaicin or protons, which operate through ligand-gated ion channels (Type I), the membrane response is slow. This presumably reflects the time-course of the biochemical events that follow receptor occupation.

In nodose ganglion cells, bradykinin produces a different kind of excitatory effect, associated with the inhibition of a long-lasting spike AHP (Fig. 3.2). The slow-AHP following a single action potential, or a short train, produces a state of inexcitability, which limits the number of action potentials that can be produced in response to a single depolarizing event (Weinreich 1986; Weinreich & Wonderlin 1987). Inhibition of the slow-AHP by bradykinin therefore allows the cell to fire more action potentials when it is depolarized, a mechanism which could account for the observed sensitization. This response to bradykinin appears to be secondary to prostaglandin formation, as it is completely prevented by cyclooxygenase inhibition (Weinreich 1986), and can be mimicked by applying various prostaglandins to the cells. The slow-AHP does not seem to occur in the soma of dorsal root ganglion neurons, so the relevance of this effect of bradykinin to nociception is uncertain.

In sensory neurons (Fig. 3.5), the main biochemical pathway through which bradykinin acts involves the G protein-mediated activation of phospholipase C, which generates two intracellular second messengers, 1,4,5-inositol-trisphosphate (IP3) and diacylglycerol (DAG) by cleavage of membrane phospholipids (Thayer et al 1988; Burgess et al 1989a; Gammon et al 1989). IP3 leads to the release of intracellular calcium, and a rise in the free calcium concentration within the cell (Thayer et al 1988). The main effect of diacylglycerol is to activate protein kinase C, leading to the phosphorylation of various intracellular proteins (Shearman et al 1989).

Burgess et al (1989a) showed that the depolarization, and associated calcium entry, caused by bradykinin could be reduced or abolished by inhibition or down-regulation

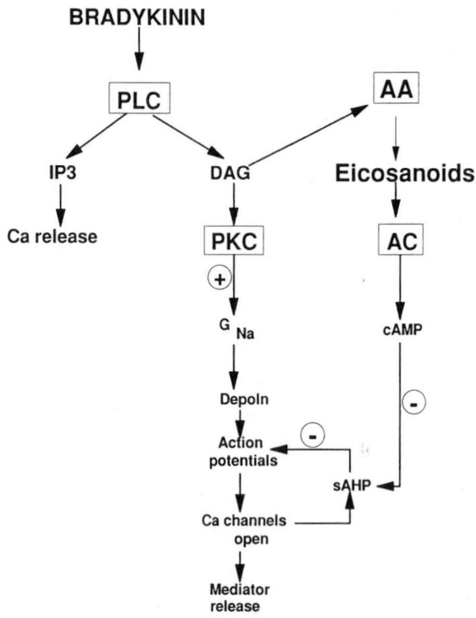

Fig. 3.5 Scheme illustrating the actions of bradykinin on sensory neurons. Activation of G-protein coupled bradykinin B_2 receptors depolarizes the neuron mainly by increasing membrane sodium permeability. Depolarization may activate voltage dependent calcium influx. Receptor activation stimulates several different biochemical pathways: 1. Phospholipase C to generate diacylglycerol (DAG) and inositol trisphosphate (IP3) from membrane phospholipids. IP3 stimulates a rise in intracellular calcium and this may increase calcium-activated potassium current leading to membrane hyperpolarization and a reduced excitability. Calcium may also induce a release of mediators. DAG activates protein kinase C (PKC) which can regulate ion channel protein and thereby alter membrane excitability as well as regulate other cellular processes. 2. Bradykinin also stimulates the production of arachidonic acid (AA) either via DAG in sensory neurons or via PLA_2 in surrounding tissues. Prostanoids (especially PGE_2 and PGI_2), produced mainly from AA metabolism, induce sensitization via activation of adenylate cyclase (AC), generation of cAMP and activation of kinase A. These change the activity of membrane ion channel proteins, e.g. calcium dependent potassium channels.

of protein kinase C, and could be mimicked by phorbol esters, which activate protein kinase C. They concluded that this enzyme played a key role in the excitatory effect. Staurosporine, a protein kinase C inhibitor, was also shown to inhibit afferent fibre stimulation by bradykinin in the rat skin (Dray et al 1992). Staurosporine did not, however, inhibit the bradykinin-evoked depolarization of the central terminals of afferent fibres in the spinal cord (Dunn & Rang 1991). Protein kinase C activation is therefore unlikely to be the only mechanism involved in the excitatory effect of bradykinin.

One puzzling observation is that bradykinin may inhibit voltage-gated calcium currents in sensory neurons, this effect being ascribed to activation of PKC (Ewald et al 1989; Boland et al 1991). This is hard to reconcile with the ability of bradykinin to evoke neuropeptide release from sensory neurons (see below), and to augment electrically-evoked release (Andreeva & Rang 1993).

The release of intracellular calcium by IP3 seems to have relatively little effect in sensory neurons. Calcium-activated potassium channels also show a low susceptibility to opening by intracellular calcium. Indeed, calcium-dependent effects of bradykinin on sensory neurons, such as neuropeptide release (Geppetti et al 1990) and generation of cGMP (Burgess et al 1989b), require the presence of extracellular calcium; the release of intracellular stores in these cells therefore appears to be a much less effective stimulus than calcium entry through voltage-activated channels.

Sensory neurons generate arachidonic acid and prostanoids in response to bradykinin, through an indirect mechanism initiated by activation of phospholipase C (Gammon et al 1989; Allen et al 1992). In many other types of cell (Farmer & Burch 1992), bradykinin can activate phospholipase A2 directly to generate prostaglandins. Thus the excitatory actions of bradykinin on sensory neurons are mediated partly through the release of prostaglandins from other tissues. In keeping with this, cyclooxygenase inhibitors reduce the excitatory effect of bradykinin on nociceptors (Lembeck & Juan 1974; Mizumura et al 1987). The mechanisms by which prostaglandins accentuate the excitatory actions of other algogenic substances are described below.

5-Hydroxytryptamine (5-HT)

5-HT is released from platelets and mast cells during tissue damage and can act in several ways on sensory neurons. Application of 5-HT to a human blister base causes a mild and transient pain (Richardson et al 1985). Two mechanisms for sensory neuron excitation have been reported. The first involves an action on 5-HT_3 receptors found on some small-diameter, capsaicin-sensitive neurons (Bevan & Robertson 1991). This may be the major mechanism of excitation as the pain produced by 5-HT application to a human blister base can be inhibited by a specific 5-HT_3 antagonist (Richardson et al 1985). Molecular cloning experiments have shown that the 5-HT_3 binding site is part of membrane protein that forms a cation (Na^+) selective ion channel (Maricq et al 1991), which when opened depolarizes and activates the neuron. 5-HT can also act on 5-HT_2 receptors. In this case the effect is indirect as 5-HT_2 receptors are linked via G-proteins to closure of potassium channels which are open in the resting membrane. This results in membrane depolarization and neuronal firing (Todorovic & Anderson 1990). The precise biochemical pathways that underlie this second type of excitation have not been established.

Sensitization.

Sensitization by 5-HT is known to lower the threshold of primary afferent nociceptors to other noxious stimuli

(Beck & Handwerker 1974; Taiwo & Levine 1992; Rueff & Dray 1992). There is experimental evidence for the involvement of both 5-HT_1-like and 5-HT_2 receptors in this process but 5-HT_3 agonists and antagonists were without effect against hyperalgesia in animals (Taiwo & Levine 1992; Rueff & Dray 1992). However, in the human blister base, 5-HT produces a marked enhancement of the pain evoked by bradykinin and this is blocked by the 5-HT_3 antagonist ICS 205.930 (Richardson et al 1985). Moreover this antagonist inhibits the hyperalgesia, but not the oedema, associated with experimental carrageenan-induced inflammation (Eschalier et al 1989) suggesting that 5-HT_3 receptors are also involved in hyperalgesia. Since ICS 205.930 blocks 5-HT_4 receptors (Boeckart et al 1990) it is possible that this receptor subtype, normally linked to adenylate cyclase system, rather than 5HT_3-receptors is involved in 5-HT-mediated hyperalgesia.

The sensitization produced by 5-HT is likely to be a direct effect on sensory neurons. Thus sympathectomy and depletion of polymorphonuclear leucocytes has no effect on 5-HT mediated hyperalgesia in animals (Taiwo & Levine 1992). Furthermore, indomethacin does not appear to affect 5-HT-mediated sensitization (Rueff & Dray 1992; Taiwo & Levine 1992), which suggests that cyclooxygenase products are not involved in this process. In contrast, sensitization can be blocked by Rp-cAMPS, an inhibitor of cAMP dependent kinase, and augmented by a phosphodiesterase inhibitor (Taiwo et al 1992). Collectively these observations suggest that a cAMP mediated phosphorylation process is required for sensitization by 5-HT. A possible ionic basis for 5-HT sensitization is a reduction of the slow inhibitory afterpotential that follows the action potential in some sensory neurons (Christian et al 1989). This inhibition is due to a cAMP-mediated reduction in a K^+ current. The overall effect is to increase the likelihood that the neuron will respond to a relatively weak stimulus with a train of action potentials rather than with a single spike.

Histamine

Histamine is released from mast cells and acts through sensory neurons to evoke the sensations of itch and pain (Broadbent 1955). In general it is thought that low concentrations of histamine induce itch while higher concentrations (or larger experimental injection volumes) cause pain (Simone et al 1991). Little is known of the mechanisms by which histamine exerts its effects. Some sensory neurons express histamine H_1 receptors (Ninkovic & Hunt 1985) and H_1 receptor activation increases membrane calcium permeability in trigeminal ganglion and DRG neurons (Tani et al 1990) and releases both tachykinins and CGRP (Saria et al 1988; Vedder & Otten 1991). Further complex interactions are therefore possible since, for example, substance P released from the sensory nerve terminals may produce mast cell degranulation and further histamine release. Histamine release is also stimulated by interleukin-1 (IL-1), which in turn can potentiate the stimulatory effects of histamine on the release of prostaglandins and monohydroxyeicosatetraenoic acids (HETEs) from endothelial cells (Falus & Meretey 1992).

Arachidonic acid metabolites

Products of both the cyclooxygenase and lipoxygenase pathways have been reported to either excite nociceptors or, more usually, to sensitize them to other stimuli and thus contribute to peripheral hyperalgesia.

Prostanoids

Inflamed tissues, such as the joints of patients suffering from rheumatoid arthritis and animals with experimentally induced arthritis, contain high concentrations of prostaglandins (Trang et al 1977; Higgs & Salmon 1979). A reduction in the levels of prostanoids by inhibition of cyclooxygenase is believed to be the basis for the analgesic actions of nonsteroidal antiinflammatory drugs (NSAIDs)(Moncada et al 1975; Bombaderie et al 1981).

A major effect of prostaglandins is to sensitize afferent neurons to noxious chemical agents, to heat, and to mechanical stimulation (Handwerker 1975; Chahl & Iggo 1977; Birrell et al 1991). It has been suggested that cyclic AMP stimulation is involved (Ferreira & Nakamura 1979) since agents that elevate cyclic AMP produce hyperalgesia by a direct action of cyclic AMP on the afferent neuron (Taiwo et al 1989; Taiwo & Levine 1991a). The ionic mechanism that underlies this sensitization has not been fully elucidated, but for visceral neurons in rabbits prostaglandins D_2 and E_2 increase excitability via cyclic AMP-mediated inhibition of a slow after-hyperpolarization (Fig. 3.2).

Although prostaglandins rarely activate cutaneous nociceptive afferents directly (Chahl & Iggo 1977) and do not evoke pain when injected intradermally into human skin (Crunkhorn & Willis 1971), PGE_1 and prostacyclin (PGI_2) were shown to increase the activity of nociceptors in rat articular nerves (Schaible & Schmidt 1988; Birrell et al 1991; Schepelmann et al 1992). These findings raise the possibility that prostanoids could contribute directly to the activation of afferent neurons in inflammatory conditions such as arthritis. Studies of rat isolated sensory (DRG) neurons have shown that application of PGE_2 can evoke excitation in some neurons. The depolarizing current was carried, at least in part, by Na^+ (Puttick 1992) and could be the basis for any direct neuronal activation by prostanoids.

Lipoxygenase products

Intradermal injection of either leukotriene B_4 (a product of the 5-lipoxygenase pathway) or 8R,15S-diHETE (a product of the 15-lipoxygenase pathway) decreases the mechanical and thermal thresholds for nociception (Levine et al 1985, 1986; Bisgaard & Kristensen 1985). There appears to be a high degree of overlap, if not identity, between the nerve fibres sensitized by LTB_4 and PGE_2, which suggests a common mode of action (Martin et al 1987). The action of LTB_4 appears to be indirect; though it is unaffected by block of cyclooxygenase activity, it requires the presence of polymorphonuclear leucocytes (PMNLs) (Levine et al 1985). Thus LTB_4 releases another agent, which has been tentatively identified as 8R,15S-diHETE, from PMNLs (Levine et al 1985). 8R,15S-diHETE itself decreases the mechanical and thermal thresholds of C-fibre mechanonociceptors (Martin 1990) and produces mechanical hyperalgesia which, like the hyperalgesia induced by LTB_4, can be inhibited by the isomer 8S,15S-diHETE (Levine et al 1986). Furthermore, repetitive injections of the related hydroxyacid, 15-HETE, produce a persistent hyperalgesia in rats (Follenfant et al 1990).

LTD_4 can also sensitize sensory neurons indirectly (Rackham & Ford-Hutchinson 1983). In inflamed tissues LTD_4 stimulates the synthesis and release of eicosanoids, as well as the production of diacylglycerol and inositol phosphates in cells such as macrophages and basophils (Crook et al 1989). Further, lipoxin A_4 has been shown to stimulate capsaicin sensitive nerves in airways (Manzini & Meini 1991) although an effect on cutaneous or articular nerves has not been reported.

The mechanisms that mediate the effects of the leukotrienes and hydroxyacids on nociceptors are unclear. Activation of protein kinase C (Rang & Ritchie 1988) would be consistent with the findings that H-7, an inhibitor of PKC, can reduce 15-HETE induced hyperalgesia in rats (Follenfant et al 1990) and that lipoxin A_4 and other eicosanoids can activate PKC (Hannson et al 1986). Another possible mode of excitation or sensitization is by inhibition of membrane potassium permeability. This has been described for a related hydroperoxyacid in invertebrates (Piomelli & Greengard 1990).

Nitric oxide (NO)

Several important mediators of inflammatory hyperalgesia, including substance P and bradykinin stimulate vascular endothelial cells to release the vasodilator nitric oxide (Moncada et al 1991). NO is an unstable molecule considered to be important in intercellular communication in peripheral tissue and in the nervous system (Moncada et al 1991), including nociceptive pathways. NO is formed from L-arginine following the activation of nitric oxide synthase (NOS) by calcium and other cofactors (Moncada et al 1991). NO then alters cellular processes via the activation of guanylate cyclase and the production of cGMP.

DRG neurons are able to make NO and an increase in cGMP has been measured in DRG satellite cells following stimulation with an NO donor such as nitroprusside (Morris et al 1992). There is little evidence for direct activation of sensory neurons by NO (McGehee et al 1992), but NO alters their excitability indirectly. For example, the tachyphylaxis seen in the excitatory effect of bradykinin on sensory neurons in culture can be prevented by NO (McGehee et al 1992). In vivo, however, NO donors have been postulated to activate cerebral sensory fibres and to release CGRP which then produces vasodilation via guanylate cyclase stimulation (Wei et al 1992). In addition, systemic administration of L-arginine analogues which are inhibitors of NOS produced antinociceptive activity against neuropathic (Meller et al 1992a) and chemically-induced pain (Moore et al 1991; Haley et al 1992). In these latter situations it is likely that the effects were mediated centrally and can be explained by the inhibition of NO-induced activation of NMDA receptors (Meller et al 1992b). Paradoxically a number of NOS-inhibitors prevented the peripheral antinociceptive action of acetylcholine and morphine (Duarte et al 1990; Ferreira et al 1991).

So far it is rather unclear how NO is involved in nociception and whether this molecule is relevant for the actions of bradykinin and substance P in peripheral hyperalgesia, or for glutamate in central hyperalgesic mechanisms. During inflammation a calcium-independent form of NOS can be induced in macrophages (Moncada et al 1991). Further studies in models of inflammation are required to see whether the large amount of NO that is generated by induced NOS affects nociceptors.

Mechanotransduction and hypertonic medium

Both C polymodal nociceptive fibres and a subpopulation of Aδ-fibres are responsive to noxious mechanical stimuli and the sensitivity of both classes of nociceptor increases after injury and inflammation (Guilbaud et al 1985; Grubb et al 1991). Products of both cyclooxygenase and lipoxygenase pathways of arachidonic acid metabolism are responsible for an increase in mechanosensitivity of the nerve terminals (see above) although the extent to which this reflects an effect on the primary transduction mechanism rather than action potential discharge is unknown. Mechanical factors may also be of importance in some conditions, for example, intraarticular pressure may increase during joint inflammation.

The mechanisms that underlie the initial steps in mechanotransduction of primary afferents are unknown.

Ion channels that are activated by mechanical stimuli have been reported for a wide range of cell types (French 1992) but information on their properties in nociceptive neurones is lacking.

Raising the tonicity of the external medium is a consistent excitatory stimulus for polymodal nociceptors but seldom induces discharges in rapidly adapting mechanoreceptors (Kumazawa & Mizumura 1980; Kumazawa et al 1987). The basis for this excitation is unclear but it may be related to the mechanisms involved in the transduction of noxious mechanical stimuli in these neurons.

CYTOKINES AND NEUROTROPHIC FACTORS

Cytokines

A variety of cytokines (interleukins, interferons, tumour necrosis factor) are released by phagocytic and antigen-presenting cells of the immune system. These molecules act as important inflammatory agents and can also influence the activity of sensory neurons, probably by indirect routes that involve products of other cell types. IL-1β, IL-6 and IL-8 have all been reported to induce hyperalgesia in animals (Ferreira et al 1988; Follenfant et al 1990; Cunha et al 1991, 1992). Injection of these agents into a rat paw causes a hyperalgesia that develops over about 1 hour, but the basis for this effect may differ between these cytokines. The nociceptive effects of IL-8 but not IL-1β are blocked by β-adrenoceptor and dopamine (D_1) antagonists, and the sympathetic neuron blocking drug, guanethidine, suggesting that the effects of IL-8 involve sympathetic nerves (Cunha et al 1991). Furthermore, α-melanocyte stimulating hormone and tripeptides, related to Lys-D-Pro-Thr, are able to block the effects of IL-1β and IL-6 but the tripeptides do not antagonize IL-8 induced hyperalgesia (Ferreira et al 1988; Follenfant et al 1990; Cunha et al 1991). One suggestion is that IL-1β and IL-6, but not IL-8, evoke the release of prostaglandins from cells such as mononuclear leucocytes and fibroblasts and that the prostaglandins in turn act on sensory nerves (Ferreira et al 1988; Schweizer et al 1988; Cunha et al 1991, 1992). However the importance of cyclooxygenase products in IL-1β-induced hyperalgesia has been questioned (Follenfant et al 1990).

Tumour necrosis factor (TNF-α) also induces hyperalgesia which can be attenuated by antisera to IL-1, IL-6 and IL-8 (Cunha et al 1992). Furthermore the effect of TNF-α is antagonized by Lys-D-Pro-Thr, indomethacin and a β-adrenergic receptor antagonist. Significantly, carrageenan-induced hyperalgesia is reduced by TNF-α antiserum suggesting that this cytokine may be an important mediator of inflammatory hyperalgesia and that TNF-α production initiates a cascade involving the release of other cytokines.

Nerve growth factor (NGF)

The neurotrophic factor, NGF, is produced in limited amounts by a range of cell types (e.g. fibroblasts, Schwann cells) in peripheral tissues (Bandtlow et al 1987) and acts on a neural membrane receptor (trk A: Type III), which has tyrosine kinase activity. The bound NGF is internalized and transported to the cell soma where it acts to regulate the expression of certain genes. Although it is essential for the survival of sensory, as well as sympathetic, neurons in the early stages of development, NGF is not required for survival of adult sensory neurons in culture (Lindsay 1988). However, recent evidence has indicated that exposure to different levels of NGF can influence the properties of sensory neurons. The full repertoire of phenotypic effects exerted by NGF remains to be catalogued, but it is already clear that the expression of a number of important proteins is regulated by NGF. For example, the presence of NGF results in an increased synthesis, axoplasmic transport and neuronal content of substance P and CGRP (Lindsay & Harmar 1989; Donnerer et al 1992). Furthermore NGF regulates the levels of at least two types of ion channel in DRG neurons; the capsaicin receptor/ion channel (Winter et al 1988) and the TTX-resistant Na^+ channel (Aguayo & White 1992). In both cases, exposure to NGF promotes channel expression while removal of the growth factor results in a large reduction or complete loss of the channel. NGF may also modify sensory neuron properties by promotion of axonal sprouting, thereby increasing the peripheral receptive field (Diamond et al 1992). Such a phenomenon could also occur at the central terminals of nociceptive neurons exposed to abnormally high levels of NGF. If so, it would explain the increased strength of synaptic connections between sensory and dorsal horn neurons after experimental elevation of NGF in vivo (Lewin et al 1992) although other mechanisms such as release of increased amounts of neuropeptides (e.g. substance P) could play an important role.

The available evidence suggests that NGF may be of considerable relevance in inflammatory pain. The levels of NGF in synovial fluid from patients with rheumatoid arthritis are elevated (Aloe et al 1992), which may well lead to an increased or altered expression of important neuronal proteins associated with increased chemosensitivity, responsiveness or synaptic efficacy. Such clinical findings are consistent with animal studies which have shown that injection of NGF leads to increased sensitivity to noxious stimuli while animals exposed to antibodies to NGF have a reduced response to painful and inflammatory stimuli (Otten 1991; Lewin et al 1993).

There is likely to be a subtle interplay between the nerves, invasive inflammatory cells and resident tissues cells at sites of tissue damage (Fig. 3.1). NGF stimulates the release of histamine as well as lipid mediators (LTC_4) from human basophils (Bischoff & Dahinden 1992) and histamine, at least, can act directly on sensory nerves (see above). The synthesis of NGF is stimulated by cytokines such as IL-1β and TNFα (Gadient et al 1990; Yoshida & Gage 1992) which are produced during inflammation. The production of these and other cytokines is, in turn, upregulated by substance P released from the sensory nerves (Hartung & Toyaka 1983; Lindholm et al 1987; Lotz et al 1988). Thus, a positive feedback loop between neuropeptides, cytokines and NGF can be activated in chronic inflammation.

In addition to the long-term effects of NGF mediated by changing gene expression, it has been reported that some short-term effects in damaged tissue are due to an amino terminal octapeptide cleaved from NGF by an endogenous endopeptidase. This peptide can produce a concentration-dependent, short-lasting (<2 hours) mechanical hyperalgesia after injection into chloroform-treated rat paw (Taiwo et al 1991). The basis for this hyperalgesia is unclear, although the finding that the response is abolished by sympathectomy implies an interaction between sensory and sympathetic nerves (McMahon 1991 and this volume).

Table 3.4 Neuropeptides found in small sensory neurons

Peptide	% Cells	Co-localization	Size	Projection
Substance P	12–38	CGRP Somatostatin/galanin	S-M	Skin, muscle Joint, viscera
Somatostatin	5–15	Substance P CGRP/βFGF	S-M	
Calcitonin gene-related peptide (CGRP)	28–50	Substance P CCK/dynorphin	S-L	Skin, muscle Joint, viscera
Bombesin	0–8	CGRP/substance P	S	
Vasoactive intestinal peptide	0–5	CGRP/substance P	S	Viscera
Galanin	0–5	Substance P	S	
Dynorphin	0–3	Substance P/CGRP CCK	S	Skin/viscera
β-Fibroblast Growth Factor (βFGF)		Somatostatin	S	
Cholecystokinin	8	Substance P/CGRP	S	Viscera/skin

Some cells contain only one peptide whereas in other cells peptides are colocalized L = 40–75 μm; M = 20–50 μm; S = < 20 μm
(References in Willis & Coggeshall 1991 and Lawson 1992.)

NEUROCHEMISTRY OF SENSORY NEURONS

Sensory neurons are capable of elaborating a variety of substances (amino acids, neuropeptides etc) which perform a multiplicity of functions (neurotransmitter, neuroeffector, neurotrophic) by acting on central or peripheral tissues. We do not propose to present an exhaustive neurochemical description of sensory neurons nor to review the specific cellular actions of substances released into the spinal cord: this has been addressed by others (Willis & Coggeshall 1991; Scott 1992). Rather, we have highlighted some of the mechanisms which control the release of sensory neurochemicals and have indicated the functions of these substances following their release in the periphery, giving emphasis to those substances which have received the greatest attention in recent years.

Neuropeptides

A multitude of neuropeptides have been identified in small sensory neurons (Willis & Coggeshall 1991; Lawson 1992) (Table 3.4) and attempts have been made to correlate peptide expression with the peripheral organ innervated. These findings have indicated some specificity in the patterns of peptidergic neuron innervation to skin, muscle and viscera (e.g. Gibbins et al 1987; Molander et al 1987). Interestingly the expression of neuropeptide may be changed when sensory fibres innervate inappropriate tissues (McMahon & Gibson 1987; Hogan & van der Kooy 1992) or after lesions of peripheral rather than central axons (Henken et al 1990). This suggests that the cell phenotype and peptide synthesis can be regulated by target organ factors for which there are specific receptors (e.g. trk A for NGF) on sensory nerve terminals.

Sensory neurons also contain a number of other biochemical markers such as enzymes or cell surface molecules (Willis & Coggeshall 1991; Lawson 1992) which distinguish different neural populations but the correlation of these with function is still unclear. In some cases, however, the expression of specific proteins (e.g. GAP 43) following tissue injury is related to neural regeneration (Van der Zee et al 1989).

Most small (capsaicin sensitive) primary sensory neurons terminate in the superficial dorsal horn but some fibres also project to the contralateral dorsal horn (Culbertson et al 1979). Since a significant portion of these afferents contain SP (Ogawa et al 1985) it is possible that ipsilaterally stimulation of fine afferents may induce contralateral excitability changes in the spinal cord.

Neuropeptide release from primary afferent neurons in the spinal cord has been studied by a number of methods (push pull cannulae, microdialysis) (Maggi et al 1993). However studies with specific antibody-coated microprobes are able to show some temporal relationship between the release and distribution of different neuropeptides. Substance P release was detected only after noxious thermal and mechanical stimuli and the peptide was confined to the spinal dorsal horn (Duggan et al 1988). Some spontaneous release of neurokinin-A was found but an increased release could be evoked by noxious stimuli during which the increase in peptide level persisted far beyond the duration of stimulation and spread to more distant parts of the spinal cord (Duggan et al 1990). Differences in peptide inactivation may partly explain these findings. However, during inflammation of the joint, passive movements of the leg also evoked neuropeptide release whereas no release occurred when an uninflamed joint was manipulated (Schaible et al 1990). These observations suggest that the release and distribution of neurokinins, and possibly other neuropeptides, may occur over large distances in the spinal cord and that the pattern of peptide release is significantly altered during inflammation. In addition there is some evidence that different modalities of noxious stimulation affect the type of peptide released. For example somatostatin was only released during heat or chemical stimulation whereas substance P was released by a pressure stimulus (Kuraishi et al 1985). Such data lend further support to the possible functional heterogeneity of nociceptive afferents.

The peptide content and expression of specific neuropeptides in sensory neurons can be profoundly affected by injury or by peripheral inflammation (Dubner & Ruda 1992). Transection or damage to peripheral afferents leads to a loss of fibres and a reduction in the content of neurokinins, CGRP and their respective mRNAs in sensory ganglia. On the other hand such injuries provoke an expression of neuropeptide Y, not normally detected in sensory neurons, and an increase in the expression of galanin (Villar et al 1989). Conversely inflammation produces an increase in mRNA for neurokinins and CGRP together with an increased content of the respective peptides (Kuraishi et al 1989). Attempts have been made to correlate functional changes with changes in peptide expression. This has been difficult since the time-course of the changes in sensory neuropeptide mRNA differ from observable changes in function. For example the changes in sensory neuron mRNA for substance P does not parallel the hyperalgesia seen with carrageenan-induced inflammation (Dubner & Ruda 1992).

Regulation of excitability and transmitter release at central primary afferent terminals

The central terminals of primary afferent fibres express a number of receptors for different transmitters, which are normally released from intrinsic spinal neurons or projection neurons. The effect of these transmitters is usually an inhibition of excitation-secretion coupling and transmitter release. In most cases the effect is due to an inhibition of voltage-gated (HVA) calcium channels via activation of a G-protein. This may occur either through a direct link between G-protein and calcium channel or via an intracellular second messenger, although the precise mechanisms of channel inhibition are unknown (Dolphin 1990; Scott et al 1991; Cox & Dunlap 1992). The list of agents that can inhibit HVA calcium channels includes adenosine, dopamine, GABA, neuropeptide Y, noradrenaline, opioids, 5-HT and somatostatin (Table 3.3). Although activation of the same types of receptors can inhibit transmitter release via modulation of voltage-gated potassium channels in other cell types (Brown 1990; Armstrong & White 1992), there is little evidence that such a mechanism operates widely in sensory neurons. A possible exception to this general assertion is that opioids can potentiate a voltage-gated potassium current (I_K), at least under some experimental conditions (Crain & Shen 1990; Shen & Crain 1990). The additional potassium current shortens the action potential and diminishes the presynaptic calcium current. Another possible mechanism to reduce the amount of transmitter release from primary afferent terminals is by opening Cl^- channels, for example by activation of $GABA_a$ receptors. This conductance pathway reduces the amplitude of the action potential in the terminal, which in turn results in a smaller calcium influx.

Neuropeptide effects in the periphery

The release of neuropeptides from the endings of peripheral sensory nerves has been well characterized. An important function here is related to efferent or trophic activities (Holzer 1988).

A number of sensory neuropeptides have an important role in inflammation and the accompanying hyperalgesia. However a more extensive function in the regulation of immune cell activity has also been proposed (Weihe et al 1991). During inflammation there is a sprouting of peptidergic peripheral fibres and an increased content of peptide, with many fibres showing coexistence of SP and CGRP. Peptide-containing fibres are often seen existing in close proximity to immune cells, particularly macrophages and mast cells (Weihe et al 1991). Several possible roles for released neuropeptides have been proposed. Substance P release can stimulate NO synthesis from vascular endothelium, thereby causing vasodilation. In addition SP-induced contraction of endothelial cells induces plasma extravasation (Holzer 1988) to allow other substances (bradykinin, ATP, 5-HT, histamine) to gain access to the site of tissue injury and the afferent nerve terminals. Mast-cell degranulation by substance P has been considered an important factor in neurogenic inflammation due to the release of other inflammatory mediators such as histamine and 5-HT and the release of proteolytic enzymes which catalyse the production of bradykinin. However, doubts about the pathophysiological relevance of this have been expressed since very high concentrations of substance P appear to be required. Consequently it has been proposed that SP may be a primer for degranulation of mast cells by other agents. Interestingly CGRP does not produce plasma extravasation but is a powerful vasodilator and also acts synergistically with substance P and other inflammatory mediators to enhance plasma extravasation (Gamse & Saria 1985; Brain & Williams 1985; Green et al 1992). On the other hand, galanin and somatostatin reduce substance P release from sensory fibres during neurogenic inflammation (Gazelius et al 1981; Green et al 1992). These mechanisms may be important in some pathological situations for it has been suggested that substance P plays a critical role in the aetiology of rheumatoid arthritis (Levine et al 1984) in which pain relief can be obtained by injections of somatostatin into the joint (Matucci & Marabini 1988). Substance P, NKA and CGRP also cause a hyperalgesia which can be induced by repetitive intradermal injection (Nakamura-Craig & Gill 1991). Presently, it is not clear whether this results from indirect mechanisms involving sympathetic nerve fibres or the release of substances from the vasculature (Green et al 1992).

Stimulation or recruitment of inflammatory cells is also an important contributory role of substance P in inflammation. There are several aspects to this: stimulation of chemotaxis (Marasco et al 1981); enhancement of lymphocyte proliferation (Payan et al 1983); stimulation of macrophages and monocytes (Wagner et al 1987). Indeed lymph organs are innervated by capsaicin-sensitive fibres containing substance P and CGRP (Popper et al 1988; Weihe et al 1989). Moreover there is a reduced immune response to antigen challenge in capsaicin pretreated rats, which can be restored by exogenously administered neurokinins (Eglezos et al 1991).

Excitatory amino acids in sensory neurons

Many types of sensory neuron make excitatory amino acids, particularly glutamate and aspartate. It is significant though that a population of small DRG neurons contain both glutamate and neurokinins (Battaglia & Rustioni 1988) suggesting that glutamate is involved in the nociceptive pathway both at the stage of the primary afferent and in subsequent neural circuitry within the spinal cord and projecting systems. In keeping with this capsaicin-evoked release of glutamate and aspartate has been demonstrated from sensory neurons (Jeftinija et al 1991). In addition capsaicin-sensitive afferent nerve terminals express amino-acid receptors but these appear to differ from those seen on spinal neurons being more sensitive to the analogues kainate and domoate and rather insensitive to NMDA (Huettner 1990). The function of EAA receptors on C-fibre afferents is presently unclear though these findings have raised the question about a function for EAA at the peripheral sensory nerve terminal. Surprisingly (because glutamate is inactivated rather rapidly) repeated daily injection of glutamate into the rat paw has been shown to induce a state of peripheral hyperalgesia (Follenfant & Nakamura-Craig 1992).

Finally, acute administration of exogenous opioids is known to reduce peptide release from sensory neurons in the viscera and to reduce the plasma extravasation following peripheral nerve stimulation (Holzer 1988). Such peripheral effects are not normally involved in opioid- induced antinociception. However, during inflammation, opioids exhibit peripheral antinociceptive and antiinflammatory activity. Thus endogenous opioid peptides are expressed and released by immune cells during inflammation (Stein 1991). From this it is levident that opioid receptors, expressed on sensory and sympathetic nerve fibres by the inflammatory challenge are involved in regulating neuronal excitability and thereby the release of proinflammatory mediators (Taiwo & Levine 1991b).

Sympathetic fibres and afferent fibre excitability

It is well established that substance P mediates the slow depolarization of sympathetic ganglion cells following the stimulation of visceral afferent fibres or distension of hollow organs (de Groat 1989). These effects are evoked following noxious stimulation but similar processes regulate normal visceral reflexes.

In somatic regions, direct interactions of sympathetic nerves or sympathetic transmitter with afferent fibres have not been easy to demonstrate (Lang et al 1990) except after peripheral nerve damage or inflammation. Recent studies show that sympathetic nerve stimulation and noradrenaline (via an α_2-receptor) directly excited some C-fibre afferents in a partially injured sensory nerve trunk (Sato & Perl 1991). During inflammation, however, afferent fibres are most often sensitized by the release of prostanoids following stimulation of sympathetic fibres (Koltzenburg & McMahon 1991). Sympathetic fibres also make important contributions to plasma extravasation since sympathectomy reduced plasma extravasation induced by noxious stimulation (Coderre et al 1989; Donnerer et al 1992). Indeed both sympathetic transmitters including noradrenaline and neuropeptide Y reduced plasma extravasation in the knee joint (Green et al 1992). It is possible that these effects were due to an inhibition of sensory neuropeptide release since both noradrenaline and NPY inhibit calcium currents in sensory neurons (Ewald et al 1988).

REFERENCES

Aguayo L G, Weight F F, White G 1991 TTX-insensitive action potentials and excitability of adult sensory neurons cultured in serum and exogenous nerve growth factor-free medium. Neuroscience Letters 121: 88–92

Aguayo L G, White G 1992 Effects of nerve growth factor on TTX- and capsaicin-sensitivity in adult rat sensory neurones. Brain Research 570: 61–67

Allen A C, Gammon C M, Ousley A H, McCarthy K D, Morell P 1992 Bradykinin stimulates arachidonic acid release through the sequential actions of an sn-1 diacylglycerol lipase and a monoacylglycerol lipase. Journal of Neurochemistry 58: 1130–1139

Aloe L, Tuveri M A, Carcassi U, Levi-Montalcini R 1992 Nerve growth factor in the synovial fluid of patients with chronic arthritis. Arthritis and Rheumatism 35: 351–355

Andreeva L, Rang H P 1993 Effect of bradykinin and prostaglandins on the release of calcitonin gene-related peptide immunoreactivity from the rat spinal cord in vitro. British Journal of Pharmacology 168: 185–190

Andrews P V, Helm R D, Thomas K L 1989 NK_1 receptor mediation of neurogenic plasma extravasation in the rat skin. British Journal of Pharmacology 97: 1232–1238

Armstrong D L, White R E 1992 An enzymatic mechanism for potassium channel stimulation through pertussis-toxin-sensitive G proteins. Trends in Neurosciences 15: 403–408

Asghar A U R, McQueen D S, Macdonald A E 1992 Absence of effect of adenosine on the discharge of articular mechanoreceptors in normal and arthritic rats. British Journal of Pharmacology 105: 309P

Bandtlow C E, Heumann R, Schwab M E, Thoenen H 1987 Cellular localization of nerve growth factor synthesis by in situ hybridization. EMBO Journal 6: 891–899

Battaglia G, Rustioni A 1988 Co-existence of glutamate and substance P in dorsal root ganglion neurons of the rat and monkey. Journal of Comparative Neurology 277: 302–310

Bean B, Williams C A, Ceelen P W 1990 ATP-activated channels in rat and bullfrog sensory neurons: current-voltage relation and single-channel behavior. Journal of Neuroscience 10: 11–19

Beck P W, Handwerker H O 1974 Bradykinin and serotonin effects on various types of cutaneous nerve fibers. Pflügers Archives 347: 209–222

Bevan S, Robertson B 1991 Properties of 5-hydroxytryptamine$_3$ receptor-gated currents in adult rat dorsal root ganglion neurones. British Journal of Pharmacology 102: 272–276

Bevan S, Szolcsanyi J 1990 Sensory neuron-specific actions of capsaicin: mechanisms and applications. Trends in Pharmacological Sciences 11: 330–333

Bevan S, Yeats J 1991 Protons activate a cation conductance in a sub-population of rat dorsal root ganglion neurones. Journal of Physiology 433: 145–161

Bevan S, Hothi S, Hughes G et al 1992 Capsazepine: a competitive antagonist of the sensory neurone excitant capsaicin. British Journal of Pharmacology 197: 544–552

Bevan S, Forbes C A, Winter J 1993 Protons and capsaicin activate the same ion channels in rat isolated dorsal root ganglion neurones. Journal of Physiology 459: 401P

Birrell G J, McQueen D S, Iggo A, Coleman R A, Grubb B D 1991 PGI_2-induced activation and sensitization of articular mechanonociceptors. Neuroscience Letters 124: 5–8

Bischoff S C, Dahinden C A 1992 Effect of nerve growth factor on the release of inflammatory mediators by mature human basophils. Blood 79: 2662–2669

Bisgaard H, Kristensen J K 1985 Leukotriene B_4 produces hyperalgesia in humans. Prostaglandins 30: 791–797

Bleehen T, Keele C A 1977 Observations on the algogenic actions of adenosine compounds on the human blister base preparation. Pain 3: 367–377

Boeckart J, Sebben M, Dumuis A 1990 Pharmacological characterization of 5-hydroxytryptamine$_4$ (5-HT_4) receptors positively coupled to adenylate cyclase in adult guinea pig hippocampal membranes: effect of substituted benzamide derivatives. Molecular Pharmacology 37: 408–411

Bombaderie S, Cattani P, Crabattoni G et al 1981 The synovial prostaglandin system in chronic inflammatory arthritis: differential effects of steroidal and non-steroidal anti-inflammatory drugs. British Journal of Pharmacology 73: 893–902

Brain S D, Williams T J 1985 Inflammatory oedema induced by synergism between calcitonin gene related peptide and mediators of increased vascular permeability. British Journal of Pharmacology 86: 855–860

Broadbent J L 1955 Observations on histamine-induced pruritus and pain. British Journal of Pharmacology 10: 183–185

Brown D A 1990 G-proteins and potassium currents in neurons. Annual Review of Physiology 52: 215–242

Burgess G M, Mullaney J, McNeil M, Dunn P, Rang H P 1989a Second messengers involved in the action of bradykinin on cultured sensory neurones. Journal of Neuroscience 9: 3314–3325

Burgess G M, Mullaney I, McNeill M, Coote P R, Minhas A, Wood J N 1989b Activation of guanylate cyclase by bradykinin in rat sensory neurones is mediated by calcium influx: possible role of the increase in cyclic GMP. Journal of Neurochemistry 53: 1212–1218

Buzzi M G, Moskowitz M A, Peroutka S J, Byun B 1991 Further characterization of the putative 5-HT receptor which mediates blockade of neurogenic plasma extravasation in rat dura mater. British Journal of Pharmacology 103: 1421–1428

Chahl L A, Iggo A 1977 The effects of bradykinin and prostaglandin E1 on rat cutaneous nerve activity. British Journal of Pharmacology 59: 343–347

Cherniak N S, Runold M, Prabhakar N R, Mitra J 1987 Effect of adenosine on vagal sensory pulmonary afferents. Federation Proceedings 46: 825

Christian E P, Taylor G E, Weinreich D 1989 Serotonin increases excitability of rabbit C-fibre neurons by two distinct mechanisms. Journal of Applied Physiology 67: 584–591

Coderre T J, Basbaum A I, Levine J D 1989 Neural control of vascular permeability; interaction between primary afferents, mast cells, and sympathetic efferents. Journal of Neurophysiology 62: 48–58

Connor J A, Stevens C F 1971 Prediction of repetitive firing behaviour from voltage clamp data on an isolated neurone soma. Journal of Physiology 213: 31–52

Cook N S 1990 Potassium channels: structure, classification, function and therapeutic potential. Ellis Horwood, Chichester

Corbe S M, Poole-Wilson P A 1980 The time of onset and severity of acidosis in myocardial ischaemia. Journal of Molecular and Cellular Cardiology 12: 745–760

Cox D H, Dunlap K 1992 Pharmacological discrimination of N-type from L-type calcium current and its selective modulation by transmitters. Journal of Neuroscience 12: 906–914

Crain S M, Shen K-F 1990 Opioids can evoke direct receptor-mediated excitatory effects on sensory neurons. Trends in Pharmacological Sciences 11: 77–81

Crook S T, Mattern M, Sarau H M et al 1989 The signal transduction system of the leukotriene D_4 receptor. Trends in Pharmacological Sciences 10: 103–107

Crunkhorn P, Willis A L 1971 Cutaneous reaction to intradermal prostaglandins. British Journal of Pharmacology 41: 49–56

Culbertson J L, Haines D E, Kimmel D L, Brown P B 1979 Contralateral projection of primary afferent fibers to mammalian spinal cord. Experimental Neurology 64: 83–97

Cunha F Q, Lorenzetti B B, Poole S, Ferreira S H 1991 Interleukin-8 as a mediator of sympathetic pain. British Journal of Pharmacology 104: 765–767

Cunha F Q, Poole S, Lorenzetti B B, Ferreira S H 1992 The pivotal role of tumor necrosis factor α in the development of inflammatory hyperalgesia. British Journal of Pharmacology 107: 660–664

De Groat WC 1989 Neuropeptides in pelvic afferent pathways. In: Polak J M (ed) Regulatory peptides. Birkhhauser Verlag, Basel, 334–361

Devor M, Keller C H, Deerinck T J, Levinson S R, Ellsmann M H 1989 Na^+ channel accumulation on axolemma of afferent endings in nerve end neuromas in Apteronotus. Neuroscience Letters 102: 149–154

Diamond J, Holmes M, Coughlin M 1992 Endogenous NGF and nerve impulses regulate the collateral sprouting of sensory axons in the skin of the adult rat. Journal of Neuroscience 12: 1454–1466.

Dickenson A H, Dray A 1991 Selective antagonism of capsaicin by capsazepine: evidence for a spinal receptor site in capsaicin-induced antinociception. British Journal of Pharmacology 104: 1045–1049
Dolphin A 1990 Ionic channels and their regulation by G protein subunits. Annual Review of Physiology 52: 197–213
Donnerer J, Schuligoi R, Stein C 1992 Increased content and transport of substance P and calcitonin gene-related peptide in sensory nerves innervating inflamed tissue: evidence for a regulatory function of nerve growth factor in vivo. Neuroscience 49: 693–698
Dray A, Perkins M 1993 Bradykinin and inflammatory pain. Trends in Neurosciences 16: 99–104
Dray A, Bettaney J, Forster P 1990 Actions of capsaicin on peripheral nociceptors of the neonatal rat spinal cord-tail in vitro: dependence of extracellular ions and independence of second messengers. British Journal of Pharmacology 101: 727–733
Dray A, Patel I A, Perkins M N, Rueff A 1992 Bradykinin-induced activation of nociceptors: receptor and mechanistic studies on the neonatal rat spinal cord-tail preparation in vitro. British Journal of Pharmacology 107: 1129–1134
Duarte I D G, Lorenzetti B B, Ferreira S H 1990 Peripheral analgesia and activation of the nitric oxide-cyclic GMP pathway. European Journal of Pharmacology 186: 289–293
Dubner R, Ruda M A 1992 Activity-dependent neuronal plasticity following tissue injury and inflammation. Trends in Neurosciences 15: 96–103
Duggan A W, Morton C R, Hendry I A, Hutchison W D, Zhao Z Q 1988 Cutaneous stimuli releasing immunoreactive substance P in the dorsal horn of the cat. Brain Research 451: 261–273
Duggan A W, Hope P J, Jarrott B, Schaible H-G, Fleetwood-Walker S M 1990 Release, spread and persistence of immunoreactive neurokinin A in the dorsal horn of the cat following noxious cutaneous stimulation: studies with antibody microprobes. Neuroscience 35: 195–202
Dunn P M, Rang H P 1990 Bradykinin-induced depolarisation of primary afferent nerve terminals in the neonatal rat spinal cord in vitro. British Journal of Pharmacology 100: 656–660
Eglezos A, Andrews P V, Boyd R L, Helme R D 1991 Tachykinin-mediated modulation of the primary antibody response in rats: evidence for mediation by NK2 receptor. Journal of Neuroimmunology 32: 11–18
Eschalier A, Kayser V, Gilbaud G 1989 Influence of specific 5-HT_3 antagonists on carageenan-induced hyperalgesia in the rat. Pain 36: 249–255
Evans R H, Evans S J, Pook P C, Sunter D C 1987 A comparison of excitatory amino acid antagonists acting at primary afferent C fibers and motoneurones of the isolated spinal cord of the rat. British Journal of Pharmacology 91: 531–537
Ewald D A, Matthies J G, Perney T M, Walker M W, Miller R J 1988 The effect of down regulation of protein kinase C on the inhibition of dorsal root ganglion neuron Ca^{2+} currents by neuropeptide Y. Journal of Neuroscience 8: 2447–2451
Falus A, Meretey K 1992 Histamine: an early messenger in inflammatory and immune reactions. Immunology Today 13: 154–156
Farmer S G, Burch R M 1992 Biochemical and molecular pharmacology of kinin receptors. Annual Review of Pharmacology 32: 511–536
Ferreira S H, Nakamura M 1979 I. Prostaglandin hyperalgesia. A cAMP/Ca^{2+}- dependent process. Prostaglandins 18: 179–190
Ferreira S H, Lorenzetti B B, Bristow A F, Poole S 1988 Interleukin 1β as a potent hyperalgesic agent antagonized by a tripeptide analogue. Nature 334: 698–700
Ferreira S H, Duarte I D G, Lorenzetti B B 1991 The molecular mechanism of action of morphine analgesia: stimulation of the cGMP system via nitric oxide. European Journal of Pharmacology 201: 121–122
Follenfant R L, Nakamura-Craig M, Henderson B, Higgs G A 1989 Inhibition by neuropeptides of interleukin-1β-induced, prostaglandin-independent hyperalgesia. British Journal of Pharmacology 98: 41–43
Follenfant R L, Nakamura-Craig M, Garland L G 1990 Sustained hyperalgesia in rats evoked by 15-hydroperoxyeicosatetraenoic acid is attenuated by the protein kinase inhibitor H-7. British Journal of Pharmacology 99: 298P
Follenfant R L, Nakamura-Craig M 1992 Glutamate induces hyperalgesia in the rat paw. British Journal of Pharmacology 106: 49P
Fowler J C Greene R, Weinreich D 1985 Two calcium-sensitive spike after-hyperpolarizations in visceral sensory neurones of the rabbit. Journal of Physiology 365: 59–75
French A S 1992 Mechanotransduction. Annual Review of Physiology 54: 135–152
Gadient R A, Cron K C, Otten U 1990 Interleukin 1β and tumor necrosis factor-α synergistically stimulate nerve growth factor (NGF) release from cultured rat astrocytes. Neuroscience Letters 117: 335–340
Gammon C M, Allen A C, Morell P 1989 Bradykinin stimulates phosphoinositide hydrolysis and mobilisation of arachidonic acid in dorsal root ganglion neurons. Journal of Neurochemistry 53: 95–101
Gamse R, Saria A 1985 Potentiation of tachykinin-induced plasma protein extravasation by calcitonin gene-related peptide. European Journal of Pharmacology 114: 61–66
Gazelius B, Brodin E, Olgart L Panopoulos P 1981 Evidence that substance P is a mediator of antidromic vasodilatation using somatostatin as a release inhibitor. Acta Physiologica Scandinavica 113: 155–159
Geppetti P, Tramontana M, Santicolli P, Del Bianco E, Giulani S, Maggi C A 1990 Bradykinin-induced release of CGRP from capsaicin-sensitive nerves in guinea-pig atria: mechanism of action and calcium requirements. Neuroscience 38: 687–692
Gibbins I L, Furness J B, Costa M 1987 Pathway specific patterns of coexistence of substance P, calcitonin gene-related peptide, cholecystokinin and dynorphin in neurons of the dorsal root ganglia of the guinea pig. Cell and Tissue Research 248: 417–437
Green P G, Basbaum A I, Levine J D 1992 Sensory neuropeptide interactions in the production of plasma extravasation in the rat, Neuroscience 50: 745–749
Grubb B D, Birrell G J, McQueen D S, Iggo A 1991 The role of PGE_2 in the sensitization of mechanoreceptors in normal and inflamed ankle joints of the rat. Experimental Brain Research 84: 383–392
Guilbaud G, Iggo A, Tegner N 1985 Sensory receptors in ankle joint capsules of normal and arthritic rats. Experimental Brain Research 58: 29–40
Haley J E, Dickenson A H, Schachter M 1992 Electrophysiological evidence for a role of nitric oxide in prolonged chemical nociception in the rat. Neuropharmacology 31: 251–258
Handwerker H O 1975 Influence of prostaglandin E2 on the discharge of cutaneous nociceptive C-fibers induced by radiant heat. Pflügers Archives 355: 116–121
Handwerker H O 1976 Influence of algogenic substances and prostaglandins on discharges of unmyelinated cutaneous nerve fibers identified as nociceptors. In: Bonica, J J, Albe-Fessard D G (eds), Advances in pain research and therapy vol 1. New York, Raven Press, p 41–51
Hannson A, Serhan C N, Haeggstroem J et al 1986 Activation of protein kinase C by lipoxin A and other eicosanoids. Intracellular action of oxygenation products of arachidonic acid. Biochemical and Biophysical Research Communications 134: 1215–1222
Harper A A, Lawson S N 1985 Electrical properties of rat dorsal root ganglion neurones with different peripheral nerve conduction velocities. Journal of Physiology 359: 47–63
Hartung H P, Toyaka K 1983 Activation of macrophages by substance P: induction of oxidative burst and thromboxane release. European Journal of Pharmacology 89: 301–305
Henken D B, Battisti W P, Chesselet M F, Murray M, Tessler A 1990 Expression of β preprotachykinin mRNA and tachykinins in rat dorsal root ganglion cells following peripheral or central axotomy. Neuroscience 39: 733–742
Hess J F, Borkowski J A, Young G S, Starder C D, Ransom R W 1992 Cloning and pharmacological characterization of a human bradykinin (BK-2) receptor. Biochemical and Biophysical Research Communications 184: 260–268
Hess P 1990 Classes of calcium channels in vertebrate cells. Annual Review of Neuroscience 13: 337–356
Higashi H, Morita K, North R A 1984 Calcium-dependent after-potentials in visceral afferent neurones of the rabbit. Journal of Physiology 355: 479–492

Higgs G A, Salmon J A 1979 Cyclooxygenase products in carrageenin-induced inflammation. Prostaglandins 17: 737–746
Hille B 1991 Ionic channels of excitable membranes. Sinauer, Sunderland, Mass
Hock F J, Wirth K, Albus U, Linz W et al 1991 Hoe 140: a new potent and long-acting bradykinin antagonist: in vitro studies. British Journal of Pharmacology 102: 769–773
Hogan K, van der Kooy 1992 Visceral target specific calcitonin gene-related peptide and substance P enrichment in trigeminal afferent projections. Journal of Neuroscience 12: 1135–1143
Hokfelt T, Elde R, Johansson P, Luft R, Nilsson G, Arimura A 1976 Immunohistochemical evidence for separate populations of somatostatin-containing and substance P containing primary afferent neurons in the rat. Neuroscience 1: 131–136
Holzer P 1988 Local effector functions of capsaicin-sensitive sensory nerve endings: involvement of tachykinins, calcitonin gene-related peptide, and other neuropeptides. Neuroscience 24: 739–768
Huettner J E 1990 Glutamate receptor channels in rat DRG neurons: activation by kainate and quisqualate and blockade of desensitization by Con A. Neuron 5: 255–266
Hunt S P, Kelly J S, Emson P C, Kimmel J R, Miller R J, Wu J-Y 1981 An immunohistochemical study of neuronal populations containing neuropeptides or γ-aminobutyrate within the superficial layers of the rat dorsal horn. Neuroscience 6: 1883–1898
Ishida M, Shinozaki H 1991 Novel kainate derivatives: potent depolarizing actions on spinal motoneurones and dorsal root fibers in newborn rats. British Journal of Pharmacology 104: 873–878
Jacobus W E, Taylor G J, Hollis D P, Nunally R L 1977 Phosphorus magnetic resonance of perfused working rat heart. Nature 265: 756–758
Jeftinija S, Jeftinija K, Liu F et al 1991 Excitatory amino acids are released from primary afferent neurons in vitro. Neuroscience Letters 125: 191–194
Ju G, Hokfelt T, Brodin E et al 1987 Primary sensory neurons of the rat showing calcitonin gene-related peptide immunoreactivity and their relation to substance P, somatostatin-, galanin-, vasoactive intestinal polypeptide- and cholecystokinin-immunoreactive ganglion cells. Cell and Tissue Research 247: 417–431
Kanaka R, Schaible H-G, Schmidt R F 1985 Activation of fine articular afferent units by bradykinin. Brain Research 327: 81–90
Kandel E, Jessell T M, Schwartz J H 1991 Principles of Neural Science. Arnold, London
Kasai H, Kameyama D, Yamaguchi K, Fukuda J 1986 Single transient K-channels in mammalian sensory neurons. Biophysical Journal 49: 1243–1247
Koerber H R, Mendell L M 1992 Functional heterogeneity of dorsal root ganglion cells. In: Scott S A (ed) Sensory neurons: diversity, development and plasticity. Oxford University Press, New York
Koltzenburg M, McMahon S B 1991 The enigmatic role of the sympathetic nervous system in chronic pain. Trends in Pharmacological Sciences 12: 399–402
Konnerth A, Lux H D, Morad M 1987 Proton-induced transformation of calcium channels in chick dorsal root ganglion cells. Journal of Physiology 386: 603–633
Kostyuk P G, Veselovsky N S, Tsyndrenko A Y 1981a Ionic currents in the somatic membrane of rat dorsal root ganglion neurons. I. Sodium currents. Neuroscience 6: 2423–2430
Kostyuk P G, Veselovsky N S, Fedulova S A, Tsyndrenko A Y 1981b Ionic currents in the somatic membrane of rat dorsal root ganglion neurons. III. Potassium currents. Neuroscience 6: 2439–2444
Krishtal O A, Pidoplichko V I 1980 A receptor for protons in the membrane of sensory neurons. Neuroscience 5: 2325–2357
Krishtal O A, Marchenko S M, Obukhov A G 1988 Cationic channels activated by extracellular ATP in rat sensory neurons. Neuroscience 27: 995–1000
Kumazawa T, Mizumura K 1980 Chemical responses of polymodal receptors of scrotal contents in dogs. Journal of Physiology 299: 219–231
Kumazawa T, Mizumura K, Sato J 1987 Response properties of polymodal receptors studied using in vitro testis superior spermatic nerve preparations of dogs. Journal of Neurophysiology 57: 702–711
Kuraishi Y, Hirota N, Sato Y, Hino Y, Satoh M, Takagi H 1985 Evidence that substance P and somatostatin transmit separate information related to pain in the spinal dorsal horn. Brain Research 325: 294–298
Kuraishi Y, Nanayama T, Ohmo H et al 1989 Calcitonin gene-related peptide increases in the dorsal root ganglia of adjuvant arthritic rat. Peptides 10: 447–452
Lam F Y, Ferrell W R 1991 Specific neurokinin receptors mediate plasma extravasation in the rat knee joint. British Journal of Pharmacology 103: 1263–1267
LaMotte R H, Lundberg L E R, Torebjörk H E 1992 Pain, hyperalgesia and activity in nociceptive C units in humans after intradermal injection of capsaicin. Journal of Physiology 448: 749–764
Lang E, Nowak A, Reeh P, Handwerker H O 1990 Chemosensitivity of fine afferents from rat skin in vitro. Journal of Neurophysiology 63: 887–901
Lawson S N 1992 Morphological and biochemical cell types of sensory neurons. In: Scott S A (ed) Sensory neurons: diversity, development and plasticity. Oxford University Press, New York, p 27–59
Lembeck F, Juan H 1974 Interaction of prostaglandins and indomethacin with algogenic substances. Naunyn-Schmiedebergs Archives of Pharmacology 285: 301–313
Lembeck F, Popper H, Juan H 1976 Release of prostaglandins by bradykinin as an intrinsic mechanism of its algesic effect. Naunyn-Schmiedebergs Archives of Pharmacology 294: 69–73
Lembeck F, Donnerer J, Bartho L 1982 Inhibition of neurogenic vasodilatation and plasma extravasation by substance P antagonists, somatostatin and [D-met^2, pro^5] enkephalinamide. European Journal of Pharmacology 85: 171–176
Lembeck F, Griesbacher T, Eckhard M et al 1991 New, long-acting, potent bradykinin antagonists. British Journal of Pharmacology 102: 297–304
Levine J D, Clark R, Devor M et al 1984 Intraneuronal substance P contributes to the severity of experimental arthritis. Science 226: 547–549
Levine J D, Gooding J, Donatoni, P, Borden L, Goetzl E J 1985 The role of the polymorphonuclear leukocytes in hyperalgesia. Journal of Neuroscience 5: 3025–3029
Levine J D, Lam D, Taiwo Y O, Donatoni P, Goetzl E J 1986 Hyperalgesic properties of 15-lipoxygenase products of arachidonic acid. Proceedings of the National Academy of Sciences USA 83: 5331–5334
Levitan I B, Kaczmarek L K 1991 The neuron: cell and molecular biology. Oxford University Press, New York
Lewin G R, Winter J, McMahon S B 1992 Regulation of afferent connectivity in the adult spinal cord by nerve growth factor. European Journal of Neuroscience 4: 700–707
Lewin G R, Ritter A M, Mendell L M 1993 Nerve growth factor-induced hyperalgesia in the neonatal and adult rat. Journal of Neuroscience 13: 2136–2148
Lindahl O 1962 Pain: a chemical explanation. Acta Rheumatologica Scandinavica 8: 161–169
Lindholm D, Neumann R, Meyer M, Thoenen H 1987 Interleukin-1 regulates synthesis of nerve growth factor in non-neuronal cells of the rat sciatic nerve. Nature 330: 658–659
Lindsay R M 1988 Nerve growth factors (NGF, BDNF) enhance axonal regeneration but are not required for survival of adult sensory neurons. Journal of Neuroscience 8: 2394–2405
Lindsay R M, Harmar A J 1989 Nerve growth factor regulates expression of neuropeptide genes in adult sensory neurons. Nature 337: 362–364
Lindstrom P, Lindblom U 1987 The analgesic effect of tocainide in trigeminal neuralgia. Pain 28: 45–50
Lotz M, Vaughan J H, Carson D A 1988 Effect of neuropeptides on production of inflammatory cytokines by human monocytes. Science 241: 1218–1221
Maggi C A 1992 Therapeutic potential of capsaicin-like molecules: studies in animals and humans. Life Sciences 51: 1777–1781
Maggi C A, Meli A 1988 The sensory-efferent function of capsaicin-sensitive neurons. General Pharmacology 19: 1–43
Maggi C A, Patacchini R, Rovero P, Giachetti A 1993 Tachykinin receptors and tachykinin receptor antagonists. Journal of Autonomic Pharmacology (in press)
Manning D C, Raja S N, Meyer R A, Campbell J N 1991 Pain and hyperalgesia after intradermal injection of bradykinin in humans. Clinical Pharmacology and Therapeutics 50: 721–729

Mantyh P W, Catton M D, Boehmer C G et al 1989 Receptors for sensory neuropeptides in human inflammatory diseases: implications for the effector role of sensory neurons. Peptides 10: 627–647

Manzini S, Meini S 1991 Involvement of capsaicin-sensitive nerves in the bronchomotor effects of arachidonic acid and mellitin: a possible role for lipoxin A_4. British Journal of Pharmacology 103: 1027–1032

Marasco W A, Showell H L, Becker E L 1981 Substance P binds to formyl peptide chemotaxis receptor on the rabbit neutrophil. Biochemical and Biophysical Research Communications 99: 1065–1072

Marceau F, Lussier A, Regoli D, Giroud J P 1983 Pharmacology of kinins and their relevance to tissue injury and inflammation. General Pharmacology 14: 209–229

Maricq A V, Peterson A S, Brake A J et al 1991 Primary structure and functional expression of the 5HT3 receptor, a serotonin-gated ion channel. Science 254: 432–437

Martin H A 1990 Leukotriene B_4 induced decrease in mechanical and thermal thresholds of C-fiber mechanonociceptors in rat hairy skin. Brain Research 509: 273–279

Martin H A, Basbaum A I, Kwiat G C, Goetzl E J, Levine J D 1987 Leukotriene and prostaglandin sensitization of cutaneous high threshold C- and A-delta mechanoreceptors in the hairy skin of rat hindlimbs. Neuroscience 22: 651–659

Matucci C, Marabini S 1988 Somatostatin treatment for pain in rheumatoid arthritis: a double blind versus placebo study in knee involvement. Medical Science Research 16: 223–234

Mayer M L, James M H, Russell R J, Kelly J S, Pasternak C A 1986 Changes in excitability induced by herpes simplex viruses in rat dorsal root ganglion neurons. Journal of Neuroscience 6: 391–402

Mayer M L, Westbrook G L 1983 A voltage-clamp analysis of inward (anomalous) rectification in mouse spinal sensory ganglion neurones. Journal of Physiology 340: 19–45

McCobb D P, Beam K 1991 Action potential waveform voltage-clamp commands reveal striking differences in calcium entry via low and high voltage-activated calcium channels. Neuron 7: 119–127

McEachern A E, Shelton E R, Bhakta S et al 1991 Expression cloning of a rat B_2 bradykinin receptor. Proceedings of the National Academy of Sciences USA 88: 7724–7728

McFarlane S, Cooper E 1991 Kinetics and voltage dependence of A-type currents in neonatal rat sensory neurons. Journal of Neurophysiology 66: 1380–1391

McGehee D S, Goy M F, Oxford G S 1992 Involvement of the nitric oxide-cyclic GMP pathway in the desensitization of bradykinin responses of cultured rat sensory neurons. Neuron 9: 315–324

McLean M J, Bennett P B, Thomas R M 1988 Subtypes of dorsal root ganglion neurons based on different inward currents as measured by whole-cell voltage clamp. Molecular and Cellular Biochemistry 80: 95–107

McMahon S B 1991 Mechanisms of sympathetic pain. British Medical Bulletin 47: 584–600

McMahon S B, Gibson S 1987 Peptide expression is altered when afferent nerves reinnervate inappropriate tissue. Neuroscience Letters 73: 9–15

Meller S T, Pechman P S, Gebhart G F, Maves T J 1992a Nitric oxide mediates the thermal hyperalgesia produced in a model of neuropathic pain in the rat. Neuroscience 50: 7–10

Meller S T, Dykstra C, Gebhart G F 1992b Production of endogenous nitric oxide and activation of soluble guanylate cyclase are required for N-methyl-D-aspartate-produced facilitation of the nociceptive tail-flick reflex. European Journal of Pharmacology 214: 93–96

Mense S, Meyer H 1988 Bradykinin-induced modulation of the response behaviour of different types of feline group III and IV muscle receptors. Journal of Physiology 398: 49–63

Mizumura K, Sato J, Kumazawa T 1987 Effects of prostaglandins and other putative chemical intermediaries on the activity of canine testicular polymodal receptors studied in vitro. Pflügers Archives 408: 565–572

Molander C, Ygge J, Dalsgaard C-J 1987 Substance P-, somatostatin- and calcitonin gene-related peptide like immunoreactivity and fluoride resistant acid phosphatase-activity in relation to retrogradely labeled cutaneous, muscular and visceral primary sensory neurons in the rat. Neuroscience Letters 74: 37–42

Moncada S, Ferreira S H, Vane J R 1975 Inhibition of prostaglandin biosynthesis as the mechanism of analgesia of aspirin-like drugs in the dog knee joint. European Journal of Pharmacology 31: 250–260

Moncada S, Palmer R M, Higgs E A 1991 Nitric oxide: physiology, pathophysiology and pharmacology. Pharmacological Reviews 43: 109–142

Moore P K, Oluyomi A O, Babbedge P, Wallace P, Hart S L 1991 L-N^G-nitro arginine methyl ester exhibits antinociceptive activity in the mouse. British Journal of Pharmacology 102: 198–202

Morris R, Southam E, Braid D J, Garthwaite J 1992 Nitric oxide may act as a messenger between dorsal root ganglion neurones and their satellite cells. Neuroscience Letters 137: 29–32

Nakamura-Craig M, Gill B K 1991 Effect of neurokinin A, substance P and calcitonin gene related peptide in peripheral hyperalgesia in the rat paw. Neuroscience Letters 124: 49–51

Naruse K, McGehee D S, Oxford G S 1992 Differential responses of Ca-activated K channels to bradykinin in sensory neurons and F-11 cells. American Journal of Physiology 262: C453–C460

Ninkovic M, Hunt S P 1985 Opiate and histamine H_1 receptors are present on some substance P-containing dorsal root ganglion cells. Neuroscience Letters 53: 133–137

Nowycky M 1992 Voltage-gated ion channels in dorsal root ganglion neurons. In: Scott S A (ed) Sensory neurons: diversity, development and plasticity. Oxford University Press, New York

Ogawa T, Kanazawa I, Kimura S 1985 Regional distribution of substance P, neurokinin α and neurokinin β in rat spinal cord, nerve roots and dorsal root ganglia, and the effects of dorsal root section or spinal transection. Brain Research 359: 152–157

Otten U 1991 Nerve growth factor: a signalling protein between the nervous and the immune systems. In: Basbaum A I, Besson J M (eds) Towards a new pharmacotherapy of pain. John Wiley, Chichester, p 353–363

Otten U Lorez H P, Businger F 1983 Nerve growth factor antagonizes the neurotoxic action of capsaicin on primary afferent neurones. Nature 301: 515–517

Payan D G, Brewster D R, Goetzl E J 1983 Specific stimulation of human T-lymphocytes by substance P. Journal of Immunology 131: 1613–1615

Payan D G, Levine J D, Goetzl E J 1984 Modulation of immunity and hypersensitivity by sensory neuropeptides. Journal of Immunology 132: 1601–1604

Perkins M N, Campbell E, Dray A 1993 Anti-nociceptive activity of the B_1 and B_2 receptor antagonists desArg^{9}Leu^{8}Bk and HOE 140, in two models of persistent hyperalgesia in the rat. Pain 53: 191–197

Perney T M, Hirning L D, Leeman S E, Miller R J 1986 Multiple calcium channels mediate transmitter release from peripheral neurons. Proceedings of the National Academy of Sciences USA 83: 6656–6659

Piomelli D, Greengard P 1990 Lipoxygenase metabolites of arachidonic acid in neuronal transmembrane signalling. Trends in Pharmacological Sciences 11: 367–373

Popper P, Mantyh C R, Vigna S R, Maggio J E, Mantyh P W 1988 The localization of sensory nerve fibers and receptor binding sites for sensory neuropeptides in canine mesenteric lymph nodes. Peptides 9: 257–267

Proud D, Kaplan A P 1988 Kinin formation: mechanisms and role in inflammatory disorders. Annual Review of Pharmacology 6: 49–84

Puttick R M 1992 Excitatory action of prostaglandin E_2 on rat neonatal cultured dorsal root ganglion cells. British Journal of Pharmacology 105: 133P

Rackham A, Ford-Hutchinson A W 1983 Inflammation and pain sensitivity: effects of leukotrienes D_4, B_4 and prostaglandin E_1 in the rat paw. Prostaglandins 25: 193–203

Rang H P, Dale M M 1991 How drugs act: molecular aspects. In: Rang H P, Dale M M (eds) Pharmacology. Churchill Livingstone, Edinburgh

Rang H P, Ritchie J M 1988 Depolarization of nonmyelinated fibers of the rat vagus nerve produced by activation of protein kinase C. Journal of Neuroscience 8: 2606–2617

Rang H P, Bevan S, Dray A 1991 Chemical activation of nociceptive peripheral neurones. British Medical Bulletin 47: 534–548

Richardson B P, Engel G, Donatsch P, Stadler P A 1985 Identification of serotonin M-receptor subtypes and their specific blockade by a new class of drugs. Nature 316: 126–131

Rogawski M A 1985 The A-current: how ubiquitous a feature of excitable cells is it? Trends in Neurosciences 5: 214–219

Rueff A, Dray A 1992 5-hydroxytryptamine-induced sensitization and activation of peripheral fibers in the neonatal rat are mediated via different 5-hydroxytryptamine receptors. Neuroscience 50: 899–905

Santicolli P, Del Bianco E, Tramontana M, Geppetti P, Maggi C A 1992 Release of calcitonin gene-related peptide-like immunoreactivity induced by electrical field stimulation from rat spinal afferents is mediated by conotoxin-sensitive calcium channels. Neuroscience Letters 136: 161–164

Saria A, Martling C R, Yan Z, Theodorssen-Northeim E, Gamse R, Lundberg J M 1988 Release of multiple tachykinins from capsaicin-sensitive sensory nerves in the lung by bradykinin, histamine, dimethylphenyl piperazinium, and vagal nerve stimulation. American Review of Respiratory Disease 137: 1330–1335

Sato J, Perl E R 1991 Adrenergic excitation of cutaneous pain receptors induced by peripheral nerve injury. Science 251: 1608–1610

Schaible H-G, Schmidt R F 1988 Excitation and sensitization of fine articular afferents from cat's knee joint by prostaglandin E_2. Journal of Physiology 403: 91–104

Schaible H-G, Jarrott B, Hope P J, Duggan A W 1990 Release of immunoreactive substance P in the spinal cord during development of acute arthritis in the knee joint of the cat: study with antibody microprobes. Brain Research 529: 214–223

Schepelman K, Messlinger K, Schaible H-G, Schmidt R F 1992 Inflammatory mediators and nociception in the joint: excitation and sensitization of slowly conducting afferent fibers of cat's knee by prostaglandin I_2. Neuroscience 50: 237–247

Schroeder J E, Fischbach P S, Moma M, McCleskey E W 1990 Mu opioids inhibit two transient calcium currents inactivated by voltage but spare a current inactivated by calcium ions. Society for Neuroscience Abstracts 16: 634

Schweizer A, Feige U, Fontana A, Muller K, Dinarello C A 1988 Interleukin-1 enhances pain reflexes. Mediation through increased prostaglandin E_2 levels. Agents and Action 25: 246–251

Scott R H, Pearson H A, Dolphin A C 1991 Aspects of vertebrate neuronal voltage-activated calcium currents and their regulation. Progress in Neurobiology 36: 485–520

Scott S A 1992 Sensory neurons: diversity, development and plasticity. Oxford University Press, New York

Scroggs R S, Fox A P 1992 Calcium current variation between acutely isolated adult rat dorsal root ganglion neurons of different sizes. Journal of Physiology 445: 639–658

Shearman M S, Sekiguchi K, Nishizuka Y 1989 Modulation of ion channel activity: a key function of the protein kinase C enzyme family. Pharmacological Reviews 41: 211–237

Shen K-F, Crain S M 1990 Dynorphin prolongs the action potential of mouse sensory ganglion neurons by decreasing a potassium conductance whereas another specific kappa opioid does so by increasing a calcium conductance. Neuropharmacology 29: 343–349

Simone D A, Alrejo M, LaMotte R H 1991 Psychophysical studies of the itch sensation and itchy skin ('allokinesis') produced by intracutaneous injection of histamine. Somatosensory and Motor Research 8: 271–279

Steen K H, Reeh P W, Anton F, Handwerker H O 1992 Protons selectively induce lasting excitation and sensitization to mechanical stimuli of nociceptors in rat skin, in vivo. Journal of Neuroscience 12: 86–95

Stein C 1991 Peripheral analgesic actions of opioids. Pain and Symptom Management 6: 119–124

Stephan M, Agnew W S 1991 Voltage-sensitive Na^+ channels: motifs, modes and modulation. Current Opinion in Cell Biology 3: 676–684

Steranka L R, Manning D C, Dehaas J R et al 1988 Bradykinin as a pain mediator: receptors are localised to sensory neurones and antagonists have analgesic actions. Proceedings of the National Academy of Sciences USA 85: 3245–3249

Sylven C 1989 Angina pectoris. Clinical characteristics, neurophysiological and molecular mechanisms. Pain 36: 145–167

Szallasi A, Blumberg P M 1989 Resiniferatoxin, a phorbol-related diterpene, acts as an ultrapotent analog of capsaicin, the irritable constituent of red pepper. Neuroscience 30: 515–520

Szallasi A, Blumberg P M 1990 Specific binding of resiniferatoxin, an ultrapotent capsaicin analog, by dorsal root ganglion membranes. Brain Research 524: 106–111

Szolcsanyi J, Jansco-Gabor A 1975 Sensory effects of capsaicin congeners. I. Relationship between chemical structure and pain-producing potency of pungent agents. Arzneimittel-Forschung 25: 1877–1881

Taiwo Y O, Levine J D 1990 Direct cutaneous hyperalgesia induced by adenosine. Neuroscience 38: 757–762

Taiwo Y O, Levine J D 1991a Further confirmation of the role of adenyl cyclase and of cAMP-dependent protein kinase in primary afferent hyperalgesia. Neuroscience 44: 131–135

Taiwo Y O, Levine J D 1991b κ- and δ-opioids block sympathetically dependent hyperalgesia. Journal of Neuroscience 11: 928–932

Taiwo Y O, Levine J D 1992 Serotonin is a directly-acting hyperalgesic agent in the rat. Neuroscience 48: 485–590

Taiwo Y O, Bjerknes L K, Goetzl E J, Levine J D 1989 Mediation of primary afferent hyperalgesia by the cAMP second messenger system. Neuroscience 32: 577–580

Taiwo Y O, Levine J D, Burch R M, Woo J E, Mobley W C 1991 Hyperalgesia induced in the rat by the amino-terminal octapeptide of nerve growth factor. Proceedings of the National Academy of Sciences USA 88: 5144–5148

Tanelian D L, Brose W G 1991 Neuropathic pain can be relieved by drugs that are use-dependent sodium channel blockers: lidocaine, carbamazepine and mexilitine. Anesthesiology 74: 949–951

Tani E, Shiosaka S, Sato M, Ishikawa T, Tohyama M 1990 Histamine acts directly on calcitonin gene-related peptide- and substance P-containing trigeminal ganglion neurons as assessed by calcium influx and immunocytochemistry. Neuroscience Letters 115: 171–176

Thayer S A, Perney T M, Miller R J 1988 Regulation of calcium homeostasis in sensory neurons by bradykinin. Journal of Neuroscience 8: 4089–4097

Todorovic S, Anderson E G 1990 5-HT2 and 5-HT3 receptors mediate two distinct depolarizing responses in rat dorsal root ganglion neurons. Brain Research 511: 71–79

Trang L E, Grantstrom E, Lovgren O 1977 Levels of prostaglandin F2 alpha and thromboxane B2 in joint fluid in rheumatoid arthritis. Scandinavian Journal of Rheumatology 6: 151–154

Van der Zee C E E M, Nielander H B, Vos J P et al 1989 Expression of growth-associated protein B-50 (GAP43) in dorsal root ganglia and sciatic nerve during regenerative sprouting. Journal of Neuroscience 9: 3505–3512

Vedder H, Otten U 1991 Biosynthesis and release of tachykinins from rat sensory neurons in culture. Journal of Neuroscience Research 30: 288–299

Villar M J, Cortes R, Theodorsson E et al 1989 Neuropeptide expression in rat dorsal root ganglion cells and spinal cord after peripheral nerve injury with special reference to galanin. Neuroscience 33: 587–604

Waddell P J, Lawson S N 1990 Electrophysiological properties of subpopulations of rat dorsal root ganglion neurons in vitro. Neuroscience 36: 811–822

Wagner F, Fink T, Hart R, Dancygier H 1987 Substance P enhances interferon-γ production by human peripheral blood mononuclear cells. Regulatory Peptides 19: 355–364

Ward T, Steigbigel R T 1978 Acidosis of synovial fluid correlates with synovial fluid leukocytosis. American Journal of Medicine 64: 933–936

Wei P, Moskowitz M A, Boccalini P, Kontos H A 1992 Calcitonin gene-related peptide mediates nitroglycerin and sodium nitroprusside-induced vasodilatation in feline cerebral arterioles. Circulation Research 70: 1313–1319

Weihe E, Muller S, Fink T, Zentel H-J 1989 Tachykinins, CGRP and neuropeptide Y in nerves of the mammalian thymus: interactions with mast cells in autonomic and sensory neuroimmunomodulation? Neuroscience Letters 100: 77–82

Weihe E, Nohr A, Muller S D, Buchler M, Friess H, Zentel H-J 1991 The tachykinin neuroimmune connection in inflammatory pain. Annals of the New York Academy of Sciences 632: 283–295

Weinreich D 1986 Bradykinin inhibits a slow spike after-hyperpolarization in visceral sensory neurons. European Journal of Pharmacology 132: 61–63

Weinreich D, Wonderlin W F 1987 Inhibition of calcium-dependent spike after-hyperpolarization increases excitability of rabbit visceral sensory neurones. Journal of Physiology 394: 415–427

Whalley E T, Clegg S, Stewart J M, Vavrek R J 1987 The effect of kinin agonists and antagonists on the pain response of the human blister base. Naunyn-Schmiedebergs Archives of Pharmacology 336: 652–655

White G, Lovinger D M, Weight F F 1989 Transient low-threshold Ca^{2+} current triggers burst firing through an afterdepolarizing potential in an adult mammalian neuron. Proceedings of the National Academy of Sciences USA 86: 6802–6806

Willis W D, Coggeshall R E 1991 Sensory mechanisms of the spinal cord. Plenum Press, New York

Winter J, Forbes C A, Sternberg J, Lindsay R M 1988 Nerve growth factor (NGF) regulates adult rat cultured dorsal root ganglion neuron responses to the excitotoxin capsaicin. Neuron 1: 973–981

Winter J, Dray A, Wood J N, Yeats J C, Bevan S 1990 Cellular mechanism of action of resiniferatoxin: a potent sensory neuron excitotoxin. Brain Research 520: 131–140

Yoshida K, Gage F H 1992 Cooperative regulation of nerve growth factor synthesis and secretion in fibroblasts and astrocytes by fibroblast growth factor and other cytokines. Brain Research 569: 14–25

4. The pathophysiology of damaged peripheral nerves

Marshall Devor

INTRODUCTION

Prevailing attitudes concerning the relative importance of the peripheral versus the central nervous system (PNS, CNS) in the aetiology of chronic pain have changed radically in recent years. In the 1930s, 40s and 50s major emphasis was placed on mechanisms associated with peripheral nerves (e.g. Lewis 1942). Since the early 60s, and particularly since the introduction of Melzack & Wall's (1965) gate control concept, research interest has shifted strongly to spinal and other CNS mechanisms. Today, although it is widely conceded that both peripheral and central processes play an essential role, the subtlety and variety of possible PNS contributions are not widely appreciated. For example, when sensitization of primary sensory endings can be ruled out as a cause of pain, it is often assumed that the abnormality must be central. The aim of this chapter is to summarize the state of knowledge on pathophysiological processes in the PNS, with special emphasis on those that are significant for an understanding of clinical symptomatology.

THE PRIMARY SENSORY NEURON

Afferent axons run uninterrupted from their peripheral sensory ending in innervated tissue (skin, muscle, etc.) to their central synaptic endings in the CNS. The cell body lies along this path, in the dorsal root or cranial nerve ganglion. Normally, each neuron constitutes an independent channel of sensory communication whose job is to report to the CNS on stimulus events that occur in the periphery.

The axon has three distinct functions: to *encode*, to *conduct* and to *relay* sensory messages. Each of these functions places particular design demands on the sensory neuron in response to which evolution has provided it with a high degree of regional specialization (Waxman & Foster 1980; Calvin 1980). Consider a myelinated afferent innervating skin of the fingertip. The distal few tens of microns are specialised for translating (transducing and encoding) a mechanical or thermal stimulus into an impulse train that is interpretable centrally. The mid-axon part is specialized for conducting this signal rapidly and accurately without missing impulses or adding extra ones. The terminal arbor with its synaptic endings is specialized for relaying the sensory message into the CNS.

The electrical properties of the three parts of the axon must be optimised and maintained. If sensory endings underwent uncontrolled changes in their sensitivity, for example, the CNS would have no way of telling from the incoming impulse train what the original stimulus really was. Nor is it trivial to maintain stability over extended periods of time. Nerve fibre endings are embedded in soft elastic tissue and in normal use are constantly being heated and cooled, stretched and squeezed, pinched and abraided. As we shall see, failure to adequately regulate regional axon properties on injury or disease can lead to sensory dysfunction and pain.

'NORMAL' VERSUS 'PATHOPHYSIOLOGIC' PAIN

Normally, pain is felt when impulses reach a conscious brain along fine myelinated (Aδ) and/or unmyelinated (C) nociceptive afferents. It is the match between the high threshold of the afferent endings in the periphery and the interpretation (pain) assigned by the brain to the impulses they carry that makes this an effective signalling system. Pain is 'normal' ('nociceptive') when it results from the activity of healthy nociceptive afferents aroused by intense stimuli, assuming baseline sensitivity of the sensory system. By this standard even chronic pain would be 'normal' if it were evoked by maintained or repeated noxious stimuli that did not change baseline system sensitivity.

'Pathophysiologic' pain, in contrast, results from a *change* in baseline somatosensory sensitivity. There are at least three types of change. First the sensitivity of nociceptor endings may increase. This is 'peripheral sensitization'. Weak, previously non-noxious stimuli now activate nociceptors, and elicit pain. Second, pathophysiologic pain can arise when otherwise normal PNS axons begin to produce impulses at abnormal (ectopic) locations along their course, for example at sites of injury. Finally, pain is pathophysiologic when it results from increased gain in central processing circuits ('central sensitization') including spontaneous impulse initiation. In the presence of central sensitization, input via non-nociceptive Aβ-afferents may trigger pain (e.g. Campbell et al 1988).

Changes in baseline sensitivity do not necessarily indicate a disease state. Indeed, they may represent a useful somatosensory adaptation. For example, in the event of a mild burn, substances are released in the skin which sensitize nociceptor endings (bradykinin, histamine, etc.). Likewise, impulses evoked by such injuries might trigger central sensitization. Both changes make the burned area feel tender for a time and therefore encourage the individual to protect it, avoiding further injury. They are therefore adaptive and desirable. However, since both set the sensory system temporarily into an abnormal state, they are grouped here within the spectrum of pathophysiologic changes. In principle, pathophysiologic pain states could be subdivided into those that are adaptive, and those that are maladaptive.

In this chapter I will deal only in passing with peripheral and central sensitization. These subjects are discussed in detail elsewhere in this textbook (Chs 1–3 and 5). Rather, I will focus on the second category of the pathophysiologic change noted above, ectopic impulse generation in injured and diseased nerves. It will be seen that there is a striking resemblance between the abnormal electrical behaviour of sensory axons in experimental models of nerve injury and the sensory symptoms that occur in various clinical pain syndromes. This resemblance encourages the hypothesis that the pathophysiologic changes in injured nerves constitute a principal cause of postinjury chronic pain.

MECHANISMS OF IMPULSE GENERATION (ELECTROGENESIS)

To fully understand pathophysiologic pain associated with abnormal impulse generation it is important to be fluent with the fundamentals of electrogenesis in normal excitable cells, and especially peripheral sensory endings. What follows is a brief and qualitative refresher. For a detailed, quantitative discussion the reader is referred elsewhere (Loewenstein 1971; Jack et al 1983; Sachs 1986; Hille 1992).

TRANSDUCTION AND ENCODING

Sensory impulse generation typically begins when a stimulus causes an increase in the permeability of the membrane of sensory endings to various ions, particularly Na^+. For mechanoreceptors, stretching triggers the opening of the transmembrane pore of specific pore-containing proteins called 'stretch-activated (SA-) channels' (Sachs 1986). NA^+ ions, among others, then flow through the channels following their electrical and concentration gradient (generator current) producing partial depolarization of the sensory ending (generator potential). For a given stimulus strength the magnitude of the generator current depends both on the amount of stretch transmitted through the viscoelastic tissue surrounding the sensory ending, and on the number and sensitivity of its SA-channels. The transduction molecules underlying thermal sensitivity have not yet been identified.

Sensory endings also contain a second class of pore-containing proteins: 'voltage-sensitive ion-channels'. These respond to transmembrane voltage rather than to stretch. At rest, the most important of these, the voltage-sensitive Na^+-channels, are closed. Stretch induces a slowly rising depolarization which triggers the most sensitive Na^+-channels to open. This lets a stream of Na^+ ions into the sensory ending, depolarizing the ending even more. Now more Na^+ channels open, letting in still more Na^+ and so forth. The result of this cascade is a depolarizatory explosion, the action potential. Notice the dual process:

1. A slowly rising generator potential triggers
2. An explosive action potential (nerve impulse).

Having opened, Na^+-channels rapidly close again, and the membrane potential drifts back towards its initial resting level. Often this repolarization is accelerated by the transient opening of K^+-selective channels. When prolonged, the opening of K^+-channels produces after-hyperpolarization, making the ending temporarily refractory, and delaying, for a time, the generation of the next action potential (Hille 1992).

THRESHOLD FOR IMPULSE INITIATION

It is obviously inappropriate to have nerve impulses set off by infinitesimally small stimuli, and this does not happen. The reason is straightforward. As soon as depolarization begins, an electromotive gradient for K^+ ions is created and K^+ begins to flow out of the sensory ending. This outward K^+ current tends to neutralize the inward Na^+ current, preventing further depolarization. Thus, at the beginning of the excitation process, there are two opposing forces at work. If the stretch-evoked generator current plus the action potential current it triggers are large, the depolarizatory chain reaction will proceed, and an action potential (spike) will be set off; if small, the depolarization will be damped out before a spike is initiated. The *threshold* for impulse initiation lies somewhere in-between. Note that threshold is not a fixed value; it is a dynamic equilibrium.

THRESHOLD FOR REPETITIVE FIRING

The individual action potential is the basic unit of neural signalling. In practice, however, sensory communication depends on repetitive impulse firing. Many cells can produce single action potentials but do not fire repetitively even when a stimulus is maintained. Repetitive firing capability depends on two factors. The first is the presence of a maintained generator potential. Even when the stimulus is constant the resulting generator potential may fade, yielding rapid or slow receptor 'adaptation'. The second has to do with the intrinsic electrical properties of the fibre's membrane (i.e. its 'encoding' or 'pacemaker' properties). Some cells fire rapidly with minimal depolarization. Others will not fire repetitively even with intense depolarization. Slowly adapting sensory neurons, which specialize in translating stimulus intensity into a frequency code, take the middle ground. Below some defined level of generator potential no rhythmic firing is produced. But once *threshold* is reached, sustained rhythmogenesis begins with a sudden jump to a relatively high 'minimum rhythmic firing frequency' (mRFF, Fig. 4.1). From this point on firing frequency varies smoothly with stimulus intensity (encoding or f-I function; Stein 1967; Calvin 1975; Matzner & Devor 1992). As we shall see, the pronounced non-linear jump in the f-I function at threshold is important for ectopic neural discharge.

Notice the difference between the concepts of *threshold for impulse initiation* and *threshold for repetitive firing*. Ignoring adaptation, a prolonged stimulus may well be strong enough to evoke a single action potential but too weak (subthreshold) to produce repetitive firing. Both thresholds depend on specific membrane proteins, particularly Na^+- and K^+-channels. The sensory neuron must strictly control these as they determine whether the ending will be a low-threshold touch fibre or a high-threshold nociceptor. Sensitizing agents (e.g. bradykinin) are usually assumed to act by adding to the generator potential. However, some agents act by enhancing the opening of Na^+-channels or suppressing the opening of K^+-channels (Strichartz et al 1987; Kirchoff et al 1992). Disruption of the processes that normally regulate these proteins can alter threshold, causing receptor hypersensitivity and/or ectopic impulse generation. There is an accumulating body of evidence suggesting that exactly this kind of regulatory abnormality underlies much chronic pain.

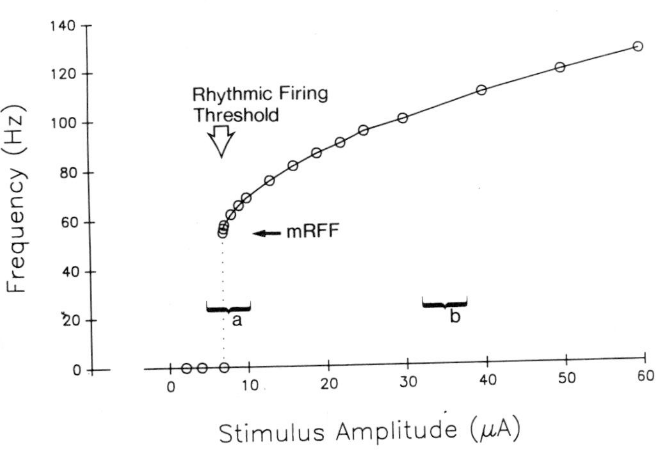

Fig. 4.1 Relationship between stimulus intensity (amplitude) and firing frequency based on computer simulations of the squid giant axon (Matzner & Devor 1992). Note the discontinuous 'threshold' (open arrow) at which discharge frequency jumps from zero to the minimum rhythmic firing frequency (mRFF). A change in stimulus intensity equivalent to bracket (a) produces a much larger change in firing frequency than does the identical stimulus (b).

ECTOPIC DISCHARGE ORIGINATING AT SITES ON NERVE INJURY

NERVE INJURY, REGENERATION AND NEUROMA FORMATION

When an axon is cut across the proximal stump, the part still connected to the cell body, seals off and forms a terminal swelling or 'endbulb'. It may also die back for up to a few millimetres and the myelin sheath near the cut end is invariably disrupted (Cajal 1928; Morris et al 1972; Fawcett & Keynes 1990; Fried et al 1991). In neonates, most axotomized cells die. In adults, however, the majority survive, and within a short time many fine processes (axonal 'sprouts') emerge from the retracted endbulb and begin to elongate. Under optimal conditions one of these regenerating sprouts reaches peripheral target tissue. Growth then stops, peripheral receptor function is restored and excess sprouts are culled. When forward growth is blocked, terminal endbulbs persist and sprouts either turn back on themselves or form a tangled mass. This structure is a 'neuroma'.

Regeneration is often ideal if the nerve has been crushed or frozen. But whenever the nerve sheath (perineurium) is breached a neuroma is created. This is true even if the neuroma does not swell to proportions that can be easily palpated, and even if there is no associated pain. 'Nerve-end neuromas', for example, *always* form after limb amputation. If the ends of a cut nerve are reapproximated, some fibres cross the gap and proceed to elongate. Even in the most favourable cases, however, many (usually most) are trapped near the suture line in a 'neuroma-in-continuity' (Horch & Lisney 1981a; Ashur et al 1987). Sprouts that do begin to regenerate may get caught up subsequently, forming disseminated 'microneuromas' scattered along the distal nerve trunk, its branches and its target tissue. Nerve injury also triggers the 'collateral sprouting' of nearby intact afferents (Devor et al 1979).

ENDBULBS AND SPROUTS ARE A SOURCE OF ECTOPIC FIRING

In 1974 Wall & Gutnick reported the presence of massive spontaneous impulse discharge in lower lumbar dorsal roots in rats in which an experimental neuroma had been made by cutting the sciatic nerve. Firing was also affected by mechanical and chemical stimulation of the neuroma (Wall & Gutnick 1974a, 1974b). These data lent support to conclusions based on clinical observations, that abnormal neural activity generated at ectopic locations in the PNS could trigger neuropathic dysaesthesias and pain (Kugelberg 1946).

It was clear from Wall & Gutnick's study that many of the impulses originated in the neuroma because pressing on it augmented the discharge and anaesthetising it reduced the discharge. However, since the active roots also contained afferents from nerves that had not been cut, some of the recorded activity undoubtedly originated in intact proprioceptive and thermosensitive fibres, and in sensory cell somata in dorsal root ganglia (DRGs) (Kirk 1974). To resolve this ambiguity Govrin-Lippmann & Devor (1978), and subsequently several other groups (e.g. Wiesenfeld & Lindblom 1980; Scadding 1981; Blumberg & Janig 1984; Burchiel 1984a; Meyer et al 1985; Brewart & Gentle 1985; Welk et al 1990), repeated these experiments but recorded from the nerve itself just proximal to the neuroma (Fig. 4.2). This change of recording locus confirmed that the neuroma is a major site of ectopic discharge in both myelinated (A-) and unmyelinated (C-) axons. By exploring the neuroma surface with fine probes, it was possible to locate the hyperexcitability to tiny mechanosensitive 'hotspots' clustered in the 3 mm, and especially the 300 μm, closest to the cut nerve end. Since this is the zone richest in neuroma endbulbs and sprouts (Fried et al 1991), these structures are strongly implicated as the source of the ectopia. Figure 4.3 illustrates neuroma endbulbs labelled by anterograde transport from the cell soma. Endbulbs, and the fine sprouts they often bear, are difficult to see in routine nerve histology and are easily missed if special preparative techniques are not used (also see Fig. 4.12).

ECTOPIC ELECTROGENESIS AFTER DEMYELINATION AND IN PERIPHERAL NEUROPATHIES

Axons that have been demyelinated locally, but are otherwise in continuity, may also become hyperexcitable. This is reflected in spontaneous impulse discharge, mechanosensitivity, and sustained rhythmic afterdischarge in response to electrical or mechanical stimulus pulses (Calvin et al 1977; Rasminsky 1978; Smith & McDonald 1980; Burchiel 1980; Calvin et al 1982; Baker & Bostock 1992). The prevalence of hyperexcitability tends to be lower than

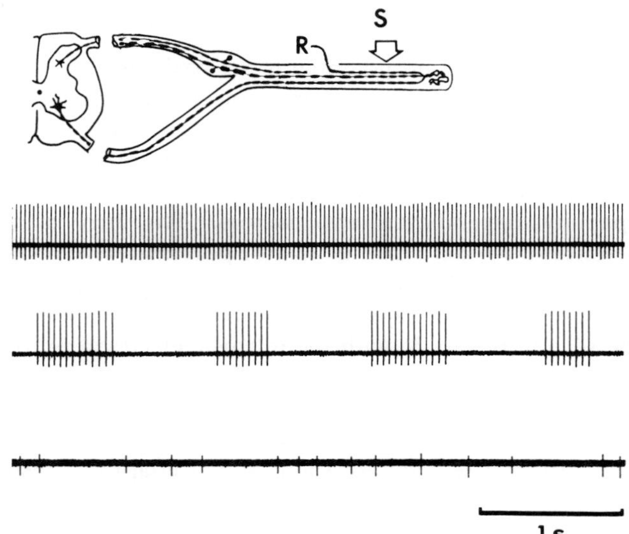

Fig. 4.2 Sketch showing the typical experimental setup for recording ectopic impulse activity from individual chronically injured axons. Recordings are made from teased fibre bundles at R, while stimulus pulses used to determine conduction velocity are delivered at S. The upper two traces show tonic and bursty activity characteristic of neuroma A-fibres. The bottom trace shows the slow, irregular discharge pattern characteristic of neuroma C-fibres.

in neuromas, but discharge patterns (see below) are remarkably similar. Since severed axons always undergo some degree of demyelination, part of the activity normally ascribed to neuroma endbulbs and sprouts could in fact originate in patches of demyelination.

Demyelination per se is expected to reduce fibre excitability to the extent of causing conduction block. This is the major cause of morbidity in demyelinating diseases such as multiple sclerosis. However, secondary reorganization of membrane electrical properties in a subset of axons (see below) can induce hyperexcitability and associated positive sensory symptoms including pain (Rasminsky 1981).

The peripheral neuropathies (e.g. diabetic neuropathy, heavy metal neuropathies, etc.) are an obvious and inviting group of conditions in which to investigate abnormal PNS electrogenesis. In many of them there is clear histological evidence of demyelination and disseminated axonal interruption and sprouting, and a diversity of positive sensory symptoms including pain (Dyck et al 1976 and various chapters in Dyck et al 1984). Abnormal spontaneous neural discharge has been observed in animal models of diabetic polyneuropathy (Burchiel et al 1985), and methylmercury intoxication (Delio et al 1992).

QUANTITATIVE ASPECTS: TYPES OF FIBRE AND PATTERNS OF DISCHARGE

In the clinical setting partial, incomplete nerve trauma or disease is the general rule. In these patients sources of

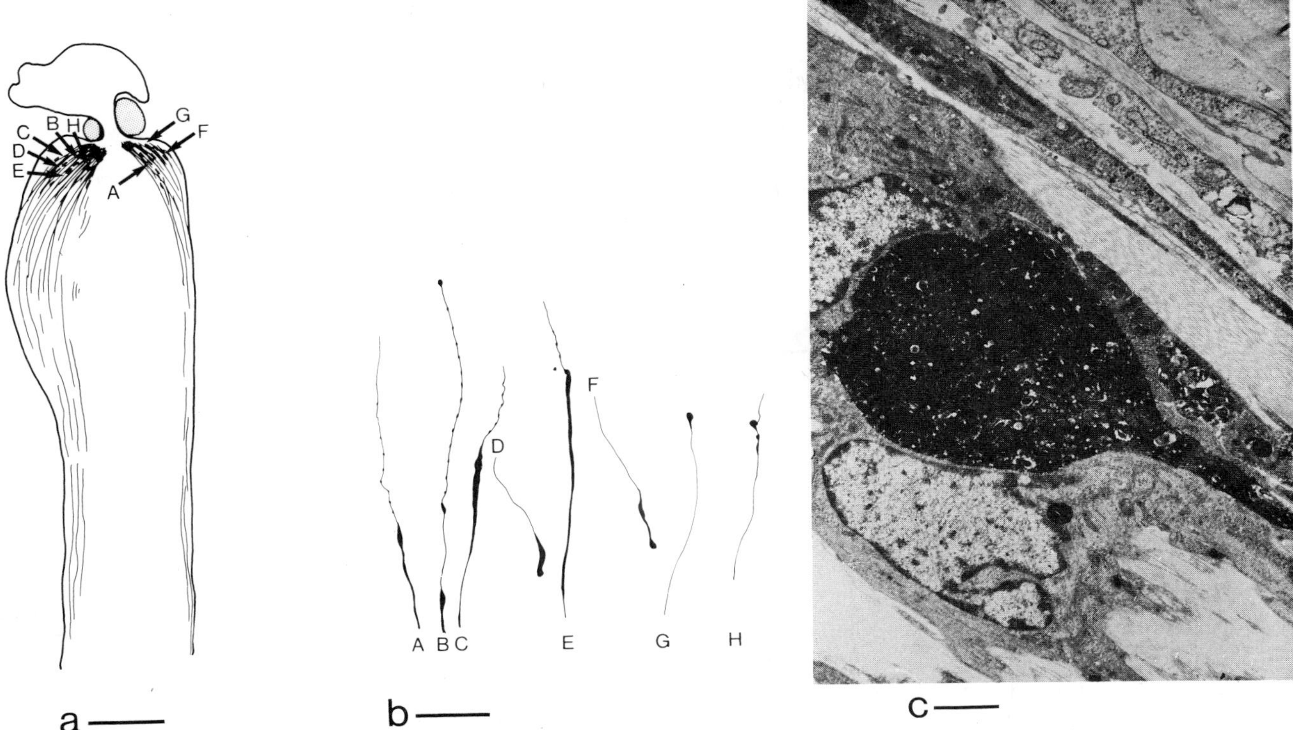

Fig. 4.3 Neuroma endbulbs visualized by anterograde transport of WGA-HRP from the DRG. (a) Camera lucida drawing showing numerous afferents as they approach the cut nerve end (15 days postinjury). Letters A–H mark the location of several endbulbs that are shown at higher magnification in (b). (c) Ultramicrograph of a single labelled endbulb (7 days postinjury). Scalebars: (a) 1 mm (b) 100 μm (c) 3 μm. (From Fried & Devor 1988; Fried et al 1991.)

ectopic firing are likely to be disseminated. For uniformity, animal studies aimed at characterizing ectopia quantitatively have favoured complete nerve injury preparations such as the nerve end neuroma. The results, however, have implications beyond the particular case of amputees.

Recordings from dorsal versus ventral roots, nerves that are purely cutaneous and mixed nerves following deefferentation, indicate that the great bulk of spontaneous ectopic activity is generated in sensory, rather than motor fibres. Measurements of axon conduction velocity in rat neuromas show that Aαβ- and Aδ-afferents are represented roughly according to their numbers in the nerve; afferent C-fibres are somewhat underrepresented at short postoperative times and somewhat overrepresented at long postoperative times (references above; Fig. 4.4). Different sensory receptor types contribute unequally to the overall neuroma barrage (Devor et al 1990; Koschorke et al 1991; Johnson & Munson 1991).

Most spontaneously active neuroma A-afferents (about 90% in rats) discharge rhythmically with highly regular intervals between adjacent impulses within a train (Fig. 4.2). This is the firing pattern expected of intrinsic electrogenesis at a single active pacemaker site ('autorhythmicity'). Interspike interval for individual fibres usually falls within the range of 65–35 ms, which translates to an instantaneous discharge rate in the range of 15–30 Hz. Such rates represent a substantial sensory stimulus in normal nerve. In just over a third of autorhythmic fibres the discharge is interrupted by silent pauses, resulting in a 'bursty', on-off pattern ('interrupted autorhythmicity', Fig. 4.2). The remaining A-fibres have a slow irregular firing pattern (0.1–10 Hz). Curiously, nearly all spontaneously active C-fibres, in rat neuromas at least, fire slowly and irregularly (Fig. 4.2). This implies an interesting and perhaps exploitable difference in the mechanism of electrogenesis in A- versus C-fibres.

VARIABILITY IN THE AMOUNT OF SPONTANEOUS NEUROMA DISCHARGE

Quantitative differences from preparation to preparation shed light on the underlying mechanism. In rat sciatic nerve, for example, there is virtually no discharge for the first day or two after nerve section, although emerging mechanosensitivity can be detected within about 4 hours (Govrin-Lippmann & Devor 1978; Koschorke et al 1991). Activity in A-fibres then rises to high levels for about 2 weeks, subsequently falling back to a relatively low, but sustained plateau (Fig. 4.4, top). During the period of peak activity (3–16 days postoperative) an average of

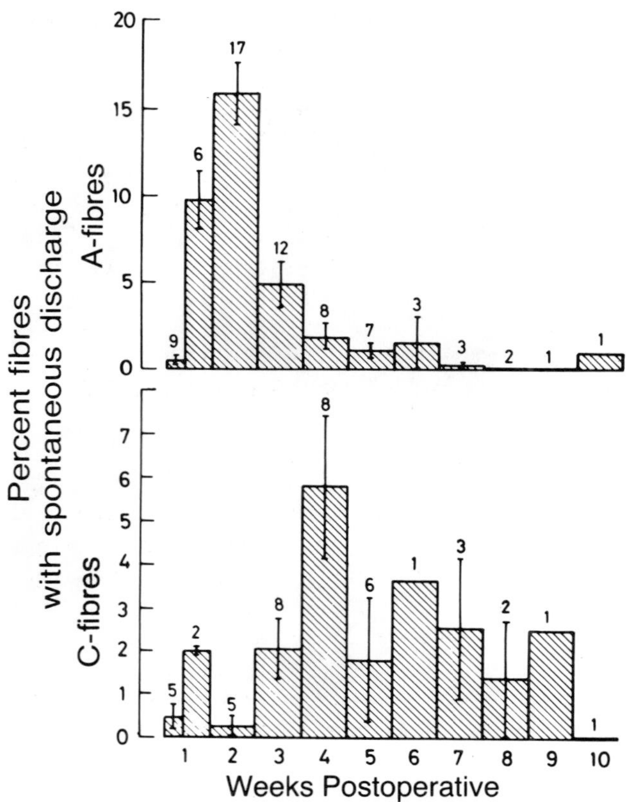

Fig. 4.4 The incidence (mean ± SD) of spontaneously active myelinated (A-) and unmyelinated (C-) fibres in experimental neuromas in the sciatic nerve of Sabra-strain rats during the first 10 weeks after nerve section. The number of experiments performed at each time interval is indicated over the bars. (From Devor & Govrin-Lippman 1985.)

nearly 17% of all fibres fire spontaneously. Since only about 65% of sciatic nerve A-fibres are afferents, this means that ≈ 25% of all injured sensory axons are spontaneously active during this period, a massive barrage by any standard. For C-fibres the natural history of spontaneous activity is different, with substantial discharge emerging only as activity in A-fibres begins to decline (Fig. 4.4, bottom). Beyond the first postoperative month C-fibre activity predominates (Blumberg & Janig 1984; Devor & Govrin-Lippmann 1985).

The figures just quoted (Fig. 4.4) are means obtained in recordings from a standardized experimental preparation in rats of uniform age, sex and strain. Averaging obscures substantial animal-to-animal variability. Moreover, moving to a different nerve, or even the same nerve fibres at a different location, may yield quantitatively different results (Papir-Kricheli & Devor 1988; Tal & Devor 1992). One of the most striking sources of variability is genetic. Following behavioural clues, we examined neuromas of different rat strains. In Lewis-strain rats there was much less ectopic hyperexcitability on average, than there was in Sabra-strain rats (Devor et al 1982). Moreover, first-

Table 4.1 Autotomy and spontaneous ectopic neuroma discharge in Sabra and Lewis strain rats, and in their F_1 offspring. Autotomy score and per cent (myelinated) fibres with spontaneous discharge are group means ± standard deviation (Data from Devor et al 1982)

	Sabra	Lewis	Lewis ♂ × Sabra ♀	Lewis ♀ × Sabra ♂
Autotomy				
Number of rats	47	25	22	23
Autotomy score (35 days p.o.)	2.7±1.2	0	0.3 ± 0.5	0.3 ± 1.3
% rats ⩾ score 2 (35 days p.o.)	40	0	0	4
Autotomy score (70 days p.o.)	5.0 ± 1.5	0	0.4 ± 0.5	0.4 ± 1.7
% rats ⩾ score 2 (70 days p.o.)	60	0	4	9
Spontaneous ectopic discharge				
Number of nerves	14	12	2	2
% fibres with spontaneous discharge (3–16 days p.o.)	16.6 ± 7.6	4.8 ± 4.1	5.8 ± 0.1	6.6 ± 2.5

generation offspring of Sabra × Lewis parents revealed low levels of activity resembling the Lewis parent (Table 4.1). Together, these observations, and related behavioural ones (see below), suggest that susceptibility to neuropathic sensory abnormalities may be in part heritable. This conclusion has obvious implications for the gross variability of neuropathic symptoms in the human patient population.

The natural history of afferent neuroma activity in CBA-strain mice is similar to that of Sabra strain rats (Scadding 1981). Random bred cats, on the other hand, show a very different pattern, with no early A-fibre peak, and overall activity increasing gradually over months (Blumberg & Janig 1984). Rabbits are said to produce little or no ectopic neuroma discharge (S J W Lisney, J Diamond, personal communication). A priori it is not obvious which of these animal models most closely resembles the situation in man (see below).

MECHANO-, THERMO- AND CHEMOSENSITIVITY

Ongoing discharge is a convenient baseline parameter for comparing ectopic activity in different experimental preparations. But hyperexcitability is also reflected in abnormal sensitivity to a broad range of presumably depolarizing stimuli. For example, as already noted, virtually all spontaneously active fibres, and many previously silent ones as well, are excited by mechanical probing (references above). The evoked discharge is sometimes limited to a short burst at the moment of stimulus onset and/or release (i.e. rapidly adapting), or it may last for the duration of force application (slowly adapting). Sometimes discharge continues for an extended period of time after the end of the stimulus ('mechanical afterdischarge', see Figs. 4.6, 4.8).

By analogy to normal mechanoreceptive nerve endings (Loewenstein 1971; Erxleben 1989; Swerup et al 1991), ectopic mechanosensitivity presumably results from the opening of SA-channels and the induction of a generator potential in endbulbs and sprouts. In man, mechanosensitivity is reflected in the Tinel sign, and in tender neuromas and in-continuity trigger points. Locations where nerves run adjacent to tendon and bone (e.g. carpal tunnel), or where small branches cross over tough fascial planes (low back pain, fibromyalgia?), are particularly at risk for developing consistently located mechanosensitive tender spots.

Temperature has a paradoxical effect on ectopic pacemaker firing. In myelinated neuroma fibres, the rate of spontaneous discharge increases with warming and additional, previously silent fibres are recruited. Cooling suppresses firing. Unmyelinated axons, in contrast, tend to be suppressed by warming and excited by cooling (Matzner & Devor 1987). This behaviour may be related to 'cold-intolerance' and cold hyperalgesia in amputees and other nerve injured patients.

In addition to physical stimuli, metabolic and chemical factors that influence membrane potential can excite ectopic discharge. Examples include ischaemia, changes in blood gases and ion concentrations, catecholamines, peptides and various other endogenous neuroactive substances, pharmacological blockade of K^+ conductances and so forth (e.g. Wall & Gutnick 1974b; Scadding 1981; Korenman & Devor 1981; Devor 1983a; Blumberg and Janig 1984, Low 1985; Zimmermann et al 1987; Devor et al 1992b) Endings of damaged nerve fibres are likely to come into contact with inflammatory mediators, both at the injury site and during regeneration into injured and inflamed tissue. These substances (e.g. histamine, prostaglandins) are known to excite injured C-fibres selectively (Zimmermann et al 1987; Devor et al 1992b).

SYMPATHETIC-SENSORY COUPLING

A particularly significant mediator, and one not readily predictable a priori, is sympathetic efferent activity. In experimentally injured afferent A- and C-fibres ongoing discharge is often evoked or enhanced by systemic or close arterial injection of adrenaline or noradrenaline, and by electrical stimulation of postganglionic sympathetic efferents (Fig. 4.5). The use of receptor-selective pharmacological agents has shown that these responses are

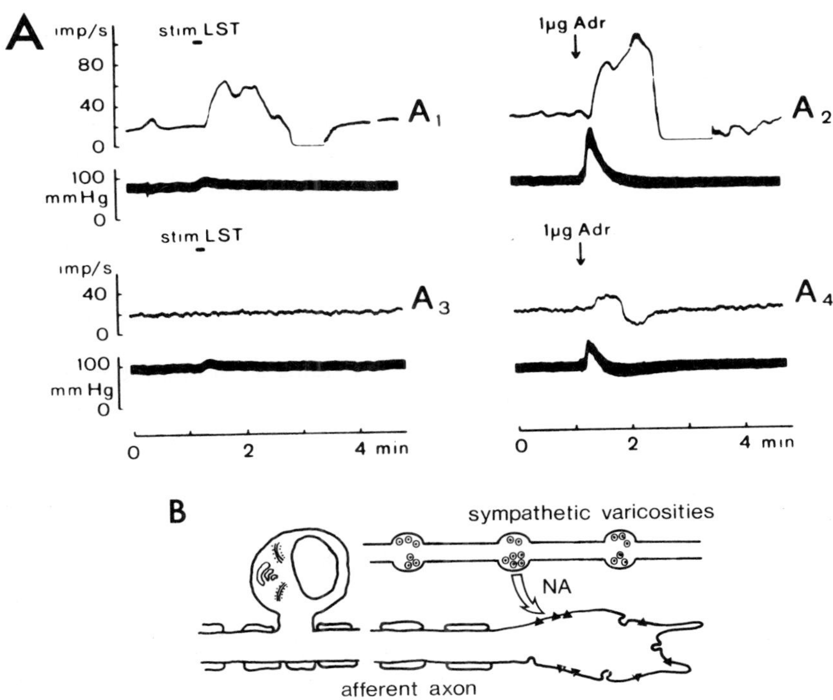

Fig. 4.5 Sympathetic-sensory coupling. The upper panel (**A**) shows excitation of a spontaneously active neuroma afferent following stimulation of sympathetic efferent fibres in the lumbar sympathetic trunk (LST, A_1), and following systemic injection of adrenaline (A_2). Both responses are attenuated by the α-adrenoreceptor antagonist phentolamine (10 μg i.v., A_3 and A_4). Simultaneous arterial pressure records are also shown. (From Devor & Janig 1981.) The lower panel **B** illustrates a model of the underlying mechanism: noradrenaline (NA) released from nearby sympathetic efferent fibres binds to α-adrenoreceptors (filled triangles) on the injured afferent evoking depolarization and ectopic firing.

mediated by α-adrenoreceptors (Wall & Gutnick 1974b; Korenman & Devor 1981; Devor & Janig 1981; Habler et al 1987; Sato & Perl 1991). This sympathetic-sensory coupling is not due to vasoconstriction-induced ischemia (Korenman & Devor 1981). Rather, it is thought to reflect a direct action of α-agonists on endbulb and/or sprout α-adrenoreceptors (Devor 1983b). The alternative possibility of indirect coupling involving intervening mediators (notably prostaglandins) has also been proposed (Levine et al 1986).

Afferent excitation by sympathetics forms the basis for a specific hypothesis for neuropathic pain in those conditions that are related to sympathetic outflow, such as reflex sympathetic dystrophy (RSD). According to this hypothesis (Fig. 4.5 bottom; Wall & Gutnick 1974a, 1974b; Devor 1983b), sympathetic activity releases noradrenaline from endings in the nerve trunk or target tissue. This activates injured sensory afferents, both touch fibres and nociceptors, that have developed ectopic α-adrenergic chemosensitivity. Circulating adrenaline may also contribute. The resulting depolarization may be sufficient to evoke repetitive firing and hence spontaneous pain. But even if not, it brings the afferent ending closer to its rhythmic firing threshold yielding hyperalgesia to mechanical and thermal stimuli. If central sensitization is present, adrenoreceptor-evoked firing limited to Aβ touch fibres may be sufficient to trigger pain (Campbell et al 1988).

The sympathetic-sensory coupling hypothesis provides a rationale for the effectiveness of chemical and surgical sympathectomy in RSD (e.g. Hannington-Kiff 1974). It also inspired the use of systemically injected phentolamine (an α-antagonist) as a diagnostic test for sympathetic dependent pain states (Arner 1991; Raja et al 1991).

ECTOPIC ELECTROGENESIS IN DORSAL ROOT GANGLIA

The development of ectopic firing capability in afferent fibres is a pathophysiological change. In contrast, sensory cell somata in DRGs and cranial nerve ganglia are intrinsically rhythmogenic. For example, even in intact animals, many DRG cells fire repetitively on direct depolarization, and are sensitive to mechanical probing (Fig. 4.6) and to various chemical mediators including circulating adrenergic agonists and sympathetic efferent activity (Howe et al 1977; Dunlap & Fischbach 1978; Wall & Devor 1983; Burchiel 1984b; Puil & Spigelman 1988; Devor et al 1991b). Mechanosensitivity, at least, is normally latent since DRGs are protected within a solid bony cavity. However, it is probably an important substrate for pain in cases of disc herniation and other injuries which apply traction or compressive forces to ganglia.

A small percentage of DRG neurons fire spontaneously, sending a low level A- and C-fibre barrage orthodromically into the CNS and antidromically into the periphery (Figs 4.6, 4.11; Wall & Devor 1983; Burchiel 1984b). The magnitude of this discharge is significantly augmented by chronic nerve injury, including nerve transection and nerve constriction (Kirk 1974, De Santis & Duckworth 1982; Wall & Devor 1983; Burchiel 1984; Kajander et al 1992). Long associated with painful disorders of the vertebral column, DRGs may prove to play a role in a much broader spectrum of neuropathic pain disorders.

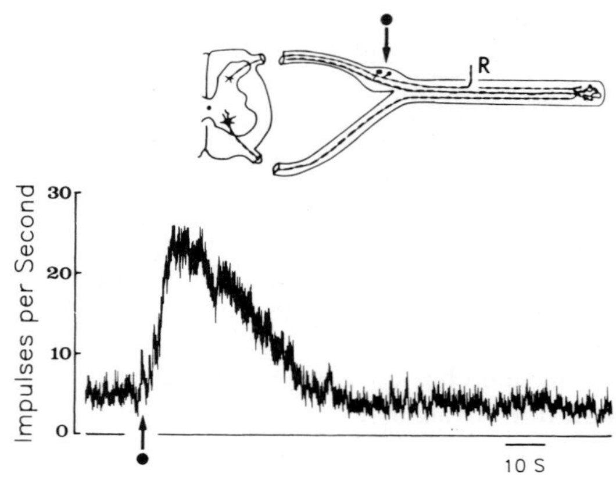

Fig. 4.6 Prolonged afterdischarge of an afferent axon following momentary (0.5 s) indentation of the DRG using a 150 mg von Frey hair (arrow). The sciatic nerve had been cut 11 days previously.

The reasons for rhythmogenesis in DRGs deserve some comment. Protected from stimulation and containing virtually no synapses, the DRG is usually assumed to be a nutritive depot with no involvement in signal processing (Lieberman 1976). Why, then, did DRG neurons evolve repetitive firing capability in the first place? There are two likely explanations. First, the centrifugal and/or centripedal impulse activity generated in the DRG may serve some hitherto unsuspected function, such as providing an afferent 'background', the sensory equivalent of sympathetic tone. Second, DRG excitability may have no adaptive purpose, and merely be an unavoidable 'flaw' in the design of sensory neurons. Consider an action potential propagating centrally along a sensory axon and approaching the T-junction in the DRG. Part of the longitudinal current needed to trigger the downstream axon is necessarily shunted into the T-stem branch and attached cell soma. Such shunting threatens conduction failure (Ito & Takahashi 1960; Parnas & Segev 1979). One way to overcome the problem is to counterbalance the shunt by providing extra inward Na^+ current at the DRG cell's initial segment (Devor & Obermeyer 1984; Matsumoto & Rosenbluth 1985). However, the extra Na^+-channels needed for this tend to create an ectopic impulse *generating* capability (Matzner & Devor 1992). Thus, an unavoidable bit of biophysics may render sensory ganglion cells sadly susceptible to abnormal firing.

BEHAVIOURAL CORRELATES OF ECTOPIC NEURAL ACTIVITY IN ANIMALS

As expected, palpating neuromas in rats evokes struggling and distress vocalization. In addition, the ectopic discharge that arises spontaneously, and as a result of mechanical stimulation of the neuroma (and DRG ?) during movement, undoubtedly triggers dysaesthesias referred to the denervated limb. In 1979 Wall et al described a behavioural syndrome of compulsive scratching and biting of the denervated paw that they proposed reflects this unpleasant sensation (anaesthesia dolorosa). The syndrome was termed ‘autotomy’. The correlation of autotomy behaviour with the amount and timing of ectopic PNS activity, and its response to various drugs and manipulations effective in the treatment of neuropathic pain, generally supports the inference that autotomy models denervation pain (Wiesenfeld & Lindblom 1980; Levitt 1985, Coderre et al 1986; Blumenkopf & Lipman 1991; Seltzer et al 1991). Ultimately, however, it is impossible to know for certain what a rat is feeling, so caution is in place.

More recently, several groups have investigated various forms of *partial* denervation in which the animal develops a marked and long-lasting hyperalgesia to thermal and/or mechanical stimuli (Markus et al 1984; Bennett & Xie 1988; Seltzer et al 1990; Kim & Chung 1992). This hypersensitivity, together with associated postural and tissue changes, recalls certain clinical neuropathic conditions. Like complete nerve section, partial injury triggers pathophysiological changes in the CNS, and this has prompted the speculation that the resulting hyperalgesia is primarily of central origin. However, even when the precipitating injury involves only gentle nerve compression (Bennett & Xie 1988), massive in-continuity neuroma formation occurs along with substantial ectopic PNS discharge (Xie & Xiao 1990; Carlton et al, 1991; Basbaum et al 1991; Kajander et al 1992). The relative contribution of PNS versus CNS changes to pain in these models is not known yet, but several authors have proposed that the two are synergistic, with the peripheral ectopia:

1. Contributing direct sensory input
2. Maintaining CNS circuits in a sensitized state (Devor et al 1991a).

Together, the autotomy model and the partial nerve injury models are powerful new tools for the analysis of chronic pain mechanisms. An example of their promise is the new light shed recently on the issue of variability in neuropathic pain symptoms. Autotomy varies greatly from rat to rat even when each has undergone an identical nerve lesion. By selective breeding of individuals with high versus low autotomy scores, Devor & Raber (1990) developed genetically isolated lines of animals that consistently expressed very high (HA) or very low (LA) levels of autotomy (Fig. 4.7). This proves that the trait is heritable. Moreover, subsequent hybridization and backcross experiments indicated that autotomy is transmitted by a single autosomal recessive gene.

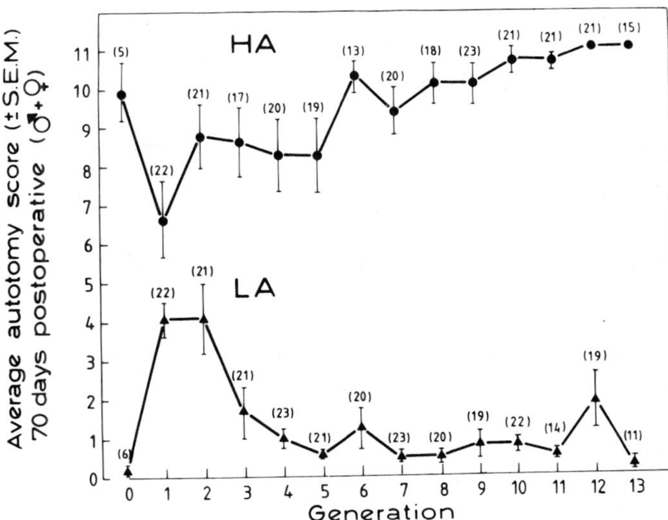

Fig. 4.7 Genetic selection of rats for high (HA) versus low (LA) levels of autotomy. Number in parentheses is number of animals tested. (From Devor & Raber 1990.)

AMPLIFICATION MECHANISMS ASSOCIATED WITH ECTOPIC RHYTHMIC FIRING CAPABILITY

THE SIGNIFICANCE OF ‘THRESHOLD FOR RHYTHMIC FIRING’

As noted above, neurons capable of discharging repetitively have marked *threshold* properties. Below their ‘rhythmic firing threshold’ they are silent, but as threshold is reached firing begins at a substantial ‘minimum rhythmic firing frequency’ (Fig. 4.1). Threshold provides amplification for two reasons. First, for pacemaker sites resting just below threshold, weak depolarizing influences (chemical, physical or metabolic) can trigger a disproportionate jump in firing frequency. Identical stimuli have a much smaller effect on firing when the cell is operating elsewhere within its normal encoding region (Fig. 4.1). Second, not only do such stimuli drive the cell, but they bring it into a domain of autonomous firing where activity may persist even after the stimulus is withdrawn (afterdischarge). The converse, of course, holds for suppressive influences, opening a window for therapeutic intervention (see below).

AFTERDISCHARGE, SILENT PERIODS AND REFRACTORINESS

Afterdischarge amplification is illustrated in Figure 4.8. The sensory neuron in Figure 4.8B did not fire spontaneously. However, when probed mechanically, or when stimulated with single electrical pulses, it produced 2–10 impulses in addition to the single response expected. The neuron illustrated in Figure 4.8C responded to single stimulus pulses with an afterdischarge lasting about 20 s and including about 500 extra spikes. In other cases much longer responses have been observed. Afterdischarge at ectopic pacemaker sites bears a striking resemblance to paroxysmal triggering and hyperpathic aftersensations seen in certain neuralgias (Noordenbos 1959).

After delivering a prolonged high frequency burst, many ectopic pacemaker sites fall silent, with baseline firing (if any) returning only gradually (Fig. 4.5). The reasons for this behaviour have not been determined directly, although there are several obvious possibilities. Silent periods can usually be evoked artificially by stimulating the active nerve fibre at high frequency (Fig. 4.8D). This implies that the silencing mechanism is intrinsic to the neuron itself, and is use- (i.e. activity-) dependent. Intrinsic, use-dependent suppression is well known in mammalian neurons (Hille 1992). One common mechanism involves Na^+ pumping. During high frequency firing Na^+ ions enter the cell. This activates the Na^+ pump (Na^+–K^+ATPase) which transiently hyperpolarizes the neuron, suppressing firing. A second example involves a specific type of delayed K^+ channel. During activity Ca^{++} ions enter the neuron. This activates Ca^{++} dependent K^+–channels and as a result the cell is hyperpolarized and suppressed. Both Na^+–K^+ATPase and Ca^{++} dependent K^+–channels are known to exist in peripheral sensory neurons. The silencing of ectopia following prolonged high frequency firing is a potential mechanism of TENS analgesia independent of spinal gating or the release of endogenous opioids.

When they fall silent after high frequency bursts, ectopic pacemaker sites typically become refractory to further stimulation. For example, when the neuron in Figure 4.8C was rested, single stimulus pulses always evoked an afterdischarge burst. In the wake of a burst, however, rhythmogenesis was suppressed. By delivering test pulses once every 10 s we showed that excitability took about 60 s to recover (Fig. 4.8C). This type of behaviour could account for the brevity of paroxysmal pain bursts in trigeminal neuralgia, for example, and for post-attack refractoriness (Kugelberg & Lindblom 1959).

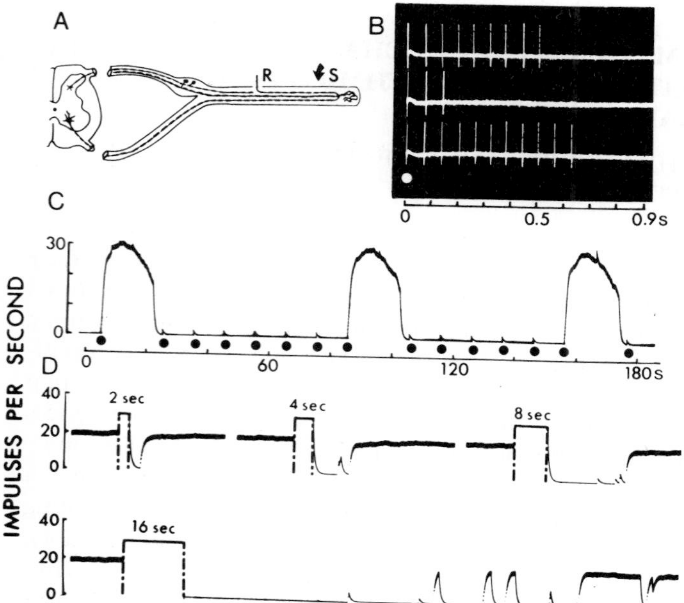

Fig. 4.8 Afterdischarge and silent periods in injured sciatic nerve afferents. **A** shows the experimental setup. **B** Single electrical stimulus pulses (S, 1 per sec) evoked a rhythmic afterdischarge of 2–10 spikes whenever stimulus intensity was above threshold for the axon (see Lisney & Devor 1987). **C** A second fibre, when rested, produced an afterdischarge of about 500 spikes in response to a single stimulus pulse. However, for nearly a minute following each such burst the afterdischarge mechanism was refractory, and single stimuli (black dots) evoked only single spikes. Brief mechanical stimuli triggered similar bursts which were also followed by periods of refractoriness. **D** This neuroma fibre fired spontaneously at about 20 impulses per second. High frequency stimulation (100 Hz) silenced it for periods which increased with increasing stimulus duration.

AMPLIFICATION BY 'EXTRA SPIKES'

Calvin et al (1977) proposed an additional mode of afterdischarge. They pointed out that if the duration of a propagating action potential were to increase, it might outlast the absolute refractory period of the axon, re-excite the membrane it had just passed over, and thus generate an 'extra spike'. Knowing that demyelination has just such an impulse broadening effect, the authors sought and found 'extra spike' production in experimentally demyelinated axons. Production of the occasional 'extra spike' does not, in itself, yield important amplification. However, if there were multiple sites of demyelination along a single axon, a brief stimulus might trigger reverberating cascades of 'extra spikes'. Calvin et al (1977) proposed this as a mechanism of pain in trigeminal neuralgia.

A related, and perhaps more realistic, scenario is based on the intrinsic rhythmogenicity associated with the 'depolarizing afterpotential (DAP)'. In some PNS axons each impulse is followed by a small membrane depolarisation (Raymond 1979; Barrett & Barrett 1982). This does not normally reach threshold. However, if the axon were injured and hyperexcitable, DAPs could transform individual spikes into doublets, triplets, or longer bursts.

CROSS-EXCITATION IN THE PNS

In healthy nerves individual afferents conduct impulses essentially independent of one another. For this reason when sensation is observed to spread beyond the site stimulated, and when pain is evoked by activation of low threshold Aβ afferents, the cause is usually ascribed to a

CNS abnormality. This conclusion ignores several different forms of cross-excitation now known to occur in the PNS.

ELECTRICAL (EPHAPTIC) CROSSTALK

The most widely known, if not necessarily the most important, form of PNS cross-excitation is ephaptic crosstalk. In the mid-1940s Granit & Skoglund (1945) discovered that acute transection short-circuits the insulation between neighbouring axons in a nerve permitting current from the cut end of one fibre to directly excite neighbours. This acute ephaptic coupling decays and vanishes within minutes of injury and is therefore unlikely to be of much functional significance. However, it has recently been found that several weeks later ephapsis develops again, now in an enduring form (Selzer & Devor 1979; Blumberg & Janig 1982; Lisney & Pover 1983; Meyer et al 1985). Ephaptic crosstalk in a neuroma is illustrated in Figure 4.9. Similar behaviour has been documented in regenerating nerve far distal to the site of injury (Seltzer & Devor 1979, 1980), and in patches of demyelination (Rasminsky 1980). In each case it is thought to result from close apposition between adjacent axons in the absence of the normal glial insulation (Fig. 4.10; Rasminsky 1980; Devor & Bernstein 1982; Bernstein & Pagnanelli 1982). Since coupled fibres are frequently of different types, this is a mechanism whereby nociceptors might be activated by low-threshold afferents or even efferents.

Electrical coupling may also occur in DRGs. Mayer and collaborators (1986) showed that infection by certain strains of herpes simplex virus can cause DRG cells to become electrically linked in a syncytium. Such coupling would tend to amplify both ectopically and naturally generated impulse activity (see below). Pathophysiologic behaviour of this sort could underlie sensory abnormalities in conditions such as postherpetic neuralgia.

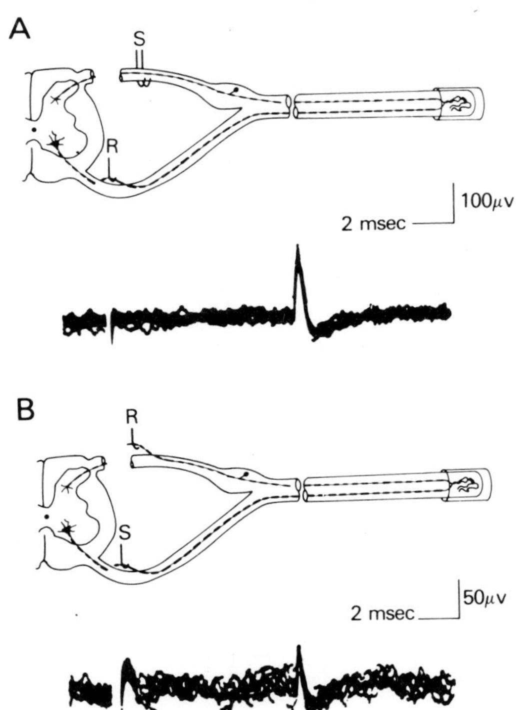

Fig. 4.9 Bidirectional ephaptic coupling between a pair of fibres ending in an experimental neuroma. **A** First a fibre was found in the L5 ventral root that responded (R) at fixed latency to electrical stimulation (S) of the ipsilateral dorsal roots. **B** Then, stimuli were applied to the ventral root filament containing the responding fibre. One fibre, in the L4 dorsal root, was found that responded to this stimulation. Note that the response latency for conduction in the two directions is identical. (Modified from Seltzer & Devor 1979.)

CROSSED AFTERDISCHARGE AT SITES OF NERVE INJURY

The signature of ephaptic crosstalk is high safety-factor, bidirectional coupling where a single impulse in an active fibre evokes a single impulse in its neighbour. Lisney & Devor (1987) first demonstrated a completely different form of cross-excitation called 'crossed afterdischarge'. Here, single impulses have no effect, but repetitive activity excites passive neighbours to repetitive *autonomous* firing. In contrast to ephapsis, crossed afterdischarge develops soon after nerve injury, is less dependent on close axonal apposition, and comes to involve a much larger proportion of afferents. The most likely mechanism is that repetitive activity releases gradually accumulating amounts of a chemical mediator within the nerve (see below). This depolarizes ectopic pacemaker sites evoking autorhythmic afterdischarge. Activity in Aβ fibres readily evokes crossed afterdischarge in Aδ fibres. However, for reasons that are still not clear, C-fibres are less affected, in the rat, at least (Amir & Devor 1992).

CROSSED AFTERDISCHARGE IN DRGs

As at sites of nerve injury, activation of sensory neurons within DRGs can asynchronously cross-excite their passive neighbours. Moreover, this can occur in animals in which the peripheral nerve is intact, or in which nerve injury is only partial (Devor & Wall 1990). A striking consequence is that afferent activity evoked by natural stroking of the skin can cross-activate DRG neurons that were not stimulated directly (Fig. 4.11), including ones serving tissue away from the area stroked. Activity spreads readily from Aβ to Aδ neurons, although once again, neurons with C-fibres appear to be relatively protected. DRG crossed afterdischarge could yield hyperpathic symptoms such as sensory spread, aftersensation and allodynia (Noordenbos 1959) even in the absence of CNS abnormalities.

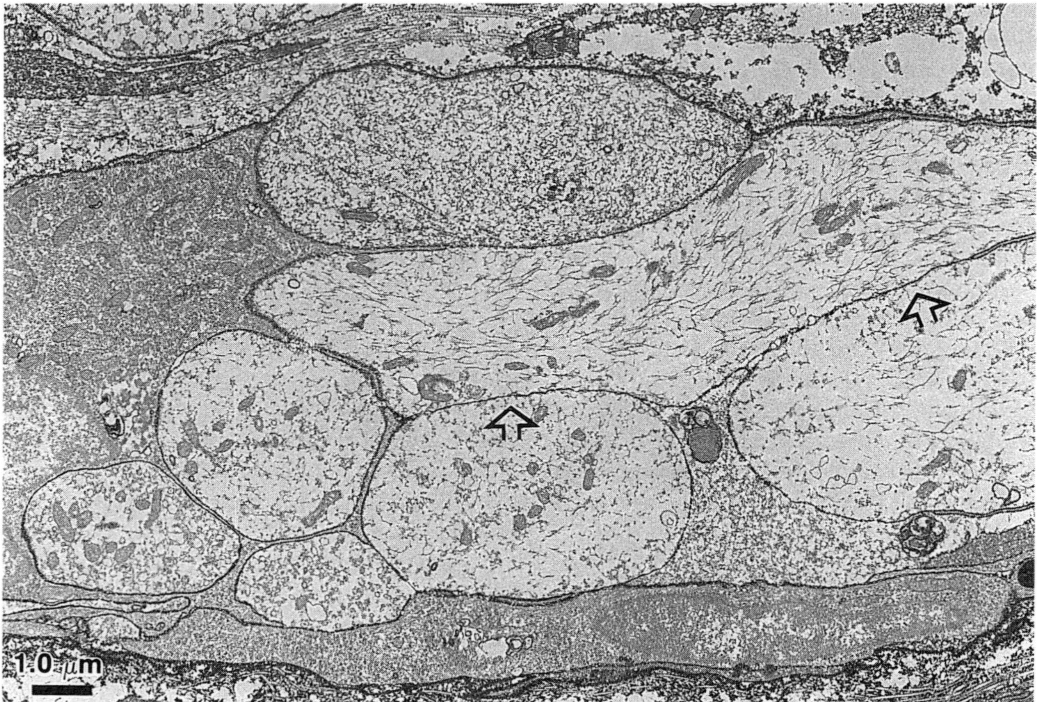

Fig. 4.10 Arrows show regions of close apposition between neighbouring demyelinated neuroma axons, in the absence of an intervening glial (Schwann cell) process. Other axons are compartmentalised by (dark) Schwann cell cytoplasm as in normal nerves (lower left). Rat sciatic nerve end neuroma, 25 days postinjury. The separation between cell profiles is emphasised by preincubation in ruthenium red. Scalebar: 1μm.

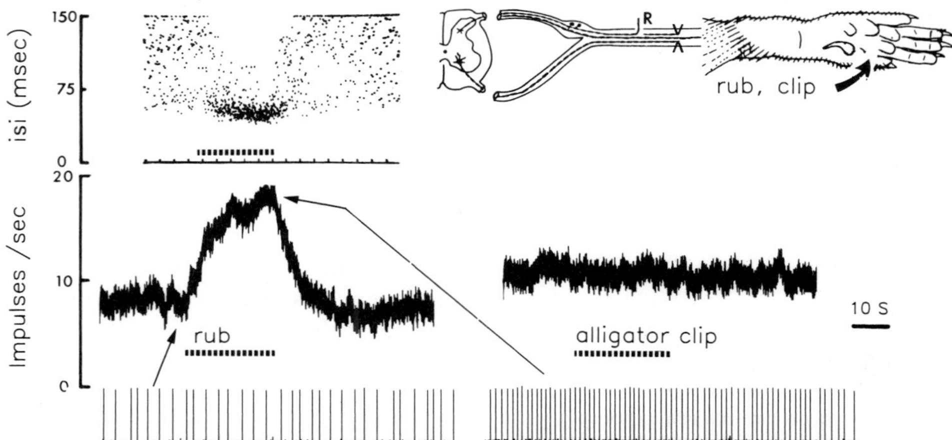

Fig. 4.11 DRG cross-excitation. The neuron illustrated had spontaneous discharge originating in the DRG. Gentle rubbing of the plantar foot activated neighbouring DRG neurons whose activity cross-excited the recorded afferent. Noxious mechanical, thermal and chemical stimuli were ineffective. The cross-excited neuron did not respond directly to cutaneous stimulation as its axon was cut at the recording site (R). (From Devor & Wall 1990.)

In vivo, crossed afterdischarge can be evoked in most DRG neurons that fire spontaneously (>80%) but only in a few previously silent ones (Devor & Wall 1990). However, intracellular recordings in vitro show that, in fact, subthreshold membrane depolarization occurs in most silent neurons as well (Utzschneider et al 1992). If an injury or disease process were to strongly reduce rhythmic firing threshold, DRG cross-excitation might come to involve a majority of DRG neurons with correspondingly drastic sensory consequences.

What causes the crossed afterdischarge? Utzschneider et al (1992) recently showed that stimuli that cross-excite DRG neurons release substantial quantities of K^+ within the interstitial space of the ganglion. This is expected to trigger Nernstian depolarization of DRG neurons, and hence cross-excitation. An alternative hypothesis is based on the fact that repetitive stimulation can release various neurotransmitter candidates within DRGs. Since DRG neurons are known to have corresponding receptors, cross-excitation could be mediated by neurotransmitters in a non-synaptic mode (references in Devor & Wall 1990). K^+ and neurotransmitter mediation are also candidate mechanisms for crossed afterdischarge in neuromas.

SYMPATHETIC-SENSORY COUPLING

The excitation of ectopic neural pacemaker sites by sympathetic efferent activity and by circulating adrenaline was discussed above in relation to sympathetic dependent neuropathic pain. This is, in effect, an example of PNS cross-excitation mediated by neurotransmitters (endogenous α-adrenoreceptor agonists). Non-adrenergic mediation has also been implicated, especially in the case of very long-standing injury (Janig 1990). In addition to neuroma endings, distally trapped regenerating sprouts and target tissue innervated by partly injured nerves, sympathetic-sensory coupling is also known to occur in DRGs (Devor et al 1991).

CROSSTALK AMONG AFFERENT TERMINALS IN THE SPINAL CORD

Afferent impulses conducted into the spinal terminals of sensory axons partially depolarise the terminals of their neighbours (PAD) (Lloyd 1952). A small minority are so intensely depolarised that they reach threshold and generate propagated action potentials (the dorsal root reflex, DRR). Calvin et al (1977) proposed that this form of cross-excitation among primary afferents might contribute to pain in trigeminal neuralgia. However, the observation that PAD and DRR are substantially *reduced* following peripheral nerve trauma mitigates against this hypothesis (Wall & Devor 1981; Horch & Lisney 1981b).

MECHANISM OF ABNORMAL RHYTHMOGENESIS IN INJURED NERVE

Unlike the sensory ending, the midnerve part of normal afferent axons is poorly adapted for impulse generation. External pressure does not trigger repetitive firing nor does direct depolarization through an intraaxonal micropipette. Even stretching axons, or cutting them across, usually produces at most a brief injury discharge (Gray & Richie 1954; Julian & Goldman 1962; Wall et al 1974; Ruiz et al 1981; Devor & Bernstein 1982). And yet the endbulbs and sprouts that form at midnerve are strongly rhythmogenic. Why?

MEMBRANE REMODELLING

As noted above, pacemaker capability depends on the distribution, and kinetics of transmembrane ion channels. An account of abnormal electrogenesis should therefore detail the mechanisms that control regional channel content, and describe changes that take place as a consequence of nerve injury. Although a comprehensive account of this sort is not yet available, recent studies on simple invertebrate and tissue culture systems, as well as on mammalian nerve fibres in situ, have shown that injury triggers extensive remodelling of the axon membrane. Three types of change are particularly significant:

1. Growth cones of developing and regenerating axons tend to have a relative overabundance of Ca^+-channels (Anglister et al 1982; Cohan et al 1985; MacVicar and Llinas 1985; Belardetti et al 1986).
2. Likewise, at the end of cut and growing axons there is an accumulation of voltage-sensitive $Na+$-channels (Fig. 4.12; Strichartz et al 1984; Lombet et al 1985; Belardetti et al 1986; Devor et al 1989; Gilly et al 1990; Fried et al 1991; Devor et al 1993). In vertebrates these are located on preterminal segments of demyelinated axolemma, on neuroma endbulbs and on sprouts (Fig. 4.12). Loss of myelin, even in the absence of axotomy, is also followed by the appearance of Na^+-channels in membrane regions normally nearly devoid of them (Bostock & Sears 1978; Rasminsky et al 1981; Foster et al 1980; Ritchie 1982; England et al 1991; Moll et al 1991; Black et al 1991).
3. There are hints that the sensitivity of ectopically located channels (channel opening kinetics) may be abnormal. Also, some nerve membranes are thought to contain latent channels that only become expressed under special circumstances such as injury or growth (e.g. Cohan et al 1985).

Ca^{++}-channels probably do not play an important role in ectopic electrogenesis as topical application of various Ca^{++}-channel blockers does not much affect neuroma discharge (Matzner 1990). Perhaps they are involved in

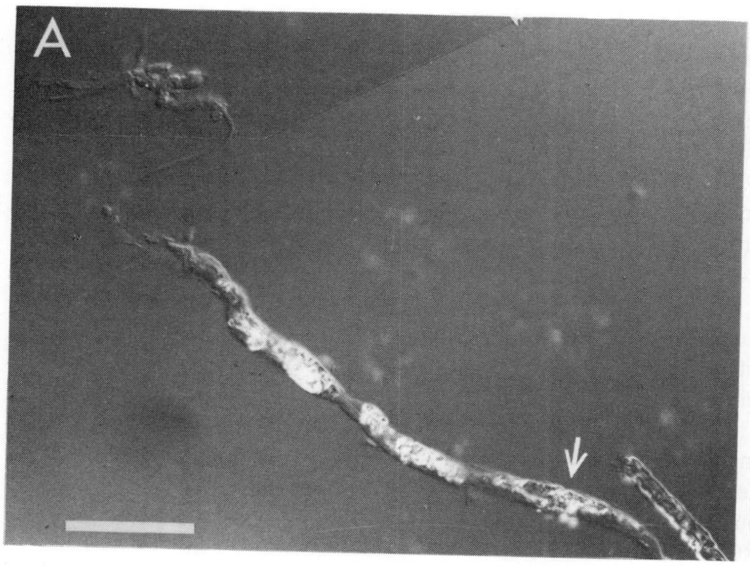

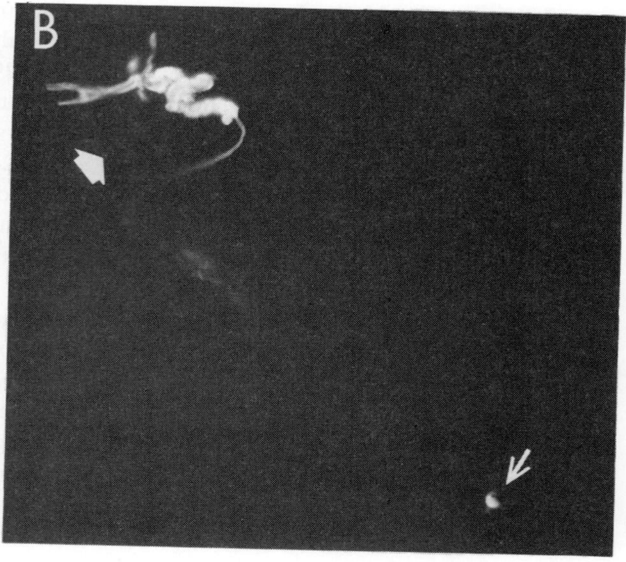

Fig. 4.12 **A** Nomarski differential interference contrast image of a chronically injured afferent axon from the lateral line nerve of *Apteronotus*. The arrow marks the location of a node of Ranvier. **B** Same axon immunolabelled with an antibody that recognizes voltage-sensitive Na^+-channels. Note the accumulation of Na^+-channels on the demyelinated preterminal axon, the endbulb and sprouts (thick arrow). Scalebar: 100μm. (From Devor et al 1989.)

axon growth (Kater & Mills 1991). The remodelling of Na^+ channels, on the other hand, appears to be of crucial importance. First, from computer simulations of the repetitive firing process we know that the addition of extra Na^+-channels, with no other change in active or passive membrane properties, is sufficient to render an axon hyperexcitable, and even to shift it from a state of silence to a state of spontaneous firing (Matzner & Devor 1992). Second, a range of pharmacological agents that block the opening of Na^+-channels (lidocaine, TTX, carbamazepine, phenytoin) suppress ectopic electrogenesis, while those that enhance Na^+-channel opening (veratridine) augment the discharge (Yaari & Devor 1985; Burchiel 1988; Chabal et al 1989a; Matzner 1990; Devor et al 1992a). The role of altered channel kinetics in ectopic neuropathic discharge has not yet been investigated.

Once an ectopic pacemaker capability is in place there are many possible sources of generator current to activate it. These include passive membrane leak (hence spontaneous discharge), and generator current passing through SA-channels, α-adrenoreceptor channels, ion channels activated by inflammatory mediators, etc.

A WORKING HYPOTHESIS

The new data on membrane remodelling, together with existing knowledge on normal cellular housekeeping processes, form the basis for the working hypothesis illustrated in Figure 4.13. Briefly, it is proposed that the proteins responsible for ectopic PNS hyperexcitability (Na^+-channels, SA-channels, etc.) are:

1. Synthesised on ribosomes in the DRG cell soma.
2. Inserted into the membrane of intracytoplasmic vesicles within the Golgi apparatus.
3. Conveyed down the axon by fast axoplasmic transport (Lombet et al 1985; Schmidt and Catterall 1986; Gilly et al 1990; Wonderlin and French 1991).
4. They are then inserted into the membrane of endbulbs, sprouts and demyelinated axolemma by exocytotic vesicle fusion (Heuser & Reese 1973; Villegas and Villegas 1981; Hammerschlag and Stone 1982; Fried et al 1991).
5. The turnover cycle is closed by internalization of excess membrane (endocytosis) and reuse or degradation of the membrane-bound proteins (Lentz 1983).

Membrane proteins typically undergo constant turnover; the half-life of Na^+-channels is only about 1–3 days (Schmidt & Catterall 1986; Brismar & Gilly 1987). This means that in the normal course of things the axon membrane is in a constant state of remodelling. The development of hyperexcitability does not require a de novo process; a quantitative shift in the normal equilibrium of channel insertion and reuptake is sufficient.

In injured nerve a combination of *permissive* and *promotional* factors underlie such equilibrium shifts. Injury-induced myelin stripping, and endbulb and sprout formation permit the insertion of Na^+-channels into axolemma; the presence of even a few layers of myelin is enough to prevent it (Waxman & Ritchie 1985; England et al 1991; Black et al 1991; Devor et al 1993). Axotomy also *promotes* membrane remodelling. In the normal economy of axons, large numbers of Na^+-channels are transported along the axon to subserve turnover downstream. This is particularly so for afferents, especially slowly adapting afferents,

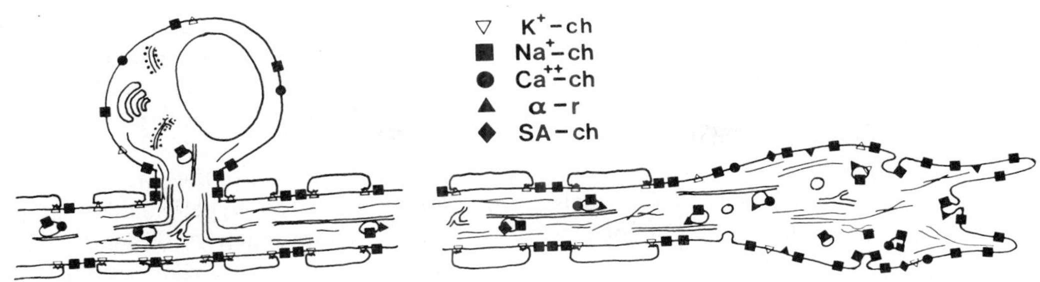

Fig. 4.13 Working hypothesis of the mechanism of hyperexcitability of injured axons. Various ion channels and receptors, notably Na^+ channels, are transported anterogradely along the axon and incorporated in excess into the axon membrane near the injury site. K^+-ch = potassium channels; Na^+-ch = sodium channels; Ca^{++}- ch = calcium channels; α-r = α-adrenoreceptors; SA-ch = stretch activated channels. (Modified from Devor 1983.)

that have the extra burden of maintaining a Na^+-channel-rich impulse encoder at their peripheral sensory ending (Katz 1950; Quick et al 1980; Seidel et al 1990; Matzner & Devor 1992). Following axotomy, many of these downstream targets no longer exist, and as a result in-transit channels are shunted into whatever membrane remains that is competent to receive them, notably endbulbs and sprouts.

Sites upstream of the injury might also receive some of the now excess channel protein. This might include the cell soma, a change that could account for the hyperexcitability of axotomized DRG cells (Wall & Devor 1983; Burchiel 1984; Titmus & Faber 1990; but see Gilly et al 1990). It has yet to be determined whether the expression of Na^+-channel genes in DRGs, or those for SA-channels, α-adrenoreceptors etc. is up- (or down-) regulated following axotomy. However, proliferating Schwann cells at the site of nerve injury and distally release large quantities of NGF (Heumann et al 1987) and this is known to promote the upregulation of Na^+-channel expression on outgrowing neurites (Pollock et al 1990).

NERVE PATHOPHYSIOLOGY AND CHRONIC PAIN IN MAN

Ectopic hyperexcitability in injured afferents has long been implicated in some clinical pain phenomena (e.g. the Tinel sign; Kugelberg 1946). However, the abundance of novel PNS pathophysiological processes recently discovered in animal preparations raises anew the question of their relevance to pain patients. The following section considers direct evidence of PNS ectopia in man, and indirect evidence based on treatment efficacy.

ECTOPIC ELECTROGENESIS AND PAIN IN MAN

The method of percutaneous microneurographic recording from single nerve fibres in conscious man (Vallbo et al 1979) permits a direct comparison of abnormal neural discharge and abnormal sensation. Practitioners have been justifiably reluctant to insert electrodes into problematic nerves in humans for essentially experimental purposes. If certain individuals are indeed predisposed to developing ectopic neural discharge, patients with neuropathic pain are at risk a priori. Nonetheless, a small number of such studies has appeared (Torebjork et al 1979; Ochoa & Torebjork 1980; Nystrom & Hagbarth 1981; Ochoa et al 1982; Nordin et al 1984; Cline et al 1989). In each, a striking correlation was found between spontaneous and evoked discharges, and neuropathic paraesthesias and pain.

For example, Nystrom & Hagbarth (1981) documented ongoing discharge in the peroneal nerve in a lower extremity amputee. The patient had ongoing phantom foot pain which was augmented by percussion of the neuroma. The same percussion elicited an intense burst of spike activity, mostly in slow-conducting axons. This was eliminated, along with the evoked pain, by local anaesthetic block of the neuroma. Interestingly, most of the ongoing discharge persisted. This is an indication that it arose upstream, perhaps in the DRG, and reached the recording electrode by propagating antidromically. In a related study, dysaesthesias referred to the foot were triggered by straight-leg lifting (Lasegue's sign) in a patient with radicular pain related to surgery for disk herniation. This manoeuvre evoked ectopic bursts in the sural nerve, the intensity of which waxed and waned in close correlation with the abnormal sensation (Nordin et al 1984). Once again, nerve blocks suggested that the ectopic source was in the injured root or DRG. Corresponding data were obtained in patients with positive sensory signs associated with nerve entrapment, and multiple sclerosis.

Another line of direct clinical evidence is sensory change evoked by the injection of test substances at foci of neuropathic pain. Animal studies, for example, predict that adrenaline, or K^+-channel blockers injected into a neuroma should augment ectopia and evoke pain, while the injection of Na^+-channel blockers (e.g. lidocaine) should suppress it. These predictions have recently been verified in man (Chabal 1989b, 1992b). Likewise, α-adrenoreceptor agonists evoke pain when injected into skin in RSD patients whose hyperalgesia was previously relieved by treatments, sympatholysis or topical clonidine, designed to reduce endogenous sympathetic drive (Wallin et al 1976; Torebjork 1989; Davis et al 1991). This implies that in RSD, afferents are abnormally adrenosensitive. The same conclusion is also supported by the observation that direct electrical stimulation of sympathetic efferent fibres in man evokes pain, but only in patients with RSD (Walker & Nulsen 1948; White & Sweet 1969).

AVENUES FOR THE MEDICAL CONTROL OF ABNORMAL NEURAL DISCHARGE

A corollary of the working hypothesis is that different chronic pain conditions are caused by misregulation of different membrane proteins. Thus, for example, upregulation of α-adrenoreceptors is expected to yield sympathetic dependent pain (even if there were no increase in sympathetic outflow), upregulation of SA-channels is expected to yield touch-evoked allodynia, hyperalgesia and mechanosensitive trigger points, and upregulation of receptors for inflammatory mediators is expected to yield inflammatory pain.

Such upregulation in itself, however, is not the whole story. Notice that each of these membrane proteins acts by contributing to the depolarizing generator potential. Thus, they could elicit or augment neural firing near a patch of membrane with repetitive firing capability, at a sensory ending in skin or in the DRG for example, but not elsewhere. In order to account for ectopic firing at other PNS locations, in the skin central to the sensory ending for example, or at midnerve, the upregulation of these proteins would have to be accompanied by an ectopic increase in membrane rhythmogenicity, e.g. brought about by Na^+-channel accumulation.

Indeed, increased rhythmogenesis in mid-nerve, in DRGs or at sensory endings is sufficient to yield hypersensitivity even if there were no change in the underlying generator potential. This is because the intrinsic threshold for rhythmic firing is reduced at locations of Na^+-channel accumulation (Matzner & Devor 1992). Na^+-channel accumulation *in and of itself* is expected to cause hyperalgesia and abnormal spontaneous firing. This would be augmented by concurrent accumulation of stimulus-specific receptors. Although each pathophysiologic pain condition may have its own molecular signature, they share the common denominator of ectopic hyperexcitability.

These insights into the peripheral neuropathic process provide a rationale for a number of effective but poorly understood therapeutic modalities, and a starting point for the rational design of new ones. For one, the model suggests that pain might ultimately be managed by controlling the expression of the relevant genes directly. Short of that, however, it indicates four ways in which painful discharge in the PNS could be attacked medically using currently available technology. These are:

1. *The stimulus underlying the generator potential.* The stimulus that drives hyperexcitable afferents could be attenuated. Approaches range from shielding mechanosensitive sites from percussion, surgical or chemical sympatholysis, reduction of noradrenaline release (e.g. using the α2-adreno-receptor agonist clonidine (Davis et al 1991) or treatment with nonsteroidal antiinflammatory drugs (NSAIDs) or corticosteroids to reduce local concentrations of inflammatory mediators.

2. *The receptor molecule underlying the generator potential.* Offending receptor molecules can be selectively blocked using appropriate pharmacological agents. For example, as noted above, the α-adrenoreceptor antagonist phentolamine suppresses sympathetic dependent pain (Arner 1991; Raja et al 1991). Likewise, gadolinium ions block SA-channels and reduce mechanoreceptor responsiveness (Swerup et al 1991). Gadolinium's effect on mechanosensation has not been tested yet.

3. *The pacemaker: normal and ectopic rhythmogenic capability.* Potentially the most powerful approach is to suppress the final common pathway of repetitive firing, i.e. normal or ectopic pacemaker capability. Since pacemaker capability is essential for repetitive neural firing no matter what the stimulus, pacemaker suppression is expected to be a general rather than a disease-specific analgesic strategy. Moreover, the effects of this approach should be additive with those that target the generator potential.

As noted, repetitive firing capability in afferents appears to depend on Na^+-channels. There are three classes of Na^+-channel blockers ('membrane stabilizers') in common clinical use (Catterall 1987). These are: local anaesthetics (e.g. lidocaine), some anticonvulsants (phenytoin, carbamazepine), and some antiarrhythmics (mexiletine). Each of these is known to suppress ectopic PNS discharge in experimental preparations (Wall & Gutnick 1984a, 1984b; Yaari & Devor 1985; Burchiel 1988; Chabal et al 1989a; Tanelian & MacIver 1991; Devor et al 1992a) and to provide relief in a broad range of clinical neuropathic conditions (Swerdlow 1984, 1988; Dejgard et al 1988; Chabal et al 1992a). Effective doses for suppression of ectopia and for achieving clinical analgesia are similar, and well below those required to blunt transduction in normal sensory endings, or to block nerve conduction, and cardiac function. These drugs are therefore capable of providing relatively selective reversal of neuropathic discharge. Furthermore, since the blood-nerve barrier collapses at injury sites associated with ectopia, and is non-existent in DRGs (Jacobs et al 1976; Sparrow & Kiernan 1981; Rechthand & Rapoport 1987), drug delivery is favourable.

Historically, phenytoin and later, carbamazepine, were adopted in the treatment of trigeminal neuralgia for their ability to suppress CNS seizures (Fromm et al 1984). Ever since, the efficacy of systemically injected Na^+-channel blockers has been presumed to be related to this central action. But is this correct? The CNS effect of these drugs derives from the same mechanism as their PNS effect, namely Na^+-channel blockade (Catterall 1987). Therefore, systemic efficacy in these cases does not indicate site of action. However, some anticonvulsants act synaptically and do not affect PNS ectopia (e.g. barbiturates). Significantly, these tend to be ineffective in trigeminal and other neuralgias (Fromm et al 1984). For several major anticonvulsants the mode of action and/or effects on PNS ectopia have not yet been determined (e.g. valproate). If indeed the primary analgesic action of the Na^+-channel blockers is in the PNS, it might be possible to obtain their benefits without their unwanted central side-effects (sedation, vertigo, etc.) by developing derivatives that do not cross the blood-brain barrier.

Corticosteroids also stabilize neuronal membranes. It is possible that this, rather than their antiinflammatory action, accounts for their ability to suppress ectopic discharge in experimental preparations (Devor et al 1985) and pain in humans when injected into trigger points (Travell & Simons 1984). Other approaches might also be pursued. For example, augmentation of K^+-channel action might be equivalent to Na^+-channel suppression. Appropriate compounds are available, although only for experimental use.

4. *The process of membrane remodelling*. In principle, the axoplasmic transport and insertion of channels and receptors could be interrupted by applying transport blockers (antimitotics such as colchicine, vinblastine and vincristine) to the nerve just central to the tender site. In experimental preparations this eliminates ectopic firing (Devor & Govrin-Lippmann 1983; see also Koschorke et al 1991). However, even though the local injection of these substances central to a nerve-end neuroma carries few if any risks, to the best of my knowledge this approach has never been tested in the clinical setting. Systemic and transcutaneous application of antimitotics has been claimed to produce analgesia (Knyihar-Csillik et al 1982; Meek et al 1985).

RELATION OF PNS PATHOPHYSIOLOGY TO CNS PATHOPHYSIOLOGY

Although this chapter has focused on pathophysiological processes in the periphery, the tight interrelationship between PNS changes and CNS changes makes it perilous to consider the one divorced from the other (Devor et al 1991a). In addition to evoking PNS pathophysiology, peripheral injury also triggers a broad range of physiological, biochemical and structural changes in the spinal cord and brainstem. For example, if nerve injury were to depress normal CNS inhibitory mechanisms, then the effect of ectopic PNS firing would be augmented. The basically serial relationship of PNS followed by CNS processing means that this ambiguity will always be present when pain is the endpoint being measured.

Not only are the various PNS and CNS changes set into motion by peripheral injury additive, but they may be mutually interdependent. Indeed, it has become clear in recent years that pathophysiological changes in the PNS can actually induce changes in the CNS. Such induction is mediated either by:

1. Trophic and metabolic influences
2. By afferent impulse traffic itself.

Injury to PNS axons, for example, triggers changes in gene expression in axotomized DRG neurons which may result in long-lasting increases or decreases in the delivery of putative neurotransmitter and trophic molecules to afferent terminals in the spinal cord (see Chs 3 and 5 in this volume). Such changes can alter the metabolism and function of second order, intrinsic spinal cord neurons (Dubner & Ruda 1992). An example of mediation by afferent impulses is the sensitisation of spinal wide-dynamic range neurons following a burst of nociceptor input (Cook et al 1987). This effect is relatively short-lasting (minutes to hours). However, in the presence of ongoing noxious input due to PNS pathophysiology, it might be maintained indefinitely. Under such circumstances, bringing the abnormal PNS firing under control would provide twin benefits: it would reduce noxious input and it would reverse central sensitization.

Finally, CNS changes triggered by PNS injury can act back out in the PNS. For example, Blumberg and Janig (1985) showed that spinal sympathetic reflexes can be altered, and even reversed in sign, by peripheral nerve injury. The altered CNS reflex patterns are expected to modify long-term sympathetic efferent activity impinging on peripheral tissues. This could play a role in sympathetically dependent pain states, and in the slow trophic tissue changes characteristic of some chronic pain syndromes (e.g. RSD).

SUMMARY

The last 25 years have witnessed an impressive accumulation of information about spinal and brainstem mechanisms of pain, and a general appreciation of their complexity and subtleness. By contrast, there remains little change in the common conception of peripheral nerves as elements that either propagate or, if injured, fail to propagate action potentials. This chapter has reviewed pathophysiological changes through which damaged nerves can come to contribute actively to chronic pain both by injecting abnormal discharge into the nervous system, and by amplifying and distorting naturally generated signals.

Data reviewed suggest that the crucial pathophysiological process triggered by nerve injury is an increase in neuronal excitability. This probably results from remodelling of membrane electrical properties. Normal nerves are capable of generating rhythmic discharge only at specialized terminal structures; damaged nerves acquire this capability at ectopic sites. Once ectopic pacemaker capability has been established, there may be spontaneous discharge, and abnormal sensitivity to a broad range of depolarising stimuli: mechanical, chemical, physical and metabolic. A working hypothesis was presented which attempts to explain the development of ectopic rhythmogenesis in terms of the fundamental processes of protein synthesis, axoplasmic transport and membrane turnover. Different chronic pain syndromes can be understood in terms of faulty regulation of different membrane proteins.

Associated with abnormal impulse generation in damaged nerves are several processes that can amplify normal or pathophysiological impulse discharge. There are also several mechanisms that can lead to cross-excitation among neighbouring sensory neurons within the injured nerve trunk and in sensory ganglia. Such cross-excitation can account for the spread of sensation in time (afterdischarge) and space, and for pain in response to normally innocuous stimuli, all without reference to any CNS pathology.

Injury-evoked changes in the PNS rarely occur without concurrent changes in the CNS. Indeed, the entire repertoire of peripheral pathophysiological processes can act to trigger and then to maintain sensitization of CNS circuits. Therefore, in the presence of injury or disease, it is essential to consider both PNS and CNS mechanisms, and the interplay between them. For the clinician, the frequent primacy of PNS processes, and the greater accessibility of peripheral nerves to therapeutic intervention, motivate increased awareness of PNS pathophysiology.

Acknowledgement

The support of the United States-Israel Binational Science Foundation, and the German-Israel Foundation for Research and Development (GIF) is gratefully acknowledged. I wish to thank W H Calvin and P D Wall for their contribution to many of the ideas developed in this chapter, and Z Seltzer for useful comments on the manuscript.

REFERENCES

Amir R, Devor M 1992 Axonal cross-excitation in nerve-end neuromas: comparison of A- and C-fibers. Journal of Neurophysiology 68: 1160–1166

Anglister L, Farber I C, Shahar A, Grinvald A 1982 Localization of voltage-sensitive calcium channels along developing neurites: their possible role in regulating neurite elongation. Developmental Biology 94: 351–365

Arner S 1991 Intravenous phentolamine test: diagnostic and prognostic use in reflex sympathetic dystrophy. Pain 46: 17–22

Ashur H, Vilner Y, Finsterbush A et al 1987 Extent of fiber regeneration after peripheral nerve repair: silicone splint vs. suture, gap repair vs. graft. Experimental Neurology 97: 365–374

Baker M, Bostock H 1992 Ectopic activity in demyelinated spinal root axons of the rat. Journal of Physiology (London) 451: 539–552

Barrett E F, Barrett J N 1982 Intracellular recording from vertebrate myelinated axons: mechanism of the depolarizing afterpotential. Journal of Physiology (London). 323: 117–144

Basbaum, A I, Gautron M, Jazat, F, Mayes M, Guilbaud G 1991 The spectrum of fiber loss in a model of neuropathic pain in the rat: an electron microscopic study. Pain 47: 359–367

Belardetti F, Schachner S, Siegelbaum S A 1986 Action potentials, macroscopic and single channel currents recorded from growth cones of *Aplysia* neurons in culture. Journal of Physiology (London) 374: 289–313

Bennett G, Xie Y-K 1988 A peripheral mononeuropathy in rat that produces disorders of pain sensation like those seen in man. Pain 33: 87–107

Bernstein J J, Pagnanelli D 1982 Long-term axonal apposition in rat sciatic nerve neuroma. Journal of Neurosurgery 57: 632–684

Black J A, Felts P, Smith K J, Kocsis J D, Waxman S G 1991 Distribution of sodium channels in chronically demyelinated spinal cord axons: immuno-ultrastructural localization and electrophysiological observations. Brain Research 544: 59–70

Blumberg H, Janig W 1982 Activation of fibers via experimentally produced stump neuromas of skin nerves—Ephaptic transmission or retrograde sprouting? Experimental Neurology 76: 468–482

Blumberg H, Janig W 1984 Discharge pattern of afferent fibers from a neuroma. Pain 20: 335–353

Blumberg H, Janig W 1985 Reflex patterns in postganglionic vasoconstrictor neurons following chronic nerve lesions. Journal of the Autonomic Nervous System 14: 157–180

Blumenkopf B, Lipman J J 1991 Studies in autotomy: its pathophysiology and usefulness as a model of chronic pain. Pain 45: 203–210

Bostock H, Sears T A 1978 The internodal axon membrane: electrical excitability and continuous conduction in segmental demyelination. Journal of Physiology (London) 280: 273–301

Brewart J, Gentle M J 1985 Neuroma formation and abnormal afferent discharges after partial beak amputation (beak trimming) in poultry. Experientia 41: 1132–1134

Brismar T, Gilly W F 1987 Synthesis of sodium channels in the cell bodies of squid giant axons. Proceedings of the National Academy of Sciences (USA) 84: 1459–1463

Burchiel K J 1980 Ectopic impulse generation in focally demyelinated trigeminal nerve. Experimental Neurology 69: 423–429

Burchiel K J 1984a Effects of electrical and mechanical stimulation on two foci of spontaneous activity which develop in primary afferent neurons after peripheral axotomy. Pain 18: 249–265

Burchiel K J 1984b Spontaneous impulse generation in normal and denervated dorsal root ganglia: sensitivity to alpha-adrenergic stimulation and hypoxia. Experimental Neurology 85: 257–272

Burchiel K J 1988 Carbamazepine inhibits spontaneous activity in experimental neuromas. Experimental Neurology 102: 249–253

Burchiel K J, Russell L C, Lee R P, Sima A A 1985 Spontaneous activity of primary afferent neurons in diabetic BB/Wistar rats: a possible mechanism of chronic diabetic neuropathic pain. Diabetes 34: 1210–1213

Cajal S, Ramon Y 1928 Degeneration and regeneration of the nervous system. (1968, trans R M May) Hafner, New York

Calvin W H 1975 Generation of spike trains in CNS neurons. Brain Research 84: 1–22

Calvin W 1980 Some design features of axons and how neuralgias may defeat them. In: Bonica J J, Albe-Fessard D, Liebeskind J C (eds)

Advances in pain research and therapy. Raven Press, New York, vol 3 p 297–309

Calvin W H, Howe J F, Loeser J D 1977 Ectopic repetitive firing in focally demyelinated axons and some implications for trigeminal neuralgia. In: Anderson D, Matthews B (eds) Pain in the trigeminal region. Elsevier/Amsterdam

Calvin W H, Devor M, Howe J 1982 Can neuralgias arise from minor demyelination? Spontaneous firing, mechanosensitivity and afterdischarge from conducting axons. Experimental Neurology 75: 755–763

Campbell J N, Raja S N, Meyer R A, MacKinnon S E 1988 Myelinated afferents signal the hyperalgesia associated with nerve injury. Pain 32: 89–94

Carlton S M, Dougherty P M, Pover C M, Coggeshall R E 1991 Neuroma formation and numbers of axons in a rat model of experimental peripheral neuropathy. Neuroscience Letters 131: 88–92

Catterall W A 1987 Common modes of drug action on Na^+ channels: local anaesthetics, antiarrhythmics and anticonvulsants. Trends in Pharmacological Sciences 8: 57–65

Chabal C, Russell L C, Burchiel K J 1989a The effect of intravenous lidocaine, tocainide, and mexiletine on spontaneously active fibers originating in rat sciatic neuromas. Pain 38: 333–338

Chabal C, Jacobson L, Burchiel K J 1989b Pain responses to perineuromal injection of normal saline, gallamine, and lidocaine in humans. Pain 36: 321–325

Chabal C, Jacobson L, Mariano A, Chaney E, Britell C W 1992a The use of oral mexiletine for the treatment of pain after peripheral nerve injury. Anesthesiology 76: 513–517

Chabal C, Jacobson L, Russell L C, Burchiel K J 1992b Pain responses to perineuromal injection of normal saline, epinephrine, and lidocaine in humans. Pain 49: 9–12

Cline M A, Ochoa J, Torebjörk H E 1989 Chronic hyperalgesia and skin warming caused by sensitized C nociceptors. Brain 112: 621–647

Coderre T J, Grimes R W, Melzack R 1986 Deafferentation and chronic pain in animals: an evaluation of evidence suggesting autotomy is related to pain. Pain 26: 61–84

Cohan C S, Haydon P G, Kater S B 1985 Single channel activity differs in growing and nongrowing growth cones of isolated identified neurons of Helisoma. Journal of Neuroscience Research 13: 285–300

Cook A J, Woolf C J, Wall P D, McMahon S B 1987 Dynamic receptive field plasticity in rat spinal cord dorsal horn following C-primary afferent input. Nature (London) 325: 151–153

Davis K D, Treede R D, Raja S N, Meyer R A, Campbell J N 1991 Topical application of clonidine relieves hyperalgesia in patients with sympathetically maintained pain. Pain 47: 309–317

Dejgard A, Peterson P, Kastrup J 1988 Mexiletine for treatment of chronic painful diabetic neuropathy. Lancet 29: 9–11

Delio D A, Reuhl K R, Lowndes H E 1992 Ectopic impulse generation in dorsal root ganglion neurons during methylmercury intoxication: an electrophysiological and morphological study. Neurotoxicology 13: 527–540

De Santis M, Duckworth J W 1982 Properties of primary afferent neurons from muscles which are spontaneously active after a lesion of their peripheral process. Experimental Neurology 75: 261–274

Devor M 1983a Potassium channels moderate ectopic excitability of nerve-end neuromas in rats. Neuroscience Letters 40: 181–186

Devor M 1983b Nerve pathophysiology and mechanisms of pain in causalgia. Journal of the Autonomic Nervous System 7: 371–384

Devor M, Bernstein J J 1982 Abnormal impulse generation in neuromas: electrophysiology and ultrastructure. In: Ochoa J, Culp W (eds) Abnormal nerves and muscles and impulse generators. Oxford University Press, Oxford, p 363–380

Devor M, Govrin-Lippmann R 1983 Axoplasmic transport block reduces ectopic impulse generation in injured peripheral nerves. Pain 16: 73–85

Devor M, Govrin-Lippmann R 1985 Spontaneous neural discharge in neuroma C-fibers in rat sciatic nerve. Neuroscience Letters suppl.22: S32

Devor M, Janig W 1981 Activation of myelinated afferents ending in a neuroma by stimulation of the sympathetic supply in the rat. Neuroscience Letters 24: 43–47

Devor M, Obermeyer M-L 1984 Membrane differentiation in rat dorsal root ganglia and possible consequences for back pain. Neuroscience Letters 51: 341–346

Devor M, Raber P 1990 Heritability of symptoms in an experimental model of neuropathic pain. Pain 42: 51–67

Devor M, Wall P D 1990 Cross excitation among dorsal root ganglion neurons in nerve injured and intact rats. Journal of Neurophysiology 64: 1733–1746

Devor M, Schonfeld D, Seltzer Z, Wall P D 1979 Two modes of cutaneous reinnervation following peripheral nerve injury. Journal of Comparative Neurology 185: 211–220

Devor M, Inbal R, Govrin-Lippmann R 1982 Genetic factors in the development of chronic pain. In: Lieblich, I (ed) Genetics of the brain. Elsevier, Amsterdam

Devor M, Govrin-Lippmann R, Raber P 1985 Corticosteroids suppress ectopic neuronal discharge originating in experimental neuromas. Pain 22: 127–137

Devor M, Keller C H, Deerinck T J, Ellisman M H 1989 Na^+ channel accumulation on axolemma of afferent endings in nerve end neuromas in *Apteronotus*. Neuroscience Letters 102: 149–154

Devor M, Keller C H, Ellisman M H 1990 Spontaneous discharge of afferents in a neuroma reflects original receptor tuning. Brain Research 517: 245–250

Devor M, Basbaum A I, Bennett G J et al 1991a Group Report: Mechanisms of neuropathic pain following peripheral injury. In: Basbaum A I, Besson J-M (eds) Towards a new pharmacotherapy of pain. Dahlem Konferenzen, Wiley, Chichester pp 417–440

Devor M, Wall P D, Janig W 1991b Cross-excitation of dorsal root ganglion neurons in nerve injured rats by neighboring afferents and by postganglionic sympathetic efferents. Society for Neuroscience Abstracts 17: 439

Devor M, Wall P D, Catalan N 1992a Systemic lidocaine silences ectopic neuroma and DRG discharge without blocking nerve conduction. Pain 48: 261–268

Devor M, White D M, Goetzl E J, Levine J D 1992b Eicosanoids, but not tachykinins, excite C-fibre endings in rat sciatic nerve-end neuromas. Neuroreport 3: 21–24

Devor M, Govrin-Lippmann R, Angelides K 1993 Na+ channel immunolocalization in peripheral mammalian axons and changes following nerve injury and neuroma formation. Journal of Neuroscience 13: 1976–1992

Dubner R, Ruda M A 1992 Activity-dependent neuronal plasticity following tissue injury and inflammation. Trends in Neuroscience 15: 96–103

Dunlap K, Fischbach G D 1978 Neurotransmitters decrease the calcium component of sensory neurone action potentials. Nature (London) 276: 837–839

Dyck P J, Lambert E H, O'Brien P C 1976 Pain in peripheral neuropathy related to rate and kind of fibre degeneration. Neurology 26: 466–471

Dyck P J, Thomas P K, Lambert E H, Bunge R (eds) 1984 Peripheral neuropathy, 2nd edn. W B Saunders, Philadelphia

England J D, Gamboni F, Levinson S R 1991 Increased numbers of sodium channels form along demyelinated axons. Brain Research 548: 334–337

Erxleben C 1989 Stretch-activated current through single ion channels in the abdominal stretch receptor organ of the crayfish. Journal of General Physiology 94: 1071–1083

Fawcett J W, Keynes R J 1990 Peripheral nerve regeneration. Annual Review of Neuroscience 13: 43–60

Foster R E, Whalen C C, Waxman S G 1980 Reorganisation of the axon membrane in demyelinated peripheral nerve fibers: morphological evidence. Science 210: 661–663

Fried K, Devor M 1988 End-structure of afferent axons injured in the peripheral and central nervous system. Somatosensory and Motor Research 6: 79–99

Fried K, Govrin-Lippmann R, Rosenthal F, Ellisman M, Devor M 1991 Ultrastructure of afferent axon endings in a neuroma. Journal of Neurocytology 20: 682–701

Fromm G H, Terrence C F, Maroon J C 1984 Trigeminal neuralgia: current concepts regarding etiology and pathogenesis. Archives of Neurology 41: 1204–1207

Gilly W F, Lucero M T, Horrigan F T 1990 Control of the spatial

distribution of sodium channels in giant fiber lobe neurons of the squid. Neuron 5: 663–674
Govrin-Lippmann R, Devor M 1978 Ongoing activity in severed nerves: source and variation with time. Brain Research 159: 406–410
Granit R, Skoglund C R 1945 Facilitation, inhibition and depression at the 'artificial synapse' formed by the cut end of a mammalian nerve. Journal of Physiology (London) 103: 435–448
Gray J A B, Ritchie J M 1954 Effects of stretch on single myelinated nerve fibers. Journal of Physiology (London) 124: 84–99
Habler H-J, Janig, W, Koltzenburg M 1987 Activation of unmyelinated afferents in chronically lesioned nerves by adrenaline and excitation of sympathetic efferents in the cat. Neuroscience Letters 82: 35–40
Hammerschlag R, Stone G C 1982 Membrane delivery by fast axonal transport. Trends in Neuroscience Jan: 12–15
Hannington-Kiff J G 1974 Pain relief. Lippincott, Philadelphia
Heumann R, Lindholm D, Bandtlow C et al 1987 Differential regulation of mRNA encoding nerve growth factor and its receptor in rat sciatic nerve during development, degeneration and regeneration: role of macrophages. Proceedings of the National Academy of Sciences (USA) 84: 8735–8739
Heuser J E, Reese T S 1973 Evidence for recycling of synaptic vesicle membrane during transmitter release at the frog neuromuscular junction. Journal of Cell Biology 57: 315–344
Hille B 1992 Ionic channels of excitable membranes, 2nd edn. Sinauer, Sunderland, Mass.
Horch K W, Lisney S J W 1981a On the number and nature of regenerating myelinated axons after lesions of cutaneous nerves in the cat. Journal of Physiology (London) 313: 287–299
Horch K W, Lisney S J W 1981b Changes in primary afferent depolarization of sensory neurones during peripheral nerve regeneration in the cat. Journal of Physiology (London) 313: 287–299
Howe J F, Loeser J D, Calvin W H 1977 Mechanosensitivity of dorsal root ganglia and chronically injured axons: a physiological basis for radicular pain of nerve root compression. Pain 3: 25–41
Ito M, Takahashi I 1960 Impulse conduction through spinal ganglion. In: Katsuki Y (ed) Electrical activity of single cells. Igakushoin, Tokyo
Jack J J B, Noble D, Tiens R W 1983 Electric current flow in excitable cells. Clarendon, Oxford
Jacobs J M, MacFarland R M, Cavanagh J B 1976 Vascular leakage in the dorsal root ganglia of the rat studied with horseradish peroxidase. Journal of the Neurological Sciences 29: 95–107
Janig W 1990 Activation of afferent fibers ending in an old neuroma by sympathetic stimulation in the rat. Neuroscience Letters 111: 309–314
Johnson R D, Munson J B 1991 Regenerating sprouts of axotomized cat muscle afferents express characteristic firing patterns to mechanical stimulation. Journal of Neurophysiology 66: 2155–2158
Julian F J, Goldman D E 1962 The effects of mechanical stimulation on some electrical properties of axons. Journal of General Physiology 46: 297–313
Kajander K C, Wakisaka S, Bennett G J 1992 Spontaneous discharge originates in the dorsal root ganglion at the onset of a painful peripheral neuropathy in the rat. Neuroscience Letters 138: 225–228
Kater S B, Mills L R 1991 Regulation of growth cone behaviour by calcium. Journal of Neuroscience 11: 891–899
Katz B 1950 Depolarization of sensory terminals and the initiation of impulses in the muscle spindle. Journal of Physiology (London) 111: 261–282
Kim S H, Chung J M 1992 An experimental model for peripheral neuropathy produced by segmental spinal nerve ligation in the rat. Pain 50: 355–363
Kirchoff C, Leah J D, Jung S, Reech P W 1992 Excitation of cutaneous sensory nerve endings in the rat by 4-aminopyridine and tetraethylammonium. Journal of Neurophysiology 67: 125–131
Kirk E J 1974 Impulses in dorsal spinal nerve rootlets in cats and rabbits arising from dorsal root ganglia isolated from the periphery. Journal of Comparative Neurology 2: 165–176
Knyihar-Csillik E, Szucs A, Csillik B 1982 Ionophoretically applied microtubule inhibitors induce transganglionic degenerative atrophy of primary central nociceptive terminals and abolish chronic autochthonous pain. Acta Neurologica Scandinavica 66: 401–412
Korenman E M D, Devor M 1981 Ectopic adrenergic sensitivity in damaged peripheral nerve axons in the rat. Experimental Neurology 72: 63–81
Koschorke G M, Meyer R A, Tillman D B, Campbell J N 1991 Ectopic excitability of injured nerves in monkey: entrained responses to vibratory stimuli. Journal of Neurophysiology 65: 693–701
Kugelberg E 1946 'Injury activity' and 'trigger zones' in human nerves. Brain 69: 310–324
Kugelberg E, Lindblom U 1959 The mechanism of the pain in trigeminal neuralgia. Journal of Neurology, Neurosurgery and Psychiatry 22: 36–43
Lentz T L 1983 Cellular membrane reutilization and synaptic vesicle recycling. Trends in Neuroscience Feb: 47–53
Levine J D, Taiwo Y O, Collins S D, Tam J K 1986 Noradrenalin hyperalgesia is mediated through interaction with sympathetic postganglionic neurone terminals rather than activation of primary afferent nociceptors. Nature (London) 323: 158–169
Levitt M 1985 Dysesthesias and self-mutilation in humans and subhumans: a review of clinical evidence and experimental studies. Brain Research Reviews 10: 247–290
Lewis T 1942 Pain. MacMillan, New York
Lieberman A R 1976 Sensory ganglia. In: Landon D N (ed) The peripheral nerve. Chapman & Hall, London, p 188–278
Lisney S J W, Devor M 1987 Afterdischarge and interactions among fibers in damaged peripheral nerve in the rat. Brain Research 415: 122–136
Lisney S J W, Pover C M 1983 Coupling between fibers involved in sensory nerve neuromata in cats. Journal of the Neurological Sciences 59: 255–264
Lloyd D P C 1952 Electrotonus in dorsal roots. Cold Spring Harbor Symposia on Quantitative Biology 17: 203–219
Loewenstein W R 1971 Mechano-electric transduction in Pacinian corpuscle. Initiation of sensory impulses in mechanoreceptors. In: Iggo A (ed) Handbook of sensory physiology, vol I. Springer, New York, p 267–290
Lombet A, Laduron P, Mourre C, Jacomet Y, Lazdunski M 1985 Axonal transport of the voltage-dependent Na^+ channel protein identified by its tetrodotoxin binding site in rat sciatic nerves. Brain Research 345: 153–158
Low P A 1985 Endoneurial potassium is increased and enhances spontaneous activity in regenerating mammalian nerve fibers – implications for neuropathic positive symptoms. Muscle and Nerve 8: 27–33
Markus H, Pomerantz B, Krushelnychy D 1984 Spread of saphenous somatotopic projection map in spinal cord and hypersensitivity of the foot after chronic sciatic denervation in adult rat. Brain Research 296: 27–39
Matsumoto E, Rosenbluth J 1985 Plasma membrane structure at the axon hillock, initial segment and cell body of frog dorsal root ganglion cells. Journal of Neurocytology 14: 731–747
Matzner O 1990 Ionic mechanisms of spontaneous impulse discharge in nerve end neuromas. PhD thesis, Hebrew University of Jerusalem
Matzner O, Devor M 1987 Contrasting thermal sensitivity of spontaneously active A- and C-fibers in experimental nerve-end neuromas. Pain 30: 373–384
Matzner O, Devor M 1992 Na^+ conductance and the threshold for repetitive neuronal firing. Brain Research 597: 92–98
Mayer M L, James M H, Russell R J, Kelly J S, Pasternak C A 1986 Changes in excitability induced by herpes simplex viruses in rat dorsal root ganglion neurons. Journal of Neuroscience 6: 391–402
Meek J B, Giudice V W, McFadden J W, Key J D, Enrick N L 1985 Colchicine highly effective in disc disorders. Journal of Neurological and Orthopedic Medicine and Surgery 6: 211–218
Melzack R, Wall P D 1965 Pain mechanisms: a new theory. Science 150: 971–978
Meyer R A, Raja S N, Campbell J N, Mackinnon S E, Dellon A L 1985 Neural activity originating from a neuroma in the baboon. Brain Research 325: 255–260
Moll C, Mourre C, Lazdunski M, Ulrich J 1991 Increase of sodium channels in demyelinated lesions of multiple sclerosis. Brain Research 556: 311–316
Morris J H, Hudson A R, Weddell G A 1972 A study of degeneration and regeneration in the divided rat sciatic nerve based on electron

microscopy. I, II, III, IV. Zeitschrift fur Zellforschung und Microskopische Anatomie 124: 76–203

Noordenbos W 1959 Pain. Elsevier, Amsterdam

Nordin M, Nystrom B, Wallin U, Hagbarth K-E 1984 Ectopic sensory discharges and paresthesiae in patients with disorders of peripheral nerves, dorsal roots and dorsal columns. Pain 20: 231–245

Nystrom B, Hagbarth K E 1981 Microelectrode recordings from transected nerves in amputees with phantom limb pain. Neuroscience Letters 27: 211–216

Ochoa J, Torebjörk H E 1980 Paraesthesiae from ectopic impulse generation in human sensory nerves. Brain 103: 835–854

Ochoa J, Torebjörk H E, Culp W L, Schady W 1982 Abnormal spontaneous activity in single sensory nerve fibers in humans. Muscle and Nerve 5: 574–577

Papir-Kricheli D, Devor M 1988 Abnormal impulse discharge in primary afferent axons injured in the peripheral versus the central nervous system. Somatosensory and Motor Research 6: 63–77

Parnas I, Segev I 1979 A mathematical model for conduction of action potentials along bifurcating axons. Journal of Physiology (London) 295: 323–343

Pollock J D, Krempin M, Rudy B 1990 Differential effects of NGF, FGF, EGF, cCAMP and dexamethasone on neurite outgrowth and sodium channel expression in PC12 cells. Journal of Neuroscience 10: 2626–2637

Puil E, Spigelman I 1988 Electrophysiological responses of trigeminal root ganglion neurons in vitro. Neuroscience 24: 635–646

Quick W, Kennedy W R, Poppele R E 1980 Anatomical evidence for multiple sources of action potentials in the afferent fibers of muscle spindles. Neuroscience 5: 109–115

Raja S N, Treede R-D, Davis K D, Campbell J N 1991 Systemic alpha-adrenergic blockade with phentolamine: a diagnostic test for sympathetically maintained pain. Anesthesiology 74: 691–698

Rasminsky M 1978 Ectopic generation of impulses and cross-talk in spinal nerve roots of 'dystrophic' mice. Annals of Neurology 3: 351–357

Rasminsky M 1980 Ephaptic transmission between single nerve fibers in the spinal nerve roots of dystrophic mice. Journal of Physiology (London) 305: 151–169

Rasminsky, M 1981 Hyperexcitability of pathologically myelinated axons and positive symptoms in multiple sclerosis. In: Waxman S G, Ritchie J M (eds) Demyelinating diseases: basic and clinical electrophysiology. Raven Press, New York p 289–297

Raymond S A 1979 Effects of nerve impulses on threshold of frog sciatic nerve fibers. Journal of Physiology (London) 290: 273–303

Rechthand E, Rapoport S I 1987 Regulation of the microenvironment of peripheral nerve: role of the blood-nerve barrier. Progress in Neurobiology 28: 303–343

Ritchie J M 1982 Sodium and potassium channels in regenerating and developing mammalian myelinated nerves. Proceedings of the Royal Society of London (Series B) 215: 273–287

Ruiz J A, Kocsis J D, Preson R J 1981 Repetitive firing characteristics of mammalian myelinated axons: an intra-axonal analysis. Society for Neuroscience Abstracts 7: 904–35

Sachs F 1986 Biophysics of mechanoreception. Membrane Biochemistry 6: 173–192

Sato J, Perl E R 1991 Adrenergic excitation of cutaneous pain receptors induced by peripheral nerve injury. Science 251: 1608–1610

Scadding J W 1981 Development of ongoing activity, mechanosensitivity, and adrenalin sensitivity in severed peripheral nerve axons. Experimental Neurology 73: 345–364

Schmidt J W, Caterrall W A 1986 Biosynthesis and processing of the α subunit of the voltage-sensitive sodium channel in rat brain neurons. Cell 46: 437–445

Seidel W M, Popper A N, Chang J S 1990 Spatial and morphological differentiation of trigger zones in afferent fibers to the teleost utricle. Journal of Comparative Neurology 302: 629–642

Seltzer Z, Devor M 1979 Ephaptic transmission in chronically damaged peripheral nerves. Neurology 29: 1061–1064

Seltzer Z, Devor M 1980 Formation of a neuroma in-continuity by sensory fibers that fail to regenerate after sciatic nerve cut and suture. Society for Neuroscience Abstracts 6: 859

Seltzer Z, Dubner R, Shir Y 1990 A novel behavioral model of neuropathic pain disorders produced in rats by partial sciatic nerve injury. Pain 43: 205–218

Seltzer Z, Paran Y, Eisen A, Ginzburg R 1991 Neuropathic pain behavior in rats depends on the afferent input from nerve-end neuroma including histamine-sensitive C-fibers. Neuroscience Letters 128: 203–206

Smith K J, McDonald W I 1980 Spontaneous and mechanically evoked activity due to a central demyelinating lesion. Nature (London) 286: 154–156

Sparrow J R, Kiernan J A 1981 Endoneurial vascular permeability in degenerating peripheral nerves. Acta Neuropathologica (Berlin) 53: 181–188

Stein R B 1967 The frequency of nerve action potentials generated by applied currents. Proceedings of the Royal Society of London (Series B) 167: 64–86

Strichartz G R, Small R S, Pfenninger K H 1984. Components of the plasma membrane of growing axons III. Saxitoxin binding to sodium channels. Journal of Cell Biology 98: 1444–1452

Strichartz G, Rnado T, Wang G K 1987 An integrated view of the molecular toxinology of sodium channel gating in excitable cells. Annual Review of Neuroscience 10: 1502–1507

Swerdlow M 1984 Review: anticonvulsant drugs and chronic pain. Clinical Neuropharmacology 7: 51–82

Swerdlow M 1988 Review: The use of local anaesthetics for relief of chronic pain. The Pain Clinic 2: 3–6

Swerup C, Purali N, Rydqvist B 1991 Block of receptor response in the stretch receptor neuron of the crayfish by gadolinium. Acta Physiologica Scandinavica 143: 21–26

Tal M, Devor M 1992 Ectopic discharge in injured nerves: comparison of trigeminal and somatic afferents. Brain Research 579: 148–151

Tanelian D L, MacIver M B 1991 Analgesic concentrations of lidocaine suppress tonic A-delta and C-fiber discharges produced by acute injury. Anesthesia 74: 934–936

Titmus M J and Faber D S 1990 Axotomy-induced alterations in the electrophysiological characteristics of neurons. Progress in Neurobiology 35: 1–51

Torebjörk E 1989 Clinical and neurophysiological observations relating to pathophysiological mechanisms in reflex sympathetic dystrophy. In: Stanton-Hicks M, Janig W, Boas R A (eds) Reflex sympathetic dystrophy. Kluver, Boston, p 71–80

Torebjörk H E, Ochoa J L, McCann F V 1979 Paraesthesiae: abnormal impulse generation in sensory nerve fibers in man. Acta Physiologica Scandinavica 105: 518–520

Travell J G, Simons D G 1984 Myofacial pain and dysfunction: the trigger point manual. Williams & Wilkins, Baltimore

Utzschneider D, Kocsis J, Devor M 1992 Mutual excitation among dorsal root ganglion neurons in the rat. Neuroscience Letters 146: 53–56

Vallbo A B, Hagbarth K E, Torebjörk H E, Wallin B G 1979 Somatosensory, proprioceptive, and sympathetic activity in human peripheral nerves. Physiological Review 59: 919–957

Villegas R, Villegas G M 1981 Nerve sodium channel incorporation in vesicles. Annual Review of Biophysics and Bioengineering 10: 387–419

Walker A E, Nulsen F 1948 Electrical stimulation of the upper thoracic portion of the sympathetic chain in man. Archives of Neurology and Psychiatry (Chicago) 59: 559–560

Wall P D, Devor M 1981 The effect of peripheral nerve injury on dorsal root potentials and on transmission of afferent signals into the spinal cord. Brain Research 209: 95–111

Wall P D, Devor M 1983 Sensory afferent impulses originate from dorsal root ganglia as well as from the periphery in normal and nerve-injured rats. Pain 17: 321–339

Wall P D, T Gutnick M 1974a Properties of afferent nerve impulses originating from a neuroma. Nature (London) 248: 740–743

Wall P D Gutnick M 1974b Ongoing activity in peripheral nerves: the physiology and pharmacology of impulses originating from a neuroma. Experimental Neurology 43: 580–593

Wall P D, Waxman S, Basbaum A I 1974 Ongoing activity in peripheral nerve: injury discharge. Experimental Neurology 45: 576–589

Wall P D, Devor M, Inbal F R et al 1980 Autotomy following

peripheral nerve lesions: experimental anaesthesia dolorosa. Pain 7: 103–113

Wallin G, Torebjörk E, Hallin R 1976 Preliminary observations on the pathophysiology of hyperalgesia in the causalgic pain syndrome. In: Zotterman Y (ed) Sensory functions of the skin in primates. Pergamon, New York, p 489–502

Waxman S G, Foster R E 1980 Ionic channel distribution and heterogeneity of the axon membrane in myelinated fibers. Brain Research Review 2: 205–234

Waxman S G, Ritchie J M 1985 Organization of ion channels in the myelinated nerve fiber. Science 228: 1502–1507

Welk E, Leah J D, Zimmerman M 1990 Characteristics of A- and C-fibers ending in a sensory nerve neuroma in the rat. Journal of Neurophysiology 63: 759–766

White J C, Sweet W H 1969 Pain and the neurosurgeon. Thomas, Springfield, p 93

Wiesenfeld Z, Lindblom U 1980 Behavioural and electrophysiological effects of various types of peripheral nerve lesions in the rat: a comparison of possible models for chronic pain. Pain 8: 285–298

Wonderlin W F, French R J 1991 Ion channels in transit: voltage-gated channels in axoplasmic organelles of the squid *Loligo pealei.* Proceedings of the National Academy of Sciences (USA) 88: 4391–4395

Xie Y-K, Xiao W-H 1990 Electrophysiological evidence for hyperalgesia in the peripheral neuropathy. Science in China (B) 33: 663–667

Yaari Y, Devor M 1985 Phenytoin suppresses spontaneous ectopic discharge in rat sciatic nerve neuromas. Neuroscience Letters 58: 117–122

Zimmermann M, Koschorke G-M, Sanders K 1987 Response characteristics of fibers in regenerating and regenerated cutaneous nerves in cat and rat. In: Pubols S M, Sessle B J *(eds)* Effects of injury on trigeminal and spinal somatosensory systems. Liss, New York, p 93–106

5. The dorsal horn: state-dependent sensory processing and the generation of pain

Clifford J. Woolf

Our sensory experiences, including that of pain, are determined both by the capacity of our nervous systems to extract particular features from the stimuli that impinge upon our bodies, and by the active processing of the neural input. Feature extraction is initiated by the highly specialized transduction properties of primary sensory neurons; sensory processing is performed by neurons within the central nervous system (CNS), the first stage of which occurs for the somatosensory system in the dorsal horn of the spinal cord or its homologue in the medulla, the spinal nucleus of the trigeminal. The dorsal horn essentially consists of the central terminals of primary sensory neurons, intrinsic dorsal horn neurons and inputs from and outputs to the rest of the CNS arranged in a pattern of bewildering complexity (Tables 5.1–5.4). Although considerable effort has been devoted to the study of the structure and function of the dorsal horn, we still do not understand the actual principles of its organization in terms of what specific neural elements operate together to form functional processing units, transferring particular types of afferent input to particular output elements of the system. An enormous amount of information is available

Table 5.1 Organization of the dorsal horn: I. Inputs

Primary afferent	
Low threshold	
Cutaneous mechanoreceptor	
Stimulus:	skin deformation, indentation, vibration, movement of hairs
Signal:	displacement – slowly adapting velocity – rapidly adapting transients – vibration
$A\beta$	(except $A\delta$ down hair afferents)
Cutaneous thermoreceptor	
Cold:	$A\delta$
Warm:	C
Joint mechanoreceptor	
Movement of joint:	$A\beta$
Visceral mechanoreceptor	
Distension:	$A\delta$
High threshold	
Cutaneous nociceptors	
Mechanoreceptors:	$A\delta$
Thermoreceptors:	$A\delta$/C
Polymodal (incl. chemoreceptors):	$A\delta$/C
Silent:	C
Muscle nociceptors	
Mechanoreceptors:	$A\delta$/C
Chemoreceptors:	C
Joint nociceptors	
Mechanoreceptors:	$A\delta$/C
Silent:	
Visceral nociceptors	$A\delta$/C
Mechanical:	$A\delta$/C
Polymodal:	C
Descending	
Major	
Raphe spinal:	inhibitory
Reticulospinal:	inhibitory and excitatory
Corticospinal:	excitatory
Minor	
(Locus coeruleus/subcoeruleus, parabrachial nuclei, vestibular, hypothalamic, red nucleus, solitary nucleus, pretectal nuclei)	

(Derived from Willis & Coggeshall 1991.)

Table 5.2 Organization of the dorsal horn: II. Intrinsic neurons

- Projection neurons
  - Spinothalamic
  - Spinoreticular
  - Spinomesencephalic
  - Spinocervical
  - Postsynaptic dorsal column
- Propriospinal neurons
- Local interneurons

Table 5.3 Organization of the dorsal horn: III. Outputs

- To the brain
  - Thalamus
  - Reticular formation
  - Parabrachial nuclei/periaqueductal grey/tectal nuclei
  - Lateral cervical nucleus
  - Dorsal column nuclei
- To the ventral horn
- Local segmental – intralaminar
  - interlaminar
  - contralateral
- Intersegmental

Table 5.4 Central termination sites of primary afferent neurons

Low threshold mechanoreceptors	Termination site
Hair follicle afferent Aβ	$\mathrm{II_i}$, III, IV
Hair follicle afferent Aδ	$\mathrm{II_i}$, III
Rapidly adapting afferent Aβ	III, IV, V
Slowly adapting afferent Aβ	IV, V, VI
Pacinian corpuscle Aβ	III, IV, V, VI
High threshold nociceptors	
Cutaneous mechanoreceptor Aδ	I, $\mathrm{II_o}$, V
Deep mechanoreceptor Aδ	I, V
Cutaneous C nociceptor C	I, II
Visceral C nociceptor C	I, II, IV, V, X

(Derived from: Brown et al 1977, 1978; Light & Perl 1979; Brown et al 1980; Ralston et al 1984; Semba et al 1985; Sugiura et al 1986; Woolf 1987; Mense & Craig 1988; Hoheisel & Mense 1989; Sugiura et al 1989; Shortland et al 1989; Brown et al 1991).

on the morphology of primary afferent central terminals, dorsal horn neurons and descending systems, together with their chemical neuroanatomy, synaptic arrangements, transmitter systems, and functional properties. A review of this literature is beyond the scope of this chapter, which will be devoted instead to an analysis of the general roles of the dorsal horn in nociception. For further detailed information the reader is advised to refer to the excellent monograph of Willis & Coggeshall (1991) and the review by Besson & Chaouch (1987).

Key to understanding the role of the dorsal horn in pain mechanisms has been the appreciation that the sensory response generated by the somatosensory system to a defined input is not fixed or static. A stimulus that generates an innocuous sensation on one occasion may produce pain on another. Essentially what this means is that the somatosensory system operates in a number of different states or modes (Fig. 5.1). One state is that which is

DORSAL HORN STATES

MODE 1	Control State
MODE 2	Suppressed State
MODE 3	Sensitized State
MODE 4	Reorganized State

Fig. 5.1 The four modes of the dorsal horn.

present when non-injurious stimuli are applied to healthy tissue, the situation that holds under what we could call normal or control situations. Another state would be that which occurs when similar stimuli are applied to a site of previous tissue damage, and a third when peripheral stimuli are applied in the presence of damage to some component of the somatosensory system itself. Changes in the dorsal horn contribute to, or are responsible for, the changes in the state of the somatosensory system (Chs 10 and 11). These changes therefore represent an essential aspect of the operating performance of the system, particularly with regard to the generation of pain. It is no longer adequate to study the system in one state, say the control situation, and then attempt to use this information to fully explain the mechanisms that come into play in another state or mode, such as those which operate in a patient suffering from intractable pain following damage to a peripheral nerve.

A highly simplified analysis of the different states of the somatosensory system is presented in Figures 5.1–5.10. In the control, normal or physiological situation a low intensity stimulus of sufficient energy to only activate low-threshold primary afferent neurons will produce a sensation which is always interpreted as being innocuous (Fig. 5.2). Under these conditions a high-intensity

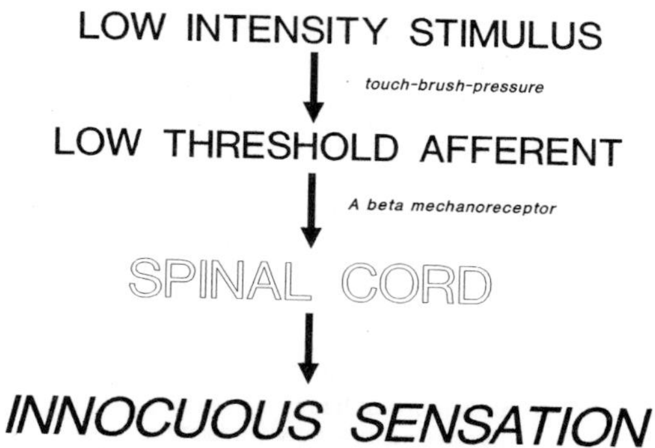

Fig. 5.2 Sensory processing of low-intensity stimuli in the control or physiological state of the dorsal horn, Mode 1.

stimulus sufficient to activate high-threshold primary afferent nociceptors produces pain provided that the rest of the CNS is in a pain permitting mode (Fig. 5.3). Until recently, the information we had on the functional organization of the dorsal horn had only been obtained from an analysis of the system in this physiological state, which I have called Mode 1 (Fig. 5.1).

Mode 2 represents that situation where transmission in

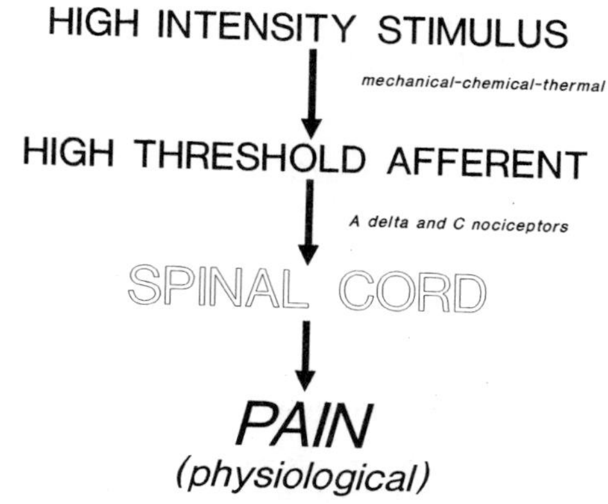

Fig. 5.3 Sensory processing of high-intensity stimuli in the control or physiological state of the dorsal horn, Mode 1.

the somatosensory system is suppressed as a result of the activation of segmental and descending inhibitory mechanisms operating on the spinal cord (Fig. 5.4). Under these conditions a high intensity stimulus, activating nociceptors, may fail to result in the sensation of pain. These

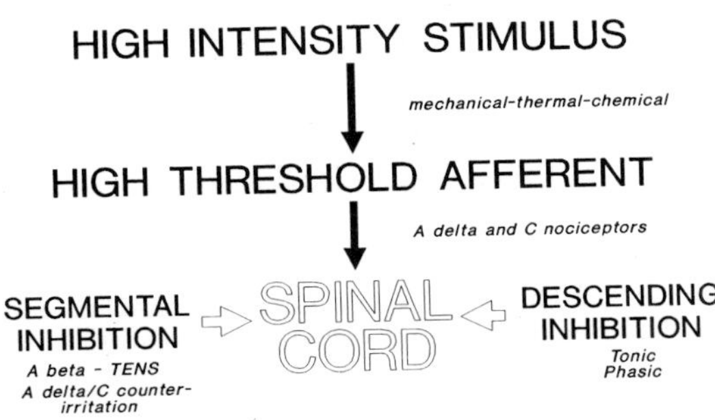

Fig. 5.4 Failure of high-intensity stimuli to produce pain in the suppressed state of the dorsal horn, Mode 2.

powerful inhibitory processes contribute to the analgesia produced by transcutaneous electrical nerve stimulation (TENS), counterirritation, including acupuncture, as well as that related to the analgesic actions of placebo, suggestion, hypnosis distraction and other high-order brain functions.

Mode 3 is that state of the dorsal horn where its excitability is increased, and its response to sensory inputs is augmented or facilitated, where it has become hypersensitive or sensitized. A low-intensity stimulus in this mode can, acting via low-threshold afferents, generate pain, the phenomenon of allodynia (Fig. 5.5). This needs to be

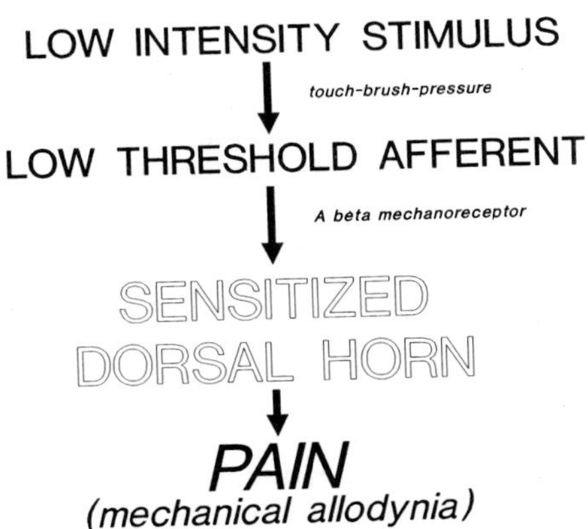

Fig. 5.5 Sensitization of the dorsal horn (Mode 3) results in low-threshold afferents gaining the capacity to evoke the sensation of pain, the phenomenon of mechanical allodynia.

differentiated from the situation which operates when the transduction properties of high-threshold afferents are changed so that their threshold falls (peripheral sensitization) (Fig. 5.6 and see Ch. 1). The sensitization of the dorsal horn can occur following peripheral tissue injury,

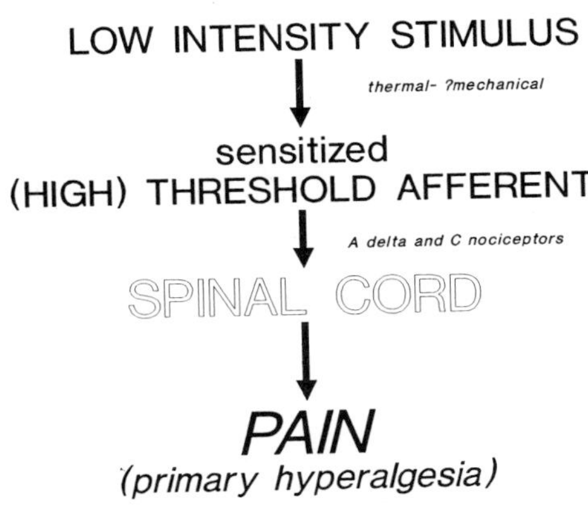

Fig. 5.6 Peripheral sensitization, manifesting as a reduction in the threshold of high-threshold nociceptors, results in low-intensity stimuli becoming capable of generating pain via activation of nociceptors.

peripheral inflammation and damage to the peripheral and central nervous systems. In addition to the reduction in the threshold of stimuli required to elicit pain in Mode 3, the response to suprathreshold high-intensity stimuli is exaggerated (Fig. 5.7). Mode 3 essentially represents an increase in the gain of the dorsal horn, in contrast to Mode 2, which

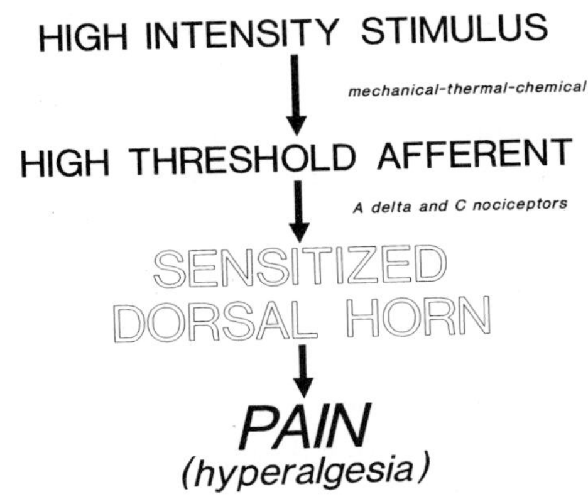

Fig. 5.7 Sensitization of the dorsal horn (Mode 3) results both in mechanical allodynia (Fig. 5.5) and an exaggeration in the response to activation of high-threshold afferents, the phenomenon of hyperalgesia.

reflects a decrease in gain (Fig. 5.8). Some of the mechanisms responsible for the change in the gain of the dorsal horn from Mode 1 to Mode 2 or from Mode 1 to Mode 3 are briefly reviewed later in the chapter (Figs 5.11 and 5.12).

The last mode of the dorsal horn, Mode 4, differs from the first three in that it represents a potentially irreversible, or at the least prolonged, reorganization of the synaptic circuitry of the system. The first three modes reflect a system operating in a range of states of excitability, from suppressed to hypersensitive, determining the sensation produced by defined stimuli. Mode 4, in contrast, is that state which occurs when there is degeneration of elements of the system, or the formation of novel inputs. Such changes have been documented after injury to the nervous

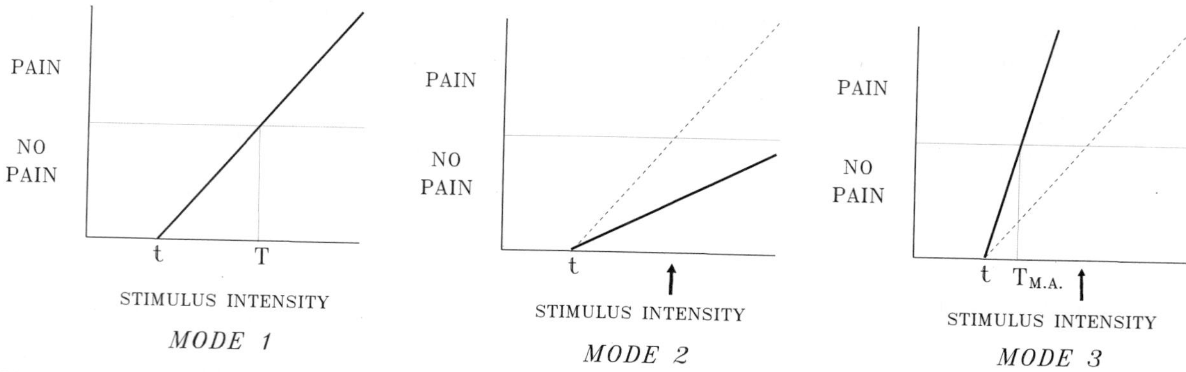

Fig. 5.8 Theoretical stimulus-response relationships in Modes 1, 2 and 3 of the dorsal horn. In Mode 1, increasing stimulus strength from a very low level results in the threshold for detection of the stimulus being reached (t). Further increases in stimulus intensity result in an increased innocuous sensation until the pain threshold is exceeded (T). Beyond this level, stimuli produce painful sensations. In Mode 2 the slope of the stimulus-response relationship is shifted to the right (solid line). Although the detection threshold remains unchanged, stimuli beyond where the pain threshold normally lies (arrow) continue to produce innocuous sensations. In Mode 3 the slope of the stimulus-response curve is shifted to the left. The threshold for pain (T_{MA}) is reached by an intensity of the stimulus well below than in the control situation (arrow). Because stimuli at this intensity activate low-threshold mechanoreceptors, the new pain threshold is actually the threshold for mechanical allodynia. Together these graphs illustrate how a change in the gain of sensory processing in the dorsal horn in its different modes can produce different sensations from identical stimuli in different situations.

system, both peripheral and central, leading to a range of sensory abnormalities including neuropathic pain.

Figure 5.9 presents a summary of the state-dependent processing of low- and high-intensity sensory stimuli according to the different modes of the dorsal horn. The normal clear distinction between a low-intensity stimulus-innocuous sensation and a high intensity stimulus-painful sensation is only present in Mode 1, the control state. In these circumstances the system operates to enable contact with a large range of external stimuli without initiating either withdrawal reflexes or the sensation of pain. However, if a stimulus of an intensity sufficient to threaten damage to the system is applied to a body part, this initiates a protective withdrawal response together with a feeling of discomfort or pain (Fig. 5.10). This system operates, therefore, as an early warning device protecting from or eliminating contact with potentially dangerous stimuli.

SENSORY PROCESSING - STATE-DEPENDENCY

MODE	INPUT	SENSATION
1	L.I.S. H.I.S.	Innocuous Pain
2	L.I.S. H.I.S.	Innocuous Innocuous
3	L.I.S. H.I.S.	Pain Hyperalgesia
4	L.I.S. H.I.S.	Pain Hyperalgesia

L.I.S = low intensity stimulus
H.I.S = high intensity stimulus

Fig. 5.9 A summary of state-dependence of sensory processing in the spinal cord illustrating the different sensory responses evoked by low or high intensity stimuli in the different modes (see Fig. 5.1) of the dorsal horn.

STATE-DEPENDENT PROCESSING IN THE DORSAL HORN – CLINICAL SYNDROMES

MODE	SYNDROME
1	Physiological Sensitivity
2	Hyposensitivity
3	Postinjury Hypersensitivity Inflammatory Pain Peripheral Neuropathic Pain
4	Peripheral Neuropathic Pain Central Neuropathic Pain

Fig. 5.10 A summary of the different clinical sensory disturbances that can manifest in the different modes or states of the dorsal horn.

The suppressed state in Mode 2 permits the individual to operate in the presence of nociceptor input without initiating withdrawal or escape responses or the sensation of pain. This can have a tremendous survival value enabling flight or fight reactions in the presence of substantial injury. The exploitation of the body's own inbuilt inhibitory mechanisms, either by ritualized treatment strategies such as acupuncture or by the controlled activation of inhibitory processes, e.g. TENS or dorsal column stimulation, is discussed in a number of chapters in this book.

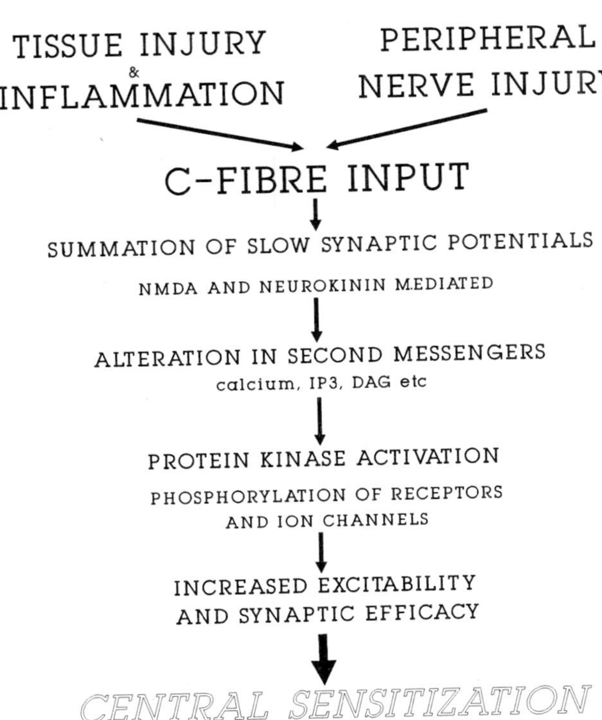

Fig. 5.11 A simple model of the pathogenesis of central sensitization by C-fibre input generated by tissue injury/inflammation or following peripheral nerve injury.

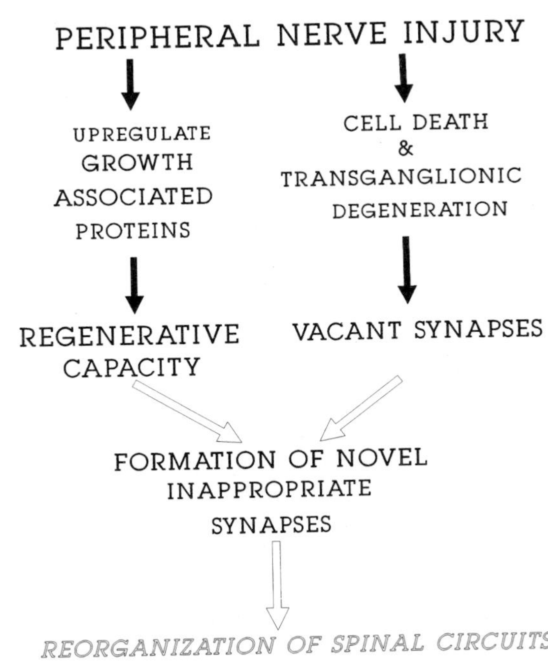

Fig. 5.12 A model of the sequence of events that can lead to a reorganization of spinal circuits following peripheral nerve injury.

Mode 3, representing a state of hypersensitivity also has survival value in some circumstances. The state of central sensitization is triggered by certain types of nociceptor afferent input which will occur with tissue damage, peripheral inflammation and following nerve injury where injury discharge and spontaneous activity occur (Fig. 5.11). A state of excessive sensitivity, such that low-intensity stimuli begin to initiate pain, can help to protect injured body parts from further injury while recuperation or healing occurs. The survival advantages of the activity-dependent facilitation of the pain system is such that it is present early in evolution in some animals, including invertebrates (Woolf & Walters 1991). Sensitization is not always adaptive, however, and when it is produced in situations where the initial damage has healed or following nerve injury, it can result in pain of no apparent benefit to the sufferer.

Modes 1, 2 and 3 reflect the capacity of the nervous system for functional plasticity, the dynamic alteration in the performance of the system in response to changing situations. Mode 4 is qualitatively quite different. In this situation cells die, axon terminals degenerate or atrophy, new axon terminals may appear, and the structural contact between cells at the synapses may be considerably modified (Fig. 5.12). This mode represents true pathology of the system and its contribution to neuropathic and central pain disorders is only just beginning to become apparent.

The rationale for discussing the dorsal horn in the context of its ability to operate in different modes or states is simply that treating a sensory disorder merely on the basis of the sensation experienced is not sufficient. I have illustrated how pain can be experienced in a number of quite different states by low- as well as high-intensity stimuli and this is summarized in Figures 5.9 and 5.10. A particular stimulus can clearly not be used as a predictor of the sensation that will be elicited, without knowing what mode the system is in, and the reverse is also true. The rational, as opposed to empirical, treatment of different pain conditions requires more than a study of the input to the system and the final output generated; the mode must be known.

In the rest of this chapter I will briefly survey the processes that appear to operate in the control situation and the mechanisms that change its sensory processing capacity.

MODE 1, PHYSIOLOGICAL, CONTROL OR NORMAL STATE

In this mode low-intensity stimuli never normally produce pain while a readily detectable pain threshold to intense mechanical and thermal stimuli can be measured, with a progressive increase in the pain experienced with increasing stimulus strength until tissue damage is produced (Fig. 5.8). In general terms there is a good correlation between sensation and the functional specialization of primary afferents, particularly for low-threshold afferents (e.g. Torebjörk et al 1987). The high degree of specialization of the afferents resides not only in their transduction properties but also in their central termination patterns in the spinal cord.

The central terminals of primary afferents occupy highly ordered spatial locations in the dorsal horn. In the dorsoventral or laminar plane this order reflects the modality and threshold sensitivity of the afferents, with specific termination sites for different afferent types (Table 5.4). From the perspective of nociception, high-threshold nociceptors terminate predominantly in laminae I and II, with some contribution to lamina V.

The rostrocaudal and mediolateral location of the central terminals of primary afferents encodes the location of the afferents' peripheral receptive field, generating a somatotopic map of the body surface in the horizontal plane of the dorsal horn. At the level of individual nerve territories the map is organized such that neighbouring peripheral fields occupy contiguous parts of the spinal cord (Swett & Woolf 1985; Woolf & Fitzgerald 1986; LaMotte et al 1991; Rivero-Mellin & Grant 1991; Maslany et al 1991).

Intraaxonal staining of individual fibres has enabled the central terminal axon of primary afferents to be studied at exquisite detail. What has become apparent is that different afferents possess distinct morphological patterns of central terminals which have been particularly well described for the large myelinated mechanoreceptor (e.g. see Brown et al 1977; Semba et al 1985; Woolf 1987a). The number of Aδ- and C-fibres labelled in this way has been limited because of the technical difficulty (Light & Perl 1979; Sugiura et al 1986; Sugiura et al 1989; Hoheisel & Mense 1989). Beyond the precisely mapped somatotopically organized terminals, some myelinated afferents extend long branches for many segments outside the normal termination site and whose function remains to be discovered (Wall & Shortland 1991).

SYNAPTIC STRUCTURE

The ultrastructure of synaptic boutons of identified primary afferents have begun to be studied (Maxwell & Rethelyi 1987). This has enabled the analysis of the pre- and postsynaptic arrangement of synaptic terminations, the transmitter content of the central terminals of identified primary afferents and the pattern of axoaxonic or dendroaxonic connections. This approach has only been applied to low-threshold mechanoreceptors and the synaptic neuropil of Aδ- and C-fibres has not yet been studied at the single cell level in identified neurons. Nevertheless from more general ultrastructural studies, it is clear that the neuropil organization of laminae I and II is extremely complex (Willis & Coggeshall 1991).

The first synaptic connection in the dorsal horn between primary afferent terminals and dorsal horn neurons is governed by structural presynaptic features – location, density and distribution of synaptic boutons. Postsynaptic structure is clearly also important; which neurons do particular types of afferent fibres contact, where are these contacts, on the distal or proximal dendrite, or on the soma? Further complicating the arrangement are the presynaptic axoaxonic and dendroaxonic control elements on axon terminals. In the simplest form of neural networking, if one assumed that all boutons were active – which may not be the case – then, with a knowledge of the distribution of the central terminals of primary afferents and information about the dendritic architecture of dorsal horn neurons, one should be able to predict the location, size and response properties of the receptive fields of dorsal horn neurons. Unfortunately this turns out not to be the case. Both for cells in the superficial dorsal horn (Light & Perl 1979; Woolf & Fitzgerald 1983; Rethelyi et al 1989) and in the deep laminae of the dorsal horn (Maxwell et al 1983; Bennett et al 1984; Ritz & Greenspan 1985; Egger et al 1986; Woolf & King 1987), no correlation between receptive field and dendritic architecture has been found. While a purely geometrical organization reflecting the structure and position of input and output elements may have some role in establishing receptive field properties for certain cells (Brown et al 1980; Brown & Noble 1982), the relative positions of primary afferent terminals and a dorsal horn neuron's dendrite is only a part of the processing picture. The reason for this lies in the convergence of multiple inputs onto dorsal horn neurons, from primary afferent and from local interneurones. These latter will themselves receive some afferent input, so that the way in which a given cell responds to a peripheral input will be determined by network related factors, including inhibitory as well as excitatory influences.

A single cell in the dorsal horn has, therefore, a limited role by itself, in the function of the entire system. The dorsal horn is characterized by a wide range of cells of different sizes and morphological appearance. Unlike some parts of the brain, such as the cerebellar cortex, hippocampus or cerebral cortex, morphological criteria by themselves have not been particularly useful in identifying the type of cell or its functional properties (Willis & Coggeshall 1991). Based on the projection of their axons dorsal horn neurons can be divided into three classes: projecting neurons, propriospinal neurons and local interneurons (Table 5.2). Although the projecting neurons transfer sensory information from the spinal cord to the brain, they represent only a tiny minority of the total number of cells (Chung et al, 1984).

SYNAPTIC PATHWAYS

Projection neurons transfer information from the spinal cord to the brain, which can result in a conscious awareness of a sensation, alter the state of arousal, initiate autonomic responses, modify mood, lead to learned behaviour or complex cognitive responses. How these responses are generated and which particular projection pathways are responsible remains the topic of intense study and debate. While many projection neurons can be activated by afferent activity in nociceptors, spinothalamic tract neurons remain likely to have a prime role in initiating the sensation of pain (Mayer et al 1975; Dubner et al 1989; Kenshalo et al 1989; Simone et al 1991) but this may not be exclusive. One role of projection neurons appears to be the activation of descending control systems which in turn control the gain of dorsal horn neurons (Schaible et al 1991). Propriospinal neurons transfer inputs from one segment of the spinal cord to another; their role in nociception is poorly understood but they appear to be able to act as a multisynaptic pathway that transfers information to the brain in some circumstances. The vast majority of intrinsic dorsal horn neurons are, however, local interneurons which send their axons for only a short distance within the spinal cord.

Although the importance of interneurons is well recognized, acting to transfer information directly (excitatory interneurons) or modulate transmission pre- or postsynaptically (inhibitory interneurons), the local circuitry of the dorsal horn is not, however, actually known. Which interneurons feed on to which projection neurons, what afferent inputs drive different interneurons, which types of afferent input are subject to particular forms of inhibition, the role of descending pathways in controlling the activity of interneurons, the importance of feedforward and feedback circuits are not yet fully understood. A part of the problem is the necessity of electrophysiological studies to investigate the properties of one cell at a time, without any information on the activity generated in the thousands of cells feeding directly or indirectly on to that cell. Alternatively, histochemical analyses that reveal groups of neurons that express a common chemical phenotype, be it a transmitter, cell surface marker or immediate early gene, tell us nothing about the function of the cells. The actual role of the neurons in the superficial dorsal horn (substantia gelatinosa) in modulating or controlling sensory inflow remains, for example, speculative at best, in spite of numerous investigations and the elaboration of complex models.

SYNAPTIC TRANSMISSION

Apart from structural factors, synaptic transfer of information is governed by the nature and amount of the transmitter released by different primary afferents, the density and identity of postsynaptic receptors, the coupling of the receptors directly or indirectly to ion channels, the kinetics of receptor activation and ion-channel opening and closing, and the factors responsible for the removal or breakdown of the transmitter. Each of these factors is subject to modulatory influences, some anterograde (from the axon terminal to the postsynaptic element), some retrograde (from the postsynaptic cell to the axon terminal) and some activity dependent (both pre- and postsynaptic). Synaptic transmission occurs over a range of time epochs from tens of milliseconds for fast transmitters such as the excitatory amino acid glutamate acting on AMPA receptors, hundreds of milliseconds, glutamate acting on NMDA receptors (Gerber & Randic 1989a, 1989b), to tens of seconds, tachykinins acting on neurokinin receptors. Simultaneous release of glutamate and neuropeptides from the same afferent means that both fast and slow synaptic currents are generated concurrently. The former seem to be responsible for signalling information related to the location, intensity and duration of peripheral stimuli by reflecting the information content in the trains of action potentials arriving at the axon terminal, while the latter provide the opportunity for integrating input both temporally and spatially (Thompson et al 1990). The actions of transmitters may not be limited to the site of release and may spread through the extracellular space to distant neurons (volume transmission); this appears to be particularly true for neuropeptides. The capacity of transmitters to modify second messenger systems means that phosphorylation of proteins including ion-channels can occur (Woolf 1987; Chen & Huang 1992) as well as the induction of gene-expression (Hunt et al 1987; Menetry et al 1989). What this means is that any analysis of the function of the dorsal horn has to be performed over a time-domain that outlasts the arrival of afferent input and the immediate changes in membrane potential. Modulation of synaptic efficacy in the dorsal horn is of fundamental importance for its operation. Unfortunately we still do not know how it occurs in specific circumstances so that the strength of a synaptic contact may vary from, at one extreme, failing to produce any postsynaptic response (an ineffective or silent synapse) to a situation where a single excitatory postsynaptic current is sufficient to generate an action potential in the target neuron. It is likely that under normal circumstances most synapses operate to produce subthreshold responses of varying amplitude and action potentials in postsynaptic cells are generated by multiple inputs (Woolf & King 1989, 1990). This offers the possibility of increasing or decreasing the strength of synaptic inputs in a range of different ways. Essentially this is how the state of the spinal cord can be rapidly changed, modifying sensory processing (the interconvertibility of modes 1, 2 and 3).

CELLULAR ANALYSIS

Conventional analysis of the function of the dorsal horn has been performed by analysing the receptive field properties of individual neurons. With extracellular analysis, cells with receptive fields responsive to high or low stimuli or combinations of both have been found. While the capacity of a cell to encode intensity must contribute to the sensory analysis of stimuli, it is important to recognize that single cells are unlikely by themselves to carry information that would lead directly to any sensation. A prominent feature of the receptive fields of dorsal horn neurons is the large number of cells with a wide dynamic range, responding to low- and high-intensity peripheral stimuli (Willis & Coggeshall 1991). More surprising is the demonstration indicating that it is these wide dynamic range cells, rather than those cells that are activated solely by intense or damaging peripheral stimuli (nociceptive specific cells), which are likely to be responsible for the conscious appreciation of pain (Dubner et al 1989). Classifying the functional class of a cell in terms of its receptive field is difficult, however, when a considerable part of its response may normally be subthreshold. Nevertheless, the fundamental question remains why do multiconvergent cells in the control or physiological situation appear to contribute to the generation of pain, when low-intensity stimuli which activate the cells only produce innocuous sensations (Le Bars et al 1986).

FUTURE PROSPECTS

There is no direct answer to this at present and a solution would represent a major breakthrough in our understanding of the operation of the dorsal horn. Nevertheless, there are some suggestions. One is that while activity in wide dynamic range spinothalamic tract neurons is necessary and sufficient to produce pain, pain only occurs with activation above a certain frequency in a critical number of these cells – essentially a 'threshold' theory (Melzack & Wall 1965; Mayer et al 1975; Willis 1992). An alternative theory is that it is a contrast signal reaching the thalamus that determines whether pain is experienced rather than activity in a small specified pathway (Le Bars et al 1986; Walker et al 1989). It is possible that the generation of the sensation of pain involves both the activation of a specific subset of neurons projecting through the anterolateral quadrant and a comparison at high levels of the brain between this activity and that carried in the dorsal column–medial lemniscal pathways and in ascending pathways from nociceptive specific cells. When there is a high degree of activity in the spinothalamic tract and the dorsal column–medial lemniscal pathways, an innocuous sensation may be experienced but when the activity in the spinothalamic tract is accompanied by high levels of activity in ascending nociceptive pathways, or the absence of activity in the dorsal column pathway, pain might result. Whether single or multiple pathways carry the 'pain' signal, the nature of the signal and why it cannot normally be driven by low-threshold mechanoreceptors remains unknown.

What we do have considerable information on, are the receptive field properties of individual cells located in different parts of the dorsal horn, their thresholds, size, responsiveness to a range of different stimuli, and the contribution of different types of afferents, Aβ, Aδ and C, to the response profiles (Besson & Chaouch 1987; Willis & Coggeshall 1991). What are also well described are the powerful inhibitory components of the receptive field generated both by local segmental and by descending pathways. Inhibition can occur pre- and postsynaptically and involves a range of transmitters, GABA, glycine, 5-HT, noradrenaline and the opioids, operating in a number of different ways over different time courses. Table 5.1 details some of the major and minor descending inputs to the dorsal horn. Note that not all are inhibitory.

The dorsal horn in Mode 1, the control or physiological state, is stable in the sense that the processing of information normally occurs in a highly reproducible and predictable way. The state of the dorsal horn can, however, shift such that its output to defined inputs becomes dramatically altered. For the remainder of this chapter, I will very briefly review some of the data available on how these mode shifts occur.

SHIFTING FROM MODE 1 TO MODE 2: SUPPRESSING SENSORY OUTFLOW

As discussed earlier, a threshold theory of nociception would hold that activity in the spinothalamic tract or similar neurons above a certain critical level, both in terms of frequency and number of cells active, will lead to the sensation of pain. Normally, according to such a theory, low-intensity stimuli activating low-threshold mechanoreceptors cannot drive the projection neurons sufficiently to cross this threshold, but the activity generated in nociceptors by high-intensity stimuli can. If the activity elicited by high-intensity stimuli is suppressed by inhibitory mechanisms, such that insufficient output is generated by projection neurons to exceed a critical threshold, then pain will not be experienced. A great deal of information is now known about endogenous pain control mechanisms (Ch. 12) in terms of their anatomy and pharmacology. What is less well understood are the precise ways in which such endogenous control mechanisms are activated and exactly how they suppress the sensation of pain. Nevertheless, mimicking these mechanisms either pharmacologically by the administration of opioids or α_2-adrenergic agonists, or by attempting to directly activate the control mechanisms with peripheral or central stimulation, remains a valuable therapeutic approach.

SHIFTING FROM MODE 1 TO MODE 3: THE GENERATION OF CENTRAL SENSITIZATION

The possibility that the hyperalgesia and allodynia following peripheral tissue injury has a central component was hotly disputed by Lewis and by Hardy and colleagues 40–50 years ago. The first direct evidence that the afferent input generated by tissue damage increased the excitability of neurons in the spinal cord appeared more recently (Woolf 1983). Since then data from a number of laboratories have repeatedly demonstrated that dorsal horn neurons including spinothalamic tract neurons can be 'sensitized' following activity in nociceptors. This manifests as a reduction in the threshold, an increase in the responsiveness, the expansion of the extent and the recruitment of novel inputs to receptive fields (Cook et al 1987; Hoheisel & Mense 1989; Hylden et al 1989; Woolf & King 1990; Neuberger & Schaible 1990; Simone et al 1991; Hu et al 1992). The changes in receptive field properties seem to be due to the recruitment of previously subthreshold components of the receptive field as a result either of increased synaptic output or increased excitability of the postsynaptic cell (Woolf 1991). The temporal summation of slow synaptic potentials (Thompson et al 1990) leading to alteration in second messenger systems (Woolf 1987) and the phosphorylation of receptors (Chen & Huang 1992) seem to be a key feature of the induction of central sensitization. Blockade of the slow potentials either with NMDA receptor antagonists or neurokinin antagonists prevents the establishment of central sensitization (Haley et al 1990; Coderre & Melzack 1991; Woolf & Thompson 1991; Xu et al 1991).

While it is now clear that during and immediately following inputs in nociceptors the excitability of a sizeable fraction of dorsal horn neuron increases and that this is almost certainly responsible for mechanical allodynia and secondary hyperalgesia (Torebjörk et al 1992), what is less certain is the extent to which such sensitization plays a role in the sensory abnormalities accompanying chronic pain states. Acute tissue damage and inflammatory states will directly and indirectly lead to the activation of nociceptors which will induce central sensitization. On recovery from the damage or inflammation, the source of the input during the central changes is removed and the hyperalgesia and allodynia commonly disappear within several hours or days. Neuropathic pain, in contrast, is typically persistent and intractable (Ch. 10). One explanation may be that a constant drive of input from axotomized nociceptors is present (Devor 1991), which maintains the central sensitization. Another is that associated with peripheral nerve damage is the decrease in segmental inhibitory mechanisms (Wall & Devor 1981; Woolf & Wall 1982) which exaggerates the synaptic response to afferent input.

Clinical studies have revealed that Aβ afferents are involved in the allodynia associated with nerve injury (Campbell et al 1988; Price et al 1989), and in some cases at least blocking C-fibre input does not decrease the allodynia (Campbell et al 1988) but in other cases it does (Koltzenburg et al 1992; Gracely et al 1992).

The recognition that the dorsal horn can shift from its normal state to a hyperexcitable one has enormous implications for therapy, both in terms of the development of potentially new analgesics such as NMDA or neurokinin antagonists and by the appreciation that the prevention of the establishment of central sensitization may substantially eliminate the pain following surgery. Although considerable work has demonstrated increases in excitability following conditioning primary afferent input in nociceptors, similar changes may potentially occur by the blockade of inhibitory mechanisms. Disinhibition by the administration of GABA or glycine antagonists can produce touch-evoked allodynia (Yaksh 1989).

SHIFTING FROM MODE 1 TO MODE 4: STRUCTURAL REORGANIZATION OF THE DORSAL HORN

If the highly ordered structure of the dorsal horn is modified by degenerative changes, this will naturally alter the sensory processing within the dorsal horn. Peripheral nerve injury, for example, results in dorsal root ganglion cell death (Arvidsson et al 1986), the withdrawal of the central axonal terminals from lamina II (Castro-Lopes et al 1990) and degenerative changes in some of the remaining afferent terminals (Aldskogius et al 1985; Knyihar-Csillik et al 1990). While this will result in the direct uncoupling of some afferent input to dorsal horn neurons, other changes occur which result in modifications other than just a reduction in synaptic drive. These include changes in the chemical phenotype of the axotomized primary sensory neurons with the down-regulation of some transmitters/neuromodulators and the up-regulation of others, so that chemical signalling at the first synaptic relay in the dorsal horn will be changed. This, together with transynaptic alteration including the upregulation of postsynaptic receptors, denervation hypersensitivity and the decrease in segmental inhibitory mechanisms, will dramatically modify sensory processing. Recently it has become apparent that degeneration is not the only consequence of peripheral nerve injury; regenerative changes also occur. As part of the induction of an injured primary sensory neuron into a growth mode, to permit peripheral regeneration, developmentally regulated growth associated proteins are expressed (Skene 1989). These are also distributed to the central terminals of axotomized primary afferents (Woolf et al 1990; Coggeshall et al 1991), where the combination of vacant synaptic sites and axon terminals controlling the molecular machinery necessary for growth leads to the 'regenerative growth' of at least some of the central axonal terminals. Of particular interest is the finding that large myelinated afferent fibres which normally terminate in the deeper laminae of the dorsal horn, grow into lamina II, the site of C-fibre terminals (Woolf et al 1992). This may result in the formation of novel and inappropriate synapses which could dramatically alter the central processing of signals generated in low-threshold mechanoreceptors. Peripheral neuropathic pain may be an expression, therefore, of an alteration in the circuitry of the spinal cord as well as of changes due to the maintenance of central sensitization by a nociceptor drive (Ch. 10).

Central neuropathic pain, resulting from spinal cord injury, stroke and a number of central lesions may also alter the spinal cord by removing some of the descending influences originating from the brainstem that control the gain of the system. If such changes resulted in a removal of a descending inhibitory input, the consequence might be a form of sustained central sensitization due to disinhibition.

CONCLUSIONS

The dorsal horn has the capacity to operate in three modes: a control mode, a suppressed mode and a sensitized mode. These alterations in the functional performance of the cord will alter sensory processing and are likely to account both for the failure to react to tissue damage on some occasions and the generation of pain in reaction to low-intensity stimuli in others. Understanding the factors controlling or determining which mode the spinal cord is in is essential in order to understand the pathogenesis of pain. The circuitry of the dorsal horn can, however, also be permanently altered or reorganized following peripheral or CNS damage. This may result in irreversible changes in sensory processing, with persistent clinical sensory disorders.

REFERENCES

Aldskogius H, Arvidsson J, Grant G 1985 The reaction of primary sensory neurons to peripheral nerve injury with particular emphasis on transganglionic changes. Brain Research 10: 27–46

Arvidsson J, Ygge J, Grant G 1986 Cell loss in lumbar dorsal root ganglia and transganglionic degeneration after sciatic nerve resection in the rat. Brain Research 373: 15–21

Bennett G J, Nishikawa N, Lu G W, Hoffert M J, Dubner R 1984 The morphology of dorsal column postsynaptic (DCPS) spino-medullary neurons in the cat. Journal of Comparative Neurology 224: 568–578

Besson J M, Chaouch A 1987 Peripheral and spinal mechanisms of nociception. Physiology Reviews 67: 67–186

Brown A G, Noble R 1982 Connexions between hair follicle afferent fibers and spinocervical tract neurones in the cat: the synthesis of receptive fields. Journal of Physiology 232: 77–91

Brown A G, Rose P K, Snow P J 1977 The morphology of hair follicle afferent fibre collaterals in the spinal cord of the cat. Journal of Physiology 272: 779–797

Brown A G, Rose P K, Snow P J 1978 Morphology and organization of axon collaterals from afferent fibers of slowly adapting type I units in cat spinal cord. Journal of Physiology 277: 15–27

Brown A G, Rose P K, Snow P J 1980 Dendritic trees and cutaneous receptive fields of adjacent spinocervical tract neurones in the cat. Journal of Physiology 300: 429–440

Brown P B, Gladfelter W E, Culberson J L, Covalt-Dunning D, Sonty R V, Pubols L M, Millecchia R J 1991 Somatotopic organization of single primary afferent axon projections to cat spinal dorsal horn. Journal of Neuroscience 11: 289–309

Campbell J N, Raja S N, Meyer R A, McKinnon S E 1988 Myelinated afferents signal the hyperalgesia associated with nerve injury. Pain 32: 89–94

Castro-Lopes J M, Coimbra A, Grant G, Arvidsson J 1990 Ultrastructural changes of the central scalloped (C_1) primary afferent endings of synaptic glomeruli in the substantia gelatinosa Rolandi of the rat after peripheral neurotomy. Journal of Neurocytology 19: 329–337

Chen L, Huang L-Y M 1992 Protein kinase C reduces Mg^{2+} block of NMDA-receptor channels as a mechanism of modulation. Nature 356: 521–523

Chung K, Kevetter G A, Willis W D, Coggeshall R E 1984 An estimate of the ratio of propriospinal to long tract neurons in the sacral spinal cord of the rat. Neuroscience Letters 44: 173–177

Coderre T J, Melzack R 1991 Central neural mediators of secondary hyperalgesia following heat injury in rats: neuropeptides and excitatory amino acids. Neuroscience Letters 131: 71–74

Coggeshall R E, Reynolds M L, Woolf C J 1991 Distribution of the growth associated protein GAP-43 in the central processes of axotomized primary afferents in the adult rat spinal cord: presence of growth cone-like structures. Neuroscience Letters 131: 37–141

Cook A J, Woolf C J, Wall P D, McMahon S B 1987 Dynamic receptive field plasticity in rat spinal cord dorsal horn following C-primary afferent input. Nature 325: 151–153

Devor M 1991 Neuropathic pain and injured nerve: peripheral mechanisms. British Medical Bulletin 47: 619–630

Dubner R, Kenshalo D R, Maixner W, Bushnell M C, Oliveras J L 1989 The correlation of monkey medullary dorsal horn neural activity and the perceived intensity of noxious heat stimuli. Journal of Neurophysiology 62: 450–457

Egger M D, Freeman N C G, Jacquin M, Proshansky E, Semba K 1986 Dorsal horn cells in the cat responding to stimulation of the plantar cushion. Brain Research 383: 68–82

Gerber G, Randic M 1989a Excitatory amino acid-mediated components of synaptically evoked input from dorsal roots to deep dorsal horn neurons in the rat spinal cord slice. Neuroscience Letters 106: 211–219

Gerber G, Randic M 1989b Participation of excitatory amino acid receptors in the slow excitatory synaptic transmission in the rat spinal dorsal horn in vitro. Neuroscience Letters 106: 220–228

Gracely R H, Lynch S A, Bennett G J 1992 Painful neuropathy: altered central processing, maintained dynamically by peripheral input. Pain 51: 175–194

Haley J E, Sullivan A F, Dickenson A H 1990 Evidence for spinal N-methyl-D-aspartate receptor involvement in prolonged chemical nociception in the rat. Brain Research 518: 218–226

Hardy J D, Wolff H G, Goodell H 1952 Pain sensations and reactions. Williams & Wilkins, New York. Reprinted by Hafner, New York, 1967

Hoheisel U, Mense S 1989 Long-term changes in discharge behaviour of cat dorsal horn neurones following noxious stimulation of deep tissues. Pain 36: 239–247

Hu J W, Sessle B J, Raboisson P, Dallel R, Woda A 1992 Stimulation of craniofacial muscle afferents induces prolonged facilitatory effects in trigeminal nociceptive brain-stem neurones. Pain 48: 53–60

Hunt S P, Pini A, Evan G 1987 Induction of c-fos like protein in spinal cord neurons following sensory stimulation. Nature 328: 632–634

Hylden J L K, Nahin R L, Traub R J, Dubner R 1989 Expansion of receptive fields of spinal lamina I projection neurons in rats with unilateral adjuvant-induced inflammation: the contribution of central dorsal horn mechanisms. Pain 37: 229–243

Kenshalo D R Jr, Anton F, Dubner R 1989 The detection and perceived intensity of noxious thermal stimuli in monkey and man. Journal of Neurophysiology 62: 429–436

Knyihar-Csillik E, Rakic P, Csillik B 1990 Transneuronal degeneration in the rolandi substance of the primate spinal cord evoked by axotomy induced transneuronal degeneration of central sensory terminals. Cell and Tissue Research 255: 515–525

Koltzenburg M, Wahren L K, Torebjörk H E 1992 Dynamic changes of mechanical hyperalgesia in neuropathic pain states and healthy subjects depend on the ongoing activity of unmyelinated nociceptive afferents. Pflügers Archives 420: R52

LaMotte C C, Kapadia S E, Shapiro C M 1991 Central projection of the sciatic saphenous median and ulnar nerves of the rat as demonstrated by transganglionic transport of cholerogenoid-HRP (BHRP) and wheat germ agglutinin-HRP (WGA-HRP). Journal of Comparative Neurology 42: 422–435

Le Bars D, Dickenson A H, Besson J M, Villaneuva L 1986 Aspects of sensory processing through convergent neurones. In: Yaksh T L (ed) Spinal afferent processing. Plenum, New York, p 467–504

Lewis T 1942 Pain. MacMillan, New York

Light A R, Perl E R 1979 Spinal termination of functionally identified primary afferent neurons with slowly conducting myelinated fibers. Journal of Comparative Neurology 186: 133–150

Maslany S, Crockett D P, Egger M D 1991 Organization of cutaneous primary afferent fibers projecting to the dorsal horn in the rat: WGA-HRP versus B-HRP. Brain Research 569: 123–135

Maxwell D J, Réthelyi M 1987 Ultrastructure and synaptic connections of cutaneous afferent fibers in the spinal cord. Trends in Neurosciences 10: 117–122

Maxwell D J, Fyffe R E W, Réthelyi M 1983 Morphological properties of physiologically characterized lamina III neurones in the cat spinal cord. Neuroscience 10: 1–22

Mayer D J, Price D D, Becker D P 1975 Neurophysiological characterization of the anterolateral spinal cord neurons contributing to pain perception in man. Pain 1: 51–58

Melzack R, Wall P D 1965 Pain mechanisms: a new theory. Science 150: 971–979

Menétrey D, Gannon J D, Levine J D, Basbaum A I 1989 Expression of c-fos protein in interneurons and projection neurons of the rat spinal cord in response to noxious somatic, articular, and visceral stimulation. Journal of Comparative Neurology 285: 177–195

Mense S, Craig J R 1988 Spinal and supraspinal terminations of primary afferent fibers from the gastrocnemius-soleus muscle in the cat. Neuroscience 26: 1023–1055

Neugebauer V, Schaible H G 1990 Evidence for a central component in the sensitization of spinal neurons with joint input during development of acute arthritis in cat's knee. Journal of Neurophysiology 64: 299–311

Price D D, Bennett G J, Raffii M 1989 Psychological observations on patients with neuropathic pain relieved by a sympathetic block. Pain 36: 273–288

Ralston H J, Light A R, Ralston D D, Perl E R 1984 Morphology and synaptic relationships of physiologically identified low-threshold dorsal root axons stained with intra-axonal horseradish in the cat and monkey. Journal of Neurophysiology 51: 777–792

Réthelyi M, Metz C B, Lund P K 1989 Distribution of neurons expressing calcitonin gene-related peptide mRNAs in the brain stem, spinal cord and dorsal root ganglia of rat and guinea-pig. Neuroscience 29: 225–239

Ritz L A, Greenspan J D 1985 Morphological features of lamina V neurons receiving nociceptive input in cat sacrocaudal spinal cord. Journal of Comparative Neurology 238: 440–452

Rivero-Melian C, Grant G 1991 B-HRP used for studying projections of some hindlimb cutaneous nerves and plantar foot afferents to the dorsal horn and Clarke's column in the rat. Experimental Brain Research 84: 125–132

Schaible H G, Neugebauer V, Cervero F, Schmidt R F 1991 Changes in tonic descending inhibition of spinal neurons with articular input during the development of acute arthritis in the cat. Journal of Neurophysiology 66: 1021–1032

Semba K, Masaracha P, Malamed S et al 1985 An electron microscopic study of terminals of rapidly adapting mechanoreceptive afferent fibers in the cat spinal cord. Journal of Comparative Neurology 232: 229–240

Shortland P, Woolf C J, Fitzgerald M 1989 Morphology and somatotopic organization of the central terminals of hindlimb hair follicle afferents in the rat lumbar spinal cord. Journal of Comparative Neurology 289: 416–433

Simone D A, Sorkin L S, Oh U T et al 1991 Neurogenic hyperalgesia: central neural correlates in responses of spinothalamic tract neurons. Journal of Neurophysiology 66: 228–246

Skene H J P 1989 Axonal growth associated proteins. Annual Reviews of Neuroscience 12: 127–156

Sugiura Y, Lee C L, Perl E R 1986 Central projections of identified, unmyelinated (C) afferent fibers innervating mammalian skin. Science 234: 358–361

Sugiura Y, Terui N, Hosoya Y 1989 Difference in distribution of central terminals between visceral and somatic unmyelinated (C) primary afferent fibers. Journal of Neurophysiology 62: 834–840

Swett J E, Woolf C J 1985 The somatotopic organization of primary afferent terminals in the superficial laminae of the dorsal horn of the rat spinal cord. Journal of Comparative Neurology 231: 66–77

Thompson S W N, King A E, Woolf C J 1990 Activity-dependent changes in rat ventral horn neurons *in vitro*; summation of prolonged afferent evoked postsynaptic depolarizations produce a D-2-amino-5-phosphonovaleric acid sensitive windup. European Journal of Neuroscience 2: 638–649

Torebjörk H E, Vallbo A B, Ochoa J L 1987 Intraneural microstimulation in man; its relation to specificity of tactile sensation. Brain 110: 1509–1529

Torebjörk H E, Lundberg L E R, LaMotte R H 1992 Central changes in processing of mechanoreceptor input in capsaicin-induced sensory hyperalgesia in humans. Journal of Physiology 448: 765–780

Wall P D, Devor M 1981 The effect of peripheral nerve injury on dorsal root potentials and on transmission of afferent signals into the spinal cord. Brain Research 209: 95–111

Wall P D, Shortland P 1991 Long range afferents in the rat spinal cord. I. Numbers, distances and conduction velocities. Philosophical Transactions of the Royal Society of London, B, 334: 85–93

Willis W D 1989 Neural mechanisms of pain discrimination. In: Lund J S (ed) Sensory processing in the mammalian brain. Oxford University Press, New York, p 130–143

Willis W D 1992 Mechanical allodynia: A role for nociceptive tract cells with convergent input from mechanoreceptors and nociceptors? APS Journal (in press)

Willis W D, Coggeshall R E 1991 Sensory mechanisms of the spinal cord. Plenum Press, New York

Woolf C J 1983 Evidence for a central component of post-injury pain hypersensitivity. Nature 306: 686–688

Woolf C J 1987a Central terminations of cutaneous mechanoreceptive afferents in the rat lumbar spinal cord. Journal of Comparative Neurology 261: 105–119

Woolf C J 1987b Excitatory amino acids increase glycogen phosphorylase activity in the rat spinal cord. Neuroscience Letters 73: 209–214

Woolf C J, Fitzgerald M 1983 The properties of neurones recorded in the superficial dorsal horn of the rat spinal cord. Journal of Comparative Neurology 221: 313–328

Woolf C J, Fitzgerald M 1986 Somatotopic organization of cutaneous afferent terminals and dorsal horn receptive fields in the superficial and deep laminae of the rat lumbar spinal cord. Journal of Comparative Neurology 251: 517–531

Woolf C J, King A E 1987 Physiology and morphology of multireceptive neurons with C-afferent inputs in the deep dorsal horn of the rat lumbar spinal cord. Journal of Neurophysiology 58: 460–479

Woolf C J, King A E 1989 Subthreshold components of the cutaneous mechanoreceptive fields of dorsal horn neurons in the rat lumbar spinal cord. Journal of Neurophysiology 62: 907–916

Woolf C J, King A E 1990 Dynamic alterations in the cutaneous mechanoreceptive fields of dorsal horn neurons in the rat spinal cord. Journal of Neuroscience 10: 2717–2726

Woolf C J, Thompson S W N 1991 The induction and maintenance of central sensitization is dependent on N-methyl-D-aspartic acid receptor activation; implications for the treatment of post-injury pain hypersensitivity states. Pain 44: 293–299

Woolf C J, Wall P D 1982 Chronic peripheral nerve section diminishes the primary afferent A-fibre mediated inhibition of rat dorsal horn neurones. Brain Research 242: 77–85

Woolf C J, Wall P D 1986 The relative effectiveness of C primary afferent fibers of different origins in evoking a prolonged facilitation of the flexor reflex in the rat. Journal of Neuroscience 6: 1433–1443

Woolf C J, Walters E T 1991 Common patterns of plasticity contributing to nociceptive sensitization in mammals and Aplysia. Trends in Neurosciences 14: 74–78

Woolf C J, Reynolds M L, Molander C et al 1990 GAP-43, a growth associated protein, appears in dorsal root ganglion cells and in the dorsal horn of the rat spinal cord following peripheral nerve injury. Neuroscience 34: 465–478

Woolf C J, Shortland P, Coggeshall R E 1992 Peripheral nerve injury triggers central sprouting of myelinated afferents. Nature 355: 75–77

Xu X-J, Maggi C A, Wiesenfeld-Hallin Z 1991 On the role of NK-2 tachykinin receptors in the mediation of spinal reflex excitability in the rat. Neuroscience 44: 483–490

Yaksh T L 1989 Behavioural and autonomic correlates of the tactile evoked allodynia produced by spinal glycine inhibition: effects of modulatory receptor systems and excitatory amino acid antagonists. Pain 37: 111–123

6. Brain areas involved in nociception and pain

G. Guilbaud, J. F. Bernard and J. M. Besson

Peripheral and spinal mechanisms of nociception have been extensively investigated and are starting to become relatively well understood (ref. in Besson & Chaouch 1987) whereas supraspinal structures have been less explored. Indeed, nociceptive messages become more and more difficult to follow as they travel further in the central nervous system (CNS), and numerous brain areas are involved in the various components of pain. According to Melzack & Casey (1968), these components include:

1. A sensory-discriminative component that refers to the capacity to analyse location, intensity, and duration of the nociceptive stimulus.
2. A motivational component that gives rise to the unpleasant character of painful perception.
3. A cognitive and evaluative component involved in the phenomena of anticipation, attention, suggestion and past experiences.

This latter is, in addition, able to interact with the sensory-discriminative and the motivational components. In humans, clinical observations have revealed that a large majority of the ascending systems activating supraspinal structures responsible for pain sensation cross at the spinal level. Sensitivity to pain disappeared on the side opposite to a spinal cord hemisection, while it persisted on the other side. Since the turn of the century the specific section of the anterolateral quadrant (ALQ), named anterolateral cordotomy, has been promoted for alleviation of certain intractable pains. Although still useful in the relief of some pains, notably as a result of terminal cancer, this technique, due to the development of other therapeutics, is used nowadays only on rare occasions. In fact, although stimulation of the ALQ can produce painful sensations, the tract does not exclusively convey nociceptive messages. This is illustrated by the observation of Noordenbos & Wall (1976) on a patient with a section of the spinal cord sparing only the ALQ, confirming the role of this quadrant for conveying pain and temperature sensation, but also light touch and pressure sense. We will see that this observation fits well with the characteristics of spinal dorsal horn neurons at the origin of the ascending pathways contained in this quadrant. We will also see that the ascending tracts contained in the ALQ and responsible for pain sensation are multiple, and not limited to the spinothalamic tract as often thought. Finally, the ALQ is not exclusive in the transmission of nociceptive messages towards higher centres. As an example, suppression of pain is only obtained in 50% of patients after a cordotomy, and these patients are still capable of feeling a pricking pain when intense cutaneous stimuli are applied to the 'analgesic' zone (King 1957).

The complexity of the pain pathways, and therefore of the brain structures able to be involved in pain processing, have been clearly emphasized by the powerful modern anatomical tracing techniques which have allowed not only a better visualization of the 'classical' pathways (origins and terminals), but also revealed numerous 'novel' ascending tracts able to participate in pain integration. This is likely to explain the lack of success of neurosurgical lesions in various brain areas performed with the hope of relieving intractable pain and of discovering a unique pain centre.

In addition to the complexity of pain pathways and of the structures in which they terminate, numerous difficulties have hampered experimental approaches devoted to the role of brainstem and forebrain structures in the processing of nociception signals in animals. Firstly, the experimenter has to deal with ethical problems related to experiments performed in animals with an intact neuraxis, and so uses anaesthetized preparations. The general depressive effect of anaesthetics on the CNS has been known for many years, and major discrepancies between studies have arisen from the use of different anaesthetic regimes. Secondly, interspecies differences in pain pathways are often significant, and make it difficult to compare results. Lastly, but not least, there is confusion resulting from delineation and naming of supraspinal areas which often vary according to the authors.

Despite these various difficulties, physiological and anatomical data obtained in various species, mainly in the rat and monkey but also in the cat, and to a lesser extent in humans, have now progressively given some clues to the understanding of pain-processing at the supraspinal level. Studies have been concerned primarily with the structures receiving projections from spinal neurons through direct or indirect pathways which have been shown to convey noxious inputs: the spinothalamic, the spinoreticular and the spinoreticulothalamic tracts, and more recently, the spino(trigemino)pontoamygdalian tract and to a lesser extent the spinohypothalamic tract. The role of some cortical areas in the transmission and integration of noxious messages will be also considered.

SUPRASPINAL AREAS RECEIVING PROJECTIONS THROUGH THE SPINOTHALAMOCORTICAL PATHWAY

SPINOTHALAMIC TRACT (STT)

The existence of STT projections has been demonstrated in many species, e.g. fish, reptiles, birds, rabbit, opossum, rat, cat, pig, monkey and humans (refs in Willis 1989; Willis & Coggeshall 1991; Gingold et al 1991; Ralston & Ralston 1992). The location and functional characteristics of the neurons at the origin of the STT have been extensively studied in the primate by Willis and co-workers (refs in Willis 1989, Willis & Coggeshall 1991) and we will mainly refer to these investigations.

Several zones of the grey matter of the spinal cord are at the origin of STT fibres: the marginal zone of the dorsal horn (lamina I and the outer part of lamina II), laminae IV–VI of the dorsal horn, a deeper and medial zone (including the base of the dorsal horn, the intermediate zone or lamina VII, and lamina VIII in the ventral horn). The locations of ascending STT axons are relatively well localized. However, there are several controversies likely to be due mostly to different tracing techniques and species (Jones et al 1987; Apkarian & Hodge 1989; Nathan 1990; Craig & Dostrovsky 1991; Willis & Coggeshall 1991; Gingold et al 1991; Blomqvist et al 1992; Ralston & Ralston 1992), and several questions remain to be answered. To what extent do the various sites of origin participate in the final constitution of the STT? To what extent do the ascending fibres ascend in the ventrolateral, in the lateral or dorsolateral quadrant? To what extent does a particular structure receive STT terminals? In particular, the proportion of lamina I cells at the origin of STT, the location of their axon terminals either in the lateral or the medial thalamus, the part of the white matter where these axons travel seem to vary according to the species and are still sharply debated. To what extent does the importance of SST vary according to the species?

There is, however, a general agreement on the fact that most if not all STT-neurons receive noxious input, either exclusively (nociceptive specific-neurons), or not (nociceptive non-specific = wide dynamic range = multireceptive neurons). The STT neurons activated by cutaneous mechanical stimuli are in most cases equally activated by thermal nociceptive stimuli either with heat or cold. An encoding for noxious heat thermal stimuli has been repeatedly demonstrated, with a sigmoid intensity-response curve. Repetition of nociceptive stimulus induces phenomena of sensitization. Convergence of noxious cutaneous, muscular and visceral inputs has been observed in different species. In particular that of visceral inputs from various organs (thoracic, abdominal, pelvic) with somatic inputs is a common feature of the STT neurons, whether they are noxious specific or nonspecific. These data largely support the convergence projection theory of referred and projected pain (refs in Willis & Coggeshall 1991; Ness & Gebhart 1990).

Even though there are still discussions on the extent of projections in some thalamic nuclei, it is possible to distinguish:

- The lateral part, i.e. the ventrobasal (VB) complex in rat and monkey (ventroposterolateral (VPL) and ventroposteromedial (VPM)), but only the VPL shell region in cat
- The posterior nuclei (PO group) mainly in the cat, but also in monkey
- The nucleus centralis lateralis in these three species
- The nucleus submedius in the cat, and to a lesser extent in the rat.

Interestingly, STT terminal sites in humans are similar to those described in the monkey, but major projections in PO group have been especially stressed in human thalamus (Mehler 1969, 1974). Although collateralization of STT axons between different areas has been described (Giesler et al 1981) it seems possible to differentiate the projecting sites of the STT neurons according to their characteristics – location, size of their receptive field (RF). STT neurons, located in laminae I and IV–VI, with relatively limited contralateral RFs, would have more chance to project laterally, and these projections are somatotopically organized in rat and monkey (Willis & Coggeshall 1991). STT neurons located in the intermediate zone between the two horns or in ventral horn have expanded and complex RFs receiving more proprioceptive inputs would project more medially, in particular in the nucleus centralis lateralis (CL). However, it can be noted that lamina I neurons usually with extremely small RFs have been described to preferentially project to the nucleus submedius, and this nucleus contains neurons driven from large RFs (see below).

It has been shown that spinal projections (and trigeminal projections originating from the subnucleus caudalis) in the VB complex of rat (Peschanski et al 1983; Peschanski 1984) and of monkey (Ralston 1985) share a common morphology with lemniscal afferents to the same areas: large endings containing round vesicles that make asymmetric contacts, usually with the dendrites of thalamic neurons. In addition, both in rat and monkey STT terminals overlap the area which receives projections from the dorsal column nuclei (Berkley 1980; Ma et al 1986), although the STT projection is less dense. The STT actually ends in a number of focal zones that in transverse sections appear as 'bursts' or 'clusters' of terminals scattered in 'archipelagolike' fashion across the VPL nucleus, following Mehler's description (Mehler 1969; Mehler et al 1960; see ref. in Willis & Coggeshall 1991). The STT terminates in variably sized 'rodlike' areas in the VPL nucleus, suggesting the possibility that each thalamic rod that receives STT input projects to a particular cortical zone (Jones 1985). As mentioned initially, the synaptic endings of STT axons in the primate VPL nucleus are of the large, round vesicle type, as in rats (Ralston 1985, 1992), but they have a triadic relationship with thalamic relay neurons and the presynaptic dendrites of interneurons. The structural arrangement suggests that activity in STT axons would result in excitation of a relay cell and also a presynaptic dendrite, which could in turn inhibit the relay neuron.

ELECTROPHYSIOLOGICAL CHARACTERISTICS OF SUPRASPINAL NEURONS RECEIVING PROJECTIONS THROUGH STT

The thalamic ventrobasal complex, posterior group and the somatosensory cortex

The influences of experimental conditions on studies of supraspinal mechanisms of pain is well illustrated by the history of the experiments concerning the possible involvement of lateral thalamic structures. The systematic investigation of Poggio & Mountcastle (1960) was the first to show that thalamic nuclei of the PO area contained numerous neurons responsive to noxious stimuli, in cats lightly anaesthetized with barbiturates. Receptive fields of these neurons, in contrast to 'non-noxious' responsive ones, were usually large, sometimes including half of the body or a whole limb; they were bilateral in half the cases and strictly contralateral in the other half, and usually well delineated. Several subsequent studies failed to reveal a significant number of such neurons in the PO of the cat. This discrepancy may be due to the use of deeply anaesthetized animals, since Poggio & Mountcastle's results were later confirmed by two different groups (Wagman & Dong 1974; Guilbaud et al 1974, 1977) using, respectively, light barbiturate anaesthesia and hyperventilated animals. These data clearly showed that, in the cat, PO neurons can play a role in the processing of noxious input; in contrast, in this species, few if any 'noxious responsive neurons' were observed in the VB and this negative result was especially clear (Woda et al 1975; Guilbaud et al 1977) when using Rinvik's (1968) delineation of the thalamic nuclei. Such results can be compared with the anatomical studies which show that the spinothalamic tract does not project to the VB in the cat (Boivie 1971; Berkley 1980). It may be noticed that studies pointing out the presence in the VB of the cat of neurons excited by noxious muscular inputs (Kniffki & Mizumura 1983; Honda et al 1983) or from the tooth pulp stimulated by noxious electrical shock (Yokota et al 1986) are essentially located in the shell and not in the core of the VB, possibly in an area where few spinothalamic or trigeminothalamic tract terminals have been described (Craig et al 1989).

In contrast, in the rat and monkey, the VB complex seems to have a crucial role in nociception, as shown by several series of experiments. In both species there are numerous neurons activated, exclusively or not, by noxious somatic stimuli, either mechanical or thermal (Hellon & Mitchell 1975; Guilbaud et al 1980; Kenshalo et al 1980; Chung et al 1986). Interestingly, neurons with similar properties have also been found in the VB of awake monkeys (Casey 1983). These 'noxious responsive neurons' are intermingled with 'non-noxious responsive neurons', as are the terminals of the spinothalamic and the lemniscal tracts, in particular in the rat. In the rat, as in the PO of the cat, receptive fields are often bilateral, but well delineated, while in the monkey there are mainly small contralateral receptive fields. Although a strict somatotopy similar to that described for 'lemniscal' non-noxious responsive neurons (Mountcastle 1980) cannot be found for noxious responsive units, they follow a preferential distribution, rostrocaudal in the rat, lateromedial in the monkey: neurons responding to stimuli applied on the posterior part of the body are located in the rostral (rat) or lateral (monkey) region of the VB. In the caudal part of the rat VB thalamus, there are also neuronal responses to mechanical noxious orofacial stimulation (Raboisson et al 1989). In the rat VB a clear relation exists between the depth of noxious cutaneous indentation and the response intensity, and responses are enhanced over the acute phase of inflammation elicited by injection of carrageenin into the neuronal RFs (Guilbaud et al 1987b) (Fig. 6.1). With hot thermal cutaneous stimulus the activation thresholds of rat and monkey VB neurons are clearly in the noxious range (around 44–45°C) and their discharge frequency can be related to the intensity of the stimulus, to its duration, and sometimes to the area of stimulation (Peschanski et al 1980; Kenshalo et al 1980; Guilbaud et al 1987a) (Fig. 6.2). Sensitization phenomena have been observed in both species after several applications of noxious thermal stimuli, and also after an acute carrageenin-inflammation in the rat (Guilbaud et al 1986, 1987a). In both species it has been established that these VB neuronal responses to noxious stimuli are abolished after section of the ventrolateral funiculus contralateral to

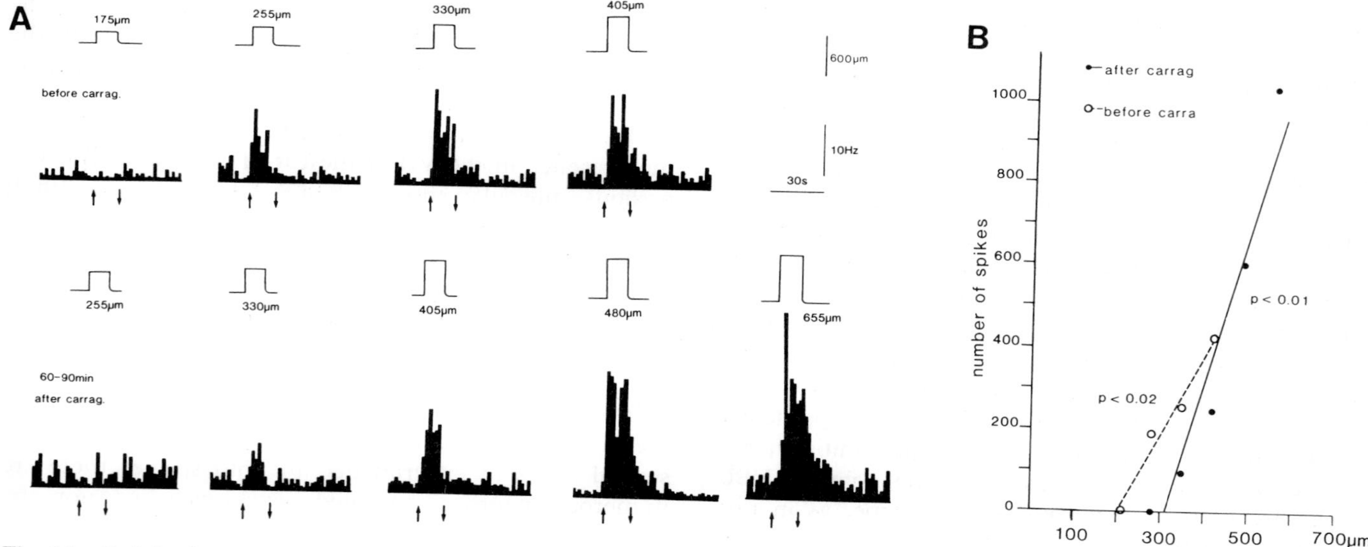

Fig. 6.1 Peristimulus histograms illustrating responses of a rat ventrobasal thalamic neuron exclusively driven by noxious stimulation, to indentations of progressively increasing depth (175–655 μm), before and after carrageenin injection. Relation between number of spikes and indentation on the right part of the figure. (From Guilbaud et al 1987b.)

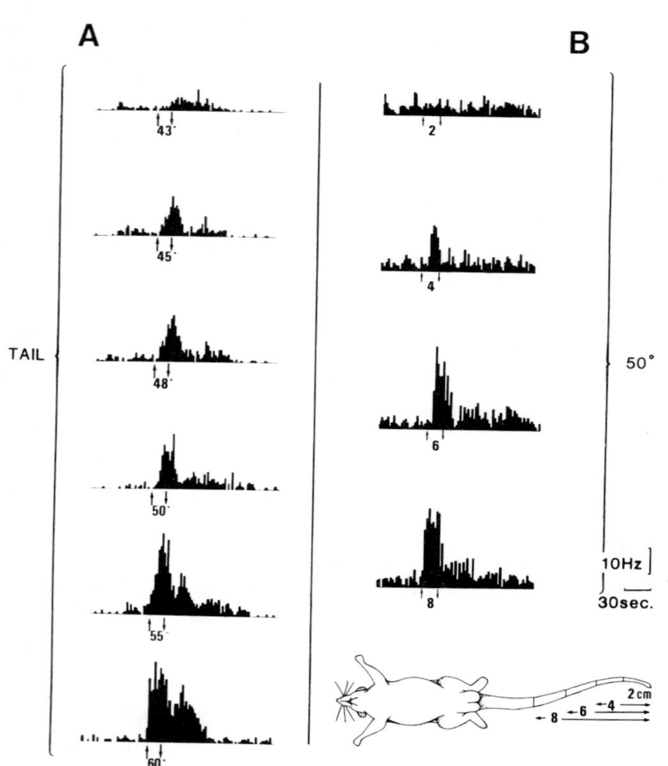

Fig. 6.2 Responses of two rat ventrobasal thalamic neurones exclusively driven by noxious stimulation to noxious heat stimuli graded in temperature (A) or applied to different surface areas (B). (From Peschanski et al 1980.)

the stimulated RFs (Kenshalo et al 1980; Peschanski et al 1985; Chung et al 1986). Finally, in the rat, low doses of morphine in the therapeutic range (0.1–1mg/kg i.v.) and other analgesics strongly depress VB neuronal responses to noxious heat or to mechanical stimuli, which give rise to nociceptive manifestations (Benoist et al 1983, 1986; Kayser et al 1983). The role of the VB complex in the sensory-discriminative aspect of pain, suggested by the ability of these neurons to encode the stimulus intensity, is also emphasized by a behavioural study which showed that the vocalization threshold to hindpaw pressure was enhanced after a neuronal lesion produced by the application of kainic acid in the part of the complex where the lumbar spinothalamic tract terminates; in the same rats the threshold for vocalization by pressing the forepaw was unchanged (Kayser et al 1985). Despite the possible role of thalamic VB complex in integration of noxious somatic messages, a large body of electrophysiological data showed that VB neurons in the rat and monkey, or neurons of the VPL shell in the cat, are additionally responsive to intense visceral stimuli arising from many visceral organs (Horie & Yokota 1990; Ness & Gebhart 1990; Chandler et al 1992; Berkley et al 1993). Due to the large convergence of somatic and visceral inputs on these neurons it is therefore possible that they might also be associated with a wider range of actions which do not necessarily involve sensory discrimination.

It is well known that thalamic structures have a dense projection to the somatosensory cortex. However, the role of the cortex in nociception and pain has long been and continues to be disputed, mainly on the basis of neurosurgical observations (see refs in White & Sweet 1969; Lamour et al 1983c). Nevertheless, several electrophysiological studies have established that numerous neurons in cat primary (SI) and the secondary (SII) somatosensory cortex are activated by electrical stimulation of the tooth pulp which contains mainly thin afferent fibres (see refs in Guilbaud et al 1989a). In addition, following the demonstrations reported above, it could be hypothetized that noxious messages reaching the rat VB are transmitted to primary somatosensory motor (SMI) cortex, since in this species, most (if not all) VB neurons are projection neurons (Saporta & Kruger 1977; Wells et al 1982; Harris & Hendrickson 1985). In the monkey more direct evidence has been obtained in that some noxious responsive VPL neurons have been antidromically activated from SI (Kenshalo et al 1980). Combining electrophysiology and anatomy Gingold et al (1991) provided further evidence that nociceptive inputs could reach the cortex in monkey. It is therefore not surprising that several studies of this cortical area in the two species have shown (Fig. 6.3) neurons responsive to noxious stimuli in the last decade (Lamour et al 1982, 1983b, 1983c; Kenshalo & Isensee 1983; Kenshalo et al 1988; Chudler et al 1990; Guilbaud et al 1992; Vin-Christian et al 1992). These neurons are located in deep cortical laminae in rats (Lamour et al 1983b) and in laminae III and IV in monkey (Chudler et al 1990). In the two species, these cortical neurons exhibit properties comparable to those of VB thalamic neurons, in particular, with regard to their ability to encode graded heat stimuli (Fig. 6.4). Several recent studies in animal models of clinical pain have provided new evidence on the role of cortex in nociceptive process (Vin-Christian et al 1992; Guilbaud et al 1992) (see below).

In summary, in the PO group and VB complex of the thalamus, and in cortical SI and/or SII areas of several species, there are neurons responding to noxious stimuli. Their characteristics, and in particular the fact that their activities reflect the various parameters of noxious stimuli, support the hypothesis that they participate in some sensory-discriminative aspects of pain. Interestingly, in the thalamus of patients with central pain unitary neuronal recordings have stressed the presence of bursting activities of high-firing rate in the ventro-caudal nucleus (Lenz et al 1987, 1989), which might be related to pain perception. In addition, and also of interest, a few data obtained in humans by using positron emission tomography (PET) tend to validate the animals' data concerning the role of the somatosensory cortex in nociception. In particular, these human studies stress the cortical representation of heat pain (Jones et al 1991; Talbot et al 1991). Combining PET with magnetic resonance imaging, Talbot et al clearly showed that a frank and durable painful heat stimulus (double pulse 47–49°C, on six spots total duration about 2 min) caused a significant activation of the contralateral anterior cingulate, and the primary and secondary somatosensory cortices. Although few, these pioneer studies allow us to

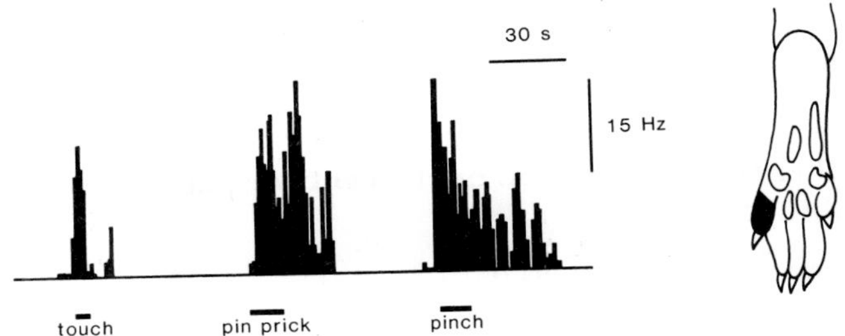

Fig. 6.3 Responses of a neuron recorded in the rat primary somatosensory cortex driven by both non-noxious and noxious stimuli. Note the intensity and the long afterdischarge of the response in the latter case. (From Lamour et al 1983c.)

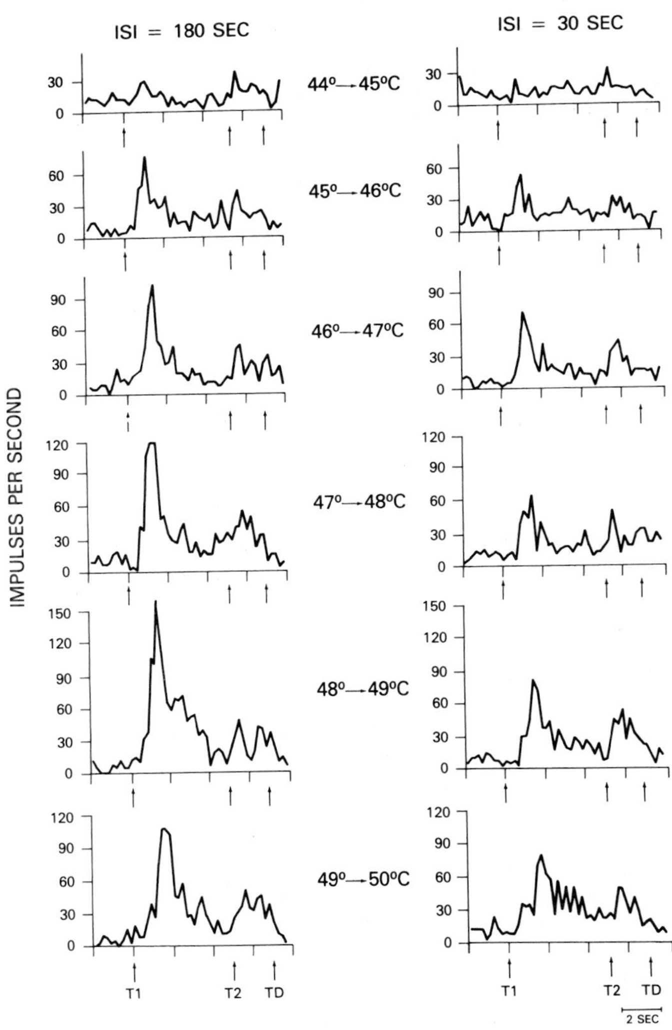

Fig. 6.4 Responses of a monkey SI neuron driven by both non-noxious and noxious mechanical stimuli to heat stimuli of graded temperature. Averaged peristimulus time histograms obtained when the interstimulus interval was 180 and 30 s. Numbers in the middle of the figure refer to the initial and final temperature presented. Binwidth 100 ms. (From Chudler et al 1990.)

expect further progress in understanding supraspinal pain processes by developing similar types of investigation.

Other thalamic nuclei: nuclei centralis lateralis and submedius

Nucleus centralis lateralis (CL)

From the anatomical studies referred to above, it has been well established that the nucleus centralis is another major site of projection for the STT (see refs in Willis 1989, Willis & Coggeshall 1991). Electrophysiological data concerning this nucleus per se are in fact much more scarce than is thought, due to the confusion between CL and other intralaminar nuclei, namely the centre median-parafascicular complex (CM–Pf) which does not receive STT terminals: indeed, the existence of spinal afferents to the parafascicular and centre median areas, although suggested in earlier studies (Bowsher 1966) is now generally denied in both past and more recent papers (Mehler 1969; Boivie 1979; Peschanski & Ralston 1985, Gingold et al 1991; ref. in Willis & Coggeshall 1991). However, the characteristics of neuronal responses seem to be similar in both the CL and CM–Pf (Dong et al 1978; Peschanski et al 1981). In particular neurons can be activated from diffuse RFs including most parts of the body (see below). In arthritic rats, however, some CL neuronal responses have comparable characteristics to those found in the VB complex (i.e. more limited RFs) (Kayser et al 1984), a fact which fits well with the collateralization of a few STT axons between the two structures (Giesler et al 1981). The distinguishing feature of the nucleus centralis, especially of its caudolateral portion receiving STT afferents (Ma et al 1987), is that it is strongly related to areas which are involved in motor activity, such as the cerebellum, and also the precentral cortex (see discussion in Mehler 1974 and Itoh & Mizuno 1977; Molinari et al 1986).

Nucleus submedius (Sm)

The presence of afferents originating in the spinal cord (and the trigeminal subnucleus caudalis) in the nucleus submedius of the medial thalamus, especially in its dorsal part, has been demonstrated by Craig & Burton (1981) in the cat, Peschanski (1984) and Ma et al (1987) in the rat, and confirmed by several anatomical studies in the former species (Craig et al 1982; Manthy 1983; Craig & Burton 1985; Ma et al 1987, Craig & Dostrovsky 1991; Blomqvist et al 1992) but questioned in rat (Dado & Giesler 1990). A systematic investigation performed in this species has clearly shown that numerous neurons in Sm were also exclusively activated by somatic stimuli, which elicited nociceptive behaviours in the freely moving animal (Dostrovsky et al 1987; Dostrovsky & Guilbaud 1988). In fact, the characteristics of its neuronal responses resemble more closely those recorded in the intralaminar nuclei, and in the medial thalamus in general (Dostrovsky & Guilbaud 1990) than those observed in the VB. In the cat, several electrophysiological data suggest that this area might play a role in some aspects of nociception and pain (Craig & Burton 1981; Craig & Kniffki 1985; Craig et al 1989) and in addition could have a role in thermal perception principally to cold (Craig & Dostrovsky 1991).

Some of the supraspinal structures described above and some of mesencephalic structures described in the next section receive noxious information through the spinocervicothalamic tract and the postsynaptic dorsal column fibre pathway. However the functional role of this pathway in nociception and pain remains poorly understood (see discussion in Besson & Chaouch 1987 and Willis & Coggeshall 1991).

SUPRASPINAL AREAS RECEIVING PROJECTIONS THROUGH THE SPINORETICULAR TRACTS

Numerous electrophysiological and behavioural studies undoubtedly favour an involvement of the reticular formation of the brain stem in the phenomena of nociception. However, data on the spinoreticular tract (SRT) are much more difficult to interpret than data on the STT. Several reasons for this emerge:

1. Unlike the relatively well circumscribed projections of the STT, the SRT projections arrive at different levels of the brainstem extending between the medulla and mesencephalon.
2. The role in nociception of certain of its components, such as those projections to the lateral reticular nucleus usually implicated in cerebellar functions, are still little understood.
3. The SRT axons are intermingled with spinothalamic and spinocerebellar axons.
4. Anatomical and electrophysiological studies indicate that STT axons can send collaterals toward bulbar and mesencephalic reticular regions. At least two components seem to make up the main spinoreticular tract, one terminating in the bulbopontine zone and another projecting to the mesencephalic level.

THE BULBOPONTINE COMPONENT AND ITS THALAMIC PROJECTIONS

In the monkey both electrophysiological and histochemical tracings have revealed the greatest concentration of spinoreticular neurons in laminae VII, VIII and X with few cells located in the dorsal horn (Willis 1989; Willis & Coggeshall 1991). After the administration of a retrograde tracer in the medullary reticular formation labelled spinal cells are frequently bilateral at the cervical level, whereas in the lumbar enlargement more labelled cells are found contralaterally. SRT cells with cutaneous receptive fields can be driven either from restricted distal cutaneous areas or from bilateral receptive fields. The great majority of spinoreticular neurons can be classified as nociceptive specific cells while others are nociceptive nonspecific.

The termination sites of the bulbopontine component are located in the nucleus gigantocellularis, the nucleus reticularis pontis caudalis and oralis, the nucleus paragigantocellularis (NGC), the subnucleus reticularis dorsalis and the nucleus subcoeruleus (see refs in Willis & Coggeshall 1991). There is no somatotopic organization. In addition dense projections of lamina I neurons have been identified on to the lateral reticular nucleus and in the adjacent A1 noradrenergic group (Menétrey et al 1992). However evidence for the involvement of the lateral reticular nucleus in pain is unclear since the nucleus is linked with the cerebellum.

The electrophysiological characteristics of neurons recorded in the bulbopontine reticular formation are extremely complex. For example, in the NGC some of them only respond to noxious stimuli (Burton 1968; Benjamin 1970) whereas others are also responsive to peripheral tapping. The hypothesis of the involvement of NGC in nociception has been strongly supported by the experiments of Casey (1971a, 1971b) who combined electrophysiological and behavioural studies in freely moving cats. By stimulating a cutaneous nerve, he showed that NGC neuronal firing reached its maximum at an intensity of stimulation high enough to elicit escape behaviour. Moreover, direct electrical stimulation of the NGC through the recording electrode induced similar escape behaviour. It is well substantiated that NGC neurons can participate in some spino-bulbospinal reflex responses, several neurons being at the origin of a reticulospinal tract (ref. in Guilbaud et al 1989a). NGC can also participate in other mechanisms of nociception and pain through its ascending projections, in particular towards medial thalamic structures, namely the nucleus CM–Pf (Bowsher 1966; Peschanski & Besson 1984).

Electrophysiological studies on CM–Pf neurons have been badly hampered by the problems which were presented in the introduction, in particular with regard to the question of anaesthesia. Indeed, in the awake monkey, Casey (1966) observed noxious responsive neurons which were no longer activated by similar stimuli after the induction of a moderate level of anaesthesia. The use of deep anaesthesia is likely to explain why some authors failed to observe tonic responses to noxious cutaneous stimuli. In contrast, in the cat and the rat, either awake or moderately anaesthetized, these neuronal responses can be repeatedly obtained and the authors agree that numerous neurons in the area are excited by noxious stimuli (see refs in Guilbaud et al 1989a). The characteristics of neuronal responses are noticeably similar to those described in NGC. Responses to graded heat stimuli have been tested in the rat (Peschanski et al 1981) and it was observed that, in contrast to VB neuronal responses, there was not a clear relationship between the temperature of the stimulus and the neuronal firing. Moreover, the mean threshold for the responses was not only much higher (between 48–50°C) than in the VB, but also higher than is generally accepted for pain sensation in humans and nocifensive reflexes in rats (Lamotte & Campbell 1978). Due to these functional characteristics – diffuse or very large receptive fields, lack of encoding of the parameters of the noxious stimulus, high threshold – it seems difficult to implicate these reticular and medial thalamic structures in some sensory-discriminative aspects of pain and nociception. However, on the basis of recent data showing that some single CM–Pf neurons discriminate changes in the intensity of noxious stimuli in awake rhesus monkey, the question of participation of medial thalamus (CM–Pf) in both discriminative and affective dimensions of pain perception was addressed (Buschnell & Duncan 1989). Nevertheless, the neuronal activation threshold was between 45–50°C, slightly higher than in the VB of anaesthetized rat (Peschanski et al 1980, Guilbaud et al 1987b) and even that of the monkey (Kenshalo et al 1980) (around 44–45°C); in addition, their activity was influenced by attention (Buschnell & Duncan 1989). Thus, even if the CM–Pf of monkey participates in the sensory discriminative component of pain, numerous ancient and more recent investigations have underlined that, due to its massive projections to striatal structures (Herkenham 1980; Bentivoglio et al 1981; ref. in Guilbaud et al 1989a), it could be involved in motor and arousal reactions which contribute to the systems of defence against nociceptive aggression (see Albe-Fessard & Besson 1973; Casey & Jones 1978; Albe-Fessard et al 1985). In fact, in a large investigation of the rat medial thalamus, including a large number of nuclei, it was shown that there are nociceptive neurons not only in the intralaminar nuclei, but also throughout the medial thalamus, including the medial dorsal nucleus, anterior medial nucleus, ventral medial nucleus, and ventral lateral nucleus (Dostrovsky & Guilbaud 1990). The response characteristics and receptive fields of all these neurons are virtually identical, suggesting that they could also be involved in mediating affective and motivational aspects of pain. Most recent anatomical studies of the striatal and cortical projection sites of intralaminar and midline thalamic nuclei in monkey and in rat provide further arguments for their participation in the affective and non-discriminative aspects of nociceptive information (Sadikot et al 1990; Berendse & Groenewegen 1991). It is even suggested that the midline and intrathalamic nuclei could prepare the striatum for an imminent cortical input or induce a time-locked initial behavioural response to be modified by the integrated cortical input (Berendse & Groenewegen 1991).

Recently a restricted region in the reticular formation of the caudal medulla, the subnucleus reticularis dorsalis (SRD) has been shown to contain numerous neurons exclusively activated by thermal and mechanical cutaneous noxious stimuli. They receive inputs from Aδ- and C-fibres (Villanueva et al 1988a). In addition, they encode the intensity of peripheral stimulation (Villanueva et al 1988b). The role of this area remains to be elucidated since some of its efferent projections descend (spinal cord) or reach the oral motor nuclei and the inferior olive (Bernard et al 1990). Nevertheless, because a marked projection ascends to the thalamus (CM–Pf and ventromedial nucleus) the SRD could be a part of the reticular formation which relays nociceptive messages in the spinoreticulothalamic pathway.

THE SPINOMESENCEPHALIC COMPONENT

Spinal cord neurons at the origin of the spinomesencephalic tract (SMT) are largely distributed in the grey matter. In the monkey they are located in laminae I and IV–VI (Willis & Coggeshall 1991) and in the rat in laminae I, V, VII, X and in the lateral spinal nucleus (Menétrey et al 1982; Willis 1989). Below the upper spinal cord, the SMT projections are predominantly contralateral. In the rat, numerous lamina I cells are at the origin of the SMT. SMT lamina I cells ascend in the dorsolateral funiculus while the others ascend in the ventrolateral white matter. The SMT terminates in numerous areas including the periaqueductal grey matter, the deep layers of superior colliculi, the parabrachial nucleus, the pretectal nuclei and the nucleus of Darkschewitsch.

The possible role of the parabrachial nucleus will be discussed in detail below. From a more general point of view it has been shown that at the level of mesencephalic tegmentum a relative high percentage of neurons have their activities affected by noxious stimulation. The importance of marginal zone projections underlines the involvement of SMT in pain mechanisms (Guilbaud et al 1989a).

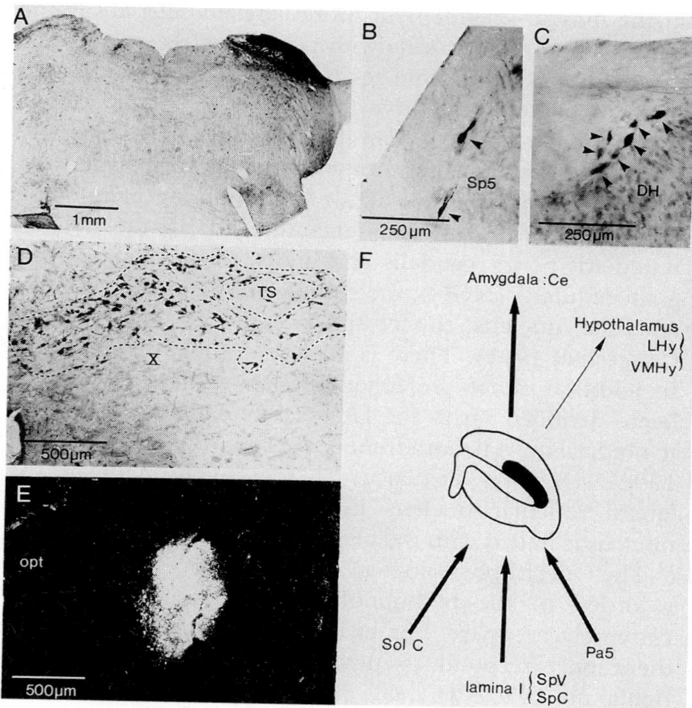

Fig. 6.5 Bright-field photomicrographs (A–D). **A** Injection site in the lateral parabrachial area. **B** Labelled cells in the marginal layer of the caudal trigeminal subnucleus. **C** Labelled cells in the lamina I of the spinal cord. **D** Labelled cells in the mediocaudal part of the nucleus of the solitary tract. Dark-field photomicrograph (E). **E** Anterograde labelling in the nucleus centralis of the amygdala. **F** Summary diagram of the connections of the subregion centered in the external portion of the lateral parabrachial area. DH = dorsal horn of the spinal cord; opt = optic tract; Pa5 = paratrigeminal nucleus; Sol C = caudal portion of the nucleus of the solitary tract; TS = tract solitary; SpC = spinal cord; SpV = trigeminal subnucleus caudalis; Sp5 = spinal trigeminal nucleus; X = dorsal motor nucleus of the vagus. (From Bernard et al 1989.)

BRAIN AREAS RECEIVING PROJECTIONS THROUGH NEWLY DESCRIBED PATHWAYS

THE SPINO(TRIGEMINO)PONTOAMYGDALOID PATHWAY

The parabrachial (PB) area is a group of cells that surrounds the brachium conjunctivum in the dorsolateral pons and runs up to the mesencephalic tegmentum. Part of this region, i.e. the lateral PB area, has recently been recognized as a major site of projection of axons originating from lamina I (Fig. 6.5) (Cechetto et al 1985; Blomqvist et al 1985; McMahon & Wall 1985; Panneton & Burton 1985) and more recently from the lateral spinal nucleus and to a lesser extent from laminae V and X of the spinal cord (Menétrey & de Pommery 1991). Lamina I neurons projecting to the PB area have been shown to be specifically driven by noxious stimuli (Hylden et al 1985, 1986; Light et al 1987).

Subsequently, in the parabrachial area, neurons backfired from the amygdala and located in a restricted region, the subnuclei external lateral (PBel) and external medial (PBem), have been shown to respond exclusively to noxious stimuli (Bernard & Besson 1988, 1990) (Fig. 6.6). Several reasons indicate that these parabrachioamygdaloid neurons convey mainly nociceptive information from different parts of the body. Numerous neurons responded to noxious mechanical and/or thermal stimuli. They are able to encode the intensity of the stimulation in the nociceptive range (44–52°C). They respond to the activation of Aδ- and/or C-fibres. The excitatory receptive fields of these nociceptive specific neurons were large for

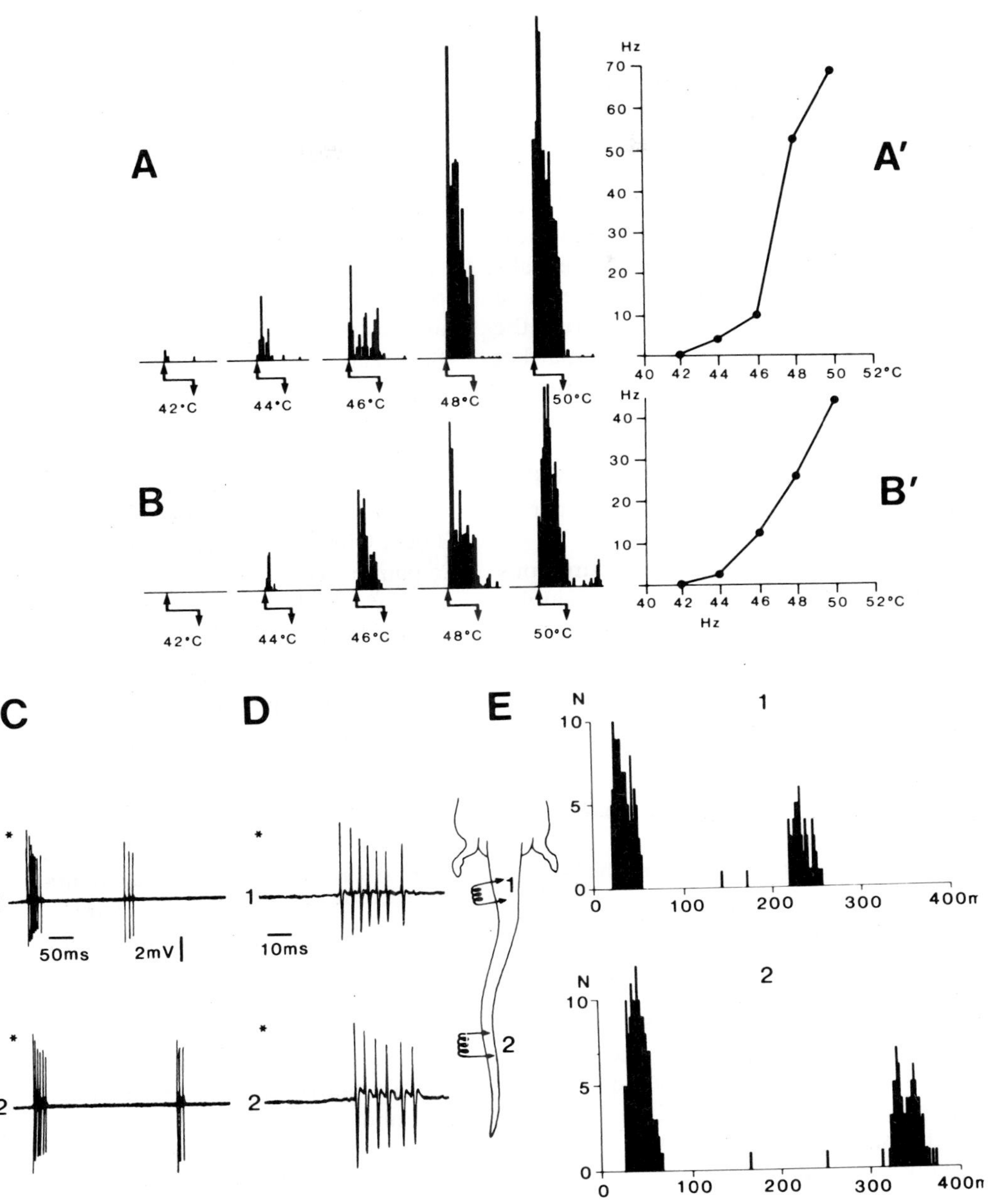

Fig. 6.6 **A–B** Encoding properties of nociceptive-specific parabrachioamygdaloid neurons to thermal stimulation. **C–E** Responses of nociceptive specific parabrachioamygdaloid neurons to percutaneous electrical stimulation of the tail. C1 and 2: single-sweep recordings of the early and late peaks evoked by stimulation of the base (C1) and the tip (C2, 50 ms apart) of the tail; D1 and 2: same response as in C1 and 2, but the scale shows detail of the early peaks. **E** Poststimulus histograms of cumulative responses (modified from Bernard & Besson 1990).

the majority (70%) of cells including several areas of the body, whilst in remaining cases (30%), it was relatively small. In numerous cases, the response due to C-fibres exhibited a wind-up phenomenon during repetitive stimulation (0.66 Hz). This phenomenon can be related to psychological observations in humans where repetitive stimulation produces an increased painful sensation.

The fact that these neurons were backfired from the amygdala is in good agreement with anatomical data showing that the PBel and PBem densely project onto the nucleus centralis of the amygdala (Ce) (Fig. 6.5) (Saper & Loewy 1980; Ottersen 1981; Fulwiler & Saper 1984; Bernard et al 1989). This is coherent with a previous electron microscopic study using double-labelling techniques where Ma & Peschanski (1988) observed synaptic contacts between spinal afferents and parabrachial neurons retrogradely labelled from the amygdala. However, despite numerous anatomical studies demonstrating the efferent projection of the parabrachial PB area to the Ce, the detailed location of terminal fibres in the Ce subregion from PB subnuclei is as yet largely unknown. Using a very sensitive and selective anterograde axonal marker, Phaseolus vulgaris leucoagglutinin (PHA-L), injected into very restricted sites it was shown that these dense projections of the PB to the Ce were topographically organized in three pathways, and two of them seem to convey nociceptive and autonomic messages, whereas the third could be involved in gustatory processes (Bernard et al 1993). By comparison, less dense but significant ascending projection of the PB has been observed at the level of the bed nucleus of the stria terminalis, the substantia innominata–globus pallidus ventralis (SI–GPv), the hypothalamus and the thalamus (see also Saper & Loewy 1980).

Eectrophysiological studies have shown that numerous neurons located in the Ce and the SI–GPv have similar properties to neurons recorded in the PBel and PBem but with larger receptive fields (Bernard et al 1992)

From the pharmacological point of view it has been shown that relatively low doses of intravenous morphine dose-dependently depress in a naloxone reversible fashion the responses induced by noxious stimuli at both the PB area and the amygdala (Bernard et al 1990; Huang et al 1993).

On the basis of the density of projection from the lamina I to the PB area and from the PB area to the CL of the amygdala, the spino(trigemino)pontoamygdaloid tract constitutes a marked anatomical and electrophysiological entity, which is implicated in the transmission of nociceptive messages. The observation of large RFs suggests that this pathway is not primarily involved in the sensory discrimination of noxious stimuli. The role of such a pathway in pain is a matter of speculation. It is proposed (see discussion in Bernard & Besson 1990) that this system could be involved in the emotional-affective (fear and memory of the aggression); behavioural (vocalization, flight, freezing, defence and offence); and autonomic (pupil dilatation, cardiorespiratory and adrenocortical responses and micturition) reactions to noxious events.

THE SPINOHYPOTHALAMIC COMPONENT

It is known that a certain number of neurons located in the hypothalamus can be activated by noxious cutaneous stimulation and visceral distension (see refs in Burstein et al 1991). This is reminiscent of the fact that these areas are involved in the regulation of autonomic, neuroendocrine, behavioural and affective responses to intense stimuli. There is general agreement that sensory information from the spinal cord ascends to the hypothalamus indirectly through multisynaptic pathways (as an example, the parabrachial area projects to several hypothalamic areas). Recently a direct spinohypothalamic projection has been described by Giesler's group (Burstein et al 1987, 1990, 1991; Cliffer et al 1991). These authors reported that 87% of spinohypothalamic neurons responded preferentially or exclusively to noxious stimuli. They are located in the superficial and deep dorsal horn and ascend in the lateral quadrant; these electrophysiological investigations were confirmed by retrograde labelling with fluorogold showing that more than 9000 spinal neurons are at the origin of this tract (Burstein et al 1990). Surprisingly a small number of hypothalamic labelled terminals have been shown with an anterograde tracing using Phaseolus vulgaris leucoagglutinin (Cliffer et al 1991) This controversy could be due at least in part to the fact that there is evidence that fluorogold can be transported avidly through fibres of passage (Dado et al 1990). Thus, without downgrading the role of the hypothalamus in pain processes, several questions remain to be answered concerning the relative importance of direct or indirect pathways reaching this area.

ELECTROPHYSIOLOGICAL STUDIES OF SOME SUPRASPINAL AREAS IN MODELS OF INFLAMMATORY AND NEUROPATHIC PAIN

Most of the experimental data reported so far involve nociception, whereas clinicians address problems of pain. The development of experimental models mimicking various clinical pain syndromes can reconcile both approaches and may eventually provide a clearer view of the real supraspinal mechanisms of pain. Several experimental models have been used for electrophysiological recordings in thalamic and cortical structures. Rats rendered arthritic by the injection of Freund's adjuvant into the tail (Pearson & Wood 1959) are commonly used as a model of inflammatory arthritic pain (ref. in Besson & Guilbaud 1988). Rats injected with Freund's adjuvant 3–4 weeks previously, at a time when arthritis is at a maximum, have been used for a systematic electrophysiological exploration of some thalamic structures (VB, CM–Pf, nuclei centralis lateralis and submedius) and the primary somatosensory cortex. As at the spinal level (Menétrey & Besson 1982; Calvino et al 1987), there are profound changes in the responses of the somatosensory neurons recorded in these areas, compared with those observed in normal animals (Gautron & Guilbaud 1982; Lamour et al 1983a; Kayser & Guilbaud 1984; Dostrovsky & Guilbaud 1988, 1990). Unlike normal rats, only a few neurons are activated by intense mechanical stimulation in arthritic rats, whereas many cells are driven by mild stimulation of the joints or adjacent cutaneous areas (light pressure, flexion or extension movement, sometimes brush) (Fig. 6.7). The functional implication of these neuronal responses is supported by the fact that

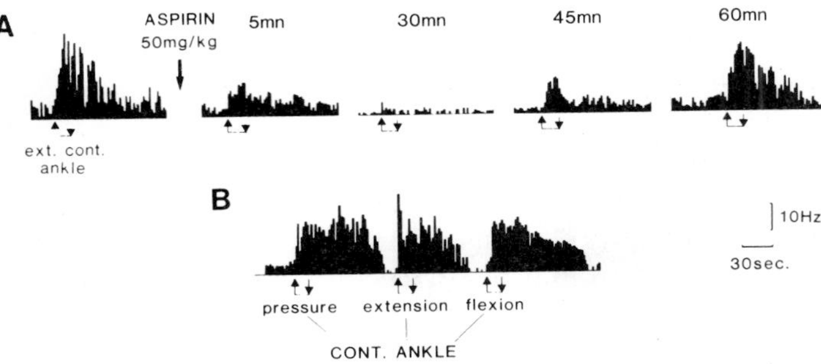

Fig. 6.7 Responses of two ventrobasal thalamic neurons recorded in arthritic rats to moderate stimulation applied to the contralateral ankle. Responses presented long afterdischarges and can be depressed by aspirin as neuron **A**. (From Gautron & Guilbaud 1982; Guilbaud et al 1982.)

they are strongly depressed by aspirin and other nonsteroidal antitinflammatory drugs (NSAIDs), well known to be particularly effective against arthritic pain (Guilbaud et al 1982; Dostrovsky & Guilbaud 1988; Attal et al 1988). The depressive effect of aspirin (Fig. 6.7) clearly reflects its peripheral action on the responses of mechanoreceptors of the inflamed ankle joint (Guilbaud & Iggo 1985). Interestingly, further observations suggest that the ascending pathways and supraspinal neuronal populations involved in the transmission of nociceptive messages from the inflamed joints differ from those influenced by noxious stimulation in the normal rat (Lamour et al 1983a, 1983b, 1983c; Guilbaud 1988).

Models of restricted inflammatory pain are also interesting. In particular, the intraplantar injection of carrageenin, a polysaccharide, commonly used to induce inflammation and hyperalgesia in several pharmacological tests of antiinflammatory and analgesic drugs, has been used over the last decade for the study of the mechanisms underlying hyperalgesia using various approaches (ref. in Besson & Guilbaud 1988). It has been clearly demonstrated that during the early phase of the inflammatory process, not only responses of cutaneous, muscular and joint nociceptors (Kocher et al 1987; Schaible & Schmidt 1988; Berberich et al 1988), but those of certain dorsal horn neurons, thalamic neurons (Schaible et al 1987; Hoheisel & Mense 1989) and thalamic SmI cortical neurons (Guilbaud et al 1986; Vin-Christian 1992), are significantly enhanced. The time-course of these modifications is similar to that of the hyperalgesia as gauged by the vocalization threshold to paw pressure (Kayser & Guilbaud 1987). In addition the enhanced neuronal responses could be depressed by the administration of antagonists of various inflammatory substances released in the exudate (histamine antagonist, 5HT antagonist, aspirin) (Neil et al 1987; Guilbaud et al 1989a).

In addition to these models of inflammatory pain, several models of neuropathic pain have been developed. One of these models (Bennett & Xie 1988), which produces a peripheral unilateral mononeuropathy in the rat by loose ligatures applied around the common sciatic nerve, has been extensively studied. Behavioural studies with the model have provided evidence of pain-related behaviours: notably hyperalgesia and allodynia to mechanical and thermal stimulus (both to heat and cold). Furthermore, the analysis and quantification of abnormal positions of the paw with the ligated sciatic provides a tool for assessing 'spontaneous' pain-related behaviours (Attal et al 1990). Electrophysiological studies performed in the VB thalamic complex and in the primary somatosensory cortex of these rats (Guilbaud et al 1990, 1992), 2–3 weeks after the nerve ligatures, when pain-related behaviours are well developed, revealed (Figs 6.8 and 6.9):

1. Exacerbated thalamic and cortical neuronal responses to mechanical and above all thermal (hot and cold) stimulation, which relate well to the modifications observed in the behavioural studies.
2. A cortical reorganization of the somatic inputs with an increase in cutaneous saphenous nerve inputs and also in joint inputs.

This latter phenomenon could reflect the abnormal paw position due to the reluctance of the rat to press the

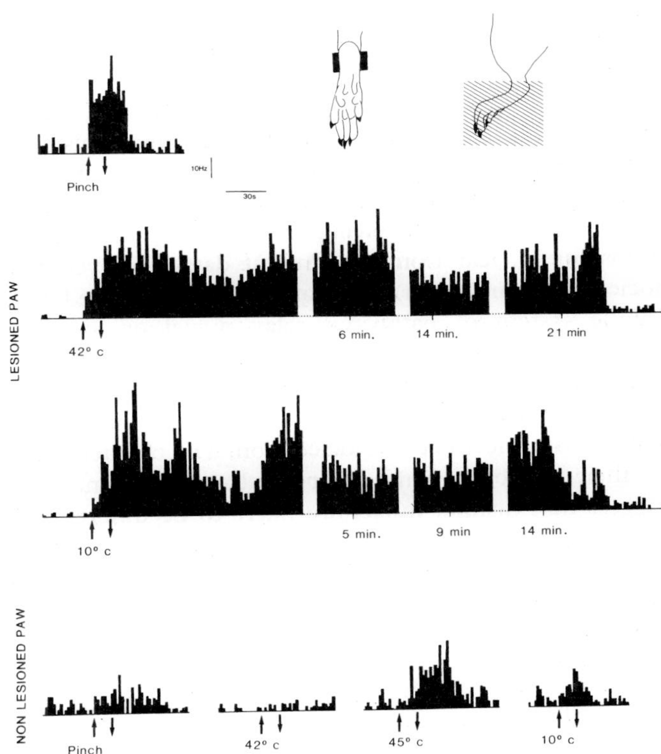

Fig. 6.8 Responses of a left ventrobasal thalamic neurone opposite to the lesioned sciatic nerve to stimulations applied to the lesioned (3 top traces) and to the intact paw (last trace). Note the afterdischarge of long duration for thermal stimuli. (From Guilbaud et al 1990.)

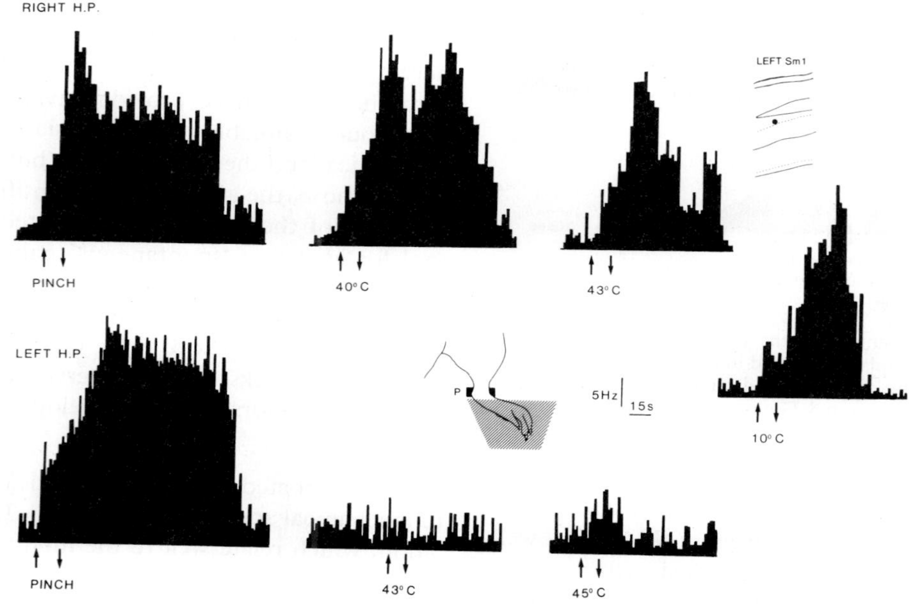

Fig. 6.9 Responses of a left SmI neuron opposite to the lesioned sciatic nerve activated by pinch applied either to the right lesioned or to the left non-lesioned paw. The 10°C waterbath was ineffective when applied to the left paw (not shown) and induced a very intense response when applied to the right lesioned paw. (From Guilbaud et al 1992.)

hindpaw normally on the floor, and/or be involved in altered non-nociceptive or nociceptive behaviours.

CONCLUSION

Experimental data relating to supraspinal mechanisms of nociception and pain are still incomplete. It must be noted that the available information essentially includes only those structures receiving direct spinal projections. It is absolutely clear from the present data, however, that nociception (and pain) are not exclusively related to a unique system of pathways, relay nuclei or 'centres'. Obviously, neurons within a number of reticular, diencephalic and cortical structures are responsive to noxious stimuli and are likely to have something to do with at least one aspect of nociception. The characteristics of their responses and their anatomical connections suggest that distinct nuclei are likely to be differentially involved in sensory-discriminative or, on the contrary, in motor, motivational and affective functions. However, these hypotheses must be considered with care, particularly when behavioural studies are lacking or contradictory. Moreover, it should be remembered that most experimental data concern nociception while clinicians address problems of pain. The development of experimental models mimicking various intractable pain syndromes should help, in future, to reconcile both approaches and give a better view of the real supraspinal mechanisms of pain. The fact that changes in neuronal activities of rat thalamic and SmI cortical neurons can account for abnormal pain-related behaviours in animals with acute or persistent inflammatory processes, or with a persistent mononeuropathy, emphasizes the roles of these structures in pain processing, as does the fact that their neuronal activities can be depressed by analgesic substances. Moreover, comparison with data obtained in normal rats and in these models has revealed an important reorganization in the various somatic inputs, with involvement of additional neuronal populations and pathways in conditions of clinical pain. There is also great hope that studies of transmitter chemistry of mammalian supraspinal structures (Hirai & Jones 1989; Jones et al 1991) and use of modern imaging techniques (Jones et al 1991; Talbot et al 1991) will shed further light on the relative roles of supraspinal regions in pain and nociception.

REFERENCES

Albe-Fessard D, Besson J M 1973 Convergent thalamic and cortical projections. The non-specific system. In: Iggo A (ed) Handbook of sensory physiology. Springer Verlag, Berlin, p 489–560

Albe-Fessard D, Berkley K J, Kruger L, Ralston H J III, Willis W D Jr 1985 Diencephalic mechanisms of pain sensation. Brain Research Review 9: 217–296

Apkarian A V, Hodge C J Jr 1989 Primate spinothalamic pathways. II. The cells of origin of the dorsolateral and ventral spinothalamic pathways. Journal of Comparative Neurology 288: 474–492

Attal N, Kayser V, Eschalier A, Benoist J M, Guilbaud G 1988 Behavioural and electrophysiological effect of a non-steroidal anti-inflammatory agent, sodium diclofenac. Pain 35: 341–348
Attal N, Kayser V, Jazat F, Guilbaud G 1990 Further evidence for 'pain-related' behaviours in a model of unilateral peripheral mononeuropathy. Pain 41: 235–251
Benjamin R M 1970 Single neurons in the rat medulla responsive to nociceptive stimulation. Brain Research 24: 525–529
Bennett G J, Xie Y K 1988 A peripheral mononeuropathy in rat that produces disorders of pain sensation like those seen in man. Pain 33: 87–107
Benoist J M, Kayser V, Gautron M, Guilbaud G 1983 Low dose of morphine strongly depresses responses of specific neurons in the ventrobasal complex of the rat. Pain 15: 333–344
Benoist J M, Kayser V, Gacel G et al 1986 Differential depressive action of two μ and δ opioid ligands on neuronal responses to noxious stimuli in the thalamic ventrobasal complex of rat. Brain Research 398: 49–56
Bentivoglio M, Macchi C, Albanese A 1981 The cortical projections of the thalamic intralaminar nuclei as studies in cat and rat with the multiple-fluorescence retrograde tracing technique. Neuroscience Letters 26: 5–10
Berberich P, Hoheisel U, Mense S 1988 Effects of carrageenin induced myositis on the discharge properties of group III and IV muscle receptors in cat. Journal of Neurophysiology 59: 1395–1409
Berendse H W, Groenewengen V H 1991 Restricted cortical termination fields of the midline and intralaminar thalamic nuclei in the rat. Neuroscience 42: 73–102
Berkley K 1980 Spatial relationship between the terminations of somatic-sensory and motor pathways in the rostral brainstem of cats and monkeys. I. Ascending somatic sensory inputs to lateral diencephalon. Journal of Comparative Neurology 193: 283–317
Berkley K J, Guilbaud G, Benoist J M, Gautron M 1993 Responses of neurons in and near the thalamus ventrobasal complex of the rat to stimulation of uterus, cervix, vagina, colon and skin. Journal of Neurophysiology 69: 557–568
Bernard J F, Besson J M 1988 Convergence d'informations nociceptives sur des neurones parabachio-amygdaliens chez le rat. Comptes Rendus de l'Académie des Sciences Ser. III-Vie, 307: 841–847
Bernard J F, Besson J M 1990 The spino(trigemino)-pontoamygdaloid pathway: electrophysiological evidence for an involvement in pain processes. Journal of Neurophysiology 63: 473–490
Bernard J F, Ma W, Besson J M, Peschanski M 1986 A monosynaptic spino-ponto-amygdalian pathway possibly involved in pain. Neuroscience Abstracts 12: 13
Bernard J F, Peschanski M, Besson J M 1989 A possible spino(trigemino)-pontoamygdaloid pathway for pain. Neuroscience Letters 100: 83–88
Bernard J F, Villanueva L, Carroue J, Le Bars D 1990 Efferent projections from the subnucleus reticularis dorsalis (SRD): A Phasoleus vulgaris leucoagglutinin study in the rat. Neuroscience Letters 122: 257–262
Bernard J F, Huang G F, Besson J M 1991 Electrophysiological evidence for an involvement of the nucleus centralis of the amygdala in nociception. 20th Annual Meeting, Society for Neuroscience, New Orleans
Bernard J F, Huang G F, Besson J M 1992 The nucleus centralis of the amygdala and the globus pallidus ventralis: electrophysiological evidence for an involvement in pain processes. Journal of Neurophysiology 68: 551–569
Bernard J F, Alden M, Besson J M 1993 The organization of the efferent projections from the pontine parabrachial area to the amygdaloid complex: a Phaseolus vulgaris leucoagglutinin (PHA-L) study in the rat. Journal of Comparative Neurology 329: 201–229
Besson J M, Chaouch A 1987 Peripheral and spinal mechanisms of nociception. Physiological Reviews 67: 67–186
Besson J M, Guilbaud G 1988 The arthritic rat as a model of clinical pain? Excerpta Medica, Amsterdam
Blomqvist A, Flink R, Westman J, Wiberg M 1985 Synaptic terminals in the ventroposterolateral nucleus of the thalamus from neurons in the dorsal column and lateral cervical nuclei: an electron microscopic study in the cat. Journal of Neurocytology 14: 869–886
Blomqvist A, Ma W, Berkley K J 1989 Spinal input to the parabrachial nucleus in the cat. Brain Research 480: 29–36
Blomqvist A, Ericson A-C, Broman J, Craig A D 1992 Electron microscopic identification of lamina I axon terminations in the nucleus submedius of the thalamus. Brain Research 585: 425–430
Boivie J 1971 The termination of the spinothalamic tract in the cat. An experimental study with silver impregnation methods. Experimental Brain Research 12: 331–353
Boivie J 1979 An anatomical reinvestigation of the termination of the spinothalamic tract in the monkey. Journal of Comparative Neurology 186: 343–370
Bowsher D 1966 Some afferent and efferent connections of the parafascicular centre median complex. In: Purpura D P, Yahr M D (eds) The thalamus. Columbia University Press, New York, p 99–108
Burstein R, Cliffer K D, Giesler G J Jr 1987 Direct somatosensory projections from the spinal cord to the hypothalamus and telencephalon. Journal of Neuroscience 7: 4159–4164
Burstein R, Cliffer K D, Giesler G J Jr 1990 Cells of origin of the spinohypothalamic tract in the rat. Journal of Comparative Neurology 291: 329–344
Burstein R, Dado R J, Cliffer K D, Giesler G J Jr 1991 Physiological characteristics of spinohypothalamic tract neurons in the lumbar enlargement of rats. Journal of Neurophysiology 66: 261–284
Burton H 1968 Somatic sensory properties of caudal bulbar reticular neurons in the cat. Brain Research 11: 357–372
Buschnell M C, Duncan G H 1989 Sensory and affective aspects of pain perception: is medial thalamus restricted to emotional issues? Experimental Brain Research 78: 415–418
Calvino B, Crepon-Bernard M O, Le Bars D 1987 Parallel clinical and behavioural studies of adjuvant-induced arthritis in the rat: possible relationship with 'chronic pain'. Behavioural Brain Research 24: 11–29
Casey K L 1966 Unit analysis of nociceptive mechanisms in the thalamus of the awake squirrel monkey. Journal of Neurophysiology 29: 727–750
Casey K L 1971a Responses of bulboreticular units to somatic stimuli eliciting escape behaviour in the cat. International Journal of Neuroscience 2: 15–28
Casey K L 1971b Escape elicited by bulboreticular stimulation in the cat. International Journal of Neuroscience 2: 29–34
Casey K L 1983 Ventral posterior thalamic neurons differentially responsive to noxious stimulation of the awake monkey thalamus. Journal of Neurophysiology 56: 370–390
Casey K L, Jones E G 1978 Supraspinal mechanisms: an overview of ascending pathways: brainstem and thalamus. Neuroscience Research Program Bulletin 16: 103–118
Cechetto, D F, Standaert, D G, Saper C B 1985 Spinal and trigeminal dorsal horn projections to the parabrachial nucleus in the rat. Journal of Comparative Neurology 240: 153–160
Chandler M J, Hobbs S F, Fu Q G et al 1992 Responses of neurons in ventroposterolateral nucleus of primate thalamus to urinary bladder distension. Brain Research 571: 26–34
Chaouch A, Menetrey D, Binder D, Besson J M 1983 Neurons at the origin of the medial component of the spinoreticular tract in the rat: an anatomical study using horseradish peroxidase retrograde transport. Journal of Comparative Neurology 214: 309–320
Chudler E H, Anton F, Dubner R, Kenshalo D R Jr 1990 Responses of nociceptive SI neurons in monkeys and pain sensation in humans elicited by noxious thermal stimulation: effect of interstimulus interval. Journal of Neurophysiology 63: 559–569
Chung I M, Lee K H, Surmeier D J et al 1986 Response characteristics of neurons in the ventral posterior lateral nucleus of the monkey thalamus. Journal of Neurophysiology 56: 370–390
Cliffer K D, Burstein R, Giesler G J Jr 1991 Distributions of spinothalamic, spinohypothalamic, and spinotelencephalic fibers revealed by anterograde transport of PHA-L in rats. Journal of Neuroscience 11: 852–868
Craig A D, Burton H 1981 Spinal and medullary lamina I projection to nucleus submedius in medial thalamus: a possible pain center. Journal of Neurophysiology 45: 443–466
Craig A D, Burton H 1985 The distribution and topographical organization in the thalamus of anterogradely-transported horseradish peroxidase after spinal injections in cat and racoon. Experimental Brain Research 58: 227–254

Craig A D, Dostrovsky J O 1991 Thermoreceptive lamina I trigeminothalamic neurons project to the nucleus submedius in the cat. Experimental Brain Research 85: 470–474

Craig A D, Kniffki K D 1985 Spinothalamic lumbosacral lamina I cells responsive to skin and muscle stimulation in the cat. Journal of Physiology 365: 197–221

Craig A D, Wiegand S J, Price J L 1982 The thalamo-cortical projection of the nucleus submedius in the cat. Journal of Comparative Neurology 206: 28–48

Craig A D, Linington A J, Kniffki KD 1989 Cells of origin of spinothalamic tract projections to the medial and lateral thalamus in the cat. Journal of Comparative Neurology 289: 568–585

Dado R J, Giesler G J Jr 1990 Afferent input to nucleus submedius in rats: retrograde labelling of neurons in the spinal cord and caudal medulla. The Journal of Neuroscience 10: 2672–2686

Dado R J, Burstein R, Cliffer K D, Giesler G J Jr 1990 Evidence that Fluoro-Gold can be transported avidly through fibers of passage. Brain Research 533: 329–333

Dong W K, Ryu H, Wagman I H 1978 Nociceptive responses of neurons in medial thalamus and their relationship to spinothalamic pathways. Journal of Neurophysiology 41: 1592–1613

Dostrovsky J O, Guilbaud G 1988 Noxious stimuli excite neurons in nucleus submedius of the normal and arthritic rat. Brain Research 460: 269–280

Dostrovsky J O, Guilbaud G 1990 Nociceptive responses in medial thalamus of the normal and arthritic rat. Pain 40: 93–104

Dostrovsky J O, Broton J G, Warma N K 1987 Functional properties of subnucleus caudalis lamina I neurons projecting to nucleus submedius. In: Schmidt R F, Schaible H-G, Vahle-Hinz C (eds) Fine afferent nerve fibers and pain. VCH Verlagsgesellschaft, Weinheim, p 358–366

Fulwiler C E, Saper C B 1984 Subnuclear organization of the efferent connections of the parabrachial nucleus in the rat. Brain Research Review 7: 229–259

Gautron M, Guilbaud G 1982 Somatic responses of ventrobasal thalamic neurones in polyarthritic rats. Brain Research 237: 459–471

Giesler G J Jr Yezierski R P, Gerhart K D, Willis W D 1981 Spinothalamic tract neurons that project to medial and/or lateral thalamic nuclei: evidence for a physiologically novel population of spinal cord neurons. Journal of Neurophysiology 46: 1285–1308

Gingold S, Greenspan J D, Apkarian A V 1991 Anatomic evidence of nociceptive inputs to primary somatosensory cortex: relationship between spinothalamic terminals and thalamocortical cells in squirrel monkey. Journal of Comparative Neurology 308: 467–490

Guilbaud G 1988 Peripheral and central electrophysiological mechanisms of joint and muscle pain. In: Dubner R, Gebhart G F, Bond M R (eds). Proceedings of the Vth World Congress on Pain. Elsevier, Amsterdam, p 201–215

Guilbaud G, Iggo A 1985 The effect of lysine acetylsalicylate or joint capsule mechanoreceptors in rats with polyarthritis. Experimental Brain Research 61: 164–168

Guilbaud G, Besson J M, Niederlender D, Benelli G, Lombard M C 1974 Responses of posterior thalamic nuclei cells to nociceptive stimulations. Proceedings of the IUSP, XXVI International Congress of Physiology and Science, New Delhi 11: 172

Guilbaud G, Caille D, Besson J M, Benelli G 1977 Single unit activities in ventral posterior and posterior group thalamic nuclei during nociceptive and non-nociceptive stimulations in the cat. Archives Italiennes de Biologie 115: 38–56

Guilbaud G, Peschanski M, Gautron M, Binder D 1980 Neurones responding to noxious stimulations in VB complex and caudal adjacent regions in the thalamus of the rat. Pain 8: 303–318

Guilbaud G, Benoist J M, Gautron M, Kayser V 1982 Aspirin clearly depresses responses of ventrobasal thalamus neurons to joint stimuli in arthritic rats. Pain 13: 153–163

Guilbaud G, Kayser V, Benoist J M, Gautron M 1986 Modifications in the responsiveness of rat ventrobasal thalamic neurons at different stages of carrageenin-produced inflammation. Brian Research 385: 86–98

Guilbaud G, Benoist J M, Neil A, Kayser V, Gautron M 1987a Neuronal response threshold to and encoding of thermal stimuli during carrageenin-hyperalgesic inflammation in the ventro-basal thalamus of the rat. Experimental Brain Research 66: 421–431

Guilbaud G, Neil A, Benoist J M, Kayser V, Gautron M 1987b Thresholds and encoding of neuronal responses to mechanical stimuli in the ventro-basal thalamus during carrageenin-induced hyperalgesic inflammation in the rat. Experimental Brain Research 68: 311–318

Guilbaud G, Peschanski M, Besson J M 1989a Experimental data related to nociception and pain at the supraspinal level. Textbook of pain. In: Melzack R, Wall PD (eds) Textbook of pain. Churchill Livingstone, Edinburgh, p 141–153

Guilbaud G, Benoist J M, Eschalier A, Gautron M, Kayser V 1989b Evidence for peripheral serotonergic mechanisms in the early sensitization after carrageenin-induced inflammation: electrophysiological studies in the ventrobasal complex of the rat thalamus using a potent specific antagonist of peripheral 5-HT receptors. Brain Research 502: 187–197

Guilbaud G, Benoist J M, Jazat F, Gautron M 1990 Neuronal responsiveness in the ventrobasal thalamic complex of rats with an experimental peripheral mononeuropathy. Journal of Neurophysiology 64: 1537–1554

Guilbaud G, Benoist J M, Levante A, Gautron M, Willer J C 1992 Primary somatosensory cortex in rats with pain-related behaviours due to a peripheral mononeuropathy after moderate ligation of one sciatic nerve: neuronal responsivity to somatic stimulation. Experimental Brain Research 92: 227–245

Harris R M, Hendrickson A E 1985 Local circuit neurons in the rat ventrobasal thalamus. Neuroscience Abstracts 11: 562

Hellon R F, Mitchell D 1975 Characteristics of neurons in the ventrobasal thalamus of the rat which respond to noxious stimulation of the tail. Journal of Physiology 250: 29–30P

Herkenham M 1980 Laminar organisation of thalamic projections to the rat neocortex. Science 207: 532–535

Hirai T, Jones E G 1989 A new parcellation of the human thalamus on the basis of histochemical staining Brain Research Review 14: 1–34

Hoheisel U, Mense S 1989 Long-term changes in discharge behaviour of cat dorsal horn neurons following noxious stimulation of deep tissues. Pain 36: 239–247

Honda C N, Mense S, Perl E R 1983 Neurons in ventrobasal region of cat thalamus selectively responsive to noxious mechanical stimulation. Journal of Neurophysiology 49: 662–673

Horie H, Yokota T 1990 Responses of nociceptive VPL neurons to intracardiac injection of bradykinin in the cat. Brain Research 516: 161–164

Huang G F, Besson J M, Bernard J F 1993 Morphine strongly depresses the transmission of noxious messages in the spino(trigemino)-ponto-amygdaloid pathway. European Journal of Pharmacology 230: 279–284

Hylden J L K, Hayashi H, Bennett G J, Dubner R 1985 Spinal lamina I neurons projecting to the parabrachial area of the cat midbrain. Brain Research 336: 195–198

Hylden J L K, Hayashi H, Dubner R, Bennett G J 1986 Physiology and morphology of the lamina I spinomesencephalic projection. Journal of Comparative Neurology 247: 505–515

Itoh K, Mizuno N 1977 Topographical arrangement of thalamocortical neurons in the contralateral nucleus (CL) of the cat, with special reference to a spino-thalamo cortical path through the CL. Experimental Brain Research 300: 471–480

Jones E G 1985 The thalamus. Plenum Press, New York

Jones M W, Apkarian A V, Stevens R T, Hodge C J Jr 1987 The spinothalamic tract: an examination of the cells of origin of the dorsolateral and ventral spinothalamic pathways in cats. Journal of Comparative Neurology 260: 349–361

Jones A K P, Brown W D, Friston K J, Qi L Y, Frackowiack R S J 1991 Cortical and subcortical localization of response to pain in man using positron emission tomography. Proceedings of the Royal Society of London 244: 39–44

Kayser V, Guilbaud, G 1984 Further evidence for changes in the responsiveness of somatosensory neurons in arthritic rats: a study of the posterior intralaminar region of the thalamus. Brain Research 323: 144–147

Kayser V, Guilbaud G 1987 Local and remote modifications of nociceptive sensitivity during carrageenin-induced inflammation in the rat. Pain 28: 99–107

Kayser V, Benoist J M, Guilbaud G 1983 Further evidence for a strong depressive effect of low doses of morphine on VB thalamic neuronal responses (a study on arthritic rats). Brain Research 267: 187–191

Kayser V, Peschanski M, Guilbaud G 1985 Neuronal loss in the ventrobasal complex of the rat thalamus alters behavioral responses to noxious stimulation. In: Fields H, Dubner R, Cervero F (eds) Advances in pain research and therapy, vol 9 Raven Press, New York, p 277–284

Kenshalo D R, Isensee O 1983 Responses of primate SI cortical neurons to noxious stimuli. Journal of Neurophysiology 50: 1479–1496

Kenshalo D R Jr, Giesler G J, Leonard R B, Wilis W D 1980 Responses of neurons in primate ventral posterior lateral nucleus to noxious stimuli. Journal of Neurophysiology 43: 1594–1614

Kenshalo D R Jr, Chudler E H, Anton F, Dubner R 1988 SI nociceptive neurons participate in the encoding process by which monkeys perceive the intensity of noxious thermal stimulation. Brain Research 454: 378–382

King R B 1957 Postchordotomy studies of pain threshold. Neurology 7: 610–614

Kniffki K D, Mizumura K 1983 Responses in VPL and VPL-VL region of the cat to algesic stimulation of muscle and tendon. Journal of Neurophysiology 49: 649–661

Kocher L, Anton F, Reeh P W, Handwerker H O 1987 The effect of carrageenin-induced inflammation on the sensitivity of unmyelinated skin nociceptors in the rat. Pain 29: 363–373

Lamotte R H, Campbell J N 1978 Comparison of responses of warm and nociceptive C fibre afferent in monkey with human judgements of thermal pain. Journal of Neurophysiology 41: 509–528

Lamour Y, Willer J C, Guilbaud G 1982 Neuronal responses to noxious stimulation in rat somatosensory cortex. Neuroscience Letters 29: 35–40

Lamour Y, Guilbaud G, Willer J C 1983a Altered properties and laminar distribution of neuronal responses to peripheral stimulation in the SmI cortex of the arthritic rat. Brain Research 273: 183–187

Lamour Y, Guilbaud G, Willer J C 1983b Rat somatosensory (SmI)-cortex: II. Laminar and columnar organization of noxious and non-noxious inputs. Experimental Brain Research 49: 46–54

Lamour Y, Willer J C, Guilbaud G 1983c Rat somatosensory (SmI) cortex: I. Characteristics of neuronal responses to noxious stimulation and comparison with responses to non-noxious stimulation. Experimental Brain Research 49: 35–45

Lenz F A, Tasker R R, Dostrovsky J O et al 1987 Abnormal single-unit activity recorded in the somatosensory thalamus of a quadriplegic patient with central pain. Pain 31: 225–236

Lenz F A, Kwan H C, Dostrovsky J O, Tasker R R 1989 Characteristics of the bursting pattern of action potentials that occurs in the thalamus of patients with central pain. Brain Research 496: 357–360

Light A R, Casale E, Sedivec M 1987 The physiology and anatomy of spinal laminae I and II neurons antidromically activated by stimulation in the parabrachial region of the midbrain and pons. In: Schmidt R F, Schaible H G, Vahle-Hinz C (eds) Fine afferent nerve fibers and pain. VCH, Weinheim, p 347–356

Ma W, Peschanski M 1988 Spinal and trigeminal projections to the parabrachial nucleus in the rat: electron-microscopic evidence of a spino-ponto-amygdalian somatosensory pathway. Somatosensory Research 5: 247–257

Ma W, Peschanski M, Besson J M 1986 The overlap of spinothalamic and dorsal column nuclei projections in the ventrobasal complex of the rat thalamus: a double anterograde labelling study using light microscopic analysis. Journal of Comparative Neurology 245: 531–540

Ma W, Peschanski M, Ralston H J III 1987 Fine structure of the spinothalamic projections to central lateral nucleus of the rat thalamus. Brain Research 414: 187–191

McMahon S B, Wall P D 1985 Electrophysiological mapping of brainstem projections of spinal cord lamina I cells in the rat. Brain Research 333: 19–26

Manthy P W 1983 The spinothalamic tract in the primate: a re-examination using wheatgerm agglutinin conjugated to horseradish peroxidase. Neuroscience 9: 847–862

Mehler W R 1969 Some neurological species differences a posteriori. Annals of the New York Academy of Sciences 167: 424–468

Mehler W R 1974 Central pain and the spinothalamic tract. In: Bonica J J (ed) Pain. Advances in Neurology 4. Raven Press, New York, p 127–146

Mehler W R, Feferman M E, Wauta W D H 1960 Ascending axon degeneration following anterolateral cordotomy. An experimental study in the monkey. Brain 83: 718–750

Melzack R, Casey K L 1968 Sensory, motivational and central control determinants of pain. In: Kenshalo D R (ed) The skin senses. C C Thomas, Springfield, p 423–443

Menétrey D, Besson J M 1982 Electrophysiological characteristics of dorsal horn cells in rats with cutaneous inflammation resulting from chronic arthritis. Pain 13: 343–364

Menétrey D, De Pommery J 1991 Origins of spinal ascending pathways that reach central areas involved in visceroception and visceronociception in the rat. European Journal of Neuroscience 3: 249–259

Menétrey D, Chaouch A, Binder D, Besson J M 1982 Neurons at the origin of the spinothalamic tract in the rat: an anatomical study using the retrograde transport of horseradish peroxidase. Journal of Comparative Neurology 206: 193–207

Menétrey D, de Pommery J, Thomasset M, Baimbridge K G 1992 Calbindin-D28K (CaBP28k)-like immunoreactivity in ascending projections. II. Spinal projections to brain stem and mesencephalic areas. European Journal of Neuroscience 4: 70–76

Molinari M, Bentivoglio M, Minciacchi D, Granato A, Macchi G 1986 Spinal afferents and cortical efferents of the anterior intralaminar nuclei; an anterograde-retrograde tracing study. Neuroscience Letters 72: 258–264

Molinari M, Hendry S H C, Jones E G 1987 Distributions of certain neuropeptides in the primate thalamus. Brain Research 426: 270–289

Mountcastle V B 1980 Medical physiology. vol 1 C V Mosby, St Louis

Nathan PW 1990 Comments on 'A dorsal spinothalamic tract in macaque monkey' by Apkarian and Hodge. Pain 40: 239–240

Neil A, Benoist J M, Kayser V, Guilbaud G 1987 Initial sensitization in carrageenin-induced rat paw inflammation is dependent on amine autacoid mechanisms: electrophysiological and behavioural evidence obtained with a quaternary antihistamine, thiazinamium. Experimental Brain Research 65: 343–351

Ness T J, Gebhart G F 1990 Visceral pain: a review of experimental studies. Pain 41: 167–234

Noordenbos W, Wall P D 1976 Diverse sensory functions with an almost totally divided spinal cord. A case of spinal cord transection with preservation of part of one anterolateral quadrant. Pain 2: 185–195

Ottersen, O P 1981 Afferent connections to the amygdaloid complex of the rat with some observations in the cat. III. Afferents from the lower brain stem. Journal of Comparative Neurology 202: 335–356

Panneton W M, Burton H 1985 Projections from the paratrigeminal nucleus and the medullary and spinal dorsal horn to the peribrachial area in the cat. Neuroscience 15: 779–798

Pearson C M, Wood F D 1959 Studies of arthritis and other lesions induced in rats by injection of mycobacterial adjuvant. I. General clinical and pathological characteristics and some modifying factors. Arthritis and Rheumatism 2: 440–459

Peschanski M 1984 Trigeminal afferents to the diencephalon in the rat. Neuroscience 12: 465–487

Peschanski M, Besson J M 1984 A spino-reticulo-thalamic pathway in the rat: an anatomical study with reference to pain transmission. Neuroscience 12: 165–178

Peschanski M, Ralston H J III 1985 Light and electron microscopic evidence of transneuronal labelling with WGA-HRP to trace somatosensory pathways to the thalamus. Journal of Comparative Neurology 236: 29–41

Peschanski M, Guilbaud G, Gautron M, Besson J M 1980 Encoding of noxious heat messages in neurones of the ventrobasal thalamic complex in the rat. Brain Research 197: 401–413

Peschanski M, Guilbaud G, Gautron M 1981 Posterior intralaminar region in rat: neuronal responses to noxious and non-noxious cutaneous stimuli. Experimental Neurology 72: 226–238

Peschanski M, Mantyh P W, Besson J M 1983 Spinal afferents to the ventrobasal complex in the rat: an anatomical study using wheatgerm agglutinin conjugated to horseradish peroxidase. Brain Research 278: 240–244

Peschanski M, Briand A, Gautron M, Guilbaud G 1985 Electrophysiological evidence for a role of the anterolateral quadrant of the spinal cord in the transmission of noxious messages to the thalamic ventrobasal complex in the rat. Brain Research 342: 77–84

Poggio G F, Mountcastle V B 1960 Study of the functional contributions of the lemniscal and spinothalamic systems to somatic sensibility. Bulletin of the Johns Hopkins Hospital 106: 266–316

Raboisson P, Dallel R, Woda A 1989 Responses of neurones in the ventrobasal complex of the thalamus to orofacial noxious stimulation after trigeminal tractotomy. Experimental Brain Research 77: 569–576

Ralston H J III 1985 Synaptic organization of spinothalamic tract projections to the thalamus, with special reference to pain. In: Kruger L, Liebeskind I C (eds) Neural mechanisms of pain. Raven Press, New York, p 183–196

Ralston H J III 1992 Local circuitry of somatosensory thalamus in the processing of sensory information. Progress in Brain Research 87: 13–28

Ralston H J III, Ralston D D 1992 The primate dorsal spinothalamic tract: evidence for a specific termination in the posterior nuclei (Po/SG) of the thalamus. Pain 48: 107–118

Rinvik E 1968 A re-evaluation of the cytoarchitecture of the ventral nuclear complex of the cat's thalamus on the basis of corticothalamic connections. Brain Research 8: 237–254

Sadikot A F, Parent A, François C 1990 The centre median and parafascicular thalamic nuclei project respectively to the sensorimotor and associative limbic striatal territories in the squirrel monkey. Brain Research 510: 161–165

Saper C B, Loewy A D 1980 Efferent connections of the parabrachial nucleus in the rat. Brain Research 197: 291–317

Saporta S, Kruger I 1977 The organisation of thalamocortical relay neurons in the rat ventrobasal complex studied by retrograde transport of horseradish peroxidase. Journal of Comparative Neurology 174: 187–208

Schaible H G, Schmidt R F 1988 Time course of mechanosensitivity changes in articular afferents during a developing experimental arthritis. Journal of Neurophysiology 60: 2180–2195

Schaible H, Schmidt R F, Willis W D 1987 Enhancement of the responses of ascending tract cells in the cat spinal cord by acute inflammation of the knee joint. Experimental Brain Research, 66: 489–99

Shibata K, Kataoka Y, Ueki S 1986 An important role of the central amygdaloid nucleus and mammillary body in the mediation of conflict behaviour in rats. Brain Research 372: 159–162

Talbot J D, Marrett S, Evanc A C et al 1991 Multiple representation of pain in human cerebral cortex. Science 251: 1355–1358

Villanueva L, Bouhassira D, Bing Z, Le Bars D 1988a Convergence of heterotopic nociceptive information onto subnucleus reticularis dorsalis neurons in the rat medulla. Journal of Neurophysiology 60: 980–1009

Villanueva L, Bing Z, Bouhassira D, Le Bars D 1988b Encoding of electrical, thermal, and mechanical noxious stimuli by subnucleus reticularis dorsalis neurons in the rat. Journal of Neurophysiology 61: 391–402

Vin-Christian K, Benoist J M, Gautron M, Levante A, Guilbaud G 1992 Further evidence for the involvement of SmI cortical neurons in nociception: Modifications of their responsiveness over the early stage of a carrageenin-induced inflammation in the rat. Somatosensory and Motor Research 9: 245–261

Wagman I H, Dong W K 1974 Effects of peripheral and dorsal column stimulation on noxious evoked responses of cells in the thalamic posterior group nuclei (PO). Proceedings of the X1th International Congress of Physiology and Science, New Delhi; p 170

Wells J, Matthews T J, Ariano M A 1982 Are there interneurons in the thalamic somatosensory projection in the rat? Neuroscience Abstracts 8: 37

White J C, Sweet W H 1969 Pain and the neurosurgeon. A forty-year experience. Charles C Thomas, Springfield, Illinois

Wiberg M, Blomqvist A 1984 The spinomesencephalic tract in the cat; its cells of origin and termination pattern demonstrated by the intraaxonal transport method. Brain Research 291: 1–18

Willis W D 1989 The origin and destination of pathways involved in pain transmission. In: Wall P D, Melzack R (eds) Textbook of pain. Churchill Livingstone, Edinburgh p 112–127

Willis W D, Coggeshall R E 1991 Sensory mechanisms of the spinal cord, 2nd edn. Plenum Press, New York

Woda A, Azerad J, Guilbaud G, Besson J M 1975 Etude microphysiologique des projections thalamiques de la pulpe dentaire chez le rat. Brain Research 89: 193–213

Yokota T, Nishikawa Y, Koyama N 1986 Tooth pulp input to the shell region of nucleus ventralis posteromedialis of the cat thalamus. Journal of Neurophysiology 56: 1380–1396

7. Mechanisms of cutaneous, deep and visceral pain

Stephen B. McMahon

The following descriptions highlight the bizarre and striking features of pain of deep origin. The first is taken from the clinical investigations of Head, on a patient with an inflamed ovary:

> Case 41. Constant pain in left loin and in abdomen below the umbilicus. At menstrual periods has pain in addition over the lower part of the abdomen and down the back of the leg. A prolapsed ovary is felt lying directly behind the uterus. It is excessively tender. Even the lightest pressure causing pain. This pain is referred to a point in the left loin corresponding roughly with the tip of the twelfth rib. It is also referred to a spot in front a little to the left of and below the umbilicus. Intense cutaneous tenderness marking out in beautiful manner the tenth dorsal area. (Head 1893).
> Head also noted that '... no pain is caused by taking a normal ovary between the fingers'.

The second description comes from an experimental study of oesophageal distension in healthy volunteers:

> ... in most of the subjects pain was felt after 15–25 cc of air had been introduced with a resulting pressure of from 80–150 mmHg. ... The sensation was usually vague and more or less widespread with a central point of maximum sensitivity ... the site of pain does not indicate any definite site for the location of the stimulus. ... If further inflation was carried out the sensation might not only be accentuated at the original site but often spread widely or appeared in new situations. For example, ... pain felt first 5 cm above the xiphoid on increased pressure radiated to both shoulder blades. The most striking feature of the referred sensations was the inability of the patient as a rule to describe them exactly. On the whole they seemed to fall under the heading of pain. ... It was difficult to define the referred sensations in relation to body surface and while the subjects pointed to a fairly definite location, either in front or back, the pain was usually described as being inside rather than superficial. (Polland & Bloomfield 1931.)

The important features illustrated by these descriptions are:

1. Direct trauma, which readily produces pain when applied to the skin, is mostly without effect in healthy visceral tissue
2. Pain which arises from deep tissues is often initially poorly localised and diffuse
3. With time, pains of deep origin are often referred to more superficial structures
4. Pain of deep origin may radiate over considerable distances
5. The site of referred pain may additionally show hyperalgesia
6. In disease states, the afflicted viscera may also become hyperalgesic.

Many of these features are not associated with cutaneous pain, and they present a challenge for those interested in understanding the neuronal processes underlying deep pain. In this respect it is important to note that experimental studies of pain mechanisms have focused overwhelmingly on the processing of stimuli applied to the skin. There are clearly several practical advantages to this, such as the accessibility of the tissue, its essentially two-dimensional structure, and the ease of maintaining its normal state and applying quantifiable and reproducible stimuli. Unfortunately, there are several reasons to believe that the experimental data and even the conceptual framework of ideas relating to pain from one tissue cannot be transferred wholesale to another.

Firstly, the skin faces primarily external threats and to these an organism can mount as a defence some avoidance behaviour. To this end, there is clearly some value in pain as an alarm signal. This consideration led Sherrington in his pioneering studies to conclude that 'pain seems the psychical adjunct to protective reflexes' (Sherrington 1900). These external threats impinge much less on the body's deep tissues, especially the viscera, which more commonly are exposed to the ravages of disease. In many cases, for instance the presence of a ureteric calculus, or the spasm of a length of gut, the protective nature of pain is less obvious, since it is not associated with any effective countermeasures or 'protective reflexes'.

A second problem arises in transferring the concept of a noxious stimulus from skin to deep tissues. Again it was Sherrington who first postulated the existence of nociceptors that detect tissue damage. Several decades later direct experimental support was forthcoming for the existence of large numbers of these receptors in skin. However, it is difficult to apply Sherrington's concept to viscera since, as discussed more fully below, many forms of tissue injury (such as neoplastic destruction of parenchymatous organs or perforation of hollow viscera) are often not painful. Moreover, pain can arise from some stimuli (such as distension of the hollow organs) which do not damage, or even threaten to damage, the tissue. The problem of defining an adequate noxious stimulus for visceral organs is further complicated by the structural complexity of some tissues. For instance, a receptor found to respond to supraphysiological levels of distension of a viscus might also respond to entirely physiological pressure changes in the associated vasculature or a nearby viscus. One cautionary example can be seen in the case of renal colic. It might at first sight appear intuitively obvious that the pain arises from the mechanical stimulation offered by the passage of a large and rough stone through the restricted lumen of a ureter. However, an alternative explanation, for which there is much evidence, is that the stone merely obstructs the ureter, leading to a distension of the entire upper urinary tract. The increased pressure, acting on receptors in the pelvis of the kidney, is likely to be the normal stimulus for renal colic (Bretland 1972).

Finally, differences in the characteristics of sensations evoked from superficial and deep tissues (discussed in the following section) suggest a need for caution in extrapolating data from one tissue to another.

THE NATURE OF PAIN FROM CUTANEOUS, DEEP AND VISCERAL STRUCTURES

Pain of cutaneous origin has distinct features. It is usually focal (that is, with well-defined boundaries) and often has a burning quality. It is well localised, even if any tactile cues are removed by block of large-diameter fibres. In contrast, pain of deep origin is usually extensive rather than focal, perceived over an area much larger than the precipitating stimulus. Deep pain has diffuse boundaries. It is frequently associated with a sense of nausea and ill-being. Visceral pain in particular can show a wave-like quality, waxing and waning with, it is assumed, contractions of smooth muscle. Autonomic and motor reflexes associated with deep pains are often extreme and prolonged. Muscle rigidity may itself form a new source of pain, although this is contested by some. The most striking feature of deep pain is its localisation. Only in exceptional circumstances is it well localised. Otherwise the localisation is at best poor and sometimes bizarre. Kellgren made extensive studies on the location of pain induced by the injection of hypertonic saline into muscle and ligaments (Kellgren 1937–38, 1938, 1939; Lewis & Kellgren 1939). From muscle, pain was felt diffusely and deep, in the neighbourhood of the muscle and at more distant sites. The distribution was generally segmental, that is, within the structures innervated by the same spinal nerve as the injected muscle. Injection of the interspinous ligaments of the vertebral columns yielded pain with similar characteristics and also localised segmentally. Figure 7.1 shows a map from Kellgren's work of the distribution of deep pain following injection of ligaments at different spinal levels. Kellgren noted that these pains took some time to develop and equally could persist for prolonged periods. This is unlike the very rapid development of pain seen with chemical stimuli of cutaneous afferents. However, it is reminiscent of the slowly developing secondary hyperalgesia that is seen surrounding focal injury in skin (see Chs 1 and 5) Kellgren found that similar segmental pains were elicited by injections of hypertonic solutions into joints (Kellgren 1939, 1940).

For visceral pain, two distinct types of localisation have been noted. Some pains, so-called 'true' visceral pains (or by early authors 'splanchnic pain', Ross 1888), are felt as arising from inside the body, in the midline. They may be perceived as anterior or posterior, and occasionally radiate over considerable distances. One example is the initial sensation perceived after myocardial infarction (Procacci et al 1986). Another is the early pain of appendicitis, which is initially felt in the midline but can then suddenly move to the lower right quadrant when parietal structures are stimulated by the inflamed or ruptured appendix.

Much visceral pain, so-called referred pain, is localised

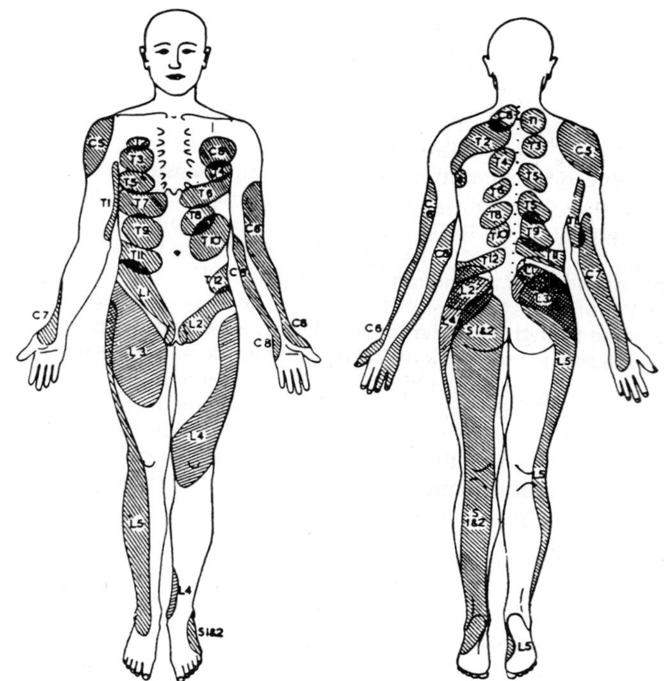

Fig. 7.1 The segmental areas of deep pain developed by the injection of hypertonic solutions into interspinous ligaments at the levels marked, as described by Kellgren. (From Lewis 1942.)

to more superficial structures, sometimes a great distance away from the site of the afflicted viscus. If intense, the referred pain often appears to radiate to involve larger areas. The area of referral is generally segmental. That is, to muscle and/or skin innervated by the same spinal nerves as the viscus giving rise to the referred sensation. A classic example is the pain that develops shortly after myocardial infarction. Although, as we have said, such pain is initially felt as deep pain felt within the chest, after a short time (measured in minutes) it is often felt in parietal structures. It is still not well localised but most often perceived as diffuse within the anterior chest and left arm. In some patients, the referred pain becomes yet more superficial with time, felt in the skin of appropriate dermatomes (Procacci et al 1986). Another example is the pain of renal colic which is felt in the iliac fossa and scrotum. This pattern of referral is consistent enough to be of much diagnostic use. However, confusion can arise from viscera which share a common segmental innervation (i.e. those within a viscerotome), for instance the heart and oesophagus. One notable feature of referred pain is that it masks the original 'true' visceral pain. Another is that the area of referral can become tender or hyperalgesic (Head 1893; Procacci et al 1986). This is true for both the pain referred to muscle and to skin. Such tenderness develops slowly, taking many minutes or even hours to become manifest and, equally, persisting for prolonged periods, measured in hours.

Descriptive studies on the nature of referred sensations in patients are sometimes confounded by the possibility that the effective stimulus moves from a visceral site to a parietal one. For instance, the rupture of an inflamed appendix is associated with the sudden appearance of a pain localised in the lower right quadrant of the abdomen (Silen 1987). Similarly, the growth of a tumour may newly involve non-visceral tissue. Stimulation of the body wall and especially its membranous linings is well recognised to give rise to poorly localised deep pain in some cases, or a more superficial referred pain in others. The surgeon Morley was a great champion of this mechanism. He made a convincing case that many forms of referred pain might conceivably be referred from deep somatic structures rather than visceral ones (Morley 1931). For instance, gall bladder pain, which is sometimes referred to the shoulder, could arise, he argued, because of traction upon, or other forms of stimulation of, the diaphragm. Similar pains are felt when a cotton swab is dragged across the diaphragm in surgery employing only local anaesthesia of the abdominal wall. Morley even maintained that the unusually well-localised pain of a gastric ulcer might arise from activation of somatically-innervated structures in the body wall, citing as evidence the fact that when the position of the underlying viscus was altered, the location of the referred pain shifted accordingly (Morley 1931). Other authors have denied that this movement occurs (Lewis 1942). It is also clear that some examples of referred pain cannot be explained on this basis, such as the pain of renal colic, angina, and in the extreme, the referred pain felt when the splanchnic nerve of conscious humans has been stimulated electrically (Foerster 1933; Leriche 1937).

MECHANISMS OF REFERRED SENSATIONS

A number of explanations have been offered for referred sensations. These are shown schematically in Figure 7.2. The first was originally proposed by Sinclair et al (1948). The suggestion is that some primary sensory neurons have bifurcating axons that innervate both somatic and visceral targets, thus leading to confusion as to the source of afferent activity, and explaining the segmental nature of referred sensations. Some electrophysiological evidence has been forthcoming in support of this idea. Bahr et al (1981) found that 18% of a limited sample of unmyelinated fibres in the lumbar splanchnic nerves could be driven by electrical stimuli applied to somatic nerves. Some of these may have been sensory neurons, but no attempts were made to identify receptive fields in peripheral tissues. Other positive results, using electrophysiological and neuroanatomical techniques and pairs of peripheral somatic nerves (Pierau et al 1982; Taylor & Pierau 1982), have been challenged on technical grounds (Devor et al 1984), and the general consensus is now that if this type of afferent exists, then it is rare. The only positive data for sensory neurons with receptive fields in two tissues come from a study by Mense et al (1981) who reported single sensory neurons with both skin and muscle fields innervating the tail of the cat. The hypothesis in any case does not explain the time delay in the evolution of referred sensations. Nor does it explain the referred hyperalgesia that frequently develops, since

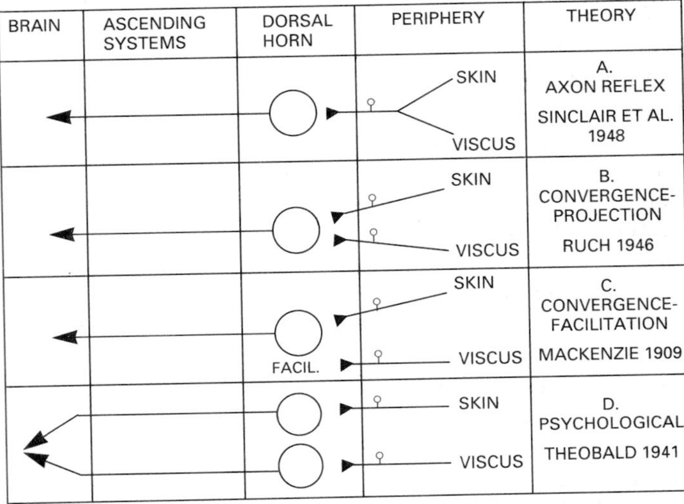

Fig. 7.2 Summary diagram illustrating the various theoretical mechanisms of referred pain. See text for details. (From Morrison 1987.)

antidromic activity (that might invade the distant branch) does not appear capable of inducing a sensitisation of peripheral terminals (Reeh et al 1986).

The second proposed mechanism of referred pain (Fig. 7.2B) is that visceral and somatic primary sensory neurons converge onto common spinal neurons. This is the projection-convergence theory, put in these terms by Ruch (1946), who adapted earlier ideas of Sturge (1883) and Ross (1888). The essence of this proposal is that the activity ascending from the spinal cord is misconstrued as originating from somatic structures because this is the normal mode of its generation. This theory is also clearly capable of explaining the segmental nature of referral, and, if one allows that intense visceral inputs recruit more and more spinal neurons, the radiation of referred pain. There is now considerable experimental evidence that somato-visceral convergence is common in spinal neurons (see below), but it should be remembered that many instances of such convergence may relate to the integration of somatic and visceral reflexes, rather than to viscerosensory processing. One limitation of this theory is that it does not adequately address the issue of referred hyperalgesia. It is possible that summation of inputs from visceral and cutaneous structures could underlie cutaneous hyperalgesia, but the theory offers no explanation of the slow evolution of referred tenderness.

A third hypothesis (Fig. 7.2C) – the convergence-facilitation theory – derives from MacKenzie (1909). He was impressed by the ideas of Sturge (1883) and Ross (1888) which led to the convergence-projection theory just described. However, MacKenzie was convinced that the viscera were wholly insensitive and therefore that activity in visceral afferent neurons never itself gave rise to pain. He claimed instead that activity in visceral afferent fibres was capable of creating an 'irritable focus' within the spinal cord, so that other, segmentally appropriate, somatic inputs could now produce abnormal and of course referred pain sensations (MacKenzie 1909). His theory did not find general acceptance, in part because it implicitly denied the existence of 'true' visceral pain. However, the theory has several redeeming features, such as the ability to explain referred hyperalgesia and the delay in the arousal of referred sensations (since the creation of an 'irritable focus' may take some time). One major problem for the theory is that it predicts that referred pain (as distinct from hyperalgesia) would depend upon ongoing activity in somatic afferents, and therefore be susceptible to local anaesthesia of the referral site. This is not universally reported to be the case. On the other hand, the concept of an irritable focus finds a strong echo in the recently described phenomenon of central sensitisation. The belief is growing that this process is of key importance in hyperalgesic states, and there is a rapid advance in our understanding of the molecular mechanisms involved (see later and Ch. 5). It is somewhat ironic that MacKenzie should, for spurious reasons, come to a view which, after the best part of a century, is gaining credence on a molecular level.

An interesting question is 'what happens to referred pain if the area of referral is anaesthetised with local anaesthetic'? The referred tenderness is of course lost. Reports are conflicting on this issue of the referred pain itself. Procacci et al (1986) have found that the referred pain of angina can be blocked and this is associated with the emergence of a new, 'true' visceral pain. Other workers have reported referred pain to be blocked, unaffected, or even to move under these conditions (Weiss & Davis 1928; Woolard et al 1932; Morley 1937; Wolf & Hardy 1943; Hockaday & Whitty 1967; see also Ruch 1965). The question is an important one since the answer has implications for the mechanism of referred pain and tenderness (see above).

A final view of referred pain is illustrated in Figure 7.2D, and suggests that interactions at supraspinal levels lead to the phenomenon. Theobold (1941) made this proposal in general terms and Lewis was in favour of it in one specific regard. He argued (Lewis 1942) that sensations were referred by default to somatic structures since the 'sensorium' contained a very large and precise representation of these structures, but a very limited and imprecise one of the viscera. Our current knowledge of somatotopic representation within sensory cortex is clearly in line with this view. However, the electrophysiological data we have (see below) do not suggest the existence of separate pathways from spinal cord to brain, as depicted in Figure 7.2D.

STIMULI THAT ELICIT SUPERFICIAL AND DEEP PAIN

In an experimental setting, a variety of intense stimuli applied to skin readily produce pain. These include mechanical and thermal stimuli that might be considered noxious (i.e. tissue damaging), as well as non-damaging events such as electrical stimuli and some chemical irritants. Pain from stronger stimuli does not usually radiate but, conversely, frequently becomes more focal. Increasing the area over which a stimulus acts causes a modest increase in perceived pain, but importantly the threshold for pain is not reduced appreciably (Price et al 1989). In the wake of strong stimuli, the skin becomes tender both at the site of damage and for some considerable distance surrounding it, and gentle mechanical stimuli can now elicit pain (see Chs 1 and 5). Deep somatic tissues, such as joint and muscle, are similarly sensitive to direct tissue-threatening stimuli. For instance, strong mechanical pressure on a muscle or distortion of a joint beyond its working range causes pain. A range of irritant chemicals can directly induce pain in muscle and joint (see Mense 1986). Frankly damaged deep somatic tissue can also exhibit hyperalgesia, as is apparent in arthritic states and after unaccustomed exercise. Lewis (1942) made extensive studies of another adequate stimulus for muscle pain – ischaemia coupled with contraction. He showed that although arresting the circulation to a limb was not itself painful, exercising the ischaemic muscles produced a severe pain that persisted when the exercise stopped, until the blood flow was restored. He concluded that a naturally occurring algogenic chemical built up with exercise. This form of stimulation may occur in the reflexly induced tonic contractions of muscle seen in some visceral pain states.

Visceral tissue exhibits a very different sensitivity. Some viscera, notably lung, liver and the parenchymatous part of the kidney, appear not to give rise to pain with any stimulus, including their gross destruction by malignant growth. The early surgeons, working under only local anaesthesia of the body wall, were surprised to find that direct trauma produced by cutting, crushing and even burning, so effective in inducing pain in somatic tissue, very rarely gave rise to any sensation when applied to visceral tissue (MacKenzie 1909; Morley 1931; Capps 1932). There are a few notable exceptions. The mesenteries are said by most authors to be sensitive to traction or clamping and it is well recognised that the trigone region of the bladder neck can give rise to pain when probed directly or stimulated by the presence of a stone.

Although most visceral organs can be subjected to the knife, clamp or cautery without producing pain, they are sensitive to other forms of stimulation. Perhaps the best described sensitivity is to distension of the hollow muscular-walled organs. Distension of the gastrointestinal (GI) tract from oesophagus to rectum, the urinary tract from kidney pelvis to bladder, and of the gall bladder, all produce pain (Hertz 1911; Polland & Bloomfield 1931; Denny-Brown & Robertson 1933a; Bentley & Smithwick 1940; Lewis 1942; Ray & Niel 1947; Nathan 1956; Goligher & Hughes 1951; Risholm 1954; Bretland 1972; Csendes & Sepulveda 1980). In healthy subjects the pain is often not severe. Its short latency suggests that indirect effects (e.g. ischaemia) are not the cause. Active contractions of smooth muscle may exacerbate pain, and indeed often result in wave-like painful sensations. The severity of labour pains is a testimony to this fact. One can readily demonstrate such pain by voluntarily checking the flow of urine, mid-stream, during micturition. When the urethral outlet is closed, a large isovolumetric contraction of the bladder follows, which, in most people, is distinctly painful. The distending pressures associated with pain are not tissue-damaging, but estimates of the threshold pressures for a particular viscus often vary considerably. One reason is that the effective stimulus is probably transmural pressure, and it is therefore important to correct for intra-abdominal pressure that will vary with posture etc. Another reason is that the area of tissue stimulated may be a crucial determinant of threshold. Unlike skin, spatial summation may drastically reduce the effective threshold for pain. This viewpoint was strongly argued by Goldscheider (1920). Given the simplicity of distending, say, various lengths of gut or oesophagus, we have remarkably little direct evidence on this point. Comparisons of different studies in man and animals suggest that spatial summation can appreciably lower the threshold for visceral pain (Lewis 1942; Peterson & Youmans 1945). Given the implications of this question for viscero-sensory processing mechanisms, it is important that more direct data should be obtained. Spatial summation may explain the failure of localised mechanical stimuli, even frankly damaging ones, to produce pain.

A second effective stimulus for visceral pain is ischaemia. The best recognised example is that of ischaemic heart disease (as detailed in Ch. 29) but it is likely that ischaemia of other visceral tissues produces pain (Lewis 1942; Poole et al 1987). With coronary occlusion there is the possibility of secondary, mechanical effects (for instance the spasm of arteries, Osler 1910) but it is frequently assumed that an important component of the stimulus is an accumulation of pain producing chemicals in the ischaemic tissue (but see Maliani 1986; Ness & Gebhart 1990). Certainly, pain can be elicited from a variety of visceral structures which are exposed to chemical stimuli. Bradykinin, as a naturally occurring agent, has been the most widely tested although other algesic chemicals are present in damaged tissue (Handwerker & Reeh 1991; Rang et al 1991). Bradykinin produces pain when infused into the abdomen (Lim et al 1967). It is less clear if it is algogenic in the heart (see Pagani et al 1985; Ness & Gebhart 1990). One complicating factor is that bradykinin may exert an indirect action via smooth muscle contraction (Floyd et al 1977). Other, non-naturally occurring chemicals have been shown to induce pain in some viscera, for instance the urinary bladder (Head 1893; Nesbit & McLellan 1939; Maggi et al 1989).

A final and clinically important circumstance where visceral pain may be triggered is in inflammatory states (Wolf 1965; Head 1893). In the urinary and alimentary tracts, inflammation is common and can be painful. In cystitis, for example, the sensations during bladder emptying often become unpleasant and painful (Nesbit & McLellan 1939; Petersén & Franksson 1955). The discomfort is not always related to the level of intravesical pressure and bouts of pain occur at the end of micturition. An important feature of inflammatory states is that the affected viscus may be hyperalgesic. Kinsella (1940) reported that direct mechanical stimulation of the inflamed, but not the healthy, appendix caused pain. A number of other anecdotal reports exist for the ureter, kidney, bladder, ovary, stomach and oesophagus (Head 1893; Hertz 1911; Hurst 1911; McLellan & Goodell 1943; Ruffin et al 1953; Petersén & Franksson 1955; Wolf

1965). In some of these cases, it has been noted that gentle mechanical stimulation of the irritated mucosa (which is not usually perceived) is painful. Quantitative studies of the increased sensitivity of inflamed viscera are few, but some data exist for patients with irritable bowel syndrome and non-cardiac chest pain (see Mayer & Raybould 1990). The altered sensibility of visceral tissue in pathological conditions such as inflammation may indicate the emergence of new neurophysiological processes, a view for which there is growing experimental evidence (see below).

PERIPHERAL PATHWAYS MEDIATING VISCERAL PAIN

Many viscera receive a dual innervation from both sympathetic and parasympathetic nerves. Afferent nerve fibres travel with both of these. It is standard textbook dogma, and all too frequently stated in even modern reviews, that visceral pain is mediated by so-called sympathetic afferents, with parasympathetic afferents playing no role. This view seems to have taken root from early reports that electrical stimulation of the vagus nerve in man did not produce pain (White & Sweet 1963). However, many abdominal viscera receive a large parasympathetic innervation from sacral segments via the pelvic nerve, and we have extensive evidence that these afferents may contribute to all types of visceral sensation. For instance, for the urinary bladder, clinicopathological investigations and studies after surgical interruption of individual nerves have determined that the pain of acute overdistension or cystitis can be signalled by primary afferents in the pelvic nerve (Head 1893; Head & Riddoch 1917; Riddoch 1921; Learmonth 1931; Denny-Brown & Robertson 1933b; Ray & Neill 1947; White et al 1952; Petersén and Franksson 1955; Bors & Comarr 1971; Gunterberg et al 1975). Indeed, for this organ, little information exists about the function of the sympathetic afferents, projecting to the thoracolumbar spinal cord. Interruption of these pathways (as today is often the case in radical retroperitoneal lymphadectomy for testicular cancer) does not appreciably interfere with bladder sensation.

The segmental pattern of referred pain suggests that afferent fibres travelling with the parasympathetic pelvic nerves are important for the appreciation of pain from a variety of visceral structures. Thus, all spinal afferents from viscera are potentially important mediators of visceral sensations, including pain.

PERIPHERAL ENCODING MECHANISMS: SUPERFICIAL AND DEEP TISSUES COMPARED

There is a great deal of functional specialisation amongst the afferent fibres innervating somatic tissues. The large myelinated afferents, with axons conducting in the Aβ range of velocities, respond to innocuous events such as light touch or limb movement. Many of the smaller diameter somatic afferents, conducting in the Aδ- and C-velocity range, are nociceptors which respond when stimulus intensities are raised so as to threaten the integrity of the tissue (see Ch. 1). In visceral nerves, there are practically no Aβ afferents. The few present appear to innervate paciniform corpuscles located in the mesenteries and are probably incapable of encoding information related to individual viscera (Jänig & Morrison 1986). This strongly suggests that both painful and non-painful sensations, and the afferent information used to regulate the mostly unconscious visceral reflexes, must be mediated by the small afferent fibres. A crucial question, about which there is still some controversy, is whether the visceral afferents, like somatic afferents, can be divided into separate groups responding to innocuous and noxious events, respectively. If so, this would be consistent with the specificity theory of pain, Figure 7.3A. The problem of transferring the concept of 'noxious' from somatic to visceral tissues has already been discussed. The result is that it is not always clear what properties one would expect from a specific nociceptor in some visceral tissues. The problem is compounded by the fact that the response properties of visceral afferents have of course been determined in animals. Even where the nature of the effective stimulus is clear, for instance in the case of distension of the hollow viscera, one must extrapolate across species as to the levels at which the stimulus becomes painful. Wary of this problem, many workers have tried to associate 'noxious' visceral stimuli with the appearance of pseudoaffective responses such as increases in blood pressure. This is certainly an unsatisfactory assumption. Where comparisons are possible, pseudoaffective responses are consistently triggered by stimuli which are not associated with any aversive behaviour in the intact animal (McMahon 1986; Ness & Gebhart 1990; see Jänig & Morrison 1986). An alternative to the specificity theory is illustrated schematically in Figure 7.3B. This is the intensity theory, which requires that individual fibres encode physiological, innocuous events, and, with higher discharge frequencies, supraphysiological, presumed noxious, ones. Considerable electrophysiological evidence has been advanced in support of this suggestion for some visceral tissues (see below). One psychophysical observation consistent with intensity encoding is the well-described way in which some acutely painful visceral stimuli, particularly distension of hollow viscera, evolve gradually from non-painful to painful, with intermediate stages which patients usually label unpleasant, but are reluctant to call pain (e.g. Polland & Bloomfield 1931).

Clearly these two theories are mutually exclusive since the specificity theory denies any contribution from other than specific nociceptors and the intensity theory requires

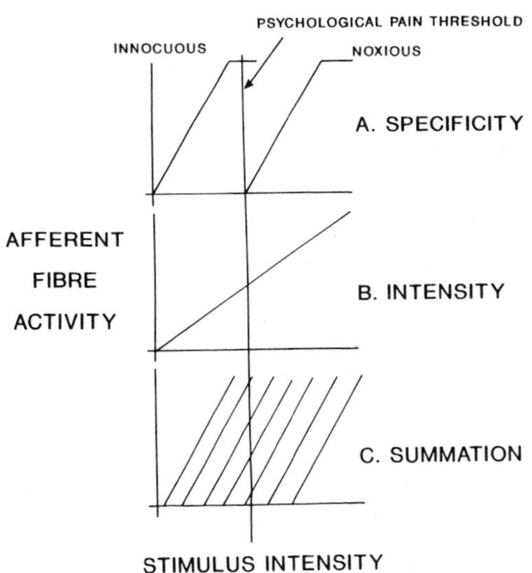

Fig. 7.3 Diagrammatic representation of three possible encoding mechanisms for noxious events by visceral afferent nerve fibres. See text for details. (Adapted from Cervero 1988.)

this contribution. Some workers have reported on afferents that appear to conform to the specificity theory, whilst others find afferents that are clearly signalling events in the physiological and supraphysiological ranges. Interestingly, for the most part, the electrophysiological data put forward by proponents of the two theories do not relate to the same viscus. A notable exception is in the case of the heart, as discussed below.

One further factor is that most visceral structures have an extremely low innervation density. The total numbers of visceral afferents, for the whole of the thoracic and abdominal organs, amounts to probably only 5–10% of all spinal afferents. One consequence, as previously mentioned, is that summation of afferent information is likely to be a necessary and important factor in viscerosensory processes. Experimental studies suggest that the stimulus-response functions of individual afferent fibres exhibit a continuum of mechanical thresholds, and so the situation depicted in Figure 7.3C may actually represent physiological reality in many cases. This form of the intensity theory is of course compatible with the existence of a subpopulation of afferents which appear to fulfil the criteria of specific nociceptors in a particular viscus (that is, the stimulus-response functions illustrated in both Figure 7.3A and B could be present amongst the afferents innervating a single viscus).

It has recently become clear that at least some viscera are supplied with appreciable numbers of afferent fibres that do not normally respond to physiological or supraphysiological forms of mechanical stimuli. Some of these afferents respond specifically to chemical stimuli and have been called 'silent' or 'sleeping' afferents. They appear ideally suited to signalling changes occurring in inflammatory states. At the onset of an experimental inflammation, some of these fibres become active and, moreover, develop a novel mechanosensitivity so that they now respond to events such as distension. The presence of these fibres serves to further reinforce the idea that mechanisms of visceral pain may change dramatically when one moves from normal healthy tissue to diseased pathological states.

The electrophysiological data derived from studies of different viscera are summarised below. In this context, the term visceral nociceptor is used to indicate a neuron that is specifically activated by stimuli which might give rise to pain.

Male reproductive organs

Kumazawa and coworkers have made extensive studies of the response properties of afferent nerve fibres in the superior spermatic nerve of the dog (Kumazawa 1986). Other than a small number (3%) of rapidly adapting low-threshold mechanoreceptors, they found that afferent fibres form a homogeneous group with polymodal receptors in testis and/or epididymis. This applied to both myelinated and unmyelinated afferents. They could be excited in a slowly adapting fashion to stimuli applied to one or more sensitive spots, each only a millimetre or so in diameter. The threshold for activation varied over a wide range but 80% of afferents responded to mechanical stimuli of less than 17 g/mm^2. The afferents were polymodal in the sense that they responded to other forms of stimulation, notably algesic chemicals and heating. Bradykinin and hypertonic saline solutions were effective stimuli for the afferents. Prostaglandins did not excite but sensitised the afferents to other stimuli. Heating the exposed testis excited afferents when stimuli exceeded about 45°C. An example of the responses of one polymodal testicular afferent is shown in Figure 7.4.

Kumazawa and colleagues correlated the response of canine testicular afferents to earlier psychophysical studies on the thresholds of testicular compression that cause pain in man (Woollard & Carmichael 1933). The testicular afferents could encode the level of compression up to several kilograms of force but most had thresholds below 50 g. Woollard & Carmichael (1933) reported that pain was felt in man with compressive forces over 200 g or so. Kumazawa concluded that these afferents, whilst similar in many respects to the polymodal fibres innervating somatic tissues, should not be regarded as polymodal *nociceptors* since they encoded innocuous and well as noxious stimuli.

Female reproductive organs

A limited number of uterine afferent fibres have been reported from cat and rat (Bower 1966; Abrahams & Teare 1969; Floyd et al 1976, 1977; Berkley et al 1988,

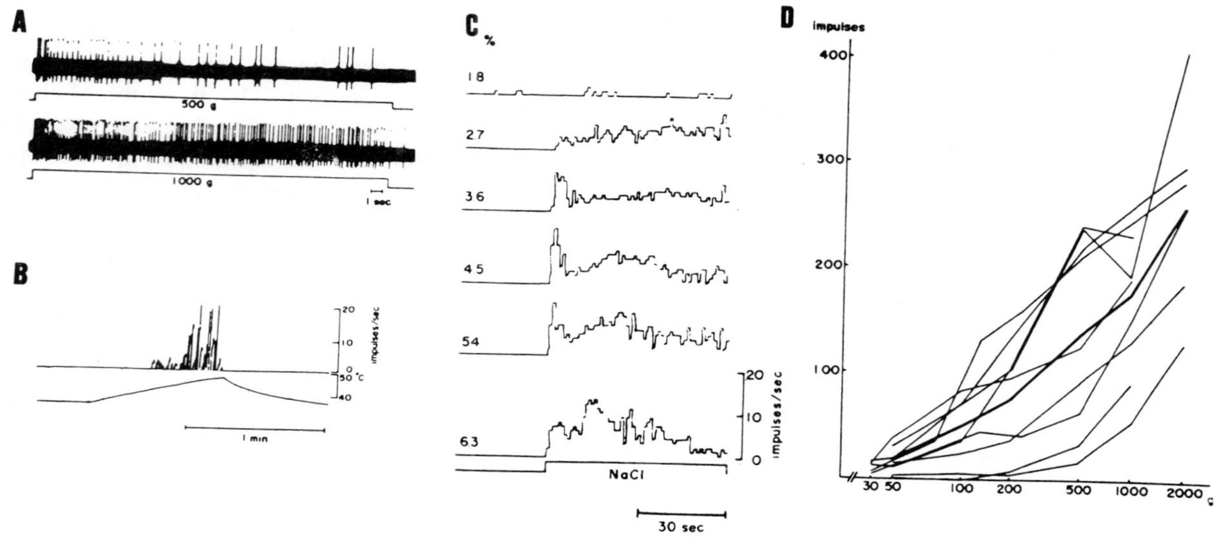

Fig. 7.4 Responses of individual testicular polymodal receptors. **A** Responses of an A-afferent to two different compressive stimuli. **B** Response of the same unit shown in **A** to heating. **C** Response of a single testicular afferent to various concentrations of hypertonic saline. **D** Stimulus-response curves for nine testicular afferents to various compressive forces. The thick line represents the mean response of these nine afferents. (From Kumazawa 1986.)

1990). These studies have described the existence of mechanosensitive fibres, conducting in the A- and C-fibre range. The fibres responded to direct probing of restricted sites along the uterine horns or in the uterine body (particularly near the cervix), vaginal canal and broad ligament of the uterus. Afferents were recorded in both pelvic (parasympathetic) and hypogastric (sympathetic) nerves. Pelvic afferents more commonly innervated the vaginal canal and cervix, whilst hypogastric afferents were mostly found to innervate the uterine horn and/or broad ligament and cervix. Afferents in both nerves responded to direct tactile stimulation, although the hypogastric afferents in the rat were found by Berkley et al (1988) to be rather unresponsive to distension with balloons and to contractions. Many sensory fibres in both nerves were strongly activated by a variety of chemical stimuli such as bradykinin, potassium chloride and 5-HT applied via the uterine artery. Ischaemia was also suggested to be an effective stimulus. Many afferents were found to exhibit ongoing activity. One interesting observation was that the sensitivity of afferents from the uterus appeared to vary with the oestrus cycle. It is possible that this was due to changes in the compliance of the tissue associated with oestrus, but it may reflect a genuine alteration in the sensitivity of afferent terminals. If so, it may be correlated with altered sensibility of uterine events in women under particular circumstances. The obvious power of uterine contractions to induce pain during parturition, but not during the Braxton-Hicks contractions occurring prior to it (Javert & Hardy 1950), may be one such example.

Whilst it is clear that many uterine afferents have the power to encode events that might give rise to pain, it is less clear if there exists a clear population that respond exclusively to such events.

Gall bladder

Distension of the gall bladder in man, both pathologically (following obstruction of the bile ducts) and experimentally, causes pain when intraluminal pressures exceed about 35–45 mmHg (Ray & Neill 1947; Newman & Northrup 1956; Csendes & Sepulveda 1980). One study on the properties of afferents innervating the biliary system of the ferret (Cervero 1982a) reports the existence of fibres with high-pressure thresholds to distension that might therefore be considered nociceptors. These afferents, travelling via the sympathetic splanchnic nerves, had no ongoing activity and responded to direct tactile stimuli applied to restricted sites in the gall bladder and its ducts. Since these afferents represent perhaps the clearest case of specific nociceptors in visceral tissue, it is unfortunate that we do not have more data relating to a range of species and experimental conditions. It is worth noting that studies on the spinal representation of biliary information disagree in some respects. Cervero (1982b, 1983) reported the existence of dorsal horn neurons with similarly high thresholds to gall bladder distension, but Ammons et al (1984a, 1984b) found in their studies that pressure thresholds were generally in the range 0–10 mmHg, well below what might be considered noxious.

Oesophagus

Another visceral structure giving rise to pain on distension is the oesophagus (Polland & Bloomfield 1931; Chapman et al 1949; Lipkin & Sleisenger 1958; Christensen & Lund 1969). At low distending pressures, an oesophageal balloon produces a sensation of fullness, located substernally. As pressure increases, the sensation evolves gradually into one of pain, and this is one reason why it has been difficult to establish a threshold pressure for painful sensations. Another is that some authors have made no allowance for tension in the wall of the distending balloon. Nonetheless, it is likely that pressures above 40 mmHg or so are generally perceived as painful in normal human subjects (Lipkin & Sleisenger 1958).

A number of workers have examined the responses of parasympathetic (vagal) or sympathetic afferent neurons innervating the oesophagus in a variety of animal species (Clerc & Mei 1983; Andrews 1986; Sengupta et al 1989, 1990). Many mechanosensitive afferents are found with fine myelinated or unmyelinated axons. The vagal afferents appear to preferentially innervate mucosa and muscle layers, and sympathetic afferents muscle and serosa (a pattern reported for other viscera, see Morrison 1987a). Many afferents have ongoing activity. Recently, the mechanosensitivity of these afferents has been carefully quantified (Sengupta et al 1989, 1990). Figure 7.5 shows a summary of the principal finding of these studies. The authors found that vagal afferents formed an approximately homogeneous population which encoded pressures from about 0–60 mmHg. The sympathetic afferents exhibited lower firing rates but encoded pressures up to more than 120 mmHg in a monotonic fashion. The authors believed that the sympathetic afferents formed two populations, one which had extrapolated pressure thresholds close to 0 mmHg, and the other, to a mean of 33 mmHg. These three populations were labelled, respectively, low-threshold mechanosensitive, wide dynamic range, and high-threshold mechanical nociceptors, by analogy with the response properties of somatosensory dorsal horn neurons. Thus, these authors apparently provide evidence for both specificity and intensity-encoding mechanisms in the same tissue. However, very different interpretations of these data are possible. Firstly, the stimulus-response relationships of vagal afferents would appear to extend clearly into the range which might be expected to cause pain in humans (certainly if step-wise distensions are considered, Sengupta 1989). One could argue that these fibres are potential contributors to an intensity coding mechanism. Secondly, the division of sympathetic afferents into two groups, with high and low thresholds, is an empirical and subjective distinction. No statistical basis for the separation is apparent. Moreover, the fibres, once divided in this fashion, show no other distinguishing features, in terms of conduction velocity, ongoing activity, maximum discharge frequency, range of pressures encoded. The individual stimulus-response functions from which these two groups were derived (shown in Fig. 7.5B) do not obviously fall into two groups, but appear to represent a continuum of responsiveness. If one considered the total afferent barrage arising from such a population of afferent fibres, one would predict a smooth increase in afferent activity as intraoesophageal pressure

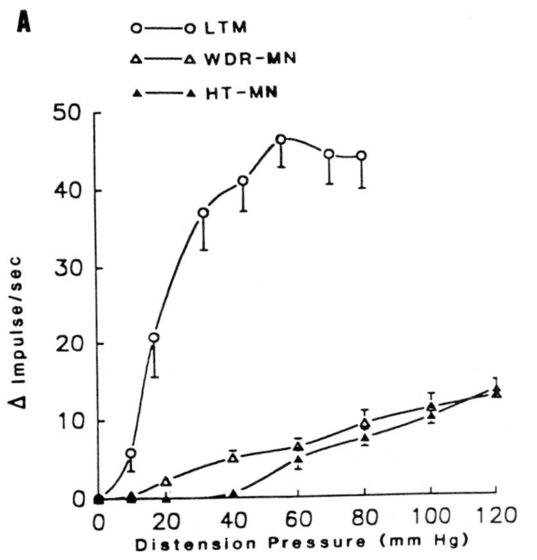

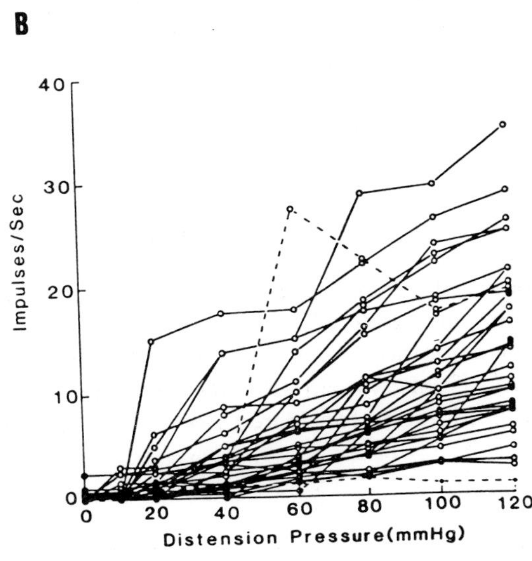

Fig. 7.5 A Average stimulus-response functions of groups of vagal and sympathetic afferents innervating oesophagus to balloon distension. The vagal population were considered low-threshold specific fibres (labelled LTM), while the sympathetic afferents were subdivided into two groups considered to be noxious specific (labelled HT-MN) and intensity coding (labelled WDR-MN). **B** Stimulus-response curves for individual sympathetic afferents, from which the average curves shown in **A** were constructed. (From Sengupta et al 1990.)

increased throughout and beyond the physiological range, with no sudden inflection with the recruitment of the 'nociceptive' population. Thus, these data do not provide clear evidence in favour of visceral pain being encoded according to the specificity theory.

Ureter

There have been only a few studies on the properties of primary afferent neurons innervating the ureter (Beacham & Kunze 1969; Floyd et al 1976; Cervero & Sann 1989). Most data have been provided by this last study, using an in vitro preparation of guinea-pig ureter. Ureteric afferents were thinly myelinated or unmyelinated, and responded to direct probing of a limited area of tissue. Two populations of afferents were distinguished by Cervero & Sann (1989). The first responded to contractions of the ureter and could also be excited by low levels of distension (average threshold 8 mmHg). They appeared to encode levels of distension throughout and beyond the physiological range. The second group did not respond to peristaltic contractions of the ureter, but they could be excited by distension with a wide range of thresholds. The average stimulus-response curves showed a monotonic rise of discharge with increasing pressure. The large majority appeared to have low levels of ongoing activity. The authors claimed that this second group of neurons could be considered a class of specific visceral nociceptor, and suggested that the ongoing activity and relatively low-pressure thresholds seen in some afferents might be due to the anoxic state of the in vitro preparation. When ureters were perfused intraluminally, higher pressure thresholds were seen, although some at least still appeared to respond to distension to only 10 mmHg (see Cervero & Sann 1989, Fig. 7.8). Therefore, as for the oesophageal afferents, it is difficult to know whether this group of fibres in vivo would show stimulus-response functions as illustrated in Figure 7.3C or behave as a group of specific nociceptors, as shown in Figure 7.3A.

The contraction-insensitive afferents were noted to respond to chemicals such as bradykinin and potassium. The urine of some rodents normally contains very high levels of potassium (Morrison 1987a). No tests were performed to determine whether these afferents might actually provide information about the composition of urine. Clearly, if this was an effective stimulus for these fibres, they could not be considered visceral nociceptors.

Urinary bladder

Graded distension of the healthy urinary bladder in humans initially gives rise to a sensation of fullness and eventually pain as volume increases and intravesical pressure exceeds about 25–35 mmHg (Denny-Brown & Robertson 1933a; Nathan 1956; Bors et al 1956; Bors & Comarr 1971; Morrison 1987a). In the inflamed bladder, the sensations during bladder emptying become unpleasant and painful. The qualitative change in the nature of sensations with cystitis suggests that new viscero-sensory mechanisms may emerge with inflammation. To address this possibility a number of animal models have been introduced in which inflammation is induced experimentally with irritant chemicals such as turpentine, xylene and mustard oil (McMahon & Abel 1987; Maggi et al 1988; Birder & de Groat 1992).

Primary sensory neurons innervating the normal urinary bladder have been repeatedly and carefully studied (Floyd et al 1976; Bahns et al 1986, 1987; Häbler et al 1988, 1990a, 1993a). Again, nearly all afferents are small myelinated or unmyelinated, and travel with sympathetic (hypogastric) or parasympathetic (pelvic) nerves. Some exhibit a low level of ongoing discharge when the bladder is empty. Distension excited mainly thin myelinated afferents, with pressure thresholds corresponding to the values where humans report the first sensation of fullness. Nearly all units were activated by the intraluminal pressures reached during normal, non-painful micturition. An example of the responses of one of these afferents, which form a homogeneous population, is shown in Figure 7.6. All myelinated afferents responded in a graded fashion to increases of the intravesical pressure throughout the innocuous and into the supraphysiological, noxious, pressure range (Floyd et al 1976; Häbler et al 1990a, 1993a). These afferents reflected the magnitude and the temporal profile of intravesical pressure changes with high fidelity.

The unmyelinated population of afferents projecting through the pelvic nerve differed markedly. Very few fibres (<2.5%) responded to changes in intraluminal pressure in normal animals, and those differed significantly in their response properties from the population of thin myelinated fibres (Häbler et al 1990b). They had pressure thresholds of 30–50 mmHg, outside, or at the top end of, the physiological range. Thus, there are only a few afferents that could be called specific nociceptors in the bladder, and which would signal only painful levels of distension. It is illuminating to estimate the magnitude of the afferent inflow arriving at the sacral spinal cord by these different afferent populations (McMahon & Koltzenburg 1993). At an intravesical pressure of 50 mmHg (painful in man and well beyond the normal physiological pressures), the total afferent discharge in the cat is about 4500 action potentials per second, of which only some 225 (around 5%) are contributed by the unmyelinated fibre population. Given the small percentage of the unmyelinated 'nociceptive' fibres and the meagre afferent barrage they generate, it is doubtful that they constitute the only (or indeed a significant) primary afferent pathway encoding visceral pain (Jänig & Koltzenburg 1990, 1992).

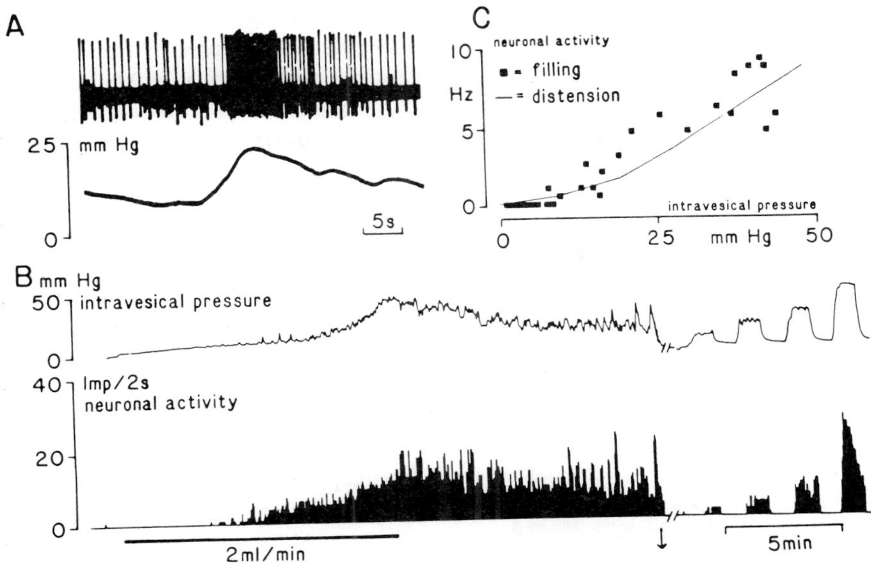

Fig. 7.6 Responses of a single myelinated (Aδ-) afferent fibre innervating the urinary bladder of the cat. In **A** the response of the unit to a small spontaneous bladder contraction (lower trace) is shown. **B** shows a ratemeter record of the firing of the same unit to slow filling of the bladder (2 ml/min) and rapid distensions. **C** plots the stimulus-response function for this afferent fibre. (From Häbler et al 1990.)

Inflammation and the recruitment of 'silent' afferents

Primary afferents have been investigated at the onset of an acute vesical inflammation induced by intraluminal injection of chemical irritants such as turpentine and mustard oil. These have been shown to produce pain-related behaviour and changes of bladder motility in unanaesthetised rats (McMahon & Abel 1987). Mechanosensitive afferents were vigorously excited by the intravesical injection of these substances, at short latencies. The afferents displayed ongoing activity once the chemicals were removed and the bladder was emptied (Häbler et al 1993b). In addition, some mechanosensitive afferents displayed a leftward shift of the stimulus-response function, indicating sensitisation to changes of intravesical pressure. An example of the response of a representative afferent is shown in Figure 7.7A. The activity of the unmyelinated fibres (that did not respond to increases of intravesical pressure) has also been studied with experimental inflammation. Following intravesical injections of irritant chemicals some 10% were excited (Häbler et al 1990b). These neurons showed an initial burst of activity which then settled to a lower level as the chemically induced inflammation progressed. Some of these initially mechanically insensitive afferents also acquired a novel mechanical sensitivity in the biologically relevant pressure range (Häbler et al 1990b) (Fig. 7.7B and C). Thus, compared to the number of unmyelinated afferents responding in the normal animal, four times as many were excited by distension at the onset of an acute inflammation. The activation of a numerically significant population of initially unresponsive afferents indicates that peripheral afferent mechanisms encoding pain from pelvic viscera are highly malleable and are strongly affected by the state of the tissue. These peripheral changes are obviously likely to be important for signalling pain and discomfort in inflammatory conditions.

Lower GI tract

The properties of afferents innervating the colon and rectum have many features in common with those innervating the urinary bladder (Morrison 1973, 1977; Floyd & Morrison 1974; Blumberg et al 1983; Haupt et al 1983; Jänig & Koltzenburg 1991). Afferents conducting in the Aδ- and C-fibre range are present in both sympathetic and parasympathetic nerves to the terminal GI tract. Many myelinated afferents respond to graded distention, with pressure thresholds in the physiological range but stimulus-response functions encoding supraphysiological pressures as well. Afferents travelling with the sympathetic nerves more frequently exhibit low levels of ongoing activity. A second group of myelinated afferents innervate the mucosa of the anal canal and respond to gentle shearing forces applied here (Jänig & Koltzenburg 1991).

Most unmyelinated afferents travelling with the pelvic nerve appear unresponsive to innocuous or noxious mechanical stimuli. The function of this numerically large

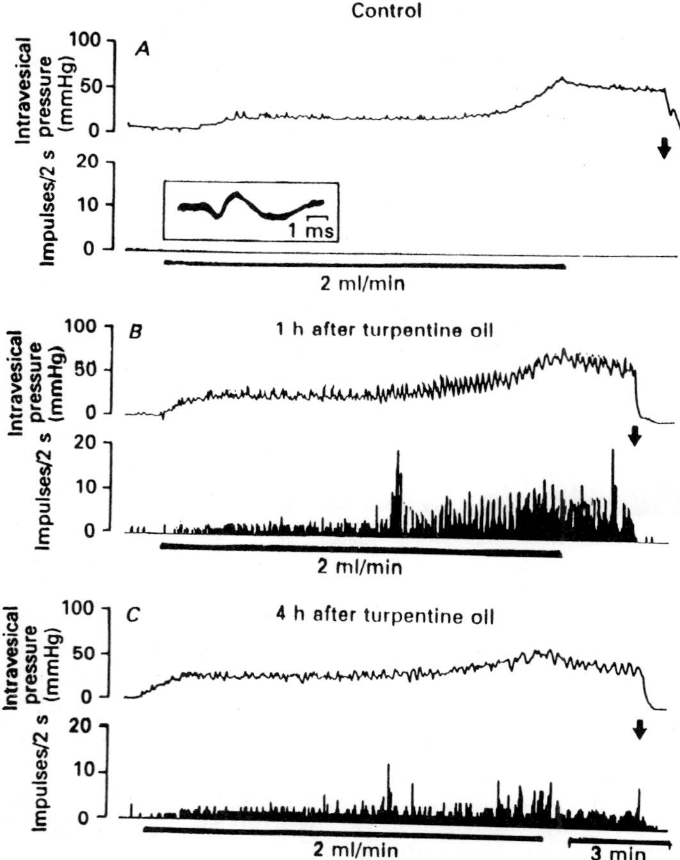

Fig. 7.7 Response of a 'silent' unmyelinated (C–) afferent fibre innervating the urinary bladder of the cat. In **A** the lack of response of this afferent to slow filling into, and beyond, the normal physiological range, is shown. After this control determination, the bladder was experimentally inflamed with turpentine. **B** and **C** show the development of novel mechanosensitivity 1 and 4 hours after the inflammatory stimulus. (From Häbler et al 1990b.)

group of afferents remains unknown, but one possibility is that some of these afferents will respond to pathophysiological states, such as inflammation, as has been reported for urinary bladder afferents (see above).

Haupt et al (1983) have reported that colonic afferents subjected to ischaemia can show an increase in their levels of ongoing and contraction-related activity. These changes took some considerable time to develop. The results suggest a chemosensitivity of these afferents, and this was directly demonstrated in some cases using bradykinin and potassium.

Heart

Many studies have been undertaken on the properties of sensory neurons innervating the ventricles and coronary vessels (see Malliani 1982). These afferents, again with thin myelinated or unmyelinated axons, travel with the sympathetic cardiac nerves. There has been some controversy as to whether these afferents could be considered specific nociceptors or not. Malliani and colleagues have found that both the Aδ- and C-fibre afferents form a homogeneous population with the following characteristics: well defined mechanosensitive receptive fields to direct probing; low levels of ongoing activity; responsiveness to physiological and innocuous events such as increases in the contractile state of the heart; and responsiveness to potentially noxious stimuli such as bradykinin. These workers therefore find no evidence for a group of specific nociceptors. Other workers have claimed that some afferents have no ongoing activity or mechanosensitivity and are recruited only when algesic chemicals are administered (Uchida & Murao 1975; Coleridge & Coleridge 1980; Baker et al 1980), and therefore might be considered nociceptive. Malliani and co-workers have provided convincing arguments that these apparent nociceptors are only seen in cases where responsiveness to innocuous stimuli is masked by inappropriate haemodynamic or other experimental conditions (see Malliani 1986).

Coronary occlusion has often been employed as an experimental noxious stimulus on the basis that cardiac ischaemia is a commonly-accepted natural cause of pain. Many afferent fibres give a robust response to such an intervention, usually with a latency of 10 or 20 seconds (suggesting a chemical mediator is involved) but occasionally with much shorter latencies. However, it has recently been emphasised that cardiac ischaemia may be neither a necessary nor sufficient cause of pain. Firstly, there are some observations in animals that the simple mechanical effects produced by occlusion or direct traction on a coronary artery (without ischaemia) may elicit aversive reactions (Osler 1910; Martin & Gordham 1938). Further, in animals with indwelling coronary cannulae, occlusion and even bradykinin injections were not associated with any aversive behaviourial responses provided that the animals had fully recovered from the surgery to implant the cannulae (Pagani et al 1985). There is also growing clinical evidence that patients experiencing transient episodes of myocardial insufficiency, whilst exhibiting electrocardiographic changes, frequently do not feel pain, especially if the ischaemic episode is short-lived. Together, these observations raise the possibility that the chemosensitivity of afferents is frequently irrelevant in the genesis of cardiac pain and pose a major challenge to the idea that cardiac pain is signalled by specific nociceptors.

SUMMARY OF PERIPHERAL PROCESSING MECHANISMS

There appear to be a number of common features of the afferent innervation of all viscera, and these differ in many respects from cutaneous afferents, and in fewer respects from other deep afferents innervating muscle and joint (Ch. 1). These are:

1. All visceral structures are predominantly innervated by afferents conducting in the Aδ- and C-fibre range.

2. Many afferent fibres have mechanosensitive endings which usually appear as a number of discrete spots.

3. Afferents travelling with the sympathetic nerves frequently terminate in muscle and serosal layers whilst those travelling with parasympathetic nerves frequently innervate muscle and mucosal layers.

4. Many mechanosensitive afferents exhibit low levels of ongoing activity.

5. Mechanosensitive afferents usually also respond to a number of chemical stimuli, some of which are algesic.

6. All the hollow muscular-walled organs (which give rise to pain with distension) have some afferent fibres which encode levels of distension both in the physiological (innocuous) range and in the supraphysiological (presumed noxious) range.

There are also a number of afferent features which have been reported for particular viscera, as follows:

7. Some afferents, particularly mucosal afferents projecting through the pelvic nerve, appear to be chemosensitive, and activated in pathophysiological states such as inflammation. They have been identified in the urinary bladder and may form a numerically large population in other pelvic viscera.

8. There are some afferent fibres responsive to distension, which might be considered specific nociceptors. The clearest example is seen in the biliary system where these fibres apparently are relatively numerous. They may exist in smaller numbers in the urinary bladder and oesophagus.

This final point has led some authors to the conclusion that visceral pain conforms to the specificity theory in particular viscera. However, these 'nociceptors' may form the tail-end of a distribution in which afferents exhibit a continuum of thresholds, as depicted in Figure 7.3C. For many other viscera, there is no evidence for a significant population of specific nociceptors. Together, the evidence suggests that for most viscera, pain may be encoded according to the intensity theory.

CENTRAL PROCESSING OF VISCERAL INFORMATION

The routing and processing of afferent information in the central nervous system (CNS) has been studied extensively for cutaneous inputs (see Ch. 5) but much less for deep and visceral ones. The available data demonstrate some clear points of correspondence and difference between these systems. The experimental evidence also throws considerable light on the likely mechanisms of referred pain and hyperalgesia. One problem in interpreting experimental data is that visceral afferent information is utilised not solely for viscerosensory processes, but also in the coordination of reflex function, much of which proceeds subconsciously. One solution, or at least partial solution, to this problem has been to study central neurons implicated in sensory processes (e.g. spinothalamic tract neurons).

Terminations of somatic and visceral afferents

This subject is reviewed in Chapter 5. A few essential differences between somatic and visceral afferents should be noted. Very few visceral afferents project in the dorsal columns, as might be expected given the relative rarity of Aβ-fibres innervating viscera. Visceral afferent fibres course with sympathetic and parasympathetic nerves. They penetrate the CNS at the same levels as the autonomic efferents. Thus, the spinal projections of visceral afferents are largely restricted to thoracic, upper lumbar and sacral segments (Ness & Gebhart 1992). The dorsal roots of lumbar and cervical enlargements do not carry any substantial visceral inputs. However, individual visceral afferents appear to have a more widespread rostrocaudal distribution than cutaneous afferents, and the extensive divergence of these afferents may partially compensate for their relative paucity (Sugiura 1989). This widespread distribution means, for instance, that some visceral afferent terminations from pelvic nerves (which enter over sacral roots) are found within the dorsal horn of the lumbar enlargement (Morrison 1987b).

Within the dorsal horn, visceral afferent terminations have patterns distinct from cutaneous afferents. Figure 7.8 compares the terminations of cutaneous, deep and visceral afferents. The incoming afferents give off collaterals which pass up and down the cord in Lissauer's tract. These then penetrate into the grey matter to terminate in lamina I or form two so-called collateral pathways that travel laterally and medially around the edge of the dorsal horn and give off terminals to lamina V, the grey matter around the central canal (lamina X) and the intermediolateral column (Morgan et al 1981; Cervero & Connell 1984; Kuo & DeGroat 1985; DeGroat 1986). Thus, in the dorsal horn, terminations are concentrated in laminae I and V, and largely avoid lamina II, which receives such a massive input from fine cutaneous afferents.

These termination patterns have been demonstrated with transganglionic tracing techniques and using the fact that some neuronal markers, such as VIP and the enzyme nitric oxide synthase, occur predominantly in visceral rather than somatic afferents (Kawatani et al 1986; Aimi et al 1991; see also Morrison 1987b).

Dorsal horn cell responses

Given the small number of visceral afferents, one might expect that, other than neurons associated with the

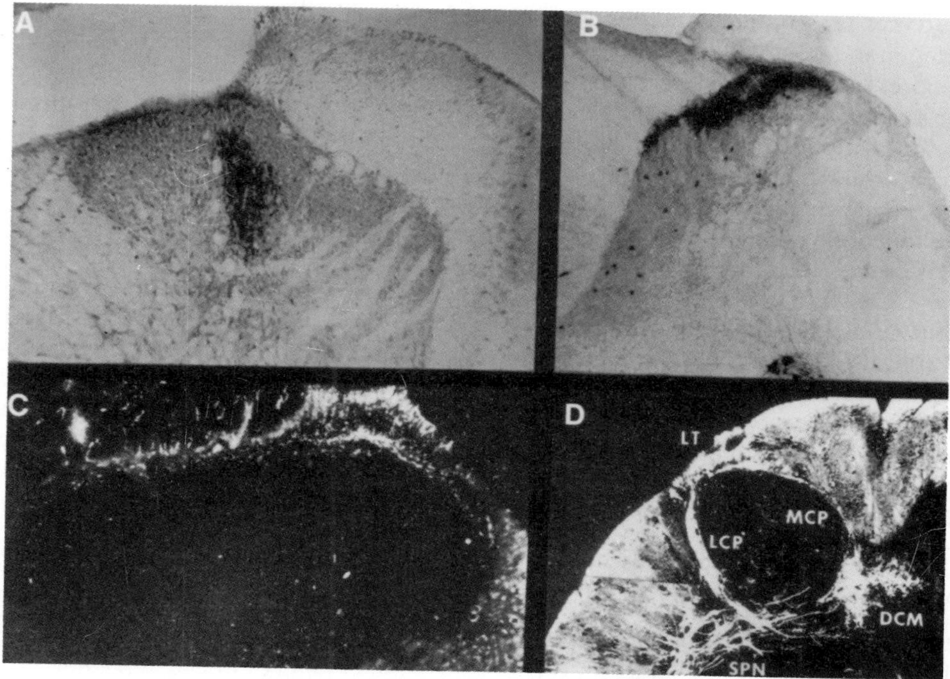

Fig. 7.8 Comparison of the central termination patterns of afferent fibres innervating skin, muscle and viscera. All the panels show photomicrographs of transverse sections of spinal cord, following anterograde labelling of various peripheral nerves. In **A**, cholera B toxin subunit had been applied to the skin of the ankle. This marker is carried predominantly in large-diameter afferents, and the central termination pattern of the cutaneous Aβ-fibres are seen heavily concentrated in the deep laminae of the dorsal horn, largely avoiding I and II. In **B**, WGA-HRP had been applied to the sciatic nerve. Most of the labelling seen is in fine cutaneous afferents, which terminate heavily in laminae I and II. (Courtesy of Dr G Lewin.) **C** shows the staining resulting from HRP labelling of the muscle gastrocnemius nerve. Dorsal horn labelling is sparse, but concentrated in lamina I. (From Craig & Mense 1984.) **D** shows the staining resulting from labelling of cat pelvic nerve with HRP. In addition to preganglionic neurons and their axons, afferent terminations are seen in laminae I and V, and in the dorsal commissure (DCM). The afferent fibres leave Lissauer's tract and form a lateral and medial collateral pathway running around the edge of the dorsal horn (labelled LCP and MCP, respectively). (From Morgan et al 1981.)

autonomic outflow (for instance, those in the intermediolateral cell column), relatively few spinal neurons would be excited by their activation. However, as we have said, the visceral afferents appear to ramify extensively within the spinal cord, and when large numbers of afferents are simultaneously activated, by electrical stimulation, a disproportionate number of spinal neurons respond. Thus, Cervero & Tattersall (1986) found that electrical stimulation of the splanchnic nerve in the cat (which contributes only some 10% of the total thoracic input) is capable of exciting about 75% of thoracic spinal neurons. Electrical stimulation is not an ideal stimulus, since it activates a wide spectrum of afferents, often from more than one viscus, and of course produces a highly unnatural synchronous afferent barrage which may reveal weak and normally ineffective synaptic inputs. Nonetheless, even when so-called natural stimuli are used (for instance, distension), a surprisingly high proportion of postsynaptic neurons appear to be responsive. Foreman and colleagues have recorded from spinothalamic tract neurons, and then asked how many respond to stimulation of individual viscera. They found, for example, that 39% of STT neurons in sacral segments were excited by bladder distension (Milne et al 1981), and, in upper thoracic segments, 36% of STT neurons were excited by gall bladder distension (Ammons et al 1984a) and 75% of similar neurons were excited by chemical stimulation of cardiac afferents (Blair et al 1982). These percentages also suggest that many individual neurons exhibit convergent inputs from more than one viscus, and this is in fact frequently observed when tested directly (Fields et al 1970; McMahon & Morrison 1982; Garrison 1992). Such multivisceral convergence may contribute to the vagueness of many visceral sensations, but it also raises something of a paradox as to how specific visceral reflexes arise. It is possible that the widespread representation of visceral information may be a feature particular to the conditions used experimentally, and that some weak inputs would normally be physiologically repressed in the intact awake animal.

There does not appear to be a set of spinal neurons exclusively dedicated to processing visceral information. This is true in two different ways. Firstly, visceral information is encoded by cells of many recognised ascending spinal pathways. For instance, the spinothalamic, spinoreticular and spinomesencephalic tracts all contain some neurons which respond to visceral stimulation. We have said that there are very few Aβ visceral afferents and it is therefore not surprising that the dorsal column pathway carries little visceral information. The spinocervical tract, prominent in the cat, may not receive visceral input (Cervero & Iggo 1978). Secondly, individual neurons responding to activation of visceral afferents in almost all cases receive a convergent somatic input (see summary in Ness & Gebhart 1990). The somatic receptive fields can be in skin and/or muscle, and are generally centred on the spinal segment of study. Cutaneous receptive fields are reported to be larger in the neurons showing viscerosomatic convergence, than for non-convergent ones (Cervero & Tattersall 1985). Cutaneous receptive fields usually, but not always, have high-threshold components, either exclusively or in combination with low-threshold inputs. That is, from the perspective of the somatic inputs alone, these neurons would usually be classified as wide dynamic range or nociceptive specific. The segmental nature, and common occurrence, of viscerosomatic convergence provides clear support for the convergence-projection theory of referred pain (Ruch 1946). The rationale is that activity in postsynaptic cells induced by visceral afferents is misinterpreted as arising from the convergent somatic inputs and therefore felt as arising in the appropriate somatic tissue. Given the extremely common occurrence of viscerosomatic convergence (generally reported to be more than 95%), it is perhaps more surprising that not all visceral pains are referred. It is also unclear why referred pain should mask a 'true' visceral pain.

Spinal responses to 'natural' stimulation of healthy visceral tissue

In experimental studies the most frequently used visceral stimulus is distension of the hollow organs. For many of these studies it is not clear whether the stimulus might be considered noxious. However, a number of general features emerge from these different studies, and, by way of example, we will here consider colorectal distension in the rat, which has been intensively examined by Gebhart and colleagues in anaesthetised and awake animals (Ness & Gebhart 1987a, 1987b, 1988a, 1988b, 1989a, 1989b). These workers have used an 8 cm balloon to distend most of the descending colon and rectum. They have shown that in awake animals, distending pressures of 40 mmHg or above act as an aversive stimulus in a conditioned avoidance behaviour task. Pseudoaffective reflex responses (cardiovascular and tensing of abdominal wall muscles) were seen with pressures above 20–30 mmHg.

The responses of spinal neurons to an identical form of stimulation have been determined in anaesthetised or spinalised animals, at both T13–L2 and L6–S2 spinal levels (the segments receiving input from afferents travelling with the sympathetic and parasympathetic nerves, respectively). Most neurons were excited by distension. They encoded colorectal distension monotonically up to distending pressures of at least 100 mmHg. The neurons were located predominantly in laminae V and X but some appeared to be located in lamina I. Some of the cells had long ascending projections destined for supraspinal structures. Cells excited by colorectal distension had convergent input from somatic structures. Mostly, somatic receptive fields were found in skin, where they frequently contained a high-threshold component. Less commonly, somatic receptive fields were located in muscle or joint. The somatic fields were ipsilateral and varied in size from a fraction of one dermatome to several dermatomes, centred on skin somatotopically appropriate to the recording site.

The neurons excited by colorectal distension appeared to form two subpopulations, according to presence of afterdischarges to pressure stimuli. Those without afterdischarges had pressure thresholds that extrapolated to about 0 mmHg, whilst those with afterdischarges extrapolated to about 15 mmHg, on average. Examples of the response of these neurons are shown in Figure 7.9, along with the stimulus-response functions for a sample of cells. These curves are reminiscent of those seen for primary afferent neurons, and appear to exhibit a spectrum of thresholds. Given the behavioural data obtained with this stimulus, it does not appear that either of these groups of spinal neurons encodes specifically noxious levels of distension. Rather, both groups are suited to encoding distension in an intensity dependent fashion.

A smaller number of spinal neurons inhibited by colorectal distension were found in these studies. In other respects (ascending axons, somatic inputs) these neurons were similar to those excited by distension. However, they had pressure thresholds of around 40 mmHg, at or above the levels of distension that are likely to be noxious. Some neurons of this type were observed in spinalised animals suggesting that, in these cases at least, the inhibitory mechanism resided in the spinal cord. The possibility that these inhibitory responses may be analogous to the so-called 'diffuse noxious inhibitory control' (DNIC) described using heterosegmental noxious somatic stimuli (see Chs 5 and 11), is considered in a later section.

Studies utilising distension of other hollow viscera have produced qualitatively very similar results when recordings have been made from spinal segments receiving a projection from the viscus of interest (reviewed in Ness & Gebhart 1990). Neurons recorded in distant spinal

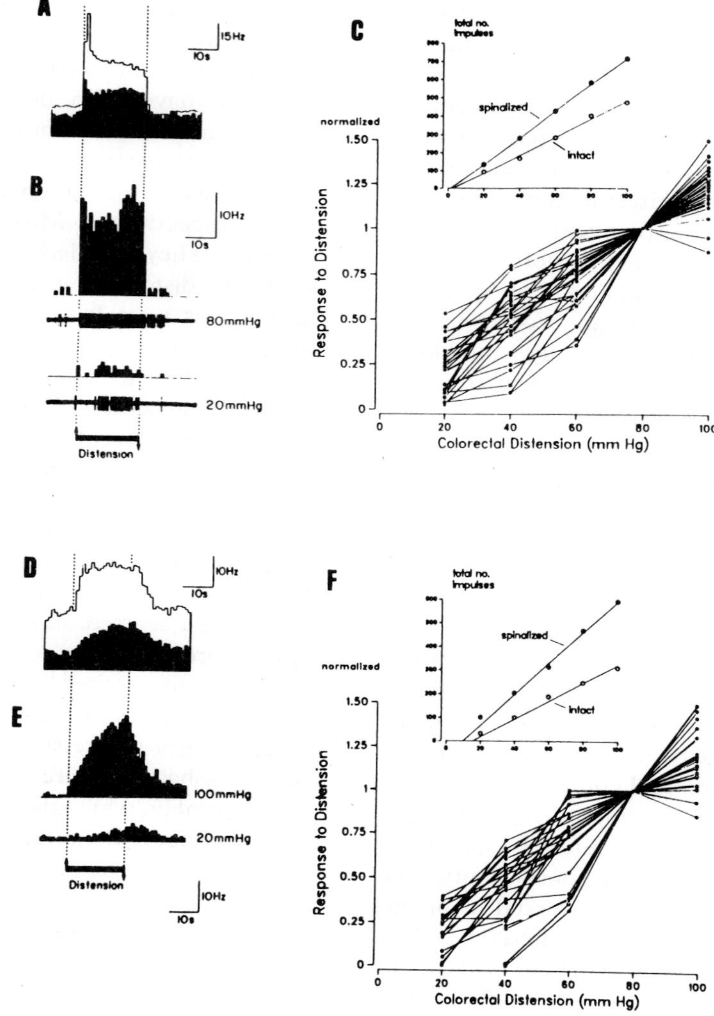

Fig. 7.9 Responses of spinal neurons to graded balloon distension of the colorectum in the rat. The responses shown in **A**–**C** are from neurons classified as 'short latency abrupt' on the basis of the rapid return to baseline firing after removal of the distending stimulus. **D**–**F** are from neurons classified as 'short latency sustained' because they showed afterdischarges lasting 4–50 s after removal of distension. **A** and **D** show ratemeter records of individual units to distension to supraphysiological levels (80 mmHg) in both the intact (solid bars) and spinalised state (open bars). **B** and **E** show ratemeter records of single neurons to graded distension, and **C** and **F** show stimulus-response curves for individual and groups of neurons. (Modified from Ness & Gebhart 1988a.)

segments frequently show inhibitory responses, as described below in the section on modulation of visceral inputs. There are some additional features that have been reported in other studies. For instance, multivisceral convergence from structures in the same viscerotome has been frequently observed when looked for. Thus, many cells in upper thoracic segments respond to stimulation of both heart and oesophagus (Garrison et al 1992), and in the sacral cord, to both urinary bladder and colon (McMahon & Morrison 1982). In cases of multivisceral convergence, neurons can exhibit an excitatory field in one viscus and an inhibitory one in another. Whilst such convergence may be enigmatic as far as sensory processing is concerned, such patterns are to be expected in some neurons regulating motility. For instance, since bladder motility is depressed by colonic stimulation, one would predict that appropriate response properties would arise in some neuronal pools.

The effects of inflammation

A number of reasons have been given to suggest that

viscerosensory mechanisms may be altered in pathological states, particularly inflammatory states. Irritant chemicals have been used to induce an acute inflammation in a number of visceral tissues. In the urinary bladder, turpentine or xylene-induced inflammation produces a number of sensory and reflex changes which are similar to those seen in cystitis in humans (McMahon & Abel 1987; Maggi et al 1988). Firstly, bladder motility increases and small distensions produce greater than normal rises in intravesical pressure. The threshold for micturition is also reduced. This hyperreflexia develops within 1 hour of the stimulus and persists for 1 or 2 days. Unanaesthetised animals excessively lick abdominal skin, and show decreased thresholds to noxious stimuli applied to the segmentally appropriate skin areas. That is, the animals' behaviour suggests the presence of referred pain and hyperalgesia.

Dorsal horn neurons in the rat lumbosacral cord that responded to electrical stimulation of the pelvic nerves were studied before and during the onset of bladder inflammation by McMahon (1988). A number of changes in response properties of these cells were observed during the development of the inflammation. Many neurons showed a progressive increase in the level of their ongoing activity and about 50% showed increased responses to bladder distension. In some cases this took the form of a leftward shift in the normal stimulus-response function, whilst in others it was seen as the development of an entirely novel mechanosensitivity. An example is shown in Figure 7.10. These changes are reminiscent of those seen in primary afferent fibres but they are likely to involve at least a component of central change. This is because in the presence of inflammation, the neurons showed enhanced responses to electrical stimuli applied to the pelvic nerves (stimuli which bypass the peripheral terminals of the afferents and provide a constant input volley) (see Fig. 7.10B). Additional evidence for a central sensitisation comes from the observation that the somatic receptive fields of some neurons are enlarged or show reduced thresholds. The somatic afferents forming these receptive field components are, of course, unaffected by the intravesical irritants.

Acute experimental inflammations of other visceral tissues such as the colon and oesophagus (Ness & Gebhart 1990; Garrison et al 1992) are reported to induce similar central excitability changes.

Thus, there is evidence for a slowly developing and maintained increase in the excitability of central neurons in inflammatory states. The most likely trigger for this change is the afferent barrage induced in the peripheral C-fibres innervating the inflamed organ. In the case of the urinary bladder, this is suggested by the observation that hyperexcitable states are not seen after impairment of C-fibres with capsaicin (Abelli et al 1988). Additionally, in a number of somatic tissues, very similar central sensitisations are induced by stimuli that specifically activate C-afferent fibres. (see Chs 5 and 11). The ionic basis of these central sensitisations is now becoming clear. Both myelinated and unmyelinated afferents appear to use excitatory amino acids as their fast neurotransmitters. In the normal state, the receptive fields of most dorsal horn neurons depend upon the released excitatory amino acids

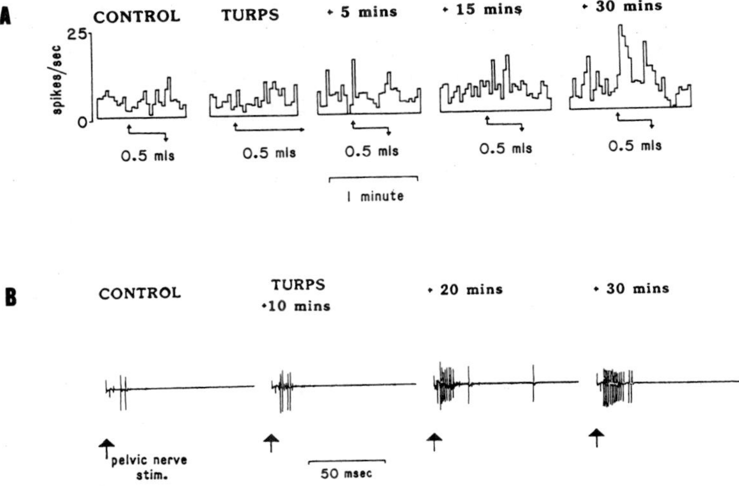

Fig. 7.10 A Ratemeter record of the discharges of a sacral cord neuron to distension of rat urinary bladder before, and at various times after, inducing an experimental inflammation with turpentine. Note the emergence of mechanosensitivity after inflammation in this unit. At least part of this enhanced responsiveness arises from a process of central rather than peripheral sensitisation. This is shown by the increased responses of the neuron to supramaximal electrical stimulation of the pelvic nerve, after inflammation **B**. (From McMahon 1988.)

acting on a particular class of postsynaptic receptor, the AMPA receptor (Dougherty et al 1992). Although postsynaptic cells possess an alternative excitatory amino acid receptor (the NMDA receptor), this does not normally carry much synaptic current and therefore contributes only modestly if at all to the receptive field (Dougherty et al 1992; Lopez-Garcia & King 1993). The unmasking of the NMDA receptor allows the postsynaptic cell to produce much larger responses than normal to an input, and to express previously weak or relatively ineffective inputs. This unmasking appears to be a crucial factor in the generation of central sensitisation. The NMDA receptor can be blocked by physiological concentrations of Mg^{+} ions, and this block is voltage-dependent and can be relieved by depolarisation of the cell. Many of the neuropeptides present in the unmyelinated afferents, and released with activity, produce slow depolarisations of dorsal horn neurons (Murase & Randic 1984). Additionally, some neuropeptides, such as substance P, appear to directly modulate the NMDA receptor ion-channel, making it more available to agonist activation (Randic et al 1990; O'Malley et al 1991). Thus, particularly in inflamed tissue, the recruitment and tonic firing of unmyelinated afferents is capable of maintaining an increased state of responsiveness to fast neurotransmitters in postsynaptic neurons.

The sensitisation of dorsal horn neurons following inflammation of visceral tissues provides a ready explanation for the phenomenon of referred tenderness or hyperalgesia that is seen in animal models and in many patients with visceral disorders. The process of central sensitisation can be viewed as an electrophysiological equivalent of the 'irritable focus' proposed by MacKenzie. Thus, the convergence-facilitation model (Fig. 7.2C) may provide the most appropriate context in which to consider referred pain and hyperalgesia associated with persistent, and clinically relevant, visceral pain states.

Modulation of viscerosensory processes

The spinal representation of visceral information is subject to a number of controls arising in distant body tissues and brainstem, and conversely, events occurring in the visceral domain can exert distant effects on other sensory inputs. There are close parallels between visceral and somatic systems in these respects.

The effects of activating descending systems from, particularly, the periaqueductal grey matter (PAG) and ventromedial medulla (including the nucleus raphe magnus), have been extensively studied (reviewed in Ch. 7). Electrical stimulation at these sites, or microinjection of opiates, is capable of producing an antinociceptive effect on the behaviour of the animal to noxious somatic stimulation. It is generally believed that these antinociceptive effects are mediated, at least in part, by descending inhibitory pathways that modulate the nociceptor-evoked activity in dorsal horn neurons, and there is a wealth of evidence that such inhibitions can occur. Several workers have claimed that stimulus-produced descending inhibition is selective for the nociceptive inputs to convergent neurons. The pharmacology of the spinal inhibitions has also been intensively studied, with the general conclusion that enkephalinergic, noradrenergic and serotonergic mechanisms may all be engaged by activation of descending pathways.

Reports of descending effects on visceral inputs have yielded similar conclusions. The behaviourial effects of hypertonic solutions given intraperitoneally (the 'writhing' response) are reduced by stimulation of the PAG in rats (Giesler & Liebeskind 1976), although the usefulness of this model of visceral pain is questionable since such injections may activate somatic afferents in the abdominal wall or peritoneum. Foreman and colleagues (Ammons et al 1984b; Chapman et al 1985) have characterised the inhibitory effects of raphe magnus stimulation on the responses of spinothalamic tract cells to cardiac inputs, and Ness & Gebhart (1987b) have directly compared the inhibition of cutaneous stimuli (noxious skin heating) and visceral stimuli (colorectal distension) to brainstem stimulation. In this latter study, it was found that the inhibition of neuronal responses to both forms of stimuli was indistinguishable, occurring at the same brainstem sites at comparable intensities of stimulation. They found, however, that the inhibition of responses to visceral stimulation operated over the entire range of stimulus pressures tested (25–100 mmHg). That is, no evidence for a selective inhibition of noxious, rather than innocuous, stimuli was found. Similar descending inhibition of other visceral inputs to dorsal horn neurons has been noted (Cervero et al 1985; Tattersall et al 1986; Cervero & Lumb 1988). Less commonly, excitatory effects have been induced in spinal neurons by activation of descending systems, for both somatic and visceral inputs (Cervero et al 1985; McMahon & Wall 1988; Cervero & Lumb 1988).

In addition to these stimulus-produced effects, a number of workers have studied tonic descending influences on spinal neurons. Many dorsal horn neurons along the entire length of the spinal cord appear to be under tonic descending inhibitory control, and show enhanced responses to both visceral and somatic inputs following spinalisation. Some neurons, in the deeper spinal laminae VII and VIII of the thoracic cord, show reduced responses to visceral stimulation on spinalisation (Cervero et al 1985; Tattersall et al 1986; Cervero & Lumb 1988). These neurons may have their visceral receptive fields mediated by an excitatory spino-bulbo-spinal loop.

The descending inhibitions operating on both visceral and somatic inputs appear to have a similar pharmacology. For instance, in one study which compared responses to colorectal distension and noxious skin heating, both inputs were similarly affected by morphine and the adrenergic agent, clonidine, although the morphine and clonidine effects differed from each other in a number of respects (Ness & Gebhart 1989b).

Another well-studied inhibitory effect results from noxious counterstimulation. In the somatic system, noxious stimulation of one body site inhibits the behavioural effects of a noxious stimulus to another site. Similarly, these so-called diffuse noxious inhibitory controls (DNIC) operate to inhibit the noxious-induced responses of convergent dorsal horn neurons, and there is considerable evidence that part of this effect operates by triggering activity in descending pathways originating in the raphe magnus (see Besson & Chaouch 1987). In their original report, Le Bars et al (1979) showed that intraperitoneal injections of bradykinin could trigger DNIC in neurons in the lumbar cord.

Subsequently, a number of other, more controlled, visceral stimuli have been found capable of inhibiting heterosegmental convergent neurons (i.e. in spinal segments outside that supplying the viscus stimulated). One example is shown in Figure 7.11, in which graded distension of the urinary bladder inhibits the response of a neuron in the lumbar enlargement with a receptive field on the hindpaw. Since in the somatic system, DNIC is only seen when noxious stimuli are applied, such experiments may give an alternative measure as to what levels of visceral stimuli might be considered noxious. In the case of the urinary bladder, the threshold for inhibitory effects was about 25 mmHg (Lumb 1986). Heterosegmental inhibition from abdominal and thoracic visceral afferents has also been reported by Foreman et al (1988). In this study, much of the inhibition survived spinalisation, suggesting a relay through the raphe magnus was not normally used. In this respect it should be remembered that some heterosegmental inhibitions from somatic structures are seen in spinal animals. Any difference between visceral and somatic systems may be qualitative rather than quantitative in this respect.

Vagal stimulation is now also clearly established to produce strong inhibitory effects on behaviour and the response of spinal neurons in lower cervical, thoracic, lumbar and sacral cords (see Fu et al 1992). It is even claimed that the antinociceptive effect of systemic morphine is reduced by vagotomy (Steinman et al 1986). Ren et al (1988) studied the stimulation parameters necessary to inhibit tail-flick reflexes in the rat. They found that maximal inhibition occurred with high frequency (20 Hz) stimulation at intensities that were sufficient to activate C-fibres in the vagus. However, the threshold stimuli for inhibitory effects occurs with stimulus parameters that are likely to activate only A-fibres, and several studies have found that even lower intensities of stimulation sometimes produce facilitatory effects. If vagally-induced inhibition is analogous to other counterstimuli, it would suggest that the stimulus was noxious. However, it is traditionally assumed that vagal afferents cannot give rise to pain. It remains to be established what functional group of vagal afferents are capable of inducing these inhibitions.

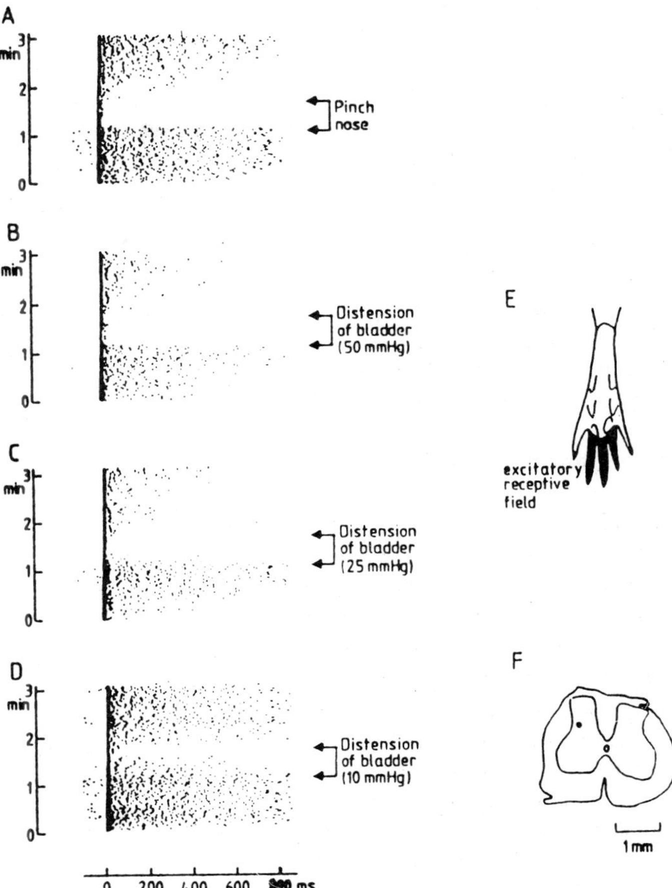

Fig. 7.11 A–D Raster dot display showing successive responses (bottom to top) of a lumbar dorsal horn neurone to repeated electrical stimulation of its receptive field (shown in **E**). Arrows indicate the period of application of noxious somatic (**A**) and of visceral (**B–D**) conditioning stimuli. The recording site is shown in **F**. (From Lumb 1986.)

SUMMARY OF SPINAL PROCESSING MECHANISMS

A number of general features are apparent in the central processing of visceral information:

1. In experiments on anaesthetised animals, afferents from individual viscera appear to excite a surprisingly large number of spinal neurons. These neurons are mostly located in spinal segments receiving the appropriate afferent projection, or nearby segments.

2. The stimulus-response functions of neurons activated by the distension of the hollow viscera are

usually monotonic with components in the innocuous pressure range and in the supraphysiological, presumably noxious, range.

3. Where tested, most spinal neurons activated by visceral mechanical stimuli are also responsive to chemical stimuli.

4. There are no private ascending spinal pathways dedicated to the signalling of visceral events. Rather, the viscera are represented in many well-recognised somatosensory pathways.

5. Somato-visceral convergence is very common, and the somatic receptive fields often include nociceptive components. The segmental nature of such common somatovisceral convergence is likely to underlie the phenomenon of referred pain.

6. Inflammation of visceral organs can induce central sensitisation of dorsal horn neurons, in which visceral and somatic inputs are facilitated. This process, which appears mechanistically similar to central sensitisation induced by somatic stimuli, is likely to be of importance in the phenomenon of referred hyperalgesia.

7. The central processing of visceral information is under descending controls that appear very similar to those operating on somatic inputs. Visceral afferent activity can trigger heterosegmental inhibitions that are also similar to those seen from somatic sources.

REFERENCES

Abelli L, Conte B, Somma V et al 1988 The contribution of capsaicin-sensitive sensory nerves to xylene-induced visceral pain in conscious, freely moving rats. Naunyn-Schmiedebergs Archives of Pharmacology 337: 545–551

Abrahams V C, Teare J L 1969 Peripheral pathways and properties of uterine afferents in the cat. Canadian Journal of Physiology and Pharmacology 47: 576–577

Aimi Y, Fujimura M, Vincent S R, Kimura H 1991 Localisation of NADPH-diaphorase containing neurones in sensory ganglia of the rat. Journal of Comparative Neurology 306: 382–392

Ammons W S, Foreman R D 1984a Cardiovascular and T2–T4 dorsal horn cell responses to gall bladder distension in the cat. Brain Research 321: 267–277

Ammons W S, Blair R W, Foreman R D 1984b Raphe magnus inhibition of primate T1–T4 spinothalamic cells with cardiopulmonary visceral input. Pain 20: 247–260

Ammons W S, Blair R W, Foreman R D 1984c Responses of primate T1–T5 spinothalamic neurons to gall bladder distension. American Journal of Physiology 247: R995–R1002

Andrews P L R 1986 Vagal afferent innervation of the gastrointestinal tract. In: Cervero F, Morrison J F B (eds) Visceral sensation. Progress in Brain Research 67. Elsevier, Amsterdam, p 65–86

Bahns E, Ernsberger U, Jänig W, Nelke A 1986 Functional characteristics of lumbar visceral afferent fibers from the urinary bladder and the urethra in the cat. Pflügers Archives 407: 510–518

Bahns E, Halsband U, Jänig W 1987 Responses of sacral visceral afferents from the lower urinary tract, colon and anus to mechanical stimulation. Pflügers Archives 410: 296–303

Bahr R, Blumberg H, Jänig W 1981 Do dichotomizing fibers exist which supply visceral organs as well as somatic structures? A contribution to the problem of referred pain. Neuroscience Letters 24: 25–28

Baker D G, Coleridge H M, Coleridge J C G, Nedrum T 1980 Search for a cardiac nociceptor: stimulation by bradykinin of sympathetic afferent nerve endings in the ear of the cat. Journal of Physiology 306: 519–536

Beacham W S, Kunze D L 1969 Renal receptors evoking a spinal vasomotor reflex. Journal of Physiology 201: 73–85

Bentley F H, Smithwick R H 1940 Visceral pain produced by balloon distension of the jejunum. Lancet i–ii: 389–391

Berkley K J, Robbins A, Sato Y 1988 Afferent fibers supplying the uterus in the rat. Journal of Neurophysiology 59: 142–163

Berkley K J, Hotta H, Robbins A, Sato Y 1990 Functional properties of afferent fibers supplying the reproductive organs and other pelvic organs in pelvic nerve of female rat. Journal of Neurophysiology 63: 256–272

Besson J M, Chaouch A 1987 Peripheral and spinal mechanisms of nociception. Physiological Reviews 67: 67–186

Birder L A, de Groat W C 1992 Increased c-fos expression in spinal neurones after irritation of the lower urinary tract in the rat. Journal of Neuroscience 12: 4878–4889

Blair R W, Weber R N, Foreman R D 1982 Responses of thoracic spinothalamic neurons to intracardiac injections of bradykinin in the monkey. Circulation Research 51: 83–94

Blumberg B, Haupt P, Jänig W, Köhler W 1983 Encoding of visceral noxious stimuli in the discharge patterns of visceral afferent fibers from the colon. Pflügers Archives 398: 33–40

Bors E, Comarr A E 1971 Neurological urology: physiology of micturition, its neurological disorders and sequelae. Karger, Basel

Bors E, Ma K T, Parker R B 1956 Observations on some modalities of bladder sensation. Journal of Urology 76: 566–575

Bower E A 1966 The characteristics of spontaneous and evoked action potentials recorded from the rabbit's uterine nerve. Journal of Physiology 183: 730–747

Bretland P M 1972 Acute ureteric obstruction. Butterworths, London

Capps J A 1932 An experimental and clinical study of pain in the pleura, pericardium and peritoneum. Macmillan, New York

Cervero F 1982a Noxious intensities of visceral stimulation are required to activate viscerosomatic multireceptive neurons in the thoracic spinal cord of the cat. Brain Research 240: 350–352

Cervero F 1982b Afferent activity evoked by natural stimulation of the biliary system in the ferret. Pain 13: 137–151

Cervero F 1983 Somatic and visceral inputs to the thoracic spinal cord of the cat: effects of noxious stimulation of the biliary system. Journal of Physiology (London) 337: 51–67

Cervero F, Connell L A 1984 Distribution of somatic and visceral primary afferent fibers within the thoracic spinal cord of the cat. Journal of Comparative Neurology 230: 88–98

Cervero F, Iggo A 1978 Natural stimulation of urinary bladder afferents does not affect transmission through lumbosacral spinocervical tract neurones in the cat. Brain Research 156: 375–379

Cervero F, Lumb B M 1988 Bilateral inputs and supraspinal control of viscerosomatic neurones in the lower thoracic cord of the cat. Journal of Physiology (London) 403: 221–237

Cervero F, Sann H 1989 Mechanically evoked responses of afferent fibers innervating the guinea-pig's ureter: an in vitro study. Journal of Physiology 412: 245–266

Cervero F, Tattersall J E H 1985 Cutaneous receptive fields of somatic and viscerosomatic neurones in the thoracic spinal cord of the cat. Journal of Comparative Neurology 237: 325–332

Cervero F, Tattersall J E H 1986 Somatic and visceral sensory integration in the thoracic spinal cord. In: Cervero F, Morrison J F B (eds) Visceral sensation. Progress in Brain Research 67. Elsevier, Amsterdam, p 189–206

Cervero F, Lumb B M, Tattersall J E H 1985 Supraspinal loops that mediate visceral inputs to thoracic spinal cord neurones in the cat: involvement of descending pathways from raphe and reticular formation. Neuroscience Letters 56: 189–194

Chapman C D, Ammons W S, Foreman R D 1985 Raphe magnus inhibition of feline T1–T4 spinoreticular tract cell responses to visceral and somatic inputs. Journal of Neurophysiology 53: 773–785

Chapman W P, Herrera R, Jones C M 1949 A comparison of pain produced experimentally in lower esophagus, common bile duct, and upper small intestine with pain experienced by patients with diseases of biliary tract and pancreas. Surgery, Gynecology and Obstetrics. 89: 573–582

Christensen J, Lund G F 1969 Esophageal responses to distension and electrical stimulation. Journal of Clinical Investigation 48: 408–419

Clerc N, Mei N 1983 Thoracic esophageal mechanoreceptors connected with fibers following sympathetic pathways. Brain Research Bulletin 10: 1–7

Coleridge H M,Coleridge J C G 1980 Cardiovascular afferents involved in the regulation of peripheral vessels. Annual Review of Physiology 42: 413–427

Csendes A, Sepulveda A 1980 Intraluminal gallbladder pressure measurements in patients with chronic or acute cholecystitis. American Journal of Surgery 139: 383–384

DeGroat W C 1986 Spinal cord projections and neuropeptides in visceral afferent neurons. In: Cervero F, Morrison J F B (eds) Visceral sensation. Progress in Brain Research 67. Elsevier, Amsterdam, p 165–187

Denny-Brown D, Robertson E G 1933a On the physiology of micturition. Brain 56: 149–190

Denny-Brown D, Robertson E G 1933b The state of the bladder and its sphincters in complete transverse lesions of the spinal cord and cauda equina. Brain 56: 397–463

Dougherty P M, Palecek J, Paleckova V, Sorkin L S, Willis W D 1992 The role of NMDA and non-NMDA excitatory amino acid receptors in the excitation of primate spinothalamic tract neurones by mechanical, chemical, thermal and electrical stimuli. Journal of Neuroscience 12: 3025–3041

Devor M, Wall P D, McMahon S B 1984 Dichotomizing somatic nerve fibers exist in rats but they are rare. Neuroscience Letters 49: 187–192

Fields H L, Partridge L D Jr, Winter D L 1970 Somatic and visceral receptive field properties of fibers in ventral quadrant white matter of the cat spinal cord. Journal of Neurophysiology 33: 827–837

Floyd K, Morrison J F B 1974 Splanchnic mechanoreceptors in the dog. Quarterly Journal of Experimental Physiology 59: 361–366

Floyd K, Hick V E, Morrison J F B 1976 Mechanosensitive afferent units in the hypogastric nerve of the cat. Journal of Physiology (London) 259: 457–471

Floyd K, Hick V E, Koley J, Morrison J F B 1977 The effects of bradykinin on afferent units in intra-abdominal sympathetic nerve trunks. Quarterly Journal of Experimental Physiology 52: 19–25

Foerster O 1933 Dermatomes in man. Brain 56: 1–39

Foreman R D, Hobbs S F, Oh U-T, Chandler M J 1988 Differential modulation of thoracic and lumbar spinothalamic tract cell activities during stimulation of cardiopulmonary sympathetic afferents fibers in the primate. In: Dubner R, Gebhart G F, Bond M R (eds) Proceedings of the Vth World Congress on Pain. Elsevier, Amsterdam, p 227–231

Fu Q-G, Chandler M J, McNeill D L, Foreman R D 1992 Vagal afferent fibers excite upper cervical neurons and inhibit activity of lumbar spinal neurons in the rat. Pain 51: 91–100

Garrison D W, Chandler M J, Foreman R D 1992 Viscero-somatic convergence onto feline spinal neurons from esophagus, heart and somatic fields: effects of inflammation. Pain 49: 373–382

Giesler G J Jr, Liebeskind J C 1976 Inhibition of visceral pain by electrical stimulation of the periaqueductal gray matter. Pain 2: 43–48

Goldscheider A 1920 Das Schmerzproblem. Springer, Berlin

Goligher J C, Hughes E S R 1951 Sensibility of the rectum and colon: its role in the mechanism of anal continence. Lancet i–ii: 543–548

Gunterberg B, Norlén L, Stener B, Sundin T 1975 Neurologic evaluation after resection of the sacrum. Investigative Urology 13: 183–188

Häbler H-J, Jänig W, Koltzenburg M 1988 A novel type of unmyelinated chemosensitive nociceptor in the acutely inflamed urinary bladder. Agents and Actions 25: 219–221

Häbler H-J, Jänig W, Koltzenburg M 1990a Properties of myelinated sacral afferents responding to filling and distension of the urinary bladder. Pflügers Archives 415: R104

Häbler H-J, Jänig W, Koltzenburg M 1990b Activation of unmyelinated afferent fibers by mechanical stimuli and inflammation of the urinary bladder in the cat. Journal of Physiology (London) 425: 545–562

Häbler H-J, Jänig W, Koltzenburg M 1993a Myelinated primary afferents of the sacral spinal cord responding to slow filling and distension of the cat urinary bladder. Journal of Physiology (in press)

Häbler H-J, Jänig W, Koltzenburg M 1993b Receptive properties of myelinated primary afferents innervating the inflamed urinary bladder of the cat. Journal of Physiology (in press)

Handwerker H O, Reeh P W 1991 Pain and inflammation. In: Bond M R, Charlton J E, Woolf C J (eds) Proceedings VIth World Congress on Pain. Elsevier, Amsterdam, p 59–70

Haupt P, Jänig W, Köhler W 1983 Response pattern of visceral afferent fibers, supplying the colon, upon chemical and mechanical stimuli. Pflügers Archives 398: 41–47

Head H 1893 On the disturbances of sensation with especial reference to the pain of visceral disease. Brain 16: 1–133

Head H, Riddoch G 1917 The autonomic bladder, excessive sweating and some other reflex conditions, in gross injuries of the spinal cord. Brain 40: 188–263

Hertz A F 1911 The sensibility of the alimentary tract in health and disease. Lancet 1: 1051–1056

Hockaday J M, Whitty, C W M 1967 Patterns of referred pain in the normal subject. Brain 90: 481–496

Hurst J 1911 The Goulstonian lectures on the sensibility of the alimentary canal. Frowde, Hodder & Stoughton, London

Jänig W, Koltzenburg M 1990 On the function of spinal primary afferent fibers supplying colon and urinary bladder. Journal of the Autonomic Nervous System 30: S89–S96

Jänig W, Koltzenburg M 1991 Receptive properties of sacral primary afferent neurons supplying the colon. Journal of Neurophysiology 65: 1067–1077

Jänig W, Koltzenburg M 1992 Pain arising from the urogenital tract. In: Maggi C A (ed) Nervous control of the urogenital system. Harwood, London (in press)

Jänig W, Morrison J F B 1986 Functional properties of spinal afferents supplying abdominal and pelvic organs, with special emphasis on visceral nociception. In: Cervero F, Morrison J F B (eds) Visceral sensation. Progress in Brain Research 67. Elsevier, Amsterdam, p 87–114

Javert C T, Hardy J D 1950 Measurement of pain intensity in labor and its physiologic, neurologic and pharmacologic implications. American Journal of Obstetrics and Gynecology 60: 552–563

Kawatini M, Nagel J, DeGroat W C 1986 Identification of neuropeptides in pelvic and pudendal nerve afferent pathways to the sacral spinal cord of the cat. Journal of Comparative Physiology 249: 117–132

Kellgren J H 1937–38 Observations on referred pain arising from muscle. Clinical Science 3: 175–190

Kellgren J H 1938 A preliminary account of referred pains arising from muscle. British Medical Journal 1: 325–337

Kellgren J H 1939 On distribution of pain arising from deep somatic structures with charts of segmental pain areas. Clinical Science 4: 35–46

Kellgren J H 1940 Somatic simulating visceral pain. Clinical Science 4: 303–309

Kinsella V J 1940 Sensibility in the abdomen. British Journal of Surgery 27: 449–463

Kumazawa T 1986 Sensory innervation of reproductive organs. In: Cervero F, Morrison J F B (eds) Visceral sensation. Progress in Brain Research 67. Elsevier, Amsterdam, p 115–132

Kuo D C, DeGroat W C 1985 Primary afferent projections of the major splanchnic nerve to the spinal cord and gracile nucleus of the cat. Journal of Comparative Neurology 231: 421–434

Learmonth J R 1931 Neurosurgery in the treatment of disorders of the urinary bladder: I. Anatomic and surgical considerations. Journal of Urology 25: 531–549

Le Bars D, Dickenson A, Besson J M 1979 Diffuse noxious inhibitory controls (DNIC). I. Effects on dorsal horn convergent neurones in the rat. Pain 6: 283–304

Leriche R 1937 Des douleurs provoquées par l'excitation du bout central des grands splanchniques (douleurs cardiaques, douleurs pulmonaires) au cours des splanchnicotomies. Presse Medicale 45: 971–972

Lewis T 1942 Pain. MacMillan, New York

Lewis,T, Kellgren J H 1939 Observations relating to referred pain, viscero-motor reflexes and other associated phenomena. Clinical Science 4: 47–71

Lim R K S, Miller D G, Guzman F et al 1967 Pain and analgesia evaluated by the intraperitoneal bradykinin-evoked pain method in man. Clinical Pharmacology and Therapeutics 8: 521–542

Lipkin M, Sleisenger M H 1958 Studies of visceral pain: measurements of stimulus intensity and duration associated with the onset of pain in esophagus, ileum and colon. Journal of Clinical Investigation 37: 28–34

Lopez-Garcia J A, King A E 1993 The role of amino acid receptor subtypes in synaptic transmission from cutaneous afferents onto rat dorsal horn neurones in vitro. Journal of Physiology 459: 219P

Lumb B M 1986 Brainstem control of visceral afferent pathways in the spinal cord. In: Cervero F, Morrison J F B (eds) Visceral sensation. Progress in brain research 67. Elsevier, Amsterdam, p 279–293

MacKenzie J 1909 Symptoms and their interpretation. Shaw, London

McLellan A M, Goodell H 1943 Pain from the bladder, ureter, and kidney pelvis. Research Publications – Association for Research in Nervous and Mental Disease 23: 252–262

McMahon S B 1986 Sensory-motor integration in urinary bladder function. In: Cervero F, Morrison J F B (eds) Visceral sensation. Progress in Brain Research 67. Elsevier, Amsterdam, p 245–253

McMahon S B 1988 Neuronal and behavioural consequences of chemical inflammation of rat urinary bladder. Agents and Actions 25: 231–233

McMahon S B, Abel C 1987 A model for the study of visceral pain states: chronic inflammation of the chronic decerebrate rat urinary bladder by irritant chemicals. Pain 28: 109–127

McMahon S B, Koltzenburg M 1993 Changes in the afferent innervation of the inflamed urinary bladder. In: Mayer E, Raybould H (eds) Basic and clinical aspects of chronic abdominal pain. Pain Research and Clinical Management, vol 9. In press

McMahon S B, Morrison J F B 1982 Two groups of spinal interneurones that respond to stimulation of the abdominal viscera of the cat. Journal of Physiology (London) 322: 21–34

McMahon S B, Wall P D 1988 Descending excitation and inhibition of spinal cord lamina I projection neurones. Journal of Neurophysiology 59: 1204–1219

Maggi C A, Abelli L, Giuliani S et al 1988 The contribution of sensory nerves to xylene-induced cystitis in rats. Neuroscience 26: 709–723

Maggi C A, Barbanti G, Santicioli P et al 1989 Cystometric evidence that capsaicin-sensitive nerves modulate the afferent branch of micturition reflex in humans. Journal of Urology 142: 150–154

Malliani A 1982 Cardiovascular sympathetic afferent fibers. Review of Physiology Biochemistry and Pharmacology 94: 11–70

Malliani A 1986 The elusive link between transient myocardial ischemia and pain. Circulation 73: 201–204

Martin S J, Gordham L W 1938 Cardiac pain: an experimental study with reference to the tension factor. Archives of Internal Medicine 62: 840–852

Mayer E A, Raybould H E 1990 Role of visceral afferent mechanisms in functional bowel disorders. Gastroenterology 99: 1688–1704

Mense S, Light A R, Perl E R 1981 Spinal terminations of subcutaneous high-threshold mechanoreceptors. In: Brown A G, Rethelyi M (eds) Spinal cord sensation. Scottish Academic Press, Edinburgh

Mense S 1986 Slowly conducting afferent fibers from deep tissues: Neurobiological properties and central nervous actions. Progress in Sensory Physiology 6: 139–219

Milne R J, Foreman R D, Giesler G J Jr, Willis W D 1981 Convergence of cutaneous and pelvic visceral nociceptive inputs onto primate spinothalamic neurons. Pain 11: 163–183

Morgan C, Nadelhaft I, DeGroat W C 1981 The distribution of visceral primary afferents from the pelvic nerve to Lissauer's tract and the spinal gray matter and its relationship to the sacral parasympathetic nucleus. Journal of Comparative Neurology 201: 415–440

Morley J 1931 Abdominal pain. Livingstone, Edinburgh

Morley J 1937 Visceral pain. British Medical Journal 2: 1270–1273

Morrison J F B 1973 Splanchnic slowly adapting mechanoreceptors with punctate receptive fields in the mesentery and gastrointestinal tract of the cat. Journal of Physiology (London) 233: 349–361

Morrison J F B 1977 The afferent innervation of the gastrointestinal tract. In: Brooks F P, Evers P W (eds) Nerves and the gut. Slack, New Jersey, p 297–322

Morrison J F B 1987a Sensations arising from the lower urinary tract. In: Torrens M, Morrison J F B (eds) The physiology of the lower urinary tract. Springer-Verlag, Berlin, p 89–132

Morrison J F B 1987b Neural connections between the lower urinary tract and the spinal cord. In: Torrens M, Morrison J F B (eds) The physiology of the lower urinary tract. Springer-Verlag, Berlin, p 53–85

Murase K, Randic M 1984 Actions of substance P on rat spinal dorsal horn neurones in vitro. Journal of Physiology 346: 203–217

Nathan P W 1956 Sensations associated with micturition. Journal of Urology 28: 126–131

Nesbit R M, McLellan F C 1939 Sympathectomy for the relief of vesical spasm and pain resulting from intractable pain infection. Surgery Gynecology and Obstetrics 68: 540–546

Ness T J, Gebhart G F 1987a Characterization of neuronal responses to noxious visceral and somatic stimuli in the medial lumbosacral spinal cord of the rat. Journal of Neurophysiology 57: 1867–1892

Ness T J, Gebhart G F 1987b Quantitative comparison of inhibition of visceral and cutaneous spinal nociceptive transmission from the midbrain and medulla in the rat. Journal of Neurophysiology 58: 850–865

Ness T J, Gebhart G F 1988a Colorectal distension as a noxious visceral stimulus: physiologic and pharmacologic characterization of pseudaffective reflexes in the rat. Brain Research 450: 153–169

Ness T J, Gebhart G F 1988b Characterization of neurons responsive to noxious colorectal distension in the T13–L2 spinal cord of the rat. Journal of Neurophysiology 60: 1419–1438

Ness T J, Gebhart G F 1989a Characterization of superficial T13–L2 dorsal horn neurons encoding for colorectal distension in the rat: comparison with neurons in deep laminae. Brain Research 486: 301–309

Ness T J, Gebhart G F 1989b Differential effects of morphine and clonidine upon visceral and cutaneous nociceptive transmission in the rat. Journal of Neurophysiology 62: 220–230

Ness T J, Gebhart G F 1990 Visceral pain: a review of experimental studies. Pain 41: 167–234

Newman H F, Northrup J D 1956 Intraluminal pressure and electrical excitability of the human gall bladder. Journal of Applied Physiology 9: 121–129

O'Malley P J, Calligaro D O, Monn J A 1991 Substance P and polyamines modulate the NMDA receptor operated ion channel by similar mechanisms. Society of Neurosciences Abstract 17: 613.5

Osler W 1910 The Lumleian lectures on 'angina pectoris' II. Lancet 1: 839

Pagani M, Pizzinelli P, Furlan R et al 1985 Analysis of the pressor sympathetic reflex produced by intracoronary injections of bradykinin in conscious dogs. Circulation Research 56: 175–183

Petersén I, Franksson C 1955 The sensory innervation of the urinary bladder. Urology International 2: 108–119

Peterson C G, Youlmans W B 1945 The intestino-intestinal inhibitory reflex: threshold variations, sensitization and summation. American Journal of Physiology 143: 407–412

Pierau Fr-K, Taylor D C M, Abel W 1982 Dichotomizing peripheral fibers revealed by intracellular recording from rat sensory neurones. Neuroscience Letters 31: 123–128

Polland W S, Bloomfield A L 1931 Experimental referred pain from the gastrointestinal tract. I. The esophagus. Journal of Clinical Investigation 10: 435–452

Poole J W, Sammartano R J, Boley S J 1987 Haemodynamic basis of the pain of chronic mesentric ischaemia. Annals of Internal Medicine 153: 171–180

Price D D, McHaffie J, Larson M 1989 Spatial summation of heat induced pain: influence of stimulus area and spatial separation of stimuli on perceived sensation intensity and unpleasantness. Journal of Neurophysiology 62: 1270

Procacci P, Zoppi M, Maresca M 1986 Clinical approaches to visceral sensation. In: Cervero F, Morrison J F B (eds) Visceral sensation. Progress in Brain Research 67. Elsevier, Amsterdam, p 21–28

Randic M, Hecimovic H, Ryu P D 1990 Substance P modulates glutamate-induced currents in acutely isolated rat spinal dorsal horn neurones. Neuroscience Letters 117: 74–80

Rang H P, Bevan S, Dray A 1991 Chemical activation of nociceptive peripheral neurones. British Medical Bulletin 47: 534–548

Ray B S, Neill C L 1947 Abdominal visceral sensation in man. Annals of Surgery 126: 709–724

Reeh P W, Kocher L, Jung S 1986 Does neurogenic inflammation alter the sensitivity of unmyelinated nociceptors in the rat? Brain Research 384: 42–50

Ren K, Randich A, Gebhart G F 1988 Vagal afferent modulation of a nociceptive reflex in rats: involvement of spinal opioid and monoamine receptors. Brain Research 446: 285–294

Riddoch G 1921 Conduction of sensory impulses from the bladder by the inferior hypogastrics and the central afferent connections of these nerves. Journal of Physiology (London) 54: 134P–135P

Risholm L 1954 Studies on renal colic and its treatment by posterior splanchnic block. Acta Chirurgica Scandinavica Suppl. 184: 1–64

Ross J 1888 On the segmental distribution of sensory disorders. Brain 10: 333–361

Ruch T C 1946 Visceral sensation and referred pain. In: Fulton J F (ed) Howell's textbook of physiology, 15th edn. Saunders, Philadelphia, p 385–401

Ruch T C 1965 Pathophysiology of pain. In: Ruch T C, Patton H D, Woodbury J W, Towe A L (eds) Neurophysiology 2nd edn. W B Saunders, Philadelphia, p 345–363

Ruffin J M, Baylin G J, Legerton C W Jr, Texter E C Jr 1953 Mechanisms of pain in peptic ulcer. Gastroenterology 23: 252–264

Sengupta J N, Kauvar D, Goyal R K 1989 Characteristics of vagal esophageal tension-sensitive afferent fibers in the opossum. Journal of Neurophysiology 61: 1001–1010

Sengupta J N, Saha J K, Goyal R K 1990 Stimulus-response function studies of esophageal mechanosensitive nociceptors in sympathetic afferents of opossum. Journal of Neurophysiology 64: 796–812

Sherrington C S 1900 Cutaneous sensation. In: Shafer E A (ed) Textbook of physiology, vol 2. Pentland, London, p 920–1001

Silen W 1987 Cope's early diagnosis of the acute abdomen 17th edn. Oxford University Press, New York

Sinclair D C, Weddell G, Feindel W H 1948 Referred pain and associated phenomena. Brain 71: 184–211

Steinman J L, Faris P L, Olney J W 1986 Further evidence for vagal involvement in the peripheral peptidergic modulation of nociception. Society of Neuroscience Abstract 12: 149.0

Sturge W A 1883 The phenomena of angina pectoris and their bearing upon the theory of counter-irritation. Brain 5: 492–510

Sugiura Y, Terui N, Hosoya Y 1989 Differences in distribution of central terminals between visceral and somatic unmyelinated (C) primary afferent fibers. Journal of Neurophysiology 62: 834–840

Tattersall J E H, Cervero F, Lumb B M 1986 Viscerosomatic neurons in the lower thoracic spinal cord of the cat: excitations and inhibitions evoked by splanchnic and somatic nerve volleys and by stimulation of brain stem nuclei. Journal of Neurophysiology 56: 1411–1423

Taylor D C M, Pierau Fr-K 1982 Double fluorescent labelling supports electrophysiological evidence for dichotomizing peripheral sensory nerve fibers in rats. Neuroscience Letters 33: 1–6

Theobald G W 1941 Referred pain: a new hypothesis. Times of Ceylon, Colombo

Uchida Y, Murao S 1975 Acid-induced excitation of afferent cardiac sympathetic nerve fibers. American Journal of Physiology 228: 27–33

Weiss S, Davis D 1928 Significance of afferent impulses from skin in mechanism of visceral pain: skin infiltration as a useful therapeutic measure. American Journal of Medical Science 176: 517–536

White J C, Sweet W H 1963 Pain and the neurosurgeon: a 40 year experience. Thomas, Springfield, Illinois, p 525–589

White J C, Smithwick R H, Simeone F A 1952 The autonomic nervous system: anatomy, physiology and surgical application. Macmillan, New York

Wolf S, Hardy J D 1943 Studies in pain; observations on pain due to local cooling and on factors involved in 'cold pressor' effect. Research Publications – Association for Research in Nervous and Neural Disease 23: 123–142

Wolf S 1965 Gastric sensibility. In: Wolf S (ed) The stomach. Springer-Verlag, New York, p 88–99

Woollard H H, Carmichael E A 1993 The testis and referred pain. Brain 56: 293–303

Woollard H H, Roberts J E H, Carmichael E A 1932 Inquiry into referred pain. Lancet 1: 337–338

8. Neurobiology of fetal and neonatal pain

Maria Fitzgerald

INTRODUCTION

Increasing recognition of the importance of pain in infancy and childhood has focused attention on the basic neurobiology of developing pain pathways. Advances in the general field of developmental neuroscience, particularly at the level of brain organization have shown that the infant nervous system is not simply an immature adult nervous system undergoing step-by-step construction. Complex changes at the molecular, cellular and organizational levels result in a series of transient functional stages throughout development until the adult pattern is achieved. To understand the development of pain processing we must therefore appreciate the changing nature of the fetal and neonatal central nervous system (CNS).

This chapter begins with a review of the emergence of pain behaviour in developing mammals and then examines the mechanisms underlying this behaviour, concentrating on the development of peripheral and central neural connections related to pain pathways and the maturation of chemical signalling within the CNS.

1. THE DEVELOPMENT OF PAIN BEHAVIOUR

A) PRENATAL PAIN BEHAVIOUR

To study the development of pain behaviour we need to consider the reactions of the fetal nervous system to sensory stimuli and the extent to which different modalities of stimuli, e.g. tactile versus noxious can be distinguished by different reflex responses. These responses are not evidence of pain perception or 'feeling' pain as such but do provide information about the sensitivity of the fetal and neonatal nervous system to nociceptive stimuli. Prenatally, studies have concentrated on the onset of sensitivity to somatic stimulation and studies of responses to noxious stimuli begin postnatally.

Reflex responses to somatic stimuli begin at 7.5 weeks in the human fetus (see Bradley & Mistretta 1975) and 15 days (E15, where gestation is 21.5 days) in the rat fetus (Narayanan et al 1971). The first area to become sensitive is the perioral region which, when touched, results in contralateral bending of the head. In the human, the palms of the hands are sensitive to stroking at 10.5 weeks; at E16 the rat forepaws are similarly sensitive. By 13.5–14 weeks in the human and E17 in the rat, the sensitive area has spread over the body and down to the hindlimbs. The feet and tail regions are the last to become responsive at E18–19. At the same time as the onset of evoked reflexes, the fetus begins to move spontaneously in the absence of any obvious external stimulation. Real time ultrasound recording of human fetuses in utero has revealed a complex variety of movements including stretching, hand to face contact, startle and sucking which build up over 7.5–15 weeks gestation and continue into postnatal life (De Vries et al 1982). Analogous spontaneous movements begin in the rat at E15 (Narayanan et al 1971).

It is important to emphasize that movements evoked at this stage are of a reflex or spontaneous nature only, even if they involve extensive body regions and therefore intersegmental and brainstem connections. The cortex is not a functional unit at this stage (see section 2) and therefore any discussion of 'perception' or of 'conscious' reaction to stimuli is inappropriate. Prechtl, who has made an extensive study of fetal behaviour, has a warning which is particularly apt when considering the emotive subject of fetal sensation and pain.

> There have been attempts to suggest intentional behaviour . . . even in the foetus, e.g. 'the foetus is exploring the uterine wall with its hand.' Such interpretations go beyond the available evidence. The same holds true for the claim of precocious sensory capabilities and learning in the fetus. The foetus does show, at an early age, a series of movement patterns which do not have a specific function before postnatal life, e.g. smiling. This anticipation of later functions must not be interpreted other than as evidence of the primacy of the motor system. Even if in later life some of these patterns acquire reflex character and become connected to specific stimuli and emotional situations, their generation in the foetus is frequently independent of the sensory triggers present in later life. (Prechtl 1985.)

B) POSTNATAL PAIN BEHAVIOUR

The somatosensory reflexes that appear in fetal life are still prominent at birth but change considerably over the postnatal period. In the neonate a prick on the hind foot may bring about 'a whole body movement' involving wriggling, rolling, and simultaneous responses from fore and hindlimbs but as it matures the response becomes more individuated and restricted to an isolated leg or foot movement. Coghill (1930) stressed the importance of individuation of specific out of larger, more diffuse behaviour patterns, but it is clear that, in mammals, this pattern should not be overemphasized. Isolated responses can be observed from birth and, even late in life, intensely painful stimuli can still bring about chaotic responses. Far more convincing is the perceptive proposal of Angulo y Gonzalez (1932) that 'individuation seems not to be achieved through disintegration or breaking up of the total patterns, but by an inhibitory process, whereby total patterns tend to go into the background, where they remain in a seemingly dormant stage, but from which they may be aroused at any time later on appropriate stimulation'. This issue of individuation through inhibition is not simply of historical interest; when applied to sensory inputs it is fundamental to our understanding of the development of pain. The idea of suppression or inhibition of neural pathways or mechanisms during development, which may be uncovered later in adult life, perhaps under certain pathological conditions, is as important today as it was in the 1930s.

A further feature of cutaneous reflexes in the newborn rat, kitten and human is that they are exaggerated compared to the adult (Ekholm 1967; Stelzner 1971; Issler & Stephens 1983; Fitzgerald & Gibson 1984). Thresholds are lower and the reflex muscle contractions more synchronized and long-lasting. Repeated skin stimulation results in considerable hyperexcitability or sensitization with generalized movements of all limbs. Ekholm (1967) detected that in young kittens the elicitation of a flexor reflex response often did not require a painful stimulus as in the adult but only light touch. A comparative study of the flexor reflex in newborn human infants, premature and full term, and rat pups has confirmed this (Fitzgerald et al 1988). Flexor reflex thresholds are very low in preterm infants and newborn rat pups but increase with postconceptional age (PCA). Furthermore, the sensitization caused by repeated stimulation is found to be present in both species but becomes much less pronounced after 29–35 weeks (PCA) in the human and postnatal day 8 (P8) in the rat.

Other reflex studies have concentrated specifically on nociceptive stimuli (Guy & Abbott 1992). Formalin injections into the rat hindpaw cause flexion of the injected limb from day 1 but the same response can also be evoked with saline injection and is overwhelmed by the very intense whole-body reactions and agitation observed at this age. Up until day 10, the responses are predominantly such 'non-specific' whole body movements, while the 'specific' flexion reflex and shaking and licking the paw predominates from then on. In the adult, the response to formalin injection has a classic biphasic pattern, whereby the early response (5–20 min) is followed by a reduced response and then a reappearance of a longer lasting response for 5–15 min that declines over the next hour (Dubuisson & Dennis 1977). Interestingly this biphasic response is not apparent in the rat pup until P15, coinciding with the depression in the overall response (Guy & Abbot 1992). This seems likely to result from the postnatal development of central inhibitory processes discussed above and in section 2C and D.

Thresholds to tail flick, hot plate, paw pinch and ophthalmic administration of capsaicin has been studied over the period of 10 days to 12 weeks (Hammond & Ruda 1991). In agreement with earlier reports, mechanical thresholds increase substantially over that period whereas hot plate and eye wipe thresholds decrease slightly with age. The same pattern is seen even more clearly if the tests are performed from day 1 (Webb et al 1993).

C) SUMMARY AND CONCLUSIONS TO SECTION 1

The rat fetus displays clear reflex responses to cutaneous stimuli which continue into the postnatal period. While these are often generalized, whole-body movements in the very young pup, localized isolated reflexes are also present becoming predominant as the animal matures. Immature cutaneous reflexes are highly exaggerated and the flexor reflex can be evoked to a lesser extent by non-noxious as well as noxious stimulation. The emergence of specific nociceptive responses that cannot be evoked by low-intensity stimuli occurs postnatally coinciding with a depression of the overall response. This suggests that developing inhibitory mechanisms, both local, segmental and descending from the brain, play a part in producing specific pain behaviour.

2. THE DEVELOPMENT OF PERIPHERAL AND CENTRAL CONNECTIONS RELATED TO PAIN

A) PERIPHERAL CONNECTIONS – ANATOMICAL STUDIES

In the rat hindlimb, peripheral nerves reach the base of the limb bud by embryonic day E13 and then gradually grow distally to reach the toes by E19 (Reynolds et al 1991). Skin innervation appears to occur in advance of muscle innervation, beginning at E14 in the proximal thigh and reaching the toes by E21. Such data are obtained from general axonal staining and it is not clear what the relative contribution of large-diameter afferents versus small-diameter C-afferents is at this stage. Since the large, light dorsal root ganglion cells giving rise to future A-fibres are born in advance of small dark cells giving rise to C-fibres (Lawson et al 1974) and have central projections that reach the spinal cord before those C-fibres (Fitzgerald 1978b), it seems logical to suppose that these are also the first to reach the skin. The cues used by cutaneous afferents to reach their appropriate skin targets is a subject of some research (see Davies 1987 for review) and it appears likely that one or more chemotropic factors are released that attract specific innervation. This is unlikely to be nerve growth factor (NGF), however, since NGF is not produced in the epidermis until after the arrival of cutaneous nerves (Davies et al 1987) and occurs independently of innervation (Rohrer et al 1988). NGF is likely to be important for maintenance of sensory nerves once they arrive in the skin. NGF receptor is markedly upregulated when first axons arrive at their target (Wyatt et al 1990) and levels of NGF in target tissue do correlate with, although are not responsible for, final innervation density (Harper & Davies 1990). Recent evidence shows that NGF is especially importanty for maintenance of C- rather than A-fibres (Ruit et al 1992) and since immature peripheral C-fibres are hard to detect, the true role of NGF in peripheral innervation pattern may have been missed so far.

Once peripheral nerves have penetrated the skin, the process of terminal elaboration is a prolonged one, and again is likely to be influenced by local growth factors (Martin et al 1989). Before the appearance or innervation of specific terminal end organs, the sensory axons in the rat form a dense and organized terminal plexus that penetrates right to the surface of the fetal epidermis perhaps encouraged by the growing epidermis (M.J.T. Fitzgerald 1966). This plexus gradually withdraws as end organs appear and the epidermis becomes thinner, leaving a major subepidermal plexus, with a few axons penetrating up into the epidermis as seen in the adult (M.J.T. Fitzgerald 1966; Reynolds et al 1991). In the rat hindlimb, these changes take place in the late fetal and early neonatal period. Merkel cells do not begin to appear and be innervated until birth in rat (English et al 1980) whereas hindlimb hair follicle innervation does not begin until postnatal day 7 (28 weeks in humans) (Payne et al 1991) and a few days earlier in mystacial skin (Munger & Rice 1986). Meissner's corpuscles do not appear in the rat until P8 (Zelena et al 1990) and early in the third trimester in primates (Renehan & Munger 1990).

As mentioned above, little is known of the development of skin innervation by C-fibres. Our knowledge depends on the use of selective markers such as substance P or somatostatin, whose expression may well be regulated by the target innervation itself. The development of these and other signalling molecules is discussed in section 3. Over the postnatal period there appears to be considerable loss of nearly 50% of axons from peripheral nerves from birth to adulthood which cannot be explained by neuron cell death (Jenq et al 1986). As yet it is not clear what contribution this makes to the final innervation pattern.

B) PERIPHERAL CONNECTIONS – PHYSIOLOGICAL STUDIES

In view of the prolonged anatomical maturation of skin innervation, recording the functional properties of single primary sensory afferents in fetal and neonatal rats has provided particularly important data with respect to the general sensory and nociceptive information arriving from the periphery at this time.

Recordings from individual embryonic rat DRG cells in vivo over this period show that cutaneous receptive fields on the hindfoot are first observed at E17, i.e. from the time the skin is first innervated (Fitzgerald 1987a). Frequency of firing and total number of impulses per stimulus are low compared to the adult, but increase with embryonic age. Even at this early stage, afferents fall into two clear categories, rapidly adapting units responding with a brief burst of impulses (200–500 ms) to skin pressure of >0.3 g and slowly adapting units capable of producing a more maintained response (up to 10 s) to pressure of >0.8 g. Examples of both receptor types are found that respond to noxious heating and chemical stimulation. One day later, at E18, a third category of low-threshold, rapidly adapting mechanoreceptor emerges, responding to light touch or brushing the skin, analogous to adult hair or touch mechanoreceptors (Lynn & Carpenter 1982). These do not respond to thermal or chemical stimuli. Similar recordings of the receptive field properties of individual DRG cells in vivo in the neonatal rat shows how the various adult receptor types differentiate functionally (Fitzgerald 1987c). At birth, the fetal pressure receptors described above are still prominent in both fast and slow conduction groups, but gradually disappear by P14. They may represent a transient population of afferents functional only during early development or, alternatively, simply be immature low-threshold mechanoreceptors. In addition, all the broad functional cutaneous afferent types found in the adult rat are found in the rat hindlimb at birth, although their maturity depends on receptor type (Fitzgerald 1987c).

Polymodal nociceptors, which have C-fibre axons in the adult, responding to mechanical, thermal and chemical noxious stimuli, are fully mature in their thresholds, pattern and frequency of firing at birth. High-threshold mechanoreceptors, which have Aδ-fibres in the adult and respond maximally to noxious mechanical rather than chemical and thermal stimulation, can also be distinguished, but their peak firing frequencies are lower at 5–8 Hz rising to 8–20 Hz at P7–14. Low-threshold mechanoreceptors responding to touch or brush with brief, rapidly adapting bursts of spikes are, relatively, the most immature at birth. At P0, typical responses are bursts of 2–6 spikes, peak 20 Hz; at P14, 8–25 spikes, peak 200 Hz. Similar observations on the postnatal maturation of low-threshold mechanoreceptors have been made in kittens, although these are more mature at birth than rat pups (Ekholm 1967; see Rowe 1982; Ferrington et al 1984).

The early maturation of C-fibre afferent receptor properties is not paralleled by their efferent function. Neurogenic extravasation, an inflammatory reaction produced by C-fibres, cannot be evoked in rat hindlimb skin before the second postnatal week (Fitzgerald & Gibson 1984). This may be due to slow development of the appropriate transmitters and their receptors, as discussed in section 3.

C) DEVELOPMENT OF SPINAL CORD CONNECTIONS

(i) Primary afferent central terminals

In the rat lumbar cord, large-diameter dorsal root afferents arrive at the spinal cord from E12 onwards but do not penetrate the grey matter for some days. Instead they travel rostocaudally in the bundle of His until E15 when the first main wave of collaterals begin to grow into the dorsal grey (Fitzgerald et al 1991). This pattern of events is also seen in the chick (Mendelson et al 1992) and the primate (Csillik & Knyhar-Csillik 1984) and it seems likely that the growth of collaterals into the grey matter is triggered by the innervation of the skin and other targets in the periphery (Fitzgerald et al 1991). Cutaneous afferents grow directly into the dorsal horn apparently avoiding the ventral horn, perhaps due to release of an inhibitory factor from that area (Fitzgerald et al 1993a) and terminal elaboration and characteristic U-shaped collaterals of hair-follicle afferents can be seen at E19 (Beal et al 1988; Fitzgerald et al 1993b). Some synapses with interneurones leading to reflex pathways are clearly made early on, since polysynaptic responses from ventral roots can be evoked from dorsal root stimulation in rat lumbar cord at E15.5, and electrical stimulation of the distal hindlimb evokes spikes in dorsal horn cells at E17. However, natural skin stimulation from defined receptive fields on the hindpaw does not evoke spike activity in the dorsal horn or reflex muscle activity until E19 (Fitzgerald 1991), suggesting that early synaptic connections may not be sufficient to produce activity in pathways projecting up to the brain. Connections between Ia afferents and motoneurons develop later than cutaneous connections in dorsal horn and the first Ia afferents reach the motoneuron pool at E17 coinciding with first recordings of a Ia reflex (Ziskind-Conhaim 1990).

C-fibres grow into the spinal cord considerably later than A-fibres, at E19 onwards (Fitzgerald 1987b) and many chemical markers associated with C-fibres and small dark DRG cells are not apparent in the spinal cord until the perinatal period (see section 3). C-type afferent terminals within synaptic glomeruli are not observed at EM level until P5 (Pignatelli et al 1989).

The growth of both A- and C-fibres into the cord is somatotopically specific, in the sense that afferents from a given skin region, e.g. the sciatic nerve field, grow directly into that part of the cord which, in the adult, is restricted to sciatic nerve terminals (Fitzgerald & Swett 1983; Fitzgerald 1987b). This presumably follows from early fetal organizational within the DRG themselves (Wessels et al 1990). This specificity is not apparent for growth into appropriate laminae, however. While in the adult, Aβ-afferents are restricted to laminae III & IV, in the fetus and neonate their terminals extend dorsally right up into laminae II & I to reach the surface of the grey matter. This is followed by a gradual withdrawal from the superficial laminae over the first 3 postnatal weeks (Fitzgerald et al 1993b). C-fibres on the other hand appear restricted to superficial laminae I and II from the outset and for a considerable postnatal period these laminae are occupied by both A- and C-fibre terminals (Fitzgerald et al 1993b). C-fibre synaptic maturation is involved in this withdrawal of A-fibres from laminae I and II, since administration of neonatal capsaicin which destroys the majority of C-fibres leaves A-fibre terminals permanently located in more superficial laminae than normal (Shortland et al 1990).

(ii) Spinal cord cell development

The spinal cord developes ventrodorsally: motoneurons are born first, followed by intermediate neurons, deep dorsal horn neurons and finally neurons of substantia gelatinosa (laminae I & II) (Nornes & Das 1974; Altman & Bayer 1984). There are also indications that axon outgrowth and synapses mature in the same direction; the first synapses occurring between interneurons and motoneurons followed by primary afferents and interneurons (Vaughn & Grieshaber 1973; Fitzgerald et al 1991). This retrograde development is by no means absolute. We have discussed the late development of Ia versus cutaneous reflexes and after the early stages of neurogenesis and axon outgrowth, cord maturation becomes highly complex and not obviously polarized.

Within the dorsal horn itself, there is good evidence that projection neurons develop in advance of local interneurons, in terms of axodendritic maturation (Bicknell & Beal 1984). This is consistent with functional evidence suggesting that some inhibitory mechanisms commonly attributed to interneuronal activity in the dorsal horn are absent in the newborn (see Fitzgerald 1990 for review). Synaptogenesis in the dorsal horn is at its maximum in the first postnatal weeks. The expression of NT75, a nerve terminal protein related to development of synaptic contacts is concentrated in deep dorsal horn at P4–5 and in laminae II at P7–9 (Cabalka et al 1990). In the human cord, neurons of laminae I are mature by 25 weeks of age (Rizvi et al 1986). The development of appropriate spinal cord connections is likely to be dependent on growth factors. Both low- and high-affinity NGF receptor levels are very high in developing spinal cord (Marchetti et al 1991) and changes in the levels of BDNF, NT3 and NGF are found over the relevant developmental period (Ernfors & Persson 1991).

(iii) Development of functional connections within the dorsal horn

Physiological studies demonstrating the onset of functional central primary afferent connections have been largely undertaken in vitro in isolated spinal cord preparations. Stimulation of the L4 dorsal root in the embryonic rat begins to produce long-latency (presumably polysynaptic) reflexes in the L4 ventral root (Saito 1979; Kudo & Yamada 1987) and long-latency excitatory postsynaptic potentials (EPSPs) in L4 motoneurons (Ziskind-Conhaim 1990) between E15.5 and E16. Neither presumptive monosynaptic reflexes nor Ia EPSPs are observed until E17.5–18.5. A similar sequence of events is observed in the chick (Lee et al 1988). The longer latency polysynaptic reflexes are presumably evoked from large-diameter cutaneous afferents as well as possible Group Ib and II muscle afferents.

Direct investigation of the development of cutaneous afferent central synaptic connections has come from recording the activity of lumbar dorsal horn cells in rat embryos in vivo (Fitzgerald 1991a). The synchronous input provided by electrical stimulation evokes spikes in dorsal horn cells at E17, but it is several days before cutaneous afferents are capable of producing suprathreshold excitation under physiological conditions. Natural stimulation of the hindpaw evokes a spike discharge in dorsal horn cells at E19. Initially this is evoked by high-intensity skin stimulation only, but by E20 dorsal horn cells are easily excited by low-intensity brush and touch of the skin.

Recording the activity of dorsal horn cells in the newborn shows that in the first postnatal week they have very unusual properties (Fitzgerald 1985). The synaptic linkage between afferents and dorsal horn cells is still weak but single stimuli can often evoke long-lasting excitation lasting minutes. Repeated stimuli can build up considerable background activity in the cells. The receptive fields of the dorsal horn cells are large in the newborn and gradually diminish over the first 2 postnatal weeks. The result of these properties is that otherwise weak cutaneous inputs are made more effective centrally. It has been proposed that this is a result of the immaturity of dorsal horn interneurons and lack of inhibitory control over inputs at this age. This proposal might explain the exaggerated cutaneous reflexes observed in the neonatal rat and human, as well as the long afterdischarges and large receptive fields of neurons in the newborn rat dorsal horn. All of these characteristics become less pronounced with increasing postnatal age in parallel with increasing segmental control and the development of descending inhibition (see below). There is evidence in a number of developing sensory systems that local inhibitory control develops secondarily to the initial excitatory afferent connections, e.g. in the olfactory system (Mair et al 1982). Not all segmental inhibition is absent in the newborn rat cord. Renshaw cell inhibition (Naka 1984) and some contralateral inhibitory mechanisms (Fitzgerald 1985) are well developed at birth. Nevertheless the maturation of interneurons in substantia gelatinosa, which appear to be particularly important for control of sensory processing, is largely postnatal (Bicknell & Beal 1984). Interestingly, it coincides with the arrival of afferent C-fibres in the dorsal horn and the two events may be causally linked. Animals treated at birth with the neutrotoxin capsaicin, which destroys afferent C-fibres, retain large receptive fields in the dorsal horn and cortex perhaps due to inadequate interneuron function (see Fitzgerald 1983).

(iv) C-fibre connections in the dorsal horn

Stimulation of a dorsal root at C-fibre intensities or noxious stimulation of the tail produces a long-latency (2–5 s), long-lasting (30 s) potential that can be recorded from the ventral root (Akagi et al 1983). It is blocked by substance P antagonists, the C-fibre neurotoxin capsaicin, and is reduced by morphine and other opioids in a naloxone reversible manner (Yanagisawa et al 1985). This slow potential is particularly prominent in the newborn rat can be evoked from many neighbouring dorsal roots. It appears to result from a widespread depolarization of spinal cord cells in response to release of substance P and other neurochemicals from C-fibre terminals rather than a specific synaptically mediated C-fibre evoked excitation. The widespread substance P receptor distribution within the spinal cord of the newborn rat (see section 3) may also be responsible (Charlton & Helke 1986). The specific C-fibre evoked synchronous long-latency bursts of action potentials seen in the adult dorsal horn do not develop until the second week of life in the rat (Fitzgerald 1985; Fitzgerald 1988). Consistent with this is the absence of a long-latency burst of activity on the ventral root after stimulation of C-fibres in the dorsal root or cutaneous nerve during the first postnatal week (Hori & Watanabe 1987; Fitzgerald et al 1987). This is in contrast to brisk A-fibre evoked mono- and polysynaptic responses that can be recorded in the dorsal horn and from the ventral root from birth (Saito 1979; Fitzgerald et al 1987). Furthermore, stimulation of the hindlimb skin with mustard oil, a specific C-fibre irritant, while exciting

C-fibre receptors in the newborn rat skin, does not evoke a clear flexion withdrawal of the limb until P10 (Fitzgerald & Gibson 1984), persumably because of the lack of sufficient C-fibre-evoked activity in the spinal cord before that time.

D) DESCENDING CONNECTIONS

Descending connections from the brainstem and higher centres to the spinal cord are an important feature of the somatosensory system. Their development is largely a postnatal event in the rat (Fitzgerald 1991b).

Animals given a mid-thoracic spinal cord transection before P15 are markedly less affected than those transected at older ages (Weber & Stelzner 1977). Concentrating here on sensory reflexes, rather than posture and movement, it is clear that in spinalized rats below 15 days of age, tactile and noxious stimuli continue to evoke withdrawal responses as well as less specific wriggling movements that are similar to those observed in intact rats. Older animals show severely depressed reponses for several days and then recover flexor responses to cutaneous stimuli with decreased duration.

These behavioural results are consistent with physiological studies of the development of descending inhibition of dorsal horn cells by brainstem neurons. Descending axons from these neurons grow down the spinal cord in the dorsolateral funiculus (DLF) early in fetal life (Leong et al 1984), although they may not extend collaterals into the dorsal horn and form connections for some time. Electrophysiological recording from adult rat dorsal horn neurons shows a clear inhibition of afferent evoked activity produced by stimulating these descending axons in the DLF. However, this descending inhibition is not apparent in the neonate until P10, and does not resemble that seen in the adult until P19. This delay in functional inhibition from the brainstem, despite the anatomical presence of the pathway may be partly due to the slow postnatal maturation of interneurones discussed above but is more likely to result from low levels of the appropriate neurotransmitters, 5-HT and noradrenaline (see section 3).

Stimulation of the periaqueductal grey (PAG) also activates the descending pathway in the DLF resulting in analgesia in a variety of species. Such PAG stimulation is ineffective in producing analgesia in rat pups, however, until the third week of life, being absent at P14 and clear at P21 (van Praag & Frenk 1991). Even at P21, higher stimulus intensities are required compared to the adult.

E) DEVELOPMENT OF CONNECTIONS IN HIGHER CENTRES

Much less is known of the maturation of projection pathways, thalamic and cortical connections in relation to pain processing compared to events in the periphery and spinal cord.

In the rat, dorsal horn projection cells begin to grow axons prenatally (Bicknell & Beal 1984; Fitzgerald et al 1991) and afferents reach the thalamus at E19. The earliest thalamic axons reach the cortical plate also at E19 and by PO there is a plexus of growth-cone tipped axons in the cortical plate and a few thalamic axons have reached the marginal zone (Erzurumlu & Jhaveri 1990). In the human, thalamocortical fibres penetrate the cortical plate at 26–34 weeks (Mrzljak et al 1988). These anatomical findings correlate well with functional studies. Evoked potentials from the forepaw develop the adult form in the rat somatosensory cortex by P12 (Thairu 1971) and in the equivalent potentials in humans begin to mature at 29 weeks PCA (Klimach & Cooke 1988).

Electrophysiological analysis of cortical cells at P7 shows them to be organized in columns as in the adult but to have larger receptive fields, suggesting a lack of inhibition as discussed above for the spinal cord (Amstrong-James 1975). The delayed maturation of inhibitory processes occurring several weeks after excitatory connections have been established has been observed in the neonatal rat hippocampus (Michelson & Lothman 1989) and may be a general pattern in developing cortex.

The rodent cortex remains immature for up to 6 weeks after birth and the human cortex for many years. The complex developmental processes taking place over this period are beyond the scope of this chapter. The development of attention and memory, and the many important cognitive factors contributing to the cortical perception of pain in infants and children are reviewed in McGrath (1990).

F) SUMMARY AND CONCLUSION TO SECTION 2

By the time a rat is born, the basic sensory connections in the periphery and spinal cord are in place. Nevertheless, enormous changes take place over the early postnatal period coinciding with the final trimester and early neonatal period in man (Fitzgerald 1991b). The maturation of C-fibre synaptic connections in the dorsal horn, interneuronal development in substantia gelatinosa and functional development of descending inhibition from the brainstem all take place postnatally in the rat. These important parts of the pain pathway display late maturation compared to the basic excitatory connections from low-threshold inputs. The effect of this is that while the newborn nervous system does mount a clear response to painful stimuli, this response is not always predictable or organized. Lack of inhibition means that responses to all sensory inputs, low and high threshold, are exaggerated and generalized and specific pain responses may require convergent inputs building up over time to become apparent. As concluded in section 1, the onset of inhibitory processes is a crucial part of the emergence of specific pain responses.

3. THE DEVELOPMENT OF NEUROTRANSMITTERS AND OTHER SIGNALLING MOLECULES RELATED TO PAIN

A) THE CHEMISTRY OF DEVELOPING PRIMARY AFFERENTS

(i) L-glutamate

L-glutamate has recently become a focus of great attention to pain neuroscientists, since its actions via the NMDA receptor are clearly very important in the production of C-fibre induced changes in central excitability and central components of hyperalgesia (see Chs 5 and 9). Glutamate-NMDA activity takes on a further interesting dimension here in view of its general role in development and plasticity of connections in the immature CNS (see Garthwaite 1989). In the adult cord NMDA receptor binding is restricted to substantia gelatinosa but at postnatal day 7 it is distributed throughout the cord. Affinity and density appears the same as in the adult but the restricted distribution is not achieved until P28 (Kalb & Hockfield 1991). In the immature hippocampus, where a similar situation occurs, NMDA EPSPs are much greater in amplitude and significantly less sensitive to Mg^{2+} (Morrisett et al 1990) although glycine modulation appears the same as in the adult (Boje & Skolnick 1992). These results suggest that NMDA-mediated slow EPSPs, wind-up and central excitability evoked by C-fibre stimulation in the adult spinal cord may be even more apparent in the neonatal cord. Furthermore this may be an important mechanism for establishing C-fibre connections with the developing spinal cord. Polysynaptic slow EPSPs evoked in motoneurons by dorsal root stimulation at E16 are blocked by the NMDA antagonist AVP indicating that initially synaptic transmission to motoneurons is mediated solely by NMDA receptors (Ziskind-Conhaim 1990). Onset of shorter latency EPSPs at E17 corresponded to an increase in glutamate sensitivity and these were mediated by both NMDA and non-NMDA receptors. Motoneurons are sensitive to glutamate, NMDA and kainate before the formation of synapses.

(ii) Substance P and other peptides

Substance P terminals, attributable to primary afferents first appear in the substantia gelatinosa of the rat at E18–19 and at 11 weeks in the human fetus (Senba et al 1982; Marti et al 1987). CGRP and somatostatin appear at about the same time. Cell bodies positive for these peptides are apparent in the dorsal root ganglia from E17 onwards. VIP immunoreactivity is detected much later than other primary afferent associated peptides in both rat, chick and human (Charnay et al 1985; New & Mudge 1986; Marti et al 1987). Despite the early appearance of these peptides, it should be emphasized that levels are very low at first and increase throughout fetal life showing a marked increase perinatally to approach adult levels by P14.

(iii) Activity related enzymes

Thiamine monophosphatase (TMP) and other acid phosphatases may play a role in purinergic transmission mechanisms. Acid phosphatases appear in the rat dorsal root ganglia very early at E13–E15 (Shoenen 1978) but are not seen in central C-fibre terminals until 24 hours after birth (Coimbra et al 1986; Gyulai 1988).

B) THE CHEMISTRY OF DEVELOPING CENTRAL CIRCUITS

(i) Opioid peptides

Opioid peptides appear in the rat brain before their receptors. β-endorphin, met-enkephalin and dynorphin are all found at E11.5, followed by μ-receptor binding at E12.5, κ-receptor binding at E14.5 and δ-receptor binding at P0 (Rius et al 1991). High-affinity opioid receptor binding increases three-fold in the first 2 postnatal weeks correlating with a 40-fold increase in opioid analgesic properties (Zhang & Pasternak 1981). At brainstem and spinal levels, however, enkephalin is not expressed in dorsal horn neurons, midbrain raphe or reticular formation until E20–P1 (Pickel et al 1982; Senba 1982; Marti et al 1987). Enkephalin containing fibres are seen in the human spinal cord at 10 weeks PCA but there is a marked increase in labelling in superficial cord from 25 weeks (Charnay et al 1984).

Physiological studies show that β-endorphin, D-ala and morphine all depress the dorsal root potential in the newborn spinal cord (Suzue & Jessell 1980) but their effect on afferent evoked activity with the dorsal horn of newborn pups has not been investigated.

Both morphine, a μ-agonist, and ketocyclazocine, a κ-agonist, induce naloxone-reversible analgesia to limb withdrawal and tail-flick tests of mechanical and thermal nociception between 3 and 5 days of age (Barr et al 1986; Giordano & Barr 1987). Ketocyclazocine-produced analgesia precedes morphine's effects by several days, such that the former produces robust analgesia between 7 and 10 days, while the latter effects do not peak until day 14.

(ii) Monoamines

Noradrenaline-containing terminals first appear in the rat dorsal horn at P4 and achieve the adult pattern by the 2nd–3rd postnatal week, although they appear in the ventral horn well before that (Commissiong 1983). Peak noradrenergic receptor development in rat spinal cord occurs at around P12; this is consistent with the analgesic effects of intrathecal noradrenaline and the α_2 agonist, clonidine, in P10 rat pups (Hughes & Barr 1988).

5-HT develops considerably later than other neurotransmitters. It has not been detected at all in fetal or neonatal spinal cord in humans and is thought to develop some time after the first 6 postnatal weeks (Marti et al 1987). The first few fibres are detected after birth in the rat spinal cord and adult concentrations are not reached until P14 (Loizou 1972; Bregman 1987). There also is evidence of a transient over expression of 5-HT in the spinal cord in the postnatal period (Bregman 1987).

(iii) Subtance P and other peptides

The appearance of the various neuropeptides in the dorsal horn of the spinal cord in rat pups and human fetuses has been reviewed by Marti et al (1987). Somatostatin is one of the first to be expressed at E16 (10 weeks in man), followed by CGRP, galanin, and substance P at E17–18. VIP develops later at P1 in rat pups and 20 weeks in man. All these peptides are found in cell bodies in fetal life but only in axons later after birth, the number of peptide-containing cells declining with postnatal age. HPLC analysis of tachykinins suggests a real change in their biosynthesis at the time and it is paralleled by a similar increase in receptor binding (see Jonakait et al 1991 for review).

Up to P15 substance P receptors are diffusely distributed over the spinal cord grey matter but they are progressively more defined to specific nuclei as the rat matures (Charlton & Helke 1986). Substance P binding decreases with age so that at P60 the cord has one-sixth of the binding sites present at P11. In the newborn, the superficial laminae have very few SP receptors. They are concentrated in deeper laminae and the high density observed in the adult substantia gelatinosa is not apparent until the second week of life (Charlton & Helke 1986).

Vasopressin receptors are transiently expressed in several areas associated with pain pathways during development, such as raphe nuclei, locus coerulus, spinal trigeminal nucleus and grey matter of the spinal cord. They appear at E16 and are lost completely in the adult but electrophysiological studies show them to be functionally active in the neonate (Tribollet et al 1991).

(iv) GABA

The appearance of GABA in the developing spinal cord has not been examined. Transient expression of GABAergic neurons in the deep dorsal horn and ventral horn has recently been reported in the developing rat spinal cord. The normal distribution of GABA, restricted to substantia gelatinosa is seen after one postnatal week (Ma et al 1992). The transient expression of GABA and its receptors by subplate zone neurons in developing cortex (Meinecke & Rakic 1992) may also occur in the spinal cord. However, bicuculline sensitive dorsal root potentials can be recorded at E17.5 and bicuculline affects dorsal root evoked potentials in motoneurons in rat embryos in a dose-dependent manner (Seno & Sato 1985). GABA and noradrenaline also inhibit secretion of peptides via a G-protein mediated inhibition of voltage dependent Ca channels in embryonic chick dorsal root ganlgia (Holz et al 1989).

C) GENE EXPRESSION IN DEVELOPING PAIN PATHWAYS

The c-fos gene, one member of a large class of 'immediate early' genes is induced in P1 neonatal rat dorsal horn cells by subcutaneous capsaicin and formalin injections. Cutaneous application of mustard oil, however, has no effect (Williams et al 1990). This finding is consistent with c-fos induction by high-threshold afferents as shown in the adult but immaturity of central C-fibre connections in the newborn leads to mustard oil being less effective.

Application of molecular biological techniques to look at gene function in the whole animal are likely to lead to great advances in the near future in our understanding of the developing nervous system (see Rosant 1990 for review). In relation to the somatosensory system and pain pathways much may be learnt from 'loss of function' studies where transfection in the early embryo allows mutation of a selected gene and subsequent study of changes in CNS development allows one to isolate the normal function of such a gene. Many such mutants die within 24 hours of birth but a recent mutant lacking low affinity NGF receptor is viable and has shown important changes in pain processing. The skin of these animals lacks SP- and CGRP-containing nerves and gradually becomes ulcerated with epidermal thinning. Furthermore, pain thresholds on hot plate testing are very high (Lee et al 1992). Another approach involves 'gain of function' studies where the relevant gene construct is introduced into transgenic mice together with a selective promoter which allows 'over expression' of the gene in the resulting phenotype.

SUMMARY AND CONCLUSION TO SECTION 3

Many neurotransmitters and signalling molecules involved in pain pathways are expressed early on in the developing nervous system but do not reach adult levels for a considerable period. More importantly, receptors are frequently transiently overexpressed or expressed in areas during development where there they are not seen in the adult. Low levels of neurotransmitter will, of course, mean reduced function but widespread and high-density receptor distribution will result in nonspecific or quite different function in the neonate compared to the adult. This will have important consequences on pain behaviour in the newborn and the effects of analgesics in controlling infant pain.

REFERENCES

Akagi H, Konishi S, Yanagisawa M, Otsuka M 1983 Effects of capsaicin and a substance P antagonist on a slow reflex in the isolated rat spinal cord. Neurochemical Research 8: 795–796

Altman J, Bayer S A 1984 The development of the rat spinal cord. Advances in Anatomy, Embryology and Cell Biology 85: 1–166

Angulo y Gonzalez A W 1932 The prenatal development of behaviour in the albino rat. Journal of Comparative Neurology 55: 395–442

Armstrong-James M 1975 The functional status and columnar organization of single cells responding to cutaneous stimulation in neonatal rat somatosensory cortex SI. Journal of Physiology 246: 501–538

Barr G A, Paredes W, Erickson K L et al 1986 K-opioid receptor mediated analgesia in the developing rat. Developmental Brain Research 29: 145–152

Beal J A, Knight D S, Nandi K N 1988 Structure and development of central arborizations of hair follicle primary afferent fibers. Anatomy and Embryology 178: 271–279

Bicknell H R, Beal J A 1984 Axonal and dendritic development of substantia gelatinosa neurons in the lumbosacral spinal cord of the rat. Journal of Comparative Neurology 226: 508–522

Boje K M, Skolnick P 1992 Ontogeny of glycine-enchanced [^{3}H] MK-801 binding to N-methyl-D-aspartate receptor coupled ion channels. Developmental Brain Research 65: 51–56

Bradley R M, Mistretta C M 1975 Fetal sensory receptors. Physiological Reviews 55: 352–382

Bregman B S 1987 Development of serotonin immunoreactivity in the rat spinal cord and its plasticity after neonatal spinal cord lesions. Developmental Brain Research 34: 245–263

Cabalka L M, Ritchie T C, Coulter J D 1990 Immunolocalization of a novel nerve terminal protein in spinal cord development. Journal of Comparative neurology 295: 83–91

Charlton C G, Helke C J 1986 Ontogeny of substance P receptors in rat spinal cord: quantitative changes in receptor number and differential expression in specific loci. Developmental Brain Research 29: 81–91

Charnay Y, Paulin C, Dray R et al 1984 Distribution of enkephalin in human fetus and infant spinal cord: an immunofluorescence study. Journal of Comparative Neurology 223: 415–423

Charnay Y, Chayvaille J-A, Said S I et al 1985 Localization of vasoactive intestinal peptide immunoreactivity in human foetus and newborn infant spinal cord. Neuroscience 14: 195–205

Coghill G E 1930 Individuation versus integration in the development of behaviour. Journal of General Psychology 3: 431–435

Coimbra A, Ribeiro-da-Silva A, Pignatelli D 1986 Rexed's laminae and the FRAP-band in the spinal cord of the neonatal rat. Neuroscience Letters 71: 131–137

Commissiong J W 1983 The development of catecholaminergic nerves in the spinal cord of the rat. II. Regional development. Developmental Brain Research 11: 75–92

Csillik B, Knyihar-Csillik E 1984 The protean gate. Akadémaiai Kiadó, Budapest

Davies A M 1987 Molecular and cellular aspects of patterning sensory neurone connections in the vertebrate nervous system. Development 101: 185–208

Davies A M, Bandtlow C, Heumann R et al (1987) Timing and site of nerve growth factor synthesis skin in developing skin in relation to innervation and expression of the receptor. Nature 326: 353–358

De Vries J I P, Visser G H A, Prechtl, H F R 1982 The emergence of foetal behaviour. I. Qualitative aspects. Early Human Development 12: 301–322

Dubuisson D, Dennis S G 1977 The formalin test: a quantitative study of the analgesic effects of morphine, meperidine and brain stimulation in rats and cats. Pain 4: 161–174

Ekholm J 1967 Postnatal changes in cutaneous reflexes and in the discharge pattern of cutaneous and articular sense organs. Acta Physiologica Scandinavica Suppl. 297: 1–130

English K B, Burgess P R, Van Norman K D 1980 Development of rat Merkel cells. Journal of Comparative Neurology 194: 475–496

Ernfors P, Persson H 1991 Developmentally regulated expression of HDNF/NT-3 mRNA in rat spinal cord motoneurones and expression of BDNF mRNA in embryonic dorsal root ganglion. European Journal of Neuroscience 3: 953–961

Erzurumlu R S, Jhaveri S 1990 Thalamic axons confer a blueprint of the sensory periphery onto the developing rat somatosensory cortex. Developmental Brain Research 56: 229–234

Ferrington D G, Hora M O H, Rowe M J 1984 Functional maturation of tactile sensory fibres in the kitten. Journal of Neurophysiology 52: 74–85

Fitzgerald M 1983 Capsaicin and sensory neurones – a review. Pain 15: 109–130

Fitzgerald M 1985 The postnatal development of cutaneous afferent fibre input and receptive field organization in the rat dorsal horn. Journal of Physiology 364: 1–18

Fitzgerald M 1987a Spontaneous and evoked activity of fetal primary afferents 'in vivo'. Nature 326: 603–605

Fitzgerald M 1987b Prenatal growth of fine-diameter primary afferents into the rat spinal cord: a transganglionic tracer study. Journal of Comparative Neurology 261: 98–104

Fitzgerald M 1987c Cutaneous primary afferent properties in the hindlimb of the neonatal rat. Journal of Physiology 383: 79–92

Fitzgerald M 1988 The development of activity evoked by fine diameter cutaneous fibres in the spinal cord of the newborn rat. Neuroscience Letters 86: 161–166

Fitzgerald M 1991a A physiological study of the prenatal development of cutaneous sensory inputs to dorsal horn cells in the rat. Journal of Physiology 432: 473–482

Fitzgerald M 1991b The developmental neurobiology of pain. In: Bond M R, Charlton J E, Woolf C J (eds) Proceedings of VIth World Congress on Pain, 1991. Elsevier, Amsterdam, p 253–261

Fitzgerald M 1991c The development of descending brainstem control of spinal cord sensory processing. In: Hanson M (ed) Fetal and neonatal brainstem: developmental and clinical issues. Cambridge University Press, Cambridge, p 127–136

Fitzgerald M, Gibson S 1984 The physiological and neurochemical development of peripheral sensory C fibers. Neuroscience 13: 933–944

Fitzgerald M, Swett J W 1983 The termination pattern of sciatic nerve afferents in the substantia gelatinosa of neonatal rats. Neuroscience Letters 43: 149–154

Fitzgerald M, King A E, Thompson S W N, Woolf C J 1987 The postnatal development of the ventral root reflex in the rat: a comparative 'in vivo' and 'in vitro' study. Neuroscience Letters 78: 41–45

Fitzgerald M, Shaw A, McIntosh N 1988 Postnatal development of the cutaneous flexor reflex: comparative study of preterm infants and newborn rat pups. Developmental Medicine and Child Neurology 30: 520–526

Fitzgerald M, Reynolds M L, Benowitz L I 1991 GAP-43 expression in the developing rat lumbar spinal cord. Neuroscience 14: 187–199

Fitzgerald M, Kwiat G, Middleton J M, Pini A 1993a Ventral spinal cord inhibition of neurite outgrowth from embryonic rat dorsal root ganglia. Development 117: 1377–1384

Fitzgerald M, Butcher T, Shortland P S 1993b Developmental changes in the laminar organization of large cutaneous sensory afferents in the rat spinal cord dorsal horn. (Submitted)

Fitzgerald M J T 1966 Perinatal changes in epidermal innervation in rat and mouse. Journal of Comparative Neurology 126: 37–42

Garthwiate 1989 NMDA receptors, neuronal development and neurodegeneration. In: Watkins J C, Collinridge G L (eds) The NMDA receptor. IRL Press, Oxford, p 187–205

Giordano J, Barr G A 1987 Morphine- and ketocyclazocine-induced analgesia in the developing rat: differences due to type of noxious stimulus and body topography. Developmental Brain Research 32: 247–253

Guy E R, Abbott F V 1992 The behavioural response to formalin pain in preweanling rats. Pain 51: 81–90

Gyulai F 1988 Ontogenesis of two genuine marker enzymes of primary sensory neurons in the rat. Zellforschung mikroskopie-anatomie Forschung 102: 423–436

Hammond D L, Ruda M A 1991 Developmental alterations in nociceptive threshold, immunoreactive calcitonin-gene related peptide and substance P, and fluoride-resistant acid phosphatase in neonatally capsaicin-treated rats. Journal of Comparative Neurology 312: 436–450

Harper S, Davies A M 1990 NGF mRNA expression in developing cutaneous epithelium related to innervation density. Development 110: 515–519

Holz G G, Kream R M, Spiegel A, Dunlap K 1989 G-proteins couple α-adrenergic and $GABA_{\beta}$ receptors to inhibition of peptide secretion from peripheral sensory neurons. Journal of Neuroscience 9: 657–666

Hori Y, Watanabe S 1987 Morphine sensitive late components of the flexion reflex in the neonatal rat. Neuroscience Letters 78: 91–96

Hughes H E, Barr G A 1988 Analgesic effects of intrathecally applied noradrenergic compounds in the developing rat: differences due to thermal vs mechanical nociception. Developmental Brain Research 41: 109–120

Issler H, Stephens J A 1983 The maturation of cutaneous reflexes studied in the upper limb in man. Journal of Physiology 335: 643–654

Jenq C-B, Chung K, Coggeshall R E 1986 Postnatal loss of axons in normal rat sciatic nerve. Journal of Comparative Neurology 244: 445–450

Jonakait G M, Ni L, Walker P D et al 1991 Development of substance P (SP)-containing cells in the central nervous system: consequences of neurotransmitter co-localization. Progress in Neurobiology 36: 1–21

Kalb R G, Hockfield S 1991 The distribution of spinal cord N-methyl D-aspartate receptors is developmentally regulated. Society for Neuroscience Abstracts 17: 1534

Kitazawa T, Saito K, Ohga A 1985 Effects of catecholamines on spinal motoneurones and spinal reflex discharges in the isolated spinal cord of the newborn rat. Developmental Brain Research 19: 31–36

Klimach V J, Cooke R W I 1988 Mutaration of the neonatal somatosensory evoked response in preterm infants. Developmental Medicine and Child Neurology 30: 208–214

Kudo N, Yamada T 1987 Morphological and physiological studies of the development of the monosynaptic reflex pathway in the rat lumbar spinal cord. Journal of Physiology 389: 441–459

Lawson S N, Caddy K W T, Biscoe T J 1974 Development of rat dorsal root ganglion neurones. Cell and Tissue Research 153: 399–413

Lee K-F, Li E, Huber L J, Landis S C et al 1992 Targeted mutation of the gene encoding the low affinity NGF receptor P75 leads to deficits in the peripheral sensory nervous system. Cell 69: 737–749

Lee M T, Koebbe M J, O'Donovan M J 1988 The development of sensorimotor synaptic connections in the lumbosacral cord of the chick embryo. Journal of Neuroscience 8: 2530–2543

Leong S K, Sheih J Y, Wong W C 1984 Localizing spinal cord projecting neurons in neonatal and immature albino rats. Journal of Comparative Neurology 228: 18–23

Loizu L A 1972 The postnatal ontogeny of monoamine albino containing neurones in the central nervous system of the rat. Brain Research 40: 395–418

Lynn B, Carpenter S E 1982 Primary afferent units from the hairy skin of the rat hindlimb. Brain Research 238: 29–43

Ma W, Behar T, Barker J L 1992 Transient expression of GABA immunoreactivity in the developing rat spinal cord. Journal of Comparative Neurology 325: 271–290

Mair R G, Gellman R L, Gesteland R C 1982 Postnatal proliferation and maturation of olfactory bulb neurons in the rat. Neuroscience 7: 3105–3116

Marchetti D, Haverkamp L J, Clark R C et al 1991 Ontogeny of high and low affinity nerve growth factor receptors in the lumbar spinal cord of the developing chick embryo. Developmental Biology 148: 306–313

Marti E, Gibson S J, Polak J M et al 1987 Ontogeny of peptide- and amine-containing neurones in motor, sensory and autonomic regions of rat and human spinal cord, dorsal root ganglia and rat skin. Journal of Comparative Neurology 266: 332–359

Martin P, Khan A, Lewis J 1989 Cutaneous nerves of the embryonic chick wing do not develop in regions denuded of ectoderm. Development 106: 335–346

McGrath P 1990 Pain in children. The Guilford Press, New York

Meinecke D L, Rakic P 1992 Expression of GABA and $GABA_A$ receptors by neurons of the subplate zone in developing primate occipital cortex: evidence for transient local circuits. Journal of Comparative Neurology 317: 91–101

Michelson A B, Lothman E W 1989 An in vivo electrophysiological study of the ontogeny of excitatory and inhibitory processes in the rat hippocampus. Developmental Brain Research 47: 113–122

Mendelson B, Koerber H R, Frank E 1992 Development of cutaneous and proprioceptive afferent projections in the chick spinal cord. Neuroscience Letters 138: 72–76

Morrisett R A, Mott D D, Lewis D V et al 1990 Reduced sensitivity of the N-methyl-D- aspartate component of synaptic transmission to magnesium in hippocampal slices from immature rats. Development Brain Research 56: 257–262

Mrzljak L, Uylings H B M, Kostovic I, van Eden C G 1988 Prenatal development of neurons in prefrontal cortex: a qualitative Golgi study. Journal of Comparative Neurology 271: 355–386

Munger B L, Rice F L 1986 Successive waves of differentiation of cutaneous afferents in rat mystacial skin. Journal of Comparative Neurology 252: 404–414

Myklebust B M, Gottlieb G L, Agarwal G C 1986 Stretch reflexes of the normal infant. Developmental Medicine and Child Neurology 28: 440–449

Naka K I 1984 Electrophysiology of the fetal spinal cord. II. Interaction among peripheral inputs and recurrent inhibition. Journal of General Physiology 47: 1023–1038

Narayanan C H, Fox M V, Hamburger V 1971 Prenatal development of spontaneous and evoked activity in the rat. Behaviour 40: 100–134

New H V, Mudge A W 1986 Distribution and ontogeny of SP, CGRP, SOM and VIP in chick sensory and sympathetic ganglia. Developmental Biology 116: 337–346

Nornes H O, Das G H 1974 Temporal pattern of neurogenesis in spinal cord of rat. I. An autoradiographic study-time and sites of origin and migration and settling patterns of neuroblasts. Brain Research 73: 121–138

Payne J, Middleton J M, Fitzgerald M 1991 The pattern and timing of cutaneous hair follicle innervation in the rat pup and human fetus. Developmental Brain Research 61: 173–182

Pickel V M, Sumal K K, Miller R J 1982 Early prenatal development of substance P and enkephalin containing neurons in the rat. Journal of Comparative Neurology 210: 411–422

Pignatelli D, Ribeiro-da-Silva A, Coimbra A 1989 Postnatal maturation of primary afferent terminations in the substantia gelatinosa of the rat spinal cord. An electron microscope study. Brain Research 491: 33–44

Prechtl H F R 1985 Ultrasound studies of human foetal behaviour. Early Human Development 12: 91–98

Renehan W E, Munger B L 1990 The development of Meissner corpuscles in primate digital skin. Developmental Brain Research 51: 35–44

Reynolds M L, Fitzgerald M, Benowitz L I 1991 GAP-43 expression in developing cutaneous and muscle nerves in the rat hindlimb. Neuroscience 41: 201–211

Rius R A, Barg J, Bern W T et al 1991 The prenatal developmental profile of expression of opioid peptides and receptors in the mouse brain. Developmental Brain Research 58: 237–241

Rizvi T A, Wadha S, Mehra R D et al 1986 Ultrastructure of marginal zone during prenatal development of human cord. Experimental Brain Research 64: 483–490

Rohrer H, Heumann R, Thoenen H 1988 The synthesis of nerve growth factor (NGF) in developing skin is independent of innervation. Developmental Biology 128: 240–244

Rosant J 1990 Manipulating the mouse genome: implications for neurobiology. Neuron 2: 323–334

Rowe M J 1982 Development of mammalian somatosensory pathways. Trends in Neurosciences 5: 408–411

Ruit K G, Elliot J L, Osborne P A, Yan Q, Snider W D 1992 Selective dependence of mammalian dorsal root ganglion neurons on nerve growth factor during embryonic development. Neuron 8: 573–587

Saito K 1979 Development of spinal reflexes in the rat fetus studied in vitro. Journal of Physiology 294: 581–594

Sakatani K, Hassan A Z, Chester M 1991 GABA-sensitivity of dorsal column axons: an in vitro comparison between adult and neonatal rat spinal cords. Developmental Brain Research 61: 139–142

Senba E, Shiosaka S, Hara Y et al 1982 Ontogeny of the peptidergic system in the rat spinal cord. Journal of Comparative Neurology 208: 54–66

Seno N, Ito S, Ohga A 1984 The development of responsiveness to substance P and glutamate in the spinal motoneurones of rat fetuses. Brain Research 298: 366–369

Seno N, Sato K 1985 The development of the dorsal root potential and the responsiveness of primary afferent fibres to γ-aminobutyric acid in the spinal cord of rat fetuses. Developmental Brain Research 17: 11–16

Shoenen J 1978 Histoenzymology of the developing rat spinal cord. Neuropathology and Applied Neurobiology 4: 37–46

Shortland P, Molander C, Woolf C J, Fitzgerald M 1990 Neonatal capsaicin treatment induces invasion of the substantia gelatinosa by the terminal arborizations of hair follicle afferents in the rat dorsal horn. Journal of Comparative Neurology 296: 23–31

Smith C L 1983 The development and postnatal organization of primary afferent projections to the rat thoracic spinal cord. Journal of Comparative Neurology 220: 29–43

Stelzner D J 1971 The normal postnatal development of synaptic end-feet in the lumbosacral spinal cord and of responses in the hindlimbs of the albino rat. Experimental Neurology 31: 337–357

Suzue T, Jessell T 1980 Opiate analgesics and endorphins inhibit rat dorsal root potential in vitro. Neuroscience Letters 16: 161–166

Tempel A, Habas J, Paredes W 1988 Morphine induced downregulation of μ-opioid receptors in neonatal rat brain. Developmental Brain Research 41: 129–133

Thairu B K 1971 Postnatal changes in the somaesthetic evoked potentials in the albino rat. Nature 231: 30–31

Tribollet E, Goumaz M, Raggenbas M, Dubois-Dauphin M, Dreifuss J-J 1991 Early appearance and transient expression of vasopressin receptors in the brain of rat fetus and infant. An autoradiographical and electrophysiological study. Developmental Brain Research 58: 13–24

Van Praag H, Frenk H 1991 The development of stimulation-produced analgesia (SPA) in the rat. Developmental Brain Research 64: 71–76

Vaughn J E, Grieshaber J A 1973 A morpological investigation of an early reflex pathway in developing rat spinal cord. Journal of Comparative Neurology 220: 29–43

Webb G, Perkins M, Dickenson A H, Fitzgerald M 1993 Developmental changes in nociceptive thresholds in normal and capsaicin treated neonates. (In preparation)

Weber E D, Stelzner D J Behavioural effects of spinal cord transection in the developing rat. Brain Research 125: 241–255

Wessels W J T, Feirabend H K P, Marani E 1990 Evidence for a rostrocaudal organization in dorsal root ganglia during development as demonstrated by intra-uterine WGA-HRP injections into the hindlimb of rat fetuses. Developmental Brain Research 54: 273–281

Williams S, Evan G, Hunt S P 1990 Spinal c-fos induction by sensory stimulation in neonatal rats. Neuroscience Letters 109: 309–314

Wu W-L, Ziskind-Conhaim L 1991 Age dependent effects of bicuculline and strychnine on dorsal root evoked potentials. Society for Neuroscience Abstracts 17: 465

Wyatt S, Shooter E M, Davies A M 1990 Expression of the NGF receptor gene in sensory neurons and their cutaneous targets prior to and during innervation. Neuron 2: 421–427

Yanagisawa M, Murakoshi T, Tamai S, Otsuka M 1985 Tail pinch method in vitro and the effects of some antinociceptive compounds. European Journal of Pharmacology 106: 231–239

Zelena J, Jirmanova I, Nitatori T 1990 Enforcement and regeneration of tactile lamellar corpuscles of rat after postnatal crush. Neuroscience 39: 513–522

Zhang A Z, Pasternak G W 1981 Ontogeny of opioid pharmacology and receptors: high and low affinity site differences. European Journal of Pharmacology 73: 29–40

Ziskind-Conhaim L 1990 NMDA receptors mediate poly- and monosynaptic potentials in motoneurones of rat embryos. Journal of Neuroscience 10: 125–135

9. Central pharmacology of nociceptive transmission

Tony L. Yaksh and Annika B. Malmberg

INTRODUCTION

THE PAIN STATE

Strong thermal or mechanical stimuli, or molecules elaborated by such stimuli from damaged tissue, applied acutely to the skin, muscle or viscera of the unanaesthetized animal will evoke a constellation of well-defined behaviours and characteristic changes in autonomic function. The composition of the behavioural profile may vary with the species and the age of the organism, but will typically include signs of agitation, (vocalization), coordinated efforts to escape (lift or withdrawal of the paw) or attenuate the magnitude of the stimulus (i.e. lick the paw). For example, placing a rat on a hot surface (greater than 48–50°C) reveals an initial increase in behavioural activity, a shifting of the weight back and forth between the hind paws and shortly a characteristic licking of the hind paw. Should the rat be left for longer periods on the surface, the animal will typically display vocalization, efforts to jump or other adaptive behaviours. Similarly, the delivery of an irritant such as formalin or capsaicin into the paw will acutely evoke grooming/licking of the paw and a shaking/flinching of the injected paw. All of the above described tests employ an acute pain stimuli and thus models have formed the basis of investigating the behavioural components of the animal's response to a noxious stimulus.

In the last 5 years, it has become increasingly appreciated that in addition to the acute component, protracted afferent drive for periods lasting minutes can evoke pronounced changes in pain behaviour, suggesting an augmented processing of the nociceptive response, i.e. a hyperalgesic state. Thus, the injection of an irritant, such as formalin, into the skin will lead to an acute barrage followed by a protracted ongoing low level of C-fibre acitivity (Heapy et al 1987). In the animal so treated, one observes a multiphase component of behaviour in which the first phase reflects the acute afferent barrage, followed, after a brief period of quiescence, in a powerful second phase of agitation (Dubuisson & Dennis 1977; Wheeler-Aceto et al 1990). In man, corresponding with the increased activity in the afferent, the psychophysics of the acute pain state has emphasized an increasing pain report as a function of the intensity of an acute thermal or mechanical stimulus, or the concentration of certain agents such as bradykinin or K^+ to a blister base (Raja et al 1988). Yet, like the animal models, it is now apparent that the pain state induced by a relatively brief afferent barrage evoked by an irritant stimulus (such as intradermal capsaicin) will lead to a pronounced and relatively long-lasting state of secondary hyperalgesia and hyperaesthesia, referred to a skin area that is considerably greater than that area originally affected by the stimulus (Torebjörk et al 1992; LaMotte et al 1992). It would seem reasonable that in fact these states of secondary hyperalgesia may well constitute an important component of most post-injury pain states in humans and that the management of clinical pain will reflect the properties governing the origin and maintenance of such states of facilitated processing.

An essential goal is to understand the mechanisms that mediate these behavioural phenomena. It is currently appreciated that the behaviour evoked by the appropriate physical stimulus reflects the activation of specific populations of sensory afferents which in turn serves to induce activity in a complex of dorsal horn neurons which project an excitatory outflow via long tracts, typically in the ventrolateral quadrant into the brainstem and diencephalon. The forward flow of information and the tracts by which such information flow occurs have been reviewed in detail elsewhere (see Ch. 5). Of equal importance in assessing the functional organization of these projection systems, is the appreciation that the movement of excitatory input through the dorsal horn and into the brainstem is highly regulated by local circuits which by actions pre- and postsynaptic to the afferent pathway may regulate the excitability of the synapse and control the excitability of the postsynaptic neurons. As noted above, the behavioural data clearly suggest that sensitivity to afferent input may be both augmented or reduced.

An important insight into the understanding of the

processing of this afferent traffic within the central nervous system (CNS) is the identification of the pharmacology of these systems. Advances in histochemistry and receptor autoradiography, coupled with increasingly sophisticated pharmacological tools make it possible to define the nature of pathways which are activated by the respective afferent stimulus. Thus, it is possible to show that transmitter X or its synthetic enzymes are present in a given neuron and that X is released upon stimulation. The application of X to the cell body/terminals postsynaptic to the cell containing X should produce an appropriate response with characteristics similar to that observed when the neuron containing X is stimulated. Conversely, the effects of agent X and the physiological actions produced when the neuronal system containing agent X is activated should be blocked by the local application of antagonists for X. Such a conceptual approach provides a powerful tool for identifying the transmitters and the systems relevant to a given function. In the present context, examining the anatomical elements that are known to play a role in the afferent processing of nociceptive information has served to identify certain transmitter/receptor systems. Local administration of the putative agonists and antagonists for these several receptor systems into the terminal regions of the respective cells have frequently shown them to produce anticipated effects on neuronal function. Such observations permit detailed analysis of the pharmacology and membrane effects of these several transmitter networks.

BIOASSAYS OF NOCICEPTION AND ANTINOCICEPTION

An important caveat to the interpretation of the data generated by electrophysiological and biochemical studies is the relevance of these observations to *pain* processing. Such interpretation presumes that we know the functional significance of the activity evoked in that cell by noxious stimulation. To define the role of a given receptor in the dorsal horn in modulating the 'pain state', we must ultimately assess the role of the manipulation of the respective systems in the bioassay which defines a pain state; i.e. the behaviour of the unanaesthetized and intact animal. Thus, combining the various pain states induced by specific and well-defined stimuli, with specific efforts to assess the pharmacology of the receptors that exist in the terminal regions of the several links in the tracts through which information generated by such high-intensity stimuli project, the behavioural relevance of those systems to pain processing can be defined. Such focal pharmacological manipulation in the intact and unanaesthetized animal is achieved through the ability to deliver drugs in a reliable, delimited manner into specific regions of the CNS. In brain, the placement of intracerebroventricular cannulae permits assessment of a central action, but there is little ability to define the drug effect in specific brain regions. The stereotactic placement of microinjection cannulae and the concurrent use of small injection volumes permit a local influence on anatomically limited volumes of brain tissue. At the spinal level, the placement of chronic catheters or the use of percutaneous injections (Hammond 1988) has permitted the examination of the pharmacology of spinal systems that alter nociceptive transmission in a variety of species. Factors governing the degree of localization of drug action after intracerebral or intrathecal injection have been intensively reviewed elsewhere (Herz & Teschemacher 1971; Yaksh & Rudy 1978; Yaksh et al 1988b).

An important consideration in the bioassay of the nociceptive state is that different models may reflect upon the manifestation of different components of the pain processing systems. As noted above, an acute high-intensity stimulus may yield a reliable escape response with no evident changes in the subsequent responsiveness of these system. Tests, such as the hot plate or paw pressure, define substrates which are activated by an acute high-intensity stimulus. On the other hand, as noted above, protracted afferent input, as generated by an injury state, may lead to a prominent hyperalgesia. Models, such as the formalin test, or threshold responses following inflammation, appear to define systems which are brought into play by such ongoing afferent input. Such multiple test systems, in combination with the use of focal delivery techniques and the application of the pharmacology of the transmitter/receptor system under study provides an experimental methodology whereby the organization and pharmacology of systems regulating pain processing can be defined.

EXCITATORY TRANSMITTERS IN THE AFFERENT COMPONENTS OF NOCICEPTIVE PROCESSING

Consideration of the connectivity of the central systems activated by high-threshold afferent stimuli suggests that an important component of the organization is the primary afferent projections into the dorsal horn and the subsequent projections via crossed and uncrossed tracts into the brainstem and diencephalon (see Chs 5 and 6). The following sections will consider the pharmacology of the systems that subserve the rostral flow of information generated by small afferent input.

PRIMARY AFFERENTS

Postsynaptic effects of primary afferents

Two principal properties characterize the nature of the neurotransmitters that are involved in the sensory afferent. First, single unit recording has indicated that stimulation of the primary afferent will result in a powerful excitation of dorsal horn neurons. Dating from some of the earliest systematic studies (Hongo et al 1968), there has been no reported evidence that primary afferents induce a monosynaptic inhibition in the dorsal horn (see for example reviews of dorsal horn function by Willis & Coggeshall, 1991; Light 1992). This property suggests that putative afferent transmitters should largely be characterized by their ability to evoke excitatory postsynaptic potentials (EPSPs) in the second order dorsal horn neurons. Second, stimulation of nerve filaments at intensities which activate small, slowly conducting afferents typically reveals the existence of at least two populations of EPSPs that are believed to be monosynaptic:

1. Fast and of brief duration
2. Delayed and of extended duration (Urban & Randic 1984; Schneider & Perl 1988; King et al 1988; Yoshimura & Jessell 1989; Gerber & Randic 1989a).

While the presence of different EPSPs on the same membrane may reflect monosynaptic input from two different families of axons and/or the presence of interneurons contributing to the slow EPSP, such multiple EPSP morphologies may also reflect the presence of at least two distinct classes of neurotransmitters acting on the dorsal horn neuron including excitatory amino acids (Jessell et al 1986; Schneider & Perl 1988; Gerber & Randic 1989a, 1989b) and peptides (Ryu et al 1988; Murase et al 1989).

Afferent transmitters

At present, histochemical analysis of the marginal layers and gelatinosa of the dorsal horn (regions where small afferents are known to terminate) and the small ganglion cells of the dorsal root (considered to be the cells of origin of small, unmyelinated afferent axons) has revealed the presence of a large number of possible transmitter candidates. The properties, where studied, of these agents are summarized in Table 9.1.

As discussed elsewhere (Ju et al 1987; Hökfelt 1991), electron microscopy frequently has shown the presence of morphologically distinct (small open versus large dense core) populations of vesicles in the dorsal horn. Such distinction is consistent with the broader appreciation in neurobiology that such distinct vesicles reflect upon the co-containment of distinct classes of releasable neurotransmitter within the same terminal (De Biasi & Rustioni 1988). Examination of the distribution of glutamate indicates that it is likely to be contained in the small open core vesicles while dense core vesicles are believed to contain peptides (Hökfelt 1991). Given the ability of glutamate, acting through receptor-gated Na^+ or Ca^{2+} channels, to produce a rapid EPSP, and peptides to decrease K^+ conductance to yield slow EPSPs (Table 9.1), such co-containment provides support for a composite of postsynaptic events to be evoked by a single terminal. With regard to the dense core vesicles, it is certain that distinct populations of afferents may be defined on the basis of peptide contents. Thus, histochemical analysis of dorsal root ganglion cells has revealed that 50% contains calcitonin gene-related peptide (CGRP) and 30% contains substance P (sP); 96% of the CGRP positive cells also showed sP immunoreactivity (Ju et al 1987). The role of such distinctive populations of phenotypically definable terminals remains to be determined, but suggests an important mechanism of afferent encodement. Important characteristics of these agents are their ability to be released into the extracellular milieu following depolarization of the primary afferent terminals. In vivo, following activation of C-fibre afferents, the release of sP (Yaksh et al 1980; Kuraishi et al 1989), CGRP (Saria et al 1986; Morton & Hutchinson 1990), vasoactive intestinal peptide (VIP) (Yaksh et al 1982a), somatostatin (Morton et al 1988) and glutamate (Skilling et al 1988) has been shown.

Effects of intrathecal transmitter agonists and antagonists

The potential role of the several primary afferent transmitters in pain processing resolves around their postsynaptic action. As noted in Table 9.1, these agents have the ability to produce both acute and prolonged membrane depolarization of dorsal horn neurons known to receive afferent input from C-fibres. The role of the respective receptors acted upon by the several agents on pain behaviour has been investigated by the effects of the intrathecal delivery of these agonists on the pain behaviour of the unanaesthetized rat. Conceptually, the direct activation of the postsynaptic receptor should yield evidence of behaviour consistent with the activation of small afferents, vocalization, irritability and scratching or biting at the dermatome at which the spinally delivered drug is acting. As indicated in Table 9.1, modest indices of pain behaviour have been reported to occur in a dose-dependent fashion after the intrathecal injection of several of the peptides and excitatory amino acids. Given the paucity of specific peptide antagonists which have been examined in this model, it is not always possible to define the nature of the receptors acted upon by all agents. For the several tachykinin sites, it appears, based on the effects of agonists and antagonist studies, that neurokinin (NK)-1 and NK-2 receptors are of most importance in nociception (Fleetwood-Walker et al 1988a; Laneuville et al 1988). Intrathecal injections of glutamate receptor agonists have emphasized the ability of both N-methyl-D-aspartate (NMDA), and nonNMDA sites (Sun & Larson 1991; Malmberg & Yaksh 1992a; but see also Aanonsen & Wilcox 1987; Coderre & Melzack 1992) to produce powerful algogenic behaviour. Given the likelihood that an excitatory amino acid and a peptide such as sP might be co-released, concurrent spinal injec-

Table 9.1 Summary of receptor mediated effects of afferent transmitter candidates on spinal function

Candidate	Receptor classes	DRG type	Location (binding or immunoreactivity)	Membrane effects	IT agonist (in vivo)	IT antagonist (in vivo)
Tachykinins	NK1	small[1]	D>V[1]	SD[2,3]	PB, HY[4,5]	BHY[6], BAP[7]
	NK2	small[1]	D>V[1]	SD[2]	PB, HY[4,5]	?
	NK3	small[1]	D>V[1]	?	NE[5], BAP[4]	?
CGRP		small and medium[8]	D>V[8]	SD[9]	HY[5]	?
Bombesin		small[10]	D>V[11,12]	HP[13]	PB[11]	?
Somatostatin		small[14]	D>V[14]	HP[15]	NE[16], BAP[17]	BHY[18]
VIP		small and medium[19]	D>V[12]	SD[20]	NE[21]	?
Glutamate	NMDA	small[22]	D>V[23]	SD[24]	PB[25], HY[5,25]	BHY[26]
	Kainate		D>V[23]	FD[24]	PB[25], NE[5]	?
	AMPA		D>V[23]	FD[24]	PB[25], NE[5]	NE[5], BHY[27]
Nitric Oxide (NO)	(activate guanylate cyclase)	medium[28] (NO synthase)	D>V[29]	?	?	BHY[30,31] (enzyme inhibition)

Abbreviations: BAP = blocks acute pain behaviour (e.g. thermal such as hot plate, tail flick); BHY = blocks hyperalgesia as evoked by peripheral injection of irritants (i.e. formalin test, phase 2); FD = fast depolarization; HP = hyperpolarization; HY = evokes hyperalgesia (i.e. reduced nociceptive thresholds or response latencies); NE = produces no effect; PB = evokes pain behaviour (i.e. scratching/biting); SD = slow depolarization; ? = unknown

References: [1]Helke et al 1990a, 1990b; [2]Urban & Randic 1984; [3]De Koninck & Henry 1991; [4]Laneuville et al 1988; [5]Coderre & Melzack 1991; [6]Yamamoto & Yaksh 1991; [7]Fleetwood-Walker et al 1990; [8]Pohl et al 1990; [9]Woodley & Kendig, 1991; [10]Panula et al 1983; [11]O'Donohue et al 1984; [12]Yaksh et al 1988a; [13]De Koninck & Henry 1989; [14]Hökfelt et al 1976; [15]Murase et al 1982; [16]Gaumann et al 1989; [17]Mollenholt et al 1988; [18]Ohkubo et al 1990; [19]Gibson et al 1984; [20]Jeftinija et al 1982; [21]Seybold et al 1982; [22]Battaglia & Rustioni 1988; [23]Jansen et al 1990; Mitchell & Anderson 1991; [24]Davies & Watkins 1983; [25]Aanonsen & Wilcox 1987; [26]Yamamoto & Yaksh 1992; [27]Malmberg, unpublished observations; [28]Aimi et al 1991; [29]Mizukawa et al 1989; [30]Meller et al 1992; [31]Malmberg & Yaksh 1993a

tion of sP and glutamate have been reported to produce a significant mutual augmentation of the algogenic effect as compared to the injection of either alone (Yaksh 1986; Mjellem-Jolly et al 1991; but see also Aanonsen & Wilcox 1987).

At present an important unresolved aspect of the transmitter pharmacology of the primary afferent is the absence of definitive data indicating that any of the antagonists given spinally can prevent the appearance of pain behaviour otherwise acutely evoked by high-threshold thermal (hot plate, tail flick) mechanical (paw pressure) or chemical (formalin) stimuli. Thus, while spinally administered antagonists for the respective agonists will prevent the appearance of pain behaviour in animals receiving the agonists, these agents typically will not produce a clearly defined thermal or mechanical analgesia. As will be discussed below, an important property of small afferent input is the evocation of a hyperesthetic/hyperalgesic state. It appears that several of these receptors may play a role in initiating this afferent-evoked condition.

ASCENDING AFFERENT TRACTS

Postsynaptic effects of primary afferents

As reviewed elsewhere (see Ch. 6) the intervening link between the spinal cord and higher order (supraspinal) processing is the long tracts which project into the brainstem and diencephalon. Single unit recording suggests that the primary monosynaptically (or short latency) effect of spinobulbar activity is excitation (Chung et al 1986; Sinclair et al 1991). Failure thus far to see evidence of supraspinal inhibition of course does not exclude such possibilities in all systems. It seems certain that an important component of the spinobulbar message is encoded in the context of excitation.

Afferent transmitters

Immunohistochemical investigations examining the content of dorsal horn neurons which are labelled after the injection of retrogradely transported label into various brainstem sites have demonstrated spinal neurons containing cholecystokinin-like immunoreactivity (LI), dynorphin 1–8, somatostatin; bombesin vasoactive intestinal peptides and sP, have been shown to project into the bulbar reticular formation (Nahin 1987, 1988; Leah et al 1988). Spinofugal cells containing cholecystokinin (CCK) and dynorphin-LI labelling have been found in and around the central canal. Ascending tract cells located in lamina I, projecting into the spinomesencephalic pathways were shown to contain dynorphin and vasoactive intestinal polypeptide, while lamina V cells projecting in a spinoreticular component contained somatostatin (Leah et al 1988). sP-labelled cells are sparsely found within the dorsal horn. sP-positive neurons or neurons containing message for preprotachykinin projecting into the thalamus were found to originate in lamina I and in lamina V and around the central canal (Battaglia & Rustioni 1992; Battaglia et al 1992; Noguchi & Ruda 1992). Glutamate has also been identified in trigeminothalamic projections suggesting the probable role of that excitatory amino acid (Magnusson et al 1987). Substance P containing fibres arising from brainstem sites have been shown to project to the parafascicular and central medial nuclei of the thalamus (Sim & Joseph 1992). Given the importance of these extraspinal terminals, the relative absence of precise information currently available on the transmitters in spinofugal pathways projecting to specific supraspinal regions is surprising. Future studies are likely to provide important insights into the identity of the long-tract spinofugal systems and thus the supraspinal organization of the afferent input.

Effects of focally injected transmitter agonists and antagonists

The presence of projecting neurons containing these materials gives rise to the likelihood that they may serve as neurotransmitters released into the supraspinal projection regions of these cells. Given the importance of this ascending linkage, there is surprisingly little information at the present time on the nature of the unconditioned pain behaviour evoked by the microinjection of these agonists into the vicinity of these terminals. In unanaesthetized animals, the microinjection of glutamate in the vicinity of the terminals of ascending pathways, notably within the mesencephalic central grey, evoked spontaneous pain-like behaviour with vocalization and vigorous efforts to escape. Examination of the pharmacology of these effects revealed the ordering of activity to be: NMDA = kainate > quisqualate ≥ D-glutamate. The effects of NMDA were reversed by MK-801 and 2-amino-5-phosphonovalorate, emphasizing the presence of at least an NMDA site mediating the behavioural effects produced by NMDA in this region (Jensen & Yaksh 1992). These effects of local glutamate in generating a pain behaviour are consistent with the extensive literature which indicates that stimulation in the central grey can evoke signs of significant agitation (Schmitt & Karli 1974; Kiser et al 1978; Fardin et al 1984). The failure to observe significant pain behaviour following injection of glutmate into either the thalamus or, modestly so, in the medulla, is surprising in view of early work emphasizing that electrical stimulation in this area is able to evoke prominent escape behaviour (Casey 1971; see Bowsher 1976 for review of early literature) and given that afferent evoked excitation of thalamic cells is inhibited by NMDA and nonNMDA antagonists (Salt 1986).

It should be emphasized that studies examining the behavioural effects arising from the direct activation of supraspinal systems must consider carefully the possibility that complex species-specific behavioural patterns, not necessarily related to pain-evoked behaviour, are being activated. Many of the complex behaviour patterns evoked by focal activation, for example within the mesencephalon, have substantial parallels with activities associated with operationally defined states of fear and anxiety in the so-called defence reaction (Bandler et al 1991). As will be discussed below, states of emotionality impact upon pain behaviour evoked by a noxious stimulus. In the context of the work discussed above, this raises the complication of attempting to define what is a link in the afferent pathways which process nociceptive information and those which govern the unconditioned behaviour of the animal in a given environment. This subtlety is likely to be an important feature of future studies in the behavioural syndromes associated with the pain state in animal models.

MODULATION OF THE AFFERENT ENCODING OF ACTIVITY EVOKED BY HIGH-INTENSITY STIMULI

It is a useful simplification to consider the pharmacology of the transmitters and receptors that subserve the forward movement of excitatory information to rostral centres, as was done in the preceding section. However, a dominant principle of the organization of this excitatory drive evoked by the release of excitatory transmitters is that at all levels it is subject to pharmacological influences which increase and decrease these excitatory influences. Psychophysical studies have shown that the reported intensity of a given physical stimulus can be significantly increased or decreased by several manipulations, producing a state of hyper- or hypoalgesia, respectively. In the following sections, components of the spinal and supraspinal systems that underlie such regulatory influences will be considered.

SPINAL DORSAL HORN RECEPTOR SYSTEMS

Characteristics of modulation of afferent-evoked excitation of dorsal horn neurons

Several lines of evidence make it clear that the response properties of the dorsal horn neuron are not simply defined by the nature of the local excitatory afferent input, but reflect a series of active encoding events. An example of this is the ability to modify the response characteristics of a common class of spinal neuron: the wide dynamic range neuron that lies within the dorsal horn and receives strong monosynaptic excitatory input from large (Aβ, low-threshold tactile) and small (C, high-threshold polymodal nociceptor) primary afferents projecting to the respective segment (Light 1992; Ch. 5 this volume). The receptive field of these cells is typically complex with dermatomal regions responding to low-threshold input overlapping with regions where the effective stimulus is a high-intensity thermal or mechanical stimulus. The response properties of such cells are, however, not simply defined by the nature of the afferent connectivity, but also by the influence of a number of pharmacologically distinct neuronal systems which serve to modify the reaction of the cell to its afferent input. Two examples of the response properties of these cells which are regulated in both a positive and negative fashion by convergent neuronal influences will be considered below.

Neuronal receptive field size. The effective receptive field of a dorsal horn cell is not invariant. Section of the lateral Lissauer tract (an intrasegmental projection system arising in part from the substantia gelatinosa) or the topical application of strychnine (a glycine receptor antagonist) will increase the size of the dermatome in primate (Denny-Brown et al 1973). Prior iontophoretic delivery of glycine and gamma-amino butyric acid (GABA) antagonists will similarly increase the receptive field size of dorsal horn neurons (Zieglgänsberger & Herz 1971). Repetitive activation of high-threshold afferent input will lead to a significant increase in the size of the receptive field of a given dorsal horn neuron and lead to a nociceptive component to input generated by otherwise low-threshold afferent input (Mendell 1966; Dickenson & Sullivan 1990; Woolf & King 1990). In contrast, other systems may serve to decrease the size or components of the receptive field of a given dorsal horn neuron. Mu opioid agonists diminish the size of the high-threshold (C-fibre) component of the receptive field, but have little or no effect upon the low-threshold component (Yaksh 1978a).

Neuronal response to afferent input. The magnitude of the response to a given noxious stimulus may be altered in the absence of a change in the magnitude of the stimulus. Thus, as noted above, repetitive activation of C-fibres will lead to an augmented response to subsequent C-fibre input, a phenomenon referred to as 'wind-up' (Mendell 1966). Conversely, the activation of bulbospinal pathways has been shown to diminish the slope of the response (frequency of discharge) versus stimulus intensity curve of dorsal horn neurons, as well as shift the 'X'-intercept of the stimulus-response curve to the left, indicating a reduction in the threshold stimulus intensity necessary to evoke activity in the cell (Gebhart et al 1983, 1984). As will be reviewed below, considerable evidence points to a complex set of modulatory substrates, some intrinsic to the spinal cord and some which are part of bulbospinal systems, typically shown to contain and release monoamines such as noradrenalin and serotonin. Based on the effects of receptor selective agonists, it can be shown that certain receptor classes such as those for the mu, delta opioid; alpha-2 and the 5-HT receptor will produce a powerful suppression of the excitation of those cells produced by the activation of populations of small afferents (see Table 9.2). In addition to modifying the magnitude of the response to a given noxious stimulus, the local application of glycine or GABA antagonists will prominently augment the response of the dorsal horn wide dynamic range (WDR) neuron to low-threshold (AB) afferent input (Khayyat et al 1975; Yokota et al 1979).

Facilitation of the excitatory efficacy of afferent input

As noted above, the encoding of afferent input is subject to influences that may exaggerate the response of the processing systems to a given stimulus. In the following section, two examples of such modulatory substrates will be considered.

Afferent evoked facilitation

Repetitive C-, but not A-fibre input will yield a highly augmented response to a subsequent C-fibre stimulus (Mendell & Wall 1965; Mendell 1966; Woolf & King, 1987). This 'wind-up' has been shown to be mediated in large part by a glutamate receptor of the NMDA subtype (Davies & Watkins 1983; Dickenson & Sullivan 1990; Woolf & Thompson 1991). Given that electrophysiological studies indicate that NMDA antagonists cannot block the monosynaptic afferent-evoked activity in dorsal horn neurons, it has been suggested that the NMDA sites do not lie immediately on postsynaptic sites to the primary afferent and may reflect upon the intervening role of a glutamate releasing interneuron (Davies & Watkins 1983), which itself is activated by the primary afferent excitatory input. Similarly, the administration of antagonists for the NK-1 tachykinin receptor has been shown to block the initiation of wind-up (De Koninck & Henry 1991).

The behavioural effects of activating these several systems suggest that they may play a role in facilitating the organized response of the animal to a given noxious stimulus. Thus, direct activation of spinal glutamate and tachykinin receptors with intrathecal agonists will induce an augmented response to a noxious thermal stimulus (i.e. a hyperalgesia: Moochhala & Sawynok 1984; Cridland & Henry 1986; Aanonsen & Wilcox 1987; Malmberg & Yaksh 1992a). Conversely, the observation that repetitive small afferent stimulation yields an exaggerated activation of dorsal horn neurons has been shown to have particular behavioural correlates. The injection of an irritant such as formalin into the paw will result in an initial burst of small afferent activity, followed by a prolonged low level of afferent discharge (Heapy et al 1987). Behaviourally, the animal displays an initial transient phase of flinching and licking of the injected paw (phase 1), followed after a brief period of quiescence by a second prolonged phase of licking and flinching of the injected paw. Significantly, the spinal delivery of NMDA and NK-1 antagonists have little effect upon the first phase, but will significantly diminish the magnitude of the second phase response (Yamamoto & Yaksh, 1991, 1992; Coderre & Melzack 1992). Physiological parallels to this behaviour have been observed in which NMDA antagonists have little effect upon acute excitation of dorsal horn neurons (Headley et al 1987; Sher & Mitchell 1990), but will significantly reduce the elevated ongoing activity evoked by the induction of a peripheral injury state (Haley et al 1990; Sher & Mitchell 1990; Schaible et al 1991).

Of equal importance, delivery of NMDA and NK-1 antagonists after the first phase of the formalin test results in a loss of their ability to alter the second phase response (Yamamoto & Yaksh 1991, 1992; Coderre & Melzack, 1992). These observations indicate that the magnitude of the second phase response is dependent upon processes which were initiated by the activation of NMDA and NK-1 sites during the first minutes after the injection of the formalin, but these sites are not required for the sustenance of the second phase activity and occur independently of these sites.

The mechanisms of this augmented responsiveness induced by repetitive C-fibre input and the activation of NMDA and sP are not completely understood. However, several intervening mechanisms have been identified. It is presently believed that depolarization of the neurons and/or the activation of the NMDA receptor will lead to an increase in intracellular Ca^{2+} (MacDermott et al 1986). This initiates a cascade of biochemical events which alter the responsivity of the cell to subsequent depolarizing stimuli. Two elements of this cascade are considered below.

Prostaglandins. One result of increased intracellular Ca^{2+} is the activation of phospholipase A_2, leading to increases in intracellular arachidonic acid and the subsequent formation of cyclooxygenase and lipoxygenase products (Leslie & Watkins 1985). Perfusion studies have shown that afferent stimulation or the direct activation of spinal neurons with NMDA will result in an increase in the extracellular levels of prostanoids in spinal cord (Ramwell et al 1966; Coderre et al 1990; Sorkin 1992). These extracellular lipidic acids can then exert powerful effects on adjacent neuronal elements. Prostaglandins have been shown to increase Ca^{2+} conductance in dorsal root ganglion cells and increase the secretion of primary afferent peptides, such as sP (Nicol et al 1992). Such a scenario leads to an augmented release in response to subsequent stimulation. Intrathecal prostaglandins delivered in the unanaesthetized rat evoke behavioural hyperalgesia (Yaksh 1982; Taiwo & Levine 1986; Uda et al 1990), while spinal cyclooxygenase inhibitors suppress the thermal hyperalgesia induced by spinally injected sP or NMDA (Malmberg & Yaksh 1992a), and the behavioural hyperalgesia resulting from peripheral tissue injury (Malmberg & Yaksh 1992b). These observations suggest a role for cyclooxygenase products in the regulation of spinal nociceptive processing, leading to a centrally mediated hyperalgesia and that cyclooxygenase inhibitors exert a role in the modulation of hyperalgesia by a spinal site of action.

Nitric oxide synthase. A second event known to occur in certain neuronal systems secondary to increased intracellular Ca^{2+} is the synthesis of a novel second messenger, nitric oxide (NO). In hippocampus, this increase has been demonstrated to be induced by NMDA receptor-mediated increases in Ca^{2+} (Garthwaite et al 1988). As indicated above, activation of spinal NMDA receptors can augment nociceptive processing and produce a hyperalgesic state. This hyperalgesia can be blocked by spinal injection of an inhibitor of NO synthesis (Meller et al 1992; Malmberg & Yaksh 1993a). Moreover, peripheral injection of an irritant, such as formalin, produces a behavioural defined hyperalgesia and electrophysiologically a prolonged discharge in WDR neurons, both of which can be suppressed by spinal NO synthesis inhibition (Haley et al 1992; Malmberg & Yaksh, 1993a). NO synthase, the enzyme responsible for NO synthesis, has been found to occur in areas important for nociceptive transmission, such as the dorsal horn (Mizukawa et al 1989; Anderson 1992) and in dorsal root ganglion cells (diaphorase positive type B ganglion cells: Aimi et al 1991; Morris et al 1992). Because NO has the ability to readily penetrate cell membranes it has been proposed as a likely candidate for a retrogradely acting messenger on presynaptic terminals (Schuman & Madison, 1991; O'Dell et al 1991).

While the studies outlined above reflect the probable role of glutamate and sP, the large number of afferent transmitters strongly suggests that a variety of these candidate transmitters may subserve roles similar to those defined above for excitatory amino acids and sP, the organization of which is outlined schematically in Figure 9.1.

Suppression of the excitatory efficacy of afferent input

It is widely appreciated that a number of spinal systems, some with cell bodies intrinsic to the spinal cord and some originating from supraspinal sources, can serve to reduce afferent evoked excitation. Several of these systems are summarized in Table 9.2. In most cases, as reviewed, agonists for such agents applied by iontophoresis, topically to the surface of the spinal cord or by systemic delivery in spinal transected animals, serve to reduce the magnitude of the response evoked by high-threshold afferent stimulation. In the case of agents such as those of the opioid class, considerable data emphasize that these agents serve to reduce the slope of the intensity–response curve (Yaksh 1978b) and diminish the magnitude of the response evoked by small, high-threshold afferent input, with

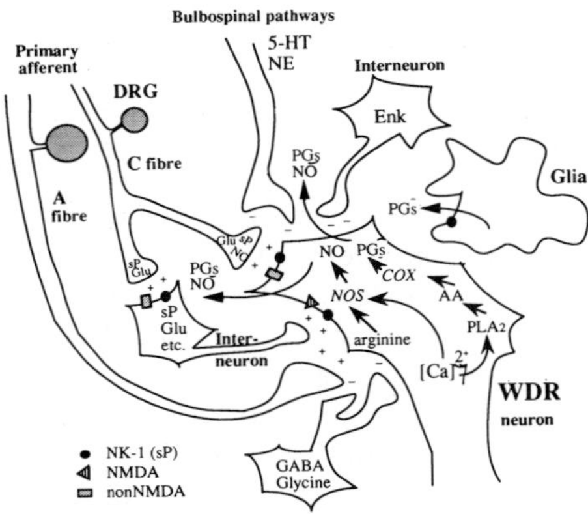

Fig. 9.1 Schematic diagram of dorsal horn facilitatory pharmacology. This cartoon presents a schematic summary of the functional organization of elements in the dorsal horn which impact upon the processing of afferent input. Such an organization reflects the response to acute stimulation, development of the hyperalgesic state induced by repetitive small afferent stimulation and the development of anomalous pain states secondary to large afferent stimulation.

1. The primary afferent C-fibres contain and release both peptide (e.g. sP/CGRP/etc.) and excitatory amino acid (Glu) products. Small dorsal root ganglion cells (DRG) as well as postsynaptic elements are diaphorase positive, suggesting that they contain NO synthase (NOS) and are thus able upon depolarization to synthesize and release NO.
2. These peptides and excitatory amino acids, acting transsynaptically can evoke excitation in second order neurons. For glutamate, it is believed that the excitation is medicated by nonNMDA receptors.
3. Under the appropriate circumstances, interneurons excited by the afferent barrage evoke excitation in the second order neurons by an action mediated by an NMDA receptor. This leads to a marked increase in intracellular Ca^{2+} and the activation of a number of kinases and phosphorylating enzymes. In this scenario, based on the effects of various enzyme inhibitors, it is believed that cyclooxygenase (COX) products (prostaglandins: PGs) and NO are formed and released. These agents move extracellularly to subsequently facilitate transmitter release from primary and nonprimary afferent terminals.
4. Intervening products, such as the prostanoids, may arise from nonneuronal structures, such as glia by the action of sP (Marriott et al 1990)
5. In certain instances, second order neurons also receive excitatory input from large afferents. Based on the effects of various inhibitory amino acid antagonists, it appears that the excitatory effects of large afferents is under a $GABA_A$/glycine modulatory control, removal of which results in an allodynia.
6. Interneurons containing peptides such as enkephalin, or bulbospinal pathways containing monoamines (norepinephrine, serotonin) and peptides (enkephalin, NPY), may be activated by afferent input and 'reflexly' exert a modulatory influence upon the release of C-fibre peptides and postsynaptically to hyperpolarize projection neurons.

minimal effects upon that excitation produced by low-threshold afferents (see Table 9.2 for references).

The mechanism of this reduction in the response evoked by high-intensity stimulation is multiple. However, examination of the data suggests several common insights. First, where examined, the majority of these agents shows predominance in binding in the dorsal horn (DH) of the spinal cord. As indicated in Table 9.2, for several families of receptors system this binding appears to be in part located on primary afferents in view of the significant reduction that is induced by rhizotomy. In specific instances, as with the opioids, treatment with capsaicin is known to be neurotoxic to small, unmyelinated primary afferents. The reduction in binding under such circumstances leads to the conclusion that a proportion of those sites are located on the terminals of the C-fibre. Physiologically, those agents with receptors thought to be located preterminally on C-fibres have been shown to reduce the depolarization-evoked release of peptides thought to be contained in these unmyelinated fibre systems. Such a correlation has for example been demonstrated with mu, delta, and alpha-2 receptors (see Table 9.2 for references). Some agents, such as baclofen, have been shown to have presynaptic binding, but fail to significantly alter the release of peptides such as sP (Go & Yaksh 1987; Sawynok et al 1982). This suggests that this binding may be on terminals which do not contain the respective transmitter. In addition to the afferent terminal actions of some classes of agent, virtually all of the compounds listed have been shown to have potent effects upon the excitation evoked by the local application of an excitatory amino acid, such as glutamate. Such postsynaptic effects have been described for mu, delta, kappa, $GABA_B$, adenosine, and several serotonin sites. The mechanism of this postsynaptic inhibition has not been defined for all agents. However, for receptors such as those of the mu, and alpha-2 type intracellular studies in several neuronal systems have emphasized that they may hyperpolarize the membrane by a G-protein coupled increase in K^+ conductance (North et al 1987).

Influence of intrinsic modulatory systems on pain behaviour

Processing of high-intensity stimuli

The extensive presence of endogenous systems that regulate afferent-evoked excitation (see Table 9.2; see discussions above) lead to the speculation that several of these systems may serve to regulate in a tonic fashion the ongoing processing of nociceptive afferent input. Consider for example that opioids and adrenoceptor agonists have been shown to exert powerful effects upon pain behaviour. Receptors and the endogenous ligands for these several systems are found within the dorsal horn (see Table 9.2). Measurement of release has indicated that these systems following direct stimulation, as in the activation of bulbospinal pathways (Sorkin et al 1992; Hammond et al 1985), or local depolarization as with enkephalin (Yaksh & Elde 1981; Cesselin et al 1984) will result in increases in the spinal extracellular levels of these several agents. Under normal conditions, these levels are typically low, but measurable. However, it has been shown that consequent to the activation of high-threshold (C-afferents), but not low (A-afferents) input, there is a reflexly evoked increase in the release of several agents (e.g. enkephalin:

Table 9.2 Summary of nonafferent spinal receptor systems which can modulate nociceptive processing

Endogenous ligand/origin	Receptor	Location of spinal binding		Spinal effects SP release	WDR	Prototypical agonist/antagonist
Opioid						
Enkephalin (Intrinsic BS project)	mu	Pre/post[1,2]	D>V[3]	⇓[4]	⇓[5,6]	Morphine/naloxone Sufentanil/CTAP
	delta	Pre/post[1,2]	D>V[3]	⇓[4]	⇓[5,6]	DPDPE/naltrindole DADL/ICI174816
Dynorphin (Intrinsic)	kappa	Pre/post[1,2]	D>V[3]	⇔[4]	⇓[5,6]	U50488H/norBNI
Adrenergic						
Noradrenaline (BS projections)	$alpha_1$	?	?	⇔[4]	⇔[10]	Methoxamine/prazocin
	$alpha_2$	Pre/post[7]	D>V[8]	⇓[4,9]	⇓[10]	Medetomidine/yohimbine Clonidine/atipamezole (nonA?) ST-91/prazocin
Dopamine						
Dopamine	D_2	?	D>V[11]	⇓[12]		Dopamine/sulpiride
Serotonin						
Serotonin (BS project)	5-HT			⇔[4]	⇓[15]	5-HT
	5-HT_{1A}	Pre/post[12]	D>V[13,14]	?	⇓[15]	8-OH-DPAT/methiothepin
	5-HT_{1B}	?	D>V[14]	?	⇓[15]	RU-24969, DOI/ketanserin
	5-HT_2	?	D>V[16]	?	⇔[15]	a-methyl-5-HT
	5-HT_3	Pre/post[16]	D>V[17]	⇑[18]	⇓[19]	2-methyl-5-HT
Adenosine						
Adenosine (Intrinsic; PA)	A_1/A_2	Post[20]	D>V[21]	⇔[22]	⇓[23]	L-PIA/theophylline
GABA						
GABA (Intrinsic)	A	Pre/post;	D>V[24]	⇓[4]	⇓[19]	Muscimol, THIP/bicuculine
	B	Pre/post;	D>V[25]	⇔[4]	⇓[26]	Baclofen/phaclofen
Cholinergic						
ACh (BS project)	M_1/M_2	Pre/post[27]	D ≈ V[28]	?	⇓[29]	Oxotremorine/atropine
	Nicotinic	?	D ≈ V[28]			
Neuropeptide Y						
NPY1–36 (BS project, PA)		Pre/post;	D>V[30]	⇓[31]	?	NPY 1–36, NPY 18–36
Neurotensin						
NT1–13 (Intrinsic)		?	D>V[32]	?	⇑[33]	NT 1–13
Glutamate						
Glutamate (BS project; PA; DH neurons)	NMDA	? (Post[34])	D>V[35]	?	⇑[36]	NMDA/MK-801
	nonNMDA					AMPA/CNQX Kainate

Abbreviations: Origin of ligand: Intrinsic = cell bodies in the spinal cord; PA = primary afferents; BS project = spinopetal pathways originating in the brainstem. Location of binding in spinal cord: D = dorsal; V = ventral horn; pre = binding presynaptic on primary afferent; post = binding postsynaptic (not on primary afferent); spinal effect = SP release = ⇓ depression, ⇑ increase or ⇔ no effect by agonist of the release of substance P from spinal cord; WDR = ⇓ agonist depresses, ⇑ facilitate or ⇔ do not change the discharge of WDR neuron in spinal dorsal horn; agonist/antagonist = representative competitive agonists and antagonists of the receptor.

References: [1]LaMotte et al 1976; [2]Gamse et al 1979; [3]Morris & Herz 1987; [4]Go & Yaksh 1987; 5 Fleetwood-Walker et al 1988a; [6]Hope et al 1990; [7]Howe et al 1987; [8]Pascual et al 1992; [9]Ono et al 1991; [10]Fleetwood-Walker et al 1985; [11]Wamsley et al 1989; [12]Fleetwood-Walker et al 1988b; [13]Daval et al 1987; [14]Pazos & Palacios 1985; [15]El-Yassir et al 1988; [16]Pazos et al 1985; [17]Hamon et al 1989; [18]Saria et al 1990; [19]Alhaider et al 1991; [20]Geiger et al 1984; [21]Braas 1986; [22]Vasko et al 1986; [23]Salter & Henry 1987; [24]Todd & Mckenzie 1989; [25]Price et al 1987; [26]Dickenson et al 1985; [27]Gillberg & Wiksten 1989; [28]Gillberg et al 1988; [29]Myslinski & Randic 1977; [30]Kar & Quirion 1992; [31]Duggan et al 1991; [32]Faull et al 1989; [33]Miletic & Randic 1979; [34]Davies & Watkins 1983; [35]Miller et al 1988; [36]Schnieder & Perl 1985

Yaksh & Elde 1981; Cesselin et al 1982; Le Bars et al 1987; norepinephrine and serotonin: Tyce & Yaksh 1981).

The potential role of such endogenous activity in regulating afferent processing can be assessed by the examination of the effects on pain behaviour produced by antagonists of the respective receptor and alterations in the disposition of endogenous agent through alterations in metabolism or reuptake. Table 9.3 summarizes the effects of antagonizing several spinal receptor systems on the thermally evoked spinal reflex (tail flick) and the responses to a light tactile stimulus applied to the lower back of the unanaesthetized rat. As indicated, these observations suggest that, aside from the opioid receptor (naloxone) and the alpha-2 adrenoceptor (yohimbine), there is little effect of antagonizing the receptors of a variety of spinal receptor systems on the thermally evoked nociceptive response. These data, though reflecting the results obtained in a single laboratory, typically reflect the relatively modest changes in baseline response latencies observed across several laboratories (see for example references cited in Table 9.3, viz. the respective agonists). These results thus suggest that at best these several

Table 9.3 Effects of spinal agents upon tail flick response latency and agitation response evoked by light touch in the unanaesthetized rat

Receptor class	Spinal antagonist (dose)	Behaviour: Tail flick	Behaviour: Touch evoked agitation
Opioid[1]	Naloxone (30 μg)	↓	0
Adrenergic[1]			
α_1	Prazocine (30 μg)	0	0
α_2	Yohimbine (30 μg)	⇓	0
β	Propranolol (30 μg)	0	0
Serotonin[2]			
5-HT_{1A}	Methiothepin (30 μg)	0	0
5-HT_{1B}	RU-24969 (30 μg)	0	0
5-HT_2	Methysergide (15 μg)	0	0
Adenosine[3]			
A_1/A_2	Theophylline (20 μg)	0	0
Cholinergic[4]			
Muscarinic	Atropine (30 μg)	0	0
Nicotinic	Mecamylamine (30 μg)	0	0
GABA[1,5]			
A	Bicuculine (5 μg)	↓	⇑⇑
B	Phaclofen (30 μg)	0	0
Glycine[1]	Strychnine (5 μg)	↓	⇑⇑

Abbreviations: 0 = No change; ↓ = less than 10% decrease in baseline latency; ⇓ = greater than 10% decrease in baseline latency; ⇑= incidence of tactile evoked hyperaesthesia (allodynia; see Yaksh 1989)
References: [1]Yaksh & Rudy 1977; [2]Ware & Yaksh, unpublished observations; [3]Sosnowski & Yaksh 1989; [4]Naguib & Yaksh, unpublished observations; [5]Yaksh 1989, unpublished observations.

receptor systems, though clearly able to modify pain behaviour following their activation by spinal agonists (Table 9.3), exert a relatively modest ongoing modulation of nociceptive processing. Such observations do not exclude the possibility that other stimulus conditions might lead to an increasing activation of these several systems. Thus, vaginal probing has been shown to elevate the nociceptive threshold (Komisaruk & Whipple 1986). Cervical probing alone will elevate the release of norepinephrine and serotonin from spinal cord in anaesthetized rats and the antinociceptive effects are diminished by intrathecal adrenoceptor and serotonin antagonism (Steinman et al 1983). Similarly, an extensive literature involving a variety of stressors, including cold water swim and foot shock (Watkins & Mayer 1986; Bodnar 1986, 1991) has shown potent effect on pain behaviour mediated by the activation of endogenous monoamine and opioid receptor systems. Foot shock evoked antinociception in rats is reversed in part by spinal noradrenergic and serotonergic antagonists (Watkins et al 1984). Histamine has been shown to play a role in supraspinal regulation of pain behaviour (see below) and histamine antagonists have been shown to reverse both opioid and opioid-mediated stress induced antinociception (Robertson et al 1988).

If these systems play a role in modulating endogenous nociceptive processing, then reducing their clearance by altering their respective antagonism should result in an augmentation of their endogenous modulation.

Metabolism of enkephalin. Enkephalinase inhibitors have been shown to increase the levels of enkephalin released from spinal cord (Yaksh & Chipkin 1989; Suh & Tseng 1990) and depress the firing of dorsal horn neurons (Dickenson et al 1988). The systemic, intracerebral and intrathecal injection of enkephalinase inhibitors has been shown to increase the response latency on thermal nociceptive endpoints (Dickenson et al 1988; Oshita et al 1990; Al-Rodhan et al 1990; Suh & Tseng 1990). These effects are typically reversed by naloxone, emphasizing an opioid receptor-mediated physiological effect.

Monoamines. The administration of amine uptake blockers or monoamine oxidase inhibitors has been shown to increase in an acute, dose-dependent fashion nociceptive response latencies and threshold in animals (Spiegel et al 1983; Bodnar et al 1988; Ardid et al 1991; Ardid & Guilbaud 1992), depress spontaneous pain behaviour in animals (Seltzer et al 1989), reduce nociceptive evoked reflexes in man (Coquoz et al 1991) and to potentiate the antinociceptive effects of opiates (Kellstein et al 1988; Fialip et al 1989; Ventafridda et al 1990). Addition of uptake inhibitors, indeed, act to increase the morphine-evoked release of spinal serotonin, an effect consistent with the potentation of opiate induced analgesia by these agents (Puig et al 1991).

Acetylcholine. The inhibition of spinal cholinesterase has been shown to produce acute dose-dependent increase in response latencies on nociceptive tests in animals (Zhuo & Gebhart 1991, 1992; Naguib & Yaksh, unpublished observation) and these effects are antagonized by atropine, indicating an augmentation in the activation of muscarinic receptors, an effect consistent with the effect of exogenous cholinergic agonists (Table 9.7).

Importantly, it might be anticipated that those systems in which altering metabolism results in an analgesic action would be those systems in which the antagonist alone would yield an exaggerated response. In the case of virtually all of the systems examined, it can be seen that the several classes of receptor preferring antagonists have in fact minimal effects at best on the response to acute pain stimuli in the normal animal. Such observations would suggest that the effects of endogenous acetylcholine, for example, do not represent a particularly active endogenous 'anti-pain system'. In contrast, it seems probable, based on the observation that protracted afferent stimulation results in pronounced system activation (see above) and that these systems may display a significant regulatory activity in models where there is an ongoing stimulus. As will be seen below, for input generated by low-threshold input, a surprisingly effective moment to moment encoding of the afferent message appears in effect.

Processing of low-intensity stimuli

While several of these systems appear to be at least modestly influential in modifying the processing evoked by acute high-intensity thermal input, such studies as shown in Table 9.3 indicate that low-threshold afferent stimuli, typically ineffective in producing evidence of escape behaviour, in fact were able to evoke a powerful pain behaviour after the spinal antagonism of GABA and glycine receptors (Yaksh 1989). Such observations are in concert with studies on the activity of trigeminal single units, where the local application of strychnine was shown to induce a powerful facilitation of the response of wide dynamic range neurons to low thresholds, otherwise innocuous mechanical stimuli (Khayyat et al 1975; Yokota et al 1979). Conversely, iontophoretic delivery of glycine and GABA are able to diminish the size of the cutaneous receptive field (Zieglgänsberger & Herz 1971). Such observations, though limited in scope, raise the likelihood that the encoding of low-threshold mechanical stimuli as innocuous, depends completely upon the presence of a tonic activation of intrinsic glycine and/or GABAergic neurons that are known to exist within the spinal dorsal horn (Todd & Sullivan 1990; Carlton et al 1992) and the presence of high levels of glycine (Zarbin et al 1981; Basbaum 1988) and GABA (Singer & Placheta 1980) binding in the dorsal horn. Importantly, these GABA-containing terminals are frequently presynaptic to the large central afferent terminal complexes and form reciprocal synapses (Barber et al 1978; Carlton & Hayes 1990). GABAergic axosomatic connections on spinothalamic cells have also been identified (Carlton et al 1992).

Several lines of evidence substantiate the relevance of these dorsal horn inhibitory amino acids in regulating the behaviour generated by low-threshold afferent transmission. Thus, genetic variants such as the poll Hereford calf (Gundlach et al 1988) and the spastic mouse (White & Heller 1982) have been shown to display particular sensitivity to even modest stimulation and these models show up to a ten-fold decrease in glycine binding. Secondly, in humans, strychnine intoxication is characterized by a hypersensitivity to light touch (Arena 1970) and the role of such interneurons in the encoding of afferent input has been suggested as an important mechanism involved in the allodynia and hyperaesthesia evoked following spinal cord ischaemia (Hao et al 1992a, 1992b; Marsala & Yaksh 1992) and peripheral nerve injury (Yaksh et al 1992).

SUPRASPINAL RECEPTOR SYSTEMS

In the preceding section, it was emphasized that significant regulation of the processing of afferent input occurred at the spinal cord level. In the present section, attention will be focused on certain supraspinal aspects of systems which regulate the animal's response to noxious stimuli. The integrated nature of these systems makes it difficult to extract a single system out of context. However, considerable evidence has evolved related to the mechanisms of actions of certain neurotransmitter/receptor systems located in specific brain regions which exert a powerful influence upon the organized response of the unanaesthetized animal.

Because of the extensive insights garnered regarding the role of the opioid receptor, the following section is principally focused on the organization of the supraspinal systems with which they are affiliated. As will be seen, it is possible to consider many of the complexities of supraspinal processing with these opioid associated systems as the organizing substrate.

Opioid receptor systems

In the preceding section, opioids with an action limited to the spinal cord can evoke an analgesic effect as assessed by a variety of endpoints. Systematic studies have emphasized that opioids in addition may exert a powerful effect upon pain behaviour by a supraspinal action. The following sections will review those sites, their pharmacology and the considered mechanisms.

Sites of opioid action

Microinjection mapping of the brain in animals prepared with stereotactically placed guide cannulae has revealed that opioid receptors are functionally coupled to the regulation of the animal's response to strong and otherwise noxious mechanical, thermal and chemical stimuli which excite small primary afferents. The following will summarize several of the characteristics of sites which have been principally identified. Table 9.4 summarizes several of the characteristics of the sites of action as they have been identified in the rat.

Mesencephalic central grey. The early studies of Tsou & Jiang revealed in 1964 that the local action of morphine in the periventricular grey would block thermally evoked hind limb reflexes in the unanaesthetized rabbit. Subsequent work revealed a similar potent effect in the rat (Sharpe et al 1974; Jacquet & Lajtha 1976; Yaksh et al 1976; Lewis & Gebhart 1977; Jensen & Yaksh 1986c), mouse (Criswell 1976), cat (Ossipov et al 1984), dog (Wettstein et al 1982) and primate (Pert & Yaksh 1974, 1975, see below). Importantly, these effects were routinely reversed by low doses of naloxone given either systemically or into the microinjection site. These studies confirmed the generality of this site of opiate action across a wide range of species. As indicated in Table 9.5, these effects of periaqueductal grey (PAG) morphine is manifested on both spinal reflexes and upon supraspinally organized responses. Also of interest is the observation that the unilateral injection of morphine into the PAG results in antinociceptive effects which are somatotopically organized. Thus, Yaksh et al (1976) noted a rostral caudal distribution such that sites in the caudal PAG evoked a whole body reduction in the pinch response, while those located rostrally tended towards an effect which was focused on the fore paw and face. A somatotopic organization to the response evoked by PAG morphine has also been reported by Kasman & Rosenfeld (1986).

The pharmacology of the actions of opioids in the PAG have been systematically examined. As indicated in Table 9.4, based on the relative activity of several receptor agonists and antagonists, the effects appear to be mediated by mu, but not delta or kappa classes of receptors. Thus, agents such as [D-Ala^2,Me-Phe^4,Gly(ol)^5] enkephalin (DAGO), sufentanil and morphine are able to produce a powerful, dose dependent antinociception with the ordering of potency being: sufentanil (mu) $\geqslant$ DAGO (mu) > morphine (mu) $\gg$ U50488 (kappa) $\ggg$ [D-Pen^2-D-Pen^5 1 enkephalin (DPDPE) (delta) (Yaksh et al 1988a). In addition, binding studies focusing on the PAG have identified a single high-affinity mu site for which delta and kappa agonists have low affinity and which is coupled to a G-protein (Fednyshyn et al 1989; Fednyshyn & Lee 1989).

Table 9.4 Summary of characteristics of actions of intracerebral opiates given into various sites in the unanaesthetized rat

Microinjection sites	Antinociceptive actions (tail flick/jaw jerk)	(hot plate/paw pressure)	Pharmacology (opioid receptor type)	References
Forebrain/diencephalon				
amygdala (corticomedial)	(–)	II-B	mu ?	1
nucleus accumbens	I		mu ?/epsilon	2
Mesencephalon				
periaqueductal grey	I	I	mu ≫ delta = kappa = 0	3
mesencephalic reticular formation	II-B	II-B	mu ?	4
substantia nigra	II-B	II-B	mu ≫ delta = kappa = 0	4
Lower brainstem				
medial medulla	II	II	mu = delta > 0	5
Spinal cord	I	I	mu = delta > kappa > 0	6

Abbreviations: Dose range for morphine sulphate to produce a comparable near maximum effect in the rat: B = bilateral injection; Effective dose range I = 1–5 ug; II = 5–15 µg; (–) = inactive or prominent side-effects occur at the dose
References:[1]Rodgers 1977; Yaksh et al 1976; [2]Tseng & Wang 1992; [3]Jensen & Yaksh 1986c; Smith et al 1988; Sanchez-Blazquez & Garzon 1989; [4]Haigler & Spring 1978; [5]Jensen & Yaksh 1986c; Bodnar et al 1988; [6]Drower et al 1991; Malmberg & Yaksh 1992c; Yaksh et al 1986; Schmauss & Yaksh 1984.

Table 9.5 Ability of intrathecal antagonists to reverse the effects of morphine given into several brainstem sites on spinal reflex activity[a]

Receptor	Spinal antagonist	Microinjection site (morphine) Periaqueductal grey	Raphe magnus	Medullary reticular form
α	Phentolamine	⇓[1,2,3]	⇓[2]	⇓[2]
α_1	Corynanthine	0[1]		
α_2	Yohimbine	⇓[1]		
α_2 nonA	(Prazocin)	⇓[1]		
β	Propranolol	0[1]		
Dopamine	cis-flupentixol Haloperidol	0[1]	0[2]	0[2]
Opioid	Naloxone	0[1]	↓[2]	↓[2]
5-HT$_2$	Methysergide	⇓[1,2,3]	⇓[2]	0[2]

Abbreviations: a ⇓ = significant reversal of tail flick inhibition; ↓ = modest reversal of tail flick; 0 = reversal of tail flick.
References: [1]Camarata & Yaksh 1985; [2]Jensen & Yaksh 1986b; [3]Yaksh 1979

Mesencephalic reticular formation. Microinjection studies have shown that bilateral injection of morphine into the mesencephalic reticular formation (adjacent anatomically to active regions of the PAG) are able to significantly increase hot plate response latency with relatively more modest effects upon spinal reflexes (Haigler & Spring 1978).

The pharmacology of these systems has not been systematically addressed, though the action of morphine clearly implicates a mu site.

Medulla. Microinjection mapping studies have suggested that there are two distinct distributions of opiate-sensitive sites within the caudal medulla medial sites overlapping the region of the cell bodies of the nucleus raphe (Levy & Proudfit 1979; Dickenson et al 1979); Prado & Roberts 1984; Jensen et al 1986a), and lateral sites which correspond grossly to the region of the nucleus gigantocelluaris (Takagi et al 1977, 1978; Akaike et al 1978; Azami et al 1982; Satoh et al 1983; Jensen et al 1986a). Microinjections of opiates into the medulla will increase in a dose-dependent fashion the response latencies on both spinal and supraspinally mediated endpoints (see Table 9.4).

The pharmacology of these systems has been examined in some detail. Based on structure–activity relationships attained after intracerebral injection, it appears that both mu and delta sites exist within the caudal medulla (Takagi et al 1977, 1978; Jensen et al 1986c).

Substantia nigra. Baumeister and colleagues have demonstrated that the bilateral microinjection of opioids into the substantia nigra will evoke a dose-dependent, naloxone reversible, increase in the tail flick and hot-plate response latencies in rats without evidence of significant motor impairment or change in the response to nonnoxious stimuli (Baumeister et al 1987, 1990). Unilateral injections failed to alter spinal reflex responses but, following unilateral injection, rats were more likely to lick the contralateral paw.

Examination of the agonist and antagonist pharmacology of this nigral action reveals the role of mu, but not delta or kappa receptors (Baumeister 1991).

The mechanisms of this opioid nigral effect are not clear. However, over half of the cells in the pars compacta and reticularis respond complexly to noxious stimuli (Pay & Barasi 1982; Schultz & Romo, 1987), while others display an inhibition (Tsai et al 1980). Electrical stimulation of the substantia nigra inhibits the response of dorsal horn nociceptors to peripheral stimulation (Barnes et al 1979). Alternately, while the effect of nigral opiates appears limited to the noxious component, catecholamine lesions of the nigra striatal pathways have been shown to produce an ipsilateral sensory inattention (Siegfried & Bures 1978), and this effect is mimicked by the nigral injection of a $GABA_A$ agonist (Houston et al 1980). The role of such changes in sensory evoked awareness remains to be determined.

Nucleus accumbens/ventral forebrain. In rats and rabbits, the injection of morphine into the ventral forebrain, notably the nucleus accumbens, preoptic and arcuate nuclei, has been shown to be able to block spinal nociceptive reflexes (Tseng & Wang 1992; Ma & Han 1992).

The pharmacology of these systems appears regionally complex. In rats, Tseng and colleagues have shown that in the preoptic and arcuate regions, both β-endorphin and morphine yield a dose-dependent, naloxone reversible increase in tail-flick latencies. In the nucleus accumbens, β-endorphin displays significant activity but morphine does not. The likelihood that morphine and β-endorphin act in this model on discriminable subclasses of receptors (mu and epsilon, respectively) is hypothesized on the basis of the observation that morphine's actions are reversed by β-endorphin 1–27, a reported antagonist of the epsilon site, while the effects of morphine are reversed by D-Phe-Cys-Tyr-D-Tyr-Orn-Thr-Pen-Thr-NH_2, a mu preferring antagonist (Tseng & Wang 1992).

Amygdala. Early studies emphasized the effects of morphine given into the basolateral amygdala in altering hot-plate, but not tail-flick response latencies (Yaksh et al 1976; Rodgers 1977). Changes in the response appear to depend upon concurrent bilateral opioid agonist activity. Extensive studies on the pharmacology of the amygdala have not been reported, but mu opioid agonists have been indicated to be active and these effects are naloxone reversible (Rodgers 1977; Yaksh et al 1976; 1988a).

Other regions. While several microinjection mapping studies of opiate action have failed to observe activity following thalamic injections (Pert & Yaksh 1974; Yaksh et al 1977; Prado 1989) reported that microinjection of morphine into the anterior pretectal region of the rat, but not adjacent nuclei resulted in an inhibition of the tail flick.

Mechanisms of antinociception following supraspinal manipulations

It is clear given the diversity of sites that it is unlikely that all of the mechanisms whereby opiates act within the brain to alter nociceptive transmission are identical. Currently, it seems likely that within the brainstem there are several mechanisms whereby opiates may act to alter nociceptive transmission.

Bulbospinal projections. In the original work, it was shown that the action of morphine in the brainstem was able to inhibit or increase the latency of spinal nociceptive reflexes. Recording from dorsal horn neurons, it has been shown that the microinjection of morphine into the PAG, the locus coeruleus/subcoeruleus region and into raphe magnus will significantly reduce the increase in activity evoked by noxious stimuli (Bennett & Mayer 1979; Gebhart et al 1984; Gebhart & Jones 1988). These effects are in accord with a variety of studies in which pharmacological enhancement of spinal monoamine activity will lead to an inhibition of the magnitude of flexor reflex-evoked ventral-root reflex activity (Anden et al 1966). Support for the probable role of bulbospinal pathways in controlling spinal sensory processing in general and for their role in the actions of opioid receptor-linked systems in particular is based on four sets of observations:

a) Supraspinal activation of bulbospinal terminals: The microinjection of morphine into the brainstem, notably the PAG or medulla, will increase the release or turnover of 5-hydroxytriptamine (5-HT) and/or noradrenaline at the spinal cord level (Yaksh & Tyce 1979; Takagi et al 1979). These observations are in accord with the effects produced when the bulbospinal pathways are directly stimulated (Hammond et al 1985) and emphasize that the actions of morphine in the PAG are in fact associated with an increase in spinofugal outflow (i.e. as opposed to a reduction in a descending excitatory drive). Importantly, considerable data have in fact shown the presence of bulbospinal aminergic pathways in a variety of species, including primate (Helke et at 1990b; Carlton et al 1991; Proudfit & Clark 1991).

b) Spinal antagonism of effects of supraspinal actions: The effects of morphine given into the brainstem on spinal reflexes should be reversed by the spinal delivery of the appropriate receptor antagonists. Thus, the spinal delivery of phentolamine and/or methysergide is able to produce a significant reversal of the inhibition of the nociceptive reflex otherwise evoked by the microinjection of morphine into the PAG (Yaksh 1979; Camarata & Yaksh 1985). Importantly, the antagonist pharmacology appears to be similar whether the spinal reflex inhibition is evoked by morphine within the PAG or by the direct stimulation with an excitatory amino acid (Jensen & Yaksh 1984a) or by focal electrial stimulation (Hammond & Yaksh 1984), again emphasizing that the effect of supraspinal morphine is to evoke net increase in spinopetal outflow.

c) Physiological mimicry by exogenous spinal agonists: If bulbospinal pathways serve to regulate different facets of spinal nociceptive processing, then the direct activation of those receptors by the spinal delivery of the respective agonists should in fact provide a mimicry of supraspinal action of morphine. As indicated in Table 9.7, the intrathecal injection of alpha-2-adrenoceptor agonists, 5-HT, dopamine (apomorphine) and muscarinic agonists can produce a powerful, dose-dependent regulation of pain behaviour in several species. Of particular interest, these observations on the pharmacology of spinal regulatory systems have provided insights into the possible utility of these systems in humans. Thus, the spinal delivery of clonidine, an alpha-2-adrenoceptor agonist in man, has been shown to exert a powerful analgesic effect in post-operative and chronic cancer pain in humans (Eisenach et al 1989a, 1989b, see below).

d) Comparability of spinal antagonist pharmacology for the supraspinal stimulus versus exogenous agonist: If the effects of bulbospinal pathways activated by the supraspinal action of morphine are mediated by specific receptors that are acted upon by the respective exogenous agonists, the antagonist pharmacology for the effects of supraspinal morphine and the spinally-delivered exogenous agonists should be the same. To this end, as noted above, in a variety of studies employing brainstem stimulation, glutamate and morphine, the effects of intrathecal 5-HT are reversed by methysergide and the effects of noradrenaline are reversed by phentolamine and yohimbine, suggesting the potential role of 5-HT_2 and alpha-2-adrenoceptor agonists, respectively. Importantly, the effects of supraspinal morphine are readily antagonized by prazocine (Camarata & Yaksh 1985). While this agent is typically considered to be an alpha-1 antagonist, it has been argued more recently that this agent is an antagonist at an alpha-2 non-A subclass of sites and recent studies on the pharmacology of the adrenoceptor system have shown the possible role of alpha-2 non-A sites in the spinal cord mediated analgesia (Takano & Yaksh 1992; Takano et al 1992).

Several points should be considered with regard to the question of the role of bulbospinal systems.

First, it seems apparent that the net effects of supraspinal opioids on spinal pathways must reflect a net activation of an inhibition (as opposed to the withdrawal of a facilitation). This is emphasized by several observations:

1. Supraspinal opioids increase the release of the several transmitters at the spinal cord level
2. The effects of morphine in the PAG and medulla are mimicked by electrical stimulation and/or by the microinjection of glutamate (Jensen & Yaksh 1984a; Hammond & Yaksh 1984)

In general, such observations are consistent with the notion that opioid receptor occupancy may, through the respective circuitry, induce an excitatory outflow from the mesencephalic central grey to both the hind brain (and as will be discussed below) and into the forebrain. Similarly, other sites of opiate action, such as the medulla, appear to induce activation of bulbospinal projections by intermediate projections to cell systems possessing the appropriate neurotransmitter (such as noradrenaline) (Proudfit & Clark 1991).

Secondly, it seems apparent based on the pharmacology of the spinal antagonists that several systems are involved in the spinal modulation induced by brainstem opioids. As summarized in Table 9.5, the mesencephalic and medullary sites of action may both serve to activate a variety of bulbospinal systems that regulate spinal reflex activities. Moreover, it appears likely that these descending mechanisms may be accessed by more rostral systems (such as the nucleus accumbens; Yu & Han 1989).

Thirdly, it is clear that a variety of sites may be involved in the mechanisms whereby bulbospinal pathways are activated. Thus, as noted in Table 9.4, the actions of opioids in regions as diverse as the medulla, the PAG, the mesencephalon and the forebrain are able to alter spinal nociceptive reflexes. While naloxone-sensitive excitatory effects of opiates have been reported (Huang 1992), in the brainstem, opioids have largely been shown to exert a suppressive effect upon neuronal function (Gebhart 1982); it seems reasonable, as was suggested earlier (Yaksh et al 1976) that the net outflow evoked by morphine from any given region must reflect an inhibition of an inhibition. The powerful role of GABAergic neurons within the medulla (Drower & Hammond 1988; Heinricher & Kaplan 1991) and the antinociceptive effects generated by the injection of GABA antagonists into the PAG (Moreau & Fields 1987), provide some insight into this system. Intracellular unit recording in ex vivo brainstem slices indeed reveals that $GABA_A$-receptor antagonism will evoke significant depolarization of PAG neurons (Behbehani et al 1990). (For detailed discussion of the microcircuitry involved in these brainstem actions of opiates see Fields et al (1991) and Ch. 12.) Pharmacological studies have implicated the role of excitatory amino acid (Aimone & Gebhart 1986, 1988), serotonin (Aimone & Gebhart 1988), neurotensin (Fang et al 1987) and alpha-1 receptors (Hammond et al 1980; Haws et al 1990) in mediating the excitatory interlink between the outflow of the several regions where opiates are thought to act and the monoaminergic projection neurons.

Fourthly, it is possible that all of the structures may channel into a single spinopetal system that modulates small afferent input. Indeed, as will be noted below, there are strong reciprocal relations between the PAG and the forebrain as well as the more caudal brainstem from which these bulbospinal fibre systems originate. If activity in a particular region were to inhibit spinal processing in a manner which was pharmacologically distinct from a second, then it could be argued that these two systems might not be serially organized. Two examples suggesting such *nonserial* bulbospinal linkages may be provided.

1. van Praag & Frenk (1990) reported that the effects of morphine on the tail flick in the rat were antagonized by the microinjection of nonNMDA glutamate receptor antagonists into the raphe magnus. However, the effects of excitatory amino acids given into the PAG was not, suggesting alternative linkages through the caudal brainstem.

2. Tseng and colleagues have shown that the effects of β-endorphin in the accumbens will block spinal reflexes. This effect is reversed by the spinal release of enkephalin and accordingly the effects upon spinal reflexes are reversed by the spinal delivery of naloxone (Tseng & Fujimoto 1985; Tseng & Tang 1990; Tseng et al 1990; Tseng & Wang, 1992).

As noted in Table 9.5, the effects of receptor occupancy by morphine in the PAG is sensitive to spinal monoamine antagonists, but not to naloxone.

Finally, as emphasized above, intrathecal antagonism of these bulbospinal systems will significantly diminish the antireflexive effects of supraspinal morphine. However, concurrent examination of the supraspinally mediated response reveals that the animal typically continues to display a clear analgesia as defined by both the hot-plate response latency and the response to pinch (supraspinally organized responses) (Yaksh 1979; Camarata & Yaksh 1985). Similarly, lesions made just caudal to the PAG significantly diminished the effects of PAG electrical stimulation on the tail flick (a spinal reflex), but not the hot-plate test (a supraspinally organized endpoint) (Morgan et al 1989). Such observations, at the least, emphasize that other systems must be superimposed on the descending modulation to account for the effects of supraspinal opiates on the organized response to a strong cutaneous stimulus. At the extreme, these observations argue the possibility that bulbospinal inhibition may play only a minor role in actually modulating the animal's supraspinally organized response to a strong stimulus following supraspinal opiate receptor occupancy. It should in fact be emphasized that several laboratories fail to see significant inhibitory influence of opiates given into the PAG on the evoked response of dorsal horn nociceptive neurons (Clarke et al 1983; Dickenson & Le Bars 1987).

Brainstem–brainstem indirect inhibition of afferent traffic. Spinomedullary and spinal mesencephalic projections have been described and are thought to play a role in the generation of the message evoked by high-threshold stimuli (see Ch. 12). While not systemically examined, previous work has shown that stimulation within the PAG can result in an inhibition of neurons in the nucleus reticulogigantocellularis (Mohrland & Gebhart 1980). More recent work by Fields and colleagues has shown powerful mesencephalic influences upon medullary cell populations. It seems probable, based on known effect projections of these systems that some of these cells may represent projection neurons that contribute to the rostral movement of nociceptive information (Fields et al 1991). Thus, 'local' descending control of input though the linkages in these regions, inhibiting activity in projection neurons, could serve to modify the content of the ascending message generated by a high-intensity stimulus.

Direct inhibition of brainstem afferent traffic. In contrast to indirect modulation of afferent processing, it is believed possible that opiates in the brainstem may directly alter the excitatory input into the brainstem core. This possibility is based on several observations. First, it is known that many spinobulbar neurons are directly sensitive to opioids delivered in the spinal cord (see above). Based on the likelihood that receptors synthesized in the cell body will be transported to the distal terminals (Atweh et al 1978; Laduron 1984), then it is accordingly likely that opioid sites would be presynaptic on the brainstem terminals of spinobulbar neurons. Second and more direct, it has been shown that cervical hemisection will result in a significant reduction in the levels of 3H dihydromorphine in the medulla and PAG/mesencephalic reticular formation (MRF) ipsilateral to the cord hemisection (Ramberg & Yaksh 1989). Significantly, many of the regions in which opioids are known to exert their effects, particularly within the mesencephalon and medulla, are known to receive significant input either from direct spinobulbar projections or collaterals from spinodiencephalic projections (Boive 1971; Kerr & Lippman 1974, Zhang et al 1990a; see Ch. 6). These observations thus provide support for the hypothesis the locally administered opiates might alter nociceptive processing though a presynaptic action on spinofugal terminals, thereby reducing the excitation otherwise evoked by the spinofugal projections in brainstem systems relevant to the organization of the response to the noxious event (Bowsher 1976; Zemlan & Behbehani 1988).

It is interesting to note that populations of cell bodies in the substantia gelatinosa have been shown to project into the ventrolateral reticular formation (Lima & Coimbra 1991). Given that significant numbers of gelatinosa neurons contain glycine and GABA (see above), these observations raise the possibility that outflow from the dorsal horn generated by afferent input may result in an inhibitory projection into the regions receiving afferent input. Further studies of such intrinsically organized systems are clearly required.

Forebrain mechanisms modulating afferent input. While there is ample evidence suggesting that opiates may interact with the mesencephalon to alter input by a variety of direct and indirect systems, the behavioural sequelae of opioids possess a significant component that reflects upon the affective component of the organism's response to the pain state. As will be discussed below, several forebrain sites may well reflect that component of the action of the opioid agonists. Nevertheless, there are significant rostral projections that connect the PAG with forebrain systems that are know to influence motivational and affective components of behaviour. Thus, while current interest has focused on the role of caudally projecting 5-HT and noradrenegic systems, the raphe dorsalis lying in proximity to the ventral medial PAG sends 5-HT projections rostrally into a variety of rostral sites, including the the nucleus accumbens, amygdala and lateral thalamus (Ma et al 1991; Westlund et al 1990; Ma & Han 1992). Similarly, the locus coeruleus has ample projections into the limbic forebrain and thalamus (Amaral & Sinnamon 1977; Westlund et al 1990). Both 5-HT and noradrenergic systems have been implicated in emotionality and maintenance of consciousness. Early work with lesions of the raphe dorsalis revealed a significant diminution of the antinociceptive effects of morphine (Samanin et al 1970; Yaksh et al 1977). Depletion of serotonin by treatment with p-chlorphenylalanine, for example, has been classically known to produce rats that were particularly irritable (Tenen 1968).

More recent studies have emphasized the probable role of a forebrain circuit which can alter nociceptive responsiveness. Thus, the microinjection of morphine into the accumbens can alter nociceptive responding and this effect is reported to be blocked by lesions of the arcuate nucleus or by the injection of naloxone or β-endorphin antisera into the PAG (Yu & Han 1989). Conversely, microinjections of morphine into the PAG evoked an increase in the release of β-endorphin and met-enkephalin-like immunoreactivity in the nucleus accumbens. Though there are differences, Tseng and colleagues have similarly emphasized the probable role of forebrain to brainstem projections modulating afferent transmission though an input into the mesencephalic central grey (Tseng & Wang 1992). The organization of these caudally projecting systems is not clear. Behbehani et al (1988) have shown that glutamate microinjected into the lateral hypothalamus will increase firing in the PAG (and elevate spinal reflex latencies). Whether the excitatory effects of such forebrain stimulation are direct is not known. Thus, opiocortin-containing projections from the ventral forebrain, particularly the arcuate nucleus, have been demonstrated (Sim & Joseph 1989). The injection of NMDA receptor agonists into the arcuate evokes a significant increase in the release of β-endorphin-like immunoreactivity into ventriculocisternal perfusates (Bach & Yaksh 1992). The likelihood of an inhibition into the vicinity of the raphe might suggest a feedback inhibition on raphe fugal cells, or conversely, as in the PAG, these opioid inputs may mediate an inhibition of acitivity in GABA-containing interneurons and thus serve to increase raphe outflow (note the effects of GABA agonists/antagonists in the caudal brainstem: Drower & Hammond 1988).

Other systems. In addition to those systems outlined above, substantial evidence has evolved to suggest that opiates may act though a number of neurochemical systems to alter pain behaviour. The precise mechanisms of such interaction are not clear.

a) Histamine. Hough and colleagues have shown in a line of studies that brain systems releasing histamine may serve to mediate the processing of nociceptive information

(Hough 1988). Thus, morphine has been shown to increase histamine release from the PAG (Barke & Hough 1992) and the effects of systemic morphine can be attenuated by the systemic or PAG injection of histamine antagonists, particularly of the H_2 type (Gogas et al 1989; Hough & Nalwalk 1992).

b) Adenosine. Sawynok and colleagues have characterized the role of adenosine in a number of spinal and supraspinal systems that modulate nociceptive processing (see Sawynok & Sweeny 1989). Their work has suggested that many of the opioid effects may have as a common mechanism the release of a purine.

At the spinal cord level, morphine has been shown to increase the release of adenosine and this effect is mediated by a pertussis toxin sensitive mechanism (Sawynok et al 1990). Based on the effects of prior treatment with capsaicin, it is believed that the adenosine release originates from primary afferent terminals (Sweeny et al 1989). Intrathecal adenosine has been shown to increase the nociceptive threshold (Sawynok et al 1989, 1991a; Sosnowski et al 1989).

In the brain, the antinociceptive effects of morphine in the PAG are antagonized by the adenosine receptor antagonists, 8-phenyltheophylline. The role of bulbospinal projections in this action is suggested by the observation that intraventricular morphine will release adenosine in the spinal cord (Sweeny et al 1991). The role of bulbospinal pathways in this effect is consistent with the observation that serotonin will release adenosine in spinal cord (Sweeny et al 1990).

INTERACTIONS BETWEEN SUPRASPINAL AND SPINAL SYSTEMS

Based on even a cursory analysis of the preceding section, it is evident that multiple entities can alter afferent processing by a diversity of mechanisms. It is of interest to consider the linearity with which these several systems may interact. In fact, only a few of the many potential combinations have been considered and yet fewer have been systematically studied. In the following section several representative anatomically linked examples will be considered.

Brainstem–spinal cord

Opiate given systemically can produce a powerful and selective effect upon pain behaviour. As outlined above, opioids with an action limited to the spinal cord and to the brainstem are able each to produce a powerful alteration in nociceptive processing. Yet, in early studies, it was shown that the delivery of an opioid antagonist into the cerebral ventricles (Tsou 1963; Vigouret et al 1973) or into the lumbar intrathecal space (Yaksh & Rudy 1978) could produce a complete antagonism of the effects of the systemic opioid agonist. This led to the hypothesis that the effects of opiate receptor occupancy in brain must synergize with the effects produced by the concurrent occupancy of spinal receptors (Yaksh & Rudy 1978). With high occupancy (as produced when the drugs are delivered focally), the systems were able independently to produce a significant change in pain processing. Yeung & Rudy (1980) demonstrated the validity of the hypothesis by showing that the concurrent administration of morphine spinally and supraspinally would lead to a prominent synergy, as indicated by hyperbolic isobolograms. Similar results have been observed in mice (Roerig & Fujimoto 1989; see Tallarida et al 1989, for discussion of analysis of synergic interactions).

Supraspinal–supraspinal

As reviewed in the above sections, it is clear that there are multiple points at which receptor occupancy may induce a potent antinociceptive effect. There are relatively few studies which have sought to investigate the interaction that may occur between these several links. Two efforts that have been reported are considered briefly below.

PAG and locus coeruleus

Bodnar and colleagues (Bodnar et al 1991) have examined the effects of concurrent actions of microinjections into the PAG and locus coeruleus. Though systematic examinations were not performed, ethyketocyclazocine (reported to have mu agonist properties) was found to be without effect when administered alone in either site, at any dose. Concurrent delivery, at doses which together were less than injected in either site alone, produced a significant, naloxone-reversible increase in response latency. These observations were argued to reflect a synergic interaction between these two anatomically distinct systems.

PAG and nucleus reticularis gigantocellularis

Xia and colleagues (Xia et al 1992) examined the effects of concurrent delivery of met-enkephalin into the PAG and into the nucleus reticularis gigantocellularis of the medulla. In these studies, single unit activity in the trigeminal nucleus was examined along with response to noxious stimulation. Injection in both regions depressed escape behaviour and evoked neuronal activity. Conjoint delivery appeared to have only a simple additive interaction.

Spinal cord–spinal cord

Consistent with the powerful nonlinear interaction between spinal and supraspinal opiates, and given the considered role of bulbospinal systems in mediating some of the supraspinal actions of opiates, it has been shown that the concurrent spinal delivery of alpha-2 and opioid agonists would also reveal a powerful synergy (Table 9.6).

The mechanisms of this synergy are not known. It may be of significance that one class of agents that routinely appears to show a nonlinear interaction at the spinal level are those that interact presynaptically with primary afferents to diminish release (e.g. mu, delta and alpha-2) (see Table 9.2). Based on our current understanding of mechanisms, neither adenosine nor kappa agonists are thought to have a potent effect upon the release of afferent transmitter (see Table 9.2). A second class of agents that appears to show significant spinal synergy with the opioids are the cyclooxygenase inhibitors. Given the presumed role outlined in preceding sections for the release of prostaglandins by afferent input and the probable role played by cyclooxygenase products in evoking a facilitated state of spinal processing, the synergy observed in the formalin test might be anticipated. Potent synergy has indeed been shown between these two classes of agents (Table 9.6) (Malmberg & Yaksh 1993b).

Aside from the synergic interactions that may occur between several receptor systems, there is increasing evidence that certain endogenous systems may serve to diminish the activity of receptor systems that modulate nociceptive transmission. Two examples of this interaction may be considered.

Cholecystokinin

A number of groups have reported that cholecystokinin (CCK), particularly the octapeptide CCK-8, may diminish the antinociceptive effects of morphine (Faris et al 1983; Wiertelak et al 1992) and reverse the inhibition of dorsal horn neurons produced by morphine (Kellstein et al 1991). Given the presence and release of CCK from spinal cord (Yaksh et al 1982a, 1982b), this peptide could serve as an endogenous opioid antagonist. Support for this hypothesis is provided by the observation that CCK antagonists (particularly of the A-type) can augment the effects of morphine (O'Neill et al 1989; Kellstein et al 1991). The nature and specificity of this interaction remains to be defined (Baber et al 1989). Thus, Tseng & Collins (1992), reported that intrathecal CCK would antagonize the effects of intraventricular β-endorphin.

Dynorphin

Fujimoto and colleagues have demonstrated that spinal dynorphin (Dyn 1–17) in low doses is able to antagonize the effects of intrathecal opiates (Fujimoto et al 1990). This effect does appear to be produced by Dyn 1–17, but not by other dynorphin analogues (Rady et al 1991) and is not mediated by a kappa receptor. Again, the presence of dynorphin in the spinal neurons as well as its upregulation following inflammation (Iadarola et al 1988) provides evidence for its possible role as an endogenous 'antialgesic' agent.

ROLE OF MODULATORY SUBSTRATES IN PAIN BEHAVIOUR

The above sections emphasize that the output of the spinal cord in response to a strong stimulus is subject to a pronounced modulation by a variety of neurotransmitter/receptor systems in the spinal cord. Given the reasonable presumption that the content of the message

Table 9.6 Summary of the characteristics of the interaction of different classes of receptor agonists following intrathecal delivery

Spinal agonist pairing[1]	Species	Test[2]	Interaction[3]	References
Mu-delta	Rat	HP	Synergistic	Malmberg & Yaksh (1992c)
	Rat	TF	Synergistic	Larson et al (1980)
	Mouse	TF	Additive	Porreca et al (1987)
Mu-alpha$_2$	Rat	HP	Synergistic	Monasky et al (1990)
	Rat	HP	Additive	Ossipov et al (1990a)
	Rat	TF	Synergistic	Ossipov et al (1990a, 1990b)
Mu-local anaesthetics	Rat	TF	Synergistic	Maves & Gebhart (1992)
	Rat	HP	Synergistic	Penning & Yaksh (1992)
Mu-cyclooxygenase inhibitor	Rat	FOR	Synergistic	Malmberg & Yaksh (1993b)
Delta-alpha$_2$	Rat	TF	Synergistic	Ossipov et al (1990b)
Kappa-alpha$_2$	Rat	TF	Synergistic	Ossipov et al (1990b)
Kappa-cyclooxygenase inhibitor	Rat	FOR	Additive	Malmberg & Yaksh (1993b)
Alpha-2-cyclooxygenase inhibitor	Rat	FOR	Synergistic	Malmberg & Yaksh (1993b)
L-PIA-cyclooxygenase inhibitor	Rat	FOR	Additive	Malmberg & Yaksh (1993b)
NMDA antagonist-cyclooxygenase	Rat	FOR	Additive	Abram & Yaksh (unpublished)

Abbreviations: [1]All analyses employed either an isobolographic analysis or multiple dose combinations with a fixed additive dose (Tallarida et al 1989); [2]HP = hot plate; TF = Tail flick; FOR = formalin test; [3]Synergistic indicates that isobologram deviated significantly from linearity or that the left shift in the dose-response curve observed in the presence of the added drug was statistically greater than that predicted on the basis of simple effects-additivity.

transmitted to higher centres by long tracts in part defines the sensory–discriminative component of the pain state, these intrinsic systems as outlined provide mechanisms whereby the content of the projected message may be associated with a response which is: i) greater than would be anticipated for a given stimulus, ii) inappropriate for the stimulus which generates the message or, iii) less than would be anticipated given the magnitude of the physical stimulus. These three conditions intuitively correspond to the behavioural states of hyperalgesia, hyperaesthesia (or allodynia) and hypoalgesia (analgesia). These states and aspects of the central pharmacology that may underlie these states of altered afferent encoding will be considered below.

STATES OF ALTERED PAIN PROCESSING

Hyperalgesia

Hyperalgesia indicates a pain behaviour which is in excess of the magnitude of the pain behaviour (normoalgesia?) which would be anticipated in the presence of a given stimulus evoking a given afferent barrage. This might be evidenced by a decrease in response latency or increase in response magnitude otherwise evoked by a given aversive stimulus. As noted above, the generation of a modestly protracted afferent barrage by the injection of an irritant into the skin or the generation of a state of inflammation will evoke an acute pain state, followed by a profound hyperalgesia. Models such as the formalin test in the rat have been shown to be associated with a two-phased response, with the magnitude of the second-phase behaviour being in excess of that anticipated on the basis of the afferent activity measured in the peripheral afferent at the corresponding time points (Heapy et al 1987; Wheeler-Aceto et al 1990). Similarly, other models of hyperalgesia involving chronic inflammatory states may well be involved in such states of facilitated processing (though if the increased pain behaviour reflects upon a greater sensitivity of the peripheral nerve to the stimulus, then this hyperalgesia might reflect a model mediated by a peripheral mechanism). The spinal delivery of certain afferent transmitters, such as sP or NMDA will evoke a prominent decrease in the thermal nociceptive threshold of the unanaesthetized rat, corresponding to the presumed mechanisms set into play by repetitive afferent input. In man, the focal activation of cutaneous C-fibres by the subcutaneous injection of capsaicin results in a prominent acute pain behaviour followed by a profound hyperalgesia over an area of skin that greatly exceeds the focal site of the original stimulus. Importantly, this secondary hyperalgesia appears centrally mediated, for (as with the formalin test) if the acute afferent barrage is blocked by local anaesthetic, the secondary phase does not occur (Torebjörk et al 1992).

Hyperaesthesia

The evocation of pain behaviour in response to light touch, referred to as allodynia, can be induced by the intrathecal delivery of low doses of glycine and $GABA_A$ antagonists (Yaksh 1989). Importantly, this effect does not appear to be a simple exaggeration of all input as the response latency to noxious thermal stimuli is little affected (Yaksh 1989; Yamamoto & Yaksh 1993). These behavioural effects produced by spinal amino acid antagonists correspond to the prominent hypersensitivity that is associated with genetic models where low levels of spinal glycine binding have been observed, such as in the poll Hereford (Gundlach et al 1988) and in the spastic mouse (White & Heller 1982). In man, strychnine intoxication is reportedly associated with prominent hypersensitivity to innocuous stimuli (Arena 1970). Similarly, tactile allodynia has been reported in models of focal (Hao et al 1991a) and global (Marsala & Yaksh 1992) spinal ischaemia. Animal models of chronic peripheral nerve compression have shown (Bennett & Xie 1988; Shir & Seltzer 1990; Kim & Chung 1992) the development of allodynia. An allodynic state following nerve and spinal cord injury is well described in man (Chs 10, 11 and 38). While the mechanisms of these hyperaesthetic states are not known, both peripheral nerve injury and incomplete spinal ischaemia are typically associated with prominent changes in the morphology of small interneurons (Kapadia & La Motte 1987), presumably similar to those which have been identified in the spinal dorsal horn and known to contain glycine and GABA (Todd & Sullivan 1990).

Hypoalgesia

A reduction in the magnitude of the pain state generated by a given stimulus is the state sought in the management of ongoing pain states. If there is no facilitated state of processing then we might precisely define such a hypoalgesia as analgesia, i.e. the animal's threshold for evocation of a response is elevated to above that which we would normally encounter in an untreated, unconditioned population of animals. As normoalgesia is a state which must be defined by exclusion of other states, it seems reasonable that analgesia would be reflected by the increased intensity required to produce a given response to an acute stimulus. Thus, in the absence of inflammation or injury, an animal exposed to a given thermal or mechanical stimulus will display escape behaviour with a certain latency or threshold. Agents which interact with a variety of specific receptors have been shown to produce a potent, dose-dependent increase, the response latency to the maximum that will be applied. If a mechanism yielding augmented/altered processing is brought into play, then an agent may yield a state of normoalgesia and thus be antihyperalgesic, or antihyperaesthetic.

CLASSES OF RECEPTORS WHICH YIELD A STATE OF NORMOALGESIA AND ANALGESIA

Based on the commentary in the preceding section, it is reasonable to presume that agents may act to produce a reduction in the response evoked by a given noxious stimulus (and thus be an analgesic) or serve to normalize the pain behaviour evoked by an otherwise nonnoxious stimulus (i.e. antihyperaesthetic) or noxious (antihyperalgesic) stimulus. Behavioural assessment of these pain states may be considered by the examination of the effects of spinally delivered agents on tests of an acute pain stimulus (as in the hot plate or paw pressure) or a hyperalgesic state (as in the phase 2 of the formalin test) or an allodynia, as defined by the action of agents on the behaviour evoked by tactile stimuli in rats having received low doses of intrathecal strychnine (strychnine test). Table 9.7 presents a summary of data to date, with the respective literature references, considering the spinal actions of a number of classes of agents which have been implicated in the modulation of spinal function. Based on these results, several points may be extracted.

Hypoalgesia and acutely evoked pain behaviour

On acute pain tests such as the hot plate, tail flick and visceral stimulation tests, intrathecal agents such as mu, delta opioid, alpha-2-adrenoceptor agonists and NPY typically produce an increase in the response latency or the threshold stimulus intensity. At the stimulus intensities typically employed, these agents can produce, in a dose-dependent, naloxone reversible fashion, an elevation in the measured nociceptive endpoint to the maximum measurable effect and this blockade is achieved in the absence of motor dysfunction. The selective antinociceptive effects of opiates have in fact been demonstrated across a wide range of species, including frog (Stevens 1991), mouse (Hylden & Wilcox 1983), rat (Yaksh & Rudy 1976), rabbit (Yaksy & Rudy 1976), cat (Yaksh 1978b; Tung & Yaksh 1982); dog (Sabbe et al 1989; Tiseo et al 1991) and nonhuman primate (Yaksh & Reddy 1981).

In contrast to the selective analgesia across a wide range of stimuli and doses, agonists such at those for adenosine, $GABA_A$ or $GABA_B$ receptors appear to produce only a modest effect at doses which do not produce motor impairment (see Table 9.7). As reviewed above, the first group of agents are thought to exert their effects upon spinal nociceptive-evoked processing by a concurrent presynaptic effect upon C-fibre transmitter release and postsynaptic effect upon WDR neurons. Thus, even though they may exert an effect in the ventral horn (based on single unit studies and the presence of the respective binding in the ventral horn), these agents, by their joint presynaptic effect upon C-afferent input and a hyperpolarization of the postsynaptic neurons, exert a powerful effect upon nocisponsive behaviour at doses which only modestly influence motor horn function (or the excitation evoked in dorsal horn neurons by large afferents which presumably do not possess significant opioid receptor binding).

In contrast, $GABA_B$ and adenosine agonists may act to inhibit the firing of WDR neurons, probably through an increase in K^+ conductance (North et al 1987). These agents, however, do not appear to exert an effect on C-fibre transmitter release (Table 9.2). Therefore, we suspect that at concentrations which induce hyperpolarization of WDR neurons, there are concurrent direct effects within the motor horn and this results in a low therapeutic ratio.

The failure of cyclooxygenase/NO synthase inhibitors to alter the acutely evoked behaviours indicates that these systems are not brought into play by such acute stimulation. Similarly, while glutamate and sP may be neurotransmitters released by the action of high-threshold afferents, the inability of NMDA, nonNMDA or NK-1 antagonists to produce a potent effect upon these acutely evoked responses, suggests at the least that they alone do mediate the transfer of information relevant to the response evoked by these acute stimuli (Table 9.7).

Hyperalgesic behavioural states

Activity-dependent hyperalgesia

On the formalin test, agents which serve to block C-fibre evoked wind-up (such as agents which serve as antagonists at the NMDA/NK-1 site) fail to have a significant action on phase 1, but significantly, reduce the magnitude of phase 2. The effect upon phase 2, while dose-dependent, displays a plateau effect. In this model of hyperalgesia, the inhibition of spinal cyclooxygenase or NO synthase will similarly produce a dose-dependent, but incomplete reduction in the magnitude of the second phase response (Malmberg & Yaksh 1992b, 1993a). These results, with the several antagonists, are consistent with the hypothesis that the acute afferent barrage generated by the formalin will evoke an initial pain state and this barrage will subsequently evoke the release of NO and prostanoids in part by an NMDA- and NK-1-sensitive mechanism (Malmberg & Yaksh 1992a, 1993a). The failure of NMDA or NK-1 antagonists to alter significantly phase 1 is consistent with the failure of these agents to act upon the acute pain tests. The observation that NK-1 and NMDA antagonists given between phase 1 and phase 2 have little effect upon phase 2 supports the argument that these receptors systems serve to initiate, but not sustain the facilitated component of the second phase (Coderre & Melzack 1991, 1992; Yamamoto & Yaksh 1991, 1992). These agents, as described, thus serve as antihyperalgesics and, to the degree that a pain state is augmented by these processes, those classes of agents will serve to normalize the facilitated pain state.

Table 9.7 Antinociceptive effects of spinally delivered receptor selective agents in the rat*

	Antinociceptive measure						
	HP[a]	TF[b]	Visceral[c]	Formalin test[d] Phase 1	Formalin test[d] Phase 2	Thermal HY[e] (nerve comp.)	Strychnine[f] (allodynia)
Agonists							
Opioid							
mu	++[1]	++[1]	++[2]	++[3]	++[3]	+[4]	(+)[5]
delta	++[1]	++[1]	++[2]	?	++[6]	+[4]	(+)[5]
kappa	(+)[1]	(+)[1]	?	0[7]	+[7]	0[4]	0[5]
Alpha adrenergic							
2_A	++[8]	++[9]	++[10]	++[7]	++[7]	+[4]	0[5]
$2_{non\text{-}A}$	++[8]	?	?	?	?	?	?
Serotonin							
$5\text{-}HT_{1A}$	+[11]	+[12]	++[14]	?	?	?	?
$5\text{-}HT_{1B}$	+[11]	+[12]	++[14]	?	?	?	?
$5\text{-}HT_2$	0/+?[11]	+[12,13]	++[14]	?	?	?	?
$5\text{-}HT_3$	+[15]	+[15]	++[14]	?	?	?	?
Adenosine							
A_1/A_2	+[16]	+[16]	+[16]	0[7]	+[7]	+[4]	++[17]
GABA							
A	0[18]	0[18]	?	?	?	++[4]	
B	+[19]	+[19]	?	?	?	++[4]	+[5]
Benzodiazepine	+[20,21]						
Cholinergic							
M_1/M_2	++[22]	++[23]	?	?	?	?	?
Dopamine							
D_2	++[24]	++[25]	?	?	?	?	?
Neuropeptide Y	++[26]	?	?	?	?	?	?
Antagonists							
Glutamate							
NMDA	0[27]	0[27]	?	(+)[3]	+[3]	++[4]	++[5]
NonNMDA	+[27]	+[27]	?	+[27,28]	+[27,28]	0[4]	+[5]
Tachykinin							
NK-1	0[29]	0[29]	?	(+)?[30]	+[30]	?	?
NK-2	+[31]	+[31]	?	?	?	?	?
Enzyme inhibitors							
Cholinesterase (muscarinic)	++[32]	+[33]	?	?	?	?	?
Cyclooxygenase	0[34,35]	0[35]	?	(+)[34]	+[34]	0[29]	?
NO synthase	0[36]	?	?	(+)[36]	+[36]	?	?
Enkephalinase (opioid)	+[37]	+[37]		?	?	?	?

*The confidence with which any receptor is affiliated with the specific changes in pain behaviour depends upon the use of receptor preferring agonists and antagonists. In the case of agents such as NPY, specific antagonists do not at present exist. For the 5-HT antagonists, there is controversy as to the selectivity of the agonists/antagonists and specific receptor designations must be considered as tentative. In the case of agents such as cholinesterase and enkephalinase inhibitors, the use of selective antagonists are used to define the site acted upon by the augmented levels of endogenous transmitter produced by the enzyme inhibitors.

Abbreviations: [a]HP 52.5°C hot plate; [b]TF = tail flick; [c]Distention of the bowel with balloon, examination of the behavioural or blood pressure response; [d]Injection of dilute formalin into one hindpaw; assessment of licking/flinching during the first phase 5–10 min or second phase 10–60 min after formalin; [e]Loose or partial compression of the sciatic nerve and examination of the thermal response latency; [f]Intrathecal injection of the glycine antagonist strychnine evoked tactile evoked agitation (allodynia) or increase in blood pressure.

References: [1]Schmauss & Yaksh 1984; [2]Ness & Gebhart 1988; [3]Yamamoto & Yaksh 1992; [4]Yamamoto & Yaksh 1991; [5]Yaksh 1989; [6]Murray & Cowan 1991; [7]Malmberg & Yaksh 1993b; [8]Takano & Yaksh 1992; [9]Reddy et al 1980; [10]Danzebrink & Gebhart 1990; [11]Ware & Yaksh, unpublished observations; [12]Eide & Hole 1991; [13]Solomon & Gebhart 1988; [14]Danzebrink & Gebhart 1991; [15]Glaum et al 1990; [16]Sosnowski et al 1989; [17]Sosnowski & Yaksh 1989; [18]Hammond & Drower 1984; [19]Aran & Hammond 1991; [20]Yanez et al 1990; [21]Edwards et al 1990; [22]Yaksh et al 1985; [23]Gillberg et al 1989; [24]Jensen & Yaksh 1984b; [25]Liu et al 1992; [26]Hua et al 1991; [27]Näsström et al 1992; [28]Malmberg & Yaksh, unpublished observations; [29]Yamamoto & Yaksh, unpublished observations; [30]Yamamoto & Yaksh 1991; [31]Fleetwood-Walker et al 1990; [32]Naguib & Yaksh, unpublished observations; [33]Gordh et al 1989; [34]Malmberg & Yaksh 1992b; [35]Yaksh 1982; [36]Malmberg & Yaksh 1993a; [37]Oshita & Yaksh 1990.

In contrast, agents such as the opioids on the formalin test serve as analgesics by blocking the afferent input responsible for evoking behaviour (as in phase 1 of the formalin test and the acute response on the hot-plate or tail-flick test). In addition, it is possible that because such agents block the afferent input, presumably by diminishing the release of the appropriate neurotransmitters, such agents might in addition block the development of the hyperalgesic state. Supporting evidence for this arises from studies in which it has been shown that pretreatment with intrathecal morphine will block phase 1. The injection of naloxone between phase 1 and phase 2 in an animal pretreated with morphine will continue to display a highly significant reduction in the phase 2 response.

This presumably reflects the ability of the mu agonists to block the release of materials which lead to the hyperalgesic state manifested during the phase 2 response. Importantly, it is conceivable that agents which act postsynaptic to the primary afferent might suppress the appearance of behaviour, i.e. agents may be analgesic, but might *not* be able to correspondingly block the initiation of the hyperalgesic state. Thus rats which are anaesthetized with a volatile anaesthetic during phase 1 and allowed to awaken during phase 2, will continue to show a significant phase 2 response (Abram & Yaksh 1993). Failure of a general anaesthetic to block the evolution of the hyperalgesic state in the formalin test is consistent with the fact that most studies examining the electrophysiology of wind-up or the release of neurotransmitters from the spinal cord have been carried out under a general anaesthetic regimen (see Fraser et al 1992 and Go & Yaksh 1987, respectively).

Nerve injury evoked hyperalgesia

With regard to the thermal hyperalgesia induced by peripheral nerve compression (Bennett & Xie 1988), the intrathecal injection of mu and alpha-2 agonists has been shown to produce a dose-dependent elevation in the thermal-evoked withdrawal response of both the normal paw and the hind paw rendered hyperalgesic with a surgical compression of the ipsilateral sciatic nerve (Table 9.7). Importantly, the dose-response curve for the hyperalgesic paw is displaced in a parallel fashion to the right, as compared to that curve obtained with the normal paw, with the maximum latency allowed being achieved with both normal and hyperalgesic paws with these agents. In contrast, intrathecal agents such as the NMDA antagonists have no effect upon the normal paw latency, but will result in a dose-dependent increase in the latency of the hyperalgesic paw to normal (nonhyperalgesic) response latencies. In this sense, as with those agents which block in a limited, but dose-dependent fashion, phase 2 of the formalin test, such agents might also be classified as being antihyperalgesic.

Comparability of hyperalgesic pain states

While there are certain parallels between the systems which underlie the mechanisms of the hyperalgesia observed in the formalin test and that in nerve injury, consideration of Table 9.7 emphasizes that the pharmacology of these two measured end-points are not the same. Thus, for the nerve injury evoked hyperalgesia, NK-1 antagonists and cyclooxygenase inhibitors are not active. Moreover, it is not known if the spinal substrates through which the NMDA antagonists act to alter the two hyperalgesic states are the same. Thus heterogeneous spinal mechanisms may be involved in the different pain states. Still, at present it is not clear that all agents which block the hyperalgesic component observed following nerve lesion will block the facilitated component of phase 2 of the formalin test.

Hyperaesthetic pain states

In the strychnine model of tactile allodynia, intrathecal opiates and alpha-2 agonists appear to be only modestly active and not significantly different from baclofen. In contrast, NMDA antagonists are extremely effective in diminishing this allodynic state. While speculative, it has been suggested that this differentiation reflects upon the fact that the allodynia is mediated by low-threshold mechanoreceptors (Yaksh 1989). Based on the binding studies and on the failure of the analgesic agents which C-fibres release to be particularly effective, it is believed that C-fibre input lacks a role in this pain state. Importantly, in deafferentation syndromes, dorsal horn neurons, some of which are likely to represent projection neurons which had been originally activated by high-threshold input, become spontaneous active. These cells under normal circumstances have a low spontaneous activity and the nociceptive evoked activity is readily suppressed by morphine. The increased spontaneous activity occurring in the deafferentiated states is considerably less sensitive to the actions of morphine, supporting the conclusion that the inhibition of the firing of these cells occurs normally by an effect upon afferent input and upon an effect postsynaptic to the primary afferent (Lombard & Besson 1989). The potent actions of the NMDA-receptor antagonists clearly indicate an important intermediate role for generating this exaggerated state. These observations, excluding the role of C-fibres in the facilitated state, are further emphasized by the failure of the NK-1 antagonists to alter the strychnine evoked allodynia. The particular activity of spinal adenosine receptor agonists is unexpected, but has been said to reflect the reported ability of adenosine to block the release of glutamate (Sosnowski & Yaksh 1989).

ANALGESIC ACTIONS OF CENTRALLY DELIVERED DRUGS IN PRIMATES AND HUMANS

In the preceding sections, it has been shown that a variety of spinal manipulations can serve to alter pain behaviour. As a majority of these studies have been carried out in rodents, it is important to consider to what degree the pharmacology as outlined in rodent models reflects upon more complex pain models, notably those in nonhuman and human primates.

Spinally delivered agents

Systematic studies in the primate have emphasized that

several classes of spinally administered agents can produce a powerful dose-dependent analgesia as measured on a number of endpoints including the operand controlled shock titration and the thermal escape threshold evoked by tail dip (Yaksh 1983; Yaksh & Rathbun unpublished observations). The microinjection of opiates into the medullary dorsal horn of the trigeminal nucleus is similarly able to increase the thermal escape threshold in the unanaesthetized primate (Oliveras et al 1986a, 1986b).

The pharmacology of these effects has been systematically examined on the shock titration endpoints, as well as thermal escape paradigms. In these models, as outlined in Table 9.8, the ordering of activity has been shown to be mu > delta ≫ kappa (i.e. DAGO, morphine, sufentanil > DPDPE ≫U-50488 = 0) (Table 9.8). The effects of DAGO and morphine are reversed by naloxone, but not the delta preferring antagonists naltrindole. In contrast, the effects of DPDPE are reversed by both naloxone and naltrindole (Yaksh unpublished observations). Such observations emphasize a spinal mu and delta opioid receptor and are consistent with the absence of cross tolerance between morphine and the delta preferring agent DADL in animals made tolerant to morphine (Yaksh 1983).

In humans, the delivery of opioids by the intrathecal or epidural route produces a powerful analgesia in a variety of acute postoperative (Abboud 1988; Sandler 1990; Tobias et al 1990; Shafer & Donnelly 1991) and chronic pain states (Payne 1987; Iacono et al 1988; Arner et al 1988). While there are few systematic studies on the pharmacology of the spinally administered opioids, considerable clinical experience (Table 9.8) has indicated involvement of a mu opioid site with regard to relative potency (lofentanil > sufentanil > morphine > meperidine). With regard to other receptors, limited experience has shown that the delta preferring agonist DADL is efficacious following spinal delivery (Moulin et al 1985), suggesting that a delta receptor may also be present. Butorphanol is reputed to have kappa-preferring activity and it has been shown to have a mild action following epidural delivery. With regard to antagonism it has been shown that relatively low doses of naloxone (10 µg/kg/h) can produce an approximate 50% reduction in the antinociceptive effects of epidural morphine. (Rawal et al 1986). These data thus jointly offer support for the presence of a mu opioid site and the data are suggestive of the presence of a delta and kappa opioid site. Further work is clearly required to further define the pharmacology of the human spinal cord.

Supraspinal actions of opiate action in primates and humans

Systematic microinjection studies in the primates examining their effect upon the supraspinally organized

Table 9.8 Effects of selected spinal agents on the pain behaviour in nonhuman and human primates

Drug class	Nonhuman primates Shock titration[a,1] (Intrathecal JMAD, mg)[d]		Tail dip escape latency[b,2] (Intrathecal JMAD, mg)[d]		Humans Postoperative/cancer pain[c] (Epidural dose, mg)	
Opiates						
mu	Meperidine	(5.0)[d]			Meperidine	(50–100)[3]
	Methadone	(1)			Methadone	(5–9)[4]
	Morphine	(1)	Morphine	(1)	Morphine	(4)[5]
	Alfentanil	(0.3)			Alfentanil	(0.3)[6]
	β-endorphin	(0.001)			β-endorphin	(3)[7]
	DAGO	(0.05)	DAGO	(0.1)		
	Sufentanil	(0.05)	Sufentanil	(0.1)	Sufentanil	(0.05)[8]
					Buprenorphine	(0.18)[9]
	Lofentanil	(0.002)			Lofentanil	(0.003–0.10)[10]
delta	DADL	(0.25)	DADL	(0.3)	DADL	(1–2)[11,e]
	DPDPE	(12)	DPDPE	(8)		
kappa	U50488	(>10)	U50488	(>10)		
	Butorphanol	(>10)			Butorphanol	(2–4)[12]
Alpha$_2$-adrenergic						
	ST-91	(4)	ST-91	(2)		
	Clonidine	(2)			Clonidine	(0.4–0.8)[13]
			Dexmedtomidine	(0.03)		

Abbreviations: [a]Operant shock titration: 25 step, 3 s discrete trial, foot shock (Yaksh 1983); [b]Tail dip = escape latency evoked by immersion of tail in 48°C water. Baseline response latency 3.4 ± 0.6 s in absence of drug; cut off time in absence of response equals 12 s. [c]Human pain states are those found in either postoperative pain states or in cancer pain patients. Does reflects that which when given spinally (I: intrathecally/E: epidurally) produces an 'adequate' analgesic effect. [d]JMAD = just maximally analgesic doses; dose in mg which produces a just maximal increase in response latency or a just maximal increase in the shock titration threshold. [e]Intrathecal delivery, morphine-treated cancer patients.

References: [1]Yaksh & Reddy 1981; Yaksh 1983; Yaksh et al 1982b; Yaksh & Harty, unpublished observations; [2]Yaksh, unpublished observations; [3]Perriss et al 1990; [4]Martin et al 1990; [5]Pybus & Torda 1982; Nordberg 1984; [6]Chauvin et al 1985; [7]Oyama et al 1982; [8]Whiting et al 1988; Graf et al 1991; Dottrens et al 1992; [9]Simpson et al 1988; [10]Albert van Steenberge, personal communication; [11]Moulin 1985; [12]Palacios et al 1991; Camann et al 1992; [13]Eisenach et al 1989a, 1989b; Huntoon et al 1992.

operant shock titration response have revealed a distribution of sites which correspond closely with those systems that have been reported in the rodent. Active sites were distributed in at least two discriminative loci: the first is found to correspond to the periventricular/PAG axis of the mesencephalon; the second distribution is in sites distributed more caudally in the lower brainstem, corresponding to the medial and lateral aspects of the medulla (Pert & Yaksh 1974, 1975; Yaksh et al 1988a). Notably absent in activity was the thalamus, though a distribution of sites lying along the dorsal aspect of the PAG and ventral aspect of the thalamus was described. These sites, notably those within the medial brainstem cores along the mesencephalic central grey correspond closely with those reported in all other species examined. The lateral distribution of sites would appear to correspond to those identified in the lateral aspects of the medullary reticular formation in the rat. With regard to pharmacology, there are unfortunately little comparative data. All that can be said in the primate is that the effects were readily antagonized by naloxone and were stereospecific (Pert & Yaksh 1974).

In humans, microinjection studies have not been carried out. However, intracerebroventricular injection of opioids, such as morphine and β-endorphin, have been shown to produce a powerful analgesic effect in patients suffering from pain secondary to head and neck cancer (Lazorthes 1988; Lee et al 1990; Sandouk et al 1991; Schultheiss et al 1992). Given the potent effects of morphine in the regions immediately surrounding the PAG in all models including primates, it seems a reasonable hypothesis that a similar site of action explains the potent analgesia resulting from the actions of opiates delivered intracranially in man.

With regard to the primate literature, while the parallels with the extensive preclinical literature in rodents are important, it should be stressed that the mechanisms of these effects in humans can only be hypothesized. Thus, for example, the prominent role of bulbospinal pathways defined in the rodent can be indirectly inferred on the basis of the action of adrenoceptor agonists in both human and nonhuman primates. On the other hand, the important observation that supraspinal morphine blocks spinal reflexes has not been reported in either primate model.

PHARMACOLOGY OF AFFECTIVE COMPONENTS OF PAIN BEHAVIOUR

THE INFLUENCE OF AFFECTIVE VARIABLES IN PAIN BEHAVIOUR

In the preceding sections, principal emphasis has been placed upon systems which can serve to alter the encoding of high-intensity afferent input in a fashion which is behaviourally relevant. As noted, the recognition of the states of hyperalgesia, hyperaesthesia and allodynia, implies that there is not a perfect correlation between the nature of the stimulus and the measured response. Clearly, changes in the processing of the afferent information leading to alterations in the content of the ascending message is clearly one important variable which can define those states of altered responsiveness. Certainly the widespread impressions gained from the actions of spinal agents emphasize the ability to alter many pain states by changing the content of the afferent processing.

There is equally a wide recognition that situational and environmental variables which do not apparently impact upon the sensory message generated by a high-intensity stimulus can induce changes in changes response evoked by that stimulus. In humans, the affective–motivational component of the pain state is widely appreciated (Melzack & Casey 1968; Melzack & Wall, 1973; see Chs 17 and 18 this volume). In humans, perceptual components such as exaggerated depression (Turner & Romano 1984; Romano & Turner 1985; Kremer et al 1983) or anxiety (Beecher 1969; Katon 1984) can alter the response to a given noxious stimulus. Positive mood states diminish the reported severity of a pain condition. Conversely, negative mood factors such as depression or aversion may augment the reported severity of the state (Chapman 1985) and correlate with lower indices of satisfaction and higher indices of the pain state Chapman (1985; Taenzer et al 1986). Mechanistically, several classes of agents are well known to exert a potent effect upon mood states and accordingly have a powerful effect upon pain behaviour in man.

While great strides have been made in defining the mechanisms which alter afferent processing, notably when we have focused upon spinal processing, there is less appreciation of the mechanism whereby supraspinal systems impact upon the affective component. This is in part due to the fact that in nonverbal animals we are committed to the assessment of the pain behaviour generated by characteristic stimuli. It is probable, for example, that stressors that may cause a change in the affective state of the organism, represented definitionally as fear or anxiety, may enhance the response of the animal to a given stimulus by altering the organized response by the animal to the stimulus. Alternately these stressors may result in the operation of the myriad of modulatory systems that are found within the CNS to directly alter the afferent input. A second problem that faces the investigator is the issue of defining the component of the drug's action on motivational components of behaviour that are relevant to its organization of the organism's response to the strong stimulus. Thus, drugs may be reinforcing, but is their reinforcing component relevant to their affect-altering properties impacting on pain behaviour? Because of the difficulty in assessing the affective component in an animal model, the role of central drug-induced changes in affective state on pain behaviour remains largely unspecified. As noted prevously, for example, the organizational role of central systems such as the PAG is really unknown.

Clearly opiates may exert a local effect in this region increasing hot plate and response latencies and thermal and shock titration escape thresholds, and the local injection of glutamate may evoke pain behaviour, but there is equally persuasive thinking that emphasizes their influence on affect. It may be quite significant that overlap between pathways traditionally considered to be related to changes in affective behaviour are being shown to exert correlated effects upon the organized response of the animal to an ongoing painful stimulus (Bandler et al 1985, 1991; Franklin 1989).

CLASSES OF MOOD ALTERING DRUGS AND THEIR EFFECTS UPON PAIN STATES

A variety of agents may be considered as a function of their respective pharmacology. In the following sections, several of these major classes will be briefly considered.

Opioids

While the current emphasis upon the mechanisms of opioid action reflects upon their actions in activating modulatory substrates, the perceptual and anxiolytic effects of the agents after systemic administration are widely appreciated as important components of their clinical action (Lasagna et al 1955; Kaiko et al 1981).

Considerable attention has been focused upon the rewarding effects of opioids. Microinjection studies have demonstrated the particular importance of the ventral tegmental area and the nucleus accumbens in the rewarding properties of these agents (see Wise 1989).

Antidepressants

The potential significance of even modest alterations in mood on pain states is readily borne out by the utility of antidepressants (such as tricyclic antidepressants). While some of these agents may exert their effect directly upon the processing of sensory information (for example, by interactions with bulbospinal noradrenergic pathways, see above), such agents can exert their effect at doses which alone do not produce a significant relief of reported pain. Thus, while the precise role of such drug-induced alterations in mood and aspects of changes in perceptual bias remains to be adequately described, the current evidence clearly supports a contributory role of such changes in ameliorating the reported impact of the pain state (Forrest et al 1977; Kaiko et al 1987; Ward et al 1984, 1985; Bonica et al 1990).

Psychomotor stimulants (such as amphetamine or caffeine)

A variety of psychomotor stimulants have been shown to augment the analgesic effects of opioids in man (Forrest et al 1977; Kaiko et al 1987; Bonica et al 1990). Interestingly, caffeine represents a widely used adjuvant in man and has been shown to modestly, but significantly, facilitate the analgesic effects of a variety of classes of agents including opiates and nonsteroidal antiinflammatory agents (Sawynok & Yaksh 1993). In humans caffeine resembles the effects seen after other psychomotor stimulants, including amphetamine and fenfluramine (Chait et al 1987; Chait & Johanson 1988), at low doses inducing mildly positive mood states and stimulant-like effects (Chait & Johanson 1988; Griffiths & Woodson 1988a, 1988b, 1988c). Given the positive impact of caffeine on mood, it is a reasonable speculation that caffeine may contribute to analgesia (as opposed to an antinociceptive) by virtue of these positive changes in the affective state. The importance of such psychological variables to the behavioural syndrome observed in the presence of an ongoing pain state (as opposed to a reflex function) remains, however, to be systematically examined in a well-defined animal model. Mechanistically, a variety of studies have implicated the mesolimbic dopamine system in psychomotor stimulation by centrally active agents (Swerdlow et al 1986). Depletion of brain catecholamines reduces stimulation of motor activity by caffeine (Finn et al 1990). Lesions to the nucleus accumbens inhibit motor stimulation by amphetamine, cocaine and methylphenidate (Kelly & Iversen 1976). Such lesions, however, do not alter the effect of caffeine (Joyce & Koob 1981). Thus, while catecholamine systems are implicated in the stimulant action of caffeine, the neurotransmitters and specific pathways involved remain to be determined (Sawynok & Yaksh 1993).

CONCLUDING COMMENTS

As noted above, considerable advances have been made over the past 10 years in our appreciation of the pharmacology of the systems which process nociceptive information. The systematic characterization of the pharmacology of the CNS systems that are involved in regulating the organism's response to a strong stimulus has provided direct insight into the complexity of the systems that are involved in controlling the throughput of such information. It is possible now to at least begin to define states of hyperalgesia, hyperaesthesia and allodynia in terms of distinct receptor substrates. The appreciation that in the presence of an acute afferent stimulus certain systems are acutely activated has been an important observation. However, the current appreciation that repetitive input can in fact generate profound changes in afferent processing has led to alterations in the way we think of the postinjury pain state and this in turn provides suggestions as to the merits of modulating the afferent input evoked by high-threshold stimuli, even when the patient is in a state of anaesthesia induced by a volatile anaesthetic. The differential pharmacology which reflects upon these several pain states emphasizes that the facilitated state of processing is a phenomenon evoked by, but distinct from, the pain state generated by the acute stimulus. The appreciation that florid changes in the response to light touch are induced by the mere blockade of a single class of inhibitory amino acids (glycine or GABA) not only suggests that these may be targets for degenerative processes that occur following nerve injuries leading to allodynic states, but also from a theoretical perspective that light touch itself possesses a nonnoxious characteristic, only because of a very effective ongoing inhibition.

The final section of this review, though brief, probably reflects the next important advances in our understanding of the processing of nociceptive information. Supraspinal components that reflect upon the affective state of the animal are clearly of theoretical and practical relevance. The interpretation of the powerful effect of opiates on perceptual processes is in part complicated because of the complicated and efficacious mechanisms by which this family of agents also control afferent processing. Perhaps more insight into the future of these classes of agents is provided by the simple drug caffeine which, while it seems to have little effect upon pain processing per se, appears to exert its effects though subtle changes in affect. One would anticipate that as our ability to ask increasingly subtle questions of the animal models, the pharmacology and mechanisms of the affective components of pain processing will acquire an importance equal to that which we place on the systems that modulate the afferent message.

Lastly, these advances in our understanding of the pharmacology of systems which process normally nonnoxious and noxious information are ultimately important as they provide the direct venue by which the various pain conditions may be differentially diagnosed. Selective modulation of various components of afferent processing by the use of specific agents targeted at the relevant receptor and anatomical systems promises to provide the essential tools for the management of the human pain state.

REFERENCES

Aanonsen L M, Wilcox G L 1987 Nociceptive action of excitatory amino acids in the mouse: effects of spinally administered opioids, phencyclidine and sigma agonists. Journal of Pharmacology and Experimental Therapeutics 243: 9–19

Abboud T K 1988 Epidural and intrathecal administration of opioids in obstetrics. Acute Care 12 (suppl 1): 17–21

Abram S, Yaksh T L 1993 Morphine, but not inhalation anesthesia, blocks post injury facilitation: The role of preemptive suppression of afferent transmission. Anesthesiology (in press)

Aimi Y, Fujimura M, Vincent S R, Kimura H 1991 Localization of NADPH-diaphorase-containing neurons in sensory ganglia of the rat. Journal of Comparative Neurology 306: 382–392

Aimone L D, Gebhart G F 1986 Stimulation produced spinal inhibition from the brainstem in the rat is mediated by an excitatory amino acid transmitter in the medial medulla. Journal of Neuroscience 6: 1803–1813

Aimone L D, Gebhart G F 1988 Serotonin and/or an excitatory amino acid in the medial medulla mediates stimulation-produced antinociception from the lateral hypothalamus in the rat. Brain Research 450: 170–180

Akaike A, Shibata T, Satoh M, Takagi H 1978 Analgesia induced by microinjection of morphine into and electrical stimulation of the nucleus reticulartis gigantocellularis of rat medulla oblongata. Neuropharmacology 17: 775–778

Alhaider A A, Lei S Z, Wilcox G L 1991 Spinal 5-HT3 receptor-mediated antinociception: possible release of GABA. Journal of Neuroscience 11: 1881–1888

Al-Rodhan N, Chipkin R, Yaksh T L 1990 The antinociceptive effects of SCH-32615, a neutral endopeptidase (enkephalinase) inhibitor, microinjected into the periaqueductal, ventral medulla and amygdala. Brain Research 520: 123–130

Amaral D G, Sinnamon H M 1977 The locus coereuleus: neurobiology of a central noradrenergic nucleus. Progress in Neurobiology 9: 147–196

Anden N-E, Jukes G M, Lundberg A, Vyklicky L 1966 The effects of L-DOPA on the spinal cord. Acta Physiologica Scandinavica 67: 373–386

Anderson C R 1992 NADPH diaphorase-positive neurons in the rat spinal cord include a subpopulation of autonomic preganglionic neurons. Neuroscience Letters 139: 280–284

Aran S, Hammond D L 1991 Antagonism of Baclofen-induced antinociception by intrathecal administration of phaclofen or 2-hydroxy-saclofen, but not delta-aminovaleric acid in the rat. Journal of Pharmacology and Experimental Therapeutics 257: 360–368

Ardid D, Guilbaud G 1992 Antinociceptive effects of acute and 'chronic' injections of tricyclic antidepressant drugs in a new model of mononeuropathy in rats. Pain 49: 279–287

Ardid D, Eschalier A, Lavarenne J 1991 Evidence for a central but not a peripheral analgesic effect of clomipramine in rats. Pain 45: 95–100

Arena, J M 1970 Poisoning: toxicology, symptoms, treatments, 4th edn. C C Thomas., Springfield, Illinois

Arner S, Rawal N, Gustafsson L L 1988 Clinical experience of long-term treatment with epidural and intrathecal opioids – a nationwide survey. Acta Anaesthesiologica Scandinavica 32: 253–259

Atweh S F, Murrin L C, Kuhar M J 1978 Presynaptic localization of opiate receptors in the vagal and accessory optic system: an autoradiographic study. Neuropharmacology 17: 65–71

Azami J, Llewelyn M B, Roberts M H T 1982 The contribution of nucleus reticularis gigantocellularis and nucleus raphe magnus to the analgesia produced by systematically administered morphine investigated with the microinjection technique. Pain 12: 229–246

Baber N S, Dourish C T, Hill D R 1989 The role of CCK caerulein, and CCK antagonists in nociception. Pain 39: 307–328

Bach F W, Yaksh T L 1992 Release of B-endorphin-IR from brain is regulated by a hypothalamic NMDA receptor. Anesthesiology (suppl) 77: A733

Bandler R, McCulloch T, McDougall A, Prineas S, Dampney R 1985 Midbrain neural mechanisms mediating emotional behaviour. International Journal of Neurology 19: 40–58

Bandler R, Carrive P, Zhang S P 1991 Integration of somatic and autonomic reactions within the midbrain periaqueductal grey, viscerotopic, somatotopic and functional organization. Progress in Brain Research 87: 269–305

Barber R P, Vaughn J E, Saito K, McLaughlin B J, Roberts E 1978 GABAergic terminals are presynaptic to primary afferent terminals in the substantia gelatinosa of the rat spinal cord. Brain Research 141: 35–55

Barke K E, Hough L B 1992 Morphine-induced increases of extracellular histamine levels in the periaqueductal grey in vivo: a microdialysis study. Brain Research 572: 146–153

Barnes C D, Fung S J, Adams W L 1979 Inhibitory effects of substantia nigra on impulse transmission from nociceptors. Pain 6: 207–215

Basbaum A I 1988 Distribution of glycine receptor immunoreactivity in the spinal cord of the rat: Cystochemical evidence for a differential glycinergic control, of Lamina I and Lamina V neurons. Journal of Comparative Neurology 278: 330–336

Battaglia G, Rustioni A 1988 Coexistence of glutamate and substance P in dorsal root ganglion neurons of the rat and monkey. Journal of Comparative Neurology 277: 302–312

Battaglia G, Rustioni A 1992 Substance P innervation of the rat and cat thalamus. II Cells of origin in the spinal cord. Journal of Comparative Neurology 315: 473–486

Battaglia G, Spreafico R, Rustioni A 1992 Substance P innervation of the rat and cat thalamus. I. Distribution and relation to ascending spinal pathways. Journal of Comparative Neurology 315: 457–472

Baumeister A A 1991 The effects of bilateral intranigral microinjection of selective opioid agonists on behavioural responses to noxious thermal stimuli. Brain Research 557: 136–145

Baumeister A A, Hawkins M F, Anticich T G et al 1987 Bilateral intranigral microinjection of morphine and opioid peptides produces antinociception in rats. Brain Research 411: 183–186

Baumeister A A, Nagy M, Hebert G, Hawkins M F, Vaughn A, Chatellier M O 1990 Further studies of the effects of intranigral morphine on behavioural responses to noxious stimuli. Brain Research 525: 115–125

Beecher H K 1969 Anxiety and pain. Journal of the American Medical Association 209: 1080–1083

Behbehani M M, Park M R, Clement M E 1988 Interactions between the lateral hypothalamus and the periaqueductal gray. Journal of Neuroscience 8: 2780–2787

Behbehani M M, Jiang M R, Chandler S D, Ennis M 1990 The effect of GABA and its antagonists on midbrain periaqueductal gray neurons in the rat. Pain 40: 195–204

Bennett G J, Mayer D J 1979 Inhibition of spinal cord interneurons by narcotic microinjection and focal electrical stimulation in the periaqueductal gray matter. Brain Research 172: 243–257

Bennett G J, Xie Y K 1988 A peripheral mononeuropathy in rat that produces disorders of pain sensation like those seen in man. Pain 33: 87–107

Bodnar R J 1986 Neuropharmacological and neuroendocrine substrates of stress-induced analgesia. Annals of the New York Academy of Sciences 467: 345–360

Bodnar R J 1991 Effects of opioid peptides on peripheral stimulation and "stress"-induced analgesia in animals. Critical Reviews in Neurobiology 6: 39–49

Bodnar R J, Williams C L, Lee S J, Pasternak G W 1988 Role of mu 1-opiate receptors in supraspinal opiate analgesia: a microinjection study. Brain Research 447: 25–34

Bodnar R, Paul D, Pasternak G W 1991 Synergistic analgesic interactions between the periaqueductal gray and the locus coeruleus. Brain Research 558: 224–230

Boive J 1971 The termination of the spinothalamic tract in the cat. An experimental study with silver impregnation methods. Experimental Brain Research 12: 331–353

Bonica J J, Ventafridda V, Twycross R G 1990 Cancer pain. In: Bonica J J (ed) The management of pain. Lea & Febiger, Philadelphia, p 400–460

Bowery N G, Hudson A L, Price G W 1987 $GABA_A$ + $GABA_B$ receptor site distribution in the cat central nervous system. Neuroscience 20: 365–383

Bowsher D 1976 Role of the reticular formation in response to noxious stimuli. Pain 2: 361–378

Braas K S, Newby A L, Wilson V S, Snyder S H 1986 Adenosine containing neurons in the brain localized by immunocytochemistry. Journal of Neuroscience 6: 1952–1961

Camann W R, Loferski B L, Fanciullo G J, Stone M L, Datta S 1992 Does epidural administration of butorphanol offer any clinical advantage over the intravenous route? A double-blind, placebo-controlled trial. Anesthesiology 76: 216–220

Camarata P J, Yaksh T L 1985 Characterization of the spinal adrenergic receptors mediating the spinal effects produced by the microinjection of morphine into the periaqueductal gray. Brain Research 336: 133–142

Carlton S M, Hayes E S 1990 Light microscopic and ultrastructural analysis of GABA immunoreactive profiles in the monkey spinal cord. Journal of Comparative Neurology 300: 162–182

Carlton S M, Honda C N, Willcockson W S et al 1991 Descending adrenergic input to the primate spinal cord and its possible role in modulation of spinothalamic cells. Brain Research 543: 77–90

Carlton S M, Westlund K N, Zhang D, Willis W D 1992 GABA-immunoreactive terminals synapse on primate spinothalamic tract cells. Journal of Comparative Neurology 322: 528–537

Casey K L 1971 Escape elicited by bulbospinal stimulation in the cat. International Journal of Neuroscience 2: 29–34

Cesselin F, Oliveras J L, Bourgoin S et al 1982 Increased levels of met-enkephalin-like material in the CSF of anaesthetized cats after tooth pulp stimulation. Brain Research 237: 325

Cesselin F, Bourgoin S, Artaud F, Hamon M 1984 Basic and regulatory mechanisms of in vitro release of met-enkephalin from the dorsal zone of the rat spinal cord. Journal of Neurochemistry 43: 763

Chait L D, Johanson C E 1988 Discriminative stimulus effects of caffeine and benzphetamine in amphetamine-trained volunteers. Psychopharmacology 96: 302–308

Chait L D, Uhlenhuth E H, Johanson C E 1987 Reinforcing and subjective effects of several anorectics in normal human volunteers. Journal of Pharmacology and Experimental Therapeutics 242: 777–783

Chapman C R 1985 Psychological factors in postoperative pain and their treatment. In: Smith G, Covino B G (eds) Acute pain. Butterworths, London

Chauvin M, Salbaing J, Perrin D, Levron J C, Viars P 1985 Clinical assessment and plasma pharmacokinetics associated with intramuscular or extradural alfentanil. British Journal of Anaesthesia 57: 886–891

Chung J M, Lee K H, Surmeier D J, Sorkin L S, Kim J, Willis W D 1986 Response characteristics of neurons in the ventral posterior lateral nucleus of the monkey thalamus. Journal of Neurophysiology 56: 370–390

Clarke S L, Edeson R O, Ryall, R W 1983 The relative significance of spinal supraspinal actions in the antinociceptive effect of morphine in the dorsal horn: an evaluation of the microinjection technique. British Journal of Pharmacology 79: 807–818

Coderre T J, Melzack R 1991 Central neural mediators of secondary hyperalgesia following heat injury in rats: neuropeptides and excitatory amino acids. Neuroscience Letters 131: 71–74

Coderre T J, Melzack R 1992 The contribution of excitatory amino acids to central sensitization and persistent nociception after formalin-induced tissue injury. Journal of Neuroscience 12: 3665–3670

Coderre T J, Gonzales R, Goldyne M E, West M E, Levine J D 1990 Noxious stimulus-induced increase in spinal prostaglandin E2 is noradrenergic terminal-dependent. Neuroscience Letters 115: 253–258

Coquoz D, Porchet H C, Dayer P 1991 Central analgesic effects of antidepressant drugs with various mechanisms of action: desipramine, fluvoxamine and moclobemide. Schweizerische Medizinische Wochenschrift. Journal Suisse de Medecine 121: 1843–1845

Cridland R A, Henry J L 1986 Comparison of the effects of substance P, neurokinin A, physalaemin and eledoisin in facilitating a nociceptive reflex in the rat. Brain Research 381: 93–99

Criswell H D 1976 Analgesia and hypereactivity following morphine microinjections into mouse brain. Pharmacology, Biochemistry and Behavior 4: 23–26

Danzebrink R M, Gebhart G F 1990 Antinociceptive effects of intrathecal adrenoceptor agonists in a rat model of visceral nociception. Journal of Pharmacology and Experimental Therapeutics 253: 698–705

Danzebrink R M, Gebhart G F 1991 Evidence that spinal 5-HT_1, 5-HT_2 and 5-HT_3 receptor subtypes modulate responses to noxious colorectal distention in the rat. Brain Research 538: 64–75

Daval G, Verge D, Basbaum A I, Bouroin S, Hamon M 1987 Autoradiographic evidence of serotonin-1 binding sites on primary afferent fibres in dorsal horn of the rat spinal cord. Neuroscience Letters 83: 71–81

Davies J, Watkins J C 1983 Role of excitatory amino acids receptors in mono- and polysynaptic excitation in the cat spinal cord. Experimental Brain Research 49: 280–290

De Biasi S, Rustioni A 1988 Glutamate and substance P coexist in primary afferent terminals in the superficial laminae of spinal cord. Proceedings of the National Academy of Sciences USA 85: 7820–7824

De Koninck Y, Henry J L 1989 Bombesin, neuromedin B and neuromedin C selectively depress superficial dorsal horn neurones in the cat spinal cord. Brain Research 498: 105–117

De Koninck Y, Henry J L 1991 Substance P-mediated slow excitatory postsynaptic potential elicited in dorsal horn neurons in vivo by noxious stimulation. Proceedings of the National Academy of Sciences USA 88: 11344–11348

Denny-Brown D, Kirk E J, Yanagisawa N 1973 The tract of Lissauer in relation to sensory transmission in the dorsal horn of spinal cord in the Macaque monkey. Journal of Comparative Neurology 151: 175–200

Dickenson A H, Le Bars D 1987 Supraspinal morphine and descending inhibitions acting on the dorsal horn of the rat. Journal of Physiology 384: 81–107

Dickenson A H, Sullivan A F 1990 Differential effects of excitatory amino acid antagonists on dorsal horn nociceptive neurons in the rat. Brain Research 506: 31–39

Dickenson A H, Oliveras J-L, Besson J-M 1979 Role of the nucleus raphe magnus in opiate analgesia as studied by the microinjection technique in the rat. Brain Research 170: 95–111

Dickenson A H, Brewer C M, Hayes N A 1985 Effects of topical baclofen on C fibre-evoked neuronal activity in the rat dorsal horn. Neuroscience 14: 557–562

Dickenson A H, Sullivan A F, Roques B P 1988 Evidence that endogenous enkephalins and a delta opioid receptor agonist have a common site of action in spinal antinociception. European Journal of Pharmacology 148: 437–439

Dottrens M, Rifat K, Morel D R 1992 Comparison of extradural administration of sufentanil, morphine and sufentanil–morphine combination after caesarean section. British Journal of Anaesthesia 69: 9–12

Drower E J, Hammond D L 1988 GABAergic modulation of nociceptive threshold: effects of THIP and bicuculline microinjected in the ventral medulla of the rat. Brain Research 450: 316–324

Drower E J, Stapelfeld A, Rafferty M F, de Costa B R, Rice K C, Hammond D L 1991 Selective antagonism by naltrindole of the antinociceptive effects of the delta opioid agonist cyclic [D-penicillamine2-D-penicillamine5] enkephalin in the rat. Journal of Pharmacology and Experimental Therapeutics 259: 725–731

Dubuisson D, Dennis S G 1977 The formalin test: a quantitative study of analgesic effects of morphine, meperidin, and brain stem stimulation in rats and cat. Pain 4: 161–174

Duggan A W, Hope P J, Lang C W 1991 Microinjection of neuropeptide Y into the superficial dorsal horn reduces stimulus-evoked release of immunoreactive substance P in the anaesthetized cat. Neuroscience 44: 733–740

Edwards M, Serrano J M, Gent J P, Goodchild C S 1990 On the mechanism by which midazolam causes spinally mediated analgesia. Anesthesiology 73: 273–277

Eide P K, Hole K 1991 Different role of 5-HT_{1A} and 5-HT_2 receptors in spinal cord in the control of nociceptive responsiveness. Neuropharmacology 30: 727–731

Eide P K, Joly N M, Hole K 1990 The role of spinal cord 5-HT_{1A} and 5-HT_{1B} receptors in the modulation of a spinal nociceptive reflex. Brain Research 536: 195–200

Eisenach J C, Lysak S Z, Viscomi C M 1989a Epidural clonidine analgesia following surgery: phase I. Anesthesiology 71: 640–646

Eisenach J C, Rauck R L, Buzzanell C, Lysak S Z 1989b Epidural clonidine analgesia for intractable cancer pain: phase I. Anesthesiology 71: 647–652

El-Yassir N, Fleetwood-Walker S M, Mitchell R 1988 Heterogeneous effects of serotonin in the dorsal horn of the rat: the involvement of 5-HT_1 receptors subtypes. Brain Research 456: 147–158

Fang F G, Moreau J L, Fields H L 1987 Dose dependent antinociceptive action of neurotensin microinjected into the rostroventral medulla of the rat. Brain Research 420: 171–174

Fardin V, Oliveras J L, Besson J M 1984 A re-investigation of the analgesic effects induced by stimulation of the periaqueductal gray matter in the rat. II. Differential characteristics of the analgesia induced by ventral and dorsal PAG stimulation. Brain Research 306: 125–139

Faris P L, Komisaruk B, Watkins L R, Mayer D L 1983 Evidence for the neuropeptide cholecystokinin as an antagonist of opiate analgesia. Science 219: 310–312

Faull R L, Villiger J W, Dragunow M 1989 Neurotensin receptors in the human spinal cord: a quantitative autoradiographic study. Neuroscience 29: 603–613

Fedynyshyn J P, Lee N M 1989 Mu type opioid receptors in rat periaqueductal gray-enriched P2 membrane are coupled to G-protein-mediated inhibition of adenylyl cyclase. FEBS Letters 253: 23–27

Fedynyshyn J P, Kwiat G, Lee N 1989 Characterization of high affinity opioid binding sites in rat periaqueductal gray P2 membrane. European Journal of Pharmacology 159: 83–88

Fialip J, Marty H, Makambila M C, Civiale M A, Eschalier A 1989 Pharmacokinetic patterns of repeated administration of antidepressants in animals. II. Their relevance in a study of the influence of clomipramine on morphine analgesia in mice. Journal of Pharmacology and Experimental Therapeutics 248: 747–751

Fields H L, Heinricher M M, Mason P 1991 Neurotransmitters in nociceptive modulatory circuits. Annual Review of Neuroscience 14: 219–245

Finn I B, Iuvone P M, Holtzman S G 1990 Depletion of catecholamines in the brain of rats differentially affects stimulation of locomotor activity by caffeine, D-amphetamine, and methylphenidate. Neuropharmacology 29: 625–631

Fleetwood-Walker S M, Mitchell R, Hope P J, Molony V, Iggo A 1985 An alpha-2 receptor mediates the selective inhibition by noradrenaline of nociceptive responses of identified dorsal horn neurones. Brain Research 334: 243–254

Fleetwood-Walker S M, Hope P J, Mitchell R, El-Yassir N, Molony V 1988a The influence of opioid receptor subtypes on the processing of nociceptive inputs in the spinal dorsal horn of the cat. Brain Research 451: 213–226

Fleetwood-Walker S M, Hope P J, Mitchell R 1988b Antinociceptive actions of descending dopaminergic tracts on cat and rat dorsal horn somatosensory neurones. Journal of Physiology 399: 335–348

Fleetwood-Walker S M, Mitchell R, Hope P J, El-Yassir N, Molony V, Bladon C M 1990 The involvement of neurokinin receptor subtypes in somatosensory processing in the superficial dorsal horn of the cat. Brain Research 519: 169–182

Forrest W H, Byron B W, Brown C R et al 1977 Dextroamphetamine with morphine for the treatment of postoperative pain. New England Journal of Medicine 296: 712–715

Franklin K B J 1989 Analgesia and the neural substrate of reward. Neuroscience and Biobehavioral Reviews 13: 149–154

Fraser H M, Chapman V, Dickenson A H 1992 Spinal local anaesthetic actions on afferent evoked responses and wind-up of nociceptive neurones in the rat spinal cord: combination with morphine produces marked potentiation of antinociception. Pain: 33–41

Fujimoto J M, Arts K S, Rady J J, Tseng L F 1990 Spinal dynorphin A (1–17): possible mediator of antianalgesic action. Neuropharmacology 29: 609–617

Gamse R, Holzer P, Lembeck F 1979 Indirect evidence for presynaptic location of opiate receptors in chemosensitive primary sensory neurones. Naunyn-Schmiedeberg's Archives of Pharmacology 308: 281–285

Garthwaite J, Charles S L, Chess-Williams R 1988 Endothelium-derived relaxing factor release on activation of NMDA receptors suggests role as intracellular messengers in the brain. Nature 336: 385–388

Gaumann D M, Yaksh T L, Post C, Wilcox G L, Rodriguez M 1989 Intrathecal somatostatin in cat and mouse – studies on pain, motor behaviour, and histopathology. Anesthesia and Analgesia 68: 623–632

Gebhart G F 1982 Opiate and opioid peptide effects on brain stem neurons: relevance to nociception and antinociceptive mechanisms. Pain 12: 93–140

Gebhart G F, Jones S L 1988 Effects of morphine given in the brainstem on the activity of dorsal horn nociceptive neurons. Progress in Brain Research 77: 229–243

Gebhart G F, Sandkuhler J, Thalhammer J G, Zimmermann M 1983 Quantitative comparison of inhibition in spinal cord of nociceptive information by stimulation in periaqueductal gray or nucleus raphe magnus of the cat. Journal of Neurophysiology 50: 1433–1444

Gebhart G F, Sandkuhler J, Thalhammer J, Zimmerman M 1984 Inhibition in spinal cord of nociceptive information by electrical stimulation and morphine microinjections at identical sites in midbrain of the cat. Journal of Neurophysiology 51: 75–89

Geiger J D, Labella F S, Nagy J I 1984 Characterization and localization of adenosine receptors in rat spinal cord. Journal of Neuroscience 4: 2303–2310

Gerber G, Randic M 1989a Excitatory amino acid-mediated components of synaptically evoked input from dorsal roots to deep dorsal horn neurons in the rat spinal cord slice. Neuroscience Letters 106: 211–219

Gerber G, Randic M 1989b Participation of excitatory amino acid receptors in the slow excitatory synaptic transmission in the rat spinal dorsal horn in vitro. Neuroscience Letters 106: 220–228

Gibson S J, Polak J M, Anand P et al 1984 The distribution and origin of VIP in the spinal cord of six mammalian species. Peptides 5: 201–207

Gillberg P-G, Wiksten B 1989 Effects of spinal cord lesions and rhizotomies on cholinergic and opiate receptor binding sites in rat spinal cord. Acta Physiologica Scandinavica 126: 575–582

Gillberg P-G, d'Ardy R, Aquilonius S M 1988 Autoradiographic distribution of 3H-acetylcholine binding sites in the cervical spinal cord of man and some other species. Neuroscience Letters 90: 197–202

Gillberg P-G, Gordh T Jr, Hartvig P, Jansson I, Pettersson J, Post C 1989 Characterization of the antinociception induced by intrathecally administered carbachol. Pharmacology and Toxicology 64: 340–343

Glaum S R, Proudfit H K, Anderson E G 1990 5-HT_3 receptors modulate spinal nociceptive reflexes. Brain Research 510: 12–16

Go V L W, Yaksh T L 1987 Release of substance P from the cat spinal cord. Journal of Physiology 391: 141–167

Gogas K R, Hough L B, Eberle N B et al 1989 A role for histamine and H2-receptors in opioid antinociception. Journal of Pharmacology and Experimental Therapeutics 250: 476–484

Gordh T, Jansson I, Hartvig P, Gillberg P G, Post C 1989 Interactions between noradrenergic and cholinergic mechanisms involved in spinal nociceptive processing. Acta Anaesthesiologica Scandinavica 33: 39–47

Graf G, Sinatra R, Chung J, Frasca A, Silverman D G 1991 Epidural sufentanil for postoperative analgesia: dose-response in patients recovering from major gynecologic surgery. Anesthesia and Analgesia 73: 405–409

Griffiths R R, Woodson, P P 1988a Reinforcing effects of caffeine in humans. Journal of Pharmacology and Experimental Therapeutics 246: 21–29

Griffiths R R, Woodson P P 1988b Reinforcing properties of caffeine: studies in humans and laboratory animals. Pharmacology, Biochemistry and Behaviour 29: 419–427

Griffiths R R, Woodson P P 1988c Caffeine physical dependence: a review of human and laboratory animal studies. Psychopharmacology 94: 437–451

Gundlach A L, Dodd P R, Grabara Watson W E J et al 1988 Deficits of spinal cord glycine/strychnine receptors in inherited myoclonus of poll Hereford calves. Science 241: 1807–1810

Haigler H J, Spring D D 1978 A comparison of the analgesic and behavioural effects of [D-Ala^2] met-enkephalinamide and morphine in the mesencephalic reticular formation of rats. Life Sciences 23: 1229–1240

Haley J E, Sullivan A F, Dickenson A H 1990 Evidence for spinal N-methyl-D-aspartate receptor involvement in prolonged chemical nociception in the rat. Brain Research 518: 218–226

Haley J E, Dickenson A H, Schachter M 1992 Electrophysiological evidence for a role of nitric oxide in prolonged chemical nociception in the rat. Neuropharmacology 31: 251–258

Hammond D L 1988 Intrathecal administration: methodological considerations. Progressive Brain Research 77: 313–320

Hammond D L, Drower E J 1984 Effects of intrathecally administered THIP, Baclofen and Muscimol on nociceptive threshold. European Journal of Pharmacology 103: 121–125

Hammond D L, Yaksh T L 1984 Antagonism of stimulation-produced antinociception by intrathecal administration of methysergide or phentolamine. Brain Research 298: 329–337

Hammond D L, Levy R A, Proudfit H K 1980 Hypoalgesia following microinjection of noradrenergic antagonists in the nucleus raphe magnus. Pain 9: 85–101

Hammond D L, Tyce G M, Yaksh T L 1985 Efflux of 5-hydroxytrptamine and noradrenaline into spinal cord superfusates during stimulation of the rat medulla. Journal of Physiology 359: 151–162

Hamon M, Gallissot M C, Menard F, Gozlan H, Bourgoin S, Verge D 1989 5-HT3 receptor binding sites are on capsaicin-sensitive fibres in the rat spinal cord. European Journal of Pharmacology 164: 315–322

Hao J X, Xu X J, Aldskogius H, Seiger A, Wiesenfeld-Hallin Z 1991a Allodynia-like effects in rat after ischaemic spinal cord injury photochemically induced by laser irradiation. Pain 45: 175–185

Hao J X, Xu X J, Yu Y X, Seiger A, Wiesenfeld-Hallin Z 1991b Hypersensitivity of dorsal horn wide dynamic range neurons to cutaneous mechanical stimuli after transient spinal cord ischemia in the rat. Neuroscience Letters 128: 105–108

Hao J X, Xu X J, Yu Y X, Seiger A, Wiesenfeld-Hallin Z 1992a Transient spinal cord ischemia induces temporary hypersensitivity of dorsal horn wide dynamic range neurons to myelinated, but not unmyelinated, fiber input. Journal of Neurophysiology 68: 384–391

Hao J X, Xu X J, Yu Y X, Seiger A, Wiesenfeld-Hallin 1992b Baclofen reverses the hypersensitivity of dorsal horn wide dynamic range neurons to mechanical stimulation after transient spinal cord ischemia, implications for a tonic GABAergic inhibitory control of myelinated fiber input. Journal of Neurophysiology 68: 392–396

Haws C M, Heinricher M M, Fields H L 1990 Alpha-adrenergic receptor agonists, but not antagonists, alter the tail-flick latency when microinjected into the rostral ventromedial medulla of the lightly anesthetized rat. Brain Research 533: 192–195

Headley P M, Parson C G, West D C 1987 The role of N-methylaspartate receptors in mediating responses of rats and cat neurones to defined sensory stimuli. Journal of Physiology 385: 169–188

Heapy C G, Jamieson A., Russell N J W 1987 Afferent C-fibre and A-delta activity in models of inflammation. British Journal of Pharmacology 90: 164P

Heinricher M M, Kaplan H J 1991 GABA-mediated inhibition in rostral ventromedial medulla: role in nociceptive modulation in the lightly anesthetized rat. Pain 47: 105–113

Helke C J, Krause J E, Mantyh P W, Couture R, Bannon M J 1990a Diversity in mammalian tachykinin peptidergic neurons: multiple peptides, receptors, and regulatory mechanisms. FASEB Journal 4: 1606–1615

Helke C J, Thor K B, Sasek C A 1990b Distribution and coexistence of neuropeptides in bulbospinal and medullary autonomic pathways. Annals of the New York Academy of Sciences 579: 149–159

Herz A, Teschemacher H 1971 Activities and sites of adrenociceptive action of morphine-like analgesics and kinetics of distribution following intravenous, intracerebral and intraventricular application. Advances in Drug Research 6: 79–119

Hökfelt T 1991 Neuropeptides in perspective. Neuron 7: 867–879

Hökfelt T, Elde R, Johansson O, Luft R, Nilsson G, Arimura A 1976 Immunohistochemical evidence for separate populations of somatostatin-containing and substance P containing primary afferent neurons in the rat. Neuroscience 1: 131–136

Hongo T, Jankowska E, Lundberg A 1968 Post synaptic excitation and inhibition from primary afferents in neurones of the spinocervical tract. Journal of Physiology (London) 199: 569–592

Hope P J, Fleetwood-Walker S M, Mitchell R 1990 Distinct antinociceptive actions mediated by different opioid receptors in the region of laminae I and laminae III-V of the dorsal horn of the rat. British Journal of Pharmacology 101: 477–483

Hough L B 1988 Cellular localization and possible functions for brain histamine: recent progress. Progress in Neurobiology 30: 469–505

Hough L B, Nalwalk J W 1992 Modulation of morphine antinociception by antagonism of H2 receptors in the periaqueductal gray. Brain Research 588: 58–66

Houston J P, Nef B, Papadoupolous G, Welzl H 1980 Activation and lateralization of sensorimotor field and perioral biting reflex by intranigral GABA agonist and by systemic apomorphine in the rat. Brain Research Bulletin 5: 745–749

Howe J R, Yaksh T L, Go V L W 1987 The effect of unilateral dorsal root ganglionectomies or ventral rhizotomies on alpha-2-adrenoceptor binding to, and the substance P, enkephalin, and neurotensin content of, the cat lumbar spinal cord. Neuroscience 21: 385–394

Hua X-Y, Boublik J H, Spicer M A, Rivier J E, Brown M R, Yaksh T L 1991 The antinociceptive effects of spinally administered neuropeptide Y in the rat: systematic studies on structure-activity relationship. Journal of Pharmacology and Experimental Therapeutics 258: 243–248

Huang L-Y M 1992 The excitatory effects of opioids. Neurochemistry International 20: 463–468

Huntoon M, Eisenach J C, Boese P 1992 Epidural clonidine after cesarean section. Appropriate dose and effect of prior local anesthetic. Anesthesiology 76: 187–193

Hylden J L K, Wilcox G L 1983 Pharmacological, characterization of substance P induced nociception in mice: modulation by opioid and noradrenergic agonists at the spinal level. Journal of Pharmacology and Experimental Therapeutics 226: 398–404

Iacono R P, Linford J, Sandyk R, Consroe P, Ryan M R, Bamford C R 1988 Intraspinal opiates for treatment of intractable pain in the terminally ill cancer patient. International Journal of Neuroscience 38: 111–119

Iadarola M J, Brady L S, Draisci G, Dubner R 1988 Enhancement of dynorphin gene expression in spinal cord following experimental inflammation: stimulus specificity, behavioural parameters and opioid receptor binding. Pain 35: 313–326

Jacquet Y F, Lajtha A 1976 The periaqueductal gray site of morphine analgesia and tolerance as shown by 2-way cross-tolerance between systemic and intracerebral injections. Brain Research 103: 501–513

Jansen K L R, Faull R L M, Dragunow M, Waldvogel H 1990 Autoradiographic localization of NMDA, quisqualate and kainic acid receptors in human spinal cord. Neuroscience Letters 108: 53–57

Jeftinija S, Murase K, Nedeljkov V, Randic M 1982 Vasoactive intestinal polypeptide excites mammalian dorsal horn neurons both in vivo and in vitro. Brain Research 243: 158–164

Jensen T S, Yaksh T L 1984a Spinal monoamine and opiate system pathways mediate the antinociceptive effects produced by glutamate at brainstem sites. Brain Research 321: 287–297

Jensen T S, Yaksh T L 1984b Effects of an intrathecal dopamine agonist, apomorphine, on thermal and chemical evoked noxious responses in rats. Brain Research 296: 285–293

Jensen T S, Yaksh T L 1986a I. Comparison of antinociceptive action of morphine in the periaqueductal gray, medial and paramedial medulla in rat. Brain Research 363: 99–113

Jensen T S, Yaksh T L 1986b II. Examination of spinal monoamine receptors through which brain stem opiate-sensitive systems act in the rat. Brain Research 363: 114–127

Jensen T S, Yaksh T L 1986c III. Comparison of the antinociceptive action of mu and delta opioid receptor ligands in the periaqueductal gray matter, medial and paramedial ventral medulla in the rat as studied by the microinjection technique. Brain Research 372: 301–312

Jensen T S, Yaksh T L 1992 Brainstem excitatory amino acid receptors in nociception: Microinjection mapping and pharmacological characterization of glutamate-sensitive sites in the brainstem associated with algogenic behaviour. Neuroscience 46: 535–547

Jessell T M, Yoshioka K, Jahr C E 1986 Amino acids receptor mediated transmission at primary afferent synapses in rat spinal cord. Journal of Experimental Biology 124: 239–258

Joyce E M, Koob G F 1981 Amphetamine-, scopolamine- and caffeine-induced locomotor activity following 6-hydroxydopamine lesions in the mesolimbic dopamine system. Psychopharmacology 73: 311–313

Ju G, Hökfelt T, Brodin E et al 1987 Primary sensory neurons of the rat showing calcitonin gene-related peptide immunoreactivity and their relation to substance P-, somatostatin, galanin-, vasoactive intestinal polypeptide- and cholecystokinin-immunoreactive ganglion cells. Cell and Tissue Research 247: 417–431

Kaiko R F, Wallenstein S L, Rogers A G, Grabinski P Y, Houde R W 1981 Analgesic and mood effects of heroin and morphine in cancer patients with postoperative pain. New England Journal of Medicine 304: 1501–1505

Kaiko R F, Kanner R, Foley K M et al 1987 Cocaine and morphine interaction in acute and chronic cancer pain. Pain 31: 35–45

Kapadia S E, LaMotte C C 1987 Deafferentation-induced alterations in rat dorsal horn: I Comparison of peripheral nerve injury vs rhizotomy effects on presynaptic, post-synaptic and glial processes. Journal of Comparative Neurology 266: 183–197

Kar S, Quirion R 1992 Quantitative autoradiographic localization of [^{125}I]neuropeptide Y receptor binding sites in rat spinal cord and the effects of neonatal capsaicin, dorsal rhizotomy and peripheral axotomy. Brain Research 574: 333–337

Kasman G S, Rosenfeld J P 1986 Opiate microinjections into midbrain do not affect the aversiveness of caudal trigeminal stimulation but produce somatotopically organized peripheral hypoalgesia. Brain Research 383: 271–278

Katon W 1984 Panic disorder and somatization. Review of 55 cases. American Journal of Medicine 77: 101–106

Kellstein D E, Malseed R T, Ossipov M H, Goldstein F J 1988 Effect of chronic treatment with tricyclic antidepressants upon antinociception induced by intrathecal injection of morphine and monoamines. Neuropharmacology 27: 1–14

Kellstein D E, Price D D, Mayer D J 1991 Cholecystokinin and its antagonist lorglumide respectively attenuate and facilitate morphine-induced inhibition of C-fibre evoked discharges of dorsal horn nociceptive neurons. Brain Research 540: 302–306

Kelly P H, Iversen S D 1976 Selective 6-OHDA induced destruction of mesolimbic dopamine neurons: abolition of psychostimulant induced locomotor activity in rats. European Journal of Pharmacology 40: 45–56

Kerr F W L, Lippman H H 1974 The primate spinothalamic tract as demonstrated by anterolateral cordotomy and commisural myelotomy. Advances in Neurology 4: 147–156

Khayyat G F, Yu Y J, King R B 1975 Response patterns to noxious and non-noxious stimuli in rostral trigeminal relay nuclei. Brain Research 97: 47–60

Kim S H, Chung J M 1992 An experimental model for peripheral neuropathy produced by segmental spinal nerve ligation in the rat. Pain 50: 355–363

King A E, Thompson S W, Urban L, Woolf C J 1988 An intracellular analysis of amino acid induced excitations of deep dorsal horn neurons in the rat spinal cord slice. Neuroscience Letters 89: 286–292

Kiser R S, Leibowitz R M, German D C 1978 Anatomic and pharmacological differences between two types of aversive midbrain stimulation. Brain Research 155: 331–342

Komisaruk B R, Whipple B 1986 Vaginal stimulation-produced analgesia in rats and women. Annals of the New York Academy of Sciences 467: 30–39

Kremer E F, Block A, Atkinson J H 1983 Assessment of pain behaviour: factors that distort self-report. In: Melzack R (ed) Pain management and assessment. Raven Press, New York, p 165–171

Kuraishi Y, Hirota N, Sato Y, Hanashima N, Takagi H, Satoh M 1989 Stimulus specificity of peripherally evoked substance P release from the rabbit dorsal horn in situ. Neuroscience 30: 201–205

Laduron P M 1984 Axonal transport of opiate receptors in capsaicin-sensitive neurones. Brain Research 294: 157–160

LaMotte C, Pert C B, Snyder S H 1976 Opiate receptor binding in primate spinal cord: distribution and changes after dorsal root section. Brain Research 112: 407–412

LaMotte R H, Lundberg L E, Torebjörk H E 1992 Pain, hyperalgesia and activity in nociceptive C units in humans after intradermal injection of capsaicin. Journal of Physiology 448: 749–764

Laneuville O, Dorais J, Couture R 1988 Characterization of the effects produced by neurokinins and three agonists selective for neurokinin receptor subtypes in a spinal nociceptive reflex of the rat. Life Sciences 42: 1295–1305

Laporte A M, Koscielniak T, Ponchant M, Verde D, Hamon M, Gozlan H 1992 Quantitative autoradiographic mapping of 5-HT3 receptors in the rat CNS using [^{125}I]iodo-zacopride and [^{3}H]zacopride as radioligands. Synapse 10: 271–281

Larson A A, Vaught J L, Takemori A E 1980 The potentiation of spinal analgesia by leukine enkephalin. European Journal of Pharmacology 61: 381–383

Lasagna L, Von Felsinger J M, Beecher H K 1955 Drug-induced mood changes in man. I. Observations on healthy subjects, chronically ill patients, and 'postaddicts.' Journal of the American Medical Association 157: 1006–1020

Lazorthes Y 1988 Intracerebroventricular administration of morphine for control of irreducible cancer pain. Annals of the New York Academy of Sciences 531: 123–132

Leah J, Menetrey D, de Pommery J 1988 Neuropeptides in long ascending spinal tract cells in the rat: evidence for parallel processing of ascending information. Neuroscience 24: 195–207

Le Bars D, Bourgoin S, Clot A M, Hamon M, Cesselin F 1987 Noxious mechanical stimuli increase the release of met-enkephalin-like material heterosegmentally in the rat spinal cord. Brain Research 402: 188–192

Lee T L, Kumar A, Baratham G 1990 Intraventricular morphine for intractable craniofacial pain. Singapore Medical Journal 31: 273–276

Leslie J B, Watkins W D 1985 Eicosanoids in the central nervous system. Journal of Neurosurgery 63: 659–668

Levy R A, Proudfit H K 1979 Analgesia produced by microinjection of baclofen and morphine at brainstem sites. European Journal of Pharmacology 57: 43–55

Lewis V A, Gebhart G F 1977 Evaluation of the periaqueductal central gray (PAG) as a morphine specific locus of action and examination of morphine-induced and stimulation produced analgesia at coincident PAG loci. Brain Research 124: 283–303

Light A R 1992 The organization of nociceptive neurons in the spinal grey matter. In Light A L (ed), The initial processing of pain and its descending control: spinal and trigeminal system. Karger, Basel, p 109–168

Lima D, Coimbra A 1991 Neurons in the substantia gelatinosa rolandi (Lamina II) project to the caudal ventrolateral reticular formation of the medulla oblongat in the rat. Neuroscience Letters 132: 16–18

Liu Q S, Qiao J T, Dafny N 1992 D2 dopamine receptor involvement in spinal dopamine-produced antinociception. Life Sciences 51: 1485–1492

Lombard M C, Besson J M 1989 Attempts to gauge the relative importance of pre- and postsynaptic effects of morphine on the transmission of noxious messages in the dorsal horn of the rat spinal cord. Pain 37: 335–435

Ma Q P, Han J S 1992 Neurochemical and morphological evidence of an antinociceptive neural pathway from nucleus raphe dorsalis to nucleus accumbens in the rabbit. Brain Research Bulletin 28: 931–936

Ma Q P, Yin G F, Ai M K, Han J S 1991 Serotonergic projections from the nucleus raphe dorsalis to the amygdala in the rat. Neuroscience Letters 134: 21–24

MacDermott A B, Mayer M L, Westbrook G I, Smith S J, Barker J L 1986 NMDA-receptor activation increases cytoplasmic calcium concentrations in cultured spinal cord neurones. Nature 321: 519–522

Magnusson K R, Clements J R, Larson A A, Madl J E, Beitz A J 1987 Localization of glutamate in trigeminothalamic projection neurons: a combined retrograde transport-immunohistochemical study. Somatosensory Research 4: 177–190

Malmberg A B, Yaksh T L 1992a Hyperalgesia mediated by spinal glutamate or SP receptor blocked by spinal cyclooxygenase inhibition. Science 257: 1276–1279

Malmberg A B, Yaksh T L 1992b Antinociceptive actions of spinal non-steroidal anti-inflammatory agents on the formalin test in the rat. Journal of Pharmacology and Experimental Therapeutics 263: 136–146

Malmberg A B, Yaksh T L 1992c Isobolographic and dose response analyses of the interaction between intrathecal mu and delta agonists: effects of naltrindole and its benzofuran analog NTB. Journal of Pharmacology and Experimental Therapeutics 263: 264–275

Malmberg A B, Yaksh T L 1993a Spinal nitric oxide synthase inhibition blocks NMDA induced thermal hyperalgesia and produces antinociception in the formalin test in rats. Pain (in press)

Malmberg A B, Yaksh T L 1993b Pharmacology of the spinal action of ketorolac, morphine, ST-91, U50488H and L-PIA on the formalin test and an isobolographic analysis of the NSAID interaction. Anesthesiology (in press)

Marriott D, Wilkin G P, Coote P R, Wood J N 1990 Eicosanoid synthesis by spinal cord astrocytes is evoked by substance P, possible implications for nociception and pain. In: Samuelsson B et al (eds) Advances in prostaglandin, thromboxane and leukotriene research 21. Raven Press, New York, p 739–741

Marsala M, Yaksh T L 1992 Reversible aortic occlusion in rats: post-reflow hyperesthesia and motor effects blocked by spinal NMDA antagonism. Anesthesiology (suppl) 77: A664

Martin C S, McGrady E M, Colquhoun A, Thorburn J 1990 Extradural methadone and bupivacaine in labour. British Journal of Anaesthesia 65: 330–332

Maves T J, Gebhart G F 1992 Antinociceptive synergy between intrathecal morphine and lidocaine during visceral and somatic nociception in the rat. Anesthesiology 76: 91–99

Meller S T, Dykstra C, Gebhart G F 1992 Production of endogenous nitric oxide and activation of soluble guanylate cyclase are required for N-methyl-D-aspartate-produced facilitation of the nociceptive tail-flick reflex. European Journal of Pharmacology 214: 93–96

Melzack R, Casey K L 1968 Sensory, motivational, and central control determinants of pain: A new conceptual model. In: Kenshalo, D (ed) The skin senses. C C Thomas, Springfield, Illinois, p 423–443

Melzack R, Wall P D 1973 The puzzle of pain Basic Books, New York

Mendell L M 1966 Physiological properties of unmyelinated fibre projections to the spinal cord. Experimental Neurology 16: 316–332

Mendell L M, Wall P D 1965 Responses of single dorsal cord cells to peripheral cutaneous unmyelinated fibers. Nature 206: 97–99

Miletic V, Randic M 1979 Neurotensin excites cat spinal neurones located in laminae I-III. Brain Research 169: 600–604

Miller K E, Clements J R, Larson A A, Beitz A J 1988 Organization of glutamate-like immunoreactivity in the rat superficial dorsal horn: light and electron microscopic observations. Synapse 2: 28–36

Mitchell J, Anderson K J 1991 Quantitative autoradiographic analysis of excitatory amino acid receptors in the cat spinal cord. Neuroscience Letters 124: 269–272

Mizukawa K, Vincent S R, McGeer P L, McGeer E G 1989 Distribution of reduced-nicotinamide-adenine-dinucleotide-phosphate diaphorase-positive cells and fibers in the cat central nervous system. Journal of Comparative Neurology 279: 281–311

Mjellem-Joly N, Lund A, Berge O-G, Hole K 1991 Potentiation of a behavioural response in mice by spinal coadministration of substance P and excitatory amino acid agonists. Neuroscience Letters 133: 121–124

Mohrland S, Gebhart G 1980 Effects of focal electrical stimulation and morphine microinjection in the periaqueductal gray of the rat mesencephalon on neuronal activity in the medullary reticular formation. Brain Research 201: 23–37

Mollenholt P, Post C, Rawal N, Freedman J, Hökfelt T, Paulsson I 1988 Antinociceptive and "neurotoxic" actions of somatostatin in rat spinal cord after intrathecal administration. Pain 32: 95–105

Monasky M S, Zinsmeister A R, Stevens C W, Yaksh T L 1990 Interaction of intrathecal morphine and ST-91 on antinociception in the rat: dose-response analysis, antagonism and clearance. Journal of Pharmacology and Experimental Therapeutics 254: 383–392

Moochhala S M, Sawynok J 1984 Hyperalgesia produced by intrathecal substance P and related peptides: desensitization and cross desensitization. British Journal of Pharmacology 82: 381–388

Moreau J-L, Fields H L 1987 Evidence for GABA involvement in midbrain control of medullary neurons that modulate nociceptive transmission. Brain Research 397: 37–46

Morgan M M, Sohn J H, Liebeskind J C 1989 Stimulation of the periaqueductal gray matter inhibits nociception at the supraspinal as well as spinal level. Brain Research 502: 61–66

Morris B J, Herz A 1987 Distinct distribution of opioid receptor types in rat lumbar spinal cord. Naunyn-Schmiedeberg's Archives of Pharmacology 336: 240–243

Morris R, Southam E, Braid D J, Gathwaite J 1992 Nitric oxide may act as a messenger between dorsal root ganglion neurones and their satellite cells. Neuroscience Letters 137: 29–32

Morton C R, Hutchinson W D, Hendry I A 1988 Release of immunoreactive somatostatin in the spinal dorsal horn of the cat. Neuropeptides 12: 189–197

Morton C R, Hutchinson W D 1990 Morphine does not reduce the intraspinal release of calcitonin gene-related peptide in the cat. Neuroscience Letters 117: 319–324

Moulin D E, Max M B, Kaiko R F, Inturrisi C E, Maggard J, Yaksh T L, Foley K M 1985 The analgesic efficacy of intrathecal D-Ala^2-D-Leu^5-enkephalin in cancer patients with chronic pain. Pain 23: 213–221

Murase K, Nedeljkov V, Randic M 1982 The actions of neuropeptides on dorsal horn neurons in the rat spinal cord slice preparation: an intracellular study. Brain Research 234: 170–176

Murase K, Ryu P D, Randic M 1989 Tachykinins modulate multiple ionic conductances in voltage-clamped rat spinal dorsal horn neurons. Journal of Neurophysiology 61: 854–865

Murata K, Nakagawa I, Kumeta Y, Kitahata L M, Colins J G 1989 Intrathecal clonidine suppresses noxious evoked activity of spinal wide dynamic range neurons in cat. Anesthesia and Analgesia 69: 185–191

Murray C W, Cowan A 1991 Tonic pain perception in the mouse: differential modulation by three receptor-selective opioid agonists. Journal of Pharmacology and Experimental Therapeutics 257: 335–341

Myslinski N R, Randic M 1977 Responses of identified spinal neurones to acetylcholine applied by micro-electrophoresis. Journal of Physiology 269: 195–219

Nahin R L 1987 Immunocytochemical identification of long ascending peptidergic neurons contributing to the spinoreticular tract in the rat. Neuroscience 23: 859–869

Nahin R L 1988 Immunocytochemical identification of long ascending peptidergic lumbar spinal neurons terminating in either the medial or lateral thalamus in the rat. Brain Research 443: 345–349

Nässtrom J, Karlsson U, Post C 1992 Antinociceptive actions of different classes of excitatory amino acid receptor antagonists in mice. European Journal of Pharmacology 212: 21–29

Ness T J, Gebhart G F 1988 Colorectal distension as a noxious visceral stimulus: physiologic and pharmacologic characterization of pseudoaffective reflexes in the rat. Brain Research 450: 153–169

Nicol G D, Klingberg D K, Vasko M R 1992 Prostaglandin E2 increases calcium conductance and stimulates release of substance P in Avian sensory neurons. Journal of Neuroscience 12: 1917–1927

Noguchi K, Ruda M A 1992 Gene regulation in an ascending nociceptive pathway: inflammation-induced increase in preprotachykinin mRNA in rat lamina I spinal projection neurons. Journal of Neuroscience 12: 2563–2572

Nordberg G 1984 Pharmacokinetic aspects of spinal morphine analgesia. Acta Physiologica Scandinavica (suppl) 79: 7–37

North R A, Williams J T, Suprenant A, Christie M J 1987 μ and ∂ receptors belong to a family of receptors that are coupled to potassium channels. Proceedings of the National Academy of Sciences USA 84: 5487–5491

O'Dell T J, Hawkins R D, Kandel E R, Arancio O 1991 Tests of the roles of two diffusible substances in long-term potentiation: evidence for nitric oxide as a possible early retrograde messenger. Proceedings of the National Academy of Sciences USA 88: 11285–11289

O'Donohue T L, Massari V J, Pazoles C J et al 1984 A role for bombesin in sensory processing in the spinal cord. Journal of Neuroscience 4: 2956–2962

Ohkubo T, Shibata M, Takahashi H, Inoki R 1990 Roles of substance P and somatostatin on spinal transmission of nociceptive information induced by formalin in spinal cord. Journal of Pharmacology and Experimental Therapeutics 252: 1261–1268

Oliveras J-L, Maixner W, Dubner R et al 1986a Dorsal horn opiate administration attenuated the perceived intensity of noxious heat stimulation in the behaving monkey. Brain Research 371: 368–371

Oliveras J-L, Maixner W, Dubner R et al 1986b The medullary dorsal horn: a target for the expression of opiates effects upon the perceived intensity of noxious heat. Journal of Neuroscience 6: 3086–3093

O'Neill M F, Dourish C T, Iversen S D 1989 Morphine induced analgesia in the rat paw pressure test is blocked by CCK and enhanced by the CCK antagonist MK-329. Neuropharmacology 28: 243–248

Ono H, Mishima A, Ono S, Fukuda H, Vasko M R 1991 Inhibitory effects of clonidine and tizanidine on release of substance P from slices of rat spinal cord and antagonism by alpha-adrenergic receptor antagonists. Neuropharmacology 30: 585–589

Oshita S, Yaksh T L, Chipkin R 1990 The antinociceptive effects of intrathecally administered SCH32615, an enkephalinase inhibitor in the rat. Brain Research 515: 143–148

Ossipov M H, Goldstein F J, Malseed R T 1984 Feline analgesia following central administration of opioids. Neuropharmacology 23: 925–929

Ossipov M H, Harris S, Lloyd P, Messineo E, Lin B S, Bagley J 1990a Antinociceptive interaction between opioids and medetomidine: systemic additivity and spinal synergy. Anesthesiology 73: 1227–1235

Ossipov M H, Lozito R, Messineo E, Green J, Harris S, Lloyd P 1990b Spinal antinociceptive synergy between clonidine and morphine, U69593, and DPDPE: isobolographic analysis. Life Sciences 47: 71–76

Oyama T, Fukushi S, Jin T 1982 Epidural β-endorphin in treatment of pain. Canadian Anaesthetists Society Journal 29: 24–26

Palacios Q T, Jones M M, Hawkins J L et al 1991 Post-caesarean section analgesia: a comparison of epidural butorphanol and morphine. Canadian Journal of Anaesthesia 38: 24–30

Panula P, Hadjiconstantinou M, Yang H-Y T, Costa E 1983 Immunohistochemical localization of bombesin/gastrin-releasing peptide and substance P in primary sensory neurons. Journal of Neuroscience 3: 2021–2029

Pascual J, del Arco C, Gonzalez A M, Pazos A 1992 Quantitative light microscopic autoradiographic localization of alpha-2 receptors in the human brain. Brain Research 585: 116–127

Pay S, Barasi S 1982 A study of the connections of nociceptive substantia nigra neurons. Pain 12: 75–89

Payne R 1987 Role of epidural and intrathecal narcotics and peptides in the management of cancer pain. Medical Clinics of North America 71: 313–327

Pazos A, Palacios J M 1985 Quantitative autoradiographic mapping of serotonin receptors in the rat brain. I. Serotonin-1 receptors. Brain Research 346: 205–230

Pazos A, Cortés R, Palacios J M 1985 Quantitative autoradiographic mapping of serotonin receptors in the rat brain. II. Serotonin-2 receptors. Brain Research 346: 231–249

Penning J P, Yaksh T L 1992 Interaction of intrathecal morphine with bupivacaine and lidocaine in the rat. Anesthesiology 77: 1186–1200

Perriss B W, Latham B V, Wilson I H 1990 Analgesia following extradural and i.m. pethidine in post-caesarean section patients. British Journal of Anaesthesia 3: 355–357

Pert A, Yaksh T L 1974 Sites of morphine induced analgesia in the primate brain: relation to pain pathways. Brain Research 80: 135–140

Pert A, Yaksh T L 1975 Localization of the antinociceptive action of morphine in primate brain. Pharmacology, Biochemistry and Behavior 3: 133–138

Pohl M, Benoliel J J, Bourgoin S et al 1990 Regional distribution of calcitonin gene-related peptide-, substance P-, cholecystokinin-, met^5-enkephalin-, and dynorphin A (1–8)-like material in the spinal cord and dorsal root ganglia of adult rats: effects of dorsal rhizotomy and neonatal capsaicin. Journal of Neurochemistry 55: 1122–1130

Porreca F, Heyman J S, Mosberg H I, Omnaas J R, Vaught J L 1987 Role of mu and delta receptors in the supraspinal and spinal analgesic effects of [D-Pen2, D-Pen5] enkephalin in the mouse. Journal of Pharmacology and Experimental Therapeutics 241: 393–400

Prado W A 1989 Antinociceptive effect of agonists microinjected into the anterior pretectal nucleus of the rat. Brain Research 493: 145–154

Prado W A, Roberts M H T 1984 Antinociception from a stereospecific action of morphine microinjected into the brainstem: a local or distant site of action. British Journal of Pharmacology 82: 877–882

Price G W, Wilkin G P, Turnbull M J, Bowery N G 1984 Are baclofen-sensitive $GABA_B$ receptors present on primary afferent terminals of the spinal cord? Nature 307: 71–73

Price G W, Kelly J S, Bowery N G 1987 The location of $GABA_B$ receptor binding sites in mammalian spinal cord. Synapse 1: 530–538

Proudfit H K, Clark F M 1991 The projections of locus coeruleus neurons to the spinal cord. Progress in Brain Research 88: 123–141

Puig S, Rivot J P, Besson J M 1991 In vivo electrochemical evidence that the tricyclic antidepressant femoxetine potentiates the morphine-induced increase in 5-HT metabolism in the medullary dorsal horn of freely moving rats. Brain Research 553: 222–228

Pybus D A, Torda T A 1982 Dose effect relationships of extradural morphine. British Journal of Anaesthesiology 54: 1259–1262

Rady J J, Fujimoto J M, Tseng L F 1991 Dynorphins other than dynorphin A(1–17) lack spinal antianalgesic activity but do act on dynorphin A(1–17) receptors. Journal of Pharmacology and Experimental Therapeutics 259: 1073–1080

Raja S N, Meyer R A, Campbell J N 1988 Peripheral mechanisms of somatic pain. Anesthesiology 68: 571–590

Ramberg D A, Yaksh T L 1989 Effects of cervical spinal hemisection of dihydromorphine binding in brainstem and spinal cord in cat. Brain Research 483: 61–67

Ramwell P W, Shaw J E, Jessup R 1966 Spontaneous and evoked release

of prostaglandins from frog spinal cord. American Journal of Physiology 211: 998–1004
Rawal N, Schott U, Dahlström B et al 1986 Influence of naloxone infusion on analgesia and respiratory depression following epidural morphine. Anesthesiology 64: 194–201
Reddy S V R, Maderdrut J L, Yaksh T L 1980 Spinal cord pharmacology of adrenergic agonist-mediated antinociception. Journal of Pharmacology and Experimental Therapeutics 213: 525–533
Robertson J A, Hough L B, Bodnar R J 1988 Potentiation of opioid and nonopioid forms of swim analgesia by cimetidine. Pharmacology, Biochemistry and Behaviour 31: 107–112
Rodgers R J 1977 Elevation of aversive threshold in rats by intraamygdaloid injection of morphine sulfate. Pharmacology, Biochemistry and Behaviour 6: 385–390
Roerig S C, Fujimoto J M 1989 Multiplicative interaction between intrathecally and intracerebroventricularly administered mu opioid agonists but limited interactions between delta and kappa agonists for antinociception in mice. Journal of Pharmacology and Experimental Therapeutics 249: 762–768
Romano J M, Turner J A 1985 Chronic pain and depression: does the evidence support a relationship? Psychopharmacology Bulletin 97: 18–26
Ryu P D, Gerber G, Murase K, Randic M 1988 Actions of calcitonin gene-related peptide on rat spinal dorsal horn neurons. Brain Research 441: 357–361
Sabbe M, Mjanger E, Hill H, Yaksh T L 1989 Epidural sufentanil in dogs: analgesia versus plasma concentration. Anesthesia and Analgesia 68: S243
Salt T E 1986 Mediation of thalamic sensory input by both NMDA receptors and non-NMDA receptors. Nature 322: 263–265
Salter M W, Henry J L 1987 Evidence that adenosine mediates the depression of spinal dorsal horn induced by peripheral vibration in the cat. Neuroscience 22: 631–650
Samanin R, Gumulka W, Valzelli L 1970 Reduced effect of morphine in midbrain raphe lesioned rats. European Journal of Pharmacology 10: 339
Sanchez-Blazquez P, Garzon J 1989 Evaluation of delta receptor mediation of supraspinal opioid analgesia by in vivo protection against the beta-funaltrexamine antagonist effect. European Journal of Pharmacology 159: 9–23
Sandler A N 1990 Epidural opiate analgesia for acute pain relief. Canadian Journal of Anaesthesia 3733–3739
Sandouk P, Serrie A, Urtizberea M, Debray M, Got P, Scherrmann J M 1991 Morphine pharmacokinetics and pain assessment after intracerebroventricular administration in patients with terminal cancer. Clinical Pharmacology and Therapeutics 49: 442–448
Saria A, Gamse R, Petermann J, Fischer J A, Theodorsson-Norheim E, Lundberg J M 1986 Simultaneous release of several tachykinins and calcitonin gene-related peptide from rat spinal cord slices. Neuroscience Letters 63: 310–314
Saria A, Javorsky F, Humpel C, Gamse R 1990 5-HT receptor antagonism inhibits sensory neuropeptide release from the rat spinal cord. Neuroreport 1: 104–106
Satoh M, Oku R, Akaike A 1983 Analgesia produced by microinjection of L-glutamate into the rostral ventromedial bulbar nuclei of the rat and its inhibition by intrathecal α-adrenergic blocking agents. Brain Research 261: 361–364
Sawynok J, Sweeney M I 1989 The role of purines in nociception. Neuroscience 32: 557–569
Sawynok J, Yaksh T L 1993 Caffeine as an analgesic adjuvant. A review of pharmacology and mechanisms of action. Pharmacological Reviews (in press)
Sawynok J, Kato N, Navilicek V, Labella F S 1982 Lack of effect of baclofen on substance P and somatostatin release from the spinal cord in vitro. Naunyn-Schiemedberg's Archives of Pharmacology 319: 78–81
Sawynok J, Sweeney M I, White T D 1989 Adenosine release may mediate spinal analgesia by morphine. Trends in Pharmacological Sciences 10: 186–189
Sawynok J, Sweeney M, Nicholson D, White T 1990 Pertussis toxin inhibits morphine-induced release of adenosine from the spinal cord. Progress in Clinical and Biological Research 328: 397–400
Sawynok J, Reid A, Nance D 1991a Spinal antinociception by adenosine analogs and morphine after intrathecal administration of the neurotoxins capsaicin, 6-hydroxydopamine and 5,7-dihydroxytryptamine. Journal of Pharmacology and Experimental Therapeutics 258: 370–380
Sawynok J, Espey M J, Reid A 1991b 8-Phenyltheophylline reverses the antinociceptive action of morphine in the periaqueductal gray. Neuropharmacology 30: 871–877
Schaible H-G, Grubb B D, Neugebauer V, Oppmann M 1991 The effects of NMDA antagonists on neuronal activity in cat spinal cord evoked by acute inflammation in the knee joint. European Journal of Neuroscience 3: 981–991
Schmauss C, Yaksh T L 1984 In vivo studies on spinal opiate receptor systems mediating antinociception. II. Pharmacological profiles suggesting a differential association of mu, delta and kappa receptors with visceral chemical and cutaneous thermal stimuli in the rat. Journal of Pharmacology and Experimental Therapeutics 228: 1–12
Schmitt P, Karli F E P 1974 Etudes des systèmes de reforcement négatif et de reforsement positiv au niveau de la substance grise centrale chez le rat. Physiology and Behavior 12: 271–279
Schneider S P, Perl E R 1985 Selective excitation of neurones in the mammalian spinal dorsal horn by aspartate and glutamate in vitro: correlation with location and excitatory input. Brain Research 360: 339–343
Schneider S P, Perl E R 1988 Comparison of primary afferent and glutamate excitation of neurons in the mammalian spinal dorsal horn. Journal of Neuroscience 8: 2062–2073
Schulthesis R, Schramm J, Neidhardt J 1992 Dose changes in long- and medium-term intrathecal morphine therapy of cancer pain. Neurosurgery 31: 664–669
Schultz W, Romo R 1987 Response of nigra striatal dopamine neurons to high intensity somatosensory stimulation in the anesthetized monkey. Journal of Neurophysiology 57: 210–217
Schuman E M, Madison D V 1991 A requirement for the intracellular messenger nitric oxide in long-term potentiation. Science 254: 1503–1506
Seltzer Z, Tal M, Sharav Y 1989 Autonomy behavior in rats following peripheral deafferentation is suppressed by daily injections of amitriptyline, diazepam and saline. Pain 37: 245–250
Seybold V S, Hylden J L K, Wilcox G L 1982 Intrathecal substance P and somatostatin in rats: behaviours indicative of sensation. Peptides 3: 49–54
Shafer A L, Donnelly A J 1991 Management of postoperative pain by continuous epidural infusion of analgesics. Clinical Pharmacy 10: 745–764
Sharpe L G, Garnett J E, Cicero T J 1974 Analgesia and hyperreactivity produced by intracranial microinjections of morphine into the periaqueductal gray matter of the rat. Behavioural Biology 11: 303–313
Sher G, Mitchell D 1990 N-methyl-D-aspartate mediates responses of rat dorsal horn neurons to hind limb ischemia. Brain Research 522: 55–62
Shir Y, Seltzer Z 1990 A-fibers mediate mechanical hyperesthesia and allodynia and C-fibers mediate thermal hyperalgesia in a new model of causalgia from pain disorders in rats. Neuroscience Letters 115: 62–67
Siegfried B, Bures, B J 1978 Asymmetry of EEG arousal in rats with unilateral 6-hydroxydopamine lesions of substantia nigra: quantification of neglect. Experimental Neurology 62: 173–190
Sim L J, Joseph S A 1989 Opiocortin and catecholamine projections to raphe nuclei. Peptides 10: 1019–1025
Sim L J, Joseph S A 1992 Serotonin and substance P afferents to parafascicular and central medial nuclei. Peptides 13: 171–176
Simpson K H, Madej T H, McDowell J M, MacDonald R, Lyons G 1988 Comparison of extradural buprenorphine and extradural morphine after caesarean section. British Journal of Anaesthesia 60: 627–631
Sinclair R J, Sathain K, Burton H 1991 Neuronal responses in ventroposterolateral nucleus of thalamus in monkeys (Macaca mulatta) during active touch of gratings. Somatosensory and Motor Research 8: 293–300
Singer E, Placheta P 1980 Reduction of 3H-muscimol binding sites in

rat dorsal spinal cord after neonatal capsaicin treatment. Brain Research 202: 484–487

Skilling S R, Smulling D H, Beitz A J, Larson A A 1988 Extracellular amino acid concentrations in the dorsal spinal cord of freely moving rats following veratridine and nociceptive stimulation. Journal of Neurochemistry 51: 127–132

Smith D J, Perrotti J M, Crisp T, Cabral M E, Long J T, Scalzitti J M 1988 The mu opiate receptor is responsible for descending pain inhibition originating in the periaqueductal gray region of the rat brain. European Journal of Pharmacology 156: 47–54

Solomon R E, Gebhart G F 1988 Mechanisms of effects of intrathecal serotonin on nociception and blood pressure in rats. Journal of Pharmacology and Experimental Therapeutics 245: 905–912

Sorkin L S 1992 Release of amino acids and PGE_2 into the spinal cord of lightly anesthetized rats during development of an experimental arthritis: enhancement of C-fiber evoked release. Society of Neuroscience Abstracts 429: 10

Sorkin L S, McAdoo D J, Willis W D 1992 Stimulation in the ventral posterior lateral nucleus of the primate thalamus leads to release of serotonin in the lumbar spinal cord. Brain Research 581: 307–310

Sosnowski M, Yaksh T L 1989 Role of spinal adenosine receptor in modulating the hyperesthesia produced by spinal receptor antagonism. Anesthesia and Analgesia 69: 587–592

Sosnowski M, Stevens C W, Yaksh T L 1989 Assessment of the role of A_1/A_2 adenosine receptors mediating the purine antinociception, motor and autonomic function in the rat spinal cord. Journal of Pharmacology and Experimental Therapeutics 250: 915–922

Spiegel K, Kalb R, Pasternak W 1983 Analgesic activity of tricyclic antidepressants. Annals of Neurology 13: 462–465

Steinman J L, Komisaruk B R, Yaksh T L, Tyce G M 1983 Spinal cord monoamines mediate the antinociceptive effects of vaginal stimulation in rats. Pain 16: 155–166

Stevens C W 1991 Intraspinal opioids in frogs: a new behavioral model for the assessment of opioid action. Nida Research Monograph 105: 561–562

Suh H H, Tseng L L 1990 Intrathecal administration of thiorphan and bestatin enhances the antinociception and release of Met-enkephalin induced by beta-endorphin intraventricularly in anesthetized rats. Neuropeptides 16: 91–96

Sun X, Larson A A 1991 Behavioral sensitization to kainic acid and quisqualic acid in mice: comparison to NMDA and substance P responses. Journal of Neuroscience 11: 3111–3123

Sweeney M I, White T D, Sawynok J 1989 Morphine, capsaicin and K+ release purines from capsaicin-sensitive primary afferent nerve terminals in the spinal cord. Journal of Pharmacology and Experimental Therapeutics 248: 447–454

Sweeney M I, White T D, Sawynok J 1990 5-Hydroxytryptamine releases adenosine and cyclic AMP from primary afferent nerve terminals in the spinal cord in vivo. Brain Research 528: 55–61

Sweeney M I, White T D, Sawynok J 1991 Intracerebroventricular morphine releases adenosine and adenosine 3',5'-cyclic monophosphate from the spinal cord via a serotonergic mechanism. Journal of Pharmacology and Experimental Therapeutics 259: 1013–1008

Swerdlow N R, Vaccarino, F J, Amalric M, Koob G F 1986 The neural substrates for the motor activating properties of psychostimulants: a review of recent findings. Pharmacology, Biochemistry and Behaviour 25: 233–248

Taenzer P, Melzack R, Jeans M E 1986 Influence of psychological factors on postoperative pain, mood and analgesic requirements. Pain 24: 331–342

Taiwo Y O, Levine J D 1986 Indomethacin blocks central nociceptive effects of PGF2a. Brain Research 373: 81–84

Takagi H, Satoh M, Akaike A, Shibata T, Kuraishi Y 1977 The nucleus reticularis gigantocellularis of the medulla oblongata is a highly sensitive site in the production of morphine analgesia in the rat. European Journal of Pharmacology 45: 91–92

Takagi H, Satoh M, Akaike A, Shibata T, Yajima H, Ogawa H 1978 Analgesia by enkephalins injected into the nucleus reticularis gigantocellularis of rat medulla oblongata. European Journal of Pharmacology 49: 113–116

Takagi H, Shiomi H, Kuraishi Y, Fukui K, Ueda H 1979 Pain and the bulbospinal noradrenergic system: pain-induced increase in normetanephrine content in the spinal cord and its modification by morphine. European Journal of Pharmacology 54: 99–107

Takano M, Takano Y, Yaksh T L 1993 Release of calcitonin gene-related peptide (CGRP), substance P (SP), and vasoactive intestinal polypeptide (VIP) from rat spinal cord: modulation by alpha-2 agonists. Peptides (in press)

Takano Y, Yaksh T L 1992 Characterization of the pharmacology of intrathecally administered alpha-2 agonists and antagonist in rats. Journal of Pharmacology and Experimental Therapeutics 261: 764–772

Takano Y, Takano M, Yaksh T L 1992 The effect of intrathecally administered imiloxan and WB4101: possible role of α-2-adrenoceptor subtypes in the spinal cord. European Journal of Pharmacology 219: 465–468

Tallarida R J, Porreca F, Cowan A 1989 Statistical analysis of drug–drug and site–site interactions with isobolograms. Life Sciences 45: 947–961

Tenen S S 1968 Antagonism of the analgesic effect of morphine and other drugs by p-chlorophenylalanine, a serotonin depletor. Psychopharmacology 12: 278

Tiseo P J, Sabbe M B, Yaksh T L 1991 Epidural and intrathecal administration of sufentanil, alfentanil and morphine in the dog: a comparison of analgesic effects and the development of tolerance. Nida Research Monograph 105: 560

Tobias J D, Deshpande J K, Wetzel R C, Facker J, Maxwell L G, Solca M 1990 Postoperative analgesia. Use of intrathecal morphine in children. Clinical Pediatrics 29: 44–48

Todd A J, McKenzie J 1989 GABA-immunoreactive neurons in the dorsal horn of the spinal cord. Neuroscience 31: 799–806

Todd A J, Sullivan A C 1990 Light microscopic study of the coexistence of GABA-like and glycine-like immunoreactivities in the spinal cord of the rat. Journal of Comparative Neurology 296: 496–505

Torebjörk H E, Lundberg L E, LaMotte R H 1992 Central changes in processing of mechanoreceptive input in capsaicin-induced secondary hyperalgesia in humans. Journal of Physiology 448: 765–780

Tsai C, Nakamura S, Iwama K 1980 Inhibition of neuronal activity of the substantia nigra by noxious stimuli and its modification by the caudate nucleus. Brain Research 195: 299–311

Tseng L F, Collins K A 1992 Cholecystokinin administered intrathecally selectively antagonizes intracerebroventricular beta-endorphin-induced tail-flick inhibition in the mouse. Journal of Pharmacology and Experimental Therapeutics 260: 1086–1092

Tseng L F, Fujimoto J M 1985 Differential actions of intrathecal naloxone on blocking the tail flick inhibition induced by intraventricular β-endorphin and morphine in the rats. Journal of Pharmacology and Experimental Therapeutics 232: 74–79

Tseng L F, Tang R 1990 Different mechanisms mediate beta-endorphin- and morphine-induced inhibition of the tail-flick response in rats. Journal of Pharmacology and Experimental Therapeutics 252: 546–551

Tseng L F, Wang Q 1992 Forebrain sites differentially sensitive to beta-endorphin and morphine for analgesia and release of Met-enkephalin in the pentobarbital-anesthetized rat. Journal of Pharmacology and Experimental Therapeutics 261: 1028–1036

Tseng L L, Tang R, Stackman R, Camara A, Fujimoto J M 1990 Brainstem sites differentially sensitive to beta-endorphin and morphine for analgesia and release of met-enkephalin in anesthetized rats. Journal of Pharmacology and Experimental Therapeutics 253: 930–937

Tsou K 1963 Antagonism of morphine analgesia by the intracerebral microinjection of nalorphine. Acta Physiologica Sinica 26: 332–337

Tung A S, Yaksh T L 1982 In vivo evidence for multiple opiate receptors mediating analgesia in the rat spinal cord. Brain 247: 75–83

Turner J A, Romano J M 1984 Review of prevalence of coexisting chronic pain and depression. In: Benedetti, C, Moricca G, Chapman C R (ed). Advances in pain research and therapy. Raven Press, New York, p 123–130

Tyce G M, Yaksh T L 1981 Monoamine release from cat spinal cord by somatic stimuli: an intrinsic modulatory system. Journal of Physiology (London) 314: 513–529

Uda R, Horiguchi S, Ito S M, Hayaishi O 1990 Nociceptive effects by intrathecal administration of prostaglandin D2, E2 or F2 a to conscious mice. Brain Research 510: 26–32

Urban L, Randic M 1984 Slow excitatory transmission in rat dorsal horn: possible mediation by peptides. Brain Research 290: 336–341

Van Praag H, Frenk H 1990 The role of glutamate in opiate descending inhibition of nociceptive reflexes. Brain Research 524: 101–105

Vasko M R, Cartwright S, Ono H 1986 Adenosine agonists do not inhibit the K+ stimulated release of substance P from rat spinal cord slices. Society of Neuroscience Abstracts 12: 799

Ventafridda V, Bianchi M, Ripamonti C et al 1990 Studies on the effects of antidepressant drugs on the antinociceptive action of morphine and on plasma morphine in rat and man. Pain 43: 155–162

Vigouret J, Tesechemacher H, Albus K, Herz A 1973 Differentiation between spinal and supraspinal sites of action of morphine when inhibiting the hind limb flexor reflex in rabbits. Neuropharmacology 12: 111–121

Wamsley J K, Gehlert D R, Filloux F M, Dawson T M 1989 Comparison of the distribution of D-1 and D-2 dopamine receptors in the rat brain. Journal of Chemical Neuroanatomy 2: 119–137

Ward N, Bokan J A, Phillips M, Benedetti C, Butler S, Spenpler D 1984 Antidepressants in concomitant chronic back pain and depression: doxepin and desipramine compared. Journal of Clinical Psychiatry 45: 54–57

Ward N, Bokan J A, Ang J, Butler S 1985 Differential effects of penfluramine and dextroamphetamine on acute and chronic pain. In: Fields H L, Dubner R, Cevero F (eds). Advances in pain research and therapy, vol 9. Raven Press, New York, p 753–760

Watkins L R, Mayer D J 1986 Multiple endogenous opiate and non-opiate analgesia systems: evidence of their existence and clinical implications. Annals of the New York Academy of Sciences 467: 273–299

Watkins L R, Johannessen J N, Kinscheck I B, Mayer D J 1984 The neurochemical basis of footshock analgesia: the role of spinal cord serotonin and norepinephrine. Brain Research 290: 107–117

Westlund K N, Sorkin L S, Ferrington D G et al 1990 Serotoninergic and noradrenergic projections to the ventral posterolateral nucleus of the monkey thalamus. Journal of Comparative Neurology 295: 197–207

Wettstein J G, Kamerling S G, Martin W R 1982 Effects of microinjections of opioids into and electrical stimulation (ES) of the canine periaqueductal gray (PAG) on electrogenesis (EEG), heart rate (HR), pupil diameter (OPD), behavior and analgesia. Neuroscience Abstracts 8: 229

Wheeler-Aceto H, Porreca F, Cowan A 1990 The rat paw formalin test: comparison of noxious agents. Pain 40: 229–238

White W F, Heller A H 1982 Glycine receptor alteration in the mutant mouse spastic. Nature 298: 655–657

Whiting W C, Sandler A N, Lau L C et al 1988 Analgesic and respiratory effects of epidural sufentanil in patients following thoracotomy. Anesthesiology 69: 36–43

Wiertelak E P, Maier S F, Watkins L R 1992 Cholecystokinin antianalgesia: safety cues abolish morphine analgesia. Science 256: 830–833

Willis W D, Coggeshall R E 1991 Sensory mechanisms of the spinal cord. 2nd edn. Plenum Press, New York

Wise R A 1989 Opiate reward: sites and substrates. Neuroscience and Biobehavioral Reviews 13: 129–133

Woodley S J, Kendig J J 1991 Substance P and NMDA receptors mediate a slow nociceptive ventral root potential in neonatal rat spinal cord. Brain Research 559: 17–21

Woolf C J, King A E 1987 Physiology and morphology of multireceptive neurons with C-afferent fibre inputs in the deep dorsal horn of the rat lumbar spinal cord. Journal of Neurophysiology 58: 460–479

Woolf C J, King A E 1990 Dynamic alterations in the cutaneous mechanoreceptive fields of dorsal horn neurons in the rat spinal cord. Journal of Neuroscience 10: 2717–2726

Woolf C J, Thompson W N 1991 The induction and maintenance of central sensitization is dependent on N-methyl-D-aspartic acid receptor activation: implications for the treatment of post-injury pain hypersensitivity states. Pain 44: 293–299

Xia L Y, Huang K H, Rosenfeld J P 1992 Behavioural and trigeminal neuronal effects of rat brainstem-nanoinjected opiates. Physiology and Behaviour 52: 65–73

Yaksh T L 1978a Inhibition by etorphine of the discharge of dorsal horn neurons: effects upon the neuronal response to both high- and low-threshold sensory input in the decerebrate spinal cat. Experimental Neurology 60: 23–40

Yaksh T L 1978b Analgetic actions of intrathecal opiates in cat and primate. Brain Research 153: 205–210

Yaksh T L 1979 Direct evidence that spinal serotonin and noradrenaline terminals mediate the spinal antinociceptive effects of morphine in the periaqueductal gray. Brain Research 160: 180–185

Yaksh T L 1982 Central and peripheral mechanisms for the analgesic action of acetylsalicylic acid. In: Barett H J M, Hirsh J, Mustard J F (eds) Acetylsalicylic acid: new uses for an old drug. Raven Press, New York, p 137–151

Yaksh T L 1983 In vivo studies on spinal opiate receptor systems mediating antinociception. Mu and delta receptor profiles in the primate. Journal of Pharmacology and Experimental Therapeutics 226: 303–316

Yaksh T L 1986 The central pharmacology of primary afferents with emphasis on the disposition and role of primary afferent substance P. In: Yaksh T L (ed) Spinal afferent processing. Plenum Press, New York, p 65–196

Yaksh T L 1989 Behavioural and autonomic correlates of the tactile evoked allodynia produced by spinal glycine inhibition: effects of modulatory receptor systems and excitatory amino acid antagonists. Pain 37: 111–123

Yaksh T L, Chipkin R E 1989 Studies on the effect of SCH-34826 and thiorphan on [Met⁵]enkephalin levels and release in rat spinal cord. European Journal of Pharmacology 167: 367–373

Yaksh T L, Elde R P 1981 Factors governing release of methionine enkephalin-like immunoreactivity from mesencephalon and spinal cord of the cat in vivo. Journal of Neurophysiology 46: 1056–1075

Yaksh T L, Reddy S V R 1981 Studies in the primate on the analgetic effects associated with intrathecal actions of opiate, α-adrenergic agonists and baclofen. Anesthesiology 54: 451–467

Yaksh T L, Rudy T A 1976 Analgesia mediated by a direct spinal action of narcotics. Science 192: 1357–1358

Yaksh T L, Rudy T A 1977 Studies on the direct spinal action of narcotics in the production of analgesia in the rat. Journal of Pharmacology and Experimental Therapeutics 202: 411–428

Yaksh T L, Rudy T A 1978 Narcotic analgesics: CNS sites and mechanisms of action as revealed by intracerebral injection techniques. Pain 4: 299–359

Yaksh T L, Tyce G M 1979 Microinjection of morphine in the periaqueductal gray evokes the release of serotinin from spinal cord. Brain Research 171: 176–181

Yaksh T L, Yeung J C, Rudy T A 1976 Systematic examination in the rat of brain sites sensitive to the direct application of morphine. Observation of differential effect within the periaqueductal gray. Brain Research 114: 83–103

Yaksh T L, Plant R L, Rudy T A 1977 Studies on the antagonism by raphe lesions of the antinociceptive actions of systemic morphine. European Journal of Pharmacology 41: 399–408

Yaksh T L, Jessell T M, Gamse R, Mudge R, Leeman S E 1980 Intrathecal morphine inhibits substance P release from mammalian spinal cord in vivo. Nature 286: 155–156

Yaksh T L, Abay E O, Go V L W 1982a Studies on the location and release of cholecystokinin and vasoactive intestinal peptide in the rat and cat spinal cord. Brain Research 242: 279–290

Yaksh T L, Gross K E, Li C H 1982b Studies on the intrathecal effect of β-endorphin in primate. Brain Research 241: 261–269

Yaksh T L, Dirksen R, Harty G J 1985 Antinociceptive effects of intrathecally injected cholinomimetic drugs in the rat and cat. European Journal of Pharmacology 117: 81–88

Yaksh T L, Noueihed R Y, Durant P A C 1986 Studies of the pharmacology and pathology of intrathecally administered 4-anilinopiperidine analogues and morphine in rat and cat. Anesthesiology 64: 54–66

Yaksh T L, Al-Rodhan N R F, Jensen T S 1988a Sites of action of opiates in production of analgesia. Progress in Brain Research 77: 371–394

Yaksh T L, Michener S R, Bailey J E et al 1988b Survey of distribution of substance P, vasoactive intestinal polypeptide, cholecystokinin, neurotensin, met-enkephalin, bombesin and PHI in the spinal cord of cat, dog, sloth and monkey. Peptides 9: 357–372

Yaksh T L, Yamamoto T, Myers R R 1992 Pharmacology of nerve compression-evoked hyperesthesia. In: Willis W D (ed) Hyperalgesia and allodynia. Raven Press, New York, p 245–258
Yamamoto T, Yaksh T L 1991 Stereospecific effects of a nonpeptidic NK1 selective antagonist, CP,96–345: antinociception in the absence of motor dysfunction. Life Sciences 49: 1955–1963
Yamamoto T, Yaksh T L 1992 Comparison of the antinociceptive effects of pre and post treatment with intrathecal morphine and MK801, an NMDA antagonist on the formalin test in the rat. Anesthesiology 77: 757–763
Yamamoto T, Yaksh L 1993 Effects of intrathecal strychnine and bicuculline on nerve compression-induced thermal hyperesthesia and selective antagonism by MK801. Pain (in press)
Yanez A, Sabbe M B, Stevens C W, Yaksh T L 1990 Interaction of midazolam and morphine in the spinal cord of the rat. Neuropharmacology 29: 359–364
Yeung J C, Rudy T A 1980 Multiplicative interaction between narcotic agonism expressed at spinal and supraspinal sites of antinociceptive action as revealed by concurrent intrathecal and intracerebroventricular injections of morphine. Journal of Pharmacology and Experimental Therapeutics 215: 633–642
Yokota T, Nishikawa N, Nishikawa Y 1979 Effects of strychnine upon different classes of trigeminal subnucleus caudalis neurons. Brain Research 168: 430–434
Yoshimura M, Jessell T M 1989 Primary afferent evoked synaptic response and slow potential generation in rat substantia gelatinosa neurons in vitro. Journal of Neurophysiology 622: 96–108
Yu L C, Han J S 1989 Involvement of arcuate nucleus of hypothalamus in the descending pathway from nucleus accumbens to periaqueductal grey subserving an antinociceptive effect. International Journal of Neuroscience 48: 71–78
Zarbin M A, Wamsley J K, Kuhar M J 1981 Glycine receptor: light microscopic autoradiographic localization with [^{3}H]strychnine. Journal of Neuroscience 1: 532–547
Zemlan F P, Behbehani M M 1988 Nucleus cuneiformis and pain modulation: anatomy and behavioural pharmacology. Brain Research 453: 89–102
Zhang D X, Carlton S M, Sorkin L S, Willis W D 1990a Collaterals of primate spinothalamic tract neurons to the periaqueductal gray. Journal of Comparative Neurology 296: 277–290
Zhang S P, Bandler R, Carrive P 1990b Flight and immobility evoked by excitatory amino acid microinjection within distinct parts of the subtentorial midbrain periaqueductal gray of the cat. Brain Research 520: 73–82
Zhuo M, Gebhart G F 1991 Tonic cholinergic inhibition of spinal mechanical transmission. Pain 46: 211–222
Zhuo M, Gebhart G F 1992 Inhibition of a cutaneous nociceptive reflex by a noxious visceral stimulus is mediated by spinal cholinergic and descending serotonergic systems in the rat. Brain Research 585: 7–18
Zieglgänsberger W, Herz A 1971 Changes of cutaneous receptive fields of spino-cervical-tract neurons and other dorsal horn neurons by microelectrophoretically administered amino acids. Experimental Brain Research 13: 111–126

10. Neuropathic pain

Gary J. Bennett

INTRODUCTION

Pain is a normal consequence of tissue injury. Afterwards, the injury site and the region surrounding it become a source of ongoing pain and tenderness. This pain and tenderness are what we expect to encounter; it is 'normal pain'. It is our common experience that the pain and tenderness gradually diminish as healing progresses and disappear when healing is complete.

I focus here on the exceptions to common experience – people who suffer injury to the nervous system and develop pain that persists for months, years or even decades after the injury has healed. These unfortunate people have trauma- or disease-evoked damage affecting the peripheral nerves, posterior roots, spinal cord or certain regions in the brain. I will refer to all of the abnormal pain conditions that result from such damage as 'neuropathic pain'. In addition, some cases present with similar or identical symptoms following injury that does not produce detectable damage to the nervous system (for example, reflex sympathetic dystrophy following a sprained ankle). The similarity of symptoms, the persistence of the pain long after healing, our imperfect ability to detect subtle kinds of nervous system damage and our suspicion of an underlying neural dysfunction, suggest that the diagnosis of neuropathic pain is also appropriate for these cases.

Neuropathic pain syndromes are difficult to treat. Several drugs are known to have limited efficacy, but complete pain control is rarely achieved and the incidence of disabling side-effects is high. Many patients obtain no relief from any medication. Various surgical procedures have been employed. The outcome is sometimes satisfactory, but relief is often temporary and there is a definite risk that the procedure will fail or even worsen the pain.

TERMINOLOGY

Abnormal pain syndromes are traditionally classified according to the disease or event that precipitated them. Thus, we speak of postherpetic neuralgia following an attack of shingles, causalgia following partial damage to a major nerve or central pain following a thalamic infarct. Many of these diagnostic categories have distinguishing features; for example, diabetic neuropathy typically presents as a burning pain in the feet. However, this tradition has tended to obscure the fact that there are many different abnormalities of pain sensation. The different kinds of abnormality occur singly or, more often, in a wide variety of combinations. Few, if any, of these abnormalities, or their combinations, are unique to any diagnostic category (Noordenbos 1959; Lindblom 1985; Leijon et al 1989; Tasker 1990; Price et al 1989, 1992a).

Tasker (1991) has proposed that the term 'deafferentation' pain is appropriate for all the conditions that I refer to here as 'neuropathic' pain. Deafferentation is a confusing term unless care is taken to specify what is being deafferented. For example, median nerve section deafferents part of the hand, while dorsal root section deafferents neurons in the spinal cord dorsal horn. Pathology that results in the death of primary afferent neurons (e.g. herpes zoster) gives both a peripheral and a central deafferentation. Central deafferentation can occur at multiple levels. For example, spinal cord injury deafferents neurons in the somatosensory thalamic nuclei, while a thalamic lesion deafferents neurons in the somatosensory cortex. There is certainly some justification for Tasker's suggestion; as detailed here, it is probable that different syndromes share at least some of a large number of different pathological mechanisms. However, the term obscures what seems to be a fundamental distinction between lesions that deafferent peripheral tissues (peripheral neuropathies) and those that deafferent the central nervous system (central pain). The fact that some, perhaps even many, syndromes (e.g. postherpetic neuralgia) are likely to have features of both peripheral and central deafferentation is not a sufficient reason for ignoring this distinction. In addition, as Bonica (1991) has pointed out, what are traditionally considered to be peripheral neuropathies and central pain syndromes have some very clear differences, most notably the long delay in the appearance of pain in many cases of central injury. In the framework presented here, one would suggest that some neuropathic mechanisms may contribute to both peripheral neuropathies and to central pain, whereas other mechanisms may contribute to only one.

ON THE RELATION BETWEEN NORMAL AND NEUROPATHIC PAIN

If we review the list of neuropathic pain symptoms given below, we see that there are several symptoms that are also found following ordinary tissue injury. In particular, an ordinary injury is associated with spontaneous (or ongoing) pain, hyperalgesia, and allodynia. What is the relationship between these symptoms and the symptoms that we call neuropathic?

We have known for a long time that increased sensitivity in primary afferent nociceptors innervating injured tissue contributes to normal postinjury pain and tenderness. More recently it has become clear that tissue injury is also normally followed by changes in the responsiveness of central pain processing neurons in the spinal cord and, perhaps, in other regions of the central nervous system (CNS) (see Ch. 11). Both of these phenomena, primary afferent sensitization and central hyperexcitability, are fundamentally involved in the pain and tenderness that normally follows tissue damage. The following sections discuss recent evidence that suggests that some (but certainly not all) kinds of neuropathic pain may be dysfunctional expressions of these normal processes.

As a practical matter, it is of great importance to keep in mind that there is no reason why normal pain due to ongoing tissue injury or inflammation and neuropathic pain cannot be present simultaneously. For example, a failed lumbar disc might lead to neuropathic pain due to compression injury to the spinal nerve or root, normal pain due to the activation of periosteal nociceptors in the facet joints and additional normal pain due to activation of the nociceptors innervating the nerve sheath (Asbury & Fields 1984). The result would be a complex mixture of normal and neuropathic pains – pain felt in the back, down the sciatic nerve ('sciatica') and in the lower limb. Similarly, the patient with a traumatic injury of the spinal column may suffer from neuropathic pain due to the damage to the spinal cord and dorsal roots, and essentially normal pain due to the attendent injury to bone and the paravertebral muscles and ligaments (Davidoff & Roth 1991). Coexistent normal and neuropathic pain is of great significance in patients with cancer. Tumours can produce essentially normal pain by activating nociceptors in muscle, viscera and bone secondary to mechanical compression and distension. The same mechanical insults may yield neuropathic pain when nerve, plexus, root or spinal cord are involved (Brose & Cousins 1991).

Lastly, it is clear that our ability to understand the pathophysiology of neuropathic pain is severely constrained by our limited understanding of normal pain.

THE SYMPTOMS: DIFFERENT KINDS OF NEUROPATHIC PAIN SENSATION

Most investigations of neuropathic pain have paid little attention to the details of the sensory symptoms. This has been largely due to two factors: a conception of neuropathic pain as a unitary phenomenon, and the difficulties encountered in a detailed sensory examination. The difficulties are many, but two are especially important. First, a thorough sensory examination causes the patient considerable pain, which is distressing for both patient and physician. Second, there is a problem of language. There are few connoisseurs of pain sensations and thus many patients are incapable (or unwilling) of analysing their pain and describing it carefully. Even those with the ability to do so often report a difficulty: they say that their neuropathic pain is unlike any normal pain that they have ever experienced.

A catalogue of the different kinds of neuropathic pain sensations is given below. It should be noted that many of the items on this list have not been studied carefully and that the incidence of each type of abnormality in any particular diagnostic category is unknown.

SPONTANEOUS PAIN, CONTINUOUS AND PAROXYSMAL

Many patients appear to have continuous pain without any detectable relation to intentional or incidental stimulation. It is commonly said that the pain is always present, although its intensity may wax and wane. Continuous spontaneous pain appears to be especially prominent in patients with central pain and in certain peripheral neuropathies, especially causalgia, reflex sympathetic dystrophy (RSD) and painful phantoms. It is important to note that continuous spontaneous pain is not present in all patients. For example, some patients with postherpetic neuralgia and trigeminal neuralgia (tic douloureux) are pain-free if they avoid the stimulation that evokes their pain. Both patients with continuous spontaneous pain and those without it report that stimulus-evoked pain, especially if severe or repeated frequently, will leave behind a lingering soreness that may last for hours. Conceptually, it is preferable to refer to this as 'ongoing pain' and to distinguish it clearly from spontaneous pain, but in practice this may be impossible; for example, in the patient who refuses to avoid the daily activities that cause incidental stimulus-evoked pains.

Continuous spontaneous pain is described as being felt in the skin, muscles and/or bones. It is noteworthy that there are few documented cases of spontaneous neuropathic pain (or any other kind of neuropathic pain) that the patient describes as arising from viscera. The exceptions are a few case reports of phantom pain after anorectal or bladder excisions (Ovesen et al 1991). When the pain is felt to lie in muscle or bone, it is generally described with words like 'cramping, aching, throbbing, crushing'. When it is felt to arise from the skin, the reports are usually of 'burning, cutting, pricking and stabbing'. Superficial and deep pain may occur singly or together.

In addition to spontaneous continuous pain, many patients suffer from apparently spontaneous paroxysmal pain. Episodic paroxysmal pain may be the patient's only form of spontaneous pain or it may present together with continuous pain. The episodic pain generally has a short duration (seconds), and it is often described as 'shooting, electric shock-like'. These paroxysmal pains appear to be particularly common in patients with central pain, but they also appear in patients with peripheral nerve damage, for example, postherpetic neuralgia. They are characteristic of tic douloureux. However, tic patients also typically have an evoked-pain abnormality with the same paroxysmal characteristics and it is unclear whether their attacks are truly spontaneous or evoked by subtle incidental stimuli.

Spontaneous dysaesthetic sensations are also reported – 'itching, tingling, raw, tight, numb'. Their presence in combination with frankly painful sensations may account for at least some of the 'strangeness' of the patient's experience.

ABNORMAL EVOKED-PAINS: ALLODYNIA AND HYPERALGESIA

Allodynia refers to the situation where a normally innocuous stimulus produces a sensation of pain whose quality is inappropriate for the stimulus, for example, when lightly touching the skin with a wisp of cotton or an ice cube produces a burning pain sensation (Merskey 1986). Allodynic sensations following the cutaneous application of mechanical, warming and cooling stimuli have been demonstrated to exist in various neuropathic pain syndromes. I know of no clear demonstration that neuropathic pain patients experience allodynic sensations following normally innocuous stimulation of muscles, joints or viscera. Although this may reflect the absence of suitable testing, it is possible that neuropathic allodynia is exclusively a disorder of cutaneous sensibility. In contrast, allodynic sensations from deep tissues are commonplace after ordinary tissue injury; for example, the slightest movement of a gouty toe is painful. Allodynic sensations are among the most debilitating symptoms of neuropathic pain syndromes. Mechanical stimuli as insignificant as contact with clothing or bed linen may cause intense pain. Mechano-allodynia, warm-allodynia and cool-allodynia may exist singly or in any combination.

Hyperalgesia refers to a painful sensation of abnormal severity following noxious stimulation (Merskey 1986). As with allodynia, the abnormality may be found with the cutaneous application of mechanical, heat or cold stimuli. I know of no clear demonstrations of neuropathic hyperalgesic sensations arising from stimulation of deep tissues, but here again this may be due to inadequate testing. In contrast, hyperalgesic sensations from deep tissues are commonplace following ordinary tissue injury. Mechano-hyperalgesia, heat-hyperalgesia and cold-hyperalgesia may occur singly or in various combinations.

Allodynia and hyperalgesia are very common symptoms. They may occur, singly or in various combinations, in any of the peripheral neuropathies and in patients with central pain. Patients with a completely transected spinal cord obviously do not have evoked pain from below the level of the lesion, but abnormal evoked pain may be present near the dermatomal border of the lesion. The conceptual difference between allodynia and hyperalgesia is straightforward, but it must be admitted that in practice it is often difficult or impossible to differentiate the two (Hansson & Lindblom 1992).

HYPERPATHIA

It is not uncommon for abnormal evoked pains to be present despite any degree of sensory loss short of anaesthesia. Hyperpathia is the term given to this condition: abnormal pain evoked from an area where there is an increased threshold for sensory detection (Merskey 1986). Hyperpathic pain can be evoked by normally innocuous stimuli, by normally noxious stimuli, or by both. The pain is often felt after a remarkable delay and it may only appear after repeated stimulation (Noordenbos 1959). Hyperpathic pain is described as having an 'explosive' onset and a greatly exaggerated severity. A personal experience with an experimental, hyperpathia-like condition is illustrative. Capsaicin was applied repeatedly to the volar skin of my forearm for 3 days, in order to test its desensitizing effect on C-fibre-mediated sensations. The efficacy of the treatment was assessed with a psychophysical examination of the heat–pain threshold using a small contact thermode and brief (3 s) heat pulses. As expected, the treatment blunted the sensation of gradually increasing warmth that precedes noxious temperatures and elevated the pain threshold beyond my normal value of about 44°C. Heat stimuli of ascending intensity were applied in sets of three. I did not feel the 45°C and 46°C stimuli or the first two applications of 47°C, but the third 47°C stimulus evoked extraordinary sensations. There was a delay of several seconds and then a sudden burning pain of great intensity. The burning sensation quickly acquired an aching and stabbing quality and the pain spread from the stimulation site to include the entire upper arm and shoulder. The pain abated slowly and disappeared after

10–15 minutes. The normal response to this stimulus is an easily tolerated superficial burning pain that is localized to the stimulation site and lasts for less than 20 seconds.

Hyperpathic pain clearly has unique characteristics, but it is not clear whether it is a separate kind of abnormality. It may be more appropriate to consider it as a special case where allodynia and/or hyperalgesia coexist with a marked reduction in the amount of afferent activity that reaches the generator(s) of the abnormal sensation.

PAROXYSMAL EVOKED-PAIN

Some patients have stimulus-evoked pains with qualitative and spatial characteristics different from those described above. In these cases, there is a discrete focus (sometimes several) that when stimulated produces a pain that is usually described as 'shooting, electric shock-like'. These foci are sometimes called 'trigger points', but it is conceptually important to distinguish between these foci and the trigger points of myofascial pain syndromes.

In tic douloureux, there is sometimes a focus (or foci) where normally innocuous stimulation evokes paroxysmal pain that is felt at a separate location, without any pain in the area between the focus and the site where the pain is felt (e.g. Dubner et al 1987). This appears to be unique to tic, as is the refractory (postictal) period which follows such an attack. Tic patients may also have a focus where normally innocuous stimulation evokes paroxysmal pain in the immediately surrounding area. In several peripheral neuropathies, stimulation of the focus produces pain with an electric shock-like quality that travels ('shoots') into a distal extremity or thoughout a contiguous region. These patterns are discussed in more detail below.

SPATIOTEMPORAL ABNORMALITIES OF STIMULUS-EVOKED NEUROPATHIC PAIN

As noted above, allodynic, hyperalgesic and hyperpathic pains are all characterized by their abnormal severity. Both the clinical and experimental literature have generally ignored a separate analysis of the principal components of pain severity: intensity, duration and area. Thus, for example, it is usually not known whether a patient's hyperalgesic response to a 45°C heat stimulus is abnormally severe because the intensity of the pain is too great, or whether the intensity is normal but the pain lasts too long, or whether both the intensity and the duration of the pain are normal, but the pain spreads too far.

Abnormal pain duration?

Investigations of this question have just begun, but preliminary data suggest there may be separable abnormalities of pain intensity and duration. For example, Figure 10.1 shows records of the time course of continuous sensory intensity ratings for pain evoked by brief pulses of noxious heat administered to symptomatic and normal skin of a patient with a posttraumatic neuropathy affecting one arm. The peak intensity ratings for a 47°C stimulus were at the maximal scale value on both the normal and symptomatic sides, so there is no information here about a possible abnormality of pain intensity (but on other tests this patient was shown to have no more than a minor degree of heat-hyperalgesia). However, the duration of the pain evoked on the symptomatic side is unequivocally abnormal.

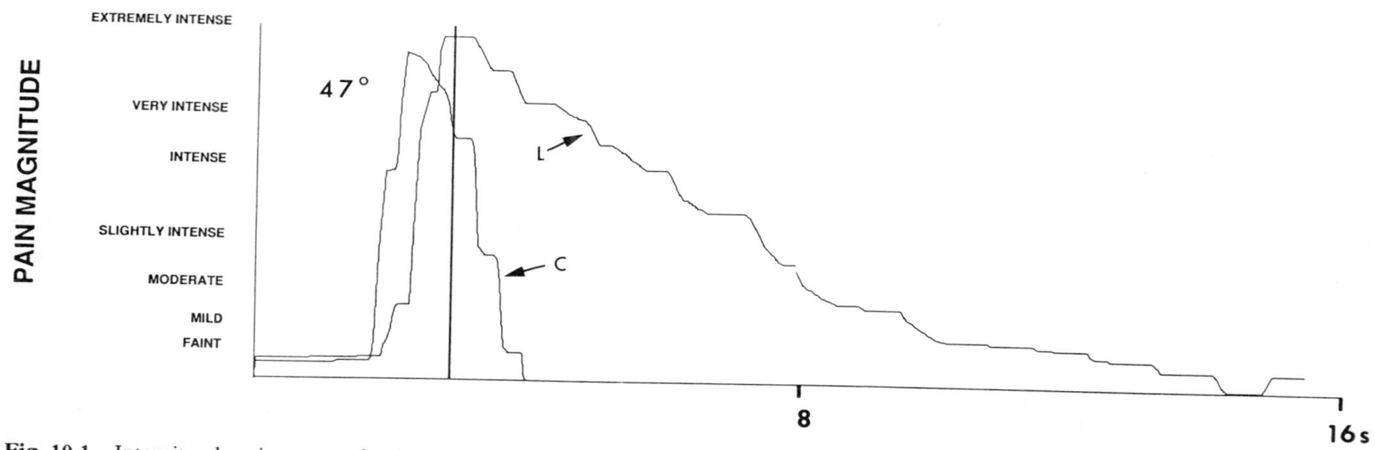

Fig. 10.1 Intensity–duration curves for the pain evoked by identical 47°C heat pulses applied to the forearm on the control (C) side and the nerve lesioned side (L) of a patient with a posttraumatic neuropathy. The vertical line marks the off-set of the 5 seconds heat pulse. The patient sat before a computer screen that showed a visual analogue scale (VAS), i.e. a pain 'thermometer', graduated with the verbal descriptors of pain intensity shown on the ordinate. Movement of a track-ball altered the height of the thermometer column. The VAS ratings were stored for subsequent display of the intensity ratings versus time curve. Note that the duration of the heat-evoked pain is grossly abnormal on the nerve injured side. Similar results were obtained with other painful temperatures. (From Gracely et al, unpublished results, with permission.)

Pain radiation

Although the subject has received little study, we know that in the normal case a punctate noxious stimulus applied to skin or muscle gives rise to pain that is felt to come from a discrete focus and that this sensation radiates outwards into the surrounding region. As the intensity of the stimulus increases, the region that is felt to be painful increases (Price et al 1978, 1992b). Similarly, in the normal case, the hyperalgesia and allodynia that develop around a punctate noxious stimulus, such as an intradermal injection of capsaicin, spread outwards from the stimulation site, with the amount of spread increasing as the intensity of the initiating pain increases (Fig. 10.2C), which can be shown, for example, by increasing the concentration of capsaicin (LaMotte et al 1991).

There is little information on whether the normal relation between the intensity of evoked-pain (of the nonparoxysmal type) and the amount of spatial radiation is disturbed in the neuropathic case. However, patients do recount that an evoked-pain sensation will give rise to a lingering soreness in a large region surrounding the site of stimulation, and this may be due to exaggerated radiation, i.e. an abnormality of the normal process that governs the spatial discrimination of pain stimuli.

As noted above, patients with tic douloureux have evoked paroxysmal pain that is triggered by stimulation at a distant point. This is often called 'referred pain', but this is a potentially confusing term because the phenomenon is distinctly different from the referred pain that is triggered by noxious stimulation of viscera but felt in distant skin and muscle, e.g. the sore arm that follows cardiac ischaemia. The 'referred' pain in tic also radiates outwards.

Referred pain

The referral of pain and hyperalgesic/allodynic tenderness to skin when there is pain in deep tissues (muscle, bone and viscera) is a normal phenomenon (Bonica 1992). The magnitude and area of the pain and tenderness referred to the skin is roughly proportionate to the severity of the deep pain (Kellgren 1938; Torebjörk et al 1984; Ness et al 1990). Electrophysiological studies in animals have repeatedly demonstrated the convergence of nociceptor input from deep and cutaneus tissues on to the same somatosensory spinal neurons (Cervero & Tattersall 1987; Milne et al 1981; Cervero et al 1992).

The importance of referred pain for neuropathic pain sensations is poorly understood; indeed, it is rarely even considered (but see Torebjörk et al 1984). Potentially important implications are obvious. For example, viscerosomatic convergence may be involved in the production of RSD in an upper limb following an episode of cardiac pain (Bonica 1990). In addition, referred pain may play a role in the peculiar interplay between abnormal deep and superficial pain that has been described following nerve transection (Denny-Brown 1965).

Wind-up

In normal skin, repeating a stimulus that activates C-fibre nociceptors causes burning pain sensations whose perceived intensity increases with each successive stimulus, provided that the stimuli are presented no more than 3 seconds apart. This perceptual phenomenon (pain summation) has an exact parallel in an electrophysiological effect known as wind-up: an increased response of spinal dorsal horn neurons to repeated C-fibre input. Wind-up is not produced by each stimulus in the train evoking larger and larger C-fibre afferent volleys; in fact, with noxious heat pulses the size of the C-fibre volley decreases with each stimulus. Wind-up appears to be due to a central process; spinal cord neurons that receive the C-fibre volleys respond with increasingly greater discharges when the input arrives with intervals of 3 seconds or less (Price 1988).

Recent work indicates that there is an abnormal wind-up-like effect in some patients with RSD. As discussed in more detail below, these patients have mechano-allodynia that is mediated by the activation of Aβ low-threshold mechanoreceptors, afferents whose activation is normally followed by tactile sensations. Price and his colleagues (1989, 1992a) have shown that repeated Aβ-strength stimuli produce burning pain sensations of increasing intensity, but only if the stimuli are, as in wind-up, presented at intervals of 3 seconds or less (Fig. 10.3B). Thus, low-threshold mechanoreceptors appear to have gained access to the central mechanism underlying wind-up, a mechanism that is normally accessed only by C-nociceptor input. It is not known whether these patients also have an abnormality of C-nociceptor-evoked pain summation.

Shooting pain

In some patients with peripheral neuropathies (other than tic), stimulation of a focus evokes pain at the focus and an electric shock-like pain that 'shoots' throughout an extremity. Unlike the paroxysmal pains of the tic patient, where electric shock-like pains jump (refer) to a distant location, the shooting pain of these patients travels through contiguous areas and there is no evidence for the existence of a refractory period. This type of evoked paroxysmal pain is encountered in patients with painful phantoms, where it is triggered by pressing on the stump neuroma and the pain is felt to shoot into the missing limb. It is also encountered in some posttraumatic neuropathies, and here also the trigger site may be a neuroma (Gracely et al 1992).

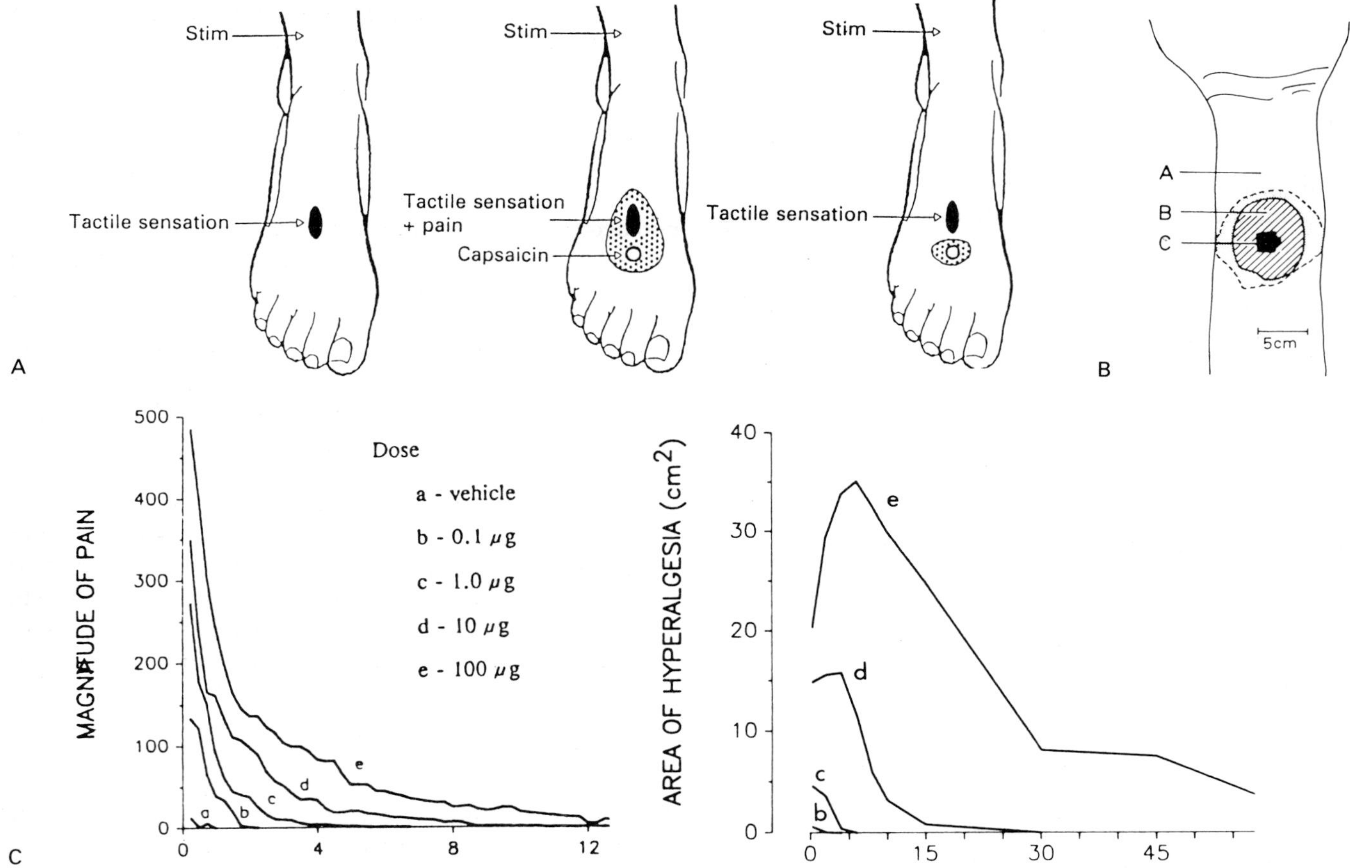

Fig. 10.2 Neuropathic pain-like sensations in normal human subjects treated with capsaicin. **A** Evidence that input from AβLTMs mediates dynamic mechano-allodynia following intradermal capsaicin injection in man. Left: Prior to injection, intraneural microstimulation (Stim) at the ankle produces an innocous tactile sensation that is referred to a small area on the dorsum of the foot. Middle: After intradermal injection of capsaicin (open circle), an area of dynamic mechano-allodynia (stippled) develops and overlaps the area of referred sensation. Microstimulation at the same intensity as before the injection now produces two coexistent sensations: the original tactile sensation and a sensation of burning pain. Right: With time, the capsaicin-evoked allodynic area shrinks. When it no longer overlaps the area of referred sensation, microstimulation evokes only the original tactile sensation. (From Torebjörk et al 1992 with permission.)
B Spatial distribution of abnormal pain sensations in a normal human subject after 30 minutes of topical capsaicin application to the volar forearm. The blackened region corresponds to the area exposed to capsaicin. There are three overlapping zones of altered sensibility. Within the largest zone (shaded region), a von Frey hair of moderate stiffness evoked hyperalgesia. The normal response to this von Frey hair is a 'sharp' or 'pricking' sensation that is variously described as dysaesthetic or barely painful. This sensation is believed to be similar to the 'static' allodynia or 'high-threshold' allodynia of Ochoa et al (1989) and Price et al (1992a). Stroking the skin with a cotton wisp within the second zone (horizontal lines) evoked a burning pain ('dynamic' allodynia). The dynamic mechano-allodynia disappeared during a tourniquet block at the same time as normal touch sensation. The dynamic allodynia is similar to what is seen in patients with peripheral neuropathies (Ochoa et al 1989; Price et al 1989, 1992a). Stimulation of the innermost region (blackened) with a blunt pressure probe evoked pain with stimulus intensities that were normally innocuous. This allodynia was unaffected by a tourniquet block at the time that Aβ- and Aδ-mediated sensations (touch and cooling) were blocked, and it was thus dependent on C-fibre activity. The C-fibre-mediated allodynia in this case may be due to C-nociceptors sensitized by the capsaicin and/or to C-nociceptor-evoked central hyperexcitability. This single individual presents evidence for the simultaneous presence of at least three kinds of mechano-allodynia: AβLTM-mediated dynamic allodynia, C-nociceptor mediated allodynia and the static allodynia evoked by punctate stimuli that is not due to AβLTM input. (From Koltzenburg et al 1993 with permission.)
C Magnitude estimations of the pain evoked by several doses of intradermally injected capsaicin in normal subjects (left-hand graph) and the area of brush-evoked (cotton wisp) pain in the area surrounding the injection. Note that increasing the dose increases the initial pain magnitude and produces a larger and longer-lasting mechano-allodynia. Ordinates are minutes postinjecton. The pain produced by the injection of capsaicin is due to C-nociceptor activation. The brush-evoked allodynia is believed to be due to AβLTM input that acts on hyperexcitable processing centres in the CNS. (From Simone et al 1989 with permission.)

THE QUALITY OF NEUROPATHIC PAIN SENSATIONS

Abnormal pain of normal quality

Although many patients report that there is a strangeness about their neuropathic pain, they are usually able to recognize familiar qualities in their sensations (burning, stabbing, aching, etc.). In normal people, noxious stimulation of the skin and muscles can give rise to sensations with distinctly different qualities. Selective activation of cutaneous C-fibre nociceptors is followed by a sensation of superfical burning pain. Activation of both C-fibre and Aδ

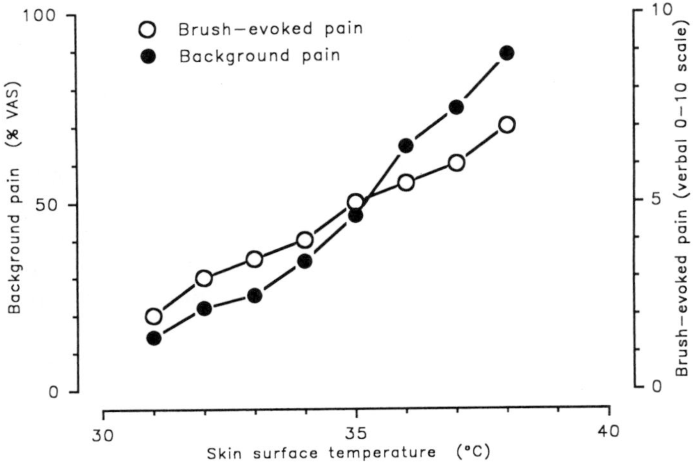

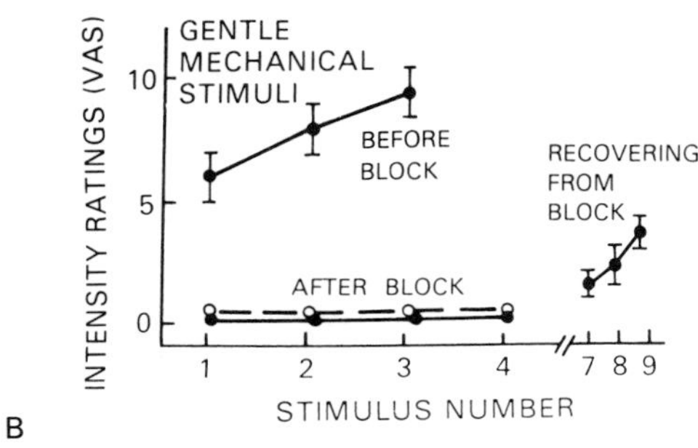

Fig. 10.3 Evidence for the modulation of neuropathic pain by a dynamically maintained central abnormality. **A** Pain intensity ratings (visual analogue scale, VAS) of a patient with a peripheral neuropathy. The patient was asked to rate the intensity of his ongoing pain (left-hand ordinate) and the pain evoked by a standard gentle brushing stimulus (right-hand ordinate). Increasing the symptomatic skin's temperature with a heating lamp increased the ongoing pain's intensity and this was significantly correlated with the intensity of the brush-evoked pain. (From Koltzenburg et al 1992 with permission.) **B** Pain intensity ratings from a patient with a sympathetically-maintained peripheral neuropathy. Before a local anaesthetic block of the sympathetic ganglia, gently brushing symptomatic skin (filled circles, solid line) with a cotton gauze pad evoked pain that summated when the stimuli were repeated once every 3 seconds ('wind-up'). After the ganglionic block, the patient's spontaneous pain disappeared and gentle brushing did not evoke pain in the previously symptomatic skin. As expected, brushing produced only an innocous tactile sensation when the same area was brushed on the opposite side (open circles, broken line). As the block faded and spontaneous pain began to return, brushing once again produced pain, but only when the stimulus was repeated at least seven times. The hypothesis put forward by Gracely et al (1992) suggests that this patient has an ongoing pain that is maintained and modulated by activity in the sympathetic system; the ongoing pain maintains an abnormality of central processing that accounts for the AβLTM- evoked allodynia produced by brushing. (From Price et al 1989 with permission.)

nociceptors by a brief noxious electrical or heat stimulus is followed by a two component pain experience – an initial pain that is felt to have a sharp, pricking quality and a second pain with a burning quality. Several lines of evidence indicate that the initial pain follows the arrival of impulses from Aδ nociceptors and that the second, burning pain follows the delayed arrival of C-nociceptor input (Price 1988). In contrast, activation of the nociceptors in muscle gives rise to a sensation of aching or cramping and these sensations have been shown to be present even in the absence of actual muscle contraction (Torebjörk et al 1984; Simone et al 1992). Anatomically, we know that cutaneous and deep nociceptors, as well as cutaneous C-fibre and Aδ nociceptors, terminate with different patterns in different regions of the spinal grey matter (Cervero & Connell 1984; Cervero & Tattersall 1987; Sugiura et al 1989). The presence of distinct pain qualities from normal skin and muscle, and the anatomical distinctions between their central terminations, raises the question of whether the different qualities of neuropathic sensations are due to abnormalities in different kinds of primary afferents or in their associated central encoding circuits. For example, we know that spontaneous discharges arise in primary afferents whose axons have been cut: does spontaneous discharge in the C-fibre nociceptors that had innervated skin produce a sensation of superficial burning pain, while spontaneous discharge in nociceptors that had innervated muscle result in deep aching pain?

Abnormal pain of abnormal quality: electric shock-like pain

A significant number of neuropathic pain sensations are described as 'shooting' and 'like an electric shock'. I have asked patients who report this type of pain if they have ever experienced an actual electric shock and nearly all have replied that they have, usually an accidental painful exposure to household current (60 Hz, 110 V). Most insist that their symptomatic pain is very similar or identical to a real shock.

Electrical stimulation of the skin or transcutaneous stimulation of a somatosensory nerve in normal subjects, or direct stimulation of an exposed nerve in surgical patients without neuropathy, reliably produces distinct sensations that vary with the frequency and intensity of the shocks (Collins et al 1960; Price 1988). Low-intensity shocks produce tactile sensations. At low frequencies these feel like taps. At progressively higher frequencies, the taps merge into an unnatural buzzing or tingling sensation, which many people find to be distinctly dysaesthetic, but not painful. The sensation produced by low-intensity stimulation occurs when the activation of Aβ fibres is detected in the neurogram (i.e. the sensory evoked potential). When the intensity is increased such that the neurogram shows the activation of Aδ fibres, the tactile sensations are joined by a sensation of sharp or stabbing pain. Increasing the intensity still further, such that C-fibres are recruited, adds another sensation – a burning pain that appears with a distinct delay (especially noticeable with stimulation of the distal extremities). When the electrical stimulus is delivered directly to the skin, each of the sensations evoked by increasingly strong shocks is felt to originate at or around the site of stimulation. But when a nerve is stimulated, the sensations are felt distally, in the territory of the nerve.

The sensations evoked by electrical stimulation are due to unnatural and highly synchronized afferent volleys. It is possible that the paroxysmal electric shock-like sensations of some neuropathic conditions are also due to such volleys. An approximately simultaneous activation of abnormally sensitive sprouts in a neuroma ought to produce the same unnatural, massive and highly synchronized volley as an electric shock to the nerve. In the experiments of Chabal et al (1992), where norepinephrine was injected into stump neuromas, eight of nine subjects described the sensation as 'shooting', 'shocks' or 'shocking' pain in their phantoms. In a patient whom I have examined, pressing on the neuroma of a surgically interrupted superficial peroneal nerve caused electric shock-like pain to shoot down the leg and into the toes. These examples suggest that electric shock-like pain may be diagnostic for pathological mechanisms that yield large, synchronous volleys in primary afferent neurons. However, as described below, electric shock-like pain might also be due to paroxysmal discharge in neurons in the central somatosensory system.

SUMMARY

The existence of multiple kinds of abnormal pain sensations in multiple combinations suggests that each abnormality may be due to a more or less separate pathophysiological mechanism. As discussed below, there is the additional possibility that any particular kind of abnormal pain sensation (e.g. mechanoallodynia) may arise from more than one mechanism. The sections that follow describe pathophysiological mechanisms that may be responsible for neuropathic pain sensations. Most of the evidence at hand is from experiments using animals or normal human volunteers, but in a several cases we have direct evidence of clinical relevance.

PATHOLOGICAL MECHANISMS IN THE PRIMARY AFFERENT NEURON

ABNORMAL NOCICEPTOR SENSITIZATION

An ordinary tissue injury changes the response characteristics of primary afferent nociceptors. In the normal case these afferents are silent in the absence of stimulation and respond to stimuli that are frankly or potentially noxious. Following injury and in the presence of an ongoing inflammatory state, they are sensitized and acquire an ongoing ('spontaneous') discharge, a lowered threshold for activation and an increased response to suprathreshold stimuli.

Ochoa and his colleagues have presented cases where C-fibre nociceptor sensitization appears to be expressed pathologically, i.e. in the absence of acute tissue injury or ongoing inflammation (Ochoa 1986; Cline et al 1989). Their most thoroughly studied case is a man who experienced 14 months of pain in the hand following a sunburn. The hand was hyperalgesic to noxious heat and mechanoallodynia was evoked by gently brushing the skin. Warmth aggravated the pain and cold relieved it. The symptomatic skin was hotter than normal. Microneurographic recordings from the nerve supplying the painful area revealed C-fibre afferents with exaggerated responsiveness (Fig. 10.4).

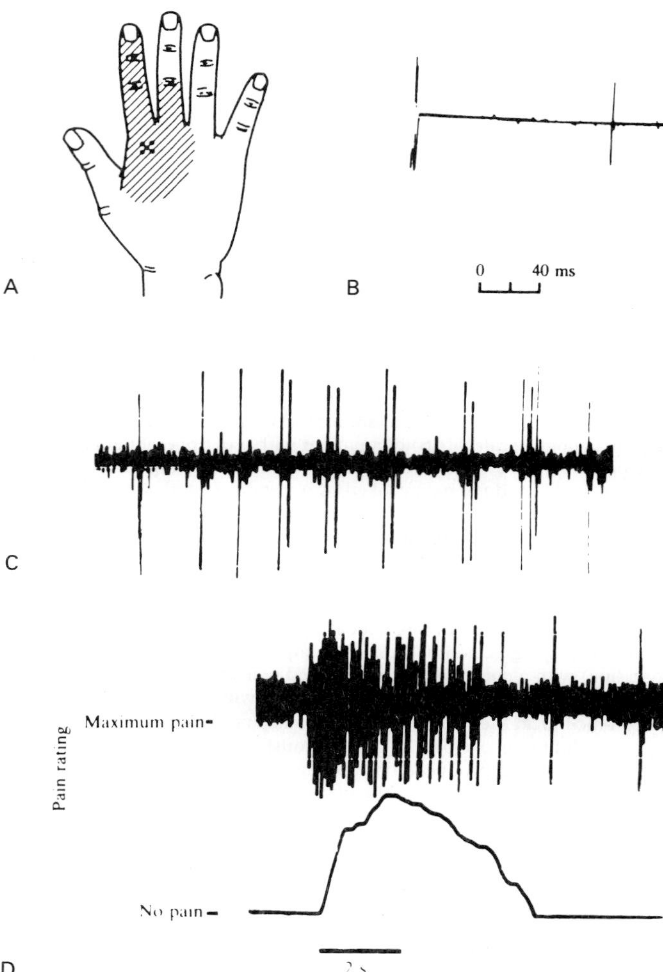

Fig. 10.4 Evidence for abnormal C-nociceptor sensitization. Single unit recording with an intraneural microelectrode of a C-fibre nociceptor with a receptive field: **A** marked with an X within the area of allodynic skin; **B** Electrical stimulation shows that the unit's conduction velocity is appropriate for an unmyelinated axon; **C** The afferent's response to nine light touch stimuli; **D** The top trace shows the afferent's response to continuous gentle stroking across its receptive field. The bottom trace shows the simultaneously obtained record of the patient's pain intensity ratings on a scale marked 'no pain' to 'maximum pain' for the period of stimulation. (From Cline et al 1989 with permission.)

The most likely interpretation of this case is that the patient's C-fibre nociceptors had failed to return to normal following the sensitization that can be presumed to have been evoked by the sunburn. The hyperalgesia and allodynia are what one expects to find in the presence of sensitized C-fibre nociceptors, as is the relief afforded by cold, which is known to counteract sensitization, and the exacerbation by warmth, which is known to amplify it (Lewis 1942; Kumazawa et al 1987). The elevation of the temperature of the symptomatic skin is also congruent with the hypothesis. C-fibre nociceptor discharge promotes cutaneous vasodilatation via the release of neuropeptides. However, this patient did not have continuous pain as a marked symptom, and the painful area was not swollen. The absence of continuous pain is compatible with a relatively minor degree of nociceptor sensitization. The absence of oedema may be related to the condition's chronicity. As the authors note, this patient's condition is very closely mimicked by the topical application of capsaicin to the skin of a normal human subject (Culp et al 1989); capsaicin selectively excites and sensitizes C-fibre nociceptors.

It should be noted that the cutaneous vasodilatation associated with C-fibre nociceptor sensitization can be masked by the vasoconstriction produced by a pain-evoked sympathetic reflex (Ochoa et al 1993). It should also be noted that it is unclear whether sensitized C-nociceptors are hyperresponsive to mechanical stimuli; Culp et al (1989) have suggested that such hyperresponsiveness may only be apparent when the skin is warm. Tissue injury also sensitizes cutaneous Aδ nociceptors, and both Aδ and C-nociceptors in deep tissue. There is no evidence as yet that abnormal sensitization of these afferents contributes to neuropathic pain.

NOCICEPTOR SENSITIZATION AND THE SYMPATHETIC NERVOUS SYSTEM

This topic is reviewed in detail in Chapter 38, but a few points need to be stressed here. Evidence from animal experimentation suggests that there may be an interaction between sensitization of the C-fibre cutaneous nociceptor terminal and the sympathetic nervous system; there is no comparable evidence for nociceptors innervating deep structures or for cutaneous Aδ nociceptors. C-fibre nociceptors with an ongoing discharge due to a sensitization-evoking tissue injury acquire an excitatory response to sympathetic stimulation and norepinephrine (Hu & Zhu 1989). In the absence of an ongoing discharge and sensitization, sympathetic stimulation has a suppressive effect on C-fibre nociceptor evoked activity. Cutaneous C-fibre nociceptors that survive a partial nerve injury acquire noradrenergic sensitivity and are subsequently more easily sensitized by tissue injury (Sato & Perl 1991). Additional evidence suggests that the sympathetic effector terminal is responsible for a chemical mediator that is necessary for the induction of nociceptor sensitization (Levine et al 1986), although evidence to the contrary has also been found (Meyer et al 1992). Lastly, a recent report indicates that selective damage to sympathetic efferents evokes the acquistion of noradrenergic sensitivity in C-fibre nociceptors (Bossut & Perl 1992). Although much more work is required to fully characterize the interaction between the activity of sympathetic efferents and nociceptor sensitization, it is already of clear importance for our understanding of pain mechanisms in peripheral neuropathies. For example, it may be that abnormal nociceptor sensitization contributes to the pain of patients with causalgia and RSD and in patients with subtotal damage to sympathetic effector axons (e.g. diabetic neuropathy and postherpetic neuralgia).

NORMAL AND SENSITIZED NOCICEPTOR DISCHARGE DUE TO OCCULT INJURY

It is possible that there are many conditions where pain is due to the activity of normal or sensitized nociceptors responding to an occult, ongoing tissue injury; such conditions might masquerade as neuropathic pain. For example, the burning pain of at least some cases of erythromelalgia (Lewis 1942) appears to be a response to vascular thrombi associated with excessive platelet production (Kurzock & Cohen 1989).

It is also possible that normally activated nociceptors are secondarily involved in peripheral neuropathies associated with vasomotor abnormalities (e.g. diabetic neuropathy). In these cases, vascular insufficiency might lead to noxious tissue conditions (e.g. hypoxia, acidosis) sufficient to activate and sensitize nociceptors. Although this is a reasonable hypothesis with a long history (Leriche 1939; Livingston 1943), there are still few data to support it.

DAMAGED PRIMARY AFFERENT AXONS AND ECTOPIC DISCHARGE

This topic is reviewed in detail in Chapter 4 and so this section will emphasize only a few selected points. Most of our information on these phenomena comes from work on neuromas following complete nerve transection. However, it is important to note that primary afferent sprouts (and their associated abnormal cell bodies) are known, or suspected, to be present in many other conditions. In diabetes and other dying-back neuropathies, sprouts are present (especially in the distal nerves) as the underlying metabolic disorder causes degeneration of the distal portion of the axon followed by attempted regeneration. The acute phase of a herpes zoster eruption causes substantial axonal damage within the nerve (directly from the virus-evoked neurolysis and indirectly from inflammation). When viral replication subsides, regenerating sprouts attempt to reinnervate and they are likely to become trapped in intraneural scars to form neuromas-in-continuity. Neuromas-in-continuity are also likely to be present in cases of subtotal nerve trauma, for example, in crush and stretch injuries. Moreover, preliminary studies suggest that small fascicles of regenerating axons may form intracutaneous microneuromas when their advance is thwarted by postherpetic scars (Bennett et al, unpublished observations).

Following peripheral axotomy, the regenerating sprouts of primary afferent nociceptors and low-threshold mechanoreceptors acquire several abnormalities that produce ectopic discharge. In animals, spontaneous ectopic discharge is seen within days of the lesion in myelinated afferents and after about 2 weeks in unmyelinated afferents. In at least some cases it is probable that this discharge is literally spontaneous, due to an inherent electrical instability of the neuronal membrane. The sprouts also acquire abnormal sensitivity to mechanical, noradrenergic, thermal and ionic stimulation and it is thus possible that some 'spontaneous' discharge is actually ongoing discharge initiated by subtle stimuli; for example, by basal levels of circulating catecholamines or by the pulsations of a nearby artery.

Spontaneous and evoked ectopic discharge in nociceptors is likely to produce the same effect as a normally evoked nociceptor discharge – a sensation of pain. Spontaneous ectopic discharge in low-threhold mechanoreceptors is likely to produce nonpainful sensations. However, the discharge will lack its normal patterning and stimulus specificity and will therefore have an abnormal quality. This abnormal quality may be paraesthetic or dysaesthetic, like the 'buzzing' or 'tingling' sensation that one experiences with a mild electric shock or recovery from a period of limb ischaemia (Ochoa & Torebjörk 1980). The combination of spontaneous ectopic discharge in nociceptors and low-threshold mechanoreceptors is likely to produce a painful sensation with a bizarre dysaesthetic component.

The sensory consequences of the abnormal stimulus-evoked ectopic discharge of sprouts has been tested in amputees with a stump neuroma. Microneurographic recordings from such a neuroma show ongoing and evoked discharge. Nyström & Hagbarth (1981) have described two patients with phantom pain and sensitive stumps in whom tapping the neuroma produced an immediate sharp pain that was followed by an accentuation of the patients' ongoing pain. Simultaneous recordings showed an initial discharge in myelinated axons followed by discharge in C-fibres. Injection of lidocaine into the neuroma blocked the tap-evoked pains and the tap-evoked neural discharges. However, spontaneous pain and spontaneous discharges were not eliminated by blocking the neuroma. This may be due to the generation of ectopic discharge in the dorsal root ganglion (see below), in which case the spontaneous discharge that they recorded would consist of impulses propagating antidromically. Injection of a potassium channel blocker, which in animals is known to greatly exacerbate a sprout's ongoing discharge, is intensely painful in patients with stump neuromas (Chabal et al 1989). Injections of norepinephrine (NE) into stump neuromas are also intensely painful, confirming the noradrenergic sensitivity of human sprouts (Chabal et al 1992). It is important to note that the painfulness of injections of a potassium channel blocker or NE was found in several cases that were of more than 20 years' duration, which indicates that abnormal primary afferent properties in humans are far more persistent than the work in animals might lead us to believe.

CROSSED AFTERDISCHARGE

The sprouts of primary afferent neurons with damaged peripheral axons can be made to discharge at high frequencies by the discharge of other afferents (Lisney & Devor 1987; Devor & Dubner 1988). The evoked discharge lacks the tight coupling of ephaptic connections (see below), often requires massive or repetitive neighbourhood discharge for initiation and often long outlasts the precipitating discharge. Devor and his colleagues have named the phenomenon 'crossed afterdischarge'. The effect is seen in both myelinated and unmyelinated afferents. One would expect that crossed afterdischarge would be clinically significant if it involved the near simultaneous excitation of a large number of afferents. Since this would involve afferents of various classes, one would predict that the resulting sensation would be a paroxysmal electric shock-like pain.

THE DORSAL ROOT GANGLIA (DRGs) OF AXOTOMIZED PRIMARY AFFERENT NEURONS

The abnormalities detected in the sprouts of damaged primary afferent neurons are also expressed at the level of their cell bodies in the DRG (see Ch. 4). For example, in rats with a chronic constriction injury to the sciatic nerve, spontaneous ectopic discharge originates in the DRG within hours of the injury, with spontaneous discharge from the sprouts appearing several days later (Kajander & Bennett 1992; Kajander et al 1992). The presence of two sites of abnormal activity, the sprout and the cell body, creates a significant problem in differentiating between peripheral and central pathogenesis. For example, in the past it has seemed reasonable to suppose that abnormal pain sensations that were not eliminated by excising or locally anaesthestizing a neuroma must represent a central pathophysiology; it is now clear that continued (or even de novo) ectopic discharge from the DRG is an alternative explanation.

Devor et al (1992) have recently shown that the DRG

ectopic generator(s) is 4–5 times more sensitive to the blocking action of low doses (i.e. doses well below those that block impulse conduction) of systemic local anaesthetics than are the ectopic generator(s) at the level of the sprout. Thus, challenge with low systemic doses of local anaesthetic might be diagnostic for ectopic discharge of DRG origin. However, pathological mechanisms in the CNS might also be sensitive to low doses of local anaesthetic. A CNS effect may explain the often noted prolongation of pain relief after a conduction block (Arnér et al 1990; Marchettini et al 1992).

EPHAPSES

There is an extensive literature from animal experiments that shows the formation of abnormal electrical connections between adjacent axons that have been demyelinated (Jänig 1988). These connections, 'ephapses', produce a very reliable transfer of impulse discharge from one fibre to its neighbour. Ephaptic cross-talk would be clinically relevant if there were large numbers of ephapses linking nociceptors with one another or linking low-threshold mechanoreceptors with nociceptors. Because there is no more than a crude somatotopic organization within many regions of nerves and roots, ephapses between afferents with different receptive fields (RFs) would be expected to result in a variety of stimulus mislocalizations. Similary, because ephapses occur between many different kinds of afferent, one would also expect to encounter instances of stimulus misidentifications. For example, gently stroking the pad of the first finger might produce an additional sensation of burning pain on the second finger. If ephapses were commonly of significance in neuropathic pain patients, one would expect that such strange phenomena would be reported frequently. In fact, I know of only one patient where this has been described (Raymond & Rocco 1990).

REFLECTED IMPULSES

Animal experiments also show that focally demyelinated axons give rise to extra ('reflected') impulses (Calvin et al 1982). The passage of an impulse through a demyelinated region leaves behind a lingering depolarization that is sufficient to initiate a new impulse as soon as the axon recovers from its refractory period; this new impulse will propagate both ortho- and antidromically. The sensory consequences of such a process would probably be trivial. However, it has been shown that repeated stimulation can produce a prolonged and high frequency discharge of 'reflected' impulses. If this were to happen in a person it would likely produce a dysaesthetic 'buzzing' sensation (from activity in Aβ low-threshold mechanoreceptors) and/or a 'stinging' pain sensation (from myelinated nociceptors). Focally demyelinated axons also have spontaneous discharge. The clinical significance of reflected impulses is unknown.

COLLATERAL SPROUTS

An area that has been completely denervated by nerve transection will receive a collateral innervation due to invading sprouts from undamaged primary afferents that innervate adjacent territories. It is possible, but not documented, that collateral sprouts also occur when there is a partial denervation (if it does, the collaterals might come from intact afferents in the damaged nerve or from afferents from undamaged nerves). Animal experiments (Markus et al 1984; Kingery & Vallin 1989; Vallin & Kingery 1991) show that skin innervated by collateral sprouts is hyperalgesic and allodynic for mechanical stimuli (responses to heat and cold have not been reported). It is nearly certain that collateral sprouting occurs in humans and that the skin innervated by sprouts is sometimes the source of painful or dysaesthetic sensations (Inbal et al 1987). The mechanisms underlying collateral hyperaesthesia are unclear. It is possible that collateral sprouts have some of the same abnormal discharge properties that are found in neuroma sprouts. It is also possible that collateral hyperalgesia is due to central pathophysiology.

PATHOLOGICAL MECHANISMS IN CNS NEURONS

It is apparent that pathological mechanisms in damaged primary afferent neurons contribute to the pain of peripheral neuropathies. Recent evidence suggests that primary afferent pathophysiology may, in turn, evoke central pathophysiology. It has been hypothesized that some conditions may initially be due mostly or completely to primary afferent pathology and gradually evolve so that the primary or sole cause of the pain is due to central pathology (Noordenbos & Wall 1981; Bennett 1991; Gracely et al 1992). In contrast, it is nearly certain that at least some cases of central pain (e.g. those following a thalamic infarct) are due entirely to pathological mechanisms in CNS neurons. The relationship between the central mechanisms operating in cases of central pain and the central mechanisms produced as a consequence of primary afferent pathology is unknown.

There is a long list of anatomical and neurochemical changes that take place in the CNS after peripheral nerve injury. The intraspinal terminal arbors of axotomized primary afferents sprout and invade new territories within the dorsal horn (Snow & Wilson 1989; LaMotte et al 1989; Woolf et al 1992). Axotomized afferents cease making their normal neuropeptides (e.g. substance P (sP) and calcitonin gene-related peptide (CGRP)) and begin making different ones, such as neuropeptide Y, galanin, and vasoactive intestinal polypeptide (Bennett et al 1989; Wakisaka et al 1992). There is a dramatic upregulation of early immediate gene regulation (e.g. c-fos) in intrinsic spinal neurons that suggests a dramatic and prolonged response of second order neurons to changes in their input (Basbaum et al 1992). One such change is known to be a large increase in the production of the endogenous opioid, dynorphin (Kajander et al 1990). The significance of the anatomical and neurochemical changes that follow peripheral nerve injury is unknown, but their presence suggests that all cases of nerve damage may have central consequences that are of potential pathophysiological importance.

MECHANO-ALLODYNIA: DYNAMIC AND STATIC

There is a large body of evidence showing that activity in Aβ low-threshold mechanoreceptors (AβLTMs), which normally gives rise only to innocuous tactile sensations, may give rise to a burning pain sensation due to abnormal CNS processing. The evidence from peripheral neuropathy patients (mostly posttraumatic cases) comes from several observations (Campbell et al 1988; Price et al 1989; Gracely et al 1992). Touch-evoked pain disappears during a tourniquet block of the symptomatic limb at the same time as normal tactile sensations, which in turn corresponds to the blockade of the Aβ potential in the neurogram. With a local anaesthetic block of a peripheral nerve that innervates the symptomatic area, touch-evoked pain is present at the time when conduction in Aβ-fibres and tactile sensations are present, but Aδ and C-fibre conduction and sensations of pain, warmth and cold are blocked. The reaction time to an Aβ-strength pain-evoking electrical pulse applied transcutaneously to symptomatic skin is too fast to include an afferent C-fibre limb and thus must be due to input from myelinated, probably Aβ, afferents.

In patients who experience pain when hairs are moved or when a cotton swab is gently drawn across the skin, transcutaneous stimulation of a nerve supplying a symptomatic limb evokes two coexistent sensations. As the intensity is increasing gradually from values that evoke no sensation to the value that first elicits any type of sensation, the detection-level sensations are described as a normal tactile sensation (tap or 'buzz', depending on whether single pulses or short high-frequency pulse trains are used) and an abnormal pain that is usually described as burning. The patients report that the burning pain is similar or identical to their touch-evoked pain. Electrical stimulation that is at threshold for detection is known to be of an intensity that excites only Aβ-fibres.

In other posttraumatic neuropathy patients, Price and his colleagues (1992a) have shown that transcutaneous electrical stimulation of a nerve supplying symptomatic skin gives rise first to a normal tactile sensation and then, at intensities about double the detection level, to an abnormal burning pain sensation. In the normal case, this intensity gives rise to a strong but still nonpainful tactile sensation. This higher-threshold abnormal pain occurs in patients who do not experience pain when a cotton swab is gently drawn across the skin, but these patients do experience pain when exposed to normally innocuous punctate stimuli (von Frey hairs of moderate stiffness). This distinction has been noted previously, where the designations of 'dynamic' and 'static' have been applied (Ochoa et al 1989). The 'static' (punctate stimuli) allodynia does not appear to depend on activation of AβLTMs. In patients, it survives tourniquet block that differentially interrupts conduction in myelinated fibres (Ochoa et al 1989).

In normal human volunteers, an intradermal injection of capsaicin produces a change in the sensations evoked by innocuous mechanical stimuli applied to a large area surrounding the injection. Lightly stroking the skin with a cotton wisp produces a sensation that is described as 'burning', 'like a sunburn' or 'raw'. This mechano-allodynia also appears to be the result of activity in AβLTMs (Torebjörk et al 1992; Koltzenburg et al 1992; Gracely et al 1993). Some of the evidence for this is shown in Figure 10.2. The touch-evoked pain following capsaicin injection may be similar, or even identical, to the touch-evoked pain of some peripheral neuropathy patients. However, it is important to note that many patients experience pain following activation of the AβLTMs that innervate hair follicles; hair movement is not painful in the skin surrounding a capsaicin injection.

Normal human volunteers who receive an intradermal injection or topical application of capsaicin also experience 'static' allodynia (LaMotte et al 1991; Koltzenburg et al 1992). Stimulation with pin prick or a moderately stiff von Frey hair, which normally evokes a sensation described as 'sharp' that may or may not be considered 'barely painful', evokes an exceptionally strong 'stinging' pain. This abnormal sensation is distinct from the AβLTM-mediated pain following stimulation with a cotton wisp. It can be evoked from a larger area and it lasts for much longer, e.g. following an intradermal injection of 100 μg of capsaicin, the cotton wisp-evoked pain lasts for about 2 hours, the abnormal pain evoked by a punctate stimulus lasts for more than 24 hours (LaMotte et al 1991). Treede & Cole (1993) have recently tested a man who had a profound loss of Aβ fibres, but with Aδ- and C-fibres intact (the loss followed a viral infection that left the man with multiple disabilities, but not with pain). Following an intradermal injection of capsaicin, he developed the abnormal pin-prick pain, but not the pain that usually follows stroking with a cotton wisp.

In summary, data from patients and from normal human volunteers in the capsaicin experiments suggest that 'dynamic' mechano-allodynia involves AβLTMs while 'static' mechano-allodynia involves Aδ- and/or C-fibres (presumably nociceptors). The capsaicin experiments suggest that these two abnormalities can coexist; the data from patients suggest that they may exist separately or together (Price et al 1992a). 'Static' and 'dynamic' mechano-allodynia are most probably dependent on different central mechanisms. It is tempting to invoke a generalized central hyperexcitability mechanism, such as that proposed for spinal wide-dynamic-range (WDR) neurons (Roberts 1986), to explain these symptoms. But the problem is not so easily solved. A generalized hyperexcitability of some central pain-signalling neurons would render the cells more responsive to all of their inputs. If this were present in a patient, or a subject receiving capsaicin, one would expect to find heat-hyperalgesia, mechano-hyperalgesia, and mechano-allodynia (static and dynamic) occurring all together. However, patients very often have one symptom without the other and the subjects in the capsaicin experiments have abnormal mechanically-evoked pains but no heat-hyperalgesia.

C-FIBRE NOCICEPTOR-EVOKED CENTRAL HYPEREXCITABILITY

Animal experiments have shown that the arrival of input from C-fibre nociceptors evokes a plastic change in the responsiveness of spinal cord dorsal horn neurons. With a small initiating input, the central change is fleeting, but with a sufficiently large input the central change persists for periods of at least hours without additional nociceptor input (Cervero et al 1984; Woolf & Wall 1986; Woolf & Thompson 1991). Nocireceptive dorsal horn neurons (both nociceptive specific and WDR types) become more responsive to all of their inputs; for example a WDR neuron will have an increased discharge when its RF is stimulated with pinch or gentle brushing (Simone et al 1991). In addition, the size of the cell's RF is enlarged (McMahon & Wall 1984; Cook et al 1987; Hylden et al 1989; Cervero et al 1992). One would expect these physiological changes to be accompanied by altered pain sensations. In animals, these changes are associated with exaggerated nocifensive withdrawal reflexes that are indicative of perceptual hyperalgesia.

The onset of many peripheral neuropathies is likely to be accompanied, or preceded, by C-nociceptor barrages. For example, partial or complete nerve transections will be accompanied by the injury discharge that is emitted by newly severed axons. The acute phase of postherpetic neuralgia is very painful due to the neuritic and cutaneous inflammation. RSD is generally precipitated by a soft tissue injury, although the injury sometimes appears to be of trivial severity. It is highly suggestive that the injuries leading to RSD are very often injuries to the musculoskeletal system (sprains, fractures, orthopaedic surgery), while strictly cutaneous injuries (lacerations, burns, abrasions) are relatively rare precedents. In animals, volleys in musculoskeletal C-fibres evoke a more pronounced and longer-lasting central hyperexcitability than that evoked by comparable volleys in cutaneous C-fibres. Aδ nociceptor discharge appears to evoke a relatively weak central hyperexcitability (Woolf & Wall 1986).

DISINHIBITION: HYPEREXCITABILITY DUE TO EXCITOTOXICITY

As noted above, C-nociceptor discharge in animals produces a central state of hyperexcitability. There is a growing body of evidence that shows that this hyperexcitability involves activity at glutaminergic synapses of the N-methyl-D-aspartate (NMDA) type for its initiation and for its maintenance (Woolf & Thompson 1991). Experimental models of epilepsy and stroke show that high levels of activity at NMDA synapses in the hippocampus and cerebral cortex produce an excitotoxic insult in certain neurons. It has been hypothesized that a similar excitotoxic phenomenon takes place in the spinal cord following peripheral nerve injury (Sugimoto et al 1990). The phenomenon is detected anatomically by the appearance of transsynaptic degenerative changes in small to medium size spinal neurons in dorsal horn laminae I–III. Cells showing these changes have been named 'dark neurons'; they have an increased chromophilia (for toluidine blue) in both cytoplasm and nucleoplasm and irregular, ruffled nucleoplasmic and cytoplasmic membranes that suggest that the cell has shrivelled. It is not known whether dark neurons die or whether they completely or partially recover. Following nerve injury, the incidence of dark neurons is greatly increased if the animal is given subconvulsive doses of strychnine, a procedure that does not produce dark neurons by itself. Strychnine blocks postsynaptic inhibitory potentials and would thus be expected to exacerbate an excitotoxic mechanism. It has been proposed that dark neurons appear secondary to the high incidence of ectopic discharge in injured primary afferent neurons and that the affected cells include inhibitory interneurons (Sugimoto et al 1990; Kajander & Bennett 1992). If the altered appearance of dark neurons indicates that the cells have at least some degree of functional impairment, then one would expect to see a decrease in the inhibitory processes that are normally triggered by primary afferent input. Electrophysiological evidence for such disinhibition has been obtained in animal models (Wall & Devor 1981; Woolf & Wall 1982; Laird & Bennett 1992). Moreover, one would predict that the behavioural consequences of this disinhibition would be exacerbated by strychnine and inhibited by NMDA-receptor blockade. A rapidly growing body of evidence from experiments in animals with neuropathic pain supports these predictions (Davar et al 1991; Mao et al

1992b, 1992c, 1993; Yamamoto & Yaksh 1992a, 1992b, 1993; Tal & Bennett 1993a).

ALTERED CENTRAL PROCESSING DYNAMICALLY MAINTAINED BY ONGOING NOCICEPTOR INPUT

A recent hypothesis suggests that once initiated, central hyperexcitability might be dynamically maintained and modulated by a source of ongoing nociceptor discharge (Gracely et al 1992). Evidence for this hypothesis comes from experiments on patients who have one or more foci of unusually great sensitivity and areas of allodynic and hyperalgesic skin that are spatially remote from the focus. As shown in Figure 10.5, gentle palpation of such a focus, which may lie near the original site of injury or near a subsequent surgical exploration, produces an intense pain that shoots throughout the entire affected limb. Local anaesthesia of the focus eliminates the patient's ongoing pain and eliminates the allodynia and hyperalgesia in the spatially remote areas. Importantly, the elimination of the remote allodynia and hyperalgesia is not accompanied by any change in the thresholds for sensation; the only change is a normalization of sensibility.

A key feature of this hypothesis is that multiple mechanisms might produce the maintaining nociceptor drive. For example, in sympathetically-maintained pain the nociceptors may themselves be driven by activity in sympathetic efferents, while in sympathetically-independent pain the nociceptor discharge might be due to spontaneous ectopic discharge from nociceptor sprouts in a neuroma or to an essentially normal nociceptor input from poorly healed tissue damage. In the cases tested by Gracely et al (1992), the source of maintaining input was focal. However, a maintaining input that was spatially disseminated might serve as well, for example, noradrenergically-sensitive nociceptor terminals throughout the skin, as suggested by the experiments of Bossut & Perl (1992) and Davis et al (1991). The hypothesis suggests a parsimonious explanation for both the similarities and the differences of several kinds of painful peripheral neuropathy. The similarity is the underlying dynamically-maintained central abnormality; the differences are due to the multiplicity of mechanisms that can sustain the maintaining nociceptor input.

Recent evidence indicates that the intensity of the peripheral input that maintains abnormal central processing modulates the severity of the associated symptoms. Patients often note that the severity of their stimulus-evoked pains increases when their ongoing pain level is increased (Gracely et al 1992). In experiments with patients with painful peripheral neuropathies, Koltzenburg and his colleagues (1993) showed that there is a very strong positive correlation between the intensity of the patient's ongoing pain (manipulated by holding skin temperature at various levels) and the intensity of allodynic pain produced by lightly touching the skin (Fig. 10.3A). They demonstrated the same phenomenon in normal subjects who had received a cutaneous application of capsaicin.

CENTRAL HYPEREXCITABILITY AFTER PERIPHERAL NERVE INJURY

In rats with a chronic constriction injury to the sciatic nerve (Bennett & Xie 1988), a subset of spinal neurons (including spinothalamic tract neurons) in the affected segments acquire abnormal responses (Palecek et al 1992; Laird & Bennett 1993). Rats with this nerve injury have behavioural signs of spontaneous pain (or dysaesthesia), hyperalgesia and allodynia. The spinal neurons discharge spontaneously at abnormally high frequencies. Many have no peripheral RFs, although they often respond to input from the neuroma (as do many of the neurons that retain RFs). When an RF is present, these neurons have abnormally prolonged afterdischarges following brief noxious stimulation of the skin or the neuroma. In behavioural studies, rats with this nerve injury appear to have stimulus-evoked pain sensations of unusually long duration. Similar abnormal responses in spinothalamic tract neurons have been found in monkeys with a peripheral neuropathy created by interruption of two lumbar spinal nerves (Kim & Chung 1992; Palecek et al 1993). It is of interest to note that in their analysis of the Kim & Chung model, Palecek et al (1993) found a significantly higher incidence of neurons with abnormal properties in the segments adjacent to those innervated by the injured spinal nerves. Both studies of the Bennett & Xie model (Palecek et al 1992; Laird & Bennett 1993) recorded only from the segments at the heart of the injured nerve's territory.

Abnormal responses are also present in the thalamus and cortex of rats with the chronic constriction injury (Guilbaud et al 1990; Guilbaud 1992). Ventrobasal thalamic neurons in these rats exhibit several abnormalities, including increased spontaneous discharge frequency, spontaneous paroxysmal discharges, lowered thresholds and increased responses to noxious heat, cold and mechanical stimuli, and prolonged afterdischarges. The majority of the abnormally responsive neurons were in the thalamus contralateral to the side of the nerve injury, but some were in the ipsilateral thalamus. Some rats with this nerve injury develop signs of neuropathic pain in the paw opposite to the nerve injury (Attal et al 1990) and these mirror-image pains, which are also noted in human causalgiaform neuropathies, may be associated with the unexpected abnormalities in the ipsilateral thalamus. Neurons in the hind paw representation in the somatosensory cerebral cortex (SM1; equivalent to the human postcentral gyrus) were also markedly abnormal, demon-

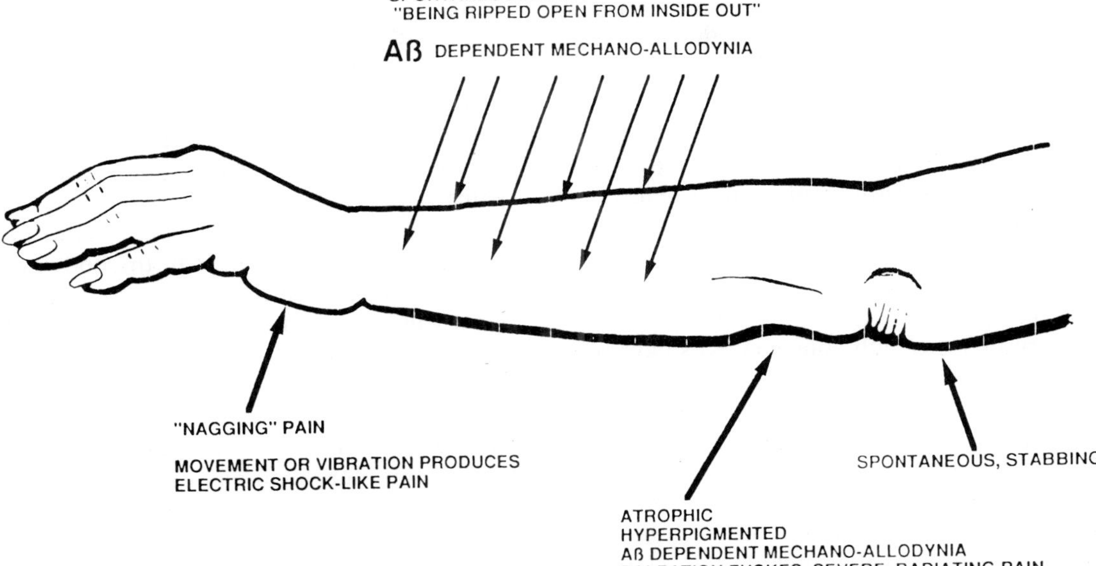

A

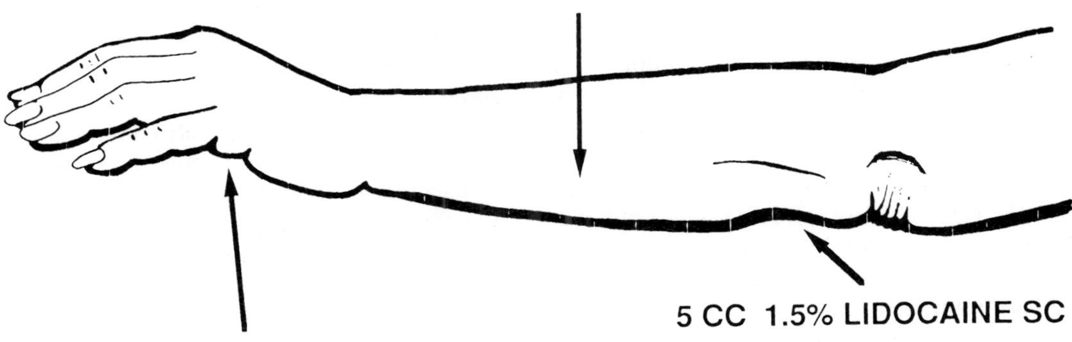

B

Fig. 10.5 A patient with a painful peripheral neuropathy subsequent to surgery (transposition of the ulnar nerve 18 months previously due to paraesthesiae and weakness indicative of ulnar entrapment). **A** The patient experienced AβLTM-mediated allodynia over the forearm, an episodic 'stabbing' pain at the elbow and a 'nagging' pain in the hand. An atrophic and hyperpigmented region just distal to the elbow developed postsurgically. Palpation of this region evoked severe 'shooting' pain that spread throughout the arm and hand. **B** Lidocaine was injected into the pain focus (the region of extreme sensitivity to palpation); this completely numbed the overlying skin and eliminated the palpation-evoked shooting pain. Within minutes the patient's spontaneous pain abated and all of the stimulus-evoked pains disappeared from the forearm and hand. Careful sensory testing showed that there was no sensory deficit in the previously allodynic areas; the only effect of blocking the pain focus was a normalization of sensibility. The abnormal spontaneous and stimulus-evoked pains returned when the local anaesthetic block of the painful focus wore off. (Adapted from Gracely et al 1992.)

strating spontaneous paroxysmal discharges, prolonged afterdischarges, lowered thresholds and increased responses to noxious and normally innocuous stimuli. It is not known whether the thalamocortical abnormalities are passive reflections of abnormal input from spinal neurons or whether there is contribution from an intrinsic pathophysiology. In contrast to the enlarged RFs seen in the spinal cord after complete nerve transection, and in the human thalamus after cord or brainstem injury (see below), the RFs of the thalamic and cortical neurons of these rats appeared to be normal.

Increased RF size

Spinal dorsal horn neurons with abnormal RFs have been noted by some authors following a complete transection of a peripheral nerve, but not after partial nerve injury (Hylden et al 1987; Snow & Wilson 1989; Palecek et al 1992; Laird & Bennett 1993). Acutely, dorsal horn neurons within the region of the spinal somatotopic map innervated by the transected nerve have no RFs, but with time some acquire 'new' RFs that include skin along the border of the denervated area. These neurons retain their synaptic connections to the severed nerve (as can be shown by their response to nerve shocks or neuroma stimulation), thus these new RFs are analogous to an enlarged RF with a silent core.

It is possible that enlarged RFs contribute to abnormal evoked-pain sensations following nerve injury. One can easily imagine that they might contribute to abnormally great pain radiation. It is also possible that they contribute to abnormal pain intensity, if perceived intensity is a function of the number of neurons responding to a stimulus (Dubner 1991). The hypothesis that pain intensity may be coded by the recruitment of larger and larger numbers of nocireceptive spinal neurons has gained considerable support from recent animal experiments (Coghill et al 1991; Mao et al 1992a). It is noteworthy that 'new' RFs are also seen in spinal dorsal horn neurons after dorsal rhizotomies and in thalamic neurons after lesions to the spinal cord and brainstem (see below).

Pathophysiology in the CNS and the spatial distribution of pain in peripheral neuropathies

One of the most puzzling features of the spontaneous and stimulus-evoked pains of peripheral neuropathies is that they are sometimes found in the territory of apparently healthy nerves. This is seen in patients with postherpetic neuralgia, where the pain is sometimes present outside of the scarred area that marks the territories of the affected nerves, and in causalgia and RSD, where the pain may have a glove- or stocking-like distribution. Mirror-image pain (i.e. the appearance of pain in the limb contralateral to the original injury) in causalgia and RSD is another example. Pain that does not respect the borders of nerve territories is not likely to be due to pathophysiology in primary afferent neurons. Cross-talk amongst afferent cell bodies in the DRGs might be advanced as an alternative to this assertion, but, as discussed above, cross-talk is likely to produce paroxysmal electric shock-like pain. In many patients, the 'extra-territorial' pain of peripheral neuropathies is not electric shock-like. In addition intraganglionic cross-talk cannot explain mirror-image pains.

The RFs of individual neurons form, in the aggregate, separate somatotopic maps of the body in the spinal cord dorsal horn, thalamus, and cortex. A central pain mechanism will be present in neurons distributed within one or more of these maps. Nerve territory borders are invisible within the somatotopic maps (there are minor exceptions, e.g. the dorsal and ventral midlines in the spinal map). For example, the RFs of dorsal horn neurons often include input from more than one major nerve. This is especially common for the large RFs of the WDR neurons of the deeper laminae, but even the small RFs of nociceptive-specific lamina I neurons sometimes straddle the border between major nerves. We would thus predict that pain due entirely or in part to a central mechanism might be felt to arise from body areas corresponding to the location of the RFs of the abnormal neurons within a particular somatotopic map, rather than from the territory of the damaged nerve. Recent experimental work (Tal & Bennett 1993b) supports this prediction. Rats with a chronic constriction injury to the sciatic nerve (Bennett & Xie 1988) have mechano-allodynia and mechano-hyperalgesia in the territory of the injured sciatic nerve and in the territory of the adjacent healthy saphenous nerve, i.e. they have mechanically-evoked neuropathic pain with a stocking-like distribution. At 18 days after the constriction injury, the sciatic or saphenous nerve was completely transected in different groups of rats; 2 days after cutting the sciatic nerve, the sciatic territory on the mid-plantar paw was anaesthetic, but the allodynia and hyperalgesia in the territory of the saphenous nerve was unaffected. Conversely, after cutting the saphenous nerve, the hyperaesthesia in the sciatic territory was unaffected, while the saphenous territory was rendered anaesthetic. These lesion studies show that the allodynic and hyperalgesic responses evoked from the saphenous territory were due to activity conveyed to the spinal cord by afferents in the undamaged nerve, rather than by afferents from the damaged sciatic nerve whose RFs overlapped the saphenous territory. It is very probable that the stocking-like distribution of neuropathic pain seen in the rats is due to AN abnormal central mechanism. Rats with the chronic constriction injury sometimes have mirror-image pain, specifically, hyperalgesia in the contralateral hind paw (Attal et al 1990), and this also implicates a central mechanism.

DIFFERENTIAL LOSS OF Aβ AFFERENTS

Nerve trauma and disease do not necessarily affect all types of primary afferent axons equally. Noordenbos (1959) suggested that a deafferentation that included a disproportionate number of Aβ low-threshold mechanoreceptors might be the basis of some painful peripheral neuropathies. The gate control theory of Melzack & Wall (1965) refined and extended this idea and proposed a model of sensory processing in the spinal cord dorsal horn that would mediate neuropathic pain via the loss of inhibition mediated by Aβ low-threshold mechanoreceptors. As discussed above, there is evidence that nerve damage leads to the loss of primary afferent-mediated inhibition, but there is no evidence that this requires *differential* damage to Aβ fibres.

DIFFERENTIAL LOSS OF Aδ FIBRES

There is evidence that a neuropathic pain sensation, cold allodynia, is mediated by a differential loss of one type of afferent – the Aδ cold-specific fibre (Yarnitsky & Ochoa 1989; Ochoa & Yarnitsky 1990). In normal humans, cold pain is produced by temperatures of 5–10°C (the exact value depends strongly on the size of the area that is cooled). The normal cold pain sensation has an aching quality together with a feeling of cold. Blocking impulse conduction in myelinated afferents with a tourniquet results in an impairment of the ability to feel small cooling stimuli, but a decrease in the threshold for cold pain (i.e. pain is produced by smaller drops in temperature). When the ability to detect all cold sensation is lost, the threshold for cold-evoked pain is 15–20°C and the pain is felt as hot and burning. The change in the quality of the sensation is remarkable; if the subject is not allowed to see what is being done, he will be convinced that the stimulus is hot. The threshold for the sensation is also remarkable; in some individuals it can approximate ordinary room temperature, which means that mere contact with the objects in the room will produce a temperature-evoked burning pain.

This phenomenon is reasonably ascribed to a central interaction between the cold-evoked activities of Aδ cold-specific afferents and cold-sensitive C-fibre nociceptors (Yarnitsky & Ochoa 1989). In the normal case, the Aδ input produces the cold sensation that overlies cold pain, and inhibits the responses to the input from the C-nociceptors. This inhibition is lost when Aδ conduction is blocked and the threshold for the C-fibre evoked sensation is thus decreased; the quality of the sensation is appropriate to the C-fibre input, burning pain, and lacks the concommitant Aδ-mediated cold sensation.

The experimental situation would be duplicated by nerve damage that had a disproportionate effect on Aδ axons while sparing C-fibres. Such patients have been described (Ochoa & Yarnitsky 1990). Their ability to detect innocuous cooling stimuli is impaired or absent, their cold pain threshold is decreased and they feel cold-evoked pain as hot and burning.

Hypothetically, there are several other mechanisms that might yield cold allodynia or cold hyperalgesia (Frost et al 1988). For example, some AβLTM afferents discharge to cooling (this phenomenon is thought to underlie a somatosensory illusion – the colder of two equal weights feels heavier). Cold-evoked discharge would be expected to produce a burning pain in patients with Aβ low-threshold mechanoreceptor-mediated allodynia (see above).

CENTRAL DEAFFERENTATION-EVOKED HYPERRESPONSIVENESS

One might expect to find spontaneous pain and abnormal stimulus-evoked pains whenever CNS neurons that normally contribute to pain sensations become spontaneously active and hyperresponsive to stimulation. Experimental evidence in animals and direct evidence from neuropathic pain patients indicate that central deafferentation can produce spontaneous discharge and hyperresponsiveness in CNS neurons. It is far from certain that the neurons that express these changes participate in the elaboration of pain sensations under normal conditions, but it is reasonable to suspect that the abnormal activity of at least some of them is related to neuropathic pain. The central deafferentation-evoked changes have some features in common with the central effects of peripheral nerve injury (peripheral deafferentation), but there are also important differences (Bonica 1991). For example, C-nociceptor-evoked hyperexcitability has a very rapid onset, but central deafferentation-evoked hyperresponsiveness takes weeks or months to develop. In addition, after dorsal root lesions the primary afferent intraspinal terminal arbors degenerate; this does not necessarily happen after peripheral nerve injury. For clarity's sake, I will refer to the phenomena evoked by central deafferentation as 'hyperresponsiveness'.

DEAFFERENTATION OF SPINAL NEURONS: DORSAL ROOT DAMAGE

Interruption of a dorsal root deafferents spinal cord neurons. Clinically, this is usually the result of trauma (avulsions or vertebral fracture) and damage to the spinal cord itself is also present. The death of primary afferent neurons also deafferents spinal neurons (e.g. as occurs after the eruption of herpes zoster or after a nerve section close to the ganglion). Single cell recordings from anaesthetized experimental preparations have shown that spinal neurons that have been extensively deafferented via multiple surgical rhizotomies are clearly abnormal

(Basbaum & Wall 1976; Lombard & Besson 1991; Albe-Fessard & Rampin 1991).

Deafferented spinal neurons acquire an abnormal spontaneous discharge (Loeser & Ward 1967; Lombard & Larabi 1983). The discharge is of high frequency and appears in one of two patterns – long trains of fairly regular discharge and paroxysmal burst discharges. The spontaneous discharge has been found in cells in both the superficial and deep laminae of the spinal grey. It has been found as early as 6 hours after root section, but its incidence clearly increases for several weeks after the lesion and thereafter declines over a course of several months. In animals, the incidence of cells with these abnormal discharges is significantly correlated with the incidence of postrhizotomy pain-related behaviours (Lombard et al 1979b; Lombard & Besson 1991). Importantly, Loeser and his colleagues (1968) have obtained recordings of spinal neuron activity in a man whose dorsal roots were lesioned by trauma to the cauda equina 19 months previously. The patient suffered from spontaneous burning pain in regions rendered anaesthetic by the lesion. High-frequency regular discharge and paroxysmal bursting discharge were seen; responses essentially identical to those seen in the experimental preparations (Fig. 10.6).

Relatively little is known of the stimulus-evoked responses of spinal neurons following rhizotomies. Basbaum & Wall (1976) have shown that some dorsal

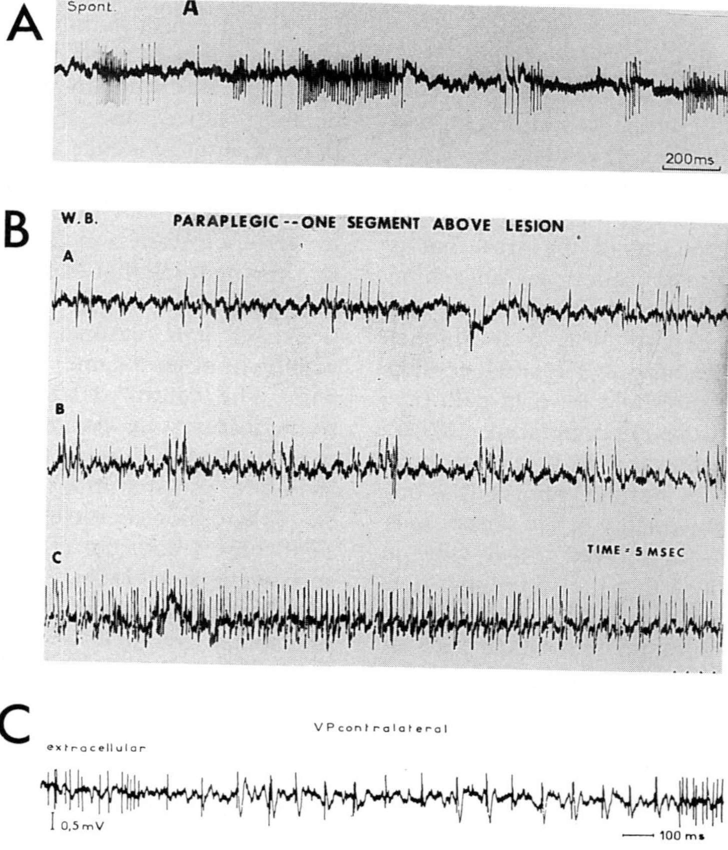

Fig. 10.6 Spontaneous paroxysmal discharges from neurons in the spinal cord dorsal horn and the ventrobasal thalamus after dorsal root lesions in man and animals (note different time scales). **A** Neuron in spinal segment C7 of a rat with rhizotomies of C5 to T1. Note the high frequency bursting discharges. (From Lombard & Larabi 1983 with permission.) **B** Three neurons in the spinal cord (segments T11 to L1) of a man whose lumbosacral dorsal roots had been crushed by an injury to the cauda equina. Note spontaneous paroxysmal discharges in the top two neurons and the abnormal high-frequency spontaneous discharge in the bottom trace. (From Loeser et al 1968 with permission.) **C** Spontaneous discharges in a neuron in the thalamic nucleus ventralis posterior (VP) of a rat with multiple cervical dorsal rhizotomies. Note the paroxysmal bursts at the beginning and end of the trace with the normal regular 10 Hz discharge in between. (From Lombard et al 1979b with permission.)

horn neurons within the deafferented segments of the cat's spinal cord acquire 'new' RFs that encompass skin along the borders of the area innervated by the cut roots. As with the 'new' RFs that appear after nerve section, it may be appropriate to think of these new RFs as enlarged RFs with silent cores. The cells with new RFs are maximally responsive to innocuous tactile stimuli; very few respond to noxious stimulation.

One might expect that the abnormal spontaneous firing of deafferented spinal neurons would appear also in the thalamic and cortical neurons that are activated by spinal input and that this would be an adequate explanation for the spontaneous pain of a patient with dorsal roots lesions. The presence of spontaneous bursting discharge in neurons of the somatosensory thalamus and cortex has been confirmed in both anaesthetized and unanaesthetized animals with multiple dorsal root transections (Lombard et al 1979a; Albe-Fessard & Lombard 1983; Albe-Fessard & Rampin 1991). In the thalamus the spontaneous bursting discharge is found interspersed with the normal 10 Hz rhythmic activity (Fig. 10.6) (Albe-Fessard & Lombard 1983). The abnormal thalamic activity is most pronounced in those parts of the somatotopic map that are deafferented by the rhizotomies, but it is also evident in adjacent regions and it is even found in the contralateral thalamus. In addition, the thalamic abnormalities appear to be expressed considerably later than the spinal phenomena, and the cortical abnormalities appear to begin later than those in the thalamus. This temporal progression suggests an evolution of pathological mechanisms, with the possibility that the spinal pathology causes that seen in the thalamus, which in turn causes that seen in the cortex. Thus it is possible that the thalamocortical abnormalities are partly a passive reflection of the abnormal input that they receive from the spinal neurons and partly due to factors initiated by the rhizotomies but elaborated secondarily in the thalamus and cortex.

Clinical evidence supports the hypothesis that an important thalamocortical pathophysiology is initiated by root damage, but subsequently becomes independent of input from the spinal cord. Lesions of spinal tracts, hemicord lesions, and even complete spinal transections have a poor record of success in the treatment of pain following dorsal root lesions (Tasker 1990). For example, the patient examined by Loeser et al (1968) was treated by removing the deafferented segments of spinal cord immediately after the single cell recordings were made; this had no effect on the patient's spontaneous pain.

Patients with dorsal root injury experience both spontaneous and evoked abnormal pain. When the patient has an area of complete anaesthesia due to extensive root damage, pain is evoked by stimulation around the borders of the anaesthetic area; when a totally anaesthetic area is absent, pain is evoked from areas whose sensibility may range from apparently normal to severely hypoaesthetic. One might therefore expect to find abnormal stimulus-evoked activity in spinal neurons in segments adjacent to the rhizotomized region. There are very few studies of abnormal stimulus-evoked activity in such spinal neurons (Brinkhus & Zimmermann 1983).

Mechanisms of postrhizotomy central hyperresponsiveness in spinal neurons

There are several hypotheses, but little supporting evidence, about the cause(s) of the abnormal spontaneous discharge of spinal neurons following root lesions. It has been proposed that the loss of primary afferent input evokes a denervation supersensitivity to primary afferent transmitters. Release of transmitter by intact afferents would thereby have an exaggerated effect. Although this would seem to be a mechanism pertinent only to abnormal evoked pain, the persistence and spread of certain transmitters, particularly primary afferent neuropeptides, in the extracellular space (Duggan et al 1989) suggest a possible connection to 'spontaneous' pain. It is known that rat spinal neurons become supersensitive to sP following dorsal root section (Roberts & Reeves 1991).

Spinal neurons are known to be under tonic descending control from modulating systems in the brainstem. A deficit in such control would be expected to yield a state of central hyperresponsiveness. Experiments in animals with dorsal root lesions have detected evidence of such a deficit in descending control (Zimmermann 1991). Indeed, Hodge et al (1983) have found that stimulation of the descending control systems originating in the locus coeruleus and raphe nuclei, which generally inhibit the activity of spinal neurons, frequently excited neurons in rhizotomized segments. Spinal neurons are also known to be under descending control of cortical origin. Rampin & Morain (1987) have shown that cortical influences on spinal neurons are greatly exaggerated after dorsal root lesion in rats.

ABNORMAL PAIN FOLLOWING CNS INJURY

Abnormal spontaneous and evoked pains, and dysaesthesia, appear after injury to the spinal cord, brainstem, thalamus and (rarely) cortex (Tasker 1990). Careful sensory testing and, more recently, improved diagnostic imaging techniques have led to the generally accepted conclusion that there is a common feature to all patients with central pain – damage to some part of the classical spinothalamic system (Cassinari & Pagni 1969; Boivie et al 1989; Leijon et al 1989). The pain is typically located in and around the area that the injury renders anaesthetic or hypoaesthetic, and there is often a very remarkable delay of months or even years between the time of injury and the appearance of the abnormal sensations. There is good reason to believe that CNS injuries produce similar or identical abnormal sensations in monkeys and other animals (Levitt 1991a, 1991b; Xu et al 1992).

Oddly, most of our knowledge about neuronal activity following CNS injury to components of the spinothalamic system comes from recording and stimulation studies in man (mostly brainstem and spinal cord injuries), rather than animals. The recordings are obtained in conscious patients with microelectrodes that are used to physiologically confirm thalamic borders prior to the placement of therapeutic lesions or chronic stimulating electrodes. Similar physiological mapping is required in patients being treated for movement disorders (without somatosensory abnormalities) and the results from these patients serve as a useful control (Lenz et al 1987; Tasker 1990; Lenz 1991).

Neurons in the ventrobasal thalamus of control ('normal') patients have RFs that form a well-organized map of the body. In the normal case, thalamic neurons have a spontaneous regular discharge of approximately 10 Hz. Microstimulation in the normal patient usually produces a nonpainful paraesthetic/dysaesthetic sensation that is felt at or near to the RFs of the adjacent neurons.

In the patients with central pain, neurons in that part of the body map representing the patient's anaesthetic area do not have any detectable RFs. Neurons whose RFs lie around the border of the anaesthetic area have RFs that are larger than normal. Many of the patient's thalamic neurons (both those with and without RFs) have spontaneous high-frequency burst discharges, a rare finding in the normal patient. Microstimulation in the vicinity of neurons without RFs frequently produces painful sensations that are felt to arise from the anaesthetic area. Microstimulation near neurons that have RFs along the border of the anaesthetic area frequently produces pain that is also felt to arise from the anaesthetic area. The quality of the microstimulation-evoked pain is often similar or identical to the patient's clinical pain.

In the 'normal' case, stimulation of thalamic regions medial to the ventrobasal complex and stimulation of the adjacent rostromedial midbrain (excluding the periaqueductal grey) does not evoke any sensation with stimulus intensities that are suprathreshold for evoked sensations in nearby regions (e.g. the medial lemniscus). However, in patients with central pain, stimulation of these medial sites evokes a somatotopographically organized pain that may closely resemble the patient's clinical pain (Tasker et al 1983; Tasker 1990). In addition, epileptiform electroencephalogram (EEG) activity has been recorded in the rostromedial midbrain of a patient with central pain (Nashold & Wilson 1966). The medial sites are known to be innervated by the ascending spinoreticulothalamic system. Tasker (1990) has proposed that the central pain patient's lesion to the spinothalamic system has disinhibited the actions of the spinoreticulothalamic system.

CONCLUSIONS

Animal and human research has revealed a large number of neural injury-evoked abnormalities in the peripheral and central nervous systems. We have very good evidence that some of them are of clinical significance for the production of neuropathic pain sensations. There does not appear to be any reason to ignore the possibility that a given patient might have two or more pathophysiological mechanisms simultaneously, with each producing different symptoms, or even with multiple mechanisms producing the same symptom. For example, there is reason to believe that mechano-allodynia can be produced by at least five different mechanisms:

1. Abnormal C-nociceptor sensitization
2. AβLTM-mediated 'dynamic' allodynia subsequent to C-nociceptor-evoked central hyperexcitability
3. Aδ/C-fibre mediated 'static' allodynia via a different C-nociceptor-evoked hyperexcitability mechanism
4. A second 'dynamic' allodynia mediated by Aβ fibres innervating hair follicles (seen in patients, but not in the capsaicin experiments)
5. An allodynia due to central deafferentation-evoked hyperresponsiveness (central pain).

The existence of multiple mechanisms, some related to the primary afferents, others to dysfunction in the CNS, yields a very complicated picture. But the complexity may be even more profound. Evidence is accumulating that the initial injury may produce one pathogenic mechanism, which in turn may produce others, so that the cause of the patient's pain changes over time. There are two lines of evidence for this. First, animal experiments suggest that ectopic primary afferent discharge may injure spinal inhibitory neurons via an excitotoxic mechanism akin to what is seen in epilepsy. The excitotoxic damage contributes to a state of spinal hyperexcitability due to disinhibition. Second, animal and human data indicate that dorsal root damage evokes a slowly evolving abnormality in spinal cord neurons, which in turn generates an abnormality in the responsiveness of thalamic neurons, which in turn may generate dysfunction in the cerebral cortex. The evidence suggests that with time these higher-level abnormalities may become independent of the lower-level abnormalities that generated them.

REFERENCES

Albe-Fessard D, Lombard M-C 1983 Use of an animal model to evaluate the origin of and protection against deafferentation pain. In: Bonica J J, Lindblom U, Iggo A (eds) Advances in pain therapy and research, vol 5. Raven Press, New York, p 691–700

Albe-Fessard D, Rampin O 1991 Neurophysiological studies in rats deafferented by dorsal root sections. In: Nashold B S, Ovelmen-Levitt J (eds) Deafferentation pain syndromes: pathophysiology and treatment. Raven Press, New York, p 125–139

Arnér S, Lindblom U, Meyerson B A, Molander C 1990 Prolonged relief of neuralgia after regional anesthetic blocks. A call for further experimental and systematic clinical studies. Pain 43: 287–297

Asbury A K, Fields H L 1984 Pain due to peripheral nerve damage: an hypothesis. Neurology 34: 1587–1590

Attal N, Jazat F, Kayser V, Guilbaud G 1990 Further evidence for 'pain-related' behaviours in a model of unilateral peripheral mononeuropathy. Pain 41: 235–251

Basbaum A I, Wall P D 1976 Chronic changes in the responses of cells in adult dorsal horn following partial deafferentation: the appearance of responding cells in a previously non-responding region. Brain Research 116: 181–204

Basbaum A I, Chi S-I, Levine J D 1992 Peripheral and central contribution to the persistent expression of the c-fos proto-onogene in spinal cord after peripheral nerve injury. In: Willis W D (ed) Hyperalgesia and allodynia. Raven Press, New York, p 295–304

Bennett G J 1991 Evidence from animal models on the pathogenesis of painful peripheral neuropathy, and its relevance for pharmacotherapy. In: Basbaum A I, Besson J-M (eds) Towards a new pharmacotherapy of pain. John Wiley, Chichester, p 365–379

Bennett G J, Xie Y-K 1988 A peripheral mononeuropathy in rat that produces disorders of pain sensation like those seen in man. Pain 33: 87–107

Bennett G J, Kajander K C, Sahara Y, Iadarola M J, Sugimoto T 1989 Neurochemical and anatomical changes in the dorsal horn of rats with an experimental painful peripheral neuropathy. In: Cervero F, Bennett G J, Headley P M (eds) Processing of sensory information in the superficial dorsal horn of the spinal cord. Plenum Press, New York, p 463–471

Boivie J, Leijon G, Johansson I 1989 Central post-stroke pain – a study of the mechanisms through analyses of the sensory abnormalities. Pain 37: 173–185

Bonica J J 1990 Causalgia and other reflex sympathetic dystrophies. In: Bonica J J (ed) The management of pain, 2nd edn. Lea & Febiger, Philadelphia, p 220–256

Bonica J J 1991 Introduction: semantic, epidemiologic, and educational issues. In: Casey K L (ed) Pain and central nervous system disease: the central pain syndromes. Raven Press, New York, p 13–29

Bonica J J 1992 Clinical importance of hyperalgesia. In: Willis W D (ed) Hyperalgesia and allodynia. Raven Press, New York, p 17–43

Bossut D F, Perl E R 1992 Sympathectomy induces novel adrenergic excitation of cutaneous nociceptors. Society for Neuroscience Abstracts 18: 287

Brinkhus H B, Zimmermann M 1983 Characteristics of spinal dorsal horn neurons after partial chronic deafferentation by dorsal root transection. Pain 15: 221–236

Brose W G, Cousins M J 1991 Subcutaneous lidocaine for treatment of neuropathic cancer pain. Pain 45: 145–148

Calvin W H, Devor M, Howe J 1982 Can neuralgias arise from minor demyelination? Spontaneous firing, mechanosensitivity, and afterdischarge from conducting axons. Experimental Neurology 75: 755–763

Campbell J N, Raja S N, Meyer R A 1988 Painful sequelae of nerve injury. In: Dubner R, Gebhart G F, Bond M R (eds) Pain research and clinical management, vol 3. Elsevier, Amsterdam, p 135–143

Cassinari V, Pagni C A 1969 Central pain: a neurological survey. Harvard University Press, Boston

Cervero F, Connell L A 1984 Distribution of somatic and visceral primary afferent fibers within the thoracic spinal cord of the cat. Journal of Comparative Neurology 230: 88–98

Cervero F, Tattersall J E H 1987 Somatic and visceral inputs to the thoracic spinal cord of the cat: marginal zone (lamina I) of the dorsal horn. Journal of Physiology (London) 388: 383–395

Cervero F, Shouenborg J, Sjölund B H, Waddell P J 1984 Cutaneous inputs to dorsal horn neurones in adult rats treated at birth with capsaicin. Brain Research 301: 47–57

Cervero F, Laird J M A, Pozo M A 1992 Selective changes of receptive field properties of spinal nociceptive neurones induced by noxious visceral stimulation in the cat. Pain 51: 335–342

Chabal C, Jacobson L, Russell L C, Burchiel K J 1989 Pain responses to perineuromal injection of normal saline, gallamine, and lidocaine in humans. Pain 36: 321–325

Chabal C, Jacobson L, Russell L C, Burchiel K J 1992 Pain responses to perineuromal injection of normal saline, epinephrine, and lidocaine in humans. Pain 49: 9–12

Cline M A, Ochoa J, Torebjörk H E 1989 Chronic hyperalgesia and skin warming caused by sensitized C nociceptors. Brain 112: 621–647

Coghill R C, Price D D, Hayes R L, Mayer D J 1991 Spatial distribution of nociceptive processing in the rat spinal cord. Journal of Neurophysiology 65: 133–140

Collins W F, Nulsen F E, Randt C T 1960 Relation of peripheral nerve fibre size and sensation in man. Archives of Neurology 3: 381–385

Cook A J, Woolf C J, Wall P D, McMahon S B 1987 Dynamic receptive field plasticity in rat spinal cord dorsal horn following C-primary afferent input. Nature (London) 325: 151–153

Culp W J, Ochoa J, Cline M, Dotson R 1989 Heat and mechanical hyperalgesia induced by capsaicin: cross modality threshold modulation in human C nociceptors. Brain 112: 1317–1331

Davar G, Hama A, Deykin A, Vos B, Maciewicz R 1991 MK-801 blocks the development of thermal hyperalgesia in a rat model of experimental painful neuropathy. Brain Research 553: 327–330

Davidoff G, Roth E J 1991 Clinical characteristics of central (dysesthetic) pain in spinal cord injury patients. In: Casey K L (ed) Pain and central nervous system disease: the central pain syndromes. Raven Press, New York, p 77–83

Davis K D, Treede R D, Raja S N, Meyer R A, Campbell J N 1991 Topical application of clonidine relieves hyperalgesia in patients with sympathetically maintained pain. Pain 47: 309–317

Denny-Brown D 1965 The release of deep pain by nerve injury. Brain 88: 725–738

Devor M, Dubner R 1988 Centrifugal activity in C-fibers influences the spontaneous afferent barrage generated in nerve-end neuromas. Brain Research 446: 396–400

Devor M, Wall P D, Catalan N 1992 Systemic lidocaine silences ectopic neuroma and DRG discharge without blocking nerve conduction. Pain 48: 261–268

Dubner R 1991 Neuronal plasticity and pain following peripheral tissue inflammation or nerve injury. In: Bond M R, Charlton J E, Woolf C J (eds) Pain research and clinical management, vol 4. Elsevier, Amsterdam, p 263–276

Dubner R, Sharav Y, Gracely R H, Price D D 1987 Idiopathic trigeminal neuralgia: sensory features and pain mechanisms. Pain 31: 23–33

Duggan A W, Morton C R, Hendry I A, Hutchinson W D 1989 Peripheral stimuli releasing neuropeptides in the dorsal horn of the cat. In: Cervero F, Bennett G J, Headley P M (eds) Processing of sensory information in the superficial dorsal horn of the spinal cord. Plenum Press, New York, p 347–363

Frost S A, Raja S N, Campbell J N, Meyer R A, Khan A A 1988 Does hyperalgesia to cooling stimuli characterize patients with sympathetically maintained pain (reflex sympathetic dystrophy)? In: Dubner R, Gebhart G F, Bond M R (eds) Pain research and clinical management, vol 3. Elsevier, Amsterdam, p 151–156

Gracely R H, Lynch S A, Bennett G J 1992 Painful neuropathy: altered central processing, maintained dynamically by peripheral input. Pain 51: 175–194

Gracely R H, Lynch S A, Bennett G J 1993 Evidence for Aβ-low-threshold mechanoreceptor-mediated mechano-allodynia and cold hyperalgesia following intradermal injection of capsaicin in the foot dorsum. Abstracts – 7th World Congress on Pain, p 372

Guilbaud G 1992 Neuronal responsivity at supra-spinal levels (ventrobasal thalamus complex and SMI cortex) in a rat model of mononeuropathy. In: Besson J-M, Guilbaud G (eds) Lesions of primary afferent fibers as a tool for the study of clinical pain. Excerpta Medica, Amsterdam, p 219–232

Guilbaud G, Benoist J M, Jazat F, Gautron M 1990 Neuronal responsiveness in the ventrobasal thalamic complex of rats with an experimental peripheral mononeuropathy. Journal of Neurophysiology 64: 1537–1554

Hansson P, Lindblom U 1992 Hyperalgesia assessed with quantitative sensory testing in patients with neurogenic pain. In: Willis W D (ed) Hyperalgesia and allodynia. Raven Press, New York, p 335–343

Hodge C J, Apkarian A V, Owen M P, Hanson B S 1983 Changes in the effects of stimulation of locus coeruleus and nucleus raphe magnus following dorsal rhizotomy. Brain Research 299: 325–329

Hu S, Zhu J 1989 Sympathetic facilitation of sustained discharges of polymodal nociceptors. Pain 38: 85–90

Hylden J L K, Nahin R L, Dubner R 1987 Altered responses of nociceptive cat lamina I spinal dorsal horn neurons after chronic sciatic neuroma formation. Brain Research 411: 341–350

Hylden J L K, Nahin R L, Traub R J, Dubner R 1989 Expansion of receptive fields of spinal lamina I projection neurons in rats with unilateral adjuvant-induced inflammation: the contribution of dorsal horn mechanisms. Pain 37: 229–243

Inbal R, Rousso M, Ashur H, Wall P D, Devor M 1987 Collateral sprouting in skin and sensory recovery after nerve injury in man. Pain 28: 141–154

Jänig W 1988 Pathophysiology of nerve following mechanical injury in man. In: Dubner R, Gebhart G F, Bond M R (eds) Pain research and clinical management, vol 3. Elsevier, Amsterdam, p 89–108

Kajander K C, Bennett G J 1992 The onset of a painful peripheral neuropathy in rat: a partial and differential deafferentation and spontaneous discharge in Aβ and Aδ primary afferent neurons. Journal of Neurophysiology 68: 734–744

Kajander K C, Sahara Y, Iadarola M J, Bennett G J 1990 Dynorphin increases in the dorsal spinal cord in rats with a painful peripheral neuropathy. Peptides 11: 719–728

Kajander K C, Wakisaka S, Bennett G J 1992 Spontaneous discharge originates in the dorsal root ganglion at the onset of a painful peripheral neuropathy in rat. Neuroscience Letters 138: 225–228

Kellgren J H 1938 Observations on referred pain arising from muscles. Clinical Science 3: 175–190

Kim S H, Chung J M 1992 An experimental model for peripheral neuropathy produced by segmental spinal nerve ligation in the rat. Pain 50: 355–363

Kingery W S, Vallin J A 1989 The development of chronic mechanical hyperalgesia, autotomy, and collateral sprouting following sciatic nerve section in rat. Pain 38: 321–332

Koltzenburg M, Lundberg L E R, Torebjörk H E 1992 Dynamic and static components of mechanical hyperalgesia in human hairy skin. Pain 51: 207–219

Koltzenburg M, Torebjörk H E, Wahren L K 1993 Nociceptor modulated central plasticity causes mechanical hyperalgesia in acute chemogenic and chronic neuropathic pain. Pain (in press)

Kumazawa T, Mizumura K, Sato J 1987 Thermally potentiated responses to algesic substances of visceral nociceptors. Pain 28: 255–264

Kurzrock R, Cohen P R 1989 Erythromelalgia and myeloproliferative disorders. Archives of Internal Medicine 149: 105–109

Laird J M A, Bennett G J 1992 Dorsal root potentials and afferent input to the spinal cord in rats with an experimental peripheral neuropathy. Brain Research 548: 181–190

Laird J M A, Bennett G J 1993 An electrophysiological study of dorsal horn neurons in the spinal cord of rats with an experimental peripheral neuropathy. Journal of Neurophysiology 69: 2072–2085

LaMotte C C, Kapadia S E, Kocol C M 1989 Deafferentation-induced expansion of saphenous terminal field labelling in the adult rat dorsal horn following pronase injection of the sciatic nerve. Journal of Comparative Neurology 288: 311–325

LaMotte R H, Shain C N, Simone D A, Tsai E-F P 1991 Neurogenic hyperalgesia: psychophysical studies of underlying mechanisms. Journal of Neurophysiology 66: 190–211

Leijon G, Boivie J, Johansson I 1989 Central post-stroke pain – neurological symptoms and pain characteristics. Pain 36: 13–25

Lenz F A 1991 The thalamus and central pain syndromes: human and animal studies. In: Casey K L (ed) Pain and central nervous system disease: the central pain syndromes. Raven Press, New York, p 171–182

Lenz F A, Tasker R R, Dostrovsky J O 1987 Abnormal single unit activity recorded in the somatosensory thalamus of a quadriplegic patient with central pain. Pain 31: 225–236

Leriche R 1939 The surgery of pain. Williams & Wilkins, Baltimore

Levine J D, Taiwo Y O, Collins S D, Tam J K 1986 Noradrenaline hyperalgesia is mediated through interaction with sympathetic postganglionic neurone terminals rather than activation of primary afferent nociceptors. Nature (London) 323: 158–160

Levitt M 1991a The behavioral syndrome of deafferentation dysesthesias. In: Nashold B S, Ovelmen-Levitt J (eds) Deafferentation pain syndromes: pathophysiology and treatment. Raven Press, New York, p 209–215

Levitt M 1991b Chronic dysesthesias of central neural origin in subhuman primates. In: Nashold B S, Ovelmen-Levitt J (eds) Deafferentation pain syndromes: pathophysiology and treatment. Raven Press, New York, p 229–238

Lewis T 1942 Pain. MacMillan, London, p 57–95

Lindblom U 1985 Assessment of abnormal evoked pains in neurological pain patients and its relation to spontaneous pain: a descriptive and conceptual model with some analytic results. In: Fields H L, Dubner R, Cervero F (eds) Advances in pain research and therapy, vol 9. Raven Press, New York, p 409–423

Lisney S J W, Devor M 1987 Afterdischarge and interactions among fibers in damaged peripheral nerve in the rat. Brain Research 415: 122–136

Livingston W K 1943 Pain mechanisms: A physiological interpretation of causalgia and its related states. Macmillan, New York

Loeser J D, Ward A A 1967 Some effects of deafferentation on neurons of the cat spinal cord. Archives of Neurology 17: 629–635

Loeser J D, Ward A A, White L E 1968 Chronic deafferentation of human spinal cord neurons. Journal of Neurosurgery 29: 48–50

Lombard M-C, Besson J-M 1991 Behavioral and physiopharmacological aspects of the deafferentation syndrome due to dorsal rhizotomy in the rat. In: Besson J-M, Guilbaud G (eds) Lesions of primary afferent fibers as a tool for the study of clinical pain. Elsevier, Amsterdam, p 83–99

Lombard M-C, Larabi Y 1983 Electrophysiological study of cervical dorsal horn cells in partially deafferented rats. In: Bonica J J, Lindblom U, Iggo A (eds) Advances in pain research and therapy, vol 5. Raven Press, New York, p 147–154

Lombard M-C, Nashold B S, Albe-Fessard D, Salman N, Sukr C 1979a Deafferentation hypersensitivity in the rat after dorsal rhizotomy: a possible animal model of chronic pain. Pain 6: 163–174

Lombard, M-C, Nashold B S, Pelissier T 1979b Thalamic recordings in rats with hyperalgesia. In Bonica J J, Liebeskind J C, Albe-Fessard D G (eds) Advances in pain research and therapy, vol 3. Raven Press, New York, p 767–772

McMahon S B, Wall P D 1984 The receptive fields of rat lamina I projection cells move to incorporate a nearby region of injury. Pain 19: 235–247

Mao J, Price D D, Coghill R C, Mayer D J, Hayes R L 1992a Spatial patterns of spinal cord [^{14}C]-2-deoxyglucose metabolic activity in a rat model of painful peripheral mononeuropathy. Pain 50: 89–100

Mao J, Price D D, Hayes R L, Lu J, Mayer D J 1992b Differential roles of NMDA and non-NMDA receptor activation in induction and maintenance of thermal hyperalgesia in rats with painful peripheral mononeuropathy. Brain Research 598: 271–278

Mao J, Price D D, Mayer D J, Lu J, Hayes R L 1992c Intrathecal MK 801 and local nerve anesthesia synergistically reduce nociceptive behaviors in rats with experimental peripheral mononeuropathy. Brain Research 576: 254–262

Mao J, Price D D, Hayes R L, Lu J, Mayer D J, Frenk H 1993 Intrathecal treatment with dextrorphan or ketamine potently reduces pain-related behaviours in a rat model of peripheral mononeuropathy. Brain Research 605: 164–168

Marchettini P, Lacerenza M, Marangoni C, Pellegata G, Sotgiu M L, Smirne S 1992 Lidocaine test in neuralgia. Pain 48: 377–382

Markus H, Pomeranz B, Krushelnycky D 1984 Spread of saphenous somatotopic projection map in spinal cord and hypersensitivity of the foot after chronic sciatic denervation in adult rat. Brain Research 296: 27–39

Melzack R, Wall P D 1965 Pain mechanisms: a new theory. Science 150: 971–979

Merskey H (ed) 1986 Classification of chronic pain: description of chronic pain syndromes and definitions of pain terms. Pain (suppl. 3): 216–221

Meyer R A, Davis K D, Raja S N, Campbell J N 1992 Sympathectomy does not abolish bradykinin-induced cutaneous hyperalgesia in man. Pain 51: 323–327

Milne R J, Foreman R D, Giesler G J, Willis W D 1981 Convergence of cutaneous and pelvic visceral nociceptive inputs onto primate spinothalamic neurons. Pain 11: 163–183

Nashold B S, Wilson W P 1966 Central pain: observations on man with chronic implanted electrodes in the midbrain tegmentum. Confinia Neurologica 27: 30–44

Ness T J, Metcalf A M, Gebhart G F 1990 A psychophysical study in humans using phasic colonic distension as a noxious visceral stimulus. Pain 43: 377–386

Noordenbos W 1959 Pain. Elsevier, Amsterdam

Noordenbos W, Wall P D 1981 Implications of the failure of nerve resection and graft to cure chronic pain produced by nerve lesions. Journal of Neurology, Neurosurgery and Psychiatry 44: 1068–1073

Nyström B, Hagbarth K E 1981 Microelectrode recordings from transected nerves in amputees with phantom limb pains. Neuroscience Letters 27: 211–216

Ochoa J 1986 The newly recognized painful ABC syndrome: thermographic aspects. Thermology 2: 65–107

Ochoa J L, Torebjörk H E 1980 Paraesthesiae from ectopic impulse generation in human sensory nerves. Brain 103: 835–853

Ochoa J L, Yarnitsky D 1990 Triple cold ["CCC"] painful syndrome. Pain (suppl 5): S278

Ochoa J L, Roberts W J, Cline M A, Dotson R, Yarntisky D, 1989 Two mechanical hyperalgesias in human neuropathy. Society for Neuroscience Abstracts 15: 472

Ochoa J L, Yarnitsky D, Marchettini P, Dotson R, Cline M 1993 Interactions between sympathetic vasoconstrictor outflow and C nociceptor induced antidromic vasodilatation. Pain (in press)

Ovesen P, Krøner K, Ørnsholt J, Bach K 1991 Phantom-related phenomena after rectal amputation: prevelance and clinical characteristics. Pain 44: 289–291

Palecek J, Paleckovà V, Dougherty P M, Carlton S M, Willis W D 1992 Responses of spinothalamic tract cells to mechanical and thermal stimulation of skin in rats with experimental peripheral neuropathy. Journal of Neurophysiology 67: 1562–1573

Palecek J, Dougherty P M, Paleckovà V et al 1993 Responses of spinothalamic tract neurons to mechanical and thermal stimuli in an experimental model of peripheral neuropathy in primate. Journal of Neurophysiology 68: 1951–1966

Price D D 1988 Psychological and neural mechanisms of pain. Raven Press, New York, p 76–149

Price D D, Hayes R L, Ruda M A, Dubner R 1978 Spatial and temporal transformations of input to spinothalamic tract neurons and their relation to somatic sensations. Journal of Neurophysiology 41: 933–947

Price D D, Bennett G J, Rafii A 1989 Psychophysical observations on patients with neuropathic pain relieved by a sympathetic block. Pain 36: 237–288

Price D D, Long S, Huitt C 1992a Sensory testing of pathophysiological mechanisms of pain in patients with reflex sympathetic dystrophy. Pain 49: 163–173

Price D D, McHaffie J G, Stein B E 1992b The psychophysical attributes of heat-induced pain and their relationships to neural mechanisms. Journal of Cognitive Neuroscience 4: 1–14

Rampin O, Morain P 1987 Cortical involvement in dorsal horn cell hyperactivity and abnormal behavior in rats with dorsal root section. Somatosensory and Motor Research 4: 237–251

Raymond S A, Rocco A G 1990 Ephaptic coupling of large fibers as a clue to mechanisms in chronic neuropathic allodynia following damage to dorsal roots. Pain (suppl 5): S276

Roberts M H T, Reeves H 1991 Denervation supersensitivity in the central nervous system: possible relation to central pain syndromes. In: Casey K L (ed) Pain and central nervous system disease: the central pain syndromes. Raven Press, New York, p 219–231

Roberts W J 1986 A hypothesis on the physiological basis for causalgia and related pain states. Pain 24: 485–504

Sato J, Perl E R 1991 Adrenergic excitation of cutaneous pain receptors induced by peripheral nerve injury. Science 251: 1608–1610

Simone, D A, Baumann, T K, LaMotte R H 1989 Dose-dependent pain and mechanical hyperalgesia in humans after intradermal injection of capsaicin. Pan 38: 99–107

Simone D A, Sorkin L S, Oh U et al 1991 Neurogenic hyperalgesia: central neural correlates in responses of spinothalamic tract neurons. Journal of Neurophysiology 66: 228–246

Simone D A, Caputi G, Marchettini P, Ochoa J L 1992 Cramping pain and deep hyperalgesia following intramuscular injection of capsaicin. Society for Neuroscience Abstracts 18: 134

Snow P J, Wilson P 1989 Denervation induced changes in somatotopic organization: the ineffective projections of afferent fibers and structural plasticity. In: Cervero F, Bennett G J, Headley P M (eds) Processing of sensory information in the superficial dorsal horn of the spinal cord. Plenum, New York, p 285–306

Sugimoto T, Bennett G J, Kajander K C 1990 Transsynaptic degeneration in the superficial dorsal horn after sciatic nerve injury: effects of a chronic constriction injury, transection, and strychnine. Pain 42: 205–213

Sugiura Y, Terui N, Hosoya Y, Kohno K 1989 Distribution of unmyelinated primary afferent fibers in the dorsal horn. In: Cervero F, Bennett G J, Headley P M (eds) Processing of sensory information in the superficial dorsal horn of the spinal cord. Plenum, New York, p 15–27

Tal M, Bennett G J 1993a Dextrorphan relieves neuropathic heat-evoked hyperalgesia. Neuroscience Letters 151: 107–110

Tal M, Bennett G J 1993b Mechano-hyperalgesia and -allodynia in the territory of the saphenous nerve in rats with an injured sciatic nerve. Abstracts – 7th World Congress on Pain, p 31

Tasker R R 1990 Pain resulting from central nervous system pathology (central pain). In: Bonica J J (ed) The management of pain. Lea & Febiger, Philadelphia, p 264–283

Tasker R R 1991 Deafferentation pain syndromes: introduction. In: Nashold B S, Ovelman-Levitt J (eds) Deafferentation pain syndromes: pathophysiology and treatment. Raven Press, New York, p 241–257

Tasker R R, Tsuda R, Hawrylyshyn P 1983 Clinical neurophysiological investigation of deafferentation pain. In: Bonica J J, Lindblom U, Iggo A (eds) Advances in pain research and therapy, vol 5. Raven Press, New York, p 713–738

Torebjörk H E, Ochoa J L, Schady W 1984 Referred pain from intraneural stimulation of muscle fascicles in the median nerve. Pain 18: 145–156

Torebjörk H E, Lundberg L E R, LaMotte R H 1992 Central changes in processing of mechanoreceptive input in capsaicin-induced secondary hyperalgesia in humans. Journal of Physiology (London) 448: 765–780

Treede R-D, Cole J D 1993 Dissociated secondary hyperalgesia in a subject with a large fibre sensory neuropathy. Pain 53: 169–177

Treede R-D, Raja S N, Davis K D, Meyer R A, Campbell J N 1991 Evidence that peripheral α-adrenergic receptors mediate sympathetically maintained pain. In: Bond M R, Charlton J E, Woolf C J (eds) Pain research and clinical management, vol 4. Elsevier, Amsterdam, p 377–382

Vallin J A, Kingery W S 1991 Adjacent neuropathic hyperalgesia in rats: a model for sympathetic independent pain. Neuroscience Letters 133: 241–244

Wakisaka S, Kajander K C, Bennett G J 1992 Effects of peripheral nerve injuries and tissue inflammation on the levels of neuropeptide Y-like immunoreactivity in rat primary afferent neurons. Brain Research 598: 349–352

Wall P D, Devor M 1981 The effects of peripheral nerve injury on dorsal root potentials and transmission of afferent signals into the spinal cord. Brain Research 209: 95–111

Woolf C J, Thompson S W N 1991 The induction and maintenance of central sensitization is dependent on N-methyl-D-aspartic acid receptor activation: implications for the treatment of post-injury pain hypersensitivity states. Pain 44: 293–299

Woolf C J, Wall P D 1982 Chronic peripheral nerve section diminishes the primary A-fibre mediated inhibition of rat dorsal horn neurons. Brain Research 242: 77–85

Woolf C J, Wall P D 1986 Relative effectiveness of C primary afferent fibers of different origins in evoking a prolonged facilitation of the flexor reflex in the rat. Journal of Neuroscience 6: 1433–1442

Woolf C J, Shortland P, Coggeshall R E 1992 Peripheral nerve injury triggers central sprouting of myelinated afferents. Nature (London) 355: 75–78

Xu X-J, Hao J-X, Aldskogius H, Seiger A, Wisenfeld-Hallin Z 1992 Chronic pain-related syndrome in rats after ischemic spinal cord lesion: a possible animal model for pain in patients with spinal cord injury. Pain 48: 279–290

Yamamoto T, Yaksh T L 1992a Studies on the spinal interaction of morphine and the NMDA antagonist MK-801 on the hyperesthesia observed in a rat model of sciatic mononeuropathy. Neuroscience Letters 135: 67–70

Yamamoto T, Yaksh T L 1992b Spinal pharmacology of thermal hyperesthesia induced by constriction injury of sciatic nerve. Excitatory amino acid antagonists. Pain 49: 121–128

Yamamoto T, Yaksh T L 1993 Effects of intrathecal strychnine and bicuculline on nerve compression induced thermal hyperalgesia and selective antagonism by MK-801. Pain 54: 79–84

Yarnitsky D, Ochoa J L 1989 Release of cold-induced burning pain by block of cold-specific afferent input. Brain 113: 893–902

Zimmermann H 1991 Central nervous mechanisms modulating pain-related information: do they become deficient after lesions of the peripheral or central nervous system? In: Casey K L (ed) Pain and central nervous system disease: the central pain syndromes. Raven Press, New York, p 183–199

11. Spinal dorsal horn plasticity following tissue or nerve injury

Ronald Dubner and Allan I. Basbaum

INTRODUCTION

The 1970s was the decade of the nociceptor in the study of sensory coding mechanisms in pathways transmitting information about pain. The discovery that tissue damage sensitizes nociceptors led to the rapid but premature conclusion that nociceptor sensitization was the sole basis of hyperalgesia following tissue injury and inflammation. The earlier proposal by Hardy (1950) that hyperexcitability in the spinal dorsal horn was important in hyperalgesia was virtually ignored until Woolf (1983) demonstrated that facilitation of the flexion reflex in the rat by natural or electrical stimulation could only be explained by alterations in excitability in the spinal cord. These findings, however, were not directly relevant to changes that might underlie more persistent pains that last for hours, days or longer. It has taken a series of studies of injury-evoked molecular, biochemical and physiological changes that are associated with pain to establish that tissue injury leads to prolonged functional changes in the nervous system (Dubner 1991). These increases in neuronal activity also occur during learning and development and appear to be an outcome of an increased neural barrage originating from sensory receptors in peripheral tissues. These changes are mediated by an activity-dependent neuronal plasticity (Dubner & Ruda 1992).

Both tissue and nerve injury can produce prolonged changes in the nervous system. Tissue damage results in an increased sensitivity of nociceptors at the site of injury. The nociceptors are spontaneously active, have lowered thresholds and increased responsiveness to noxious stimuli. The increased nociceptor activity leads to functional changes in the spinal cord and possibly elsewhere, ultimately contributing to hyperalgesia and spontaneous pain. Similarly, nerve damage can lead to increased activity, at the site of neuroma formation, in the dorsal root ganglion (DRG), or at demyelinated zones of the peripheral nerve. The result again is altered processing in the central nervous system (CNS) contributing to hyperalgesia and spontaneous pain. This chapter will focus on the peripheral and central changes that follow tissue and nerve injury.

Our increased knowledge of injury-induced changes in the CNS was spurred by the development of animal models of tissue and nerve injury leading to persistent pain (see Ch.15). Examples include the injection of formalin or the injection of an inflammatory agent, such as complete Freund's adjuvant (CFA) or carrageenan into the foot pad of a rat. The inflammatory agents produce an intense hyperalgesia and oedema that is limited to the injected paw. The hyperalgesia can be assessed by exposing the limb to a thermal or mechanical stimulus and measuring the threshold or latency of paw withdrawal. The reduction in paw withdrawal latency as compared to control animals or the contralateral limb is used as a measure of hyperalgesia. CFA-induced hyperalgesia peaks within 4–6 hours, and can persist for 10–14 days. There is no change in the latency of withdrawal of the contralateral paw compared to control animals, so that the noninjected paw can be used as a control. Models of tissue injury are important not only because they produce persistent pain that mimics clinical conditions, but also because they are influenced by analgesic agents that have no effect on phasic, acute pain (see below). Similarly, models of nerve injury mimic clinical conditions such as causalgia and reflex sympathetic dystrophy. Recent models (see Ch. 15 and below) on nerve injury produce mechanical and thermal hyperalgesia which can be assessed by the methods described above.

PERIPHERAL NERVOUS SYSTEM CHANGES FOLLOWING INJURY

Although traditional textbooks teach that peripheral injury to tissue or nerve does not result in significant biochemical or morphological reorganization of the cell bodies in the DRG or of the central terminals of the injured primary afferents, there is now considerable evidence that both short- and long-term changes are, in fact, readily demonstrable. To date most studies have used one of three peripheral manipulations to study these changes: peripheral tissue inflammation, peripheral nerve section and ligation (resulting in neuroma formation) and peripheral nerve constriction. Several of these manipulations result in a profound allodynia and hyperalgesia; the neuroma model has been used to study the changes that contribute to neuropathic pains in humans. Although nerve crush has also been studied, the changes observed in this model are far less profound.

PERIPHERAL INFLAMMATION

Peripheral inflammation can be produced in many ways, most commonly with formalin, carrageenan or CFA, as mentioned above. In these inflammatory models the hyperalgesia is produced in large part through the production of prostaglandin and leukotriene products of arachidonic acid metabolism (see Ch. 2). The latter sensitize the peripheral terminals of primary afferent nociceptors, resulting in an increase in spontaneous activity of nociceptors and a lowering of the threshold for their activation. By contrast, few changes are observed in the firing of larger diameter myelinated afferents.

Under conditions of inflammation, peptide levels in primary afferent cell bodies and terminals are typically increased (Lembeck et al 1981), as is the release of neurotransmitter in the spinal cord dorsal horn (Oku et al 1987). Based on these observations it has been proposed that the increased activity of the primary afferents triggers gene transcription in the DRG cells of small-diameter primary afferents. Most recently, Smith and colleagues (1992) reported that both substance P (SP) and calcitonin gene-related peptide (CGRP) are increased (69 and 204%, respectively) ipsilateral to an inflamed joint. In light of the evidence for contralateral consequences of unilateral nerve injury (Woolf 1983) it was of interest that these authors found no change in peptide levels in the DRG contralateral to the inflamed paw. Other studies demonstrated enhanced expression of the preprotachykinin gene (the precursor for SP) in DRG from rats with experimental arthritis (Minami et al 1989). In related studies, Noguchi et al (1988) reported that noxious stimulation (viz. formalin injection into the paw) also increased preprotachykinin mRNA in ipsilateral DRG cells, as early as 3 hours after the formalin injection. Note that the pain behaviour produced by formalin injection is typically resolved within 2 hours. In this model, therefore, the increase in neurotransmitter expression may be secondary to the depletion of neurotransmitter that resulted from the massive stimulation. As a result, the changes in peptide levels are more likely to influence *subsequent* responses to noxious stimulation rather than the behaviour produced by the stimulus. Indeed there is evidence that both SP and N-methyl-D-aspartate (NMDA) contribute to the prolonged central sensitization that is produced by noxious stimulation (see below and Dougherty & Willis 1992; Rusin et al 1992).

On the other hand, there is evidence that increased neural activity is not the only critical factor. Donnerer and colleagues (1992) demonstrated that administration of antisera to nerve growth factor (NGF) blocked the inflammation-provoked increase in tachykinin expression; this was true for the DRG, the peripheral nerve and in the dorsal horn. Most importantly, injections of NGF resulted in increases of SP *in the absence of peripheral inflammation*. These data strongly argue that although the afferent barrage produced by noxious stimulation may contribute to enhanced neurotransmitter expression, it is neither necessary nor sufficient.

PERIPHERAL NEUROMA MODEL

In the neuroma model (see Ch. 4) a peripheral nerve (usually the sciatic) is transected and ligated, preventing regeneration. Within a few days myelinated fibres that have been severed become spontaneously active and show a bursting pattern of activity (Wall & Gutnick 1974). At later times injured unmyelinated afferents express this hyperactivity (Scadding 1981; Matzner & Devor 1987). Furthermore, the injured afferents become sensitive to local or systemic administration of adrenergic agents. These properties (and the correlated observation of autotomy in these rats (Basbaum 1974; Devor 1991)) led to the suggestion that the changes that occur in the neuroma provide a model for studying neuropathic pain that may follow peripheral nerve injury in humans. An important difference between the neuroma model and the inflammation model, of course, is that after complete transection, neither hyperalgesia nor allodynia can be demonstrated. The existence of a neuropathic pain state is, thus, inferred. Although there is strong correlative evidence that the rats indeed experience some abnormal sensation that drives the autotomy behaviour (Basbaum 1974; Devor 1991; Ch. 15), other studies suggest that the autotomy behaviour may be directed at an insensate limb (Rodin & Kruger 1984).

Since increased activity of primary afferents is a feature of both the neuroma and the inflammation model, it is of interest to compare the changes in neurotransmitter expression under the two conditions. It was originally reported that DRG derived neurotransmitter compounds (e.g. neuropeptides) are reduced after nerve section (Jessell et al 1979). This is most marked for SP and related tachykinins and for fluoride-resistant acid phosphatase (FRAP) (Knyihar & Csillik 1976), a marker of a large population of unmyelinated primary afferent fibres. The reduction of staining is detectable in the DRG and in the dorsal horn terminals of primary afferents. The extent to which CGRP, which coexists with SP in many small-diameter primary afferents, is downregulated is not clear;

some laboratories find no consistent change (Villar et al 1991), others find a decrease that parallels the SP change (Noguchi et al 1993).

A reduction in neurotransmitter compounds is, however, not uniform. Thus, in constrast to the decrease in SP, the levels of primary afferent derived galanin and vasoactive intestinal polypeptides (VIP) significantly increase after peripheral nerve section (Villar et al 1991). Galanin levels increase in the DRG cells of injured somatic afferents; VIP increase after section of either somatic or visceral afferents (Anand et al 1990). Of particular interest are studies of Doughty et al (1991) which demonstrated that the increase in VIP occurred in neurons that were previously CGRP-positive. Nonpeptide containing neurons (e.g. the FRAP positive population) did not begin to synthesize VIP after nerve injury. In other studies, Wakisaka et al (1991) reported that 14 days after sciatic nerve section, the levels of the neurotransmitter neuropeptide Y (NPY), which is normally not detectable in DRG cells, increases dramatically. The change could also be detected in the dorsal horn. Parallel increases in mRNA for NPY have also been demonstrated after sciatic nerve section (Noguchi et al 1993). These results indicate that nerve section not only results in changes in the level of neurotransmitters normally synthesized by DRG cells, but also that the phenotype of a given DRG cell (and its central terminal) can change after nerve section.

The fact that the level of some peptides decreases after nerve section while others increase, indicates that factors other than the increased spontaneous activity of the injured afferents must contribute to the changes. Indeed it may be that the alterations in the biochemistry of primary afferent neurons are more related to the many structural changes that occur after nerve section, including cell death in the DRG, atrophy and regeneration of injured primary afferent terminals (Knyihar & Csillik 1976; Knyihar-Csillik et al 1987; however, see Klein et al 1991) and sprouting of intact primary afferents into areas normally innervated by the injured primary afferents (Woolf et al 1992). Also of interest are studies demonstrating that 20% of all cells in the L5 DRG neurons in the adult rat die after sciatic nerve section (Himes & Tessler 1989) and that the levels of the growth associated protein, GAP-43, increase in DRG and dorsal horn after nerve injury (Coggeshall et al 1991; Knyihár et al 1992). At early postoperative time points, the increase in GAP-43 is predominantly in the cell bodies of unmyelinated axons. By 14 days, however, cell bodies of the large myelinated axons also showed increased GAP-43 expression. In these studies it is assumed that the increase in GAP-43 is associated with regenerative features of the primary afferents. The fact that in the neuroma model the increased spontaneous activity in myelinated afferents precedes that in unmyelinated afferents, but that the reverse is true for the increase in GAP-43, provides further evidence that the induction of genes is not directly related to the activity within the particular fibre.

PERIPHERAL NERVE CONSTRICTION MODEL

The model of Bennett & Xie (1988) is produced by applying several loose ligatures that barely constrict the sciatic nerve. This produces a compression injury to the nerve. Within 2 days of nerve ligature, the rats display a profound thermal and mechanical hyperalgesia and behaviour indicative of spontaneous pain (see Ch. 15). Although the first anatomical descriptions of the nerve emphasized the loss of large myelinated fibres, subsequent electron microscopic studies revealed a very large, distal loss of both myelinated and unmyelinated axons (Basbaum et al 1991; Carlton et al 1991). In fact, up to 80% of the unmyelinated axons degenerate distal to the ligatures over time. Increased spontaneous discharge in the constriction model has to date only been recorded in myelinated axons, proximal to the ligature placement at early time points of up to 3 days (Kajander & Bennett 1992). As in the neuroma model, there is evidence that a part of the generator for the increased activity lies in the dorsal root ganglia (Kajander et al 1992).

Since there is such a profound injury to the peptide containing unmyelinated axons, it is not surprising that cytochemical changes observed in primary afferents in the constriction model are very similar to those seen after total peripheral nerve transection. Thus, SP and CGRP levels decrease significantly and markers of regenerative changes in primary afferents, including GAP-43 and two growth associated lectins, RL-29 and soybean agglutinin, increase (Cameron et al 1991). Based on these comparisons, it appears that at least with respect to the changes that occur in the primary afferent fibres, similar mechanisms operate in the neuroma and constriction models.

Conceivably, the peripheral changes in constriction are an attenuated form of the neuroma model. The fact that SP levels are only minimally changed after nerve crush also argues that the constriction model is more similar to nerve section than to the nerve crush situation, despite the fact that there is regeneration in both the crush and constriction models. The relationship of these two models to the Selzer et al (1990) model of neuropathic pain which is produced by partially cutting across the sciatic nerve of the rat is unclear; cytochemical studies have not been performed in this model.

SPINAL DORSAL HORN HYPEREXCITABILITY AFTER TISSUE OR NERVE INJURY

The increased peripheral barrage of impulses arising from nociceptors and from ectopic generators in nerves and the DRG lead to hyperexcitability of dorsal horn neurons. One indication of CNS hyperexcitability is the enlargement of the receptive field (RF) of neurons. Inflammatory agents or repeated tissue injury lead to expansion of the RFs of spinal dorsal horn neurons (McMahon & Wall 1984; Calvino et al 1987; Hylden et al 1989; Laird & Cervero 1989; Hu et al 1992). The response properties of neurons in the superficial laminae and the neck of the dorsal horn have been studied following the administration of CFA (Hylden et al 1989; Ren et al 1992b). In control animals, cutaneous RFs to noxious stimuli include one or more digits of the hind limb (Fig. 11.1), spontaneous activity is minimal and there are no responses to joint movement. By 5 days after CFA, many neurons exhibit an enlargement of their RFs in response to cutaneous noxious stimuli (Fig. 11.1). Some fields include the entire surface of the foot; others have discontinuous

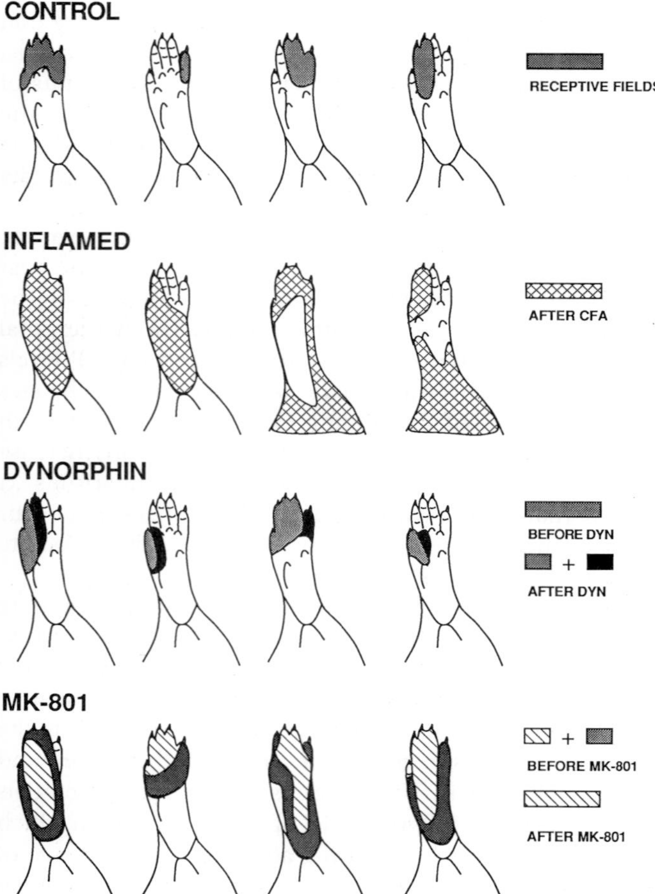

Fig. 11.1 Changes in the receptive fields (RFs) of superficial dorsal horn neurons following inflammation and drug manipulations. The first row illustrates examples of the small RFs found in control animals. The second row shows examples of enlarged RFs after inflammation induced by complete Freund's adjuvant (CFA). The third row illustrates the enlargement of the normal RFs following the application of dynorphin peptide to the surface of the spinal cord. The fourth row illustrates that MK-801 given systemically in rats with CFA-induced inflammation reduces RF size. The findings suggest that the large RFs found in rats with inflamed paws are a result of multiple neurochemical influences. (From Dubner & Ruda 1992.)

fields; other neurons respond to joint movement. In addition, there is a significant increase in the number of cells exhibiting spontaneous activity. When the responses of these neurons are studied between 4 and 8.5 hours after CFA administration, the changes in RF size parallel the development of the behavioural hyperalgesia. Neurons studied at early time points before 6-hours post-CFA have RFs that resemble those in control animals; by 6–8-hours post-CFA, the fields are similar to those found at 5 days post-CFA. A few neurons were studied for over 2 hours in this time period and their RFs increased from a few digits to almost the entire foot (Fig. 11.2).

How does the expansion of the RFs of nociceptive neurons lead to hyperalgesia? One hypothesis is that expanded RFs will result in greater overlap of RFs and will therefore lead to a greater number of neurons activated by a stimulus than the number activated in the absence of RF expansion (Dubner 1991). The increase in neuronal activity may ultimately be perceived as more intense pain. Definitive proof that expanded RFs are partially responsible for behavioural hyperalgesia is lacking. The correlation of the time of occurrence of RF expansion with the onset of the hyperalgesia is evidence supporting the hypothesis. In addition, pharmacological manipulations that reduce the behavioural hyperalgesia such as the administration of NMDA antagonists also reduce RF size (Ren et al 1992b).

Other measures of hyperexcitability of dorsal horn neurons after inflammation have been examined. There are reports of decreases in the thresholds of dorsal horn neurons to mechanical stimulation (Menétrey & Besson 1982; Calvino et al 1987; Woolf & King 1990) as well as evidence that neurogenic inflammation (produced by the intradermal injection of capsaicin) results in enhanced responses to suprathreshold stimuli (Simone et al 1991) and that responses to joint stimulation are enhanced (Schaible et al 1987; Dougherty et al 1992). All of these changes will lead to increased neuronal activity at supraspinal sites and may contribute to pain sensations.

These increases in excitability at the dorsal horn level could represent increased sensitivity of peripheral nociceptors or altered processing in the CNS. There is considerable evidence that peripheral nociceptors exhibit enhanced responsiveness following tissue injury (see above and Dubner & Bennett 1983). Hylden et al (1989) tested whether the increases in RF size of dorsal horn neurons could be explained by peripheral sensitization or by physical changes of the oedematous paw. The effects of physical changes leading to distant mechanical activation of nociceptors were ruled out by showing that the enlarged fields were sensitive to electrical and thermal stimuli. Enhanced responses to electrical stimulation of the nerve proximal to the receptor region indicated that the effects were due to altered excitability in the dorsal horn and not due to activation of 'silent' primary afferent fibres (see

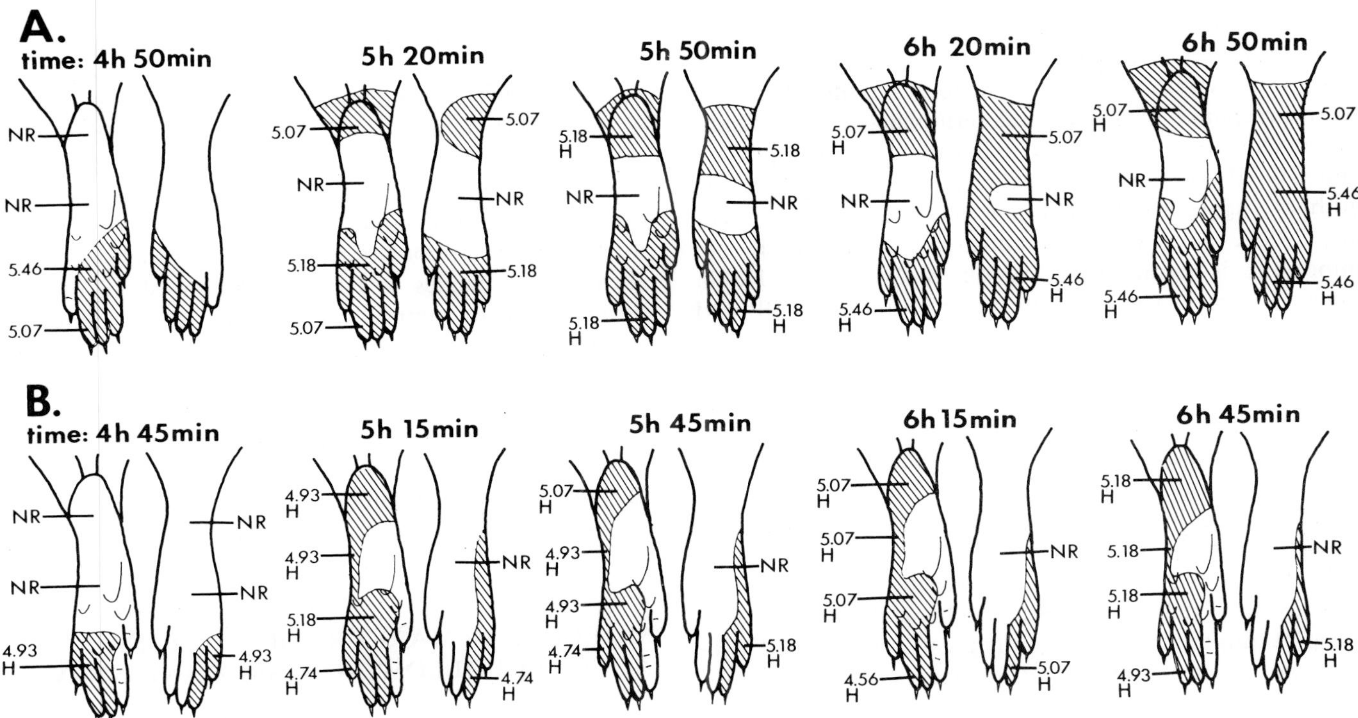

Fig. 11.2 The receptive fields (RFs) of two lamina I spinal neurons (**A** and **B**) observed for over 2 hours approximately 5–7 hours after complete Freund's adjuvant (CFA) injection. Each pair of sketches of the hind paw represents a dorsal (right) and ventral (left) view of the injected hind paw. The apparent RF to mechanical and thermal stimuli at each time point is shaded. Mechanical thresholds were determined with von Frey filaments and are indicated by the numbers near the shaded regions (values are expressed as log $_{10}$ [10 × force in mg]). H = response to radiant heat; NR = no response. (From Hylden et al 1989.)

below). Finally, local anaesthetization of parts of the RF did not alter the hyperexcitability, suggesting that central summation of activity from spontaneously active sensitized nociceptors was not responsible for the changes. Therefore, RF expansion following inflammation appears to involve altered processing in the dorsal horn.

Following complete transection of the peripheral nerve and neuroma formation there also is an expansion of the RFs of nociceptive neurons (Devor & Wall 1981a, 1981b; Hylden et al 1989). After chronic sciatic nerve transection, the normal RFs on the toes or toe pads of rats are lost and cells with more proximal RFs appear in the medial as well as the lateral part of the superficial dorsal horn. This shifting of RFs represents an expansion of the RF of these neurons to skin territories not innervated by the sciatic nerve. The expansion is seen as a shift because of the absence of the normal RF of the neuron. The normal field can be revealed by electrical stimulation of the proximal end of the transected nerve. The nerve constriction model developed by Bennett & Xie (1988) does not result in changes in the size of RFs of nociceptive neurons (Palecek et al 1992; Laird & Bennett 1993) but other changes are seen suggestive of dorsal horn hyperexcitability. These changes parallel the hyperalgesia produced in this model of neuropathic pain and include both an increase in spontaneous activity of the neurons and abnormally prolonged discharges.

RELATIVE CONTRIBUTIONS OF DEEP AND SUPERFICIAL TISSUE

To this point we have made no distinction between the consequences of injury to skin, muscle or viscera or to stimulation of nerves innervating different tissues. In fact, important differences in the central changes provoked by injury to different tissues have been identified. Specifically, conditioning stimulation to a muscle nerve at C-fibre intensities produced a much more prolonged facilitation of the hamstring flexor withdrawal reflex than did stimulation of cutaneous afferents (Wall & Woolf 1984; Woolf & Wall 1986). Intraarticular injection of mustard oil produced the most prolonged facilitation. Since electrical stimulation of the cutaneous (sural) nerve is likely to have activated a larger number of C-fibres than stimulation of the muscle nerve, the authors concluded that the size of the afferent volley did not mediate the difference in duration of the facilitation. In other studies it was shown that cross anastomosis of the sural and gastronemius nerves reversed the effects of nerve stimulation (McMahon & Wall 1989). That is, when a muscle nerve that innervates skin is stimulated, it now evokes a facilitation equivalent to that produced by a cutaneous nerve that innervates skin. Apparently the target organ of the innervated nerve contributes to the magnitude of the response of the central terminals of the afferent fibres. On the other hand, since intrathecal injection of SP and CGRP synergistically facilitates the flexor reflex, the authors' suggestion that differences in the peptide content on C-fibre afferents innervating skin and muscle are important is paradoxical (Woolf & Wiesenfeld-Hallin 1986). There is a much higher concentration of SP and CGRP in cutaneous than in muscle nerves. An alternative explanation is that differences in the central termination of cutaneous and muscle afferents are critical. Conceivably the subliminal fringes of interneurons that drive flexor motoneurons are more directly influenced by C-afferents originating in muscle than skin.

The observation that intraarticular C-fibre stimulation produced particularly potent central changes is consistent with studies of Schaible and colleagues (1987) which demonstrated that nonnoxious mechanical stimulation of the joint resulted in a significantly greater response of wide dynamic range (WDR) and nociceptive-specific (NS) spinal neurons after inflammation of the joint was established. In some cases the RF of the spinal neuron expanded into regions outside of the area of inflammation, including the contralateral joint. Taken together with the fact that discharges of greater magnitude and duration were also produced by the same intensity of electrical stimulation to articular nerves, this indicates that sensitization of peripheral afferents was not the sole contribution to the changes observed. Central changes must have been induced (Neugebauer & Schaible 1990). Using reversible cold block before and after inflammation was established, the authors also demonstrated that during inflammation there is an *enhancement* of the tonic descending inhibitory influences that are normally exerted upon spinal nociceptive neurons (Schaible et al 1991). The latter results indicate that the central changes provoked by inflammation (and probably by increases in C-afferent barrages by other means) are, in fact, somewhat attenuated by a compensatory increase in descending control. It follows that any event that *decreases* descending control in the setting of injury might produce particularly severe conditions of hyperalgesia. For example, the neuropathic pains that are relatively insensitive to control by opioids might result in part from a reduction in the opioid-mediated descending inhibitory controls that are normally activated under conditions of injury and pain.

Although a comparison of the relative effects of stimulating visceral with cutaneous, joint or muscle afferents has not been made, there is considerable evidence that activity produced by noxious stimulation of viscera can also evoke prolonged changes in the CNS. Of particular interest is the evidence that many unmyelinated primary afferents that innervate viscera are 'silent', i.e. although activated by electrical stimulation, these fibres have no response to adequate stimulation under normal conditions (Cervero 1991). Originally described in the joint (Grigg et al 1986; McMahon & Koltzenburg 1990), these fibres develop a response to natural stimulation under conditions of inflammation. It follows that the properties of dorsal horn neurons under conditions of inflammation are influenced by a population of afferents which are usually silent. The changes in RF size and threshold of dorsal horn nociceptive neurons after visceral inflammation may, therefore, be dependent on the sensitization of the silent fibres as well as the long-term changes in spinal dorsal horn hyperexcitability that take place secondary to large afferent C-fibre barrages. Since it has been estimated that a majority of C-afferents innervating viscera are silent, it is likely that reorganization of spinal neurons which respond to visceral stimulation would be particularly susceptible under conditions of inflammation and/or nerve injury.

MOLECULAR MARKERS OF NEURONAL ACTIVITY FOLLOWING TISSUE AND NERVE INJURY

Recent studies have reported significant changes in the spinal cord neuronal expression of immediate early genes (IEGs), so-called because they are among the first genes to be induced when a neuron is stimulated, and because protein synthesis is not required for their induction. The most studied IEGs are the c-*fos* and c-*jun* protooncogenes, cellular homologues of viral oncogenes (Morgan & Curran 1989). Neuropeptides and proteins in the nervous system are coded by specific genes in the cell nucleus. These genes transcribe mRNA which is then released into the cytoplasm and translated into precursor molecules (proteins) that contain active neuropeptide sequences. These proteins are then enzymatically cleaved to yield the active peptide products. The Fos and Jun protein products of c-*fos* and c-*jun* are translocated to the nucleus of the neurons where they can be identified immunocytochemically. Although it is known that the Fos and Jun proteins are transcriptional factors that regulate the expression of a host of other genes, their precise function in postmitotic neurons has not been established.

Of importance to this review is that peripheral inputs induce expression of the c-*fos* and c-*jun* genes in spinal cord neurons. Therefore, by monitoring the distribution of neurons which express these genes, it has been possible to map large populations of spinal cord neurons which are presumed to be active. The first studies used natural stimulation and demonstrated that many neurons in regions that contain nociceptive neurons (e.g. laminae I, II, V, VII, VIII and X) express the Fos protein within minutes of stimulation (Hunt et al 1987). In fact, the c-*fos* message is induced within 5 minutes and the protein can be detected within 15–30 minutes. Thus, a typical experiment involves administering a noxious stimulus and killing the rat 1 hour later. The tissue is then processed by either in situ hybridization methods to demonstrate the c-*fos* mRNA, or immunocytochemistry, to demonstrate the Fos protein in sections of spinal cord.

Recent results demonstrated that the pattern of Fos expression is greater when studies are performed in the awake rat (Menétrey et al 1989). This approach also permits one to correlate the pattern of Fos protein expression with pain behaviour using the formalin test (Dubuisson & Dennis 1977) in the awake rat. Figure 11.3 illustrates the pattern of Fos protein expression after formalin injection into the paw of the rat. Importantly, the number of Fos-positive neurons correlates very highly with the pain behaviour provoked by the stimulus (Gogas et al 1991). Furthermore, analgesia-producing electrical stimulation of the medullary raphe region significantly reduces heat-evoked Fos protein expression (Jones & Light 1990) and morphine dose-dependently blocks pain behaviour and Fos protein expression (Presley et al 1990). In the latter study morphine was administered 20 minutes prior to injection of the formalin. It was found that analgesia was best correlated with the inhibition of Fos expression in more ventral laminae, VII and X. By contrast, although systemic morphine significantly reduced the expression of Fos protein in the superficial laminae I and II, it was possible to render the rats completely analgesic without completely eliminating the expression of Fos protein in these regions. Whether the reduction in the superficial laminae was sufficient to eliminate the expression more ventrally (i.e. whether there is a cascade of activity that originates dorsally) could not be discerned from this study. In subsequent studies, however, it was shown that intracerebroventricular administration of the mu-selective opioid DAMGO also blocked formalin-evoked Fos protein expression in the spinal cord. However, significant analgesia could be produced at doses that were without effect on Fos protein expression in the superficial dorsal horn (Gogas et al 1991). Only at the highest doses tested was Fos protein expression in the latter regions reduced. These data indicate that different factors may induce Fos protein expression (and by inference, induce firing) in the different populations of nociceptive neurons in the spinal cord.

Not all neurons express the Fos protein, however, and thus this approach does not provide a complete picture of the patterns of activity produced by noxious stimulation or nerve injury. Alternate approaches have been used, in

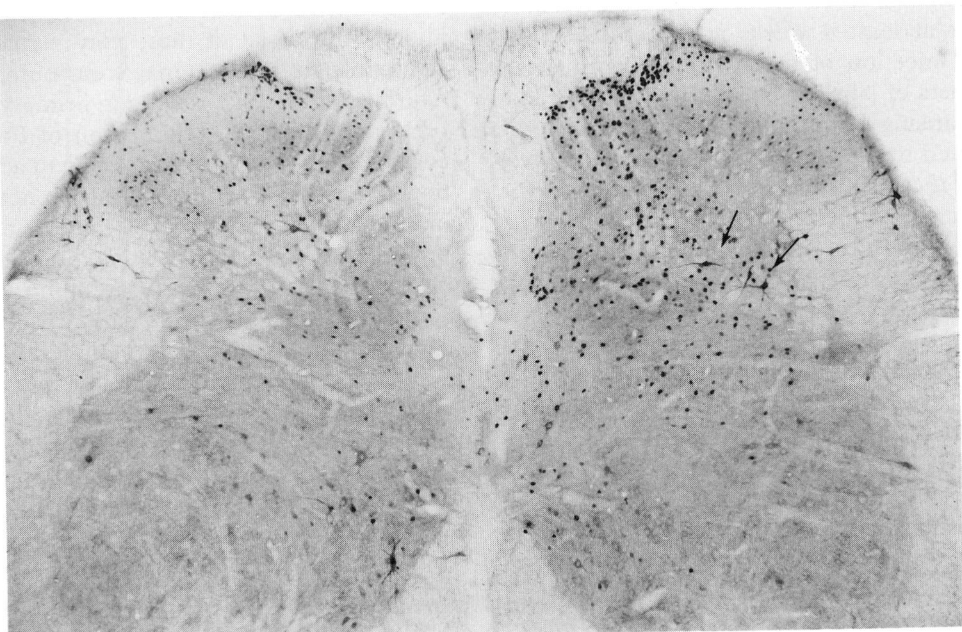

Fig. 11.3 This photomicrograph through the L5 spinal segment of the rat illustrates the pattern of Fos protein-like immunoreactivity produced by formalin injection into the right hind paw. The densest labelling is in the medial half of the ipsilateral superficial dorsal horn (laminae I and II), which is the region of termination of small-diameter afferents from the hind paw. There is also considerable labelling in the neck of the dorsal horn and around the central canal. Bilateral labelling is also notable in lamina VIII of the ventral horn. This particular rat had also received an injection of the retrograde tracer, Fluorogold, into the medullary reticular formation, so that the distribution of Fos protein-immunoreactive projection neurons to this region could be studied. Some of the projection neurons are illustrated by arrows. Double labelled neurons can only be appreciated at higher power or with colour photomicrography.

particular, the 2-deoxyglucose (2DG) methods which provide a better global measure of glucose utilization (which is activity dependent) (Price et al 1991; Mao et al 1992b), but do not provide the cellular resolution that is possible using Fos protein immunoreactivity as a marker.

Of interest to the present discussion are those studies which monitored the expression of protooncogenes under conditions of persistent inflammation or nerve injury. Note that the half-life of the Fos protein is about 2 hours and thus persistence of the Fos protein in spinal cord neurons is indicative of continuous afferent drive or of the development of spontaneous activity/central hyperexcitability of neurons secondary to peripheral injury. For example, Abbadie & Besson (1992) recently reported on the temporal pattern of Fos protein expression in the spinal cord of the polyarthritic rat. Although acute stimulation produces maximal activation in the superficial laminae, 3 weeks after induction of arthritis the densest staining was found in the neurons of laminae V–VII, suggesting that activity in these regions contributes to the hyperalgesia that characterizes this chronic pain model.

Other studies followed the expression of the Fos protein in the neuroma model, produced by sciatic nerve section and ligation (Basbaum et al 1992). Not surprisingly, the greatest number of cells was found within 2 hours of nerve section. In contrast to the short-lived expression after tissue inflammation, high levels of staining were present in laminae I–VII for at least 4 weeks after nerve section. Local anaesthetic injection of the neuroma significantly reduced the numbers of labelled neurons, suggesting that abnormal activity arising from the injured afferents in the neuroma contributed to the increased Fos protein expression. Injection of the anaesthetic in the dorsum of the neck, to control for a systemic action of the drug, however, also reduced Fos protein expression, particularly at longer postoperative times, suggesting that a central (i.e. spinal) action of the local anaesthetic may have contributed to the reduced Fos protein expression. That observation was consistent with other studies which demonstrated that abnormal activity of spinal cord neurons could occur independent of persistent activity resulting from neuroma formation and that the increased firing of 'sensitized' dorsal horn neurons is readily inhibited by very low doses of systemically administered local anaesthetics (Woolf & Wiesenfeld-Hallin 1985).

Persistent Fos protein expression in the spinal cord has also been observed in the constriction injury model (Kajander et al 1990b), indicating that both complete transection and partial nerve injury are associated with persistent activity of populations of dorsal horn neurons. In other studies, Leah and colleagues (1992) demonstrated that the extent of IEG immunostaining ipsilateral to a noxious stimulus is significantly greater than normal, if the contralateral side of the body had previously been exposed to a noxious stimulus. These data suggest that central hyperexcitability can indeed contribute to enhanced expression of these genes and raise the possibility that the induction of IEGs contributes to the central hyperexcitability that is observed in electrophysiological studies. To some extent the differences among the different studies could be explained by the fact that some experiments were performed in anaesthetized animals, which significantly reduces the expression of IEGs in the spinal cord.

It is of interest that although both the Fos and Jun proteins are readily expressed in spinal cord neurons, only the Jun protein can be demonstrated in DRG cells. In fact, Jun protein expression is dramatically upregulated in DRG neurons after peripheral nerve section or after blockade of axoplasmic transport by colchicine or vinblastine (Leah et al 1991). Moreover, the enhanced Jun protein expression persisted until the peripheral nerve regeneration was complete, presumably until signals from target organs reached the DRG neurons. This indicates that induction of the gene in DRG cells is probably not indicative of increased activity, but rather is a response to the biochemical changes that follows nerve injury. To what extent peripheral nerve injury-induced persistence of Fos protein expression in dorsal horn neurons is dependent on growth factors remains to be determined. As described above, various growth-related proteins are upregulated in the spinal cord after peripheral nerve injury. Any or all of these may regulate transcription of IEGs; the latter in turn may contribute to the alterations in neurotransmitter expression in primary afferents.

By monitoring the expression of Fos protein in spinal cord neurons, it has been possible to address the contribution of injury discharge to the prolonged hyperexcitability of dorsal horn neurons. The latter is characterized by the presence of wind-up, i.e. enhanced discharge to subsequent stimuli, as well as to development and persistence of spontaneous activity of dorsal horn neurons independent of maintained activity of peripheral nociceptors. Local anaesthetic injection of the sciatic nerve prior to its being sectioned prevents the injury discharge and significantly reduces the prolonged expression of Fos protein (Basbaum et al 1992). The reduction, however, was only apparent in the superficial laminae of the dorsal horn (I and II); the numbers of labelled cells in laminae V–VII was unaffected. This result provides evidence that the 'activity' of neurons in the superficial laminae can, at least partly, be dissociated from that of neurons located more ventrally. A similar result was reported in studies of the effects of intrathecal injection of MK-801, an NMDA receptor antagonist, on formalin-evoked Fos protein expression. Specifically, MK-801, at doses that were not antinociceptive, reduced Fos protein expression in the superficial laminae by about 30%, without affecting the Fos protein expression in deeper laminae (Kehl et al 1991). The fact that NMDA has been implicated in the injury-induced wind-up and central hyperexcitability (Woolf & Thompson 1991) suggests that the nerve injury-induced Fos protein expression in superficial laminae is also mediated by glutamate action at the NMDA receptor. Activity at the NMDA receptor allows Ca^{2+} to flow into the neuron and increased intracellular Ca is a critical contributor to Fos protein induction (Pompidou et al 1987). It is likely that primary afferent-derived SP, which enhances the action at the NMDA receptor, also contributes to the induction of IEGs in dorsal horn neurons. It should be pointed out that other laboratories found no effect of NMDA antagonists on noxious stimulus-evoked Fos protein expression in the dorsal horn (Tölle et al 1990).

CHANGES IN OPIOID GENE EXPRESSION AND PEPTIDE SYNTHESIS FOLLOWING TISSUE DAMAGE AND NERVE INJURY

As described above, peripheral inflammation can be induced by the injection of an inflammatory agent like CFA into the paw or the ankle joint. In these situations the hyperalgesia and oedema is limited to the injected paw. The injection of CFA into the rat's tail results in polyarthritis after 2–3 weeks and involves all four limbs (see Ch. 15). Both models are associated with an increase in dynorphin peptide levels in the spinal dorsal horn (Millan et al 1986, 1988; Iadarola et al 1988a, 1988). Unilateral inflammation has been shown to produce an increase in messenger RNA that codes for the dynorphin percursor protein (Iadarola et al 1988a, 1988b). The increase in dynorphin message is present as early as 4 hours with a peak eight-fold increase occurring between 2 and 5 days and returning to control levels by 10–14 days. Thus, the change in dynorphin gene expression parallels the development and the time course of behavioural hyperalgesia produced by the inflammatory agent. The increase in dynorphin peptide content occurs later; it is apparent by 2 days and a three-fold increase can be found by 4–5 days after inflammation is induced (Millan et al 1986; Iadarola et al 1988b). An increase in enkephalin message is also induced by inflammation with the same time course, but the elevation is only 50% above control levels (Iadarola et al 1988a). The changes in dynorphin and enkephalin message and dynorphin peptide levels only occur in that part of the spinal cord receiving input from the inflamed limb after injection of the paw.

With histochemical methods, the neurons showing increases in dynorphin mRNA can be localized in the dorsal horn (Ruda et al 1988). There is approximately a three-fold increase in the number of cells with a higher intensity of labelling on the experimental side compared with the control side. The increase in labelling is concentrated in the medial part of the superficial laminae of the dorsal horn and the neck of the dorsal horn, the areas that receive innervation from the inflamed paw. Using immunocytochemical methods, dynorphin peptide is observed ipsilateral in the same regions (Ruda et al 1988). Therefore, the neurons that exhibit increases in dynorphin synthesis and peptide levels are located in the two regions of the dorsal horn that contain projection neurons and local circuit neurons and convey nociceptive information. These are also the same zones of the spinal dorsal horn where expanded RFs are induced by CFA.

Similar to the changes seen in models of inflammation, the nerve constriction model results in a large increase in dynorphin gene expression that peaks at 5 days, coincident with the peak of hyperalgesia seen in this nerve injury model (Draisci et al 1991). The increase in dynorphin peptide peaks at 10 days (Kajander et al 1990a). The increases in dynorphin peptide are localized to the superficial laminae and the neck of the dorsal horn.

Neurons expressing enkephalin message also can be localized in the spinal cord. Inflammation induces minor increases in enkephalin message that is concentrated in the superficial laminae and the neck of the dorsal horn (Noguchi et al 1992). Similar increases in enkephalin expression are induced by formalin injection or by electrical stimulation (Nishimori et al 1989; Noguchi et al 1989).

As discussed above, noxious stimulation results in the activation of IEGs including c-*fos*. Following inflammation, the level of c-*fos* message in the dorsal horn increases within 30 minutes, there is a peak elevation by 2 hours, and a nearly complete recovery by 8 hours after injection into the hind limb (Draisci & Iadarola 1989). The protein product of c-*fos* is localized to the superficial laminae and the neck of the dorsal horn following inflammation. Thus, neurons exhibiting Fos protein are located at the same sites as the neurons exhibiting increased dynorphin and enkephalin message. Fos protein and either dynorphin or enkephalin message have been colocalized in spinal dorsal horn neurons using double-labelling methods (Naranjo et al 1991; Noguchi et al 1991, 1992). Double-labelled neurons are found in the superficial laminae and the neck of the dorsal horn on the side receiving input from the inflamed hind paw. Very few double-labelled neurons are found on the side contralateral to the inflamed hind paw. Over 80% of the neurons showing increased expression of the dynorphin and enkephalin genes also contain Fos protein. The high percentage of dynorphin and enkephalin message colocalized with Fos and Fos-related proteins suggests that Fos phosphoprotein signalling may be coupled to dynorphin and enkephalin transcription following inflammation. Fos protein binds cooperatively in a heterodimer with Jun protein at a DNA recognition site called the AP-1 site, located in the promotor region of some genes (Morgan & Curran 1989). Such binding is thought to regulate transcription of target genes. Recently, AP-1-like binding sites have been located in the promotor region of the dynorphin gene and appear to regulate transcription (Iadarola et al 1991; Naranjo et al 1991).

Evidence has been presented above that the alterations in dynorphin gene expression and the changes in RF size of dorsal horn neurons are both closely related to the development of behavioural hyperalgesia. The effects of dynorphin or a nonpeptidergic kappa-opioid agonist on dorsal horn RFs were directly examined (Hylden et al 1991a). Spinally-administered dynorphin produced an expansion of the RFs of one-third of neurons tested. The average increase in RF size was about 50% (Fig. 11.1). RF expansion in one-third of cells also occurred after the administration of the kappa-opioid agonist U50,488H. The kappa-opioid agonist also produced enhanced responses to noxious thermal and mechanical stimuli in about one-third of the neurons. These effects were not reversed by naloxone. The dose of the kappa agonist was important, since increasing doses resulted in suppression of activity to noxious mechanical and thermal stimuli. These results suggest that dynorphin and kappa-opioid agonists have dual effects in the spinal dorsal horn. At low doses, they produce expanded RFs of some neurons accompanied often by increased sensitivity to mechanical and thermal stimuli; there is a suppression of responsiveness that often occurs at higher doses. Other studies have reported facilitation or inhibition of dorsal horn neuronal activity after the administration of kappa-opioid agonists (Knox & Dickenson 1987; Caudle & Issac 1988). The two types of response may represent activation of different populations of neurons or, alternatively, the two responses may reflect interaction at different types of receptors. Recent data show that in models of inflammation, kappa-opioid agonists produce analgesia that is opioid-mediated (Millan & Colpaert 1991). The facilitatory effect of dynorphin or kappa-opioid agonists may involve nonopioid or opioid mechanisms. Dynorphin-induced facilitation appears to involve NMDA receptor sites (Caudle & Isaac 1988) and in vitro studies indicate that dynorphin displaces glutamate binding to the NMDA receptor (Massardier & Hunt 1989). Recently, mu-opioid agonists have been reported to increase NMDA activation via second messenger systems (Chen & Huang 1991). Finally, dynorphin-induced potentiation of dorsal horn responsivity could involve disinhibitory mechanisms (Stewart & Isaac 1991; Dubner & Ruda 1992) similar to observations in the hippocampus (Swearengen & Chavkin 1987).

Unilateral inflammation and polyarthritis in rats result in enhanced analgesic effects to systemically-administered opioid agonists (Kayser & Guilbaud 1983; Neil et al 1986; Stein et al 1988). These effects have been attributed to an action at peripheral receptor sites within inflamed tissue (Joris et al 1987; Stein et al 1988). However, recent evidence indicates that an increase in sensitivity to opioid agonists takes place also at the spinal level (Hylden et al 1991b). Such enhanced sensitivity following inflammation suggests that spinal cord neuronal plasticity following inflammation may involve biochemical changes at the receptor level.

ROLE OF OTHER CHEMICAL MEDIATORS IN DORSAL HORN HYPEREXCITABILITY

Excitatory amino acids such as glutamate and aspartate act at nonNMDA and NMDA receptors in the spinal cord dorsal horn. NMDA receptors appear to be involved in activation of nociceptive neurons. The phenomenon of 'wind-up' (see above) is prevented by the administration of NMDA antagonists (Davies & Lodge 1987; Dickenson & Sullivan 1990). The hyperexcitability of dorsal horn nociceptive neurons produced by formalin or inflammatory agents is blocked by NMDA antagonists (Haley et al 1990; Ren et al 1992b). The expanded RFs of dorsal horn neurons following inflammation and hyperalgesia is reduced by MK-801, a noncompetitive NMDA antagonist (Fig. 11.1). MK-801 also significantly attenuates the inflammatory hyperalgesia (Ren et al 1992a). NMDA antagonists also significantly attenuate the hyperalgesia induced by the nerve constriction model of partial nerve injury (Mao et al 1992a; Yamamoto & Yaksh 1992b). The hypersensitivity of the rat flexion reflex following electrical stimulation or mustard oil administration is blocked or eliminated by NMDA antagonists (Woolf & Thompson 1991) and presumably reflects alterations in dorsal horn activity. It appears that dorsal horn neuronal plasticity and hyperexcitability following tissue or nerve injury involve the release of excitatory amino acids and their action at NMDA receptor sites.

The action of excitatory amino acids in the spinal dorsal horn is enhanced presynaptically and postsynaptically by the neuropeptides SP and CGRP (Murase et al 1989; Randic et al 1990; Kangrga & Randic 1990). When the dorsal root is stimulated, these neuropeptides potentiate the release of glutamate and aspartate from spinal cord slices. The co-release of excitatory amino acids and neuropeptides facilitates dorsal horn excitability. The responses of spinothalamic tract neurons of the monkey to NMDA are enhanced by SP and these responses are blocked by an NMDA antagonist (Dougherty & Willis 1991). These effects may be important in the strengthening of synaptic connections in the spinal cord and are likely to participate in the hyperexcitability following inflammation and hyperalgesia.

NMDA antagonists are an interesting class of drugs which may have potential utility as analgesics (Dubner 1991; Woolf & Thompson 1991; Ren et al 1992b). They have no effect in the absence of tissue or nerve injury. This is in contrast to opioid analgesics which reduce responsiveness to noxious stimulation in the presence and in the absence of persistent tissue or nerve injury. As previously mentioned, opioid effects are enhanced following inflammation. Recent studies suggest that NMDA antagonists and opioids may be useful drug combinations for analgesia, particularly following persistent tissue or nerve injury (Chapman & Dickenson 1992; Yamamoto & Yaksh 1992a). Such a combination takes advantage of the sensitivity of the enhanced spinal cord neuronal plasticity to NMDA antagonists and opioids.

CONTRIBUTION OF THE SYMPATHETIC NERVOUS SYSTEM

Among the many factors which contribute to peripheral sensitization, and somewhat indirectly to central sensitization, is the sympathetic nervous system. In recent years several theories have been proposed to account for the clinical observation that pains arising from injury to peripheral nerves are exacerbated by sympathetic activity and can be relieved by chemical or surgical sympathectomy. Based on the observation that sprouting fibres in a neuroma become sensitive to circulating catecholamines, Wall & Gutnick (1974) first proposed that receptors for adrenergic agents (norepinephrine and epinephrine) are upregulated in injured afferent fibres. More recently, Sato & Perl (1991) used a partial peripheral nerve injury model and provided evidence that the upregulation was in fact in the *intact* afferents. The latter observation was of interest since it is generally very difficult to demonstrate activation of uninjured afferent fibres by sympathetic stimulation. Other studies, however, suggest that even under normal conditions, sympathetics can directly or indirectly influence the discharge of uninjured primary afferents (Roberts & Foglesong 1988a, 1988b). This, in turn, would regulate the firing and presumably the hyperexcitability of second order nociceptive neurons in the spinal cord.

Most recently, McGaughlin & Janig (unpublished observations) reported that after a sciatic nerve section and neuroma formation, there is a dramatic increase in the number of glyoxylic-acid induced cathecholamine fluorescent nerve fibres surrounding cell bodies of the DRG. These were presumably cell bodies of axons which were injured. This observation raises the possibility that when peripheral afferents and/or sympathetic afferents are injured, there is an increase in the sympathetic regulation of the afferent drive to the spinal cord, *via an action in the DRG*. This conclusion is consistent with results of earlier studies which reported abnormal discharges in DRG neurons after peripheral nerve injury, either complete (Wall & Devor 1983) or partial (Kajander et al 1992). The fact that sympathectomy by peripheral injection of guanethidine is effective for sympathetically maintained pains, however, indicates that a more distal sympathetic hyperactivity must also contribute to the pain that is observed and to any sympathetically maintained central reorganization. Guanethidine would not destroy sympathetic postganglionic terminals innervating the DRG, yet it is effective in some of the neuropathic pain models in the rat (Neil et al 1991; Shir & Seltzer 1991). In fact, Levine et al (1986) concluded that the target of the noradrenaline is the sympathetic terminal, not the primary afferent. They provide evidence that the sympathetic contribution is via regulation of prostaglandin synthesis and release from the terminals of the sympathetic postganglionic fibres. Until it is unequivocally established that the target of the upregulated sympathetic activity is indeed the primary afferent (for example, by in situ hybridization of the adrenergic receptor), we cannot exclude any of the foregoing explanations for the contribution of the sympathetic nervous system.

COMPARISON OF CHANGES FOLLOWING TISSUE OR NERVE INJURY

The results from models of tissue and nerve injury permit several conclusions to be drawn concerning the factors that induce changes in neurotransmitter expression in the peripheral nervous system and the relationship between these changes and the development of hyperalgesia. First, increased activity alone cannot account for the neurochemical changes that are observed following tissue or nerve injury. Second, at least with respect to the changes in the primary afferent, the nerve constriction model is more similar to the nerve transection model than to the chronic inflammation models. If follows that the magnitude of the change in gene and peptide expression in primary afferents cannot be the contributor to the development of hyperalgesia. This is, of course, consistent with the observation that the hyperalgesia in inflammatory models is sensitive to blockers of cyclooxygenase; that produced in the constriction model, and for that matter the autotomy that characterizes the transection model, is probably not responsive. These differences are certainly related to the transduction mechanisms operating in the two systems. When the nociceptor is intact but hyperactive (i.e. under conditions of inflammation), the terminal is readily sensitized in the presence of inflammatory mediators (prostaglandins, etc). When the nerve is injured, there is probably a disruption of the normal membrane distribution of receptors for these mediators so that they are less responsive, even though inflammatory mediators may be present in the neuroma. On the other hand, changes in the chemical (ionic) milieu of the neuroma may depolarize sprouts in the neuroma, resulting in hyperactivity and increased mechanical sensitivity. Ephaptic connections between injured sprouts may also contribute to ongoing discharges. Importantly, injury to the nerve also sets up abnormal discharges at the level of the DRG.

On the other hand, there are important *central* changes

produced in these different models which suggest that the ultimate basis for the hyperalgesia and central hyperexcitability that are observed in the inflammation and constriction models are similar. Among the most profound changes in both the inflammation and constriction models is a dramatic increase in the expression of dynorphin in dorsal horn neurons and a similar increase in enkephalin expression. By contrast, total nerve transection produces a much smaller change in opioid expression.

What drives the increase in dynorphin expression in the inflammation and constriction models is, however, almost certainly different. Since SP and CGRP immunoreactive terminals are located presynaptic to dynorphin neurons of the dorsal horn, and since SP and CGRP levels are increased in the inflammation models, it has been proposed that the increase in dynorphin expression in the inflammation models is driven by the increased activity of peptide containing unmyelinated afferents. Unfortunately, since SP and CGRP expression are reduced in the constriction model, this attractive hypothesis cannot account for the upregulation of dynorphin gene expression in the constriction model. Since there is an almost total loss of myelinated fibres distal to the ligatures in the constriction model, it is possible that the increase of activity centrally reflects a loss of *inhibitory* control exerted by large-diameter afferents, rather than increased afferent drive over unmyelinated primary afferents. Although there is some spontaneous activity of injured large-diameter fibres, this may not be sufficient to bring in the inhibitory processes normally present. Another possibility has been proposed, namely that the constriction injury produces a selective loss of inhibitory local circuit neurons in the dorsal horn, due to excessive excitability (i.e. hyperexcitability of dorsal horn nociceptive neurons). Excessive neuronal depolarization leads to a pathological state by promoting excitotoxicity and neuronal dysfunction (Dubner & Ruda 1992). Neurons most sensitive to this excitotoxicity are small local circuit neurons that probably are inhibitory. Small neurons in the rat dorsal horn, in fact, exhibit morphological changes suggestive of dysfunction following partial nerve injury (Sugimoto et al 1990). Such dysfunction could lead to a loss of inhibitory mechanisms that would further contribute to dorsal horn hyperexcitability. Taken together these results indicate that the constriction model is an unusual hybrid; it has features that are characteristic of both the complete nerve transection *and* the tissue inflammation models. These data suggest that central changes common to the inflammation and constriction models, not changes in the primary afferents, are critical to the development of hyperalgesia under those conditions.

It should be pointed out that very effective agents for reducing the behavioural hyperalgesia produced by partial nerve injury or tissue injury in rats are either competitive on noncompetitive NMDA antagonists (Mao et al 1992a; Yamamoto & Yaksh 1992a; Ren et al 1992a, 1992b). Similarly, both models are sensitive to opioid administration (Attal et al 1990; Hylden et al 1991b). All of these findings suggest that central hyperexcitability is precipitated by the release of excitatory amino acids and their interactive effects with various neuropeptides, including opioids as well as nonopioids, on NMDA and probably nonNMDA receptors.

A SUMMARY OF CONTEMPORARY THEORIES ON MECHANISMS OF PERSISTENT PAIN FOLLOWING INJURY AND THEIR CLINICAL IMPLICATIONS

The prevailing theories regarding mechanisms of persistent pain following injury are based on either peripheral nervous system or CNS changes, or both. The hypotheses based solely on peripheral mechanisms are of two general types. The first involves peripheral sensitization. After tissue injury, nociceptors exhibit lower thresholds to noxious stimuli, increased response to suprathreshold stimuli and the presence of spontaneous activity. These signs of receptor sensitization are thought to account for lower pain thresholds, increased magnitude of pain, and spontaneous pain following tissue damage (Dubner & Bennett 1983). Similarly, chemical sensitization of damaged as well as intact nerves following nerve injury provides a possible explanation for the increased adrenergic sensitivity and sympathetic nervous system involvement in neuropathic pain conditions (Meyer et al 1992). This general hypothesis of peripheral sensitization cannot readily account for some of the characteristics of persistent pain such as pain produced by innocuous mechanical stimulation of A-beta afferents, summation of pain with repeated stimulation and various types of referred pain.

An alternative hypothesis based on peripheral mechanisms is the model of cross-excitation in the DRG and associated ectopic discharges resulting from damage to nerves (Devor 1989). In this hypothesis, increased neuronal activity, arising from neuromas, DRG or demyelinated zones of peripheral nerves, results in excitation of undamaged neurons in DRG which spreads through the ganglion as the activity summates. Cross-excitation between large myelinated low-threshold mechanoreceptors and small-fibre nociceptors could explain the finding that light touch stimulation produces pain in neuropathic conditions. Such cross-excitation will theoretically lead to pain produced by innocuous stimulation, spontaneous pain, and summation of pain with increased peripheral neuronal activity. This hypothesis, especially in combination with the peripheral sensitization hypothesis, is attractive. Its weakness is that the somatotopic organization of the ganglion does not easily account for referred pain to regions of the body innervated by adjacent DRGs. In addition, cross-excitation should result in mislocation of sensation, which is rarely found. The cross-excitation hypothesis also is not supported by evidence on the clinical effectiveness of drugs such as tricyclic antidepressants and anticonvulsants agents such as carbamazepine, phenytoin and baclofen. The predominant effect of these drugs is CNS-related. Their delayed effectiveness argues against a peripheral action which should occur rapidly and not build up over time.

Proposals that CNS changes account for persistent pain after injury are of two general types: those that hypothesize that there is an increase in excitability of populations of neurons that transmit messages about tissue and nerve injury and those that postulate a loss of inhibitory mechanisms leading to an increase in CNS hyperexcitability (see Dubner 1991 for references). These proposals are mainly based on studies at the level of the spinal and medullary dorsal horns. Of course, similar mechanisms can take place at other levels of the neuraxis. For example, after nerve injury, there is a rapid loss of the large fibres mediating dorsal root potentials (Wall & Devor 1981; Laird & Bennett 1992), which correlate with presynaptic inhibitory controls in the dorsal horn.

The disinhibition hypothesis is based on studies showing that nerve injury leads to a loss of segmental inhibitory mechanisms. The blocking of inhibitory transmission by picrotoxin or strychnine produces an increase in dorsal horn excitability. As mentioned above, one effect of dynorphin in the dorsal horn may be to inhibit the activity of inhibitory local circuit neurons that normally decrease excitability.

It has been postulated that the WDR neuron of the dorsal horn is critically involved in neuronal hyperexcitability (Roberts 1986; Dubner et al 1987). The RFs of WDR neurons have extensive gradients of sensitivity. The central zone evokes activity in the WDR that is proportional to stimulus intensity; pinch produces a greater discharge than does pressure or brushing. Surrounding this zone is an area that responds only to more intense stimuli such as pressure or pinch. Activation of this surround zone also results in an increase in surround inhibitory mechanisms via activation of inhibitory local circuit neurons (Hillman & Wall 1969). Roberts (1986) proposed that increased low-threshold input to WDR neurons would result in their increased discharge leading to pain. However, firing frequency alone of WDR neurons cannot explain the transformation in sensory experience that takes place since WDR neurons participate in the encoding of pain over a wide range of discharge frequences (Dubner et al 1989). It has been postulated that expansion of the low-threshold portions of the RFs of WDR neurons seen following tissue or nerve injury underlies the pain triggered by innocuous stimuli (Dubner et al 1987). This expansion may be due to direct excitation or removal of the surrounding inhibitory mechanisms. Following this expansion, a touch stimulus will activate a larger number of WDR neurons in the peripheral zone of their RFs due to both the expansion and the greater overlap of fields. Since the temporal and spatial profile of neural activity after injury will mimic that produced by noxious stimulation of the peripheral RF zones of the WDR RF, this will be perceived centrally as pain. A punctuate tactile stimulus will now be misperceived as a pinprick stimulus or a sharp, localized, throbbing sensation.

Although the terms allodynia and hyperalgesia are often used interchangeably (because they often occur together in the clinical situation), it is important to recognize that they are very different behavioural phenomena which probably have a different physiological basis. Most importantly, allodynia, which is the induction of pain by a previously innocuous stimulus, may arise from nonnoxious stimulation of sensitized nociceptors, or of normal A-beta mechanoreceptors. By contrast, hyperalgesia, namely the phenomenon characterized by exaggerated pain to a noxious stimulus, is likely to arise from activation of nociceptors with or without the presence of a background of central sensitization. Indeed hyperalgesia can be produced in normal individuals by blocking conduction in large-diameter afferents; under these conditions all noxious stimuli (pin-prick, cold or pinch) are perceived as burning pain, presumably secondary to the loss of some inhibitory control in the dorsal horn that is normally exerted by the large-diameter afferents.

It is evident that a parsimonious model must incorporate both peripheral and central changes as contributing to persistent pain following injury. A model has been proposed that takes into account the increased nociceptive input arising from the site of tissue or nerve injury and central changes consequent upon that injury. Taken together these changes produce dorsal horn hyperexcitability and persistent pain (Dubner 1991; Dubner & Ruda 1992). Nerve injury leads to ectopic spontaneous activity and increased chemical sensitivity of peripheral nerve fibres arising from neuromas, from the DRG and from demyelinated zones. Tissue injury results in a sensitization of peripheral nociceptors and increased spontaneous and evoked activity. Both produce an increased neuronal barrage that reaches the CNS albeit via different mechanisms. The sequence of events is diagrammed in Figure 11.4. Increased neuronal activity from the site of injury will lead to increased excitation via an action at NMDA receptor sites. This increase in excitation is facilitated by neuropeptide release (SP, CGRP and dynorphin). The result is an expansion of RFs and other forms of hyperexcitability leading to an increase in pain. This hyperexcitability, if excessive, may lead to a pathological state by promoting excitotoxicity, cell dysfunction and a loss of inhibitory mechanisms. The combined effects of

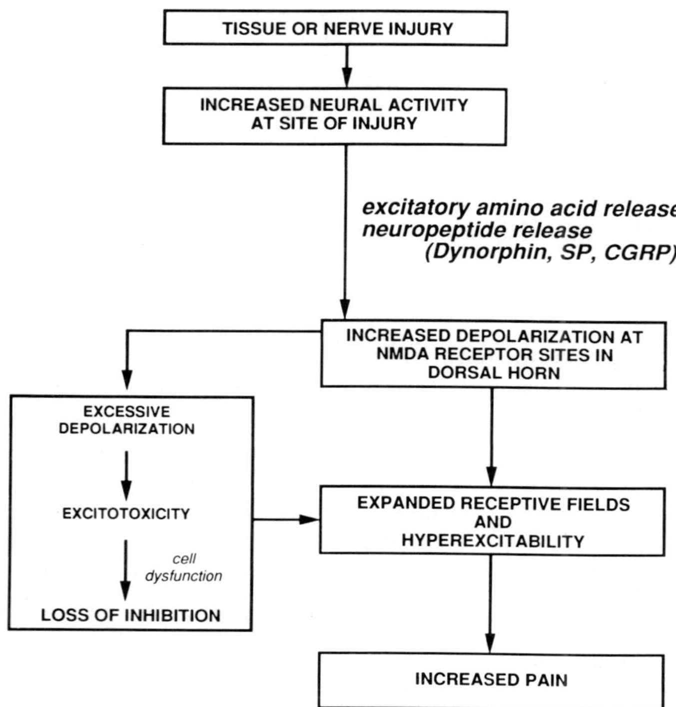

Fig. 11.4 Sequence of events that may occur following peripheral tissue inflammation or peripheral nerve injury. (Adapted from Dubner 1991.)

excessive excitation and loss of inhibition would further exacerbate the hyperexcitability resulting in even greater and more prolonged pain.

The identification of the mechanisms that underlie injury-evoked changes in the spinal cord have led to the development of new treatment strategies to reduce or prevent the neural barrage that arises from the site of injury (Wall 1988; Tverskoy et al 1990). Attention has mainly been directed at the use of pre-emptive local anaesthesia for the treatment of postoperative pain. Local anaesthetics are administered before surgery under general anaesthesia in order to prevent the development of hyperexcitability in the dorsal horn, i.e. to prevent the spinal cord from 'experiencing' the injury and to prevent the laying down of a 'memory' trace of the injury. A similar approach can be used to reduce or eliminate the pain associated with nerve injury (Bach et al 1988). Neural activity that originates from neuromas or DRG can be blocked by local anaesthetics administered as soon as possible and for the first few days after a traumatic nerve injury. The strategy is less useful when the nerve injury is caused by metabolic or viral disease and the onset of the neuropathy is insidious. In such instances, drugs that reduce CNS hyperexcitability, including anticonvulsants and/or NMDA antagonists, should also be effective treatment strategies.

REFERENCES

Abbaidie C, Besson J M 1992 C-fos expression in rat lumbar spinal cord during the development of adjuvant-induced arthritis. Neuroscience 48: 985–994

Anand P, Gibson S J, Scaravilli F, et al 1990 Studies of vasoactive intestinal polypeptide expression in injured peripheral neurons using capsaicin, sympathectomy and mf mutant rats. Neuroscience Letters 118: 61–66

Attal N, Jazat F, Kayser V, Guilbaud G 1990 Further evidence for "pain-related" behaviours in a model of unilateral peripheral mononeuropathy. Pain 41: 235–251

Bach S, Noreng M F, Tjéllden N U 1988 Phantom limb pain in amputees during the first 12 months following limb amputation, after preoperative lumbar epidural blockade. Pain 33: 297–301

Basbaum A I 1974 Effects of central lesions on disorders produced by multiple dorsal rhizotomy in rats. Experimental Neurology 42: 490–501

Basbaum A I, Gautron M, Jazat F, Mayes M, Guilbaud G 1991 The spectrum of fiber loss in a model of neuropathic pain in the rat:. Pain 47: 359–367

Basbaum A I, Chi S-I, Levine J D 1992 Peripheral and central contribution to persistent expression of the c-fos proto-oncogene in spinal cord after peripheral nerve injury. In: Willis W D (ed): Hyperalgesia and allodynia. Raven Press, New York, p 295–304

Bennett G J, Xie Y-K 1988 A peripheral mononeuropathy in rat that produces disorders of pain sensation like those seen in man. Pain 33: 87–107

Calvino B, Villanueva L, LeBars D 1987 Dorsal horn (convergent) neurons in the intact anaesthetized arthritic rat. I. Segmental excitatory influences. Pain 28: 81–98

Cameron A A, Cliffer K D, Dougherty P M, Willis W D, Carlton S M 1991 Changes in lectin, GAP-43 and neuropeptide staining in the rat superficial dorsal horn following experimental peripheral neuropathy. Neuroscience Letters 131: 249–252

Carlton S M, Dougherty P M, Pover C M, Coggeshall R E 1991 Neuroma formation and numbers of axons in a rat model of experimental peripheral neuropathy. Neuroscience Letters 131: 88–92

Caudle R M, Isaac L 1988 Influence of dynorphin (1–13) on spinal reflexes in the rat. Journal of Pharmacology and Experimental Therapeutics 246: 508–513

Cervero F 1991 Mechanisms of acute visceral pain. British Medical Bulletin 47: 549–560

Chapman V, Dickenson A H 1992 The combination of NMDA antagonism and morphine produces profound antinociception in the rat dorsal horn. Brain Research 573: 321–323

Chen L, Huang L-Y M 1991 Sustained potentiation of NMDA receptor-mediated glutamate responses through activation of protein kinase C by a mu opioid. Neuron 7: 319–326

Coggeshall R E, Reynolds M L, Woolf C J 1991 Distribution of the growth associated protein GAP-43 in the central processes of axotomized primary afferents in the adult rat spinal cord; presence of growth cone-like structures. Neuroscience Letters 131: 37–41

Davies S N, Lodge D 1987 Evidence for involvement of N-methylasparate receptors in 'wind-up' of class 2 neurons in the dorsal horn of the rat. Brain Research 424: 402–406

Devor M 1989 The pathophysiology of damaged peripheral nerves. In: Wall P D, Melzack R (eds) Textbook of pain, 2nd edn Churchill Livingstone, Edinburgh, p 63–81

Devor M 1991 Sensory basis of autotomy in rats. Pain 45: 109–110

Devor M, Wall P D 1981a Plasticity in the spinal cord sensory map following peripheral nerve injury in rats. Journal of Neuroscience 1: 679–684

Devor M, Wall P D 1981b Effect of peripheral nerve injury on receptive fields of cells in the cat spinal cord. Journal of Comparative Neurology 199: 277–291

Dickenson A H, Sullivan A F 1990 Differential effects of excitatory amino-acid antagonists on dorsal horn nociceptive neurons in the rat. Brain Research 506: 31–39

Donnerer J, Schuligoi R, Stein C 1992 Increased content and transport of substance P and calcitonin gene-related peptide in sensory nerves innervating inflamed tissue: evidence for a regulatory function of nerve growth factor in vivo. Neuroscience 49: 693–698

Dougherty P M, Willis W D 1991 Enhancement of spinothalamic neuron responses to chemical and mechanical stimuli following combined microiontophoretic application of N-methyl-D-aspartic acid and substance P. Pain 47: 85–93

Dougherty P M, Willis W D 1992 Enhanced responses of spinothalamic tract neurons to excitatory amino acids accompany capsaicin-induced sensitization in the monkey. Journal of Neuroscience 12: 883–894

Doughty S E, Atkinson M E, Shehab S A 1991 A quantitative study of neuropeptide immunoreactive cell bodies of primary afferent sensory neurons following rat sciatic nerve peripheral axotomy. Regulatory Peptides 35: 59–72

Draisci G, Iadarola M J 1989 Temporal analysis of increases in c-fos, preprodynorphin and preproenkephalin mRNAs in rat spinal cord. Molecular Brain Research 6: 31–37

Draisci G, Kajander K C, Dubner R, Bennett G J, Iadarola M J 1991 Up-regulation of opioid gene expression in spinal cord evoked by experimental nerve injuries and inflammation. Brain Research 560: 186–192

Dubner R 1991 Neuronal plasticity and pain following peripheral tissue inflammation or nerve injury. In: Bond M R, Charlton J E, Woolf C J (eds) Proceedings of the VIth World Congress on Pain. Elsevier, Amsterdam, pp 264–276

Dubner R, Bennett G J 1983 Spinal and trigeminal mechanisms of nociception. Annual Review of Neuroscience 6: 381–418

Dubner R, Ruda M A 1992 Activity-dependent neuronal plasticity following tissue injury and inflammation. Trends in Neurosciences 15: 96–103

Dubner R, Sharav Y, Gracely R H, Price D D 1987 Idiopathic trigeminal neuralgia: sensory features and pain mechanisms. Pain 31: 23–33

Dubner R, Kenshalo D R Jr, Maixner W, Bushnell M C, Oliveras J-L 1989 The correlation of monkey medullary dorsal horn neuronal activity and the perceived intensity of noxious heat stimuli. Journal of Neurophysiology 62: 450–457

Dubuisson D, Dennis S G 1977 The formalin test: a quantitative study of the analgesic effects of morphine, meperidine, and brain stem stimulation in rats and cats. Pain 4: 107–126

Gogas K R, Presley R W, Levine J D, Basbaum A I 1991 The antinociceptive action of supraspinal opioids results from an increase in descending inhibitory control: correlation of nociceptive behaviour and c-fos expression. Neuroscience 42: 617–628

Grigg P, Schaible H-G, Schmidt R F 1986 Mechanical sensitivity of group III and IV afferents from posterior articular nerve in normal and inflamed cat knee. Journal of Neurophysiology 55: 1–9

Haley J E, Sullivan A F, Dickenson A H 1990 Evidence of spinal N-methyl-D-aspartate receptor involvement in prolonged chemical nociception in the rat. Brain Research 518: 218–226

Hardy J D, Wolff H G, Goodell H 1950 Experimental evidence on the nature of cutaneous hyperalgesia. Journal of Clinical Investigation 29: 115–140

Hillman P, Wall, P D 1969 Inhibitory and excitatory factors influencing the receptive fields of lamina 5 spinal cord cells. Experimental Brain Research 9: 284–306

Himes B T, Tessler A 1989 Death of some dorsal root ganglion neurons and plasticity of others following sciatic nerve section in adult and neonatal rats. Journal of Comparative Neurology 284: 215–230

Hu J W, Sessle B J, Raboisson P, Dallel R, Woda A 1992 Stimulation of craniofacial muscle afferents induces prolonged facilitatory effects in trigeminal nociceptive brain-stem neurons. Pain 48: 53–60

Hunt S P, Pini A, Evan G 1987 Induction of c-fos-like protein in spinal cord neurons following sensory stimulation. Nature (London) 328: 632–634

Hylden J L K, Nahin R L, Traub R J, Dubner R 1989 Expansion of receptive fields of spinal lamina I projection neurons in rats with unilateral adjuvant-induced inflammation: the contribution of dorsal horn mechanisms. Pain 37: 229–243

Hylden J L K, Nahin R L, Traub R J, Dubner R 1991a Effects of spinal kappa-opioid receptor agonists on the responsiveness of nociceptive superficial dorsal horn neurons. Pain 44: 187–93

Hylden J L K, Thomas D A, Iadarola M J, Nahin R L, Dubner R 1991b Spinal opioid analgesic effects are enhanced in a model of unilateral inflammation/hyperalgesia: possible involvement of noradrenergic mechanisms. European Journal of Pharmacology 194: 135–143

Iadarola M J, Brady L S, Draisci G, Dubner R 1988a Enhancement of dynorphin gene expression in spinal cord following experimental inflammation: stimulus specificity, behavioural parameters and opioid receptor binding. Pain 35: 313–326

Iadarola M J, Douglass J, Civelli O, Naranjo J R 1988b Differential activation of spinal cord dynorphin and enkephalin neurons during hyperalgesia: evidence using cDNA hybridization. Brain Research 455: 205–212

Iadarola M J, Mojdehi G, Gu J, Yeung C L, Levens D, Dubner R 1991 A protein complex differing from the fos/jun complex binds at an AP-l variant sequence in the dynorphin promoter and is induced in spinal cord by peripheral inflammation. Society of Neuroscience Abstracts 17: 905 (abstract)

Jessell T, Tsunoo A, Kanazawa I, Otsuka M 1979 Substance P: depletion in the dorsal horn of rat spinal cord after section of the peripheral processes of primary sensory neurons. Brain Research 168: 247–259

Jones S L, Light A R 1990 Electrical stimulation in the medullary nucleus raphe magnus inhibits noxious heat-evoked fos protein-like immunoreactivity in the rat lumbar spinal cord. Brain Research 530: 335–338

Joris J L, Dubner R, Hargreaves K M 1987 Opioid analgesia at peripheral sites: a target for opioids released during stress and inflammation. Anesthesia and Analgesia 66: 1277–1281

Kajander K, Bennett G J 1992 Onset of a painful peripheral neuropathy in rat: a partial and differential deafferentation and spontaneous discharge in A-beta and A-delta primary afferent neurons. Journal of Neurophysiology 68: 734–744

Kajander K C, Sahara S, Iadarola M J, Bennett G J 1990a Dynorphin increases in the dorsal spinal cord in rats with a painful peripheral neuropathy. Peptides 11: 719–278

Kajander K C, Wakisaka S, Draisci G, Iadarola M J 1990b Labeling of Fos protein increases in an experimental model of peripheral neuropathy in the rat. Society of Neuroscience Abstracts 16: 1281

Kajander K C, Wakisaka S, Bennett G J 1992 Spontaneous discharge originates in the dorsal root ganglion at the onset of a painful peripheral neuropathy in the rat. Neuroscience Letters 138: 225–228

Kangrga I, Randic M 1990 Tachykinins and calcitonin gene-related peptide enhance release of endogenous glutamate and aspartate from the rat spinal dorsal horn slice. Journal of Neuroscience 10: 2026–2038

Kayser V, Guilbaud G 1983 The analgesic effects of morphine, but not those of the enkephalinase inhibitor thiorphan, are enhanced in arthritic rats. Brain Research 267: 131–138

Kehl L J, Gogas K R, Lichtblau L, et al 1991 The NMDA receptor antagonist MK801 reduces noxious stimulus-evoked FOS expression in the spinal dorsal horn. Pain Research and Clinical Management 4: 307–312

Klein C M, Guillamondegui O, Krenek C D, La F R, Coggeshall R E 1991 Do neuropeptides in the dorsal horn change if the dorsal root ganglion cell death that normally accompanies peripheral nerve transection is prevented? Brain Research 552: 273–282

Knox R J, Dickenson A H 1987 Effects of selective and non-selective kappa-opioid receptor agonists on cutaneous C-fiber-evoked responses of rat dorsal horn neurons. Brain Research 415: 21–29

Knyihár C E, Csillik B 1976 Effect of peripheral axotomy on the fine structure and histochemistry of the Rolando substance: degenerative atrophy of central processes of pseudounipolar cells. Experimental Brain Research 26: 73–87

Knyihár C E, Csillik B, Oestreicher A B 1992 Light and electron microscopic localization of B-50 (GAP43) in the rat spinal cord during transganglionic degenerative atrophy and regeneration. Journal of Neuroscience Research 32: 93–109

Knyihar-Csillik E, Rakic P, Csillik B 1987 Transganglionic degenerative atrophy in the substantia gelatinosa of the spinal cord after peripheral nerve transection in rhesus monkeys. Cell and Tissue Research 247: 599–604

Laird J M A, Bennett G J 1992 Dorsal root potentials and afferent input to the spinal cord in rats with an experimental peripheral neuropathy. Brain Research 584: 181–190

Laird J M A, Bennett G J 1993 An electrophysiological study of dorsal horn neurons in the spinal cord of rats with an experimental peripheral neuropathy. Journal of Neurophysiology (in press)

Laird J M A, Cervero F 1989 A comparative study of the changes in receptive-field properties of multireceptive and nocireceptive rat dorsal horn neurons following noxious mechanical stimulation. Journal of Neurophysiology 62: 854–863

Leah J D, Herdegen T, Bravo R 1991 Selective expression of Jun proteins following axotomy and axonal transport block in peripheral nerves in the rat: evidence for a role in the regeneration process. Brain Research 566: 198–207

Leah J D, Sandkuhler J, Herdegen T, Murashov A, Zimmermann M 1992 Potentiated expression of FOS protein in the rat spinal cord following bilateral noxious cutaneous stimulation. Neuroscience 48: 525–532

Lembeck F, Donnerer J, Colpaert F C 1981 Increase of substance P in primary afferent nerves during chronic pain. Neuropeptides 1: 175–180

Levine J D, Taiwo Y, Collins S, Tam J 1986 Noradrenaline hyperalgesia is mediated through interaction with sympathetic postganglionic neurone terminals rather than activation of primary afferent nociceptors. Nature 323: 158–159

McMahon S B, Koltzenburg M 1990 Novel classes of nociceptors: beyond Sherrington. Trends in Neurosciences 13: 199–201

McMahon S B, Wall P D 1984 Receptive fields of rat lamina I projection cells move to incorporate a nearby region of injury. Pain 19: 235–247

McMahon S B, Wall P D 1989 Changes in spinal cord reflexes after cross-anastomosis of cutaneous and muscle nerves in the adult rat. Nature (London) 342: 272–274

Mao J, Price D D, Mayer D J, Lu J, Hayes R L 1992a Intrathecal MK-801 and local nerve anesthesia synergistically reduce nociceptive behaviors in rats with experimental peripheral mononeuropathy. Brain Research 576: 254–262

Mao J, Price D D, Coghill R C, Mayer D J, Hayes R L 1992b Spatial patterns of spinal cord [14C]-2-deoxyglucose metabolic activity in a rat model of painful peripheral mononeuropathy. Pain 50: 89–100

Massardier D, Hunt P F 1989 A direct non-opiate interaction of dynorphin (1–13) with the N-methyl-D-aspartate (NMDA) receptor. European Journal of Pharmacology 170: 125–126

Matzner O, Devor M 1987 Contrasting thermal sensitivity of spontaneously active A- and C-fibers in experimental nerve-end neuromas. Pain 30: 373–384

Menétrey D, Besson J-M 1982 Electrophysiological characteristics of dorsal horn cells in rats with cutaneous inflammation resulting from chronic arthritis. Pain 13: 343–364

Menétrey D, Gannon A, Levine J D, Basbaum A I 1989 Expression of c-fos protein in interneurons and projection neurons of the rat spinal cord in response to noxious somatic, articular, and visceral stimulation. Journal of Comparative Neurology 285: 177–195

Meyer R A, Treede R-D, Raja S N, Campbell J N 1992 Peripheral versus central mechanisms for secondary hyperalgesia: is the controversy resolved. American Pain Society Journal 1: 127–131

Millan M J, Colpaert F C 1991 Opioid systems in the response to inflammatory pain: sustained blockade suggests role of κ- but not μ-opioid receptors in the modulation of nociception, behavior and pathology. Neuroscience 42: 541–553

Millan M J, Millan M H, Czonkowski A et al 1986 A model of chronic pain in the rat: response of multiple opioid systems of adjuvant-induced arthritis. Journal of Neuroscience 6: 899–906

Millan M J, Czonkowski A, Morris B et al 1988 Inflammation of the hind limb as a model of unilateral, localized pain: influence on multiple opioid systems in the spinal cord of the rat. Pain 35: 299–312

Minami M, Kuraishi Y, Kawamura M et al 1989 Enhancement of preprotachykinin A gene expression by adjuvant-induced inflammation in the rat spinal cord: possible involvement of substance P-containing spinal neurons in nociception. Neuroscience Letters 98: 105–110

Morgan J I, Curran T 1989 Stimulus-transcription coupling in neurons: role of cellular immediate-early genes. Trends in Neurosciences 12: 459–462

Murase K, Ryu P D, Randic M, 1989 Excitatory and inhibitory amino acids and peptide-induced responses in acutely isolated rat spinal dorsal horn neurons. Neuroscience Letters 103: 56–63

Naranjo J R, Mellström B, Achaval M, Sassone-Corsi P 1991 Molecular pathways of pain: fos/jun-mediated activation of a noncanonical AP-1 site in the prodynorphin gene. Neuron 6: 607–617

Neil A, Attal N, Guilbaud G 1991 Effects of guanethidine on sensitization to natural stimuli and self-mutilating behaviour in rats with a peripheral neuropathy. Brain Research 565: 237–246

Neil A, Kayer V, Gacel G, Besson J-M, Guilbaud G 1986 Opioid receptor types and antinociceptive activity in chronic inflammation: both κ- and μ-opiate agonistic effects are enhanced in arthritic rats. European Journal of Pharmacology 130: 203–208

Neugebauer V, Schaible H G 1990 Evidence for a central component in the sensitization of spinal neurons with joint input during development of acute arthritis in cat's knee. Journal of Neurophysiology 64: 299–299

Noguchi K, Morita Y, Kiyama H, Ono K, Tohyama M 1988 A noxious stimulus induces the preprotachykinin-A gene expression in the rat dorsal root ganglion: a quantitative study using in situ hybridization histochemistry. Molecular Brain Research 4: 31–35

Noguchi K, Kowalski K, Traub R, Solodkin A, Iadarola M J, Ruda M A 1991 Colocalization of dynorphin and Fos proteins in spinal cord neurons following inflammation induced hyperalgesia. Molecular Brain Research 10: 227–233

Noguchi K, Dubner R, Ruda M A 1992 Preproenkephalin mRNA in spinal dorsal horn neurons is induced by peripheral inflammation and is co-localized with Fos and Fos-related proteins. Neuroscience 46: 561–570

Noguchi K, De Leon M, Nahin R L, Senba E, Ruda M A 1993 Quantification of axotomy-induced alteration of neuropeptide mRNAs in dorsal root ganglion neurons with a special reference to neuropeptide Y mRNA and the effects of neonatal capsaicin treatment. Journal of Neuroscience Research, 35: 54–66

Oku R, Satoh M, Takagi H 1987 Release of substance P from the spinal dorsal horn is enhanced in polyarthritic rats. Neuroscience Letters 74: 315–319

Palecek J, Palecekova V, Dougherty P M, Carlton S M, Willis W D 1992 Responses of spinothalamic tract cells to mechanical and thermal stimulation of skin in rats with an experimental peripheral neuropathy. Journal of Neurophysiology 67: 1562–1573

Pompidou A, Corral M, Michel P, Defer N, Kruh J, Curran T 1987 The effects of phorbol ester and Ca ionophore on c-fos and c-myc expression and on DNA synthesis in human lymphocytes are not directly related. Biochemical and Biophysical Research Communications 148: 435–442

Presley R W, Menétrey D, Levine J D, Basbaum A I 1990 Systemic morphine suppresses noxious stimulus-evoked Fos protein-like immunoreactivity in the rat spinal cord. Journal of Neuroscience 10: 323–335

Price D D, Mao J, Coghill R C, et al 1991 Regional changes in spinal cord glucose metabolism in a rat model of painful neuropathy. Brain Research 564: 314–318

Randic M, Hecimovic H, Ryu P D 1990 Substance P modulates glutamate-induced currents in acutely isolated rat spinal dorsal horn neurons. Neuroscience Letters 117: 74–80

Ren K, Williams G M, Hylden J L K, Ruda M A, Dubner R 1992a The intrathecal administration of excitatory amino acid receptor antagonists selectively attenuated carrageenan-induced behavioural hyperalgesia in rats. European Journal of Pharmacology 219: 235–243

Ren K, Hylden J L K, Williams G M, Ruda M A, Dubner R 1992b The effects of a non-competitive NMDA receptor antagonist, MK-801, on behavioural hyperalgesia and dorsal horn neuronal activity in rats with unilateral inflammation. Pain 50: 331–344

Roberts W J 1986 A hypothesis on the physiological basis for causalgia and related pains. Pain 24: 297–311

Roberts W J, Foglesong M E 1988a I. Spinal recordings suggest that wide-dynamic-range neurons mediate sympathetically maintained pain. Pain 34: 289–304

Roberts W J, Foglesong M E 1988b II. Identification of afferents contributing to sympathetically evoked activity in wide-dynamic-range neurons. Pain 34: 305–314

Rodin B E, Kruger L 1984 Deafferentation in animals as a model for the study of pain: an alternative hypothesis. Brain Research Reviews 7: 213–228

Ruda M A, Iadarola M J, Cohen L V, Young W S III 1988 In situ hybridization histochemistry and immunocytochemistry reveal an increase in spinal dynorphin biosynthesis in a rat model of peripheral inflammation and hyperalgesia. Proceedings of the National Academy of Science (USA) 85: 622–626

Rusin K I, Ryu P D, Randic M 1992 Modulation of excitatory amino acid responses in rat dorsal horn neurons by tachykinins. Journal of Neurophysiology 68: 265–286

Sato J, Perl E R 1991 Adrenergic excitation of cutaneous pain receptors induced by peripheral nerve injury. Science 251: 1608–1610

Scadding J W 1981 Development of ongoing activity, mechanosensitivity, and adrenaline sensitivity in severed peripheral nerve axons. Experimental Neurology 73: 345–364

Schaible H-G, Schmidt R F, Willis W D 1987 Enhancement of the responses of ascending tract cells in the cat spinal cord by acute inflammation of the knee joint. Experimental Brain Research 66: 489–499

Schaible H G, Neugebauer V, Cervero F, Schmidt R F 1991 Changes in tonic descending inhibition of spinal neurons with articular input during the development of acute arthritis in the cat. Journal of Neurophysiology 66: 1021–1031

Seltzer Z, Dubner R, Shir Y 1990 A novel behavioral model of neuropathic pain disorders produced in rats by partial sciatic nerve injury. Pain 43: 205–218

Shir Y, Seltzer Z 1991 Effects of sympathectomy in a model of causalgiform pain produced by partial sciatic nerve injury in rats. Pain 45: 309–320

Simone D A, Sorkin L S, Oh U et al 1991 Neurogenic hyperalgesia: central neural correlates in responses of spinothalamic tract neurons. Journal of Neurophysiology 66: 228–246

Smith G D, Harmar A J, McQueen D S, Seckl J R 1992 Increase in substance P and CGRP, but not somatostatin content of innervating dorsal root ganglia in adjuvant monoarthritis in the rat. Neuroscience Letters 137: 257–260

Stewart P, Isaac L 1991 Dynorphin-induced depression of the dorsal root potential in rat spinal cord: a possible mechanism for potentiation of the C-fiber reflex. Journal of Pharmacology and Experimental Therapeutics 259: 608–613

Sugimoto T, Bennett G J, Kajander K C 1990 Transsynaptic degeneration in the superficial dorsal horn after sciatic nerve injury: effects of a chronic constriction injury, transection, and strychnine. Pain 42: 205–213

Swearengen E, Chavkin C 1987 NMDA receptor antagonist D-APV depresses excitatory activity produced by normorphine in rat hippocampal slices. Neuroscience Letters 78: 80–84

Tölle T R, Castro L J, Coimbra A, Zieglgänsberger W 1990 Opiates modify induction of c-fos proto-oncogene in the spinal cord of the rat following noxious stimulation. Neuroscience Letters 111: 46–51

Tverskoy M, Cozacov C, Ayache M, Bradley E L, Kissin I 1990 Postoperative pain after inguinal herniorrhaphy with different types of anesthesia. Anesthesia and Analgesia 70: 29–35

Villar M J, Wiesenfeld H Z, Xu X J, Theodorsson E, Emson P C, Hökfelt T 1991 Further studies on galanin-, substance P-, and CGRP-like immunoreactivities in primary sensory neurons and spinal cord: effects of dorsal rhizotomies and sciatic nerve lesions. Experimental Neurology 112: 29–39

Wakisaka S, Kajander K C, Bennett G J 1991 Increased neuropeptide Y (NPY)-like immunoreactivity in rat sensory neurons following peripheral axotomy. Neuroscience Letters 124: 200–203

Wall P D 1988 The prevention of postoperative pain. Pain 33: 289–290

Wall P D, Devor M 1981 The effect of peripheral nerve injury on dorsal root potentials and on transmission of afferent signals into the spinal cord. Brain Research 209: 95–111

Wall P D, Devor M 1983 Sensory afferent impulses originate from dorsal root ganglia as well as from the periphery in normal and nerve injured rats. Pain 17: 321–339

Wall P D, Gutnick M 1974 Properties of afferent nerve impulses originating from a neuroma. Nature (London) 248: 740–743

Wall P D, Woolf C J 1984 Muscle but not cutaneous C-afferent input produces prolonged increases in excitability of the flexion reflex in the rat. Journal Physiology (London) 356: 443–458

Woolf C J 1983 Evidence for a central component of post-injury pain hypersensitivity. Nature 306: 686–688

Woolf C J, King A E 1990 Dynamic alterations in the cutaneous mechanoreceptive fields of dorsal horn neurons in the rat spinal cord. Journal of Neuroscience 10: 2717–2726

Woolf C J, Thompson S W M 1991 The induction and maintenance of central sensitization is dependent on N-methyl-D-aspartic acid receptor activation: implications for the treatment of post-injury pain hypersensitivity states. Pain 44: 293–299

Woolf C J, Wall P D 1986 Relative effectiveness of C primary afferent fibers of different origins in evoking a prolonged facilitation of the flexor reflex in the rat. Journal of Neuroscience 6: 1433–1442

Woolf C J, Wisenfeld-Hallin Z 1985 The systemic administration of local anesthetics produces a selective depression of C-afferent fibre evoked activity in the spinal cord. Pain 23: 361–374

Woolf C, Wiesenfeld-Hallin Z 1986 Substance P and calcitonin gene-related peptide synergistically modulate the gain of the nociceptive flexor withdrawal reflex in the rat. Neuroscience Letters 66: 226–230

Woolf C J, Shortland P, Coggeshall R E 1992 Peripheral nerve injury triggers central sprouting of myelinated afferents. Nature (London) 355: 75–78

Yamamoto T, Yaksh T L 1992a Studies on the spinal interaction of morphine and the NMDA antagonist MK-801 on the hyperalgesia observed in a rat model of sciatic mononeuropathy. Neuroscience Letters 135: 67–70

Yamamoto T, Yaksh T L 1992b Spinal pharmacology of thermal hyperesthesia induced by constriction injury of sciatic nerve. Excitatory amino acid antagonists. Pain 49: 121–128

12. Central nervous system mechanisms of pain modulation

Howard L. Fields and Allan I. Basbaum

INTRODUCTION

The perception of pain is evoked by stimuli that are sufficient or nearly sufficient to produce tissue damage and, at least in human psychophysical studies, there is a direct relationship between stimulus intensity and reported pain intensity. This relationship can be highly variable, particularly in clinical situations. The variability depends on both peripheral and central nervous system (CNS) factors. For example, pain thresholds to mechanical stimulation can be dramatically lowered in an area of inflammation by the sensitization of primary afferents (see Ch. 2). Long-lasting increases in excitability of nociresponsive dorsal horn neurons may also contribute to the lowering of pain threshold. In addition to the plasticity of afferent pain pathways that is induced by prolonged or repeated noxious stimuli, factors such as arousal, attention and emotional stress, which clearly involve CNS mechanisms, profoundly alter responses to noxious stimuli. For example, traumatic injuries sustained during athletic competitions or combat are often initially reported as being relatively painlesss (Melzack et al 1982). In other circumstances, these same injuries are extremely painful (Beecher 1959). The weight of evidence indicates that changes in pain responses due to arousal, attention and stress result from the action of modulatory networks that control the transmission of nociceptive messages in the CNS. This chapter will describe the properties of pain modulatory networks in the CNS.

There are inherent problems in studying modulatory networks. In contrast to sensory and motor systems, there may be no subjective or behavioural consequence of activating a modulatory network. Thus electrical stimulation of a motor pathway produces movement, stimulation of a sensory pathway sensation. In contrast, without a noxious stimulus, the activity of a pain modulatory pathway may have no overt behavioural or subjective consequence. Furthermore, the complexity of some factors, such as arousal and attention, which engage pain modulatory networks, makes it difficult to study the activity of their constituent neurons under physiological conditions (Oliveras et al 1990). Nonetheless, significant progress has been made; an anatomically distinct and physiologically selective CNS pain modulating network has been identified. This network has links in the hypothalamus and brainstem, controls nociresponsive dorsal horn neurons and is sensitive to opioids. It is unlikely that this is the only pain modulating network in the CNS, but it is the most extensively studied and will be the primary focus of this chapter.

DESCENDING MODULATORY CONTROL

As early as 1911 Head & Holmes explicitly postulated modulatory influences on pain. They proposed that the thalamus is the centre for the perception of pain and that the neocortex, the discriminative perception centre, continuously modulates the responses of the thalamus to noxious stimuli. According to their hypothesis, modulation of pain is a necessary part of the on-going process of discriminative sensation.

Clearcut examples of centrifugal control of sensory transmission were subsequently described. Hagbarth & Kerr (1954) provided the first direct evidence that supraspinal sites control ascending (presumably sensory) pathways, and Carpenter et al (1965) demonstrated descending control of sensory input to ascending pathways. The existence of a specific *pain* modulatory system was, however, first clearly articulated in 1965 by Melzack & Wall in 'the Gate Control theory of pain'. Supraspinal influences on the 'gate' were proposed but there was limited evidence for the existence of descending control of nociception. In 1967, Wall reported that cells in lamina V of the dorsal horn of decerebrate cats are more responsive to noxious stimuli when the spinal cord is blocked, thus showing that structures in the brainstem tonically inhibit nociresponsive neurons in the spinal cord. The hypothesis that descending systems contribute to pain modulation was strongly supported by the discovery of the phenomenon of stimulation-produced analgesia (SPA) (Reynolds 1969; Mayer & Liebeskind 1974). SPA is a highly specific suppression of responses to noxious stimuli produced by electrical stimulation of discrete brain sites. During SPA, animals remain alert and active and, although their responses to most environmental stimuli are unchanged, responses to noxious stimuli such as orientation, vocalization, escape and defaecation are absent. Thus, in animals, SPA is a powerful, highly selective and robust phenomenon. Importantly, SPA is associated with the inhibition of reflex responses to noxious stimulation, such as the tail flick, which are mediated by intraspinal connections. This implicates descending pathways to the spinal cord in the antinociceptive action of periaqueductal grey (PAG) stimulation.

The significance of SPA was confirmed by its demonstration in human subjects with chronic pain (Boivie & Meyerson 1982; Baskin et al 1986). This analgesia is produced without eliciting any movement or consistent positive sensation. The specificity of the analgesia and the fact that it is consistently elicited from discrete brain sites that are homologous in a variety of species including humans is powerful evidence for a specific pain-modulating system.

Shortly after SPA was discovered, two of its important features were established. First, nociresponsive cells in the spinal cord dorsal horn are selectively inhibited by stimulation at analgesia-producing brainstem sites (Guilbaud et al 1973). Second, discrete lesions of the spinal cord dorsolateral funiculus (DLF) block the inhibition by brainstem neurons of behavioural responses to noxious stimuli (Basbaum et al 1976). These observations demonstrated that there is a descending limb of the nociceptive modulatory system. In fact, our most extensive knowledge of pain modulation concerns those systems that descend to the spinal cord in the DLF (Mayer & Price 1976; Basbaum & Fields 1978, 1984; Fields et al 1991).

Figure 12.1 illustrates the major CNS structures which have been implicated in supraspinal control of spinal nociceptive transmission. This chapter will focus on the periaqueductal grey (PAG), the rostral ventromedial medulla (RVM), the dorsolateral pontine tegmentum (DLPT) and the spinal cord.

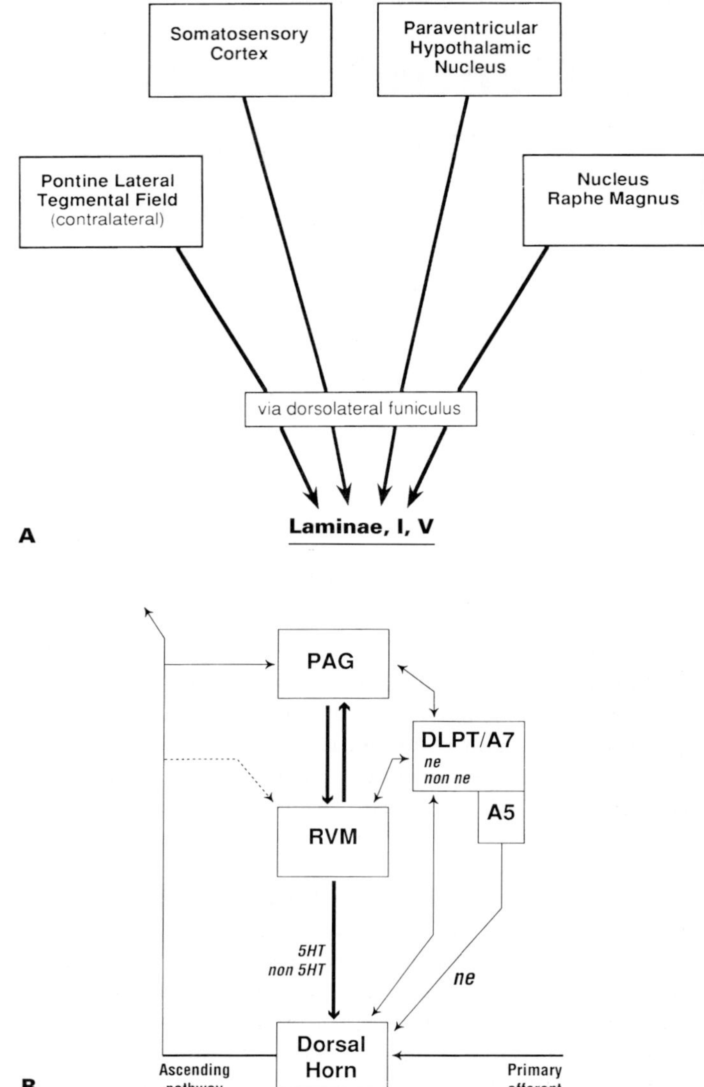

Fig. 12.1 **A** Diagram of the major inputs from supraspinal sites to laminae I and V of the dorsal horn. Each of these locations contains neurons that are potentially capable of modulating the firing of nociceptive projection neurons. **B** Diagram of connectivity of brainstem structures implicated in nociceptive modulation. PAG = midbrain periaqueductal grey; DLPT = dorsolateral pontine tegmentum which is rostrally contiguous with the nucleus cuneiformis and caudally with the medullary A5 noradrenergic group; RVM = the rostral ventromedial medulla which is the major serotonergic input to the dorsal horn.

PERIAQUEDUCTAL GREY (PAG)

Anatomical studies emphasize that the PAG is cytoarchitectonically and chemically heterogeneous and that different subdivisions of the PAG differ in their contribution to analgesia (Cannon et al 1982). Inputs to PAG from more rostral brain centres are apparently critical for initiating the powerful descending control systems that act on spinal nociresponsive neurons. In addition, the presence of projections from PAG to medial thalamus and orbital frontal cortex raises the possibility of ascending control of nociception (Coffield et al 1992). A major source of afferents to the PAG is the hypothalamus (Beitz 1982b; Reichling & Basbaum 1990) and electrical stimulation of certain hypothalamic regions produces analgesia (Rhodes & Liebeskind 1978). Other important forebrain inputs to PAG arise from frontal granular and insular cortex (Hardy & Leichnetz 1981) and from the amygdala (Gray & Magnuson 1992). Whether the cortical inputs to PAG contribute to analgesia is unknown. Analgesia, however, can be elicited by stimulation of the amygdala and lesions of the amygdala reduce the analgesia associated with fear (Fanselow 1991) or systemically administered opiates (Calvino et al 1982).

Major brainstem inputs to the PAG arise from the adjacent nucleus cuneiformis, the pontomedullary reticular formation, the locus coeruleus and other brainstem catecholaminergic nuclei (Herbert & Saper 1992). The PAG is also reciprocally connected with neurons in the rostral medulla that give rise to the bulk of pain-modulatory fibres that project directly to the dorsal horn. Finally, the PAG and adjacent nucleus cuneiformis receive a major projection from the spinal cord dorsal horn. This projection arises from lamina I nociresponsive neurons (Hylden et al 1986; Menétrey et al 1982).

THE ROSTRAL VENTROMEDIAL MEDULLA (RVM)

This includes the midline nucleus raphe magnus (NRM) and the adjacent reticular formation that lies ventral to the nucleus reticularis gigantocellularis. The RVM includes the nucleus reticularis magnocellularis (RMC) in the cat and the nucleus reticularis paragigantocellularis (RPG) in the rat. Electrical stimulation or microinjection of opioids or excitatory amino acids into the RVM produces analgesia.

The PAG and the adjacent nucleus cuneiformis are the major source of inputs to the RVM. There is evidence that glutamate and/or aspartate are excitatory transmitters in the PAG to RVM connection (Aimone & Gebhart 1986). Although the PAG contains a large number of enkephalin, substance P (SP) and gamma-aminobutyric acid (GABA)ergic neurons (Hökfelt et al 1977a, 1977b; Moss et al 1983) these neurons appear not to project to the RVM (Prichard & Beitz 1981; Reichling & Basbaum, 1990). The RVM does, however, receive an input from serotonin (5-HT)-containing neurons of the dorsal raphe (Beitz 1982a). There is also a significant noradrenergic input to RVM that derives from the A5 and A7 cell groups of the rostral medulla and dorsolateral pons, respectively (Clark et al 1991). Direct spinal projections to the RVM are sparse but the RVM does receive a projection from the adjacent medullary nucleus reticularis gigantocellularis which in turn receives a large projection from nociceptive spinoreticular neurons (Fields et al 1977a).

The RVM is the major brainstem source of axons that project to the spinal cord via the DLF. The terminals of these descending axons are most dense in the superficial layers of the dorsal horn and in the region of lamina V. These same regions are targets of small-diameter primary afferents and contain large numbers of nociresponsive neurons (Basbaum et al 1978). Electrical stimulation of the RVM selectively inhibits nociresponsive dorsal horn neurons, an effect that is blocked by DLF lesions (Fields et al 1977b; Willis et al 1977). Since there are few direct PAG-spinal projections, it is likely that the descending pain-modulating action of the PAG is relayed through the RVM. This hypothesis is supported by the observations that lesions of, or local anaesthetic injections into, RVM abolish the analgesia produced by stimulation of PAG (Behbehani & Fields 1979; Aimone & Gebhart 1986) and that opioid injections into PAG produce concomitant analgesia and activation of putative pain-inhibitory neurons in RVM (Cheng et al 1986).

DORSOLATERAL PONTOMESENCEPHALIC TEGMENTUM (DLPT)

This region also plays a critical role in pain modulation (Haws et al 1989). The DLPT includes the nucleus cuneiformis which is adjacent to the ventrolateral PAG and shares many of its anatomical features, including an input from lamina I of the dorsal horn and a major projection to the RVM. The DLPT also includes areas around the brachium conjunctivum including the subcoerulear and parabrachial nuclei which project to the RVM and via the DLF directly to the spinal cord dorsal horn. The DLPT also includes the A7 region of noradrenaline (NA)-containing neurons, many of which project to the dorsal horn (Clark & Proudfit 1991b; Kwiat & Basbaum 1992). The A7 region is reciprocally connected to the RVM (Clark & Proudfit 1991a; Drolet et al 1992; Paice & Proudfit 1992). Electrical stimulation throughout the DLPT inhibits nocifensor spinal reflexes (Haws et al 1989) and dorsal horn nociresponsive neurons (Carstens et al 1980). It is of interest that recent studies have shown that electrical stimulation of this region can relieve clinically significant chronic pain (Young et al 1992).

In summary, there is a network that extends from frontal cortex and hypothalamus through the PAG to the RVM and then via the DLF to the dorsal horn of the spinal cord. Neurons in the DLPT are linked to this network by their reciprocal connection with the RVM. The DLPT also provides a parallel direct projection to the spinal cord dorsal horn. Activation of the PAG, RVM or DLPT by either opioids or electrical stimulation reduces the firing of nociresponsive dorsal horn neurons and produces behavioural antinociception.

NEUROTRANSMITTER SYSTEMS IN PAIN MODULATION

BIOGENIC AMINES

There is evidence that both norepinephrine (NE) and 5-HT containing brainstem neurons contribute to pain modulation. For example, the analgesia produced by PAG injection of morphine can be antagonized completely only when a combination of 5-HT and NE antagonists is coadministered at the level of the cord (Yaksh 1979). Furthermore, iontophoresis of either NE or 5-HT inhibits the firing of spinal cord nociresponsive neurons (see below).

SEROTONIN (5-HT)

An extensive body of evidence implicates bulbospinal serotonergic projections in pain modulation (Le Bars 1988). The analgesic action of systemic opiates can be at least transiently reduced by depletion of 5-HT by inhibiting its synthesis (Tenen 1968), by neurotoxic destruction of spinal 5-HT terminals with 5,7-dihydroxytryptamine (Vogt 1974) or by lesions of medullary regions which contain 5-HT neurons (Roberts 1988). The analgesia produced by intracerebral morphine can be partially blocked by intrathecal methysergide, a nonselective 5-HT antagonist (Yaksh 1979). Iontophoresis of 5-HT inhibits the response of dorsal horn neurons to noxious stimulation (Randic & Yu 1976; Headley et al 1978; Jordan et al 1979) and when 5-HT is applied directly to the spinal cord it produces analgesia (Hylden & Wilcox 1983; Schmauss et al 1983; Solomon & Gebhart 1988).

Of particular interest are recent studies demonstrating differential effects of ligands with selectivity for different 5-HT receptor subtypes. For example, there is evidence that 5-HT_2 receptors in the spinal cord mediate the antinociceptive effects of 5-HT (Crisp et al 1991). In other studies, Alhaider et al (1991) reported that intrathecal injection of a selective 5-HT_3 receptor agonist (2-methyl 5-HT) is antinociceptive in both behavioural and electrophysiological studies. Moreover, the 'pain' behaviour produced by both N-methyl-D-aspartate (NMDA) and SP were blocked by 2-methyl 5-HT which indicates that a postsynaptic action mediates the antinociceptive effect. The complexity of the 5-HT contribution, however, is underscored by other studies which demonstrate that, acting via the 5-HT_{1A} receptor, 5-HT may produce either a *facilitatory* (Zemlan et al 1983; Alhaider et al 1990) or an *inhibitory* (Eide et al 1990) action on spinal nociceptive processing.

Spinally projecting brainstem noradrenergic neurons are also critical to the regulation of transmission of nociceptive messages (Proudfit 1988). Powerful antinociceptive actions can be evoked by electrical stimulation of the locus coeruleus and, as described above, the A5 and A7 noradrenergic cell groups of the rostral medulla and pons. Glutamate injection into several of these sites produces a comparable antinociceptive effect. In general, noradrenergic controls are mediated at the spinal level by the action at the α-2-adrenergic receptor (Yeomans et al 1992).

RVM neurons contribute to the activation of the descending noradrenergic controls. There are direct projections from the RVM to noradrenergic cell groups which project to the spinal cord (Clark & Proudfit 1991a; Kwiat & Basbaum 1992). Furthermore, electrical stimulation of the RVM evokes the release of both 5-HT and NE in the spinal cord cerebrospinal fluid (CSF) and the analgesia produced by this stimulation is blocked by combinations of 5-HT and NE antagonists (Fields & Besson 1988).

Although questions have been raised as to the relative importance of spinal 5-HT and NE to *endogenous* antinociceptive control mechanisms, there is no clear answer. Indeed, it appears that the two are concurrently activated by opioids administered supraspinally (Tseng & Tang 1989). Moreover, there is considerable evidence that interactions occur in the dorsal horn at the level of the 5-HT and NE terminal (Archer et al 1986; Eide & Hole 1991). From a clinical perspective, however, noradrenergic controls may be more relevant. Thus intrathecal injection of α-2-adrenergic agonists produces a profound analgesia, that may synergize with that produced by opioids.

Finally, it must be emphasized that although 5-HT and NE are the major contributors to descending antinociceptive controls, many of the spinally projecting 5-HT and NE neurons contain other neurotransmitters. Among these are the peptides, enkephalin, SP and thyrotrophin-releasing hormons (TRH). Although the raphe neurons which cocontain 5-HT and SP predominantly target the ventral horn and the preganglionic sympathetic neurons of the intermediolateral cell column, it is likely that some of the neurons which cocontain enkephalin and 5-HT project to nociceptive neurons of the dorsal horn. Studies are clearly needed which are directed at the questions of corelease of the peptide and the amine at the level of the cord and how such release might influence nociceptive transmission.

ENDOGENOUS OPIOID PEPTIDES

The discovery of endogenous opioid peptides was one of the most important keys to our understanding of CNS pain modulating circuits. The existence of an endogenous morphine-like compound was suspected based on the observations that narcotic analgesics, such as morphine, act in the CNS and that binding sites with opiate receptor characteristics were found to be associated with brain membranes. Using a gut smooth muscle preparation as a sensitive bioassay, Hughes and his colleagues (1975) isolated the first opioid peptides from the pig brain: the pentapeptides leucine (Leu)- and methionine (Met)-enkephalin (Enk). Since that discovery, several other opioid peptides have been characterized; most mimic narcotic analgesics in bioassay and analgesia tests (Miller 1981). Importantly, the significance of the contribution of endogenous opioid peptides to pain modulation has been confirmed by the observations that SPA in animals and humans, some forms of stress-induced analgesia in animals and placebo analgesia in humans with postoperative pain can all be reduced by the narcotic antagonist naloxone (Watkins & Mayer 1982; Fields 1988).

Among the opioid peptides, one of the most potent for analgesia is β-endorphin (BE), a 31-amino acid peptide, the N-terminal of which is identical to Met-enkephalin. Two other opioid peptides with N-terminal Leu-enkephalin have been isolated; dynorphin, a 17-amino acid peptide, and the decapeptide α-neoendorphin (see Table 12.1; Goldstein et al 1979; Weber et al 1981).

Peptide transmitters and hormones are derived by cleavage of larger, usually inactive, precursor polypeptides. Met- and Leu-enkephalin are derived from a common precursor, pro-enkephalin, each molecule of which generates multiple copies of Met-enkephalin and one of Leu-enkephalin (Comb et al 1982). Met- and Leu-enk are found in numerous cell groups throughout the neuraxis. Consistent with their having a common precursor, Leu- and Met-enk have completely overlapping distributions. The distribution of Met- and Leu-enk is not restricted to pain modulating circuits. In fact, their densest concentration within the brain is in the striatum. On the other hand, most of the CNS structures associated with pain modulation do have significant amounts of Met- and Leu-enk (Table 12.2). This includes the PAG, RVM and superficial dorsal horn.

BE is cleaved from a larger precursor, pro-opiomelanocortin, which also gives rise to adrenocorticotropic hormone (ACTH) and several copies of melanocyte-stimulating hormone (MSH) (Mains et al 1977). There is only one copy of BE in each pro-opiomelanocortin molecule. Most BE is derived from cells in the anterior and intermediate pituitary. Although the intermediate lobe contains more BE than the anterior lobe, much of the intermediate lobe BE is acetylated at its N-terminal or shortened at its C-terminal, modifications which block its analgesic potency. In addition to pituitary BE there are discrete populations of neurons in the ventromedial hypothalamus which contain BE (Watson & Akil 1980). These neurons may have a role in pain modulation (see below).

Two copies of dynorphin (A and B) and α-neoendorphin are cleaved together from still another precursor molecule. Although some brain areas contain dynorphin and the enkephalins, considerable segregation of these two systems is present. For example, although dynorphin is the predominant opioid peptide in the substantia nigra, it overlaps considerably with enkephalin in the dorsal horn and PAG.

PAG

This contains significant quantities of all families of endogenous opioid peptides. Opioid peptides present in the PAG include Leu- and Met-enk, BE and dynorphin.

Table 12.1 Sequences of endogenous opioid peptides involved in pain modulation

Leucine-enkephalin	Tyr-Gly-Gly-Phe-Leu-OH
Methionine-enkephalin	Tyr-Gly-Gly-Phe-Met-OH
β-Endorphin	*Tyr-Gly-Gly-Phe-Met*-Thr-Ser-Glu-Lys-Ser-Gln-Thr-Pro-Leu-Val-Thr-Leu-Phe-Lys-Asn-Ala-Ile-Val-Lys-Asn-Ala-His-Lys-Gly-Gln-OH
Dynorphin	*Tyr-Gly-Gly-Phe-Leu*-Arg-Arg-Ile-Arg-Pro-Lys-Leu-Lys-Tyr-Asp-Asn-Gln-OH

Table 12.2 Opioid peptides and analgesia: anatomical relationships

Anatomical site	β-Endorphin, enkephalin or dynorphin	Opiate receptor	Opiate microinjection analgesia	Stimulation-produced analgesia	Local naloxone blocks analgesia
Amygdala	+	+	+[1]	+	?
Periventricular diencephalon	+	+	+	+	?
Periaqueductal grey	+	+	+	+	+
Rostral ventromedial medulla	+	+	+	+	+
Dorsal horn	+	+	+	0	+

+ = present; 0 = not demonstrated, or very low; ? = unknown.
[1]Rodgers R J 1977 Elevation of aversive threshold in rats by intra-amygdaloid injection of morphine sulphate. Pharmacology, Biochemistry and Behavior 6: 385–390

Unlike BE, which derives exclusively from cells in the hypothalamus, enkephalin and dynorphin cell bodies are intrinsic to the PAG. A major unanswered question concerns the relative contribution of each of the different opioid peptides to the analgesia produced by electrical stimulation. Studies by Millan and his colleagues (1986, 1987) suggest a predominant contribution of BE.

RVM

Many RVM neurons contain enkephalin and the region is rich in enkephalin-containing terminal fields. Some BE terminals and dynorphin-immunoreactive somata and terminals are also present in RVM. There is evidence for μ-opioid binding sites in the RVM (Bowker et al 1988); however, this is not a particularly dense pattern. Nevertheless, microinjection of μ-opioids in RVM produces potent analgesia.

In summary, there are at least three biochemically and anatomically distinct populations of opioid-containing cells. Each is present in neural somata or terminal fields in brainstem locations linked to pain modulation.

SPINAL CORD CIRCUITS UNDERLYING MODULATION OF NOCICEPTIVE TRANSMISSION

A full understanding of the neural mechanisms through which brainstem neurons control nociceptive transmission requires a detailed map of relevant dorsal horn circuitry. Projections to the dorsal horn from brainstem nuclei involved in modulation of nociceptive transmission terminate densely in laminae I and II and in laminae IV, V, VI and X. Small-diameter primary afferents, including all classes of primary nociceptors, terminate densely in laminae I and II. Neurons of both laminae respond to noxious stimulation. There are also direct projections to deeper laminae from both myelinated primary afferent nociceptors and brainstem nuclei involved in nociceptive modulation. It is also important to point out that the modulatory circuitry in laminae I and II may have relevance to the control of nociceptive neurons in deeper laminae since lamina II contains dendrites of some nociceptive neurons in deeper laminae (e.g. wide-dynamic-range (WDR) laminae V cells), and some laminae II neurons connect to neurons in deeper laminae (Light & Kavookjian 1988) (Fig. 12.2).

A variety of cell types are found in the superficial dorsal horn. Many lamina I neurons are projection neurons; in fact, in primates lamina I is the largest source of spinothalamic tract axons. In contrast, most substantia gelatinosa (SG) (lamina II (outer)) cells are locally connecting interneurons. Some of the SG interneurons that send their axons into lamina I respond to both noxious and nonnoxious input (Bennett et al 1979). Since these SG neurons are activated at shorter latency than overlying lamina I cells, it has been suggested that they are excitatory interneurons that relay inputs from primary afferents to marginal neurons. Direct primary afferent connections to lamina I cells also exist, but these constitute a relatively small percentage of the total marginal cell input (Ralston & Ralston 1979).

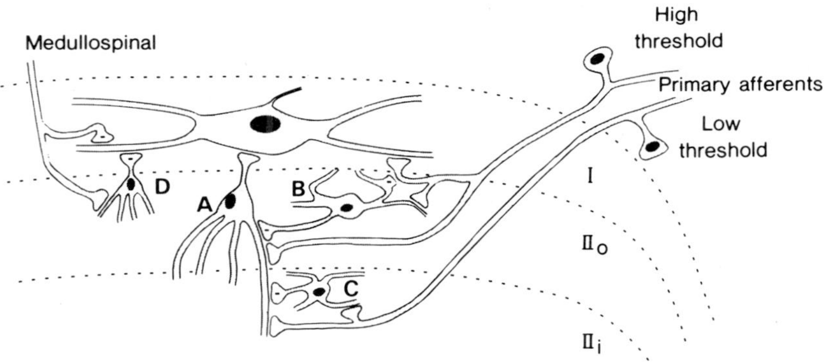

Fig. 12.2 Local circuitry in the superficial dorsal horn. Schematic illustration of afferent terminals and local circuitry within the superficial dorsal horn of the spinal cord. Nociceptive inputs, transmitted via high-threshold, primary afferent fibres, excite the nociceptive projection neurons of the marginal zone, lamina I. The same afferents excite dendrites of stalk cell excitatory interneurons (A) and inhibitory islet interneurons (B) of lamina IIo. The stalk cell input results in further excitatory drive on to marginal projection neurons; the input to the islet cell interneuron (B) in lamina IIo provides a circuit that generates an inhibitory, feedforward control of marginal neurons by nociceptive inputs.

Low-threshold primary afferent fibres provide a nonnociceptive input to marginal neurons via their excitatory connections with dendrites of stalk cell (A) in lamina IIi. In contrast, the nonnociceptive input to islet cell interneurons of lamina IIi (C) may contribute to the inhibitory control of nociceptive marginal neurons.

The schema also illustrates some possible descending control mechanisms. These may be exerted directly upon dorsal horn projection neurons. Alternatively, descending bulbospinal axons (some of which are 5-HT-containing) may excite inhibitory interneurons (e.g. enkephalin-containing stalk (D) or islet cells), which in turn postsynaptically control the nociceptive projection neurons. Another possibility, not illustrated, is that the descending systems inhibit the excitatory stalk cell (A).

Other interneurons in SG and lamina I are likely to have an inhibitory action on projection neurons. This conclusion is based largely on immunocytochemical evidence that subpopulations of neurons in these laminae contain inhibitory neurotransmitters (e.g. GABA and enkephalin) and are the likely source of the inhibitory transmitters in afferents to projection neurons (see below).

ACTIONS OF PUTATIVE BRAINSTEM PAIN MODULATORY NEURONS UPON SPINAL CIRCUITRY

The control of spinal nociceptive transmission by brainstem neurons may involve a number of parallel actions. As described above, the largest projection from the brainstem to the dorsal horn arises from the RVM. RVM axon terminals directly contact both thalamic relay cells and local circuit neurons in the dorsal horn. The synapses made by the dorsal horn terminals of RVM neurons are axodendritic and axosomatic but not axoaxonic; thus there is no evidence that they directly exert conventional presynaptic control of primary afferent terminals (Ruda et al 1986; Basbaum et al 1986b; Light & Kavookjian 1988). On the other hand, there is recent evidence that the spinal terminals of nociceptive primary afferents are postsynaptic to GABA-containing synapses (Alvarez et al 1992). This provides a potential mechanism for descending control of the terminals of primary afferent nociceptors.

Direct control of projection neurons

There are several possible circuits involving a postsynaptic action by RVM neurons that could account for inhibition of nociceptive transmission in the dorsal horn. One possibility is that brainstem neurons monosynaptically inhibit rostrally projecting nociceptive dorsal horn cells (Fig. 12.2). In fact, electrical stimulation in RVM produces a monosynaptic inhibitory postsynaptic potential in spinothalamic tract (STT) neurons (Giesler et al 1981). Furthermore, because the RVM is the primary source of 5-HT terminals in the dorsal horn, the demonstration that STT neurons receive a large 5-HT input provides a substrate for direct postsynaptic control by brainstem neurons. Similarly, there is a direct catecholaminergic innervation of primate STT neurons which most likely derives from brainstem neurons (Westlund et al 1990).

Inhibition of an excitatory dorsal horn interneuron

As described above, there is evidence that lamina II interneurons provide a major excitatory input from C-fibres to lamina I projection cells. In favour of a role in pain modulation for supraspinal inhibition of an excitatory interneuron, Light & Kavookjian (1988) have described a population of nociceptive lamina II cells that is inhibited by RVM stimulation. Some of these interneurons have been shown to make asymmetric, presumably excitatory, synapses on to neurons in deeper laminae of the dorsal horn.

Excitation of an inhibitory interneuron (Fig. 12.2A)

The superficial dorsal horn contains large numbers of neurons with immunoreactivity for the inhibitory neurotransmitters GABA (Ruda et al 1986; Magoul et al 1987; Todd & McKenzie, 1989) and enkephalin (Glazer & Basbaum 1981; Ruda et al 1986). Some of these neurons are immunoreactive for both (Todd et al 1992). Furthermore, there is a population of neurons in the superficial dorsal horn that is excited by antinociceptive PAG stimulation (Millar & Williams 1989). The existence of such a population of neurons is required by the hypothesis that supraspinal pain modulation neurons produce inhibition by exciting an inhibitory interneuron. In view of the dense projection of RVM serotonergic neurons to the superficial dorsal horn and the evidence implicating 5-HT in pain modulation (LeBars 1988) it is important that there is a population of superficial dorsal horn neurons that is excited by iontophoresis of 5-HT (Todd & Millar 1983). Furthermore, the inhibition of dorsal horn neurons produced by some 5-HT agonists (5-HT_3) is blocked by a GABA antagonist, suggesting that the 5-HT effect involves a GABAergic interneuron (Alhaidar et al 1991).

Opioid interneurons are also implicated in descending control. Although there are direct projections to the spinal cord from enkephalin-containing RVM neurons (Hökfelt et al 1979), the vast majority of opioid terminals in the dorsal horn are derived from local interneurons. Both enkephalin and dynorphin terminals and cells are present in superficial dorsal horn (Glazer & Basbaum 1981; Cruz & Basbaum 1985), as are dense concentrations of opiate receptor (Atweh & Kuhar 1977). There are differences between the distribution of enkephalin and dynorphin. The enkephalin distribution includes nociceptive, e.g. laminae I, outer II and V, as well as nonnociceptive regions, inner laminae II and III. In contrast, dynorphin cells and terminals are almost exclusively found in laminae I and V. Interestingly, a component of the dynorphin but not enkephalin terminal staining in lamina I originates in primary afferents (Basbaum et al 1986a).

Enkephalin-immunoreactive neurons in laminae I and II are directly contacted by serotonergic terminals (Glazer & Basbaum 1984; Miletic et al 1984) which are most likely derived from the RVM. Furthermore, there are enkephalin immunoreactive contacts upon STT neurons in laminae I and V (Ruda et al 1984; Priestly & Cuello 1989). Spinal application of opioids produces analgesia (see Ch. 9) and there is an extensive body of evidence demonstrating that opioid iontophoresis inhibits dorsal horn nociceptive neurons (Duggan & North 1984; Fleetwood-Walker et al 1988). Intrathecal naloxone reduces the antinociceptive action of electrical stimulation of RVM (Zorman et al 1982; Aimone et al 1987) or supraspinal opioid administration (Levine et al 1982). Furthermore, intrathecal administration of drugs that block enkephalin degrading enzymes produces behavioural antinociception (Oshita et al 1990) and inhibits nociceptive dorsal horn neurons (Dickenson et al 1987).

PHYSIOLOGY OF MODULATORY NETWORKS

PAIN MODULATION IS BIDIRECTIONAL

Early research focused on the antinociceptive actions of pain-modulating networks. Recent work, however, has demonstrated facilitatory actions on nociceptive transmission elicited by activating pain-modulating regions of the brainstem (Fields 1992; Zhou & Gebhart 1992). In attempting to understand this bidirectional control, studies in awake primates have been particularly instructive. Duncan et al (1987) recorded the activity of nociceptive trigeminal dorsal horn neurons, including some that project to the thalamus. These primates were trained to press a button in response to a light cue. Pressing the button initiated a trial during which the animal had to discriminate between two noxious thermal stimuli. Some neurons underwent abrupt increases or decreases in their activity that were time locked to the light cue or the button press. Importantly, these 'task-related' changes in activity occurred *prior to the onset of the thermal stimulus.* These experiments show that the activity of dorsal horn nociceptive neurons can be increased or decreased by a context-specific modulatory signal that originates in the CNS. The presence of facilitatory modulation of dorsal horn nociresponsive neurons raises the intriguing possibility that pain could be produced by centrally originating drive of dorsal horn nociceptive neurons without activation of primary afferent nociceptors.

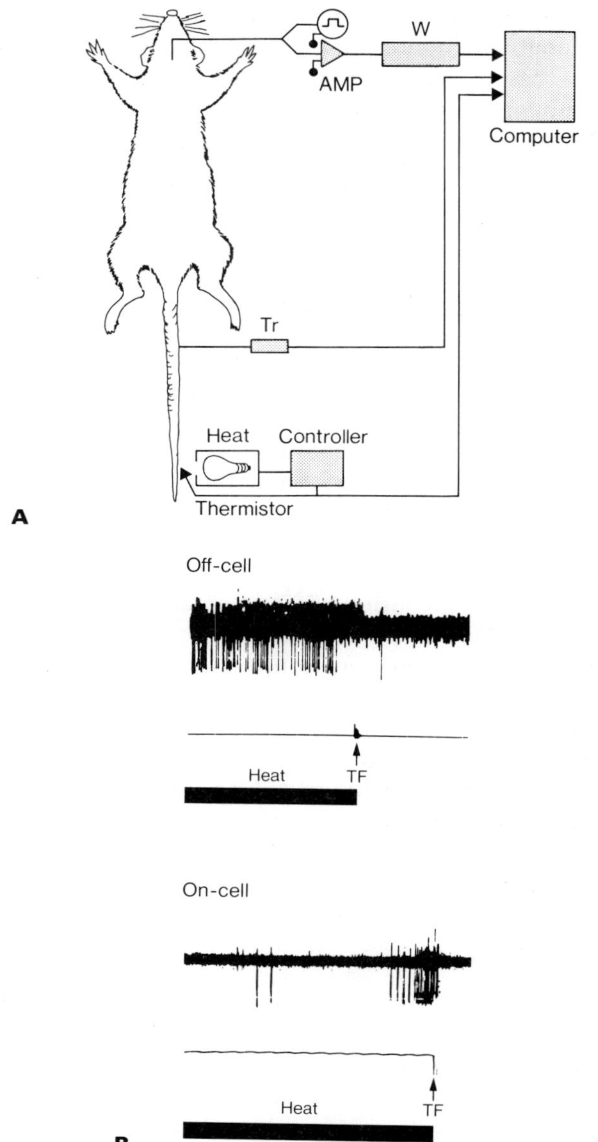

Fig. 12.3 Properties of proposed medullary pain modulating neurons. **A** Experimental set up. A microelectrode for single unit recording is placed in the region of the rostral medulla that projects to the dorsal horn. Heat was applied to the tail and recorded with a thermistor while recording both the neuronal activity and the time of occurrence of the tail flick with a force transducer (Tr). **B** Top trace illustrates the firing pattern of an off-cell in RVM, which pauses starting just prior to a withdrawal movement (TF = tail flick) from noxious heat. The on-cell demontrates a firing pattern reciprocal to that of the off-cell.

BRAINSTEM PAIN-MODULATING NEURONS

We have recorded from cells in RVM while monitoring the tail-flick reflex produced by noxious heat. In addition, we used microstimulation through the recording electrodes to map low-threshold sites for SPA. Using this approach we found three classes of cell in low-threshold SPA sites: those which discharge just prior to occurrence of a tail-flick (on-cells), those which shut off just prior to a tail-flick occurrence (off-cells) and those showing no consistent changes in activity correlated to withdrawal reflexes (neutral-cells; Fields & Heinricher 1985). Figure 12.3 illustrates the firing patterns of on- and off-cells. On-cells are consistently excited by noxious stimuli over most of the body surface. Most off-cells are inhibited by the same stimuli. Neutral-cells show variable responses or are unresponsive to noxious stimuli. A significant proportion of neurons of each class of RVM cell projects to the spinal cord. On- and off-cells are excited by electrical stimulation of PAG; however, only the off-cell is excited by morphine (Fields & Heinricher 1985). Thus, activity of the off-cell is most consistently related to suppression of nociceptive transmission. On-cells are inhibited by systemic, PAG or RVM opioid administration (Fields et al 1991; Heinricher et al 1992). Furthermore, during acute opioid abstinence, when there is enhancement of withdrawal reflexes (Kim et al 1990) and dorsal horn responses to noxious stimuli (Kaplan & Fields 1991), there is a marked increase in firing of RVM on-cells (Bederson et al 1990). Thus on-cells are likely to facilitate nociceptive transmission at the level of the dorsal horn. Although the role of the neutral-cell in nociceptive modulation is presently obscure, a subset of neutral cells contains 5-HT, suggesting that they have a role in nociceptive modulation (Potrebic et al 1992). In addition to the RVM, these three classes of neurons are also present in the PAG (Heinricher et al 1987) and the DLPT (Haws et al 1989). This may point to a common neural mechanism for opioid actions in these sites to produce antinociception.

OPIOID ANALGESIA AND DESCENDING PAIN MODULATORY NETWORKS

Administration of exogenous opioids is the most reliable way to activate pain modulating circuits and it provides insight into the possible contribution of endogenous opioids to antinociception. The opioid sensitive CNS sites and the receptor classes involved in analgesia are discussed in detail in Chapter 9. Importantly, microinjection of opioids into either the PAG or the RVM produces behavioural antinociception.

Although there has been controversy about whether supraspinal opioids produce analgesia by inhibiting dorsal horn neurons (Gebhart & Jones 1988) this issue has recently been addressed using a new technique to study the activity of large populations of neurons (Gogas et al 1991). The approach involves immunostaining for the presence of the Fos protein product of the c-*fos* protooncogene, which is induced in neurons when they are active. The procedure is particularly useful to study neurons in the spinal cord of awake rats, because basal levels of expression of the gene are quite low. Furthermore, since the animals are awake their behaviour can be correlated with the pattern of expression of the gene (Hunt et al 1987; Menétrey et al 1989). Different types of noxious stimulation evoke characteristic patterns of expression of the gene. We found that there was a significant correlation between suppression of pain behaviour by opioids and suppression of Fos staining in dorsal horn laminae containing nociresponsive neurons (Tolle et al 1990; Presley et al 1990; Gogas et al 1991; Hammond et al 1992).

Consistent with the hypothesis that the analgesia produced by opioids involves activation of descending inhibitory controls, injection of [D-Ala, N-Me-Phe^4, Gly^5-ol] enkephalin (DAMGO), a μ-opioid receptor selective agonist, into the third ventricle, produces a parallel dose-dependent inhibition of both pain behaviour and Fos expression. Furthermore, bilateral lesions of the spinal DLF block the DAMGO inhibition of both pain behaviour and Fos expression (Gogas et al 1991).

LOCAL CIRCUIT ACTIONS OF OPIOIDS

Clearly, supraspinal opioid administration activates descending antinociceptive controls. An important issue is how opioids produce this effect. One important point is that opioids can act concurrently and synergistically at multiple CNS sites involved in pain modulation including the medulla and midbrain. One possibility is that the synergy results from interactions within a distributed interconnected network of opioid sensitive neurons. In fact, in addition to their direct actions when applied within RVM, opioids applied into the PAG change the firing of putative pain-modulating neurons in the RVM (Morgan et al 1992).

Opioid actions in the RVM

How do opioids act upon pain modulatory neurons? Our knowledge of opioid actions is most extensive for the RVM. As described above RVM off-cells are activated, on-cells inhibited and neutral-cells unaffected by opioids. Since there is strong evidence that off-cells inhibit and on-cells facilitate nociceptive transmission, opioid actions on these two classes of RVM neuron are likely to contribute to analgesia. There are two direct actions of μ-opioid receptor ligands upon neurons: one, a hyperpolarization due to increased potassium conductance and, two, reduced transmitter release secondary to inhibition of a voltage dependent calcium conductance. Since both of these direct actions are inhibitory, it is not surprising that local iontophoretic application of morphine inhibits on-cells (Heinricher et al 1992). It is also significant that off- and neutral-cells are unaffected by iontophoresis of opioids. In vitro studies indicate that the direct effect of opioids on RVM neurons (presumably on-cells) is to hyperpolarize them through an increase in K^+ conductance (Pan et al 1990). It is likely that the activation of off-cells by opioids is an indirect effect, secondary to inhibition of an inhibitory input. In fact, the weight of evidence indicates that opioids inhibit a GABAergic input to off-cells (Mason et al 1990; Heinricher et al 1991). The simplest arrangement is illustrated in Figure 12.4. According to this model, opioids inhibit a subset of GABAergic on-cells leading to disinhibition of off-cells. Consistent with this hypothesis, the $GABA_A$ receptor antagonist, bicucculine, has an antinociceptive action when microinjected into either the PAG (Moreau & Fields 1986; Depaulis et al 1987) or the RVM (Drower & Hammond 1988; Heinricher & Kaplan 1991). Furthermore, RVM on-cells receive a significantly greater density of enkephalin-immunoreactive contacts than either off- or neutral-cells (Mason et al 1992). That these

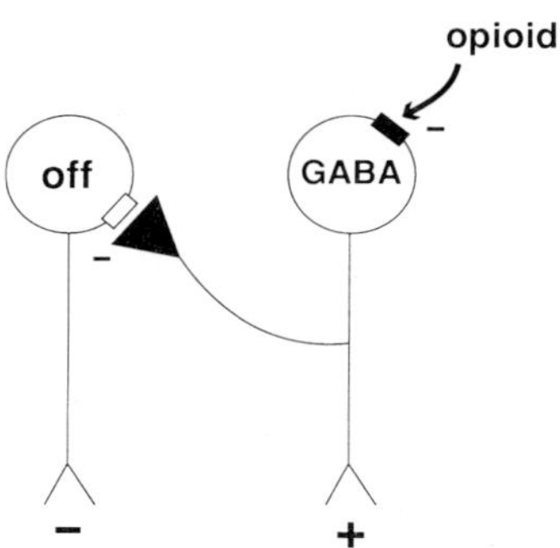

Fig. 12.4 Disinhibition model for opioid action in the RVM. The direct actions of opioids on neurons are predominantly inhibitory, yet when given systemically or locally by microinjection they excite RVM off-cells. This figure illustrates our proposed model in which opioids excite the off-cell indirectly by inhibiting a GABAergic inhibitory neuron that contacts the off-cell. The simplest arrangement is that the inhibitory input to off-cells derives from a subset of GABAergic on-cells.

enkephalinergic contacts to on-cells contribute to pain modulation is consistent with the observation that microinjection of an enkephalinase inhibitor into the RVM produces analgesia (Al-Rodhan et al 1990).

PHYSIOLOGICAL FUNCTION OF PAIN MODULATING NETWORKS

The evidence outlined in this chapter demonstrates that there are networks that control nociceptive transmission, that brainstem to spinal cord projections are crucial to their operation, that endogenous opioid peptides are involved in their function and that they may be called into play in some patients with clinically significant pain. Despite these advances in our understanding, major gaps in our knowledge remain. For example, it has been difficult to identify how the system functions on a moment to moment basis in awake unrestrained animals or even to understand with any degree of precision and certainty how pain modulatory systems contribute to survival.

One approach to these unresolved issues is to study the responses of putative nociceptive modulating neurons under different conditions and to try to correlate their activity with behaviour. Another approach is to determine how sensory stimuli or behavioural variables alter 'pain' behaviours or the activity of nociceptive transmission neurons.

That expectation and attentional factors can reliably alter perceived pain intensity is well established. For example, Miron and colleagues (1989) trained human subjects to make either a visual or noxious thermal discrimination. Prior to each discrimination trial they received a cue indicating whether they would be required to make a visual or noxious thermal discrimination. They consistently rated the noxious thermal stimulus as less intense when they received an 'incorrect' cue indicating that they would be required to make a visual discrimination. In experiments in monkeys in a very similar task, the responses of nociceptive dorsal horn neurons to the same noxious thermal stimulus was greater during performance of a noxious thermal discrimination task than when the monkey was carrying out a visual discrimination (Hayes et al 1981). Furthermore, under conditions of correct cuing of a thermal discrimination task, monkeys have shorter response latencies for signalling their detection of the increase in skin temperature, from which it was inferred that they perceive the stimulus as more intense (Bushnell et al 1985). These studies suggest that there is a centrally generated component to the 'response' of dorsal horn neurons to noxious thermal stimulation and that this centrally generated increment adds to the perceived intensity of pain. Although the modulatory networks underlying these discharges are unknown, these studies demonstrate the importance to pain perception of centrally originating modulatory signals related to expectation, attention and arousal (Fields 1992).

THE ACTIVITY OF PUTATIVE PAIN MODULATING NEURONS

The properties of putative pain modulating neurons in RVM, PAG and the DLPT were described above. It is worth emphasizing that these neurons have very large, virtually total body 'receptive fields' (RFs). Furthermore, in awake rats RVM neurons that resemble on-cells respond briskly to light touch and to sudden sound (Oliveras et al 1990). Anatomical studies indicate that individual RVM neurons project diffusely to multiple levels of the neuraxis including the trigeminal dorsal horn and multiple spinal levels. Furthermore, many RVM neurons have axons that are highly collateralized within the RVM itself (Mason & Fields 1989) and, at least in anaesthetized rats, cells of the same physiological class tend to fire at the same time (Heinricher et al 1989). This organization suggests that the network functions as a unit and exerts global, rather than topographically discrete control over dorsal horn pain transmission neurons. These anatomical and physiological properties would be consistent with a function of this system in arousal and attention.

DOES PAIN INHIBIT PAIN? MULTIPLE PAIN-MODULATING NETWORKS

Noxious stimuli activate on-cells and inhibit off-cells. Since RVM neurons have total body RFs and since on-cells facilitate and off-cells inhibit nociceptive transmission, one would expect noxious stimuli in one part of the body to enhance nociceptive transmission in other parts of the body. Although this may occur under some circumstances (Ramirez & Vanegas 1989), noxious input is, paradoxically, a reliable way to activate the systems that produce analgesia. In fact, acupuncture and many other traditional pain therapies based on counterirritation may operate through such a mechanism (Le Bars et al 1979a, 1979b). Thus, biting your lip, banging your head against the wall, mustard plasters, cupping and other manipulations have been proposed to work by activation of pain-modulating systems.

Consistent with these largely anecdotal observations, noxious stimuli in one part of the body inhibit dorsal horn nociceptive neurons in spinal segments innervating distant body parts. For example, primate STT neurons excited by noxious stimuli on the left foot can be inhibited by noxious stimuli on the face or the contralateral foot (Gerhart et al 1981). Since this inhibition largely survives spinal cord transection it must involve propriospinal connections and not the pain modulatory network that includes the PAG and RVM.

These results also help explain the paradox that noxious stimuli, which activate pain facilitating on-cells, often inhibit neural and behavioural responses to noxious stimulation (Watkins & Mayer 1982; Watkins et al 1983). Thus noxious stimuli activate multiple CNS networks, some of which have an antinociceptive effect while others are pronociceptive. Whether responses to noxious stimuli are enhanced or suppressed will depend on stimulus location, duration, the environment in which the stimulus is applied and the behavioural state of the animal (Watkins et al 1982). In anaesthetized rats the diffuse inhibitory effect produced by noxious somatic stimuli (which does not involve the RVM) (Morgan and Fields 1992; Bouhassira et al 1993) appears to override the potential facilitatory action of RVM on wide dynamic range neurons activated by the same stimulus.

WHAT SIGNALS ACTIVATE THE PAG–RVM–SPINAL PAIN MODULATING NETWORK? STRESS-INDUCED ANALGESIA

Since noxious stimuli reliably engage antinociceptive mechanisms but through pathways that largely bypass the PAG–RVM network, we are left with the problem of the biological significance of this pathway. One clue is that involvement of the PAG–RVM network in an antinociceptive effect may depend on whether endogenous opioids are involved (Watkins & Mayer 1982; Fanselow 1991). In fact, a variety of signals are capable of activating an opioid-mediated analgesic effect. These signals have been called stressors and the analgesic effect called stress-induced analgesia.

Noxious stimuli can induce the release of enkephalin-like immunoreactivity (Yaksh & Elde 1981; Cesselin et al 1982). Duration is an important variable for this effect; the opioid antagonist, naloxone, enhances reflex responses to noxious stimulation but only when prolonged noxious stimuli are used to elicit responses (Jacob et al 1974). In humans, naloxone has little effect on relatively brief experimental pains (El-Sobky et al 1976) but significantly increases the reported intensity of prolonged clinical pains such as postoperative pain (Levine et al 1979).

Under certain circumstances, a noxious stimulus can lead to an opioid-mediated analgesic effect that involves the PAG–RVM network. Stimulus location may be an important factor. For example, using relatively brief (90 s) shock, Watkins and her colleagues (1982) showed that fore paw shock analgesia is completely blocked by naloxone and by RVM lesions. In contrast, the antinociceptive action of hind paw shock was resistant to naloxone and spinal transection, indicating that nonopioid propriospinal networks were involved.

DEFENSIVE BEHAVIOURS, FEAR AND CONDITIONED ANALGESIA

When placed in threatening situations such as proximity to a predator, many animals freeze and become unresponsive to noxious stimulation (Fanselow 1991). These responses are part of a repertoire of 'fear' behaviours that presumably promote survival by helping the animal escape detection. Similar responses can be learned. Thus analgesia can be conditioned either to a light or tone contingently paired with foot shock or to the environment in which the foot shock is received. The analgesia that accompanies these 'fear' situations is blocked by lesions of the amygdala as well as the RVM and DLF. It is also blocked by naloxone administered systemically or into the PAG (Watkins & Mayer 1982; Fanselow 1991).

Interestingly, it appears that 'safety' signals can reverse the analgesia that would be expected in a conditioned fear situation (Wiertelak et al 1992). Thus when rats are placed in an environment where they previously received a noxious electric shock, the expected analgesia can be blocked if they are given a cue indicating that the shock will not occur. The 'antianalgesic' effect of this safety signal appears to involve the release of the neuropeptide cholecystokinin (CCK).

These experiments on conditioned analgesia and antianalgesia are particularly interesting and valuable because they link antinociceptive actions to specific, biologically relevant environmental conditions and to specific neural networks and transmitter systems.

SUMMARY AND CONCLUSIONS

This chapter has presented an overview of pain modulation with an emphasis on a brainstem–spinal cord network. This network exerts bidirectional control over dorsal horn nociceptive transmission neurons. Endogenous opioid peptide immunoreactivity is present in neural somata and/or terminal fields in each component nucleus of this pain-modulating network and each site is sensitive to the antinociceptive actions of exogenous opioids. There is good evidence that this network is reliably activated in situations characterized by threat of injury. There are clearly other neural pathways without opioid links that can produce antinociceptive actions. Their behavioural significance and the neurotransmitter systems that underly their action is presently unknown.

The discovery of pain-modulatory systems and of the neurotransmitters that mediate their action has provided us with a preliminary mechanistic understanding of the variability of subjective responses to noxious stimuli. This greater understanding offers the promise of rationally developed treatments based on manipulation of psychological variables, counterirritation and new, more selective drugs. These improvements in treatment will depend on further progress in elucidating the anatomy, neurotransmitter content and behavioural context for activation of the neural circuits involved in pain modulation.

REFERENCES

Aimone L D, Gebhart G 1986 Stimulation-produced spinal inhibition from the midbrain in the rat is mediated by an excitatory amino acid neurotransmitter in the medial medulla. Journal of Neuroscience 6: 1803–1813

Aimone L D, Jones S L, Gebhart G F 1987 Stimulation-produced descending inhibition from the periaqueductal gray and nucleus raphe magnus in the rat: mediation by spinal monoamines but not opioids. Pain 31: 123–136

Alhaider A A, Kitto K F, Wilcox G L 1990 Nociceptive modulation by intrathecally administered 5-HT_{1A} and 5-HT_{1B} agonists in mice. Federation of American Societies of Experimental Biology Journal 4: A988

Alhaider A A, Lei S Z, Wilcox G L 1991 Spinal 5-HT_3 receptor-mediated antinociception: possible release of GABA. Journal of Neuroscience 11: 1881–1888

Al-Rodhan N, Chipkin R, Yaksh T L 1990 The antinociceptive effects of SCH-32615, a neutral endopeptidase (enkephalinase) inhibitor, microinjected into the periaqueductal gray, ventral medulla and amygdala. Brain Research 520: 123–130

Alvarez F J, Kavookjian A M, Light A R 1992 Synaptic interactions between GABA-immunoreactive profiles and the terminals of functionally defined myelinated nociceptors in the monkey and cat spinal cord. Journal of Neuroscience 12: 2901–2917

Archer T, Jonsson G, Minor B G, Post C 1986 Noradrenergic–serotonergic interactions and nociception in the rat. European Journal of Pharmacology 120: 295–308

Atweh S F, Kuhar M J 1977 Autoradiographic localization of opiate receptors in rat brain. I Spinal cord and lower medulla. Brain Research 124: 53–67

Basbaum A I, Fields H L 1978 Endogenous pain control mechanisms: review and hypothesis. Annals of Neurology 4: 451–462

Basbaum A, Fields H L 1984 Endogenous pain control systems: brain-stem spinal pathways and endorphin circuitry. Annual Review of Neuroscience 7: 309–338

Basbaum A, Clanton C H, Fields H L 1976 Opiate and stimulus-produced analgesia: functional anatomy of a medullospinal pathway. Proceedings of the National Academy of Sciences (USA) 73: 4685–4688

Basbaum A I, Clanton C H, Fields H L 1978 Three bulbospinal pathways from the rostral medulla of the cat. An autoradiographic study of pain modulating systems. Journal of Comparative Neurology 178: 209–224

Basbaum A I, Cruz L, Weber E 1986a Immunoreactive dynorphin B in sacral primary afferent fibers of the cat. Journal of Neuroscience 6: 127–133

Basbaum A I, Ralston D D, Ralston H J III 1986b Bulbospinal projections in the primate: a light and electron microscopic study of a pain modulating system. Journal of Comparative Neurology 250: 311–323

Baskin D S, Mehler W R, Hosobuchi Y, Richardson D E, Adams J E, Flitter M A 1986 Autopsy analysis of the safety, efficacy and cartography of electrical stimulation of the central gray in humans. Brain Research 371: 231–236

Bederson J B, Fields H L, Barbaro N M 1990 Hyperalgesia during naloxone-precipitated withdrawal from morphine is associated with increased on-cell activity in the rostral ventromedial medulla. Somatosensory and Motor Research 7: 185–203

Beecher H K 1959 The measurement of subjective responses. Oxford University Press, New York

Behbehani M M, Fields H L 1979 Evidence that an excitatory connection between the periaqueductal grey and nucleus raphe magnus mediates stimulation produced analgesia. Brain Research 170: 85–93

Beitz A J 1982a The sites of origin of brain stem neurotensin and serotonin projections to the rodent nucleus raphe magnus. Journal of Neuroscience 2: 819–824

Beitz A J 1982b The organisation of afferent projections to the midbrain periaqueductal grey of the rat. Neuroscience 7: 133–159

Bennett G J, Hayashi H, Abdelmoumene M, Dubner R 1979 Physiological properties of stalked cells of the substantia gelatinosa intracellularly stained with horseradish peroxidase. Brain Research 164: 285–289

Bouhassira D, Bing Z, Le Bars D 1993 Studies of the brain structures involved in diffuse noxious inhibitory controls in the rat: the rostral ventromedial medulla. Journal of Physiology (London) 463: 667–687

Boivie J, Meyerson B A 1982 A correlative anatomical and clinical study of pain suppression by deep brain stimulation. Pain 13: 113–126

Bowker R M, Abbott L C, Dilts R P 1988 Peptidergic neurons in the nucleus raphe magnus and the nucleus gigantocellularis: their distribution, interrelationships, and projections to the spinal cord. In: Fields H L, Besson J-M (eds) Pain modulation. Elsevier, Amsterdam, p 95–127

Bushnell M C, Duncan G H, Dubner R, Jones R L, Maixner W 1985 Attentional influences on noxious and innocuous cutaneous heat detection in humans and monkeys. Journal of Neuroscience 5: 1103–1110

Calvino B, Levesque G, Besson J-M 1982 Possible involvement of the amygdaloid complex in morphine analgesia as studied by electrolytic lesions in rats. Brain Research 233: 221–226

Cannon J T, Prieto G J, Lee A, Liebeskind J C 1982 Evidence for opioid and non-opioid forms of stimulation-produced analgesia in the rat. Brain Research 243: 315–321

Carpenter D, Engberg I, Lundberg A 1965 Differential supraspinal control of inhibitory and excitatory actions from the FRA to ascending spinal pathways. Acta Physiologica Scandinavica 63: 103–110

Carstens E, Klumpp D, Zimmerman M 1980 Differential inhibitory effects of medial and lateral midbrain stimulation on spinal neuronal discharges to noxious skin heating in the cat. Journal of Neurophysiology 43: 332–342

Cesselin F, Oliveras J L, Bourgoin S et al 1982 Increased levels of met-enkephalin-like material in the CSF of anaesthetized cat after tooth pulp stimulation. Brain Research 237: 325–338

Cheng Z-F, Fields H L, Heinricher M M 1986 Morphine microinjected into the periaqueductal gray has differential effects on 3 classes of medullary neurons. Brain Research 375: 57–65

Clark F M, Proudfit H K 1991a Projections of neurons in the ventromedial medulla to pontine catecholamine cell groups involved in the modulation of nociception. Brain Research 540: 105–115

Clark F M, Proudfit H K 1991b The projection of noradrenergic neurons in the A7 catecholamine cell group to the spinal cord in the rat demonstrated by anterograde tracing combined with immunocytochemistry. Brain Research 547: 279–288

Clark F M, Yeomans D C, Proudfit H K 1991 The noradrenergic

innervation of the spinal cord: differences between two substrains of Sprague-Dawley rats determined using retrograde tracers combined with immunocytochemistry. Neuroscience Letters 125: 155–158

Coffield J A, Bowen K K, Miletic V 1992 Retrograde tracing of projections between the nucleus submedius, the ventrolateral orbital cortex, and the midbrain in the rat. Journal of Comparative Neurology 321: 488–499

Comb M, Seeburg P H, Adelman J, Eiden L, Herbert E 1982 Primary structure of the human met- and leu-enkephalin precursor and its mRNA. Nature 295: 663–666

Crisp T, Stafinsky J L, Spanos L J, Uram M, Perni V C, Donepudi H B 1991 Analgesic effects of serotonin and receptor-selective serotonin agonists in the rat spinal cord. General Pharmacology 22: 247–251

Cruz L, Basbaum A I 1985 Multiple opioid peptides and the modulation of pain: immunohistochemical analysis of dynorphin and enkephalin in the trigeminal nucleus caudalis and spinal cord of the cat. Journal of Comparative Neurology 240: 331–348

Depaulis A, Morgan M M, Liebeskind J C 1897 GABAergic modulation of the analgesic effects of morphine microinjected in the ventral periaqueductal gray matter of the rat. Brain Research 436: 223–228

Dickenson A H, Sullivan A F, Fournie-Zaluski M C, Roques B P 1987 Prevention of degradation of endogenous enkephalins produces inhibition of nociceptive neurones in rat spinal cord. Brain Research 408: 185–191

Drolet G, Van Bockstaele E J, Aston-Jones G 1992 Robust enkephalin innervation of the locus coeruleus from the rostral medulla. Journal of Neuroscience 12: 3162–3174

Drower E J, Hammond D L 1988 GABAergic modulation of nociceptive threshold: effects of THIP and bicuculline microinjected in the ventral medulla of the rat. Brain Research 450: 316–324

Duggan A W, North R A 1984 Electrophysiology of opioids. Pharmacology Review 35: 219–281

Duncan G H, Bushnell M C, Bates R, Dubner R 1987 Task related responses of monkey medullary dorsal horn neurons. Journal of Neurophysiology 57: 289–310

Eide P K, Hole K 1991 Interactions between serotonin and substance P in the spinal regulation of nociception. Brain Research 550: 225–230

Eide P K, Joly N M, Hole K 1990 The role of spinal cord 5-HT1A and 5-HT1B receptors in the modulation of a spinal nociceptive reflex. Brain Research 536: 195–200

El-Sobky A, Dostrovsky J O, Wall P D 1976 Lack of effect of naloxone on pain perception in humans. Nature 263: 783–784

Fanselow M 1991 The midbrain periaqueductal gray as a coordinator of action in response to fear and anxiety, In: Depaulis A, Bandler R (eds) The midbrain periaqueductal gray matter. Plenum Press, New York, p 151–173

Fields H L 1988 Sources of variability in the sensation of pain. Pain 33: 195–200

Fields H L 1992 Is there a facilitating component to central pain modulation? American Pain Society Journal 1: 139–141

Fields H L, Besson J-M 1988 Pain modulation. Elsevier, Amsterdam

Fields H L, Heinricher M M 1985 Anatomy and physiology of a nociceptive modulatory system. Philosophical Transactions of the Royal Society of London B 308: 361–374

Fields H L, Clanton C H, Anderson S D 1977a Somatosensory properties of spinoreticular neurons in the cat. Brain Research 120: 49–66

Fields H L, Basbaum A I, Clanton C H, Anderson S D 1977b Nucleus raphe magnus inhibition of spinal cord dorsal horn neurons. Brain Research 126: 441–453

Fields H L, Heinricher M M, Mason P 1991 Neurotransmitters in nociceptive modulatory circuits. Annual Review of Neuroscience 14: 219–245

Fleetwood-Walker S M, Hope P J, Mitchell R, El-Yassir N, Molony V 1988 The influence of opioid receptor subtypes on the processing of nociceptive inputs in the spinal dorsal horn of the cat. Brain Research 451: 213–226

Gebhart G F, Jones S L 1988 Effects of morphine given in the brain stem on the activity of dorsal horn nociceptive neurons. In: Fields L H, Besson J-M (eds) Pain modulation. Elsevier, Amsterdam, p 229–243

Gerhart K D, Yezierski R P, Giesler G J 1981 Inhibitory receptive fields of primate spinothalamic tract cells. Journal of Neurophysiology 46: 1309–1325

Giesler G J, Gerhart K D, Yezierski R P, Wilcox T K, Willis W D 1981 Postsynaptic inhibition of primate spinothalamic neurons by stimulation in nucleus raphe magnus. Brain Research 204: 184–188

Glazer E J, Basbaum A I 1981 Immunohistochemical localization of leucine-enkephalin in the spinal cord of the cat: enkephalin-containing marginal neurons and pain modulation. Journal of Comparative Neurology 196: 377–389

Glazer E J, Basbaum A I 1984 Axons which take up [^{3}H]serotonin are presynaptic to enkephalin immunoreactive neurons in cat dorsal horn. Brain Research 298: 386–391

Gogas K R, Presley R W, Levine J D, Basbaum A I 1991 The antinociceptive action of supraspinal opioids results from an increase in descending inhibitory control: correlation of nociceptive behavior and c-fos expression. Neuroscience 42: 617–628

Goldstein A, Tachibana S, Lowney L I, Hunkapiller M, Hood L 1979 Dynorphin (1–13), an extraordinarily potent opiod peptide. Proceedings of the National Academy of Sciences (USA) 76: 6666–6670

Gray T S, Magnuson D J 1992 Peptide immunoreactive neurons in the amygdala and the bed nucleus of the stria terminalis project to the midbrain central gray in the rat. Peptides 13: 451–460

Guilbaud G, Besson J M, Oliveras J L, Liebeskind J C 1973 Suppression by LSD of the inhibitory effect exerted by dorsal raphe stimulation on certain spinal cord interneurons in the cat. Brain Research 61: 417–422

Hagbarth K E, Kerr D I B 1954 Central influences on spinal afferent conduction. Journal of Neurophysiology 17: 295–307

Hammond D L, Presley R, Gogas K R, Basbaum A I 1992 Morphine or U-50, 488 suppresses fos protein-like immunoreactivity in the spinal cord and nucleus tractus solitarii evoked by a noxious visceral stiimulus in the rat. Journal of Comparative Neurology 315: 244–253

Hardy S G P, Leichnetz G R 1981 Cortical projections to the periaqueductal gray in the monkey: a retrograde and orthograde horseradish peroxidase study. Neuroscience Letters 22: 97–101

Haws C M, Williamson A M, Fields H L 1989 Putative nociceptive modulatory neurons in the dorsolateral pontomesencephalic reticular formation. Brain Research 483: 272–282

Hayes R L, Dubner R, Hoffman D S 1981 Neuronal activity in medullary dorsal horn of awake monkeys trained in a thermal discrimination task. II. Behavioral modulation of responses to thermal and mechanical stimuli. Journal of Neurophysiology 46: 428–443

Head H, Holmes G 1911 Sensory disturbances from cerebral lesions. Brain 34: 102–254

Headley P M, Duggan A W, Griersmith B T 1978 Selective reduction by noradrenaline and 5HT of nociceptive responses of cat dorsal horn neurons. Brain Research 145: 185–189

Heinricher M M, Kaplan H J 1991 GABA-mediated inhibition in rostral ventromedial medulla: role in nociceptive modulation in the lightly anesthetized rat. Pain 47: 105–113

Heinricher M M, Cheng Z-F, Fields H L 1987 Evidence for two classes of nociceptive modulating neurons in the periaqueductal gray. Journal of Neuroscience 7: 271–278

Heinricher M M, Barbaro N M, Fields H L 1989 Putative nociceptive modulating neurons in the rostral ventromedial medulla of the rat: firing of on- and off-cells is related to nociceptive responsiveness. Somatosensory and Motor Research 6: 427–439

Heinricher M M, Haws C M, Fields H L 1991 Evidence for GABA-mediated control of putative nociceptive modulating neurons in the rostral ventromedial medulla: iontophoresis of bucuculline eliminates the off-cell pause. Somatosensory and Motor Research 8: 215–225

Heinricher M M, Morgan M M, Fields H L 1992 Direct and indirect actions of morphine on medullary neurons that modulate nociception. Neuroscience 48: 533–543

Herbert H, Saper C R 1992 Organization of medullary adrenergic and noradrenergic projections to the periaqueductal gray matter in the rat. Journal of Comparative Neurology 314: 34–52

Hökfelt R, Elde R, Johansson O, Terenius L, Stein L 1977a The distribution of enkephalin-immunoreactive cell bodies in the rat central nervous system. Neuroscience Letters 5: 25–31

Hökfelt T, Ljungdahl A, Terenius L, Elde R, Nilsson G 1977b Immunohistochemical analysis of peptide pathways possibly related to

pain and analgesia: enkephalin and substance P. Proceedings of the National Academy of Sciences (USA) 74: 3081–3085
Hökfelt T, Terenius T, Kuypers H G J M, Dann O 1979 Evidence for enkephalin immunoreactive neurons in the medulla oblongata projecting to the spinal cord. Neuroscience Letters 14: 55–60
Hughes J, Smith T W, Kosterlitz H W, Fothergill L A, Morgan B A, Morris H R 1975 Identification of two related pentapeptides from the brain with potent opiate agonist activity. Nature 258: 577–579
Hunt S P, Pini A, Evan G 1987 Induction of c-fos-like protein in spinal cord neurons following sensory stimulation. Nature 328: 632–634
Hylden J L K, Wilcox G L 1983 Intrathecal serotonin in mice: analgesia and inhibition of a spinal action of substance P. Life Sciences 33: 789–795
Hylden J L K, Hayashi H, Bennett G J 1986 Physiology and morphology of the lamina I spinomesencephalic projection. Journal of Comparative Neurology 247: 505–515
Jacob J J, Tremblay E C, Colombel M-C 1974 Facilitation de réactions nociceptives par la naloxone chez la souris et chez le rat. Psychopharmacologia 37: 217–223
Jordan L M, Kenshalo D R Jr, Martin R T, Willis W D 1979 Two populations of spinothalamic tract neurons with opposite responses to 5HT. Brain Research 164: 342–346
Kaplan H, Fields H L 1991 Hyperalgesia during acute opioid abstinence: evidence for a nociceptive facilitating function of the rostral ventromedial medulla. Journal of Neuroscience 11: 1433–1439
Kim D H, Barbaro N M, Fields H L 1990 Morphine analgesia and dependence: immediate onset of two opposing, dose related processes. Brain Research 516: 37–40
Kwiat G C, Basbaum A I 1992 The origin of brainstem noradrenergic and serotonergic projections to the spinal cord dorsal horn in the rat. Somatosensory and Motor Research 9: 157–173
Le Bars D 1988 Serotonin and pain. In: Osborne N M, Hamon M (eds) Neuronal serotonin. John Wiley, New York, p 171–226
LeBars D, Dickenson A H, Besson J-M 1979a Diffuse noxious inhibitory controls (DNIC). I. Effects on dorsal horn convergent neurones in the rat. Pain 6: 283–304
LeBars D, Dickenson A H, Besson J-M 1979b Diffuse noxious inhibitory controls (DNIC). II. Lack of effect on non-convergent neurons, supraspinal involvement and theoretical implications. Pain 6: 305–327
Levine J D, Gordon N C, Fields H L 1979 Naloxone dose dependently produces analgesia and hyperalgesia in postoperative pain. Nature 278: 740–741
Levine J D, Lane S R, Gordon N C, Fields H L 1982 A spinal opioid synapse mediates the interaction of spinal and brain stem sites in morphine analgesia. Brain Research 236: 85–91
Light A R, Kavookjian A M 1988 Morphology and ultrastructure of physiologically identified substantia gelatinosa (lamina II) neurons with axons that terminate in deeper dorsal horn laminae (III-V). Journal of Comparative Neurology 267: 172–189
Magoul R, Onteniente B, Geffard M, Calas A 1987 Anatomical distribution and ultrastructural organization of the GABAergic system in the rat spinal cord. An immunocytochemical study using anti-GABA antibodies. Neuroscience 20: 1001–1009
Mains R E, Eipper B A, Ling N 1977 Common precursor to corticotrophin and endorphins. Proceedings of the National Academy of Sciences of the United States of America 74: 3014–3018
Mason P, Fields H L 1989 Axonal trajectories and terminations of on- and off-cells in the lower brainstem of the cat. Journal of Comparative Neurology 288: 185–207
Mason P, Skinner K, Cho H J, Basbaum A I, Fields H L 1990 Anatomical evidence for GABAergic control of physiologically identified off-cells in the rostral ventromedial medulla. In: Bond M R (ed) Proceedings of the VIth International Congress of IASP. Elsevier, Amsterdam, p 331–335
Mason P, Back S A, Fields H L 1992 A confocal laser microsopic study of enkephalin-immunoreactive appositions on to physiologically identified neurons in the rostral ventromedial medulla. Journal of Neuroscience 12: 4023–4036
Mayer D J, Liebeskind J C 1974 Pain reduction by focal electrical stimulation of the brain: an anatomical and behavioural analysis. Brain Research 68: 73–93
Mayer D J, Price D D 1976 Central nervous system mechanisms of analgesia. Pain 2: 379–404
Melzack R, Wall P D 1965 Pain mechanisms: a new theory. Science 150: 971–979
Melzack R, Wall P D, Ty T C 1982 Acute pain in the emergency clinic. Pain 14: 33–43
Menétrey D A, Chaouch A, Binder D, Besson J M 1982 The origin of the spinomesencephalic tract in the rat: an anatomical study using the retrograde transport of horseradish peroxidase. Journal of Comparative Neurology 206: 193–207
Menétrey D, Gannon A, Levine J D, Basbaum A I 1989 Expression of c-fos protein in interneurons and projection neurons of the rat spinal cord in response to noxious somatic, articular, and visceral stimulation. Journal of Comparative Neurology 285: 177–195
Miletic V, Hoffert M J, Ruda M A, Dubner R, Shigenaga Y 1984 Serotoninergic axonal contacts on identified cat spinal dorsal horn neurons and their correlation with nucleus raphe magnus stimulation. Journal of Comparative Neurology 228: 129–141
Millan M H, Millan M J, Herz A 1986 Depletion of central β- endorphin blocks midbrain stimulation-produced analgesia in the freely-moving rat. Neuroscience 18: 641–649
Millan M J, Czlonkowski A, Millan M H, Herz A 1987 Activation of periaqueductal grey pools of beta-endorphin by analgetic electrical stimulation in freely moving rats. Brain Research 407: 199–203
Millar J, Williams G V 1989 Effects of iontophoresis of noradrenaline and stimulation of the periaqueductal gray on single-unit activity in the rat superficial dorsal horn. Journal of Comparative Neurology 287: 119–123
Miller R J 1981 Peptides as neurotransmitters: focus on the enkephalins and endorphins. Pharmaceutical Therapy 12: 73–108
Miron D, Duncan G H, Bushnell M C 1989 Effects of attention on the intensity and unpleasantness of thermal pain. Pain 39: 345–352
Moreau J-L, Fields H L 1986 Evidence for GABA involvement in midbrain control of medullary neurons that modulate nociceptive transmission. Brain Research 397: 37–46
Morgan M M, Fields H L 1992 Comparison of the noxious-evoked activity of dorsal horn multireceptive neurons and paw withdrawal latency in the lightly anesthetized rat. Society for Neuroscience Abstracts 18: 291 (130.9)
Morgan M M, Heinricher M M, Fields L H 1992 Circuitry linking opioid-sensitive nociceptive modulatory systems in periaqueductal gray and spinal cord with rostral ventromedial medulla. Neuroscience 47: 863–871
Moss M S, Glazer E J, Basbaum A I 1983 The peptidergic organization of the cat periaqueductual grey. I. The distribution of enkephalin-containing neurons and terminals. Journal of Neuroscience 3: 603–616
Oliveras J-L, Gilles M, Montagne J, Vos B 1990 Single unit activity at ventromedial medulla level in the awake, freely moving rat: effects of noxious heat and light tactile stimuli onto convergent neurons. Brain Research 506: 19–30
Oshita S, Yaksh T L, Chipkin R 1990 The antinociceptive effects of intrathecally administered SCH32615, an enkephalinase inhibitor, in the rat. Brain Research 515: 143–148
Paice J A, Proudfit H K 1992 The antinociception produced by stimulation of the dorsolateral pontine tegmentum is mediated in part by neurons in the ventromedial medulla. Society for Neuroscience Abstracts 18: 684 (290.2)
Pan Z Z, Williams J T, Osborne P B 1990 Opioid actions on single nucleus raphe magnus neurones from rat and guinea pig in vitro. Journal of Physiology 427: 519–532
Potrebic S, Fields H L, Mason P 1992 Serotonin immunocytochemistry of physiologically identified neurons in the rat rostral ventromedial medulla. Society for Neuroscience Abstracts 18: 683
Presley R W, Menetrey D, Levine J D, Basbaum A I 1990 Systemic morphine supresses noxious stimulus-evoked Fos protein-like immunoreactivity in the rat spinal cord. Journal of Neuroscience 10: 323–335
Prichard S M, Beitz A J 1981 The localisation of brainstem enkephalinergic and substance P neurons which project to the rodent nucleus raphe magnus. Society of Neuroscience Abstracts 7: 59
Priestley J V, Cuello A C 1989 Ultrastructural and neurochemical

analysis of synaptic input to trigemino-thalamic projection neurones in laminae I of the rat: a combined immunocytochemical and retrograde labelling study. Journal of Comparative Neurology 285: 467–486

Proudfit H K 1988 Pharmacological evidence for the modulation of nociception by noradrenergic neurons. In: Fields H L, Besson J-M (eds) Pain modulation. Elsevier, Amsterdam, p 357–370

Ralston H J, Ralston D D 1979 The distribution of dorsal root axons in laminae I, II and III of the macaque spinal cord: a quantitative electron microscopy study. Journal of Comparative Neurology 184: 643–684

Ramirez F, Vanegas H 1989 Tooth pulp stimulation advances both medullary off-cell pause and tail flick. Neuroscience Letters 100: 153–156

Randic M, Yu H H 1976 Effects of 5-hydroxytryptamine and bradykinin in cat dorsal horn neurones activated by noxious stimuli. Brain Research 111: 197–203

Reichling D B, Basbaum A I 1990 Contribution of brainstem GABAergic circuitry to descending antinociceptive controls. I. GABA-immunoreactive projection neurons in the periaqueductal gray and nucleus raphe magnus. Journal of Comparative Neurology 302: 370–377

Reynolds D V 1969 Surgery in the rat during electrical analgesia induced by focal brain stimulation. Science 164: 444–445

Rhodes D L, Liebeskind J C 1978 Analgesia from rostral brain stem stimulation in the rat. Brain Research 143: 521–532

Roberts M H T 1988 Pharmacology of putative neurotransmitters and receptors: 5-hydroxytryptamine. In Fields H L, Besson J-M (eds) Pain modulation. Elsevier, Amsterdam, p 329–338

Ruda M A, Coffield J, Dubner R 1984 Demonstration of postsynaptic opioid modulation of thalamic projection neurons by the combined techniques of retrograde horseradish peroxidase and enkephalin immunocytochemistry. Journal of Neuroscience 4: 2117–2132

Ruda, M A, Bennett G J, Dubner R 1986 Neurochemistry and neural circuitry in the dorsal horn. Progress in Brain Research 66: 219–268

Schmauss C, Hammond D L, Ochi J W, Yaksh T L 1983 Pharmacological antagonism of the antinociceptive effects of serotonin in the rat and spinal cord. European Journal of Pharmacology 90: 349–357

Solomon R E, Gebhart G F 1988 Mechanisms of effects of intrathecal serotonin on nociception and blood pressure in rats. Journal of Pharmacology and Experimental Therapeutics 245: 905–912

Tenen S S 1968 Antagonism of the analgesic effect of morphine and other drugs by p-chlorophenylalanine, a serotonin depletor. Psychopharmacologia 12: 278–285

Todd A J, McKenzie J 1989 GABA-immunoreactive neurons in the dorsal horn of the rat spinal cord. Neuroscience 31: 799–806

Todd A J, Millar J 1983 Antagonism of 5-hydroxytryptamine-evoked excitation in the superficial dorsal horn of the cat spinal cord by methysergide. Neuroscience Letters 48: 167–170

Todd A J, Spike R C, Johnston H M 1992 Immunohistochemical evidence that Met-enkephalin and GABA coexist in some neurones in rat dorsal horn. Brain Research 584: 149–156

Tölle T R, Castro L J, Coimbra A, Zieglgènsberger W 1990 Opiates modify induction of c-fos proto-oncogene in the spinal cord of the rat following noxious stimulation. Neuroscience Letters 111: 46–51

Tseng L L, Tang R 1989 Differential actions of the blockade of spinal opioid, adrenergic and serotonergic receptors on the tail-flick inhibition induced by morphine micro-injected into dorsal raphe and central gray in rats. Neuroscience 33: 93–100

Vogt M 1974 The effect of lowering the 5-hydroxytryptamine content of the rat spinal cord on analgesia produced by morphine. Journal of Physiology 236: 483–498

Wall P D 1967 The laminar organisation of dorsal horn and effects of descending impulses. Journal of Physiology 188: 403–423

Watkins L R, Mayer D J 1982 Organization of endogenous opiate and nonopiate pain control systems. Science 216: 1185–1192

Watkins L R, Cobelli D A, Mayer D J 1982 Classical conditioning of front paw and hind paw footshock induced analgesia (FSIA): naloxone reversibility and descending pathways. Brain Research 243: 119–132

Watkins L R, Young E G, Kinscheck I B, Mayer D J 1983 The neural basis of footshock analgesia: the role of specific ventral medullary nuclei. Brain Research 276: 305–315

Watson S J, Akil H 1980 α-MSH in rat brain: occurrence within and outside of β-endorphin neurons. Brain Research 182: 217–223

Weber E, Roth K A, Barchas J D 1981 Colocalisation of α-neo-endorphin and dynorphin immunoreactivity in hypothalamic neurons. Biochemical and Biophysical Communications 103: 951–958

Westlund K N, Carlton S M, Zhang D, Willis W D 1990 Direct catecholaminergic innervation of primate spinothalamic tract neurons. Journal of Comparative Neurology 299: 178–186

Wiertelak E P, Maier S F, Watkins L R 1992 Cholecystokinin antianalgesia: safety cues abolish morphine analgesia. Science 256: 830–833

Willis W D, Haber L H, Martin R F 1977 Inhibition of spinothalamic tract cells and interneurons by brain stem stimulation in the monkey. Journal of Neurophysiology 40: 968–981

Yaksh T L 1979 Direct evidence that spinal serotonin and noradrenaline terminals mediate the spinal antinociceptive effects of morphine in the periaqueductal grey. Brain Research 160: 180–185

Yaksh T L, Elde R P 1981 Factors governing release of methionine-enkephalin-like immunoreactivity from mesencephalon and spinal cord of cat in vivo. Journal of Neurophysiology 46: 1056–1075

Yeomans D C, Clark F M, Paice J A, Proudfit H K 1992 Antinociception induced by electrical stimulation of spinally projecting noradrenergic neurons in the A7 catecholamine cell group of the rat. Pain 48: 449–461

Young R F, Tronnier V, Rinaldi P C 1992 Chronic stimulation of the Kölliker-Fuse nucleus region for relief of intractable pain in humans. Journal of Neurosurgery 76: 979–985

Zelman F P, Kow L-M, Pfaff D W 1983 Spinal serotonin receptor subtypes and nociception. Journal of Pharmacology and Experimental Therapeutics 226: 477–485

Zhuo M, Gebhart G F 1992 Characterization of descending facilitation and inhibition of spinal nociceptive transmission from the nuclei reticularis gigantocellularis and gigantocellularis pars alpha in the rat. Journal of Neurophysiology 67: 1599–1614

Zorman G, Belcher G, Adams J E, Fields H L 1982 Lumbar intrathecal naloxone blocks analgesia produced by microstimulation of the ventromedial medulla in the rat. Brain Research 236: 77–84

Psychological

13. Emotional aspects of pain

Kenneth D. Craig

Emotions are distinctive features of the complex subjective experience of pain. For people suffering from painful injuries or diseases, emotional distress provides the most salient, disruptive and undesirable qualities of the experience. This emotional aspect of all pain experiences may vary in severity from unpleasant or annoying feelings to agonizing or excruciating distress. In addition, a broad range of emotions accompanies pain of all types to provide a context for the experience itself. These commonly include fear, anxiety, depression and anger, but may also include guilt, frustration, subservience or even sexual arousal. In the absence of negative affect and related fears, including physical harm, mutilation or death, people in pain could not reasonably be described as 'suffering'.

Emotional distress often provides the most striking evidence of pain. To communicate their distress, people readily offer dramatic affective language, describing pain in terms of personal misery, fear and physical malaise. Expressions describing terrifying, frustrating and sickening experiences (Melzack & Torgerson 1971) are accompanied by paralinguistic vocalizations such as changes in voice quality, moaning and crying, and non-verbal signs in the form of facial grimaces and protective or awkward movements (Craig et al 1992; Keefe & Dunsmore 1992).

HISTORICAL NOTES

Reflecting the integral role of emotions in painful experiences, throughout most of recorded history pain was characterized as an affective feeling state rather than a sensation (Dallenbach 1939; Keele 1957). To the ancient Greeks, it was an essential emotional component of the human spirit – the negative counterpart of pleasure. Aristotle was responsible for the enduring idea that pain is an affect, a 'passion of the soul', distinct from the classic five senses. The enduring concept recognized pain as an affective experience, like sadness or bitterness, signalling something to be avoided or terminated, but not as a sense, because it was not referrable to any specific quality of external objects (Hardy 1952).

The contrasting sensory model gradually became accepted, beginning with Descartes' concept of pain in the the 17th century. He proposed that sensory nerves conduct non-corporeal copies of the objects perceived to the brain. By the end of the 19th century, sensory models of pain had been placed in juxtaposition to the older emotion theory and there was widespread disagreement as to whether pain should be construed as an emotion or a sensation. Marshall (1984) illustrated the argument with his statement that 'pleasures and pains can in no proper sense be classed with sensations'. There were also historical precedents for the current position that both affective and sensory qualities are interactive components of the pain experience. For example, Strong (1895) asserted 'that physical pain is not a compound of an indifferent sensation with a feeling of displeasure, but itself a sensation which calls forth displeasure'.

Rapid advances in basic medical knowledge in the 19th and early 20th centuries led to an emphasis on sensory systems conveying messages of pain to the brain. The emphasis on sensory processes as primary and emotions as secondary led to studies of the psychophysical properties of pain. Cognitive and affective processes were treated as if they were 'contaminants' or sources of experimental error that needed to be controlled. Affective dimensions were relegated to secondary importance. The meaning of pain and suffering remained a preoccupation of philosophers (Buytendijk 1961; Bakan 1971) and the issues were central to religious and spiritual understandings of the human predicament. Reductionistic biophysical concepts came to dominate practitioner-oriented approaches to pain management.

Exploration of peripheral and central pain-transmitting pathways yielded exciting discoveries, but central processing mechanisms in the spinal cord and brain that integrate sensory qualities of pain with affective and cognitive dimensions remained poorly understood and largely unexplored until the mid-20th century (Melzack & Wall 1965). It became clear that surgical and pharmaceutical treatments designed to prevent peripheral transmission of noxious sensory input were insufficient to control all forms of pain. Hence, exploration of central nervous system plasticity and the substrates of perceptual, affective and cognitive processes became necessary. Of particular interest were discoveries that cortical and other central mechanisms could exert descending inhibitory or facilitory control over sensory input and that the brain produces substances with potent analgesic and algesic effects (Fields 1987).

Toward the mid-20th century, the emotional component of pain came to be characterized as a reaction to the more fundamental sensory component of pain (Hardy et al 1952; Beecher 1959). This formulation attracted attention to the emotional consequences of pain, but it did not recognize that emotions were integral to the painful experience or that preexisting emotions, such as depression or anxiety, influence pain. Emotions were seen as subject to control by means other than those designed to control the more fundamental problem of pain itself. Treating emotional distress such as depression, anger or traumatic stress reactions could be seen as leaving the more fundamental cause of the distress untouched. While this perspective is no longer accepted (Leventhal & Everhart 1979; Wall 1979), characterizing emotions as reactions to the more fundamental sensory qualities of pain again favoured sensory-specificity and biophysical models of pain and supported medical intervention (e.g. analgesic medication and surgery) to eliminate pain as a sensation and ignored innovative practices that focus on affective mechanisms themselves.

Fortunately, alternative, comprehensive theoretical models have emerged which recognize affective qualities as integral and essential to the experience. They not only may be a consequence of pain, but also may have been instigated in advance of the experience and always arise as a component of the experience. Melzack & Wall (1965) and Melzack & Casey (1968) developed a model of pain in which tissue damage concurrently activates affective – motivational and sensory – discriminative components of pain. The nature and severity of pain then become consequences of affective and cognitive mechanisms as well as sensory events deriving from tissue damage. This formulation has been accepted in part because traditional medical intervention has only been partially successful, leaving a large residue of patients who suffer prolonged pain. Exclusively sensory models of pain neglected major affective, cognitive and behavioural processes that are amenable to other forms of control. These psychological processes have parallels in the descending neural and hormonal systems that modulate the biological substrates of pain experiences. In gate control theory (Melzack & Wall 1965), sensory neurons trigger central control systems in the brain which inhibit or facilitate input. Central messages reflecting cognitive, attentional and emotional factors descend from the brain through the spinal cord and influence nociceptive messages coming from the periphery.

The broadening constructs are consistent with nontechnological, religious and philosophical world views of pain. In a classic monograph, Keele (1957) observed that non-Western cultures assign greater weight to the emotional qualities of pain. For example, he stated: 'Though recognizing pain as a sensation, Buddha, and indeed Hindu thought in general, attached more significance to the emotional level of experience'. The cultural-specificity of concepts of emotion in pain and the importance of alternative orientations toward pain in the traditions of non-Western cultures have been described by Tu (1980). In Western culture, unidimensional sensory formulations of pain have yielded to multidimensional concepts that assign importance to cognitive and emotional dimensions as well as sensory components (Melzack & Casey 1968). The concept of suffering has also reemerged to encompass the broad range of thoughts and feelings provoked by major, traumatic and ongoing crises and the meaning this has for the person (Szasz 1957; Buytendijk 1961; Fordyce 1988).

CONCEPTUAL ISSUES

Fine-grained analyses of the role of emotion in pain are complicated by the difficult task of tapping subjective experiences. The dynamic, often turbulent, and intimate flow of feelings, images and thoughts is not readily reduced to descriptive language. Lewis (1942) observed that 'pain, like similar subjective feelings, is known to us by experience and described by illustration'. The language used to describe pain often refers metaphorically to physical properties of the external environment (e.g. cutting, dull or hot), rather than to the more elusive qualities of subjective feeling states. Melzack & Dennis (1980) take note of the vague and diffuse feelings associated with pain and observe: 'The affective dimension is difficult to express – words such as exhausting, sickening, terrifying, cruel, vicious and killing come close but are often inadequate descriptions of the affective experience of the pain of cancer or causalgia'.

Judgemental and decision-making demands on observers who must understand subtle qualities of another person's pain are no less complex than reporting on the experience itself. Numerous, often idiosyncratic sources of information must be integrated, including the observer's formal understanding of pain, memories of personal experiences and contacts with other people experiencing similar distress. Individual differences in the experience of pain (Craig 1983) and variability among painful conditions (Dubuisson & Melzack 1976) complicate the task. Thus, clinicians and others find it difficult to genuinely understand or empathize with another person's painful distress.

Patients may not only have difficulty describing painful experiences, but they may also be unwilling or reluctant to confide these feelings of distress. In consequence, onlookers pay attention to nonverbal expressions that communicate qualities of emotional distress and pain (LeResche & Dworkin 1988; Craig et al 1992). Clinicians and others in the nonclinical social environment usually are sensitively attuned to the facial and bodily activity of people in pain and often attach greater importance to nonverbal messages than to verbal report (Poole & Craig 1992). While voluntary control can be used to suppress or exaggerate the expression of pain (Craig et al 1991), nonverbal expression is less subject to purposeful misrepresentation (Craig 1992).

While emotional aspects of pain may be difficult for patients to describe, they can be discriminated from sensory qualities at the level of experience and they are differentially sensitive to social and therapeutic influences. This is consistent with observations that they have at least partially separate neuroanatomical substrates (Fields 1987). Through introspective analysis, people experiencing pain are able to report separately on the sensory and affective dimensions (Johnson & Rice 1974; Craig et al 1978; Price et al 1980; Wade et al 1990) and emotional qualities differ dramatically across different forms of clinical pain and within individuals over time (Price et al 1987). For some time, it was believed that analgesic interventions moderated the severity of affective distress leaving sensory qualities relatively unaffected (Barber 1959; Johnson & Rice 1974; Martelli et al 1987).

Current evidence indicates that pharmaceutical and psychological interventions have different effects on either sensory, affective or both qualities of the experience. The narcotic fentanyl reduces the sensory intensity but not the unpleasantness of painful tooth pulp sensations (Gracely et al 1982). In contrast anxiolytics such as diazepam reduce affective discomfort rather than sensory-intensity qualities of the experience (Gracely et al 1978). Similarly, placebo medication has an impact on unpleasantness rather than on sensory qualities of painful events. Price et al (1980) found that advance warnings of noxious events selectively influenced affective discomfort. Martelli et al (1987) found that emotion-focused interventions for patients who undergo oral surgery reduce affective discomfort. They propose 'that behavioural stress-management procedures have similar action and thus may be a viable alternative to antianxiety medications for reducing pain and anxiety in health care settings'. Melzack & Perry (1975) found that a combination of alpha biofeedback and hypnotic suggestion yielded significant decreases in sensory and affective components of pain, but the affective dimension showed the largest decrease. Melzack et al (1981) observed that labour pain ranked among the most intense pains recorded with the McGill Pain Questionnaire. Prepared childbirth training yielded lower scores on both sensory and affective dimensions of pain for mothers delivering their first child. Unfortunately, chronic pain patients have difficulty discriminating qualities of their experience, rendering focal treatments more difficult. They are not as adept in scaling judgements of pain as healthy people, with judgements of unpleasantness even less reliable than those of intensity (Urban et al 1984).

Emotional distress appears most conspicuous when renewed or increased pain is anticipated. Impending threats can precipitate dispassionate preparation or serious distress in the form of disorganized, hysterical behaviour, inappropriate avoidance strategies and substantial physiological arousal. Moderate preoperative fear based on foreknowledge can trigger the use of coping skills that reduce postoperative distress. A variety of preparatory procedures for patients confronting painful medical and dental care have been developed (Melamed & Siegel 1980). In contrast, unreasonable apprehension of severe pain can have serious debilitating effects. For example, a pattern of 'catastrophizing', or excessive self-alarming thoughts, has been observed in patients with unrestrained pain displays, substantial emotional behaviour, somatic preoccupation, dependency on the health care system and behavioural disorganization (Rosenstiel & Keefe 1983; Reesor & Craig 1988; Keefe et al 1989; Sullivan & D'Eon 1990). The relationship between emotional distress and pain-related behaviour appears curvilinear. Lesser levels mobilize attention towards threat and lead to effective action. Increases beyond some optimal level lead to disorganized, inefficient action.

Efforts to protect oneself during pain increase in proportion to affective discomfort. The affective component of pain is intimately related to its motivational properties. For example, Philips (1982) noted that among headache patients, the stronger the affective distress, the more the complaints and pill-taking. Many people genuinely dread the prospect of pain and work steadfastly to avoid it, even to their disadvantage. Bond (1980) has suggested that Western cultures have erred in promoting the belief that medicine can make people's lives painfree. Sternbach (1974) has noted tendencies in patients to anticipate that increases in pain will accelerate with time despite evidence that increases are usually within a tolerable range. As Fordyce (1986) notes, hurt does not necessarily signal harm. Confusion of the two appears to precipitate distress that unduly prolongs disability.

Clinical practitioners willing to attribute the origins of pain complaints to emotional distress regrettably often do this through 'diagnosis by exclusion'. In the absence of organic pathology, they conclude that emotional factors are causal. Fortunately, techniques for the psychological assessment of the pain patient have improved to the extent that emotional states such as anxiety, depression and defensive personality styles can now be identified (Turk & Melzack 1992). It is also clear that many patients experiencing pain with a substantial organic basis suffer serious psychological distress. Indeed, Benjamin et al (1988) found that pain patients with diagnosable organic diseases had significantly higher ratings for the severity of psychiatric symptoms and they rejected the assumption that there is a simple dichotomy between patients with physical and mental illnesses.

Diagnostic techniques for identifying signs and symptoms that are medically incongruent (i.e. could not have a basis in physical pathology) have been developed (Waddell et al 1989). Patients who present with a high incidence of medically incongruent signs and symptoms are more likely to display dysfunctional behaviour, thoughts and feelings (Reesor & Craig 1988; Hadjistavropoulos & Craig 1992). Given that these patients are less likely to benefit from conventional medical intervention (Flor & Turk 1984), strategies designed to deal directly with dysfunctional behavioural, cognitive and affective processes are in order.

INTERACTIONS BETWEEN EMOTIONAL DISTRESS AND PAIN

Emotional distress serves not only as a component of pain, but it may be a consequence of pain, a cause of pain, or a concurrent problem with independent sources. All possibilities deserve the attention of clinicians (Feuerstein & Skjei 1979). These distinctions have not always been made clear and there has been debate and confusion concerning whether emotional processes should be conceptualized as causes or consequences of pain (Beutler et al 1986). The challenge is considerable and important when it is recognized that a substantial subgroup of chronic pain patients can be characterized as 'dysfunctional' because of a consistent pattern of higher than average levels of pain severity, affective distress, life interference and lower than average levels of life control and activity (Turk & Rudy 1990). Clarification is to be found in conceptualizing both pain and emotion as multidimensional and sometimes overlapping processes with reciprocal influences on each other. Gamsa (1990) provides a critical literature review and a study of chronic pain patients indicating that pain is more likely to cause emotional disturbances than to be precipitated by them.

EMOTIONAL DISTRESS AS A CONSEQUENCE OF PAIN

Consideration of the temporal qualities of pain suggests that three different forms of pain can be distinguished (Melzack & Dennis 1980). Distinct affective states appear to be associated with each.

Phasic pain

Short-duration phasic pain reflects the immediate impact of the onset of injury. With some exceptions, traumatic injuries such as lacerations or burns provoke vigorous reflexive withdrawal, protective movements, and stereotyped patterns of verbal and nonverbal expressive behaviour recognizable as pain to onlookers (Craig et al 1992). The reaction pattern is evident even in both preterm and fullterm newborns subjected to heel lancing to provide a blood sample (Grunau & Craig 1987; Craig et al 1993). The urgency of the actions suggests that subjective distress motivates efforts to escape the source of pain.

However, pain may not be the inevitable, immediate consequence of traumatic injury. Substantial numbers of people who sustain injuries report that pain emerged some time after the injury itself (Wall 1979). The most common sources of persistent pain arising from motor vehicle accidents, soft tissue neck and low-back injuries, only infrequently provoke immediate pain. When it is reported, clinicians suspect earlier injuries or that the patient is exaggerating.

The primary biological function of pain may be to trigger recuperative behaviour rather than to signal physical threat or danger. Wall (1979) proposed that pain promotes actions directed at healing rather than defensive avoidant behaviour. Bolles & Fanselow (1980) similarly hypothesized that perception of traumatic threat, including physical pain, motivates fear and concerted defensive, self-preservative efforts. At the moment of injury, pain-instigated recuperative activity in the form of passivity and rest would be maladaptive; hence fear rather than pain would be the more adaptive reaction to injury. Stress can activate endogenous analgesic systems in emergency conditions when pain suppression would be adaptive (Frenk et al 1986). After the danger has passed and fear has dissipated, recuperative behaviours such as resting and immobilization would be appropriate. Anecdotal evidence is strong that people involved in activities that would be disrupted by pain sustain injuries without complaints. Wounds and injuries are often ignored by soldiers on the battlefield, athletes on the playing field, people engaged in masochistic erotic activities, and even the weekend gardener who ignores a blistered thumb. Thus, even the immediate reaction to physical insult is subject to modulation contingent upon the biological, physical and social context in which it occurs.

Acute pain

Acute pain is provoked by tissue damage and comprises both phasic pain and a tonic state which persists for a variable period of time until healing takes place. The perception of traumatic injury or the precipitous onset of disease tends to provoke fear and anxious concern for one's well-being. Often, as a result of fear of pain, the anticipation may be more severe than the experience itself (Arntz et al 1991; Gross 1992). The clinical observation that the greater the anxiety the greater the perception of events as painful appears warranted (Weisenberg 1977; Sternbach 1986b). Postoperative anxiolytics are frequently prescribed because clinicians perceive their patients to be in emotional distress as well as suffering from pain (Taenzer 1983). More anxious patients report greater pain and require more analgesic medication following surgery (Taenzer et al 1986). In addition, anxiety disorders in children and adults are accompanied by an increased incidence of somatic symptoms and pain complaints (Beidel et al 1991).

Nevertheless, a clear empirical basis for the simple proposition that anxiety increases pain is not available. Arntz et al (1991) reviewed studies that varyingly indicated that anxiety enhances, relieves, or has no impact on pain. Similarly, once phasic pain and the immediate perception of life-threatening danger have passed, acute pain may not be associated with high levels of anxiety, as in the case of acute back pain patients (Philips & Grant 1991). Contradictions in findings concerning the relationship between pain and anxiety may reflect difficulties in clearly defining and measuring both pain and anxiety, response biases as people become less or more willing to complain of pain when anxious (Malow et al 1989) and the moderating role that attention has on both anxiety and pain (Arntz et al 1991). There is also the issue of the direction of causality. Does the high level of anxiety make the experience of pain more severe or does a high level of pain provoke high levels of anxiety? Pain and resulting anxiety also can contribute to further deterioration in a vicious cycle, even contributing further to physical decompensation and psychophysiological disorders.

While anxiety has conventionally been associated with acute pain, it is also recognized as a component of the constellation of emotional reactions to chronic pain. Thus, depression, somatic anxiety and anger frequently interact with each other in chronic pain syndromes (Blumer & Heilbronn 1982) and anxious chronic pain patients can be distinguished from those that are depressed (Krishnan et al 1985; Chaturvedi 1987).

Chronic pain

The psychological impact and behavioural course of painful conditions vary. The injury or the onset of disease alone may create emotional turmoil. Many pain patients display substantial emotional, behavioural and social disruption during the earliest stages of their illness (Hadjistavropoulos & Craig 1992). For many chronic pain patients, the long-term problem may be best conceptualized as persistence of the acute presentation (Philips & Grant 1991). Persistence of pain also can have a profoundly debilitating effect. In any of its recurrent, persistent or progressive forms, pain may dramatically impair the individual's social, vocational and psychological well-being (International Association for the Study of Pain 1986). There may be deprivation from customary roles at work, in the family or in social and leisure settings. This may be accompanied by the realization that neither one's own best efforts to promote healing nor the highly respected, best interventions of health care professionals have been effective. Challenges to the legitimacy of complaints can also represent a major source of stress. Recognition that pain and a disrupted lifestyle may have to be long endured takes its toll and despondency and a sense of hopelessness become likely outcomes. The emotional and behavioural disturbances provoked by chronic pain have been well-documented (Bonica 1979; Sternbach 1986a), but they can be missed during diagnostic assessments when the focus is on pain and pathophysiological processes rather than on psychological well-being (Doan & Wadden 1989).

Deterioration over time is not inevitable. A recent follow-up study of chronic pain patients from family practice and specialty pain clinic settings indicated that over 2 years a substantial proportion no longer experienced pain and, of those who continued to experience pain, it had become intermittent and emotional distress and demands on the health care system had strikingly diminished (Crook et al 1989). Indeed, rather than having to accept that their pain will go on for the rest of their lives, many patients can expect the pain to disappear or become intermittent.

Chronic pain is frequently associated with depression that may be relatively minor, as in dysthymia, or severe. The common diagnostic criteria for depression include depressed mood, loss of pleasure or interest, appetite disturbance, sleep disturbance, loss of energy, psychomotor agitation or retardation, excessive guilt, concentration difficulties and suicidal ideation (Sullivan et al 1992). Depression appears to intensify pain. Affleck et al (1991) found that depression predicted pain severity in rheumatoid arthritis patients over a long sequence of days, independent of disease activity or disability. Doan & Wadden (1989) found that the severity of depressive symptoms predicted the number and severity of pain complaints.

Estimates of the prevalence of mood disorders in chronic pain patients vary considerably, reflecting both the shortcomings of the measures and diagnostic procedures used and variations in the populations studied (Romano & Turner 1985). Not all chronic pain patients display evidence of debilitating depression. Pilowsky et al (1977) observed that only 10% of a continuous series of chronic pain patients presenting to a pain clinic displayed the symptoms of depressive disorders and their sample's mean depression score was low relative to a psychiatric patient sample. Magni et al (1990) concluded on the basis of a large-scale population-based survey of pain and depression in the United States that 18% of people suffering from chronic pain could be classified as depressed using a stringent psychiatric criterion, whereas 8% of the population who did not suffer chronic pain satisfied this criterion. A recent literature review (Sullivan et al 1992) led to the conclusion that the prevalence of major depression among patients suffering chronic low back pain was approximately three to four times higher than that in the general population. The highest incidence appears likely to be seen in specialty pain clinics. While the actual incidence reported appears to vary with the group sampled and the criteria applied, it is clear that a greater proportion of chronic pain patients are depressed than there are depressed people in the population at large. But it is also noteworthy that a larger proportion of people with chronic pain are not depressed. Chronic pain and depression exist as separate phenomena and, despite their capacity for mutual influence, they are best seen as independent processes (Garron & Leavitt 1983; Kerns et al 1983).

Attention has been devoted to the causal direction of the relationship between pain and depression. Does pain lead to depression or vice versa? Stressful life events may also be implicated, perhaps accounting for the concurrent development of the two disorders simultaneously. This is the case for about 50% of all patients with pain and depression (Romano & Turner 1985). Atkinson et al (1988) note that those chronic low back pain patients who become depressed are likely to experience untoward life events and ongoing life difficulties.

A variety of theories has been applied to the problem of the causal relationship between pain and depression (Romano & Turner 1985), along with empirical studies utilizing causal modelling statistical procedures. Fordyce (1976) proposed a role for the severe reduction in activity levels at work, home and in recreational pursuits. The loss of control over one's health and life activities may lead to thoughts of helplessness and despair. Crisson & Keefe (1988) found that patients who view events in their lives as primarily due to circumstances beyond their control, such as chance, fate or luck, are more likely to use maladaptive pain coping strategies and may report more psychological distress than patients who believe they have control. Rudy et al (1988) found that depression was the consequence of the extent to which increases in pain severity interfered with important life activities, thereby limiting social rewards and reducing the patient's sense of self-control or personal mastery. Brown's (1990) study of depression in rheumatoid arthritis patients provided support for a causal model in which pain predicts depression, but only after an extended period of time (1 year in this study). Certain recursive, vicious cycles are possible. Pain, by increasing unpleasant affect, promotes access to memories of unpleasant events. The negative memories and thoughts, in turn, intensify the unpleasant affect and help perpetuate pain (Eich et al 1990).

From a psychodynamic perspective, chronic pain patients and depressed patients share an inability to modulate or express intense, unacceptable feelings (Beutler et al 1986). This position would also be consistent with findings that adults and children frequently moralize about the meaning of pain, experiencing guilt and construing pain as punishment (Gaffney & Dunne 1987; Eisendrath et al 1986). Biomedical theories derive from the observation that pain and depression have common biological systems that subserve both processes (Beutler et al 1986; Magni 1987). It has been observed that antidepressants may reduce chronic pain, leaving depression untouched (France et al 1984). Often overlooked is the possibility that commonplace treatment recommendations for patients with persistent pain may have depressive effects; withdrawal from work and other activities, prolonged bed-rest, lapsing into the dependent sick role, and analgesics and medications may provoke or exacerbate depression. For example, Aronoff et al (1986) reviewed evidence that benzodiazepines can increase depression, hostility, anger and pain.

While some patients display distress and depression, others maintain a dispassionate attitude and do not become heavy consumers of health care services (Zitman et al 1992). Well-adjusted patients with chronic pain appear to have either strong personal or social resources or the pain disorder provides a focus in life that enables them to ignore stressful life-challenges, thereby controlling depression or resentment. In this paradoxical manner, pain can provide a means of coping with an unsatisfactory existence. Patients who voluntarily inflict self-injury in the interests of instigating medical care and hospitalization, or to escape an intolerable setting (e.g. prison or marital distress), provide extreme illustrations.

A small portion of chronic pain patients become angry, demanding and manipulative in the course of their illness. Factor analyses of pain and personality measures from patients with chronic pain syndromes led Timmermans & Sternbach (1974) to conclude that variability on a factor of interpersonal alienation and manipulativeness was a central characteristic of chronic pain patients. Wade et al (1990) found that pain patients reported higher levels of frustration than any other negative emotion. Anxiety and frustration as well predicted the overall unpleasantness of pain, and anger was an important concomitant of the depression that pain patients experienced. Persistently angry patients impose special demands on health professionals. Special management programmes using explicit treatment contracts have been devised for patients who become angry, demanding and manipulative (Sternbach 1974).

It should be noted that because psychological and social dysfunction are highly probable outcomes of persistent pain, it is a mistake to use global evidence of emotional and behavioural problems to diagnosis so called 'psychogenic pain'. Psychological dysfunction is as great or more severe among those with diagnosable disease as among those for whom physical pathology cannot be identified (Woodforde & Merskey 1971; Benjamin et al 1988). Heaton et al (1982) observed that a group of patients with objective physical findings obtained higher scores than those without objective physical findings on measures of psychosocial factors which exacerbate and maintain chronic pain problems. Roberts & Reinhardt (1980) report that even those patients with an objective basis for their chronic pain disability responded well to an operant pain management programme. Clearly, psychological processes cannot be ignored even if there is an organic basis for pain disorders.

EMOTIONAL DISTRESS AS A CAUSE OF PAIN

Evidence supporting the argument that severe emotional distress can trigger new pain or reinstigate old pain in the absence of physical pathology does not extend beyond clinicians' reports. Nevertheless, complaints of pain may be precipitated or exacerbated by emotional and social crises rather than tissue insult. For example, in the couvade syndrome, the precipitating event for a husband's complaints of aches and pains characteristic of pregnancy and labour appears to be the wife's complaints. Similarly, injured children occasionally do not become alarmed or display pain until they observe that the injury has upset a parent. These complaints appear to represent genuine distress rather than purposeful attempts to derive benefit or avoid activities.

Merskey (1968) described two forms of pain that appear to derive exclusively from psychological factors: pain during hallucinations, as observed in schizophrenics, and pain associated with conversion hysteria. The International Association for the Study of Pain description of chronic pain syndromes and definitions of pain terms (1986) acknowledges pain of psychological origin that may be attributed to specific delusional or hallucinatory causes. These syndromes are estimated to have a prevalence of less than 2% in patients with chronic pain without lesions. Similarly, certain painful conditions are believed to have hysterical or hypochondriacal origins, in the sense that the pain is attributable to remarkable thinking, emotions or personality factors. Patients diagnosed as hypochondriacal tend to have excessive fears of their symptoms, to engage in unrealistic interpretations of physical signs or sensations and to have a conviction that disease is present despite thorough investigations and reassurance.

Blumer & Heilbronn (1982) proposed that chronic pain without an organic basis is a variant of affective disorder and is best conceptualized as a syndrome within the spectrum of depressive disorders. An empirical basis for this concept does not exist (Turk & Salovey 1984; Romano & Turner 1985; Ahles et al 1987). The hypothesis proposes that an affective disorder underlies the chronic pain even when there is no manifest evidence of depression. Tangible support is evident in findings that some patients fail to recognize affective distress and, instead, somatize their complaints using both pain and non-pain somatic complaints (Katon et al 1982). France et al (1987) have established biological bases for distinguishing between patients with chronic pain without depression, patients with chronic pain and depression and patients with depression and no pain complaints. It would appear that chronic pain and depression are best construed as independent phenomena that have potential for reciprocal influences at both the biological and psychological levels of analysis.

Stressful events can enhance or perpetuate pain, or reduce the individual's capacity to tolerate pain (Sternbach 1974; Weisenberg 1977). Stressful events include major life trauma (e.g. disasters, loss of position, death of a loved one) and life's daily 'hassles'. Sternbach (1986b) reported that life's daily 'hassles' (e.g. upsetting incidents at home or work) are strongly associated with increased pain. Leavitt et al (1980) observed that low-back pain patients who were psychologically disturbed had a higher incidence of recent stressful events than patients who were not. Feuerstein et al (1985) similarly found environmental stressors such as family conflict and major life events to be more common among chronic low-back pain patients.

Emotional stress may increase pain by precipitating activity in psychophysiological systems that are also activated by noxious events. Anxiety, depression, anger and other emotions provoke substantial autonomic, visceral and skeletal activity. The interactions among these biological systems are well illustrated by the 'pain–anxiety–tension' cycle that has been proposed to account for some forms of acute and chronic pain. This vicious cycle has frequently been observed in disorders involving the musculoskeletal system. Pain provokes anxiety which in turn induces prolonged muscle spasm at the pain location and at trigger points, as well as vasoconstriction, ischaemia and release of pain-producing substances (Keefe & Gil 1986). The cycle may then repeat itself (Dolce & Raczynski 1985). Flor et al (1985) found accelerated lumbar electromyogram (EMG) reactivity in chronic back pain patients when they discussed personal stress. Tension headaches have been assumed to be the result of sustained contraction of muscles of the face, scalp and neck in the absence of permanent structural change, usually as a reaction to life stress. However, Philips (1982) has observed that diagnoses of tension headache are most often made on the basis of exclusion of other diagnostic possibilities rather than by demonstrating excessive tension in head and neck muscles. Numerous studies now suggest that patients with tension headaches do not always display sustained or elevated levels of EMG activity (Philips 1982). Similarly, pain during labour contractions in childbirth is reported to be magnified by skeletal muscle tension and self-induced relaxation is assumed to interrupt vicious cycles of tension and pain. Again, the model lacks empirical support and is probably oversimplistic. For example, women's concerns about their ability to bear the child and the baby's health all contribute to the distress experienced (Beck & Siegel 1980). In general, more support is needed for the proposition that muscle tension provides a basis for chronic pain (Turner & Chapman 1982).

Exaggerated or persistent pain behaviour can also be maintained by fear of pain. Pain behaviours, including high levels of self-report, reduced activity and other observable expressions of pain, may persist because of their past success in averting pain, even though tissue damage has healed (Fordyce 1976). Anxiety and fear of renewed pain persist and strengthen avoidance behaviour (Lethem et al 1983; Philips 1987a; McCracken et al 1992). Avoidance behaviour may also contribute to a disuse syndrome including loss of muscular strength, loss of mobility and weight gain.

Several studies have suggested that positive emotional states may diminish pain. Horan & Dellinger (1974) observed enhanced tolerance to cold-pressor pain in experimental subjects encouraged to use 'emotive imagery', defined as classes of images producing positive feelings such as self-assertion, pride or mirth. Other investigators have observed that self-controlled distraction by pleasant images yielded greater pain tolerance (Chaves & Barber 1974).

Emotional distress may produce diseases with lesions that are painful themselves. The autonomic and neuroendocrine changes provoked by psychological stress have been associated with diseases in cardiovascular, digestive, respiratory and eliminative systems (Selye 1976). Distressing events are capable of contributing to the initiation and exacerbation of a large number of painful diseases, including angina pectoris, painful menstruation, rheumatoid arthritis, gastric ulcer, duodenal ulcer, regional enteritis and ulcerative colitis (American Psychiatric Association 1987). Clearly illustrating the impact of stress would be the result of the unrelieved severe pain during myocardial infarction, which evokes abnormal reflex responses that may produce complications and death. Recent evidence indicates that stress may inhibit the capacity of the immune system to deal with pathogens that lead to painful diseases (Beutler et al 1986).

EMOTIONAL DISTURBANCES CONCURRENT WITH PAIN PROBLEMS

Pain symptoms have been identified as generally prevalent in psychiatric patients, particularly among those suffering anxiety disorders and exogenous depression (Merskey 1986). Merskey (1986) found pain to be less frequently associated with schizophrenia or endogenous depression. About 50% of all patients with pain and depression develop the two disorders simultaneously (Romano & Turner 1985). Philips & Hunter (1982) found tension headaches to be no more prevalent in psychiatric than in general practice populations, but reported pain intensity in the psychiatric population to be substantially higher.

Unfortunately, physical diagnoses in psychiatric populations are difficult to make because these patients tend to use pain language in a relatively indiscriminate and diffuse manner. Atkinson et al (1982) concluded that pain language is not accurate for medical diagnoses in patients who suffer affective disturbances.

Emotional distress may also precipitate pain complaints because these provide a legitimate, less stigmatized access to medical care. Patients suffering from anxiety or depression-based disorders may exaggerate painful complaints as they are more socially acceptable. Pain patients frequently disavow personal and interpersonal distress, despite conspicuous evidence, and emphasize their somatic problems. This pattern is associated with poor outcome from conventional medical care (Wilfling et al 1973; Sternbach 1974) and better outcome when the psychological distress is addressed (Blendis et al 1978). Clinicians sensitive to the multiple determinants of pain symptoms may detect presenting complaints as diagnostic of psychological distress, expressed in a socially acceptable manner, and provide suitable care.

Variations in emotional distress during pain

Clinicians benefit from close attention to the nuances of patients' verbal complaints, but only recently have there been concerted efforts to describe different pain disorders in terms of their sensory, affective and evaluative qualities.

Analyses of a number of major pain syndromes have led to interesting conclusions concerning the role of affect in pain. Melzack (1975) observed that pain due to cancer lesions has a high value on the sensory dimension, but affective intensity is no higher than for menstrual discomfort, despite the dramatic difference in the two disorders as threats to survival. In contrast, Kremer et al (1982) observed that high-intensity chronic back pain and cancer pain were associated with particularly high affective loadings. Similarly, Price et al (1987) found high affective-distress ratings to be associated with cancer pain and other forms of chronic pain which were associated with a high degree of threat to health or life. Reading (1980) noted that pain sensation appeared to be a relatively minor component of episiotomy pain when it was most severe just after childbirth but that affective distress was particularly salient. Reading & Newton's (1979) analyses of pain from intrauterine devices (IUD) and dysmenorrhoea disclosed a larger sensory component with IUD users, whereas with dysmenorrhoea the affective component predominated. The latter was attributed to the influence of culture, upbringing and attitudes, whereas the IUD pain was believed to have a more prominent sensory component because there was a tangible pain stimulus giving rise to pain sensations. Hunter & Philips (1981) found that tension and migraine headaches could be distinguished on a variety of sensory and affective scales of the McGill Pain Questionnaire.

Social influences on emotional distress

Social contextual factors that determine the nature and severity of the pain experience and the manner in which it is expressed have received attention. A developmental perspective has been instructive. The newborn infant's reaction to tissue damaging events appears relatively stereotyped and includes reflexive withdrawal, crying, body tension and facial grimaces. This reflects a genetically determined reflex that has social communication value and soon comes to be influenced by the social environment. Painful distress is strikingly visible in the facial expressions of newborns experiencing tissue damaging events from the first days of life (Grunau & Craig 1987; Grunau et al 1990). The grimace resembles that observed in older children, but, in the absence of the as yet undeveloped capacity to attach meaning to the situation, it is perhaps best interpreted as one of raw emotional distress.

Studies of infants' facial expressions during painful immunization injections have been informative about emotional aspects of pain. Until about 7 or 8 months, infants' reactions largely appear limited to pain, but thereafter their faces display fearful anticipation when they see needles being prepared, followed by pain as an immediate reaction to injection, and anger shortly thereafter (Izard et al 1980). The pain reaction evident in the younger infants decreases in severity, with anger dominating at about 19 months (Izard et al 1983). Craig et al (1984) noted that in the first year of life infants' behavioural reactions to needle injections appeared reflexive and diffuse, but, in the second year, the reactions were more localized, protective and socially responsive, as the babies carefully watched the nurse prior to and after the injection, attempted to protect themselves by pulling away and communicated a range of feelings and sentiments to their mothers.

Early in life, emerging capacities to interact with and control the social environment transform innately communicative reactions into patterns of behaviour that conform to social norms. The frequent and inevitable crises of childhood lead to frequent bouts of pain. These are powerful instigators of action in parents and others who fear for the child's safety and impose their expectations as to how children should avoid dangerous situations and respond when they have been hurt. Children also have numerous opportunities to observe how others react when hurt. Witnessing another person's reaction to a painful event has a powerful impact on the onlooker in terms of emotional reactions, disruptions in activity and behavioural reactions (Craig 1986). For example, children and adults exposed to others who display intense protracted pain appear to become vulnerable to atypical patterns of pain behaviour. In this manner, familial and cultural expectations and patterns of pain complaint become the standard for children and patterns of pain experience and expression, including the symptoms important to patients, come to conform to family belief systems and popular or folk models (Katon et al 1982; Sargent 1984; Craig & Wyckoff 1987). In addition, dysfunctional family experiences, for example physical or sexual abuse, have the capacity to predispose people to pain complaints without a pathophysiological basis (Sherry et al 1991; Reiter et al 1991).

Social support can play a restorative or destructive role with patients. A substantial portion of chronic pain patients experience interpersonal distress as a result of viewing their family and significant others as nonsupportive (Turk & Rudy 1990). Jamison & Virts (1990) report that chronic pain patients who enjoy a high level of support are more active, display less psychological distress and demand less pain medication. In contrast, other patients who report satisfaction with perceived levels of social support show high levels of pain behaviour when asked to perform simple tasks such as sitting, walking or reclining (Gil et al 1987). Discrepancies among the studies may reflect whether the support was provided for being ill or for maintaining a healthy lifestyle.

Cognitive appraisal and emotional aspects of pain

Emotional qualities of pain are influenced by the individual's appraisal of the event (Weisenberg 1977; Turk et al 1983). A vigorous search for information is usually dictated by the onset of pain because it may dictate efforts to avoid pain. Beecher (1959) attracted attention to the role of cognitive appraisal with his observations that soldiers wounded during battle complain far less than civilians comparably injured during accidents, presumably because the soldiers were relieved that they had escaped from the battlefield and expected to return home, whereas the civilians evaluated the injury as a threat to comfortable, established lives. Contrasting findings indicate that people who 'catastrophize', or self-alarm by focusing negatively upon their distress, desperately trying to escape and, anticipating the worst, suffer higher levels of anxiety, are the most disabled and benefit the least from conventional medical care. Depressed chronic low back pain patients have also been found to misinterpret or distort the nature and significance of their dilemma (LeFebvre 1981). Cognitive errors of catastrophizing, overgeneralization (assuming similar outcomes of different experiences) and selective abstraction (selectively attending to negative aspects of experience) are particularly prominent when depressed low-back pain patients focus on their disorder. Smith et al (1986) found the pattern of cognitive distortion in depressed chronic low back patients to be stronger in those who display general distress than in those who somatize their distress.

The availability of personal or external resources to control pain influences its emotional impact, a finding consistent with evidence that self-appraisals of power or potency are major determinants of emotional states (Russell 1978). Substantial individual differences exist in the coping strategies people use to modulate pain. In children, coping strategy use, perceived self-efficacy and frequency of catastophizing thoughts significantly predict postoperative pain, affective distress and physical recovery (Bennett-Branson & Craig 1993).

The broad categories of attentional diversion, cognitive restructuring and self-relaxation serve as coping strategies for some people (Turk et al 1983; Lawson et al 1990). Distraction alone appears insufficient as an analgesic technique, probably also requiring substantive changes in mood or the meaning of the experience (Leventhal 1992; McCaul et al 1992). Peoples' judgements of self efficacy, or their ability to use self-control strategies (Bandura et al 1987), determines whether these strategies are actually applied to clinical pain (Manning & Wright 1983; Holroyd et al 1984). Loss of control is undoubtedly important in chronic pain. As patients pursue rounds of health practitioners, failure to find lasting relief contributes to feelings of hopelessness, helplessness, despair and pessimism. Patients with strong feelings of helplessness have higher levels of psychological distress (Keefe et al 1990). It is exceedingly difficult for people to abandon efforts to achieve control over chronic pain and the risks of vicious circles are considerable. Anxiety about pain directs attention to pain which leads to stronger pain responses (Arntz et al 1991). Thus, ever more desperate measures carry the risk of compounding the initial problem.

Clinical implications

The central role of affect in pain argues for the further development of assessment and treatment strategies that have emotional processes as their target. While it may be convenient for both patients and health care professionals to ignore emotional aspects of pain in the search for an anatomical explanation, to do so can prolong pain and suffering. The severity of emotional distress has been shown to be an important predictor of treatment outcome (Wade et al 1990). A range of procedures can effectively reduce stress during noxious medical procedures (Ludwick-Rosenthal & Neufeld 1988). Meta-analysis of the outcome of some 48 studies providing psychologically-based treatments for chronic pain confirmed that anxiety and depression were reduced to a greater extent than measures of pain intensity and duration of pain episodes (Malone & Strube 1988). Reductions in anxiety, depression and hostility may also be associated with reduced demands on the health care delivery system (Caudill et al 1991).

Interventions designed to alter emotional aspects of pain are in order as failure to target them directly will delay recovery (Blanchard et al 1982). Sullivan et al (1992) conclude that the treatment of depression has not become a major component of the therapeutic management of chronic pain patients, despite evidence that cognitive/behavioural and antidepressant medication interventions work. Doan & Wadden (1989) observed that depressed chronic pain patients were more likely to be prescribed narcotics than antidepressants. Treatment failures in chronic pain rehabilitation programmes often may reflect inadequate attention to depression.

Therapeutic interventions designed to alleviate and control pain may be targeted to a number of components of the response. Broad band approaches such as the operant behavioural approach (Fordyce 1976) and the cognitive behavioural approach (Turk et al 1983) can be expected to have an impact on affective mechanisms. Changing social and environmental contingencies to reduce the frequency of excessive dependence on bed-rest, family members and medication can be expected to provoke anger in some patients prior to salutary effects. In contrast, providing social reinforcement for adaptive, healthy behaviour can be gratifying for patients. Similarly the cognitive–behavioural approach to helping patients understand the relationship of their pain to cognitive, affective and physiological variables and instruction in skills designed to cope more effectively has an impact on affective distress. For example, Philips (1987b) reported that a cognitive–behavioural treatment package (relaxation, exercise, activity pacing and cognitive interventions) had a substantial impact on mood, affective reactions to pain, self-efficacy, avoidance behaviour, drug intake and exercise capacity, which largely continued to improve a full year later.

Early identification of emotional problems and the introduction of early intervention programmes may be of benefit. Hadjistavropoulos & Craig (1993) noted that a substantial number of acute back pain patients present with unfavourable emotional distress and a high incidence of 'medically incongruent signs' that alone are prognostic of unfavourable outcome from conventional medical treatment. Linton et al (1989) found that a prevention programme comprising physical and behavioural interventions was a highly effective strategy for nurses with back pain, who were at risk for chronic problems. It reduced pain, pain behaviour, psychological distress, helplessness and fatigue. Given that a substantial proportion of the general population is at risk for the development of chronic pain (Von Korff et al 1988, 1990), there is a substantial need for prevention programmes.

There is also a range of more specific analgesic interventions designed to change emotional qualities such as fear, anxiety and depression, in addition to sensory qualities. Opioids can affect both sensory and emotional qualities of pain. In some instances, they induce elevated mood or euphoric states and in others they are distinctively aversive and dysphoric (Shippenberg et al 1988). Many psychoactive drugs reduce emotional distress rather than sensory qualities. Time-contingent analgesic medication should reduce the anticipatory distress produced by on-demand schedules of medication. Relaxation training reduces both the sensory and affective dimensions of pain and relieves pain intensity (Philips 1988). Instruction in imagery, distraction strategies and biofeedback disrupt the pain–anxiety–tension cycle and enhance perceived self-efficacy (Keefe et al 1986). Hypnosis and alpha feedback relieve both sensory and affective qualities of pain (Melzack & Perry 1975). Recognizing the potential role of anger and frustration in the problems encountered by pain patients (Wade et al 1990) should lead to the introduction of treatment techniques that target frustration and anger. There is reason to believe that encouraging patients to recognize the emotional dimensions of their illness may facilitate treatment (Large 1985). Elsewhere in this volume, there are descriptions of the growing armamentarium of behavioural and cognitive intervention strategies that have as their target changes in the affective component of pain experience and behaviour.

REFERENCES

Affleck G, Tennen H, Urrows S, Higgins P 1991 Individual differences in the day-to-day experience of chronic pain: a prospective daily study of rheumatoid arthritis patients. Health Psychology 10: 419–426

Ahles T A, Yunus M B, Masi A T 1987 Is chronic pain a variant of depressive disease? Pain 29: 105–112

American Psychiatric Association 1987 Diagnostic and statistical manual of mental disorders, 3rd edn (Revised). American Psychiatric Association, Washington, DC

Arntz A, Dreessen L, Merckelbach H 1991 Attention, not anxiety, influences pain. Behaviour Research and Therapy 29: 41–50

Aronoff G M, Wagner J M, Spangler A S 1986 Chemical interventions for pain. Journal of Consulting and Clinical Psychology 54: 769–775

Atkinson J H, Kremer E F, Ignelzi R J 1982 Diffusion of pain language with affective disturbance confounds differential diagnosis. Pain 12: 375–384

Atkinson J H, Slater M A, Grant I, Patterson T L, Garfin S R 1988 Depressed mood in chronic low back pain: relationship with stressful life events. Pain 35: 47–55

Bakan D 1971 Disease, pain and sacrifice: toward a psychology of suffering. Beacon Press, Chicago

Bandura A, O'Leary A, Taylor C B, Gauthier J, Gossard D 1987 Perceived self-efficacy and pain control: opioid and nonopioid mechanisms. Journal of Personality and Social Psychology 53: 563–571

Barber T X 1959 Towards a theory of pain: relief of chronic pain by prefrontal leucotomy, opiate, placebos and hypnoses. Psychological Bulletin 56: 430–460

Beck N C, Siegel L J 1980 Preparation for childbirth and contemporary research on pain, anxiety and stress reduction: a review and critique. Journal of Psychosomatic Research 24: 429–447

Beecher H K 1959 Measurement of subjective responses: quantitative effects of drugs. Oxford University Press, New York

Beidel D C, Christ M A G, Long P J 1991 Somatic complaints in anxious children. Journal of Abnormal Child Psychology 19: 659–670

Benjamin S, Barnes D, Berger S, Clarke I, Jeacock J 1988 The relationship of chronic pain, mental illness and organic disorders. Pain 32: 185–195

Bennett-Branson S M, Craig K D 1993 Postoperative pain in children: Developmental and family influences on spontaneous coping strategies. Canadian Journal of Behavioural Science (in press)

Beutler L E, Engle D, Oro-Beutler M E, Daldrup R, Meredith K 1986 Inability to express intense affect: a common link between depression and pain. Journal of Consulting and Clinical Psychology 54: 752–759

Blanchard E B, Andrasid F, Neff D et al 1982 Biofeedback and relaxation training with three kinds of headaches: treatment effects and their prediction. Journal of Consulting and Clinical Psychology 50: 562–565

Blendis L M, Hill O W, Merskey H 1978 Abdominal pain and the emotions. Pain 5: 179–191

Blumer D, Heilbronn M 1982 Chronic pain as a variant of depressive disease. Journal of Nervous and Mental Disease 170: 381–414

Bolles R C, Fanselow M S 1980 A perceptual–defensive–recuperative model of fear and pain. Behavioural and Brain Sciences 3: 291–323

Bond M R 1980 The suffering of severe intractable pain. In: Kosterlitz H W, Terenius L Y (eds) Pain and society. Verlag Chemie, Weinheim, p 53

Bonica J J 1979 Important clinical aspects of acute and chronic pain. In: Beers R E, Bassett E C (eds) Mechanisms of pain and analgesic compounds. Raven Press, New York, p 183

Brown G K A 1990 Causal analysis of chronic pain and depression. Journal of Abnormal Psychology 99: 127–137

Buytendijk F J J 1961 Pain. Greenwood Press, Westport, Connecticut

Caudill M, Schnable R, Zuttermeister P, Benson H, Friedman R 1991 Decreased clinic use by chronic pain patients: response to behavioral medicine intervention. Clinical Journal of Pain 7: 305–310

Chaturvedi S K 1987 A comparison of depressed and anxious chronic pain patients. General Hospital Psychiatry 9: 383–386

Chaves J F, Barber T X 1974 Cognitive strategies, experimenter modeling, and expectation in the attenuation of pain. Journal of Abnormal Psychology 83: 356–363

Craig K D 1983 Modeling and social learning factors in chronic pain. In: Bonica J J (ed) Advances in pain research and therapy. Raven Press, New York, p 813–827

Craig K D 1986 Social modelling influences: pain in context. In: Sternbach R A (ed) The psychology of pain, 2nd edn. Raven Press, New York, p 67–96

Craig K D 1992 The facial expression of pain: better than a thousand words? American Pain Society Journal 1: 153–162

Craig K D, Wyckoff M G 1987 Cultural factors in chronic pain management. In: Burrows G D, Elton D, Stanley G (eds) Handbook of chronic pain management. Elsevier, Amsterdam, p 99–108

Craig K D, Best H, Best J A 1978 Self-regulatory effects of monitoring sensory and affective dimensions of pain. Journal of Consulting and Clinical Psychology 46: 563–564

Craig K D, McMahon R H, Morrison J, Zaskow C 1984 Pain expression in infants during immunization injections. Social Science and Medicine 19: 1331–1337

Craig K D, Hyde S A, Patrick C J 1991 Genuine, suppressed and faked facial behavior during exacerbation of chronic low back pain. Pain 46: 161–172

Craig K D, Prkachin K M, Grunau R V E 1992. The facial expression of pain. In Turk D C, Melzack R (eds). Handbook of pain assessment. Guilford Press, New York p 255–274.

Craig K D, Whitfield M F, Grunau R V E, Linton J, Hadjistavropoulos H D 1993. Pain in the preterm neonate: behavioural and physiological indices. Pain 52: 287–299

Crisson J E, Keefe F J 1988 The relationship of locus of control to pain coping strategies and psychological distress in chronic pain patients. Pain 35: 147–154

Crook J, Weir R, Tunks E 1989 An epidemiological follow-up survey of persistent pain sufferers in a group family practice and speciality pain clinic. Pain 36: 49–61

Dallenbach K M 1939 Pain: history and present status. American Journal of Psychology 52: 331–347

Doan B D, Wadden N P 1989 Relationship between depressive symptoms and descriptions of chronic pain. Pain 36: 75–84

Dolce J J, Raczynski J M 1985 Neuromuscular activity and electromyography in painful backs: psychological and biomechanical models in assessment and treatment. Psychological Bulletin 97: 502–520

Dubuisson D, Melzack R 1976 Classification of clinical pain descriptors by multiple group discriminant analysis. Experimental Neurology 51: 480–487

Eich E, Rachman S, Lopatka C 1990 Affect, pain, and autobiographical memory. Journal of Abnormal Psychology 99: 174–178

Eisendrath S J, Way L W, Ostroff J W, Johanson C A 1986 Identification of psychogenic abdominal pain. Psychosomatics 27: 705–712

Feuerstein M, Skjei E 1979 Mastering pain. Bantam Books, New York

Feuerstein M, Salt S, Houle M 1985 Environmental stressors and chronic low back pain: life events, family and work environment. Pain 22: 295–307

Fields H L 1987 Pain. McGraw-Hill, New York

Flor H, Turk D C 1984 Etiological theories and treatments for chronic back pain. I. Somatic models and interventions. Pain 19: 105–122

Flor H, Turk D C, Birbaumer N 1985 Assessment of stress-related psychophysiological reactions in chronic back pain patients. Journal of Consulting and Clinical Psychology 53: 354–364

Fordyce W E 1976 Behavioural methods for chronic pain and illness. C V Mosby, St Louis, Missouri

Fordyce W E 1986 Learning process in pain. In: Sternbach R A (ed) The psychology of pain, 2nd edn. Raven Press, New York, p 49–65

Fordyce W E 1988 Pain and suffering: a reappraisal. American Psychologist 43: 276–283

France R D, Houpt J L, Ellinwood E H 1984 Therapeutic effects of antidepressants in chronic pain. General Hospital Psychiatry 6: 55–63

France R D, Krishnan K R R, Traunor M, Pelton S 1987 Chronic pain and depression. IV. DST as a discriminator between chronic pain and depression. Pain 28: 39–44

Frenk H, Cannon J T, Lewis J W, Liebeskind J C 1986 Neural and neurochemical mechanisms of pain inhibition. In: Sternbach R A (ed) The psychology of pain, 2nd edn. Raven Press, New York, p 25–48

Gaffney A, Dunne E A 1987 Children's understanding of the causality of pain. Pain 29: 91–104

Gamsa A 1990 Is emotional disturbance a precipitator or a consequence of chronic pain. Pain 42: 183–195

Garron D C, Leavitt F 1983 Chronic low back pain and depression. Journal of Clinical Psychology 30: 486–493

Gil K M, Keefe F J, Crisson J E, Van Dalfsen P J 1987 Social support and pain behavior Pain 29: 209–217

Gracely R H, McGrath P, Dubner R 1978 Validity and sensitivity of ratio scales of sensory and affective verbal pain descriptors. Pain 5: 19–29

Gracely R H, Dubner R, McGrath P A 1982 Fentanyl reduces the intensity of painful tooth pulp sensations: controlling for detection of active drugs. Anesthesia and Analgesia 61: 751–755

Gross P R 1992 Is pain sensitivity associated with dental avoidance. Behaviour Research and Therapy 30: 7–13

Grunau R V E, Craig K D 1987 Pain expression in neonates: facial action and cry. Pain 28: 395–410

Grunau R V E, Johnston C C, Craig K D 1990 Facial activity and cry to invasive and noninvasive tactile stimulation in neonates. Pain: 42: 295–305

Hadjistavropoulos H D, Craig K D 1993 Acute and chronic low back pain: cognitive, affective and behavioural dimensions. (Submitted for publication)

Hardy J, Wolff H, Goodell H 1952 Pain sensations and reactions. Williams & Wilkins, Baltimore

Heaton R K, Getto C J, Lehman A W, Fordyce W E, Brauer E, Groban S E 1982 A standardized evaluation of psychosocial factors in chronic pain. Pain 12: 165–174

Holroyd K A, Penzien D B, Hursey K G et al 1984 Change mechanisms in EMG biofeedback training: cognitive changes underlying improvements in tension headache. Journal of Consulting and Clinical Psychology 52: 1039–1053

Horan J A, Dellinger D K 1974 'In vivo' emotive imagery: a preliminary test. Perceptual and Motor Skills 39: 359–362

Hunter M, Philips C 1981 The experience of headache: an assessment of the qualities of tension headache pain. Pain 10: 209–219

International Association for the Study of Pain 1986 Classification of chronic pain: descriptions of chronic pain syndromes and definitions of pain terms. Pain (suppl 3): 1–222

Izard C E, Heubner R R, Resser D, McGinnes G C, Dougherty L M 1980 The young infant's ability to produce discrete emotion expressions. Developmental Psychology 16: 132–140

Izard C E, Hembree E A, Dougherty L M, Spizziri C C 1983 Changes in facial expressions of 2 to 19-month-old infants following acute pain. Developmental Psychology 19: 418–426

Jamison R N, Virts K L 1990 The influence of family support on chronic pain. Behaviour Research and Therapy 28: 283–287

Johnson J E, Rice V H 1974 Sensory and distress components of pain. Nursing Research 23: 203–209

Katon W, Kleinman A, Rosen G 1982 Depression and somatization: a review (parts 1 and 2). American Journal of Medicine 72: 127–247

Keefe F J, Dunsmore J 1992 Pain behavior: concepts and controversies. American Pain Society Journal 1: 92–100

Keefe F J, Gil K M 1986 Behavioral concepts in the analysis of chronic pain syndromes. Journal of Consulting and Clinical Psychology 54: 776–783

Keefe F J, Wilkins R H, Cook W A, Crisson J E, Muhlbaier L H 1986 Depression, pain, and pain behavior. Journal of Consulting and Clinical Psychology 54: 665–669

Keefe F J, Brown, G K, Wallston K A, Caldwell D S 1989 Coping with rheumatoid arthritis pain: catastrophizing as a maladaptive strategy. Pain 37: 51–56

Keefe F J, Crisson J, Urban B J, Williams D A 1990 Analyzing chronic low back pain: the relative contribution of pain coping strategies. Pain 40: 293–301

Keele K D 1957 Anatomies of pain. C C Thomas, Springfield, Illinois

Kerns R D, Turk D C, Holzman A D 1983 Psychological treatment for chronic pain: a selective review Clinical Psychology Review 3: 15–26

Kremer E F, Atkinson J H Jr, Ignelzi R J 1982 Pain measurement: the affective dimensional measure of the McGill pain questionnaire with a cancer population. Pain 12: 153–163

Krishnan K R R, France R D, Pelton S, McCann U D, Davidson J, Urban B J 1985 Chronic pain and depression. II. Symptoms of anxiety in chronic low back pain patients and their relationship to subtypes of depression. Pain 22: 289–294

Large R G 1985 Self-concepts and illness attitudes in chronic pain. A repertory grid study of a pain management program. Pain 23: 113–119

Lawson K, Ressor K A, Keefe F J, Turner J A 1990 Dimensions of pain-related cognitive coping: cross-validation of the factor structure of the Coping Strategy Questionnnaire. Pain 43: 195–204

Leavitt F, Carron D C, Bieliauskas L A 1980 Psychological disturbance and life event differences among patients with low back pain. Journal of Consulting and Clinical Psychology 48: 115–116

LeFebvre M F 1981 Cognitive distortion and cognitive factors in depressed psychiatric and low back pain patients. Journal of Consulting and Clinical Psychology 49: 517–525

LeResche L, Dworkin S F 1988 Facial expressions of pain and emotions in chronic TMD patients. Pain 35: 71–78

Lethem J, Slade P D, Troup J D G, Bentley G 1983 Outline of a fear-avoidance model of exaggerated pain perception – I. Behaviour Research and Therapy 21: 401–408

Leventhal H 1992 I know distraction works even though it doesn't. Health Psychology 11: 208–209

Leventhal H, Everhart D 1979 Emotions, pain and physical illness. In: Izard C E (ed) Emotions in personality and psychopathology. Plenum Press, New York, p 261–299

Lewis T 1942 Pain. MacMillan, London

Linton S J, Bradley, L A, Jensen, E, Spangfort E, Sundell L 1989 The secondary prevention of low back pain: a controlled study with follow-up. Pain 36: 197–207

Ludwick-Rosenthal R, Neufeld R W J 1988 Stress management during noxious medical procedures: an evaluative review of outcome studies. Psychological Bulletin 104: 326–342

McCaul K D, Monson N, Maki R H 1992 Does distraction reduce pain-produced distress among college students? Health Psychology 11: 210–217

McCracken L M, Zayfert C, Gross R T 1992 The Pain Anxiety Symptoms Scale: development and validation of a scale to measure fear of pain. Pain 50: 67–73

Magni G 1987 On the relationship between chronic pain and depression when there is no organic lesion. Pain 31: 1–21

Magni C, Caldieron C, Rigatti-Luchini S, Merskey H 1990 Chronic musculoskeletal pain and depressive symptoms in the general population. An analysis of the first National Health and Nutrition Examination Survey data. Pain 43: 299–307

Malone M D, Strube M J 1988 Meta-analysis of non-medical treatments for chronic pain. Pain 34: 231–244

Malow R M, West J A, Sutker P B 1989 Anxiety and pain response changes across treatment: sensory decision analysis. Pain 38: 35–44

Manning M M, Wright T L 1983 Self-efficacy expectancies, outcome expectancies, and persistence of pain control in child birth. Journal of Personality and Social Psychology 45: 421–431

Marshall H R 1894 Are there special nerves for pain? Journal of Nervous and Mental Disease 21: 71–94

Martelli M F, Auerbach S M, Alexander J, Mercuri L G 1987 Stress management in the health care setting: matching interventions with patient coping styles. Journal of Consulting and Clinical Psychology 55: 201–207

Melamed B G, Siegel L J 1980 Behavioural medicine: practical applications in health care. Springer, New York

Melzack R 1983 The McGill pain questionnaire. In: Melzack R (ed) Pain measurement and assessment. Raven Press, New York, p 41–48

Melzack R, Casey K L 1968 Sensory, motivational and central control determinants of pain: a new conceptual model. In: Kenshalo D L (ed) The skin senses. C C Thomas, Springfield, Illinois, p 423

Melzack R, Dennis S G 1980 Phylogenetic evolution of pain expression in animals. In: Kosterlitz H W, Terenius L Y (eds) Pain and society. Verlag Chemie, Weinheim, p 13

Melzack R, Perry C 1975 Self-regulation of pain: the use of alpha feedback and hypnotic training for the control of chronic pain. Experimental Neurology 46: 452–469

Melzack R, Torgerson W S 1971 On the language of pain. Anesthesiology 34: 50–59

Melzack R, Wall P D 1965 Pain and mechanisms: a new theory. Science 150: 971–979

Melzack R, Taenzer P, Feldman P, Kinch R A 1981 Labour is still painful after prepared childbirth training. Canadian Medical Association Journal 125: 356–363

Melzack R, Abbott F V, Zackon W, Mulder D S, Davis M W L 1987 Pain on a surgical ward: a survey of the duration and intensity of pain and the effectiveness of medication. Pain 29: 67–72

Merskey H 1968 Psychological aspects of pain. Postgraduate Medical Journal 44: 297–306

Merskey H 1986 Psychiatry and pain. In: Sternbach R A (ed) The psychology of pain. Raven Press, New York, p 97–120

Philips C 1982 The nature and treatment of chronic tension headache. In: Craig K D, McMahon R J (eds) Advances in clinical behaviour therapy. Brunner/Mazel, New York, p 211–231

Philips H C 1987a Avoidance behavior and its role in sustaining chronic pain. Behaviour Research and Therapy 25: 273–279

Philips H C 1987b The effects of behavioural treatment on chronic pain. Behaviour Research and Therapy: 25: 365–377

Philips H C 1988 Changing chronic pain experience. Pain 32: 165–172

Philips H C, Grant L 1991 The evolution of chronic back pain problems: a longitudinal study. Behaviour Research and Therapy 29: 435–441

Philips H C, Hunter M 1982 Headache in a psychophysical population. Journal of Nervous and Mental Disease 170: 1–12

Pilowsky I, Chapman C R, Bonica J J 1977 Pain, depression and illness behaviour in a pain clinic population. Pain 4: 183–192

Poole F D, Craig K D 1992 Judgements of genuine, suppressed and faked facial expression of pain. Journal of Personality and Social Psychology 63: 797–805

Price D D, Barrell J J, Gracely R H 1980 A psychophysical analysis of experimental factors that selectively influence the affective dimension of pain. Pain 8: 137–150

Price D D, Harkins S W, Baker C 1987 Sensory-affective relationships among different types of clinical and experimental pain. Pain 28: 297–308

Reading A E 1980 A comparison of pain rating scales. Journal of Psychosomatic Research 24: 119–124

Reading A E, Newton J R 1979 A card sort method of pain assessment. Journal of Psychosomatic Research 22: 503–509

Reesor K A, Craig K D 1988 Medically incongruent back pain: physical restriction, suffering, and ineffective coping. Pain 32: 35–45

Reiter R C, Shakerin L R, Gambone J C, Milburn A K 1991 Correlation between sexual abuse and somatization in women with somatic and nonsomatic chronic pelvic pain. American Journal of Obstetrics and Gynecology 165: 104–109

Roberts A H, Reinhardt L 1980 The behavioural management of chronic pain: long-term follow-up with comparison groups. Pain 8: 151–162

Romano J M, Turner J A 1985 Chronic pain and depression: does the evidence support a relationship? Psychological Bulletin 97: 18–34

Rosensteil A, Keefe F J 1983 The use of coping strategies in chronic low back pain patients: relationship to patient characteristics and adjustment. Pain 17: 33–43

Rudy T E, Kerns R D, Turk D C 1988 Chronic pain and depression: toward a cognitive-behavioral mediation model. Pain 35: 129–140

Russell J A 1978 Evidence of convergent validity on the dimensions of affect. Journal of Personality and Social Psychology 36: 1152–1168

Sargent C 1984 Between depth and shame: dimensions of pain in Bariba culture. Social Science and Medicine 19: 1299–1304

Selye H 1976 The stress of life. McGraw-Hill, New York

Sherry D D, McGuire T, Mellins E, Salmonson K, Wallace C A, Nepom B 1991 Psychosomatic musculoskeletal pain in childhood: clinical and psychological analyses of 100 children. Pediatrics 88: 1093–1099

Shippenberg T S, Stein C, Huber A, Millan M J, Herz A 1988 Motivational effects of opioids in an animal model of prolonged inflammatory pain. Pain 35: 179–186

Smith T W, Aberger E W, Follick M J, Ahern D K 1986 Cognitive distortion and psychological distress in chronic low back pain. Journal of Consulting and Clinical Psychology 54: 573–575

Sternbach R 1974 Pain patients: traits and treatment. Academic Press, New York

Sternbach R A 1986a Clinical aspects of pain. In: Sternbach R A (ed) The psychology of pain, 2nd edn. Raven Press, New York, p 223–239

Sternbach R A 1986b Pain and 'hassles' in the United States: findings of the Nuprin pain report. Pain 27: 69–80

Strong C A 1895 The psychology of pain. Psychological Review 2: 329–354

Sullivan M J L, D'Eon J L 1990 Relation between catastrophizing and depression in chronic pain patients. Journal of Abnormal Psychology 99: 260–263

Sullivan M J L, Reesor K, Mikail S, Fisher R 1992 The treatment of depression in chronic low back pain: review and recommendations. Pain 50: 5–13

Szasz T S 1947 Pain and pleasure. New York, Basic Books

Taenzer P 1983 Postoperative pain: relationships among measures of pain, mood and narcotic requirements. In: Melzack R (ed) Pain measurement and assessment. Raven Press, New York, p 111–118

Taenzer P, Melzack R, Jeans M E 1986 Influence of psychological factors on postoperative pain, mood and analgesic requirement. Pain 24: 331–342

Timmermans G, Sternbach R A 1974 Factors of human chronic pain: an analysis of personality and pain reaction variables. Science 184: 806–808

Tu W 1980 A religiophilosophical perspective on pain. In: Kosterlitz H W, Terenius L Y (eds) Pain and society. Verlag Chemie, Weinheim, p 63

Turk D C, Melzack R 1992 Handbook of pain assessment. Guilford, New York

Turk D C, Rudy T E 1990 The robustness of an empirically derived taxonomy of chronic pain patients. Pain 43: 27–35

Turk D C, Salovey P 1984 'Chronic pain as a variant of depressive disease': a critical reappraisal. Journal of Nervous and Mental Disorders 1972: 398–404
Turk D C, Meichenbaum D H, Genest M 1983 Pain and behavioural medicine: theory, research and clinical guide. Guilford, New York
Turner J A 1991 Coping and chronic pain. In: Bond M R, Charlton J E, Woolf C J (eds). Proceedings of the VIth World Congress of Pain, Elsevier, Amsterdam, p 219–228
Turner J A, Chapman C R 1982 Psychological interventions for chronic pain: a critical review. II. Operant conditioning, hypnosis, and cognitive-behavioral therapy. Pain 12: 23–46
Urban B J, Keefe F J, France R D 1984 A study of psychophysical scaling in chronic pain patients. Pain 20: 157–168
Von Korff M, Dworkin S F, LeResche L, Kruger A 1988 An epidemiologic comparison of pain complaints. Pain 32: 173–183
Von Korff M, Dworkin S F, LeResche L 1990 Graded chronic pain status: an epidemiologic evaluation. Pain 40: 293–301
Waddell G, Pilowsky I, Bond M R 1989 Clinical assessment and interpretation of abnormal illness behaviour in low back pain. Pain 39: 41–53
Wade J B, Price D D, Hamer R M, Schwartz S M, Hart R P 1990 An emotional component analysis of chronic pain. Pain 40: 303–310
Wall P D 1979 On the relation of injury to pain. Pain 6: 253–264
Weisenberg M 1977 Pain and pain control. Psychological Bulletin 84: 1008–1044
Wilfling F J, Klonoff H, Kokan P 1973 Psychological, demographic and orthopaedic factors associated with prediction of outcome of spinal fusion. Clinical Orthopaedics 90: 153–160
Woodforde J M, Merskey F G 1971 Some relationships between subjective measures of pain. Journal of Psychosomatic Research 16: 173–178
Zitman F G, Linssen C G, Van H R L 1992 Chronic pain beyond patienthood. Journal of Nervous and Mental Disease 180: 97–100

14. Cognitive aspects of pain

Matisyohu Weisenberg

INTRODUCTION

The past decade has witnessed an enormous growth in the use of cognitive theory and techniques for the treatment of pain. Cognition is 'a generic term embracing the quality of knowing, which includes perceiving, recognizing, conceiving, judging, sensing, reasoning and imagining' (Stedman's Medical Dictionary 1976). Generally, cognitive interventions are part of a total multidisciplinary package offered by pain clinics. Examples of the problems to which the cognitive or cognitive-behavioural approach has been applied include low back pain (Nicholas et al 1992), rheumatoid arthritis (McCracken 1991), cancer (Syrjala et al 1992), headache (Holroyd et al 1991), temporomandibular joint dysfunction (Wilson et al 1992), preparation for treatment (Jay et al 1991), pain of the upper limbs (Spence 1991) and as part of a multidisciplinary programme (Peters & Large 1990).

The word 'cognitive' has had a long history in the study of human development with a growing literature on pain in children (McGrath 1990). To understand the experience of children more clearly and to plan interventions that are meaningful for the child, there has been an attempt to correlate the child's pain experience with his level of cognitive development. Thus, for example, Lavigne et al (1986) tried to correlate the child's reaction to the pain experience according to the Piagetian stages of cognitive development. At the early ages (2–6), the preoperational stage, the pain may be seen as external with causal explanations tending to contain a magical element. Unrelated events are seen as causally related. When these children reach the age of kindergarten, they tend to see illness as caused by some concrete action or lack of action. Pain may be seen as punishment for his/her acts. The cognitive developmental approach also has had an influence on pain assessment in children (Thompson & Varni 1986). For those who work with children, adequate communication and appropriate treatment require a knowledge of cognitive development.

As used in most research and treatment, cognitive approaches are concerned with the way the person perceives, interprets and relates to his pain rather than with the elimination of the pain per se. Because pain patients often suffer from stress, anxiety or depression, it is likely that cognitive interventions affect pain directly as well as indirectly, by reducing the stress or the emotional disturbance (Sternbach 1986; Malone & Strube 1988; Rudy et al 1988; Tyrer et al 1989; Gamsa & Vikis-Freibergs 1991; Dworkin et al 1992b).

This chapter reviews the theoretical and experimental bases of cognitive approaches to pain control. The applied aspects are found in other chapters.

THEORETICAL APPROACHES

COGNITIVE THEORIES: COPING AND BELIEVING

Theoretically, the basic cognitive concepts can be traced to Ellis (1962), Beck et al (1979, 1985, 1990), Roskies & Lazarus (1980), Lazarus & Folkman (1984), Meichenbaum (1977, 1985), Bandura (1977, 1984, 1989) Freeman et al (1990) and Kendall et al (1991). Applications to pain control also can be traced to these authors (Meichenbaum & Turk 1976; Turk 1978; Turk & Rudy 1992).

Coping has been conceptualized as 'the person's cognitive and behavioural efforts to manage (reduce, minimize, master or tolerate) the internal and external demands of the person–environment transaction that is appraised as taxing or exceeding the person's resources' (Folkman et al 1986a). According to Roskies & Lazarus (1980) and Lazarus & Folkman (1984), the way a person copes with a stressful situation depends on his view of the situation. This cognitive evaluation, referred to as appraisal, is a dynamic process that changes according to the person's perception of the consequences of an event, its importance to his well-being, and the resources he has to cope with the threat. The appraisal process also changes as events change (Folkman et al 1986b).

Coping has been classified according to the mode of action used (direct action, action inhibition, information search, intrapsychic processes) as well as the function it serves: problem-oriented (or problem-focused) coping or palliative regulation of the emotional response (that is, emotion-focused coping). Most individuals use both modes of coping (problem-focused or emotion-focused) at various times. However, there are circumstances where one or the other mode is preferable. For example, Forsythe & Compas (1987) examined the relationships among the individual's appraisal of a situation as controllable or not, the mode of coping used and the psychological distress. Problem-focused coping was associated with lower levels of distress in situations perceived as controllable, and higher distress in situations perceived as uncontrollable. The opposite results were obtained with emotion-focused coping.

Individual differences in coping preferences have been shown to affect coping success. Heyneman et al (1990) assessed the untrained, preferred-coping behaviours of subjects undergoing cold-pressor stimulation. During this baseline trial, subjects were asked to verbalize their thoughts while experiencing cold-pressor pain. Subjects were then classified as catastrophizers (use of a large number of negative self-statements or negative thoughts about the future) or noncatastrophizers. After random assignment, subjects were trained in either self-statement, self-instructional training (SI) or attention diversion (AD) coping strategies. The training more closely matched or mismatched the subject's untrained, preferred way of reacting to cold-pressor pain. Noncatastrophizers showed higher pain tolerance under AD than SI, while catastrophizers showed a greater increase in tolerance under SI than under AD. Interventions that matched the spontaneous preferences were more successful. In a similar fashion, Rokke & Absi (1993) were able to demonstrate the effectiveness for coping with cold-pressor pain by matching intervention strategy with the preferred mode of coping as determined by means of a standardized coping questionnaire, the Cognitive Coping Strategy Inventory. The emphasis on and the importance of identifying coping strategies have led to the development of a number of measures, which will be discussed later.

According to Beck et al (1979, 1985, 1990), coping involves what a person does as well as what he thinks and says to himself. Cognitive processes and structures (schemata) include the assumptions, beliefs, commitments and meanings that influence the way the person perceives and reacts to the world. These processes and structures help the person identify stimuli quickly, categorize them, fill in missing information, select a strategy for obtaining more information, solve a problem or reach a goal. Stressful events can trigger schemata that prime the person to respond in a given way. Distorted underlying assumptions and errors in information processing can serve to maintain emotional disturbance.

Cognitive therapeutic techniques are designed to help the person identify and correct distorted conceptualizations. The patient is taught how to monitor negative, automatic thoughts, to recognize the connections between cognition, affect, and behaviour, to examine evidence for and against his distorted automatic thoughts, to substitute reality-oriented interpretations and to recognize dysfunctional or irrational beliefs that predispose him to distort experiences (Ellis 1962; Meichenbaum 1977, 1985; Beck et al 1979; 1985, 1990). Interventions could involve changing the patient's thoughts, moods or behaviour.

Meichenbaum (1985) discusses the need to provide the patient with a variety of coping strategies. These include use of relaxation techniques, teaching problem-solving skills (D'Zurilla & Goldfried 1971; Turk et al 1983), cognitive restructuring to correct cognitive errors or distortions, behavioural and imaginal rehearsal, self-monitoring, self-reinstruction and self-reinforcement of effort to change.

Meichenbaum & Turk (1976), Meichenbaum (1977, 1985) and Turk (1978) developed a technique called stress-inoculation training. It deals with individual differences by offering subjects a variety of strategies and skills. Subjects choose those strategies they feel most capable of using. There is a period of training prior to exposure to the pain situation. During the education phase, subjects are told of the different components of pain as described in the gate-control theory of pain (Melzack & Wall 1965) and subjects are provided with coping strategies such as relaxation, attention-diversion and imagery manipulations. Prior to actual confrontation with the pain stimuli, they are given the opportunity to practise using different strategies while imagining they feel pain. Subjects are also asked to role-play at giving advice to a new subject. In the Meichenbaum & Turk study (1976), dealing with preparations for muscle ischaemic pain, the entire training procedure took about 1 hour. Subjects then underwent a submaximal-effort muscle-ischaemic test. Compared to a pretest duration of 17 minutes, posttraining tolerance increased to 32 minutes. In a later study reported by Turk (1978), the training was increased to $3\frac{1}{2}$ hours. Expanded training was provided in relaxation, imagery rehearsal, attentional focusing and exposure to a novel stressor. The results confirmed the earlier study and also demonstrated generalization of effects to a novel stressor. Stress inoculation in general has been found to be effective in a variety of stress and anxiety situations. What is not always clear, however, is exactly which and how much of the described ingredients are necessary for treatment (Kendall et al 1991).

In general, as cognitive approaches are applied to treatment for pain, patients are taught to become actively involved in their treatment. Cognitive–behavioural techniques are normally used as part of a more comprehensive programme to teach the relationships between thoughts, feelings, behaviour, environmental stimuli and pain. Patients with chronic pain, for example, may have negative expectations regarding their ability to exert any control over their pain and may see themselves as helpless. This could lead to demoralization, inactivity and a tendency to overreact to pain. If the pain is interpreted as due to increasing tissue damage or to a life-threatening situation, it could produce greater suffering than pain of the same or even a higher intensity. In the cognitive approach, there is an emphasis on replacing helplessness and hopelessness with resourcefulness and hope. Patients also are taught a variety of coping strategies and skills to deal with the pain and the circumstances surrounding it. These include relaxation, imagery, cognitive restructuring, self-statements and attention diversion (Turk et al 1983; Turk & Fernandez 1990; Turk & Rudy 1992).

Turk & Rudy (1992), using the taxonomy developed by Ingram & Kendall (1986), categorized cognitive constructs into three major groups:

1. *Cognitive schemata* that include general beliefs, appraisals and expectations about pain
2. *Cognitive processes* that refer to the mental processes used in pain control attempts
3. Specific *cognitive content* concerning patient circumstances and attempts to cope with pain.

Several studies show that these constructs are related to pain status.

Cognitive schemata

Cognitive schemata or beliefs can influence the willingness of the patient to accept treatment and to adhere to treatment recommendations as well as his perceptions of disability (Williams & Thorn 1989; Slater et al 1991). Philips (1987a) has argued that chronic pain patients adopt an avoidance strategy based on the belief that increased physical activity would cause harm to their fragile status, whereas for chronic, benign pain, the opposite is recommended for treatment and rehabilitation. As a consequence of a cognitive–behavioural treatment intervention for a group of 40 chronic pain patients, Philips (1987b) was able to demonstrate a significant reduction of avoidance behaviour and a major shift in attitude regarding the perceived control over their pain in comparison to a waiting-list control group. Philips (1989) developed the 48-item Cognitive Evaluation Questionnaire (CEQ) to permit the systematic assessment of patient expectations and beliefs. The 15-item Pain and Impairment Relationship Scale (PAIRS) is another example of a recently developed operational measure of the relationship of beliefs and schemata to impairment from chronic pain (Slater et al 1991). Using the PAIRS permits the identification of beliefs associated with impairment, as opposed to disease severity, that may impede functioning to capacity and decrease compliance with rehabilitation efforts. These beliefs become a direct target of treatment.

Cognitive processes

Cognitive processes relate to how the individual utilizes the information that he encounters. It is here that such things as automatic thinking, cognitive distortion and catastrophizing become very relevant, especially for chronic pain. In a study of 138 low back patients, Smith et al (1986) used the CEQ to assess cognitive distortions. This instrument, based on reactions to 48 vignettes, measures the cognitive errors of overgeneralization, catastrophizing, personalization and selective abstraction. Cognitive distortion was found to be related to disability. Especially noteworthy was overgeneralization that could lead to restriction of activity and may be a type of spread-of-disability effect. Gil et al (1990) developed the 33-item Negative Thoughts in Response to Pain (INTRP) questionnaire. They were able to show a relationship between pain flare-ups and negative thoughts, with high numbers of negative thoughts being associated with high levels of pain.

Cognitive content

This includes the methods people use to control their emotional arousal and reactions to a pain episode. Several measures have been used to assess how individuals react when faced with pain. One example is the Cognitive Strategies Questionnaire (CSQ), a 42-item measure of different strategies used by pain patients that includes diverting attention, coping self-statements, praying or hoping, increased behavioural activities, reinterpretation of pain sensations, ignoring pain sensations and catastrophizing (Rosenstiel & Keefe 1983; Lawson et al 1990). Turner & Clancy (1986) used the CSQ to assess a cognitive or behavioural intervention for low-back pain. They reported that increased use of praying and hoping strategies and less catastrophizing were associated with lower pain intensity. Keefe et al (1990) using the CSQ found that the helplessness factor accounted for 50% of the variance in psychological distress and 46% of the depression among chronic low back pain patients.

Brown & Nicassio (1987) argued that despite the specific content, coping can be considered to be adaptive or active, or maladaptive or passive in coping with pain. They developed a 27-item questionnaire to measure these dimensions of coping called the Vanderbilt Pain Management Inventory (VPMI). It was tested with rheumatoid arthritis patients to demonstrate adaptive or maladaptive coping. Smith & Wallston (1992) developed a model of adaptation of rheumatoid arthritis patients, based on the Lazarus & Folkman (1984) conceptualization of appraisal and coping. They utilized the Brown & Nicassio measure to show that helplessness appraisal, passive coping with pain and impairment were associated with maladaptation to rheumatoid arthritis.

Catastrophizing

Catastrophizing has been singled out in several studies and reviews as particularly important in predicting reaction to pain and treatment even though Lawson et al (1990) reported that it appears to be separate from other factors on the CSQ. For example, Keefe et al (1989) were able to predict 6 months later the pain intensity and functional impairment of 223 rheumatoid arthritis patients as found on the Arthritis Impact Measurement Scale on the basis of prior scores on the catastrophizing scale of the CSQ. Zautra & Manne (1992), after reviewing 10 years of coping research among rheumatoid arthritis patients, concluded that catastrophizing and wishful thinking were associated with poorer outcomes while attempts to restructure thoughts to be more positive were associated with positive outcomes. Reesor & Craig (1988) found more catastrophizing and less of a sense of control to typify chronic low back patients for whom the symptomatology was not congruent with the physical findings, had poorer outcomes to treatment and rehabilitation and used health care resources excessively.

Catastrophizing as it relates to pain refers to negative self-statements and overly negative thoughts and ideas about the future. As such, it is undoubtedly related to some of the negative thought measures described earlier. Several researchers have suggested that reduction of negative thoughts may be more important for adaptive coping than enhancing positive thoughts (Kendall 1985, 1992; Turk & Rudy 1992). Newton & Barbaree (1987), in a study of headache patients treated with stress-inoculation training compared to a no-treatment waiting-list group, examined patients' thoughts during and immediately after a headache. The treated group, compared to the controls, exhibited a significant shift toward positive thinking and more problem-focused thinking. Complaints of more intense pain were found to be associated with more negative appraisal of headache episodes, more frequent cognitive avoidance, and greater negative affect. Treated subjects reported a reduction in pain intensity and in headache frequency. The increased use of coping strategies, however, was not found to be significantly related to pain reduction. The authors postulate that the reduction in negative appraisal was the key change mechanism.

Coping strategies

Williams & Keefe (1991) used a combined assessment of the CSQ and the Pain Beliefs and Perceptions Inventory (PBAPI) of Williams & Thorn (1989). They were able to identify patients who were more or less likely to use cognitive coping strategies. Patients who believed that pain was enduring or mysterious were less likely to use cognitive coping strategies and were more likely to catastrophize than patients who believed their pain to be understandable and of short duration.

It is clear that the various cognitive aspects of pain have a strong association with the reactions to pain. After reviewing the literature on coping with chronic pain, Jensen et al (1991a) concluded that beliefs and coping have a strong relationship to adjustment to chronic pain. Patients who believe they can control their pain, who avoid catastrophizing, and who believe that they are not severely disabled function better than those who do not. It is important, however, to note that much of the current data are correlational. As Kendall et al (1991) point out about cognitive theories in general, many of the beliefs measured at different stages of treatment may reflect a state of mind rather than a personality trait. Cause and effect are not always clear.

Self-efficacy

It is important to emphasize that effective coping depends on a person's assessment of his competence. It is not enough to possess the relevant skills. The person must *believe* that he has them and that he is capable of applying them as needed. This concept has been labelled 'self-efficacy' by Bandura (1977). A person's belief in his own effectiveness determines whether he tries to cope with or avoid a situation that is viewed as beyond his ability. Efficacy expectations can also determine how much effort a person will invest and how long he will persist in the face of aversive experiences. Lack of perceived self-efficacy leading to faulty appraisal of coping abilities can produce anxiety and behavioural dysfunction. Perceived self-efficacy is seen as influencing how an individual will behave, think and react emotionally in a challenging or stressful situation. Recent research has even shown that perceived self-efficacy could affect the body's endogenous opiate and immune systems (Bandura et al 1987, 1988; Wiedenfeld et al 1990). It is important to note that perceived self-efficacy is a changeable commodity. Bandura (1977) has referred to four major sources by which self-efficacy can be influenced. They are: performance experiences, vicarious experiences, verbal or social persuasion, and emotional or physiological arousal. One of the most potent influences on self-efficacy is the mastery experience acquired through actual performance. In the pain area, self-efficacy has been shown to be a basic concept both in laboratory and clinical studies. Subjects who possess higher self-efficacy are willing to tolerate higher levels of pain. Manipulation of self-efficacy also appears to be causally related to the outcome (Vallis &

Bucher 1986; Litt 1988; Williams & Kinney 1991). In a laboratory study using cold-pressor pain, Dolce et al (1986a) found that self-efficacy expectancies were the best predictors of pain tolerance. They also found that setting of quotas contributed to increased pain tolerance, perhaps via the raising of self-efficacy expectations. The laboratory research was followed up with clinical application and study. Dolce et al (1986b) utilized a quota system for exercise with chronic pain patients. After three baseline sessions, exercises were introduced on an increasing quota basis. Patients demonstrated an increase in self-efficacy for the physical activity. The authors conceptualize the approach as a desensitization of the avoidance behaviour associated with the faulty belief that activity is associated with harm and pain increase. Self-efficacy was increased at the same time as worry and concern over activity decreased.

The success of cognitive strategies depends to a great extent on motivational factors as has become increasingly recognized (Weisenberg 1984, 1989; Turk & Rudy 1990, 1991). The self-efficacy concept has been found to play a key motivational role in pain control. For example, Holroyd et al (1984) told a group of patients that they had achieved high control over tension or relaxation of frontalis muscles in order to induce a high sense of self-efficacy so that they could abort or reduce headache intensity. The actual amount of physiological change was found to be unrelated to headache activity. Perceived self-efficacy was the determining factor. Several studies with chronic pain patients have since reported that a key predictor of patient success at the conclusion of treatment was perceived self-efficacy (Council et al 1988; Kores 1990; Jensen et al 1991b).

PAIN THEORIES

Conceptually, the gate control theory (Melzack & Wall 1965; Melzack 1986) is still the most comprehensive and relevant for an understanding of the cognitive aspects of pain. There are gaps in the theory, the details of which are currently being filled in by others. According to gate control theory, pain phenomena are viewed as consisting of sensory–discriminative, motivational–affective and cognitive–evaluative components. More than any other theoretical approach, gate control theory emphasizes the tremendous role of psychological variables and how they affect the reaction to pain. Especially with chronic pain, successful pain control often involves changing the cognitive–motivational components while the sensory component remains intact. Hypnosis, anxiety reduction, desensitization, attention distraction and other behavioural approaches can be effective alternatives and supplements to pharmacology and surgery in the control of pain. Their effect is felt mostly on the cognitive–motivational components of pain (see Weisenberg 1977, 1980, 1983, 1987 for a more extensive review of psychological factors in pain control).

Recently, other theoretical statements have attempted to fill in the pieces of gate control or to introduce new concepts that have not appeared in gate control theory. Some of them were formulated to explain or understand results of clinical practice (Turk & Flor 1987; Turk & Rudy 1992), while others were formulated to explain the place of key concepts such as depression, emotional disturbance or other psychological phenomena of chronic pain (Rudy et al 1988; Gamsa & Vikis-Freibergs 1991).

The functional theory of pain (Algom 1992) stresses the sensory component of pain. It has grown out of the psychophysiological laboratory and the question of how several aversive stimuli interact with one another. This is an area that will likely become more important as the limitations of dealing with the cognitive–motivational components are clarified and reached.

Dworkin et al (1992a) presented a theoretical, biobehavioural model designed to show the importance of epidemiological concepts for understanding chronic pain. Cognitive concepts are given a prominent place in the model. The authors argue that no single dimension is adequate to understand chronic pain. Proper understanding requires examination of pain over time as well as the interaction of biological, psychological and social factors. Chronic pain involves both extrinsic and intrinsic factors. There is a dynamic interaction of nociception, pain perception, pain appraisal and behavioural responses to pain (intrinsic), as well as social contexts of family, workplace and the health care system (extrinsic). Chronic pain can be dysfunctionally minimized (e.g. excessive stoicism) or maximized (e.g. catastrophizing). These processes are in a dynamic flux. Working with chronic pain patients requires taking the various elements into account. The theory is not in conflict with gate control. It, too, fills in areas not specified in gate control.

Differences between chronic and acute pain have been emphasized by Melzack & Dennis (1978) and Melzack (1986). With acute pain, there is usually a well-defined cause and a characteristic time course in which the pain disappears after healing. However, with chronic pain, the pain may continue even after healing has occurred. Melzack & Dennis (1978) note that, after lesions of the peripheral or central nervous system (CNS), prolonged bursting activity occurs that can be modulated by somatic, visceral and autonomic inputs as well as by inputs from emotional and personality mechanisms by means of the activation of descending inhibitory input. Memories of previous pain experiences at spinal or supraspinal levels can also trigger abnormal firing patterns. In the absence of clear, detectable lesions, it would be easy to diagnose such an individual as a person with hysterical-like pain. Once the pain is under way, central processes are of prime importance. The role of neuromas, nerve injury or other physical damage becomes less important. What is needed is therapy to affect the pattern-generating mechanisms in the CNS.

The dimensions of pain as seen in gate control have been reflected in the development of the McGill Pain Questionnaire (MPQ) (Melzack & Torgerson 1971; Melzack 1975). They have also been used as the conceptual model around which cognitive-behavioural interventions have been structured (Turk et al 1983; Turk & Rudy 1986). The MPQ groups pain descriptors into three main classes reflecting the underlying dimensions of pain:

1. Sensory words that describe pain in terms of temporal, spatial, pressure, thermal and other properties
2. Affective words that describe the pain in terms of tension, fear and autonomic properties
3. Evaluative words that describe the intensity of the total pain experience.

The study of Hackett & Horan (1980) can be used as an illustration of how these dimensions have been used by the cognitive approach. Hackett & Horan used the three dimensions (sensory, affective, evaluative) to conceptualize the active ingredients in a coping-skills approach to pain control. Against the sensory–discriminative dimension of pain, relaxation training was taught. To counteract the motivational–affective dimension of pain in which anxiety and helplessness were seen as critical, simple distraction such as mental arithmetic, focusing on painful bodily sensations, changing the context of pain via imagery and in vivo emotive imagery were used. Emotive imagery relies on classes of images that produce feelings of pride, self-assertion etc. Against the cognitive evaluative dimension, subjects were provided with self-instructional training (Meichenbaum 1977, 1985) consisting of coping statements. Subjects were taught self-talk for four stages of stimulus presentation:

1. Preparing for the stressor
2. Confronting the pain
3. Dealing with feelings at critical moments
4. Self-reinforcement for having successfully coped.

Each of the coping skills related to the three pain dimensions was provided separately or in various combinations in nine different groups. A total of 81 female subjects were tested using cold-pressor pain. Results indicated that relaxation training produced an increased pain tolerance, while the distraction and imagery training resulted in a higher threshold score. Self-statements did not result in any significant effect and in fact reduced the effectiveness of distraction and imagery use. The failure of the self-statement group may have been due to its lack of subject acceptance or outcome expectancies as a method to reduce pain.

Attentional processes have been postulated as playing a key role in the effectiveness of cognitive coping strategies (Fernandez & Turk 1989). As postulated by gate control, Fernandez & Turk view attentional processes as possibly being accompanied by descending cortical influences that inhibit transmission of pain signals.

RESEARCH SUPPORT

Much of the earlier work on the use of cognitive techniques was designed to identify the basic strategies (Weisenberg 1984, 1989). The basic coping techniques have been catagorized. Tan (1982) used six basic descriptive categories that include:

1. Imaginative inattention whereby the subject is to ignore the pain by use of incompatible imagery, e.g. enjoying a pleasant day at the beach.

2. Imaginative transformation of pain requires the subject to interpret what he is feeling as something other than pain.

3. Imaginative transformation of context requires the person to change the context of the stimulation, e.g. being chased by enemy agents.

4. Attention–diversion (external) asks the person to focus on physical characteristics of the environment, e.g. counting ceiling tiles.

5. Attention–diversion (internal) requires the subject to use self-generated thoughts, e.g. doing mental arithmetic.

6. Somatization requires the person to focus upon the part of the body being stimulated in a detached manner.

On the basis of multidimensional scaling, Wack & Turk (1984) classified the basic variety of coping strategies into 10 groups. Subsequently Fernandez & Turk (1989) used a six-category classification to examine study outcomes via meta-analysis. The six groups included:

1. External focus of attention such as slides of landscapes
2. Neutral imagery, i.e. imagery that was neither pleasant or unpleasant
3. Dramatized coping involving reconstructing the context of the nociception such as a football game
4. Rhythmic cognitive activity which refers to cognitive activity of a repetitive or systematized nature such as counting backwards from 100 by threes
5. Pain acknowledging, involving a reappraisal of the nociception in terms of objective sensations
6. Pleasant imagery, such as imagining oneself sitting comfortably and listening to music.

The meta-analysis, based on 51 studies, showed a significant advantage to the cognitive strategies as compared to the control groups or to placebo expectancy groups. No significant differences were obtained for the relative advantage of one strategy over the other. However, it seems that imagery strategies were most effective, while the repetitive cognitions or acknowledgement of sensations were least effective.

The accumulated studies of the cognitive control of pain demonstrate that changing how a person thinks about the pain stimulus and attends to it can lead to an increase in pain tolerance. Several points would be worth noting. Choosing a specific strategy must fit the context and the person (Weisenberg 1984, 1989). What is acceptable and relaxing to one person may be aversive to another. It is also important to realize that motivational processes can be a vital key to determining the effectiveness of a given strategy and the willingness of a person to use it. Cognitive strategies have not always been effective with stimuli to which the person has had prior exposure before learning the strategy (Berntzen 1987) nor does generalization from one situation to another necessarily occur (Hackett et al 1979; Klepac et al 1981). When using distraction, the more the distraction can gain a person's attention, the more effective it is (McCaul & Malott 1984). Distraction was found to be more effective for stimuli of low intensity while sensation redefinition was more effective for intense pain. Several studies also have shown that specifying a given time limit for the pain ('tolerate this for 15 minutes', as opposed to 'last as long as you can') has increased the pain tolerance and the effectiveness of the cognitive strategies (Williams & Thorn 1986; Thorn & Williams 1989).

PERCEIVED CONTROL

Control as a variable has been shown to be important in clinical and laboratory settings for both acute and chronic pain (Thompson 1981; Chapman & Turner 1986). Attribution of control to internal rather than to external factors has become a key factor in the clinical treatment of pain, especially for chronic pain (Jensen et al 1991a). Patients with chronic pain often exhibit learned helplessness as a result of their disability which tends to become reinforced by frequent medication and dependency on others. Patients, therefore, are taught self-regulation rather than drug regulation for dealing with their problems as part of a comprehensive treatment programme (McArthur et al 1987). Several studies have shown that an internal locus of control was associated with better coping with pain while a chance, external orientation to control of pain was associated with maladaptive coping (Crisson & Keefe 1988; Harkapaa et al 1991). The locus of control measure assesses the individual's perception that things are under a person's control (not that the person giving the rating necessarily can exert that control) rather than due to chance or luck. Spinhoven & Linssen (1991), reporting on their low-back pain sample, suggested that at 6-month follow-up after treatment, the perception of control may be more important for pain reduction than the specific coping strategy used. In a recent study, Elliot (1992) reported that perceived ineffective personal control, a measure that reflects the extent to which the individual can regulate emotional reactions during problem-solving, was associated with higher levels of premenstrual and menstrual pain. Jensen & Karoly (1991), in a study of chronic pain patients, found that patients' belief in control over pain, as well as the cognitive strategies used, were related to well-being and to activity level. In some instances this was valid only for a low level of pain severity. Affleck et al (1987) reported that patients' perceived control over the course of treatment for rheumatoid arthritis was associated with positive mood and global adjustment.

After Keeri-Szanto (1979) first described the technique of patient-controlled analgesia (PCA), it became a standard procedure in many clinical settings. It started as a means of avoiding many of the negative aspects of pain–drug administration. The prescription must be written, the nurse must be convinced that the patient is 'really' in pain, and the drug must be signed out of the locked cabinet. The time it takes for the drug to be absorbed after injection must also be included. By the time the patient begins to feel the effect of the medication, the pain level for which relief was originally requested has intensified. By contrast, with PCA, the drug is received immediately, few patients have abused the drug and the overall level of drug use may be less with at least the same level of drug effectiveness (Hill et al 1990), an effect that may be attributed to patients' enhanced sence of control.

A substantial number of studies have been performed to assess the use of PCA. The general conclusion is that it is safe, efficient, does not always lead to better levels of pain control but is often preferred by patients. Some of the areas for which PCA has been used successfully include postoperative pain (Hecker & Albert 1988), bone marrow transplantation (Hill et al 1986, 1990), cancer patients (Bruera et al 1991), gynaecological procedures (Johnson et al 1989) and shock wave lithotripsy of gallstones (Schelling et al 1992). Recent research has focused on patient characteristics such as locus of control status (Johnson et al 1989) or whether the patient has a previous history of chronic pain, in which case PCA is less effective (Magnani et al 1989). PCA effectiveness also has been assessed in terms of the type of PCA instrument (Hecker & Albert 1988) or the drug used. Hill et al (1992), for example, found that morphine has three times the potency of alfentanil when used in PCA.

Numerous laboratory studies have indicated that providing subjects with some degree of control over pain stimulation can reduce stress and increase pain tolerance (Weisenberg 1984,1989). Several researchers have tried to relate the positive effects of control to predictability (Staub et al 1971). Uncertainty increases anxiety and results in less pain tolerance, while reduction of uncertainty increases tolerance. However, control and predictability can be separated from each other (Miller 1981). Controllability refers to what the person can do about the event. Control can refer to changing the aversive stimulus itself or to changing one's response to it. The expectation of control can lead to improved performance even under conditions of learned helplessness (Mikulincer 1986).

When predictability is kept constant, Miller (1980) has suggested the minimax hypothesis to account for the effects of perceived control. This hypothesis views control as based upon an internal, stable attribution, e.g. the person's own response. When the situation is not controllable by the person himself, external attributions must be considered, e.g. the experimenter, chance, etc. The external factor may or may not be able to guarantee the low maximum level of aversiveness the person would be willing to have. Miller has suggested, with some empirical support, that an individual would be willing to hand over control to someone else when the person doubts his own ability to perform a given action in dealing with a threat, when the action to reduce the threat is unclear or when the person perceives another to have more skill or expertise in dealing with the threat. Weisenberg et al (1985), in a laboratory study, found unexpectedly that a condition in which the experimenter exerted control yielded the lowest pain reaction among subjects with high perceived self-efficacy for pain control, but a high pain reaction in subjects with low perceived self-efficacy for pain control. These results raise questions for the clinical situation. When would giving control to a competent other person reduce or increase distress? In the clinic, for a person who perceives himself as lacking control, does giving control to a health care provider make him feel more out of control? These questions have not yet been answered.

In terms of predictability, Matthews et al (1980), after reviewing the literature, concluded that for every study that reports positive outcomes for predictability, there is a conflicting report showing no effect or a negative effect. They conclude that the only thing to be said about the effects of predictability 'is that they are unpredictable'. Abbott et al (1984) and Abbott & Badia (1986) conclude that unpredictable shocks are physiologically more stressful than predictable shocks when there are firstly, one or only a few sessions and secondly, the stress is severe. However, when the experiment is conducted over several days and the stress is less severe, predictable shocks can be more stressful than unpredictable shocks. It is possible that this may be due to the greater habituation that occurs when shock is unpredictable because of the need to be on guard for a longer time – chronic physiological arousal. With the predictable shocks, the subject can relax between stressors and as a consequence adapt more gradually.

Predictability is usually achieved by means of a warning signal. One issue that arises is the time gap between the warning and stimulation. In a laboratory study using electric shock (a quick, sharp, short-acting stimulus), Mittwoch et al (1990) reported that a warning signal of 5 or 30 seconds was less aversive than one of 60 or 180 seconds. With a longer-acting, repeated stimulus such as cold-pressor pain, Weisenberg et al (1992) found that the longer 180-second interval was less aversive. It seems that subjects prefer having the extra time to recover from the previous stimulus.

The accuracy of prediction of pain intensity can influence subsequent behaviour of the person. Rachman & Lopatka (1988) examined the predicted pain of chronic arthritis patients while they performed a series of physiotherapy exercises. After overpredictions of pain, the next assessment of predicted pain was lower, while after underpredictions of pain the predicted assessment of anticipated pain was raised. The match–mismatch approach could affect subsequent escape and avoidance behaviour as seen in cases of fear. In a series of laboratory studies, Arntz et al (1991) examined the effects of match–mismatch of shock intensity. Subjects were provided with a cue to signal the intensity of the subsequent shock level. For several of the trials the cue either under- or overestimated the shock intensity. The largest effect on pain response and on anticipatory responses was obtained for the underestimation. These subjects did not differ on the pain ratings, but showed a slower physiological recovery. In addition, the anticipated pain level and fear level were also higher for the upcoming shock. Examining the discrepancies between expectations of dental patients to anticipated treatments and the treatments themselves, Arntz et al (1990) found that, unlike the laboratory, simple over- or underprediction of pain did not lead to decreased or increased fear. Instead the more trait-like rating of anxiety was more relevant. Anxious dental patients expected more pain and anxiety than they actually experienced and needed more experiences before their predictions became accurate. The data indicate the importance of dealing with anxiety and helping the patient disconfirm his expectations of treatment. Dentist credibility should play a key role as will be seen in studies of preparation for treatment.

STRESS-INOCULATION THERAPY

The past 6 years were characterized by more clinical than laboratory studies in assessing the application of cognitive–behavioural treatment of pain. Earlier work had shown the effectiveness of stress-inoculation therapy for pain. It has been applied successfully to such areas as pain in adult burn patients (Wernick et al 1981) as well as burn pain in children aged 5–12 (Elliott & Olson 1983), preparation for surgery (Wells et al 1986; Zastowny et al 1986), headaches (McGrath 1987; Newton & Barbaree 1987) and chronic pelvic pain (Kames et al 1990).

The effectiveness of stress-inoculation often requires the presence of the therapist (Elliott & Olson 1983; Hayes & Wolf 1984). Another important point demonstrated by D'Eon & Perry (1984) is that the type of coping strategy was less important than providing the subjects with the choice of strategy.

As previously mentioned, stress-inoculation involves three basic phases of treatment (Meichenbaum 1985): the educational reconceptualization of pain, acquisition of skills and practice of what is taught. The coping strategies often include such things as relaxation, deep breathing, use of pleasant images, use of positive self-statements and self-reinforcement for having coped. In general, it appears that stress-inoculation training can be beneficial in tolerating the stress of pain. However, as with other cognitive procedures it is still not clear exactly what the critical ingredients are and which of them are absolutely essential (Horan et al 1977; Vallis 1984; Moses & Holandsworth 1985).

RELAXATION

One of the prominent coping strategies used in cognitive treatment is relaxation. Quite a few studies have been done to show the impact of relaxation in and of itself on cognition and pain. Peveler & Johnston (1986), in a laboratory study, reported that relaxation affected overall arousal and also reduced negative cognitions. Relaxation produced by mindfulness meditation is said to produce an attentional stance of detached observation by which the sensory component is detached from the affective and evaluative components of pain. In a 4-year follow-up of 225 chronic pain patients who were taught mindfulness meditation, Kabat-Zinn et al (1987) found that 60–72% of patients reported moderate or great improvement in their pain status despite the fact that the pain rating index tended to revert to preintervention levels.

Philips (1988) reported that a group of chronic pain patients who were taught progressive relaxation, compared to a similar group of patients not so taught, rated significant reductions of their pain on both their sensory and affective experience. The overall intensity of pain also was reduced.

The successful treatment of headache pain has been obtained using only relaxation procedures. Richter et al (1986) compared relaxation training, cognitive coping involving restructuring of dysfunctional thoughts and a placebo control condition. Compared to the placebo control, both interventions were equally successful in reducing overall headache activity even at the 16-week follow-up. In a series of 6-weekly sessions of relaxation training of ulcerative colitis patients, Shaw & Ehrlich (1987) found that, compared to an attention control condition, there was a reduction in pain and distress ratings as well as less drug use. Tobin et al (1988) compared relaxation alone and relaxation plus cognitive–behavioural therapy for headache treatment. The cognitive intervention included stress management skills such as problem-solving and cognitive restructuring. The average reduction in the headache index for the relaxation group was 36% but it was 76% for the combined treatment. The researchers suggest that the cognitive–behavioural intervention is especially helpful for patients who report a high pretreatment headache level and for patients with high daily stress.

PREVENTION

One important area that has begun to receive attention is the prediction and prevention of acute pain from becoming chronic. Philips et al (1991) studied 117 acute, back pain patients and followed them for 6 months. The patients that still had pain reported more negative cognitive reactions to pain, higher anxiety and a greater impact of the pain on their everyday life. The researchers found that they were able to predict which patients would have difficulty with pain 6 months later. Dworkin et al (1992b), in their 12-month study of acuted herpes zoster, found that disease conviction, pain intensity and state anxiety were able to predict the development of chronic herpes zoster pain.

Linton et al (1989) designed an intervention programme for a group of nurses who suffered from back pain. The 5-week programme consisted of physical therapy and cognitive–behavioural therapy that included relaxation as well as other coping methods. Subjects were followed for 6 months. Compared to control group, the treated group showed improvement in pain control, sleep and fatigue ratings, observed pain behaviour, activities and helplessness. The study is an example of what a potential intervention might be, using cognitive–behavioural techniques to prevent an acute situation from becoming chronic. Practical widespread application of such a programme would require that it be made cheaper, as the investment required in the above illustration appeared to be quite high.

PREPARATION FOR TREATMENT

Many studies have been conducted dealing with the effects of preparing patients for stressful medical or dental procedures. Reviews of the literature almost uniformly point to the benefits of prior preparation (Reading 1979; Kendall & Watson 1981, Mumford et al 1982; Melamed 1984; Guggenheim 1986; Auerbach 1989). Although it is not always clear which ingredients are most important, some of the most recent studies have begun to test more specific components and their effects. Studies of repeated surgeries are also beginning to appear.

As is true with many other clinical studies, it is not always clear what is being manipulated: information, cognitive skills or other coping skills. Often there is a combined approach that is tested. Control groups remain problematic. Many times what is compared is the 'usual' routine that remains unspecified. Process variables are still quite difficult to measure (Auerbach 1989); that is, if a specific coping skill is said to be taught, to what extent was it really taught and to what extent was it actually used?

The early work of Janis (1958) emphasized an optimal relationship between the amount of suffering expected and the amount obtained which seems conducive to inoculation and a feeling of mastery of a difficult situation and to speed of recovery. The optimal degree of worry or anxiety prior to stressful surgery is best reached when the patient receives realistic information and is able to listen to and accept what is being told to him. This occurs when the patient experiences a moderate level of anxiety. The credibility of the practitioner is enhanced and the patient is helped to prepare for the event. Without the 'work of worrying', there is little anticipatory fear. When the inevitable postsurgical pain is experienced, the patient feels victimized.

The emphasis of Janis on fear and a moderate anxiety level has not always received support (Melamed 1984). Wilson (1981) found that surgical patients who claimed that they used high levels of denial actually required less analgesia and left the hospital earlier. Cohen & Lazarus (1973) have emphasized the importance of coping strategies in dealing with the stress of surgery. When the outcome of surgery was likely to be successful, they reported the best results with an avoidance strategy.

Although the exact relationship of presurgical anxiety and outcome still remains unclear, there is enough evidence to point to the importance of considering anxiety, especially trait-anxiety status, when preparing for surgery. Thus, it would be appropriate to use any strategies that are usually successful in dealing with elevated anxiety (Johnston 1986). Jamison et al (1987) studied 50 women undergoing elective laparoscopic surgery as ambulatory patients. They found that presurgical fear and anxiety was predictive of later postoperative complications. Boeke et al (1991), in a study of 111 patients with gallstones, found that preoperative anxiety did not predict postoperative pain, but did predict length of hospitalization. Taenzer et al (1986) in a study of 40 gallbladder patients, found that trait anxiety and neuroticism were the most important factors that predicted postsurgical pain levels. Situational anxiety, measured the night before surgery, was not predictive of postsurgical pain level. Thus, it appears that although there is little support for a curvilinear relationship of anxiety and surgical outcome, there is support for the importance of presurgical anxiety in determining postsurgical outcomes. It is not always clear, however, whether situational anxiety is as important as trait anxiety.

Although a period of advance notice with prior information and coping techniques does help patients, it is not always clear as to the amount of detail, the temporal spacing of information and how the personality of the subject affect the outcome (Andrew 1970; DeLong 1970; Melamed 1984). Copers (those who attempt to deal with stress) and those called nonspecific defenders (those who use both coping and avoiding strategies) seem to be able to accept more detailed information than avoiders (those who try to deny or avoid dealing with stress) (DeLong 1970). Similarly, Miller (1988) reported that gynaecological patients who are monitors (those who use an active coping style) do better with a high level of information as opposed to blunters (those who use a passive, distancing coping style) who do better with less information. Gattuso et al (1992) also reported that monitors did worst with endoscopy when provided with little information while blunters did most poorly when provided with procedural information. Scott & Clum (1984) concluded that avoiders might be better off without any information.

Faust & Melamed (1984) compared groups of children who were to have surgery the same day or the following day. Older children were able to retain more of the information provided. The preparation resulted in less physiological arousal for children who were to be operated on the next day, but greater arousal for children to be operated on the same day. Same-day patients may be better off with a distraction-type of preparation (Fowler-Kerry & Lander 1987). Faust et al (1991), however, found that children (aged 4–10) prepared for the same-day surgery showed lower arousal than the control condition. They compared participant modelling (in which a filmed model asked them to practise coping skills) with or without the presence of the mother, and a control that received the standard hospital preparation (tell–show–do in which the children could manipulate the operating room equipment). The most successful condition was the participant modelling without the presence of the mother and the least successful condition was the standard hospital preparation.

The effects of prior information, however, are not always consistent. Dworkin et al (1984) compared subjects who were provided with high or low levels of information on how nitrous oxide works to increase analgesia. Subjects were given tooth-pulp stimulation along with nitrous oxide. High- as compared to low-information subjects yielded higher sensation and pain tolerance thresholds. Wallace (1985), on the other hand, found that if the preparation leads to a greater expectation of pain, there is a more intense report of pain postsurgery. Scott et al (1983) reported that without any specific kind of preparation, higher levels of information were associated with higher levels of pain and more analgesics taken. Twardosz et al (1986) reported that when a videotape is used to prepare patients, the addition of the personal contact of a nurse increased the effectiveness of the preparation for surgery.

Information regarding sensations to be experienced seems to be more effective than information regarding the procedures to be used (Johnson 1973; Johnson &

Leventhal 1974). For example, Johnson et al (1975), in a study of cast removal, found that children exposed to a brief tape-recording, which included the sound of the saw and a description of the sensations of heat and flying chalk, showed less distress and resistance to the procedure compared with a group who were only told of the procedure or not told at all. However, the results are not clearcut. Positive results were obtained for cholecystectomy but not for herniorrhaphy patients (Johnson et al 1978). The results of the intervention, therefore, remain somewhat unclear.

Litt et al (1992a), in a study of oral surgery patients undergoing third molar extractions, used a dismantling design to test the relative contributions of the addition of cognitive elements to the preparation. The cognitive elements included information and cue exposure, decreased arousal, self-control attributions and enhanced self-efficacy. Four treatment groups were created into which patients were randomly assigned. Each treatment group added another of the four cognitive elements. The groups were:

1. Standard treatment (providing information, cue exposure)
2. Oral premedication (information, cue exposure, decreased arousal)
3. Relaxation only (information, cue exposure, decreased arousal, self-control attributions)
4. Relaxation plus self-efficacy (information, cue exposure, decreased arousal, self-control attributions, enhanced self-efficacy).

The information and cue exposure were given to the patient by the dentist 1–4 weeks before surgery while the other manipulations took place about $1\frac{1}{2}$ hours before surgery. The results indicated that the relaxation and the relaxation plus self-efficacy groups showed less distress than the other groups. The least distress was obtained for the relaxation plus self-efficacy group.

In a follow-up oral surgery study, Litt et al (1992b) tested the effects of self-efficacy enhancement as a function of dispositional style. Overall, they replicated their previous findings in that the relaxation plus self-efficacy enhancement yielded the lowest distress. However, they found that high blunters did best with the standard surgical preparation. They concluded that providing patients with a sense of control and raising their self-efficacy or confidence is effective in preparing patients for oral surgery. However, patients whose dispositional style involves distraction or ignoring of threat, may benefit more from noninvolving interventions.

In one of the few studies of multiple surgeries, Croog et al (1992) prepared patients for two periodontal surgeries. The positive affect enhancement (PAE) intervention was designed to stress positive feelings and benefits as an outcome of the surgery. The self-efficacy enhancement (SEE) intervention was designed to present information to promote the patient's sense of control of the sequelae of the periodontal surgery. A third group combined the two interventions (PAA-SEE). The control condition presented to patients a review of oral hygiene and dental care. The results indicated that after surgery I the SEE group tended to yield lower pain scores. The superiority of the SEE group became stronger after surgery II in comparison to the control group and even in comparison to the combined PAE-SEE group in terms of pain reduction. This result takes on added importance in that, by contrast to the laboratory studies that have shown a tendency for cognitive techniques to be less effective with repeated stimuli, the emphasis on self-efficacy and self-control in this study showed stronger results with the repeated surgery.

An added point to note before concluding this section concerns the preparation of children. Wolfer & Visitainer (1975), Melamed (1984) and Fradet et al (1990) underscore the importance of age differences among children. Children aged 3–6 compared to those aged 7–14 showed greater upset behaviour. The patient's age should also be considered in terms of the timing of the preparation. Less time in advance is desirable for younger children. Reducing parental feelings of anxiety has also been found to have a positive effect on the child patient.

CONCLUDING COMMENT

There is little doubt that the cognitive approach has become part of the standardized approach to treating pain. The results of many studies have demonstrated that the various cognitive techniques are effective in reducing the reactions to pain. Most often, however, these techniques are applied as part of a comprehensive programme in which the cognitive approach is only one ingredient in the treatment. Such multidisciplinary programmes have been shown to be beneficial as inpatient, outpatient or home-management treatments (Peters & Large 1990; Maruta et al 1990, Cott et al 1990; Kames et al 1990; Flor et al 1992). At times the success of treatment is likely to be indirect, as a consequence of the treatment of depression or some other emotional concomitant of the pain. What appears to be quite clear is the need to consider the motivational issues as an integral part of treatment. That is, more important than the effectiveness of one technique over the other, is the perception on the part of the patient that he is capable of carrying out the tasks required of him and that this will control the pain effectively. In general, as Turk & Rudy (1990, 1991) have indicated, it is necessary to take into account motivational factors when treating pain. This is also appropriate in the use of cognitive techniques. However, whatever the shortcomings, there is little doubt that cognitive aspects of pain are significant in pain perception and control.

REFERENCES

Abbott B B, Badia P 1986 Predictable versus unpredictable shock conditions and physiological measures of stress: a reply to Arthur. Psychological Bulletin 100: 384–387

Abbott B B, Schoen L S, Badia P 1984 Predictable and unpredictable shock: behavioral measures of aversion and physiological measures of stress. Psychological Bulletin 96: 45–71

Affleck G, Tennen H, Pfeiffer C, Fifield J 1987 Appraisals of control and predictability in adapting to a chronic disease. Journal of Personality and Social Psychology 53: 273–279

Algom D 1992 Psychophysical analysis of pain: a functional perspective. In: Geissler H G, Link S W, Townsend J T (eds) Cognition, information processing, and psychophysics: basic issues. Erlbaum, Hillsdale, New Jersey, p 267

Andrew J M 1970 Recovery from surgery with and without preparatory instruction for three coping styles. Journal of Personality and Social Psychology 15: 223–226

Arntz A, vanEck M, Heijmans M 1990 Predictions of dental pain: the fear of any expected evil is worse than the evil itself. Behaviour Research and Therapy 28: 29–41

Arntz A, Vandenhout M A, Vandenberg G, Meijboom A 1991 The effects of incorrect pain expectations on acquired fear and pain responses. Behaviour Research and Therapy 29: 547–560

Auerbach S M 1989 Stress management and coping research in the health care setting: an overview and methodological commentary. Journal of Consulting and Clinical Psychology 57: 388–395

Bandura A 1977 Self-efficacy: toward a unifying theory of behavioral change. Psychological Review 84: 191–215

Bandura A 1984 Recycling misconceptions of perceived self-efficacy. Cognitive Therapy and Research 8: 231–255

Bandura A 1989 Human agency in social cognitive theory. American Psychologist 44: 1175–1184

Bandura A, O'Leary A, Taylor C B, Gauthier J, Gossard D 1987 Perceived self-efficacy and pain control: opioid and nonopioid mechanisms. Journal of Personality and Social Psychology 53: 563–571

Bandura A, Cioffi D, Taylor C B, Brouillard H E 1988 Perceived self-efficacy in coping with cognitive stressors and opioid activation. Journal of Personality and Social Psychology 55: 479–488

Beck A T, Rush A J, Shaw B F, Emory G 1979 Cognitive therapy of depression. Guilford Press, New York

Beck A T, Emory G, Greenberg R L 1985 Anxiety disorders and phobia. Basic Books, New York

Beck A T, Freeman A and Associates 1990 Cognitive therapy of personality disorders. Guilford Press, New York

Berntzen D 1987 Effects of multiple cognitive coping strategies on laboratory pain. Cognitive Therapy and Research 11: 613–623

Boeke S, Duivenvoorden H J, Verhage F, Zwaveling A 1991 Prediction of postoperative pain and duration of hospitalization using two anxiety measures. Pain 45: 293–297

Brown G K, Nicassio P M 1987 Development of a questionnaire for the assessment of active and passive coping strategies in chronic pain patients. Pain 31: 53–64

Bruera E, MacMillan K, Hanson J, MacDonald R N 1991 The Edmonton injector: a simple device for patient-controlled subcutaneous analgesia. Pain 44: 167–169

Chapman C R, Turner J A 1986 Psychological control of acute pain in medical settings. Journal of Pain and Symptom Management 1: 9–20

Cohen F, Lazarus R S 1973 Active coping process, coping dispositions and recovery from surgery. Psychosomatic Medicine 35: 375–389

Cott A, Anchel H, Goldenberg W M, Fabich M, Parkinson W 1990 Non-institutional treatment of chronic pain by field management: an outcome study with comparison group. Pain 40: 183–194

Council J R, Ahern D K, Follick M J, Kline C L 1988 Expectancies and functional impairment in chronic low back pain. Pain 33: 323–331

Crisson J E, Keefe F J 1988 The relationship of locus of control to pain coping strategies and psychological distress in chronic pain patients. Pain 35: 147–154

Croog S H, Baume R, Nalbandian J 1992 Psychological preparation for surgery: self-efficacy and positive affect enhancement. Unpublished manuscript, University of Connecticut Health Center, Farmington, Connecticut

DeLong R D 1970 Individual differences in patterns of anxiety arousal, stress-relevant information and recovery from surgery. Unpublished doctoral dissertation, University of California, Los Angeles, California

D'Eon J L, Perry C W 1984 The role of imagery and coping cognitions in response to pressure pain as moderated by choice of pain control strategy. Paper presented at the annual meeting of the American Psychological Association, Toronto, Canada

Dolce J J, Doleys D M, Raczynski J M, Lossie J, Poole L, Smith M 1986a The role of self-efficacy expectancies in the prediction of pain tolerance. Pain 27: 261–272

Dolce J J, Crocker M F, Moletteire C, Doleys D M 1986b Exercise quotas, anticipatory concern and self-efficacy expectancies in chronic pain: a preliminary report. Pain 24: 365–372

Dworkin S F, Chen A C N, Schubert M M, Clark D W 1984 Cognitive modification of pain: information in combination with NO_2. Pain 19: 339–351

Dworkin S F, von Korff M R, LeResche L 1992a Epidemiologic studies of chronic pain: a dynamic-ecologic perspective. Annals of Behavioral Medicine 14: 3–11

Dworkin R H, Hartstein G, Rosner H L, Walther R R, Sweeney E W, Brand L 1992b A high-risk method for studying psychosocial antecedents of chronic pain: the prospective investigation of herpes zoster. Journal of Abnormal Psychology 101: 200–205

D'Zurilla T J, Goldfried M R 1971 Problem-solving and behavior modification. Journal of Abnormal Psychology 78: 107–126

Elliott C H, Olson R A 1983 The management of children's distress in response to painful medical treatment for burn injuries. Behaviour Research and Therapy 21: 675–683

Elliott T R 1992 Problem-solving appraisal, oral contraceptive use, and menstrual pain. Journal of Applied Social Psychology 22: 286–297

Ellis A 1962 Reason and emotion in psychotherapy. Lyle Stuart, New York

Faust J, Melamed B G 1984 Influence of arousal, previous experience, and age on surgery preparation of the same day of surgery and in-hospital pediatric patients. Journal of Consulting and Clinical Psychology 52: 359–365

Faust J, Olson R, Rodriguez H 1991 Same day surgery preparation: reduction of pediatric patient arousal and distress through participant modeling. Journal of Consulting and Clinical Psychology 59: 475–478

Fernandez E, Turk D C 1989 The utility of cognitive coping strategies for altering pain perception: a meta-analysis. Pain 38: 123–135

Flor H, Fydrich T, Turk D C 1992 Efficacy of multidisciplinary treatment centers: a meta-analytic review. Pain 49: 221–230

Folkman S, Lazarus R S, Gruen R J, DeLongis A 1986a Appraisal, coping, health status and psychological symptoms. Journal of Personality and Social Psychology 50: 571–579

Folkman S, Lazarus R S, Dunkel-Schetter C, DeLongis A, Gruen R J 1986b Dynamics of a stressful encounter: cognitive appraisal, coping, and encounter outcomes. Journal of Personality and Social Psychology 50: 992–1003

Forsythe C J, Compas B E 1987 Interaction of cognitive appraisals of stressful events and coping: testing the goodness of fit hypothesis. Cognitive Therapy and Research 11: 473–485

Fowler-Kerry S, Lander J R 1987 Management of injection pain in children. Pain 30: 169–175

Fradet C, McGrath P J, Kay J, Adams S, Luke B 1990 A prospective survey of reactions to blood tests by children and adolescents. Pain 40: 53–60

Freeman A, Pretzer J, Fleming B, Simon K M 1990 Clinical application of cognitive therapy. Plenum Press, New York

Gamsa A, Vikis-Freibergs V 1991 Psychological events are both risk factors in, and consequences of, chronic pain. Pain 44: 271–277

Gattuso S M, Litt M D, Fitzgerald T E 1992 Coping with gastrointestinal endoscopy: self-efficacy enchancement and coping style. Journal of Consulting and Clinical Psychology 60: 133–139

Gil K M, Williams D A, Keefe F J, Beckham J C 1990 The relationship of negative thoughts to pain and psychological distress. Behavior Therapy 21: 349–362

Guggenheim F G 1986 Psychological aspects of surgery. In: Wise T N (ed) Advances in psychosomatic medicine, volume 15. Karger, Basel

Hackett G, Horan J J 1980 Stress inoculation for pain: what's really going on? Journal of Counseling Psychology 27: 107–116

Hackett G, Horan J J, Buchanan J, Zumoff P 1979 Improving exposure generalization potential of stress inoculation for pain. Perceptual and Motor Skills 48:1132–1134

Harkapaa K, Jarvikoski A, Mellin G, Hurri H, Luoma J 1991 Health locus of control beliefs and psychological distress as predictors for treatment outcome in low-back pain patients: results of a three-month follow-up of a controlled intervention study. Pain 46: 35–41

Hayes S C, Wolf M R 1984 Cues, consequences and therapeutic talk: effects of social context and coping statements on pain. Behaviour Research and Therapy 22: 385–392

Hecker B R, Albert L 1988 Patient-controlled analgesia: a randomized, prospective comparison between two commercially available PCA pumps and conventional analgesic therapy for postoperative pain. Pain 35: 115–120

Heyneman N E, Fremouw W J, Gano D, Kirkland F, Heiden L 1990 Individual differences and the effectiveness of different coping strategies for pain. Cognitive Therapy and Research 14: 63–77

Hill H F, Saeger L C, Chapman C R 1986 Patient-controlled analgesia after bone marrow transplantation for cancer. Postgraduate Medicine: A Special Report August 28: 33–40

Hill H F, Chapman C R, Kornell J A, Sullivan KM, Saeger L C, Benedetti C 1990 Self-administration of morphine in bone marrow transplant patients reduces drug requirement. Pain 40: 121–129

Hill H F, Coda B A, Mackie A M, Iverson K 1992 Patient-controlled analgesic infusions: alfentanil versus morphine. Pain 49: 301–310

Holroyd K A, Penzien D B, Hursey K G et al 1984 Change mechanism in EMG biofeedback training. Journal of Consulting and Clinical Psychology 52: 1039–1053

Holroyd K A, Nash J M, Pingel J D, Cordingley G E, Jerome A 1991 A comparison of pharmacological (Amitriptyline HCL) and nonpharmacological (cognitive-behavioral) therapies for chronic tension headaches. Journal of Consulting and Clinical Psychology 59: 387–393

Horan J J, Hacket G, Buchanan J D, Stone I, Demchik-Stone D 1977 Coping with pain: a component analysis of stress inoculation. Cognitive Therapy and Research 1: 211–221

Ingram R E, Kendall P C 1986 Cognitive clinical psychology: implications of an information processing prospective. In: Ingram R E (ed) Information processing approaches to clinical psychology. Academic Press, New York, p 3

Jamison R N, Parris W C V, Maxson W S 1987 Psychological factors influencing recovery from outpatient surgery. Behaviour Research and Therapy 25: 31–37

Janis I 1958 Psychological stress. John Wiley, New York

Jays S M, Elliot C H, Woody P D, Siegel S 1991 An investigation of cognitive-behavior therapy combined with oral valium for children undergoing painful medical procedures. Health Psychology 10: 317–322

Jensen M P, Karoly P 1991 Control beliefs, coping efforts, and adjustment to chronic pain. Journal of Consulting and Clinical Psychology 59: 431–438

Jensen M P, Turner J A, Romano J M, Karoly P 1991a Coping with chronic pain: a critical review of the literature. Pain 47: 249–283

Jensen M P, Turner J A, Romano J M 1991b Self-efficacy and outcome expectancies: relationship to chronic pain coping strategies and adjustment. Pain 44: 263–269

Johnson J E 1973 Effects of accurate expectations about sensations of the sensory and distress components of pain. Journal of Personality and Social Psychology 27: 261–275

Johnson J E, Leventhal H 1974 Effects of accurate expectations and behavioral instructions on reactions during a noxious medical examination. Journal of Personality and Social Psychology 29: 710–718

Johnson J E, Kirchoff K T, Endress M P 1975 Deferring children's distress behavior during orthopaedic cast removal. Nursing Research 75: 404–410

Johnson J E, Fuller S S, Endress M P, Rice V H 1978 Altering patients' responses to surgery: an extension and replication. Research in Nursing and Health 1: 111–121

Johnston L R, Magnani B, Chan V, Ferrante F M 1989 Modifiers of patient-controlled analgesia efficacy. I. locus of control. Pain: 39: 17–22

Johnston M 1986 Preoperative emotional states and postoperative recovery. Advances in Psychosomatic Medicine 15: 1–22

Kabat-Zinn J, Lipworth L, Burney R, Sellers W 1987 Four-year follow-up of a meditation-based program for the self-regulation of chronic pain: treatment outcomes and compliance. The Clinical Journal of Pain 2: 159–173

Kames L D, Rapkin A J, Naliboff B D, Afifi S, Ferrer-Brechner T 1990 Effectiveness of an interdisciplinary pain management program for the treatment of chronic pelvic pain. Pain 41: 41–46

Keefe F J, Brown G K, Wallston A, Caldwell D S 1989 Coping with rheumatoid arthritis pain: catastrophizing as a maladaptive strategy. Pain 37: 51–56

Keefe F J, Crisson J, Urban B J, Williams D A 1990 Analyzing chronic low back pain: the relative contribution of pain coping strategies. Pain 40: 293–301

Keeri-Szanto M 1979 Drugs or drums: what relieves postoperative pain? Pain 6: 217–230

Kendall P C 1985 Cognitive processes and procedures. In: Wilson G T, Franks C M, Brownell K D, Kendall P C (eds) Annual review of behavior therapy: theory and practice, vol 10. Guilford Press, New York, p 123

Kendall P C 1992 Healthy thinking. Behavior Therapy 23: 1–11

Kendall P C, Watson D 1981 Psychological preparation for stressful medical procedures. In: Prokop C K, Bradley L A (eds) Medical psychology: contributions to behavioral medicine. Academic Press, New York, p 197

Kendall P C, Vitousek K B, Kane M 1991 Thought and action in psychotherapy: cognitive-behavioral approaches. In: Hersen M, Kazdin A E, Bellack A S (eds) The clinical psychology handbook. Pergamon Press, Elmsford, p 596

Klepac R K, Hauge G, Dowling J, McDonald M 1981 Direct and generalized effects of three components of stress inoculation for increased pain tolerance. Behavior Therapy 12: 417–424

Kores R C, Murphy W D, Rosenthal T L, Elias D B, North W C 1990 Predicting outcome of chronic pain treatment via a modified self-efficacy scale. Behaviour Research and Therapy 28: 165–169

Lavigne J V, Schulein M J, Hahn Y S 1986 Psychological aspects of painful medical conditions in children. I. Developmental aspects and assessment. Pain 27: 133–146

Lawson K, Reesor K A, Keefe F J, Turner J A 1990 Dimensions of pain-related cognitive coping: cross-validation of the factor structure of the Coping Strategy Questionnaire. Pain 43: 195–204

Lazarus R S, Folkman S 1984 Stress appraisal and coping. Springer, New York

Linton S J, Bradley L A, Jensen I, Spangfort E, Sundell L 1989 The secondary prevention of low back pain: a controlled study with follow-up. Pain 36: 197–207

Litt M 1988 Self-efficacy and perceived control: cognitive mediators of pain tolerance. Journal of Personality and Social Psychology 54: 149–160

Litt M D, Horswell B B, Nye C K, Shafer D M 1992a Perceptions of self-efficacy and control in coping with oral surgery. Unpublished manuscript, University of Connecticut School of Dental Medicine, Farmington, Connecticut

Litt M, Nye C, Shafer D 1992b Distraction from information in coping with oral surgery. Unpublished manuscript, University of Connecticut School of Dental Medicine, Farmington, Connecticut

McArthur D L, Cohen M J, Gottlieb H J, Naliboff B D, Schandler S L 1987 Treating chronic low back pain. I. Admission to initial follow-up. Pain 29: 1–22

McCaul K D, Malott J M 1984 Distraction and coping with pain. Psychological Bulletin 95: 516–533

McCracken L 1991 Cognitive-behavioral treatment of rheumatoid arthritis: a preliminary review of efficacy and methodology. Annals of Behavioral Medicine 13: 57–65

McGrath P A 1987 The multidimensional assessment and management of recurrent pain syndromes in children. Behaviour Research and Therapy 25: 251–262

McGrath P A 1990 Pain in children: nature, assessment, treatment. Guilford Press, New York

Magnani B, Johnson L R, Ferrante F 1989 Modifiers of patient-controlled analgesia efficacy. II. Chronic pain. Pain 39: 23–29

Malone M D, Strube M J 1988 Meta-analysis of non-medical treatments for chronic pain. Pain 34: 231–244

Maruta T, Swanson D W, McHardy M J 1990 Three-year follow-up of patients with chronic pain who were treated in a multidisciplinary pain management center. Pain 41: 47–53

Matthews K A, Scheier M F, Brynson B I, Carducci B 1980 Attention, unpredictability and reports of physical symptoms: eliminating the benefits of predictability. Journal of Personality and Social Psychology 38: 525–537

Meichenbaum D 1977 Cognitive behavior modification. Plenum Press, New York

Meichenbaum D 1985 Stress inoculation training. Pergamon Press, New York

Meichenbaum D, Turk D 1976 The cognitive-behavioral management of anxiety, anger, and pain. In: Davidson P O (ed) The behavioral management of anxiety, depression and pain. Brunner/Mazel, New York, p 1

Melamed B G 1984 Health intervention: collaboration for health and science. In: Hammonds B L, Scheirer C J (eds) Psychology and health: the master lecture series, vol 3. American Psychological Association, Washington, DC

Melzack R 1975 The McGill pain questionnaire: major properties and scoring methods. Pain 1: 277–299

Melzack R 1986 Neurophysiological foundations of pain. In: Sternbach R A (ed) The psychology of pain. Raven Press, New York, p 1

Melzack R, Dennis S G 1978 Neurophysiological foundations of pain. In: Sternbach R A (ed) The psychology of pain. Raven Press, New York, p 1

Melzack R, Torgerson W S 1971 On the language of pain. Anesthesiology 34: 50–59

Melzack R, Wall P D 1965 Pain mechanisms: a new theory. Science 150: 971–979

Mikulincer M, 1986 Attributional processes in the learned helplessness paradigm: the behavioral effect of globality attributions. Journal of Personality and Social Psychology 51: 1248–1256

Miller S M 1980 Why having control reduces stress: if I can stop the roller coaster, I don't want to get off. In: Garber J, Seligman M E P (eds) Human helplessness: theory and applications. Academic Press, New York, p 71

Miller S M 1981 Predictability and human stress: toward a clarification of evidence and theory. In Berkowitz L (ed) Advances in experimental social psychology, vol 14. Academic Press, New York, p 203

Miller S M 1988 The interacting effects of coping styles and situational variables in gynecologic settings: implications for research and treatment. Journal of Psychosomatic Obstetrics and Gynecology 9: 23–34

Mittwoch T, Weisenberg M, Mikulincer M 1990 The influence of warning signal timing and cognitive preparation on the aversiveness of electric shock. Pain 42: 373–381

Moses A N III, Holandsworth J G 1985 Relative effectiveness of education alone versus stress inoculation training in the treatment of dental phobia. Behavior Therapy 16: 531–537

Mumford E, Schlesinger H G, Glass G V 1982 The effects of psychological intervention on recovery from surgery and heart attacks: an analysis of the literature. American Journal of Public Health 72: 141–151

Newton C R, Barbaree H E 1987 Cognitive changes accompanying headache treatment: the use of a thought-sampling procedure. Cognitive Therapy and Research 11: 635–651

Nicholas M K, Wilson P H, Goyen J 1992 Comparison of cognitive-behavioral group treatment and an alternative non-psychological treatment for chronic low back pain. Pain 48: 339–347

Peters J L, Large R G 1990 A randomized control trial evaluating in- and outpatient pain management programmes. Pain 41: 283–293

Peveler R C, Johnston D W 1986 Subjective and cognitive effects of relaxation. Behaviour Research and Therapy 24: 413–419

Philips H C 1987a Avoidance behaviour and its role in sustaining chronic pain. Behaviour Research and Therapy 25: 273–279

Philips H C 1987b The effects of behavioral treatment on chronic pain. Behaviour Research and Therapy 25: 365–377

Philips H C 1988 Changing chronic pain experience. Pain 32: 165–172

Philips H C 1989 Thoughts provoked by pain. Behaviour Research and Therapy 27: 469–473

Philips H C, Grant L, Berkowitz J 1991 The prevention of chronic pain and disability: a preliminary investigation. Behaviour Research and Therapy 29: 443–450

Rachman S, Lopatka C 1988 Accurate and inaccurate predictions of pain. Behaviour Research and Therapy 26: 291–296

Reading A E 1979 The short-term effects of psychological preparations for surgery. Social Science and Medicine 13A: 641–654

Reesor K A, Craig K D 1988 Medically incongruent chronic back-pain: physical limitations, suffering and ineffective coping. Pain 32: 35–45

Richter I L, McGrath P J, Humphreys P J Goodman J T, Firestone P, Keene D 1986 Cognitive and relaxation treatment of paediatric migraine. Pain 25: 195–203

Rokke P D, Al Absi M 1993 Matching pain coping strategies to the individual: a prospective validation of the cognitive coping strategy inventory. Journal of Behavioral Medicine (in press)

Rosenstiel A K, Keefe F J 1983 The use of coping strategies in chronic low back pain patients: relationship to patient characteristics and current adjustment. Pain 17: 33–44

Roskies E, Lazarus R S 1980 Coping theory and the teaching of coping skills. In: Davidson P O, Davidson S M (eds) Behavioral medicine: changing health lifestyles. Brunner/Mazel, New York, p 38

Rudy T E, Kerns R D, Turk D C 1988 Chronic pain and depression: toward a cognitive behavioral mediation model. Pain 35: 129–140

Schelling G, Mendl G, Weber W et al 1992 Patient-controlled analgesia for extracorporeal shock wave lithotripsy of gallstones. Pain 48: 355–359

Scott L E, Clum G A 1984 Examining the interaction effects of coping style and brief interventions in the treatment of postsurgical pain. Pain 20: 279–291

Scott L E, Clum G A, Peoples J B 1983 Preoperative predictors of postoperative pain. Pain 15: 283–293

Shaw L, Ehrlich A 1987 Relaxation training as a treatment for chronic pain caused by ulcerative colitis. Pain 29: 287–293

Slater M A, Hall H F, Atkinson H, Garfin S R 1991 Pain and impairment beliefs in chronic low back pain: validation of the Pain and Impairment Relationship Scale (PAIRS). Pain 44: 51–56

Smith C A, Wallston K A 1992 Adaptation in patients with chronic rheumatoid arthritis: application of a general model. Health Psychology 11: 151–162

Smith T W, Follick M J, Ahern D K, Adams A 1986 Cognitive distortion and disability in chronic low back pain. Cognitive Therapy and Research 10: 201–210

Spence S H 1991 Cognitive-behavioural therapy in the treatment of chronic occupational pain of the upper limbs: a two-year follow-up. Behaviour Research and Therapy 29: 503–509

Spinhoven P, Linssen A C G 1991 Behavioral treatment of chronic low back pain. I. Relation of coping strategy use to outcome. Pain 45: 29–34

Staub E, Tursky B, Schwartz G E 1971 Self-control and predictability: their effects on reactions to aversive stimulation. Journal of Personality and Social Psychology 18: 157–162

Stedman's Medical Dictionary 1976, 23rd edn. Williams & Wilkins, Baltimore

Sternbach R A 1986 Pain and 'hassles' in the United States: findings of the Nuprin Pain Peport. Pain 27: 69–80

Syrjala, K L, Cummings C, Donaldson G W 1992 Hypnosis or cognitive behavioral training for the reduction of pain and nausea during cancer treatment: a controlled clinical trial. Pain 48: 137–146

Taenzer P, Melzack R, Jeans M E 1986 Influence of psychological factors on postoperative pain, mood, and analgesic requirements. Pain 24: 331–342

Tan S Y 1982 Cognitive and cognitive-behavioral methods for pain control: a selective review. Pain 12: 201–228

Thompson K L, Varni J W 1986 A developmental cognitive-biobehavioral approach to pediatric pain assessment. Pain 25: 283–296

Thompson S C 1981 Will it hurt less if I can control it? A complex answer to a simple question. Psychological Bulletin 90: 89–101

Thorn B E, Williams G A 1989 Goal specification alters perceived pain

intensity and tolerance latency. Cognitive Therapy and Research 13: 171–183
Tobin D L, Holroyd K A, Baker A, Reynolds R V C, Holm J E 1988 Development and clinical trial of a minimal contact, cognitive-behavioral treatment for tension headache. Cognitive Therapy and Research 12: 325–339
Turk D C 1978 Cognitive-behavioral techniques in the management of pain. In: Foreyt J P, Rathjen D P (eds) Cognitive behavior therapy: research and application. Plenum Press, New York, p 199
Turk D C, Fernandez E 1990 On the putative uniqueness of cancer pain: do psychological principles apply? Behavioural Research and Therapy 28: 1–13
Tuk D C, Flor H 1987 Pain > pain behaviors: the utility and limitations of the pain behavior construct. Pain 31: 277–295
Turk D C, Rudy T E 1986 Assessment of cognitive factors in chronic pain: a worthwhile enterprise? Journal of Consulting and Clinical Psychology 54: 760–768
Turk D C, Rudy T E 1990 Neglected factors in chronic pain treatment outcome studies–referral patterns, failure to enter treatment, and attrition. Pain 43: 7–25
Turk D C, Rudy T E 1991 Neglected topics in the treatment of chronic pain patients – relapse, noncompliance, and adherence enhancement. Pain 44: 5–28
Turk D C, Rudy T E 1992 Cognitive factors and persistent pain: a glimpse into Pandora's Box. Cognitive Therapy and Research 16: 99–122
Turk D C, Meichenbaum D, Genest M 1983 Pain and behavioral medicine: a cognitive-behavioral perspective. Guilford Press, New York
Turner J A, Clancy S 1986 Strategies for coping with chronic low back pain: relationships to pain and disability. Pain 24: 355–364
Twardosz S, Weddle K, Borden L, Stevens E 1986 A comparison of three methods of preparing children for surgery. Behavior Therapy 17: 14–25
Tyrer S P, Capon M, Peterson D M, Charlton J E, Thompson J W 1989 The detection of psychiatric illness and psychological handicaps in a British pain clinic population. Pain 36: 63–74
Vallis T M 1984 A component analysis of stress inoculation for pain tolerance. Cognitive Therapy and Research 8: 313–329
Vallis T M, Bucher B 1986 Self-efficacy as a predictor of behavior change: interaction with type of training for pain tolerance. Cognitive Therapy and Research 10: 79–94
Wack J T, Turk D C 1984 Latent structure of strategies used to cope with nociceptive stimulation. Health Psychology 3: 27–43
Wallace L M 1985 Surgical patients' expectations of pain and discomfort: does accuracy of expectations minimize postsurgical pain and distress? Pain 22: 363–373
Weisenberg M 1977 Pain and pain control. Psychological Bulletin 84: 1008–1044
Weisenberg M 1980 Understanding pain phenomena. In: Rachman S (ed) Contributions to medical psychology, vol 2. Pergamon Press, Oxford, p 79
Weisenberg M 1983 Pain and pain control. In: Daitzman R (ed) Diagnosis and intervention in behavior therapy and behavioral medicine. Springer, New York, p 90
Weisenberg M 1984 Cognitive aspects of pain. In: Wall P D, Melzack R (eds) Textbook of pain, 1st edn. Churchill Livingstone, Edinburgh, p 162
Weisenberg M 1987 Psychological intervention for the control of pain. Behaviour Research and Therapy 25: 301–312
Weisenberg M 1989 Cognitive aspects of pain. In: Wall P D, Melzack R (eds) Textbook of pain, 2nd edn. Churchill Livingston, Edinburgh, p 231
Weisenberg M, Wolf Y, Mittwoch T, Mikulincer M, Aviram O 1985 Subject versus experimenter control in the reaction to pain. Pain 23: 187–200
Weisenberg M, Tepper I, Mikulincer M 1992 The influence of warning signal timing and cognitive preparation on the aversiveness of cold-pressor pain. Unpublished manuscript, Bar-Ilan University, Ramat-Gan, Israel
Wells J K, Howard G S, Nowlin W F, Vargas M J 1986 Presurgical anxiety and postsurgical pain and adjustment: effects of a stress inoculation procedure. Journal of Consulting and Clinical Psychology 54: 831–835
Wernick R L, Jaremko M E, Taylor P W 1981 Pain management in severly burned adults: a test of stress inoculation. Journal of Behavioral Medicine 4: 103–109
Wiedenfeld S A, O'Leary A, Bandura A, Brown S, Levine S, Raska K 1990 Impact of perceived self-efficacy in coping with stressors on components of the immune system. Journal of Personality and Social Psychology 59: 1082–1094
Williams D A, Keefe F J 1991 Pain beliefs and the use of cognitive-behavioral coping strategies. Pain: 46: 185–190
Williams D A, Thorn B E 1986 Can research methodology affect treatment outcome? A comparison of two cold pressor test paradigms. Cognitive Therapy and Research 10: 539–545
Williams D A, Thorn B E 1989 An empirical assessment of pain beliefs. Pain 36: 351–358
Williams S L, Kinney P J 1991 Performance and nonperformance strategies for coping with acute pain: the role of perceived self-efficacy, expected outcomes and attention. Cognitive Therapy and Research 15: 1–19
Wilson J F 1981 Behavioral preparation for surgery: benefit or harm? Journal of Behavioral Medicine 4: 79–102
Wilson L, Massoth D, Dworkin S F et al 1992 Evaluation of an early cognitive–behavioral treatment for temporomandibular disorder pain. Paper presented at the annual meeting of the Society of Behavioral Medicine, New York
Wolfer J A, Visitainer M A 1975 Pediatric surgical patients' and parents' stress responses and adjustments. Nursing Research 24: 244–255
Zastowny T R, Kirschenbaum D S, Meng A L 1986 Coping skills training for children: effects on distress before, during and after hospitalization for surgery. Health Psychology 5: 231–247
Zautra A J, Manne S L 1992 Coping with rheumatoid arthritis: a review of a decade of research. Annals of Behavioral Medicine 14: 31–39

Measurement

15. Methods of assessing pain in animals

Ronald Dubner

This chapter will review methods of assessing pain in animals in which the goal of the studies is to explore the phenomenon of pain itself. A major purpose of such studies is to provide knowledge that can ultimately be applied to the management of acute and chronic pain conditions in humans and animals. Although scientists engaged in these studies feel morally justified in conducting such experiments in animals, there is a need to demonstrate a continuing responsibility in the proper treatment of the animals that participate in these experiments. The animals should be exposed to the minimal pain necessary to carry out the experiment (Dubner 1983). Thus, both scientific and ethical considerations require that methods of assessing pain in animals be developed.

MINIMIZING PAIN IN ANIMAL EXPERIMENTATION

A committee of the International Association for the Study of Pain has defined pain in humans as an 'unpleasant sensory and emotional experience associated with actual or potential tissue damage, or described in terms of such damage' (Mersky 1979). Although animals lack the ability to verbally communicate, they exhibit the same motor behaviours and physiological responses as humans in response to pain. Such behaviours include simple withdrawal reflexes, more complex unlearned behaviours such as vocalization or escape, and learned behaviours such as pressing a bar to avoid further exposure to noxious stimulation. From these behaviours we can infer that an animal is experiencing pain. An important concept in animal studies of pain is that experimental animals should not be exposed to pain greater than humans themselves would tolerate (Bowd 1980). Another way of stating this concept is that we should apply principles used in human studies to studies of pain in animals. Human subjects are exposed only to painful stimuli that they can tolerate and they can remove a painful stimulus at any time. Thus, they establish the acceptable level of pain under which the experiment is performed.

The tolerance for pain needs to be clearly distinguished from the threshold for pain. Stimuli near-threshold produce minimal aversive reactions and are well-tolerated by human subjects and animals. It is only when the intensity of the stimulus approaches tolerance levels that our behaviour is dominated by attempts to avoid or escape it. Therefore, it is critical that the experimenter determine the level of pain produced by stimuli whose intensity cannot be controlled by the animal.

How does an investigator decide which is the appropriate method to minimize pain? Although the scientific merit of each method needs to be decided on an individual basis, Table 15.1 presents a list of approaches based on ethical considerations. As one proceeds down the list, the control of pain becomes more difficult and more procedures are necessary to ensure that the animal is exposed to minimal pain.

Most experiments are performed on anaesthetized animals. There are no ethical concerns about such experiments as long as sufficient anaesthetic is provided. This can be accomplished by the monitoring of pupillary size, stability of heart rate and blood pressure and electroencephalographic activity. Alternatives to anaesthetic agents are surgical lesions such as those that produce a functional decerebration, thus eliminating all possibility of conscious sensation. Another approach is to study pain

Table 15.1 Methods for eliminating or minimizing pain

Anaesthesia
Pharmacological
Surgical
Analgesia
Pharmacological
Surgical
Awake with stimulus control
Restraint
Minimal or no restraint
Awake with no stimulus control
Minimum pain established

mechanisms in awake animals that have received analgesic agents. Experiments on pain mechanisms in animals that were administered anaesthetics or analgesics are of limited usefulness since the procedures suppress the very neurobiological processes that are under study. Nevertheless, important lines of inquiry can be pursued with such methods and they can be useful in the study of neural processes minimally affected by such agents. For example, anaesthetics that act in the central nervous system (CNS), such as barbiturates, can be employed in the study of primary afferent nociceptor activity.

Many studies of pain today are concerned with the relationship between behaviour related to pain and neurobiological processes. Such studies require that animals be exposed to actual or potential tissue damage with electrical, thermal, mechanical or chemical stimuli. Most investigations utilize techniques in which the animal has control over the intensity and duration of the stimulus. This ensures that the animal is not exposed to intolerable levels of stimulation and can escape stimulation by appropriate motor behaviour. A simple example of such a method is a withdrawal reflex produced by stimulating a paw or the tail of an animal. In unlearned tasks utilizing reflex measures, animals often need to be placed under considerable restraint. This unfortunately may produce unwanted levels of stress that can influence the outcome of the experiment (Dubner & Bennett 1983). Such stress is minimized in animals trained to perform pain detection and discrimination tasks (Dubner 1985). These studies employ operant conditioning procedures and most closely mimic conditions under which humans participate in experimental pain studies: the animals choose to participate by initiating trials, they determine the levels of stimulation they will accept by escaping intolerable stimuli and they can withdraw from the experiment by ceasing to initiate new trials.

It is difficult to minimize pain in studies in which the animals cannot control the pain magnitude (Table 15.1). In such experiments it is important that the investigator infer the level of pain by carefully monitoring the animal's general behaviour. Does the animal engage in normal activity? Does it feed properly and exhibit normal social adjusment when placed in a cage with other animals of the same species? Does it maintain its weight as compared to controls? Is its sleep/waking cycle normal? Significant changes from the normal state suggest that the magnitude of pain may be above tolerable levels. Therefore, it is necessary to determine whether the experiment can be performed with lower levels of pain.

GENERAL PROPERTIES OF PAIN ASSESSMENT METHODS

An ideal behavioural model for assessing pain should have the following characteristics (Dubner et al 1976; Vierck & Cooper 1984; Dubner 1985):

1. It should distinguish between responses to innocuous and noxious stimuli.
2. The behavioural response or responses to be measured should vary in magnitude with changes in stimulus intensity over a range from threshold to tolerance.
3. Multiple threshold and suprathreshold behavioural measures should be used to infer pain.
4. The model should be susceptible to behavioural and pharmacological manipulations that alter the perceived intensity of noxious stimuli.
5. The modification of behavioural responses by nonsensory variables such as attention, motivation and motoric ability should be distinguishable from effects on sensory capacities.
6. There should be little or no tissue damage with repetitive stimulation.

The selection of an appropriate noxious stimulus in a behavioural model is also of considerable importance (Table 15.2). It should be a natural, quantifiable stimulus that has a rapid onset and termination. Pain threshold and tolerance levels should be comparable across species so that inferences about pain mechanisms can be made between species and animal models. The stimulus should excite a restricted group of primary afferent fibres and activate only receptors preferentially sensitive in the noxious range. Finally, the noxious stimulus chosen should not produce tissue damage over the pain sensitivity range.

Noxious thermal stimuli (temperatures of 45°C or greater) appear to meet these requirements although they

Table 15.2 Selection of an appropriate noxious stimulus

Requirements	Thermal	Electrical	Mechanical
Natural quantified stimulus that can be varied between threshold and tolerance	++	–	+
Rapid onset and termination	+	++	++
Threshold and tolerance levels comparable across species	++	–	+
Stimulation activates a restricted group of nociceptors	++	–	–
Stimulation activates only nociceptors in the pain sensitivity range	++	–	–
Stimulus quality is constant across pain sensitivity range in humans	++	–	++
Stimulation does not produce tissue damage	+/–	++	+/–

++ = Fully satisfactory; + = minimally satisfactory; – = unsatisfactory.
From Dubner 1985.

tend to produce tissue damage with repeated stimulation near tolerance levels. The two most common methods of applying heat stimuli are the heat-radiation technique used successfully by Opppel & Hardy (1937) and the contact thermode method described by Kenshalo et al (1967) and modified by Darian-Smith et al (1973) and Dubner et al (1975). In the radiation method, the light from a projection lamp is focused through a lens and directed to an area of skin that is often blackened to enhance heat absorption. The thermal energy can be determined by a radiometer placed in the beam or, alternatively, a thermocouple placed over the skin can measure the stimulus temperature. In both instances, the stimulus energy can be fed back to the heating device through electronic circuitry to produce predetermined temperature levels with minimal overshoot. There are some disadvantages in this method: it is difficult to hold the rate of rise of temperature constant for different final temperatures, the baseline temperature cannot be easily varied and the skin temperature returns to baseline slowly. These factors influence the activity of thermally-sensitive skin receptors and presumably the sensations perceived by the animals. Furthermore, the slow termination of the heat can be a problem in behavioural studies in which the animals are escaping the stimulus. Laser devices that provide very rapid changes in skin temperature overcome some of these disadvantages (Mor & Carmon 1975).

The contact probe method avoids most of these difficulties. A Peltier device (Kenshalo et al 1967) provides both cooling and heating, but has a slow rise time of approximately 2°C per second. The device designed by Darian-Smith et al (1973) and modified by Dubner et al (1975) employs a contact thermode consisting of a cylindrical cold sink cooled by 4°C water and covered by thermally conductive epoxy in which is embedded a spiral nichrome wire. The probe surface is usually a thin copper sheet in which a thermistor is embedded. The thermistor senses the surface temperature and, through a feedback circuit, controls the nichrome wire heater voltage and maintains or changes the surface temperature. The rate of temperature change can be as high as 20°C per second depending on the size of the probe face. Similar devices are now commercially available. Contact probes have the disadvantage of activating mechanoreceptors innervating the skin underneath the probe and care must be taken not to confuse such sensory input with that provided by the thermal stimulus.

Although electrical stimulation is favoured by some (Vierck & Cooper 1984), it does not meet the stimulus requirements outlined in Table 15.2 as well as heat stimulation. In addition, electrical stimulation produces synchronous activation of all primary afferent neurons at high intensity, thereby distorting the temporal pattern of discharge produced by natural stimuli. Electrical stimulation of the skin appears to bypass receptor activation and can be useful in differentiating peripheral receptor effects from more central mechanisms when used in conjunction with heat or mechanical natural stimuli.

Tooth pulp electrical stimulation is a favourite stimulus of some investigators because it is thought that pain is the only sensation produced by such stimuli. Recent findings suggest that this is not the case and that large A-beta fibres that do not produce pain under normal circumstances are activated by tooth pulp electrical stimuli (Sessle 1979; McGrath et al 1983). Tooth pulp electrical stimulation, therefore, may have disadvantages similar to cutaneous electrical stimuli.

METHODS OF ASSESSING PAIN

Animal studies on pain employ behavioural measures that are of two types: simple withdrawal reflexes and more complex voluntary and intentional behaviours that are unlearned or learned (Chapman et al 1985).

SIMPLE REFLEX MEASURES

These include the tail-flick test, the limb-withdrawal reflex and the jaw-opening reflex. In most cases latency measures are used to assess reflex responses. In the tail-flick reflex, a radiant heat stimulus is focused on the blackened area of the tail and the animal flicks its tail to escape the stimulus. The technique was introduced by D'Armour & Smith (1941) to demonstrate analgesia. The effectiveness of analgesic agents in this model is highly correlated with their effectiveness in relieving pain in humans (Grumbach 1966). More recently, it has been used to assess pain produced by brain stimulation, stress or the microinjection of opioids or other chemical mediators (Dubner & Bennett 1983). In the limb-withdrawal test, thermal or electrical stimuli are typically employed and the latency of a brisk motor response is used as the behavioural endpoint (Bonnett & Peterson 1975). Limb-withdrawal and tail-flick responses can also be investigated by immersion of the appendage into a waterbath at 47°C (Coderre & Melzack 1985). The jaw-opening reflex (Mitchell 1964) is elicited by electrical stimulation of a tooth and electromyographic recordings from jaw muscles are used to assess the behaviour. These simple reflex measures permit the animal to have control over stimulus magnitude and thus ensure that the animal can control the level of pain. There are minimal ethical concerns about the use of these measures in conscious animals. The tail-flick reflex has the added advantage that it can be elicited under light anaesthesia (Fields et al 1983; Sandkuhler & Gebhart 1984). The tail-flick latency is faster in the lightly anaesthetized state than in the awake animal.

Reflex responses suffer from a number of limitations as measures of pain behaviour (Chapman et al 1985). They are a measure of reflex activity and not pain sensation.

The tail-flick reflex, for example, can be elicited in spinalized animals. Although analgesia in humans and tail-flick latencies are highly correlated, reflex activity in humans produced by noxious stimulation can be dissociated from pain sensation produced by the same stimulus (Willer et al 1979; McGrath et al 1981). Changes in reflex activity can result from alterations in motor as well as sensory processing. Drugs that effect motoneuron or muscle function will alter reflex latencies in a manner similar to analgesic drugs. Reflex latencies also are not easily related to stimulus intensity. In fact, most investigators empirically choose a convenient endpoint and normalize distributions to avoid the problem of baseline variability in a large group of animals.

ORGANIZED UNLEARNED BEAVIOURS

More complex organized unlearned behaviours are often used as measures of pain because they involve a voluntary purposeful act requiring supraspinal sensory processing (Chapman et al 1985). A commonly used method is the rodent hot-plate test in which a rat or mouse is placed on a plate preheated to 50–55°C. A paw-licking response, usually of the hind paws, is measured. A variant of the hot-plate reaction is the face-rubbing escape response in which rats are exposed to facial heat stimuli (Rosenfeld et al 1983).

A method has been devised in which rats receive radiant heat stimuli through a glass plate while they stand unrestrained in a plastic chamber. The rats withdraw their limb reflexively but also exhibit more complex organized behaviours such as paw-licking and guarded behaviour of the limb (Hargreaves et al 1987). A paw withdrawal latency measure and the withdrawal duration (how long the limb remains off the glass plate) can be used to infer pain. This method appears to be particularly useful in assessing hyperalgesia following inflammation or partial nerve injury (Hargreaves et al 1987; Bennett & Xie 1988). Figure 15.1 shows the effect of the radiant heat stimulus used in this method on the cutaneous temperature of inflamed and saline-treated rat paws. The inflamed paws have greater initial paw temperatures than the saline-injected paws. In addition, stimulation of the inflamed paws results in shorter pain-withdrawal latencies than stimulation of the saline-treated paws, and this shorter latency corresponds to a lower threshold temperature. Figure 15.2 compares withdrawal latencies using this model to more complex organized behaviours such as withdrawal duration and paw-licking. The onset of change in these behaviours following the induction of inflammation appears similar to the reflex measure, paw-withdrawal latency, but the duration of the effects outlast the reflex measure for a considerable time period. The ability to assess multiple measures that can be used to infer pain increases the reliability of this model.

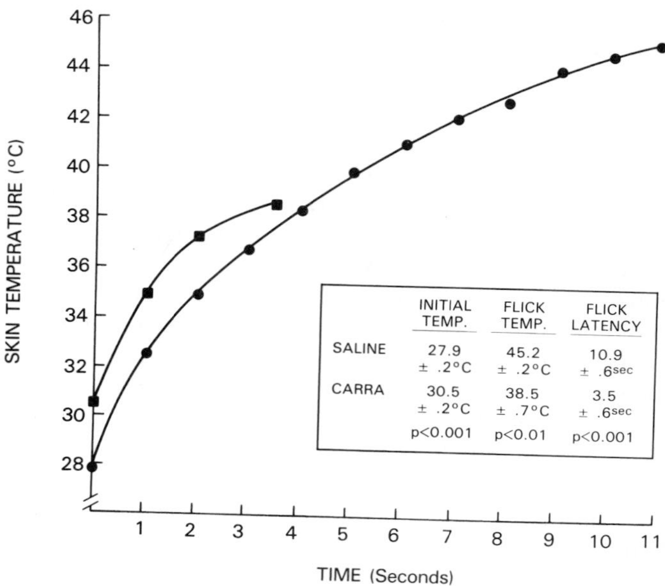

Fig. 15.1 Effect of radiant heat on cutaneous temperature of rat hind paws after saline administration and after carrageenan (carra)-induced inflammation. Animals are unrestrained in an enclosed plastic chamber and the radiant heat stimulus was positioned under the glass floor directly beneath the hind paw. The inset shows the mean initial temperature and the mean temperature when the rats withdrew their hind paws (flick temperature) under both conditions. Mean withdrawal latencies are also shown. (From Hargreaves et al 1988.)

Recently, a model of visceral pain has been developed which utilizes a natural, reproducible stimulus (colorectal distension) in awake, unrestrained rats (Ness & Gebhart 1988; Ness et al 1991). Colorectal distension produces aversive behaviour measured in a passive-avoidance task. Latencies in the task vary monotonically with graded distensions above 30 mmHg (Fig. 15.3). This visceral stimulus also produces a vigorous pressor response and tachycardia that also grade with increasing intensities of colorectal distension. The rats also demonstrate a visceromotor response consisting of contraction of the abdominal and hind limb musculature. Modulators of nociception such as morphine and capsaicin affect responses to the stimulus in a fashion consistent with the conclusion that the responses to colorectal distension are due to the noxious nature of the stimulus (Ness et al 1991). Psychophysiological studies indicate that this same stimulus is noxious to human subjects (Ness et al 1990).

All of the above organized behaviours provide the animal with control of the intensity or duration of the stimulus since the behaviour results in removal of the aversive stimulus. In contrast, there are assessment methods in which the animal does not have control of stimulus intensity or duration. For example, the writhing response is produced in rodents by injecting pain-producing chemical substances intraperitoneally. The acute peritonitis resulting from the injection produces a response characterized by internal rotation of one foot,

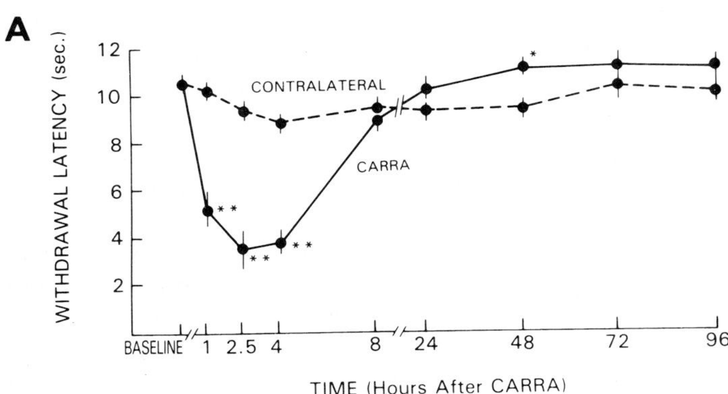

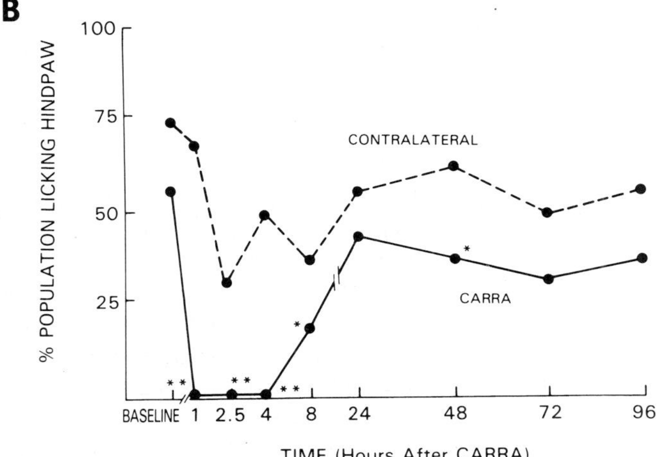

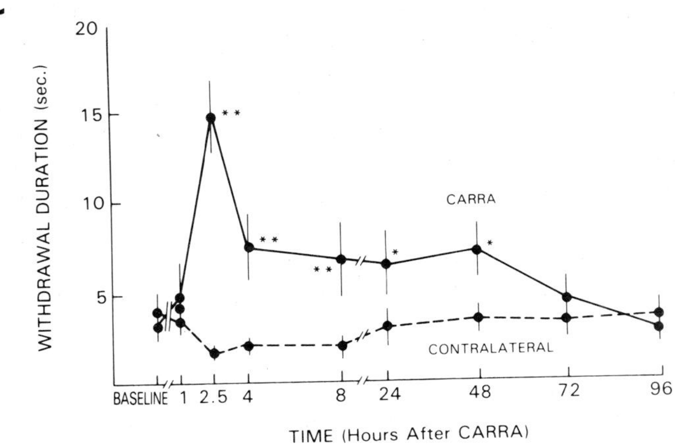

Fig. 15.2 Different behavioural measures of hyperalgesia in the carrageenan-induced inflammation model. Carrageenan was injected into the hind paw of 16 rats and the responses of the inflamed paw were compared to the contralateral untreated paw. **A** Effects of carrageenan on paw withdrawal latency. **$p<0.01$. **B** Effects of carrageenan on postwithdrawal paw-licking behaviour. *$p<0.05$; **$p<0.01$. **C** Effects of carrageenan on the duration of paw withdrawal from the glass floor. *$p<0.05$; **$p<0.01$. (From Hargreaves et al 1988.)

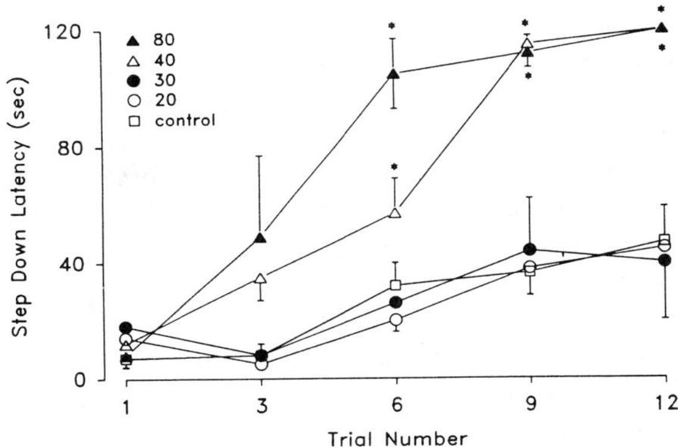

Fig. 15.3 The effect of graded colorectal distension on passive-avoidance behaviour in rats. The latency to step down from a platform was measured. When intraluminal colorectal distension pressures were either 40 or 80 mmHg, rats avoided colorectal distension by remaining on the paltform. At pressures of 20 or 30 mmHg, experimental rats did not behave differently from the control rats that received no distension or distension in a different environment. Asterisks indicate significant differences between experimental and control rats at the $p<0.05$ level. Vertical bars indicate Standard error of the mean. (From Ness et al 1991.)

arching of the back, rolling on one side and accompanying abdominal contractions. The writhing response is considered a model of visceral pain (Vyklický 1979). In addition to the lack of stimulus control offered to the animal with this method, the experimenter cannot control the duration of the stimulus. Vocalization is another commonly used, unlearned reaction to painful stimuli (Kayser & Guilbaud 1987). The stimulus intensity necessary to elicit a vocal response from the animal is determined. The stimulus can be applied to any part of the body. The animals cannot control the intensity or duration of the stimulus.

TISSUE INJURY MODELS OF PERSISTENT PAIN

The methods described above produce phasic increases in stimulus intensity that are very short-lasting (with the exception of the writhing response). Recent attempts have been made to develop models of tissue injury and inflammation that produce responses that mimic human clinical pain conditions in which the pain lasts for longer periods of time. In one test, formalin is injected beneath the footpad of a rat or cat (Dubuisson & Dennis 1977 see review by Tjølsen et al 1992). The chemical produces complex response patterns that last for approximately 1 hour. The behavioural state of the animal can be graded numerically as the effect wears off; initially the animals elevate the limb and do not place it on the cage floor, but during the ensuing 60–90 minutes they begin to use it as a weight-bearing limb.

Models of inflammation that produce more persistent pain include the injection of carrageenan or complete Freund's adjuvant (CFA) into the footpad (Iadarola et al 1988) or into the joint of the limb (Schaible et al 1987).

These models result in rapid, short-lasting, acute pain responses, similar in duration to the formalin method; higher doses of the irritants can produce more persistent pain that mimics the time course of postoperative pain or even arthritis. In the inflammation model elicited by injection of CFA into the footpad, the cutaneous inflammation appears within 2 hours and peaks within 6–8 hours. Hyperalgesia and oedema are present for approximately 1 week to 10 days. The physiological and biochemical effects are limited to the affected limb (Iadarola et al 1988a) and there are no signs of systemic disease. It is obvious that the animal cannot control the pain associated with these inflammation models. Therefore, it is important to determine that the levels of pain are below the tolerance level of the animals. Iadarola et al (1988b) observed that rats with adjuvant or carrageenan-induced inflammation exhibit minimal reductions in weight and show normal grooming behaviour. Exploratory motor behaviour is normal and no significant alterations occur in an open-field locomotion test. Thus, the impact of the inflamed limb on the rat's behaviour is minimal and the rats will use the limb for support, if necessary.

A model of neurogenic inflammation similar to one utilized in human subjects is the use of intradermal capsaicin to produce hyperalgesia (LaMotte et al 1991). The intradermal injection of capsaicin produces primary hyperalgesia at the site of injection and a surrounding area of secondary hyperalgesia to light touch. A flare reaction extends into the zone of secondary hyperalgesia. This model has been used in monkeys to study changes in nociceptor activity and changes in the responses of spinal dorsal horn neurons induced by the neurogenic inflammation (Simone et al 1991).

Other methods have been developed which attempt to mimic human conditions of persistent or chronic pain. Included are models of polyarthritis in which CFA is injected into the rat's tail (De Castro Costa et al 1981). The adjuvant results in a delayed hypersensitivity reaction with inflammation and hyperalgesia of multiple joints occurring after 10 days to 3 weeks. Pain is inferred from scratching behaviours, reduced motor activity by the animal, weight loss, vocalization when the effected limbs are pinched and a reduction in these behaviours following the administration of opioids. It should be noted that this is a systemic disease of the animal that includes skin lesions, destruction of bone and cartilage, impairment of liver function and a lymphadenopathy (Coderre & Wall 1987). These systemic lesions make it more difficult to associate the animal's behaviour with pain as opposed to generalized malaise and debilitation. The likely presence of CNS changes associated with the alterations in immune function also question the use of this model to correlate neural activity and neurochemical alterations with behaviour presumably related to pain. Other models of arthritis have been developed in which sodium urate crystals are injected into the ankle joint of rat or cat (Okuda et al 1984; Coderre & Wall 1987). The arthritis is fully developed within 24 hours. These animals reduce the weight placed on the treated hind limb and exhibit quarded movement of the limb. In the rat, touch, pressure and thermal stimuli applied to the affected paw result in a decrease in responsiveness, presumably due to the pain associated with the movement. There are no signs of systemic disease in the urate arthritis model other than joint pathology secondary to tissue oedema and the infiltration of polymorphonuclear leucocytes (Coderre & Wall 1987). Acute arthritis can also be induced by the injection of carrageenan and kaolin into the cat or monkey knee joint just below the patella (Schaible et al 1987; Dougherty et al 1992). Changes in joint receptor and spinal dorsal horn neuronal activity begin as soon as 1–2 hours following injection and build up for several hours. Behavioural studies related to this model have not been performed.

NERVE INJURY MODELS OF PERSISTENT PAIN

Approximately 2 weeks after complete sectioning of the sciatic nerve in the rat with encapsulation, the rats engage in self-mutilation of the denervated area that begins with chewing of the toe nails and is followed by a progressive degree of amputation of the digits and the foot. The validity of this model as a suitable model of chronic pain has been debated (Sweet 1981; Rodin & Kruger 1984; Coderre et al 1986) and redebated (Devor 1992; Kruger 1992). The critical issue is whether the self-mutilation is a response to abnormal sensations attributable to the deafferented limb, or simply a response to an insensate appendage which the animal considers a foreign body and is trying to remove. Blumenkopf & Lipman (1991) have recently provided evidence that chronic nerve block with lidocaine does not result in self-mutilation of the limb, suggesting that rats do not self-mutilate an insensate limb.

Recently developed models indicate that partial nerve injury in the rat results in signs of hyperalgesia and spontaneous pain. In one model, loose ligatures are placed around the sciatic nerve with resultant demyelination of the large fibres and destruction of some unmyelinated axons (Bennett & Xie 1988). In another model, ligation and severing of the dorsal half to one-third of the sciatic nerve produces similar behavioural changes (Seltzer et al 1990). Both models mimic the clinical conditions of painful neuropathy with evidence of allodynia, hyperalgesia and spontaneous pain. Although both models exhibit evidence of thermal hyperalgesia (Fig. 15.4), Bennett & Xie (1988) did not report mechanical hyperalgesia. A subsequent paper by Attal et al (1990) did find mechanical hyperalgesia, however. Bennett & Xie (1988) reported cold allodynia whereas Seltzer et al (1990) did not. There also may be differences in sympathetic nervous system

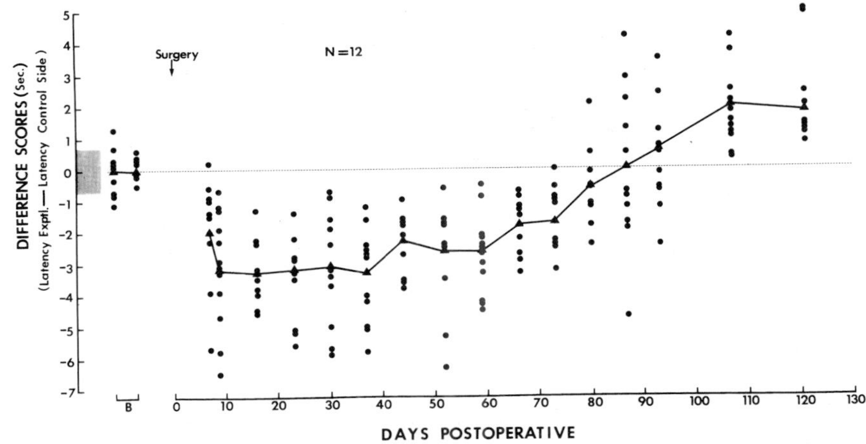

Fig. 15.4 Time course of thermal hyperalgesia produced by tying loose ligatures around the sciatic nerve of the rat. Hyperalgesia was measured using the noxious heat-evoked paw-withdrawal method described in Figures 15.1 and 15.2. Negative difference scores indicate a lowered nociceptive threshold on the side of the sciatic nerve ligation. Filled circles indicate difference scores of individual rats and the filled triangles and solid line show the group mean difference scores. (From Bennett & Xie 1988.)

involvement in the two models (Bennett 1991; Shir & Seltzer 1991). It should be noted that signs of nerve injury in diabetic rats have been reported earlier (Birchiel et al 1985). In addition, a number of papers have recently appeared describing mechanical allodynia following spinal nerve injury (Kim & Chung 1991), laser radiation induced ischaemia of the spinal cord (Hao et al 1991) and intrathecal administration of spinal inhibitory transmitter antagonists (Yaksh 1989). These models of allodynia are particularly useful for examining CNS changes responsible for pain behaviours and the role of excitatory amino acids and neuropeptides in these effects.

All of the above nerve injury models which attempt to mimic human conditions of chronic or persistent pain produce pain that the animal cannot control. Therefore, it is important that investigators assess the level of pain in these animals and provide analgesic agents when it does not interfere with the purpose of the experiment. Pain in these studies can be inferred from on-going behavioural variables such as feeding and drinking, sleep–waking cycle, grooming and social behaviour (Sternbach 1976). Significant deviation from normal behaviour suggests that the animal is in severe and possibly intolerable pain.

ORGANIZED LEARNED BEHAVIOURS

Learned or operant responses are a separate category of behaviours from which pain has been inferred in animals. The most common and simplest method involves an animal escaping a noxious stimulus by initiating a learned behaviour such as crossing a barrier or pressing a bar. For example, electric shock can be delivered to a grid floor in a cage and the animal can be trained to jump over a barrier partition to escape the stimulus. The latency of escape is usually measured. Vierck & Cooper (1984) have developed a sophisticated version of this type of model in monkeys in which there are multiple measures of the animal's escape behaviour. Another operant procedure used with electrical stimulation is the shock titration method (Weiss & Laties 1963). The animals press a bar to reduce the intensity of a continuously increasing stimulus. The animals tend to titrate the stimulus intensity at or near the noxious level. However, this method tends to assess avoidance rather than escape behaviour and it is extremely difficult to determine whether the animals are titrating the stimulus in the noxious range or below it.

Other more complex methods include reaction time

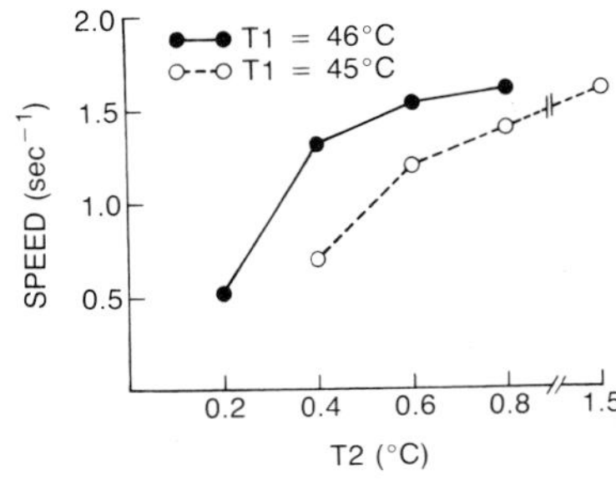

Fig. 15.5 Behavioural detection latencies in a noxious heat detection task. Latency is expressed as speed of reaction, the reciprocal of latency, and is plotted as a function of second temperature shifts (T2) from either 45° or 46°C first temperature shifts (T1). Each point represents the mean obtained from 40 trials. Speed of reaction is monotonically related to intensity and is a function of the first temperature level. Speed of reaction is an indirect measure of the perceived intensity of the stimulus and correlates very highly with magnitude estimation in humans. (From Maixner et al 1986.)

Table 15.3 Pain assessment methods and their characteristics

Characteristics of pain assessment methods	Reflex measures			Unlearned organized behaviours								Learned behaviours			
	Tail-flick	Limb-withdrawal	Jaw-opening	Hot plate	Models of inflammation	Writhing response	Vocalisation	Formalin test	Models of arthritis	Complete deafferentation	Partial deafferentation	Escape	Shock titration	Reaction time conflict task	Detection task
1. Distinguish between responses to innocuous and noxious stimuli				x	x	x		x	x		x			x	x
2. Response varies with stimulus intensity								x				x		x	x
3. Multiple behavioural measures available					x				x		x	x		x	x
4. Susceptible to behavioural and pharmacological manipulations	x	x	x	x	x	x	x	x	x	x	x	x	x	x	x
5. Distinguishes nonsensory variables from sensory effects														x	x
6. Little or no tissue damage	x	x	x	x			x*					x	x	x	x
Animal has control over stimulus intensity and/or duration	x	x	x	x	x							x	x	x	x

X indicates which properties are met by each assessment method
*Depends on the stimulus employed

experiments in which the animal detects or discriminates a noxious stimulus. In conflict paradigms (Vierck et al 1971; Dubner et al 1976), animals learn to perform a task to receive a reward, but also are exposed to noxious stimulation during the task. The animals must choose between receiving a reward or escaping the aversive stimulus on each trial. This method produces escape rather than avoidance behaviour in the animals. When monkeys and humans perform such a task with noxious heat stimuli, they exhibit similar escape thresholds (Dubner et al 1976). Correlative behavioural and neural studies using this model have established that the activity of myelinated mechanothermal nociceptors is sufficient to account for correct performance in such a task (Dubner et al 1977).

Reaction time tasks have been developed in which monkeys are trained to detect stimuli in the noxious heat range (Dubner 1985). This task can be designed so that the detection involves stimuli only in the noxious heat range and no cues are provided by preceding innocuous warming stimuli. Another advantage of this behavioural task is that it can be used in conjunction with the detection of innocuous stimuli. A comparison of the effects of drug manipulations on innocuous versus noxious stimuli rules out the possibility that the drug is altering attentional, motivational or motoric aspects of the animal's behaviour intead of influencing the perceived intensity of the noxious stimuli (Oliveras et al 1986). Figure 15.5 shows the behavioural detection latencies (expressed as speed of reaction) to increases in temperature in the noxious heat range from first temperature increases of 45 and 46°C. Monkeys are capable of detecting 0.1–0.2° increases in temperature from 46 or 47°C first temperature increases and wide-dynamic-range neurons participate in the encoding process by which the monkeys perceive these sensations (Maixner et al 1986).

As with unlearned behaviours related to pain, all of the above operant procedures provide only indirect measures of pain such as the latency or the probability of a motor response. However, they have the advantage over simpler unlearned behaviours in that the magnitude of the behavioural change varies with stimulus intensity, providing more reliable evidence that the change in behaviour reflects the perception of a noxious stimulus rather than a change in motor performance. Sophisticated operant tasks in animals also allow the experimenter to rule out that changes in performance are related to attentional and motivational variables rather than changes in sensory perception. It also should be recalled that these operant procedures give the animal control over the stimulus and other parameters of the experiment to a degree comparable to that found in human studies of experimental pain.

Table 15.3 lists some of the pain assessment methods discussed above and shows how they meet the criteria described for an ideal pain assessment method. In addition, Table 15.3 identifies the methods in which the animals have control over the levels of pain that they will tolerate. Such methods ensure that the animals are exposed to minimal pain and should be considered similar to the use of anaesthetics and analgesics in the control of pain. Investigators should establish the minimal pain necessary to perform studies using those methods where the animals do not control the levels of pain that they are exposed to.

REFERENCES

Attal N, Jazat F, Kayser V, Guilbaud G 1990 Further evidence for 'pain-related' behaviours in a model of unilateral peripheral mononeuropathy. Pain 41: 235–251

Bennett G J 1991 The role of the sympathetic nervous system in painful peripheral neuropathy. Pain 45: 221–223

Bennett G J, Xie Y 1988 A peripheral mono-neuropathy in rat that produces disorders of pain sensation like those seen in man. Pain 33: 87–107

Birchiel K J, Russell L C, Lee R P, Sima A A F 1985 Spontaneous activity of primary afferent neurons in diabetic BB/wistar rats. Diabetes 34: 1210–1213

Blumenkopf B, Lipman J J 1991 Studies in autotomy: its pathophysiology and usefulness as a model of chronic pain. Pain 45: 203–209

Bonnett K A, Peterson K E 1975 A modification of the jump-flinch technique for measuring pain sensitivity in rats. Pharmacology, Biochemistry & Behaviour 3: 1–47

Bowd A D 1980 Ethics and animals experimentation. American Psychologist 35: 224–225

Casey K L, Morrow T J 1983 Nocifensive responses to cutaneous thermal stimuli in the cat: stimulus-response profiles, latencies and afferent activity. Journal of Neurophysiology 50: 1497–1515

Chapman C R, Casey K L, Dubner R, Foley K M, Gracely R H, Reading A E 1985 Pain measurement: an overiew. Pain 22: 1–31

Coderre T J, Melzack R 1985 Increased pain sensitivity following heat injury involves a central mechanism. Brain Research 15: 259–262

Coderre T J, Wall PD 1987 Ankle joint urate arthritis (AJUA) in rats: an alternative animal model of arthritis to that produced by Freund's adjuvant. Pain 28: 379–393

Coderre T J, Grimes R W, Melzack R 1986 Deafferentation and chronic pain in animals: an evaluation of evidence suggesting autotomy is related to pain. Pain 26: 61–84

D'Amour F E, Smith D 1941 A method for determining loss of pain sensation. Journal of Pharmacology and Experimental Therapeutics 72: 74–79

Darian-Smith I, Johnson K O, Dykes R 1973 'Cold' fibre population innervating palmar and digital skin of the monkey: responses to cooling pulses. Journal of Neurophysiology 36: 325–346

De Castro Costa M, De Sutter P, Gybels J, Van Hees J 1981 Adjuvant-induced arthritis in rats: a possible animal model of chronic pain. Pain 10: 173–185

Devor M 1992 Autotomy sense and nonsense. Reply to L. Kruger. Pain 49: 156

Dougherty P M, Sluka K A, Sorkin L S, Westlund K N, Willis W D 1992 Neural changes in acute arthritis in monkeys. I. Parallel enhancements of responses of spinothalamic tract neurons to mechanical stimulation and excitatory amino acids. Brain Research Review 17: 1–13

Dubner R 1983 Pain research in animals. Annals of the New York Academy of Sciences 406: 128–132

Dubner R 1985 Specialization in nociceptive pathways: sensory discrimination, sensory modulation, and neural connectivity. In: Fields H L, Dubner R, Cervero F (eds) Advances in pain research and therapy, vol 9. Raven Press, New York, p 111–137
Dubner R, Bennett G J 1983 Spinal and trigeminal mechanisms of nociception. Annual Review of Neuroscience 6: 381–418
Dubner R, Sumino R, Wood W I 1975 A peripheral 'cold' fiber population responsive to innocuous and noxious thermal stimuli applied to monkey's face. Journal of Neurophysiology 38: 1373–1389
Dubner R, Beitel R E, Brown F J 1976 A behavioural animal model for the study of pain mechanisms in primates. In: Weisenberg M, Tursky B (eds) Pain: new perspectives in therapy and research. Plenum, New York, p 155–170
Dubner R, Price D D, Beitel R E, Hu J W 1977 Peripheral neural correlates of behavior in monkey and human related to sensory-discriminative aspects of pain. In: Anderson D J, Matthews B (eds) Pain in the trigeminal region. Elsevier, Amsterdam, p 57–66
Dubuisson D, Dennis S G 1977 The formalin test: a quantitative study of the analgesic effects of morphine, meperidine and brain-stem stimulation in rats and cats. Pain 4: 161–174
Fields H, Bry J, Hentall I, Zorman G 1983 The activity of neurons in the rostral medulla of the rat during withdrawal from noxious heat. Journal of Neuroscience 3: 545–552
Grumbach L 1966 The prediction of analgesic activity in man by animal testing. In: Knighton R S, Dumke P R (eds) Pain. Little, Brown, Boston, p 163–182
Hao J-X, Xu X-J, Aldskogius H, Seiger Å, Wiesenfeld-Hallin Z 1991 Allodynia-like effects in rat after ischaemic spinal cord injury photochemically induced by laser irradiation. Pain 45: 175–185
Hargreaves K, Dubner R, Brown F, Flores C, Joris J 1987 A new and sensitive method for measuring thermal nociception in cutaneous hyperalgesia. Pain 32: 77–88
Iadarola M J, Douglass J, Civelli O, Naranjo J R 1988a Differential activation of spinal cord dynorphin and enkephalin neurons during hyperalgesia: evidence using cDNA hybridization. Brain Research 455: 202–212
Iadarola M J, Brady L S, Draisci G, Dubner R 1988b Enhancement of dynorphin gene expression in spinal cord following experimental inflammation: stimulus specificity, behavioural parameters and opioid receptor binding. Pain 45: 313–326
Kayser V, Guilbaud G 1987 Local and remote modifications of nociceptive sensitivity during carrageenin-induced inflammation in the rat. Pain 28: 99–107
Kenshalo D R, Duncan D G, Weymark C 1967 Thresholds for thermal stimulation of the inner thigh, footpad, and face of cats. Journal of Comparative Physiology and Psychology 63: 133–138
Kim S H, Chung J M 1991 Sympathectomy alleviates mechanical allodynia in an experimental animal model for neuropathy in the rat. Neuroscience Letters 134: 131–134
Kruger L 1992 The non-sensory basis of autotomy in rats: a reply to the editorial by Devor and the article by Blumenkopf and Lipman. Pain 49: 153–155
LaMotte R H, Shain C N, Simone D A, Tsai E-F P 1991 Neurogenic hyperalgesia: psychophysical studies of underlying mechanisms. Journal of Neurophysiology 66: 190–211
McGrath P A, Sharav Y, Dubner R, Gracely R H 1981 Masseter inhibitory periods and sensations evoked by electrical tooth pulp stimulation. Pain 10: 1–17
McGrath P A, Gracely R H, Dubner R, Heft M W 1983 Non-pain and pain sensations evoked by tooth pulp stimulation. Pain 15: 377–388
Maixner W, Dubner R, Bushnell M C, Kenshalo D R Jr, Oliveras J-L 1986 Wide-dynamic-range dorsal horn neurons participate in the encoding process by which monkeys perceive the intensity of noxious heat stimuli. Brain Research 374: 385–388
Mersky H (Chairman) 1979 Pain terms: a list with definitions and notes on usage. Pain 6: 249–252
Mitchell C L 1964 A comparison of drug effects upon the jaw jerk response to electrical stimulation of the tooth pulp in dogs and cats. Journal of Pharmacology and Experimental Therapeutics 146: 1–6
Mor J, Carmon A 1975 Laser emitted radiant heat for pain research. Pain 1: 233–237
Ness T J, Gebhart G F 1988 Colorectal distension as a noxious visceral stimulus: physiologic and pharmacologic characterization of pseudaffective reflexes in the rat. Brain Research 450: 153–169
Ness T J, Metcalf A M, Gebhart G F 1990 A psychophysiological study in humans using phasic colonic distension as a noxious visceral stimulus. Pain 43: 377–386
Ness T J, Randich A, Gebhart G F 1991 Further behavioral evidence that colorectal distension is a 'noxious' visceral stimulus in rats. Neuroscience Letters 131: 113–116
Okuda K, Nakahama H, Miyakawa H, Shima K 1984 Arthritis induced in cats by sodium urate: a possible animal model for chronic pain. Pain 18: 287–297
Oliveras J-L, Maixner W, Dubner R et al 1986 The medullary dorsal horn: a target for the expression of opiate effects on the perceived intensity of noxious heat. Journal of Neuroscience 6: 3086–3093
Oppel T W, Hardy J D 1937 Studies in temperature sensations. I. A comparison of the sensation produced by infra-red and visible radiation. II. The temperature changes responsible for the stimulation of the heat end organs. Journal of Clinical Investigation 16: 517–531
Rodin B E, Kruger L 1984 Deafferentation in animals as a model for the study of pain: an alternative hypothesis. Brain Research Review 7: 213–228
Rosenfeld P J, Pickrel C, Broton J G 1983 Analgesia for orofacial nociception produced by morphine microinjection into spinal trigeminal complex. Pain 15: 145–155
Sandkühler J, Gebhart G F 1984 Characterization of inhibition of a spinal nociceptive reflex by stimulation medially and laterally in the midbrain and medulla in the pentobarbital-anesthetized rat. Brain Research 305: 67–76
Schaible H-G, Schmidt R F, Willis W D 1987 Enhancement of the responses of ascending tract cells in the cat spinal cord by acute inflammation of the knee joint. Experimental Brain Research 66: 498–499
Seltzer Z, Dubner R, Shir Y 1990 A novel behavioral model of neuropathic pain disorders produced in rats by partial sciatic nerve injury. Pain 43: 205–218
Sessle B J 1979 Is the tooth pulp a 'pure' source of noxious input? In: Bonica J J, Liebeskind J C, Albe-Fessard D G (eds) Advances in pain research and therapy, vol 3. Raven Press, New York pp 245–260
Shir Y, Seltzer Z 1991 Effects of sympathectomy in a model of causalgiform pain produced by partial sciatic nerve injury in rats. Pain 43: 309–320
Simone D A, Sorkin L S, Oh U et al 1991 Neurogenic hyperalgesia: central neural correlates in responses of spinothalamic tract neurons. Journal of Neurophysiology 66: 228–246
Sternbach R A 1976 The need for an animal model of chronic pain. Pain 2: 2–4
Sweet W H 1981 Animal models of chronic pain: their possible validation from human experience with posterior rhizotomy and congenital analgesia. Pain 10: 275–295
Tjølsen A, Berge O-G, Hunskaar S, Rosland J H, Hole K 1992 The formalin test: an evaluation of the method. Pain 51: 5–17
Vierck C J Jr, Cooper B Y 1984 Guidelines for assessing pain reactions and pain modulation in laboratory animal subjects. In: Kruger L, Liebeskind J C (eds) Advances in pain research and therapy, vol 6. Raven Press, New York, 305–322
Vierck C J Jr, Hamilton D M, Thornby J I 1971 Pain reactivity of monkeys after lesions to the dorsal and lateral columns of the spinal cord. Experimental Brain Research 13: 140–158
Vyklický L 1979 Techniques for the study of pain in animals. In: Bonica J J, Liebeskind J C, Albe-Fessard D G (eds) Advances in pain research and therapy, vol 3. Raven Press, New York, p 727–745
Wall P D, Devor M, Inbal R et al 1979 Autotomy following peripheral nerve lesions: experimental anesthesia dolorosa. Pain 7: 103–113
Weiss B, Laties V G 1963 Characteristics of aversive thresholds measured by a titration schedule. Journal of Experimental Analysis of Behavior 6: 563–572
Willer J C, Boureau F, Albe-Fessard D 1979 Supraspinal influences on nociceptive flexion reflex and pain sensation in man. Brain Research 179: 61–68
Yaksh T L 1989 Behavioural and autonomic correlates of the tactile evoked allodynia produced by spinal glycine inhibition: effects of modulatory receptor systems and excitatory amino acids antagonists. Pain 37: 111–123

16. Measurement and assessment of paediatric pain

Patrick J. McGrath and Anita M. Unruh

INTRODUCTION

There have been major advances in the measurement of pain in children in recent years and, generally, appropriate research attention is being paid to the reliability and validity of paediatric pain measures. However, these measures are not yet widely used in clinical situations.

Pain is a subjective, private event that can be measured only indirectly by one of three strategies. It is agreed that the 'gold standard' for measuring pain should be what children report about their experience (self-report measures). In addition, pain can be measured by the way children react in response to pain (behavioural measures). Finally, how children's bodies respond to pain (biological measures) can be used. Unfortunately, neonates, preverbal children and handicapped children cannot describe their experiences and thus behavioural and biological measures must be used.

Even with verbal children, measurement by self-report may be hampered by several factors. Young children have relatively limited cognitive ability to understand what is being asked of them in pain measurement, and they may have difficulty in articulating descriptions of their pain. Furthermore, our limited understanding of the developmental psychology of pain in children may prevent us from asking questions in a developmentally appropriate fashion. Finally, the preconceptions many professionals and lay persons hold about children's pain may preclude children being asked about their pain.

Behavioural and biological reactions to pain may also be considerably influenced by the age and health of the child. As young children develop, their behavioural responses to pain change. Neonates, in particular, may have substantially different biological responses than older children. In addition, seriously ill neonates and children may have substantially different behavioural and biological responses than healthy individuals of the same age.

MEASUREMENT AND ASSESSMENT

The distinction between measurement and assessment in pain research has not always been clearly drawn. Measurement refers to the application of some metric to a specific aspect, usually intensity, of pain. Assessment is a much broader endeavour which should encompass the measurement of the interplay of different factors on the total experience of pain. Measurement is like using a ruler or scale to determine the height or weight of something whereas assessment is deciding whether it is height, weight, volume, density or tensile strength that is important to measure.

While measurement of pain in children has become increasingly sophisticated, assessment has lagged behind. At least four groups have developed standardized paediatric pain assessment packages (Varni et al 1987; Savedra & Tesler 1989; McGrath 1990; Abu-Saad 1990) that are modelled on the McGill Pain Questionnaire (MPQ; Melzack 1975). Each package measures location and intensity of pain and some factors that may be related to the pain. Although useful as basic instruments, they have not been guided by an explicit conceptual model.

The lack of a theoretical model to address the assessment of pain has left the clinician with no guide for clinical thinking and decision-making. Pain problems are more than just the physiological transmission of nociceptive impulses (even when modulated by psychological inputs). They are complex social-physiological-behaviourial puzzles that require assessment on different levels. As a result, models of pain transmission alone cannot sufficiently guide the clinician in assessment and management.

THE WHO MODEL OF PAIN ASSESSMENT

The model that we (McGrath et al 1991) have proposed is a variant of the World Health Organization's (WHO) International Classification of Impairments, Disabilities and Handicaps (World Health Organization 1980). This classification provides a model of the consequences of

Table 16.1 The World Health Organization model of the consequences of disease as applied to migraine

	Jon	Bill	Mary
Disease/disorder	Migraine	Migraine	Migraine
Impairment	Weekly headache	Weekly headache, nausea	Weekly headache, photophobia
Disability	Inability to concentrate	Can't play hockey	No disability
Handicap	School absence	No handicap	Social isolation

disease conceptualized as occurring in four planes or levels. The first plane is that of the occurrence of an abnormality (disease). The second plane (impairment) occurs when the affected individual becomes aware of the abnormality or develops a symptom. The third plane, disability, occurs when there is a restriction or lack of ability to perform an activity in the normal way. The fourth plane, handicap, occurs when the individual's experience is socialized. Handicaps are concerned with the social disadvantages experienced by the individual as a result of impairments and disabilities. Table 16.1 illustrates the relationship between these four planes with three fictitious children who suffer from migraine.

Extensive impairment may or may not result in disability. Similarly, disability may not cause a handicap. In addition, impairment may directly result in handicap with little or no intervening disability. The causal chain may be parallel or reversed. In the parallel case, disability in one area may thwart development of new abilities or mask their expression. In the reverse situation, the effect may be from handicap to disability or impairment. That is, a handicap may cause impairment or disability. For example, a child who becomes socially isolated and bedridden (handicap) because of reflex sympathetic dystrophy may exacerbate the underlying problem by increasing muscle atrophy and bone demineralization.

When applying the model to pain, disease refers to the cause of the pain, such as sickle cell disease. Impairment refers to the pain itself. The WHO classification system uses pain as one example of an impairment and the detail is probably insufficient for everyday use with clinical pain problems.

DISCORDANCE IN PAIN ASSESSMENT

Concordance and discordance in pain measures and assessments can occur both within and between planes or levels. Few problems are caused by concordance, so we will focus our attention on discordance. Usually a discordance in which a child functions beyond the level that is expected is not only accepted, but may be seen as admirable, and the child's behaviour may be reinforced. Such discordance can be a problem, however, if a child's lack of disability or handicap and subsequent activity exacerbate damage from the disease.

Generally, the most problematic discordance occurs when the child has more disability or handicap than expected on the basis of his underlying disease or disorder. A common reaction to this discordance is the 'leap to the head' (Wall 1989), in which malingering or psychogenicity is assumed.

Discordance within levels may occur across behaviours, settings or time. Discordance between the child's self-report of pain and observers' evaluations of the child's pain based on his behaviour are not unusual. For example, children who report moderate levels of pain when asked, may be observed to be playing and seem to be unaffected. This can best be seen as a normal way for a child to cope with pain.

Discordance between levels can also be confusing to the clinician and researcher. For example, a parent or health professional may expect a low level of pain based on the amount of tissue damage suffered from an injection, but the child may exhibit and report severe pain. Conversely, a child may exhibit very little pain behaviour at the same time as reporting high levels of pain in a situation where one might expect severe pain (e.g. postoperatively) (Beyer et al 1990).

A clinician faced with conflicting information about the amount of pain a child is suffering may have difficulty deciding on a course of action. Should a clinician administer an analgesic when a child is not reporting pain but is behaving in a way that seems to indicate pain? Similarly, should an analgesic be given when pain report is high but pain behaviour cannot be observed? It is not unusual for clinicians to view discordance with alarm or as evidence of malingering or psychogenicity. This is unwarranted but discordant findings indicate the need for further assessment. At this time, we do not have ways to routinely resolve discordances. Clinical problem solving is required.

PSYCHOMETRICS OF PAIN MEASUREMENT

If measures of pain lack reliability or validity they will be of little use to clinicians or researchers. Reliability refers to the consistency of a measure. Consistency may be across situations, across time or across raters. If pain actually varies over time or situation, then reliability of scores on a measure is not important. However, if pain is stable and the measure is not, there is a major problem. Validity of an instrument refers to whether or not the scale measures the construct that is intended. That is, a pain scale measures pain, not depression or anxiety. Scales may be valid or reliable in one situation or population and not in another. It is important to determine the psychometric properties of a measure in a situation and with a sample that is similar to that being evaluated.

The utility of a measure refers to its usefulness. One aspect of utility is ease of use, another is versatility. A measure that requires a trained observer is less useful than an equally reliable and valid measure that can be done by anyone in a few seconds. Versatile measures have the advantage of being used in several different situations (e.g. across a wide age range or in both acute and chronic pain). Versatility is convenient and allows for comparisons across different situations. Whereas utility and versatility are desirable, reliability and validity are prerequisites for use.

Some pain measures are used in research settings but may be too expensive or too demanding in terms of skills or time needed for clinical use. Moreover, some pain measures may not be precise enough for making specific clinical decisions. In addition, some clinical measures may lack the precision needed for particular research questions.

STRATEGIES OF PAIN MEASUREMENT

The three most frequently considered aspects of pain are the subjective (measured by self-report), the behavioural (measured by observation and coding or rating of behaviour) and the biological (measured by sampling of physiological or electrical potentials and assaying body fluids or other biological responses). Not only are there multiple aspects but for each there may be several different measurement strategies.

SELF-REPORT MEASURES OF PAIN

Self-report measures depend on the child's own report of his or her subjective pain experience. This can include descriptions of pain-relevant feelings, statements and images, as well as information about the quality, intensity and temporal/spatial dimensions of the child's pain. Self-report measures, when they can be obtained, should be regarded as the 'gold standard'. Indeed, the International Association for the Study of Pain (Merskey 1986) emphasizes 'pain is always subjective'. There are two major problems with self-report measures. First of all, they require the child to have a level of cognitive and linguistic development that excludes all preverbal children and may exclude many other young children. The level of cognitive and language development depends on the type of question asked. Children at the earliest levels of language development may be able to respond to the least demanding questions, such as those about the existence of pain.

The second problem is that all self-report measures are open to bias because of the demand characteristics of the specific situation. Eland & Anderson (1977) report that following surgery children may deny having pain when they are asked because they fear that if they say they have pain they will get a needle. Ross & Ross (1988) have shown that the reason given to a child for asking a question about pain and the person asking the question make a substantial difference in the child's response. For example, if children are asked to describe pain to their mothers they will give different answers than if they are asked to describe pain to a doctor. In addition, the type of question and the response options (for example, open-ended versus a checklist) may also substantially alter the child's answers (Ross & Ross 1988). Clearly, demand and other contextual characteristics cannot be eliminated from the measurement of pain. We must, however, be aware that a change in context can substantially influence the measurement of pain.

The methods used to measure self-report of pain include: direct questioning, pain adjective descriptors, self-rating scales, numerical rating scales and nonverbal methods.

DIRECT QUESTIONING

Spontaneous reports (e.g. 'My tummy hurts') or direct questioning about pain can be useful with verbal preschoolers and school-age children. However, reliance on spontaneous reports is likely to seriously underestimate pain; some children may not spontaneously report pain because they want to be brave or because they do not know that anything can be done about it. Direct questioning may include:

- asking the child to make comparisons with previous pain experiences ('Is this pain like the stomach ache you had last week?')
- providing the child with temporal anchors for measuring the duration of pain ('Has the pain been going on since you woke up?')
- facilitating communication through the use of objects and gestures ('How much pain do you have, a little bit or a lot').

Ross & Ross (1988) suggest using questions that are open-ended rather than those with forced-choice answers.

Although direct questioning is clinically useful, several shortcomings have been observed. To a great extent, questions such as 'How is your pain today?' are more conversational gambits than pain measures. Because of their unstructured nature these methods may be particularly open to bias due to demand characteristics. As well, they lack an associated metric (i.e. there are no numbers associated with the answers) and may be biased by inaccurate memory or the recall of a previous experience. Even if specific questions are asked about pain frequency, intensity and duration, retrospective questions are likely to be inaccurate.

The typical clinical strategy is to ask the child's mother how much pain her child has been experiencing. This is similar to asking parents if they remember whether or not their child had recently appeared to have a fever. In some cases, this strategy, whether it is related to fever or pain, produces sufficient information to guide diagnosis and treatment. It is, however, likely to be insufficient in more complex situations such as those where pain is of unknown origin or where there is serious discordance within or across planes or levels. More precise measures of pain are likely to be obtained by the child using prospective, well-validated measures.

PAIN ADJECTIVE DESCRIPTORS

Pain adjective lists, such as the MPQ (Melzack 1975) have been used successfully with older adolescents to measure the sensory, affective and evaluative dimensions of pain. A major strength of this type of scale is that it is not restricted to the intensity dimension of pain but also measures affective and evaluative aspects of pain. Experience in several different laboratories has shown that children are able to select simple adjectives from word lists to describe their pain. For example, Savedra, Tesler and their colleagues have examined children's language of pain in a series of studies (e.g. Savedra et al 1990; Savedra & Tesler 1990; Wilkie et al 1990). They have developed and tested lists of words that include sensory, affective and evaluative words that can be completed by children over 8 years. A 56-item word list that measures sensory, affective and evaluative components of pain has been developed and evaluated for reliability and validity. Similar work has been undertaken in the Dutch language by Abu-Saad (1990) and by P. A. McGrath (1990) and Varni et al (1987) in English. As yet, the meaning of different patterns of words has not been determined. Pain descriptors rely on advanced linguistic competence and may not be appropriate for some children. Although these methods are appealing because the richness of the pain experience is described, they have not yet been shown to be superior to simpler methods that focus on the intensity of pain.

Self-rating scales of intensity of pain vary according to the type and number of anchor points provided and may be categorized into three types: visual analogue scales, category rating scales, and numerical rating scales.

Visual analogue scales

Visual analogue scales (VAS) consist of either a vertical or horizontal line with verbal or pictorial anchors indicating a continuum from no pain to severe pain at each end. Children are asked to indicate on the line how much pain they are experiencing. Studies have shown that for children over 5 years, VAS are reliable and valid measures of pain. Children's ratings of their pain on VAS correlate with parents', nurses', and physicians' ratings (O'Hara et al 1987; Varni et al 1987; McGrath et al 1990). Ratings on VAS also correlate with behaviourial measures of pain (McGrath et al 1985; Maunuksela et al 1987). Figure 16.1 provides an example of a visual analogue scale.

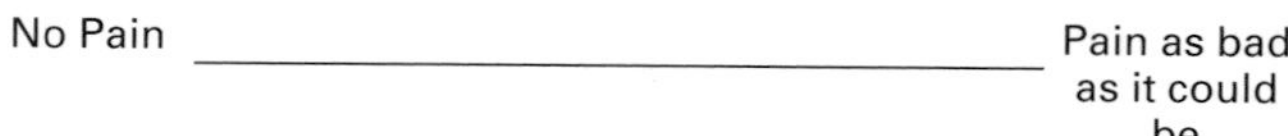

Fig. 16.1 Visual analogue scale.

Some authors have suggested that a vertical scale is more appropriate than a horizontal scale because children may find it easier to conceptualize the notion of greater or lesser intensity of pain with up and down rather than left or right. The VAS is versatile as it allows one to measure different dimensions such as intensity ('How bad is the pain?') and affect ('How bad do you feel about the pain?'). However, the child must have the cognitive ability necessary to translate the pain experience into an analogue format and to understand proportionality. Care must be taken when repeatedly xeroxing the scale to ensure that the process does not alter the length of the line and thus confound scoring. Maunuksela et al (1987) developed and validated a variant of a VAS in the form of a 50-cm red and white wedge.

Category rating scales

Category scales consist of a series of words along a continuum of increasing value (e.g. no pain, mild pain, medium pain, severe pain). Category rating scales may be difficult to interpret because descriptors may have different meanings for different children (Ross & Ross 1988). However, Wilkie et al (1990) have recently provided data suggesting that a category scale may be valid and useful with children.

The Poker Chip Tool (Hester 1979), a derivative of the category scales, is a concrete measure requiring the child to evaluate the intensity of pain by choosing one to four poker chips, representing the 'pieces of hurt' experienced. This method is appropriate for younger children between the ages of 4 and 8 years. Children's ratings correlate with overt behaviour during immunization (Hester 1979). A recent study comparing child, nurse and parental ratings of pain demonstrated adequate convergent validity and partial support for discriminant validity of this tool (Hester et al 1990). It would appear that the Poker Chip Tool is the most appropriate measure for 4- and 5-year-old children.

Face scales, another form of category scale, consist of faces expressing varying amounts of distress. Each face is assigned a numerical value reflecting its order within a series of facial expressions. Several variants of face scales have been used to measure children's level of pain. However, if the scales do not approach being ratio scales, the numerical values assigned to each face may be deceiving.

The Oucher scale (Beyer 1984) is a variant of the face scale and is designed to measure pain intensity in children aged 3–12 years. The scale is displayed in a poster format and consists of a vertical numerical scale (0–100) on the

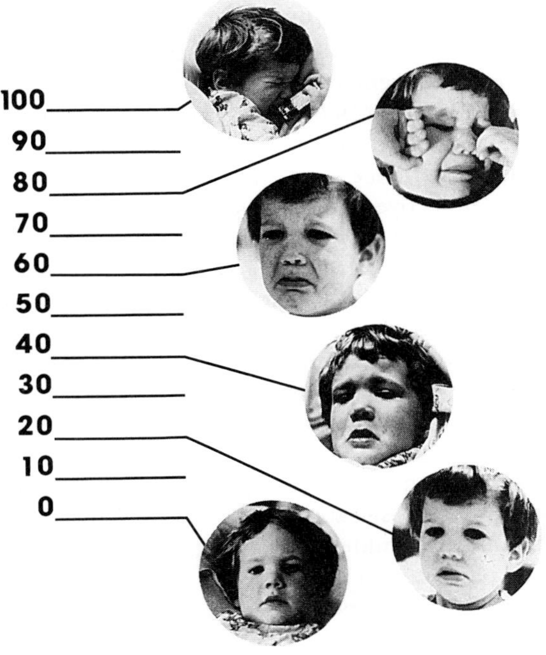

Fig. 16.2 The Oucher Scale. (From Beyer 1984 with permission.)

left and six photographs of children in varying degress of pain positioned vertically to the right (Fig. 16.2).

Validity studies indicate that children are able to classify the pictures in the correct sequence and that scores correlate highly with visual analogue scores and results from the Poker Chip measure (Beyer & Aradine 1987). Although the scale has been criticized for confounding intensity and affective measures (P A McGrath 1987), it correlates poorly with measures of fear (Beyer & Aradine 1987), suggesting that it does indeed tap into the pain-intensity dimension. Moreover, scores on the Oucher scale are sensitive to analgesia-caused reduction in pain. The Oucher remains the most thoroughly validated scale and has good psychometric properties.

A recent study (Bieri et al 1990) focused on the development of a face scale to assess pain intensity in children aged 6–8 years. A unique feature of this measure is that the drawings used in the scale's development were derived from those generated by the children themselves. In addition, the faces were drawn to be reflective of the facial response to pain. Further, strong agreement was demonstrated among children on the rank ordering of the faces according to pain severity as well as their perception of the faces as representing equal intervals. Finally, the scale demonstrated adequate test-retest reliability over a 2-week period. The scale is presented in Figure 16.3. Other face scales have been developed (Whaley & Wong 1987; Kuttner & Lepage, 1989) and there is no clear

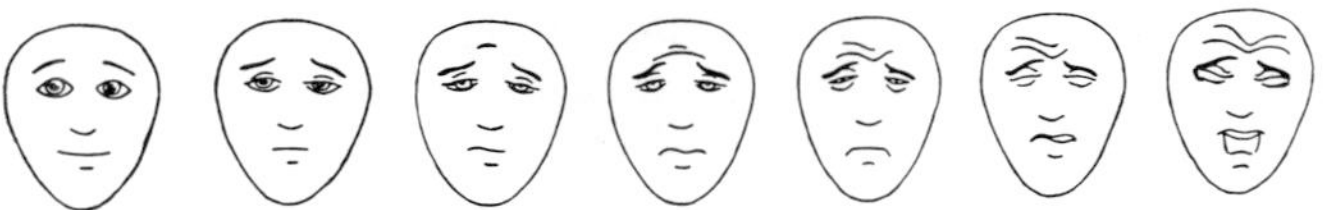

Fig. 16.3 Faces scale. (From Bieri et al 1990 with permission.)

evidence that one scale is more accurate than another. In summary, face scales are easily understood by children. They are inexpensive and several have excellent psychometric characteristics.

Numerical rating scales

These scales use numbers (i.e 0–5, 0–10 or 0–100) to reflect increasing degrees of pain. Children must understand number concepts in order to use this type of scale. The intervals along the scale cannot be assumed to be equal and a change between 0 and 3 is not necessarily the same as a change between 6 and 9. Although there has not been careful work on the psychometric properties of numerical rating scales, they have a place in the clinical setting. From a practical perspective, since they require no materials, are readily understood by health care professionals and are so easy to chart (e.g. 'James rated his pain as 7 out of 10'), numerical scales have distinct advantages.

Pain thermometers consist of a vertical numerical rating scale ranging between 0–10 or 0–100 superimposed on a visual analogue scale. Anchors at each endpoint indicate no hurt and most hurt possible. The child is asked to point to the place on the thermometer that represents the intensity of his pain. Scores on the pain thermometer correlate with scores on other rating scales as well as predicted changes in pain associated with burns (Szyfelbein et al 1985).

Diaries are a specific type of numerical rating scale in which repeated ratings of pain are taken. Pain diaries have been used for the measurement of headache, abdominal pain and limb pain. In a typical format, ratings range from 0–5 and each number corresponds to a verbal description of pain severity. The scale requires a minimum of instruction and has satisfactory interrater reliability when comparisons are made between parent and child ratings (Richardson et al 1983; Andrasik et al 1985). Pain diaries may be particularly useful with older children and adolescents as they encourage self-management strategies and consequently foster a sense of mastery and increased self-esteem (Ross & Ross 1988). Figure 16.4 presents a diary used in our clinical and research work.

Nonverbal methods

Primarily nonverbal methods have also been used to measure the subjective component of pain. These methods include asking children to describe the colour of

Introduction Week 1
Headache Diary

Fill in this form at breakfast, lunch, dinner and bedtime each day

Name: ______________________ **Week beginning:** ____________

Day	Time	Intensity Rating	Other Symptoms	Medication	Possible Cause
	Breakfast				
	Lunch				
	Dinner				
	Bedtime				
	Breakfast				
	Lunch				
	Dinner				
	Bedtime				
	Breakfast				
	Lunch				
	Dinner				
	Bedtime				
	Breakfast				
	Lunch				
	Dinner				
	Bedtime				
	Breakfast				
	Lunch				
	Dinner				
	Bedtime				
	Breakfast				
	Lunch				
	Dinner				
	Bedtime				
	Breakfast				
	Lunch				
	Dinner				
	Bedtime				

Intensity Ratings

0 – No headache.
1 – Headache – I am only aware of it if I pay attention to it.
2 – Headache – but I can ignore it at times.
3 – Headache – I can't ignore it but I can do my usual activities
4 – Headache – It is difficult for me to concentrate; I can only do easy activities.
5 – Headache – such that I can't do anything.

Fig. 16.4 Pain diary.

their pain or to draw pictures of their pain. Children are reported typically to describe severe pain as being red or black (Eland 1974; Jeans 1983; Unruh et al 1983; Kurylyszyn et al 1987). Unfortunately, no validation of colour scales or their utility in clinical situations has been done. Red and black appear to be the preferred colours for all pain drawings, even for drawings of low intensities of pain (Kurylyszyn et al 1987). Children's pain drawings are rich in detail, are emotively powerful and provide a basis for discussion about pain. Although they can be reliably classified by raters (Unruh et al 1983) and may show developmental differences (Jeans 1983), it is not clear that drawings can tell us much about the intensity or origin of the child's pain. Kurylyszyn et al (1987) found that drawings of different intensity of headache could not be well discriminated on the basis of overall ratings of intensity or by examination of specific features of the drawings. However, drawings provide valuable information about the location of pain. Several studies have shown that children over 6 years of age can locate their pain on a pain drawing or body outline and that these markings correspond to clinical observations and records (Varni et al 1987; Savedra & Tesler 1989).

Projective techniques have not been shown to be effective in the measurement of intensity of pain in children. For example, Eland (1974) found no relationship between responses to cartoons in which an animal was subjected to a painful experience and the child's own response. However, projective approaches may be of some use in a more broad-based assessment of children's attitudes to painful experiences, perceptions of family response to pain and coping strategies. Lollar et al (1982) developed a projective pain scale that used 24 pictures to determine how children perceive pain experienced by themselves and their parents. This scale has not been used in clinical pain measurement. The Charleston Pain Pictures (Belter et al 1988) are 17 cartoon pictures of a young child of indeterminate sex in scenes of medical, play and home situations. The scales depict situations that have been assessed by experts and by children as being no pain, low pain, moderate pain or high pain.

In summary, self-report measures of pain are the 'gold standard' when they can be obtained. Several well-designed methods that can be easily used in clinical situations have been developed. However, they cannot be used with developmentally delayed or preverbal children.

BEHAVIOURIAL MEASURES OF PAIN

The second component of pain that can be measured is pain behaviour. Behaviours such as vocalization, facial expression and body movement are typically associated with pain. Behaviourial responses are invaluable for inferring pain in children who cannot rate their pain. There is, however, the ever-present challenge of distinguishing behaviour due to other forms of distress, such as hunger, thirst and anxiety, from behaviour due to pain. The best evidence for reliability and validity of behaviourial measures is based on studies of short, sharp pain such as that from needle procedures such as venipuncture, heelstick or bone marrow aspirations. For example, Fradet et al (1990) found that child self-report correlated significantly with a measure of discrete pain behaviours ($r = 0.54$) and also with global estimates by nurses ($r = 0.52$) and global measures by parents ($r = 0.42$).

Some of the most interesting work on behavioural measures has been carried out with neonates. Grunau & Craig (1987) developed the Neonatal Facial Action Coding System which consisted of 10 facial actions that trained coders could indentify from review of videotapes. Facial movements observed in response to heel lance (the 'pain face') were: brow bulge, eye squeeze, nasolabial furrow, lip part, taut tongue, stretch mouth and chin quiver. Results indicated that facial response to heel lance was also state dependent, with increased facial responding observed in babies who were quiet and awake compared to babies who were sleeping. In a subsequent study, Grunau et al (1990) found that facial expression (especially brow bulging, eyes squeezed shut, deepening of the nasolabial furrow and open mouth) combined with a short-latency cry and long-duration first-cry cycle is the most typical (but not uniform) response to short, sharp, invasive stimuli.

Barr (1992) has sounded a note of caution about the assumption that the 'pain face' necessarily means pain. He points out that there is considerable overlap in facial response between babies experiencing stimuli assumed to be painful and those experiencing nonpainful stimuli. Similarly, in a study of babies with colic and pain-free controls, there was no uniformity of facial action but some indication that children with a 'pain face' were more likely to be regarded as being in pain by adults.

Facial expressions are interesting because they are relatively free of learning biases and may represent the infant's innate response to pain. To date, the facial coding systems have been used primarily for short, sharp pain in a research context. They require video-recording and time-consuming scoring of responses. As a result, these methods are not appropriate for routine clinical use. In addition, facial action may be difficult to record in sick babies who often have their faces obstructed due to medical interventions.

Others (Craig et al 1984; Johnston & Strada 1986; Pigeon et al 1989) have observed more gross body movements associated with pain in infants and young children. Commonly observed behaviours include: general diffuse movements in newborns, withdrawal of the affected limb in 6-month-old infants, and touching the affected area in 12-month-old infants (McGraw 1945). Kicking and thrashing of limbs, tensing of limbs and a rigid, tense torso have also been observed in response to immunization (Craig et al 1984; Johnston & Strada 1986). The Infant Pain Behaviour Rating Scale (Craig et al 1984), a time-sampling scale, rates expressive body responses (rigidity, kicking) as well as vocalizations and facial expressions in infants and young children. The scale has satisfactory interrater reliability for most of the items, as well as validity. Franck (1986) used photogrammetric techniques to quantify infants' body responses to heel lance. In a survey of neonatal nurses' perceptions of pain, similar behaviours were identified as indicative of pain in neonates but there was essentially no relationship between the various behaviours and pain intensities (Pigeon et al 1989).

The Procedural Behavioral Rating Scale (Katz et al 1980) and the Observational Scale of Behavioral Distress (Jay et al 1983) were developed to measure distress in paediatric oncology patients due to bone-marrow aspirations and lumbar punctures. Behaviours include crying, screaming, physical restraint, verbal resistance, requests for emotional support, muscular rigidity, verbal pain expression, flailing, nervous behaviour and information seeking. The scales have satisfactory interrater reliability, and distress behaviours on the Observational Scale of Behavioral Distress correlate with children's self-report of pain and anxiety scores (Jay et al 1983).

A particular behaviour that has received considerable attention as a pain measure is crying. Investigators have attempted to differentiate the pain cry in infants in terms of its psychoacoustic properties (Johnston & Strada 1986; Grunau & Craig 1987). Johnston (1989) reported that a high-pitched, tense, nonvoiced, intense cry is typical in very stressed states. Grunau & Craig (1987) found that both gender and psychological state affected crying behaviour. Specifically, in response to heel lance, boys cried sooner and had more crying cycles than girls. Also, sleeping babies cried less quickly than alert babies. Although some characteristic cry patterns have been identified during medical procedures (Johnston 1989), a cry pattern or cry template unique to painful stimuli has not been identified. Grunau et al (1990) have discussed the methodological difficulties in cry research.

Behavioural measures of longer-lasting pain are less well developed and it appears that the scales to measure short-term pain may not be valid for longer-term pain. Three scales have been developed for measuring postoperative pain in children. All have been validated in the immediate postoperative period. The Children's Hospital of Eastern Ontario Pain Scale (CHEOPS) (McGrath et al 1985) is a behaviourial rating scale developed with children in the recovery room to measure postoperative pain. It consists of six behaviours (crying, facial expression, verbal expression, torso position, touch position and leg position). The scale has interrater reliability above 0.80 and independent pain ratings by nurses provide evidence for concurrent validity. Also, the scale is sensitive to changes in behaviour due to intravenous analgesic medication. It has excellent measurement characteristics with needle pain (Fradet et al 1990). However, Beyer et al (1990) have shown that the CHEOPS is insensitive to pain outside the immediate postoperative situation.

Norden et al (1991) developed the Objective Pain Scale, which has five areas of observation including blood pressure, crying, movement, agitation and verbal evaluation or body language. This scale correlates from between 0.89 and 0.98 with the CHEOPS. Unfortunately, evaluation of the scale has only been presented in abstract form.

Tarbell et al (1992) recently published a seven-item Toddler-Preschool Postoperative Pain Scale that includes items on vocal pain expression, facial pain expression and bodily pain expression. The scale has good reliability and validity data but, like the CHEOPS and the Objective Pain Scale, it has not been shown to be valid outside the immediate postoperative period. These three scales are valid for measuring pain in the recovery room but are probably not valid for measuring pain in children several hours after surgery. Beyer et al (1990) established that gross behaviours such as grimacing and body movements occur very rarely in children suffering from postoperative pain once they are out of the recovery room.

As we have noted, there is little work on longer-lasting pain. Gauvain-Piquard et al (1987) developed a 15-item behaviourial rating scale for paediatric oncology patients between the ages of 2 and 6 years. The scale consists of three sub-scales:

1. Pain behaviours such as protective behaviours toward the affected area
2. Psychomotor alterations such as slowing down and withdrawal
3. Anxiety behaviours such as nervousness and irritability.

The scale appears to have adequate sensitivity between patients and satisfactory interrater reliability (Gauvain-Piquard et al 1987). Validity studies are ongoing and the scale is being used with other groups such as paediatric burn patients (Gauvain-Piquard & Rodary 1989).

In summary, there has been extensive work on measures of short, sharp pain and extremely limited work on long-term pain. The scales range from measures of gross behaviour to measures of small changes in facial response. The behavioural measurement of long-term pain and the development of measures for special populations such as the handicapped and the sick neonate should be of highest priority.

BIOLOGICAL MEASURES

Biological measures of pain in children suffer from many of the same problems as behavioural measures. In particular, it is often difficult to determine if the perturbation being measured is due to causes other than pain such as hunger. Some authors (Porter 1993) have argued that the discrimination between pain and other distress may be meaningless for infants and that a search for a pain-specific measure in this age group should be abandoned in favour of a biological measure of distress. Much like behavioural measures of pain, it appears that biological indices of pain habituate in the face of longer-term pain.

There are sufficient data on heart rate, transcutaneous oxygen, sweating and the stress response to argue for their validity as measures of pain in some circumstances. There is less evidence for using endorphins, respiration and blood pressure. However, further research may elucidate their validity.

Heart rate is the most widely used biological measure of pain in infants and children. In general, heart rate increases in response to more invasive procedures. However, depending on the length of period sampled, there may be a slowing of the heart rate as the first response to pain (Johnston & Strada 1986). There appear to be major differences between healthy and ill neonates, and full-term and premature neonates, with generally weaker, more variable, disorganized responses in ill and premature babies (Field & Goldson 1984; Porter 1993). Porter (1993) has described the use of vagal tone as a direct measure of parasympathetic control and a possible index of pain and distress. However, there have been no studies to demonstrate the superiority of this measure to simple heart rate. Indeed, no studies have adequately attempted to evaluate heart rate as a measure of longer-term pain although it is clear that heart rate is not substantially elevated by postoperative pain in older children (O'Hara et al 1987).

Transcutaneous oxygen is reduced during painful procedures such as circumcision (Rawlings et al 1980; Williamson & Williamson 1983), lumbar punctures (Porter 1993) and intubation (Kelly & Finer 1984), but this also occurs during nonpainful handling of neonates. Transcutaneous oxygen is widely used in anaesthesia and critical care monitoring and is a frequently available measure in the Intensive Care Unit (ICU). Transcutaneous oxygen may, however, be influenced by factors other than pain and may not be responsive in infants who have mechanically supported ventilation.

Harpin & Rutter (1983) demonstrated that, in full-term babies (but not in preterm babies), palmar sweating, as measured by an Evaporimeter, was a sensitive index of pain from heel lance. Gedaly-Duff (1989) has reviewed the use of a simpler measure, the palmar sweat index, that measures the number of active sweat glands rather than the extent of sweating. Palmar sweating has been primarily used as a measure of distress rather than pain.

Surgery or trauma triggers the release of stress hormones (corticosteroids, catecholamines, glucagon and growth hormone). This leads to a cascade of events that may have positive effects of facilitating healing but, in the sick neonate, can have disastrous results. Anand and his colleagues (Anand et al 1987a, 1987b; Anand 1993) have detailed the stress response of premature and full-term infants to surgery. The response generally consists of marked increases in plasma catecholamines, glucagon and corticosteroids and a suppression of insulin secretion, leading to hyperglycaemia and lactic acidosis. The response in neonates is generally greater, particularly with regard to increases in plasma epinephrine, glucagon, growth hormone, blood glucose, blood lactate and other gluconeogenic substrates. In addition, infants tend to have a uniphasic cortisol response which is smaller than the biphasic response of adults. The stress response in neonates is blunted by appropriate anaesthesia, probably by dampening input to the hypothalamus, by lessening the hypothalamic response to neural input and by altering synaptic transmission within the hypothalamus (Anand

1993). The reaction to anaesthesia indicates the validity of the measures but it is clear that the stress response is more than a measure of pain. Although useful in the research context, these measures have limited use as clinical pain measures in individual patients.

Cortisol release has been widely studied in adults and quite frequently examined in infants and children (Gunnar 1986). Cortisol release is not specific to pain and occurs with many aversive situations. Changes in cortisol level from a resting baseline are significant in response to circumcision (Gunnar et al 1981). However, sick premature babies may have very unstable levels. Thus, small perturbations from specific painful procedures may not be detectable.

Lewis & Thomas (1990), in their cross-sectional study of healthy infants who were 2, 4 and 6 months, provide insight into the complexity of the response even in healthy infants at different ages. They used the diphtheria-pertussis-tetanus inoculation as a standard stimulus and found that the strongest increase in cortisol levels, as measured by salivary assay, occurred with the 2-month-old children. These was little change in cortisol level in the 4-month-old children and only moderate response in the 6-month-old children. The age differences in cortisol response were eliminated if behavioural response was used as a covariate. In addition, baseline levels of cortisol were important in interpreting cortisol response to painful stimulation.

Biological methods of measuring pain provide important information about the body's response to insult. These measures are particularly important to the clinician when they provide warning about responses affecting the medical stability of the child. However, biological measures are not specific to pain and sometimes are not available in the clinical setting.

IMPLEMENTATION OF MEASURES

The major impediment to the measurement of pain in children is the failure to implement what is already known. All children who are at risk for pain, including children who have had surgery and children who are in the active phase of potentially painful diseases or disorders such as cancer, sickle cell disease, migraine headache or juvenile arthritis, should have their pain routinely monitored. Hospitalized children's pain should be recorded on pain flow sheets on a regular basis every few hours (McGrath & Unruh 1987). Stevens (1990) has shown that this will decrease pain by improving pain management. Pain diaries, completed by the child or by the parent, can be used with children who are at risk for significant recurrent pain. Routine measurement should be used in quality assurance programmes to ensure the adequacy of pain control in hospitals. Adequate paediatric pain measurement is an ethical imperative that all health care professionals are obligated to implement.

DISABILITY DUE TO PAIN

Disability (the restriction in ability to perform an activity) because of pain has received little systematic attention. Both Varni's pain assessment questionnaire (Thompson & Varni 1986; Varni et al 1987) and Patricia McGrath's (1990) assessment tool contain a measure of disability. However, the validity of the measures or the extent of disability in populations is unknown. Recently, Walker & Greene (1991) have developed and validated the Functional Disability Inventory. The measure was carefully developed and shows excellent construct, concurrent and predictive validity. The instrument was stable over time and also sensitive to medical treatment. Instruments such as the Functional Disability Inventory will allow further investigation of disability due to various childhood pains.

HANDICAP DUE TO PAIN

The major social roles of children are as peers and as students. Consequently, handicaps include educational and social handicap. Although there are limited data on the topic, it appears that handicap due to pain is relatively rare in children. School failure is the most relevant measure of educational handicap. However, no studies have examined school failure resulting from pain. School absence could serve as a proxy measure and absence due to pain has been examined in one study. Collin et al (1985) examined the amount of school time that children between 5 and 14 years of age missed because of headache. They recorded both absence from school and attendance at sick bay. During two 12-week periods, school absence was 0.05%, which amounted to about 1% of all absences, with 85% of absences of less than 1 day. Attendance at sick bay was also low and rarely resulted in leaving school.

Pain is a frequent complaint by the child who has a phobia toward school. However, the pain symptom is usually so transparent that it is quite readily (and quite appropriately) given little attention.

The prevalence of handicap due to pain in children is clearly lower than that found in adults. However, those children who are handicapped are particularly troubling to the health-care system and appropriate assessment may lead to more effective treatment. Little work has been done on the correlates of handicap. In a small study, we (Dunn-Geier et al 1986) found that the mothers of adolescents who were missing school because of pain became over-involved when supervising an exercise task that might elicit pain in their adolescent.

SUMMARY AND CONCLUSIONS

This chapter reviews the measurement of pain in infants and children and proposes the adoption of the WHO model of the consequences of disease for the assessment of pain. We have examined the way such a model could facilitate pain assessment and have recast existing measures in terms of the model. Our review of the existing measures of pain has highlighted the significant advances that have been made in the area and has pinpointed the deficiencies that exist. Although much research remains to be done, measures are now sufficiently developed and validated to call for the routine measurement of pain in all clinical situations where pain is likely to occur. Such measurement is likely to improve the comfort and pain management of our young patients.

REFERENCES

Abu-Saad H H 1990 Toward the development of an instrument to assess pain in children: Dutch study. In: Tyler D C, Krane E J (eds) Advances in pain research and therapy: pediatric pain. Raven Press, New York, p 101–106

Andrasik F, Burke E J, Attanasio V et al 1985 Child, parent, and physician reports of a child's headache pain: relationships prior to and following treatment. Headache 25: 421–425

Anand K J S 1993 The applied physiology of pain. In: Anand K J S, McGrath P J (eds) Pain in the neonate. Elsevier, Amsterdam (in press)

Anand K J S, Sippell W G, Aynsley-Green A 1987a Randomized trial of fentanyl anaesthesia in preterm babies undergoing surgery: effects on the stress response. Lancet 1: 243–248

Anand K J S, Sippell W G, Schofield N M et al 1987b Does halothane anaesthesia decrease the stress response of newborn infants undergoing operation? British Medical Journal 296: 668–672

Barr R G 1992 Is this infant in pain? Caveats from the clinical setting. American Pain Society Journal 1: 187–190

Belter R W, McIntosh J A, Finch A J et al 1988 Preschoolers' ability to differentiate levels of pain: relative efficacy of three self-report measures. Journal of Clinical Child Psychology 17: 329–335

Beyer J E 1984 The Oucher: a user's manual and technical report. The Hospital Play Equipment Co., Evanston, Illinois

Beyer J E, Aradine C R 1987 Patterns of pediatric pain intensity: a methodological investigation of a self-report scale. Clinical Journal of Pain 3: 130–141

Beyer J E, McGrath P J, Berde C 1990 Discordance between self report and behavioral pain measures in 3–7 year old children following surgery. Journal of Pain and Symptom Management 5: 350–356

Bieri D, Reeve R A, Champion G D et al 1990 The faces pain scale for the self-assessment of the severity of pain experienced by children: development, initial validation, and preliminary investigation for ratio scale properties. Pain 41: 139–150

Collin C, Hockaday J M, Waters W E 1985 Headache and school absence. Archives of Disease in Childhood 60: 245–247

Craig K D, McMahon R J, Morison J D et al 1984 Developmental changes in infant pain expression during immunization injections. Social Science in Medicine 19: 1331–1337

Dunn-Geier B J, McGrath P J, Rourke B P et al 1986 Adolescent chronic pain: the ability to cope. Pain 26: 23–32

Eland J M 1974 Children's communication of pain. Master's Thesis, University of Iowa

Eland J, Anderson J 1977 The experience of pain in children. In: Jacox A (ed) A source book for nurses and other health professionals. Little, Brown, Boston, p 453–476

Field T, Goldson E 1984 Pacifying effects of nonnutritive sucking on term and preterm neonates during heelstick procedures. Pediatrics 74: 1012–1015

Fradet C, McGrath P J, Kay S et al 1990 A prospective survey of reactions to blood tests by children and adolescents. Pain 40: 53–60

Franck L S 1986 A new method to quantitatively describe pain behavior in infants. Nursing Research 35: 28–31

Gauvain-Piquard A, Rodary C 1989 Evaluation de la douleur. In: Pichard-Leandri E, Gauvain-Piquard A (eds) La douleur chez l'enfant. Medsi/McGraw-Hill, New York, p 38–59

Gauvain-Piquard A, Rodary C, Rezvani A et al 1987 Pain in children aged 2–6 years: a new observational rating scale elaborated in a paediatric oncology unit – preliminary report. Pain 31: 177–188

Gedaly-Duff V 1989 Palmar sweat index use with children in pain research. Journal of Pediatric Nursing 4: 3–8

Grunau R V E, Craig K D 1987 Pain expression in neonates: Facial action and cry. Pain 28: 395–410

Grunau R V E Johnston C C, Craig K D 1990 Neonatal facial and cry responses to invasive and non-invasive procedures. Pain 42: 295–305

Gunnar M E, Fisch R O, Korsvik S et al 1981 The effects of circumcision on serum cortisol and behaviour. Psychoneuroendocrinology 6: 269–275

Gunnar M R 1986 Human developmental phoneuroendocrinology: a review of research on neuroendocrine response to challenge and threat in infancy and childhood. In: Lamb M E, Brown S L, Rogoff B (eds) Advances in developmental psychology, vol 9. Erlbaum, Hillsdale, New Jersey, p 51–103

Harpin V A, Rutter N 1983 Making heel pricks less painful. Archives of Disease in Childhood 58: 226–228

Hester N K 1979 The pre-operational child's reaction to immunization. Nursing Research 28: 250–255

Hester N K, Foster R, Kristensen K 1990 Measurement of pain in children: generalizability and validity of the pain ladder and the poker chip tool. In: Tyler D C, Krane E J (eds) Advances in pain research and therapy: pediatric pain. Raven Press, New York, p 79–84

Jay S M, Ozolins M, Elliott C et al 1983 Assessment of children's distress during painful medical procedures. Journal of Health Psychology 2: 133–147

Jeans M E 1983 Pain in children: a neglected area. In: Firestone P, McGrath P J, Feldman W (eds) Advances in behavioral medicine for children and adolescents. Erlbaum, Hillsdale, New Jersey, p 23–38

Johnston C C 1989 Pain assessment and management in infants. Pediatrician 16: 16–23

Johnston C C, Strada M E 1986 Acute pain response in infants: a multidimensional description. Pain 24: 373–382

Katz E R, Kellerman J, Seigel S E 1980 Distress behavior in children with cancer undergoing medical procedures: developmental considerations. Journal of Consulting and Clinical Psychology 48: 356–365

Kelly M A, Finer N N 1984 Nasotracheal intubation in the neonate: Physiologic responses and effects of atropine and pancuronium. Journal of Pediatrics 105: 303–309

Kurylyszyn N, McGrath P J, Cappelli M et al 1987 Children's drawings: what can they tell us about intensity of pain? Clinical Journal of Pain 2: 155–158

Kuttner L, Lepage T 1989 Faces scales for the assessment of pediatric pain: a critical review. Canadian Journal of Behavioral Science 21: 198–209

Lewis M, Thomas D 1990 Cortisol release in infants in response to inoculation. Child Development 61: 50–59

Lollar D J, Smits S J, Patterson D L 1982 Assessment of pediatric pain: an empirical perspective. Journal of Pediatric Psychology 7: 267–277

McGrath P A 1987 An Assessment of children's pain: a review of behavioral, physiological and direct scaling techniques. Pain 31: 147–176

McGrath P A 1990 Pain in children: nature, assessment, treatment. Guilford, New York

McGrath P J, Unruh A M 1987 Pain in children and adolescents. Elsevier, Amsterdam

McGrath P J, Johnson G, Goodman J T et al 1985 The CHEOPS: A behavioral scale to measure post operative pain in children. In: Fields H L, Dubner R, Cervero F (eds) Advances in pain research and therapy. Raven Press, New York, p 395–402

McGrath P J, Hsu E, Cappelli M et al 1990 Pain from pediatric cancer: a survey of an outpatient oncology clinic. Journal of Psychosocial Oncology 8: 109–124

McGrath P J, Mathews J, Pigeon H 1991 Assessment of pain in children: a systematic psychosocial model. In: Bond M R, Charlton K E, Woolf C J (eds) Proceedings of the VIth World Congress on Pain. Pain research and clinical management, vol 5. Elsevier, Amsterdam, p 505–521

McGraw M B 1945 The neuromuscular maturation of the human infant. Hafner, New York

Maunuksela E L, Olkkola K T, Korpela R 1987 Measurement of pain in children with self-reporting and behavioral assessment. Clinical Pharmacology and Therapeutics 42: 137–141

Melzack R 1975 The McGill pain questionnaire: major properties and scoring methods. Pain 1: 227–299

Merskey H 1986 Classifications of chronic pain: descriptions of chronic pain syndromes and definitions of pain terms. Pain (suppl 3)

Norden J, Hannallah R, Getson P et al 1991 Concurrent validation of an objective pain scale for infants and children. Anesthesiology 75: A934

O'Hara M, McGrath P J, D'Astous J et al 1987 Oral morphine versus injected meperidine (Demerol) for pain relief in children after orthopedic surgery. Journal of Pediatric Orthopedic Surgery 7: 78–82

Pigeon H, McGrath P J, Lawrence J et al 1989 Nurses' perceptions of pain in the neonatal intensive care unit. Journal of Pain Symptom Management 4: 179–183

Porter F 1993 Pain assessment in children: infants. In: Schechter N L, Berde C B, Yaster M (eds) Pain in infants, children and adolescents. Williams & Wilkins, Baltimore, p 87–96

Porter F, Miller J P, Marshall R E 1987 Local anesthesia for painful medical procedures in sick newborns. Pediatric Research 21: 374

Rawlings D J, Miller P A, Engel R R 1980 The effect of circumcision on transcutaneous Po_2 in term infants. American Journal of Diseases of Children 13: 676–678

Richardson G M, McGrath P, Cunningham S J et al 1983 Validity of the headache diary for children. Headache 23: 184–187

Ross D M, Ross S A 1988 Childhood pain: current issues, research and management. Urban & Schwarzenberg, Baltimore

Savedra M C, Tesler M D 1989 Assessing children's and adolescents' pain. Pediatrician 16: 24–29

Savedra M C, Tesler M D, Holzemer W L, Wilkie D J, Ward J A 1990 Testing a tool to assess postoperative pediatric and adolescent pain. In: Tyler D C, Krane E J (eds) Advances in pain research and therapy: pediatric pain. Raven Press, New York, p 85–93

Stevens B 1990 Development and testing of a pediatric pain management sheet. Pediatric Nursing 16: 543–548

Szyfelbein S K, Osgood P F, Carr D B 1985 The assessment of pain and plasma beta-endorphin immunoactivity in burned children. Pain 22: 173–182

Tarbell S E, Cohen T, Marsh J L 1992 The Toddler-Preschool Postoperative Pain Scale: an observational scale for measuring postoperative pain in children aged 1–5. Preliminary report. Pain 50: 273–280

Thompson K L, Varni J W 1986 A developmental cognitive-biobehavioral approach to pediatric pain assessment. Pain 25: 283–296

Unruh A, McGrath P J, Cunningham S J et al 1983 Children's drawings of their pain. Pain 17: 385–392

Varni J W, Thompson K L Hanson V 1987 The Varni/ Thompson pediatric pain questionnaire. 1. Chronic musculo-skeletal pain in juvenile rheumatoid arthritis. Pain 28: 27–38

Walker L S, Greene J W 1991 The Functional Disability Inventory: measuring a neglected dimension of child health status. Journal of Pediatric Psychology 16: 39–58

Wall P D 1989 Introduction. In: Wall P D, Melzack R (eds) Textbook of pain, 2nd edn. Churchill Livingstone, Edinburgh, p 1–18

Whaley L, Wong D L 1987 Nursing care of infants and children, 3rd edn. Mosby, St. Louis

Wilkie D J, Holzemer W L, Tesler M D et al 1990 Measuring pain quality: validity and reliability of children's and adolescents' pain language. Pain 41: 151–159

Williamson P S, Williamson M L1983 Physiologic stress reduction by a local anesthetic during newborn circumcision. Pediatrics 71: 36–40

World Health Organization 1980 International Classification of Impairments, Disabilities and Handicaps. World Health Organization, Geneva

17. Studies of pain in normal man

Richard H. Gracely

INTRODUCTION

Studies of pain can be divided into three types: clinical studies in patients, research using laboratory animals and laboratory investigations using pain-free 'normal' human subjects. The two companion chapters in this section document the large body of knowledge that has been derived from clinical studies with patients in pain and from basic research using laboratory animals (see Chs 16 and 18). These approaches are indispensable and yet also limited. Clinical studies must contend with a 'stimulus' of often uncertain origin which can be neither controlled nor measured. Animal experiments are limited by interspecies differences and the difficulty of measuring the ultimate variable of interest – the amount of pain experienced by the organism. In addition, both animal and clinical studies are limited by ethical concerns. Studies must demonstrate an adequate 'suffering–benefit ratio' which balances expected pain and likely scientific or clinical benefit.

There is clearly a strong scientific and ethical need for studies of pain mechanisms in normal pain-free individuals. Such studies allow precise control of experimental stimulation, experimental interventions and increasingly sophisticated measurement techniques. They take full advantage of the human ability to subjectively evaluate both perceptual and conceptual magnitude.

This chapter will review the essential features of studies that use volunteer subjects to provide information relevant to the field of pain. Most, but not all, administer experimentally controlled somatic stimuli and measure a verbal, behavioural or physiological response. Some, such as studies of pain memory or those classifying pain descriptors, may involve pain concepts rather than pain sensations. Specific adaptations of experimental methods to clinical pain assessment also will be addressed in this chapter.

Many reviews of experimental pain methods begin with a consideration of the methods used to evoke and measure experimental pain stimulation. Sections on pain stimuli and response methods may be followed by examples of how these methods are used. This organization logically first describes the building blocks and then how they are assembled into pain experiments. Unfortunately, this approach may lead to an experimental myopia in which measurement tools are emphasized over the questions which are addressed by specific tools.

This chapter will emphasize the questions which can be investigated by studies in normal individuals. These problems can be divided into at least five overlapping categories:

1. Measurement development and validation
2. Assessment of analgesic efficacy
3. Evaluation of the underlying mechanisms of pain and pain control
4. Studies of psychological variables and constructs involved in pain experience and pain report
5. Use of experimental methods as an adjunct to clinical pain assessment.

These goals will be followed by sections on the properties of an ideal pain measure and an ideal pain stimulus, methods of experimental pain stimulation, and how these methods address ideal properties.

PAIN PROBLEMS STUDIED IN NORMAL INDIVIDUALS

MEASUREMENT DEVELOPMENT AND VALIDATION

Early measures of threshold and tolerance

Early investigations of pain sensation in pain-free volunteers focused on the pain threshold – the minimum amount of stimulation that reliably evoked a report of pain. These measures were later supplemented by measures of a pain tolerance – the time that a continuous stimulus is endured or the maximally tolerated stimulus intensity.

Threshold and tolerance measures are attractive because of their simplicity for both the administrator and the subject. In addition, the response is expressed in physical units of stimulus intensity or time, avoiding the subjectivity of a psychological scale of pain. These methods are still useful for many situations today, especially for the evaluation of sensory function in the clinic. However, the extensive use of these methods has revealed several limitations. Both threshold and tolerance are single measures usually associated with time or increasing intensity. A subject can easily be biased to respond sooner or later or to a lower or higher intensity. In addition, threshold measures only assess the very bottom of the pain sensory range and change in threshold may not reflect suprathreshold changes (e.g. hyperpathia, characterized by a raised threshold and increased suprathreshold sensitivity). Tolerance of a painful stimulus has been shown to be related to a separate endurance factor which is not associated with sensory intensity (Wolff 1971; Timmermans & Sternbach 1974).

The evolution of measurement methods from these simple threshold and tolerance procedures can be divided into three categories:

1. Methods that treat pain as a single dimension and that assess the range from pain threshold to intense pain levels
2. Separation of the single dimension of pain into two dimensions of sensory intensity and unpleasantness
3. Multidimensional assessment of the many attributes of pain sensation including its intensive, qualitative and aversive aspects.

Pain as a single dimension

Many, if not most, methods treat pain as a single dimension varying in magnitude, much like varying sound level by turning the volume knob on a radio. Pain magnitude has been assessed by both sophisticated measures of pain threshold and by classical indirect and direct psychophysical scaling methods. Pain magnitude also has been evaluated by novel scaling methods developed specifically for pain evaluation and by application of recent advances in subjective measurement.

Pain threshold

For practically all stimulus modalities (e.g. heat, pressure, electrical skin stimulation) increasing stimulus intensity results in a detection of a nonpainful sensation (detection threshold), followed by a range of prepain sensation and then a level at which this prepain sensation becomes painful (pain threshold). The pain threshold can be determined by the classical (Engen 1971a) Method of Limits (ascending and descending trials), Method of Adjustment (subject adjusts stimulus intensity) and Method of Constant Stimuli (set of fixed stimuli presented several times in a random sequence). The result of each method is a specific magnitude of stimulus intensity which is always an approximation since:

1. the pain threshold is not a discrete event but rather a probability function; the probability of attaining the threshold increases over a range of stimulus intensities and the probability function is evaluated directly by the Method of Constant Stimuli
2. the subjective criteria used to attach the label of pain to a specific sensation vary between, and within, individuals.

There have been simple and sophisticated applications of threshold methodology to pain assessment. The simplest methods use a modification of the Method of Limits. A good example is the Marstock method described by Fruhstorfer et al (1976). A thermal stimulus slowly increases or decreases from a neutral baseline and subjects indicate either warm or cool detection threshold, or heat or cold pain threshold, by a button-press which also either returns the stimulus to baseline or initiates a stimulus excursion in the opposite direction. Although this method lacks rudimentary psychophysical controls, it is very adequate for the large changes in threshold observed in neuropathic pain conditions.

In striking contrast to the detection of large changes by the simple Marstock method, other procedures use sophisticated judgment models to evaluate pain-scaling behaviour. The powerful methods of sensory decision theory (SDT) have been applied to the analysis of both pain thresholds and to category responses of suprathreshold pain sensations. This method yields not one but two parameters. The beta, or response criterion, parameter is a direct measure of the subjective criteria used to attach the label of pain. For example, the criteria may be stoical, labelling only clearly painful (or greater) sensations as pain. The second SDT parameter (classically called d′) is a measure of discrimination – that is, the ability to distinguish between two stimuli. The interpretation of discrimination as a measure of pain sensitivity (Clark & Yang 1983) has been controversial (Chapman 1977; Rollman 1977). One issue is the role of extraneous components of discrimination, since measures such as d′ are influenced by sensory variability and variability in choosing labels to describe sensations (Coppola & Gracely 1983). Thus, changes in discrimination do not necessarily indicate analgesia, although unchanged discrimination is evidence that pain sensitivity has not changed (Clark & Clark 1980).

The use of staircase or stimulus titration procedures is a third application/modification of threshold methods to pain assessment. These methods, described below, track threshold interactively; a positive response lowers the intensity of the next stimulus to be delivered while a negative response increases the intensity of the next stimulus.

Scaling suprathreshold pain sensation: response-dependent methods

Tolerance measures and the threshold procedures described above can be considered to be 'stimulus-dependent' methods since the dependent variable is an amount of stimulus intensity (or time) corresponding to a fixed response of pain threshold. In contrast, many of the suprathreshold scaling procedures can be classified as 'response-dependent' methods. These methods deliver a series of discrete stimuli of varying but fixed intensity in random sequence. The dependent variable is some measure of subjective response. These methods assume that subjects can meaningfully quantify the evoked sensation on a psychological scale of pain magnitude. These response-dependent methods vary in both the type of response and the analysis of these responses. Common responses include both discrete numerical (1–10) or verbal (mild, moderate, severe) categorical scales, continuous response dimensions such as the visual analogue scale (VAS) and the psychophysical scaling techniques of magnitude estimation and cross-modality matching.

Simple category scales such as the four-point 'none, mild, moderate and severe' or the common 1–10 numerical scale can be scored in several ways. The simplest, 'The Method of Equal Appearing Intervals', assigns successive integers to verbal categories or uses numerical categories directly (Engen 1971b). The more complex 'Method of Successive Categories' (Thurstone 1959) determines specific category values depending on the proportions of responses to each stimulus intensity. An additional approach (described below) determines specific numerical values for each category in a separate session. Subjects used several types of scaling methods to quantify the magnitude implied by each response category.

The VAS consists usually of a 10 cm line labelled at the anchor points with 'no pain' and 'most intense pain imaginable' or similar descriptions. Subjects indicate their pain magnitude by marking the line at the appropriate point. The ease of administration and scoring has contributed to the popularity of this method.

VAS and category scales have been compared in terms of sensitivity, distribution of responses and preference. Results of these studies appear equivocal. For example, the VAS has been described as superior in one study because it was more sensitive than a category scale (Joyce et al 1975) and superior in another study because it was less sensitive (Ohnhaus & Adler 1975). The reliability of both methods has been demonstrated repeatedly and they both generally produce equivalent results (Harms-Ringdahl et al 1986; M D Jensen et al 1986).

Both VAS and category scales are 'bounded', that is, they provide a limited range of measurement confined by fixed endpoints. When using these scales to describe a range of painful stimuli, subjects typically spread out their responses to cover the entire range of possible responses. In the extreme case, this tendency results in the same scale for any stimulus set. In most cases it makes VAS, category and other bounded scales very sensitive to stimulus range, spacing and frequency (Beck & Shaw 1965; Parducci 1974). This effect would tend to reduce the sensitivity of a scale to a pain-control intervention, since subjects would use the same responses before and after the manipulation. This effect has been demonstrated in pain assessment for a simulated analgesic (Gracely et al 1984) but it has not been investigated in any detail. Despite these theoretical limitations, VAS scales have been used successfully for assessment of the sensory intensity and unpleasantness of experimental pain sensations, and for the evaluation of the mechanisms and efficacy of both pharmacological and nonpharmacological interventions (Price 1988; Price & Harkins 1992). Use of longer VAS scales (Price 1988) and specific instructions appear to avoid many of the problems of bounded scales.

Many modern psychophysical scaling methods avoid the problem of bounded scales by the use of scales with an unbounded response range. The most widely used example is the method of magnitude estimation (ME) in which subjects describe the magnitude of the sensation evoked by the first stimulus with a number and then assign numbers to subsequent stimuli in proportion to this judgment (Engen 1971b). If the second sensation is judged twice as great as the first, the number given is twice that made to the first sensation. The first stimulus may be either arbitrary or fixed (the standard) and the first response value may be either arbitrary or fixed (the modulus). These methods theoretically result in ratio scales with a true zero point that allow multiplicative statements such as 'the pain is one-third of what it was before the analgesic'. Price and colleagues have also provided evidence that VAS scales also provide ratio-level measurement (Price 1988). Although the ratio properties of these various methods have been debated in both the psychophysical and pain literature (Gracely & Dubner 1981), these methods at least provide information about the spacing between response categories not found in conventional categorical scales. They also may be less sensitive to the biases associated with the bounded response range of VAS and category scales. ME has been used to assess both continuously increasing pain sensations (Hilgard 1975) and sensations evoked by discrete stimuli presented in random sequence (Fernandes de Lima et al 1982; Meyer et al 1985).

ME is actually a subset of a class of direct-ratio scaling techniques termed cross-modality matching (CMM). With these methods, subjects use any adjustable modality, such as the length of a line, duration of a tone or brightness of a light, to indicate perceptual magnitude of another modality. These methods have been used to scale pain sensation both directly (Gracely 1979) and indirectly. Duncan et al (1988b) have used an indirect CMM procedure, termed magnitude matching, to measure group differences in pain perception. Subjects used ME to scale the intensity of both painful thermal stimuli and the brightness of interspersed visual stimuli. Assuming the eccentric use of numbers would be expressed equally in ratings of the two stimulus sets, the data set is reduced to an indirect CMM function by expressing the response to the thermal stimuli in terms of brightness. The CMM method increased the assay sensitivity of the comparison of the two different groups (Duncan et al 1988b).

Another variant of CMM has been used to quantify verbal descriptors subsequently used for pain measurement (Tursky 1976; Gracely et al 1978a, 1978b). This approach presents a greater number of categories (e.g. 12) than typically used in a category scale, often in a random order. Subjects choose descriptors that best describe their sensation and the previously determined numbers are used for analysis. These scales result in a psychophysical function similar to that produced by CMM methods yet, unlike other scales, each judgment is anchored to a subjective descriptor standard, providing an absolute scale of measurement that may increase the validity of comparisons between groups. These methods have been used to assess the action of opioid analgesic and nonopioid agents such as nitrous oxide and amitriptyline in both laboratory and clinical settings (Heft et al 1978; Gracely et al 1979, 1982; Max et al 1987; Kaufman et al 1992). Verbal descriptors also permit random presentation of response choices, which requires a cognitive task that is uniquely different from other methods which require matching to a response space. Randomized response lists force responses based on the meaning of the descriptor rather than its spatial location in a list. Although possibly difficult for the subject, this method may be a particularly effective means of minimizing rating biases (e.g. spreading responses over the scale) found with bounded spatial scales.

Other suprathreshold scaling methods have combined verbal and VAS scales into graphic rating scales, which place descriptors in appropriate locations on an analogue continuum (Gracely et al 1978a; Heft & Parker 1984; Gracely 1991a). These and VAS scales have been incorporated into automated systems which can provide continuous measures of a pain sensation. Such measures can indicate pathological states, such as abnormally prolonged sensations, which are not evaluated by ordinary scaling methods (Cooper et al 1986; Gracely 1991a).

There have also been a few applications of more sophisticated methods of pain assessment. Two similar methods, functional measurement and conjoint measurement, require a single response to not one stimulus, but rather to an integrated impression of two or more stimuli. These stimuli can both be painful (Jones 1980; Heft & Parker 1984) or subjects can respond to a combination of pain evoked by somatosensory stimulation and pain implied by a verbal descriptor (Gracely & Wolskee 1983). These stimulus-integration methods provide more information than that available from single-stimulus, single-response designs. They simultaneously evaluate subjective magnitude and, in addition, evaluate each subject's ability to perform the scaling task.

Item response theory methods have also recently been applied to the analysis of categorical pain scales (McArthur et al 1989). These promising procedures examine the discriminative ability of each response category, providing a scientific basis for scale improvement.

Scaling suprathreshold pain sensation: stimulus-dependent methods

Stimulus-dependent methods are simply defined as procedures which use a physical measure of the stimulus as a dependent measure. While commonly used to measure pain threshold, these methods have been adapted to the assessment of suprathreshold pain sensation. In these methods, an interactive computer program continuously adjusts the intensity of stimuli so that some fall within specific response categories such as 'mild' and 'moderate' or 'moderate' and 'intense'. The algorithm for this adjustment can be based on either staircase rules (Gracely 1988; Gracely et al 1988b; Gracely & Gaughan 1991; Greenspan & Winfield 1992; Messinides & Naliboff 1992) or probability estimates (Duncan et al 1992). These stimulus-dependent scaling procedures may possess several advantages over commonly used response-dependent scales; they automatically equalize the psychological range of stimulus-evoked sensations, ensuring that all subjects receive a similar sensory experience. Equalization after administration of an analgesic intervention minimizes extraneous cues (e.g. reduced stimulus range) that perception has been altered. The response is expressed in units of stimulus intensity, avoiding assumptions about psychological magnitude and allowing comparison of effects across different experiments. The methods can also track the time course of an analgesic effect and provide information about scaling consistency.

This brief description of unidimensional pain measurement indicates how conventional measures like ME, or procedures such as randomized verbal descriptors, magnitude-matching, or stimulus-dependent scaling methods are adapted to the measurement of suprathreshold pain magnitude. These methods may control for specific biases such as those associated with spreading responses to cover the range of a scale. However, they do not address another important issue in subjective pain assessment: the measurement of all of the relevant dimensions of the pain experience.

Dual dimensions of sensory intensity and unpleasantness

The dual nature of pain has been recognized throughout philosophical and scientific history. Pain is both a somatic sensation and a powerful feeling state which evokes behaviours that minimize bodily harm and promote healing (Wall 1979). Single measures of pain magnitude blur this distinction and create confusion since the underlying meaning of either a pain magnitude or change in magnitude is not known.

This confusion may be minimized by scales which essentially ask, 'how intense is your sensation, and how much does it bother you?' There is a precedent for such scales, since the sensation of pain is not uniquely endowed with motivational characteristics. The chemical senses (taste, olfaction) and the thermal senses (warm, cool) can also be characterized by a sensory intensity and a feeling state. Studies with these modalities have demonstrated different psychophysical functions for scales of sensory intensity and 'hedonic' scales of pleasantness-unpleasantness. In addition, manipulation of internal state (core temperature, hunger) has been shown to shift the hedonic responses without altering judgments of sensory intensity (Gracely et al 1978b).

The applications of intensity and hedonic scales to pain assessment fall into three classes. The first uses different kinds of scale to measure the two dimensions, showing for example that preparatory information about expected postsurgical pain reduces unpleasantness, but not intensity ratings of postoperative pain (Johnson 1973). While this is probably valid, these methods confound the different dimensions with the type of scale; thus the results could be due to method variance and not to a differential effect of pain dimension (Gracely et al 1978b).

The second and third classes use the same type of scale to assess both dimensions. The second class establishes magnitude values for verbal descriptors of sensory intensity and unpleasantness, and uses the values to quantify descriptor choices (Gracely et al 1978a; Luu et al 1988, Tursky 1976; Duncan et al 1988b). The authors of these verbal scales have postulated a number of advantages, including the reduction of rating biases and the anchoring of each judgment to a subjective standard. The authors also point out that, unlike the senses of temperature, taste and smell, the hedonic dimension of pain is univalent, an unpleasantness growing monotonically with sensory intensity. Thus it may be more difficult to discriminate between the intensity and unpleasantness of pain sensations. The use of language specific to a dimension is assumed to facilitate the discrimination of these dimensions.

The validity and utility of verbal descriptor scales have been demonstrated in a number of studies (Duncan et al 1989; Gracely 1979, 1989, 1991b), including a demonstration that skin conductance responses classically conditioned to either intensity or unpleasantness descriptors using 100 db white noise would be evoked by additional descriptors from the same dimension, but not by descriptors from the other dimension (Jamner & Tursky 1987).

The third class has used VAS scales to separately assess pain intensity and unpleasantness. The results of several studies (Price 1988) suggest that the combination of instructions to the subject and the labels on a VAS scale ('the most intense pain sensation imaginable', 'the most unpleasant feeling imaginable') are sufficient for discrimination of intensity and unpleasantness. These results suggest that the increased complexity of verbal methods is not needed and problems of verbal methods, such as use with different languages, can be avoided by using VAS scales. On the other hand, studies which have directly compared verbal and VAS scales have shown greater discriminative power with the verbal methods (Gracely 1979; Gracely et al 1978b; Duncan et al 1989). The ability of subjects to describe these dimensions with each method, and the role of instructions and training, are obvious topics for future research.

The nonsensory aspect of pain experience has been termed the reaction component, the emotional component, the affective component, the evaluative component and other terms such as discomfort, distress and suffering. The number and structure of these components have not been firmly established, although recent proposals included both an immediate unpleasantness component similar to the feelings associated with other senses and a secondary affective component which includes emotions and feelings of distress mediated through cognitive appraisals (Wade et al 1990; Price & Harkins 1992; Gracely 1991a, 1992). These types of studies and those described in the next section, should continue to clarify the feeling and emotional components of pain sensation.

Two points are relevant in comparisons of dual scales of sensory intensity and unpleasantness to the multidimensional scales and scaling methods described below. First, separate scales of sensory intensity and unpleasantness, and derivatives of such scales, assess dimensions common to all types of pain, whether chronic, acute or experimental. These scales provide a common language useful in describing and comparing the variety of pain experience. In contrast, multidimensional scales emphasize the differences between pain sensations, the distinguishing features which separate various pain syndromes. Second, sensory intensity and unpleasantness scales are a priori scales in the sense that they assume two significant dimensions of pain. In contrast, multidimensional methods empirically determine the number and character of relevant dimensions. They do not make a priori assumptions about the structure of pain experience.

Multiple pain dimensions

Our own experience verifies the variety of pain qualities. Pain can be deep or superficial, pricking, burning, throbbing, aching or shooting. This breadth of pain experience is evaluated in normal individuals by three types of study:

1. Multidimensional scaling of experimentally-evoked pain sensation to determine scale dimensions
2. Multidimensional scaling of verbal descriptor items to construct a scale or verify the structure of an existing scale
3. Use of existing scales to assess experimentally-evoked pain sensations.

Examples of the first type are provided by multidimensional scaling of sensations evoked by electrical or thermal stimulation (Clark et al 1986). Ten-point similarity judgments of sensations evoked by all possible stimulus pairs could be characterized by two dimensions. The predominant dimension was related to sensory intensity, while a secondary dimension appeared to be related to the 'painfulness' of the stimulus-evoked sensations (Clark et al 1986; Janal et al 1991).

Examples of the second type include several studies which have examined the structure of the McGill Pain Questionnaire (MPQ), which is the most widely-used multidimensional instrument. This instrument and related studies are discussed in Chapter 18. The questionnaire was developed from a study by Melzack & Torgerson (1971) in which a large number of pain descriptors were classified into ultimately 20 categories describing sensory qualities, affective qualities and an evaluative dimension. A total of 78 descriptors appear in the present instrument, with two to six descriptors per category. Subsequent studies have replicated this method, or derived a structure by use of multidimensional scaling methods (Kwilosz et al 1983; Reading et al 1982; Boureau & Paquette 1988). Results of these experiments confirm the two main dimensions of sensory intensity and affect/unpleasantness, but have resulted in different category assignments and variations in the overall organizational scheme of hierarchical categories (Kwilosz et al 1983). The most recent and extensive of these studies has been performed by Torgerson and colleagues (Torgerson et al 1988), who have developed the ideal type model which rates each descriptor on an intensity continuum and, in addition, quantifies 'quality' in terms of a number of primary ideal qualities or types. The number of primary qualities and the degree to which each of them contributes to a specific descriptor are specified, much like the primary components of a colour mixture. The MPQ, in contrast, assigns only one quality to each descriptor. A review of all of these descriptor structures reveals many commonalities. Pain sensation is described by thermal qualities, by temporal patterning, by location or changing location (superficial or deep, spreading, moving) and by a series of mechanical qualities such as punctate, traction and compression pressure. New analyses have made finer distinctions. For example, the ideal type model places 'pricking' and 'stabbing' in a class separate from 'drilling' and 'boring', distinguished by the rotational character of the latter class. The most variability appears in the affective components of pain, with dimensions that describe unpleasantness, suffering, fear, autonomic reactions and fatigue. A more extensive treatment of these dimensions can be found in Chapter 18.

The third class uses multidimensional scales to assess the magnitude and quality of pain sensations produced by experimental stimulation. Few such studies have been performed since these scales are used predominantly in clinical evaluations. An early study compared the responses of both patients and normal subjects receiving painful electrical skin stimulation (Crockett et al 1977). A factor analysis identified five common factors, emphasizing the utility of assessing common dimensions of experimental and clinical pain. Another experiment by Klepac et al (1991) assessed high or low levels of either cold pressor pain or electrical tooth pulp pain in a 2 × 2 factorial design. Overall intensity scores differentiated the two types of stimulation, which also resulted in qualitatively different responses. The authors noted the problems of statistically evaluating quality differences by chi-square analyses and single-item tests.

Nonverbal measures

Mistrust of verbal judgments has motivated the development of physiological and behavioural 'objective measures' of pain magnitude that should be relatively insensitive to biasing factors and the psychological demands associated with requests for introspective reports (Craig & Prkachin 1983). In addition, these methods are the only measures available for pain assessment in animals and in infants or in adults with poorly developed language skills.

Although arguments have been made for exclusive use of nonverbal methods, these procedures also can be influenced by extraneous factors. In addition, nonverbal methods lack the face validity of verbal report. They use similarity to verbal report to establish concurrent validity, suggesting that verbal measures are preferable if available.

Generally, arguments for the superiority of one method over another often reflect the tendency of research laboratories to specialize in a single measurement method. The resulting differences have sparked lively debates, identified important measurement flaws and generally improved the technology of pain assessment. However, more effective pain assessment may ultimately result from an approach that integrates information from these separate, yet complementary sources of information (Luu et al 1988; Cleeland 1989; Craig 1989; Boureau et al 1991).

Behavioural measures

It is well known that pain elicits stereotypical behaviours in both man and animals. Grimace, vocalization, licking, limping and rubbing are often elicited by a painful stimulus. Both these naturally-occurring reactions and trained operant behaviours (such as manipulating a bar to escape a painful stimulus) have been used to assess magnitude of stimulus-evoked pain sensation. Many have been used more extensively for assessment of clinical pain syndromes (Keefe & Block 1982; Craig & Prkachin 1983; Keefe & Dolan 1986; McDaniel et al 1986). Recent exceptions include studies of facial expression evoked by experimental stimulation (Craig & Patrick 1985; Patrick et al 1986) or analysis of pain expressions from photographs (LeReshe 1982).

The behavioural measure of reaction time latency to pain produced by a contact thermode has been shown to be monotonically related to stimulus intensity, permitting the use of reaction time, in controlled conditions, as a measure of pain magnitude (Gracely et al 1987; Kenshalo et al 1989).

Physiological measures

The search for a physiological pain measure more objective than verbal report has a long and largely fruitless history. Autonomic measures such as heart rate, skin conductance and temperature have been correlated with painful stimulation. Although influenced by painful stimulation, these responses habituate quickly and respond nonspecifically to nonpainful stressing or novel stimulation (Bromm & Scharein 1982). Measures of cortical-evoked potentials have been studied extensively and under certain conditions correlate with both stimulus intensity and verbal report (Fernandes de Lima et al 1982; Chudler & Dong 1983; Hill & Chapman, 1989). Cortical activity has also been assessed recently by analysis of noncontingent electroencephalogram (EEG) (Chen et al 1989; Veerasarn & Stohler 1992) and by nuclear magnetic resonance (NMR) techniques (Hari et al 1985).

Two issues are pertinent in the evaluation of these and other nonverbal methods. The first is the relationship between the measure and subjective reports of pain. In the case of brain activity, reports of good agreement are counterbalanced by examples of dissociation in which the amplitudes of evoked potentials do not covary with pain reports (Chapman et al 1981; Chudler & Dong 1983; Benedetti et al 1984; Willer et al 1987; Klement et al 1992). This dissociation does not condemn their utility for pain measurement, but rather defines the boundaries within which measurement is acceptable. Dissociation is also beneficial for the second issue, the use of these methods for evaluation of mechanisms of pain and analgesia. This issue is discussed in the following section on mechanisms of pain and pain-control interventions.

Willer and others (Chan & Tsang 1985; DeBroucker et al 1989; Willer et al 1989) have used measures of reflex activity (e.g. blink, H and nociceptive reflex) as objective measures of pain sensation. Results with these measures are similar to those with measures of brain activity. Reflex amplitude has correlated with stimulus intensity and verbal report and has been altered appropriately by a number of pharmacological and nonpharmacological interventions. However, these measures have also been dissociated, possibly defining both conditions for acceptable pain measurement and a means of analysing pain mechanisms (Bromm & Treede 1980; Luu et al 1988; Price 1989; Campbell et al 1991).

Neurophysiological recording methods commonly employed in animal research have been used to investigate peripheral mechanisms in unanaesthetized normal volunteers (Vallbo & Hagbarth 1968). Human microneurography is a powerful tool which can:

1. Compare intervening primary afferent activity to both the evoking stimulus and the resulting sensation
2. Stimulate through the recording electrode and evaluate the resulting sensation and projected sensory field (location of evoked pain sensation).

These techniques can identify all classes of primary afferent fibres and have verified the association of specific sensations with type of fibre stimulated (Torejörk & Hallin 1970; Van Hees & Gybels 1972). The recent use of microneurography in experimental studies of neuropathic pain mechanisms is described below.

ASSESSMENT OF ANALGESIC EFFICACY

The evaluation of analgesic efficacy has been a classical goal of studies using experimental stimulation (Beecher 1959; Gracely 1991b). A validated technique promised to avoid the uncontrolled and highly variable nature of the pain 'stimulus' associated with clinical syndromes, and its report. The pioneering studies enjoyed an initial success, followed by criticism and repeated failures. Methodological improvements resulted in renewed success with the demonstration of opioid analgesia, which is routinely observed in present experiments (Gracely 1991b).

Many of the important features of present methods evolved from these early studies. Initially, successful methods used the pain threshold to thermal stimuli as the dependent measure in uncontrolled studies. Positive effects vanished with the introduction of double-blind placebo controls, but reappeared with the use of severe, long-lasting pain sensations produced by the continuous, increasing pain of the tourniquet ischaemia technique (Beecher 1959; Smith et al 1966) or by the use of discrete stimuli to stimulate an increasing, continuous pain sensation (Parry et al 1972). The demonstration of opioid analgesia with these stimulus modalities was attributed to their severity, which was deemed sufficient to evoke a sufficient 'reaction component', an affective component associated with clinically significant pain but not usually found with brief discrete stimuli. Present evidence suggests that this success was not due to the reaction component but rather to the use of suprathreshold stimulation. A wide range of discrete suprathreshold stimuli (e.g. thermal stimuli from a contact thermode or laser), double-blind placebo controls and several response methods have repeatedly demonstrated significant effects of both pharmacological and nonpharmacological pain control interventions. Nonetheless, the reaction component has remained an influential concept in pain measurement and treatment.

Presently, experimental demonstrations of opiate analgesia are practically taken for granted. A recent review cited 34 reports showing analgesia to pain evoked by thermal, electrical, cold pressor and tourniquet ischaemia (Gracely 1991b). These studies have now moved beyond the mere establishment of an effect to demonstrations of dose response (Price et al 1985b; Gracely 1988), effects of infusion rate (Gracely et al 1988a), effects of real or simulated potentiation (Price et al 1985a; Gracely & Gaughan 1991), influence of central summation mechanisms (Gracely et al 1987; Price 1988; Brennum et al 1991, 1992) and relationship between subjective report and neurophysiological measures (Willer & Bussel 1980; Willer 1985; Luu et al 1988; Bromm 1989).

Studies of weaker analgesics have been performed less frequently and the results are less consistent. The weak opiate codeine has been shown to be analgesic both in older studies by Wolff et al using electrical stimulation (1969) and in recent experiments using cold pressor (Garcia de Jalon et al 1985) and tourniquet ischaemia (Posner 1984). Peripherally acting nonsteroidal anti-inflammatory drugs (NSAIDs), such as aspirin or ibuprofen, have significantly reduced measures of experimental pain in some studies (Bromm & Seide 1982; Smith & Beecher 1969; Chen & Chapman 1980; Rohdewald et al 1982; Forster et al 1988) but not others (Posner 1984; Garcia de Jalon et al 1985; Telekes et al 1987; Jones et al 1988). These conflicting results could be due to a number of factors, including experimental error, weak potency and the use of an inadequate stimulus. This variability may reflect the mechanism of action (see next section). The NSAID class of drugs is presumed to have a peripheral site of action and experimental pain stimuli showing analgesia (pressure but not cold-pressor pain) may preferentially activate mechanisms which can be modulated by NSAID action. However, positive results with electrical skin stimulation also implicate central modes of NSAID action since the effect of electrical stimulation, which is assumed to directly activate primary afferent axons, should not be influenced by peripheral agents acting at the receptor level. A central NSAID effect is supported by a recent study by Willer and colleagues, discussed under reflex activity below.

Methods using experimental pain stimulation in normal individuals have also been used to assess the effects of other drugs, including positive, but modest, effects with nitrous oxide (thermal skin stimulation, electrical tooth pulp stimulation), ketamine (tourniquet ischaemia) and imipramine (electrical skin stimulation) (Gracely 1991b; Kaufman et al 1992).

The efficacy of nonpharmacological treatments has been assessed in a number of studies in normal subjects. Somatic treatments such as acupuncture or transcutaneous electrical nerve stimulation (TENS) have been investigated by several stimulation methods. Recent studies have shown no effect of laser acupuncture in either normal volunteers (Brockhaus & Elger 1990) or patients (Haker & Lundeberg 1990). Analgesic effects of needle acupuncture have been demonstrated in several experimental studies, although the relative roles of central, segmental and peripheral mechanisms have not been firmly established (Mayer et al 1977; Chapman et al 1983; Price et al 1984; Ernst & Lee 1985; Yan & Zonglian 1989; Moret et al 1991).

Studies of TENS in normal volunteers have produced variable results, varying over types of pain stimulation and TENS parameters. Positive effects have been observed with cold-pressor pain (greatest at TENS frequency of 40 Hz) and tourniquet ischaemia, and with thermal pain thresholds but only with high TENS stimulation currents (Eriksson et al 1985; Sjölund & Eriksson 1985; Johnson et al 1989).

Psychological treatments include methods such as hypnosis and meditation. A large number of studies have been performed evaluating hypnotic modification of painful stimuli, many with cold-pressor pain (Hilgard 1975; Spanos 1986; Houle et al 1988; Walther & Gracely 1988; Moret et al 1991). Hypnosis has also modified pain sensations evoked by thermal stimulation (Price & Barber 1987; Walther & Gracely 1988), electrical tooth pulp stimulation (Barber & Mayer 1977; Houle et al 1988) and radio-frequency heating of the chest cavity (Reeves et al 1983).

Meditation exercises, in comparison to relaxation procedures, have reduced ratings of painful cold-pressor or heat stimuli when performed by either experienced (Mills & Farrow 1981) or naive subjects trained for 6 weeks (Gaughan et al 1990). Both of these studies found greater effects with scales of pain unpleasantness than with scales of pain sensory intensity.

Relevance

Studies that assess analgesic efficacy by experimental methods have been criticized for being clinically irrelevant. Critics rightfully point out that laboratory administration of experimentally painful stimuli cannot duplicate the physiological features of an acute or chronic pain condition, or the accompanying psychological features such as anxiety, uncertainty, suffering and foreboding. However, this inability to exactly duplicate clinical pain syndromes only imposes modest limits on the inferential utility of these methods. The consistent results with opiates suggest that the antinociceptive efficacy of opioid agonists or antagonists can be evaluated using laboratory procedures. It is likely that any intervention which shows experimental efficacy will also show clinical efficacy. The important issues may relate to whether does and potency relationships established experimentally predict clinical findings and whether the models are developed sufficiently to predict accurately poor clinical analgesic action.

The usefulness of experimental models naturally extends beyond the measurement of *if* an analgesic works to *why* it works, to the identification of mechanisms of analgesic action. The next section describes experimental investigations of the mechanisms of pain and pain control.

EVALUATION OF THE MECHANISMS OF PAIN AND PAIN CONTROL

Laboratory methods with normal individuals provide a powerful tool for the investigation of mechanisms of pain and interventions which relieve pain. Examples are identified below, progressing from the receptor level to central processes.

Peripheral mechanisms

Burning a toe results in two pain sensations: an immediate sharp pricking pain, followed after about 1 second by a dull, diffuse, burning pain. The mechanisms of these first and second pain sensations have been identified and explored by studies using trains of intense heat or electrical stimuli (Price et al 1977, 1985b; Cooper et al 1986; Gracely et al 1987). These experiments reveal that the first pain sensation is mediated by the thinly myelinated Aδ nociceptor afferents, while the second pain sensation is mediated by the unmyelinated C-fibre nociceptor afferents. If the stimuli are repeated every 3 seconds or less, the first pain sensation is quickly suppressed via a peripheral mechanism and the magnitude of the second pain increases via a central summation mechanism. Opiates selectively attenuate second pain and second pain summation, although a small effect has also been observed for first pain sensations.

Neurophysiological measures have also identified responses specific to primary afferent fibre classes. Many studies of cerebral-evoked potentials, nociceptive reflexes and nerve conduction evoke pain sensation by electrical stimulation of the skin surface. At pain-evoking intensities, this stimulus activates all fibre classes, so that measures such as evoked potential amplitudes contain a contribution from nonpain-related inputs, including those from the large-diameter Aβ fibres mediating tactile sensation (Dowman 1991). The effect of this Aβ component is reported to be minimized by use of an electrocutaneous stimulus applied beneath the skin surface (Bromm & Meier 1984) or avoided by the use of laser thermal stimulation (Bromm 1989).

In many studies, nociceptive components that elicit the cerebral-evoked potential appear to be evoked by the thinly myelinated Aδ afferents which mediate first-pain sensation. Blocking Aδ-mediated pain abolished this component (Harkins et al 1983), resulting in either no response using electrical stimuli and conventional averaging techniques or revealing a late C-fibre mediated component if laser stimuli and single trial or power analyses are used (Bromm & Treede 1987; Arendt-Nielsen 1990).

The section below on evaluation of experimental and clinical neuropathic pain describes how the methods of microneurography can be used to identify both peripheral and central mechanisms.

Reflex activity

Several measures of reflex activity, such as the H reflex, the nociceptive reflex and the blink reflex have been investigated in human subjects. The results of several studies suggest that these reflexes can serve as a physiological correlate of subjective pain. These measures have been attenuated by opiates such as morphine, have demonstrated stress-produced changes antagonized by naloxone and have been correlated with other physiological parameters such as cerebral-evoked potentials or concentration of circulating opioids (Willer 1977, 1985; Willer & Bussel 1980; Willer et al 1981, 1982; Facchinetti et al 1984; Chan & Tsang 1985; McMilan & Moudy 1986; Dowman 1991). These reflex measures have been shown to correlate with verbal report, although recent studies have demonstrated nonlinear relationships at high intensities of radiant heat stimuli (Campbell et al 1991) or dissociations of reflex and subjective measures, either between patient and pain-free volunteers (Boureau et al 1991) or after low doses of morphine (Luu et al 1988). The dissociations may provide an informative tool for the localization of analgesic actions, separating spinal from supraspinal processes.

An example of identifying the location of analgesic actions is provided by recent studies of reflex responses, cortical-evoked potentials and microneurography. NSAIDs have been presumed to act peripherally by mechanisms such as inhibition of prostaglandin production associated with inflammation. However, recent studies suggest a central action for NSAID-class drugs. Aspirin has been observed to attenuate late cerebral potentials, an effect associated with central processing (Chen & Chapman 1980). Zompirac has been shown to reduce the magnitude of pain sensations evoked by direct intraneural stimulation, bypassing any possible peripheral mechanisms (Schady & Torebjörk 1984). Willer et al (1989) found that the NSAID, ketoprofen, altered the nociceptive reflex evoked by electrical skin stimulation in normals but not in paraplegic patients. This intriguing finding implicates a central site of NSAID action and indicates that this central effect is mediated by descending inhibition of spinal activity.

Neural mechanisms of peripheral neuropathic pain syndromes

Anyone who has had a sunburn has encountered a clinical condition in which the skin is spontaneously painful and both innocuous stimuli and previously subthreshold noxious stimuli evoke pain sensations. These symptoms are present in neuropathic pain syndromes such as reflex sympathetic dystrophy and causalgia. Patients experience both spontaneous pain, usually in an extremity, and often exhibit mechano-allodynia: lightly brushing or touching the skin evokes sharp, stinging and burning pain sensations. They may also exhibit hyperalgesia, in which the pain of noxious stimulation is enhanced. These syndromes result in severe pain and functional limitations; patients zealously guard the affected limb, avoiding contact with bed sheets or clothes. These problematic conditions resist conventional analgesic treatments. Even large doses of powerful opiates offer little relief.

The recent development of an experimental human model of these neuropathic syndromes is an excellent example of the usefulness of pain studies in normal subjects. Intradermal injection of 100 μg of capsaicin, the active ingredient in chili pepper, into the skin of the volar forearm immediately evokes a profound, burning, stinging, primary pain sensation. The correspondence between the features of this experimental model and those of clinical syndromes is dramatic; patients and experimental volunteers use the same language to describe abnormal sensations evoked by similar stimuli (Gracely et al, unpublished observations).

The effects of a capsaicin injection are examined by administration of painful, and especially nonpainful, stimuli. Touch sensation, mediated by Aβ low-threshold mechanoreceptors (Aβ-LTMs), is often assessed by graded nylon monofilaments (von Frey hairs) or cotton wisps, which usually produce a faint tactile sensation at levels near detection threshold. Mechano-allodynia is indicated when detection-level stimulation evokes a painful sensation. However, pain evoked by these mechanical stimuli does not indicate the fibre types mediating allodynia since this pain could occur from either activation of Aβ-LTMs or sensitized nociceptors. Low-intensity electrical stimuli similarly produce tactile sensations at detection threshold and pain at detection also indicates allodynia. The results with electrical stimulation, however, can indicate that these pain sensations are mediated by Aβ-LTMs. The effects of electrical stimulation are especially informative because, at detection, this stimulus is always an Aβ-LTM stimulus. This exclusivity is due to the fact that:

1. Electrical stimulation activates afferent axons directly, bypassing receptors (and is thus independent of receptor processes such as sensitization)
2. The largest fibres (Aβ-LTMs) are the most sensitive to electrical stimulation and are the only fibres activated at detection threshold levels of stimulation.

Nonpainful thermal stimuli play an important role in these sensory assessments by indirectly monitoring the functional capacity of nociceptor subclasses. For example, the sensation of cool is mediated by the thinly myelinated Aδ fibres and altered cool sensation threshold (during differential blocks or in disease processes) can be used to infer Aδ nociceptive afferent function. Similarly, warmth detection, mediated by C-fibres, can be used in the same manner to infer the functioning or involvement of C-fibre nociceptors.

The activity of specific fibres may also be monitored, or evoked, by microneurographic recordings of primary afferent nerves in human subjects (Torebjörk et al 1992).

The application of these methods to the capsaicin experiments has revealed underlying neural mechanisms. They essentially duplicate the procedures used in the historic studies by Lewis (1936) and Hardy et al (1952) and more recent experiments using experimental burns (Raja et al 1984). An intradermal injection of capsaicin produces four concentric areas of altered sensation which surround the injection site and persist for varying amounts of time. The smallest area is an analgesic bleb at the injection site (Simone et al 1989; LaMotte et al 1991), surrounded by an area of primary hyperalgesia, which testing with painful and nonpainful thermal stimuli indicates is probably mediated by C-fibres. This area of primary hyperalgesia is surrounded by an area of mechano-allodynia, which testing with electrical stimuli indicates is probably mediated by Aβ–LTMs (Gracely et al 1993; Koltzenberg et al 1992). Aβ–LTM mechano-allodynia is confirmed by a recent study which also demonstrates the usefulness of microneurography (Torebjörk et al 1992). Electrical intraneural stimulation at levels which normally evoked only touch sensations evoked painful sensations when these sensations were located in an area of allodynia resulting from the capsaicin injection. In addition, the threshold for painful intraneural stimulation, usually much higher than the threshold for nonpainful detection, was reduced to the nonpainful detection level during the capsaicin-produced allodynia. The fourth and largest area is characterized by secondary hyperalgesia; the pain from a light pin prick is dramatically pronounced.

The sensory tests used in capsaicin studies have played a major role in clinical studies of peripheral neuropathic pain syndromes. (These results are presented briefly here since they depend on common experimental methodologies.) These experiments have identified a few cases in which mechano-allodynia may be mediated by sensitized nociceptors (Cline et al 1989) and many cases in which it is mediated by Aβ–LTMs. Aβ–LTM involvement is based on five lines of evidence from studies using experimental stimulation:

1. As discussed above, electrical stimuli at detection threshold are painful (Price et al 1989; Gracely et al 1992).
2. Reaction times to electrical or mechanical stimuli are consistent with Aβ–LTM conduction velocities (Lindblom & Verrillo 1979; Fruhstorfer & Lindblom 1984; Campbell et al 1988; Gracely et al 1992).
3. During differential local anaesthetic blocks, touch and mechano-allodynia return while cool and warm fibres (and hence nociceptors) are still blocked (Dubner et al 1987; Campbell et al 1988; Gracely et al 1992).
4. During ischaemic or pressure blocks, touch and mechano-allodynia are abolished while cool and warm sensation, and thus activity in Aδ and C-fibre nociceptors, is not blocked (Wallin et al 1976; Meyer et al 1985; Campbell et al 1988; Gracely et al 1992).
5. Exclusive stimulation of Aβ–LTMs through microneurographic electrodes is painful (Torebjörk et al 1992).

With these methods, parallel studies in patients and in normal volunteers receiving capsaicin indicate that Aβ–LTM mechano-allodynia is mediated by a central process which is dynamically maintained by ongoing input from peripheral activity in nociceptive afferents (Gracely et al 1992; LaMotte et al 1992; Torebjörk et al 1992).

Central transmission and modulation

The above studies indicate that peripheral neuropathic pain involves both peripheral generators and central, probably spinal, mechanisms. Several types of experimental pain studies have provided information about spinal processing of nociceptive input. While many laboratories specialize in one stimulation method, Brennum et al (1991, 1992) have administered a large number of stimulus modalities in investigations of the effects of epidural infiltrations in normal subjects. They found that 4 mg of epidural morphine raised the pain threshold for slowly increasing stimulation by pressure, heat pain (and cooling) and increased the tolerance to pressure, thermal and electrical stimulation. Ratings of pain evoked by brief, discrete electrical (1 ms), mechanical (20 ms) and laser (200 ms) stimuli were not altered by morphine. Using the same stimuli in a different study, these investigators found that epidural lidocaine had the opposite effect, attenuating the ratings of the brief discrete stimuli with little effect on the other measures. The authors concluded that morphine inhibits central integration of prolonged stimuli, with little effect on brief stimuli, while lidocaine is effective for brief stimuli, but is partially countered by central integration mechanisms.

The role of spinal integration mechanisms has been investigated in studies by Price et al (1977, 1985b). Human psychophysical studies are consistent with physiological results in primates showing that brief thermal stimuli produce summation in second-order wide-dynamic-range (WDR) neurons if these stimuli are administered at rates of 0.3 Hz or faster. More recent studies show that patients with mechano-allodynia who showed temporal summation to light mechanical stimuli at these frequencies also reported greater spontaneous pain magnitude (Price et al 1992). This correspondence suggests that spinal summation mechanisms may contribute to the magnitude of ongoing pain in these patients.

Spinal projection neurons have also been investigated in a study that measured pain evoked by direct stimulation of spinal neurons (Mayer et al 1975). This study varied the intrapair interval of electrical pulse pairs applied to the exposed spinal (anterolateral quadrant) cord in patients undergoing cordotomy for relief of intractable pain. This technique places the second pulse of the pair in or out of the relative refractory period of the axons of the specific neuronal populations, resulting in either one or two action potentials per pulse pair from that population. The transition from one to two potentials results in increased pain; in this case the increase was noted with intrapair intervals corresponding to axons with refractory periods similar to those of WDR neurons identified in the monkey (Price & Mayer 1975). The properties of anterolateral quadrant neurons have also been assessed in man by using percutaneous electrodes to record the averaged potentials evoked by skin stimulation (Campbell & Lipton 1983).

The central consequences of experimental painful stimulation

Measures of spontaneous and evoked EEG have been used to construct brain surface maps that localize the central activity produced by experimental painful stimulation. Recently, two laboratories have published three-dimensional images of brain activity derived from positron emission tomography (PET) measures during painful stimulation. Talbot et al (1991) showed pain-related activity in SI, SII and anterior cingulate cortex. This pain-specific activity was determined by subtracting activity from warm 41–42°C stimulation of six spots on the forearm from activity following painful thermal stimuli of 49–49°C applied to the same spots. Jones et al (1991), using a similar method but stimulating only one spot with 46–47°C, also found activity in the anterior cingulate cortex and, in addition, activity in lateral thalamus and basal ganglia. These initial findings suggest that the anterior cingulate cortex may be involved in processing the affective components of pain. This hypothesis is consistent with clinical pain relief produced after surgical ablation of the anterior portion of the cingulate cortex (Gybels & Sweet 1989). Further imaging studies will hopefully explore this concept and also reconcile differences between these two studies.

Experimental painful and nonpainful stimuli have also been used in a recent series of experiments by Lenz and colleagues (Seike et al 1991; Lenz et al 1993). Using a specially developed verbal scale to quickly measure pain quality, Lenz trained patients to rate sensations evoked by a wide range of mechanical and thermal stimuli. During a subsequent brain operation for motor abnormalities, Lenz repeated this procedure while recording from the principal sensory nucleus of the thalamus (Vc) and also used the scale to measure sensations evoked by thalamic microstimulation. Preliminary findings indicate that preoperative training facilitates the discrimination of intraoperative pain qualities – for example, revealing that both thermal and pain sensation can be evoked by microstimulation posterior and inferior to Vc.

Experimental methodology has also been applied to patients with central pain syndromes, which are particularly difficult to evaluate and treat. The diagnosis is often based on central nervous system damage from either a hamorrhage or infarct or other conditions such as tumour metastasis. These patients often present with a profound disturbance of pain and temperature sensibility (Boivie et al 1989; Leijon et al 1989; Holmgren et al 1990; Greenspan & Winfield 1992). Experimental stimulation with mechanical, electrical and thermal stimuli applied to both the affected and unaffected areas has verified that the spontaneous pain is associated with lesions in the spinothalamic tract, with few differences observed between lesions at different levels (Cassinari & Pagni 1969). Application of recent techniques may improve the evaluation of these syndromes (Gracely 1991a). For example, cortical-evoked potentials of electrical and thermal stimuli may distinguish between lemniscal and spinothalamic mechanisms (Treede & Bromm 1991).

Mechanism of nonpharmacological treatments

Studies of hypnotic analgesia and the effects of relaxation and meditation exercises have identified factors involved in the production and assessment of pain reduction. Several studies have found that experimental analgesia can be predicted by individual differences in hypnotic responsiveness. A novel method of radio-frequency heating of the chest cavity showed that analgesic effects were correlated with hypnotic susceptibility (Reeves et al 1983). Another experiment found that susceptibility was associated with analgesia assessed by the cold-pressor method, which is easily simulated (Gracely 1991b), but not to analgesia assessed by a thermal staircase method which is less easily simulated (Walther & Gracely 1988).

The recent development of dual scales of pain intensity and unpleasantness may further clarify the effects of susceptibility. Price & Barber (1987) found that hypnotic attenuation of thermal pain sensations was modestly correlated with standard measures of susceptibility ($r = 0.4$), with a greater association at higher stimulus intensities. The authors also observed a powerful reduction of pain unpleasantness which was not associated with susceptibility. Using highly susceptible subjects, Malone et al (1989) found that specific suggestion of analgesia reduced verbal descriptor responses of sensory intensity of painful sensations evoked by electrical skin stimulation, with nonsignificant reductions of unpleasantness responses. Specific suggestions of relaxation showed an opposite effect, reducing unpleasantness but not sensory intensity responses. The influence of susceptibility was not reported. In contrast, Houle et al (1988) found similar effects of relaxation and hypnosis but a differential effect of stimulation method: hypnosis and relaxation reduced both the intensity and unpleasantness of pain evoked by electrical tooth pulp stimulation, but only unpleasantness ratings of pain evoked by the cold pressor method. Hypnotic susceptibility was not related to the effects. The previously mentioned studies of meditation have also shown greater effects on measures of pain unpleasantness (Mills & Farrow 1981; Gaughan et al 1990).

The mechanisms of hypnotic analgesia have also been investigated in studies comparing subjective reports and evoked cortical potentials to painful stimuli. Arendt-Nielsen et al (1990) found that suggestions of analgesia and hyperaesthesia produced corresponding changes in both subjective ratings and cerebral potentials evoked by a laser stimulus in highly susceptible subjects. In contrast, Meier et al (1993) found that suggestions of either analgesia or hyperaesthesia produced expected changes in subjective ratings made to electrocutaneous stimuli in highly susceptible subjects, but no change in evoked potentials. Scores on the MPQ indicated that the major change in response was in the choice of affective-evaluative words and not in the sensory dimensions. The authors concluded that the hypnotic effect was thus primarily on the unpleasantness component of pain assessed by these measures and not on the sensory dimension assessed either by the evoked potentials or the sensory dimensions of the MPQ.

These studies show that nonpharmacological interventions such as hypnosis may be mediated via independent effects on sensory intensity and unpleasantness, effects which also may, or may not, be reflected in evoked measures of brain activity. The conditions under which these putative different mechanisms are evoked, and their subjective and neurophysiological consequences, are topics for further research.

Modulation of experimental pain sensation.

Many studies have investigated physiological factors that may modulate pain sensitivity, such as diurnal rhythm, menstrual and ovulatory cycles, age and gender (Goolkasain 1980; Hapidou & DeCatanzaro 1988; Feine et al 1991; Gibson 1991a; Levine & DeSimone 1991). Variations in blood pressure have been inversely associated with pain sensitivity (Zamir & Shuber 1980; Maixner et al 1991; Bruehl et al 1992), supporting a model linking hypertension as an adaptive response to stress (Randich & Maixner 1984).

These types of study suggest that the variability of subjective pain reports may be controlled in part by evaluating physiological factors such as blood pressure. Additional studies, described below, also implicate several psychological factors that can contribute to this variability.

PSYCHOLOGICAL FACTORS IN PAIN EXPERIENCE AND REPORT

A number of recent studies have assessed the influence of baseline or induced mood on subjective and physiological responses to experimental stimulation. Baseline (Gaughan & Gracely 1989) and induced (Cornwall & Donderi 1988) anxiety have been shown to increase pain ratings to thermal or pressure pain, while an experimentally induced depressive mood (induced by presentation of text with depressing themes) decreased tolerance to cold pressor pain (Zelman et al 1991). Messinides & Naliboff (1992) found that patients diagnosed with either major depression or adjustment disorder with depressed mood by DSM-IIIR criteria produced more reliable responses to thermal pain sensations using the multiple random staircase method, and had significantly higher tolerance scores than a normal control group. Interestingly, scores on the Beck Depression Inventory were related to pain sensitivity only in the normal group.

Extraversion had no effect on VAS ratings of sensory intensity and unpleasantness of thermal pain sensations, while high neuroticism scores were associated with increased VAS ratings of unpleasantness (Harkins et al 1989).

Manipulation of the subject's attention away from the painful stimulus has been shown to decrease both discrimination and subjective ratings of sensory intensity and unpleasantness of thermal stimuli (Miron et al 1989). Hodes et al (1990) found that the distraction of mental arithmetic decreased intensity ratings but not tolerance to cold pressor stimulation.

Providing accurate information about expected sensation has reduced the unpleasantness, but not the intensity, of clinical pain sensations and of experimental sensations evoked by contact heat (Johnson 1973; Price et al 1980).

Pain memory processes have been investigated using experimental painful stimulation. Cold pressor pain reduced the memorization of positive verbal stimuli, while increasing the recall of negative stimuli (Seltzer & Yarczower 1991). In another study, recall of words was greater under the conditions during which they were exposed (either warm water or cold pressor stimulation), favouring a state-dependent learning hypothesis (Pearce et al 1990). These studies provide experimental examples of how the experience of chronic pain can exert subtle influences on cognitive processes and mood.

The power, and problem, of suggestion was amply demonstrated in an experiment (Bayer et al 1991) in which, following instructions of an expected headache after electrical stimulation, 50% of the subjects reported pain after sham electrical stimulation and 25% reported pain after receiving the additional knowledge that the stimulator was not connected!

Taken together, these studies have identified psychological factors which may play an important role in pain perception or explain a portion of the variance in subjective pain reports. One important issue is the relevance of these findings for clinically significant acute and chronic pain. Like experimental measures of analgesic efficacy, these types of experiment ultimately must be cross-validated in the clinic (see Ch. 18). Several of the above studies (Harkins et al 1989; Pearce et al 1990) employed groups of patients and volunteers or delivered experimental stimuli to pain patients. The use of experimental stimuli in the clinic, the focus of the next section, provides an important bridge between the laboratory and the clinic.

EXPERIMENTAL PAIN ADJUNCTS TO CLINICAL PAIN ASSESSMENT

The use of experimental pain stimulation to augment clinical pain assessments can be divided into two areas:

1. Psychophysical adjuncts
2. Modulation of experimental pain perception.

Psychophysical adjuncts

In these methods, patients use verbal descriptors or visual analogue scales to rate both clinical pain magnitude and the magnitude of brief sensations evoked by stimuli of differing intensity presented in random sequence. They also match the magnitude of their clinical pain to that of the experimental pain stimulus by one of several matching methods. This method results in two measures of clinical pain magnitude, one from direct rating and one from the combination of experimental pain rating and matching. Results from acute dental pain, chronic low back pain or from myofascial pain syndromes show that these two scales agree (Gracely 1979; 1984; Heft et al 1980; Price et al 1984). This result indicates that subjects can do all three procedures, providing further evidence for the accuracy of subjective pain reports under controlled conditions. Methods that assess reporting accuracy may be useful for identifying noncompliant research subjects and for assessing the veracity of clinical pain reports.

Modulation of experimental pain perception

The second class of adjuncts explores the possibility that the modulation of experimental pain perception by clinical pain may be used as an indirect measure of clinical pain sensation (Gibson et al 1991b). These studies are detailed in recent reviews by Boureau et al (1991) and Naliboff & Cohen (1989). Generally the effects of ongoing clinical pain include increased detection threshold, increased suprathreshold pain ratings, a reduction in pain tolerance and a decrement in the ability to discriminate between sensations. However, there is considerable variability and these effects are not always observed; thus the eventual utility of these measures is not yet known.

Related studies have found differences between chronic pain patients and normal subjects in perceptual studies that do not involve painful stimulation. Chronic pain patients reliably quantify the magnitude of meaning implied by sensory intensity pain descriptors, but have difficulty with unpleasantness descriptors (Urban et al 1984). Chronic pain also degrades psychophysical assessments of two-point discrimination (Seltzer & Seltzer 1986).

PROPERTIES OF AN IDEAL PAIN MEASURE

The previous examples emphasize the multiple goals of experimental pain studies with normal subjects. Specific pain measurement methods may be more useful only for specific goals. An ideal method useful for all applications would include the following properties (Gracely 1983):

1. PROVIDE SENSITIVE MEASUREMENT FREE OF BIASES INHERENT IN DIFFERENT ASSESSMENT METHODS

Biases can include the expectations of both the subject and the experimenter, the influence of extraneous clues such as drug side-effects and psychophysical scaling biases. Identifying and reducing these biases is a major goal of many pain studies.

2. PROVIDE IMMEDIATE INFORMATION ABOUT ACCURACY AND RELIABILITY

As with psychometric assessment methods, the sensitivity and validity of experimental pain measures may be improved by identifying individuals who, by choice or ability, perform well or poorly in an assessment procedure.

3. SEPARATE THE SENSORY-DISCRIMINATIVE ASPECTS OF PAIN FROM ITS HEDONIC QUALITIES

The distinction between the unpleasantness and intensity of pain sensations has been emphasized in both philosophy and present pain research. These separate components of pain experience vary independently among individuals and can be affected differently by pain control interventions.

4. ASSESS EXPERIMENTAL AND CLINICAL PAIN WITH THE SAME SCALE, PERMITTING COMPARISONS BETWEEN THE TWO

Experimental pain scales with this property can be used to evaluate clinical pain mechanisms and as adjuncts to clinical pain assessments.

5. PROVIDE ABSOLUTE, RATHER THAN RELATIVE, SCALES THAT ALLOW ASSESSMENT OF PAIN BETWEEN GROUPS AND WITHIN GROUPS OVER TIME

'Absolute' refers to the assessment of a sensation in comparison to an internal or external standard. Absolute assessment should not be influenced by the sensory context, such as the level and frequency of other stimulus-evoked sensations presented in the same session. Relative measurement refers to the judging of the magnitude of a sensation in comparison to other sensations. Many pain assessment procedures require only relative measurement. They measure either the differences in sensation evoked by different stimuli or assess change in pain following an intervention, conditions in which many scales will yield satisfactory results. Measures that involve assessment between groups, such as pain experienced by different cultural groups or postoperative pain after two different procedures, must be made on an absolute level since there is no baseline or preintervention pain for comparison. Pain measurement in these situations requires scales providing absolute and not relative measurement. Absolute measurement is also important for longitudinal assessments.

These five properties are meant to serve as an initial framework for the development and evaluation of pain scales. Future studies may address new properties; for example, McArthur et al (1989) propose two more:

1. Provide a method of predicting an individual's future pain response
2. Provide estimates of the confidence of such predictions.

The first is similar to properties 1 and 5 above, and the second is similar to property 2 above. The difference is that these new proposals apply to the prediction of the future rather than the assessment of the present.

PROPERTIES OF AN IDEAL PAIN STIMULUS

Many of the several goals of studies of pain in normal man involve the production of experimentally evoked pain sensations. Many types of experimental pain stimulation are in use and available to the investigator. Choice of a particular stimulus should be made by considering both general properties and goal-specific requirements.

Beecher (1959) described 10 properties of an ideal pain stimulus: it should:

1. be applied to body parts exhibiting minimal neurohistological variation between individuals
2. provide minimal tissue damage
3. show a relationship between stimulus and pain intensity
4. provide information about discrimination between stimuli
5. result in repeatable stimulation without temporal interaction
6. be applied easily and produce a distinct pain sensation.
7. allow a quantifiable determination of pain quality.
8. be sensitive
9. show analgesic dose relation
10. be applicable to both man and animals.

Additional requirements have emerged as the scope of pain research broadened from the demonstration of experimental analgesia (Gracely 1984, 1985). These include:

1. RAPID ONSET

Rapid and controllable stimulus onset is required for studies in which the stimulus event must be timed precisely, such as studies using averaged measures of cortical or muscle activity.

2. RAPID TERMINATION

Rapid termination is required for stimuli administered at fast rates, such as one every 1–3 seconds. As described above, these stimulus parameters result in the suppression of the first, Aδ-mediated pain sensation, and summation of the second, C-fibre-mediated pain sensation. This dissociation cannot be easily demonstrated with methods such as radiant heating that have a slow stimulus offset.

3. NATURAL

Electrical stimulation provides reliable, easily controlled stimuli with instantaneous onset and offset. However, it excites afferent axons directly and synchronously, resulting in afferent volleys with unnatural spatial and temporal characteristics. Unlike the other methods, electrical stimuli cannot be used to assess pain or analgesic mechanisms at the receptor level or to infer analgesia in natural states. Almost all other stimulus modalities provide natural stimulation which can range from the extremely controllable stimulation produced by lasers to the relatively uncontrollable pain evoked by topically or intradermally administered capsaicin.

4. REPEATABLE WITH MINIMAL TEMPORAL EFFECTS

Repetitive or continuous stimulation can result in either an increase or decrease in perceived sensation. An increase in sensory intensity may result from sensitization of pain receptors (nociceptors) at the periphery (LaMotte et al 1982; Meyer et al 1985), or temporal summation of afferent activity at spinal or higher levels (Price et al 1977). Decreases in perceived sensation may result from suppression of nociceptors output (Price et al 1977) or more central processes (Ernst et al 1986). The influence of stimulation on the perception of subsequent stimuli varies widely among the pain-production methods. The choice of stimulus and stimulus parameters can either maximize the effects of sensitization, suppression and summation for experimental study or minimize them in experiments in which reproducible stimulation is required.

5. OBJECTIVITY: SIMILAR SENSITIVITIES IN DIFFERENT INDIVIDUALS

Many studies compare only pain sensitivity, not change in pain sensitivity following an intervention. These experiments are valid only with methods such as thermal or electrical stimulation of the skin that produces consistent effects across the populations studied.

6. EXCITE A RESTRICTED GROUP OF PRIMARY AFFERENTS

Specific Aδ and C-fibre primary afferent fibre systems signal nociceptive information. The large A fibres mediating touch, vibration and position usually do not convey nociceptive information. Certain stimulation methods, such as heat applied to the skin, electrical stimulation of intact teeth or application of capsaicin, activate predominantly nociceptive fibres. Other methods nonselectively activate several fibre systems. Mechanical stimuli can activate low-threshold cutaneous pressure afferents as well as deeper receptor systems. Electrical stimuli may activate all fibre types and bypass receptor transduction mechanisms to directly stimulate afferent axons. These methods evoke a collage of separate sensations, many unrelated to nociception. Recent methods using intraelectrocutaneous stimulation may minimize the contribution of nonnociceptive primary afferents (Bromm & Meier 1984).

METHODS OF SENSORY STIMULATION IN STUDIES WITH NORMAL INDIVIDUALS

Mechanical pressure has been used to produce pain sensations by deformation of the skin by von Frey hairs and needles, by application of gross pressure to the fingers or mastoid process and by distention of the oesophagus or bile duct (Beecher 1959). Present studies often use pressure to a finger joint (Whipple & Komisurak 1985) or to muscles (K Jensen et al 1986; Reeves et al 1986; Brennum et al 1989; Jensen et al 1992). Mechanical methods produce a wide range of pain intensities and durations. However, stimulus control is difficult since tissue elasticity, stimulating area, rate and degree of compression can influence results (Wolff 1984; K Jensen et al 1986; Greenspan & McGills 1991).

Chemical stimulation has been applied to punctured or blistered skin, to the gastric mucosa or gastric ulcers, to the nasal mucosa, to teeth, or injected intramuscularly (Beecher 1959; Ahlquist et al 1985; Foster & Weston 1986; Kobal & Hummel 1990; Veerasarn & Stohler 1992). Chemical stimuli activate unique pain processes not evoked by other methods. The degree of stimulus control is generally less, although the method developed by Kobal and coworkers allows precise delivery of CO_2 to the nasal mucosa, resulting in orderly responses assessed by electrical brain activity (Kobal & Hummel 1990) or by psychophysical judgments (Anton et al 1992)

The use of topical or intradermal capsaicin, the pungent ingredient in chilli pepper, is a special case in which the primary pain of the application is of less interest than the secondary phenomena of primary heat hyperalgesia, allodynia and secondary mechanical hyperalgesia (Simone et al 1989)

Ischaemic pain is produced by arresting blood flow in an arm by a tourniquet and exercising the hand by isometric or isotonic contractions (Smith et al 1966; Fox et al 1979; Moore et al 1979; Sternbach 1983). This method produces a severe, continuous and increasing pain. It is still used extensively as a pain stimulus and as an experimental stressor.

Cold pressor pain is produced by immersion of a limb in very cold water (Garcia de Jalon et al 1985). It produces a severe pain that increases quickly and is tolerated for a much shorter time than ischaemic pain.

Electrical stimulation is applied to the skin (Tursky 1974; Bromm & Meier 1984) and teeth (Matthews et al 1974; Fernandes de Lima et al 1982; McGrath et al 1983), and directly to peripheral (Vallbo & Hagbarth 1968; Torebjörk & Hallin 1970; Van Hees & Gybels 1972) and central (Mayer et al 1975; Campbell & Lipton 1983; Lenz et al 1993) neurons. Stimulus current is often used as the independent variable and current ranges for pulsed stimuli are usually 0–30 mA for the skin (depending on pulse density) and 0–100 μA for teeth.

Heat pain has been produced by contact with hot water or objects to the skin or alimentary canal, although most studies use radiant heating (Hardy et al 1952). An infrared light source is focused on a skin site usually blackened to improve absorption. Stimulus intensity is determined by lamp voltage and stimulus duration by a mechanical shutter. Modern adaptations employ a laser stimulus source and assess cutaneous temperature by radiation emitted by the skin (Meyer et al 1976; Bromm & Treede 1987; Arendt-Nielsen 1990; Gibson et al 1991b).

PROPERTIES OF STIMULATION METHODS

The relationship between research goals and types of experimental pain stimulus is shown in Table 17.1. It is apparent that specific pain-production methods satisfy some but not all criteria of an ideal pain stimulus. For example, electrical tooth pulp stimulation provides a controllable, repeatable sensation with minimal temporal effects, excites a relatively restricted group of primary afferent fibres and exhibits a precise onset and termination. Thus, it is an ideal stimulus for many investigations. However, it is an inappropriate stimulus for studies that compare sensitivities between groups, since the range of intensities required to elicit pain sensations varies widely between individuals, probably as a consequence of individual tooth geometry. Electrical tooth pulp stimulation also bypasses receptor mechanisms to produce a synchronous barrage of afferent activity and resultant unnatural sensation. Electrical stimulation of the skin also produces unnatural sensations, but sensitivities are similar between individuals, permitting between-group comparisons. However, sensations evoked by electrical skin stimulation contains a powerful Aβ-mediated pressure–vibration component. The evoked sensation can

Table 17.1 Properties of experimental pain stimulation methods. Stimulation requirements are shown for electrical toothpulp and electrical skin stimulation, thermal stimulation by contact or radiant heat, pressure stimulation, ischaemic pain produced by exercising a limb in which circulation has been occluded by a tourniquet, cold pressor stimulation achieved by immersion of a limb in cold water and chemical stimulation of the skin, teeth or mucosa. Asterisks indicate that the method satisfies the requirement, question marks indicate that the method may satisfy the requirement under specific conditions.

Type of stimulus

Requirement	Electrical		Thermal		Pressure	Ischaemic	Cold press	Chemical
	Pulp	Skin	Contact	Radiant				
Fast onset	*	*	?	*	?			?
Fast offset	*	*	*					
Natural			*	*	*	*	*	*
Repeatable	*	*						?
Objective		*	*	*	?	?	?	?
Severe, constant	?	?	?	?	?	*	*	*
Few afferents	*		*	*				*

be felt as an aversive intense stab or vibration without actually being painful. The contribution of Aβ stimulation may be reduced by stimulus preparation (Bromm & Meier 1984) or minimized by stimulating teeth. Although Aβ fibres have been identified in the tooth pulp, the majority of the afferent fibres are nociceptive afferents conducting in the Aδ and C-fibre range (Dong et al 1985). The sensation evoked by electrical tooth pulp stimulation contains a measurable prepain component (Chatrian et al 1982; McGrath et al 1983) at near threshold levels. Suprathreshold stimulation results in a distinct pain sensation without the significant nonpain qualities found with electrical skin stimulation. Radiant heat stimulation produces similar sensations in different individuals, allowing comparison of pain sensitivities across groups. It excites a restricted group of primary afferents and onset is rapid. Termination is slow, however, and thus these methods are less appropriate for studies in which stimulation must be repeated quickly. Contact heat stimulation has a fast termination and can be used for such studies. It excites a restricted group of primary afferent fibres but also activates slowly adapting mechanoreceptors. Laser stimulation contains all the advantages of a radiant source. The return to baseline temperature is faster due to the small area stimulated. Laser stimuli have been used to identify C-fibre-mediated brain potentials (Bromm & Treede 1987). This small area may not be adequate for studies of summation or warmth which require variable or large surface stimulation. The chemical methods range from very controllable (CO_2 applied to nasal mucosa) to moderately (pH buffers) and minimally controllable (application of capsaicin or mustard oil). Stimulation is natural and, in the case of capsaicin or mustard oil, is capable of mimicking many of the significant features of a clinical syndrome.

It is obvious from these examples that the choice of pain stimulus depends on experimental criteria other than familiarity or availability. Unfortunately, many methods are used inappropriately and the requirements shown in Table 17.1 must be kept in mind when planning or evaluating experimental pain research.

CONCLUSION

Pain studies in normal man were once focused on the experimental evaluation of analgesic agents and rightfully regarded with some suspicion by clinical investigators. The methodology of these early experiments has evolved into a broad array of stimulation and assessment procedures. Experimental pain assessments now reveal many relevant features of an analgesic intervention. Moreover, the goals of studies in normal man are not confined to measurement of analgesic efficacy, but also include studies of pain measurement and studies of the mechanisms of pain and pain control.

A complete review of the relevant studies requires a book-length volume and several such books have been published in the last decade (Melzack 1983; Bromm 1984; Price 1988; Chapman & Loeser 1989; Turk & Melzack 1992) as well as numerous reviews (Procacci & Zoppi 1979; Chapman et al 1985; Gracely 1991a, 1991b; Fernandez & Turk 1992; Price & Harkins 1992). This chapter could not cite all of the relevant work, much of which is referenced in the cited articles. It emphasizes the larger perspective of experimental studies, presenting a framework in which the various methods can be organized. This organization stresses the applications of the methods rather than details of the methods themselves. This is where an experimenter should begin, by first formulating the experimental questions, and then choosing the tools best suited to find an answer. Too often questions are chosen to fit the tools at hand.

Acknowledgments

The author thanks Wendy B. Smith for her technical assistance and Gary J. Bennett for his comments on the manuscript.

REFERENCES

Ahlquist M L, Franzen O G, Edwall L G A, Fors U G, Haegerstam G A T 1985 In: Fields H L, Dubner R, Cervero F (eds) Advances in pain research and therapy, vol 9. Raven Press, New York

Anton F, Euchner I, Handwerker O 1992 Psychophysical examination of pain induced by defined CO_2 pulses applied to nasal mucosa. Pain 49: 53–60

Arendt-Nielsen L 1990 Second pain event related potentials to argon laser stimuli: recording and quantification. Journal of Neurology, Neurosurgery and Psychiatry 53: 405–410

Arendt-Nielsen L, Zachariae R, Bjerring P 1990 Quantitative evaluation of hypnotically suggested hyperaesthesia and analgesia by painful laser stimulation. Pain 42: 243–251

Barber J, Mayer D 1977 Evaluation of the efficacy and neural mechanism of a hypnotic analgesia procedure in experimental and clinical dental pain. Pain 4: 41–48

Bayer T L, Baer P E, Early C 1991 Situational and psychophysiological factors in psychologically induced pain. Pain 44: 45–50

Beck J, Shaw W A 1965 Magnitude of the standard numerical value of the standard and stimulus spacing in the estimation of loudness. Perceptual and Motor Skills 21: 151–156

Beecher H K 1959 Measurement of subjective responses. Oxford University Press, New York

Benedetti C, Colpitts Y, Kaufman E, Chapman C R 1984 Effects of methanol on evoked potentials elicited by painful dental stimuli. Pain (suppl 2): 162

Boivie J, Leijon G, Johansson I 1989 Central post-stroke pain – a study of the mechanisms through analyses of the sensory abnormalities. Pain 37: 173–185

Boureau F, Paquette C 1988 Translated versus reconstructed McGill Pain Questionnaires: a comparative study of two French forms: In: Dubner R, Gebhart G F, Bond, M R (eds) Proceedings of the Vth World Congress on Pain. Elsevier, Amsterdam, p 395–402

Boureau F, Luu M, Doubrère J F 1991 Study of experimental pain measures and nociceptive reflex in chronic pain patients and normal subjects. Pain 44: 131–138

Brennum J, Kjeldsen M, Jensen K, Jensen T S 1989 Measurements of human-pain thresholds on fingers and toes. Pain 38: 211–217

Brennum J, Horn A, Jensen T S, Arendt-Nielsen L, Secher N H 1991 Differential sensory effect of spinal opioid receptors. Scandinavian Association for the Study of Pain 15: 18 (abstract)

Brennum J, Arendt-Nielsen L, Secher N H, Jensen T S, Bjerring P 1992 Quantitative sensory examination during epidural anesthesia in man: Effects of lidocaine. Pain 51: 27–34

Brockhaus A, Elger C E 1990 Hypalgesic efficacy of acupuncture on experimental pain in man. Comparison of laser acupuncture and needle acupuncture. Pain 43: 181–185

Bromm B (ed) 1984 Neurophysiological correlates of pain. Elsevier, Amsterdam

Bromm B, 1989 Laboratory animal and human volunteer in the assessment of analgesic efficacy. In: Chapman C R, Loeser J D (eds) Advances in pain research and therapy: issues in pain measurement, vol 12. New York, Raven Press, p 117–143

Bromm B, Meier W 1984 The intracutaneous stimulus: a new pain model for algesimetric studies. Methods and Findings in Experimental and Clinical Pharmacology 87: 431–440

Bromm B, Scharein E 1982 Response plasticity of pain evoked potentials in man. Physiology and Behaviour 28: 109–116

Bromm B, Seide K 1982 The influence of tilidine and prazepam on withdrawal reflex, skin resistance reaction and pain ratings in man. Pain 12: 247–258

Bromm B, Treede R-D 1980 Withdrawal reflex, skin resistance reaction and pain ratings due to electrical stimuli in man. Pain 9: 339–354

Bromm B, Treede R-D 1987 Human cerebral potentials evoked by CO_2 laser stimuli causing pain. Experimental Brain Research 67: 153–162

Bruehl S, Carlson C R, McCubbin J A 1992 The relationship between pain sensitivity and blood pressure in normotensives. Pain 48: 463–467

Campbell I G, Carstens E, Watkins L R 1991 Comparison of human pain sensation and flexion withdrawal evoked by noxious radiant heat. Pain 45: 259–268

Campbell J A, Lipton S 1983 Somatosensory evoked potentials recorded from within the anterolateral quadrant of the human spinal cord. In: Bonica J J, Lindblum U, Iggo A (eds) Advances in pain research and therapy, vol 5. Raven Press, New York

Campell J N, Raja S N, Meyer R A, MacKinnon S E 1988 Myelinated afferents signal the hyperalgesia associated with nerve injury. Pain 32: 89–94

Cassinari V, Pagni C 1969 Central pain: a neurosurgical survey. Harvard University Press, Cambridge, Massachusetts

Chan C W Y, Tsang H H 1985 A quantitative study of flexion reflex in man: relevance to pain research. In: Fields H L, Dubner R, Cervero F (eds) Advances in pain research and therapy, vol 9. New York, Raven Press

Chapman C R 1977 Sensory decision theory methods in pain research: a reply to Rollman. Pain 3: 295–305

Chapman C R, Loeser J D (eds) 1989 Advances in pain research and therapy: issues in pain measurement, vol 12. New York, Raven Press .

Chapman C R, Colpitts Y H, Mayeno J K, Gagliardi G J 1981 Rate of stimulus repetition changes evoked potential amplitude: dental and auditory modalities compared. Experimental Brain Research 43: 246–252

Chapman C R, Benedetti C, Colpitts Y H, Gerlach R 1983 Naloxone fails to reverse pain thresholds elevated by acupuncture: acupuncture analgesia reconsidered. Pain 16: 13–31

Chapman C R, Casey K L, Dubner R, Foley K M, Gracely R H, Reading A E 1985 Pain measurement: an overview. Pain 22: 1–31

Chatrian G E, Fernandes de Lima V M, Lettich E, Canfield R C, Miller R C, Soso M J 1982 Electrical stimulation of tooth pulp in humans. II. Qualities of sensations. Pain 14: 233–246

Chen A C N, Chapman C R 1980 Aspirin analgesia evaluated by event-related potentials in man: possible central action in brain. Experimental Brain Research 39: 359–364

Chen A C N, Dworkin S F, Haug J, Gehrig J 1989 Human responsivity in a tonic pain model: psychological determinants. Pain 37: 143–160

Chudler E H, Dong W K 1983 The assessment of pain by cerebral evoked potentials. Pain 16: 221–224

Clark W C, Clark S B 1980 Pain response in Nepalese porters. Science 209: 410–411

Clark W C, Yang J C 1983 Applications of sensory decision theory to problems in laboratory and clinical pain. In: Melzack R (ed) Pain measurement and assessment. Raven Press, New York

Clark W C, Carroll J D, Yang J C, Janal M N 1986 Multidimensional scaling reveals two dimensions of thermal pain. Journal of Experimental Psychology (Human Perception) 12: 103–107

Cleeland C S 1989 Measurement of pain by subjective report. In: Chapman C R, Loeser J D (eds) Advances in pain research and therapy: issues in pain measurement, vol 12. New York, Raven Press, p 391–403

Cline M A, Ochoa J, Torebjörk H E 1989 Chronic hyperalgesia and skin warming caused by sensitized C nociceptors. Brain 112: 621–647

Cooper B Y, Vierck C J Jr, Yeomans D C 1986 Selective reduction of second pain sensation by systemic morphine in humans. Pain 24: 93–116

Coppola R, Gracely R H 1983 Where is the noise in SDT pain assessment? Pain 17: 257–266

Cornwall A, Donderi D C 1988 The effect of experimentally induced anxiety on the experience of pressure pain. Pain 35: 105–113

Craig K D 1989 Clinical pain measurement from the perspective of the human laboratory. In: Chapman C R, Loeser J D (eds) Advances in Pain Research and Therapy: Issues in Pain Measurement laboratory. vol 12, New York, Raven Press.

Craig K D, Patrick C J 1985 Facial expression during induced pain. Journal of Personality and Social Psychology 48: 1080–1091

Craig K D, Prkachin K M 1983 Nonverbal measures of pain. In: Melzack R (ed) Pain measurement and assessment. Raven Press, New York.

Crockett D J, Prakchin K M, Craig K D 1977 Factors of the language of pain in patient volunteer groups. Pain 4: 175–182

DeBroucker T, Willer J C, Bergeret S 1989 The nociceptive reflex in humans: a specific and objective correlate of experimental pain. In:

Chapman C R, Loeser J D (eds) Advances in pain research and therapy: issues in pain measurement, vol 12. Raven Press, New York, p 337–352

Dong W K, Chudler E H, Martin R F 1985 Physiological properties of intradental mechanoreceptors. Brain Research 334: 389–395

Dowman R 1991 Spinal and supraspinal correlates of nociception in man. Pain 45: 269–281

Dubner R, Sharav Y, Gracely R H, Price D D 1987 Idiopathic trigeminal neuralgia: sensory features and pain mechanisms. Pain 31: 23–33

Duncan G H, Bushnell M C, Lavigne G J, Duquette P 1988a Le développement d'une échelle descriptive verbale francaise pour mesurer l'inensité et l'aspect désagréable de la douleur. Douleur et Analgesie 1: 121–126

Duncan G H, Feine J S, Bushnell M C, Boyer M 1988b Use of magnitude matching for measuring group differences in pain perception. In Dubner R, Gebhart G R, Bond M R (eds) Proceedings of the Vth World Congress on Pain. Elsevier, Amsterdam

Duncan G H, Bushnell M C, Lavigne G J 1989 Comparison of verbal and visual analogue scales for measuring the intensity and unpleasantness of experimental pain. Pain 37: 295–303

Duncan G H, Miron D, Parker S R 1992 Yet another adaptive scheme for tracking threshold. Meeting of the International Society for Psychophysics, July 1992, Stockholm

Engen T 1971a Psychophysics I: discrimination and detection. In: Kling J W, Riggs L A (eds) Experimental psychology, 3rd edn. Holt, New York

Engen T 1971b Psychophysics II: scaling methods. In: Kling J W, Riggs L A (eds) Experimental psychology, 3rd edn. Holt, New York

Eriksson M B E, Rosen I, Sjolund B 1985 Thermal sensitivity in healthy subjects is decreased by a central mechanism after TNS. Pain 22: 235–242

Ernst M, Lee M H M 1985 Sympathetic vasomotor changes induced by manual and electrical acupuncture of the Hoku point visualized by thermography. Pain 21: 25–34

Ernst M, Lee M H M, Dworkin B, Zaretsky H H 1986 Pain perception decrement produced through repeated stimulation. Pain 26: 221–231

Facchinetti F, Sandrini G, Petraglia F, Alfonsi E, Nappi G, Genazzani A R 1984 Concomitant increase in nociceptive flexion reflex threshold and plasma opioids following transcutaneous nerve stimulation. Pain 19: 295–303

Feine J S, Bushnell M C, Miron D, Duncan G H 1991 Sex differences in the perception of noxious heat stimuli. Pain 44: 255–262

Fernandes de Lima V M, Chatrian G E, Lettich E, Canfield R C, Miller R C, Soso M J 1982 Electrical stimulation of tooth pulp in humans. I. Relationships among physical stimulus intensities, psychological magnitude estimates, and cerebral evoked potentials. Pain 14: 207–232

Fernandez E, Turk D C 1992 Sensory and affective components of pain: separation and synthesis. Psychological Bulletin 112: 205–217

Forster C, Anton F, Reeh P W, Weber E, Handwerker H O 1988 Measurement of the analgesic effects of aspirin with a new experimental algesimetric procedure. Pain 32: 215–222

Foster R W, Weston K M 1986 Chemical irritant algesia assessed using the human blister base. Pain 25: 269–278

Fox C D, Steger H G, Jennison J H 1979 Ratio scaling of pain perception with the submaximum effort tourniquet technique. Pain 7: 21–29

Fruhstorfer H, Lindblom U 1984 Sensibility abnormalities in neuralgic patients studied by thermal and tactile pulse stimulation. In: von Euler C, Franzen O, Lindblom U, Ottoson D (eds.), Somatosensory mechanisms. Wenner-Gren International Symposium, vol 41. Macmillan, London p 353–361

Fruhstorfer H, Lindblom U, Schmidt W G 1976 Method for quantitative estimation of thermal thresholds in patients. Journal of Neurology, Neurosurgery and Psychiatry 39: 1071–1075

Garcia de Jalon P D, Harrison F J J, Johnson K I, Kozma C, Schnelle K 1985 A modified cold stimulation technique for the evaluation of analgesic activity in human volunteers. Pain 22: 183–189

Gaughan A M, Gracely R H 1989 A somatization model of repressed negative emotion: defensiveness increases affective ratings of thermal pain sensations. Society of Behavioural Medicine Abstracts

Gaughan A M, Gracely R H, Friedman R 1990 Pain perception following regular practice of meditation, progressive muscle relaxation and sitting. Pain (suppl 5)

Gibson S J, Gorman M M, Helme R D 1991a Assessment of pain in the elderly using event-related potentials, In: Bond M R, Charlton J E, Woolf C J (eds) Proceedings of the VIth World Congress on Pain. Elsevier, Amsterdam

Gibson S J, LaVasseur S A, Helme R D 1991b Cerebral event-related responses induced by CO_2 laser stimulation in subjects suffering from cervico-brachial syndrome. Pain 47: 173–182

Goolkasian P 1980 Cyclic changes in pain perception: an ROC analysis. Perception and Psychophysics 27: 499–504

Gracely R H 1979 Psychophysical assessment of human pain. In: Bonica J J, Liebeskind J C, Able-Fessard D G (eds) Advances in pain research and therapy, vol 3. Raven Press, New York

Gracely R H 1983 Pain language and ideal pain assessment. In: Melzack R (ed) Pain measurement and assessment. Raven Press, New York

Gracely R H 1984 Subjective quantification of pain perception. In: Bromm B (ed) Neurophysiological correlates of pain. Elsevier, Amsterdam

Gracely R H 1985 Pain psychophysics. In: Manuk S, Katkin E (eds) Advances in behavioural medicine, vol 1. JAI Press, New York

Gracely R H 1988 Multiple random staircase assessment of thermal pain perception. In: Dubner R, Bond M, Gebhart G (eds) Proceedings of the Vth World Congress on Pain. Elsevier, Amsterdam, p 391–394

Gracely R H 1989 Pain psychophysics. In: Chapman C R, Loeser J D (eds) Advances in pain research and therapy: issues in pain measurement, vol 12. Raven Press, New York, p 211–229

Gracely R H 1991a Theoretical and practical issues in pain assessment in central pain syndromes. In: Casey K L (ed) Pain and central nervous system disease. Raven Press, New York, p 85–101

Gracely R H 1991b Experimental pain models. In: Max M, Portenoy R, Laska E (eds) Advances in pain research and therapy: the design of analgesic clinical trials, vol 18. Raven Press, New York, p 33–47

Gracely R H 1992 Affective dimensions of pain: how many and how measured? APS Journal 1: 243–247

Gracely R H, Dubner R 1981 Pain assessment in humans: a reply to Hall. Pain 11: 109–120

Gracely R H, Gaughan A M 1991 Staircase assessment of simulated opiate potentiation. In: Bond M R, Charlton J E, Woolf C J (eds) Proceedings of the VIth World Congress on Pain. Elsevier, Amsterdam, p 547–551

Gracely R H, Wolskee P J 1983 Semantic functional measurement of pain: integrating perception and language. Pain 15: 389–398

Gracely R H, McGrath P A, Dubner R 1978a Ratio scales of sensory and affective verbal pain descriptors. Pain 5: 5–18

Gracely R H, McGrath P, Dubner R 1978b Validity and sensitivity of ratio scales of sensory and affective verbal pain descriptors: manipulation of affect by diazepam. Pain 5: 19–29

Gracely R H, Dubner R, McGrath P A 1979 Narcotic analgesia: fentanyl reduces the intensity but not the unpleasantness of painful tooth pulp sensation. Science 203: 1261–1263

Gracely R H, Dubner R, McGrath P A 1982 Fentanyl reduces the intensity of painful tooth pulp sensations: controlling for detection of active drugs. Anesthesia and Analgesia 61: 751–755

Gracely R H, Taylor F, Schilling R M, Wolskee P J 1984 The effect of a simulated analgesic on verbal descriptor and category responses to thermal pain. Pain (suppl 2): 173

Gracely R H, Dubner R, Walther D, Wolskee P J, Lota L 1987 Opiates increase reaction time latency to first and second pain sensations. Neuroscience Abstracts 13: 189

Gracely R H, Gaughan A M, Meister B M, Dionne R A, Hargreaves K M, Dubner R 1988a Staircase assessment of opiate analgesia time-course: effect of infusion rate and naloxone antagonism. American/Canadian Pain Society SS-5d (abstract)

Gracely R H, Lota L, Walther D J, Dubner R 1988b A multiple random staircase method of psychophysical pain assessment. Pain 32: 55–63

Gracely R H, Lynch S A, Bennett G J 1992 Painful neuropathy: altered central processing maintained dynamically by peripheral input. Pain 51: 175–194

Gracely R H, Lynch S A, Bennett G J 1993 Evidence for Aβ low-threshold mechanoreceptor-mediated mechano-allodynia and cold hyperalgesia following intradermal injection of capsaicin into the foot dorsum. Pain supplement (in press)

Greenspan J D, McGillis S L B 1991 Stimulus features relevant to the perception of sharpness and mechanically evoked cutaneous pain. Somatosensory and Motor Research 8: 137–147

Greenspan J D, Winfield J A 1992 Reversible pain and tactile deficit associated with a cerebral tumor compressing the posterior insula and parietal operculum. Pain 50: 29–39

Gybels J M, Sweet W H 1989 Neurosurgical treatment of persistent pain. Karger, Basel

Haker E, Lundeberg T 1990 Laser treatment applied to acupuncture points in lateral humeral epicondylagia: a double-blind study. Pain 43: 243–247

Hapidou E G, DeCatanzaro D 1988 Sensitivity to cold pressor pain in dysmenorrheic and non-dysmenorrheic women as a function of menstrual cycle phase. Pain 34: 277–283

Hardy J D, Wolff H G, Goodell H 1952 Pain sensation and reactions. Williams & Wilkins, Baltimore

Hari R, Kaukoranta E, Kobal G 1985 Neuromagnetic evoked responses and acute laboratory pain. In: Fields H L, Dubner R, Cervero F (eds) Advances in pain research and therapy, vol 9. Raven Press, New York

Harkins S W, Price D D, Katz M A 1983 Are cerebral evoked potentials reliable indices of first or second pain? In: Bonica J J, Lindblum U, Iggo A (eds) Advances in pain research and therapy, vol 5. Raven Press, New York

Harkins S W, Price D D, Braith J 1989 Effects of extraversion and neuroticism on experimental pain, clinical pain, and illness behavior. Pain 36: 209–218

Harms-Ringdahl K, Carlsson A M, Ekholm J, Raustorp A, Svensson T, Toresson H G 1986 Pain assessment with different intensity scales in response to loading of joint structures. Pain 27: 401–412

Heft M W, Parker S R 1984 An experimental basis for revising the graphic rating scale. Pain 19: 153–161

Heft M W, Gracely R H, McGrath P, Dubner R 1978 Effect of nitrous oxide and oxygen on the perception of electrical tooth pulp stimulation. Journal of Dental Research 57A: 91

Heft M W, Gracely R H, Dubner R, McGrath P A 1980 A validation model for verbal descriptor scaling of human clinical pain. Pain 9: 363–373

Hilgard E R 1975 The alleviation of pain by hypnosis. Pain 1: 213–231

Hill H F, Chapman C R 1989 Brain activity measures in assessment of pain and analgesia. In: Chapman C R, Loeser J D (eds) Advances in pain research and therapy: issues in pain measurement, vol 12. Raven Press, New York, p 231–247

Hodes R L, Howland E W, Lightfoot N, Cleeland C S 1990 The effects of distraction on responses to cold pressor pain. Pain 41: 109–114

Holmgren H, Leijon G, Boivie J, Johansson I, Ilievska L 1990 Central post-stroke pain – somatosensory evoked potentials in relation to location of the lesion and sensory signs. Pain 40: 43–52

Houle M, McGrath P A, Moran G, Garrett O J 1988 The efficacy of hypnosis- and relaxation-induced analgesia on two dimensions of pain for cold pressor and electrical tooth pulp stimulation. Pain 33: 241–251

Jamner J D, Tursky B 1987 Discrimination between intensity and affective pain descriptions: a psychophysiological evaluation. Pain 30: 271–283

Janal M N, Clark W C, Carroll J D 1991 Multidimensional scaling of painful and innocuous electrocutaneous stimuli: reliability and individual differences. Perception and Psychophysics 50: 108–116

Jensen K, Anderson H O, Olesen J, Lindblom U 1986 Pressure-pain threshold in human temporal region. Evaluation of a new pressure algometer. Pain 25: 313–323

Jensen M D, Koroly P, Braver S 1986 The measurement of clinical pain intensity: a comparison of six methods. Pain 27: 117–126

Jensen R, Rasmussen B K, Pedersen B, Lous I, Olesen J 1992 Cephalic muscle tenderness and pressure pain threshold in a general population. Pain 48: 197–203

Johnson J E 1973 Effects of accurate expectations about sensations on the sensory and distress components of pain. Journal of Personality and Social Psychology 27: 261–275

Johnson M I, Ashton C H, Bousfield D R, Thompson J W 1989 Analgesic effects of different frequencies of transcutaneous electrical nerve stimulation on cold induced pain in normal subjects. Pain 39: 231–236

Jones A K P, Brown W D, Friston K J, Qi L Y, Frackowiak R S J 1991 Cortical and subcortical localization of response to pain in man using positron emission tomography. Procceedings of the Royal Society, London (Biol) 244: 39–44

Jones B 1980 Algebraic models for integration of painful and nonpainful electric shocks. Perception and Psychophysics 28: 572–576

Jones S F, McQuay H J, Noore R A, Hand C W 1988 Morphine and ibuprofen compared using the cold pressor test. Pain 34: 117–122

Joyce C R B, Zutshi D W, Hrubes V, Mason R M 1975 Comparison of fixed interval and visual analogue scales for rating chronic pain. European Journal of Clinical Pharmacology 8: 415–420

Kaufman E, Chastain D C, Gaughan A M, Gracely R H 1992 Staircase assessment of the magnitude and timecourse of 50% nitrous oxide analgesia. Journal of Dental Research 71: 1598–1603

Keefe F J, Block A R 1982 Development of an observation method for assessing pain behaviour in chronic low back pain patients. Behavior Therapy 13: 363–375

Keefe F J, Dolan E 1986 Pain behavior and pain coping strategies in low back pain and myofascial pain dysfunction. Pain 24: 49–56

Kenshalo D R Jr, Anton F, Dubner R 1989 The detection and perceived intensity of noxious thermal stimuli in monkey and in human. Journal of Neurophysiology 62: 429–436

Klement W, Medert H A, Arndt J O 1992 Nalbuphine does not act analgetically in electrical tooth pulp stimulation in man. Pain 48: 269–274

Klepac R K, Dowling J, Hauge G 1981 Sensitivity of the McGill Pain Questionnaire to intensity and quality of laboratory pain. Pain 10: 199–207

Kobal G, Hummel T 1990 Brain responses to chemical stimulation of the trigeminal nerve in man. In: Green B G, Mason J R, Kare M R (eds) Chemical senses: irritation, vol 2. Marcel Decker, Burlington, Vermont, p 123–136

Koltzenburg M, Lundberg L E R, Torebjörk H E 1992 Dynamic and static components of mechanical hyperalgesia in human hairy skin. Pain 51: 207–219

Kwilosz D M, Green B F, Torgerson W S 1983 Qualities of hurting: the language of pain. American Pain Society Abstracts

LaMotte R H, Thalhammer J G, Torebjörk H E, Robinson C J 1982 Peripheral neural mechanisms of cutaneous hyperalgesia following mild injury by heat. Journal of Neuroscience 2: 765–781

LaMotte, R H, Shain C N, Simone D A, Tsai E-F P 1991 Neurogenic hyperalgesia: psychophysical studies of underlying mechanisms. Journal of Neurophysiology 66: 190–211

LaMotte R H, Lundberg L E R, Torebjörk H E 1992 Pain, hyperalgesia and activity in nociceptive C units in humans after intradermal injection of capsaicin. Journal of Physiology 448: 749–764

Leijon G, Boivie J, Johansson I 1989 Central post-stroke pain – neurological symptoms and pain characteristics. Pain 36: 13–25

Lenz F A, Seike M, Richardson R T et al 1993 Thermal and pain sensations evoked by microstimulation in the area of human ventrocaudal nucleus (Vc). Journal of Neurophysiology (in press)

LeReshe L 1982 Facial expression in pain: a study of candid photographs. Journal of Nonverbal Behavior 7: 46–56

Levine F M, DeSimone L L 1991 The effects of the experimenter gender on pain report in male and female subjects. Pain 44: 69–72

Lewis T 1936 Experiments relating to cutaneous hyperalgesia and its spread through somatic nerves. Clinical Science 2: 373–421

Lindblom U, Verrillo R T 1979 Sensory functions in chronic neuralgia. Journal of Neurology, Neurosurgery and Psychiatry 42: 422–435

Luu M, Bonnel A M, Boureau F 1988 Multidimensional experimental pain study in normal man: combining physiological and psychological indices. In Dubner R, Bond M, Gebhart G (eds) Proceedings of the Vth World Congress on Pain. Elsevier, Amsterdam, p 375–382

McArthur D L, Cohen M J, Schandler S L 1989 A philosophy for measurement of pain. In: Chapman C R, Loeser J D (eds) Issues in pain measurement. Raven Press, New York

McDaniel L K, Anderson K O, Bradley L A et al 1986 Development of an observation method for assessing pain behaviour in rheumatoid arthritis patients. Pain 24: 159–163

McGrath P A, Gracely R H, Dubner R, Heft M W 1983 Non-pain and pain sensations evoked by tooth pulp stimulation. Pain 15: 377–388

McMillan J A, Moudy A M 1986 Differences in nociception during voluntary flexion and extension. Pain 26: 329–336

Maixner W 1991 Interactions between cardiovascular and pain modulatory systems: physiological and pathophysiological implications. Journal of Cardiovascular Electrophysiology (suppl 2): 3–12

Malone M D, Kurts R M, Strube M J 1989 The effects of hypnotic suggestion on pain report. American Journal of Clinical Hypnosis 31: 221–230

Matthews B, Horiuchi H, Greenwood F 1974 The effects of stimulus polarity and electrode area on the threshold to monopolar stimulation of teeth in human subjects with some preliminary observations on the use of a bipolar pulp tester. Archives of Oral Biology 19: 35–42

Max M B, Culnane M, Schafer S C et al 1987 Amitriptyline relieves diabetic neuropathy pain in patients with depressed or normal mood. Journal of Neurology 37: 589–596

Mayer D J, Price D D, Becker D P 1975 Neurophysiological characterization of the anterolateral spinal cord neurons contributing to pain perception in man. Pain 1: 51–58

Mayer D J, Price D D, Rafii A 1977 Antagonism of acupuncture analgesia in man by the narcotic antagonist naloxone. Brain Research 121: 368–372

Meier W, Kolszynski M, Soyka D, Bromm B 1993 Hypnotic hypo- and hyperalgesia: divergent effects on pain ratings and pain-related cerebral potentials. Pain (in press)

Melzack R (ed) 1993 Pain measurement and assessment. Raven Press, New York

Melzack R, Torgerson W S 1971 On the language of pain. Anesthesiology 34: 50–59

Messinides L, Naliboff B D 1992 The impact of depression on acute pain perception in chronic back pain patients. American Pain Society Abstracts

Meyer R A, Walker R E, Mountcastle V B 1976 A laser stimulator for the study of cutaneous thermal pain sensation. IEEE Transaction on Biomedical Engineering 23: 54–60

Meyer R A, Campbell J N, Raja S N 1985 Peripheral neural mechanisms of cutaneous hyperalgesia. In: Fields H L, Dubner R, Cervero F (eds) Advances in pain research and therapy, vol 9. Raven Press, New York

Mills W M, Farrow J T 1981 The transcendental meditation technique and acute experimental pain. Psychosomatic Medicine 43: 157–164

Miron D, Duncan G H, Bushnell M C 1989 Effects of attention on the intensity and unpleasantness of thermal pain. Pain 39: 345–352

Moore P A, Duncan G H, Scott D S, Gregg J M, Ghia J N 1979 The submaximal effort tourniquet test: its use in evaluating experimental and chronic pain. Pain 6: 375–382

Moret V, Forster A, Laverrière M-C et al 1991 Mechanism of analgesia induced by hypnosis and acupuncture: is there a difference? Pain 45: 135–140

Naliboff B D, Cohen M J 1989 Psychophysical laboratory methods applied to clinical pain patients. In: Chapman C R, Loeser J D (eds) Advances in pain research and therapy: issues in pain measurement, vol 12. New York, Raven Press p 365–386

Ohnhaus E E, Adler R 1975 Methodological problems in the measurement of pain: a comparison between the verbal rating scale and the visual analog scale. Pain 1: 379–384

Parducci A 1974 Contextual effects: a range-frequency analysis. In: Carterette E C, Friedman M P (eds) Handbook of perception, vol 2. Academic Press, New York

Parry W L, Smith G M, Denton J E 1972 An electric-shock method of inducing pain responsive to morphine in man. Anesthesia and Analgesia 51: 573–578

Patrick C J, Craig K D, Prkachin K M 1986 Observer judgments of acute pain: facial action determinants. Journal of Personality and Social Psychology 50: 1292–1298

Pearce S A, Isherwood S, Hrouda D, Richardson P H, Erskine A, Skinner J 1990 Memory and pain: tests of mood congruity and state dependent learning in experimentally induced and clinical pain. Pain 43: 187–193

Posner J A 1984 Modified submaximal effort tourniquet test for evaluation of analgesics in healthy volunteers. Pain 19: 143–151

Price D D 1988 Psychological and neural mechanisms of pain. Raven Press, New York

Price D D 1989 Nociceptive reflexes and pain. In: Chapman C R, Loeser J D (eds) Advances in pain research and therapy: issues in pain measurement, vol 12. Raven Press, New York

Price D D, Barber J 1987 An analysis of the factors that contribute to the efficacy of hypnotic analgesia. Journal of Abnormal Psychology 96: 46–51

Price D D, Harkins S W 1992 The affective–motivational dimension of pain: a two stage model. APS Journal 1: 229–239

Price D D, Mayer D J 1975 Neurophysiological characterization or the anterolateral quadrant neurons subserving pain in Mulatta. Pain 1: 59–72

Price D D, Hu J W, Dubner R, Gracely R H 1977 Peripheral suppression of first pain and central summation of second pain evoked by noxious heat pulses. Pain 3: 57–68

Price D D, Barrell J J, Gracely R H 1980 A psychophysical analysis of experiential factors that selectively influence the affective dimension of pain. Pain 8: 137–149

Price D D, Rafii, A, Watkins L R, Buckingham B 1984 A psychophysical analysis of acupuncture analgesia. Pain 19: 24–42

Price D D, Von der Gruen A, Miller J, Rafii A, Price C 1985a Potentiation of systemic morphine analgesia in humans by proglumide, a cholecystokinin antagonist. Anesthesia and Analgesia 64: 801–806

Price D D, Von der Gruen A, Miller J, Rafii A, Price C 1985b A psychophysical analysis of morphine analgesia. Pain 22: 261–269

Price D D, Bennett G J, Rafii A 1989 Psychophysical observations on patients with neuropathic pain relieved by a sympathetic block Pain 36: 237–288

Price D D, Long S, Huit C 1992 Sensory testing of pathophysiological mechanisms of pain in patients with reflex sympathetic dystrophy. Pain 49: 163–173

Procacci P, Zoppi M, Maresca M 1979 Experimental pain in man. Pain 6: 123–140

Raja S N, Campbell J N, Meyer R A 1984 Evidence for different mechanisms of primary and secondary hyperalgesia following heat injury to the glabrous skin. Brain 107: 1179–1188

Randich A, Maixner W 1984 Interactions between cardiovascular and pain regulatory systems. Neuroscience and Biobehavioral Review 8: 343–367

Reading A E, Everitt B S, Sledmere 1982 The McGill Pain Questionnaire: a replication of its construction. British Journal of Clinical Psychology 21: 339–349

Reeves J L, Jaeger B, Graff-Radford S B 1986 Reliability of the pressure algometer as a measure of myofascial trigger point sensitivity. Pain 24: 313–321

Reeves J R, Redd W H, Minagawa R Y, Storm F K 1983 Hypnosis in the control of pain during hyperthermia treatment of cancer. In: Bonica J J, Lindblom U, Iggo A (eds) Advances in pain research and therapy, vol 5. Raven Press, New York, p 857–861

Rohdewald P, Derendorf H, Drehsen G, Elgar C E, Knoll O 1982 Changes in cortical evoked potentials as correlates of the efficacy of weak analgesics. Pain 12: 329–341

Rollman G B 1977 Signal detection theory measurement of pain: a review and critique. Pain 3: 187–211

Schady W, Torebjörk H E 1984 Central effects of zomepirac on pain evoked by intraneural stimulation in man. Journal of Clinical Pharmacology 24: 429–435

Seike M, Lenz F A, Lin Y C, Baker F H, Gracely R H, Richardson R T 1991 Neurons in human Vc respond to noxious heat stimuli. Society for Neuroscience Abstracts 17: 294

Seltzer S F, Seltzer J L 1986 Tactual sensitivity of chronic pain patients to non-painful stimuli. Pain 27: 291–295

Seltzer S F, Yarczower M 1991 Selective encoding and retrieval of affective words during exposure to aversive stimulation. Pain 47: 47–51

Simone D A, Baumann T K, LaMotte R H 1989 Dose-dependent pain and mechanical hyperalgesia in humans after intradermal injection of capsaicin. Pain 38: 99–107

Sjölund B, Eriksson M 1985 Relief of pain by TENS. John Wiley, New York

Smith G M, Beecher H K 1969 Experimental production of pain in man: sensitivity of a new method to 600 mg of aspirin. Clinical Pharmacology and Therapeutics 10: 213–216

Smith G M, Egbert L D, Markowitz R A, Mosteller F, Beecher H K 1966 An experimental pain method sensitive to morphine in man: the submaximum effort tourniquet technique. Journal of Pharmacological and Experimental Therapeutics 154: 324–332

Spanos N 1986 Hypnotic behavior: a social-psychological interpretation of amnesia, analgesia and 'trance logic'. Behavioural and Brain Sciences 9: 449–502

Sternbach R A 1983 The tourniquet pain test. In: Melzack R (ed) Pain measurement and assessment. Raven Press, New York

Talbot J D, Marrett S, Evans A C, Meyer E, Bushnell M C, Duncan G H 1991 Multiple representations of pain in human cerebral cortex. Science 251: 1355–1358

Telekes A, Holland R L, Peck A W 1987 Indomethacin: effects on cold-induced pain and the nervous system in healthy volunteers. Pain 30: 321–328

Thurstone L I 1959 The measurement of values. University of Chicago Press, Chicago

Timmermans G, Sternbach R A 1974 Factors of human chronic pain: An analysis of personality and pain reaction variables. Science 184: 806–808

Torebjörk H E, Hallin R G 1970 C fiber units recorded from human sensory nerve fascicles in situ. Acta Societatis Medicorum Upsaliensis 75: 81–84

Torebjörk H E, Lundberg L E R, LaMotte R H 1992 Central changes in processing of mechanoreceptive input in capsaicin-induced secondary hyperalgesia in humans. Journal of Physiology 448: 765–780

Torgerson W S, BenDebba M, Mason K J 1988 Varieties of pain. In: Dubner R, Gebhart G F, Bond M R (eds) Proceedings of the Vth World Congress on Pain. Elsevier, Amsterdam, p 368–374

Treede R-D, Bromm B 1991 Neurophysiological approaches to the study of spinothalamic tract function in humans. In: Casey K L (ed) Pain and central nervous system disease. Raven Press, New York, p 117–127

Turk D C, Melzack R 1992 Handbook of pain assessment. Guilford Press, New York

Tursky B 1974 Physical physiological and psychological factors that affect pain reaction to electric shock. Psychophysiology 11: 95–112

Tursky B 1976 The development of a pain perception profile: a psychological approach. In: Weisenberg M, Tursky B (eds) Pain: new perspectives in therapy and research. Plenum Press, New York

Urban B J, Keefe F J, France R D 1984 A study of psychophysical scaling in chronic pain patients. Pain 20: 157–168

Vallbo A B, Hagbarth K E 1968 Activity from skin mechanoreceptors recorded percutaneously in awake human subjects. Experimental Neurology 21: 270–289

Van Hees J, Gybels J M 1972 Pain related to single afferent C fibers from human skin. Brain Research 48: 397–400

Veerasarn P, Stohler C S 1992 The effect of experimental muscle pain on the background electrical brain activity. Pain 49: 349–360

Wade J B, Price D D, Hamer R M, Schwartz S M, Hart R P 1990 An emotional component analysis of chronic pain. Pain 40: 303–310

Wall P D 1979 On the relation of injury to pain. Pain 6: 253–264

Wallin B G, Torebjörk E, Hallin R G 1976 Preliminary observations on the pathophysiology of hyperalgesia in the causalgic pain syndrome. In: Zotterman Y (ed) Sensory functions of the skin of primates with special reference to man. Pergamon Press, Oxford, p 489–499

Walther D J, Gracely R H 1988 Choice of psychophysical procedure determines hypnotic hypalgesia. American/Canadian Pain Society SS-5e

Whipple B, Komisurak B R 1985 Elevation of pain threshold by vaginal stimulation in women. Pain 21: 357–367

Willer J C 1977 Comparative study of perceived pain and nociceptive flexion reflex in man. Pain 3: 69–80

Willer J C 1985 Studies on pain. Effects of morphine on a spinal nociceptive flexion reflex and related pain sensation in man. Brain Research 331: 105–114

Willer J C, Bussel V 1980 Evidence for a direct spinal mechanism in morphine-induced inhibition of nociceptive reflexes in humans. Brain Research 187: 212–215

Willer J C, Dehen H, Cambier J 1981 Stress-induced analgesia in humans: endogenous opioids and naloxone reversible depression of pain reflexes. Science 212: 689–690

Willer J C, Roby A, Boulu P, Boureau F 1982 Comparative effects of electroacupuncture and transcutaneous nerve stimulation on the human blink reflex. Pain 14: 267–278

Willer J C, DeBroucker T, Barranquero A, Kahn M F 1987 Brain evoked potentials to noxious sural nerve stimulation in sciatalgic patients. Pain 30: 47–58

Willer J C, De Borucker T, Bussel B et al 1989 Central analgesic effect of ketoprofen in humans: electrophysiological evidence for a supraspinal mechanism in a double-blind cross-over study. Pain 38: 1–7

Wolff B B 1971 Factor analysis of human pain responses: pain endurance as a specific pain factor. Journal of Abnormal Psychology 78: 292–298

Wolff B B 1984 Methods of testing pain mechanisms in normal man. In: Wall P D, Melzack R (eds) Textbook of pain. Churchill Livingstone, Edinburgh

Wolff B B, Kantor T G, Jarvik M E, Laska E 1969 Response of experimental pain to analgesic drugs. III. Codeine, aspirin, secobarbital and placebo. Clinical Pharmacology and Therapeutics 10: 217–228

Yan Z, Zonglian H 1989 The peripheral pathway of afferent impulses in traditional acupuncture analgesia. Schmerz/Pain/Douleur 10: 15–18

Zamir N, Schuber E 1980 Altered pain perception in hypertensive humans, Brain Research 201: 471–474

Zelman D C, Howland E W, Nichols S N, Cleeland C S 1991 The effects of induced mood on laboratory pain. Pain 46: 105–111

18. Pain measurement in persons in pain

Ronald Melzack and Joel Katz

INTRODUCTION

Pain research and therapy during the past century evolved from Descartes' concept of pain as a direct transmission system from 'pain receptors' in the body tissues to a 'pain centre' in the brain. Injury or other pathology is assumed to lead inevitably to pain. As a result, the early history of pain measurement is focused on the psychophysical relationship between the extent of injury and perceived pain. Various stimuli such as electric shock or radiant heat were applied to the skin and subjects in the laboratory provided estimates of pain intensity. Elegant psychophysical power functions were generated and all studies of pain measurement up to the time of publication of the gate control theory of pain (Melzack & Wall 1965) concentrated exclusively on the measurement of pain intensity.

The gate control theory, together with the increasing emphasis on pain as a major clinical problem (Livingston 1943; Bonica 1953; Noordenbos 1959), led to the recognition that pain rarely has a one-to-one relationship to a 'stimulus'. Acute pain is sometimes proportional to the extent of injury, but the contribution of psychological factors reveals complex relationships that are profoundly influenced by fear, anxiety, cultural background and the meaning of the situation to the person (Melzack & Wall 1988). Chronic pain presents an even greater problem for the Cartesian psychophysical concept: backaches often occur without any discernible organic cause; postherpetic neuralgia persists long after peripheral nerve regeneration and healing of all tissue.

The new emphasis on the varieties of clinical pain and their variability led to new concepts of pain measurement. Instead of using stimuli such as radiant heat to obtain psychophysical standards to measure clinical pain (Hardy et al 1952), it became necessary to measure the subjective experience of pain as such, without reference to external causes.

People suffering acute or chronic pain provide valuable opportunities to study the mechanisms of pain and analgesia. The measurement of pain is therefore essential to determine the initial intensity, perceptual qualities and time-course of the pain so that the differences among different pain syndromes can be ascertained and investigated. Furthermore, measurement of these variables provides valuable clues that help in the differential diagnosis of the underlying causes of the pain. They also help determine the most effective treatment (such as the types of analgesic drugs or other therapies) necessary to control the pain and are essential to evaluate the relative effectiveness of different therapies. The measurement of pain, then, is important:

1. to determine pain intensity, quality and duration
2. to aid in diagnosis
3. to help decide on the choice of therapy
4. to evaluate the relative effectiveness of different therapies.

DIMENSIONS OF PAIN EXPERIENCE

Research on pain, since the beginning of this century, has been dominated by the concept that pain is purely a sensory experience. Yet pain also has a distinctly unpleasant affective quality. It becomes overwhelming, demands immediate attention and disrupts ongoing behaviour and thought. It motivates or drives the organism into activity aimed at stopping the pain as quickly as possible. To consider only the sensory features of pain and ignore its motivational–affective properties is to look at only part of the problem. Even the concept of pain as a perception, with full recognition of past experience, attention and other cognitive influences, still neglects the crucial motivational dimension.

These considerations led Melzack & Casey (1968) to suggest that there are three major psychological dimensions of pain: sensory–discriminative, motivational–affective, and cognitive–evaluative. They proposed, moreover, that these dimensions of pain experience are subserved by physiologically specialized systems in the brain: the sensory–discriminative dimension of pain is influenced primarily by the rapidly conducting spinal systems; the powerful motivational drive and unpleasant affect characteristic of pain are subserved by activities in reticular and limbic structures that are influenced primarily by the slowly conducting spinal systems; neocortical or higher central nervous system processes, such as evaluation of the input in terms of past experience, exert control over activity in both the discriminative and motivational systems.

It is assumed that these three categories of activity interact with one another to provide *perceptual information* on the location, magnitude and spatiotemporal properties of the noxious stimuli; *motivational tendency* toward escape or attack, and *cognitive information* based on past experience and probability of outcome of different response strategies (Melzack & Casey 1968). All three forms of activity could then influence motor mechanisms responsible for the complex pattern of overt responses that characterize pain.

THE LANGUAGE OF PAIN

Clinical investigators have long recognized the varieties of pain experience. Descriptions of the burning qualities of pain after peripheral nerve injury, or the stabbing, cramping qualities of visceral pains frequently provide the key to diagnosis and may even suggest the course of therapy. Despite the frequency of such descriptions, and the seemingly high agreement that they are valid descriptive words, studies of their use and meaning are relatively recent.

Anyone who has suffered severe pain and tried to describe the experience to a friend or to the doctor often finds himself at a loss for words. The reason for this difficulty in expressing pain experience, actually, is not because the words do not exist. As we shall soon see, there is an abundance of appropriate words. Rather, the main reason is that, fortunately, they are not words which we have occasion to use often. Another reason is that the words may seem absurd. We may use descriptors such as splitting, shooting, gnawing, wrenching or stinging, but there are no external objective references for these words. If we talk about a blue pen or a yellow pencil we can point to an object and say 'that is what I mean by yellow', or 'this color of the pen is blue'. But what can we point to to tell another person precisely what we mean by smarting, tingling, or rasping? A person who suffers terrible pain may say that the pain is burning and add that 'it feels as if someone is shoving a red-hot poker through my toes and slowly twisting it around.' These 'as if' statements are often essential to convey the qualities of the experience.

If the study of pain in man is to have a scientific foundation, it is essential to measure it. If we want to know how effective a new drug is, we need numbers to say that the pain decreased by some amount. Yet, while overall intensity is important information, we also want to know whether the drug specifically decreased the burning quality of the pain or if the especially miserable, tight, cramping feeling is gone.

RATING SCALES

VISUAL ANALOGUE SCALES (VAS)

Until recently, the methods that were used for pain measurement treated pain as though it were a single unique quality that varies only in intensity (Beecher 1959). These methods included the use of verbal rating scales (VRS) (e.g. mild, moderate, severe), numerical rating scales (1–100) and VAS (Huskisson 1974; Joyce et al 1975). These simple methods have all been used effectively in hospital clinics and have provided valuable information about pain and analgesia.

VAS provide simple, efficient and minimally intrusive measures of pain intensity which have been used widely in clinical and research settings where a quick index of pain is required and to which a numerical value can be assigned. The most common VAS consists of a 10 cm horizontal (Huskisson 1983) or vertical (Sriwatanakul et al 1983) line with the two endpoints labelled 'no pain'and 'worst pain ever' (or similar verbal descriptors). The patient is required to place a mark on the 10 cm line at a point which corresponds to the level of pain intensity he or she presently feels. The distance in centimetres from the low end of the VAS to the patient's mark is used as a numerical index of the severity of pain.

The VAS is sensitive to pharmacological and nonpharmacological procedures which alter the experience of pain (Bélanger et al 1989; Choinière et al 1990) and correlates highly with pain measured on verbal and numerical rating scales (Ohnhaus & Adler 1975; Kremer & Atkinson 1983; Ekblom & Hansson 1988). Instructions to patients to rate the amount or percentage of pain relief using a VAS (e.g. following administration of a treatment designed to reduce pain) may introduce unnecessary bias (e.g. expectancy for change and reliance on memory) which reduces the validity of the measure. It has been suggested (Carlsson 1983), therefore, that a more appropriate measure of change may be obtained by having patients rate the absolute amount of pain at different points in time such as before and after an intervention (but see Ekblom & Hansson 1988).

A major advantage of the VAS as a measure of sensory pain intensity is its ratio scale properties (Price et al 1983; Price 1988). In contrast to many other pain measurement tools, equality of ratios is implied, making it appropriate to speak meaningfully about percentage differences between VAS measurements obtained either at multiple points in time or from independent samples of subjects. Other advantages of the VAS include:

1. its ease and brevity of administration and scoring (Jensen et al 1986)
2. minimal intrusiveness
3. providing that adequately clear instructions are given to the patient, its conceptual simplicity (Huskisson 1983; Chapman et al 1985).

The major disadvantage of the VAS is its assumption that pain is a unidimensional experience (Melzack 1975). Although intensity is, without a doubt, a salient dimension of pain, it is clear that the word 'pain' refers to an endless variety of qualities that are categorized under a single linguistic label, not to a specific, single sensation that varies only in intensity. Each pain has unique qualities. The pain of a toothache is obviously different from that of a pin-prick, just as the pain of a coronary occlusion is uniquely different from the pain of a broken leg. To describe pain solely in terms of intensity is like specifying the visual world only in terms of light flux without regard to pattern, colour, texture and the many other dimensions of visual experience.

THE McGILL PAIN QUESTIONNAIRE (MPQ)

Development and description

Melzack & Torgerson (1971) developed the procedures to specify the qualities of pain. In the first part of their study, physicians and other university graduates were asked to classify 102 words, obtained from the clinical literature, into small groups that describe distinctly different aspects of the experience of pain. On the basis of the data, the words were categorized into three major classes and 16 subclasses (Fig. 18.1). The classes are:

1. Words that describe the *sensory qualities* of the experience in terms of temporal, spatial, pressure, thermal and other properties
2. Words that describe *affective qualities* in terms of tension, fear and autonomic properties that are part of the pain experience
3. *Evaluative* words that describe the subjective overall intensity of the total pain experience.

Each subclass, which was given a descriptive label, consists of a group of words that were considered by most subjects to be qualitatively similar. Some of these words are undoubtedly synonyms, others seem to be synonymous but vary in intensity, while many provide subtle differences or nuances (despite their similarities) that may be of importance to a patient who is trying desperately to communicate to a physician.

The second part of the Melzack & Torgerson (1971) study was an attempt to determine the pain intensities implied by the words within each subclass. Groups of physicians, patients and students were asked to assign an intensity value to each word, using a numerical scale ranging from least (or mild) pain to worst (or excruciating) pain. When this was done, it was apparent that several words within each subclass had the same relative intensity relationships in all three sets. For example, in the spatial subclass, 'shooting' was found to represent more pain than 'flashing', which in turn implied more pain than 'jumping'. Although the precise intensity scale values differed for the three groups, all three agreed on the positions of the words

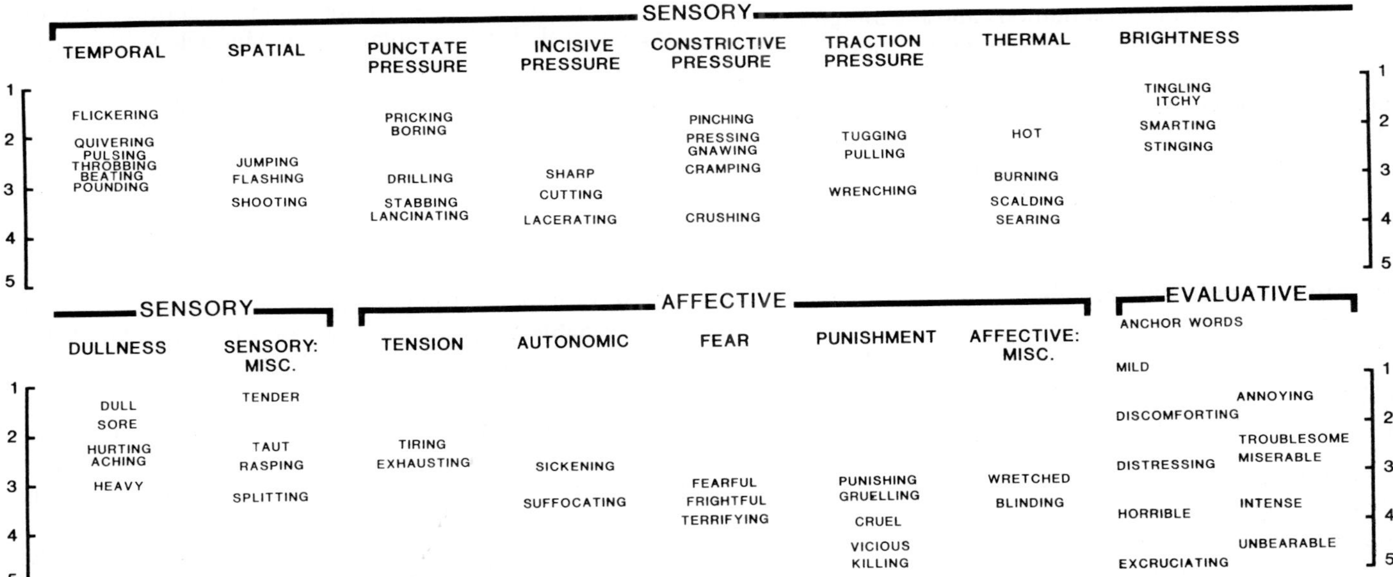

Fig. 18.1 Spatial display of pain descriptors based on intensity ratings by patients. The intensity scale values range from 1 (mild) to 5 (excruciating).

relative to each other. The scale values of the words for patients, based on the precise numerical values listed in Melzack & Torgerson (1971), are shown in Figure 18.1.

Because of the high degree of agreement on the intensity relationships among pain descriptors by subjects who have different cultural, socioeconomic and educational backgrounds, a pain questionnaire (Fig. 18.2) was developed as an experimental tool for studies of the effects of various methods of pain management. In addition to the list of pain descriptors, the questionnaire contains line drawings of the body to show the spatial distribution of the pain, words that describe temporal properties of pain and descriptors of the overall present pain intensity (PPI). The PPI is recorded as a number from 1–5, in which each number is associated with the following words: 1, mild; 2, discomforting; 3, distressing; 4, horrible; 5, excruciating. The mean scale values of these words, which were chosen from the evaluative category, are approximately equally far apart (Melzack & Torgerson 1971) so that they represent equal scale intervals and thereby provide 'anchors' for the specification of the overall pain intensity.

In a preliminary study, the pain questionnaire consisted of the 16 subclasses of descriptors shown in Figure 18.1, as well as the additional information deemed necessary for the evaluation of pain. It soon became clear, however, that many of the patients found certain key words to be absent. These words were then selected from the original word list used by Melzack & Torgerson (1971), were categorized appropriately and ranked according to their mean scale values. A further set of words (cool, cold, freezing) was used by patients on rare occasions but was indicated to be essential for an adequate description of some types of pain. Thus, four supplementary (or 'miscellaneous') subclasses were added to the word lists of the questionnaire (Fig. 18.2). The final classification, then, appeared to represent the most parsimonious and meaningful set of subclasses without at the same time losing subclasses that represent important qualitative properties. The questionnaire, which is known as the 'McGill Pain Questionnaire' (Melzack 1975), has become a widely used clinical and research tool (Melzack 1983; Reading 1989; Wilkie et al 1990).

Measures of pain experience

The descriptor-lists of the MPQ are read to a patient with the explicit instruction that he or she choose only those words which describe his or her feelings and sensations at that moment. Three major indices are obtained:

1. The pain rating index (PRI) based on the rank values of the words. In this scoring system, the word in each subclass implying the least pain is given a value of 1, the next word is given a value of 2 etc. The rank values of the words chosen by a patient are summed to obtain a score separately for the sensory (subclasses 1–10), affective (subclasses 11–15), evaluative (subclass 16) and miscellaneous (subclasses 17–20) words, in addition to providing a total score (subclasses 1–20). Figure 18.3 shows MPQ scores (total score from subclasses 1–20) obtained by patients with a variety of acute and chronic pains.
2. The number of words chosen (NWC).
3. The PPI, the number-word combination chosen as the indicator of overall pain intensity at the time of administration of the questionnaire.

Recently several additional scoring procedures have been suggested. Hartman & Ainsworth (1980) have proposed transforming the data into a pain ratio or fraction: the 'pain ratio was calculated for each session by dividing the postsession rating by the sum of the pre- and postsession ratings'. Kremer et al (1982) suggested dividing the sum of the obtained ranks within each dimension by the total possible score for a particular dimension, thus making differences between the sensory, affective, evaluative and miscellaneous dimensions more interpretable.

A final form of computation (Melzack et al 1985) may be useful since it has been argued (Charter & Nehemkis 1983) that the MPQ fails to take into account the true relative intensity of verbal descriptors since the rank-order scoring system loses the precise intensity of the scale values obtained by Melzack & Torgerson (1971). For example, Figure 18.1 shows that the affective descriptors generally have higher scale values than the sensory words. This is clear when we consider the fact that the words 'throbbing' and 'vicious' receive a rank value of 4, but have scale values of 2.68 and 4.26 respectively, indicating that the latter descriptor implies considerably more pain intensity than the former. A simple technique was developed (Melzack et al 1985) to convert rank values to weighted rank values which more closely approximate the original scaled values obtained by Melzack & Torgerson (1971). Use of this procedure may provide enhanced sensitivity in some statistical analyses (Melzack et al 1985). The weights for each descriptor category are presented in Table 18.1.

Usefulness of the MPQ

The most important requirement of a measure is that it be valid, reliable, consistent and, above all, useful. The MPQ appears to meet all of these requirements (Melzack 1983; Chapman et al 1985; Reading 1989; Wilkie et al 1990) and provides a relatively rapid way of measuring subjective pain experience (Melzack 1975). When administered to a patient by reading each subclass, it can be completed in about 5 minutes. It can also be filled out by the patient in a more leisurely way as a paper-and-pencil test, though the scores are somewhat different (Klepac et al 1981).

Since its introduction in 1975, the MPQ has been used

McGill Pain Questionnaire

Patient's Name ______ Date ______ Time ______ am/pm

PRI: S ______ (1-10) A ______ (11-15) E ______ (16) M ______ (17-20) PRI(T) ______ (1-20) PPI ______

1 FLICKERING	11 TIRING	BRIEF
QUIVERING	EXHAUSTING	MOMENTARY
PULSING	12 SICKENING	TRANSIENT
THROBBING	SUFFOCATING	RHYTHMIC
BEATING	13 FEARFUL	PERIODIC
POUNDING	FRIGHTFUL	INTERMITTENT
2 JUMPING	TERRIFYING	CONTINUOUS
FLASHING	14 PUNISHING	STEADY
SHOOTING	GRUELLING	CONSTANT
3 PRICKING	CRUEL	
BORING	VICIOUS	
DRILLING	KILLING	
STABBING	15 WRETCHED	
LANCINATING	BLINDING	
4 SHARP	16 ANNOYING	
CUTTING	TROUBLESOME	
LACERATING	MISERABLE	
5 PINCHING	INTENSE	
PRESSING	UNBEARABLE	
GNAWING	17 SPREADING	
CRAMPING	RADIATING	
CRUSHING	PENETRATING	
6 TUGGING	PIERCING	
PULLING	18 TIGHT	
WRENCHING	NUMB	
7 HOT	DRAWING	
BURNING	SQUEEZING	
SCALDING	TEARING	
SEARING	19 COOL	
8 TINGLING	COLD	
ITCHY	FREEZING	
SMARTING	20 NAGGING	
STINGING	NAUSEATING	
9 DULL	AGONIZING	
SORE	DREADFUL	
HURTING	TORTURING	
ACHING	PPI	
HEAVY	0 NO PAIN	
10 TENDER	1 MILD	
TAUT	2 DISCOMFORTING	
RASPING	3 DISTRESSING	
SPLITTING	4 HORRIBLE	
	5 EXCRUCIATING	

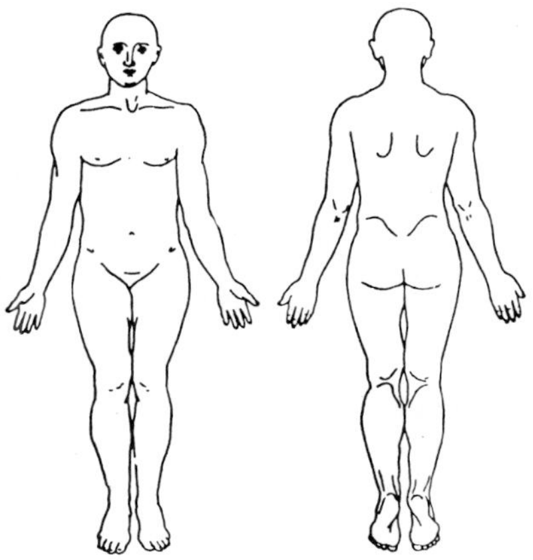

E = EXTERNAL

I = INTERNAL

COMMENTS:

Fig. 18.2 McGill Pain Questionnaire. The descriptors fall into four major groups: sensory, 1–10; affective, 11–15; evaluative, 16; and miscellaneous, 17–20. The rank value for each descriptor is based on its position in the word set. The sum of the rank values is the pain rating index (PRI). The present pain intensity (PPI) is based on a scale of 0 to 5.

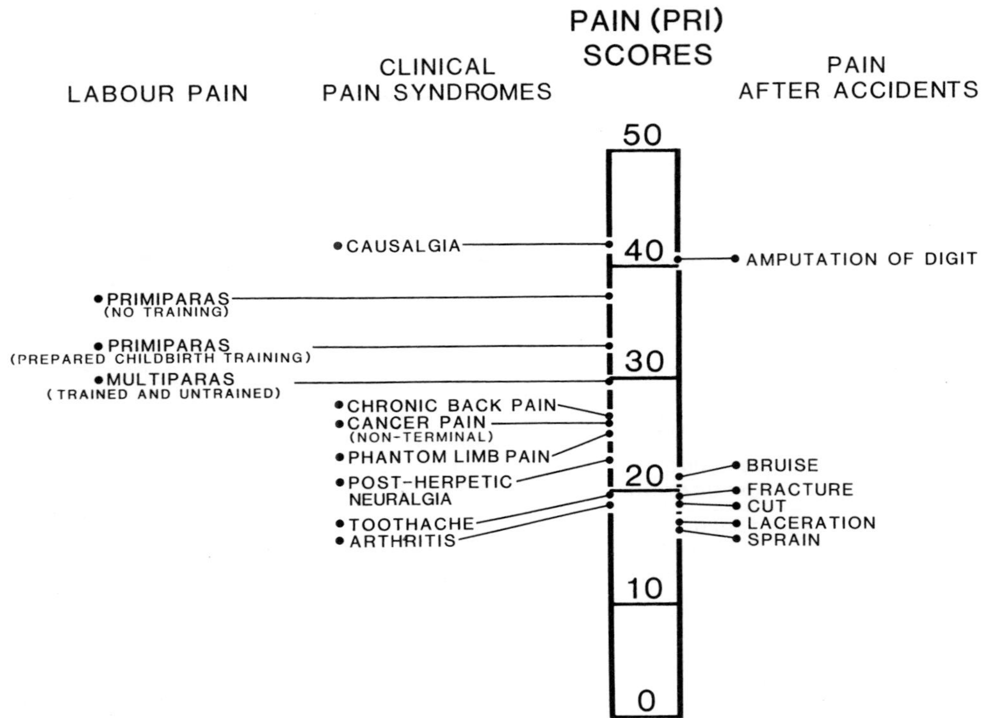

Fig. 18.3 Comparison of pain scores using the McGill Pain Questionnaire, obtained from women during labour (Melzack et al 1981), from patients in a general hospital pain clinic (Melzack 1975) and an emergency department (Melzack et al 1982). The pain score for causalgic pain is reported by Tahmoush (1981).

in over 100 studies of acute, chronic and laboratory produced pains. It has been translated into several languages and has also spawned the development of similar pain questionnaires in other languages (Table 18.2).

Because pain is a private, personal experience, it is impossible for us to know precisely what someone else's pain feels like. No man can possibly know what it is like to have menstrual cramps or labour pain. Nor can a psychologically healthy person know what a psychotic patient is feeling when he says he has excruciating pain (Veilleux & Melzack 1976). But the MPQ provides us with an insight into the qualities that are experienced. Recent studies indicate that each kind of pain is characterized by a distinctive constellation of words. There is a remarkable consistency in the choice of words by patients suffering the same or similar pain syndromes (Van Buren & Kleinknecht 1979; Graham et al 1980; Melzack et al 1981; Grushka & Sessle 1984; Katz & Melzack 1991; Katz 1992).

Reliability and validity of the MPQ

Reading et al (1982) investigated the reliability of the groupings of adjectives in the MPQ by using different methodological and statistical approaches. Subjects sorted each of the 78 words of the MPQ into groups that described similar pain qualities. The mean number of groups was 19 (with a range of 7–31), which is remarkably close to the MPQ's 20 groups. Moreover, there were distinct subgroups for sensory and affective–evaluative words. Since the cultural backgrounds of subjects in this study and in Melzack & Torgerson's (1971) were different, and the methodology and data analysis were dissimilar, the degree of correspondence is impressive. More recently, Gaston-Johansson et al (1990) reported that subjects with diverse ethnic-cultural and educational backgrounds use similar MPQ adjectives to describe commonly used words such as 'pain', 'hurt' and 'ache'. Nevertheless, interesting differences between the studies were found which suggest alternative approaches for future revisions of the MPQ.

Evidence for the stability of the MPQ was recently provided by Love et al (1989) who administered the MPQ to patients with chronic low back pain on two occasions (separated by several days) prior to receiving treatment. Their results show very strong test-retest reliability coefficients for the MPQ PRI as well as for some of the 20 categories. The lower coefficients for the 20 categories may be explained by the suggestion that many clinical pains show fluctuations in quality over time yet they still represent the 'same' pain to the person who experiences it.

Studies of the validity of the three-dimensional framework of the MPQ are numerous and have recently been

Table 18.1 Sample MPQ responses and scoring using the weighted rank method[1]

MPQ category	Weight (W_i)	Descriptor chosen	Rank score	Weighted rank score
1	0.69	Pulsing	3	2.07
2	1.38	—	0	0.00
3	0.93	Stabbing	4	3.72
4	1.59	Sharp	1	1.59
5	0.81	—	0	0.00
6	1.19	Wrenching	3	3.57
7	1.28	Hot	1	1.28
8	0.70	Smarting	3	2.1
9	0.72	Aching	4	2.88
10	0.95	Tender	1	0.95
			PRI-S = 20	18.16
11	1.74	Exhausting	2	3.48
12	2.22	Sickening	1	2.22
13	1.87	Frightful	2	3.74
14	1.32	Vicious	4	5.28
15	2.33	Wretched	1	2.33
			PRI-A = 10	17.05
16	1.01	Intense	4	4.04
			PRI-E = 4	4.04
17	1.22	—	0	0.00
18	0.82	Numb	2	1.64
19	1.0	Cool	1	1.0
20	1.15	Agonizing	3	3.54
			PRI-M = 6	6.09
			PRI-T = 40	45.34

[1] The rank score of each descriptor chosen by the patient is multiplied by the weight (W_i) for that category to obtain the corresponding weighted rank score. These scores are summed to obtain a score for each of the pain rating index (PRI) subclasses: PRI-S = sensory; PRI-A = affective; PRI-E = evaluative; PRI-M = miscellaneous; PRI-T = total score.

reviewed by Reading (1989). Generally, the distinction between sensory and affective dimensions has held up extremely well, but there is still considerable debate on the separation of the affective and evaluative dimensions. Nevertheless, several excellent studies (Reading 1979; Prieto et al 1980; McCreary et al 1981; Holroyd et al 1992) have reported a discrete evaluative factor. The different factor-analytic procedures that were used undoubtedly account for the reports of four factors (Reading 1979; Holroyd et al 1992), five factors (Crockett et al 1977), six factors (Burckhardt 1984) or seven factors (Leavitt et al 1978). The major source of disagreement, however, seems to be the different patient populations that are used to obtain data for factor analyses. The range includes brief laboratory pains, dysmenorrhoea, back pain and cancer pain. In some studies relatively few words are chosen, while large numbers are selected in others. It is not surprising, then, that factor-analytic studies based on such diverse populations have confused rather than clarified some of the issues.

Table 18.2 Pain questionnaires in different languages based on the McGill Pain Questionnaire

Language	Authors
Arabic	Harrison (1988)
Chinese	Hui & Chen (1989)
Czech	Solcovä et al (1990)
Dutch (Flemish)	Vanderiet et al (1987)
	Verkes et al (1989)
Finnish	Ketovuori & Pöntinen (1981)
French	Boureau et al (1984, 1992)
German	Kiss et al (1987)
	Radvila et al (1987)
	Stein & Mendl (1988)
Italian	De Benedittis et al (1988)
	Ferracuti et al (1990)
	Maiani & Sanavio (1985)
Japanese	Satow et al (1990)
Norwegian	Strand & Wisnes (1991)
Polish	Sedlak (1990)
Slovak	Bartko et al (1984)
Spanish	Bejarano et al (1985)
	Laheurta et al (1982)

A recent study by Turk et al (1985) examined the internal structure of the MPQ by using techniques that avoided the problems of most earlier studies and confirmed the three (sensory, affective and evaluative) dimensions. Still more recently, Lowe et al (1991) again confirmed the three-factor structure of the MPQ, using elegant statistical procedures and a large number of subjects. Finally, a recent paper by Chen et al (1989) presents data on the remarkable consistency of the MPQ across five studies using the cold pressor task and Pearce & Morley (1989) provided further confirmation of the construct validity of the MPQ using the Stroop colour naming task with chronic pain patients.

Discriminative capacity of the MPQ

One of the most exciting features of the MPQ is its potential value as an aid in the differential diagnosis between various pain syndromes. The first study to demonstrate the discriminative capacity of the MPQ was carried out by Dubuisson & Melzack (1976), who administered the questionnaire to 95 patients suffering from one of eight known pain syndromes: postherpetic neuralgia, phantom limb pain, metastatic carcinoma, toothache, degenerative disc disease, rheumatoid arthritis or osteoarthritis, labour pain and menstrual pain. A multiple group discriminant analysis revealed that each type of pain is characterized by a distinctive constellation of verbal descriptors (Fig. 18.4). Further, when the descriptor set for each patient was classified into one of the eight diagnostic categories, a correct classification was made in 77% of cases. Table 18.3 shows the pain descriptors that are most characteristic of the eight clinical pain syndromes in the Dubuisson & Melzack (1976) study.

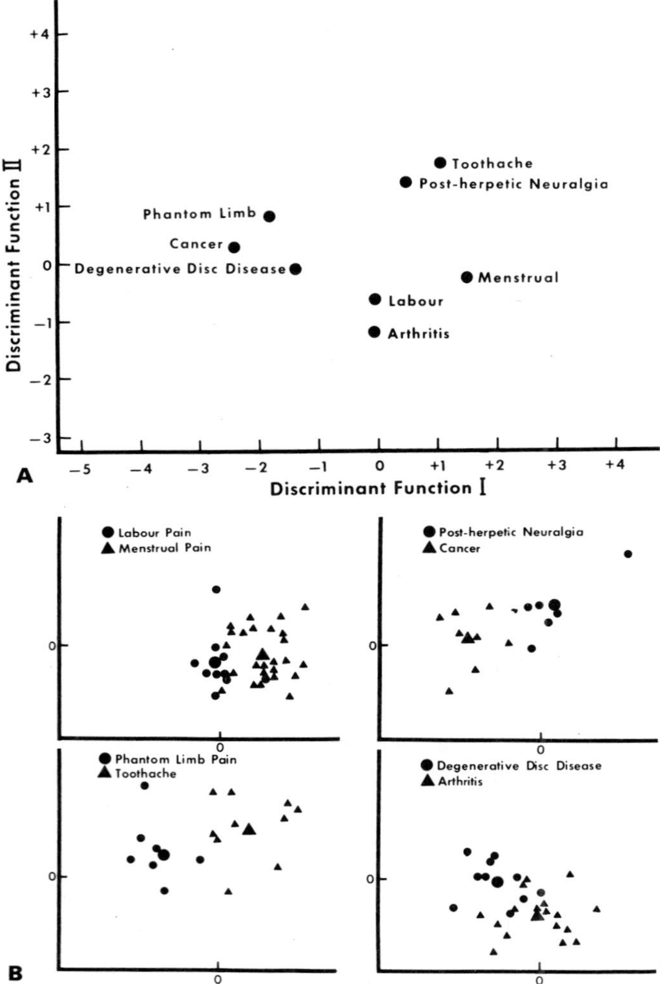

Fig. 18.4 (**A**) Centroids of eight diagnostic groups in the space of the first two discriminant functions reported by Dubuisson & Melzack (1976). (**B**) Individual patients' scores on the first two discriminant functions, for each diagnostic group. Large circle or triangle represents group centroid; small circles and triangles represent individual scores.

Descriptor patterns can also provide the basis for discriminating between two major types of low back pain. Some patients have clear physical causes such as degenerative disc disease, while others suffer low back pain even though no physical causes can be found. Using a modified version of the MPQ, Leavitt & Garron (1980) found that patients with physical ('organic') causes use distinctly different patterns of words from patients whose pain has no detectable cause and is labelled as 'functional'. A concordance of 87% was found between established medical diagnosis and classification based upon the patients' choice of word patterns from the MPQ. Along similar lines, Perry et al (1988, 1991) report differences in the pattern of MPQ subscale correlations in patients with and without demonstrable organic pathology.

Further evidence of the discriminative capacity of the MPQ was furnished by Melzack et al (1986) who differentiated between the pain of trigeminal neuralgia and atypical facial pain. A thorough neurological examination was given to 53 patients which led to a diagnosis of either trigeminal neuralgia or atypical facial pain. Each patient rated his or her pain using the MPQ and the scores were submitted to a discriminant analysis. Of these patients, 91% were correctly classified using seven key descriptors. To determine how well the key descriptors were able to predict either diagnosis, the discriminant function derived from the 53 patients was applied to MPQ scores obtained from a second, independent validation sample of patients with trigeminal neuralgia or atypical facial pain. The results showed a correct prediction for 90% of the patients.

Specific verbal descriptors of the MPQ have also been shown recently to discriminate between reversible and irreversible damage of the nerve fibres in a tooth (Grushka & Sessle 1984), and between leg pain caused by diabetic neuropathy and leg pain arising from other causes (Masson et al 1989). Jerome et al (1988) further showed that the MPQ discriminates between cluster headache pain and other vascular (migraine and mixed) headache pain. Cluster headache is more intense and distressing than the others and is characterized by a distinct constellation of descriptors.

It is evident, however, that the discriminative capacity of the MPQ has limits. High levels of anxiety and other psychological disturbance, which may produce high affective scores, may obscure the discriminative capacity (Kremer & Atkinson 1983). Moreover, certain key words that discriminate among specific syndromes may be absent (Reading 1982). Nevertheless, it is clear that there are appreciable and quantifiable differences in the way various types of pain are described and that patients with the same disease or pain syndrome tend to use remarkably similar words to communicate what they feel.

The short-form McGill Pain Questionnaire (SF-MPQ)

The short-form MPQ (Melzack 1987; Fig. 18.5) was developed for use in specific research settings when the time to obtain information from patients is limited and when more information is desired than that provided by intensity measures such as the VAS or PPI. The SF-MPQ consists of 15 representative words from the sensory (n = 11) and affective (n = 4) categories of the standard, long-form (LF-MPQ). The PPI and VAS are included to provide indices of overall pain intensity. The 15 descriptors making up the SF-MPQ were selected on the basis of their frequency of endorsement by patients with a variety of acute, intermittent, and chronic pains. An additional word (splitting) was added because it was reported to be a key discriminative word for dental pain (Grushka & Sessle 1984). Each descriptor is ranked by the patient on an

Table 18.3 Descriptions characteristic of clinical pain syndromes[1]

	Menstrual pain (n = 25)	Arthritic pain (n = 16)	Labour pain (n = 11)	Disc disease pain (n = 10)	Toothache (n = 10)	Cancer pain (n = 8)	Phantom limb pain (n = 8)	Postherpetic pain (n = 6)
Sensory	Cramping (44%) Aching (44%)	Gnawing (38%) Aching (50%)	Pounding (37%) Shooting (46%) Stabbing (37%) Sharp (64%) Cramping (82%) Aching (46%)	Throbbing (40%) Shooting (50%) Stabbing (40%) Sharp (60%) Cramping (40%) Aching (40%) Heavy (40%) Tender (50%)	Throbbing (50%) Boring (40%) Sharp (50%)	Shooting (50%) Sharp (50%) Gnawing (50%) Burning (50%) Heavy (50%)	Throbbing (38%) Stabbing (50%) Sharp (38%) Cramping (50%) Burning (50%) Aching (38%)	Sharp (84%) Pulling (67%) Aching (50%) Tender (83%)
Affective	Tiring (44%) Sickening (56%)	Exhausting (50%)	Tiring (37%) Exhausting (46%) Fearful (36%)	Tiring (46%) Exhausting (40%)	Sickening (40%)	Exhausting (50%)	Tiring (50%) Exhausting (38%) Cruel (38%)	Exhausting (50%)
Evaluative		Annoying (38%)	Intense (46%)	Unbearable (40%)	Annoying (50%)	Unbearable (50%)		
Temporal	Constant (56%)	Constant (44%) Rhythmic (56%)	Rhythmic (91%)	Constant (80%) Rhythmic (70%)	Constant (60%) Rhythmic (40%)	Constant (100%) Rhythmic (88%)	Constant (88%) Rhythmic (63%)	Constant (50%) Rhythmic (50%)

[1]Only those words chosen by more than one-third of the patients are listed and the percentages of patients who chose each word are shown below the word.

intensity scale of 0 = none, 1 = mild, 2 = moderate, 3 = severe.

The SF-MPQ correlates very highly with the major pain rating indices (sensory, PRI-S; affective, PRI-A; total, PRI-T) of the LF-MPQ (Melzack 1987; Dudgeon et al 1992) and is sensitive to clinical change brought about by various therapies– analgesic drugs (Melzack 1987; Harden et al 1991), epidurally or spinally administered agents (Melzack 1987; Harden et al 1991; Serrao et al 1992), transcutaneous electrical nerve stimulation (Melzack 1987) and low-power light therapy (Stelian et al 1992). In addition, concurrent validity of the SF-MPQ was recently reported in a study of patients with chronic pain due to cancer (Dudgeon et al 1992). On each of three occasions separated by at least a 3-week period, the PRI-S, PRI-A and PRI-T scores correlated highly with scores on the LF-MPQ.

Preliminary results from a study designed to examine the qualities of pain experienced by patients in a physical rehabilitation hospital indicate that the sensory dimension of the SF-MPQ correlates highly with analgesic use among a subgroup of patients with high pain scores (Katz & Vadnais 1990). The SF-MPQ has also recently been used in studies of chronic pain of diverse aetiology (Grönblad et al 1990; Guieu et al 1991; Dudgeon et al 1992) and to evaluate discomfort in response to internal mammary artery injections during coronary angiography (Miller & Knox 1992). Furthermore, initial data (Melzack 1987) suggest that the SF-MPQ may be capable of discriminating among different pain syndromes, which is an important property of the LF-MPQ. A Czech version of the SF-MPQ has been recently developed (Solcovä et al 1990).

Multidimensional pain experience

Turk et al (1985) and, more recently, Holroyd et al (1992) evaluated the theoretical structure of the MPQ using

SHORT-FORM McGILL PAIN QUESTIONNAIRE
RONALD MELZACK

PATIENT'S NAME: ____________________ DATE: __________

	NONE	MILD	MODERATE	SEVERE
THROBBING	0) ____	1) ____	2) ____	3) ____
SHOOTING	0) ____	1) ____	2) ____	3) ____
STABBING	0) ____	1) ____	2) ____	3) ____
SHARP	0) ____	1) ____	2) ____	3) ____
CRAMPING	0) ____	1) ____	2) ____	3) ____
GNAWING	0) ____	1) ____	2) ____	3) ____
HOT-BURNING	0) ____	1) ____	2) ____	3) ____
ACHING	0) ____	1) ____	2) ____	3) ____
HEAVY	0) ____	1) ____	2) ____	3) ____
TENDER	0) ____	1) ____	2) ____	3) ____
SPLITTING	0) ____	1) ____	2) ____	3) ____
TIRING-EXHAUSTING	0) ____	1) ____	2) ____	3) ____
SICKENING	0) ____	1) ____	2) ____	3) ____
FEARFUL	0) ____	1) ____	2) ____	3) ____
PUNISHING-CRUEL	0) ____	1) ____	2) ____	3) ____

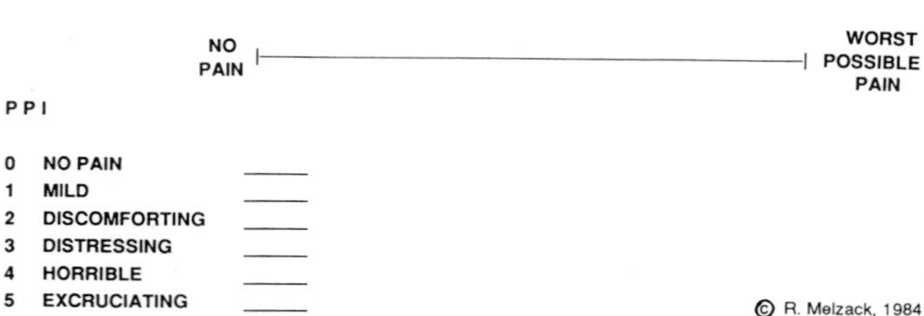
NO PAIN |————————————————| WORST POSSIBLE PAIN

PPI

0 NO PAIN ____
1 MILD ____
2 DISCOMFORTING ____
3 DISTRESSING ____
4 HORRIBLE ____
5 EXCRUCIATING ____

Fig. 18.5 The short-form McGill Pain Questionnaire. Descriptors 1–11 represent the sensory dimension of pain experience and 12–15 represent the affective dimension. Each descriptor is ranked on an intensity scale of 0 = none, 1 = mild, 2 = moderate, 3 = severe. The present pain intensity (PPI) of the standard long-form McGill Pain Questionnaire and the visual analogue scale are also included to provide overall pain intensity scores.

factor analytic methods to analyse their data. Turk et al concluded that the three-factor structure of the MPQ (sensory, affective and evaluative) is strongly supported by the analyses; Holroyd's 'most clearly interpretable structure' was provided by a four-factor solution obtained by oblique rotation in which two sensory factors were identified in addition to an affective and an evaluative factor.

Like most others who have used the MPQ, Turk et al (1985) and Holroyd et al (1992) find high intercorrelations among the factors. However, these authors then argue that because the factors measured by the MPQ are highly intercorrelated, they are therefore not distinct. They conclude that the MPQ does not discriminate among the factors and according to Turk et al only the PRI-T should be used. It is fallacious and potentially misleading to argue that the MPQ lacks discriminative capacity and clinical utility because factor-analytic studies reveal significant intercorrelations among the identified factors (Gracely 1992). There is, in fact, considerable evidence that the MPQ is effective in discriminating among the three factors despite the high intercorrelations.

First, Gracely (1992) has convincingly argued that factor-analytic methods may be inappropriate for assessing the factor structure of the MPQ although they provide useful information about patient characteristics. Torgerson (1988) distinguished between semantic meaning (how the MPQ descriptors are arranged) and associate meaning (how patients arrange the MPQ descriptors) to emphasize that factor analysis provides a context-dependent structure of the latter – that is, the outcome depends on how specific patient samples make use of the MPQ descriptors. Gracely (1992) elaborates further on the difference between semantic and associative meaning and concludes that factor-analytic techniques do not 'directly evaluate the semantic structure of the questionnaire'.

Second, a high correlation among variables does not necessarily imply a lack of discriminant capacity. Traditional psychophysics has shown repeatedly that, in the case of vision, increasing the intensity of light produces increased capacity to discriminate colour, contours, texture and distance (Kling & Riggs 1971). Similarly, in the case of hearing, increases in volume lead to increased discrimination of timbre, pitch and spatial location (Kling & Riggs 1971). In these cases, there are clearly very high intercorrelations among the variables in each modality. But this does not mean that we should forget about the differences between colour and texture, or between timbre and pitch just because they intercorrelate highly. This approach would lead to the loss of valuable, meaningful data (Gracely 1992).

Third, many papers have demonstrated the discriminant validity of the MPQ. Reading & Newton (1977) showed, in a comparison of primary dysmenorrhoea and intrauterine device (IUD) related pain, that the 'pain intensity scores were reflected in a larger sensory component with IUD users, whereas with dysmenorrhoea the affective component predominated'. In a later study, Reading (1982) compared MPQ profiles of women experiencing chronic pelvic pain and postepisiotomy pain and showed that 'acute-pain patients displayed greater use of sensory word groups, testifying to the pronounced sensory input from the damaged perineum. Chronic pain patients used affective and reaction subgroups with greater frequency.'

In a study of hypnosis and biofeedback, Melzack & Perry (1975) found that 'there were significant decreases in both the sensory and affective dimensions, as well as the overall PRI, but that the affective dimension shows the largest decrease'. In studies on labour pain, Melzack and his colleagues (Melzack et al 1981, 1984) found that distinctly different variables correlate with the sensory, affective and evaluative dimensions. Prepared childbirth practice, for example, correlates significantly with the sensory and affective dimensions but not the evaluative one. Menstrual difficulties correlate with the affective but neither the sensory nor evaluative dimension. Physical factors, such as mother's and infant's weight, also correlate selectively with one or another dimension.

Similarly, a study of acute pain in emergency ward patients (Melzack et al 1982) has 'revealed a normal distribution of sensory scores but very low affective scores compared to patients with chronic pain'. Finally, Chen et al (1989) have consistently identified a group of pain-sensitive and pain-tolerant subjects in five laboratory studies of tonic (prolonged) pain. Compared with pain-tolerant subjects, pain-sensitive subjects show significantly higher scores on all PRIs except the sensory dimension. Atkinson et al (1982) are undoubtedly right that high affect scores tend to diminish the discriminant capacity of the MPQ so that, at high levels of anxiety and depression, some discriminant capacity is lost. However, the MPQ still retains good discriminant function even at high levels of anxiety.

A recent study is of particular interest because it examines laboratory models of phasic (brief) and tonic (prolonged) pain and compares them by using the MPQ. Chen & Treede (1985) found a very high sensory loading for phasic pain and relatively few choices of affective and evaluative words. In contrast, tonic pain was characterized by much higher scores in the affective and evaluative dimensions. Furthermore, they found that when tonic pain is used to inhibit the phasic pain, 'the sensory component is reduced by 32%, whereas the affective component vanishes almost completely'.

In summary:

1. High intercorrelations among psychological variables do not mean that they are all alike and can therefore be lumped into a single variable such as intensity; rather, certain biological and psychological variables can covary to a high degree yet represent distinct, discriminable entities.
2. The MPQ has been shown in many studies to be capable of discriminating among the three component factors.

THE DESCRIPTOR DIFFERENTIAL SCALE (DDS)

Recently, simple but sophisticated psychophysical techniques have been applied to the development of pain measurement instruments which have been used to assess clinical and experimentally induced pain (Gracely & Dubner 1981; Hall 1981; Gracely & Kwilosz 1988; Price 1988; Gracely 1989a, 1989b). The psychophysical approach uses cross-modality matching (CMM) procedures to determine the relative magnitudes of verbal descriptors of pain (Gracely et al 1978a).

DDS (Gracely & Kwilosz 1988) was developed by Gracely et al (1978a) to remedy a number of deficiencies associated with existing pain measurement instruments. The DDS was designed to reduce bias, assess separately the sensory intensity and 'unpleasantness' (hedonic) dimensions of pain and provide quantification by ratio-scaling procedures (Gracely 1983). The DDS consists of two forms that measure separately the sensory intensity and unpleasantness qualities of pain. Each form consists of 12 verbal descriptors, in which each descriptor is centred over a 21-point scale with a minus sign at the low end and a plus sign at the high end. The patients rate the magnitude of the sensory intensity or unpleasantness of the pain they are experiencing. The magnitude of pain endorsed by the patient in relation to each descriptor is assigned a score of 0 (minus sign) to 20 (plus sign) where a score of 10 represents pain intensity or unpleasantness equal to the magnitude implied by the descriptor. Total mean scores may be obtained for the sensory intensity and unpleasantness dimensions by averaging the patient's scores on each 12-item form.

The DDS, derived from CMM procedures, has been demonstrated to be differentially sensitive to pharmacological interventions that alter the sensory or unpleasantness dimensions of pain (Gracely et al 1978b, 1979, 1982). Recent results point to the importance of using multidimensional measures of pain with clear instructions to rate separately the sensory intensity and unpleasantness aspects of pain as opposed to the 'painfulness' of the experience (Gracely & Dubner 1987). When used in conjunction with CMM techniques, the DDS has been shown to be a reliable and valid instrument with ratio scale properties (Gracely et al 1978a, 1978b).

More recently, Gracely & Kwilosz (1988) assessed the psychometric properties of the DDS for use as a clinical pain measure among a sample of 91 dental patients after third molar extraction. Sensory intensity and unpleasantness DDS forms were administered to all patients 1 hour and 2 hours after surgery. Total scores on both forms showed high test-retest reliability coefficients as did scores derived from individual items. Correlation coefficients between individual items and the total score revealed a high degree of internal consistency for both forms of the DDS. One of the most useful features of the DDS is the potential to define a measure of scaling consistency that can be used to identify invalid patient profiles obtained by inconsistent responding. Elimination of invalid profiles improved reliability and internal consistency of the DDS.

BEHAVIOURAL APPROACHES

Recent research into the development of behavioural measures of pain has produced a wide array of sophisticated observational techniques and rating scales designed to assess objective behaviours that accompany pain experience (Keefe 1989; Turk & Melzack 1992). Techniques that have demonstrated high reliability and validity are especially useful for measuring pain in infants and preverbal children who lack language skills (McGrath & Unruh 1987; Ross & Ross 1988; McGrath 1990), adults who have a poor command of language (Reading 1989) or when mental clouding and confusion limit the patient's ability to communicate meaningfully (Cleeland 1989). Under these circumstances, behavioural measures provide important information that is otherwise unavailable from patient self-report. Moreover, when administered in conjunction with a subjective, patient-rated measure, behavioural measures may provide a more complete picture of the total pain experience. However, behavioural measures of pain should not replace self-rated measures if the patient is capable of rating his or her subjective state and such administration is feasible.

The subjective experiences of pain and pain behaviours are, presumably, reflections of the same underlying neural processes. However, the complexity of the human brain indicates that although experience and behaviour are usually highly correlated, they are far from identical. One person may be stoic so that his calm behaviour belies his true subjective feelings. Another patient may seek sympathy (or analgesic medication or some other desirable goal) and in so doing exaggerate his complaints without also eliciting the behaviours that typically accompany pain complaints of that degree. Concordance between patients' self ratings of pain and ratings of the same patients by nurses or other medically trained personnel may be modestly low (Teske et al 1983; Cleeland 1989; Loeser 1989; Van der Does 1989; Choinière et al 1990), but even in the presence of a significant correlation between physician and patient ratings of patient pain, physicians significantly underestimate the degree of pain the patients reported experiencing (Sutherland et al 1988). Moreover, when health care providers observe a discordance between nonverbal pain behaviour and the patient's verbal complaint of pain, the discrepancy often is resolved by disregarding the patient's self-report (Craig & Prkachin 1983; Craig 1989). These studies point to the importance of obtaining multiple measures of pain and should keep us aware that since pain is a subjective experience, the patient's self-report is the most valid measure of that experience.

PHYSIOLOGICAL APPROACHES

Profound physiological changes often accompany the experience of pain, especially if the injury or noxious stimulus is acute (Cousins 1989). Physiological correlates of pain may serve to elucidate mechanisms that underlie the experience and thus may provide clues which may lead to novel treatments (Chapman et al 1985; Price 1988). Physiological correlates of pain experience that are frequently measured include heart rate, blood pressure, electrodermal activity, electromyogram (EMG) and cortical-evoked potentials. Despite high initial correlations between pain onset and changes in these physiological responses, many habituate with time despite the persistence of pain (Gracely 1989b). In addition, these responses are not specific to the experience of pain per se, and occur under conditions of general arousal and stress. Recent studies that examined the general endocrine-metabolic stress response to surgical incision indicate that under certain conditions it is possible to dissociate different aspects of the stress response and pain (Kehlet 1986, 1988). Severe injury to a denervated limb produces a significant adrenocortical response (Kehlet 1988), but use of general anaesthesia clearly eliminates the conscious experience of pain in response to surgical incision without altering the subsequent rapid rise in plasma cortisol levels (Brandt et al 1976; Christensen et al 1982). These studies indicate that although there are many physiological events which occur concurrently with the experience of pain, many appear to be general responses to stress and are not unique to pain.

SUMMARY

Pain is a personal, subjective experience influenced by cultural learning, the meaning of the situation, attention and other psychological variables. Approaches to the measurement of pain include verbal and numeric self-rating scales, behavioural observation scales, and physiological responses. The complex nature of the experience of pain suggests that measurements from these domains may not always show high concordance. Because pain is subjective, the patient's self-report provides the most valid measure of the experience. The VAS and the MPQ are probably the most frequently used self-rating instruments for the measurement of pain in clinical and research settings. The MPQ is designed to assess the multidimensional nature of pain experience and has been demonstrated to be a reliable, valid and consistent measurement tool. The SF-MPQ is available for use in specific research settings when the time to obtain information from patients is limited and when more information than simply the intensity of pain is desired. The DDS was developed using sophisticated psychophysical techniques and is designed to measure separately the sensory and unpleasantness dimensions of pain. It has been shown to be a valid and reliable measure of pain with ratio scale properties and has recently been used in a clinical setting. Behavioural approaches to the measurement of pain also provide valuable data. Further development and refinement of pain measurement techniques will lead to increasingly accurate tools with greater predictive powers.

REFERENCES

Atkinson J H, Kremer E F, Ignelzi R J 1982 Diffusion of pain language with affective disturbance confounds differential diagnosis. Pain 12: 375–384

Bartko D, Kondos M, Jansco S 1984 Slovak version of the McGill-Melzack's Questionnaire on pain. Ceskoslovenska Neurologie a Neurochirurgie 47: 113–121

Beecher H K 1959 Measurement of subjective responses. Oxford University Press, New York

Bejarano P F, Noriego R D, Rodriguez M L, Berrio G M 1985 Evaluación del dolor: Adaptatión del cuestionario del McGill (Evaluation of pain: Adaptation of the McGill Pain Questionnaire) Revista Columbia Anestesia 13: 321–351

Bélanger E, Melzack R, Lauzon P 1989 Pain of first-trimester abortion: a study of psychosocial and medical predictors. Pain 36: 339–350

Bonica J J 1953 The management of pain. Lea & Febiger, Philadelphia

Boureau F, Luu M, Doubrère J F, Gay C 1984 Elaboration d'un questionnaire d'auto-évaluation de la douleur par liste de qualicatifs (Development of a self-evaluation questionnaire comprising pain descriptors). Thérapie 39: 119–129

Boureau F, Luu M, Doubrère J F 1992 Comparative study of the validity of four French McGill Pain Questionnaire (MPQ) versions. Pain 50: 59–65

Brandt M R, Kehlet H, Binder C, Hagen C, McNeilly A S 1976 Effect of epidural analgesia on the glucoregulatory endocrine response to surgery. Clinical Endocrinology 5: 107–114

Burckhardt C 1984 The use of the McGill Pain Questionnaire in assessing arthritis pain. Pain 19: 305–314

Carlsson A M 1983 Assessment of chronic pain. I. Aspects of the reliability and validity of the visual analogue scale. Pain 16: 87–101

Chapman C R, Casey K L, Dubner R, Foley K M, Gracely R H, Reading A E 1985 Pain measurement: an overview. Pain 22: 1–31

Charter R A, Nehemkis A M 1983 The language of pain intensity and complexity: new methods of scoring the McGill Pain Questionnaire. Perceptual and Motor Skills 56: 519–537

Chen A C N, Dworkin S F, Haug J, Gerhig J 1989 Human pain responsivity in a tonic pain model: psychological determinants. Pain 37: 143–160

Chen A C N, Treede R D 1985 McGill Pain Questionnaire in assessing the differentiation of phasic and tonic pain: behavioral evaluation of the 'pain inhibiting pain' effect. Pain 22: 67–79

Choinière M, Melzack R, Girard N, Rondeau J, Paquin M J 1990 Comparisons between patients' and nurses' assessments of pain and medication efficacy in severe burn injuries. Pain 40: 143–152

Christensen P, Brandt M R, Rem J, Kehlet H 1982 Influence of extradural morphine on the adrenocortical and hyperglycaemic response to surgery. British Journal of Anaesthesia 54: 23–27

Cleeland C S 1989 Measurement of pain by subjective report. In: Chapman C R, Loeser J D (eds) Issues in pain measurement (Advances in pain research and therapy, vol 12). Raven Press, New York, p 391–401

Cousins M 1989 Acute and postoperative pain. In: Wall P D, Melzack R (eds) Textbook of pain, 2nd edn. Churchill Livingstone, Edinburgh, p 284–305

Craig K D 1989 Clinical pain measurement from the perspective of the human laboratory. In: Chapman C R, Loeser J D (eds) Issues in pain measurement (Advances in pain research and therapy, vol 12). Raven Press, New York, p 433–442

Craig K D, Prkachin K M 1983 Nonverbal measures of pain. In: Melzack R (ed) Pain measurement and assessment. Raven Press, New York, p 173–182

Crockett D J, Prkachin K M, Craig K D 1977 Factors of the language of pain in patients and normal volunteer groups. Pain 4: 175–182

De Benedittis G, Massei R, Nobili R, Pieri A 1988 The Italian pain questionnaire. Pain 33: 53–62

Dubuisson D, Melzack R 1976 Classification of clinical pain descriptors by multiple group discriminant analysis. Experimental Neurology 51: 480–487

Dudgeon D, Ranbertas R F, Rosenthal S 1992 The Short-Form McGill Pain Questionnaire in chronic cancer pain. Journal of Pain and Symptom Management (submitted)

Ekblom A, Hansson P 1988 Pain intensity measurements in patients with acute pain receiving afferent stimulation. Journal of Neurology, Neurosurgery and Psychiatry 51: 481–486

Ferracuti S, Romeo G, Leardi M G, Cruccu G, Lazzari R 1990 New Italian adaptation and standardization of the McGill Pain Questionnaire. Pain (suppl 5): S300

Gaston-Johansson F, Albert M, Fagan E, Zimmerman L 1990 Similarities in pain descriptors of four different ethnic-culture groups. Journal of Pain and Symptom Management 5: 94–100

Gracely R H 1983 Pain language and ideal pain assessment. In: Melzack R (ed) Pain measurement and assessment. Raven Press, New York, p 71–78

Gracely R H 1989a Methods of testing pain mechanisms in normal man. In: Wall P D, Melzack R (eds) Textbook of pain, 2nd edn. Churchill Livingstone, Edinburgh, p 257–268

Gracely R H 1989b Pain psychophysics. In: Chapman C R, Loeser J D (eds) Issues in pain measurement (Advances in pain research and therapy, vol 12). Raven Press, New York, p 211–229

Gracely R H 1992 Evaluation of multi-dimensional pain scales. Pain 48: 297–300

Gracely R H, Dubner R 1981 Pain assessment in humans – a reply to Hall. Pain 11: 109–120

Gracely R H, Dubner R 1987 Reliability and validity of verbal descriptor scales of painfulness. Pain 29: 175–185

Gracely R H, Kwilosz D M 1988 The descriptor differential scale: applying psychophysical principles to clinical pain assessment. Pain 35: 279–288

Gracely R H, McGrath P A, Dubner R 1978a Ratio scales of sensory and affective verbal pain descriptors. Pain 5: 5–18

Gracely R H, McGrath P A, Dubner R 1978b Validity and sensitivity of ratio scales of sensory and affective verbal pain descriptors: manipulation of affect by diazepam. Pain 5: 19–29

Gracely R H, McGrath P A, Dubner R 1979 Narcotic analgesia: fentanyl reduces the intensity but not the unpleasantness of painful tooth pulp sensations. Science 203: 1361–1379

Gracely R H, Dubner R, McGrath P A 1982 Fentanyl reduces the intensity of painful tooth pulp sensations: controlling for detection of active drugs. Anesthesia and Analgesia 61: 751–755

Graham C, Bond S S, Gerkovitch M M, Cook M R 1980 Use of the McGill Pain Questionnaire in the assessment of cancer pain: replicability and consistency. Pain 8: 377–387

Grönblad M, Lukinmaa A, Konttinen Y T 1990 Chronic low-back pain: intercorrelation of repeated measures for pain and disability. Scandinavian Journal of Rehabilitation Medicine 22: 73–77

Grushka M, Sessle B J 1984 Applicability of the McGill Pain Questionnaire to the differentiation of 'toothache' pain. Pain 19: 49–57

Guieu R, Tardy-Gervet M F, Roll J P 1991 Analgesic effects of vibration and transcutaneous electrical nerve stimulation applied separately and simultaneously to patients with chronic pain. Canadian Journal of Neurological Sciences 18: 113–119

Hall W 1981 On 'ratio scales of sensory and affective verbal pain descriptors'. Pain 11: 101–107

Harden R N, Carter T D, Gilman C S, Gross A J, Peters J R 1991 Ketorolac in acute headache management. Headache 31: 463–464

Hardy J D, Wolff H G, Goodell H 1952 Pain sensations and reactions. Williams & Wilkins, Baltimore

Harrison A 1988 Arabic pain words. Pain 32: 239–250

Hartman L M, Ainsworth K D 1980 Self-regulation of chronic pain. Canadian Journal of Psychiatry 25: 38–43

Holroyd K A, Holm J E, Keefe F J et al 1992 A multi-center evaluation of the McGill Pain Questionnaire: results from more than 1700 chronic pain patients. Pain 48: 301–311

Hui Y L, Chen A C 1989 Analysis of headache in a Chinese patient population. Ma Tsui Hsueh Tsa Chi 27: 13–18

Huskisson E C 1974 Measurement of pain. Lancet 2: 1127–1131

Huskisson E C 1983 Visual analogue scales. In: Melzack R (ed) Pain measurement and assessment. Raven Press, New York, p 33–37

Jensen M P, Karoly P, Braver S 1986 The measurement of clinical pain intensity: a comparison of six methods. Pain 27: 117–126

Jerome A, Holroyd K A, Theofanous A G, Pingel J D, Lake A E, Saper J R 1988 Cluster headache pain vs. other vascular headache

pain: differences revealed with two approaches to the McGill Pain Questionnaire. Pain 34: 35–42
Joyce C R B, Zutshi D W, Hrubes V, Mason R M 1975 Comparison of fixed interval and visual analogue scales for rating chronic pain. European Journal of Clinical Pharmacology 8: 415–420
Katz J 1992 Psychophysical correlates of phantom limb experience. Journal of Neurology, Neurosurgery and Psychiatry 55: 811–821
Katz J, Melzack R 1991 Auricular TENS reduces phantom limb pain. Journal of Pain and Symptom Management 6: 73–83
Katz J, Vadnais M 1990 A survey of pain and analgesic use in a physical rehabilitation hospital. Canadian Pain Society Abstracts 30
Keefe F J 1989 Behavioural measurement of pain. In: Chapman C R, Loeser J D (eds) Issues in pain measurement (Advances in pain research and therapy, vol 12). Raven Press, New York, p 405–424
Kehlet H 1986 Pain relief and modification of the stress response. In: Cousins M J, Phillips G D (eds) Acute pain management. Churchill Livingstone, New York, p 49–75
Kehlet H 1988 Modification of responses to surgery by neural blockade: clinical implications. In: Cousins M J, Bridenbaugh P O (eds) Neural blockade in clinical anesthesia and management of pain, 2nd edn. J B Lippincott, Philadelphia, p 145–188
Ketovuori H, Pöntinen P J 1981 A pain vocabulary in Finnish – the Finnish pain questionnaire. Pain 11: 247–253
Kiss I, Müller H, Abel M 1987 The McGill Pain Questionnaire – German version. A study on cancer pain. Pain 29: 195–207
Klepac R K, Dowling J, Rokke P, Dodge L, Schafer L 1981 Interview vs. paper-and-pencil administration of the McGill Pain Questionnaire. Pain 11: 241–246
Kling J W, Riggs L A 1971 Experimental psychology. Holt, Rinehart & Winston, New York
Kremer E, Atkinson J H 1983 Pain language as a measure of affect in chronic pain patients. In: Melzack R (eds) Pain measurement and assessment. Raven Press, New York, p 119–127
Kremer E, Atkinson J H, Ignelzi R J 1982 Pain measurement: the affective dimensional measure of the McGill Pain Questionnaire with a cancer pain population. Pain 12: 153–163
Lahuerta J, Smith B A, Martinez-Lage J L 1982 An adaptation of the McGill Pain Questionnaire to the Spanish language. Schmerz 3: 132–134
Leavitt F, Garron D C 1980 Validity of a back pain classification scale for detecting psychological disturbance as measured by the MMPI. Journal of Clinical Psychology 36: 186–189
Leavitt F, Garron D C, Whisler W W, Sheinkop M B 1978 Affective and sensory dimensions of pain. Pain 4: 273–281
Livingston W K 1943 Pain mechanisms. Macmillan, New York
Loeser J D 1989 Pain relief and analgesia. In: Chapman C R, Loeser J D (eds) Issues in pain measurement (Advances in pain research and therapy, vol 12). Raven Press, New York, p 175–182
Love A, Leboeuf D C, Crisp T C 1989 Chiropractic chronic low back pain sufferers and self-report assessment methods. Part I. A reliability study of the Visual Analogue Scale, the pain drawing and the McGill Pain Questionnaire. Journal of Manipulative and Physiological Therapeutics 12: 21–25
Lowe N K, Walker S N, McCallum R C 1991 Confirming the theoretical structure of the McGill Pain Questionnaire in acute clinical pain. Pain 46: 53–60
Maiani G, Sanavio E 1985 Semantics of pain in Italy: the Italian version of the McGill Pain Questionnaire. Pain 22: 399–405
McCreary C, Turner J, Dawson E 1981 Principal dimensions of the pain experience and psychological disturbance in chronic low back pain patients. Pain 11: 85–92
McGrath P A 1990 Pain in children: nature, assessment, and treatment. Guilford Press, New York
McGrath P J, Unruh A 1987 Pain in children and adolescents. Elsevier, Amsterdam
Masson E A, Hunt L, Gem J M, Boulton A J M 1989 A novel approach to the diagnosis and assessment of symptomatic diabetic neuropathy. Pain 38: 25–28
Melzack R 1975 The McGill Pain Questionnaire: major properties and scoring methods. Pain 1: 277–299
Melzack R 1983 Pain measurement and assessment. Raven Press, New York
Melzack R 1987 The short-form McGill Pain Questionnaire. Pain 30: 191–197
Melzack R, Casey K L 1968 Sensory, motivational, and central control determinants of pain: a new conceptual model. In: Kenshalo D (ed) The skin senses. C C Thomas, Springfield, Illinois, p 423–443
Melzack R, Perry C 1975 Self-regulation of pain: the use of alpha-feedback and hypnotic training for the control of chronic pain. Experimental Neurology 46: 452–469
Melzack R, Torgerson W S 1971 On the language of pain. Anesthesiology 34: 50–59
Melzack R, Wall P D 1965 Pain mechanisms: a new theory. Science 150: 971–979
Melzack R, Wall P D 1988 The challenge of pain. Basic Books, New York
Melzack R, Taenzer P, Feldman P, Kinch R A 1981 Labour is still painful after prepared childbirth training. Canadian Medical Association Journal 125: 357–363
Melzack R, Wall P D, Ty T C 1982 Acute pain in an emergency clinic: latency of onset and description patterns related to different injuries. Pain 14: 33–43
Melzack R, Kinch R, Dobkin P, Lebrun M, Taenzer P 1984 Severity of labour pain: influence of physical as well as psychologic variables. Canadian Medical Association Journal 130: 579–584
Melzack R, Katz J, Jeans M E 1985 The role of compensation in chronic pain: analysis using a new method of scoring the McGill Pain Questionnaire. Pain 23: 101–112
Melzack R, Terrence C, Fromm G, Amsel R 1986 Trigeminal neuralgia and atypical facial pain: use of the McGill Pain Questionnaire for discrimination and diagnosis. Pain 27: 297–302
Miller R M, Knox M 1992 Patient tolerance of ioxaglate and iopamidol in internal mammary artery arteriography. Catheterization and Cardiovascular Diagnosis 25: 31–34
Noordenbos W 1959 Pain. Elsevier, Amsterdam
Ohnhaus E E, Adler R 1975 Methodological problems in the measurement of pain: a comparison between the Verbal Rating Scale and the Visual Analogue Scale. Pain 1: 374–384
Pearce J, Morley S 1989 An experimental investigation of the construct validity of the McGill Pain Questionnaire. Pain 39: 115–121
Perry F, Heller P H, Levine J D 1988 Differing correlations between pain measures in syndromes with or without explicable organic pathology. Pain 34: 185–189
Perry F, Heller P H, Levine J D 1991 A possible indicator of functional pain: poor pain scale correlation. Pain 46: 191–193
Price D D 1988 Psychological and neural mechanisms of pain. Raven Press, New York
Price D D, McGrath P A, Rafii A, Buckingham B 1983 The validation of visual analogue scales as ratio scale measures for chronic and experimental pain. Pain 17: 45–56
Prieto E J, Hopson L, Bradley L A et al 1980 The language of low back pain: factor structure of the McGill Pain Questionnaire. Pain 8: 11–19
Radvila A, Adler R H, Galeazzi R L, Vorkauf H 1987 The development of a German language (Berne) pain questionnarie and its application in a situation causing acute pain. Pain 28: 185–195
Reading A E 1979 The internal structure of the McGill Pain Questionnaire in dysmenorrhea patients. Pain 7: 353–358
Reading A E 1982 A comparison of the McGill Pain Questionnaire in chronic and acute pain. Pain 13: 185–192
Reading A E 1989 Testing pain mechanisms in persons in pain. In: Wall P D, Melzack R (eds) Textbook of pain, 2nd edn. Churchill Livingstone, Edinburgh, p 269–283
Reading A E, Newton J R 1977 On a comparison of dysmenorrhea and intrauterine device related pain. Pain 3: 265–276
Reading A E, Everitt B S, Sledmere C M 1982 The McGill Pain Questionnaire: a replication of its construction. British Journal of Clinical Psychology 21: 339–349
Ross D M, Ross S A 1988 Childhood pain: current issues, research, and management. Schwartzenberg, Baltimore
Satow A, Nakatani K, Taniguchi S, Higashiyama A 1990 Perceptual characteristics of electrocutaneous pain estimated by the 30-word list and Visual Analog Scale. Japanese Psychological Review 32: 155–164
Sedlak K 1990 A Polish version of the McGill Pain Questionnaire. Pain (suppl 5): S308

Serrao J M, Marks R L, Morley S J, Goodchild C S 1992 Intrathecal midazolam for the treatment of chronic mechanical low back pain: a controlled comparison with epidural steroid in a pilot study. Pain 48: 5–12

Solcovä I, Jacoubek B, Sÿkora J, Hnïk P 1990 Characterization of vertebrogenic pain using the short form of the McGill Pain Questionnaire. Casopis Lekaru Ceskych 129: 1611–1614

Sriwatanakul K, Kelvie W, Lasagna L, Calimlim J F, Weis O F, Mehta G 1983 Studies with different types of visual analog scales for measurement of pain. Clinical Pharmacology and Therapeutics 34: 234–239

Stein C, Mendl G 1988 The German counterpart to McGill Pain Questionnaire. Pain 32: 251–255

Stelian J, Gil I, Habot B et al 1992 Improvement of pain and disability in elderly patients with degenerative osteoarthritis of the knee treated with narrow-band light therapy. Journal of the American Geriatric Society 40: 23–26

Strand L I, Wisnes A R 1991 The development of a Norwegian pain questionnaire. Pain 46: 61–66

Sutherland J E, Wesley R M, Cole P M, Nesvacil L J, Daley M L, Gepner G J 1988 Differences and similarities between patient and physician perceptions of patient pain. Family Medicine 20: 343–346

Tahmoush A J 1981 Causalgia: redefinition as a clinical pain syndrome. Pain 10: 187–197

Teske K, Daut R L, Cleeland C S 1983 Relationships between nurses' observations and patients' self-reports of pain. Pain 16: 289–296

Torgerson W S 1988 Critical issues in verbal pain assessment: multidimensional and multivariate issues. American Pain Society Abstracts, Washington, D C

Turk D C, Melzack R (eds) 1992 Handbook of pain assessment. Guilford Press, New York

Turk D C, Rudy T E, Salovey P 1985 The McGill Pain Questionnaire reconsidered: confirming the factor structures and examining appropriate uses. Pain 21: 385–397

Van Buren J, Kleinknecht R 1979 An evaluation of the McGill Pain Questionnaire for use in dental pain assessment. Pain 6: 23–33

Van der Does A J W 1989 Patients' and nurses' ratings of pain and anxiety during burn wound care. Pain 39: 95–101

Vanderiet K, Adriaensen H, Carton H, Vertommen H 1987 The McGill Pain Questionnaire constructed for the Dutch language (MPQ-DV). Preliminary data concerning reliability and validity. Pain 30: 395–408

Veilleux S, Melzack R 1976 Pain in psychotic patients. Experimental Neurology 52: 535–563

Verkes R J, Van der Kloot W A, Van der Meij J 1989 The perceived structure of 176 pain descriptive words. Pain 38: 219–229

Wilkie D J, Savedra M C, Holzemier W L, Tesler M D, Paul S M 1990 Use of the McGill Pain Questionnaire to measure pain: a meta-analysis. Nursing Research 39: 36–41

Clinical aspects of diseases in which pain predominates

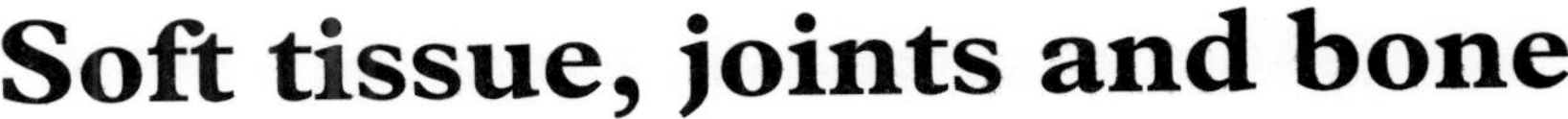

Soft tissue, joints and bone

19. Acute and postoperative pain

Michael Cousins

BACKGROUND AND HISTORICAL PERSPECTIVE

It is an indictment of modern medicine that an apparently simple problem such as the reliable relief of postoperative pain remains largely unsolved (Editorial, British Medical Journal 1978).

Despite substantial advances in knowledge of acute pain mechanisms and in treatment, acute pain is generally not effectively treated. This is partly a reflection of the emphasis in medicine on diagnosis and treatment of causative factors rather than on symptomatic treatment. In the case of acute pain, a cause is usually rapidly determined and its treatment reduces or relieves pain after a period of time. This relegates the relief of acute pain, in the minds of many doctors and nurses, to a minor level of priority. Diagnosis and treatment of the cause of acute pain due to trauma and acute medical and surgical conditions is the first priority. However, this should never preclude the use of appropriate effective methods of symptomatic pain relief. A well controlled study of patients with acute abdominal pain reported that the diagnosis was not altered in a single patient by the relief of acute pain with sublingual buprenorphine, even though there were minor changes in physical signs in 12% of patients receiving pain relief, compared to a control group (Zolte & Cust 1986).

Recognition of acute pain as a major problem has been unacceptably slow in view of repeated documentation of the inadequacies of its treatment. In a study of acute pain of various causes, Marks & Sacher (1973) reported that three-quarters of the patients who received narcotics for severe pain continued to experience pain. These findings have been confirmed in adults by Cohen (1980) and in children by Mather & Mackie (1983). In the USA alone 23 million patients undergo surgery every year and the majority of these experience postoperative pain (Acute Pain Management 1992).

Trauma produced by accidents ranks third as the cause of death in industrialised societies, being surpassed only by cardiovascular disease and cancer. Trauma causes more deaths in young people between the ages of 15 and 24 years than all other causes combined. In a single year in the USA, at least 17 million civilians sustained injuries requiring hospitalisation. The overall cost of all injuries in 1977 was $62 billion (Accident Facts 1978). Most of these injured patients eventually experience pain that requires management.

It is likely that all forms of acute pain are poorly managed: postoperative, posttrauma, following burns, acute medical diseases (e.g. pancreatitis, myocardial infarction), obstetric pain (Melzack et al 1981; Bonica 1985; Cousins & Phillips 1986). The effective relief of labour pain with epidural block in more than 95% of patients gives hope that other types of acute pain can also be relieved (Cousins & Bridenbaugh 1988). This does not imply that neural blockade is 'the answer' to acute pain – it is one of the answers. A wide range of pharmacological, physical and psychological treatments for acute pain is now available.

Improved understanding of peripheral and central mechanisms of pain offers new treatment options. Pain treatment techniques depend, for their effective use, on overcoming financial, administrative and logistical hurdles (Cousins & Phillips 1986). Educational programmes need to be developed and implemented for nursing, medical and other staff. Much of this depends on a close collaboration between medical, nursing and administrative staff. The regimens chosen for each institution must be appropriate to the resources and range of expertise in that setting. A powerful aid to improving acute pain treatment would be the use of a 'pain control audit'. In some hospitals, pain is now charted, along with temperature and pulse, and orders for treatment are based on a pain score, obtained with a visual analogue scale or other techniques described in Chapter 18. Audit of the efficacy of pain control becomes feasible if a record of this type is a routine part of the medical record. Acute pain in children is a special case requiring urgent attention. This is because of the fallacious dogma that children suffer less pain than do adults. Techniques developed in adults can be applied in children; however, problems in implementation need to be overcome.

In addition to humanitarian reasons for improving acute pain treatment, there is now convincing evidence that unrelieved acute pain may result in harmful physiological and psychological effects. These adverse effects may result in significant morbidity and even mortality (Yeager et al 1987; Kehlet 1988; Scott & Kehlet 1988; Cousins 1989).

Evidence of shortened hospital stay, decreased morbidity and mortality, and increased patient satisfaction have been reported in association with effective relief of acute pain (Modig 1976; Brandt et al 1978; Modig et al 1983; Rawal et al 1984; Cullen et al 1985; Yeager et al 1987). This has increased medical and public interest in acute pain as an important problem. In some institutions it has resulted in the setting up of 'acute pain services', sometimes in association with a comprehensive unit managing both acute and chronic pain.

The US Department of Health and Human Services recently took the unprecedented step of publishing a clinical practice guideline for acute pain management, which is based upon a detailed analysis of several thousand scientific publications, examining the efficacy and safety of different methods of acute pain control. Based upon this analysis, strong recommendations are made for the organisation, delivery and monitoring of acute pain services (Acute Pain Management 1992).

A summary of the major elements and goals of an acute pain service is outlined in Table 19.1. The scientific basis for the various treatment options for acute pain management, as recently evaluated in the Clinical Practice Guideline, is summarised in Table 19.2. It is apparent that a major impetus has now been provided to improve the treatment of acute pain on the basis of substantially increased scientific knowledge and by setting up 'acute pain services' (Ready et al 1988; Cousins 1989).

Table 19.1 Clinical practice and acute pain: guidelines and major goals

Guidelines	A collaborative, interdisciplinary approach to pain control, including all members of the health care team and input from the patient and the patient's family, when appropriate. An individualised proactive pain control plan developed preoperatively by patients and practitioners (since pain is easier to prevent than to treat)
	Assessment and frequent reassessment of the patient's pain
	Use of both drug and nondrug therapies to control and/or prevent pain
	A formal, institutional approach, with clear lines of responsibility
Major goals	Reduce the incidence and severity of patients' postoperative or post-traumatic pain
	Educate patients about the need to communicate regarding unrelieved pain, so they can receive prompt evaluation and effective treatment
	Enhance patient comfort and satisfaction
	Contribute to fewer postoperative complications and, in some cases, shorter stays after surgical procedures

BIOLOGICAL FUNCTIONS OF ACUTE PAIN

Religious, philosophical and other connotations have been ascribed to acute pain. However, it is clear that pain usually signals impending or actual tissue damage and thus permits the individual to avoid harm. It is interesting to examine the evidence of studies in patients with congenital insensitivity to pain. Such individuals appear to have shortened life expectancy because of unrecognised trauma and associated complications (Sternbach 1963).

Pain may also prevent harmful movement, for example, in the case of a fracture; this may be viewed as a protective role. For a finite period of time reduced mobility associated with acute pain may aid healing. However, evidence is emerging that the organism benefits only briefly from this effect and its prolongation results in an adverse outcome (Bonica 1985; Cousins & Phillips 1986; Kehlet 1988).

Pain also initiates complex neurohumoral responses (see below) that help initially to maintain homeostasis in the face of an acute disease or injury; if these changes are excessive or unduly prolonged, they may cause morbidity or mortality (Cousins & Phillips 1986; Kehlet 1988). Psychological responses to acute pain may initially be helpful in coping with the physical insult; however, if excessively severe or prolonged, they may become deleterious. In the medical context, acute pain alerts the patient to the need for medical help and helps the medical practitioner to pinpoint the location and cause of the problem. However, there is a substantial error rate in the diagnosis of some forms of acute pain. This is particularly so for acute visceral pain; for example, over 20% of diagnoses of acute appendicitis are in error. Knowledge of mechanisms of acute pain may aid clinical diagnosis and reduce this error rate, thereby supporting a more positive biological role for acute pain.

PHYSIOLOGICAL RESPONSES TO TISSUE INJURY AND ACUTE PAIN

The response to tissue damage is similar regardless of whether it results from surgical incision, traumatic injury such as a fracture of the bony skeleton or crush to soft tissue, burns, or disease of internal organs. It would be expected that very major trauma would produce a greater response than rather minor degrees of tissue trauma and, at this gross level, this appears to be true. However, there is now impressive evidence of an enormous individual

Table 19.2 Scientific evidence for interventions to manage pain in adults (for references see Acute Pain Management 1992). Insufficient scientific evidence is available to provide specific recommendations regarding the use of hypnosis, acupuncture, and other physical modalities for relief of postoperative pain. In this table 'Expert opinion' refers to evidence obtained from expert committee reports or opinions and/or clinical experiences of respected authorities.

Intervention	Type of evidence	Comments
Pharmacological		
NSAIDs		
Oral (alone)	At least one randomised, controlled trial Expert opinion	Effective for mild to moderate pain. Begin preoperatively. Relatively contraindicated in patients with renal disease and risk of or actual coagulopathy. May mask fever.
Oral (adjunct to opioid)	Meta-analysis of randomised, controlled trials Expert opinion	Potentiating effect resulting in opioid sparing. Begin preoperatively. Cautions as above.
Parenteral (ketorolac)	At least one randomised, controlled trial Expert opinion	Effective for moderate to severe pain. Expensive. Useful where opioids contraindicated, especially to avoid respiratory depression and sedation. Adjunct to opioid.
Opioids		
Oral	Expert opinion	As effective as parenteral in appropriate doses. Use as soon as oral medication tolerated. Route of choice.
Intramuscular	At least one randomised, controlled trial Expert opinion	Has been the standard parenteral route, but injections painful and absorption unreliable. Hence, avoid this route when possible.
Subcutaneous	At least one randomised, controlled trial Expert opinion	Preferable to intramuscular for low volume continuous transfusion. Injections painful and absorption unreliable. Avoid this route for long-term repetitive dosing.
Intravenous	At least one randomised, controlled trial Expert opinion	Parenteral route of choice after major surgery. Suitable for titrated bolus or continuous administration (including patient-controlled analgesia), but requires monitoring. Significant risk of respiratory depression with inappropriate dosing.
PCA (systemic)	Meta-analysis of randomised, controlled trials Expert opinion	Intravenous or subcutaneous routes recommended. Good, steady level of analgesia. Popular with patients but requires special infusion pumps and staff education. See cautions about opioids above.
Epidural and intrathecal	Meta-analysis of randomised, controlled trials Expert opinion	When suitable, provides good analgesia. Significant risk of respiratory depression, sometimes delayed in onset. Requires careful monitoring. Use of infusion pumps requires additional equipment and staff education.
Local anaesthetics		
Epidural and intrathecal	Meta-analysis of randomised, controlled trials Expert opinion	Limited indications. Expensive if infusion pumps employed. Effective regional anaesthesia. Opioid sparing. Addition of opioid to local anaesthetic may improve anaglesia. Risks of hypotension, weakness, numbness. Use of infusion pump requries additional equipment and staff.
Peripheral nerve block	Meta-analysis of randomised, controlled trials Expert opinion	Limited indications and duration of action. Effective regional analgesia. Opioid sparing.
Nonpharmacological		
Simple relaxation (begin preoperatively)		
Jaw relaxation Progressive muscle relaxation Simple imagery	Meta-analysis of randomised, controlled trials At least one well-designed, controlled study without randomisation. At least one other type of well-designed quasi-experimental study Expert opinion	Effective in reducing mild to moderate pain and as an adjunct to analgesic drugs for severe pain. Use when patients express an interest in relaxation. Requires 3–5 minutes of staff time for instructions.
Music	At least one randomised, controlled trial At least one well-designed, controlled study without randomisation Expert opinion	Both patient-preferred and 'easy listening' music are effective in reducing mild to moderate pain.
Complex relaxation (begin preoperatively)		
Biofeedback	At least one randomised, controlled trial At least one well-designed, controlled study without randomisation Expert opinion	Effective in reducing mild to moderate pain and operative site muscle tension. Requires skilled personnel and special equipment.

Table 19.2 *(contd)*

Intervention	Type of evidence	Comments
Imagery	At least one randomised, controlled trial At least one well-designed, controlled study without randomisation At least one other type of well-designed quasi-experimental study Expert opinion	Effective for reduction of mild to moderate pain. Requires skilled personnel.
Education/instruction (begin preoperatively)	Meta-analysis of randomised, controlled trials At least one well-designed controlled study without randomisation At least one other type of well-designed quasi-experimental study Expert opinion	Effective for reduction of pain. Should include sensory and procedural information and instruction aimed at reducing activity-related pain. Requires 5–15 minutes of staff time.
TENS (transcutaneous electrical nerve stimulation)	Meta-analysis of randomised, controlled trials At least one well-designed, controlled study without randomisation Well-designed nonexperimental, descriptive, such as comparative, correlational and case studies Expert opinion	Effective in reducing pain and improving physical function. Requires skilled personnel and special equipment. May be useful as an adjunct to drug therapy.

variability in response to tissue trauma which probably relates to both physiological and psychological factors (see Wall 1979; Dubner et al 1981; also Introduction to this volume). Because of this individual variability, there is no clear relationship between the amount of tissue injury and the pain experienced by the patient (Melzack & Scott 1957; Beecher 1959; Carlen et al 1978; Wall 1979; Clark & Clark 1980; Melzack et al 1982). In acute pain, as in chronic pain, it is important to recognise the contribution of psychological factors. Indeed, the definition of pain is equally applicable to acute and chronic pain: 'Pain is an unpleasant sensory and emotional experience associated with actual or potential tissue damage, or described in terms of such damage' (Merskey 1986).

Many people report pain in the absence of tissue damage or any likely pathophysiological cause. There is usually no way to distinguish their experience from that due to tissue damage if we take the subjective report. On the other hand, some individuals with apparently extensive tissue damage do not report pain or have a very delayed experience of pain (Beecher 1959; Carlen et al 1978; Melzack et al 1982). It is likely that individual differences in the experience of pain following acute trauma relate to a multitude of psychological factors which influence pain (see Peck 1986; Melzack 1988 and also Chs 16–18). Individual differences in physiological responses to tissue injury are also likely to play a part both in the response to tissue trauma and in the subjective report of pain. However, this is an area which is in the early stages of investigation (Wall 1979; Dubner et al 1981). In theory, one would expect substantial variation among individuals when one considers the powerful descending modulation that was brought to general attention by the publication of the gate control theory (Melzack & Wall 1965). Also, there are diverse opportunities of differences in response at a peripheral level when one considers the possibility of differences in release of algogenic substances and the powerful potentiating effect of noradrenaline and prostanoids such as the prostaglandins (Yaksh 1988; Cousins 1989, 1991) (Fig. 19.1).

Peripheral responses

The chemistry of peripheral sensory nerve fibres has recently been greatly clarified. Of clinical significance, the 'triple response' described by Lewis (1942) is now known to be a fairly consistent result of high intensity thermal or mechanical stimuli. The response includes a flush at the site of the stimulus, accompanied by a wheal resulting from widespread arterial dilatation and local oedema secondary to increased vascular permeability. This state of inflammation is often accompanied by a local decrease in the magnitude of the stimulus required to elicit a pain response. This state is termed primary hyperalgesia. The region of primary hyperalgesia is often surrounded by a much larger region of secondary hyperalgesia. There is now strong evidence that these phenomena are partly mediated by a peripheral mechanism (Coderre & Melzack 1987; Yaksh 1988).

Peripheral mechanisms of pain and the injury response have assumed great importance because it is increasingly recognised that peripheral aspects of the injury response may be associated with some of the adverse effects on outcome after surgery or trauma. Also, increased knowledge of the injury response holds new promise for developing peripherally acting pharmacological agents which are potent and which potentially avoid some of the problems of centrally acting drugs. The events of the

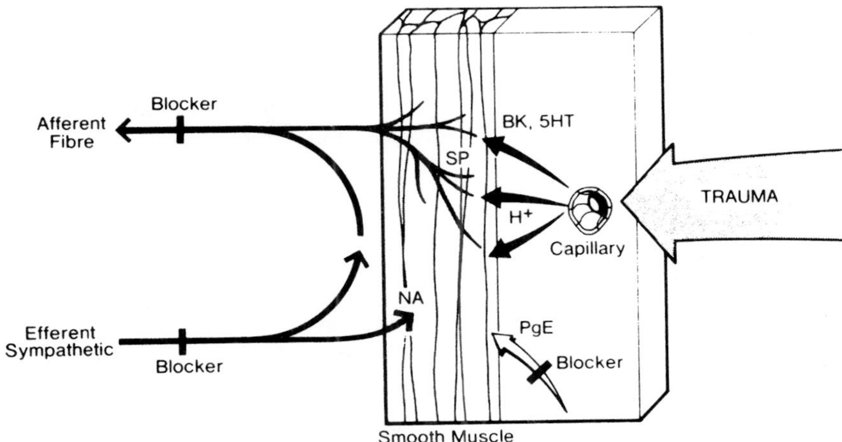

Fig. 19.1 Acute trauma and pain: simplified schema of some proposed mechanisms. Tissue trauma evokes nociceptive afferent activity which travels back to spinal cord. Action potentials also travel antidromatically, by axon collaterals into the surrounding vascular bed to release substance P (SP) which is proposed to cause vasodilation and increased vascular permeability. The latter results in local oedema and also permits the release of potentially algogenic agents from the circulation, e.g. bradykinin (BK). Some algogenic agents may be derived from traumatised tissue, e.g. potassium (see text). The algogenic agents sensitise sensory afferent terminals, producing a state of hyperalgesia. Prostaglandins (PgE) have a facilitating effect on the algogenic agents. Note also that noradrenaline (NA) release may increase nociceptor sensitivity, further increasing afferent input to spinal cord and initiating reflex increases in sympathetic activity. A vicious circle is signified by the circular arrow from efferent to afferent fibre (this is not a direct neural connection). Increased sympathetic activity may cause vasoconstriction, local tissue ischaemia, increased hydrogen ion (H^+) concentration and further increases in nociceptor sensitivity. Some possible sites of modification of peripheral nociception are depicted by the notation 'Blocker': e.g. afferent fibre blockade by local anaesthetics or modification of local nociceptive activity by depletion of substance P and diverse other options (see text); PgE synthesis blockade by aspirin-like drugs, and efferent sympathetic blockade at the level of sympathetic fibre by local anaesthetics, or at sympathetic terminals by depletion of NA (e.g. guanethidine). From Cousins & Phillips 1986.

injury response are summarised in Figures 19.2 and 19.3, showing the potential for developing vicious circles which could play an important part in the development of severe pain following surgery or trauma. Preemptive use of peripherally acting drugs seems attractive in order to avoid the foregoing changes and thus enhance analgesia.

Peripheral nerves, nerve roots and dorsal root ganglia

As discussed in Chapter 4, damaged nerves and also possibly dorsal root ganglia are capable of generating nociceptive impulses upon appropriate stimulation. Furthermore, the introductory chapter to this text shows that there is a diversity of conditions which may lead to the development of persisting pain following trauma, due to abnormal impulse generation in damaged peripheral nerves, nerve roots and dorsal root ganglia.

Segmental spinal reflexes

There is evidence from studies in animals and man that

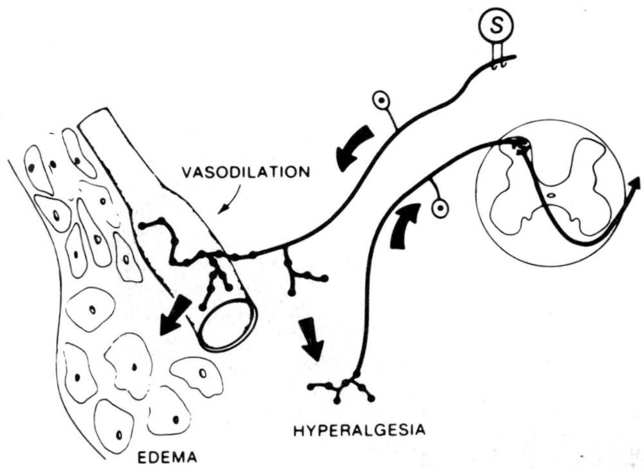

Fig. 19.2 Effect of antidromic impulses in primary afferents. Stimulating (S) the peripheral cut end of a primary afferent results in impulses being conducted in an antidromic direction (opposite of normal; in this case outward toward the peripheral terminals). The antidromic impulses cause vasodilatation (flare) and oedema (wheal), and sensitise nociceptor terminals (hyperalgesia). (From Fields 1987 with permission.)

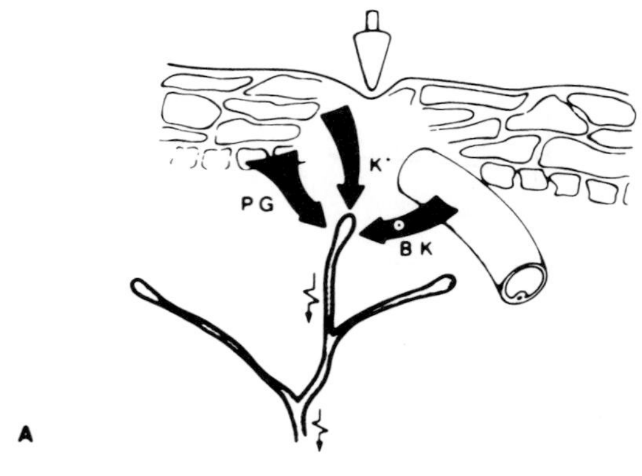

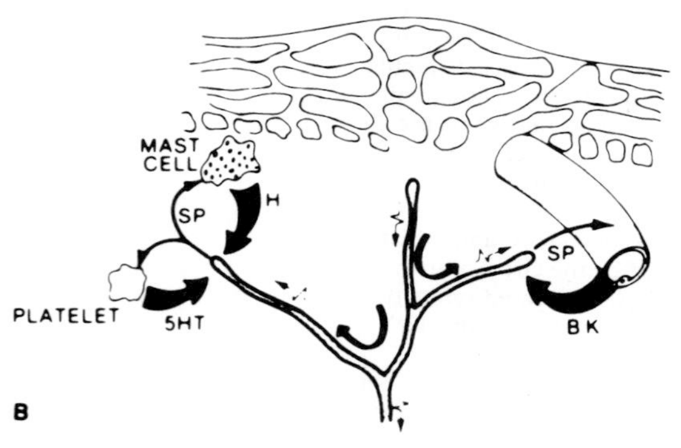

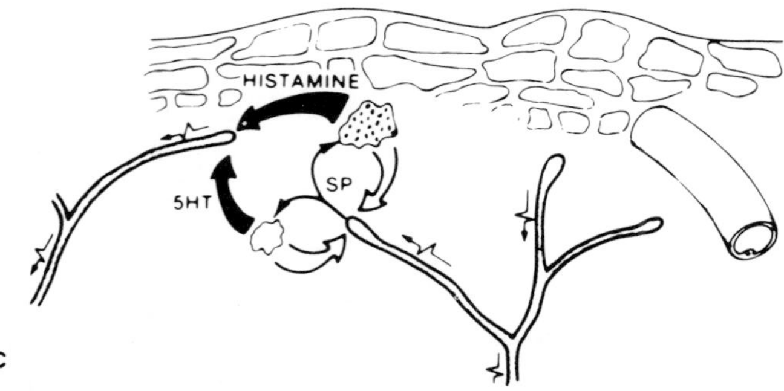

Fig. 19.3 Physiological responses to injury: peripheral events. **A** Direct tissue trauma results in K^+ release and synthesis of bradykinin (BK) and prostaglandins (PG), as well as leukotrienes and thromboxanes, in the area of damaged tissue. K^+ and BK activate, and PG sensitises nociceptors with resultant activation of primary afferent nerve fibres. **B** Antidromic impulses (travelling back along nerve fibres) reach adjacent primary afferent nerve terminals, resulting in release of substance P (SP), which in turn increases blood flow (vasodilatation flare) and increased vascular permeability, permitting release of BK. Note the vicious circle where BK stimulates primary afferent with release of more SP. SP also stimulates release of histamine (H) from mast cells and serotonin (5-HT) from platelets. H and 5-HT activate primary afferent with further release of SP, and so a further vicious circle is initiated. H also increases vascular permeability further increasing BK release. **C** In surrounding areas, increases in histamine and 5-HT activate nearby nociceptors thus initiating the chain of events described above. This is one reason for hyperalgesia in areas surrounding the initial injury (secondary hyperalgesia). (From Fields 1987 with permission.)

noxious input to the spinal cord results in reflex activation of the intermediolateral cell column, resulting in reflex increases in sympathetic activity. This is associated with increases in peripheral resistance, heart rate and stroke volume, which cause an increased workload for the heart and thus increased myocardial oxygen consumption.

Sympathetic hyperactivity is also associated with regional vasoconstriction in various organs. Sphincter tone is increased in the urinary bladder and gut. Reflex increases in activity of anterior horn cells result in increased *skeletal* muscle tension which may in turn increase nociception at the periphery and thus generate positive feedback loops or vicious circles (Fig.19.4).

Suprasegmental spinal reflexes

Nociceptive input to cardiovascular and respiratory control centres in the medulla may result in stimulatory effects on ventilation and circulation. Nociceptive input to hypothalamic centres such as the autonomic and neuroendocrine control centres may result in diverse neuroendocrine responses characterised by the 'stress response' (see below).

Response of higher centres

The perception of pain as an unpleasant sensation is usually associated with various psychological responses which include anxiety, apprehension and fear (Peck 1986). It is likely that these are mediated or enhanced by hypothalamic activity which feeds into important control centres in the nucleus raphe magnus. It is important to recognise that anxiety by itself may initiate a diversity of hypothalamic endocrine responses (the stress response) which can be of a greater magnitude than those responses caused directly by nociceptive impulses. An extensive literature now attests to the potent effect of anxiety and stress in evoking changes in immune function, blood viscosity and clotting time, fibrinolysis and platelet aggregation (Kehlet 1988).

PATHOPHYSIOLOGY WITHIN THE NERVOUS SYSTEM

Much previous research has attempted to define the extent of pathophysiological changes in systems 'outside' the nervous system, such as cardiovascular, respiratory and endocrine systems. It is now apparent that certain surgical and traumatic stimuli may result in pathophysiology within the nervous system at the level of the spinal cord (Woolf 1983, 1989; Wall & Woolf 1984, 1986; Woolf & Wall 1986). There is also evidence that, in the presence of nerve damage, noxious stimuli may result in abnormal activity in neurons of the ventrobasal region of the thalamus, which far outlasts the stimulus (Guilbaud et al 1990).

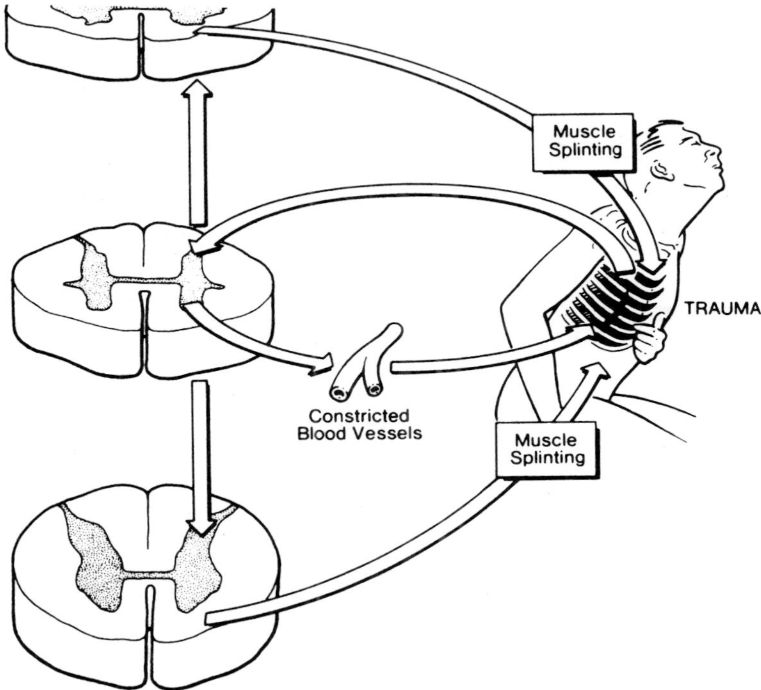

Fig. 19.4 Some effects of postoperative pain. Surgery or trauma may result in a vicious circle of pain–muscle spasm – increased sympathetic activity and other reflex changes. Note that interneuronal activity increases several segments above and below pain stimulus. This may result in widespread increase in motor and sympathetic activity. Increased motor activity results in muscle spasm, causing further stimulus at the site of pain stimulus and more pain. Increased sympathetic activity releases norepinephrine, which sensitises pain receptors. Local microcirculatory vasospasm results in changes in local pH and release of algogenic substances, further increasing pain. These vicious circles can be broken by peripheral (intercostal) or epidural neural blockade. From Cousins & Phillips 1986.

In 1983 Woolf examined noxious skin stimuli which were sufficiently intense to produce tissue injury in rats (Woolf 1983). Such stimuli usually generate prolonged poststimulus sensory disturbances including continuous pain, increased sensitivity to noxious stimuli (hyperalgesia) and pain following innocuous stimuli (allodynia). Woolf reported marked increases in excitability of the injury-induced flexor reflex. Electrophysiological analysis showed that this hyperexcitability in part arises from changes in activity of the spinal cord (Woolf 1983): i.e. spinal dorsal horn neurons effectively 'light up' (Fig. 19.5). This important study thus confirmed that long-term consequences of noxious stimuli result from central as well as peripheral changes. Subsequent work confirmed these findings (Coderre & Melzack 1987). In his review Woolf discusses the prolonged consequences of 'acute pathologic pain' which is associated with acute tissue damage, pain and inflammation resulting in disturbance of the normal functioning of the somatosensory system (Woolf 1989). Such changes occur not only with reference to the area of damage (primary hyperalgesia), but also in undamaged adjacent areas (secondary hyperalgesia and referred pain).

Subsequent basic studies by Woolf, Wall and their group have great relevance to 'preventive' treatment of postoperative pain:

1. Brief stimulation of peripheral unmyelinated afferent fibres can produce substantial and prolonged changes in the cutaneous receptive fields of dorsal horn neurons (Cook et al 1987; Kinman et al 1990). The key aspect of this study was the demonstration that stimulus–response profiles of dorsal horn neurons are partly determined by the 'history' of their previous noxious and other afferent inputs, again pointing to the value of 'preemptive' treatment of noxious input'.

2. Repetitive peripheral stimulation results in a progressive increase in response of spinal dorsal horn neurons (so-called 'wind up') and also in continued firing after the stimulus ('afterdischarge') which may be quite long-lasting. Up to 12–14 days after peripheral nerve section, stimuli applied to the central end of the nerve evoke a much larger response in the corresponding spinal cord motor neurons associated with the nociceptive flexor response. Also, repetitive stimulation produces

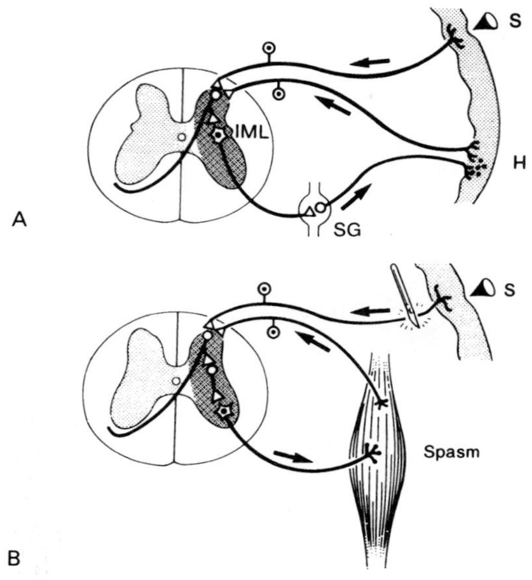

Fig. 19.5 Depiction of increased spinal neuron activity (hyperactivity) in response to various stimuli. **A** Nociceptive stimuli at skin surface activate dorsal horn neurons which in turn activate reflex sympathetic efferent responses. As described in the text, peripheral injury is associated with progressive increase in spinal neuron activity, depicted by the shaded area of the spinal cord, as if the spinal neurons 'light up' with hyperactivity, so that they respond even to non-noxious stimuli. IML = intermediolateral cells (sympathetic); S = nociceptive stimulus; SG = sympathetic ganglion; H = area of hyperalgesia. **B** Section of a peripheral nerve (e.g. during surgery) results in very pronounced and long-lasting increases in spinal cord activity (see text). In the presence of tissue injury, noxious stimulation in muscle results in very marked and prolonged increases in spinal neuron activity, causing further activation of anterior horn cells, muscle spasm and further increase in noxious input from muscles. (Modified from Fields 1987.)

'afterdischarge' which is four times longer than that produced by stimulation of the intact nerve (Wall & Woolf 1986). Postsynaptic spinal cord morphological changes are also reported (Sugimoto et al 1987). Sunderland, in his text *Nerves and Nerve Injuries*, describes a range of different degrees of injury beginning at mild stretching and proceeding to complete disruption of the nerve (Sunderland 1978). The effects of such different degrees of injury on spinal neuron response remain to be studied. However, it is clear that at least major nerve injury in surgical patients can result in profound and long-lasting changes in the response of spinal neuron (Fig. 19.5).

3. In the presence of an intact nervous system noxious C-afferent input usually does not produce prolonged excitability of the flexion reflex in the rat. However, Wall & Woolf (1984) reported that noxious muscle stimulation does produce prolonged changes in nociceptive flexion reflex. This finding is of great potential relevance to the surgical patient who has muscle trauma and muscle spasm which in turn produce local ischaemia and other inflammatory changes. It is now clear that changes at a spinal level can lead to the development of a vicious circle of enhanced muscle spasm and progressive increases in pain and injury response (Woolf 1989) (Fig. 19.5). Again, the importance of preemptive treatment is self-evident, to prevent the development of such significant factors in postoperative pain and associated pathophysiology as abdominal muscle spasm and inability to cough, leading to pneumonia (Cousins 1989).

4. Woolf & Wall have reported that large doses of morphine are required to suppress established hyperexcitability of spinal neurons. However, if a small dose of morphine is given before noxious stimulation, the triggered central hyperexcitability never occurs (Woolf & Wall 1986).

The mechanism(s) of long-lasting changes in excitability of spinal neurons seem to relate at least partially to N-methyl-D-aspartic acid (NMDA) receptors, with second messengers such as calcium, cyclic AMP and diacylglycerol (DAG) triggering prolonged changes (Woolf 1989).

Recent studies indicate that prolonged changes in nociceptive response of dorsal horn neurons may be associated with induction of 'third messengers' such as the protooncogene *c-fos*, permitting genetic encoding of an altered pattern of enhanced responsiveness of dorsal horn neurons. Of great importance is the finding that 'preemptive' use of morphine suppresses the *fos* protein-like immunoreactivity in the rat spinal cord evoked by noxious stimuli (Presley et al 1990), suggesting the potential to prevent long-lasting or persistent postsurgical pain.

Following surgery and trauma, some patients will manifest the hitherto unexplained phenomenon of allodynia, that is perception of pain in response to a stimulus that is not normally noxious. Woolf et al have now demonstrated that the central terminals of deafferented primary myelinated afferent neurons undergo structural reorganisation, with sprouting into lamina 2 of the dorsal horn (Woolf et al 1992). This study provides the first clear evidence for a direct connection between normal sensory input into the spinal cord and ongoing nociceptive activity.

Much research is now aimed at pharmacological intervention with drugs which act directly or indirectly on NMDA and associated receptors, with the aim of determining whether such agents can prevent the phenomena of hyperpolarisation, wind-up, long-term potentiation, genetic changes and anatomical reorganisation. The emphasis has now shifted quite strongly towards a 'preventive' approach to treatment of acute pain.

Pharmacological options for preventive treatment

A summary of some, but not all, of the wide array of potential pharmacological treatments is given in Fig. 19.6. Even at the present time effective peripherally active agents are available. Local anaesthetics are currently the most potent inhibitors of pain and also the injury

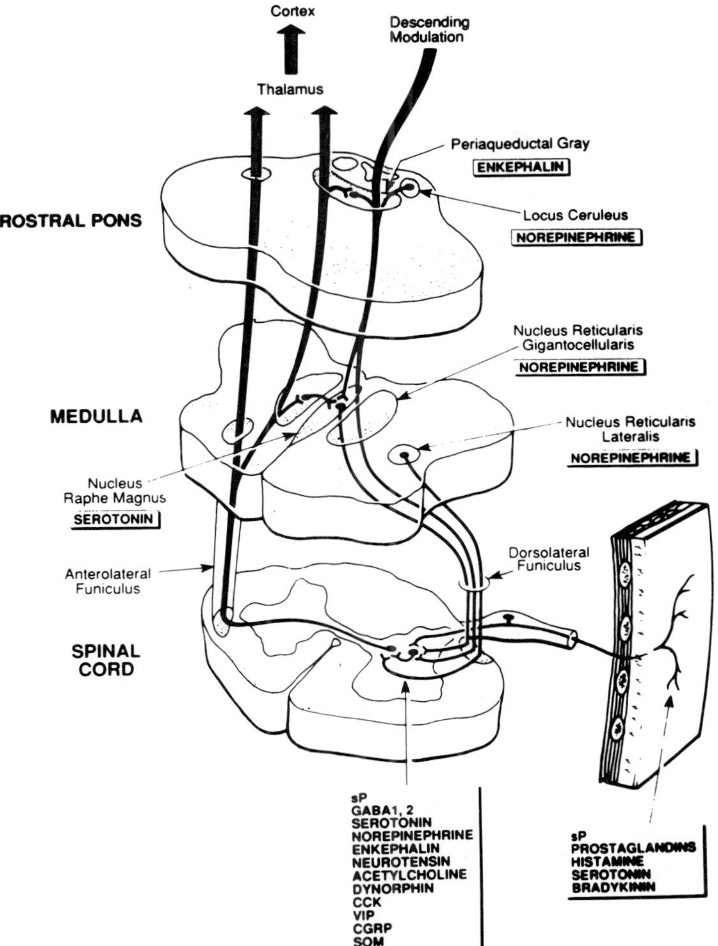

Fig. 19.6 Sites used at present for prevention and treatment of acute pain. GABA – γ-aminobutyric acid, sP = substance P. Broadly, the major targets are brain, spinal cord neurons, dorsal root and peripheral nerve axons, and peripheral nociceptors/inflammatory response mediators. Brain targets: many potential preventive measures probably act predominantly via descending modulation at the level of various undefined brain sites (e.g. cortex and limbic system, midbrain, medulla, etc.). Included are patient preparation; relaxation techniques; transcutaneous nerve stimulation; acupuncture; preemptive use of drugs such as opioids, tricyclic antidepressants, α_2-agonists. Spinal cord targets: some of the potential options for pharmacological manipulation in the dorsal horn are the endogenous neurochemical mediators of nociception and descending modulation listed in the figure (see also text). Dorsal root and peipheral nerve axons: (see text). Peripheral nocicpetors: only some of the endogenous mediators of peripheral nociception in skin surface and of the 'injury response' are shown (see text). (From Presley & Cousins 1993 with permission.)

response. Nonsteroidal antiinflammatory drugs, acting via cyclooxygenase, and also other peripherally active agents, acting on various aspects of the injury response e.g. via substance P, serotonin, bradykinin, histamine, leukotrienes and even peripheral opiate receptors, are useful.

At the axonal target in peripheral nerves and dorsal nerve roots, the local anaesthetics are extraordinarily effective (Bowler et al 1986). At the level of the dorsal horn of the spinal cord, the options are potentially very great and include opioid and nonopioid agents (Cullen et al 1985; Cousins et al 1988).

Opioid receptors are distributed pre- and postsynaptically and have been shown to have significant effects in modifying the activity of the NMDA receptor. Alpha-2 receptors are also located pre- and postsynaptically. A limited number of studies of acute and also chronic pain management have indicated a favourable analgesic effect of the combination of an opiate and an alpha-2 agonist. In a basic study, morphine and clonidine were synergistic over a narrow range of doses (Plummer et al 1992).

Potential options for opioid and nonopioid drugs at a spinal level have recently been reviewed (Smart & Cousins 1993). Such data point to the desirability of combined therapy approaches, to maximise analgesia and to hopefully minimise side-effects.

Many pharmacological and other approaches produce at least some of their analgesic effects at the level of the brain; opiates probably produce analgesia at least partly at brain level. Noradrenergic and serotonergic central actions of tricyclic antidepressant drugs are held to be involved in their analgesia; however, this is unproven.

Nevertheless, such drugs produce analgesia and are powerful coanalgesics, or analgesic adjuvants, in the treatment of cancer pain; such an option needs exploration with respect to prevention and treatment of postoperative pain. The vast array of pharmacological options shown in Figure 19.6 provide opportunities for many different types of combined therapy. Investigation of the efficacy of such combinations in preventing pain and the injury response is only now beginning (see below).

A recent clinical study has provided convincing evidence that preemptive local anaesthesia with bupivacaine reduces the requirement for postoperative opiate treatment, provides superior early postoperative analgesia and substantially reduces hyperalgesia even 10 days following surgery for inguinal hernia (Tverskoy et al 1990). The efficacy of a preemptive approach using a combined regimen of preoperative opiate and nonsteroidal drug, combined with intraoperative local anaesthetic and opiate given spinally, was demonstrated by pain scores close to zero, even during vigorous coughing, in patients who had undergone upper abdominal surgery (Schulze et al 1988). However, the definition of preemptive or preventive analgesia is subject to interpretation. In two well controlled studies, patients undergoing surgery under general anaesthesia received a regional anaesthetic either immediately before surgery or at the end of surgery. In neither of these studies was there any difference in analgesia, either at rest or during vigorous activity. (Dahl et al 1992a; Dierking et al 1992). On the other hand, physical heat injury to the skin results in allodynia inside and outside the area of injury. Preinjury infiltration with lignocaine reduces the development of mechanical allodynia outside the injury more effectively than does postinjury blockade (Dahl et al 1993).

Clinical evidence of hyperexcitability of spinal neurons following surgery has been provided by a study of nociceptive reflex excitability in patients studied before and after lower abdominal surgery (Dahl et al 1992b).

It may be that the concept of preemptive analgesia has been applied too literally. Most general anaesthetic regimens now include an opiate given pre- and intraoperatively and these effects are added to those of the other anaesthetic agents administered. While there may be other benefits provided by intraoperative use of potent methods of decreasing nociception, such as epidural blockade, it is obviously difficult to demonstrate these benefits in terms of pain control in the immediate postoperative period, provided the potent method of pain control is at least instituted at the end of surgery prior to the patient emerging from the general anaesthetic. In this sense, the potent method of analgesia is still being applied on a preventive basis and it may be splitting hairs to argue whether it is best to give it at the start or end of the operation. It would appear much more important to ensure that the analgesia continues from the intraoperative period well into the postoperative period.

PSYCHOLOGICAL FACTORS AND ACUTE PAIN

Psychological response

Severe pain can cause a number of changes in an individual's behaviour, including increased self-absorption and concern, withdrawal from interpersonal contact, and an increased sensitivity to external stimuli such as light and sound. Fear and anxiety are the major emotional concomitants of acute pain and are especially pronounced when associated with fear of death. When pain is prolonged and unrelieved, the sufferer may express a range of emotions including anger and resentment, especially if it is believed that pain relief is being withheld. It is important to recognise that severe acute pain which remains unrelieved for days on end may lead of depression and helplessness as a result of patients experiencing a loss of control over their environment (Fig. 19.7). It is now generally agreed that unrelieved severe acute pain exacerbates premorbid tendencies for anxiety, hostility, depression or preoccupation with health. In a few cases, the inability to cope with pain may create an acute psychotic reaction (Peck 1986). Acute pain is one of the important factors contributing to the development of delirium in the intensive care unit. Intensive care units and surgical high dependency wards can introduce a number of factors which may increase patients' susceptibility to acute pain (Cousins & Phillips 1986): sleep deprivation and abnormal sleep patterns; excessive noise (peak levels approximating those of heavy traffic); disturbing sounds; unguarded conversations; lack of communication; preoccupation of staff with equipment; lack of windows and associated deprivation of day–night cycles; deprivation of information on seasonal and weather conditions; disturbances of visual and auditory vigilance; inability to concentrate; increased boredom, and depression. Reporting a case of postoperative psychosis following massive facial surgery, Cranin & Sher (1979) observed: 'when one is undiverted, pain hurts more, fear becomes more intense, the usual conscious control mechanisms fall away'.

It should be acknowledged that much of the literature on the psychological response to acute pain has been

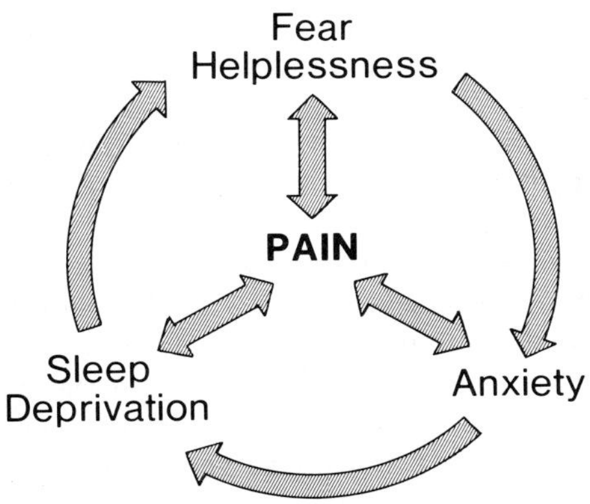

Fig. 19.7 Vicious circle of pain, anxiety, fear, helplessness, sleep deprivation. If pain persists unrelieved for several days, anger and depression also begin to contribute to the vicious circle as patients become demoralised and lose confidence in the ability (and motivation) of their medical attendants to relieve their pain. Sleeplessness compounds the problem.

gained from the experimental laboratory using various types of experimental pain. An important challenge remains for more clinical psychologists to come into the clinical setting where various types of acute pain are experienced by patients.

Psychological factors affecting the acute pain response

In both the clinical setting and the laboratory, large individual differences in responsiveness to noxious stimuli are well documented. Psychological factors affecting pain response are summarised in Table 19.3. The clinical observations by Beecher (1946) of wounded soldiers were the first clear description of individual differences in pain response to acute injury. He reported that 65% of soldiers who were severely wounded in battle felt little or no pain. He attributed this to the positive meaning of the situation, since being wounded meant that the individual was still alive and would be taken back to the safety of a hospital and then possibly sent home. The meaning of the situation may also be important in civilian surgery. For example, civilian surgical teams visiting developing countries comment on the lack of requirement for postoperative pain medication in many patients who are treated by these teams. Presumably this is because the opportunity to have corrective surgery is viewed by the patients in a very positive sense. However, in developed parts of the world it has also been documented that approximately 20% of civilians who undergo major surgery feel very little pain after the operation (quoted in Peck 1986). In a study of patients in an emergency unit, 30% did not feel pain at the time of injury and some experienced delays of up to 9 h before the onset of pain. Melzack et al (1982) concluded: 'Clearly the link between injury and pain is highly variable: injury may occur without pain and pain without injury'.

Table 19.3 Physchological factors affecting pain response

Cultural differences
Observational learning (modelling)
Cognitive appraisal (meaning of pain)
Fear and anxiety
Neuroticism and extroversion
Perceived control of events
Coping style
Attention/distraction

There is now considerable evidence that a substantial proportion of the variance in pain response is due to psychological factors. As indicated in Table 19.3, many factors have some effect on the experience of acute pain, such as the anxiety state of the patient, which seems to be particularly important in patients who were inadequately prepared psychologically and who experience a great deal of uncertainty and fear (Averill 1973). Unfortunately, the majority of studies have investigated the effect of differences in patients' characteristics on acute pain response. The effects of situational or environmental variables have been shown to be important, as exemplified by the powerful effect of anxiety and perceived control over the situation (Peck 1986). Another important area of investigation has been the interaction between individual and situational variables, such as the interaction between coping style and the control the patient has over the situation (Andrew 1970).

A detailed analysis of the psychological factors affecting acute pain response (Table 19.3) has been made by Peck (1986). She observes that anxiety is the psychological variable which is most reliably related to high levels of pain. Fear of death and general anxiety about bodily well-being are probably the most pervasive and intense emotions known to mankind. Circumstances associated with acute postoperative pain, trauma pain and other situations of acute pain are probably some of the most potent in aggravating such fears. Fear of the unknown is also a major component of the general anxiety which patients experience. The routine of a postoperative ward or intensive therapy unit will continue to be stressful to patients (Cousins & Phillips 1986). Hospitalisation itself produces many threats, including possible disability, loss of life, coping with a new situation, loss of normal freedom and separation from one's family and normal routine (Johnson 1980). Some patients may interpret the use of sophisticated monitoring equipment as implying that their situation is one of imminent disaster (Cousins 1970). The anxiety experienced by family members is often transferred directly to the patient and serves to reinforce or reactivate his or her own fears.

Some important implications for treatment have arisen from knowledge of psychological factors affecting acute pain response:

Table 19.4 Psychological methods for reducing pain

Placebo and expectation
Psychological support
Procedural and instructional information
Sensory information
Filmed modelling
Relaxation training
Cognitive coping strategies
Stress inoculation

1. Measures to reduce anxiety levels have an important bearing on the acute pain experienced by patients and their need for pain treatment (Egbert et al 1964; Fortin & Kirovac 1976; Chapman & Cox 1977; Peck 1986).
2. Approaches which give patients more control are likely to be successful in reducing anxiety and decreasing the requirement for pain and medication. Patient-controlled analgesia (PCA) is a highly successful example.
3. The relief of acute pain is likely to reduce the risks of unwanted psychological sequelae, such as depression, poor motivation to return to normal activities, antipathy towards further surgical procedures and, in some situations, psychotic reactions.

Psychological methods for reducing pain have been discussed by Peck (1986) and Melzack (1988). Some of these methods are summarised in Table 19.4. It is worth emphasising that placebo and expectation effects can sometimes play a very powerful role. One aspect of these effects is the patient's confidence and belief that the health care professional will be able to provide pain relief, and clearly such a placebo response is augmented by a positive doctor–patient or nurse–patient relationship (Dimatteo & DiNicola 1982). Studies suggest that the initial relief experienced in a new situation may be an important determinant of future relief, since the patient's expectations may be conditioned at that time. On the other hand, inadequate relief may condition a negative expectation which could adversely affect later pain control. This indicates the importance of providing adequate pain control as quickly as possible and conveying the expectation that the pain control procedures will continue to provide effective pain relief (Voudoris & Peck 1985).

PATHOPHYSIOLOGY AND COMPLICATIONS OF UNRELIEVED ACUTE PAIN

In general, severe acute pain results in abnormally enhanced versions of the physiological and psychological responses described above. Such responses set up pronounced reflex changes which result in so-called vicious circles with progressively increasing pathophysiology. If this situation is allowed to continue, it may result in significant dysfunction in a substantial number of organ systems which may progress to organ damage and even failure. We must also now include pathophysiology in the nervous system itself leading to severe persistent pain (see Fig. 19.5). Thus it is possible for acute severe unrelieved pain to result in significant morbidity and even mortality.

Treatment should be instituted before or during the period of functional impairment resulting from the pathophysiology of acute severe pain. Clearly, there is a critical time interval, before morbidity such as atelectasis or pneumonia ensues (see below). Most of the information concerning the pathophysiology of acute pain has been obtained in patients following surgery. However, the information is also applicable to patients who have been injured in motor vehicle accidents and other situations of acute trauma.

Respiratory system

After surgery or trauma to the chest or abdominal region, respiratory dysfunction is the most common and most important result of the pain that is associated with such situations. Involuntary spinal reflex responses to the noxious input from the injured area result in reflex muscle spasm in the immediate region of the tissue injury, as well as in muscle groups cephalad and caudad to the injury site. This is not surprising when one considers that nociceptive afferents commonly travel two to three segments above or below their site of entry into the tract of Lissauer before synapsing in the dorsal horn. The patient's appreciation of pain may also result in voluntary reduction of muscle movement in the thorax and abdominal area. The end result is often described in the clinical setting as 'muscle splinting', which means muscle contraction on either side of the injured area in an attempt to 'splint' the area to prevent movement, comparable to the way one would apply an external splint to a fractured bone (Fig. 19.4). This splinting is often associated with partial closure of the glottis, which produces a 'grunting' sound during breathing. The glottic closure is probably part of a primitive response which permits an increase in intra-abdominal and intrathoracic pressure, associated with muscle spasm, to brace the individual against an impending injury.

Such a response becomes totally inappropriate in a patient who has received corrective surgery, or whose trauma has been effectively treated. The pattern of ventilation is illustrated in Figure 19.8, where the small tidal volume and high inspiratory and expiratory pressures are seen in association with acute pain. In addition to decreased tidal volume, there are decreases in vital capacity, functional residual capacity (FRC) and alveolar ventilation. FRC may become less than the volume at which small airway closure occurs. The potential for this problem is exaggerated in elderly patients, smokers and those with respiratory disease. This situation progresses to

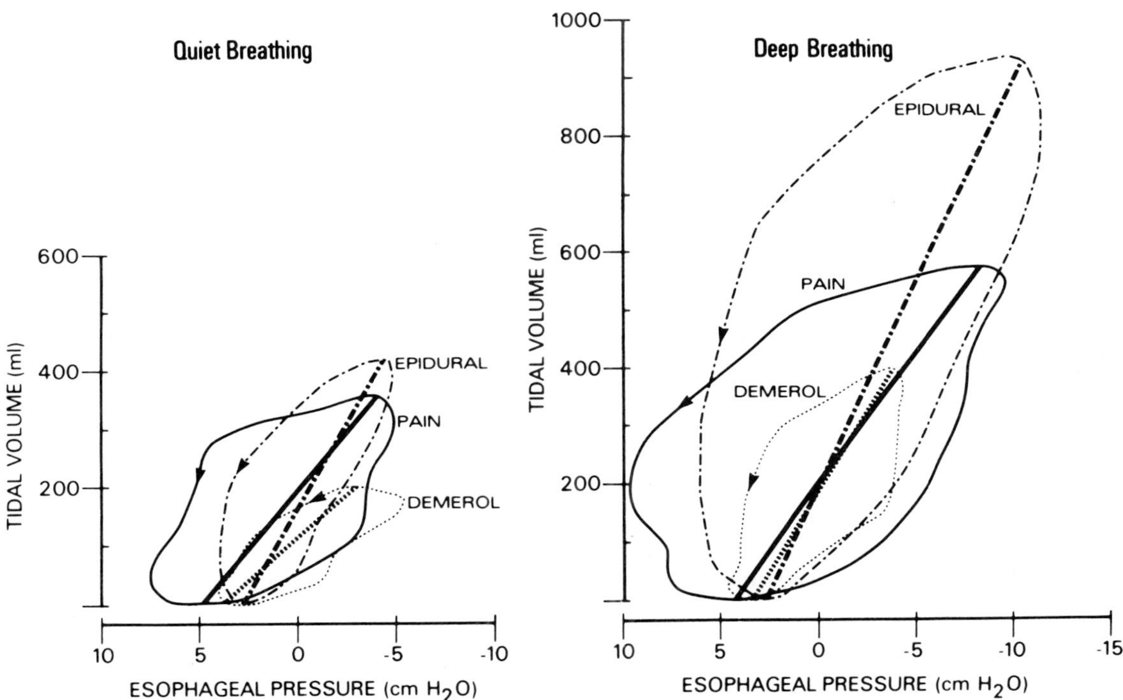

Fig. 19.8 Effect of pain and analgesia on thoracic pressure–volume relationships. Pressure–volume loops are shown 2–6 h after cholecystectomy during quiet breathing and deep breathing. Pain is associated with decreased tidal volume, which is marked when deep breathing is attempted. During expiration there is high positive pressure, particularly during deep breathing. Such high pressure would be associated with glottic closure, abdominal splinting, and grunting type of respiration. Demerol decreases tidal volume but also decreases the high pressure during expiration, thus grunting diminishes, an apparent and deceptive improvement. Epidural blockade increases tidal volume, particularly during deep breathing. This is achieved with much lower positive pressure during expiration, and would be accompanied by elimination of grunting and abdominal splinting. A tidal volume of close to 1000 ml would be associated with effective coughing. From Bromage 1978.

regional lung collapse (atelectasis), associated with considerable impairment of pulmonary gas exchange as a result of alteration of the relationship between ventilation and perfusion of the lung (V/Q inequality) leading to hypoxaemia. The low volume of ventilation also causes hypercarbia and contributes to the hypoxaemia. As a result of the muscle splinting, the patient is unable to cough and clear secretions, and this contributes to lobular or lobar collapse (Craig 1981). Infection often follows this situation, leading to pneumonia. Inability to cooperate with chest physiotherapy further complicates treatment and greatly prolongs the course of pulmonary complications and in turn prolongs hospital stay.

It is not commonly recognised that elderly patients and those in poor general condition may suffer pulmonary complications following lower abdominal and peripheral limb surgery, as a result of unrelieved severe pain which causes them to become immobile, resulting in a hypostatic pneumonia, initially at the base of the lung. This was demonstrated by Modig (1976) who reported on a group of elderly patients following total hip replacement. Those patients who were managed with routine intramuscular opioids had low tidal volumes and high respiratory rates associated with hypoxaemia. It seemed likely that the hypoxaemia was due to immobility and other adverse reflexes due to pain, since patients who were managed with epidural analgesia and were completely pain-free did not show these abnormalities in pulmonary function (Fig. 19.8).

Recent basic and clinical studies have demonstrated a 'viscerosomatic' reflex involving the diaphragm, with changes in amplitude and pattern of diaphragm activity in response to noxious visceral stimuli. This can be blocked by epidural bupivacaine (Mankikian et al 1988).

The classic clinical picture of the patient with unrelieved severe pain and impending respiratory failure is as follows: obvious splinting of abdominal and thoracic muscles; grunting on expiration, and small tidal volume and very rapid respiratory rate. Unfortunately, this is a very inefficient and energy-consuming method of respiration and may result in a high oxygen consumption which is not matched by an increase in cardiac output. This may cause excessive desaturation of mixed venous blood which will contribute to hypoxaemia (Bowler et al 1986). Impressive correction of the majority of these abnormalities in pulmonary function can be obtained with effective pain relief associated with epidural block (Bowler et al 1986; Scott 1988).

Cardiovascular system

It is generally agreed that severe acute pain results in sympathetic overactivity with increases in heart rate, peripheral resistance, blood pressure and cardiac output. The end result is an increase in cardiac work and myocardial oxygen consumption. Because heart rate is greatly increased, diastolic filling time is decreased and this may result in reduced oxygen delivery to the myocardium. Thus an imbalance results between myocardial oxygen demand and oxygen supply, with a resultant risk of hypoxaemia. Also, it is now known that alpha receptors in the coronary vasculature may respond to intense sympathetic stimulation by producing coronary vasoconstriction. The end result of this pathophysiology may be myocardial ischaemia associated with anginal pain and even myocardial infarction. The potential for this situation is increased in patients with preexisting coronary artery disease (Bowler et al 1986; Scott 1988). Anginal pain is associated with increased anxiety, further increases in circulating catecholamines and further potential for coronary artery constriction.

The effects of postoperative pain on cardiovascular variables have been demonstrated by Sjögren & Wright (1972) and are summarised in Figure 19.9. That the cardiovascular changes were predominantly due to noxious stimuli is illustrated by the effect of epidural analgesia in preventing and reversing these abnormalities (Sjögren & Wright 1972; Hoar & Hickey 1976; Kumar & Hibbert 1984). There is impressive evidence from animal studies that noxious stimulation results in coronary artery vasoconstriction and potential for myocardial ischaemia.

Prevention of these noxious stimuli with thoracic epidural analgesia greatly improves the oxygen supply to

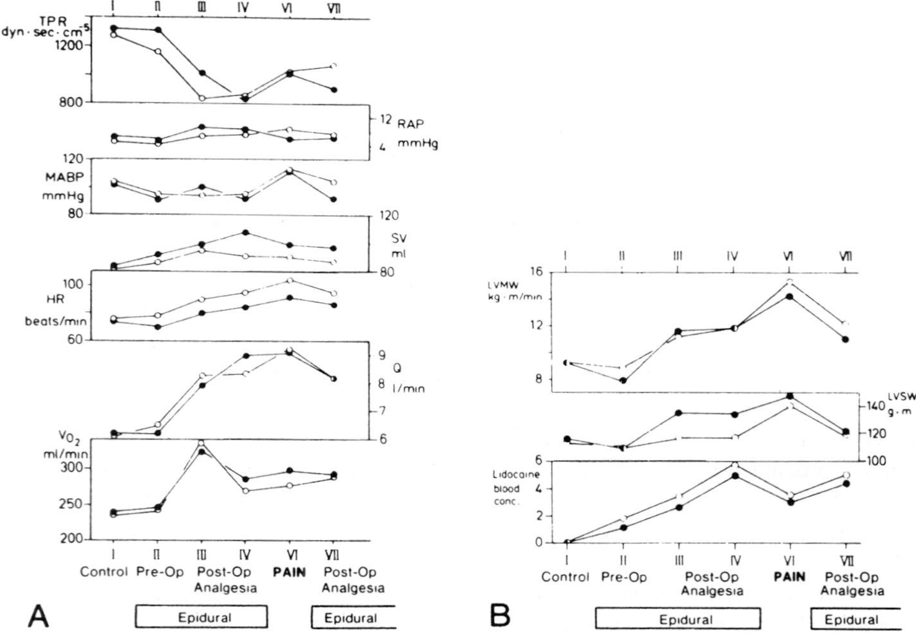

Fig. 19.9 Effect of epidural block on cardiovascular sequelae of severe pain. I = Period of control cardiovascular measurements; II = 30 min after epidural injection of 2% lidocaine either in the lumbar region (15 ml) (open circles) or thoracic region (8 ml) (closed circles); III = 1 h after cholecystectomy, analgesia maintained with 0.4% lidocaine drip; IV = on the morning after surgery, after 17 h of continuous pain relief by epidural; V (not shown) = pain returning, when epidural drip ceased for 30–60 min; VI = 60–90 min after epidural drip ceased, severe pain present; VII = 90 min after pain relief reestablished by epidural drip. In both A and B: open circles = lumbar epidural, closed circles = thoracic epidural. **A** Changes in total peripheral resistance (TPR); right atrial pressure (RAP); mean arterial blood pressure (MABP); stroke volume (SV); heart rate (HR); cardiac output (Q); oxygen uptake (VO_2). **B** Changes in left ventricular minute work (LVMW); left ventricular stroke work (LVSW); and lidocaine venous blood concentrations. Note: in **A** and **B**, pain is associated with increased TPR, MABP, HR and Q. As well as increased LVMW and LVSW. Pain relief by the thoracic epidural route restored all these variables to levels close to those prior to the emergence of pain. From Sjögren & Wright 1972.

the myocardium and reduces the myocardial ischaemic insult (Vik-Mo et al 1978; Klassen et al 1980). These findings have recently been supported by evidence in man of a lesser incidence of myocardial ischaemic episodes intraoperatively when noxious stimuli are impeded by epidural blockade (Reiz et al 1982). There is a decreased incidence of postoperative cardiovascular complications when effective pain relief is provided by epidural block (Yeager et al 1987). In this study by Yeager et al there was an overall decrease in mortality associated with effective pain relief produced by epidural blockade compared with conventional and less effective methods of pain relief. Acute anginal pain in nonsurgical patients can be relieved with thoracic epidural block and, at the same time, blood flow in 'at risk' myocardium is improved by increasing the diameter of stenosed coronary artery segments (Blomberg et al 1990).

In the peripheral circulation, acute pain is associated with decreased limb blood flow and this can be particularly serious in patients undergoing vascular grafting procedures. Relief of pain with epidural blockade results in a reversal of reductions in blood flow associated with surgical trauma and acute pain (Cousins & Wright 1971), and in an improved outcome (Tuman et al 1991). Severe postoperative pain and high levels of sympathetic activity may be associated with reduced arterial inflow and decreased venous emptying (Modig et al 1980). In association with changes in blood coagulability and immobility of patients, this may lead to venous thrombosis and pulmonary embolism (Modig et al 1983). Although increased sympathetic activity due to pain would be expected to reduce renal blood flow and also hepatic blood flow, data documenting such changes in patients with pain have not been obtained.

Musculoskeletal system

As noted above, segmental and suprasegmental motor activity in response to pain results in muscle spasm which may further increase pain, thus setting up a vicious circle. This vicious circle may also activate marked increases in sympathetic activity, which further increases the sensitivity of peripheral nociceptors. This situation can result in widespread disturbances, even in patients with relatively localised nociceptive foci in the long bones or other areas of the bony skeleton. Recent data indicate that persistent postoperative pain and limitation of movement may be associated with marked impairment of muscle metabolism, muscle atrophy and significantly delayed normal muscle function. These changes appear to be due to pain and reflex vasoconstriction, and possibly reflex responses which can be at least partly reversed by relief of pain with epidural analgesia. Patients managed in this manner appear to have a much quicker return to normal function (Bonica 1985).

Gastrointestinal and genitourinary systems

Increased sympathetic activity increases intestinal secretions and smooth muscle sphincter tone, whereas it decreases intestinal motility. Gastric stasis and even paralytic ileus may occur. These changes are at least partly related to severe pain and a resultant increase in sympathetic activity. However, recent data indicate that administration of opioid analgesic drugs may also make a significant contribution to delayed gastric emptying (Nimmo 1984). There is some evidence that pain relief with neural blockade may reduce the transit time of X-ray contrast media through the gut, from up to 150 h in a control group to 35 h in a group receiving epidural analgesia (Ahn et al 1987).

There is also evidence that the pain-related impairment of intestinal motility may be relieved by epidural local anaesthetic but not by epidural opioid (Scheinin et al 1987; Thoren et al 1987; Wattwil et al 1989; Thorn et al 1992).

Increased sympathetic activity also results in increased urinary sphincter activity which may result in urinary retention. Once again the precise role of pain in this situation is difficult to assess, since administration of opioid analgesic drugs may result in a significant incidence of urinary retention.

General stress response to acute injury

The responses to surgical and other trauma may be divided into two phases.

The initial acute 'ebb' or 'shock phase' is characterised by a hypodynamic state, a reduction in metabolic rate and depression of most physiological processes. With surgical trauma this phase is either absent or very transient during the operative period.

The second phase is the hyperdynamic or 'flow phase', which may last for a few days or weeks depending on the magnitude of the surgical or traumatic insult or on the occurrence of complications. Characteristically in this phase, metabolic rate and cardiac output are elevated (Kehlet 1988). There is some evidence that nociceptive impulses play an important part in the ebb phase and in the early part of the flow phase. However, there are a substantial number of other factors which contribute to initiation of the stress response (Table 19.5) and it seems likely that these play an increasingly important part in the flow phase. This is an important area for investigation since clinical experience indicates that the major benefits from the relief of severe postoperative pain with potent techniques may be obtained in the first 48 h following surgery (Cousins & Phillips 1986).

A summary of the endocrine and metabolic changes which are elicited by surgical trauma is given in Table 19.6. It should be emphasised that it is assumed that

Table 19.5 Activation of stress response*

Emotional factors: anxiety, fear
Noxious impulses from wound
Temperature changes
Hypovolaemia, ischaemia + acidosis
Starvation + dehydration
Infection, hypoxia, prolonged bedrest
? Wound hormones: (e.g. prostaglandins, interleukin-1)

* Also initiated by large doses of some drugs, including general anaesthetics

Table 19.6 Neuroendocrine and metabolic responses to surgery

Endocrine	
Catabolic	
Due to increase in	ACTH, cortisol, ADH, GH, catecholamines, renin, angiotensin II, aldosterone, glucagon, interleukin-1
Anabolic	
Due to decrease in	Insulin, testosterone
Metabolic	
Carbohydrate	Hyperglycaemia, glucose intolerance, insulin resistance
Due to increase in	Hepatic glycogenolysis (epinephrine, glucagon) — gluconeogenesis (cortisol, glucagon, growth hormone, epinephrine, free fatty acids)
Due to decrease in	Insulin secretion/action
Protein	Muscle protein catabolism, increased synthesis of acute phase proteins
Due to increase in	Cortisol, epinephrine, glucagon, interleukin-1
Fat	Increased lipolysis and oxidation
Due to increase in	Catecholamines, cortisol, glucagon, growth hormone
Water and electrolyte flux	Retention of H_2O and Na^+, increased excretion of K^+, decreased functional extracellular fluid with shifts to intracellular compartments
Due to increase in	Catecholamines, aldosterone, ADH, cortisol, angiotensin II, prostaglandins and other factors

nociceptive stimuli originating from the surgically traumatised area are partly responsible for these responses. However, it is almost certain that other factors, such as those presented in Table 19.5, contribute. Although the precise contribution of pain has not been defined, it is clear that the changes in energy metabolism and substrate flow are predominantly determined by the injury response. The intensity of the stress response to surgery is in general related to the degree to tissue trauma (but see above). Thus procedures of short duration on the body surface and other minor procedures evoke a slight and transient response, whereas procedures involving the thorax and abdominal cavity elicit a more pronounced response in which the flow phase may last up to several days or weeks if there are complications. A detailed description of the endocrine metabolic response to surgery and trauma has been provided by Kehlet (1988) and Wilmore (1983). The role of different factors in modifying the stress response is also reviewed by Kehlet (1988).

The specific role of nociceptive stimuli in initiating the injury response was first raised by the hypothesis of anociassociation, which suggested that disruption of nociceptive stimuli by neural blockade might favourably affect posttraumatic outcome (Crile 1910). In contrast to this proposal was the demonstration by Cannon (1939) of the importance of the sympathetic nervous system in maintaining homeostasis in response to a variety of stresses such as fluid deprivation, haemorrhage and cold. The theory of anociassociation was supported by experimental studies which demonstrated that spinal anaesthesia given before injury reduced the mortality due to blunt hind limb trauma (O'Shaughnessey & Slome 1934). This was supported by classic studies by Hume & Egdahl (1959) demonstrating the importance of the peripheral as well as the central nervous system in mediating the adrenocortical responses to trauma.

More recently a large amount of data has indicated that blockade of noxious impulses by local anaesthetic and opioid neural blockade may produce a powerful modification of the responses to surgical injury (see Kehlet 1988, 1989). Neural blockade with local anaesthetics may diminish a predominant part of the physiological response to surgical procedures in the lower abdomen and to procedures on the lower extremities (Table 19.7). This usually occurs in situations where postoperative pain is completely alleviated. The inhibitory effect is much less pronounced during and following major abdominal and thoracic procedures, possibly because of the difficulty in obtaining sufficient afferent neural blockade by the currently available techniques. In order to obtain a pronounced reduction of the surgical stress response, it is necessary to maintain pain relief with continuous epidural analgesia for at least 48–72 h postoperatively (Kehlet 1988, 1989).

Current data indicate that pain relief by epidural or intrathecal administration of opioids is less efficient in reducing the stress response (Cousins et al 1988) (Fig. 19.10). However, studies of mixtures of local anaesthetics and opioids indicate that this combination may be capable of a more potent modification of the stress response. A convincing demonstration of the efficacy of pain relief with epidural blockade in modifying stress response is the significant improvement in cumulative nitrogen balance that is obtained when pain relief is provided both intra- and postoperatively with continuous epidural neural blockade (Brandt et al 1978) (Fig. 19.11).

Changes in coagulation and fibrinolysis associated with major surgery may be partly modified by pain relief with neural blockade (Jorgensen et al 1991). However, interpretation of these results is complex since factors other than pain may be involved. Also the absorption of local anaesthetics associated with neural blockade may result in an anthithrombotic effect (Kehlet 1988). Changes in immunocompetence and acute phase proteins are well documented in association with surgical trauma. Pain relief with neural blockade has a mild influence on various

Table 19.7 Influence of regional (spinal/epidural) anaesthesia on the endocrine response to lower abdominal (gynaecological) surgery or procedures on the lower extremities*

	Intraoperative response	Postoperative response
Prolactin	↓	↓
Growth hormone	↓	↓
ACTH	↓	↓
ADH	↓	↓
TSH	?	?
FSH	→	↘
LH	→	↘
Beta-endorphin	↓	?
Cortisol	↓	↓
Aldosterone	↓	↓
Renin	↓	↓
Adrenalin	↓	↓
Norepinephrine	↓	↓
Insulin	↘	↘
C-peptide	↘	↘
Glucagon	?	?
T_3	→	→
T_4	→	→
Testosterone	?	?
Oestradiol	?	?
Glucose	↓	↓
Glucose tolerance	↑	→
Free fatty acids	↓	?
Sodium balance		→
Potassium balance		↑
Water balance		→
Nitrogen balance		↑
Creatinine phosphokinase		↓
Acute phase proteins		→
Oxygen consumption		↓

* Continuous epidural analgesia only.
?– No data, ↑ – improvement or normalisation (nitrogen balance, glucose tolerance), ↘ –slight inhibition, ↓ – inhibition of response, → – no effect on response,
ACTH – adrenocorticotropic hormone, ADH – antidiuretic hormone, TSH – thyroid-stimulating hormone, FSH – follicle-stimulating hormone, LH – luteinising hormone, T_3 – triiodothyronine, T_4 – tetraiodothyronine.
Data from Kehlet 1982, 1984

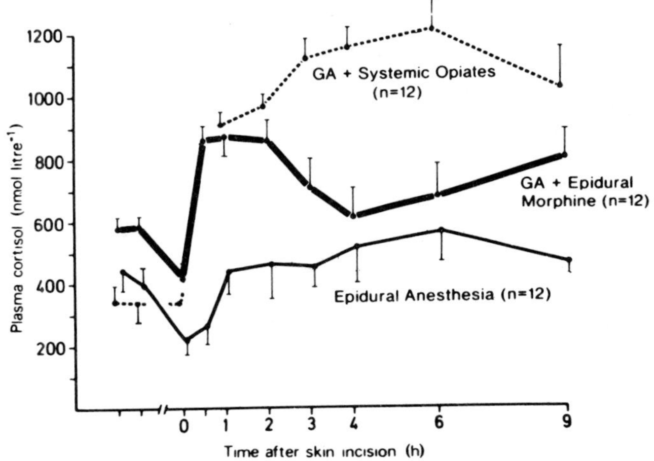

Fig. 19.10 Plasma cortisol: comparison of systemic opiates with epidural local anaesthesia or morphine. In patients receiving general anaesthesia followed by systemic opiates: during surgery (0–2 h), there is a large increase in plasma cortisol which continues into the postoperative period (2–9 h). In patients receiving general anaesthesia followed by epidural morphine: during surgery there is only slight modification of cortisol response; postoperatively cortisol response is modified but not to normal levels. In patients receiving epidural local anaesthesia intra- and postoperatively: plasma cortisol remains unchanged. From Christensen et al 1982.

aspects of the surgically induced impairment of immunocompetence. The mechanism has not been completely elucidated but may be partly explained by the concomitant inhibition of various endocrine metabolic responses. It is currently not clear if the mechanism of this effect is predominantly due to blockade of nociception. Elucidation of this mechanism is important because posttraumatic immunodepression has been impossible to modulate by other therapeutic measures (Kehlet 1988).

Adverse effects of unrelieved pain are likely to manifest themselves in failure in more than one system, particularly in high-risk surgical patients. This question was examined by Yeager et al (1987) in a controlled study of high-risk patients undergoing major surgery. Patients were randomly assigned to receive general anaesthesia and epidural local anaesthetic during surgery followed by epidural opioid after surgery, or general anaesthesia alone during surgery followed by parenteral opioid postoperatively. The results of the study showed a striking difference in morbidity in several systems and in mortality between the two groups. Although the number of patients studied was rather small, the results are so consistently in favour of the group receiving epidural analgesia, that it is unlikely that a Type I error resulted, particularly in view of the powerful randomised, controlled design. Of further interest was the substantial reduction in cost of treatment for the group receiving epidural analgesia. The precise role of pain relief in producing these more favourable results with epidural analgesia is not certain from the results of the study. Intraoperatively, epidural local anaesthesia permitted a reduction in doses of anaesthetic agents and resulted in *efferent* sympathetic blockade, in addition to blockade of nociceptive afferents. Postoperatively, however, it is likely that the effects of epidural opioids were predominantly due to pain relief. Unfortunately, corroborative evidence of reduced morbidity and mortality following potent methods of pain relief is hard to find (Scott & Kehlet 1988).

PATHOPHYSIOLOGICAL CHANGES AND OTHER FORMS OF ACUTE PAIN

Tissue trauma usually, but not always, results in immediate sharp pain, probably associated with the rapidly conducting A-delta-fibres. 'Second' pain then follows, partly due to more slowly arriving impulses in

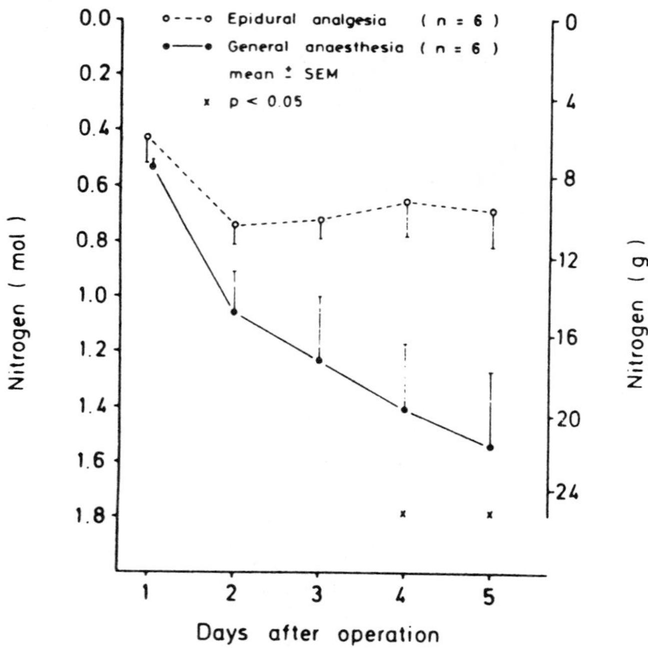

Fig. 19.11 Nitrogeen balance: comparison of urinary nitrogen excretion during the initial 5 days after abdominal hysterectomy in patients under general anaesthesia with halothane, or continuous epidural analgesia for 24 h with intermittent injections of plain bupivacaine 0.5%. Sensory level of analgesia was held from T4 to S5. During the 5-day postoperative period, both groups received a hypocaloric oral intake amounting to 20 g of nitrogen and about 2900 calories. Patients receiving epidural analgesia had no intraoperative and postoperative increase in plasma cortisol and glucose, and concomitantly, urinary nitrogen excretion was significantly reduced. From Brandt et al 1978.

C-fibres, but also due to the complex neurochemical events associated with the inflammatory response (Fig. 19.1). In the case of musculoskeletal pain, mechanical factors such as physical distension of joints or fascial compartments may contribute, as may ischaemia. In acute visceral trauma, distension, obstruction, ischaemia, chemical irritation from rupture of viscera into the peritoneal cavity, infection and other factors may also play a part.

Patients with multiple trauma often need assessment and treatment by a number of different specialities because they have pain and injury in different systems. However, their resuscitation, pain relief and overall care is frequently coordinated by specialists in emergency medicine or intensive care; indeed it is often most appropriate for such specialists to maintain knowledge and expertise in pain relief for critically ill patients. There have been major developments in pain management in these settings which have been reviewed by Cousins & Phillips (1986).

Patients with more localised and minor trauma were studied by Melzack et al (1982). The patients presented to an emergency department with simple fractures, dislocations, strains, sprains, lacerations and bruises. Of the 138 patients studied, 37% did not feel pain at the time of injury; of 46 patients with injuries limited to the skin, 53% had a pain-free period, whereas of 86 patients with deep-tissue injuries (e.g. fractures, sprains, amputation, bruises, stabs and crushes) only 28% had a pain-free period. Delay periods varied from a few minutes up to several hours (Melzack et al 1982).

Using the McGill Pain Questionnaire, it was found that the sensory scores were similar to those of patients with chronic pain, but the affective scores were lower. The descriptions used were very similar for the types of injury: 'hot' or 'burning' characterised fractures, cuts and bruises; cuts and lacerations had a 'throbbing' or 'beating' quality; sprains or fractures and bruises had a 'sharp' quality (Melzack et al 1982).

In the case of pain following major trauma, it is likely that the injury and pathophysiological response is almost identical to that of postoperative pain. However, there has been only a moderate degree of investigation of this important area. Because of the lack of preparation, suddenness of the injury and associated severe psychological responses, anxiety levels are usually very high; segmental, suprasegmental and cortical responses are extreme and initiate pronounced versions of the changes in various body systems that have been described above (Hume & Egdahl 1959; Wilmore et al 1976; Wilmore 1983). It has been claimed that excessive vasoconstriction may result in splanchnic ischaemia with hypoxic damage, particularly to the gut region; continued pain may result in further vasoconstrictor activity and further initiation of nociceptive impulses. It is hypothesised that toxic peptides with vasoactive properties may be released from the gut region and may be responsible for cardiovascular depression. The role of severe unrelieved pain in initiating these postulated events is currently unproven (Bonica 1985).

Acute pancreatitis is an example of an acute medical condition which may be accompanied by severe pain and pronounced abnormal reflex responses. The abdominal pain is usually accompanied by severe abdominal muscle spasm, with resultant decrease in diaphragmatic movement, and progressive hypoventilation with a potential for hypoxaemia and hypercarbia. Release of pancreatic enzymes and other substances into the peritoneal cavity is associated with severe pain. It is also possible that depressant toxic substances are released which may result in cardiovascular depression and shock. Once again, the precise role of pain in contributing to these events is unclear. There are clinical reports of the relief of pain of acute pancreatitis with epidural local anaesthetics or opioids and an associated improvement in the overall condition of the patient (Cousins & Phillips 1986).

Myocardial infarction produces a disruption of the usual reciprocal relationship between sympathetic and parasympathetic control of cardiac function, frequently with overactivity of both systems. It is likely that these changes are substantially induced by haemodynamic alterations associated with myocardial infarction. However, it is possible that pain and associated increases in sympathetic activity, as well as increases in vagal activity, may contribute to the problem. Sudden changes in vagal activity may result in severe bradycardia, atrioventricular block, peripheral vasodilatation (faint response) and severe hypotension that may progress to cardiogenic shock. As indicated above, experimental evidence in animals (Vik-Mo et al 1978; Klassen et al 1980) and in man (Reiz et al 1982; Yeager et al 1987; Blomberg et al 1990) indicate that epidural neural blockade may substantially modify these adverse effects. It is not known how much of this effect is due to blockade of efferent sympathetic activity and how much is due to blockade of afferent nociceptive impulses from the myocardium. It has recently been reported that the pain of myocardial infarction can be relieved by spinal administration of opioids (Pasqualucci et al 1980), thus it should be possible to dissect out the relative role of pain relief and efferent sympathetic blockade (see also Blomberg et al 1990).

CLINICAL SYNDROMES OF ACUTE PAIN: IMPLICATIONS FOR DIAGNOSIS AND TREATMENT

As indicated above there is a wide variety of situations that may produce acute pain. These include pain following surgery; posttraumatic pain, burns and various acute medical and surgical emergencies, such as myocardial infarction, acute pancreatitis and renal and biliary colic. It should also be recognised that a number of conditions which are usually regarded as being chronic in nature may have acute exacerbations which are associated with acute pain. Prominent in this respect is the patient with cancer who is subject to acute episodes of pain as a result of pathological fractures of long bones, acute intestinal obstructions and other problems. It would be quite wrong to regard this type of pain in the same category as other forms of chronic cancer pain. Patients with chronic occlusive vascular disease may also suffer acute episodes of pain during an exacerbation of their condition in winter months. Another chronic condition that may present with acute episodes of pain is the acquired immune deficiency syndrome (AIDS). The special problems of pain associated with labour and acute pain in children are discussed in other chapters.

Acute pain may arise from cutaneous, deep somatic or visceral structures. Careful mapping of the precise area of the pain is important. In the case of pain arising entirely from cutaneous structures, it is helpful to determine which dermatomes or superficial nerves are involved in the pain. In the case of deep somatic or visceral pain, some guidance as to the source of pain can be obtained by reference to classic viscerotome regions and also to superficial areas to which visceral pain is referred (Fig. 19.12). There is considerable overlap in the viscerotomes for various body organs, which undoubtedly results in a high error rate in the diagnosis of acute visceral pain. It is important to be aware of the spinal cord segments which are associated with nociceptive input from the various viscera (Table 19.8).

There are a number of general differences between visceral and somatic pain and these are summarised in

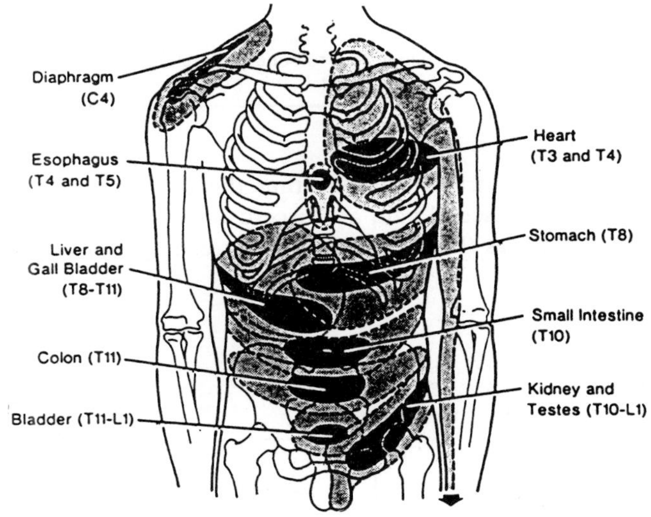

Fig. 19.12 Viscerotomes. Approximate superficial areas to which visceral pain is referred, with related dermatomes in brackets. The dark areas are those most commonly associated with pain in each viscus. The grey areas indicate approximately the larger area that may be associated with pain in that viscus. From Cousins 1987.

Table 19.8 Viscera and their segmental nociceptive nerve supply

Viscus	Spinal segments of visceral nociceptive afferents*
Heart	T1–T5
Lungs	T2–T4
Oesophagus	T5–T6
Stomach	T6–T10
Liver and gallbladder	T6–T10
Pancreas and spleen	T6–T10
Small intestine	T9–T10
Large intestine	T11–T12
Kidney and ureter	T10–L2
Adrenal glands	T8–L1
Testis, ovary	T10–T11
Urinary bladder	T11–L2
Prostate gland	T11–L1
Uterus	T10–L1

* These travel with sympathetic fibres and pass by way of sympathetic ganglia to the spinal cord. However, they are not sympathetic (efferent) fibres. They are best referred to as visceral nociceptive afferents. Note: Parasympathetic afferent fibres may be important in upper abdominal pain (vagal fibres, coeliac plexus)

Table 19.9 Visceral pain compared with somatic pain

	Somatic	Visceral
Site	Well localised	Poorly localised
Radiation	May follow distribution of somatic nerve	Diffuse
Character	Sharp and definite	Dull and vague (may be colicky, cramping, squeezing, etc.)
Relation to stimulus	Hurts where the stimulus is: associated with external factors	May be referred to another area; associated with internal factors
Time relations	Often constant (sometimes periodic)	Often periodic and builds to peaks (sometimes constant)
Associated symptoms	Nausea usually only with deep somatic pain owing to bone involvement	Often nausea, vomiting, sickening feeling

Table 19.9. Further complicating the differentiation of somatic and visceral pain are viscerosomatic and somatovisceral reflexes (Fig. 19.13). A classic example of various neural pathways associated with acute pain is acute appendicitis. During the early phases of inflammation of the appendix, pain is conveyed by visceral nociceptive afferents arising from the appendix and conveyed to the T10 segment of the spinal cord. As indicated in Figure 19.12 this viscerotome is represented centrally around the umbilical area. The inflammation associated with the appendicitis spreads to the parietal peritoneum in the region of the right iliac fossa and pain becomes localised in this region, as somatic nociceptive afferents in the T10 and L1 region become involved. However there may be wide variations in this pattern as the result of anatomical placement of the appendix, the initiation of viscerovisceral and viscerosomatic reflexes and other factors (Fig. 19.13).

Clear delineation of the neural pathways involved in acute pain may be important for treatment, particularly if neural blockade techniques are contemplated. Extensive somatic and visceral nociceptive afferent blockade may be required to relieve acute pain associated with some types of major surgery. For example, the following pathways may need to be blocked for pain associated with thora-

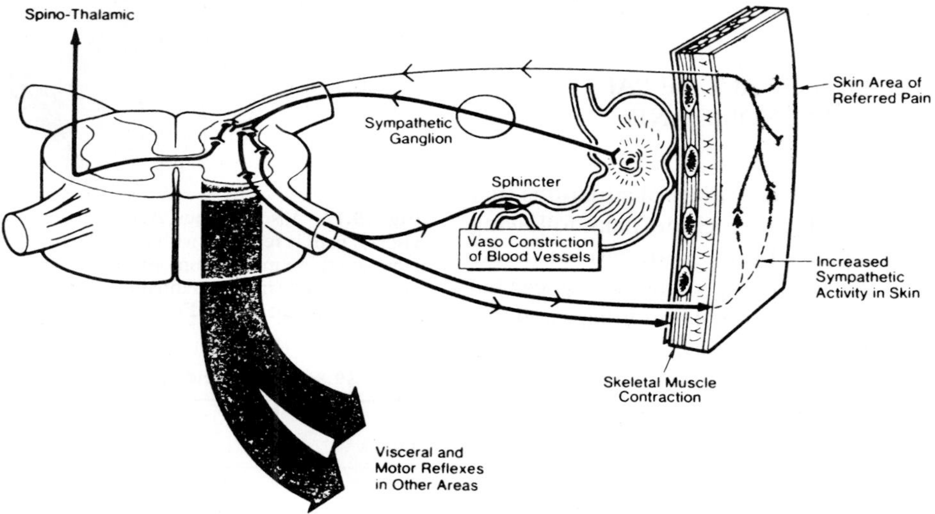

Fig. 19.13 Visceral pain: convergence of visceral and somatic noncipeptive afferents. Visceral sympathetic afferents converge on the same dorsal horn neuron as do somatic nociceptive afferents. It is possible that visceral afferents activate interneurons that synapse at a deeper level than for somatic afferents. Viceral noxious stimuli are then conveyed, together with somatic noxious stimuli, by means of the spinothalamic pathways to the brain. Notes: 1. Referred pain is felt in the cutaneous area corresponding to the dorsal horn neuron upon which visceral afferents converge. This is accompanied by allodynia and hyperalgesia in this skin area. 2. Reflex somatic motor activity results in muscle spasm, which may stimulate parietal peritoneum and initiate somatic noxious input to dorsal horn. 3. Reflex sympathetic efferent activity may result in spasm of sphincters of viscera over a wide area, causing pain remote from the original stimulus. 4. Reflex sympathetic efferent activity may result in visceral ischaemia and further noxious stimulation. Also, visceral nociceptors may be sensitised by norepinephrine release and microcirculatory changes (see also Fig. 19.1). 5. Increased sympathetic activity may influence cutaneous nociceptors (see Fig. 19.1), which may be least partly responsible for referred pain. 6. Peripheral visceral afferents branch considerably, causing much overlap in the territory of individual dorsal roots. Only a small number of viceral afferent fibres converge on dorsal horn neurones compared with somatic nociceptor fibres. Also, visceral afferents converge on the dorsal horn over a wide number of segments. Thus dull, vague visceral pain is very poorly localised. This is often called 'deep visceral pain'. Form Cousins & Phillips 1986.

coabdominal oesophagectomy with anastomosis of the oesophagus and bowel in the cervical region: C3–C4 and T2–T12 sensory nerves (somatic structures in neck, thorax and abdomen); C8–T4 cervicothoracic sympathetic chain and coeliac plexus (intrathoracic and abdominal viscera), and C3, C4 phrenic nerve sensory afferents (pain from incision in central diaphragm referred to shoulder tip). Also neural pathways associated with acute gynaecological pain have generally not been well understood (Cousins 1987).

In the diagnosis and treatment of acute pain associated with medical emergencies or acute trauma, a clear definition of the involvement of visceral and/or somatic structures may play an important part in deciding upon the treatment of the underlying cause of the pain. Quite clearly, diagnosis and treatment of the causes of the pain must take precedence over the symptomatic relief of pain. However, the availability of a wide range of clinical diagnostic techniques can now supplement the clinical history and physical examination, in which the patient's report of pain and response to examination is an important part. The availability of opioid drugs with rapid onset and offset of action when given intravenously, makes it possible to provide periods of pain relief for the patient, while still permitting reassessment at a later time. The use of intravenous boluses or controlled intravenous infusions of rapidly acting drugs such as fentanyl and alfentanil permits a more humanitarian approach to the early relief of acute pain.

In differentiating between the various causes of acute pain, the following are of particular importance: onset, time relations after onset, characteristics and intensity of pain, site and radiation, and symptoms associated with the pain. Usually, but not always, it is possible to determine whether the pain has a somatic or visceral origin by reference to the factors outlined in Table 19.9. In the case of visceral pain, a rapid onset suggests mechanisms such as rupture of an organ or arterial occlusion due to embolus. More gradual onset is suggestive of inflammation or infection. Constant pain may be associated with ischaemia or inflammation, whereas intermittent pain may be associated with periodically increased pressure in hollow organs due to obstruction.

An important example of referred pain is provided by the life-threatening situation of a torn spleen, with bleeding under the diaphragm which results in stimulation of phrenic afferent fibres (C3 and C4) and thus referral of pain to the shoulder tip region. In the thoracic region, pain due to acute trauma in the apical region of the lung may activate somatic afferents in the brachial plexus (C5–T1), resulting in pain on the outer aspect of the arm and shoulder and radiation into other regions of the arm. Pain emanating from trauma to the mediastinum may be diffusely located over the retrosternal area but may also radiate into the neck and abdomen. Because of the involvement of sympathetic afferent fibres which may involve segments from at least C8–T5, it is possible for pain to be referred into one or other arm. The pain of acute gallbladder and bile duct disease is usually located either diffusely in the upper abdomen or the right upper quadrant and may radiate to the back near the right scapula. This is often a colicky pain which is related to eating and may be relieved by vomiting. Acute pain involving the liver is also located diffusely in epigastrium and right upper quadrant. It may be a constant dull pain and have a sickening component. Acute pancreatitis pain is usually located high in the upper abdomen or left upper quadrant and radiates directly through to the back in the region of the first lumbar vertebra to the left of this area or to the interscapular region. The pain is usually described as being very severe, constant and dull.

Pain from the kidney usually radiates from the region of the loin to the groin and sometimes to the penis if the ureter is also involved, for example due to a stone in the ureter (renal colic). It seems likely that reflex increase in sympathetic activity associated with renal colic may intensify the pain and set up a vicious circle, which prevents the passage of the stone due to intense spasms of the ureter. Relief of such pain with continuous epidural block will sometimes not only result in highly effective pain relief, but also the passage of the stone (Scott 1988).

Following surgery, the treatment of acute pain cannot be carried out without reference to the cause of the pain. This is so because of different requirements for drug treatment of somatic and visceral pain; also, as indicated above, the use of neural blockade techniques may be greatly influenced by neural pathways involved in the pain. 'Incident pain' is pain occurring other than at rest, such as during deep breathing and coughing or during ambulation. This pain usually, not unexpectedly, has a higher requirement for analgesia. Another cause of apparently increased levels of pain is opioid tolerance in patients treated with opioids for 7–10 days or more before surgery. Of particular importance, pain of certain patterns may be indicative of the development of postoperative complications which require surgical correction rather than pressing on blindly with the treatment of pain. A sudden increase in the requirements for intravenous opioid infusion, epidural administration of opioids or local anaesthetics should be carefully examined bearing in mind the possibility that a new event has occurred (Fig. 19.14). A similar situation exists in patients treated in a critical care unit following trauma and who have been stabilised initially on an analgesic regimen. In the experience of this author, the development of an important complication is frequently associated with pain which will break through an analgesic regimen which was previously successful (Cousins & Phillips 1986).

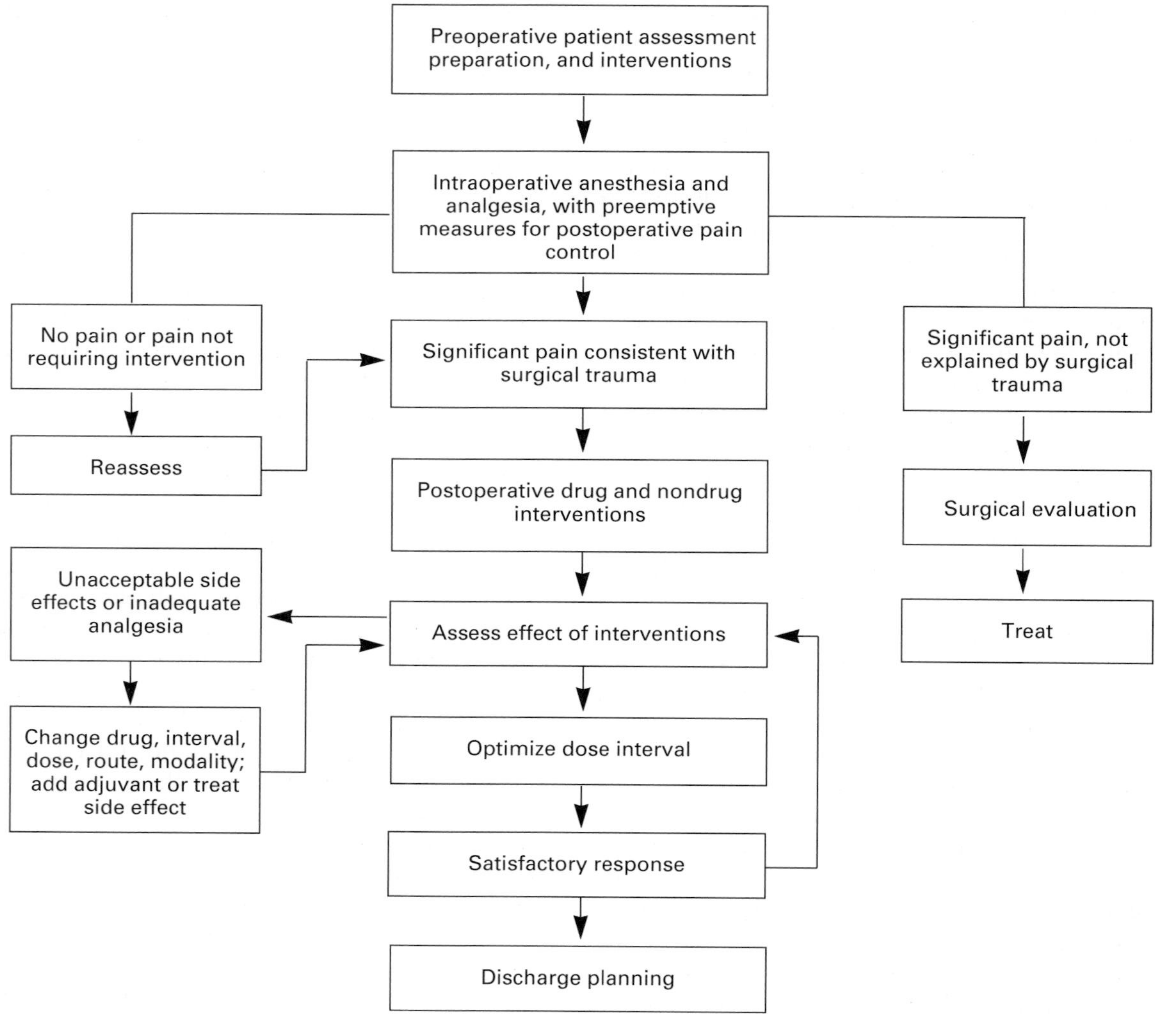

Fig. 19.14 Postoperative pain management: a brief flow chart

LONG-TERM EFFECTS OF SURGICAL INCISION AND ACUTE TISSUE TRAUMA

It might be assumed that surgical incision would be followed by a rather orderly healing process with minimal residual potential for continuing pain. However, surgical incision is inevitably complicated by the division of small peripheral nerves and sometimes larger nerves, in addition to a variable amount of tissue trauma, retraction and compression of tissues, and other factors. Interestingly, there is no convincing evidence that pain problems are less frequent after elective surgical incision and associated tissue trauma compared to traumatic injuries.

The subject of continuing pain following traumatic injury is a very large one and is considered in many other chapters in this book. Important examples are the following: stump pain, phantom limb pain, causalgia, reflex sympathetic dystrophy, trigeminal neuralgia secondary to trauma, occipital neuralgia due to trauma, cervical sprain or whiplash syndrome, acute postmastectomy pain, postthoracotomy pain, abdominal cutaneous nerve entrapment syndrome, and a large variety of postoperative neuralgias involving peripheral nerves such as the iliohypogastric, ilioinguinal, genitofemoral, lateral femoral cutaneous, obturator, femoral, sciatic and ulnar nerves. The specific features, associated symptoms and diagnostic criteria for all of these syndromes will not be repeated here, since they are well described in the classification of chronic pain (Merskey 1986). Rather, the reader is directed to some important chapters in the basic section of this text which explain the underlying mechanisms of these disorders and to chapters in the clinical section and treatment section which discuss diagnosis and management.

Effects of injury to nerves

As pointed out by Wall in the Introduction to this volume,

there are inevitable primary, secondary and tertiary effects of injury to nerve terminals. Although the immediate effects in generating impulses in A-delta- and C-fibres are generally understood, it is often forgotten that powerful secondary changes occur due to release of chemicals from nerves, from damaged cells and as a result of the release of enzyme products. Even more neglected is an appreciation of the tertiary phase with invasion of the injured area by phagocytes and fibroblasts. It is of great significance that damaged nerve endings and capillaries 'sprout' and infiltrate into the area. The sprouting nerves include sensory, sympathetic and motor fibres. The C-fibres are involved in detecting or 'tasting' the altered chemical environment and perhaps transporting abnormal chemicals to the area. Clinically, this tertiary phase probably coincides with the beginning of formation of reparative scar tissue. It is a critical time for close observation of the patient, since early detection of continuing pain at this stage is a signal for early intervention to prevent the development of some of the very difficult postincisional and posttraumatic pain syndromes (Cousins 1989, 1991).

The majority of long-term effects of incision and trauma appear to begin with damage to axon terminals, axon sheaths or dorsal root ganglia. This has been covered extensively in this book (Ch. 4) by Devor, who proposes that there is normal and pathological pain. Normal pain results from activity in nociceptive afferents aroused by intense stimuli. Pain produced in any other way is said to be pathological. There is a considerable number of possibilities for the development of pathological pain (Wall & Devor 1978). Briefly, abnormalities may occur at the periphery, due to sensitisation of nociceptors or damaged axons, permitting abnormal (ectopic) locations for excitation, or from abnormal activity originating within the central nervous system itself (Lindblom 1970; Tasker et al 1983). As discussed in the section below on clinical syndromes, neuroma formation may sometimes be the dominant mechanism of the pain, reflex increases in sympathetic activity may be prominent at other times and, more rarely, loss of sensory input from a substantial area (deafferentation) may be the basis of the problem.

An important aspect of understanding persistent pain following surgical incision and trauma is the process of wallerian degeneration and regeneration of nerves. The process is summarised in Fig. 19.15. It is not commonly recognised that the formation of a neuroma is inevitable whenever peripheral nerves are cut. These are the fibres that failed to reach end organs. Substantial nerve-end neuromas always form after limb amputation. Axons trapped in suture lines will form tangled sprouts which result in a neuroma in continuity along the course of the nerve. After partial injury, regions of external regeneration may be arrested, forming microneuromas.

Neuromas, whether at a cut nerve ending or along the course of an axon, are capable of spontaneous discharge, have greatly enhanced and prolonged discharges in response to stimuli and show minimal accommodation to stimuli. In animal experiments, and also in the clinical setting, the sensitivity of neuromas appears to be related to the time since nerve injury. It seems to be most intense within the first 2 weeks of neuroma development, but then continues at a lesser but sustained level. Clinically, this situation is recognised by the production of intense radiating pain in response to tapping on the neuroma (Tinel's sign) and in extreme tenderness to palpation of the neuroma region. This situation may be accompanied by allodynia (pain due to a stimulus which does not normally provoke pain) and hyperalgesia (an increased response to a stimulus which would normally only provoke minimal pain). Of clinical importance in the treatment of neuroma pain is the finding that neuroma activity is enhanced by a number of chemical mediators, including noradrenaline, and thus can be decreased by noradrenaline depletion with agents such as guanethidine or bretylium. It should also be recognised that damage to axon sheaths may produce demyelination, resulting in an area which is capable of generating abnormal nerve impulses. This state of hyperexcitability results in paroxysms of pain and the afferent activity may initiate reflex motor activity causing muscle spasm.

Although it has not been possible to confirm that events occurring in damaged axons in animals are directly applicable to man, evidence is accumulating and this may be the case. In keeping with animal studies, Nystrom & Hagbarth (1981) found that spontaneous discharge and phantom pain associated with stump neuromas could not be blocked with local anaesthetic injection of stump neuromas. This implies a central as well as peripheral abnormality. Thus, although there may be initially an abnormality which is predominantly of a peripheral nature, this rapidly involves more central portions of axons, dorsal root ganglia and cells in dorsal horn. Increased sympathetic activity enhances peripheral nociception, and ephaptic 'cross-talk' between high and low threshold sensory channels may contribute to the problem. The underlying problem in all situations appears to be increased nerve excitability. Considerable recent progress in treatment has resulted from the early use of sympathetic nerve blocks, if sympathetic hyperactivity is a predominant part of the problem.

Even more promising has been recent evidence that the systemic administration of drugs acting on the sodium channel may switch off excitable cells and attack the problem at all of the major sites of abnormality. The prototype drugs in this treatment are the local anaesthetic drugs (Boas et al 1982), such as lidocaine and its longer-acting congeners, tocainide, mexiletine and flecainide, and the antiepileptics such as sodium valproate and carbamazepine. There is evidence that systemic administration of the local anaesthetics produces a rather selective depression of C-afferent fibre-evoked activity in the spinal

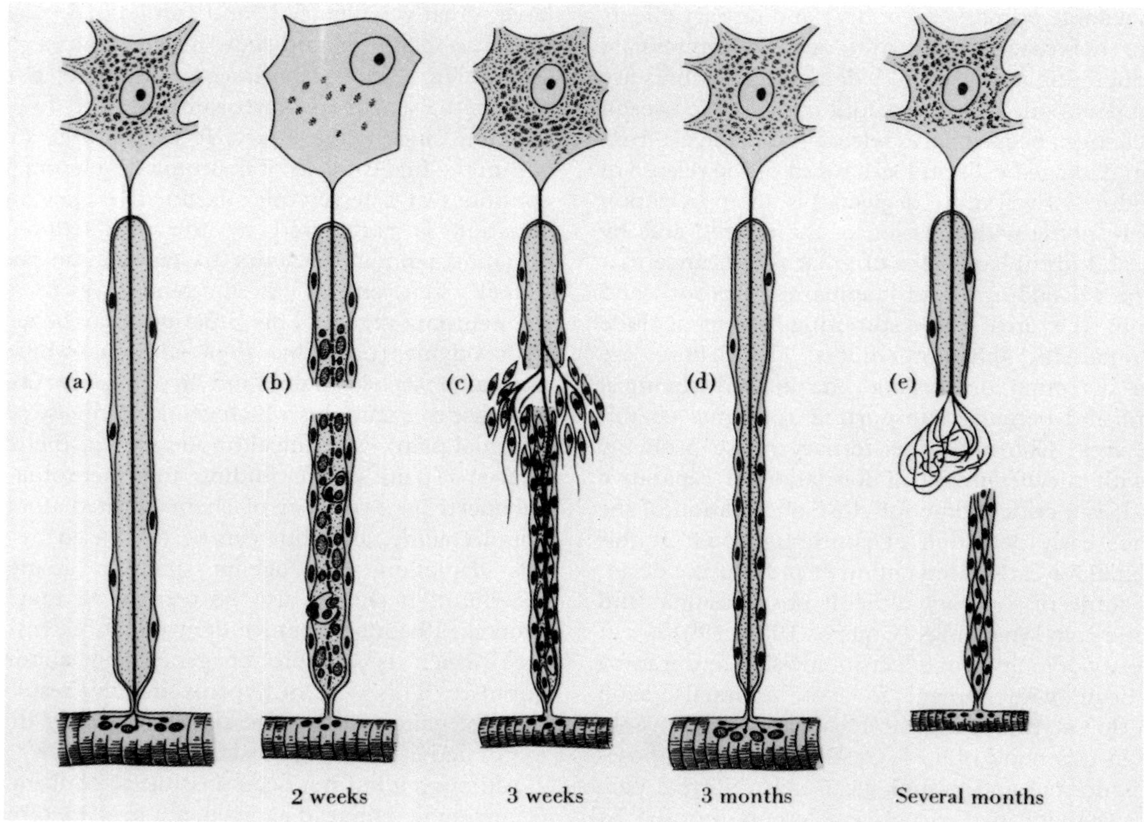

Fig. 19.15 Major changes associated with nerve fibre regeneration. **(a)** Normal nerve fibre with its perikaryon and its effector cell (striated skeletal muscle). The axon is surrounded by myelin generated by Schwann cells. **(b)** When the fibre is injured, the neuronal nucleus moves to the periphery and Nissel bodies in the perikaryon become greatly reduced in number. The nerve fibre distal to the injury degenerates along with its myelin sheath – wallerian degeneration. The blood–nerve barrier is damaged, and debris is phagocytised by macrophages. **(c)** By 3 weeks the muscle fibre shows a pronounced disuse atrophy. Schwann cells proliferate, forming a compact cord through which an axon may grow. The axon grows at a rate of 1 mm/day. **(d)** In this example, the nerve fibre has regenerated successfully 3 months after inury. **(e)** In other cases, however, the axon may not successfully find its original and organ if growth is impeded by mechanical obstacles or is unorganised for other reasons. It is almost invariably the case that some axons form neuromas, which then gradually recede. However if a number of axons have their path obstructed, a large tangled mass of neuroma may form. From Ross & Reigh 1985.

cord (Woolf & Wiesenfield-Hallin 1985). This opens the way for the development of drugs which have a very selective and safe effect in reducing the abnormal neuronal excitability associated with nerve damage following surgical incision and traumatic injury. Another finding of possible significance to treatment of pain associated with neuromas is the report that corticosteroids suppress ectopic neural discharge originating in experimental neuromas (Devor et al 1985). Pathophysiology at a spinal level undoubtedly plays a part in the genesis of pain following nerve injury (Woolf 1983, 1989; Woolf et al 1992).

Clinical pain syndromes following incision

The precise incidence of persistent pain following surgical incision and trauma is difficult to determine. However, in this author's experience, it is seen in at least 10% of surgical operations. There is strong evidence from animal studies that there is a genetic predisposition to development of spontaneous activity in neuromas. This evidence is supported by observations that patients who develop neuromas and incisional pain frequently have similar problems if an attempt is made to remove the neuroma tissue surgically. Such patients tend to have similar problems when operations on other parts of the body are carried out. Thus, the preceding history of the patient is important and may point to the need for careful surveillance and the early use of appropriate treatment measures.

Surgical textbooks discuss factors in wound healing such as gentleness of handling tissues, different methods of suturing, use of appropriate suture material, avoidance of haematoma and infection and other factors (Sabiston 1982). However, there appears to have been only limited investigation of factors that have a significant influence on the development of various pain syndromes following surgical incision. It is generally held that incisions which cut across muscle fibres cause more postoperative pain than those that separate fibres. One of the few studies to test this hypothesis compared a dorsal approach to the kidney (muscle-separating) with the classic flank approach (muscle-cutting). The former was associated with a lesser requirement for postoperative analgesia and shorter hospital stay (Freiha & Zeineh 1983). Unfortunately patients were not followed up to determine the comparative incidence of postincisional pain.

Clinical observation suggests that the following operations are particularly prone to be associated with long-term pain in or near the surgical incision: lateral thoracotomy; cholecystectomy; nephrectomy (flank incision); radical mastectomy; vein-stripping (especially long saphenous because of proximity to saphenous nerve); inguinal herniorrhaphy; episiotomy; various operations on the arm and hand; facial surgery (Litwin 1962; White & Sweet 1962; Applegate 1972; Lindblom 1979; Tasker et al 1983; Kitzinger 1984). However, there are few data to indicate which surgical factors are important in the genesis of postincisional pain. Patient factors such as genetic makeup (Inbal et al 1980), middle to old age (Tasker et al 1983) and the presence of unrelieved pain prior to surgery may be important (Melzack 1971). The latter is supported in animal studies, where injury prior to denervation of a limb by neurectomy resulted in increased self-mutilation (autotomy) compared to animals who were not injured prior to neurectomy (Coderre et al 1986). The study suggests that tissue damage and unrelieved pain prior to surgery may predispose to persistent pain problems following surgery. This is supported by the clinical observation that patients with pain due to occlusive vascular disease have a lower incidence of postamputation pain if their pain is relieved by neurolytic sympathectomy (Cousins et al 1979) or by epidural block (Bach et al 1988) prior to amputation.

The long-term effects of surgical incision can be considered in three broad categories: the postoperative neuralgias, reflex sympathetic dystrophies and causalgia, and deafferentation syndromes.

Postoperative neuralgias

The postoperative neuralgias may involve numerous peripheral nerves, as indicated above. A classic example is postthoracotomy neuralgia which presents as pain that either recurs or persists along a thoracotomy scar, characterised by a change from the usual aching sensation to a burning, dysaesthetic component. The skin may sometimes but not always show hyperaesthesia. In this situation it is most likely that neuroma formation has occurred, but it is also possible for the syndrome to follow stretching or scarring of intercostal nerves, following either incisional trauma or infection.

If treated early, this condition may sometimes respond to transcutaneous electrical nerve stimulation, but may require a number of other modalities, including nerve blocks of both distal and proximal tissues with local anaesthetic, sympathetic blocks, intravenous local anaesthetic infusion, oral membrane stabilising drugs, and the use of centrally acting drugs such as the tricyclic antidepressant drugs, anticonvulsants and phenothiazines.

Reflex sympathetic dystrophies and causalgia

The reflex sympathetic dystrophies present as continuous pain in a portion of an extremity after surgery or trauma which does not include a major nerve, but clinical signs of sympathetic hyperactivity are associated. The pain is described as burning, continuous, and exacerbated by movement, cutaneous stimulation or stress. The onset is usually weeks after the injury or surgery.

In contrast to this is causalgia, which is defined as burning pain, allodynia and hyperpathia, usually in the hand or foot, after partial injury of a nerve or one of its major branches. In this case the onset is usually immediately after partial nerve injury but may sometimes be delayed for some months. In other respects the features and signs of causalgia are rather similar to reflex sympathetic dystrophy, except that they are more severe.

The many factors involved in the genesis of causalgia and reflex sympathetic dystrophy have been extensively reviewed (Sunderland 1978; Bonica 1979; Roberts 1986; Schott 1986). The nerves most commonly involved are the median, the sciatic and its two main branches, and the brachial plexus. Sunderland proposes that these nerves are most at risk since they carry the bulk of the sensory fibres and postganglionic supply to the hand and foot respectively (Sunderland 1978). However, causalgia and reflex sympathetic dystrophy can involve other nerves. There seems to be a particular risk of reflex sympathetic dystrophy following surgery of the hand.

It is also important to recognise that in some cases early forms of reflex sympathetic dystrophy may present with an appearance of sympathetic hypoactivity, increase in skin temperature congestion and swelling of the extremity. The pain is diffuse but localised to the hand or other region and the skin is usually warm, dry and pink. This picture often changes with time and manifests the features of sympathetic overactivity with cold, sweaty, cyanosed skin. Trophic changes then follow in the skin and nails.

The critical aspect of the treatment of causalgia and reflex sympathetic dystrophy is early recognition and the use of sympathetic blocking techniques with local anaesthetics, intravenous sympathetic techniques (e.g. guanethidine) or systemic-acting sympathetic drugs in combination with vigorous physical therapy and rehabilitation (Sunderland 1978; Bonica 1979; Bonelli et al 1983; Hannington-Kiff 1984; Horowitz 1984; Holder & Mackinnon 1984).

Deafferentation syndromes

The third major category, the deafferentation syndromes (Lindblom 1979; Tasker et al 1983), are less common and usually only occur after major surgery, such as extensive back surgery. These syndromes usually present clinically with a substantial area of sensory loss. However, sometimes there is a less noticeable area of sensory loss, for example following thoracotomy, where only one intercostal nerve was cut or traumatised (Tasker et al 1983). The pathophysiology is complex, but is at least partly due to loss of normal sensory input and consequent reduction in normal modulatory mechanisms (Wall 1983; Woolf et al 1992). Treatments such as transcutaneous and dorsal column stimulation are based on this concept. However, as the syndrome progresses clinically, more complex mechanisms seem to operate and treatment often involves the use of centrally-acting drugs such as the tricyclic antidepressants and phenothiazines. Severe forms of this problem, such as brachial plexus avulsion, are usually the result of trauma. There is some evidence that an important part of the pathophysiology in this situation is in disturbed activity in the region of the dorsal horn. The treatment of dorsal root entry zone (DREZ) lesion is based on this assumption and initial results have shown considerable promise.

The unfortunate consequence of some extensive and repeated back surgeries has been the development of large areas of sensory denervation. It is important to document this area of sensory loss since it is often a vital guide to treatment. In general such problems are not responsive to treatment with the usual analgesic drugs such as nonsteroidal antiinflammatory drugs and opioids.

Evidence of pathophysiology and neuroanatomical reorganisation in the dorsal horn of the spinal cord, following nerve trauma, has raised the possibility of treatment aimed at the NMDA receptor, or associated receptors. Thus there are some anecdotal reports now appearing of patients with severe neuropathic pain which has persisted following surgery and which has been responsive to the epidural or intrathecal administration of opioids, with or without the addition of drugs such as clonidine. At this early stage, there is no indication of how effective such treatment will prove to be in the long term, nor is it clear how long such treatment would be required before it could be discontinued without reappearance of the pain.

CONCLUSION

Acute pain has emerged as an important issue because of humanitarian aspects, associated morbidity and mortality, and important financial consequences. Substantial progress in understanding peripheral, spinal cord and brain mechanisms involved in acute pain has been made in the past decade. Diagnosis and treatment of the cause of acute pain must always have high priority. However, new methods of pain relief have sufficient flexibility to provide early pain relief while still permitting reassessment of patients. Management of acute pain now focuses on important issues such as preparation of patients, preventive measures, careful surveillance to identify important acute pain syndromes which may lead to persisting pain, and the application of greatly improved methods of treatment. The current situation, in which acute pain is unrelieved in 50–70% of patients, can be rapidly changed so that the majority of patients have relief of acute pain. To achieve this result will require a substantial educational effort to apply the knowledge and methodology that is now available. If this is achieved, we will truly be able to enter a new era of acute pain management.

REFERENCES

Accident Facts 1978 National Safety Council, Chicago

Acute Pain Management operative or medical procedures and trauma. Clinical practice guidelines 1992 AHCPR Pub No. 92-0032. Agency for Health Care Policy and Research, Public Health Service, US Department of Health and Human Services, Rockville, MD

Ahn H, Andaker L, Bronge A et al 1988 Effect of continuous epidural analgesia on gastro-intestinal motility. British Journal of Surgery 75: 1176–1178

Andrew J 1970 Recovery from surgery with and without preparation instruction, for three coping styles. Journal of Personality and Social Psychology 15: 233

Applegate W V 1972 Abdominal cutaneous nerve entrapment syndrome. Surgery 71: 118

Averill J R 1973 Personal control over aversive stimuli and its relationship to stress. Psychological Bulletin 80: 286

Bach S, Noreng M F, Tjellden N U 1988 Phantom limb pain in amputees during the first 12 months following limb amputation, after preoperative lumbar epidural blockade. Pain 33: 297–301

Beecher H K 1946 Pain in men wounded in battle. Annals of Surgery 123: 96

Beecher H K 1959 Measurement of subjective response. Oxford University Press, New York

Blomberg S et al 1990 Effects of thoracic epidural anaesthesia on coronary arteries and arterioles in patients with coronary artery disease. Anesthesiology 73: 840

Boas R A, Covino B G, Shahwarian A 1982 Analgesic response to iv lidocaine. British Journal of Anaesthesia 54: 501

Bonelli S, Conoscente F, Movilia P G et al 1983 Regional intravenous guanethidine vs stellate ganglion block in reflex sympathetic dystrophyies: a randomized trial. Pain 16: 297–307

Bonica J J 1979 Causalgia and other reflex sympathetic dystrophies. In: Bonica J J, Liebeskind J C, Albe-Fessard D (eds) Advances in pain research and therapy, vol 3 Raven Press, New York p 141–166

Bonica J J 1985 Biology, pathophysiology and treatment of acute pain. In: Lipton S, Miles J (eds) Persistent pain. vol 5 Grune & Stratton, Orlando, p 1–32

Bowler G, Wildsmith J, Scott D B 1986 Epidural administration of local anaesthetics. In: Cousins M J, Phillips G D (eds) Acute pain management. Churchill Livingstone, New York, p 187–236

Brandt M R, Fernandes A, Mordhorst R, Kehlet H 1978 Epidural anaglesia improves postoperative nitrogen balance. British Medical Journal 1: 1106–1108

British Medical Journal 1978 Editorial: Post-operative pain. British Medical Journal 2: 517

Bromage P R 1978 Epidural analgesia, W B Saunders, Philadelphia

Cannon W B 1939 The wisdom of the body. Norton, New York

Carlen P L, Wall P D, Nadvorna H, Steinbach T 1978 Phantom limbs and related phenomena in recent traumatic amputations. Neurology 28: 211

Chapman C R, Cox G B 1977 Anxiety, pain and depression surrounding elective surgery: a multivariate comparison of abdominal surgery patients with kidney donors and recipients. Journal of Pyschosomatic Research 21: 7

Christensen P, Brandt M R, Rem J et al 1982 Influence of extradural morphine on the adrenocortical and hyperglycaemic response to surgery. British Journal of Anaesthesia 54: 24

Clark W C, Clark S B 1980 Pain responses in Nepalese porters. Science 209: 410

Coderre J J, Melzack R 1987 Cutaneous hyperalgesia, contributions of the peripheral and central nervous systems to the increase in pain sensitivity after injury. Brain Research 404: 95–106

Coderre T, Grimes R W, Melzack R 1986 Autonomy after nerve section in the rat is influenced by tonic descending inhibition from locus coeruleus. Neuroscience Letters 67: 81–86

Cohen F L 1980 Postsurgical pain relief: patients' status and nurses' medication choice. Pain 9: 265

Cook A J, Woolf C J, Wall P D, McMahon S B 1987 Synaptic receptive field plasticity in rat spinal cord dorsal horn following c-primary afferent input. Nature 325: 151–153

Cousins M J, 1987 Visceral pain. In: Andersson S, Bond M, Mehta M, Swerdlow M (eds) Chronic non-cancer pain: assessment and practical management. MTP Press, Lancaster

Cousins M J 1989 Acute pain and the injury response: immediate and prolonged effects. Regional Anaesthesia 14: 162–178

Cousins M J 1991 Prevention of postoperative pain. In: Bond M R, Charlton J E, Woolf C J (eds) Proceedings of the VIth World Congress on Pain. Elsevier, Amsterdam, p 41–52

Cousins M J, Bridenbaugh P O (eds) 1988 Neural blockade in clinical anaesthesia and management of pain, 2nd edn. J B Lippincott, Philadelphia

Cousins M J, Wright C J 1971 Graft, muscle and skin blood flow after epidural block in vascular surgical procedures. Surgery, Gynecology and Obstetrics 133: 59

Cousins M J, Phillips G D (eds) 1986 Acute pain management. Churchill Livingstone, Edinburgh

Cousins M J, Reeve T S, Glynn C J, Walsh J A, Cherry D A 1979 Neurolytic lumbar sympathetic blockade: duration of denervation and relief of rest pain. Anaesthesia and Intensive Care 7: 121–135

Cousins M J, Cherry D A, Gourlay G K 1988 Acute and chronic pain: use of spinal opioids. In: Cousins M J, Bridenbaugh P O (eds) Neural blockade in clinical anaesthesia and management of pain, 2nd edn. J B Lippincott, Philadelphia, p 955–1029

Cousins N 1970 Anatomy of an illness as perceived by the patient. Norton, New York

Craig D B 1981 Postoperative recovery of pulmonary function. Anesthesia and Analgesia 60: 46

Cranin A N, Sher J 1979 Sensory deprivation. Oral Surgery 47: 416

Crile G W 1910 Phylogenetic association in relation to certain medical problems. Boston Medical and Surgical Journal 103: 893

Crile G W, Lower W E 1914 Anoci-association. W B Saunders, Philadelphia, p 223–225

Cullen M L, Staren E D, el Ganzouri A, Logas W G, Ivankovitch A D, Economov S G 1985 Continuous epidural infusion for analgesia after major abdominal operations; a randomized, prospective double blind study. Surgery 98: 718

Dahl J B, Hansen B L, Hjortso N C, Erichsen C J, Moiniche S, Kehlet H 1992a Influence of timing on the effect of continuous extradural analgesia and bupivacaine and morphine after major abdominal surgery. British Journal of Anaesthesia 69: 4–8

Dahl J B, Fuglsang-Frederiksen A, Kehlet H 1992b Pain sensation and nociceptive reflex excitability in surgical patients and human volunteers. British Journal of Anaesthesia 69: 117–121

Dahl J B, Brennan J, Nielsen L A, Jensen T, Kehlet H 1993 The effect of pre versus post injury infiltration with lidocaine on thermal and mechanical allodynia after heat injury to skin. Pain

Devor M, Govrin-Lippmann R, Raber P 1985 Corticosteroids suppress ectopic neural discharge originating in experimental neuromas. Pain 22: 127

Dierking G W, Dahl J B, Kanstrup J, Dahl A, Kehlet H 1992 Effect of pre versus postoperative inguinal field block on postoperative pain after herniorrhaphy. British Journal of Anaesthesia 68: 344–348

Dimatteo M R, Di Nicola D D 1982 Achieving patient compliance: the psychology of the medical practitioner's role. Pergamon Press, New York

Dubner R, Hoffman D S, Hayes R L 1981 Neuronal activity in medullar dorsal horn of awake monkeys trained in a thermal discrimination task. III Task-related responses and their functional role. Journal of Neurophysiology 46: 444–464

Egbert L D, Battit G E, Welch C E et al 1964 Reduction of postoperative pain by encouragement and instruction of patients. New England Journal of Medicine 270: 825

Fields H L 1987 Pain. McGraw Hill, New York

Fortin F, Kirovac S 1976 A randomized controlled trial of pre-operative patient education. Educational Journal of Nursing Studies 13: 11

Freiha F, Zeineh S 1983 Dorsal approach to upper urinary tract. Urology 21: 15–16

Guilbaud G, Benoist J M, Jazat F, Gautron M 1990 Neuronal responsiveness in the ventrobasal thalamic complex of rats with experimental peripheral mononeuropathy. Journal of Neurophysiology 64: 1537–1554

Hannington-Kiff J G 1984 Pharmacologic target blocks in hand surgery and rehabilitation. Journal of Hand Surgery 9: 29–36

Hoar P F, Hickey R F 1976 Systemic hypertension following myocardial revascularization: a method of treatment using epidural anesthesia. Journal of Thoracic and Cardiovascular Surgery 71: 859

Holder L E, Mackinnon S E 1984 Reflex sympathetic dystrophy in the hands: clinical and scintigraphic criteria. Radiology 152: 517–522

Horowitz S H 1984 Iatrogenic causalgia: clarification, clinical findings and legal ramifications. Archives of Neurology 41: 819–824

Hume D M, Egdahl R H 1959 The importance of the brain in the endocrine response to injury. Annals of Surgery 150: 697

Inbal R, Devor M, Tuchendler O, Lieblich L 1980 Autonomy following nerve injury: genetic factors in the development of choronic pain. Pain 9: 327–337

Johnson M 1980 Anxiety in surgical patients. Psychological Medicine 10: 145

Jorgensen L, Rasmussen L, Nielsen A, Leffers A, Albrecht-Beste E 1991 Antithrombotic efficacy of continuous extradural analgesia after knee replacement. British Journal of Anaesthesia 66: 8–12

Kehlet H 1982 The modifying effect of general and regional anesthesia on the endocrine–metabolic response to surgery. Regional Anesthesia 7: 538

Kehlet H 1984 The stress response to anaesthesia and surgery: release mechanisms and modifying factors. Clinical Anaesthesiology 2: 315

Kehlet H 1988 Modification of responses to surgery by neural blockade: clinical implications. In: Cousins M J, Bridenbaugh P O (eds) Neural blockade in clinical anesthesia and management of pain, 2nd edn. J B Lippincott, Philadelphia, p 145–188

Kehlet H 1989 Surgical stress: the role of pain and analgesia. British Journal of Anaesthesia 63: 189–195

Kinman E, Aldskogius H, Wiesenfeld-Hallin Z, Johansson O 1990 Expansion of sensory innervation after peripheral nerve injury. Pain (suppl 5): S22

Kitzinger S 1984 Episiotomy pain. In: Wall P D, Melzack R (eds) Textbook of pain, 1st edn. Churchill Livingstone, Edinburgh, p 293–303

Klassen G A, Bramwell P R, Bromage R S, Zborawska-Sluis D T 1980 Effect of acute sympathectomy by epidural anesthesia on the canine coronary circulation. Anesthesiology 52: 8–15

Kumar B, Hibbert G R 1984 Control of hypertension during aortic surgery using lumbar extradural blockade. British Journal of Anesthesia 56: 797

Lewis T 1942 Pain. MacMillan, New York

Lindblom U 1979 Sensory abnormalities in neuralgia. In Bonica J J, Liebeskind J C, Albe-Fessard D L (eds) Advances in pain research and therapy, vol 3, Raven Press, New York, p 111–120

Litwin M S 1962 Postsympathectomy neuralgia. Archives of Surgery 84: 591–595
Mankikian B et al 1988 Improvement of diaphragmatic dysfunction by extradural blockafter upper abdominal surgery. Anesthesiology 68: 379–386
Marks R M, Sacher E J 1973 Undertreatment of medical patients with narcotic analgesics. Annals of Internal Medicine 78: 173
Mather L E, Mackie J 1983 The incidence of postoperative pain in children. Pain 15: 271
Melzack R 1971 Phantom limb pain. Anesthesiology 35: 409
Melzack R 1988 Psychological aspects of pain, implications for neural blockade. In: Cousins M J, Bridenbaugh P O (eds) Neural blockade in clinical anesthesia and management of pain, 2nd edn. J B Lippincott, Philadelphia, p 845–860
Melzack R, Scott T H 1957 The effects of early experiences on the response to pain. Journal of Comparative Physiology and Psychology 50: 155
Melzack R, Wall P D 1965 Pain mechanisms a new theory. Science 150: 971–980
Melzack T, Taenzer P, Feldman P, Kinch R A 1981 Labour is still painful after prepared childbirth training. Canadian Medical Association Journal 125: 357
Melzack R, Wall P D, Ty T C 1982 Acute pain in an emergency clinic: latency of onset and description patterns. Pain 14: 33
Merskey H 1986 Classification of chronic pain. Descriptions of chronic pain syndromes and definition of pain terms. Pain (suppl) 3: S1–S225
Modig J 1976 Respiration and circulation after total hip replacement surgery: a comparison between parenteral analgesics and continuous lumbar epidural block. Acta Anaesthesiologica Scandinavica 20: 225–236
Modig J, Malmberg P, Karlstom G 1980 effect of epidural versus general anesthesia on calf blood flow. Acta Anaesthesiologica Scandinavica 24: 305
Modig J, Borg T, Karlstom G, Maripuu E, Sahlstedt B 1983 Thromboembolism after hip replacement: role of epidural and general anesthesia. Anesthesia and Analgesia 62: 174–180
Nimmo W S 1984 Effect of anaesthesia on gastric motility and emptying. British Journal of Anaesthesia 56: 29–37
Nystrom B, Hagbarth K E 1981 Microelectrode recordings from transected nerves in amputees with phantom limb pain. Neuroscience Letters 27: 211–216
O'Shaughnessey L, Slome D 1934 Aetiology of traumatic shock. British Journal of Surgery 22: 589
Pasqualucci V, Moricca G, Solinas P 1980 Intrathecal morphine for the control of the pain of myocardial infarction. Anaesthesia 35: 68
Peck C 1986 Psychological factors in acute pain management. In: Cousins M J, Phillips G D (eds) Acute pain management. Churchill Livingstone, Edinburgh, p 251–274
Plummer J L, Cmielewski P L, Gourlay G K, Owen H, Cousins M J 1992 Antinociceptive and motor effects of intrathecal morphine combined with intrathecal clonidine, noradrenaline, carbachol or midazolam in rats. Pain 49: 145–152
Presley R W, Cousins M J 1993 Current concepts of chronic pain management. Current Therapeutics
Presley R W, Mentrey D, Levine J D, Basbaum A I 1990 Systemic morphine suppresses noxious stimulus-evoked fos protein-like immunoreactivity in the rat spinal cord. Journal of Neuroscience 10: 323–335
Rawal N, Sjostrand U, Christoffersson E, Dahlstrom B, Avril A, Raymond H 1984 Comparisons of intramuscular and epidural morphine for postoperative analgesia in the grossly obese: influence on postoperative ambulation and pulmonary function. Anesthesia and Analgesia 63: 583–592
Ready L B, Oden R, Chadwick H S, et al 1988 Development of an anesthesiology-based postoperative pain service. Anesthesiology 68: 100–106
Reiz S, Balfors E, Sorensen M R et al 1982 Coronary hemodynamic effects of general anesthesia and surgery. Regional Anesthesia 7 (suppl): S8–S18
Roberts W J 1986 An hypothesis on the physiological basis for causalgia and related pains. Pain 24: 297–311
Ross M H, Reigh E J 1985 Histology. J B Lippincott, Philadelphia
Sabiston D C 1982 Davis Christopher textbook of surgery: the biological basis of modern surgical practice, 2nd edn. W B Saunders, Philadelphia, p 265–286
Scheinin B et al 1987 The effect of bupivacaine and morphine on pain and bowel function after colonic surgery. Acta Anaesthesiologica Scandinavica 31: 161–164
Schott G D 1986 Mechanisms of causalgia and related clinical conditions: the role of the central and of the sympathetic nervous systems. Brain 109: 717–738
Schulze S, Roikjaer O, Hasseistrom L, Jensen N H, Kehlet H 1988 Epidural bupivacaine and morphine plus systemic indomethacin eliminates pain but not systemic response and convalescence after cholecystectomy. Surgery 103: 321–327
Scott D B 1988 Acute pain management. In: Cousins M J, Bridenbaugh P O (eds) Neural blockade in clinical anesthesia and management of pain, 2nd edn. J B Lippincott, Philadelphia, p 861–864
Scott N, Kehlet H 1988 Regional anaesthesia and surgical morbidity. British Journal of Surgery 75: 199–204
Sjögren S, Wright B 1972 Circulatory changes during continuous epidural blockade. Acta Anaesthesiologica Scandinavica (suppl) 46: 5
Smart N, Cousins M J, Mather L E 1993 The spinal route of analgesia: opioids and future options. Anesthesiology (in press)
Sternbach R A 1963 Congenital insensitivity to pain: a critique. Physiological Bulletin 60: 252–264
Sugimoto T, Takemura M, Sakai A, Ishimaru M 1987 Rapid transneuronal destruction following peripheral nerve transection. Pain 30: 385–394
Sunderland S 1978 Nerves and nerve injuries, 2nd edn. Churchill Livingstone, Edinburgh
Tasker R R, Tsuda T, Hawrylyshyn P 1983 Clinical neurophysiological investigation of deafferentation pain. In: Bonica J J, Lindblom U, Iggo A (eds) Advances in pain research and therapy, vol 5 Raven Press, New York, p 713–738
Thoren T et al 1989 Effects of epidural bupivacaine and epidural morphine on bowel function and pain after hysterectomy. Acta Anaesthesiologica Scandinavica 33: 181–195
Thorn S E et al 1992 Post-operative epidural morphine but not epidural bupivacaine, delays gastric emptying on the first day after cholecystectomy. Regional Anesthesia 17 (in press)
Tuman K J, McCarthy R J, March R J et al 1991 Effects of epidural anesthesia and analgesia on coagulation and outcome after major vascular surgery. Anesthesia and Analgesia 73: 696–704
Tverskoy M, Cozacov C, Ayache M, Bradley E I, Kissin I 1990 Postoperative pain after inguinal herniorrhaphy with different types of anesthesia. Anesthesia and Analgesia 70: 29–35
Vik-Mo H, Ottsen S, Renck H 1978 Cardiac effects of thoracic epidural analgesia before and during acute coronary artery occlusion in open-chest dogs. Scandinavian Journal of Clinical and Laboratory Investigation 38: 737–746
Voudoris N, Peck C 1985 Conditional placebo responses. Journal of Personality and Social Psychology 48: 47
Wall P D 1979 On the relation of injury to pain. Pain 6: 253–264
Wall P D 1983 Alterations in the central nervous system after deafferentation. In: Bonica J J, Lindblom U, Iggo A (eds) Advances in pain research and therapy, vol 5. Raven Press, New York p 677–689
Wall P D, Devor M 1978 Physiology of sensation after peripheral nerve injury, regeneration and neuroma formation. In: Waxman S G (ed) Physiology and pathobiology of axons. Raven Press, New York
Wall P D, Gutnick M 1974 Ongoing activity in peripheral nerves: 2. The physiology and pharmacology of impulses originating in a neuroma. Experimental Neurology 43: 580–593
Wall P D, Woolf C J 1984 Muscle but not cutaneous c-afferent input produces prolonged increases in the excitability of the flexion reflex in the rat. Journal of Physiology (London) 356: 443–488
Wall P D, Woolf C J 1986 The brief and the prolonged facilitory effects of unmyelinated afferent input on the rat spinal cord are independently influenced by peripheral nerve section. Neuroscience 17: 1199–1205
Wattwil M et al 1989 Epidural analgesia with bupivacaine reduces post-operative paralytic ileus after hysterectomy. Anesthesia and Analgesia 68: 353–358
White J C, Sweet W H 1962 Pain and the neurosurgeon. C C Thomas, Springfield, Illinois, p 11–49

Wilmore D W 1983 Alterations in protein, carbohydrate and fat metabolism in injured and septic patients. Journal of the American College of Nutrition 2: 3

Wilmore D W, Long J M, Mason A D, Pruitt B A 1976 Stress in surgical patients as a neurophysiologic reflex response. Surgery, Gynecology and Obstetrics 142: 257

Woolf C J 1983 Evidence for a central component of post injury pain hypersensitivity. Nature 306: 686–688

Woolf C J 1989 Recent advances in the pathophysiology of acute pain. British Journal of Anaesthesia 63: 139–146

Woolf C J, Wall P D 1986 A dissociation between the analgesic and antinociceptive effects of morphine. Neuroscience Letters 64: 238

Woolf C J, Wiesenfield-Hallin Z 1985 The systemic administration of local anaesthetics produces a selective depression of c-afferent fiber evoked activity in the spinal cord. Pain 23: 361–374

Woolf C J, Shortland P, Coggeshall R E 1992 Peripheral nerve injury triggers central sprouting of myelinated afferents. Nature 355: 75–78

Yaksh T L 1988 Neurologic mechanisms of pain. In: Cousins M J, Bridenbaugh P O (eds) Neural blockade in clinical anesthesia and management of pain, 2nd edn. J B Lippincott, Philadelphia, p 791–844

Yeager M P, Glass D D, Neff R K, Brinck-Johnson T 1987 Epidural anesthesia and analgesia in high risk surgical patients. Anesthesiology 66: 729–736

Zolte N, Cust M D 1986 Analgesia in the acute abdomen. Annals of the Royal College of Surgeons of England 68: 209–210

20. Osteoarthritis

Conor McCarthy, Janet Cushnaghan and Paul Dieppe

INTRODUCTION

Osteoarthritis (OA) is the commonest of all the rheumatic diseases, and causes symptoms and disability in a large proportion of elderly people (Wood 1976; Felson 1990; Dieppe 1991). It presents a special challenge in the study of pain for several reasons:

1. It is a very common cause of severe, chronic, disabling and intractable pain. OA is one of the most frequent causes of referral to pain clinics.
2. Whereas some patients with advanced joint damage due to OA have considerable pain, others with destroyed joints remain asymptomatic.
3. It is a condition whose main target tissue is the articular cartilage, a structure devoid of nerves. The causes of the pain experienced by some people with OA remain ill understood.

This chapter is divided into three parts. Section one contains a brief general description of OA, including the definition and pathogenesis of the disorder, its epidemiology and clinical features, and general principles of management. The second section concentrates on the causes, effects and treatment of pain in OA, including an outline of some specific investigations into pain mechanisms. The final section provides a brief introduction to some of the recent advances in OA and current avenues of research that might help elucidate the causes and treatment of pain in this disorder.

Pain in OA was the subject of a recent comprehensive review (Altman et al 1989).

PART ONE: OSTEOARTHRITIS

WHAT IS OSTEOARTHRITIS?

Osteoarthritis is a disorder of synovial joints with a pathological basis for its definition. It is characterised by local areas of destruction of the articular cartilage and remodelling of the subchondral bone (Howell et al 1979; Gardner 1992). When joint damage is extensive, this pathology results in the radiographic changes used to define it in clinical practice. In some cases these pathological and/or radiographic changes are accompanied by clinical features that can be attributed to the resulting changes in joint anatomy and function.

The pathological changes include focal areas of fibrillation and thinning of the articular cartilage, sclerosis and cyst formation in the underlying bone, and the formation of cartilagenous and bony spurs at the joint margins (osteophytosis). There is a patchy, mild chronic inflammatory synovitis, accompanied by fibrotic thickening of the joint capsule (Gardner 1992). Destruction of the cartilage matrix is the focus of most current research into the OA process. The chondrocytes control both synthesis and degradation of the matrix; in OA cartilage they increase in number and synthetic activity and form 'brood capsules'. Similarly there is an increase in the cellular activity and blood flow to the subchondral bone. Thus much of the pathology of OA is seen as either an attempted or an aberrant repair reaction. If these pathological changes become sufficiently advanced, they are reflected by the characteristic radiographic changes of joint space narrowing, osteophytes, sclerosis and cyst formation (Table 20.1, Fig. 20.1). The plain radiograph is the only technique used to diagnose the presence of OA in most epidemiological and clinical studies, in spite of its known insensitivity to pathological change (Rogers et al 1990). This is because there are no other simple, noninva

Table 20.1 Relationship between pathological and radiographic features of osteoarthritis

Pathological features	Radiological features
Focal areas of loss of articular cartilage	Asymmetrical loss of inter-bone distance ('joint space narrowing')
Marginal lipping and overgrowth	Osteophytosis of bone
Remodelling of subchondral bone	Sclerosis and cysts in subchondral bone, altered bony contour
Capsular thickening and mild chronic synovitis	

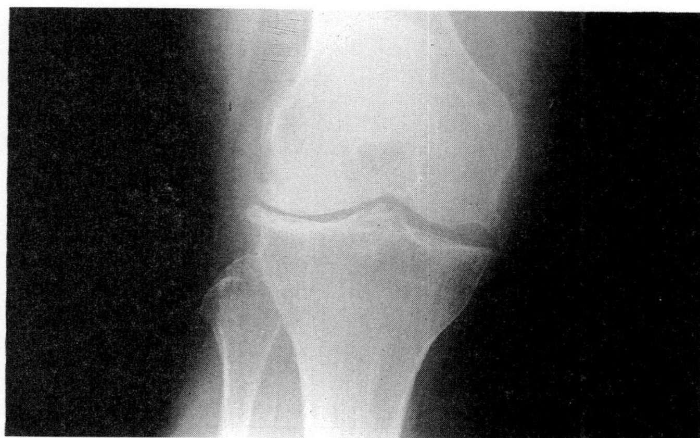

Fig. 20.1 Radiograph of the knee joint showing typical features of osteoarthritis in the lateral compartment of the tibiofemoral joint, including narrowing of the joint space, subchondral bone sclerosis and osteophytes.

sive tests that can detect the presence of the condition; conventional blood tests, for example, are normal, and only invasive techniques such as arthroscopy provide a direct view of the condition.

The main joints to be affected by OA include some of the small joints of the hands (mainly the distal interphalangeal joints and thumb base), the knees, hips and apophyseal joints of the cervical and lumbar spine. Almost any joint can be affected, although involvement of the ankles and shoulders is relatively uncommon (Cushnaghan & Dieppe 1991). When it results in clinical problems, OA most often causes use-related pain, joint stiffness after inactivity and difficulty in using the affected joints. The results of severe OA of the lower limb joints can be particularly disabling.

The definitions and nomenclature used to describe OA continue to cause problems. Terms such as 'degenerative joint disease' have become inappropriate since the dynamic, active nature of the process has been recognised; it is now clear that the term covers several disorders with a similar end point, rather than a specific disease entity. Some authors now regard OA as 'joint failure', analogous to cardiac or renal failure (Dieppe 1991); for them the disorder is the pathophysiological changes seen in the joint. Others argue that OA is a clinical entity which should only be diagnosed in the presence of symptoms. For example the American College of Rheumatology (ACR) defines OA as: 'a heterogenous group of conditions that lead to joint symptoms and signs which are associated with defective integrity of cartilage in addition to the related changes in the underlying bone and at the joint margin' (Altman et al 1986). It has been suggested that the term 'osteoarthrosis' could be used to describe the pathology, and 'osteoarthritis' the clinical condition, using the analogy of diverticulosis and diverticulitis. However, clinical definitions remain elusive and recent attempts by the ACR to provide diagnostic criteria have been criticised (McAlindon & Dieppe 1989).

THE AETIOPATHOGENESIS OF OA

Two main types of risk factor have been identified: general, systemic factors, such as age, sex, race and heredity; and local, biomechanical factors, such as joint injury, selected activities or altered joint shape (Felson 1990). The main aetiological factors, and the way in which they may interact to cause OA, are illustrated in Figure 20.2. In clinical practice OA is often classified as 'secondary' if a clear causative factor can be identified, such as a previous fracture through the affected joint; or 'primary' when the aetiology is not known. However, this distinction is not clear cut, there being a complex and varying interaction of systemic predisposition and local factors at the different joint sites affected. It is also clear that many different types of disorder can cause OA: in some the major aetiological factors involve too much mechanical stress on relatively normal tissues, whereas in others, abnormal tissues may fail with normal biomechanics.

The OA process involves a mixture of degradation, attempted repair and mild inflammation, and all tissues in the joint are involved. The outcome of this process includes changes in both the anatomy and physiology of the joint, which may lead to symptoms and disability. Social and psychological factors may affect the clinical outcome. The impact of OA includes an immense burden of pain and disability, as well as extensive socioeconomic consequences.

THE EPIDEMIOLOGY OF OA

It is widely quoted that OA is a disorder that has affected man and other beasts throughout history. However, most of the change seen in ancient skeletons is osteophytosis, which can occur in the absence of OA. Although it is clear that OA is and has been common in man for centuries (Rogers et al 1981), there is also recent evidence that it may be changing in frequency and distribution with time (Rogers & Dieppe 1992). Another common misapprehen-

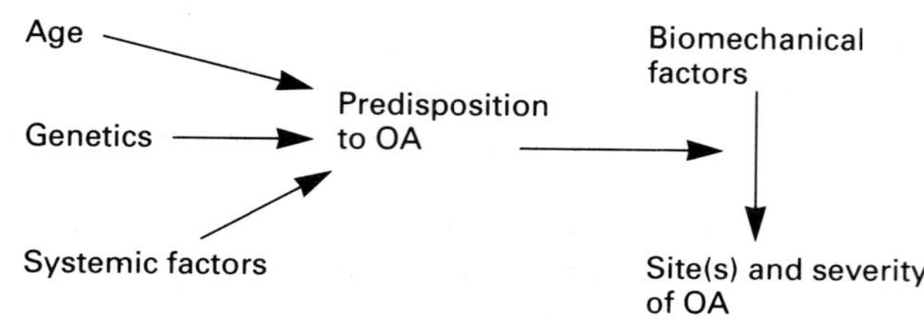

Fig. 20.2 Hypothetical scheme of the aetiopathogenesis of osteoarthritis (OA).

sion is that OA is the inevitable consequence of aging, that will affect us all given time. Sokoloff (1980) has estimated that we would have to live to be 200 years old before aging alone would cause OA; furthermore, only some 10% of the adult population is affected and only some of their joints have OA.

Most of the population-based epidemiology of OA has used a system of radiographic scoring described by Kellgren & Lawrence (1957). These radiographic surveys emphasise the association with age and the high frequency of hand, knee and spinal involvement. OA is relatively uncommon until middle age and has a similar frequency in men and women until the age of about 50 years. In young adults the hip is one of the joints most likely to be involved, especially in men. After the age of 50, there is a steep increase in prevalence in women, the knees and hands being the principal joint sites affected. There are differences in the frequency with which OA is seen at different joint sites in different parts of the world. For example, in Asia, knee disease is common, but OA of the hip is rare in comparison to the experience of Caucasian populations (Felson 1988).

The main associations of OA revealed by these epidemiological surveys, other than age and sex, vary according to the joint site involved. Obesity is a major risk factor for knee OA, severe obesity increasing the risk by 4–7 times normal in women (Felson et al 1988). Certain occupations have also been implicated, including farming for hip OA (Croft et al 1992), and occupations involving squatting and loading for knee disease (Felson et al 1991). Joint injury and surgery increase the risk of OA greatly, but are relatively uncommon causes in the population at large.

CLINICAL FEATURES OF OA

One of the most important observations concerning OA is that radiographic evidence of joint damage does not correlate well with symptoms. This discordance has been remarked on by many authors, including Lawrence et al (1966) who said that 'it is evident that...osteoarthritis is a predisposing factor rather than a cause of symptoms in the corresponding region'. Kellgren (1983) and Acheson (1983) have both explored this dilemma, the latter calling OA 'the mystery crippler'; and more recently Hadler (1992) has written an article with the title 'Knee pain is the malady – not osteoarthritis'. It is clear that the clinical entity of OA must be separated from the pathological disorder.

There are very few population-based surveys of OA in which clinical features have been recorded and most of the clinical descriptions of the disorder are from hospital-based populations, which may not be representative (Huskisson et al 1979; Cushnaghan & Dieppe 1991). These clinical surveys describe patient groups with an average age of disease onset of about 55 years, and in which women outnumber men by two or three to one. Isolated hip disease is seen in younger men, a combination of knee and hand involvement in middle-aged women and a more polyarticular disease in the elderly. Obesity is common, particularly in those with knee disease.

Pain, particularly use-related pain, is the main symptom of the disease. Stiffness, or 'gelling' of the joints in the morning, or after inactivity, is also common. On examination, 'bony' swelling at the joint margin is usually apparent (Fig. 20.3). There may also be some soft tissue swelling or a moderate effusion. In contrast to rheumatoid arthritis, the joints are rarely so overtly inflamed, although some warmth and small effusions are common, and redness of affected interphalangeal joints can occur. In advanced, long-standing disease, the joints may become unstable and there is often wasting and weakness of muscles acting on the affected joints. The range of motion of the joint is generally reduced, with exacerbation of pain on movement, particularly at the end of the range. Joint movement usually results in palpable crepitus. Associated changes in the periarticular tissues, such as an enthesopathy or bursitis, are not uncommon.

Relatively little is known about the natural history of OA. Recent data suggest that it may be a phasic disease, with episodes of relatively rapid change (several months or a few years) being interrupted by long periods of inactivity, in which the anatomy of the joint can remain much the same for many years (Massardo et al 1989; Spector et al 1991; Dieppe & Cushnaghan 1992). In many cases the condition seems to stabilise and symptoms may improve. A minority show evidence of anatomical healing. However, a significant proportion develop severe joint damage and symptoms or disability that are so intrusive that a joint replacement is undertaken. The determinants of this variable outcome are not known.

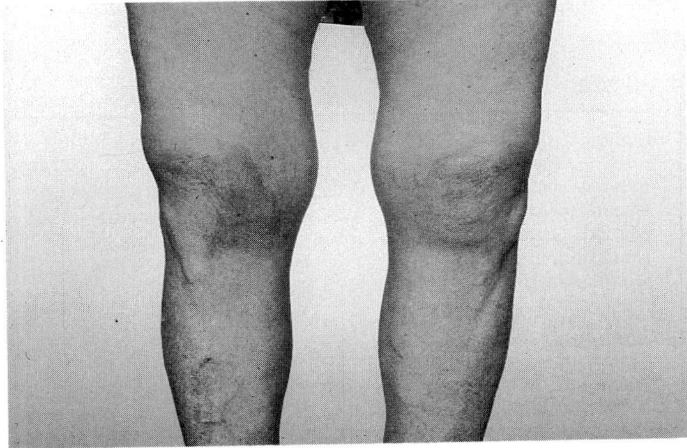

Fig. 20.3 Knee joints of a patient with osteoarthritis, showing swelling at the joint margins and weakness of the quadriceps muscles.

THE MANAGEMENT OF OA

The general objectives and modalities used in the treatment of OA are listed in Table 20.2. The management of disorders such as OA can be divided into prevention (either primary or secondary), effective treatment of an established disease or salvage (Hutton 1990). In the case of OA, strategies for prevention are only just beginning to emerge, and possible disease-modifying drugs are only now being developed and tested; no proven preventative strategy or curative medication is available. The general management of OA is therefore limited to the three objectives listed:

1. the treatment of symptoms such as pain, anxiety and depression
2. to maximise joint function and reduce the disability and handicap that might result from OA to a minimum
3. to try to prevent further joint damage.

The main modalities available to achieve these aims include education, physical therapy, drugs, surgery and psychosocial interventions, including the alterations of function and environment that can be achieved with the help of social workers and occupational therapists.

Education is valuable. A positive attitude to outcome is warranted, in view of the fact that the condition often stabilises and improves symptomatically. Recent work has shown that educational support and group exercise therapy can be of great value in pain reduction (Kovar et al 1992). Physical therapy should be used to keep muscles strong around affected joints and to maintain as good a range of motion as possible. In addition impact loading and abnormal stresses on the affected joints should be minimised. The use of shock-absorbing insoles may reduce symptoms, as can a walking stick, for those with lower limb OA. The obese may benefit from losing weight. Local applications such as heat may reduce pain, and other physical therapy, such as hydrotherapy, can be of great benefit, particularly in the rehabilitation of disabled patients. Disability can also be reduced by a number of other measures dependent on physiotherapists and occupational therapists. Unstable joints may be helped by splints or orthoses and by regimens to ensure joint protection. Suitable periods of rest and activity can be helpful and numerous modifications to the environment, such as raising toilet seats, or providing bath aids, can be invaluable to those disabled by damaged joints (Dieppe 1993).

Table 20.2 The Management of osteoarthritis

Objectives	Modalities used
1. Relief of symptoms	1. Education
2. Maximise function	2. General exercise therapy
Minimise handicap	3. Specific physical therapies
3. Limit progression of joint damage	4. Aids to reduce joint loading (e.g. sticks, insoles)
	5. Aids to improve function
	6. Systemic drugs
	7. Local applications
	8. Intra- and periarticular injections
	9. Psychosocial intervention
	10. Occupational therapy
	11. Surgery

Drug treatment is controversial (McAlindon & Dieppe 1990). Simple analgesics, used regularly or on demand, can be of value. In the UK, as in many other countries, nonsteroidal antiinflammatory drugs have become popular for symptomatic treatment of OA. However, their advantages over simple analgesics have not been established and recent work has questioned their value, particularly in view of the fact that the risk of toxicity is highest in elderly women, the group most in need of pain relief because of OA (Bradley et al 1991). Rubrefacients are used widely, although it is not clear to what extent the physical aspect of their use, as opposed to any active medication that they might contain, is of importance. Local steroid injections have a limited role in the treatment of OA. Their effect on the knee joint, for example, is short-lived and only slightly superior to the excellent response achieved with placebo injections (Dieppe et al 1980; Friedman & Moore 1980). In contrast, thumb base OA may benefit particularly well and for a longer time period, a single injection of a long-acting steroid preparation often resulting in relief of pain for months. The other indications for the use of steroid injections include complications such as a flare of an acute crystal induced synovitis on top of preexisting OA, and secondary periarticular syndromes such as bursitis or an enthesopathy. Finally, several drugs are now being tested for possible slow-acting symptomatic value, or disease-modifying effects in OA, including, for example, injections of high molecular weight hyaluronate. Some of these agents are of proven value in animal models of OA and it seems likely that specific drug therapy for this condition will soon be available.

Surgical management of OA has been an enormous growth industry over the last 20 years. The greatest advances have been in the use of hip and knee prostheses for the salvage of patients with destroyed joints and intractable symptoms. Other valuable procedures include osteotomy, which can lead to healing of the joint cartilage and subchondral bone, as well as pain relief, and the lavage and debridement of joints with earlier stages of OA. The main indication for most surgical procedures in OA is intractable pain.

PART TWO: PAIN AND OSTEOARTHRITIS

THE PAIN EXPERIENCED BY THOSE WITH OSTEOARTHRITIS

Pain is the major symptom of OA. It is generally insidious in onset, localised and not associated with any systemic disturbance (Moskowitz 1981). OA often 'creeps up' on people, with a gradually increasing awareness of a mild discomfort and stiffness of joints slowly turning into an aching sensation, and finally to more clear cut painful experience, over a period of months or years. Hart (1974) has described six types of pain in OA, which have some relationship to the gradual evolution of the disorder:

1. Aching of joints: the first sensation is often a mildly unpleasant aching sensation when the joints are at rest; it may be relieved by massage and movement.
2. Use-related pain: this is the major form of pain sensation that arises as the disorder develops; it may be particularly severe on initiation of movement or weight-bearing.
3. Pain at the end range of movement: this is a sensation of discomfort and stiffness, accompanied by pain as the joint comes to the end of its limited range of movement; it may be related to contraction of the capsule limiting movement.
4. Inflammatory pain: synovitis causes pain that is present at rest as well as on movement and is associated with severe morning stiffness as well as localised signs of joint inflammation.
5. Pain due to joint trauma: OA joints may become unstable due to a combination of ligamentous damage and muscle weakness. They become vulnerable to trauma which may produce an acute injury to periarticular or articular structures, resulting in a self-limiting episode of posttraumatic pain.
6. Pain amplification: some patients with OA may have pain aggravated by the fibrositis or pain amplification syndrome, leading to more widespread pain, without the usual localisation to affected joints, nor any clear relationship to joint use.

Patients with established OA record pain which is as severe as that recorded on a visual analogue scale by patients with rheumatoid arthritis (Huskisson et al 1979) and use similar adjectives to describe the pain. However, the diurnal rhythm is different from that seen in the inflammatory arthropathies (Bellamy et al 1990). The pain of OA is worse in the evenings rather than the morning. In addition to this diurnal rhythm, Bellamy and colleagues have shown that there is considerable day-to-day variation in pain severity, with the pain being most likely to be severe at the weekends. The symptoms can also be weather-dependent, as shown by Hollander & Yeostros (1963), who found that a fall in barometric pressure was associated with an exacerbation of the pain experienced by patients with OA and other arthropathies.

Cushnaghan has reported a comprehensive study of symptoms in 500 patients with established OA of limb joints (1991). Use-related pain was recorded in 89% of the subjects, compared with 59% who experienced pain at night, and only 44% who reported pain at rest. In patients with hand and knee OA, pain at night or at rest was hardly ever recorded in the absence of exacerbations of pain on use; however, use-related pain was not so apparent with hip disease. As described by other workers, women with OA appeared to experience more pain than men with similar severity of joint disease. Pain severity was also dependent on age and the joint site affected. There was a significant increase in pain severity with increasing age of the patients ($p<0.05$) and hand disease caused less pain than hip or knee disease. Analysis of patients with OA of a single site, such as the knee, showed that pain severity was associated with the severity of radiographic change, as well as age, sex and the degree of disability, but these variables only accounted for a small percentage of the variation in pain experience, suggesting that other variables are important determinants of pain in OA.

Cushnaghan also recorded other symptoms, including stiffness. Early morning stiffness of joints was recorded by 68.8% of patients, with a mean duration of 30 min (only 20.7% of patients had early morning stiffness lasting longer than 30 min). Stiffness after inactivity was present in 82.8%, with a mean duration of 7.4 min (over 5 min in 18.1%). Only 6% of patients reported early morning stiffness in the absence of inactivity stiffness and the latter is generally the more prominent symptom.

WHY ARE OA JOINTS SOMETIMES PAINFUL?

Lynn & Kellgren have indicated that three different questions need to be asked when considering the causes of articular pain (1986). First the anatomical source of the pain should be ascertained; secondly the pathophysiological processes involved – both local and central – need to be considered; finally the psychosocial factors that may influence both its genesis and tolerance must be addressed.

The anatomy of pain in OA

The innervation of joints has been described by Wyke (1981) and more recently by Kidd et al (1991). The capsule, ligaments and their insertions are the areas most richly innervated, but there is also a generous nerve supply to the periosteum close to joint margins and the blood vessels that penetrate into the synovium and subchondral bone. Of the four types of receptor described by Wyke, it is the noncorpuscular type IV nerve endings which are responsible for the sensation of pain. These unmyelinated receptors are present as interstitial and perivascular plexiform arrangements and also as free nerve endings in the capsule, synovium and articular fat pads. These receptors are normally inactive and only stimulated by the development of high tensions in the joint or by exposure to chemical irritants such as lactic acid, histamine, kinins, prostaglandins and neuropeptides. According to Wyke, joint pain may therefore by considered as either mechanical or chemical in origin, or a combination of both.

The possible anatomical origins of the pain in OA include the subchondral bone, synovium, capsule, ligaments, enthesis, marginal bone and periosteum and periarticular structures. The lack of nerve endings in the articular cartilage, the main target tissue of OA, may help explain the lack of pain in many patients, especially those with relatively mild disease, when the degree of pathology of other tissues may be relatively mild. Clinical examination, as well as the symptoms reported, may help clinicians to ascertain which of the possible structures is responsible for pain in any individual patient (Dieppe & McCrae 1987). For example, periarticular tender spots over capsular or ligamentous insertions may be present and there may be signs of ligamentous damage or joint inflammation.

The pathophysiology of pain in OA

Acute joint pain, in response to mechanical or chemical insults, may well have an important protective function, leading to avoidance behaviour. However, prolonged pain, as in OA, can lead to abnormal persistence of the nociceptive process, with changes in the dorsal horn synapse, as well as the joint (Alexander & Black 1992). Increased activity of the pronociceptive afferents causes persistent alterations in the projection neurones of the dorsal horn (Wilcox 1991). At the local level there may be a persistent increase in the sensitivity of the nerve endings, resulting in a lowering of the pain threshold at the joint level, as well as centrally.

Much of the local stimulus to pain in OA probably results from mechanical stimuli. The anatomy of the joint is abnormal, leading to mechanical stresses on the capsule, ligaments and periarticular tissues. The fibrosis of the capsule, and growth of marginal osteophytes, stretching the periosteum, may also contribute. Some inflammation also occurs in OA, allowing release of chemical pain stimuli, as discussed further below.

Psychosocial aspects of the pain in OA

Depression is a common feature of any disorder causing chronic pain (Gershon 1986). The importance of such psychological variables in the pain experience of OA patients has been highlighted by the work of Summers et al (1988). They found that pain severity was strongly associated with both anxiety and depression scores; this may help explain why Cushnaghan (1991) and others have found that the severity of jont pathology does not explain much of the variation in pain recorded by different patients.

EXPERIMENTAL STUDIES OF PAIN AND PAIN RELIEF IN OA

Three aspects of pain pathogenesis and management have attracted special attention: synovial inflammation, bone pain and periarticular syndromes. The following paragraphs detail some of the published work in these areas.

Synovitis and crystal deposition

Synovitis is a feature of OA and an important potential cause of pain. Synovial inflammation could cause chemical stimulation of nerve endings, as well as leading to increased intraarticular pressure. Early work in this area emphasised the possible role of cartilage fragments and other 'joint debris' in the genesis of secondary inflammatory synovitis (George & Chrisman 1968). More recent work has concentrated on the possible role of calcium-containing crystals, including basic calcium phosphates, and calcium pyrophosphate dihydrate (Dieppe et al 1976; McCarty 1976; Schumacher et al 1981). Attacks of crystal-induced synovitis (especially pseudogout due to pyrophosphate crystals) are an important, not uncommon, complication of OA and respond well to antiinflammatory therapy. The more general theory that inflammation is a key factor in the pathogenesis of OA and in its symptoms is less well substantiated by clinical or experimental evidence.

Clinical evidence of synovitis in OA is common, heat and redness of some involved joints being described by many authors (Kellgren & Moore 1952; Ehrlich 1975; Huskisson et al 1979). The synovial fluid is usually described as noninflammatory, because the cell content is much lower than that seen in rheumatoid arthritis, and consists mainly of mononuclear cells, in contrast to the intense polymorphonuclear cell infiltrate seen in rheumatoid disease. However, moderately large effusions are not uncommon in OA (Fig. 20.4) and the number of mononuclear cells is significant. The most striking evidence of synovial inflammation in OA comes from synovial biopsies (Goldenberg et al 1982). Direct inspection of the synovium with arthroscopy may be the most sensitive way of detecting areas of synovial inflammation, particularly as they may be patchy, and appear to be particularly common in the synovium adjacent to areas of joint damage (Linblad 1989).

Many of the treatments used in OA are directed towards suppressing inflammation or synovitis. It is clear that drugs that inhibit prostaglandin synthesis, such as the nonsteroidal antiinflammatory agents, do reduce pain in OA. However, as outlined above, it is unclear how much better they are than a simple analgesic (Doyle et al 1981; Parr et al 1985; Bradley et al 1991). Transcutaneous administration of nonsteroidal agents has become fashion-

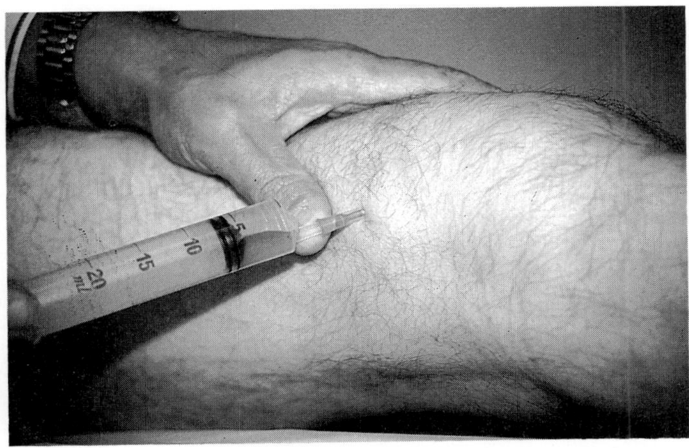

Fig. 20.4 Synovial fluid being withdrawn from a knee joint with osteoarthritis. Synovitis, with raised intraarticular pressure, is one possible cause of pain.

able in the treatment of OA, and has efficacy (Shamzad et al 1986; Doogan 1989), but it is not clear whether this is due to an effect on the synovium or on the periarticular tissues. Intraarticular steroids also produce some pain relief (Dieppe et al 1980, Friedman & Moore 1980), but it is not clear which patients will benefit most, or why. One of the problems with all the drug studies reported is the heterogeneity of the disease. It seems likely that the inflammatory component of OA varies in different patients and in the same joint over time. The process probably waxes and wanes and may be more apparent in some joints, and at certain times, than in others. However, because it is difficult to measure the synovitis of OA, this dimension is lacking from most trials.

Other therapeutic techniques aimed at the synovial element of OA include synovectomy. Surgical synovectomy has been reported to be of limited value in OA, the best results being achieved when it is combined with lavage and joint debridement (Gschwend 1981); the procedure cannot be recommended. Medical synovectomy, achieved with the intraarticular injection of radiocolloids such as yttrium-90 may be of some benefit. Doherty & Dieppe (1981) found that this procedure produced lasting symptomatic relief in patients with advanced OA associated with pyrophosphate deposition. External radiation therapy does not appear to be of value (Gibson et al 1973).

Joint lavage has become popular again in recent years and is made easier by the introduction of small arthroscopes, allowing the procedure to be done under local anaesthetic. One of the rationales for this way of treating patients with painful OA joints is that it reduces the secondary synovitis induced by crystals or joint debris. Many authors have reported pain relief lasting for many months, but the mechanisms for this benefit are unclear, and it is difficult to conduct any form of controlled trial of this procedure.

Bone pain in OA

The bony changes at the joint margin and beneath focal areas of damaged cartilage are probably major causes of pain in OA. The marginal tissue proliferation, first with the formation of new cartilage (the 'chondrophyte'), which subsequently forms bone (the osteophyte) is thought to cause pain (Kellgren 1983), perhaps via periosteal elevation. It has also been suggested that the formation of cysts in subchondral bone is associated with pain, although studies to determine a relationship between radiographic evidence of cysts and pain have proved negative (Danielsson 1964; Lawrence et al 1966).

Increased intraosseous pressure has been detected in OA, and there is extensive evidence to link this with the generation of pain, particularly pain at rest. Arnoldi and colleagues (1972, 1975) demonstrated that patients with hip OA develop venous stasis and intraosseous hypertension and described the 'intraosseous engorgement pain syndrome' (Lempberg & Arnoldi 1978), characterised by a dull aching pain, worst at the end of the day and present at rest. In more extensive studies, using scintigraphy and phlebography, they were able to correlate the raised pressure with rest pain, irrespective of the degree of radiographic change (Arnoldi et al 1980). More recent work indicates that the same mechanism probably operates at the knee joint.

Osteotomy provides rapid relief of pain in OA (Insall et al 1974). It has been suggested that the mechanism is by relief of intraosseous pressure. The fact that simple fenestration of the bone can also relieve pain would support this theory (Astrom 1975; Hietala & Astrom 1977).

Studies with bone scans have reemphasised the early nature and general importance of increased activity of the subchondral bone in OA (McCrae et al 1992). Pain shows some correlation with scan evidence of bone activity, as well as being predictive of outcome. In view of these and other studies, some treatments designed to alter bone turnover are being experimented with in OA, such as the use of calcitonin.

Periarticular pain in OA

Periarticular tender spots are common in patients with OA (Dixon 1965). There are three likely causes of these (Lynn & Kellgren 1986). First there may be bursitis, tendonitis or an enthesopathy around an affected joint; secondly, referred tender spots may be present; finally, the fibrositis or pain amplification syndrome may lead to tender spots which do not correspond to sites of pathology (Smythe 1979). Tender spots due to underlying pathology usually give rise to sharper, more severe pain than referred tender areas, but the distinction may be difficult (Fig. 20.5).

Bursitis is common around OA joints, the trochanteric bursa around the hip and anserine bursa at the medial

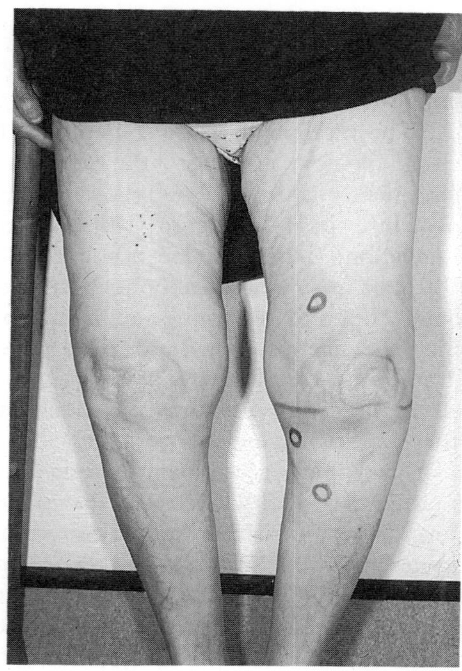

Fig. 20.5 This patient with knee osteoarthritis had discrete tender spots in the areas shown. The spot just below the medial joint line (marked by a horizontal line) may be caused by periarticular disease secondary to joint deformity (anserine bursitis or medial ligament). The other areas are not easily explained on anatomical grounds and may represent referred tenderness.

tibial margin of the knee being common examples. Local steroid injections may provide excellent, lasting pain relief. Minor degrees of instability or muscle weakness can lead to enthesopathies, with damage and inflammation at the insertions of capsules and ligaments. The knee collateral ligaments are frequently involved; again, local injection therapy may be valuable.

Rubrefacients are also used in the treatment of OA and, as mentioned above, can be helpful in pain relief. A recent development has been the introduction of capsaicin. Early trials suggest that rubbing capsaicin-containing creams on painful OA joints results in valuable pain relief (McCarthy & McCarty 1992). Capsaicin depletes substance P from C-fibres and any action in OA is presumably due to an effect on periarticular nerves, including those emerging from the joint and subchondral bone.

PART 3: RECENT DEVELOPMENTS IN OA

OA has been a difficult disorder to study for two main reasons: firstly, its evolution is very slow, with a time course of years, and secondly, there is no easy way of measuring or recording the presence of the disease processes. However, recent advances in technology are bringing new insights, and may well open the door to a wave of new approaches to an old disease.

Imaging

For years, the plain radiograph has been the gold standard for diagnosis and staging of severity in OA. Its insensitivity to pathology (Rogers et al 1990) and inaccuracies (Fife et al 1991) have now been revealed, but more importantly, new imaging technology is providing more sensitive and informative data on anatomical changes and the pathophysiology of joints (Cobby et al 1991). For example, magnetic resonance imaging has shown changes in the subchondral bone and soft tissues that cannot be imaged by the radiograph and scintigraphy has indicated the phasic nature of the disease activity. In addition, new ways of taking and assessing radiographs has led to much better means of following disease progression (Dacre & Huskisson 1989; Adams & Wallace 1991).

Biochemical markers

Conventional blood tests are normal in OA and the synovial fluid, until recently, was considered to be near normal and uninformative. Recent developments in the biology of cartilage have led to methods of detecting minute quantities of the products of normal and abnormal turnover of the cartilage matrix. Products of synthesis, such as collagen propeptides, and of degradation, such as fragments of proteoglycans, can now be assayed in the synovial fluid, blood and urine, providing a new technology for the detection, assessment and measurement of therapeutic responses in OA (Hardingham & Caterson 1991; Lohmander et al 1992). Although biochemical markers specific to OA have yet to be found, this area of research is helping to link the huge progress in the biochemistry of the disease to the clinical problem.

Disease outcome

There have also been major advances in techniques for measuring disease outcome. A number of indices have been designed for use specifically in OA, such as the WOMAC (Bellamy et al 1988) and Lequesne (Lequesne et al 1987) indices. These instruments combine measures of pain with assessment of the disability and psychosocial consequences of the disorder. In combination with other advances in the general approach to the assessment of disease progression and outcome (Kirwan 1992), and in the clinical techniques used to assess an OA joint (Cushnaghan et al 1990), these instruments are allowing accurate patient documentation to be linked to modern biochemical and imaging technology.

CONCLUSIONS

In the past OA has been considered to be a degenerative, inevitable 'wear-and-tear' condition. It is now thought to be an important, interesting, dynamic set of disease processes that can lead to a final common pathway of joint failure, but is potentially reversible. The technology to explore it is now available. However, pain remains the main consequence of the disorder and the causes of the pain, and adequate ways of controlling it, have yet to be discovered. OA is a fascinating and important model disease for those interested in pain and pain control to study.

REFERENCES

Acheson R M 1983 Osteoarthritis – the mystery crippler. Journal of Rheumatology 10: 174–176

Adams M E, Wallace C J 1991 Imaging of osteoarthritis. Seminars in Arthritis and Rheumatism 20: 26–39

Alexander J, Black A 1992 Pain mechanisms and the management of neuropathic pain. Current Opinion in Neurology and Neurosurgery 5: 228–234

Altman R, Asch E, Bloch D et al 1986 Development of criteria for the classification and reporting of osteoarthritis. Classification of osteoarthritis of the knee. Arthritis and Rheumatism 29: 1039–1049

Altman R D, Gottlieb N L, Howell D S (eds) 1989 Pain in osteoarthritis. Seminars in Arthritis and Rheumatism 18: 4(suppl 2)

Arnoldi C C, Linderholm H, Mussbichler H 1972 Venous engorgement and intraosseous hypertension in osteoarthritis of the hip. Journal of Bone and Joint Surgery 54B: 409–421

Arnoldi C C, Lempberg R K, Linderholm H 1975 Intraosseous hypertension and pain in the knee. Journal of Bone and Joint Surgery 57B: 360–363

Arnoldi C C, Djurhuus J C, Heerfordt J, Karte A 1980 Intraosseous phlebography, intraosseous pressure measurements and ^{99m}Tc polyphosphate scintigraphy in patients with various painful conditions in the hip and knee. Acta Orthopaedica Scandinavica 51: 19–28

Astrom J 1975 Preoperative effect of fenestration upon intraosseous pressure in patients with osteoarthritis of the hip. Acta Orthopaedica Scandinavica 46: 963–967

Bellamy N, Buchanan W W, Goldsmith C H, Campbell J, Stitt L W 1988 Validation study of WOMAC: a health status instrument for measuring clinically important patient relevant outcomes to anti-rheumatic drug therapy in patients with osteoarthritis of the hip or knee. Journal of Rheumatology 15: 1833–1840

Bellamy N, Sothern R B, Campbell J 1990 Rhythmic variations in pain perception in osteoarthritis of the knee. Journal of Rheumatology 17: 364–372

Bradley J D, Brandt K D, Katz B P, Kalasinski L A, Ryan S I 1991 Comparison of an anti-inflammatory dose of ibuprofen, an analgesic dose of ibuprofen and acetaminophen in treatment of patients with osteoarthritis of the knee. New England Journal of Medicine 325: 87–91

Cobby M, Watt I, Dieppe P 1991 Imaging in osteoarthritis. In: Russell R G G, Dieppe P A (eds) Osteoarthritis: current research and prospects for pharmacological intervention. IBC Technical Services, London, p 34–50

Croft P, Coggon D, Cruddas M, Cooper C 1992 Osteoarthritis of the hip: an occupational disease in farmers. British Medical Journal 304(6837): 1269–72

Cushnaghan J 1991 Osteoarthritis: A clinical and radiological study. MSc thesis, University of Bristol

Cushnaghan J, Dieppe P 1991 Study of 500 patients with limb joint osteoarthritis. I. Analysis by age, sex and distribution of symptomatic joints sites. Annals of the Rheumatic Diseases 50: 8–13

Cushnaghan J, Cooper C, Dieppe P, Kirwan J, McAlindon T, McCrae F 1990 Clinical assessment of osteoarthritis of the knee. Annals of the Rheumatic Diseases 49: 768–770

Dacre J E, Huskisson E C 1989 The automatic assessment of knee radiographs in osteoarthritis using digital image analysis. British Journal of Rheumatology 28: 506–510

Danielsson L G 1964 Incidence and prognosis of coxarthrosis. Acta Orthopaedica Scandinavica (suppl) 66: 9–61

Dieppe P A 1991 Osteoarthritis: The scale and scope of the clinical problem. In: Russell R G G, Dieppe P A (eds) Osteoarthritis: current research and prospects for pharmacological intervention. IBC Technical Services, London, p 4–23

Dieppe P A 1993 Treatment of osteoarthritis. In: Klippel J, Dieppe P (eds) Rheumatology. Gower Medical Publishing, London

Dieppe P, Cushnaghan J 1992 The natural course and prognosis of osteoarthritis. In: Moskowitz R W, Howell D S, Goldberg V M, Mankin J H (eds) Osteoarthritis: diagnosis and management. Saunders, Philadelphia, p 399–412

Dieppe P, McCrae F 1987 Pain and pain relief in osteoarthritis. Hospital Update: 904–913

Dieppe P A, Huskisson E C, Crocker P, Willoughby D A 1976 Apatite deposition disease: a new arthropathy. Lancet 1: 266–268

Dieppe P A, Sathapatayavongs B, Jones H E, Bacon P A, Ring E F J 1980 Intra-articular steroids in osteoarthritis. Rheumatology and Rehabilitation 19: 212–217

Dixon A St J (ed) 1965 Progress in clinical rheumatology. J A Churchill, London, p 313–329

Doherty M, Dieppe P A 1981 Effect of intra-articular yttrium-90 on chronic pyrophosphate arthropathy of the knee. Lancet 2: 1243–1246

Doogan D P 1989 Topical non-steroidal anti-inflammatory drugs. Lancet 2: 1270–1271

Doyle D V, Dieppe P A, Scott J, Huskisson E C 1981 An articular index for the assessment of osteoarthritis. Annals of the Rheumatic Diseases 40: 75–78

Ehrlich G E 1975 Osteoarthritis beginning with inflammation definitions and correlations. JAMA, 232: 157–159

Felson D T 1988 Epidemiology of hip and knee osteoarthritis. Epidemiological Review 10: 1–28

Felson D T 1990 Osteoarthritis. Rheumatic Diseases Clinics of North America 16: 499–512

Felson D, Anderson J J, Naimark A et al 1988 Obesity and knee osteoarthritis. The Framingham Study. Annals of Internal Medicine 109: 18–24

Felson D T, Hannan M T, Naimark A et al 1991 Occupational physical demands, knee bending and knee osteoarthritis: Results from the Framingham Study. Journal of Rheumatology 18: 1587–1592

Fife R S, Brandt K D, Brainstein E M et al 1991 Relationship between arthroscopic evidence of cartilage damage and radiographic evidence of joint space narrowing in early osteoarthritis of the knee. Arthritis and Rheumatism 34: 377–382

Friedman D M, Moore M E 1980 The efficacy of intra-articular steroids in osteoarthritis: a double blind study. Journal of Rheumatology 7: 850–856

Gardner D L 1992 Pathological basis of the connective tissue diseases. Edward Arnold, London p 842–923

George R C, Chrisman O D 1968 The role of cartilage polysaccharides in osteoarthritis. Clinical Orthopaedics 57: 259

Gershon S 1986 Chronic pain: hypothesized mechanism and rationale for treatment. Neuropsychobiology 15 (suppl 1): 22–27

Gibson T, Winter P J, Grahame R 1973 Radiotherapy in the treatment of osteoarthrosis of the knee. Rheumatology and Rehabilitation 12: 42–46

Goldenberg D L, Egan M S, Cohen A S 1982 Inflammatory synovitis in degenerative joint disease. Journal of Rheumatology 9: 204–209

Gschwend N 1981 Synovectomy. In: Kelly W N, Harris E D, Ruddy S, Sledgre C B (eds) Textbook of rheumatology. W B Saunders, Philadelphia

Hadler N M 1992 Knee pain is the malady – not osteoarthritis. Annals of Internal Medicine 116(7): 598–599

Hart F A 1974 Pain in osteoarthrosis. Practitioner 212: 244–250

Hardingham T E, Caterson B 1991 Biochemistry of articular cartilage and joint disease. In: Russell R G G, Dieppe P A (eds) Osteoarthritis. IBC Technical Services, London, p 51–64

Hietala S O, Astrom J 1977 The effect of fenestration on intraosseous

drainage in osteoarthritis of the hip. Acta Orthopaedica Scandinavica 48: 80–85
Hollander J L, Yeostros S J 1963 The effect of simultaneous variations of humidity and barometric pressure on arthritis. Bulletin of the American Meteorological Society 44: 489–494
Howell D S, Woessner J F, Jimenez S, Seda H, Schumacher H R 1979 A view on the pathogenesis of osteoarthritis. Bulletin on the Rheumatic Diseases 29: 996–1000
Huskisson E C, Dieppe P A, Tucker A K, Cannell L B 1979 Another look at osteoarthritis. Annals of the Rheumatic Diseases 38: 423–428
Hutton C W 1990 Treatment, pain and epidemiology of osteoarthritis. Current Opinion in Rheumatology 2(5): 765–769
Insall J, Shoji H, Mayer V 1974 High tibial osteotomy. A 5-year evaluation. Journal of Bone and Joint Surgery 56A: 1397–1405
Kellgren J H 1983 Pain in osteoarthritis. Journal of Rheumatology 10 (suppl 9): 108–109
Kellgren J H, Lawrence J S 1957 Radiological assessment of osteo-arthrosis. Annals of the Rheumatic Diseases 16: 494–502
Kellgren J H, Moore R 1952 Generalised osteoarthritis and Heberden's nodes. British Medical Journal 1: 181–184
Kidd B L, Gilson S J, Mapp P I et al 1991 Neuropeptides as mediators of inflammation and chronic pain. European Journal of Rheumatology and Inflammation 11: 47–65
Kirwan J R 1992 A theoretical framework for process, outcome and prognosis in rheumatoid arthritis (editorial). Journal of Rheumatology 19: 333–336
Kovar P A, Allegrante J P, Mackenzie C R, Peterson M G, Gutin B, Charlson M E 1992 Supervised fitness walking in patients with osteoarthritis of the knee. A randomized, controlled trial. Annals of Internal Medicine 116: 529–534
Lawrence J S, Bremner J M, Bier F 1966 Osteoarthrosis. Prevalence in the population and relationship between symptoms and x-ray changes. Annals of the Rheumatic Diseases 25: 1–24
Lempberg R K, Arnoldi C C 1978 The significance of intraosseous pressure in normal and diseased states with special reference to the intraosseous engorgement – pain syndrome. Clinical Orthopaedics and Related Research 136: 143–156
Lequesne M, Mery C, Samson M et al 1987 Indexes of severity for osteoarthritis of the hip and knee. Validation. Value in comparison with other assessment tests. Scandinavian Journal of Rheumatology (suppl 65): 85–89
Lindblad S 1989 Arthroscopic and synovial correlates of pain in osteoarthritis. Seminars in Arthritis and Rheumatism 18 (suppl 2): 91–93
Lohmander L S, Lark M W, Dahlberg L, Walakovits L A, Roos H 1992 Cartilage matrix metabolism in osteoarthritis: markers in synovial fluid, serum and urine. Clinical Biochemistry 25: 167–174
Lynn B, Kellgren J H 1986 Pain. In: Scott J T (ed) Copeman's textbook of the rheumatic diseases, 6th edn. Churchill Livingstone, p 143–160
Massardo L, Watt I, Cushnaghan J, Dieppe P 1989 An eight year prospective study of osteoarthritis of the knee joint. Annals of the Rheumatic Diseases, 48: 893–897
McAlindon T, & Dieppe P 1989 Osteoarthritis: Definitions and criteria. Annals of the Rheumatic Diseases 48: 531–532
McAlindon T, Dieppe P 1990 The medical management of osteoarthritis of the knee; An inflammatory issue? British Journal of Rheumatology 29: 471–473
McCarty D J 1976 Calcium pyrophosphate dihydrate crystal deposition disease. Arthritis and Rheumatism 19: 295
McCrae F, Shouls J, Dieppe P, Watt I 1992 Scintigraphic assessment of osteoarthritis of the knee joint. Annals of the Rheumatic Diseases 51: 938–942
McCarthy G, McCarty D J 1992 Effect of topical capsaicin in the therapy of painful osteoarthritis of the hands. Journal of Rheumatology 19: 604–607
Moskowitz R W 1981 Management of osteoarthritis. Bulletin on the Rheumatic Diseases: 31: 31–35
Moskowitz R W 1992 Osteoarthritis symptoms and signs. In: Moskowitz R W, Howell D S, Goldberg V M, Mankin J H (eds) Osteoarthritis: diagnosis and management, 2nd edn. Saunders, Philadelphia p 255–263
Parr G, Darekar B, Fletcher A, Bulpitt C J 1985 Joint pain and quality of life; results of a randomised trial. British Journal of Clinical Pharmacology 27: 235–242
Rogers J, Dieppe P 1992 Prevalence of hip and knee osteoarthritis (OA) in the past: is tibio-femoral knee OA a new disease? Osteoarthritis and Cartilage 1: 17 (abstract)
Rogers J, Dieppe P, Watt I 1981 Arthritis in Saxon and medieval skeletons. British Medical Journal 283: 668–671
Rogers J, Watt I, Dieppe P 1990 A comparison of the visual and radiographic detection of bony changes at the knee joint. British Medical Journal 300: 367–368
Schumacher H R, Cherian P V, Reginato A J, Bardin T, Rothfuss S 1983 Intra-articular apatite crystal deposition. Annals of the Rheumatic Diseases 42 (suppl 1): 54–59
Shamzad M, Perkal M, Golden E L, Marlin R L 1986 Two double blind comparisons of a topically applied salicylate cream and orally ingested aspirin in the relief of chronic musculoskeletal pain. Current Therapeutic Research 39: 470–479
Smythe H A 1979 Fibrositis as a disorder of pain modulation. Clinics in Rheumatic Diseases 5: 823–832
Sokoloff L 1980 The pathology of osteoarthrosis and the role of aging. In: Nuki G (ed): The aetiopathogenesis of osteoarthrosis. Pitman Medical, London, p 1–15
Spector T D, Dacre J E, Harris P A, Huskisson E C 1991 The radiological progression of OA: An 11 year follow-up study of the knee. British Journal of Rheumatology 30 (suppl 2): 72 (abstract)
Summers M N, Haley W E, Reveille J D, Alarcón G S 1988 Radiographic assessment and psychologic variables as predictors of pain and functional impairment in osteoarthritis of the knee or hip. Arthritis and Rheumatism 31: 204–209
Wilcox G L 1991 Excitatory neurotransmitters and pain. In: Bond M, Charlton E, Woolf C J (eds). Proceedings of VIIth World Congress on Pain. Elsevier, Amsterdam, p 97–112
Wood P H N 1976 Osteoarthrosis in the community. Clinics in Rheumatic Diseases 2: 495–507
Wyke B 1981 The neurology of joints: a review of general principles. Clinics in Rheumatic Diseases 7: 233–239

21. Rheumatoid arthritis

D. M. Grennan and M. I. V. Jayson

AETIOLOGY

The exact aetiology of rheumatoid arthritis is unknown but current hypotheses suggest that both genetic and microbiological factors may be important.

Genetic factors

An increased familial aggregation for the disease, and a greater concordance in monozygotic and diyzygotic twins, shows that rheumatoid arthritis has a genetic predisposition (Lawrence 1970), but unknown environmental factors are also necessary for the disease to develop. The best documented genetic marker for rheumatoid arthritis is the Class II major histocompatibility complex (MHC) antigen, HLA-DR4 (Panayi et al 1978) which appears as a risk marker for the disease in most caucasoid populations. Class II antigens are expressed as receptors on B lymphocytes and macrophages and present antigenic peptide to T cell alpha-beta receptors on T helper cells during an immune response, so that changes in Class II antigen configuration are thought to be associated with the immune response. In patients who have developed rheumatoid arthritis, variation in HLA-DR genotype influences the severity of the arthritis, whilst genes within the HLA region but outside the HLA-DR locus influence the risk of an individual's developing extraarticular features of rheumatoid disease (Hillarby et al 1991). Any part of the genetic contribution to rheumatoid disease susceptibility can be accounted for by genes within the HLA region, so that genes outside HLA also influence susceptibility to the disease although these non-HLA genes have still to be identified (Grennan & Sanders 1988).

Microbiological factors

Despite many years' work by many centres no one infectious agent has been shown to cause rheumatoid arthritis in man. Clinical infection by mycoplasmas and by a whole range of agents (e.g. rubella, hepatitis B, arboviruses) may be followed by acute arthropathies which rarely become chronic (Denman 1975). Although mycoplasmas have been isolated from rheumatoid joint fluids by some workers, it is extremely difficult to exclude contaminant organisms and these findings have not been confirmed by the majority. Recently it has been shown that a peptidoglycan component of bacterial cell walls is arthritogenic in rats and it has been suggested that bacterial cell wall products absorbed from the gut may cause arthritis in man (Bennett 1978).

Recent speculations into a possible viral aetiology for rheumatoid arthritis have been stimulated by the concept that slow viruses may produce disease many years after initial infection and require special techniques for their detection. Genetically determined susceptibility may be essential to permit such viruses becoming established in host tissues.

PATHOLOGY

The normal synovial lining of a diarthrodial joint is a delicate tissue consisting of a cavity lining layer up to three cells thick and a loosely arranged stroma with connective tissue, microvasculature and lymphatics. In early active disease the synovium becomes swollen and hypertrophic. Microscopically the stroma is invaded by lymphocytes and plasma cells. Fibrin deposition may occur on the surface of the hypertrophic synovium (Fassbender 1975). The synovial stroma is replaced by proliferation of local connective tissue cells by the process of mesenchymoid transformation. The destructive phase of the disease is associated with production of a chronic granulation tissue or pannus from this transformed tissue which spreads over the articular cartilage surface. Cartilage destruction appears on the deep surface of the pannus and is seen as loss of joint space on X-ray. Bone erosions usually appear first at the joint margins at the point of normal synovial reflection and where bone is relatively unprotected by cartilage. Neutral proteolytic enzymes (Barrett &

Saklatvala 1981), secreted by macrophages in the pannus, and acidic lysosomal enzymes, secreted by polymorphonuclear leucocytes in the synovial fluid, both play a part in bone and cartilage destruction. In severe forms of the disease continued bone and cartilage destruction are associated with irreversible deformity and, particularly in weight-bearing joints, secondary osteoarthritis may occur.

CLINICAL FEATURES

Severe forms of the disease may be associated with both articular and extraarticular features and all the symptoms and signs of a systemic disease process. These include general malaise and lassitude, weight loss and low-grade pyrexia. The disease onset is insidious in up to 70% of patients but may be acute and associated with systemic upset and fever.

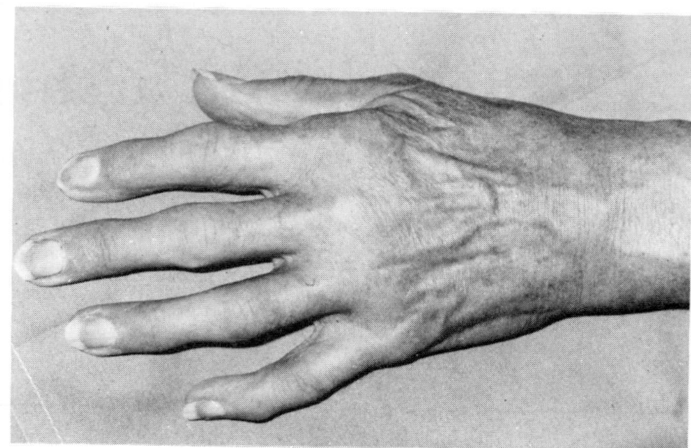

Fig. 21.1 Early rheumatoid inflammation of the proximal interphalangeal and metacarpophalangeal joints of the hand.

ARTICULAR CLINICAL FEATURES

Established rheumatoid disease is typically a symmetrical peripheral polyarthritis which most often involves the small joints of the hands and feet, the wrists, ankles, knees and cervical spine. The shoulders and elbows may be involved and the hips are frequently spared. In severe forms of the disease however any synovial joint may be affected.

In early active rheumatoid disease there is pain, soft-tissue swelling and stiffness. The pain and stiffness of active inflammation are typically worse in the early morning and improve with activity during the day although many patients develop further symptoms when they become tired in the early evening. 'Gelling' or stiffening of the joints with rest or inactivity during the day is also typical of inflammatory disease. On examination the soft-tissue swelling of active rheumatoid arthritis may be associated with synovial hypertrophy and synovial effusions and is warm and tender. Muscle wasting appears rapidly around painful swollen joints and there is sometimes periarticular inflammatory oedema.

In late-stage destructive rheumatoid arthritis problems of deformity and loss of function predominate with relatively little active inflammation.

Hands

Early active disease typically is associated with involvement of the proximal interphalangeal joints producing spindling of the fingers and synovitis of the metacarpophalangeal joints (Fig. 21.1). Synovial hypertrophy may also involve the flexor tendon sheaths of the fingers producing diffuse swelling of the palmar aspects of the fingers and contributing to impaired finger movement and poor grip. Synovitis of the wrists may lead to compression of the median nerve beneath the flexor retinaculum and produce features of the carpal tunnel syndrome. These include paraesthesiae and numbness of the fingers, which are worse at night. They may occur as a presenting feature of the disease. Severe forms of carpal tunnel syndrome are associated with wasting of the thenar eminence and sensory loss in a median nerve distribution. Such wasting should be distinguished from generalised muscle wasting due to disuse with active joint disease. Synovitis of the extensor aspect of the wrist may rupture the extensor tendons, particularly the extensor pollicis longus.

The deformities of chronic rheumatoid arthritis in the hands are produced by chronic synovial inflammation and swelling, giving rise to stretching and rupture of capsules surrounding ligaments and tendons (Swezey 1971). They include the following:

1. Swan-neck deformity of the fingers with hyperextension of the proximal interphalangeal joints and flexion at the distal interphalangeal joints.
2. The boutonnière or buttonhole deformity (Fig. 21.2) is associated with hyperflexion at the proximal interphalangeal joint, stretching or rupture of the central slip of the extensor and buttonholing of the joint between the lateral extensor tendon slips.
3. Continued inflammation at the metacarpophalangeal joints produces flexion deformity and ulnar deviation (Fig. 21.3).
4. The more frequent deformity of the thumb is the Z thumb or Nalebuff type 1 deformity associated with continued inflammation at the first metacarpophalangeal joint. This deformity consists of flexion at the metacarpophalangeal joint produced by volar displacement of the long extensor and hyperextension at the distal joints. Other thumb deformities may result from chronic inflammation at the first metacarpal joint resulting in abduction of the

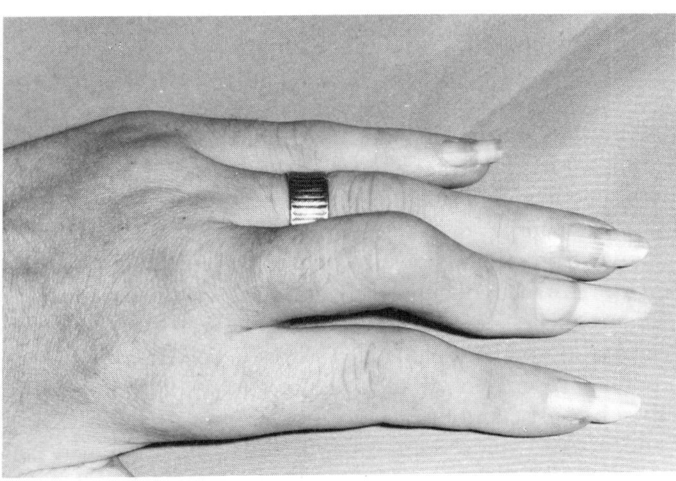

Fig. 21.2 The boutonnière, or buttonhole, deformity of the middle finger.

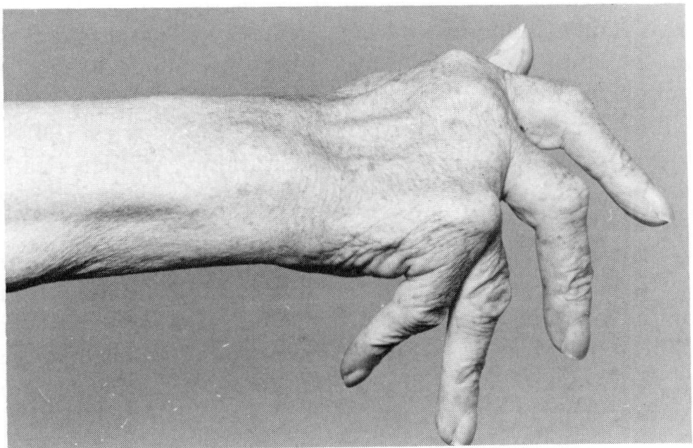

Fig. 21.3 Ulnar deviation of the fingers.

thumb and hyperextension of either the distal or proximal phalanx (Swezey 1971).

5. Dorsal subluxation of the ulnar head at the wrist ('caput ulnae') is associated with a high risk of rupture of fourth and fifth extensor tendons and 'dropped fingers' (Fig. 21.4). Prophylactic surgical resection of the ulnar head with synovectomy usually prevents this complication.

Feet and ankles

Foot involvement is an important but often neglected aspect of the disease. Both active synovitis and radiological changes are most frequent at the metatarsophalangeal joints (Vidigal et al 1975) and may be detected by the presence of swelling and tenderness around the joints. Erosions of the metatarsophalangeal joints are common even in the absence of symptoms and may be found in over 80% of rheumatoid patients admitted to hospital (Dixon 1969; Vidigal et al 1975). Active synovitis may also produce symptoms in ankles, subtalar and midtarsal joints. Synovial hypertrophy may produce symptoms laterally as a result of peroneal tendon sheath involvement and medially as a result of flexor tendon sheath involvement.

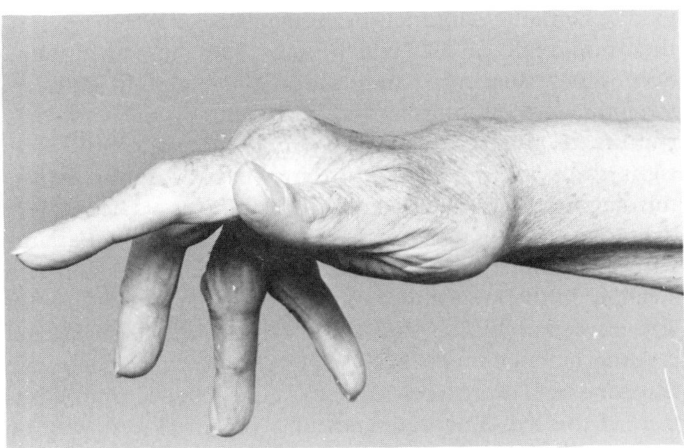

Fig. 21.4 Rupture of extensor tendons with 'dropped fingers'.

The most frequent rheumatoid foot deformity is associated with subluxation at the metatarsophalangeal joints and displacement of the normally weight-bearing fat pad distally. The subluxated metatarsal heads may be felt in the sole and are often associated with callosities. Patients with this deformity often complain of a feeling like 'walking on stones'. Other toe deformities found in rheumatoid arthritis include hallux valgus and cock-up toes.

Chronic synovitis in the midtarsal and subtalar regions may cause destruction of the ligaments supporting the longitudinal and transverse arches of the feet. This results in broadening and flattening of the foot and production of the characteristic pes planovalgus deformity. Uncommonly a pes varus deformity may be produced but it has been suggested that such patients have had a preexisting pes cavus (Vidigal et al 1975).

Other foot symptoms may result from rheumatoid nodules in weight-bearing regions. Rheumatoid disease may also cause symptoms in the region of the plantar fascia and Achilles tendon insertion with the calcaneus, although these features are more typical of ankylosing spondylitis and other seronegative arthritides.

Knees

Active synovitis in the knees is associated with soft-tissue swelling and effusions, which are often visible around the knee itself and in the suprapatellar pouch. Quadriceps muscle-wasting commonly accompanies inflammation of the joint. Effusions of the joint may be associated with a gastrocnemius – semimembranous bursa or Baker's cyst in the popliteal fossa, which may be uncomfortable. Sometimes this cyst extends down the calf to produce swelling and discomfort and this joint or the cyst may rupture to give acute pain, swelling and tenderness. The signs and symptoms of rupture may exactly mimic and be misdiagnosed as deep venous thrombosis. The correct diagnosis can often be made on clinical grounds. Patients with a ruptured cyst may previously have noted pain and swelling in the knee and popliteal fossa which decreases in size immediately the pain in the calf begins. Cyst rupture is often associated with physical activity whilst deep vein thrombosis is more likely to occur after rest or immobilisation of the leg. The diagnosis of a ruptured cyst may be confirmed by an arthrogram when dye is seen extravasating into the calf. Treatment of ruptured cyst is by rest and local injection of steroid into the knee. Rarely ruptured cysts and deep vein thrombosis occur together. However, in general, anticoagulants should be given to rheumatoid patients with calf pain only if thrombosis has been proven by venography.

Chronic synovitis of the knee may produce instability of the joint by destruction of cruciate or medial and lateral ligaments.

Elbows

Synovial effusions in the elbows may produce limitation of extension of the joint and be detected clinically as a bulge felt on either side of the olecranon as the joint is extended. Pronation and supination may be affected if the superior radioulnar joint is involved.

Cervical spine

Pain on movement of the neck is a common feature of active rheumatoid arthritis. Radiological abnormalities of the cervical spine are often asymptomatic, however, and may be found in up to 80% of patients (Bland et al 1963; Conlon et al 1966). They include osteoporosis, apophyseal joint erosions, erosions of the vertebral end plates, loss of disc space without osteoporosis, atlantoaxial and subaxial subluxations and erosions of the odontoid peg.

Both anterior atlantoaxial and subaxial subluxations may be associated with neurological complications. Subluxations at the atlantoaxial region occur in about 25% of rheumatoid patients seen in hospital (Conlon et al 1966; Mathews 1974) although only a minority have features of neurological involvement. This deformity is caused by destruction within the network of ligaments which normally maintains the odontoid peg in apposition to the posterior aspect of the anterior arch of the atlas during movements of the head and neck. This ligamentous framework includes the transverse ligament, which forms part of the cruciate ligament, the apical ligament of the odontoid peg, the alar ligaments and posterior longitudinal ligament. Anterior atlantoaxial subluxation is demonstrated by lateral X-ray of the cervical spine with the neck in flexion, when the gap between odontoid peg and anterior arch of the atlas should not become greater than 3 mm. Vertical subluxation of the odontoid peg may also occur and is diagnosed when the tip of the odontoid peg is seen more than 3 mm above McGregor's line, drawn from the posterior edge of the hard palate to the margin of the occipital curve. Less common forms of atlantoaxial subluxation include lateral and posterior subluxations (Brunton et al 1978).

The presence of gross forms of atlantoaxial subluxation may be suspected because of peculiar posture of the head and neck. Typical symptoms include upper cervical pain which may radiate to the occiput or retroorbital areas. Cervical cord compression may result from both atlantoaxial and subaxial subluxation. Clinical features of neurological involvement include weakness in arms and legs which is out of proportion to the degree of articular involvement, bladder or bowel symptoms, shooting pains in the arms and sometimes symptoms suggestive of a peripheral neuropathy. There is a risk that a subsequent fall or accident may convert a minor neurological deficit into complete quadriplegia. Uncommonly, sudden death has occurred after vertical subluxation of the odontoid peg into the foramen magnum.

Pain or minor neurological symptoms resulting from cervical spine involvement may respond to immobilisation of the neck in a Plastazote fitted collar. Severe pain or neurological features which fail to respond to conservative measures may require immobilisation of the cervical spine by surgery.

Other

Any synovial joint may become involved by the more severe forms of rheumatoid arthritis. Pain in the shoulder may be due to periarticular involvement and synovitis of the glenohumeral or acromioclavicular joints. A minority of patients are seen who develop severe destructive changes of the glenohumeral joint and if such patients also have elbow disease they may have severe functional difficulties. Hip joint involvement may occur occasionally. Both bilateral and unilateral forms of temporomandibular involvement may occur and affect chewing and mouth opening. Occasionally more unusual joints are affected, such as the cricoarytenoid, which produces difficulty on swallowing, and the joints of the middle ear with production of hearing difficulties.

EXTRAARTICULAR CLINICAL FEATURES

Extraarticular features are found particularly in patients with the most severe forms of articular disease. The pathogenesis of many of the systemic features, such as vasculitis and nodules, are thought to be related to the local deposition of circulating immune complexes containing IgM and possibly IgG rheumatoid factors.

Nodules

Rheumatoid nodules are found most frequently in subcutaneous regions subject to recurrent mechanical stress. Common sites include the subcutaneous borders of the forearms, the olecranon, often in association with an olecranon bursa, and also over sites such as the tips of the fingers and sacrum. Rheumatoid nodules in these sites are firm, nontender and larger and less transient than the small nodules of rheumatic fever. In certain areas, such as over the sacrum, nodules may ulcerate and become infected bedsores. They can form a potential focus for systemic infections.

The histology of the rheumatoid nodule is almost diagnostic for rheumatoid arthritis and consists of a central area of fibrinoid necrosis which is surrounded by a palisade layer of fibroblasts and peripherally by a zone of loose connective tissue (Fassbender 1975). Rheumatoid nodules may have an adverse prognostic as well as diagnostic significance. Although most frequently found in the subcutaneous regions, these nodules may also occur as intracutaneous nodules and within other tissues such as the sclera, lung, pleura and myocardium.

Vasculitis

This is an uncommon but potentially fatal complication found in the most severe forms of the disease. All sizes of blood vessels may become affected. Cutaneous vasculitis is most often seen as nailfold haemorrhages in the fingers. Patients with these lesions do not always develop the more serious forms of vasculitis although they are at increased risk of doing so. More serious forms of cutaneous vasculitis may be associated with persistent cutaneous ulceration which often appears in the lower leg and may prove resistant to healing. Medium or large blood vessels may become involved and present clinically with gangrene of the fingers, small bowel infarction or perforation and pulmonary hypertension. Small vessel vasculitis is thought to underline many of the other extraarticular disease features such as peripheral neuropathy and probably nodule formation.

The histological changes found in rheumatoid vasculitis range from intimal hyperplasia to an inflammatory reaction affecting all layers of the vessel wall and sometimes associated with necrosis (Fassbender 1975). Immunological tests often show high titres of circulating IgM rheumatoid factors, antinuclear antibodies and evidence of circulating immune complex activity, such as reduced serum complement levels and sometimes circulating cryoglobulins (Ansell & Loewi 1977).

Patients with severe forms of vasculitis are medical emergencies and often require aggressive treatment with corticosteroids and immunosuppressive drugs.

Haematological

The anaemia of rheumatoid arthritis is similar to that found in other chronic disorders such as malignancy, chronic infections and uraemia. This anaemia is usually normocytic normochromic, but may be hypochromic and, less commonly, macrocytic (Bennett 1977). The degree of anaemia in rheumatoid disease roughly correlates with the erythrocyte sedimentation rate (ESR). Typically the serum iron and total iron binding capacity are reduced and serum ferritin is elevated. The anaemia is associated with an increased affinity of the reticuloendothelial system for iron and bone marrow iron stores are plentiful. The anaemia of rheumatoid disease is to be distinguished from the iron deficiency which commonly results from gastrointestinal blood loss produced as a side-effect of nonsteroidal antiflammatory drug therapy. In an iron deficiency anaemia serum iron is low but the total iron binding capacity is elevated and the bone marrow iron stores are reduced. The two types of anaemia may coexist and factors which might suggest that iron deficiency is contributing to anaemia include a history of melaena or recent dyspepsia, a sudden drop in haemoglobin or a haemoglobin value much lower than 9 g/dl. Unless there is coincidental iron deficiency, oral iron therapy does not improve the anaemia of rheumatoid arthritis. Parenteral iron is occasionally used but the main treatment of this anaemia consists of measures directed at suppressing the underlying disease process.

The major factor associated with the pathogenesis of rheumatoid anaemia is the high affinity of the reticuloendothelial system for iron which is then sequestered in a nonutilisable form. Other factors which may contribute include ineffective erythropoiesis and haemolysis and possibly inadequate erythropoietin production (Bennett 1977). Serum folate levels may be low as a nonspecific feature of inflammation but folate therapy is usually unhelpful.

Felty's syndrome is the association of rheumatoid arthritis with splenomegaly and leucopenia. Other features of the syndrome may include normocytic normochromic anaemia, thrombocytopenia, lymphadenopathy, cutaneous ulceration and pigmentation. The major hazard of the condition is recurrent major or minor infection. Patients with Felty's syndrome tend to have more severe forms of articular disease and on serological testing usually have high titres of IgM rheumatoid factor and antinuclear factors.

The leucopenia of Felty's syndrome usually lies between 800 and 2500 cells per mm^3 and is associated with a fall in granulocyte number. Occasionally a leucopenia of less than 800/m³ is seen. The most frequent bone marrow abnormality found is granulocyte maturation arrest. The pathogenesis of Felty's syndrome is multifactorial and includes both an increased peripheral destruction partly attributable to circulating immune complexes as well as depression of granulopoiesis by a splenic humoral factor (Bennett 1977). Some recent leucokinetic studies have suggested that excessive margination of leucocytes in the peripheral circulation may account for some of the apparent fall in circulating cell counts.

Treatment of Felty's syndrome is only indicated if the leucopenia is associated with significant recurrent infection. Although corticosteroid therapy may increase the peripheral white cell count it also increases the susceptibility to infection and is of uncertain value in the treatment of Felty's syndrome. Gold or penicillamine therapy can be very effective but these drugs must be used carefully because of their own potentially toxic effects on the bone marrow. A proportion of patients with this condition respond to splenectomy, although the operation itself is associated with significant postoperative mortality. Rarely, despite a rise in the peripheral white cell count after splenectomy, susceptibility to infection does not improve and patients die of fulminating septicaemia. Removal of splenic factors normally helpful in the defence against infecion may be responsible.

Thrombocytosis or increase in the circulating platelet count may be seen in active rheumatoid disease and probably represents a nonspecific effect of inflammation. This thrombocytosis is not usually clinically significant.

Sjögren's syndrome

Sjögren's syndrome is the association of keratoconjunctivitis sicca (KCS) and/or xerostomia with rheumatoid arthritis or other connective tissue disorders. Dysfunction of lacrimal and salivary glands is associated with lymphocytic infiltration which may progress to fibrosis and complete loss of acinar tissue. This is distinguished from the gland dysfunction due to simple atrophy in old age. Clinical evidence of Sjögren's syndrome may be found in up to 15% of rheumatoid patients (Williamson 1976).

The symptoms of KCS are of a gritty feeling or irritation of the eyes and as the lysozyme content of tears is also reduced the eyes may be subject to recurrent infection. The diagnosis of KCS is best confirmed with a slit lamp, when absence of the normal tear film will be noted. In addition, thick strands of mucus may be seen sticking to the conjunctiva and cornea. Two drops of 1% rose bengal instilled into the eye can be used to show up the mucus strands and abnormal epithelium of the dry conjunctiva. In the absence of a slit lamp the reduction in tear secretion may be demonstrated by the Schirmer tear rest. A strip of filter paper is hooked over the lower lid at the junction of the middle and outer thirds and wetting of less than 15 mm of the paper over a 5-minute period is considered abnormal. The symptoms of KCS are usually relieved by the regular instillation of artificial tear drops into the affected eyes. Occasionally, tarsorrhaphy or lacrimal canal ablation is indicated.

The xerostomia may be associated with recurrent salivary gland swelling. A clinical diagnosis of xerostomia may be made if the patient complains of a dry mouth and on examination there is no salivary pool in the floor of the mouth. Again it is advisable to consider other nonspecific factors such as drug therapy and anxiety before attributing all complaints of mouth dryness to this condition. Biopsy of minor salivary glands from the lip may be used to confirm the diagnosis. Other investigations which have been used in the formal assessment of xerostomia include measurement of salivary flow rate following cannulation of the parotid, duct, sialography and radioisotope imaging of the salivary glands. Treatment of the xerostomia of Sjögren's syndrome is unsatisfactory. Dental hygiene is important, as patients with the condition are susceptible to dental caries. Local radiotherapy to the involved glands is not helpful and increases the risk of these patients developing lymphoma to which they already have an increased susceptibility (Zulman et al 1978).

Secretions from other endothelial surfaces may also be affected so that other features of the condition may include dysphagia, dyspareunia and dryness of the skin. Sjögren's syndrome may be associated with a number of immunological symptoms including renal tubular acidosis and autoimmune thyroid disease. Sjögren's patients may also have an increased risk of drug hypersensitivity (Whaley et al 1973).

Ophthalmic

Keratoconjunctivitis sicca is the most frequent eye feature of rheumatoid disease. Scleritis (Jayson & Jones 1971) is less common but is potentially more serious. It may occur in diffuse or nodular forms. Rarely, a severe necrotising form of scleritis is seen. The complications of untreated scleritis include perforation of the sclera, glaucoma and cataract. Systemic steroids in dosages of around 60 mg daily, and sometimes immunosuppressive drugs, may be required for the treatment to this condition. Occasionally, milder attacks may respond to treatment with nonsteroidal antiinflammatory drugs.

Respiratory

Pleurisy and pleural effusions are the most common form of pulmonary involvement by the disease. Rheumatoid pleural effusions particularly show lymphocytosis and reduced glucose content in the absence of infection. Sometimes macrophages containing IgM inclusions (ragocytes) are present and immunological tests for antinuclear antibodies and IgM rheumatoid factor may be positive. The histology of the underlying pleura often shows nonspecific changes of chronic inflammation, but occasionally rheumatoid nodule formation is seen.

Interstitial fibrosis (fibrosing alveolitis) may occur uncommonly as the cause of progressive breathlessness in seropositive, nodular rheumatoid disease (Turner-Warwick & Evans 1977). The associated features found in the idiopathic condition are also found in the form associated with rheumatoid disease and these include finger clubbing, coarse pleural crepitations and widespread pulmonary shadows on chest X-ray. Treatment with corticosteroid drugs is usually disappointing but occasionally immunosuppressive drugs appear to help. Asymptomatic impairment of carbon monoxide diffusion capacity in the absence of radiological change is common in rheumatoid disease, as in other forms of connective tissue disease, and usually does not progress to symptomatic interstitial fibrosis.

Rheumatoid nodules may appear in the lungs as nodules of varying size and need to be differentiated from other causes of pulmonary shadowing such as neoplasms and tuberculosis.

Seropositive rheumatoid arthritics who are coal miners or are exposed to industrial dusts may develop gross forms of pulmonary fibrosis and nodules. Caplan (1953) originally described such lesions in coal miners.

Destructive airways disease has been shown to be more frequent in rheumatoid arthritis patients than in controls matched for smoking habits (Geddes et al 1977). A rare and progressively fatal form of obstructive bronchiolitis has also been described in a group of rheumatoid patients (Geddes et al 1977).

Cardiovascular

Pericardial effusions may be detected by echocardiography in up to 55% of rheumatoid patients (Bacon & Gibson 1974). They are frequently asymptomatic, and rarely cardiac tamponade may result from massive effusions.

Clinical forms of rheumatoid disease affecting the myocardium or cardiac valve structures are rare. However postmortem studies have shown nonspecific valvulitis in up to 30% of rheumatoid patients (Iveson et al 1975). Rheumatoid granulomata of the myocardium have also been noted in postmortem studies. Rheumatoid disease is an uncommon cause of chronic valve malfunction but granulomata have been frequently noted in the aortic and mitral valves in patients receiving cardiac valve surgery (Iveson et al 1975).

Neurological

Peripheral nerve symptoms in rheumatoid patients may arise from entrapment neuropathies, rheumatoid peripheral neuropathies and cervical myelopathy. Symptoms of entrapment neuropathy can usually be relieved by appropriate decompression. The sites of entrapment include compression of the median nerve at the wrist (carpal tunnel syndrome), compression of the posterior tibial nerve at the ankle (tarsal tunnel syndrome) and ulnar nerve compression at the elbow.

Rheumatoid peripheral neuropathies fall into two pain groups – severe sensorimotor neuropathy and milder sensory neuropathy (Chamberlain & Bruckner 1970). The former is associated with a sudden loss of motor and sensory function and often picks out isolated nerves in a mononeuritis multiplex pattern. It is associated with the more severe forms of seropositive nodular disease and there is often evidence of vasculitis elsewhere. Nerve conduction tests usually show features of muscle denervation and the condition is thought to be produced by vasculitis of the vasa nervorum. The sensory type of neuropathy usually occurs as a glove-and-stocking pattern of sensory loss, and if motor signs to occur they are usually minor. Nerve conduction tests may be normal or may show slowing of motor and sensory conduction.

Cervical myelopathy from atlantoaxial or subaxial subluxation of the cervical spine may mimic a peripheral neuropathy and has been discussed earlier.

Renal

Slight impairment of renal function is common in rheumatoid patients (Bury 1972). The most frequent histological abnormalities found on biopsy are interstitial nephritis and amyloidosis (Brun et al 1965). Interstitial nephritis may result from chronic bacterial infection or antiinflammatory analgesic drug therapy. Renal papillary necrosis is a less common renal side-effect of drugs but in man probably only results from chronic ingestion of compound analgesics containing both phenacetin and aspirin. A more frequent cause of drug-induced renal disease is gold and penicillamine therapy, both of which may induce an immune complex-associated glomerulonephritis. Occasionally, in vasculitic forms of rheumatoid disease, a mild form of disease-associated glomerulonephritis may occur (Bury 1972).

Hepatic

Liver enlargement is found clinically in about 11% of rheumatoid patients (Whaley & Webb 1977). Liver biopsies in these patients are often normal but otherwise show nonspecific fatty change or mild lymphocytic infiltration of portal tracts. Asymptomatic increases in serum alkaline phosphatase are also common in rheumatoid patients and sometimes reflect hepatotoxicity from salicylates and other antiinflammatory drugs.

Septic arthritis

This severe and potentially fatal complication is found particularly in patients with the most severe forms of rheumatoid disease. Presentation may be acute, with one disproportionately painful and inflamed joint and pyrexia. At other times septic arthritis may present in a more obscure fashion such as felling unwell or even with an apparent flare of the disease. Fever and leucocytosis may be absent in the debilitated and steroid-treated patients most prone to develop this condition (Mitchell et al 1976). *Staphylococcus aureus* is the organism most frequently isolated. Prompt diagnosis and treatment are essential both in order to minimise joint damage and to preserve life.

LABORATORY FINDINGS

The diagnosis of rheumatoid arthritis is made mainly on clinical grounds but laboratory investigations may help. They provide objective measurements of disease activity and sometimes have prognostic value. The anaemia of rheumatoid disease has been discussed. In active disease the ESR and acute phase reactants such as C-reactive protein are elevated and provide a rough guide to disease activity. Also as a nonspecific feature of chronic inflammation serum albumin may be reduced and alpha$_2$ and gamma globulin elevated on protein electrophoresis. All the immunoglobulin components (IgG, IgA and IgM) may be elevated or sometimes just IgG is increased.

The serological tests for IgM rheumatoid factor become positive in 75% of patients with rheumatoid arthritis. However the higher the titre of rheumatoid factor and the earlier in the disease course that the test becomes positive, the worse the prognosis tends to be. Antinuclear antibodies are also found in a proportion of patients and again tend to be associated with extraarticular disease. Neither of these autoantibodies is specific for rheumatoid arthritis and they may be found in association with other autoimmune diseases. They may be of some help in diagnosis. Significant titres of rheumatoid factor would be in keeping with a diagnosis of rheumatoid arthritis while high titres of antinuclear antibodies in association with low or absent titres of IgM rheumatoid factor suggest systemic lupus erythematosus.

PROGNOSIS

The natural history of rheumatoid arthritis is variable. A high proportion of patients with the disease have a mild illness with a good prognosis. In a 10-year follow-up of a group of rheumatoid patients who were treated fairly conservatively by present-day practices, Duthie and colleagues found that over 50% had an eventual satisfactory outcome whilst only 11% became completely disabled (Duthie et al 1955). The following are adverse prognostic factors: development of erosions within 1 year of onset, poor functional capacity early in the disease course, the presence of extraarticular disease features, a persistently high ESR and failure to respond to nonsteroidal antiinflammatory drugs. Some studies also suggest that the histocompatibility antigen DR4 may be associated with severe disease (McMichael et al 1977; Roitt et al 1978).

THERAPY

Decisions on effective treatment depend on the stage and activity of the disease. When there is early active inflammation the emphasis is on suppression of inflammation by general measures and antirheumatic drugs. In the late stages when destructive disease and secondary osteoarthritis predominate, the emphasis of management shifts towards relief of pain by provision of simple analgesics, improving joint function and reconstructive surgery. The prognosis in the majority of patients is reasonable and the aim of treatment is to suppress the disease process to prevent the development of erosions and the development of deformities and disabilities.

General measures

The long-term management of patients with rheumatoid arthritis is undertaken by a management team which includes not only rheumatologists but also orthopaedic surgeons, physiotherapists, occupational therapists, social workers, disablement resettlement officers and nurses. The programme includes advice and education about the nature of the disease and the aims and limitations of treatment. During phases of active disease many patients require an extra rest period during the day. Physiotherapists and occupational therapists can help by designing exercises to maintain or restore muscle function and range of joint movement, providing splints to prevent or reduce deformity and by providing aids to improve function. During major disease exacerbations short periods in bed, together with splinting of particularly inflamed joints, are helpful. Individual inflamed joints may be controlled by aspirating synovial effusions and injection of slow-release corticosteroids under strict aseptic conditions.

Drug therapy

The drugs used in the treatment of rheumatoid arthritis can be considered under the following headings:

1. simple analgesics
2. nonsteroidal antiinflammatory drugs
3. second-line antirheumatic drugs
4. Immunosuppressives and corticosteroids.

Simple analgesics

These include paracetamol, often in mixtures with codeine, dextropopoxyphene and others, which act on the central nervous system. They are not very effective in relieving the pain of acute inflammation and are of more use for the pain of secondary osteoarthritis and for a top-up effect in patients in whom the nonsteroidal antiinflammatory drugs prove inadequate. These drugs do not have the gastrointestinal effects of the nonsteroidal antiinflammatory agents which are discussed in detail in Chapter 48. Narcotic analgesics are virtually never required for rheumatoid arthritis.

Nonsteroidal antiinflammatory drugs

Drugs in this group provide symptomatic relief of pain and stiffness. However they do not alter the natural history of the disease and are inadequate on their own for patients who show signs of progressive joint damage. These agents may be adequate for a large proportion of rheumatoid patients. Soluble aspirin was the prototype of this type of drug but is now largely replaced by newer agents such as the propionic acid derivatives. These are better tolerated but are not significantly more effective.

There is some evidence from studies of osteoarthritis that some antiinflammatory drugs such as indomethacin may actually exacerbate damage to articular cartilage. All these drugs may cause gastrointestinal ulceration and bleeding in susceptible patients. If a patient suffers from dyspepsia it may be possible to administer the drug successfully as a suppository, as it is then absorbed more slowly and lower peak levels occur in the peripheral blood. Other alternatives include the prophylactic use of antiulcer drugs or the use of prodrugs, such as benoxaprofen, in which the agent is taken in an inactive form and only activated after absorption through the intestinal muscosa. Both the antiinflammatory properties and the gastrointestinal adverse toxicity of these agents are in part due to their abilities to inhibit the cyclooxygenase enzymes involved in prostaglandin synthesis.

Second-line antirheumatic drugs

Active rheumatoid arthritis is now treated aggressively in most units and the second-line antirheumatic drugs are instituted rapidly if there is continued articular inflammation despite nonsteroidal antiinflammatory drug therapy. These drugs are all given on a long-term basis and all have a delay from the start of treatment until the onset of action of commonly 2 or 3 months.

Sulphasalazine This agent is effective in causing remission of rheumatoid arthritis. The usual regimen is to start with 0.5 g of the enteric-coated form daily and increase by weekly increments to a maximum of 1 g three times per day. Gastrointestinal side-effects such as nausea may occur but more serious problems such as blood dyscrasias are rare. Sulphasalazine may uncommonly cause hepatotoxicity and in males a fall in sperm count.

Antimalarials Chloroquine and hydroxychloroquine have definite disease-suppressing properties. There is a small risk of producing retinopathy and visual impairment but this is minimised if the daily dosage is kept as low as possible and the eyes are monitored by an ophthalmologist. Gastrointestinal problems are uncommon and these agents lack the haematological and renal side-effects which are found in many more potent antirheumatic drugs.

Gold therapy Gold salts have been used in the treatment of rheumatoid arthritis since the 1930s. Intramuscular sodium aurothiomalate (Myocrisin) is the gold salt most commonly used in the UK although an oral preparation has also been introduced. In a commonly used regimen, after incremental test doses, the drug is given as 50 mg weekly by intramuscular injections to a maximum of 1 g or until there is disease remission or toxicity. Once remission has occurred and maximum benefit appears to have been achieved, it is usual to lengthen the intervals between injections and reduce the dose to a monthly maintenance regimen. If there has been no response to the gold after a cumulative dose of 1 g has been given, most physicians withdraw the drug but it is possible to try increasing the weekly injection dose (Rothermick et al 1976).

Possible side-effects of gold therapy include minor skin rashes, itching, exfoliative dermatitis, stomatitis, renal problems, blood dyscrasias, hepatotoxicity and pneumonitis. All patients receiving gold therapy will require regular monitoring of the skin, blood and urine.

D-Penicillamine This drug was initially used as a chelating agent in the treatment of Wilson's disease. It is given orally but otherwise has indications and side-effects similar to gold salts. The usual starting dose is 125 mg or 250 mg daily and it is important to take this drug well away from food as it can combine with food nutrients. Some patients respond to doses as low as this but if there is no improvement the dosage is slowly increased by similar amounts, at intervals, to a maximum of 750 mg daily. Most commonly however the final dose is around 375 mg per day. Adverse effects include skin rashes, blood dyscrasias and renal problems. Rare side-effects include immunological syndromes such as myasthenia gravis and drug-induced systemic lupus erythematosus. Regular monitoring of the skin, blood and urine for toxicity is essential with penicillamine, as with gold therapy.

Immunosuppressives and corticosteroids

Immunosuppressive agents, and in particular methotrexate, are more frequently used for patients with severe persistent disease not controlled by more conservative measures. Methotrexate is a folic acid antagonist with immunosuppressive properties. It is given in a weekly dose, starting at 5 mg and then increasing usually to a maximum of 15 mg per week. It appears much more effective than the second-line antirheumatic agents (Ward 1985). The onset of benefit commonly does not start for at least a month after initiating treatment. Adverse effects are uncommon but may affect the blood, liver and lungs and the drug is contraindicated in patients with a high alcohol intake. Careful monitoring of the blood and liver function is essential.

Alternative immunosuppressive agents such as cyclophosphamide are used for very severe individual cases and are sometimes given as bolus infusions. They are particularly reserved for patients with complications such as severe forms of vasculitis and for patients who have failed to respond to more conservative therapy.

Oral corticosteroids such as prednisolone have dramatic effects in relieving symptoms. Unfortunately once patients have started on steroids it is commonly very difficult, if not impossible, to withdraw them. Patients receiving steroid therapy over a number of years frequently develop severe adverse effects such as osteoporosis, hypertension, dermal atrophy, etc. and in the long run these may outweigh the benefits in relieving the arthritis symptoms. The decision to start corticosteroids is a major one and should only be taken after very careful consideration.

Surgery

Surgery is indicated for the relief of pain and prevention of loss of function when medical measures prove inadequate. The programme is best planned in a combined clinic held jointly by the rheumatologist and the orthopaedic surgeon.

In early disease synovectomy may be helpful symptomatically when synovial swelling is localised to one or two joints and before erosions have appeared. Tenosynovectomy may help when synovial hypertrophy has involved tendon sheaths and is affecting hand function or threatening tendon rupture. Decompression may be required for the relief of nerve entrapment syndromes.

In advanced cases, joint replacements are now available for a variety of joints and are continually being improved. Hip and knee replacements are commonplace and are the most successful. Replacements are available for the shoulder, and elbow and ankle replacements are currently being designed.

Other surgical procedures may be appropriate such as excision arthroplasty, fusion and repair of ruptured tendons.

REFERENCES

Ansell B M, Loewi G 1977 Rheumatoid arthritis – general features. Clinics in Rheumatic Diseases 3: 385–401

Bacon P A, Gibson D G 1974 Cardiac involvement in rheumatoid arthritis. An echocardiographic study. Annals of the Rheumatic Diseases 33: 20–24

Barrett A J, Saklatvala H 1981 Proteinases in joint disease. In: Kelley W N, Harris E D, Ruddy S F, Sledge C B (eds) Textbook of rheumatology. W B Saunders, Philadelphia, p 195–209

Bennet J C 1978 The infectious aetiology of rheumatoid arthritis. New consideration. Arthritis and Rheumatism 21: 530–538

Bennett R M 1977 Haematological changes in rheumatoid disease. Clinics in Rheumatic Diseases 3: 433–465

Bland J H, David P H, London M G, Van Buskirk F W, Duarte E G 1963 Rheumatoid arthritis of cervical spine. Archives of Internal Medicine 122: 892–898

Brun C, Olsen T S, Raaschou F, Sorenson A W S 1965 Renal biopsy in rheumatoid arthritis, Nephron 2: 65–81

Brunton R W, Grennan D M, Palmer D G, de Silva R T A 1978 Lateral subluxation of the atlas in rheumatoid arthritis. British Journal of Radiology 51: 963–967

Bury H C 1972 Reduced glomerular function in rheumatoid arthritis. Annals of the Rheumatic Diseases 31: 65–68

Caplan A 1953 Certain unusual radiological appearances in the chest of coalminers suffering from rheumatoid arthritis. Thorax 8: 29–37

Chamberlain M A, Bruckner F E 1970 Rheumatoid neuropathy. Clinical and electrophysiological features. Annals of the Rheumatic Diseases 29: 609–616

Conlon P W, Isdale I C, Rose B S 1966 Rheumatoid arthritis of the cervical spine. Annals of the Rheumatic Diseases 25: 120–126

Denman A M 1975 The viral theory of connective tissue diseases: a review. Medical Biology 53: 67–84

Dixon A St J 1969 The rheumatoid foot. Proceedings of the Royal Society of Medicine 63: 677–679

Duthie J J R, Thompson M, Wier M M, Fletcher W B 1955 Medical and social aspects of the treatment of rheumatoid arthritis with special reference to factors affecting prognosis. Annals of the Rheumatic Diseases 14: 133–149

Fassbender H G 1975 Rheumatoid arthritis in pathology of rheumatic diseases Springer Verlag, Berlin, p 70–210

Geddes D M, Corris B, Brewerton D A, Davies R J, Turner-Warwick M 1977 Progressive airway obstruction in adults and its association with rheumatoid disease. Quarterly Journal of Medicine 46: 427–444

Grennan D, Sanders A 1988 Rheumatoid arthritis. Baillières Clinical Rheumatology 2: 585–601

Hill H F H 1977 Treatment of rheumatoid arthritis with penicillamine. Seminars in Arthritis and Rheumatism 6: 361–388

Hillarby M, Clarkson R, Grennan D M et al 1991 Immunogenetic heterogeneity in rheumatoid disease characterised by different MHC association (DQ, Dw, and C4) in articular and extra-articular subsets. British Journal of Rheumatology 30: 5–9

Iveson J M I, Thadani U, Ionesou M, Wright V 1975 Aortic valve incompetence and replacement in rheumatoid arthritis. Annals of the Rheumatic Diseases 354: 312–320

Jayson M I V, Jones D E P 1971 Scleritis and rheumatoid arthritis. Annals of the Rheumatic Diseases 30: 343–347

Lawrence J S 1970 Rheumatoid arthritis – nature or nurture. Annals of the Rheumatic Diseases 29: 357–379

McMichael A J, Sasazuki T, McDevitt H O, Payne R D 1977 Increased frequency of HLA-Cw3 and HLA-Dw4 in rheumatoid arthritis. Arthritis and Rheumatism 20: 1037–1042

Marks J S, Power B J 1979 Is chloroquine obsolete in treatment of rheumatic disease? Lancet 1: 371–373

Mathews J A 1974 Atlanto-axial subluxation in rheumatoid arthritis – a 5 year follow-up. Annals of the Rheumatic Diseases 33: 526–531

Mitchell W S, Brooks P M, Stevenson R D, Buchanan W W 1976 Septic arthritis in patients with rheumatoid disease: a still under-diagnosed complication. Journal of Rheumatology 3: 124–133

Panayi G S, Wooley P H, Batchelor J R 1978 Genetic basis of rheumatoid disease. HLA antigens, disease manifestations and toxic reactions to drugs. British Medical Journal 1326–1328

Roitt I M, Corbett M, Festenstein H et al 1978 HLA-DR4 and prognosis in rheumatoid arthritis. Lancet 1: 990

Rothermick N O, Philips V K, Bergen W, Rhomas M H 1976 Chrysotherapy. A prospective study. Arthritis and Rheumatism 19: 1321–1327

Swezey R L 1971 Dynamic factors in deformity of the rheumatoid arthritic hand. Bulletin on the Rheumatic Diseases 22: 649–656

Turner-Warwick M, Evans R C 1977 Pulmonary manifestations of rheumatoid disease. Clinics in Rheumatic Diseases 3: 549–562

Vidigal E, Jacoby R K, Dixon St J, Ratuff A H, Kirkup J 1975 The foot in chronic rheumatoid arthritis. Annals of the Rheumatic Diseases 34: 292–297

Ward T 1985 Historical perspective on the use of methotrexate for the treatment of rheumatoid arthritis. Journal of Rheumatology Suppl 12: 3–6

Whaley K, Webb J 1977 Liver and kidney disease in rheumatoid arthritis. Clinics in Rheumatic Diseases 3: 527–547

Whaley J, Webb J, McAvory B A et al 1973 Sjögren's syndrome in clinical associations and immunological phenomenon. Quarterly Journal of Medicine 42: 513

Williamson J 1976 Ocular hazards in connective tissue diseases. In: Buchanan W W, Dick W C (eds) Recent advances in rheumatology 1. Churchill Livingstone, Edinburgh, p 146–165

Zulman J, Jaffe R, Ralal R 1978 Evidence that the malignant lymphoma of Sjögren's syndrome is a monoclonal B-cell neoplasm. New England Journal of Medicine 299: 1215–1220

22. Orthopaedic pain after trauma

D. A. H. Yates and M. A. Smith

The management of injuries to bones and soft tissues following trauma accounts for an increasing proportion of the medical workload in this country. There are significant economic consequences with regard both to the loss of working hours and, later, in litigation. Fortunately, there is a relatively low mortality, but there is a significant morbidity which can be caused by the inadequate management of the acute pain, which can then go on to become a chronic problem. It should be emphasised that pain is a symptom and not a diagnosis and it follows therefore that the underlying cause of any pain must be established before effective treatment and with it, relief of pain, can take place. However, if there is a delay, either in making that diagnosis or instituting treatment, then the treatment of the pain itself should become a priority.

Pain has several functions in that it prevents use of the injured part, thereby reducing further damage, and aids in the diagnosis; but it can also be harmful, leading to morbidity as a persistent symptom with stress and psychological consequences. This latter aspect is found commonly in certain types of injury, notably those involving sport, industry and war casualties.

Pain intensity following injury during acute physical stress may be greatly modified. Under conditions of war or competitive sport the subject may be able to continue to participate since the pain, stiffness and loss of function may only be apparent after the conflict ceases. However the subject cannot disguise instability if, for example, weight-bearing is impossible or the upper limb cannot be elevated. Then fracture of one of the long bones, dislocation of a joint or gross muscle or tendon rupture may have occurred.

PAIN FOLLOWING TRAUMA

Immediate

The distortion of subcutaneous, perivascular and periarticular nerve plexuses will give rise to immediate sharp nociceptive pain. Certain severe injuries, e.g. crushed hand, may be followed by a period of relative freedom from pain, particularly if there is marked associated mental stimulation or shock.

Delayed

After a variable interval deep, boring, persistent pain begins and increases. This may be the result of physical distension of the joint capsule or fascial compartments by blood or tissue fluid transudate. If pressure continues to build up within relatively rigid fascial compartments then secondary impairment of blood supply may cause pain due to chronic ischaemia. The pain also arises from tissue damage liberating transmitter substances which activate the kinin and prostaglandin systems.

At a later stage extravasated blood or necrotic tissue will initiate phagocytosis. This will be accompanied by a sterile (nonbacterial) inflammatory response consisting of local vasodilation causing reddening and heat and increased transudation producing swelling. Secondary release of transmitter substances may produce persistent pain. A typical example of prolonged pain after injury is with subperiosteal bruising occurring over the sacrum or tibia.

Once the immediate effects of the injury have subsided the persistence of pain at rest may indicate the persistence of an inflammatory reaction. This is exemplified by pain at the shoulder where normal movements set up chronic inflammatory changes in the subacromial bursa, secondary to degenerative changes in the rotator cuff. Chronic rest pain may disturb sleep for several years.

Typically, musculoskeletal pain is brought on by use or weight-bearing and is relieved by rest. Chronic recurrence of pain suggests instability of the structure. Particularly in athletes, recurrence can arise with persistent overuse, especially if the technique is faulty, as in tennis elbow, surfer's knee or jogger's heel.

The perception of pain after musculoskeletal injury follows the stimulation of peripheral nociceptors (Lynn 1975; Zimmerman 1976). Pain receptors in the skin and nerve tissues are all free nerve endings (Bonica et al 1979)

In addition there are nociceptors which are responsive to mechanical stress or damage (Casey 1973). There is some evidence that there may be a chemical intermediary between the stimulation of the nociceptor and its activation. The delayed pain often found in musculoskeletal trauma is related to the inflammatory process described above with prostaglandins being the chemical intermediary (Terenius 1981). Local control of the pain is often directed towards reducing the inflammation, with aspirin and other nonsteroidal antiinflammatory agents being effective, partly due to inhibition of prostaglandin synthesis (Vane 1978). This complements its inhibitory effect on the pain-producing actions of bradykinin. Following stimulation of the nociceptors it is unmyelinated C-fibres and the small myelinated A-delta fibres that transmit the sensory impulses to the dorsal horn of the spinal cord (Meyer & Campbell 1981). Local anaesthetic infiltration is a most effective way of blocking the transmission. Benzoic acid derivatives (notably procaine) are widely used, as is bupivacaine, one of the newer, longer-acting local anaesthetics. Local anaesthetics block the transmembrane sodium channels during depolarisation, thus preventing it from taking place. Fibre size plays a part: smaller fibres are affected more. Thus, by utilising a suitable concentration of the local anaesthetic the smaller A-delta and C-fibres can be blocked, sparing the larger alpha and beta fibres responsible for motor function, touch and pressure. Local anaesthetics are very attractive as they have a very rapid onset of activity, and are completely reversible without damaging the affected nerve. These local agents can also be used for regional blocks of larger named nerves, or at the spinal level by epidural or intraspinal block.

The sensory input in the dorsal horn is modified prior to transmission of the impulses in the lateral and ventral spinothalamic tracts. Regions in the medulla and thalamic nuclei process this information before it is finally assimilated in the somatosensory areas found in the postcentral area and certain posterior parietal areas. For the central control of severe acute pain the opiate analgesic drugs remain the drugs of choice. Clinicians often have great reservations about the use of opiates owing to their fear of the patient becoming drug-dependent. However, provided the drug is given for pain and the pain is relatively short-lived, there is no clinical reason for withholding the use of this most effective means of pain control. By being aware of both the anatomy and physiology of pain and knowing the site of origin of the pain, the attending physician is then in an ideal position not only to prescribe the most appropriate drug but also to decide on the best route for its administration. In addition, the environment may play a major factor in influencing the patient's perception and response to pain following injury. During war, casualties have been shown to require inordinately large doses of narcotic analgesics in order to control pain (Jowitt & Knight 1983). Conversely there may be a latent period between the time of injury and the appreciation by the victim of that pain, particularly during times of acute physical stress such as in war or competitive sport.

SEGMENTAL REFERENCE

Hilton (1863) first emphasised that a joint receives its innervation from the same spinal segments as the skin over the joint and the muscles that act on the joint. His teaching was derived mainly from experience with severe infection of joints and in the absence of antibiotics he stressed the desirability of rest in treatment. Nowadays this concept is of more interest in appreciating where pain from affected joints may be referred.

Inaccuracies over terminology can give rise to confusion in diagnosis.

Dermatome is the area of skin predominantly innervated by a single spinal segment, e.g. the C5 dermatome overlies the deltoid region.

Myotome refers to those muscles innervated by a single spinal segment (Gray 1973). The majority of skeletal muscles receive their motor innervation from several spinal segments, but in each group one segment predominates, e.g. the C5 myotome consists mainly of the periscapular muscles, deltoid, infraspinatus, teres and brachioradialis. These muscles also receive some innervation from C6 so that if the C5 root is interrupted there will be incomplete paralysis.

The *sclerotome* comprises all the tissues of embryonic mesodermal origin: muscle, fascia and connective tissue innervated by a spinal segment, although here again there is considerable overlap.

Pain arising from root compression or from soft tissue injuries is often incorrectly described as being referred within the affected dermatome. However, referred pain is felt not only in the skin but in the deeper tissues within the affected sclerotome. Hence, this term would be more correctly used. The more intense the pain the further distally the pain tends to be experienced. For example, the pain of mild subacromial bursitis, a C5 structure, is felt at the insertion of deltoid. The intense pain associated with acute calcific subacromial bursitis radiates down the forearm within the C5 sclerotome.

Musculoskeletal injuries can be classified according to their aetiology or the tissues involved. Where an injury occurs as the result of an extrinsic cause, such as a direct blow, there will be sudden damage to the bones and soft tissues. There is usually a direct correlation between the severity and intensity of that force and the resultant injury and tissue damage. The application of that force is usually short-lived and the pain caused by the tissue damage. A notable exception follows crush injuries. Intrinsic injuries, on the other hand, appear to occur without an identifiable cause, usually arising spontaneously as a result of overload or physical stress. This is seen most commonly in sport-associated injuries and in children where the immature skeleton may be exposed to excessive load. Such intrinsic injuries are often precipitated in those patients who involve themselves in inappropriate activities following inadequate preparation, using poor technique and often inadequate equipment (Williams 1976). Alternatively, the injuries can be categorised anatomically according to the tissue or organ injured:

1. skeletal injury
2. joint injury
3. periarticular tissue injury
4. muscle tendon complex injury
5. hand injury.

HISTORY

A careful clinical history will give much useful information about the lesion. An assessment of the intensity of the trauma will indicate whether normal bones, ligaments and tendons could be excepted to have parted under the stress. If the tissue failure seems excessive for the stress this might indicate an underlying deficiency, which in bone would include osteoporosis, osteomalacia, Paget's or malignant deposits as possible causes. Lax joints, as seen in the various hypermobility syndromes, are more prone to minor repetitive injury: the Achilles tendon which gives way may have been the site of preliminary central degeneration. Appreciating such tissue deficiencies is important in planning repair and rehabilitation and may indicate necessity for corrective treatment, such as calcium and vitamin D replacement in osteomalacia.

The immediate response to injury is a useful index of the severity, since the majority of patients will be unable to walk on a fractured limb. Rapid swelling suggests bleeding within the joint, which may need early aspiration if blood coagulation is normal or can be corrected. Slow swelling indicates a traumatic synovitis, which if it persists should respond to intraarticular steroid injection. Persistent pain at rest indicates distension of tissues, inflammatory hyperaemia and synovitis.

The mechanism of the injury will often indicate what has happened. A severe valgus injury of the knee is likely to damage the medial ligament, whereas twisting on a loaded knee is likely to injure the medial meniscus and often the anterior cruciate ligament. A patient must be asked about his job, sports and recreations, since any of these may produce chronic repetitive trauma or overuse, particularly in older people. Accurate assessment and localisation are relatively easy after acute trauma. In chronic lesions localisation necessitates a systematic anatomical examination. In the limbs where pain may be referred distally it is usually necessary to examine the articulations proximal to the painful structure, for example in chronic shoulder pain it is advisable to examine the neck to see whether sustained movements reproduce the pain in the shoulder (Yates 1986). If a tendon or ligamentous lesion is postulated and steroid injection is planned, then a small quantity of dilute local anaesthetic can be mixed with it and infiltrated. Rapid relief of pain tends to confirm that that is the affected structure. However, there are exceptions to this in painful lesions over the shoulder and hip girdle. Spinal pain may produce referred painful trigger spots which can be suppressed by local injection. However, the more peripheral the lesion the more likely it is that relief of pain by local anaesthetic injection will indicate the true site.

MANAGEMENT

While the primary aim in the management of musculoskeletal trauma is the early restoration of normal function, initial management may involve appropriate splintage with elevation in order to rest the injured part, so that aggravation of the injury and possible complications can be avoided, and also to maintain reduction of any fracture. These simple measures often result in the dramatic relief of pain, but often they may have to be augmented by the use of suitable analgesics. The use of a particular analgesic and its method of administration will depend on many factors, including the age of the patient, the site and severity of the pain, the presence of other injuries, particularly to the cardiothoracic, respiratory or central nervous systems, and whether or not other drugs have been administered. Acute pain following accidental trauma, once the diagnosis has been made and appropriate first aid or definitive treatment initiated, serves no very useful purpose in the acute stages other than increasing the morbidity; its persistence may increase the likelihood of chronic pain developing. Thus, in those patients where treatment of the underlying condition is either delayed or fails to relieve the pain, the management of the pain can and should become the primary therapeutic goal. While the aim should be the adequate relief of pain, in achieving this care must be taken to avoid any complications, both local and systemic, such as respiratory depression; the attending physician should be aware of potential complications that may be disguised by analgesia. The analgesics can be administered in one of four ways.

Oral analgesia

An enormous range of analgesics is available but, unfortunately, the more potent the agent the more side-effects there are. Those with a combined analgesic and anti-inflammatory effect, e.g. aspirin and indomethacin, are prone to cause gastric irritation, bleeding and even peptic ulceration; these, therefore, are not particularly appropriate to the intense skeletal pain following trauma. The

Table 22.1 Oral analgesics

	Strength (length of action)	Nausea	Intestinal suppression
Paracetamol (Panadol)	Weak (short)	–	–
Dihydrocodeine (DF 118)	Moderate	±	+
Dextropropoxyphene (Co-proxamol)	Moderate	±	±
Meptazinol (Meptid)	Moderate	±	±
Nefopam (Acupan)	Moderate	±	±
Buprenorphine (Temgesic)	Moderate	+	+
Dipipanone (Diconal)	Strong	±	±
Dextromoramide (Palfium)	Strong	+	+
Methadone (Physeptone)	Strong*	±	±
Pentazocine (Fortral)	Strong* (short)	+	+
Pethidine	Strong* (short)	+	±
Phenazocine (Narphen)	Strong*	+	+
Morphine (MST)	Strong*	+	+

*Risk of dependence

stronger, purer analgesics tend to produce nausea, vomiting and constipation and the strongest carries the theoretical and serious risk of dependence if used over long periods. The relative merits and demerits of some of the current and more popular preparations are presented in Table 22.1. In practice the clinician will often have to tailor the analgesic to each patient since the severity of the pain and the patient's response to that pain differ widely.

Systemic analgesia

Certainly in more major injuries this is the preferred method of pain control. Following major trauma, intravenous administration is usually the mode of choice because of its rapid effect and ease of control, particularly if an infusion is used. If an infusion is set up, it must be under close medical supervision. The intramuscular route is contraindicated in patients where there is blood loss and poor tissue perfusion, owing to delay and consequent uncertainty in the timing of action of the analgesic. In the main, narcotic analgesics are used. These are contraindicated in patients with head injuries; if there is any injury to the respiratory system or history of respiratory disease, narcotic analgesics should be used with caution.

Inhalational analgesics

Nitrous oxide is the most commonly used and is normally the gas of choice. It is often given mixed with oxygen in a 50:50 mixture. The administration is simple and mostly effective. Nitrous oxide is contraindicated where there is respiratory depression or head injury, as it is known to raise intracranial pressure. It is available in most casualty departments and in some ambulances.

Local and regional blocks

Peripheral injuries can be well controlled by local nerve blocks or regional anaesthesia; these may also be used as the definitive anaesthetic for any surgical treatment, either open or closed, that may be indicated. Such forms of analgesia are also useful in the postoperative period, particulary in the lower limb. If more extensive analgesia is required, epidural or spinal anaesthesia can be used. Local blocks can be performed in certain injuries to the trunk, particularly rib injuries where a local block can often permit the early return of normal respiratory function which was previously depressed owing to pain. Local infiltration to the site of injury can also be used. Where there is any danger of complications, especially vascular or neurological, such as in fractures of the tibia, distal humerus or forearm with compartment compression syndromes, or where a plaster has been applied and there may be loss of reduction of the fracture or pressure areas, regional blocks are contraindicated.

PHYSICAL TREATMENT

There is debate over the real value of physical treatment, both immediate and later, after minor trauma. The patient, particularly if he or she is a professional athlete, is usually overwrought and anxious for rapid relief and repair. Professional and amateur sporting organisations invest large sums in physicians, trainers, physiotherapists and equipment in the hopes of reducing morbidity. Theory and enthusiasm often overshadow careful scientific assessment of the efficacy of treatments.

The various modalities, including heat, cold, diathermy, ultrasound, short-wave and laser therapy, massage and muscle reeducation, are discussed in other chapters. After trauma, pain and swelling can be reduced by support and elevation augmented by physical methods when available. However, it must be emphasised that when tissues have been damaged the natural processes of removal of debris followed by repair can at best be only mildly enhanced. In order to avoid recurrence and morbidity the physician must remember that fibroblastic repair is inevitably slow and often incomplete.

STEROID INJECTIONS

Various microcrystalline suspensions of insoluble corticosteroid are available for injection and have a useful but limited role in the treatment of traumatic soft tissue lesions. It is postulated that their effect is exerted in suppressing or dispersing the chronic granulomatous response in traumatised tissue.

Preparations in common use are hydrocortisone acetate 25 mg/ml, methyl prednisolone 40 mg/ml and triamcinolone hexacetonide 40 mg/ml. Soluble preparations are less painful but are rapidly dispersed and less effective. However, there are drawbacks. In the suspension there may be microcrystals which are sufficiently small (5-10 μm) to be phagocytosed and to produce a local gout-like reaction. Severe pain may result for several days but can be modified by prescribing an oral antiinflammatory, such as indomethacin 25 mg, starting with four doses daily and reducing over 4 days. Some of the crystals persist at the injection site for several weeks and will tend to suppress fibroblastic repair. In elderly degenerative tendons, rupture may follow repeated injections Where synovitis is the result of chronic instability of ligaments, repeated intraarticular steroid injections are obviously contraindicated.

A detailed description of factures and soft tissue injuries is inappropriate to the purpose of this book. It is sufficient to outline here the general principles related to diagnosis, treated and prognosis.

FRACTURES

Pain is the principal symptom of a fracture and arises mainly from two sources: the periosteum and the surrounding damaged soft tissues. The pain immediately following a fracture is sharp and severe. This can be aggravated by movement and any stimulus that might precipitate reflex muscle spasm. Conversely, certain movements may relieve the spasm and the pain. Traction in the long axis of the fractured bone, which may be the definitive treatment of the fracture, will almost immediately overcome muscle spasm and relieve most of the pain. Further, in restoring the anatomical alignment other potential complications, notably neurovascular, can be avoided. Nerve or vascular injury can be the direct consequence of the trauma or may arise as the result of a compartment compression syndrome. Often neurological and vascular involvement occur together and, while this may aggravate already existing pain, complete nerve damage may have the contrary effect of obliterating pain. In order to avoid unnecessary movement of the injured limb, temporary splintage may be indicated. Splints must be applied with care as their injudicious use can cause further damage and may give a false sense of security. Manipulation in order to apply a splint, unless performed by an experienced physician, should not be undertaken. If pneumatic splints are used, the vascular state of the limb must be well documented and regularly monitored.

There are always delays before fractures are treated in hospital, arising from transport, examinations, X-rays and treatment for other injuries. Throughout this period first aid measures must be applied and pain controlled. The pain following a fracture, although temporary, can be severe and will require narcotic analgesia. Certain precautions must be taken, as the majority of fractures occur after car or motorcycle accidents and the patient may have other injuries. In cases of head injury narcotics are contraindicated. If the fracture is compound or there are multiple fractures there may be considerable blood loss, which can also occur in certain closed fractures, such as of the pelvis. In such patients the analgesics must be given intravenously in small doses and the patient must be carefully observed to monitor the effectiveness of the analgesia and to prevent complications.

The definitive treatment of a fracture will depend on many factors, including the type of fracture, the age of the patient and the presence of other injuries. Management can be summarised as follows:

Reduction: if the fracture is displaced
Maintenance of the reduction: if the fracture is unstable splintage may be external (cast or traction) or internal (plating)
Treatment of the soft tissues: initially rest and elevation to reduce soft tissue swelling followed by early rehabilitation of the injured limb

The stabilising of a fracture will result in the rapid diminution of pain so that within 48 hours the residual discomfort can be controlled by nonnarcotic oral analgesia.

In the control of pain in the acute period systemic analgesics are often preferred to local blocks or regional anaesthesia, owing to the possibility of local complication in the early stages following injury. However, certain fractures lend themselves to local blocks, by virtue of their site and lack of associated complications, either vascular or neurological. Fractures around the ankle can be well controlled by peripheral nerve blocks or regional anaesthesia, which can also be used as a definitive anaesthetic for any surgical management. Such control of pain is also useful in the postoperative period. In the upper limb certain fractures are amenable to local infiltration, notably Colles' fracture, while pain from injuries to the digits in both the hands and feet can be well controlled by ring blocks. The persistence of pain or the development of further pain may signal the onset of local complications.

Complications

Immediate

Haemorrhage
Neurovascular damage
Compartment syndrome

Delayed

Skin breakdown
Infection
Loss of reduction

Late

Delayed union of the fracture
Nonunion of the fracture
Failure of the fixation, e.g. broken plate
Soft tissue contracture
Reflex sympathetic dystrophy
Refracture
Myositis ossificans

It is difficult to distinguish the pain of a fracture from the pain caused by immediate complications. The attending physician must always be aware, therefore, of the possible associated injuries and complications. Comminuted and compound fractures of the tibia and fibula and the distal humerus have a high incidence of associated neurovascular injury. Conversely, closed injuries to the same sites are particularly associated with compression syndromes. The fascial compartments in the forearm, and particularly the deep posterior and anterolateral compartments in the lower leg, are most prone to compression syndrome (Matsen 1975). These are described as early complications since the onset is immediate although the symptoms may take several hours to develop. Pain is the earliest symptom which is well localised to the affected compartment and increases in intensity. It is a constant rather than a throbbing pain. Hypoaesthesia of the skin or loss of the arterial pulse distally occurs late and is an indication for immediate fasciotomy. The acute syndrome is in contrast to the chronic and milder form seen in athletes – mostly long-distance runners.

A high index of suspicion is necessary in diagnosing the later complications of a fracture that may give rise to pain following splintage. Infection is always a danger following a compound fracture. Where a rigid cast is used for immobilisation, skin breakdown over pressure points or loss of reduction should be suspected and looked for, if further pain should develop. Towards the end of treatment the occurrence of pain may signal the failure of a fixation device. If there is a recent history of local injury with pain, the limb should be examined for evidence of refracture.

Reflex sympathetic dystrophy (Thompson 1979) as opposed to causalgia after nerve injury (Tahmoush 1981) is an uncommon but serious complication of distal trauma to the upper and lower limbs. Early treatment, which includes sympathetic block, is essential if early return of function to the affected part is to be excepted. Recently this condition has been recognised in children, but is of a milder form with a correspondingly good prognosis (Ruggeri et al 1982).

A fractured long bone in a child, while it may be complete, is more often incomplete (greenstick). The deformity and swelling can be minimal. Pain may be a minor feature unless the affected part is stressed and the child may be too young to express himself. Commonly the major sign is loss of function, as in the case of a child who will not walk or limps as the result of an undisplaced greenstick fracture of the tibia. Radiographs may be difficult to interpret and the incomplete fracture may be difficult to see. Care must be taken in the management of greenstick fractures. The physician should bear in mind the possibility of parental injury.

SOFT TISSUE INJURIES

Tendon lesions

Sudden stress may rupture a tendon, particularly if it is already affected by degenerative change. Severe pain is followed by loss of movement, sometimes with extravasation of blood. The Achilles tendon usually ruptures just above the os calcis where a gap can be felt. Plantar flexion is weakened but can still be achieved through the long flexors of the toes. It is necessary to repair the tendon surgically and the lower leg is immobilised in serial plasters for 6 weeks. The Achilles tendon does not have a true sheath but a paratenon which can be inflamed by poorly fitting running shoes. Steroid injection into the tendon should be avoided as there is a risk of accelerating rupture, but the paratenon can be injected.

Partial tendon tears at the tenoperiosteal junction are often caused by repetitive overuse. Common sites are at the insertions of supraspinatus and infraspinatus in the rotator cuff at the shoulder; the anterior and posterior tibial tendon in a valgus, flat foot; the musculotendinous origins of the common extensor and flexor muscles at the wrists (tennis and golfer's elbows). There is a marked local tenderness at the insertion and the pain is sharply exacerbated on resisted static contraction of the affected muscle. Local friction massage and ultrasonic therapy may produce slow benefit. Injection of steroid, which may be mixed with local anaesthetic, is quicker and more predictable. The underlying mechanical cause should be analysed and modified to achieve lasting benefit.

Tendon sheaths become inflamed by repetitive use, particularly over bony promontories. The tendency is increased by inflammatory thickening in rheumatoid, psoriatic and gouty arthritis or xanthomatous deposition in diabetes. There is exquisite tenderness on local pressure and painful crepitus is produced on passive movement. Common sites are the extensor tendons of the tumb and the flexor tendons of the fingers over the metacarpal heads. Usually good relief is produced by careful steroid injection of the sheath, taking care not to penetrate the tendon.

Extraarticular ligaments

Acute and chronic painful lesions can arise from trauma. There is marked local tenderness over the insertion and pain is produced by strong stressing of the ligament. Common sites are at the wrist, knee and ankle. Friction, massage and ultrasound may hasten relief but, providing the ligament is predominantly intact, local steroid injection is more quickly effective. The calcaneal end of the long plantar ligament (policeman's heel) is more difficult and painful to inject and relief may be achieved by sponge supports and elevating the heel. Inflammatory plantar fasciitis is a common feature of spondyloarthritis in ankylosing spondylitis and Reiter's syndrome.

Joints

Pain arising from a joint may be the consequence of either direct or indirect trauma. A direct blow to a joint, while acutely painful, will often result in relatively minor trauma. A force applied indirectly will frequently result in serious joint injury; this is seen in the knee following skiing accidents and after soccer injury. The resultant ligamentous injury, if it is a complete disruption, may be surprisingly painless. Thus, the pain following a joint injury may not be a reliable guide to the severity of the damage to that joint. Further, the acute pain will be masked in many instances by the pain of any subsequent effusion. An effusion is a very reliable indicator of intraarticular pathology and with trauma will be one of two types – synovial effusion or, more commonly, haemarthrosis. Taking a history will help to differentiate between the two and where there is any doubt, and particularly if the effusion is very tense and therefore painful, the affected joint should be aspirated under sterile conditions. If a ligamentous injury is suspected the aspiration must be carried out under general anaesthetic and a careful examination of the ligaments performed at the same time. Where indicated an immediate repair should be undertaken (Fowler 1980).

While the majority of haemarthroses are posttraumatic, patients with severe haemophilia may have spontaneous bleeding into a joint. The joints most commonly affected are the knee and elbow. These become painful very quickly, but usually the first symptom of an intraarticular bleed is a disturbed sensation rather than a frank pain. Home treatment by the prompt injection of factor VIII in sufficient dosage has helped to minimise the severity of the bleeding episodes and their consequences. This has reduced the need for analgesia in these patients, since it was necessary to administer narcotics in the past with the inevitable incidence of addiction. Recent advances in the surgical management of haemophilic arthropathy have helped to reduce further the incidence of spontaneous haemorrhage in severe haemophiliacs and reduce the pain of the arthropathy (Smith et al 1981).

When a joint is dislocated there is usually an obvious deformity with acute and severe pain that is aggravated by any movement. The most common joints affected are the shoulder, hip and elbow. Prompt and unforced reduction is essential to ensure the early return of joint function and to avoid possible complications. There may be complications as a result of the injury, e.g. injury to the median or ulnar nerves in association with shoulder dislocation. These can be aggravated or precipitated by forced manipulation in attempting to reduce the dislocation. It is advisable, therefore, in the hospital environment, to reduce dislocations under general anaesthetic and have facilities available to proceed to an open reduction where necessary.

Reduction of the dislocated joint will be followed by almost complete relief of pain. There will be some residual discomfort from the damaged articular and periarticular structures. It is for this reason, and to avoid redislocation, that all joints following reduction should be splinted, either on traction in the case of a hip or in a sling with the shoulder and elbow. Persistence of a significant pain implies a failure of reduction or the presence of a complication such as a fracture. It is very important when examining a patient with an obvious or suspected dislocation to look carefully for other injuries or complications of the dislocation. Adequate radiographs must be taken prior to initiating treatment both to confirm the diagnosis and to confirm or exclude an associated fracture. The presence of a fracture may influence the method of reduction and the subsequent splintage of the joint.

Recurrence of pain may be caused by redislocation or may indicate instability secondary to a ligamentous deficit. Intraarticular ligamentous injuries are always the consequence of trauma and the joint most often involved and most commonly misdiagnosed is the knee. Pain in a knee with swelling from an effusion must always be fully investigated. This occurs most often on the soccer field and the ski slope after a twisting injury. If there is evidence of a significant ligamentous injury then an examination of the injured knee must be performed under anaesthetic. Partial tears of ligaments are locally painful and will heal without surgical intervention. Temporary splintage helps to reduce the pain and minimise swelling. This should be followed by active exercising and a specialised physiotherapy programme to rehabilitate and reactivate those muscles responsible for controlling and stabilising the joint. Return of muscle control is fundamental to the restoration of normal joint function. This type of intensive rehabilitation applies particularly to those joints with complete ligamentous disruption which have undergone surgical repair or reconstruction.

The menisci may be damaged, either in isolation or in association with ligamentous injuries to the knee. A torn meniscus characteristically produces the features of a loose body in the joint. There is intermittent pain which is commonly at the joint line and may be localised. The knee may be locked and cannot be fully extended, though it can be fully flexed. Usually there is a small effusion. Further investigation is indicated and should include a contrast arthrogram or arthroscopy, the latter having the advantage of being a tool both for diagnosis and treatment.

Joint disruption or dislocation is not always caused by trauma and may not be painful. Dislocations may be congenital and the most common joints affected are the hip and proximal radioulnar joints. Gross joint distruption may be surprisingly painless and in such cases an underlying pathology such as diabetes, syringomyelia, tabes dorsalis, congenital indifference to pain and repeated intraarticular injections of steroid must be considered.

Intraarticular injuries in children are relatively rare. Injuries to the epiphysis and epiphyseal plate are most common. They must be reduced promptly and accurately to minimise the danger of future deformity and growth discrepancy. Locking of the knee does occur, often after trauma. However, meniscal tears are uncommon and other causes are a congenital discoid meniscus or a loose body arising from osteochondritis dissecans, which can also affect the elbow, ankle and hip.

MUSCLE

The prognosis of muscle trauma depends on the extent of damage to the muscle fibres. Quite large haematomata in lax compartments, such as the thigh, gradually resolve without residue. When a significant number of muscle fibres have been torn pain and recovery are prolonged. Massage may reduce fibrous adhesions. Local anaesthetic injection may reduce persistent pain in the tear but steroid injection is inadvisable in case repair is impaired. In the relatively restricted anterior fascial compartments of the forearm and shin, extensive crush injuries of muscle may become ischaemic due to the build-up of pressure of extravasated blood and oedema. If unrelieved, calcification in necrotic tissue (myositis ossificans) may occur.

BURSAE

In numerous sites of the body bursae are developed as lubricating cushions over bony promontories or interposed between bony structures. The synovial lining secretes a thin lubricating film and can react to acute or chronic trauma by granulomatous thickening. It is surprising how such a reaction can give rise to chronic persistent pain, particularly at rest. The most common site is the subacromial bursa, the floor of which is formed by the rotator cuff of the shoulder which can be roughened and even contain calcific plaques. This abrades against the under-surface of the acromion whenever the arm is used. Physical treatments are normally ineffectual but fortunately steroid injection into the subacromial region usually produces sustained relief.

CHILDREN

The type of trauma that effects children differs from adults, as does the response of children to that trauma. Extrinsic injuries tend to result in fractures, usually incomplete greenstick fractures with angular deformity as opposed to displacement. While displacement may occur this is often not so severe as in the adult. Further, in the child where the epiphyses are still open, the epiphyseal plate is a weak link in the skeleton and is particularly susceptible to injury with fracture and displacement. This is particularly relevant in the longer term with regard to future growth and possible deformity and therefore early and accurate reduction are essential to minimise complications. Pain as a result of these injuries is often acutely severe but with rest is surprisingly painless. Suitable centrally-acting analgesics with a sedative effect, such as the narcotics, are indicated in order to settle pain, certainly in lower limb injuries, to permit the application of traction. In the older child local nerve blocks, providing the patient is cooperative, not only result in early pain relief but also may provide suitable analgesia in order to permit the reduction and application of an appropriate splint. Certain types of fracture, notably the supracondylar fracture of the humerus, must be watched carefully because of possible neurological and vascular complications. Local blocks in those types of fracture are contraindicated. With control of the acute fracture, pain relief can often be provided by oral preparation. In the younger child elixirs of paracetamol are appropriate.

A significant soft tissue injury is relatively uncommon in the child from extrinsic cause. More commonly, they are intrinsic and associated with excessive stress, often at musculotendinous insertions. The traction osteochondritides are common causes of pain in the growing child. Where tendons are inserted into apophyses, such as the patellar tendon on to the tibial tubercle and the tendo Achilles on to the base of the os calcis, an *osteochondritis* may develop. These all occur as a consequence of excessive use or load, usually traction, or less commonly a local blow, resulting in local pain on activity, tenderness and sensitivity and sometimes swelling. The two common examples are Osgood-Schlatter's osteochondritis of the tibial tubercle and Sever's osteochondritis of the os calcis. These are both self-limiting and, following ossification of the apophyses at maturity, symptoms subside. Swelling may persist, however, but is of no pathological significance. In the younger, immature patient immediate rest will relieve most cases, but occasionally temporary splintage to rest the painful limb may be indicated. Analgesia in order to permit continuing abuse is contraindicated.

There are other conditions often associated with trauma. Notable amongst these is infection. Thus, persistent pain that fails to improve after 48 hours should be looked on with suspicion in the young child, because of the danger of developing infection. Early recognition of this condition is essential to prevent complications. Thus, even where there is recognised trauma, if the injury does not clear as the natural history would suppose the clinician must be aware of possible complications such as developing sepsis. Another disturbing development occurring with increasing frequency in the paediatric clinics is the development of persistent pain often precipitated by injury in a sporting context but potentiated by psychological overtones. This often reflects the increasing pressures children are exposed to in order to succeed. These pressures are in part from their peers but also come from parents and overzealous coaches. Sometimes in order to disguise failure to make the grade, an injury can be a convenient excuse. In those instances it is essential that the clinician looks beyond the pain for the root cause to the problem.

SOFT TISSUE INJURY TO THE CERVICAL SPINE

The term 'whiplash' is not a diagnosis. It is hardly a medical term. Although used first by Crowe in 1928 in a talk on neck injuries in rear end automobile collisions, it is with reference to the medicolegal aspects of this condition that the term 'whiplash' has increasingly come to be associated (Breck & Van Norman 1971). As judged by current case reports in the legal literature, the term 'whiplash' is a most convenient legal peg on which to hang one's case, as the word seems to be synonymous with a generous financial settlement. It is often stated that litigation has a deleterious effect on outcome and may prolong the natural history of the condition. The evidence for this is unconvincing, despite claims to the contrary in various medicolegal reviews (Mendelson 1982).

The term 'whiplash' should be removed from the medical dictionary. Instead, the injury to the neck should be accurately described and, where known, the pathology. Excluded are fractures, fracture dislocations and dislocations, herniated discs and congenital anomalies.

Pathology

There is surprisingly little direct or experimental evidence in the literature to support the idea that it is a soft tissue injury. There is a preliminary and incomplete report by McNab (1964) based on experiments carried out on monkeys that were strapped to seats and dropped from various heights. He described widespread soft tissue injury, muscle contusion and stressed that the principal injury was an anterior longitudinal ligament tear with separation of the discs from the vertebral end plate anteriorly. Also, he postulated a cervical sympathetic injury when the longus colli muscles were involved. He noted bruising of the oesophagus. In this preliminary report he concluded that it was a hyperextension injury as a result of a sudden deacceleration force. Roaf (1974) on the other hand, concluded from his studies on in vitro cadaveric cervical spines, that the anterior longitudinal ligament could not be ruptured by an extension force alone; there had to be a rotational element in addition to the flexion/ extension force.

In a further study MacNab (1973) reported results of a series of experiments on animals in tracked vehicles, in which he showed damage to the longus colli muscles and widespread soft tissue contusion throughout the neck, of a variable pattern. The cervical sympathetic nerves were also, but not inevitably, involved.

Marar (1975) in his paper on proven hyperextension injury to the cervical spine in patients with tetraplegia following cord involvement, described the autopsy findings and the levels involved, which were C3, C4 and C5. In a cadaveric study reported in the same paper, hyperextension forces resulted in fractures at C4, C5 and C6. Interestingly, these correspond with the levels found to be involved by McNab and Roaf in their studies.

Mechanism of injury

The majority of cases, in excess of 90%, result from motor vehicle accidents, either involving cars or motor cycles (Balla 1984); other examples inlude sporting injuries. The classical description is of the driver, or passenger, sitting in a stationary vehicle which is hit from behind. This causes an acceleration of the trunk, with the head being left behind relative to the body, producing a hyperextension injury of the neck. Because of the spread of movement there is no time for the normal protective muscle reflex contraction to occur, which would ordinarily protect against such a hyperextension injury. Provided there is a head rest, the degree of hyperextension can be limited. Without that physical restraint there is nothing to stop the head until it hits the midscapular region of the back. Following this initial movement, the trunk is then held either by the safety belt or steering wheel and the head and neck now flex forward. The degree of flexion is limited physically by the chin hitting the chest. It is well established that the degree of damage to the vehicle bears little relationship to the size of force applied, both to the neck and also the head (McKenzie & Williams 1971).

It must be stressed at this point that there may well be concomitant cerebral contusion, a factor that is often overlooked, because of what appear to be overwhelming symptoms arising from the cervical spine.

Age and sex

This is a condition affecting adults and is extremely rare in the under 20s and over 60s. (Balla 1984; Pearce 1989). There is evidence that increasing age is associated with more severe and more prolonged symptoms (Radanov et al 1991).

The male:female incidence ratio is 1:3, as reported by Hohl (1974) and confirmed by Balla (1984). This is remarkable as there is a male predominance in all other motor vehicle injuries.

History

A total of 20–30% of patients attending hospital after a motor vehicle accident complain of some form of neck pain. The incidence rises with particular injuries, notably rear and, to a lesser extent, front-impact motor vehicle accidents. Gargan & Bannister (1990) describe 88% of patients being involved in rear-end collisions with less than 10% presenting as a result of side-on collisions.

In a recent review (Pearce 1989), hyperextension–flexion mechanisms of injury were emphasised.

Symptoms

These can be divided into cervical and central/cranial (Hohl 1975). However, most, if not all, of the symptoms attributed to the central/cranial injury can be caused by cervical injury (Braaf & Rosner 1975; Tamura 1989).

Cervical

Cervical symptoms may present as:

1. Neck ache/pain. The onset may be delayed for up to 48 h. This is usually a dull ache which may become pain, radiating from the midcervical spine up to the occiput. It may spread laterally in relation to the trapezius muscles. There is often a sensitivity in the midcervical spine to local pressure.
2. Shoulder ache/pain. Again, this may be uni- or bilateral and associated with a heaviness of the shoulders. Movement and any physical effort tend to aggravate this.
3. Radiation of neck pain. The pain may spread up to the occiput and can go across the scalp to the eyes. There may be midscapular referral. Paraesthesiae or aching pain in one or both arms are described, but are seldom referrable to any identifiable dermatome.
4. Difficulty in swallowing. This is a very rare, but definitely described, symptom in a small proportion of patients.

The neck, shoulder and radiating neck pain symptoms tend to be aggravated by movement, tension and prolonged static positioning, such as reading or typing.

Central/cranial

Central/cranial symptoms may present as:

1. Headaches. These are in various sites, most commonly occipital or frontal and perioribital. They tend to be chronic and unremitting and seldom respond to simple analgesics
2. Dizziness
3. Tinnitus
4. Visual disturbances
5. Mood change.

These symptoms can occur singularly or together and usually fluctuate in severity. There is a huge disparity in both the severity and the duration of the symptoms following what may appear, on initial presentation, an uncomplicated soft tissue injury to the neck.

Cranial symptoms after cervical injury are well described. The Barre–Lieou syndrome, first described in 1926, is a series of symptoms including headache, vertigo, tinnitus and ocular problems in association with posttraumatic disc prolapse at the C3/4 level. Mechanical derangement of the disc complex, disturbances of the craniocervical sympathetic and the vertebral vessels, have all been reported as possible causes (Braaf & Rosner 1975). Nonneurogenic referred pain from cervical spine structures and radiating down both arms is well recognised. Stimulation of the annulus during discography (Cloward 1959) and the injection of hypotonic saline into cervical muscles and ligaments (Feinstein et al 1954) all give a pattern of referred pain down the arm without direct neurological involvement.

Signs

There are very few reliable reports of the findings on initial examination following hyperextension–flexion cervical spine soft tissue injuries. Farbman (1973) reported that 86% of 136 patients had no physical findings, 8% had questionable objective signs and only 6% had definite objective signs. More recently, Norris & Watt (1983) reported 61 patients with neck injuries resulting from rear end vehicle collisions in which 27 had no signs, 24 had some form of reduction in range of cervical movement and only 10 of the 61 patients had definite physical signs.

Swelling is seldom, if ever, seen. Cervical muscle spasm may be present in association with a reduction in range of cervical movements, although rotation is relatively well preserved, as most of this takes place at the one level, above the level of injury. It is exceedingly rare to find a central neurological deficit and only occasionally are there peripheral neurological signs. Definite peripheral neurological signs imply a more significant injury and possibly a disc prolapse which automatically excludes the patient from this particular grouping.

On general examination, associated injuries in these patients are uncommon.

Investigations

Plain radiographs are the single most common investigation. These continue to be done mainly for medicolegal reasons rather than strictly on medical grounds. An anteroposterior view, lateral in flexion and extension, plus oblique views and a 'through the mouth' view of the odontoid peg, should be done where indicated. By this means preexisting pathology can be excluded, plus any significant bony injury, subluxation, or dislocation. Norris & Watt (1983) have described an abnormal curve pattern on the lateral X-ray with a loss of cervical lordosis and even a reversal of the curve. This is usually associated with spasm of the paravertebral musculature and is neither a fixed nor structural deformity. Cervical spondylosis should be noted as this is associated with more severe and prolonged symptoms.

More recently, magnetic resonance imaging has been performed in an attempt to show soft tissue pathology. There have only been two reviews to date, in which a total of 19 patients have been reported (Van Meydam et al 1986; Maimaris 1989). All the scans were normal. Evidence of soft tissue injury on X-ray is singularly lacking; there is one reported example of retrophalangeal swelling in the literature (Gotten 1956). If a prolapsed disc is suspected on clinical grounds, then enhanced computed tomography is probably the investigation of choice in the cervical spine. Where there is evidence of radicular damage, electrodiagnosis may be helpful.

Management

The literature is lacking in reliable information on the management of soft tissue extension–flexion injuries to the cervical spine. There is no reliable or reproducible test to diagnose the injury. The natural history has not yet been established. The majority of reports to date concerning the management of these patients have, with one exception, been poorly designed, retrospective and incomplete. There has been one prospective trial comparing two forms of treatment, but there were no controls. A multitude of different conservative treatments have been reported with, not surprisingly, conflicting results.

In an attempt to establish the prognostic significance of presenting symptoms and signs, and thereby some insight into the natural history, Norris & Watt (1983) subdivided a group of patients with soft tissue injuries of the cervical spine into three groups. The first group had symptoms, but no physical signs and normal neurology; the second group had symptoms, a decrease in one or more of the cervical movements and normal neurology, and in the third group there were symptoms, decreased cervical movements and neurological signs.

There appeared to be a correlation between the severity of the condition on presentation and the time off work and duration of symptoms. Unfortunately, the long-term follow-up of these same patients, as reported by Gargan & Bannister (1990), was incomplete and there was little reference to the original groupings.

There is some evidence from the literature that certain forms of conservative treatment are harmful, exacerbating symptoms and prolonging their duration.

Cervical collars, both soft and hard, do not appear to help and the patient can become dependent on the collar. Vigorous range of movement exercises are contraindicated, as is manipulative therapy. In the past, traction has been advocated in the early stages (Breck & Van Norman 1971). Early active mobilisation has been shown to be superior to splinting in a collar (Mealy et al 1986) in one of the few prospective studies on treatment. There is no evidence that nonsteroidal antiinflammatory agents help. Surgery has little or no part to play in the management of the acute condition (Fleming 1973).

Rest, without splintage, appropriate analgesics, local heat and gentle massage would appear to be not only the safest, but the most beneficial of initial treatments.

Factors other than the apparent severity of the soft tissue injury to the cervical spine seem to influence the outcome. Farbman (1973) listed four elements that prolonged symptoms: emotional factors, previous medical history, the type of treatment and current litigation. The effect of litigation would appear to have a significant influence, but again the evidence is inconclusive and often conflicting. In addition to Farbman, Schutt & Dohan (1968) and DePalma & Subin (1965) all stated that litigation prolonged and increased the severity of symptoms. In contrast, Hirschfield & Behan (1963) and Mendelson (1982) stated that litigation had no effect. Unfortunately, these papers are all uncontrolled, incomplete and retrospective reviews. In a prospective study, psychosocial stress was found not to affect either the severity of the symptoms or the recovery following hyperextension–flexion injury to the cervical spine (Radanov et al 1991), which contradicts a previous report (Mills & Horne 1986).

Prognosis

There is an enormous variation in the numbers of patients having symptoms more than 6 months after the accident. Deans et al (1987) reported that 26% had intermittent pain 1 year after the accident, while 4% had continuous pain. Hohl (1975) reported 43% as having permanent disability after 5 years. MacNab (1964) described 45% as having important symptoms 2 years after the accident. Gargan & Bannister (1990) in their incomplete review reported only 12% as symptom-free, with 12% being severely incapacitated, at 8–12 years following the accident.

A more precise definition of the condition and a continuity of method of recording and controls would help to clarify the wide discrepancy in these reports.

WHIPLASH SYNDROME

Those patients with significant symptoms persisting for more than 6 months following the injury fall into the category of the late whiplash syndrome, recently reviewed by Pearce (1989). The majority of patients complain of neckache and neck stiffness and headache, with a significant number suffering from anxiety, irritability and symptoms of depression. Arm pain is relatively uncommon, while tinnitus/dizziness affects up to 15% of patients.

The symptoms are often complex in their nature. It is difficult to elucidate them and to decide whether they originate from the neck, or centrally. The results of physical examination, apart from a possibly painful and limited range of movement in the cervical spine, are usually normal.

Physical and pharmacological treatments on their own are usually inappropriate. Where there are definite physical signs attributable to the cervical spine, notably neck stiffness, then appropriate physiotherapy treatments may be tried, but at this late stage they are usually unsuccessful. Symptoms of pain seldom respond to pharmacological agents alone. Local infiltration and cervical epidurals have been tried, but with mixed success.

Where symptoms are significant and are interfering with day-to-day activities and work, referral to a pain management team is probably indicated.

REFERENCES

Balla J I 1984 Report to the Motor Accidents Board of Victoria on whiplash injuries. Headache and Cervical Disorders 10: 256–269

Bonica J J, Linblóm U, Iggo A (eds) 1979 Proceedings of the Second World Congress on Pain. Raven Press, New York

Braaf M M, Rosner S 1975 Trauma of cervical spine as a cause of headache. Journal of Trauma 15(5): 441–446

Breck L W, Van Norman R W 1971 Medicolegal aspects of cervical spine sprain. Clinical Orthopaedics and Related Research 74: 124–128

Casey K L 1973 Pain: a current view of neural mechanisms. American Scientist 61: 194

Cloward R B 1959 Cervical discography – a contribution to the aetiology and mechanism of neck, shoulder and arm pain. Annals of Surgery 150: 1052–1056

Crowe H D 1958 Whiplash injuries of the cervical spine. In: Proceedings of the section of insurance, negligence and compensation law. American Bar Association, Chicago, p 176–184

Deans D T, Majalliard J N, Kerr M, Rutherford W H 1987 Neck sprains – a major cause of disability following car accidents. Injury 18: 10–12

DePalma A F, Subin D K 1965 A study of the cervical syndrome. Clinical Orthopaedics and Related Research 38: 135–142

Farbman A A 1973 Neck sprain – associated factors. Journal of the American Medical Association 223: 1010–1015

Feinstein B, Layton J N K, Jameson R M, Schiller F 1954 Experiments on pain referred from deep somatic tissue. Journal of Bone and Joint Surgery 36A: 981–983

Fleming J F R 1973 Whiplash syndrome II. Clinical Neurosurgery 20: 232–242

Fowler P J 1980 The classification and early diagnosis of knee joint instability. Clinical Orthopaedics and Related Research 147: 5–21

Gargan M F, Bannister G C 1990 Long-term prognosis of soft tissue injuries of the neck. Journal of Bone and Joint Surgery 72B: 901–903

Gotten N 1956 Survey of 100 cases of whiplash injury after settlement of litigation. Journal of the American Medical Association 162: 865–867

Gray J R, Abbott K H 1953 Common whiplash injuries of the neck. Journal of the American Medical Association 152: 1698–1702

Gray's anatomy 1973 Williams P L, Warwick R (eds). Churchill Livingstone, Edinburgh

Hilton J 1963 The influence of mechanical and physiological rest. Bell, London

Hirschfield A H, Behan R C 1963 The accident process. Journal of the American Medical Association 186: 300–306

Hohl M 1974 Soft tissue injuries of the neck in automobile accidents. Journal of Bone and Joint Surgery 56A: 1675–1682

Hohl M 1975 Soft tissue injuries of the neck. Clinical Orthopaedics and Related Research 109: 42–49

Inman V T, Sanders J B de C M 1944 Referred pain from skeletal structures. Journal of Nervous and Mental Disease 99: 660–662

Jowitt M D, Knight R G 1983 Anaesthesia during the Falklands campaign. Anaesthesia 38: 776–783

Lynn B 1975 Somatosensory receptors and their CNS connections. Annual Review of Physiology 37: 105

McKenzie J A, Williams J F 1971 The dynamic behavior of the head and cervical-spine during whiplash. Journal of Biomechanics 4: 477–490

MacNab I 1964 Acceleration injuries of the cervical spine. Journal of Bone and Joint Surgery 46A: 1797–1799

MacNab I 1973 Whiplash syndrome I. Clinical Neurosurgery 20: 232–242

Maimaris C 1989 Neck sprains after car accidents. British Medical Journal 299: 123

Marar B C 1975 Hyperextension injuries of the cervical spine. Journal of Bone and Joint Surgery 56A(8): 1655–1663

Matsen F A 1975 Compartmental syndrome. Clinical Orhopaedics and Related Research 113: 8–14

Mealy K, Brennan H, Fenelon G C C 1986 Early mobilisation of acute whiplash injuries. British Medical Journal 292: 656–657

Mendelson G 1982 Not 'cured by a verdict'. Effect of legal settlement on compensation claimants. Medical Journal of Australia 1: 132–134

Meyer R A, Campbell J N 1981 Evidence for two distinct classes of unmyelinated nociceptive afferents in monkeys. Brain Research 224: 149–152

Mills H, Horne G 1986 Whiplash – man-made disease? New Zealand Medical Journal 99: 373–374

Norris S H, Watt I 1983 The prognosis of neck injuries resulting from rear-end vehicle collisions. Journal of Bone and Joint Surgery 65B: 608–611

Pearce J M S 1989 Whiplash injury – a re-appraisal. Journal of Neurology, Neurosurgery and Psychiatry 52: 1329–1331

Radanov B P, Di Stefano G, Schnidrig A, Ballinari P 1991 Role of psychosocial stress in recovery from common whiplash. Lancet 338: 712–715

Roaf R 1974 A study of the mechanics of the spinal injuries. Journal of Bone and Joint Surgery 42: 810–814

Ruggeri S B, Athraya B H, Doughty R, Gregg J R, Das M M 1982 Reflex sympathetic dystrophy in children. Clinical Orthopaedics and Related Research 163: 225–230

Schutt C H, Dohan F C 1968 Neck injuries to women in auto accidents. A metropolitan plague. Journal of the American Medical Association 206: 2689–2692

Smith M A, Urquhart D R, Savidge G F 1981 The surgical management of varus deformity in haemophilic arthropathy of the knee. Journal of Bone and Joint Surgery 63B: 261–265
Tahmoush A J 1981 Causalgia; redefinition as a clinical pain syndrome. Pain 10: 187–197
Tamura T 1989 Cranial symptoms after cervical injuries. Journal of Bone and Joint Surgery 71B: 283–287
Terenius L 1981 Biochemical mediators in pain. Triangle 20: 19–26
Thompson J E 1979 The diagnosis and management of post-traumatic pain syndromes (causalgia). Australian and New Zealand Journal of Surgery 49: 299–304
Van Meydam K, Sehlen S, Schlenkoff D, Kiricuta J C, Beyer H K 1986 Kernspintomographische Befunde beim Halswirbelsaulentrauma. Fortschritte auf dem Roentgenstrahlen 145: 657–660
Vane J R 1978 The mode of action of aspirin-like drugs. Agents and Actions 8: 430–431
Williams J G P 1976 Injury in sport. In: Williams J G P, Sperry P N (eds) Sports medicine. Edward Arnold, London, p 243–250
Yates D A H 1986 The neck and shoulder. In: Scott J T (ed) Copeman's textbook of the rheumatic diseases, 5th edn. Churchill Livingstone, Edinburgh
Zimmerman M 1976 Neurophysiology of nociception. International Review of Physiology 10: 179

23. Skeletal muscle pain

D. J. Newham, R. H. T. Edwards and K. R. Mills

Most individuals will have experienced skeletal muscle pain; usually it is clearly associated with trauma or exercise and is of a temporary nature. There are, however, a considerable number of people who complain of muscle pain which, by its severity or chronicity, causes them to seek advice. A wide variety of pathological conditions may also give rise to myalgia. This chapter commences by considering the structures responsible for the perception of muscle pain.

MUSCLE NOCICEPTORS

At the turn of the century Sherrington (1900) thought that specific afferent nerve fibres did not exist for the transmission of noxious stimuli from skeletal muscle and that 'adequate' stimulation of muscle spindles and tendon organs would elicit pain. Later workers have shown that, as in the skin, the thin myelinated (group III or A delta) and unmyelinated (group IV or C) fibres are responsible for transmitting muscular nociceptive impulses (Knighton & Dumke 1966). Group I and II fibres from muscle spindles and tendon organs do not transmit noxious information from skeletal muscle, since electrical stimulation of Group I fibres (which elicit the H-reflex) is not at all painful and known algesic agents such as bradykinin do not excite Group I or II muscle afferent units (Mense 1977).

The unencapsulated, freely branching endings of these afferents are found throughout skeletal muscle with particularly dense projections in the region of tendons, fascia and aponeuroses (Stacey 1969). Experimental access to these endings is complicated by their intimate connections with surrounding tissue, but despite technical difficulties the receptors of muscular Group III (Paintal 1960; Bessou & Laporte 1961) and IV (Iggo 1961) fibres have been shown to be activated by a variety of noxious stimuli. Physiological mechanisms of pain in the musculoskeletal system are reviewed by Zimmermann (1988).

Two major types of muscle pain receptor have been demonstrated and termed chemonociceptors and mechanonociceptors. The former are responsive to chemical stimuli and the latter to mechanical changes in their environment. The receptive properties of these units indicate that they are a heterogeneous group; some may respond to a single chemical substance while others are polymodal and respond to a variety of chemical, mechanical and thermal stimuli (Kumazawa & Mizumura 1977; Mense & Schmidt 1977).

The most effective substances for activation of these receptors are bradykinin, 5-hydroxytryptamine (serotonin), histamine, potassium and hydrogen ions. Aspirin has been shown to reduce the increased activity in Group III and IV muscle afferents which is induced by bradykinin, but not by 5-hydroxytryptamine (Mense 1982).

In addition to transmitting nociceptive information, these muscle afferents play a role in the cardiovascular and respiratory adjustments occurring during exercise. Electrical stimulation produces changes similar to those during exercise (Coote & Perez-Gonzales 1971). Nerve-blocking techniques established that the reflex responses to exercise are mediated by muscle Group III and IV afferents (Kalia et al 1972; McCloskey & Mitchell 1972). Afferent units fulfilling this function have been termed 'ergoreceptors', but they are not a distinct population, as many afferents have both nociceptive and ergoreceptive properties (Kniffki et al 1978).

Recent evidence indicates that thick myelinated afferents may transmit information which is perceived as pain in some circumstances. Thus the conventional classification of nociceptors and nociception may be misleading (McMahon & Koltzenburg 1990).

MUSCLE PAIN AND EXERCISE

In normal healthy subjects there is usually a clear association between muscle pain and exercise but two very different time courses may occur. In one case, pain occurs *during* the exercise and rapidly increases in intensity until the contractions stop and blood flow is restored, whereupon the pain disappears very rapidly, within seconds or a few minutes. This is termed ischaemic muscle pain. Alternatively, the pain may occur with a delayed onset of some hours *after* exercise and may persist for days.

Ischaemic muscle pain

Intermittent claudication and angina pectoris are two well-known clinical presentations of this type of pain. It occurs in muscles whose blood supply is compromised: a situation which occurs in normal muscle as the result of the increase in intramuscular pressure during muscular activity. In normal subjects it disappears within seconds of the contractions stopping and the circulation being restored, leaving no residual effects.

Hypoxia was thought to cause this type of pain but a preliminary period of hypoxia does not reduce the time for which ischaemic contractions can be performed (Park & Rodbard 1962). It is now accepted that accumulation of metabolites is, at least in part, responsible for ischaemic pain although the metabolic stimulus, or combination of stimuli, is not clear. Lactic acid was thought by many to be the prime algesic substance but it has been eliminated from this role by the finding that patients with myophosphorylase deficiency (McArdle's syndrome) experience particularly severe ischaemic muscle pain during exercise, despite an inability to produce lactic acid (Schmid & Hammaker 1961). Recent data, acquired by magnetic resonance spectroscopy, have shown that clearance of intramuscular lactic acid at the end of exercise or vascular occlusion is slower than the disappearance of pain. Possible agents, acting alone or in combination, are currently thought to include histamine, acetylcholine, serotonin and bradykinin. Potassium (Lendinger & Sjogaard 1991) and adenosine (Sylven et al 1988) are currently receiving considerable attention in this respect.

Ischaemic muscle pain also has mechanical determinants and the effects of contraction force and frequency have been investigated by many workers. The repetition rate of intermittent contractions has a marked effect, the onset and severity of pain increasing with increasing contraction frequency (Park & Rodbard 1962; Rodbard & Pragay 1968; Mills et al 1982a).

Delayed onset muscle pain

Heavy or unaccustomed exercise has long been associated with muscle pain which has a delayed onset of about 8 hours and persists for days. Asmussen (1956) was the first to establish that it is particularly associated with unaccustomed eccentric contractions – those in which the active muscle is lengthened by external forces. This observation has since been confirmed by many workers (Newham 1988, Stauber 1989). Eccentric contractions generate a higher force per active fibre (Katz 1939; Abbott et al 1952) and have a lower metabolic cost per unit force than other types of muscle activity (Curtin & Davies 1973; Menard et al 1991). Thus delayed onset muscle pain is likely to be caused by mechanical, rather than metabolic, factors and differs from ischaemic pain in time course as well as underlying mechanisms.

Delayed onset pain is associated with considerable muscle damage, as shown by structural (Newham et al 1983b; Friden 1984; Jones et al 1986; Newham 1988), biochemical (Newham et al 1988; Stauber 1989) and radioisotopic changes. The damage is presumably initiated by the high forces generated in active fibres during eccentric contractions, but none of these damage markers follow the same time course as the pain (Jones et al 1986; Newham et al 1986b), the cause of which remains unknown. Indirect evidence indicates connective tissue. Affected muscles are tender and often feel swollen. Increased intramuscular pressures have been reported in muscles in noncompliant compartments (Friden et al 1986), but not in others (Newham & Jones 1985), and the increased pressure precedes pain.

There is conflicting evidence about the effect of steroidal and nonsteroidal antiinflammatory agents on delayed onset pain.

CLINICAL MYALGIA

Signs and symptoms

The vocabulary of patients presenting with myalgia is relatively restricted. Common terms for the symptom are stiffness, soreness, aching, spasms or cramps. Tenderness is a common self-reported sign. The symptom of stiffness usually means discomfort on muscle movement, rather than a change of compliance.

Muscle pain is most often reported as having a dull, aching quality. Sharp, lancinating pain is relatively rare, although acute tenderness from a 'trigger point' (Travell & Simons 1992) may occur. Even severe cramps have a relatively dull quality compared with pain arising from superficial structures. Muscle pain is usually exacerbated by voluntary contraction, although rarely the opposite may be the case.

The terms cramp, contracture, spasm and tetanus or tetany have precise definitions but are often used inaccurately. Cramps are strong, involuntary contractions of rapid onset which are extremely painful and are associated with electromyographic signals similar to those of a normal voluntary contraction. A contracture is an extremely rare form of involuntary contraction due to depletion of muscle adenosine triphosphate (ATP) and is electrically silent. It is a sign of rare metabolic disorders (e.g. myophosphorylase deficiency) and only occurs in healthy individuals as rigor mortis because force fatigue prevents ATP depletion. Spasm usually implies a reflex contraction of the muscles surrounding an injured or inflamed structure and is seen in the abdominal muscles during visceral inflammation or obstruction. Tetany is an involuntary contraction, often in carpopedal muscles, and is usually associated with hypocalcaemia or hypocapnia (Layzer & Rowland 1971).

Less common are myotonia and dystonia. The former is a prolongation of muscle contraction and delayed relaxation; it is most often associated with dystrophia myotonica. Dystonia is an involuntary contraction of muscles acting over the same joint, but which have opposing actions and may be described as either spasm or cramp.

Associated signs and symptoms

Patients with myalgia often complain of weakness, fatigability or exercise intolerance (discussed under 'Investigation of muscle pain').

Swelling of painful muscles is often reported, but rarely substantiated. If it is, it almost always implies serious underlying pathology and occurs in polymyositis, dermatomyositis, myophosphorylase and phosphofructokinase deficiencies and acute alcoholic myopathy.

Enquiry should be made about alcohol, diet and fasting. A drinking bout in an alcoholic may precipitate acute alcoholic myopathy and even myoglobinuria (Penn 1980). A diet deficient in vitamin D is associated with osteomalacia, causing bone and muscle pain (Smith & Stern 1967). Attacks of pain and weakness occur in carnitine palmityltransferase deficiency, particularly during prolonged exercise after fasting or after a high fat, low carbohydrate diet or meal (Di Mauro & Di Mauro 1973; Bank et al 1975). Fasting may be used as a provocative test for this condition (Carroll et al 1979).

Both muscle pain and dyskinesia are associated with poor sleep patterns, although it is not known which is the primary event (Lavigne et al 1991).

Differentiation of muscle pain from pain in other tissues

Pain localisation is poor in skeletal muscle and patients may also be unable to differentiate it from pain arising from tendons, ligaments and bones, as well as from joints and their capsules. Several conditions (e.g. systemic lupus erythematosus) involve both muscles and joints. It is obviously important to distinguish the painful tissue but this may be very difficult due to poor localisation and referred pain; that from an arthritic hip may be referred to the thigh muscles or knee joint, from a carpal tunnel syndrome to the forearm muscles or that from cervical spondylosis to the arm muscles.

Pain from joints and their capsules tends to be more localised than myalgia and arthralgia is often worsened by passive joint movement. Capsular pain may be present only in specific joint positions (e.g. painful arc syndrome in the shoulder). Bone pain also tends to be poorly localised but, unlike myalgia, usually has a deep, boring quality. Furthermore, bone pain is usually worse at night and tends to be unaffected by either movement or muscle activity.

Myalgia, exercise and rest

Many patients presenting with myalgia describe a relationship between exercise and muscle pain which has one of the two time courses found in normal subjects. Others find no relationship or that their pain is relieved by moderate exercise.

The paradigm of exercise-related muscle pain is intermittent claudication in which pain occurs in the calf muscles during exercise then disappears after a period of rest. This is a pathological form of ischaemic muscle pain caused by stenosis of the feeding artery and is experienced distal to the stenosis. Thus thrombosis of the terminal aorta leads to pain in the buttocks (Leriche's syndrome), narrowing of the axillary artery by a cervical rib gives rise to forearm pain and arteritis of cranial arteries may result in pain in the muscles of mastication during chewing. Reduced blood supply can also occur due to increased blood viscosity (e.g. Waldenström's macroglobulinaemia). Ischaemia can also arise with a normal blood flow if the oxygen-carrying capacity of blood is reduced, as in anaemia.

Other conditions in which myalgia is clearly related to exercise involve an impaired energy supply to a contracting muscle; the machanism is presumably the same as ischaemic muscle pain. Myophosphorylase deficiency (Schmid & Mahler 1959), glycolytic disorders of muscle (McArdle 1951) and phosphofructokinase deficiency (Tarui et al 1965) all present as exercise-related myalgia with cramps and contracture. Contracture is a potentially serious event since it leads to irreversible muscle breakdown and the release of large amounts of myoglobin may lead to renal cast formation and failure. A clear association between exercise and myalgia is also found in several of the mitochondrial myopathies (Land & Clark 1979) and in carnitine palmityltransferase deficiency (Bank et al 1975).

In those individuals where failure of energy or blood supply has been eliminated, the relationship of pain to exercise or rest appears to have no diagnostic or prognostic value (Mills & Edwards 1983).

AETIOLOGY (Table 23.1)

Trauma and sports injuries

Direct trauma to muscle, varying from intramuscular injections to severe crush injuries, is an obvious cause of

Table 23.1 Principal medical conditions associated with myalgia

Trauma and sports injuries
Primary infective myositis
Inflammatory myopathies
Polymyositis
Dermatomyositis
Polymyositis or dermatomyositis in association with connective tissue disease
Viral myositis
Polymyalgia rheumatica
Myalgia of neurogenic origin
Muscle cramp
Impaired muscle energy metabolism
Cytosolic enzyme defects
Lipid storage myopathies
Mitochondrial myopathies
Drug-induced myalgia
Myalgic encephalomyelitis
Muscle pain of uncertain cause

muscle pain. If sufficient tissue is damaged, life is threatened by hypercalcaemia and acute renal failure from myoglobinuria. Sports injuries, from minor muscle sprains to complete rupture (e.g. hamstring rupture) may include direct trauma. They are increasingly common in exercise-conscious cultures (Renstrom 1991).

Traumatic muscular damage is invariably associated with muscle pain, which may have a gradual or immediate onset. It may also be detected by imaging techniques, blood biochemistry and the immunohistochemical (Fechner et al 1991) and routine histochemical examination of tissue samples as described in this chapter. The combination of damage and immobilisation (Appell 1990) results in considerable weakness and wasting which may only be reversed by relatively long periods of rehabilitation.

In many cases the cause of injury is obvious and associated with a forced lengthening of an active muscle, but spontaneous ruptures of many muscle groups, particularly the hamstrings and pectoralis major (Kretzler & Richardson 1989), occur frequently. Muscle ruptures and tears of limb muscle may mimic a compartment syndrome, while those of the abdominal musculature may cause groin pain. They are commonly associated with muscle spasms, which in turn give rise to additional muscle pain. Myositis ossificans is a potentially disabling complication of muscle trauma which may be confused with a sarcoma (Booth & Westers 1989)

Activity-related compartment syndromes occur in muscle groups within a relatively inextensible fascial sheath, such as the anterior tibial muscles (Allen 1990). Pain occurs during exercise and increases in intensity as the blood supply to the active tissue is inadequate. Symptoms include pain and cramp-like sensations, very similar to the symptoms of intermittent claudication. They usually disappear at rest but tenderness may persist. Weakness, paralysis and numbness may occur in acute cases, which tend to result in continued symptoms and raised intramuscular pressures at rest (Martens & Moeyersoons 1990).

Great emphasis has been placed on the ability of training to protect against injury in sports (Safran et al 1989). Nevertheless, it is currently accepted that for many athletes overtraining in itself can produce a wide variety of symptoms, both physical and psychological (Fry et al 1991). There appears to be a considerable individual variation in the susceptibility to sports-related injuries which is little understood and may be caused by a combination of physical and psychological factors (Taimela et al 1990).

Primary infective myositis

Direct infection of muscle with bacteria is uncommon. Tropical myositis (Taylor et al 1976) is an infection with staphylococcus aureus, probably secondary to a viral myositis. It affects children and young adults in the tropics and is characterised by fever, muscle pains (often severe and localised to a single limb) and deep intramuscular abscesses. It usually responds to antibiotics and surgical drainage.

Parasitic infections of muscle that cause muscle pain and tenderness include trichinosis (Gould 1970), sparganonosis (Wirth & Farrow 1961), sarcosporidosis (Jeffrey 1974) and cysticercosis. Infection with *Trichinella spiralis*, usually by eating undercooked pork, is common in many parts of the world, especially the United States, but many cases are asymptomatic. The disease is ushered in with fever and periorbital oedema. Later myalgia and muscle weakness develop to reach a peak at 3 weeks. The prognosis depends on the heaviness of the infection; 2–10% of cases are fatal. Treatment with thiabendazole and steroids has been successful.

Inflammatory myopathies

Polymyositis and dermatomyositis

The idiopathic inflammatory myopathies, polymyositis and dermatomyositis, classified by Bohan & Peter (1975a, 1975b) and Carpenter & Karpati (1981), have been reviewed by Currie (1981), Mastaglia (1988) and Dalakas (1988). In a few cases muscle pain may be a prominent feature but usually the presentation is with muscle weakness. It was originally thought that the two diseases represented part of the same spectrum with skin lesions being present in dermatomyositis but not in polymyositis. This view has now been challenged and there are both clinical and pathological distinctions between them. Dermatomyositis presents more commonly in the female with acute or subacute onset of limb girdle weakness, dysphagia, muscle tenderness and skin involvement.

There is often involvement of other systems, such as the lungs and heart and in 20% of cases there may be an associated carcinoma. Pathologically in dermatomyositis, there is evidence of a microangiopathy with immunoglobulin deposits on vessel walls which lead to microinfarcts. On muscle biopsy there may be striking perivascular atrophy. Polymyositis on the other hand presents equally in males and females, has a chronic course, respiratory muscle involvement is unusual and muscle tenderness infrequent. There is no skin involvement or involvement of other systems. Pathologically, muscle biopsy shows endomysial lymphocyte infiltration and cytotoxic T cells predominate.

Diagnosis rests on the findings of:

1. a muscle biopsy showing muscle cell necrosis, lymphocyte infiltration, phagocytosis, variation in size of both fibre types and basophilic fibres reflecting regeneration
2. EMG showing brief, small amplitude polyphasic potentials and fibrillations
3. plasma creatine kinase (CK) which is raised in the acute phase but may be normal in 30% of cases
4. a raised erythrocyte sedimentation rate in 60% of cases.

Treatment remains controversial. Despite widespread clinical use of high dose corticosteroids, no well-controlled trial has been performed. Nevertheless, the clinical usefulness of steroid therapy is a widely held view and the complications of long-term steroid therapy are said to be uncommon (Riddoch & Morgan-Hughes, 1975; Currie, 1981), although they must always be borne in mind (Edwards et al 1981). Other immunosuppressive drugs such as azathioprine, cyclophosphamide, methotrexate and cyclosporin, immunoglobulin infusions, whole body irradiation and plasmapheresis have all been tried but the results and the benefits are not clear cut. Estimates of prognosis and mortality in polymyositis vary; in the 20 cases studied by Riddoch & Morgan-Hughes over a 5-year period, eight patients died and only four improved. De Vere & Bradley (1975) reported 25–30% mortality over 5 years. The prognosis of dermatomyositis is rather better, with many patients showing full recovery of muscle function; although the disease will eventually burn itself out, this may take several years.

Muscle pain is not a feature of inclusion body myositis (Lotz et al 1989).

Polymyositis in association with connective tissue disease

Polymyositis may be seen in association with systemic lupus erythematosus (Tsokos et al 1991), progressive systemic sclerosis, mixed connective tissue disease, rheumatoid disease (Haslock et al 1970), Sjögrens syndrome, polyarteritis nodosa and, occasionally, myasthenia gravis. In polyarteritis nodosa muscle changes are probably due to infarction, but in the other conditions findings are similar to those in idiopathic polymyositis, although the changes of steroid myopathy are often superimposed.

Viral polymyositis

Myalgia is a feature of several acute viral infections; in the vast majority of cases, influenza virus A or B or coxsackie virus A or B are the agents involved. Coxsackie B virus is the agent responsible for epidemic myalgia (Bornholm disease) in which there is fever, headache and muscle pain in the chest and abdomen. The disease is rapidly self-limiting as is benign acute childhood myositis which can follow influenza A or B virus infection. In these conditions, the CK may be raised and in the few patients who have been tested, the EMG may show myopathic features. A syndrome of muscle cramps, aching and fatigability following an influenza-like illness, has been described and designated 'benign post-infectious polymyositis' (Schwartz et al 1978). The symptoms may persist for 2 years after the initial febrile episode. Occasionally, a viral infection is thought to precipitate idiopathic polymyositis or dermatomyositis and it has recently been suggested that inclusion body myositis may be a slow mumps virus infection (Chou 1988).

Polymyalgia rheumatica

This condition affects patients over the age of 55 and is characterised by pain and stiffness of the proximal muscles especially the shoulder girdle (Hamrin 1972). There may be mild anaemia, weight loss and malaise. The erythrocyte sedimentation rate is typically over 50 mm in the first hour, but CK, muscle biopsy and EMG are normal. Occasional cases show arthritic change within muscle and there appears to be a close relationship between this condition and temporal, cranial or giant cell arteritis. The response to steroids is usually immediate and dramatic (Bird et al 1979), most authorities advising a high initial dose of 40–60 mg per day.

Myalgia of neurogenic origin

Pain which appears to be localised to muscle may be a predominant feature in a number of neurogenic diseases. Cervical radiculopathy with pain radiating into the myotomal distribution of the roots, or nerve compression (e.g. carpel tunnel syndrome), may produce pain radiating into the forearm or upper arm muscles. Peripheral neuropathies may produce pain especially when they affect small fibres, but this is usually distinguishable on its peripheral and superficial characteristics. Spasticity of any origin can give rise to flexor 'spasms' which can be very distressing. Treatment is difficult but diazepam and baclofen can be tried.

Muscle cramps

Apart from the benign 'ordinary' muscle cramps experienced by most individuals, cramps are also seen in glycolytic disorders (see below), in dehydration, in uraemia, with certain drugs such as salbutamol, phenothiazine, vincristine, lithium, cimetidine and bumetanide (Lane & Mastaglia 1978), after haemodialysis and in tetanus.

The 'stiff man' syndrome, first described by Moersch & Woltman (1956) and reviewed by Gordon et al (1967) is characterised by continuous board-like stiffness of muscles, paroxysms of intense cramp, abolition of muscle stiffness during sleep and a normal motor and sensory examination. Stiffness treatment with diazepam, often in very large doses, has been reported.

Neuromyotonia (Isaacs' syndrome) features widespread fasciculation, generalised stiffness, excessive sweating and continuous motor unit activity, which persist during sleep and anaesthesia (Isaacs 1961; Newsom-Davis & Mills 1992). A family with cramps in the distal muscles with fasciculation (Lazaro et al 1981), and a muscular pain and fasciculation syndrome (Hudson et al 1978), have also been reported. In all the above conditions the defect is thought to be in the spinal cord or motor axons.

Impaired muscle energy metabolism

Cytosolic enzyme defects

Myophosphorylase deficiency (McArdle's disease). In 1951 McArdle first described a patient with exercise-induced muscle pain and contractures, and postulated a defect in muscle glycolysis. Myophosphorylase deficiency was demonstrated by Mommaerts et al (1959) and Schmid & Mahler (1959) in further cases. The symptoms usually begin in early adolescence with painful muscle stiffness, cramps, contractures and muscle weakness induced by vigorous exercise. The symptoms disappear after a period of rest but contractures may persist for several hours. Moderate exercise may be performed for long periods without symptoms developing but if they do, further exercise may result in resolution of the pain. This is the 'second wind' phenomenon (Pernow et al 1967), thought to be due to a combination of increased muscle blood flow and the mobilisation of free fatty acids and glucose from the liver. The condition has a relatively benign course, symptoms becoming less troublesome after the age of 40 years. Patients often have no physical signs at rest, although quadriceps weakness may be demonstrated by quantitative testing. CK is elevated at rest and reaches very high values as contractures resolve. EMG may be normal or show myopathic changes, but the definitive investigation is muscle biopsy showing excessive glycogen deposition and a reduction or absence of myophosphorylase. Biopsy in an acute attack may, in addition, show muscle cell necrosis.

Phosphofructokinase (PFK) deficiency. This condition was described initially by Tarui et al (1965). The symptoms are very similar to those of McArdle's disease but may begin early in childhood and contractures are less frequent. The second wind phenomenon has also been reported (Layzer et al 1967). Diagnosis is achieved by the demonstration of the absence of phosphofructokinase (PFK) activity and of glycogen accumulation in muscle. CK is elevated between attacks of pain and, as in McArdle's disease, there is no rise in venous lactate on the ischaemic exercise test. PFK is also present as an isoenzyme in erythrocytes and patients with the deficiency have mild haemolysis with a raised reticulocyte count.

Other cytosolic enzyme defects. A number of other enzyme deficiencies have been reported which cause exercise intolerance, exercise-induced muscle pains and muscle fatigue. Phosphoglycerate kinase deficiency (type 9 glycogenesis) (Di Mauro et al 1983), phosphoglycerate mutase deficiency (type 10 glycogenesis) (Di Mauro et al 1982) and lactate dehydrogenase deficiency (Kanno et al 1980) have been reported in only a few cases.

Lipid storage myopathies

Transport of long-chain fatty acids to the interior of the mitochondrion depends on the enzyme carnitine palmityltransferase (CPT) located on the innner membrane and the carrier molecule carnitine. Deficiency of either would be expected to lead to a block in energy supply once intramuscular glycogen stores were depleted. Syndromes due to carnitine palmityltransferase deficiency, to carnitine deficiency and to both have been described.

Systemic carnitine deficiency, in which both muscle and plasma carnitine are low, presents in childhood with episodes of nausea, vomiting, encephalopathy and muscle weakness (Karpati et al 1975). Muscle carnitine deficiency (Willner et al 1979), in which plasma carnitine is normal, presents in young adults with proximal muscle weakness and pain. CK is usually raised and the EMG myopathic. Muscle biopsy shows lipid accumulation beneath the plasma membrane and between myofibrils, and low levels of carnitine. Response to treatment with carnitine (Angelini et al 1976; Carroll et al 1980) has been variable, possibly indicating heterogeneity in the disease.

CPT deficiency usually presents in adolescence with attacks of muscle pain, weakness and myoglobinuria precipitated by prolonged exercise, especially after fasting or after a low carbohydrate, high fat diet (Bertorini et al 1980). CK is usually normal between attacks but rises markedly during and after attacks of pain. Muscle biopsy at the height of an attack may show lipid accumulation and/or muscle cell necrosis and assay for CPT shows very low levels. Management with a high carbohydrate, low fat diet has achieved some increase in exercise tolerance. Ionasescu et al (1980) have described a mother and son who had attacks of muscle cramp and myoglobinuria and whose muscle biopsies showed deficiency of both carnitine and CPT.

Mitochondrial myopathies

This is a heterogeneous group of conditions, often presenting with muscle weakness and/or exercise-induced pain, and distinguished by the finding, usually on electron microscopy, of mitochondria of abnormal size, shape or numbers, often with crystalline inclusions. Many patients may have 'ragged red fibres' on the modified Gomori trichrome stain. With increasingly sophisticated biochemical investigations, metabolic abnormalities isolated to particular segments of the cytochrome chain can now be distinguished (Petty et al 1986; Morgan-Hughes et al 1987). For example, patients have been described with cytochrome B deficiency (Morgan-Hughes et al 1979), with NADH cytochrome B reductase deficiency (Land et al 1979), and cytochrome B deficiency (complex 3) (Hayes et al 1984). Several other mitochondrial cytopathies have been associated with a bewildering number of other abnormalities: deafness, myoclonus, encephalopathy, ophthalmoplegia, growth retardation and retinitis pigmentosa (Kearns–Sayre syndrome), as reviewed by Petty et al (1986).

Drug-induced myalgia

A large number of agents have now been catalogued as the cause of muscle pain (Lane & Mastaglia 1978). A polymyositis can be produced by D-penicillamine, with myopathic features on EMG, muscle cell necrosis and an inflammatory infiltrate on muscle biopsy samples. A severe acute rhabdomyolysis with myoglobinuria and the threat of renal failure can be induced by diamorphine, amphetamine, phencyclidine and alcohol.

Myalgic encephalomyelitis (ME)/chronic fatigue syndrome

This well-publicised syndrome commonly presents with diffuse muscle pain, which is exacerbated by muscle activity, marked exercise intolerance, weakness and fatigability. Other symptoms include loss of concentration and sleep disturbance. A proportion of cases relate the onset of symptoms to a viral illness, giving rise to the term postviral (fatigue) syndrome. The multiplicity of possible symptoms often makes diagnosis difficult and a consensus has recently been agreed on diagnostic criteria (Dawson 1990). It may occur sporadically or in epidemics and is most common in young and middle-aged women (Behan & Bakheit 1991). Currently there is much debate about whether the aetiology is physical or psychological (Wessely 1990). Irrespective of the underlying mechanisms, the symptoms affect a large number of individuals, some of whom will recover over a few months or years, while others are transformed into chronic invalids (Wessely & Newham 1992). A recent publication presents a series of expert reviews on the diagnosis, aetiology, clinical findings and management of the syndrome (Behan et al 1991).

There is a lack of agreement about whether the patients show immunological indications of chronic viral infections. Hyperventilation is reported as being a common finding, which when treated brings symptomatic improvement. There is neurophysiological evidence of attentional deficits and slowed information processing (Prasher et al 1990). There appears to be an increased incidence of phychiatric disorder in these patients, compared to normal individuals and those with muscle disease (Wessley & Powell 1989; Wood et al 1991).

On objective muscle testing there is no evidence of muscle wasting, weakness or abnormal fatigability, due to either central or peripheral mechanisms (Stokes et al 1989; Edwards et al 1991; Lloyd et al 1991; Rutherford & White 1991). Neither are there consistent histochemical or metabolic changes, other than the nonspecific changes associated with immobility. Blood levels of skeletal muscle cytoplasmic enzymes (e.g. CK), usually raised with muscle damage, are normal.

Muscle pain of uncertain cause

Vague muscle aches and pains commonly form part of the symptomatology in depressive illness and in individuals with a neurotic or obsessive personality disorder. However, care must be taken not to dismiss these symptoms; the depression may be secondary to an organic muscle abnormality.

In large studies a group of patients always appears who complain of muscle pain, in whom no abnormality can be found despite exhaustive investigation (Serratrice et al 1980; Mills & Edwards 1983). Rational criteria to filter out those patients with organic abnormalities appear to be the measurement of erythrocyte sedimentation rate and CK. If either of these is abnormal, then muscle biopsy, EMG, exercise and strength testing should be performed. However, there exists a considerable group of patients with muscle pain in whom no definite muscle abnormality can be found. Undoubtedly, a number of specific muscle abnormalities remain to be characterised.

The term 'repetitive strain injury' has recently gained popularity as a catch-all term for pain developing as the consequence of some repetitive occupation. Although changes in muscle biopsy specimens have been reported (Fry 1986), there has been no firm confirmation of any neurological or rheumatological abnormality (Barton et al 1992).

Primary fibromyalgia (Bengtsson 1986) or 'fibrositis' (Bennett 1981) is a disorder in which histological abnormalities have been detected (Bartels & Danneskiold-Samsöe 1986; Bengtsson et al 1986a), as have reduced high energy phosphate levels (Bengtsson et al 1986b), although the clear definition of the syndrome remains controversial.

INVESTIGATION OF MUSCLE PAIN

Muscle biopsy

This is often the definitive investigation in the management of a patient with myalgia. Percutaneous muscle biopsy is suitable for histological, histochemical, electron microscopic and metabolic characterisation (Fig. 23.1).

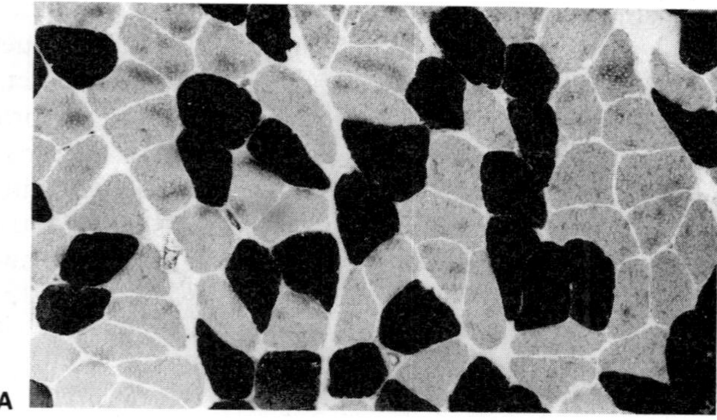

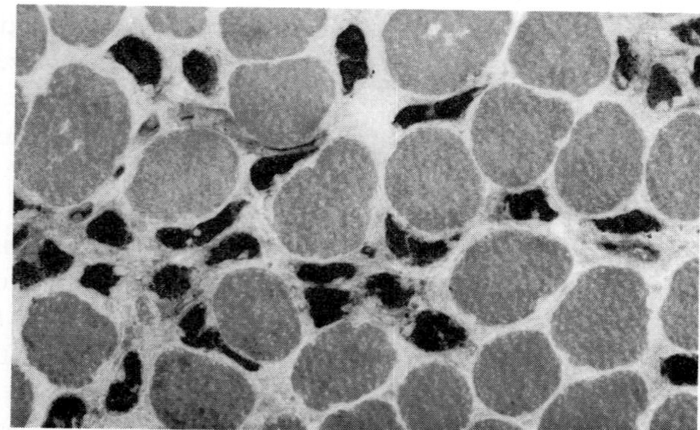

Fig. 23.1 Needle biopsy from a human gastrocnemius muscle, with Type II, fast twitch fibres staining dark. **A** No histochemical abnormalities. **B** Inflammatory changes (rounded fibres with increased extracellular fluid and infiltration of white cells) typical of an inflammatory myopathy and also Type II fibre degeneration. The samples were taken from the same normal individual 4 (A) and 12 (B) days after eccentric exercise. On day 4 they had severe delayed-onset muscle pain which disappeared by day 12. ATPase stain at pH 9.4. Original magnification ×100.

With needle biopsies (Edwards et al 1980) all these procedures may be performed, despite the fact that only a small quantity (100–300 mg) of tissue is obtained. The conchotome technique allows the percutaneous removal of larger tissue samples (Dietrichson et al 1987). These procedures are relatively atraumatic and can be used serially for following progress.

Muscle biopsy can be useful in the diagnosis of inflammatory myopathies with demonstration of muscle cell necrosis and inflammatory cell infiltrate. There is, however, a poor correlation between muscle morphology and myalgia. Where the pain is of neurogenic origin, fibre type grouping may be found. In the case of metabolic disorders, histochemical staining techniques reveal the absence or reduction of enzymes such as myophosphorylase. Direct measurement can be made of enzymes such as carnitine palmityltransferase and mitochondrial activity.

Muscle biopsy is essential in the analysis of mitochondrial myopathies in which there is a defect in either mitochondrial substrate transport or in electron transport. The defective components of the electron transport chain can be identified on relatively small biopsy samples obtained by needle biopsy (Gohil et al 1981).

Open biopsy is still commonly practised and may have advantages in 'patchy' diseases such as focal polymyositis or in arthritic diseases (e.g. polyarteritis nodosa). In the majority of primary investigations of myalgia we consider it unnecessary and unethical.

Biochemical markers of muscle damage

Myoglobinuria and myoglobinaemia

Myoglobinuria is an important sign of muscle disease and has many causes (Rowland et al 1964; Penn 1980). It may be the presenting complaint in a number of conditions with exercise-induced muscle pain or may be a concomitant of severe polymyositis, viral myositis or alcoholic myopathy.

Myoglobin is a muscle protein involved in oxygen storage and transport (Penn 1980); when muscle fibres degenerate, myoglobin leaks out into the plasma and is a sufficiently small molecule (molecular weight 17 500) to pass into the urine. This is important to recognise because of the potentially fatal complication of oliguric renal failure due to acute tubular necrosis (Paster et al 1975). Myoglobinuria can also occur in normal individuals after prolonged strenuous exercise, especially when performed at high ambient temperatures (Demos et al 1974). Although patients may report 'muddy' coloured urine after exercise, the pigment may only be detectable by appropriate testing of the urine. Myoglobinaemia may be seen in up to 74% of patients with myositis and may precede elevation of creatine kinase in relapses.

Creatine kinase

Creatine kinase (CK) is the enzyme responsible for catalysing the breakdown and synthesis of phosphoryl creatine and plays a central role in the metabolism of muscle contraction. It is present as three isoenzymes, MM, MB and BB; the MB and BB isoenzymes are not generally found much in normal skeletal muscle. Probably because of the regeneration of immature muscle fibres in various myopathies, all three isoenzymes may occasionally be seen. However, in most muscle diseases the MM isoenzyme, which comprises 95–99% in muscle, is predominantly elevated. It has been suggested that the MB fraction which emanates from heart muscle can be used as an indicator of cardiac involvement in polymyositis. However, this enzyme can be elevated in as many as 28% of patients with polymyositis uncomplicated by cardiac disease.

Leakage of the enzyme into plasma is usually taken as evidence of muscle damage, but this must be seen in perspective since it is known that moderate exercise in normal individuals will cause a rise in CK (Thomson et al 1975; Brooke et al 1979) and that CK is higher in outpatients with a higher level of habitual activity than inpatients (Griffiths 1966). Intramuscular injection and electromyographic investigation are also known to cause a rise in CK.

CK is many times higher than normal in the muscular dystrophies, especially Duchenne dystrophy, and may be elevated in spinal muscular atrophy, motor neurone disease, postpoliomyelitis muscular atrophy, hypothyroidism and toxic muscle damage. In acute rhabdomyolysis, CK can reach very high values and is then associated with myoglobinuria. CK can nevertheless be used as a screening test in painful myopathies of less dramatic onset, since it may be elevated in asymptomatic periods between attacks. In McArdle's disease, for example, CK is usually 5–15 times the upper limit of normal with habitual daily activity, but may rise to 100 times this level during and after a painful cramp or contracture. CK is said to be elevated in myoadenylate deaminase deficiency (Fishbein et al 1978), but is normal between attacks of muscle pain in carnitine palmityltransferase deficiency (Morgan-Hughes 1982). In polymyositis and dermatomyositis, CK is usually elevated but even in acute myositis it may be normal. Only in 3% of patients does the CK remain persistently normal throughout the entire clinical course of polymyositis. It has been reported to be of use in following the course of polymyositis (Bohan & Peter 1975b), rising 5–6 weeks before a relapse and decreasing 3–4 weeks before an improvement in muscle strength. CK is usually normal in polymyalgia rheumatica.

3-Methylhistidine

Myofibrillar protein contains the amino acid 3-methylhistidine; when protein is broken down, this amino acid is not reutilised but is excreted in the urine unchanged and may therefore, if related to the total excretion of creatinine (generally taken as an index of total muscle mass), be used as an indicator of muscle breakdown (McKeran et al 1977). However, although muscle contains the largest amount of 3-methylhistidine, other actin-containing tissues such as skin and gut may turn over 3-methylhistidine much faster and thus there are uncertainties in using 3-methylhistidine excretion as an indicator of muscle breakdown.

Erythrocyte sedimentation rate (ESR)

Inflammatory myopathies, particularly polymyalgia rheumatica, cause a rise in ESR. This simple investigation is useful as a screening test for active disease and in following the progress of treatment.

Magnetic resonance (MR) techniques

Spectroscopy (MRS)

Phosphorus MRS of skeletal muscle enables muscle metabolism to be monitored by the determination of the amount of the phosphocreatine (PCr), inorganic phosphate (Pi) and ATP. Intramuscular pH can also be calculated. It is assumed that the volume sampled equates to the muscle of interest, but this may not be the case where relatively large coils are used over small muscles, as in the forearm, and this is particularly important in exercise studies (Fleckenstein et al 1989a).

Patients with the metabolic disorders of myophosphorylase deficiency (Ross et al 1981; Radda et al 1984) and phosphofructokinase deficiency (Chance et al 1982; Edwards et al 1982a; Cady et al 1985, 1989) usually have normal spectra at rest, as do patients with an alcoholic myopathy (Bollaert et al 1989). Exercise causes unusually large metabolic changes, with the exception of the internal pH in myophosphorylase deficiency which shows no or little change.

Mitochondrial myopathies are associated with excessive changes in pH, Pi and PCr during exercise. Abnormal amounts of these metabolic markers may also be found in unexercised, resting muscle (Gadian et al 1981; Narayana et al 1989; Matthews et al 1991a, 1991b). Similar findings occur in numerous neuromuscular diseases (Barany et al 1989). Patients with peripheral vascular disease (PVD) often show signs of excessive metabolism at rest (Hands et al 1986) as do those with hypothyroidism (Kaminsky 1992). In PVD patients the metabolic abnormalities are greater in those with rest pain (Hands et al 1990). Vascular surgery eliminates symptoms and abolishes the metabolic abnormalities (Hands et al 1986).

MRS has failed to detect metabolic abnormality in the tender points of patients with fibromyalgia (De Blecourt et al 1991).

Normal individuals with delayed onset muscle pain have an unusually high Pi concentration in resting muscle (Aldridge et al 1986; McCully et al 1988). However, this metabolic abnormality precedes the onset of pain. It is also found in some patients with primary muscle diseases (Barany et al 1989) which are not usually painful. This may be a nonspecific finding which has no direct relationship with myalgia (Newham & Cady 1990).

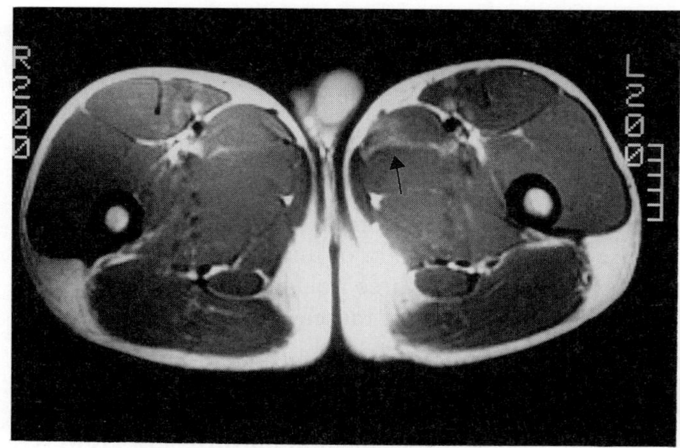

Fig. 23.2 Magnetic resonance image (T2 weighted) from a footballer presenting with pain in the left groin. The image shows a tear with resolving haematoma in the belly of the left adductor longus muscle. (Courtesy of Professor Graham Whitehouse, University department of Radiodiagnosis and Magnetic Resonance Research Centre, University of Liverpool.)

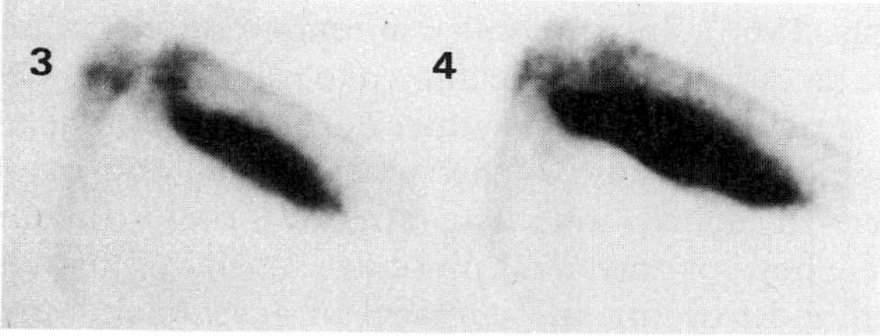

Fig. 23.3 Lateral views of the lower limb showing an abnormal increase of radioisotope (technetium-99m pyrophosphate) uptake in the calf muscles. The scans were taken 3 and 4 days after eccentric exercise by a normal individual, when the muscles were painful. Note greater area of increased uptake on day 4. The biopsy sample taken from the gastrocnemius muscle on day 4 is shown in Fig. 23.1A.

Imaging

Magnetic resonance imaging (MRI) techniques have the advantage of allowing tissue visualisation which is precise enough for differentiating one tissue from another. Individual muscle groups and also their relative composition of fat and water can be seen, enabling sensitive monitoring of therapies (Fleckenstein et al 1991b). In patients presenting with muscle pain, intramuscular masses (Turner et al 1991), abscesses (Stephenson et al 1991) and anomalous muscles (Paul et al 1991; Sanger et al 1991) have been identified.

Valuable information can be obtained for differential diagnosis and also in cases of referred pain (Chevalier et al 1991). MRI can determine the aetiology of shoulder (Fritz et al 1992) and foot pain (Kier et al 1991) with greater accuracy than either computerised tomographic arthrography or ultrasonography (Nelson et al 1991) and conventional radiographs (Kier et al 1991). Myositis ossificans circumspecta (pseudomalignant osseous soft tissue tumour) may be differentiated from malignant neoplasms (Ehara et al 1991). Imaging techniques may be combined with spectroscopy to study tumour site, size and metabolic characteristics (Zlatkin et al 1990).

In patients with an existing diagnosis of primary skeletal muscle disease, the distribution and severity of individual muscle involvement can be determined (Lamminen 1990; Fleckenstein et al 1991b). Exercise testing may reveal further abnormalities (Amendola et al 1990; Fleckenstein et al 1991a).

Traumatic and sports injuries are readily visualised (Fig. 23.2) (Fleckenstein et al 1989b; Greco et al 1991; Farley et al 1992) and may be accompanied by haemorrhage (De Smet et al 1990).

As with other investigations, the technique to be used should be chosen with care (Erlemann et al 1990; Greco et al 1991), and both the operator and obesity of the subject may affect accuracy (Nelson et al 1991).

Radioisotope scanning

This technique also allows the indentification of individual muscles, showing abnormal isotopic uptake and the extent and distribution of abnormality in affected muscles (Fig. 23.3). An excessive uptake of radioisotope-labelled complexes into muscle has been shown in a variety of muscle diseases, the majority of which are pain-free (Bellina et al 1978; Giraldi et al 1979). It has been suggested that the extent of uptake in patients with polymyositis and dermatomyositis has prognostic value (Buchpiguel et al 1991).

These techniques allow the affected bone and soft tissues to be identified in cases of trauma and sports injuries (Elgazzar et al 1989; Rockett & Freeman 1990). Muscular involvement may be identified in cases of ischaemic damage (Yip et al 1990; Rivera-Luna & Spiegler 1991) and peripheral vascular disease (Sayman & Urgancioglu 1991).

Increased muscle uptake of isotope has been observed after exercise in normal, pain-free individuals (Matin et al 1983; Valk 1984). When the pectoral muscles are involved there is the possibility of a false diagnosis of exercise-induced left ventricular dysfunction (Campeau et al 1990). Similar findings occur in those with delayed onset muscle pain (Jones et al 1986; Newham et al 1986b). Serial studies show that the time course of changes in muscle uptake parallel the changes in blood levels of CK (Jones et al 1986; Newham et al 1986b) and both presumably reflect changes in the integrity of the sarcolemma. The mechanism of increased isotope uptake is unclear (for review, see Brill 1981) and it appears that different mechanisms may be involved in different situations.

Exercise testing

The energy supply for muscle contraction is held in essentially three pools:

1. Creatine phosphate interacts with ADP to reform ATP, which forms an instantly available energy buffer but which can sustain energy supply for only a very short time.
2. Glycogen stores within muscle provide an intermediate energy supply system. Glycogen is a large glucose polymer linked by means of α_{1-4} linkages with α_{1-6} linkages at each branch point. Myophosphorylase cleaves glucose molecules from glycogen which is then degraded to provide ATP, with lactate produced as a by-product. Phosphofructokinase is the controlling enzyme in this metabolic sequence.
3. Long-term energy supply to muscle is provided by carbohydrate and fat. This energy supply is used in long-term, endurance-type exercise. The degree to which carbohydrate oxidation and fat oxidation are used to provide energy depends on the duration of the exercise and the availability of oxygen.

It can be seen that the energy supply to muscle is complex and exercise testing needs to be tailored to test specific aspects of the system.

There is a large literature on the response to exercise of normal individuals and in many disease categories exercise testing may be revealing (Jones et al 1975). Performance of whole-body exercise, such as cycle ergonometry, stresses not only the neuromuscular system but also the cardiovascular and respiratory systems and is of course dependent on the motivation of the subjects. The technique may be useful not only for assessing the overall work fitness of an individual, but can also provoke symmptoms in patients with muscle pain which can then be analysed further. Exercise testing can also be useful in the management of patients, in that they can be reassured that they can perform adequately without producing excessive pain.

Many protocols for progressive exercise tests on a cycle ergometer are available (Jones et al 1975). The aim is to assess the cardiovascular, respiratory and metabolic responses to exercise; blood pressure, heart rate, ventilation and blood lactate and pyruvate may be measured during and after the exercise. Submaximal exercise tests are usually performed at a work rate that is a fixed proportion of the previously determined maximal rate and continue for a fixed time with regular and frequent monitoring. Exercise testing is useful in patients with muscle pain when a metabolic muscle disease is suspected. In many mitochondrial myopathies (see below) there is a raised resting lactate which rises markedly after moderate exercise.

The prolonged exercise test (Brooke et al 1979) attempts to measure the individual's ability to switch to fatty acid oxidation once glycogen in muscle has been depleted.

Ischaemic forearm exercise tests (McArdle 1951; Munsat 1970; Sinkeler et al 1986) are designed to test the phosphorylase system in muscle. Essentially, a catheter is placed in a superficial vein and, with the arm rendered ischaemic by a cuff, the patient performs hand grips once a second for 1 minute. A workload of between 4 and 7 kg is required and blood is sampled at intervals for lactate. In normal subjects, lactate rises to between three and five times the resting level at 3 minutes. In McArdle's disease and phosphofructokinase deficiency, there is no rise in lactate. The tests should be performed with care since it is invasive and can also produce contractures in myophosphorylase-deficient patients.

Electromyography (EMG)

Electrical activity can be recorded from muscles, either with surface electrodes or with intramuscular recording needles. With the former, activity from a large volume of tissue can be recorded and this can be useful in the study of abnormalities in the gross pattern of muscle activation (e.g. kinaesiological studies) and in the study of fatigue. The electrical properties of the skin, however, effectively filter out diagnostic information from the muscle signal. For diagnostic purposes, needle EMG is required. Conventional concentric EMG needles record from a tissue volume of 1 mm radius and therefore sample from a large number of fibres, but only from a small proportion of the fibres belonging to one motor unit. EMG is useful in distinguishing primary muscle diseases from those conditions associated with abnormalities of the anterior horn cell or motor axons. In primary muscle disease, motor unit potentials recorded with a conventional concentric needle electrode consist of brief, small amplitude potentials. These summate to form a crowded recruitment pattern when the muscle is moderately activated. In contrast, in muscle which has undergone denervation followed by reinnervation, motor unit potentials of high amplitude and broad simple waveform are seen and, even when the muscle is producing its maximal force, they occur as discrete potentials repeating at high rates. In primary muscle disease, motor unit potentials may have maximal amplitude of 0.5–1 mV, whereas in chronic reinnervation due to a neurogenic process, motor unit potentials may be up to 20 mV in amplitude.

Healthy muscle at rest is electrically silent. Spontaneous muscle fibre potentials (fibrillations) are most characteristically seen in acute denervating processes, but may also be seen in muscular dystrophies and inflammatory muscle diseases.

Apart from this major function in distinguishing primary muscle and neurogenic diseases, EMG may also be useful in the investigation of muscle pain in other situations. It can detect myotonia when clinical myotonia is absent, and can distinguish the electrically silent contracture of McArdle's disease from the excessive motor unit activity of a muscle cramp. Combined with nerve conduction studies, EMG can be used to assess the distribution of muscles affected by denervation, and may help to provide information about which nerve or nerve roots are involved. EMG may also be useful in deciding which muscle is active in focal dystonia prior to botulinum toxin injection and can be helpful in selecting the appropriate muscle for biopsy, although clearly the site of needle entry should be avoided.

Measurements of muscle force

The two most common force-related symptoms are weakness and excessive fatigability. The two should be differentiated; weakness is a failure to achieve the expected force, while fatigue is an excessive loss of force generation during or after activity.

Measurements of maximal voluntary force generation, using either strain-gauge systems or dynamometers ranging from simple hand-held devices to expensive dynamic systems, provide information about the presence and distribution of weakness, as well as about longitudinal changes in strength (Edwards 1982; Edwards et al 1980, 1983). Percutaneous electrical stimulation, either through the motor nerve or its intramuscular nerves, can provide useful information about abnormalities in muscle contractile properties, i.e. force–frequency characteristics, relaxation rate and fatigability (Edwards et al 1977).

Patients with both myalgia and weakness are likely to have a specific muscle problem. The distribution may be informative, e.g. pain and weakness in the forearm and fingers may simply be a nerve entrapment syndrome whereas weakness of proximal muscles is often associated with primary muscle disease.

Muscle weakness and wasting are associated with, and may be the main presenting symptom of, both neuropathic and myopathic conditions, the former usually being pain-free. Electromyographic studies and clinical examination enable the two to be distinguished. Myopathies are subdivided into the atrophic and destructive forms. Atrophic myopathies may cause muscle pain (hypothyroid, osteomalacia) but others are not (steroid, Cushing's). The destructive myopathies are further subdivided into those of a destructive nature (the muscular dystrophies) and inflammatory (poly- and dermatomyositis). In both categories the relationship with pain is very variable and does not appear to correlate well with any findings. When muscular discomfort is reported it is usually described as aching, especially on activity but sometimes at rest, and also as muscle tenderness.

Muscle weakness and pain are reported by some, but not all, former victims of poliomyelitis. The underlying mechanism is unclear (Agre et al 1991).

In unilateral conditions the extent of weakness may be estimated by comparison of the muscle strength on the affected and unaffected sides. There is also a substantial body of literature on the strength of a number of muscle groups in healthy individuals in a wide age range.

With measurements of voluntary force there is always the possibility that poor motivation or central fatigue is preventing the generation of the maximal force of the muscle. The superimposition of electrical stimulation on a voluntary contraction determines if it is maximal or not (Fig. 23.4) (Belanger & McComas 1981; Rutherford et al 1986), since additional force is generated only if the voluntary contraction is submaximal. Furthermore, the true strength of the muscle can be estimated when the voluntary contraction is not maximal (Bigland-Ritchie et al 1983). Interestingly, patients with primary myopathy and myalgia rarely show central fatigue (Rutherford et al 1986). In contrast, mechanical joint damage which may be completely pain-free is strongly associated with an inability to produce a maximally activated voluntary contraction (Newham et al 1989).

Peripheral fatigue is a failure of force generation despite the muscle being fully activated by either a voluntary or electrically stimulated contraction. Undue fatigability of this type is seen without pain in myasthenia gravis and myotonic disorders (Wiles & Edwards 1977; Ricker et al 1978). Fatigability and pain are found in mitochondrial myopathies (De Jesus 1974; Edwards et al 1982b).

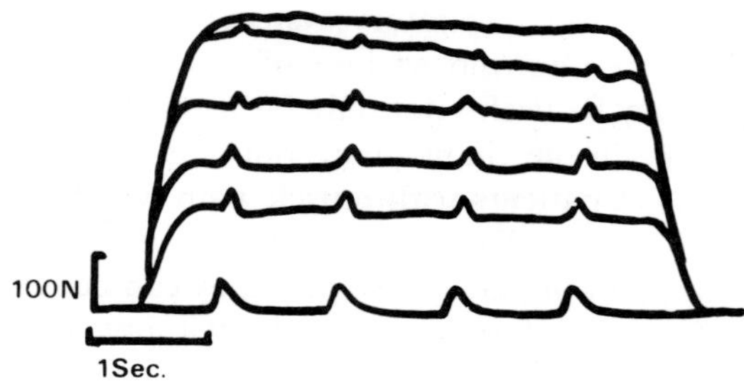

Fig. 23.4 Force traces from human muscle stimulated electrically with single impulses at 1 Hz. The muscle was stimulated at rest and during a series of voluntary contractions at varying forces up to maximum (top trace). Additional force is generated by electrical stimulation only when the voluntary contraction is submaximal and increases in amplitude as the level of voluntary activation decreases.

Using motor nerve stimulation, simultaneous measurements of force and the compound muscle action potential allow the investigation of excitation and activation. These techniques have revealed that the excessive peripheral fatigue in myophosphorylase deficiency is mainly due to a failure of muscle membrane excitation (Wiles et al 1981; Linssen et al 1990).

TREATMENT

Specific drug therapy for a specific disease is rarely attainable and even when the diagnosis is clear, treatment may be either unknown or controversial. In polymyositis, for example, steroid therapy may contribute to the pathological changes by superimposing a steroid myopathy (Edwards et al 1980).

A number of drugs are available for myalgia. Aspirin and many other steroidal and nonsteroidal anti-inflammatory drugs (e.g. ibuprofen, flurbiprofen, naproxen, indomethacin) may be used but no single preparation has been shown to be superior. Diazepam and other benzodiazepines may be effective for muscle 'spasm', as may baclofen or dantrolene sodium, although the latter may impair force generation.

Quinine sulphate has long been used to treat night cramps and those associated with haemodialysis. In the latter case the drug appears to reduce the frequency but not severity (Kaji et al 1976). Verapamil has helped some patients with exertional muscle pain (Lane et al 1986).

A wide range of physical therapies is used, particularly in the case of trauma and sport and traumatic injuries. The repertoire includes ice, transcutaneous nerve stimulation and a variety of electrical treatments. Despite the high incidence of these conditions, the effectiveness of these therapies in any particular situation has rarely been compared (Renstrom 1991). Both immobilisation and mobilisation are considered important at different stages (Lehto & Jarvinen 1991; Renstrom 1991). Immobilisation results in marked muscle atrophy which, although reversible, may delay full rehabilitation (Appell 1990).

Surgical intervention is indicated in cases of severe or complete muscle tears, severe haematomas and compartment syndromes.

Patients with myalgia of unknown aetiology may be offered a variety of treatments as part of behavioural therapy. Elimination of serious underlying pathology may be of reassurance. Those with diffuse myalgia may be profoundly unfit as a result of inactivity and some may have a degree of postural hypotension (Newham & Edwards 1979). A logical approach is to provide a well-supervised exercise programme (Edwards 1986) although the individual response to this is very variable. Most patients with ME report their symptoms to be increased by excessive exercise, although a carefully graded programme may be beneficial.

Dietary supplementation of essential fatty acids in ME (Behan et al 1990) and protein in McArdle's syndrome (Jensen et al 1990) has been reported to improve symptoms.

Occasionally, patients with mitochondrial cytopathies have been reported to respond to vitamins. The best documented example (Eleff et al 1984) is a patient with complex III deficiency in whom vitamins K_3 and C (which might be expected to bypass the metabolic defect) resulted in rapid clinical improvement.

REFERENCES

Abbott B C, Bigland B, Ritchie J M 1952 The physiological cost of negative work. Journal of Physiology 117: 380–390

Agre J C, Rodriquez A A, Tafel J A 1991 Late effects of polio: a critical review of the literature on neuromuscular function. Archives of Physical Medicine and Rehabilitation 72: 923–931

Aldridge R, Cady E B, Jones D A, Obletter G 1986 Muscle pain after exercise is linked with an inorganic phosphate increase as shown by 31P NMR. Bioscience Reports 6: 663–667

Allen M J 1990 Compartment syndromes of the lower limb. Journal of the Royal College of Surgeons of Edinburgh 35: S33–36

Amendola A, Rorabeck C H, Vellett D, Vezina W, Rutt B, Nott L 1990 The use of magnetic resonance imaging in extertional compartment syndromes. American Journal of Sports Medicine 18: 29–34

Angelini C, Luke S, Cantarutti F 1976 Carnitine deficiency of skeletal muscle: report of a treated case. Neurology 26: 633–637

Appell H J 1990 Muscular atrophy following immobilisation. A review. Sports Medicine 10: 42–58

Asmussen E 1956 Observations on experimental muscular soreness. Acta Rheumatologica Scandinavica 2: 109–116

Bank W J, Di Mauro S, Bonilla E, Capuzzi D M, Rowland L P 1975 A disorder of muscle lipid metabolism and myoglobinuria. Absence of carnitine palmityl transferase. New England Journal of Medicine 292: 443–449

Barany M, Siegel I M, Venkatasubrananian P N , Mok E, Wilbur A C 1989 Human leg neuromuscular diseases: P-31 MR spectroscopy. Radiology 172: 503–508

Bartels E M, Danneskiold-Samsöe B 1986 Histological abnormalities in muscle from patients with certain types of fibrositis. Lancet 1: 755–757

Barton N J, Hooper G, Noble J, Steel W M 1992 Occupational causes of disorders in the upper limb. British Medical Journal 304: 309–311

Behan P O, Bakheit A M O 1991 Clinical spectrum of postviral fatigue syndrome. In: Behan P O, Goldberg D P, Mowbray J F (eds) Postviral fatigue syndrome. British Medical Bulletin 47: 793–809

Behan P O, Behan W M, Horrobin D 1990 Effects of high doses of essential fatty acids on the postviral fatigue syndrome. Acta Neurologica Scandinavica 82: 209–216

Behan P O, Goldberg D P, Mowbray J F (eds) 1991 Postviral fatigue syndrome. British Medical Bulletin 47(4)

Belanger A Y, McComas A J 1981 Extent of voluntary unit activation during effort. Journal of Applied Physiology 51: 1131–1135

Bellina C R, Biachi R, Bombardini S et al 1978 Quantitative evaluation of ^{99m}Tc pyrophosphate muscle uptake in patients with inflammatory and non-inflammatory muscle diseases. Journal of Nuclear Medicine 22: 89–96

Bengtsson A 1986 Primary fibromyalgia. A clinical and laboratory study. Linkoping University Dissertation no. 224

Bengtsson A, Henriksson K-G, Jarson J 1986a Muscle biopsy in primary fibromyalgia. Light microscopical and histochemical findings. Scandinavian Journal of Rheumatology 15: 1–6

Bengtsson A, Henriksson K-G, Jarson J 1986b Reduced high energy phosphate levels in painful muscle in patients with primary fibromyalgia. Arthritis and Rheumatism 29: 817–821

Bennett R M 1981 Fibrositis: misnomer for a common rheumatic disorder. Western Journal of Medicine 134: 405–413

Bertorini T, Yeh Y Y, Trevisan C, Standlan E, Sabesin S, Di Mauro S 1980 Carnitine palmityltransferase deficiency: myoglobinuria and respiratory failure. Neurology 30: 263–271

Bessou P, Laporte Y 1961 Some observations on receptors of the soleus muscle innervated by group III afferent fibers. Journal of Physiology 155: 19P

Bigland-Ritchie B, Jones D A, Hosking G P, Edwards R H T 1978 Central and peripheral fatigue in sustained maximum voluntary contractions of human quadriceps muscle. Clinical Science and Molecular Medicine 54: 609–614

Bigland-Ritchie B, Furbush F, Woods J J 1986 Neuromuscular transmission and muscular activation in human post-fatigue ischaemia. Journal of Physiology 337: 76P

Bird H A, Esselinck W, Dixon A St J, Mowat A G, Wood P H N 1979 An evaluation of the criteria for polymyalgia rheumatica. Annals of the Rheumatic Diseases 38: 424–439

Bohan A, Peter J B 1975a Polymyositis and dermatomyositis: part 1. New England Journal of Medicine 292: 344–347

Bohan A, Peter J B 1975b Polymyositis and dermatomyositis: part 2. New England Journal of Medicine 292: 402–407

Bollaert P E, Robin-Lherbier B, Escanye J M, et al 1989 Phosphorus nuclear magnetic resonance evidence of abnormal skeletal muscle metabolism in chronic alcoholics. Neurology 39: 821–824

Booth D W, Westers B M 1989 The management of athletes with myositis ossificans traumatica. Canadian Journal of Sport Science 14: 10–16

Brill D R 1981 Radionuclide imaging of non-neoplastic soft tissue disorders. Seminars in Nuclear Medicine 11: 277–288

Brooke M H 1986 A clinician's view of neuromuscular diseases, 2nd. edn. Williams & Wilkins, Baltimore

Brooke M H, Carroll J E, Hagberg J M 1979 The prolonged exercise test. Neurology 29: 636–643

Buchpiguel C A, Roizenblatt S, Lucena-Fernandes M F et al 1991 Radioisotopic assessment of peripheral and cardiac muscle involvement and dysfunction in polymyositis/dermatomyositis. Journal of Rheumatology 18: 1359–1363

Bunch T W, Worthington J W, Combs J J, Ilstrup D M, Engel A G 1980 Azathioprine with prednisone for polymyositis. Annals of Internal Medicine 92: 365–369

Cady E B, Griffiths R D, Edwards R H T 1985 The clinical use of nuclear magnetic resonance spectroscopy for studying human muscle metabolism. International Journal of Technological Assessment in Health Care 1: 631–645

Cady E B, Jones D A, Lynn J, Newham D J 1989 Changes in force and intracellular metabolites during fatigue of human skeletal muscle. Journal of Physiology 418: 311–325

Campeau R J, Garcia O M, Correa O A, Mace J E 1990 Pectoralis muscle uptake of thallium-201 after arm exercise ergometry. Possible confusion with lung thallium-201 activity. Clinical Nuclear Medicine 15: 303–306

Carpenter S, Karpati G 1981 The major inflammatory myopathies of unknown cause, Pathological Annual 16: 205–237

Carpenter J R, Bunch T W, Angel A G, O'Brien P C 1977 Survival in polymyositis: corticosteroids and risk factors. Journal of Rheumatology 4: 207–214

Carroll J E, De Vivo D C, Brooke M H, Planner G J, Hagberg J H 1979 Fasting as a provocative test in neuromuscular diseases. Metabolism 28: 683–687

Carroll J E, Brooke M H, De Vivo D C et al 1980 Carnitine 'deficiency': lack of response to carnitine therapy. Neurology 30: 618–626

Chance B, Eleff S, Bank W, Leigh J R, Warnell R 1982 ^{31}P NMR studies of control of mitochondrial function in phosphofructokinase deficient human skeletal muscle. Proceedings of the National Academy of Sciences 79: 7714–7718

Chevalier X, Wrona N, Avouac B, Larget B 1991 Thigh pain and multiple osteonecrosis: value of magnetic resonance imaging. Journal of Rheumatology 18: 1627–1630

Chou S M 1988 Viral myositis. In Mastaglia F L (ed) Inflammatory diseases of muscle, 1st edn. Blackwell, Oxford, p 125–153

Coote J H, Perez-Gonzales J F 1971 The reflex nature of the pressure response to muscular exercise. Journal of Physiology 215: 789–804

Currie S 1981 Inflammatory mypathies. Polymyositis and related disorders. In: Walton J N (ed) Disorders of voluntary muscle, 4th edn. Churchill Livingstone, Edinburgh, p 525–568

Curtin N A, Davies R E 1973 Chemical and mechanical changes during stretching of activated frog muscle. Cold Spring Harbor Symposia on Quantitative Biology 37: 619–626

Dalakas M C (ed) 1988 Polyositis and dermatomyositis. 1st edn. Butterworths, Boston

Daube J R 1981 Quantitative EMG in nerve-muscle disorders. In: Stålberg E, Young R R (eds) Neurology 1: Clinical neurophysiology. Butterworths, London

Dawson J 1990 Consensus on research into fatigue syndrome. British Medical Journal 300: 832

De Blecourt A C, Wolf R F, van Rijswijk M H et al 1991 In vivo ^{31}P magnetic resonance spectroscopy (MRS) of tender points in patients with primary fibromyalgia syndrome. Rheumatology International 1: 51–54

De Jesus P V 1974 Neuromuscular physiology in Luft's syndrome. Electroencephalography and Clinical Neurophysiology 14: 17–27

Demos M A, Gitlin E L, Kagen L 1974 Exercise myoglobinuria and acute exertional rhabdomyolysis. Archives of Internal Medicine 134: 669–673

De Smet A A, Fischer D R, Heiner J P, Keene J S 1990 Magnetic resonance imaging of muscle tears. Skeletal Radiology 19: 283–286

Desmedt J E (ed) 1983 Computer aided electromyography. Progress in clinical neurophysiology, vol 10. Karger, Basle

De Vere R, Bradley W G 1975 Polymyositis: its presentation, morbidity and mortality. Brain 98: 637–666

Dietrichson P, Oakley J, Smith P E M, Griffiths R D, Helliwell T R, Edwards R H T 1987 Conchotome and needle percutaneous biopsy of skeletal muscle. Journal of Neurology, Neurosurgery and Psychiatry 50: 1461–1476

Di Mauro S, Di Mauro P M 1973 Muscle carnitine palmityltransferase deficiency and myoglobinuria. Science 182: 929–931

Di Mauro S, Miranda A F, Olarte M, Friedman R, Hays A P 1982 Muscle phosphoglycerate mutase (GAM) deficiency: a new metabolic myopathy. Neurology 32: 584–591

Di Mauro S, Dalakas M, Miranda A F 1983 Phosphoglycerate kinase deficiency: another cause of recurrent myoglobinuria. Annals of Neurology 13: 11–19

Douglas J G, Ford M J, Innes J A, Munro J F 1979 Polmyalgia arteritica: a clinical review. European Journal of Clinical Investigation 9: 137–140

Edwards R H T 1982 Weakness and fatigue of skeletal muscles. In: Sarner M (ed) Advanced medicine 18. Pitman Medical, London, p 100–119

Edwards R H T 1986 Muscle fatigue and pain. Acta Medica Scandinavica (suppl) 711: 179–188

Edwards R H T, Young A, Hosking G P, Jones D A 1977 Human skeletal muscle function: description of tests and normal values. Clinical Science and Molecular Medicine 52: 283–290

Edwards R H T, Young A, Wiles C M 1980 Needle biopsy of skeletal muscle in diagnosis of myopathy and the clinical study of muscle function and repair. New England Journal of Medicine 302: 261–271

Edwards R H T, Isenberg D A, Wiles C M, Young A, Snaith M L 1981 The investigation of inflammatory myopathy. Journal of the Royal College of Physicians 15: 19–24

Edwards R H T, Dawson M J, Wilkie D R, Gordon R E, Shaw D 1982a Clinical use of nuclear magnetic resonance in the investigation of myopathy. Lancet 1: 725–731

Edwards R H T, Wiles C M, Gohil K, Krywawych S, Jones D A 1982b Energy metabolism in human myopathy. In: Schotland D C (ed) Disorders of the motor unit. Wiley, London, p 715–728

Edwards R H T, Wiles C M, Mills K R 1983 Quantitation of human muscle function. In: Dyck P, Thomas P K, Lambert E H (eds) Peripheral neuropathy. W B Saunders, Philadelphia, p 1093–1102

Edwards R H T, Newham D J, Peters T J 1991 Muscle biochemistry and pathophysiology in postviral fatigue syndrome. In: Behan P O, Goldberg D P, Mowbray J F (eds) Postviral fatigue syndrome. British Medical Bulletin 47: 826–837

Ehara S, Nakasato T, Tamakawa Y et al 1991 MRI of myositis ossificans circumscripta. Clinical Imaging 15: 130–134

Eleff S, Kennaway N G, Buist N R M et al 1984 ^{31}P–NMR studies of improvement of oxidative phosphorylation by vitamins K3 and C in a patient with a defect in electron transport and complex III in skeletal muscle. Proceedings of the National Academy of Sciences USA 81: 3529–3533

Elgazzar A H, Malki A A, Abdel-Dayem H M, et al 1989 Indium-111 monoclonal anti-myosin antibody in assessing skeletal muscle damage in trauma. Nuclear Medicine Communications 10: 661–667

Engel A G, Sieckert R G 1972 Lipid storage myopathy responsive to prednisone. Archives of Neurology 27: 174–181

Erlemann R, Vassallo P, Bongartz G et al 1990 Musculoskeletal neoplasm: fast low-angle shot MR imaging with and without Gd-DTPA. Radiology 176: 489–495

Farley T E, Neumann C H, Steinbach L S, Jahnke A J, Petersen S S1992 Full-thickness tears of the rotator cuff of the shoulder: diagnosis with MR imaging. American Journal of Roentgenology 158: 347–351

Fechner G, Hauser R, Sepulchre M A, Brinkman B 1991 Immunohistochemical investigations to demonstrate vital direct damage of skeletal muscle. International Journal of Legal Medicine 104: 215–219

Fishbein W N, Armbrustmacher K W, Griffin J L 1978 Myoadenylate deaminase deficiency: a new disease of muscle. Science 200: 545–548

Fleckenstein J L, Bertocci L A, Nunnally R L, Parkey R W, Peshock R M 1989a Exercise-enhanced MR imaging of variations in forearm muscle anatomy and use; importance in MR spectroscopy. American Journal of Roentgenology 153: 693–698

Fleckenstein J L, Weatherall P T, Parkey R W, Payne J A, Peshock R M 1989b Sports-related muscle injuries: evaluation with MR imaging. Radiology 172: 793–798

Fleckenstein J L, Haller R G, Lewis S F et al 1991a Absence of exercise-induced MRI enhancement of skeletal muscle in McArdle's disease. Journal of Applied Physiology 71: 961–969

Fleckenstein J L, Weatherall P T, Bertocci L A et al 1991b Locomotor system assessment by muscle magnetic resonance imaging. Magnetic Resonance Quarterly 7: 79–103

Friden J 1984 Muscle soreness after exercise: implications of morphological changes. International Journal of Sports Medicine 5: 57–66

Friden J, Sfakianos P N, Hargens A R 1986 Delayed muscle soreness and intramuscular fluid pressure: comparison between eccentric and concentric load. Journal of Applied Physiology 61: 2175–2179

Fritz R C, Helms C A, Steinbach L S, Genant K K 1992 Suprascapular nerve entrapment: evaluation with MR imaging. Radiology 182: 437–444

Fry H J H 1986 Overuse syndrome of the upper limb in musicians. Medical Journal of Australia 144: 182–185

Fry R W, Morton A R, Keast D 1991 Overtraining in athletes. An update. Sports Medicine 12: 32–65

Gadian D G, Radda G K, Ross B D et al 1981 Examinations of a myopathy by phosphorus nuclear magnetic resonance. Lancet 2: 774–775

Giraldi C, Marciani G, Molla N, Rossi B 1979 99m Tc-pyrophosphate muscle uptake in four subjects with Becker's disease. Journal of Nuclear Medicine 23: 45–47

Gohil K, Jones D A, Edwards R H T 1981 Analysis of muscle mitochondrial function with techniques applicable to needle biopsy samples. Clinical Physiology 1: 195–207

Gordon E E, Januszko D M, Kaufman L 1967 A critical survey of stiff-man syndrome. American Journal of Medicine 42: 582–599

Gould S E (ed) 1970 Trichinosis in man and animals. C C Thomas, Springfield, Illinois, p 147–189

Greco A, McNamara M T, Escher R M, Trifilio G, Parienti J 1991 Spin-echo and STIR imaging of sports related injuries at 1.5 T. Journal of Computer Assisted Tomography 15: 994–999

Griffiths P D 1966 Serum levels of ATP and creatine phosphotranferase (creatine kinase). The normal range and effect of muscular activity. Clinica Chimica Acta 13: 413–420

Hamrin B 1972 Polymyalgia rheumatica. Acta Medica Scandinavica (suppl) 553: 1–131

Hands C J, Bone P J, Galloway G, Morris P J, Radda G K 1986 Muscle metabolism in patients with peripheral vascular disease investigated by ^{31}P nuclear magnetic resonance spectroscopy. Clinical Science 71: 283–290

Hands L J, Sharif M H, Payne G S, Morris P J, Radda G K 1990 Muscle ischaemia in peripheral vascular disease studied by 31P-magnetic resonance spectroscopy. European Journal of Vascular Surgery 4: 637–642

Haslock D I, Wright V, Harriman D G F 1970 Neuromuscular disorders in rheumatoid arthritis. A motor-point muscle biopsy study. Quarterly Journal of Medicine 39: 335–358

Hayes D J, Lecky B R F, Landon D N, Morgan-Hughes J A, Clark J B 1984 A new mitochondrial myopathy: biochemical studies revealing a deficiency in the cytochrome b-c_1 complex (complex III) of the respiratory chain. Brain 107: 1165–1177

Hayward M, Willison R G 1973 The recognition of myogenic and neurogenic lesions by quantitative EMG. In: Desmedt J E (ed) New developments in electromyography and clinical neurophysiology, vol 2. Karger, Basle p 448–453

Headley S A, Newham D J, Jones D A 1986 The effect of prednisolone on exercise induced muscle pain and damage. Clinical Science 70: 85P

Hudson J, Brown W F, Gilbert J J 1978 The muscular pain–fasciculation syndrome. Neurology 28: 1105–1109

Iggo A 1961 Non-myelinated afferent fibers from mammalian skeletal muscle. Journal of Physiology 155: 52–53P

Ionasescu V, Hug G, Hoppel C 1980 Combined partial deficiency of muscle carnitine palmityltransferase and carnitine with autosomal dominant inheritance. Journal of Neurology, Neurosurgery and Psychiatry 43: 679–682

Isaacs H 1961 A syndrome of continuous muscle fibre activity. Journal of Neurology, Neurosurgery and Psychiatry 24: 319–325

Itoi E, Tabata S 1992 Conservative treatment of rotator cuff tears. Clinical Orthopaedics 275: 165–173

Janssen E, Kuipers H, Venstrappen F T J, Costill D L 1983 Influence of an anti-inflammatory drug on muscle soreness. Medicine and Science in Sports and Exercise 15: 165

Jeffrey H C 1974 Sarcosporidosis in man. Transactions of the Royal Society of Tropical Medicine and Hygiene 68: 17–29

Jensen K E, Jakobsen J, Thomsen C, Henriksen O 1990 Improved energy kinetics following high protien diet in McArdle's syndrome. A 31P magnetic resonance spectroscopy study. Acta Neurologica Scandinavica 81: 499–503

Jones D A, Newham D J, Round J M, Tolfree S E J 1986 Experimental human muscle damage: morphological changes in relation to other indices of damage. Journal of Physiology 375: 435–448

Jones N L, Campbell E J M, Edwards R H T, Robertson D G 1975 Clinical exercise testing. W B Saunders, Philadelphia

Kaji D M, Ackad A, Nottage W G, Stein R M 1976 Prevention of muscle cramps on haemodialysis patients by quinine sulphate. Lancet 2: 66–67

Kalia M, Serapati B P, Panda A 1972 Reflex increase in ventilation by muscle receptors with non-modulated fibers (C-fibers). Journal of Applied Physiology 32: 189–193

Kaminsky P, Robin Lherbier B, Brunotte F, Escanye J M, Walker P 1992 Energetic metabolism in hypothyroid skeletal muscle, as studied by phosphorus magnetic resonance spectroscopy. Journal of Clinical Endocrinology and Metabolism 74: 124–129

Kanno T, Sudo K, Takeuchi I et al 1980 Hereditary deficiency of lactate dehydrogenase M subunit. Clinica Chimica Acta 108: 267–276

Karpati G, Carpenter S, Engel A et al 1975 The syndrome of systemic carnitine deficiency. Neurology 25: 16–24

Katz B 1939 The relation between force and speed in muscular contraction. Journal of Physiology 96: 46–64

Kier R, McCarthy S, Dietz M J, Rudicel S 1991 MR appearance of painful conditions of the ankle. Radiographics 11: 401–414

Kniffki K D, Mense S, Schmidt R F 1978 Response of group IV afferent units from skeletal muscle to stretch, contraction and chemical stimulation. Experimental Brain Research 31: 511–522

Knighton R S, Dumke P R 1966 Pain. Little, Brown, Boston
Kretzler H H Jr, Richardson A B 1989 Rupture of the pectoralis major muscle. American Journal of Sports Medicine 17: 453–458
Kuipers H, Kieren H A, Venstrappen F T J, Costill D L 1983 Influence of a prostaglandin inhibiting drug on muscle soreness after eccentric work. Journal of Sports Medicine 6: 336–339
Kumazawa T, Mizumura K 1977 Thin fibre receptors responding to mechanical, chemical and thermal stimulation in the skeletal muscle of the dog. Journal of Physiology 273: 179–194
Lamminen A E 1990 Magnetic resonance imaging of primary skeletal diseases: patterns of distribution and severity of involvement. British Journal of Radiology 63: 946–950
Land J M, Clark J B 1979 Mitochondrial myopathies. Biochemical Society Transactions 7: 231–245
Lane R J M, Mastaglia F L 1978 Drug-induced myopathies in man. Lancet 2: 562–566
Lane R J M, Turnbull D M, Welch J L, Walton J 1986 A double blind placebo controlled cross-over study of verapamil on exertional muscle pain. Muscle and Nerve 9: 635–641
Layzer R B 1986 Muscle pain, cramps and fatigue. In: Engel AG (ed) Myology, 1st edn. McGraw Hill, New York, p 1907–1922
Layzer R B, Rowland L P 1971 Cramps. New England Journal of Medicine 285: 31–40
Layzer R B, Rowland L P, Ranney H M 1967 Muscle phosphofructokinase activity. Archives of Neurology 17: 512–523
Lavigne G J, Velly-Miguel A M, Montplaisir J 1991 Muscle pain, dyskinesia and sleep. Canadian Journal of Physiology and Pharmacology 69: 678–682
Lazaro R P, Rollinson R D, Fenichez G M 1981 Familial cramps and muscle pain. Archives of Neurology 38: 22–24
Lehto M U, Jarvinen M J 1991 Muscle injuries, their healing processes and treatment. Annales Chirurgiae et Gynaecologiae 80: 102–108
Lendinger M I, Sjogaard G 1991 Potassium regulation during exercise and recovery. Sports Medicine 11: 382–401
Linssen W H, Jacobs M, Stegman D F, Joosten E M, Moleman J 1990 Muscle fatigue in McArdle's disease. Muscle fibre conduction velocity and surface EMG frequency spectrum during ischaemic exercise. Brain 113: 1779–1793
Lloyd A R, Gandevia S C, Hales J P 1991 Muscle performance, voluntary activation, twitch properties and perceived effort in normal subjects and patients with the chronic fatigue syndrome. Brain 114: 85–98
Lotz B P, Enger A G, Nishino H, St Evens J C, Litchy W J 1989 Inclusion body myositis. Observations on 40 cases. Brain 122: 727–747
McArdle B 1951 Myopathy due to a defect in muscle glycogen breakdown. Clinical Science 10: 13–33
McCloskey D I, Mitchell J H 1972 Reflex cardiovascular and respiratory responses originating in exercising muscle. Journal of Physiology 224: 173–186
McCully K K, Argov Z, Boden B A, Brown R L, Blank W J, Chance B 1988 Detection of muscle injury in humans with 31P magnetic resonance spectroscopy. Muscle and Nerve 11: 212–216
McKeran R O, Halliday D, Purkiss D 1977 Increased myofibrillar protein catabolism in Duchenne muscular dystrophy measured by 3-methylhistidine excretion in the urine. Journal of Neurology, Neurosurgery and Psychiatry 40: 979–981
McMahon S, Koltzenburg M 1990 The changing role of afferent neurones in pain. Pain 43: 269–272
Martens M A, Moeyerssoons J P 1990 Acute and recurrent effort-related compartment syndrome in sports. Sports Medicine 9: 62–68
Mastaglia F L (ed) 1988 Inflammatory diseases of muscle, 1st edn. Blackwell, Oxford
Matthews P M, Allaire C, Shoubridge E A, Karpati G, Carpenter S, Arnold D L 1991a In vivo muscle magnetic resonance spectroscopy in the clinical investigation of mitochondrial disease. Neurology 41: 114–120
Matthews P M, Berkovic S F, Shoubridge E A, et al 1991b In vivo magnetic resonance spectroscopy of brain and muscle in a type of mitochondrial encephalomyopathy (MERRF). Annals of Neurology 29: 435–438
Marinacci A A 1965 Electromyography in the diagnosis of polymyositis. Electromyography 5: 255–268
Matin P, Lang G, Ganetta R, Simon G 1983 Scintiographic evaluation of muscle damage following extreme exercise. Journal of Nuclear Medicine 24: 308–311
Menard M R, Penn A M, Lee J E, Dusik L A, Hall L D 1991 Relative metabolic efficiency of concentric and eccentric exercise determined by 31P magnetic resonance spectroscopy. Archives of Physical Medicine and Rehabilitation 72: 976–983
Mense S 1977 Nervous outflow from skeletal muscle during chemical noxious stimulation. Journal of Physiology 267: 75–88
Mense S 1982 Reduction of the bradykinin induced activation of feline group III and IV muscle receptors by acetylsalicylic acid. Journal of Physiology 376: 269–283
Mense S, Schmidt R F 1977 Muscle pain: which receptors are responsible for the transmission of noxious stimuli? In: Clifford Rose F (ed) Physiological aspects of clinical neurology. Blackwell, Oxford, p 265–278
Middleton P J, Alexander R M, Szymanski M T 1970 Severe myositis during recovery from influenza. Lancet 2: 532
Mills K R, Edwards R H T 1983 Investigative strategies for muscle pain. Journal of the Neurological Sciences 58: 73–88
Mills K R, Willison R G 1987 Quantification of EMG on volition. In: The London Symposia (electroencephalography and clinical neurophysiology, suppl 39). Elsevier, Amsterdam, p 27–32
Mills K R, Newham D J, Edwards R H T 1982a Force, contraction frequency and energy metabolism as interactive determinants of ischaemic muscle pain. Pain 14: 149–154
Mills K R, Newham D J, Edwards R H T 1982b Severe muscle cramps relieved by transcutaneous nerve stimulation. Journal of Neurology, Neurosurgery and Psychiatry 45: 539–542
Millward D J, Bates P C, Grimble G K, Brown J G, Nathan M, Rennie M J 1980 Quantitative importance of non-skeletal muscle sources of N^T methylhistidine in urine. Biochemical Journal 190: 225–228
Moersch F P, Woltman H W 1956 Progressive fluctuating muscular rigidity and spasm ('stiff man' syndrome): report of a case and some observations in 13 other cases. Proceedings of the Staff Meetings of the Mayo Clinic 31: 421–427
Mommaerts W F H M, Illingworth B, Pearson C M, Guillory R J, Seraydarian K 1959 A functional disorder of phosphorylase. Proceedings of the National Academy of Sciences 45: 791–797
Morgan-Hughes J A 1982 Defects of the energy pathways of skeletal muscle. In: Matthews W B, Glaser G H (eds) Recent advances in clinical neurology 3. Churchill Livingstone, Edinburgh, p 1–46
Morgan-Hughes J A, Darveniza P, Landon D N, Land J M, Clark J D 1979 A mitochondrial myopathy characterised by a deficiency of reducible cytochrome B. Brain 100: 617–640
Morgan-Hughes J M, Cooper J M, Schapira A H V, Hayes D J, Clark J B 1987 The mitochondrial myopathies. Defects of the mitochondrial respiratory chain and oxidative phosphorylation system. In: Ellingson J R, Murray N M F, Halliday A M (eds). The London Symposia (electroencephalography and clinical neurophysiology, suppl 39). Elsevier, Amsterdam, p 103–114
Munsat T L 1970 A standardised forearm ischaemic test. Neurology 20: 1171–1178
Narayana P A, Slopis J M, Jackson E F, Jazle J D, Kulkarni M V, Butler I J 1989 In vivo muscle magnetic resonance spectroscopy in a family with mitochondrial cytopathy. A defect in fat metabolism. Magnetic Resonance Imaging 7: 33–39
Nelson M C, Leather G P, Nirschl R P, Pettrone F A, Freedman M T 1991 Evaluation of the painful shoulder. A prospective comparison of magnetic resonance imaging, computerized tomographic arthrography, ultrasonography and operative findings. Journal of Bone and Joint Surgery 73A: 707–716
Newham D J 1988 The consequences of eccentric contractions and their relation to delayed onset muscle pain. European Journal of Applied Physiology 57: 353–359
Newham D J, Cady E B 1990 A 31P study of fatigue and metabolism in human skeletal muscle with voluntary, intermittent contractions at different forces. NMR in Biomedicine 3: 211–219
Newham D J, Edwards R H T 1979 Effort syndromes. Physiotherapy 65: 52–56
Newham D J, Jones D A 1985 Intramuscular pressure in the painful human biceps. Clinical Science 69: 27P

Newham D J, Jones D A, Edwards R H T 1983a Large and delayed plasma creatine kinase changes after stepping exercise. Muscle and Nerve 6: 36–41

Newham D J, McPhail G, Mills K R, Edwards R H T 1983b Ultrastructural changes after concentric and eccentric contractions. Journal of Neurological Science 61: 109–122

Newham D J, Mills K R, Quigley B M, Edwards R H T 1983c Pain and fatigue after eccentric contractions. Clinical Science 64: 55–62

Newham D J, Jones D A, Edwards 1986a Plasma creatine changes after eccentric and concentric contractions. Muscle and Nerve 9: 59–63

Newham D J, Jones D A, Tolfree S E J, Edwards R H T 1986b Skeletal muscle damage: a study of isotope uptake enzyme efflux and pain after stepping exercise. European Journal of Applied Physiology 55: 106–112

Newham D J, Hurley M V, Jones D W 1989 Ligamentous knee injuries and muscle inhibition. Journal of Orthopaedic Rheumatology 2: 163–173

Newsom-Davies J M, Mills K R 1992 Immunological associations in acquired neuromyotonia (Isaacs' syndrome): report of 5 cases and literature review. Brain 116: 453–469

Paintal A S 1960 Functional analysis of group III and IV afferent fibers of mammalian muscle. Journal of Physiology 152: 250–270

Park S R, Rodbard S 1962 Effects of load and duration of tension on pain induced by muscular tension. American Journal of Physiology 203: 735–738

Paster S B, Adams D I, Hollenberg N K 1975 Acute renal failure in McArdle's disease and myoglobinuric states. Radiology 114: 567–570

Paul M A, Imanse J, Golding R P, Koomen A R, Meijer S 1991 Accessory soleus muscle mimicking a soft tissue tumour. Acta Orthopaedica Scandinavica 62: 609–611

Pearson C M, Bohan A 1977 The spectrum of polymyositis and dermatomyositis. Medical Clinics of North America 61: 349–357

Penn A S 1980 Myoglobin and myoglobinuria. In: Vinken P J, Bruhn G W (eds) Handbook of clinical neurology. Elsevier, Amsterdam

Perkoff G T, Hardy P, Velez-Garcia E 1966 Reversible acute muscular syndrome in chronic alcoholism. New England Journal of Medicine 274: 1277–1285

Pernow B B, Havel R J, Jennings D B 1967 The second wind phenomenon in McArdle's syndrome. Acta Medica Scandinavica (suppl) 472: 294–307

Petty R K H, Harding A E, Morgan-Hughes J A 1986 The clinical features of mitochondrial myopathy. Brain 109: 915–938

Prasher D, Smith A, Findley L 1990 Sensory and cognitive event-related potentials in myalgic encephalomyelitis. Journal of Neurology, Neurosurgery and Psychiatry 53: 247–253

Radda G K, Bone P J, Rajagoplan B 1984 Clinical aspects of ^{31}P NMR spectroscopy. British Medical Bulletin 40: 155–159

Renstrom P 1991 Sports traumatology today. A review of common sports injury problems. Annales Chirugiae et Gynaecologiae 80: 81–93

Ricker K, Haass A, Hertel G, Mertens H G 1978 Transient muscular weakness in severe recessive myotonia congenita. Journal of Neurology 218: 253–262

Riddoch J, Morgan-Hughes J A 1975 Prognosis in adult polymyositis. Journal of the Neurological Sciences 26: 71–80

Rivera-Luna H, Spiegler E J 1991 Incidental rectus abdominis muscle visualization during bone scanning. Clinical Nuclear Medicine 16: 523–527

Rockett J F, Freeman B L 1990 3D scintigraphic demonstration of pectineus muscle avulsion injury. Clinical Nuclear Medicine 15: 800–803

Rodbard S, Pragay E B 1968 Contraction frequency, blood supply and muscle pain. Journal of Applied Physiology 24: 142–145

Ross B D, Radda G K, Gadian D G, Rolker G, Esiri M, Falloner-Smith J 1981 Examination of a case of suspected McArdle's syndrome with ^{31}P nuclear magnetic resonance. New England Journal of Medicine 304: 1338–1342

Rowland L P, Tahn S, Hirschberg E, Harter D H 1964 Myoglobinuria. Archives of Neurology 10: 537–562

Rutherford O M, Jones D A, Newham D J 1986 Clinical and experimental application of the switch superimposition technique for the study of human muscle activation. Journal of Neurology, Neurosurgery and Psychiatry 49: 1288–1291

Rutherford O M, White J 1991 Human quadriceps strength and fatigability in patients with post-viral syndrome. Journal of Neurology, Neurosurgery and Psychiatry 54: 961–964

Safran M R, Seaber A V, Garrett W E Jr 1989 Warm-up and muscular injury prevention. An update. Sports Medicine 8: 239–249

Sanger J R, Krasniak C L, Matloub H S, Yousif N J, Kneeland J B 1991 Diagnosis of an anomalous superficialis muscle in the palm by magnetic resonance imaging. Journal of Hand Surgery (America) 16: 98–101

Sayman H B, Urgancioglu I 1991 Muscle perfusion with technetium-MIBI in lower extremity peripheral arterial diseases. Journal of Nuclear Medicine 32: 1700–1703

Schmid R, Hammaker L, 1961 Hereditary absence of muscle phosphorylase (McArdle's syndrome). New England Journal of Medicine 264: 223–225

Schmid R, Mahler R 1959 Chronic progressive myopathy with myoglobinuria: demonstration of a glycogenolytic defect in muscle. Journal of Clinical Investigation 38: 2044–2058

Schwartz M S, Swash M, Gross M 1978 Benign post-infection polymyositis. British Medical Journal 2: 1256–1257

Serratrice G, Gastaut J L, Schiand A, Pellissier J F, Carrelet P 1980 A propos de 210 cas de myalgies diffuses. Semaine des Hopitaux de Paris 56: 1241–1244

Sherrington C S 1900 Cutaneous sensations. In Schäfer's textbook of physiology. Y J Pentland, London, vol 2, p 920–1001

Shumate J B, Katnik R, Ruiz M et al 1979 Myoadenylate deaminase deficiency. Muscle and Nerve 2: 213–216

Sinkeler S P, Wevers R A, Joosten E M et al 1986 Improvement of screening of exertional myalgia with a standardised ischaemic forearm test. Muscle and Nerve 9: 731–737

Smith R, Stern G 1967 Myopathy, osteomalacia and hyperparathyroidism. Brain 90: 593–602

Stacey M J 1969 Free nerve endings in skeletal muscle of the cat. Journal of Anatomy 105: 231–254

Stälberg E 1980 Macro EMG, a new recording technique. Journal of Neurology, Neurosurgery and Psychiatry 43: 475–482

Stauber W 1989 Eccentric action of muscles: physiology, injury and adaptation. In: Pandolf K B (ed) Exercise and sports sciences reviews, vol 17. Williams & Wilkins, Baltimore, p 157–186

Stephenson C A, Seibert J J, Golladay E S et al 1991 Abscess of the iliopsoas muscle diagnosed by magnetic resonance imaging and ultrasonography. Southern Medical Journal 84: 509–511

Stokes M, Cooper R, Edwards R H T 1988 Normal strength and fatigability in patients with effort syndrome. British Medical Journal 297: 1014–1018

Stout A P 1946 Rhabdomyosarcoma of the skeletal muscles. Annals of Surgery 123: 447–472

Sylven C, Jonzon B, Fredholm B B, Kaijser L 1988 Adenosine injection into the brachial artery produces ischaemia-like pain or discomfort in the forearm. Cardiovascular Research 22: 674–678

Taimela S, Kujala U M, Osterman K 1990 Intrinsic risk factors and athletic injuries. Sports Medicine 9: 205–215

Tarui S, Okuno G, Ikura Y, Tanaka T, Suda M, Nishikawa M 1965 Phosphofructokinase deficiency in skeletal muscle: a new type of glycogenosis. Biochemical and Biophysical Research Communications 19: 517–523

Taylor J F, Fluck D, Fluck D 1976 Tropical myositis: ultrastructural studies. Journal of Clinical Pathology 29: 1081–1084

Thomson W H S, Sweetin J C, Hamilton I J D 1975 ATP and muscle enzyme efflux after physical exertion. Clinica Chimica Acta 59: 241–245

Travell J 1976 Myofascial trigger points: clinical review. In: Bonica J J, Albe-Fessard D (eds) Advances in pain research and therapy. Raven Press, New York, p 916–926

Travell J G, Simons D G 1992 Myofascial pain and dysfunction. Williams & Wilkins, Baltimore.

Tsokos G C, Moutsopoulos H M, Steinberg A D 1981 Muscle involvement in systemic lupus erythematosus. Journal of the American Medical Association 246: 766–768

Turner R M, Peck W W, Prietto C 1991 MR of soft tissue chloroma in a patient presenting with left pubic and hip pain. Journal of Computer Assisted Tomography 15: 700–702

Valk P 1984 Muscle localisation of Tc 99m MDP after exertion. Clinics in Nuclear Medicine 492–494

Wessley S 1990 Old wine in new bottles: neurasthenia and ME. Psychological Medicine 20: 35–53

Wessely S, Newham D J 1993 Virus syndromes and chronic fatigue. In: Vaeroy H, Merskey H (eds) Progress in fibromyalgia and myofascial pain. Elsevier, Amsterdam, (in press)

Wessley S, Powell R 1989 Fatigue syndromes: A comparison of postviral fatigue with neuromuscular and affective disorders. Journal of Neurology, Neurosurgery and Psychiatry 52: 940–948

Wiles C M, Edwards R H T 1977 Weakness in myotonic syndromes. Lancet 2: 598–601

Wiles C M, Jones D A, Edwards R H T 1981 Fatigue in human metabolic myopathy. In: Porter R, Whelan J (eds) Human muscle fatigue: physiological mechanisms. Ciba Foundation symposium 82. Pitman, London, p 264–282

Willison R G 1971 Quantitative electromyography. In: Licht S (ed) Electrodiagnosis and electromyography, 3rd edn. Elizabeth Licht, New Haven, Connecticut, p 390–411

Willner J, Di Mauro S, Eastwood A, Hays A, Roohi R, Lovelace R 1979 Muscle carnitine deficiency: genetic heterogeneity. Journal of the Neurological Sciences 41: 235–246

Wirth W A, Farrow C C 1961 Human sparganosis. Case report and review of the subject. Journal of the American Medical Association 177: 6–9

Wood G C, Bentall R P, Gopfert M, Edwards R H T 1991 A comparative psychiatric assessment of patients with chronic fatigue syndrome and muscle disease. Psychological Medicine 21: 619–628

Yip T C, Houle S, Hayes G, Forrest I, Nelson L, Walker P M 1990 Quantitation of skeletal muscle necrosis using 99Tc pyrophosphate with SPECT in a canine model. Nuclear Medicine Communications 11: 143–149

Zimmermann M 1988 Physiological mechanisms of pain in the musculo-skeletal system. In: Emre M, Mathies H (eds) Muscle spasms and pain. Parthenon Publishing, Carnforth, p 7–17

Zlatkin M B, Leninski R E, Shinkwin M et al 1990 Combined MR imaging and spectroscopy of bone and soft tissue tumours. Journal of Computer Assisted Tomography 14: 1–10

24. Low back pain: epidemiology, anatomy and neurophysiology

John M. Cavanaugh and James N. Weinstein

EPIDEMIOLOGY

Low back pain is a health problem with major medical and societal costs. In the United States back problems constitute 25% of all disabling occupational injuries and cause a loss of 1400 working days per 1000 workers per year. About 12 million people have low back impairment and 5 million disability (Boachie-Adjei 1988). About 2% of the workforce have compensatable back injuries each year for a total of over 400 000 injuries. National statistics from European countries reveal that 10–15% of all sickness absence is due to back pain, with rising absolute numbers of lost working days per worker. The 1-year prevalence is 25–45% and chronic back pain is present in 3–7% of the adult population. It is the most frequent cause of activity limitation in people below the age of 45 years, the second most frequent reason for physicians' visits, the fifth most frequent for hospitalisation, and the third-ranking reason for surgical procedures. The overall or lifetime prevalence of back pain exceeds 70% in all industrial countries.

Sciatica and/or accompanying leg pain is present in about one-quarter of those with back problems. Sickness absence for workers with sciatica greatly exceeds that for back pain alone. An estimated $7 billion was spent in compensation and medical costs in 1984 (Frymoyer & Cats-Baril 1987). The total annual cost attributable to low back pain ranges from 16 to 60 billion dollars per year. This includes lost earnings and productivity (Frymoyer et al 1989). Low back pain can be divided into three groups based on duration of symptoms: acute (7 days or less); subacute (1 week to 3 months), and chronic (longer than 3 months) (Mooney 1989).

The prevalence of herniated lumbar disc ranges from 1–3% of those with low back pain or in the general population. The number of operations for herniated lumbar disc varies between countries and it is estimated that the rate per 100 000 is 100 in Great Britain; 200 in Sweden; 350 in Finland, and between 450 and 900 in the United States. Of these operations, 90+% are done at the L4–L5 levels. The mean age of these patients is 40–45 years and males are operated on twice as often as females.

Occupational factors are difficult to research because of the uncertainty of exposure. The healthy worker is difficult to assess compared to the 'unhealthy worker' and injury mechanisms remain unclear. Disability may be related to work factors, individual factors and medical, legal or social factors. Known work factors include heavy lifting, static work postures, bending and twisting, and exposure to vibration, all being associated with increased risk of back pain. Psychosocial and psychological factors in the workplace include work dissatisfaction as an important risk factor in low back disability.

Gender appears to be of little importance with respect to low back symptoms, although women seem to have an increased prevalence postmenopausally. Posture is only a risk factor when clearly abnormal and anthropometric data are contradictory. Parenthetically, there appears to be no relationship between height, weight, body build and low back pain. Physical fitness on the other hand is also not a predictor for acute low back pain but physically fit patients have a lesser risk of chronic low back pain and often have a more rapid recovery following a back pain episode (Andersson 1991; Praemer et al 1992).

According to the Arthritis Foundation, 40% of all visits to neurosurgeons and orthopaedists are for complaints of back pain. As an estimated 70% or more of the population experiences low back pain sometime during adulthood, by inference, the longer one lives, the greater one's chances of developing back pain. Despite the frequency of this complaint, back pain is notoriously difficult to diagnose and treat, partly because of the complex structure of the spine. Only 10–15% of patients with low back pain complaints have a known cause (Frymoyer et al 1989). Symptoms do not always correspond with the severity of the disorder. Relatively minor, self-limiting injury can produce incapacitating pain, whereas extensive pathology may initially cause mild symptoms. Thus, the only rule that can be stated with confidence is: clinical manifestations do not necessarily reflect the cause or severity of disease.

POSSIBLE SOURCES OF LOW BACK PAIN: CLINICAL STUDIES

Despite the enormity of this problem, the causes of low back pain remain largely obscure. In the last 50 years much of the focus has been on the ruptured or herniated intervertebral disc. Other suspected sources of low back pain include the nerve roots, the lumbar facet joints, the paraspinal muscles and the posterior longitudinal ligament.

Just what are the tissues involved in the generation of low back pain and sciatica? Kuslich et al (1991) over the past decade have reported on nearly 200 consecutive patients studied prospectively. The authors used progressive regional anaesthesia in 193 consecutive patients undergoing decompression for a herniated disc or lumbar spinal stenosis. In their cases the lumbar fascia could be touched or even cut without anaesthetic. The supraspinous ligament, however, did produce some level of low back pain. The muscles never produced pain in response to gentle pressure. Forceful stretching, on the other hand, at the base of the muscles, especially at the site of blood vessels or nerves or the attachment of bone, usually produced a localised low back pain. It was felt that the pain was probably derived from the local vessels and nerves rather than from the muscle bundles themselves. The normal nerve root, uncompressed or unstretched, was generally completely insensitive to pain. Retraction over a long period of time, however, did result in mild paraesthesias, but again, never in any significant pain. On the other hand, stimulation of a compressed or stretched nerve root consistently produced the same sciatic distribution of pain as the patient had experienced prior to surgical intervention. In their series they were never able to reproduce the patient's sciatica except by finding and stimulating a stretched, compressed or swollen nerve root. In this case, sciatica could be reproduced by either pressure or stretch on the caudal dura, the nerve root sleeve, the ganglion, or the nerve distal to the ganglion, depending on the site of compression. The ganglion was somewhat more tender than other parts of the nerve root and in general, the closer the stimulation was to the site of compression or tension, the greater was the response to pain. The pain was always eliminated with the injection of 0.5 cm 1% Xylocaine via a 30 gauge needle beneath the nerve sheath proximal to the site of compression.

In patients who had undergone prior surgery the authors always found perineural fibrosis. The scar itself, however, was never tender while the nerve root itself was frequently very sensitive. The scar, it was hypothesised, may actually increase the sensitivity or pain by fixing the nerve now sensitive to compression and/or tension. In about two-thirds of their patients the outer annulus when stimulated produced back pain of a nature similar to the preoperative pain. Again local anaesthetic would obliterate this pain. Buttock pain was reproduced only by simultaneous application of pressure on the nerve root and the outer annulus. In a combined herniated disc and/or stenosis population the outer annulus was differentially sensitive in the patients studied, one-third being exquisitively tender, one-third being moderately tender and one-third being insensitive. This difference may be due to the presence of more neural tissues in certain patients; an increased sensitivity in certain disease processes with an altered threshold, or other factors responsible for the different sensitivities in different patients, some of which had the same pathology.

What about referral of pain? It was clear from the work of Kuslich and colleagues (1991) that the central annulus and posterior longitudinal ligament (PLL) produced central back pain. Stimulation to the right or the left centre of the PLL directed pain to the side being stimulated. The PLL, as we know, is intimately connected to the posterior central portion of the annulus and frequently produces central low back pain upon stimulation.

What about the vertebral end plates? It appeared that pressure and/or curettement resulted in deep rather than superficial low back pain, and was often more severe than the preoperative symptoms. The facet joints during surgical exposure produced sharp pain, localised to the region of dissection. The quality of this pain was not consistent with preoperative symptoms, which were more likely to be perceived as deep and dull. To relieve this pain it was never necessary to inject the joint itself but periarticular injections always blocked the pain around the facet joint. Neither the facet synovium nor articular cartilage were tender. Other tissues in and around the functional spinal unit such as the ligamentum flavum, epidural fat, posterior dura, nucleus, lamina or spinous processes were insensitive to local mechanical stimulation. Spinous processes, lamina and facet bone could be removed with surgical rongeurs without the use of anaesthetic.

Anterior elements in low back pain

The intervertebral disc and nerve roots

Mooney (1987) reviewed much of the current knowledge on low back pain and concluded that the disc may be the primary source in the production of low back pain, but the mechanisms of pain production are uncertain. Hirsch et al (1963) reported that 0.3 ml of (11%) hypertonic saline injected into the disc produced severe pain, 'identical to a real lumbago', that could not be localised but that was described as a deep aching across the low back. Kuslich et al, in 1991, demonstrated that of 144 patients whose central lateral annulus was stimulated, 71% had pain by this procedure and 30% experienced significant pain. The work of Kuslich et al (1991) has already been described. In this study, 18 spine tissue sites were stimulated with blunt surgical instruments or electrical current of low voltage. Significant pain was reported by 90% of patients upon stimulation of compressed nerve roots, by 30% of patients upon stimulation of central lateral annulus, and by 15% upon central annulus stimulation. Normal-looking nerve roots caused significant pain in only 9% of cases.

Posterior elements in low back pain

Facet joints

The facet joint capsule is richly innervated (Hirsch et al 1963; Jackson et al 1966; Wyke 1980; Ozaktay et al 1991) and can undergo extensive stretch under physiological loading (El-Bohy et al 1987). The facet can 'bottom out' or 'impinge' on the lamina below during spinal extension (Yang et al 1984). Is pain from the facet joint due to capsular deformation (pinch or strain) bony impingement or a combination thereof?

Hirsch et al (1963) and Mooney & Robertson (1976) produced a typical low back syndrome including radiation of pain into the posterior thigh, by injection of hypertonic saline into the facet joint capsules. Similar findings are reproduced with injection into the intervertebral disc. Ghormley (1933), Mooney & Robertson (1976) and Shealy (1976) have suggested that facet joint pathology plays an important role in low back pain. Shealy reported on the results of facet denervation using percutaneous radiofrequency coagulation of the facet joint (1976) in 234 patients. After a minimum 6-month follow-up, 82% of primary low back pain patients had benefited significantly, while only 40% of those with previous surgery and 29% of those with previous fusion showed improvement. Bogduk & Long (1980) reported that previous techniques of others would not reliably denervate the medial branch of the dorsal ramus, which innervates the facet joints, and they reported a more refined technique for medial branch neurotomy.

A review of the literature shows that facet block has a 50–60% success rate and facet rhyzolysis has similar results (Helbig & Lee 1988). Placebo effects, and a lack of a definitive set of diagnostic criteria for facet syndrome, may contribute to the mixed success rate of these treatment modalities. Lilius et al (1989), in a clinical trial of 109 patients with unilateral low back pain, found no statistical difference in the treatment outcomes of those who received facet injections with a corticosteroid and analgesic compared to those injected with normal saline. Pain scores showed significant improvement at 1 hour, 2 weeks and 6 weeks after injection with either treatment. Jackson et al (1988) performed facet injections on 454 patients without root tension signs and in whom conservative therapy had failed. A clinical facet syndrome or a set of variables to select patients responsive to the injections could not be identified. Helbig & Lee (1988) developed numerical selection criteria for facet syndrome. The scoring system was: back pain with groin or thigh pain (30 points), well-localised paraspinal tenderness (20 points), reproduction of pain with extension–rotation (30 points), corresponding radiological changes (20 points) and pain below the knee (–10 points). Of 22 patients, all seven patients with scores of 60 or greater experienced prolonged pain relief after facet injection with corticosteroid. Of the remaining 15 patients, seven experienced prolonged relief, six temporary relief and five no relief.

Sacroiliac joints

Despite a widespread perception that the sacroiliac (SI) joints are involved in at least some cases of low back pain, scientific evidence of this is limited (Pope et al 1982). The SI joints are innervated by posterior primary rami. Factors supporting a primary role for SI joints in low back pain include:

1. Portions of the joint contain hyaline cartilage and synovial lining, thus making this tissue susceptible to degenerative and inflammatory processes.
2. Age-related degeneration is seen in radiographs and is increased when there is a history of trauma.
3. Displacement of the SI joint is palpable and can be seen using biplanar radiography.

Overall, the role of the SI joint in low back pain is controversial except in the case of the spondyloarthropathies (Frymoyer et al 1989).

Back muscles

The most common diagnosis for low back pain is acute or chronic lumbosacral sprain or strain. However, the scientific evidence for low back pain of muscle origin is lacking (Andersson et al 1989). Some patients with palpable abnormalities in their back muscles had increased myeloelectric activity (Denslow & Clough 1941; Elliot 1944; Arroyo 1966; Fisher & Chang 1985) while Kraft et al (1968) found no increase in activity in areas of muscle spasm. The role of muscles and musculoskeletal pain is discussed further in Chapter 58.

NEUROANATOMY OF THE FUNCTIONAL SPINAL UNIT

The innervation of the lumbar spine is illustrated in Fig. 24.1. The spine can be divided into dorsal and ventral compartments (separated by the intervertebral foramen)

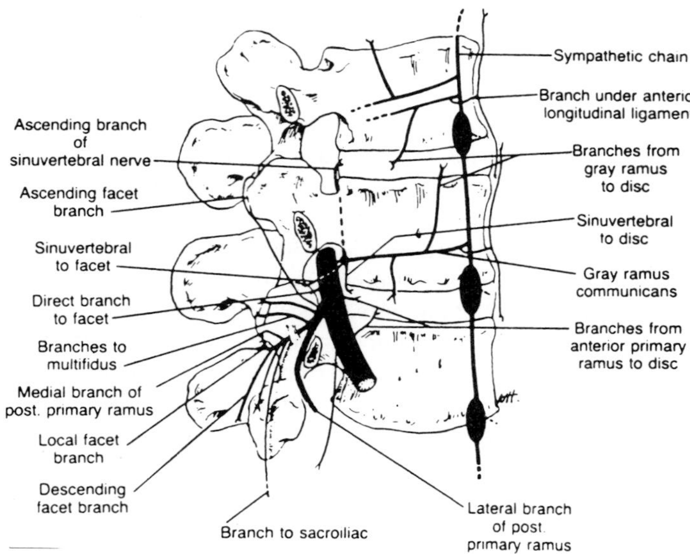

Fig. 24.1 Segmental innervation of the lumbar spine. Disc innervation: Branches from the sympathetic chain innervate the lateral and anterior portions of the disc above and below. The recurrent sinuvertebral nerve which is formed from the grey ramus communicans and mixed spinal nerves innervates the posterior and posterolateral portions of the disc at two levels inside the spinal canal. The ventral ramus sends small branches to the disc at the level of nerve exit. Facet and erector spinae muscles: The posterior primary ramus sends medial branches to the facet at the level of nerve exit and to the facet below. According to some investigators there is also a branch to the facet above (as shown). There are also medial branches to multifidus muscle. Intermediate erector spinae muscle (longissimus) is innervated by the intermediate branches of posterior primary rami. Lateral erector spinae (iliocostalis) is innervated by lateral branches of posterior primary rami, which also innervate cutaneous tissue. (From Paris 1983.)

and laterally by the transverse processes and intertransverse ligaments. The ventral compartment contains ventral dura, intervertebral disc, posterior longitudinal ligament, anterior longitudinal ligament and prevertebral muscle (psoas major, psoas minor, quadratus lumborum and lateral intertransverse muscles). The dorsal compartment contains the neural arches and their joints and ligaments. These structures includes the lamina, the facet joints and their capsules, ligamentum flavum, supraspinous and interspinous ligaments and the intrinsic back muscles. The intrinsic back muscles can be divided into medial (rotatores, multifidus), intermediate (longissimus) and lateral (iliocostalis) groups, which are innervated by the medial, intermediate and lateral branches of the dorsal ramus, respectively (Bogduk 1983). The lateral branch of the dorsal ramus is also the cutaneous supply to the back.

Anatomical studies indicate that the facet joint, annulus of the disc, supraspinous and interspinous ligaments and other ligaments contain free and encapsulated nerve endings (Stillwell 1956; Hirsch et al 1963; Jackson et al 1966). Free nerve endings can serve as pain receptors while encapsulated nerve endings largely serve as pressure, position or motion detectors. Free nerve endings are not necessarily for pain transmission, as it has been demonstrated that some free nerve endings are temperature detectors. Others may serve as low threshold mechanoreceptors. Thus the presence of free nerve endings in spinal tissue suggests that these are sources of pain but do not prove or demonstrate it.

Nerve supply to anterior elements

Sinuvertebral nerve

The sinuvertebral nerve (SVN) supplies the skeletal elements of the ventral compartment of the lumbar spine. At each ventral level, the SVN is formed by the union of a nerve branch from the ventral ramus and an autonomic root from the grey ramus communicans. The SVN may actually be observed as a series of fine filaments rather than an actual nerve trunk. The SVN innervates the ventral aspect of the dural sac, PLL, annulus fibrosus, blood vessels of the ventral compartment and vertebral bodies. The SVN surrounds the blood vessels it innervates and accompanies blood vessels into the vertebral bodies. The branches of the SVN go *only* into structures of the spinal canal. Transverse and descending branches supply the PLL and intervertebral disc at the level of nerve entry into the canal. An ascending branch goes to the next higher level and overlaps the innervation of the SVN above. The lateral and anterior annuli fibrosi are not innervated by the SVN, but rather by nerves from ventral rami and grey rami communicans. The anterior longitudinal ligament is supplied by grey rami communicans or by a branch from the sympathetic chain (Bogduk 1983).

Nerve endings in the disc

For pain or sensation to originate from the disc, the disc must have nerve endings. Hirsch et al (1963), Jackson et al (1966) and Jung & Brunschwig (1932) found nerve endings in the PLL and superficial annulus. Roofe (1940), Wiberg (1947), Ikari (1954) and Pedersen et al (1956) found no nerve endings within the intervertebral disc. Earlier studies which reported nerve endings were corroborated by Malinsky (1959), Yoshizawa et al (1980) and Bogduk et al (1981). Nerve endings were found as deep as one-third of the depth of the annulus in cadaveric specimens and one-half of the depth in surgically removed specimens.

The types of nerve endings are various. Hirsch et al and Jackson et al found only simple free nerve endings. Yoshizawa et al found not only simple free nerve endings, but complex sprays and convoluted tangles. Malinsky found five types of free nerve endings in the outer annulus: lone, simple, free; simple, branching; shrubby; mesh-like loops, and clusters running in parallel. On the external lateral surfaces of the annulus, Malinsky also found encapsulated and partially encapsulated nerve endings.

Regional anatomy around the intervertebral disc

The posterior longitudinal ligament is well innervated, with both complex encapsulated nerve endings and numerous poorly myelinated free nerve endings. The lateral expansion of the PLL covers all of the dorsal and most of the dorsolateral aspects of the disc. Disc protrusions may elevate these well-innervated PLL attachments, possibly producing low back pain. Blikra (1969) has shown that the ventral dura, particularly at the L4–L5 level can be fixed to the ventral surface of the spinal canal. The protruding nucleus pulposus can actually, although rarely, rupture this dura. The damage or stress produced could cause pain (transmitted by the meningeal branches of the sinuvertebral nerve).

The ligaments of Hoffmann connect the anterior dura to the PLL and vertebral periosteum. It has been hypothesised that posterior displacement of the dural sac and/or nerve roots may apply traction through the ligaments of Hoffmann to the PLL and vertebral periosteum, producing low back pain. Disc herniations may displace the dura and nerve roots posteriorly, applying traction to the PLL and periosteum, which may produce low back pain. Disc surgery or chymopapain treatment may, in fact, work by decreasing tension on these nociceptive ligaments.

Posterior elements

The facet joint is innervated by the medial branch of the dorsal ramus from two levels: the branch exiting the intervertebral foramen at the same level as the facet joint and the branch exiting the foramen one level above the facet joint. As in other synovial joints, the facet joint contains encapsulated, unencapsulated and free nerve endings. Recent silver impregnation studies in human cadaver joint capsules support these findings (Ozaktay et al 1991). Ashton et al (1992) demonstrated immunoreactivity for substance P, calcitonin gene-related peptide (CGRP) and vasoactive intestinal peptides (VIP) in surgically removed human facet joint capsule. Immunoreactivity was not seen in the ligamentum flavum.

The pinching of facet synovial folds might play a role in low back pain if the folds contain nociceptive innervation. It has been suggested that the synovial folds lack innervation (Wyke 1980), but more recent work demonstrates the contrary. Using silver and gold impregnation, Giles & Taylor (1987) reported nerves in capsular tissue and synovial folds (plical tissue). Gronblad et al (1991a, 1991b) reported nerves in close apposition to blood vessels and fat cells in synovial folds from surgically removed human specimens but most of these did not demonstrate immunoreactivity to substance P, or galanin. They suggested that plical folds contain nerves involved in vasoregulation but not in sensory innervation. This is suggested by the sparse neuropeptide immunoreactivity.

THE DORSAL ROOT GANGLION

Anatomical studies indicate that a dorsal root ganglion (DRG) can readily be trapped between a herniated disc and the facet (Lindblom & Rexed 1948; Weinstein 1992). Neurophysiological data show that pressure on the DRG causes excitation of afferent fibres. Howe et al (1977) demonstrated that in anaesthetised cats, minor compression of DRG produced repetitive firing lasting several minutes and occasionally up to 25 minutes. The chronically damaged dorsal root also responded to mechanical stimuli, but discharges did not last as long as with DRG stimulation. The normal root did not fire in response to mechanical stimulation. Devor & Obermayer (1984) using a ferric ion-ferrocyanide staining procedure on rat DRG, reported that the initial segment of the stem axon and a variable portion of the cell body stained heavily, suggesting that these were areas of high sodium channel content and elevated electrical excitability. These authors suggested that the elevated excitability of the DRG is a design compromise: it contributes to reliable afferent impulse propagation past the ganglion, but makes the system a likely site of ectopic impulse generation, which can lead to dysaesthesias and pain. Wall & Devor (1983) reported that 4.75% of myelinated and 4.4% of unmyelinated neurons recorded from anaesthetised rats contained impulses generated within the DRG. Devor & Wall (1990) reported that spontaneous DRG firing increased substantially with tetonic (repetitive) stimulation of neighbouring axons, a phenomenon which could contribute to sensory abnormalities including spatial effects, such as referred pain, and temporal effects, such as after-sensation and wind-up. The failure of C-fibres to exhibit crossexcitation limits the significance in pain states.

The cells of the dorsal root ganglion are largely divided into two classes according to their diameters (Lieberman 1976). The large diameter cells give rise to the large myelinated A-beta fibres, while the small diameter cells are thought to give rise to the unmyelinated C-fibres and finally myelinated A-delta fibres. The central terminations of these primary afferent fibres, derived from the small ganglion cells, are primarily, but certainly not exclusively, in the substantia gelatinosa or laminae I and II of the spinal cord dorsal horn.

The dorsal root ganglion manufactures several neurogenic peptides, including calcitonin gene-related peptide and substance P. Calcitonin gene-related peptide is the most abundant peptide discovered to date (Gibson et al 1981).

Spinal nerve roots proximal to the DRG have a peculiar structure, different from the arrangements in peripheral nerves (Yoshizawa et al 1991). The root is surrounded by cerebrospinal fluid (CSF) infiltrating the endoneural space through the thin nerve root sheath. The dorsal root ganglion, including not only nerve fibres but also abundant nerve cells, is located at the border between the nerve root and the peripheral nerve, initially called the spinal nerve, and is also influenced by the CSF.

A great deal of information is available on blood supply to the spinal cord, but little has been written about the blood supply to the dorsal root ganglion (Bergmann & Alexander 1941; Yoshizawa et al 1991). Its vascular supply, venous and arterial, must play a significant role in its function. Bergmann & Alexander (1941) suggest the aging and concomitant vascular changes of the dorsal root ganglion are associated with degeneration and changes in vibratory sensation. The DRG has its own nutrient arteries branching directly from the spinal segmental artery, and has more abundant intrinsic vessels than the nerve root, consisting of not only continous but also fenestrated capillaries, meaning that the blood–nerve-barrier is not as tight in the dorsal root ganglion as it is in the peripheral nerve.

The blood supply of the nerve roots themselves depends on the ascending distal radicular arteries and the descending proximal radicular arteries. There is no hypovascular region in the nerve root, although there exists a so-called 'watershed' of bloodstream in the radicular artery itself.

Yoshizawa et al (1991) suggest that mechanical compression of the extradural nerve root, commonly seen with degenerative conditions of the spine, disturbs the blood flow in the proximal part of the nerve root more than in the distal part. Blocking the CSF around the nerve root on the distal side of the compression, however, provokes reduction of the blood flow to a certain extent, not only in the distal part of the nerve root but also in the dorsal root ganglion, suggesting that clinical symptoms derived from the dorsal root ganglion may exist even when it is not compressed directly.

Because of the ganglion's vascular supply and tight capsule, Rydevik and associates (1981) have suggested that compression of the ganglion may result in intraneural oedema and a subsequent decrease in cell body blood supply, accounting for abnormal dorsal root ganglion activity in pain. In the spinal stenosis model of Delamarter, neurogenic claudication appears to begin with venous congestion of the nerve roots and dorsal root ganglion distal to the induced constriction (Delamarter et al 1990).

Another source of pain may be epineurium itself. Nervi nervorum, located on the dorsal root ganglion as well as peripheral nerves, are mechanically sensitive nociceptors themselves. Therefore, the epineurium of the dorsal root ganglion may be directly activated by compression or mechanical stimulation of these receptors. These epineurally-located receptors appear to respond in a way similar to cutaneous nociceptors in the peripheral nervous system (Shantha & Evans 1972).

One of the issues the present authors have studied is the role of the dorsal root ganglion in modulating the pain response associated with discography, a commonly performed diagnostic procedure prior to spinal surgery (Weinstein et al 1988a). Discography is thought to be highly specific (Walsh et al 1990); however the question remains as to the relevance of an abnormal or painful discogram. A second study suggests the DRG as a potential modulator of disc-related nociception. The study was performed to investigate changes in substance P and vasoactive intestinal peptides (VIP) following discography in normal and abnormal canine lumbar intervertebral discs. Data from this study suggested that dorsal root ganglion substance P and VIP are indirectly affected by manipulations of the intervertebral disc. The present authors ask if neurochemical changes within the intervertebral disc may be expressed by sensitised (injured) annular nociceptors and if, in part, this expression is modulated by dorsal root ganglion neurotransmitters. Therefore it may be (as hypothesised) that an abnormal discogram image, accompanied by an abnormal pain response, may in part be related to the chemical environment within the intervertebral disc and the sensitised state of its annular nociceptors. Immunohistochemically, substance P (SP), vasoactive intestinal peptide (VIP), and calcitonin gene-related peptide (CGRP) were identified in the outer annulus and quantitated DRG neuropeptide levels (SP, VIP, CGRP) were indirectly stimulated by discal interventions i.e. discography (Weinstein et al 1988a). Clearly more work is needed to establish the significance of this clinically used diagnostic test.

THE LUMBAR NERVE ROOTS

Smyth & Wright (1958) placed nylon threads into various lumbar tissue sites during operations on the spine. The threads exited from the surgical sites and were pulled upon in the postoperative period to determine pain sensitivity at the suture sites in the affected spinal tissue(s). The nerve roots were the most common pain site. Nerve roots, compressed by disc or bony impingement, were thought to be the cause of sciatica and were painful and sensitive. With normal nerve or uninvolved roots, there was much less pain. Greenbarg et al (1988) reported that compressed and inflamed nerve roots were sensitive to mechanical manipulation in patients undergoing laminectomy under epidural anaesthesia. As previously stated Kuslich et al (1991) reported similar findings in the back pain patients undergoing progressive local anaesthesia. Stimulation of stretched, compressed or swollen nerve roots caused significant pain in 90% of patients and was the only tissue site which, upon stimulation, reproduced the patient's sciatica. Only 9% of cases of normal nerve root stimulation produced significant pain.

In an electrophysiological study in anaesthetised cats Janig & Koltzenburg (1991) reported 14 mechanosensitive units with conduction velocities in the C-fibre range, whose receptive fields were on sacral (S2) ventral roots and whose afferent projections were to sacral dorsal roots at the same level. These findings demonstrate a pain pathway through excitation of nervi nervorum on ventral roots and suggest this as a possible mechanism of radicular pain.

NEUROPHYSIOLOGY OF THE POSTERIOR ELEMENTS

In the neurophysiology of sensory nerve fibres, the nerve is assigned to one of four groups (I, II, III, IV) based on conduction velocity (Guyton 1981). Group IV are the unmyelinated C-fibres and Group III the thinly myelinated A-delta fibres (see Table 24.1). Pain fibres generally belong to groups III and IV, but not all group III and IV fibres are pain fibres.

The neurophysiology of muscle pain

Mense & Meyer (1985) reported on the activity of group III and IV muscle units in the triceps surae muscle or calcaneal tendon of anaesthetised cats. Group III included units that were low threshold pressure-sensitive (44%), nociceptive (33%) and contraction-sensitive (23%). Group IV units included nociceptive (43%), low threshold pressure-sensitive (19%), contraction-sensitive (19%) and thermosensitive (19%) units. In these small diameter afferents, nonnociceptive units outnumbered nociceptive units 62% to 38%.

Nonneurogenic pain mediators excite muscle units. Bradykinin, a nonapeptide, has been shown to be excitant of muscle group III and IV afferent fibres (Franz & Mense 1977; Mense 1977). Prostaglandin E_2 and 5-HT enhance this action (Mense 1981). Carrageenan-induced myositis caused an increase in the background activity of group III and IV units in inflamed leg muscle and a lowering of threshold of group IV units (Berberich et al 1988).

The raised discharge frequency could account for the spontaneous pain in tissue inflammation and lowered thresholds could account for the tenderness to movement in inflamed tissue.

Table 24.1 Classification and function of sensory nerve fibres

Group	Function	Diameter (μm)	Conduction velocity(m/s)
Group Ia	Muscle spindle, primary ending	13–20	80–120
Group Ib	Golgi tendon organs	12–18	70–110
Group II	Muscle spindle, secondary ending	5–12	20–70
Group III (A-delta)	Pricking pain Temperature Crude touch	1–5	2.5–20
Group IV (C-fibres)	Pain Itich Temperature Crude touch	0.5–2	0.5–2.5

Neurophysiology of 'facet' joint pain

A large percentage of low back pain is deemed 'idiopathic' and in many cases the source of the pain may be in and/or around the facet joint, joint capsule, musculotendinous junctions or ligaments. This pain may have an inflammatory component and is sometimes treated with a local or epidural injection of a steroidal antiinflammatory drug and/or a local anaesthetic (i.e. celestone, lidocaine).

Neurophysiology of joint inflammation

Several neurophysiological investigations have demonstrated that inflammation makes nerves in joints more sensitive to movement than normal joints and also increases the background neural discharge in joints. These studies demonstrate scientifically a likely mechanism for pain production in inflamed joints. Carrageenan and kaolin are often used to produce joint inflammation. These substances activate the contact activation system (Kozin & Cochrane 1988) resulting in the production of bradykinin, which causes inflammation and hyperalgesia. Carrageenan is a seaweed product and kaolin a mineral product containing silica. These substances, when injected into joints, produce oedema, fibrin formation and infiltration of leucocytes to the inflamed area. At least part of their action appears to be due to their negative surface charges.

The ankle joint (Iggo 1985), knee joint (Coggeshall et al 1983; Schaible & Schmidt 1985; Grigg et al 1986) and lumbar facet joint (Cavanaugh et al 1990) have been studied using such inflammation models. Schaible & Schmidt (1985), in a neurophysiological study of inflammation of the cat knee joint induced by kaolin and carrageenan, reported that units in the inflamed joint were not decreased in von Frey threshold compared to controls, but were more sensitive to stretch and had higher resting discharge rates than controls. A similar study by Grigg et al (1986) of units of the posterior articular nerve (PAN) innervating the posterior knee joint capsule of the cat, found that group IV units were much more readily activated by normal joint movements in the inflamed joint than in the normal joint. Guilbaud et al (1985) demonstrated increased sensitivity of group III and IV units in the ankle joint of rats after inflammation with Freund's adjuvant.

Neurophysiology of the lumbar facet joint

A series of neurophysiological studies were undertaken in anaesthetised rats and New Zealand White rabbits to characterise the neuronal response of joints and surrounding tissue of the lumbar spine (Cavanaugh et al 1989, 1990; Yamashita et al 1990, 1992; Avramov et al 1992). The studies have focused on the facet joint and adjacent musculotendinous junctions. The results of these studies indicate the following:

1. The facet joint capsule contains low and high threshold mechanoreceptors, the low threshold receptors probably being proprioceptors, and the high threshold probably nociceptors (pain receptors).
2. The surrounding deep back musculotendinous units contain the same type of receptors, with a higher proportion of proprioceptors.
3. In addition to being mechanosensitive as described above, neurons of these spinal tissues are chemosensitive:
   a. when inflamed with carrageenan and kaolin, the facet joint and surrounding muscles produce ongoing neuronal discharge
   b. localised injection of synthetic substance P, a neuromodulator of the pain pathway, activates nociceptors and proprioceptors of the facet joints and deep back muscles
   c. injection of bradykinin and serotonin, chemical mediators of inflammation, activate units of the facet joint and spinal canal.
4. In an in vitro spine preparation, loading the spine activates three types of units: low threshold units which may signal position sense, high threshold units which may signal pain and phasic units which may signal motion.
5. Spine loading or mechanical stimulation, even in the clearly noxious range, does not maintain the discharge of putative nociceptors. Chemical mediators, on the other hand, do maintain the discharge of putative nociceptors in the posterior elements in this model.

In control animals, facet joint and muscle units were identified (Yamashita et al 1990). A total of 24 mechanosensitive units have been identified at the facet joint and 12 others in the muscles and tendons near their insertion into the facet. Of the 24 units at the facet joint, 10 were in the capsule, 12 in the border regions between capsule and muscle or tendon, and two in the ligamentum flavum. Two units (8%) had conduction velocities less than 2.5 m/s (group IV); 15 units (63%) had conduction velocities of 2.5–20 m/s (group III) and seven units (29%) had conduction velocities greater than 20 m/s. Seven units had thresholds greater than 6.0 g, 13 units had thresholds less than 6.0 g, and four units were not examined (Fig. 24.2). Seven units responded to facet joint movement caused by pulling on the isolated L5 lamina. Five of these were in the medial aspect of the facet joint. These units were most responsive to caudal-to-rostral stretch. The two units in the ligamentum flavum were most responsive to ventral-to-dorsal stretch. These data suggest that units with thresholds greater than 6.0 g, particularly those in areas of high tissue strain, could be the source of facet pain.

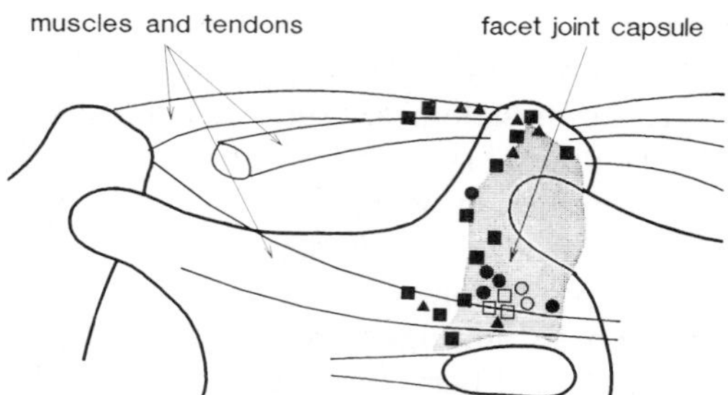

Fig. 24.2 Receptive fields characterised in the facet joint and adjacent muscles of the New Zealand White rabbit. Squares denote units with thresholds less than 6 g, circles denote units with thresholds greater than 6.0 g and triangles denote units for which thresholds could not be determined. If the unit responded to stretch the symbol is hollow. (From Yamashita et al 1990).

Facet joint and musculotendinous units in inflamed tissue

In seven anaesthetised adult male New Zealand White rabbits (Cavanaugh et al 1990) the L5/L6 or L6/L7 left facet joint was injected with 0.1 ml of 2% carrageenan and 0.1 ml of 4% kaolin. In these rabbit studies, units were found in multifidus, rotatory and intermamillary muscle, or in the facet joint capsule and border regions at the junction of capsule and muscle tendon insertions. Spontaneous discharge rates (SDRs) were monitored for 21 units in inflamed animals and 21 units in controls. The average SDR was 18.1 units/s (range 0–50) in the inflamed joints and 9.3 units/s (range 0–28) in the controls. In the inflamed tissue there was generally a high spontaneous discharge rate which increased with stimulation (Fig. 24.3A). The inflamed units often showed vigorous multiunit response to stretch by moving the facet joint approximately 1 mm in caudal-rostral, ventral-dorsal and lateral-medial directions (Fig. 24.3B). Lidocaine and hydrocortisone applied to the receptive fields and to the dorsal roots caused a large decrease in discharge rate from the inflamed tissue (Fig. 24.4A–C).

NEUROPHYSIOLOGICAL STUDIES IN SPINAL LOADING AND LUMBAR CANAL TISSUE STIMULATION

Response of units to spine loading

An in vitro procedure was undertaken in 24 rabbits

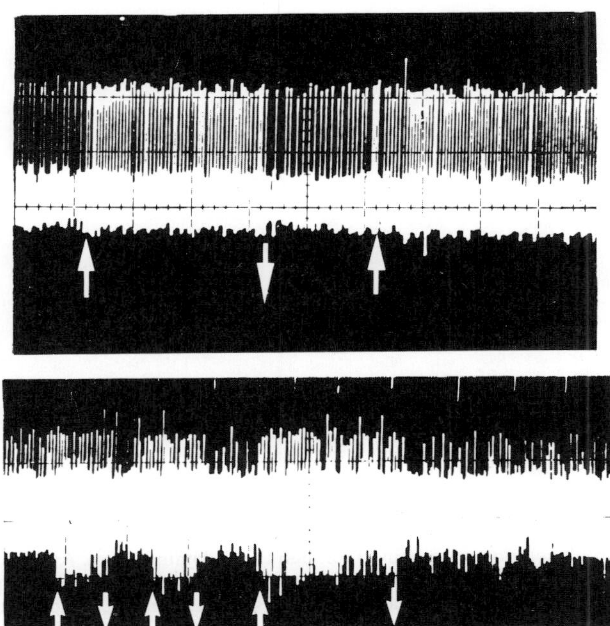

Fig. 24.3 Responses from facet joints inflamed with kaolin and carrageenan. **A** Increased discharge with 2 g von Frey hair applied to receptive field in multifidus muscle. The baseline discharge rate is already high in this inflamed tissue. **B** Multiunit response to ventral-to-doral pull on the facet joint. (↑ = onset of pull; ↓ = offset of pull; sweep speed = 1 s per division.)

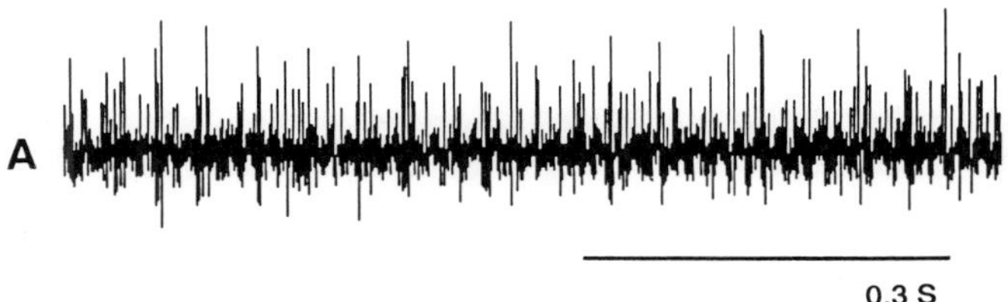

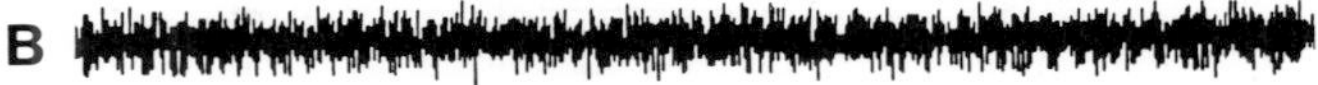

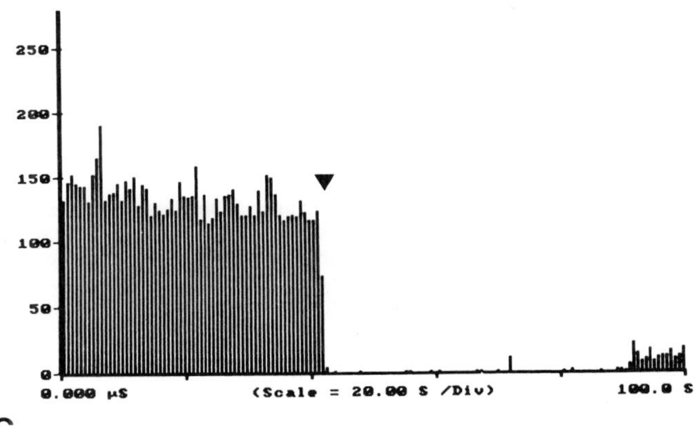

Fig. 24.4 Time course–effect of application of 5 mg hydrocortisone succinate to dorsal roots. **A** Dorsal root multiunit activity. **B** Cessation of activity immediately after hydrocortisone application. **C** Histogram showing discharge rate on the vertical axis. Arrowhead indicates time of hydrocortisone application.

(Avramov et al 1992). In this series of experiments the abdominal aorta of anaesthetised New Zealand White rabbits was cannulated and perfused with Kreb's solution. The lumbar spine was removed with bone rongeurs and placed in a loading chamber, perfused in Kreb's solution, and bubbled with 95% oxygen–5% carbon dioxide. The experimental chamber is illustrated in Fig. 24.5.

A constant finding during these experiments was a vigorous multiunit response to loading. Characteristically, units with spontaneous activity were excited, as well as units that were silent before loading was initiated. A portion of the load-activated units could be characterised by their conduction velocities and von Frey thresholds (Fig. 24.6A–C). Some units not located on or adjacent to the facet joint were presumed to be around the disc, ligaments or muscle tissue. It was possible to characterise the type of response of these units. Three patterns were observed:

1. Phasic type mechanoreceptors responded to movement, regardless of direction or initial position; response did not outlast the movement phase of loading. Firing rates of these units did not change with the amount of the load applied to the spine and appeared to increase with increased rate of loading.

2. Slowly-adapting, low threshold mechanoreceptors tended to respond to loads exceeding 0.3–0.5 kg with immediate and sustained increase in the firing rate. As load decreased, rate of firing decreased. The preload rate of firing was usually reached within 1 minute after initial spinal position was restored. A total of 16 units responding to such loading were identified.

3. Slowly adapting high threshold mechanoreceptors could not be activated until a threshold load ranging from 3 to 5.5 kg was exceeded. They did not demonstrate any phasic response and responded to suprathreshold loads by irregular bursts of activity that increased in frequency and duration with increased loads.

Initial studies of neural activity within the lumbar spinal canal

Cavanaugh et al (1992) reported activation of units recorded from dorsal roots of anaesthetised New Zealand White rabbits after mechanical manipulations and application of algesic substances to the lumbar spinal canal. Only occasionally did probing into disc or posterior longitudinal ligament evoke neural discharge. However pulling the ventral dura with forceps caused multiunit activation. It is not known whether those units were in the dura itself or in the tissue that receives traction when the dura is pulled. Applications of bradykinin into the intervertebral foramen

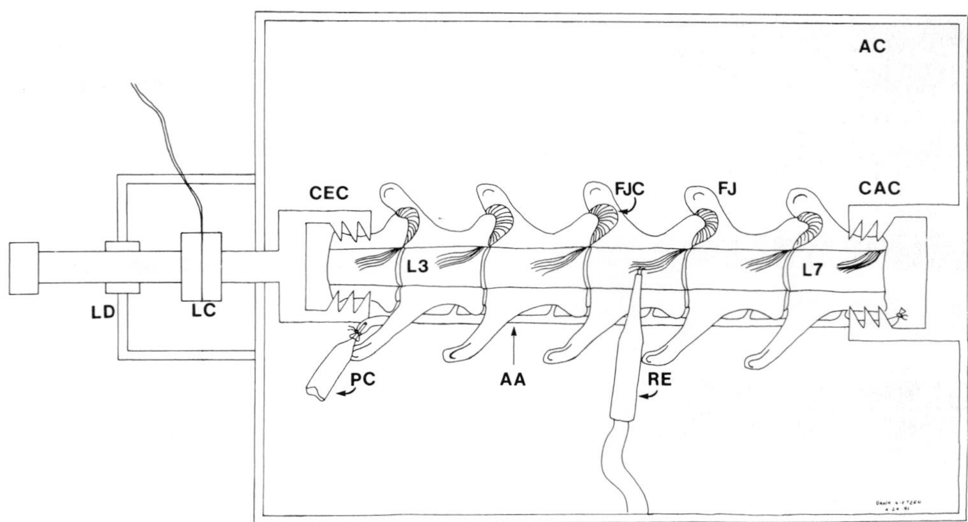

Fig. 24.5 Diagram of rabbit spinal specimen in loading chamber. Oxygenated Kreb's solution was perfused through the abdominal aorta. Axial load, measured by a load cell, was recorded simultaneously with neuronal discharge recorded from dorsal rootlets, using a bipolar recording electrode. (AA = abdominal aorta; AC = acrylic chamber, filled with Kreb's solution; CAC = caudal clamp; CEC = cephalad clamp; FJ = facet joint; FJC = facet joint capsule; LC = load cell; LD = loading device; L3 = third lumbar vertebra; L7 = seventh lumbar vertebra; PC = perfusing catheter; RE = recording electrode.) (From Avramov et al 1992.)

and serotonin to the ventral portion of the lumbar spinal canal caused vigorous neural discharges of over 20 per second. These sometimes occurred after latencies of several minutes. Conduction velocities were obtained from 40 units in the spinal canal. The majority of these were in the A-delta and A-beta fibre range. Most of these could not be mechanically evoked.

CHEMICAL MEDIATORS OF NOCICEPTION

Non-neurogenic mediators

The mediators of inflammation include the amines (histamine, 5-hydroxytryptamine), the kinins (including bradykinin), arachidonic acid derivatives (prostaglandins and leukotrienes), the kinin-forming enzymes (kallikrein, plasmin), products of the complement system and components of polymorphonuclear leucocytes. The major pain-producing substances involved in inflammatory reactions appear to be bradykinin, 5-hydroxytryptamine (serotonin), and prostaglandin E_1 (PGE_1).

Bradykinin, a nonapeptide, has been shown to be an excitant of muscle group III and IV afferent fibres (Franz & Mense 1975; Mense 1977). Prostaglandin E_2 and 5-HT enhance this action. (Mense 1981). In a study on human volunteers, intradermal injection of histamine and bradykinin produced short-lasting pain, but prolonged oedema and erythema (Ferreire 1972). Subdermal infusions of PGE_1 with histamine or bradykinin produced more intense pain than with these agents alone. In areas made hyperalgesic with PGE_1, infusion of bradykinin or histamine produced strong to intense pain, bradykinin being more effective. Aspirin, which blocks synthesis of prostaglandins, may produce analgesia by preventing the sensitisation of pain receptors by prostaglandins. Although high levels of prostaglandins were required to produce overt pain, only minute amounts were required to cause sensitisation to chemical and mechanical stimulation (Ferreire 1972).

Hyperalgesia is related to lipoxygenation of arachidonic acid: a dihydroxyeicosatetraenoic acid (diHETE), a 15-lipoxygenase product; and leukotriene B_4, a 5-lipoxygenase product. Leukotriene B_4 is chemotactic for polymorphonuclear leucocytes that accumulate at locations of inflammation to destroy antigens (Ford-Hutchinson et al 1980). Leukotriene injected interdermally into the rat paw sensitises C nociceptors to mechanical stimulation and produces hyperalgesia. This hyperalgesia is apparently dependent upon the presence of the polymorphonuclear leucocytes (Kumazawa & Mizumura 1977). It is important to remember that the hyperalgesia produced from these substances is not affected by nonsteroidal antiinflammatory drugs that normally block the cyclooxygenation of arachidonic acid (Levine et al 1985). Levine and his colleagues have demonstrated that diHETE injected interdermally into the rat produces a hyperalgesia similar to that produced by leukotriene B_4, bradykinin or prostaglandin E_2. Phospholipase A_2 activity may play an important role in the presence of a chemical radiculopathy associated with a herniated nucleus pulposus (Saal et al 1989).

Neurogenic mediators

Substance P has been identified immunohistochemically

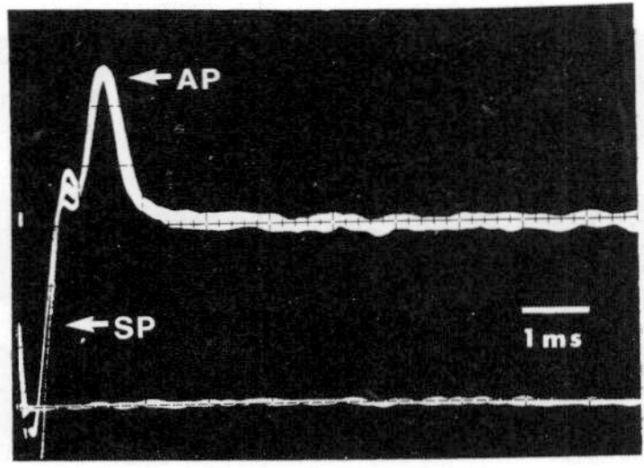

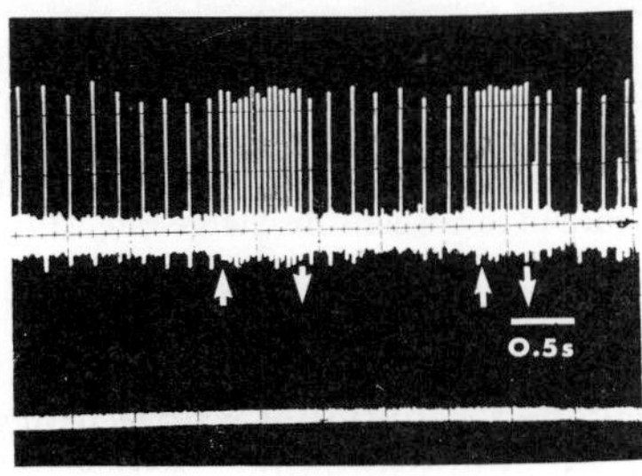

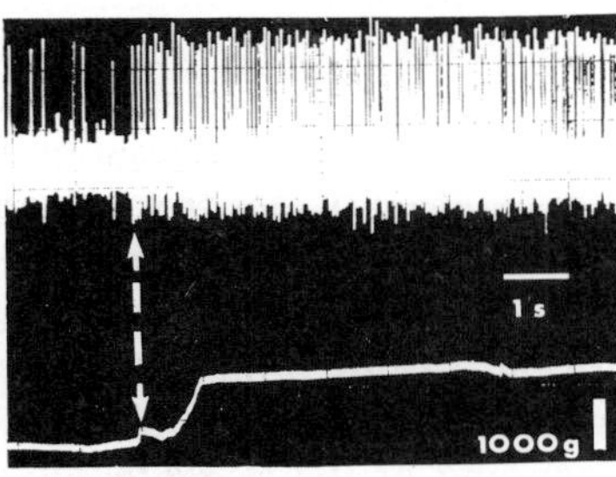

Fig. 24.6 **A** Electrically evoked potential from a unit at tip of rabbit facet joint. Conduction velocity was calculated by dividing the distance between the locus of stimulation and the recording electrode (in millimetres) by the onset latency (in milliseconds). Lower tracing shows zero load from the load cell. (AP = action potential; SP = stimulus pulse.) **B** Stimulation of the receptor field with a von Frey hair. The von Frey threshold is described as the thinnest hair capable of activating the unit, in this case 0.93 g. (↑ = onset of stimulus; ↓ = offset of stimulus.) Lower tracing shows zero load from the load cell. **C** Simultaneous recording of neuronal discharge (upper trace) and load as measured by the load cell (lower trace). An initial peak load of 350 g at the double arrow activated the low threshold mechanoreceptor. (From Avramov et al 1992.)

in various regions of the peripheral and central nervous system. Its presence in the outer laminae of the spinal dorsal horn, which receive nociceptive afferent fibres, suggests that it may play a role in transmission of pain signals (Hokefelt et al 1975; Cuello et al 1976). Iontophoretic application of substance P causes excitation of nociceptive dorsal horn neurons (Henry 1976 Randic & Miletic 1977; Zieglgansberger & Tulloch 1979). The release of substance P from the dorsal horn is reported to increase during acute noxious mechanical stimuli (Kurahashi et al 1985) and in the polyarthritic state (Oku et al 1987). Thus, many studies have suggested that substance P may be a neurotransmitter or a neuromodulator of nociceptive sensation. In addition, Pioro et al (1984) have found immunoreactivity to substance P in the nucleus dorsalis of the spinal cord, which receives mainly afferent fibres from the lower trunk and extremities related to proprioception, touch and pressure.

Identification of substance P in lumbar spinal tissues

Substance P may make a contribution to transmission of pain sensation from lumbar spinal tissues, acting perhaps as a transmitter or modulator of excitability of nociceptive units. Korkala et al (1985) found substance P-immunofluorescent nerves in the posterior longitudinal ligament of the human lumbar spine and suggested that they have nociceptive function. El Bohy et al (1988) identified substance P in the facet joint capsules of rabbits (Fig. 24.7A–C). In this study indirect immunofluorescence techniques were used to identify substance P-like-immunoreactive (SPLI) and neurofilament protein-immunoreactive (NFIR) fibres in the facet joint capsule and supraspinous ligament of the New Zealand White rabbit. There was a larger population of NFIR fibres and these were sometimes co-localised with the smaller population of SPLI fibres. The SPLI fibres tended to be in the

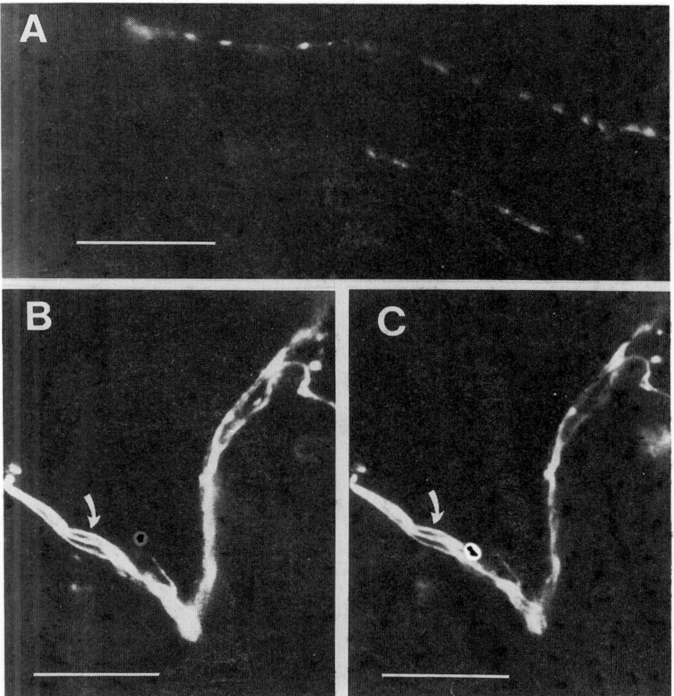

Fig. 24.7 **A** Photomicrograph at the lumbar supraspinous ligament showing substance P-like immunoreactive (SPLI) fibres. **B** Fibres stained positive for SPLI in the rabbit lumbar facet joint. **C** The same fibres stained for neurofilament protein, a more general marker of nerve tissue. (From El-Bohy et al 1988.)

smaller axons, suggesting that they were a subpopulation that may be involved in pain transmission.

The sensitising effect of substance P on peripheral nerve endings has not been fully resolved. Fitzgerald & Lynn (1976) reported only weak excitation of cutaneous receptors in cats and rabbits by synthetic substance P. On the other hand, Nakamura-Craig & Smith (1989) reported that multiple injections of subthreshold doses of SP in the rat paw caused long-lasting hyperalgesia. The threshold to produce hyperalgesia was 10 ng per pad. In 15 rabbits a study was undertaken to examine how substance P affects the mechanosensitive afferent units identified in the lumbar facet joint and adjacent tissues of the rabbit (Yamashita et al 1993). Synthetic substance P (10 μg in 0.1 ml of 0.9% NaCl) was applied to the receptive fields of the units by means of injection with a 27 gauge needle and afferent activity of the units was recorded from dorsal root filaments. Changes of afferent discharge rates and von Frey thresholds were measured sequentially after the application of substance P.

Most of the units (83.3%) showed an increase in spontaneous discharge rates after the application of substance P; 54.2% of the units showed immediate onset and 29.2% of the units showed slow onset of the excitation (Fig. 24.8A–F). One-third of the units showed decreased von Frey thresholds after the application of substance P. Substance P had an excitatory effect on 81.8% of the units, with thresholds greater than 5.0 g and conduction velocities less than 30 m/s, that may serve as nociceptors, and on 84.6% of the units, with thresholds less than 2.0 g, which may serve as proprioceptors. These results suggest that substance P may contribute in transmission of both nociceptive and proprioceptive sensations in the primary afferent units in the lumbar facet joint and adjacent tissues.

Recently it has been demonstrated that aging and/or degeneration of the lumbar spine may be in part related to neurogenic mediators secondary to vibration (Weinstein et al 1988b; Frymoyer et al 1989). Animal-based paradigms and techniques for experimentally creating accelerated aging and/or degeneration within the functional spinal unit, have established that low frequency vibration causes changes in the amounts of substance P and vasoactive intestinal peptides within the dorsal root ganglion. The results of preliminary studies have led to the development of a model to help explain chronic functional spinal unit degeneration that supports causal links between environmental factors (e.g. vibration) and degeneration, mediated by biological events. The model proposes that neuropeptides released from the dorsal root ganglion, induced by environmental and structural factors such as vibration, mediate a progressive degeneration of the functional spinal unit by stimulating the synthesis of inflammatory agents (e.g. prostaglandin E_2) and various degradative enzymes (e.g. proteases).

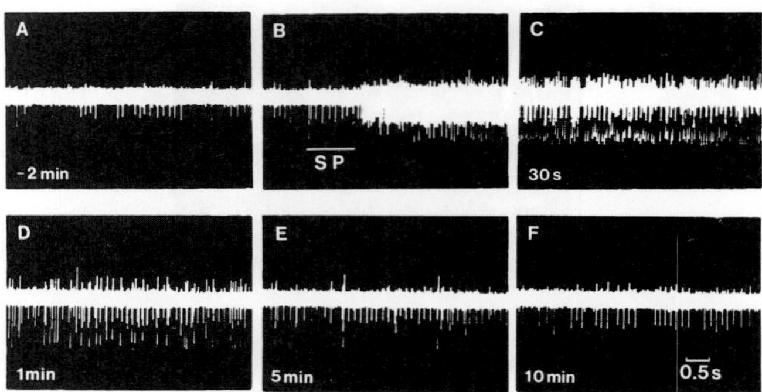

Fig. 24.8 Excitation of multiple units in the facet joint in response to the application of substance P (SP, 0.1 ml, 100 μg/ml). **A** Discharges 2 min before SP application. **B** SP application at horizontal bar. **C-F** Discharges at 30 s, 1 min, 5 min and 10 min after SP application. In (F) the larger unit returned to baseline discharge rate. (From Yamashita et al 1993.)

The now weakened functional spinal unit has increased susceptibility to environmental factors which in turn, lowers the threshold necessary to stimulate neuropeptide activity, thereby perpetuating a degenerative spiral (Fig. 24.9) (Weinstein 1992).

In studies by Levine and by Lotz, arthritis was produced by infusion of substance P and decreased or inhibited by substance P antagonists (Levine et al 1985; Lotz et al 1987). If substance P is released in and around the functional spinal unit, it is, in theory, capable of stimulating or activating various proteases that, in effect, will degrade collagen. Thus, this rationale is important for further understanding of the degenerative 'aging' spiral. Furthermore, the aforementioned nonneurogenic mediators, such as prostaglandins (PGE_1 or E_2), bradykinin, serotonin, histamine and leukotrienes, appear to play a significant role in pain, hyperalgesia and puritis. Prostanglandins are known to enhance the C fibre response. Bradykinin and serotonin are known to enhance the heat-sensitive response of C fibres as well as their mechanosensitivity. Leukotriene B_4 is chemotactic as stated, and is necessary to sensitise C nociceptors.

It is obviously important to keep in mind the interrelationships between these neurogenic and nonneurogenic mediators in the injury and repair process when considering the degenerative spiral or aging of osteoarthritis. Recently, paradigms have been proposed that suggest cytokines may leak from a degenerated facet joint and may, in and of themselves, be injurious to nerve tissue. In an experimental model, cytokines appear to impair nerve impulse conduction of rat sciatic nerves (Wehling et al 1989).

SUMMARY

While indications for surgical intervention for a patient with a herniated disc are relatively clear, those for back

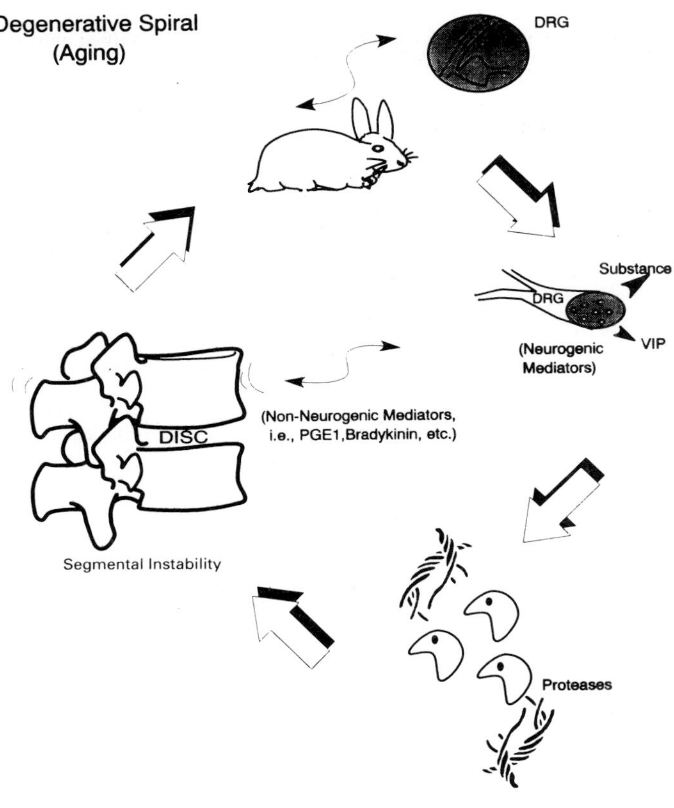

Fig. 24.9

and/or neck pain, accompanied by incidential spondylosis, are not. To further understand the pathophysiology of spinal pain and interventions thereof, our treatment should be directed to controlling, where possible, not only pain but also the degenerative 'aging' spiral.

In the classic model of disease, patients often have symptoms and present with significant pathology. However, more often than not, patients present with many symptoms and little pathology, or a great deal of pathology and few symptoms. How can we, therefore, explore these complicated issues? Can we use animal models to stimulate the herniated disc or spinal stenosis and objectively measure function and/or monitor pain behaviours? Can we measure changes associated with the clinical and the neurophysiological responses to injury and repair and can we assess the cellular response to injury and repair?

Despite our scientific efforts to understand the physical properties of spinal pain and degenerative arthritis, we have numerous untravelled roads to explore. Many of these roads will be dead-ends, which makes for a tortuous journey for the uninterested. Those who care to pursue the path of further understanding should not be discouraged by our scientific limitations. Textbooks are filled with knowledge about pain impulses travelling from the spine to the dorsal horn and into the spinal cord. Yet we still do not understand our most important processes as they relate to the perception of pain or how these perceptions interact in the development and manifestation of arthritis and/or spondylosis. Today, in the United States, one family in three contains someone suffering from pain and we, as investigators interested in studying the spine and its causes of pain, must call upon our colleagues from various scientific disciplines – biological, neurochemical, immunological, psychological and biomechanical – to acheive a better understanding in the diagnosis and treatment of spinal disease. Until these disciplines and others are united in this common goal, our individual domains will remain unable to understand back pain.

REFERENCES

Andersson G 1991 The epidemiology of spinal disorders. In: J W Frymoyer (ed) The adult spine: principles and practice, Raven Press, New York ch 7, p 107–146

Andersson G, Bogduk N, DeLuca C et al 1989 Muscle, part A: clinical perspective. In: Frymoyer J W, Gordon S L (eds) New perspectives on low back pain. American Academy of Orthopaedic Surgeons, Park Ridge, Illinois, 293–334

Arroyo P 1966 Electromyography in the evaluation of reflex muscle spasm. Journal of the Florida Medical Association 53: 29–31

Ashton I K, Ashton B A, Gibson S J, Polak J M, Jaffray D C, Eisenstein S M 1992 Morphological basis for back pain: the demonstration of nerve fibers and neuropeptides in the lumbar facet joint capsule and not in ligamentum flavum. Journal of Orthopaedic Research 10: 72–78

Avramov A, Cavanaugh J M, Ozaktay A C, Getchell T V, King A I 1992 Effects of controlled mechanical loading on group II, III, and IV afferents from the lumbar facet joint and surrounding muscle: an in vitro study. Journal of Bone and Joint Surgery (in press)

Berberich P, Hoheisel U, Mense S 1988 Effects of carrageenan-induced myositis on the discharge properties of Group III and IV muscle receptors in the cat. Journal of Neurophysiology 59: 1395–1409

Bergmann L, Alexander L 1941 Vascular supply of spinal ganglia. Archives of Neurology 46: 761–782

Blikra G 1969 Intradural herniated lumbar disc. Journal of Neurosurgery 31: 676–679

Boachie-Adjei O 1988 Evaluation of the patient with low back pain. Postgraduate Medicine 84: 110–119

Bogduk N 1983 The innervation of the lumbar spine. Spine 8: 286–293

Bogduk N, Long D M 1980 Percutaneous lumbar medial branch neurotomy: a modification of facet denervation. Spine 5: 193–200

Bogduk N, Tynan W, Wilson A S 1981 The innervation of the human lumbar intervertebral discs. Journal Anatomy 132: 39–56

Cavanaugh J M, El-Bohy A A, Hardy W H, Getchell T V, Getchell M L, King A I 1989 Sensory innervation of soft tissues of lumbar spine in the rat. Journal of Orthopaedic Research 7: 389–397

Cavanaugh J M, Yamashita T, Ozaktay A C, King A I 1990 An inflammation model of low back pain. Proceedings of the International Society for the Study of the Lumbar Spine, Boston, p 46

Cavanaugh J M, Avramov A, Ozaktay A C, Blagoev D, King A I 1992 Initial electrophysiological studies of neurons of the lumbar spinal canal. Proceedings of the International Society for the Study of the Lumbar Spine, May 20–24, Chicago

Coggeshall R E, Hong K A P, Langford L A, Schaible H G, Schmidt R F 1983 Discharge characteristics of fine medial articular afferents at rest and during passive movements of inflamed knee and joints. Brain Research 272: 185–188

Cuello A C, Polak J M, Pearse A G E 1976 Substance P: a naturally occuring transmitter in human spinal cord. Lancet 2: 1054–1056

Delamarter R, Bohlman H, Dodge L, Biro C 1990 Experimental lumbar spinal stenosis. Journal of Bone and Joint Surgery 72: 110–120

Denslow J S, Clough G H 1941 Reflex activity in the spinal extensors. Journal of Neurophysiology 1: 430–437

Devor M, Obermeyer M 1984 Membrane differentiation in rat dorsal root ganglia and possible consequences for back pain. Neuroscience Letters 51: 341–346

Devor M, Wall P D 1990 Cross-excitation in dorsal root ganglion of nerve-injured and intact rats. Journal of Neurophysiology 64: 1733–1746

El-Bohy A A, Goldberg S J, King A I 1987 Measurement of facet capsular stretch. Biomechanics symposium. 1987 Conference of the American Society of Mechanical Engineers, Cincinnati, Ohio, vol 84, p 161–164

El-Bohy A A, Cavanaugh J M, Getchell M L, Bulas T, Getchell T V, King A I 1988 Localization of substance P and neurofilament immunoreactive fibers in the lumbar facet joint capsule and supraspinous ligament of the rabbit. Brain Research 460: 379–382

Elliot F A 1944 Tender muscles in sciatica: electromyographic studies. Lancet 1: 47–49

Ferreira S H 1972 Prostaglandins, aspirin-like drugs and analgesia. Nature 240: 200–203

Fisher A A, Chang C H 1985 Electromyographic evidence of paraspinal muscle spasm during sleep in patients with low back pain. Clinical Journal Pain 1: 147–154

Fitzgerald M, Lynn B 1976 The weak excitation of some cutaneous receptors in cats and rabbits by synthetic substance P. Journal of Physiology 265: 549–563

Ford-Hutchinson A W, Bray M A, Doig M V et al 1980 Leukotriene B, a potent chemokinetic and aggregating substance released from polymorphonuclear leukocytes. Nature 286: 264–265

Franz M, Mense S 1975 Muscle receptors with group IV afferent fibers responding to application bradykinin. Brain Research 92: 369–383

Frymoyer J W, Cats-Baril W 1987 Predictors of low back pain disability. Clinical Orthopaedics and Related Research 221: 89–98

Frymoyer J, Akeson W, Brandt K, Goldenberg D, Spencer D 1989 Posterior support structures, part A: clinical perspective. In: Frymoyer J W, Gordon S L (eds) New perspectives in low back pain. American Academy of Orthopaedic Surgeons, ch 6, p 217–248

Ghormley R K 1933 Low back pain with special reference to the articular facets, with presentation of an operative procedure. Journal of the American Medical Association 17: 73

Gibson S J, Polak J M, Bloom S R et al 1981 The distribution of nine peptides in rat spinal cord with special emphasis on the substantia gelatinosa and on the area around the central canal lamina ten. Journal Comparative Neurology 201: 65–79

Giles G F, Taylor J R 1987 Human zygapophyseal joint capsule and synovial fold innervation. British Journal of Rheumatology 26: 93–98

Greenbarg P E, Brown M D, Pallares V S, Tompkins J S, Mann N H 1988 Epidural anesthesia for lumbar spine surgery. Journal of Spinal Disorders 1: 139–143

Grigg P, Schaible H G, Schmidt R F 1986 Mechanical sensitivity of group III and IV afferents from posterior articular nerve in normal and inflamed cat knee. Journal of Neurophysiology 55: 635–643

Gronblad M, Korkala O, Konttinen Y T et al 1991a Silver impregnation and immunohistochemical study of nerves in lumbar facet joint plical tissue. Spine 16: 34–38

Gronblad M, Weinstein J N, Santavirta S 1991b Immunohistochemical observations on spinal tissue innervation. A review of hypothetical mechanisms of back pain. Acta Orthopaedica Scandinavica 62: 614–622

Guilbaud G, Iggo A, Tegner R 1985 Sensory receptors in ankle joints of normal and arthritic rats. Experimental Brain Research 58: 29–40

Guyton A C 1981 Sensory receptors and their basic mechanisms of action. In: Guyton A C (ed) Textbook of medical physiology, 6th edn. W B Saunders, Philadelphia, p 588–596

Helbig T, Lee C K 1988 The lumbar facet syndrome. Spine 13: 61–64

Henry J L 1976 Effects of substance P on functionally identified units in cat spinal cord. Brain Research 114: 439–451

Hirsch C, Ingelmark B E, Miller M 1963 The anatomical basis for low back pain. Acta Orthopaedica Scandinavica 33: 1–17

Hokefelt T, Kellerth J O, Nilsson G, Pernow B 1975 Experimental immunohistochemical studies on the localization and distribution of substance P in cat primary sensory neurons. Brain Research 100: 235–252

Howe J F, Loeser J D, Calvin W H 1977 Mechanosensitivity of dorsal root ganglia and chronically injured axons: a physiological basis for the radicular pain of nerve root compression. Pain 3: 25–41

Iggo A 1985 Sensory receptors in inflamed tissues. Advances in Inflammation Research 10: 352–355

Ikari C 1954 A study of the mechanism of low back pain. The neurohistological examination of the disease. Journal of Bone and Joint Surgery 36A: 195

Jackson H C, Winkelmann R K, Bickel W H 1966 Nerve endings in the human spinal column and related structures. Journal of Bone and Joint Surgery 48A: 1272–1281

Jackson R P, Jacobs R R, Montesano P X 1988 Facet joint injection in low back pain: a prospective statistical study. Spine 13: 966–971

Janig W, Koltzenburg M 1991 Receptive properties of pial afferents. Pain 45: 77–85

Jung A, Bruschwig A 1932 Recherches histologique des articulations des corps vertebraux. Presse Medicale 40: 316–317

Korkala O, Gronblad M, Liesi P, Karaharju E 1985 Immunohistochemical demonstration of nociceptors in the ligamentous structures of the lumbar spine. Spine 10: 156–157

Kozin F, Cochrane C G 1988 The contact activation system of plasma: biochemistry and pathophysiology. In: Gallin J I, Goldstein I M, Snyderman R, (eds) Inflammation: basic principles and clinical correlates. Raven Press, New York, ch 7, p 101–120

Kraft G H, Johnson E W, Laban M M 1968 The fibrositis syndrome. Archives of Physical Medicine and Rehabilitation 49: 155–162

Kumazawa T, Mizumura K 1977 The polymodal receptors in the testes of dogs. Brain Research 136: 553–558

Kurahashi Y, Hirota N, Sato Y, Hino Y, Satoh M, Takagi H 1985 Evidence that substance P and somatostatin transmit separate information related to pain in the spinal dorsal horn. Brain Research 325: 294–298

Kuslich S D, Ulstrom C L, Micheal C J 1991 The tissue origin of lowback pain and sciatica: a report of pain response to tissue stimulation during operation on the lumbar spine using local anesthesia. Orthopedic Clinics of North America 22: 181–187

Levine J D, Gooding J, Donatoni P et al 1985 The role of polymorphonuclear leukocytes in hyperalgesia. Journal of Neuroscience 5: 3025–3029

Lewin T, Moffett B, Viidik A 1962 The morphology of the lumbar synovial intervertebral joints. Acta Morphologica Neurologica Scandinavica 4: 299–319

Lewis T, Kellgren J H 1939 Observations relating to referred pain, visceromotor reflexes and other associated phenomena. Clinical Science 4: 47–71

Lieberman A R 1976 Sensory ganglion. In: London D N (ed) The peripheral nerve. Chapman & Hall, London p 188–278

Lilius G, Laasonen E M, Myllynen P, Harilainen A, Gronlund G 1989 Lumbar facet syndrome: a randomised clinical trial. Journal of Bone and Joint Surgery 71B: 681–684

Lindblom K, Rexed B 1948 Spinal nerve injury in dorsolateral protrusion of lumbar discs. Journal of Neurosurgery 5: 413

Lotz M, Carson D A, Vaughan J H 1987 Substance P activation of rheumatoid synoviocytes: Neural pathway in the pathogenesis of arthritis. Science 235: 893–895

Malinsky J 1959 The ontogenetic development of nerve terminations in the intervertebral discs of man. Acta Anatomica 38: 96–113

Mense S 1977 Nervous outflow from skeletal muscle following chemical noxious stimulation. Journal of Physiology 267: 75–88

Mense S 1981 Sensitization of group IV muscle receptors to bradykinin by 5-hydroxytryptamine and prostaglandin E_2. Brain Research 225: 95–105

Mense S, Meyer H 1985 Different types of slowly-conducting afferent

units in cat skeletal muscle and tendon. Journal of Physiology 363: 403–417
Mooney V 1987 Where is the pain coming from? Spine 12: 754–759
Mooney V 1989 The classification of low back pain. Annals of Medicine 21: 321–325
Mooney V 1991 The classification of low back pain. In: Mayer T G, Mooney V, Gatchell R J (eds) Contemporary conservative care for painful spinal disorders. Lea & Febiger, Philadelphia
Mooney V, Robertson J 1976 The facet syndrome. Clinical Orthopaedics and Related Research 115: 149–156
Nakamura-Craig M, Smith T W 1989 Substance P and peripheral inflammatory hyperalgesia. Pain 38: 91–98
Oku R, Satoh M, Takagi H 1987 Release of substance P from the spinal dorsal horn is enhanced in polyarthritic rats. Neuroscience Letters 74: 315–319
Ozaktay A C, Yamashita T, Cavanaugh J M, King A I 1991 Fine nerve fibers and endings in the fibrous capsule of the lumbar facet joint. Proceedings of the 37th Annual Meeting of the Orthopedic Research Society, Anaheim, California, vol 16, section 2, p 353
Paris S V 1983 Anatomy as related to function and pain. In: Symposium on evaluation and care of lumbar spine problems. Orthopedic Clinics of North America 14: 475–489
Pedersen H E, Blunck C F J, Gardner E 1956 The anatomy of lumbosacral posterior rami and meningeal branches of spinal nerves (sinuvertebral nerves). Journal of Bone and Joint Surgery 38A: 377–391
Pioro E, Hughes J T, Cuello A C 1984 Demonstration of substance P immunoreactivity in the nucleus dorsalis of human spinal cord. Neuroscience Letters 51: 61–65
Pope M, Wilder D, Booth J 1982 The biomechanics of low back pain. In: White A A III, Gordon S L (eds) Symposium on idiopathic low back pain. American Academy of Orthopedic Surgeons. C V Mosby, St. Louis p 252–295
Praemer A, Furner S, Rice D 1992 Musculoskeletal conditions in the United States. American Academy of Orthopaedic Surgeons, Park Ridge, Illinois
Randic M, Miletic V 1977 Effect of substance P in cat dorsal horn neurons activated by noxious stimuli. Brain Research 128: 164–169
Roofe P G 1940 Innervation of annulus fibrosus and posterior longitudinal ligament. Archives Neurology Psychiatry 44: 100–103
Rydevik B, Lundborg G, Bagge U 1981 Effects of greater compression on interneural blood flow: an in vivo study on rat tibial nerve. Journal of Hand Surgery 6: 3–12
Saal J D, Dobrow R, White A H et al 1989 Biochemical evidence of inflammation in discogenic lumbar radiculopathy. Presented at International Society for the Study of the Lumbar Spine Meeting, May 1989, Kioto, Japan
Schaible H G, Schmidt R F 1985 Effects of an experimental arthritis on the sensory properties of fine articular afferent units. Journal of Neurophysiology 54: 1109–1122
Shantha T R, Evans J A 1972 The relationship of epidural anesthesia to neuromembranes and arachnoid villi. Anesthesiology 37: 543–557
Shealy C N 1976 Facet denervation in the management of back pain and sciatic pain. Clinical Orthopaedics and Related Research 115: 157–164
Smyth M J, Wright V 1958 Sciatica and the intervertebral disc: an experimental study. Journal of Bone and Joint Surgery 40A: 1401–1418
Stillwell D L 1956 The nerve supply of the vertebral column and its associated structures in the monkey. Anatomical Records 125: 139–169
Wall P D, Devor M 1983 Sensory afferent impulses originate from dorsal root ganglia as well as from the periphery in normal and nerve injured rats. Pain 17: 321–339
Walsh T, Weinstein J N, Aprill C, Montgomery W 1990 Lumbar discography in normal subjects: a controlled prospective study. Journal of Bone and Joint Surgery 72A: 1081–1088
Wehling P, Bandara G, Evans C H 1989 Synovial cytokines impair the function of the sciatic nerve in rats: a possible element in the pathophysiology of radicular syndromes. Neuro-Orthopedics 7: 55–59
Weinstein J N 1992 The role of neurogenic and non-neurogenic mediators as they relate to pain in the development of osteoarthritis. (A clinical review.) Spine 17 (10S). Special Edition Cervical Spine Research Society
Weinstein J N, Claverie W, Gibson S 1988a The pain of discography. Spine 13: 1344–1348
Weinstein J N, Pope M, Schmidt R, Seroussi R 1988b Neuropharmacologic effects of vibration on the dorsal root ganglion and the model model. Spine 13: 521–525
Wiberg G 1947 Back pain in relation to the nerve supply of the intervertebral disc. Acta Orthopaedica Scandinavica 19: 211–221
Wiesel S W, Feffer H L, Rothman R H 1984 Industrial low back pain: A prospective evaluation of a standardized diagnostic and treatment protocol. Spine 9: 199–203
Wyke B 1980 The neurology of low back pain. In: Jayson M I V (ed) The lumbar spine and back pain, 2nd Edn. Pitman Medical London, p 265–339
Yamashita T, Cavanaugh J M, El-Bohy A, Getchell T V, King A I 1990 Mechanosensitive afferent units in the lumbar facet joint. Journal of Bone and Joint Surgery 72A: 865–870
Yamashita T, Cavanaugh J M, Ozaktay A C, Avramov A, Getchell T V, King A I 1993 Effects of substance P on the mechanosensitive units in the lumbar facet joint and adjacent tissue. Journal of Orthopaedic Research 11: 205–214
Yang K H, King A I 1984 Mechanism of facet load transmission as a hypothesis for low back pain. Spine 9: 557–565
Yoshizawa H, O'Brien J P, Smith W T, Trumper M 1980 The neuropathology of intervertebral discs removed for low back pain. Journal of Pathology 132: 95–104
Yoshizawa H, Kobayashi S, Hachiya Y 1991 Blood supply of nerve roots and dorsal root ganglia. Orthopedic Clinics of North America 22: 195–211
Zieglgansberger W, Tulloch I F 1979 Effects of substance P on neurones in the dorsal horn of the spinal cord of the cat. Brain Research 166: 273–282

25. Upper extremity pain

Anders E. Sola

EVALUATION OF THE PATIENT PRESENTING WITH UPPER EXTREMITY PAIN

Upper extremity pain can be an enigma to physicians because it may be related to many different conditions: degeneration of cervical spine processes, degeneration of the affected joint, trauma to the cervical spine or affected joint, vascular compromise, nerve impingement, thoracic or abdominal pathology or any combination of these elements. Further, pain which emanates from a joint area may involve muscle, ligaments, tendons or the capsule. Therefore unless the aetiology of pain is obvious, the clinical management of upper extremity pain begins with a determination, through history and examination, of whether the pain is intrinsic to the shoulder area, extrinsic, or of combined aetiologies (Table 25.1)(DePalma 1973; Bateman 1978; Calliet 1981)

Intrinsic shoulder pain

Intrinsic pain is most often caused by acute trauma, minor chronic trauma (overuse or strain), arthritides (osteoarthritis is fairly common; rheumatoid arthritis is less common), local infection or tumour, infectious arthritis and capsulitis in association with any condition that causes splinting. When the supraspinatus tendon, acromioclavicular joint, sternoclavicular joint, or anterior subacromial area is implicated as the source of pain, the specific structure will be exquisitely sensitive to touch (Steindler 1959; DePalma 1973). Examination for trigger points (TPs) requires more diligence and pressure to identify the cause of pain referral (Travell & Simons 1983).

Extrinsic shoulder pain

Cervical radiculopathy affecting the C5–T1 roots is a common neurological cause of shoulder pain; however, cervical lesions may cause multilevel nerve root irritation without radiculitis (Bateman 1978). Other neurological

Table 25.1 Causes of shoulder pain

Intrinsic causes
The joint
Acromioclavicular separation
Acute with instability
Chronic with degenerative joint disease
Adhesive capsulitis (idiopathic, secondary)
Glenohumeral instability (capsular laxity, labrum tear)
Periarticular
Myofascial syndromes
Bursitis, tendinitis (supraspinatus, infraspinatus, bicipital)
Impingement (subacromial)
Rotator cuff tear
Other
Fracture (proximal humerus, scapula, clavicle)
Myofascial trigger points in interscapular, periscapular muscles
Tumour (metastatic, primary)
Extrinsic causes of shoulder pain
Elbow or wrist pathology (carpal tunnel syndrome)
Cervical or thoracic nerve root irritation; spondylosis; herniated disc
Injuries to the brachial plexus
Myofascial trigger points in the trapezii, levator scapulae, scalenae, pectoralis muscles
Thoracic outlet syndrome (cervical rib, scalenus anticus)
Somatic disorders (free air under diaphragm)
Visceral disorders (gallstones, cholecystitis, hepatitis, myocardial infarction, pneumonitis or tumours of lung/spinal cord)

Adapted from Gerhart et al 1985

disorders affecting the shoulder are pathology in the cervical roots, the brachial plexus, and the axillary, suprascapular or other peripheral nerves (Gerhart et al 1985).

Additional causes of extrinsic pain are myofascial trigger points in the muscles of the neck and shoulder, severe temporomandibular joint disease, cervicodorsal ligamental sprains, thoracic outlet syndromes, injuries to the brachial plexus and referred pain from visceral disorders, such as gallstones, cholecystitis, hepatitis, myocardial infarction, pneumonitis or tumours of the lung or spinal cord (Bonica 1990). When pain is referred to the shoulder, a common site of pain is the anterior-superior portion of the shoulder.

Three clues suggest exclusively extrinsic causes:

1. virtual absence of objective findings in the shoulder joint
2. normal active and passive range of movement (ROM) without pain
3. absence of point tenderness with direct pressure on the bicipital tendon, supraspinatus tendon, and the clavicular joints.

Pain referred from the shoulder is rarely felt beyond the insertion of the deltoid; therefore a primary or secondary extrinsic cause is suggested when the extremities are affected.

Pain of combined intrinsic and extrinsic aetiology increases with aging; i.e. in older patients shoulder pain is more likely to be complicated by spondylosis or multiple involvement of nerve root and degeneration of the joint, particularly of muscles of the rotator cuff. Myofascial disorders are often present as a secondary disorder in conjunction with acute or nonacute trauma and degenerative conditions.

Finally, there are a number of factors that may contribute to the aetiology and intensity of a painful event. These include stressors, either physical or psychological, latent trigger points from previous injuries and the patient's physical and psychological 'interpretation' of the pain and its importance.

Important elements of the history

The first purpose of the history is to determine whether the pain experienced in the upper extremity actually originates in the structures of the neck, shoulder, forearm or wrist. Observation of the total patient is important. Does the patient appear ill? Is he or she feverish or reporting recent illness? What is the patient's age and general health status? Does the patient appear tense or report unusual stresses?

Pertinent data can usually be elicited from the patient by asking what the patient thinks the problem is. If it is necessary to lead the patient, the examiner should ask what has happened recently, if the patient has been involved in a motor vehicle accident in the past or whether there has been any change in work or recreational activities.

Always using the vocabulary of the patient, the history-taker should question him or her closely about the chronological development of the symptoms and the onset and nature of the pain. Where is it felt? Does it feel superficial or deep, such as bone pain? What does it feel like? 'Pins and needles', 'burning sensations' and 'shooting pains' are terms easily understood. Does the patient experience a 'grating feeling' when turning the head or neck? Does he or she experience electric-like pain on flexion or extension of the neck? Has the patient experienced any arthritis/gout/rheumatic problems? Does the patient have other aches and pains? Difficulty in swallowing? Does the patient have unusual sensations into the hand or fingers? Has the patient had the same problem before? If so, what was the diagnosis and treatment?

It is wise to also question the effects of the pain. Is there anything the patient normally does that he or she cannot do because of pain? Does riding in a car aggravate the condition? Does pain result in limitation of movements or weakness? Is it worse at night? Does it interfere with sleep or result in the patient's assuming different sleeping positions?

The history should also include recent medical care and medication or drug use. Has the patient been treated recently by another physician? Were any X-rays taken? Has the patient been hospitalised, particularly because of injury to the back or upper extremity? Is the patient taking any drugs, antibiotics? Heavy alcohol consumption may be a significant clue and exposure to industrial chemicals may play a part in upper extremity pain. (See also Scadding (Ch. 37 in this book) for a discussion of peripheral neuropathies caused by diabetes or thyroid disease, nutritional deficiencies, metabolic disorders, viral infections and other entities.)

Examination

Head, neck, and cervical spine

A thorough screening to determine the probable aetiology of upper extremity pain usually begins with at least a routine evaluation of head, neck and cervical spine. The few procedures outlined below are adequate to eliminate these structures as the probable source of pain in the initial assessment.

1. Visual inspection, looking for deformities, atrophy, loss of normal contour
2. Palpation of spinous and transverse processes, thyroid gland and carotid pulse
3. Range of movement of head and neck, with rotation right-to-left, flexion/extension, and lateral bending
4. Distraction or evaluation of the effect of cervical traction by placing hands on occiput and under chin
5. Compression: if neural foramina are compromised, this may produce or intensify pain
6. Valsalva manoeuvre to determine if straining with holding the breath reproduces pain
7. Lhermitte's sign: flexion or extension of the head and neck causes lancinating or 'electric' shock radiating from neck into hands (Brody & Wilkins 1969)
8. Adson's test: in the modified Adson's test, the patient's arm is abducted to 90° and externally rotated with the elbow flexed. The patient turns the head toward the abducted arm, takes a deep breath, and

coughs. The test is positive if the radial pulse is reduced or absent. This may indicate compression of the subclavian artery. (Adson 1951)

Testing for radiculitis is based on radiation of symptoms such as sensory changes, weakness and loss of reflexes. If the symptoms are aggravated by cervical tests that stretch the nerve roots, increase intraspinal pressure (Valsalva manoeuvre) or decrease the spinal formina (head compression), the diagnosis is implied.

Cervical spondylosis, which results in gradually increasing clinical signs, may present multiple levels of nerve root irritation and contribute to confusion of diagnosis, particularly in patients over 55 years of age. In younger age groups, single nerve root involvement due to cervical herniation is more common (see Chs 40 and 55).

A summary of neurological levels relating to the upper extremity is shown in Table 25.2. Weakness in any of these extremity structures calls for further evaluation of the cervical spine in addition to assessment of the extremity itself.

Local structures

The shoulder joint has the most complex motions of the body (Saha 1961; Post 1987). They are possible because the shoulder girdle is composed of three joints (the sternoclavicular, acromioclavicular and glenohumeral) which work with the scapulothoracic articulation in a synchronised pattern to provide extension, flexion, abduction, adduction, internal and external rotation. ROM in any of the three joints may be inhibited because of pain, neurological deficit or skeletal or soft tissue pathology. Both extremities should be tested for active and passive ROM to characterise the pain pattern and compared. ROM should also be tested against resistance. If any weakness is noted, a thorough muscle test and grading should be done.

Pain upon abduction between 60–120° suggests supraspinatus tendinitis; pain with forward flexion up to 90° with internal rotation suggests rotator cuff involvement due to impingement; pain at 140–180° of abduction suggests acromioclavicular joint pain. In testing ROM, the first 30–40° involve only glenohumeral motion, and patients may compensate for restriction in this area with scapulothoracic motion.

Observations of joint noises, crepitation or loss of normal gliding motion suggest that degenerative changes and intrinsic injury must be ruled out. A not uncommon condition is friction rub secondary to exostoses either on the scapula or rib, causing pain, although ROM may be normal. When this is suspected, special thoracic and scapular X-ray views are required.

Point tenderness examination of the two clavicular joints, supraspinatus tendon, bicipital tendon and anterior subacromial region (for impingement syndrome) will usually be sufficient to identify local pathology. Figure 25.1 provides a review of shoulder structures with common points of tenderness. Palpation must be done gently, as excessive pressure will be painful and may irritate sensitive tissues. To palpate the bicipital groove, the arm is rotated externally (Yergason's test). The groove lies between the medial lesser tuberosity and the more lateral greater tuberosity. Passive extension of the shoulder will allow examination of the bursa and the cuff as it moves these structures forward; the insertion of the subscapularis is not palpable. Swelling and unusual warmth should be noted. Careful examination may reveal abnormal masses or thickening. Fluid can never be palpated in a normal synovial joint and its presence is a sign of joint pathology. If a ligament is tender or painful on palpation, the ligament has been injured or there is pathology at the joint. Palpation of muscle will identify sensitive trigger points that may be the primary or secondary cause of pain.

Table 25.2 Summary of neurological levels relating to upper extremity pain and/or dysfunction

	Motor	Sensory	Reflex
C5	Shoulder abduction, deltoids, biceps	Lateral aspect, arm (C5 axillary nerve)	Biceps
C6	Wrist extension	Lateral forearm, musculocutaneous	Brachioradialis
C7	Wrist flexion Finger extension	Middle finger	Triceps
C8	Finger flexion	Medial forearm	Finger flexion Hand intrinsics
T1	Finger abduction	Medial arm	Hand intrinsics

Supporting diagnostic procedures

Often careful history-taking, palpation and range of motion will establish a clear aetiology for upper extremity pain on the initial visit. However, with more complex problems or combined aetiologies, two or three evaluation visits may be necessary and it may be helpful to utilise supporting diagnostic procedures such as special roentgenographs or electromyograms (EMG) with peripheral nerve conduction studies.

Diagnostic radiographic studies

Radiographic studies are done on joints as indicated by the initial work-up. In any situation where diagnosis is difficult, these studies should include anterior/posterior and lateral views of the neck in extended, neutral and flexed positions and also oblique views to visualize the neuroforamina. Routine shoulder films include anterior and posterior views, and abduction, axillary, and bicipital

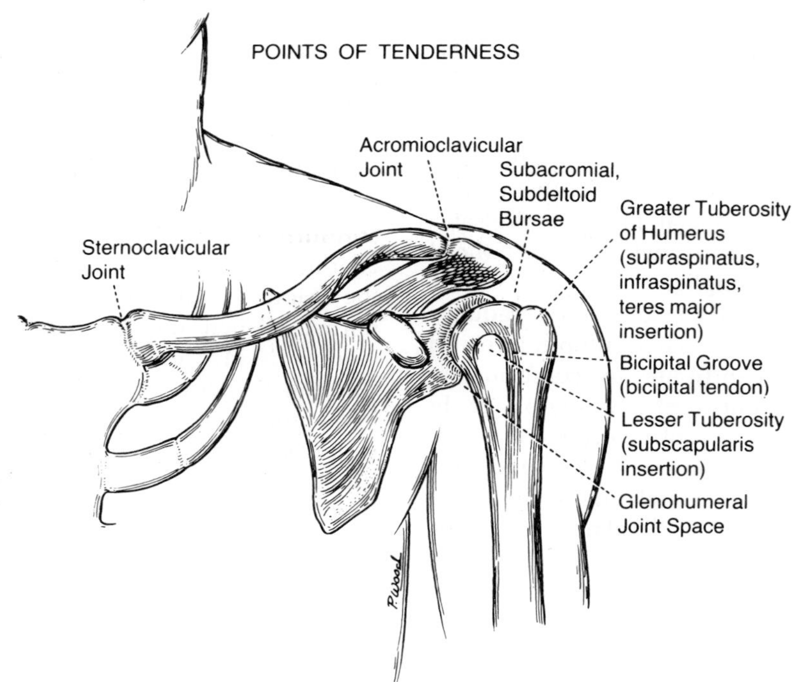

Fig. 25.1 Shoulder joint pain can arise from the greater tuberosity, the lesser tuberosity, the subacromial bursa, the subdeltoid bursa, bicipital groove and the long head of the biceps, the glenohumeral joint and the acromioclavicular joint. When degenerative changes interact with clinical findings, severe pain, dysfunction or loss of range of movement may result. Poor muscle tone, often associated with ageing, tends to exacerbate shoulder lesions.

groove views. Note that negative findings do not rule out pathology. Even positive findings do not necessarily explain the cause of pain or other symptoms.

High resolution ultrasonography is particularly helpful as a noninvasive procedure to rule out rotator cuff tears. If there is any question, or a tear is suspected, it is most easily confirmed by arthrography. Magnetic resonance imaging (MRI) holds great promise for evaluation and diagnosis of soft tissue injuries. The technology is particularly valuable in diagnosing damage to tendons, ligaments and fibrocartilage and tears in the rotator cuff or glenoid labrum.

EMG and peripheral nerve conduction studies

EMG is particularly valuable for identifying peripheral neuropathies and for eliminating cervical lesions, discogenic disease and nerve root entrapment as probable contributors to pain and dysfunction in the upper extremity. It is the only reliable tool for identifying peripheral neurocervical radiculitis.

ROTATOR CUFF INJURIES

Tendinitis

Tendinitis is generally a nontraumatic lesion which occurs as the result of gradual degenerative changes in the rotator cuff. These changes may or may not be accompanied by calcium deposits in the tendon. A mild ache or discomfort may be present for months. In calcific tendinitis the ache may suddenly develop into an intolerable, unremitting pain, usually referred to the top or lateral aspect of the shoulder. The patient will usually hold the arm immobile against the body. Deep breathing may increase the pain. This acute episode may be associated with acute bursitis as a result of calcium, which may form in the tendon in response to injury, penetrating into the bursal sac. Since the condition is related to degenerative changes, it is more common after the fifth decade of life (Calliet 1981).

Signs and symptoms

It is usually possible to arrive at a working diagnosis of shoulder tendinits through phsycial examination including resisted range of motion. With involvement of the supraspinatus tendon, pain is often localised at the greater tuberosity of the humerus. The patient may be unable or unwilling to move the arm but full passive range of motion is possible. Pain upon resisted abduction is an indication of supraspinatus tendinitis. Infraspinatus involvement is also associated with pain localised at the greater tuberosity, but it is resisted external rotation which exacerbates the pain. Tendinitis of teres minor results in pain at the greater tuberosity which is aggravated by resisted external rotation. Pain experienced locally at the lesser tuberosity may be tendinitis of the subscapularis. This will be further confirmed if the pain is associated with resisted medial rotation. Bicipital tendinitis most frequently involves the long head of the biceps muscle. Pain is experienced locally in the bicipital groove and at its attachment at the superior rim of the glenoid fossa.

Treatment course and prognosis

Calcific tendinitis in the acute stage may require immobilisation of the arm in a sling, the use of cold packs, medication with oral antiinflammatory and nonsteroidal antiinflammatory products, local anaesthetic and steroid injections. Some patients may require the use of a narcotic for several days. If this treatment course is not successful, some physicians prefer to aspirate the joint. Milder cases usually respond to conservative treatment. The most important aspect of treatment is early mobilisation of the shoulder starting with passive pendular exercises. These are followed by active pendular exercises as soon as tolerated.

Bursitis

Unfortunately the term 'bursitis' is often used inappropriately for any painful shoulder. Specifically, bursitis is an acute inflammatory response usually associated with the deposition of calcific material. The bursa swells and impinges upon surrounding structures, causing excruciating pain. Primary bursitis is an uncommon entity, but it does occur. Inflammation of the bursa is more likely to occur secondarily to a tear or inflammation of adjacent tendon or muscle, or to direct trauma. It is essentially a disease of middle-age, being associated with degenerative changes of tendon, muscle or the rotator cuff, although it is occasionally seen in a young patient.

Signs and symptoms

Subdeltoid bursitis is characterised by painful passive arc. Passive abduction is limited by pain at approximately 70 through 110–115°, after which point the pain disappears. The pain is usually sharp and localised. Abduction and external rotation increase the pain dramatically, although any motion can cause pain. Pain seems to be aggravated at night.

Roentgenograms may confirm the presence of calcific deposits. It is important to note, however, that only 35% of patients with X-ray evidence of calcium develop symptoms. Symptoms usually accompany calcium deposits greater than 1.5 cm.

Treatment course and prognosis

Treatment for bursitis is much the same as for calcific tendinitis. An unfortunate sequela of bursitis is adhesive capsulitis, particularly without proper treatment to ensure range of motion.

Bicipital tendinitis

The long head of the big tendon passes through the bicipital groove across the shoulder joint and is attached to the superior rim of the glenoid cavity. As result of degenerative changes, chronic irritation may occur over the anterior aspect of the shoulder. This is often related to repetitious movement. This condition is frequently misdiagnosed as bursitis because of the similarity of location of pain.

Signs and symptoms

Bicipital tendinitis should be suspected if there is pain and tenderness to pressure over the bicipital groove. Yergason's sign (increased pain on resistance to supination) is a positive indicator as is a palpable, swollen tendon. The pain of bicipital tendinitis may occur after heavy lifting and is associated with unusual athletic activity in young adults.

Treatment course and prognosis

Most of these patients respond to conservative treatment of resting the arm in a sling and providing analgesics for pain. Some clinicians advise local injections of steroids, but this writer has seen several cases in which treatment by steroid injection has resulted in rupture of the tendon. Range of motion must be maintained during treatment to prevent 'frozen shoulder' or adhesive capsulitis. This is usually done passively until pain is adequately controlled, at which time active exercises are introduced.

Rotator cuff tears

The rotator cuff is a band of tendinous-fibrous tissue composed of the tendons of the subscapularis, supraspinatus, infraspinatus, and teres minor muscles, which fuse around the anatomic neck of the humerus where it inserts with the joint capsule. This part of the cuff is characterised by a marginal blood supply, which contributes to early degeneration, which in turn is associated with minor tears from normal activities.

Tears of the rotator cuff should be considered in conjunction with injuries sustained while working with arms overhead, with falls involving striking the shoulder or breaking the force of the fall with an outstretched hand and with fractures or dislocations of the shoulder and greater tuberosity of the humerus. Residual pain subsequent to an earlier injury with loss of range of motion should also suggest rotator cuff tear. Degenerative cervical disease is a predisposing factor. Small tears may not require treatment. It has been reported that 30% of cadavers have rotator cuff tears.

Signs and symptoms

Rotator cuff tears are associated with pain at the anterolateral margin of the acromion. They are rare in patients under 40 years with the exception of those using the joint heavily. The patient, most often a labourer between the ages of 40 and 65, reports feeling a tear or snap in the shoulder, followed by severe pain if the tear is extensive. With less severe tears, the pain may increase in intensity, reaching a peak after 48 hours and remaining in an acute stage for several days. Shoulder motion increases the pain, which is usually felt first in the shoulder joint but may spread to the posterior scapular area and to the deltoid and forearm. Frequently the pain is described as a deep, throbbing sensation, and it may interfere with sleep.

Physical findings may include exquisite tenderness on pressure over the greater tuberosity, reduced abduction or pain on resisted abduction and weakness on forward flexion or pain on internal rotation. Scapulohumeral dysrhythm may be present. The patient may be unable to control lowering of the arm to his side, and it may drop freely. This is a useful guide for rotator cuff tears, but it should be noted that injuries to the suprascapular and axillary nerves, as well as fifth cervical root lesions, produce the same clinical sign. Atrophy of the ratator cuff suggests an injury several weeks old which involves the supraspinatus or infraspinatus muscles.

To rule out a diagnosis of rotator cuff impingement, 5 ml of local anaesthethic is injected laterally into the subacromial bursa just underneath the acromial arch. Relief of pain and improved strength around the shoulder joint following injection confirm rotator cuff impingement syndrome.

Treatment course and prognosis

Suspected lesions must be confirmed by contrast radiography, ultrasonography or MRI. Minor tears respond to nonsurgical treatment and usually heal within 2 months. Since tears are often associated with some degree of degenerative process, they tend to be a chronic problem. Severe tears should be evaluated by an orthopaedic surgeon for possible repair (Neviaser 1975; Post 1987) (Table 25.3).

Adhesive capsulitis

Adhesive capsulitis affects the glenohumeral joint. Adhesions form as result of an inflammatory response which produces saturation with a serofibrinous exudate. It is a common finding secondary to heavy use, immobilisation, injury, tendonitis, fractures about the shoulder, infections, neoplasms, general surgery and heart attacks. Bicipital tenosynovitis is also reported as a frequent cause.

Table 25.3 Shoulder pain: clinical findings and treatment

Differential diagnosis	Key findings	Key tests	Treatment
Impingement syndrome	Acromial pain on humeral forward flexion beyond 90°; tenderness on anterior insertion of supraspinatus tendon	Reduced pain with subacromial lidocaine	NSAID; subacromial steroid injection (× 3 max); cuff-strengthening exercises; acromioplasty
Rotator cuff tear	Weak external rotation; supraspinatus atrophy; painful arc 60–120°; difficulty initiating abduction; usually more painful at night; uncommon in patients under 40 years	Drop-arm test positive; subacromial dye extravasation on arthrogram	Cuff-strengthening exercises for small tears; surgery for large tears
Supraspinatus tendinits	Point tenderness; pain with external rotation	Calcification on X-ray	NSAID; acromioplasty
Biceps tendinitis	Positive Yergason's test; tender bicipital groove; anterior shoulder pain	None	NSAID; restricted activity; surgery
Frozen shoulder	Diffuse pain and tenderness; decreased passive glenohumeral motion	Reduced capsular space on arthrogram	Range of movement exercises
Glenohumeral arthritis	Increased pain with activity; barometric sensitivity	X-rays	NSAID; arthroplasty
AC joint arthritis	AC joint tenderness and pain with adduction 140–180°	X-ray; injection of lidocaine into AC joint decreases pain	NSAID; AC joint steroid injection (×3 max); distal clavicle resection

AC = acromioclavicular; NSAID = nonsteroidal antiinflammatory drug.
Adapted from Lippert & Teitz 1987

McLaughlin (1961) maintains that a shoulder which is put through the full range of movement a few times daily will not develop adhesive capsulitis, indicating that prolonged dependency is the initiating factor. The condition is unusual in patients under 40 years of age.

Signs and symptoms

The patient may report pain with a gradual onset without any known injury. It is often seen in sedentary persons who have recently begun to participate in an activity involving the upper extremities, such as golf, tennis or bowling (Neer & Welsh 1977). The patient will have difficulty putting on a shirt, combing hair, or placing the hand in a back pocket. There may be little pain on palpation, but it will be aggravated by both external and internal rotation. Pain may seem to localise in the deltoid, particularly at its insertion, and frequently causes suffering at night.

A tentative diagnosis of adhesive capsulitis must be confirmed with arthrography to differentiate a simple stiff shoulder from the inflammatory condition. Neviaser (1975) classifies patients according to how much of the injected dye is accepted into the capsule and what the patient's range of passive abduction indicates. Abduction to more than 90° and dye acceptance of more than 10 ml indicates a mild form. Moderate involvement includes patients who cannot abduct over 90° and whose capsular joint space measures from 5–10 ml. A third classification is severe capsulitis, which is usually seen only after proximal humerus fracture in patients with osteoporosis or following severe shoulder dislocation.

Treatment course and prognosis

The best treatment for adhesive capsulitis is prevention with regular, daily range of movement exercises. Fortunately, many cases respond to a conservative treatment programme consisting mainly of steroid therapy and pain management in conjuction with an aggressive physical therapy programme carried out by a qualified physical therapist. The judicious use of steroids injected into the rotator cuff and intraarticular space may be helpful when used in combination with intensive physical therapy (Sheon et al 1987).

Local anaesthetics may be adequate to facilitate therapy; however, local nerve block, particularly of the suprascapular nerve, may be indicated. Muscle relaxants are sometimes of help. Trigger points can be injected with either lidocaine or procaine to reduce the possibility of a pain cycle. Manipulation is frequently used.

When the degree of involvement is greater, manipulation may require anaesthesia. The arm may be positioned in 90° abduction during a period of 2 weeks bed rest, followed by a 3–6 month therapy programme usually leading to full recovery. The use of narcotics is not recommended over an extended period of time. Depression is not uncommon in these patients, and it should be recognised and treated as necessary.

BICIPITAL LESIONS

Bicipital subluxation

The same type of degenerative process that precipitates tendonitis can predispose older patients toward subluxation of the tendon. In younger individuals this condition may be associated with sports activities.

Signs and symptoms

When the transverse ligament is torn, local tenderness is normally experienced. The clinician may be able to feel the muscle 'snap' in and out of the groove upon passive rotation of the arm in the abducted position.

Treatment course and prognosis

When subluxation occurs in a young active person, surgery is indicated. Bicipital subluxation can lead to chronic tenosynovitis. In the older individual, restriction of activity may be the preferable course unless the patient is experiencing severe pain.

Bicipital rupture

Bicipital rupture is another condition which is usually related to degenerative changes in the biceps tendon or muscle. It may be a painless condition in which the biceps has completely separated between the muscle belly and the tendon or away from the supraglenoid fossa.

Signs and symptoms

Complete separation can usually be visualised. The flaccid biceps muscle bulges.

Treatment course and prognosis

In younger patients surgical repair is indicated. In older patients, if decrease of upper extremity strength would not impair lifestyle, no treatment is required although it may be desirable for cosmetic reasons.

ACROMIOCLAVICULAR JOINT LESIONS

Lesions of the acromioclavicular joint are one of the most overlooked causes of shoulder and arm pain. The joint is subject to arthritic involvement, to various injuries including sprains, contusions and separations, and to tumours, although these are rare (DePalma 1957).

Signs and symptoms

Pain associated with the acromioclavicular joint is usually local without referral. It is aggravated by shrugging the shoulder and by full passive adduction of the arm across the chest. X-rays are not particularly useful for diagnostic purposes if the aetiology is an arthritic process, but they will rule out separation of the joint. Separation usually involves pain over the entire shoulder, often accompanied by weakness of all shoulder movements and loss of function. Palpation of the clavicular attachment may reveal subluxation, in which the clavicle usually displaces upward.

The symptoms of degenerative arthritis include tenderness, swelling, and/or warmth over the joint.

Treatment course and prognosis

In the case of mild injury of the joint, a shoulder elbow strap is used for immobilisation for 1–2 weeks as needed. If the injury is more severe (subluxation) the strap is worn for up to 5–6 weeks. Surgery may be necessary if immobilisation is not successful. The shoulder joint must be passively put through the range of movement as tolerated by pain. In addition, appropriate measures to prevent disabilities to the hand, wrist and elbow must be taken.

ARTHRITIS

The shoulder joint has only minimal susceptibility to arthritis, probably because it is not a weight-bearing joint and only under certain conditions is it a power-bearing joint. To a great extent it escapes the destructive degenerative changes of repeated pressure and trauma. The major exception to this is athletes, particularly those who load the joint 'in bursts'. Osteoarthritis is moderately common among persons who play baseball and overhead racquet sports, skiers and musicians, being activity-related rather than disease-related. However, osteoarthritis and traumatic arthritis do occur in other patients and symptoms of painful, swollen, warm joints should suggest a systematic work-up for arthritic involvement. Other arthritides, including rheumatoid arthritis, are discussed elsewhere in this book.

HEMIPLEGIA

Shoulder pain is a common complaint of people with hemiplegia. It can be so severe that it interferes with the rehabilitation programme that is so crucial immediately after 'stroke'. Appropriate splinting to prevent capsular stretching and resultant subluxation of the glenohumeral joint is necessary early in therapy, and should help to prevent the complication of pain.

Treatment of the pain is comparable to that used in other painful shoulder conditions: injections of steroids, local anaesthetics, suprascapular nerve block and oral medications consistent with the medical status of the patient. These patients should be managed by medical personnel trained in rehabilitation or by a health care team which includes a physical therapist.

PAIN OF COMBINED AETIOLOGIES

Myofascial disorders

An understanding of myofascial disorders, their pain patterns, incidence, origins and proper treatment is absolutely essential in treatment of upper extremity pain (Travell & Rinzler 1952; Sola & Kuitert 1955; Sola et al 1955; Sola & Williams 1956; Kraft et al 1968; Simons 1975, 1976; Travell 1976; Sola 1984; Travell & Simons 1984; Bonica 1990; Roberts & Hedges 1991).

Like the lower back, the shoulder and neck region are commonly the 'storehouse' of numerous latent points that, when challenged by physical (and, to some degree, emotional) stressors can cause pain. The mechanism of pain can be described as follows: from an initiating stimulus such as trauma, fatigue, or stress, a physiological response is generated and a particular trigger point begins to send distress signals to the central nervous system. Muscles associated with the triger point become tense, and soon muscle fatigue is experienced. Local ischaemia occurs, leading to change in the extracellular environment of the affected cells, including release of algesic agents. These feed into a cycle of increasing motor and sympathetic activity and other trigger points 'flare up' contributing to the cycle (Zimmerman 1980). Thus a painful event may be magnified far out of proportion to its precipitating challenge (Fig. 25.2). Furthermore, once established as a cycle, a painful event may sustain itself in spite of control of the stimulus which originally initiated the cycle. Thus, proper and adequate treatment of a local injury may not provide alleviation of pain.

Trigger-point syndromes affect virtually everyone, either in a primary role of translating stress responses into pain or in a secondary role in which activation intensifies or prolongs pain from another stimulus. Trigger-point pain varies from slight discomfort to severe unrelenting pain and is described as either sharp or dull. It can also simulate the pain of visceral disorders which are referred to the shoulder area.

The 'injury pool' concept

Trigger points (TPs) seem to be involved in a phenomenon by which the body 'remembers' previous injury.

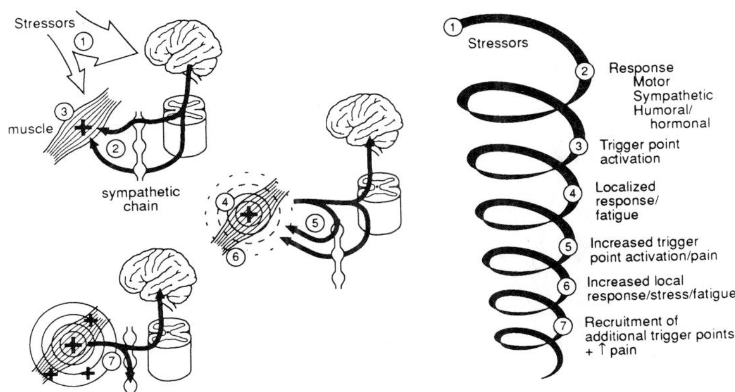

Fig. 25.2 The pain cycle. The individual, subjected to the physical and emotional stresses of daily living (1), responds with defence mechanisms (2) that include various physiological changes, such as splinting and bracing of muscles, vasomotor changes, increased sympathetic discharge, and hormonal and other humoral changes in the plasma and extracellular fluids. A particular point in a braced, stressed muscle or fascia that is more sensitive than the surrounding tissue, perhaps due to previous injury or genetic mandate, fatigues and begins to signal its distress to the central nervous system (3). A number of responses may result. The most readily understood involves the motor reflexes. Various muscles associated with the trigger point become more tense and begin to fatigue. Sympathetic responses lead to vasomotor changes within and around the trigger point. Local ischaemia after vasoconstriction or increased vascular permeability after vasodilation may lead to changes in the extracellular environment of the affected cells, release of algesic agents (bradykinins, prostaglandins), osmotic changes and pH changes, all of which may increase the sensitivity or activity of nociceptors in the area. Sympathetic activity may cause smooth muscle contraction in the vicinity of nociceptors, increasing their activity (4), which contributes to the cycle by increasing motor and sympathetic activity. This in turn leads to increased pain (5). The pain is shadowed by growing fatigue, adding an overall mood of distress to the patient's situation and feeds back to the cycle (6). As tense muscles in the affected area begin to fatigue in an environment of sympathetic stimulation and local biochemical change, latent trigger points within these muscles may also begin to fire, adding to the positive feedback cycle and spreading the pain to these adjacent muscle groups. The stress of pain and fatigue, coupled with both increased muscle tension and sympathetic tone throughout the body (conceivably with ipsilateral emphasis through the sympathetic chain) may lead to flare ups or trigger points in other muscles remote from the initial area of pain (7).

Tissues that were affected by an earlier injury become prone to react to a new challenge. Each new insult may provide additional TPs that become a part of an 'injury pool'. These 'pooled' TPs may in turn be recruited into the pain cycle in response to a later injury (Fig. 25.3). Thus a painful stimulus in a young person may be painful in direct proportion to the damage with little or no myofascial involvement in the pain process. However, in an individual with an established 'pool' of repeated injuries (generally an older individual), an injury may well be accompanied by myofascial pain and muscle involvement out of proportion to the insult (Sola 1984).

Many physicians are only now becoming aware of TPs and their significance. Most of the scapular muscles can cause shoulder pain, including the cuff muscles (infraspinati, supraspinati, subscapularis, teres minor), pectoralis major and minor, teres major and trapezii (Fig. 25.4). The erector spinii are often overlooked as a frequent source of TPs. Posterior and anterior strap muscles can also refer pain to the shoulder, and TPs present in the lumbar–gluteal region can activate TPs in the shoulder girdle.

It is important to note that although trigger-point pain can affect both sides of the body it is commonly confined to one side and is often associated with ipsilateral hypersensitivity in muscles seemingly quite removed from the reported problem. For example, pain in the neck and shoulder is commonly associated with gluteal TPs that are exquisitely sensitive to pressure even though the patient may not report overt pain in these muscles. In such cases

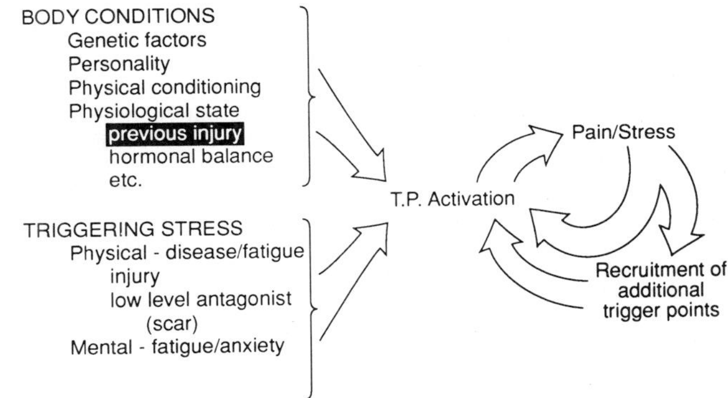

Fig. 25.3 Injury pool. A variety of stress-inducing stimuli may be implicated in the onset of myofascial pain. The power of these stimuli to induce pain is moderated by the genetics, personality, conditioning and physiological state of a particular individual. Once established, however, a painful event may sustain itself despite control or elimination of the initiating stimuli.

treatment must involve the remote ipsilateral TPs as well as those in the painful area (see Fig. 25.5).

Treatment course and prognosis

An injection of local anaesthetic or physiological saline into the TPs is often adequate to break the pain cycle (Bray & Sigmond 1941; Frost et al 1980; Tfelt-Hansen et al 1980). The use of vasocoolants, such as fluoromethane spray, has been shown to be a useful technique by Travell

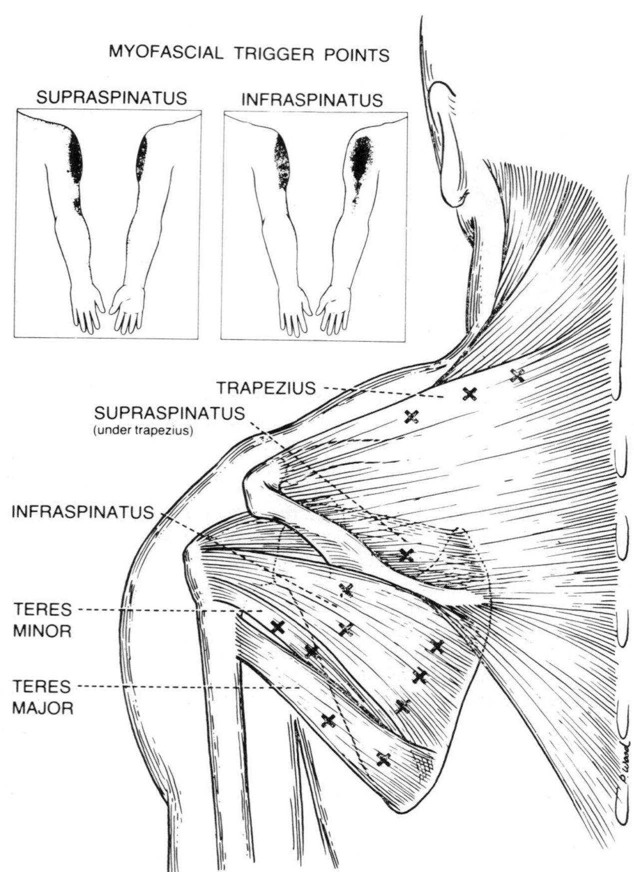

Fig. 25.4 Trigger points tend to concentrate in groups of muscles, such as the shoulder. When activated, adjacent muscle groups may become involved. The scapular muscles refer pain to the posterior or lateral surface of the shoulder girdle. The trapezius usually has local pain at the trigger points and refers to the posterior scalp and neck. Myofascial pain from the shoulder area can be reflected to the proximal arm, wrist or hand and symptoms may include weakness of grip, paraesthesia and hyperhydrosis.

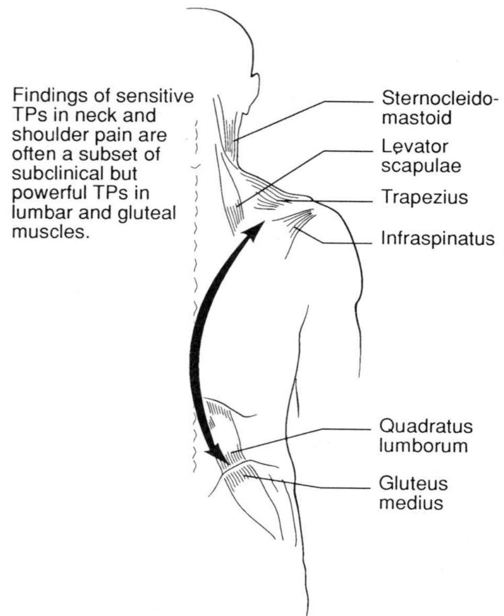

Fig. 25.5 Ipsilateral pain, a diagnostic key to treatment of refractory local pain. An ipsilateral pattern of pain is very common, with simultaneously active painful trigger points in the neck and shoulder, quadratus lumborum and gluteal muscles. The patient may not be aware of pain in the lumbar gluteal region but may confirm aching or stiffness in the hip area, sciatica-like pain or fatigue in the lower back and extremities. Hyperactive trigger points (TPs) in the lumbar gluteal muscles must be treated before positive results can be expected from treatment of TPs in head, neck or extremities.

(Travell & Daitz 1990). The insertion of thin solid needles alone (dry needling as described by Gunn) (Gunn 1989) has been found to be as effective as injection without subjecting the patient to the added tissue disruption caused by edged hypodermic needles. When the pain is secondary to another stimulus, particularly nerve root lesions or nerve compression, the treatment is never more than moderately successful in relieving pain. Therefore this procedure is useful as a differential diagnostic tool, as it interrupts the pain cycle and allows exposure of the underlying disorder. Periosteal stimulation reportedly enhances the effectiveness of TP injection, reducing myofascial pain (Lawrence 1978).

REFLEX DYSTROPHY-LIKE SYNDROMES

Reflex dystrophies are part of the group of sympathetic disorders whose features may include throbbing, burning or aching pain, hyperaesthesia, hyperalgesia and oedema, and/or erythema. These are serious, painful and disabling disorders. Onset may be triggered by coronary ischaemia, hemiplegia, adhesive capsulitis, bicipital tendinitis, trauma or even simple bruises or sprains. In a study of 140 patients with reflex dystrophy, 40% of the cases occurred following soft tissue injury, 25% following fractures, 20% were postoperative, 12% followed myocardial infarction and 3% followed CVA. It was also noted that 37% of these patients had significant emotional disturbances at the time of onset. Thus elements of the process include CNS involvement and the entire myofascial pain cycle of stressors, trigger point activation, pain and sympathetic involvement (Fig. 25.2) (Pak et al 1970). Treatment must be instituted immediately, and includes injection of the affected trigger points with an anaesthetic – corticosteroid mixture and physical therapy. If this provides no relief, one must resort to sympathetic blocks, oral corticosteroids and, finally, sympathectomy. Early treatment of the affected TPs has shown great promise in breaking this cycle.

SHOULDER–HAND SYNDROME

Signs and symptoms

The disease has several stages. Onset is usually insidious. The patient may present with a burning pain involving the shoulder and vasomotor changes in the hand and fingers. This phase may last several months. After this initial phase, shoulder pain may ease but trophic changes appear: atrophy of the muscles in the affected extremity, thickening of palmar fascia, demineralisation and atrophy of the nails. By the time these trophic changes have occurred, it is extremely difficult to reverse the disease process despite aggressive treatment and the end result is flexion deformities of the fingers. At this stage vasomotor changes are absent.

Treatment course and prognosis

This condition requires aggressive treatment. Residual damage is usually irreversible; surgery has not proven successful in restoring function. The pain associated with shoulder–hand syndrome can be excruciating, and the patient will normally require narcotics for pain management. Phenobarbital should not be given; however, other sedatives may be used. Sympathetic blocks done early in the course of the disease may be helpful, as well as corticosteroid therapy. Injection of local anaesthetics into hypersensitive areas of the shoulder or the suprascapular nerve may also be helpful. From the outset treatment must be accompanied by an intensive physical therapy programme to maintain function.

OVERUSE SYNDROMES

Although a given action or set of actions may be well within the body's capabilities, excessive repetition may, through interference with circulation, repeated microinjury, build-up of waste products, or any of these and other factors, stress a tissue beyond its anatomical or physiological limits. The stressor may be either dynamic as in the case of repetitive movement, or static as in the case of prolonged bracing or maintenance of a particular posture. In 1990 the US Bureau of Statistics reported that more than 180 000 workers suffered overuse injuries. Workers who performed more than 2000 manipulations per hour were particularly vulnerable. Those performing highly repetitive, forceful jobs were most at risk (LaDou 1990).

One should suspect an overuse syndrome when a patient reports that he or she:

1. performs a repetitive task
2. maintains a fixed posture for long periods of time
3. lifts above or below a mechanically strainful height
4. performs a tedious or monotonous task.

Furthermore it should be suspected when numerous other workers or participants have been disabled performing the same tasks. Such a finding would suggest that an evaluation of the ergonomics of the workplace would be in order (Sheon et al 1987).

The repeated movements of certain sports such as tennis, swimming and baseball, and extended periods of wrist pressure involved in cycling are well-documented sources of overuse injury. So to are certain occupations. For example, musicians are particularly vulnerable to a variety of overuse phenomena. Pianists, clarinettists, and oboists may suffer carpal tunnel syndrome or de Quervain's tenosynovitis (both dynamic stressor-related), while string and wind players frequently have shoulder problems (static stressor-related), especially impingement syndrome, subdeltoid and subacromial bursitis and bicipital tendinitis, and may also demonstrate dynamic problems in the hand or wrist such as carpal tunnel syndrome. Inflammation is rarely apparent on physical examination in patients with overuse syndrome and it is often not clear if the injured structure is tendon, muscle, ligament, joint capsule or a combination of these (Sataloff et al 1990).

CARPAL TUNNEL SYNDROME

Carpal tunnel syndrome is the second most common industrial injury in the United States, surpassed only by low back pain. Workers in occupations which require heavy wrist activity, such as data entry operators, grocery checkers, pipefitters, tool workers, carpenters, secretaries and pianists, are considered most at risk for this syndrome. Recent findings suggest that the condition is exacerbated by psychological stressors such as boredom, insecurity or the stress of other painful processes. Furthermore, recent studies of the wrist using computerised tomography suggest that workers with carpal tunnel syndrome tend to have carpal bones of a smaller cross-sectional area (Bleecker 1987). This suggests a potential for screening for those most at risk.

Carpal tunnel syndrome is caused by pressure on the median nerve; this may be due to increased synovial hypertrophy, as it occurs in rheumatoid arthritis, gout, hypothyroidism, diabetes, ganglion tumours or lipomas, pregnancy and trauma. Biomechanical studies have shown that intracarpal pressure is particularly increased with flexon and ulnar deviation. Rosenbaum & Ochoa (1993) suggest that Phalen's wrist flexion test is more reliable than Tinel's nerve stimulation of the median nerve at the wrist in diagnosis of carpal tunnel syndrome.

Signs and symptoms

This syndrome causes paraesthesias and dysthaesias along the median nerve into the hand and wrist. The pain may be localised at the wrist, but may also show retrograde spread to the elbow or shoulder. Shaking or moving the hand may relieve symptoms, suggesting a pressure gradient involving the lymphatic or circulatory system. However, if such shaking causes increased pain, cervical radiculitis should be suspected. Thenar atrophy may be present.

Treatment course and prognosis

Conservative treatment measures include splinting, cortisone injections, rest and/or change in activities. Treatment of trigger points in the forearm, shoulder, neck and, often, gluteal region may help relieve both the pain and dystrophy-like syndromes. In difficult cumulative disorders the patient should ideally begin a 'work hardening' programme under the supervision of trained hand, occupational or physical therapists to develop strength and endurance. When other treatments are not effective, surgical release is recommended. Although Silverstein et al (1987) have reported that 58% of surgically treated patients return to their former job, none of these returned to jobs that required forceful repetitive motion.

OTHER PERIPHERAL ENTRAPMENT SYNDROMES

Among the most puzzling pains of the extremity are the peripheral neuropathies (Fig. 25.6). The causes are obscure and differential diagnosis is not easy, especially since cervical nerve root irritation must be considered (Kopell & Thompson 1973; Dyck et al 1976). There is evidence that radiculitis increases the susceptibility of nerve entrapment (Upton & McComas 1973; Bland 1987). Table 25.4 gives some guidelines to differentiate between entrapment and peripheral radiculopathy (Dawson et al 1983, 1990). Peripheral radiculopathy must also be differentiated from cervical spondylosis and other less common entities that cause cervical root irritation, such as tumours, infection, osteophytes, prolapsed disc, fractures and epidural abscess, all of which have been considered in Chapter 40 in this book. Note that patients can usually distinguish between pain that radiates from the hand to the shoulder and pain that originates in the neck or shoulder and spreads to the hand. The only definitive way to diagnose peripheral neuropathy is by electromyography and nerve conduction studies in addition to routine radiological studies.

Any one of the entrapment syndromes can cause hand, forearm, and shoulder pain which is not consistent in character. Generally, there is some local pain at the area of entrapment, but muscles distal to the entrapment may or

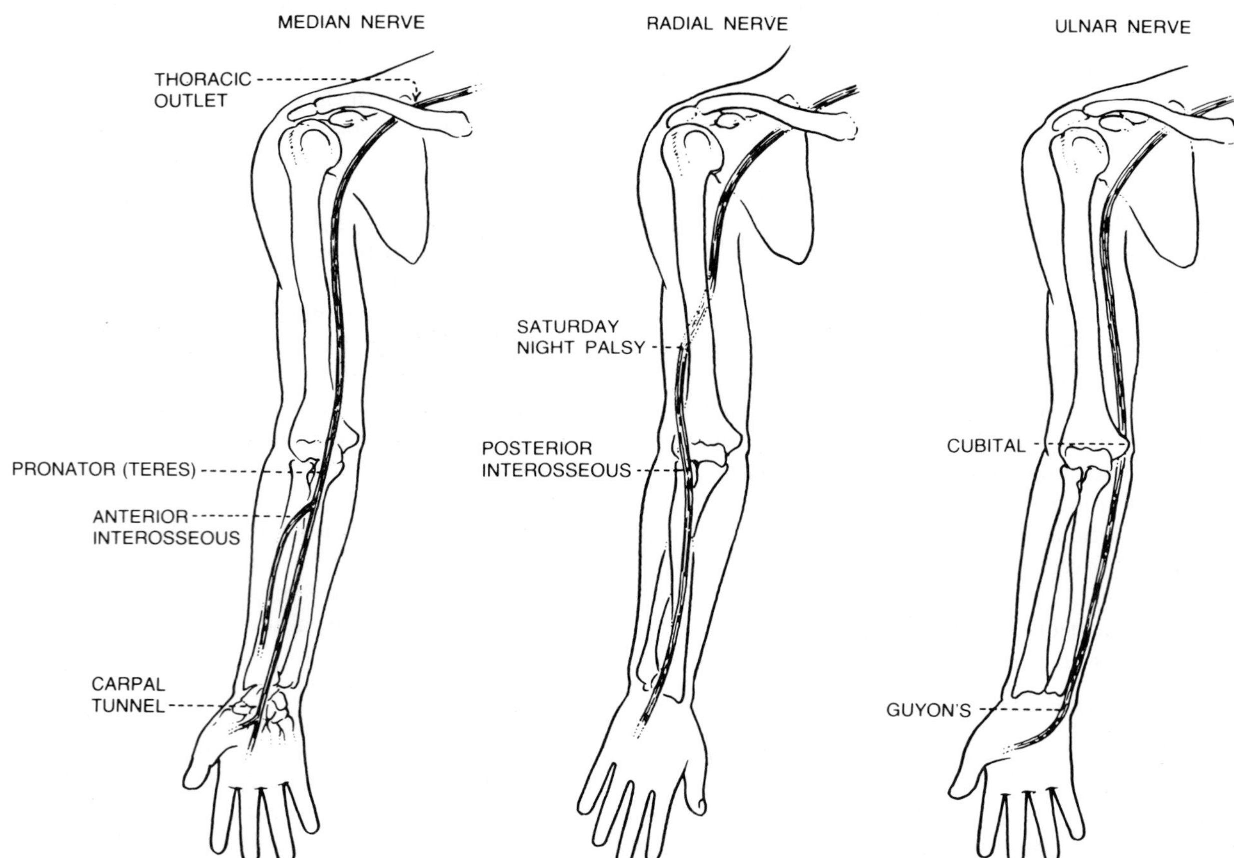

Fig. 25.6 Common neurovascular and peripheral entrapment syndromes. There are four thoracic outlet syndromes: scalenus anticus, costoclavicular syndrome, cervical rib syndrome and hyperabduction syndrome. Peripheral entrapment syndromes affect the radial, ulnar or median nerves and can cause pain at the area of entrapment and in muscles distal to the entrapment. These are often inconsistent or intermittent pains.

Table 25.4 Differentiating between radiculopathy and entrapment syndromes

Radiculopathy	Entrapment
Involves posterior division of cervical root; radiation along medial border of scapula	Signs uncommon with entrapment
Pain with coughing, sneezing, Valsalva manoeuvre, highly specific for radiculopathy when present	Signs not associated with entrapment
Pain increases with use of hand	Carpal tunnel syndrome pain is relieved by massage, shaking hand, immersion of hand in water, changing positions
Muscle weakness rarely severe. Most easily identified: deltoid, infraspinatus (C5); biceps, wrist extensors (C6); triceps, long finger flexors, finger extensors (C7); intrinsic muscles of hand and wrist flexors (C8); arm and when testing muscle	Not a diagnostic feature
Electrophysiological studies Nerve conduction studies almost always normal with uncomplicated radiculopathy. EMGs done on a number of arm muscles may show changes in a radicular pattern. Paraspinus muscles may be denervated, confirming nerve root damage. Myelography/computerized tomography delineates lateral disc protrusion	*Electrophysiological studies* Local changes may be present
Treatment Successful response to several weeks of conservative treatment (traction, cervical collar, local massage and analgesics) confirms diagnosis	*Treatment* In early stages is likely to respond to conservative treatment: splinting, cortisone, rest. More advanced may require surgical release

may not have pain involvement. Frequently the pain experienced is intermittent, low-grade and worse at night. Scapulocostal irritation and myofascial disturbances tend to distort the pain patterns to peripheral nerve compression. Carpal tunnel syndrome is the most common of the nerve compression syndromes affecting the median nerve. Two other conditions related primarily to median nerve compression are pronator teres syndrome and anterior interosseous nerve syndrome. Conditions affecting the radial nerve are radial palsy and posterior interosseous syndrome. Ulnar nerve compression is associated with cubital tunnel syndrome and Guyon's canal compression. In addition to the conditions described below, compression of the suprascapular nerve can cause dull, deep pain in the rhomboid area, and dorsal scapular nerve syndrome can cause pain particularly in the posterolateral aspect of the shoulder.

Treatment course and prognosis

Treatment for these syndromes follows much the same pattern as treatment for carpal tunnel syndrome and includes splinting, cortisone injections, rest and/or change in activities, as well as treatment of trigger points in the affected and related areas to help relieve both the pain and dystrophy-like syndromes.

PRONATOR TERES SYNDROME

This syndrome occurs when the median nerve is trapped as the nerve passes below the two heads of the muscle. Pain and paraesthesias occur in flexor muscles of the forearm and in the thenar muscles. There is associated weakness in the muscles.

ANTERIOR INTEROSSEOUS NERVE SYNDROME

This nerve supplies the flexor pollicis longus, the flexor digitorus profundus and the pronator quadratus muscle. Pressure causes weakness or paralysis in the index and middle fingers. When the elbow is flexed, the pronator teres will be weak; the pronator quadratus will be weak in pronation.

RADIAL PALSY

Radial palsy occurs because of excessive pressure over the spiral groove. This affects all muscles of the forearm supplied by the radial nerve. This condition is usually painless, but frequently hyperparaesthesia is present.

POSTERIOR INTEROSSEOUS SYNDROME

Posterior interosseous nerve syndrome describes compression of the radial nerve, where the nerve penetrates the supinator. The patient is able to extend the wrist but unable to extend metacarpophalangeal joints of the fingers, unable to abduct the thumb and unable to extend the distal joint of the thumb.

CUBITAL TUNNEL SYNDROME

Cubital tunnel syndrome describes a condition of pressure on the ulnar nerve as it passes under the medial epicondyle. The patient may experience pain along the ulnar border of the forearm, weakness of intrinsic muscles of the hand and hyperaesthesias.

GUYON'S CANAL COMPRESSION

Guyon's canal compression is impingement on the ulnar nerve where it enters the hand through the canal of Guyon, between the pisiform and hamate bones. The condition is associated with fractures or aneurysm of the small artery. The patient may experience local pain and numbness in the ulnar distribution of the fourth and fifth fingers.

TENNIS ELBOW OR EPICONDYLITIS

Signs and symptoms

The patient complains of severe pain in the elbow, frequently radiating to wrist or shoulder. Any grasping movements are painful, and the patient may drop things from the hand. The pain is usually described as 'deep'. Pressure applied over the lateral condyles causes extreme pain. Dorsiflexion of the wrist may be painful. This clinical picture of pain is usually accompanied by a history of overuse of the extensors and supinators of the wrist in sports such as tennis and golf and in occupations requiring similar motions such as hammering. It can also be associated with excessive hand-shaking. In older patients, this lesion is more likely to be a chronic condition unrelated to a specific activity and much less amenable to treatment. Chronic inflammation of periosteal nerves and blood vessels may contribute to the pain.

Treatment course and prognosis

When a clear association with activity is not present from the history, X-rays may be indicated to eliminate the possibility of fracture or pathological bone formations. Treatment depends on the structures involved. Common extensor and flexor tendons will usually respond to steroids and local anaesthetic. When the extensor carpi radialis tendon is involved, the pain may originate with muscle rather than on the epicondyle and a local anaesthetic may be indicated. Muscle involvement is uncommon at the supracondylar ridge. Joint dysfunction at any of the three elbow joints can cause pain simulating tennis elbow. These are treated by manipulation. Refractory cases of tennis elbow are frequently treated by surgery. Trigger points may occur in any of the muscles around the elbow joint and these frequently respond to injection therapy. Trigger points in the scalenus anticus muscle can frequently refer pain to this area (Zohn & Mennell 1976).

OLECRANON BURSA

Signs and symptoms

The olecranon bursa, which lies over the bony olecranon process, is frequently injured by constant mechanical pressure. Clinically, the bursa sac area becomes red and swollen, warm to the touch and tender on palpation. Occasionally it may become infected. Patients who have gout and rheumatoid arthritis are prone to this disorder.

Treatment course and prognosis

Pain and swelling usually subside if a cushioning ring is used around the area of irritation to prevent further mechanical pressure. If pain persists, fluid can be aspirated from the bursal sac and examined for evidence of infection and/or to differentiate between aetiologies. If the condition is persistent or recurrent, surgical excision may be the treatment of choice.

LIGAMENTAL INJURIES

Ligamental injuries are common at the wrist. Diagnosis is made on the basis of local pain and tenderness. The most frequent of these injuries is sprain of the ulnar collateral ligament, which is characterised by pain on radial deviation. When the radial ligament is sprained or torn, pain is present on ulnar deviation. The ulnar-capitate sprain is also quite common. With flexion of the wrist, pain is felt at the dorsal aspect.

Treatment course and prognosis

Local management with steroid injection treatment is usually effective for ligamental injuries. Ruptures may require surgical intervention.

GANGLION CYST

Signs and symptoms

Ganglia are the most common tumours of the hand and wrist. They are most frequently found on the dorsal aspect of the wrist joint, and occasionally on the volar aspect of the wrist. The cystic swelling is found near, and often attached to, a tendon sheath, and it is believed that the cyst may be derived from these structures. Ganglia are often painless; however they can be locally tender and painful.

Treatment course and prognosis

Ganglia are known to disappear spontaneously. However, the usual treatment is puncture of the cyst and aspiration of its contents. Some clinicians inject a corticosteroid into the cyst after aspiration.

DE QUERVAIN'S DISEASE (CONSTRICTIVE TENOSYNOVITIS)

Signs and symptoms

De Quervain's disease may have slow or acute onset precipitated by an injury to the wrist which causes swelling in tendons thickened by the disease process. The patient will present with pain in the wrist and thumb area and weakness of grip. In the acute state, there may be local swelling with symptoms similar to wrist sprain. Examination will reveal marked tenderness to pressure over the styloid process and over the tendons, abductor pollicis longus and extensor pollicis brevis.

The pain is related to thickening and stenosis of the sheath surrounding the tendons. It is most commonly seen in female workers doing heavy hard work, such as cooks and dressmakers who lift heavy material. Diagnosis of de Quervain's disease is affirmed by holding the patient's thumb in flexion and abducting the wrist. This will elicit a pain response.

Treatment course and prognosis

Immobilisation is recommended, and the area is injected with long-acting anaesthetic. Injectable steroid therapy is also appropriate. In one study, symptoms of infectious arthritis were present in one-quarter of the patients with this condition.

TRIGGER FINGER

As result of injury, small tears in the flexor tendon curl into a ball and form a nodule, usually at the proximal end of the tendon sheath. This nodule interferes with normal gliding motion and abnormal tension is required to force it through the tendon sheath, causing the finger to snap in extension. Palpation of the tendon sheath will usually be painful.

Treatment is the same as for de Quervain's disease: immobilisation, steroid injection and surgical release if necessary.

IMPINGEMENT SYNDROMES

Diagnosis of shoulder pain is facilitated by an understanding of impingement syndromes, which are common in athletes and persons doing heavy physical labour. Impingement is diagnosed by point tenderness over the anterior insertion of the supraspinatus tendon and positive findings on forward flexion with internal rotation. The critical test is relief of symptoms with use of local anaesthetic injected into the anterior acromial process (coracoid acromial ligament).

Tendinitis, rotator cuff tears and adhesive capsulitis may all be components of a degenerative process beginning with impingement. When impingement syndromes are present in young persons, they are almost always associated with racquet sports, swimming, baseball, football and repetitive overhead motions (Moseley 1969; Post 1987; Nichols & Hershman 1990).

Neer & Welsh (1977) have suggested three stages:

- Stage I is characterised by oedema and/or inflammation and usually occurs in patients between the ages of 15 and 30 years. Treatment at this stage is conservative; restriction of shoulder movement, antiinflammatory medications and ice packs. Occasionally steroid injections are given if these measures do not provide relief.
- Stage II is characterised by fibrosis and thickening of the rotator cuff which further compromises subacromial mechanisms. If the patient does not respond to conservative treatment, and cuff tear has been ruled out, a partial anterior acromioplasty and sectioning of the coracoid acromial ligament may be necessary.
- Stage III is usually associated with patients over the age of 40 years, when further degeneration has taken place, and it may include partial tears of the rotator cuff and bony changes. Surgery may be necessary to correct the condition, particularly if tears are involved (Post 1987). The diagnosis can be confirmed by an arthrogram (see Table 25.3).

THORACIC OUTLET SYNDROME

Thoracic outlet syndrome (TOS) involves discomfort caused by compression or irritation of the neurovascular bundle by the scalene muscles, rib, clavicle or pectoralis minor muscle. Most commonly, it is the inferior portion of the brachial plexus which is involved, affecting the ulnar and, sometimes, the medial nerves. In a small percentage of cases the subclavian vein may also be compressed.

Signs and symptoms

In this condition, there is a gradual increase in discomfort until the patient experiences pain involving the upper extremity, lower neck region, shoulder and arm. The pain tends to be intermittent and is associated with movement, particularly with lifting objects overhead. The patient may describe a 'pins and needles' sensation in the forearm and wrist and may experience weakness or numbness in the fourth or fifth finger. Symptoms are usually worse in the morning than later in the day. The condition is seen most often in young adult patients with poor posture and is reported more frequently in women.

Palpation or percussion during examination may indicate tenderness of the brachial plexus. A confirming test for TOS is to have the patient assume the 'Hold up' position for 3 minutes while slowly opening and closing the hands. If radial pulses remain strong, but the patient experiences the usual symptoms, the test is positive for TOS. (The 'Hold up' position consists of sitting with both arms elevated to 90° abduction with external rotation. The elbows are maintained somewhat behind the frontal plane.)

Treatment course and prognosis

Insofar as TOS may be related to poor posture, a conservative approach is to recommend posture-related therapy and mild exercise to strengthen shoulder muscles. If the problem can be associated with a particular type of activity or position during sleeping, these should be modified. Medication for muscle relaxation may be indicated. However, all of these measures are limited if the condition has progressed to the extent that only surgical procedures can provide decompression. Surgery will establish the presence of congenital fibromuscular bands which could not be identified by X-ray. When these bands are present, they usually affect both sides of the body.

CERVICAL SPRAIN

The rapid acceleration of the neck into hyperextension and/or flexion in classic 'whiplash' type of injury can cause cord damage but most commonly is associated with some trauma to the supporting muscles, tendons and ligaments. Common sources of such injury include automobile or other transportation accidents, falls or high velocity sports injuries. It may also be associated with damage or functional compromise of the cervical nerve roots either directly or through the pressures of subsequent muscle spasm (Bland 1987; Bonica 1990).

The short-term signs of cervical sprain include stiffness and pain in the neck and shoulder girdle, hoarseness or dysphagia (in anterior damage), headache and various sympathetic dystrophy-like symptoms. A normal neurological examination with no swelling or apparent trauma to the neck may be taken as a good indication that there is no spinal or cord damage. Even if the injury appears minimal, the patient must be carefully followed for several days following the incident. Muscles and ligaments heal within 4–6 weeks, whereas intervertebral discs heal slowly because they have no blood supply. If there is any suspicion of damage to the cervical spine or cord, one must obtain a trans-table lateral view of the entire cervical spine.

If spinal injury has been ruled out, immediate treatment includes applying a soft cervical collar, mild cervical traction and physical therapy and administration of nonsteroidal antiinflammatory medications. Injury may well involve the scalene, sternocleidomastoid and posterior cervical muscles. Spasm and TPs in these muscles may affect nerve roots as low as T7 (see Fig. 25.7). Related pain in the muscles of the lower back, becoming apparent at some time after the injury, is also quite common. The application of vasocoolant sprays, injection or dry needling of trigger points in the neck, shoulder girdle and lower back may help to relieve muscle spasm and interrupt the potential for the establishment of a long-term pain cycle precipitated by the injury (see Fig. 25.2). The sternocleidomastoid in particular in a source of such

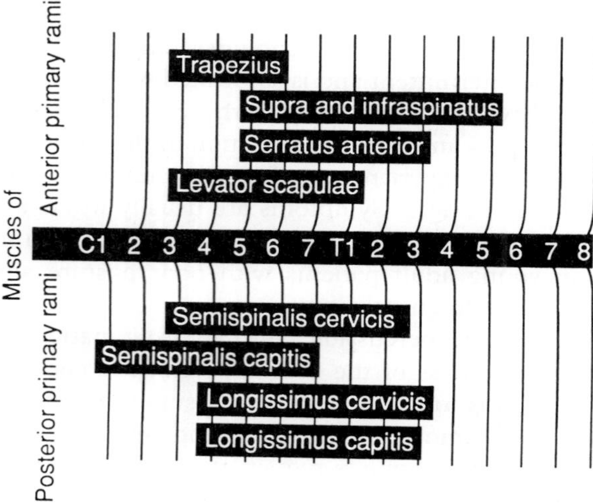

Fig. 25.7 This schematic illustration gives examples of upper extremity muscles supplied by the anterior primary rami of the cervical spine. Note the length of the muscles supplied by the posterior rami shown for the same cervical region. Activation of trigger points (TPs) that exist along the entire length of a muscle can cause or intensify pain felt in muscles supplied by any common nerve segment. Therefore, pain experienced along a muscle such as the semispinalis capitis can contribute to shoulder pain. Injection treatment of posterior primary rami muscles beginning at T6 is indicated if hypersensitive TPs are found in the muscles.

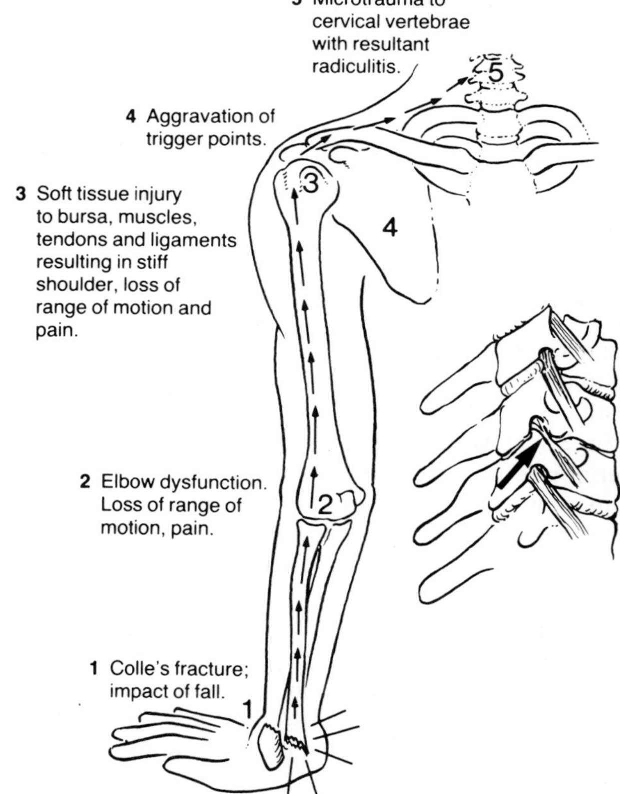

Fig. 25.8 Even a relatively minor force applied to a distal extremity can cause injury at any of these points on the shock pathway, or can cause flare up of residual sequelae which were not identified at the time of an earlier injury. Minimal changes of EMG can reflect presence of radiculitis (Gunn 1980).

long-term, low intensity TPs. Usually 85% of those injured have returned to their jobs at the end of 3 months. About 75% of accident cases do not involve litigation. When pain persists beyond 6 months, these cases are labelled as chronic. Posttraumatic syndromes are frequent with those patients who have, in addition, residual injuries, socioeconomic stresses, depression, anger and the complicating problem of litigation (Bland 1987).

MULTIPLE UPPER EXTREMITY LESIONS

One of the problems in managing upper extremity pain is that several lesions may be contributing to it. This is particularly true in the case of a middle-aged or older patient who sustains an injury as result of a fall in which the first contact was made by his or her outstretched hand, an elbow or shoulder (Fig. 25.8). The initial contact injury may be a fracture, contusion, ligamental sprain or muscle/soft tissue injury. After successful treatment, the patient experiences residual pain, dysfunction or limitation of movement.

When this is the history, the first accessory injury site to be considered is the cervical region, especially if cervical spondylosis is present. Slight injuries can occur at the nerve roots, involving nerve fibres in the root sleeves. When these are injured, they set up a radiculitis which continues to feed impulses to the original injury site (Gunn & Milbrandt 1978; Sola 1984). Unrelieved or persistent pain following seemingly satisfactory healing of the point of injury should always suggest further evaluation for potential cervical problems. In treating cervical radiculitis it is important to remember that it takes several months of treatment with traction and supportive physical therapy for recovery of damaged nerves.

Further assessment should also include examination of the shoulder for hypersensitive TPs, which, as stated before, may be perpetuating a pain cycle even though the initial stimulus has been negated. The elbow should be examined to rule out joint dysfunction and painful hypersensitive TPs.

If cervical and myofascial pain sources have been eliminated, further evaluation of tendons, bursae, rotator cuff and joint capsule should be carried out to eliminate the possibility of undiagnosed injuries along the path of shock absorption. Any injury site has the potential for setting up a dystrophy-like syndrome, a possibility which must be recognised and prevented. An extremity which has residual sequelae from a previous injury is much more vulnerable to pain and dysfunction following another injury to the same extremity. It is unfortunate for the patient if the clinician overlooks these sequelae, since they can usually be treated effectively and the pain can be eliminated.

REFERENCES

Adson A W 1951 Cervical ribs: symptoms, differential diagnosis and indications for section of the insertion of the scalenus anticus muscle. Journal of the International College of Surgeons 16: 546

Bateman J E 1978 The shoulder and neck, 2nd edn. W B Saunders, Philadelphia

Bland J H 1987 Disorders of the cervical spine: diagnosis and medical management. W B Saunders, Philadelphia, chs 13, 20

Bleecker M L 1987 Medical surveillance for carpal tunnel syndrome and workers. Journal of Hand Surgery 12A: 845

Bonica J J 1990 The Management of pain, 2nd edn. Lea & Febiger, Philadelphia, chs 21, 40, 47, 52

Bray E A, Sigmond H 1941 The local and regional injection treatment of low back pain and sciatica. Annals of Internal Medicine 15: 840–852

Brody I A, Wilkins R H 1969 Lhermitte's sign. Archives of Neurology 21: 338

Calliet R 1981 Shoulder pain, 2nd edn. F A Davis, Philadelphia

Dawson D M, Hallet M, Millender L H 1983 Entrapment neuropathies. Little, Brown, Boston, Massachusetts

Dawson D M, Hallet M L, Millender L H 1990 Entrapment neuropathies, 2nd edn. Little, Brown, Boston

DePalma A F 1957 Degenerative changes in sternoclavicular and acromioclavicular joints in various decades. C Thomas, Springfield, Illinois

DePalma A F 1973 Surgery of the shoulder, 2nd edn. J B Lippincott, Philadelphia

Dyck P J, Lambert E H, O'Brien P C 1976 Pain in peripheral neuropathy related to rate and kind of nerve fiber degeneration. Neurology 26: 466–477

Frost F A, Jeason B, Siggaard-Anderson J A 1980 A controlled, double-blind comparison of mepivacaine injection versus saline injection for myofacial pain. Lancet 1: 499–501

Gerhart T N, Dohlman L E, Warfield C A 1985 Clinical diagnosis of shoulder pain. Hospital Practice 134–141

Gunn C C 1980 'Prespondylosis' and some pain syndromes following denervation supersensitivity. Spine 5: 185–192

Gunn C C 1989 Treating myofascial pain: intramuscular stimulation (IMS) for myofascial pain syndromes of neuropathic origin. Health Sciences Center for Educational Resources, Univeristy of Washington, Seattle

Gunn C C Milbrandt W E 1978 Tennis elbow and the cervical spine. Canadian Medical Association Journal 114: 803–809

Kraft G H, Johnson E W, LaBan M M 1968 The fibrositis syndrome. Archives of Physiological Medicine and Rehabilitation 49: 155–162

Kopell H P, Thompson W 1973 Peripheral entrapment neuropathies. Williams & Wilkins, Baltimore

LaDou J 1990 Occupational medicine. Appleton & Lange, Hoaglund, Maryland

Lawrence R M 1978 New approach to the treatment of chronic pain: combination therapy. American Journal of Acupuncture 6: 59–62

Lippert F G III, Teitz C C 1987 Diagnosing musculoskeletal problems – a practical guide. Williams & Wilkins, Baltimore

McLaughlin H L 1961 The 'frozen shoulder'. Clinical Orthopedics 20: 126–131

Moseley H F 1969 Shoulder lesions, 3rd edn. E & S Livingstone, Edinburgh, p 75–81, 243–292

Neer C S II, Welsh R P 1977 The shoulder in sports. Orthopedic Clinics of North America 8: 583–591

Neviaser J S 1975 Arthrography of the shoulder: the diagnosis and management of the lesions visualized. C C Thomas, Springfield, Illinois

Nichols J A, Hershman E B 1990 The upper extremity in sports medicine. C V Mosby, St Louis

Pak T J, Martin G M, Magnes J L, Kavanaugh G J 1970 Reflex sympathetic dystrophy. Minnesota Medical 53: 507–512

Post M 1987 Physical examination of the musculoskeletal system. Year Book Medical Publishers, Chicago

Roberts J R, Hedges J R 1991 Clinical procedures in emergency medicine, 2nd ed. W B Saunders, Philadelphia, ch 64
Rosenbaum R B, Ochoa J L 1993 Carpal tunnel syndrome and other disorders of the median nerve. Butterworth-Heinemann, New York
Saha A K 1961 Theory of shoulder mechanism. C C Thomas, Springfield, Illinois
Sataloff R T, Brandfonbrenner A G, Lederman R J 1990 Textbook of performing arts medicine. Raven Press, New York
Sheon R P, Moskowitz R W, Goldberg V M 1987 Soft tissue rheumatic pain, 2nd edn. Lea & Febiger, Philadelphia
Silverstein B, Fine L, Stetson, D 1987 Hand-wrist disorders among investment casting plant workers. Journal of Hand Surgery 12A: 838
Simons D G 1975 Muscle pain syndromes. Part I. American Journal of Physical Medicine 54: 289–311
Simons D G 1976 Muscle pain syndromes. Part II. American Journal of Physical Medicine 55: 15–42
Sola A E 1981 Myofascial trigger point therapy. Resident Staff Physicians 38–48
Sola A E 1984 Treatment of myofascial pain syndromes. In Benedetti C et al (eds) Advances in pain research and therapy. Raven Press, New York, p 13
Sola A E, Kuitert J H 1955 Myofascial trigger point pain in the neck and shoulder girdle: 100 cases treated by normal saline. Northwest Medicine 54: 980–984
Sola A E, Williams R L 1956 Myofascial pain syndromes. Neurology 6: 91–95
Sola A E, Rodenberg M L, Getty B B 1955 Incidence of hypersensitive areas in posterior shoulder muscles. American Journal of Physical Medicine 34: 585–590
Steindler A 1959 Lectures on the interpretation of pain in orthopedic practice. C C Thomas, Springfield, Illinois
Tfelt-Hansen P et al 1980 Lignocaine versus saline in migraine pain. Lancet 1: 1140
Travell J 1976 Myofascial trigger points. In: Bonica J J (ed) Advances in pain research and therapy. Raven Press, New York
Travell J, Daitz B 1990 Myofascial pain syndromes: the Travell trigger point tapes. Williams & Wilkins Electronic Media, Baltimore
Travell J, Rinzler S H 1952 The myofascial genesis of pain. Postgraduate Medicine 11: 425–434
Travell J, Simons D G 1983 Myofascial pain and dysfunction: the trigger point manual. Williams & Wilkins, Baltimore
Upton A R M, McComas A J 1973 The double crush syndrome in nerve entrapment syndromes. Lancet 2: 359
Zimmermann M 1980 Physiological mechanisms in chronic pain. In: Pain and society. Report of Dahlem workshop
Zohn D A, Mennell J M 1976 Musculoskeletal pain: diagnosis and physical treatment. Little, Brown, Boston

26. Fibromyalgia and myofascial pain syndromes

Glenn A. McCain

INTRODUCTION

Musculoskeletal pain syndromes which have no readily identifiable cause have perplexed medical investigators for centuries. These conditions are characterized by chronic pain for which no abnormality can be demonstrated either in histological sections or in the physiology of the affected tissues. Fibromyalgia syndrome (FMS) and myofascial pain syndrome (MPS) are two such complex conditions which have only recently been studied with acceptable scientific rigour. Experimental evidence using current epidemiological techniques has allowed for the development of classification criteria which, at least in the case of FMS, can be used at the bedside for diagnostic purposes. These clinical criteria have enabled investigators to identify more homogeneous groups of patients for study and have resulted in a better understanding of the overlap between these two conditions as well as their relationship to other chronic pain syndromes. These efforts have led to the view that FMS and MPS can be classified using the positive features of the patient's illness, obviating the need to perform an exhaustive number of laboratory tests or procedures to exclude other clinical conditions. Diagnosis using the positive rather than the negative features of the patient's illness, therefore, can be accomplished even in the absence of knowledge of well-defined pathological processes. Furthermore such an approach can lead to useful treatment strategies which can be tested using the appropriate scientific methods.

This chapter will focus on recent advances in the diagnosis, treatment and classification of FMS and MPS. Only those studies which have conformed to the principles of the scientific method will be cited. Subexperimental and uncontrolled studies will be indicated, allowing the reader to make an informed decision about the information presented.

Historical perspective

These conditions cannot be understood without an appreciation of the historical development of our understanding of the pathophysiology of chronic musculoskeletal pain syndromes. The earliest reports of the latter have been elegantly catalogued by Simons (1975, 1976b) and first appeared in German medical literature between 1850 and 1900. They contain descriptions of patients with a host of clinical presentations characterised by chronic pain of unidentifiable cause. Some patients had localised pain complaints while others had a more diffuse and generalised pain syndrome. The characteristic physical finding linking these conditions to each other was thought to be an easily identifiable muscle hardness or *Muskelharten*, which was also tender to palpation and hence thought to be responsible for the patients' clinical complaints. Indeed, vigorous palpation often reproduced pain in the area of complaint. These reports undoubtedly contained descriptions of what we now call 'trigger points' (Travell & Simons 1983) or taut bands in muscle. Modern day therapies of local injection and 'stretch and spray' which have been popularised by Travell & Simons (1983) evolved from these initial reports. Using the recent classification of the International Association for the Study of Pain (IASP) (Merskey 1986), such localised disease would be termed 'specific myofascial pain syndrome'.

These reports also contain descriptions of patients who would fulfil present day criteria for FMS, which is also called 'fibrositis' or 'diffuse myofascial pain syndrome' in the IASP classification. In fact the term 'fibrositis' has been used erroneously in the past to include both myofascial pain syndrome and fibromyalgia syndrome. This stems from the use of 'fibrositis' by Gowers in 1904 to indicate the then generally held belief that these varied clinical conditions were the result of a proliferation or inflammation of subcutaneous and muscular tissue. 'Fibrositis' has persisted in the literature despite the failure of several authors to show reproducible and consistent anatomical changes in the structure of these connective tissues.

Real progress in putting the classification of these conditions on a firm physiological basis came with Kellgren's observations on the nature of pain emanating from deep connective tissue structures (Kellgren 1938, 1939; Kellgren et al 1944). His studies showed that irritation of different anatomical areas like fascia, tendon and muscle produced pain which differed not only in quality but also in its distribution of radiation. Subsequent work elucidated trigger points and zones of radiating pain as well as the taut bands in muscle so characteristic of MPS (Simons & Travell 1983; Travell & Simons 1983; Simms et al 1988a). Similarly, Smythe & Moldofsky can be credited with describing the concept of fibrositic tender points and the sleep disturbance common to patients with FMS (Moldofsky et al 1975, Moldofsky & Scarisbrick 1976, Smythe & Moldofsky 1977).

More recently, the Fibromyalgia Multicenter Criteria Committee, working under the auspices of the American College of Rheumatology, has developed criteria acceptably sensitive and specific for use at the bedside (Wolfe et al 1990). These criteria are described in Table 26.1, and are generally known as the American College of Rheumatology Classification Criteria for Fibromyalgia. Fibromyalgia, therefore, can be distinguished with certainty and differentiated from other chronic musculoskeletal pain syndromes which are also of uncertain cause. These criteria have also allowed for the construction of a more rational approach to investigations into the cause and treatment of this condition.

Clinical criteria have been proposed for MPS but have not been tested in multicentre trials, so that no estimate of their sensitivity or specificity can be made. These criteria are outlined in Table 26.2.

FIBROMYALGIA SYNDROME

Fibromyalgia syndrome is a common clinical pain disorder in which a reproducible physical finding, the presence of palpable fibrositic tender points, is associated with characteristic symptoms of generalised muscular aching, stiffness, fatigue and nonrestorative sleep.

CLINICAL PRESENTATION

Fibromyalgia can be viewed as consisting of a central set of core features,which are essential for diagnosis, superim-

Table 26.1 The American College of Rheumatology 1990 criteria for the classification of fibromyalgia syndrome

1. History of widespread pain	Definition: pain is considered widespread when all of the following are present: pain in the left side of the body, pain in the right side of the body, pain above the waist, pain below the waist. In addition, axial skeletal pain (cervical spine or anterior chest or thoracic spine or low back) must be present. In this definition shoulder and buttock pain is considered as pain for each involved side. Low back pain is considered lower segment pain.
2. Pain in 11 of 18 tender point sites on digital palpation	Definition. Pain on digital palpation must be present in a least 11 of the following 18 tender point sites: Occiput: bilateral, at the suboccipital muscle insertion Low cervical: bilateral, at the anterior aspect of the intertransverse spaces at C5–C7 Trapezius: bilateral, at the midpoint of the upper border Supraspinatus: bilateral, at origins above the medial border of the scapular spine Second rib: bilateral, upper surfaces just lateral to the costochondral junctions Lateral epicondyle: bilateral, 2 cm distal to the epicondyles Gluteal: bilateral, in upper outer quadrants of buttocks in anterior fold of muscle Greater trochanter: bilateral, posterior to the trochanteric prominence Knee: bilateral, at the medial fat pad proximal to the joint line Digital palpation should be performed with a force of 4 kg. For a tender point to be considered 'positive' the subject must state that the palpation was painful; 'tender' is not to be considered 'painful'.

Note: For classification purposes, patients will be said to have fibromyalgia if both criteria are satisfied. Widespread pain must have been present for at least 3 months. The presence of a second clinical disorder does not exclude the diagnosis of fibromyalgia.

Table 26.2 Clinical criteria for the diagnosis of myofascial pain syndrome

Major criteria	1. Regional pain complaint 2. Pain complaint or altered sensation in the expected distribution of referred pain from a myofascial trigger point 3. Taut band palpable in an accessible muscle 4. Exquisite spot tenderness at one point along the length of the taut band 5. Some degree of restricted range of motion, when measurable
Minor criteria	1. Reproduction of clinical pain complaint, or altered sensation, by pressure on the tender spot 2. Elicitation of a local twitch response by transverse snapping palpation at the tender spot or by needle insertion into the tender spot in the taut band 3. Pain alleviated by elongation (stretching) the muscle or by injecting the tender spot

posed on a variable number of ancillary manifestations, often seen in association with, but not integral to, final diagnosis of the condition. The core features are generalised pain and widespread tenderness over discrete anatomical areas known as fibrositic tender points (FTPs). Ancillary features are of two types:

1. those which can be considered almost characteristic since they occur in over 75% of individuals, such as fatigue, a nonrestorative sleep pattern and morning stiffness
2. those which are less common, occurring in perhaps 25% of cases, such as irritable bowel syndrome, Raynaud's phenomenon, headache, subjective swelling, nondermatomal paraesthesiae, psychological distress and marked functional disability.

Pain

Widespread pain, best described by the term 'chronic muscular aching', is the central dominating feature of FMS and is considered essential to the diagnosis. In published series widespread chronic muscular aching, which by definition should be longer than 3 months in duration, accounts for more than half of the variance in disease severity. Table 26.3 summarises the percentage of fibromyalgia patients reporting pain in various body regions in four different clinical settings (Campbell et al 1983; Wolfe et al 1984a, 1984b, Hudson et al 1985; Wolfe et al 1985; Dinerman et al 1986, Wolfe 1986, Yunus & Kalyan-Raman 1989). This shows that the sites of chronic muscular aching and stiffness in a large population of patients are varied. As a rule muscular aching and stiffness are more proximal than distal even though the patient 'hurts all over'. Even though symptoms may be reported fancifully with many subjective overtones, the hallmark historical findings are chronicity, persistence and the

Table 26.3 Percentage of fibromyalgia patients reporting pain in various body regions

	Wolfe et al (1985)	Leavitt et al (1986)	Yunus et al (1981)	McCain & Scudds (1988b)
Low back	95	80	65	66
Neck	90	65	35	34
Shoulders	90	75	55	54
Hips	80	70	35	38
Hands	75	65	55	52
Knees	70	70	68	66
Chest wall	70	30	—	—
Feet	70	50	18	18
Elbows	65	52	22	24
Ankles	55	55	20	22
Wrists	55	55	15	14

Table 26.4 Percentage frequency of symptoms in patients with fibromyalgia and rheumatoid arthritis compared with healthy controls

Symptoms	Fibromyalgia	Rheumatoid arthritis	Healthy controls
Pain	94	79	0
Fatigue	85	62	10
Stiffness	76	66	0
Anxiety	72	47	31
Poor sleep	62	32	9
Generalised aching	60	40	0
Mental stress	60	33	25
Swelling	40	56	5
Depression	37	26	9
Paraesthesia	36	9	2

absence of a migratory pattern of symptomatology. As such, there is a general tendency towards the recurrence and invariability of complaints.

The preponderance of chronic muscular aching as a presenting sympton has been brought into relief in a recent study by Yunus et al (1989) in which the clinical features of FMS were compared with those of patients with rheumatoid arthritis as well as with healthy controls. Table 26.4 shows that patients with fibromyalgia not only complain of pain more often than patients in the comparative groups, but also that some anatomical areas, particularly those of the axial skeleton, are involved much more frequently.

There is also reason to believe that patients with fibromyalgia experience more severe pain than those with other painful disease states (Carette et al 1986; Tunks et al 1988; Scudds et al 1989a). Patients with fibromyalgia use a larger number of more charged words in describing their painful experiences than do patients with rheumatoid arthritis and healthy controls (Leavitt et al 1986). Scudds et al (1987) have demonstrated that fibromyalgia patients have diminished pain thresholds not only over FTPs but also over control points, which are not generally tender in rheumatoid arthritis patients and normal controls. The American College of Rheumatology Multicenter Criteria Committee reported lower pain thresholds over control sites in fibromyalgia patients, compared with consecutive outpatient controls suffering from other painful localised and nonlocalised rheumatic disease syndromes (Wolfe et al 1990). These data are in accord with patient self-reports, which show that fibromyalgia patients consistently score lower on visual analogue pain scales and, hence, report greater present pain intensity than comparable pain groups. These findings, taken together, suggest that fibromyalgia patients experience significantly more pain over a larger body area than do patients with other chronic pain syndromes.

Fibrositic tender points (FTPs)

Local tenderness elicited at known FTPs is considered the

hallmark physical finding in fibromyalgia and distinguishes it from other diseases in the broad category of soft tissue rheumatism (Wolfe et al 1990). FTPs are areas of mild tenderness in normal individuals, but palpation of these sites in fibromyalgia patients often causes extreme pain and withdrawal from the examiner's hand. It is best to begin palpation of FTPs by firm pressure over a neutral area such as the middle of the forehead. This gives the examiner an appreciation of the individual's pain threshold. About 80% of that effort is then used to apply direct pressure over areas known to be FTPs. For practical purposes this technique will yield palpation pressures of approximately 4 kg/cm^2. Lighter palpation pressures are likely to result in a failure to elicit higher threshold FTPs. Using this technique tender points can be discretely localised (McCain et al 1988b). For example, the midpoint of the muscle belly of the trapezius, or insertion of the common extensor tendons at the lateral epicondyle of the elbow, can be demonstrated to be quite tender while areas 1 or 2 cm distant in any direction show no tenderness.

Even though a large number of tender points have been described by several authors, only those outlined in the American College of Rheumatology Classification Criteria are useful for diagnosis (see Table 26.1). This reflects the fact that these particular tender points have withstood the scrutiny of scientific study and possess the intrarater and interrater reliability necessary for them to be used with acceptable sensitivity and specificity in a wide variety of patients with chronic pain. They consist of a series of nine paired, anatomically discrete sites. Tenderness is defined as the report by the individual of distinct pain of mild or greater degree upon digital palpation of the tender point by the examiner. When 11 of 18 tender points are so elicited in conjunction with the criterion of widespread muscular aching, a sensitivity of 88.4% and a specificity of 81.1% is achieved (Wolfe et al 1990).

Care must be taken here to distinguish FTPs from 'trigger points'. Palpation of a fibrositic tender point causes pain localised to the area of palpation. The pain does not radiate to adjacent or trigger areas and no pain is experienced at sites proximal or distal to the examining finger. Furthermore, no muscle hardness or induration is palpable. Trigger points, on the other hand, do indeed refer pain, usually in a typical pattern, throughout the soma. This zone of radiation of pain is predictable for each trigger point and Simons & Travell (Travell & Simons 1983; Simons & Travell 1983; Simons 1988) have produced elegant maps describing these radiations from empirical observations. Trigger points are felt to be specific for myofascial pain syndrome. However no data are available on the frequency of trigger points in FMS. Scudds et al (1989b) have shown increased pain sensitivity, analogous to FTPs, in muscles affected by myofascial pain. This is the only study which has addressed the question of how frequently tender points occur in patients with MPS. In the absence of corroborating data the prevalence of tender points in myofascial pain remains presently unresolved. It may be of more than academic interest since many FTPs occur in close anatomical relation to trigger points, suggesting that these tender sites may be indicative of the same aetiological phenomenon. Table 26.5 shows the differences between myofascial trigger points and FTPs. These differences have led to the clinical axiom: 'FTPs are to fibromyalgia as trigger points are to myofascial pain'.

Table 26.5 Some differences between fibromyalgia and myofascial pain syndromes

	Fibromyalgia	Myofascial pain
Sex	Female/male 10:1	Male/female 2:1
Tender point pain	Local	Referred
Tender point distribution	Widespread	Regional
Tender point anatomy	Muscle–tendon junction	Muscle belly
Stiffness	Widespread	Regional
Fatigue	Debilitating	Usually absent
Treatment	Drugs	Local injection. Stretch and spray therapy
Prognosis	Seldom cured	Usually good

Ancillary features

While widespread pain and multiple FTPs are core diagnostic features in FMS, constellations of other seemingly nonspecific symptoms occur frequently enough to warrant their use as adjunctive characteristics. Fig. 26.1 shows the relative frequency of these ancillary symptoms in reported studies. The most commonly reported symptoms are morning stiffness, fatigue and sleep disturbance, occurring in over 75% of cases (Wolfe 1986, 1989). Sleep disturbance usually takes the form of a nonrestorative sleep pattern in which the patient wakes each morning unrefreshed, feeling as if he or she has not gone to bed. This may be so despite reports of undisturbed sleep. There is commonly an overwhelming sense of fatigue and tiredness with marked stiffness which abates as the morning passes. These symptoms may be the result of alpha–delta sleep which has been shown to occur in a large number of such patients (see below). Morning stiffness, fatigue, nonrestorative sleep and, indeed, the alpha-delta sleep abnormality may be seen in other rheumatic diseases, most notably rheumatoid arthritis. The frequency of these complaints is significantly lower, however, compared to fibromyalgia.

Some other complaints also appear more commonly in fibromyalgia patients but not to the extent that they can be

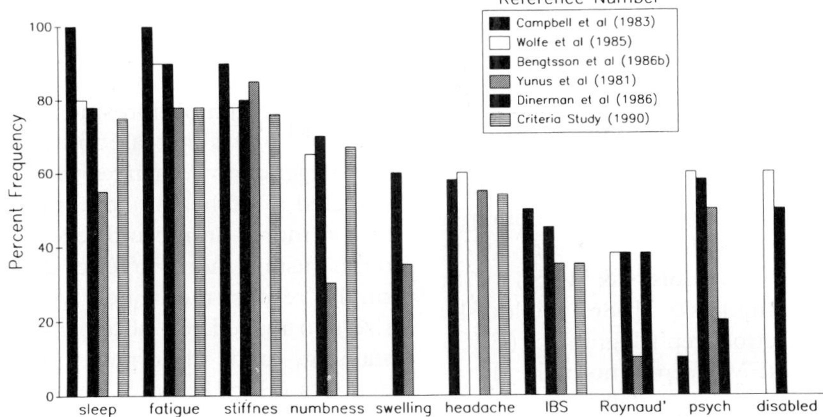

Fig. 26.1 Percentage of fibromyalgia patients reporting 'characteristic' and 'common' symptoms in clinical studies. (IBS – irritable bowel syndrome; psych – psychological distress; disabled – functional disability.)

considered integral to diagnosis. These symptoms should be considered as a group since 25% of cases will have at least one of the following: nondermatomal paraesthesiae, subjective swelling in joint and interjoint areas, both migrainous and nonmigrainous headache, irritable bowel syndrome and Raynaud-like symptoms of bluish discoloration or whiteness of the fingertips (Yunus et al 1981; Wolfe 1986, 1989; Wolfe et al 1990). True Raynaud's phenomenon is uncommon in fibromyalgia and occurred in only 12% of cases in the American College of Rheumatology Multicenter Criteria Study (Wolfe et al 1990). Primary dysmenorrhoea may be more common in fibromyalgia when compared with other chronic pain control groups (Yunus et al 1989).

PREVALENCE AND DEMOGRAPHIC CHARACTERISTICS

The true prevalence of fibromyalgia is unknown. However, recent estimates have placed this condition among the most common in musculoskeletal practice. In rheumatic disease clinics estimates of its prevalence have ranged from 3.7 to 20% (Yunus et al 1981; Wolfe & Cathey 1983). In one study a prevalence of 3.7% rose to 13.6% when patients with other known rheumatic diseases were excluded and to 14.6% when patients with concomitant fibromyalgia were included (Wolfe & Cathey 1983). Another study reported a prevalence of 7.5% in a hospital-based inpatient population (Muller 1987). In a family practice clinic 2.1% of patients were diagnosed as having fibromyalgia. This rose to 5.7% in those similarly classified in a general medical clinic outpatient population (Hartz & Kirchdoerfer 1987). Wolfe has estimated that 13% of patients attending general medical and rheumatic disease clinics may have fibromyalgia (Wolfe 1989). The number of individuals in a general medical setting is expected to be correspondingly lower, perhaps in the range of 2–3%. Unfortunately, no study to date has established the prevalence of fibromyalgia symptoms within the community, but some have suggested that it may rival the 15% quoted for symptoms of irritable bowel syndrome.

Most researchers report that patients with fibromyalgia are women in the third to fifth decade. These demographic features are commonly reported in studies of different methods of treatment but may simply reflect the referral bias or enrolment suitability of the particular cohort. One study reported on 81 patients seen in a midwestern private practice outpatient clinic: the mean age was 52.9 years; 90% were women; 89% had at least a high school education; 83.4% were married and with a mean family income of $29 000 (1985 US$) (Cathey et al 1986). Overall about 73% of patients in published studies, from whatever venue, are women between 30 and 55 years of age (Wolfe 1989). It should be pointed out, however, that fibromyalgia may present at any age and is quite common in rheumatological practice not only among adolescents but also in the geriatric population. It is likely that reported age of onset is artificially high as firstly, patients presenting to general medical and rheumatic disease clinics are usually older, and secondly, fibromyalgia commonly occurs with other medical conditions. Fibromyalgia, therefore, should be suspected in an individual of any age group or socioeconomic class who presents with typical clinical features.

PATHOPHYSIOLOGY

The pathophysiology of fibromyalgia is unknown. Even though a significant amount of research has been undertaken in this area, no unified hypothesis has emerged to explain the mechanisms underlying this condition. Theories about its aetiology fall into four main categories: sleep disturbance, muscle abnormalities, neuropeptide changes and immune system alterations.

Sleep disturbance

Waking each morning unrefreshed, fatigued and tired are extremely common symptoms in patients with fibromyalgia (Wolfe et al 1990). This complaint has been termed the nonrestorative sleep pattern (NRSP). Moldofsky and his colleagues were the first to discover that the physiological correlate of NRSP was an abnormality in stage IV nonrapid eye movement (NREM) sleep (Moldofsky et al 1975; Moldofsky & Scarisbrick 1976; Moldofsky & Warsh 1978; Moldofsky & Lue 1980; Moldofsky 1986; Moldofsky 1989a, 1989b, 1989c). Electroencephalographic (EEG) recording during stage IV NREM sleep in normal individuals is characterised by a series of slow delta waves oscillating at a frequency of 0.5–2.0 Hz (cycles per second). Patients with fibromyalgia, however, show the frequent intrusion of a faster alpha wave with a frequency of 7.5–11.0 Hz. This phenomenon known as 'alpha–delta' sleep was simulated in a group of volunteers who were deprived of stage IV sleep by hand or buzzer arousal. Within a few days these volunteers developed not only alpha intrusion in sleep EEG recordings, but also muscular fatigue and tenderness over FTPs, thus suggesting a pivotal role for a sleep abnormality in the aetiology of FMS. An important finding was that rapid eye movement (REM) sleep deprivation was not associated with self-reported malaise and point tenderness, indicating that symptoms of a fibromyalgia-like syndrome occurred only after the deprivation of NREM sleep. Alpha intrusion, however, was not relegated to delta sleep but was also demonstrable in other sleep stages (Moldofsky et al 1975). Hence the pattern identified in fibromyalgia patients was termed the alpha EEG NREM sleep anomaly. This anomaly has been demonstrated in more than 100 patients with fibromyalgia in whom the alpha rhythm intrudes upon nearly 60% of NREM sleep, compared with only 25% in normal controls, insomniacs and dysthymics (Saskin et al 1986; Gupta & Moldofsky 1986). A number of other groups have now confirmed these data indicating that the alpha EEG sleep anomaly is at least of diagnostic importance in fibromyalgia and may play an important role in the onset or maintaining of fatigue, muscular aching and point tenderness (Campbell & Bennett 1986; Molony et al 1986, Ware et al 1986; Schakel & Horne 1987; Simms et al 1988b). The major question remains of whether alpha intrusion is the primary defect in fibromyalgia and represents an endogenous arousal system or whether the observed abnormalities are simply the consequence of chronic pain.

Muscle abnormalities

The first reports of muscle abnormalities in fibromyalgia claimed to find inflammatory changes in tissue sections of biopsies from painful muscle (Gowers 1904; Stockman 1904). Recent investigators have reported more sophisticated changes. Brendstrup et al (1987) found oedema and elevated numbers of mast cells in a proportion of biopsies taken from painful fibrositic nodules. Similarly, Mielke et al (1960) found increased interstitial fluid and fat content and degenerative changes in muscle. Fassbender (1985) detected a motheaten appearance and swollen mitochondria in more chronic and severe cases. Two recent laboratories using more precise diagnostic criteria obtained similar results: motheaten type I fibres, variation in fibre size and ragged red fibres under haematoxylin and eosin staining, and abnormal mitochondria and glycogen deposits (Henriksson & Bengtsson 1982; Bengtsson et al 1986a, 1986b, 1989; Yunus et al 1986; Yunus & Kalyan-Raman 1989). Other observers have demonstrated a pattern of 'rubber band morphology', wherein muscle fibres were compressed at intervals by band-like structures which were in turn connected to each other by what appeared to be elastic or reticular fibres (Bartels & Danneskiold-Samsöe 1986). These histological abnormalities have not been replicated by independent investigators. Similarly it is not clear whether all patients fulfilled criteria for FMS in these various studies. At present there is little consensus about histological abnormalities and none are felt to be characteristic for FMS.

Bengtsson and Henriksson (Henriksson & Bengtsson 1982; Bengtsson et al 1986b; Bengtsson & Henriksson 1989) have theorised that pain in the muscles of individuals with fibromyalgia is the result of muscle hypoxia. They suggest that subtle alterations in the handling of high energy phosphates results in an energy deficit in resting and exercising muscle. This results in hypoxia, microscopic tissue damage and pain. In support of this view these authors have demonstrated abnormally low intramuscular levels of adenosine triphosphate (ATP), adenosine diphosphate (ADP) and phosphocreatine (PS), and increases in adenosine monophosphate (AMP) and creatine in fibromyalgia patients, but not in sedentary controls (Bengtsson & Henriksson 1989). These authors have also demonstrated compromised capillary blood flow isolated to the trapezius tender point in patients with FMS but not in controls (Bengtsson & Henriksson 1989). Other authors have also shown decreased oxygenation of the trapezius and brachioradialis tender points in some patients and explained this on the basis of decreased microcirculatory flow (Lund et al 1986).

The observation that capillary density was normal in fibromyalgia muscle (Bengtsson et al 1986a) prompted Bennett et al (1989) to look at regulatory mechanisms in local blood flow. They had previously observed that exercising fibromyalgia patients exhibited lower than expected maximum oxygen uptake (VO_2 max) during heavy exercise. This was unlikely to be the result of lactic acidosis or a defect in mitochondrial oxidative enzymes.

The evidence for this was a low respiratory quotient at maximal exercise and a normal ventilatory threshold compared to normal individuals. This corroborated previous work showing no evidence for lactic acidosis after ischaemic forearm exercise in individuals with fibromyalgia (Valen et al 1988). Exercising blood flow in the anterior tibialis muscle, measured by the method of xenon-133 clearance, however, was markedly below that of normal sedentary controls (Bennett et al 1989). This conflicted with a previous study showing normal flow in resting muscle (Valen et al 1988), suggesting that the pain of fibromyalgia might result from subtle abnormalities in the regulation of microcirculatory blood flow during activity leading to tissue hypoxia and histological change. In this view muscle energy deficits could be considered secondary to reduced blood flow.

Yunus & Kalyan-Raman (1989) speculated that ischaemic injury might be a consequence of clinically undetectable microspasm of the musculature. However, others found either fragmentary evidence of EMG abnormality (Bengtsson et al 1986b) or no differences between tonic and phasic EMG muscle tension when fibromyalgia patients were compared with matched controls (Sveback 1989, personal communication). Muscle weakness was reported by Jacobsen & Danneskiold-Samsöe (1987), who found that a sample of fibromyalgia patients manifested a 60% reduction in isometric and isokinetic muscle strength when their performance on a Cybex II dynamometer was compared to that of normal individuals.

At present there are no conclusive data to establish abnormalities of muscle blood flow, tissue hypoxia or metabolic defects in energy handling as important mechanisms in the generation of FMS. It remains possible that the observations catalogued above are the consequence of chronic pain, which leads to sedentary activity and subsequent loss of aerobic work capacity or 'detraining' of muscle. Future studies must control for the confounding effects of detraining which most assuredly takes place in painful muscles. McCain (1986) has shown that patients with fibromyalgia are capable of high levels of aerobic exercise and that no untoward alterations in muscle result. Furthermore, physical fitness training and specifically, aerobic exercise, leads to an improvement in self-reports of present pain intensity, and a decrease in the number of FTPs as well as the degree of tenderness elicited over them (McCain et al 1988, 1990). These observations suggest that some muscle abnormality may indeed be at the root of FMS, but do not clearly identify a physiological mechanism which is at fault.

Neuropeptide changes

Researchers have attempted to explain the chronic pain and point tenderness of fibromyalgia as a disorder of the pain-sensing pathways in the nervous system. The relevance of some of the neurotransmitters known to be important in pain transmission has been the subject of recent study in FMS.

Serotonin, or 5-hydroxytryptamine, is a central nervous system neurotransmitter which is converted from the essential amino acid, tryptophan, after crossing the blood–brain barrier. An inverse relationship between serum levels of tryptophan and self-reported pain in fibromyalgia has been observed in patients with FMS (Moldofsky & Warsh 1978). Russell et al also found low concentrations of tryptophan as well as of six other amino acids in the serum of their patients (Russell et al 1989). These data were consistent with clinical studies showing the usefulness of amitriptyline and other tricyclic antidepressants (TCAs) which are known to block the reuptake of serotonin at the synaptic cleft, thereby making it more available for transmission along serotonin-dependent pathways (see below). One such pathway has recently been described, originating in an area rich in serotonin-containing neurones, known as the nucleus raphe magnus. This pathway terminates in the Rexed laminae of the dorsal horn of the spinal cord, an area known to be responsible for modulation of nociceptive impulses from the periphery. Presumably, TCAs exert some of their analgesic properties through potentiating these inhibitory neuronal circuits as a direct result of the increased bioavailability of serotonin. It is also noteworthy that the raphe magnus is known to be involved in sleep architecture in laboratory animals (Morgane 1981).

Furthermore, depletion of serotonin in humans results in a decrease of NREM sleep and an increase in somatic complaints, depression and perceived pain (Moldofsky 1982; Russell et al 1986). Relative serotinin deficiency may, therefore, play a role in the NREM sleep anomaly described above. Recent studies, showing low levels of serum serotonin and upregulation of imipramine binding sites on peripheral blood platelets in fibromyalgia patients, have supported this concept (Russell et al 1987). It also remains possible that TCAs exert some salutary effects through their anticholinergic actions, since amitriptyline, the most useful drug in treatment of this condition, possesses the least serotoninergic effects of the TCAs studied so far. Furthermore, large oral doses of tryptophan have been shown to have no effect on reported pain intensity and sleep in patients with fibromyalgia (Moldofsky & Lue 1980).

Russell et al (1989) implicated catecholamines in this syndrome, reporting higher urinary norepinephrine levels in 14 patients. These norepinephrine levels correlated with pain over tender points and ratings of anxiety but not of depression. Substance P levels in cerebrospinal fluid (CSF) have been reported to be higher in fibromyalgia than in normal subjects (Vaeöry et al 1988). This elevation contrasted with a previous study which showed that other individuals with organic and nonorganic pain syndromes had low or normal levels (Almay et al 1988). Low substance P levels in CSF were negatively correlated in this study with visual analogue scale measurements of sadness, inner tension, concentration difficulties, pain and memory disturbance. When fibromyalgia patients were compared to normal controls, levels of beta-endorphin were not elevated either in serum (Almay et al 1978) or in CSF (Vaeöry et al 1988).

These studies leave the impression that abnormalities or changes in central nervous system neuropeptides may play a role in the generation or maintaining of fibromyalgia. However these studies, while provocative, have not been independently corroborated, with the result that no theory unifying these observations has emerged.

Immune system alterations

Fibromyalgia commonly accompanies autoimmune rheumatic and nonrheumatic diseases like rheumatoid arthritis, Sjögren's syndrome, Raynaud's phenomenon and hypothyroidism. This has led to speculation about a possible link with immune system abnormalities (Goldenberg 1987). More specifically, a pattern of reticular skin discoloration resembling livedo reticularis, a condition usually seen in conjunction with immune-mediated neurovascular injury in systemic lupus erythematosus and some forms of vasculitis, has often been observed in fibromyalgia patients. Skin biopsies from areas exposed to the sun have revealed abnormal serum immunoglobulin deposits at the dermal–epidermal junction in fibromyalgia (Burda 1984; Caro 1984; Caro et al 1984; Dinerman et al 1985; Caro 1986, 1989). These studies often conflict with one another but show a prevalence of immune deposits ranging between 12 and 86%. This may reflect sampling bias as well as differences in the staining techniques used by different investigators. Goldenberg et al (1986) have reported on a group of 118 patients in which only 11% showed immunoflourescent abnormalities on initial biopsy. After a 30-month follow-up, no patient had developed a systemic disease, thus suggesting little support for the autoimmune hypothesis. Wallace and his colleagues (1988, 1989) have reported most extensively on immune abnormalities. One other laboratory has reported similar results (Russell et al 1988a, 1988b). The alterations observed in cellular subsets of T cells and natural killer cells, however, have been minor and not found consistently by different investigators. Furthermore, it is difficult to assess whether observed abnormalities occur in a majority, or only in a minority, of patients. These studies indicate an apparent lack of interlaboratory support for the general hypothesis of immune system involvement.

However, a second line of inquiry has led to renewed support for the theory that immune mechanisms are implicated in fibromyalgia. Recent work by Goldenberg and Komaroff (Goldenberg 1989a; Goldenberg et al 1989; Komaroff & Goldenberg 1989) has shown that between 60 and 70% of patients with chronic fatigue and immune dysfunction syndrome (CFIDS) fulfil the recently validated criteria for fibromyalgia. It has also been shown that CFIDS patients have an elevated number of tender points compared with normal controls (Moldofsky 1989b). Immune system dysfunction is frequently seen in CFIDS so that it appears that some individuals with these conditions may manifest findings indicating immune system dysfunction or recent immune system activation. Abnormalities of immune function that have been described in CFIDS patients include: partial hypogammaglobulinaemia; elevated serum antibodies to some viruses; abnormal levels of circulating immune complexes; increased leucocyte 2'5'-oligoadenylate synthetase; Epstein–Barr virus (EBV)-related T lymphocyte dysfunction; monocyte dysfunction; a decrease in natural killer cell activity, and enhanced skin test reactivity to food and inhaled antigen (Morag et al 1982; Hamblin et al 1983; Straus et al 1985; Tosato et al 1985; Borysiewicz et al 1986; Calder et al 1987; Caligiuri et al 1987; Read et al 1988; Linde et al 1988; Murdoch 1988; Lloyd et al 1989; Prieto et al 1989; Klimas et al 1990; Lloyd et al 1990). It has been suggested that both fibromyalgia and CFIDS may result from an acute infectious process which leads to chronic disturbances in both the functioning of the immune system and the mechanisms of sleep regulation. This has been supported by one study which demonstrated that eight CFIDS patients manifested fibromyalgia-like disturbances in sleep architecture (delayed sleep onset, nocturnal wakefulness, alpha EEG sleep anomaly in NREM sleep) which could not be accounted for by psychological factors alone (Moldofsky 1989a). Further indirect evidence of a link between immune system function and fibromyalgia has come from research demonstrating that the immune system is influenced by sleep–wake cycles (Krueger & Karnovsky 1987); that administration of interferon produces sleepiness (Horning et al 1982) and that injection of interleukin-2 has produced a distinctive set of fibromyalgia-like symptoms in cancer patients (Wallace et al 1988).

PSYCHOLOGICAL CONSIDERATIONS

Psychological disturbances form an integral part of the fibromyalgia syndrome. Controlled studies, however, have shown that only a minority of patients suffer from major psychiatric disorders. Furthermore, these studies suggest that observed psychological distress is likely to be the result, rather than the cause, of chronic pain (Leavitt & Garron 1979; Clarke et al 1985a; Wolfe et al 1984b; Hawley et al 1988). Initial studies used psychological tests which included items on the patient self-report inventories which were heavily weighted toward somatic complaints, so that raw scores were erroneously higher than population means. This was particularly true for items in the Minnesota Multiphasic Personality Inventory (MMPI) (Rook et al 1981; Smythe 1984; Lamping 1985). A slightly more consistent relationship has been noted between fibromyalgia and negative affect. One study reported that current and past diagnoses of depression were far more common among fibromyalgia patients (71%) than among rheumatoid patients (13%) or controls (12%). A similar pattern was found for anxiety disorders: 26% of fibromyalgia patients experienced anxiety disorders compared with none in either of the other two groups. Depression was also more prevalent among first-degree relatives of fibromyalgia patients than those of rheumatoid patients and normal controls (Hudson et al 1985). A similar study found that fibromyalgia patients manifested a higher level of symptom reporting and help-seeking behaviours than patients with rheumatoid arthritis (Kirmayer et al 1988). Four out of five subsequent studies, however, reported no differences in either anxiety or depression measurements between fibromyalgia and rheumatoid patients (Payne et al 1982; Wolfe et al 1984a; Clark et al 1985a; Ahles et al 1987; Scudds et al 1989a). Although the available research suggests a relationship between psychological distress and fibromyalgia, the connection remains elusive. It may be more profitable to consider psychological malaise as an integral consequence of the fibromyalgia experience rather than as a marker of the syndrome.

TREATMENT

The long-term treatment of fibromyalgia remains problematical since the natural history of this condition appears to be one of continuous and unremitting pain. One current report has shown that only 5% of individuals sustained remission of all symptoms during a 3-year follow-up. (Felson & Goldenberg 1986). Over 60% of patients continued to complain of significant fatigue and nonrestorative sleep despite the fact that over 85% received medication during the study period. Even though some of these therapies have been studied with acceptable scientific rigour, no definitive treatment strategy has emerged. Two studies have asked patients about the effectiveness of their previous treatment regimens. Cathey et al (1986) surveyed 81 patients about medication use during the previous year of their illness. They noted that the average patient used 4.7 drugs during the year and that they were taking 3.8 medications at the year's end. Of the 50% of patients taking amitriptyline or cyclobenzaprine only one-third improved sufficiently to report moderate or great improvement. Interestingly, analgesics were reported to be equally as effective as these two medications. Goldenberg (1989b) reported similar results after following 87 patients treated over a 3-year period. These observations indicated that over 50% of patients failed to respond to numerous pharmacological and nonpharmacological therapies. This indicates that fibromyalgia patients present difficult treatment problems and that the average patient will require multiple methods of treatment over the natural course of their disease, often with limited success.

A list of therapies believed to be beneficial in fibromyalgia is shown in Table 26.6. Treatments for fibromyalgia can be divided into those based on pharmacological and nonpharmacological principles.

Pharmacological treatments

Acceptable clinical trials have now been completed showing that both amitriptyline (Carette et al 1986; Goldenberg et al 1986; Scudds et al 1989a; Jaeschke et al 1991) and cyclobenzaprine (Bennett et al 1988; Quimby et al 1989; Reynolds et al 1991) are effective in fibromyalgia. The recommended dose of these drugs (10–50 mg of amitriptyline and 10–30 mg of cyclobenzaprine) is much smaller than the dose used in the treatment of depression. In fact, even low doses of these drugs are often poorly tolerated in fibromyalgia as a result of what seems to be extreme sensitivity to their central nervous system and anticholinergic side-effects. Common side-effects are drowsiness, agitation and gastrointestinal upset. Jaeschke

Table 26.6 Treatment of the fibromyalgia syndrome

	Effective	Ineffective
Pharmacological	Amitriptyline Cyclobenzaprine	Imipramine Fenfluramine Doxepin
	Alprazolam	
	Zopiclone	Prednisone
	Dothiepin	Naproxen (alone)
	S-adenosyl-methionine Regional sympathetic block	
Nonpharmacological	Cardiovascular fitness training	Transcutaneous electrical nerve stimulation Interferential current
	EMG biofeedback	Local injection Postisometric relaxation
	Cognitive behavioural therapy	Laser therapy Massage Hypnosis Acupuncture Local ice/heat

et al (1991) have reported on amitriptyline using the new method of 'N-of-1' trials. About one-third of patients who initially were thought to be eligible for entry into these studies benefited from amitriptyline. This corroborates a clinical observation that amitriptyline may be quite useful in selected patients, but that these are usually in the minority. No N-of-1 trials have been reported for cyclobenzaprine. One study has correlated EEG sleep recordings in 12 patients taking cyclobenzaprine in a double-blind, placebo-controlled, crossover design (Reynolds et al 1991). While improvements were noted in evening fatigue and total sleep time during cyclobenzaprine treatment, present pain intensity, pain thresholds over FTPs and mood ratings did not change. The most striking finding was that alpha EEG NREM sleep anomaly was unchanged in patients taking cyclobenzaprine.

Alprazolam (a triazalobenzodiazepine) has been approved for the treatment of anxiety and the depression associated with anxiety. Its antidepressant activity is comparable to imipramine, amitriptyline and doxepin. One report has compared alprazolam, alone or in combination with ibuprofen, in a placebo-controlled, randomised, double-blind protocol (Russell et al 1991). Over half of the patients treated with alprazolam plus ibuprofen showed a greater than 30% improvement, which was considered clinically significant. The authors remarked on the greater than expected drop-out rate (>30%) and the fact that, while alprazolam showed good effects at 8 weeks, improvements were slow to occur and required up to 16 weeks of treatment for some patients.

Several other medications have been shown to have little or no effect on the symptoms and signs of fibromyalgia. Imipramine, for example, was found to be ineffective in one report (Wysenbeek et al 1985). Doxepin and fenfluramine have also had anecdotal success in treatment, but no controlled trials have been carried out that specifically studied these compounds. Similarly, phenothiazines have not been well studied but have been shown to be of limited usefulness, because of the unacceptable incidence of side-effects (Moldofsky & Warsh 1978). They do, however, lead to a predictable improvement in sleep disturbance. Dothiepin has been reported to be superior to placebo in one study, when given as a single dose of 75 mg at bedtime (Caruso et al 1987). Bengtsson & Bengtsson (1988) have also reported on the beneficial effects of regional sympathetic blockade in fibromyalgia. Antiinflammatory medications have shown disappointing results in clinical trials. In properly controlled randomised trials, prednisone, 20 mg per day (Clark et al 1985b), and naproxen, 500 mg per day (Goldenberg et al 1986) were no more effective than placebo. A novel compound, s-adenosyl-methionine (SAMe) which has both antidepressant and antiinflammatory properties, has been found to be more effective than placebo in one report (Tavoni et al 1987). Zopiclone, a nonbenzodiazepine hypnotic, has been reported to improve subjective sleep complaints but not pain-reporting behavior in FMS (Drewes et al 1991).

Nonpharmacological treatments

It is apparent from the foregoing discussion that drug therapy alone is often insufficient for patients with fibromyalgia. Medicinal therapies are, therefore, often relegated to an adjunctive role and it is often necessary to include a number of nonmedical modalities of treatment for patients with this disorder. Note that, so far, only a minority of such treatments has been studied using acceptable scientific methods. At present, these treatments are used with little rationale, often haphazardly, and rarely in conjunction with pharmacological therapies. To date, preliminary evidence exists only for three forms of such treatment: cardiovascular fitness training (McCain 1986; McCain et al 1988, 1990; McCain 1989); EMG biofeedback training (Furaccioli et al 1987) and cognitive behavioural therapy (Nielson et al 1992).

Cardiovascular fitness training

A recent study reported the effects of cardiovasular fitness training on the manifestations of primary fibromyalgia. A total of 42 patients were randomised to a 20-week programme of either cardiovascular fitness training or flexibility training (McCain et al 1988). Enhanced cardiovascular fitness was attained in 83% of those randomised to the cardiovascular fitness group. Significant improvements in pain threshold measurements over fibrositic tender points was noted in those receiving cardiovascular fitness training when compared with patients treated with flexibility exercises alone. Both physician and patient global assessment scores were also improved in the cardiovascular-treated group. However, no significant differences were found between the groups in present pain intensity scores as measured by visual analogue scale, the percentage of total body area involved, or in hours per night or nights per week of disturbed sleep. Psychological profiles were no different in the two groups before and after treatment. The authors concluded that cardiovascular fitness training improved objective and subjective measurements of pain in primary fibromyalgia.

EMG biofeedback training

Only one controlled study of the effects of biofeedback training in primary fibromyalgia has been reported (Furaccioli et al 1987). This study consisted of an open trial of 15 patients who underwent 15 sessions of EMG biofeedback over a 5-week observation period. Nine patients had improvement in the number of fibrositic tender points and present pain intensity as measured by visual analogue scores and morning stiffness. These improvements persisted up to 6 months after EMG biofeedback had ceased. A follow-up study, randomising a further 12 patients to a similar regimen of EMG biofeedback or sham biofeedback showed a significant improvement in visual analogue pain scores, morning stiffness and number of fibrositic tender points in the true EMG biofeedback group. Again, these differences were significant both at 5 weeks and 5 months after treatment. Another report by the same authors indicated that EMG biofeedback reduces plasma ACTH and beta endorphin levels during treatment, indicating an opioid and/or neuroendocrine basis for some of the observed beneficial effects in fibromyalgia (Molina et al 1987).

Cognitive behavioural therapy

Cognitive behavioural therapy for chronic pain has been proved useful in a number of clinical settings, such as low back pain, headache, temporomandibular joint pain and rheumatoid arthritis. This multidisciplinary approach has recently been applied to fibromyalgia (Nielson et al 1992). A total of 30 consecutive patients attending a rheumatic diseases unit were assessed 5 months before, at admission to, and at discharge from, a 3-week, inpatient, multidisciplinary, cognitive behavioural treatment programme. The programme included medical, psychological, social work, physiotherapy, occupational therapy and nursing interventions, based on the cognitive behavioural model. The primary goal of the programme was to assist patients in developing an active, resourceful, self-management approach to coping with their fibromyalgia. Cognitive techniques were used in conjunction with aerobic exercise, physiotherapy, biofeedback training and relaxation therapy.

Outcome measures were primarily psychological in nature and showed significant improvements in perceived pain severity, affective distress (depressed mood, irritability and tension) and the extent to which pain interfered with normal activities. Sense of control and mastery over life circumstances were also enhanced in comparison to preadmission status. This study provided no follow-up data on how long these good effects persisted, but did show improvements over the short-term which were very significant statistically. No data were provided regarding the effect of cognitive behavioural therapy on specific disease-related outcome measures like pain threshold over FTPs, pain palpation scores or degree of morning stiffness. There was an improvement, however, in functional abilities such as time spent out of bed and activity level. Cognitive behavioural therapy, therefore, may be of benefit to selected patients when administered in the proper setting by trained personnel.

MYOFASCIAL PAIN SYNDROME

DIAGNOSTIC CRITERIA

Diagnostic criteria and treatment modalities for myofascial pain syndrome (MPS) have not been tested as rigorously as those for FMS. Most studies in the MPS literature are descriptive in nature and rely heavily on anecdotal evidence from single investigators which has not been corroborated by multicentre studies. Nevertheless present knowledge has allowed for the emergence of empirically based clinical criteria which can be used to determine not only differences between MPS and other pain syndromes but also to devise rational treatment strategies.

Suggested diagnostic features have been divided into major and minor criteria (see Table 26.2). MPS is said to be present when all five major criteria and at least one minor criterion are satisfied (Simons 1990). It should be pointed out, however, that while these diagnostic criteria possess some validity they have not been rigorously tested against other pain syndromes and that no useful estimates of their sensitivity and specificity can be made given our present state of knowledge.

CLINICAL PRESENTATION

The principal diagnostic feature of MPS is that pain and tenderness are usually localised to one or a few discrete muscles. In this respect patients with FMS can be readily distinguished from those with MPS because the former is a generalised pain syndrome, characterised by widespread muscular aching. The patient with MPS, however, usually complains of pain in one quadrant of the body or more often at one anatomical site, which localises the problem to one or a few muscle groups. Palpation of the muscles in the affected quadrant reveals an area of localised tenderness often within one or several muscle bellies or their tendon attachments. The tenderness is discrete and lies within a structure known as the 'taut band'. A taut band is defined as an area of increased consistency or hardness which is usually linear, but sometimes nodular, in shape and runs parallel to the direction of the muscle fibres at that point in the muscle. The localised tenderness within the taut band is known as a 'trigger point'.

Palpation of the trigger point results in a number of phenomena which are considered essential to diagnosis. The most commonly observed feature is the elicitation of a zone of radiating pain which is quite stereotypical for the individual muscle. This pain is described as a localised, subcutaneous ache with slightly blurred edges that projects well beyond the originating tender point. Simons & Travell (Simons 1975, 1976b; Travell & Simons 1983) have mapped trigger points and their respective zones of radiating pain for the entire soma. Their work shows that any one muscle may have several trigger points each exhibiting a uniquely distributed zone of referred pain. Most trigger points refer pain distally rather than proximally but are not restricted to a segmental or peripheral nerve root distribution. Some muscles, like the deltoid, gluteus maximus and serratus posterior inferior, characteristically refer to a zone in the immediate vicinity of the trigger point. Others, like the infraspinatus and tensor fascia lata muscles, refer pain to adjacent joints and may therefore be confused with articular diseases like arthritis. Still others, like the serratus posterior superior, refer pain deep into the chest and may mimic visceral disease. Sensations other than pain may be referred in typical distribution patterns from trigger points. For example, trigger points may refer hypoaesthesia or anaesthesia instead of pain, but always do so in a stereotypical geographic zone of radiation that is constant for each muscle-derived trigger point. The fifth major criterion stipulates that trigger points and taut bands must be associated with shortening as evidenced by restricted range of motion in an affected muscle. This criterion may be omitted when range of motion is not measurable in an affected muscle.

Three minor criteria have been suggested to further aid in the diagnosis of MPS.

1. Palpation of a trigger point should reproduce the clinical pain complaint or lead to altered sensation in the zone of referral.
2. A local twitch response may be elicited in the affected muscle by transverse snapping palpation at the trigger point or by needle insertion into the trigger point within the taut band. A twitch response is seen as an involuntary contraction of the affected muscle, akin to a deep tendon reflex, but localised only to the affected muscle (Fig. 26.2).
3. Alleviation of pain by elongation or stretching of the muscle, or after injection of the trigger point with saline, local anaesthetic, steroid or dry needling.

Trigger points may also be said to be latent. Latent trigger points are incidental findings in muscles which are not areas of clinical pain but which, when palpated, give rise to a zone of radiating pain typical for the muscle involved. It is at present unclear whether latent trigger points represent evolving true trigger points, or whether they indicate a more generalised abnormality in pain perception similar to that seen in FMS.

PREVALENCE AND DEMOGRAPHIC FEATURES

Few controlled studies have been published on the prevalence of this condition. There appears to be a female predominance with the highest estimates in the range of 3:1, a ratio much lower than that of FMS. Anecdotal evidence from expert examiners suggests that MPS is a very common condition, particularly in industry where it is a frequent cause of disability after trauma. It is also seen as a major component of the whiplash syndrome which occurs as a consequence of injury from motor vehicle accidents (Teasell & McCain 1992). Only one study has attempted to determine the prevalence of muscle tenderness in asymptomatic adults. Sola et al (1955) palpated the shoulder and neck girdle musculature of 100 male and 100 female new recruits in the US Air Force. They found one or more tender areas in 49.5% of subjects. While trigger points were not catalogued in this study referred pain similar to that seen after palpation of trigger points was seen in 12.5% of individuals. More than one tender area was found in more than 65% of subjects. Just four muscles, the trapezius, levator scapulae, infraspinatus and scalenes, accounted for 84.7% of the tender points observed. These data suggest that trigger points may be seen in normal individuals free of pain complaints. No properly controlled epidemiological study has explored this possibility in the general population.

PATHOPHYSIOLOGY

The mechanisms that produce the symptoms of MPS are also largely speculative. Travell & Simons (1983) have proposed that initial changes may be precipitated by such factors as local trauma, fatigue of the muscles from repeated overuse, chronic postural imbalance and psychological distress. These stressors give rise to a physiological contracture at the level of the sarcomere. The physiological contracture would lead to stimulation of group III and group IV muscle afferents, which respond more readily to serotonin, histamine and bradykinin, to produce a dull, aching pain. Prolonged pain leads to subsequent contracture of the muscles which then leads to restriction of range of joint movement. Concurrent local and distal autonomic changes may also be present under these circumstances. There is some support for these events from animal studies which have shown that pain arising in muscle travels in the unmyelinated group IV fibres after stimulation of nociceptors by serotonin, histamine, potassium and bradykinin (Fock & Mense 1976).

Muscle biopsies have been taken from tender muscles of patients with MPS. In general, few abnormalities have been found. Frequent observations include: disruption of myofibrillar structure; increased amounts of ground substance and mucopolysaccharides; multifocal loss of selected oxidative enzymes, and occasional 'ragged red' fibres, suggestive of mitochondrial damage (Bennett 1990). One recent study showed a decreased level of high energy phosphates in muscle biopsies taken from the trapezius muscle in MPS (Larsson et al 1988). These findings are identical to those observed in patients with FMS.

A possible explanation for taut bands is the presence of a localised area of muscle spasm. This idea originated with Kellgren's observation of palpable muscle spasm within paracervical muscles after hypotonic saline injections were

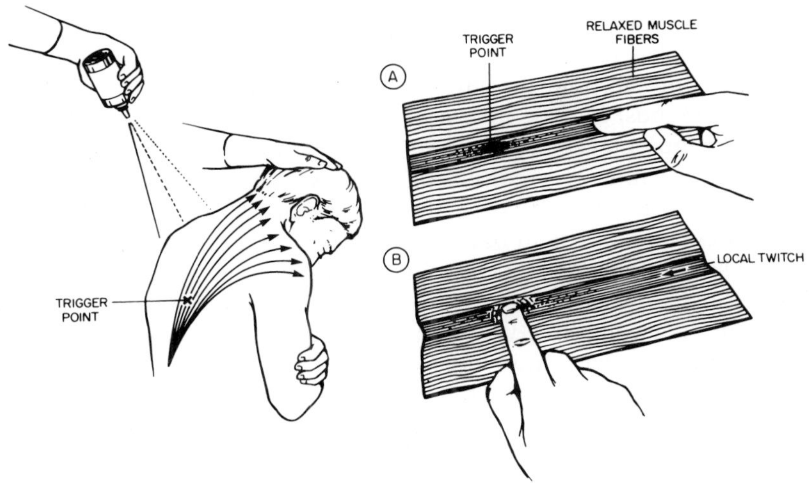

Fig. 26.2 Trigger points occur within taut bands which run parallel to the orientation of fibres in an affected muscle. **A** shows that the taut band may be palpated as a linear (or nodular) zone of increased consistency within the surrounding relaxed normal muscle. **B** Digital palpation using a plucking motion (like that used to pluck a violin string) results in the local twitch response which is seen as an immediate contraction of the taut band and adjacent normal muscle. The twitch response is quite similar to the movement elicited in the deep tendon reflex. Stretch and spray therapy is directed at the trigger point (X) and its associated taut band. The trigger point is isolated by palpation and marked visually. A vapocoolant spray is administered to the skin overlying the affected muscle through long continuous sweeps in the direction of orientation of the prevailing muscle fibres while the muscle undergoes a simultaneous passive stretch. This procedure may be repeated several times during each treatment session. Permanent eradication of trigger points may require several treatment sessions.

given into the intraspinous ligaments (Kellgren 1938). EMG studies, however, have shown such areas to be electrically silent (Raft et al 1968; Simons, 1976a; Fricton et al 1985a). On the other hand, stimulation of trigger points, either by dry needling or manual snapping of the involved muscle, has been shown to result in motor unit action potentials of 0.2 seconds at 500 μV (Simons 1976a; Bennett 1990). At present there is no convincing evidence that taut bands or trigger points are associated with electrophysiological abnormalities at rest and the significance of their excitability after mechanical stimulation is unknown.

Sleep studies have been performed in patients with MPS. One study reported that 42% of 164 patients with MPS involving the head and neck reported poor sleep (Fricton & Kroening 1982). A subsequent study reported finding the alpha–delta sleep anomaly in some patients with posttraumatic myofascial pain (Saskin et al 1986). In this respect, patients with MPS resemble those with FMS.

Few studies have assessed psychological factors in MPS. Fricton studied 164 patients with MPS of the head and neck and noted that anxiety, depression and anger occurred in about one-quarter (Fricton & Kroening 1982). Another study compared patients with MPS to patients with low back pain (Fricton et al 1985b). This study showed high scores for somatisation, obsessive–compulsive tendencies, depression, anxiety and hostility which were not significantly different between these two groups.

A recent study showed a decrease in pain and a concomitant increase in range of motion after injection of trigger points with 0.25% bupivacaine (Fine et al 1988). The affect was reversed by pretreatment with intravenous naloxone and suggested that local injection therapies might harness the endogenous opioid system with resultant decrease in pain and improved range of motion.

PROGNOSIS

MPS is a chronic disease. Although no long-term studies have been done to determine the natural history of this condition it is accepted that most patients receive multiple modalities of treatment usually over many years with only limited benefit. In one study of 164 individuals the mean duration of complaint was 5.8 years for males and 6.9 years for females (Fricton & Kroening 1982). In another study of 102 patients with orofacial pain in which 59.8% had MPS the mean duration of pain was 6.0 years (Fricton 1990). These studies documented numerous treatment modalities and physician contacts indicating that MPS patients are significant users of the health care facilities (Aronoff et al 1983).

TREATMENT

Since only limited studies on outcome of specific modalities of therapy have been reported any discussion on treatment must remain strictly anecdotal. However some general treatment strategies can be enunciated on empirical grounds and are amenable to future study. Management of MPS must take into account the chronic nature of the disease process and must include measures to eradicate muscular trigger points, prevent their recurrence and deal with possible aggravating or predisposing factors. This approach necessarily involves treating the whole patient and fits into our current paradigm of multidisciplinary treatment for chronic pain syndromes in general.

Inactivation of trigger points is accomplished through counterstimulation coupled with active and passive stretching which may include postural rehabilitation (Travell & Simons 1983). The goal is to restore the muscle to normal length, posture and full range of motion. Preventing the redevelopment of trigger points includes maintenance of an exercise programme with concomitant control of predisposing contributing factors. Counterstimulation may be achieved by a number of measures which, although widely used, have not been thoroughly tested in well controlled studies. These measures include massage, acupressure, ultrasound, moist heat, ice packs, fluorimethane spray and diathermy. Transcutaneous nerve stimulation, electroacupuncture and direct current stimulation have also been used. Acupuncture and trigger point injections with saline, steroid or alcohol cause mechanical disruption of trigger points. It is generally acknowledged that counterstimulation can provide short-term relief from pain but that long-term management by a regular muscle stretching and strengthening programme is also important. Postural contributing factors, whether behavioural or biological, perpetuate trigger points if not corrected (Glyn 1971; Fricton & Kroening 1982; Simons & Travell 1983). One study of 164 head and neck MPS patients found poor sitting/standing posture in 96%, forward head in 84.7%, rounded shoulders in 82.3%, lower tongue position in 67.7%, abnormal lordosis in 46.3%, scoliosis in 15.9% and leg length discrepancy in 14% of patients (Fricton & Kroening 1982). Muscles held in sustained contraction, either in a normal position or in an abnormal shortened position, are more prone to redevelop trigger points. Mechanical abnormalities like spinal scoliosis or leg length discrepancy, therefore, should be corrected with orthotics and other devices whenever possible. Similarly, unusual or repetitive movements in the workplace or at the work station should be simplified to allow for stretching and use of alternative muscle groups.

Special care must be taken to address psychological contributing factors, such as those associated with litigation and long-term disability, which lead to uncertainty about future employability. Loss of self-esteem is the consequence of the anxiety surrounding these issues and should be dealt with through patient education and practical guidance regarding money issues when necessary. Learned illness behaviours which detract from an adaptive, coping style are best remedied with a cognitive–behavioural approach. These psychological factors may be the source of the greatest morbidity in both FMS and MPS. Attention to details in this area may often yield the most success when return of function is the endpoint of treatment.

These principles are outlined in Table 26.7 which describes an approach that can be tailored not only to severity but also to the impact of MPS on the functional abilities of the individual patient. The evidence for efficacy of two commonly used counterstimulation techniques, namely stretch and spray therapy and trigger point injections, is discussed below.

Stretch and spray therapy

Stretch and spray therapy involves passive stretching of an affected muscle while simultaneously administering a vapocoolant spray, such as fluorimethane, to the overlying skin. The technique (see Fig. 26.2) involves directing a fine stream of fluorimethane spray from a calibrated nozzle toward the skin directly overlying the muscle with the trigger point. The spray is directed over the reference zone to which pain has radiated on previous palpation of the trigger point. After a few initial sweeps over the reference zone the affected muscle is passively stretched with enough force to elicit pain and discomfort. The muscle is then put on progressive passive stretch while the vapocoolant stream is directed to the skin at an acute angle from 30–50 cm away. The spray is applied in one direction, from the trigger point toward its reference zone, in slow, even, parallel sweeps over the whole muscle at a rate of about 10 cm/s. This sequence can be repeated four times, with care being taken not to freeze the underlying skin, a condition which may aggravate the trigger point. The endpoint is the eradication of pain and point tenderness over the trigger point, as well as an improvement in the range of active and passive movement. Despite its great popularity, only one study has shown that trigger point tenderness, as measured by pressure algometry and visual analogue pain rating scales was reduced after stretch and spray therapy (Jaeger & Reeves 1986). Referred pain was also reduced after stretch and spray therapy in this study.

Trigger point injections

Trigger point injections have been shown to reduce pain, increase range of motion, increase exercise tolerance and increase circulation in muscles (Dorigo et al 1979; Lewit 1979; Hameroff et al 1981; Jaeger & Skootsky 1987). The pain relief may last from minutes to many months depending on the chronicity and severity of the trigger point. The critical factor in needling is the mechanical disruption of the trigger point rather than the solution

Table 26.7 Treatment of myofascial pain (adapted from Fricton 1990)

	Clinical characteristics	Treatment
Acute onset with rapid resolution	Onset less than 2 months No previous treatment Simple psychological and/or behavioural factors Few trigger points, unilateral No other symptoms Prognosis excellent	3 months Fluorimethance spray and stretch (office) Home exercises: stretching and posture exercises for affected muscle groups Control of contributing factors Reduce muscle tension habits Evaluate for other perpetuating factors
Subacute onset with good response	Onset within 2–6 months Minimal previous treatment Some psychological and/or behavioural factors Numerous trigger points bilaterally No other symptoms Prognosis good	6 months Fluorimethane spray and stretch (office and home) Home exercises: stretching and posture exercises for affected muscle groups Stabilisation splints for craniofacial pain Nonsteroidal anti-inflammatory drugs optional Control of contributing factors Reduce tension-producing habits Reduce contributing postural habits Behavioural therapy to include relaxation techniques, biofeedback, pacing skills If not successful, use physical therapy, trigger point injections, or acupuncture, or reevaluate perpetuating factors
Chronic pain syndrome with slow response	Onset within more than 6 months Many previous unsuccessful therapies and medications Many psychological, behavioural and social factors Many muscles with trigger points Other symptoms: diminished sensation dizziness, tinnitus, flushing, migraine Prognosis is guarded for long-term reduction of pain and improved function and is dependent on patient compliance	1 year Physical therapy: mobilisation with heat, ultrasound or other modalities Home stretching and postural exercises Eliminate medications, except short-term antidepressants for sleep disturbance Tryptophan for sleep disturbance only Control of contributing factors Improve postural habits Behaviour therapy with biofeedback, stress management, pacing skills training Education and control of social factors Management of depression if present Management of drug dependency Consider injection of trigger points, reevaluation of contributing factors, and consider the need for a chronic pain programme and cognitive-behavioural approach

used during injection. Therefore, precision in needling the exact trigger point is the most important factor in trigger point inactivation. Fine et al (1988) used a double-blind, crossover study design to determine whether analgesia after trigger point injection was reversed with naloxone and, thus, mediated by activation of the endogenous opioid system. The short-term analgesic effect of injections was reversed with naloxone compared to placebo, suggesting that the antinociceptive effect of injection of trigger points is in part mediated by the opioid system. This does not explain the long-term analgesia often seen after such injections.

Trigger point injections with local anaesthetic agents are preferred to dry needling or injecting other substances because they are inherently less painful. The use of local anaesthetics such as 3% chlorpromazine (short-acting) and 5% procaine (medium-acting), without vasoconstrictors is suggested (Fricton 1990). Hamerhoff et al (1981) compared injection of bupivacaine, etidocaine and saline and found the former two anaesthetics superior to saline. One study compared dry needling, injection of saline or procaine and placebo skin injection in a double-blind design. These authors found that reduction in trigger point tenderness was dependent on penetration of the trigger point with the needle. Reduction of referred pain was greater with injection of either saline or procaine than with dry needling or placebo. Only one other study looked at the short- and long-term effects of dry needling of trigger points and found immediate improvement in 86.8% of patients and permanent improvement in 29.8% (Lewit 1979).

The following considerations are important for trigger point injection. The patient must be positioned in a comfortable, relaxed posture so that the location of the exact trigger point can be accomplished. Proper aseptic skin preparation is required. The needle must be inserted quickly through the skin for maximum comfort and placed directly and precisely within the trigger point with the taut band of muscle at the tip of the needle. The 'local twitch response' or contraction of the band containing the trigger point, as well as the intensification of dull pain over the muscle or in the zone of reference, will indicate when the trigger point has been 'needled'. It is at this point that aspiration and slow injection of the local anaesthetic can be accomplished. Repeated probing of the taut band without removal of the needle may isolate satellite trigger points which can also be injected. Pain relief should be seen within a few minutes. Immediate full range manual stretching of the muscle is then required to restore the muscle to normal resting length and to determine whether additional trigger points are present. Shortening activation or a reactive spasm may occasionally occur due to shortening of an antagonist muscle that also contains a trigger point. This may cause a slight increase in pain 2–5 hours after injection. Failure to eradicate pain beyond this period is probably the result of inexact needling of the isolated trigger point. Trigger point injection should not be attempted in the acute phase after muscle trauma or in patients with bleeding diatheses, allergy to anaesthetic agents or with cellulitis of the injection area.

OVERLAP BETWEEN FMS AND MPS

A careful reading of the literature on FMS and MPS suggests some major similarities between these two conditions. There are at least two studies which have addressed the possibility that FMS and MPS may be different manifestations of the same phenomenon (Wolfe et al 1992; Tunks et al 1992). In one study four myofascial pain experts performed trigger point examinations and four fibromyalgia experts performed tender point examinations on three groups of patients: eight with FMS; eight with MPS, and eight normal individuals (Wolfe et al 1992). The examiners were unaware of the diagnosis and individual group membership. Myofascial pain experts had difficulty agreeing with one another on the presence of active trigger points, taut bands and the local twitch response, whereas fibromyalgia tender points were elicited with excellent intrarater and interrater agreements. Local tenderness was more likely to be elicited by myofascial pain experts and occurred in 82% of their examinations. Despite these limitations, active trigger points were seen in 18% of examinations of FMS and MPS patients. When a more liberal definition of trigger point was used, requiring only local tenderness and referred pain, a 38 and 23% positive rate was seen among FMS and MPS patients respectively. Taut bands and local twitch responses were common (50 and 30% respectively) and noted equally in all three diagnostic groups.

Tunks et al (1991) performed a similar study in which patients with FMS, MPS, localised mechanical or arthritic pain and normal controls underwent a standardised medical examination which included specific search for tender points and trigger points. Expert examiners unaware of patient diagnosis were able to agree with acceptable rater reliability on the presence of tenderness at specific fibromyalgia and myofascial pain tender points. Poor agreements were noted for the presence or absence of taut bands, twitch responses and the zone of radiating pain. Furthermore, patients with myofascial pain complaints which were localised to a single body quadrant showed tenderness (by pressure algometer readings and palpation scores) in other body quadrants in 66.7% of cases.

These data suggest that patients with FMS and MPS may be more alike than dissimilar when only tenderness is considered. They also indicate that some aspects of the examination of patients with MPS, such as the presence of taut bands and local twitch response, may not be sufficiently reproducible to warrant inclusion in future diagnostic criteria.

SUMMARY

FMS and MPS are common clinical conditions which present not only diagnostic challenges but also therapeutic hurdles for physicians and other therapists interested in the treatment of chronic pain. The last decade has seen major changes in our thinking and in strategies to deal with these conditions. The application of sound scientific principles to future studies in this area will lead to fewer anecdotal reports and to the study of more homogeneous patient populations. We can look forward to a clearer understanding of these complex conditions.

REFERENCES

Ahles T A, Yunus M B, Masi AT 1987 Is chronic pain a variant of depressive disease? The case of primary fibromyalgia syndrome. Pain 29: 105

Almay B G L, Johansson F, Von Knorring L, Terenius L, Wahlstrom A 1978 Endorphins in chronic pain: differences in CSF endorphin levels between organic and psychogenic pain syndromes. Pain 5: 153

Almay B G L, Johansson F, Von Knorring L, Le Greves P, Terenius L 1988 Substance P in CSF of patients with chronic pain syndromes. Pain 33: 3

Aronoff G M, Evans W O, Enders P L 1983 A review of follow-up studies of multidisciplinary pain units. Pain 16(1): 1

Bartels E M, Danneskiold-Samsöe B 1986 Histological abnormalities in muscle in patients with certain types of fibrositis. Lancet 1: 755

Bengtsson A, Bengtsson M 1988 Regional sympathetic blockade in primary fibromyalgia Pain 33: 161

Bengtsson A, Henriksson K G 1989 The muscle in fibromyalgia: a review of the Swedish studies. Journal of Rheumatology 16 (suppl 19): 144

Bengtsson A, Henriksson K G, Jorfeldt L 1986a Primary fibromyalgia: a clinical and laboratory study of 55 patients. Linkoping University Medical Dissertation 224: 1

Bengtsson A, Henriksson K G, Jorfeldt L, Kadedal B, Lennmarken C,

Lindstrom F 1986b Primary fibromyalgia: a clinical and laboratory study of 55 patients. Scandinavian Journal of Rheumatology 15: 340

Bennett R M 1990 Myofascial pain syndromes and fibromyalgia pain syndrome: A comparative analysis. In: Fricton J R, Awad E A (eds) Advances in pain research and therapy, vol 17. Myofascial pain and fibromyalgia. Raven Press, New York, p 43

Bennett R M, Gatter R A, Campbell S M, Andrews R P, Clark S R, Scarlo J A 1988 A comparison of cyclobenzaprine and placebo in the management of fibrositis. Arthritis and Rheumatism 31: 1535

Bennett R M, Clark S R, Goldberg L et al 1989 Aerobic fitness in the fibrositis syndrome: a controlled study of respiratory gas exchange and 133 xenon clearance from exercise in muscle. Arthritis and Rheumatism 32: 454

Borysiewicz L K, Haworth S J, Cohen J, Mundin J, Rickinson A, Sissons J G 1986 Epstein–Barr virus specific immune defects in patients with persistent symptoms following infectious mononucleosis. Quarterly Journal of Medicine 58: 111

Brendstrup P, Jesperson K, Asbol-Hansen G 1987 Morphological and chemical tissue changes in fibrositic muscles. Annals of Rheumatic Diseases 16: 438

Burda C D 1984 Immunoglobulin-G deposits at the dermal–epidermal junction in secondary (traumatic) fibromyalgia syndrome (letter). Clinical and Experimental Rheumatology 2: 195

Calder B D, Warnock P J, McCartney R A, Bell E J 1987 Coxsackie B virus and the post-viral syndrome: a prospective study in general practice. Journal of the Royal College of General Practioners 37: 11

Caligiuri M, Murray C, Buchwald D et al 1987 Phenotypic and functional deficiency of natural killer cells in patients with chronic fatigue syndrome. Journal of Immunology 139: 3306

Campbell S M, Bennnett R M 1986 Fibrositis. Disease-a-Month 11: 653

Campbell S M, Clark S R, Tindall E A, Forehand M E, Bennett R M 1983 Clinical characteristics of fibrositis. I. A 'blinded' controlled study of symptoms and tender points. Arthritis and Rheumatism 26: 817–824

Carette S, McCain G A, Bell D A, Fam A G 1986 Evaluation of amitriptyline in primary fibrositis. A double-blind, placebo-controlled study. Arthritis and Rheumatism 29: 655

Caro X J 1984 Immunofluorescent detection of IgG at the dermal-epidermal junction in patients with apparent primary fibrositis syndrome. Arthritis and Rheumatism 27: 1174

Caro X J 1986 Immunofluorescent studies of skin in primary fibrositis syndrome. American Journal of Medicine 81 (suppl 3A): 43

Caro X J 1989 Is there an immunologic component to fibrositis syndrome? Rheumatic Diseases Clinics of North America 15: 169

Caro X J, Wolfe F, Johnston W H, Smith A L 1984 A controlled and blinded study of immunoreactant deposition at the dermal–epidermal junction in patients with primary fibrositis syndrome. Arthritis and Rheumatism 27: abstract S76

Caruso I, Sarzi Puttini P C, Boccassini L et al 1987 Double blind study of dothiepin versus placebo in the treatment of primary fibromyalgia syndrome. Journal of Internal Medicine Research 15: 154

Cathey M A, Wolfe F, Kleinheksel S M, Hawley D J 1986 Socioeconomic impact of fibrositis: a study of 81 patients with primary fibrositis. American Journal of Medicine 81 (suppl 3A): 78

Clark S R, Campbell S M, Forehand M E, Tindall E A, Bennett R M 1985a Clinical characteristics of fibrositis. II. A blinded controlled study using standard psychological tests. Arthritis and Rheumatism 28: 132

Clark S R, Tindall E A, Bennett R A 1985 A double-blind crossover trial of prednisone versus placebo in the treatment of fibrositis. Journal of Rheumatology 12: 980

Dinerman H, Felson D T, Goldenberg D L, Solomon J 1985 Lupus band test and antinuclear antibodies in fibromyalgia. Arthritis and Rheumatism 28: abstract S53

Dinerman H, Goldenberg D L, Felson D T 1986 A prospective evaluation of 118 patients with the fibromyalgia syndrome: prevalence of Raynaud's phenomenon, sicca symptoms, ANA, low complement, and Ig deposition at the dermal–epidermal junction. Journal of Rheumatology 13: 368

Dorigo B, Bartoli V, Grisillo D, Beconi D 1979 Fibrositic myofascial pain in intermittent claudication. Effect of anesthetic block of trigger points on exercise tolerance. Pain 6: 183

Drewes A M, Andreasen A, Jennum P, Nielsen K D 1991 Zopiclone in the treatment of sleep abnormalities in fibromyalgia. Scandinavian Journal of Rheumatology 20: 288

Fassbender H G 1985 Pathology of rheumatic diseases, Springer, New York

Felson D T, Goldenberg D L 1986 The natural history of fibromyalgia. Arthritis and Rheumatism 29: 1522

Fine P G, Milano R, Hare B D 1988 The effects of myofascial trigger point injections are naloxone reversible. Pain 32: 15

Fock S, Mense S 1976 Excitatory effects of 5-hydroxytryptamine, histamine and potassium ions on muscular group IV afferent units: a comparison with bradykinin. Brain Research 105: 459

Fricton J R 1990 Management of myofascial pain syndrome. In: Fricton J R, Awad E A (eds) Advances in pain research and therapy, vol 17. Myofascial pain and fibromyalgia. Raven Press, New York, p 325

Fricton J R, Kroening R 1982 Practical differential diagnosis of chronic craniofacial pain. Oral Surgery 54: 628

Fricton J R, Auvinen M D, Dykstra D, Schiffman E 1985a Myofascial pain syndrome: electromyographic changes associated with local twitch response. Archives of Physical Medicine and Rehabilitation 66: 314

Fricton J R, Kroening R, Haley D, Siegert R 1985b Myofascial pain syndrome of the head and neck: a review of clinical characteristics of 164 patients. Oral Surgery, Oral Medicine, Oral Pathology 60: 615

Furaccioli G, Chirelli L, Scita F et al 1987 EMG-biofeedback training in fibromyalgia syndrome. Journal of Rheumatology 14: 820

Glyn J H 1971 Rheumatic pains: some concepts and hypotheses. Proceedings of the Royal Society of Medicine 64: 354

Goldenberg D L 1987 Fibromyalgia syndrome: an emerging but controversial condition. Journal of the American Medical Association 257: 2782

Goldenberg D L 1989a Fibromyalgia and its relation to chronic fatigue syndrome, viral illness and immune abnormalities. Journal of Rheumatology 16 (suppl 19): 91

Goldenberg D L 1989b Treatment of fibromyalgia syndrome. Rheumatic Diseases Clinics of North America 15: 61

Goldenberg D L, Felson D T, Dinerman H 1986 A randomized, controlled trial of amitriptyline and naproxen in the treatment of patients with fibromyalgia. Arthritis and Rheumatism 29: 1371

Goldenberg D L, Simms R W, Geiger A G, Komaroff A L 1989 Most patients with chronic fatigue syndrome have fibromyalgia. Arthritis and Rheumatism 32: abstract S47

Gowers W R 1904 Lumbago: its lessons and analogues. British Medical Journal 1: 117

Gupta M, Moldofsky H 1986 Dysthymic disorder and rheumatic pain modulation disorder (fibrositis syndrome): a comparison of symptoms and sleep physiology. Canadian Journal of Psychiatry 31: 608

Hamblin T J, Hussain J, Aklsar A N, Tang Y C, Smith J L, Jones D B 1983 Immunological reason for chronic ill health after infectious mononucleosis. British Medical Journal 267: 85

Hameroff S R, Crago B R, Blitt C D, Womble J, Kanel J 1981 Comparison of bupivacaine, etidocaine, and saline for trigger point therapy. Anesthesia and Analgesia 60: 752

Hartz A, Kirchdoerfer E 1987 Undetected fibrositis in primary care practice. Journal of Family Practice 25: 365

Hawley D J, Wolfe F, Cathey M A 1988 Pain, functional disability and psychological status: a 12 month study of severity in fibromyalgia. Journal of Rheumatology 15: 1551

Henriksson K G, Bengtsson A 1982 Muscle biopsy findings of possible diagnostic importance in primary fibromyalgia (fibrositis, myofascial syndrome). Lancet 2: 1395

Horning S J, Levine J D, Miller R A 1982 Clinical and immunologic effects of recombinant leukocyte A interferon in eight patients with advanced cancer. Journal of the American Medical Association 247: 1718

Hudson J I, Hudson M S, Pliner L F, Goldenberg D L, Pope H G Jr 1985 Fibromyalgia and major depressive disorder: a controlled phenomenology and family history study. American Journal of Psychiatry 142: 441

Jacobsen S, Danneskiold-Samsöe B 1987 Isometric and isokinetic muscle strength in patients with fibrositis syndrome. Scandinavian Journal of Rheumatology 16: 61

Jaeger B, Reeves J L 1986 Quantification of changes in myofascial trigger point sensitivity with the pressure algometer following passive stretch. Pain 27: 203

Jaeger B, Skootsky S A 1987 Male and female chronic pain patients categorized by DSM-III psychiatric criteria. Pain 29: 263

Jaeschke R, Adachi J, Guyatt G, Keller J, Wong B 1991 Clinical usefulness of amitriptyline in fibromyalgia: the results of 23 N-of-1 randomized controlled trials. Journal of Rheumatology 18: 447

Kellgren J H 1938 Observations on referred pain arising from muscle. Clinical Science 3: 175

Kellgren J H 1939 On the distribution of pain arising from deep somatic structures with charts of segmental pain areas. Clinical Science 4: 35

Kellgren J H, McGowan A J, Hughes E S R 1944 On deep hyperalgesia and cold pain. Clinical Science 7: 13

Kirmayer L J, Robbins J M, Kapusta M A 1988 Somatization and depression in fibromyalgia syndrome. American Journal of Psychiatry 145: 950

Klimas N G, Salvato F R, Morgan R, Fletcher M A 1990 Immunological abnormalities in the chronic fatigue syndrome. Journal of Clinical Microbiology 26: 1403

Komaroff A L, Goldenberg D L 1989 The chronic fatigue syndrome: definition, current studies and lessons for fibromyalgia research. Journal of Rheumatology 16 (suppl 16): 23

Kruger J M, Karnovsky M L 1987 Sleep and the immune response. New York Academy of Sciences 496: 517

Lamping D L 1985 Assessment in health psychology. Canadian Journal of Psychology 26: 187

Larsson S E, Bengtsson A, Bodegard L, Henriksson K G, Larsson J 1988 Muscle changes in work related chronic myalgia. Acta Orthopaedica Scandinavica 59: 552

Leavitt F, Garron D C 1979 Psychological disturbance and pain report differences in both organic and non-organic low back pain patients. Pain 7: 187

Leavitt F, Katz R S, Golden H E, Glickman P B, Layfer L F 1986 Comparison of pain properties in fibromyalgia patients and rheumatoid arthritis patients. Arthritis and Rheumatism 29: 775

Lewit K 1979 The needle effect in the relief of myofascial pain. Pain 6: 83

Linde A, Hammerstrom L, Smith C I E 1988 IgG subclass deficiency in chronic fatigue syndrome. Lancet 1: 885

Lloyd A R, Wakefield D, Boughton C R, Dwyer J M 1989 Immunological abnormalities in the chronic fatigue syndrome. Medical Journal of Australia 151: 122

Lloyd A, Hickie I, Wakefield D, Boughton C, Dwyer J 1990 A double-blind, placebo controlled trial of intravenous immunoglobulin therapy in patients with chronic fatigue syndrome. American Journal of Medicine 89: 561

Lund N, Bengtsson A, Thorborg P 1986 Muscle tissue oxygen pressures in primary fibromyalgia. Scandinavian Journal of Rheumatology 15: 165

McCain G A 1986 Role of physical fitness training in the fibrositis/fibromyalgia syndrome. American Journal of Medicine 81 (suppl 3A): 73

McCain G A, 1989 Non-medicinal treatments in fibromyalgia. Rheumatic Diseases Clinics of North America 15: 73

McCain G A, Scudds R A 1988 The concept of primary fibromyalgia (fibrositis): clinical value, relation and significance to other musculoskeletal pain syndromes. Pain 33: 273

McCain G A, Bell D A, Mai F, Halliday P D 1988 A controlled study of the effects of a supervised cardiovascular fitness training program on the manifestations of primary fibromyalgia. Arthritis and Rheumatism 31: 1135

McCain G A, Bell D A, Mai F M, Halliday P D 1990 A controlled study of the effects of a supervised cardiovascular fitness program on the manifestations of the primary fibromyalgia syndrome. Arthritis and Rheumatism Primary Care Review 2: 1

Merskey H 1986 International Association for the Study of Pain Subcommittee on taxonomy, chronic pain syndromes and definition of pain terms. Pain (suppl 3): S1

Mielke K, Schulze G, Eger W 1960 Klinische und experimentelle untersichungen zum fibrositissyndrom. Zeitschrift für Rheumatologie 19: 310

Moldofsky H 1982 Rheumatic pain modulation disorder: the relationships between sleep, CNS serotonin and pain. In Critchley M, Friedman A (eds) Headache: physiopathological and clinical concepts. Raven Press, New York, p 51

Moldofsky H 1986 Sleep and musculoskeletal pain. American Journal of Medicine 81 (suppl 3A): 85

Moldofsky H 1989a Sleep and fibrositis syndrome. Rheumatic Diseases Clinics of North America 15: 91

Moldofsky H 1989b Non-restorative sleep and symptoms after a febrile illness in patients with fibrositis and chronic fatigue syndrome. Journal of Rheumatology 16 (suppl 19): 150

Moldofsky H 1989c Sleep-wake mechanisims in fibrositis. Journal of Rheumatology 16 (suppl 19): 47

Moldofsky H, Lue F A 1980 The relationship of alpha and delta EEG freqencies to pain and mood in 'fibrositis' patients treated with chlorpromazine and L-tryptophan. Electroencephalography and Clinical Neurophysiology 50: 71

Moldofsky H, Scarisbrick P 1976 Induction of neurasthenic musculoskeletal pain syndrome by selective sleep stage deprivation. Psychosomatic Medicine 38: 35

Moldofsky H, Warsh J J 1978 Plasma trytophan and musculoskeletal pain in nonarticular rheumatism. Pain 5: 65

Moldofsky H, Scarisbrick P, England R, Smythe H A 1975 Musculoskeletal symptoms and non-REM sleep disturbance in patients with 'fibrositis syndrome' and healthy subjects. Psychosomatic Medicine 37: 341

Molina E, Cecchettin M, Fontana S 1987 Failure of EMG-BF after sham BF training in fibromyalgia. Federation Proceedings 46: 1357

Molony R R, MacPeek D M, Schiffman P L et al 1986 Sleep, sleep apnea and the fibrositis syndrome. Journal of Rheumatology 13: 797

Morag A, Toby M, Ravid Z et al 1982 Increased (2'5')-oligo-A synthetase activity in patients with prolonged illness associated with serological evidence of persistent Epstein–Barr virus infection. Lancet 1: 744

Morgane P J 1981 Serotonin twenty five years later: monoamine theories of sleep. Psychopharmacology Bulletin 17: 13

Muller W 1987 The fibrositis syndrome: diagnosis, differential diagnosis and pathogenesis. Scandinavian Journal of Rheumatology 65: 40

Murdoch J C 1988 Cell mediated immunity in patients with myalgic encephalomyelitis syndrome. New Zealand Medical Journal 101: 511

Nielson W R, Walker C, McCain G A 1992 Cognitive behavioural treatment of fibromyalgia syndrome: preliminary findings. Journal of Rheumatology 19: 98

Payne T C, Leavitt D C, Garron D C et al 1982 Fibrositis and psychologic disturbance. Arthritis and Rheumatism 25: 213

Peter J B, Wallace D J 1988 Abnormal immune regulation in fibromyalgia. Arthritis and Rheumatism 31: abstract S24

Prieto J, Subira M L, Castilla A, Serrano M 1989 Naloxone reversible monocyte dysfunction in patients with chronic fatigue syndrome. Scandinavian Journal of Immunology 30: 13

Quimby L G, Gratwick G M, Whitney C A, Block S R 1989 A randomized trial of cyclobenzaprine for the treatment of fibromyalgia. Journal of Rheumatology 16 (suppl 19): 140

Raft G H, Johnson E W, LaBan M M 1968 The fibrositis syndrome. Archives of Physical Medicine and Rehabilitation 49: 155

Read R, Spickett G, Harvey J 1988 IgG1 subclass deficiency in patients with chronic fatigue syndrome. Lancet 1: 241

Reynolds W J, Moldofsky H, Saskin P, Lue F A 1991 The effects of cyclobenzaprine on sleep physiology and symptoms in patients with fibromyalgia. Journal of Rheumatology 18: 452

Rook J C, Pesch R N, Keeler E C 1981 Chronic pain and the questionable use of the Minnesota Multiphasic Personality Inventory. Archives of Physical Medicine and Rehabilitation 62: 373

Russell I J 1989 Neurohormonal aspects of the fibromyalgia syndrome. Rheumatic Diseases Clinics of North America 15: 149

Russell I J, Vipraio G A, Morgan W M, Bowden C L 1986 Is there a metabolic basis for fibrositis syndrome? American Journal of Medicine 81 (suppl 3A): 50

Russell I J, Bowden C L, Michalek J E, Fletcher E, Hester G A 1987 Imipramine receptor density on platelets of patients with fibrositis syndrome: Correlation with disease severity and response to therapy. Arthritis and Rheumatism 30: abstract S56

Russell I J, Vipraio G A, Michalek J E 1988a Abnormal T cell populations in fibrositis syndrome. Arthritis and Rheumatism 31: abstract S98

Russell I J, Vipraio G A, Tovar Z, Michalek J E, Fletcher E 1988b Abnormal natural killer cell activity in fibrositis syndrome is responsive to in vitro IL-2. Arthritis and Rheumatism 31: abstract S24

Russell I J, Michalek J E, Vipraio G A, Fletcher E M, Wall K 1989 Serum amino acids in fibrositis/fibromyalgia syndrome. Arthritis and Rheumatism 32: abstract S47

Russell I J, Fletcher E M, Michalek J E, McBroom P C, Hester G G 1991 Treatment of primary fibrositis/fibromyalgia syndrome with ibuprofen and alprazolam: A double-blind, placebo-controlled study. Arthritis and Rheumatism 34: 552

Saskin P, Moldofsky H, Lue F A 1986 Sleep and rheumatic pain modulation disorder (fibrositis syndrome). Psychosomatic Medicine 48: 319

Schakel B S, Horne J A 1987 The alpha sleep anomaly and related phenomena. Sleep Restoration 16: 432

Scudds R A, Rollman G B, Harth M, McCain G A 1987 Pain perception and personality measures as discriminators in the classification of fibrositis. Journal of Rheumatology 14: 563

Scudds R A, McCain G A, Rollman G B, Harth M 1989a Improvements in pain responsiveness in patients with fibrositis after successful treatment with amitriptyline. Journal of Rheumatology 16 (suppl 19): 113

Scudds R A, Trachsel L C E, Luckhurst B A, Percy J S 1989b A comparitive study of pain, sleep quality and pain responsiveness in fibrositis and myofascial pain syndrome. Journal of Rheumatology 16 (suppl 19): 120

Simms R W, Goldenberg D L, Felson D T, Mason J H 1988a Tenderness in 75 anatomic sites. Distinguishing fibromyalgia patients from controls. Arthritis and Rheumatism 31: 182

Simms R W, Gunderman J, Howard F, Goldenberg D L 1988b The alpha–delta sleep anomaly in fibromyalgia. Arthritis and Rheumatism 31: 100

Simons D G 1975 Muscle pain syndromes – Part I. American Journal of Physical Medicine 54: 289

Simons D G 1976a Advances in pain research and therapy, vol 1. Raven Press, New York

Simons D G 1976b Muscle pain syndromes – Part II. American Journal of Physical Medicine 55: 15

Simons D G 1988 Myofascial pain syndromes: Where are we? Where are we going? Archives of Physical Medicine and Rehabilitation 69: 207

Simons D 1990 Muscular pain syndromes In: Fricton J R, Awad E A (eds) Advances in pain research and therapy, vol 17. Myofascial pain and fibromyalgia. Raven Press, New York, p 1

Simons D G, Travell J G 1983 Myofascial origins of low back pain. 1. Principles of diagnosis and treatment. Postgraduate Medicine 73: 68

Smythe H A 1984 Problems with the MMPI. Journal of Rheumatology 11: 417

Smythe H A, Moldofsky H 1977 Two contributions to an understanding of the 'fibrositis' syndrome. Bulletin on the Rheumatic Diseases 28: 928

Sola A E, Rodenberger M L, Gettys B B 1955 Incidence of hypersensitive areas in posterior shoulder muscles: a survey of two hundred young adults. American Journal of Physical Medicine 34: 585

Stockman R 1904 The causes, pathology and treatment of chronic rheumatism. Edinburgh Medical Journal 15: 107

Straus S E, Tosato G, Armstrong G et al 1985 Persisting illness and fatigue in adults with evidence of Epstein–Barr virus infection. Annals of Internal Medicine 102: 7

Tavoni A, Vitali C, Bombardieri S 1987 Evaluation of S-adenosyl-methionine in primary fibromyalgia. American Journal of Medicine 83 (suppl 5A): 107

Teasell R W, McCain G A 1992 Clinical spectrum and management of whiplash injuries. In: Tollison C D, Satterthwaite J R (eds) Painful cervical trauma. Williams & Wilkins, Baltimore, p 292

Tosato G, Straus S, Henle W, Pike S E, Blaese R M 1985 Characteristic T cell dysfunction in patients with chronic active Epstein–Barr virus infection (chronic infectious mononucleosis). Journal of Immunology 134: 3082

Travell J G, Simons D G 1983 Myofascial pain and dysfunction. The trigger point manual. Williams & Wilkins, Baltimore

Tunks E, Crook J, Norman G, Kalaher S 1988 Tender points in fibromyalgia. Pain 34: 11

Tunks E, McCain G A, Hart L E et al 1991 The reliability of physical findings in patients with fibromyalgia and myofascial pain syndromes. Arthritis and Rheumatism 34: S190 (abstract)

Tunks E, McCain G A, Hart L E et al 1992 An investigation into the reliability of physical findings in patients with fibromyalgia and myofascial pain syndromes. Arthritis and Rheumatism, in press

Vaeöry H, Helle R, Förre O, Koss E, Terenius L 1988 Elevated CSF levels of substance P and high incidence of Raynaud's phenomenon in patients with fibromyalgia: new features for diagnosis. Pain 32: 21

Valen P A, Flory W, Powell M, Wortman R 1988 Forearm ischemic exercise testing and plasma ATP degredation products in primary fibromyalgia. Arthritis and Rheumatism 31: abstract C115

Wallace D J, Margolin K, Waller P 1988 Fibromyalgia and interleukin-2 therapy for malignancy. Annals of Internal Medicine 108: 909

Wallace D J, Bowman R L, Wormsley S B, Peter J B 1989 Cytokines and immune regulation in patients with fibrositis (letter). Arthritis and Rheumatism 32: 1334

Ware J C, Russell J, Campos E 1986 Alpha intrusions into the sleep of depressed and fibromyalgia syndrome (fibrositis) patients. Sleep Research 15: 210

Wolfe F 1986 The clinical syndrome of fibrositis. American Journal of Medicine 81: 7

Wolfe F 1989 Fibromyalgia: the clinical syndrome. Rheumatic Diseases Clinics of North America 15: 1

Wolfe F, Cathey M A 1983 Prevalence of primary and secondary fibrositis. Journal of Rheumatology 10: 965

Wolfe F, Cathey M A, Kleinheksel S M 1984a Fibrositis (fibromyalgia) in rheumatoid arthritis. Journal of Rheumatology 11: 814

Wolfe F, Cathey M A, Kleinheksel S M et al 1984b Psychological status in primary fibrositis and fibrositis associated with rheumatoid arthritis. Journal of Rheumatology 11: 500

Wolfe F, Hawley D J, Cathey M A, Caro X, Russell I J 1985 Fibrositis: symptom frequency and criteria for diagnosis. An evaluation of 291 rheumatic disease patients and 598 normal individuals. Journal of Rheumatology 12: 1159

Wolfe F, Smythe H A, Yunus M B et al 1990 The American College of Rheumatology 1990 criteria for the classification of fibromyalgia. Report of the Multicenter Criteria Committee. Arthritis and Rheumatism 33: 160

Wolfe F, Simons D G, Fricton J R et al 1992 The fibromyalgia and myofascial pain syndromes: a preliminary study of tender points and trigger points in persons with fibromyalgia, myofascial pain syndrome and no disease. Journal of Rheumatology, in press

Wysenbeek A J, Nor F, Lurie T, Weinburger A 1985 Imipramine for the treatment of fibrositis: a therapeutic trial. Annals of Rheumatic Diseases 44: 752

Yunus M B, Kalyan-Raman V P 1989 Muscle biopsy findings in primary fibromyalgia and other forms of nonarticular rheumatism. Rheumatic Diseases Clinics of North America 15: 115

Yunus M B, Masi A T, Calabro J J, Miller K A, Feigenbaum S L 1981 Primary fibromyalgia (fibrositis): clinical study of 50 patients with matched normal controls. Seminars in Arthritis and Rheumatism 11: 151

Yunus M B, Kalyan-Raman V P, Kalyan-Raman K, Masi A T 1986 Pathologic changes in muscle in primary fibromyalgia syndrome. American Journal of Medicine 81 (suppl 3A): 38

Yunus M B, Masi A T, Aldag J C 1989 A controlled study of primary fibromyalgia syndrome: clinical features and association with other functional syndromes. Journal of Rheumatology 16(suppl 19): 62

27. Headache

Jean Schoenen and Alain Maertens de Noordhout

INTRODUCTION

Headache is the most common pain syndrome. It is also the most frequent symptom in neurology, where it may be a disease in itself or indicate an underlying local or systemic disease. Many excellent textbooks on headache have been published in recent years (see bibliography). We felt therefore that a comprehensive synthesis would be more useful to the reader than detailed descriptions of the various headache types. We decided to follow the new headache classification (Cephalalgia 1988), which was elaborated by a Committee of the International Headache Society (IHS) chaired by J Olesen, and to emphasise tables rather than phrases. For each of the most common types of headache this chapter will summarise present knowledge on diagnosis, epidemiology, pathogenesis and therapy.

It is well known that the brain parenchyma itself is insensitive to pain. Nociceptive input can be generated from cranial sinuses and veins, proximal parts of cerebral arteries, dura mater mainly in the vicinity of the large vessels, cranial nerves and upper cervical roots, as well as from extracranial structures. Headache must be due to excessive nociceptive input from these intra- or extracranial sites, a disturbed central control of these inputs or a combination of both. Many classifications of headache have been proposed. One can schematically distinguish primary and secondary headaches. Primary (or idiopathic) headaches are autonomous diseases, or syndromes, in which there is a transient or permanent functional disorder without a structural lesion. These are by far the most frequent headache types, comprising migraine, tension headache and cluster headache. Secondary (or symptomatic) headaches are due to a local organic lesion or to a systemic disease. In several headache types, however, such a simplistic distinction is not applicable.

The IHS Headache Classification is hierarchically constructed and based on operational diagnostic criteria for all headache disorders. The hierarchical system coding with up to four digits makes it possible to use the classification at different levels of sophistication. Table 27.1 represents the headings of the various headache groups and subgroups. Codes 1–4 comprise most of the so-called primary headaches. Although this classification grades headaches and not patients, it represents a major advance in headache research because it offers a common denominator allowing for better comparison of clinical data between centres. Several large field trials have tested the IHS classification and found excellent scores for sensitivity, specificity and interrater reproducibility. Nonetheless a modified version of the classification is expected in the near future with improved diagnostic criteria for some headache types. Because of space limitations, we will cover only the primary and the most frequent secondary headaches, leaving aside some very common but generally obvious causes of pain in head or face, such as systemic infections (code 9), metabolic disorders (code 10), eye disorders (code 11.3) or nose and sinus diseases (code 11.5).

1. MIGRAINE

Diagnosis and clinical features

Migraine is a multifaceted disorder, of which the head pain is only one component. It is an autonomous disease, but in some instances it may occur for the first time in close temporal relation to one of the disorders listed in groups 5–11 of Table 27.1, e.g. to head trauma (Weiss et al 1991). Migraine is characterised by attacks which are separated by symptom-free intervals. In 10–15% of patients premonitory symptoms (or prodromes) may precede the migraine attack by hours or by a day or two (Blau 1980). These consist of symptoms which are unspecific, but often reproducible in a given patient such as sudden mood changes, repetitive yawning or craving for special foods. At the other end of the spectrum, the migraine attack can be followed by so-called 'postsyndromes', such as fatigue. The clinical diagnosis of migraine is based on the characteristics of the attack. The

Table 27.1 Classification and diagnostic criteria for headache disorders, cranial neuralgias and facial pain (Cephalalgia 1988)

1. Migraine
- 1.1 Migraine without aura
- 1.2 Migraine with aura
  - 1.2.1 Migraine with typical aura
  - 1.2.2 Migraine with prolonged aura
  - 1.2.3 Familial hemiplegic migraine
  - 1.2.4 Basilar migraine
  - 1.2.5 Migraine aura without headache
  - 1.2.6 Migraine with acute onset aura
- 1.3 Ophthalmoplegic migraine
- 1.4 Retinal migraine
- 1.5 Childhood periodic syndromes that may be precursors to or associated with migraine
  - 1.5.1 Benign paroxysmal vertigo of childhood
  - 1.5.2 Alternating hemiplegia of childhood
- 1.6 Complications of migraine
  - 1.6.1 Status migrainosus
  - 1.6.2 Migrainous infarction
- 1.7 Migrainous disorder not fulfilling above criteria

2. Tension-type headache
- 2.1 Episodic tension-type headache
  - 2.1.1 Episodic tension-type headache associated with disorder of pericranial muscles
  - 2.1.2 Episodic tension-type headache unassociated with disorder of pericranial muscles
- 2.2 Chronic tension-type headache
  - 2.2.1 Chronic tension type headache associated with disorder of pericranial muscles
  - 2.2.2 Chronic tension-type headache unassociated with disorder of pericranial muscles
- 2.3 Headache of the tension type not fulfilling above criteria

3. Cluster headache and chronic paroxysmal hemicrania
- 3.1 Cluster headache
  - 3.1.1 Cluster headache periodicity undetermined
  - 3.1.2 Episodic cluster headache
  - 3.1.3 Chronic cluster headache
    - 3.1.3.1 Unremitting from onset
    - 3.1.3.2 Evolved from episodic
- 3.2 Chronic paroxysmal hemicrania
- 3.3 Cluster headache-like disorder not fulfilling above criteria

4. Misellaneous headaches unassociated with structural lesion
- 4.1 Idiopathic stabbing headache
- 4.2 External compression headache
- 4.3 Cold stimulus headache
  - 4.3.1 External application of a cold stimulus
  - 4.3.2 Ingestion of a cold stimulus
- 4.4 Benign cough headache
- 4.5 Benign exertional headache
- 4.6 Headache associated with sexual activity
  - 4.6.1 Dull type
  - 4.6.2 Explosive type
  - 4.6.3 Postural type

5. Headache associated with head trauma
- 5.1 Acute posttraumatic headache
  - 5.1.1 With significant head trauma and/or confirmatory signs
  - 5.1.2 With minor head trauma and no confirmatory signs
- 5.2 Chronic posttraumatic headache
  - 5.2.1 With significant head trauma and/or confirmatory signs
  - 5.2.2 With minor head trauma and no confirmatory signs

6. Headache associated with vascular disorders
- 6.1 Acute ischaemic cerebrovascular disease
  - 6.1.1 Transient ischaemic attack (TIA)
  - 6.1.2 Thromboembolic stroke
- 6.2 Intracranial haematoma
  - 6.2.1 Intracerebral haematoma
  - 6.2.2 Subdural haematoma
  - 6.2.3 Epidural haematoma
- 6.3 Subarachnoid haemorrhage
- 6.4 Unruptured vascular malformation
  - 6.4.1 Arteriovenous malformation
  - 6.4.2 Saccular aneurysm
- 6.5 Arteritis
  - 6.5.1 Giant cell arteritis
  - 6.5.2 Other systemic arteritides
  - 6.5.3 Primary intracranial arteritis
- 6.6 Carotid or vertebral artery pain
  - 6.6.1 Carotid or vertebral dissection
  - 6.6.2 Carotidynia (idiopathic)
  - 6.6.3 Postendarterectomy headache
- 6.7 Venous thrombosis
- 6.8 Arterial hypertension
  - 6.8.1 Acute pressor response to exogenous agent
  - 6.8.2 Phaeochromocytoma
  - 6.8.3 Malignant (accelerated) hypertension
  - 6.8.4 Preeclampsia and eclampsia
- 6.9 Headache associated with other vascular disorder

7. Headache associated with nonvascular intracranial disorder
- 7.1 High cerebrospinal fluid pressure
  - 7.1.1 Benign intracranial hypertension
  - 7.1.2 High pressure hydrocephalus
- 7.2 Low cerebrospinal fluid pressure
  - 7.2.1 Postlumbar puncture headache
  - 7.2.2 Cerebrospinal fluid fistula headache
- 7.3 Intracranial infection
- 7.4 Intracranial sarcoidosis and other noninfectious inflammatory diseases
- 7.5 Headache related to intrathecal injections
  - 7.5.1 Direct effect
  - 7.5.2 Due to chemical meningitis
- 7.6 Intracranial neoplasm
- 7.7 Headache associated with other intracranial disorder

8. Headache associated with substances or their withdrawal
- 8.1 Headache induced by acute substance use or exposure
  - 8.1.1 Nitrate/nitrite-induced headache
  - 8.1.2 Monosodium glutamate-induced headache
  - 8.1.3 Carbon monoxide-induced headache
  - 8.1.4 Alcohol-induced headache
  - 8.1.5 Other substances
- 8.2 Headache induced by chronic substance use or exposure
  - 8.2.1 Ergotamine-induced headache
  - 8.2.2 Analgesic abuse headache
  - 8.2.3 Other substances
- 8.3 Headache from substance withdrawal (acute use)
  - 8.3.1 Alcohol withdrawal headache (hangover)
  - 8.3.2 Other substances
- 8.4 Headache from substance withdrawal (chronic use)
  - 8.4.1 Ergotamine withdrawal headache
  - 8.4.2 Caffeine withdrawal headache
  - 8.4.3 Narcotics abstinence headache
  - 8.4.4 Other substances
- 8.5 Headache associated with substances but with uncertain mechanism
  - 8.5.1 Birth control pills or oestrogens
  - 8.5.2 Other substances

9. Headache associated with noncephalic infection
- 9.1 Viral infection

Table 27.1 (*contd*)

- 9.1.1 Focal noncephalic
- 9.1.2 Systemic
- 9.2 Bacterial infection
  - 9.2.1 Focal noncephalic
  - 9.2.2 Systemic (septicaemia)
- 9.3 Headache related to other infection

10. Headache associated with metabolic disorders
- 10.1 Hypoxia
  - 10.1.1 High altitude headache
  - 10.1.2 Hypoxic headache
  - 10.1.3 Sleep apnoea headache
- 10.2 Hypercapnia
- 10.3 Mixed hypoxia and hypercapnia
- 10.4 Hypoglycaemia
- 10.5 Dialysis
- 10.6 Headache related to other metabolic abnormality

11. Headache or facial pain associated with disorder of cranium, neck, eyes, ears, nose, sinuses, teeth, mouth or other facial or cranial structures
- 11.1 Cranial bone
- 11.2 Neck
  - 11.2.1 Cervical spine
  - 11.2.2 Retropharyngeal tendinitis
- 11.3 Eyes
  - 11.3.1 Acute glaucoma
  - 11.3.2 Refractive errors
  - 11.3.3 Heterophoria or heterotropia
- 11.4 Ears
- 11.5 Nose and sinuses
  - 11.5.1 Acute sinus headache
  - 11.5.2 Other diseases of nose or sinuses
- 11.6 Teeth, jaws and related structures
- 11.7 Temporomandibular joint disease

12. Cranial neuralgias, nerve trunk pain and deafferentation pain
- 12.1 Persistent (in contrast to tic-like) pain of cranial nerve origin
  - 12.1.1 Compression or distortion of cranial nerves and second or third cervical roots
  - 12.1.2 Demyelinisation of cranial nerves
    - 12.1.2.1 Optic neuritis (retrobulbar neuritis)
  - 12.1.3 Infarction of cranial nerves
    - 12.1.3.1 Diabetic neuritis
  - 12.1.4 Inflammation of cranial nerves
    - 12.1.4.1 Herpes zoster
    - 12.1.4.2 Chronic postherpetic neuralgia
  - 12.1.5 Tolosa–Hunt syndrome
  - 12.1.6 Neck-tongue syndrome
  - 12.1.7 Other causes of persistent pain of cranial nerve origin
- 12.2 Trigeminal neuralgia
  - 12.2.1 Idiopathic trigeminal neuralgia
  - 12.2.2 Symptomatic trigeminal neuralgia
    - 12.2.2.1 Compression of trigeminal root or ganglion
    - 12.2.2.2 Central lesions
- 12.3 Glossopharyngeal neuralgia
  - 12.3.1 Idiopathic glossopharyngeal neuralgia
  - 12.3.2 Symptomatic glossopharyngeal neuralgia
- 12.4 Nervus intermedius neuralgia
- 12.5 Superior laryngeal neuralgia
- 12.6 Occipital neuralgia
- 12.7 Central causes of head and facial pain other than tic douloureux
  - 12.7.1 Anaesthesia dolorosa
  - 12.7.2 Thalamic pain
- 12.8 Facial pain not fulfilling criteria in groups 11 or 12

13. Headache, nonclassifiable

diagnostic criteria for *migraine without aura* (code 1.1) (formerly common migraine) are illustrated in Table 27.2. In *migraine with aura* (code 1.2) the headache phase is immediately preceded by focal neurological symptoms (Table 27.3).

Visual disturbances are the most common aura symptoms, occurring in 90% of patients. Aura symptoms of sensory, motor or speech disturbances seldom occur without preexisting visual symptoms (Rasmussen & Olesen 1992).

In *migraine with prolonged aura* (code 1.2.2) all the criteria for migraine with typical aura (code 1.2.1) are fulfilled but at least one symptom lasts more than 60 min and less than a week. Compared to migraine without aura, migraine with aura is characterised on average by headache of lower intensity and shorter duration. The headache may even be completely absent (code 1.2.5). Many patients have both attacks of migraine with and migraine without aura. In so-called 'early morning' migraine, it is impossible to ascertain whether the attack was preceded by an aura or not.

In *basilar migraine* (code 1.2.4) two or more aura symptoms are of the following types: visual symptoms in both the temporal and nasal fields of both eyes, dysarthria, vertigo, tinnitus, decreased hearing, double vision, ataxia, bilateral paraesthesias, bilateral pareses, decreased level of consciousness. The differential diagnosis between *migraine with acute onset aura* (code 1.2.6) and thromboembolic transient ischaemic attacks may be difficult.

In children below the age of 12 years, migraine attacks often last less than 4 h and the duration criterion of

Table 27.2 Migraine without aura (code 1.1): diagnostic criteria

A. At least five attacks fulfilling criteria B–D

B. Headache attacks lasting 4–72 hours (untreated or unsuccessfully treated)

C. Headache has at least two of the following characteristics:
1. Unilateral location
2. Pulsating quality
3. Moderate or severe intensity (inhibits or prohibits daily activities)
4. Aggravation by walking stairs or similar routine physical activity

D. During headache at least one of the following:
1. Nausea and/or vomiting
2. Photophobia and phonophobia

E. At least one of the following:
1. History and physical and neurological examinations do not suggest one of the disorders listed in groups 5–11
2. History, and/or physical and/or neurological examinations do suggest such disorder, but it is ruled out by appropriate investigations
3. Such disorder is present, but migraine attacks do not occur for the first time in close temporal relation to the disorder

Table 27.3 Migraine with aura (code 1.2): diagnostic criteria

A. At least two attacks fulfilling criterion B

B. At least three of the following four characteristics:
1. One or more fully reversible aura symptoms indicating focal cerebral cortical and/or brainstem dysfunction
2. At least one aura symptom develops gradually over more than 4 min or two or more symptoms occur in succession
3. No aura symptom lasts more than 60 min. If more than one aura symptom is present, accepted duration is proportionally increased
4. Headache follows aura with a free interval of less than 60 min. (It may also begin before or simultaneously with the aura.)

C. As criterion E in migraine without aura (Table 27.2)

Table 27.2 does not apply. It remains controversial whether *childhood periodic syndromes* (code 1.5), such as cyclical vomiting, abdominal pains or benign vertigo, are precursors of adulthood migraine and of similar pathophysiology. It has been reported in some studies that childhood somnambulism is frequently found in the history of adult migraineurs (Pradalier et al 1987).

The two major complications of migraine are *status migrainosus* (code 1.6.1) and *migrainous infarction* (code 1.6.2). In the former the headache lasts more than 72 h without interruption, despite treatment, or headache-free intervals do not exceed 4 h. To qualify for migrainous infarction, a neurological deficit has to occur during a migraine attack that is typical of those previously experienced by a patient, to last more than 7 days and/or to be associated with ischaemic infarction in the relevant area on neuroimaging techniques. Moreover, other causes of infarction have to be ruled out by appropriate investigations.

Epidemiology

The results of epidemiological studies performed in various countries are remarkably consistent. The prevalence of migraine is around 15% whatever the study design: 15% in a cross-sectional epidemiological survey of the Danish population aged between 25 and 64 years, and diagnosed following to a structured interview as well as a neurological examination (Rasmussen et al 1991); 12% in a nationwide survey performed by mailed questionnaire in a representative sample of French residents aged 15 years or older (Henry et al 1992) and 23.3% in a study using a self-administered questionnaire sent to a sample of 15 000 US households (Stewart et al 1992). In Third World countries, prevalence of migraine is similar to that found in western Europe and North America. Migraine presents therefore with a uniform worldwide distribution.

Migraine without aura is almost twice as frequent as migraine with aura in population-based studies. In many patients both types of attack may coexist. Female preponderance is a characteristic feature of migraine, but also of other nonsymptomatic headache. Male–female ratios vary between studies. A ratio of 1:7 has been reported in migraine without aura and a ratio of 1:2 in migraine with aura (Rasmussen & Olesen 1992). Although the prevalence of migraine is as high in children as in adults, boys and girls are affected in the same proportions (Bille 1962; Chu & Shinnar 1991). This suggest that migraine attacks may disappear in boys after puberty.

More than 50% of migraineurs have less than two attacks per month. The most common precipitating (or trigger) factors of attacks are mental stress, menstruation and alcohol (Amery & Vandenbergh 1987). It remains controversial whether other dietary factors can consistently precipitate attacks in certain patients. The majority of female migraineurs report occurrence of attacks in the perimenstrual period. In less than 10% however attacks occur exclusively at this stage of the ovarian cycle and this corresponds to ‘menstrual migraine’ (MacGregor et al 1990).

Pathophysiology

The exact pathogenesis of migraine is still unknown. Many theories have been elaborated, but none can account for all the clinical features or for all the pathophysiological aspects demonstrated in recent years. The pendulum has been swinging between vascular (Wolff 1963) and neurogenic (Sicuteri 1986) theories, with brief peripheral blood excursions (Hannington et al 1981). In recent years, however, a general consensus has been emerging that in migraine both vascular and neural components are relevant and most probably interrelated (Lance et al 1983; Welch 1987; Olesen 1991).

Tables 27.4 and 27.5 list some recent pathophysiological data obtained in migraineurs during attacks and in headache-free intervals with modern biochemical, neurophysiological, blood flow and metabolic methods.

The trigeminovascular system. Experimental studies in animals suggest that the trigeminovascular system is the final common pathway where migraine headache is generated (Moskowitz 1984). Activation of trigeminal sensory fibres surrounding large cerebral or dural vessels, via antidromic impulses or an axon reflex, produces local release of neuropeptides leading to neurogenic inflammation and vasodilatation. The latter are accompanied by platelet as well as mast cell activation and result in sensitisation and stimulation of trigeminal nociceptive fibres. Pain is referred to the peripheral territory of the first division of the trigeminal nerve and the superior cervical roots because of convergence of visceral and somatic afferents in the brain stem. The elevation of neuropeptides such as calcitonin gene-related peptide (CGRP) in the external jugular vein blood during migraine attacks (Goadsby et al 1989) could support the trigeminovascular theory, but this could be common to all so-called vascular

Table 27.4 Migraine: pathophysiology of the attack

Data	Methods	Authors	Hypotheses
Spreading oligaemia by hyperaemia (migraine with aura)	SPECT	Olesen et al 1990	Spreading followed depression
Severe focal oligaemia (migraine with aura)	SPECT	Olesen et al 1987	Focal ischaemia
Hyperaemia (migraine without aura)	SPECT	Bès et al 1990	Vasodilatation
DC shifts, long-lasting depressions (migraine with and ? without aura)	Magneto -EEG	Barkley et al 1990	Spreading depression
Unilateral depression of α power (migraine with and without aura)	Topographic EEG mapping	Schoenen et al 1987a, 1987b	Cerebral dysfunction initiates both types of migraine
Reduction of organic phosphates, normal pH (migraine with aura)	NMR spectroscopy	Welch et al 1989	Not in favour of ischaemia
Reduction of flow velocity and increased pulsatility in middle cerebral artery (migraine without aura)	Transcranial doppler	Thie et al 1990 Friberg et al 1991 Caekebeke et al 1992	Vasodilatation of large calibre cerebral arteries (reversed by sumatriptan)
Increase of CGRP in external jugular vein	Radioimmunoassay system, as in	Goadsby et al 1987, 1991	Neurogenic inflammation in the trigeminovascular animal model (Moskowitz 1991), reversed by sumatriptan
5-HT decreased in platelets, increased in plasma	Biochemistry	Anthony & Lance 1975 Ferrari et al 1989	Increased release from platelets, or reduced turnover of 5-HT

CGRP = calcitonin gene-related peptide; SPECT = single photon emission computerized tomography.

Table 27.5 Migraine: interictal pathophysiology

Data	Methods	Authors	Hypotheses
Decreased cerebral magnesium	NMR spectroscopy	Ramadan et al 1989	Hypersensitivity of NMDA receptors favouring spreading depression
Increased excitatory amino acids in plasma and platelets	HPLC	Ferrari et al 1990 D'Andrea et al 1991	
Disturbed energy metabolism in brain and muscle	NMR spectroscopy	Barbiroli et al 1992	Mitochondrial abnormality reducing energy reserve
Increased visual evoked potential	Neurophysiology	Kennard et al 1978 Diener et al 1989	Cortical hyperexcitability
Increased contingent negative variation normalised by beta-blockade (migraine without aura)	Neurophysiology	Schoenen et al 1985, 1986	Hyperreactivity of central catecholamine pathways
Plasma noradrenaline and dopamine-β-hydroxylase increased or decreased	Biochemistry	Schoenen & Maertens (1988)	Sympathetic instability, stress sensitivity
5-HT increased in platelets, decreased in plasma	Biochemistry	Anthony & Lance 1975 D'Andrea et al 1989 Ferrari et al 1989	Reduced platelet release or increased systemic 5-HT turnover

HPLC = high performance liquid chromatography; NMDA = N-methyl-D-aspartate

headaches, since it is also found in cluster headache. Moreover, it has been demonstrated that drugs that are highly effective in treating migraine (and cluster headache) attacks, such as ergot alkaloids or sumatriptan, can block the neurogenic plasma extravasation into the dura of the rat produced by electrical stimulation of the trigeminal ganglia. It remains to be determined whether these drugs exert their therapeutic action through an effect on 5-HT_1 receptors, located presynaptically on perivascular trigeminal peptidergic fibres, as suggested by laboratory experiments (Moskowitz 1991; Buzzi & Moskowitz 1992) and some clinical data (Goadsby et al 1990), or via a direct effect on vessels, as suggested by pharmacology (Humphrey 1991) and some human studies using the transcranial doppler (Friberg et al 1991, Caekebeke et al 1992). It must be pointed out that the trigeminal vascular system is the final common pathway not only for migraine, but for many other types of presumably vascular head pain, including the headaches of vasculitis, arteriovenous malformation, ischaemic cerebrovascular disease, subarachnoid haemorrhage, posttraumatic vascular headaches and possibly analgesic withdrawal headaches.

Cerebral blood flow. Changes in cerebral blood flow depend on the pattern of the attack and on the timing of the recording. The most convincing cerebral blood flow changes have been reported in migraine with aura (Olesen 1992). In the early phase of the attack a focal hypoperfusion can be recorded over the cortical area which is responsible for the aura symptoms. This hypoperfusion may precede and outlast the aura symptoms. The degree varies between patients and attacks, but probably reaches the threshold for ischaemia in some patients. Spreading of hypoperfusion from posterior to more anterior parts of the hemisphere has been observed with the intracarotid regional cerebral blood flow (rCBF) method. In the later stages of the attack, cerebral hyperperfusion may appear, but this is not chronologically related to the headache. Rapid oscillations between hypo- and hyperperfusion have been found in some patients. In migraine without aura some investigators have reported normal cerebal blood flow (Olesen 1992), while others have found diffuse or focal hyperperfusion not related to headache intensity or localisation (Bès & Fabre 1992).

Cortical spreading depression. There is indirect evidence that migraine aura is the clinical manifestation of cortical spreading depression rather than of ischaemia (Lauritzen 1992). Indeed, the clinical aura symptoms progress at a pace (Lashley 1941) similar to that of the wave of cortical spreading depression in the animal brain (Leão 1944; Leão & Morrison 1945) and spreading depression can produce cerebral blood flow changes similar to those observed during migraine with aura (Olesen et al 1981). Spreading depression however, although easily elicited in animals, has been recorded only in the hippocampus and caudate nucleus of man (Bures et al 1974). It remains to be demonstrated whether the DC shifts and activity reductions observed with magneto-electroencephalography (Barkley et al 1990), or the unilateral reductions of alpha power shown with topographical EEG mapping during attacks of migraine with or without aura (Schoenen et al 1987a, 1987b), may be related to the phenomenon of cortical spreading depression.

Abnormal functioning of the migrainous brain. During the headache-free interval, an abnormal functioning of the migrainous brain can be demonstrated by neurophysiological and metabolic studies. Neurophysiological methods indicate hyperactivity or hyperreactivity in several neural pathways (Schoenen 1992). For instance, visual and event-related potentials such as contingent negative variation, are increased in migraine and tend to normalise after treatment with beta-blockers. Metabolic studies using nuclear magnetic resonance spectroscopy have suggested reduction of magnesium (Ramadan et al 1989) and a low phosphorylation potential (Barbiroli et al 1992) in the brain of patients affected by migraine with aura. The former, which might be related to the decrease of erythrocyte magnesium reported in both types of migraine (Schoenen et al 1991a), could increase the excitability of N-methyl-D-aspartate (NMDA) receptors; the latter could be due to a mitochondrial abnormality, and lessen the ability of the migrainous brain to handle energy demands. It remains to be demonstrated whether the increased incidence in migraine with aura of patchy white matter lesions on magnetic resonance imaging (Ferbert et al 1991) is the result of repetitive hypoxic-ischaemic phenomena.

Peripheral blood. Furthermore, various modifications of neurotransmitters (Ferrari 1992) or platelets (Ollat & Gurruchaga 1992) in the peripheral blood have been described in migraine between and during attacks. It is still not clear whether these peripheral changes contribute to the pathophysiology of migraine or are just an epiphenomenon of the central migrainous process.

In summary, more scientific data are clearly needed before the pathophysiological pieces of the migraine patchwork can be assembled into a comprehensive and definite pathogenetic model. In the meantime, migraine, both with and without aura, can be regarded as a constitutional, perhaps genetically determined, hypersensitivity of the brain and the trigeminovascular system to internal or external stimuli (Welch 1987; Edmeads 1992; Lance 1992).

Treatment

Any therapeutic regimen in migraine has to be tailored to the individual patient, taking into account his demands, disability, previous medical history and psychosocial profile. Some general therapeutic rules can nonetheless be defined. Therapy can be divided into acute treatment of the attack and prophylactic treatment. Figures 27.1 and 27.2 are tentative algorithms which may guide the decision process in treating migraine patients.

Whenever possible, precipitating factors should be avoided or treated. Strategies for coping with stress, or dietary measures, can be advised. Attacks occurring during the perimenstrual period can sometimes be prevented by treatment with transdermal oestradiol and/or a nonsteroïdal antiinflammatory drug (NSAID) such as naproxen.

Although ergotamine tartrate is the reference drug for acute migraine treatment, many migraine attacks can be effectively treated with high doses of aspirin, paracetamol or NSAIDs. Because of the gastrointestinal symptoms that accompany the attack, all these drugs are more effective when administered by the rectal or parenteral route and usually need to be associated with an antiemetic such as metoclopramide or domperidone. At present, one of the most effective drugs for interrupting a migraine attack is the 5-HT_1D agonist sumatriptan. Its major advantages are its rapid and high efficacy with acceptable side-effects; its major disadvantage is its high cost. All the acute treatments of migraine are more effective if combined with a short resting period or a nap.

Prophylactic antimigraine treatment should be considered when attacks are frequent and/or disabling. On average the long-term efficacy of prophylactic treatments does not exceed 60–70%. Drugs effective for preventing migraine attacks include: beta-blockers devoid of intrinsic sympathomimetic activity (Massiou & Bousser 1992); calcium channel blockers, especially flunarizine (Montastruc & Senard 1992); serotonin antagonists such as methysergide or pizotifen (Ollat 1992), and sodium

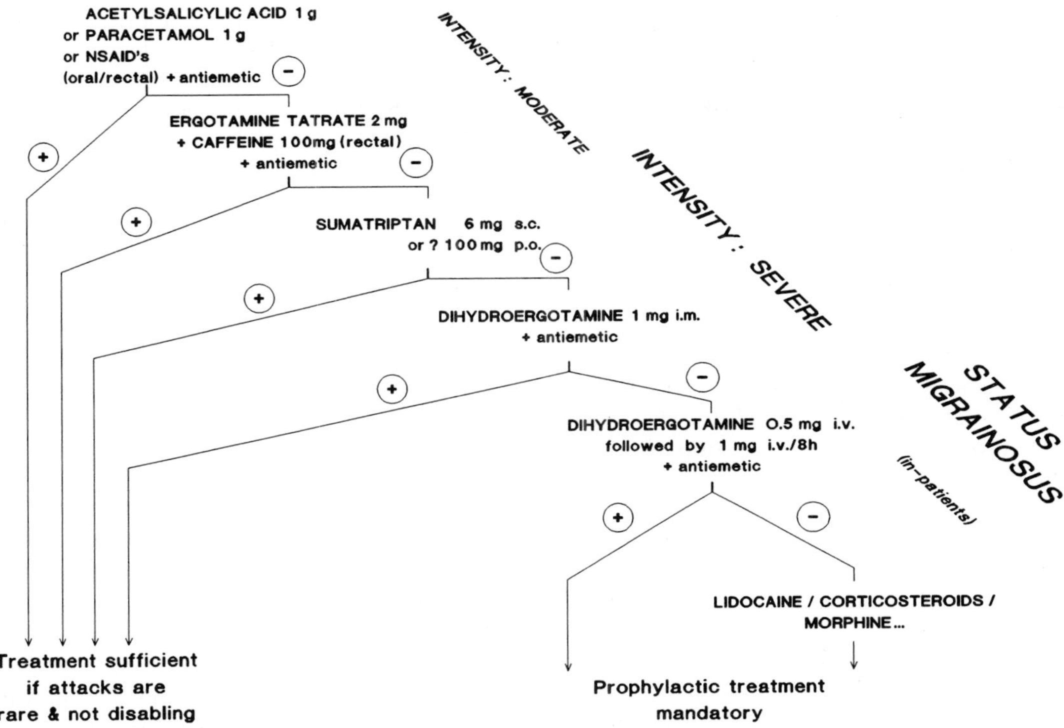

Fig. 27.1 An algorithm for acute migraine treatment. Circles with plus signs, ⊕, – disappearance of migraine within 2 h and absence of unpleasant side-effects.

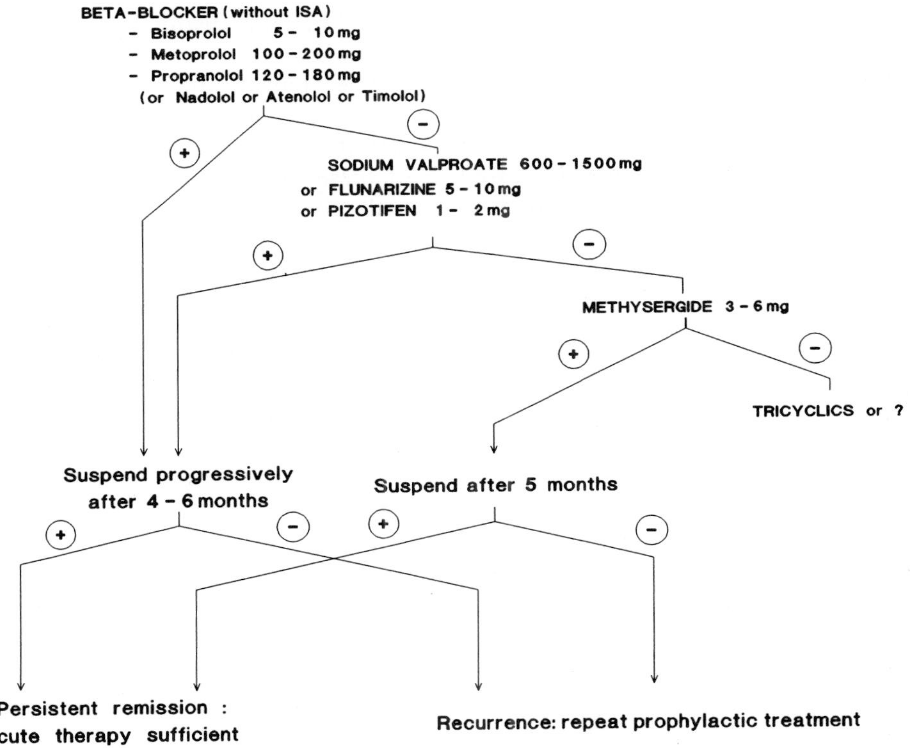

Fig. 27.2 An algorithm for prophylactic migraine treatment. Circles with plus signs, ⊕, – reduction by at least 50% of attack frequency and intensity, without unpleasant side-effects.

valproate (Hering & Kuritzky 1992). In some patients tricyclics may be useful as an adjuvant therapy.

Among the nondrug treatments of migraine, behavioural therapies, such as relaxation and biofeedback, have proved their efficacy in many studies (Holroyd et al 1984) and acupuncture has been found effective in a few reports.

2. TENSION-TYPE HEADACHE

Diagnosis and clinical features

The headaches formerly described as 'muscle contraction', 'psychogenic', 'stress' or 'essential' are classified in this group. It is thus a heterogeneous group which can appear controversial and may undergo modifications in the future. The term 'tension-type' has been chosen in order to offer a new heading, underlining the uncertainties about the precise pathogenesis, but indicating nevertheless that some kind of mental or muscular tension may play a causative role.

The diagnostic criteria of *episodic tension-type headache* (code 2.1) are listed in Table 27.6. In *chronic tension-type headache* (code 2.2) the average headache frequency is equal to, or greater than, 15 days per month or 180 days per year. The characteristics of the headache are similar to that of episodic tension-type headache except that nausea can be accepted as an isolated associated symptom.

The third digit code number reflects the existence of two kinds of tension-type headache: associated and unassociated with disorder of the pericranial muscles. Such a disorder is supposed to be present when pericranial muscles are excessively tender by manual palpation or pressure algometer measurements or when increased electromyographic (EMG) levels can be recorded in pericranial muscles at rest or during physiological tests. Although pericranial tenderness and pericranial muscle activity vary greatly between patients, there is at present no conclusive evidence that patients with higher levels of these differ from those with normal findings in clinical presentation, pathogenesis of pain or response to therapy (Schoenen et al 1991b).

The single episode of tension-type headache is the least distinct of all headache types since clinical diagnosis is chiefly based on negative features, e.g the absence of symptoms that characterize other idiopathic or symptomatic headache. These include the absence of unilaterality, pulsatility, aggravation by physical activity and associated symptoms. Moreover, as demonstrated in recent population-based studies (Rasmussen et al 1991), a substantial proportion of patients may present with atypical symptoms such as unilateral pain (10%), aggravation by routine activity (27.7%), anorexia (18.2%), photophobia (10.6%) or nausea (4.2%). Episodic tension-type headache can therefore be difficult to distinguish from migraine without aura (code 1.1) or from organic brain disease (see below). The diagnosis of chronic tension-type headache is straightforward in most cases. In addition, it can be confirmed by a neurophysiological abnormality, i.e. reduction or abolition of the late exteroceptive suppression period of temporalis muscle. This neurophysiological test has a very high sensitivity and specificity in distinguishing chronic tension-type headache from migraine (Schoenen et al 1987c) (Table 27.7), but this distinction is rarely a problem in clinical practice.

The fourth digit code number for tension-type headache gives an indication of the most probable causative or precipitating factors. In many patients several of these factors may be associated, as described in the pathophysiology section.

Table 27.6 Episodic tension-type headache (code 2.1): diagnostic criteria

A. At least 10 previous headache episodes fulfilling criteria B–D listed below. Number of days with such headache < 180/year (< 15/month)

B. Headache lasting from 30 min to 7 days

C. At least two of the following pain characteristics:
   1. Pressing/tightening (nonpulsating) quality
   2. Mild or moderate intensity (may inhibit, but does not prohibit activities)
   3. Bilateral location
   4. No aggravation by walking stairs or similar routine physical activity

D. Both of the following:
   1. No nausea or vomiting (anorexia may occur)
   2. Photophobia and phonophobia are absent, or one but not the other is present

E. As criterion E in migraine without aura (Table 27.2)

Table 27.7 Diagnostic usefulness of second temporalis exteroceptive suppression (ES_2) in primary headaches. (Percentages as shown; other figures represent numbers of patients)

	Stimulation	
ES_2 duration	0.1 Hz (cut-off 32 ms)	2 Hz (cut-off 16 ms)
Chronic tension-type headache		
ES_2 reduced	21	14
ES_2 normal	4	11
Migraine without aura		
ES_2 reduced	0	1
ES_2 normal	20	19
Sensitivity	84%	56%
Specificity	100%	95%
Predictive value	100%	93%

Epidemiology

In many epidemiological studies the prevalence of muscle contraction headache or psychogenic headache has been found to be equal to, or greater than that of migraine. At present there has been only one population-based epidemiological survey which has used the new concept of 'tension-type headache' and applied the diagnostic criteria of the IHS classification (Rasmussen et al 1991). In this Danish study the lifetime prevalence of tension-type headache was 66% for the episodic form and 3% for the chronic form. Since most patients with episodic tension-type headache do not consult a doctor, the proportion of patients with chronic tension-type headache is much higher in specialised headache or pain centres than in the general population (Table 27.8). In this selected patient population, coexistence of migraine and tension-type headache is also frequently found, which may give the impression that both headache types have a common pathophysiological denominator (Olesen 1991) and that they are at the opposite ends of a disease spectrum. On the contrary however, recent population-based epidemiological studies demonstrate that tension-type headache is not significantly more prevalent in migraineurs than in nonmigraineurs (Rasmussen et al 1992), supporting the contention that these types of headache are distinct entities.

Pathophysiology

The unanswered questions regarding the pathophysiology of tension-type headache are manifold. As far as the chronic form is concerned, there is little doubt that increased activity in pericranial or nucal muscles per se is not causing the pain. Indeed half of EMG studies have yielded normal results (Pikoff 1984). In studies which found increased mean EMG levels, only a minority of patients taken individually had EMG levels which significantly exceeded normative levels and all these increases remained modest (Schoenen et al 1991c). There is no relation between headache intensity and level of EMG activity during long-term ambulatory recordings (Schoenen 1993a). Tenderness of pericranial myofascial tissues is increased in tension-type headache according to a population-based study (Jensen et al 1993). Pressure-pain thresholds were, on average, decreased in patients with chronic tension-type headache recruited from a specialised headache clinic, but taken individually, less than 40% of patients had a significantly abnormal pressure-pain threshold (Schoenen et al 1991d). In the latter study, the average pressure-pain threshold over the Achilles tendon was also lower, which could indicate a general disturbance of pain control systems. As mentioned above, the most consistent abnormality in chronic tension-type headache is reduction or abolition of the second exteroceptive suppression period of temporalis muscle (ES2) (Schoenen et al 1991b; Schoenen 1993b). ES2 changes are not correlated with headache intensity, with EMG levels or with pain thresholds. They point towards a central nervous system dysfunction, probably a disturbance of the limbic control of those brainstem centres (e.g. periaqueductal grey matter, raphe magnus, lateral reticular nucleus) which control the excitability of medullary ES2 inhibitory interneurons, via serotonergic and presumably opioid mechanisms (Schoenen 1993c).

In episodic tension-type headache EMG levels may be modestly increased, but this increase is far too small to explain muscle pain on the basis of ischaemia due to muscle contraction. Muscle tenderness on pericranial palpation is exaggerated, more so during an actual headache (Jensen et al 1993). Temporalis ES2 may be normal in a substantial proportion of patients with episodic tension-type headache (Wallasch et al 1990).

As a working hypothesis, tension-type headache, which is likely to be multifactorial in origin, can be regarded as the result of a complex and dynamic interplay between myofascial nociception, pericranial muscle activity and descending (limbic) control of nociceptive brainstem neurones (Olesen & Schoenen 1993) (Fig. 27.3). The relative importance of these factors may vary from one patient to another and in the same patient from one headache episode to the other. In episodic tension-type headache muscle strain could be an important pathogenetic factor, but pain will preferentially develop in those individuals where excitability of brainstem nociceptors is increased because of modified limbic input due to mental strain. Repetitive episodes of headache may lower the threshold for new episodes, perhaps through changes in myofascial tissues, but especially through central changes of nociceptive neurons and their descending control systems. In chronic tension-type headache a

Table 27.8 Clinical diagnoses in 596 outpatients of the University of Liège Headache Clinic 1/92–6/92

	Number	%
Migraine	186	31
Without aura	166	28
With aura	20	3
Tension-type headache	137	23
Drug abuse headache	60	10
Initially migraine	25	4
Initially tension-type	28	5
Initially not defined	7	1
Cluster headache	38	6
'Cervicogenic' headache	60	9
Others	160	27

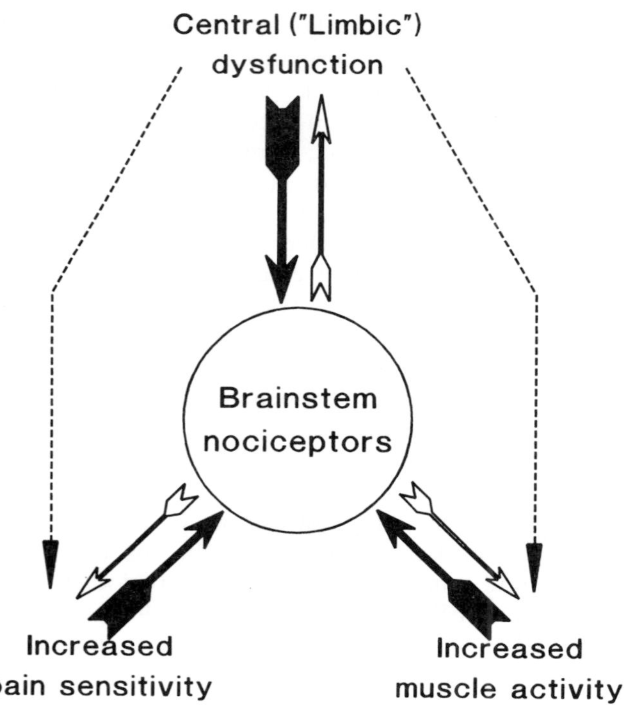

Fig. 27.3 Tension-type headache: model of potential mechanisms.

central dysfunction would therefore become the predominant causal mechanism, which is important for therapeutic strategies.

Treatment

Nondrug treatments

Nondrug treatments are of primary importance in the management of patients suffering from tension-type headache. Strategies for coping with stress, physical therapies and physical activities are most useful and may be sufficient in patients with occasional episodic tension-type headache.

Behavioural strategies such as relaxation therapy with EMG biofeedback are effective even in the long-term (Holroyd et al 1984; Diamond 1984; Blanchard et al 1987). Although their objective is to reduce EMG activity in pericranial muscles, they probably act via a central, cognitive–emotional mechanism (Kroener-Herwig & Weich 1989). The latter may explain why temporalis exteroceptive suppression is protracted in patients after biofeedback therapy (Schoenen 1989).

Drug treatments

Little progress has been made recently in the drug therapies of tension-type headache. For the acute headache episode, simple analgesics or NSAIDs are useful. The latter should be preferred because of the risk of chronic headache induced by overconsumption of analgesic preparations (see section 8.2).

Antidepressants such as amitryptiline, clomipramine or mianserin are effective as prophylactic treatments of chronic tension-type headache at doses which are usually below those used in the treatment of depression. In resistant cases, monoamine-oxidase (MAO) inhibitors can be used as well as a combination of behavioural and drug therapies.

3. CLUSTER HEADACHE AND CHRONIC PAROXYSMAL HEMICRANIA

Cluster headache and chronic paroxysmal hemicrania share common features such as location of pain and associated autonomic symptoms, but differ by sex preponderance, frequency and duration of attacks and drug effects.

Diagnosis and clinical features of cluster headache

The diagnostic criteria of cluster headache are listed in Table 27.9.

A most typical feature of cluster headache is, as suggested by the term itself, the temporal clustering of attacks during periods usually lasting between 2 weeks and 3 months, separated by remissions of at least 14 days, but usually of several months. This is the temporal profile of *episodic cluster headache* (code 3.1.2.). When onset of the disease is too recent to determine periodicity, the headache is coded 3.1.1. *Chronic cluster headache* (code 3.1.3) is characterised by absence of remissions of at least 14 days for more than 1 year. This may be the case from onset (primary chronic, code 3.1.3.1.) or an evolution over time from the episodic form (code 3.1.3.2).

Table 27.9 Cluster headache (code 3.1): diagnostic criteria

A. At least five attacks fulfilling criteria B–D

B. Severe unilateral orbital, supraorbital and/or temporal pain lasting 15–180 min untreated

C. Headache is associated with at least one of the following signs which have to be present on the side of the pain:
   1. Conjunctival injection
   2. Lacrimation
   3. Nasal congestion
   4. Rhinorrhoea
   5. Forehead and facial sweating
   6. Miosis
   7. Ptosis
   8. Eyelid oedema

D. Frequency of attacks: from one every other day to eight per day

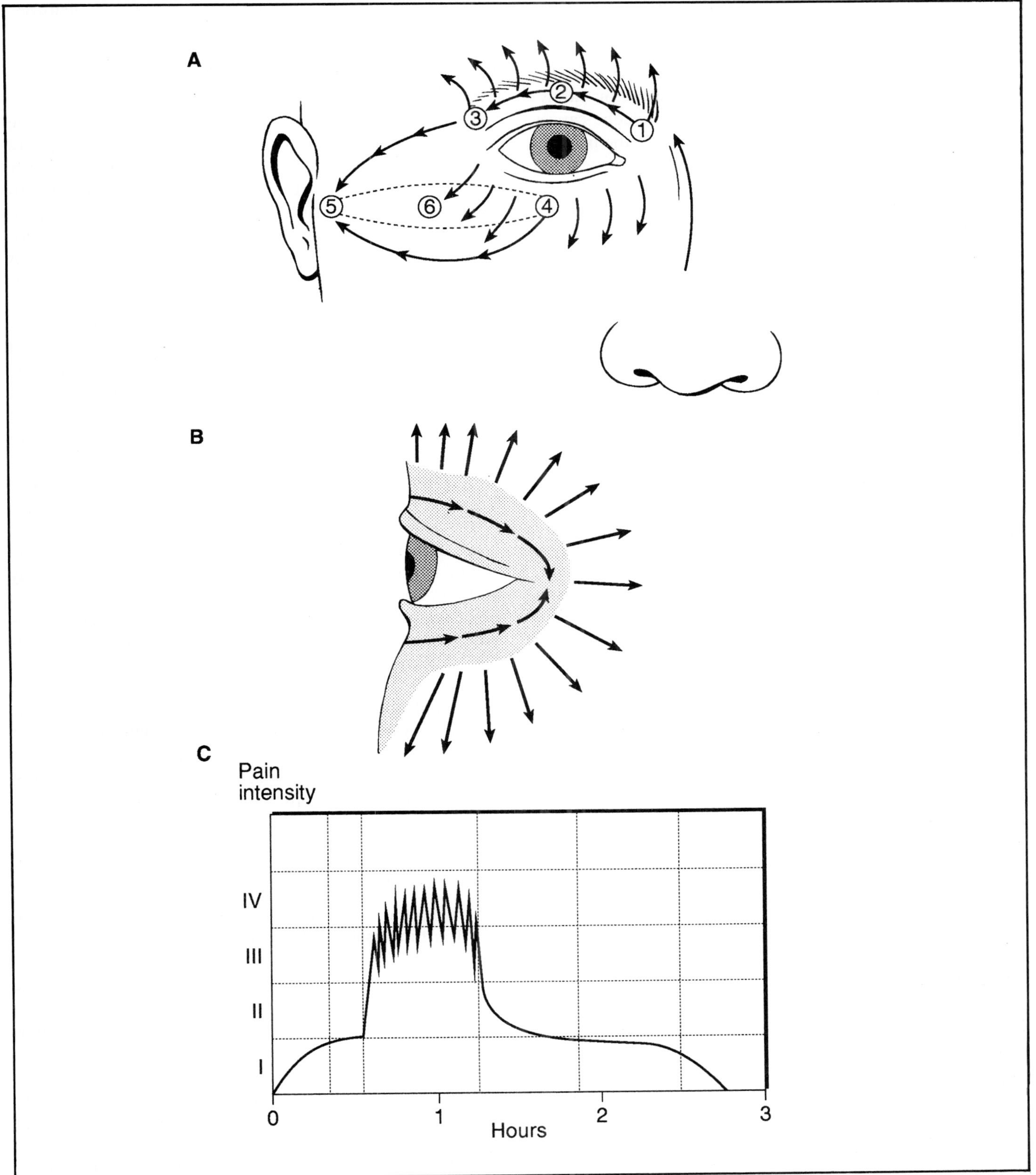

Fig. 27.4 A patient's drawing of the topographic and temporal patterns of an attack of cluster headache. Patient's comments: **A** 1 = initial pain; 2–6 = successive spread of pain; the most intense pain is located within the 1–3–4 triangle; slight pain in areas 4, 5 and 6 may outlast the attack. **B** Pain is most intense in the shaded area. **C** Grading of pain intensity: I = slight, II = moderate, III = violent, IV = excruciating.

Although pain is maximal periorbitally, it may spread in some patients to other regions of the face or the cranium on the same side (Fig. 27.4). Attacks recur on the same side of the head during a cluster period. In some patients, pain may shift sides from one cluster to another or, rarely, in the midst of a cluster period. Cluster headache causes the most intense and excruciating pain among the primary nonsymptomatic headaches. Patients tend to be agitated and to pace the floor which is clearly different from migraine where patients seek rest. Other features distinguishing the cluster headache attack from the migraine attack are shorter duration, presence of autonomic symptoms and absence of gastrointestinal disturbances. During a cluster period attacks can be provoked by alcohol (or histamine or nitroglycerin) and tend to occur in the evening or during sleep. In the general population, and among general practitioners, cluster headache is most often confused with trigeminal neuralgia (see section 12.2) from which it is clearly different by duration of attacks, associated symptoms and temporal profile.

Cluster migraine is a variant of migraine not sufficiently validated, but characterised by unilateral autonomic features, such as conjunctival injection or tearing, accompanying an otherwise typical migraine attack. A very rare syndrome is the so-called cluster-tic syndrome where periods of cluster headache attacks can alternate with episodes of trigeminal neuralgia. There are a few reports in the literature linking cluster headache attacks to an organic lesion, e.g. pituitary adenoma, upper cervical meningioma or cerebral arteriovenous malformations (Sjaastad 1986a). In 16% of patients, the onset of cluster headache can be preceded by (even minor) head trauma (Turkewitz et al 1992).

Epidemiology of cluster headache

Epidemiological surveys of cluster headache are rare and/or controversial. Comparing various studies, the overall prevalence is around 0.04–0.09% (Sjaastad 1986a). The relative incidence of the chronic form (code 3.1.3.) in various published series of cluster headache patients is, on average, 10% (Ekbom 1986). There is a clear preponderance of the male sex in all large series with an average male-to-female ratio of 5:1. Cluster headache may begin at any age, but most often the first attack occurs between 20 and 40 years.

Some familial cases of cluster headache have been described, but genetic influences seem to be much less pronounced than in migraine.

Pathophysiology of cluster headache

There is at present no pathogenetic theory of cluster headache that accounts for all aspects of this disorder, i.e. the pain location and characteristics, autonomic features, temporal profile of attacks and clusters and the male preponderance. Several pathophysiological abnormalities have been demonstrated both during and between attacks. For instance, corneal indentation pulse, intraocular pressure and corneal temperature are increased during the attack. Abnormal sweating, lacrimation, salivation and pupillometric patterns have been demonstrated not only on the symptomatic side, but also, to a lesser degree, on the nonsymptomatic side (see review Sjastad 1992). There is compelling evidence from transcranial doppler, angiographic and magnetic resonance imaging studies that at the maximum of the pain the internal carotid artery is constricted, which has been considered as a reflex activation of sympathetic efferents (Hannerz & Greitz 1992), and that the ophthalmic artery is dilated on the affected side. Heart rate changes and even cardiac rhythm disturbances may accompany attacks probably due to a central disturbance in autonomic function. Neuroendocrinological tests have indicated disturbances of circadian secretory rhythmicity of various substances such as melatonin, beta-endorphin or beta-lipotropin (Nappi & Savoldi 1985). The significance of reduced choline levels in erythrocytes is not clear, while the lowering of testosterone plasma levels in some patients may be secondary to the pain.

The hypothesis that supersensitivity of the carotid body and oxygen desaturation might trigger the attack lacks objective proof. A satisfactory explanation for the peripheral pain and autonomic features could be a pathophysiological focus in the superior pericarotid cavernous sinus plexus, involving sympathetic, parasympathetic and trigeminal fibres (Moskowitz 1988). However, the cause of this dysfunction remains to be determined and neuroendocrinological data as well as the temporal rhythms of the disorder point towards a dysfunctioning of the 'biological clock' in the hypothalamus.

Treatment of cluster headache

To abate the single attack inhalation of 100% oxygen (7–10 l/min) using a face mask is effective within 10–15 minutes in 60–70% of cases. Because of its delayed effectiveness orally or rectally administered ergotamine tartrate is rarely useful, unless attacks are of long duration. In contrast, intranasal application of dihydroergotamine is effective in about 50% of patients.

At present, subcutaneous injection of sumatriptan, an agonist of $5HT_1$ D serotonin receptors also effective in migraine, is the most efficient treatment of cluster headache attacks. At a dose of 6 mg, it alleviates the attacks within 15 min in more than 80% of patients without tachyphylaxis in the long term. Studies investigating the potential prophylactic effect of sumatriptan are in progress.

There is no general agreement on a standard prophylactic therapy for cluster headache.

Lithium carbonate is an effective treatment at doses inducing plasma levels between 0.7 and 1 mmol/l. The effectiveness of lithium may decrease during successive clusters. Lithium may be more effective in the chronic form.

Methysergide has been used with success in cluster headache for many years. Daily dosage should be as low as possible, preferably 3–4 mg. Methysergide has to be interrupted every 5–6 months for 1 month to avoid retroperitoneal fibrosis.

Calcium antagonists such as verapamil or nicardipine have recently been found effective prophylactics.

In some patients, it can be helpful to combine two of the above mentioned substances. Other drugs like pizotifen or indomethacin may have an effect in selected patients. The recently reported benefits of sodium valproate need to be confirmed.

Ergotamine tartrate given orally at bedtime may be useful to prevent nocturnal attacks.

Corticosteroids at high doses are able to interrupt a cluster in many patients. However, their use should be restricted to incapacitated and resistant patients with the episodic form. Tapering or interruption of cortisone treatment is indeed frequently followed by recurrence of attacks.

Suboccipital injection of corticosteroids, associated or not with a local anaesthetic, is used as an adjuvant therapy in some centres. By itself, this may interrupt a cluster in a few patients, but whether this is due to a systemic or to a local effect of the drug remains to be determined.

Various surgical treatments have been tried in cluster headache: alcoholisation, radiofrequency lesions or glycerol injections of the Gasserian ganglion; cryosurgery, or resection of the sphenopalatine ganglion. None of these procedures gives consistent long-lasting relief and they should therefore not be considered before failure of a full trial of medical therapy. At present, percutaneous alcoholisation of the sphenopalatine ganglion appears to be one of the most effective and least invasive procedures used in experienced centres.

Diagnosis and clinical features of chronic paroxysmal hemicrania (CPH)

The diagnostic criteria for chronic paroxysmal hemicrania are listed in Table 27.10.

Attacks of CPH resemble those of cluster headache, but they last for a shorter time; are more frequent; have no nocturnal preponderance; occur mostly in females, and are absolutely responsive to indomethacin. The mean duration of attacks is around 15 min. The frequency of attacks may be as high as 40 per 24 h, with a mean of about 12. In some patients, attacks can be mechanically precipitated, for instance by certain movements of the head. Frequency, duration and severity of attacks may vary. The chronic stage, which characterises most reported cases, may be preceded by an episodic, 'preCPH', stage.

Table 27.10 Chronic paroxysmal hemicrania (code 3.2): diagnostic criteria

A. At least 50 attacks fulfilling criteria B–E

B. Attacks of severe unilateral orbital, supraorbital and/or temporal pain, always on the same side, lasting 2–45 min

C. Attack frequency: above five a day for more than half of the time (periods with lower frequency may occur)

D. Pain is associated with at least one of the following signs/symptoms on the side of the pain:
1. Conjunctival injection
2. Lacrimation
3. Nasal congestion
4. Rhinorrhoea
5. Ptosis
6. Eyelid oedema

E. Absolute effectiveness of indomethacin (150 mg/d or less)

Short-lasting, unilateral, neuralgiform headache attacks with conjunctival injection, tearing, sweating and rhinorrhoea, the so-called SUNCT syndrome, may be a new entity which has similarities with cluster headache and CPH (Sjaastad et al 1989). SUNCT is characterised by a multiplicity of short (usually less than 120 s) paroxysms of moderate to severe intensity with massive autonomic symptoms in the eye. Only a few cases have been described in the literature up to now; so far all of them are males.

Epidemiology of CPH

CPH is a rare disorder, affecting adult females almost exclusively. The disorder was first described by Sjaastad & Dale (1974). In 1986 information was available about 44 cases, of which only eight were males (Sjaastad 1986b). The number of cases reported in the literature is constantly increasing.

Pathophysiology of CPH

The exact pathogenesis of CPH is not known. Various abnormalities (e.g. corneal indentation or temperature changes, intraocular pressure changes) are similar to those reported in cluster headache. Several symptomatic cases occuring with sellar or parasellar neoplasms have been reported.

Treatment of CPH

The absolute responsiveness of CPH to indomethacin is

part of the diagnostic criteria. It is not known why this disorder is selectively responsive to indomethacin. The effective dosage of indomethacin varies between patients. Doses up to 150 mg or more per day may be necessary. Attacks disappear within hours or a few days when the effective dosage of indomethacin is attained. On discontinuation of the drug attacks frequently reappear, but long-lasting remissions have been observed in some patients. Recently other NSAIDs, such as ketoprofen, have been found effective in a few patients.

4. MISCELLANEOUS HEADACHES UNASSOCIATED WITH STRUCTURAL LESION

This section comprises several rather characteristic headaches which are benign in nature. Pathophysiologically, they are triggered by stimulation of the trigeminal nerve territory or changes in intracranial pressure. Some of them have been more frequently reported in migraineurs.

Idiopathic stabbing headache (code 4.1), previously called ice-pick pains or 'jabs and jolts', is characterised by short-lasting pains, in the distribution of the first division of the trigeminal nerve, occurring at irregular intervals. It was found in 2% of the general population (Rasmussen & Olesen 1992) and is significantly more prevalent in migraineurs. If treatment is necessary, indomethacin or other NSAIDs are usually effective.

External compression headache (code 4.2), also called 'swim-goggle headache', is a dull constant pain felt in an area of the scalp subjected to prolonged pressure. Up to 4% of the population may present with such a headache (Rasmussen & Olesen 1992), preferentially individuals suffering also from migraine.

Cold stimulus headache (code 4.3) includes headaches developing during external exposure to cold (subzero weather, cold water) or during ingestion of a cold food or drink (previously called 'ice-cream headache'). This type of headache seems to be frequent in the general population, affecting 15% of individuals in the Danish study; it is also more frequent in migraineurs.

Benign cough headache (code 4.4) and *benign exertional headache* (code 4.5) are rare (1% of the population) and not associated with migraine or tension-type headache (Rasmussen & Olesen 1992). Exertional headache can be prevented in some patients by the ingestion of indomethacin before exercise. Ergotamine tartrate, methysergide and propranolol have also been used.

Headache associated with sexual activity (code 4.6) may present under three different forms: a dull pain in the head and neck that intensifies as sexual excitement increases (code 4.6.1); a sudden severe, explosive, headache occurring at orgasm (code 4.6.2) or a postural headache resembling that of low cerebrospinal fluid pressure developing after coitus (code 4.6.3). Benign headaches in these categories affected only 1% of subjects in the population-based study by Rasmussen & Olesen (1992). When a sudden severe headache occurs for the first time during sexual activity or exertion, an intracranial aneurysm has to be excluded (see section 6.4).

5. HEADACHE ASSOCIATED WITH HEAD TRAUMA

Diagnosis and clinical features

The diagnostic criteria for *acute posttraumatic headache* (code 5.1) are listed in Table 27.11. In the *chronic form* (code 5.2) the headache continues for more than 8 weeks after regaining consciousness or after trauma, if there has been no loss of consciousness.

Acute posttraumatic headache is often moderate to severe, throbbing in quality, with accompanying nausea, vomiting, photo- and phonophobia, memory impairment, irritability or drowsiness, or vertigo. It is usually exacerbated by physical exercise, described as incapacitating by the patient, and bears many similarities to migraine, except the attack pattern.

Although the quality of chronic posttraumatic headache is not characteristic, it is usually a generalised headache, almost permanent like chronic tension-type headache, but aggravated by physical effort and mental strain. The pain may be focused on the area that the patient believes to have been damaged and which tends to be tender. Migrainous features, such as a pulsating quality or nausea, may occur.

Many patients with chronic posttraumatic headache fulfil DSM-III-R criteria for posttraumatic stress disorder (Hickling et al 1992). Depressive features are common

Table 27.11 Acute posttraumatic headache (code 5.1): diagnostic criteria

With significant head trauma and/or confirmatory signs (code 5.1.1)

A. Significance of head trauma documented by at least one of the following:
   1. Loss of consciousness
   2. Posttraumatic amnesia lasting more than 10 min
   3. At least two of the following exhibit relevant abnormality: clinical neurological examination, X-ray of skull, neuroimaging, evoked potentials, spinal fluid examination, vestibular function test, neuropsychological testing

B. Headache occurs less than 14 days after regaining consciousness (or after trauma, if there has been no loss of consciousness)

C. Headache disappears within 8 weeks after regaining consciousness (or after trauma, if there has been no loss of consciousness)

With minor head trauma and no confirmatory signs (code 5.1.2)

A. Head trauma that does not satisfy 5.1.1. criterion A

B. Headache occurs less than 14 days after injury

C. Headache disappears within 8 weeks after injury

and decreased amplitude of contingent negative variation has been reported (Schoenen & Timsit-Berthier 1993).

As mentioned elsewhere, migraine or cluster headache may appear de novo after a head trauma. The incidence of posttraumatic migraine was as high as 3% in one study (Kelly 1986). Worsening of preexisting headache is coded according to preexisting headache form.

Epidemiology and pathophysiology

Headache is a major factor in the symptomatology of head trauma. It is obvious however that the severity of trauma has little relationship to the intensity or duration of the headache. There is even some evidence that the incidence of posttraumatic headache is inversely related to the severity of head injury (Kay et al 1971). In a recent study severe posttraumatic headache was found in 72% of mildly injured and 33% of severely injured patients, despite the fact that cervical X-ray and CT scan abnormalities were more frequent in the latter group (Yamaguchi 1992).

Acute posttraumatic headache is very common. The incidence of chronic posttraumatic headache varies between studies from 15–40% (Jensen & Nielsen 1990). Patients suffering from headache before the trauma are no more at risk of having traumatic headache than patients who did not suffer from headache before the trauma. For an unexplained reason, posttraumatic headache is, like many other headaches, reported by more women than men (Jensen & Nielsen 1990).

Russell (1932) and Cook (1972) observed that persistence of posttraumatic symptoms and duration of absence from work were longer in patients claiming financial compensation from the employer or insurance company. In a long-term follow-up of over 800 patients with the chronic posttraumatic syndrome Kelly (1986) found that only 0.06% of patients had not already returned to work before settlement of their claim for litigation and that for this subgroup of patients it was unusual to return to work after the case had come to settlement irrespective of whether the latter was favourable or not.

Treatment

Treatment of acute posttraumatic headache is part of the general management of the cerebral concussion syndrome: physical and mental rest in a supine position and simple analgesics or antiinflammatory drugs. After the immediate acute stage, the practitioner has frequently to deal with the other symptoms of the postconcussion syndrome such as memory impairment, mood and personality changes and social dysfunctioning.

Treatment of chronic posttraumatic headache is difficult because of the complex interrelation between organic and psychosocial factors. Daily consumption of analgesics can lead to chronic drug-induced headaches (see section 8.2). Moreover, there is often an outstanding claim for compensation from the employer (when trauma occurred at work) or from insurance companies (for traffic accidents) and, until this claim is settled, a complete failure of any proposed treatment may be observed. The first, and possibly major, step is to recognise that the condition does exist and is not always a 'figment of the patient's cupidity' (Kelly 1986). Once this is accepted, therapeutic strategy has to be planned for each patient individually. In patients who have migrainous features, prophylactic antimigraine drugs can be useful (see above). Behavioural treatments, such as biofeedback, have provided persistent relief in some patients. In many of them antidepressants, tricyclics or MAO inhibitors, are necessary. In all cases of resistant posttraumatic headache, psychosocial guidance is the cornerstone of management with the objective of helping the patient to recover progressively his social and professional status.

6. HEADACHE ASSOCIATED WITH VASCULAR DISORDER

All headaches coded to this group fulfil the following criteria: symptoms and/or signs of vascular disorder; appropriate investigations indicate the vascular disorder and headache as a new symptom or of a new type occurring in close temporal relation to onset of vascular disorder.

As previously, worsening of preexisting headache is coded according to preexisting headache form.

Acute ischaemic cerebrovascular disease (code 6.1)

Although it has been repeatedly emphasised for many years, the importance of headache as a symptom of occlusive cerebrovascular disease is still neglected by many physicians. Comprehensive reviews have recently been undertaken by Edmeads (1986) and Mitsias & Ramadan (1992). Their major conclusions can be summarised as follows:

1. The incidence of headache accompanying transient ischaemic attacks (TIAs) or strokes varies from 15–65% between studies, with an average incidence of 30%. The literature suggests that headache is more likely to occur in patients with posterior circulation ischaemia, independent of mechanism.

2. The headache can precede the ischaemic event in about 10% of patients ('sentinel headache').

3. The headache is usually on the side of the affected artery when the carotid circulation or the posterior cerebral artery are involved and in most cases its location is frontal. In basilar artery or vertebral occlusion or stenosis the headache is most often occipital and nonlateralised; sometimes it is occipitofrontal and lateralised.

4. The quality of headache in ischaemic cerebrovascular disease varies widely among patients. The headache

may be continuous or throbbing. It is usually of moderate intensity.

5. Headache at the onset of the ischaemic stroke does not help to distinguish embolic from atherothrombotic stroke. Headache may be less frequent in lacunar infarcts.

Whether or not migraine is an independent risk factor for ischaemic stroke is still debated. Recent surveys suggest that it is not, except possibly in young females who smoke.

Intracranial haematoma (code 6.2)

The overall incidence of headache as a major symptom in various series of *intracerebral haemorrhages* (code 6.2.1.) ranges from 36–66% (Edmeads 1986). Impaired consciousness or aphasia can prevent patients from complaining of headache. In all the published series there is nevertheless a proportion of noncomatose, nonaphasic patients, ranging from 10% in putamenothalamic to 30% in lobar haemorrhages, who do not have headaches. The occurrence, acuity and severity of headache will depend largely on the location, rate of evolution and size of the haemorrhage.

Headache is a useful and common indicator of the late development of an acute *epidural* (code 6.2.3) or *subdural* (code 6.2.2) haematoma in patients who have recovered consciousness and subsequently appear to deteriorate. It may be similar to that due to raised intracranial pressure (see section 7.1). Subdural haematomata can sometimes produce a characteristic paroxysmal headache that returns on and off irregularly throughout the day, lasts only minutes and is accompanied by generalised sweating and an increase in the pulse rate (Kelly 1986). The headache is usually frontal, but when the subdural haematoma is in the posterior fossa, it is likely to be occipital. Occipital headache associated with neck stiffness may indicate the onset of cerebellar pressure coning from the presence of an unrelieved supratentorial bilateral subdural haematoma.

Subarachnoid haemorrhage (code 6.3)

The headache of subarachnoid haemorrhage is typically abrupt in onset and incapacitating in severity. Time from onset to maximal pain intensity is less than 60 min in the case of ruptured aneurysm and less than 12 h if it is an arteriovenous malformation. The headache is diffuse, often posterior and radiating into the neck. It can be accompanied by blunting of consciousness, vomiting, stiff neck and sometimes subhyaloid haemorrhages. The diagnosis is confirmed by CT scan, which may be normal in 10% of cases, and CSF examination.

Unruptured vascular malformation (code 6.4)

About one-quarter of patients with an intracranial aneurysm present prerupture manifestations. The most frequent of these is the so-called 'sentinel headache' (or 'premonitory headache', 'minibleeds' or 'warning leaks'), suggesting that an aneurysm might leak intermittently into the subarachnoid space (Edmeads 1986). Fortunately, every severe global headache of abrupt onset, the so-called 'thunderclap' headache, is not the first symptom of an *intracranial aneurysm* (code 6.4.1). Two recent studies have shown that patients struck by 'thunderclap' headache, who have normal CT scan and lumbar puncture results, do not subsequently develop subarachnoid haemorrhage (Wijdicks et al 1988; Markus 1991). Consequently, the following guidelines may be helpful in patients with an abrupt 'worst headache of my life' thunderclap, and a normal neurological examination: perform CT scan; if normal, perform lumbar puncture; if normal, the patient can be reassured and the headache considered to be benign (but it may recur in some patients). If any aspect of the CT scan or lumbar puncture is abnormal, an angiography is required.

Arteriovenous malformations (code 6.4.1), which account for 6% of all subarachnoid haemorrhages (Edmeads 1986), often cause focal seizures or neurological deficits. Although the relationship of migraine and other headaches to unruptured arteriovenous malformation (AVM) is poorly substantiated, there are several case reports in the literature of AVMs mimicking attacks of migraine with aura. Possible diagnostic clues are symptom localisation being always on the same side; absent family history for migraine; absence of visual aura symptoms and atypical auras.

Arteritis (code 6.5)

Giant cell arteritis (code 6.5.1)

Diagnosis and clinical features. In the IHS classification, the diagnostic criteria for giant cell arteritis (temporal arteritis or Horton's disease) are the presence of typical histopathological features on temporal artery biopsy, and one or more of the following: swollen and tender scalp artery; elevated erythrocyte sedimentation rate, and disappearance of headache within 48 h of steroid therapy.

Other clinical characteristics, however, may be helpful for the diagnosis at an earlier stage. For instance, giant cell arteritis is a disease of the elderly. Its prevalence increases after the age of 50 years and was found to be 78.1 per 100 000 in the ninth decade in some studies (Ross Russell 1986). In two recent series the mean age was over 65 years and women predominated by 2:1 (Berlit 1992; Chmelewski et al 1992). The headache is usually temporal, of variable severity, of a constant boring quality and temporarily relieved by analgesics such as aspirin. Pulsation in branches of the superficial temporal artery or the facial artery may be absent. Symmetrical arthralgia–

myalgia in pectoral or pelvic girdle areas ('polymyalgia rheumatica') frequently accompanies this systemic disease as well as general malaise, anorexia or mild fever. Early morning large joint stiffness may be the only manifestation of polymyalgia rheumatica. Typical complications are claudication of jaw muscles and visual loss due to ischaemia of the optic nerve and retina. The frequency of visual loss has been variously reported to be between 7 and 60% (Ross Russell 1986). Visual disturbances require immediate and energetic treatment, because the prognosis for recovery of vision lost for more than a few hours' duration is poor. Stroke due to involvement of cerebral arteries may occur in exceptional cases.

Pathology. Temporal artery biopsy confirms the diagnosis of a granulomatous arteritis, but it may be normal in a minority of patients. Treatment should nevertheless be undertaken if the clinical and biological picture of the disease is suggestive (Berlit 1992). Although reported otherwise in some series, bilateral temporal artery biopsy does not increase the incidence of positive results (Chmelewski et al 1992).

Treatment. The first choice treatment of giant cell arteritis is corticosteroids. Initial steroid dosage ranges from 40–90 mg/d prednisone. The clinical response to treatment is rapid and severe headache disappears within 48 h. Whenever necessary, corticosteroid treatment can be initiated before temporal artery biopsy is performed since this does not appear immediately to suppress diagnostic histopathologic abnormalities.

Once symptoms are controlled, doses of steroids should gradually be reduced over a period of weeks to months. The erythrocyte sedimentation rate is a helpful guide at this stage for determining the lowest effective dose. With doses of steroids below 20 mg of prednisone, as many as 30% of patients may have a relapse. Unfortunately, in these elderly patients the long-term side-effects of prednisone are manifold and troublesome. It is therefore recommended that the prednisone dosage should be brought down to 10–15 mg/d by the third month, while monitoring the erythrocyte sedimentation rate value as the first, early indication of potential relapse. If side-effects of corticosteroids are severe, it may be possible to control the arteritis with immunosuppressive drugs such as azathioprine.

Carotid or vertebral artery pain (code 6.6)

Ipsilateral headache and/or cervical pain may be the only manifestation of *carotid or vertebral dissection* (code 6.6.1) or accompany the neurological symptoms (Biousse et al 1992). *Carotidynia* (code 6.6.2) is a controversial entity. Its is doubtful whether an idiopathic form of carotidynia exists, but there is clear evidence that a number of diseases of the carotid artery or of the neck are able to produce symptoms suggestive of carotidynia, such as tenderness, swelling and increased pulsation of the carotid artery.

Postendarterectomy headache (code 6.6.3) is defined as an ipsilateral headache beginning within 2 days of carotid endarterectomy, in the absence of carotid occlusion or dissection. Recent studies suggest that these criteria are not satisfactory and that endarterectomy headache may be multifactorial. In a prospective study of 50 patients, 62% reported headache, which occurred in the first 5 days after surgery in 87% of cases. The headache was mostly bilateral (74%), mild or moderate (78%) and requiring no treatment (77%). In this series only five patients met the IHS criteria for postendarterectomy headache (Tehindrazanarivelo et al 1992).

Venous thrombosis (code 6.7)

Headache is the most frequent symptom in cerebral venous thrombosis and most often the first one. It is more frequently diffuse than localised and more often subacute than acute. Its intensity is highly variable. Associated neurological signs (focal deficit or seizures), and/or raised intracranial pressure causing papilloedema, are present in the majority of cases. Headache can however occasionally be the only symptom of cerebral venous thrombosis. This is thus another reason why recent, persisting headache should prompt appropriate investigations including CT scan, magnetic resonance imaging and, if necessary, angiography.

Arterial hypertension (code 6.8)

There is convincing evidence from several epidemiological studies that chronic hypertension of mild or moderate degree does not cause headache. Arterial hypertension is considered to be the cause of headache in four conditions which are not usually difficult to diagnose: acute pressor response to exogenous agent (code 6.8.1); phaeochromocytoma (code 6.8.2); malignant hypertension and hypertensive encephalopathy (code 6.8.3) and preeclampsia and eclampsia (code 6.8.4).

7. HEADACHE ASSOCIATED WITH NONVASCULAR INTRACRANIAL DISORDER

In the IHS classification this category comprises mainly headaches associated with changes in intracranial pressure. Some of the disorders, such as intracranial infections, need no further comment, as their diagnosis is usually straightforward. Others have to be considered in more detail, because they are frequent and/or because their diagnosis is difficult at a stage when headache is the only symptom. This is the case for benign intracranial hypertension, postlumbar puncture headache and headache associated with brain tumour.

High cerebrospinal fluid pressure (code 7.1)

Benign intracranial hypertension (code 7.1.1)

Diagnosis and clinical features. The diagnostic criteria for *benign intracranial hypertension*, also called pseudotumour cerebri or idiopathic intracranial hypertension, are listed in Table 27.12.

The headache accompanying this condition may mimic that of chronic tension-type headache: it is generalised, nonthrobbing and of low or moderate intensity. It is usually increased, however, on suddenly jolting or rotating the head. In the recent study by Wall (1990) the following features were found to be characteristic for the diagnosis: predominant occurrence in young obese women (93%); the most severe headache ever experienced by the patient (93%); pulsatile character (83%); nausea (57%); vomiting (30%); orbital pain (43%); transient visual obscuration (71%); diplopia (38%) and visual loss (31%). Papilloedema, without neuroradiological abnormalities (except for a possible 'empty sella'), is pathognomonic for this condition, but may be lacking in a small subgroup of patients (Marcelis & Silberstein 1991). The resting spinal pressure varies from 220–600 mmH_2O. CSF cytology is normal, but protein content may be low. Computerised axial tomography may show narrow, 'slit-like' ventricles.

Pathogenesis. Pathogenetic factors which may be associated with benign intracranial hypertension include, in addition to intracranial venous occlusion, menstrual dysfunction, deficiency of the adrenals, corticosteroid therapy, hypoparathyroidism, vitamin A intoxication, insecticides (e.g. kepone) and administration of tetracycline in infants (Dalessio 1989). In many cases no precise cause is found.

Treatment. The treatment of elevated intracranial pressure syndromes depends on the underlying cause. If the diagnosis is benign intracranial hypertension, secondary causes should be sought and if possible eliminated. The headache has been reported to respond to standard headache treatment, including beta-adrenergic blockers, calcium channel antagonists, antidepressants, MAO inhibitors, anticonvulsants, analgesics and ergotamine preparations. If such therapy is unsuccessful, then a 4–6-week trial of furosemide or a potent carbonic anhydrase inhibitor (acetazolamide) should be given. The use of high dose corticosteroid is controversial, but may be effective in benign intracranial hypertension. Lumbar puncture typically relieves headache, but the long-term usefulness of repeated lumbar puncture is uncertain.

Careful ophthalmological follow-up is necessary in all patients. Surgical treatment has been directed toward preventing visual loss secondary to papilloedema. Optic nerve sheath fenestration can produce improvement of headache as a felicitous side-effect. Ventriculoperitoneal shunts can be performed successfully in selected patients.

Table 27.12 High cerebrospinal fluid pressure (code 7.1): diagnostic criteria

A. Patient suffers from benign intracranial hypertension fulfilling the following criteria:
   1. Increased intracranial pressure (> 200 mm of water) measured by epidural or intraventricular pressure monitoring or by lumbar puncture
   2. Normal neurological examination except for papilloedema and possible sixth nerve palsy
   3. No mass lesion and no ventricular enlargement on neuroimaging
   4. Normal or low protein concentration and normal white cell count in CSF
   5. No clinical or neuroimaging suspicion of venous sinus thrombosis

B. Headache intensity and frequency related to variations of intracranial pressure with a time lag of less than 24 h.

High pressure hydrocephalus (code 7.1.2)

High pressure hydrocephalus may not cause headache when it develops progressively. The acute increase in intracranial pressure which occurs for example with ventricular obstruction or shunt malfunction in a treated hydrocephalic usually causes severe headache followed by visual disturbance.

Low cerebrospinal fluid pressure (code 7.2)

Diagnosis and clinical features

The clinical hallmark of low CSF pressure headache is that the pain is aggravated by upright position and relieved with recumbency ('orthostatic headache'). The headache may be frontal, occipital or diffuse. The pain is severe, dull or throbbing in nature and not usually relieved with analgesics. Other symptoms include anorexia, nausea, vomiting, vertigo and tinnitus. The pain is aggravated by head shaking and jugular compression. Physical examination may show mild neck stiffness and a slow pulse rate, but is most often normal. Spinal fluid pressure usually ranges from 0–30 mmH_2O in the lateral supine position.

Aetiology

The most frequent cause of low CSF pressure is lumbar puncture. Theories concerning pathogenesis of *postlumbar puncture headache* (code 7.2.1) have nonetheless been contradictory. Although the weight of the evidence supports the view that it is related to a loss of CSF secondary to leakage through the dural hole, other factors may favour the syndrome: for instance, postlumbar puncture headache, the prevalence of which may be as high as 40–50% in some studies, is more frequent in young, healthy, female patients with low body mass and in subjects who have a history of previous headaches (Göbel & Schenkl 1989; Kuntz et al 1992).

There are many other causes of low pressure headache syndrome like posttraumatic, postoperative or idiopathic *cerebrospinal fluid leak* (code 7.2.2) or systemic illnesses such as dehydration, diabetic coma, hyperpnoea or uraemia. Moreover, a syndrome of spontaneous intracranial hypotension has been described (Rando & Fishman 1992).

Treatment

The incidence of postlumbar puncture headache may be lower when small-diameter needles are used (20 or 22 G), but this hypothesis lacks definite proof (Kuntz et al 1992). Contrary to previous belief, recommendation of a resting period in the supine position after the procedure makes no difference to the incidence (Vilming et al 1988).

Treatment of postlumbar puncture headache and spontaneous intracranial hypotension is similar. It begins with noninvasive therapeutic modalities of bed rest and, eventually, an abdominal binder. If there is no improvement, intravenous or oral caffeine may produce significant relief, possibly associated with the use of corticosteroids for a short period if necessary. If the patient continues to be symptomatic after a noninvasive medical approach for 2 weeks, an epidural blood patch is indicated. If the headache of intracranial hypotension recurs, an epidural blood patch can be repeated or a continuous intrathecal saline infusion may be attempted (Silberstein & Marcelis 1992).

Intracranial neoplasm (code 7.6)

Headache occurs at presentation in approximately 36–50% of adult patients with brain tumours and develops in the course of the disease in 60% (Silberstein & Marcelis 1992). The headache is usually generalised, of the dull, deep aching type. It is usually intermittent and relieved by simple analgesic. If there is any variation in intensity during the 24-hour cycle, it is worse in the early morning and it may be ameliorated by breakfast. Elevation of intracranial pressure is not necessary for its production. It is said to be more prominent with rapidly growing tumours than with those of slower growth, but this has been challenged in some studies. Headache is a rare initial symptom in patients with pituitary tumours, craniopharyngiomas or cerebellopontine angle tumours.

In 30–80% of patients the headache overlies the tumour. Some general rules concerning headache as an aid to localisation in patients with brain tumour have been proposed by Dalessio (1989):

1. Although the headache of brain tumour may be referred from a distant source it approximately overlies the tumour in about one-third of all patients
2. If the tumour is above the tentorium, the pain is frequently at the vertex or in the frontal region
3. If the tumour is below the tentorium, the pain is occipital and cervical muscle spasms may be present
4. Headache is always present with posterior fossa tumour
5. If the tumour is midline, it may be increased with cough or strain or sudden head movement
6. If the tumour is hemispheric, the pain is usually felt on the same side of the head
7. If the tumour is chiasmal, at the sella, the pain may be referred to the vertex.

Headache may be a more common symptom of brain tumour in children (over 90%). The following characteristics were found to occur frequently in children with brain tumour headache: headache awakening the child from sleep or present on arising; increased severity or frequency of headache, and increased frequency of vomiting. The majority of children presenting with headache because of a brain tumour have abnormal signs on neurological examination.

In specialised headache or pain clinics, brain tumours account for less than 1% of cases. There is significant overlap between the headache of brain tumour and migraine and tension-type headache. The following clues indicate that a thorough neuroradiological examination is recommended: any headache of recent onset; a headache that has changed in character; a focalised headache not resembling one of the vascular headaches, and morning or nocturnal headache, associated with vomiting, in a nonmigraineur.

8. HEADACHE ASSOCIATED WITH SUBSTANCES OR THEIR WITHDRAWAL

A new headache including migraine, tension-type headache or cluster headache, in close temporal relation to substance use or substance withdrawal is coded to this group. As usual, type of headache may be specified with the fourth digit. As stated in the IHS classification, effective doses and temporal relationships have not yet been determined for most substances. Although headache may be caused by a number of different substances, the most significant and intriguing headaches in clinical practice are those which are induced by misuse of antiheadache medications, i.e. ergotamine and analgesic compounds.

Headache induced by acute substance use or exposure (code 8.1)

General surveys suggest that a vast number of drugs can cause headaches (Askmark et al 1989). To establish however that any substance really induces headache, double-blind placebo controlled experiments are necessary.

There is evidence that headache can be produced by nitrates/nitrites ('hot dog headache') (code 8.1.1), monosodium glutamate ('chinese restaurant syndrome') (code 8.1.2), carbon monoxide (code 8.1.3) or alcohol (code 8.1.4).

Headache induced by chronic substance use or exposure (code 8.2)

Diagnosis and clinical features (Table 27.13)

It can be estimated that around 10% of the patients attending a specialised headache clinic, of whom only half originally had migraine, suffer this condition (Steiner et al 1992). Drug-induced headache is a chronic, usually daily, headache involving the whole skull, often described as a pressing helmet over the head (Henry 1992). Pain is exacerbated by physical exercise and intellectual effort and is often accompanied by asthenia, irritability, sleep and memory disturbances. The characteristics of chronic drug-induced headache are very similar to those of tension-type headache, except that nausea, photo- and phonophobia are much more frequent in drug-induced headache. Most of the time, these patients use analgesics for even the mildest headaches or even before pain appears. There is a long-lasting history of abortive drug intake, with escalation over months or years of the doses needed to provide some relief. Most patients are women, showing the general characteristics of all forms of addiction: tolerance to even-larger doses of medication and physical and emotional dependence (Henry 1992). Concomitant depression or anxiety are common, as is the tendency towards tranquilliser abuse.

Table 27.13 Headache induced by chronic substance use or exposure (code 8.2): diagnostic criteria

A. Occurs after daily doses of a substance for > 3 months
B. A certain minimum dose should be indicated
C. Headache is chronic (15 days or more a month).
D. Headache disappears within 1 month after withdrawal of the substance

Ergotamine-induced headache(code 8.2.1)
A. Is preceded by daily ergotamine intake (oral > 2 mg, rectal > 1 mg)
B. Is diffuse, pulsating and distinguished from migraine by absent attack pattern and/or absent associated symptoms

Analgesic abuse headache (code 8.2.2)
One or more of the following:
1. > 50 g of aspirin a month or equivalent of other analgesics
2. >100 tablets a month of analgesics combined with barbiturates or other nonnarcotic compounds
3. One or more narcotic analgesics

Pathophysiology

So far, headache induced by chronic use of ergotamine and analgesics has only been described when the drugs have been taken for headaches and not when they have been taken for other disorders such as chronic low back pain. It remains to be determined whether such pain syndromes as the latter might also be rendered chronic by analgesic abuse. Although some side-effects of ergotamine and analgesics are well known, many physicians still ignore the fact that use of these drugs in large amounts can induce chronic headaches. Moreover, analgesic abuse seems to nullify the effects of prophylactic drugs given for the original headache condition (Mathew et al 1990).

In the criteria of the IHS classification, the cumulative doses of ergotamine or analgesics capable of inducing chronic headaches are obviously overestimated. Individual susceptibility must play a role and like others, we have seen many otherwise typical cases of chronic drug-induced headache whose consumption was far less than reported in the classification (Schoenen et al 1989). The mechanisms of drug-abuse headache are still poorly understood. A similar clinical pattern is encountered in patients using such different drugs as analgesics, ergotamine, barbiturates or opiates. It has been hypothesised that a crucial site of action of analgesics and ergotamine might be some central neurotransmitter systems (e.g. norepinephrine, serotonin and endorphins) playing a role in the control of nociception and mood (Mathew 1987; Saper 1987).

Treatment

The only treatment of drug misuse headache is complete withdrawal of the substance(s) involved (Kudrow 1982; Dichgans et al 1984). This can be done in the ambulatory patient, but management of withdrawal reactions often requires a short hospitalisation. These reactions include nervousness, restlessness, increased headaches, nausea, vomiting, insomnia, diarrhoea, tremor, autonomic dysfunction and even seizures in the case of barbiturate or benzodiazepine abuse (Saper 1987; Mathew et al 1990). These can be alleviated by temporary prescription of neuroleptics or tranquillisers. We use infusions (100 mg/d for 8 days), or oral administration (75 mg/d) of clomipramine, followed by decreasing oral dosage for 2–3 months in association with tiapride (75–100 mg/d). Results of withdrawal in 121 patients are given in Figure 27.5. Kudrow (1982) suggests use of amitryptiline with the same beneficial effect (over two-thirds of patients were headache-free when discharged). It remains to be confirmed whether sumatriptan is useful in migraineurs with ergotamine misuse (Diener et al 1991).

Long-term prognosis primarily depends on the ability of the patient to remain free of his/her drug, on the physician's skill in prescribing efficient prophylaxis for the

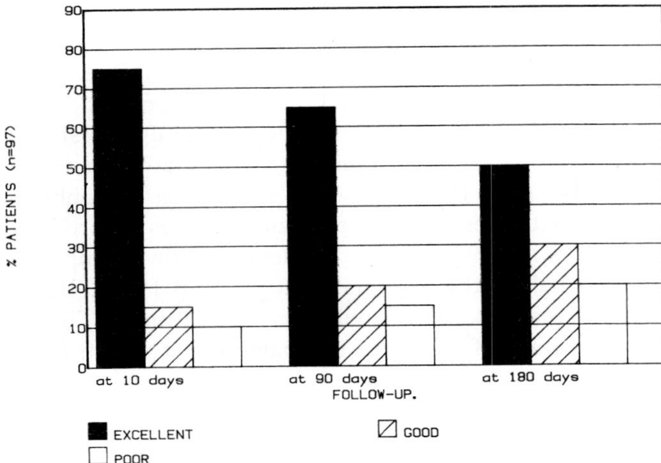

Fig. 27.5 Results at 10 days, 3 months and 6 months of abrupt withdrawal of analgesics and/or ergotamine, and substitution treatment with clomipramine, tiapride and NSAIDs and, if necessary, prophylactic therapy, in 121 patients with drug misuse headaches. Excellent = more than 75% headache reduction; good = 30–75% reduction; poor = less than 30% reduction. (From Schoenen et al 1989 with permission)

original headache condition and in providing appropriate psychological support (Henry et al 1985).

Education of patients and their physicians is obviously important in the prevention of this syndrome. Important steps include: limiting the prescription of ergotamine/analgesics; avoiding treatment with combined drugs including psychotropics, which should be replaced by NSAIDs, aspirin or paracetamol alone, and considering prophylactic therapy whenever headache is frequent and/or incapacitating (Schoenen et al 1989).

11. HEADACHE OR FACIAL PAIN ASSOCIATED WITH DISORDER OF CRANIUM, NECK, EYES, EARS, NOSE, SINUSES, TEETH, MOUTH OR OTHER FACIAL OR CRANIAL STRUCTURES

Cervical spine (code 11.2.1)

Diagnosis and clinical features

Cervicogenic headache is not well defined by the criteria shown in Table 27.14. Edmeads (1988) underlines the similarities between diagnostic criteria of migraine without aura and cervicogenic headache, an opinion partly challenged by Sjaastad et al (1990). They describe cervicogenic headache as a unilateral headache, without sideshift (unlike migraine), affecting mostly women. It can be provoked by passive movements of the neck or pressure over the ipsilateral neck region. Pain can extend to ipsilateral neck, shoulder and arm, without radicular distribution. It is usually of moderate intensity, nonthrobbing, starting in the neck, eventually spreading to anterior areas. Pain episodes vary in duration without clustering or there is fluctuating, almost continuous pain. If present, photophobia or blurred vision of the ipsilateral eye are mild to moderate. There is often a history of whiplash, but in Sjaastad's description, no overt reference is made to X-ray abnormalities described in the IHS diagnostic criteria (point D in Table 27.14).

Table 27.14 Cervical spine (code 11.2.1): diagnostic criteria

A. Pain localised to neck and occipital region. May project to forehead, orbital region, temple, vertex or ears

B. Pain is precipitated or aggravated by certain neck movements or sustained neck posture

C. At least one of the following:
   1. Resistance to, or limitation of, passive neck movements
   2. Changes in neck muscle contour, texture, tone or response to active and passive stretching and contraction
   3. Abnormal tenderness of neck muscles

D. Radiological examination reveals at least one of the following:
   1. Movement abnormalities in flexion/extension
   2. Abnormal posture
   3. Fractures, congenital abnormalities, bone tumours, rheumatoid arthritis or other distinct pathology (not spondylosis or osteochondrosis)

Pathophysiology

In many cases, pain is transiently relieved by anaesthetic blockade of the greater occipital nerve (GON) not only posteriorly but also in the supraorbital area (Bovim & Sand 1992). The latter suggests that the GON might play a role in the pathophysiology of cervicogenic headache and that pain in the area of the ophthalmic division of the trigeminal nerve might indeed be due in this condition to the projection of upper cervical root (C2–C3) fibres to the spinal trigeminal complex (Kerr 1961). However, other possibly damaged structures located in the neck area (bones, muscles and arteries) can induce pain. The actual origin of the pain remains unknown and, like tension-type headache, cervicogenic headache (although triggered initially by peripheral mechanisms) might be caused in its chronic form by dysfunction of central rather than peripheral structures.

Treatment

Pharmacological treatment of cervicogenic headache is often disappointing. Analgesics and NSAIDs can provide temporary relief, but side-effects of such drugs often preclude long-term treatment. Tricyclic antidepressants can also produce some benefit. As with tension-type headaches, physical therapy, relaxation and biofeedback can provide some relief (Graff-Radford et al 1987; Jaeger 1989). Besides anaesthesia of the GON, neurolysis of this nerve or of C2 roots had been performed, but results were short-lasting (Bovim et al 1992). Radiofrequency electrocoagulation in the GON territory has also been proposed (Blume et al 1982).

Temporomandibular joint disease (code 11.7)

Diagnosis and clinical features

Temporomandibular joint disease is a pain in the jaw, located to the temporomandibular joint and/or radiating from there, usually of mild to moderate intensity. It is often precipitated by movement and/or clenching the teeth. Range of movement of the joint is reduced, with tenderness of the capsule and noise ('click') during joint movements. Plain X-rays and/or scintigraphy of the temporomandibular joint are abnormal.

Pathophysiology

Pain from temporomandibular joints is common, but is rarely due to definable organic disease. By far the most frequent cause of temporomandibular pain is a myofascial one, due to oromandibular dysfunction and related to tension-type headache (see code 2). Patients with rheumatoid arthritis or generalised osteoarthrosis often show X-ray involvement of the temporomandibular joints but do not experience significantly more pain in that area than the normal population (Chalmers & Blair 1973, 1974). The so-called 'Costen's syndrome' includes impaired hearing, tinnitus, pain in the region of the ear and vertical or occipital headache, attributed by Costen (1934) to retroposition of the head of the mandibular condyle, causing irritation of the auriculotemporal or chorda tympani nerves. Treatment of this condition would rest on the fitting of dental prostheses, stabilisation splint or physical therapy (Schokker 1989).

However, 60 years after Costen's original description, pathological proof of the existence of this syndrome is still missing. Moreover, there is strong evidence that many patients with temporomandibular pain syndrome suffer from concomitant anxiety or depression and should be treated accordingly (Feinmann et al 1984).

12. CRANIAL NEURALGIA, NERVE TRUNK PAIN AND DEAFFERENTATION PAIN

Herpes zoster (code 12.1.4.1) and chronic postherpetic neuralgia (code 12.1.4.2)

Herpes zoster affects the trigeminal ganglion in 10–15% of patients, with particular affinity for the ophthalmic division (80% of cases). Third, fourth or sixth cranial nerve palsies are sometimes observed. Herpes zoster may also involve the geniculate ganglion, with an eruption in the external auditory meatus often associated with facial nerve palsy or acoustic symptoms.

Postherpetic neuralgia (code 12.1.4.2) is a chronic pain developing during the acute phase of infection, and persisting more than 6 months after the eruption. It is a frequent sequela of herpes zoster infection, affecting up to 50% of patients, particularly those of older age (Watson & Evans 1988). Pain is felt in the area formerly involved by the infection. It is constant, moderate to severe, often described as burning. Paraesthesia or hypoaesthesia is frequent. Treatment of postherpetic neuralgia rests on tricyclic antidepressants (amitryptiline) (Watson & Evans 1988; Max et al 1988) or, when side-effects are unbearable, other classes of antidepressants such as maprotiline (Watson et al 1992). Such treatments improve symptoms in about half of the patients (Watson et al 1991). Better outcome seems to be related to early treatment. Topical administration of capsaicin or analgesics can be tried in refractory cases.

Trigeminal neuralgia (tic douloureux) (code 12.2)

Idiopathic trigeminal neuralgia (code 12.2.1)

Diagnosis and clinical features. Trigeminal neuralgia or tic douloureux is characterised by very short-lasting (a few seconds to 2 min) attacks of intense, electric shock-like pain limited to the distribution of one or more divisions of the trigeminal nerve (Table 27.15). Idiopathic trigeminal neuralgia more often affects women than men (ratio 3:2), and usually starts after 50 years of age. Pain can often be triggered by trivial stimuli such as washing, shaving, chewing, brushing the teeth or speaking. It may also occur spontaneously. Painful episodes start and end abruptly, may recur dozens of times in a single day but interfere little with sleep. Remissions of variable duration are described. In most cases, pain is restricted to the second or third divisions of the trigeminal nerve. It never crosses the midline, but a few patients (less than 5%) have bilateral attacks. The pain often induces reflex spasms of facial muscles on the affected side, hence the name 'tic douloureux'.

Pathophysiology. It is currently believed that in many cases, so-called idiopathic trigeminal neuralgia might result from local demyelination of the trigeminal root

Table 27.15 Idiopathic trigeminal neuralgia (code 12.2.1): diagnostic criteria

A. Paroxysmal attacks of facial or frontal pain which last from a few seconds to less than 2 minutes

B. Pain has at least four of the following characteristics:
   1. Distribution along one or more divisions of the trigeminal nerve
   2. Sudden, intense, sharp, superficial, stabbing or burning in quality
   3. Pain intensity severe
   4. Precipitation from trigger areas, or by certain daily activities such as eating, talking, washing the face or cleaning the teeth
   5. Between paroxysms the patient is entirely asymptomatic

C. No neurological deficit

D. Attacks are stereotyped in the individual patient

E. Exclusion of other causes of facial pain by history, physical examination and special investigations when necessary.

entry zone due to compressions in the posterior fossa, usually by small tortuous arteries or veins (Jannetta 1970). Favouring this hypothesis, it has been shown that surgical decompression of the trigeminal root can induce prolonged remissions (Taarnhoj 1982). Thus, many cases of idiopathic trigeminal neuralgia should in fact be considered symptomatic. The painful episodes are thought to result from repetitive and aberrant electric discharges (ephaptic transmission) originating in the axons of the demyelinated segment (Loeser et al 1977).

Treatment. More than two-thirds of patients with idiopathic trigeminal neuralgia respond favourably to drug treatment with carbamazepine (200–400 mg t.i.d.) or in refractory cases, carbamazepine plus baclofen (25 mg t.i.d.) or plus clonazepam (2 mg t.i.d.) or phenytoin (200–300 mg/d) (Green & Selman 1991). For refractory cases, thermocoagulation of the Gasserian ganglion can be proposed or microsurgical decompression of the trigeminal root in the posterior fossa (Jannetta 1970). Radiofrequency thermocoagulation of the Gasserian ganglion is safe and can be performed even in very old patients. The relapse rate is variable (21–85%), depending on the duration of follow-up and the depth of anaesthesia produced (Menzel et al 1974; Siegfried 1981). Side-effects include anaesthesia dolorosa (2–3%), numbness and paraesthesia (15–50%) and corneal anaesthesia (1–8%). Posterior fossa decompression is a more serious procedure, although the reported perioperative mortality is low (1–2%) (Jannetta 1981; Apfelbaum 1982). Long-term complete relief is achieved in about 70–85% of cases, but some patients still need some drugs and a minority (4–6%) develop permanent cranial nerve palsies (usually of the 8th, but sometimes of the 4th or 7th nerves).

Symptomatic trigeminal neuralgia (code 12.2.2)

Besides microvascular compressions, several diseases can produce trigeminal neuralgia, such as acoustic neurinomas, brainstem infarcts and, chiefly, multiple sclerosis. The main differences from the idiopathic form are a younger age at onset, persistence of aching between paroxysms and signs of sensory impairment in the distribution of the corresponding trigeminal division.

Glossopharyngeal (code 12.3) and nervus intermedius (code 12.4) neuralgias

These forms of neuralgia are uncommon and their pathophysiology and treatment is similar to that of trigeminal neuralgia. The attack pattern is also similar, with very short paroxysms. Glossopharyngeal neuralgia is characterised by unilateral attacks of transient stabbing pain in the ear, base of tongue, tonsillar fossa or beneath the angle of the jaw. It is provoked by swallowing, talking and coughing. Neuralgia of the nervus intermedius is felt deeply in the ear, lasting for seconds or minutes, with a trigger zone in the posterior wall of the auditory canal.

Facial pain not fulfilling criteria in groups 11 and 12 (code 12.8)

Many patients, usually middle-aged women, complain of facial pain which cannot be put into one of the previous categories (‘atypical facial pain’). Pain is described as burning or aching, is present daily and persists for most of the day. At onset, it is confined to a limited area on one side of the face but later it may spread to the upper and lower jaws or a wider area of the face and neck. It is poorly localised and does not fit with the sensory distribution of a trigeminal branch. Clinical examination and paraclinical investigations are fully normal. Pain is often triggered by operations or injuries to the face or dental problems, but becomes chronic without any demonstrable lesion. Such patients often exhibit depressive traits (Lascelles 1966). Tricyclic antidepressants may provide some relief.

Exceptionally, unilateral facial pain mimicking atypical facial pain is due to lung cancer compressing the vagus nerve (Schoenen et al 1992).

CONCLUSIONS

The operational diagnostic criteria of the IHS Headache Classification allow a more uniform grouping of headache types for research purposes. Their usefulness in routine clinical practice is limited. When confronted with a headache patient, the practitioner first has to decide whether the headache is symptomatic of an underlying disease or whether it is a ‘primary’ headache.

With few exceptions, any headache of recent onset should, as a rule, be considered to be symptomatic. Recognising the cause needs, above all, clinical skill and an adequate choice of paraclinical investigations.

Most chronic headaches correspond to one of the primary headache types. Many, if not all, are probably biobehavioural disorders, resulting from a complex, variable interplay between neurobiological (in part genetically determined) mechanisms and behavioural processes. Treatment of these patients, besides alleviating the symptom ‘head pain’, has to be directed towards both body and mind.

REFERENCES

Amery W K, Vandenbergh V 1987 What can precipitating factors teach us about the pathogenesis of migraine? Headache 27: 146–150

Anthony M, Lance J W 1975 The role of serotonin in migraine. In: Pearce J (ed) Modern topics in migraine. Heinemann, London, p 107–123

Apfelbaum R I 1982 Microvascular decompression for tic douloureux. In: Brackman D E (ed) Neurological surgery of the ear and skull base. Raven Press, New York, p 175–180

Askmark H, Lundberg O, Olsson S 1989 Drug related headache. Headache 29: 441–444

Barbiroli B, Montagna P, Cortelli P et al, 1992 Abnormal brain and muscle energy metabolism shown by ^{31}P magnetic resonance spectroscopy in patients affected by migraine with aura. Neurology 42: 1209–1214

Barkley G L, Tepley N, Simkins R T, Moran J E, Welch K M A 1990 Neuromagnetic findings in migraine. Preliminary findings. Cephalalgia 10: 171–176

Berlit P 1992 Clinical and laboratory findings with giant cell arteritis. Journal of the Neurological Sciences 111: 1–12

Bès A, Fabre N 1992 Débit sanguin cérébral et migraine sans aura. Pathologie et Biologie 40: 325–331

Bès A, Fabre N, Soulages X, Pavy-Le-Traon A, Geraud G 1990 La migraine est-elle une maladie vasculaire? Circulation et Métabolisme du Cerveau 7: 251–266

Bille B 1962 Migraine in school children. Acta Paediatrica 51 (suppl 136): 3–151

Biousse V, Woimant F, Amarenco P, Touboul P J, Bousser M G 1992 Pain as the only manifestation of internal carotid artery dissection. Cephalalgia 12: 314–317

Blanchard E B, Appelbaum K A, Guarnieri P, Morrill B, Dentinger M P 1987 Five year follow-up on the treatment of chronic headache with biofeedback and/or relaxation. Headache 27: 580–583

Blau J N 1980 Migraine prodromes separated from the aura: complete migraine. British Medical Journal 281: 658–660

Blume H, Kakolewski R, Richardson R 1982 Radiofrequency denaturation in occipital pain: results in 450 cases. Applied Neurophysiology 45: 543–548

Bovim G, Sand T 1992 Cervicogenic headache, migraine without aura and tension-type headache. Diagnostic blockade of greater occipital and supraorbital nerves. Pain 51: 43–48

Bovim G, Fredriksen T A, Stolt-Nielsen A, Sjaastad O 1992 Neurolysis of the greater occipital nerve in cervicogenic headache. A follow-up study. Headache 32: 175–179

Bures J, Buresova O, Krivanek J 1974 The mechanism and applications of Leão's spreading depression of electroencephalographic activity. Academic Press, New York.

Buzzi G, Moskowitz M A 1992 The trigeminovascular system and migraine. Pathologie et Biologie 40: 313–317

Caekebeke J F V, Ferrari M D, Zwetsloot C P, Jansen J, Saxena P R 1992 Antimigraine drug sumatriptan increases blood flow velocity in large cerebral arteries during migraine attacks. Neurology 42: 1522–1526

Cephalagia 1988 Classification and diagnostic criteria for headache disorders, cranial neuralgias and facial pain. Cephalagia 8 (suppl 7)

Chalmers I M, Blair G S 1973 Rheumatoid arthritis of the temporomandibular joint. Quarterly Journal of Medicine 42: 369–386

Chalmers I M, Blair G S 1974 Is the temporomandibular joint involved in primary osteoarthrosis? Oral Surgery, Oral Medicine, Oral Pathology 38: 74–79

Chmelewski W L, McKnight K M, Agudelo C A, Wise C M 1992 Presenting features and outcomes in patients undergoing temporal artery biopsy: a review of 98 patients. Archives of Internal Medicine 152: 1690–1695

Chu M L, Shinnar S 1991 Headaches in children younger than 7 years of age. Archives of Neurology 49: 79–82

Cook J B 1972 The postconcussional syndrome and factors influencing after minor head injury admitted to hospital. Scandinavian Journal of Rehabilitation Medicine 4: 27–30

Costen J B 1934 A syndrome of ear and sinus symptoms dependent upon disturbed function of the temporomandibular joint. Annals of Otology Rhinology and Laryngology 43: 1–15

Dalessio D J 1989 Headache. In: Wall P D, Melzack R (eds) Textbook of pain, 2nd edn. Churchill Livingstone, Edinburgh, p 38: 386–401

D'Andrea G, Welch K M A, Riddle J M, Grunfeld S 1989 Platelet serotonin metabolism and ultrastructure in migraine. Archives of Neurology 46: 1187–1189

D'Andrea G, Cananzi A R, Joseph R et al 1991 Platelet glycine, glutamate and aspartate in primary headache. Cephalalgia 11: 197–200

Diamond S 1984 The value of biofeedback in the treatment of chronic headache: a four-year retrospective study. Headache 25: 5–18

Dichgans J, Diener H C, Gerber W D, Verspohl E J, Kukiolka H, Kluck M 1984 Analgetikainduzierter Dauerkopfsschmerz. Deutsche Medizinische Wochenschrift 109: 369–373

Diener H C, Scholz E, Dichgans J et al 1989 Central effects of drugs used in migraine prophylaxis evaluated by visual evoked potentials. Annals of Neurology 25: 125–130

Diener H C, Haab J, Peters C, Ried S, Dichgans J, Pilgrim A 1991 Subcutaneous sumatriptan in the treatment of headache during withdrawal from drug-induced headache. Headache 31: 205–209

Edmeads J 1986 Headache in cerebrovascular disease. In: Viken P J, Bruyn G W, Klawans H L (eds) Handbook of clinical neurology, vol 4(48), Rose F C (ed) Headache. Elsevier, Amsterdam, ch 18, p 273–290

Edmeads J 1988 The cervical spine and headache. Neurology 38: 1874–1878

Edmeads J 1992 Migraine – disease or syndrome? Pathologie et Biologie 40: 279–283

Ekbom K 1986 Chronic migrainous neuralgia. In: Vinken P J, Bruyn G W, Klawans H L (eds) Handbook of clinical neurology, vol 4(48), Rose F C (ed) Headache. Elsevier, Amsterdam ch 15, p 247–255

Feinmann C, Harris M, Cawley R 1984 Psychogenic facial pain: presentation and treatment. British Medical Journal 88: 436–438

Ferbert A, Busse D, Thron A 1991 Microinfarction in classic migraine? A study with magnetic resonance imaging findings. Stroke 22: 1010–1014

Ferrari M D 1992 Biochemistry of migraine. Pathologie et Biologie 40: 287–292

Ferrari M D, Odink J, Tapparelli C, Van Kempen G M J, Pennings E J M, Bruyn G W 1989 Serotonin metabolism in migraine. Neurology 39: 1239–1242

Ferrari M D, Odink J, Bos K D, Malessy M J A, Bruyn G W 1990 Neuroexcitatory plasma amino acids are elevated in migraine. Neurology 40: 1582–1586

Friberg L, Olesen J, Iversen H K, Sperling B 1991 Migraine pain associated with middle cerebral artery dilatation: reversal by sumatriptan. Lancet 338: 13–17

Goadsby P J, Edvinsson L 1987 Sumatriptan reverses the changes in calcitonin gene-related peptide seen in the headache phase of migraine. Cephalalgia (suppl 11): 3–4

Goadsby P J, Edvinsson L, Ekman R 1989 Extracerebral levels of circulating vasoactive peptides during migraine headache. Cephalalgia 9 (suppl 10): 292–293

Goadsby P J, Edvinsson L, Ekman R 1990 Vasoactive peptide release in the extracerebral circulation of humans during migraine headache. Annals of Neurology 28: 183–187

Göbel H, Schenkl 1989 Post-lumbar puncture headache: the relation between experimental suprathreshold pain sensitivity and a quasi-experimental clinical pain syndrome. Pain 40: 267–278

Graff-Radford S B, Reeves J L, Jaeger B 1987 Management of chronic head and neck pain: effectiveness of altering factors perpetuating myofascial pain. Headache 27: 180–185

Green M W, Selman J E 1991 The medical management of trigeminal neuralgia. Headache 31: 588–592

Hannerz J, Greitz D 1992 MRI of intracranial arteries in nitroglycerin induced cluster headache attacks. Headache 32: 485–488

Hannington E, Jones R J, Amess J A, Wachowicz B 1981 Migraine: a platelet disorder. Lancet 2: 720–723

Headache Classification Committee of the International Headache Society 1988 Classification and diagnostic criteria for headache disorders, cranial neuralgias and facial pain. Cephalalgia 8 (suppl 7): 9–96

Henry P 1992 Drug abuse in headache. Functional Neurology 6 (suppl 7): 5–6

Henry P, Dartigues J F, Benetier M P et al 1985 Ergotamine and analgesic induced headache. Controlled study of the use of electrical stimulation by high frequency current. In Clifford-Rose (ed) Migraine: clinical and research advances. Karger, Basle, p 195–207

Henry P, Michel P, Brochet B et al 1992 A nationwide survey of migraine in France: prevalence and clinical features in adults. Cephalalgia 12: 229–237

Hering R, Kuritzky A 1992 Sodium valproate in the prophylactic treatment of migraine: a double-blind study versus placebo. Cephalalgia 12: 81–84

Hickling E J, Blanchard E B, Silverman D J, Schwarz S P 1992 Motor vehicle accidents, headaches and post-traumatic stress disorder: assessment findings in a consecutive series. Headache 32: 147–151

Holroyd K A, Penzien D B, Holm J E, Hursey K G 1984 Behavioural treatment of tension and migraine headache: what does the literature say? Headache 24: 167–168

Humphrey P P A, Apperley E, Feniuk W, Perrin L J 1991 A rational approach to identifying a fundamentally new drug for the treatment of migraine. In: Saxena P R, Wallis D I, Wouters W, Vevan P (eds) Cardiovascular pharmacology of 5-hydroxytryptamine. Kluwer Academic, Hingham, Massachusetts, p 417–431

Jaeger B 1989 Are 'cervicogenic' headaches due to myofascial pain and cervical spine dysfunction? Cephalalgia 9: 157–164

Jannetta P J 1970 Observations on the etiology of trigeminal neuralgia, hemifacial spasm, acoustic nerve dysfunction and glossopharyngeal neuralgia: definitive microsurgical treatment and results in 117 cases. Neurochirurgia 20: 145–154

Jannetta P J 1981 Vascular decompression in trigeminal neuralgia. In: Samii M, Jannetta P J (eds) The cranial nerves. Springer, Berlin, p 331–340

Jensen O K, Nielsen F F 1990 The influence of sex and pre-traumatic headache on the incidence and severity of headache after head injury. Cephalalgia 1: 285–294

Jensen R, Rasmussen B K, Pedersen B, Olesen J 1993 Muscle tenderness and pressure pain thresholds in headache. A population study. Pain 52: 193–200

Kay D W K, Kerr T A, Lassman L P 1971 Brain trauma and the postconcussional syndrome. Lancet 2: 1052–1055

Kelly R E 1986 Post-traumatic headache. In : Vinken P J, Bruyn G W, Klawans H L (eds) Handbook of clinical neurology, vol 4(48), Rose F C (ed) Headache. Elsevier, Amsterdam, ch 26, p 383–390

Kennard C, Gawel M, Rudolph N, Clifford-Rose F 1978 Visual evoked potentials in migraine subjects. Research and Clinical Studies in Headache 6: 73–80

Kerr F W L 1961 Structural relation of the trigeminal spinal tract to upper cervical roots and the solitary nucleus in cat. Experimental Neurology 4: 134–148

Kroener-Herwig B, Weich K W 1989 Biofeedback in chronic headache: is phsyiological learning necessary for positive outcome? Cephalalgia 9 (suppl 10): 383–384

Kudrow L 1982 Paradoxical effects of frequent analgesic use. Advances in Neurology 3: 335–341

Kuntz K M, Kohmen E, Stevens J C, Miller P, Offord K P, Ho M M 1992 Post-lumbar puncture headaches: experience in 501 consecutive procedures. Neurology 42: 1884–1887

Lance J W 1992 The pathophysiology of migraine: a tentative synthesis. Pathologie et Biologie 40: 355–360

Lance J W, Lambert G A, Goadsby P J, Duckworth J W 1983 Brain-stem influences on the cephalic circulation: experimental data from cat and monkey of relevance to mechanisms of migraine. Headache 23: 258–265

Lascelles R G 1966 Atypical facial pain and depression. British Journal of Psychiatry 112: 651–659

Lashley K S 1941 Patterns of cerebral integration indicated by the scotomas of migraine. Archives of Neurology and Psychiatry 46: 331–339

Lauritzen M 1992 Spreading depression and migraine. Pathology et Biologie 40: 332–337

Leão A A 1944 Spreading depression of activity in cerebral cortex. Journal of Neurophysiology 7: 359–390

Leão A A, Morrison R S 1945 Propagation of spreading cortical depression. Journal of Neurophysiology 8: 33–35

Loeser J D, Calvin W H, Howe J F 1977 Pathophysiology of trigeminal neuralgia. Clinical Neurosurgery 24: 527–537

MacGregor E A, Chia H, Vohrah R C, Wilkinson M 1990 Migraine and menstruation: a pilot study. Cephalalgia 10: 305–310

Marcelis J, Silberstein S D 1991 Idiopathic intracranial hypertension without papilloedoma. Archives of Neurology 48: 392–399

Markus H S 1991 A prospective follow-up thunderclap headache mimicking subarachnoid haemorrhage. Journal of Neurology Neurosurgery and Psychiatry 54: 1117–1118

Massiou H, Bousser M-J 1992 Bêta-bloquants et migraine. Pathologie et Biologie 40: 373–380

Mathew N T 1987 Transformed or evolutive migraine. In: Clifford-Rose F (ed) Advances in headache research. John Libbey, London, p 241–247

Mathew N, Kurman R, Perez F 1990 Drug induced refractory headache. Headache 30: 634–638

Max B, Schafer S C, Culnane M, Smoller B, Dubner R, Gracely R H 1988 Amitriptyline, but not lorazepam, relieves post-herpetic neuralgia. Neurology 38: 1427–1432

Menzel J, Piotrowski W, Penholz H 1974 Long-term results of Gasserian ganglion electrocoagulation. Journal of Neurosurgery 42: 140–143

Mitsias P, Ramadan N M 1992 Headache in cerebrovascular disease. Part I: Clinical features. Cephalalgia 12: 269–274

Montastruc J L, Senard J M 1992 Médicaments anticalciques et prophylaxie de la migraine. Pathologie et Biologie 40: 381–388

Moskowitz M A 1984 Neurobiology of vascular head pain. Annals of Neurology 6: 157–168

Moskowitz M A 1988 Cluster headache: evidence for a pathophysiological focus in the superior pericarotid cavernous sinus plexus. Headache 28: 584–586

Moskowitz M A 1991 The visceral organ brain: implications for the pathophysiology of vascular head pain. Neurology 41: 182–186

Olesen J 1991 Clinical and pathophysiological observations in migraine and tension-type headache explained by integration of vascular, supraspinal and myofascial inputs. Pain 46: 125–132

Olesen J 1992 Cerebral blood flow in migraine with aura. Pathologie et Biologie 40: 318–324

Olesen J, Schoenen J 1993 Mechanisms of tension-type headache. Synthesis. In: Olesen J, Tfelt-Hansen P, Welch K M A (eds) The headaches. Raven Press, New York, ch 2

Olesen J, Larsen B, Lauritzen M 1981 Focal hyperemia followed by spreading oligemia and impaired activation of rCBF in classic migraine. Annals of Neurology 9: 344–352

Olesen J, Friberg L, Olsen T S et al 1990 Timing and topography of cerebral blood flow, aura, and headache during migraine attacks. Annals of Neurology 28: 791–798

Ollat H 1992 Agonistes et antagonistes de la sérotonine et migraine. Pathologie et Biologie 40: 389–396

Ollat H, Gurruchaga J M 1992 Plaquettes et migraine. Pathologie et Biologie 40: 305–312

Olsen T S, Friberg L, Larsen N A 1987 Ischemia may be the primary cause of the neurologic deficits in classic migraine. Archives of Neurology 44: 156–161

Pikoff H 1984 Is the muscular model of headache still viable? A review of conflicting data. Headache 24: 186–198

Pradalier A, Giroud M, Dry J 1987 Somnambulism, migraine and propranolol. Headache 27: 143–145

Ramadan N M, Halvorsen H, Vande-Linde A, Levine S R, Helpern J A, Welch K M A 1989 Low brain magnesium in migraine. Headache 29: 590–593

Rando T A, Fishman R A 1992 Spontaneous intracranial hypotension. Neurology 42: 481–487

Rasmussen B K, Olesen J 1992 Migraine with aura and migraine without aura: an epidemiological study. Cephalalgia 12: 221–228

Rasmussen B K, Jensen R, Schroll M, Olesen J 1991 Epidemiology of headache in a general population – a prevalence study. Journal of Clinical Epidemiology 44: 1147–1157

Rasmussen B K, Jensen R, Schroll M, Olesen J 1992 Interrelations between migraine and tension-type headache in the general population. Archives of Neurology 49: 914–918

Ross Russell R W 1986 Giant cell (cranial) arteritis. In: Vinken P J, Bruyn G W, Klawans H L (eds) Handbook of clinical neurology, vol. 4(48), Rose F C (ed) Headache. Elsevier, Amsterdam, ch 20, p 309–328

Russell W R 1932 Cerebral involvement in head injury; a study based on the examination of 200 cases. Brain 55: 549–570

Saper J R 1987 Ergotamine dependency. A review. Headache 27: 435–438

Schoenen J 1989 Exteroceptive silent periods of temporalis muscle in headache. In: Van Steenberghe D, de Laat A (eds) EMG of jaw reflexes in man. Leuven University Press, p 357–368

Schoenen J 1992 Clinical neurophysiology studies in headache: a review of data and pathophysiological hints. Functional Neurology 7: 191–204

Schoenen J 1993a Tension-type headaches: neurophysiology. In: Olesen J, Tfelt-Hansen P, Welch K M A (eds) The headaches. Raven Press, New York, ch 2

Schoenen J 1993b Exteroceptive suppression of temporalis muscle activity: methodological and physiological aspects. Cephalalgia 13: 3–10

Schoenen J 1993c Exteroceptive suppression of temporalis muscle activity in patients with chronic headache and in normal volunteers: methodology, clinical and pathophysiological relevance. Headache 33: 3–17

Schoenen J, Maertens de Noordhout A 1988 The role of the sympathetic nervous system in migraine and cluster headache. In: Olesen J, Edvinsson L (eds) Basis mechanisms of headache. Pain research and clinical management. Elsevier, Amsterdam, vol 2 ch 34, p 393–410

Schoenen J, Timsit-Berthier M 1993 Contingent negative variation: methods and potential interest in headache. Cephalalgia 13: 28–32

Schoenen J, Maertens de Noordhout A, Timsit-Berthier M, Timsit M 1985 Contingent negative variation (CNV) as a diagnostic and physiopathologic tool in headache patients. In: Clifford Rose F (ed) Clinical and research advances. Karger, Basle, p 17–25

Schoenen J, Maertens de Noordhout A, Timsit-Berthier M, Timsit M 1986 Contingent negative variation and efficacy of beta-blocking agents in migraine. Cephalalgia 6: 229–233

Schoenen J, Jamart B, Delwaide P J 1987a Topographic EEG mapping in common and classic migraine during and between attacks. In: Clifford Rose F (ed) Advances in headache research. Smith Gordon, London, p 25–33

Schoenen J, Jamart B, Delwaide P J 1987b Cartographie électroencéphalographique dans les migraines en périodes critique et intercritique. Revue d'Electroencephalographie et de Neurophysiologie Clinique 17: 259–270

Schoenen J, Jamart B, Gérard P, Lenarduzzi P, Delwaide P J 1987c Exteroceptive suppression of temporalis muscle activity in chronic headache. Neurology 37: 1834–1836

Schoenen J, Lenarduzzi P, Sianard-Gainko 1989 Chronic headaches associated with analgesics and/or ergotamine abuse: a clinical survey of 434 consecutive out patients. In: Clifford Rose F (ed) New advances in headache research. Smith Gordon, London, p 255–259

Schoenen J, Sianard-Gainko J, Lenaerts M 1991a Blood magnesium levels in migraine. Cephalalgia 11: 97–99

Schoenen J, Gérard P, De Pasqua V, Sianard-Gainko J 1991b Multiple clinical and paraclinical analyses of chronic tension-type headache associated or unassociated with disorder of pericranial muscles. Cephalalgia 11: 135–139

Schoenen J, Gérard P, De Pasqua V, Juprelle M 1991c EMG activity in pericranial muscles during postural variation and mental activity in healthy volunteers and patients with chronic tension-type headache. Headache 31: 321–324

Schoenen J, Bottin D, Hardy F, Gérard P 1991d Cephalic and extracephalic pressure pain thresholds in chronic tension-type headache. Pain 47: 145–149

Schoenen J, Broux R, Moonen G 1992 Unilateral facial pain as the first symptom of lung cancer: are there diagnostic clues? Cephalalgia 12: 178–179

Schokker P 1989 Craniomandibular disorders in headache patients. Thesis, University of Amsterdam

Sicuteri F 1986 Migraine, a central biochemical dysnociception. Headache 16: 145–149

Siegfried J 1981 Percutaneous controlled thermocoagulation of Gasserian ganglion in trigeminal neuralgia: experience with 1000 cases. In: Samii M, Jannetta P J (eds): The cranial nerves. Springer, Berlin, p 322–330

Silberstein S D, Marcelis J 1992 Headache associated with changes in intracranial pressure. Headache 32: 84–94

Sjaastad O 1986a Cluster headache. In: Vinken P J, Bruyn G W, Klawans H L (eds) Handbook of clinical neurology, vol. 4(48). Rose F C (ed). Headache. Elsevier, Amsterdam, ch 14, p 217–246

Sjaastad O 1986b Chronic paroxysmal hemicrania (CPH). In: Vinken P J, Bruyn G W, Klawans H L (eds) Handbook of clinical neurology, vol. 4(48). Rose F C (ed) Headache. Elsevier, Amsterdam ch 16, p 257–266

Sjaastad O, Dale I 1974 Evidence for a new (?) treatable headache entity. Headache 14: 105–108

Sjaastad O, Saunte C, Salvesen R et al 1989 Shortlasting, unilateral, neuralgiform headache attacks with conjunctival injection, tearing, sweating, and rhinorrhea. Cephalalgia 9: 147–156

Sjaastad O, Fredriksen T A, Pfaffenrath V 1990 Cervicogenic headache: diagnostic criteria. Headache 30: 25–26

Steiner T J, Couturier E G M, Catarci T, Hering R 1992 Social aspects of drug abuse in headache. Functional Neurology 6 (suppl 7): 11–14

Stewart W F, Lipton R B, Celentano D D, Reed M L 1992 Prevalence of migraine headache in the United States. JAMA 267: 64–69

Taarnhoj P 1982 Decompression of the posterior trigeminal root in trigeminal neuralgia: a 30 year follow-up review. Journal of Neurosurgery 57: 14–17

Tehindrazanarivelo A D, Lutz G, Petitjean C, Bousser M G 1992 Headache following carotid endarterectomy: a prospective study. Cephalalgia 12: 380–382

Thie A, Fuhlendorf A, Spitzer K, Kunze K 1990 Transcranial doppler evaluation of common and classic migraine. Part II. Ultrasonic features during attacks. Headache 30: 209–215

Turkewitz J L, Wirth O, Dawson G A, Casaly J S 1992 Cluster headache following head injury: a case report and review of the literature. Headache 32: 504–506

Vilming S T, Schrader H, Monstad I 1988 Post-lumbar puncture headache: the significance of body posture. A controlled study of 300 patients. Cephalalgia 8: 75–78

Wall M 1990 The headache profile of idiopathic intracranial hypertension. Cephalalgia 10: 331–335

Wallasch T M, Reinecke R, Langohr H D 1990 Exterozeptive Suppression der Temporalis Muskelaktivität bei Kopfschmerzen. Nervenheilkunde 9: 58–60

Watson C P N, Evans R J 1988 Post-herpetic neuralgia: 208 cases. Pain 35: 289–297

Watson C P N, Watt V R, Chipman M, Birkett N, Evans R J 1991 The prognosis with post-herpetic neuralgia. Pain 46: 195–199

Watson C P N, Chipman M, Reed K, Evans R J, Birkett N 1992 Amitriptyline versus maprotiline in post-herpetic neuralgia: a randomized, double blind, cross-over trial. Pain 8: 29–36

Weiss H D, Stern B J, Goldberg J 1991 Post-traumatic migraine: chronic migraine precipitated by minor head or neck trauma. Headache 31: 451–456

Welch K M A 1987 Migraine, a biobehavioural disorder. Archives of Neurology 44: 323–327

Welch K M A, Levine S R, D'Andrea G, Schultz L, Helpern J A 1989 Preliminary observations on brain energy metabolism in migraine studied by in vivo 31-phosphorus NMR spectroscopy. Neurology 39: 538–541

Wijdicks E F, Kerkhoff H, van Gijn J 1988 Long-term follow-up of 71 patients with thunderclap headache mimicking subarachnoid haemorrhage. Lancet 2: 68–70

Yamaguchi M 1992 Incidence of headache and severity of head injury. Headache 32: 427–431

BIBLIOGRAPHY

Blau J N (ed) 1987 Migraine: clinical, therapeutic, conceptual and research aspects. Chapman and Hall, London

Dalessio D J (ed) 1980 Wolff's headache and other head pain. Oxford University Press, New York

Ekbom K (ed) 1993 On behalf of the European Headache Federation (EHF). Migraine for general practitioners. Smith Gordon, London

Lance J W (ed) 1982 The mechanisms and management of headache, 4th edn. Butterworths, London

Lance J W (ed) 1986 Migraine and other headaches. Scribner, New York

Nappi G, Savoldi F (eds) 1985 Headache: diagnostic system and taxonomic criteria. John Libbey, London

Olesen J, Edvinsson L (eds) 1988 Basic mechanisms of headache. Pain research and clinical management, vol 2. Elsevier, Amsterdam

Olesen J, Saxena P R (eds) 1992 5-Hydroxytryptamine mechanisms in primary headaches. Frontiers in headache research, vol 2. Raven Press, New York

Olesen J, Schoenen J (eds) 1993 Tension-type headache: classification, mechanisms and treatment. Frontiers in headache research, vol 3. Raven Press, New York

Olesen J, Tfelt-Hansen P, Welch K M A (eds) 1993 The headaches. Raven Press, New York

Sjaastad O (ed) 1992 Cluster headache syndrome. Major problems in neurology, vol 23. W B Saunders, London

Wolff H G (ed) 1963 Headache and other head pain. Oxford University Press, New York

28. Pain of burns

Manon Choinière

Severe burn injuries are among the most devastating forms of trauma which require highly specialised, intensive and prolonged treatment. Burn injuries affect the victims both physically and psychologically, causing an atrocious type of pain. Hospitalised for weeks or months, burn victims must face pain every day; they suffer not only the pain of their injuries but also the pain due to the multiple therapeutic procedures that are carried out during the course of treatment. Burn pain ranges from mild to excruciating, and is difficult to manage due to wide variations in the patients' analgesic requirements. Because the adverse effects of uncontrolled pain may affect the patient's recovery, strategies to provide optimal pain control are essential. Although efforts have been made to correct deficiencies in analgesic practices, effective pain control continues to be a problem in many burn care facilities.

This chapter provides an overview of the pain problems associated with burn injuries. After a brief review of some epidemiological and clinical features of this type of injury, various components of burn pain are described. Data on the intensity, time course and aetiology of the pain are presented along with a discussion of psychological and other influencing factors. In the final section, current pain-control methods and various issues in the management of burn pain are discussed, with particular emphasis on pharmacotherapy.

BURNS: EPIDEMIOLOGICAL AND CLINICAL ASPECTS

More than 2 million burn accidents occur each year in the USA. Thermal burns (contact with hot liquids, objects or flames) are by far the most frequent, followed by electrical and chemical burns. Of these injuries, 3–5% are sufficiently severe to require hospitalisation (Artz 1979; Demling 1985; Demling & Lalonde 1989).

Burn severity is determined by the depth, extent and location of the injuries. Burn depth is classified into three degrees. First-degree burns involve the superficial layer of epidermis and heal within 1 week without scarring; they are characterised by erythema and generate pain of mild to moderate intensity. Second degree burns involve variable portions of deep epidermis and dermis, and usually take from 1–3 weaks to heal. Superficial second-degree burns are extremely painful, since the nerve endings are exposed to stimulation. In deep second-degree burns, pain is still present but less intense than in more superficial burns, since many nerve endings have been destroyed. Third-degree burns involve destruction of the entire epidermis and dermis. Since no residual epidermal cells are present for repopulation, the wounds can heal only by skin grafting or through a long process of wound contraction. Third-degree burns are usually painless because all nerve endings are destroyed. However, pain may be felt initially because the areas are surrounded by more superficial burns from which pain arises (Demling 1990; Freund & Marvin 1990).

Management of severe burn injuries can be separated into three phases: acute, subacute and rehabilitative. During the acute or resuscitation phase, which usually lasts 2–3 days, priorities are directed towards hypovolaemia management, respiratory function maintenance and infection control. The subacute phase that follows lasts until complete wound closure. This phase is focused on burn wound care and involves numerous nursing procedures, surgical debridement, skin grafting, physiotherapy and occupational therapy. Once all the wounds are closed, the patient enters the rehabilitative phase. Management is focused on functional rehabilitation, scarring control and contracture prevention, which may involve serial reconstruction surgeries. This phase covers the final period of hospitalisation and may last up to a few years (Pruitt 1979; Demling & Lalonde 1989; Waymack & Pruitt 1990).

COMPONENTS OF BURN PAIN

Burn pain is not a single entity but involves several components which cause the patient to experience one of the most severe and prolonged types of pain (Fagerhaugh

1974; Perry et al 1981; Charlton et al 1983; Ahrenholz & Solem 1987; Choinière et al 1989; Freund & Marvin 1990; Mackersie & Karagianes 1990; Kinsella & Booth 1991). The first component of burn pain is related to the injury itself and is felt at the wound site and surrounding areas. Patients report feeling this pain relatively constantly and it can be exacerbated by any movement of the affected areas or even by simple acts such as breathing. Donor sites (the areas of normal skin which have been harvested for grafting) also elicit a similar type of pain, since donor sites mimic superficial second-degree burns. Patients report that donor sites are sometimes even more painful than the burn injuries themselves (Osgood & Szyfelbein 1989; Kavanagh et al 1991).

The second component of burn pain is related to the multiple therapeutic procedures carried out during the course of treatment. These painful procedures, which occur daily or even several times a day, include dressing changes, debridement (excision of necrotic tissue in a tub or at the bedside), application of topical antimicrobial agents, hydrotherapy and physiotherapy. Other sources of pain related to treatment include the enforced immobilisation of limbs in splints and special garments, surgical debridement and grafting, and care of donor sites.

Finally, a third component of burn pain is related to the tissue regeneration and healing process. As newly regenerated skin buds emerge, pain is commonly experienced along with intense tingling or itching sensations which may be almost as unpleasant as the pain itself (Fagerhaugh 1974; Giuliani & Perry 1985; Ahrenholz & Solem 1987). Additionally, the healing process may lead to the formation of contractures and hypertrophic scars, especially in wounds that heal through granulation and in donor sites that have been harvested more than once. This healing process may continue for months or even years and pain or paraesthetic sensations may persist after completion of scar formation (Pruitt 1979; Ahrenholz & Solem 1987; Ward et al 1989; Freund & Marvin 1990; Choinière et al 1991).

Except for a few anecdotal reports (McBride 1979; Ton 1984; Lane & Hogan 1985; Racz et al 1988), the problem of chronic pain in healed wounds is poorly documented in the burn literature. Probably, cases often go undiagnosed because they coincide with postinjury depression syndrome (Marvin & Heimback 1985; Freund & Marvin 1990). Furthermore, a large number of patients are lost to follow-up care because of the long-term nature of the recovery process (Knudson-Cooper 1984). Two recent studies (Ward et al 1989; Choinière et al 1991) support the hypothesis that the prevalence of chronic pain problems in burn patients has been underestimated in the literature. In their study, Choinière et al (1991) found that more than 80% of the 104 patients interviewed 1 year or more after their accident reported paraesthesic sensations (e.g tingling, cold sensations, numbness, etc.) and 35% complained of pain at the burn injury site. Further analysis revealed that these problems may persist for many years after the accident, be present every day and interfere with the patients' daily activities such as work, sleep and social life. Since variations in the sensations were often reported to be weather-related (Ward et al 1989; Choinière et al 1991), it is possible that the prevalence of chronic sensory problems may vary in different climates. Further studies are needed to address this issue.

PAIN INTENSITY

Burn pain is described by many patients as the worst they had ever experienced (Fagerhaugh 1974; Charlton et al 1983; Mannon 1985). However, it would be erroneous to believe that burn patients suffer atrocious pain continuously. Furthermore, the most severe pain does not appear to be related to the injury itself but to intermittent trauma caused by the various therapeutic procedures. Choinière et al (1989) used the McGill Pain Questionnaire (Melzack 1975) and visual analogue scales to measure pain in a group of adult burn patients at different times of the day. Consistent with earlier clinical reports (Perry et al 1981; Szyfelbein et al 1985), this study revealed that the pain is relatively mild, on average, when the patients are at rest. In contrast, when they undergo therapeutic procedures (e.g. dressing changes), significantly more pain is experienced and its intensity can reach extremely high levels. Similar results were observed in burn children by Atchison et al (1991). In another study with burn children, Szyfelbein et al (1985) measured pain at different times during dressing changes and found wide fluctuations over the course of the procedure, ranging from mild pain (e.g. when the superficial layers of the bandage were removed) to very severe pain (e.g. when the innermost layers of gauze were detached from skin).

Choinière et al (1989) and Atchison et al (1991) have demonstrated that pain intensity varies considerably from one patient to another, especially during therapeutic procedures. This finding contrasts with earlier results (Perry et al 1981) in which procedural pain was described as severe to excruciating by most patients. This is probably due to the fact that the patients in the latter study described the greatest pain they had during procedures. In the most recent studies (Choinière et al 1989; Atchison et al 1991), pain measures were collected during or right after the therapeutic procedures. The type, duration and extent of these procedures varied among patients depending on their therapeutic needs, and this probably explains the wider variation in pain scores. Such variation means, however, that standard and inflexible doses of analgesics are quite likely to be inadequate for pain relief in burn patients.

In all the above-mentioned studies, even though most patients received analgesic medication prior to the therapeutic procedures, many of them reported intense pain levels, thereby bringing into question the adequacy of the analgesic therapy. In their study with burn children, Atchison et al (1991) denounced the fact that fixed doses of oral opioids were usually administered for procedural pain without taking into consideration the patient's weight, burn size and number of days postburn. This may also explain why the pain intensity associated with therapeutic procedures varied widely from one patient to another.

In summary, burn pain can best be described as a conditioned in which the patients experience a background pain of relatively low intensity upon which are superimposed episodes of severe pain due to treatments.

TIME COURSE OF THE PAIN

Burn pain usually begins a few minutes after the injury. However, some victims may experience a painfree period which persists from several minutes to hours. In Choinière et al's study (1989), more than one-third of the burn patients reported a painfree period after the injury. This percentage is remarkably similar to that observed by Melzack et al (1982) after other types of injury. Wall (1979) has proposed that pain may be inhibited for a period after an injury to permit other behavioural and physiological responses that have greater biological priorities for adaptation and survival. This may explain why burn victims are often seen perfoming unbelievable actions such as rescuing others, extinguishing flames with their hands or walking for miles to find help, with apparently little or no perception of pain (Fagerhaugh 1974; Beales 1983; Marvin & Heimbach 1984, 1985). Individual differences in pain onset may also be related to the fact that severe burn injuries often put the victims in a state of physiological or psychological shock which renders them less responsive to stimuli, including painful ones (Andreasen et al 1972; Watkins et al 1988). Finally, pain may also be absent or minimal at first because nerve endings have been destroyed as a result of deep injuries (Demling 1990; Freund & Marvin 1990).

Depending upon the duration of hospitalisation, the pain then persists for weeks or months. The patient is confronted with pain on a daily basis and, unlike other types of pain, such as postsurgical pain, it does not decline with time. Choinière et al (1989) measured pain in a group of hospitalised burn patients and found wide fluctuations in the pain intensity ratings from day to day with high pain levels being reported even in the late phases of treatment. No significant relationship was found between the pain scores obtained at rest and the length of time elapsed since injury. These findings have important clinical implications in terms of the patients' analgesic requirements. For various reasons, including the fear of addiction or due to a misconception about burn pain, the medical staff may be inclined to decrease the patient's medication as times goes on. However, the patient may suffer as much or more pain in the intermediate or late phases of treatment, since new sources of pain are introduced. Thus, patients may feel less pain at the injury site as healing progresses or when skin grafts are applied, but they may now have to endure other pains such as the pain associated with nerve regeneration or the pain at the donor site.

The intensity of the pain experienced during therapeutic procedures may also increase rather than decrease over time, especially during lengthy and repetitive dressing changes. Several clinical reports in burn adults and children (Andreasen et al 1972; Fagerhaugh 1974; Savendra 1977; Avni 1980; Beales 1983; Kelley et al 1984; Watkins et al 1988; Osgood & Szyfelbein 1989, 1990; Kavanagh et al 1991) suggest that many patients experience increasing discomfort during dressing changes, manifested by a decrease in pain threshold and/or pain tolerance. Various factors have been proposed to explain why the patient pain during treatment may worsen with time. These include:

1. a return of normal sensation in the burn wounds
2. an increase in apprehension and anticipatory anxiety about treatment to come
3. a gradual loss of energy and fatigue due to sleep disturbance and repetitive episodes of intense procedural pain
4. respondant and operant conditioning of pain responses.

Finally, towards the end of hospitalisation, the pain eventually decreases to reach minimal levels. As mentioned earlier, however, a certain number of patients develop postburn neuralgia at the site of injury, which can persist for variable periods of time ranging from weeks to several years (Ward et al 1989; Freund & Marvin 1990; Choinière et al 1991).

INTERINDIVIDUAL VARIABILITY

Pain perception can be greatly influenced by medical, demographic, personal, situational and psychological factors. The sources of variability in the amount of pain experienced by burn patients are not well understood and the literature provides little scientific information on this issue.

Medical factors

Contrary to common belief, burn severity does not appear to be a good predictor of the amount of pain experienced by the patients. Several studies which have measured pain or pain behaviours in adult patients (Klein & Charlton 1980; Perry et al 1981; Choinière et al 1989; Van der

Does 1989) failed to find any significant correlation between pain and various severity indices such as the size, depth or location of the burns. These negative findings may be partly due to the fact that burn severity was assessed at the time of admission while the pain measures were taken several days or often several weeks after injury without taking into account the current clinical condition of the patients' wounds. Choinière et al (1989) reanalysed their data using only the pain observations made during the first week after injury. The size of the first-degree burns was also included in the calculation of the burn surface since these superficial burns are known to be painful. The analysis revealed that burn patients with more extensive injuries tended to report significantly more pain both at rest and during therapeutic procedures. However, this relationship did not hold up after the first week after injury. After this period, patients with small injuries may report as much pain as patients with larger burns.

Szyfelbein et al (1985) and Atchison et al (1991) conducted two studies on burn children in which they examined whether pain intensity during dressing changes varied as a function of burn size. A significant correlation was found between the measures; children with larger burns tended to report more pain during dressing changes. The authors insisted, however, that even if pain intensity and burn size were interrelated, all patients reported a range of pain intensity from mild to severe, over the course of their treatment.

Atchison et al (1991) also found a significant relationship between the children's pain scores and the percentage of third-degree burns; the larger the area of full-thickness burn, the greater the pain reported by the children. As pointed out by the authors, this finding has important clinical implications since it can help to dispel the notion that 'third-degree burns don't hurt'. Full-thickness burns involve destruction of the nerve endings but the areas are often intermingled with and/or surrounded by more superficial burns from which pain arises. Furthermore, the clinical condition of the wounds changes over time, thereby altering pain sensations: the areas usually become more sensitive following debridement or as a result of nerve regeneration (Osgood & Szyfelbein 1989; Demling 1990; Freund & Marvin 1990; Atchison et al 1991).

None of the above studies provides information on whether first-, second- and third-degree burns differ in pain intensity. Clinically, however, superficial second-degree burns are generally recognised as being the most painful type of burns, at least in the first few days after injury (Demling 1990; Freund & Marvin 1990). In contrast, deeper burn injuries require longer hospitalisation, multiple manipulations (e.g. dressing changes) and frequent surgical interventions, all of which may contribute to increased pain sensitivity over time (Osgood & Szyfelbein 1989; Atchison et al 1991).

Sociodemographic and personal history variables

According to the results of several studies (Klein & Charlton 1980; Perry et al 1981; Choinière et al 1989; Van der Does 1989), the degree of pain or the incidence of pain behaviours in adult burn patients cannot be predicted on the basis of age, sex, ethnicity, education, occupation or socioeconomic status. In burn children, Atchison et al (1991) also failed to find any significant relationship between age and the amount of pain reported by the patients.

There is now clear evidence which refutes the myth that infants and children do not feel pain as keenly as adults (Anand & Hickey 1987; McGrafth 1990). In the field of burn pain, there is no reason to believe that the experience is different in adults and children. Studies which have measured burn pain levels in each group show similar results (Perry et al 1981; Szyfelbein et al 1985; Choinière et al 1989; Atchison et al 1991). In a large survey of USA burn unit staff (Perry & Heidrich 1982), the respondents also felt that the degree of pain experienced by adults and children is comparable. Some clinical observations suggest, however, that the two groups may differ in their behavioural expression of pain, the incidence of pain behaviours (screaming, noncompliance, etc.) probably being higher in children (Fagerhaugh 1974; Savedra 1977; Klein & Charlton 1980). Fagerhaugh (1974) proposed that sociological factors such as attitude of the medical staff towards pain expression as well as the support and pressure of the patient group are probably more efficient in controlling pain expression in adults than in children. Other variables such as history of drug abuse, alchoholism or psychiatric antecedents do not significantly influence the degree of pain or the incidence of pain behaviours in burn adults (Klein & Charlton 1980; Perry et al 1981).

Anxiety and anticipation of pain

Pain and anxiety have been described by Wall (1979) as two indissoluble reactions or aspects of the same phenomenon triggered by severe tissue injury. That anxiety is a cardinal feature in the recovery process of burn patients (adults and children) is well documented in the literature. As in other acute pain states (Wall 1979), burn patients experience anxiety about the past (circumstances of the injury, blame, guilt, etc.), present anxiety about the treatment in progress and anxiety about the future (survival, prolonged suffering, appearance, ability to work, etc.) (Andreasen et al 1972; Steiner & Clark 1977; Watkins et al 1988, 1992; Osgood & Szyfelbein 1989; Konigova 1992).

Of particular interest is the anxiety about treatment. Without effective analgesic medication, considerable pain may be experienced during therapeutic procedures. As a result, the patient becomes fearful and anxious about treatment. Expectation of pain, in turn, increases the amount of pain experienced during therapeutic procedures and creates a vicious cycle in which pain is increased by anxiety and vice versa (Andreasen et al 1972; Watkins et al 1988, 1992). In burn children, several authors (Beales 1983; Kavanagh 1983a, b; Osgood & Szyfelbein 1989) have described how anticipation of the dressing changes often elicits fear and anxiety that undoubtedly magnify the child's pain perception during the event and lead to disruptive behaviours which render pain management extremely difficult.

Unfortunately, however, few systematic studies have evaluated the relationship between anxiety and pain levels in burn patients. Charlton et al (1983) administered the State-Trait Anxiety Inventory (STAI) (Spielberger et al 1970) to a group of burn adults. State anxiety levels were comparable to those seen in general medical/surgical patients, but the few patients with very high state anxiety scores presented pain problems which were difficult to manage. In a more recent study, Choinière et al (1989) analysed the relationship between anxiety levels in burn patients and the pain felt at rest and during therapeutic procedures, using the McGill Pain Questionnaire, the STAI and visual analogue scales. The results confirmed that anxiety and pain are interrelated in burn patients: the more anxious the patients were, the more pain they tended to report at rest. Surprisingly, however, high levels of anxiety were not necessarily associated with high pain scores during therapeutic procedures.

Other psychological factors

To be severely burned is a devastating experience, not only from a physical but also from a psychological point of view. The injury itself is frightening and, during hospitalisation, the patient must face helplessness, pain, dependency and the possibility of disfigurement, deformity and death. Many burn patients experience various forms of psychological distress during their hospitalisation. These reactions can take the form of a normal process of psychological adaptation to the injury (e.g. sadness, depression, sleep disturbance, anger, frustration, fear, anxiety, dread) or degenerate into frank psychiatric disorders (e.g. delirium, adjustment disorders, major depression, posttraumatic stress disorder). Preexisting psychopathology may also complicate the situation (Andreasen et al 1972; Steiner & Clark 1977; Watkins et al 1988, 1992; Bernstein et al 1992; Konigova 1992). Several authors have divided the process of psychological adaptation after burn injury into phases or stages, each one characterised by different types of psychological reactions. Comprehensive reviews of these reactions are provided by Avni (1980), Steiner & Clark (1977) and Watkins et al (1988).

Few systematic studies have examined the interrelationship between psychological disturbances in burn patients and the pain experience itself. The literature on this issue is mainly based on clinical observations and anecdotal reports. Several authors (Andreasen et al 1972; Steiner & Clark 1977; Watkins et al 1988, 1992) have noted that prolonged, intense suffering is a central feature in many of the acute psychological disturbances observed in burn patients. These reactions are expressed by hostile, dependent, apathetic or depressive attitudes and behaviours which are centered around the issue of pain. Kavanagh (1983a, 1983b) has presented evidence that intolerable pain contributes to the emotional responses of the burn child, including severe anxiety, depression, aggression and regression.

Conversely, negative emotional states engendered by the burn injuries, such as anxiety or depression, may directly increase the amount of pain the patient perceives, Several authors (Andreasen et al 1972; Avni 1980; Watkins et al 1988, 1992) have related the decrease in the patient's pain threshold and tolerance observed in the second phase of hospitalisation to the amount of anxiety or depression usually experienced during this period.

Choinière et al (1989) measured depression levels in a group of burn patients and found small but significant correlations with their pain scores: high depression levels were associated with greater pain. A similar relationship was observed with anxiety levels (see previous section). These authors and Charlton et al (1983) also found that patients who had been in the hospital for a longer time tended to be more depressed or anxious. These findings suggest that psychological interventions aimed at controlling anxiety, depression and pain would benefit patients if they were introduced relatively early in the course of treatment so as to prevent the acceleration of these problems.

Only one other study examined the relationship between acute psychiatric complications and pain. Perry et al (1987) compared hospitalised burn patients with and without a diagnosis of acute posttraumatic stress disorder (PTSD), and found that those patients with PTSD symptoms reported significantly more intense pain during treatment (debridement) and at rest; however, they also had larger burns than the other group. Such results must be interpreted with caution, mainly because their correlational nature does not allow any inference of a causal link between psychiatric complications and pain. The same is true for the remaining literature on this issue. Whether acute psychological disturbances predispose burn patients to heightened sensitivity to pain or vice versa is unknown and requires further investigation.

PAIN-GENERATING MECHANISMS

Several neural and chemical pain-generating mechanisms are involved in burn injuries. The immediate pain following the burn is due to damage to skin nerve endings, which gives rise to a high-frequency burst of impulses transmitted to the brain. Then, the nerve endings which have been completely destroyed become silent until they regenerate and become exposed to stimulation. In contrast, the nerve endings which are intact or only partially damaged continue to generate impulses (Melzack & Wall 1982; Woolf 1989).

Soon after the burn injury, there is an inflammatory response which involves the release of chemical substances such as histamine, bradykinin and prostaglandins. These substances sensitise the nociceptors, producing pain in and around the injured sites. Peripheral and central mechanisms have also been suggested to explain the spread of pain to surrounding areas (Melzack & Wall 1982; Woolf 1989).

Laboratory studies with humans and animals (Meyer & Campbell 1981; Campbell et al 1984; Coderre & Melzack 1985, 1987) further suggest that thermal injuries produce hyperalgesia in the damaged site and surrounding unburned areas. Hyperalgesia is characterised by a decrease in pain threshold and by spontaneous pain. This may result from sensitisation of A-fibre nociceptor afferents at the injury site (Meyer & Campbell 1981) and from changes in the central nervous system (e.g. spinal cord hyperexcitability), leading to a facilitation of afferent signals (Coderre & Melzack 1987; Wall 1988; Woolf 1989; Katz et al 1991). Considering that any manipulation of the burn injury site (e.g. movement, dressing changes, debridement) also triggers the previously described neural and chemical mechanisms, it is not surprising that more pain is felt during treatment than at rest and that pain sensitivity may increase over time.

Some animal and human studies (Szyfelbein et al 1985; Osgood et al 1987; Deitch et al 1988) further suggest that endogenous opioid substances (beta-endorphins) may also modulate pain perception after a burn injury and thereby account for some of the variability in pain perception among inviduals and even in the same patient from day to day (Levine 1984; Osgood & Szyfelbein 1989, 1990).

Recently, other clinical observations (Atchison et al 1991; Jonsson et al 1991) have suggested that some components of burn pain may, to an extent, resemble neuropathic pain, especially if the injury is deep or extensive. These may develop several days or weeks after the injury and may frequently persist as a chronic pain syndrome. Neuropathic-like pain must be distinguished from pain arising in other damaged tissue and must be treated differently (Atchison et al 1991; Ready & Edwards 1992). Clinical experience reveals cases of severely burned patients whose pain is relatively refractory to opioids, even in very high doses (Wermeling et al 1986; Osgood & Szyfelbein 1989). Because severe burns damage nerve receptors and fibres, this may, at least in part, account for the opioid-resistant quality of the pain similar to that observed in neuropathic pain (Casey 1988). This interesting hypothesis merits further study considering its relevance for analgesic therapy.

Chronic sensory problems in the healed wounds may also be related to damage to underlying nerve structures. Paraesthesic and/or painful sensations may persist as a result of abnormalities in regenerated nerve endings or deficiencies in the reinnervation of the scarred tissue (Pontén 1960; Pruitt 1979; Terzis 1976; Hermanson et al 1986). This phenomenon has been observed in other types of injury of peripheral nerves (Melzack & Wall 1982; Devor 1989; Levitt 1990). Central mechanisms may be involved as well. Some studies (Devor & Wall 1981; Wall & Cusick 1984; Katz et al 1991) suggest that peripheral nerve lesions trigger changes in spinal, subcortical and cortical pathways that may modify sensory information. The mechanisms involved in postburn neuralgia are far from being understood. The possible resemblance to neuropathic pain and the interesting idea of a parallel between phantom limb pain and 'phantom skin' evoked by Atchison et al (1991) need to be explored.

PAIN MANAGEMENT

Local treatment

The various nursing and surgical techniques used to treat burn wounds affect the patient's pain experience. In the immediate postburn period, prompt cooling of the wound may reduce the pain (Davies 1982). Then, covering the burn wounds with dressings (closed method) may also provide some pain relief but the frequent dressing changes which must be performed several times a day cause considerable discomfort to the patient. In some burn centres, the wounds are first treated by exposure to dry warm air (open method). Burns treated with this method are generally believed to be more painful than those which are immediately covered with dressings (Demling 1985; Hurt & Eriksson 1986).

Early surgical debridement and skin grafting can also minimise pain in burn patients. This approach obviates the need for long, painful and debilitating sessions of bedside debridement and may result in improvement in long-term function by minimising hypertrophic scarring (Helm et al 1982; Demling & Lalonde 1989; Waymack & Pruitt 1990). The use of splints and external pressure (garments) may further help to control the development of hypertrophic scars and contractures (Parks et al 1978; Larson et al 1979) and, thereby, may reduce the chances of developing long-term pain and paraesthesia problems.

Pharmacological treatment

Problems and deficiencies in analgesic therapy for burn patients

Pharmacotherapy occupies a central place in the management of pain in burn patients. However, wide variations exist in analgesic practices and major deficiencies have been pointed out. The fact that analgesic requirements are often underestimated in burn patients is well documented in the literature (Heidrich et al 1981; Perry et al 1981; Perry & Heidrich 1982; Perry 1984; Choinière et al 1989, 1990; Osgood & Szyfelbein 1990; Atchison et al 1991). Various factors contribute to this problem.

Owing to lack of research, the choice and use of a given pain-control method is primarily based on the personal bias of the prescribing physicians and the nurses who administer the medication. Because routine measurements of pain levels are lacking in most clinical settings, the only assessment which is made of the patient's pain is based on the opinion of medical staff. Several studies have shown discrepancies between the way the medical staff and patients rate the severity of burn pain or the degree of pain relief obtained with medication (Walkenstein 1982; Iafrati 1986; Van der Does 1989; Choinière et al 1990). As a result, requirements for analgesics are not assessed properly and, in many cases, are underestimated.

The fear of addiction to opioids also contributes to undermedication in burned patients. Interestingly, not one case of iatrogenic addiction has been documented in a nationwide survey of 93 burn centres which had treated more than 10 000 patients (Perry & Heidrich 1982). Nevertheless, insufficient amounts of opioids continue to be prescribed (Choinière et al 1989; Atchison et al 1991) and, even when adequate doses are ordered, burn patients may receive less than one-half of the prescribed daily dose (Marvin & Heimbach 1984). Heidrich et al (1981) observed that nurses' concern about addiction leads to a fear of using opioids at sufficient frequency or by an effective route of administration. In a more recent study, Atchison et al (1991) also noticed that the type or amount of analgesic drug prescribed for dressing changes was not adjusted over time and little compensation was made for the patient's changing condition or for the tolerance that may develop in patients receiving opioids for a prolonged period of time.

Another factor which may influence prescribing habits is the belief that the patient who develops tolerance to opioids will also become psychologically dependent on the drug. However, tolerance should not be equated with psychological addiction (Jaffe 1985). When tolerance does occur, it can be treated safely and effectively by increasing the dose as there appears to be no limit to the development of tolerance (Portenoy et al 1986; Foley 1989, 1991). Awareness of this phenomenon should alert the clinician to make upward adjustments in dosage of opioids as long as there continues to be uncontrolled pain (Osgood & Szyfelbein 1989, 1990; Freund & Marvin 1990). However, the complexity of the problem of tolerance must be kept in mind. The literature on cancer pain indicates that the development of tolerance varies greatly among patients and most of them do not require an escalation of their dose of opioids for pain control (Twycross 1974; Portenoy et al 1986; Foley 1989, 1991). In burn patients, no experimental data exist on this issue. Anecdotal evidence and clinical experience (Osgood & Szyfelbein 1989; Freund & Marvin 1990; Atchison et al 1991) suggest that dose escalation usually occurs when opioids are administered over an extended period of time to burn patients. Occasionally, the required dose for alleviating pain during a dressing change may escalate sharply (Wermeling et al 1986; Osgood & Szyfelbein 1989). However, it is not known whether increased doses of opioids are needed because true tolerance occurs or because more pain is felt as a result of the healing process (e.g. of third-degree burns). Alternatively, some component of the pain may depend upon mechanisms which are known to respond poorly to opioid therapy (e.g. neuropathy) and, thereby, require a different treatment strategy (Atchison et al 1991; Ready & Edwards 1992). It is clear that further research is needed to study the effects of long term opioid therapy in burn patients.

Long-term administration of opioids usually produces physical dependence which should not be equated with psychological addiction (Jaffe 1985). Furthermore, physical dependence is not a significant problem in burn patients since withdrawal symptoms can be prevented by gradually reducing the dose over a number of days when the patient no longer needs the medication. As pointed out by Osgood & Szyfelbein (1989), burn patients at this stage often accept the end of their reliance on opioids as a welcome milestone on the road to recovery.

The fear that drug metabolism is altered in burn patients may also make medical staff reluctant to use high doses of opioids. Although this concern may be justified during the immediate postinjury phase (Martyn 1990), it is not warranted during the later phases of treatment, as suggested by several reports on the pharmacokinetics of morphine (Perry & Inturrisi 1983; Cederholm et al 1990; Furman et al 1990), meperidine (Bloedow et al 1986), sufentanyl (Gregoretti & Vinik 1986) and methadone (Denson et al 1990) in burn patients. Cederholm et al (1990) examined the metabolism of morphine in a burn child who was administered high doses of morphine for more than 30 days. Pharmacokinetics values for morphine were normal and no complications occurred despite high-dose, long-term therapy with the drug. In a recent critical review of the literature on drug therapy in burn patients, Martyn (1990) concludes that, although more studies are necessary, the administration of opioids does not appear to be harmful to burn patients. These patients are known to be hypermetabolic and resistant to many drugs used in anaesthetic practice. They are also known to require high doses of opioids to achieve adequate pain relief. Whether this is due to pharmacokinetic or pharmacodynamic alterations in the drug has not been completely established. Neuronal and hormonal mediators may also be involved

(Kim & Martyn 1987; Martyn 1990). Finally, the possibility that large doses of opioids are appropriate for the severity of the pain that these patients experience should not be excluded (Furman et al 1990).

A further factor which may be responsible for the problem of undermedication in burn patients is the fear of inducing respiratory depression when administering high doses of opioid analgesics. All opioids are capable of producing respiratory depression. However, this complication is rarely a problem in the presence of severe pain since the pain stimulates respiration and thereby acts as a natural antidote to counteract the respiratory depressant effects of opioids (Jaffe & Martin 1985). Therefore, when the drug is carefully titrated to the patient's needs, the risk of respiratory depression is considerably reduced and should not prevent the administration of effective dosages to burn patients. If serious respiratory depression occurs, it can be reversed by naloxone, a specific opioid antagonist (Jaffe & Martin 1985).

In order to correct prejudices and mistaken notions, education programmes on pain and on the clinical pharmacology of opioids should be obligatory for nurses as well as the prescribing physicians who treat burn patients. Continuing education sessions should also be given on a regular basis to provide updated information on various pharmacological issues related to pain management.

Basic considerations in analgesic pharmacotherapy for burn patients

There is ample evidence in the burn literature that current analgesic practices need to be reevaluated in order to provide burn patients with adequate pain relief. Various approaches have been suggested over the past 10 years (Perry et al 1981; Marvin & Heimback 1984, 1985; Martyn 1986) but only recently has the need for more aggressive analgesic intervention been stressed (Choinière et al 1989; Osgood & Szyfelbein 1989, 1990; Freund & Marvin 1990; Markersie & Karagianes 1990; Atchinson et al 1991; Kinsella & Booth 1991). The importance of the adverse physical effects of pain is increasingly recognised. Severe, persistent pain can be devastating; it can affect sleep and appetite and may thus impede recovery from injury and, in a weakened individual like a burn patient, it may perhaps make the difference between life and death, as pointed out by Melzack (1990).

With increased sophistication in the management of burn injuries, health care professionals have intensified the search for the best means of providing optimal analgesia for their patients. However, there is no general agreement on this issue, mainly due to a lack of research.

Strong opioids continue to be the mainstay for pain management in burn patients. In many cases, morphine remains the drug of choice for burn adults or children: it is effective for moderate to severe pain; it is available in different forms (e.g. sustained vs instant release), and it is not expensive compared to other opioid analgesics. Meperidine is also a popular drug for treating pain in burn patients but is of limited usefulness because it cannot be administered for long periods. Repeated doses of meperidine result in the accumulation of normeperidine, an active metabolite of meperidine which is a central nervous system stimulant that produces neurotoxic reactions (Kaiko et al 1983). For this reason, meperidine should not be used chronically and its oral preparation has been listed as 'not recommended' in two recent publications (AHCPR 1992; APS 1992). Methadone, a long-acting opioid, is often used to provide a sustained level of analgesia. In contrast, synthetic opioids, with a more rapid onset of action and a shorter duration of effect (e.g. fentanyl), may be helpful for therapeutic procedures. Synthetic oral compounds that have both agonist and antagonist properties can also be employed but it should be pointed out that mixed agonist–antagonists may precipitate withdrawal symptoms in patients who have previously received pure agonists (e.g. morphine). Finally, mild opioids (codeine) and nonopioids (e.g. acetaminophen) can be part of the panoply of medication used in the later phases of treatment for burn patients.

Opioids are preferentially administered in burn patients by using the intravenous (i.v.) or oral route (Osgood & Szyfelbein 1989, 1990; Freund & Marvin 1990; Martyn 1990). Intramuscular (i.m.) administration is generally avoided, not only on account of poor absorption, but because the pain associated with the injections makes this route impractical for prolonged pain (Austin et al 1980; Osgood & Szyfelbein 1989, 1990; Freund & Marvin 1990; APS 1992). The i.v. route has the advantage of rapid effect and ease of titration. As soon as this is no longer required, the oral route should be employed since opioid tolerance may develop more rapidly when the drug is administered parenterally (Foley & Inturrisi 1987).

Whatever the type of drug used and the route of administration, several key principles to optimise pharmacological treatment of pain have recently been summarised in several excellent practical guides (AHCPR 1992; APS 1992; Ready & Edwards 1992). The same principles obviously apply to the management of burn pain but some unique characteristics of this pain syndrome call also for specific strategies to maximise the efficacy of the pharmacotherapy:

Burn pain is not a single entity but involves two major components that must be treated separately. The most intense pain results from the therapeutic procedures but most patients also experience pain when they are at rest. Each type of pain (background and procedural) has its own characteristics and therefore requires distinct and effective treatment strategies.

Flexibility in dosing is essential to account for the wide variation in the analgesic requirements of burn patients. Burn pain is extremely variable from one patient to the other and it undergoes wide fluctuations over time. Prescriptions of analgesics must be highly individualised and frequently adjusted according to the changing nature of the patient's pain during the different phases of treatment.

Systematic procedures to assess pain and success of analgesia must be instituted. As with any type of therapeutic intervention, the effects of analgesic therapy must be closely monitored, both for efficacy and for side-effects. Separate measurements should be obtained for the pain felt at rest and at times of treatment. Simple rating scales can be used for this purpose and the information charted in the patient's file can provide a documented rationale to adjust the medication for each type of pain.

The role of fear, anxiety and depression must be carefully assessed at each phase of treatment. Most burn patients experience various forms of psychological distress over the course of treatment and pain may influence or be influenced by these factors. Careful psychological assessment of the patients is essential since it will underpin the judicious use of antianxiety and/or antidepressant medication in conjunction with the analgesic therapy.

Pharmacotherapy for pain at rest

As mentioned earlier, in the immediate postinjury phase, analgesic needs may be reduced or even absent in some burn patients. However, most patients will require prompt and effective pain medication. During the acute phase of resuscitation, small but frequent doses of i.v. opioid narcotics are recommended. Other routes of administration should be avoided during this phase because decreased blood flow to organs and tissues may delay drug absorption and lead to respiratory depression, especially if high dosages have been administered to overcome poor absorption (Martyn 1990). The role of anxiety and fear must be carefully assessed at this stage since the patient's agitation may be interpreted as a pain response. Reassurance and information may help considerably in managing agitation while anxiolytic medication may contribute to reducing the analgesic needs (Andreasen et al 1972; Steiner & Clark 1977; Watkins et al 1988; Ready & Edwards 1992).

Once the initial resuscitation phase is over, sufficient analgesia should be given for the pain felt at rest. The discomfort resulting from the burns may affect sleep and mood and this may in turn limit pain tolerance at times of treatment. The primary goal of therapy is, therefore, to provide adequate baseline analgesia.

The mainstay of analgesia for continuous background pain is opioids administration. Physicians usually prescribe intermittent i.v. boluses, but continuous i.v. infusions are gaining increasing acceptance. Continuous infusions permit careful titration, ensure more stable opioid blood levels and thus may provide a sustained background of analgesia (Portenoy et al 1986; AHCPR 1992). Recent preliminary reports and single-case studies show successful results with continuous i.v. infusions of morphine (Cederholm et al 1990; Osgood & Szyfelbein 1990) or methadone (Concilus et al 1989) for controlling background pain in burn adults and children.

Patient-controlled analgesia (PCA) represents another useful technique for background pain. This drug delivery system allows the patient to self-administer small doses of i.v. opioids within limits prescribed by the physician. Since the patient can titrate his medication according to his own needs, the wide variations in patients' analgesic requirements can be overcome (White 1988a). In the burn literature, some open trials and a single-case study suggest that PCA can provide good quality analgesia in burn adults (Wermeling et al 1986; Kinsella et al 1988) and children (Gaukroger et al 1991). Recently, Choinière et al (1992) used a double-blind controlled design to assess the safety and efficacy of PCA compared to conventional analgesic therapy consisting of intermittent i.v. morphine injections. Their results suggest that PCA is a safe, effective method for controlling burn pain. It offers good pain relief and individualised treatment in burn patients who are stable, alert and able to understand how to use the pump. The authors suggest, however, that the PCA approach may not suffice for the intense pain levels felt during therapeutic procedures. On these occasions, an i.v. bolus administered prior to the procedure may be necessary to supplement the PCA regimen.

In patients who can take medication by mouth, oral opioids with a long duration of action (e.g. MS Contin, methadone) are useful in providing stable analgesia when the patient is at rest (Osgood & Szyfelbein 1989; Freund & Marvin 1990). Preliminary results confirm the efficacy and safety of sustained-release morphine formulations in burn patients (Wilson & Tomlinson 1988; Heinle et al 1989) while recent pharmacokinetic data also support the use of the product in this population of patients (Herman et al 1992).

Invasive routes of administration (spinal or epidural) are generally not recommended in burn patients due to the risk of infection. The presence of hypotension with or without sepsis may also preclude the use of these routes for pain control (Freund & Marvin 1990; Kinsella & Booth 1991; AHCPR 1992). Except for one anecdotal report which suggests that regional analgesia may have some role in the management of peripheral burns (Wilson & Tomlinson 1988), no studies have been published on the use of spinal, epidural or regional analgesia for controlling burn pain. However, the therapeutic merit of these techniques deserves more careful assessment in selected categories of patients. If the burn is located in the lower part of the body and the region of the spinal column is not involved, continuous epidural techniques could be helpful in providing stable baseline analgesia for hours or even days. The same could be true for analgesia of skin graft donor sites (Wilson & Tomlinson 1988; Freund & Marvin 1990; Kinsella & Booth 1991). The presence of sepsis or the development of coagulopathies however, are major obstacles to the use of these techniques in burn patients (Kinsella & Booth 1991; AHCPR 1992).

A possibly useful technique to improve background analgesia in burn patients is the use of topical anaesthetics, but this is a relatively uninvestigated area of research. Brofeldt et al (1989) conducted an open trial in which they applied high doses of topical lidocaine cream (5%) to burn wounds; their results suggest improved pain relief without associated systemic effects. Freund & Marvin (1990) reported preliminary results suggesting that lidocaine spray (1%) provides superior analgesia than does a placebo solution, when used under dressings on hand burns. In a recent randomised controlled study, Owen & Dye (1990) showed that the addition of 2% lidocaine gel to dressings applied to skin graft donor sites resulted in significantly more pain relief during the first week without interfering with wound healing. The authors recommend the routine use of this technique in patients with normal renal and hepatic function, provided very large burn areas are not involved since systemic toxicity can occur. More extensive trials on the safety and efficacy of topical analgesia are needed but the results are promising, especially for skin graft donor sites.

As mentioned earlier, when persistent burn pain cannot be adequately controlled despite increasing the dose of opioids, other diagnoses such as the presence of a neuropathic pain component should be considered. Drugs that are effective for this type of pain, such as tricyclic antidepressants, anticonvulsants and/or membrane-stabilising drugs may be indicated for controlling burn pain (Ready & Edwards 1992). Some recent results reported by Jonsson et al (1991) suggest that continous infusion of low doses of lidocaine, which is known to alleviate neuropathic pain in other settings, may be a valuable additional option for pain control in burn patients. Because these results may have important clinical implications for the treatment of burn pain, further studies using larger samples and randomised controlled designs are needed to replicate these findings.

When the background pain is mild and less persistent, weak opioids (e.g. codeine), nonopioids (e.g. acetaminophen) or combined preparations of analgesics (e.g. codeine plus acetaminophen) may be sufficient to make the patient comfortable. The same is true during the last phase of treatment when the wounds are all healed. At this point, opioids therapy is rarely necessary and can easily be discontinued by using an appropriate weaning schedule. However, some patients develop postburn neuralgia problems during this phase and these may persist for variable periods of time (Ward et al 1989; Choinière et al 1991). For relieving intense itching sensations at the injury sites, antihistamines are commonly prescribed (Gordon 1988). However, the treatment for painful or paraesthesic sensations in healed wounds is poorly understood and may involve experimenting with a variety of medications including opioids or drugs that are employed for neuropathic pain.

Finally, since fear and anxiety are almost universal responses to burn injury, anxiolytics (e.g. benzodiazepines) may be useful supplements to the analgesic medication given to the resting patient. Many patients are anxious when they are in pain but are calm once the pain is relieved. If the anxiety persists, for reasons other than anticipation of painful treatments, anxiolytics may be used. (See next section for treatment of anticipatory anxiety.) These drugs and/or hypnotics can also be given at bedtime to favour optimal sleep (Steiner & Clark 1977; Watkins et al 1988, 1992; APS 1992). Antidepressant drugs may also be necessary in burn patients who are hospitalised for prolonged periods of time and who develop problems of depression. Antidepressant drugs are helpful not only in elevating mood but they may also relieve pain and improve sleep and appetite (Steiner & Clark 1977; APS 1992; Watkins et al 1992).

Pharmacotherapy for pain due to therapeutic procedures

The burn literature provides a variety of methods for alleviating the pain associated with therapeutic procedures but there is no general agreement as to the optimum method of analgesia in these circumstances. In a large survey of USA burn units, Perry & Heidrich (1982) found that, in roughly two-thirds of the burn units, morphine or meperidine were used with or without psychotropics for debridement and dressing changes. However, dosages varied widely, with up to a 35-fold difference when route and relative potency were considered. Other respondents reported using milder opioids, nonopioid analgesics, psychotropics, anaesthetic agents or even no medication at all during painful therapeutic procedures. Another striking finding in this study was that children were four times more likely than adults to receive no analgesics at all for dressing changes, even though their pain was judged to be comparable. Schechter (1985) made similar observations in a large teaching hospital: burn children received an average of 1.3 doses of opioids per day whereas adults with burns of similar size received 3.6 doses.

Some modifications of analgesic practices are clearly needed. Given that therapeutic procedures produce intense pain, a conscientious and thoughtful approach to pain management is essential. Strong opioids such as morphine or fentanyl are typically required to bring the pain under control for dressing changes and debridement both in adults and children (Osgood & Szyfelbein 1989, 1990; Freund & Marvin 1990; Mackersie & Karagianes 1990; Kinsella & Booth 1991). Doses must be increased and adjusted according to the needs of each patient. Flexible doses of drugs coupled with frequent evaluation of the resulting analgesia are necessary. The need to administer drugs, such as morphine, far enough in advance of treatment to be maximally effective must also be taken into account. Other clinicians (Osgood & Szyfelbein 1989, 1990; Freund & Marvin 1990) have pointed out the potential usefulness of synthetic opiates with a more rapid onset of action. The idea is to provide analgesia which does not leave the patient oversedated when the procedure is over. Thus, short-acting agents such as fentanyl can offer some advantage, but this may depends upon the duration of the procedure as many doses may be needed for a long dressing change. In such a case, morphine will most probably prove to be easier to use and it is cheaper than fentanyl. In burn children, oral preparations such as Percocet (oxycodone plus acetaminophen) continue to be commonly used for dressing changes since nearly all children prefer the oral route for drug administration. However, several authors (Osgood & Szyfebein 1989, 1990; McGrath 1990; Atchison et al 1991) have pointed out the inadequacy of this medication for controlling severe pain during dressing changes. Oral preparations of short-acting morphine are more likely to be effective and can easily be administered in the form of a solution or tablet. If the pain is severe and requires rapid titration to achieve effect, the drug should be given parentally.

Depending upon the patient's anxiety level, opioids can be administered alone or in combination with a benzodiazepine before the therapeutic procedure. Since under-medication for pain can escalate anxiety, optimal control of pain for the first procedure is necessary in order to minimise anxiety for future procedures (Choinière et al 1989; AHCPR 1992; Watkins et al 1992). This helps to prevent the continual use of benzodiazepines for controlling anticipatory anxiety. As pointed out by Watkins et al (1992), once the patient has learned to associate burn treatment with agonising pain, even massive increases in opioids will fail to provide adequate pain relief. In such a case, the addition of a benzodiazepine (e.g. lorazepam, midazolam) can be most beneficial (Steiner & Clark 1977; Freund & Marvin 1990; Watkins et al 1992).

In patients who require extensive dressing changes and wound debridement, analgesic regimens may call for anaesthetic agents. Self-administration of inhalational agents such as nitrous oxide (Baskett 1972; Filkins et al 1981) provides successful analgesia for dressing changes in burn adults and children. However, there is some controversy in the burn literature with respect to the potential toxicity of these agents. Based on a review of various studies on the use of nitrous oxide in burn patients, Freund & Marvin (1990) concluded that this agent is safe except in the presence of pulmonary disorders. Considering the various adverse effects of nitrous oxide which have been reported, especially those on bone marrow, several other authors (Osgood & Szyfelbein 1989, 1990; Kinsella & Booth 1991; AHCPR 1992) have stressed the increased risk of these side-effects in burn patients who are repeatedly exposed to nitrous oxide over prolonged periods of time.

Ketamine is another popular anaesthetic agent which is commonly used with burn patients. Several studies (Slogoff et al 1974; Demling et al 1978; White et al 1982; Gordon 1987) indicate that subanaesthetic doses of ketamine can provide effective analgesia for burn dressings and wound debridement. Ketamine has several advantages: it can be administered by the i.v. or i.m. route; there is no need to withhold food or fluid for long periods before or after the procedure, and it does not depress respiration when used in subanaesthetic doses (Freund & Marvin 1990, Martyn 1990). However, some adverse effects of ketamine have also been reported. These include a very rapid development of tolerance to the product, a relatively prolonged recovery and hallucinogenic reactions upon emergence from anaesthesia (Slogoff et al 1974; Demling et al 1978, Martyn 1990). However, two case reports (Shetty et al 1986; Cederholm et al 1990) question the problem of rapid tolerance to ketamine. Cederholm et al (1990) administered ketamine infusion to a burn child for more than 30 days and noticed no tachyphylaxis. Psychological sequelae were not observed either, possibly because of the concomitant administration of midazolam. Freund & Marvin (1990) also maintain that unpleasant reactions associated with ketamine administration can be minimised with suitable premedication and pretreatment explanations.

Perhaps a more promising tool to provide sedation for painful procedures with burn patients is propofol, a recently introduced i.v. anaesthetic agent which offers several advantages: its dosage can be accurately titrated for sedation or total anaesthesia; recovery after its use is rapid, and emergence after a single bolus or short infusion is free of the 'hangover' associated with the use of most other i.v. anaesthetic drugs (Aitkenhead 1989; White 1988b). However, limited information is available regarding the safety of propofol for sedation in different clinical settings, including burn units. Galizia et al (1987) conducted a comparative study on the use of ketamine and propofol for dressing changes in two groups of burn adults. A significantly greater incidence of transient apnoea was observed after induction with propofol (9/24 patients: 37%). Periods of tachypnoea were also more frequent with this agent probably because, unlike ketamine, it does not have any analgesic activity. However, propofol had particular advantages over ketamine: patients in the propofol group were more rapidly oriented upon recovery, and did not suffer psychomotor agitation or hallucinogenic reactions as had been found with ketamine. More recently, Noe et al (1991) reported the results of a preliminary study on the repeated administration of propofol for 'bedside procedures' in nonintubated burn patients. They observed ventilatory depression in one-third of the instances of propofol administration, but only after induction. The authors attribute this effect to the induction dose and speed of propofol administration since no further episodes of apnoea were observed during maintenance of anaesthesia. Recovery from anaesthesia was quick and no psychotic reactions were observed. Finally, Mills & Lord (1992) reported the use of propofol for repeated dressing changes in a severely burned and psychologically disturbed child. Fentanyl was used concomitantly and no periods of apnoea were noticed in any of the procedures. Furthermore, there was no tachyphylaxis with propofol, the amount used being proportional to the time taken for the procedure. Considering the rapid recovery with propofol and its lack of negative sequelae, the authors stress the potential usefulness of this agent for repeated burn dressings. Although all characteristics of propofol may make this drug a valuable innovative tool in the treatment of burn patients, well-controlled drug trials and pharmacokinetic studies are still needed to substantiate its efficacy and safety.

Finally, in extreme cases where pain cannot be tolerated by the awake or sedated patient, general anaesthesia may be the only choice for extensive dressing changes and wound debridement. Considering the various adverse side-effects of anaesthetic agents, there is an obvious reluctance to repeatedly expose burn patients to general anaesthesia (Osgood & Szyfelbein 1989, 1990; Martyn 1990; Kinsella & Booth 1991). A study carried out by Reyneke et al (1989) suggests that propofol may overcome some of the drawbacks associated with general anaesthesia in burn patients. However, a major disadvantage remains regardless of the type of drug used. The repeated administration of anaesthetic agents requires the withholding of food prior to each intervention and for some time afterwards, thereby interrupting the intensive nutritional support so important for the recovery of burn patients.

Considering the disadvantages and adverse side-effects of anaesthetic agents, there is some consensus in the burn literature that these approaches are best reserved for difficult, refractory cases or for major surgical interventions involving massive wound debridement and skin grafting.

Other treatment methods

It is well known that burn patients frequently show signs of anxiety, fear, depression or acute grief reactions and that these may influence pain. Therefore, psychological interventions can also be helpful in the treatment of burn pain. In a review of the literature, Patterson et al (1987) concluded that most published reports support the efficacy of hypnotherapy to reduce pain in burn patients; however, little else can be concluded because of the poor descriptions of the patients or methods and procedures in most articles (Patterson et al 1987; Van der Does & Van Dyck 1989). Most of the published reports are anecdotal and only one study included a control group (Wakeman & Kaplan 1978). Additional well-designed studies are needed, as well as information about which types of patient are most likely to benefit from hypnotherapy and at what stages of burn care this technique will be helpful. More research must also be conducted to determine the practicality and cost-effectiveness of hypnotherapy compared with other interventions (e.g. use of opioids plus benzodiazepines) (Patterson et al 1987; Van der Does & Van Dyck 1989; Patterson 1992).

A variety of other types of psychological technique have been used with varying degrees of success in burn adults (see reviews by Freund & Marvin 1990; Patterson 1992) and burn children (see reviews by Osgood & Szyfelbein 1989, 1990; McGrath 1990). These approaches, which have been used alone or in combination, include relaxation training (breathing exercises, progressive muscle relaxation), biofeedback, behaviour modification (respondant and operant techniques), desensitisation, stress inoculation training, cognitive behavioural strategies (guided imagery, distraction techniques, coping skills training) and group or individual psychotherapy. Unfortunately, many of these studies, like those on hypnosis, suffer from methodological deficiencies or generalisations may not be made from them because of small sample sizes. Nevertheless, several well-designed studies on the use of behaviour modification (Varni et al 1980; Kelley et al 1984) and stress reduction techniques (Knudson-Cooper 1981; Wernick et al 1981; Tobiasen & Hiebert 1985) have shown promising results in some burn patients (children or adults). Significant improvement with these approaches was observed on various measures including the amount of pain felt and observed during therapeutic procedures; the incidence of maladaptive pain behaviours; requests for analgesic medication; compliance with hospital routine; manifest and self-reported anxiety; sense of well-being and control, and length of hospitalisation.

Although the above studies need to be replicated, they suggest that burn patients can be helped to control their pain and anxiety through behavioural and stress reduction techniques. All these techniques can help the patient to relax and maintain a sense of control. They can be particularly useful if introduced early in the course of the patient's treatment so as to prevent the development of a pain–anxiety–pain cycle (Tobiasen & Hiebert 1985; Osgood & Szyfelbein 1989, 1990; Freund & Marvin 1990; Patterson 1992; Ready & Edwards 1992; Watkins et al 1992).

Considering the severity of burn pain, it is very unlikely that psychological techniques alone can provide complete pain relief. Furthermore, hospitalised burn patients are often too fatigued, disoriented or sick to engage in psychological interventions that require time and discipline (Patterson 1992). This does not mean, however, that psychological techniques cannot serve as useful adjuncts to opioids in burn-pain control. Coupled with adequate and effective medication, psychological interventions can be helpful in optimising pain relief in selected categories of patients (Osgood & Szyfelbein 1989, 1990; Freund & Marvin 1990; McGrath 1990; Patterson 1992).

More research is needed to identify the patients who will be most responsive to particular pain-control methods. Clinical studies must be conducted to evaluate critically the efficacy of the available interventions and to develop more clear-cut guidelines for their application, according to the burn severity, age group, attitudes and coping abilities of the patients. Burn-pain management is most likely to be maximally effective if individualised strategies are employed. The search for the best means of providing and maintaining optimal analgesia in burn patients represents a challenge for both researchers and clinicians alike. This challenges lies in the changing pattern of pain that the patient experiences over time and in response to treatment interventions and the natural healing process.

REFERENCES

Agency for Health Care Policy and Research (AHCPR) 1992 Acute pain management: operative or medical procedures and trauma, part 2. Clinical Pharmacy 11: 391–413

Ahrenholz D H, Solem L D 1987 Management of pain after thermal injury. Advances in Clinical Rehabilitation 1: 215–229

Aitkenhead A R 1989 Analgesia and sedation in intensive care. British Journal of Anaesthesia 63: 196–206

American Pain Society (APS) 1992 Principles of analgesic use in the treatment of acute pain and cancer pain. American Pain Society, Skokie, Illinois

Andreasen N J C, Noyes R, Hartford C E, Brodland G, Proctor S 1972 Management of emotional reactions in seriously burned adults. New England Journal of Medicine 286: 65–69

Anand K J S, Hickey P R 1987 Pain and its effects in the human neonate and fetus. New England Journal of Medicine 317: 1321–1329

Artz C P 1979 Epidemiological causes and prognosis. In: Artz C P, Moncrief J A, Pruitt B A (eds) Burns, a team approach. W B Saunders, Philadelphia, p 17–22

Atchison N E, Osgood P F, Carr D B, Szylfelbein S K 1991 Pain during burn dressing change in children: relationship to burn area, depth and analgesic regimens. Pain 47: 41–45

Austin K L, Stapelton J V, Mather L W 1980 Multiple intramuscular injections: a major source of variability in analgesic response to meperidine. Pain 8: 47–62

Avni J 1980 Severe burns. In: Freyberger H, Reichsman F (eds) Advances in psychosomatic medicine: psychotherapeutic interventions in life-threatening illness. Karger, New York, p 57–77

Baskett P J F 1972 Analgesia for dressing of burns in children: a method using neuroleptanalgesia and entonox. Postgraduate Medical Journal 48: 138–142

Beales J G 1983 Factors influencing the expectation of pain among patients in a children's burn unit. Burns 9: 187–192

Bernstein N R, O'Connell K, Chedekel D 1992 Patterns of burn adjustment. Journal of Burn Care and Rehabilitation 13: 4–12

Bloedow D C, Goodfellow L A, Marvin J, Heimback D 1986 Meperidine disposition in burned patients. Research Communications in Chemical Pathology and Pharmacology 54: 87–99

Brofeldt B T, Cornwell P, Doherty D, Batra K, Gunther R A 1989 Topical lidocaine in the treatment of partial-thickness burns. Journal of Burn Care and Rehabilitation 10: 63–68

Campbell J N, Meyer R A, Raya S N 1984 Hyperalgesia: new insights. Pain (suppl 2): abstract 3

Casey K L 1988 Towards a rationale for the treatment of painful neuropathies. In: Dubner R, Gebhart G F, Bond M R (eds) Proceedings of the Vth World Congress on Pain. Elsevier, Amsterdam, p 165–174

Cederholm I, Bengtsson M, Bjorkman S, Choonara I, Rane A 1990 Long-term high dose morphine, ketamine, and midazolam infusion in a child with burns. British Journal of Clinical Pharmacology 30: 901–905

Charlton J E, Klein R, Gagliardi G, Heimbach D M 1983 Factors affecting pain in burned patients – a preliminary report. Postgraduate Medical Journal 59: 604–607

Choinière M, Melzack R, Rondeau J, Girard N, Paquin M J 1989 The pain of burns: characteristics and correlates. Journal of Trauma 29: 1531–1539

Choinière M, Melzack R, Girard N, Rondeau J, Paquin M J 1990 Comparisons between patients' and nurses' assessment of pain and medication efficacy in severe burn injuries. Pain 40: 13–152

Choinière M, Melzack R, Papillon J 1991 Pain and paraesthesia in patients with healed burns: an exploratory study. Journal of Pain and Symptom Management 6: 437–444

Choinière M, Grenier R, Paquette C 1992 Patient-controlled analgesia: a double-blind study in burned patients. Anaesthesia 47: 467–472

Coderre T, Melzack R 1985 Increased pain sensitivity following heat injury involves a central mechanism. Behavioural Brain Research 15: 259–262

Coderre T, Melzack 1987 Cutaneous hyperalgesia: contributions of the peripheral and central nervous systems to the increase in pain sensitivity after injury. Brain Research 404: 95–106

Concilus R, Denson D D, Knarr D, Warden G, Raj P 1989 Continuous intravenous infusion of methadone for control of burn pain. Journal of Burn Care and Rehabilitation 10: 406–409

Davies J W L 1982 Prompt cooling of burned areas: a review of benefits and the effector mechanisms. Burns 9: 1

Deitch E A, Dazhong X, Bridges R M 1988 Opioids modulate human neutrophil and lymphocyte function: thermal injury alters plasma β-endorphin levels. Surgery 104: 41–48

Demling R H 1985 Burns. New England Journal of Medicine 313: 1389–1398

Demling R H 1990 Pathophysiological changes after cutaneous burns and approach to initial resuscitation. In: Martyn J A J (ed) Acute management of the burned patient. W B Saunders, Philadelphia, p 12–24

Demling R H, Lalonde C 1989 Burn trauma. Thieme, New York

Demling R H, Ellerbee S, Jarrett F 1978 Ketamine anesthesia for tangential excision of burn eschar: a burn unit procedure. Journal of Trauma 18: 269–270

Denson D D, Concilus R R, Warden G, Raj P 1990 Pharmacokinetics of continuous intravenous infusion of methadone in the early post-burn period. Journal of Clinical Pharmacology 30: 70–75

Devor M 1989 The pathophysiology of damaged peripheral nerves. In: Wall P D, Melzack R (eds) Textbook of pain, 2nd edn. Churchill Livingstone, Edinburgh, p 63–81

Devor M, Wall P D 1981 Effect of peripheral nerve injury on receptive fields of cells in the cat spinal cord. Journal of Comparative Neurology 199: 227–291

Fagerhaugh S Y 1974 Pain expression and control on a burn care unit. Nursing Outlook 22: 645–650

Filkins S A, Cosgrave P, Marvin J A, Engrav L, Heimbach D M 1981 Self administered anesthetic: a method of pain control. Journal of Burn Care and Rehabilitation 2: 33–34

Foley K M 1989 Controversies in cancer pain: medical perspectives. Cancer 63: 2257–2265.
Foley K M 1991 Clinical tolerance to opioids. In: Basbaum A I, Besson J M (eds) Towards a new pharmacology of pain. John Wiley, Chichester, p 181–203
Foley K M, Inturrisi C E 1987 Analgesic drug therapy in cancer pain: principles and practice. Medical Clinics of North America 71: 207–233
Freund P R, Marvin J A 1990 Postburn pain. In: Bonica J J (ed) The management of pain 2nd edn. Lea & Febiger, Philadelphia, p 481–489
Furman W R, Munster A M, Cone E J 1990 Morphine pharmacokinetics during anesthesia and surgery in patients with burns. Journal of Burn Care and Rehabilitation 11: 391–394
Galizia J P, Cantineau D, Selosse A, Crepy A, Scherpereel P H 1987 Essai comparatif du propofol et de la kétamine au cours de l'anesthésie pour bain des grands brûlés. Annales Françaises d'Anesthésie et de Réanimation 6: 320–323
Gaukroger P B, Chapman M J, Davey R B 1991 Pain control in paediatric burns – the use of patient-controlled analgesia. Burns 17: 396–399
Giuliani C A, Perry G A 1985 Factors to consider in the rehabilitation aspect of burn care. Physical Therapy 65: 619–623
Gordon M D 1987 Burn care protocols: administration of ketamine. Journal of Burn Care and Rehabilitation 8: 146–149
Gordon M D 1988 Pruritus in burns. Journal of Burn Care and Rehabilitation 9: 305–311
Gregoretti S, Vinik H R 1986 Sufentanyl pharmacokinetics in burned patients undergoing skin grafting. Anesthesia and Analgesia 65: S64
Heidrich G, Perry S, Amand R 1981 Nursing staff attitudes about burn pain. Journal of Burn Care and Rehabilitation 2: 259–261
Heinle J, Kealy G P, Hauer M 1989 Breakthrough pain control in burn patients. Proceedings of the American Burn Association, New Orleans, abstract 50
Helm P A, Kevorkian C G, Lushbaugh M, Pullium G, Head M D, Cromes G F 1982 Burn injury: rehabilitation management in 1982. Archives of Physical Medicine and Rehabilitation 63: 6–16
Herman R A, Veng-Pedersen P, Kealy G P 1992 Clearance of morphine sulphate oral solution and sustained release (MS Contin) in burn patients. Proceedings of the American Burn Association, Salt Lake City, Abstract 55
Hermanson A, Jonsson C E, Lindblom U 1986 Sensibility after injury. Clinical Physiology 6: 507–521
Hurt A, Ericksson E 1986 Management of the burn wound. Clinics in Plastic Surgery 13: 57–67
Iafrati N S 1986 Pain on the burn unit: patient vs. nurse perception. Journal of Burn Care and Rehabilitation 7: 413–416
Jaffe J H 1985 Drug addiction and drug abuse. In: Gilman A G, Goodman L S, Rall T W et al (eds) The pharmacological basis of therapeutics, 7th edn. McMillan, New York, p 535–584
Jaffe J H, Martin W R 1985 Opioids analgesics and antagonists. In: Gilman A G, Goodman L S, Rall T W et al (eds) The pharmacological basis of therapeutics, 7th edn. McMillan, New York, p 491–531
Jonsson A, Cassuto J, Hanson B 1991 Inhibition of burn pain by intravenous lignocaine infusion. Lancet 338: 151–152
Kaiko R F, Foley K M, Grabinski P Y et al 1983 Central nervous system excitatory effects of meperidine in cancer patients. Annals of Neurology 13: 180–185
Katz J, Vaccarino A, Coderre T J, Melzack R 1991 Injury prior to neurectomy alters the pattern of autotomy in rats. Anesthesiology 75: 876–883
Kavanagh C T 1983a A new approach to dressing change in the severely burned child and its effect on burn-related psychopathology. Heart and Lung 12: 612–619
Kavanagh C T 1983b Psychological intervention with the severely burned child: Report of an experimental comparison of two approaches and their effects on psychological sequelae. Journal of the American Academy of Child Psychiatry 2: 145–153
Kavanagh C T, Lasoff E, Eide Y et al 1991 Learned helplessness and the pediatric burn patient: dressing change behaviour and serum cortisol and β-endorphin. Advances in Pediatrics 38: 335–363
Kelley M L, Jarvie G J, Middlebrook J L, McNeer M F, Drabman R S 1984 Decreasing burned children's pain behaviour: impacting the trauma of hydrotherapy. Journal of Applied Behavior Analysis 17 : 147–158
Kim C, Martyn J 1987 Altered pharmacology in burned patients. Baillière's Clinical Anaesthesiology 1: 649–661
Kinsella J, Booth M G 1991 Pain relief in burns: James Laing Memorial Essay 1990. Burns 17: 391–395
Kinsella J, Glavin R, Reid W H 1988 Patient-controlled analgesia for burned patients: a preliminary report. Burns 14: 500–503
Klein R M, Charlton J E 1980 Behavioural observation and analysis of pain behavior in critically burned patients. Pain 9: 27–40
Knudson-Cooper M 1981 Relaxation and biofeedback training in the treatment of severely burned children. Journal of Burn Care and Rehabilitation 2: 102–109
Knudson-Cooper M 1984 What are the research priorities in the behavioral areas for burned patients? Journal of Trauma 24 (suppl): 197–200
Konigova R 1992 The psychological problems of burned patients – The Rudy Hermans Lecture 1991. Burns 18: 189–199
Lane P R, Hogan D J 1985 Chronic pain and scarring from cement burns. Archives of Dermatology 121: 368–369
Larson D, Huang T, Linares H, Dubrovsky M, Baur P, Parks D 1979 Prevention and treatment of scar contracture. In: Artz C P, Moncrief J A, Pruitt B A (eds) Burns, a team approach. W B Saunders, Philadelphia, p 466–491
Levine J 1984 What are the functions of endorphins following thermal injury? Journal of Trauma 24(S): 168–172
Levitt M 1990 The theory of chronic deafferentation dysesthesias. Journal of the Neurosurgical Sciences 34:71–98
McBride M 1979 The fire that would not die. ETC Publications, Palm Springs
McGrath P 1990 Pain in children. Guilford Press, New York, p 223–228
Mackersie R C, Karagianes T G 1990 Pain management following trauma and burns. Critical Care Clinics 6: 433–449
Mannon J M 1985 Caring for the burned: life and death in a hospital burn center. C C Thomas, Springfield, Illiois
Martyn J A J 1986 Clinical pharmacology and drug therapy in the burned patient. Anesthesiology 65: 67–75
Martyn J A J 1990 Clinical pharmacology and therapeutics in burns. In: Martyn J A J (ed) Acute management of the burned patient. W B Saunders, Philadelphia, p 180–200
Marvin J A, Heimbach D M 1984 Pain management. In: Fisher S V, Helm P A (eds) Comprehensive rehabilitation of burns. Williams & Wilkins, Baltimore, p 311–329
Marvin J A, Heimbach D M 1985 Pain control during the intensive care phase of burn care. Critical Care 1: G1–G6
Melzack R 1975 The McGill pain questionnaire: major properties and scoring methods. Pain 1: 277–297
Melzack R 1990 The tragedy of needless suffering. Scientific American 262: 27–33
Melzack R, Wall P D 1982 The challenge of pain. Basic Books, New York
Melzack R, Wall P D, Ty T C 1982 Acute pain in an emergency clinic: latency of onset and descriptor patterns related to different injuries. Pain 14: 33–43
Meyer R A, Campbell J N 1981 Myelinated nociceptive afferents account for the hyperalgesia that follows a burn to the hand. Science 213: 1527–1529
Mills D C, Lord W D 1992 Propofol for repeated burn dressings in a child: a case report. Burns 18: 58–59
Noe L M, De Gasperi A, Prosperi M, Santandrea E 1991 Propofol anaesthesia for bedside dressings in burned patients. In: Prys-Roberts C, Grundy E, Yate P (eds) Focus on infusion. Current Medical Literature, London, p 199–201
Osgood P F, Szyfelbein S K 1989 Management of burn pain in children. Pediatric Clinics of North America 36: 1001–1013
Osgood P F, Szyfelbein S K 1990 Management of pain. In: Martyn J A J (ed) Acute management of the burned patient. W B Saunders, Philadelphia, p 201–216

Osgood P F, Murphy J L, Carr D B, Szyfelbein S K 1987 Increases in plasma beta-endorphine and tail-flick latency in the rat following burn injury. Life Sciences 40: 547–554
Owen T D, Dye D 1990 The value of topical lignocaine gel in pain relief on skin graft donor sites. British Journal of Plastic Surgery 43: 480–482
Parks D H, Evans E B, Larson D L 1978 Prevention and correction of deformity after severe burns. Surgical Clinics of North America 58: 1279–1289
Patterson D R 1992 Practical applications of psychological techniques in controlling burn pain. Journal of Burn Care and Rehabilitation 13: 13–18
Patterson D R, Questad K A, De Lateur B J 1987 Hypnotherapy as a treatment in patients with burns: research and clinical considerations. Journal of Burn Care and Rehabilitation 8: 263–268
Perry S 1984 Undermedication for pain on a burn unit. General Hospital Psychiatry 6: 308–316
Perry S, Heidrich G 1982 Management of pain during debridement: a survey. Pain 13: 267–280
Perry S, Inturrisi C E 1983 Analgesia and morphine disposition in burned patients. Journal of Burn Care and Rehabilitation 4: 276–279
Perry S, Heidrich G, Ramos E 1981 Assessment of pain by burned patients. Journal of Burn Care and Rehabilitation 2: 322–326
Perry S, Cella D F, Falkenberg J, Heidrich G, Goodwin C 1987 Pain perception in burned patients with stress disorders. Journal of Pain and Symptom Management 2: 22–33
Pontén B 1960 Grafted skin. Acta Chirurgica Scandinavica 257 (suppl): 1–78
Portenoy R K, Moulin D E, Rogers A, Inturrisi C E, Foley K M 1986 IV infusions of opioids for cancer pain: clinical review and guidelines for use. Cancer Treatment Reports 70: 575–581
Pruitt B A 1979 The burn patient. II. Later care and complications of thermal injury. Current Problems in Surgery 16: 1–95
Racz G B, Browne T, Lewis R 1988 Peripheral stimulator implant for the treatment of causalgia caused by electrical burns. Texas Medicine 84: 45–50
Ready L B, Edwards W T 1992 Management of acute pain: a practical guide. IASP Publications, Seattle, p 26–33
Reyneke C J, James M F M, Johnson R 1989 Alfentanyl and propofol infusions for surgery of the burn patient. British Journal of Anaesthesia 63: 418–422
Savedra M 1977 Coping with pain: strategies of severely burned children. The Canadian Nurse 73: 28–29
Schechter N L 1985 Pain and pain control in children. Current Problems in Pediatrics 15: 1–67
Shetty G K, Kelsall P G, Ryan D W 1986 Long-term ketamine infusion. Anaesthesia 41: 1262–1263
Slogoff S, Allen G W, Wessels J V, Cheney D H 1974 Clinical experience with subanesthetic ketamine. Anesthesia and Analgesia 53: 354–360
Spielberger C D, Gorsush R L, Lushene R E 1970 Manual for the state–trait anxiety inventory. Consulting Psychologist Press, Palo Alto, California
Steiner H, Clark W R 1977 Psychiatric complications of burned adults: a classification. Journal of Trauma 17: 134–143
Szyfelbein S K, Osgood P F, Carr D B 1985 The assessment of pain and plasma β-endorphin immunoactivity in burned children. Pain 22: 173–182
Terzis J K 1976 Functional aspects of reinnervation of free skin grafts. Plastic and Reconstructive Surgery 58: 142–146
Tobiasen J M, Hiebert J M 1985 Burns and adjustment to injury: do psychological coping strategies help? Journal of Trauma 25: 1151–1155
Ton T E 1984 The flames shall not consume you. David C Publishing, Elgin
Twycross R G 1974 Clinical experience with diamorphine in advanced malignant disease. Journal of Clinical Pharmacology and Therapeutics 9: 184–198
Van der Does A J 1989 Patients' and nurses' ratings of pain and anxiety during burn wound care. Pain 39: 95–101
Van der Does A J, Van Dyck R 1989 Does hypnosis contribute to the care of burned patients. General Hospital Psychiatry 11: 119–124
Varni J W, Bessman C A, Russo D S, Catalo M E 1980 Behavioral management of chronic pain in children: a case-study. Archives of Physical Medicine and Rehabilitation 61: 275–379
Wakeman R, Kaplan J 1978 An experimental study of hypnosis in painful burns. American Journal of Clinical Hypnosis 21: 3–12
Walkenstein M 1982 Comparison of burned patients' perception of pain with nurses' perception of patient pain. Journal of Burn Care and Rehabilitation 3: 233–236
Wall J T, Cusick C G 1984 Cutaneous responsiveness in primary somatosensory (S–I) hindpaw cortex before and after hindpaw deafferentation in adult rats. Journal of Neurosciences 4: 1499–1515
Wall P D 1979 On the relationship of injury to pain. Pain 6: 253–264
Wall P D 1988 The prevention of post-operative pain. Pain 33: 289–290
Ward R S, Jeffrey P T, Saffle R, Schnebly A, Hayes-Lundy C, Reddy R 1989 Sensory loss over grafted areas in patients with burns. Journal of Burn Care and Rehabilitation 10: 536–538
Watkins P N, Cook E L, May R, Ehleben C M 1988 Psychological stages in adaptation following burn injury: a method for facilitating psychological recovery of burn victims. Journal of Burn Care and Rehabilitation 9: 376–384
Watkins P N, Cook E L, May R, Still J M 1992 The role of the psychiatrist in the team treatment of the adult patient with burns. Journal of Burn Care and Rehabilitation 13: 19–27
Waymack J P, Pruitt B A 1990 Burn wound care. In: Tompkins R K (ed) Advances in surgery, vol 23. Year Book Medical Publishers, Chicago, p 261–289
Wermeling D P, Record K E, Foster T S 1986 Patient-controlled high dose morphine therapy in a patient with electrical burns. Clinical Pharmacy 5: 832–835
Wernick R L, Jarenko M E, Taylor P W 1981 Pain management in severely burned patients: a test of stress inoculation. Journal of Behavioral Medicine 4: 103–109
White P F 1988a Use of patient-controlled analgesia for management of acute pain. Journal of the American Medical Association 259: 243–247
White P F 1988b Propofol: pharmacokinetics and pharmacodynamics. Seminars in Anesthesia 7(S): 4–20
White P F, Way W L, Trevor A J 1982 Ketamine – its pharmacology and therapeutic uses. Anesthesiology 56: 119–136
Wilson G R, Tomlinson p 1988 Pain relief in burns – how we do it. Burns 14: 331–332
Woolf C J 1989 Recent advances in the pathophysiology of acute pain. British Journal of Anaesthesia 63: 139–146

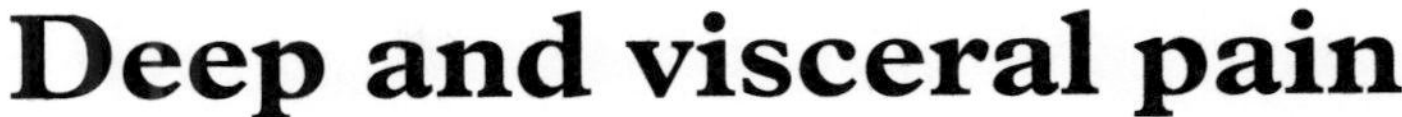

Deep and visceral pain

29. Heart and vascular pain

Paolo Procacci, Massimo Zoppi and Marco Maresca

INTRODUCTION

The main diagnostic problem for a clinician who sees a patient suffering from chest pain is whether he is affected by heart disease. Particular attention is focussed on exploring for possible cardiac ischaemia. We have, however, to remember that many diseases cause chest pain. Apart from angina pectoris and myocardial infarction, there is pain in the early phases of mitral stenosis (Teodori & Galletti 1962) and pain in pericarditis. Many thoracic diseases may cause chest pain that often resembles pain from the heart, including:

1. some diseases of the aorta, such as dissection and atherosclerotic aneurysms
2. some diseases of the lungs, such as pulmonary embolism, infarction, pneumonia, neoplasm and pneumothorax
3. pleuritis
4. diseases of the oesophagus, such as alterations of motility and inflammation.

Chest wall pain may also accompany or follow herpes zoster, chest injury or Tietze's syndrome (i.e. discomfort localised in swelling of the costochondral and costosternal joints, which are painful to palpation).

Differential diagnosis between chest pain from visceral organs and that from somatic diseases, such as cervicodorsal arthritis and fibrositis of the thoracic muscles, may often be difficult. The diagnosis is even more complex when there are intricate problems, i.e. algogenic summation and/or interaction from different structures, such as those observed in cholecystocardiac syndromes, in vertebrocoronary syndromes and in the association of hiatus hernia or peptic ulcer with ischaemic cardiopathies. We recommend lastly that great care should be taken not to make a diagnosis of functional painful disease when organic alterations are not observed.

We think that a careful investigation of the characteristics of pain, of other sensory disturbances and of accompanying symptoms should not be neglected, because, together with laboratory and instrumental examinations, they are of fundamental importance for a correct diagnosis.

This chapter will attempt a wide study of the clinical aspects of chest pain, particularly from the heart, referring the reader to other textbooks for laboratory and instrumental investigations (Julian 1977; Braunwald 1988).

HISTORICAL NOTES ON CARDIAC PAIN

In a historical review on heart pain (Procacci & Maresca 1985a) the first term found for cardiac pain is *passio cardiaca propria* used by Caelius Aurelianus, a fifth-century Roman physician (published 1722). The phrase was translated from the Greek physician Soranus of Ephesus who lived in the second century. After the Dark Ages, many scientists, such as Castelli (1598), Morgagni (1765), Lieutaud (1759) and Van Swieten (1768), mentioned pain in the chest referred to the heart. The term 'angina pectoris' was introduced by Heberden in 1768 in a lecture to the Royal College of Physicians of London (published in 1772) to designate a very distinctive 'disorder of the breast' attended with 'a sense of strangling and anxiety'. Heberden probably read this term in Celsus' works and adopted it because of the similarity of the symptoms to those of the inflammatory diseases of the throat, accompanied by a feeling of choking and strangling, for which ancient Greek and Latin writers such as Celsus and Aretaeus used the term 'angina'. The word derives from the Indo-European root *agh* and, nasalised, *angh*, which means 'to choke, to oppress, to suffer'. Hence the Sanskrit *agha*, the Greek ἀγχειν (*ànchein*) and the Latin *angere*, *angina*. In English, from the same root we have *ake* (Middle English), *ache*, *anguish*, *anger* and *anxious* (Skeat 1882; Procacci & Maresca 1985b).

Heberden (1772) observed the typical relationship between effort and the onset of pain. He wrote that the patients suffering from angina pectoris

> ... are seized, while they are walking, and more particularly when they walk soon after eating, with a painful and most

> disagreeable sensation in the breast which seems as if it would take their life away if it were to increase or to continue: the moment they stand still, all this uneasiness vanishes. ...

In the *Commentarii*, translated into English from the original Latin and published by Heberden's son in 1802, the localisation of pain is carefully described:

> ... the pain is sometimes situated in the upper part, sometimes in the middle, sometimes at the bottom of the *os sterni*, and often more inclined to the left than to the right side. It likewise very frequently extends from the breast to the middle of the left arm.

Heberden differentiated between angina pectoris and other forms of chest pain which were assembled under the heading of *dolor pectoris*. He observed that angina pectoris was often accompanied by anguish of the mind (*angor animi*).

A few years after Heberden's description, Fothergill (1776), Jenner (mentioned by Parry 1799), Parry (1799), Burns (1809) and Testa (1810) discovered that the severity of angina, often leading to sudden death, was due to a severe sclerosis (ossification) of the coronaries.

Good descriptions of anginal pain were given by Laënnec (1826) and by Trousseau (1861), who observed the radiation of pain to the thoracic muscles, clearly indicating the deep parietal component of pain, and the radiation to the internal surface of the arm, interpreted as heart neuralgia.

Other important contributions in this field were: the discovery by Brunton (1867) that inhaled amyl nitrite relieved the anginal pain; the clear separation of myocardial infarction from angina pectoris by Herrick (1912) and the description of electrocardiographic changes during attacks of angina pectoris by Bousfield (1918) and Fiel & Siegel (1928).

GENERAL CONSIDERATIONS ON PAIN FROM ISCHAEMIC HEART DISEASE

Pain from ischaemic heart disease is a symptom well known to every physician, for it is frequently observed. However, descriptions in textbooks and personal experience give the impression of a wide variety of symptoms because of different areas of reference, different kinds of pain in the same area and involvement of areas far away from the heart. This pain, therefore, seems not to follow any rules. We believe that for this reason the attention of the physician is given less to an exact observation of the pain and more to laboratory and instrumental investigations which often do not suggest the right diagnosis. However, serious angina pectoris and even myocardial infarction may be diagnosed with careful observation of the characteristics of the pain, when laboratory signs are negative.

The absence of rules for cardiac pain is only apparent if we examine in detail the various types of pain perceived by the patient. Indeed, it is not enough to investigate where pain is felt, but it is also necessary to distinguish between true visceral pain and referred pain and to determine whether pain is referred in deep or superficial parietal structures. Only an adequate and careful investigation of the patient can give us such information. Consequently, we think that the description of cardiac pain should be preceded by a few clinical concepts on the characteristics of visceral pain.

The subsequent discussion on pain from the heart and from other chest organs is mainly based on observations made in the Medical School in Florence over the last 50 years (Teodori & Galletti 1962; Procacci & Zoppi 1983; Procacci et al 1986).

CLINICAL CHARACTERISTICS OF VISCERAL PAIN

The qualities of true visceral pain are clearly different from those of deep pain or of cutaneous pain. Visceral pain is dull, aching or boring; it is not well-localised and is described differently by the patient. It is always accompanied by a sense of malaise and of being ill. It is associated with strong autonomic reflexes, such as diffuse sweating, vasomotor responses, changes of arterial pressure and heart rate and with an intense alarm reaction. This deep pain was defined as 'splanchnic pain' by Ross (1887) and as 'direct pain of viscera' (*'direkter Schmerz der Eingeweide'*) by Hansen & Schliack (1962).

When an algogenic process affecting a viscus recurs frequently or becomes more intense and prolonged, the location is more exact, and pain is gradually felt in more superficial structures, even, sometimes, far from the site of origin. This phenomenon is usually called 'referred pain' in English, whereas German authors use the less common but, in our opinion, more appropriate term 'transferred pain' (*übertragener Schmerz*).

1. *Deep referred pain.* This pain shows a segmental pattern. It is felt in bones (sclerotomes) and muscles (myotomes).
2. *Superficial referred pain.* This pain is felt in the skin within the dermatomes related to the affected viscus.

Both deep and superficial referred pain may be accompanied by autonomic reflexes. Cutaneous hyperalgesia and zones of muscular tenderness are often present.

With unpleasant visceral feelings, the patient often declines to apply the word pain, selecting words such as pressure, tightness or squeezing. Between the lack of sensory symptoms and the true pain we have a continuum of intensity and unpleasantness. For these intermediate sensations, which are unpleasant but not painful, we can use the term proposed by Keele & Armstrong (1964): 'metaesthesia'. These sensations should be carefully investigated before defining a visceral disease as 'silent'.

PAIN IN MYOCARDIAL INFARCTION

This pain arises with various modalities, at times suddenly during more or less stressful activities, or after a large meal, or during rest or sleep. Occasionally, in 20–50% of cases, it is preceded by a vague feeling of chest discomfort, or slight dyspnoea, or unpleasant gastric sensations described as fullness of the stomach or indigestion. The patient has often experienced previous paroxysm of angina pectoris. The early pain is deep, central, anterior and sometimes also posterior; it lasts from a few minutes to a few hours, showing the characteristics of the true visceral pain. It is defined by most patients as pressing, constricting or squeezing, or with phrases such as 'a band across the chest'. This kind of pain is present in about 80% of patients. It is central, often behind the lower sternum, less frequently on the epigastrium, or in both these sites. In about 15% of patients, anterior pain is concomitant with central back pain; in 1% of cases the pain is only posterior (Fig. 29.1). Pain is often accompanied by nausea and vomiting and by diffuse sweating. This pain is very intense and often accompanied by a strong alarm reaction with sometimes a feeling of impending death.

In a following phase, after a period which varies from 10 minutes to a few hours, the pain reaches the parietal structures, assuming the characteristics of deep referred pain. In about 14% of patients this is the first perceived pain. This pain is often defined as pressing or constricting and tends to radiate. The spatial localisation is more exact than for visceral pain; it is often accompanied by sweating and rarely by nausea and vomiting. This pain is often referred beneath the sternum or in the precordial area, sometimes spreading to both sides of the anterior chest and, in a few cases, only to the right. The radiation is accompanied by feelings such as numbness, cramp or squeezing of the elbow or wrist. Frequently the pain radiates to the whole left arm or to both arms, or involves the left forearm and hand; in a few cases it radiates only to the right arm. Another uncommon radiation is to the neck, jaw and temporomandibular joint on both sides simultaneously. In rare cases a posterior pain is felt in the interscapulovertebral region and may radiate to the ulnar aspect of the left arm. In patients not treated with drugs, the duration of this parietal pain varies from half an hour to 12 or more hours. It always lasts longer than true visceral pain.

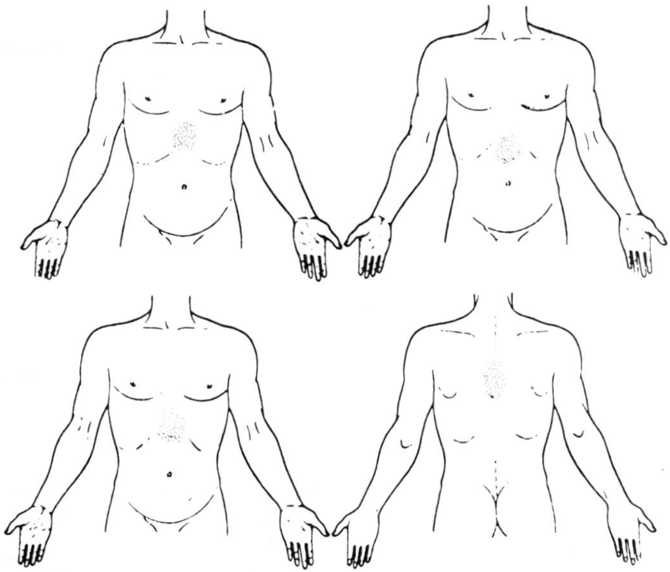

Fig. 29.1 Areas of deep visceral pain in myocardial infarction and in unstable angina.
(From Teodori & Galletti 1962 with permission.)

Muscular tenderness follows the onset of this pain after a delay that varies from a few hours to half a day. It mainly involves the pectoralis major, the deep muscles of the interscapular region, the muscles of the forearm and, less frequently, the trapezius and deltoid muscles (Fig. 29.2).

In 20% of patients a superficial referred pain arises. This pain is localised by the patient within the dermatomes C8–T1, that is, on the ulnar side of the arm and forearm. This pain is rarely the only starting symptom. It lasts from half an hour to 6 hours. It is intense, stabbing or lancinating. In the areas of reference cutaneous hyperalgesia is often found (Fig. 29.3). There are no clear correlations between the type of infarction (inferior, anterior, transmural, nontransmural) and the pattern of pain.

PAIN IN ANGINA PECTORIS

The pain is generally referred, often deep, more rarely superficial, with the same qualities and radiations as those described in myocardial infarction, but the intensity and duration are less. Pain is not accompanied by a feeling of impending death and is seldom accompanied by nausea and vomiting. The alarm reaction with the accompanying symptoms is less intense than in myocardial infarction. In these patients deep muscular tenderness is found in the same areas as in infarction and is constant and independent of pain attacks.

The deep referred pain with muscular tenderness in many cases does not replace, but only inhibits the perception of true visceral pain. In patients suffering from angina of effort Procacci & Zoppi (1983) observed that pain during stress-testing was referred anteriorly on the chest wall. These patients had areas of deep tenderness on the chest wall which were blocked with a local anaesthetic. After the block, during stress-testing and at S–T segment displacement in the electrocardiogram, the patients experienced a new type of pain or a general discomfort which had never been felt before. The new pain was substernal or epigastric, with the characteristics of true visceral pain.

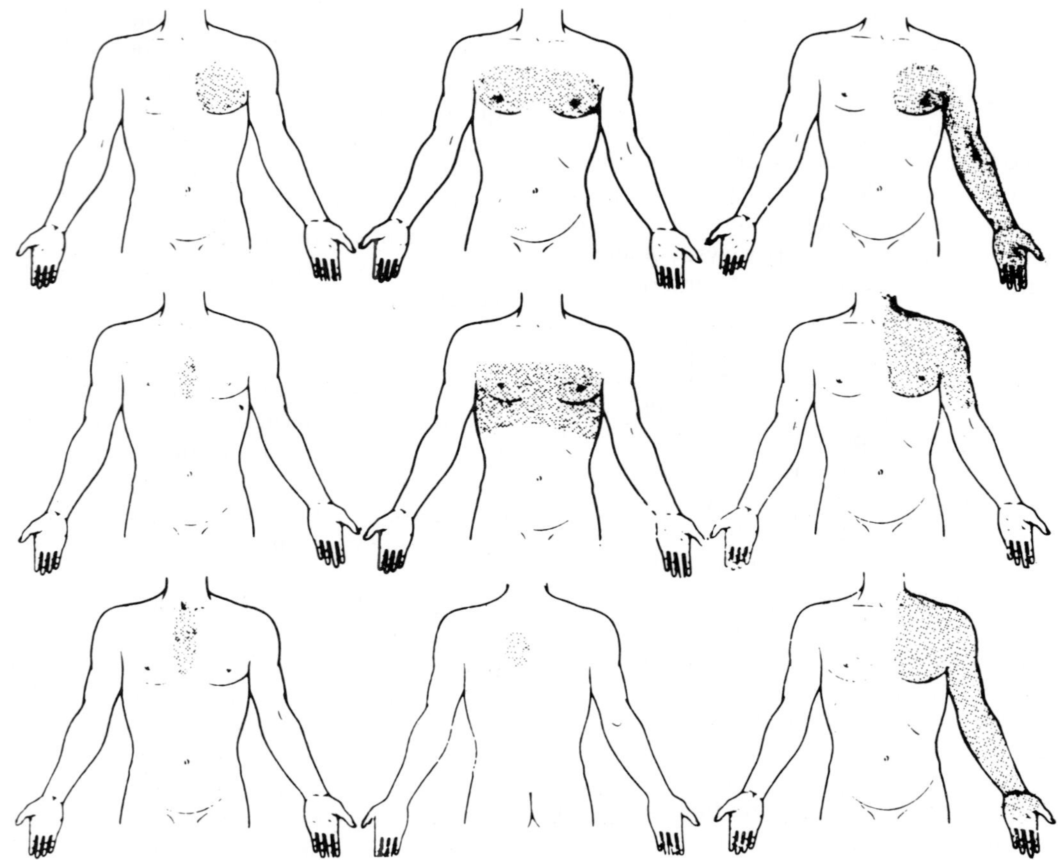

Fig. 29.2 Areas of deep referred pain in myocardial infarction and in angina. (From Teodori & Galletti 1962 with permission.)

In recent classifications of angina pectoris, the following anginal syndromes are distinguished: stable angina, unstable angina and variant (Prinzmetal's) angina (Rutherford et al 1988; Willerson 1988).

Stable angina

Patients with stable angina usually have angina with effort or exercise or during other conditions in which myocardial oxygen demand is increased. The quality of sensation is sometimes vague and may be described as a mild pressure-like discomfort or an uncomfortable numb sensation. Anginal 'equivalents' (i.e. symptoms of myocardial ischaemia other than angina) such as breathlessness, faintness, fatigue and belching have also been reported (Rutherford et al 1988). A classical feature of stable angina is the disappearance of pain after the use of nitroglycerine or the inhalation of amyl nitrite.

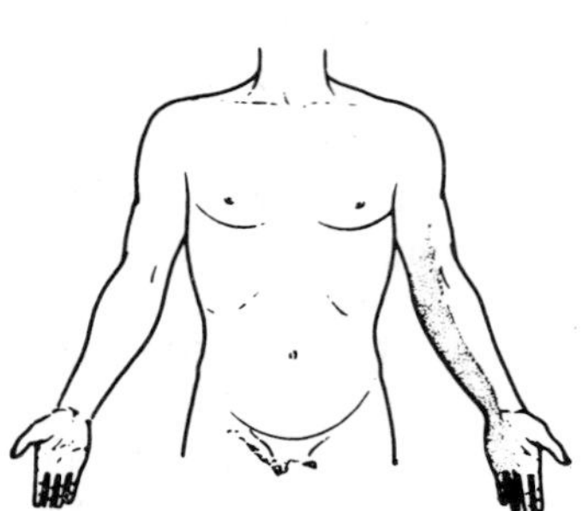

Fig. 29.3 Superficial referred pain in myocardial infarction and in angina. (From Teodori & Galletti 1962 with permission.)

Unstable angina

The term 'unstable angina', previously also known as preinfarction angina, acute coronary insufficiency and intermediate coronary syndrome, indicates the following syndromes:

1. crescendo angina (more severe, prolonged or frequent) superimposed on a preexisting pattern of relatively stable, exertion-related angina pectoris
2. angina pectoris at rest as well as with minimal exertion
3. angina pectoris of new onset (usually within 1 month), which is brought on by minimal exertion.

In unstable angina the chest discomfort is similar in quality to that of chronic stable angina, although it is usually more intense, is usually described as pain, may persist for as long as 30 minutes and occasionally awakes the patient from sleep. When it lasts more than 30 minutes, an infarction should be suspected. One of the characteristics of this pain is that its intensity varies greatly, from very slight to (more frequently) intermediate, sometimes reaching maximal intensity, like that described in infarction.

Several clues should alert the physician to a changing anginal pattern. These include an abrupt reduction in the threshold of physical activity which provokes angina; an increase in the frequency, severity and duration of angina; radiation of the discomfort to a new site; onset of new features associated with the pain, such as nausea and decreased relief of pain afforded by nitroglycerine (Rutherford et al 1988). Some authors recently held that the natural history of stable angina and that of unstable angina are in many cases different; except that in some patients stable angina evolves into unstable angina, whereas unstable angina almost never evolves into stable angina (Poggesi et al 1992). Moreover, recent studies suggest that the increase of plasma fibrinopeptide-A levels and the lymphocyte activation in patients with active, unstable angina indicate that the outbursts of unstable angina appear to be an acute, transient inflammatory phase, repeatedly occurring only in a subgroup of the patients with coronary atherosclerotic disease (Neri Serneri et al 1992).

Variant angina

Variant (Prinzmetal's) angina is an unusual syndrome of cardiac pain that occurs almost exclusively at rest, usually is not precipitated by physical exertion or emotional stress and is associated with S–T segment elevations on the electrocardiogram (Prinzmetal et al 1959). This syndrome has been demonstrated convincingly to be due to coronary artery spasm. However, in arteriographic studies Maseri et al (1978) observed that in many patients the coronary vasospasm occurring during an anginal attack was associated with S–T segment elevation or depression, blurring the distinction between variant (Prinzmetal's) angina and unstable angina.

SYNDROME X AND INCREASED CARDIAC SENSITIVITY

Kemp (1973) described a 'syndrome X', consisting of chest pain, angiographically normal coronary arteries and ischaemic-appearing S–T segment responses with exercise tests. It was proposed that patients with syndrome X have a patchily distributed abnormal constriction of coronary prearteriolar vessels not involved in metabolic autoregulation of flow. The term became a label for patients with normal coronary angiograms, who present with angina pectoris or at least chest discomfort (Maseri et al 1991).

It is interesting that a high percentage of these patients show a typical anginal pain or a chest discomfort (Shapiro et al 1988; Cannon et al 1990) during:

1. catheter manipulation in cardiac angiography
2. pacing at various stimulus intensities
3. intracoronary injection of contrast medium.

These patients probably have a heightened cardiac pain sensitivity. Whether this phenomenon represents an abnormal activation of receptors within the heart or an abnormal processing of visceral afferent neural impulses is unknown.

THE PROBLEM OF PAINLESS CORONARY HEART DISEASES

It is well known that myocardial infarction has been found in electrocardiographic studies or at postmortem examinations in patients in whom there was no history of a well defined episode of chest pain. The occurrence of painless infarctions has not been correlated with the location, size or age of the infarction, nor with the age of the patient (Rinzler 1951; Friedberg 1956; Teodori & Galletti 1962). During long-term follow-up in the Framingham study one-quarter of patients had 'unrecognised' myocardial infarction, detected only on routine 2-yearly electrocardiogram, and of these approximately half of the episodes were truly silent (Kannel & Abbott 1984). Other population studies suggest that between 20 and 60% of nonfatal myocardial infarctions are unrecognised by the patient and are discovered only on subsequent routine electrocardiographic or postmortem examination (Pasternak et al 1988). These differences are partly due to the use of different methods of investigating and understanding the symptoms. If indeed we assemble an accurate history of patients in whom a diagnosis of asymptomatic previous myocardial infarction is suspected in the course of routine examination, we would find a transient episode of chest discomfort, or sudden and unusual thoracic paraesthesias (tingling, pricking, numbness) radiating to the left arm, or a slight pain which was judged unimportant by the patient, or an episode of nausea and vomiting interpreted as due to gastric fullness or indigestion (Procacci et al 1976). The history should be very accurate, since often these episodes are underestimated and have been forgotten by patients. Taking into account these factors, the frequency of asymptomatic myocardial infarction is greatly reduced.

Recently the term and concept of 'silent myocardial ischaemia' have been introduced to indicate all forms of painless myocardial ischaemia documented with ambulatory electrocardiogram, exercise testing, arteriography or when an extensive coronary artery obstruction not accompanied by symptoms evolves into myocardial infarction. Furthermore, in many patients with angina, ambulatory electrocardiographic monitoring showed that most episodes of ischaemia were asymptomatic (Rutherford et al 1988; Cohn 1989). According to Chierchia et al (1983) all ischaemic attacks lasting less than 3 minutes or associated with increases in left ventricular filling pressure of less than 7 mmHg are painless. Above this level, clinical, haemodynamic, electrocardiographic and angiographic studies could not differentiate between painful and painless ischaemic episodes (Maseri et al 1985). Central transmission or perception, or both, of potentially painful stimuli is likely to play a major role in determining the presence or absence of cardiac pain, particularly in patients who have both painful and painless episodes of apparently similar severity (Maseri 1987). The frequency of silent myocardial ischaemia is higher in patients with diabetes, probably because of neuropathy involving the visceral afferent fibres.

PAINFUL COMPLICATIONS OF MYOCARDIAL INFARCTION

Angina may evolve into myocardial infarction. After myocardial infarction, stable or unstable angina may develop.

Left scapulohumeral periarthritis, giving a picture of 'frozen shoulder', with pain, stiffness and marked limitation of motion of the shoulder joint, may complicate some cases of long-lasting angina and 5% of cases of myocardial infarction. In some cases, 3–6 weeks after myocardial infarction, progressive dystrophy of the left arm begins. It mainly involves the shoulder, the wrist and the hand (shoulder–hand syndrome). The evolution may be very severe and includes advanced stages of osteoporosis, muscular and cutaneous atrophy, glossy skin, loss of hair and vasomotor changes etc. As in other reflex dystrophies, it often improves with blocks of the stellate ganglion.

Persistent pain after myocardial infarction, especially transmural, may be due to pericarditis. It is important to diagnose the chest pain of pericarditis accurately, since failure to appreciate it may lead to the erroneous diagnosis of recurrent ischaemic pain and/or extension of the infarction and to the inappropriate use of anticoagulants, nitrates, beta-adrenergic blocking agents or narcotics.

Pleuropericardial chest pain with fever may begin in a few cases 1–6 weeks after myocardial infarction. This postmyocardial infarction syndrome (or Dressler's syndrome) is thought to be due to an autoimmune pericarditis, pleuritis and pneumonitis (Dressler 1956). The pain can often be distinguished from that of an extending infarction by its characteristic pericardial pattern: the pain is relieved by leaning forward, and exacerbated by deep breathing. The syndrome usually benefits from treatment with aspirin-like agents or corticosteroids. Since effusions associated with Dressler's syndrome may be haemorragic, anticoagulants should be discontinued if they are being administered.

PAIN IN CARDIAC NEUROSIS

Patients with chest pain and without instrumental signs of ischaemic heart disease are frequently observed. A precordial pain, often radiating, with characteristics that resemble those of angina, worries most of these patients, who then frequently undergo medical visits and examinations, the normality of which reassures them for only a short while.

Pain is variously described as stabbing, piercing, burning, dull, squeezing, annoying, slight, intense, variable and synchronous with the cardiac beats etc. First of all, the physician must consider other causes of chest pain.

Some characteristics of this pain distinguish it from true angina: the duration varies from a few moments to some days; it is often not related to exertion; the patient is restless and nervous, while during an attack of angina he remains relatively immobile. The behaviour of patients often differs when they are asked where they feel pain: the patient with angina puts an open hand on the sternum, the neurotic patient touches, with his index finger, the left submammary region or other zones of the precordial area.

In spite of these differences we should be very cautious in diagnosing cardiac neurosis, because to differentiate between angina and neurosis is often difficult. It occurs too frequently that tiresome patients, dismissed too soon and labelled as neurotics, die suddenly from an acute myocardial infarction. An investigation carried out on patients with a typical chest pain showed that many of these patients, during atrial pacing, had electrocardiographic, haemodynamic and metabolic signs of myocardial ischaemia. In these patients the coronary arteriography was normal and the standard effort test gave dubious results (Daubert et al 1975). It appears, thus, that the criteria of a normal coronary arteriography and a negative or insignificant effort test are insufficient to discard the diagnosis of myocardial ischaemia in cases of pain habitually considered as nonorganic.

DIAGNOSIS OF ISCHAEMIC HEART PAIN

We shall limit the description to the criteria based on the characteristics of the pain. The duration of pain is usually a few minutes in stable angina, variable but not exceeding 30 minutes in unstable angina and longer in infarction: pain of myocardial infarction is often accompanied by a feeling of impending death. Other symptoms, such as nausea and vomiting, are often present in infarction, but rarely in angina. The importance of other characteristics of pain and their limits for diagnosis have been previously explained.

Some acute diseases of abdominal organs, such as peptic

ulcer, acute cholecystitis and pancreatitis, may simulate heart pain, just as heart pain may simulate those diseases.

Among the diagnostic criteria which should be mentioned are the use of nitroglycerine and antacids. Nitroglycerine interrupts pain in stable angina, has a variable effect in unstable angina and is ineffective in myocardial infarction. Antacids induce pain relief in peptic ulcer but not in infarction. The value of these diagnostic criteria is not absolute.

OTHER CAUSES OF CHEST PAIN (FROM THE HEART)

Aortic stenosis

Angina pectoris has been noted in about 50% of cases of symptomatic aortic stenosis. Angina pectoris occurs more frequently in aortic stenosis than in other valvular lesions. The pain is usually a typical angina of effort. The excruciating persistent variety seen in myocardial infarction is rarely observed. Patients with severe chronic aortic stenosis tend to be free of cardiovascular symptoms until relatively late in the course of the disease. Once patients become symptomatic the average survival is 2–3 years (Frank et al 1973). Obviously the course of this disease changes after cardiac surgery or angioplasty. The pain is generally related to a coronary narrowing or to myocardial hypertrophy with increased oxygen demand.

Aortic insufficiency

It is well known that angina pectoris has long been regarded as a symptom of aortic insufficiency. According to Friedberg (1956), angina pectoris is uncommon in uncomplicated aortic insufficiency, but it may occur because of coronary atherosclerosis or because superimposed calcification of the aortic valve leads to stenosis of the coronary arteries.

Mitral stenosis

In the course of mitral stenosis the patient may have a posterosuperior pain on the left side of the chest, which is sometimes deep and sometimes superficial. Hope (1832) wrote that pain in the course of mitral stenosis is a rather frequent event. Vaquez (1922) identified a myalgic spot on the left interscapulovertebral region which is particularly evident in the phase of mitral stenosis that precedes heart failure. More recently, it has been pointed out that about 15% of patients suffering from mitral stenosis have a pain with the same characteristics as that of angina pectoris (Reichek et al 1973).

We think, instead, on the basis of studies at our school in Florence, that the clinical characteristics of pain in the course of mitral stenosis differ from those of angina (Teodori & Galletti 1962): pain in mitral stenosis is indeed located in the left interscapulovertebral area, while in angina this location is rare. The pain in mitral stenosis is deep and crushing. It is accompanied by deep and/or superficial tenderness in the same area, i.e. within the metameres T2–T4. The evolution is typical: it starts together with an increase of atrial pressure when the compliance of the atrial wall is still unchanged, i.e. during the initial phases of the disease, and decreases and disappears when the compliance of the atrial wall is progressively reduced. Subsequently, when the posterosuperior pain has disappeared, a new pain may be felt on the precordium together with laboratory signs of right strain. In some cases of severe mitral stenosis with very high pulmonary hypertension, pain is similar to that of angina pectoris. The observation of pain in mitral stenosis is now rare, after the development of cardiac surgery.

Mitral valve prolapse

Mitral valve prolapse is an anatomical and clinical entity, characterised by systolic bowing in the left atrium of one or both mitral leaflets and by typical auscultatory findings (midsystolic clicks and late systolic murmurs) (Barlow et al 1963; Braunwald 1988). Chest pain is sometimes reported. In some cases, in which mitral valve prolapse is associated with coronary heart disease, a typical anginal pain is present. Maresca et al (1989) carefully examined a group of patients with mitral valve prolapse in whom association with any other valvular or heart disease had been ruled out. A characteristic which did emerge was that most of them suffered a typical myofascial pain of the muscles of the chest.

Inflammatory diseases of the heart

Pain can occur in all inflammatory diseases of the heart, i.e. pericarditis, myocarditis and endocarditis. Pain is however more frequent in pericarditis than in myocarditis or in endocarditis; consequently we shall describe only the pain from pericarditis.

In acute pericarditis the onset of pain often coincides with fever or it may follow a shivering chill.

Chronic pericarditis is often painless, but on careful questioning the patient may report a deep, dull, slight pain or sensation of heaviness or fullness in the chest. Pain in pericarditis is, however, less frequent than in pleurisy, so when pain is present, pleural involvement should be suspected. For these reasons the pericardium is considered to be less sensitive to pain than the pleura (Teodori & Galletti 1962).

Pain in pericarditis is often deep and substernal, usually involving the upper two-thirds of the sternum, less commonly precordial; it is continuous and lasts from a few hours to 3 days. It may appear repeatedly, always for brief periods. It is aggravated by deep inspiration, cough and lateral movements of the chest. Pain is reduced by sitting up and leaning forward.

In about half the cases, together with this deep pain, there is a superficial referred pain. The pain may radiate to the left shoulder, scapula and arm, to the neck and to the epigastrium. It may appear during exertion, resembling angina. This characteristic is probably due to the inflammatory involvement of the aorta and periaortic tissues. Pain is often accompanied by tenderness of the subclavicular fossa, of the superior ridge of the trapezius muscle and of the coracoid process, and more rarely of the left chest base.

We must remember that in systemic vasculitis (giant cell arteritis, Takayasu's syndrome) angina pectoris and myocardial infarction are sometimes observed.

Cor pulmonale

In many cases of acute cor pulmonale (pulmonary embolism) a true visceral pain is observed that has the same qualities and radiation of myocardial infarction, including a strong alarm reaction.

Some patients suffering from chronic cor pulmonale have pain that shows great similarities with that of angina. The pain may be present in all diseases in which pulmonary hypertension is present – chronic cor pulmonale, mitral stenosis, some congenital heart diseases and idiopathic pulmonary hypertension. Anginal pain in patients with pulmonary hypertension is similar to that of angina pectoris: both types of pain have the same location, radiation, quality and intensity. A careful analysis, however, will show that during spontaneous or exertional pain in pulmonary hypertension the severity of cyanosis increases (*angor coeruleus*), whereas in coronary angina the patient is pale (*angor pallidus*). The duration of pain in pulmonary hypertension is often longer than in heart angina; it may last some hours, and afterwards gradually disappears. In some cases the pain worsens during inspiration, and this does not happen in heart angina. This phenomenon is probably due to an increase of pulmonary pressure during this phase of the breathing.

CAUSES OF CHEST PAIN (FROM ORGANS OTHER THAN THE HEART)

Diseases of the aorta

Aneurysms

The aneurysms that give rise to chest pain are those of the thoracic aorta, while aneurysms of the abdominal aorta are often asymptomatic but are sometimes accompanied by abdominal and low back pain.

Pain in thoracic aortic aneurysms is probably due to compression and erosion of adjacent musculoskeletal structures and to the excitation of aortic end-organs. It is usually steady and boring and occasionally may be pulsating.

Aortic dissection

According to Eagle & De Sanctis (1988) by far the commonest presenting symptom of aortic dissection is severe pain, which is found in over 90% of cases. In fact, those patients without pain have usually suffered some disturbances of consciousness that render them unable to perceive pain. The pain of dissection is often unbearable, forcing the patient to writhe in agony or to pace restlessly in an attempt to gain some measure of relief. Pain resembles that of myocardial infarction but several features of the pain may arouse suspicion of aortic dissection. The quality of the pain as described by the patient is often remarkably appropriate to the actual event. Adjectives such as 'tearing', 'ripping' and 'stabbing' are frequently used. Another characteristic of the pain of aortic dissection is its tendency to migrate from the point of its origin to other sites, following the path of the dissecting haematoma as it extends through the aorta. Pain felt maximally in the anterior thorax is more frequent with proximal dissection, whereas pain that is most severe in the interscapular area is much more common with a distal site of origin. Nausea and vomiting, diffuse sweating, fainting and hiccup, resistant to drugs and to manoeuvres which would ordinarily stop it, can frequently accompany the pain.

Syphilitic aortitis

Syphilitic aortitis is generally an asymptomatic lesion. The symptoms attributed to it are probably due to its complications: coronary ostial stenosis, aortic insufficiency or aneurysm.

Diseases of the lungs

Thoracic or thoracobrachial pain is present in many patients with lung diseases, always in pulmonary infarction and very often in pneumonia. Marino et al (1986), in 164 patients with nonmetastatic cancer of the lungs, observed that pain was present in 40% of the patients. Pain was always deep, referred on the chest anteriorly or posteriorly, with a good correlation between its location and the site of the pulmonary lesion.

Pleurisy

Chest pain is frequently observed in the course of pleurisy because the pain sensitivity of the pleura is very high. The pain shows a more exact spatial localisation than in diseases of the lung. Its onset is more frequently sudden than progressive, often preceding other symptoms such as fever, dyspnoea and cough, and lasts a few days.

The location of pain varies according to the location and extent of the inflammation.

1. In effusive pleurisy it is frequently referred to the submammary area
2. In diaphragmatic pleurisy, pain is often felt on the trapezius ridge and on the base of the affected side of the chest
3. In apical pleurisy, pain is in the interscapulovertebral region.

Almost always, in effusive pleurisies, pain is steady, aggravated by deep inspiration, cough, movements of the chest and by lying on the affected side. Shoulder pain with diaphragmatic pleurisy and interscapulovertebral pain with apical pleurisy are less localised, constrictive, and not aggravated by movement, cough or deep inspiration. Pain is very intense in effusive pleuritis, especially when it is located in the submammary area, in empyema, in pleurisy that follows a pulmonary or subdiaphragmatic abscess and in pleurisy that complicates pneumonia or cancer of the lung. Pain is often associated with superficial and/or deep hyperalgesia and with slight contraction of the hyperalgesic muscles.

Diseases of the oesophagus

Experimental and spontaneous oesophageal pain shows the typical characteristics of visceral pain: it is poorly localised, is accompanied by autonomic reflexes and by emotions and becomes referred.

The fundamental algogenic stimuli for the oesophagus are :

1. Strong mechanical stimulation from oesophageal stenosis and motor disorders, such as achalasia, diffuse oesophageal spasm, nutcracker oesophagus (symptomatic peristalsis) and aspecific motor disorders (Clouse et al 1983).

2. Inflammation. In patients with oesophagitis, pain was experimentally induced with the introduction of liquids at 5°C and 30°C (Teodori & Galletti 1962). These individuals felt a very unpleasant, deep, burning pain behind the sternum, mainly at the level of the xiphoid process. This pain is felt by patients with oesophagitis, gastrooesophageal reflux and peptic ulcer of the oesophagus.

The areas of reference of oesophageal pain are the higher sternum for the diseases of the proximal third of the oesophagus and lower sternum for diseases of the distal third. Diseases of the intermediate third give rise to pain referred to one or other areas. The zones to which pain radiates are many and may be the same for diseases of the upper and lower oesophagus. The more frequently observed are: the interscapular and central dorsal areas at the level of the sixth and seventh thoracic vertebrae, the neck, the ear, the jaw, the precordium, the shoulders, the upper limbs and the epigastrium.

Oesophageal pain can mimic that of myocardial ischaemia. Discomfort is often relieved by nitroglycerine, sometimes by calcium antagonists, but unlike angina, by milk or antacids.

Gastrooesophageal reflux is often associated with hiatus hernia, which can be diagnosed radiographically. In this disorder, postprandial distress is more marked in the recumbent position and this feature helps to differentiate it from angina pectoris.

COMPLEX PROBLEMS

Frequently heart pain is mingled with pain arising from other structures (*angors coronariens intriqués*) (Froment & Gonin 1956). For instance, a myocardial ischaemia may be accompanied by cervicothoracic osteoarthritis (vertebrocoronary syndrome), by chest fibromyalgias, or by many diseases of the gastrointestinal tract, such as diseases of the oesophagus, hiatus hernia, gastroduodenitis, peptic ulcer, calculus and noncalculous cholecystitis (cholecystocoronary syndrome). In these cases algogenic summation from different organs probably occurs. We should also consider the consequence of induced reflexes. Pain may vary from typical angina pectoris to chest pain with different patterns.

MECHANISMS OF CARDIAC PAIN

The mechanisms of cardiac pain seem to be partly similar to those of visceral and partly similar to those of skeletal muscles. For instance, a solution of NaCl 5%, a well known algogenic stimulus for the skeletal muscles, injected in the left ventricular wall of the cat induces a powerful discharge of A-delta afferent fibres from the heart (Brown 1967). A spasm of the coronaries during painful attacks was shown in patients with unstable angina (Maseri et al 1975).

Aviado & Schmidt (1955) advanced the hypothesis that the adequate stimuli in the heart for the onset of pain and of reflex phenomena were the following:

1. reduced coronary arterial pressure distal to an occlusion, acting on coronary arterial pressoreceptors
2. ischaemia, stimulating the myocardial pressoreceptors
3. release of chemical substances formed by tissue breakdown or platelet disintegration
4. myocardial ischaemia stimulating visceral pain receptors.

To these mechanisms Teodori & Galletti (1962) added the distension of the cardiac chambers and possibly of the large vessels. This mechanism probably prevails for posterior chest pain in early phases of mitral stenosis and may be important for pain in the course of other clinical conditions accompanied by enlargement of cardiac ventricles (cor pulmonale, aortic valve diseases, etc.)

The first mechanism, a localised hypotension, finds experimental support in Brown's experiments on the cat (1967): the pseudoaffective reaction, an indirect sign of pain, begins in fact only 1 second after experimental coronary occlusion, too short a time for the release and/or activation of pain-producing substances (Iggo 1974). This mechanism could therefore be prevalent in early phases of cardiac pain.

These findings were supported by research in the cat which showed an increased discharge of the afferent C-fibres from the left ventricle following mechanical and biochemical stimuli. Silent, afferent, myelinated or unmyelinated fibres were not found (Malliani & Lombardi 1982). The discharge increased after powerful stimuli, such as the intracoronary injection of bradykinin. The fact that silent fibres from the resting heart were not found suggests that a specific receptive apparatus for pain does not exist in the heart . When algogenic stimuli are applied, the discharge increases in fibres connected with receptors which during rest probably behave as mechanoreceptors. These can be considered as low threshold polymodal receptors. Echocardiography showed that during an attack of angina pectoris there is a localised hypokinesia, akinesia or dyskinesia of the ventricular wall. At this level a massive stretching may induce a particular pattern of impulses giving rise to pain.

When a volley of impulses in C-fibres, from deep tissue but not from skin, arrives in the spinal cord there is initially a short phase of facilitation of dorsal horn cells. Following this there is a second phase of massive facilitation with a latency of many minutes and a very long duration. During the second period cells which were previously nociceptive-specific respond to light pressure (Wall & Woolf 1984). It seems reasonable to propose that there are cells in the upper thoracic cord with a convergent input from skin and the heart and that these cells become facilitated during angina attacks. These observations can explain some mechanisms of referred pain.

Together with mechanical factors the biochemical components of cardiac pain in ischaemic heart disease should be considered. These arise from increase of lactic acid, release of potassium ions and production of kinins and of other pain-producing substances. In the present authors' opinion, it is probable that a group of pain-producing substances act in concert. Whatever the pain-producing substances could be, the metabolic disturbance during angina pectoris induces changes in peripheral microenvironment, and is responsible for pain which shows similarities to pain from fibrositis of skeletal muscles. Keele & Armstrong (1964) suggested a parallel between the biochemical and algogenic phenomena of myocardial infarction and those of myonecrosis of skeletal muscles, as observed in idiopathic myoglobinuria, in Haff disease and in sea-snake poisoning. In both infarction and myonecrosis, the release of pain-producing substances from the necrotic tissue could be the fundamental stimulus for the severe, long-lasting pain characteristic of these afflictions.

We believe that another important mechanism is the development of an ischaemic neuropathy of heart nerves. Such a neuropathy is present in atherosclerotic arterial disease of the legs with *claudicatio intermittens* in which, according to Lewis (1942), pain resembles that of angina (*claudicatio cordis*).

The various mechanisms for cardiac pain intermingle, one or other being prevalent in different conditions and in different patients (Procacci & Zoppi 1983; Procacci et al 1986).

THERAPY

Pain in angina pectoris is relieved by a group of drugs which are ineffective in other types of pain. The first drugs used were amyl nitrite (Brunton 1867) and, a few years later, nitroglycerine. The relief of pain with nitrates is often dramatic. Other drugs are used to prevent ischaemic attacks, such as beta-blocking agents, long-lasting organic nitrates and calcium antagonists. The mechanism of these drugs is as controversial as is the mechanism of pain.

The drug of choice in myocardial infarction is morphine, which generally induces relief of pain and good sedation. Morphine in myocardial infarction not only relieves pain but also centrally interrupts reflexes that may worsen the cardiovascular state or induce life-threatening arrhythmias.

We should also mention the useful association of antianginal drugs with aspirin which contributes to the elimination of the algogenic summation from myalgic spots, often present in patients with angina. This latent afferent input may assume an important role in reflexes which facilitate the attacks of angina. Aspirin is also useful for its antithrombotic effect, due to inhibition of platelet aggregation.

In myocardial infarction intracoronary thrombolysis with streptokinase, urokinase and other drugs is useful in the first hours after the onset of symptoms. When intracoronary thrombolysis cannot be performed, intravenous thrombolysis is used.

The treatment of ischaemic heart disease with drugs or surgery is rapidly developing and the interested reader is referred to specialised journals and textbooks.

In cardiac surgery, it is well known that some patients with angina have good relief of pain after coronary angioplasty or aortocoronary bypass. The disappearance of pain is generally related to an improvement of coronary flow. It should however be considered that during the operation of aortocoronary bypass some of the cardiac afferent fibres running in sympathetic nerves are cut. This denervation may be relevant to the relief of heart pain.

VASCULAR PAIN

Vascular pain is a complex area. It may be divided into three sections: arterial pain; pain due to lesion or dysfunction of the microvessels (metarterioles, capillaries, small venules) and venous pain.

Obviously many traumas, frequent in daily life, can damage the vascular tree with different consequences.

Vascular pain due to haemorrhage in the brain is described in Chapter 46.

Arterial pain

Pain originating in coronary vessels and in the aorta has been treated in previous sections of this chapter.

Arterial pain is due to different diseases such as atherosclerosis and/or thrombosis of the arterial bed; arteritis or arteriolitis, and dysfunction of the arterioles.

Atherosclerosis and/or thrombosis of arterial bed

Atherosclerosis and/or thrombosis in the coronary vessels gives rise to the pain of angina pectoris and of myocardial infarction. In arterial occlusive diseases of the limbs it gives rise to intermittent claudication or to rest pain. Leriche's syndrome is due to isolated aortoiliac occlusive arterial disease, which produces a characteristic clinical picture: intermittent claudication of the low back, buttocks and thigh or calf muscles, impotence, atrophy of the limbs and pallor of the skin of the feet and legs. In rare cases, when the same pathological processes involve abdominal vessels, the patient suffers from *angina abdominis*. There is usually intermittent dull or cramping midabdominal pain, characteristically beginning 15–30 minutes after eating and lasting for 1–2 hours. The arteriographic studies of angina abdominis demonstrate occlusion or high grade stenosis of the superior or inferior mesenteric artery or of the coeliac axis.

A 'coeliac compression syndrome' has also been described. This syndrome is characterised by recurrent abdominal pain due to the narrowing of the coeliac axis alone compressed by the median arcuate ligament of the diaphragm. In some cases, however, the stenosis has been reported to be due to neurofibrous tissue of the coeliac ganglion or to intimal narrowing of the vessel itself. The validity of this syndrome is a matter of considerable controversy (Osmundson & Bernatz 1980; Grendell 1988).

The congenital coarctation of the aorta is painless. The acquired coarctation of the aorta, which is generally due to extensive atherosclerosis with or without thrombosis, may produce symptoms of arterial insufficiency, such as intermittent claudication or coldness of the lower extremities.

Arteritis or arteriolitis

Some diseases, such as thromboangiitis obliterans, Takayasu's syndrome and systemic giant cell arteritis, are well known.

Thromboangiitis obliterans (Bürger's disease) is an obstructive arterial disease caused by segmental inflammatory and proliferative lesions of the medium and small arteries and veins of the limbs (Kontos 1988). The symptoms result mainly from impairment of arterial blood supply to the tissues and to some extent from local venous insufficiency. The symptoms are: intermittent claudication; rest pain when severe ischaemia of tissues has developed; pain from ulcerations and gangrene, and pain from ischaemic neuropathy, which must be considered an important component. Raynaud's phenomenon and migratory superficial thrombophlebitis are common.

Takayasu's syndrome is due to arteritis and arteriolitis of the vessels of the upper part of the body as far as the arterioles of the eye. In a prodromic phase about two-thirds of the patients complain of malaise, fever, limb-girdle stiffness and arthralgia; this prodromic phase is similar to that seen in giant cell arteritis, rheumatic diseases and systemic lupus erythematosus. In many instances this is soon followed by local pain over the affected arteries, erythema nodosum and erythema induratum. In some cases the disease evolves in angina pectoris or myocardial infarction.

Systemic giant cell arteritis is an inflammation of medium and large arteries. It characteristically involves one or more branches of the carotid artery, particularly the temporal artery, hence the name 'cranial' or 'temporal arteritis'. Headaches are often intense and almost unbearable. Headache typically occurs over involved arteries, usually the temporal arteries, but occasionally in the occipital region. A typical tenderness and induration along the vessels is observed. The area around arteries is exquisitely sensitive to pressure. Claudication in the jaw muscles while chewing occurs in up to two-thirds of patients. Giant cell arteritis is considered a systemic disease and can involve arteries in multiple locations (Fauci 1991). The patient often describes an illness that begins like a 'flu syndrome', with severe malaise, slight fever and myalgia. The muscle pain progresses and may become severe, involving mainly the neck, shoulder girdle and pelvic girdle and also the trunk and the distal limbs to a lesser degree; the involvement is bilateral but not necessarily equal in severity. This syndrome is considered strictly related to polymyalgia rheumatica and consequently it is classified with connective tissue diseases. The borderline between Takayasu's syndrome and giant cell arteritis is often not clear. Today they are both considered connective tissue diseases. Wolff (1988) classifies cranial or temporal arteritis and Takayasu's arteritis as subgroups of giant cell arteritides.

Dysfunction of arterioles

Raynaud's phenomenon is characterised by episodes of intense pallor of the fingers and toes (ischaemic phase), generally followed by rubor and cyanosis. The patients usually feel an intense burning or throbbing pain during the ischaemic phase and a less intense pain together with paraesthesias (tingling, pricking or numbness) during the cyanotic phase. This condition may be classified as primary or idiopathic Raynaud's phenomenon (Raynaud's disease) and as Raynaud's phenomenon secondary to diseases, trauma or drugs. Raynaud's phenomenon is due to a sudden arteriolar constriction, followed by a paralytic phase. In Raynaud's disease, different alterations of the arterioles, characteristic of different kinds of arteriolitis, have been described. Adrenergic-blocking drugs are considered the specific therapy for Raynaud's phenomenon (Creager & Dzau 1991).

Erythromelalgia (erithermalgia) is a syndrome characterised by the following symptoms in the extremities: red discoloration and increased temperature of the skin, deep and superficial burning pain, often accompanied by tingling and pricking and in many cases, oedema. The symptoms simultaneously involve the distal part of the lower limbs and, less frequently, of the upper limbs as well. The attacks of erythromelalgia are induced by increased temperature, either in the environment or locally and are aggravated by a dependent position. The duration of attacks varies from a few minutes to hours. Erythromelalgia may be primary or secondary to disorders such as polycythemia vera and hypertension (Creager & Dzau 1991). A role has recently been attributed to prostaglandins; in fact, aspirin may induce relief (Jørgensen & Søndergard 1978). It is pertinent to ask whether erythromelalgia could be classified with reflex sympathetic dystrophies. As a matter of fact, excellent results, with complete disappearance of the symptoms, were observed with local anaesthetic blocks of the sympathetic chain (Zoppi et al 1985).

Mechanisms of arterial pain

The mechanisms of pain in arterial diseases are many and often intermingle.

1. Ischaemia per se. The most evident examples of diseases due to this mechanism are: angina at rest, pain occurring in arterial embolism and Raynaud's phenomenon. Ischaemia can give rise to a continuous pain in the limb when:

a. the ischaemia is very severe

b. myalgic spots with the characteristics of trigger points are present in the limbs (Dorigo et al 1979)

c. a reflex sympathetic dystrophy arises which contributes to pain and dystrophy through different mechanisms: vasomotor changes; fast and slow changes in permeability of microvessels and tissue imbibition; release of active substances; direct control of some enzymatic reactions, and direct modulation of sensory receptors (Procacci 1969; Maresca et al 1984).

2. Ischaemia occurring during muscular exercise because of a discrepancy between the supply and demand of oxygen carried to muscles. This mechanism, according to Lewis (1942), is typical of effort angina pectoris (stable chronic angina) (see page 544) and intermittent claudication of the limbs. Typical myalgic spots are found in many patients with intermittent claudication and are a component of pain (Procacci 1969; Dorigo et al 1979; Maresca et al 1984).

3. Ischaemia plus inflammation and/or metabolic disorders, typical of thromboangiitis obliterans, of inflammatory arteriolitis and of diabetic arteriolitis.

The process of vascular thrombosis is generally considered a common arrival point of different pathways. However, in many vascular diseases the two mechanisms, thrombosis and inflammation, are in part overlapping, as is clear from clinical observations, e.g. in thromboangiitis obliterans or in angina or infarction that sometimes occur in giant cell arteritis and in thrombophlebitis.

Pain due to dysfunction of microvessels

Pain originating from microvessels must be distinguished from classical arterial and venous pain for pathophysiological and clinical reasons.

First of all, both arterial and venous vessels are involved in some classic syndromes, such as Raynaud's phenomenon, pernio (chilblains) and erythromelalgia (erythermalgia) (Kontos 1988; Creager & Dzau 1991). Obviously, in these cases an alteration of capillary filtration is also present, with changes in the microenvironment important for the onset of pain, as stated by Zimmermann (1979) and Jänig (1988). Many substances may be active in inducing pain. Only some of these have been identified: histamine, 5-hydroxytryptamine, kinins and substance P. The temporal relationships involved in the release of active substances in different cases are unknown. Neurogenic inflammation probably plays a role in many diseases of microvessels; certainly neurogenic phenomena are important in Raynaud's phenomenon and erythromelalgia. It must be noted that Raynaud's phenomenon is often induced by cold, applied not on the hands but on the face: a disorder of the hypothalamic centres of thermoregulation may be considered a possibility.

Venous pain

A typical venous pain is observed in thrombophlebitis. In superficial thrombophlebitis the vein may be apparent as a red, tender cord. Pain at rest is often observed. In deep vein thrombophlebitis about one-half of the patients may be asymptomatic. Tenderness to palpation and pain on the voluntary dorsiflexion of the foot can be observed (Kazmier & Juergens 1980; Kontos 1988; Creager & Dzau 1991). Many factors are active in inducing pain: biochemical factors and mechanical factors, especially venous stasis. Much more than in arterial pain, in venous pain perivascular tissues, muscles and tendons are involved in inflammation and hence are painful. The importance of these additional factors is demonstrated by the fact that, when thrombophlebitis is resolved, a postphlebitis pain often remains in the limbs. The authors have observed that in many cases pain originates not only from the vein which remains painful, but also from myalgic spots, often accompanied by skin hyperalgesia. In conclusion, a postphlebitic fibrositis is observed, which often responds to aspirin-like drugs.

In every vascular disease, as well as in myocardial infarction, a reflex sympathetic dystrophy can arise. In this case skin dystrophy (glossy skin), muscle atrophy, osteoporosis and clear vasomotor and sudomotor phenomena are observed in the limbs. The classical treatment of reflex sympathetic dystrophies with sympathetic blocks can be opportune (Procacci & Maresca 1987).

REFERENCES

Aviado D M, Schmidt C F 1955 Reflexes from stretch receptors in blood vessels, heart and lungs. Physiological Reviews 35: 247–300

Barlow J B, Pocock W A, Marchand P, Denny M 1963 The significance of late systolic murmurs. American Heart Journal 66: 443–452

Bousfield G 1918 Angina pectoris: changes in the electrocardiogram during paroxysm. Lancet 2: 457

Braunwald E (ed) 1988 Heart disease, 3rd edn. W B Saunders, Philadelphia

Brown A M 1967 Excitation of afferent cardiac sympathetic nerve fibers during myocardial ischaemia. Journal of Physiology 190: 35–53

Brunton T L 1867 On the use of nitrite of amyl in angina pectoris. Lancet 2: 97

Burns A 1809 Observations on diseases of the heart. Murray & Callow, London

Caelius Aurelianus 1722 De morbis acutis et chronicis. Wetseniana, Amsterdam

Cannon R O, Quyyumi A A, Schenke W H et al 1990 Abnormal cardiac sensitivity in patients with chest pain and normal coronary arteries. Journal of the American College of Cardiology 16: 1359–1366

Castelli B 1598 Lexicon medicum graeco-latinum ex Ippocrate et Galeno desumptum. Breae, Messanae

Chierchia S, Lazzari M, Freedman S B, Brunelli C, Maseri A 1983 Impairment of myocardial perfusion during painless myocardial ischemia. Journal of the American College of Cardiology 1: 924–930

Clouse R E, Staiano A, Landau D W, Schlachter J L 1983 Manometric findings during spontaneous chest pain in patients with presumed esophageal 'spasm'. Gastroenterology 85: 395–402

Cohn F P 1989 Silent myocardial ischemia and infarction. Dekker, New York

Creager M A, Dzau V J 1991 Vascular diseases of the extremities. In: Wilson J D, Braunwald E, Isselbacher K J et al (eds) Harrison's principles of internal medicine, 12th edn. McGraw-Hill, New York, p 1018–1026

Daubert J C, Rouxel P, Feuillu A, Pony J C, Gouffault J 1975 Douleurs thoraciques litigieuses à coronaires saines. Archives des Maladies du Coeur et des Vaisseaux 68: 607–618

Dorigo B, Bartoli V, Grisillo D, Beconi D 1979 Fibrositic myofascial pain in intermittent claudication. Effect of anesthetic block of trigger points on exercise tolerance. Pain 6: 183–190

Dressler W 1956 Post-myocardial infarction syndrome; preliminary report of a complication resembling idiopathic, recurrent, benign pericarditis. Journal of the American Medical Association 160: 1379–1383

Eagle K A, De Sanctis R W 1988 Diseases of the aorta. In: Braunwald E (ed) Heart disease, 3rd edn. W B Saunders, Philadelphia, p 1546–1576

Fauci A S 1991 The vasculitis syndromes. In: Wilson J D, Braunwald E, Isselbacher K J et al (eds) Harrison's principles of internal medicine, 12th edn. McGraw-Hill, New York, p 1456–1463

Fiel H, Siegel M L 1928 Electrocardiographic changes during attacks of angina pectoris. American Journal of Medical Sciences 175: 255–259

Fothergill J 1776 Further account of the angina pectoris. Medical Observer and Inquiry 5: 252–281

Frank S, Johnson A, Ross J Jr 1973 Natural history of valvular aortic stenosis. British Heart Journal 35: 41–46

Friedberg C K 1956 Disease of the heart, 2nd edn. W B Saunders, Philadelphia

Froment R, Gonin A 1956 Les angors coronariens intriqués. Expansion Scientifique Française, Paris

Grendell J H 1988 Vascular diseases of the intestine. In: Wyngaarden J B, Smith L H (eds) Cecil's textbook of medicine, 18th edn. W B Saunders, Philadelphia, p 760–765

Hansen K, Schliack H 1962 Segmentale Innervation. Thieme, Stuttgart

Heberden W 1772 Some account of a disorder of the breast. Medical Transactions of the Royal College of Physicians of London 2: 59–67

Heberden W 1802 Commentarii de morborum historia et curatione. Payne, London

Herrick J B 1912 Clinical features of sudden obstruction of the coronary arteries. Journal of the American Medical Association 72: 2015–2021

Hope J 1832 A treatise on the diseases of the heart. Kidd, London

Iggo A 1974 Pain receptors. In: Bonica J J, Procacci P, Pagni C A (eds) Recent advances on pain. C C Thomas, Springfield, Illinois, p 3–35

Jänig W 1988 Pathophysiology of nerve following mechanical injury. In: Dubner R, Gebhart G, Bond M R (eds) Proceedings of the Vth World Congress on Pain. Elsevier, Amsterdam, p 89–108

Jørgensen H P, Søndergard J 1978 Pathogenesis of erythromelalgia. Archives of Dermatology 114: 112–114

Juergens J L, Lofgren K A 1980 Chronic venous insufficiency. In: Juergens J L, Spittell J A, Fairbairn J F (eds) Peripheral vascular diseases. W B Saunders, Philadelphia, p 809–821

Julian D G (ed) 1977 Angina pectoris. Churchill Livingstone, Edinburgh

Kannel W B, Abbott R D 1984 Incidence and prognosis of unrecognized myocardial infarction. New England Journal of Medicine 311: 1144–1147

Kazmier F J, Juergens J L 1980 Venous thrombosis and obstructive diseases of the veins. In: Juergens J L, Spittell J A, Fairbairn J F (eds) Peripheral vascular diseases. W B Saunders, Philadelphia, p 731–755

Keele C A, Armstrong D 1964 Substances producing pain and itch. Arnold, London

Kemp H G 1973 Left ventricular function in patients with the anginal syndrome and normal coronary arteriograms. American Journal of Cardiology 32: 375–376

Kontos H A 1988 Vascular diseases of the limbs. In: Wyngaarden J B, Smith L H (eds) Cecil's textbook of medicine, 18th edn. W B Saunders, Philadelphia, p 375–389

Laënnec R T H 1826 Traité de l'auscultation médiate, 2nd edn. Broffon & Chaude, Paris

Lewis T 1942 Pain. Macmillan, New York
Lieutaud J 1759 Précis de médecine pratique. Vincent, Paris
Malliani A, Lombardi F 1982 Considerations of fundamental mechanisms eliciting cardiac pain. American Heart Journal 103: 575–578
Maresca M, Nuzzaci G, Zoppi M 1984 Muscular pain in chronic occlusive arterial diseases of the limbs. In: Benedetti C, Chapman C R, Moricca G (eds) Recent advances in the management of pain. Raven Press, New York, p 521–527
Maresca M, Galanti G, Castellani S, Procacci P 1989 Pain in mitral valve prolapse. Pain 36: 89–92
Marino C, Zoppi M, Morelli F, Buoncristiano U, Pagni E 1986 Pain in early cancer of the lungs. Pain 27: 51–55
Maseri A 1987 Role of coronary artery spasm in symptomatic and silent myocardial ischemia. Journal of the American College of Cardiology 9: 249–262
Maseri A, Mimmo R, Chierchia S, Marchesi C, Pesola A, L'Abbate A 1975 Coronary artery spasm as a cause of acute myocardial ischemia in man. Chest 68: 625–633
Maseri A, Severi S, Nes M D et al 1978 'Variant' angina: one aspect of a continuous spectrum of vasospastic myocardial ischemia. Pathogenetic mechanisms, estimated incidence and clinical and coronary arteriographic findings in 138 patients. American Journal of Cardiology 42: 1019–1035
Maseri A, Chierchia S, Davies G, Glazier J 1985 Mechanisms of ischemic cardiac pain and silent myocardial ischemia. American Journal of Medicine 79 (suppl 3A): 7–11
Maseri A, Crea F, Kaski J C, Crake T 1991 Mechanisms of angina pectoris in syndrome X. Journal of the American College of Cardiology 17: 499–506
Morgagni G B 1765 De sedibus et causis morborum per anatomen indagatis. Remondini, Padua
Neri Serneri G G, Abbate R, Gori A M et al 1992 A transient intermittent lymphocyte activation is responsible for the instability of the angina. Circulation 86: 790–797
Osmundson P J, Bernatz P E 1980 Occlusive disease of abdominal visceral arteries. In: Juergens J L, Spittell J A, Fairbairn J F (eds) Peripheral vascular diseases. W B Saunders, Philadelphia, p 295–325
Parry C H 1799 An inquiry into the symptoms and causes of the syncope anginosa, commonly called angina pectoris. Murray & Callow, London
Pasternak R C, Braunwald E, Sobel B E 1988 Acute myocardial infarction. In: Braunwald E (ed) Heart disease, 3rd edn. W B Saunders, Philadelphia, p 1222–1313
Poggesi L, Balli E, Comeglio M et al 1992 Comparative natural history of unstable and effort angina. Thrombosis Research 65 (suppl 1): S71
Prinzmetal M, Kennamer R, Merliss R, Wada T, Bor N 1959 A variant form of angina pectoris. American Journal of Medicine 27: 375–388
Procacci P 1969 A survey of modern concepts of pain. In: Vinken P J, Bruyn G W (eds) Handbook of clinical neurology, vol 1. North-Holland, Amsterdam, p 114–146
Procacci P, Maresca M 1985a Historical considerations of cardiac pain. Pain 22: 325–335
Procacci P, Maresca M 1985b A philological study on some words concerning pain. Pain 22: 201–203
Procacci P, Maresca M 1987 Reflex sympathetic dystrophies and algodystrophies: historical and pathogenic considerations. Pain 31: 137–146
Procacci P, Zoppi M 1983 Pathophysiology and clinical aspects of visceral and referred pain. In: Bonica J J, Lindblom U, Iggo A (eds) Proceedings of the Third World Congress on Pain. Raven Press, New York, p 643–658
Procacci P, Zoppi M, Padeletti L, Maresca M 1976 Myocardial infarction without pain. A study of sensory function of the upper limbs. Pain 2: 309–313
Procacci P, Zoppi M, Maresca M 1986 Clinical approach to visceral sensation. In: Cervero F, Morrison J F B (eds) Visceral sensation. Elsevier, Amsterdam, p 21–28
Reichek N, Shelburne J C, Perloff J R 1973 Clinical aspects of rheumatic heart disease. Progress in Cardiovascular Diseases 15: 491–537
Rinzler S H 1951 Cardiac pain. C C Thomas, Springfield, Illinois
Ross J 1887 On the segmental distribution of sensory disorders. Brain 10: 333–361
Rutherford J D, Braunwald E, Cohn P F 1988 Chronic ischemic heart disease. In: Braunwald E (ed) Heart disease, 3rd edn. W B Saunders, Philadelphia, p 1314–1378
Shapiro L M, Crake T, Poole-Wilson P A 1988 Is altered cardiac sensation responsible for chest pain in patients with normal coronary arteries? Clinical observation during cardiac catheterization. British Medical Journal 296: 170–171
Skeat W W 1882 Etymological dictionary of the English language. Clarendon Press, Oxford
Teodori U, Galletti R 1962 Il dolore nelle affezioni degli organi interni del torace. Pozzi, Roma
Testa A G 1810 Delle malattie di cuore. Loro cagioni, specie, segni e cure. Lucchesini, Bologna
Trousseau A 1861 Clinique médicale de l'Hôtel-Dieu de Paris. Baillière, Paris
Van Swieten G B 1768 Commentaria in omnes aphorismos Hermani Boerhaave, de cognoscendis et curandis morbis. Remondini, Venice
Vaquez H 1922 Malattie del cuore. UTET, Turin
Wall P D, Woolf C J 1984 Muscle but not cutaneous C-afferent input produces prolonged increases in the excitability of the flexion reflex in the rat. Journal of Physiology 356: 443–458
Willerson J T 1988 Angina pectoris. In: Wyngaarden J B, Smith L H (eds) Cecil's textbook of medicine, 18th edn. W B Saunders, Philadelphia, p 323–329
Wolff S M 1988 The vasculitic syndromes. In: Wyngaarden J B, Smith L H (eds) Cecil's textbook of medicine, 18th edn. W B Saunders, Philadelphia, p 2025–2028
Zimmermann M 1979 Peripheral and central nervous mechanisms of nociception, pain and pain therapy: facts and hypotheses. In: Bonica J J, Liebeskind J C, Albe-Fessard D G (eds) Proceedings of the Second World Congress on Pain. Raven Press, New York, p 3–32
Zoppi M, Zamponi A, Pagni E, Buoncristiano U 1985 A way to understand erythromelalgia. Journal of the Autonomic Nervous System 13: 85–89

30. Eye pain

R. A. Hitchings

In this chapter the mechanisms of eye pain are considered. Firstly symptoms and signs are described, then aetiology and therapy are discussed. In so doing, an attempt is made to set out a rational approach to this particular symptom of eye disease.

Pain in or around the eye usually arises from disease of the eyeball; it may also be referred pain from contiguous structures. Referred pain may come from teeth, jaw, neck or sinuses; it may have a vascular cause – migraine, arteritis and aneurysm – or a neurogenic one – trigeminal neuralgia, postherpetic neuralgia, tension head- and-face pain, and finally it may come from inflammatory pseudotumour of the orbit and occur with the Tolosa–Hunt syndrome. Surfacing above this multitude of extraocular causes of eye pain, in terms of frequency, if not severity, are those pains caused by eye disease. It is the purpose of this chapter to describe eye pain caused by ocular disease.

Eye pain from ocular disease conveniently subdivides into three major types. With little overlap between these groups they can conveniently be discussed in turn. These types are:

1. superficial or corneal pain
2. deep or inflammatory pain
3. pain from excess retinal illumination.

SUPERFICIAL OR CORNEAL PAIN

Symptoms and aetiology

Typically pain from superficial corneal disease is sharp, stabbing and severe. It is located beneath the upper lid

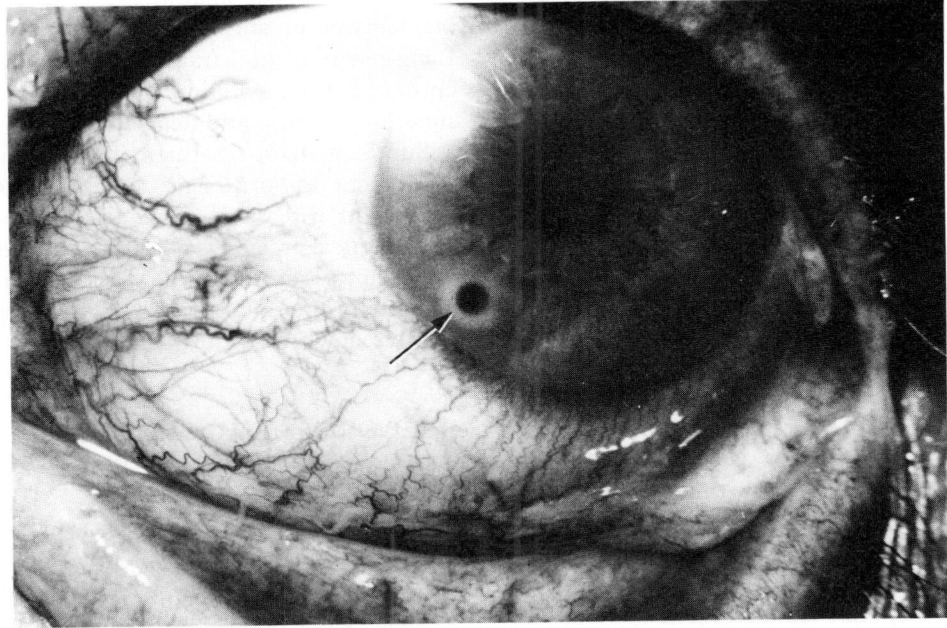

Fig. 30.1 Corneal foreign body. This diffuse illumination photograph shows superficially placed foreign body (arrow), sited for maximum stimulation of the superficial corneal nerve endings.

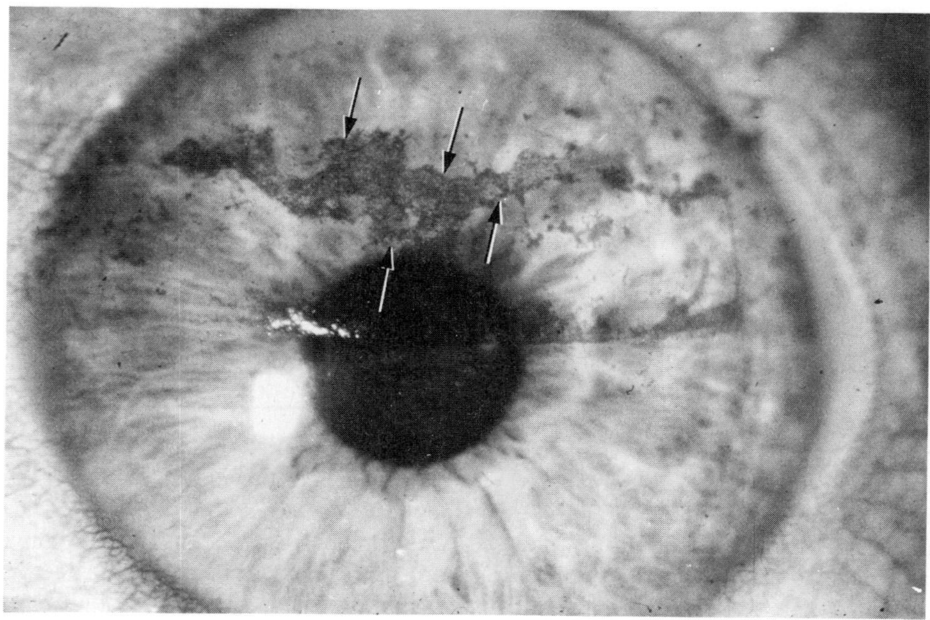

Fig. 30.2 Corneal erosion. Rose bengal stain has been used to outline the area of corneal epithelial loss with exposure of the superficial corneal nerve fibres (arrows).

and associated with photophobia, blepharospasm and lacrimation. It arises from an external stimulus which irritates the superficial (sensory) corneal plexus. This is most often a subtarsal foreign body, a corneal foreign body (Fig. 30.1) or a superficial corneal erosion (Fig. 30.2). In these cases the history is short, the symptoms acute and the cause easily found. There may be a history of something striking ('entering') the eye. Eversion of the upper lid and/or torchlight examination of the cornea will usually reveal the foreign body.

Less commonly a bullous keratopathy (Fig. 30.3) will be the cause. In this case there will be a long history of corneal (eye) disease, the symptoms will be long-standing and recurrent and the corneal surface will show irregular scarring.

Mechanism

The symptoms develop following stimulation of the sensory nerve endings in the cornea. The ophthalmic division of the fifth cranial nerve sends long ciliary nerves through the sclera which end as an anterior (subepithelial) and posterior (midstromal) plexus (Fig. 30.4) (Lim & Ruskell 1978). These nerves carry pain stimuli and any lesion of the superficial cornea may stimulate the nerve endings.

Stimulation of these pain fibres results in antidromic impulses which produce lacrimation. This reflex is a necessary protective response for the cornea. Persistent stimulation produces chemosis and lid swelling; lacrimation induces rhinorrhoea. In time similar impulses cause iris muscle stimulation, associated with miosis and release of substance P (Bill et al 1979) resulting in iritis and chemical induction of additional pain (see below).

Treatment

While removal of the foreign body is the most important aspect of treatment, this must often be preceded by application of a local anaesthetic to the cornea to reduce blepharospasm and allow a proper ocular examination. Long-term administration of topical anaesthetics for chronic corneal irritation is not wise, for it can damage the superficial cornea and delay healing.

Supplementary treatment includes a topical antibiotic to prevent opportunistic infection and a mydriatic for coincident iritis and miosis (see below). The healing of large corneal erosions is hastened by patching the eye, but this is not performed in the presence of overt infection, as bacteria proliferate more easily in the warm moist conditions created under the patch.

DEEP OR INFLAMMATORY PAIN

Symptoms and aetiology

A dull, frequently severe, occasionally throbbing pain centred within the eyeball and referred to any of the surrounding structures is a characteristic symptom. Typically, it is persistent, often fluctuating, occasionally severe enough to prevent sleep, and differing markedly in character from the stabbing pain of corneal irritation.

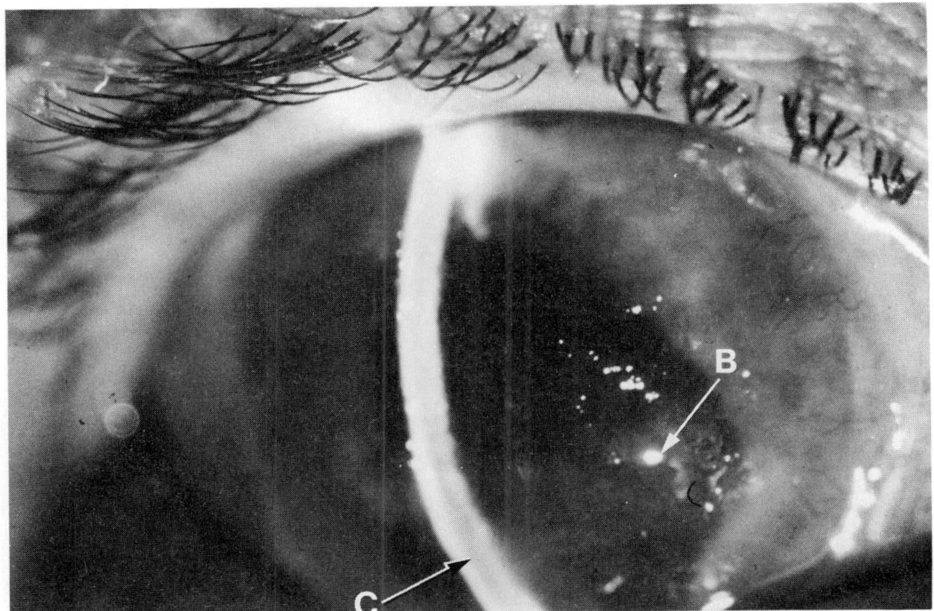

Fig. 30.3 Bullous keratopathy. Gross corneal oedema following loss of the dehydrating function of the corneal endothelial layer allows waterlogging of the cornea. Accumulation of water within and beneath the corneal epithelium produces bullae formation with the stimulation of the corneal nerve endings. (B = light reflected from bullae; C = thickened cornea on slit illumination.)

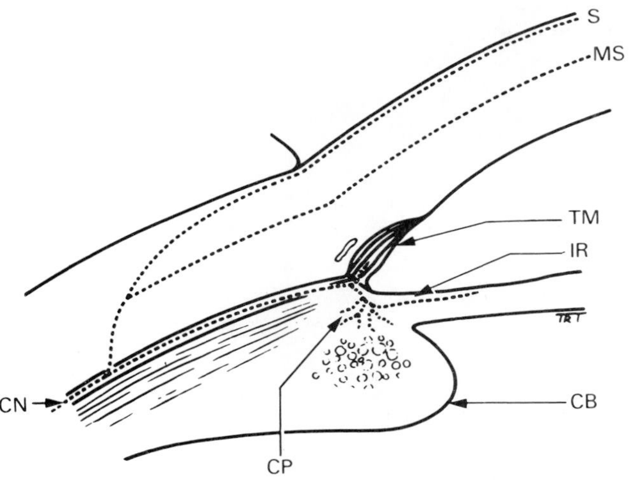

Fig. 30.4 Distribution of the fifth cranial nerve in the anterior segment of the eye. S = superficial corneal plexus; MS = midstromal corneal plexus; TM = trabecular meshwork; IR = iris root; CB = ciliary body; CP = ciliary plexus; CN = ciliary nerve. (Reproduced by permission of *Transactions of the Ophthalmological Societies of the United Kingdom*).

This pain arises secondarily to inflammation of the anterior segment. Thus the deeper cornea, anterior sclera, iris or ciliary body may be involved: as keratitis (Fig. 30.5), scleritis (Fig. 30.6), iritis or iridocyclitis. In addition acute (angle closure) glaucoma (Fig. 30.7) and thrombotic glaucoma may also cause this symptom. The pain may be severe enough in acute angle closure glaucoma for the patient to vomit, become dehydrated and produce symptoms which distract attention from the original aetiology. Patients with acute angle closure glaucoma have been suspected as suffering from intestinal obstruction and cholecystitis as well as from ruptured intracranial aneurysm and cerebrovascular accident. The presence of a red eye with an ipsilateral fixed pupil in this type of patient should alert the internist that the apparent general medical problem originates within the eye!

Whatever the cause, ocular examination reveals signs of inflammation: injection, tenderness to palpation and swelling (chemosis). Other signs helping to identify the correct aetiology will also be present and have been summarised in Table 30.1.

Mechanism

Pain fibres within the eye also are distributed along the course of the fifth cranial nerve (Fig. 30.4). They reach the paralimbal sclera, iris root and ciliary body (Bergmansson 1977). These fibres would be stimulated by mechanical, thermal and chemical injury, causing the sensation of pain. Pain would appear to be the only sensation to originate from disease of deep structures within the anterior segment.

Whatever the initiating stimuli, they share a final common pathway: a breakdown of the blood–aqueous barrier, with release of kinins and prostaglandins from leucocytes, while substance P and other polypeptides are released from the iris itself. These chemicals stimulate

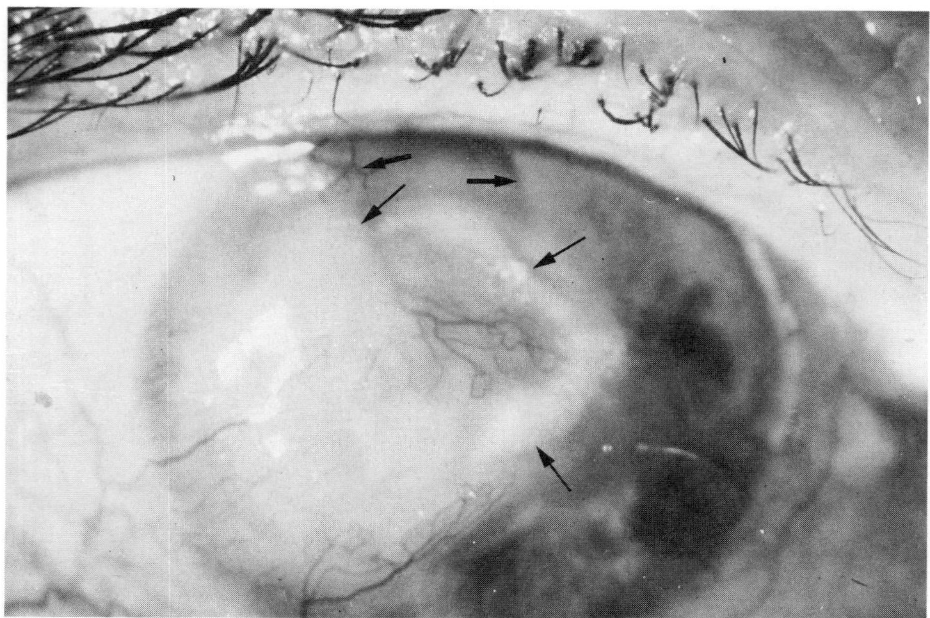

Fig. 30.5 Keratitis showing a focal opacification of the cornea abutting on to the limbal sclera (thin arrows). This patient has previously had a sector iridectomy (thick arrows).

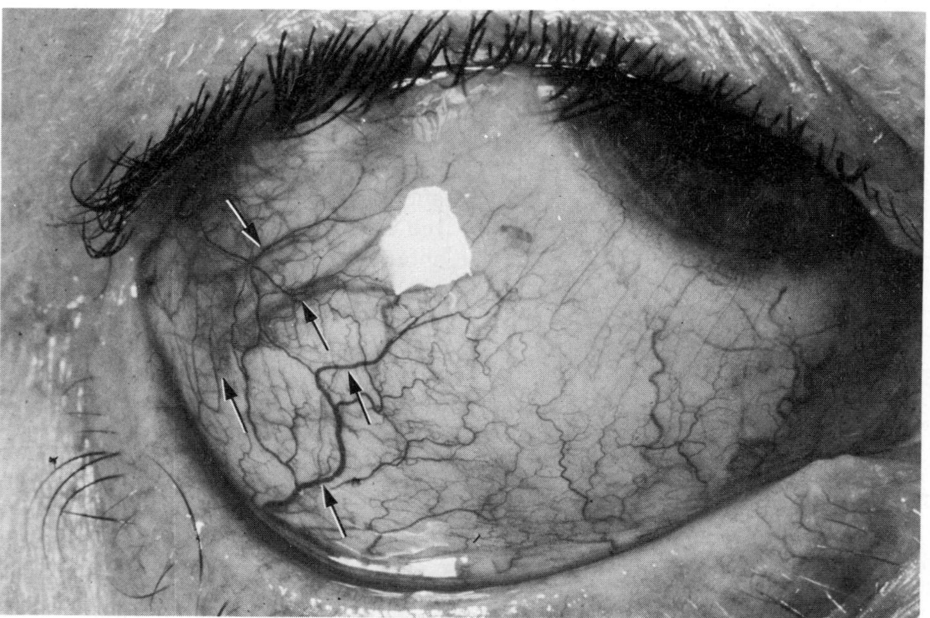

Fig. 30.6 Scleritis. A deep 'brawny' swelling of the equatorial sclera with dilated episcleral blood vessels (arrows).

receptors within the ciliary body nerve plexus and probably also cause miosis (Cole & Unger 1973; Unger et al 1974).

Additional factors are inportant in acute angle closure glaucoma. Here the intraocular pressure increase causes iris infarction with release of chemical mediators and production of the signs of inflammation. Additionally the midstromal corneal plexus seems to act as a stretch receptor, as the acute rise in intraocular pressure (seen for example after provocative testing) may be associated with a feeling of 'ocular discomfort'. Many glaucoma patients notice the same symptom and seem to be aware when their intraocular pressure is raised above normal.

The variations in pupil size seen in the conditions listed in Table 30.1 need explanation. The normal pupillary response to inflammation is miosis; the pupil is small and

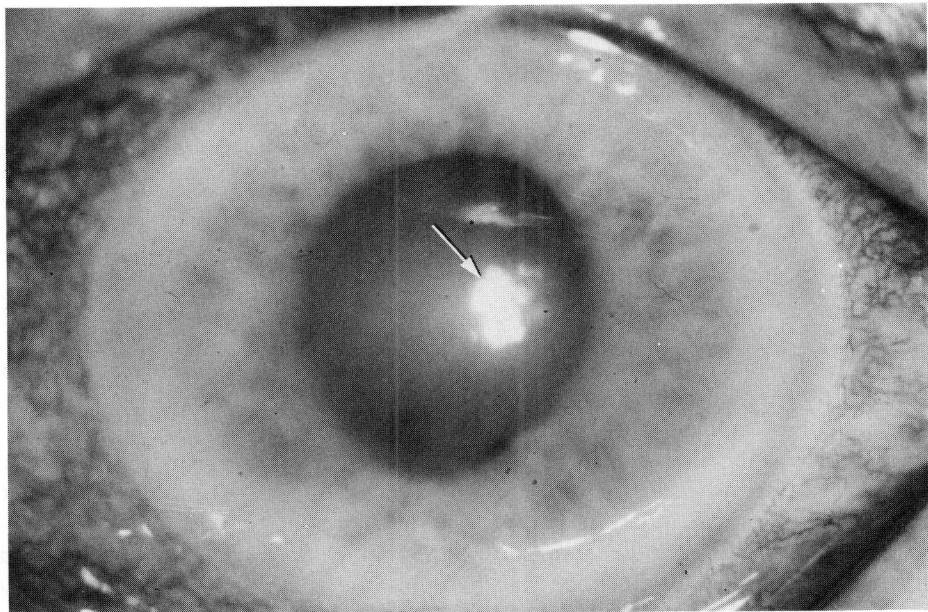

Fig. 30.7 Acute glaucoma. Diffuse ocular congestion associated with a semidilated, vertically oval pupil and corneal oedema (shown by the irregular light reflection (arrow)).

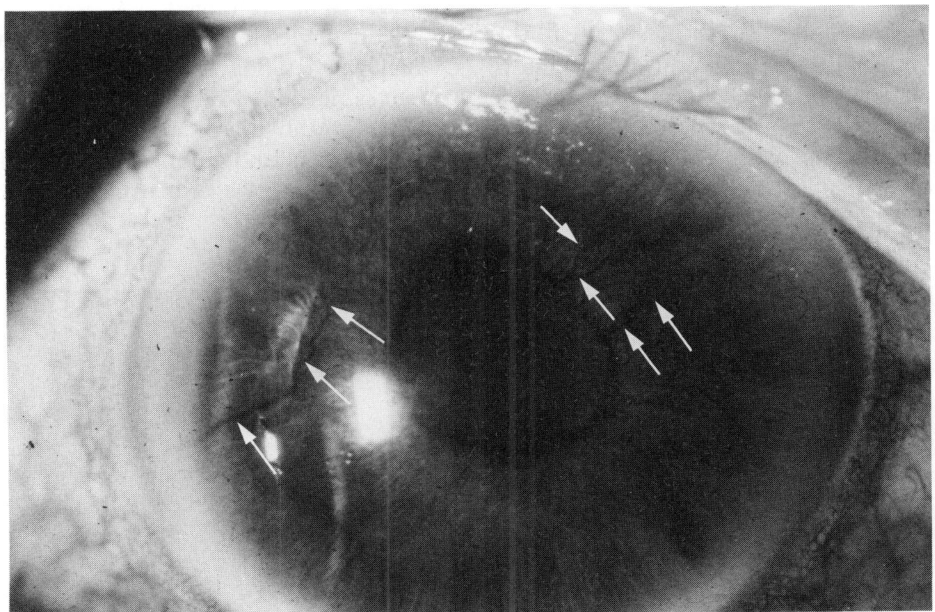

Fig. 30.8 Thrombotic glaucoma. In this instance dilated vessels may be seen on the anterior iris surface indicative of the neovascular membrane which exists in this condition (arrows).

round. If the pupil in the inflamed eye becomes adherent to the lens then it becomes small, fixed and irregular.

Acute angle closure glaucoma may be precipitated by low light levels with resultant mydriasis. The high intraocular pressure causes relative iris ischaemia, affecting the sphincter muscle more than the dilator muscle. The pupil remains dilated while the intraocular pressure remains high. Should (segmental) infarction of the iris sphincter muscle occur then the pupil becomes oval in shape as well as semidilated.

Thrombotic glaucoma is associated with a proliferating fibrovascular membrane on the anterior iris surface. This contracts and, being tethered at the limbus, causes pupillary mydriasis with ectropion pupillae.

Other less common causes of deep-seated pain also involve stimulation of the same nerve endings. Topical

Table 30.1 Characteristic factors seen in eyes with ocular pain and inflammation

	Vision	Congestion	Cornea	Intraocular tension	Pupil
Keratitis and scleritis	Normal or reduced	+	Clear or focal opacity	Normal or raised	Normal or miosed
Iridocyclitis	Usually reduced	+	Clear	Normal, raised or lowered	Miosed and often fixed
Acute glaucoma	Reduced (often ≤ CF)	+	Cloudy	Raised	Fixed and oval, semidilated
Thrombotic glaucoma	Reduced (often ≤ HM)	+	Cloudy	Raised	Fixed and dilated

CF = visual acuity of 'counting fingers'; HM = visual acuity of 'hand movements'.

pilocarpine can, when first used, induce quite severe brow ache, probably from traction of the ciliary muscle upon the scleral spur with distortion of the ciliary nerve plexus. Laser photocoagulation of the trabecular meshwork is painless, but accidental burns of the adjacent iris root are painful – again from stimulation of an adjacent nerve. Laser iridotomy does not last long enough to generate the heat required to produce pain, but the resultant shock may induce a dull sensation of being hit 'like a blow' (Unger 1977).

Treatment

It may not be easy to identify the cause of inflammatory pain. Iritis and scleritis have associated systemic inflammatory conditions, e.g. inflammatory arthritides, but these do not usually come with a specific aetiology. Treatment therefore is directed towards suppressing the inflammation and steroids are the mainstay of therapy. Cycloplegic agents and nonsteroidal antiinflammatory drugs are also used.

The intensity of steroid treatment is titrated against the perceived level of inflammation. It can range from topically applied prednisolone drops 3–4 times a day for a mild attack of iritis, through intensive drops 1–2 hourly, to pulsed steroids in 1 g doses for severe scleritis. Cycloplegic agents remove ciliary muscle spasm. Nonsteroidal antiinflammatory agents are a useful alternative or supplement to topical steroids, particularly if the duration of treatment is likely to be prolonged.

Acute angle closure glaucoma is a cause of deep pain for which the aetiology is known and for which specific treatment is needed. The intraocular pressure is lowered with carbonic anhydrase inhibitors, hyperosmotics, topical beta-blockers and miotics. Topical steroids are the only antiinflammatory agents usually required.

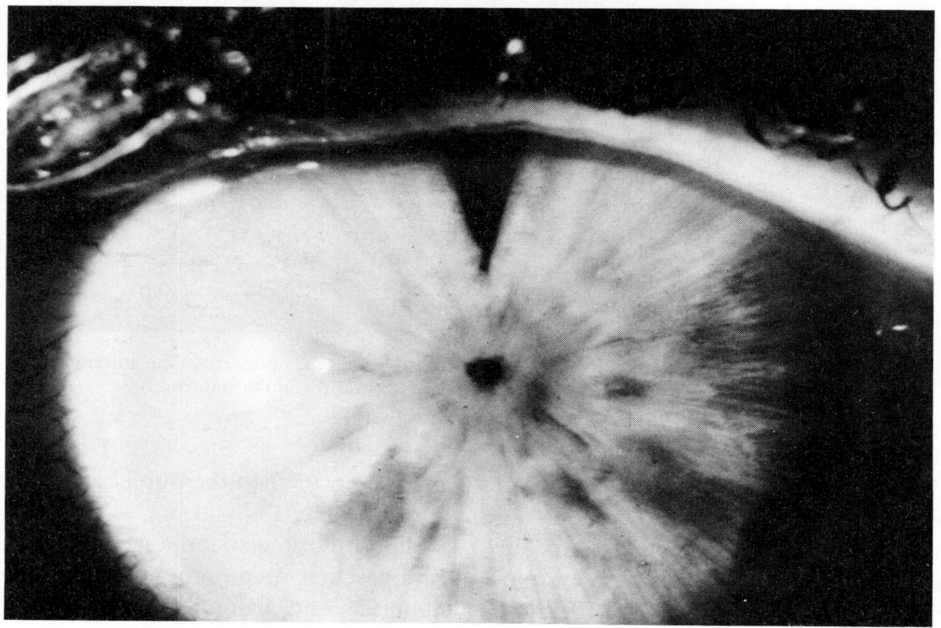

Fig. 30.9 Effect of pilocarpine on the sphincter pupillae muscle. This patient had severe visual restriction because of the intense miosis induced by pilocarpine. This example shows how retinal illumination may be severely reduced by excess miosis.

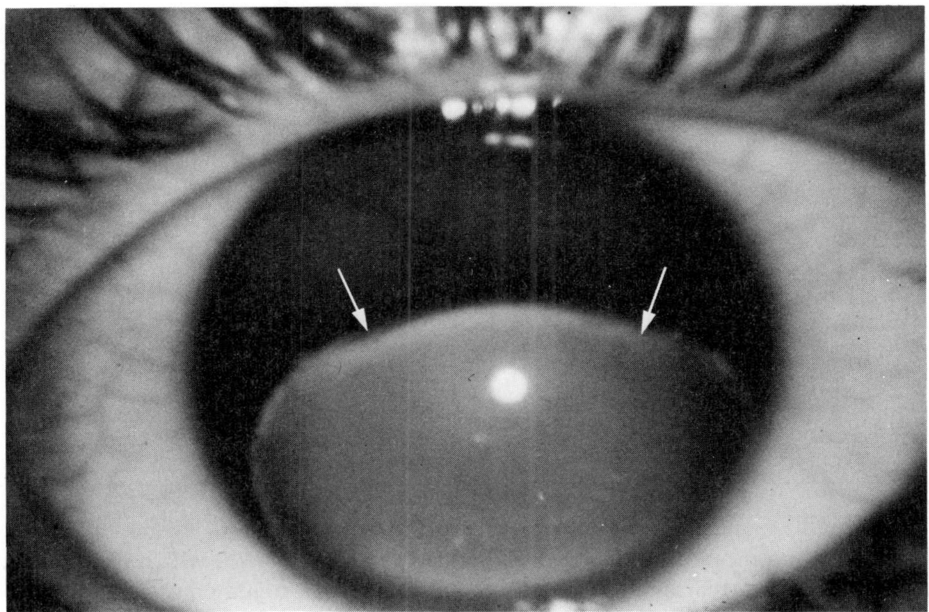

Fig. 30.10 Sector iridectomy. A surgically induced iris coloboma, with resulting decrease in the ability to regulate retinal illumination. (Arrows outline cut iris pillars of the iridectomy.)

EXCESS RETINAL ILLUMINATION

Ocular discomfort which follows retinal illumination may be classified as 'glare' or 'photophobia'. Under normal conditions retinal illumination is regulated by light-induced reflex changes in pupil size. Age-related miosis (following the reduced action of the dilator pupillary muscle (Weale 1971)), miotic drops (Fig. 30.9) and increasing lens sclerosis (pigmentation) combine to further reduce retinal illumination.

Glare is the discomfort produced by a strong fierce light, when the normal reflex miosis is inadequate. A

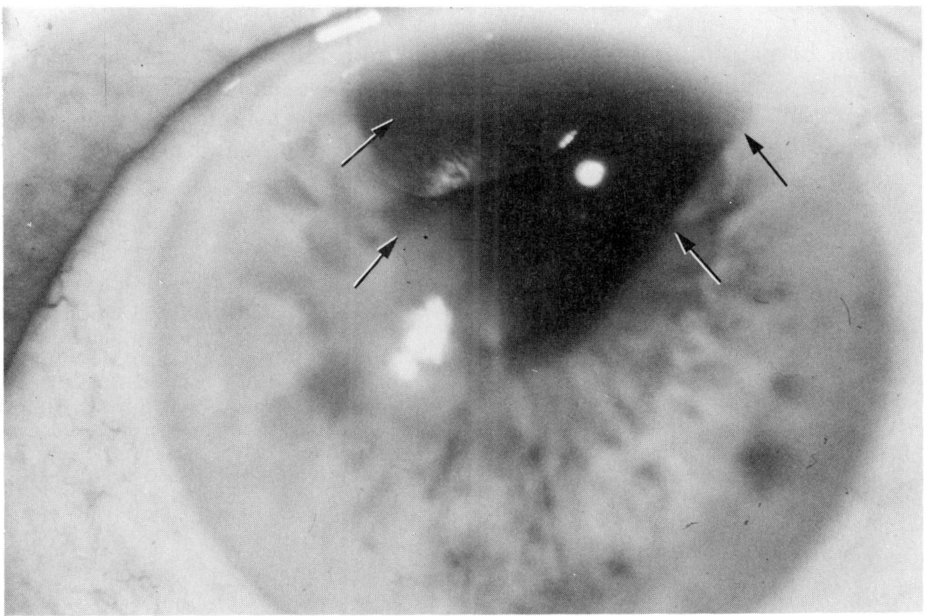

Fig. 30.11 Anirida. The red reflex seen in this photograph shows total lack of visible iris. No regulation of retinal illumination by iris sphincter action may occur. (This patient also had a dislocated lens (arrows)).

Table 30.2 Conditions producing photophobia

Group	Condition	Category	Mechanism	Severity of pain
1.	Superficial corneal lesion, e.g. foreign body	Inflammation	Light-induced miosis and coinciding anterior segment inflammation	May be severe
1.	Iritis	Inflammation	Directly stimulating ciliary body plexus	
2.	Iris coloboma Surgical iridectomy (Fig. 30.10) Anirida (Fig. 30.11) Mydriatics	Reduced iris sphincter action	Insufficient retinal-induced light respose on pupil to limit retinal illumination	Discomfort
2.	Albinism	Transiris light pathway increase	Lack of iris pigment epithelium	
3.	Albinism	Altered retinal response	Lack of retinal pigment delays light absorption Heightened retinal reflectivity	Discomfort
3.	Chronic glaucoma	Altered retinal response	Marked intolerance to normal light levels. Often associated with moderate cataract and may reflect an inability to manage lens-induced light scatter	Marked intolerance, some discomfort
4.	Altered central response	Mental state	Light intolerance reflecting heightened central sensitivity	May be severe

special variant would be the discomfort that occasionally follows the use of laser light in the treatment of chorioretinal disease; under these conditions the normal ocular mechanism for regulating retinal illumination has been bypassed.

Photophobia is 'fear of light', a symptom produced by retinal illumination of normal (physiological) levels. There will be overlap between these two conditions; indeed the pain-producing mechanism may be the same in some cases. Both may produce ocular discomfort sufficient to register as pain. Such pain is light-induced, monocular or binocular, localised to the eye and relieved by reducing retinal illumination.

Mechanism

There do not appear to be pain fibres in the posterior segment of the eye. The stimulus from excess retinal illumination may either stimulate the long ciliary nerves directly or pass along the optic nerve. The former run forward to the anterior segment of the eye, carrying antidromic impulses which in turn cause chemical release from the iris together with muscle spasm. Alternatively, for the optic nerve, an intense sensation of light produces a centrally mediated reflex protective response which, to be effective, is registered as pain.

Undue sensitivity to normal levels of retinal illumination may occur in four separate states; ocular inflammation, a failure of the normal iris sphincter, an alteration in the retinal response to ambient light and a heightened central response. These conditions have been grouped, together with possible mechanisms, in Table 30.2. In each case the patient's own pain threshold and coexistent stoicism will play a large part in the degree of pain experienced.

CONCLUSION

From the above discussion it may be seen that the pain from eye disease exists in three basic types, each with specific symptoms, aetiology and mechanisms. Recognition of the type allows diagnosis and rational treatment.

REFERENCES

Bergmanson J P G 1977 The ophthalmic innervation of the uvea in monkeys. Experimental Eye Research 24: 225–240

Bill A, Stjernschantz J, Mandahl A, Brodin Nilsson G 1979 Substance P: release on trigeminal nerve stimulation, effects in the eye. Acta Physiologica Scandinavica 106: 371–373

Cole D F, Unger W G 1973 Prostaglandins as mediators for the responses of the eye to trauma. Experimental Eye Research 17: 357–368

Lim C H, Ruskell G L 1987 Corneal nerve access in monkeys. Journal of Comparative Neurology 208: 15–23

Unger W G, Perkins C S, Bass M S 1974 The response of the rabbit eye to laser irradiation of the iris. Experimental Eye Research 19: 367–377

Unger W G, Brown N A P, Edwards J 1977 Response of the human eye to laser irradiation of the iris. Experimental Eye Research 61: 148–153

Weale R A 1971 The aging eye. The Scientific Basis of Medicine Annual Review: 244–260

31. Orofacial pain

Yair Sharav

INTRODUCTION

Diagnosis and treatment of orofacial pain are complicated by the density of anatomical structures in the area, mechanisms of referred pain and the important psychological meaning attributed to the face and the oral cavity.

The most prevalent pain in the orofacial region originates from the teeth and their surrounding structures. This is dealt with in detail in the section on oral pain, subdivided into dental, periodontal, gingival and mucosal pain, and is summarised in Table 31.1. The temporomandibular pain and dysfunction syndrome is another prevalent entity of orofacial pain, which affects up to 15% of the population. Its controversial aetiology, diagnosis and treatment are thoroughly discussed. Modern concepts, associated with possible relationships with

Table 31.1 Differential diagnosis of oral pain

	History				Physical examination		Radiography	
Source of pain	Ability to locate	Character of pain	Pain intensified by	Pain intensity	Associated signs	Pain duplicated by	Bite-wing	Periapical
Dental								
Dentinal	Poor	Evoked, does not outlast stimulus	Hot, cold, sweet, sour	Mild to moderate	Caries, defective restorations, exposed dentine	Hot or cold application, scratching dentine	Interproximal caries, defective restorations	NA
Pulpal	Very poor	Spontaneous, explosive, intermittent	Hot, cold, sometimes chewing	Usually severe	Deep caries, extensive restoration	Hot or cold, caries probing, sometimes percussion	Deep caries and deep restoration with no secondary dentine	Limited use, sometimes early periapical change
Periodontal								
Periapical	Good	For hours on same level, deep, boring	Chewing	Moderate to severe	Periapical swelling and redness, tooth mobility	Percussion, palpation of periapical area	Limited use, deep caries and deep restorations	Sometimes periapical changes
Lateral	Good	For hours on same level, boring	Chewing	Moderate to severe	Periodontal swelling, deep pockets with pus exudating, tooth mobility	Percussion, palpation of periodontal area	Sometimes alveolar bone resorption	Very useful when X-rayed with probe inserted into pocket
Gingival	Good	Pressing, annoying	Food impaction, tooth-brushing	Mild to severe	Acute gingival inflammation	Touch, percussion	NA	NA
Mucosal	Usually good	Burning, sharp	Sour, sharp and hot food	Mild to moderate	Erosive or ulcerative lesions, redness	Palpation of lesion	NA	NA

NA = not applicable.

Table 31.2 Differential diagnosis of orofacial pain

	Dental	TMP	TMJ (ID)	Salivary glands	Vascular (migraine)	Vascular (cluster)	Neuralgic	Atypical
Location	Mouth, ear, jaws, cheek	Temple, angle of mandible, jaw, teeth	TMJ, ear	Area of gland	Upper jaw, infraorbital	Periorbital, maxillary	Nerve distribution	Diffuse, deep, may cross midline
Localisation	Poor, radiating, does not cross midline	Diffuse, deep, but usually unilateral	Localised, usually good	Usually good	Usually good, unilateral	Usually good, unilateral	Fair to good	Poor, diffuse, may change location
Duration	Minutes to hours	Weeks to years	Weeks to years	Hours to days	1–2 days	0.5–2 h	Seconds	Weeks to years
Character of pain	Intermittent sharp, paroxysmal	Dull continuous, annoying	Deep, boring	Drawing, pulling	Throbbing, deep, continuous	Paroxysmal in clusters	Lancinating, paroxysmal	Dull, boring, continuous
Pain intensity	Mild to severe	Mild to moderate	Mild to moderate	Moderate to severe	Moderate to severe	Severe	Severe	Mild to severe
Precipitating factors	Hot and cold foods	Yawning, chewing	Yawning, chewing	Eating	Menopause	Alcohol	Touch, vibration, cold wind	Stress, fatigue
Associated signs	Caries	Limited mouth opening	Click in TMJ, deviation of mouth opening	Salivary gland swelling, blockage of salivary glands	Cheek swelling and redness	Lacrimation, injected eye, nasal discharge	Facial tic	None
Pain duplication	Cold and hot application	Masticatory muscle palpation	TMJ palpation	Pressure to gland, citric acid to tongue	Unknown	Nitroglycerine	Touch of trigger point	Unknown
Sleep association	May disturb	Does not disturb	May disturb	May disturb	Disturbs usually toward morning	Disturbs, 'REM-locked'	Does not disturb	Does not disturb
Aetiological factors	Caries	Parafunction (?), stress-related	TMJ derangment	Saliva retention, ascending infection	Vasomotor inflammation (?)	Vasomotor	Idiopathic	Depression, nerve injury
Treatment	Endodontic tooth restoration	Physiotherapy, behavioural, antidepressants	Biteguard, NSAID, transquillisers	Antibiotics, blockage removal	*Prophylactic*: Amitriptyline, beta- or Ca-channel blockers *Abortive*: Ergot, NSAID	*Prophylactic*: Methysergide, lithium carbonate *Abortive*: Ergot, sumatriptan, oxygen	Carbamazepine, baclofen, nerve block, neurosurgery	Tricyclic antidepressants, clonazepam, behavioural

ID = internal derangement; NSAID = nonsteroidal antiinflammatory durgs; REM = rapid eye movement; TMP = temporomandibular pain; TMJ = temporomandibular joint.

headache mechanisms and fibromyalgia are examined. Ill-defined atypical oral and facial pain is discussed next, possible mechanisms are reviewed and suggested therapies are indicated. The 'burning mouth' syndrome (BMS) is considered in detail.

To conclude, the differential diagnosis of orofacial pain is discussed. It is subclassified into pain associated with defined local injury and pain not related to defined injury and is summarised in Table 31.2.

ORAL PAIN

Oral pain is primarily associated with the teeth and their supporting structures, i.e. the periodontium. Most frequently, dental pain is a sequela of dental caries. Initially, when the carious lesion is confined to the dentine, the tooth is sentitive both to changes in temperature and to sweet substances, but pain is not spontaneous. As the lesion penetrates deeper into the tooth, the pain produced by these stimuli becomes stronger and lasts longer. Eventually, when the carious lesion invades the tooth pulp, an inflammatory process develops (pulpitis) associated with acute, intermittent spontaneous pain. If microorganisms and products of tissue disintegration invade the area around the root apex (periapical periodontitis), the tooth becomes very sensitive to chewing, touch and percussion. At that stage the explosive, intermittent pain acquires a continuous boring nature and the tooth is no longer sensitive to changes in temperature. In clinical practice the demarcation between these various stages is sometimes indistinct; for example, the tooth may be sensitive simultaneously to temperature changes and to chewing. Other sources of oral pain are associated with direct insult to the tissues surrounding the teeth resulting in lateral periodontal or gingival pain. Pain arising from the oral mucosa can be localised and associated with a detectable erosive or ulcerative lesion or be of a diffuse nature resulting from widespread irritation of the oral mucosa. It is important to realise that there is no correlation between the amount of tissue damage to dental or other oral tissues and reported presence or absence of pain. Pain alone is an insufficient diagnostic tool for oral disease and must be validated by other diagnostic procedures for each individual case.

DENTAL PAIN

Dentinal pain

The pain originating in dentine is described as a sharp, deep sensation that is usually evoked by an external stimulus and subsides within a few seconds. Natural external stimuli are normally produced by food and drinks when hot, cold, sweet, sour and sometimes salty changes are produced. Although extreme changes in temperature (e.g. hot soup followed by ice cream) may cause pain in intact, nonaffected teeth, in most cases pain evoked by natural stimuli indicates a hyperalgesic state of the tooth. The pain is poorly localised, often only to an approximate area within two or three teeth adjacent to the affected tooth. Frequently, the patient is unable to distinguish whether the pain originates from the lower or the upper jaw. However, patients rarely make localisation errors across the midline, and posterior teeth are more difficult to localise than anterior ones (Friend et al 1968). A wide two-point discrimination threshold is believed to exist when teeth are electrically stimulated (Van Hassel & Harrington 1969).

Duplication of pain produced by controlled application of cold or hot stimuli to various teeth in the suspected area can aid in identifying the affected, hyperalgesic tooth. Most frequently this hyperalgesic state is associated with dental caries, which can be found by means of direct observation and probing with a sharp dental explorer. The 'bite-wing' intraoral dental radiograph (Fig. 31.1) is a very useful diagnostic aid in these cases. Defective restorations and any other cavity, e.g. abrasion and erosion of the enamel or roots exposed due to gingival recession, are other causes for pain. In these instances, scratching the exposed dentine with a sharp probe can evoke pain and aid in locating the source of pain.

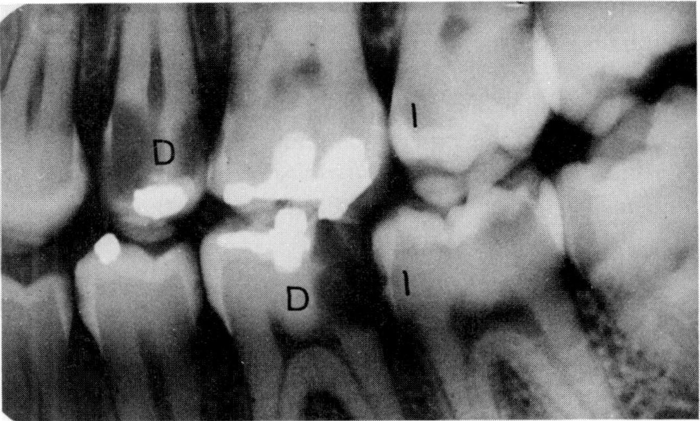

Fig. 31.1 Bite-wing radiograph demonstrating the coronal parts of the posterior teeth on the left. I – initial caries associated with dentinal pain; D – deep caries associated with pulpal pain.

In addition to these symptoms, the patient may also complain of a sharp pain, elicited by biting, that ceases immediately when pressure is removed from the teeth. Localisation of the source of pain is not precise, although the affected area can often be limited to two or three adjacent teeth. The patient complains of pain and discomfort associated with cold and hot stimuli in the area. These complaints indicate that there may be a crack in the dentine, the so-called 'cracked tooth syndrome' (Cameron 1976; Goose 1981). Although the diagnosis is frequently difficult because the affected tooth is not readily localised and radiographs are unhelpful, diagnosis and localisation of the affected tooth can be achieved by the following:

1. percussing the cusps of the suspected teeth at different angles
2. asking the patient to bite on individual cusps using a fine wooden stick
3. probing firmly around margins of fillings and in suspected fissures
4. applying cold stimuli to various areas of the suspected tooth.

Other possible additional diagnoses include occlusal abrasion with exposed dentine or a cracked filling. However, these can be detected visually with the aid of a sharp explorer.

Treatment

Dentinal pain due to caries is best treated by removal of the carious lesion and restoring the tooth by a filling.

Sensitivity usually disappears within a day. Treatment of the 'cracked tooth' consists of covering the crown of the tooth with a crown. Treatment of exposed, hypersensitive dentine is somewhat controversial (Seltzer 1978). It has been the author's experience that good oral hygiene is essential in reducing the sensitivity of dentine exposed at the root surface and that acidic foods and beverages will enhance dentinal sensitivity.

Pulpal pain

Pain associated with pulp disease is spontaneous, strong, often throbbing and is exacerbated by temperature change, sweet foods and pressure on the carious lesion. When pain is evoked it outlasts the stimulus (unlike stimulus-induced dentinal pain) and can be excruciating for many minutes. Similarly to dentinal pain, localisation is poor and seems to be even poorer when pain becomes more intense (Mumford 1982). Pain tends to radiate or refer to the ear, temple and cheek but does not cross the midline (Fig. 31.2). Pain may be described by patients in different ways and a continuous dull ache can be periodically exacerbated (by stimulation or spontaneously) for short (minutes) or long (hours) periods.

Pain may increase and throb when the patient lies down, and in many instances wakes the patient from sleep (Sharav et al 1984). The pain of pulpitis is frequently not continuous and abates spontaneously; the precise explanation for such abatement is not clear (Seltzer 1978). This interrupted, sharp, paroxysmal, nonlocalised pain may lead to the misdiagnosis of idiopathic trigeminal neuralgia.

The initial aim of the diagnostic process is to identify the affected tooth and then to assess the state of the tooth pulp in order to determine treatment. Localisation of the affected tooth is achieved through the same methods detailed in the previous section on dentinal pain. The application of heat and cold to the teeth should be done very carefully because these can cause excruciating pain. Percussion aids in localising the affected tooth. The state of the pulp cannot be judged from one single sympton and should be based on the combination of several signs and symptoms (Seltzer & Bender 1975).

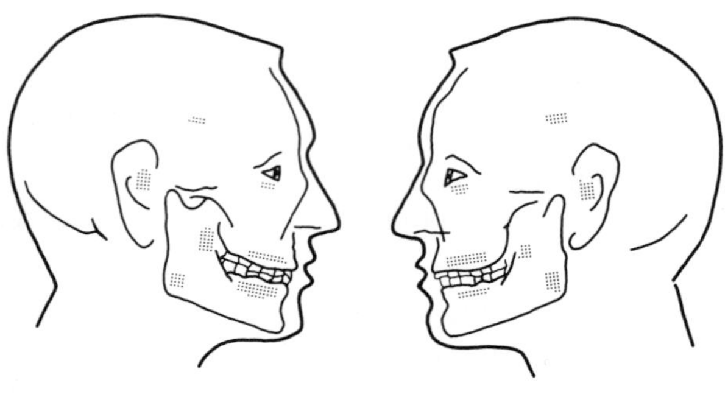

Fig. 31.2 The distribution of pain in the face from dental and periodontal sources. Each dot represents a painful area pointed to by the patient. There is a considerable overlap in pain reference locations for maxillary and mandibular sources.

Although pain is the most common symptom of a diseased pulp, no correlation exists between specific pain characteristics and the histopathological status of the pulp (Seltzer et al 1963; Tyldesley & Mumford 1970).

Treatment

Depending on the prognosis of the pulp, treatment may aim at conserving the pulp, extirpating it or extracting the tooth. Pulpal pain normally disappears immediately after treatment.

MECHANISMS OF DENTAL SENSITIVITY AND PAIN

Recently erupted human teeth with uncompleted roots are often insensitive to tooth-pulp stimulation (Tal & Sharav 1985). This cannot be explained by the absence of innervation, as nerve fibres are already present at the time of eruption (Avery 1971). Tal & Sharav (1985) demonstrated that masseteric reflex activity could be evoked in the absence of sensation when teeth were electrically stimulated in children. They proposed that segmental reflex connections appear to be established before the cortical sensory projections are functional.

It is agreed that under certain conditions of tooth-pulp stimulation sensations other than pain can be evoked (Sessle 1979). Recent studies address the question of whether nonpain and pain sensations are mediated by two distinct populations of afferents (McGrath et al 1983; Brown et al 1985; Virtanen et al 1987). When temporal summation stimuli were employed it was suggested by McGrath et al (1983) that nonpain sensations are mediated by a distinct population of afferents. Brown et al (1985), utilising spatial summation techniques, favoured the hypothesis of a single modality innervation for both nonpain and pain sensations. Based upon their temporal summation experiments, Virtanen et al (1987) concluded that 'prepain' and painful sensations from electrical tooth-pulp stimulation are both evoked by the same A-fibre populations.

The mechanisms of dentinal sensitivity and pain have been extensively reviewed and deal with the problems of pain conduction in a noninnervated, yet very sensitive, dentine (Anderson et al 1970; Dubner et al 1978; Seltzer 1978; Brannstrom 1979; Närhi 1985; Olgart 1985). Morphologically, nerve fibres may penetrate into the dentine as far as 150–200 μm only (Byers & Kish 1976). Furthermore, the concept that the odontoblast has a role as a sensory receptor of the dentine has not been substantiated (Byers et al 1982).

Experimentally induced pain was produced by applying various stimuli to exposed dentine, i.e. drying by application of absorbent paper or a blow of air, mechanical stimulation (e.g. cutting, scratching, probing) and changes in osmotic pressure, pH or temperature. However, the application of various pain-inducing substances, such as potassium chloride, acetylcholine, 5-hydroxytryptamine (5-HT), bradykinin and histamine to exposed dentine does not evoke pain (Anderson & Naylor 1962; Brannstrom 1962). All these substances can produce pain when placed on a blister base on the skin (Armstrong et al 1953). The limited distribution of nerve fibres in dentine and the fact that neuroactive chemical agents fail to stimulate or anaesthetise dentine led to the proposal of the hydrodynamic mechanism by Brannstrom (1963). The movement of the extracellular fluid that fills the dentinal tubules will, according to Brannstrom's hypothesis, distort the pain-sensitive nervous structure in the pulp and predentinal area and activate mechanoreceptors to produce pain (Brannstrom 1979). Mumford & Newton (1969) and Horiuchi & Matthews (1973) could detect, however, an electrical potential across the dentine of extracted teeth to which hydrostatic pressure was applied. It is not clear whether these currents would be sufficient to excite nerves in the pulp (Greenwood et al 1972).

Many possible pain mechanisms have been suggested for pulpal pain. These have been summarised by Seltzer (1978), Mumford (1982) and Olgart (1985), are related to pulp inflammation and include a host of mediators found in the pulp, such as cholinergic and adrenergic neurotransmitters (probably the most important among these is 5-HT), prostaglandins and cyclic adenosine monophosphate (cAMP). Most of these are hypothetical mechanisms, suggested only because such agents produce pain in other parts of the body (Keele & Armstrong 1968). Recent studies do confirm, however, the effect of some substances, such as prostaglandins (probably PGE_2) and serotonin, on tooth-pulp nerve excitability. It is suspected that, unlike pulpal C-fibres, A-fibres are relatively insensitive to inflammatory mediators (Olgart 1985). It has recently been found, however, that leukotriene B_4 can sensitise pulpal A-delta fibres (Madison et al 1992).Other factors to be considered are lowered oxygen tension and impaired microcirculation associated with increased intrapulpal pressure.

PERIODONTAL PAIN

Pain originating in the structures surrounding the teeth is readily localised; the affected teeth are very tender to pressure. Periodontal pain usually results from an acute inflammatory process of the gingiva, the periodontal ligament and alveolar bone due to bacterial infection. Aetiologically, two modes of affection are possible:

1. a sequela of pulp infection and pulp necrosis which results in periapical inflammation
2. gingival and periodontal infection and pocket formation that result in a lateral periodontal involvement.

Although pain characteristics, ability to localise and pain-producing situations are similar in both cases (see Table 31.1), treatment differs for aetiological reasons and these categories are therefore discussed separately.

Acute periapical periodontitis

Pain associated with acute periapical inflammation is spontaneous and moderate to severe in intensity for long periods of time (hours). Pain is exacerbated by biting on the tooth and, in more advanced cases, even by closing the mouth and bringing the affected tooth into contact with the opposing teeth. In these cases, the tooth feels highly extruded and is very sensitive to touch. Frequently the patient reports that pulpal pain preceded the pain originating from the periapical area. The latter, although of a more continuous nature, is usually better tolerated than the paroxysmal and excruciating pulpal pain. Localisation of pain originating from the periapical area is usually precise and the patient is able to indicate the affected tooth. In this respect periodontal pain differs from the poorly localised dentinal and pulpal pain. The improved ability to localise the source of pain may be attributed to the proprioreceptive and mechanoreceptive sensibility of the periodontium (Harris 1975; Van Steenberghe 1979) that is lacking in the pulp. However, although localisation of the affected tooth is usually precise, in approximately half the cases the pain is diffuse and spreads into the jaw on the affected side of the face (Sharav et al 1984).

During examination the affected tooth is readily located by means of tooth percussion. The periapical vestibular area is usually tender to palpation. The pulp of the affected tooth is nonvital, i.e. it does not respond to thermal changes or to electrical pulp stimulation. However, as mentioned above, in clinical practice pulpitis may not be sharply distinguished from acute periapical periodontitis and pulpal as well as periapical involvement could occur at the same time. In these cases, although the periapical area has been invaded by endogenous pain-producing substances due to pulp tissue damage (e.g. 5-HT, histamine, bradykinin) and exogenous pain-producing substances (e.g. bacterial toxins) the pulp has not yet completely degenerated and can still react to stimuli such as temperature changes. These instances are fairly common (Mumford 1982). In more severe, purulent cases, swelling of the face associated with cellulitis is sometimes present and can be associated with fever and malaise. The affected tooth may be extruded and mobile. Usually, when swelling to the face occurs, pain diminishes in intensity due to rupture of the periostium of the bone around the affected tooth and the decrease in pus pressure.

The radiographic picture is of limited use in the diagnosis of acute periapical periodontitis as no periapical radiographic changes are detected in the early stages. If a radiographic periapical rarifying osteitis is noticed in a tooth that is sensitive to touch and percussion, the condition is then classified as reacutisation of chronic periapical periodontitis. Many times, however, such a rarifying osteitis lesion is present in an otherwise symptomless situation. This lack of correlation between pain and the radiographic picture is also true for pain and the type of periapical inflammation and infection present (Block et al 1976; Langeland et al 1977).

Treatment

While the pain originates from the periodontal periapical tissues, the source of insult and infection usually lies within the pulp chamber and the root canal. The primary aim of treatment is to eliminate the source of irritation. The pulp chamber is opened and the root canal cleansed. Grinding the tooth to prevent contact with the opposing teeth also relieves pain. If cellulitis, fever and malaise are present, systemic administration of antibiotics is recommended. Incision and drainage are very effective when a fluctuating abscess is present. Pain usually subsides within 24–48 hours.

Lateral periodontol abscess

Pain characteristics of the lateral periodontal abscess are very similar to those of acute periapical periodontitis. The pain is continuous, moderate to severe in intensity and is exacerbated by biting on the affected tooth. The pain is well-localised. During examination swelling and redness of the gingiva may be noticed, usually located more gingivally than in the case of the acute periapical lesion. The affected tooth is sensitive to percussion and is often mobile and slightly extruded. In more severe cases, cellulitis, fever and malaise may occur. A deep periodontal pocket is usually located around the tooth; once probed there is pus exudation and subsequent relief from pain. The tooth pulp is usually vital, i.e. it reacts normally to temperature changes and electrical stimulation. The pulp may occasionally be slightly hyperalgesic in these cases and sometimes pulpitis and pulpal pain may develop due to retrograde infection (Fig. 31.3). Abscess formation usually results from a blockage of drainage from a periodontal pocket, and is frequently associated with a deep infrabony pocket and teeth with root furcation involvement (Fig. 31.3).

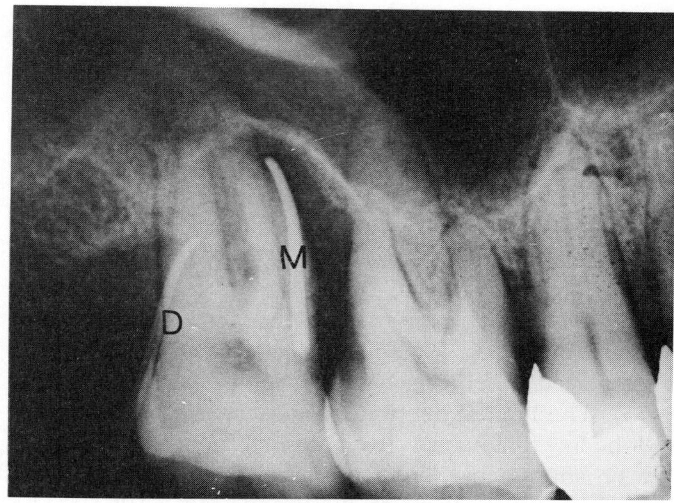

Fig. 31.3 Periapical radiograph of the molar area in the right maxillary region. Radiopaque probes were inserted into mesial (M) and distal (D) periodontal pockets of the second molar to demonstrate the depth of these pockets. Lateral periodontal and pulpal pain were both present. Pulpal pain in this case was not associated with caries but with 'retrograde' infection of the pulp through the deep mesial pocket.

Treatment

Gentle irrigation and curettage of the pocket should be performed. The tooth is ground in order to avoid contact with the opposing teeth. When cellulitis, fever and malaise are present, systemic antibiotic administration is recommended. Direct incision and drainage are recommended when the abscess cannot be approached through the pocket and it is ripe for incision.

Pain usually subsides within 24 hours of treatment.

GINGIVAL PAIN

Gingival pain may occur as a result of mechanical irritation, due to acute inflammation associated with a gingival pocket, or as a result of infection when specific underlying factors prevail.

Food impaction

The patient complains of localised pain that develops between two teeth after meals, especially when food is fibrous (e.g. meat, celery). The pain is associated with a feeling of pressure and discomfort that is very annoying. The patient reports that the pain may gradually disappear until evoked again at the next meal or the pain may be relieved immediately by removing the food impacted between the teeth. Upon examination, a faulty contact between two adjacent teeth is noticed so that food is usually trapped between these teeth; the gingival papilla is tender to touch and bleeds easily. The two adjacent teeth are usually sensitive to percussion. The cause of the faulty contact between the teeth is often a carious lesion, and restoring the tooth will eliminate pain.

Pericoronitis

Pain, which may be severe, is usually located at the distal end of the arch of teeth in the lower jaw. Pain is spontaneous and may be exacerbated by closing the mouth. In more severe cases, pain is aggravated by swallowing and trismus may occur. Acute pericoronal infections are common in teeth that are incompletely erupted and are partially covered by flaps of gingival tissue.

Upon examination, the flap of gingiva is acutely inflamed, red and oedematous. Frequently, an indentation of the opposing tooth can be seen imprinted on the oedematous gingival flap. Occasionally, fever and malaise are associated with this infection.

Treatment includes irrigation of debris between the flap and the affected tooth and eliminating trauma by the opposing tooth (by grinding or extraction). Systemic antibiotic administration is commonly recommended, especially when trismus occurs.

Acute necrotising ulcerative gingivitis

Soreness and pain are felt at the margin of the gums. Pain is intensified by eating and brushing the teeth; these activities are usually accompanied by gingival bleeding. In the early stages some patients may complain of a feeling of tightness around the teeth. Metallic taste is sometimes experienced and usually there is a foetid smell from the mouth. Pain is fairly well-localised to the affected areas, but in cases when lesions are spread all over the gums pain is experienced all over the mouth. Fever and malaise are sometimes present. Upon examination necrosis and ulceration are noticed on the marginal gingiva with different degrees of gingival papillary destruction. An adherent greyish slough represents the so-called pseudomembrane that is present in the acute stage of the disease.

Swabbing this slough is associated with pain and bleeding. Although basically a bacterial disease that responds dramatically to antibiotics, it is not clear whether the bacteria actually initiate the disease or are merely secondary to some underlying factors. Local as well as systemic factors are suggested as possible underlying factors. These include, locally, gross neglect of oral hygiene, heavy smoking and mouth-breathing. Systemically, any underlying debilitating factors are suggested, but there is no doubt that these are secondary to the more important local factors (Burket & Greenberg 1977).

Treatment includes swabbing and gentle irrigation of the ulcerative lesions, preferably with an oxidising agent (hydrogen peroxide), and scaling and cleaning the teeth. Systemic antibiotics are recommended when fever and malaise are present.

INTENSITY AND LOCATION OF ACUTE ORAL PAIN

Acute dental and periodontal pain is frequently rated as moderate to severe in intensity or from 60–100 on a 100 mm visual analogue scale (Sharav et al 1984). Pain is conceived of as deep and unpleasant. In about 60% of cases pain is not localised only at the affected site but spreads into remote areas in the head and face (Fig. 31.2). There is a considerable overlap in pain reference locations for maxillary and mandibular sources (Fig. 31.2). Pain spread is correlated positively with pain intensity and unpleasantness (Fig. 31.4). Two factors which may be important for this pain spread are the large receptive fields of wide-dynamic-range neurons with extensive gradient sensitivity and the somatotopic organisation (Sharav et al 1984).

MUCOSAL PAIN

Pain originating from the oral mucosa can be either localised or of a more generalised diffuse nature. The localised pain is usually associated with a detectable erosive or ulcerative lesion; the diffuse pain may be associated with a widespread infection, a systemic underlying deficiency disease or other unknown factors.

The localised pain that is associated with a detectable lesion results from physical, chemical or thermal trauma, viral infection or lesions of unknown origin. Pain is usually mild to moderate but may become quite severe when there

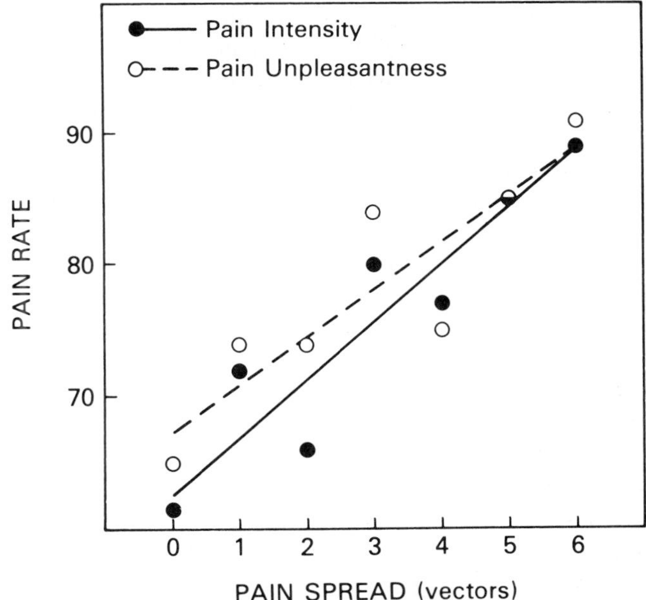

Fig. 31.4 Pain spread in the face, from dental and periodontal sources, as a function of pain intensity and pain unpleasantness ratings. Pain spread is rated as the number of pain reference locations (vectors). Pain intensity and pain unpleasantness are visual analogue scale ratings.

is irritation, mechanically or by sour, spicy or hot foods. This exacerbation of pain may last for some minutes. Detailed descriptions of the various lesions of the oral mucosa are beyond the scope of this chapter and only the most common lesion (recurrent aphthous stomatitis) will be described briefly. Presumably of autoimmune nature, and aggravated by stress, recurrent aphthous stomatitis is characterised by a prodromal burning sensation from 2–48 h before an ulcer appears. Although small in diameter (0.3–1.0 cm) this lesion may be quite painful (Greenberg 1977). In the mild form, healing occurs within 10 days and pain is usually mild to moderate in severity. In the more severe forms (major aphthous ulcers), deep ulcers occur which may be confluent, are extremely painful and interfere with speech and eating. Such lesions may last for months, heal slowly and leave scars. Treatment is mostly symptomatic, including the application of a topical protective emollient for the mild form and the use of topical corticosteroids and tetracycline to decrease healing time for the severe form.

When a generalised diffuse pain occurs in the oral mucosa, it usually has a burning nature and may be accompanied by a change in taste, predominantly of a bitter metallic quality. This pain may result from a direct insult to the tissues due to bacterial, viral or fungal infection, which can be identified by the characteristic appearance of the oral mucosa. Diagnosis is aided by microbiological laboratory examinations. In cases of chronic fungal infection (candidiasis), possible underlying aetiological factors such as prolonged broad spectrum antibiotic therapy, immunodeficiencies and other debilitating factors should be investigated. Radiation therapy to the head and neck region may result in acute mucositis with severe generalised mucosal pain (Kolbinson et al 1988). Decreased salivary flow is a later sequela that may result in chronic pain and discomfort of the oral mucosa.

Burning sensation of the oral mucosa, particularly the tongue, may result from systemic deficiency disease, such as chronic iron-deficiency anaemia. This is usually associated with observable atrophic changes, in particular that of the filiform and fungiform papillae of the tongue. However, there is a large proportion of patients, mostly women between the ages of 50–70 years, who complain of a burning sensation in the mouth and the tongue, with no observable changes in the oral mucosa and with no detectable underlying systemic changes. This group of patients is discussed further in the section on the burning mouth syndrome.

TEMPOROMANDIBULAR MYOFASCIAL PAIN AND DYSFUNCTION

This prevalent entity of orofacial pain and mandibular dysfunction (Helkimo 1979) has acquired more than a dozen names (De Boever 1979) since it was first described by Costen in 1934. In addition to a variety of names, a variety of diferent criteria have been used for defining this disorder (Rugh & Solberg 1979). Indeed, the criteria for the syndrome were such that they encompassed disorders which under today's concepts would be diagnosed differently (Eversole & Machado 1985). By the 1950s it was becoming obvious that many of these patients suffered from a masticatory muscle disorder apparently unrelated to the temporomandibular joint TMJ. However it was only during the last decade that, with the aid of modern TMJ imaging techniques (Dolwick et al 1983), we began to understand that there was also a temporomandibular disorder of the joint proper that justified separate classification. The definition of internal derangements of the TMJ finally dissociated the temporomandibular joint from this 'syndrome', and the justification for a separate entity of temporomandibular myofascial pain as opposed to the 'general' myofascial pain dysfunction (MPD) syndrome was further questioned. Indeed, the 1986 International Association for the Study of Pain (IASP) classification combines temporomandibular pain and dysfunction and tension headache under the same category of 'craniofacial pain of musculoskeletal origin'. The segregation of temporomandibular myofascial pain and dysfunction (TMPD) form other myofascial pain disorders of a more generalised type, such as primary fibromyalgia, has recently been questioned by others (Widmer 1991). The question whether TMPD is a localised symptom of a more generalised condition or a discrete entity will be addressed in more detail later.

TMPD will be discussed as two distinct entities: one is associated primarily with pain and dysfunction of myofascial origin, and will be referred to as temporomandibular pain (TMP); the other is due to internal derangement (ID) of the TMJ.

TEMPOROMANDIBULAR PAIN (TMP)

Patients usually describe a poorly localised, dull, continuous ache, typically around the ear, the angle of the mandible and the temporal area. However pain has also been described in the jaws, teeth and diffusely throughout one side of the face (Campbell 1958; Bell 1989). Pain may also occur bilaterally; there is some evidence that bilateral pain is more commonly associated with underlying psychogenic factors (Gerschman et al 1990). The temporal pain pattern varies considerably, with some patients experiencing the most intense pain in the morning or late afternoon and others having no fixed pattern (Perry 1968; Laskin 1969). Duration can be from weeks to several years, but fortunately the pain rarely wakes the patient from sleep. Pain may be aggravated during function with transient spikes of pain occurring spontaneously or induced by jaw movements (Bell 1989).

In addition to pain there may be deviation of the mandible on opening, fullness of the ear, dizziness and soreness of the neck (Travell 1955; Schwarz 1959; Molin 1973; Gelb & Tarte 1975; Block 1976; Sharav et al 1978; Blasberg & Chalmers 1989). Dizziness has been associated with pain in the sternomastoid muscle (Travell 1955; Sharav et al 1978) and ear stuffiness with spasm of the medial pterygoid (Block 1976).

Examination may reveal limited mouth opening (less than 40 mm, interincisal). Masticatory and neck muscles are tender to palpation (Butler et al 1975; Gelb & Tarte 1975; Sharav et al 1978) and pain often refers (Travell 1960; Bell 1989). Trigger points in the muscles may also be detected (Krauss 1970; Travell & Simons 1983). Diagnosis is usually based on the history and clinical examination of the patient. However clinical signs are difficult to measure with consistency (Kopp & Wenneberg 1983; Carlsson et al 1980); moreover interrater reliability for some signs of MPD is not good (Dworkin et al 1990b).

Neurophysiological studies

Numerous physiological investigations have been performed in temporomandibular pain patterns (Dubner et al 1978; Yemm 1979; Lund et al 1991). It has been shown that these patients have a substantially reduced biting force compared to controls, which has been attributed to muscle pain and tenderness (Molin 1972). In 1971 Bessette et al reported that the interruption of sustained electromyographic (EMG) activity of the masseter by a tap to the chin (the so called 'silent period'), was longer in patients than in controls. This was later confirmed by some (Wildmalm 1976; Baily et al 1977), but not by others (Zulqarnain et al 1989). Subject selection and experimental methodological variations could account for some of these differences. Sharav et al (1982) found that masseteric inhibitory periods were shorter in patients than in controls when evoked by electrical tooth-pulp stimulation. Shorter inhibitory periods were also described in patients in response to tooth tapping (De Latt et al 1985; Zulqarnain et al 1989). Sharav et al (1982) suggested that there was an increase in excitability of the central motor neuron pool in these patients and muscle hyperactivity was suggested by De Latt et al (1985). A further demonstration of an association between hyperactivity of masticatory muscles and temporomandibular disorders is that EMG inhibitory responses following initial tooth contact are either absent or reduced and that EMG activity, not normally detected when the mouth is open, is found in 50% of temporomandibular patients (Munro 1975). Several other studies report that patients with TMP have higher resting masseter and temporalis EMG activity than nonpatients (Glaros et al 1989). No difference was found in the duration of the masseteric inhibitory period between the painful and the nonpainful sides (Sharav et al 1982). Comparison of the bilateral activity in the anterior temporalis and the masseter muscles during clenching showed, however, that patients with muscle pain demonstrate asymmetrical recruitment of these muscles in contrast to the more symmetrical recruitment seen in normal individuals (Nielsen et al 1990).

Epidemiology

Temporomandibular pain and dysfunction disorders are recognised as the most common chronic orofacial pain condition (Dworkin et al 1990a). However information on the prevalence of TMPD signs and symptoms was based mainly on studies of patients seeking treatment (Greene & Marbach 1982). A further major problem is the definition of inclusion and exclusion criteria (Rugh & Solberg 1979). Moreover, given poor interrater reliability, comparing data seems perilous. The advent of the diagnosis of internal derangement (ID) of the TMJ certainly questions the validity of much of the epidemiological research done before this diagnostic entity was defined. In the available epidemiological studies of the general population, TMPD signs and symptoms appear to be equally distributed between the sexes (Helkimo 1979; Christensen 1981) or the differences are minor (Locker & Slade 1988). In Agerberg & Carlsson's classic cross-sectional study (1972) about half of the 15–44-year-old population had at least one symptom of dysfunction and one-third had two or more symptoms. Reporting symptoms in a population over 18 years old, Locker & Slade (1988) describe a prevalence of 48.8% while the percentage of those needing treatment was estimated at 3.5–9.7%. Of much interest in this respect is the study of Wanmann & Agerberg (1986a) who reported a prevalence of 20% in a study group of 17-year-olds. They followed up this group for 2 years and found that although the incidence was 8% there was no general increase in the severity or number of symptoms in this study period; the explanation offered was that new symptoms appear as often as old ones disappear (Wanman & Agerberg 1986b). Thus, spontaneous remission seems to be quite prevalent in this disorder.

While signs and symptoms of TMPD are equally distributed between the sexes in the general population, the majority of patients who seek treatment (up to 80%) are females (Perry 1968; Butler et al 1975; Sharav et al 1978; Helkimo 1979; Rugh & Solberg 1985). Signs and symptoms of mandibular dysfunction have been found in all age groups (Helkimo 1979; Nielsen et al 1990), with a tendency to increase with age (Rugh & Solberg 1985; Tervonen & Knuuttila 1988). Dworkin et al (1990) report that TMJ pain however is less common among the elderly. Signs of mandibular dysfunction have been described in children and adolescents with a higher prevalence than was previously suspected (Perry 1973; Nielsen et al 1989).

The syndrome occurs also in edentulous patients (Carlsson 1976; Agerberg 1988).

Aetiological factors

Bruxism and occlusal derangement

The association between TMP, the teeth and dental occlusion stems back to Costen (1934), who believed that overclosure of the mandible due to loss of teeth was responsible for TMJ pain. More recent theories consider occlusal disturbances a prerequisite for the development of dysfunction and pain. Whilst the extent of the occlusal 'interference' may be minute, the important fact is that such interference can upset proprioceptive feedback and thus cause bruxism and spasm of masticatory muscles (Krogh-Poulsen & Olsson 1966). These assumptions were recently refuted by Rugh et al (1984) who demonstrated that occlusal discrepancies, produced experimentally, tend to reduce bruxism rather than enhance it. Furthermore, data by Thomson (1971), Solberg et al (1972), Clarke (1982) and presented in Greene & Marbach's review (1982) indicate that there are no significant differences between the occlusal relationship in patients and in asymptomatic controls.

Bruxism is no longer perceived as related to occlusal 'disharmonies' but rather as a physiological behaviour that may sometimes be associated with TMP (Rugh & Harlan 1988). Clark et al (1980) suggest that bruxism is stress-related. They demonstrated a positive relationship between increased urinary epinephrine and high levels of nocturnal masseter muscle activity. The forces exerted during nocturnal tooth grinding are quite high and were found to exceed maximal conscious clenches (Clarke et al 1984). However, the association between bruxism and TMP is not entirely clear. Bruxism is viewed as an arousal phenomenon (Satoh & Harada 1973) or as a sleep parasomnia (American Sleep Disorder Association 1990). Some preliminary results suggest that a majority of patients with bruxism have pain levels and sleep quality comparable with TMP patients (Lavigne et al 1991). On the other hand patients having bruxism without muscle pain did not show differences in any of the sleep variables compared to matched controls (Velly-Miguel et al 1991).

A specific relationship between bruxism and TMP is based on the vicious cycle theory where an occlusal interference or a painful lesion of a muscle is supposed to induce a spasm in the affected muscle, which in turn leads to ischaemia because of the compression of blood vessels. Ischaemic contractions are painful and activate muscle nociceptors; by this mechanism the vicious cycle is closed. However, this concept is not supported by experimental data (Mense 1991). If muscle hyperactivity, presumably associated with stress and bruxism, is not the cause of pain but rather a 'pain-adaptation' response (Lund et al 1991) then bruxism can no longer be considered as a specific aetiological mechanism of pain in TMP.

Psychosocial correlates

Early studies emphasise the contribution of psychological factors to TMP (Moulton 1955; Schwatz 1959). Lascelles (1966) described a background of depressive illness in the majority of his 93 facial pain patients and a significantly larger number of Fine's (1971) TMP patients were depressed compared to controls. However, on the basis of an extensive literature review, Rugh & Solberg (1979) concluded that there was little evidence suggesting that TMP is related to any specific personality trait. Thus, Marbach et al (1978) found no significant difference in either state-anxiety or trait-anxiety between patients with intractable facial pain and groups of general dental and general medical patients. In a later study Marbach & Lund (1981) found no difference in depression and anhedonia between TMP patients and a normal, nonpatient group. Salter et al (1983) challenge the idea that TMP patients represent a population whose pain results form their emotional state. They found that the comparison of TMP patients and patients with facial pain and lesions or pathophysiological disorders showed little evidence of neuroticism in either group. Furthermore, examining the premorbid characteristics of TMP patients did not reveal abnormal parental bonding attitudes in this group (Salter et al 1983) nor did they show any other measures of previous premorbid personality traits (Merskey et al 1987). Sharav et al (1987) found that only two out of 32 patients with chronic facial pain were cortisol non-suppressors on the dexamethasone suppression test (DST). In a recent study Schnurr et al (1990) classified their TMPD patients according to the diagnostic criteria of Eversole & Machado (1985), enabling a separate comparison of myogenic (TMP) and of TMJ facial pain to nonfacial injury 'pain controls' and healthy controls. The results of Schnurr et al (1990) suggested that TMP and TMJ pain patients do not appear to be significantly different from other pain patients or healthy controls in personality type, response to illness, attitudes toward health care or ways of coping with stress.

Vascular mechanisms and headache

Muscle tenderness is a frequent finding in headache patients (Raskin & Appenzeller 1980), and the distribution may be distinctly similar to that in TMP patients (Butler et al 1975; Sharav et al 1978; Tafelt-Hansen et al 1981; Clarke et al 1987). Patients with signs of TMP report a significantly higher incidence of tension headache than controls (Magnusson & Carlsson 1978; Watts et al 1986); indeed epidemiological data suggest great similarity and possible overlap between patients suffering from headache and TMP (Magnusson & Carlsson 1978). The sex ratio is similar – about 75% females in both groups; age distribution and contributing psychophysiological mechanisms are also shared (Rugh & Solberg 1979; Raskin & Appenzeller 1980). It seems therefore that two of the fundamental symptoms of TMP, i.e. pain of daily occurrence and tenderness of muscles to palpation, fail to properly differentiate between tension-type headache and TMP patients. As previously mentioned, the 1986 IASP classification combines these two under 'craniofacial pain of musculoskeletal origin'. However, most TMP patients have pain and muscle tenderness on palpation unilaterally (Butler et al 1975; Sharav et al 1978) while tension-type headache causes pain bilaterally.

The association between migraine and temporomandibular dysfunction was studied by Watts et al (1986). A total of 50 patients with mixed headache syndromes were compared to 50 TMP patients. The authors stated that the rate of migraine in the TMP group did not differ from that in the general population, and concluded that TMP and migraine patients are two segregated groups. That TMP and vascular headache are two distinct entities can also be inferred from studies of sleep physiology. Bruxism, associated with TMP (Lavigne 1991) occurred mostly in non-rapid eye movement (REM) stages of sleep (Satoh & Harada 1973; Wieselman et al 1986; Rugh & Harlan 1988), while vascular headache is REM 'locked' (Dexter & Weizman 1970). Recently, however a severe tooth destructive form of bruxism has been found in REM sleep (Ware & Rugh 1988), which may suggest that in some cases vascular mechanisms could be associated with TMP.

Fibromyalgia

Much controversy exists in the medical literature concerning muscle tenderness and its diagnosis in specific cases. The boundaries between fibromyalgia (FM) and myofascial pain dysfunction (MPD) are at times poorly demarcated although specific criteria have been established (Scudds et al 1989). In the light of the possibility that on the one hand FM may begin as a localised pain disorder and later become widespread, and on the other hand that persistent MPD may involve multiple sites and cause systemic symptoms (Wolfe 1988; Bennet 1986), some authors believe that all local 'syndromes' of myofascial pain should be conflated to form one entity. Thus it is claimed by Widmer (1991) that when the symptoms of FM patients are compared with those of patients with temporomandibular disorders, without joint pathology, no symptoms are specific to TMP. TMP seems to be a localised condition but the evidence needs to be examined carefully. Blasberg & Chalmers (1989) retrospectively reviewed a series of TMP patients for evidence of generalised musculoskeletal pain. They conclude that there are great similarities between these and primary fibromyalgia (PFM) patients. Eriksson et al (1988) studied eight patients with PFM and found that six had severe signs of mandibular dysfunction using the Helkimo Anamnestic Dysfunction Index, thus promoting the hypothesis that a connection may exist between these entities.

These conclusions should be viewed very carefully; PFM, by definition, is characterised by a widespread pain on both sides of the body and in both the upper and the lower parts of the body in 97.6% of PFM patients (Henriksson & Bengtsson 1991), whereas TMP is mostly a local, unilateral, pain syndrome (Sharav et al 1978; Bell 1989).

TMJ damage

Theoretically, trauma or noxious stimulation of TMJ tissues can produce a sustained excitation of masticatory muscles that may serve to protect the masticatory system from potentially damaging movements and stimuli (Sessle & Hu 1991). However, injection into the TMJ of algesic chemicals resulted in sustained reflex increase in EMG activity of jaw-opening muscles; excitatory effects were also seen in jaw-closing muscles but were generally weaker (Broton & Sessle 1988). While such effects might be related to clinically-based concepts of myofascial dysfunction (e.g. splinting, myospastic activity and trigger points), the weak effects in muscles that are invoked clinically to show such dysfunction (jaw-closing) and the stronger effects in antagonist muscles (jaw-opening) suggest associations more in keeping with protective, withdrawal-type reflexes (Sessle & Hu 1991). Based upon the present available data it seems that pain originating in the TMJ contributes minimally to the development of TMP.

Conclusions

Bruxism and TMJ derangements do not seem to be primary aetiological factors of TMP. The role that vascular mechanisms, related to other craniofacial pains (e.g. migraine, cluster headache, paroxysmal hemicrania), play in TMP is not entirely clear. Whilst the importance of vascular mechanisms may not yet be fully appreciated, one should not dismiss their contribution to TMP. Some data (Ware & Rugh 1988) point to a REM-locked destructive form of bruxism that may link certain forms of TMP with vascular mechanisms. Recent findings strongly suggest that neurogenic inflammation may play the major role in vascular headache (Moskowitz et al 1989). In view of the cardinal role of the trigeminal system in conveying vascular headache (Dostrovsky et al 1991), the possibility of interrelated central mechanisms of headache and facial pain cannot be discounted. Research in the area of TMP should concentrate more on central generators of pain mechanisms rather than peripheral inputs such as occlusal interferences and 'muscle hyperactivity' (Lund et al

1991). One attractive way to understand TMP better is to study the role of trigeminal neurogenic inflammation and the contribution of the sympathetic nervous system (Basbaum & Levine, 1991) regarding the pain mechanisms of TMP.

Differential diagnosis

TMP should be differentiated from pain due to TMJ derangement and other specific TMJ disease (e.g. psoriasis, rheumatoid arthritis). Of particular importance are instances where TMP can mask underlying malignancies such as nasopharyngeal carcinoma (Sharav & Feinsod 1977; Roistacher & Tanenbaum 1986).

Treatment

Like other chronic pain syndromes, TMP is a complex entity associated with behavioural changes, secondary psychological gains, changes in mood and attitudes to life and drug abuse. While alleviation of pain and dysfunction remain the primary goals of therapy, restoring the patient's attitudes by modelling behavioural changes and controlling drug abuse should also be achieved. Often reassurance of the patient, combined with simple muscle exercises for masticatory and neck muscles, will result in pain alleviation and restored mandibular function (Schwarz 1959; Krauss 1970; Selby 1985). Muscle tenderness may be treated with vapocoolant sprays and injections of local anaesthetics into identified trigger points (Travell & Simons 1983). Diazepam is significantly more effective than placebo in the relief of pain, while ibuprofen has had minimal therapeutic benefit in TMP patients (Singer et al 1987). Sharav et al (1987) demonstrated the beneficial effect of low doses of amitriptyline (less than 30 mg/day) in patients with chronic facial pain of myofascial origin. The efficacy of amitriptyline in relieving chronic facial pain, such as TMP, is through a direct analgesic effect not associated with the antidepressive effect of the drug (Sharav et al 1987). Occlusal splint therapy is a widely used mode of treatment (Clarke et al 1984), and may be associated with the reduction of nocturnal bruxism (Clark et al 1979). Some investigators found occlusal splint therapy to be superior to relaxation procedures (Okeson et al 1983).

It is widely believed that chronic pain patients lack psychological insight and therefore do not respond to psychodynamic interpretation (Sternbach 1978). Consequently other psychological interventions such as relaxation training, biofeedback and cognitive behaviour approaches (Carlsson & Gale 1976; Stem et al 1979) would be more appropriate for these patients.

Prognosis in the majority of patients is good and remission of pain and dysfunction is readily achieved for long periods.

INTERNAL DERANGEMENT OF THE TEMPOROMANDIBULAR JOINT

Internal derangement (ID) of the TMJ is defined as an abnormal relationship of the articular disc to the mandibular condyle, fossa and articular eminence. Usually the disc is displaced in an anteromedial direction (Dolwick & Riggs 1983). In addition to pain, limited mouth-opening, or deviation of mouth-opening, patients complain of clicking in the TMJ. Clicking refers to a distinct cracking, snapping sound associated with opening and closing of the mouth. Farrar (1971) introduced the term 'reciprocal clicking' to describe patients with opening and closing clicks. Reciprocal click is considered pathognomonic to internal derangement. Patients may report an increase in the intensity of the pain prior to the click with relief after the click occurs. Pain is usually limited to the TMJ area. The TMJ will generally be tender to palpation and the muscles of mastication may sometimes be tender. Crepitus and multiple scraping sounds are best detected with the aid of a stethoscope placed over the TMJ while the patient opens and closes the mouth. Crepitus frequently indicates a distruption of the disc or its posterior attachment and heralds more advanced disease. The final, definitive diagnosis of ID is made by arthrography of the TMJ using radiopaque contrast material injected into the joint space, usually the lower one (Katzberg et al 1979). On the basis of clinical signs and arthrographic findings, ID of the TMJ has been further classified (Dolwick & Riggs 1983; Eversole & Machado 1985; Roberts et al 1985). This classification includes:

1. disc displacement with reduction
2. disc displacement with intermittent locking
3. disc displacement without reduction
4. disc displacement with perforation.

Clinical signs and arthrographic findings are usually in good agreement (Roberts et al 1985).

Anatomical studies on nerve fibre distribution in the joint disclose the fact that the adult joint possesses no nerve endings within the disc. Specialised and free nerve endings are located in the retrodiscal tissues (Griffin & Harris 1975). Unlike rheumatoid arthritis, ID of the TMJ is not associated with an inflammatory cell reaction in the joint capsule. However, deposits of extravasated erythrocytes and altered composition of the connective tissue are present. The presence of these pain-initiating breakdown products and that of nerve fibres trapped in the posterior disc attachment, which become compressed during movement, may be responsible for TMJ arthralgia (Isacsson et al 1986). There are no proved aetiological factors for IDs of the TMJ. Proposed aetiological factors include jaw trauma, muscle hyperactivity and hyperextension of the mandible.

Recent findings may challenge the relationship between TMJ pain dysfunction and the concept of disc displacement (Westesson et al 1989; Nitzan et al 1991a). Westesson et al (1989) demonstrated that 15% of healthy asymptomatic volunteers were radiographically abnormal with displacement of the disc; Nitzan & Dolwick (1991) showed that more than 50% of patients in a most advanced stage of ID (closed-locked) had normally shaped discs. Although in both studies there may be a sample selection bias, they still indicate that factors other than disc position may be considered, at least in some patients, for the genesis of pain and dysfunction associated with the TMJ. These may include decreased volume of synovial fluid with high viscosity or a 'vacuum effect' (Nitzan et al 1991, 1992).

Treatment

Conservative treatment modalities recommended for MPD are utilised for ID of the TMJ. Unfortunately, as has long been known, the elimination of joint sounds is the single most resistant feature in most studies dealing with these patients (Eversole & Machado 1985). Interocclusal anterior repositioning splints are of value in eliminating clicks, but are of short-term benefit with no known long-term effect (Lundh et al 1985). In more advanced cases which do not respond to nonsurgical treatment, surgery is recommended (Dolwick & Riggs 1983). However, long-term evaluation of nonsurgical treatment of advanced cases demonstrated favourable results (Yoshimura et al 1982). In selected cases, arthrographic surgery or rinsing and lavage seems to be the treatment of choice (Nitzan et al 1991). On the basis of current data one is unable to conclusively recommend any specific treatment modality.

ATYPICAL ORAL AND FACIAL PAIN

This ill-defined category includes a variety of pain descriptions such as phantom tooth pain (Marbach 1989), atypical odontalgia (Rees & Harris 1979; Brooke 1980), atypical facial neuralgia (Marbach et al 1982), sore mouth (Brooke & Seganski 1977) and the syndrome of oral complaint (Lowental & Pisanti 1978). Chronic pain, usually at a constant intensity, is a common feature of all the above. The pain has a burning quality which occasionally intensifies to produce a throbbing sensation. The pain is not triggered by remote stimuli, but may be intensified by stimulation of the painful area itself. Autonomic phenomena are usually not seen. Grushka et al (1987a) demonstrated that pain in the burning mouth syndrome was comparable in intensity to toothache and was more severe than has previously been suggested. The pain does not usually wake the patient from sleep. The location is ill-defined. Although the pain usually starts in one quadrant of the mouth, it often spreads across the midline to the opposite side. Frequently, the pain changes location, which may result in extensive dental work, alcohol nerve blocks and surgery; this does not usually alleviate the pain. Unfortunately, it has been the author's experience and that of others (Marbach et al 1982) to see patients who have had more than 70 (!) operations performed in their mouth (e.g. pulp extirpation, apicoectomy, tooth extraction) for the relief of this type of pain.

Typically in most of these patients there is a lack of objective signs and all other tests are negative. The age range of these patients is wide (20–82 years), but the mean age of patients with atypical odontalgia is around 45 years (Marbach 1978; Rees & Harris 1979; Brooke 1980), and of patients with sore mouth and other oral complaints (e.g. burning sensation) around 55 years (Brooke & Seganski 1977; Lowental & Pisanti 1978; Grushka et al 1987a). All reports indicate an overwhelming majority of females (82–100%) in the series of atypical oral and facial pain studied.

There is no identified uniform aetiology of atypical oral and facial pain (Loeser 1985). Several underlying mechanisms have been proposed. A number of reports have suggested that atypical facial pain is a psychiatric disorder (Engel 1951; Lascelles 1966; Feinmann et al 1984; Remick & Blasberg 1985). Depression is considered the most likely diagnosis and is explained on the basis of the catecholamine hypothesis of affective disorders (Rees & Harris 1979). However, Sharav et al (1987) showed that only two of their 28 patients were cortisol nonsuppressors on the dexamethasone suppression test and that half the patients were not depressed at all. Grushka et al (1987a) conclude that the personality characteristics of patients with burning mouth syndrome are similar to those seen in other chronic pain patients, and that these personality disturbances tend to increase with increased pain. Marbach (1978) postulates that phantom tooth pain associated with previous trauma such as tooth extraction and tooth pulp extirpation interferes with central nervous system pain modulatory mechanisms. This idea is supported by the observation that experimental tooth extraction produces lesions in the trigeminal nucleus caudalis (Westrum et al 1976; Gobel & Binck 1977). Recently it was found that more extensive tooth-pulp injury is associated with greater excitatory changes of central trigeminal neurons (Hu et al 1990). Although far from proven, a deafferentation associated with peripheral nerve injury may be responsible for some types of atypical facial pain.

Vascular changes are other possible underlying mechanisms for atypical facial pain (Reik 1985). Rees & Harris (1979) and Brooke (1980) found a history of migraine in about a third of their patients.

Atypical facial pain should be differentiated from pains associated with a causative lesion. Chronic atypical facial pain can be a presenting symptom of a slow-growing cerebellopontine angle tumour (Nguyen et al 1986).

While various treatment modalities are used for atypical oral and facial pain, the predominant trends are clear. All authors firmly recommend against any surgical or dental interventions for the relief of pain (Loeser 1985). Since such interventions usually exacerbate the condition, reassurance, psychological counselling and the use of antidepressants, particularly from the tricyclic group, have been found to be a very promising mode of therapy. Recently two double-blind controlled studies demonstrated that tricyclic antidepressive drugs were superior to placebo in reducing chronic facial pain (Feinmann et al 1984; Sharav et al 1987). Furthermore, Sharav et al (1987) showed that amitriptyline was effective in a daily dose of 30 mg or less and that the relief of pain was independent of the antidepressive activity.

THE BURNING MOUTH SYNDROME

The burning mouth syndrome (BMS) is an intraoral pain disorder that is unaccompanied by clinical signs. Its vague definition and unknown aetiology warrant its inclusion under atypical oral and facial pain. Inclusion criteria of patients with BMS may differ in different studies, e.g. the presence of systemic disorders may or may not be an exclusion criterion (Grushka 1987; Van der Ploeg et al 1987). Numerous names have been given to this disorder, such as: glossodynia, glossopyrosis, oral dysaesthesia, oral galvanism or the more widely accepted name 'burning mouth syndrome' (Hampf et al 1987; Zilli et al 1989; Cekic-Arambasin et al 1990; Grushka & Sessle 1991).

The prevalence of BMS is in the range of 1.5–2.5% of the general population but may be as high as 15% in women over 40 years of age (Grushka & Sessle 1991).

Clinical features

Burning pain often occurs at more than one oral site, with the anterior two-thirds of the tongue, the anterior hard palate and the mucosal aspect of the lower lip most frequently affected (Grushka et al 1987a; Main & Basker 1983). The pain is intense and quantitatively similar to toothache pain but differs from toothache in quality. While toothache was mostly described as annoying and sharp, BMS pain was most commonly described as burning (Grushka et al 1987a). Burning pain is constant throughout the day or begins by mid-morning and reaches maximum intensity by early evening, but is not usually present at night and does not disturb sleep (Gorsky et al 1987; Grushka 1987). Many studies indicate, however, that BMS patients have difficulty falling asleep (Grushka 1987; Lamey & Lamb 1988; Zilli et al 1989). Grushka (1987) reported no significant difference between BMS and controls in any clinical oral features including number of teeth, oral mucosal conditions, presence of *Candida* and parafunctional habits.

Psychophysical assessment

There is evidence for taste dysfunction in BMS, especially in those individuals with self-reported dysgeusia (Grushka et al 1987). Sweet thresholds were significantly higher for BMS than control subjects. At suprathreshold concentrations, perception intensity was significantly higher for the BMS cases than for controls for sweet tastes, and for sour at some of the lower suprathreshold concentrations (Grushka & Sessle 1991). No differences were found between BMS and control subjects in somatosensory modalities such as two-point discrimination, temperature perception and stereognostic ability at any of eight intraoral and facial sites tested (Grushka et al 1987b). Grushka et al (1987b) did, however, find that heat pain tolerance was significantly reduced at the tongue tip of BMS subjects and suggested as an explanation the possibility that hyperalgesia in these patients may depend on prolonged temporal or spatial central summation.

Aetiology

Many possible aetiologies have been suggested and include local, intraoral factors as well as general, systemic ones.

Local factors. These include galvanic currents, denture allergy and mechanical irritation and decreased salivary secretion or change in saliva composition. No difference was found in electric currents, potential or energy capacity in the dental metallic restorations between BMS patients and controls (Hampf et al 1987). Most studies have not supported an allergic or mechanical irritation cause for BMS (Grushka & Sessle 1991). Most salivary flow rate studies have not demonstrated a significant decrease in salivary, stimulated or unstimulated output (Glick et al 1976; Syrjanen et al 1984; Lamey & Lamb 1988). On the other hand, some studies found significant alterations in salivary components such as proteins, immunoglobulins and phosphates as well as differences in saliva pH buffering capacity (Glick et al 1976; Syrjanen et al 1984; Hampf et al 1987; Grushka & Sessle 1991). Whether these alterations in salivary composition are a causal or a coincidental event in BMS is unknown (Grushka & Sessle 1991).

Systemic factors. Among these are menopause and hormonal imbalance, nutritional deficiencies and psychogenic factors.

A wide range of prevalence rates (18–80%) was given to BMS during menopause or after oophorectomy (Storer 1965; Ferguson et al 1981; Wardrop et al 1989) pointing to different definition criteria and possibly to various sampling methods. In a recent study Wardrop et al (1989) found significantly more oral discomfort in menopausal women. The oral discomfort was not associated with any of the vasomotor symptoms of menopause nor did it show any relationship to mucosal health. The presence of oral discomfort bore no relationship to follicle-stimulating hormone (FSH) or oestradiol levels measured in menopausal women, but hormone replacement therapy was accompanied with a significant reduction in oral discomfort (Wardrop 1989). However, as no control group was utilised it was difficult to asses how much of this reduction was due to a placebo effect. In spite of the conflicting data on the effect of menopause and oestrogen replacement therapy on oral discomfort, the high frequency of oral complaints in menopausal women clearly indicates a significant, although poorly understood, association between menopause and BMS (Grushka & Sessle 1991).

Iron serum deficiency was observed in 40% of patients with BMS (Brooke & Seganski 1977) but no control group was used. Lamey et al (1986) did not find any deficiency in A, C, D or E vitamins but did observe deficiency of vitamins B_1, B_2 and B_6. With appropriate replacement therapy Lamey et al (1986) produced clinical resolution of symptoms in most cases but no lasting effect in nonvitamin-deficient BMS subjects. It is difficult to draw conclusions from this study since a double-blind cross-over design was not used and a double-blind placebo-controlled study (Hugoson & Thorstensson 1991) could not demonstrate any effect of B_1, B_2 and B_6 vitamin replacement therapy in vitamin-deficient BMS patients. Recently serum zinc levels were found to be significantly lower in BMS patients than in matched controls (Maragou & Ivanyi 1991). However only nine out of 30 BMS patients demonstrated zinc levels less than the minimum normal levels. There is certainly a need for more controlled studies in order to determine the role of these nutrient elements in BMS.

Numerous studies have used psychological questionnaires and psychiatric interviews to demonstrate psychological disturbances such as depression, anxiety and irritability in patients with BMS (Grushka et al 1987a; Van der Ploeg et al 1987; Hammaren & Hugoson 1989; Zilli et al 1989). BMS patients showed elevation in certain personality characteristics which were similar to those seen in other chronic pain patients (Grushka et al 1987a). Zilli et al (1989) indicate that psychiatric illness, especially depression, may play an important role in BMS. However, most investigators cannot say whether depression and other personality characteristics are causative or the result of the pain (Grushka et al 1987a; van der Ploeg et al 1987; Zilli et al 1989; Grushka & Sessle 1991).

In conclusion, no clear aetiology is available today and it is possible that a further subclassification of this 'syndrome' is needed. A more rigorous definition of inclusion and exclusion criteria may help in future studies of aetiology and possible therapy.

Treatment

Before treatment is instigated, local and systemic underlying factors should be ruled out and treated. Thus, faulty irritating prosthetic devices should be corrected and underlying diseases, such as diabetes or anaemia, should be treated. Unfortunately, as noted above, in many instances these corrections may not improve the burning sensation and oral discomfort. Symptomatic treatment with psychotropic drugs, such as armitriptyline or clonazepam, may be of some benefit, but no good controlled studies are available to demonstrate a real effect of these drugs.

DIFFERENTIAL DIAGNOSIS OF OROFACIAL PAIN

PAIN AND DEFINED LOCAL INJURY

Diagnosis of pain in the orofacial region is complicated by the density of anatomical structures, rich innervation and the high vascularity of the area, and the important psychological meaning that is attributed to the face and the oral cavity. Most prevalent is pain in the area that results from local injury to fairly well-defined anatomical structures. Injury can result from trauma, infection and neoplasia. Pain in these cases can be defined and described in terms of anatomical structures and thus originates from the oral cavity, the jaws, salivary glands, paranasal sinuses or the TMJ.

Oral pain has been extensively reviewed above and can be divided into dental, periodontal and mucosal pain. These have been summarised in Tables 31.1 and 31.2.

Pain from the jaws can be associated with acute infection, malignancies and direct trauma. Unless infected, cysts, retained roots or impacted teeth are usually not responsible for pain in the jaws. Radiation therapy to this area may result in severe pain due to infection and osteomyelitis associated with osteoradionecrosis. Odontogenic and other benign tumours of the bone do not normally produce pain in the jaws except for the osteoid osteoma, which is known to be associated with severe pain. However, this tumour is extremely rare in the jaws (Shafer et al 1974). Malignant tumours, both primary and those metastasised to the jaws, usually produce deep, boring pain, associated with paraesthesia (Massey et al 1981).

Pain from salivary glands is localised to the affected gland, may be quite severe and is intensified by increased saliva production, such as that occurring before meals. The salivary gland is swollen and extremely sensitive to palpation. Salivary flow from the affected gland is usually reduced and sometimes abolished completely. Pain may be associated with fever and malaise. In children, the most common causes are acute recurrent parotitis and mumps. In adults, pain from salivary glands usually results from blockage of a salivary duct by calculus or mucin plug formation. Pain results from salivary retention, resulting in pressure, and sometimes ascending infection. In acute parotitis, mouth-opening exerts pressure on the gland by the posterior border of the mandible, resulting in severe pain.

Pain from the maxillary sinus is deep, boring and may become quite severe. Usually the maxillary posterior teeth on the affected side are tender to pressure and percussion. Pain is commonly felt all over the maxillary sinus. In some cases, the infraorbital nerve on the affected side is very sensitive to pressure and there is hyperaesthesia in the area supplied by this nerve. Pain is intensified by either moving the head rapidly or by lowering the head. Pain may be associated with fever and malaise.

Pain from the TMJ is usually intensified by movement of the mandible; the joint is tender when palpated via the external auditory meatus. Pain may result from acute infection, trauma, rheumatoid arthritis or primary or secondary malignant tumours. When acutely inflamed the joint may be swollen and warm to touch. A splinting protective mechanism by the masticatory muscles may result in muscle spasm, producing secondary pain.

PAIN NOT RELATED TO DEFINED INJURY

Pain in the orofacial area can result from mechanisms other than local injury described above. Thus, pain may be due to muscle spasm related to the temporomandibular pain and dysfunction syndrome previously described. Pain may also be generated by vascular, neuralgic, referred and psychogenic mechanisms.

Vascular pain in the orofacial area can be migrainous, both the acute, cluster type and the chronic type. The former may mimic dental pain (Brooke 1978). The classical syndrome has been described in detail by Horton et al (1939) and reviewed extensively by Ekbom (1970). The pain is severe, unilateral and sited mainly around the orbit and temple. Pain onset is rapid, frequently waking the patient from sleep. Pain usually lasts from 30 minutes to 2 hours and is associated with redness of the eye on the affected side, lacrimation and nostril congestion. Occasionally there is ptosis and miosis. The cluster of attacks occurs for 6–12 weeks, after which there is complete remission from months to years. A chronic variant has been described and reviewed by Pearce (1980). Methysergide is recommended for the periodic type of this syndrome and lithium carbonate for the chronic type.

Pain in the facial area may also be associated with occlusive vascular disease, such as temporal arteritis (Paine 1977). External carotid occlusive disease has been described as a cause of facial pain (Herishanu et al 1974) and carotid system arteritis is an important entity in the differential diagnosis of facial pain (Troiano & Gaston 1975).

Neuralgic pain is primarily expressed in the facial area as idiopathic trigeminal neuralgia, also known as tic douloureux. Classical features are: paroxysmal pain which lasts only seconds; pain produced by nonnoxious stimuli applied to a trigger zone; pain confined to the trigeminal nerve and unilateral in any one paroxysm; the patient is pain free between attacks, and there is no accompanying sensory loss. (Dubner et al 1987). A rare form of facial neuralgia pain associated with sweet food intake was recently described (Sharav et al 1991). Neuralgia pain of a completely different type may be associated with herpes zoster, which is a boring, burning pain of long duration and high intensity. Postherpetic neuralgia may develop in some of these cases.

Referred pain is a frequent feature in the facial area: pain may refer from teeth to remote areas in the head and face (Sharav et al 1984) and muscle pain from both neck and masticatory muscle is referred to the oral and facial areas (Travell 1960). Pain in the teeth may also be referred from the ear (Silverglade 1980). Of special interest is pain due to cardiac ischaemia that is referred to the orofacial area (Tzukert et al 1981).

Psychogenic pain in the orofacial area is associated with many emotional disorders; however, depression is apparently the most frequent disorder (Lascelles 1966; Harris 1974; Remick & Blasberg 1985). Psychogenic pain overlaps many of the features of atypical oral and facial pain that have been described previously. It is possible that apparent atypical oral and facial pain is often psychogenic in nature.

The differential diagnosis of orofacial pain should also include pain of central origin and a host of syndromes (Jurgens & Jurgens 1977).

Some of the most important disgnoses of orofacial pain have been briefly summarised in Table 31.2.

REFERENCES

Agerberg G 1988 Mandibular function and dysfunction in complete denture wearers – a literature review. Journal of Oral Rehabilitation 15: 237–249

Agerberg G, Carlsson G E 1972 Functional disorders of the masticatory system. Distribution of symptoms accordings to age and sex as judged from investigation by questionnaire. Acta Odontologica Scandinavica 30: 597–613

American Sleep Disorder Association 1990 International clssification of sleep disorders: diagnosis and coding manual. American Sleep Disorder Association, Rochester, Minnesota, p 181–185

Anderson D J, Naylor M N 1962 Chemical excitants of pain in human dentine and dental pulp. Archives of Oral Biology 7: 413

Anderson D J, Hannam A G, Matthews B 1970 Sensory mechanisms in mammalian teeth and their supporting structures. Physiological Review 50: 171

Armstrong D, Dry R M L, Keele C A, Harkham J N 1953 Observations of chemical excitants of cutaneous pain in man. Journal of Physiology 120: 326

Avery J K 1971 Structural elements of the young normal human pulp. Oral Surgery 32: 113

Baily J O, McCall W D, Ash M M Jr 1977 Electromyographic silent periods and jaw motion parameters; quantitative measures of temporomandibular joint dysfunction. Journal of Dental Research 56: 249

Basbaum A I, Levine J D 1991 The contribution of the nervous system to inflammation and inflammatory disease. Canadian Journal of Physiology and Pharmacology 69: 647–651

Bell W E 1989 Orofacial pains: classification, diagnosis, management, 4th edn. Year Book Medical Publishers, Chicago, p 239–284

Bennet R M 1986 Current issues concerning management of the fibrositis/fibromyalgia syndrome. American Journal of Medicine (suppl 3A): 1–115

Bessette R W, Bishop B, Mohl N 1971 Duration of masseteric silent period in patient with TMJ syndrome. Journal of Applied Physiology 30: 864

Blasberg B, Chalmers A 1989 Temporomandibular pain and dysfunction syndrome associated with generalized musculoskeletal pain: a retrospective study. Journal of Rheumatology (suppl 19): 87–90

Block S L 1976 Possible etiology of ear stuffiness (barohypoacusis) in MPD syndrome. Journal of Dental Research 55: B250 abstract 752

Block R M, Bushel A, Rodrigues H, Langeland K 1976 A histological, histobacteriologic and radiographic study of periapical endodontic surgical specimens. Oral Surgery 42: 656

Brannstrom M 1962 The elicitation of pain in human dentine and pulp by chemical stimuli. Archives of Oral Biology 7: 59

Brannstrom M 1963 Dentine sensitivity and aspiration of odontoblasts. Journal of the American Dental Association 66: 366

Brannstrom M 1979 The transmission and control of dentinal pain. In: Crossman L I (ed) Mechanism and control of pain. Masson, New York, p 15

Brooke R I 1978 Periodic migrainous neuralgia: a cause of dental pain. Oral Surgery 46: 511

Brooke R I 1980 Atypical odontalgia. Oral Surgery 49: 196

Brooke R I, Seganski D P 1977 Aetiology and investigation of the sore mouth. Journal of the Canadian Dental Association 10: 504

Broton J G, Sessle B J 1988 Reflex excitation of masticatory muscles induced by algesic chemicals applied to the temporomandibular joint of the cat. Archives of Oral Biology 33: 741–747

Brown A C, Beeler W J, Kloka A C, Fields E W 1985 Spatial summation of pre-pain and pain in human teeth. Pain 21: 1

Burket L W, Greenberg M S 1977 Disease primarily affecting the gingiva. In: Lynch M A (ed) Burket's oral medicine, 7th edn. J B Lippincott, Philadelphia, p 175

Butler J H, Folke L E, Brandt C L 1975 A descriptive survey of signs and symptoms associated with the myofascial pain-dysfunction syndrome. Oral Surgery 90: 635

Byers M R, Kish S J 1976 Delineation of somatic nerve endings in rat teeth by radioautography of axon-transported protein. Journal of Dental Research 55: 419

Byers M R, Neuhaus S J, Gehirg J D 1982 Dental sensory receptor structure in human teeth. Pain 13: 221

Cameron C E 1976 The cracked tooth syndrome: additional findings. Journal of the American Dental Association 93: 971

Campbell J 1958 Distribution and treatment of pain in temporomandibular arthroses. British Dental Journal 105: 393

Carlsson G E 1976 Symptoms of mandibular dysfunction in complete denture wearer. Journal of Dentistry 4: 265

Carlsson G E, Gale E N 1976 Biofeedback treatment for muscle pain associated with the temporomandibular joint. Journal of Behavioural Therapeutic Experimental Psychiatry 7: 383

Carlsson G E, Egermark-Eriksson I, Magnusson T 1980 Intra- and inter-observer variation in functional examination of the masticatory system. Swedish Dental Journal 4: 187–194

Cekic-Arambasin A, Vidas I, Stipetic-Mravak M 1990 Clinical oral test for the assessment of oral symptoms of glossodynia and glossopyrosis. Journal of Oral Rehabilitation 17: 495–502

Christensen L V 1981 Facial pains and the jaw muscles: a review. Journal of Oral Rehabilitation 8: 193

Clark G T, Beemsterboer P L, Solberg W K, Rugh J D 1979 Nocturnal electromyographic evaluation of myofascial pain dysfunction in patients undergoing occlusal splint therapy. Journal of the American Dental Association 99: 607–611

Clark G T, Rugh J D, Handelman S L 1980 Nocturnal masseter muscle activity and urinary acid catecholamine levels in bruxers. Journal of Dental Research 59: 1571–1576

Clark G T, Green E M, Dornan M R, Flack V F 1987 Craniocervical dysfunction levels in a patient sample from a temporomandibular joint clinic. Journal of the American Dental Association 115: 251–256

Clarke N G 1982 Occlusion and myofascial pain dysfunction: is there a relationship? Journal of the American Dental Association 85: 892

Clarke N G, Townsend G C, Carey S E 1984 Bruxing patterns in man during sleep. Journal of Oral Rehabilitation 11: 123–127

Costen J B 1934 Syndrome of ear and sinus symptoms dependent upon disturbed function of the temporomandibular joint. Annals of Otorhinolaryngology 43: 1

De Boever J A 1979 Functional disturbances of the temporomandibular joint. In: Zarb G A, Carlsson G E (eds) Temporomandibular joint. Munksgaard, Copenhagen, p 193

De Laat A, Van der Glas, H W, Weytjens J L F, Van Steenberghe D 1985 The masseteric post-stimulus electromyographic-complex in poeple with dysfunction of the mandibular joint. Archives of Oral Biology 30: 177

Dexter J D, Weizman E D 1970 The relationship of nocturnal headaches to sleep stage patterns. Neurology 20: 513–518

Dolwick M D, Riggs R R 1983 Diagnosis and treatment of internal derangements of the temporomandibular joint. Dental Clinics of North America 27: 561

Dolwick M F, Katzberg R W, Helms C A 1983 Internal derangements of the temporomandibular joint: fact or fiction? Journal of Prosthetic Dentistry 49: 415

Dostrovsky J O, Davis K D, Kawakita K 1991 Central mechanisms of vascular headaches. Canadian Journal of Physiology and Pharmacology 69: 652–658

Dubner R, Sessle B J, Storey A T 1978 The neural basis of oral and facial function. Plenum, New York

Dubner R, Sharav Y, Gracely R H, Price D D 1987 Idiopathic trigeminal neuralgia: sensory features and pain mechanisms. Pain 31: 23–33

Dworkin S F, Huggins K H, LeResche L et al 1990a Epidemiology of signs and symptoms in temporomandibular disorders: clinical signs in cases and controls. Journal of the American Dental Association 120: 273–281

Dworkin S F, LeResche L, DeRouen T, Von-Kroff M (1990b) Assessing clinical signs of temporomandibular disorders: reliability of clinical examiners. Journal of Prosthetic Dentistry 63: 574–579

Ekbom K 1970 A clinical comparison of cluster headache and migraine. Acta Neurologica Scandinavica 46: (suppl 41): 7

Engel G L 1951 Primary atypical facial neuralgia. An hysterical conversion symptom. Psychosomatic Medicine 13: 375

Eriksson P O, Lindmen R, Stal P, Bengtsson A 1988 Symptoms and signs of mandibular dysfunction in primary fibromyalgia syndrome (PSF) patients. Swedish Dental Journal 12: 141

Eversole L R, Machado L 1985 Temporomandibular joint internal derangements and associated neuromuscular disorders. Journal of the American Dental Association 110: 69

Farrar W 1971 Diagnosis and treatment of anterior dislocation of the articular disc. New York Journal of Dentistry 41: 348

Feinmann C, Harris M, Cawley R 1984 Psychogenic facial pain: presentation and treatment. British Medical Journal 288: 436

Ferguson M M, Carter J, Boyle P et al 1981 Oral complaints related to climacteric symptoms in oophorectomized women. Journal of the Royal Society of Medicine 74: 492

Fine E W 1971 Psychological factors associated with non-organic temporomandibular joint pain dysfunction syndrome. British Dental Journal 131: 402

Friend L A, Glenwright H D 1968 An experimental investigation into the localisation of pain from the dental pulp. Oral Surgery 25: 765

Gelb H, Tarte J 1975 A two-year dental clinical evaluation of 200 cases of chronic headache: craniocervical-mandibular syndrome. Journal of the American Dental Association 91: 1230

Gerschman J A, Reade P C, Hall W, Wright J, Holwill B 1990 Lateralization of facial pain, emotionality and affective disturbance. Pain (suppl, 5): S42

Glaros A G, McGlynn F D, Kapel L 1989 Sensitivity, specificity and the predictive value of facial electromyographic data in diagnosing myofascial pain-dysfunction. Cranio 7: 189–193

Glick D, Ben Aryeh H, Gutman D et al 1976 Relation between idiopathic glossodynia and salivary flow rate and content. International Journal of Oral Surgery 5: 161

Gobel S, Binck J M 1977 Degenerative changes in primary trigeminal axons and in neurons in nucleus caudalis following tooth pulp extirpations in the cat. Brain Research 132: 347

Goose D H 1981 Cracked tooth syndrome. British Dental Journal 2: 224

Gorsky M, Silverman S Jr, Chinn H 1987 Burning mouth syndrome: A review of 98 cases. Journal of Oral Medicine 42: 7

Greenberg M S 1977 Ulcerative, vesicular and bullous lesions. In: Lynch M A (ed) Burket's oral medicine, diagnosis and treatment, 7th edn. J B Lippincott, Philadelphia, p 33

Greene C S, Marbach J J 1982 Epidemiologic studies of mandibular dysfunction: a critical review. Journal of Prosthetic Dentistry 48: 184–190

Greenwood F, Horiuchi H, Matthews B 1972 Electrophysiological evidence on the types of nerve fibres excited by electrical stimulation of teeth with a pulp tester. Archives of Oral Biology 17: 701

Griffin C J, Harris E 1975 Innervation of the temporomandibular joint. Australian Dental Journal 20: 78

Grushka M 1987 Clinical features of burning mouth syndrome. Oral Surgery 63: 30

Grushka M, Sessle B J 1991 Burning mouth syndrome. Dental Clinics of North America 35: 171

Grushka M, Sessle B J, Howely T P 1987 Taste dysfunction in burning mouth syndrome (BMS). Annals of the New York Academy of Sciences 510: 321

Grushka M, Sessle B J, Miller R 1987a Pain and personality profiles in burning mouth syndrome. Pain 28: 155

Grushka M, Sessle B J, Howley T P 1987b Psychophysical assessment of tactile pain and thermal sensory functions in burning mouth syndrome. Pain 28: 169

Hammaren M, Hugoson A 1989 Clinical psychiatric assessment of patients with burning mouth syndrome resisting oral treatment. Swedish Dental Journal 13: 77–88

Hampf G, Ekholm A, Salo T et al 1987 Pain in oral galvanism. Pain 29: 301

Harris R 1975 Innervation of the human periodontinum. In: Griffin C J, Harris R (eds) The temporomandibular joint syndrome. Monographs in oral science. Karger, Basel p 27

Harris S M 1974 Psychogenic aspects of facial pain. British Dental Journal 136: 199

Helkimo M 1979 Epidemiological surveys of dysfunction of the masticatory system. In: Zarb G A, Carlsson G E (eds) Temporomandibular joint. Munksgaard, Copenhagen, p 175

Henriksson K G, Bengtsson A 1991 Fibromyalgia – a clinical entity? Canadian Journal of Physiology and Pharmacology 69: 672–677

Herishanu Y, Bendheim P, Dolberg M 1974 External carotid occlusive disease as a cause of facial pain. Journal of Neurology, Neurosurgery and Psychiatry 8: 963

Horiuchi H, Matthews B 1973 In-vitro observations on fluid flow through human dentine caused by pain-producing stimuli. Archives of Oral Biology 18: 275

Horton B T, MacLean A R, Graig W M 1939 A new syndrome of vascular headache: results of treatment with histamine: preliminary report. Mayo Clinic Proceedings 14: 257

Hu J W, Sharav Y, Sessle B J 1990 Effect of one- or two-stage deafferentation of mandibular and maxillary tooth pulps on the functional properties of trigeminal brainstem neurons. Brain Research 516: 271–279

Hugoson A, Thorstensson B 1991 Vitamin B status and response to replacement therapy in patients with burning mouth syndrome. Acta Odontologica Scandinavica 49: 367–375

Isacsson G, Isberg A, Johansson A-S, Larson D 1986 Internal derangement of the temporomandibular joint: radiographic and histologic changes associated with severe pain. Journal of Maxillofacial Surgery 44: 771

Jurgens E H, Jurgens P E 1977 Syndromes involving facial pain. In: Alling C C III, Mahan P E (eds) Facial pain, 2nd edn. Lea & Febiger, Philadelphia, p 227

Katzberg R W, Dolwick M F, Bles D J, Helms C A 1979 Arthrography of the temporomandibular joint: new technique and preliminary observations. American Journal of Roentgenology 132: 949

Keele C A, Armstrong D 1968 Mediators of pain. In: Lim R D S, Armstrong D, Pardo E G (eds) Pharmacology of pain. Pergamon, Oxford, p 3–24

Kolbinson D A, Schubert M M, Flournoy N, Truelove E L 1988 Early oral changes following bone marrow transplantation. Oral Surgery, Oral Medicine and Oral Pathology 66: 130–138

Kopp S, Wenneberg B 1983 Intra- and interobserver variability in the assessment of signs of disorder in the stomatognathic system. Swedish Dental Journal 7: 239–246

Krauss H 1970 Clinical treatment of back and neck pain. McGraw Hill, New York

Krogh-Poulsen W E, Olsson A 1966 Occlusal disharmonies and dysfunction of the stomatognathic system. Dental Clinics of North America, November: 627–635

Lamey P J, Hammond A, Allam B F, McIntosh W B 1986 Vitamin status of patients with burning mouth syndrome and the response to replacement therapy. British Dental Journal 160: 81

Lamey P J, Lamb A B 1988 Prospective study of aetiological factors in burning mouth syndrome British Medical Journal 296: 1243

Langeland K, Block R M, Grossman L I 1977 A histopathologic and histobacteriologic study of 35 periapical endodontic surgical specimens. Journal of Endodontics 3: 8

Lascelles R G 1966 Atypical facial pain and psychiatry. British Journal of Psychiatry 112: 654

Laskin D M 1969 Etiology of the pain dysfunction syndrome. Journal of the American Dental Association 79: 147

Lavigne G J, Velly-Miguel A M, Montplaisir J 1991 Muscle pain, dyskinesia, and sleep. Canadian Journal of Physiology and Pharmacology 69: 678–682

Locker D, Slade G 1988 Prevalence of symptoms associated with temporomandibular disorders in a Canadian population. Community Dental and Oral Epidemiology 16: 310–313

Loeser J D 1985 Tic douloureux and atypical facial pain. Journal of the Canadian Dental Association 12: 917

Lowental U, Pisanti S 1978 The syndrome of oral complaints: etiology and therapy, Oral Surgery 46: 2

Lund J P, Donga R, Widmer C G, Stohler C S 1991 The pain adaptation model: a discussion of the relationship between chronic musculoskeletal pain and motor activity. Canadian Journal of Physiology and Pharmacology 69: 683–694

Lundh H, Westesson P-L, Kopp S, Tillström B 1985 Anterior repositioning splint in the treatment of temporomandibular joints with reciprocal clicking: comparison with a flat occlusal splint and untreated control group. Oral Surgery 60: 131

McGrath P A, Gracely R H, Dubner R, Heft M 1983 Non-pain and pain sensations evoked by tooth pulp stimulation. Pain 15: 377

Madison S, Whitsel E A, Suarez-Roca H, Maixner W 1992 Sensitizing effects of leukotriene B_4 on intradental primary afferents. Pain 49: 99

Magnusson T, Carlsson G E 1978 Comparison between two groups of patients in respect of headache and mandibular dyfunction. Swedish Dental Journal 2: 85–92

Main D M G, Basker R M 1983 Patients complaining of a burning mouth. British Dental Journal 154: 206

Maragou P, Ivanyi L 1991 Serum zinc levels in patients with burning mouth syndrome. Oral Surgery Oral Medicine and Oral Pathology 71: 447–450

Marbach J J 1978 Phantom tooth pain. Journal of Endodontics 4: 362

Marbach J, Lund P 1981 Depression, anhedonia and anxiety in temporomandibular joint and other facial pain syndromes. Pain 11: 73–84

Marbach J, Lipton J, Lund P et al (1978) Facial pains and anxiety levels: considerations for tretament. Journal of Prosthetic Dentistry 40: 434–437

Marbach J J, Hulbrock J, Hohn C, Segal A G 1982 Incidence of phantom tooth pain: a typical facial neuralgia. Oral Surgery 53: 190

Massey E W, Moore J, Schold S C 1981 Dental neuropathy from systemic cancer. Neurology 31: 1227

Mense S 1991 Considerations concerning the neurobiological basis of muscle pain. Canadian Journal of Physiology and Pharmacology 69: 610–616

Merskey H, Lau C L Russel E S et al 1987 Screening for psychiatric morbidity. The pattern of psychological illness and premorbid characteristics in four chronic pain populations. Pain 30: 141–157

Molin C 1972 Vertical isometric muscle forces of the mandible. A comparative study of subjects with and without manifest mandibular pain dysfunction syndrome. Acta Odontologica Scandinavica 30: 485

Molin C 1973 Studies in mandibular pain dysfunction syndrome. Swedish Dental Journal 66 (suppl 4): 1

Moskowitz M A, Buzzi M G, Sakas D E, Linik M D 1989 Pain mechanisms underlying vascular headaches. Revue Neurologique (Paris) 145: 181–193

Moulton R 1955 Psychiatric considerations in maxillofacial pain. Journal of the American Dental Association 51: 408

Mumford J M 1982 Orofacial pain, 3rd edn, Churchill Livingstone, Edinburgh

Mumford J M, Newton A V 1969 Transduction of hydrostatic pressure to electric potential in human dentine. Journal of Dental Research 48: 226

Munro R 1975 Electromyography of the masseter and anterior temporalis muscles in the open-close-clench cycle in temporomandibular joint dysfunction. In: Griffin C J, Harris R (eds) The temporomandibular joint syndrome. Monographs in oral sciences. Karger, Basel, p 117

Närhi M V O 1985 The characteristic of intradental sensory units and their responses to stimulation. Journal of Dental Research 64: 564

Nguyen M, Maciewicz R, Bouckoms A, Poletti C, Ojemann R 1986 Facial pain symptoms in patients with cerebellopontine angle tumors: a report of 44 cases of cerebellopontine angle meningioma and review of the literature. Clinical Journal of Pain 2: 3

Nielsen L L, McNeil C, Danzig W, Goldman S, Levy J, Miller A J 1990 Adaptation of craniofacial muscles in subjects with craniomandibular disorders. American Journal of Orthodontics and Dentofacial Orthopedics

Nitzan D W, Dolwick M F 1991 An alternative explanation for the genesis of closed-lock symptoms in the internal derangement process. Journal of Oral and Maxillofacial Surgery 49: 810–815

Nitzan D W, Dolwick M F, Martinez G A (1991) Temporomandibular joint arthrocentesis: A simplified treatment for severe, limited mouth opening. Journal of Oral and Maxillofacial Surgery 49: 1163–1167

Nitzan D W, Mahler Y, Simkin A 1992 Intra-articular pressure measurements in patients with suddenly developing severely limited mouth opening. Journal of Maxillofacial Surgery 50: 1038

Okeson J P, Moody P M, Kemper J T, Haley J V 1983 Evaluation of occlusal splint therapy and relaxation procedures in patients with temporomandibular disorders. Journal of the American Dental Association 107: 420

Olgart L M 1985 The role of local factors in dentine and pulp in intradental pain mechanisms. Journal of Dental Research 64: 572

Paine R 1977 Vascular facial pain. In: Alling C C III, Mahan P E (eds) Facial pain, 2nd end. Lea & Febiger, Philadelphia, p 57

Pearce M S 1980 Chronic migrainous neuralgia, a variant of cluster headache. Brain 103: 149

Perry H T 1968 The symptomatology of temporomandibular joint disturbance. Journal of Prosthetic Dentistry 19: 288

Perry H T 1973 Adolescent temporomandibular dysfunction. American Journal of Orthodontics 63: 517

Ramfjord S S, Ash M M 1966 Occlusion. W B Saunders, Philadelphia

Raskin N H, Appenzeller O (1980) Headache. W B Saunders, Philadelphia, p 132–136

Rees R T, Harris M 1979 Atypical odontalgia. British Journal of Oral Surgery 16: 212

Reik L 1985 Atypical facial pain: a reappraisal. Headache 25: 30

Remick R A, Blasberg B 1985 Psychiatric aspects of atypical facial pain. Journal of the Canadian Dental Association 12: 913

Roberts C A, Tallents R H, Espeland M A, Handelman S L, Katzberg R W 1985 Mandibular range of motion versus arthrographic diagnosis of the temporomandibular joint. Oral Surgery 60: 244

Roistacher S L, Tanenbaum D 1986 Myofascial pain associated with oropharyngeal cancer. Oral Surgery 61: 459

Rugh J D, Harlan J 1988 Nocturnal bruxism and temporomandibular disorders. Advances in Neurology 49: 329–341

Rugh J D, Solberg W K 1979 Psychological implications in temporomandibular pain and dysfunction. In: Zarb G A, Carlsson G E (eds) Temporomandibular joint. Munksgaard, Copenhagen, p 239

Rugh J D, Solberg W K 1985 Oral health status in the United States: temporomandibular disorders. Journal of Dental Education 49: 398–405

Rugh J D, Barghi N, Drago C J 1984 Experimental occlusal discrepancies and nocturnal bruxism. Journal of Prosthetic Dentistry 51: 548

Salter M, Brooke R L, Merskey H et al 1983 Is the temporomandibular pain and dysfunction syndrome a disorder of the mind? Pain, 17: 151–166

Satoh T, Harada Y 1973 Electrophysiological study on tooth grinding during sleep. Electroencephalography and Clinical Neurophysiology 35: 267–275

Schnurr R F, Brooke R I, Rollman G B 1990 Psychosocial correlates of temporomandibular joint pain and dysfunction. Pain 42: 153–165

Schwarz C 1959 Disorders of the temporomandibular joint. W B Saunders, Philadelphia

Scudds R A, Trachsel L C, Luckhurst B J, Percy J S 1989 A comparative study of pain, sleep quality and pain responsiveness in fibrositis and myofascial pain syndrome. Journal of Rheumatology Suppl 19: 120–126

Selby A 1985 Physiotherapy in the management of temporomandibular disorders. Australian Dental Journal 30: 273–280

Seltzer S 1978 Pain control in dentistry – diagnosis and management. J B Lippincott, Philadelphia

Seltzer S, Bender I B 1975 The dental pulp, 2nd edn. J B Lippincott, Philadelphia, p 203

Seltzer S, Bender I B, Ziontz M 1963 The dynamics of pulp inflammation: correlation between diagnostic data and actual histologic findings in the pulp. Oral Surgery 16: 846

Sessle B 1979 Is the tooth pulp a 'pure' source of noxious input? Advances in Pain Research and Therapy 3: 245

Sessle B J, Hu J W 1991 Mechanisms of pain arising from articular tissues. Canadian Journal of Physiology and Pharmacology 69: 617–626

Shafer W G, Hine M K, Levy B M 1974 A textbook of oral pathology, 3rd edn. W B Saunders, Philadelphia, p 152

Sharav Y 1977 The myofascial pain dysfunction syndrome, a common expression to various etiologies. Israel Journal of Dental Medicine 26: 11

Sharav Y, Feinsod M 1977 Nasopharyngeal tumor manifested as myofascial pain dysfunction syndrome. Oral Surgery 44: 54

Sharav Y, Tzukert A, Refaeli B 1978 Muscle pain index in relation to pain dysfunction and dizziness associated with myofascial pain-dysfunction syndrome. Oral Surgery 46: 742

Sharav Y, McGrath P A, Dubner R, Brown F 1982 Masseteric inhibitory periods and sensations evoked by electric tooth-pulp stimulation in patients with oral-facial pain and mandibular dysfunction. Archives of Oral Biology 27: 305

Sharav Y, Leviner E, Tzukert A, McGrath P A 1984 The spatial distribution intensity and unpleasantness of acute dental pain. Pain 20: 363

Sharav Y, Singer E, Schmidt E, Dionne R A, Dubner R 1987 The analgesic effect of amitriptyline on chronic facial pain. Pain 31: 199

Sharav Y, Benoliel R, Schnarch A, Greenberg L (1991) Idiopathic trigeminal pain associated with gustatory stimuli. Pain 44: 171–174

Silverglade D 1980 Dental pain without dental etiology: a manifestation of referred pain from otitis media. Journal of Dentistry for Children 47: 358

Singer E J, Sharav Y, Dubner R, Dionne R A 1987 The efficacy of diazepam and ibuprofen in the treatment of the chronic myofascial orofacial pain. Pain (suppl 4): 583

Solberg W K, Flint R T, Brantner J P 1972 Temporomandibular joint pain and dysfunction: a clinical study of emotional and occlusal components. Journal of Prosthetic Dentistry 28: 412

Stem P G, Mothersill K J, Brooke R I 1979 Biofeedback and a cognitive behavioral approach to treatment of myofascial pain dysfunction syndrome. Behavioural Therapy 10: 29

Sternbach R A 1978 Clinical aspects of pain. In: Sternbach R S (ed) The psychology of pain. Raven, New York, p 241

Storer R 1965 The effects of the climacteric and of aging on prosthetic diagnosis and treatment planning. British Dental Journal 119: 340–354

Syrjanen S, Piironen P, Yli-Urpo A 1984 Salivary content of patients with subjective symptoms resembling galvanic pain. Oral Surgery 58: 387

Tafelt-Hansen P, Lous I, Olesen J 1981 Prevalence and significance of muscle tenderness during common migraine attacks. Headache 21: 49–54

Tal M, Sharav Y 1985 Development of sensory and reflex responses to tooth-pulp stimulation in children. Archives of Oral Biology 30: 467

Thomsom H 1971 Mandibular dysfunction syndrome. British Dental Journal 130: 187

Travell J 1955 Referred pain from skeletal muscle, the pectoralis major syndrome of breast pain and soreness and the sternomastoid syndrome of headache and dizziness. New York State Journal of Medicine 55: 331

Travell J 1960 Temporomandibular joint pain referred from muscles of head and neck. Journal of Prosthetic Dentistry 10: 475

Travell J, Simons D 1983 Myofascial pain and dysfunction: the trigger point manual. Williams & Wilkins, Baltimore, p 165–182

Troiano M F, Gaston G W 1975 Carotid system arteritis: an overlooked and misdiagnosed syndrome. Journal of the American Dental Association 91: 589

Tyldesley W R, Mumford J M 1970 Dental pain and the histological condition of the pulp. Dental Practice and Dental Research 20: 333

Tzukert A, Hasin Y, Sharav Y 1981 Orofacial pain of cardiac origin. Oral Surgery 51: 484

Van der Ploeg, H M, Van der Wal N, Ejkman M A J et al 1987 Psychological aspects of patients with burning mouth syndrome. Oral Surgery 63: 664

Van Hassel H J, Harrington G W 1969 Localization of pulpal sensation. Oral Surgery 28: 753

Van Steenberghe D 1979 The structure and function of periodontal innervation. Journal of Periodontal Research 14: 185

Velly-Miguel A, Montplaisir J, Lavigne G 1991 Nocturnal bruxism, jaw movements and sleep parameters: a controlled pilot study. Journal of Dental Research 70 (abstract): 1970

Virtanen A S J, Huopaniemi T, Nahri M V O, Perovaara A, Wallgren K 1987 The effect of temporal parameters on subjective sensations evoked by electrical tooth stimulation. Pain 30: 361

Wanman A, Agerberg G 1986a Mandibular dysfunction in adolescents. I. Prevalence of symptoms. Acta Odontologica Scandinavica 44: 47–54

Wanman A, Agerberg G 1986b Two year longitudinal study of symptoms of mandibular dysfunction in adolescents. Acta Odontologica Scandinavica 44: 321–331

Wardrop R W, Hailes J, Burger H et al 1989 Oral discomfort at menopause. Oral Surgery 67: 535

Ware J C, Rugh J D (1988) Destructive bruxism: sleep state relationship. Sleep 11: 172–181

Watts P G, Peet K M, Juniper R P 1986 Migraine and the temporomandibular joint: the final answer? British Dental Journal 161: 170–173

Westesson P L 1982 Double contrast arthrography and internal derangement of the temporomandibular joint. Swedish Dental Journal 13 (suppl): 1–57

Westesson P L, Eriksson L, Kurita K 1989 Reliability of negative clinical temporomandibular joint examination: Prevalence of disc displacement in asymptomatic temporomandibular joints. Oral Surgery, Oral Medicine and Oral Pathology 68: 551–554

Westrum L E, Canfield R C, Black R G 1976 Transganglionic degeneration in the spinal trigeminal nucleus following removal of tooth pulps in adult cats. Brain Research 101: 137

Widmer C G 1991 Introduction III. Chronic muscle pain syndromes: an overview. Canadian Journal of Physiology and Pharmacology 69: 659–661

Wieselmann G, Permann R, Korner E 1986 Distribution of muscle activity during sleep in bruxism. European Neurology 25 (suppl 2): 111–116

Wildmalm S E 1976 The silent period in the masseter muscle of patients with TMJ dysfunction. Acta Odontologica Scandinavica 34: 43–52

Wolfe F 1988 Fibrositis, fibromyalgia, and musculoskeletal disease: the current status of the fibrositis syndrome. Archives of Physical Medicine and Rehabilitation 69: 527–531

Yemm R 1979 Neurophysiologic studies of temporomandibular joint dysfunction. In: Zarb G A, Carlsson G E (eds) Temporomandibular joint. Munksgaard, Copenhagen, p 215

Yoshimura Y, Yoshida Y, Oka M, Miyoshi M, Uemura S 1982 Long-term evaluation of non-surgical treatment of osteoarthrosis of temporomandibular joint. International Journal of Oral Surgery 11: 7

Zilli C, Brooke R I, Lau C L et al 1989 Screening for psychiatric illness in patients with oral dysaesthesia by means of the General Health Questionnaire – twenty-eight item version (GHQ-28) and the Irritability, Depression and Anxiety Scale (IDA). Oral Surgery 67: 384

Zulqarnain B J, Furuya R, Hedegard B, Magnusson T 1989 The silent period in the masseter and the anterior temporalis muscles in adult patients with mild or moderate mandibular dysfunction symptoms. Journal of Oral Rehabilitation 16: 127–137

32. Abdominal pain

Laurence M. Blendis

The symptom of pain in the abdomen is one of the most common presenting complaints in family practice. Yet, in the vast majority of patients, no physical cause is apparent, and in most of these, the symptoms are short-lived. In the minority, the pain persists or recurs and yet usually, even after investigation, no cause is found, suggesting that the pain is psychogenic in origin. With many causes of pain there are both organic and nonorganic elements, with one or other factor dominating. Thus, although we classify abdominal pain as organic or nonorganic, this only refers to the precipitating cause, whereas even nonorganic pain can often be shown to have a clear-cut physical mechanism.

THE ACUTE ABDOMEN

Sudden onset of abdominal pain is a very common surgical diagnostic problem, since the surgeon must often decide whether or not the patient requires an operation (Botsford & Wilson 1969; Silen 1979). Less than 5% of young people presenting with this symptom are admitted to hospital for observation and even fewer undergo surgery (Stevenson 1985). One helpful approach is to divide the abdomen into four quadrants and to discuss the differential diagnosis for each quadrant.

Right lower quadrant pain

Acute appendicitis

Pain is the right lower quadrant is common and the main differential diagnosis is that of acute appendicitis. The pain often starts in the periumbilical area and moves to the right lower quadrant after some hours, often associated with a slight temperature of up to 38°C with or without frequency of bowel action or micturition. The patient is usually exquisitely tender in the right lower quadrant except for patients with retrocaecal appendix, and there may be a sensation of a mass. The patient is also tender in the right side on rectal examination. Abdominal X-rays are unlikely to show any diagnostic features other than a faecolith in 25% of cases in young children. Blood tests usually reveal a polymorphonuclear leucocytosis (Longino et al 1958) and urinalysis shows increased white cells. The 10% incidence of negative surgical explorations can be more than halved in uncertain cases by a simple 24-hour observation period, during which more than 60% will be found to have an infection not requiring surgery (Wenham 1982).

However, the clinical challenge is also to make the correct diagnosis of appendicitis early enough to prevent complications such as perforation with increased morbidity (Malt 1986). To this end, additional technologies have been incorporated into the diagnostic workup, such as ultrasonography, with the abdomen compressed. With this technique, no patients were operated upon unnecessarily for a normal appendix (100% specificity) but the sensitivity was only 75% (Puylaert et al 1987).

Mesenteric lymphadenitis

This differential diagnosis is a large one, and is among the more common disorders shown in Table 32.1. In children and young adolescents, who are at the commonest age of presentation of acute appendicitis, mesenteric lymphadenitis is a likely alternative. This usually occurs in a setting of an 'epidemic' or contact history of virus infections, usually of the upper respiratory tract. Symptomatically, the patients closely resemble those with acute appendicitis. One helpful differentiating point is that in mesenteric lymphadenitis, the white blood count is usually normal with a relative lymphocytosis, although it may be surprisingly high. Despite this, many young people with this condition have a normal appendix removed.

Acute distal ileitis

Patients with distal ileitis due to *Yersinia* very often give a history of swimming in a lake or drinking possibly contaminated water. Serial serological studies for *Yersinia*

Table 32.1 Some common causes of the acute abdomen: differential diagnosis

Right lower quadrant
Acute appendicitis
Mesenteric lymphadenitis
Infective distal ileitis
Crohn's disease
In females, tuboovarian disorders, e.g:
Ectopic pregnancy
Rupture of ovarian cyst
Acute salpingitis
Renal disorders, e.g:
Right ureteric calculus
Acute pyelonphritis
Acute cholecystitis
Acute rheumatic fever,
Pyogenic sacroiliitis
Right upper quadrant
Acute cholecystitis
Biliary colic
Acute hepatic distension or inflammation
Perforated duodenal ulcer
Central abdominal pain
Gastroenteritis
Small intestinal colic
Acute pancreatitis
Left upper quadrant
Perisplenitis
Splenic infarct
Disorders of splenic flexure
Left lower quadrant
Acute diverticulitis
Pyogenic sacroiliitis

antibodies should be performed and the faeces should be examined for the organism. The diagnosis may be confirmed by small bowel enema. However, many of these patients also have a normal appendix removed. In contrast, elevated *Yersinia* antibody titres occur in over 30% of patients with acute appendicitis (Attwood et al 1987), indicating that *Yersinia* may be an important aetiological factor in that condition.

Crohn's disease (Kirsner & Shorter 1980)

In contrast, patients with Crohn's disease usually, but not always, give a past history of abdominal symptoms such as intermittent discomfort with distension and alteration in bowel habit and weight loss, with or without other systemic manifestations. On examination, the most important differential diagnostic sign is that of a mass in the right lower quadrant. Barium radiographs are diagnostic in patients with Crohn's disease, but they are inadvisable in a patient with acute appendicitis who is about to undergo surgery. Instead, noninvasive techniques such as an abdominal flat plate, ultrasonography and computed axial tomography scan may provide further diagnostic support (Weill 1982).

Ovarian tubular disorders

In young women in the third and fourth decades, ovariotubal disorders become more important. Thus, it is extremely important to obtain a complete menstrual history. A period of amenorrhoea suggests the possibility of an ectopic pregnancy, whereas a history of promiscuity would suggest the possibility of acute salpingitis. However, this is usually bilateral. These conditions usually give rise to tenderness on vaginal examination.

Renal ureteric pain

Renal pain is usually due to acute renal colic caused by a ureteric calculus. In this condition, the calculus passes from the renal pelvis into the ureter where it causes obstruction and the pain results from increasing peristaltic contractions as the calculus is forced distally toward the bladder. Colicky pain characteristically comes in waves which gradually build up in intensity, causing the patient to sweat and to feel nauseated. As the wave of pain recedes, the patient feels considerable relief, although he may feel a residual soreness until the next wave. The symptoms are similar, regardless of the source of colicky pain, but the sites are different. Thus, with renal colic, the pain starts in either flank and radiates around and down into the groin. The patient will often be tender in the loin or flank of the painful side.

Pyogenic sacroiliitis

Pyogenic sacroiliitis commonly presents in the second and third decades with a history of about 1-week of gluteal pain on walking. There is then acute onset of right or left lower quadrant pain and fever, and pain also when the patient is examined with the leg extended or flexed and externally rotated or abducted at the hip. The commonest predisposing factors are intravenous drug abuse, trauma and skin injections. The diagnosis is made by the aspiration of sacroiliac joint fluid (Cohn & Schoetz 1986).

Right upper quadrant pain

Biliary colic

Biliary colic usually starts in the right upper quadrant and radiates around to the back with or without referred pain to the right shoulder tip. Such patients are often tender in the right upper quadrant, particularly on deep inspiration. In contrast, in acute inflammation of the gallbladder or cholecystitis without the passage of a gallstone, the pain is constant and the patient is exquisitely tender in the right upper quadrant. At least two other conditions have to be considered in acute right upper quadrant pain: acute duodenal ulcer perforation and acute hepatic congestion.

Acute duodenal ulcer perforation

Acute perforation of a duodenal ulcer produces pain. Acute ulcers are often precipitated by stress. The sudden onset of severe pain in the region is followed by symptoms and signs of peritonism with 'boardlike' rigidity of the anterior abdominal wall and 'guarding'. A straight abdominal radiograph may show a telltale gas shadow outside the duodenal lumen under the right diaphragm.

Acute hepatic congestion (enlargement)

The major organ in the right upper quadrant, the liver, occasionally causes acute pain which is usually associated with acute enlargement and stretching of the hepatic capsule, due either to inflammation, as in acute viral hepatitis, or to acute congestion secondary to acute heart failure or hepatic vein obstruction (the Budd–Chiari syndrome). All conditions result in a variable degree of jaundice and an acute release into the blood stream of hepatic enzymes, especially the transaminases with levels rising from less than 50 to greater than 1000 iu/l. Clinical examination should reveal the presence of heart failure.

If acute Budd–Chiari syndrome is suspected, a liver–spleen radionuclide scan may show the characteristic pattern of hepatic 'wipe-out' with sparing of the caudate lobe due to its drainage directly into the inferior vena cava. The diagnosis must be confirmed by hepatic venography to demonstrate the blockage (Reynolds & Peters 1982).

Central abdomen

Colic of the small intestine

The third type of colic is intestinal and is most commonly due to acute inflammation of the bowel, such as acute gastroenteritis, in which the patient suffers from acute nausea, with or without vomiting, and crampy or colicky abdominal pain, repeatedly relieved by defaecation of loose or watery stools. The infection is either viral, usually by contact during an epidemic, or bacterial from contaminated food. In contrast, intestinal colic may be secondary to intestinal obstruction, the cause of which will depend on the site, and on the age of the patient. Table 32.2 shows some of the conditions that can cause gastrointestinal colic. In contrast to infection, this is associated with partial or complete constipation and abdominal distension. Vomiting occurs in relation to the site of the obstruction; the more proximal the lesion, the more likely the associated vomiting.

Noninvasive techniques are most useful in the diagnosis of colicky conditions. A flat plate of the abdomen may reveal a calcified stone in the ureter, gallbladder or bile duct, whereas a noncalcified stone may be seen on ultrasonography (Weill 1982). With intestinal obstruction, a supine and erect film will show distension of the bowel-proximal to the obstruction whilst the erect film will show multiple air-fluid levels.

Table 32.2 Some common causes of intestinal obstruction

Age group	Stomach	Small intestine	Large intestine
Neonates	Pyloric stenosis	Congenital lesions Cystic fibrosis	Imperforate anus
Infants			Intussuception
Young adults	Duodenal ulcer	Crohn's disease Coeliac syndrome Pseudoobstruction	Crohn's disease
Middle-aged adults and elderly		Crohn's disease	Carcinoma of colon Diverticular disease Faecal impaction

Acute pancreatitis

One of the few pains to begin in the centre of the abdomen is pancreatic. Acute pancreatitis is one of the severest of all pains and has a number of causes (Table 32.3). This central pain is constant in nature and commonly bores through to the back so that relief may be attained by the patient sitting forward hugging his knees. If the diagnosis is considered from a suggestive history, it cannot be made by examination but by estimation of the pancreatic enzymes, serum amylase or lipase which are greatly elevated, the amylase rising from less than 200 to over 1000 iu.

Abdominal angina

Central abdominal pain associated with large as opposed to small meals, may be due to intestinal ischaemia. The diagnosis can only be made by angiographic demonstration of narrowed coeliac or superior mesenteric vessels and confirmed by the demonstration of a pressure difference across the stricture.

Left upper quadrant

Splenic pain

The left side of the abdomen is an uncommon site of acute

Table 32.3 Some common causes of acute pancreatitis

Alcohol
Gallstones
Drugs, e.g. thiazides, frusemide, the Pill
Metabolic: parathyroidism, hyperlipidaemia
Local inflammation: gastric or duodenal ulcer
Postoperative

abdominal pain. The left upper quadrant is occupied by the spleen, which rarely causes pain except following a splenic infarct or when involved in a serositis, as in familial Mediterranean fever. Much more commonly, the spleen causes discomfort or a dragging sensation when it becomes enlarged due to any cause.

Splenic flexure of colon

The splenic flexure of the colon may cause pain if distended acutely, for example in patients with toxic megacolon secondary to ulcerative colitis, although this usually occurs in the transverse or descending colon. It is a common site of involvement in elderly patients with ischaemic colitis and secondary stricture formation may occur in the area.

Miscellaneous

Pain originating from the stomach due to distension or ulceration, or from the tail of an inflamed pancreas, may radiate to this area.

Left lower quadrant

Acute diverticulitis

The left lower quadrant is the classical site of pain in elderly patients with acute diverticulitis. Characteristically, they suffer from fever, pain and either bloody stools or constipation. On examination, they will have a painful, sometimes 'hot' mass in this area and a polymorphonuclear leucocytosis on the blood film.

Nonspecific ulcerative colitis

The commonest site of pain in patients with ulcerative colitis is the left lower quadrant, since the commonest site of involvement is the distal colon. The patient is often tender over the descending colon. The diagnosis is made by observing the classical characteristics of the colonic and rectal muscosa on sigmoidoscopy. However, this condition, by spreading proximally, can involve any amount of the colon and thus cause pain and tenderness over the surface markings of the colon, especially in patients with toxic megacolon (Kirsner & Shorter 1980).

Peritonitis

This can present either as acute or chronic abdominal pain. Acute peritonitis usually occurs secondarily to perforation of a viscus or from direct involvement with an inflamed organ, such as the pancreas (Table 32.4). The pain is usually generalised, although it may start in the area of the perforated organ. The patient learns to lie very still, since any movement of the abdomen increases the pain. Thus, on examination, the abdomen is still and the anterior abdominal wall is not involved in respiration. It feels 'boardlike' on palpation as the anterior abdominal wall muscles 'guard' the inflamed mucosa underneath. The secondary effect of peritonitis is a loss of bowel sounds as the bowel becomes paralysed by contact with the inflammation and an ileus develops. Abdominal radiographs show large dilated loops of both large and small bowel.

Table 32.4 Some common causes of peritonitis

Acute
Infectious
Appendicitis
Diverticulitis
Toxic megacolon in inflammatory bowel disease
Perforated duodenal ulcer
Postoperative
Spontaneous peritonitis in cirrhosis
Noninfectious
Familial Mediterranean fever
Biliary: perforated gallbladder
Pancreatic: acute haemorrhagic pancreatitis
Chronic
Tuberculosis

From the clinical viewpoint, the physician has to make the following decisions. Is the cause surgical (e.g. perforation) or medical, infectious or just inflammatory? Then, clearly, the cause will determine the management.

Acute abdominal pain in general medical conditions

All physicians must be aware of the possibility of a generalised medical condition presenting as acute abdominal pain.

Collagen vascular disorders (mesenteric arteritis)

Abdominal pain is a feature of juvenile rheumatoid arthritis or Still's disease. However, it does not lead to complications or major problems in management. In contrast, acute abdominal pain may be the presenting feature in patients with polyarteritis nodosa. The pain may be due to intestinal perforation or infarction resulting in significantly higher mortality rates (Jacobsen et al 1985) The pain may also be associated with a purpuric rash, arthralgia and nephritis, or Henoch–Schonlein purpura (Martinez-Frontanilla et al 1984).

Diabetes mellitus

These patients, usually young, can present with acute abdominal pain. Commonly, the diabetes is poorly controlled, with ketoacidosis. The pain may be associated with hyperamylasaemia, but in the majority of cases they do not have acute pancreatitis. Alternatively, it may be associated with an autonomic neuropathy.

Tabes dorsalis

One of the symptoms of this condition is acute abdominal pain known as a tabetic crisis. This should rarely be confused with an acute surgical abdomen.

Sickle cell anaemia

The onset of acute abdominal pain in a black person should always make the clinician think of sickle cell anaemia. Undergoing a sickle cell crisis (sickling of red cells in small blood vessels) is thought to be the cause of this, precipated by dehydration, hypoxia, infection, etc. (Diggs 1965). The diagnosis is made by observing sickling.

Acute intermittent porphyria

Colicky acute abdominal pain is a cardinal presenting symptom of this inherited disorder of haem synthesis. The pain may be extremely severe, colicky and either localised to the epigastrium or right lower quadrant or generalised and associated with mild tenderness, vomiting and constipation. It may be associated with an autonomic neuropathy and a cutaneous photodermatitis and precipitated by drugs metabolised by microsomal cytochrome P_{450} enzymes such as phenobarbitone, anticonvulsants and alcohol. The diagnosis is made by detecting urinary porphyrins.

Opiate withdrawal

Opiate withdrawal can give rise to severe abdominal pains.

Lead poisoning

Lead poisoning most commonly occurs in children as the result of sucking lead-painted toys or other objects. The diagnosis, if considered, can be confirmed by detecting a black 'lead line' on the gingival margins, basophilic stippling of erythrocytes and elevated blood lead levels.

Acute rheumatic fever

Epigastric or right lower quadrant pain with anorexia, nausea and vomiting may be an early presentation. However, 50% have a history of sore throat and associated symptoms include fever, migratory arthritis, erythema marginatum, heart murmur and an inappropriate tachycardia for the height of the fever.

Jogger's pain

With the recent popularity of physical exercise, it has become apparent that intense physical exertion even in extremely fit individuals can result in acute severe abdominal pain and vomiting, possibly due to acute splanchnic ischaemia. The relationship of the pain to exercise should suggest the diagnosis.

Abdominal migraine

This is characterised by episodic attacks of abdominal pain and vomiting, often in the absence of headaches (Lundberg 1975). It is commoner in male children and the symptoms often respond to antimigraine therapy, usually giving way to the more typical headaches as the individual grows older (Kunkel 1986).

Chemotherapeutic enterocolitis (neutropenic enteropathy)

This condition occurs in cancer patients on chemotherapy. It presents with acute abdominal pain and neutropenia, fever greater than 37.8°C, with or without diarrhoea or melaena and diffuse or localised tenderness. The symptoms usually resolve with antibiotic therapy (Starnes et al 1986).

Diagnosis of difficult cases of acute abdominal pain

When the diagnosis of acute abdominal pain is in doubt and the question of laparotomy is being considered, there are a number of diagnostic prelaparotomy tests that can be used to help with the decision. These include simple paracentesis (Baker et al 1967), peritoneal lavage (Evans et al 1975) and peritoneoscopy (Sugarbaker et al 1975). More recently, a new method of fine catheter aspiration cytology was described by Stewart et al (1986). Cytological specimens were prepared by the cytosieve technique and the number of neutrophils per 500 cells counted. Of 27 patients, 25 had a successful test. Prelaparotomy diagnosis was correct in 14 patients before the test compared to 20 after the test.

CHRONIC ABDOMINAL PAIN

Chronic abdominal wall pain

Before discussing the causes of chronic visceral pain it is important to exclude the above condition. This is done first and foremost by considering this diagnosis and then looking for the characteristics indicated in Table 32.1. The most likely explanation for this pain is entrapment and stretching of the anterior cutaneous branch of the thoracoabdominal nerve, and the treatment is by local anaesthetic injection.

Organic causes of chronic abdominal pain

Gastric ulcer

Patients with gastric ulcer complain of upper abdominal pain over a fairly large area, often that covered by a hand placed on the upper abdomen. The pain is frequently related to meals and occurs soon after the patient starts eating. The pain may radiate in any direction and is usually relieved to some extent by antacid medication. The pain is usually periodic in nature, at least at the onset, with painfree periods of several weeks. Other gastric symptoms such as nausea and vomiting are uncommon. Gastric ulcer patients may lose a little weight in association with decreased food intake.

Gastric cancer

The major differential diagnosis of a gastric ulcer is whether it is benign or malignant. Malignant ulcers are usually associated with atypical pain, i.e. not periodic but rather constant in nature and not related to meals. They are often associated with anorexia and considerable weight loss. Associated symptoms will be caused by variation in the site of the cancer. Fundic cancer causes dysphagia and regurgitation whereas prepyloric lesions will cause gastric outlet obstruction with vomiting. The malignant ulcers differ in their appearance of heaped-up edges and nodular involvement of the gastric wall and should be diagnosed by biopsy or brush cytology.

Duodenal ulcer

In contrast to gastric ulcer, patients with duodenal ulcer are often able to localise the pain with one finger to the epigastrium, the most common sites being to the right of the midline or very high up in the epigastrium in the midline. The pain is also characteristically associated with the fasting state, often waking the patient in the early hours of the morning, and is then relieved by eating or drinking or antacid medication. The pain commonly does not radiate or else radiates through to the back. Duodenal ulcer pain is also periodic in nature at first, the most common times of exacerbation being in the spring and the autumn.

Nausea, abdominal distension or bloating and vomiting are uncommon symptoms; the last two especially are usually associated with gastric outlet obstruction due to pylorospasm, oedema or even fibrosis. These patients do not usually lose weight and may actually gain weight due to eating frequently to relieve the pain.

The mechanism of pain in peptic ulcer disease remains controversial; suggestions include smooth muscle spasm and low intraluminal pH. Recently, intravenous boluses of adenosine produced typical epigastric pain in duodenal ulcer patients (Watt et al 1987), possibly through both mechanisms.

Diagnosis. The diagnosis of peptic ulcer disease can now be made with confidence by upper gastrointestinal endoscopy, which is the investigation of choice.

Treatment. Once the diagnosis has been made, the patient can be treated symptomatically with antacids in sufficient doses, i.e. 15–30 ml every 2 hours. However, many randomised controlled trials have shown the benefit of the H_2 receptor antagonists in accelerating the healing of a significantly higher number of duodenal ulcers than with antacids or controls. The evidence for patients with gastric ulcer is less convincing. There is an alternative therapy of sucralphate, an aluminium salt of a sulphated disaccharide. This coats the ulcer crater, thus providing a protective coating. There is probably little difference in the efficacy of these two preparations for duodenal ulcer or prepyloric gastric ulcers (Martin et al 1982). However, for ulcers in the body of the stomach, sucralphate may turn out to be the drug of choice (Mayberry et al 1978). In patients with ulcers resistant to therapy and in Zollinger–Ellison syndrome, the new proton pump inhibitor, omeprazole, is the treatment of choice.

Carcinoma of the pancreas

Carcinoma of the pancreas often presents painlessly, with a variety of symptoms related to its position. The associated pain is usually central abdominal, deep and radiating through to the back. Unrelated to meals, it is characteristically severe and requires powerful analgesics. Once the diagnosis is suspected, abdominal computed tomography scan is the test of choice, showing pancreatic enlargement. This can be confirmed by endoscopic retrograde cholangiopancreatography (ERCP) examination. Unfortunately, only a small percentage of such cancers are operable.

Mesenteric panniculitis (sclerosing mesocolitis, Weber–Christian disease)

This is characterised by recurrent episodes of moderate to severe, generalised or focal, abdominal pain, associated with intermittent nausea, vomiting, malaise, low grade fever and occasionally weight loss. On examination, a tender, central abdominal mass is commonly found, with or without chylous ascites. Barium small bowel radiographs show irregularity, nodularity, thickening and strictures. The principal differential diagnosis is malignant disease, particularly abdominal lymphoma, the diagnosis being made by laparotomy and biopsy (Steely & Gooden 1986). The final diagnosis may be of retractile mesenteritis with or without retroperitoneal fibrosis (Tedeschi & Botta 1962).

Nonorganic or psychogenic pain

The criteria for psychogenic abdominal pain were reviewed by Glaser & Engel (1977).

1. The location, distribution, timing, quality and intensity of the pain do not relate to established pathophysiological patterns.
2. There is often a marked discrepancy between the severity of the pain and the patient's behaviour.
3. The patient usually has or has had multiple pains in many other parts of the body which may have been fully investigated without any obvious abnormality being discovered. In other words, the patient is 'pain-prone'.
4. The onset of pain may bear an obvious temporal relationship to stress. This is particularly the case with bereavement, where the onset may coincide with the death of a close relative or friend in whom abdominal pain may have been a major symptom.

The abdomen is the third commonest site of pain in psychiatric patients (Spear 1967), whereas in patients suffering from chronic pain the abdomen is the second commonest site (Merskey 1965). Of a large unselected series of children 1–15% complained of abdominal pain (Apley & Naish 1958). The high incidences of parents with abdominal pain, large sibships and bereavement (Hill & Blendis 1967) have all been described in association with nonorganic abdominal pain and the relationship of pain to the emotions has been previously reviewed (Blendis et al 1978).

Gaseous distension

The major stimulus of normal gut is stretch and tension receptors have been demonstrated electrically in series with muscle cells.

Gas is a normal constituent of the gastrointestinal tract, being found in nearly half of all newborn babies and in the other half by 2–3 hours (Boreadis & Gershon-Cohen 1956). However, no obvious function has as yet been ascribed to it. The main sources of gas are swallowed air (oxygen and nitrogen) and endogenous production. The latter is due to diffusion from the blood into the bowel lumen (carbon dioxide), acidification of bicarbonate from biliary and pancreatic secretion by gastric juice in the duodenum (carbon dioxide) and bacterial fermentation (carbon dioxide, hydrogen and methane) (Calloway 1968; Levitt & Bond 1970).

Thus, oxygen is found only in small quantities in the upper gastrointestinal tract and is due to the swallowing of small amounts of air (2–3 ml) with each mouthful of food, but especially after swallowing liquids. Carbon dioxide and nitrogen may be found both in the small and large intestine, and therefore in flatus, whilst hydrogen is normally found only in the caecum and colon. There it is formed by the bacterial fermentation of nonabsorbable carbohydrate and protein (Calloway 1966); Levitt et al 1974). Certain foods, such as broad beans, produce more gas than others, related to the oligosaccharides, stachyose and raffinose (Steggerda 1968). The bacteria include coliform and bacteroides. Surprisingly, some individuals appear to be unable to produce hydrogen and this may vary from 2–20% (Bond & Levitt 1977; Gilat et al 1978). Since hydrogen will readily diffuse across the colonic mucosa into the portal bloodstream and then, by way of the systemic circulation, to the lungs and into the expired air, luminal hydrogen production can readily be measured by gas chromatography from samples of expired air (Calloway & Murphy 1968; Levitt 1969).

In contrast, methane is produced by only about one-third of the population (Levitt & Bond 1970) who have methane bacteria in their colon; the ability to produce methane appears to be inherited from the mother (Levitt & Bond 1970). But other constitutional and ethnic factors may also play a role, since methane production was found to be commoner in white females than in males and commoner in Orientals and Indians (Pitt et al 1980). As with hydrogen production, methane production will vary from day to day and may increase with ingestion of unabsorbed carbohyrate (Pitt et al 1980).

Gaseous distension syndromes

Aerophagy

Aerophagy or excessive air-swallowing is due to both organic and nonorganic causes. Organic conditions are those that cause pain or discomfort of the pharynx and oesophagus and include acute pharyngitis and peptic oesophagitis. The patient experiences relief of discomfort momentarily by swallowing air since, presumably, this results in a 'cushion' of air separating the inflamed surfaces.

The nonorganic and far more common causes of aerophagy include anxiety and depression. Again, in these cases, the patient presumably gains some comfort from it or swallows air at the same time as taking deep sighs. Also, anxious people tend to eat more quickly and take in excessive amounts of air whilst swallowing food. Gradually the air builds up in the fundus of the stomach until, at a certain critical level, it starts to produce discomfort and eventually pain throughout the gastrointestinal tract by stimulation of stretch receptors in the wall of the viscera. The patient will then gain temporary relief by belching the air out and the process is repeated.

The amount of air required to produce symptoms in the stomach is unknown, although insufflation of approximately 200 ml of air via a gastroscope reproduced symptoms in patients presenting with nonorganic upper abdominal pain (Hill & Blendis 1967). Normally, there is up to 150 ml of gas in the entire gastrointestinal tract at any one time, although ten times this amount may pass through in 24 hours (Danhot 1978).

In a study of a number of consecutive patients, it was found that pain was constant rather than periodic, as in peptic ulcer patients; that it could not be localised with one finger, nor did it radiate through to the back, and yet it never woke the patients at night, unlike duodenal ulcer pain. It was variably related to meals, commonly associated with abdominal distension, nausea (but rarely vomiting), flatulence and borborygmi as the air passed down the bowel. It was unrelieved by antacids. Most patients were tender in the upper abdomen. By definition, all investigations were negative. Most of the patients had suffered for years. There was a high incidence of bereavement and of a family history of the symptoms, or of a close friend who had died with abdominal pain. Of interest was the fact that the patients came from families with significantly larger sibships than a control hospital population. In a small group of these patients, the pain responded to antidepressant therapy (Hill & Blendis 1967).

Carbohydrate maldigestion and malabsorption

Small intestinal

It has been known for centuries that certain foods, such as beans, produce more gas than others; for example, that 5 g indigestible carbodydrate via colonic bacterial fermentation could produce 1000 ml carbon dioxide, 400 ml methane (in methane producers) and 200 ml hydrogen (Hightower 1977). However, the whole science of gastrointestinal gas production was stimulated by the American space programme where it was essential for the astronauts to produce as little flatus as possible in their confined space. The research led to detailed tables of gas-producing foods and the development of no-gas (or faecal) low residue 'elemental' diets (Murphy 1964).

Hypolactasia

However, patients with certain carbohydrate maldigestion or malabsorption syndromes will still produce excessive amounts of gas even with low-residue carbohydrates such as disaccharides. The best example of this is patients with disaccharidase deficiency, the commonest form of which is hypolactasia (Bond & Levitt 1977). Lactases are situated at the tips of the jejunal villi and, in many parts of the world, the population normally loses lactase activity in infancy.

In contrast, caucasians in Europe and the United States retain lactase activity throughout life. However, diseases of the jejunum, resulting in atrophy of the villi, will result in loss of lactase activity, for example, coeliac syndrome, tropical sprue and postgastroenteritis enteropathy. The result is that on drinking milk or eating certain dairy foods, lactose malabsorption occurs. The lactose passes down to the colon where it undergoes fermentation to several gases, including hydrogen and organic acids. The patient will then complain of crampy abdominal pain over the colon and diarrhoea and excessive flatus. The diagnosis is made by sampling expired air before and at half-hourly intervals after ingestion of 50 g lactose as a drink (Bond & Levitt 1977). In those with normal lactase activity, breath hydrogen concentrations rarely increase by more than 10 parts per million. In patients with lactase deficiency the concentrations increase by more than 20 and, in some cases, by more than 50 parts per million (Metz et al 1975). Management consists of treating any underlying pathology such as coeliac syndrome, in this case with a gluten-free diet, and then putting the patient on a lactose-free diet. Alternatively, if the patient needs or likes milk and dairy foods, these can be given together with synthetic lactases.

Hyposucrasia

Because of their position further down the villi and their greater number and quantity, other disaccharidase deficiencies are either extremely rare or never occur. For example, there are only a few case reports of sucrase deficiency. The patients present in the same way after eating foods containing sucrose, are diagnosed by the sucrose hydrogen breath test (Metz et al 1976a) and are treated by the elimination of sucrose from the diet.

Stagnant loop syndrome (Donaldson 1973)

Carbohydrate maldigestion may also occur in patients who have bacterial colonisation of the small intestine. Normally, the upper small intestine is only significantly colonised after meals and the bacteria are 'swept downstream' with the food. In patients with certain pathologies of the small intestine, luminar contents stagnate and become colonised. Examples of this are: jejunal diverticulosis; systemic sclerosis of the duodenum and jejunum; fistulae producing a blind loop, such as Crohn's disease, and incomplete obstruction, such as radiation enteropathy. These conditions are grouped under the heading of 'stagnant loop syndrome' and, if the abnormality is proximal enough, monosaccharide fermentation may even occur, leading to increased hydrogen production from glucose (Metz et al 1976b). The symptomatology is similar but the site of the crampy pain is central or periumbilical over the area of the small intestine. The diagnosis in this group requires anatomical demonstration of the lesion by barium X-rays and then appropriate therapy.

Colonic

Colonic 'maldigestion' of carbohydrate occurs normally if the diet contains large amounts of indigestible carbohydrate (Hickey et al 1972). These can be classified as cereal fibres such as wheat bran, gums from certain beans, such as guar, and pectins from citrus fruits. It has already been noted that 5 g of such carbohydrate can produce more than 1500 ml of gas. Providing the individual has a regular bowel action, as a result of adequate amounts of cereal fibre in the diet, the gas will either be absorbed or be passed as flatus.

Constipation

In constipated individuals, increasing amounts of faecal material and gas build up in the colon, causing crampy pain. This may occur in the absence of any colonic pathology or, commonly, in association with diverticular disease of the colon. This diagnosis is made by barium enema examination and treatment consists of normalising the bowel action with a combination of diet and laxatives.

Irritable bowel syndrome

Definition

As indicated at the beginning of the chapter, most people at some time or other suffer from a bout of nonorganic abdominal pain associated with stress or after a bout of gastroenteritis. However, in the majority, the symptoms gradually disappear. Therefore, in children, irritable bowel syndrome (IBS) has been classified as symptoms lasting for longer than 3 months (Apley & Naish 1958) and a similar period seems reasonable for adults. Thus, IBS may be defined as symptoms of abdominal pain and disturbance of bowel action of more than 3 months' duration without any organic cause.

Incidence (Krag 1985)

A recent study in the United States indicates that from 1.5–3% of the population suffer from IBS at any one point in time (Sandler 1990). IBS affects females more commonly than males, with ratios in published series varying from 1.5:1 (Waller & Misiewicz 1969) to 5.2:1 (Keeling & Fielding 1975). A recent study found that in up to 44% of women presenting with IBS, there is a history of sexual and physical abuse (Drossman et al 1990). The peak age of onset is in the third decade, although it also affects children and old people (Hislop 1971).

Clinical features

Abdominal pain is predominantly periumbilical in children (Stone & Barbero 1970) whereas in adults it tends to occur over the surface markings of the colon with the commonest site in the left lower quadrant (Waller & Misiewicz 1969). Occasionally, it may be in either the right or left upper quadrant over the hepatic or splenic flexures. The pain varies from a dull ache to attacks of excruciating severity requiring powerful analgesic injections. It may last from minutes to several hours. Often the pain lasts all day, but it rarely prevents the patient from sleeping through the night. 'Meteorism' is due to 'air-trapping' in which segmental accumulation of gas occurs.

Alterations of bowel habit occur in up to 90% of the patients and vary from diarrhoea to constipation or both (Chaudhary & Truelove 1962). A classical history is that on waking, the patient immediately has a loose bowel action and then three or four more watery bowel actions during the morning. After midday, the patient may not have any further bowel actions, or may have a normally formed stool later in the day. In the constipated patient, the patient passes 'rabbity' small, hard stools irregularly. In about half the patients, defaecation may relieve the pain, whereas it is often aggravated by eating. However, the patient's appetite is rarely affected and therefore a history of significant weight loss (i.e. more than 3.5 kg) is unusual and should raise suspicions of an alternative diagnosis.

As in patients with nonorganic upper abdominal pain, nausea without vomiting is a frequent associated symptom, as well as dyspepsia (Watson et al 1976), urinary symptoms (especially dysuria) (Fielding 1977), gynaecological symptoms (especially dysmenorrhea) and headache. Approximately 50% of women attending gynaecological clinics with pelvic pain had symptoms suggestive of IBS (Prior & Whorwell 1989) and 40% having elective hysterectomy, compared to 32% of age-matched controls (Longstreth et al 1990). Thus, these patients fit another of the criteria of nonorganic pain by being multisymptomatic and prone to pain. They frequently have a past history of appendicectomy for 'chronic appendicitis' and dilation and curettage for dysmenorrhoea (Waller & Misiewicz 1969). Cancer phobia is another frequent observation in these patients.

Several authors have attempted to identify symptom complexes that will reliably distinguish IBS patients. Manning et al (1978) identified four such symptoms: pain onset with loose bowel movement; pain relieved by bowel movement; increased bowel movements with pain, and bloating. More recently Talley and coworkers (1989) described the following cluster of symptoms: more than one episode of pain per week; of greater than 2 hours' duration; diffuse localisation; associated with eating, and bowel disturbance. Finally, Whitehead et al (1990) in a factor analysis of 23 symptoms found a cluster of four: relief of pain with defaecation; looser stools with pain onset; more frequent stools with pain, and symptoms with eating, thus verifying at least three of Manning's four.

Although control patients and individuals identified as having abdominal pain but not having sought medical advice, have similar symptoms, in patients with IBS abdominal pain occurred six times more frequently (Heaton et al 1991).

Psyche

Historical evidence of an affective disorder is common. Continuous fatigue is almost universal, some patients waking up tired after a full night's sleep, although insomnia may also be a problem. Alternatively, they may feel depressed and frequently close to tears (Hislop 1971). Occasionally, the patient may be suicidal. On formal testing, patients scored higher for anxiety, neuroticism and introversion than normal controls and patients with ulcerative colitis (Esler & Goulston 1973). Their neurosis score may lie midway between normal and frank neurosis (Palmer et al 1974). However, more recent studies indicate that the psychological abnormalities undoubtedly found in IBS are secondary to their patient status and not primary factors causing IBS (Drossman et al 1988, Talley et al 1990; Kumar et al 1990). Indeed, as with organic disease, they were the determinants of health care seeking (Smith et al 1990).

Examination

On examination, there is usually a disparity between the severity of the patient's symptoms and his or her physical condition. Far from looking ill, they look well, often slightly or moderately overweight. The main finding is in the abdomen where the patient will be tender over an area of the colon, most commonly the descending colon, which is also palpable, and less commonly over the transverse colon or the entire colon. Some patients are exquisitely tender on rectal examination. Sigmoidoscopic examination is usually normal but it is extremely difficult to proceed beyond the rectosigmoid junction with a rigid scope because of spasm and pain. The patients may also have mucosal hyperalgesia to light touch via the sigmoidoscope. Routine blood tests, including sedimentation rate, should be normal.

Investigations

Any evidence of anaemia, leucocytosis, etc. should be further investigated to exclude other disease such as inflammatory bowel disease. Although it is important psychologically not to overinvestigate these patients, most of them eventually have a barium enema, which is normal apart from a variable amount of spasm, usually in the descending or sigmoid colon, which should be relieved by intravenous antispasmodics. A small but significant number of patients with IBS may have lactose intolerance.

Motility studies

Intestinal motility has frequently been shown to be abnormal in IBS patients. Initially, all the studies were on the colon, hence the name 'spastic colon' but more recent studies on the upper gastrointestinal tract, including the oesophagus, have shown abnormalities and hence 'irritable gut' or 'gastrointestinal tract syndrome' would be more appropriate (Watson et al 1976).

Using a mediotelemetering capsule, attacks of pain were shown to correlate with pressure peaks in both small and large intestine (Holdstock et al 1969. Using balloons and open-ended tubes, distension of the appropriate area of intestine reproduced the pain (Swarbrick et al 1980), particularly with distension of the rectum and sigmoid colon (Kendall 1985), but not distension using the introduction and retention of ice water (Whitehead et al 1990). It was also shown that the pain threshold in IBS patients from distension of the sigmoid colon was much lower than that of normal volunteers (Ritchie 1973). Furthermore, pain did not originate from hypercontractions (Trotman & Misiewicz 1988).

Other manometric studies have shown a variety of motility abnormalities. One of the best studies separated the patients into the diarrhoeal types in which colonic motor activity was increased and disordered and the constipation type in which it was significantly reduced (Chaudhary & Truelove 1961). Another characteristic finding is that of decreased resting activity in the fasting state (Connell et al 1965) with an exaggeration of the colonic motor response to eating (Connell et al 1965). Recent motility studies have confirmed that the whole gut is affected in IBS (Moriarty & Dawson 1982; Kumar & Wingate 1985); that decreased lower oesophageal sphincter pressure and disordered oesophageal motility (Whorwell et al 1981) leads to gastroesophageal reflux with oesophagitis (Smart et al 1986), and that superficial gastritis is a frequent finding (Fielding & Doyle 1982). In addition it has been found that small bowel motility is disordered (Kingham et al 1984), with clusters of jejunal pressure activity and ileal propulsive waves (Kellow & Phillips 1987) and excessive responses to infusions of cholecystokinin (Kellow et al 1988), leading to slowing of transit (Cann et al 1983) particularly in the constipation group (Nielsen et al 1986); and with the use of technetium bran scans, that ileocaecal valve clearance is slower, especially in patients with bloating (Trotman & Price 1986).

Gastrointestinal hormones

One explanation for these later findings could be abnormalities in gastrointestinal hormones. Both gastrin and cholesystokinin (Harvey & Read 1973) increase colonic and small intestinal motor activity and some IBS patients have an exaggerated response to these hormones. It is conceivable, therefore, that IBS patients could have either abnormalities of excretion of these or other gastrointestinal hormones, or increased sensitivity to them, as previously shown for neostigmine (Chaudhary & Truelove 1961).

Treatment (Thompson 1986)

The essence of treatment of IBS is a sympathetic physician who is prepared to spend time discussing the patient's symptoms, the pathogenesis of IBS as far as it is known, and who is willing to try various therapeutic regimes without growing impatient. The basis of therapy is a high fibre diet using cereal fibre such as natural bran. This appears to normalise abnormal transit time, whether too rapid or too slow (Harvey et al 1978). As in normal subjects, abdominal symptoms occur frequently in IBS patients following the ingestion of fructose and sorbitol due to malabsorption (Rumessen and Gudmand-Hoyer 1988; Nelis et al 1990). Therefore, it may be worth attempting to exclude these carbohydrates, in the form of confectionery and soft drinks, from the diet. In addition, stool-softening agents such as diocyte sodium 100 mg twice daily can be given. Antispasmodic agents with or without sedatives have been tried with some success but lack of control trials makes interpretation difficult. In contrast, in a control trial of diphenylhydantoin versus a placebo, no significant difference was found (Greenbaum et al 1973). Other control trials with dicyclomine (Page & Dirnberger 1981), domperidone (Fielding 1982) and cimetropium bromide (Dobrilla et al 1990) have shown efficacy despite a placebo response of greater than 50%. Recently a controlled trial of psychotherapy and relaxation showed a significant improvement over standard medical therapy (Guthrie et al 1991). However, in a recent extensive review, Klein (1988) was unable to find any convincing evidence that any study showed effective therapy.

Prognosis

Irritable bowel syndrome is considered a chronic pain condition lasting for many years. However, in a recent report of the aggressive use of high fibre diets and bulking agents, nearly 70% of patients were reported to be painfree at 5 years (Harvey et al 1987).

Postsurgical pain

In a significant number of patients pain may recur following a surgical operation. This may follow the removal of a normal organ or one showing mild chronic inflammation only, as with an appendix or gallbladder. Other pains may result from a complication of surgery such as ulcer surgery. Some patients complain of obscure abdominal pain following surgery, such as hysterectomy or trauma. Balloon insufflation of the rectum or sigmoid colon may reproduce their pain (Kendall 1985).

Postcholecystectomy syndrome (Spiro 1977)

This is a fairly well defined entity of right upper quadrant pain which occurs usually after a 3–6 month latent period. The pain often resembles the patient's preoperative pain although it is frequently more severe and persistent. The patient is often tender in the right upper quadrant but all routine investigations may be normal and an ERCP examination must be performed to exclude retained stones in the bile duct or a stricture. However, if normal, a characteristic finding is reproduction of the pain on ERCP examination when contrast material is injected under pressure. This is an important observation since it enables the physician to discuss the mechanism of the pain with the patient even though medical therapy is disappointing. Recently anecdotal information suggests that ursodeoxycholic acid may be helpful symptomatically in such patients.

Postgastrectomy pain

Postgastrectomy pain, when associated with rapid satiety on eating and a feeling of distention, is usually due to 'small stomach syndrome' and is managed by small frequent meals.

A more severe pain with easily localised tenderness may indicate a stomal ulcer and requires maximum antiulcer therapy with either cimetidine or sucralfate.

Thus, there are many causes of abdominal pain which present the physician with one of his commonest and most difficult diagnostic problems. Management of abdominal pain is one of the best examples of the importance of a full, carefully taken history as well as clinical examination. The interrelationships of the physical and the psychological have been probed but a great deal more investigation is required to understand the mechanisms of abdominal pain.

REFERENCES

Apley J, Naish N 1958 Recurrent abdominal pains; a field survey of 1000 school children. Archives of Disease in Childhood 33: 165–167

Attwood S E A, Mealy K, Cafferkey M T et al 1987. *Yersinia* infection and acute abdominal pain. Lancet 1: 529–533

Baker W N W, Mackie D R, Newcombe J F 1967 Diagnostic paracentesis in the acute abdomen. British Medical Journal 3: 393–398

Blendis L M, Hill O W, Merskey H 1978 Abdominal pain and the emotions. Pain 5: 179–191

Bond J H, Levitt M D 1977 Use of breath hydrogen (Hc) in the study of carbohydrate absorption. American Journal of Digestive Diseases 22: 379–382

Boreadis A G, Gerson-Cohen J 1956 Aeration of the respiratory and gastrointestinal tracts during the first minute of neonatal life. Radiology 67: 407–409

Botsford T W, Wilson R E 1969 The acute abdomen. W B Saunders, Philadelphia

Calloway D H 1966 Respiratory hydrogen and methane as affected by consumption of gas forming foods. Gastroenterology 51: 383–389

Calloway D H 1968 Gas in the alimentary canal. In: Code C F (ed) Handbook of physiology, section 6: Alimentary canal, vol 5. Waverly Press, Baltimore, p 2839–2859

Calloway D H, Murphy E L 1968 The use of expired air to measure intestinal gas information. Annals of the New York Academy of Sciences 150: 82–95

Cann P A, Read N W, Brown C, Hobson N, Holdsworth C D 1983 Irritable bowel syndrome; relationship of disorders in the transit of a single solid meal to symptom patterns. Gut 24: 405–411

Chaudhary N A, Truelove S C 1961 Human colonic motility 1. Resting patterns of motility. Gastroenterology 40: 1–17

Chaudhary N A, Truelove S C 1962 The irritable colon syndrome. A study of the clinical features, predisposing causes and prognosis in 130 cases. Quarterly Journal of Medicine 31: 307–322

Cohn S M, Schoetz D J 1986 Pyogenic sacroillitis: another imitator of the acute abdomen. Surgery 100: 95–98

Connell A M, Jones F A, Rowlands E N 1965 Motility of the pelvic colon. Part IV. Abdominal pain associated with colonic hypermotility after meals. Gut 6: 105–112

Danhot I 1978 The clinical gas syndromes, a pathophysiologic approach. Annals of the New York Academy of Sciences 150: 127–130

Diggs L W 1965 Sickle cell crises. American Journal of Clinical Pathology 44: 1–19

Dobrilla G, Imbimbo B P, Piazzi L, Bensi G 1990 Longterm treatment of irritable bowel syndrome with cimetropium bromide. Gut 31: 351–358

Donaldson R M 1973 The blind loop syndrome. In: Sleisinger M H, Fordtran J S (eds) Gastrointestinal disease. W B Saunders, Philadelphia, p 927

Drossman D A, McKee D C, Sandler R S et al 1988 Psychosocial factors in the irritable bowel syndrome. Gastroenterology 95: 701–708

Drossman D A, Leserman J, Nachman G et al 1990 Sexual and physical abuse in women with functional or organic gastrointestinal disorders. Annals of Internal Medicine 113: 828–833

Esler M D, Goulston K J 1973 Levels of anxiety in colonic disorders. New England Journal of Medicine 288: 16–20

Evans C, Rashid A, Rosenberg I L, Pollock A V 1975 An appraisal of peritoneal lavage in the acute abdomen. British Journal of Surgery 62: 119–120

Fielding J F 1977 The irritable bowel syndrome. Clinics in Gastroenterology 6: 60–622

Fielding J F 1982 Domperidone treatment in the irritable bowel syndrome. Digestion 23: 125–127

Fielding J F, Doyle G D 1982 The prevalence and significance of gastritis in patients with lower intestinal irritable bowel (irritable colon) syndrome. Journal of Clinical Gastroenterology 4: 507–510

Gilat T, Ben-Hur H, Gelman-Malachi E, Terdiman R, Peled Y, 1978 Alterations of the colonic flora and their effect on the hydrogen breath test. Gut 19: 602–605

Glaser J P, Engel G L 1977 Psychodynamics, psychophysiology and gastrointestinal symptomatology. Clinics in Gastroenterology 6: 507–531

Greenbaum D S, Ferguson R K, Kater L A, Kuiper D H, Rosen L W 1973 A controlled therapeutic study of the irritable bowel syndrome. New England Journal of Medicine 288: 13–16

Guthrie E, Creed F, Dawson D, Tomenson B 1991 A controlled trial of psychological treatment for the irritable bowel syndrome. Gastroenterology 100: 450–457

Harvey R F, Read A E 1973 Effect of cholecystokinin on colonic motility and symptoms in patients with irritable bowel syndrome. Lancet 1: 1–3

Harvey R F, Pomare E W, Heaton K W 1973 Effects of increased dietary fiber on intestinal transit. Lancet 1: 1278–1280

Harvey R F, Mauad E C, Brown A M 1987 Prognosis in the irritable bowel syndrome: a 5 year prospective study. Lancet 1: 963–965

Heaton K W, Ghosh S, Braddon F E M 1991 How bad are the symptoms of patients with irritable bowel syndrome? Gut 32: 73–79

Hickey C A, Calloway D H, Murphy E 1972 Intestinal gas production following ingestion of fruits and fruit juices. American Journal of Digestive Diseases 17: 383–389

Hightower N C 1977 Intestinal gas and gaseousness. Clinics in Gastroenterology 6: 597–606

Hill O W, Blendis L M 1967 Physical and psychological evaluation of non-organic abdominal pain. Gut 8: 221–229

Hislop I G 1971. Psychological significance of the irritable colon syndrome. Gut 12: 452–457

Holdstock D J, Misiewicz J J, Waller S L 1969 Observation on the mechanism of abdominal pain. Gut 10: 19–31

Jacobsen S E H, Petersen P, Jenson P 1985. Acute abdomen in rheumatoid arthritis due to mesenteric arteritis. Danish Medical Bulletin 32: 191–193

Keeling P W N, Fielding J F 1975 The irritable bowel syndrome. A review of 50 consecutive cases. Journal of the Irish College of Physicians and Surgeons 4: 91–94

Kellow J E, Phillips S F 1987 Altered small bowel motility in irritable bowel syndrome is correlated with symptoms. Gastroenterology 92: 1885–1893

Kellow J E, Phillips S F, Miller L J, Zinsmeister A R 1988 Dysmotility of the small intestine in irritable bowel syndrome. Gut 29: 1236–1243

Kendall G P N 1985 Visceral pain. British Journal of Surgery 72 (suppl): 64–65

Kingham J G C, Brown R, Colson R, Clark M L 1984 Jejunal motility in patients with functional abdominal pain. Gut 25: 375–380

Kirsner J B, Shorter R G 1980 Inflammatory bowel disease, 2nd edn. Lea & Febiger, Philadelphia

Klein K B 1988 Controlled treatment trials in the irritable bowel syndrome. A critique. Gastroenterology 95: 232–241

Krag E 1985 Irritable bowel syndrome: current concepts and future trends. Scandinavian Journal of Gastroenterology 20 (suppl 109): 107–115

Kumar D, Wingate D L 1985 The irritable bowel syndrome, a paroxysmal bowel disorder. Lancet 2: 973–977

Kumar D, Pfeffer J, Wingate D L 1990 Role of psychological factors in the irritable bowel syndrome. Digestion 45: 80–87

Kunkel R S 1986 Acephalgic migraine. Headache 26: 198–201

Levitt M D 1969 Production and excretion of hydrogen gas in man. New England Journal of Medicine 281: 122–127

Levitt M D, Bond J H Jr 1970 Volume composition and source of intestinal gas. Gastroenterology 59: 921–929

Levitt M D, Berggren T, Hastings J, Bond J H 1974 Hydrogen (H_2) catabolism in the colon of the rat. Journal of Laboratory and Clinical Medicine 84: 163–167

Longino L A, Holder T M, Gross R E 1958 Appendicitis in childhood. A study of 1358 cases. Pediatrics 22: 238–246

Longstreth G F, Preskill D B, Youkeles L 1990 Irritable bowel syndrome in women having diagnostic laparoscopy or hysterectomy. Digestive Disease Sciences 35: 1285–1290

Lundberg P O 1975 Abdominal migraine – diagnosis and therapy. Headache 15: 122–128

Malt R A 1986 Editorial: The perforated appendix. New England Journal of Medicine 315: 1546–1547

Manning A P, Thompson W E, Heaton K W, Morris A F 1978 Towards positive diagnosis of the irritable bowel. British Medical Journal 3: 762–763

Martin F, Farley A, Gagnon M, Bensemana D 1982 Comparison of the healing capacities of sucralfate and cimetidine in the short term treatment of duodenal ulcer. Gastroenterology 82: 401–405

Martinez-Frontanilla L A, Haase G M, Ernster J A 1984. Surgical complications of Henoch–Schonlein purpura. Journal of Pediatric Surgery 19: 434–436

Mayberry J F, Williams R A, Rhodes J, Lawrie B W 1978. A controlled clinical trial of sucralfate in the treatment of gastric ulcers. British Journal of Clinical Practice 32: 291–293

Merskey H 1965 Psychiatric patients with persistent pain. Journal of Psychosomatic Research 9: 299–309

Metz G, Jenkins D J A, Peters T J, Newman A, Blendis L M 1975 Breath hydrogen as a diagnostic method for hypolactasia. Lancet 1: 1155–1157

Metz G, Jenkins D J A, Newman A, Blendis L M 1976a Breath hydrogen in hyposucrasia. Lancet 1: 119–120

Metz G, Gassull M A, Draser B S, Jenkin D J A, Blendis L M 1976b Breath hydrogen test for small intestinal bacterial colonization. Lancet 1: 668–669

Moriarty K J, Dawson A M 1982 Functional abdominal pain: further evidence that the whole gut is affected. British Medical Journal 284: 1670–1677

Murphy E L 1964 Flatus. Conference on nutrition in space and related waste problems. Tampa, Florida. Document 8P–70, p 255–259

Nelis G F, Vermeeren M A P, Jansen W 1990 Role of fructose sorbitol malabsorption in the irritable bowel syndrome. Gastroenterology 99: 1016–1020

Nielsen O H, Gjoru P T, Christensen F N 1986 Gastric emptying rate and small bowel transit time in patients with irritable bowel syndrome. Digestive Sciences 31: 1287–1292

Page J G, Dirnberger M S 1981 Treatment of the irritable bowel syndrome with bentyl. Journal of Clinical Gastroenterology 3: 153–156

Palmer R L, Stonehill E, Crisp A H, Waller S L, Misiewicz J J 1974 Psychological characteristics of patients with the irritable bowel syndrome. Postgraduate Medical Journal 50: 416–419

Pitt P, Bruijn K M, Beeching M, Goldberg E, Blendis L M 1980 Studies on breath methane: the effect of ethnic origins and lactulose. Gut 21: 951–954

Prior A, Whorwell P J 1989 Gynecological consultation in patients with irritable bowel syndrome. Gut 30: 996–998

Puylaert J B, Rutgers P H, Lalisang R I et al 1987 A prospective study of ultrasonography in the diagnosis of appendicitis. New England Journal of Medicine 317: 666

Reynolds T B, Peters R L 1982 Budd–Chiari syndrome in diseases of the liver. In: Schiff L, Schiff E R (eds) Diseases of the liver. J B Lippincott, Philadelphia, p 1622

Ritchie J A 1973 Pain from distension of the pelvic colon by inflating a balloon in the irritable colon syndrome. Gut 14: 125–132

Rumessen J J, Gudmand-Hoyer E 1988 Functional bowel disease. Gastroenterology 95: 694–700

Sandler R S 1990 Epidemiology of irritable bowel syndrome in the United States. Gastroenterology 99: 409–415

Silen W 1979 Cope's early diagnosis of the acute abdomen. Oxford University Press, Oxford.

Smart H L, Nicholson D A, Atkinson M 1986. Gastroesophageal reflux in the irritable bowel syndrome. Gut 27: 1127–1131

Smith R C, Greenbaum D S, Vancouver J B et al 1990. Psychosocial factors are associated with health care seeking rather than diagnosis in irritable bowel syndrome. Gastroenterology 98: 293–301

Spear F G 1967 Pain in psychiatric patients. Journal of Psychosomatic Research 11: 187–193

Spiro H M 1977 Clinical gastroenterology, 2nd edn. Macmillan, New York, p 952

Starnes H F, Moore F D, Mentzer S, Osteen R T, Steele G D, Wilson R E 1986 Cancer. abdominal pain in neutropenic cancer patients 57: 616–621

Steely W M, Gooden S M 1986 Sclerosing mesocolitis. Diseases of the Colon and Rectum 29: 266–268

Steggerda F R 1968 Gastrointestinal gas following food consumption. Annals of the New York Academy of Science 150: 57–66

Stevenson R J 1985 Abdominal pain unrelated to trauma. Surgical Clinics of North America 65: 1181–1215

Stewart R J, Gupta R K, Purdie G L, Isbister W H 1986 Fine catheter aspiration cytology of peritoneal cavity in difficult cases of acute abdominal pain. Lancet 2: 1414–1415

Sugarbaker P K, Bloom B S, Sanders J H, Wilson R E 1975 Preoperative laparoscopy in diagnosis of acute abdominal pain. Lancet 1: 442–445

Stone R T, Barbero G J 1970 Recurrent abdominal pain in childhood. Pediatrics 45: 732–738

Swarbrick E T, Hegarty J E, Bat L, Williams C B, Dawson A M 1980 Site of pain from the irritable bowel. Lancet 2: 443–446

Talley N J, Phillips S F, Melton J, Wiltgen C, Zinsmeister A R 1989 A patient questionaire to identify bowel disease. Annals of Internal Medicine 111: 671–674

Talley N J, Phillips S F, Bruce B et al 1990 Relation among personality and symptoms in non-ulcer dyspepsia and the irritable bowel syndrome. Gastroenterology 99: 327–333

Tedeschi C G, Botta G C 1962 Retractile mesenteritis. New England Journal of Medicine 266: 1035–1040

Thompson W G 1986 A strategy for management of the irritable bowel. American Journal of Gastroenterology 81: 37–41

Trotman I F, Misiewicz J J 1988 Sigmoid motility in diverticular disease and the irritable bowel syndrome. Gut 29: 218–222

Trotman I F, Price C C 1986 Bloated irritable bowel syndrome defined by dynamic 99mTc brain scan. Lancet 2: 364–366

Waller S L, Misiewicz J J 1969. Prognosis in the irritable bowel syndrome. Lancet 2: 753–756

Watson W C, Sullivan S N, Corke M, Rush D 1976 Incidence of esophageal symptoms in patients with irritable bowel syndrome. Gut 17: 827A

Watt A H, Lewis D J M, Horne J J, Smith P H 1987 Reproduction of epigastric pain of duodenal ulceration by adenosine. British Medical Journal 294: 10–12

Weill F S 1982 Ultrasonography of digestive disease, 2nd edn. C V Mosby, St Louis

Wenham P W 1982 Viral and bacterial associations of acute abdominal pain in children. British Journal of Clinical Practice 36: 321

Whitehead W E, Crowell M D, Bosmajian L et al 1990 Existence of irritable bowel syndrome supported by factor analysis of symptoms in two community samples. Gastroenterology 98: 336–340

Whorwell P J, Clouter C, Smith C L 1981 Oesophageal motility in the irritable bowel syndrome. British Medical Journal 282: 1101–1103

33. Chronic gynaecological pain

R. W. Beard, K. Gangar and Shirley Pearce

INTRODUCTION

Chronic gynaecological pain, or chronic pelvic pain (CPP) can be defined as pain that has been present, either intermittently or constantly, for at least 6 months and which is severe enough to interfere with the quality of life of the woman. In Britain, it is the commonest complaint amongst women consulting a gynaecologist (Morris & O'Neil 1958) and with a prevalence of 52% is probably the commonest indication for diagnostic laparoscopy (RCOG Confidential Enquiry into Gynaecological Laparoscopy 1978). In the USA, Rapkin (1986) and Reiter (1990) have reported a prevalence of 34% and 35% respectively.

An understanding of the aetiology of CPP is important because of the damaging effect it has on women. Their lives are dominated by a pain for which neither a cause nor an effective form of treatment is available. They are unable to function as mothers, as sexual partners and as working women. CPP has long been recognised as a complaint without a diagnosis (Gooch 1831; Lawson Tait 1883) but no advance has been made in effectively treating it. It tends to occur in women of reproductive age (mean age 30 years) but is unrelated to parity, race or marital status (Reiter & Gambone 1990). These women have a high prevalence of emotional disturbance (Beard et al 1988) ranging from feelings of lassitude, depression and chronic anxiety to loss of interest in social and physical pursuits (Fry et al 1991). Their quality of life is seriously impaired.

An estimate of the prevalence of CPP in Britain has been undertaken (Davies et al 1992) using available evidence from women known to have endometriosis and pelvic congestion, but it is likely that the true prevalence is considerably underestimated using this approach. A large population survey is much needed to determine this. It was estimated that in Britain the annual incidence is 14 000 cases with a prevalence of about 350 000. The calculated cost to the National Health Service (NHS) of diagnosis and treatment of these women, at £770 per woman, is £158.4 millions per annum, or 0.6% of the total government expenditure on the NHS in 1990–91.

In recent years many factors have contributed to advances in our understanding of CPP. Foremost have been the demands of women that their quality of life and effectiveness should be improved. In addition, better investigative technologies, greater knowledge of the control of the reproductive system and a widening range of therapeutic modalities have all been important in this development. The authors of this chapter have attempted to review the present state of knowledge, accepting that there remain many areas of uncertainty and disagreement.

A description of chronic gynaecological pain, strictly speaking, should be confined to conditions originating in the female organs of reproduction. However, because of the relatively nonspecific clinical presentation of the condition, it is necessary to describe a number of nongynaecological conditions which have been grouped under the general heading of chronic pelvic pain. Abdominal wall and bowel pain are particular examples of nongynaecological pain.

Nerve supply to the lower abdomen and pelvic organs

Fig. 33.1 shows the cutaneous innervation of the lower abdomen. Damage to any of these nerves can simulate gynaecological pain (Brose & Cousins 1992). Pelvic organs have both a sympathetic and parasympathetic nerve supply. The pain impulses from the uterus, medial part of the fallopian tubes and upper part of the vagina travel through the visceral afferent nerve to Frankenhäuser's paracervical plexus. From this plexus impulses travel to the inferior, middle and superior hypogastric plexus and enter the lumbar and lower thoracic sympathetic chain. From there they enter the spinal cord through the posterior nerve root at the level of T10–L1 and to the neurons in the posterior lateral tract of Lissauer and the dorsal horn, where the impulses are subjected to various modulating influences. Some of the impulses that are transmitted pass through the spinothalamic tract to reach the sensory cortex. Sympathetic nerves from the

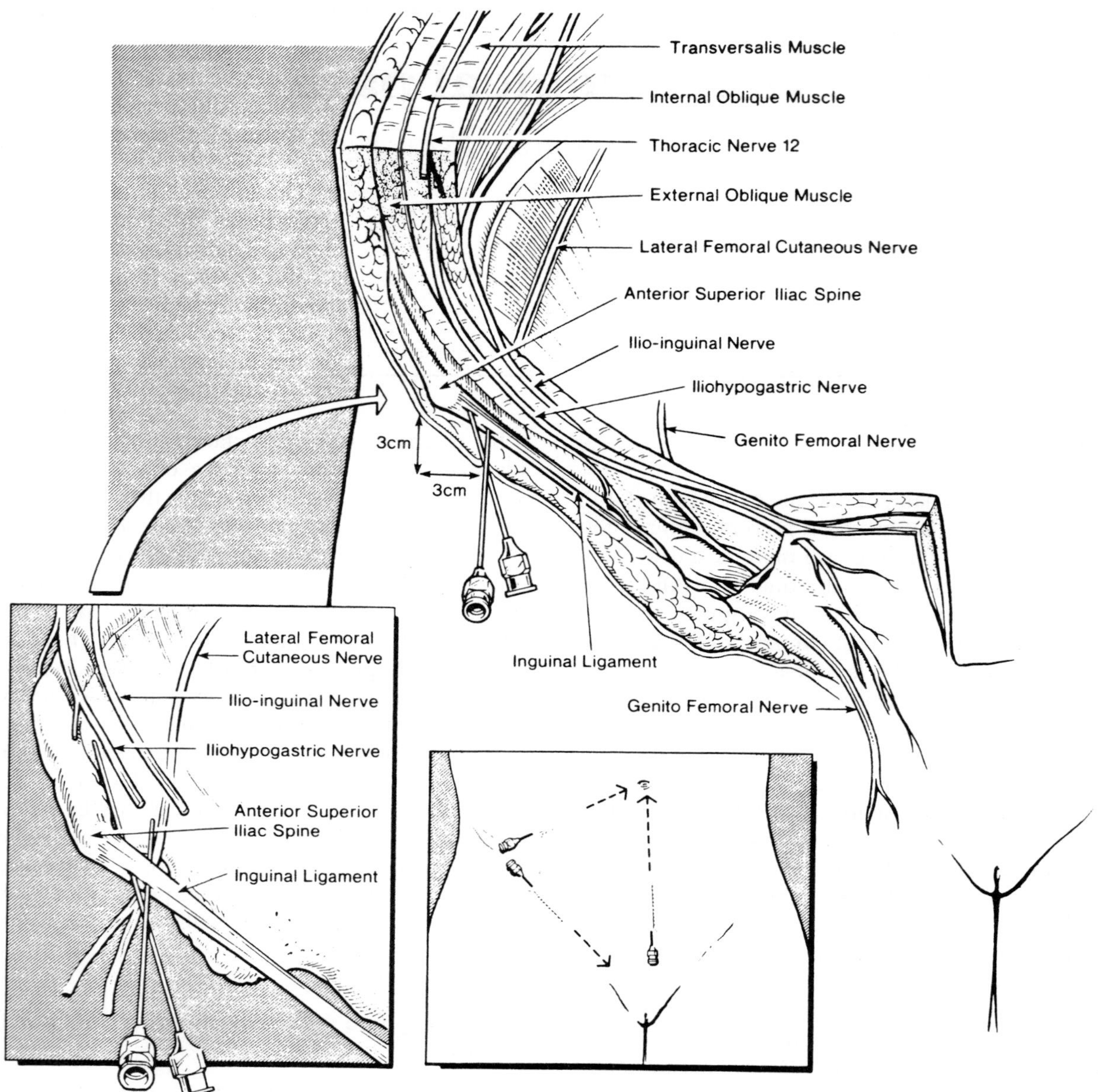

Fig. 33.1 Cutaneous innervation of the lower abdomen. The iliac crest block shown allows the simultaneous blockade of the ilioinguinal, iliohypogastric and lateral femoral cutaneous nerves. **Inset left** Bone and ligamentous landmarks in relation to the nerves. **Inset right** Superficial infiltration for right lower quadrant anaesthesia. (From Brose & Cousins 1992, with permission.)

ovary, lateral part of the fallopian tubes and from the peritoneum of the broad ligament travel along the ovarian vessels and enter the aortic plexus. The parasympathetic fibres originating from the pelvic organs travel along the pudendal nerves and enter the spinal cord at S2, S3 and S4. The dual innervation of the pelvic organs comprising the thoracolumbar and sacral visceral afferent fibres not only overlap the same organs but also have different reflex arcs that convey to the spinal cord pressure as well as pain impulses.

Pain originating from any one of these pelvic organs is also experienced by the skin areas supplied by the somatic afferent fibres of the same spinal segment. This is termed 'referred pain'. Accordingly, pain arising from the ovaries may be referred to the skin on the front of the leg. Pain in the uterus and cervix will be referred to the lower abdominal wall supplied by the 12th thoracic nerve and in the bladder and vagina will be referred to the skin area over the pubic bone and groin. In addition, pain arising from the uterus and cervix because of its dual innervation can be referred to the skin area over the dorsum of the sacrum (S2, S3 and S4).

The fact that all the pelvic organs, including the bladder, are innervated by Frankenhäuser's plexus explains the loss of function of the bladder after major surgery such as Wertheim's hysterectomy (Seski & Diokno 1979).

Pelvic vasculature

Little is known about the control of the pelvic circulation except that it is of particular importance in:

1. the regulation of the many changes occurring in the menstrual cycle
2. support of the developing fetus, placenta and uterus during pregnancy
3. vascular responses during sexual excitement and recovery.

The pelvic veins, like those draining the intestinal tract, are deficient in valves, which may well be an advantage by allowing them to accommodate the considerable fluctuations in the volume of venous blood accompanying these functions. However, the absence of valves will also increase venous pressure in the erect position due to gravity, thereby impeding venous return from the pelvis.

DYSMENORRHOEA

By definition, dysmenorrhoea is lower abdominal pain around the time of menstruation. The pain is commonly described as a continuous dull ache, although it may be colicky, and the intensity varies considerably. The study of Andersch & Milsom (1982) summarises several psychosocial and biological factors associated with dysmenorrhoea. There is undoubtedly a strong family association, with mothers of women with the condition having also suffered from it. No association with parity and smoking could be demonstrated; however an early menarche and menorrhagia were both positively associated with dysmenorrhoea. In a study conducted by Skandhan et al (1988) 305 Indian women were surveyed and it was found that those with prior knowledge of menarche viewed menstruation as a normal physiological function, whilst those without prior knowledge showed an adverse psychological response, being 'appalled' and 'horrified'. Those women with prior knowledge had higher rates of menstrual regularity, lower rates of dysmenorrhoea and earlier onset. The importance of the contribution of psychological factors to the complaint of dysmenorrhoea has been much discussed (Coppen & Kessel 1963; Hirt et al 1967; Berry & McGuire 1972). Gath et al (1987) found a high index of neuroticism amongst dysmenorrhoea sufferers. At present, it is not possible to be sure whether anxiety has a primary role in causing dysmenorrhoea or whether it is a consequence of the pain and leads to the vicious circle interaction of pain and anxiety. The latter seems more likely as, in a study looking at the reaction of women with and without dysmenorrhoea to experimentally induced pain throughout the menstrual cycle, no evidence was found that dysmenorrhoeic women have lower thresholds or more lenient response criteria for reporting certain sensations as 'pain' (Amodei & Nelson-Gray 1989). It has also been suggested that women with dysmenorrhoea have different social networks from women without dysmenorrhoea (Whittle et al 1987). Women suffering from dysmenorrhoea were found to have as many people in their social network as did the controls but reported a higher frequency of inadequate and geographically distant relationships. Whether this is an indication of causal or resultant factors in dysmenorrhoea is unknown but may be linked with higher neuroticism and somatic scores in dysmenorrhoea sufferers.

Two classifications of dysmenorrhoea are in use. The first involves the distinction between primary and secondary dysmenorrhoea, where primary dysmenorrhoea is defined as pain for which there is no obvious cause and secondary dysmenorrhoea is defined as being due to some form of clear pathology, such as endometriosis, fibroids or pelvic inflammatory disease (PID). The limitation of this classification is that an unwarranted assumption is made that in the absence of visible pelvic pathology it can be assumed that the condition is physiological (primary dysmenorrhoea) whereas when pathology is found it is the cause of the pain (secondary dysmenorrhoea). At this stage of limited knowledge of the origin of the pain, such assumptions are unjustified. The second, more pragmatic classification of dysmenorrhoea, which is used in this chapter, relates the pain to the onset of menstruation. Congestive dysmenorrhoea occurs before the onset and is usually relieved by the flow, whereas spasmodic dysmenorrhoea is pain confined to the time of menstrual flow.

The pathophysiology of spasmodic dysmenorrhoea is still not fully understood although one recent theory has suggested that painful contractions of the uterus cause the pain of dysmenorrhoea and are the product of obstruction at the uterine isthmus and cervix, which is only overcome when the intrauterine pressure is high enough (Youssef 1958a, 1958b). Akerlund (1979) has studied the origin of the pain of spasmodic dysmenorrhoea (Fig. 33.2). During menstruation, women with dysmenorrhoea usually show an increase in uterine contractility and a rise in basal tone. With each contraction, there is a marked fall in uterine blood flow which is positively correlated with the intensity of the contraction. The two main somatic factors which are likely to be the cause of the pain of dysmenorrhoea are diminished blood flow and increased myometrial activity. Prostaglandins released in response to ovarian activity and vasopressin further diminish uterine blood flow and increase myometrial contractions. Finally, the hypothalamic–pituitary axis on which normal ovarian and hence menstrual function is dependent may be disturbed by

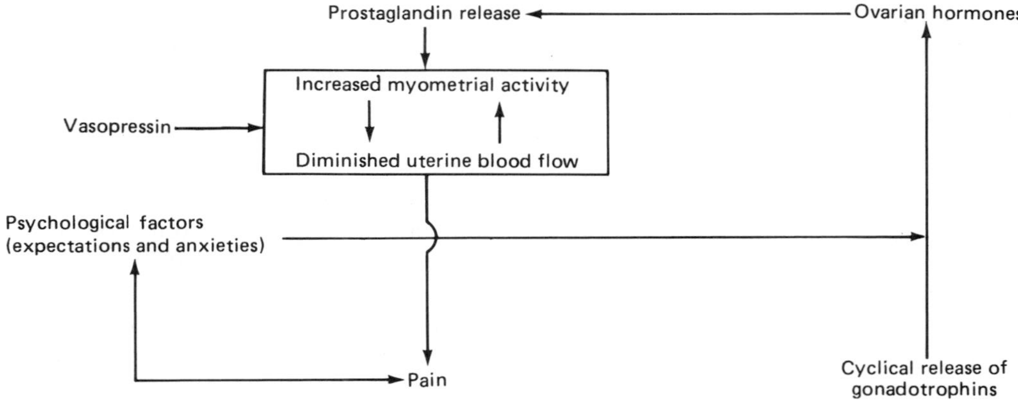

Fig. 33.2 Possible interaction of factors responsible for dysmenorrhoea. (Modified from Akerlund 1979.)

psychological factors, such as the expectations and anxieties of women concerning the pain they are likely to experience, leading to dysfunctional bleeding with associated dysmenorrhoea.

Treatment with some form of oral contraceptive usually provides relief of the pain of spasmodic dysmenorrhoea. For those who fail to respond to this form of treatment or who cannot be treated with steroid hormones, treatment with prostaglandin synthetase inhibitors such as mefenamic acid (Ponstan) usually provides satisfactory relief (Lumsden 1985). In some women treatment by these methods is often only partially successful or occasionally quite unsuccessful. For these women psychological methods have been considered. There is, however, no a priori reason why psychological methods should be considered only when physical methods have failed. Indeed, psychological methods can effectively be conducted in parallel with physical treatment as will be described later in this chapter. The main psychological strategy for dysmenorrhoea, which has consistently been found to help spasmodic dysmenorrhoea sufferers, is relaxation training (Chesney & Tasto 1975; Nicassio 1980; Amodei et al 1987). Both Chesney & Tasto and Amodei and co-workers found relaxation training ineffective for women with congestive dysmenorrhoea, in contrast to Cox & Meyer (1978) and Quillen & Denney (1982). The most recent study compared relaxation with desensitisation for both congestive and spasmodic dysmenorrhoea (Amodei et al 1987) and provided further evidence that relaxation seems more effective for spasmodic dysmenorrhoea than for congestive dysmenorrhoea, and that desensitisation adds little to treatment outcome.

The situation is less clear for congestive dysmenorrhoea, but it seems likely that the underlying pathophysiology is the same as, or similar to, pelvic congestion (see below). Exercise has been suggested as an effective treatment for dysmenorrhoea. Choi (1992) has demonstrated an association between positive mood and exercise, which has implications for reducing the distress which is part of dysmenorrhoeic symptomatology. However, Metheny & Smith (1989) in a study of 176 student nurses found a direct relationship between increased exercise and severity of menstrual symptoms. They suggest that although exercise often relieves stress it may aggravate symptoms and a balance must therefore be obtained such that the optimum level of exercise for each individual is achieved. In a survey of 88 adolescents, Wilson & Keye (1989) found most were unaware of the causes of and treatments for their symptoms of dysmenorrhoea and these authors designed a self-help model. An evaluation of its effectiveness in preventing the development of a more chronic problem would clearly be worthwhile.

ENDOMETRIOSIS

Endometriosis is a poorly understood disease with a variable clinical presentation. The commonest symptom is pelvic pain, which frequently makes it difficult to distinguish from other forms of pelvic pathology. The condition is typified by the presence of endometrium situated outside the uterine cavity. The most common sites are within the pelvis, but it can also occur in distant sites such as abdominal scars and even the lung. It is known as adenomyosis when the endometrial glands are found in the uterine wall. The clinical presentation of the condition and its management has been well reviewed by Shaw (1992).

The symptom of pelvic pain presents either in the form of dysmenorrhoea (45%), dyspareunia (16%) or rectal pain (8%) (Roddick et al 1960), or occasionally a persistent dull pelvic ache. A recent large study (Mahmood et al 1991) showed that dysmenorrhoea is significantly more common in women with endometriosis compared to those with other forms of pelvic pathology, such as pelvic adhesions, and those with a normal pelvis. However two other symptoms, deep dyspareunia and postcoital ache, are equally prevalent in women with endometriosis and pelvic adhesions. This therefore suggests that dyspareunia, postcoital ache and generalised pelvic pain are not reliable indicators of endometriosis and are more likely to be due to other pelvic pathology such as pelvic venous congestion (see below).

The condition is commonly asymptomatic, only being discovered during the course of investigations for infertility or some other condition found coincidentally at laparoscopy. The most common sites of implantation are the ovary, the pouch of Douglas, the uterosacral ligaments and the pelvic peritoneum. When it is deposited on the ovary, the altered blood from the endometriotic process can give rise to cyst formation within the ovarian tissue and cause 'chocolate cysts'. Less common sites of implantation are the large bowel and the rectum when it can present like a carcinoma of the large bowel with lower abdominal pain and rectal bleeding. Endometriotic tissue can also deposit in the rectovaginal septum and cause pain on defaecation. Endometriosis has been reported in almost every structure within the pelvis, including the bladder and the ureter.

Because endometriosis is derived from endometrium, it follows that it is only an active disease during the reproductive years. Thus it never occurs before puberty and is relieved when ovarian failure occurs at the menopause. The ectopic endometrium behaves very much like endometrium within the uterine cavity in that it responds with proliferation to oestrogen stimulation, and likewise progesterone produces typical epithelial changes with local bleeding occurring at the time of menstruation. It is believed that this bleeding leads to intense fibrosis around the endometrial deposits and is thought to be one of the reasons why women with this condition frequently suffer severe dysmenorrhoea. However, this concept does not explain why many women with sometimes widespread pelvic endometriosis have no pain with their menses. It is well recognised that there is little relationship between the extent of the endometriotic disease per se and the severity of the symptoms experienced by the patient (Wardle 1992).

Various mechanisms have been suggested to explain why endometriosis causes pain. Retrograde menstruation, which is the upward passage of menstrual blood through the fallopian tubes into the pelvic cavity, is said to be a possible cause. However, women undergoing laparoscopic sterilisation at the time of menstruation who complain of no pelvic pain are quite often found to have retrograde menstruation. Also there are reports from women having peritoneal dialysis suggesting that women commonly have some blood in the peritoneal cavity during menstruation, most of whom have no pain. Reduced mobility of the pelvic organs has also been postulated as a possible cause of pain. Severe adhesions quite often tether pelvic organs such as the ovaries into positions where they might be affected during intercourse so causing dyspareunia. It might also be possible that adhesions which reduce the mobility of pelvic organs could lead to interference with normal blood flow patterns and hence to vascular congestion. Indeed, the encapsulating active endometriotic lesions may be so extensive that there is unyielding scar tissue causing increased tension and pain around pelvic structures. Direct involvement of autonomic nerves by endometriotic tissues has been suggested as a possible mechanism. This might be an important mechanism of pain when small deposits are found in the uterosacral ligaments. Certainly, anecdotal evidence from clinical experience suggests that lesions at these sites on the uterosacral ligaments frequently seem to produce pain symptoms which are out of all proportion to their actual size. This has led to a renewal of interest in the uterosacral ligament transsection as a possible treatment for painful pelvic conditions (see below).

An alternative hypothesis to explain the variability of pain with endometriosis is based upon the presence of prostaglandins. Schmidt (1985) showed that women with endometriosis have more peritoneal fluid in the pouch of Douglas and that this fluid contains significantly greater quantities of prostaglandin E_2 (PGE_2) and $PGF_{2\alpha}$. It is possible that these compounds, which are vasoactive, give rise to vascular stasis leading to the generation of pain-producing substances. This hypothesis is supported by the knowledge that prostaglandin inhibitors are effective in relieving pain associated with endometriosis. Although the PGF content has been reported to be similar in endometriotic deposits with different morphological features and with varying degrees of pain, variations have been observed in the capacity of different *types* of implant to produce PGF. Vernon et al (1986) found that petechial or reddish implants had a greater capacity for synthesising PGF than intermediate or brown implants. The powder-burn and the black implants have the least capacity for synthesising PGF. They therefore suggested that the morphological appearance and the biochemical activity of endometriotic implants may correlate more closely with the severity of symptoms than do standard classifications. This might also be important in determining the prognosis of the disease.

Treatment of endometriosis is well reviewed by Wardle (1992). The commonest indications for treatment are pain and infertility. It is not within the scope of this chapter to discuss the management of infertility due to endometriosis, except to make the point that there is no good evidence to suggest that treatment of any kind improves fertility rates. When CPP is a dominant symptom, treatment of endometriosis has to be individualised according to factors such as the age of patient, the desire to preserve fertility and the severity of the pain and its effect on the quality of life. The site of the endometriotic deposit may also be important, as there is some evidence that chocolate cysts of the ovary respond better to surgical rather than medical treatment.

PELVIC CONGESTION

Many cases of so-called unexplained pain may be related to pelvic congestion. The word 'congestion' means 'an excessive accumulation of blood in an organ' and, in the case of venous congestion, this is due to increased venous pressure or obstruction. Lawson Tait (1883) regarded ovarian hyperaemia as a major cause of chronic pelvic pain and advocated bilateral oophorectomy as the treatment of choice regardless of age. Chronic hyperaemia and congestion of the ovary were thought to produce proliferation of the connective tissue and cortical fibrosis, leading to cyst formation (Sturmdorf 1916; Taylor 1949a, 1949b, 1949c).

In 1955, Allen & Masters described a syndrome, in women with CPP, of an enlarged, congested, frequently retroverted uterus, enlarged veins in the infundibulopelvic ligaments and a clear fluid exudate in the pouch of Douglas. They explained these changes as being due to tears in the broad ligament, from childbirth, with loss of support for pelvic blood vessels leading to congestion and pain. There is little evidence to support the pathogenesis proposed by these authors. Although defects in the broad ligament are occasionally seen at laparoscopy, they are not confined to parous women and many women with pelvic congestion do not have such tears (Renaer et al 1980; Reginald et al 1987). However, the description these authors gave fits much more with changes associated with long-standing pelvic congestion. Stearns & Sneeden (1966) further amplify the changes associated with congestion:

> The typical uterus weighed 135–150 g or more with a cavity length of 8.5–10.00 cm (normal 6–8 cm). Sections of the cervix revealed sub-epithelial pale staining bands of oedematous fibrous connective tissue containing dilated lymphatics and blood-filled vascular spaces. There was also oedema, lymphangiectasia and telangiectasia in the subserosal layer.

Recent studies

The advent of better methods for investigating women with CPP, in particular laparoscopy, pelvic venography and ultrasound, has provided a means of observing changes in the pelvis without the need to resort to laparotomy. Studies by Beard et al (1984) have shown that 84% of women, with a history of chronic pelvic pain of more than 6 months' duration with no obvious pathology on laparoscopy, have large dilated pelvic veins and vascular stasis. When this condition is present all pelvic veins appear to be involved, but particularly the ovarian veins in the infundibulopelvic ligament and the mass of veins at the hilum of the ovary. Women with pelvic congestion are nearly always in the reproductive period of life, having a mean age of 32 years, and the condition is not found in postmenopausal women.

Clinical features

The symptoms and signs of pain in women with pelvic congestion have been reported by Beard et al (1988). The duration varies from 6 months to 20 years. Typically, the pain is dull and aching, interspersed with acute episodes. It is situated, more commonly, in one or other iliac fossa but nearly always occurs occasionally on the contralateral side. These women commonly have a number of other complaints such as vaginal discharge, backache, headache and urinary symptoms. Bowel symptoms are uncommon. They may have a history of being treated on a number of occasions for PID (46%) and have often had abdominal surgery such as the removal of simple cysts of the ovary or appendicectomy (48%). Menstrual cycle defects are common (54%) and congestive dysmenorrhoea is often present. The frequency of sexual intercouse is diminished (46%) and apareunia is a frequent finding. The most usual reason given for this change in sexual activity is dyspareunia (71%) and postcoital ache (65%).

On examination the abdomen feels soft and, unless the woman is having an acute attack of pain, it is uncommon to elicit tenderness on pressure in either iliac fossa. However, deep pressure over the ovarian point (the junction of the upper and middle third of a line drawn from the umbilicus to the anterior–superior iliac spine) commonly elicits pain in the iliac fossa (77%). Vaginal examination may reveal a visibly congested vagina and eroded cervix with a blue or violet colour. If the woman is experiencing moderate or severe pain, the whole pelvis will be tender, but in a quiescent phase, typically, it is only the ovaries and sometimes the uterus which are tender on gentle compression.

Although a provisional diagnosis can be made from a good history and clinical examination, a definite diagnosis can only be made by further investigation. A full blood count is nearly always normal and investigations such as urine culture, intravenous pyelography and barium enema are only useful when urinary or bowel disturbance is complained of. Laparoscopy, ultrasound imaging and pelvic venography should be performed.

Laparoscopy is essential to exclude pelvic endometriosis and the occasional case of PID. While pelvic adhesions are an unlikely cause of chronic pelvic pain, their presence is evidence of PID. Large dilated pelvic veins on the back of the broad ligament and/or infundibulopelvic ligament with or without hyperaemia of all the structures in the pelvis, is often seen at the start of the laparoscopy but gradually disappears with head-down tilt. Careful inspection with the laparoscope commonly reveals bulky ovaries with multiple subcortical follicular cysts.

Ultrasound imaging. Figure 33.3 shows that in women with pelvic congestion it is possible to detect and measure dilated pelvic veins and to count the number of

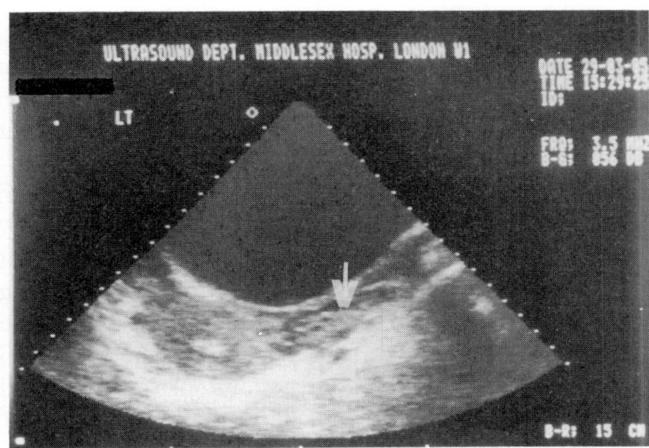

Fig. 33.3 Ultrasound picture showing dilated pelvic veins in a woman with the pelvic pain syndrome.

veins which are dilated. In women without pelvic congestion the veins are not visible. Although it is not possible as yet to quantify the severity of congestion using ultrasound, Stones et al (unpublished observations) have shown that women with pelvic pain and demonstrable congestion on venography have a significantly greater number of dilated veins than a group of women with no pain, matched for age and parity. This group also confirmed the observation made by Adams et al (1990) and Farquhar et al (1989) that women with pelvic congestion have a significantly increased incidence of ovaries with multiple cortical cysts. Doppler time-averaged velocity measurement of venous flow is at present not reliable because of poor technical reproducibility. The tortuosity of the veins also makes it difficult to confirm the angle of insonation. However, relative measurements in numerous women with pelvic congestion have shown a venous circulation which is almost static.

Pelvic venography is a technique developed by Topolanski-Sierra (1958) for directly visualising the pelvic veins and observing blood flow through those veins. A radiopaque dye is injected for 1–2 minutes into the muscle of the uterus. The passage of the dye through the parauterine, paravesical and ovarian veins is observed on a fluoroscopic screen. In a normal woman all the dye has disappeared by 20 seconds after the injection, and the diameter of the ovarian vein is less than 4 mm (Fig. 33.4). Women with pelvic pain syndrome have evidence of dilated veins, particularly the ovarian vein (range 4–15 mm), delayed disappearance and pooling of dye (Fig. 33.5). In a venographic study of women complaining of pelvic pain (Beard et al 1984), 45 had no obvious pathology at laparoscopy and eight had pathology such as endometriosis or PID. As controls, eight women who were to undergo sterilisation had a pelvic venogram done. This study showed that pelvic congestion, defined as dilated pelvic veins and vascular stasis with delayed disappearance

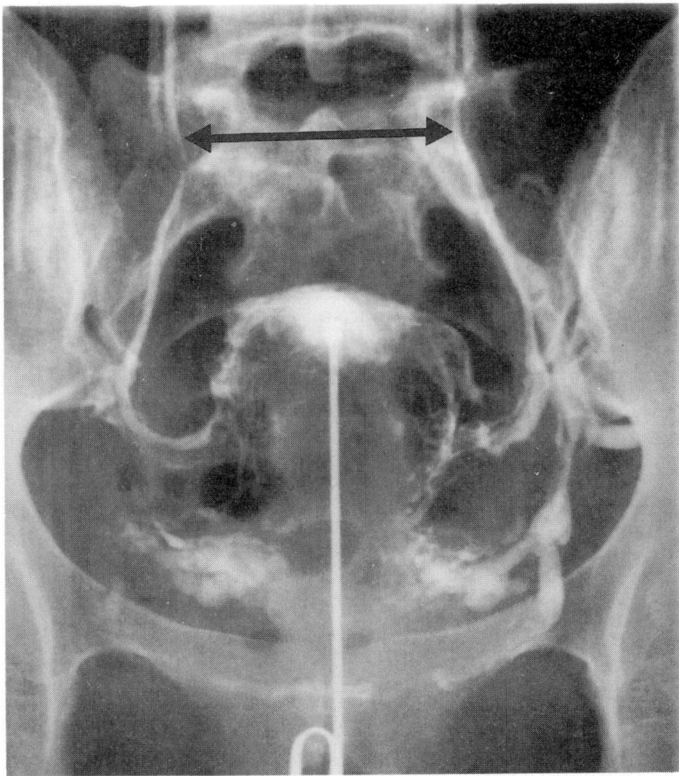

Fig. 33.4 Venogram showing normal pelvic vasculature. Arrow shows ovarian veins.

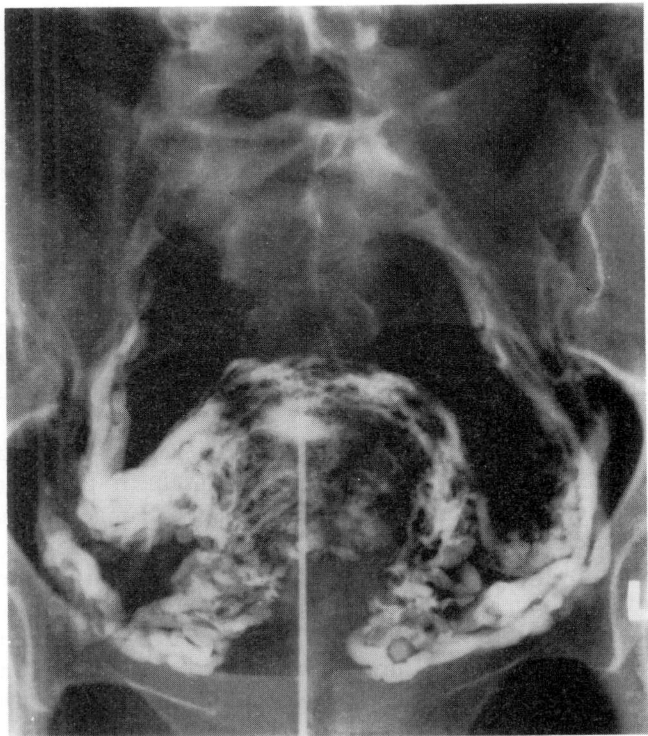

Fig. 33.5 Venogram showing dilated pelvic veins with congestion in the ovarian plexus of a woman with chronic pelvic pain syndrome.

of dye, was a common finding in the women with no apparent cause for their pelvic pain. The diagnostic sensitivity of an abnormal venogram was 91% with a specificity of 89%. The technique is only recommended if there is doubt about the diagnosis on the ultrasound imaging.

Causes of pelvic congestion

The network of veins draining the pelvis (see section on Pelvic vasculature) has certain characteristics that make it unique in the body. Hodgkinson (1953) estimated that the capacity of pelvic veins increased 60-fold by late pregnancy. These features make them vulnerable in the nonpregnant state to chronic dilatation and stasis with resultant vascular congestion. Factors which further contribute to this tendency to dilatation are weakening of the fascial supports during parturition and the vasodilating effects of cyclically fluctuating hormones (Stearns & Sneeden 1966).

If congestion is sufficiently severe then it is likely that pain will develop. Standing for long periods by increasing pelvic congestion commonly brings on pain in these women. Thomas and co-workers (1991) using electrical impedance tomography have shown that women with pelvic congestion demonstrated by venography have an increase in the area of vascular exchange when going from the supine to the erect condition as compared with normal women. This group have also shown (Thomas et al 1992) that when women with pelvic congestion change posture, pelvic blood flow is much more variable, suggesting poor vascular control.

Reginald and co-workers (1987) have shown that the intravenous administration of the selective venoconstrictor, dihydroergotamine, is followed by a 30% reduction in the diameter of dilated pelvic veins. This effect is accompanied by a visible increase in pelvic blood flow with the more rapid disappearance of dye and a reduction in pain. The delayed pain response to intravenous dihydroergotamine of 3–4 hours despite an immediate venoconstricting effect tends to support the concept that congestion is the cause of the pain, with the improvement coinciding with the clearance of pain-producing substances from the pelvic tissues.

The possibility that distension of the pelvic veins is a cause of pelvic pain cannot be dismissed. One of the most consistent symptoms in women with pelvic congestion is an increase in pain on bending forwards. In these women, compression of the ovarian vein per abdomen at the ovarian point, as it crosses the transverse processes of the second and third lumbar vertebrae, induces referred pain similar to that complained of at the site of the ovary on that side. The interpretation of these results is complicated by the known vascular changes accompanying a decrease in pelvic blood flow that occurs on standing (Beard et al 1986).

Hormonal factors

It seems likely that pelvic congestion is related in some way to the secretion of ovarian hormones because pelvic congestion is largely confined to women in their reproductive years. Stearns & Sneeden (1966) considered that a hormonal factor was the most likely cause of pelvic congestion. McCausland et al (1963) also reported a 30% increase in venous distensibility a week prior to menstruation and implicated progesterone as the cause, although the possibility that oestrogen played a part was not ruled out. Barwin & McCalden (1972) demonstrated during in vitro experiments that the contractions produced by field stimulation of the smooth muscle in the veins of humans could be blocked by 17β-oestradiol and progesterone. McCausland and co-workers (1961) showed the effect of pregnancy on venous distensibility and thought this was mediated through oestrogen and progesterone on the smooth muscle of the vessel wall. They considered that pelvic veins were particularly distensible which contributed to marked dilatation of veins draining the pregnant uterus.

Circumstantial and indirect evidence, summarised by Reginald et al (1988), suggests that ovarian hormones, and most probably oestrogen, are the cause of dilated pelvic veins in women with pelvic congestion.

Hypothesis on the cause of pain accompanying pelvic congestion

These and many other studies have led to the following formulation to explain why women with demonstrable pelvic congestion develop pain. Congestion in any part of the body leads to pain. The severity of the pain is partly determined by the extent of the venous stasis which leads to hypoxaemia and local tissue damage followed by the release of pain-producing substances. Being in the erect position for any length of time commonly exacerbates or initiates pelvic pain when pelvic congestion is present (Beard et al 1988). Relief from pain is obtained by lying down and, experimentally, by intravenous injection of the vasoconstrictor dihydroergotamine during an acute attack of pain in women (Reginald et al 1987). The probable reason why pregnant women, all of whom have dilated veins, do not often have CPP is that an adequate flow of venous blood is maintained through the pelvis by a physiological increase in circulating blood volume that normally accompanies pregnancy.

Psychological factors in unexplained pelvic pain

The failure to identify a clear organic disturbance for many women with chronic pelvic pain has led to the search for psychological disturbance in this group of women. Many early studies report mood disturbance

(Benson et al 1959; Magni et al 1984) and high levels of psychopathology (Gidro-Frank et al 1960). There are considerable problems in the interpretation of these findings since the direction of the relationship between chronic pelvic pain and psychological disturbance is unknown. Many of the studies failed to use comparison groups of patients with pain of equivalent chronicity, so that the possibility that psychological disturbance may arise from the long-term experience of pain cannot be ruled out. It is also possible that the patients who become selected for these studies represent a more disturbed group than those routinely attending gynaecological outpatient clinics for pelvic pain. In a prospective study, in which all patients attending gynaecological outpatient clinics with a complaint of chronic pelvic pain of more than 6 months' duration were assessed, no difference was observed, on measures of personality or mood, between women who later, at laparoscopy, showed clear evidence of pathology and those who did not (Pearce 1986). Global measures of psychological disturbance do not therefore seem to suggest a causal role in chronic pelvic pain. Specific differences in attitudes to illness, sexual problems and exposure to death and illness did, however, emerge. Women with pain in the absence of detectable pathology reported a greater number of deaths and illnesses among family members and close friends. It is possible that this greater exposure to illness acts in some patients to induce greater attention to health and illness and a closer monitoring of their physical state. This possibility is supported by the finding that women with pain in the absence of clear pathology score higher on the 'disease conviction' scale of the illness behaviour questionnaire (Pilowsky 1978). Hence, women in this group may be paying greater attention to physiological changes in their bodies. Their 'schema' for the perception of pelvic pain may therefore be such as to lead low levels of pelvic sensory activity to be labelled as painful. If they also have a pelvic vascular disturbance, as described in the preceding section, it is not unreasonable to suggest that their preoccupation with physiological changes leads to their attending to, and labelling as painful, afferent stimulation from pelvic congestion.

A diagrammatic representation of the possible interaction between the different psychological influences discussed above and the somatic changes identified by the venographic studies is provided in Figure 33.6. In this model it is proposed that women who have pain associated with pelvic congestion have a developed biological predisposition to pelvic blood flow responses to stress which are either greater in magnitude or take longer to return to baseline levels than normal. Hence, when exposed to psychological stressors, changes occur in the pelvic vasculature which over time contribute to the development of chronically dilated pelvic veins. Pain sensation is heightened in these women who already have anxiety as a consequence of concern about illness in general and of pelvic dysfunction in particular. This pain then leads to 'pain behaviours', particularly if these are reinforced by concerned family members (Fordyce 1976).

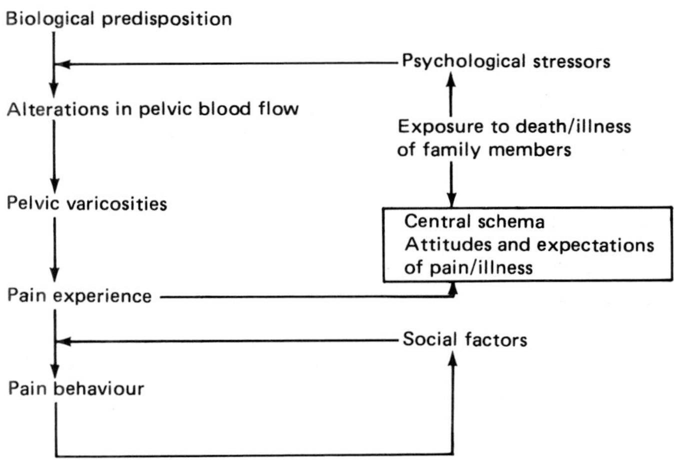

Fig. 33.6 Possible mode of interaction between psychological and somatic factors in pelvic pain associated with pelvic congestion.

Feedback loops may arise at several of these levels of pain experience. Being in pain, for example, is likely to direct further attention to the pelvis and strengthen the central schema or expectation of pain. Such a model, although based to a large extent on research findings, is clearly speculative and should give rise to experimental investigations to test some of the hypothetical links. However, it does suggest a number of potential levels of intervention. Treatment could be directed at the somatic level or at the alteration of the central schema or manipulation of expectations influencing pain perception. Alternatively, it could be directed towards altering pain behaviours and the responses to pain and attitudes of family members.

PERITONEAL ADHESIONS

It seems likely that peritoneal adhesions are occasionally responsible for abdominal pain, although they are often asymptomatic. It is a matter of considerable importance in the evaluation of the cause of pelvic pain since adhesions in the pelvis resulting from infection are a common finding. Alexander-Williams (1987) stated: 'it is a poorly substantiated myth that adhesions can cause abdominal or pelvic pain'. This is clearly not always so. For example, a single band of adhesions which is under tension is likely to cause pain in certain positions or with movement and division of the band affords immediate relief. What seems certain is that while peritoneal adhesions are usually asymptomatic, they can cause pain particularly if they are extensive and involve sensitive structures like the ovary (see section on Ovarian pain).

CHRONIC PELVIC INFLAMMATORY DISEASE

Chronic pelvic inflammatory disease is a consequence of acute pelvic infection leading to permanent damage to tissues such as the parametrium, tubes and ovaries. Peritoneal adhesions may lead to hydrosalpinges, tuboovarian masses, fixity and distortion of the pelvic organs and the 'trapped ovary' already referred to. The diagnosis of chronic pelvic inflammatory disease implies an active but subclinical infective process. There is little evidence that this is so and it is more likely that if the condition is progressive, it is due to recurrent infections.

Some women with chronic pelvic pain give a history of pain which started with an acute attack of salpingitis. Such a history is commonly the product of a diagnosis made at the time without adequate investigation. Many investigators (Murphy & Fliegner 1981; Brihmer et al 1987) have confirmed the laparoscopic findings of Stacey et al (1989), shown in Figure 33.7, which reveal that even in cases of acute pelvic pain many women have no evidence on laparoscopy of PID. Equally, women with laparoscopic evidence of chronic PID do not necessarily give a history of acute PID. For example, infection with chlamydial salpingitis is frequently asymptomatic. These observations reveal how unwise it is to make a diagnosis of such a potentially serious condition, in women with lower abdominal pain, without the diagnostic laparoscopy.

Pain due to acute PID often resolves completely after appropriate treatment, with disappearance of pelvic sepsis leaving no residual adhesion or tubal occlusion. However, some women continue to complain of pelvic pain that may be associated with tuboovarian adhesions. Cultures from the cervix or from pelvic organs are usually negative unless there is an acute attack due to reinfection. The actual cause of chronic pelvic pain in such cases is not clear. It could be due to recurrence of acute infection when the patient presents with signs and symptoms of acute salpingitis. Some women with chronic PID complain of constant unilateral pain, of bilateral pelvic pain and dyspareunia. Pelvic examination reveals generalised pelvic tenderness and thickening of adnexal tissue with or without the presence of tuboovarian mass. A standard investigative approach which includes laparoscopy, pelvic ultrasound and pelvic venography excludes conditions such as ovarian entrapment and pelvic congestion.

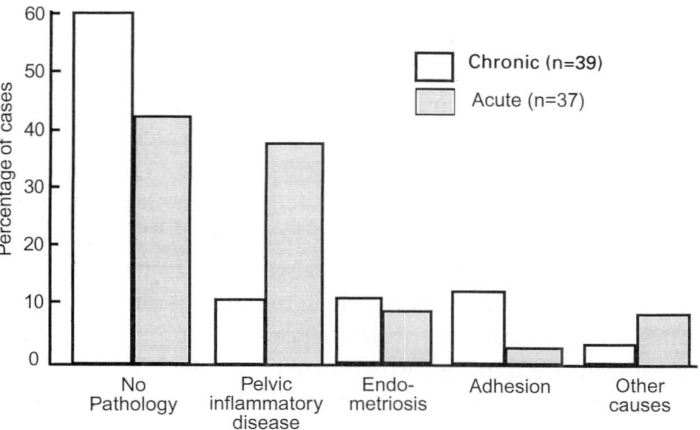

Fig. 33.7 Distribution of cases of acute and chronic pelvic pain according to diagnosis at laparoscopy. (From Stacey et al 1989.)

OVARIAN PAIN

There has been a notable reluctance on the part of British gynaecologists to consider the possibility that the ovary, which on inspection appears normal, may be the site of pelvic pain. The great gynaecologist Lawson Tait was the last surgeon to advocate oophorectomy in women with chronic pelvic pain (Lawson Tait 1883), since when the subject has not been reconsidered in depth. Randall (1963) raised the possibility that neoplastic change in an ovary was an indication for oophorectomy but concluded: 'There are no generally accepted criteria for the removal or conservation of the apparently normal ovary'.

At present the accepted view of most gynaecologists is that ovarian function should be safeguarded in women of reproductive age almost at all costs unless there is a risk of carcinoma or in acute conditions involving the ovary such as torsion. In recent years a number of publications have appeared in the American and Australian literature describing the beneficial effects of oophorectomy in women with CPP who have previously had a total hysterectomy with conservation of one or both ovaries (residual ovaries) or after oophorectomy where a fragment of ovary (ovarian remnant) was inadvertently left behind.

A residual ovary may be either macroscopically normal or abnormal in appearance, being encapsulated in adhesions ('trapped' residual ovaries). When macroscopically normal residual ovaries are found in association with CPP, it is often found that the symptoms of pain preceded the hysterectomy (Siddall-Allum et al 1993). Equally, in women with trapped ovaries there may be a history of PID or postoperative complications leading to periovarian adhesions. Christ & Lotze (1975) reported on 202 women with the residual ovary syndrome and, in a retrospective study, concluded that it occurred in about 3% of women who had had a hysterectomy. In their study 77% of the women complained of pelvic pain, chiefly deep dyspareunia. Like Grogan (1967), they noted that one or both ovaries were usually encased in dense fibrous tissue on the side wall of the pelvis near or just over the ureter. The surface of the ovary contained multiple tense ovarian cysts. The likely cause of the adhesions was preceding pelvic surgery, usually for benign conditions such as dysfunctional bleeding or fibroids. Endometriosis was only associated with residual ovaries in 14% of cases, and 64% were less than 40 years old at the time of the original surgery.

In the long term, the only reliable treatment of a trapped ovary, causing CPP, is to remove it. Ovariolysis is indicated if the woman wishes to retain her fertility or her ovaries for other reasons. Unfortunately, a return of the pain months or even years later is quite common, necessitating oophorectomy. With the advent of hormone replacement therapy (HRT), oophorectomy in women of reproductive age who have no wish to become pregnant becomes a more acceptable possibility than in the past. Serious consideration can now be given to oophorectomy at the time of hysterectomy for women with a history of CPP due to pelvic congestion, endometriosis or pelvic adhesions.

Ovarian remnant syndrome

Fragments of ovary are quite commonly left behind after a 'difficult' oophorectomy. The condition must be distinguished from the supernumerary or accessory ovary, an embryological variant of normal ovarian development, which is extremely rare (Wharton 1959; Cruikshank & van Drie 1982).

Ovarian remnant syndrome and its management has been well described by Symmonds & Pettit (1979), Steege (1987), Pettit & Lee (1988) and Webb (1989). Typically, women with this condition present with constant or cyclical pain situated on one side or the other of the pelvis. They may also complain of postcoital ache, postmicturition or postdefaecation pain. Most have a history of the removal of one or both residual ovaries for pain associated with pelvic adhesions or endometriosis pain. The history of pain is usually prolonged because of the inability of gynaecologists to find a cause and it is quite common for these women to be labelled as having psychological problems. Localised abdominal tenderness is a constant feature of the condition but frequently no mass can be felt on vaginal examination. Ultrasound scan is usually diagnostic, revealing a rounded sometimes cystic mass (Fig. 33.8). Diagnostically, administration of clomiphene citrate may be useful by increasing the size of the mass and of the pelvic pain (Kaminski et al 1990). Serum gonadotrophin concentrations are often in the premenopausal range whether or not the woman is on HRT. Treatment is surgical which, although usually difficult, is preferable to the alternative of radiotherapy (Steege 1987).

VULVODYNIA

This is a severe intractable burning pain found in the postmenopausal woman. It is made worse by lying down. Local examination often reveals nothing apart from perineal or levator ani pain occasionally. It is often confused with CPP but a careful history reveals the site of the pain being more perineal or vaginal. Unfortunately, virtually nothing is known about the condition and efforts to treat it are nearly always ineffective.

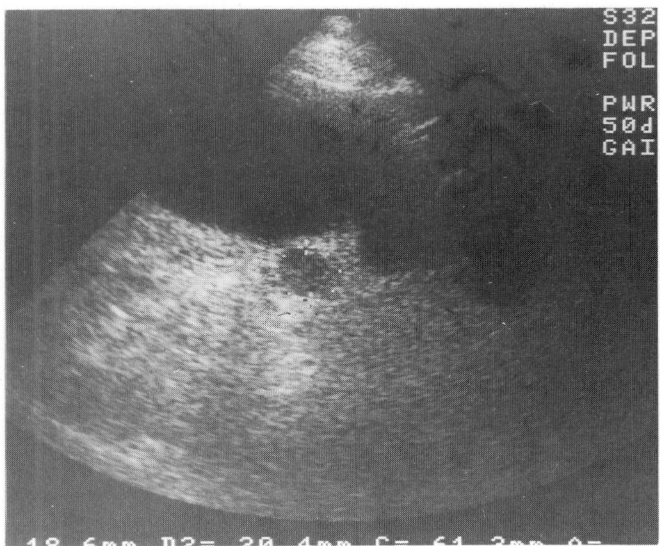

Fig. 33.8 Ultrasound picture showing an ovarian remnant.

LOWER ABDOMINAL WALL PAIN

A lesion of the lower abdominal wall may lead to CPP. It is possible to distinguish between pain arising in the abdominal wall from that originating in the viscera by getting the patient to tense her abdominal muscles by raising her head and shoulders off the couch. If tenderness persists on pressure over the site of pain complained of, then the cause is likely to be found in the abdominal wall.

Myofascial and 'trigger point' pain

Myofascial pain is a well accepted cause of chronic pain in other parts of the body. Hyperirritable spots develop in soft tissues such as muscles or ligaments that have been damaged and movement tends to prevent healing, thereby perpetuating the pain. The abdominal wall has long been recognised as an important primary site in women presenting with gynaecological pain (Adelman 1987).

Slocumb (1990) has termed tender spots in the abdominal wall 'trigger points'. He suggests that trigger points may also be present in the pelvic cavity. In a study of 131 women with chronic lower abdominal pain, Slocumb (1984) reported finding trigger points on the abdomen (89%), vaginal fornices (71%) and sacrum (25%). They may be identified by inserting a 22-gauge needle into the fat pad above the abdominal fascia. Movement of the tip of the needle reproduces the pain complained of and injection of local anaesthesia temporarily obliterates the pain. Treatment consists of hyperstimulation analgesia by stretch or cold spray, serial local anaesthetic injections or counterirritation by transcutaneous electrical nerve stimulation (TENS) or acupuncture to the trigger points, all of which are designed to prolong the central block by altering the central gate control. Among the 122 women with trigger point pain treated by Slocumb, 89% reported complete or partial relief from pain 3–36 months after treatment.

The results are impressive in clinical terms but are of little assistance in helping to determine the aetiology of the pain. Referred pain is a common phenomenon and the use of local anaesthesia to temporarily relieve the pain may be effective in the long term by the reassurance induced. While it is perfectly possible to accept that myofascial pain does occur in the lower abdomen, it would be fair to say that at present the prevalence of this condition amongst women with CPP remains uncertain.

Ilioinguinal nerve entrapment

Nerve entrapment is thought to be one of the conditions causing lower abdominal pain which may simulate gynaecological pain. The ilioinguinal nerve originates from L1–L2 nerve roots innervating the muscles of the lower abdomen, the skin over the inguinal ligament, base of the labia and inner aspect of the thigh. It passes through the abdominal muscles just medial to the anterior superior iliac spine, finally emerging through the external aponeurosis to supply the skin lateral to the pubis. It may be damaged by operations in this region, particularly herniorrhaphy, appendicectomy, and the Pfannenstiel incision (Sippo et al 1987). The pain, which is stabbing and colicky, exacerbated by exercise and relieved by rest, is almost the only symptom. It is relieved by serial injections of local anaesthesia, with or without steroids, into the aponeurosis over the site of maximum tenderness or by surgical division of the nerve. The success of nerve division in a carefully selected group of 46 women followed up for at least 1 year was claimed to be excellent or good in 41 (90%) (Hahn 1989).

The published symptomatology and criteria recommended for making a diagnosis of this condition are so similar to those of myofascial abdominal pain that it may be difficult to distinguish between them. As with so many other causes proposed for chronic lower abdominal pain, only where rigorous methodology is applied to evaluation will it be possible to determine the prevalence of the condition and how effective treatment is.

IRRITABLE BOWEL SYNDROME (IBS)

This is an example of a nongynaecological psychosomatic condition which is often confused with gynaecological causes of lower abdominal pain and, equally, is frequently mistakenly diagnosed when no gynaecological cause has been found (Hogston 1987).

The condition occurs more commonly in women, with a frequency ranging from 56–90% (Thompson & Heaton 1980; Svedlund et al 1983; Whorwell et al 1986; Harvey et al 1987). Sufferers tend to be polysymptomatic, the predominant symptoms being colicky abdominal pains and frequent loose motions alternating with bouts of constipation.

Urgency and frequency of micturition, backache and dyspareunia are common (Whorwell et al 1986), as are psychological correlates such as lassitude, fear of serious disease and palpitations and it has been suggested that individuals with IBS tend to be overanxious, highly sensitive people who complain more about minor ailments (Heaton 1983).

The condition with which IBS is most likely to be confused is pelvic congestion. The tendency to be polysymptomatic is common to both groups, but the similarity ceases there. Bowel symptoms predominate in IBS which is why the condition generally leads to referral to the gastroenterologists, whereas the absence of such symptoms is striking in women with pelvic congestion (Beard et al 1988). There is good evidence of abnormal sensitivity to distension of the large bowel with IBS (Cann et al 1983), which responds to treatment with anticholinergic drugs.

The treatment of IBS reveals the dichotomy that exists between those who regard the condition as predominantly somatic in origin and those who consider psychological factors as being of paramount importance. A controlled trial of psychotherapy for IBS which took the form of 10 1-hour sessions was reported by Svedlund et al (1983). In total, 101 men and women with IBS, on conventional treatment with bulk-forming agents and anticholinergic drugs, were randomly allocated to psychotherapy and a control group. At 15 months after completion of treatment the psychotherapy group showed a significant improvement over the control group in terms of bowel function and abdominal pain. Of interest is that the initial early improvement of the control group had tended to regress. Similar results were reported by Harvey et al (1987) from their study of the short- and long-term results of treatment with reassurance, a bulking agent and an antispasmodic drug, in 104 individuals. At 5–7 years after treatment started, 23% of these individuals had no symptoms, 45% had 'occasional minor symptoms', while the remainder were not significantly improved.

The success of a combination of pharmaco- and psychotherapy is evidence of the effective interaction of these different types of treatment and is relevant to the management of all forms of pelvic pain.

INVESTIGATION

It is only with an improved understanding of the aetiology of CPP that the history has proved helpful in making a diagnosis. Probably the major defect of the current management of women with this complaint is that, unfortunately, time is rarely available to the busy general practitioner or gynaecologist to take a careful history.

The duration of the pain and any factor that may have coincided with the onset of the pain, such as an abdominal operation (ilioinguinal nerve entrapment) or following a pregnancy (pelvic congestion), may be significant. The nature of the pain, its position and whether it is confined to one site (endometriosis) or may occasionally arise on the other side is helpful. Conditions involving the ovary often present with pain over the front of the leg. Exercise commonly exacerbates myofascial pain (Slocumb 1990) and pelvic congestion, while standing and bending commonly exacerbate the pain of pelvic congestion (Beard et al 1988). Postcoital ache, which by definition develops after intercourse, is a classical symptom associated with pelvic congestion. Trapped ovaries present with symptoms almost identical to those of pelvic congestion. In women with one or more ovarian remnants a dull ache usually develops some time after removal of the ovary or ovaries, often presenting as cyclical pain lasting several days.

Physical signs are important for discriminating between different causes of CPP. Trigger point pain is said to be commonest in the lower abdominal wall and can be distinguished from visceral pain by the persistence of tenderness and pain when the rectus abdominis muscles are tensed (Slocumb 1990). Ilioinguinal nerve entrapment typically presents as a painful area at some point along the course of the ilioinguinal nerve (Hahn 1989), which is successfully blocked by injection of local anaesthesia. Endometriosis presents variably, but usually as localised deep abdominal tenderness over the site of implantation. Pelvic congestion, trapped ovaries and ovarian remnants typically present as deep tenderness, often referred to the iliac fossa when pressure is applied over the ovarian point. Pelvic tenderness is only present on vaginal examination in the last four conditions. Endometriotic nodules are tender, particularly in the uterosacral ligament. Ovarian tenderness is a diagnostic feature of pelvic congestion, residual ovaries and ovarian remnants.

It is essential for diagnostic purposes, and the satisfaction of women complaining of pelvic pain, that further investigations are done. When trigger point and ilioinguinal nerve pain is suspected, injection of a local anaesthetic agent into the myofascial area, preceded or followed after some time by the injection of saline, determines whether or not the provisional diagnosis is correct. Laparoscopy is essential for all women with CPP unless the pain is clearly located in the abdominal wall. The presence of dilated veins in the infundibulopelvic ligament, ovarian hilum or broad ligament, combined with polycystic changes in the ovary which may only be apparent on close inspection, is diagnostic of pelvic congestion. An ultrasound scan is also valuable for revealing polycystic changes in the ovaries and dilated veins in the broad ligament and uterus (see Fig. 33.3). Ovarian remnants can be demonstrated with ultrasound scanning but this may require pretreatment with clomiphene. Most recently, magnetic resonance imaging has been used to clearly demonstrate relatively small foci of adenomyosis (Scoutt et al 1990). Pelvic venography (see Fig. 33.5) is the best way of demonstrating congestion, but is not required if the ultrasound findings are definite.

TREATMENT

It is not possible in such a wide-ranging review of CPP to provide a comprehensive account of the many forms of treatment that have been recommended. However, it is possible to propose a number of principles that are useful when deciding on the selection of effective treatment.

1. Fear of pain is the feature that makes CPP so disruptive to the quality of life. This being so, it follows that reassurance that the pain can be ameliorated is an important component of a treatment programme. Amelioration can be achieved by psychological, medical and surgical interventions. The therapist should be prepared to use all three in a variety of combinations, depending on a careful evaluation of the psychological and somatic status of the sufferer.
2. Success in the therapeutic sense is often difficult to define when treating women with CPP. If a total relief of pain is aimed for then many women will be disappointed because of the relapsing nature of CPP. If, on the other hand, a return to the quality of life the woman knew before the onset of pain is the objective, then the chances of success are likely to be greater.
3. CPP is not caused by life-threatening conditions which means that the final decision on treatment must rest with the patient.
4. Women with CPP are mostly of reproductive age which dictates the need to preserve ovarian and uterine function. Surgical intervention, which includes oophorectomy, is only justified in the treatment of CPP providing that all conservative methods have been tried and the woman (and partner) accept the loss of fertility and the requirement to take HRT for many years.
5. Women with CPP tend to be suspicious of all explanations and treatments prescribed, because of the conflicting views of many of the doctors they have seen in the past. It is essential that the therapist is able to provide a convincing explanation of the aetiology of the pain and the rationale of management. In Britain, the general practitioner knows more about the problems a woman has suffered with CPP but will often need specialist support (Woodward 1992) in the management of CPP. A clinic, in a gynaecological setting, devoted to CPP is an effective

way of providing the multidisciplinary approach recommended by Gambone & Reiter (1990).

Psychological interventions

Psychological interventions have largely been investigated for their value in the management of women with pain for which there is no obvious somatic cause. However, given the involvement of psychological processes in the perception of pain of all kinds, there is no reason why psychological interventions should be any more beneficial for women with unexplained CPP than, for example, for women with endometriosis. Strategies which help women to be distracted from the pain and encourage them to cope despite the pain, may be helpful for all forms of pelvic as well as other chronic pain conditions. In the future, it is likely that advances in pain management will involve a closer integration of pharmacological, surgical and psychological methods of pain control. To date, however, psychological approaches have been almost exclusively used for unexplained pelvic pain whilst medical and surgical approaches are used for pain when a somatic pathology is thought to be the cause. Experience suggests that neither of these approaches used independently of each other is as effective as when they are combined (Farquhar et al 1989).

One of the earliest papers to mention the use of psychological approaches to CPP was that of Beard and co-workers (1977). This paper reported that some women responded well to relaxation training. However, there was no formal evaluation of the efficacy of relaxation training and hence conclusions from this study are limited. Subsequent studies are also limited since inadequate control groups and outcome measures were used (Petrucco & Harris 1981; Pearce et al 1982).

Pearce (1986) compared stress analysis and pain analysis with a minimal intervention control group. Women allocated to the 'stress analysis' group received a form of cognitive and behavioural stress management and relaxation training. Discussion of the pain was discouraged and the focus was directed towards identifying current worries and concerns apart from the pain. Treatment started with a semistructured interview to assess potential areas of stress, such as financial, marital or housing, and the problem areas were identified. The women were also asked to keep a daily record of the main concerns they had. The therapist's aim throughout was to identify cognitive strategies used in response to identified stressors and to discuss alternative responses. In addition, the use of Jacobsonian relaxation strategies in stressful situations was encouraged. The 'pain analysis' treatment involved close monitoring of the woman's pain and associated antecedent and consequent events. Therapy was aimed, in collaboration with the patient, at identifying patterns associated with pain episodes and alternative strategies for avoiding or reducing pain episodes were discussed. These strategies were determined on an individual basis and included cognitive, behavioural and environmental manipulations. In addition, graded exercise programmes were instituted for each patient. Spouses were asked to prompt and encourage 'well behaviours' and, whenever possible, to become involved in the exercise programme. Patients allocated to the minimal intervention control group were given the same explanation as the treatment groups about the probable aetiology and frequency of their disorders and the absence of a proven medical or surgical treatment approach. A range of measures was used to assess outcome, including mood, pain intensity ratings, behavioural disruption and gynaecologists' 'blind' ratings of the extent to which the patient was affected by the pain. On all measures of outcome, women in both of the treatment groups performed significantly better than the minimal intervention control group at 6 months after starting the study.

The development of pain management programmes within obstetrics and gynaecology should be guided by the increasing knowledge about pain control that has emerged from other clinical areas. A review by Pearce & Erskine (1991) describes some practical details of these programmes. The development of pain clinics within gynaecology will need to take a multidisciplinary approach with medical staff, psychologists and, ideally, physiotherapists and occupational therapists being involved.

Medical interventions

Table 33.1 summarises some of the treatments for CPP that are widely used based on diagnostic categorisation.

The medical treatment of endometriosis (Shaw 1992) and of pelvic congestion (Beard & Reginald 1992) is essentially the same. Being primarily ovarian hormone-dependent conditions, the treatment is either ovarian suppression or blocking oestrogen receptors. Consequently when such treatment is stopped, the pain is likely to return.

Farquhar and co-workers (1989), in a randomised, controlled treatment trial of 84 women with pelvic congestion, used a 4-month course of oral medroxyprogesterone acetate (Provera) 50 mg a day. Figure 33.9 shows:

1. a mean 38% placebo response
2. that whilst on treatment with Provera, 73% had a more than 50% reduction in pain score but that 6 months after stopping treatment, there was no significant difference between the response of those treated by Provera alone compared with the control group
3. at 6 months after the end of treatment there was no significant difference between those treated with Provera and Provera plus psychotherapy. However (not shown in Fig. 33.9) 9 months after treatment had

Table 33.1 Medical (including psychological where appropriate) and surgical treatment for chronic pelvic pain based on diagnostic categorisation

	Medical	Surgical
Endometriosis	Gestinone 2.5–5.0 mg twice weekly for 6–9 months or Progestogens; Provera 50 mg per day for an indefinite period or GnRH analogue + Premarin 0.625 mg + Provera 5 mg daily Psychotherapy	Local excision after pretreatment with GnRH analogue or Laparoscopic laser coagulation of localised implants especially on uterosacral ligament or Bilateral oophorectomy + total hysterectomy with/without HRT
Pelvic congestion	Provera 50 mg for at least 4 months + Premarin 0.625 mg daily or GnRH analogue (+ Premarin 0.625 mg and Provera 5 mg daily) monthly for 4–6 months Psychotherapy	Bilateral oophorectomy + total hysterectomy followed by HRT
Residual ovary		
Not trapped	Treat as for pelvic congestion	Oophorectomy followed by HRT
Trapped	None	Oophorectomy with wide excision followed by HRT
Ovarian remnant		Surgical removal after pretreatment with clomiphene
Chronic PID/pelvic adhesions	Full investigation to exclude other causes of pain Psychotherapy	Division of adhesions with/without removal of damaged pelvic organs(s)
Abdominal wall pain		
Trigger point	Nerve block	
Myofascial	Counterirritants	
Ilioinguinal nerve entrapment	Nerve block	Division of nerve
Irritable bowel syndrome	Bulk forming agents Psychotherapy	

GnRH = gonadotrophin releasing hormone; HRT = hormone replacement therapy; PID = pelvic inflammatory disease.

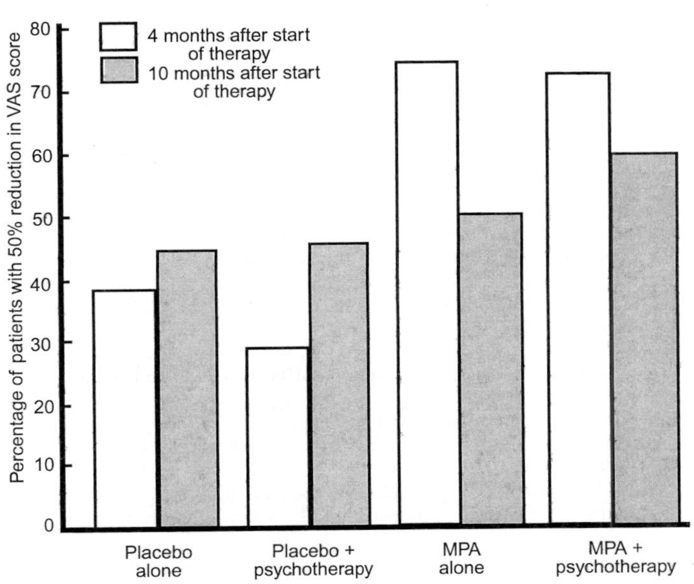

Fig. 33.9 Percentage of patients with 50% reduction in pain score (by visual analogue scale) 4 and 10 months after start of therapy. (MPA = medroxyprogesterone acetate.)

ceased there was a positive interaction between Provera and psychotherapy with 71% of women showing a continued reduction of more than 50% in pain score.

Table 33.1 also shows the recommended use of local anaesthetic agents with or without counterirritants or steroids for the treatment of lower abdominal wall conditions causing CPP, myofascial pain, trigger point pain and ilioinguinal nerve entrapment (Hahn 1989; Slocumb 1990) While these forms of treatment are clearly effective in relieving pain, there is still a need to determine the limit of their effectiveness by controlled treatment trials. The value of the combination of psychotherapy and pharmacotherapy in the effective treatment of the irritable bowel syndrome is well described in a randomised controlled trial by Svedlund et al (1983).

Surgical interventions

These are also summarised in Table 33.1. The surgical management of local deposits of endometriosis has

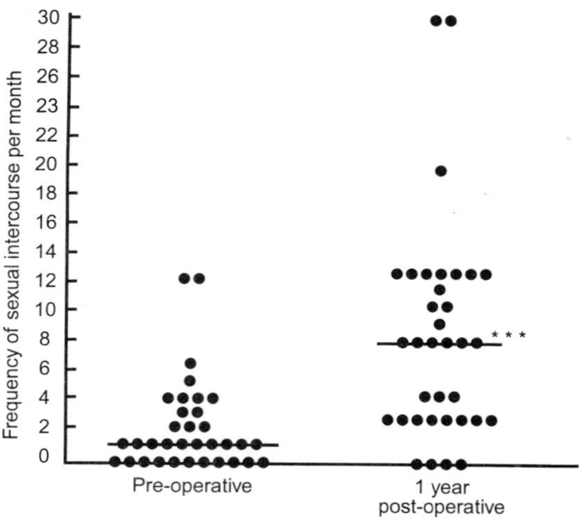

Fig. 33.10 Frequency of sexual intercourse before and after bilateral oophorectomy and hysterectomy. Median values shown by the bars; *** $p < 0.001$. (From Beard et al 1991.)

recently gained in popularity because of the advances in the use of lasers with endoscopic surgery (Sutton & Hill 1990). The effectiveness of this limited approach to treatment still needs to be demonstrated. Long-term surgical relief of pain can only be achieved reliably in both endometriosis and pelvic congestion by bilateral oophorectomy. Taylor (1949c) reported on 58 cases of pelvic congestion of whom 16 were treated by surgical methods, none of which involved oophorectomy. Only one was cured of pain, eight improved and nine showed no improvement. More recently, Slocumb (1990) has reviewed the outcome of various surgical procedures used in the treatment of CPP. He found little evidence that any form of surgery had a lasting beneficial effect.

This view has been challenged by those interested in pelvic congestion as a possible cause of CPP (Beard et al 1991). The present author and colleagues have reported on 36 women who had a bilateral oophorectomy and total hysterectomy for intractable CPP. It seemed probable that as ovarian suppression with Provera had significantly reduced CPP, oophorectomy was likely to produce a permanent cure. The accompanying hysterectomy was done to facilitate the use of HRT. By 1 year after operation not only had the visual analogue pain score fallen to zero in 33 of the 36 women, but there was a significant improvement in the monthly frequency of sexual intercourse (Fig. 33.10).

The effectiveness of HRT after oophorectomy in ensuring continued female function and conservation of skeletal bone has been shown in a follow-up to 5 years in a group of 107 women who have undergone the same form of treatment (Reid et al 1992). Clearly it would be preferable to find a less drastic form of treatment in such a young group of women, but for the time being oophorectomy combined with hysterectomy provides an effective cure when all other approaches have failed.

Finally, there is general agreement amongst gynaecological surgeons that sharp dissection must be used when the trapped residual ovary or ovarian remnant is being removed. Care must be taken to avoid leaving any ovarian tissue and to beware of damage to surrounding structures, particularly the bladder and ureter. For most gynaecologists the operation is best done with the assistance of a urological surgeon. The possibility that a mobile residual ovary is a cause of CPP can be determined by inducing ovarian suppression and this can be continued as a form of medical treatment if the woman wishes to conserve ovarian function. Bilateral oophorectomy combined with HRT provides a satisfactory alternative (Siddall-Allum et al 1993).

REFERENCES

Adams J, Reginald P W, Franks S, Wadsworth J, Beard R W 1990 Uterine size and endometrial thickness and the significance of cystic ovaries in women with pelvic pain due to congestion. British Journal of Obstetrics and Gynaecology 97: 583–587

Adelman A 1987 Abdominal pain in the primary care setting. Journal of Family Practice 25: 27–32

Akerlund M 1979 Pathophysiology of dysmenorrhea. Acta Obstetrica et Gynecologica Scandinavica 87: 27–32

Alexander-Williams J 1987 Do adhesions cause pain? British Medical Journal 294: 659–660

Allen W M, Masters W H 1955 Traumatic laceration of uterine supports. American Journal of Obstetrics and Gynecology 70: 500–513

Amodei N, Nelson-Gray R O 1989 Reactions of dysmenorrheic and non-dysmenorrheic women to experimentally induced pain throughout the menstrual cycle. Journal of Behavioral Medicine 12: 373–385

Amodei N, Nelson R O, Jarrett R B, Sigmon S 1987 Psychological treatments of dysmenorrhea: differential effectiveness for spasmodics and congestives. Journal of Behavior Therapy and Experimental Psychiatry 18: 95–103

Andersch B, Milsom I 1982 An epidemiologic study of young women with dysmenorrhea. American Journal of Obstetrics and Gynecology 144: 655–660

Barwin B N, McCalden T A 1972 The inhibitory action of estradiol-17beta and progesterone on human venous smooth muscle. Proceedings of the Physiological Society 4 P

Beard R W, Reginald P W 1992 Chronic pelvic pain. In: Shaw R W, Soutter W P, Stanton S L (eds) Gynaecology. Churchill Livingstone, London, p 777–788

Beard R W, Belsey E N, Lieberman M B, Wilkinson J C M 1977 Pelvic pain in women. American Journal of Obstetrics and Gynecology 128: 566–570

Beard R W, Highman J W Pearce S, Reginald P W 1984 Diagnosis of pelvic varicosities in women with chronic pelvic pain. Lancet 2: 946–949

Beard R W, Randall N J, Reginald P W, Sutherland I A, Wertheim D F P 1986 Postural changes in pelvic blood flow in women. Journal of Physiology 374: 9P

Beard R W, Reginald P W, Wadsworth J 1988 Clinical features of women with chronic lower abdominal pain and pelvic congestion. British Journal of Obstetrics and Gynaecology 95: 153–161

Beard R W, Kennedy R G, Gangar K F et al 1991 Bilateral oophorectomy and hysterectomy in the treatment of intractable pelvic pain associated with pelvic congestion. British Journal of Obstetrics and Gynaecology 98: 988–992

Benson R, Hanson K, Matarazzo J 1959 Atypical pelvic pain in women: gynecologic psychiatric considerations. American Journal of Obstetrics and Gynecology 77: 806–823

Berry C, McGuire F 1972 Menstrual distress and acceptance of sexual role. American Journal of Obstetrics and Gynecology: 114: 83–87

Brihmer C, Kallings I, Nord C-E, Brundin J 1987 Salpingitis; aspects of diagnosis and etiology: a 4-year study from a Swedish capital hospital. European Journal of Obstetrics, Gynecology and Reproductive Biology 24: 211–220

Brose W G, Cousins M J 1992 Physiology and relief of pain: In: Shaw R W, Soutter W P, Stanton S L (eds) Gynaecology. Churchill Livingstone, London, p 745–767

Cann P A, Read N W, Brown C, Hobson N, Holdsworth C D 1983 Irritable bowel syndrome: relationship of disorders in the transit of a single solid meal to symptom patterns. Gut 24: 405–411

Chesney M, Tasto D 1975 The effectiveness of behaviour modification with spasmodic and congestive dysmenorrhea. Behaviour Research and Therapy 19: 303–313

Choi P Y L 1992 The psychological benefits of physical exercise: implications for women and the menstrual cycle. Journal of Reproductive and Infant Psychology 10: 111–115

Christ J L, Lotze E C 1975 The residual ovary syndrome. Obstetrics and Gynecology 46: 555–566

Coppen A, Kessel N 1963 Menstruation and personality. British Journal of Psychiatry 109: 711–721

Cox D J, Meyer R G 1978 Behavioural treatment parameters with primary dysmenorrhea. Journal of Behavioral Medicine 1: 297–310

Cruikshank S H, Van Drie D M 1981 Supernumerary ovaries: update and review. Obstetrics and Gynecology 60: 126–129

Davies L, Gangar K F, Drummond M, Saunders D, Beard R W 1992 The economic burden of intractable gynaecological pain. Journal of Obstetrics and Gynaecology 12 (suppl 2): S50–S52

Farquhar C M, Rogers V, Franks S, Pearce S, Wadsworth J, Beard R W 1989 A randomised controlled trial of medroxyprogesterone acetate and psychotherapy for the treatment of pelvic congestion. British Journal of Obstetrics and Gynaecology 96: 1153–1162

Fordyce W E 1976 Behavioral methods for chronic pain and illness. C V Mosby, St Louis

Fry R P W, Crisp A H, Beard R W 1991 Patients' illness models in chronic pelvic pain. Psychotherapy and Psychosomatics 55: 158–163

Gambone J C, Reiter R C 1990 Non-surgical management of chronic pelvic pain: a multidisciplinary approach. Clinical Obstetrics and Gynecology 33: 205–211

Gath D, Osborn M, Bungay G et al 1987 Psychiatric disorder and gynaecological symptoms in middle-aged women: a community survey. British Medical Journal 294: 213–218

Gidro-Frank L, Gorton T, Taylor H C 1960 Pelvic pain and female identity. American Journal of Obstetrics and Gynecology 79: 1184–1202

Gooch R 1831 On some of the most important diseases peculiar to women. Republished by the Sydenham Society, London, 1859, p 299–331

Grogan R H 1967 Reappraisal of residual ovaries. American Journal of Obstetrics and Gynecology 97: 124–129

Hahn L 1989 Clinical findings and results of operative treatment in ilioinguinal nerve entrapment syndrome. British Journal of Obstetrics and Gynaecology 96: 1080–1083

Harvey R F, Mauad E C, Brown A M 1987 Prognosis in the irritable bowel syndrome: a 5-year prospective study. Lancet 2: 963–965

Heaton K W 1983 Irritable bowel syndrome: still in search of its identity. British Medical Journal 287: 852–853

Hirt M, Kurtz R, Ross W D 1967 The relationship between dysmenorrhea and selected personality variables. Psychosomatics 8: 350–353

Hodgkinson C P 1953 Physiology of the ovarian veins during pregnancy. Obstetrics and Gynecology 1: 26–37

Hogston P 1987 Irritable bowel syndrome as a cause of chronic pain in women attending a gynaecology clinic. British Medical Journal 294: 934–935

Kaminski P F, Sorosky J L, Mandell M J, Broadstreet R P, Zaino R J 1990 Clomiphene citrate stimulation as an adjunct in locating ovarian tissue in ovarian remnant syndrome. Obstetrics and Gynecology 76: 924–926

Lumsden M A 1985 Dysmenorrhoea. In: Studd J (ed) Progress in obstetrics and gynaecology, vol 5. Churchill Livingstone, London, p 276–292

McCausland A M, Hyman G, Winsor T, Trotter A D Jr 1961 Venous distensibility during pregnancy. American Journal of Obstetrics and Gynecology 81: 472–478

McCausland A M, Holmes F, Trotter A D Jr 1963 Venous distensibility during menstrual cycle. American Journal of Obstetrics and Gynecology 68: 640–643

Magni G, Salmi A, Leo D, Ceola A 1984 Chronic pelvic pain and depression. Psychopathology 17: 132–136

Mahmood T A, Templeton A A, Thomson L, Fraser C 1991 Menstrual symptoms in women with pelvic endometriosis. British Journal of Obstetrics and Gynaecology 98: 558–563

Metheney W P, Smith R P 1989 The relationships among exercise, stress and primary dysmenorrhea. Journal of Behavioral Medicine 12: 569–586

Morris N, O'Neill D 1958 Outpatient gynaecology. British Medical Journal 2: 1038

Murphy A, Fliegner J 1981 Diagnostic laparoscopy. Role in the management of acute pelvic pain. Medical Journal of Australia 1: 571–573

Nicassio P M 1980 Behavioural management of dysmenorrhea: an overview. In: Dan A J, Graham E A, Beecher C P (eds) The menstrual cycle: a synthesis of interdisciplinary research. Springer, New York, vol 1, p 273–282

Pearce S 1986 A psychological investigation of chronic pelvic pain in women. PhD Thesis, University of London

Pearce S, Erskine A 1991 Pain in gynaecology. In: Davis H, Fallowfield L (eds) Counselling and communication in health care. John Wiley, Chichester, ch II

Pearce S, Knight C, Beard R W 1982 Pelvic pain – a common gynaecological problem. Journal of Psychosomatic Obstetrics and Gynaecology 1: 12–17

Petrucco D M, Harris R D 1981 Pelvic pain – the disease with 20 different names. In: Dennerstein L, Burrows G D (eds) Obstetrics, gynaecology and psychiatry. York Press, Victoria, Australia, p 111–118

Pettit P D, Lee R A 1988 Ovarian remnant syndrome: diagnostic dilemma and surgical challenge. Obstetrics and Gynecology 71: 580–583

Pilowsky I 1978 Psychodynamic aspects of pain experience. In: Sternbach R A (ed) The psychology of pain. Raven Press, New York, p 203–217

Quillen M A, Denney D R 1982 Self-control of dysmenorrheic symptoms through pain management training. Journal of Behaviour Therapy and Experimental Psychiatry 13: 123–130

Randall C L 1963 Ovarian conservation. Progress in Gynecology 4: 457–464

Rapkin A J 1986 Adhesions and pelvic pain. A retrospective study. Obstetrics and Gynecology 68: 13–15

Reginald P W, Beard R W, Kooner J S et al 1987 Intravenous dihydroergotamine to relieve pelvic congestion with pain in young women. Lancet 2: 351–353

Reginald P W, Pearge S, Beard R W 1988 Pelvic pain due to venous congestion. In: Studd J (ed) Progress in obstetrics and gynaecology. Churchill Livingstone, Edinburgh, p 275–292

Reid B A, Gangar K F, Rogers V E, Stones R W, Beard R W 1992 Premature menopause and hormone replacement therapy. Are 'conventional' HRT regimens adequate? Abstract no. 70. 25th British Congress of Obstetrics and Gynaecology (Part 1). Royal College of Obstetricians and Gynaecologists, London

Reiter R C 1990 A profile of women with chronic pelvic pain. Clinical Obstetrics and Gynaecology 33: 130–136

Reiter R C, Gambone J C 1990 Demographic and historic variables in women with idiopathic chronic pelvic pain. Obstetrics and Gynecology 75: 428–432

Renaer M, Nijs P, Van Assche A, Vertommen H 1980 Chronic pelvic pain without obvious pathology in women. Personal observations and a review of the problem. European Journal of Obstetrics and Gynaecology and Reproductive Biology 10: 415–463

Roddick J W, Conkey G, Jacobs E J 1960 The hormonal response of endometrium in endometriotic implants and its relationship to symptomatology. American Journal of Obstetrics and Gynecology 79: 1173–1177

Royal College of Obstetricians and Gynaecologists 1978 Gynaecological laparoscopy. Report of the Working Party of the Confidential Enquiry into Gynaecological Laparoscopy. Chamberlain G, Brown J C (eds). RCOG, London

Schmidt C 1985 Endometriosis: a reappraisal of pathogenesis and treatment. Fertility and Sterility 44: 157–173

Scoutt L M, McCarthy S M 1990 Applications of magnetic resonance imaging to gynecology. Topics in Magnetic Resonance Imaging 2: 37–49

Seski J C, Diokno A C 1979 Bladder dysfunction after radical abdominal hysterectomy. American Journal of Obstetrics and Gynecology 128: 643–651

Shaw, R W 1992 Endometriosis. In Shaw R W, Soutter W P, Stanton S L (eds) Gynaecology. Churchill Livingstone, London, p 421–435

Siddall-Allum J, Beard R W, Witherow R O N, Rogers V, Rae T 1993 The ovarian remnant: a cause for persistent pelvic pain after hysterectomy and bilateral salpingo-oophorectomy. Presented at the Royal Society of Medicine, February 1993

Sippo W C, Burghardt A, Gomez D C 1987 Nerve entrapment after Pfannenstiel incision. American Journal of Obstetrics and Gynecology 157: 420–421

Skandhan K P, Pandya A K, Skandhan S, Mehta Y B 1988 Menarche: prior knowledge and experience. Adolescence 23: 149–154

Slocumb J C 1984 Neurological factors in chronic pelvic pain: trigger points and the abdominal pelvic pain syndrome. American Journal of Obstetrics and Gynecology 149: 536–543

Slocumb J C 1990 Chronic, somatic myofascial and neurogenic abdominal pain. Clinical Obstetrics and Gynecology 33: 145–153

Stacey C M, Munday P E, Beard R W 1989 Pelvic inflammatory disease: diagnosis and microbiology. Presented at the Silver Jubilee Congress of Obstetrics and Gynaecology, London, July 1989

Stearns H C, Sneeden U D 1966 Observations on the clinical and pathological aspects of the pelvic congestion syndrome. American Journal of Obstetrics and Gynecology 94: 718–732

Steege J F 1987 Ovarian remnant syndrome. Obstetrics and Gynecology 70: 64–67

Sturmdorf A 1916 Tracheloplastic methods and results. Surgery, Gynecology and Obstetrics 22: 93–104

Sutton C, Hill D 1990 Laser laparoscopy in the treatment of endometriosis. A 5-year study. British Journal of Obstetrics and Gynaecology 97: 178–180

Svedlund J, Ottosson J-O, Sjodin I, Doteval G 1983 Controlled study of psychotherapy in irritable bowel syndrome. Lancet 2: 589–592

Symmonds R E, Pettit P D M 1979 Ovarian remnant syndrome. Obstetrics and Gynecology 54: 174–177

Tait L 1883 The pathology and treatment of the diseases of the ovaries. William Wood, New York

Taylor H C 1949a Vascular congestion and hyperemia I: Psychologic basis and history of the concept. American Journal of Obstetrics and Gynecology 57: 211–230

Taylor H C 1949b Vascular congestion and hyperemia II: The clinical aspects of the congestion–fibrosis syndrome. American Journal of Obstetrics and Gynecology 57: 637–653

Taylor H C 1949c Vascular congestion and hyperemia III: Etiology and therapy. American Journal of Obstetrics and Gynecology 57: 654–668

Thomas D C, McArdle F J, Rogers V G, Beard R W, Brown B H 1991 Local blood volume changes in women with pelvic congestion measured by applied potential tomography. Clinical Science 81: 401–404

Thomas D C, Stones R W, Farquhar C M, Beard R W 1992 Measurement of pelvic blood flow changes in response to posture in normal subjects and in women with pelvic pain owing to congestion by using a thermal technique. Clinical Science 83: 55–58

Thompson W G, Heaton K W 1980 Functional bowel disorders in apparently healthy people. Gastroenterology 79: 283–288

Topolanski-Sierra R 1958 Pelvic phlebography. American Journal of Obstetrics and Gynecology 76: 44–52

Vernon M W, Beard J S, Graves K, Wilson E A 1986 Classification of endometriotic implants by morphological appearance and capacity to synthesize prostaglandin F. Fertility and Sterility 46: 801–805

Wardle P 1992. In: Shaw R W (ed) Conference Report: Intractable gynaecological pain – new management strategies. Royal College of Obstetricians and Gynaecologists, 1 April 1992. Journal of Obstetrics and Gynaecology 12: 355–359

Webb M J 1989 Ovarian remnant syndrome. Australian and New Zealand Journal of Obstetrics and Gynaecology 29: 433–435

Wharton L R 1959 Two cases of supernumerary ovary and one accessory ovary, with an analysis of previously reported cases. American Journal of Obstetrics and Gynecology 78: 1101–1119

Whittle G C, Slade P, Ronalds C M 1987 Social support in women reporting dysmenorrhea. Journal of Psychosomatic Research 31: 79–84

Whorwell P J, McCallum M, Creed F H, Roberts C T 1986 Non-colonic features of irritable bowel syndrome. Gut 27: 37–40

Wilson C A, Keye W R 1989 A survey of adolescent dysmenorrhea and premenstrual symptom frequency: a model program for prevention, detection and treatment. Journal of Adolescent Health Care 10: 317–322

Woodward J 1992 In Shaw R W (ed) Conference Report: Intractable gynaecological pain – new management strategies. Royal College of Obstetricians and Gynaecologists, 1 April 1992. Journal of Obstetrics and Gynaecology 12: 355–359

Youssef A E 1958a The uterine isthmus and its sphincter mechanism I. The uterine isthmus under normal conditions. American Journal of Obstetrics and Gynecology 75: 1305–1319

Youssef A E 1958b The uterine isthmus and its sphincter mechanism II. The uterine isthmus under abnormal conditions. American Journal of Obstetrics and Gynecology 75: 1320–1332

34. Labour pain

John J. Bonica

INTRODUCTION

Effective control of pain of childbirth has long been an important health and sociological issue worldwide and remains so today (Bonica 1967, 1980, 1993a). This is for several reasons. For one thing, contrary to the claims of proponents of 'natural childbirth' and 'educated childbirth' that labour and vaginal delivery can and should be painless, it has been known for a long time that labour and delivery are painful events for most women. Also misconceptions exist among the public and some physicians, nurses, midwives and other health professionals about the nature, function and effects of labour pain, and about methods for its control. Many believe that the pain has an important biological function and should not be relieved; others believe that pharmacological methods of pain relief have deleterious effects on the mother and fetus and should be avoided (Dick-Read 1933, 1953; Lamaze 1956). Finally, and most importantly, obstetric analgesia and anaesthesia has been neglected until recently by the medical profession.

Fortunately, during the past two decades, especially during the 1980s, there has been a surge of interest among anaesthetists, obstetricians, nurses and the lay public. This has prompted an expanding amount of basic and clinical research in this field, producing much new information on the physiology and pathophysiology of the mother, fetus and newborn. This has been paralleled by an ever-increasing number of anaesthetists who have a special interest in this field and in some countries the subspecialty of 'obstetric anaesthesia' has developed. The Society of Obstetric Anesthesia and Perinatology (SOAP) in the United States and Canada and the Obstetric Anaesthesia Association (OAA) in the United Kingdom are very active organisations, holding national, international and regional meetings. An impressive number of textbooks, monographs, articles, major journals and other types of communication is now available.

All of these activities have reaffirmed many of the points made in the previous edition of this chapter, including the wide recognition that pain has the important biological function of indicating to the gravida that labour is beginning. It is also recognised that once pain has served its function, it must be relieved effectively, because persistent severe pain and the associated stress response have harmful effects on the mother and possibly on the fetus and newborn. Improperly administered analgesia and anaesthesia can entail the risk of complications and contribute to maternal and perinatal morbidity and even mortality. However, there is now impressive evidence that, properly administered, they do not contribute to maternal and perinatal mortality and morbidity rates, but may help to reduce them, especially in high-risk pregnancies (Crawford 1984; Albright et al 1986; Shnider & Levinson 1987; Gabbe et al 1991; Bonica & McDonald 1993). Finally, many gravidas in developed countries, having been informed of the benefits of modern analgesia by the news media and other sources, expect effective pain relief during their labour and delivery.

The purpose of this chapter is to give a concise overview of the nature of pain of childbirth, its impact on the mother, the fetus and newborn, and the therapeutic modalities that currently are being used to relieve the pain. The material is presented under the following headings:

1. the magnitude of the problem, including a brief historical perspective and the frequency, intensity, and other characteristics of labour pain
2. the nature of labour pain, including its mechanism and the factors that influence its frequency and severity
3. the physiological, psychological and sociological effects of labour pain on the mother, the fetus, the forces of labour and the newborn, and how these can be modified by analgesia with consequent benefit to the mother and perinate
4. a summary of the current methods being used to relieve childbirth pain.

This material represents an updated summary of previously published works (Bonica 1967, 1969; Bonica & McDonald 1990, 1993) and information that can be found in other textbooks (Crawford 1984; Albright et al 1986; Shnider & Levinson 1987).

MAGNITUDE OF THE PROBLEM

The aforementioned misconceptions and confusion about the nature of labour pain and its treatment have probably been due to our lack of knowledge and, although there is much new information, the current progress in research and patient care needs to be nurtured and expanded. Many of the proponents of natural childbirth have added to the misconceptions and confusion by insisting that pain need not occur during normal labour and when it does it is the product of modern cultural and environmental factors.

The origin of this notion is not known, but among the first to mention it was Behan who stated (1914):

> Like menstruation, childbirth naturally should be a painless process. It is only as culture advances that the labour becomes painful, for in women of primitive races pain is absent. Savages of low degree of civilisation are generally little troubled by parturiency.

Later the same argument was put forth by Dick-Read (1933, 1953), by Velvovski et al (1950) who developed the technique of psychoprophylaxis in the USSR in the late 1940s and by Lamaze (1956) who did much to popularise psychoprophylaxis in the western world. In more recent years the idea that, with intensive antepartal preparation of the gravida, childbirth can be painless in most parturients has been retained by many midwives and some physicians/obstetricians. As mentioned below, the controlled studies carried out by Melzack and his associates (Melzack 1984) revealed that this is not the case and prompted him to entitle one of his publications *The Myth of Painless Childbirth*.

The claim by Dick-Read (1933, 1953) and other enthusiasts of natural childbirth that primitive women experienced no more pain in labour than the animals among which they fought for existence, is disputed by a number of studies. It is unlikely that the process of labour, and consequently the physiological stimulus of the pain associated with it, was any different in prehistoric times from what it is now.

For example, Ford (1945), who studied this and other problems of reproduction in 64 primitive societies, wrote that: 'the popular impression of childbirth in primitive society as painless and easy is definitely contraindicated in our cases. As a matter of fact, it is often prolonged and painful.' Freedman & Ferguson (1950) reported that the pain response in these groups during childbirth was similar to that observed in American and European parturients. Similar views have been expressed by others who have studied the problem of labour pain in primitive societies (Jochelson 1910). I have personally observed several dozen parturients in primitive societies in Australia and Africa, most of whom manifested severe pain behaviour (unpublished data). Mention of the prevalence and importance of pain during childbirth is found in the writings of the ancient Babylonians, Egyptians, Chinese, Hebrews and Greeks, and in the writings of many subsequent cultures and civilisations (Lévy-Strauss 1956).

Finally, a recent study by Lefebvre & Carli (1985) of parturition of 88 individuals of 29 species of captive and wild nonhuman primates, revealed that 69 (78%) manifested moderate to very severe pain, characterised by straining, stretching, arching, grimacing, writhing, shaking, doubling-up, restlessness and vocalisation. This article provides impressive evidence that while the behaviour of the monkeys varied according to environmental circumstances, the process of parturition in these animals provoked, in varying degress, what in humans we would call pain.

Prevalence and intensity of labour pain

Although it is a common observation in obstetrics that parturients vary in the amount of suffering associated with labour and vaginal delivery, well designed studies on the prevalence, intensity and quality of labour pain have been very few in number. In a study of 78 Swedish randomly selected primiparae, Nettelbladt et al (1976) found that 35% reported intolerable pain, 37% had severe pain and 28% had moderate pain during labour and delivery. Lundh (1974) published a survey of Swedish investigations which included both primiparae and multiparae, and which revealed that the incidence of intolerable severe pain ranged between 35 and 58% with the remainder having moderate pain, while Bundsen (1975) found that 77% of primiparae reported that their pain during childbirth was severe or intolerable. I have observed (and, in many cases, interviewed) 2700 parturients in 121 obstetric centres (some supporting 100–150 deliveries per day) in 35 countries on six continents, while visiting or working, demonstrating obstetric anaesthetic techniques. Their records indicated that the frequency and intensity of labour pain were as follows: 15% had little or no pain; 35% had moderate pain; 30% had severe pain, and 20% had very severe pain. The figures are similar to those noted among over 8000 American parturients to whom I have administered or supervised anaesthetic care during the past four decades (Bonica, unpublished data).

Obviously, these surveys and observations have been based on very simple numerical or verbal descriptors of pain and thus lack quantification. One of the first attempts to quantify the intensity of labour pain was made by Javert & Hardy (1950), who used the Hardy–Wolff–Goodell dolorimeter to induce experimental pain and asked the parturients to compare it to the pain of their labour. The method entailed the application of thermal heat, measured in millicalories (mcal) to 3.5 cm^2 of skin for 3 seconds, and increasing the stimulus intensity stepwise until perceptible pain (pain threshold) and eventually the greatest perceivable pain (ceiling or maximun pain) were induced. They used a pain scale that ranged from 1 pain unit or 'dol', assigned to pain threshold, to 12.5 dol, denoting maximum pain, which was produced by a stimulus of sufficient intensity to produce a third-degree burn. They studied 26 primiparae and six multiparae during the course of normal labour and delivery and found that the intensity of pain in the early part (latent phase) of the first stage was 2–3 dol (very mild) and then increased progressively to 3–4 dol at about 4 cm cervical dilatation, to 5–7 dol at 6–8 cm dilatation, to 8–9 dol at full dilatation, and ranged between 9 and 10.5 dol or maximum pain as the head dilated and stretched the perineum during the second stage.

The incidence, intensity, quality and other aspects of labour pain have been elucidated more precisely by Melzack and associates (Melzack et al 1981, 1984; Melzack & Schaffelberg 1987; Melzack & Belanger 1989) who have carried out a series of studies using the McGill Pain Questionnaire (MPQ) (1975), the most extensively tested multidimensional scale of pain measurement available. The MPQ consists of 20 sets of words describing the sensory, effective and evaluative dimension of the pain experience. In the first study (1981), labour pain was measured with the MPQ in 87 primiparae and 54 multiparae, all of whom had cervical dilatation of at least 2–3 cm and contractions at intervals of 5 minutes or less. Of the 141 parturients, 61 primiparae and 30 multiparae had received prepared childbirth training in specialised training units in hospitals or private clinics, while 26 primiparae and 24 multiparae had received no training.

It was found that the mean total pain rating index (PRI) was 34 for primiparae and 30 for multiparae, thus confirming the widely held view that labour is significantly more painful for the first birth than for later births. As might be expected, although the average intensity of labour pain was extremely high, a wide range in pain scores was observed, which Melzack (1984) divided into six groups within the range of the PRI scores recorded (range 2–62) as shown in Figure 34.1A. Assigning verbal descriptors of pain intensity to these data suggests that about 10% of primiparae and about 24% of multiparae experienced 'mild to moderate' pain; about 30% of both groups rated their pain as 'severe'; about 38% of primiparae and 35% of multiparae felt 'very severe' pain and 22% of primiparae and 11% of multiparae experienced 'horrible' or 'excruciating' pain. Melzack (1984) compared the mean total PRI scores for several pain syndromes obtained in earlier studies (Melzack 1975; Melzack et al 1982) with those of labour and noted that the scores for labour pain were 8–10 points higher than those associated with back pain, cancer pain, phantom limb pain, arthritis and postherpetic neuralgia (Fig. 34.1B).

The mean PRI score of the 61 primiparae who had received prepared childbirth training was 33 and for the 26 primiparae who received no training it was 37 (Fig. 34.1B). On the other hand, no significant difference was noted in any of the PRI scores of the 30 multiparae who had received training and 24 who had not received training.

Of the 28 parturients who were given successful epidural analgesia, the PRI scores decreased from a mean of 28 before the block to a mean of 8 and 7.6 at 30 and 60 minutes respectively, after induction of analgesia. These scores were based on the use of such words as 'numbness', 'pressing' and 'tingling' which were apparently sensations from the effects of the epidural block.

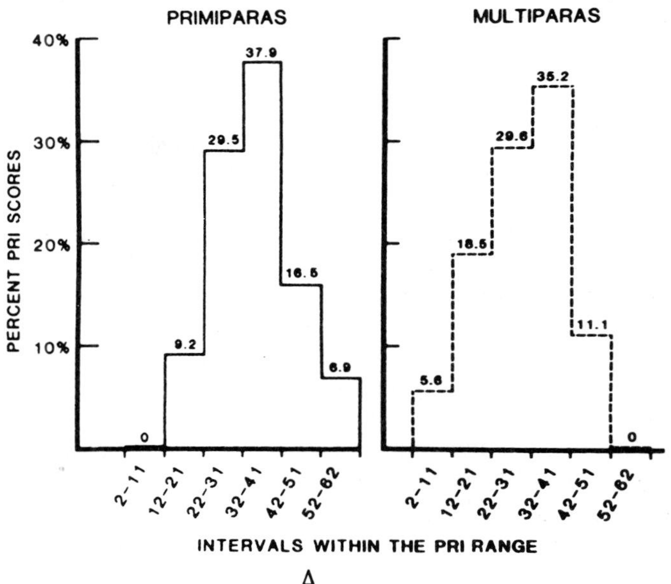

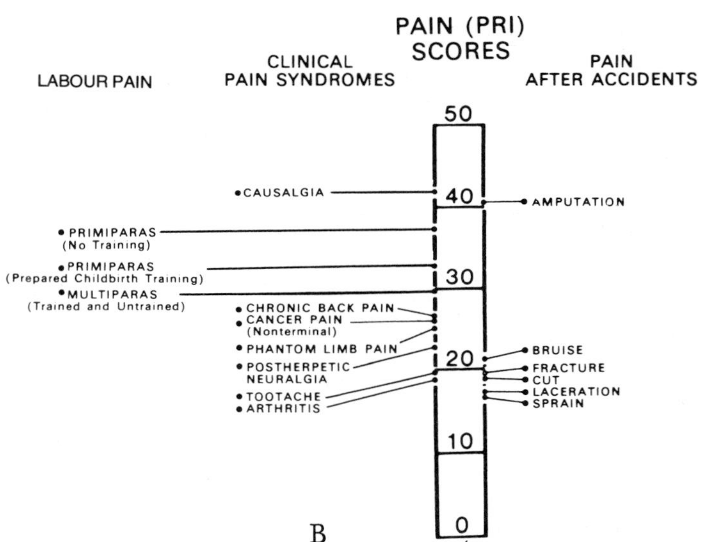

Fig. 34.1 **A** Distribution of PRI scores of primiparae and multiparae in six intervals of the total pain rating index (PRI) range. (From Melzack 1984.) **B** Comparison of the intensity of labour pain with other clinical pain syndromes. (From Melzack 1985.)

In another study, Melzack et al (1984) studied pain curves as labour progressed for both trained and untrained women. Although these curves indicated a gradually rising pain intensity, graphs of pain scores obtained from individual parturients revealed a high level of variability as labour progressed.

Similar results were reported by Gaston-Johansson and associates (1988), who studied 130 Swedish parturients, using a modified MPQ and visual analogue scale to quantitate pain during three phases of the first stage of labour: when cervical dilatation was 2–4, 5–7 and 8–10 cm. Among the 138 parturients, 80% of the primiparae and 20% of the multiparae had received prepared childbirth training. A total of 72% of primiparae and 27% of multiparae received meperidine. Despite the preparation for childbirth and systemic analgesia, most of the primiparae and over two-thirds of the multiparae reported severe pain during the first stage of labour. Primiparae reported more intense pain than multiparae, even though they consumed significantly more pain medication than did multiparae. It is of interest to note that individuals who had participated in childbirth training reported significantly higher in-labour pain scores than those who did not participate. The authors commented that prepared childbirth while providing much information may lead to unrealistic expectations about in-labour pain, and consequently patients invariably experienced much more pain than they had anticipated.

MECHANISMS, PATHWAYS AND CHARACTERISTICS OF THE PAIN OF CHILDBIRTH

To provide optimal pain relief with regional analgesia, it is essential for the obstetric team to understand the peripheral mechanisms and pathways of the pain of parturition and the factors that influence its intensity, duration and quality. Most of these factors vary during the different phases and stages of labour and are therapeutically significant, so they are considered separately.

Pain of the first stage of labour

Intrinsic mechanisms

During much of the first stage, labour pain is caused entirely by uterine contractions and their effects. The hypotheses formerly proposed to account for the pain include:

1. pressure on nerve endings between the muscle fibres of the body and the fundus of the uterus (Reynolds 1949)
2. contraction of the ischaemic myometrium and cervix consequent to expulsion of blood from the uterus during the contraction (Moir 1939), or due to vasoconstriction consequent to sympathetic hyperactivity caused by fear (Dick-Read 1953)
3. inflammatory changes in the uterine muscles (Reynolds 1949)
4. contraction of the cervix and lower uterine segment consequent to fear-induced hyperactivity of the sympathetic nervous system (Dick-Read 1953).

The evidence against these hypotheses is discussed in detail in the chapter that appeared in the second edition of this book (Bonica & Chadwick 1989). Most available data support the concept that the pain of the first stage of labour is predominantly a result of dilatation of the cervix (CX) and lower uterine segment (LUS) and of the consequent distension, stretching and tearing of these structures during contractions. An added aetiological factor is the contraction of the uterus under isometric conditions, that is, against the obstruction presented by the cervix and perineum, which is the 'adequate stimulus' for provoking pain in hollow viscera.

Peripheral neural pathways

For nearly a century, based on the results published by Head (1893) and subsequently by Cleland (1933), it was widely taught that nociceptive impulses from the body of the uterus are transmitted through T11 and T12 nerves and that pain from the LUS and CX is transmitted through the pelvic nerve to the S2, S3, and S4 spinal segments. Because my own observations were at variance with this concept, my colleagues (Akamatsu, Kohl, Kennedy and others) and I carried out a study that involved 305 parturients and 41 gynaecological patients investigated over a period of 22 years. Discrete blocks with local anaesthetics of various nociceptive pathways during the entire course of the first and second stages of labour were achieved by paravertebral blocks of two, three or four nerves of T10, T11, T12, and L1; segmental epidural block involving different segments; ascending caudal block; lumbar sympathetic block and transsacral block of one or more sacral spinal nerves (Bonica 1969, 1974, 1979). The results demonstrated conclusively that the CX and LUS are not supplied by the sensory fibres that accompany pelvic nerves (nervi erigentes), as stated in almost every modern anatomy and obstetric textbook (Gray 1973, 1980; Romanes 1972; Williams 1985). Rather, they are supplied by afferents which, like those that supply the body of the uterus, accompany the sympathetic nerves as depicted in Figure 34.2. Despite repeated publication of these results, anatomy and obstetric textbooks continue to insist that the CX is supplied by sacral segments.

The A-delta and C primary afferent fibres that supply the uterus and CX accompany the sympathetic nerves in the following sequence; the uterine and cervical plexus; the pelvic (inferior hypogastric) plexus; the middle

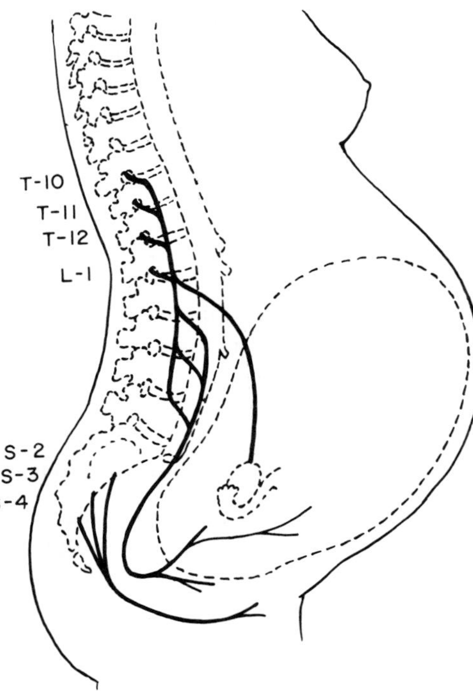

Fig. 34.2 Schema of the peripheral nociceptive pathways involved in the pain of childbirth. Note that the uterus, including the cervix, is supplied by sensory fibres that are associated with the sympathetic nerves supplied to the uterus. The course of the nociceptive fibres starting from the nerve endings in the uterus and cervix to the spinal cord pass through the uterine and cervical plexuses and then sequentially through the pelvic (inferior hypogastric) plexus, the middle hypogastric plexus or nerve and the superior hypogastric plexus; from this structure they pass to the lumbar sympathetic chain through two major nerves that lie posterior to the common iliac arteries and also through lumbar splanchnic nerves. From the lumbar sympathetic chain they proceed cephalad through the lower thoracic chain and then leave it by coursing through the white rami communicantes connected with T10, T11, T12 and L1 spinal nerves, and finally course through these nerves and their posterior roots to enter the spinal cord and make contact with dorsal horn neurons. Nociceptive fibres from the perineal structures course through the pudendal nerve and into the spinal cord through the posterior roots of S2, S3 and S4. In addition, the lower lumbar and upper sacral segments supply nerves to pelvic structures which become involved in the pain of parturition.

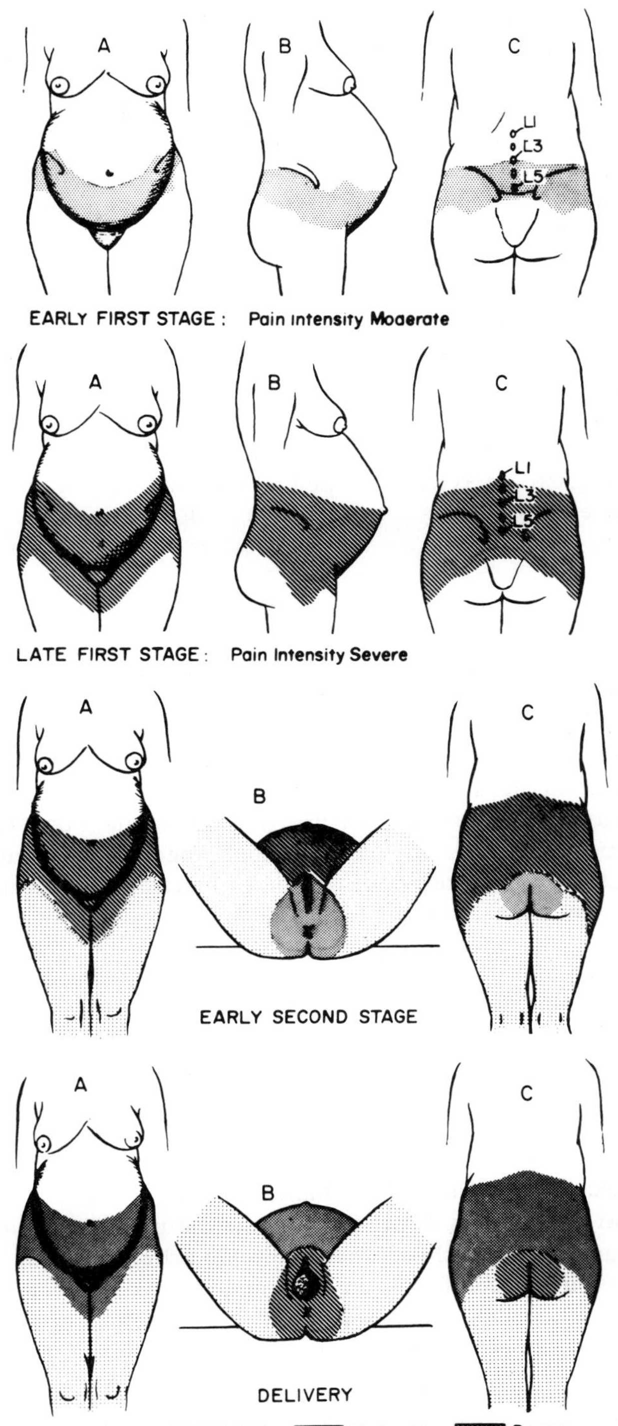

Fig. 34.3 The intensity and distribution of parturition pain during the various phase of labour and delivery. **A** anterior view; **B** lateral view; **C** posterior view. (From Bonica 1980.)

hypogastric plexus or nerve, and the superior hypogastric and aortic plexuses. The nociceptive afferents then pass to the lumbar sympathetic chain and course cephalad through the lower thoracic sympathetic chain, which they leave by way of the rami communicantes associated with the T10, T11, T12, and L1 spinal nerves. Finally, they pass through the posterior roots of these nerves to make synaptic contact with interneurons in the dorsal horn. Typically of pain arising from viscera, the pain caused by uterine contractions is referred to the dermatomes supplied by the same spinal cord segments which receive input from the uterus and CX (see Fig. 34.3, and discussion after the next section; this is followed by discussion of the pathways and mechanisms of the nociception in the neuraxis and the responses thereto).

These findings have been recently confirmed in animal experiments carried out by a number of investigators (Kawatani et al 1986; Peters et al 1987; Berkeley et al 1988, 1993a, 1993b; Berkeley & Wood 1989; Berkeley

1990). Berkeley and her associates have carried out a systematic and comprehensive series of experiments, using in vitro and in vivo electrophysiological and behavioural studies of the nerve supply of the uterus and other pelvic organs. These investigators have used mechanical and chemical stimuli of the uterine cavity including the cervix and vagina. Their findings led them to conclude that afferent fibres in the hypogastric and other sympathetic nerves are concerned with the transmission of nociceptive information. In contrast, the uterine pelvic nerve afferent fibres are capable of conveying information regarding more physiologically innocuous events that are likely to subserve a wide range of reproductive functions. These afferent fibres differ considerably from, but must somehow be coordinated with, those of the hypogastric nerve during the lifetime course of reproductive events.

Second and third stages of labour

Intrinsic mechanisms

Once the cervix is fully dilated, the amount of nociceptive stimulation arising in this structure decreases, but the contractions of the body of the uterus and distension of the lower uterine segment continue to cause pain in the same areas of reference as in the first stage of labour (Fig. 34.3, uppermost row). In addition, the progressively greater pressure of the presenting part on pain-sensitive structures in the pelvis, and the distension of the outlet and perineum, become new sources of pain. Progressively greater distension causes intense stretching and actual tearing of fascia and subcutaneous tissues and pressure on the skeletal muscles of the perineum. Like other pain caused by stimulation of superficial somatic structures, the perineal pain is sharp and well localised, predominantly in the regions supplied by the pudendal nerves, and can be eliminated by block of these nerves (see final section of this chapter) (Klink 1953; Bonica 1967).

In the late part of the first stage and during the second stage, a number of parturients develop aching, burning or cramping discomfort in the thigh and less frequently in the legs. This is presumably a result of stimulation of pain-sensitive structures in the pelvic cavity, including:

1. traction on the pelvic parietal peritoneum and the structures it envelops, including the uterine ligaments
2. stretching and tension of the bladder, urethra, and rectum
3. stretching and tension of ligaments, fascia, and muscles in the pelvic cavity
4. abnormal pressure on one or more roots of the lumbosacral plexus.

These factors usually produce mild pain referred to the lower lumbar and sacral segments; but, if the fetus is in an abnormal position with greater than usual pressure by the presenting part, the referred pain can become moderate or severe.

Neural pathways

The neural pathways for the second and third stages of labour involve the pudendal nerve and other smaller nerves which are derived from S2, S3, and S4. The pain caused by pressure on the intrapelvic structures and which is felt in the thigh and upper legs usually involves the L2–S3 spinal segments.

Patterns of distribution of pain of parturition

As noted above the pain of the first stage of labour is referred to the dermatomes supplied by the same spinal cord segments that receive nociceptive input form the uterus and cervix. During the latent (very early) phase of the first stage, the pain is felt as an ache or moderate cramp and is limited to the T11 and T12 dermatomes (Fig. 34.3, uppermost row). As labour progresses the active phase of the first stage (usually 3–4 cm cervical dilatation), and the uterine contractions, become more intense, the pain in the T11 and T12 dermatomes becomes more severe, is described as sharp and cramping and spreads to the two adjacent (T10 and L1) dermatomes (Fig. 34.3, second row).

The distribution of the T10, T11, T12 and L1 dermatomes in the back overlies the lower three lumbar vertebrae and the upper half of the sacrum. This distribution of pain during the first stage of labour has been misinterpreted as showing transmission by the lower lumbar and sacral spinal segments. However, the low back pain is the result of nociceptive transmission in the T10–L1 segments proved by the observation that epidural block limited to these four segments produces relief of the low back pain, until descent of the presenting part causes pressure on the pelvic structures that are supplied by the lower lumbar and sacral segments (see below). As previously mentioned, often the pain is not referred to the entire dermatome but can be more severe in one or more patches of varying size within a territory of one or more dermatomes. However, one can demonstrate hyperalgesia in the entire extent of the involved dermatomes.

In the late first stage and in the second stage of labour, the pain is felt most sharply in the perineum, in the lower part of the sacrum, anus and frequently, in the thighs (Fig. 34.3, second and third rows). As mentioned earlier, in the late part of the first stage, and during the second stage, aching, burning or cramping discomfort in the thighs and less frequently in the legs may develop (Fig. 34.3, third and lowermost rows).

Other factors influencing the pain of childbirth

In addition to the role played by such intrinsic factors as the intensity, duration, and pattern of contractions and related physiological and biochemical mechanisms, the extent of pain and suffering associated with childbirth is influenced by physical, physiological, psychological, emotional and motivational factors (Lundh 1974; Bundsen 1975; Nettelbladt et al 1976; Norr et al 1977; Eustace 1978; Marx 1979; Melzack et al 1981, 1984; Scott-Palmer & Skevington 1981; Kohnen 1986; Melzack & Schaffelberg 1987; Fridh et al 1988). Although different investigators found differences in the role played by each of the factors discussed below, there is a consensus that many of these play an important role in determining the incidence, intensity and quality of pain in the general parturient population.

Physical factors

Physical factors that influence the incidence, severity and duration of the pain of childbirth include the age, parity and physical condition of the parturient, the condition of the cervix at the outset of labour and the relationship of the size of the infant to the size of the birth canal. Many of these factors are interrelated. Generally, an uninformed, unmarried teenage gravida may experience more anxiety-induced pain. Moreover, older (>40 years) primiparae experience longer, more painful labours than young primiparae. The cervix of the multipara begins to soften even before the onset of labour and is less sensitive than that of the primiparae. In general, the intensity of uterine contractions in early labour tends to be higher in primiparae than in multiparae, whereas in the later phase of labour the reverse is true (Melzack et al 1981, 1984; Melzack & Schaffelberg 1987; Gaston-Johansson et al 1988).

In the presence of dystocia caused by a contracted pelvis, a large baby or abnormal presentation, the parturient experiences more pain than under normal conditions. Melzack and associates (1984) found that the heavier the primipara per unit of height, the higher the pain scores. The same variable contributed to the pain scores of multiparae and in addition, heavier mothers and those with heavier babies had higher pain scores.

There are also a number of reports cited by Kohnen (1986) that women who labour and deliver in the vertical position (sitting, standing or squatting), experience less pain and have a shorter second stage of labour. However, in a recent study by Melzack & Belanger (1989) in which they used part of the MPQ and Visual Analogue Scale to measure pain intensity, they found that in the latent and early first stage of labour, parturients had less pain in the vertical position, but in the late first stage and second stage they experienced less pain in the lateral supine position. This confirms results reported by others.

Melzack and associates (Melzack et al 1981, 1984; Melzack & Schaffelberg 1987) found that high pain scores were associated with menstrual difficulties. They also noted that menstrual pain felt in the back, but not in the front, was correlated with increasing levels of pain in the abdomen and back, during contractions and with the continuous low back pain previously mentioned. Similar relationships between menstrual pain and higher pain scores were reported by Fridh and associates (unpublished), who also noted that primiparae had more pain in the late first stage, whereas multiparae had more pain in the early first stage. Marx (1979) has presented strong evidence that women who have dysmenorrhoea produce excessive amounts of prostaglandins, which trigger uterine contractions, and that drugs that inhibit prostaglandin synthesis also diminish menstrual pain. Melzack (1984) has suggested that because of the positive correlation between menstrual pain and the pain during childbirth, it is conceivable that parturients who suffer severe labour pain may also produce excessive prostaglandins during labour.

Fatigue, loss of sleep and general debility influence a parturient's tolerance of the painful experience and increase the pain behaviour. This is particularly significant in parturients with prolonged labour.

Physiological and biochemical factors

A number of studies have demonstrated a progressive increase during labour of plasma beta-endorphin, beta-lipotropin and adrenocorticotropic hormone (ACTH) levels, all of which are derived from a common precursor (Csontos et al 1980; Goland et al 1981; Facchinetti et al 1982; Abboud et al 1983; Fettes et al 1984; Goebelsmann et al 1984). These values have been found to peak, at delivery or in the immediate postpartum period, at 4–10 times the prelabour and nonpregnant values. These findings have led to the speculation that plasma beta-endorphin might have an intrinsic analgesic role during parturition (Facchinetti et al 1982). However plasma beta-endorphins at levels considerably higher than those observed in these studies do not appear to cross the blood–brain barrier or have analgesic effects on nonpregnant humans and Foley et al (1979) cast doubt on the idea.

On the other hand, other opioid systems may play a role in raising the pain tolerance threshold. This suggestion is based on the findings of Gintzler (1980) who noted that the pain threshold in rats rises at the end of pregnancy, peaks around delivery and returns to normal nonpregnant levels within 12 hours of delivery. This 'pregnancy-induced analgesia', or more properly 'hypalgesia', is blocked by the opioid antagonists naloxone and naltrexone. This phenomenon has been observed using several noxious modalities, including response threshold to electric foot shock and tail withdrawal latencies (Gintzler et al 1983;

Sander et al 1988). Similar rises in pain threshold have been noted in studies involving humans during late pregnancy in which responses to radiant heat to dermatomes C1–S1 or intense pressure applied to the forearm were used as aversive (noxious) stimuli (Rust et al 1983; Cogan & Spinnato 1986). Gintzler et al (1983) have identified the pregnancy-induced hypalgesia as resulting from action of spinal dynorphin/kappa opioid receptor systems. These data suggest this system may be sufficient to lower the intensity and perhaps modify the quality of the pain of parturition. This phenomenon may be the factor responsible for a decrease in the minimum anesthetic concentration (MAC) of inhalation anaesthesia required by parturients (Palahniuk et al 1974).

Psychological factors

Psychological factors that can, and frequently do, affect the incidence and intensity of parturition pain include the mentation, attitude and mood of the parturient at the time of labour, and other emotional factors. Fear, apprehension and anxiety probably enhance pain perception and pain behaviour (Deutsch 1955; Zuckerman et al 1963; Brown et al 1972; Myers 1975; Wallach 1982; Reading & Cox 1985; Fridh et al 1988). One of the most frequent causes of fear and anxiety is ignorance or misinformation about the process of pregnancy and parturition and what the onset of labour signifies. An uninformed parturient, especially a primipara, can be disturbed by fear of the unknown, death, suffering, mutilation or possible complications and by concern for her condition or that of her fetus (Deutsch 1955; Gaston-Johansson et al 1988; Fridh et al 1988). Parturients who have had an unplanned or illegitimate pregnancy or have an ambivalent or negative reaction to gestation report more pain than those who do not (Nettelbladt et al 1976).

The relationship between the parturient and her spouse plays an important role in the degree of pain she experiences. Melzack (1984) reported that the effective pain scores were higher when the husband was in the labour room than when he was absent. He suggested that this may reflect genuinely higher effective pain scores or may be due to a deliberate choice of descriptors in the attempt to impress the husband or express anger at him, but in any case, the finding was not spurious. Wallach (1982) found a similar effect in an independent study. In contrast, Nettelbladt and associates (1976), Norr et al (1977) and Fridh et al (1988) found that positive feelings of the expectant father toward the pregnancy seemed to be an important factor in decreasing the mother's feelings of apprehension during pregnancy. When expectant fathers were very supportive of their mates during pregnancy and labour, the women experienced less pain during parturition. Fridh et al (1988) emphasised the need to include supportive fathers in prenatal training.

In contrast, other emotional factors such as intensive motivation and cultural influences can affect modulation of sensory transmissions and certainly can influence the effective and behavioural dimensions of pain. Moreover, cognitive intervention such as giving the parturient preparatory information about labour, thus reducing uncertainty, while focusing attention or producing distraction and dissociation from pain (all parts of an 'educated' childbirth programme) reduces pain behaviour. In a study of 134 low risk parturients at term, Lowe (1989) found that confidence in ability to handle labour was the most significant predictor of all components of pain during active labour. The greater the confidence the parturient had, the less the pain and vice versa.

Cultural and ethnic factors

Racial, cultural and ethnic factors have long been considered to be important in influencing pain tolerance and pain behaviour. Persons of Italian and other Latin cultures, or of Jewish or Mediterranean background, are said to express pain in an emotive fashion and to exaggerate their verbal report, whereas those of Anglo-Saxon origin (e.g. English, third-generation Americans), as well as Scandinavians, Irish, Asians, American Indians and Eskimos, are said to be more stoic and to manifest less pain behaviour (Wolff & Langley 1975). Experimental data and clinical observations, however, suggest that although racial, cultural and ethnic differences do exist, there appear to be differences in expressiveness consequent to underlying attitudes toward the pain, rather than differences in the sensory experience or pain perception.

True (1954) reported that Mojave Indian women experienced a great deal of pain during childbirth but avoided expressing their suffering for fear of ridicule. In an experimental study, Meehan and colleagues (1954) found no significant differences between pain tolerance of American Indians, Eskimos and whites. In a study of Turkomenian women, Preissman & Ogoulbostan-Essenova (1956) noted that they behaved calmly during childbirth and manifested no pain behaviour, but inquiry revealed that the process was very painful. Nettelbladt and associates (1976), in a study of 78 women, noted that 56% of parturients who reported intolerable pain were not rated by the midwives as having very painful deliveries. This discrepancy probably occurred because the parturients manifested less overt pain behaviour than they actually felt, which is a characteristic of Scandinavian culture. Winsberg & Greenlick (1967) examined pain behaviour in black and white parturients who were matched on such parameters as age, social class and education and found no differences in pain responses or estimated degrees of pain.

The hypothesis that cultural and racial differences can

have some influence on pain behaviour, but probably not on the pain felt by parturients, is supported by my own studies (unpublished data) of 2700 parturients in other countries and of 8000 parturients in the United States (see above: Prevalence and intensity of labour pain). In Western and Eastern Europe, Latin America, Africa, Asia, Australia, the Near East and North America, parturients who were not 'educated' and who were psychologically unprepared for childbirth manifested a similar incidence of pain behaviour, although the patterns of behaviour varied. During the contractions some women moaned, others screamed, others writhed and had facial expressions of suffering with little or no verbal expression, whole still others used incantations (said to be specific for labour pain in that particular country). Contrary to traditional belief, Asian women (including Japanese, Chinese, Malaysians, Indians, Cambodians and Thais) did not remain stoic but manifested as much pain behaviour as American and European parturients. Moreover, the large oriental population of Seattle, and the recent influx of refugees from Indochina, afforded the opportunity to observe and interview several hundred parturients from various countries in Southeast Asia. These studies revealed that the frequency and intensity of labour pain and the request for analgesia were the same as for occidental parturients living in Asia and the pain behaviour was similar to that observed among parturients in their native countries (Bonica, unpublished data).

The influence of education and psychological conditioning inherent in psychoprophylaxis and natural childbirth in modifying pain behaviour without significantly affecting pain sensation is now widely appreciated. During 5–10 day visits to obstetric centres practising psychoprophylaxis or natural childbirth in the former Soviet Union, France, Germany, Italy, The Netherlands, Sweden and the United States made over a 5-month period in 1959, I observed about 700 parturients (and interviewed many) who had received training in one of these methods, and over 85% of them manifested little or no pain behaviour during labour and delivery. When questioned the next day, however, most of them indicated that the process had been painful, but many quickly added that they were pleased to cooperate with their instructor and obstetric team. Especially impressive was the marked change in behaviour of Italian parturients in a large obstetric centre in Turin noted during two visits made 5 years apart. During the first visit, in 1954, the labour ward was a scene of cacophony caused by the screaming, pleading and praying of the nearly 50 women in labour in the same ward. In contrast, 5 years later, one heard only an occasional moan from a similar number of parturients who had undergone an intensive course of psychoprophylaxis. Most went through the entire labour and delivery with minimal pain behaviour but later stated that they had had moderate to severe pain.

Summary

It is obvious that the pain and associated responses to noxious stimulation provoked by uterine contractions and other tissue-damaging factors during labour and vaginal delivery are the net effects of highly complex interactions of various neural systems, modulating influences and psychological and cultural factors. Through the interaction of the afferent systems and neocortical processes, the parturient receives perceptual and discriminate information that is analysed and that usually activates motivational/cognitive processes. These, in turn, act on the motor system and initiate psychodynamic mechanisms of anxiety and apprehension that produce the complex physiological, behavioural and affective responses that characterise acute pain.

EFFECTS OF PARTURITION PAIN AND ITS MODIFICATION BY ANALGESIA AND ANAESTHESIA

Labour and vaginal delivery produce tissue damage and, like tissue injury from other causes, it stimulates the endings of A-delta and C nociceptive fibres that transmit the nociceptive information to neurons, primarily in laminae I, IIo and V, but also in lamina VI of the dorsal horn of the spinal cord (Fig. 34.4). Some peripheral neurons make synaptic connections with interneurons that send axons to the anterior and anterolateral horns where they synapse with somatomotor and sympathetic motor neurons, respectively. Particularly important in obstetric anaesthesia is the fact that all of the lamina V neurons that respond to visceral high threshold afferents also respond to low threshold cutaneous afferents from the area of skin supplied by the same spinal cord segments. This convergence of lamina V cells provides a neural basis for the phenomenon of referred pain that occurs during uterine contractions.

After being subjected to modulating influences, some of the nociceptive impulses from the dorsal horn pass to the anterior and anterolateral horns, while others pass to axons that make up the contralateral spinothalamic tract and other ascending systems, conveying the nociceptive information to the brainstem and brain, where it provokes suprasegmental reflex responses and the perception of pain, respectively (Fig. 34.4). These responses include marked stimulation of respiration, circulation, hypothalamic and autonomic (predominantly sympathetic) centres of neuroendocrine function, limbic structures and psychodynamic mechanisms of anxiety and apprehension, resulting in what has come to be known as the 'stress response' to injury. As a result, the parturient incurs marked increases in respiration, circulation and metabolism, and other body functions are altered. These maternal changes can have a deleterious impact on the fetus and

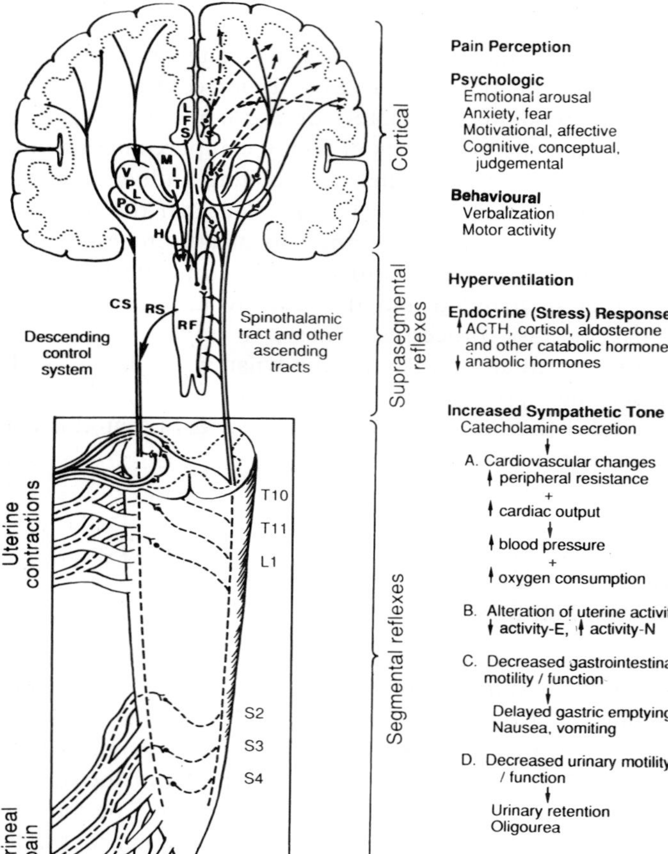

Fig. 34.4 Schematic depiction of the nociceptive input to the spinal cord, provoked by uterine contractions throughout labour and stimulation of the perineum during the second and third stages of labour. The spinothalamic tract and other ascending tracts in the neuraxis are primarily involved in central transmission of nociceptive information to the anterior and anterolateral horn cells of the spinal cord, which provoke segmental reflex responses and impulses that reach the brainstem provoking the suprasegmental responses listed on the right. The nociceptive impulses that reach the brain provoke the cortical responses that include perception of pain, initiation of psychological mechanisms and behavioural responses. On the left is a simple schematic illustration of descending pathways that convey modulating influence from the brain to the spinal cord. RF = reticular formation; RS = reticulospinal; CS = corticospinal; H = hypothalamus; PO = posterior thalamus; VPL = ventral posterolateral thalamus; MIT = medial and intralaminar thalamic nuclei; LFS = limbic forebrain structures. (Modified from Bonica 1990.)

newborn. Pain and reflex responses have a predominant role in these alterations of maternal function, because blockade of the nociceptive pathways by epidural (or other regional) analgesia with a local anaesthetic and an opioid greatly diminish or eliminate them.

The following is a summary of the impact of childbirth pain on the mother, on uterine contractility and on the fetus and newborn and how these are modified by analgesia and anaesthesia. While systemic analgesics such as opioids, sedatives and inhalation analgesia mildly dampen or slightly decrease these reflex responses, the best results are obtained with regional analgesia achieved with a local anaesthetic alone or combined with an opioid as discussed below. In recent years, properly administered continuous lumbar epidural analgesia has been shown to be the most effective method in blocking the nociceptive afferent barrage to the spinal cord (see below).

Effects on the mother

Changes in ventilation

It has long been known that pregnancy produces impressive anatomical and physiological changes involving the respiratory system, including changes in the airways, lung volumes, dynamics of breathing and, particularly, ventilation (Bonica 1973). Beginning from around the third month of gestation, there is an increase in respiratory rate and tidal volume resulting in a 50% increase in minute volume and, since the dead space remains normal, alveolar ventilation increases by 70%. The decrease in lung volumes and the increase in ventilation cause a reduction of arterial and alveolar carbon dioxide tension to an average 32 mmHg at term, and an increase in oxygen tension to about 105 mmHg (Prowse & Gaensler 1965; Bonica 1973).

The pain of childbirth is a powerful respiratory stimulus and consequently causes a further marked increase in tidal volume and minute ventilation, and an even greater increase in alveolar ventilation. This causes a fall of $P\text{aCO}_2$ from the pregnancy level of 32 mmHg to a value of 16–20 mmHg, or occasionally as low as 10–15 mmHg and a concomitant increase in pH to 7.5–7.6 (Cole & Nainby-Luxmoore 1962; Fisher & Prys-Roberts 1968; Bonica 1973; Huch et al 1977; Peabody 1979) (Fig. 34.5). This severe respiratory alkalosis, which occurs at the peak of each uterine contraction, is associated with decreases in cerebral and uterine blood flow and a shift to the left of the maternal oxygen dissociation curve. With the onset of the relaxation phase, pain no longer stimulates respiration so that the hypocapnia causes a transient period of hypoventilation that decreases the maternal $P\text{aO}_2$ by 10–50% with a mean of 25–30% (Huch et al 1977; Peabody 1979). In parturients who have received an opioid, the depressant effect of the respiratory alkalosis is enhanced by the action of the opioids. When the maternal $P\text{aO}_2$ falls below 70 mmHg, it has a significant effect on the fetus, namely a decrease in fetal $P\text{aO}_2$ and late decelerations (Fig. 34.6).

Effects of analgesia. Partial relief of labour pain with opioids or inhalation analgesia decreases the degree of hyperventilation so that $P\text{aCO}_2$ is in the 20–25 mmHg range and oxygenation improves (Marx et al 1969). However, between contractions the respiratory alkalosis combined with the depressant effects of the opioid may cause hypoventilation and hypoxaemia. Complete pain relief achieved with epidural analgesia prevents the

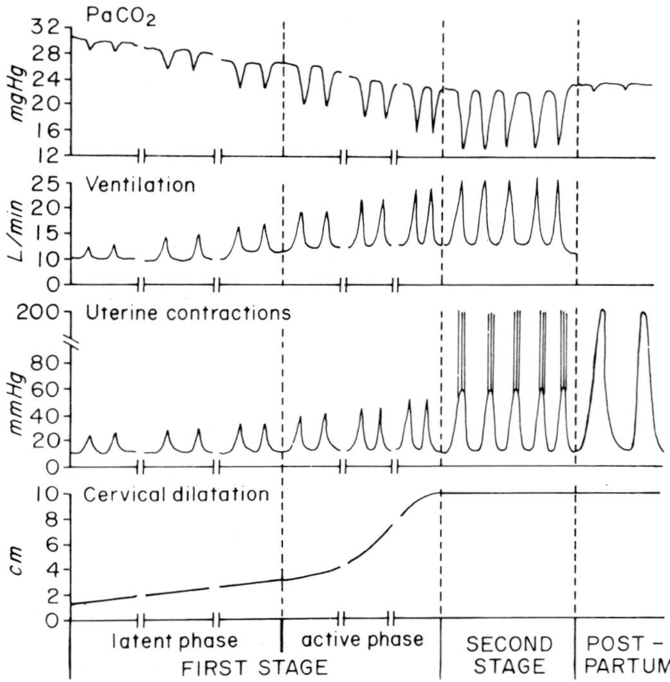

Fig. 34.5 Schematic depiction of the ventilatory changes measured during labour in an unpremedicated teenage primigravida. Early in labour uterine contractions are small and produce mild pain causing only small increases in minute ventilation and decreases in $P\text{aCO}_2$, but as labour progresses greater intensity of contraction causes greater changes in ventilation and $P\text{aCO}_2$. (Modified from Bonica 1973.)

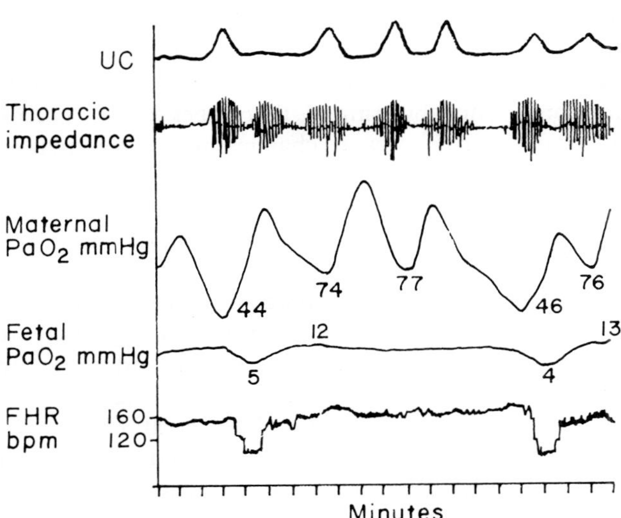

Fig. 34.6 Continuous recording of uterine contractions (UC), maternal thoracic impedance, maternal transcutaneous oxygen tension, fetal oxygen tension and fetal heart rate (FHR) in a primipara 120 min before spontaneous delivery of an infant with an Apgar score of 7. Marked hyperventilation during uterine contractions was followed by hypoventilation or apnoea in between contractions. With the parturient breathing air during and after the first and fourth periods of hyperventilation, the maternal $P\text{aO}_2$ fell to 44 and 46 mmHg with a consequent fall of fetal $P\text{aO}_2$ and variable decelerations which reflected fetal hypoxia. (Modified from Huch et al 1977.)

transient period of hyperventilation during the contraction and prevents hypoventilation during relaxation so that $P\text{aCO}_2$ remains in the range of 28–32 mmHg, and the $P\text{aO}_2$ increases to about 100 mmHg (Bonica 1973; Huch et al 1977; Peabody 1979) (Figs 34.7 and 34.8).

Neuroendocrine effects

Animal studies have shown that acute pain caused by noxious stimulation produces a significant (20–40%) increase in catecholamine levels, particularly in norepinephrine, with a consequent 35–70% decrease in uterine blood flow (Myers 1975; Jouppila 1977; Morishima et al 1978; Shnider et al 1979) (Fig. 34.9). Human studies have shown that severe pain and anxiety during active labour cause a 300–600% increase in the epinephrine (E) level, a 200–400% increase in the norepinephrine (NE) level, a 200–300% increase in the cortisol level and significant increases in corticosteroid and ACTH levels during the course of labour; these reach peak values at or after delivery (Lederman et al 1977, 1978; Falconer & Powles 1982; Ohno et al 1986).

Lederman and associates (1977, 1978) noted that during the period of active labour the E level increased by nearly 300%, the NE level by 150% and the cortisol level

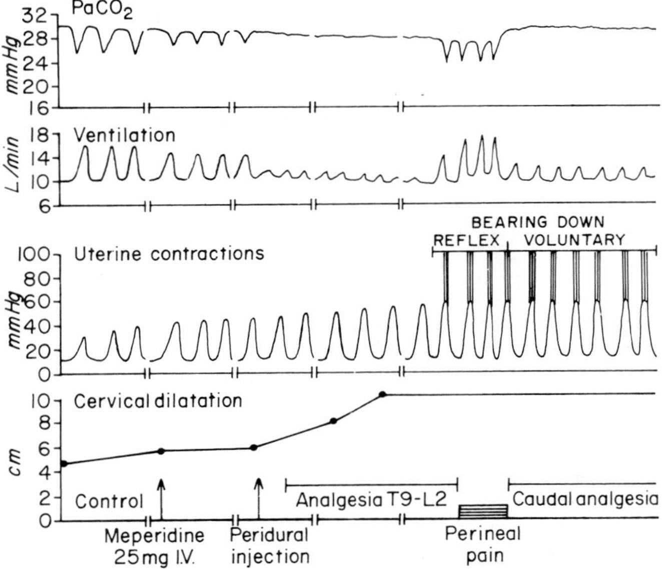

Fig. 34.7 A schematic diagram based on measurements in a primipara showing the effects of analgesia on ventilation. At 5 cm cervical dilatation, 25 mg pethidine given intravenously resulted in partial relief of pain and consequently smaller changes in ventilation and $P\text{aCO}_2$. Subsequent induction of segmental epidural analgesia produced complete pain relief which eliminated maternal hyperventilation and $P\text{aCO}_2$ changes without affecting uterine contractions. During the second stage, the onset of perineal pain and initiation of the reflex bearing-down efforts caused a concomitant increase in ventilation and slight decrease in $P\text{aCO}_2$ which were eliminated with the induction of low caudal (S1–S5) analgesia. Compare with Fig. 34.5.

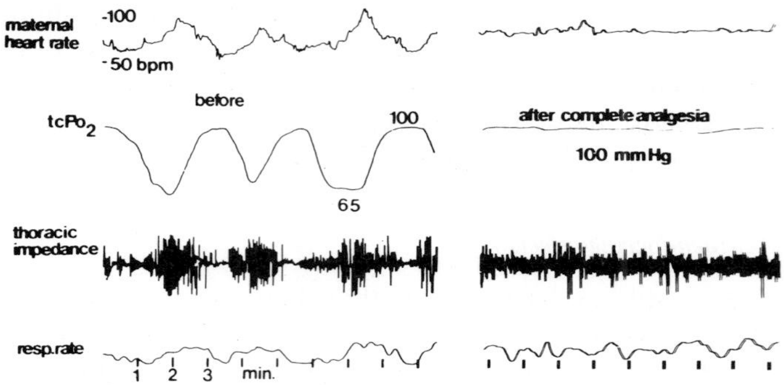

Fig. 34.8 Polygraph recording of maternal heart rate, transcutaneous oxygen tension (tcPo_2), thoracic impedance and respiratory rate during labour. Before the induction of epidural analgesia, the pain of uterine contractions caused marked hyperventilation and consequent increase in tcPo_2 to 100 mmHg (13.33 kPa), which fell to 65–70 mmHg (8.66–9.33 kPa) between contractions. After complete epidural analgesia, all curves were more regular, and tcPo_2 was maintained at a stable 100 mmHg (13.33 kPa). (From Peabody 1979, with permission.) Compare with Fig. 34.6.

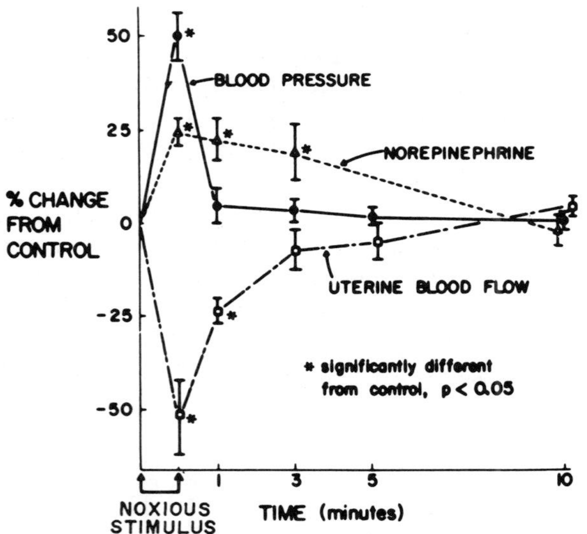

Fig. 34.9 The effects of a noxious stimulus on maternal arterial blood pressure, noradrenaline blood level and uterine blood flow. The stress was induced by application of an electric current on the skin of a ewe at term. Note that the increase in arterial pressure is very transient but the decay in noradrenaline level is more protracted and is reflected by a mirror-image decrease in uterine blood flow. (From Shnider et al 1979, with permission.)

by 200%. They noted that the higher E levels were significantly associated with uterine activity at the onset of active labour (4 cm cervical dilatation) and with longer labour during the active phase (4–10 cm cervical dilatation). Increased E and cortisol levels correlated significantly with anxiety and pain. Ohno and associates (1986) carried out a comprehensive study of catecholamines and cyclic nucleotides during labour and following delivery and noted a nearly twofold increase in the dopamine levels, a threefold increase in the E level and a twofold increase in the NE as well as a small increase in the cyclic adenosine monophosphate (cAMP) level. They noted a positive correlation between E on the one hand and heart rate and systolic blood pressure on the other, as well as a correlation between NE and cAMP during labour.

Effect of analgesia. Recent studies have provided impressive evidence that regional analgesia, especially lumbar epidural block, interrupts nociceptive input and the sympathetic efferents and thus reduces the release of catecholamines, beta-endorphins, ACTH and cortisol (Jouppila & Hollmén 1976; Buchan 1980; Abboud et al 1982; Browning et al 1983; Shnider et al 1983; Neumark et al 1985; Westgren et al 1986). This neuroendocrine lowering effect is primarily a result of relief of pain during labour. Abboud and associates (1982) noted that regional anaesthesia decreased catecholamine levels in women in labour, but did not do so in women who were not in labour. This selectivity suggests that the mechanism by which catecholamine release is decreased is relief of maternal pain.

Epidural analgesia during labour and delivery does not decrease catecholamine and beta-endorphin release in the fetus and newborn (Shnider et al 1979; Abboud et al 1982; Browning et al 1983; Raisanen et al 1986; Westgren et al 1986), and norepinephrine predominates over epinephrine (Abboud et al 1982). This response indicates that, even during uncomplicated deliveries with adequate maternal analgesia, the infant is distressed by the process of birth via vaginal delivery. A number of studies have suggested that catecholamines have an important role for neonatal adaptation to the extrauterine environment, including surfactant synthesis and release, lung liquid resorption, nonshivering thermogenesis, glucose homeostasis, cardiovascular changes and water metabolism (Abboud et al 1982).

Cardiovascular changes

Beginning at 6–8 weeks of pregnancy, the total blood, plasma and red cell volumes progressively increase, reaching a maximum at 28–32 weeks and thereafter remaining constant until parturition (Adams & Alexander 1958; Hansen & Ueland 1966; Lees et al 1970). This increase in blood volume is accompanied by a similar increase in cardiac output caused by an increase in both stroke volume and heart rate. During labour, cardiac output increases further above prelabour levels. The percentage increase in cardiac output is higher when the parturient is in the supine position than when she is in the lateral position. With the parturient in the supine position, between contractions cardiac output during the early first stage is about 15% above that of prelabour, during the late first stage it is about 30%, during the second stage about 45% and immediately after delivery 65–80% above

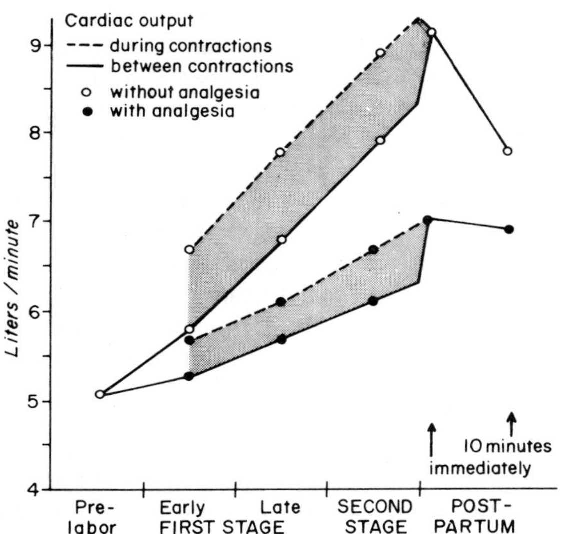

Fig. 34.10 Cardiac output during various phases of labour between contractions and during contractions. In a group of patients labouring without analgesia, the progressive increase between contractions and the further increase during each contraction were much greater than the changes in the group of patients who received continuous epidural analgesia. (Developed from data of Hendricks & Quilligan 1956; Ueland & Hansen 1969.)

prelabour (Hendricks & Quilligan 1956; Adams & Alexander 1958; Hansen & Ueland 1966). During painful uterine contraction, there is a further increase of 15–20% in cardiac output (Fig. 34.10).

With the parturient in the lateral position, cardiac output between contractions increases by approximately 5% in early labour, 10% at mid-first stage (5–7 cm cervical dilatation), 15% during late first stage, and 20% during the second stage (Robson et al 1987) (Fig. 34.11). However, the increments in cardiac output produced by uterine contractions above the level of output between contractions, during the same phases and stages of labour, are 17, 25, 35 and 40%, respectively (Robson et al 1987) (Figs 34.11 and 34.12).

Available data suggest that 40–50% of the increase during the contraction is caused by the extrusion of 250–300 ml of blood from the uterus and by increased venous return from the pelvis and lower limbs into the maternal central circulation. The rest is caused by an increase in sympathetic activity provoked by pain, anxiety, apprehension and the physical effort of labour, which contribute to the progressive rise in cardiac output as labour advances. Uterine contractions in the absence of analgesia also cause increases of 20–30 mmHg in the systolic and diastolic blood pressures (Fig. 34.13). The increase in cardiac output and systolic blood pressure leads to a significant increase in left ventricular work; this is tolerated by healthy parturients but can prove deleterious if the parturients have heart disease, pregnancy-induced hypertension (preeclampsia), essential hypertension, pulmonary hypertension or severe anaemia (Hendricks & Quilligan 1956; Hansen & Ueland 1966; Robson et al 1987).

Effect of analgesia. By decreasing the pain-induced sympathetic hyperactivity and neuroendocrine response, epidural analgesia eliminates that portion of the increase in cardiac output and blood pressure caused by pain. Figures 34.10–34.12 show that epidural analgesia decreases the progressive increase in cardiac output and its

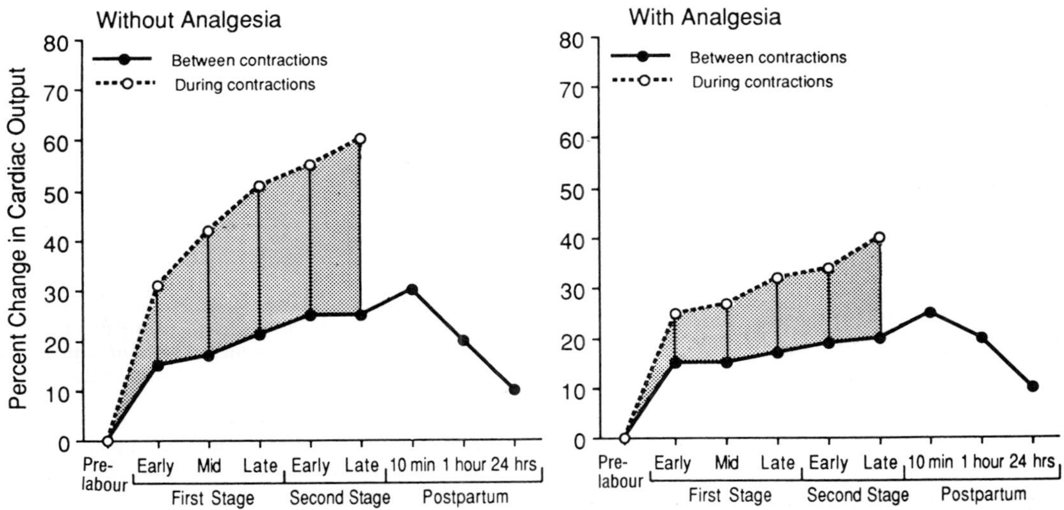

Fig. 34.11 Cardiac output during various phases of labour between contractions and during contractions measured in parturients in the lateral position. In parturients labouring without analgesia (left), the progressive increases between contractions and the further increases during each contraction were much greater than corresponding changes in a group of parturients who received continuous epidural analgesia (right). (From Bonica 1993b.)

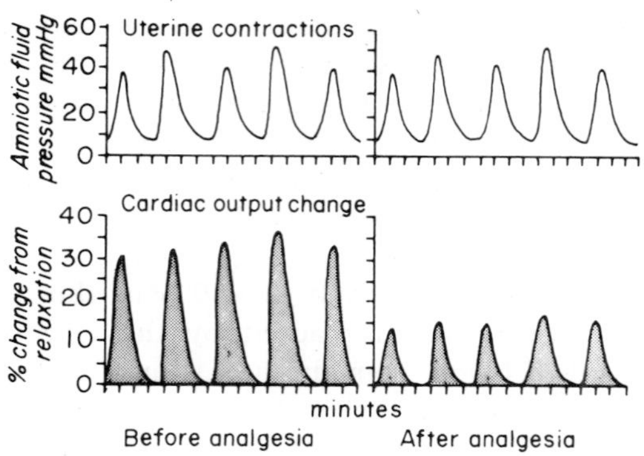

Fig. 34.12 Increases in cardiac output during each uterine contraction before and after induction of continuous epidural analgesia in a primipara. With pain relief the increases in cardiac output during contractions were about half of those before induction of analgesia.

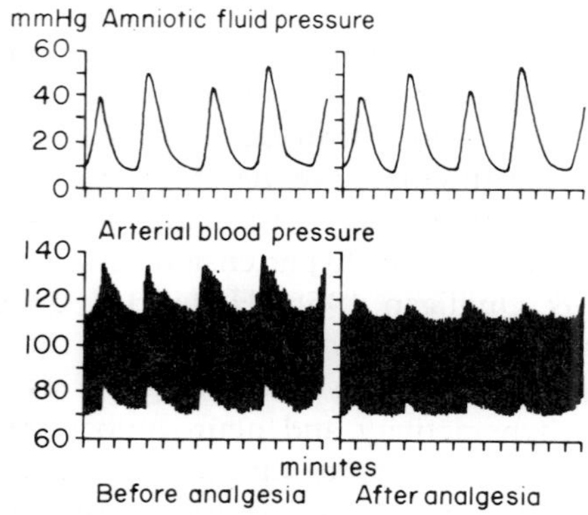

Fig. 34.13 The fluctuation in blood pressure produced by uterine contractions before and after induction of continuous epidural analgesia. Like the cardiac output changes, complete relief of pain resulted in decreasing the contraction-induced fluctuations to nearly half of the values measured before analgesia.

further increase during contractions to about 50% of that without analgesia. A similar decrease occurs in periodic increases in blood pressure (Fig. 34.13). Several studies have proved the value of epidural analgesia in dampening the increase in cardiac output, cardiac work and blood pressure in labouring parturients with heart disease, pregnancy-induced hypertension (preeclampsia) and pulmonary hypertension, provided of course that maternal hypotension is avoided (Jouppila & Hollmén 1976; Sorenson et al 1982; Lynch & Rizor 1982; Clark et al 1985).

Metabolic effects

During pregnancy, the basal metabolic rate and oxygen consumption progressively increase; at term, their values are 20% above normal (Bonica 1967, 1969, 1980; Bonica & McDonald 1990, 1993). During parturition, the metabolism and oxygen consumption increase further (Buchan 1980). During the first and second stages of labour, free fatty acids and lactate levels increase significantly, apparently as a result of pain-induced release of catecholamines and the consequent sympathetically induced lipolytic metabolism (Buchan 1980). This assumption is based on the fact that, with complete blockade of nociceptive (afferent) and efferent pathways, as achieved with epidural analgesia, only slight increases in maternal free fatty acid and lactate levels and acidosis are seen (Marx & Greene 1964). During the second stage of labour, maternal acidosis is a result of the pain and physical exertion inherent in the active bearing down (pushing) effort during contractions (Fig. 34.14).

Increased sympathetic activity caused by labour pain and anxiety also increases metabolism and oxygen consumption. The increased oxygen consumption, plus that inherent in the work of labour, together with the loss of bicarbonate from the kidney as compensation for the pain-induced respiratory alkalosis and often reduced carbohydrate intake, produce a progressive metabolic

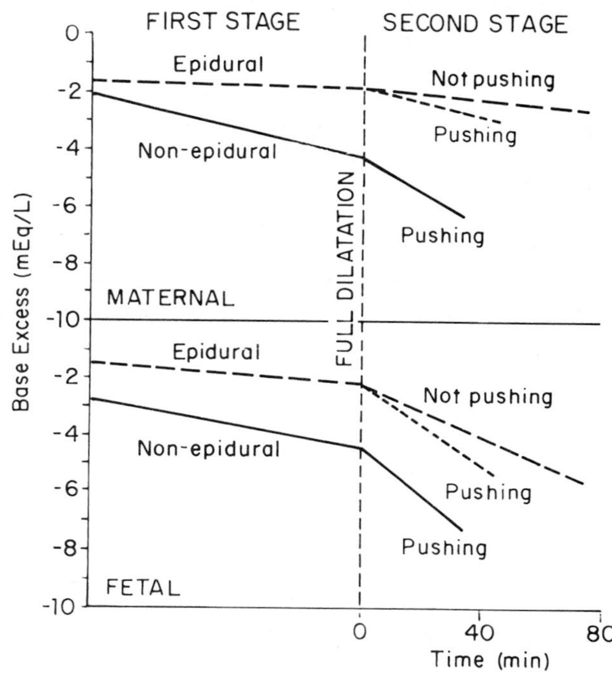

Fig. 34.14 Mean changes in extent of maternal (above) and fetal (below) metabolic acidosis, during the first and second stages of labour, in a group of parturients managed without lumbar epidural analgesia and in two similar groups managed with epidural analgesia, one of which retained the bearing down reflex while the other did not. The parturients were delivered by outlet forceps. Significant metabolic acidosis was experienced by those in the nonepidural group of parturients, whereas those given epidural analgesia experienced little or no change in their acid–base status. Fetuses born of mothers managed without epidural also developed significant metabolic acidosis during the first stage and to an even greater degree during the second stage. In contrast, fetuses of mothers given epidural analgesia had no change in acid–base status during the first stage but showed a time-dependent increase in metabolic acidosis during the second stage, due to the process of birth (see text). (From Bonica 1980, based on data from Pearson & Davies 1974.)

acidosis that is transferred to the fetus (Pearson & Davies 1973a, 1973b, 1974; Bonica & McDonald 1990). The maternal pyruvate level increases, along with an even greater increase in the lactate level and a progressive accumulation of excess lactate which is reflected by a progressive increase in base excess (Marx & Greene 1964; Pearson & Darvies 1973a, 1973b 1974).

Effects of analgesia. The relief of pain and associated anxiety with continuous epidural analgesia decreases the total work of labour, maternal metabolism and oxygen consumption. Buchan (1980) showed that, during labour, epidural analgesia reduced maternal stress by abolishing pain, thus eliminating the progressive increase in the 11-hydroxycorticosteroid levels normally seen throughout labour. Consequently, epidural analgesia significantly reduces maternal and fetal metabolic acidosis.

The superiority of epidural analgesia over parenteral opioids and other systemic analgesics in decreasing maternal work, oxygen consumption and maternal and fetal metabolic acidosis has been impressively demonstrated by a number of investigators (Marx & Greene 1964; Pearson & Davies 1973a, 1973b, 1974; Thalme et al 1974; Jouppila & Hollmén 1976; Buchan 1980). Because active pushing during the second stage of labour contributes to metabolic acidosis, epidural analgesia does not completely eliminate metabolic and fetal acidosis. Figure 34.14 demonstrates that epidural analgesia and elimination of the bearing down (pushing) effort during the second stage almost eliminates maternal metabolic acidosis. Moreover, under these conditions, it decreases but does not eliminate the degree of fetal acidosis. Undoubtedly, this is a result of the physical stress on the fetus inherent in the process of birth.

Gastrointestinal and urinary function

The pain of labour and the consequent increase in sympathetic activity also affects the function of the gastrointestinal and urinary tracts. Gastrin release is stimulated during painful labour and results in an increase in gastric acid secretion (Hayes et al 1972). Moreover, the pain and associated anxiety and emotional stress produce segmental and suprasegmental reflex inhibition of gastrointestinal and urinary motility and function, and consequently a significant delay in gastric and urinary bladder emptying. These reflex effects of nociception are aggravated by the recumbent position and by the use of opioids and other depressant drugs (Hayes et al 1972; Nimmo et al 1975; Holdsworth 1978). The combined effect of pain and depressant drugs can cause food and fluids other than water to be retained for as long as 36 hours or more. During this period, swallowed air and gastric juices accumulate progressively, with the pH of the stomach contents decreasing below the critical value of 2.5 in most parturients. Delayed gastric emptying of the acidic gastric contents increases the risk of regurgitation and pulmonary aspiration, especially during the induction of general anaesthesia. This hazard has long been and today remains one of the most common causes of maternal motality and morbidity due to anaesthesia (Tomkinson et al 1982).

Effects of analgesia. Unlike parenteral opioids, properly administered continuous epidural analgesia has no directly deleterious effects on gastrointestinal or urinary function. Moreover, by eliminating the pain-induced increased sympathetic activity, it reduces the gastrointestinal and urinary dysfunction mentioned above.

Psychological effects

Severe labour pain can produce serious long-term emotional disturbances that might impair the parturient's mental health, negatively influence her relationship with her baby during the first few crucial days and cause a fear of future pregnancies that could affect her sexual relationship with her husband (Bonica & McDonald 1990). Melzack and associates (1981, 1984), Gaston-Johansson and associates (1988), and others (Stewart 1982), reported that a significant number of women who had participated in natural childbirth had developed or had aggravation of prelabour depression, or had other deleterious emotional reactions in the postpartum period, consequent to the pain experienced during their childbirth without analgesia. Melzack et al (1981, 1984) noted that some women experienced an added burden of guilt, anger and failure when they anticipated 'a natural painless childbirth' and then were confronted with such severe pain that they required epidural analgesia. Stewart (1982) reported that such patients became miserable, depressed and even suicidal and lost interest in sex. In some cases, the husbands of women who anticipated 'natural' childbirth had to undergo psychotherapy for serious reactions after seeing their wives experience such severe pain; they themselves developed feelings of guilt and subsequent impotence and phobias.

Effects of analgesia. Properly administered epidural analgesia will relieve most of the pain and thus obviate-many of the psychological and emotional reactions to the severe pain mentioned above. Melzack has summarised the data from the studies mentioned earlier (1984). On the basis of his own studies and data from other sources, Melzack (1984) pleaded for a well-developed and well-balanced approach whereby all prospective parturients are given education and training for childbirth and, if they experience more than mild pain, to have skilfully administered epidural analgesia, because these are compatible and complementary procedures that allow the recognition of the individuality of each woman.

Effects on uterine activity and labour

Through increased secretion of catecholamines and cortisol, pain and emotional stress can either increase or decrease uterine contractility and thus influence the duration of labour. Norepinephrine increases uterine activity, whereas epinephrine and cortisol decrease it (Lederman et al 1977, 1978). Morishima and colleagues (1980) reported that, in pregnant baboons and rhesus monkeys, nociceptive stimulation increased uterine activity by about 60–65% and was associated with a decrease in fetal oxygen tension and in fetal heart rate that often was characterised by ominous signs of late decelerations. Lederman and associates (1977, 1978) noted that in some parturients severe pain and anxiety caused such an increase in epinephrine and cortisol levels that uterine activity was consequently decreased and labour was prolonged. In a small percentage of parturients, pain and anxiety produce 'incoordinate uterine contractions' manifested by a decrease in intensity coupled with an increase in frequency and uterine tonus (Moir & Willocks 1967; Bonica & Hunter 1969; Morishima et al 1980).

Effects of analgesia. By decreasing the sympathetically induced hyperactivity, sedation and effective pain relief can reduce or eliminate uterine hyperactivity or hypoactivity and can change incoordinate uterine contractions to a normal labour pattern (Moir & Willocks 1967; Bonica & Hunter 1969). Equally important is the efficacy of analgesia in reducing placental hypoperfusion and any existing deterioration in uterine blood flow, thus decreasing or even eliminating any impairment of blood gas transfer that might be a result of increased catecholamines or uterine hyperactivity (Bonica & Hunter 1969; Morishima et al 1980).

Effects on the fetus

During labour, the intermittent reduction of intervillous blood flow during the peak of a contraction leads to a temporary decrease in placental gas exchange. This impairment is often further increased by pain-induced severe hyperventilation which causes severe respiratory alkalosis (see above) and results in the following:

1. a shift (to the left) in the maternal oxygen dissociation curve, which diminishes the transfer of oxygen from mother to fetus
2. maternal hypoxaemia during uterine relaxation with consequent fetal hypoxaemia
3. a reduction in uterine blood flow which is provoked by an increase in norepinephrine and cortisol release.

These deleterious effects on the fetus have been demonstrated in several species of animals and in humans (Jouppila & Hollmén 1976; Lederman et al 1977, 1978; Morishima et al 1980). Figure 34.6 depicts the deleterious effects on fetal heart rate that were caused by marked hyperventilation during a contraction and by hypoventilation between contractions. Lederman and associates (1978) also noted that parturients who were anxious and had pain had a higher incidence of abnormal fetal heart rate patterns and their infants had lower 1- and 5-minute Apgar scores than infants of parturients who were not anxious and had good pain relief.

Under the conditions of normal labour, such a series of transient and intermittent impairments of blood gas exchange is tolerated by the normal fetus because oxygen is stored in the fetal circulation and intervillous space and is sufficient to maintain adequate fetal oxygenation during the brief period of placental hypoperfusion. Moreover, the fetus can compensate by increasing the proportion of cardiac output that is distributed to the myocardium and brain (Assali et al 1962). If the above factors are combined with an excessive increase in uterine activity, however, fetal hypoxia, hypercapnia, and acidosis develop. These might still be tolerated by the normal fetus, although its ability to withstand oxygen deprivation becomes limited. Under such conditions, any unexpected complication, such as cord around the neck at delivery, may prove deleterious to the fetus. On the other hand, if the fetus is already at risk because of obstetric or maternal complications (e.g. preeclampsia, heart disease or diabetes), the pain-induced reductions of oxygen and carbon dioxide transfer can be the critical factors that produce perinatal morbidity and could even contribute to mortality (Beard et al 1967; Morishima et al 1980). The maternal metabolic acidosis is transferred to the fetus (Marx & Greene 1964; Pearson & Davies 1973a, 1973b, 1974; Buchan 1980) making it more vulnerable to the effects of intrauterine asphyxia caused by cord compression, prolapse or other obstetric complications.

Effects of analgesia. The benefits of effective (complete) pain relief, best achieved with continuous epidural analgesia, are likely to be of value to many infants, but they are especially important to the fetus at risk (Beard et al 1967; Bonica 1967, 1969, 1980, 1993b; Pearson & Davies 1973a, 1973b, 1974; Thalme et al 1974; Jouppila & Hollmén 1976; Buchan 1980; Abboud et al 1982; Shnider et al 1983; Crawford 1984; Shnider & Levinson 1987; Bonica & McDonald 1990, 1993). It has been found to be the best method of analgesia for breech delivery and for multiple pregnancies (Bonica 1967, 1969, 1980; Crawford 1984; Shnider & Levinson 1987; Bonica & McDonald 1990). It has been shown that epidural analgesia, through its vasomotor blocking effect, increases intervillous blood flow in parturients with severe preeclampsia and probably also in those with hypertension, diabetes, and other conditions that decrease placental blood flow and function (Bonica 1967, 1969, 1980; Crawford 1984; Shnider & Levinson 1987; Bonica & McDonald 1990). Janisch and coworkers (1978) found that continuous epidural analgesia administered to preeclamptics during their last few weeks of gestation produced a 100% increase in placental blood flow. Jouppila and colleagues (1982) studied the influence of lumbar epidural analgesia that was limited to a few segments and the effect of a more extensive type of lumbar epidural block on parturients with severe preeclampsia. They found that the limited block increased intervillous blood flow by 34%, whereas the more extensive block increased it by a mean of 77%. They attributed this effect to the relief of severe vasoconstriction by the vasomotor block. Maternal hypotension must be strictly avoided by appropriate prophylactic measures (e.g. intravenous infusion of fluids, lateral displacement of the uterus) to achieve these benefits.

MANAGEMENT OF THE PAIN OF CHILDBIRTH

The primary objective of obstetric analgesia and anaesthesia is to provide the mother with optimal relief of pain with little or no risk to her and her infant. To achieve this objective requires that each member of the obstetric team adhere to certain basic principles. The type of analgesia or anaesthesia must be tailored to the needs of each mother and infant within the framework of the personnel and resources available. Each member of the obstetric team must be fully informed of the plans and possible problems of other members – conditions which require observance of the three cardinal Cs: *communication*, *coordination* and *cooperation*. The anaesthesiologist must have a thorough understanding of the physiological and pathophysiological alterations caused by pregnancy and labour and how these are affected by each type of analgesia/anaesthesia. Observation of these principles requires excellent antepartal and preanaesthetic care and proper intrapartal and intraanaesthetic management.

Preanaesthetic care

The proper preparation of the gravida and her spouse during the antepartum period is one of the most important responsibilities of the obstetric team. She and her husband should be fully informed about the physiology and psychology of pregnancy and labour and about the psychological and emotional reactions these might produce. This type of information not only helps the gravida cope with changes that occur during pregnancy but helps her to cooperate and participate actively during labour and delivery. During one of the antepartum visits, the obstetrician should bring up the matter of analgesia and anaesthesia; if the gravida indicates that she is interested, the advantages and disadvantages and limitations of each technique should be clearly explained. If the gravida delivers in hospital, it is essential that everyone who comes in contact with the patient (from the admission clerk to members of the house staff) thoroughly appreciate the importance of a friendly and reassuring attitude.

Those gravidas who indicate a desire for some form of pain relief should be seen by an anaesthesiologist either prior to or soon after admission to the hospital. Proper preanaesthetic care requires a thorough evaluation of the physical examination, assessment of the physiological and emotional status of the parturient and discussion of the various forms of analgesia and anaesthesia available. Selection of the method of analgesia to be used is made in consultation with the parturient and obstetrician.

Current methods of obstetric analgesia/anaesthesia

Currently, many drugs and techniques are available to provide relief of childbirth pain. All of these can be arbitrarily classified into four categories:

1. psychological analgesia
2. simple methods of pharmacological analgesia
3. inhalation analgesia/anaesthesia
4. regional analgesia.

For proper application, each of these methods must be evaluated on the basis of four criteria:

1. analgesic potency and other therapeutic efficacy
2. side-effects on the mother
3. side-effects on the fetus and newborn
4. side-effects on the forces of labour.

Detailed consideration of these methods is precluded by the purpose of this book, and by severe space limitations. Therefore only a few comments will be made about each method and summarised in Table 34.1.

During the past two decades, but especially since the previous editions of this book appeared, there have been significant changes in the methods used for the relief of pain of childbirth. This is suggested by four major surveys of the practice of obstetric analgesia/anaesthesia carried out in the United States during the past three decades, and two surveys which included current practice in the United Kingdom, Scandinavian countries and a number of other countries throughout the world (Bonica & McDonald 1990; Bonica 1993a). These surveys indicate that in major hospitals where obstetric services are well organised and an obstetric anaesthesia service is available, there has been a trend of increasing use of continuous lumbar epidural block with a dilute solution of local anaesthetics and opioids and a decrease in the use of paracervical block and inhalation analgesia.

About 20–30% of parturients in these institutions select psychological analgesia (see below), but eventually two-thirds of them receive lumbar epidural or other forms of regional analgesia. There has also been a trend not to use general *anaesthesia* for labour and vaginal delivery. In the

Table 34.1 Pharmacological techniques of obstetric analgesia – anaesthesia

	Analgesics		Regional analgesia – anaesthesia			General analgesia–anaesthesia
Specific drugs/ techniques	Meperidine Demerol Butorphanol Morphine	Continuous lumbar epidural (see text for technique) Infusion Segmental T10–L1 that eventually spreads to T10–S5	Subarachnoid block STB, T10–S5 SB, S1–S5	Paracervical block Pudendal block	Inhalation analgesia	Balanced anaesthesia. Preoxygenation → i.v. thiopental + muscle relaxant + cricoid pressure → intubation; maintenance with light inhalation anaesthesia + muscle relaxant + artificial ventilation
Optimal dose and route	Demerol, 100 mg i.m. Butorphanol, 2 mg i.m. Morphine, 10 mg i.m. or 1/3–1/2 dose i.v. slowly	See text	Subarachnoid block, variable amounts to produce analgesia/ anaesthesia	6–10 ml of 1% lidocaine or 0.25% bupivacaine for each nerve	50–60% of nitrous oxide in oxygen; 0.35% methoxyflurane in air; 0.35–0.5% trichloroethylene in air; 0.25–1.25% enflurane in air	
Therapeutic effects	Analgesia, sedation and decrease of anxiety due to pain relief	Greater degree of pain relief than with other techniques	STB – analgesia for labour and delivery SB – anaesthesia for delivery only	Paracervical block – good relief of uterine pain Pudendal block – fair relief of perineal pain	Satisfactory analgesia in 60–70% with nitrous oxide, methoxyflurane, trichloroethylene and enflurane, and in 90% with combination of methoxyflurane and nitrous oxide	Insures adequate oxygenation, anaesthesia, relaxation and satisfactory maintenance
Side-effects on mother	↓ Respiration between contractions, delayed gastric emptying; nausea and vomiting in some	Minimal hypotension with proper management, moderate to severe hypotension in supine position or hypovolaemia	STB – more hypotension than with 'Analgesics' group and continuous lumbar epidural SB – none	None if properly done, but sedation and toxic reaction with overdose	None with analgesic concentration except occasional amnesia and confusion	Little or none with optimal doses, hypotension with some inhalation anaesthetics, risk of regurgitation and aspiration
Effects on active labour	None; slowing if given in latent phase	None in first stage unless initiated too early → prolonged latent phase, obviated with oxytocin; bearing down reflex lost but able to push voluntarily	STB – same as with 'Analgesics' group SB – none except loss of bearing down reflex	Paracervical block – transient depression of contractions, but no effect on labour progress Pudendal block – none	None	Produces good uterine relaxation when necessary
Effects on fetus	Mild ↓ CNS ↓ BBV	Transient ↓ BBV with bolus not none with epidural infusion	STB – none unless severe and sustained hypotension leads to fetal distress SB – none	Paracervical block – frequent bradycardia ↓ BBV Pudendal block – none	None	Minimal ↓ CNS ↓ BBV
Effects on newborn	Mild ↓ CNS ↓ EEG, ENNS	None if no maternal complication occurred	None except if severe and sustained hypotension leads to neonatal depression	Paracervical block – ENNS Pudendal block – none	None or slight neonatal	Minimal ↓ CNS with optimal dose, moderate ↓ CNS with larger amounts or concentrations

Table 34.1 (*contd*)

	Analgesics		Regional analgesia – anaesthesia		General analgesia–anaesthesia	
Remarks	Effective analgesia for mild/ moderate pain in 70–80% of parturients	Effective analgesia but with intermittent injection → premature motor block → nonrotation and loss of reflex urge to bear down	Simple and rapid analgesia and perineal relaxation, but premature perineal and limb paralysis and loss of reflex → prolonged second stage and need for instrument delivery	Paracervical + pudendal block – good analgesia; can be done by obstetrician; however frequency of fetal bradycardia has markedly decreased use of paracervical block	Provide satisfactory analgesia and are simple to administer	Best method of anaesthesia in hypovolaemic/ hypotensive parturients; use limited to caeserean section and instrumental vaginal delivery

↓ = depression of; ↑ = increase in; → = leads to; BBV = beat-to-beat variability; CNS = central nervous system, CV = cardiovascular; ENNS = early neonatal behavioural scale; i.m. = intramuscular; i.v. = intravenous; STB = standard subarachnoid block; SB = true saddle block.
Reprinted by permission of Pharmacia Deltec Inc., St Paul, MN.

United Kingdom and in Scandinavian countries, inhalation *analgesia* is still being used, alone or together with the systemic opioids, in 20–50% of parturients. In the United Kingdom, there has been a steady increase in the use of continuous lumbar epidural block and the use of inhalation analgesia for the first stage of labour in a significant percentage of patients.

In developing countries, most parturients receive either no analgesia or simple methods of inhalation and local anaesthesia (Bonica & McDonald 1990; Bonica 1993b). On the basis of these data, psychological analgesia and simple techniques of inhalation and regional anaesthesia are briefly commented upon below and due emphasis is given to the use of continuous lumbar epidural analgesia/anaesthesia.

Psychological analgesia

This term is used for 'educated' (natural) childbirth, psychoprophylaxis and hypnosis because, despite the claims to the contrary by the proponents of each method, these have similar physiotherapeutic and psychophysiological bases (Bonica 1967). Early proponents of these techniques insisted that most patients can achieve 'painless' childbirth; however most current workers in the field acknowledge that in most patients pain is not eliminated but somewhat lessened (the exception is the 20–25% who can achieve hypnotic analgesia). The major benefits are a decrease in anxiety and apprehension, enhancement of the parturient's ability to cope with the entire process and to control her behaviour, the experience of a personal sense of achievement and enhancement of the early 'bonding' process by immediate visual, auditory and tactile contact between mother and her newborn.

Analysis of published data and my own observations in various countries suggest that, if psychoprophylaxis or natural childbirth is properly applied to both primiparae and multiparae, it can be expected that:

1. 5–10% experience little or no pain and will require no analgesia/anaesthesia during the entire process
2. in an additional 15–20%, the pain is decreased to a moderate degree, and the parturient will require less pharmacological analgesia/anaesthesia
3. in the remainder, the pain is not influenced but fear and anxiety will be less and the patients will manifest less pain behaviour (Bonica 1967, 1980).

While some reports indicate that prepared childbirth patients have shorter labour, fewer operative deliveries, fewer intrapartum and postpartum complications, less blood loss and better and happier babies than patients given drug-induced analgesia/anaesthesia (Hughey et al 1978), other reports (including some with proper controls) indicate no significant differences regarding these variables between prepared and unprepared (anaesthesia) groups (Davenport-Slack & Boylan 1974; Scott & Rose 1976; Melzack et al 1981). Personal observations in the former Soviet Union and in Western European and American hospitals suggest that the discrepancies are due to differences in motivation, attitude and personality of the parturient and her instructor, the practices of the obstetrician and – most importantly – the skill with which pharmacological analgesia/anaesthesia is administered.

On the basis of these observations and from long personal experience with regional analgesia, I agree with Melzack et al (1981) in recommending that prepared childbirth training should be combined with regional analgesia in order to achieve the best results for the mother and her infant.

Simple techniques of pharmacological analgesia

In many parts of the world where anaesthetists are not

available, the midwife or obstetrician must rely on the use of prepared childbirth and simple methods of drug-induced analgesia. During the early first stage, the main pain can be relieved by using suggestion and combining it with sedatives and tranquillisers, but, with the onset of the moderate pain of the active phase of labour, systemic opioids are usually required and are given either intramuscularly or in small increments intravenously or via patient-controlled analgesia (PCA). Properly administered narcotics produce adequate, albeit not complete, relief of moderate pain in 70–80% of parturients and relief of severe pain in about 35–60% (Bonica 1967, 1969). In optimal doses, they do not produce significant maternal respiratory depression but do produce neonatal depression that can be minimised. For the actual delivery, inhalation analgesia, bilateral pudendal nerve block or infiltration of the perineum may be used.

Inhalation analgesia/anaesthesia

Inhalation *analgesia* is a widely used method of relieving childbirth pain because it produces moderately effective pain relief without causing loss of consciousness or significant maternal or neonatal depression. The agents most commonly used are 40–50% nitrous oxide in oxygen, or 0.35% methoxyflurane or 0.35–0.5% trichloroethylene or 0.25–1% enflurane in either air or oxygen. Each of these agents can be administered intermittently during uterine contractions by the patient, midwife or anaesthetist. Premixed cylinders of 50% nitrous oxide and 50% oxygen (Entonox) are available in some parts of the world and greatly facilitate the use of this agent either by the parturient or midwife. For optimal results, the inhalation of the drug should begin some 10–15 seconds before the painful period of each contraction. Properly used, inhalation analgesia produces good analgesia in one-third and partial relief in another one-third of parturients.

Inhalation *anaesthesia* for the delivery is still employed because it can be rapidly induced; it affords maximum control of depth and duration of action and is rapidly eliminated at the end of the procedure. On the other hand, general anaesthesia carries the risk of maternal mortality due to difficult endotracheal intubation with consequent asphyxia (Glassenberg 1991). This, and regurgitation and pulmonary aspiration, are the two leading causes of anaesthesia-related maternal mortality in Britain and the United States. For this reason, general anaesthesia should be avoided but, if necessary, should be given only by a properly trained anaesthetist who has secured the airway by endotracheal intubation prior to induction of anaesthesia.

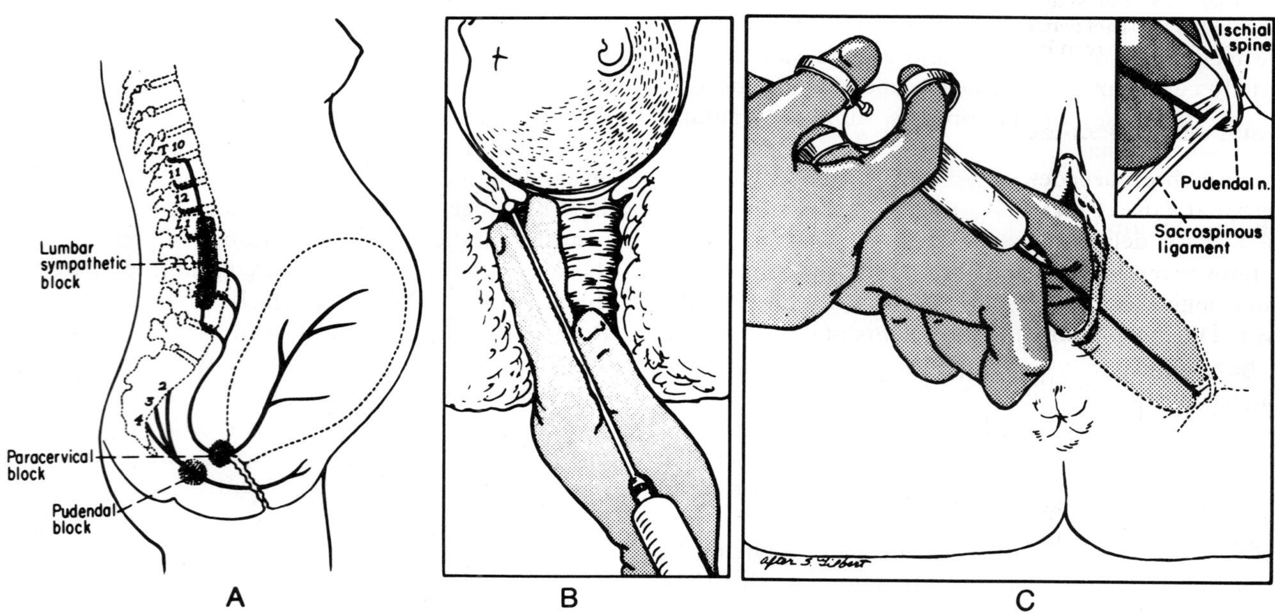

Fig. 34.15 **A** Sites of three regional techniques for obstetric analgesia. Lumbar sympathetic block is rarely used but is highly effective in relieving pain of the first stage and may be preferable to paracervical block, especially in high-risk pregnancies. **B** Schematic coronal section of vagina and lower part of the uterus containing the fetal head, showing the techniques of paracervical block. The 22-gauge needle is within a guide, with its point protruding only 5–7 mm beyond the end of the guide. This prevents insertion of the needle more than 5–7 mm beyond the surface of the mucosa. After negative aspiration, an injection of 8–10 ml of 0.25% bupivacaine at 4 and 8 o'clock of the cervical fornix will produce relief of uterine pain for several hours. **C** Transvaginal technique of blocking the pudendal nerve. The two fingers of the left hand are inserted into the vagina to guide the needle point into the sacrospinous ligament. As long as the bevel of the needle is in the ligament, there is some resistance to the injection of local anaesthetic, but as soon as the bevel passes through the ligament, there is sudden lack of resistance, indicating that the needle point is next to the nerve. (Modified from Bonica 1967.)

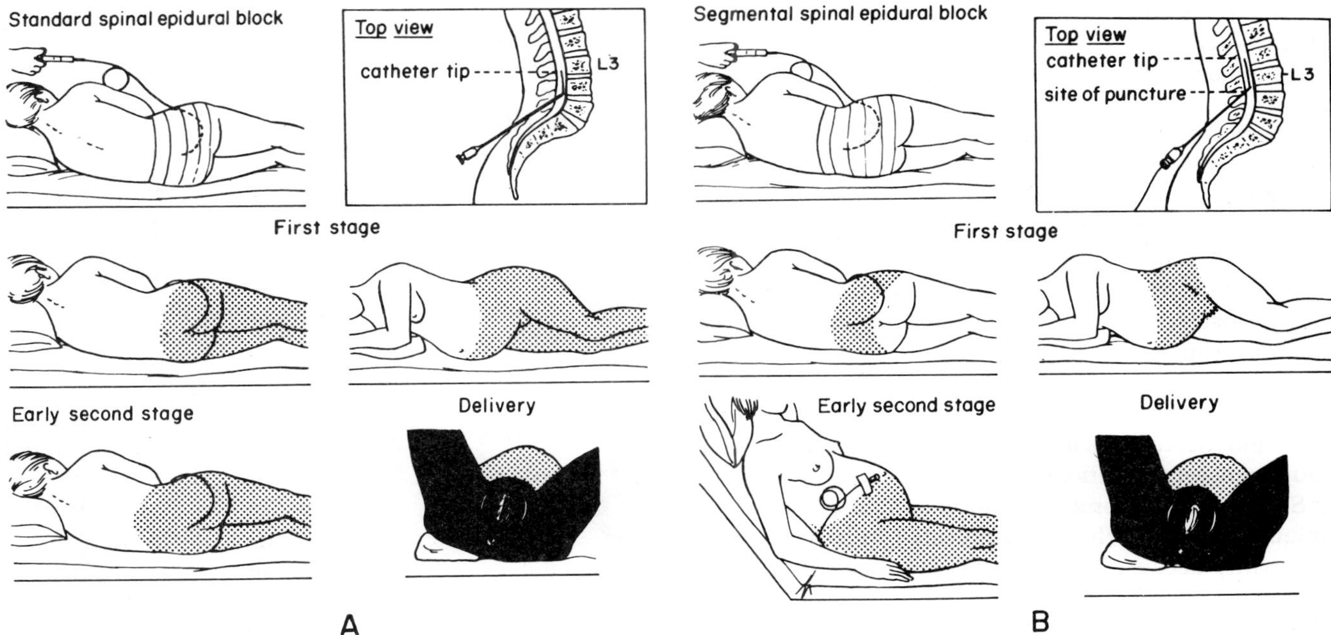

Fig. 34.16 Techniques of lumbar epidural block for labour and vaginal delivery. **A** The standard continuous technique, which is carried out as follows: after starting a preload infusion of fluid, a continuous catheter is inserted through a needle placed in the L4 interspace and advanced until its tip is at the L3 vertebra. With the onset of moderate pain, a test dose is injected and, if negative, 10–12 ml of a local anaesthetic (e.g. 0.25% bupivacaine) is injected to produce analgesia extending from T10–S5. The patient is then made to lie on her side, is given oxygen and frequently monitored, and 'top-up' analgesic doses are injected as soon as pain returns, to produce continuous analgesia. After flexion and internal rotation have occurred, a high concentration of local anaesthetic is injected with the patient in the semirecumbent position to produce perineal relaxation and anaesthesia as depicted (black) in the lower right figure. For the delivery, a wedge is placed under the right buttock to displace the uterus toward the left away from the inferior vena cava and aorta. **B** The technique of segmental epidural analgesia differs slightly from the standard technique in that the catheter is placed higher (L2) and for the first stage the dose is limited to 5–6 ml of local analgesic solution. At the onset of perineal pain, analgesia is extended to the lower lumbar and sacral segments by injecting 10–12 ml of local analgesic solution with the patient in Fowler's position.

Regional analgesia/anaesthesia

In the past three decades, there has been an impressive increase in the use of regional analgesia/anaesthesia during labour and for delivery in the United States and Britain and, more recently, in many European countries where pharmacological obstetric anaesthesia was previously avoided. The most common techniques are:

1. continuous lumbar epidural block (LEB)
2. subarachnoid (saddle) block (SAB)
3. bilateral paracervical (PCB) and/or bilateral pudendal block (PB)
4. double catheter extradural block (DCEB) – combined segmental epidural and low caudal blocks.

Advantages of regional analgesia/anaesthesia

1. In contrast to narcotic and inhalation analgesia, regional analgesia/anaesthesia can produce complete relief of pain in most parturients.

2. The hazards of inability to intubate and of pulmonary aspiration of gastric contents inherent in general anaesthesia are virtually eliminated.

3. By blocking all nociceptive pathways, it obviates the pain-induced deleterious reflex responses mentioned in the previous section.

4. With most techniques, the use of a dilute solution of local anaesthetic produces a block of nociceptive (A-delta and C) fibres with minimal or no effect on the larger somatomotor and tactile fibres.

5. Provided it is properly administered and complications are avoided, regional analgesia/anaesthesia causes no maternal or neonatal depression.

6. Administered properly, it does not have a clinically significantly effect on the progress of labour.

7. 'Continuous' epidural analgesia can be extended for delivery and may even be modified for caesarean section if this becomes necessary.

8. Regional analgesia permits the mother to remain awake and alert during labour and delivery so that she can experience the pleasure of actively participating in the birth process and promptly 'bond' with her child.

Disadvantages of regional analgesia/anaesthesia

1. It requires greater knowledge of anatomy and greater

technical skill to administer than do systemic drugs or inhalation agents.

2. Technical failures occur, although the incidence is very small in experienced hands.

3. The vasomotor block inherent in spinal, standard epidural and caudal blocks may cause significant maternal hypotension if prophylactic measures are not taken.

4. Techniques that produce perineal analgesia cause loss of the afferent limb of the reflex urge to bear down; unless the parturient is given instruction on how to bear down effectively, the second stage may be prolonged or outlet forceps may be required.

5. Techniques that produce premature perineal muscle relaxation may interfere with the mechanism of internal rotation and increase the incidence of occiput–posterior or occiput–transverse positions.

6. Spinal, caudal, lumbar epidural and double catheter techniques are relatively contraindicated in patients with coagulopathy because of risk of haemorrhage within the spinal canal.

7. Regional analgesia/anaesthesia procedures can only be carried out in a hospital.

Complications

Care must be exercised to avoid three serious complications: maternal hypotension, systemic toxic reactions and very high or total spinal anaesthesia.

1. *Maternal hypotension.* This is avoided by infusing 1 litre of fluid before inducing spinal, epidural or caudal block to compensate for the increased vascular capacitance consequent to the vasomotor blockade; it is also wise to have the parturient labour on her side to avoid the aortocaval compression inherent in the supine position.

2. *Systemic toxic reactions.* These may be prevented by avoiding excessive doses or accidental intravenous injection of therapeutic doses.

3. *Very high or total spinal anaesthesia.* This may result from accidental subarachnoid injection of a local anaesthetic dose intended for extradural block.

The latter two complications can be virtually obviated by attempting to aspirate blood or cerebrospinal fluid and injecting a test dose of 2–3 ml of solution containing 5–7.5 mg bupivacaine and 15 μg adrenalin. If the injection is accidentally subarachnoid, the parturient will develop a low (T10-S5) spinal anaesthesia which can be used instead of the extradural block, whereas if the injection is intravenous the adrenalin will produce moderate tachycardia and hypertension within 20–30 seconds of the injection and this will last 30–60 seconds (Moore & Batra 1981). Only when neither occurs should large therapeutic doses be injected.

Current use of various regional techniques

Techniques of paracervical block combined with pudendal block (Fig. 34.15), performed by an obstetrician skilled in these procedures, are very useful especially in cases where anaesthetists are not available. However, because of the frequent incidence of severe fetal bradycardia, paracervical block which was widely used a decade ago has virtually been discontinued in most centres. On the other hand, bilateral pudendal block is being used by obstetricians in those institutions where obstetric anaesthesia services are not available.

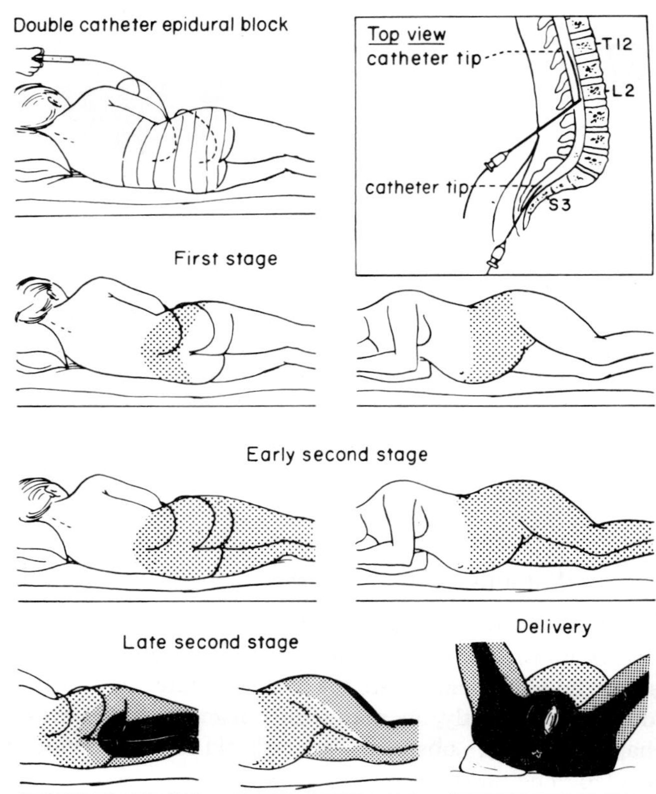

Fig. 34.17 The double catheter technique for extradural analgesia and anaesthesia for labour and delivery. It is best to introduce the two catheters during the latent phase when the patient is not too uncomfortable. The upper catheter is introduced through a needle placed in the L2 interspace and advanced untill its tip is at the T12 vertebral level. Once this is secured, a second needle is introduced through the sacral hiatus into the sacral canal and a second catheter advanced so that its tip is at the S3 vertebral level, and the patient given a preload infusion of solution. With the onset of moderate uterine pain a test dose is given and, if negative, 4–5 ml of local analgesic solution is injected through the upper catheter and 'top-up' doses are given to produce continuous uterine pain relief. With the onset of perineal pain, 5–7 ml of analgesic solution is injected through the sacral catheter. After flexion and internal rotation are completed, a high concentration of local anaesthetic (e.g. 0.5% bupivacaine or 1.5% lidocaine or 3% chloroprocaine) is injected through the sacral catheter to produce perineal muscle relaxation and anaesthesia of sacral segments only. This technique produces exquisitely specific analgesia for the various stages of labour and delivery with less drug and obviates premature numbness or weakness of the limbs or perineal relaxation. (From Bonica 1980.)

In centres with obstetric anaesthesia services, standard continuous epidural block or continuous segmental block (Fig. 34.16) were the procedures of choice for most parturients up to a decade ago.

Continuous caudal block was formerly used widely, but the increasing use of continuous lumbar epidural block has replaced it in most centres. It is still being used as part of the double catheter epidural technique considered below. Unfortunately, in the United States, the United Kingdom and other countries, there is little training in caudal block, and consequently continuous caudal analgesia used alone is employed in only a few medical centres.

Notwithstanding these comments, a depiction of the techniques (Figs 34.16 and 34.17) and a brief description of their execution is presented here for the sake of completeness.

Continuous epidural analgesia/anaesthesia

During the past four decades, with an increasing use of continuous epidural analgesia/anaesthesia for labour and vaginal delivery and for cesarean section, the technique has undergone a number of modifications. In the 1950s and 1960s, the method entailed the intermittent injection of 12–15 ml of 1–1.5% lidocaine or equianaesthetic concentrations of another local anaesthetic (LA) that usually produces analgesia/anaesthesia from T9–10 to S5 (Fig. 34.16A). While usually effective in providing pain relief throughout labour and delivery, the use of such a relatively high dose of LA increased the risk of systemic toxic reactions from accidental intravenous injection or total spinal anaesthesia from accidental subarachnoid injection leading to mild neonatal depression. Moreover, in many parturients each injection of LA produced a transitory decrease in uterine activity and the technique produced premature weakness or paralysis of the lower limbs and perineal muscles. In the lower limbs this caused discomfort and inconvenience to the patient, while premature perineal muscle weakness or paralysis diminished resistant forces essential for internal rotation of the presenting part. Sacral anaesthesia also eliminated the afferent limb of the reflex urge to bear down. All of these effects resulted in prolongation of the second stage and the need for instrumental delivery (Bonica 1967, 1969, 1980, 1993b; Bonica & McDonald 1990).

These and other concerns led to a series of modifications (Bonica 1993b). Firstly analgesia was limited to T10–11 during the first stage and then extended to the sacral segments (Fig. 34.16B). As previously mentioned, the DCEB provides an excellent form of obstetric analgesia and anaesthesia (Cleland 1949) (Fig. 34.17). The advantage of this technique is that less medication is required than with other epidural block techniques mentioned above. It causes no premature numbness or weakness of the lower limbs and no premature weakness of perineal muscles and consequently no interference with flexion and internal rotation. As mentioned above, it is not used routinely but is reserved for parturients who have maternal and/or fetal complications that require the exquisitely specific type of analgesia/anaesthesia provided by this technique (Fig. 34.17). In some obstetric centres where

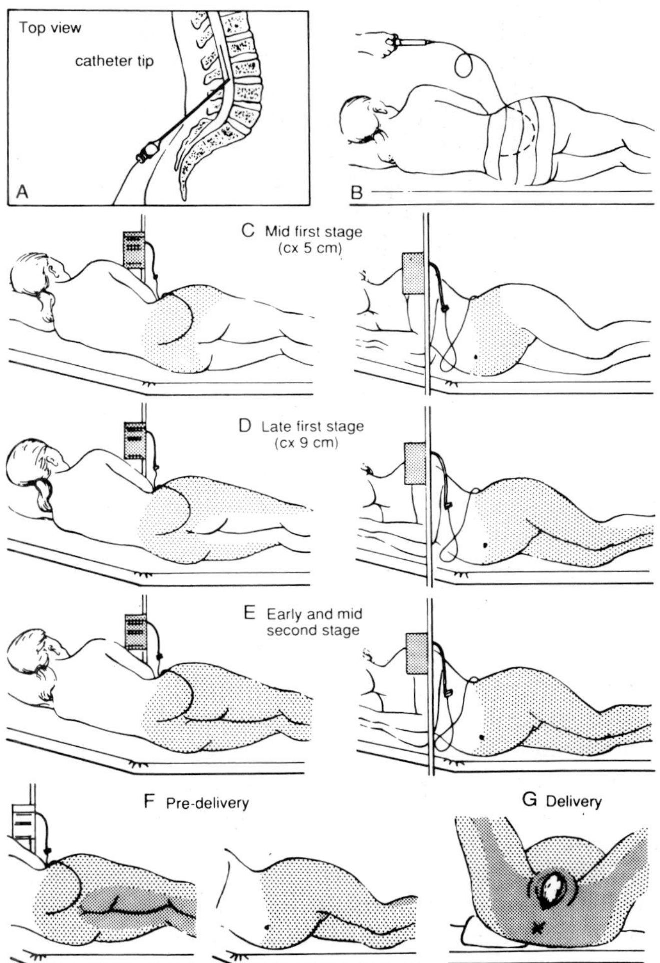

Fig. 34.18 Schematic illustration showing technique of continuous epidural analgesia and the extent and intensity of analgesia during the first and second stages of labour and for delivery. **A** The epidural needle and catheter in place. After removing the needle, the catheter is taped to the patient's back and a test dose of local anaesthetic given. **B** If after 5 min there is no sign of accidental intravenous or subarachnoid injection, a bolus of 5 ml of local anaesthetic is injected while the patient is in the lateral position. **C** After signs of epidural analgesia of T9–10 to 1–2 are noted, the catheter is connected to the continuous infusion system and the solution is administered at a rate of 10–12 ml/h with the patient in a 15–20° head-up position, lying on her side. **D** Extent of analgesia after 1.5–2 h of infusion. **E** Extent of analgesia in the early and mid-second stage. **F** After internal rotation has occurred, injection of a bolus of 10 ml of local anaesthetic solution (e.g. 1% lidocaine) produces an increase in the intensity of analgesia indicated by the more heavily shaded area involving the lower sacral segments. **G** The patient is ready for delivery. Note the wedge under the right hip and lower region to help displace the uterus to the left. (See text for details.)

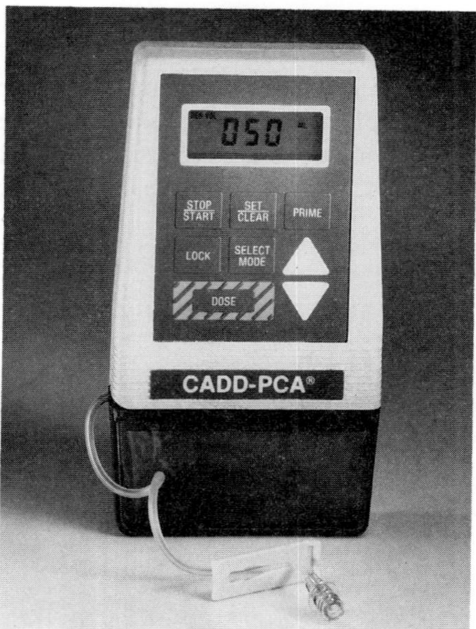

Fig. 34.19 The Pharmacia Deltec CADD-PCA® ambulatory infusion pump.

the anaesthesiologists have had extensive experience with caudal blocks as well as lumbar epidural blocks, the double catheter technique has been used in half of the parturients who required analgesia (Bonica 1993a). Another modification, given trial during the 1980s, was the use of low concentrations of local anaesthetics first injected as boluses and later administered via an infusion pump.

Over several years, the practices have become more widespread of adding opioids to the infusion solution, to enhance the analgesic efficacy of LA, and of using infusion pumps that permit more precise administration of the analgesic solution. This last technique has become very popular. In many institutions where anaesthesiologists provide an obstetric anaesthesia service, it has replaced all other regional techniques for labour and vaginal delivery because it has been shown to:

1. produce more stable levels of analgesia
2. lead to a smaller incidence of maternal hypotension
3. decrease the risk of systemic toxic reaction or accidental total spinal anaesthesia
4. have decreased and, in some instances, eliminated the incidence of motor block, thus obviating the problems mentioned above (Bonica 1993c).

The last advantage mentioned is especially important during the second stage; the incidence of lack of rotation of the presenting part is decreased and the mother can voluntarily mobilise the expulsive forces of labour to achieve spontaneous delivery if this is desired.

Technique of continuous epidural infusion

Detailed description of the technique of achieving lumbar epidural analgesia is beyond the scope of this chapter. Most clinicians use a single catheter placed with its tip in the upper lumbar epidural space. To introduce the catheter, I prefer the use of a Touhy needle via the paramedian technique (Bonica 1956). Once the catheter is fixed in place and all the monitoring and resuscitation equipment is available for immediate use, a test dose consisting of 3 ml of 0.25% bupivacaine and 1:200 000 epinephrine is injected. If no signs of intravenous or subarachnoid injection develop within 5 minutes, a single bolus of 5 ml of 0.25% bupivacaine is injected as a priming dose. This usually produces analgesia extending from T9–T10 to L1–L2 (Fig. 34.18C). As soon as this is achieved, a continuous infusion of a solution containing 0.0625% bupivacaine and 0.0002% fentanyl (2 μg/ml) is initiated at a rate of 10–12 ml/h and this is subsequently increased or decreased to maintain analgesia with the upper level at T10. Usually a total of 120 ml of solution is prepared. Some clinicians use a mixture of 30 ml of 0.25% bupivacaine, 60 μg of sufentanyl and 200 μg of epinephrine in 120 ml volume.

Many clinicians use the Pharmacia Deltec CADD-PCA® ambulatory infusion pump (Fig. 34.19). This infusion pump is preferred because once one learns how to programme it, three options are offered for drug delivery: continuous, continuous plus bolus or bolus. Moreover, it is easy to deliver precisely the needed amounts of drugs and it is small and portable so that the patient can ambulate during the early part of labour, which some obstetricians prefer because they believe that it enhances the progress of labour. A unique advantage related to portability is that it has a self-contained medication cassette with a capacity of 100 ml of solution and thus obviates the need to have a separate medication bottle that requires a pole for its suspension. It also has a number of other important advantages over most of the other infusion pumps available.

Throughout labour and until delivery, if the patient prefers to lie in bed, she is made to lie in the left or right lateral position with the upper part of the body raised about 15–20°. With each subsequent hour, the extent of cephalad level of analgesia remains fairly constant at T10, but the caudal level tends to extend. After about the third or fourth hour, analgesia usually involves all of the lumbar and sacral segments (Fig. 34.18E). In about 50–60% of the parturients, the sacral analgesia is sufficient for perineal analgesia. About 15 minutes before the anticipated delivery 10 ml of 1% lidocaine or 2% chloroprocaine are given with the patient sitting. This usually produces sufficient analgesia and perineal relaxation for the actual delivery.

REFERENCES

Abboud T K, Artal R, Henriksen E H, Earl S, Kammula R K 1982 Effects of spinal anesthesia on maternal circulating catecholamines. American Journal of Obstetrics and Gynecology 142: 252–254

Abboud T K, Sarkis F, Hung T T et al 1983 Effects of epidural anesthesia during labor on maternal plasma beta-endorphin levels. Anesthesiology 59: 1–5

Adams J Q, Alexander A M Jr 1958 Alterations in cardiovascular physiology during labour. Obstetrics and Gynecology 12: 542–549

Albright G A, Ferguson J E, Joyce T H, Stephenson D K 1986 Anaesthesia in obstetrics: maternal, fetal and neonatal aspects, 2nd ed. Butterworths, London

Assali N S, Holm I W, Sehgal N 1962 Hemodynamic changes in foetal lamb in utero in response to asphyxia, hypoxia and hypercapnia. Circulation Research 11: 423–430

Beard R W, Morris E D, Clayton S G 1967 pH of foetal capillary blood as an indication of the condition of foetus. Journal of Obstetrics and Gynaecology of the British Commonwealth 74: 812–822

Behan R J 1914 Pain. Appleton, New York

Berkley K J 1990 The role of various peripheral afferent fibers in pain sensation produced by distension of the vaginal canal in rats. Pain (suppl 5): S239

Berkley K J, Wood E 1989 Responses to varying intensities of vaginal distension in the awake rat. Society of Neuroscience Abstracts 15: 979

Berkley K J, Robbins A, Sato Y 1988 Afferent fibres supplying the uterus in the rat. Journal of Neurophysiology 59: 142–163

Berkley K J, Robbins A, Sato Y 1993a Functional differences between afferent fibres in hypogastric and pelvic nerves innervating female reproductive organs in the rat. Journal of Neurophysiology. 69: 533–544

Berkley K J, Hubscher C H, Wall P D 1993b Neuronal responses to stimulation of the cervix, uterus, colon and skin in the rat spinal cord. Pain 69: 545–556

Bonica J J 1956 Continuous peridural block. Anesthesiology 17: 626–630

Bonica J J 1960 An atlas on mechanisms and pathways of pain in labor. What's New 217: 16

Bonica J J 1967 Principles and practice of obstetric analgesia and anaesthesia, vol 1. F A Davis, Philadelphia

Bonica J J 1969 Principles and practice of obstetric analgesia and anaesthesia, vol 2. F A Davis, Philadelphia

Bonica J J 1973 Maternal respiratory changes during pregnancy and parturition. In: Marx G F (ed) Parturition and perinatology. F A Davis, Philadelphia

Bonica J J 1974 Current role of nerve blocks in the diagnosis and therapy of pain. In Advances in neurology, vol 4. (Proceedings of the International Symposium on Pain). Raven Press, New York, p 445–453

Bonica J J 1978 Effects of analgesia and anaesthesia on the mother, fetus, and newborn. In: Marcus S L, Marcus C (eds) Advances in obstetrics and gynecology. Williams & Wilkins, Baltimore

Bonica J J 1979 Peripheral mechanisms and pathways of parturition pain. British Journal of Anaesthesia 51: 3–9

Bonica J J 1980 Obstetric analgesia and anaesthesia, 2nd edn. World Federation of Societies of Anaesthesiologists, Amsterdam. University of Washington Press, Seattle

Bonica J J 1990 Postoperative pain. In: Bonica J J (ed) Management of pain, 2nd edn. Lea & Febiger, Philadelphia

Bonica J J 1993a Historical perspectives: evolution and current status of obstetric analgesia and anesthesia. In: Bonica J J, McDonald J S (eds) Principles and practice of obstetric analgesia and anesthesia, 2nd edn. Lea & Febiger, Malvern, Pennsylvania, p 1

Bonica J J 1993b The nature of the pain of childbirth. In: Bonica J J, McDonald J S (eds) Principles and practice of obstetric analgesia and anesthesia, 2nd edn. Lea & Febiger, Malvern, Pennsylvania, ch 9

Bonica J J 1993c Epidural analgesia and anesthesia. In: Bonica J J, McDonald J S (eds) Principles and practice of obstetric analgesia and anesthesia, 2nd edn. Lea & Febiger, Malvern, Pennsylvania, ch 12

Bonica J J, Chadwick H S 1989 Labour pain. In: Melzack R, Wall P D (eds) Textbook of pain, 2nd edn. Churchill Livingstone, Edinburgh, p 482

Bonica J J, Hunter C A Jr 1969 Management in dysfunction of the forces of labor. In: Bonica J J (ed) Principles and practice of obstetric analgesia and anesthesia, vol 2. F A Davis, Philadelphia, p 1188–1208

Bonica J J, McDonald J S 1990 The pain of childbirth In: Bonica J J (ed) The management of pain, 2nd edn. Lea & Febiger, Malvern, Pennsylvania, p 1313–1343

Bonica J J, McDonald J S 1993 Principles and practice of obstetric analgesia and anaesthesia, 2nd edn. Lea & Febiger, Malvern, Pennsylvania

Brown W A, Manning T, Grodin J 1972 The relationship of antenatal and perinatal variables to the use of drugs of labor. Psychosomatic Medicine 34: 119–127

Browning A J, Butt W R, Lynch S S, Shakespear R A, Crawford J S 1983 Maternal and cord plasma concentrations of beta-lipotrophin, beta-endorphin and γ-lipotrophin at delivery: effect of analgesia. British Journal of Obstetrics and Gynaecology 90: 1152–1156

Buchan P C 1980 Emotional stress in childbirth and its modification by variations in obstetric management – epidural analgesia and stress in labor. Acta Obstetricia et Gynecologica Scandinavica 59: 319–321

Bundsen P 1975 Subjectiva resultat av smärtlindring under förlossning – enkätundersökning. Läkartidningen 3: 129–136

Clark S L, Phelan J P, Greenspoon J, Aldahl D, Horenstein J 1985 Labor and delivery in the presence of mitral stenosis: central hemodynamic observations. American Journal of Obstetrics and Gynecology 152: 984–988

Cleland J G 1933 Paravertebral anesthesia in obstetrics. Surgery, Gynecology and Obstetrics 57: 51–62

Cleland J G P 1949 Continuous peridural and caudal analgesia in obstetrics. Current Researches in Anesthesia and Analgesia 28: 61–76

Cogan R, Spinnato J A 1986 Pain and discomfort thresholds in late pregnancy. Pain 27: 63–68

Cole P V, Nainby-Luxmoore R C 1962 Respiratory volumes in labour. British Medical Journal 1: 1118

Crawford J S 1984 Principles and practice of obstetric anaesthesia, 5th edn. Blackwell, Oxford

Csontos K, Rust M, Hollt V 1980 The role of endorphins during parturition. National Institute of Drug Abuse Research Monograph Series, p 164–271

Davenport-Slack B, Boylan C H 1974 Psychological correlates of childbirth pain. Psychosomatic Medicine 36: 215–223

Deutsch H 1955 Psychology of pregnancy, labour and puerperium. In: Greenhill J P (ed) Obstetrics, 11th edn. W B Saunders, Philadelphia, p 349–360

Dick-Read G 1933 Natural childbirth. Heinemann, London

Dick-Read G 1953 Childbirth without fear. Harper, New York

Eustace T D 1978 Cognitive, attitudinal and socioeconomic factors influencing parents' choice of childbirth procedure. Dissertation Abstracts International 39: 1474B

Facchinetti F, Centini G, Parrini D et al 1982 Opioid plasma levels during labour. Gynecologic and Obstetric Investigation 13: 155–163

Falconer A D, Powles A B 1982 Plasma noradrenaline levels during labor. Anesthesiology 37: 416–420

Fettes I, Fox J, Kuzniak S, Shime J, Gare D 1984 Plasma levels of immunoreactive beta-endorphin and adrenocorticotropic hormone during labor and delivery. Obstetrics and Gynecology 64: 359–362

Fisher A, Prys-Roberts C 1968 Maternal pulmonary gas exchange: a study during normal labour and extradural blockade. Anaesthesia 23: 350–355

Foley K M, Kourides I A, Inturrisi C E et al 1979 Beta-endorphin: analgesic and hormonal effects in humans. Proceedings of the National Academy of Sciences USA 76: 5377–5831

Ford C S 1945 A comparative study of human reproduction. Yale University Press, New Haven, Connecticut

Freedman L Z, Ferguson V S 1950 The question of 'painless childbirth' in primitive cultures. American Journal of Orthopsychiatry 20: 363–379

Fridh G, Kopare T, Gaston-Johansson F, Norvell K T 1988 Factors associated with more intense labor pain. Research in Nursing and Health 11: 117–124

Gabbe S G, Niebyl J R, Simpson J L 1991 Obstetrics: normal and problem pregnancies, 2nd edn. Churchill Livingstone, New York
Gaston-Johansson F, Fridh G, Turner-Norvell K 1988 Progression of labor pain in primiparas and multiparas. Nursing Research 37: 86–90
Gintzler A R 1980 Endorphin-mediated increases in pain threshold during pregnancy. Science 210: 193–195
Gintzler A R, Peters L C, Komisaruk B R 1983 Attenuation of pregnancy-induced analgesia by hypogastric neurectomy in rats. Brain Research 277: 186–188
Glassenberg R 1991 General anesthesia and maternal mortality. Seminars in Perinatology 15: 386–396
Goebelsmann U, Abboud T K, Hoffman D I, Hung T T 1984 Beta-endorphin in pregnancy. European Journal of Obstetrics, Gynaecology and Reproductive Biology 17: 77–89
Goland R S, Wardlaw S L, Start R I, Frantz A G 1981 Human plasma beta-endorphin during pregnancy, labor and delivery. Journal of Clinical Endocrinology and Metabolism 52: 74–78
Gray H 1973 Anatomy of the human body, 29th edn (American). Lea & Febiger, Philadelphia
Gray H, 1980 Gray's anatomy. Williams P L, Warwick R (eds) 36th edn (British). Churchill Livingstone, Edinburgh
Hansen J M, Ueland K 1966 The influence of caudal analgesia on cardiovascular dynamics during normal labour and delivery. Acta Anaesthesiologica Scandinavica 23 (suppl 10): 449–452
Hayes J R, Ardill J, Kennedy T L, Shanks R G, Buchanan K D 1972 Stimulation of gastrin release by catecholamines. Lancet 1: 819–821
Head H 1893 On disturbances of sensation with special reference to the pain of visceral disease. Brain 16: 1–132
Hendricks C H, Quilligan E J 1956 Cardiac output during labor. American Journal of Obstetrics and Gynecology 71: 953–972
Holdsworth J D 1978 Relationships between stomach contents and analgesia in labour. British Journal of Anaesthesia 50: 1145–1148
Huch A, Huch R, Schneider H, Rooth G 1977 Continuous transcutaneous monitoring of foetal oxygen tension during labour. British Journal of Obstetrics and Gynaecology 84 (supp 1): 1–39
Hughey M J, McElin T W, Young T 1978 Maternal and fetal outcome of Lamaze-prepared patients. Obstetrics and Gynecology 51: 643–647
Janisch H, Leodolter S, Neumark J, Phillip K 1978 Der Einfluss der kontinuierlichen Epiduralanaesthesia auf die uteroplazentare Durchblutung. Zeitschrift für Geburtshilfe und Perinatologie 182: 343–346
Javert C T, Hardy J D 1950 Measurement of pain intensity in labor and its physiologic, neurologic and pharmacologic implications. American Journal of Obstetrics and Gynecology 60: 552–563
Jochelson W 1910 The Ukaghir and the Youkaghirized Tungus. Volume XIII of the Memoirs of the American Museum of Natural History which constitutes at the same time volume IX, part I, of the Jesup North Pacific Expedition. New York and Leiden
Jouppila R 1977 The effect of segmental epidural analgesia on hormonal and metabolic changes during labour. Acta Universitatis Ouluensis, Series D, Medica No. 16, Anaesthesiologica No. 2
Jouppila R, Hollmén A 1976 The effect of segmental epidural analgesia on maternal and foetal acid-base balance, lactate, serum potassium and creatine phosphokinase during labour. Acta Anaesthesiologica Scandinavia 20: 259–268
Jouppila P, Jouppila R, Hollmén A, Koivula A 1982 Lumbar epidural analgesia to improve intervillous blood flow during labour in severe pre-eclampsia. Obstetrics and Gynecology 60: 19–29
Kawatani M, Takeshige C, Narasimhan S, De Groat W C 1986 An analysis of the afferent and efferent pathways to the uterus of the cat using axonal tracing techniques. Society of Neuroscience Abstracts 12: 1055
Klink E W 1953 Perineal nerve block: an anatomic and clinical study in the female. Obstetrics and Gynecology 1: 137–146
Kohnen N 1986 "Natural" childbirth among the Kankanaly-Igorot. Bulletin of the New York Academy of Medicine 62: 768–777
Lamaze F 1956 Qu'est-ce que l'accouchement sans douleur par la méthode psychoprophylactique? Ses principles, sa réalization, ses résultants. Savoir et Connâitre, Paris
Lederman, R P, McCann D S, Work B, Huber M J 1977 Endogenous plasma epinephrine and norepinephrine in last-trimester pregnancy and labour. American Journal of Obstetrics and Gynecology 129: 5–8
Lederman R P, Lederman E, Work B A Jr, McCann D S 1978 The relationship of maternal anxiety, plasma catecholamines, and plasma cortisol to progress in labor. American Journal of Obstetrics and Gynecology 132: 495–500
Lees M M, Scott D B, Kerr M G 1970 Haemodynamic changes associated with labour. Journal of Obstetrics and Gynaecology of the British Commonwealth 77: 29–36
Lefebvre L, Carli G 1985 Parturition pain in non-human primates: pain and auditory concealment. Pain 21: 315–327
Lévy-Strauss C 1956 Sorciers et psychanalyse. Courier de l'UNÉSCO 7–8: 808–810
Lowe N K 1989 Explaining the pain of active labor: the importance of maternal confidence. Research in Nursing and Health 12: 237–245
Lundh W 1974 Mödraundervisning, Förlossningsträning eller föräldrakunskap? PhD dissertation, Pedagogiska Institutionen, Stockholms Universitet
Lynch C III, Rizor R F 1982 Anesthetic management and monitoring of a parturient with mitral and aortic valvular disease. Anesthesia and Analgesia 61: 788–792
Marx G F, Greene N M 1964 Maternal lactate, pyruvate and excess lactate production during labor and delivery. American Journal of Obstetrics and Gynecology 90: 786–793
Marx G F, Macatangay A S, Cohen A V, Schulman H 1969 Effect of pain relief on arterial blood gas values during labor. New York Journal of Medicine 69: 819–822
Marx J L 1979 Dysmenorrhea: basic research leads to a rational therapy. Science 205: 175–176
Meehan J P, Stoll A M, Hardy J D 1954 Cutaneous pain threshold in native Alaskan Indians and Eskimos. Journal of Applied Physiology 6: 397–400
Melzack R 1975 The McGill pain questionnaire: major properties and scoring methods. Pain 1: 277–299
Melzack R 1984 The myth of painless childbirth – the John J. Bonica Lecture. Pain 19: 321–337
Melzack R, Belanger E 1989 Labour pain: correlations with menstrual pain and acute low-back pain before and during pregnancy. Pain 36: 225–229
Melzack R, Schaffelberg D 1987 Low-back pain during labor. American Journal of Obstetrics and Gynecology 156: 901–905
Melzack R, Taenzer P, Feldman P, Kinch R A 1981 Labour is still painful after prepared childbirth training. Canadian Medical Association Journal 125: 357–363
Melzack R, Wall P D, By T C 1982 Acute pain in an emergency clinic: latency of onset and descriptor patterns related to different injuries. Pain 14: 33–43
Melzack R, Kinch R, Dobkin P, Lebrun M, Laenzer P 1984 Severity of labour pain: influence of physical as well as psychological variables. Canadian Medical Association Journal 130: 579–584
Moir C 1939 The nature of the pain of labour. Journal of Obstetrics and Gynaecology of the British Empire 46: 409–424
Moir D D, Willocks J 1967 Management of incoordinate uterine action under continuous epidural analgesia. British Medical Journal 3: 396–400
Moore D C, Batra M S 1981 The components of an effective test dose prior to epidural block. Anesthesiology 55: 693–696
Morishima H O, Pedersen H, Finster M 1978 The influence of maternal psychological stress on the fetus. American Journal of Obstetrics and Gynecology 131: 286–290
Morishima H O, Pedersen H, Finster M 1980 Effects of pain on mother, labour and fetus. In: Marx G F, Bassel G M (eds) Obstetric analgesia and anaesthesia. Elsevier/North Holland, Amsterdam p 197–210
Myers R E 1975 Maternal psychological stress and fetal asphyxia: a study in the monkey. American Journal of Obstetrics and Gynecology 122: 47–59
Nettelbladt P, Fagerström C F, Uddenberg N 1976 The significance of reported childbirth pain. Journal of Psychosomatic Research 20: 215–221
Neumark J, Hammerle A F, Biegelmayer C 1985 Effects of epidural analgesia on plasma catecholamines and cortisol in parturition. Acta Anaesthesiologica Scandinavica 29: 555–559
Nimmo W S, Wilson J, Prescott L F 1975 Narcotic analgesics and delayed gastric emptying during labour. Lancet 1: 890–893

Norr K L, Block C R, Charles A, Meyering S, Meyers E 1977 Explaining pain and enjoyment in childbirth. Journal of Health and Social Behavior 18: 260–275

Ohno H, Yamashita K, Yahata et al 1986 Maternal plasma concentrations of catecholamines and cyclic nucleotides during labor and following delivery. Research Communications in Chemical Pathology and Pharmacology 51: 183–194

Palahniuk R J, Shnider S M, Eger E I II 1974 Pregnancy decreases the requirement for inhaled anesthetic agents. Anesthesiology 41: 82–83

Peabody J L 1979 Transcutaneous oxygen measurement to evaluate drug effect. Clinical Perinatology 6: 109–121

Pearson J F, Davies P 1973a The effect of continuous epidural analgesia on the acid–base status of maternal arterial blood during the first stage of labour. Journal of Obstetrics and Gynaecology of the British Commonwealth 80: 218–224

Pearson J F, Davies P 1973b The effect of continuous epidural analgesia on maternal acid–base balance and arterial lactate concentration during the second stage of labour. Journal of Obstetrics and Gynaecology of the British Commonwealth 80: 225–229

Pearson J F, Davies P 1974 The effect of continuous lumbar epidural analgesia upon fetal acid–base status of maternal arterial blood during the first stage of labour. Journal of Obstetrics and Gynaecology of the British Commonwealth 81: 975–979

Peters L C, Kristal M B, Komisaruk B R 1987 Sensory innervation of the external and internal genitalia of the female rat. Brain Research 408: 199–204

Preissman A B, Ogoulbostan-Essenova 1956 Some details of psychoprophylactic preparation for childbirth in the Turkomenian. S S R Kiev Congress 90: 66–67

Prowse C M, Gaensler E A 1965 Respiratory and acid–base changes during pregnancy. Anesthesiology 26: 381–392

Raisanen I, Paatero H, Salminen K, Laatikainen T 1986 Beta-endorphin in maternal and umbilical cord plasma at elective cesarean section and in spontaneous labor. Obstetrics and Gynecology 67: 384–387

Reading A E, Cox D N 1985 Psychosocial predictors of labor pain. Pain 22: 309–315

Reynolds S R M 1949 Physiology of the uterus, 2nd edn. Paul B Hoeber, New York

Robson S C, Dunlop W, Boys R J, Hunter S 1987 Cardiac output during labor. British Medical Journal 295: 1169–1172

Romanes G J (ed) 1972 Cunningham's textbook of anatomy, 11th edn. Oxford University Press, Oxford

Rust M, Egbert R, Gessler M et al 1983 Verminderte Schmerzempfindung wahrend Schwangerschaft und Geburt. Archives of Gynecology 235: 676–677

Sander H W, Portoghese P S, Gintzler A R 1988 Spinal κ-opiate receptor involvement in the analgesia of pregnancy: effects of intrathecal norbinal-torphimine, a κ-selective antagonist. Brain Research 474: 343–347

Scott J R, Rose N B 1976 Effect of psychoprophylaxis (Lamaze preparation) on labor and delivery in primiparas. New England Journal of Medicine 294: 1205–1207

Scott-Palmer J, Skevington S M 1981 Pain during childbirth and menstruation: a study of locus of control. Journal of Psychosomatic Research 25: 151–155

Shnider S M, Levinson G 1987 Anesthesia for obstetrics, 2nd edn. Williams & Wilkins, Baltimore

Shnider S M, Wright R G, Levinson G et al 1979 Uterine blood flow and plasma norepinephrine changes during maternal stress in the pregnant ewe. Anesthesiology 50: 524–527

Shnider S M, Abboud T K, Artal R, Henriksen E H, Stefani S J, Levinson G 1983 Maternal catecholamines decrease during labor after lumbar epidural anesthesia. American Journal of Obstetrics and Gynecology 147: 13–15

Sørenson M B, Korshin J D, Fernandes A, Secher O 1982 The use of epidural analgesia for delivery in a patient with pulmonary hypertension. Acta Anaesthesiologica Scandinavica 26: 180–182

Stewart D E 1982 Psychiatric symptoms following attempted natural childbirth. Canadian Medical Association Journal 127: 713–716

Thalme B, Belfrage P, Raabe N 1974 Lumbar epidural analgesia in labour. Acta Obstetricia et Gynecologica Scandinavica 53: 27–35

Thalme B, Belfrage P, Raabe N 1974 Lumbar epidural analgesia in labour. Acta Obstetricia et Gynecologica Scandinavica 53: 113–119

Tomkinson J et al 1982 Report on confidential enquiries into maternal death in England and Wales 1976–1978. Report on Health and Social Subjects No.16. HMSO, London

True R M 1954 Obstetrical hypoanalgesia. American Journal of Obstetrics and Gynecology 67: 373–376

Ueland K, Hansen J M 1969 Maternal cardiovascular dynamics. II. Posture and uterine contractions. American Journal of Obstetrics and Gynecology 103: 1–7

Velvovski I Z, Chougom E A, Plotitcher V A 1950 The psychoprophylactic and psychotherapeutic method in painless childbirth. Pediatriia, Akushertvo i Ginekologiia 1: 32–41

Westgren M, Lindahl S G E, Nord'en N E 1986 Maternal and fetal endocrine stress response at vaginal delivery with and without an epidural block. Journal of Perinatal Medicine 14: 235–241

Williams J W 1985 In: Prichard J A, MacDonald P C, Gant N F (eds) Obstetrics, 17th edn, Appleton-Century-Crofts, Neward, Connecticut

Winsberg B, Greenlick M 1967 Pain response in Negro and white obstetrical patients. Journal of Health and Social Behavior 8: 222–227

Wolff B B, Langley S 1975 Cultural factors and the response to pain: a review. In: Weisenberg M (ed) Pain: clinical and experimental perspectives. C V Mosby, St Louis

Zuckerman M, Nurnberger J I, Gardiner S H, Vandiveer J M, Barrett B H, den Breeijen A 1963 Psychological correlates of somatic complaints in pregnancy and difficulty in childbirth. Journal of Consulting and Clinical Psychology 27: 324–329

35. Genitourinary pain

Mostafa M. Elhilali and Howard N. Winfield

INTRODUCTION

Pain related to the genitourinary tract is a frequent presenting symptom in general as well as urological practice. The relationship between the pain and an underlying pathology which explains it is not always that simple. Patients referred for renal colic, or flank pain, particularly when the French term for back pain, *mal au rein*, is literally interpreted as 'pain in the kidney', are frequently suffering from musculoskeletal-type pain completely unrelated to the kidney. On the other hand a true renal colic or renal pain can be elusive, requiring repeated evaluation, and frequently only provocative tests will confirm its aetiology. A small stone harmlessly lodged in a lower calyx is frequently dismissed as nonobstructive, until an X-ray during a second renal colic demonstrates its mobile and obstructive nature. In the same way a ureteropelvic junction which appears patent on a urogram becomes quite obstructive when the system is challenged by a fluid overload or a diuretic. Patients presenting with pelvic or suprapubic pain can be similarly challenging to the treating physician and this may be quite frustrating to the patient. It is not always acceptable to the patient that his doctor is unable to pinpoint the disease and even less acceptable that the doctor may not be able to get rid of the pain once and for all.

Acute and chronic pelvic pain in the female is well covered in Chapter 33. We will restrict our discussion to pelvic and perineal pain in the male.

Painful micturition associated with urinary frequency can be produced by acute cystitis or acute prostatitis, which respond well to treatment. Chronic symptoms are not as easily cured and can be very disturbing. Testicular pain is no exception. It can also be straightforward, but frequently the pain is referred from other organs, in which case the diagnosis is not always clear.

In this chapter we will give a short description of the innervation of the genitourinary tract. The different types of pain related to these organs will be discussed, with descriptions of the pathophysiology, diagnosis and treatment of each type of pain.

INNERVATION OF THE GENITOURINARY TRACT

The innervation of the urinary and male genital tract is rather complex and consists mainly of autonomic nerves with somatic innervation primarily involved with the urethra and external urethral sphincter, as well as the penis.

RENAL NERVE SUPPLY

The renal plexus is formed by a group of nerve cells situated behind the origin of each renal artery at the level of T12–L2. Contributing to this plexus are branches from the coeliac ganglia, aorticorenal ganglion, the aortic plexus, the lowest thoracic nerves and finally the first lumbar splanchnic nerve. The autonomic fibres follow the renal artery into the kidney hilus supplying the vessels, glomerular structures and tubules. Afferent fibres arising in the region of the renal capsule and cortex follow the same pathway out of the kidney with most of the fibres terminating in the sympathetic system, with some following the vagus nerve. These fibres reach the spinal cord at the level of the T11–L2 segments.

Renal pain, through the autonomic innervation, is perceived in a nonspecific fashion in the region of the costovertebral angle (CVA). However, renal pain may be referred to the inguinal and thigh regions. Somatic fibres from the inguinal and thigh regions enter the spinal cord at the same level as the renal autonomic afferent fibres. Afferent sensory renal fibres which follow the course of the vagus nerve explain the nausea, vomiting and decreased peristalsis of the intestine which are frequently associated with renal colic.

URETERAL NERVE SUPPLY

The upper third of the ureter is innervated by branches from the renal and aortic plexuses, the middle third from the superior hypogastric plexus and the lower third from the hypogastric nerve and inferior hypogastric plexuses.

The visceral-type pain of the ureter may be experienced in the CVA region, radiating to the iliac fossa, groin, ipsilateral testicle and proximal thigh regions. When a renal stone reaches the intramural ureter, pain can be referred to the urinary meatus, associated with irritable vesical symptoms.

BLADDER AND URETHRA

The autonomic nervous system is primarily responsible for bladder and proximal urethral innervation. Sympathetic nerve fibres originating from the level of T11–L2 pass via the sympathetic nerve trunks to the superior hypogastric plexus into the inferior hypogastric plexus. From here, motor alpha- and beta-adrenergic fibres arise and are distributed throughout the bladder body, base and proximal urethral region, encouraging bladder relaxation (beta-adrenergic) and bladder neck closure (alpha-adrenergic). Sensory sympathetic fibres, travelling in a reverse fashion, transmit the sensation of pain, touch and temperature. The sensation of bladder muscle stretching or fullness (proprioception) is transmitted by parasympathetic nervous fibres, through the inferior hypogastric plexus to the sacral spinal cord at the levels between S2 and S4. Bladder muscle contraction and emptying are produced primarily by motor parasympathetic cholinergic innervation. The synchronisation of detrusor–sphincter activities is beyond the scope of this discussion.

Parasympathetic and sympathetic (alpha) nerves are distributed throughout the urethra. Somatic fibres from the pudendal nerve corresponding to the sacral segments S2–S4 innervate the external sphincter and distal urethra beyond the prostatomembranous region. The sensation of pain in the distal urethra is transmitted by the pudendal nerve.

PROSTATE GLAND

The prostate gland is richly supplied by sympathetic and parasympathetic innervation. The adrenergic receptors in the prostate gland are predominantly of alpha-1 type and are localised in the prostatic smooth muscle. The few alpha-2 receptors found in the prostate gland are associated specifically with the blood vessels. The beta-adrenergic receptor content of the prostatic tissue is negligible.

The muscarinic receptors are not found in the prostatic muscle but are localised to the glandular epithelium. The function of the cholinergic system is related to prostatic secretion and not to muscular contraction.

The surgical capsule surrounding the prostatic tissue is also rich in alpha-adrenergic receptors, and beta receptors are almost absent. The muscarinic receptors are abundant in the muscle of the anterior part of the surgical capsule but negligible in that of the posterior part.

TESTES AND SCROTUM

The testes originate from the genital ridge on each side of the midline between the primitive kidneys. The blood, lymph and innervation are primarily from this region. There is no somatic innervation – only autonomic fibres from the renal plexus and intermesenteric nerve fibres in the region from T12–L2. The innervation of the epididymis arises from the hypogastric and vesical plexuses. The anterior scrotal wall is innervated by branches of the genitofemoral nerve (L1–L2) and some perineal branches from the internal pudendal and posterior femoral cutaneous nerves supply the posterior scrotum.

PENIS

In recent years, the complex innervation of the penis has been more completely delineated. The autonomic innervation of the penis, emanating mainly from the sacral spinal cord (S2–S4) via the hypogastric plexus, is responsible for erections and is beyond the scope of this chapter.

Sensory somatic innervation from the glans penis, shaft of the penis, urethra and external urethral sphincter is transmitted by branches of the pudendal nerve which pass through Alcock's canal, entering into the true pelvis and terminating at the sacral spinal cord segments S2–S4. Some minor sensory fibres of the ilioinguinal nerve supply cutaneous innervation of the skin at the base of the penis.

PAIN AND THE GENITOURINARY TRACT

KIDNEY PAIN

This type of pain may be intermittently colicky or steady, boring and visceral in nature. The colicky type of pain may result from a rather acute distension of the upper collecting system due to an obstructing lesion. Its mechanism does not seem to be related to ureterohyperperistalsis. The visceral type of renal pain may be caused by inflammation of the kidneys, as in pyelonephritis, or may be caused by sudden renal ischaemia caused by an obstructing embolus or thrombus in the renal vasculature.

Renal colic

The symptoms associated with renal colic vary from intermittent aching flank pain to what is described as the 'worst pain ever experienced'– squeezing, nauseating, radiating from the costovertebral angle laterally around to the lower quadrant and into the testicle or labia. Its onset is usually sudden and often wakes the patient at night or begins while he is sitting quietly. The patient is restless, unable to find a comfortable position and frequently only narcotic analgesics can control the waves of colicky pain.

In most cases the renal colic is caused by the passage of a renal calculus causing a degree of obstruction at the ureteropelvic junction (UPJ) or passing down the ureter. However, intrinsic or extrinsic congenital UPJ obstruction, blood clots from a renal tumour (usually intrapelvic transitional cell carcinoma), sloughed papilla (from papillary necrosis as in diabetes or analgesic abusers) and fungus balls (in immunocompromised patients or diabetics) are other disease entities which must be considered.

The pain of renal colic is best explained by the sudden distension of the proximal ureter and renal pelvis. As the autonomic nervous system transmits the pain from the distended upper collecting system it is nonspecific in nature, with pathways passing through the coeliac ganglia, aorticorenal and aortic plexuses. Discomfort in the testis is referred from similar autonomic nerve pathways supplying the kidney. Associated nausea, vomiting and intestinal ileus are a result of transmission of renal afferent pain fibres through the coeliac ganglion.

Acute pyelonephritis and/or perinephric abscess

The features associated with pyelonephritis and perinephric processes are chills, dysuria, fever and CVA tenderness. From a pathological point of view the kidney is usually grossly enlarged due to the inflammation and oedema of the collecting system as well as nephric tissue extending to the renal capsule. The infection may extend through the renal capsule and form a perinephric abscess.

The pain associated with these infectious processes of the kidney is constantly aching in character and transmitted through the previously mentioned renal nervous pathways. With extension of the infectious process into the perinephric space, irritation of the psoas muscle with ilioinguinal, iliohypogastric and genitofemoral nerves may refer pain to the inguinal, genital and ipsilateral hip/thigh regions.

Renal artery embolus–renal vein thrombosis

Renal artery embolism should be suspected in an individual who develops sudden severe persistent pain in the CVA or upper abdomen, associated with nausea, vomiting and fever. It is most commonly associated with a history of cardiac disease, atrial fibrillation, mitral stenosis, artificial heart valves with embolic phenomena if not properly anticoagulated or known mural thrombus associated with a myocardial infarction. Individuals with significant atherosclerotic aortic or renal disease who have arteriography or vessel surgery, such as angioplasty, are at risk of a plaque being sloughed off and acting as an embolus. Renal vein thrombosis in the adult is often associated with the nephrotic syndrome and has associated gross haematuria, hypertension and fever. In infants it is associated with severe dehydration, often resulting in bilateral renal vein thrombosis. The pain associated with these renal vascular diseases is very severe and is caused by ischaemic tissue with resultant oedema and cellular destruction. The pain fibres are transmitted through the aorticorenal and aortic plexuses as well as the coeliac ganglia.

It has also been suggested by some authors that traction on the renal pedicle or 'vascular drag', as sometimes seen with nephroptosis, may cause significant renal pain, mimicking the other renal vascular entities.

Differential diagnosis of renal pain

The differential diagnosiss of renal pain is quite extensive and can be related to gastrointestinal or gynaecological disorders. Herpes zoster has also been associated with severe flank discomfort along the T12–L1–L2 dermatomes. The diagnosis becomes apparent once the herpetic vesicles appear. One of the most difficult diagnoses to make, and where renal pain is often mimicked, is radiculitis or costovertebral joint derangement. This has an abrupt onset of pain with exacerbation from certain body movements. Some 40% of patients with radiculitis have involvement of the 10th, 11th or 12th costovertebral joint complex, which suggests the diagnosis of renal flank pain. The disease entity should be strongly suspected in individuals who have normal urograms; the pain is accentuated by deep palpation over the costovertebral region and is augmented by movement. Films of the thoracic spine concentrating on the costotransverse joints will often demonstrate some abnormality.

In investigating the aetiology of kidney pain it is important to examine the urine carefully and, if necessary, to take a urine culture. The mainstay urological X-rays of intravenous pyelography, renal ultrasound and renal scan are invaluable. Radiolucent stones or suspected upper tract filling defects should be investigated further with urine cytology, cystoscopy and retrograde pyelogram. Pending the results of these initial tests, appropriate further investigations or treatment are instituted. Occasionally provocative tests such as diuretic urography or renography are essential for reaching a diagnosis.

URETERAL PAIN

Pain associated with the ureter is in most cases related to abrupt distension of the ureteral lumen above an obstructing process, usually a stone, but possibly a blood clot, tumour or necrosed papilla. As described in the section on ureteral nerve innervation, the pain is generally colicky in nature with radiation from the CVA region towards the ipsilateral groin and genital area. Obstructing stones in the lower uterer are also associated with bladder discomfort, urgency and frequency of micturition.

The treatment of choice for upper or midureteral calculi is extracorporeal shockwave lithotripsy or percutaneous removal. Lower ureteral stones are best removed by ureteroscopic extraction.

Ureteral tumours rarely cause pain, as the obstruction is usually slow and gradual. Pain associated with ureteral tumour may be due to sloughing of tumour tissue with distal obstruction and/or stone crystallisation with the tumour acting as a nidus. Treatment for proximal or midureteral tumours is generally total nephroureterectomy with removal of bladder cuff around the ureteric orifice. Distal ureteral tumours can be best managed by distal ureteral removal with ureterovesical reimplantation.

Appendicitis, diverticulitis and salpingitis may mimic ureteral pain and also contribute to extrinsic compression and inflammation of the mid- to distal ureter.

BLADDER PAIN

Pain in the suprapubic region is readily ascribed to the bladder. True bladder pain is frequently related to the state of bladder fullness, being most pronounced when the bladder is full and partly or totally improved by emptying the bladder. Bladder pain may be the result of distension of an inflamed bladder wall which may result from an acute or chronic nonspecific inflammation or interstitial cystitis. It may also be produced by a bladder stone, bladder tumour (particularly infiltrating tumour) or following radiotherapy. It may be less frequently associated with large diverticulum or infiltration by a peridiverticulitis, in which case intestinal symptoms should suggest the proper diagnosis.

Uninhibited bladder contractions may be interpreted by the patient as bladder pain or spasm. These contractions may be due to central lesions but may also be reflex in nature.

Interstitial cystitis, in which suprapubic pain is a relatively frequent feature, deserves more specific mention. The aetiology is still unknown although many theories have been put forward. The incidence of the full picture of Hunner's ulcer is infrequent. The incidence of early signs (such as mucosal glomerulation on bladder distension during cystoscopy) is more frequent. The suprapubic pain and frequency of micturition may become so incapacitating that bladder replacement becomes indicated.

The investigations to determine the cause of bladder pain include urine analysis and culture, cystometrogram and cystoscopy. Bladder biopsy of suspicious lesions or ulcers becomes important to confirm the diagnosis of interstitial cystitis or carcinoma in situ.

Management depends on the diagnosis. Antibiotics are indicated if significant infection is confirmed. A foreign body requires removal. Interstitial cystitis is not readily responsive to treatment: antihistamines have been tried with varying results and anticholinergics and antispasmodics have been tried with minimal success. Local bladder instillations of dimethyl sulphoxide (DMSO) with or without heparin, and oral ingestion of sodium pentosanpolysulphate (Elmiron) have been used with some favourable results. When bladder capacity is markedly reduced, removal of the bladder up to the trigone and replacement with intestinal substitutes can be undertaken.

Some dyes, such as pyridium or methylene blue, have been used nonspecifically as bladder mucosal analgesics. Their therapeutic value is quite limited and they are usually effective for a short period of time.

Management of chronic pelvic and bladder pain with neurostimulation

During the last decade, there has been a growing interest in applying long-term stimulation of the sacral nerve roots to control the spasticity of pelvic musculature that accompanies chronic pelvic pain. The exact mechanism of such neuromodulation is unknown at present; however, it is believed that the stimulation of A-delta myelinated fibres (typically, sacral roots S3 and S4) decreases the spastic behaviour of the pelvic floor and alleviates the associated pain. Such neuromodulation lessens the perceived intensity of the pain by exciting antinociceptive neuronal systems and by masking or changing the nature of the pain through the sensation of the electric stimulation.

The principle has been applied in patients presenting with urge–frequency syndrome associated with pelvic pain and/or incontinence. These patients undergo a percutaneous nerve evaluation, using an external pulse generator to stimulate S3 uni- or bilaterally. They are allowed to try such stimulation for a 3–4-day period during which time they monitor their degree of pain and other symptoms.

Following the removal of the external device, if the symptoms have shown 70% or more improvement, the patient is considered as a candidate for implantation of a permanent pulse generator.

The use of sacral nerve modulation via the implantation of either a temporary or a permanent electrode in the S3 sacral foramen is an effective therapeutic tool for the control of chronic pelvic pain.

When the pain is protracted due to infiltrating inoperable cancer or following radiotherapy, some form of denervation can be contemplated.

PAINFUL MICTURITION

Painful micturition is frequently associated with urinary frequency and nocturia and may also be accompanied by suprapubic pain. The pain referred down the urethra to the urinary meatus starts with voiding and usually subsides with the termination of urination, to start again with the next micturition. It is frequently described by the patient as burning, sharp pain or strangury.

The most frequent cause is urinary infection, whether acute or chronic, specific or nonspecific. It can be caused by acute or chronic prostatitis or urethritis. In the female 'urethral syndrome' is frequently used to describe patients presenting with painful frequent urination with sterile urine and negative physical findings. The patients are frequently postmenopausal, occasionally have associated sexual dysfunction and are usually frustrated with their problems.

In the male the equivalent of urethral syndrome is the chronic prostatitis symptom complex in the form of painful urination, frequency, nocturia, painful ejaculation and pain referred to many areas, including the suprapubic region, lower back, perineum, inguinal region and the testis. Occasionally the similarities of the two syndromes are attributed to similar anatomical distribution of the prostatic ducts and glands in the male as compared to the periurethral glands in the female. The chronic prostatitis syndrome may be associated with bacterial infection – *Chlamydia* or *Mycoplasma* – but frequently all cultures are negative and the term prostatodynia or painful sterile prostate is used to describe the complex. The patients are typically in the third or fourth decade, with a history of urethritis and a nervous personality. The prostate is frequently tender on rectal examination and a copious secretion with many white blood cells can be expressed. The symptoms are exaggerated by alcohol, spicy food and irregular sexual activity. Prolonged sitting increases the perineal pain and hot sitz baths seem to improve the symptoms.

Painful micturition may sometimes be caused by pathology in nearby organs. A stone in the lower end of the ureter may produce frequency, burning and pain referring to the tip of the penis or urinary meatus. Pathology related to the trigone usually causes pain referred to the meatus. This may be produced by a mobile bladder stone which frequently lies on the trigone, by a tumour invading the trigone or, rarely, by membranous trigonitis. A tumour invading the bladder, such as a cervical or ovarian tumour, may be associated with pain related to the bladder and painful micturition. Diverticulitis and peridiverticular abscess involving the bladder may cause similar symptoms.

Patients who have indwelling urethral catheters may present with bladder spasms, suprapubic pain and pain referring to the meatus from trigonal irritation.

Investigation of painful micturition

Following the history and physical examination, which are frequently negative, a stepwise investigation is usually necessary; this can be stopped as soon as a confirmation of the aetiology is made.

Urine analysis and culture will confirm the presence of infection.

Prostatic secretions should be investigated, with microscopic examination as well as culture, and including culture for *Chlamydia*. Urography and cystography may be indicated if the diagnosis is not clear from history, physical examination and previous investigations.

Cystoscopy is frequently indicated in resistant cases or if bladder pathology is suspected.

Treatment

Acute or chronic urinary infection is treated with appropriate antibiotics.

Chronic prostatitis, if a positive culture has been demonstrated, should be treated; this usually consists of a course of tetracycline, a quinolone such as ciprofloxacin, or a sulphonamide and trimethoprim combination. Treatment should be for at least 4–6 weeks and occasionally has to be prolonged to 3 months. In chronic nonbacterial prostatitis, if the patient is very symptomatic and rectal examination shows a tender prostate, with significant prostatic secretion findings on microscopic examination but a negative culture is obtained, this could justify a single course of empirical treatment.

The female with urethral syndrome and negative culture is occasionally improved by prolonged suppressive therapy using sulphatrimethoprim or nitrofurantoin. Oestrogen vaginal suppositories or cream are occasionally helpful. In the past some urologists have resorted to empirical treatment, such as urethral dilatation, which has no scientific explanation but occasionally results in short- or long-term improvement. Periurethral injections of steroids have been tried with variable results. Symptomatic relief can sometimes be obtained by urinary analgesics, such as pyridium or methylene blue. Occasionally these patients will improve on nonsteroidal antiinflammatory agents.

The major component of treatment of both urethral syndrome and chronic prostatitis symptom complex is proper counselling to explain the chronicity, our lack of knowledge in this area and the high rate of recurrence, to assure the patient that his or her condition is not malignant in nature and to explain that, no matter what is done, they will still occasionally have some symptoms. This is most important as these patients will usually see several physicians and are frequently never satisfied; this affects their quality of life tremendously. We cannot promise these patients long-term cure. Surgery is definitely not indicated and patients undergoing prostatectomy for prostatitis syndrome are frequently more symptomatic afterwards. Some conservative measures, such as hot sitz baths, avoidance of alcohol and spicy food and regular sexual intercourse, are frequently rewarding.

If the pain is referred, treatment of the primary pathology is of paramount importance. If there is pelvic malignancy the presence of bladder symptoms should be taken as a serious problem indicating bladder invasion.

The management of the patient with indwelling catheter and suprapubic or urethral pain with bladder spasms could include bladder irrigation to avoid catheter blockage and reduce encrustations. The use of an anticholinergic agent, such as oxybutinin hydrochloride (Ditropan) or probantheline bromide (Pro-Banthine) can be very helpful in relieving the bladder spasms. On occasion, local anaesthetic instillations may be necessary. The ideal course, if feasible, may be to dispose of the indwelling catheter and resort to alternatives such as intermittent catheterisation.

TESTICULAR–SCROTAL PAIN

Pain associated with the testicles is generally related to trauma, testicular torsion, or epididymoorchitis. In a small number of cases testicular tumours may be associated with pain. The pain is felt locally although there may be some radiation of pain along the spermatic cord into the lower abdomen or CVA region. Pain in the scrotal area, however, may be referred from the ureter, trigone or bladder neck regions. Referred scrotal pain demonstrates no local testicular tenderness on examination.

Testicular torsion may occur at any age and is most common between the ages of 12–18 years, presenting with rapid onset of testicular pain and swelling. The pain is due to the twisting of the spermatic cord, causing obstruction to the venous and arterial vessels, with resulting oedema and haemorrhage. The pain may radiate up the inguinal canal and may be associated with nausea and vomiting. In most cases the pain is continuous and well localised to the scrotal region. The diagnosis is made on the basis of clinical history and physical examination, absence of urinary symptoms or findings on urine analysis. The testicular scan is the most definitive examination, showing a 'halo sign' or region of hypoperfusion. If the torsion is not corrected surgically within 4–6 hours necrosis of the testicle is likely.

Epididymoorchitis must be differentiated from testicular torsion as an explanation for scrotal testicular pain. Acute epididymoorchitis is associated with elevated temperature, symptoms of cystitis and/or urethritis and evidence of pyuria and bacteriuria on urine analysis. Nuclear testicular scan will demonstrate a hyperfused testicle. The treatment is by antibiotics, scrotal elevation, ice compresses and analgesics. The pain localisation is to the scrotum with radiation into the groin. Other intrascrotal diseases which may be associated with pain should be considered; these include testicular tumours (20% associated with pain), hydrocoeles and spermatocoeles, torsion of testicular appendages and incarcerated or strangulated hernias.

PENIS

Pain of the penis associated with direct trauma or infection to the skin or corporal bodies of the penis is transmitted directly to the scrotal nerve roots of S2–S4 by way of the pudendal nerve. Similarly, irritation or injury of the urethra follows the same routes.

Of less frequent occurrence is priapism (persistent prolonged erections) which may become painful due to ischaemia of the corpora cavernosa which are engorged with stagnant blood. The aetiology of this relatively rare entity may be associated with sickle cell disease, leukaemia, clotting disorders, malignant infiltration of the corporal bodies themselves or compression of the internal iliac vessels. In many cases the cause is idiopathic.

In the last few years, a treatment for impotence has been the intracavernosal injection of papaverine, a smooth muscle relaxant which promotes good erections in many patients, or prostaglandin E (PGE). One of the side-effects may be prolonged erection which is usually not painful and is less frequently encountered with PGE_1, than with papaverine and Regitine.

The treatment of priapism depends on the aetiology. For idiopathic or papaverine-induced priapism, the treatment is to irrigate the corpora cavernosa with a solution of saline and noradrenaline or neosynephrine. If the cause is a malignancy, the disease must first be controlled by chemotherapy and/or radiotherapy. Sickle cell patients require fresh blood transfusions.

FURTHER READING

Chapple C R, Aubry M L, James S et al 1989 Characterization of the human prostatic adrenoreceptors using pharmacology receptors and localization. British Journal of Urology 63: 487

De Wolf W C, Fraley E E 1975 Renal pain. Urology VI: 403

Hassouna M M, Elhilali M M 1991 Role of the sacral root stimulation in voiding dysfunction. World Journal of Urology 3: 145–148

Hedlund H, Andersson A-E, Larson B 1985 Alpha adrenoreceptors and muscarinic receptors in the isolated human prostate. Journal of Urology 134: 1291

Lepor H, Baumann M, Shapiro E 1984 Characterization and localization of the muscarinic cholinergic receptor in human prostatic tissue. Journal of Urology 132: 397

Levy O M, Gittelman M C, Strashun A M, Cohen E L, Fine E J 1983 Diagnosis of acute testicular torsion using radionuclide scanning. Journal of Urology 129: 975

Llach F, Papper S, Massry S G 1980 The clinical spectrum of renal vein thrombosis: acute and chronic. American Journal of Medicine 69: 819

Meares E M Jr 1973 Bacterial prostatitis versus 'prostatosis': a clinical and bacteriological study. Journal of the American Medical Association 224: 1372

Meares E M Jr 1978 Urinary tract infections in men. In: Harrison J,

Gittes R F, Perlmutter A D, Stamey T A, Walsh P C (eds) Campbell's urology, 4th edn. W B Saunders, Philadelphia, p 509
Messing E M 1987 The diagnosis of interstitial cystitis. Urology XXIX (suppl): 4
Nashold B S J, Goldner J L, Mullen J B, Bright D S 1982 Long-term pain control by direct peripheral nerve stimulation. Journal of Bone and Joint Surgery 64A: 1–10
Olsson C A 1986 Anatomy of the upper urinary tract. In: Walsh P C, Gittes R F, Perlmutter A D, Stamey T A (eds) Campbell's urology, 5th edn. W B Saunders, Philadelphia, Vol 1, p 12–46
Parsons C L 1987 19-Sodium pentosanpolysulfate treatment in interstitial cystitis. An update. Urology XXIX (suppl): 14
Perlmutter A D, Blacklow R S 1983 Urinary tract pain, hematuria and pyuria. In: Blacklow R S (ed) MacBryde's signs and symptoms. Applied pathologic physiology and clinical interpretation, 6th edn. J B Lippincott, Philadelphia, p 181–185
Rubenstein M A, Walz B J, Bucy J G 1978 Transitional cell carcinoma of the kidney: 25 year experience. Journal of Urology 199: 594
Sant G R 1987 Intravesical 50% dimethyl sulfoxide in treatment of interstitial cystitis. Urology XXIX (suppl): 17
Sheinfeld J, Erturk E, Spataro R F, Cockett A T K 1987 Perinephric abscess: current concepts. Journal of Urology 137: 191
Sidi A A, Cameron J S, Duffy L M, Lange P H 1986 Intracavernous drug-induced erections in the management of male erectile dysfunction: experience with 100 patients. Journal of Urology 135: 704
Smith D R, Raney F L 1976 Radiculitis distress as a mimic of renal pain. Journal of Urology 116: 269
Tanagho E A 1984 Anatomy of the lower urinary tract. In: Smith D (ed) General urology (Lange series). Lange Medical Publishers, East Norwalk, Connecticut
Tanagho E A, Schmidt R A 1988 Electrical stimulation in the clinical management of the neurogenic bladder. Journal of Urology 140: 1331–1339
Tynes W V 1984 Unusual reno-vascular disorders. In: Novick A C (ed) The urologic clinics of North America, vol 2. W B Saunders, Philadelphia, p 529–542

36. Phantom pain and other phenomena after amputation

Troels Staehelin Jensen and Peter Rasmussen

INTRODUCTION

Peripheral nerve section due to loss of a body part is almost invariably followed by an awareness of the denervated part, a phenomenon noted as far back as the 15th century when the French military surgeon Ambroise Paré called attention to the strange fact that patients, long after amputation of a leg, complained of vigorous pain in the missing part (Keil 1990). While this phenomenon has been known in the literature, e.g. René Descartes, Albrect von Haller, Herman Melville and Hans Christian Andersen – and has undoubtedly been the secret knowledge of many amputees for centuries – it was not until Rhône (1842), Bell (1830), Magendie (1833), Guéniot (1861) and later Mitchell (1872) gave their detailed description of remaining limb image after amputation that this phenomenon was recognized in medical literature. According to Whitaker (1979) Mitchell termed the remaining limb image 'limbs invisible' and later 'phantom limb', a term that is still used. Phantom limb is a natural – and today an expected – consequence of amputation, which rarely presents therapeutic problems. Occasionally the phantom becomes the site of severe and excruciating pain, presenting a major obstacle to successful rehabilitation of the amputee. Although a painless and a painful part of the missing limb may be at either end of the same clinical spectrum, it seems useful from the point of view of description to distinguish between:

1. *phantom pain*: painful sensations referred to the missing limb
2. *stump pain*: pain at the site of an extremity amputation
3. *phantom limb*: any sensation of the missing limb except pain.

Despite a rather well known symptomatology of postamputation neurological sequelae, the mechanisms underlying phantom pain and related phenomena are still hypothetical. The present chapter will therefore concentrate on the symptoms and signs of postamputation sequelae and their natural course. The relationship between phantom pain and other pain syndromes associated with traumatic neuropathies will be described briefly. An understanding of the clinical aspects of amputation is a prerequisite for offering a plausible explanation of the phantom limb phenomena and for treating properly the unpleasant sensations associated with such phenomena.

SYMPTOMS AND SIGNS AND THEIR NATURAL COURSE

PHANTOM PAIN

Definition and classification

Phantom pain is defined as pain referred to a surgically removed limb or portion thereof (Merskey 1986). Phantom pain, however, is not a well defined clinical concept. It comprises – in the literature, too – some undefined, incomparable sensory phenomena. Pain localized in the amputation stump (i.e. stump pain) and limb pain experienced prior to the amputation (i.e. preamputation pain) should be distinguished from proper phantom pain. Other sensory phenomena such as paraesthesia, dysaesthesia, hyperpathia and soreness should not be included under the term 'phantom pain'.

It is also obvious that differences in pain threshold and pain tolerance both among individual amputees and their observers, together with differences in the way in which painful sensations are described and recorded, make a clinical delimitation of phantom or stump pain difficult.

Frequency of phantom pain

The difficulty in penetrating into the phantom pain problem is clearly reflected in the reported frequency of phantom pain, with figures ranging from less than 2% to nearly 100% (Table 36.1). In the literature, severe phantom pain is generally reported to occur in 0.5–5% of amputees (Ewalt et al 1947; Henderson & Smyth 1948; Melzack & Loeser 1978). Phantom pain rates based on, for example, analgesic treatment given, should be evalu-

Table 36.1 Frequency of total phantom pain among amputees in some previous studies

Authors	Year of publication	Number of amputees	Total pain (%)
Pitres	1897	30	97
Riddoch	1941	N/A	50
Herrmann & Gibbs	1945	120	6
Ewalt et al	1947	100	4
Browder & Gallagher	1948	150	34
Lunn	1948	189	57
Henderson & Smyth	1948	300	4
Sliosberg	1948	251	72.5
Cronholm	1951	122	35
Solonen	1962	1000	80
James	1973	38	62
Parkes	1973	46	61
Kegel et al	1977	134	41
Carlen et al	1978	73	67
Finch et al	1980	133	30
Abramson & Feibel	1981	2000	2
Sherman & Sherman	1983	764	85
Sherman et al	1984a	2694	78
Jensen et al	1985	58	72
Krebs et al	1985	86	52
Buchanan & Mandel	1986	716	62

N/A = not available.

ated extremely carefully. Thus, Sherman's group (Sherman & Sherman 1983, 1985; Sherman et al 1984) found that 50–75% of amputees reported phantom pain to their physicians but only 20% were offered treatment for their pain. In the studies by Sherman and coworkers many amputees with phantom pain got the impression that physicians considered their phantom pain to be pure imagination.

Onset of phantom pain

Pain is present in the first week after amputation in 50–75% of patients (Lunn 1948; Sliosberg 1948; Brown 1968; Parkes 1973; Jensen et al 1983), although it may be delayed for months or even years (Mitchell 1872; Browder & Gallagher 1948).

Pain localization

Phantom pain is mainly localized distally in the phantom limb (Lunn 1948; Sliosberg 1948; Krainick & Thoden 1976; Carlen et al 1978; Jensen et al 1983, 1985; Sherman & Sherman 1983, 1985; Sherman et al 1984; Katz & Melzack 1990). Thus, among 64 above-knee amputees with phantom pain in Lunn's series (Lunn 1948), 66% had pain in the foot or the toes, 39% also in the calves, and only 6% had additional pain in the thigh. Figure 36.1 shows the distribution of phantom pain in amputees at different time intervals after limb loss. As can be seen, there is a clear preference for distal pain localization.

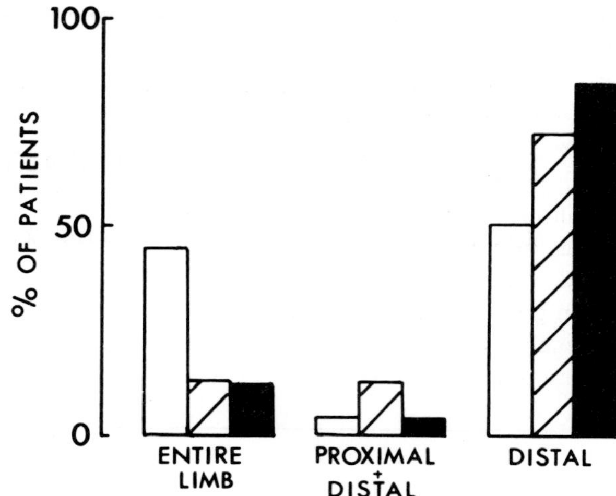

Fig. 36.1 Percentage of amputees with phantom pain localization 8 days (open bars $n = 42$), 6 months (hatched bars, $n = 33$) and 2 years (shaded bars, $n = 20$) after amputation. (From Jensen et al 1985 with permission).

Phantom pain quality

The literature contains a variety of descriptions given by amputees of their pain bearing little or no resemblance to any previous sensory experience. Some consider a painful distorted position to be typical of the phantom state (Brown 1968): a feeling as if the hand or foot is squeezed, fingers or toes clenched and the nails digging into the flesh of the hand or foot (Lunn 1948). However, only 16% of patients with phantom pain reported this type of pain. A burning, crushing or squeezing type of pain is reported by some (Jensen et al 1985; Krebs et al 1986).

The general lack of studies in which preamputation phenomena have been recorded *before* amputation makes it difficult to determine the value of information from patients with such experiences.

Time course of phantom pain

It is generally assumed that phantom pain gradually diminishes and finally vanishes within the first 1–2 postoperative years. Parkes (1973) found that 63% had severe or moderate phantom pain immediately after amputation; 13 months later 30% of patients reported this intensity of pain.

Others have reported phantom pain in 50–75% of amputees after several years (Sherman et al 1984; Krebs et al 1985). In Sherman's study covering 2694 amputees of whom 78% had current phantom pain, 51% had pain more than 6 days per month and 44% had not noted a decline of phantom pain during a 30-year period.

However, lack of prospective studies in unselected materials, together with failure to distinguish between different categories of phantom pain, make it difficult to determine the temporal course and estimate the exact incidence of persistent phantom pain. In our prospective study (Jensen et al 1985) the incidence of phantom pain 1 week, 6 months and 2 years after amputation was 72, 65 and 59%, respectively. Although the incidence of phantom pain did not decline significantly during the 2-year follow-up period, both the duration and the frequency of phantom pain attacks decreased significantly. Thus, 2 years after amputation only 21% had daily phantom pain attacks and none were in constant pain. It seems likely that persistent severe pain is only seen in a small fraction of amputees, perhaps in the order of 5–10%.

Modulating effect on phantom pain

Phantom limb experiences, whether painful or not, vary considerably among individuals and even in the same individual. Many internal and external stimuli are known to modify phantom pain. Table 36.2 shows factors reported by amputees which may alter the pain experience. The modulation effect of sensory inflow from within and outside the body is neither simple nor predictable: it may evoke pain in a previously painless phantom, relieve existing phantom pain and make the painless phantom limb experience even more vivid.

Feinstein et al (1954) showed and Noordenbos (1959) confirmed that counterirritation with hypertonic saline injected in the L4–L5 interspinous tissue first exacerbated phantom limb pain and then produced transient awareness of the whole phantom followed by a long-lasting, sometimes permanent, phantom pain relief. Spinal anaesthesia in amputees may cause appearance of phantom pain in otherwise pain free subjects (Mackenzie 1983). These findings show that the phantom limb experience is the result not of a single event but of many interacting neuronal events.

Determinant factors for the phantom limb

Great effort has been made to point out and delineate factors that might play a role for the development and persistence of phantom pain. Since many of these aspects are common both in the painless and the painful phantom, they will be considered together.

Table 36.2 Factors aggravating and relieving the painful and the non-painful phantom limb experience

Aggravating factor	Relieving factor
Attention	Rest
Emotional distress	Distraction
Stump touch or pressure	Stump movement
Weather change	Cold or heat
Autonomic reflex acts	Using a prosthesis
Stimulation of other body parts	Elevation of stump
Pain of other origin	Percussion or massage of stump
Wearing a prosthesis	

Preamputation pain

Several rather striking case reports (Mitchell 1872; Bailey & Moersch 1941; Riddoch 1941; Cronholm 1951; Nathan 1962) have suggested that postamputation pain is more likely to occur in patients who had pain in the limb prior to amputation and that the clinical feature of such pain (quality, localization, modulating effects, etc.) closely resembles the pain experienced prior to amputation. Some studies (Browder & Gallagher 1948; Cronholm 1951; Parkes 1973) but not all (Henderson & Smyth 1948) have lent support to this notion and found that phantom pain is more frequent in patients who have suffered from severe preamputation pain than in those who have not had such pain prior to amputation. In an extensive retrospective study of 68 amputees, Katz & Melzack (1990) have compared phantom pain experience reported by 44 amputees with possible preamputation pain experienced. In 25/44 patients (57%) phantom pain was found to be similar to experienced preamputation pain. In a prospective study we have concentrated on the possible role of preamputation pain for the subsequent development of phantom pain (Jensen et al 1985). A total of 98% of amputees examined prior to amputation had preamputation limb pain. Figure 36.2 shows the proportion of amputees reporting similar or changed localization and character of their preamputation pains and their subsequent phantom pains. Phantom pain and preamputation limb pain were similar in both localization and character in 36% of patients immediately after amputation, but in only 10% of patients 2 years after limb amputation. This observation shows that factors other than preamputation pain play a role in late phantom limb pain. As stated by Katz & Melzack (1990) a well-controlled prospective study is needed in order to clarify the similarity between preamputation pain and phantom limb pain.

Nervous system lesions

An already-established phantom limb experience, whether painful or not, may be dramatically changed by lesions in the brain or the spinal cord. A focal brain infarct in the posterior internal capsule made a former phantom limb experience disappear (Yarnitsky et al 1988). Transient cerebral dysfunction, such as simple or complex partial seizures, suffices to modify a phantom temporarily (Riddoch 1941). Lesions in the spinal cord may either induce or erase a phantom limb experience.

Psychological factors

The severe psychological impact of losing a limb is evident

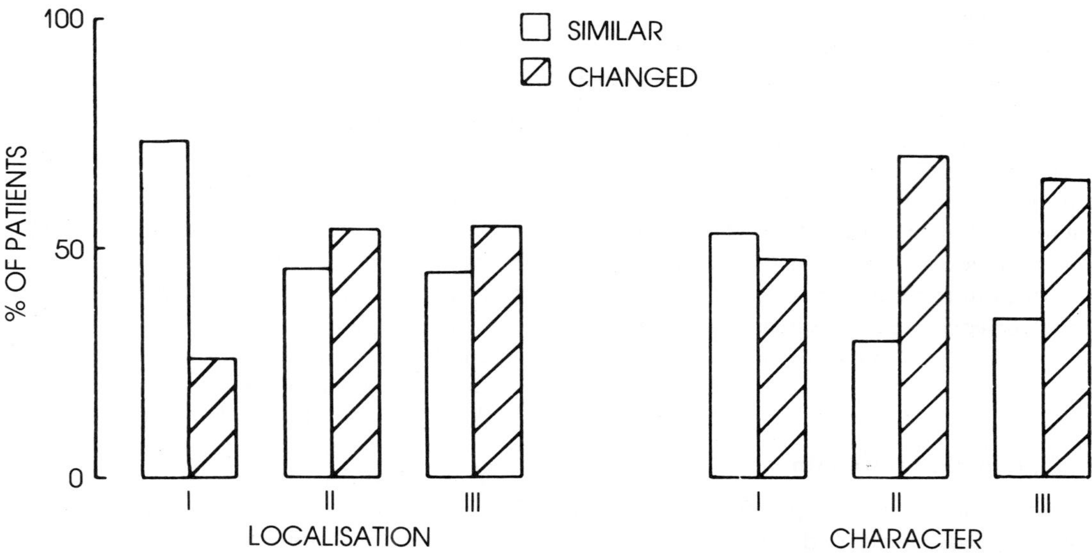

Fig. 36.2 Percentage of patients in whom preamputation pain and phantom limb pain were similar or different in localization and character 8 days (I), 6 months (II) and 2 years (III) after limb amputation. (From Jensen et al 1985 with permission.)

and various emotional disturbances such as anxiety about physical and social adjustment, depression, bitterness and self-pity are sometimes met in patients with phantom limb (Parkes 1973; Shukla et al 1982b; Lindesay 1985). It is also evident that emotional disturbances can trigger and aggravate pain. Parkes (1973) suggested that complaints of persisting pain were related to patients with a rigid, self-reliant personality and to unemployment or retirement. Although emotional factors probably play a role in the occurrence and persistence of phantom pain – as in many other chronic pain states – it remains to be seen whether emotional disturbances are the cause of such pain. The motivational–affective aspect of any chronic pain syndrome makes it difficult, of course, to determine whether emotional disorders are merely a manifestation of pain or an aetiological determinant. So far there is no obvious evidence that personality disorders are more frequent among those amputees with phantom pain than among amputees without phantom pain (Sherman et al 1987).

Other factors

The significance of amputation cause, level of amputation and particular limb removed in the development and persistence of pain remain controversial. While some studies have found phantom pain in amputees to be more common after military accidents and after proximal and upper limb amputation than after civilian accidents, distal and lower limb amputations, respectively, other studies have failed to find such differences, or even the contrary. In our studies sex, side, level of amputation, age or cause of amputation were not related to the presence of persistent phantom pain (Jensen et al 1985).

It has been claimed that sudden loss of a limb is a necessary factor for the occurrence of phantom limb (Sunderland 1968). Gradual loss of a limb, however, does not prevent the occurrence of phantom limb phenomena. Thus Price (1976) found among 42 patients with limb shortening due to leprosy that 90% reported phantom limb phenomena which occurred irrespective of whether limb shortening was due to surgical amputation or a slow manifestation of leprosy.

STUMP PAIN

The literature rarely distinguishes between pain in the stump and phantom pain. The frequency of stump pain varies: 27% (Sliosberg 1948), 13% (Cronholm 1951), 71% (Krainick & Thoden 1976), 15% (Abramson & Feibel 1981) and 17.5% (Finch et al 1980). As for painful phantom, the frequency of stump pain obviously depends on the material studied and on what one considers pain or merely 'normal discomfort'. Immediate postoperative pain follows most surgical interventions, and amputation of a limb is certainly no exception to the rule. Thus Parkes (1973), in an unselected, carefully analysed study, found that stump pain occurred in 50% of cases during the first weeks. At 3 weeks and 13 months after amputation the figures were 50 and 13%, respectively. What is of interest here is the pain that persists despite an apparently healed wound. This pain is usually described as a feeling of sore spots, a stabbing sensation or an electric current, which is strictly localized to the stump and often to its posterior aspect close to the scar (Browder & Gallagher 1948). These pains can easily be triggered by stimulating the stump with pinpricks or pressing tender neuromas. A variant of this type is what Sunderland (1978) termed 'nerve storms', with painful attacks of up to 2 days' duration. The pain is sharp, shooting and waxes and wanes from minute to minute. Browder & Gallagher (1948) considered a burning sensation of the stump, which can be triggered by light touch, to be equally characteristic of the stump pain syndrome. In these latter cases the stump may appear atrophic, cold, cyanotic and sweating.

Spontaneous movements, also known as chorea of the stump, tic douloureux, *épilepsie du moignon* or jactitation, form part of the painful phantom. These movements range from painful, hardly visible, myoclonic jerks to severe clonic contractions of the stump. Although rarely reported, Sliosberg (1948) observed it in nearly 50% of amputees and considered it to be even more common.

In our material 57% of the patients experienced stump pain immediately after amputation. At 6 months and 2 years after amputation, stump pain was reported by 22 and 21%, respectively. In the early postoperative period stump pain is usually of a sharp, sticking, pressing character which gradually changes to a more burning or squeezing type of pain. Phantom pain is significantly more frequent in those amputees with long-term stump pain than in those without stump pain (Jensen et al 1985; Sherman & Sherman 1985).

Stump pathology associated with phantom and/or stump pain

Examinations of stumps often disclose definite pathological findings which may account for the pain in the stump and/or the phantom: (i) skin pathology; (ii) circulatory disturbances; (iii) infection of the skin or underlying tissue or bone; (iv) bone spurs; (v) neuromas.

The different pathological changes will not be dealt with in detail. It is important, however, to emphasize that although phantom/stump pain is significantly more frequent in patients with obvious stump pathology than in patients without pathological findings, phantom/stump pain may occur in perfectly healed stumps. This means either that peripheral conditions are not the only factor responsible for the pain or that our ability to detect pathological changes in the periphery is insufficient. A systematic analysis of stump sensibility in amputees has not been carried out. In preliminary work we have seen that careful examination of stump sensibility reveals areas of altered sensitivity (e.g. hypalgesia, hyperalgesia, hyperpathia or allodynia) in almost all amputees. The significance of these sensory disturbances in the periphery for phantom limb phenomena is at present unknown.

PAIN AFTER NERVE INJURY

Following any nerve injury there is a potential risk for development of persisting pain in the denervated area irrespective of the aetiology and the location of the lesion. Amputation represents the most radical form of nerve injury. Mitchell (1872) introduced the term 'causalgia' for a continuous burning type of pain after large battlefield nerve injuries. Subsequently, several terms have emerged such as: reflex sympathetic dystrophy, posttraumatic pain syndrome, major and minor causalgia, Sudeck's atrophy, terms often used synonymously, but sometimes referring to different clinical conditions.

Nerve injury pain shares many of the features seen in neuropathic pain:

1. delayed onset
2. abnormal sensations usually of a burning type
3. paroxysms of lancinating stabs
4. pain in area with sensory deficit
5. pain provoked by innocuous stimuli (allodynia)
6. build-up and after-sensations following repetitive stimuli.

Table 36.3 shows some of the characteristics and distinguishing features of various types of nerve injury pain.

Figure 36.3 illustrates a patient who suffered from a brachial plexus avulsion followed by pain. As can be seen from Table 36.3 apart from sympathetic hyperactivity, the pain after amputation is almost similar to that encountered in causalgia. While some consider sympathetic hyperactivity to be a feature of causalgia, e.g. IASP classification of chronic pain (Mersky 1986), this view is not accepted by all (Schott 1986). Injuries of the median and the sciatic nerve are those injuries most often associated with causalgia while injuries of the radial nerve rarely produce causalgia (Sunderland 1978). Causalgia usually occurs after proximal lesions and typically pain is referred to distal parts of the limb. The variable involvement of the sympathetic nervous system in nerve injury pain has given rise to the terms sympathetically maintained and sympathetically independent pain (Roberts 1986).

Table 36.3 Pain characteristics of some nerve injuries

Pain	Plexus avulsion	Causalgia	Amputation	Nerve entrapment
Onset	Immediate	Immediate or delayed	Immediate or delayed	Gradually
Frequency of severe pain	90%	1–5%	5%	Variable
Type of pain	Burning + lancinating stabs	Burning + lancinating stabs	Burning or crushing	Lancinating pain
Allodynia	Always	Always	Variable	Rarely
Sympathetic hyperactivity	Variable	Always	Rarely	Rarely

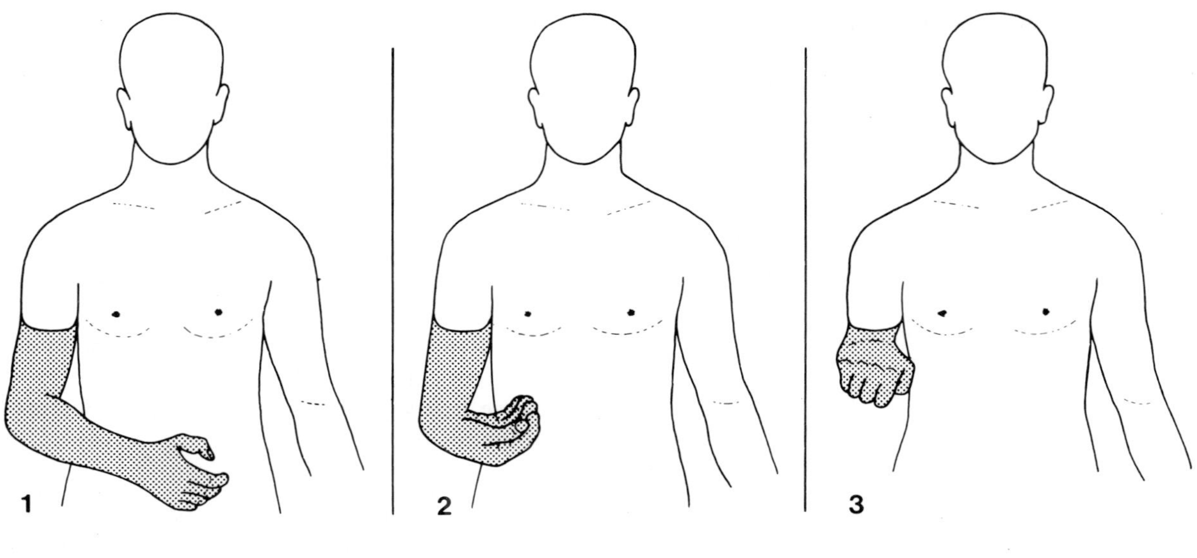

Fig. 36.3 A 34-year-old man who was injured when he drove his moped into a lamp-post in September 1980. There was a right-sided humerus fracture and a total paralysis of the entire upper extremity. The paralysed arm felt localized in the position in which it was at the time of the accident: as if the patient held the handlebars of the moped (1). After a few weeks the patient had pains in the hand and fingers and the distal third of the forearm. The pains were squeezing and of increasing intensity during the following 3 months. Simultaneously the phantom began shrinking and 6 months after the injury the hand felt as if it were localized distally to the elbow joint (2). Amputation was performed in May 1981, but it had no effect on the pains. The shrinking continued, and from December 1981 the hand felt as if placed directly on the amputation stump and clenched more tightly (3). Electrocoagulation in the cervical medulla (Lissauer) in May 1982 had no effect on the phantom pains.

PHANTOM LIMB

Phantom limb experiences vary considerably, ranging from a precise and distinct replica of the lost body part to a transient, vague, tingling sensation in parts of the limb. On the basis of the multifaceted descriptions offered by amputees, Stetter (1950) and Frederiks (1963) distinguished between phantom limb (the experience of possessing a limb that behaves in a way that the actual limb would) and phantom limb sensations (various positive sensations referred to the missing limb). This distinction is rarely made in the literature, but Lunn (1948) found that in about 10% of patients with phantom limb sensations the experience of reality of the missing limb was lacking. In our experience nearly all amputees have a sense of reality.

Frequency and onset

Previous surveys and reports indicate that 80–100% of amputees will experience phantom limb sensations at some time or other following amputation (Table 36.4) Lunn (1948) found that 71% of 142 amputees experienced phantom limb within the first 24 hours, and in only 10% was the phenomenon delayed for more than 1 month. In our material, phantom limb sensations occurred within 24 hours after amputation in 34% of patients and, in less than 10% of amputees, onset of phantom limb sensations was delayed for more than 8 days (Jensen et al 1984). Similar figures have been noted by others (Sliosberg 1948; Carlen et al 1978). Phantom limb is rarely observed in congenital amputees or in children amputated before the age of 6 years (Riese & Bruck 1950), although it has been described at an earlier age (Browder & Gallagher 1948; Weinstein & Sersen

Table 36.4 Frequency of phantom limb experience following limb amputation in some previous studies

Authors	Year of publication	Number of amputees	Number with phantom limb experience	(%)
Mitchell	1872	90	86	96
Ewalt et al	1947	100	95	95
Henderson & Smyth	1948	300	–	98
Lunn	1948	189	171	91
Sliosberg	1948	211	202	96
Cronholm	1951	122	110	90
James	1973	38	32	84
Parkes	1973	46	45	98
Krainick & Thoden	1976	52	44	85
Kegel et al	1977	134	110	82
Carlen et al	1978	73	73	100
Finch et al	1980	57	31	54
Shukla et al	1982a	72	62	86
Jensen et al	1984	58	50	84
Krebs et al	1985	86	66	77
Buchan & Mandel	1986	716	602	84

1961; Simmel 1962). Whether this lack of phantom limb sensations in the very young child is due to an immature body image at the time of amputation is not clear (Simmel 1962).

Clinical characteristics

Despite variations in phantom limb experiences certain characteristics are so common that phantom limb phenomena may be divided into the following categories:

1. Simple sensations
   a. touch
   b. temperature
   c. pressure
   d. itch
   e. other
2. Complex sensations
   a. posture
   b. length
   c. volume
3. Movements
   a. willed movements
   b. spontaneous movements
   c. associated movements.

A remarkable feature of the phantom limb experience is what L'hermitte (1951) termed 'sentiment du realité concrète'. Sometimes this sense of reality of the missing limb is so vivid that the somatic defect is forgotten. Simple and complex sensations and feelings of movements all contribute to an image of a missing limb.

Simple sensations

Various cutaneous sensations such as numbness, pins and needles, heat, cold, itch are reported by amputees and described in various terms by individuals, making a classification extremely difficult. These simple phantom sensations are usually undifferentiated and diffuse in localization.

Complex sensations

Most amputees have a sense of position, length and volume of the amputated limb. The position sensed may be one of the following: relaxed, fixed or distorted. For example, the arm may be perceived as either hanging limply along the side of the body, moving freely while walking, or as being in a fixed position, with the elbow flexed and the forearm lying across the front of the chest, assuming a position as in a supranuclear paresis (Henderson & Smyth 1948). In some patients, usually less than 10% (Lunn 1948), the phantom is experienced in a distorted, bizarre position closely resembling the one immediately prior to amputation (Mitchell 1872; Riddoch 1941).

Berger & Gerstenbrand (1981) found phantom illusions in 33 of 37 patients with spinal lesions, often with a phantom position resembling that at the time of the accident. This corresponds with our own experience in patients with lesions of the brachial plexus and spinal cord lesions. Amputation has rarely – or not at all – any effect on these complex sensations.

The phenomenon may be illustrated by a bizarre case story:

The patient was 24 years old when, in September 1946, he crashed his motorcycle and immediately suffered paralysis and sensory loss of the right upper extremity. After a few days he could make rocking movements with his fingers and the sensory loss was replaced by hypaesthesia in a limited area. Four months after the trauma the patient complained of squeezing pain of increasing intensity in his hand and fingers and of phantom sensations in the arm which felt abducted in the shoulder joint at a right angle to the body. An exploration of the brachial plexus did not reveal abnormal findings. Avulsion of the fourth to the seventh cervical roots was present. Six months after the trauma an amputation was performed high on the humerus. Amputation had no effect either on pains or on phantom sensations. The patient was still hampered by a feeling that the phantom extended at a right angle to the body, so that he had to walk sideways through narrow passages such as doorways and corridors. As blocks of sympathetic ganglia and psychotherapy (hypnosis) had no effect, a bilateral lobotomy was perfomed in 1948, after which the pain disappeared for 3 months. Five years after the accident an incision was performed on the precentral cortex. Subsequently, both phantom pain and phantom sensation faded away and only slight stump pain occurred in response to changing weather conditions. At the latest follow-up examination, 24 years after the accident and 19 years after the gyrectomy, no major complaints were present.

Immediately after amputation the amputated limb usually feels normal to the patient, as regards volume and length, but in a few patients it is felt to have shrunk. In our material the phantom was felt to be of normal volume and length in 48 and 55% of amputees, respectively, 8 days after amputation. A shrunken limb occurred in only 9% of patients immediately after amputation (Jensen et al 1984).

Movements

More than 50% of amputees have experienced movements of the phantom, more often so in arm and distal amputations than in leg and proximal amputations (Henderson & Smyth 1948; Sunderland 1978; Shukla et al 1982a). The movements may be willed, spontaneous or associated. Lunn (1948) reported willed movements in 70% of cases. These were confined to the distal joints of the limb and less complex than in the intact limbs (i.e. generally restricted to flexion and extension movements). Occasionally more complex movements like tardive dyskinesia may occur (McCalley-Whitters & Nasrallah 1983).

In our material, 36% of amputees experienced phantom movements on the 8th day after surgery, 27% 6 months later and 24% 2 years after limb loss (Jensen et al 1984).

Factors modulating the phantom limb percept

It is well known that the phantom limb feeling may be either increased or attenuated by various external and internal stimuli (yawning, micturition, defecation, ejaculation, weather change, visual attention, thinking of the phantom, emotions, etc.). Cronholm (1951) found that deep pressure produced phantom limb sensations in 46%, while touch stimuli only did so in 29% of patients. Induced sensations may be evoked not only from the stump area, but also from body parts distant from severed nerves (Katz & Melzack 1987).

Time course of phantom limb

Although the phantom limb experience may remain completely unchanged for several years (Abbatucci 1894; Browder & Gallagher 1948) the phantom as a rule undergoes important changes within the first 1–2 years of amputation.

Telescoping

This is a phenomenon originally described by Guéniot (1861) under the term 'hétérotopie subjective' and later known as 'regressive deformation' or 'telescoping' (Shukla et al 1982a); it refers to a shrinkage of the phantom, where the digits of the hand or the foot gradually and in a diffuse manner approach the stump to which they finally become attached (Fig. 36.3). The time it takes for telescoping to develop and be completed varies, but the process is generally completed within the first year. Most agree that telescoping occurs in 25–75% of cases and more commonly in arm amputees than in leg amputees (Henderson & Smyth 1948). Figure 36.4 shows the temporal characteristics of telescoping in our material of 58 amputees. Telescoping occurred within 6 months in 30% of patients – a figure that remained stable up to 2 years after amputation. The level of amputation influences neither the incidence of telescoping nor the rate at which it occurs. Distal parts of the phantom, however, retain their normal size longer than proximal parts of the phantom. This may occasionally result in the experience of a giant hand or finger attached to the stump (Fig. 36.3) or a hand tightly squeezed within a 'too small' stump (Sliosberg 1948). It is usually the painless phantom which shortens. Superadded phantom pain may prevent or retard the development of telescoping, and an already telescoped phantom may temporarily lengthen during attacks of pain (Sunderland 1978).

Fading of the phantom

Apart from this regressive deformation in size and length of the phantom, the frequency and intensity of phantom

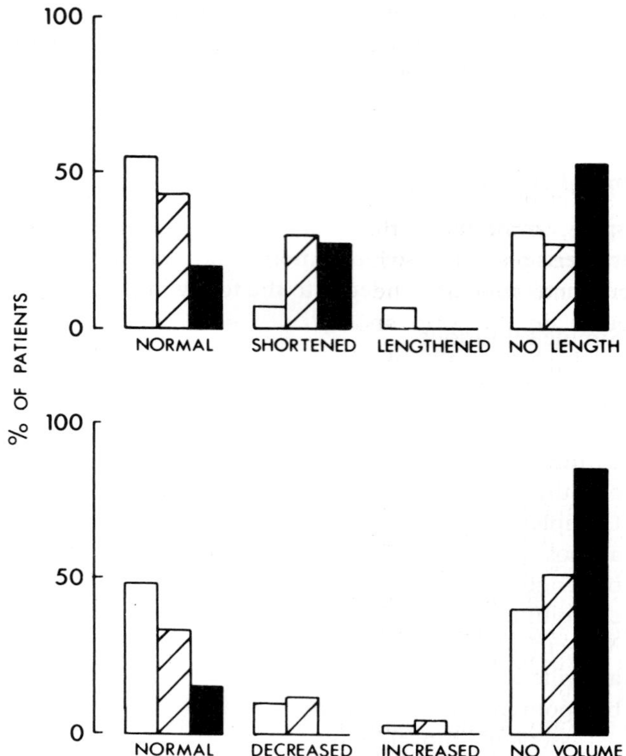

Fig. 36.4 Percentage of amputees with feeling of length (top) or volume (bottom) 8 days (open bars, $n = 49$). 6 months (hatched bars. $n = 46$) and 2 years (shaded bars, $n = 24$) after limb amputation. (From Jensen et al 1984 with permission).

limb sensations also diminish as times goes by. Again, great individual variations occur. In some patients the phantom experience is a short-lasting, vivid sensation persisting for a few weeks and then rapidly vanishing. In others this fading takes 1–2 years and in still others it may take several years. Parkes (1973) found that 70% had a marked phantom immediately after amputation and in only 39% did this intense feeling persist 3 weeks after. Lunn (1948) found that within the first month 47% had a vivid sensation of the phantom; after 1 year this figure had declined to 25%. Among patients examined more than 10 years after amputation, 29% still reported the most intense sensation of the missing limb. Likewise it was found that the clarity of the phantom in patients seen during the first postoperative year was similar to that reported by patients examined up to 3 years after amputation. The frequency of experienced phantom limb sensations takes a similar course. It therefore seems justified to conclude that after the first year the phantom is only subject to minor changes.

Peripheral parts of an amputated limb are always the most vividly and strongly felt parts (Mitchell 1872; Henderson & Smyth 1948; Krainick & Thoden 1976; Carlen et al 1978). This difference in clarity between proximal and distal phantom parts is less marked immediately after amputation.

In our studies the incidence of nonpainful phantom limb sensations 8 days, 6 months and 2 years after limb amputation was 84, 90 and 71%, respectively. Phantom limb phenomena change from a mainly proximal and distal localization to a mainly distal distribution as time goes by.

Usually only islands of the missing limb are felt. For example, in the hand, the thumb and index are the most prominent parts felt, while in the leg the great toe, the instep and heel are the most vividly felt parts. In no instance do the form and feature of the phantom limb experiences correspond to any known peripheral nerve supply or a particular segmental dermatome.

Phantom sensation without loss of limb

Phantom sensations may be experienced after amputation of body parts other than limbs, such as nose, eyeball, tongue, teeth, penis, rectum and breast. Breast phantom is experienced by approximately 25% of mastectomized women and sometimes reported to be painful (Weinstein et al 1970; Jamison et al 1979; Staps et al 1985). Krøner et al (1989) in a study of 120 women who underwent mastectomy found phantom breast syndrome in 25% of women during the first year after mastectomy. In half of these patients the phantom sensation was reported as painful. In the study by Jamison et al (1979) 58% of the patients did not report their sensations spontaneously to the attending physician. After rectal amputation painful phantom rectum is reported in 68% of patients and noted as painful in 18% (Ovesen et al 1991).

AETIOLOGY AND PATHOPHYSIOLOGICAL MECHANISMS

The aetiology and pathophysiological mechanisms underlying phantom pain and other types of nerve injury pain are still unknown, despite great efforts to explain them (Frederiks 1963; van Wirdum 1965; Melzack 1971; Melzack & Loeser 1978; Sunderland 1978; Lawrence 1980; Wall 1981; Sherman 1989). Development of chronic pain after lesions in the nervous system is not related to the pathogenesis, aetiology or any specific lesion site. Thus it is clear that trauma, infectious diseases, neoplasms, demyelinating disease and vascular lesions may all lead to chronic pain and sensory abnormalities in the painful area. Similarly, chronic pain is not linked to any specific aetiology. For example, infarction in the thalamus or the posterolateral medulla may sometimes be associated with pain and sometimes not. Pain after dorsal root avulsions may mimic the pain seen in patients with tabes dorsalis. Finally deafferentation pain may be seen at almost every level of the nervous system, where lesions directly or indirectly interfere with processing of afferent somatosensory information. Thus injuries of peripheral nerves, dorsal roots, spinal cord, brain stem, thalamus and cortex may all lead to the same pain syndrome with excruciating spontaneous chronic pain and cutaneous sensory changes. It is obvious that the phantom limb image with its complex, perceptual, emotional and cognitive qualities involves interaction of some cerebral structure(s). This, however, does not contradict the notion that neuronal mechanisms located at a much lower level in the central nervous system or in the cut peripheral nerves may furnish the brain with information necessary for creating a phantom.

The starting point in interpreting the phantom limb phenomenon, painful or not, must be that amputation of a limb causes a sudden cessation of a normal patterned afferent influx to the spinal cord. This input is substituted by an as yet unknown, but certainly different, new input to the spinal cord and to the brain. We now know that a temporal sequence of morphological, physiological and chemical events takes place in the peripheral nerve fibres, the spinal cord and in the brain following nerve injury (Wall 1981; Devor & Rappaport 1990; see also Chs 4 and 5).

A comparison of the clinical aspects of phantom pain, its related phenomena and the effects of experimental nerve sections may give clues about possible pathophysiological mechanisms involved in generating phantom limb phenomena.

PERIPHERAL MECHANISMS

Several clinical observations suggest that mechanisms in the periphery (i.e. in the stump or in central parts of sectioned primary afferents) may play a role in the phantom limb percept: (i) phantom limb sensations can be modulated by various stump manipulation; (ii) phantom limb sensations are temporarily abolished after local stump anaesthesia; (iii) stump revisions and removal of tender neuromas often reduce pain transiently; (iv) phantom pain is significantly more frequent in those amputees with long-term stump pain than in those without persistent pain; (v) although obvious stump pathology is rare, changed cutaneous sensibility in the stump is a common if not universal feature; (vi) finally, changes in stump blood flow alter the phantom limb percept.

Given these simple clinical observations it is obvious to look in the periphery for a pathophysiological mechanism. Experimentally it is known that peripheral nerve sections produce a list of anatomical, physiological and biochemical changes in cut peripheral nerves, including formation of sprouts and neuromas, spontaneous activity and increased sensitivity of such sprouts to mechanical stimuli and various neurochemicals, e.g. noradrenaline (norepinephrine) (Wall 1983; Devor & Rappaport 1990; see also Chs 4 and 5). Although the clinical significance of these experimental findings at present is unclear, they do allow some presumptions. For example, the increased sensitivity of sprouts and neuromas to noradrenaline may in part explain the exacerbation of phantom pain by stress and other emotional states associated with increased catecholaminergic activity. Nyström & Hagbarth (1981) in microelectrode recordings from transected nerves in two amputees found that tapping of neuromas induced activity in afferent fibres (some probably of C-fibre type) and that such activity was associated with increased phantom limb pain. Chabal et al (1989) recently examined the effect of a potassium channel blocker gallamine injected into neuroma of human amputees suffering from phantom pain. It was found that gallamine increased pain while saline had no effect. This suggests that ion channel permeability in neuroma do play a role in phantom pain. The chaotic reinnervation of stumps with formation of ectopic excitation sites and ephaptic synapses may contribute to the changed sensitivity of stumps and to alterations in evoked sensations (e.g. allodynia) (Devor & Rappaport 1990). Thus, various factors in the periphery may contribute to the phantom limb percept.

SPINAL CORD MECHANISMS

Spinal cord lesions and root avulsions from the plexus brachialis are sometimes associated with pain of the same character and localisation as seen in amputees with phantom pain (Bors 1951; Melzack & Loeser 1978; Wynn Parry 1980). A few previously published case reports support the notion that spinal mechanisms could play a role in the phantom limb percept. Brihaye (1958) described a patient with a right lower limb phantom which disappeared after herniation of a cervical disc causing myelopathy. After removal of the herniated disc and upon recovery from myelopathy, the phantom limb percept reappeared. Catchlove (1983) reported a case in which a paraplegic patient with a full sensory loss below Th11 had phantom limb pain after amputation of one leg. Mackenzie (1983) described the appearance of phantom limb pain during spinal anaesthesia in two amputees who formerly had not experienced phantom pains. Similar induction or reduction of phantom limb pain following spinal anaesthesia has been noted by others (Carrie & Glynn 1986; Jacobsen et al 1989). While these findings suggest that spinal cord mechanisms modulate the phantom limb percept, including pain, it is noteworthy that extramedullary processes, such as herniated discs, neurinomas, meningiomas and malignant tumours are only rarely associated with those pain types seen in phantom pain. These well known clinical experiences suggest that peripheral nerve sections induce changes in the spinal cord. Noordenbos (1959) more than 30 years ago suggested that disinhibition of dorsal horn neurons which have lost their neuronal afferent input may play a role in triggering phantom limb phenomena. Subsequent experimental work has demonstrated a cascade of morphological, physiological and neurochemical changes in the dorsal horn following peripheral nerve injury, including atrophy of primary afferent terminals, loss of several peptides in terminals of afferent fibres, changes in primary afferent depolarization, postsynaptic inhibitions and expansions of peripheral receptive fields, with the result that dorsal horn neurons that have lost their normal afferent input begin to respond to nearby intact afferent nerves (see Chs 5 and 10). The clinical significance of these experimental findings is at present incompletely understood. However, it is of interest to note that phantom limb phenomena, whether painful or not, are most vivid in the distal parts of a limb and that these sensations can be induced by stimulating the stump. One possible explanation could be that medial dorsal horn neurons in the cord, with skin receptive fields located in distal parts of a limb, show spontaneous activity and expansion of receptive fields after limb amputation with the result that these cells can be driven from areas located more proximally (e.g. stump).

SUPRASPINAL MECHANISMS

The phantom limb percept with its complex perceptual qualities and its modification by a variety of internal stimuli (e.g. attention, distraction or stress), clearly indicates that the phantom image is ultimately integrated in the brain. Some case reports suggest that cortical and thalamic structures modulate phantom limb and phantom pain. Head & Holmes (1915) noted the disappearance of a left leg phantom after a cerebral lesion in the right hemisphere. Others (Appenzeller & Bicknell 1969; Yarnitsky et al 1988) have suggested that cortical or subcortical lesions may erase a contralateral phantom limb experience. Finally, electrical stimulation of the parvocellular part of nucleus ventralis posterolateralis in thalamus is reported to reduce phantom limb and phantom pain (Merienne & Mazars 1981).

Although previous concepts (Penfield & Jasper 1954) denied any role of cortical structures in nociceptive processing, there is now evidence indicating that the cerebral cortex is involved in the sensory discriminative aspects of pain (Sweet 1981; Perl 1984). Recent electrophysiological studies have documented the existence of nociceptive specific neurons in the cerebral cortex. In view of the plasticity in nociceptive and antinociceptive systems it is reasonable to assume that amputation not only produces a cascade of events in the periphery and the dorsal horn of the spinal cord, but that these changes eventually sweep more centrally. The general arrangement of nociceptive transmitting systems, with modulatory circuits that increasingly project to rostral relays in ascending pathways, makes it difficult to document those possible supraspinal mechanisms involved in triggering and modulating phantom limb phenomena.

THERAPY

GENERAL

The treatment of chronic pain following amputation is a difficult task; with an unknown pathophysiology and aetiology it is not possible to give clear directives for pain treatment in amputees. The treatment of chronic pain in amputees – as in any other chronic pain condition – depends on the type of pain, its severity and to what extent pain incapacitates the patient. It is useful to distinguish between: (i) preoperative pain persisting after amputation; (ii) phantom pain; (iii) stump pain.

Any combination of these types of pain may be seen in individual amputees. The severity of pain and the degree of incapacitation is difficult to determine. According to the literature severe phantom pain is claimed to occur in less than 5% of amputees (see above). This figure probably represents an underestimation of the magnitude of the problem. Thus Sherman & Sherman (1985) recently reported that only 20% of amputees with phantom pain were given any treatment for their pain.

Various treatments have been and are currently in use for chronic pain after amputation. A survey of the literature in 1980 (Sherman et al 1980) identified 68 different treatment methods, of which 50 were in current use. Most studies dealing with pain treatment in amputees suffer from major methodological errors: (i) samples are small and heterogenous; (ii) studies are open; (iii) controls are often lacking; (iv) follow-up periods are short. A success rate of any previous reported treatment rarely exceeds a placebo response of 30% (Sherman & Sherman 1985). Table 36.5 shows a summary of noninvasive and invasive treatment methods and their presumed site of action. In general, treatment should be based on noninvasive techniques. Surgery on the peripheral or the central nervous system in cases of deafferentation pain always implicates further deafferentation and thereby provides an increased risk for persistent pain. However, for historical reasons some invasive treatment methods will briefly be mentioned.

Table 36.5 Previous or currently used invasive and noninvasive treatments for stump/phantom pain

Presumed site of action	Method	
	Noninvasive	Invasive
Periphery	Nonnarcotic analgesics Anticonvulsants Local anaesthetics Physiotherapy Guanethidine Electrical stimulation Biofeedback	Neurectomy Neuromectomy Stump revision Rhizotomy Ganglionectomy Sympathectomy
Spinal cord	Narcotic analgesics Baclofen Lidocaine Tricyclic antidepressants Calcitonin Anticonvulsants Peripheral electrical stimulation	DREZ lesion Dorsal column stimulation Chordotomy Epidural blockåde
Brain	Narcotic analgesics Nonnarcotic analgesics Tricyclic antidepressants Neuroleptics Peripheral electrical stimulation 'Placebo' Psychotherapy	Brain stem stimulation Thalamic stimulation Brain stem lesions Thalamic lesions Parietal lobectomy Prefontal lobotomy Cingulectomy

DREZ = dorsal root entry-zone.

NONINVASIVE TECHNIQUES

Nonmedical

Transcutaneous electrical nerve stimulation (TENS), acupuncture, relaxation training, ultrasound and hypnosis may in some cases have a beneficial effect on stump and phantom pains. Physical therapy involving massage, manipulation and passive movements may prevent trophic changes and vascular congestion in the stump. Induction of sensory inflow from the stump area by physical therapy could play a role in the ameliorating effect of such types of treatment.

TENS either on the stump or on the contralateral extremity has been used with some success in the treatment of phantom pain (Thoden et al 1979; Sherman et al 1980; Carabelli & Kellerman 1985; Lundeberg 1985). Thus Lundeberg (1985) found that in 24 patients with phantom pain given either peripheral vibratory stimulation or placebo, 75% of the patients reported pain reduction during stimulation, while 44% noted pain reduction during placebo. The advantages of peripheral nerve stimulation are the lack of side-effects and complications and the fact that the treatment can be easily repeated.

Medical

No drug treatment is specifically effective in the treatment of chronic pain in amputees. However, in a double-blind, crossover study Jaeger & Maier (1992) recently reported a beneficial effect of intravenous calcitonin on phantom limb pain. The preoperative existing persisting pains are in our experience often less intense than the genuine phantom pain, which has varying characteristics, to some extent depending on the basic disease (e.g. circulatory disturbances or a tumour). In most cases an effective preoperative pain therapy may be continued successfully after the amputation.

Persistent long-term phantom pain is often resistant to any treatment. In some cases carbamazepine has a splendid effect and can relieve the patient from pain when the membrane-stabilizing drug is administered in ordinary neuralgic doses (Elliott et al 1976; Patterson 1988). Certain antidepressants (e.g. clomipramine) may also have a beneficial effect in some patients, especially para- and tetraplegics with spinal column fractures. Used in the treatment of pain, antidepressants may be effective at doses lower than those corresponding to their antidepressant effect. In single cases the antidepressant doxepin has been reported to be effective (Iacono et al 1987). Others have found beta-blockers to be of value (Marsland et al 1982).

Permanent phantom pain should not be accepted until opioids have been tried. It is our experience (as well as that of others; Urban et al 1986) that opioids can be used safely for years with a limited risk of drug dependence.

Phantom pain is neither to be considered a manifestation of a psychological disorder nor a part of any psychiatric disease (Sherman et al 1987). Amputees are for obvious reasons often depressed, emotionally unstable and insecure about their future life, so psychological support and psychiatric aid may be necessary. Again controlled double-blind studies with carbamazepine are lacking (Patterson 1988). Educational programmes for amputees, their relatives and those health professionals dealing with cases of amputees may perhaps contribute to a reduction of chronic pain after amputation.

INVASIVE TECHNIQUES

Stump revision

Surgery on amputation neuromas and more extensive amputation have played important roles in the treatment of stump and phantom pain. By surgical stump revision Baumgartner & Riniker (1981) achieved considerable relief of both stump and phantom pain in 87 out of 100 patients.

In order to avoid the development of traumatic neuromas in amputees, others have performed encapsulation with Millipore, fascicle ligation (Battista 1979) and centrocentral anastomosis (Samii 1981). Formation of neuroma is a universal phenomenon after a peripheral nerve cut. Excision of tender neuromas in a stump usually leads to new bulbs, which are as painful as the first (Fig. 36.5). Stump revision should probably be limited to those few amputees with obvious stump pathology. Embedding tender neuromas deep into tissue and thereby protecting neuromas from mechanical compression may in some cases eliminate symptoms of increased mechanosensitivity (Herndon et al 1976). In properly healed stumps there is almost never any indication for proximal extension of the amputation because of pain.

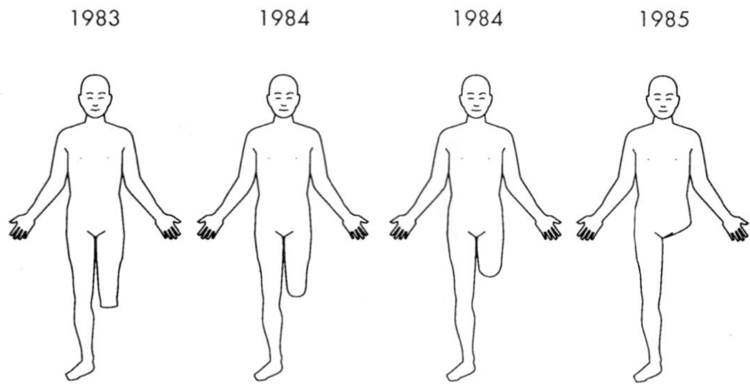

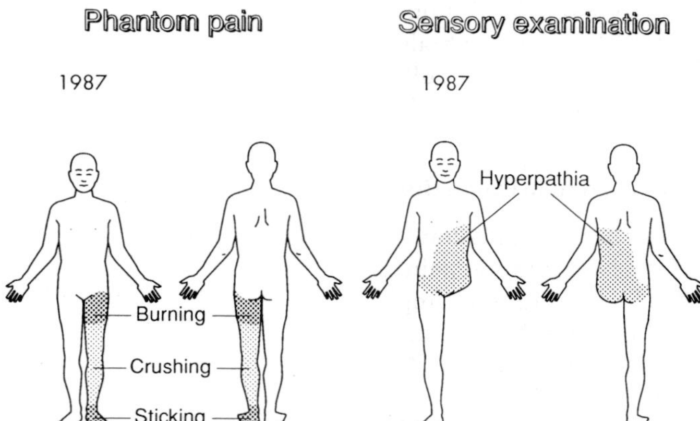

Fig. 36.5 A 54-year-old man, a former soccer player, who, since the age of 30, had suffered from bilateral knee pain. Meniscectomies were performed several times. At the age of 37, a right-sided knee arthrodesis was done because of painful osteoarthrosis. At the age of 44 a left-sided artificial knee joint was inserted because of severe painful osteoarthrosis now in the left knee. During the following 2 years he had continuous left-sided knee pain and, because of loosening of the artificial joint, this was removed in 1983 when he was 46 years old and an amputation at knee level was done. He immediately developed severe phantom pain, which was resistant to peripheral and central analgesics and membrane stabilizing agents. Palpable tender neuromas present in the stump were removed twice without effect. Reamputations at successively higher levels were performed during the following 2 years on the indication of pain, ending with left-sided hip exarticulation in 1985 (upper figurine row). When seen in 1987 he had severe constant phantom pain (lower left figurine) despite treatment with ketobemidon 90 mg daily. Sensory examination revealed hyperpathia which extended to the left Th4 dermatome (lower right figurine). Touch stimulation of left Th7–12 evoked phantom pain on the back of the leg. Touch stimulation of the right Th10–12 dermatome evoked pain on the outer aspect of the left phantom thigh. Stimulation in the S5 dermatome (anal area) evoked phantom pain in the knee.

Neurectomy/rhizotomy and sympathectomy

Denervation between the amputation stump and the spinal nerve roots was previously used in the treatment of amputation pains, but owing to the poor results it has now been almost entirely abandoned.

While both clinical and experimental findings support the notion that sympathetic activity influences phantom and/or stump pain (see above), sympathectomy has only a limited effect on stump and phantom pain. The role of chemical sympathectomy after guanethidine (see Ch. 54) in phantom pain is not yet clear.

Dorsal root entry-zone lesions

This treatment, primarily introduced for the treatment of painful brachial plexus avulsions, has also been used in the treatment of phantom pain (Nashold & Ostdahl 1979; Samii & Moringlane 1984; Saris et al 1985; Wiegand & Winkelmüller 1985; Saris et al 1988). It is generally believed that dorsal root entry-zone lesions have a limited effect on the treatment of phantom pain. Saris et al (1985) studied 22 patients with postamputation phantom/stump pain. All underwent dorsal root entry-zone lesions and were followed for 6 months to 4 years after surgery. Only 36% of the patients obtained pain relief from the operation. However, in patients suffering from phantom pain alone a good result was obtained in six patients (Saris et al 1985).

Spinal cord stimulation

Spinal cord stimulation has been widely used in the treatment of amputation pain. Krainick et al (1980) stimulated 64 patients with postamputation pain and obtained a 50–100% pain reduction in 45% of patients and a 25–50% pain reduction in 11%. At a follow-up examination 5 years later 23% still had 50–100% pain relief. Siegfried & Cetinalp (1981) analysed the material of nine authors and found that among 148 patients 51% obtained 50–100% pain relief, while 18% obtained 25–50% pain reduction.

Brain stimulation

Mundinger & Salomáo (1980) treated 32 patients with thalamic pains, persisting zoster pains, anaesthesia dolorosa and phantom pains and achieved more than 50% pain relief in 53% of the patients. Out of 14 amputees, 13 (93%) treated with a combination of deep brain stimulation and transcutaneous stimulation had a reduction of pain of more than 50% (Mundinger & Neumüller 1981).

Cordotomy

This operation was used for many years in the treatment of phantom pain (Doupe et al 1944; de Gutierrez-Mahoney 1948). In a survey, Siegfried & Cetinalp (1981) summarized the results of five small studies comprising 52 patients in whom cordotomy had been performed: 38% had a 50–100% reduction of pain, 44% had a 25–50% reduction. This treatment is exceedingly rare today.

PREVENTION

So far no treatment, whether invasive or noninvasive, has proven effective in persistent phantom pain. In a prospective study it was observed that patients with severe preamputation pain (as determined by opioid consumption) more frequently had phantom pain than did patients with less severe preamputation pain (Jensen et al 1985). This observation prompted Bach et al (1988) to investigate whether an effective preoperative blockade in patients undergoing amputation might reduce the subsequent incidence of phantom pain. They found that preoperative lumbar epidural blockade with bupivacaine and/or morphine for 3 days before amputation reduced the incidence of phantom pain in the first year but not the 2nd year after amputation. These findings may have important implications for future preoperative handling of patients undergoing limb amputation, but further studies are needed to clarify the value of preemptive treatment.

CONCLUSION

Nonpainful phantom limb and phantom pain are imaginary sensations from a limb that has been amputated. Although phantom limb phenomena are an invariable consequence of limb amputation in adults, persistent and severe phantom pain is seen in only less than 10% of amputees. The incidence of severe phantom pain is similar to other chronic pain states associated with denervation and deafferentation. Experimental studies within the last two decades have shown that a nerve cut produces a range of morphological, physiological and biochemical changes both in the peripheral and in the central nervous systems. The significance of these experimental changes observed in rodents for the chronic pain syndrome in humans after limb amputation is less clear. A fascinating but still unresolved question is whether these peripheral and central changes can be prevented.

REFERENCES

Abbatucci J 1884 Etudes psychologiques sur les hallucinations des amputés. Thesis, Bordeaux

Abramson A S, Feibel A 1981 The phantom phenomenon; its use and disuse. Bulletin of the New York Academy of Medicine 57: 99–122

Appenzeller O, Bicknell J M 1969 Effects of nervous system lesions on phantom experience in amputees. Neurology 19: 141–146

Bach S, Noreng M F, Tjéllden N U 1988 Phantom limb pain in amputees during the first 12 months following limb amputation after preoperative lumbar epidural blockade. Pain 33: 297–301

Bailey A A, Moersch F P 1941 Phantom limb. Canadian Medical Association Journal 45: 37–42
Battista A F 1979 Pain of peripheral neve origin: fascicle ligation for prevention of painful neuroma. In: Bonica J J, Liebeskind J C, Albe-Fessard D G (eds) Advances in pain research and therapy 3. Raven Press, New York
Baumgartner R, Riniker C 1981 Surgical stump revision as a treatment of stump and phantom pains. Results of 100 cases. In: Siegfried S, Zimmermann M (eds) Phantom and stump pain. Springer Verlag, Berlin, p 118–122
Bell C 1830 The nervous system of the human body. Longman, London
Berger M, Gerstenbrand F 1981 Phantom illusions in spinal cord lesions. In: Siegfried J, Zimmermann M (eds) Phantom and stump pain. Springer Verlag, Berlin, p 66–73
Bors E 1951 Phantom limbs of patients with spinal cord injury. Archives of Neurology and Psychiatry 66: 610–631
Brihaye J 1958 Extinction of phantom limb in leg amputated during medullary compression by cervical discal hernia: revival of phantom after surgical removal of hernia. Acta Neurologica Psychiatrica Belgica 58: 536
Browder J, Gallagher J P 1948 Dorsal cordotomy for pain phantom limbs. Annals of Surgery 128: 456–469
Brown W A 1968 Postamputation phantom limb pain. Diseases of the Nervous System 29: 301–306
Buchanan D C, Mandel A R 1986 The prevalence of phantom limb experience in amputees. Rehabilitation Psychology 31: 183–188
Carabelli R A, Kellerman WC 1985 Phantom limb pain: relief by application of TENS to contralateral extremity. Archives of Physical Medicine and Rehabilitation 66: 466–477
Carlen P L, Wall P D, Nadvorna H, Steinbach T 1978 Phantom limbs and related phenomena in recent traumatic amputations. Neurology 28: 211–217
Carrie L E S, Glynn C J 1986 Phantom limb pain and epidural anesthesia for cesarean section. Anesthesiology 65: 220–221
Catchlove R F 1983 Phantom pain following limb amputation in a parapelgic. A case report. Psychotherapy and Psychosomatics 39: 89–93
Chabal C, Jacobsen L, Russell L C, Burchielh K J 1989 Pain responses to perineuromal injection of normal saline, gallamine and Lidocaine in humans. Pain 36: 321–325
Cronholm B 1951 Phantom limb in amputees. Acta Psychiatrica et Neurologica Scandinavica (suppl) 72: 1–310
de Gutierrez-Mahoney C G 1948 The treatment of painful phantom limb. A follow-up study. Surgical Clinics of North America 28: 481–483
Devor M, Rappaport Z H 1990 Pain and the pathophysiology of damaged nerve. In: Fields HL (ed) Pain syndromes in neurology. Butterworths, London, p 47–83
Doupe J, Cullen C H, Chance G Q 1944 Post-traumatic pain and the causalgic syndrome. Journal of Neurology, Neurosurgery and Psychiatry 7: 33–48
Elliott F, Little A, Milbrandt W 1976 Carbamazepine for phantom limb phenomena. New England Journal of Medicine 295: 678
Ewalt J R, Randall G C, Morris H 1947 The phantom limb. Psychosomatic Medicine 9: 118–123
Feinstein B, Luce J C, Langton J N K 1954 The influence of phantom limbs. In: Klopsteg P, Wilson P (eds) Human limbs and their substitutes. McGraw-Hill, New York, p 19–138
Finch D R A, Mac-Dougal M, Tibbs D J, Morris P J 1980 Amputation for vascular disease: the experience of a peripheral vascular unit. British Journal of Surgery 67: 233–237
Frederiks J A M 1963 Occurrence and nature of phantom limb phenomena following amputation of body parts and following lesions of the central and peripheral nervous system. Psychiatria Neurologica Neurochirurgica 66: 73–97
Guéniot M 1861. D'une hallucination du toucher (ou hétérotopie subjective des extrémités) particulière a certains amputés. Journal de la Physiologie d I'Homme et des Animaux 4: 416
Head H, Holmes G 1915 Sensory disturbances from cerebral lesions. Brain 34: 102–254
Henderson W R, Smyth G E 1948 Phantom limbs. Journal of Neurology, Neurosurgery and Psychiatry 11: 88–112
Herndon J H, Eaton R G, Little J W 1976 Management of painful neuromas in the hand. Journal of Bone and Joint Surgery 58: 69–373
Herrmann L G, Gibbs E W 1945 Phantom limb pain. American Journal of Surgery 67: 168–180
Iacono R P, Sandyk R, Baumford C R, Awerbuch G, Malone J M 1987 Post-amputation phantom pain and autonomous stump movements responsive to doxepin. Functional Neurology 2: 343–348
Jacobsen L, Chabal C, Brody M C 1989 Relief of persistent postamputation stump and phantom limb pain with intrathecal fentanyl. Pain 37: 317–322
Jaeger H, Maier C 1992 Calcitonin in phantom limb pain: a double-blind study. Pain 48: 21–27
James U 1973 Unilateral above-knee amputees. Scandinavian Journal of Rehabilitation Medicine 5: 23–34
Jamison K, Wellisch D K, Katz R L, Pasnau R O 1979 Phantom breast syndrome. Archives of Surgery 114: 93–95
Jensen T S, Krebs B, Nielsen J, Rasmussen P 1983 Phantom limb, phantom pain and stump pain in amputees during the first 6 months following limb amputation. Pain 17: 243–256
Jensen T S, Krebs B, Nielsen J, Rasmussen P 1984 Non-painful phantom limb phenomena in amputees: incidence, clinical characteristics and temporal course. Acta Neurologica Scandinavica 70: 407–414
Jensen T S, Krebs B, Nielsen J, Ramussen P 1985 Immediate and long-term phantom limb pain in amputees: incidence, clinical characteristics and relationship to preamputation limb pain. Pain 21: 267–278
Katz J, Melzack R 1987 Referred sensations in chronic pain patients. Pain 28: 51–59
Katz J, Melzack R 1990 Pain 'memories' in phantom limbs: review and clinical observations. Pain 43: 319–336
Kegel B, Carpenter M L, Burgess E M 1977 A survey of lower-limb amputees: prosthesis, phantom sensations and psychosocial aspects. Bulletin of Prosthesis Research 10: 43–60
Keil G 1990 Sogenannte erstbeschreibung des phantomschmerzes von Alubroise Paré. Fortschritte der Medicine 108: 58–66
Krainick J-U, Thoden U 1976 Schmerzhänomene bei Amputierten. Neurochirurgica 19: 72–80
Krainick J-U, Thoden U, Riechert T 1980 Pain reduction in amputees by long-term spinal cord stimulation. Journal of Neurosurgery 52: 346–350
Krebs B, Jensen T S, Krøner K, Nielsen J, Jørgensen H S 1985 Phantom limb phenomena in amputees 7 years after limb amputation. In: Fields H L, Dubner R, Cervero F (eds) Advances in pain research and therapy 9. Raven Press, New York, p 425–429
Krøner K, Krebs B, Skov J, Jørgensen H S 1989 Immediate and long-term phantom breast syndrome after mastectomy: incidence, clinical characteristics and relationship to pre-mastectomy breast pain. Pain 36: 327–334
Lawrence R M 1980 Phantom pain: a new hypothesis. Medical Hypotheses 6: 245–248
Lhermitte J 1951 Les hallucinations. Clinique et physiopathologie. G Doin, Paris
Lindesay J E 1985 Multiple pain complaints in amputees. Journal of the Royal Society of Medicine 78: 452–455
Lundeberg T 1985 Relief of pain from nine phantom limbs by peripheral stimulation. Journal of Neurology 232: 79–82
Lunn V 1948 Om legemsbevidstheden. Munksgaard, Copenhagen
McCalley-Whitters M, Nasrallah H A 1983 Tardive dyskinesia in a phantom limb. British Journal of Psychiatry 142: 206–207
Mackenzie N 1983 Phantom limb pain during spinal anaesthesia. Anaesthesia 38: 886–887
Magendie F 1833 Précis élémentaires de physiologie, 3rd edn, vol 1. Masson, Paris
Marsland A R, Weekes J W N, Atkinson R L, Leong M G 1982 Phantom limb pain: a case for beta blockers? Pain 12: 295–297
Melzack R 1971 Phantom limb pain: implications of treatment of pathological pain. Anesthesiology 35: 409–419
Melzack R, Loeser J D 1978 Phantom body pain in paraplegics: evidence for a central 'pattern generating mechanism' for pain. Pain 4: 195–210
Merienne L, Mazars G 1981 Transformation of body scheme caused by

thalamic stimulation. Thalamic stimulation for painful phantom limb. Neurochirurgie 27: 121-123
Merskey H 1986 Classification of chronic pain: descriptions of chronic pain syndromes and definitions of pain terms. Pain (suppl) 3: 1–225
Mitchell S W 1872 Injuries of nerves and their consequences. J B Lippincott, Philadelphia
Mundinger F, Neumüller H 1981 Programmed transcutaneous (TNS) and central (DBS) stimulation for control of phantom limb pain and causalgia: a new method for treatment. In: Siegfried J, Zimmermann M (eds) Phantom and stump pain. Springer Verlag, Berlin, p 167–178
Mundinger F, Salomáo J F 1980 Deep brain stimulation in mesencephalic lemniscus medialis for chronic pain. Acta Neurochirurgica 30: 245–258
Nashold B S, Ostdahl R H 1979 Dorsal root entry zone lesions for pain relief. Journal of Neurosurgery 51: 59–69
Nathan P W 1962 Pain traces left in the central nervous system. In: Keele C A, Smith R (eds) The assessment of pain in man and animals. E & S Livingstone, Edinburgh, p 129–134
Nordenbos W 1959 Pain. Elsevier, Amsterdam
Nyström B, Hagbarth K E 1981 Microelectrode recordings from transected nerves in amputees with phantom limb pain. Neuroscience Letters 27: 211–216
Ovesen P, Krøner K, Ømsholt J, Bach K 1991 Phantom-related phenomena after rectal amputation: prevalence and clinical characteristics. Pain 44: 289–291
Parkes C M 1973 Factors determining the persistence of phantom pain in the amputee. Journal of Psychosomatic Research 17: 97–108
Patterson J F 1988 Carbamazepine in the treatment of phantom limb pain. Southern Medical Journal 81: 1100–1102
Penfield W, Jasper H 1954 Epilepsy and the functional anatomy of the human brain. Little, Brown, Boston, Massachusetts
Penfield W, Rasmussen T 1955 The cerebral cortex of man. Macmillian, New York
Perl E R 1984 Pain and nociception. In: Darian Smith I (ed) Handbook of physiology, vol III. American Physiological Society, Bethesda, p 915–975
Pitres A 1897 Étude sur les sensations illusoires des amputés. Annales Medico-psychologiques 55: 177–192
Price D B 1976 Phantom limb phenomena in patients with leprosy. Journal of Nervous and Mental Disease 163: 108–116
Rhône G F 1842. De sensuum mendaciis apud eos homines, quibus membrum aliquod amputatum est. Thesis, Halle
Riddoch G 1941 Phantom limbs and body shape. Brain 64: 197–222
Riese W, Bruck G 1950 Le membre fantôme chez l'enfant. Revue Neurologique 83: 221–222
Roberts W J 1986 A hypothesis on the physiological basis for causalgia and related pain. Pain 24: 297–311
Samii M 1981 Centrocentral anastomosis of peripheral nerves: a neurosurgical treatment of amputation neuromas. In: Siegfried J, Zimmermann M (eds) Phantom and stump pain. Springer Verlag, Berlin, pp 123–125
Samii M, Moringlane J R 1984 Thermocoagulation of the dorsal root entry zone for the treatment of intractable pain. Neurosurgery 15: 953–955
Saris S C, Iacono R P, Nashold B S Jr 1985 Dorsal root entry zone lesions for post-amputation pain. Journal of Neurosurgery 62: 72–76
Saris S C, Iacono R P, Nashold B S Jr 1988 Successful treatment of phantom pain with dorsal root entry zone coagulation. Applied Neurophysiology 51: 188–187
Schott G D 1986 Mechanisms of causalgia and related clinical conditions. The role of the central and of the sympathetic nervous system 109: 717–738
Sherman R 1984 Direct evidence of a link between burning phantom limb pain and stump blood flow: a case report. Orthopedics 7: 1319–1320
Sherman R A 1989 Stump and phantom limb pain. Neurologic Clinics 7: 249–264
Sherman R, Sherman C 1983 Prevalence and characteristics of chronic phantom limb pain among American veterans: results of a trial survey. American Journal of Physical Medicine 62: 227–238
Sherman R A, Sherman C J 1985 A comparison of phantom sensations among amputees whose amputations were of civilian and military origins. Pain 21: 91–97
Sherman R A, Sherman C J, Gall N G 1980 A survey of current phantom limb pain treatment in the United States. Pain 8: 85–99
Sherman R, Sherman C, Parker L 1984 Chronic phantom and stump pain among American veterans: results of a survey. Pain 18: 83–95
Sherman R A, Sherman C J, Bruno G M 1987 Psychological factors influencing chronic phantom limb pain: an analysis of the literature Pain 28: 285–295
Shukla G D, Sahu S C, Tripathi R P, Gupta D K 1982a Phantom limb: a phenomenological study. British Journal of Psychiatry 141: 54–58
Shukla G D, Sahu S C, Tripathi R P, Gupta D K 1982b A psychiatric study of amputees. British Journal of Psychiatry 141: 50–53
Siegfried J, Cetinalp E 1981 Neurosurgical treatment of phantom limb pain: a survey of methods. In: Siegfried J, Zimmermann M (eds) Phantom and stump pain. Springer Verlag, Berlin, p 148–155
Simmel ML 1962 Phantom experiences following amputation in childhood. Journal of Neurology, Neurosurgery and Psychiatry 25: 69–78
Sliosberg A. 1948 Les algies des amputés. Masson, Paris
Solonen K A 1962 The phantom phenomenon in amputated Finnish war veterans. Acta Orthopaedica Scandinavica 54 (suppl 3): 1–119
Staps T, Hoogenhout J, Woobes T. 1985 Phantom breast sensations following mastectomy. Cancer 56: 2898–2901
Stetter E 1950 Zur Phaenomenologie des Phantomgliedes. Deutsche Zeitschrift für Nervenheilkunde 163: 141–171
Sunderland S 1978 Nerves and nerve injuries. Williams & Wilkins, Baltimore
Sweet W H 1981 Cerebral localization of pain. In: Thompson R A (ed) New perspectives in cerebral localization. Raven Press, New York, p 205–240
Thoden U, Gruber R P, Krainick J-U, Huber-Mück L 1979 Langzeitergebnisse transkutaner Nervenstimulation bei chronisch neurogenen Schmerzzuständen. Nervenarzt 50: 179–184
Urban B J, France R D, Steinberger E K, Scoot D L, Maltbie A A 1986 Long-term use of narcotic/antidepressant medication in the management of phantom limb. Pain 24: 191-196
van Wirdum P 1965 A new explanation of phantom symptoms. Psychiatrica Neurologica Neurochirurgica 68: 306–313
Wall P D 1981 On the origin of pain associated with amputation. In: Siegfried J, Zimmermann M (eds) Phantom and stump pain. Springer Verlag, Berlin, p 2–14
Wall P D 1983 Alterations in the central nervous system after deafferentation: connectivity control. In: Bonica J J, Lindblom U, Iggo A (eds) Advances in pain research and therapy 5. Raven Press, New York, p 677–689
Weinstein S, Sersen E A 1961 Phantoms in cases of congenital absence of limbs. Neurology 11: 905–911
Weinstein S, Vetter R J, Sersen E A 1970 Phantoms following breast amputation. Neuropsychologia 8: 185–197
Whitaker H A 1979 An historical note on the phantom limb. Neurology 29: 273
Wiegand H, Winkelmüller W 1985 Treatment of deafferentation pain by high-frequency intervention of the dorsal root entry zone. Deutsche Medizinische Wochenschrift 100: 216–220
Wynn Parry C B 1980 Pain in avulsion lesions of the brachial plexus. Pain 9: 40–53
Yarnitsky D, Barron S A, Bental E 1988 Disappearance of phantom pain after focal brain infarction. Pain: 32: 285–287

37. Peripheral neuropathies

J. W. Scadding

The primary sensory neuron may be affected in a number of different ways by a great variety of diseases. Motor or sensory fibres may be preferentially affected, but in most neuropathies both are involved, leading to various patterns of sensorimotor deficit. Sensory neuropathies are frequently accompanied by positive sensory symptoms, which usually take the form of paraesthesiae which are not severe and which are overshadowed by the symptoms of sensory or motor deficits. However, there are neuropathies in which pain and severe paraesthesiae are typical and troublesome features. In these neuropathies, the dysaesthesiae may be the presenting and most severe continuing symptoms. This chapter is concerned with these neuropathies, which include many polyneuropathies and mononeuropathies. Experimental animal studies, trigeminal neuropathies, amputation and phantom pain, causalgia and reflex sympathetic dystrophy, and the treatment of pain due to peripheral neuropathies are topics dealt with in other chapters in this volume.

The relationship of painful symptoms to morphological and electrophysiological changes in peripheral nerves has been a subject of interest for many years, particularly since the introduction of nerve biopsy (see Thomas 1970; Stevens et al 1975), and the development of clinical electrophysiological techniques (Buchthal et al 1975; Lambert & Dyck 1975). Since it was established that the transmission of impulses in different classes of peripheral nerve fibre depended on the type of peripheral stimulus in animals and man (Adrian 1931; Lewis et al 1931; Clark et al 1935; Collins et al 1960), the early observations have been greatly expanded by single-fibre recordings in animals and man (Burgess & Perl 1973; Iggo 1977; Vallbo et al 1979; Yaksh & Hammond 1982). Wortis et al (1942) noted the similarity of the burning pain in patients with alcoholic neuropathy to the sensations that were obtained by peripheral stimulation after prolonged anoxia of a limb in normal subjects and, in the light of the observations of Gasser's group (Clark et al 1935), suggested that the burning pain in alcoholic neuropathy might be due to a predominantly C-fibre input, with loss of the normal large-fibre input.

Subsequently, Weddell et al (1948) examined nerve fibres in biopsies of hyperpathic skin, finding a decreased number of fibres in small dermal nerves with a reduced fibre density in the hyperpathic skin, and postulated that the presumed decreased afferent barrage from these areas was responsible for hyperpathia. Lourie & King (1966) also reported a decreased fibre density in hyperpathic skin and noted a preponderance of small-diameter fibres. In particular, they found that hyperpathic hairs arose from follicles innervated predominantly by small fibres. In a study of herpes zoster neuropathy, Noordenbos (1959) found a predominant loss of larger myelinated fibres in affected nerves.

These observations seemed to suggest that in situations where there was either preferential regeneration of small fibres or selective loss of large fibres, dysaesthesiae might result. This idea, and the formulation of the gate control theory (Melzack & Wall 1965), provoked great interest in the further investigation of peripheral neuropathy in man.

TYPE OF PAIN IN PERIPHERAL NEUROPATHY

Many terms may be used by patients with neuropathies to describe their painful sensations. The symptoms may be divided into those which are unprovoked (spontaneous) and those which are provoked by manoeuvres such as skin stimulation, pressure over affected nerves, changes in temperature, or emotional factors. The most commonly described spontaneous symptoms are a deep aching in the extremities and a superficial burning, stinging or prickling pain. Some patients also report paroxysmal, shock-like, lancinating pains, sometimes radiating through a whole limb (Thomas 1975, 1979; Dyck et al 1976).

Allodynia may be particularly incapacitating in some neuropathies, and accompanying hyperpathia is not uncommon (Lindblom 1979; Noordenbos 1979). In the following descriptions of the different neuropathies, the major painful complaints typical of each condition are given, but it should be emphasized that, within a single aetiological or pathological diagnostic category, considerable symptom variation occurs.

INVESTIGATION OF PERIPHERAL NEUROPATHIES

The cause of some neuropathies may become apparent after a few simple tests, and there is no need for specialized investigation. Nevertheless, as pointed out by Thomas (1975), even after extensive investigation the cause of a large minority of neuropathies remains uncertain. Detailed discussion of basic clinical diagnostic aspects of peripheral neuropathies and of the specialized investigative techniques is beyond the scope of this chapter, but some aspects of the morphological techniques are considered, with regard particularly to their limitations. Full accounts of these topics are to be found in reviews by Thomas (1970), Buchtal et al (1975), Lambert & Dyck (1975) and Stevens et al (1975).

NERVE BIOPSY

A major problem of structure–function correlation in peripheral neuropathies is the sampling error inherent in relating sensory abnormalities and whole-nerve electrophysiology to the morphology of a small fascicular nerve biopsy. To overcome this, Dyck and coworkers (Dyck et al 1971b; Lambert & Dyck 1975) took long multifascicular biopsies of sural nerve and investigated these electrophysiologically in vitro by measurement of compound action potentials, and morphologically, the main emphasis being fibre population and teased fibre studies. Biopsies from normal volunteers were compared with biopsies from patients with Friedreich's ataxia, dominantly inherited amyloidosis, hereditary motor and sensory and sensory neuropathies, and chronic relapsing inflammatory polyneuropathy. In Friedreich's ataxia, a substantial reduction of the A-alpha potential with preservation of A-delta and C potentials correlated well with the decrease in the large myelinated fibre population and with the sensory deficit of touch-pressure and two-point discrimination with preservation of pain and temperature sensation. In dominantly inherited amyloidosis, the absent C-fibre potentials, greatly reduced A-delta potential and only moderately reduced A-alpha potential correlated well both with a near absence of C-fibres and reduced small myelinated fibre population, and with the impaired pain and temperature sensation and autonomic function in this patient. Similar good correlations were found in the two types of hereditary sensory neuropathy and in uraemic neuropathy, but not in chronic relapsing inflammatory neuropathy. This was thought to be due to extensive segmental demyelination and remyelination, leading to dispersion of large-fibre action potentials, some of which were considered to have contributed to the C-fibre potential.

These observations established that a selective loss of small myelinated and unmyelinated fibres leads to impaired pain sensation in man and indicated that reasonable predictions about fibre population could be made from physiological observations, except where segmental demyelination was a prominent feature. It should be emphasized, however, that such extensive nerve biopsy and in vitro electrophysiology remain research investigations.

Some problems of standard nerve biopsy morphological observations require mention here. Examination of transverse sections by light microscopy will fail to recognize segmentally demyelinated axons and will thus underestimate the myelinated fibre population. An increase in the density of small fibres does not necessarily imply a selective loss of large fibres, since regeneration will increase the population of small fibres. By relating axonal diameter to myelin sheath thickness by electron microscopic examination and using certain criteria for differentiating the sprouts of myelinated and unmyelinated fibres, this problem can be overcome to some extent (Ochoa 1970; Morris et al 1972; Dyck 1975).

The two major pathological processes in peripheral neuropathy are axonal degeneration and segmental demyelination. The division of polyneuropathies into either of these pathological categories is somewhat artificial, since both processes are usually present, albeit in varying proportions (Thomas 1971). This has been evident since the introduction of routine examination of teased fibres (Dyck et al 1968; Thomas 1970) which permits easier recognition of demyelination, remyelination, and degenerative changes, which may be graded according to severity (Dyck et al 1971b). Single teased fibres may also subsequently be examined by electron microscopy (Dyck & Lais 1970; Spencer & Thomas 1970; Dyck 1975).

The various patterns of axonal degeneration, affecting distal parts of the axon or the cell body or both, and details of segmental demyelination, remyelination and onion bulb formation, and of pathological reactions of unmyelinated fibres are reviewed by Dyck (1975), Schroder (1975) and Ochoa (1978).

POLYNEUROPATHIES

From the point of view of understanding mechanisms of pain in human polyneuropathies, information is limited. Standard neurophysiological tests are essentially diagnostic, but tell us little about the properties which may be responsible for pain. Single fibre microneurographic recordings up to the present time have been performed almost exclusively on normal subjects, and there is little direct information in human polyneuropathies concerning the presence of the abnormal properties of ectopic impulse generation, catecholamine sensitivity and interactions between fibres, which have been so extensively studied in experimental animals (see Ch. 4). As a result of the technical limitations of neurophysiological investigation in man, the morphological changes in nerve biopsies and their correlation with nerve conduction studies have provided the only basis on which to consider the reasons for the development of pain in neuropathy.

Following the earlier indications that an imbalance between large and small fibre input might be of particular importance, fibre size distribution in different neuropathies has been a particular focus of attention. In the account of the polyneuropathies here, it is convenient to follow the subdivision of the neuropathies on this basis, both to trace the development of ideas about mechanisms of pain in neuropathy, and also as a means of showing that fibre size distribution per se is unlikely to be an important factor leading to pain. Table 37.1 lists some neuropathies important to the present discussion, divided on the basis of painfulness and fibre size distribution.

POLYNEUROPATHIES WITH SELECTIVE LOSS OF PAIN SENSATION

These comprise a rare, poorly defined group of inherited disorders in which, from an early age, an insensitivity to pain is evident. It is important to distinguish those disorders in which the peripheral and central nervous systems are intact, where the problem appears to be a lack of recognition of pain, an indifference or asymbolia, rather than an insensitivity (Schilder et al 1931), which can be explained on the basis of observed structural abnormalities. In the former group, patients are able to identify noxious stimuli and sensory thresholds are normal but they do not react behaviourally or physiologically in the expected way (Ogden et al 1959; Winkelmann et al 1962). Peripheral nerves, spinal cord and thalamus are all normal in these patients (Feindel 1953; Baxter & Olszewski 1960). Asymbolia for pain may also be acquired, recent evidence suggesting a crucial role for the insular cortex, damage to which may lead to disconnection between sensory cortex and the limbic system (Berthier et al 1988).

Table 37.1 Painful and painless polyneuropathies

Polyneuropathies with selective loss of pain sensation
Congenital analgesia with anhidrosis
Congenital analgesia with other sensory impairment
Tangier disease (familial alpha-lipoprotein deficiency)
Painful polyneuropathies with selective large-fibre loss
Isoniazid neuropathy
Pellagra neuropathy
Painless polyneuropathies with selective large-fibre loss
Friedreich's axatia
Chronic renal failure
Painful polyneuropathies with selective small-fibre loss
Diabetic neuropathy
Amyloid neuropathy
Fabry's disease
Dominantly inherited sensory neuropathy
Painful polyneuropathies with nonselective fibre loss
Alcoholic neuropathy
Myeloma neuropathy
Miscellaneous painful neuropathies
Acute inflammatory polyneuropathy
Nutritional neuropathies
Beriberi
Strachan's syndrome
Burning feet syndrome
Arsenic neuropathy

Leaving such cases aside, two major subgroups may be recognized. In congenital analgesia with anhidrosis (Swanson 1963), impairment of pain sensation predisposes to tissue-damaging injury, leading on occasion to loss of fingers (Mazar et al 1976) or severe mutilation of the tongue (Pinsky & DiGeorge 1966). Sweet (1981) reviewed reports of 15 such patients. Typically, pain, and to a lesser extent thermal sensation, are severely defective, while other sensory modalities remain intact. The associated anhidrosis may lead to episodes of hyperpyrexia. Of the 15 patients, only four were of normal intelligence, and these children mutilated themselves less severely. Pathologically, a case coming to autopsy showed evidence of a severe sensory neuropathy with a total absence of small dorsal root ganglion cells, of small fibres in dorsal roots and of Lissauer's tract, together with a reduction in size of the spinal tract of the trigeminal nerve (Swanson et al 1965).

In the second group, an insensitivity to pain is evident in childhood, accompanied by symptoms and signs of a sensory polyneuropathy, but the impairment of pain sensation is out of proportion to impairment of other modalities. 21 such cases were reviewed by Sweet (1981), in which the degree of selectivity of pain sensation impairment was variable. The case reports of a brother and sister aged 6 and $2^1/_2$ years by Haddow et al (1970) exemplify the most extreme form. Both siblings had extensive mutilating lesions of the fingers, and in the 6-year-old a pin was not painful anywhere, while there was a much milder distal loss to other modalities. The pathological peripheral nerve changes in this group range from a complete absence of myelinated fibres to a marked nonselective reduction, with normal unmyelinated fibres (Sweet 1981). It seems likely that some of these cases were examples of dominantly inherited sensory neuropathy, considered below.

Tangier disease

Tangier disease, familial alpha-lipoprotein deficiency, is an extremely rare lipid disorder in which a neuropathy occurs in at least half those affected (Pleasure 1975). The complex biochemistry of this disorder is reviewed by

Pleasure (1975). Two patients with a remarkable dissociated sensory loss of pain and temperature sensation over most of the body have been reported (Kocen et al 1967; Fredrickson et al 1972). Kocen et al (1973) reported the radial nerve biopsy features in one of these. Small myelinated fibres were selectively lost, and unmyelinated fibres were virtually absent.

PAINFUL POLYNEUROPATHIES WITH SELECTIVE LOSS OF LARGE FIBRES

Isoniazid neuropathy

Pain as a feature of polyneuropathies in which a selective large-fibre loss occurs would accord with the predictions of the gate control theory. An example is isoniazid neuropathy, which was first recognized by Pegum (1952); clinical features were described by Gammon et al (1953). Initial symptoms of distal numbness and tingling paraesthesiae are later accompanied by pain, which may be felt as a deep ache or burning. The calf muscles are often painful and tender, and the exacerbation of symptoms produced by walking may prevent the patient from walking. Spontaneous pain and paraesthesiae may be particularly troublesome at night. Examination shows signs of a sensorimotor neuropathy, often confined to the legs. Cutaneous hyperaesthesia is a frequent finding. Ochoa (1970) examined sural nerve biopsies from nine patients, reporting a primary axonal degeneration in myelinated fibres with evidence of degeneration in unmyelinated fibres and regeneration in both types, together with degeneration of regenerated myelinated fibres. Using several ultrastructural criteria Ochoa (1970) was able to distinguish as yet unmyelinated sprouts of myelinated fibres from unmyelinated fibres, and was also able to make an accurate assessment of differential myelinated fibre damage, finding that large fibres were preferentially lost. The relative resistance of unmyelinated fibres to isoniazid was shown by Hopkins & Lambert (1972) who reported preservation of the C-fibre compound action potential in severe experimental isoniazid neuropathy. Prevention and treatment with pyridoxine was described by Biehl & Vilter (1954); the biochemical pathogenesis is discussed by Victor (1975).

Pellagra neuropathy

Peripheral polyneuropahty is one of the many neurological manifestations of pellagra, due to niacin deficiency (Spillane 1947). A predominant feature of the sensorimotor neuropathy is spontaneous pain in the feet and lower legs, with tenderness of the calf muscles and cutaneous hyperaesthesia of the feet (Lewy et al 1940). There are no recent pathological studies of this neuropathy, and no ultrastructural study. Wilson (1913–1914) reported changes suggesting a predominant axonal degeneration and, in a later investigation, Aring et al (1941) observed a decreased density of myelinated fibres, with a preferential loss of larger fibres. In spinal cord, extensive degeneration was found in the dorsal and lateral tracts by Anderson & Spiller (1940) in two patients at autopsy, while others, for example Greenfield & Holmes (1939), observed degeneration mainly in the posterior columns, with less marked changes in the pyramidal tracts. Pellagra neuropathy would thus appear to be a further example of a painful neuropathy in which large fibres are selectively lost. The possibility that regenerated myelinated fibres biased the fibre population studies of Aring et al (1941) is made less likely, but is not excluded, by the overall decrease in fibre density. The spinal cord changes suggest that this is an example of a central–peripheral distal axonopathy.

Hypothyroid neuropathy

Pollard et al (1982) reported the pathological changes in sural nerve biopsies from two patients with untreated hypothyroidism. One presented with a long history of pain in the feet and progressive difficulty in walking, the other with pain and paraesthesiae in the hands. In both there were signs of a sensorimotor neuropathy. The biopsies showed a mainly axonal degeneration with occasional segmental demyelination. In both patients, myelinated fibre densities were decreased with a relative loss of large fibres, but there were regenerating myelinated fibres which may have contributed to the small-fibre bias, though probably not to a significant extent. Unmyelinated fibre densities were increased, due to small-diameter regenerating axons. Dyck & Lambert (1970) also found reduced myelinated fibre densities in two hypothyroid patients, associated with reduced A-alpha and delta potentials in vitro, with normal C-fibre potentials. Teased fibres showed more marked segmental demyelination and remyelination with less axonal degeneration than in the patients of Pollard et al (1982).

PAINLESS POLYNEUROPATHIES WITH SELECTIVE LARGE-FIBRE LOSS

In contrast to the polyneuropathies described above, there are two neuropathies in which a selective loss of large fibres is not generally associated with painful symptoms. These are Friedreich's ataxia and chronic renal failure.

Friedreich's ataxia

The physiological and pathological characteristics of the neuropathy of Friedreich's ataxia were referred to earlier (Dyck et al 1971b). Pain is only an occasional complaint in this condition and is only occasionally severe. Friedreich himself mentioned it, as did Dyck & Ohta

(1975), though others with a large experience of the condition do not report pain as an important feature (Thomas 1974, 1979). It is worth emphasizing that the selective loss of myelinated fibres occurs only in the earlier stages of the disorder, and eventually loss of all fibre sizes occurs (Dyck & Ohta 1975). The pathology is an axonal degeneration with secondary segmental demyelination (Dyck & Lais 1973). Pain might be expected as a regular feature in the earlier stages of Friedreich's ataxia, during the period of selective fibre loss, but this is not the case (Dyck & Ohta 1975).

Chronic renal failure

Chronic renal failure due to any cause may be associated with a neuropathy in which a selective loss of large fibres occurs, but which is rarely painful. A complaint of restless legs is an early symptom, followed by distal numbness and paraesthesiae, with distal weakness usually confined to the legs. The rate of progression and eventual extent of the disability are extremely variable (Asbury et al 1963; Asbury 1975). Thomas et al (1971) noted that painful symptoms were uncommon, though Asbury (1975) reported burning on the soles on the feet in some patients. Extensive pathological studies have been performed in patients coming to autopsy (Marin & Tyler 1961; Asbury et al 1963; Forno & Alston 1967) and showed axonal degeneration in distal parts of the lower limb nerves, with chromatolysis of anterior horn cells and, in one case of Asbury et al (1963) with a neuropathy of long duration, there were myelin degenerative changes in the cervical dorsal columns, suggesting that this may be a central–peripheral distal axonopathy. Demyelination and remyelination in teased fibres have caused some to take the view that the pathology is primarily a segmental demyelination (Dayan et al 1970; Dinn & Crane 1970) but the extensive studies of Thomas et al (1971) and Dyck et al (1971a) leave little doubt that it is a primary axonal degeneration.

Thomas et al (1971) observed a reduced myelinated fibre density in five of six biopsies, with selective loss of larger fibres, without significant numbers of regenerating fibres in teased fibres. This was also found by Dyck et al (1971a), who noted a nonrandom distribution of demyelination on fibres about to degenerate as a result of primary axonal pathology. None of the eight patients in the two investigations had experienced major painful symptoms. Improvement in chronic renal failure neuropathy may occur with dialysis (Thomas et al 1971) and after renal transplantation (Dyck 1982).

PAINFUL POLYNEUROPATHIES WITH SELECTIVE SMALL-FIBRE LOSS

It is perhaps surprising that small fibre neuropathies should be painful, but there are several examples, including some patients with diabetic polyneuropathy, amyloid, Fabry's disease and some hereditary neuropathies.

Diabetes

Diabetes is associated with several types of polyneuropathy of which the commonest is a symmetrical sensory polyneuropathy (Thomas 1973). Numbness and paraesthesiae are common presenting complaints, the paraesthesiae sometimes having a burning quality. In addition, some patients complain of a spontaneous deep, aching pain, and lightning pain may be reported. The prevalence of these severe dysaesthetic symptoms is not known, but in the experience of Thomas & Tomlinson (1993) pain is frequently troublesome, even when sensory and motor deficits are mild. Severe sensory neuropathy in diabetes may lead to painless perforating foot ulcers, and in such patients the upper limbs may also be involved and there may be an associated autonomic neuropathy. The pathology and biochemical factors in the sensory neuropathy due to diabetes are complex controversial topics (Thomas & Tomlinson 1993). As with other neuropathies, uncertainty as to whether the pathology is primarily an axonal degeneration of Schwann cell dysfunction leading to demyelination has been the major issue. Segmental demyelination and remyelination, sometimes leading to onion-bulb formation, has been reported (Thomas & Lascelles 1966; Ballin & Thomas 1968) but axonal loss has also been observed (Greenbaum et al 1964; Thomas & Lascelles 1966). In addition, dorsal root ganglion cell degeneration occurs (Olsson et al 1968), and loss of anterior horn cells has been reported (Greenbaum et al 1964). The characteristic marked slowing of conduction velocity in most cases of diabetic neuropathy (Gilliatt 1965) suggests that demyelination is the usual primary pathology, but it is now recognized that at times extensive demyelination may occur as a result of pathological processes primarily affecting axons (Thomas 1971). Overall, the evidence indicates that demyelination is the predominant pathology in the majority of patients and axonal degeneration in a minority. Earlier suggestions that the neuropathy might result from a diabetic microangiopathy have not been supported by more recent observations (Thomas & Tomlinson 1993), though a vascular pathology in diabetic mononeuropathy is likely.

Brown et al (1976) reported clinical and pathological findings in three patients with severe pain due to diabetic polyneuropathy. Two of the patients had shooting pains in the legs. In all three there was a distal sensory impairment, but tendon reflexes were preserved. Nerve biopsies suggested a predominant axonal degeneration affecting mainly small myelinated and unmyelinated fibres. There were also myelinated fibre sprouts, and their presence in appreciable numbers led Brown et al (1976) to suggest that the pain in these patients might have been due to abnormal impulse generation, as in sprouts forming experimental neuromas (Wall & Gutnick 1974). They also reviewed patients with diabetic polyneuropathy with attention to painfulness in relation to physical signs. Patients without pain tended to have areflexia with distal sensory loss particularly involving joint position sense, while patients with severe burning pain and hyperasthesia tended to have sensory loss with a relative preservation of position sense, intact reflexes, and more often had evidence of an accompanying autonomic neuropathy.

Said et al (1983) reported three patients similar to those of Brown et al (1976), with a striking selective loss of pain and temperature sensation, producing a pseudosyringomyelic picture. However, some of the patients with chronic sensorimotor neuropathy reported by Behse et al (1977) had pain. Nerve biopsies showed a nonselective fibre loss. A similar nonselective fibre loss, but accompanied by evidence of regeneration, characterized the nerve biopsies of the patients with the acute painful neuropathy reported by Archer et al (1983).

Britland et al (1991) report a morphometric study of sural nerve biopsies from six diabetics, four with active acute painful neuropathy and two with recent remission from this type of neuropathy. Myelinated and unmyelinated fibre degeneration and regeneration were present in all the nerves, the only discernible differences between the nerves from patients with and without pain being that those with remission from the pain had a less abnormal axon/Schwann cell calibre ratio, more successful myelinated fibre regeneration and less active myelinated fibre regeneration. However these were all differences in severity, and the authors emphasize the similarity of the pathological changes in the two groups.

Over and above the structural and physiological alterations common to many types of peripheral nerve damage which may lead to pain, two other factors may be of importance in diabetic neuropathy. Hyperglycaemia in diabetics may itself lower pain threshold and tolerance, compared with nondiabetic controls (Morley et al 1984). Further, it has been found in animal experiments that hyperglycaemia reduces the antinociceptive effect of morphine (Simon & Dewey 1981) indicating a possible effect of glucose on opiate receptors. This raises the further possibility that hyperglycaemia might modulate the abnormal properties such as ectopic impulse generation, which develop in damaged nerve.

The other factor is blood flow. Autonomic involvement in diabetic neuropathy increases peripheral blood flow. Archer et al (1984) compared peripheral blood flow and its response to sympathetic stimulation in diabetics with severe nonpainful sensory polyneuropathy, and diabetics with acute severe painful neuropathies of the type described by Archer et al (1983). High flow was present in both groups, but was reduced by sympathetic stimulation only in the group with painful neuropathy, and this reduction was accompanied by an improvement in pain. The explanation of this effect is uncertain; a decrease in temperature may be important. The observations seem to conflict with the experimental observation of an increase in ectopic impulse generation in neuromas produced by sympathetic stimulation (Devor & Janig 1981).

The primary prevention and treatment of diabetic neuropathy is good control of the diabetes (Thomas & Eliasson 1975), though neuropathies have occasionally developed soon after initiation of treatment either with insulin or oral hypoglycaemic drugs (Ellenberg 1958).

Amyloid neuropathy

A second example of a painful small-fibre neuropathy is that caused by amyloid, both the inherited and sporadic varieties (Dyck & Lambert 1969; Dyck et al 1971b; Thomas & King 1974). Patients typically present with a distal sensory loss which initially affects pain and thermal sensations, often with autonomic involvement. As the neuropathy progresses, all modalities are affected, reflexes are lost and there is motor involvement. The physiological and morphological findings of Dyck & Lambert (1969) and Dyck et al (1971b), referred to earlier, showed that small myelinated and unmyelinated fibres are selectively lost, and this was confirmed by Thomas & King (1974). It is thus a surprising but common experience that this type of polyneuropathy is often very painful, the pain usually having a deep aching quality, sometimes with superimposed shooting pains.

Fabry's disease

Fabry's disease, angiokeratoma corpus diffusum, is a rare lipid storage disorder in which a painful peripheral neuropathy is the usual presenting feature. The dermatological manifestation is telangiectasis with proliferation of keratin and epidermal cells (Wise et al 1962) and most tissues, including heart, kidneys and lungs may be involved (Brady & King 1975). There is a deficiency of ceramide trihexosidase in this sex-linked recessive disease, leading to accumulation of ceramide trihexoside in the tissues (Brady et al 1967). Typically, boys or young men present with tenderness of the feet and spontaneous burning pain in the legs, which may be extremely severe (Wise et al 1962), occasionally leading to suicide (Thomas 1974). The accompanying sensorimotor deficit is often mild. A rash is usually present early on, and this should always suggest the diagnosis of Fabry's disease in a young man. Heterozygous carrier females occasionally develop symptoms later in life (Brady & King 1975). The central nervous system is relatively spared, though patients with mental retardation have been reported (Rahman & Lindenberg 1963). Dorsal root ganglion cells are variably affected, but in peripheral nerves there is a selective loss of small myelinated fibres and a decrease in unmyelinated axons, particularly those of larger diameter (Kocen & Thomas 1970; Ohnishi & Dyck 1974). On electron microscopy the accumulated lipid appears as lamellated, often concentric inclusions known as zebra bodies.

Hereditary sensory neuropathy

The last example of a painful small-fibre neuropathy is dominantly inherited sensory neuropathy, in which symptoms develop slowly from the second decade onwards, mainly in the feet. Distal sensory impairment, particularly affecting pain and temperature sensation in the early stages, with little motor involvement and distal autonomic involvement, are the major clinical features. The selective loss of pain sensation may lead to painless penetrating foot ulcers and eventually loss of large parts of the feet (Dyck & Ohta 1975). Severe lancinating pains are well recognized in this condition, and are not related to the severity of rate of progression of the disease. In their combined electrophysiological and morphological study, Dyck et al (1971b) found a preferential reduction in A-delta and C-fibre potentials associated with a selective loss of unmyelinated and small myelinated fibres, though there was also a considerable reduction of larger myelinated fibres. It is interesting to compare this neuropathy with recessively inherited sensory neuropathy, in which touch–pressure sensation is initially preferentially impaired, though in which a painless mutilating acropathy may eventually occur. Pain is not a feature. Recordings in vitro showed absent myelinated fibre potentials with reduced C-fibre potentials, associated with a histological absence of myelinated fibres and reduced numbers of unmyelinated axons (Ohta et al 1973).

PAINFUL POLYNEUROPATHIES WITH NONSELECTIVE FIBRE LOSS

Two commonly painful polyneuropathies are associated with a nonselective fibre loss. These are alcoholic and myeloma neuropathies. They are discussed separately from the miscellaneous group of painful neuropathies that follow, since they have been extensively studied pathologically, particularly with regard to the question of differential fibre involvement.

Alcoholic neuropathy

The incidence of neuropathy in chronic alcoholism is in the region of 9% (Victor & Adams 1953), including asymptomatic patients. Of the symptomatic patients, approximately one-quarter complains of pain or paraesthesiae as the first symptom (Victor 1975). Burning pain and tenderness of the feet and legs are the characteristic complaints, the upper limbs being only rarely involved. Examination reveals a sensorimotor neuropathy, and the occurence of painful symptoms is not related to the severity of the deficit. In a pathological study, Walsh & McLeod (1970) examined sural nerve biopsies from 11 patients who were divided into those with acute and those with chronic neuropathies, and in addition their diet was assessed. Myelinated fibre densities were decreased in all the biopsies. Fibre-size histograms in five biopsies showed reduction of all fibre sizes in three, but in two there was a relative excess of small-diameter fibres. Teased-fibre preparations showed that these were regenerating sprouts. Patients presenting with an acute neuropathy and a poor diet had active axonal degeneration, whereas those with chronic neuropathies and a better diet had less degeneration, and regeneration was present. However, Walsh & McLeod (1970) did not relate this to painfulness in their patients.

In the early stages of alcoholic neuropathy in some patients, clinical evidence of large sensory fibre involvement is slight or even absent, but abnormal thermal thresholds indicate a preferential affection of unmyelinated afferent fibres. This is thus another example of a painful neuropathy with selective small fibre involvement.

Treatment of alcoholic neuropathy consists of stopping drinking and ensuring an adequate diet. An inadequate diet is a major contributory factor to the development of the neuropathy, and there are obvious clinical similarities to the neuropathies caused by specific vitamin deficiencies; pellagra has already been discussed, and some further examples are considered below. The therapeutic effect of thiamine in alcoholic peripheral neuropathy was demonstrated by Victor & Adams (1961). Vicotor (1975) drew attention to the causalgic nature of the pain in alcoholic neuropathy and reported good temporary pain relief with sympathetic blockade.

Myeloma

Both multiple and solitary myeloma may be associated with a peripheral sensorimotor neuropathy (Walsh 1971; Davis & Drachman 1972; McLeod & Walsh 1975). The neuropathy is extremely variable in severity and rate of progression, ranging from a mild, predominantly sensory neuropathy to a complete tetraplegia. Bone pain is of course a common symptom, but in addition pain attribution to the associated neuropathy occurs. In reviewing reported patients, Davis & Drachman (1972) calculated an incidence of painful symptoms of 59% in patients with neuropathy. In five sural nerve biopsies from patients with neuropathies, but without painful symptoms, Walsh (1971) found a loss of myelinated fibres of all sizes, and in teased fibres the appearances suggested a primary axonal degeneration. Unmyelinated axon counts in two patients showed a substantial decrease in numbers, without regeneration. Amyloid has only occasionally been found in nerves of patients with myeloma neuropathy, and is not the cause of the neuropathy (Davies-Jones & Esiri 1971). The neuropathy responds well to myeloma chemotherapy, or radiotherapy for solitary myeloma, and this includes resolution of the painful symptoms.

MISCELLANEOUS PAINFUL NEUROPATHIES

Some further polyneuropathies not included in the above categories and which may be painful are considered here. They have been excluded from the foregoing sections either because of inadequate pathological studies or because the primary demyelinating pathology precludes an accurate assessment of differential fibre loss.

Acute inflammatory polyneuropathy (AIP)

In AIP of the Guillain–Barré type, pain is a common early symptom, often preceding sensory impairment or weakness. It may present in a distal distribution, as generalized muscular pain, or as root pain, which sometimes leads to diagnostic difficulties. It has been suggested by Thomas (1979) that such pain may be due to local inflammation in roots, mediated by the nervi nervorum, rather than neuropathic pain due to the pathological processes involving the root fibres themselves. Pain in AIP may be severe but is usually transient. Persisting pain is more often in a distal distribution. In patients with chronic relapsing and chronic progressive inflammatory polyneuropathy, pain is not usually a prominent symptom. The pathology of AIP is demyelination, usually predominantly affecting the roots, and in the great majority of patients full recovery occurs.

Nutritional neuropathies

In addition to niacin deficiency neuropathy and nutritional factors in the pathogenesis of alcoholic neuropathy already discussed, several other painful neuropathies attributed to specific nutritional deficiencies have been described (reviewed by Victor 1975). Many accounts in the literature provide descriptions of clinical features but lack biochemical or neuropathological investigation. Other problems of aetiological differentiation are that nutritional deficiency of a single vitamin seldom occurs, and that in some cases, for example alcoholic neuropathy, a known neurotoxin is also involved. Three painful polyneuropathies of probable or possible nutritional origin are relevant here, beriberi, Strachan's syndrome (Jamaican neuropathy) and the burning feet syndrome.

Beriberi neuropathy

In beriberi, a painful sensorimotor polyneuropathy is very common. There is spontaneous pain in the feet and sometimes the hands, often with a burning character. The calf muscles may be particularly painful, and although sensory thresholds are raised, skin stimulation may produce extremely unpleasant paraesthesiae. It is likely, though not completely proven, that thiamine deficiency is the cause of this neuropathy and the associated cardiac disorder, and improvement with thiamine is well recorded (Victor 1975). In experimental studies, Swank (1940) showed peripheral nerve degeneration in thiamine-deficient pigeons, and North & Sinclair (1956) and Prineas (1970) in rats. In Swank's (1940) investigation, the large myelinated fibres degenerated before the smaller fibres and the longest fibres were preferentially affected. In man, the reported pathological studies are all in the older literature. In an extensive postmortem study, Pekelharing & Winkler (1889; quoted by Victor 1975) described degenerative changes which were most marked in the distal parts of peripheral nerves, and in the posterior columns and their nuclei. Wright (1901) observed degeneration of dorsal root ganglion cells and anterior horn cells. The animal and human pathology suggest that beriberi neuropathy is primary axonal degeneration of the central peripheral distal type. Reversal of the experimental neuropathy with thiamine was shown by Swank & Prados (1942).

Strachan's syndrome (Jamaican neuropathy)

In 1897, Strachan described 510 cases of a neuropathy observed in Jamaica. Patients presented with pain, paraesthesiae and sensory impairment in the feet and hands, together with pains proximally around the shoulder and hip girdles, visual impairment, deafness and orogenital dermatitis, in some cases resembling the lesions of pellagra. Many of the patients were ataxic, though whether this was peripheral or central in origin is not clear. More recent studies have shown that the neuropathy of Jamaican neuropathy is accompanied by features of spinal cord disease (Montgomery et al 1964) and that a pure peripheral disorder of the type described by Strachan (1897) is not now seen.

There is no evidence that the patients described by Strachan (1897) had a specific nutritional deficiency, though nutritional or toxic factors may have been important in some patients included in this clinically heterogeneous group. Those patients with spinal cord disturbances almost certainly included what is now recognized as tropical spastic paraparesis, due to HTLV1 infection (Gessain & Gout 1992).

Burning feet syndrome

This syndrome was seen in many prisoners of war during the Second World War (Cruickshank 1946; Simpson 1946; Smith & Woodruff 1951). The symptoms were severe aching or causalgic-like burning pains with unpleasant paraesthesiae, starting on the soles of the feet and sometimes spreading up the legs. The symptoms were often worse at night and were relieved by cold. Objective signs of neuropathy were not always present in these patients, some of whom also had amblyopia and orogenital dermatitis (Simpson 1946). Hyperhidrosis of the feet was sometimes a prominent feature. A single nutritional deficiency was not identified in this condition, and most patients responded to an improvement in general diet and vitamin B-rich foods.

In summary, various nutritional deficiency syndromes may involve peripheral nerves, and severe pain is a leading symptom in these neuropathies. Opportunities for further study of these fascinating neuropathies have decreased in recent years, but it is suggested that examination of animal models might be a worthwhile area of pain research.

Arsenic neuropathy

The polyneuropathy caused by arsenic may be painful, though it is as often painless. It is the commonest of the heavy metal neuropathies and presents as a pure sensory or mixed sensorimotor neuropathy (Goldstein et al 1975). Patients may complain of intense pain or painful paraesthesiae of the extremities (the feet more than the hands) with tenderness. Nerve biopsies show axonal degeneration involving fibres of all classes (Goldstein of al 1975).

CENTRAL–PERIPHERAL DISTAL AXONOPATHIES

An advance in the understanding of diseases affecting the primary sensory neuron was the recognition that some pathological processes may have differential effects on the peripheral and central axons. Several references have already been made to the process of dying back or distal axonopathy, and it seems likely that this is a common pattern in peripheral neuropathies in which axonal degeneration is the primary pathology. The process of distal axonopathy is now well established in a number of experimental neuropathies, for example those caused by triortho-cresyl phospate (Cavanagh 1954) and acrylamide (Fullerton & Barnes 1966; Prineas 1969), and the underlying cellular processes involved have been the subject of several investigations (Spencer & Schaumburg 1976; Schoental & Cavanagh 1977). In man, anatomical information concerning the central processes of primary sensory neurons is rather more difficult to obtain than the peripheral processes, but there is now physiological evidence that central processes may be selectively involved in some diseases, for example in subacute myelooptic neuropathy (SMON) due to clioquinol poisoning in Japan, and in pure hereditary spastic paraplegia (Thomas 1982). A more common pattern in distal axonopathies is probably affectation of both central and distal axons, but as pointed out by Thomas (1982), differential recovery of function in peripheral and central axons may occur, as is probably the case in SMON, where there is poor resolution of the painful symptoms after removal of the toxin, and in a patient with vitamin E deficiency, in whom differential electrophysiological recovery was documented by Harding et al (1982). The implications of differential vulnerability and recovery in relation to pain in neuropathies other than SMON are at present not clear.

MONONEUROPATHIES AND MULTIPLE MONONEUROPATHIES

Clinical and pathological observations on mononeuropathies have drawn attention to several potentially important mechanisms underlying the production of painful symptoms, which may also be relevant to pain production in some polyneuropathies. Nerve transection with neuroma formation and other types of nerve trauma are discussed in other chapters, but brief reference is made to entrapment neuropathies. The other mononeuropathies considered here include postherpetic neuralgia, diabetic mononeuropathies, ischaemic neuropathy, neuralgic amyotrophy and carcinomatous neuropathies.

Postherpetic neuralgia (PHN)

Definition and description

PHN is one of the commonest intractable conditions seen in pain clinics. There is no generally agreed definition of PHN. Pain persisting past the stage of healing of the rash, at 1 month after the onset, is the time chosen by many investigators (e.g. Hope-Simpson 1965). However, as PHN tends to diminish in severity with time and may cease to be troublesome many months or even years later (vide infra), most now accept the longer interval of 3 months after the onset of the acute eruption (Watson et al 1988).

It is unusual for shingles to be entirely painless in middle-aged or older people. Preeruptive pain for up to 3 weeks is well described (Juel-Jensen & MacCallum 1972), though pain for more than 2 days before the rash is uncommon. Acute herpetic neuralgia is often severe. There are no features of the pain unique to the acute neuralgia, and it merges into PHN. The pain is most often of two types; an ongoing pain described as burning, raw, severe aching or tearing, and superimposed paroxysmal pains, stabbing or electric shock-like. Both the ongoing and paroxysmal pains may be present throughout the whole of the affected dermatome, but commonly become concentrated particularly in one part of the dermatome, particularly after a period of more than 6 months.

The pain is frequently accompanied by a very unpleasant sensitivity of the skin, which again is often most severe in part of the dermatome. The scars themselves tend to be hypoaesthetic, but elsewhere there is hyperaesthesia, allodynia and sometimes hyperpathia (Watson et al 1988a). Allodynia may take the form of an exacerbation of the underlying ongoing pain, or the evoked dysaesthesiae may be different, often a severe itching sensation. These evoked sensations constitute the most unbearable part of PHN for many patients, usually produced by clothes contact and skin stretching with movement. The patient's emotional state (there is often associated depression), environmental temperature and fatigue may all profoundly affect the severity of the ongoing and evoked pains.

Incidence of PHN

PHN, defined as pain persisting at 1 month, has an incidence of between 9% (Ragozzino et al 1982) and 14.3% (Hope-Simpson 1975). Of these patients, the number with pain at 3 months is between 35 and 55%, and at 1 year is between 22 and 33% (Demoragas & Kierland 1957; Ragozzino et al 1982). Watson et al (1988a) draw attention to an incidence at one year of only 3%, and in a further study of 91 patients with PHN defined as pain persisting at more than 3 months (Watson et al 1988a), found that at a median of 3 years follow-up (range 3 months to 12 years), 52 patients (56%) either had no pain or pain which had decreased to the level of no longer being troublesome. More than half of these 52 patients had had PHN for longer than 1 year at the time of first being seen.

This study underlines the tendency of PHN to gradually improve in many patients even after long periods, an important fact which has often been overlooked in studies of treatment for PHN. It is also of interest that Watson et al (1988a) found that a good or bad outcome did not depend on age, sex, or affected dermatome. In a further study of prognosis of PHN, Watson et al (1991a) in general confirmed these findings, but found that those patients with longer duration PHN at the time of presentation tended to do worse, and some patients were identified whose pain appeared to gradually worsen, despite all attempts at pain relief.

The commonest sites for PHN are the mid-thoracic dermatomes and the ophthalmic division of the trigeminal nerve, but may occur in any dermatome. Women are more often affected than men, in a ratio of approximately 3 to 2 (Hope-Simpson 1975; Watson et al 1988).

Pathology and pathogenesis of pain

There have been few pathological studies in PHN. Head & Campbell (1900) were the first to document the changes in the DRG and sensory roots, but of 21 patients only one was reported to have PHN. Lhermitte & Nicholas (1924) studied a patient with acute zoster myelitis, who had acute haemorrhagic inflammatory in DRG, posterior roots and peripheral nerve, with demyelination and axonal degeneration. Denny-Brown et al (1944) observed similar changes in three patients, with marked lymphocytic infiltration at the sites of inflammation. Noordenbos (1959) found a reduction in the large myelinated fibre population in intercostal nerves. In peripheral nerves of patients biopsied early and late after the acute eruption, Zachs et al (1964) found Wallerian degeneration, followed by marked fibrotic change, leading to severe myelinated fibre depletion with preservation of small myelinated fibres only in some patients. Esiri & Tomlinson (1972) described a patient with myeloma who died in the acute phase of ophthalmic zoster. Skin, nerve and DRG all contained virus particles and the nerve showed severe degenerative changes which were unevenly distributed in nerve fascicles.

In an autopsy study of a 67-year-old man with PHN for 5 years before death in a right T7–8 distribution, Watson et al (1988b) found atrophy of the dorsal horn on the right from T4 to T8 with loss of myelin and axons. Only the T8 DRG and dorsal root were affected by fibrosis and cell loss. Markers of unmyelinated fibres (substance P levels), substantia gelatinosa neurons (opiate receptors), glial cells (glial fibrillary acidic protein) and monoaminergic descending spinal projections (dopamine beta-hydroxylase and serotonin levels) were all normal.

In a further autopsy study, Watson et al (1991b) examined spinal cords, DRG, dorsal roots and peripheral nerves from five patients, three of whom had had severe persistent PHN and two of whom had had no pain. Dorsal horn atrophy was only found in those patients with PHN. Axonal and myelin loss and fibrosis were found in one DRG from all the patients without pain. In all patients the peripheral nerve showed severe loss of myelin and axons. In these nerves, there was a relative loss of larger myelinated fibres. The dorsal roots in all patients with PHN and in one patient without pain showed loss of myelin and axons but in the other pain-free patient the dorsal root was normal. Substance P and CGRP levels were measured in two patients with PHN. Staining was absent in the affected DRG but apparently normal in the dorsal horn. Quantitative study of the unmyelinated fibres was not performed in either study, so the degree to which unmyelinated afferents were affected in patients with PHN remains uncertain. An additional finding of interest in one patient who had had PHN for 22 months prior to death was marked inflammatory change with lymphocytic infiltration bilaterally in the DRG of four adjacent segments and in the respective peripheral nerves, suggesting that an ongoing inflammatory process may result following acute zoster in some patients.

Clearly, further studies of this type are needed, in a larger number of patients, before the interpretation of the findings of Watson et al (1988a, 1988b, 1991a, 1991b) in relation to pain pathogenesis. As yet, the pathological studies have not revealed a specific change present in patients with PHN and absent in patients without pain, which might offer a clue as to the mechanism of pain. Preferential loss of larger myelinated fibres appears to be a feature common to both patients with and without PHN. Watson et al (1991a) speculate whether the persistent inflammation found in one patient at a longer interval after acute zoster might indicate continuing low-grade infection and might be a feature of those patients whose pain gradually worsens.

Prevention

Treatment options for PHN are discussed by Fields (Ch. 51). The important issue of prevention of PHN has received considerable attention. There are obvious difficulties in conducting an adequate trial of any treatment to answer this question, given the low and decreasing incidence of PHN at intervals between 3 and 12 months after the acute eruption. In a trial of 40% idoxuridine in DMSO in a fairly small group of patients, Juel-Jensen et al (1970) showed a reduction in incidence of PHN. However, subsequent widespread use of this treatment has been disappointing. Systemic corticosteroids may be effective, as suggested in two controlled trials (Eaglstein et al 1970; Keczkes & Basheer 1980), and in other studies (Appleman 1955; Elliott 1964). There is a danger of dissemination (Merselis et al 1964), though this may be confined to those patients with underlying malignancy or other serious disease leading to immune suppression. Acyclovir has been advocated as an effective preventive drug but controlled studies have not confirmed earlier hopes that this drug would substantially reduce the incidence of PHN, though some studies have shown shorter periods of acute zoster neuralgia and faster healing of the rash (Esman et al 1982; Bean et al 1982, Balfour et al 1983). Colding (1969) reported that PHN could be reduced by sympathetic blockade, but this was not a controlled study and the finding has not been confirmed by others.

Diabetic mononeuropathy and amyotrophy

Mononeuropathies occur more frequently in diabetes than in the normal population, affecting particularly the motor nerves to the extraocular muscles, but also single peripheral nerves including median, ulnar, peroneal, femoral and lateral cutaneous nerve of the thigh. It is particularly interesting that approximately half the patients with acute lesions of the third, fourth, and sixth cranial nerves have pain, which may precede the ocular palsy by a few days (Zorilla & Kozak 1967). Third nerve palsy is the most common, and is usually pupil-sparing. Pain is felt around or behind the eye and may be severe. Since there are no somatosensory fibres in these nerves, where is the pain arising? Two suggestions have been forwarded: the first is that the lesions involve the nervi nervorum producing pain (Thomas 1974), and the second is that there may be concurrent lesions of the branches of the trigeminal nerve in the cavernous sinus, in support of which Zorilla & Kozak (1967) reported discrete facial sensory impairment in some of their patients. With regard to the acute peripheral nerve lesions, pain is a common symptom, though usually transient. Thomas (1979) reported a diabetic patient with an acute radial nerve palsy which was heralded by severe pain in the upper arm, but there was no pain distally. A fascicular biopsy of the nerve in the upper arm showed only small-diameter regenerating myelinated fibres and the endoneurial vessels showed the changes of diabetic microangiopathy. This case is again suggestive of pain arising as a result of activity in nervi nervorum, also termed nerve trunk pain (Asbury & Fields 1984).

Postmortem studies of the pathology of diabetic mononeuropathy include a patient reported by Dreyfus et al (1957), who died 5 weeks after developing a unilateral third cranial nerve palsy. The nerve was swollen retro-orbitally, with degenerative changes in the central parts of nerve and wallerian degeneration distally. This lesion was considered to have a vascular cause, on the basis of arteriolar changes observed, though no vessel occlusion was seen. Raff et al (1968) reported the presence of punctate lesions in the nerve of a diabetic patient who had developed mononeuritis multiplex in the legs 6 weeks before death, which also suggested a vascular pathology. A particularly interesting patient who died a month after the onset of a third nerve palsy and who had had a contralateral transient third nerve palsy 3 years earlier was studied by Asbury et al (1970). As in the patient of Dreyfus et al (1957), the changes in the acutely affected nerve were maximal in the central parts of the nerve, though they were less severe, consisting mainly of demyelination. The contralateral previously affected nerve was structurally normal.

Diabetic amyotrophy, an asymmetrical motor neuropathy, possibly related in some patients to poor diabetic control, often of acute onset, is frequently associated with pain. Though there is some doubt as to the location of the pathology, there is evidence for motor root and peripheral nerve involvement (Thomas & Tomlinson 1993). The origin of the pain in this variety of multiple mononeuropathy is not clear, but in part may be a further example of pain mediated by nervi nervorum (Thomas 1979).

Entrapment neuropathies

Entrapment neuropathies of sensory or mixed nerves, such as carpal tunnel syndrome, are usually characterized in the early stages by paraesthesiae and pain. Morphologically, entrapment lesions cause damage to myelinated fibres in the first instance (Thomas & Fullerton 1963; Neary et al 1975; Ochoa & Noordenbos 1979), with a near absence of myelinated fibres only in severe lesions, in which there is preservation only of C-fibres. Local pain and tenderness at the site of nerve entrapment in many patients is likely to be nerve trunk pain, mediated by nervi nervorum, as discussed in relation to diabetic mononeuropathy. Paraesthesiae of nonpainful type with entrapment neuropathies presumably reflect activity in damaged myelinated fibres, as demonstrated microneurographically in experimental nerve ischaemia in man by Ochoa & Torebjork (1980).

The explanation of pain in entrapment neuropathies (other than nerve trunk pain) is more difficult. Severe pain, sometimes with a burning quality is frequently a symptom, albeit often in short-lived episodes in electrophysiologically mild carpal tunnel syndrome, in which myelinated fibre conduction is relatively mildly affected and thus it is difficult to imagine that C-fibres are damaged. Whether pain is due to activity in myelinated afferents alone in this situation remains uncertain.

Morton's neuralgia is an example of a frequently histologically severe entrapment neuropathy in which a plantar digital nerve becomes compressed in the region of the metatarsal heads in the foot. In badly affected nerves, many myelinated fibres may be distruped within the region of compression, producing a nerve which is populated almost exclusively by C-fibres. However, explanations of pain pathogenesis based on these findings have to take account of the fact that similar changes are often found in control nerves from subjects who never suffered this type of neuralgia (Scadding & Klenerman 1987).

Ischaemic neuropathy

Polyarteritis nodosa, rheumatoid arthritis and systemic lupus erythematosus may all be associated with painful peripheral mononeuropathies, which probably have a microangiopathic basis (Dyck et al 1972, Conn & Dyck 1975). In a study of nerves involved in rheumatoid arthritis, Dyck et al (1972) found degenerative changes in the central parts of fascicles in nerves from the upper arm and thigh, and postulated that these represented watershed areas in these nerves. The probable ischaemic basis for these changes is supported by the experimental ischaemic peripheral nerve lesions produced by injection of arachidonic acid in rats (Parry & Brown 1982), which produced similar central fascicular degenerative changes, in which small myelinated fibres and unmyelinated fibres were affected to a greater extent than large myelinated fibres. The effects of whole-limb ischaemia on peripheral nerves was shown by Eames & Lange (1967), who found clinical signs of sensory neuropathy in 87.5% of patients undergoing amputation for major vessel atheromatous disease, and observed loss of myelinated fibres with segmental demyelination, remyelination and wallerian degeneration in nerves from these patients. Ischaemia to the nerves of a limb may, of course, be associated with ischaemia to nonneural structures, which may be the source of pain rather than the neuropathic changes.

There is good evidence that ischaemia may precipitate or potentiate painful symptoms in nerves already damaged by other factors. Gilliatt & Wilson (1954) demonstrated an abnormally rapid onset of paraesthesiae with cuff ischaemia in patients with carpal tunnel syndrome, and Harding & LeFanu (1977) reported precipitation of symptoms of carpal tunnel syndrome in patients during haemodialysis with antebrachial arteriovenous fistulae.

Neuralgic amyotrophy

Neuralgic amyotrophy, or cryptogenic brachial plexus neuropathy, is a condition characterized by acute onset of severe pain around the shoulder girdle or in the arm, often in a root distribution, which is followed within 2 weeks by weakness in the limb. This is most frequently distributed around the shoulder girdle and upper limb but may involve distal muscle groups. A minority of patients report a minor, possibly viral, preceding illness (Tsairis et al 1972). The ensuing paralysis is extremely variable in severity and duration, but good recovery is usual within 2 years. Little is known about the pathology of the condition, or even whether the site of the initial lesion is in the roots or more distally in the brachial plexus, though the patchy distribution favours involvement of the plexus and its branches rather than the roots in the majority of patients. The time course of milder lesions suggests demyelination without axonal disruption, whereas that of severe lesions indicates that axonal degeneration probably occurs. There are similarities between neuralgic amyotrophy and the brachial neuritis which occurs in serum sickness. In the latter condition, severe lancinating pain around the shoulder girdle and in the arms is a leading symptom, tending to be more common on the side of handedness, though it may be bilateral (Doyle 1933). Pathological studies are few, but marked swelling of roots has been observed (Roger et al 1934) and it has been suggested that in some patients the swollen roots may become entrapped in the cervical exit foraminae and that this is the cause of the radicular pain (Arnason 1975).

Carcinomatous neuropathies

Neuropathies of various types are well documented as non-metastatic complications of malignant disease, the commonest being a progressive sensory neuropathy which is only occasionally painful (Croft & Wilkinson 1969). However, it was subsequently reported that causalgia may occur as a result of direct invasion of peripheral nerves by carcinoma, responding to sympathectomy (Hupert 1978).

HUMAN MICRONEUROGRAPHY

Single-fibre recordings made by microneurography in nerve damage are still few in number, but have confirmed some of the abnormal properties found in animal experiments. Ochoa et al (1982) recorded mechanical sensitivity in fibres proximal to a peroneal nerve lesion. Similarly, Nordin et al (1984) found ectopic impulse generation provoked by light mechanical stimulation over an ulnar nerve entrapped at the elbow. Perhaps the most interesting observation to date is the ongoing activity and mechanical sensitivity recorded by Nystrom & Hagbarth (1981) proximal to a median nerve neuroma in an amputee with phantom limb pain. Following local anaesthetic blockade of the nerve distal to the recording site, impulses evoked by mechanical stimulation of the neuroma were abolished, but ongoing activity at the recording site continued. It is likely that this residual activity arose from the DRG, as observed experimentally by Wall & Devor (1983). One further microneurographic observation of interest is that neuropathic pain of peripheral nerve origin can be reproduced by intraneural microstimulation of single afferent fibres (Ochoa et al 1985).

SUMMARY OF HUMAN EVIDENCE

As stated earlier, the emphasis of most investigations of human neuropathy has been on morphological correlation of fibre size distribution with nerve conduction and painfulness, but a review of the data shows that there are too many exceptions to a general hypothesis of fibre size imbalance as a cause of pain for it to be tenable. This has been recognized for some time (Thomas 1974; 1979). Dyck et al (1976) reviewed 72 patients who had had nerve biopsies, looking at the type and rate of myelinated fibre degeneration and correlating this with painfulness. There was inevitably bias in the diseases represented in this study, but it was concluded that pain was a feature of those neuropathies in which there was acute axonal degeneration, and this bore no relationship to fibre size distribution. It is interesting to note here that a recent morphological study of an animal model of hyperalgesia due to nerve injury produced by loose ligatures (Bennett & Xie 1988) has revealed very acute degenerative changes in both myelinated and unmyelinated fibres (Basbaum et al 1991).

Overall, the human evidence may be summarized as follows:

1. Pain is not related to fibre size distribution alone, if at all.
2. Those neuropathies in which there is rapid degenerative change are more likely to be painful.
3. Neuropathies involving small fibres, with or without large fibre involvement, are often painful.
4. The coexistence of degenerative and regenerative changes appears to be an important factor (e.g. in some diabetic neuropathies).
5. Some pain may be sympathetic dependent. This evidence derives from studies in traumatic mononeuropathies in man, particularly causalgia (see Ch. 36). The extent to which this is important in polyneuropathies remains uncertain.
6. Ischaemia in nerves may exacerbate paraesthesiae and pain due to peripheral damage, and, in certain circumstances, severe ischaemia is the cause of neuropathies which may be very painful.
7. Nerve trunk pain is a feature of some mononeuropathies, and this mechanism may also be important in certain polyneuropathies.

Evidence from animal experiments

The above conclusions of course leave us far short of an adequate explanation for pain in peripheral neuropathy, and we must turn to animal experiments to provide clues about other mechanisms. This evidence is discussed in detail by Devor (Ch. 4). Following a brief injury discharge in damaged nerve fibres, a chronic afferent barrage of impulses develops. There are sites of ectopic impulse generation both at the point of injury, with or without axonal disruption (demyelination is sufficient to produce this), and proximal to the injury, at the DRG. In addition, an abnormal mechanical sensitivity and noradrenalin sensitivity develop in damaged axons, both of these properties increasing the magnitude of the afferent impulse discharge. Warming tends to increase the A-fibre discharge, while cooling increases the C-fibre discharge. Ephaptic impulse transmission, from motor to sensory axons, develops in a small proportion of fibres, and another type of interaction, crossed after discharge, also develops. The ongoing activity in damaged peripheral nerve (experimental neuromas) is reduced by phenytoin and carbamazepine and by locally applied corticosteroid and glycerol.

Other than in the special case of trigeminal neuralgia in which systemic carbamazepine and local glycerol are often highly effective, the therapeutic actions of the drugs mentioned are usually disappointing in peripheral neuropathic pain, but the experimental observations do provide some evidence for a peripheral action for these agents.

It must be emphasized that central factors are also likely to be of great importance. These include reduced inhibitions and altered sensitivities of dorsal horn cells, and more rostral changes, all of which may occur following peripheral nerve damage (see Ch. 5). The identification of these peripheral and central abnormal physiological and pharmacological properties following peripheral nerve damage has opened up a new range of possible explanations of the mechanisms of peripheral neuropathic pain. However, to what extent each of the experimentally observed properties exists in different neuropathies in man remains uncertain, as do the balance and interactions of the various peripheral and central factors. This continues to be a considerable and crucial gap in our understanding of mechanisms of pain in neuropathy. However, the experimental observations provide a powerful stimulus to the further investigation of human neuropathies. This is a prerequisite to the establishment of rational and specific treatment. Clinicians who regularly deal with patients suffering from pain resulting from peripheral neuropathies are the first to admit the inadequacies and unpredictability of the present range of treatments which can be offered to this unfortunate group of patients.

REFERENCES

Adrian E D 1931 The messages in sensory nerve fibers and their interpretation. Proceedings of the Royal Society of London Series B 109: 1–18

Anderson P V, Spiller W G 1940 Pellagra, with a report of two cases with necropsy. American Journal of the Medical Sciences 141: 307–312

Appleman D H 1955 Treatment if herpes zoster with ACTH. New England Journal of Medicine 253: 693–695

Archer A G, Watkins P J, Thomas P K, Sharma A K, Payan J 1983 The natural history of acute painful neuropathy in diabetes mellitus. Journal of Neurology, Neurosurgery and Psychiatry 46: 491–499

Archer A G, Roberts V C, Watkins P J 1984 Blood flow patterns in painful diabetic neuropathy. Diabetologia 27: 563–567

Aring C D, Bean W B, Roseman E, Rosenbaum M, Spies T D 1941 Peripheral nerves in cases of nutritional deficiency. Archives of Neurology and Psychiatry 45: 772–787

Arnason B G W 1975 Neuropathy of serum sickness. In: Dyck P J, Thomas P K, Lambert E H (eds) Peripheral neuropathy. W B Saunders, Philadephia, p 1104–1109

Asbury A K 1975 Uremic neuropathy. In: Dyck P J, Thomas P K, Lambert E H (eds) Peripheral neuropathy. W B Saunders, Philadelphia, p 982–992

Asbury A K, Fields H L 1984 Pain due to peripheral nerve damage: an hypothesis. Neurology 34: 1587–1590

Asbury A K, Victor M, Adams R D 1963 Uremic polyneuropathy Archives of Neurology 8: 413–428

Asbury A K, Aldredge H, Hershberg R, Fisher C M 1970 Oculomotor palsy in diabetes mellitus: a clinico-pathology study. Brain 93: 555–556

Balfour H, Bean B, Laskin O L et al 1983 Acyclovir halts progression of herpes zoster in immunocompromised patients. New England Journal of Medicine 308: 1453

Ballin R H M, Thomas P K 1968 Hypertropic changes in diabetic neuropathy. Acta Neuropathologica 11: 93–102

Basbaum A I, Gautrum M, Jazat F, Mayes M, Guilbaud G 1991 The spectrum of fiber loss in a model of neuropathic pain in the rat: an electron microscopic study. Pain 47: 357–367

Baxter D W, Olszewski J 1960 Congenital universal insensitivity to pain. Brain 83: 381–393

Bean B, Braun C, Balfour H H 1982 Acyclovir therapy for acute herpes zoster. Lancet ii: 118–121

Behse F, Buchthal F, Carlsen F 1977 Nerve biopsy and conduction studies in diabetic neuropathy. Journal of Neurology, Neurosurgery and Psychiatry 40: 1072–1082

Bennett G J, Xie Y-K 1988 A peripheral mononeuropathy in rat that produces disorders of pain like those seen in man. Pain 33: 87–108

Berthier M, Starkstein S, Leignarda R 1988 Asymbolia for pain: a sensory-limbic disconnection syndrome. Annals of Neurology 24: 41–49

Biehl J P, Vilter R W 1954 The effect of isoniazid on vitamin B6 metabolism, and its possible significance in producing isoniazid neuritis. Proceedings of the Society for Experimental Biology and Medicine 85: 389–392

Brady R O, King F M 1975 Fabry's disease. In: Dyck P J, Thomas P K, Lambert E H (ed) Peripheral neuropathy. W B Saunders, Philadelphia, p 914–927

Brady R O, Gal A E, Bradley R M, Martensson E, Warshaw A L, Laster L 1967 Enzymatic defect in Fabry's disease: ceramidetrihexosidase deficiency. New England Journal of Medicine 276: 1163–1167

Britland S T, Young R J, Sharma A K, Clarke B F 1992 Acute and remitting painful diabetic polyneuropathy: a comparison of peripheral nerve fiber pathology. Pain 48: 361–370

Brown M J, Martin J R, Asbury A K 1976 Painful diabetic neuropathy. A morphometric study. Archives of Neurology 33: 164–171

Buchthal F, Rosenfalck A, Behse F 1975 Sensory potentials of normal and diseased nerves. In: Dyck P J, Thomas P K, Lambert E H (eds) Peripheral neuropathy. W B Saunders, Philadelphia, p 442–464

Burgess P R, Perl E R 1973 Cutaneous mechanoreceptors and nociceptors. In: Iggo A (ed) Handbook of sensory physiology, vol 2. Springer Verlag, Berlin, p 29–78

Cavanagh J B 1954 The toxic effects of tri-ortho-cresyl phosphate on the nervous system. Journal of Neurology, Neurosurgery and Psychiatry 17: 163–172

Clark D, Hughes J, Gasser H S 1935 Afferent function in the group of nerve fibers of the slowest conduction velocity. American Journal of Physiology 114: 69–76

Colding A 1969 The effect of sympathetic blocks on herpes zoster. Acta Anaesthesiologica Scandinavica 13: 113–141

Collins W F, Nulsen F E, Randt C T 1960 Relation of peripheral nerve fiber size and sensation in man. Achives of Neurology 3: 381–397

Conn D L, Dyck P J 1975 Angiopathic neuropathy in connective tissue diseases. In: Dyck P J, Thomas P K, Lambert E H (eds) Peripheral neuropathy. W B Saunders, Philadelphia, p 1149–1165

Croft P B, Wilkinson M 1969 The course and prognosis in some types of carcinomatous neuromyopathy. Brain 92: 1–8

Cruickshank E K 1946 Painful feet in prisoners of war in the Far East. Lancet ii: 369–381

Davies-Jones G A B, Esiri M M 1971 Neuropathy due to amyloid in myelomatosis. British Medical Journal 2: 444

Davis L E Drachman D B 1972 Myeloma neuropathy: successful treatment of two patients and a review of cases. Archives of Neurology 27: 507–511

Dayan A D, Gardner-Thorpe C, Down P F, Gleadle R I 1970 Peripheral neuropathy in uremia. Neurology (Minneapolis) 20: 649–658

Demoragas J M, Kierland R R 1957 The outcome of patients with herpes zoster. Archives of Dermatology 75: 193–196

Denny-Brown D, Adams R D, Fitzgerald P J 1944 Pathologic features of herpes zoster: a note on 'geniculate herpes'. Archives of Neurology and Psychiatry 77: 337–349

Dinn J J, Crane D L 1970 Schwann cell dysfunction in uraemia. Journal of Neurology, Neurosurgery and Psychiatry 33: 605–608

Doyle J B 1933 Neurological complications of serum sickness. American Journal of the Medical Sciences 185: 484–492

Dreyfus P M, Hakim S, Adams R D 1957 Diabetic ophthalmoplegia. Archives of Neurology and Psychiatry 77: 337–347

Dyck P J 1975 Pathologic alterations of the peripheral nervous system of man. In: Dyck P J, Thomas P K, Lambert E H (eds) Peripheral neuropathy. W B Saunders, Philadelphia, p 296–336

Dyck P J 1982 Current concepts in neurology: the causes, classification and treatment of peripheral neuropathy. New England Journal of Medicine 307: 283–285

Dyck P J, Lais A C 1970 Electron microscopy of teased nerve fibers:

method permitting examination of repeating structures of same fiber. Brain Research 23: 418–424

Dyck P J, Lais A C 1973 Evidence for segmental demyelination secondary to axonal degeneration in Friedreich's ataxia. In: Kakulas B A (ed) Clinical studies of myology. Excerpta Medica, Amsterdam, 253–263

Dyck P J, Lambert E H 1969 Dissociated sensation in amyloidosis. Archives of Neurology 20: 490–507

Dyck P J, Lambert E H 1970 Polyneuropathy associated with hypothyroidism. Journal of Neuropathology and Experimental Neurology 29: 631–658

Dyck P J, Ohta M 1975 Neuronal atrophy and degeneration predominantly affecting peripheral sensory neurons. In: Dyck P J, Thomas P K, Lambert (eds) Peripheral neuropathy. W B Saunders, Philadelphia, p 791–824

Dyck P J, Gutrecht J A, Bastron J A, Karnes W E, Dale A J D 1968 Histologic and teased-fiber measurement of sural nerve in disorders of lower motor and primary sensory neurons. Mayo Clinic Proceedings 43: 81–114

Dyck P J, Johnson W J, Lambert E H, O'Brien P C 1971a Segmental demyelination secondary to axonal degeneration in uremic neuropathy. Mayo Clinic proceedings 46: 400–431

Dyck P J, Lambert E H, Nichols P C 1971b Quantitative measurement of sensation related to compound action potential and number and sizes of myelinated and unmyelinated fibers of sural nerve in health, Friedreich's ataxia, hereditary sensory neuropathy and tabes dorsalis. In: Remond A (ed) Handbook of electroencephalography and clinical neurophysiology, vol. 9 Elsevier, Amsterdam, p 83–118

Dyck P J, Conn D L, Okazaki H 1972 Necrotizing angiopathic neuropathy: three-dimensional morphology of fiber degeneration related to sites of occluded vessels. Mayo Clinic Proceedings 47: 461

Dyck P J, Lambert E H, O'Brien P C 1976 Pain in peripheral neuropathy related to rate and kind of fiber degeneration. Neurology 28: 466–471

Eaglstein W H, Katz R, Brown J A 1970 The effects of early corticosteroid theraphy on the skin eruption and pain of herpes zoster. Journal of the American Medical Association 211: 1681–1683

Eames R A, Lange L S 1967 Clinical and pathological study of ischaemic neuropathy. Journal of Neurology, Neurosurgery and Psychiatry 30: 215–226

Ellenberg M 1958 Diabetic neuropathy precipitating after institution of diabetic control. American Journal of the Medical Sciences 238: 418

Elliott F A 1964 Treatment of herpes zoster with high doses of prednisolone. Lancet ii: 610–611

Esiri M M, Tomlinson A H 1972 Herpes zoster. Demonstration of virus in trigeminal nerve and ganglion by immunofluorescene and electron microscopy. Journal of the Neurological Sciences 15: 35–48

Esman V, Ipsen J, Peterslund N A et al 1982 Therapy of acute herpes zoster with acyclovir in the non-immunocompromised host. American Journal of Medicine 73: 320–325

Feindel W 1953 Note on nerve endings in a subject with arthropathy and congenital absence of pain. Journal of Bone and Joint Surgery 35B: 402–407

Forno L, Alston W 1967 Uremic polyneuropathy. Acta Neurologica Scandinavica 43: 640–654

Frederickson D S, Gotto A M, Levy R I 1972 Familial lipoprotein deficiency (abetalipoproteinemia, hypobetalipoproteinemia and Tangier disease). In: Stanbury J B, Wyngaarden J B, Fredrickson D S (eds) The metabolic basis of inherited disease. McGraw-Hill, New York, p 493–530

Fullerton P M, Barnes J M 1966 Peripheral neuropathy in rats produced by acrylamide. British Journal of Industrial Medicine 25: 210–221

Gammon G D, Burge F W, King G 1953 Neural toxicity in tuberculous patients treated with isoniazid (isonicotinic acid hydrazide). Achives of Neurology and Psychiatry 70: 64–69

Gessain A, Gout O 1992 Chronic myelopathy associated with human T-lymphotropic virus type I (HTLV-I). Annals of Internal Medicine 117: 933–946

Gilliatt R W 1965 Clinical aspects of diabetes. In: Cummings J N, Kremer M (eds) Biochemical aspects of neurological disorders, 2nd series. Blackwell, Oxford, p 117–142

Gilliatt R W, Wilson T G 1954 Ischaemic sensory loss in patients with peripheral nerve lesions. Journal of Neurology, Neurosurgery and Psychiatry 17: 104–123

Goldstein N P, McCall J T, Dyck P J 1975 Metal neuropathy. In: Dyck P J, Thomas P K, Lambert E H (eds) Peripheral neuropathy. W B Saunders, Philadelphia, p 1227–1262

Greenbaum D, Richardson P C, Salmon M V, Urich H 1964 Pathological observation on six cases of diabetic neuropathy. Brain 87: 201–214

Greenfield J G, Holmes J M 1939 A case of pellagra: the pathological changes in the spinal cord. British Medical Journal 815–819

Haddow J E, Shapiro S R, Gall D G 1970 Congenital sensory neuropathy in siblings. Pediatrics 45: 651–655

Harding A E, Le Fanu J 1977 Carpal tunnel syndrome related to antebrachial Cimmino-Brescia fistula. Journal of Neurology, Neurosurgery and Psychiatry 40: 511–513

Harding A E, Muller D P R, Thomas P K, Willison H J 1982 Spinocerebellar degeneration secondary to chronic intestinal malabsorption: a vitamin E deficiency syndrome. Annals of Neurology 12: 419–424

Head H, Campbell A W 1900 The pathology of herpes zoster and its bearing on sensory localisation. Brain 23: 353–523

Hope-Simpson R E 1965 The nature of herpes zoster: a long term study and a new hypothesis. Proceedings of the Royal Society of Medicine 58: 9–20

Hope-Simpson R E 1975 Post-herpetic neuralgia. Journal of the Royal College of General Practitioners 25: 571–575

Hopkins A P, Lambert E H 1972 Conduction in unmyelinated fibers in experimental neuropathy. Journal of Neurology, Neurosurgery and Psychiatry 35: `63–`69

Hupert C 1978 Recognition and treatment of causalgic pain occurring in cancer patients. Pain Abstracts 1:47

Iggo A 1977 Cutaneous and subcutaneous sense organs. British Medical Bulletin 33: 97–102

Juel-Jensen B E, MacCallum F O, MacKenzie A M R, Pike M C 1970 Treatment of zoster with idoxuridine in dimethyl sulphoxide. Results of two double blind controlled trials. British Medical Journal iv: 776–780

Juel-Jensen B E, MacCallum F O 1972 Herpes simplex varicella and zoster. J B Lippincott, Philadelphia

Keczkes K, Basheer A M 1980 Do corticosteroids prevent post-herpetic neuralgia? British Journal of Dermatology 102: 551–555

Kocen R S, Thomas P K 1970 Peripheral nerve involvement in Fabry's disease. Archives of Neurology 22: 81–87

Kocen R S, Lloyd J J, Lascelles P T, Fosbrooke A S, Williams D 1967 Familial alpha-lipoprotein deficiency (Tangier disease) with neurological abnormalities. Lancet i: 1341–1345

Kocen R S, King R H M, Thomas P K, Haas L F 1973 Nerve biopsy findings in two cases of Tangier disease. Acta Neuropathologica 26: 317–327

Lambert E H, Dyck P J 1975 Compound action potentials of sural nerve in vitro in peripheral neuropathy. In: Dyck P J, Thomas P K, Lambert E H (eds) Peripheral neuropathy. W B Saunders, Philadelphia, p 427–441

Lewis T, Pickering G W, Rothschild P 1931 Centripetal paralysis arising out of arrest block flow to the limb, including notes on a form of tingling. Heart 16: 1–32

Lewy F H, Spies T D, Aring C D 1940 Incidence of neuropathy in pellagra; effect of cocarboxylase upon its neurologic signs. American Journal of the Neurological Sciences 199: 840–849

Lhermitte J, Nicholas M 1924 Les lesions spinales du zona. La myelite zosterienne. Revue Neurologique 1: 361–364

Lindblom U 1979 Sensory abnormalities in neuralgia. In: Bonica J J, Liebeskind J C, Albe-Fessard D G (eds) Advances in pain research and therapy 3. Raven Press, New York, p 11–120

Lourie H, King R B 1966 Sensory and neurohistological correlates of cutaneous hyperopathia. Archives of Neurology 14: 313–320

Lynn B 1975 Somatosensory receptors and their CNS connections. Annual Review of Psysiology 37: 105–127

McLeod J G, Walsh J C 1975 Neuropathies associated with paraproteinaemias and dysproteinaemias. In: Dyck P J, Thomas P K, Lambert E H (eds) Peripheral neuropathy. W B Saunders, Philadelphia, p 1012–1029

Marin O S M, Tyler H R 1961 Hereditary interstitial nephritis associated with polyneuropathy. Neurology 111: 999–1005

Mazar A, Herold H Z, Vardy P A 1976 Congenital sensory neuropathy with anhidrosis. Orthopaedic complications and management. Clinical Orthopaedic 118: 184–187

Melzack R, Wall P D 1965 Pain mechanisms: a new theory. Science 150: 971–979

Merselis J G, Kaye D, Hook E W 1964 Disseminated herpes zoster. Archives of Internal Medicine 113: 679–686

Montgomery R D, Cruickshank E K, Robertson W B, McMenemey W H 1964 Clinical and pathological observations on Jamaican neuropathy– a report on 206 cases. Brain 87: 425–462

Morley G K, Mooradian A D, Levine A L, Morley J E 1984 Mechanisms of pain in diabetic peripheral neuropathy: effect of glucose on pain perception in humans. American Journal of Medicine 77: 79

Morris J H, Hudson A R, Weddell G 1972 A study of degeneration and regeneration in the divided rat sciatic nerve based on electron microscopy. Zeitschrift für Zellforschung und Mikroskopische Anatomie 124: 76–203

Neary D, Ochoa J, Gilliatt R W 1975 Sub-clinical entrapment neuropathy in man. Journal of the Neurological Sciences 24: 283–298

Noordenbos W 1959 Pain. Elsevier, Amsterdam

Noordenbos W 1979 Sensory findings in painful traumatic nerve lesions. In: Bonica J J, Liebeskind J C, Albe-Fessard D G (eds) Advances in pain research and therapy 3. Raven Press, New York, p 91–102

Nordin M, Nystrom B, Wallin U et al 1984 Ectopic sensory discharges and paraesthesiae in patients with disorders of peripheral nerves, dorsal roots and dorsal columns. Pain 20: 231–245

North J D K, Sinclair H M 1956 Nutritional neuropathy: chronic thiamine deficiency in the rat. Archives of Pathology 62: 341–353

Nystrom B, Hagbarth K-E 1981 Microelectrode recordings from transected nerves in amputees with phantom limb pain. Neuroscience Letters 27: 211–216

Ochoa J 1970 Isoniazid neuropathy in man. Brain 93: 831–850

Ochoa J 1978 Recognition of unmyelinated fiber disease: morphologic criteria. Muscle and Nerve 1: 375–387

Ochoa J, Noordenbos W 1979 Pathology and disordered sensation in local nerve lesions: an attempt at correlation. In: Bonica J et al (eds) Advances in pain research and therapy, Vol 3. Raven Press, New York

Ochoa J, Torebjörk H E 1980 Paraesthesiae from ectopic impulse generation in human sensory nerves. Brain 103: 835

Ochoa J L, Torebjörk H E, Culp W L et al 1982 Abnormal spontaneous activity in single sensory nerve fibers in humans. Muscle and Nerve 5: 574–577

Ochoa J L, Torebjörk H E, Marchettini P et al 1985 Mechanisms of neuropathic pain: cumulative observations, new experiments and further speculation. In: Fields H L, Dubner R, Cervero F (eds) Advances in pain research and therapy, vol 9. Proceedings of the Fourth World Congress on Pain. Raven Press, New York, p 431–450

Ogden T E, Robert F, Carmichael E A 1959 Some sensory syndromes in children: indifference to pain and sensory neuropathy. Journal of Neurology, Neurosurgery and Psychiatry 22: 267–276

Ohnishi A, Dyck P J 1974 Loss of small peripheral sensory neurons in Fabry's disease. Archives of Neurology 31: 120–127

Ohta M, Ellefson R D, Lambert E H, Dyck P J 1973 Hereditary sensory neuropathy, type II: clinical, electrophysiologic, histologic, and biochemical studies in a Quebec kinship. Archives of Neurology 29: 23–37

Olsson Y, Save-Soderbergh J, Sourander P, Angervaall L 1968 A pathoanatomical study of the central and peripheral nervous system in diabetes of early onset and long duration. Pathologia Europaea 3: 62–79

Parry G J, Brown M J 1982 Selective fiber vulnerability in acute ischaemic neuropathy. Annals of Neurology 11: 147–154

Pegum J S 1952 Nicotinic acid and burning feet. Lancet ii: 536

Pinsky L, Di George A M 1966 Congenital familial sensory neuropathy with anhidrosis. Journal of Pediatrics 68: 1–13

Pleasure D E 1975 Abetalipoproteinaemia and Tangier disease. In Dyck P J, Thomas P K, Lambert E H (eds) Peripheral neuropathy. W B Saunders, Philadelphia, p 928–941

Pollard J D, McLeod J G, Honnibal T G A, Verheijden M A 1982 Hypothyroid polyneuropathy. Clinical, electrophysiological and nerve biopsy findings in two cases. Journal of Neurological Sciences 53: 461–471

Prineas J 1969 The pathogenesis study of experimental triortho-cresyl phosphate intoxication in the cat. Journal of Neuropathology and Experimental Neurology 28: 571–597

Prineas J 1970 Peripheral nerve changes in thiamine-deficient rats. Archives of Neurology 23: 541–548

Raff M C, Sangaland V, Asbury A K 1968 Ischaemic mononeuropathy multiplex associated with diabetes mellitus. Archives of Neurology 18: 487

Ragozzino M W, Melton L J, Kurland L T et al 1982 Population based study of herpes zoster and its sequelae. Medicine 21: 310–316

Rahman A N, Lindenberg R 1963 Neuropathology of hereditary dystrophic lipidosis. Archives of Neurology 9: 373–385

Roger H, Poursines Y, Recordier M 1934 Polynevrite apres serotherapie antitetanique curative, avec participation du nevraxe et des meninges (observation anatomoclinique). Revue Neurologique 1: 1078–1088

Said G, Slama G, Selva J 1983 Progressive centripetal degeneration of axons in small fiber diabetic polyneuropathy. A clinical and pathological study. Brain 106: 791–807

Scadding J W, Klenerman L E 1987 Light and electron microscopic observations in Morton's neuralgia. Pain (suppl 4) 5: 246

Schilder P, Schmidt B J, Leon L 1931 Asymbolia for pain. Archives of Neurology and Psychiatry 25: 598–600

Schoental R, Cavanagh J B 1977 Mechanisms involved in the dying-back process – an hypothesis implicating coenzymes. Neuropathology and Applied Neurobiology 3: 145–158

Schroder J M 1975 Degeneration and regeneration of myelinated nerve fibers in experimental neuropathies. In: Dyck P J, Thomas P K, Lambert E H (eds) Peripheral neuropathy. W B Saunders, Philadelphia, p 337–362

Simon G S, Dewey W L 1981 Narcotics and diabetes. The effect of streptozotocin-induced diabetes on the antinociceptive potency of morphine. Journal of Pharmacology and Experimental Therapeutics 218: 318–323

Simpson J 1946 'Burning feet' in British prisoners of war in the Far East. Lancet i: 959–961

Smith D A, Woodruff M F 1951 Deficiency diseases in Japanese prison camps. Medical Research Council, Special Report Series 274 HMSO, London

Spencer P S, Schanmburg H H 1976 Central peripheral distal axonopathy – the pathology of dying back polyneuropathies. Progress in Neuropathology 3: 253–295

Spencer P S, Thomas P K 1970 The examination of isolated nerve fibers by light and electron microscopy with observations on demyelination proximal to neuromas. Acta Neuropathologica 16: 177–186

Spillane J D 1947 Nutritional disorders of the nervous system. Williams & Wilkins, Baltimore

Stevens J C, Lofren E P, Dyck P J 1975 Biopsy of peripheral nerves. In: Dyck P J, Thomas P K, Lambert E H (eds) Peripheral neuropathy. W B Saunders, Philadelphia, p 410–426

Strachan H 1897 On a form of multiple neuritis prevalent in the West Indies. Practitioner 59: 477–484

Swank R L 1940 Avian thiamine deficiency. Journal of Experimental Medicine 71: 683–702

Swank R L, Prados M 1942 Avian thiamine deficiency. II. Pathologic changes in the brain and cranial nerves (especially vestibular) and their relation to the clinical behaviour. Archives of Neurology and Psychiatry 47: 97–131

Swanson A G 1963 Congenital insensitivity to pain with anhidrosis. Archives of Neurology 8: 299–306

Swanson A G, Buchan G C, Alvord E C 1965 Anatomic changes in congenital insensitivity to pain. Archives of Neurology 12: 12–18

Sweet W H 1981 Animal models of chronic pain: their possible validation from human experience with posterior rhizotomy and congenital analgesia. Pain 10: 275–295

Thomas P K 1970 The quantitation of nerve biopsy findings. Journal of the Neurological Sciences 11: 285–295

Thomas P K 1971 Morphological basis for alterations in nerve conduction in peripheral neuropathy. Proceedings of the Royal Society of Medicine 64: 295–298

Thomas P K 1973 Metabolic neuropathy. Journal of the Royal College of Physicians, London 7: 154–160

Thomas P K 1974 The anatomical substratum of pain. Canadian Journal of Neurological Science 1: 92

Thomas P K 1975 Clinical features and differential diagnosis. In: Dyck P J, Thomas P K, Lambert E H (eds) Peripheral neuropathy. W B Saunders, Philadelphia, p 495–512

Thomas P K 1979 Painful neuropathies. In: Bonica J, Liebeskind J C, Albe-Fessard D G (eds) Advances in pain research and therapy 3. Raven Press, New York, p 103–110

Thomas P K 1982 The selective vulnerability of the centrifugal and centripetal axons of primary sensory neurons. Muscle and Nerve 5: S 117–121

Thomas P K, Fullerton P M 1963 Nerve fiber size in the carpal tunnel syndrome. Journal of Neurology, Neurosurgery and Psychiatry 26: 520–527

Thomas P K, King R H M 1974 Peripheral nerve changes in amyloid neuropathy. Brain 97: 395–406

Thomas P K, Lascelles R G 1966 The pathology of diabetic neuropathy. Quarterly Journal of Medicine 35: 489–509

Thomas P K, Tomlinson D R 1993 Diabetic and hypoglycaemic neuropathy. In: Dyck P J, Thomas P K, Griffin J W, Low P A, Poduslo J F (eds) Peripheral neuropathy, 3rd edn. W B Saunders, Philadelphia, p 1219–1250

Thomas P K, Hollinrake K, Lascelles R G et al 1971 The polyneuropathy of chronic renal failure. Brain 94: 761–780

Tsairis P, Dyck P J, Mulder D W 1972 Natural history of brachial plexus neuropathy: report on 99 patients. Archives of Neurology 27: 109–117

Vallbo A B, Hagbarth K E, Torebjörk H E, Wallin B G 1979 Somatosensory, proprioceptive and sympathetic activity in human peripheral nerves. Physiological Reviews 59: 919–957

Victor M 1975 Polyneuropathy due to nutritional deficiency and alcoholism. In: Dyck P J, Thomas P K, Lambert E H (eds) Peripheral neuropathy. W B Saunders, Philadelphia, p 1030–1066

Victor M, Adams R D 1953 The effect of alcohol on the nervous system. Research Publications – Association for Research in Nervous and Mental Disease 32: 526–573

Victor M, Adams R D 1961 On the aetiology of the alcoholic neurologic diseases. With special reference to the role of nutrition. American Journal of Clinical Nutrition 9: 379–397

Wall P D, Devor M 1983 Sensory afferent impulses originate from dorsal root ganglia as well as from the periphery in normal and nerve injured rats. Pain 17: 321–339

Wall P D, Gutnick M 1974 Ongoing activity in peripheral nerves: the physiology and pharmacology of impulses originating from a neuroma. Experimental Neurology 43: 580–593

Walsh J C 1971 The neuropathy of multiple myeloma. Archives of Neurology 25: 404–414

Walsh J C, McLeod J G 1970 Alcoholic neuropathy. An electrophysiological and histological study. Journal of the Neurological Sciences 10: 457–469

Watson C P N, Evans R J 1986 Post-herpetic neuralgia: a review Archives of Neurology 43: 836–840

Watson C P N, Evans R J, Watt V R, Birkett N 1988a Post-herpetic neuralgia: 208 cases. Pain 35: 289–297

Watson C P N, Morshead C, Van der Koog D, Deck J H, Evans R J 1988b Post-herpetic neuralgia: post-mortem analysis of a case. Pain 34: 129–138

Watson C P N, Watt V R Chipman M, Birkett N, Evans R J 1991a The prognosis with post-hepertic neuralgia Pain 46: 195–199

Watson C P N, Deck J H, Morshead C, Van der Koog D, Evans R J 1991b Post-herpetic neuralgia: further post-mortem studies of cases with and without pain. Pain 44: 105–117

Weddell G, Sinclair D C, Feindel W H 1948 An anatomical basis for alterations in quality of pain sensibility. Journal of Neurophysiology 11: 99–109

Wilson S A K 1913–1914 The pathology of pellagra. Proceedings of the Royal Society of Medicine 7: 31–41

Winklemann R K, Lambert E H, Hayles A B 1962 Congenital absence of pain. Archives of Dermatology 85: 325–339

Wise D, Wallace H J, Jellinek E H 1962 Angiokeratoma corporis diffusum. Quarterly Journal of Medicine 31: 177–206

Wortis H, Stein M H, Jolliffe M 1942 Fibre dissociation in peripheral neuropathy. Archives of Internal Medicine 69: 222–237

Wright H 1901 Changes in the neuronal centres in beri-beric neuritis. British Medical Journal i: 1610–1616

Yaksh T L, Hammond D L 1982 Peripheral and central substrates involved in the rostrad transmission of nociceptive information. Pain 13: 1–86

Zacks S I, Langfit T W, Elliot F A 1964 Herpetic neuritis: a light and electron in microscopic study. Neurology 14: 644–750

Zorilla E, Kozak G P 1967 Ophthalmoplegia in diabetes mellitus Annals of Internal Medicine 67: 968–976

38. Clinical manifestations of reflex sympathetic dystrophy and sympathetically maintained pain

Helmut Blumberg and Wilfrid Jänig

INTRODUCTION

The involvement of the sympathetic nervous system in the generation of pain and associated phenomena has puzzled clinicians since the turn of the century. It has become an intense focus of interest in basic and clinical research in the last ten years (see Jänig 1985; Stanton-Hicks 1990; Devor et al 1991; Jänig & Schmidt 1992). Tissue damage at the extremities with and without obvious nerve lesions is sometimes followed by diffuse burning pain and hyperalgesia which can be relieved by blockade of the (efferent) sympathetic activity to the affected extremity. Spontaneous pain and hyperalgesia may be associated with changes of blood flow and sweating, changes of active and passive movements, including increase in physiological tremor, and trophic changes in skin and subcutaneous tissues. Also, these changes are thought to be, directly or indirectly, associated with the sympathetic nervous system and may be alleviated, some with time, by blockade of the sympathetic activity (Bonica 1979, 1990). Pain syndromes of this type are called 'reflex sympathetic dystrophy' (RSD) and 'sympathetically maintained pain' (SMP). These terms were introduced by Evans (1946) and Roberts (1986), respectively.

The general problem is that no consensus exists about the clinical criteria leading to a reliable diagnosis of RSD and SMP. This is probably related, first, to the lack of systematic quantitative investigations of patients with pain in which the sympathetic nervous system is involved and, secondly, the belief that changes of blood flow, trophic changes and oedema (swelling), which are observed in patients with RSD/SMP are associated with abnormal sympathetic activity to the affected extremity and that these changes are causally related to the pain. However, most of the observed changes, including the pain, can also occur independently of the sympathetic innervation in patients who do not have RSD or SMP, and most of these changes, although correlated with the pain, may not be causally connected with the pain. Thus, any of these changes alone do not allow the diagnosis of RSD and SMP.

In this chapter we will first describe the clinical phenomenology of RSD and SMP in patients following trauma at one of the extremities, with and without nerve lesions, and then discuss briefly the pathophysiological mechanisms which may operate in these two groups of patients.

DEFINITION AND PATIENTS

DEFINITION

Recently, a consensus statement and general recommendations for diagnosis and clinical research on RSD were published (Jänig et al 1991). In this statement the following operational definition of RSD using clinical criteria was given: 'RSD is a descriptive term meaning a complex disorder or group of disorders that may develop as a consequence of trauma affecting the limbs, with or without obvious nerve lesion. RSD may also develop after visceral diseases, and central nervous system lesions or, rarely, without an obvious antecedent event. It consists of pain and related sensory abnormalities, abnormal blood flow and sweating, abnormalities in the motor system and changes in structure of both superficial and deep tissues ('trophic' changes). It is not necessary that all components are present. It is agreed that the name 'reflex sympathetic dystrophy' is used in a descriptive sense and does not imply specific underlying mechanisms'. This definition is compatible with the usage of the term as described by Bonica (1990) and others, but avoids indicating mechanisms. The description of the clinical phenomenology of RSD and SMP in the present article was made using the guidelines given in the consensus statement. The patients were primarily separated into those having RSD and those having SMP in terms of the clinical phenomenology.

PATIENTS

The description of the clinical phenomenologies is based on 203 patients (136 upper extremity, 67 lower extremity) who were investigated from 1990–92 in Freiburg by one of the authors (H.B.) and his coworkers (H. J. Griesser, U. Hoffmann, M. Hornyak). 190 patients were given the diagnosis of RSD, and eight patients the diagnosis of SMP. Five patients had both, RSD and SMP.

In 63 RSD patients (53 with spontaneous pain, 10 without) sympathetic blocks with intravenous regional guanethidine or local anaesthetics applied to paravertebral ganglia were used for diagnostic and therapeutic reasons. In the 53 patients with spontaneous pain (mean duration of RSD: 4.9 months, range: 3 days to 30 months), a diagnostic sympathetic block was performed prior to the treatment. In 51 patients the pain was either abolished (n = 47) or was markedly diminished (n = 4) directly after the block. In two patients the pain was not influenced by the block.

The treatment consisted of one (nine patients), two (11 patients) or up to 20 blocks (mean number of blocks: 4.3) over 1 day to 3 months, and was systematically documented. In 42 (82%) of the 51 patients the pain had disappeared at the end of the sympatholytic therapy, in nine patients no relief or only partial relief of pain was obtained. In the 10 patients without spontaneous pain this treatment decreased or abolished swelling and improved motor functions.

21 RSD patients with spontaneous pain, who were successfully treated with sympathetic blocks, were followed up in a clinical study over 3–18 months (mean duration of follow up: 7.7 months). Pain did not return in 18 (86%) of these patients and recurred in the other three cases.

The therapy of the other 127 RSD patients was not under the control of one of us (H.B.). These patients were treated by physiotherapy alone, or by sympathetic blocks, or else they underwent spontaneous remissions. They expressed the same clinical symptoms as did those who were treated by the controlled sympathetic blocks. In all SMP patients and all cases with combined RSD/SMP the pain was temporarily or permanently relieved by sympathetic blocks.

CLINICAL PHENOMENOLOGY OF RSD

The clinical picture of RSD is characterized by a triad of autonomic (sympathetic), motor and sensory symptoms (Blumberg 1991; Blumberg et al 1993a). These symptoms develop in the distal region of the affected extremity following a noxious event, irrespective of its type and location. They are not confined to the innervation zone of an individual nerve and show a distally generalized (quasi-polyneuropathic) distribution. They are present in tissues that are not directly affected by the preceding lesion, and the injured area itself may eventually not show any symptoms at all. The latter is most obvious in patients who develop RSD following a proximal minor lesion. Thus, there is not necessarily a spatial relationship between the site of a lesion and the occurrence of RSD symptoms.

NEUROLOGICAL FINDINGS AND THEIR EVALUATION

The procedure for the clinical investigation of RSD patients is described in detail by Blumberg (1991). The incidence of symptoms is listed in Table 38.1, separated for RSD diagnosed in the first 10 days after its onset and for RSD diagnosed later. Only patients (n = 181) with generalized symptoms are included in Table 38.1; in 121 patients the upper extremity was affected, in 60 the lower extremity was affected. Symptoms generated directly by the noxious event (e.g. neurological deficits in the zone of the lesioned nerve) are not listed.

Somatosensory functions in particular pain

Spontaneous pain is a prominent feature in 75% of the patients with RSD and absent in about 25% (see Table 38.1). The quality of the spontaneous pain varies and may be throbbing, pressing, burning, shooting or aching. In nearly all cases the pain is felt deeply inside the distal part of the affected extremity. It shows a diffuse distribution and is unrelated to the territories of individual nerves. The pain is more severe during the night, and it usually decreases when the extremity is elevated and increases when it is lowered (orthostatic component, see below).

Various kinds of evoked abnormal sensations are found in RSD (see Table 38.1). In the skin, these are mechanical hyperalgesia and hypoalgesia as well as mechanical hyperaesthesia and hypoaesthesia. Usually, these are more pronounced on the palmar/plantar side than on the dorsal

Table 38.1 Type and incidence of RSD symptoms with respect to duration of RSD (m = months)

	RSD duration	
	≤10 days (n = 24)	6.3±16m (n = 157)
Autonomic symptoms		
Distally generalized swelling	96%	96%
Warm/cold affected extremity	54/21%	61/18%
Hypohydrosis/hyperhydrosis	17/25%	55/22%
Motor symptoms		
Active movement reduced	88%	80%
Muscular strength diminished	92%	89%
Tremor (postural/action)	33%	47%
Sensory symptoms		
Deep spontaneous pain	75%	75%
Hypoalgesia/hyperalgesia	58/29%	35/41%
Hypoaesthesia/hyperaesthesia	79/04%	56/15%
Movement-related pain	33%	65%
Mechanical allodynia	0%	8%

side of the hand/foot. In about 60% of the cases pain is elicited by movements at one or more finger/hand or toe/foot joints, even when these are not affected by the preceding lesion. In severe cases, this may lead to a 'pseudoarthritic' condition. Mechanical allodynia was observed in only about 8% of the patients, showing a diffuse distribution with no spatial relationship to individual nerve territories and to the site of the preceding lesion (in contrast to allodynia in SMP, see below). Hyperpathia (pain elicited by painful stimuli that appears with a delay, outlasts the stimulus and spreads beyond the site of the stimulus) was absent in our sample of patients. However, in the literature both symptoms are reported to be a common finding in patients with RSD (see Bonica 1990).

Autonomic (sympathetic) functions

Skin blood flow is abnormal in most cases of RSD: the skin is often marbled/reddish or cyanotic. The skin temperature, measured with an infrared thermometer (Blumberg 1991), on the palmar or plantar side of the ipsi- and contralateral finger or toe tips, respectively, shows in about 80% of the patients a systematic side difference, i.e. all fingers or toes of the affected extremity being either warmer or colder when compared with the corresponding contralateral fingers or toes (see Table 38.1). The mean side difference of skin temperature in these patients is 2.46 ± 1.9°C (mean ± 1 SD, n = 141). Some 22% of the controls also exhibit a systematic side difference in skin temperature of 1.62 ± 1.32°C (mean ± 1 SD, n = 20). The sweating is also disturbed in many patients with RSD, whereby preferentially the palmar or plantar side is either hypo- or hyperhydrotic (see Table 38.1). Oedema (swelling) is a major symptom of RSD (see Table 38.1) Since it can be treated by sympathetic blocks it is considered to be a sign of a disturbed sympathetic function. Oedema occurs predominantely on the dorsal side of the hand/fingers or the foot. In cases with severe swelling it is often combined with shiny skin. Slight swelling is indicated by a loss of skin folds.

Skeletomotor functions

In most cases of RSD, muscular strength is reduced (paresis) or even absent (plegia); this often involves all muscles of the affected distal extremity (see Table 38.1), especially those exerting the strength of the hand grip (Kozin et al 1976). Active movements of the affected distal extremity are considerably reduced, in particular the ability to close the fist and to oppose the tips of thumb and fifth finger. Furthemore, in about half of the patients with an affected upper extremity, tremor (postural or action) is present (see Table 38.1). The postural tremor is an increased physiological tremor (Deuschl et al 1991). These motor disturbances, in particular the tremor, are more obvious and severe at the upper extremity than at the lower extremity. Rare cases with longstanding RSD may develop dystonia at the affected extremity (Jancovic & van der Linden 1988; Schwartzmann & Kerrigan 1990).

Trophic changes and changes in bone

In 29% of the RSD patients, trophic changes (e.g. disturbed nail growth, increased hair growth and palmar/plantar fibrosis, thin glossy skin and hyperkeratosis) are present. None of these changes was observed during the first 10 days after the onset of RSD. This also applies to the diffuse distal osteoporosis in RSD. Thus, trophic changes and osteoporosis cannot be used for early diagnosis of RSD. Whether the passive movement restrictions (stiff joints) are related to the trophic changes of joints and tendons, which are seen in cases with longstanding RSD, or to functional motor disturbances (e.g. flexor–extensor co-contractions), or to both, remains to be clarified.

MANIFESTATION OF RSD SYMPTOMS

Location of symptoms

Usually only one extremity is affected by the RSD syndrome; the relationship between affected upper and lower extremities is about 2:1. Rarely, both sides exibit symptoms of RSD (one of our cases), and, very rarely, all four extremities exhibit these symptoms (Bentley & Hameroff 1980). The distal part of an extremity is predominantly affected. There, in 96% of the patients, the symptoms show a generalized (quasipolyneuropathic) distribution with no relation to the territories of individual nerves. In 5% of the patients the symptoms of RSD are localized (Blumberg et al 1993a, 1993c). Rarely, RSD may also be present in more proximal regions, such as lower leg, knee, hip or shoulder, and in extreme cases of RSD the entire extremity may become symptomatic.

For further differentiation (see below), RSD symptoms can be divided into superficial (e.g swelling, disturbed skin blood flow, changes of skin aesthesia/algesia) and deep symptoms (e.g. deep spontaneous pain, joint pain, reduced muscular strength, osteoporosis).

Combination and variability of symptoms

The clinical picture of RSD is characterized by a combination of autonomic, motor and sensory symptoms. Such a triad is present in 91% of our sample of RSD patients. In the other cases, symptoms of only two parts of the triad are present. In each part of the triad the combination of symptoms varies from patient to patient. For example, swelling might be combined with normal skin temperature and normal sweating, normal movement ability with tremor and paresis, or absence of spontaneous or movement-related pain with cutaneous hypoaesthesia/ hypoalgesia.

The expression of RSD symptoms may vary considerably from mild to severe. In most cases, superficial and deep symptoms of RSD are about equally represented, but in some cases severe superficial symptoms (e.g. marked swelling, large differences of skin temperature, profound numbness) may be combined with less prominent deep symptoms (e.g. no spontaneous pain, no osteoporosis, little paresis) or vice versa. Thus, RSD may preferentially be expressed in the deep or the superficial somatic domain. On the other hand, patients may predominantly exhibit autonomic, motor or sensory symptoms.

The expression of symptoms, in particular those associated with the sympathetic nervous system, may also spontaneously vary in the same patient. Normal sweating may alternate with periods of strong hyperhydrosis and cold skin with warm skin when compared with the healthy side. Periods with no side difference of skin temperature may be followed by periods with large side differences. In an extreme case the maximum skin temperature side difference switched from +7°C on one day to −11°C on the next day.

Aggravation of symptoms in RSD by external interventions

Several events may aggravate the symptoms in RSD, such as swelling, pain, blood flow through skin (which is reflected in the skin temperature). These are physical load, painful movements (e.g. during physiotherapeutical sessions), environmental temperature changes, local temperature changes (e.g. by application of cold or warm water) and increase in hydrostatic pressure (e.g. in orthostasis).

TIME COURSE AND DEVELOPMENT OF SYMPTOMS

Onset and duration

For therapeutic reasons, any effort should be undertaken to diagnose RSD as early as possible. In this context it is important to know whether RSD has an acute or slow onset. Most RSDs start acutely, i.e. the cardinal symptoms may appear within minutes to hours. At the onset, the main symptoms of RSD are pain, generalized swelling and the systematic side difference of skin temperature. These early symptoms develop in areas and tissues that are not directly affected by the preceding lesion.

Swelling and pain provide valuable information for an early diagnosis of RSD: before the onset of RSD, pain is felt inside the area of the preceding lesion. With the onset of RSD, the pain is diffuse and deep inside the distal extremity and the swelling is generalized, yet the initial pain may have already disappeared. It is important to note that, in a number of cases, spontaneous diffuse pain may not be present at the onset of RSD but may develop later.

If the RSD syndrome is untreated, its symptoms, in many cases, will be present more or less continuously over months or years. In this 'permanent' form of RSD trophic changes and diffuse allodynia may occur. If the syndrome finally subsides, the swelling is reduced and severe restriction of passive movements, together with muscular atrophy, are likely to be present. In this condition, spontaneous pain may still be present or may subside.

About 30% of the patients exhibit an 'intermittent' form of RSD: the symptoms appear and disappear spontaneously or, more commonly, in relation to various kinds of strain (see above). Finally, there are spontaneous remissions of RSD, in which the symptoms disappear days and weeks after onset. The frequency of these remissions is unknown.

Symptoms in early and late RSD

When comparing the clinical picture of patients with early RSD (duration of symptoms no longer than 10 days) and those with longer lasting RSD in terms of type and incidence of symptoms, there are no relevant differences between these two groups (see Table 38.1). In other words, it should usually be possible to diagnose RSD very early. Trophic changes and, interestingly, also allodynia, are absent in early RSD, in contrast to cases with longstanding RSD (see Table 38.1, Blumberg 1991).

Staging of RSD: is it appropriate?

It has been stated in the literature that RSD, if untreated, may pass through three stages (see Bonica 1990). The first (acute) stage is characterized by the key symptoms of pain, oedema and warm skin, the second (dystrophic) stage by cold skin and trophic changes, and the third (atrophic) stage by atrophy of skeletal muscles and bone as well as contractures of joints. The duration of the first two stages is reported to be very variable, lasting from weeks to months. It is impossible to predict whether RSD patients, if untreated, will reach the second or third stage or whether spontaneous remissions will occur. Furthermore, recovery from the third stage is unlikely to occur. Symptoms which are specific for the first and the second stage do not exist.

Although perhaps of some practical value, it is generally questionable whether staging of RSD is appropriate. What is probably more important, is that patients with RSD should be graded, according to the intensity of the sensory, autonomic, motor and trophic changes, as being mild, moderate or severe (Stanton-Hicks et al 1989; Bonica 1990).

EPIDEMIOLOGICAL ASPECTS

Age and sex

The frequency of RSD with respect to age shows a normal distribution with a peak at around 50 years of age (Fig. 38.1), which agrees with previous reports (Kleinert et al 1970; Pak et al 1970). Both children and very old persons may also suffer from RSD (Olsson et al 1990; Arnér 1991). Female patients are somewhat more frequent than male patients (Fig. 38.1; Kleinert et al 1970; Pak et al 1970; but see Carron & Weller 1974).

Preceding events and incidence

The onset of RSD in almost all cases is preceded by noxious events. These include minor trauma, partial nerve lesion, bone fracture and other lesions (e.g. shoulder trauma, myocardial infarction or even a contralateral cerebrovascular lesion) (Askey 1941; Steinbrocker et al 1947; Moskowitz et al 1958; Patman et al 1973; Loh et al 1981). Thus, the symptoms of RSD occur irrespective of the type and the site of the preceding lesion (Blumberg 1991; Blumberg et al 1993a).

Reliable information about the incidence of RSD does not exist since different criteria were used for its diagnosis, and criteria for its early diagnosis were absent. A rough estimate from the clinical experience in Freiburg gives an incidence of 1:5000 persons per year.

DIAGNOSTIC AND PROGNOSTIC TESTS

The clinical symptomatology of RSD alone does not allow us to conclude whether the sympathetic nervous system is involved in the generation of pain and swelling. Therefore, special diagnostic and prognostic tests should be applied before treatment is started. Here we offer four tests, two of them being well established and two of them still being in

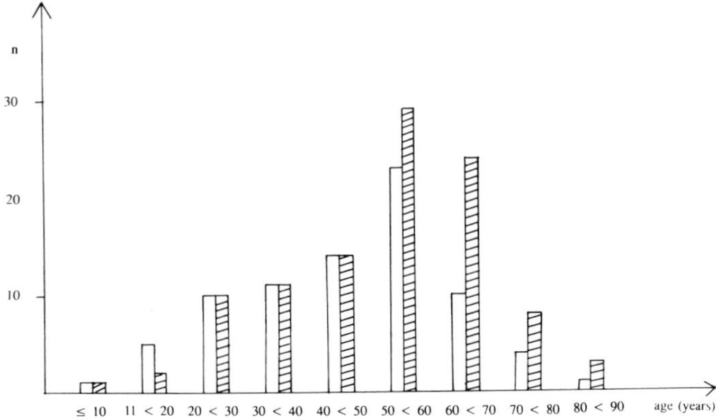

Fig. 38.1 Distribution of RSD patients with respect to age and sex. Hatched bars: females (n = 102), open bars: males (n = 79). The same sample of patients as in Table 38.1

the process of independent verification before they can be generally recommended. The relief of spontaneous pain and evoked pain (mechanical hyperalgesia and allodynia) should be measured quantitatively by using the visual analogue scale or another scale. Placebo effects should be checked by injection of NaCl solution, for example, when sympathetic ganglia are blocked or in the phentolamine test (see Arnér 1991; Price et al 1992).

Sympathetic blocks with local anaesthetics

In order to block impulse activity in sympathetic neurons to the upper or lower extremity a local anaesthetic is applied ipsilaterally to the stellate ganglion or the lumbar paravertebral sympathetic ganglia, respectively (Bonica 1990). A sufficient block is assumed when the skin temperature of ipsilateral finger- or toetips increases to ≥ 35°C. An ipsilateral Horner's sign does not prove that the sympathetic impulse transmission through the stellate ganglion to the upper extremity is blocked. Temporary relief of pain indicates that the (efferent!) sympathetic system is involved in the generation of pain. 'False positives', which may be generated by blockade of impulse activity in nociceptive afferents of adjacent nerve trunks (plexus brachialis, plexus lumbalis), can be excluded by careful clinical testing of sensory functions. Afferents projecting through the paravertebral ganglia to upper and lower extremities most likely do not exist and cannot be responsible for the pain-relieving effects of the sympathetic blocks by local anaesthetics (see Jänig 1990a).

Guanethidine test

Intravenous injection of guanethidine (1.25–30 mg in 20–50 ml saline solution, depending on the site of the cuff) into an extremity with RSD distal to a suprasystolic cuff is used for treatment of RSD (see Ch. 54; Blumberg & Hoffmann, unpublished). This procedure can also be applied to test whether the sympathetic nervous system is involved in the generation of pain. The guanethidine test is positive, first, if the injection is followed by a short-lasting (burning) pain and/or by paraesthesias (e.g., pressure, hotness), which have the same distribution as the spontaneous pain experienced by the patient and, secondly, if the spontaneous pain is relieved after opening the cuff (about 15 min after injection of the guanethidine). Both effects of the guanethidine are related to the pharmacological actions of the drug. First, it is taken up by the noradrenergic varicosities of postganglionic axons and depletes noradrenaline from its stores, leading to excitation of nociceptors. Secondly, it prevents further release of noradrenaline from the depleted postganglionic axons for up to 1–2 days. A negative test does not exclude a sympathetic–afferent coupling proximal to the cuff (see section on Pathophysiology).

Phentolamine test

Recently, the phentolamine test was introduced as a tool for the diagnosis of RSD/SMP independently by Arnér (1991) and Raja et al (1991) (see also Campbell et al 1992). Phentolamine is an alpha-adrenoceptor antagonist (alpha-1, alpha-2). The rationale of this test is that excitation of nociceptive afferent neurones by noradrenaline, which is released from postganglionic axons, is prevented by blockade of alpha-adrenoceptors. Up to 30 mg phentolamine in 100 ml saline are infused intravenously over about 20 minutes (Raja et al 1991; Campbell et al 1992) or 5–15 mg over 5–10 minutes (Arnér 1991). Pain (spontaneous pain, mechanical and cold hyperalgesia) is measured using a visual analogue scale. If pain is reduced, the sympathetic nervous system is likely to be involved in the generation of pain. Arnér (1991) has shown that patients who obtained transient pain relief during intravenous infusion of phentolamine were likely to respond favourably to treatment with intravenous regional guanethidine. However, this test needs confirmation by further independent investigation before it can be universally recommended as a diagnostic test.

Ischaemia test

Interruption of the circulation in the distal part of an RSD extremity by a suprasystolic cuff (after an Esmarch bandage or equivalent is wrapped around the hand/foot from distal to proximal up to the cuff to reduce the volume of the distal extremity) suppresses or reduces the deep diffuse pain after 1–2 min. This pain-suppressing effect has occasionally been reported in the literature (de Takats 1945; Loh et al 1981; Gracely et al 1990) and is used by one of the authors as a supplementary test for the diagnosis of RSD (Blumberg & Hoffmann 1992; Hoffmann & Blumberg 1993). The pain suppression is not due to blockade of A- or C-fibres. A positive test has a high prognostic value for pain relief generated by sympatholytic interventions in RSD. All the patients tested (n = 41, out of the patients as described in the section on Patients) and who acutely obtained pain relief by a sympathetic block (n = 39) also showed a positive test (Hoffmann & Blumberg 1993). However, these observations need independent confirmation. Preliminary results show that the test is negative in patients who have pain in the extremities which is not dependent on activity in the sympathetic nervous system (e.g. pain due to carpal tunnel syndrome; Blumberg & Hoffmann, unpublished observations). The mechanism of the pain-relieving effect of this test is unclear, but it may be related to microvascular conditions (see section on Pathophysiology).

X-ray and bone scan

Since the work of Paul Sudeck (1902) it is known that bone demineralization (osteoporosis) may develop in RSD. X-ray shows a diffuse and spotty distal distribution of osteoporosis of small bones with a periarticular dominance at the longer bones. These changes are not seen in early RSD but are likely to occur months after its onset.

In the last 20 years, the technique of three-phase bone scanning has also been used for the diagnosis of RSD. The uptake of an intravenously injected radionuclide tracer into the bone is measured at various time periods (seconds/minutes/hours) after injection of the tracer (the three phases: arterial phase/soft-tissue phase/mineral phase). For all three phases, characteristic scintigraphic findings seem to occur in RSD, i.e. a diffuse increase in uptake of tracer is found distally on the ipsilateral side in comparison with the contralateral one, indicating vascular and nonvascular changes in the bone (Holder & Mackinnon 1984; Demangeat et al 1988).

The changes seen in the bone with both techniques in RSD are interesting and assist the diagnosis of RSD. However, it is as yet unclear how specific these changes are for RSD.

SUMMARY

1. RSD develops after several types of noxious events. It is defined by a triad of sensory, autonomic and motor symptoms, which occur distally at the affected extremity in a generalized (quasi-polyneuropathic) distribution independently of type and location of the preceding trauma.

2. RSD is mostly acute in its onset and can be diagnosed early. Its clinical picture is characterized as follows:
   a. Spontaneous deep diffuse pain is present in 75% of the patients and absent in the rest of the patients. Cutaneous and deep hyperalgesia and changes of other sensations are almost regularly found. Allodynia is present in only about 8% of the patients; hyperpathia is absent.
   b. The autonomic changes consist of swelling (oedema), disturbances of blood flow through skin (side differences of skin temperature) and of sweating (hyper- and hypohydrosis).
   c. The motor changes are represented by a reduction of the range of active movement and of muscular strength and by an increase in physiological tremor of the distal extremity.
   d. Most trophic disturbances (changes of skin and its appendages; atrophy of muscles and contractures of joints) and changes in bones (osteoporosis) are late consequences of RSD.

3. If untreated, RSD may be present continuously for

months to years or may change into an intermittent form. Spontaneous remissions of RSD also occur.

4. Some tests are proposed which assist the diagnosis of RSD. These tests support the notion that the (efferent) sympathetic nervous system is involved in the generation of RSD and have a prognostic value for sympatholytic therapy.

CLINICAL PHENOMENOLOGY OF SMP

NEUROLOGICAL FINDINGS AND LOCATION OF SYMPTOMS

When defining the term SMP, Roberts (1986) specified only two symptoms as constituting the necessary diagnostic criteria: spontaneous pain and allodynia. It was also stated that these symptoms, which should be present in a primarily lesioned area, can be abolished by sympathetic blocks. Thus, SMP was originally defined as a localized pain (sensory) syndrome. Patients who fit this definition were rarely reported in the literature (Nathan 1947; Leriche 1949; Loh & Nathan 1978). Campbell and coworkers (Frost et al 1988; Meyer et al 1990; Campbell et al 1992) and others use the term for similar patients. However, the criteria for differentiating between cases with RSD and SMP remained unclear (Blumberg 1992; Blumberg et al 1993b).

Patients with SMP usually exhibit a less complex clinical picture than do patients with RSD. The cardinal symptoms of SMP are spontaneous pain, mechanical allodynia and (cold) hyperalgesia. These sensory symptoms are mostly restricted to the territory of the affected peripheral or spinal nerve (dermatome). Spontaneous and evoked pain are felt superficially and not deep inside the extremity and are not in their intensity dependent on the position of the extremity (absence of the orthostatic component), nor are they aggravated by physical exercise. The triad of sensory, autonomic and motor symptoms which extends, at the affected extremity, into territories outside of the lesioned site and which is typical for most cases with RSD, is more or less absent in SMP. Autonomic changes, if present, are usually restricted to the zone of the lesioned nerve and can be explained sufficiently by denervation and reinnervation of autonomic effector organs. None of our patients with SMP showed a systematic side difference of skin temperature. Motor changes, if at all present, are explained by lesions of motor axons. Swelling and trophic changes are either absent or very discrete. Abnormal reflexes in neurons of the sympathetic outflow have not been detected in the small number of SMP patients tested (Blumberg, unpublished results).

ONSET AND DURATION

The onset of SMP may be acute, mostly in close temporal relationship to the preceding lesion. If untreated, the syndrome may last for years without any change of symptoms. However, some SMP patients may additionally develop RSD (see below).

INCIDENCE AND PRECEDING EVENTS

No data are available about the incidence (morbidity) of SMP. However, compared with the frequency of patients with RSD, it is much less common (relation of RSD/SMP about 30:1 in Freiburg). SMP is almost always preceded by a partial lesion of a peripheral nerve.

SPECIAL DIAGNOSTIC TESTS

The pain in SMP should be alleviated by any form of sympathicolytic therapy and this is almost the only recommended therapy to treat this pain. Consequently, the guanethidine test, the phentolamine test (see Raja et al 1991) and the test with local anaesthetics (applied to paravertebral ganglia), as described above for patients with RSD, should be positive. Preliminary results show that the ischaemia test is negative in patients with SMP (Blumberg & Hoffmann, unpublished results).

RSD COMBINED WITH SMP

Sometimes RSD and SMP are present simultaneously in the same patient. In such patients, the pain syndrome may start with SMP and then develops into RSD. For example, an accidental trauma or a carpal tunnel syndrome (or its surgical treatment) may lead to spontaneous pain and allodynia inside the area of the lesioned nerve. Later, the whole hand distally may exhibit the generalized triad of sensory, autonomic and motor changes which is typical of RSD. In these patients, the pain consists of superficial spontaneous pain and evoked pain (allodynia), which is related to the lesioned nerve zone (SMP type of pain), and of deep diffuse spontaneous and movement-related pain, which is typical for RSD and which may be aggravated by various manoeuvres (orthostasis, physical exercise, thermal load) (Blumberg et al 1993b). Such patients fit the clinical description of causalgia (Bonica 1979, 1990). On the other hand, SMP occurs in addition to RSD. For example, if RSD with its typical triad has developed following a radial fracture, which is treated by a plaster cast, a partial superficial radial nerve lesion may take place secondarily. This can result in additional (superficial) spontaneous pain and allodynia, restricted to the territory of the lesioned nerve (SMP symptoms).

Diagnostic sympathetic blocks should, at least temporarily, interrupt the pain in the cases with combined RSD and SMP, as has been reported (see Bonica 1990) and was found in our five patients.

SUMMARY

SMP is a rare pain syndrome which develops in most cases after a peripheral nerve lesion. Its cardinal symptoms are spontaneous pain, (mechanical) allodynia and (cold) hyperalgesia. These sensory symptoms are preferentially restricted to the territory of the affected nerve. Generalized sensory, autonomic, motor and trophic changes at the affected extremity are absent. Sympathetic reflexes seem to be normal. Spontaneous and evoked pain are relieved by sympathetic blocks. Symptoms of SMP and RSD may be present in the same patient. The criteria for differential diagnosis of RSD and SMP are listed in Table 38.2.

COMMENTS

The classification of the patients with pain which is dependent on activity in the sympathetic nervous system into those having RSD and those having SMP is based on the clinical phenomenology and not on the peripheral and central pathophysiological mechanisms which may operate in these patients. Neither the description of the clinical phenomenology of RSD and SMP nor the usage of both terms is new. What is new here is the systematic way in which the clinical symptoms are described with the suggestion to differentiate between RSD and SMP and the finding that RSD can be diagnosed very early. In most RSD patients and in all SMP patients the pain was at least temporarily relieved by sympathetic blocks. Although not explicitly tested, it is unlikely that these pain-relieving effects are placebo effects in our patients (see also Arnér 1991; Price et al 1992).

Three caveats should be kept in mind with this classification. First, SMP patients may also develop RSD (or vice versa) and RSD may be locally restricted in some cases (Blumberg et al 1993c). Therefore, it may turn out in the future that transitory states between RSD and SMP do exist. Secondly, the diagnosis of RSD cannot be made solely on the basis of spontaneous pain. This pain is absent in about 25% of the RSD patients, but evoked abnormal sensations, such as movement-related pain and hyperalgesia (and the other symptoms of the triad, see Table 38.1), are present in some of them. Thirdly, RSD may be indistinguishable in its clinical phenomenology from posttraumatic reactions as far as pain and swelling are concerned. Thus, there may be transitions between RSD and posttraumatic pain states.

Taking these caveats into account, it should in future be possible to come to a general consensus as far as the subclassification of patients with RSD and SMP is concerned. It may, for example, be advisable to use a neutral term, such as sympathetically dependent pain, as an umbrella term for other more specific terms, which may be not only RSD and SMP.

In this chapter we have concentrated on patients with RSD and SMP at the extremities. This does not exclude that the sympathetic nervous system is also involved in the generation of other pain states which are associated with traumata, such as postherpetic neuralgia, stump pain, phantom limb pain, atypical facial pain, etc. However, this is hypothetical and requires careful clinical investigation before it can be accepted.

Table 38.2 Criteria for differential diagnosis of SMP and RSD

	SMP	RSD
Incidence	Rare	Common
Aetiology	Mostly partial nerve lesion	Any kind of lesion
Localization	Any peripheral site of the body Confined to the lesioned area (nerve zone)	Distal part of extremity Independent from the site of the lesion
Spontaneous pain	Obligatory Mostly burning Predominantly superficial No orthostatic component	Common Variable character Mostly deep, diffuse With orthostatic component
Allodynia	Obligatory	Rare (<10%)
Autonomic symptoms Motor symptoms Sensory symptoms	related to nerve lesion (injury)	>90% distally generalized (glove-like distribution)

PATHOPHYSIOLOGICAL MECHANISMS

Several observations strongly argue that the sympathetic nervous system is involved in the generation of pain and the other associated changes in patients with RSD and SMP (see Table 38.2):

First, pain is relieved following sympathetic blocks (by local anaesthetics applied to paravertebral ganglia, by regional application of guanethidine, by phentolamine injected intravenously, see above). It is irrelevant in the present context, although important from a therapeutical point of view, that the sympathetic blocks are sometimes only temporarily successful and do not lead in some cases to permanent relief of pain.

Secondly, pain is rekindled or enhanced by an alpha-adrenoceptor agonist applied to the affected extremity (e.g. iontophoretically through the skin in patients with superficial burning pain and hyperalgesia), as has been observed by Wallin et al (1976) and Davis et al (1991).

Thirdly, guanethidine injected intravenously into the affected extremity initially elicits pain which is generated by noradrenaline released from postganglionic terminals.

Fourthly, continuous electrical stimulation of decentralized thoracic sympathetic ganglia in conscious patients suffering from causalgia who underwent surgery reproducibly elicited the tingling and burning pain at latencies of 4–20 s (Walker & Nulsen 1948). White & Sweet (1969) confirmed this observation.

The following discussion will summarize pathophysiological mechanisms which might operate in RSD and SMP patients and in which the sympathetic nervous system is involved. Several reviews on this subject have been published recently (Jänig 1990a; Devor et al 1991; Jänig & Schmidt 1992; see also Chs 4 and 10).

A GENERAL HYPOTHESIS

Figure 38.2 outlines a general hypothesis which explains several phenomena observed in patients with RSD and SMP (Blumberg & Jänig 1983; Jänig 1985, 1990a). The main clinical observations (see Table 38.2) are double framed; the initiating events are at the top, the most important one being trauma with and without nerve lesions. This heuristic hypothesis consists of several components (numbers, see Fig. 38.2). Each component is fully or partially supported by experiments on animals and some by experimental investigations on humans:

1. The afferent neurons with small-diameter fibres in the affected territory, in particular the nociceptive ones, may be sensitized as a consequence of the initial trauma. They generate ongoing activity and react abnormally to mechanical, thermal and chemical stimulation. Lesioned afferent axons may generate ectopically spontaneous and evoked impulse activity (see Jänig 1988; Cervero et al 1989; Bond et al 1991; Willis 1992; see also Ch. 4).

2. Noradrenergic postganglionic neurons are coupled in some abnormal way to the peripheral afferent neurons leading to an abnormal afferent impulse traffic to the spinal cord. This coupling may occur at the site of the coupling as well as in unlesioned tissues (for reviews see Jänig & Koltzenburg 1991a, 1992; see below).

3. The decoding of nociceptive and nonnociceptive afferent information by neurons in the spinal cord (particular in the dorsal horn), including the control of transmission of nociceptive information by supraspinal systems, is changed. Neurons of the central nociceptive pathways are sensitized by a continuous input in nociceptive afferents which may originate from the primary lesioned as well as the unlesioned tissues (see Bond et al 1991; Willis 1992; Jänig & Schmidt 1992).

4. The discharge pattern in the neurons of the sympathetic outflow to the affected extremity may be changed as a consequence of the changes of nociceptive transmission in the spinal cord (Blumberg & Jänig 1985; Jänig & Koltzenburg 1991b, 1991c).

5. The discharge pattern in alpha- and gamma-motoneurons may be changed too as a consequence of the sensitization of spinal neurons.

6. In the case of nerve lesions the regulation of small blood vessels by noradrenergic (vasoconconstrictor) neurons (neurovascular transmission) may be changed following regeneration of lesioned postganglionic axons. Furthermore, blood vessels may develop adaptive super-

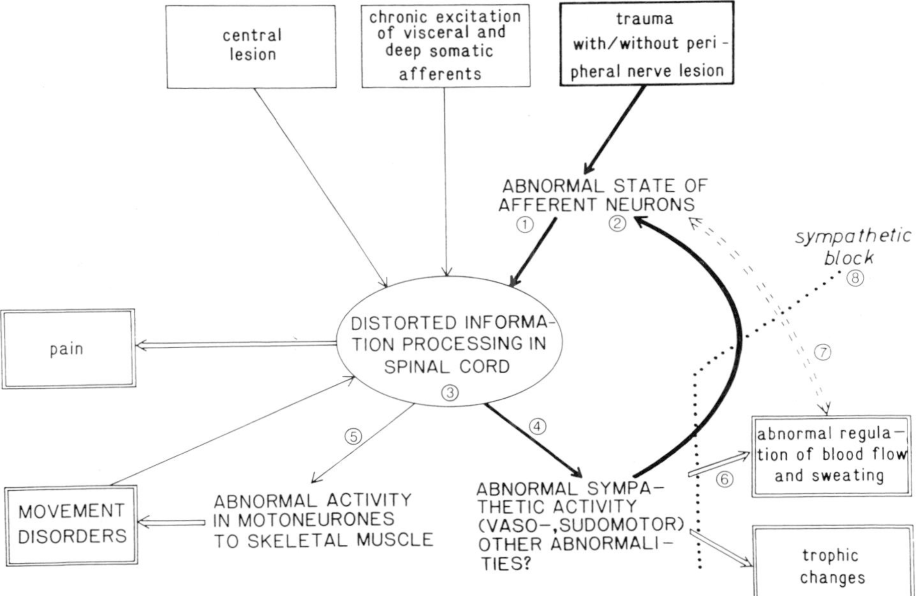

Fig. 38.2 General hypothesis about the neural mechanisms of generation of reflex sympathetic dystrophy (RSD) and sympathetically maintained pain (SMP) following peripheral trauma with and without nerve lesions, chronic stimulation of visceral afferents (e.g. myocardial infarction) and deep somatic afferents and, rarely, central trauma. The clinical observations are double framed. Note the vicious circle (arrows in bold black). An important component of this circle is the excitatory influence of postganglionic sympathetic axons on primary afferent fibres in the periphery. For details see text. The numbers refer to the text. Modified from Blumberg & Jänig (1983) and Jänig (1990).

sensitivity to circulating catecholamines and to impulses in vasoconstrictor neurons (Jänig & Koltzenburg 1991b; Jobling et al 1992).

7. Blood vessels in skin and deep somatic tissues (e.g. joint capsule) are also under afferent control. Activation of polymodal nociceptors generates precapillary vasodilatation and (in hairy skin and deep somatic tissues) postcapillary plasma extravasation. Both may be enhanced or reduced following trauma (Jänig & Koltzenburg 1991b; Jänig & Schmidt 1992).

8. This complex concerto of events may establish a vicious circle which is interrupted by blocking the sympathetic impulse traffic to the affected territory.

This heuristic hypothesis is not testable as such. Furthermore, the prevalence of the different components varies for the generation of RSD and SMP and may help to explain the different clinical phenomenologies. For example, in RSD without nerve lesion chemical sympathetic–afferent coupling may not be important. We will now concentrate mainly on components 2 and 4 which are the key issues in pain states in which the sympathetic nervous system might be involved. Component 5 will not be discussed because there is almost nothing known about its mechanisms (Deuschl et al 1991; Schott 1992). A further subject, not mentioned, is the generation of trophic changes and the involvement of the sympathetic nervous system in it. This has been extensively discussed in Jänig (1990a) and Jänig & Schmidt (1992). Components 1 and 3 are described elsewhere in this volume (see Chs 4 and 10).

SYMPATHETIC–SENSORY COUPLING IN THE PERIPHERY

Under normal conditions sympathetic neurons have little or no effect on the receptive properties of afferent neurons in mammals. However, after trauma there may be an influence of the sympathetic noradrenergic neurons on the afferent neurons in the periphery. This influence must be postulated for the reasons given above. Possible ways of coupling which may operate in the patients with RSD or SMP are summarized here in connection with Figure 38.3 (see also Jänig & Koltzenburg 1991a, 1992):

1. Direct chemical coupling between sympathetic and afferent nerve terminals following nerve lesions has been well documented (a in Fig. 38.3). The transmitter of this coupling is noradrenaline. The effect is alphadrenergic. The subtype of adrenoceptor is probably alpha-1. However, alpha-2 adrenoceptor-mediated (Sato & Perl 1991) and nonadrenergic chemical coupling (Jänig 1990b) cannot be discarded.

2. Chemical coupling may not occur only at the afferent nerve terminal in the periphery but may also

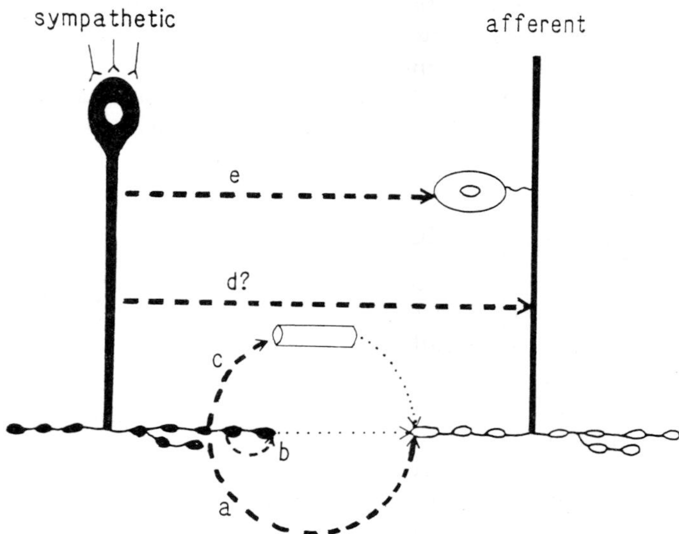

Fig. 38.3 Possible modes of coupling (interaction) between sympathetic postganglionic neurones and afferent neurons under pathological conditions. (**a**) Noradrenergic (and nonnoradrenergic?) chemical coupling in the periphery. (**b**) Indirect chemical coupling. (**c**) Indirect coupling via the vascular bed or other nonneural peripheral cells. (**d**) Interaction along the nerve. (**e**) Noradrenergic chemical coupling in the dorsal root ganglion. For details see text.

occur proximal to the nerve lesion along the nerve (d in Fig. 38.3) and in the dorsal root ganglion (e in Fig. 38.3). The latter is supported by neurophysiological and morphological experiments on rats in which the sciatic nerve was cut and ligated (Devor et al 1993; Jänig & McLachlan 1993; McLachlan et al 1993).

3. A further possibility discussed (Levine et al 1986) is that the sympathetic postganglionic fibres could modulate the excitability of the afferent receptors through an inflammatory process (b in Fig. 38.3). It is assumed that noradrenaline released by the postganglionic terminals acts presynaptically on the noradrenergic varicosities via alpha-2 adrenoceptors; this in turn leads to a release of prostanoids (e.g. prostaglandin I_2) which sensitize the nociceptors. This possibility is largely based on pharmacological experiments. It may operate in chronic inflammations (for discussion see Jänig & Koltzenburg 1991a, 1992).

4. It is possible that coupling occurs indirectly via the vascular system leading to changes of the micromilieu of the afferent receptive terminal and to its sensitization (c in Fig. 38.3). Two potential mechanisms must be discriminated: (i) changes of the neurovascular transmission of the efferent (postganglionic) signal to the blood vessels, and (ii) centrally induced changes of the activity in the sympathetic vasoconstrictor neurones leading to differential reactions of blood vessels (small resistance vessels, capacitance vessels, arteriovenous anastomoses). Both may not only be important for the generation of pain but also for

the changes of regulation of blood flow and sweating and for the generation of swelling and of trophic changes.

5. Ephaptic coupling between sympathetic terminal and afferent terminals has not been found so far (Blumberg & Jänig 1982, 1984; Häbler et al 1987).

A VICIOUS CIRCLE MAY BE ESTABLISHED BY THE SYMPATHETIC–AFFERENT COUPLING

Under physiological conditions, peripheral sympathetic pathways are distinct with respect to their target organs and somatosensory pathways are functionally distinct with respect to the peripheral receptors and the corresponding sensations. This is illustrated in Figure 38.4A. However, in RSD and SMP the situation may radically change. Now the sympathetic (efferent) and sensory channels are no longer separated (Fig. 38.4B). Activity in sympathetic neurons may lead to continuous activity in afferent nociceptive neurons. This continuous nociceptive activity generates the spontaneous pain and leads to sensitization of dorsal horn neurons (see 3 in Fig. 38.4B) resulting in various forms of allodynia and hyperalgesia (Price et al 1989, 1992; see also Ch.10). Sensitized central neurons may now be activated by stimulation of low-threshold mechanoreceptive afferents. Pathway 4 in Figure 38.4B is now open, and neurons of the nociceptive pathways are excited by activity in innocuous afferents. This could be the spinal substrate of mechanical allodynia (e.g. in patients with SMP and in some with RSD). Any type of sympathetic–afferent coupling is compatible with this model. If the sympathetic neurons were also coupled to the low threshold mechanoreceptors (see 2 in Fig. 38.4B) it is even possible that the pain is maintained via this pathway provided the central nociceptive pathways are sensitized.

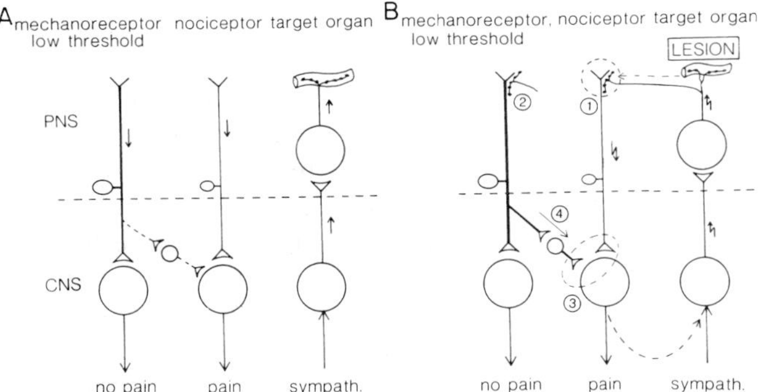

Fig. 38.4 (**A**) Separate sympathetic and somatosensory pathways associated with distinct regulation of vascular beds and other autonomic target organs and with painful as well as nonpainful sensations. The dotted lined pathway is normally not patent. Stimulation of nociceptors (with C- and A-fibres) elicits pain. Stimulation of low-threshold mechanoreceptors (associated with Aβ- and possibly some A-fibres) elicits nonpainful mechanical sensations, stimulation of thermoreceptors (with C- and A-fibres) elicits temperature sensations. Stimulation of vasoconstrictor neurones elicits vasoconstriction, etc. (**B**) Noradrenergic fibres are coupled to the afferent nociceptive (1) and to other afferent terminals (2) and maintain the afferent nociceptive input to the spinal cord. For modes of sympathetic–afferent coupling see Figure 38.3. This generates sensitization of the central nociceptive pathway with activation of the neurons of this pathway from low-threshold mechanoreceptors (3). Changes of activity and reflex pattern in sympathetic neurons may aggravate this process (4). CNS = central nervous system; PNS = peripheral nervous system.

Chemical sympathetic–afferent coupling, as worked out in animal experiments, seems to operate in patients with SMP and in some patients with RSD. Nociceptive neurones may express or uncover alpha-adrenoceptors which then react with noradrenaline which is released from the postganglionic terminals. However, to reduce RSD and SMP to an alpha-adrenoreceptor disease is problematic (see Campbell et al 1992; Jänig 1992).

This vicious circle does not principally require, for the generation of pain, that the sympathetic activity be increased or changed in its pattern. To emphasize, there is no proof that activity in sympathetic neurons is increased in patients with RSD or SMP (Blumberg 1988; Torebjörk 1990; Drummond et al 1991). However, any change in the pattern of activity in the sympathetic neurons supplying the affected extremity could aggravate pain and the associated phenomena (indicated in Fig. 38.4B by the interrupted arrow). Experiments on animals have shown that this change may occur in cutaneous vasoconstrictor neurons following nerve lesions, in particular lesions in which cutaneous afferent and efferent fibres reinnervate inappropriate target tissues (Blumberg & Jänig 1985; Jänig & Koltzenburg 1991c).

DOES A VICIOUS CIRCLE OCCUR VIA THE VASCULAR BED?

As reported above, many patients with RSD have spontaneous pain and hyperalgesia that is associated with deep somatic structures (joint, bone, fascia, skeletal muscle). These are accompanied by generalized distal swelling of the affected extremity and abnormal regulation of blood flow. Sympathetic blocks relieve pain, swelling and abnormal regulation of blood flow. The mode of sympathetic–afferent coupling in these patients is unknown. In the case of trauma with nerve lesions it may be chemical as discussed above. In other cases, in which nerve injury appears to be absent, for example, in RSD patients with radial fracture or with minor trauma, the coupling may occur more indirectly via the vascular system. This idea is favoured by one of the authors (Blumberg 1988, 1992).

The proposed model also describes a vicious circle and is a specification of the general model described above (see Fig. 38.2). A nociceptive afferent input which is generated by the trauma sensitizes spinal circuits. This sensitization also affects the spinal circuits of the sympathetic system and leads to an abnormal discharge pattern in the vasoconstrictor neurons. This in turn generates the oedema by an increased vasoconstriction on the postcapillary side with respect to the precapillary side, leading to an increased filtration pressure. The increased interstitial pressure is presumed to activate deep nociceptors in nonlesioned tissues maintaining the central sensitization process. Raising or cuffing the affected extremity would logically decrease the activity in the deep nociceptive afferents because the filtration pressure and the pulsations decrease. This could explain the almost prompt relief of pain in the ischaemia test and the orthostatic component of the pain in RSD. Furthermore, the activity in the vasoconstrictor neurones to the arteriovenous anastomoses may decrease or increase, leading to an increased/ decreased blood flow through the distal parts of the affected extremities and consequently to warm/cold hands and feet as seen in RSD.

The model is based on three assumptions which, up to now, have had only weak experimental support: first, a differential innervation and regulation of precapillary resistance and postcapillary capacitance vessels; secondly, a differential innervation and regulation of arteriovenous anastomoses and nutritional vessels; and thirdly, an impairment of thermoregulation via the sympathetic nervous system in the skin of the affected extremity (Blumberg 1988).

Theoretically, it is possible that changes of the neurovascular transmission could lead to the same phenomenology. Experimentally, it has been shown that reinnervated blood vessels exhibit stronger than normal vasoconstrictions to stimulation of the noradrenergic vasoconstrictor neurons and to circulating catecholamines, whereas the vasodilatation induced by activation of polymodal nociceptive afferents (the 'axon reflex') is decreased or absent (Jänig & Koltzenburg 1991b, 1991c). Investigation of reinnervated blood vessels in vitro has shown that the alpha-adrenoceptor mediated potentials elicited by nerve stimulation in the smooth muscle cells may increase relative to the intracellular junction potentials which are resistant to blockade by alpha- or beta-adrenoceptor antagonists (Jobling et al 1992). If the same were to occur under conditions in which the nerves are not lesioned, the whole phenomenology in RSD patients could be explained by peripheral mechanisms which require normal activity but not a distorted pattern or increased activity in sympathetic neurons. However, this does not apply to the acute development of symptoms in patients with early RSD. In summary, the phenomenology in many RSD patients cannot be explained by a simple mechanisms of sympathetic–afferent coupling. Therefore it is necessary to look for alternative models which are testable in experiments on animals and humans.

Acknowledgements

This work was supported by the Bundesministerium für Forschung und Technologie (H.B.) and by the Deutsche Forschungsgemeinschaft (W.J.). We wish to thank Dr Ulrike Hoffmann, Department of Anaesthesiology, University of Freiburg, for performing the sympathetic blocks in our patients. We also wish to thank Mrs A. Böger-Koch for her technical assistance.

REFERENCES

Arnér S 1991 Intravenous phentolamine test: diagnostic and prognostic use in reflex sympathetic dystrophy. Pain 46: 17–22

Askey J M 1941 The syndrome of painful disability of the shoulder and hand complicating coronary occlusion. American Heart Journal 22: 1–12

Bentley J B, Hameroff S R 1980 Diffuse reflex sympathetic dystrophy. Anaesthesiology 53: 256–257

Blumberg H 1988 Zur Entstehung und Therapie des Schmerzsyndroms bei der sympathischen Reflexdystrophie. Der Schmerz 2: 125–143

Blumberg H 1991 A new clinical approach for diagnosing reflex sympathetic dystrophy. In: Bond M R, Charlton J E, Woolf C J (eds) Pain research and clinical management (Proceedings of the VIth World Congress on Pain). Elsevier, Amsterdam vol 4; p 399–403

Blumberg H 1992 Clinical and pathophysiological aspects of reflex sympathetic dystrophy and sympathetically maintained pain. In: Jänig W, Schmidt R F (eds) Reflex sympathetic dystrophy. Pathophysiological mechanisms and clinical implications. VCH Verlagsgesellschaft, Weinheim, p 29–49

Blumberg H, Hoffmann U 1992 Der 'Ischämie-Test'–ein neues Verfahren in der klinischen Diagnostik der sympathischen Reflexdystrophie (Kausalgie, M Sudeck). Der Schmerz 6: 196–198

Blumberg H, Jänig W 1982 Activation of fibers via experimentally produced stump neuromas of skin nerves: ephaptic transmission or retrograde sprouting? Experimental Neurology 76: 468–482

Blumberg H, Jänig W 1983 Changes of reflexes in vasoconstrictor neurons supplying the cat hindlimb following chronic nerve lesions: a model for studying mechanisms of reflex sympathetic dystrophy? Journal of the Autonomic Nervous System 7: 399–411

Blumberg H, Jänig W 1984 Discharge patterns of afferent fibers from a neuroma. Pain 20: 335–353

Blumberg H, Jänig W 1985 Reflex patterns in postganglionic vasoconstrictor neurons following chronic nerve lesions. Journal of the Autonomic Nervous System 14: 157–180

Blumberg H, Griesser H J, Hornyak M 1993a Reflex sympathetic dystrophy – a neurological disorder? I. Preceding events, symptoms and signs, and early bedside diagnosis. Pain (submitted)

Blumberg H, Griesser H-J, Hornyak M 1993b Differential diagnosis of reflex sympathetic dystrophy and the sympathetically maintained pain syndrome. Pain (submitted)

Blumberg H, Wakhloo A K, Hoffman A U, Wokalek H 1993c Die lokalisierte Form einer sympathischen Reflexdystrophie. Der Schmerz 7: 178–181

Bond M R, Charlton J E, Woolf C J 1991 Proceedings of the VIth World Congress on Pain. Elsevier, Amsterdam

Bonica J J 1979 Causalgia and other reflex sympathetic dystrophies. In: Bonica J J, Liebeskind J C, Albe-Fessard D G (eds) Advances in pain research and therapy. Raven Press, New York, vol 3; p 141–166

Bonica J J 1990 Causalgia and other reflex sympathetic dystrophies. In: Bonica J J (ed) The management of pain, 2nd edn. Lea & Febiger, Philadelphia, p 220–243

Campbell J N, Meyer R A, Raja S N 1992 Is nociceptor activation by alpha-1 adrenoreceptors the culprit in sympathetically maintained pain? American Pain Society Journal 1: 3–11

Carron H, Weller R W 1974 Treatment of post-traumatic sympathetic dystrophy. Advances in Neurology 4: 485–490

Cervero F, Bennett G J, Headley P M (eds) 1989 Processing of sensory information in the superficial dorsal horn of the spinal cord. Nato ASI series, A: Life Sciences : 176. Plenum Press, New York

Davis K D, Treede R D, Raja S N, Meyer R A, Campbell J N 1991 Topical application of clonidine relieves hyperalgesia in patients with sympathetically maintained pain. Pain 47: 309–317

Demangeat J L, Constantinesco A, Brunot B, Foucher G, Farcot J M 1988 Three phase bone scanning in reflex sympathetic dystrophy of the hand. Journal of Nuclear Medicine 29: 26–32

De Takats G 1945 Nature of painful vasodilatation in causalgic states. Archives of Neurology and Psychiatry 53: 318–326

Deuschl G, Blumberg H, Lücking C H 1991 Tremor in reflex sympathetic dystrophy. Archives in Neurology 48: 1247–1252

Devor M, Basbaum A I, Bennett G J et al 1991 Mechanisms of neuropathic pain following peripheral injury. In: Basbaum A I, Besson J–M (eds) Towards a new pharmacotherapy of pain, Dahlem Workshop Reports. Wiley, Chichester, p 417–440

Devor M, Jänig W, Michaelis M 1993 Modulation of activity in dorsal root ganglion (DRG) neurons by sympathetic activation in nerve-injured rats. Journal of Neurophysiology (in press)

Drummond P D, Finch P M, Smythe G A 1991 Reflex sympathetic dystrophy: the significance of differing plasma catecholamine concentrations in affected and unaffected limbs. Brain 114: 2025–2036

Evans J A 1946 Reflex sympathetic dystrophy. Surgical Clinics of North America 26: 780–790

Frost S A, Raja S N, Campbell J N, Meyer R A, Khan A A 1988 Does hyperalgesia to cooling stimuli characterise patients with sympathetically maintained pain (reflex sympathetic dystrophy)? In: Dubner R, Gebhard M R, Bond M R (eds) Pain research and clinical management (Proceedings of the VIth World Congress on Pain). Elsevier, Amsterdam, vol 4, p 151–156

Gracely R H, Lynch S, Bennett G J 1990 Ischemic block of large fibre function in reflex sympathetic dystrophy: a paradox. Society of Neuroscience Abstracts 16: 1280

Häbler H-J, Jänig W, Koltzenburg M 1987 Activation of unmyelinated afferents in chronically lesioned nerves by adrenaline and excitation of sympathetic efferents in the cat. Neuroscience Letters 82: 35–40

Hoffmann U, Blumberg J 1993 The pain suppressing effect of acute regional ischemia – a new diagnostic tool for reflex sympathetic dystrophy. Pain (submitted)

Holder L E, Mackinnon S E 1984 Reflex sympathetic dystrophy in the hands: clinical and scintigraphic criteria. Radiology 152: 517–522

Jänig W 1985 Causalgia and reflex sympathetic dystrophy: in which way is the sympathetic nervous system involved? Trends in Neurosciences 8: 471–477

Jänig W 1988 Pathophysiology of nerve following mechanical injury. In: Dubner R, Gebhart G F, Bond M R (eds) Pain research and clinical management. Elsevier, Amsterdam, vol 3, p 89–109

Jänig W 1990a The sympathetic nervous system in pain: physiology and pathophysiology. In: Stanton-Hicks M (ed) Pain and the sympathetic nervous system. Kluwer Academic Publishers, Boston, p 17–89

Jänig W 1990b Activation of afferent fibers ending in an old neuroma by sympathetic stimulation in the rat. Neuroscience Letters III: 309–314

Jänig W 1992 Can reflex sympathetic dystrophy be reduced to an alpha-adrenoceptor disease? American Pain Society Journal 1: 16–22

Jänig W, Koltzenburg M 1991a What is the interaction between the sympathetic terminal and the primary afferent fibre? In: Basbaum A I, Besson J-M (eds) Towards a new pharmacotherapy of pain. Dahlem Workshop Reports, Wiley, Chichester, p 331–352

Jänig W, Koltzenburg M 1991b Sympathetic reflex activity and neuroeffector transmission change after chronic nerve lesions. In: Bond M R Charlton J E, Woolf C J (eds) (1991b) Pain research and clinical management (Proceedings of the VIth World Congress on Pain). Elsevier, Amsterdam, vol 4, p 365–371

Jänig W, Koltzenburg M 1991c Plasticity of sympathetic reflex organization following cross union of inappropriate nerves. Journal of Physiology 436: 309–323

Jänig W, Koltzenburg M 1992 Possible ways of sympathetic afferent interactions. In: Jänig W, Schmidt R F (eds) Reflex sympathetic dystrophy. Pathophysiological mechanisms and clinical implications. VCH Verlagsgesellschaft, Weinheim, p 213–245

Jänig W, McLachlan E M 1993 The role of modification in noradrenergic peripheral pathways after nerve lesions in the generation of pain. In: Fields H L, Liebeskind J C (eds) Pharmacological approaches to the treatment of pain: new concepts and critical issues. IASP Press, Seattle (in press)

Jänig W, Schmidt, F R 1992 Reflex sympathetic dystrophy. Pathophysiological mechanisms and clinical implications, VCH Verlagsgesellschaft, Weinheim

Jänig W, Blumberg H, Boas R A, Campbell J A 1991 The reflex sympathetic dystrophy syndrome: consensus statement and general recommendations for diagnosis and clinical research. In: Bond M R, Charlton J E, Woolf C J (eds) Pain research and clinical management (Proceedings of the VIth World Congress on Pain). Elsevier, Amsterdam, vol 4, p 372–375

Jancovic J, van der Linden C 1988 Dystonia and tremor induced by peripheral trauma: predisposing factors. Journal of Neurology, Neurosurgery and Psychiatry 51: 1512–1519

Jobling P, McLachlan E M, Jänig W, Anderson C R 1992 Electrophysiological responses in the rat tail artery during reinnervation following lesions of the sympathetic supply. Journal of Physiology 454: 107–128

Kleinert H E, Cole N M, Wayne L, Harvey R, Kutz J E, Atasoy E 1973 Posttraumatic sympathetic dystrophy. Orthopedic Clinics of North America 4: 917–927

Kozin F, McCarty D J, Sims J, Genant H 1976 The reflex sympathetic dystrophy syndrome. I. Clinical and histologic studies: evidence of bilateraly, response to corticosteroids and articular involvement. American Journal of Medicine 60: 321–331

Leriche R 1949 La chirurgie de la douleur, 3rd edn. Masson, Paris

Levine J D, Taiwo Y O, Collins S D, Tam J K 1986 Noradrenaline hyperalgesia is mediated through interaction with sympathetic postganglionic neurone terminals rather than activation of primary afferent nociceptors. Nature 323: 158–160

Loh L, Nathan P W 1978 Painful peripheral states and sympathetic blocks. Journal of Neurology, Neurosurgery and Psychiatry 41: 664–671

Loh L, Nathan P W, Schott G D 1981 Pain due to lesions of central nervous system removed by sympathetic block. British Medical Journal 282: 1026–1028

McLachlan E M, Jänig W, Devor M, Michaelis M 1993 Peripheral nerve injury triggers noradrenergic sprouting within dorsal root ganglia. Nature 363: 543–546

Meyer R A, Raja S N, Treede R-D, Davis K D, Campbell J N 1990 Neural mechanisms of sympathetically maintained pain. In: Jänig W, Schmidt R (eds) Reflex sympathetic dystrophy. VCH Verlagsgesellschaft, Weinheim, p 57–66

Moskowitz E, Bishop H F, Shibutani K 1958 Posthemiplegic reflex sympathetic dystrophy. Journal of American Medical Academy 167: 836–838

Nathan P W 1947 On the pathogenesis of causalgia in peripheral nerve injuries. Brain 70: 145–170

Olsson G L, Arnér S, Hirsch G 1990 Reflex sympathetic dystrophy in children. Advances in Pain Therapy 15: 323–331

Pak T J, Martin G M, Magness J M, Kavanaugh G J 1970 Reflex sympathetic dystrophy. Minnesota Medicine 53: 507–512

Patman R D, Thompson J E, Persson A V 1973 Management of post-traumatic pain syndromes: report of 113 cases. Annual Surgery 177: 780–787

Price D D, Bennett G J, Raffii A 1989 Psychophysical observations on patients with neuropathic pain relieved by a sympathetic block. Pain 36: 273–288

Price D D, Long S, Huitt C 1992 Sensory testing of pathophysiological mechanisms of pain in patients with reflex sympathetic dystrophy. Pain 49: 163–173

Raja S N, Treede R-D, Davis K D, Campbell J N 1991 Systemic alpha-adrenergic blockade with phentolamine: a diagnostic test for sympathetically maintained pain. Anesthesiology 74: 691–698

Roberts W J 1986 A hypothesis on the physiological basis for causalgia and related pains. Pain 24: 297–311

Sato J, Perl E R 1991 Adrenergic excitation of cutaneous pain receptors induced by peripheral nerve injury. Science 251: 1608–1610

Schott G D 1992 The relationship of peripheral trauma to generation of reflex sympathetic dystrophy and involuntary movements. In: Jänig

W, Schmidt R F (eds) Reflex sympathetic dystrophy. Pathophysiological mechanisms and clinical implications. VHC Verlagsgesellschaft, Weinheim, p 51–57

Schwartzman R J, Kerrigan J 1990 The movement disorder of reflex sympathetic dystrophy. Neurology 40: 57–61

Stanton-Hicks M 1990 Pain and the sympathetic nervous system. Kluwer Academic Publishers, Boston

Stanton-Hicks R J, Jänig W, Boas R A 1989 Reflex sympathetic dystrophy. Kluwer Academic Publishers, Boston

Steinbrocker O, Spitzer N, Friedman H 1948 The shoulder–hand syndrome in reflex sympathetic dystrophy of the upper extremity. Annals of Internal Medicine 29: 22–52

Sudeck P Über die akute (trophoneurotische) Knochenatrophie nach Entzündungen und Traumen der Extremitäten. Deutsche Medizinische Wochenschrift 28: 336–338

Torebjörk E 1990 Clinical and neurophysiological observations relating to psychophysiological mechanisms in reflex sympathetic dystrophy. In: Stanton-Hicks M, Jänig W, Boas R A (eds) Reflex sympathetic dystrophy. Kluwer Academic Publishers, Boston, p 71–80

Walker A E, Nulsen F 1948 Electrical stimulation of the upper thoracic portion of the sympathetic chain in man. Archives of Neurology and Psychiatry 59: 559–560

Wallin G, Torebjörk H E, Hallin R G 1976 Preliminary observations on the pathophysiology of hyperalgesia in the causalgic pain syndrome. In: Zottermann Y (ed) Sensory functions of the skin in primates. Pergamon, Oxford, p 489–499

White J C, Sweet W H 1969 Pain and the neurosurgeon. C C Thomas, Springfield

Willis W D 1992 Hyperalgesia and allodynia. Raven Press, New York

39. Tic douloureux and atypical face pain

John D. Loeser

INTRODUCTION

Tic douloureux is a unique disease, a chronic pain state readily treated by both pharmacological and surgical means. Tic is one of the most painful of human afflictions; it allows the physician to exercise diagnostic and therapeutic skills which should regularly produce symptomatic relief for the patient. Atypical face pain, which occurs in the same part of the body, is a dramatic contrast; it is not usually ameliorated by either drugs or surgery. Ironically, we still do not understand either the pathological processes or the neurophysiological basis of either tic douloureux or atypical face pain. Medical and surgical therapies have been based upon chance observations, assumptions often unsubstantiated by data, a few good guesses and the patient's willingness to trade pain for sensory loss in the face. Physicians tend to see only those aspects of the patient's problem that fit preconceived notions of pathogenesis or their limited therapeutic repertoire. Lack of knowledge of the natural history of tic and atypical face pain has led to erroneous claims for therapeutic efficacy; inadequate long-term follow-up of patients has also led to inflated claims for the efficacy of a procedure or drug. In spite of these problems, the medical literature in the past two decades has demonstrated major improvements in the diagnosis, treatment and study of tic douloureux; atypical face pain has not received as much attention and remains a poorly managed disease.

SIGNS AND SYMPTOMS

TIC DOULOUREUX

Although the classification of painful diseases of the face is often unclear, tic douloureux can be discriminated from all other painful afflictions on the basis of the patient's history and physical examination (Table 39.1). Tic is characterized by:

1. electric shock-like, brief, stabbing pains
2. painfree intervals between attacks when the patient is completely asymptomatic
3. unilateral pain during any one attack
4. pain of abrupt onset and equally abrupt termination
5. pain restricted to the trigeminal nerve distribution (rarely may involve the nervus intermedius of the facial nerve or the glossopharyngeal nerve alone or in combination with the trigeminal nerve)
6. minimal or no sensory loss in the trigeminal distribution
7. nonnociceptive triggering of pain, almost always ipsilateral to the pain and usually from the perioral region.

It is unfortunately true that the patient has not often read the texbook, and differential diagnosis may not be as easy in the examining room as it is in the literature. Deviations from the rigid diagnostic criteria proposed above can occur, but the more unusual features the patient manifests, the less likely he is to respond to either medical or surgical therapies, and the more diligently the search for alternative aetiologies should be undertaken. The most common variant is the patient who has electric shock-like pain superimposed upon a background of burning discomfort. A small amount of burning immediately after a jab of pain is not uncommon and should not cause the physician to challenge the diagnosis of tic. If the patient has had a prior nerve-damaging procedure and has an associated sensory loss on this basis, a burning or dysaesthetic component is common. In such a case it is important to ascertain that the burning, constant pain was not part of the original symptom complex. Such a patient has both tic douloureux and pain due to denervation; the latter, iatrogenic component may be much more refractory to therapy than the tic itself.

Some patients initially describe a pain which lasts for minutes or hours which is not characteristic of tic douloureux. Careful questioning may reveal that the patient is actually describing a flurry of brief attacks recurring at a rapid rate and that the intervals between each jab of pain are, in fact, free of any pain. This emphasizes the importance of a careful, detailed evaluation of the patient if an accurate diagnosis is to be established.

Table 39.1 Characteristics of facial pains

Tic douloureux	Atypical facial pain	Vascular facial pain	Myofascial or TMJ pain
Intermittent painfree intervals, abrupt on and off	Constant	Intermittent, clustered, gradual	Constant with fluctuation
Stabbing, electric shocks, sharp	Burning, aching	Throbbing, burning	Aching, radiating
Unilateral	Unilateral or bilateral	Unilateral	Unilateral
Trigeminal, rarely nervus intermedius or glossopharyngeal	Trigeminal, upper cervical	Midfacial	Lateral facial
Minimal or no sensory changes	Frequent sensory changes	No sensory changes	No sensory changes
Triggered by nonpainful stimulus, always ipsilateral, often remote from painful area	Rarely triggered; trigger in area of pain when present	No trigger	No trigger
No facial flushing, lacrimation or rhinitis	No facial flushing, lacrimation or rhinitis	Facial flushing, lacrimation, rhinitis	No facial flushing lacrimation or rhinitis
No local tenderness	Rarely local tenderness	Rarely local tenderness	Tender over TMJ muscles of mastication

Approximately 3% of patients with tic douloureux have pain on both sides of their face. I am not aware of any patient who has had simultaneous bilateral pain; usually an interval of years separates the pains on the two sides of the face. The history of bilateral pain does not support any presumed aetiology of tic, nor does it influence the likelihood of therapeutic success by medical or surgical means.

The early literature on tic douloureux suggested that women were afflicted more than men and that the right side of the face was a more common site of pain than the left (Stookey & Ransohoff 1959). Recent studies have not upheld these findings; dextral predominance is minimal, and over 45% of the patients are male. Whether this represents a true change in the incidence or extraneous factors such as access to health care is unclear. The majority of patients with tic douloureux are in the 50–70 year age group, but patients have been reported from childhood to over 90 years of age. In contrast to the old belief, the onset of tic douloureux in early years is not an indication that the disease is a symptom of multiple sclerosis; typical arterial cross-compression of the trigeminal nerve has been described in patients with the onset of tic in the second decade of life (see below). Patients whose tic douloureux started in the second or third decade of life do not usually develop other lesions suggestive of multiple sclerosis.

Although the overwhelming majority of patients with tic have pain restricted to the trigeminal nerve distribution, a small number may have pain in the glossopharyngeal or nervus intermedius or a combination of two or three of these sensory cranial nerves. Nervus intermedius involvement is suggested by pain in the ear or posterior pharynx; glossopharyngeal involvement by pain in the posterior tongue, tonsillar fossa or larynx. On rare occasions, glossopharyngeal tic is associated with syncopal attacks, presumably due to involvement of branches from the carotid sinus. When either glossopharyngeal or nervus intermedius pain is present, the third division is the most likely site of associated trigeminal pain. Tic pain most commonly involves the third (mandibular) division of the trigeminal nerve, least commonly the first (ophthalmic) division. The second (maxillary) division is involved slightly less often than the third; the combination of second and third divisions is the most frequent in many reported series. Every combination of pain sites in the trigeminal distribution can and does occur.

The triggering stimulus for tic pain is nonnoxious stimulation, almost always of the perioral or nasal region (Kugelberg & Lindblom 1959). The triggering site bears no necessary relation to the painful areas; they may be in the same division of the trigeminal nerve or may be widely separated. Many patients do not recognise a specific trigger but state that their pain is brought on by chewing, talking, swallowing, smiling, or exposure to temperature change, usually cold air. An occasional patient will describe a trigger area outside the trigeminal nerve territory; upper cervical segments are the most common sites. The trigger zone is always ipsilateral to the pain. Patients with triggering from the scalp will often refuse to brush their hair; shaving may be impossible for the man with a trigger zone in the upper lip or chin; triggering from the teeth or gingivae may preclude oral hygiene. Patients with pain triggered by chewing or swallowing may have insufficient oral intake to maintain caloric requirements adequately.

Tic douloureux can be an intermittent disease. Many patients report intervals of months or years between episodes of pain. Recurrences are usually in similar areas of the face, but it is characteristic for the regions of pain to spread to involve a wider area over time. It is common for the intervals between episodes of pain to become shorter over time. Some patients never enter remission once their pain begins; others will have episodes lasting days to months, only to have the pain stop completely; a recurrence is likely but by no means certain. In the patient with tic douloureux, emotional or physical stress usually increases the frequency of attacks and their severity.

Classical tic douloureux is so unique that it should not be confused with any other pain state. Its antithesis is atypical face pain, which appears to be more pleomorphic in its signs and symptoms.

ATYPICAL FACE PAIN

Atypical facial pain is usually described by the patient as a continuous, burning or aching pain, without painfree intervals, unrelated to a particular activity or triggering stimulus, often bilateral or extending beyond the trigeminal nerve distribution into cervical dermatomes. Atypical facial pain rarely, if ever, involves the glossopharyngeal or nervus intermedius distribution. This is a waste-basket diagnosis that contains several distinct pain syndromes. The name was coined to distinguish face pains of various types from tic douloureux, or 'typical face pain'. A neurosurgeon (Temple Fay) chose the terms on the basis of the response to lesions of the trigeminal nerve for pain relief. There is no widely accepted categorization of these pains, but my own beliefs are described below.

The most important discrimination is between unilateral and bilateral atypical facial pain. Bilateral atypical facial or intraoral pain is a plague for dentists, physicians and their patients. It occurs almost exclusively in middle-aged women who are frequently depressed and agitated. The pain is described as constant and burning; it usually is not triggered, and cutaneous stimulation is only disagreeable, not painful. There is rarely any sensory loss. Although described with great vehemence, the pain does not interrupt eating or talking. It is not paroxysmal. There are no associated autonomic abnormalities that can be detected clinically. Honest appraisal of the paranasal sinuses or teeth and gums does not reveal pathology. All imaging studies are normal; they are a waste of money for patients with this syndrome. Patients with bilateral atypical facial pain do not respond often to existing therapies.

Unilateral atypical facial pain also contains several different pain syndromes. Patients complain of constant, usually burning pain restricted to one side of the face. Sometimes there is a component of shock-like, stabbing pain superimposed upon the constant, background pain.

One cause of this type of pain is injury to a branch of the trigeminal nerve. Facial lacerations are the most common aetiology, but occasionally infection or neoplasm can be a cause. The history of trauma and the sensory loss in the distribution of the damaged nerve are tell-tale signs. Sometimes the pain ceases when nerve regeneration has occurred, but this is not always the case. This pain syndrome can occur in patients with tic douloureux who undergo denervating procedures to treat their tic pain. When their tic pain recurs, they may suffer from both the shock-like pain of tic douloureux and the constant burning pain that follows trigeminal nerve injury. It is critical to recognize that further damage to the trigeminal nerve or its peripheral branches does not often relieve this type of atypical facial pain, even when peripheral nerve blocks provide temporary pain relief. This point was again emphasized in Kuhner's review (1988).

Another type of unilateral atypical facial pain begins insidiously and increases in intensity and distribution over months. Although there may be no sensory loss initially, progressive trigeminal hypaesthesia becomes apparent. The pain is deep, aching and sometimes burning; it is rarely triggered and does not migrate about the face. The patient with this type of unilateral atypical facial pain is likely to harbour a neoplasm or infection at the base of the skull (Yonas & Jannettta 1980). Modern imaging techniques, especially the MR scan, have made early diagnosis much more likely (Tanaka et al 1987).

A third type of atypical facial pain is associated with a wide variety of autonomic changes in the face and borders on the cluster headache or vascular face pain syndromes. Whether or not it is a variant of the vascular face pains or just an example of the fact that the patients are never as clear-cut as the textbook descriptions is not known at this time.

The final type of unilateral atypical facial pain occurs without known antecedent. The patient complains of a burning, constant, usually circumscribed pain. Some report a superimposed jabbing component that may be triggered. There is no sensory loss, but touching the skin in the painful area is often very unpleasant. Such patients are again most commonly female, but usually younger than the bilateral atypical face pain sufferers. Significant behavioural and psychosocial dysfunction often predates the onset of the facial pain (Weddington & Blazer 1979). The behaviour of these patients is so different from that of sufferers from tic douloureux, that diagnostic tests such as pain drawings, Minnesota Multiphasic Personality Inventory or McGill Pain Questionnaires, as well as a brief interview that does not ask about the pain itself can allocate patients to the proper diagnostic group (Melzack et al 1986). In spite of the patient's painful behaviours, eating, talking and facial grooming are not often interrupted, as they are in patients with tic douloureux.

DIFFERENTIAL DIAGNOSIS

Vascular headache and face pain may be intermittent but consist of episodes lasting for hours with burning, dysaesthetic pain often associated with rhinitis, lacrimation, flushing and sweating. The pains may occur in clusters or may be random. They are not triggered and are not usually associated with sensory loss. A plethora of eponymous syndromes describe the variants of vascular pain; some atypical facial pain patients have a clearcut vascular component. The role of the sympathetic nervous system in such pain is unclear.

Myofascial pains originating in the muscles of mastication or temporomandibular joint (TMJ) pain may be hard to separate from each other but should not be confused with tic douloureux. The pain is lateral, is described as aching or cramping, is associated with local tenderness and may radiate up into the scalp or down into the neck. Local tenderness may mean that chewing or palpating the area causes pain; this should not be confused with triggering of pain in tic douloureux, in which the trigger site may be widely removed from the painful area. Sensory loss is never seen with TMJ or myofascial pain. Some patients diagnosed as having atypical facial pain may instead have myofascial or TMJ pain.

Local pathology in the paranasal sinuses, jaws, teeth or pharynx can cause severe pain which radiates from the region of injury. There is no sensory loss and the pain is not triggered by nonnoxious stimuli remote from the site of the pain. In contrast, a noxious stimulus causes the pain, which is usually described as throbbing, aching or burning but rarely as electric shock-like. Physical examination and appropriate imaging studies will usually reveal the pathological process causing the patient's pain. Local tenderness over the involved region with reproduction or augmentation of the pain is a helpful diagnostic sign.

LABORATORY TESTS

The patient with classical tic douloureux and no neurological abnormalities on careful examination does not need diagnostic tests to confirm the diagnosis. Patients who manifest neurological abnormalities or have some atypical features do require further assessment: magnetic resonance imaging (MRI) is by far the most valuable, but computerized tomography (CT) scanning is the next best alternative when MRI is not available. Carefully performed MR imaging can reveal the usual arterial loop impinging upon the trigeminal nerve as it exits the pons (Wong 1989; Tash 1989; Hutchins 1990; Sens 1991). The diagnosis of multiple sclerosis can also be confirmed. Other, very rare causes of tic douloureux, such as angiomas or tumours may also be detected on MRI or CT scan (Tsubaki 1989). Although the diagnosis and medical management of tic douloureux do not require an imaging study, an MRI with particular attention to the trigeminal nerve and lateral pons should be obtained prior to any surgical procedure. When indicated by the imaging study, further tests such as angiography or myelography may be appropriate.

It must be recognized, however, that even though the MRI is a very sensitive test that identifies the offending blood vessel, it is not a specific test, as approximately one-third of the patients, undergoing MRI for another diagnosis have a vessel impinging upon the trigeminal nerve (Tash 1989). At present, the major value of MRI is to identify the pathology in patients with tic douloureux.

The majority of patients with atypical facial pain have no abnormality on any diagnostic medical test. This is particularly true for the bilateral pain syndromes. MRI is the diagnostic study of choice for the evaluation of the patient with unilateral atypical facial pain. CT scanning can also be useful in the delineation of the osseous structures at the base of the skull. Psychometric and behavioural analysis and testing can be helpful in such patients and may point the way to successful therapeutic interventions.

TIME COURSE AND PROGNOSIS

The time course and prognosis of these two facial pain syndromes are distinctly different. Tic douloureux typically has an onset in older age, is intermittent, may have intervals of years between flurries of attacks and usually leads to total disruption of daily activities if untreated. Although spontaneous remissions can occur and last for years, they are not predictable and painful epochs usually become more frequent as the years go by. Medical or surgical therapy has a very high likelihood of producing complete relief of symptoms and the restoration of a healthy life pattern.

Atypical face pain usually occurs in a young or middle-aged adult. The symptoms are amazingly constant over time. Medical therapy is rarely effective; denervating operations usually make the patient's pain syndrome more severe. Over many years the patient seems to manifest less florid pain behaviour, but the somatic preoccupation, passive lifestyle and depression are long-term characteristics of these patients. Although tic patients may be depressed when they have their pain, the alleviation of their symptoms almost always results in prompt restoration of normal mood and behaviour. Atypical face pain patients are a source of great frustration to pain clinics, neurologists and neurosurgeons.

AETIOLOGY

TIC DOULOUREUX

A satisfactory explanation for the pain of tic douloureux is not possible at the present time. There are two distinct issues that must be addressed: is there any anatomical lesion, and, if so, where, and how does a structural lesion lead to the clinical phenomena that characterize tic?

Claims for the responsible anatomical lesions have ranged from the skin, dental structures, blood supply to the face and trigeminal nerve, peripheral branches of the nerve, gasserian ganglion, posterior root and brain stem nuclei of the trigeminal nerve. Mechanical compression of the gasserian ganglion by the carotid artery or bony structures has also been invoked. Several schools of thought are currently active: the structural lesion lies in the posterior root of the trigeminal nerve or pathology in the jaws irritates local nerves and leads to tic pain (Jannetta 1967; Ratner et al 1979; Roberts & Person 1979; Shaber & Krol 1980). Neither viewpoint can be proven to be the cause of all cases of tic, nor can their role be disproved in all patients. Indeed, a third viewpoint suggests that we have no identified anatomical substrates for tic douloureux (Gybels & Sweet 1989). Clinical observations have been utilized by the proponents of each school to support their viewpoints.

The observations of Jannetta and many other neurosurgeons have shown that the great majority (>85%) of patients with tic douloureux have compression of the trigeminal root adjacent to the pons, usually by an artery, occasionally a vein and rarely a small neoplasm (Jannetta 1967; Lazar & Kirkpatrick 1979; Burchiel et al 1981). When the pain is in the second or third trigeminal divisions, the usual finding is compression of the rostral and anterior portion of the nerve by the superior cerebellar artery. When first-division pain is present, the most frequent finding is cross-compression of the caudal and posterior portion of the trigeminal nerve by the anterior inferior cerebellar artery. Other vessels may occasionally be responsible for compression of the nerve (Jannetta 1976).

Surgeons have reported arteriovenous malformations in the cerebellopontine angle compressing the trigeminal nerve (Tsubaki 1989). Veins have been observed to run through and adjacent to the nerve and have been thought to be a cause of tic. A very low incidence of neurinoma or another neoplasm impinging upon or growing within the trigeminal nerve has also been reported. The lesion responsible for tic lies close to the pons, within a centimetre of the root entry-zone. Some surgeons have reported that lesions closer to Meckel's cave may be the cause of atypical facial pain, but this is not universally accepted.

Some still doubt the causal relationship between a lesion at the root entry-zone and tic douloureux. A small number of autopsy studies have been performed on patients who had tic douloureux; the findings have not been clearcut. A recent clinical and autopsy study by Hamlyn & King (1992) clarifies some of the ambiguities and, in conjunction with MRI studies, confirms the concept that vascular compression of the trigeminal root is the principal cause of tic douloureux. These authors not only carefully observed the site of compression by the vessel in their surgical patients, but also found no such indentation of the trigeminal nerve in autopsies on patients who did not have tic. When they perfused the vessels in cadavers, they could observe vessels adjacent to the nerve in 40% of their 50 specimens. This fits with the MRI observations of vessels adjacent to the nerves in about one third of patients who have had MRI studies for reasons other than face pain. However, the anatomical relationships at postmortem and during life are distinctly different. The arterial system collapses; the brain stem falls posteriorly in the supine cadaver; autopsy findings may not be relevant.

The patient with tic douloureux and multiple sclerosis has been seen to have a demyelinating plaque in the trigeminal posterior root both under the surgical microscope and in surgical specimens (Lazar & Kirkpatrick 1979). However, plaques have also been found in the descending trigeminal tract and nucleus and throughout the lemniscal system; it is not possible to state that a plaque in the root is either sufficient or necessary to cause tic douloureux. Indeed, there is no reason why a patient cannot have multiple sclerosis and an artery compressing the trigeminal nerve!

The evidence for cross-compression of the trigeminal nerve adjacent to the root entry-zone in patients with tic douloureux is overwhelming; the causal relation to tic is less clear. Very few patients without tic douloureux have a posterior fossa approach to the trigeminal nerve with opening of the arachnoid cisterns and visualisation of the nerve. Autopsy studies do not reveal anatomical relationships present during life. Changes in position of the patient's head during craniectomy can also alter anatomic relationships. Hence, we are unable at this time to ascertain if patients who do not have tic douloureux may have similar arterial cross-compression. Most of the neurosurgeons who have operated on a series of patients with tic douloureux have reported 5–10% of the patients do not have a visible lesion extrinsic to the nerve. The question of adequate exposure or interpretation of the findings can always be raised, but it seems to be true that not every patient with tic has a structural lesion in the posterior root of the trigeminal nerve. Neither do those without a structural lesion all have multiple sclerosis.

Another pathological theory invokes cavities in the jaws due to dentition loss and chronic infection as the aetiological agent. Ratner and his associates have published in the dental literature on this potential causation; questions remain about its validity (Schurmann et al 1972; Ratner 1979). Similar cavities have been described in patients who do not have any facial pain. Secondly, the response to therapy may or may not be prompt, leading to the questions of the role of spontaneous remission. Thirdly, a significant number of patients with tic douloureux do not appear to have the characteristic lesions described by Ratner. Again, the question of the adequacy of the search for the lesion can be raised. There is no question that active intraoral disease can be the site of a triggering stimulus for tic in a patient who has the disease; again, causality is not proven by this association.

None of the pathological observations explains the characteristics of the pain of tic douloureux. The neurophysiological basis of this disease remains an enigma; the lack of a good animal model hampers research on this topic. The theories for tic can be divided into 'central' and 'peripheral' aetiologies. The similarity of tic to focal epilepsy has been obvious to clinicians for many years. This led to the proposal that tic could be due to epileptiform activity in the trigeminal nucleus; the therapeutic efficacy of diphenylhydantoin seemed to support this concept of the physiological basis of tic douloureux. Studies which implicated deafferentation in the genesis of epilepsy led to the investigation of the effects of rhizotomy, neurectomy and tooth avulsion or pulpectomy upon the trigeminal system: deafferentation does lead to epileptiform firing patterns in the trigeminal descending nucleus. Chronic sensory abnormalities which look like pain, but not tic douloureux can ensue (Anderson et al 1971). Epileptogenic agents injected into the nucleus can also lead to abnormal electrical activity and pain; the resemblance to tic douloureux is a function of the agent used (Black 1970). Other studies utilizing epileptogenic agents suggested that exaggerated dorsal root reflexes and antidromic activity in the trigeminal nerve were associated with pain. Hypotheses involving concepts such as 'reverberating circuits', ephaptic connections and altered central connectivity due to deafferentation have also been proposed.

Our analysis of the phenomena to tic douloureux led us to the conclusion that both peripheral and central mechanisms were involved in the genesis of tic pain (Calvin et al 1977). As the triggering stimulus is known to be conducted by large myelinated axons and the report of pain is uniquely associated with activation of finely myelinated or unmyelinated A-delta or C-fibres, it is not possible to explain the pain on the basis of a lesion exclusively in one of these fibre systems or its central connections (Kugelberg & Lindblom 1959). Furthermore, there is a need to explain the sudden onset and cessation of pain, the separation of trigger-zone from the area of pain and the absence of sensory loss, even during the refractory period, which occurs after each jab of tic pain. We have proposed a mechanism which involves both disordered axonal function and alterations in central synaptic activity. Structural lesions affecting the trigeminal nerve begin the process; excessive attempts by the nervous system to regulate the abnormal activity result in the generation of tic pain. Human and animal experiments will be necessary to prove this or any other hypothesis; no other existing theory begins to explain the clinical phenomena. This theory does not require any one of the existing concepts of the structural pathology causing tic, nor can it be used to infer their validity.

ATYPICAL FACIAL PAIN

There have been few attempts to search for the physiological bases for the several varieties of atypical facial pain. It is likely that the several types of pain syndrome subsumed in this rubric have different mechanisms. Those unilateral pain syndromes that occur following nerve injury or secondary to nerve compression by a neoplasm (Yonas & Jannetta 1980; Tanaka 1987) suggest that axonal injury can be a cause. Yet, the majority of patients with trigeminal nerve injuries never develop atypical facial pain. Those with bilateral atypical facial pain have no evidence either from history, physical examination or laboratory testing of a neuropathic process.

It is possible that some patients with sensory changes induced by nerve injury or, perhaps, a subtle dysfunction of the nerves, may report a perturbation of sensation as 'pain' while other patients might describe the sensation as 'peculiar' but not painful. The role of such cognitive factors in chronic pain states is unclear. Obviously, therapies designed to reduce the perception of a noxious stimulation, i.e. cutting a nerve, will not help the patient who is labelling a distortion of sensation as painful.

THERAPY

PHARMACOTHERAPY

It is important to recognize that tic douloureux and atypical facial pain are central pain states, characterized by the absence of pathology in the painful area. Medications which suppress nociception, the pain due to tissue damage, do not have much value in the alleviation of tic or atypical facial pain, nor do the anticonvulsants which alleviate tic pain have any value in the management of pain due to tissue damage, such as a broken leg or abscessed tooth. Narcotics may be of short-term value during a crisis, but they are rarely adequate in the long-term management of tic or atypical facial pain. Many vitamins, tranquillizers and antidepressants have been claimed to be of value; all that is lacking is a shred of evidence of their

Table 39.2 Classification of atypical facial pains

I. Bilateral
II. Unilateral
   A. Nerve injury
   B. Nerve compression or irritation
   C. Vascular
   D. Unknown

Table 39.3 Medications useful for tic douloureux

Generic name	Brand names	Pill size	Usual dosage/day	Common side-effects
Carbamazepine	Tegretol	200 mg	600–1200 mg	Nausea, dizziness, somnolence, hepatic and haematopoetic dysfunction
Phenytoin	Dilantin Epanutin Epamin etc.	100 mg	300–500 mg	Nausea, dizziness, somnolence, ataxia, dermatitis
Chlorphenesin	Maolate	400 mg	800–2400 mg	Dizziness, somnolence
Mephenesin	Tolserol Tolseram	500 mg	5–15 g	Dizziness, nausea
Baclofen	Lioresal	10 mg	40–80 mg	Nausea, dizziness, confusion, drowsiness

efficacy. Spontaneous remissions are certainly responsible for some of these claims.

Tic douloureux

Reasonably good clinical studies have demonstrated the efficacy of two anticonvulsant drugs in the management of tic douloureux: diphenylhydantoin and carbamazepine (Crill 1973). Mephenesin and chlormephenesin may also be effective in some patients when the first two drugs cannot be tolerated or are not beneficial. Baclofen is also useful. Valproate has also been successful in a small series (Peiris et al 1980). A few other drugs have undergone limited trials: see Table 39.4.

Carbamazepine is the most likely drug to control tic douloureux; approximately 70% of patients will have significant pain relief. Although the incidence of side-effects is real, carbamazepine is not a dangerous drug, as is commonly believed. Haematological studies should be performed monthly for the first year of therapy and quarterly thereafter; a major fall in red blood count, white blood count or platelets mandates cessation of the drug; prompt restoration of normal indices can be expected. Haematosuppression usually occurs in the first 3 months of treatment; I have never seen a delayed reduction in blood elements. Carbamazepine can be a gastric irritant and should never be taken without some food or fluid. It is necessary to start at a dose of 100 mg (half a tablet) twice daily and increase by 100 mg every 2 days until a dose of 200 mg three times a day is reached. A small number of patients will get relief at a lower dose; the incremental dose should be stopped if pain relief occurs. After a week at 200 mg three times a day, if there are neither side-effects nor pain relief, the dosage is increased to 200 mg four times a day; the dose can eventually be increased to a total daily dose of 1800 mg. Higher doses have not added to the likelihood of pain relief.

Common side-effects are nausea, dizziness, slurred speech, ataxia and somnolence. If they occur in a patient who is getting good pain relief, the wisest course is to

Table 39.4 Medications for tic douloureux: recent experimental trials

	Number of patients	Controlled study	Good results	Comments
Oxcarbazepine[a]	6	No	6/6	All patients had failed CBZ and DPH
Mexiletine[b]	4	No	0/4	Two patients had failed DPH
Pimozide[c]	48	Yes	24/24	Better than CBZ
Oxcarbazepine[d]	13	No	13/13	Some intolerable side-effects
GP47779[d]	11	No	11/11	Some intolerable side-effects
Pimozide[e]	2	No	2/2	>3-year follow-up
Tocainide[f]	12	Yes	9/11	Similar to CBZ; can have lethal side-effects: NOT USED
L-Baclofen[g]	15	Yes	11/15	Better than racemic Baclofen
Tizanidine[h]	6	Yes	6/6	CBZ is better

[a]Zakrzewska 1989; [b]Pascual 1989; [c]Lechin 1989; [d]Farago 1987; [e]Lechin 1988; [f]Lindstrom 1986; [g]Fromm 1987; [h]Vilming 1986; CBZ = carbamazepine; DPH = phenytoin.

discontinue the drug completely for 24 hours and then resume therapy at a 200 mg lower dosage. About 25% of patients never get pain relief with carbamazepine; 25% get both pain relief and unacceptable side-effects. Therefore, 50% of patients with tic douloureux are successfully treated with this drug. Effective serum levels appear to be 24–43 μmol/l, although extensive data are lacking on this topic (Tomson et al 1980).

Diphenylhydantoin is the second-choice drug (Chinitz et al 1966). Approximately 25% of patients will get pain relief with therapeutic serum levels of 15–25 μg/ml. Side-effects will occur in 5–10% of the patients given this drug; somnolence, ataxia, dizziness, slurred speech and dermatitis are the most common. Diphenylhydantoin may be started at a dosage of 100 mg three times a day; after 3 weeks the serum level should be ascertained and the dosage adjusted so as to achieve a therapeutic blood level. Stable blood levels do not occur for several weeks unless a larger (1000 mg) loading dose is given; this is not usually indicated in the management of tic douloureux. When side-effects occur, the drug should be stopped completely for 24 hours and resumed at a 100 mg lower dose if it has been helpful in alleviating the tic pains.

Mephenesin and chlormephenesin have been available for over three decades; they are sometimes helpful but not as often as diphenylhydantoin or carbamazepine (King 1958). They appear to have a shorter duration of action and must be taken frequently. Side-effects are all too common. Baclofen appears to be effective against the pain of tic douloureux. A limited number of trials has been reported; side-effects have been frequent in my experience. The initial dose should be 5 mg three times a day, increasing to a maximum of 80 mg per day (Table 39.3).

Nonnarcotic analgesics and narcotics may be used during a crisis, but they should not be part of the long-term management of tic douloureux. There is no place for sedative-hypnotics, tranquillizers or antidepressants unless other conditions warrant their use. The efficacy of special diets, vitamin supplementation and other types of medications is totally unproven and their prescription is probably a waste of the patient's money and a false hope.

Nerve blocks

Local anaesthetics will temporarily block the pain of tic douloureux. Anaesthesia of either the trigger area or the painful area usually produces pain relief for the duration of the nerve block; a few patients will report long-term relief after one or more local nerve blocks. Blocking cervical and trigeminal divisions not in the painful or trigger areas will sometimes provide relief. Nerve blocks can also be used to allow the patient to experience analgesia and anaesthesia in a region of the face when neurectomy or total rhizotomy is planned; these are not usually optimal surgical strategies.

Alcohol blocks of the gasserian ganglion or peripheral branches of the trigeminal nerve have a long history in the management of tic douloureux. Highly skilled operators have reported series with good initial success and low complication rates. However, pain relief rarely lasts longer than 1 year and repeated alcohol blocks have increased morbidity and decreased success rates. The amount of hypalgesia and its distribution are difficult to control; most patients end up anaesthetic, not hypaesthetic, in the division of the ganglion or nerve injected. Alcohol injection is an out-of-date procedure when gangliolysis is available.

Tic douloureux is often thought by patients to be a disease of the part that hurts; hence they often visit medical and dental physicians and demand therapy aimed at the painful part. Ironically, pain in the nose never results in the extirpation of that portion of the face, yet pain in the teeth or jaw frequently leads to extraction of healthy teeth or needless endodontic surgery. Intraoral disease can trigger pain in the patient with tic douloureux and should be treated appropriately. Similarly, paranasal sinus drainage and surgical procedures will not cure tic.

Acupuncture is also touted by some as a method of controlling tic pain. No published study that I have seen demonstrates the efficacy of acupuncture for this disease. I believe that it is a cruel hoax to refer a patient with tic douloureux for acupuncture therapy, although no one is made worse and some patients want a trial of acupuncture before taking medicines or considering surgery.

The pharmacological management of atypical facial pain is inadequate. No drug has a significant likelihood of improving the complaint of pain, although many seem to have benefit for a small fraction of the patients. Tricyclic antidepressants (TCAs) are probably the most commonly prescribed; they may be beneficial not only because of their effect on neuropathic pains but also because of their effects on depression and sleep disturbance. The combination of a TCA and a phenothiazine (such as amitriptyline 75 mg at bedtime and fluphenazine 1 mg four times a day) has been effective for some patients. Other TCAs with different side-effects may be better tolerated in some patients. Side-effects are common and require gradual increments of medications and careful follow-up.

Mexiletine, a lidocaine-like drug that is absorbed from the gastrointestinal tract has been useful in a small number of patients. An initial dose of 150 mg once a day can be incremented to three times a day; as this is primarily an antiarrthymic drug, the patient's cardiovascular status must be monitored.

Local anaesthetics will stop the pain when the painful area is completely blocked. Repeated blocks do not give long-term success. There is no known efficacy for steroids of sympathetic blockade. The effects of a local block do not predict the long-term result of ablative surgery in patients with atypical facial pain.

SURGICAL THERAPY

Tic Douloureux

A surgical procedure is warranted for tic douloureux only when a thorough trial of pharmacological therapy has failed. However, the prudent physician should not delay offering the patient surgical means of pain relief when drugs produce unacceptable side-effects or inadequate pain relief. Surgery is very rarely helpful for atypical facial pain. Innumerable surgical strategies have been used for tic but only two remain appropriate for the initial management of tic douloureux by operative means: gangliolysis and suboccipital craniectomy with decompression of the trigeminal nerve.

Cryotherapy

One method of damaging the peripheral branches of the trigeminal nerve is cryotherapy: using a cooling probe to render the region anaesthetic. Several papers indicate that this results in pain relief that usually does not last 1 year, as well as transient sensory loss (Zakrzewska 1987; Politis 1988; Juniper 1991). Most authors report the use of a C-arm fluoroscope and a specialized stimulator-lesion maker, so the technology required is no less than that needed for gangliolysis, save for local anaesthesia versus general anaesthesia during the procedure. Since the results are far less satisfactory than gangliolysis, this procedure is probably not as useful.

Gangliolysis

Gangliolysis is the most recent development in a long series of neurodestructive procedures to alleviate tic pain (Sweet & Wespic 1974). Peripheral nerve avulsions, alcohol injections, subtemporal rhizotomy, posterior rhizotomy and descending trigeminal tractotomy have all been supplanted by gangliolysis as primary procedures. These procedures have in common the goal of producing a sensory deficit in the painful region. The major long-term complications (anaesthesia dolorosa, painful paraesthesiae and neuroparalytic keratitis) are directly related to the amount of sensory deficit produced. Gangliolysis offers the lowest rate of operative complication (less than 0.5%), the most control over the extent and density of sensory loss, good long-term pain relief and lowest cost.

This procedure is performed under fluoroscopic control utilizing brief, general anaesthesia. Atropine or glycopyrrolate are administered intravenously to block the vagal response that can occur with the introduction of a needle into foramen ovale. The cheek is cleansed and a skin wheal made with local anaesthetic 2.5 cm lateral to the corner of the mouth in the occlusal plane. Intravenous Propafol is, in my opinion, the best available short-acting anaesthetic but many have reported using hexabarbital and other medications. An insulated needle is placed through the skin wheal into foramen ovale using the fluoroscope to insure correct placement. The patient is then allowed to awaken. Stimulation with a weak electrical current at 60 Hz is used to adjust the needle tip so as to evoke paresthesiae in the region of the pain or trigger zone. When a suitable position has been achieved, the patient is again anaesthetized and a radiofrequency lesion is made using a thermistor in the electrode tip to monitor temperature precisely. The patient is again allowed to awaken and sensory testing with a pin prick is used to evaluate the extent of the lesion. Only mild difference from the contralateral side is required. The patient can be reanaesthetized and another lesion made if the first is inadequate. The entire process takes less than 1 hour in most patients and they can leave the hospital within 2 hours after the procedure has been completed.

Numerous case series and review articles have been written about radiofrequency gangliolysis in the past 18 years. It is by far the most commonly reported operation in the modern neurosurgical literature; cases presented in large series exceed 10 000 (Sweet 1988). My own experience in about 300 procedures and a review of the larger series indicates that over 80% of the patients will have at least 1 year of pain relief and at least 50% will have 5 years of pain relief; complications are less than 0.5% and mortality is nil. Aiming for a minimally adequate lesion greatly reduces the risk of painful paraesthesiae or anaesthesia dolorosa; it probably does increase the likelihood of a pain recurrence. Radiofrequency gangliolysis can be repeated whenever the pain recurs with an equally good chance of pain relief as after the first operation. A lesion involving the first division does carry the risk of corneal anaesthesia and the possibility of neuroparalytic keratitis. Patients with multiple sclerosis causing tic douloureux can expect similar results to those with vascular compression, although the recurrence rate may be somewhat higher.

A modification of gangliolysis was introduced by Hakansson: a smaller needle is introduced into the arachnoid cistern of the gasserian ganglion via foramen ovale and a small (0.1–0.3 ml) volume of glycerol instilled (Hakansson 1981). Patient cooperation is not required, unlike radiofrequency gangliolysis, and the procedure can be done under sedation or light general anaesthesia. Although Hakansson claimed wonderful results, others have not been able to obtain results as good as those with radiofrequency gangliolysis (Lundsford & Bennet 1984; Sweet & Poletti 1985; Saini 1987; Dieckmann et al 1987; Young 1988; Burchiel 1988). There remain some, however, who prefer glycerol to radiofrequency and report better results in their hands. Since glycerol is less likely to produce corneal anaesthesia than is a radiofrequency first-division lesion, some advocate glycerol for first-division pain only (Sweet 1988). A debate still rages about the efficacy and complications or glycerol gangliolysis. Perhaps some of the variance is related to the purity of the injectate.

A third method of percutaneously damaging the gasserian ganglion and its rootlets has been developed by Mullan & Lichtor: a 14 gauge needle is introduced into the gasserian ganglion via foramen ovale and a #4 Fogarty balloon catheter is passed into Meckel's cave and inflated for 1–10 minutes (Mullan & Lichtor 1983). Several hundred cases have thus far been reported with results similar to those obtained with other gangliolysis methods (Meglio et al 1987; Lobato et al 1990). This procedure requires no patient cooperation or intraoperative evaluation and is readily accomplished under general anaesthesia. The extent of the sensory loss produced is not predictable although it is usually mild. Further trials of this technique and long-term follow-up studies will be required to assess its proper place in the treatment of tic douloureux.

Gangliolysis by one method or another is particularly useful in the elderly or debilitated patient with tic douloureux. The patient's bleeding and clotting status should be ascertained and corrected preoperatively with any of the techniques. The results of surgical neurectomy or rhizotomy are not as good as those with gangliolysis and the former are more hazardous, more costly and lead to more sensory loss. It probably is not productive to argue with one's neurosurgeon as to which method of gangliolysis he or she utilizes.

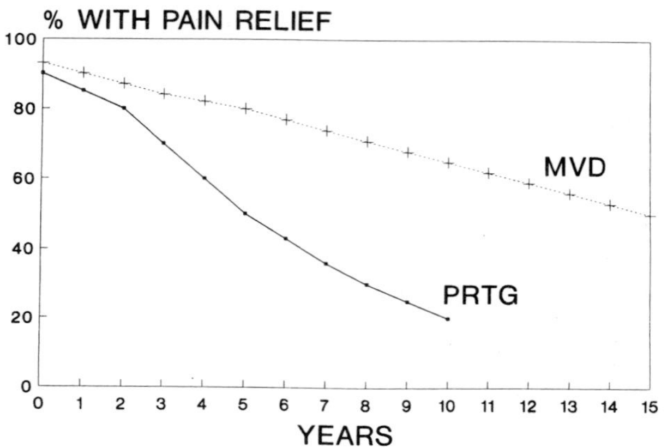

Fig. 39.1 Results of microvascular decompression (MVD) and percutaneous radio-frequency trigeminal gangliolysis (PTRG) for tic douloureux. Complete pain relief is plotted against time in years following initial surgery. Neither operation leads to permanent cure for most patients. Data derived from published reports of large series and personal experience.

Suboccipital craniotomy with microvascular decompression

Suboccipital craniotomy with microvascular decompression (MVD) of the trigeminal nerve has proven to be a highly successful operation for tic douloureux (Apfelbaum 1977; Burchiel 1988; Bederson 1989). Jannetta (1967, 1976), although not the first to observe arterial compression at the root entry zone, was the neurosurgeon who introduced this operation to modern neurosurgery. This procedure is performed under general anaesthesia via a small lateral retroauricular craniotomy or craniectomy. Using the operating microscope, the cerebellum is retracted medially and inferiorly to expose the trigeminal nerve as it courses from Meckel's cave to the pons. Greater than 90% of the patients will have clear-cut impingement on the nerve by an artery or vein, or sometimes a combination of the two. A small tumour or osseous abnormality may be found in 1–2%. Many neurosurgeons have reported that a small fraction of the patients with tic douloureux have no demonstrable pathology. The usual finding is an ectatic superior cerebellar artery that is trapped under the nerve; this leads to second- and third-division pain. Most patients with first-division pain have a loop of the anterior inferior cerebellar artery impinging upon the caudal part of the nerve. The arachnoid is opened and the nerve and vessel separated. A small pledget of muscle or synthetic fibre such as Ivalon or Dacron is placed between the nerve and the vessel to prevent recompression. Veins are usually divided, as they are harder to mobilize and usually can be sacrificed without neurological dysfunction. Prior surgical manipulations may adversely influence the outcome from this operation (Barba & Alksne 1984; Bederson & Wilson 1989).

In the small fraction of patients in whom an offending lesion is not found, a partial rhizotomy should be performed. Exactly how much of the nerve needs to be cut is unclear: The pre-MVD literature suggested that long-term cure of tic pain was best when major portions of the root were transected; however, the more sensory loss is produced, the greater the likelihood of anaesthesia dolorosa or painful paraesthesiae. If the tic pain recurs, reexploration can be undertaken. Many of the patients with a recurrence do not appear to have a new compression of the nerve and are best managed by partial rhizotomy.

The history of the risks and results of MVD is revealing, as it is typical for new surgical procedures. The 1-year success rate (success = no tic pain) is about 85%. Early reports, including prior versions of this chapter, suggested that there were no late failures. However, longer-term studies have shown that the 5-year success rate is about 80% and that there is a 2–3% failure rate per annum after that. This results in a half-life of MVD of about 15 years.

Complications for MVD are well described in many large and small series. There is little question that those who frequently operate with the microscope around the cranial nerves can expect fewer complications than those less practised. The mortality rate is about 0.5% in reported series, permanent cranial nerve complications occur in 5–10% and other significant complications in about 10% (Burchiel et al 1981; Bederson & Wilson 1989).

An excellent review of surgical treatment for tic can be found in Gybels & Sweet (1989).

Peripheral nerve avulsions

Peripheral nerve avulsions should be offered only when gangliolysis has failed and the patient cannot or will not tolerate an intracranial procedure. They result in dense sensory loss and rarely provide more than a year or two of pain relief. Repeat avulsions are even less likely to be successful. Compression or decompression of the gasserian ganglion via the subtemporal approach are outmoded; pain relief is unpredictable; surgical morbidity is as high or higher than a posterior fossa approach to the trigeminal nerve. Posterior fossa subtotal rhizotomy is the procedure of choice if a structural lesion cannot be identified; when MVD fails to provide long-term relief and reexploration does not reveal an anatomic lesion compressing the nerve, rhizotomy is the most reasonable alternative.

Patients who have failed to get pain relief with any of the above operations can be offered descending trigeminal tractotomy or trigeminal nucleotomy. These procedures result in loss of pain and temperature sensation on the ipsilateral side of the face and do not alter touch perception. They are performed under general anaesthesia via a C1–2 laminectomy; long-term statistical data are sparse for tic patients, but they have been very successful in a small number of patients in our institution and reported elsewhere.

The choice of operative procedure should be based on the patient's full understanding of the goals, risks and outcomes for each of the alternatives. Patients must have a thorough diagnostic evaluation and trial of medications before they are offered any type of surgical procedure. The intensity of tic douloureux mandates careful attention by the physician to the patient's physical and emotional state; uncontrolled pain can lead to suicide. It is important to recognize that only surgical procedures can cure tic douloureux; available medications offer only palliation. One can hope that a more reliable pharmacological method of curing this excruciating pain can be developed when the neurophysiological basis of tic is understood.

Atypical facial pain

It is prudent to avoid performing ablative surgical procedures on patients with atypical facial pain. Those operations that involve additional denervation, such as nerve avulsions, gangliolysis, and rhizotomy usually fail to relieve the existing pain and result in additional complaints about both pain and numbness. Some neurosurgeons have reported that patients with unilateral atypical facial pain have a lesion (blood vessel, rarely tumour) that is compressing the trigeminal nerve distal to the juxtapontine site of the lesion responsible for tic douloureux. Others have disputed this finding.

Some successes in patients with unilateral atypical facial pain have been reported following chronic stimulation of the gasserian ganglion as reported by Meyerson & Hakansson (1980) and Lazorthes (1987). A stimulating electrode can be introduced either percutaneously or via a temporal craniotomy and connected to a stimulus generator implanted on the chest wall. It is not clear how to select patients for this operation; about two-thirds seem to have good long-term results. Trigeminal tractotomy or nucleotomy have also been used with variable results in a small number of patients.

REFERENCES

Anderson L S, Black R G, Abraham J, Ward, A A Jr 1971 Neuronal hyperactivity in experimental trigeminal deafferentation. Journal of Neurosurgery 34: 444–452

Apfelbaum R I 1977 A comparison of percutaneous radiofrequency trigeminal neurolysis and microvascular decompression of the trigeminal nerve for the treatment of tic douloureux. Neurosurgery 1: 16–21

Apfelbaum R I 1978 Technical considerations for facilitation of selective percutaneous radiofrequency neurolysis of the trigeminal nerve. Neurosurgery 3: 396–399

Baldwin N G, Sahni K S, Jensen M E et al 1991 Association of vascular compression in trigeminal neuralgia versus other 'facial pain syndromes' by magnetic resonance imaging. Surgical Neurology 36: 447–452

Barba D Alksne J F 1984 Success of microvascular decompressions with and without prior surgical therapy for trigeminal neuralgia. Journal of Neurosurgery 60: 104–107

Bederson J B Wilson C B 1989 Evaluation of microvascular decompression and partial sensory rhizotomy in 252 cases of trigeminal neuralgia. Journal of Neurosurgery 71: 359–367

Black R G 1970 Trigeminal pain. In: Crue B L (ed) Pain and suffering. C C Thomas, Springfield, p 119–137

Burchiel K J 1988 Percutaneous retrogasserian glycerol rhizolysis in the management of trigeminal neuralgia. Journal of Neurosurgery 69: 361–366

Burchiel K J, Steege T D, Howe J F, Loeser J D 1981 Comparison of percutaneous radiofrequency gangliolysis and microvascular decompression for the surgical management of tic douloureux. Neurosurgery 9: 111–119

Burchiel K J, Clarke H, Haglund M, Loeser J D 1988 Long-term efficacy of microvascular decompression in trigeminal neuralgia. Journal of Neurosurgery 69: 35–38

Calvin W H, Loeser J D, Howe J F 1977 A neurophysiological theory for the pain mechanism of tic douloureux. Pain 3: 147–154

Chinitz A, Seelinger D F, Greenhouse A H 1966 Anticonvulsant therapy in trigeminal neuralgia. American Journal of Medical Science 252: 62–67

Crill W 1973 Carbamazepine. Annals of Internal Medicine 79: 79–80

Dieckmann G, Bockermann V, Heyer C, Henning J, Roesen M 1987a Five-and-a-half years' experience with percutaneous retrogasserian glycerol rhizotomy in treatment of trigeminal neuralgia. Applied Neurophysiology 50: 401–413

Dieckmann G, Veras G, Sogabe K 1987b Retrogasserian glycerol

injection or percutaneous stimulation in the treatment of typical and atypical trigeminal pain. Neurology Research 9: 48–49
Farago F 1987 Trigeminal neuralgia: its treatment with two new carbamazepine analogues. European Neurology 26: 73–83
Fromm G H, Terrence C F 1987 Comparison of L-baclofen and racemic baclofen in trigeminal neuralgia. Neurology 37: 1725–1728
Gybels J M, Sweet W H 1989 Neurosurgical treatment of persisting pain. Pain and headache, vol 11. Karger, Basel, p 442
Hakansson S 1981 Trigeminal neuralgia treated by injection of glycerol into the trigeminal cistern. Neurosurgery 9: 638–646
Hamlin P J, King T T 1992 Neurovascular compression in trigeminal neuralgia: a clinical and anatomical study. Journal of Neurosurgery 76: 948–954
Hutchins L G, Harnsberger H R, Jacobs J M, Apfelbaum R I 1990 Trigeminal neuralgia (tic douloureux): MR imaging assessment. Radiology 175: 837–841
Jannetta P J 1967 Arterial compression of the trigeminal nerve at the pons in patients with trigeminal neuralgia. Journal of Neurosurgery 26: 159–162
Jannetta P J 1976 Microsurgical approach to the trigeminal nerve for tic douloureux. Progress in Neurological Surgery 7: 180–200
Juniper R P 1991 Trigeminal neuralgia – treatment of the third division by radiologically controlled cryoblockade of the inferior dental nerve at the mandibular lingula: a study of 31 cases. British Journal of Oral and Maxillofacial Surgery 29: 154–158
King R B 1958 The medical control of tic douloureux. Journal of Neurosurgery 15: 290–298
King R B 1967 Evidence for a central etiology of tic douloureux. Journal of Neurosurgery (suppl) 26: 175–180
Kugelberg E, Lindblom U 1959 The mechanism of the pain in trigeminal neuralgia. Journal of Neurology, Neurosurgery and Psychiatry 22: 36–43
Kuhner A 1988 The value of destructive surgery of the trigeminal nerve in atypical facial pain. Neurochirurgia 31: 210–212
Lazar M L, Kirkpatrick J B 1979 Trigeminal neuralgia and multiple sclerosis: demonstration of the plaque in an operative case. Neurosurgery 5: 711–717
Lazorthes Y, Armengaud J P, Da Motta M 1987 Chronic stimulation of the gasserian ganglion for treatment of atypical facial neuralgia. Pacing Clinical Electrophysiology 10: 257–265
Lechin F, van der Dijs B, Amat J et al 1988 Definite and sustained improvement with pimozide of two patients with severe trigeminal neuralgia. Journal of Medicine 19: 243–256
Lechin F, van der Dijs B, Lechin M E et al 1989 Pimozide therapy for trigeminal neuralgia. Archives of Neurology 46: 960–963
Lindstrom P, Lindblom U 1987 The analgesic effect of tocainide in trigeminal neuralgia. Pain 28: 45–50
Lobato R D, Rivas J J, Sarabia R, Lamas E 1990 Percutaneous microcompression of the gasserian ganglion for trigeminal neuralgia. Journal of Neurosurgery 72: 546–553
Lundsford L D, Bennett M H 1984 Percutaneous retrogasserian glycerol rhizotomy for tic douloureux part I. Neurosurgery 14: 424–429
Meglio M, Cioni B, d'Annunzio V 1987 Percutaneous microcompression of the gasserian ganglion: personal experience. Acta Neurochirurgica (suppl 39) 142–143
Melzack R, Terrence C, Fromm G, Amsel R 1986 Trigeminal neuralgia and atypical facial pain: use of the McGill Pain Questionnaire for discrimination and diagnosis. Pain 27: 297–302
Menzel J, Piotrowski W, Penzholz H 1975 Long-term results of gasserian ganglion electrocoagulation. Journal of Neurosurgery 42: 140–143
Meyerson B A, Hakansson S 1980 Alleviation of atypical trigeminal pain by stimulation of the gasserian ganglion via an implanted electrode. Acta Neurochirurgica (suppl) 30: 303–309
Mullan S, Lichtor T 1983 Percutaneous microcompression of the trigeminal ganglion for trigeminal neuralgia. Journal of Neurosurgery 59: 1007–1012
Pascual J, Berciano J 1989 Failure of Mexiletine to control trigeminal neuralgia. Headache 29: 517–518
Peiris J B, Perera G L S, Devendra S V, Lionel N D W 1980 Sodium valproate in trigeminal neuralgia. Medical Journal of Australia 2: 278
Politis C, Adriaensen H, Bossuyt M, Fossion E 1988 The management of trigeminal neuralgia with cryotherapy. Acta Stomatologica Belgica 85: 197–205
Ratner E J, Person P, Kleinman D J, Shklar G, Socransky S S 1979 Jawbone cavities and trigeminal and atypical facial neuralgias. Oral Surgery 48: 3–20
Roberts A M, Person P 1979 Etiology and treatment of idiopathic trigeminal and atypical facial neuralgias. Oral Surgery 48: 298–308
Saini S S 1987 Retrogasserian anhydrous glycerol injection therapy in trigeminal neuralgia: observations in 552 patients. Journal of Neurology, Neurosurgery and Psychiatry 50: 1536–1538
Schurmann K, Butz M, Brock M 1972 Temporal retrogasserian resection of trigeminal root versus controlled elective percutaneous electrocoagulation of the ganglion of Gasser in the treatment of trigeminal neuralgia. Acta Neurochirurgica 26: 33–53
Sens M A A, Higer H P 1991 MRI of trigeminal neuralgia: initial clinical results in patients with vascular compression of the trigeminal nerve. Neurosurgical Review 14: 69–73
Shaber E P, Krol A J 1980 Trigeminal neuralgia – a new treatment concept. Oral Surgery 49: 286–293
Siegfried J 1977 500 percutaneous thermocoagulations of the gasserian ganglion for trigeminal pain. Surgical Neurology 8: 126–131·
Sindou M, Keravel Y 1979 Thermocoagulation percutanee du trijumeau dans le traitement de la neuralgia faciale essentielle. Neurochirurgie 25: 166–172
Stookey B, Ransohoff J 1959 Trigeminal neuralgia. Its history and treatment C C Thomas, Springfield
Stowsand D, Markakis E, Laubner P 1973 Zur Electrocoagulation des ganglion gasseri bei der idiopathischen trigeminusneuralgie.
Sweet W H 1988 Percutaneous methods for the treatment of trigeminal neuralgia and other faciocephalic pain; comparison with microvascular decompression. Seminars in Neurology 8: 272–279
Sweet W H, Poletti C E 1985 Problems with reterogasserian glycerol in the treatment of trigeminal neuralgia. Applied Neurophysiology 48: 252–257
Sweet W H, Wespic J G 1974 Controlled thermocoagulation of trigeminal ganglion and rootlets for differential destruction of pain fibres. Journal of Neurosurgery 40: 143–156
Tanaka A, Takaki T, Maruta Y 1987 Neurinoma of the trigeminal root presenting as atypical trigeminal neuralgia: diagnostic values of orbicularis oculi reflex and magnetic resonance imaging. A case report. Neurosurgery 21: 733–736
Tash R R, Sze G, Leslie D R 1989 Trigeminal neuralgia: MR imaging features. Radiology 172: 767–770
Tomson T, Tybring G, Bertilsson L, Ekbom K, Rane A 1980 Carbamazepine in trigeminal neuralgia: clinical effects in relation to plasma-concentration. Uppsala Journal of Medical Science (suppl) 31: 45–46
Tsubaki S, Fukushima T, Tamagawa T et al 1989 Parapontine trigeminal cryptic angiomas presenting as trigeminal neuralgia. Journal of Neurosurgery 71: 368–374
Vilming S T, Lyberg T, Lataste X 1986 Tizanidine in the management of trigeminal neuralgia. Cephalalgia 6: 181–182
Weddington W N, Blazer D 1979 Atypical facial pain and trigeminal neuralgia: a comparison study. Psychosomatics 20; 348–356
Wong, B Y, Steinberg G K, Rosen Larry 1989 Magnetic resonance imaging of vascular compression in trigeminal neuralgia. Journal of Neurosurgery 70: 132–134
Yonas H, Jannetta P J 1980 Neurinoma of the trigeminal root and atypical trigeminal neuralgia: their commonality. Neurosurgery 6: 273–277
Young R F 1988 Glycerol rhizolysis for treatment of trigeminal neuralgia. Journal of Neurosurgery 9: 39–45
Zakrzewska J M 1987 Cryotherapy in the management of paroxysmal trigeminal neuralgia. Journal of Neurology, Neurosurgery and Psychiatry 50: 485–487
Zakrzewska J M, Patsalos P N 1989 Oxcarbazepine: a new drug in the management of intractable trigeminal neuralgia. Journal of Neurology, Neurosurgery and Psychiatry 52: 472–476

40. Nerve root damage and arachnoiditis

David Dubuisson

It is appealing to be able to diagnose one or more sites of nerve root compression as the cause of a patient's chronic pain. The great majority of patients with root compression will be relieved of their symptoms eventually, either by simple conservative measures and passage of time, or by a decompressive operation. A large population of chronic pain sufferers fall into the category of failed back or neck surgery, and many of them may, on reinvestigation, turn out to have problems amenable to treatment. Close attention to the history, details of the neurological examination, and radiological findings will suffice in most cases to determine whether the spaces around spinal roots have been made as anatomically correct as possible. It often happens that efforts directed at a single root have led the physician to ignore relevant problems at other neighbouring levels of the spine. It is also frequent to find pain patients and their referring physicians who are too quickly convinced that something is bothering a nerve root, and if only a surgical exploration were done, everything would be solved. It is important for clinicians with special interest in chronic pain to be wary of the abuse of surgery in such patients, but at the same time to be willing to seek objective evidence of root compression. Again, the clinical history, examination, and radiology will point the way to proper care for the patient, often avoiding needless additional tests or surgery. The first half of the present chapter gives most of the salient details needed to investigate or reinvestigate possible nerve root problems.

An unfortunate and more difficult problem of pain management is the patient whose underlying condition and failed surgery have resulted in a chronic, intractable state of nerve root damage. In some instances, the condition known as arachnoiditis is present. Chronic root damage and arachnoiditis are among the most frequent, and difficult to treat, causes of severe chronic pain.

Often, pain is not the only issue at stake in cases of root damage and arachnoiditis. Muscle weakness, loss of sensation, gait disorder, or loss of bowel and bladder control may supervene and, in some instances, direct the further approach to management. The neurological examination should be carefully and repeatedly documented in these patients. Progression of neurological damage might require surgery even at a time when pain is resolving.

In the assessment, careful thought must be given to the number and location of roots involved. A common but unreliable approach is to investigate and treat as if the patient's pain were due entirely to damage of a single nerve root. In the author's practice, few patients complaining of pain in the back, neck or extremities will ultimately be shown to have an isolated root lesion as the cause of their symptoms. Clinics that treat intractable pain may see even fewer patients whose complaints result from damage of only one root. The underlying disease processes causing root compression tend, especially in the older population, to occur at multiple levels of the spine. Sometimes previous surgery or other invasive treatment measures have increased the extent of the problem. One lesson that we are learning especially well in the era of computerized imaging is that spondylosis is often far more extensive than we anticipate on first meeting a new patient with root problems.

SIGNS AND SYMPTOMS

The essential quality of pain associated with root damage is referral along the peripheral distribution of fibres in the root. In many cases but not in all, this follows one of the dermatomes down the arm or leg or around the trunk. When a patient describes pain radiating down an extremity or in a segment of the chest or abdomen, it is important to record the exact distribution of pain on several occasions when it is actually present. It is useful to do this on diagrams which do not depict peripheral nerve territories or dermatomes. Plain diagrams counteract the clinician's urge to make the findings fit neatly into his own concept of what is happening. Comparison with standard charts can be made later if necessary.

The cutaneous afferent distributions of the spinal nerves are not yet adequately defined in humans. The dermatomes are certainly not constant from individual to individual (see Foerster 1933) and no two dermatomal charts agree in all details. There is particular confusion about the cervicothoracic and lumbosacral junctions. Not all authors agree, for instance, that the second and third thoracic dermatomes involve the arm or that the fourth lumbar and second sacral dermatomes extend to the toes. Some charts show the fourth and fifth lumbar dermatomes spiralling across the anterior thigh; others place the second lumbar dermatome there (see Fig. 40.1). These issues have not been resolved. Lack of agreement of dermatomal charts, frustrating for the clinician, is due to the various methods used to define the dermatomes. Head & Campbell (1900) devised a dermatomal chart based on cutaneous eruptions in herpes zoster. It was assumed that the lesions were confined to single dorsal root ganglia, although it is now known that the lesions of herpes zoster may also involve the spinal cord (Adams 1976). Head & Campbell showed dermatomes with contiguous borders but Sherrington's (1898) studies in monkeys made it clear that extensive overlap was present. Subsequently, Foerster (1933) revised the dermatomes in accord with his examination of a series of patients in whom he had sectioned several adjacent dorsal roots, leaving a zone of remaining skin sensation. In addition, Foerster used electrical stimulation of the distal end of divided dorsal roots to produce cutaneous vasodilatation which approximated the dermatome. Like Sherrington, he found large overlapping dermatomes (Figs 40.1 and 40.2). In zones of remaining sensation, the borders for complete anaesthesia were smaller than those for analgesia with some preservation of touch sensation. Individual variations in the size and shape of isolated dermatomes were frequent. Some 60 years later, Foerster's diagrams still provide some of our best information about the extent and variability of the dermatomes in man. As pointed out by White & Sweet (1969), these experiments are not likely to be repeated by any modern surgeon because it is now appreciated that extensive deafferentation of a limb makes it useless and may add to the patient's pain.

In some instances, root compression by herniated intervertebral discs may produce distinct areas of sensory loss. On this basis, Keegan & Garrett (1948) constructed a map of the dermatomes which depicted them as sharply demarcated bands extending to the midline in front and back. In some areas, the zones of hyposensitivity to pinscratch extended much farther proximally than Foerster's maps had indicated. The precise organization of dermatomes shown by Keegan & Garrett has received little experimental confirmation. Instead, physiological studies in monkeys (Dykes & Terzis 1981) suggest that the cutaneous region served by each spinal nerve root is even wider and more variable in location than that envisaged by Sherrington or Foerster. The apparent size of an isolated dermatome also depends on the integrity of distant roots

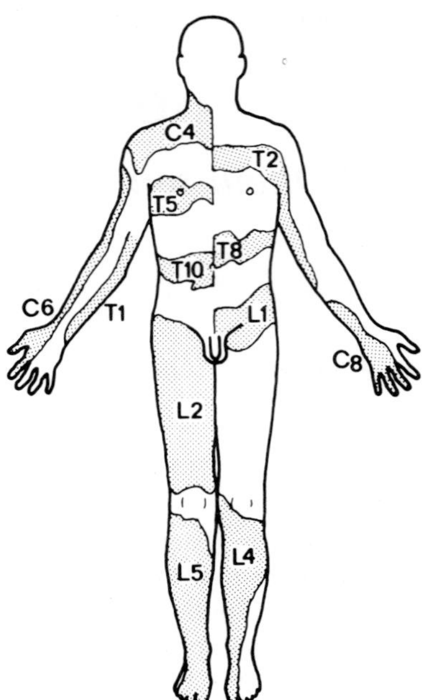

Fig. 40.1 Examples of dermatomes isolated by multiple root section: anterior aspect (after Foerster 1933).

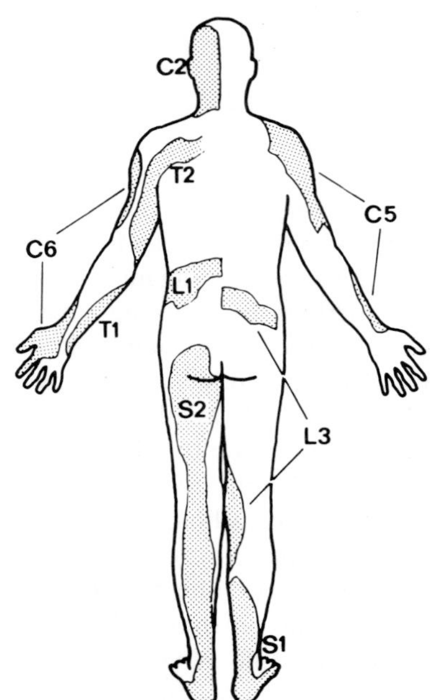

Fig. 40.2 Further examples of dermatomes isolated by multiple root section: posterior aspect (after Foerster 1933).

and of the Lissauer tract (Kirk & Denny-Brown 1970; Denny-Brown et al 1973).

The segmental distributions in muscle, fascia and joints are less well known. It is known that a radicular pattern of pain may result from disease of a spinal apophyseal (facet) joint. The pattern of pain may be difficult to interpret, since each facet joint is innervated by branches of two nerve roots. Certainly the pattern of innervation in muscles and other deep structures does not conform strictly to the overlying dermatomes. Kellgren (1939) injected hypertonic saline into the paraspinous muscles and ligaments to produce pain which was referred in segmental patterns. His map of deep segmental sensory innervations suggested that some myotomes and sclerotomes in the vicinity of the cervicothoracic and lumbosacral junctions were confined to the trunk while the corresponding dermatomes extended down the leg or arm. A clinical situation which illustrates this principle is pain referred to the anterior chest in compression of lower cervical roots (D Davis 1957). The serratus anterior and pectoral muscles are innervated by these roots while the corresponding dermatomes are restricted to the arm and hand. Charts of myotomes and sclerotomes are available (Inman & Saunders 1944) but perhaps not widely used, due to the difficulty of applying stimuli accurately to deep structures. In a clinical setting, involvement of muscle is usually detected as weakness, decreased bulk, visible fasciculation or an electromyographic change. A detailed compilation of segmental muscle innervations is given by Kendall et al (1971) in their excellent monograph on muscle function and testing.

SPECIFIC ROOT LESIONS

SEVENTH CRANIAL NERVE (NERVUS INTERMEDIUS COMPONENT)

The nervus intermedius, a component of the seventh cranial nerve, is known to contain sensory afferents whose cell bodies are located in the geniculate ganglion in the roof of the temporal bone. These axons supply part of the external auditory canal and tympanic membrane, the skin in the angle between ear and mastoid process, the tonsillar region and some other deep structures of the head and neck. The nervus intermedius may be involved in attacks of pain referred to the ear. Recurrent stabbing or shooting pain of a paroxysmal nature felt deep in the ear and sometimes in the ipsilateral face, neck or occiput suggests the possibility of *geniculate neuralgia*. The condition is not likely to be encountered in most clinical practices because of its rarity. Stimulating or cutting the nervus intermedius distinguishes the condition from glossopharyngeal neuralgia.

Patients with geniculate neuralgia are typically young or middle-aged adults. In most cases, a vesicular rash in the external ear and mastoid, typical of herpes zoster, precedes the onset of pain by several days. This has been called the Ramsay Hunt syndrome when it is accompanied by ipsilateral facial paralysis. Attacks of pain lasting seconds, minutes or sometimes hours may be entirely spontaneous. Less commonly they can be triggered by touching the external ear canal. Dull background pain may persist between attacks. Other possible symptoms include tenderness in or near the external ear, salivation, nasal discharge, tinnitus, vertigo or a bitter taste during attacks. Further details of several cases are summarised in the volume by White & Sweet (1969).

NINTH AND TENTH CRANIAL NERVES

Pain in the afferent distribution of the glossopharyngeal and vagus nerves may be felt in the larynx, base of the tongue, tonsillar region, ear and occasionally ipsilateral face, neck or scalp. Paroxysms of pain of unknown aetiology occurring in this distribution may be due to *glossopharyngeal neuralgia*, also known as vagoglossopharyngeal neuralgia in recognition of the role of the upper vagal rootlets (Robson & Bonica 1950; White & Sweet 1969). The uncommon variant known as *neuralgia of the superior laryngeal nerve* (vagus nerve neuralgia) is a syndrome of pain around the thyroid cartilage and pyriform sinus. Pure glossopharyngeal neuralgia is more likely to be felt in the tonsillar region. The attacks are usually described as stabbing, sharp, 'like a knife', 'like an electric shock', and sometimes hot or burning. Their intensity ranges from mild to severe. The attacks are probably less intense than typical bouts of trigeminal neuralgia, which is 70–100 times as common (Rushton et al 1981). Patients with glossopharyngeal neuralgia are almost always above the age of 20. Men and women are about equally affected. There is a slight predominance of left-sided cases in most large series. Attacks are bilateral in less than 2% of cases. Individual attacks commonly last seconds or minutes and rarely occur at night (Deparis 1968). Constant dull aching, burning or pressure may persist between attacks (Rushton et al 1981). It is characteristic of glossopharyngeal neuralgia that the pain is triggered by such innocuous stimuli as swallowing, yawning, coughing and chewing. Other reported triggers are laughing, touching the throat, ear or neck, turning the head or moving the arm. In unusual cases, particular tastes may trigger attacks (White & Sweet 1969).

A variety of cardiovascular and other symptoms may accompany the attacks. They include cardiac arrhythmias or cardiac arrest, hiccups, spells of intractable coughing, inspiratory stridor, excessive salivation and seizures. These accompanying symptoms can be especially troublesome during and after surgical manipulation of the tenth nerve in the posterior fossa (White & Sweet 1969; Nagashima et al 1976).

Due to overlap of the sensory territories of the seventh, ninth and tenth cranial nerves, a lesion of one does not always cause objective loss of sensation in the throat or ear. Numbness in both locations has been found following placement of a surgical lesion just dorsal to the trigeminal descending tract in the medulla (Kunc 1965) which is thought to interrupt primary afferents of the seventh, ninth and tenth nerves together.

UPPER CERVICAL ROOTS

The caudal border of the cranial nerve supply to the skin was demonstrated by Foerster (1933) who cut all of the cervical roots on one side in 12 of his patients. Typically anaesthesia included the ear but not the external auditory meatus. Also included were the submental region, the area overlying the angle of the mandible and the posterior scalp as far as the vertex. With more selective root sections, Foerster demonstrated the region innervated by the second and third cervical roots (Fig. 40.3). Posterior rootlets of the first cervical segment are not invariably present but with careful dissection at least one small filament is found in nearly all cases (Kerr 1961).

Pain at the craniocervical junction is frequently associated with disease of the upper cervical spine. When the C1, C2 or C3 roots are compressed or distorted, pain may be felt in the neck, occiput and mastoid area. It often radiates upward to the vertex and temporal region and sometimes downward to the interscapular region. The ear and the underside of the jaw are commonly involved, as one might expect from the dermatomal pattern (Fig. 40.3). The pain may be bilateral or unilateral. Unilateral symptoms are often caused by traumatic rotational injuries of the upper cervical spine (Hunter & Mayfield 1949). *Occipital neuralgia* is a syndrome of recurring pain in the distribution of the greater occipital nerve, which is almost a direct continuation of the C2 dorsal root. Attacks are rarely paroxysmal. Instead, they tend to be prolonged for hours, appearing at irregular intervals, usually worse late in the day. The pain may be aggravated by neck movements. Discrete trigger zones of the type seen in trigeminal neuralgia are rare. Direct pressure on the greater occipital nerve may be painful. It is sometimes possible to reproduce or to aggravate the patient's pain by applying firm pressure over the upper cervical spinous processes or transverse processes. This can be done with the neck extended to relax the otherwise taut ligamentum nuchae. Downward pressure on the skull vertex with the head flexed and rotated to the painful side may also reproduce the symptoms of upper cervical root compression (Dugan et al 1962). Extension of the neck is sometimes painful as well. An occasional patient will complain of pain with every kind of neck movement. Patients whose upper cervical roots are stretched by downward displacement of the medulla and cerebellar tonsils in Chiari malformation often mention sharp bilateral occipital pain radiating to the vertex with sneezing, coughing or jarring of the head. Rarely a patient will experience nuchal or suboccipital pain with simultaneous paraesthesias of the ipsilateral half of the tongue ('neck–tongue syndrome') suggesting the presence of afferents to C2–C3 through the ansa hypoglossi (Lance & Anthony 1980).

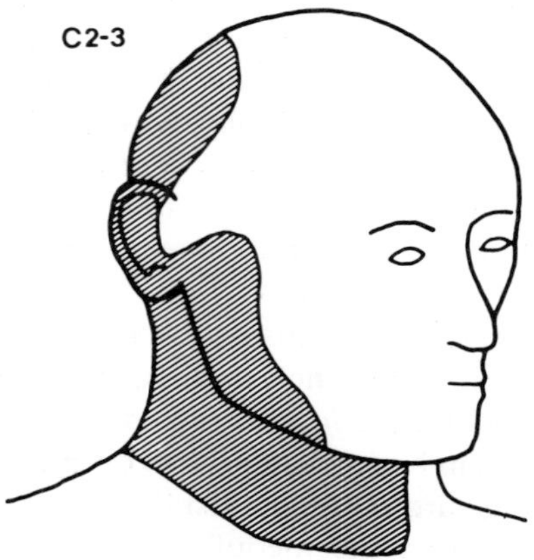

Fig. 40.3 The cutaneous field of the upper cervical roots (after Foerster 1933).

Tenderness or hyperaesthesia in the occipital or mastoid region is sometimes reported in occipital neuralgia. Tingling paraesthesias may be felt in the scalp. Blunting of pinprick sharpness is commonly found in the back of the scalp if the patient is examined carefully, but complete anaesthesia of this area is almost never seen in the absence of severe damage to more than one upper cervical root. The motor supply to neck muscles is derived from several spinal and lower cranial roots. Perhaps because of this overlap, weakness and atrophy are not frequently encountered in cases of upper cervical radiculopathy. Autonomic signs are unusual.

LOWER CERVICAL ROOTS

In nerve root lesions associated with protruded cervical intervertebral discs, certain patterns of pain are fairly constant (Murphey et al 1973). Some typical neurological signs which accompany lower cervical root pain are listed in Table 40.1. Compression of the C5 root may produce pain in the neck, shoulder, anterior chest, medial scapular region and lateral aspect of the arm. Lesions affecting the C6 or C7 root are often associated with pain in the neck, shoulder, anterior chest, scapular region, lateral aspect of the arm and dorsum of the forearm. Compression of C8 is suggested by pain in the neck, medial scapular region, somtimes in anterior chest and usually along the medial aspect of the arm and forearm. A similar pattern may be seen in damage of the first thoracic root. It is somewhat unusual to find a patient with pain in the hand due to cervical root compression (Murphey et al 1973) even though the dermatomes of C6, C7 and C8 clearly include the fingers (see Figs 40.1 and 40.2). Numbness and tingling paraesthesias ('pins and needles') are often described in a wider zone than the painful one. These innocuous but annoying sensations frequently radiate into the fingers while the pain does not. They therefore provide important clues to the level of involvement (Table 40.1).

As noted above, chest pain may be of lower cervical root origin. When it is severe, it may imitate the pain of angina or

Table 40.1 Typical findings in cervical root compression (after Murphey et al 1973)

C5 root compression (C4–C5 disc)
Pain – neck, shoulder, medial scapula, anterior chest, lateral aspect of upper arm
Numbness – sometimes lateral upper arm or area over deltoid
Weakness – deltoid, supraspinatus, infraspinatus, biceps, brachioradialis
Hyporeflexia – biceps, brachioradialis reflexes

C6 root compression (C5–C6 disc)
Pain – neck, shoulder, medial scapula, anterior chest, lateral aspect of upper arm, dorsal aspect of forearm
Numbness – thumb and index finger (sometimes absent)
Weakness – biceps (mild to moderate), extensor carpi radialis
Hyporeflexia – biceps reflex

C7 root compression (C6–C7 disc)
Pain – same as in C6 root compression
Numbness – index and middle fingers (sometimes absent)
Weakness – triceps
Hyporeflexia – triceps reflex

C8 root compression (C7–T1 disc)
Pain – neck, medial scapula, anterior chest, medial aspect of arm and forearm
Numbness – fourth and fifth fingers, occasionally middle finger
Weakness – triceps, all extensors of wrist and fingers except extensor carpi radialis; all flexors of wrist and fingers except flexor carpi radialis and palmaris longus; all intrinsic hand muscles
Hyporeflexia – triceps reflex

T1 root compression (T1–T2 disc)
Pain – same as in C8 root compression
Numbness – ulnar aspect of forearm (usually subjective)
Weakness – only intrinsic muscles of hand
Hyporeflexia – none
Miscellaneous – Horner's syndrome

myocardial infarction. Davis (1957) presented convincing histories of patients whose attacks of substernal and praecordial pain closely resembled the events of coronary insufficiency. It was shown that all of the symptoms could be reproduced by manipulations of the neck. Firm pressure over the lower cervical or uppermost thoracic vertebrae caused excruciating pain in the chest. Spine films confirmed the existence of spondylosis which was thought to be the cause of root compression.

Pain associated with cervical disc protrusions is usually constant with daily exacerbations related to activity, especially movements of the neck. Coughing, sneezing, pushing and any type of straining may severely aggravate the pain and reproduce the paraesthesias. In some cases, a Valsalva manoeuvre or bilateral jugular compression for 5–10 seconds will reproduce the pain or the paraesthesias. When the intervertebral foramina are narrowed by protruding discs and by spondylotic changes of the vertebral bodies ('osteophytes') and articular facets, the contained roots may be subject to marked compression during extension of the neck or tilting of the head to the involved side.

Chronic compression of an individual cervical root produces a continuous aching pain with sharp, shooting sensations superimposed during movements. Murphey (1968; Murphey et al 1973) performed a large number of cervical discectomies under local anaesthetic. Touching the damaged root produced severe pain in the arm, whereas touching normal cervical roots produced only electric sensations. When an involved root was blocked with local anaesthetic and retracted, it was sometimes possible to reproduce pain in the neck, shoulder, chest or scapular region by pressing on the posterior longitudinal ligament and torn annulus fibrosus. It was postulated that these stimuli activated afferents in the sinuvertebral nerves which enter the spinal canal as recurrent branches of the roots (Pedersen et al 1956).

Signs of damage to lower motor neurons are usually prominent in cervical root compression. At first weakness, and later atrophy and fasciculation may appear in muscles innervated by the damaged root. Patterns of weakness are usually consistent; loss of tendon stretch reflexes completes the picture (Table 40.1). Trophic changes of the skin and nails are rare in cervical root compression. Their presence is more typical of peripheral nerve damage. Autonomic changes are unusual, with the exception of Horner's syndrome: a small pupil, dryness of the face and ptosis may be seen on the side of T1 root compression, due to loss of sympathetic axons.

A special type of pain seen in cases of traumatic avulsion of cervical nerve roots was described in detail by Wynn Parry (1980) who found that of 108 cases of brachial plexus avulsion injury, 98 patients suffered significant pain. Pain was not a problem in 167 additional patients whose brachial plexus lesions were distal to the dorsal root ganglia. A remarkably consistent description of the pain was given which differed substantially from that of cervical disc protrusions. Pain was almost invariably felt in the hand and forearm after C6, C7, C8 or T1 root avulsions, conforming fairly well to the dermatome of the avulsed root. Some patients with avulsed C5 roots felt pain in the shoulder. Almost all of the patients used the terms 'hot' or 'burning' to describe the pain and many had a feeling that the hand was on fire or that boiling water was being poured over it. Some had a sensation of severe pressure, of pounding, or of 'electric shock'. This formed a constant background of severe pain in which, in 87 cases, additional sudden paroxysms occurred. These lasted usually for a few seconds, came without warning, and were sometimes of unbearable intensity. They radiated from the fingers to the shoulder and were described as sharp, shooting, cutting, or 'like lightning'. The paroxysms came unpredictably at intervals of 10 minutes to 1 week. Typically the patient would stop what he was doing and grip the arm or cry out. Paraesthesias were also common and almost all of the patients complained of tingling, 'pins and needles', or a feeling of electricity. Nearly all were aware of a phantom limb with sensations of movement when effort was made to use paralysed muscles. The pain of root avulsion was aggravated by worry and emotional stress. It was relieved by relaxation and by distraction. Some patients reported less pain when gripping, striking or massaging the painful limb. Others had moderate relief when moving the neck or the paralysed arm. In this series, all of the patients were young men between the ages of 18 and 30, and nearly all sustained their injuries in motorcycle accidents.

THORACIC ROOTS

Root lesions from T2 to L1 mainly involve the trunk. Radicular pain at truncal levels often appears as a discrete band around the chest or abdomen. When due to a spinal tumour, it may be constant, becoming worse at night when the patient is recumbent for hours. It may involve a single root initially, later more than one adjacent root or the contralateral root at the same level. Radicular pain of thoracic spinal tumours or disc protrusions is typically aggravated by coughing, sneezing and straining. It often has an aching, constrictive quality. When due to herpes zoster it is apt to be described as sharp, tender, tugging or pulling (Dubuisson & Melzack 1976). The skin may be exquisitely sensitive in the involved dermatome. Characteristic vesicles usually appear as viral particles are distributed along peripheral branches of the spinal nerve. Subjective numbness, tingling and other paraesthesias are common but objective loss of sensation is unusual in solitary thoracic root lesions. When present it suggests either involvement of several adjacent roots or an intramedullary lesion of the spinal cord at the equivalent level.

Weakness of the trunk muscles is not typical of solitary thoracic root lesions, or at least not clinically detectable. If several adjacent roots are damaged, weakness of the abdominal wall may give rise to visible bulging of the abdomen (Boulton et al 1984). Autonomic signs are rare. Marked tenderness over the spine at a corresponding level may signal infectious or tumorous destruction of bone. Metastatic lesions of vertebrae may announce their presence with a sudden collapse, occasionally audible to the patient, followed by abrupt radicular pain. Root pain accompanied by fever, spinal ache with local tenderness, nuchal rigidity or paraparesis is a warning of spinal epidural abscess which is most common in the thoracic region (Baker et al 1975).

LUMBOSACRAL ROOTS

This group includes two broad categories: involvement of individual roots and involvement of the cauda equina as a bundle of roots. Individual root lesions will be considered here. As with cervical root lesions, patterns of pain, numbness, weakness and loss of reflexes are fairly consistent in the lumbosacral region (Keegan & Garrett 1948; Bertrand 1975; C H Davis 1982). Pain associated with L3 root compression is usually felt in the lower back, anteromedial thigh and knee. Numbness may be reported in the anterior thigh and knee. Pain in the lower back, with radiation down the anterolateral thigh to the front of the knee or shin suggests L4 root involvement. Sometimes numbness can be detected around the medial aspect of the lower leg. An L5 root lesion characteristically produces pain in the lower back, posterolateral thigh, lateral aspect of the lower leg and sometimes lateral malleolus of the ankle or dorsum of the foot. Accompanying numbness or paraesthesias may be present in the dorsum of the foot, great toe and second or third toe. Pain of S1 lesions usually radiates from the lower back and buttock down the posterior thigh to the calf and sometimes to the heel, with tingling or numbness in the sole of the foot, lateral border of the foot, little toe and sometimes fourth toe. Continuous pain in the foot itself is not typical of lumbosacral disc protrusions (C H Davis 1982) and suggests instead some local problem of the foot. Numbness is of good localising value since it frequently extends distally in the dermatome when the pain does not. Foerster (1933) argued that the dorsal aspect of the foot was predominantly supplied by L5 while the entire plantar surface was supplied by S1. Nevertheless, the medial-lateral distinction seems more useful in distinguishing L5 from S1 root compression. Numbness along the lateral border of the foot is most consistent with an S1 lesion. Pain radiating to the groin may result from compression of any root from T12 to S1, but this is more common with upper lumbar root compression. These features are summarised in Table 40.2.

Paraesthesias consisting of subjective numbness, tingling, 'pins and needles' or a wooden sensation are often more widespread than the pain. Due to the overlap of dermatomes, zones of objective sensory loss defined by touch and pinprick are usually small or absent. Some patients show hypoaesthesia over a large part of a dermatome (Keegan & Garrett 1948).

Radicular pain associated with ordinary lumbosacral disc protrusions is described as sharp, tender and shooting by a majority of patients given a verbal questionnaire. Other descriptive terms which are commonly chosen are cramping, throbbing, aching, heavy and stabbing. Bertrand (1975) described a group of patients suffering from 'battered root', a permanent radiculopathy with severe pain and paraesthesias in the lower extremity following unsuccessful lumbar disc surgery. Pain from the 'battered root' was constant, not intermittent as with most ordinary disc protrusions. It was described as burning or 'ice-cold' by many patients and was often superimposed on a zone of residual numbness. Similar pain was sometimes reported following rhizotomy or ganglionectomy. Despite the patient's description of thermal qualities, autonomic signs were subtle or absent. This type of

Table 40.2 Typical findings in lumbosacral root compression

L3 root compression (L2–L3 disc)
Pain – low back, anterior or anteromedial thigh, anterior knee, sometimes groin
Numbness – anterior thigh, knee (sometimes absent)
Weakness – quadriceps
Hyporeflexia – knee jerk (may be normal)
Miscellaneous – positive reversal-leg-raising test

L4 root compression (usually L3–L4 disc)
Pain – low back, anterior thigh, sometimes medial aspect of lower leg, sometimes groin
Numbness – medial aspect of lower leg (may be absent)
Weakness – quadriceps, sometimes tibialis anterior
Hyporeflexia – knee jerk
Miscellaneous – positive straight-leg-raising and reversed-leg-raising test

L5 root compression (usually L4–L5 disc)
Pain – low back, buttock, posterolateral thigh, lateral aspect of lower leg, lateral malleolus, sometimes dorsum of foot, sometimes groin
Numbness – dorsum of foot, big toe, occasionally second toe or lateral aspect of lower leg
Weakness – tibialis anterior, extensor hallucis longus, extensor digitorum brevis, sometimes gluteals
Hyporeflexia – occasionally biceps femoris reflex
Miscellaneous – positive straight-leg-raising test

S1 root compression (usually L5–S1 disc)
Pain – low back, buttock, posterior thigh, calf, heel, rarely groin
Numbness – lateral border of foot, sole, heel, sometimes fourth and fifth toes
Weakness – gastrocnemius/soleus, gluteals, occasionally hamstrings
Hyporeflexia – ankle jerk
Miscellaneous – positive straight-leg-raising test

pain is distinct from the discomfort of ordinary root compression in its severity and in the terms used by the patient to describe it. It is typically more distressing to the patient than the original pain of disc protrusion.

Weakness, loss of tendon stretch reflexes, less commonly atrophy or fasciculation occur in myotomal patterns with lumbosacral root lesions (Table 40.2). Most common are: quadriceps weakness with a diminished or absent knee jerk due to damage of the L3 or L4 root; foot drop or weakness of the tibialis anterior and extensor hallucis longus with normal reflexes in L5 damage; and weakness of plantar flexion, occasional cramping in the calf and an absent ankle jerk with S1 damage. The examiner asks the patient to walk on his heels and on his toes to demonstrate weakness of dorsiflexion or of plantar flexion. Less obvious instances of S1 radiculopathy can be brought out by asking the patient to raise himself on the toes of one foot five or 10 times. The involved side fatigues more rapidly. The girth of the calf may be smaller and the gastrocnemius muscle softer with an S1 lesion. In some patients, softening or visible wasting of the extensor digitorum brevis muscle, on the dorsolateral aspect of the foot, is a clue to L5 involvement. Softening of the gluteal muscles and sagging of a gluteal fold may be seen in some cases of S1 damage.

Less objective but still valuable are the signs elicited by various postural manipulations. Bending at the waist is usually restricted in painful lumbosacral radiculopathies of any cause. If the patient is able to touch his toes comfortably from a standing position or, lying supine, to hold both heels off the examining table for some time, a mechanical lesion of the lumbosacral roots is unlikely. Passive straight-leg-raising in the supine position is almost always painful in the presence of mechanical L4–L5–S1 root lesions. This manoeuvre, which stretches the sciatic nerve and its tributaries, causes pain to radiate into the appropriate dermatome or muscles. In the apprehensive patient and in the malingerer, the same postural manipulation can often be produced without the patient's knowledge by passively extending his knee while he is seated. Passive reverse-leg-raising with the knee flexed stretches the femoral nerve and is often painful when the L3 or L4 root is involved (Dyck 1976).

LOWER SACRAL AND COCCYGEAL ROOTS

The sacrococcygeal dermatomes are known mainly from stimulation of the roots at the time of rhizotomy for painful sacral and pelvic disorders. Stimulation of S2 produces pain in the buttock, groin, posterior thigh and genitalia. Foerster (1933) mapped portions of an isolated S2 dermatome on the sole of the foot (Fig. 40.2). During stimulation of S3, pain is felt in the perianal region, rectum and genitalia. Stimulation of S4 may evoke pain in the vagina. Pain in the anus and around the coccyx is felt with stimulation of S4, S5 and coccygeal roots (Bohm & Franksson 1959; White & Sweet 1969).

Severe burning pain around the coccyx in the absence of tumour or other disease is termed *coccygodynia*. The pain can be unilateral or bilateral and usually occurs in middle-aged or elderly women. The S4, S5 and coccygeal roots are involved in some cases (White & Sweet 1969). In others, the pain may be referred from L4, L5, or S1 (Long 1982). Sensory deficits are not typical, nor are signs of bowel and bladder involvement, despite the known innervation of the bladder and anal sphincter by the S2–S4 roots. Objective loss of sensation, diminished bladder tone and loss of the bulbocavernosus reflex suggest destruction of the roots.

A particularly intractable type of pain can occur in the sacral dermatomes in association with the finding of sacral cysts. These cysts are in fact abnormal dilatations of the meninges around the sacral nerve roots, filled with cerebrospinal fluid, expanding the sacral neural canal and foramina. On surgical exploration, which the author rarely advises, the sacral roots are found to be embedded in the meningeal wall of the cyst, stretched and thinned from growth of the fluid-filled compartment. There may or may not be a visible spinal fluid communication with the rest of the subarachnoid space. Various terminology to describe this condition includes 'sacral arachnoid cyst', 'sacral meningocele', and 'sacral root sleeve diverticula'. The anatomy of the meningeal cystic anomaly varies from case to case, but the symptomatology seems to have in common some unusual and relentless, painful sensations and dysaesthesias around the saddle region, rectum or vagina. The symptoms may be positional, with bizarre-sounding descriptions of pulsation or formication in the region. The usual pertinent neurological findings can often be brought out by a thorough examination. Consultation with a urologist and, for women, a gynaecologist is usually appropriate to complete the assessment of these patients.

MULTISEGMENTAL ROOT SYNDROMES

CERVICAL SPONDYLOSIS

Cervical spondylosis sometimes declares its presence by pain in the distribution of one root, but more often the picture is multisegmental, diffuse and bilateral. A clinical hallmark of cervical spondylosis is restriction of neck motion with discomfort on attempting a complete range of movement. Multiple root constriction in the intervertebral foramina leads to symptoms of numbness in the hands and forearms, in a pattern not conforming to that of any peripheral nerve territory. Weakness and diminished reflexes point to loss of innervation of muscles. Weakness of the wrist extensors, triceps, and shoulder girdle is detectable in a typical case. Long tract signs such as upgoing plantar reflexes, difficulty maintaining balance on attempting to walk a straight line in heel-to-toe fashion, and clumsy fine movements of the toes and fingers may indicate cord compression in the spondylotic canal. In the author's practice, it has been common to find concomitant lumbar spondylosis of a degree resembling that found in the neck, so that reflex changes in the legs are unpredictable. In cases with both cervical and lumbar spondylosis, there may be loss of tendon reflexes in the lower limbs, instead of the expected hyperreflexia due to cervical cord compression. It is also undoubtedly true that in patients with documented lumbar spondylosis, studies of the cervical spine will usually reveal cervical spondylosis. Occasionally, paraesthesias such as tingling or electrical sensations can occur in the trunk and legs with cervical spondylosis, particularly during neck extension. Frank pain in the legs is rarely if ever due to cervical spondylosis; at least, this author has never seen a believable example of it. Occipital pain due to bony encroachment on the upper cervical roots may add to the confusing picture of a patient with pain and paraesthesias all over the body! The character of pain in cervical spondylosis resembles that of chronic compression of individual roots and the same aggravating factors may be present (M Wilkinson 1971). In general, patients with single lateral cervical disc protrusions of soft nucleus pulposus tend to form a younger group than patients with multiple degenerated cervical discs and extensive bony spurs and ridges.

LUMBAR SPONDYLOSIS

Pain distributed in several dermatomes of the lower extremities, often bilateral and otherwise resembling the pain of a solitary lumbar disc protrusion, may be due to widespread spondylotic changes of the lumbar spine. Regardless of whether disc protrusions are present, back pain and leg pain are prominent complaints. Weinstein et al (1977) found that 66% of patients with narrowed lumbar canals due to spondylosis suffered from back pain; 36% had unilateral leg pain and 36% had bilateral leg pain. Painful muscle spasms and cramps in the back and legs were frequent but the localization of pain was not consistent or helpful in diagnosis. Of 227 cases, pain was felt in the buttock or hip in 25, in the thigh in 23, and in the groin or genitalia in 9. In many cases, the pain was aggravated by extension of the lumbar spine. 20 cases were classified as 'neurogenic claudication', which is discussed below. Objective sensory abnormalities were present in only half of the cases and often did not obey a discrete dermatomal pattern. In a few cases, perianal or 'saddle' hypoaesthesia was noted. Muscle weakness was observed in 64% and was often most marked in the extensor hallucis longus and tibialis anterior, suggesting predominant L5 root involvement. Tendon stretch reflexes in the ankles or knees were decreased or absent in 70% of cases. In about 10% there was additional evidence of cauda equina involvement consisting of bowel or bladder incontinence, urinary retention or impotence. A positive response to straight-leg-raising was found in only 30% of the 227 cases, a useful point in distinguishing the pain of lumbar spondylosis and canal stenosis from that of simple disc protrusion.

Neurogenic claudication

A prominent caudal radiculopathy caused by lumbar spondylosis or by congenital lumbar spinal stenosis has come to be known as *neurogenic claudication*. This syndrome of the narrow spinal canal was described by Verbiest (1954). Typically there is a distinctly unpleasant sensation in the legs which can be frankly painful in some cases. It is variably described as numb, cold, burning or cramping (Weinstein et al 1977). This sensation characteristically appears after assumption of an upright posture or during prolonged extension of the lumbar spine. The symptoms may begin in the feet and spread proximally or vice versa. Paraesthesias often appear even when the patient is standing still, but they are typically brought on by walking. These points help to distinguish the syndrome from peripheral vascular claudication, in which cramps affect the leg muscles after exercise regardless of posture. A useful rule of thumb is that the patient whose intermittent claudication is due to arterial insufficiency would rather walk downhill than uphill. The reverse is true of the patient with a narrow spinal canal since the back is slightly flexed in climbing. Descending places the spine in lordosis with further constriction of the cauda equina. Objective sensory deficits are usually slight or absent in cases of neurogenic claudication, and straight-leg-raising does not usually cause pain.

ARACHNOIDITIS

There is often diffuse involvement of nerve roots in chronic spinal arachnoiditis. In recent decades, reported cases have been predominantly lumbosacral (Shaw et al 1978) but any part of the spine may be affected. Almost always, pain is the first symptom. The pain of arachnoiditis may obey a radicular pattern but more often it involves portions of two or more root distributions. In some cases, widely separated zones are involved in an irregular distribution (Whisler 1978). In others, the painful region is large with poorly demarcated borders. Pain tends to be bilateral (Elkington 1951). The low back is often a focal point from which pain seems to be distributed to both legs. The locations of painful zones in the extremities may shift over days or weeks, and so may the patient's description of his symptoms. The sensory quality of the pain is described as stinging, burning, aching or gnawing (Elkington 1951). It is continuous but worsened by movement. Jarring, straining, coughing or sneezing may aggravate the pain (Feder & Smith 1962). It may be particularly severe in the morning or after prolonged bedrest (Christensen 1942). Cramping sensations and painful muscle spasms suggest ventral root involvement later confirmed by atrophy and fasciculation. Painful spasms of the extremities may also indicate spinal cord involvement at a higher level.

With lumbosacral arachnoiditis, the straight-leg-raising test is positive on one or both sides in the vast majority of cases (French 1946). There is typically stiffness and tenderness of the paravertebral muscles and marked limitation of lumbar spine flexion. Pain in the lower extremities may be aggravated by flexing the neck. Numbness and paraesthesias are common. They are often widespread, poorly localized and inconstant from day to day. The paraesthesias may be described as dull, tingling, hot, burning, cold, constricting, or 'like pins and needles' (Rocovich 1947). Occasional patients complain of an inexorable feeling of fullness in the rectum. Tingling in the extremities can often be reproduced by flexing the neck. Objective sensory examination by touch and pinprick may be vague or entirely normal despite bizarre subjective complaints. Autonomic signs and trophic changes are not commonly found.

Like lumbosacral disc disease, to which it is related, arachnoiditis affects men more often than women in a ratio of almost 2:1. The typical age of onset is between 25 and 65 (French 1946). When extensive spondylosis or multiple disc protrusions are present it will be difficult to blame arachnoiditis for the patient's symptoms even when the myelogram shows diagnostic signs. Only the history, extent and variability of symptoms and occasional involvement of the spinal cord distinguish arachnoiditis clinically from disc protrusions and entrapment of nerve roots.

TABETIC AND PSEUDOTABETIC ROOT SYNDROMES

In tabetic neurosyphilis (tabes dorsalis), degeneration of dorsal roots and dorsal columns is associated with a clinical syndrome of lancinating pains and visceral crises. The typical patient is 40–60 years of age, because the symptoms rarely appear less than 10–20 years after the disease begins (Storm-Mathisen 1978). The most frequent complaint is of 'lightning pains'; sudden intense, fleeting pains in the legs, less often in the back or arms. The pains are described as cramping, crushing, burning, lancinating or 'like an electric shock'. They tend to occur in clusters and may shift unpredictably in location. Individual attacks last only moments in most cases, but in some, pain continues for hours or days.

Paraesthesias are variably present in the trunk or extremities. Numbness, aching and tingling sensations are described. There may be a sense of band-like constriction of the trunk or a feeling of walking on cotton. Either hyperaesthesia or diminished touch and pinprick sensation may be found. Hypersensitivity to light touch tends to appear in the hips, legs and soles of the feet. Objective sensory loss is said to occur in characteristic zones: the middle of the face, the ulnar aspect of the forearm, the nipple area, the perianal region (Storm-Mathisen 1978).

Additional signs which may be encountered are diminished vibration and position sense in the legs, swollen dislocated knees or hips (Charcot's joints), ulceration of the plantar surface of the feet, loss of tendon stretch reflexes and of muscle tone with hyperextensile joints, a stamping, ataxic gait and pupillary abnormalities. The Argyll Robertson pupil is small, sometimes irregular, does not react to light but constricts during accommodation.

Patients may also experience abdominal pains in the form of sudden excruciating crises with vomiting. Similar rectal, vesical and laryngeal crises are described. Loss of bladder tone, constipation and impotence are also common.

Diabetic pseudotabes is a posterior radiculopathy of diabetes mellitus in which brief, shooting pains occur, often in a single dermatome. There are also signs of dorsal column dysfunction with paraesthesias. Charcot's joints may develop. An irregular pupil that accommodates but reacts poorly to light is occasionally found and further confuses the clinical picture. There are usually no motor or reflex changes, but bladder disturbances may occur (Gilroy & Meyer 1975).

Another syndrome of recurrent pseudotabetic pain is that which sometimes follows laminectomy for disc protrusions. Sudden fleeting pains in the legs occur in a small subgroup of patients who undergo lumbar discectomy (Martin 1980).

MENINGEAL CARCINOMATOSIS

Multiple nerve roots may be involved at different levels by leptomeningeal metastases from solid tumours. The subject of nerve and root pain in cancer is reviewed elsewhere in this volume and will be mentioned only briefly here. The typical clinical syndrome of *meningeal carcinomatosis* consists of neurological dysfunction at several levels of the neuraxis without radiological evidence of brain metastasis or of epidural spinal metastasis. About two-thirds of the patients in one reported series were women (Wasserstrom et al 1982). Patients ranged in age from 30–74 years in this series. Breast cancer was the commonest primary source, followed by lung cancer and malignant melanoma. Spinal root infiltrates are also a common problem in leukaemic patients, who are frequently children (Neiri et al 1968).

Root symptoms, including radicular pain, may be the first sign of meningeal carcinomatosis. Olson et al (1974) found that 25% of patients whose leptomeninges were infiltrated by metastatic cancer had only root symptoms initially. Another 15% had spinal root symptoms plus symptoms of other sites of neurological damage. In a series of 90 patients with known carcinomatous invasion of the meninges, Wasserstrom et al (1982) reported that 74 had spinal symptoms and signs. Pain in a radicular pattern was a prominent feature in 19, while back pain or neck pain was present in 23. Other frequent complaints were of weakness, usually of the legs, paraesthesias in the extremities and bowel or bladder dysfunction. Seven patients had nuchal rigidity and 11 had back pain on straight-leg-raising. 30 patients had signs of cauda equina involvement. The tendency for lumbosacral root involvement has also been noted in leukaemic patients (Neiri et al 1968). It is thought to be due to the gravitation of malignant cells in the cerebrospinal fluid as well as the relatively long course of the lumbosacral roots within the subarachnoid space (Little et al 1974). Headaches are a frequent accompanying complaint. Some patients experience pain when the neck is manipulated, others show tenderness to percussion over the spine. Absence of one or more of the tendon stretch reflexes is typical, as is muscle wasting and fasciculation. Additional signs and symptoms due to systemic cancer may complicate the picture.

TIME COURSE AND PROGNOSIS

Few generalities apply to pain of root damage. Lesions of single roots are usually of recent onset in young individuals, while multiradicular syndromes are apt to be of chronic duration in an older age group. Pain of individual root origin is often due to benign mechanical lesions which compress or distort. Pain of multiradicular origin suggests a diffuse degenerative, neoplastic or inflammatory cause, frequently intradural. In general, pain due to mechanical distortion of a single root is more amenable to surgery than is pain of multiple root damage.

Possibly the great majority of root compressions due to disc protrusion are asymptomatic. In a series of 300 patients having no symptoms referrable to cervical or lumbar roots, myelography showed root–sleeve deformities and other abnormalities characteristic of disc protrusion in 110 (37%). Multiple defects were shown in 18% (Hitselberger & Witten 1968). In a similar study using computed tomography of the lumbar spine in asymptomatic individuals, there was a 35% incidence of abnormalities. In the group under 40 years of age, these were changes typical of disc protrusion in every case. In the over-40-year-old age group, there was a 50% incidence of abnormalities, including disc protrusion, facet joint degeneration and spinal stenosis (Wiesel et al 1984). It is likely that many instances of root compression by bulging discs are transient and that healing of the torn annulus takes place (C H Davis 1982). In a study of 47 patients followed prospectively for symptomatic disc herniations, without significant joint disease or stenosis, 42 patients tolerated conservative management without surgery until signs of radiculopathy subsided (Maigne et al 1992). Serial CT scans documented shrinkage of the disc herniations over periods of 1–40 months, with the largest herniations tending to decrease the most. A majority of patients who experience an episode of low back pain can be expected to be asymptomatic within a month with no treatment (Nachemson 1977). When radicular pain is also present, the percentage is less but many patients will still recover with rest. In most instances of cervical radiculopathy due to spondylosis, the symptoms will resolve over about 6 weeks (M Wilkinson 1971).

The typical patient with radicular pain due to cervical or lumbosacral disc protrusion has a history of one or more previous episodes of neck or back pain which cleared with rest. These episodes took place during preceding months or years and usually lasted several days or weeks at a time. The onset of new, severe symptoms then commenced with neck or back pain, often brought on by exercise or by some twisting movement. This improved somewhat over days or weeks but was replaced by radicular pain. In some cases, the radicular pain then spread distally in a saltatory fashion.

A few patients do not fit this pattern but instead develop

sudden severe radiating pain as the initial symptom. After a radicular pattern is established, some patients with disc protrusion still obtain relief by resting in bed but they are very susceptible to future attacks of a similar nature. More commonly the pain persists with fluctuations which are closely related to physical activity. Sudden disappearance of radicular pain is cause for concern since this might indicate destruction of the root. Increasing numbness and weakness or further diminution of tendon reflexes signal worsening of the root lesion even when the pain is improving (Murphey 1968).

In many cases, particularly when the patient is unable to function at work, the sequence of events will be interrupted by disc surgery. Spangfort (1972) concluded that complete relief of both back pain and leg pain occurs in 60% of patients undergoing discectomy on the basis of clear cut mechanical and neurological findings supported by indisputable radiological abnormalities. Many neurosurgeons would find this figure to be an underestimate of the success rate of disc surgery today. Even before the advent of microsurgical techniques, Scoville (1973) reported a 96% success rate in 779 patients undergoing 'radical' lumbar disc operations. There is a good correlation between the degree of pain relief and the degree of disc herniation which indicates the severity of root compression prior to surgery. It is among the unfortunate minority of patients failing surgery that we find cases of chronic pain associated with root damage and arachnoiditis. Some patients who are not relieved by operation may continue to experience pain because of surgical trauma to the root. In this group of patients who have prolonged pain and paraesthesias, the chronology is often difficult to follow because the patient, unhappy with his treatment, migrates from place to place seeking relief. It can become almost impossible to reconstruct the course of events, but this is what is needed in such cases. If the previous records and X-ray films are gathered and studied, one of three chronological patterns may emerge (Bertrand 1975). The sequence: *radicular pain → operation → relief for weeks or months → return of pain in the same or in a different distribution* does not usually indicate permanent root damage but rather suggests that recurrent root compression at the same level or at a different level is present. The sequence: *radicular pain → operation → no change* suggests that the cause of pain was not identified at surgery. A disc fragment may have migrated out of reach or the root may have been trapped in a hidden zone. The sequence: *radicular pain → operation → relief of pain but severe numbness* suggests surgical trauma to the root or its vascular supply. A fourth pattern might be added. The sequence: *radicular pain → operation → increased radicular pain and severe bilateral leg cramps → temporary improvement → chronic bilateral pain* suggests the development of arachnoiditis (Auld 1978). In this syndrome, severe cramps and spasms in both legs, sometimes accompanied by fever and chills, begin on the first, second or third postoperative day and last for 4–20 days. There is usually some improvement then but signs of chronic arachnoiditis develop over the following months or years with new neurological deficits and relentless bilateral back and leg pain.

The long-range prognosis of arachnoiditis is poor in that the neurological deficits tend to persist permanently. Late onset of urinary frequency, urgency or frank incontinence was noted in 23% of a group of arachnoiditis patients followed over 10–21 years (Guyer et al 1989). Of the patients in that study, 90% had undergone Pantopaque myelography and disc surgery prior to developing arachnoiditis. Progression of neurological disability did not appear to be the typical natural course of the disease. When increased neurological deficits were seen, they were most often due to surgical intervention. A majority of the patients depended on daily narcotic analgesics; alcohol abuse, depression, and two deaths by suicide were also noted.

The time course of pain due to various other forms of root damage depends on the aetiology. The pain of paroxysmal cranial neuralgias usually appears suddenly and unexpectedly in previously healthy adults and recurs at irregular but increasingly frequent intervals of months, weeks, days or hours. Attacks may appear in clusters with painfree periods lasting less than an hour. Spontaneous remissions lasting as long as 20 years were described in 161 of 217 cases of glossopharyngeal neuralgia (Rushton et al 1981). Neuralgias associated with upper cervical root lesions can also be expected to persist with repeated aggravations for months or years in the absence of treatment.

The course of radiculopathies due to fractures and other mechanical disorders is similar to that described above for disc protrusions in that there is a tendency for pain to persist as long as the root is distorted or compressed. Exacerbations are closely related to physical activity and the patient is understandably reluctant to return to work. Pain associated with cervical or lumbar spondylosis, including the syndrome of neurogenic claudication, can be considered permanent in the absence of treatment. The neurological symptoms tend to be slowly progressive over years. Generous laminectomy and decompression of the involved roots at the intervertebral foramina usually arrests the process.

Pain of spinal tumours tends to be overshadowed by signs of spinal cord or cauda equina compression during succeeding weeks or months depending on the histological nature of the tumour. Relief can be expected following surgical excision of benign masses, particularly if only a single root is involved, if a rhizotomy is done and if neighbouring roots are not traumatised.

There is a disturbing tendency of lumbosacral arachnoiditis to ascend, causing cord compression by tense, fluid-filled loculations. In a few unfortunate cases, adhesions reform at accelerating intervals despite repeated surgical lysis until the patient is paraplegic and incontinent. However, this is by no means the typical expected course of arachnoiditis. In mild cases relief is imminent for many patients within a year or two. It has not been possible to predict which patients will improve and which will deteriorate. The number of roots involved gives some indication of the severity of the process.

Diabetic root pain may also improve spontaneously in some cases, and this does not necessarily depend on rigorous control of blood sugar levels. Pseudotabetic pain after discectomy tends to improve over 3–5 years (Martin 1980). In most cases of herpes zoster, segmental pain may precede the appearance of cutaneous vesicles by 3–4 days. Healing of the skin lesions takes place over 2–3 weeks. Pain lasts an additional week or two in young patients and usually disappears leaving hypo- or hyperaesthesia. Pain persists for over 2 months in 70% of patients over 60 years of age, even though the skin lesions heal normally (Ray 1980). Intractable postherpetic neuralgia occurs mainly in elderly patients. When it has been present for 6 months or more, the prognosis for recovery is very poor (Lipton 1979).

The prognosis of meningeal carcinomatosis depends on the response to intrathecal chemotherapy and radiation as well as the tumour histology and extent of disease. The pain of root destruction by trauma, scarring, avulsion, very severe herpetic or syphilitic lesions, or advanced arachnoiditis, is usually a protracted affair with a component of deafferentation in many cases. Pain continues for years or for the rest of the patient's life unless effective treatment can be found.

AETIOLOGY AND DIAGNOSTIC STUDIES

Some conditions associated with radicular pain are listed in Table 40.3. Most of them have been mentioned already in the discussion of symptoms and prognosis. Here we are concerned with the way in which roots are damaged and the way in which pain results.

Geniculate neuralgia may appear subsequent to an attack of acute herpes zoster involving the external auditory canal (Hunt 1915). The exact role of the virus in causing this pain syndrome is not known. No animal model has been developed, and neuropathological studies in confirmed cases of geniculate neuralgia are lacking. This type of neuralgia is infrequent; some instances of lancinating pain in the ear may be due to glossopharyngeal neuralgia, in which case the herpetic prodrome is not seen.

Glossopharyngeal neuralgia resembles trigeminal neuralgia in many respects, and may indeed be confused with trigeminal neuralgia limited to the mandibular division. Both types of neuralgia may be due to focal pressure along the course of the nerve. In the case of glossopharyngeal neuralgia, the cause is sometimes a tortuous vertebral artery or posterior inferior cerebellar artery impinging on the roots of the ninth nerve (Laha & Jannetta 1977). In many cases, no definite cause is found. In others, trauma, local infection, an elongated styloid process or ossified stylohyoid ligament is responsible. The variant known as vagus nerve neuralgia has been associated with similar pathology. Partial demyelination of the

Table 40.3 Some common aetiologies of radicular pain

Lower cranial roots
Glossopharyngeal neuralgia
idiopathic
associated with vascular anomaly
Cerebellopontine angle tumour
Skull base tumour
Geniculate neuralgia
Upper cervical roots
Occipital neuralgia
idiopathic
associated with C1–C2 arthrosis
associated with rheumatoid arthritis
post-traumatic
Postherpetic neuralgia
Metastatic spine tumour
Chiari malformation
Lower cervical roots
Cervical disc protrusion
Cervical spondylosis
Metastatic spine tumour
Brachial plexus avulsion injury
Cervical spine fracture or dislocation
Intradural tumour
Thoracic roots
Postherpetic neuralgia
Intercostal neuralgia
idiopathic
following thoracotomy
associated with systemic malignancy
Thoracic disc protrusion
Metastatic spine tumour
Intradural tumour
Meningeal carcinomatosis, lymphoma, leukaemia
Spinal epidural abscess
Diabetic neuropathy
Thoracic spine fracture or dislocation
Tabes dorsalis
Lumbar and first sacral roots
Lumbar disc protrusion
Lumbar spondylosis
spinal stenosis
superior facet syndrome
Postsurgical epidural scarring
Arachnoiditis
Spondylolisthesis
Occult postoperative facet fracture
Metastatic spine tumour
Intradural tumour
Meningeal carcinomatosis, lymphoma, leukaemia
Spinal epidural abscess
Lumbar spine fracture or dislocation
Perineurial or leptomeningeal cyst
Tabes dorsalis
Sacrococcygeal roots
Coccygodynia
Metastatic sacral tumour
Meningeal carcinomatosis, lymphoma, leukaemia
Perineurial cyst

glossopharyngeal nerve has been shown postmortem in some cases, but unlike trigeminal neuralgia, glossopharyngeal neuralgia is almost never associated with multiple sclerosis (Rushton et al 1981).

The diagnosis of the cranial neuralgias can often be facilitated by finding a trigger area. Trigger areas associated with trigeminal neuralgia are typically located on the face, inside the cheeks, or around the gums. Trigger areas for glossopharyngeal neuralgia are usually found in the tonsillar region, where they may be inactivated temporarily with local anaesthetic spray (Rushton et al 1981). The trigger zone in cases of vagus nerve neuralgia is deeper in the throat, and its inactivation may require injection of local anaesthetic around the superior laryngeal nerve where it enters the larynx.

Some cases of paroxysmal pain in the trigeminal or glossopharyngeal distribution may be associated with tumours of the cerebellopontine angle. Nonparoxysmal pain in a similar distribution may originate from partial destruction of the ninth and tenth nerves by malignant tumours of the skull base. Certainly any cranial neuralgia warrants investigation with computed tomography (CT) or magnetic resonance imaging (MRI). Plain X-ray films of the skull base can also be revealing, but they can no longer be considered adequate.

Pain in the posterior scalp, occiput, above the ear, or at the angle of the jaw may be due to pathology of the upper cervical nerve roots or the peripheral branches to which they give rise. In some instances, direct trauma to scalp sensory nerves gives rise to a relentless neuralgic syndrome even in the absence of frank nerve transaction. This may take the form of anaesthesia dolorosa, or it may closely resemble the pattern of occipital neuralgia. The latter is a disorder of multiple aetiologies, having in common damage of the greater occipital nerve or the C2 dorsal root from which it originates. Following head and neck trauma, occipital pain is probably most often due to stretch injury and recurrent spasm of the posterior cervical muscles. In particular, the semispinalis capitis muscle surrounds and is penetrated by the greater occipital nerve. This muscle is a major neck extensor, sustained contraction of which may create pressure on the enclosed greater occipital nerve and on branches of the C3 dorsal root. Local scarring may lead to actual encasement of these nerves or of the C2 or C3 root (Poletti 1983). The author has encountered cases of otherwise typical occipital neuralgia which appeared for the first time after lower cervical laminectomies were performed to treat spinal stenosis. Presumably, retraction of the cervical muscles during surgery caused an injury of the posterior branches of C2 and C3. The distinction between occipital neuralgia and chronic tension (scalp muscle contraction) headache in this group of patients is seldom clear. Radiological investigations in this subgroup of patients with occipital neuralgia usually show no abnormality. Occasionally, plain films of the cervical spine in flexion will reveal an excessive separation of the spinous processes at one level, suggesting a previous hyperflexion neck injury with partial disruption of the interspinous ligament.

When there is nontraumatic posterior head and neck pain in the absence of radiological abnormalities, the possibility of postherpetic neuralgia can be raised. This diagnosis may be overlooked unless the patient is questioned about a preceding vesicular rash on the neck. Radiculopathies associated with herpes zoster are commonest in the second to fourth cervical segments, and between the second thoracic and first lumbar levels, several neighbouring roots may be affected. It has been suggested that postherpetic neuralgia and posttraumatic radicular neuralgia have in common an inflammatory reaction in the dorsal root ganglion (Forrest 1980). Inflammation and necrosis of dorsal root ganglia have been well documented in pathological reports of herpes zoster (Adams 1976), but the evidence of similar pathology following cervical root trauma is unimpressive.

There is a second group of patients will occipital neuralgia in whom radiological studies do reveal the cause. A combination of CT scanning and plain X-ray films of the upper cervical spine, including an open-mouth view of C1–C2, will often demonstrate gross pathology of the joints or foramina near the second and third cervical nerve roots. Cervical spondylosis is often present, with multiple levels of narrowing of the intervertebral foramina by osteophytes, and enlarged facet joints. The C1–C2 joint may itself be a source of pain, since it receives its sensory innervation from the C2 root. Severe arthrosis of this joint may be sufficient to provoke occipital neuralgia, which is then typically aggravated by motion of the head and neck (Ehni & Benner 1984). Other cases may result from fractures of the upper cervical spine, leading to bony callus formation and joint enlargement, with frank compression of the second cervical root. Still others may be due to inflammatory disease, usually rheumatoid arthritis, of the C1–C2 joint. Careful radiological investigations will exclude the possibility of a meningioma or Chiari malformation at the craniocervical junction, or a metastatic tumour eroding the upper cervical vertebrae or occipital bone.

At lower cervical, thoracic and lumbar levels, spinal nerve roots may be distorted in a variety of ways. Disc protrusion and the accompanying osteophytes may compress the root anteriorly, or enlarged facet joints encroach upon it posteriorly. In the event of frank disc herniation, a free fragment of the degenerated nucleus pulposus may become lodged against the root in the spinal canal or in the intervertebral foramen. Free fragments of disc material are common sources of root compression which may occasionally escape detection by all radiological studies, including myelography, CT, and MRI. In this author's experience, it is not unusual to discover occult disc fragments and other sources of mechanical root distortion in patients seeking reevaluation after failed discectomy.

Lumbar disc protrusions are most common at L5–S1 and at L4–L5, less so at L3–L4, and even less common at successively higher levels. Cervical disc protrusions are most common at C5–C6 and C6–C7, and C4–C5. Thoracic disc protrusions are seen far less often than lumbar and cervical, but when present are typically at the most caudal levels of the thoracic spine or at the thoracolumbar junction.

In the cervical and thoracic regions, the root endangered by a disc protrusion is generally the one which exits above the vertebra of the same number (i.e. the C7 root is compressed by the C6–C7 disc). This pattern does not necessarily hold true in the lumbar region since the spinal cord ends around the level of the L1–L2 disc space. Several roots may pass behind a given lumbar disc. Thus the L5 root and the S1 root may both be injured by a large protrusion of the L4–L5 disc. The S1 root alone may be injured by a posterolateral L5–S1 disc protrusion, or rarely the L5 root affected by huge osteophytes laterally at a point outside the spinal canal. It would be most unusual to see pain in the lower sacral root distribution with an L5–S1 disc protrusion, even though the S2–S5 roots pass directly behind that disc. This is so because the smaller sacral roots float freely in cerebrospinal fluid in a fairly capacious theca.

In some cases, spondylotic changes of the lumbar facet joints cause entrapment of a root as it passes caudally in the lateral recess of the spinal canal producing the 'superior facet syndrome' (Epstein et al 1972), also known as lateral recess stenosis (Figs 40.5 and 40.6). This bony entrapment of the root is not always confined to a single level. In fact, it can be a harbinger of advancing lumbar spondylosis. In severe cases, roots at nearly every level of the lumbar spine may be flattened in the lateral recesses. Radicular pain due to lateral recess stenosis is indistinguishable from that of disc protrusion. This is another common cause for the failure of discectomy to relieve pain.

Another potential cause of radicular pain following surgery is an occult fracture of the inferior articular process of a vertebra. This typically follows bone removal at the time of laminotomy and discectomy. The fracture occurs postoperatively when the patient resumes activities in an upright posture. Fractures of this type can lead to subluxation of the facet joint. The unopposed superior articular process of the vertebra below migrates upward and its tip may impinge on the nerve root in the foramen (see Fig. 40.4). Occult facet fractures were found in 25 of a series of 400 patients undergoing routine postoperative CT scans after lumbar spinal surgery (Rothman et al 1985). These fractures were usually not discernible by plain spine films, and CT images in the axial plane showed no abnormality other than slight widening of the joint space on the affected side. Sagittally reformatted CT scans demonstrated a lucent defect at the site of the fracture. Because cortical bone creates a signal void on

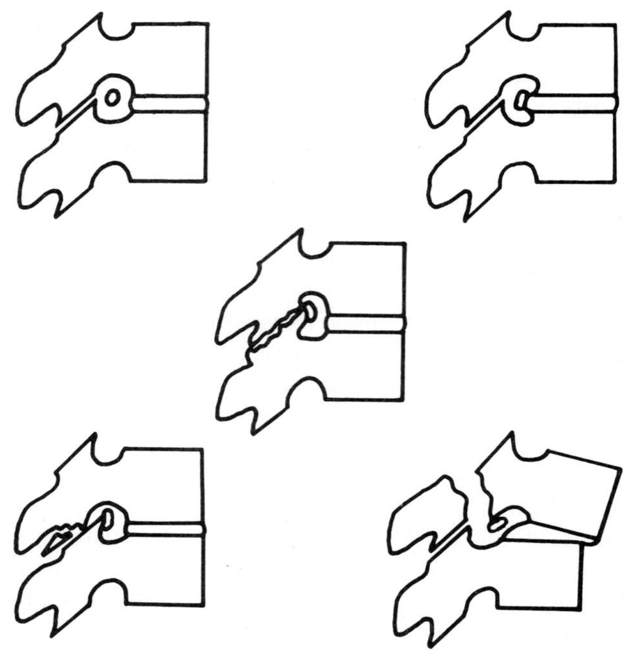

Fig. 40.4 Mechanical root lesions (lateral view). **Upper left** Normal relationship of nerve root to disc and vertebrae. **Upper right** Disc protrusion and osteophytes. **Centre** Facet joint degeneration. **Lower left** Fracture of inferior articular process. **Lower right** Spondylolysis with spondylolisthesis.

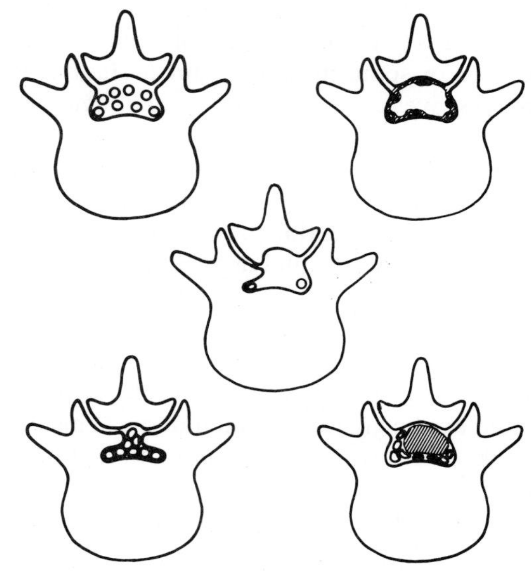

Fig. 40.5 Lumbosacral root lesions (horizontal view). **Upper left** Normal configuration of the spinal canal and cauda equina. **Upper right** Chronic adhesive arachnoiditis and atrophic roots. **Centre** Entrapment of a root descending in narrow lateral recess ('superior facet syndrome'). **Lower left** Lumbar spinal stenosis due to spondylosis. **Lower right** Intradural tumour compressing the cauda equina.

hydrogen proton magnetic resonance images, currently available MRI scanners may fail to detect facet fractures even though the images can be displayed in sagittal format.

The foregoing must be distinguished from spondylolysis, which is a congenital defect in the pars interarticularis of the vertebra sparing the articular processes. This defect is commonly associated with forward slippage (spondylolisthesis) of the upper vertebra on the one below. In severe cases, a portion of the listhetic vertebra may hook the root below (see Fig. 40.4). Further root embarassment may be due to an overgrowth of dense fibrous tissue which fills the gap in the pars interarticularis defect. These events usually take place at the L5–S1 level with bilateral L5 root entrapment, but they may occur at L4–L5 with L4 root involvement.

Other mechanical causes of root distortion include primary and metastatic tumours of the vertebrae, which encroach upon the intervertebral foramen as the pedicle is destroyed. Spinal intradural tumours may grow directly from the root (e.g. schwannoma, neurofibroma) or so close to it that compression is inevitable (e.g. meningioma, ependymoma). Vertebral metastases may occur at all levels. Meningiomas and schwannomas are commonly thoracic, while ependymomas are more likely to develop in the lumbar region. Tumours of the lumbar canal and cauda equina may produce crowding of the lumbosacral roots similar to that found in lumbar spinal stenosis (see Fig. 40.5). Benign arachnoid cysts and perineurial cysts (Tarlov 1970) may behave like tumours, causing radicular pain in the lumbosacral region, or sometimes coccygeal pain. Pelvic tumours may closely mimic spine disorders by causing compression of the lumbosacral plexus. In patients with advanced vascular disease, atherosclerotic aneurysms of the hypogastric or common iliac arteries may behave in similar fashion, producing sciatica of rather abrupt onset (Chapman et al 1964).

Focal deposits of leukaemic cells, lymphoma, or metastatic carcinoma within the cerebrospinal fluid pathways cause radicular pain. Some types of carcinoma actually infiltrate the dorsal roots, spinal nerve trunks, and dorsal root ganglia (Barron et al 1960). In addition, a syndrome of slowly progressive sensory neuropathy, which may be painful, has been described as a remote effect of carcinoma. In three autopsied cases, this syndrome was associated with inflammation and degeneration of the dorsal root ganglia and dorsal roots (Horwich et al 1977).

The pathophysiology of root dysfunction causing pain and claudication in lumbar stenosis is not known with certainty. When a narrow spinal canal is present, compression of the cauda equina when the lumbar spine is in extension may cause mechanical distortion of the roots, venous stasis and swelling of the roots, and relative ischaemia and hypoxia of the roots in the face of an increased neuronal oxygen demand during exercise (Weinstein et al 1977).

Coccygodynia is a loosely defined syndrome which undoubtedly has more than one possible aetiology. Fibrosis, inflammation and demyelination of sacral roots have been reported in some cases of coccygodynia (Bohm & Franksson 1959). In other cases, sacral root cysts or arachnoiditis have been found. Some instances of coccygodynia are thought to be referred pain from degenerative disease of the lumbosacral facet joints.

ARACHNOIDITIS

The literature regarding arachnoiditis is based largely on myelographic descriptions of filling defects in the subarachnoid space, absence of root sleeves, an irregular contrast pattern resembling 'candle drippings', arachnoid cysts, and sometimes complete obstruction of flow (Seaman et al 1953; Smith & Loeser 1972). After repeated myelograms with oil-based contrast agents, seldom used today, it was not unusual to see residual contrast material lodged permanently within arachnoid loculations and adhesions. Ironically, of the many factors contributing to the development of arachnoiditis (Table 40.4), myelographic contrast agents are probably the most often incriminated. The severe adhesive arachnoiditis which was associated with iophendylate (Pantopaque) myelography is rarely seen today since the introduction of water-soluble agents such as metrizamide and meglumine iocarmate. Nevertheless, there is still cause for concern with these

Table 40.4 Some factors predisposing to arachnoiditis

Chronic lumbosacral root compression
- Disc protrusion
- Spinal stenosis

Infection
- Bacterial meningitis, including tuberculous
- Fungal meningitis
- Cryptococcal meningitis
- Viral meningitis
- Syphilis

Haemorrhage
- From spinal vascular malformation
- Following trauma
- Following lumbar puncture
- Following surgery

Irritant chemicals
- Myelographic contrast agents
  - Iophendylate
  - meglumine iocarmate
  - methiodal
  - ? metrizamide
- Anaesthetic agents
- Amphotericin B
- Methotrexate
- ? Steroids
- Polyethylene glycol
- 2-Chloroprocaine

newer agents. Metrizamide can produce signs of meningeal irritation, including fever, nuchal rigidity, and the appearance of inflammatory cells in the cerebrospinal fluid (Junck & Marshall 1983). Methiodal myelography was shown to cause the known radiographic changes of arachnoiditis in 29% of nonoperated cases and 48% of those who had subsequent spinal surgery (Skalpe 1976). Typical adhesive arachnoiditis has been demonstrated after administration of either meglumine iocarmate or metrizamide in monkeys (Haughton et al 1977). Even though blood is known to increase the chance of arachnoiditis after myelography with iophendylate, the addition of blood to cerebrospinal fluid along with aqueous contrast agents failed to increase the incidence of experimental arachnoiditis in monkeys (Haughton & Ho 1982). Adhesive arachnoiditis was described in 15 patients who underwent lumbar radiculography with a combination of meglumine iocarmate and depository steroids. This complication may have been due partly to steroids, since patients studied with meglumine iocarmate alone did not show arachnoiditis (Dullerud & Morland 1976).

Chronically compressed lumbar nerve roots and dorsal root ganglia may develop swelling and histological signs of an inflammatory reaction inside the root sleeve (Lindahl & Rexed 1951). This should be distinguished from the dense scar formation which so often follows surgery. The latter is generally restricted to the epidural space and has been called 'pachymeningitis externa'. In chronic arachnoiditis, some or all of the lumbosacral roots may be encased by dense leptomeningeal adhesions within the dura. The final stage of this process is a lumbar canal in which the roots are bound circumferentially to the dura (see Fig. 40.5). Burton (1978) suggested the following sequence of events:

1. The pia of individual roots is inflamed, with root swelling and hyperaemia (radiculitis).
2. The roots adhere to each other and to the surrounding arachnoid trabeculae, and fibroblasts proliferate.
3. There is atrophy of the roots, which are displaced circumferentially and encased in collagen deposits.

As discussed below, myelography is now generally losing favour among clinicians. The changes characteristic of arachnoiditis can often be demonstrated by MRI or high resolution CT. The lumbar nerve roots can sometimes be shown to cluster together and to adhere to the surrounding meninges, leaving the centre of the spinal canal void. With many long-standing cases of arachnoiditis, one sees trapped radiographic contrast material of high density which may produce scattering artefacts on CT images. This is more of a problem with older CT scanners than with the current generation. Magnetic resonance imaging does accurately diagnose arachnoiditis, comparing favourably with CT myelography and plain film myelography for that purpose (Delamarter et al 1990). However, use of gadolinium during MR imaging does not reveal significant additional information about the condition (Johnson & Sze 1990).

Arachnoiditis is usually worst in the lumbosacral subarachnoid space, although it can involve any level of the spinal canal or even the intracranial cisterns. In many cases, arachnoiditis seems to result from an initial focus of inflammation such as a nerve root compressed by lumbar stenosis or disc protrusion. The presence of blood in the cerebrospinal fluid after lumbar puncture, myelography or surgery aggravates this. The additional presence of an irritating foreign substance such as iophendylate greatly augments the effect of blood in the subarachnoid space. Intrathecal drugs and infection of the meninges may also contribute. Drugs with known risk of arachnoiditis include the antifungal agent amphotericin B; methotrexate; 2-Chloroprocaine, and methylprednisolone acetate (for references, see Esses & Morley 1983). Wilkinson (1992) reviewed the literature on intrathecal methylprednisolone and concluded that most of the evidence implicating the drug in arachnoiditis was circumstantial; also, most of the complications of intrathecal steroids appeared to be related to frequent injections and large doses. All types of infectious meningitis, including viral, parasitic, cryptococcal, tuberculous and ordinary bacterial, may be followed by arachnoiditis.

The exact cause of root dysfunction in arachnoiditis is not known, but direct compression by scar encasement, arachnoid cysts and tense fluid loculations must certainly contribute. Caplan et al (1990) postulated that central spinal cord ischaemia and altered cerebrospinal fluid flow patterns associated with chronic arachnoiditis may lead to formation of cystic regions of myelomalacia in the cord, or even frank syrinx formation. Possibly the encasement of roots by collagen deposits leads to atrophy on an ischaemic basis. It is also reasonable to think that roots which are tethered by scarred meninges are no longer free to slide during flexion/extension motions of the spine and legs, so that recurring stretch injury to individual nerve fibres would be likely. In some cases, the arachnoid is known to contain chronic inflammatory cells as well as collagen deposits and hyaline material (Quiles et al 1978). Macrophages may also be found (Dujovny et al 1978). Surgical swab debris retained in the epidural space after spinal surgery was identified histologically within dense fibrous connective tissue in 55% of cases submitted to biopsies (Hoyland et al 1988). This material consists mainly of cotton fibres, originating from surgical swabs and patties. Cotton is known to produce a fibrotic reaction, so that epidural fibrosis may result. It is not known whether these extradural changes are relevant to the intrathecal events leading to arachnoiditis.

INVESTIGATIONS

The use of myelography to investigate disc protrusion, spondylosis and spinal tumour is now rapidly giving way to noninvasive imaging techniques. There is a growing consensus among radiologists, and a somewhat reluctant agreement by clinicians, that myelography is no longer the procedure of choice for investigating root symptoms. Either CT or MRI can demonstrate cervical disc protrusions, spondylotic changes, fractures, spinal tumours and cysts at almost any level of the spine. While high-resolution CT is perhaps better for demonstrating bone pathology (Fig. 40.6), MRI has the advantage of showing syringomyelic cavities and intraspinal tumours without introduction of contrast media into the cerebrospinal fluid. Nostalgia should not blind the clinician to the reality that computerised imaging has virtually no risk. Myelography, which has significant risks, should be reserved for cases in which a small root lesion cannot be demonstrated on technically satisfactory CT and MRI studies, and perhaps also those cases in which an anxious and claustrophobic patient cannot tolerate the confined space of the scanning machine.

Discography (pressure injection of radiographic contrast into the nucleus pulposus of the disc) has also lost favour in recent years. As noted above, better imaging techniques have made it unnecessary to resort to invasive procedures to diagnose root compression in most cases. Moreover, discography is not reliable. In theory, increasing the pressure within a degenerated disc should cause further root compression and an exacerbation of pain. However, the neighbouring discs are often also degenerated. Patients undergoing discography frequently complain of pain during injection of nearly every disc, so that it is seldom clear that any one of them is the culprit. After decades of clinical experimentation with discography, we still await soundly designed studies comparing the outcome of this procedure with that of less invasive tests. In the author's opinion, better methods such as CT and MRI are now available to judge the severity of disc degeneration and root compression. The degree of procedural discomfort to the patient and the acknowledged risk of disc space infection make it hard to justify discography in any case.

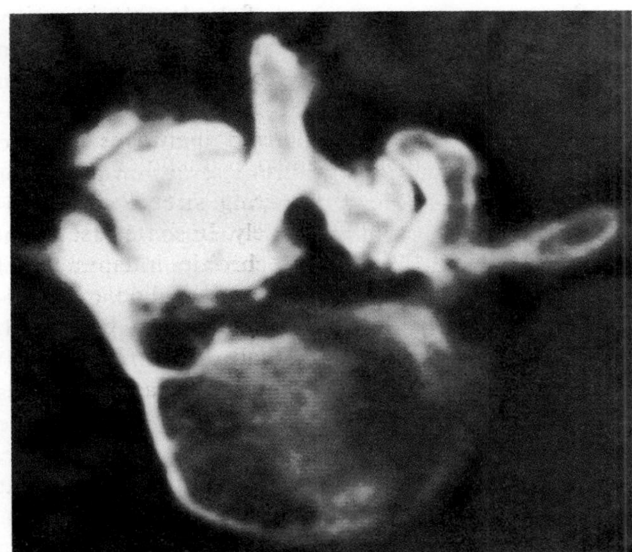

Fig. 40.6 Computed tomographic (CT) scan in horizontal plane showing severely degenerated, hypertrophic facet joint at the L4–L5 level (left side of photograph; compare this with Fig. 40.5, centre).

The technique of injecting an individual nerve root sheath with local anaesthetic (MacNab 1971; Schutz et al 1973) has not gained popularity since it was introduced. It may in fact be the only way to achieve a reasonably selective root block which does not spread to other levels, but it is very painful and risks further injury to a root which may already be damaged. Injection of local anaesthetic into the adjacent facet joints may be useful in carefully selected cases, proving that the radicular pain is referred from the joint and not the root itself. Whether it is possible to distinguish a 'facet syndrome' in the population of patients with chronic low back pain and sciatica is doubtful. Most patients with significant facet degeneration also have disc degeneration, ligamentous hypertrophy and other causes of pain, if not frank root compression.

Various electromyographic techniques are useful to identify sites of nerve root damage (Stewart 1987). In radicular pain of recent onset, signs of active denervation appear in muscles innervated by the damaged root and not in other muscles. These signs of active denervation include fibrillation potentials and positive sharp waves. In chronic lesions, active denervation is no longer seen. Instead, an increased number of polyphasic potentials may be the only evidence of root damage. Electromyogram (EMG) abnormalities tend to appear sooner in the deep paraspinous muscles than in limb muscles. Changes in the paraspinous muscle EMG may persist for 2 years after spinal surgery (See & Kraft 1975). In patients who have undergone previous root decompressions, the most valuable finding would therefore be a normal EMG (Eisen 1981).

Recordings of selective somatosensory-evoked potentials have been shown to be helpful in determining the sites of cervical and lumbosacral root lesions (Eisen & Elleker 1980; Aminoff et al 1985). Recordings of peripheral nerve and muscle responses to stimulation may serve to distinguish central damage (cord, roots or ganglia) from peripheral nerve injury. If there is a history of trauma and a paralysed, anaesthetic arm, the finding of normal sensory nerve action potentials and absence of muscle action potentials on nerve stimulation suggests that nerve roots of the brachial plexus have been avulsed from the cord (Warren et al 1969). Similar findings could occur in syringomyelia (Fincham & Cape 1968) which might also develop after spine trauma and which may mimic the segmental anaesthesia and severe pain of root avulsion.

PHYSIOLOGICAL CORRELATES OF RADICULAR PAIN

The physiological events which cause root pain are controversial. Some authors (e.g. Kelly 1956) maintain that nerve compression per se is not painful. This may be so in many cases of asymptomatic disc protrusion, as noted earlier (Hitselberger & Witten 1968). Acute mechanical injuries of nerve roots in laboratory animals cause only short (1–50 s) trains of repetitive firing in sensory axons (Wall et al 1974). Clearly this brief injury discharge is not the physiological correlate of chronic sciatica in humans.

Some of the pain associated with root compression is referred from regions of distortion of neighbouring muscle insertions, joint capsules and ligaments. Truncal pain can be produced during surgery under local anaesthesia by direct pressure on these structures, whereas pain radiating to the extremity is best reproduced by stimulation of the root itself (Frykholm 1951; Murphey 1968). Even gentle mechanical stimuli to dorsal roots, such as stroking with a probe or slight stretching, can elicit segmental pain in humans (Smyth & Wright 1958).

It is unlikely that axons in chronically compressed, ischaemic, inflamed or otherwise damaged roots would behave in normal fashion. Many of the physical events which damaged nerve roots lead to either focal loss of myelin or loss of axons. This is most likely to occur at sites between the dorsal root ganglia and the dorsal root entry zone. Ectopic impulse generation is known to occur in fibres of chronically injured nerves and in compressed dorsal root ganglia (Howe et al 1977). At least in myelinated axons, long periods (5–15 min) of repetitive firing may result. The dorsal root ganglion itself is subject to compression in some cases of disc disease (Lindblom & Rexed 1948). The ganglion is undoubtedly affected in some cases of perineurial cysts and arachnoiditis as well. Slight root movements may serve as mechanical triggers of abnormal impulse generation in mechanosensitive chronically injured roots and ganglia when they are tethered by adhesions or compressed by disc, bone or tumour. Dorsal root ganglion cells can also be a source of ectopic afferent impulses in sensory fibres after peripheral nerve damage (Wall & Devor 1983). This latter finding may be relevant to cases of so-called 'double crush' syndrome (Upton & McComas 1973), in which peripheral nerve entrapment and nerve root entrapment coexist.

An explanation of the paroxysmal pain which occurs in cranial neuralgias might include ectopic impulse generation at sites of nerve compression where there is focal demyelination, reflection of impulses at these sites and others to produce reverberation in the nerve, and recruitment of small afferent fibres by means of strong presynaptic depolarisation of their terminals (Calvin et al 1977). Another possible mechanism for recruitment of thinly myelinated and unmyelinated fibres might be ephaptic impulse transmission at sites lacking myelin, similar to that which is thought to occur in ventral roots of dystrophic mice (Rasminsky 1980).

In cases of chronic root avulsion, transection, or destruction, the resulting chronic deafferentation of spinal sensory transmission neurons might cause paroxysmal pain. Deafferented cord neurons are thought to discharge in an uncontrolled fashion (Loeser et al 1968). It follows that lesions of the dorsal horn might stop the abnormal discharge, a theory which helps to explain the success of dorsal root entry zone lesions for controlling root avulsion pain (Nashold et al 1983). Traumatic, syphilitic and herpetic lesions of the dorsal roots can sometimes involve portions of the Lissauer tract and substantia gelatinosa which are thought to be involved in the physiological mechanisms of pain suppression (Wall 1980). This suggests that some types of deafferentation pain may be due to an indirect rather than a direct disinhibition of dorsal horn transmission cells.

The quality of pain and the size of the painful region must depend on:

1. the population of fibres which are destroyed
2. the population of normally functioning afferents
3. the number and types of fibres which are discharging excessively, and
4. the interaction of impulses in the cord.

In laboratory animals, the receptive fields of individual dorsal horn neurons show marked long-term plasticity after chronic root section (Wall 1977). Sensory deficits in human patients who have undergone dorsal rhizotomy can also fluctuate, and the surface area of a gradually diminishing cutaneous sensory deficit is said to return to maximal size in some cases when the serotonin precursor tryptophan is given (King 1980). A large body of experimental work indicates that neuronal function in the dorsal horn is modulated from the brain stem by way of descending serotoninergic pathways, some of which terminate in the substantia gelatinosa. In the cat spinal cord, substantia gelatinosa neurons have variable ('amoeboid') receptive fields (Dubuisson et al 1979). These unit fields sometimes enlarge rather abruptly after stimulation of the dorsolateral funiculus (DLF) of the cord white matter, which contains descending serotoninergic axons that terminate in the dorsal horn (Dubuisson & Wall 1980). This enlargement of receptive fields is accompanied by a facilitation of activity in the same population of substantia gelatinosa units. Units of this type may show direct transsynaptic excitation by DLF stimulation (Dubuisson

1980). Since the predominant effect of descending impulses upon dorsal horn projection neurons of the spinothalamic and spinocervical tracts is an inhibitory one, one might speculate that there is a population of inhibitory interneurons near the dorsal root entry zone and that their state of activity and receptivity controls the apparent size of the dermatome.

Pain is sometimes abolished temporarily by root blocks distal to the site of root damage (Kibler & Nathan 1960), so that some 'normal' afferent impulses must play a facilitating role. Local anaesthetic block of neighbouring roots might have a similar effect, reducing the total afferent input to cord transmission neurons. Therefore the results of diagnostic nerve root blocks must be interpreted with caution. When pain is referred to the distal portion of the dermatome from a source located proximally, local anaesthetic blockade of branches to that proximal source may alleviate the referred pain. Thus, in some cases of severe lumbar facet joint degeneration, injection into the facet joint itself (facet block) may rid the patient of pain radiating down the leg. Similar phenomena undoubtedly occur when local anaesthetic is injected into trigger points in the back muscles and ligaments.

The role of the ventral rootlets in radicular pain is speculative. Ectopic efferent activity in ventral root fibres could lead to muscle spasm, which might in turn generate painful afferent activity in the associated myotome (Frykholm 1951). However, the territory of pain radiation to muscles correlates poorly with electromyographic evidence of damage to the ventral roots (Fisher et al 1978). The ventral roots do contain some unmyelinated afferent fibres (Coggeshall et al 1975). Some of these fibres loop back to reenter the dorsal root ganglion and some may innervate the leptomeninges around the ventral cord surface (Chung et al 1984). Others may possibly enter the ventral horn and terminate in the cord grey matter. Their function remains a matter of speculation. Reasons to think that they could contribute to segmental pain in some cases were put forth by Hosobuchi (1980), who favoured the use of dorsal root ganglionectomy instead of dorsal rhizotomy in order to eliminate possible ventral root afferent connections.

TREATMENT

The usual initial treatment of mechanical lesions of the spinal nerve roots is rest, mild analgesic medication, and avoidance of physical activities which increase the pain. Some patients will benefit from the use of a soft collar, intermittent cervical traction, or a lumbar brace. The author prescribes a muscle relaxant for a limited time in nearly all cases, in order to counteract the inevitable spasm of the paravertebral muscles. Orphenadrine, methocarbamol, or cyclobenzaprine usually suffices as long as the patient understands that the medication is not a simple analgesic to be taken on an occasional basis. Application of heat also helps to quell muscle spasm temporarily; some patients find ice massage more useful than heat. In cases of severe reactive muscle spasm, the author has found baclofen helpful, and has occasionally resorted to intravenous diazepam or methocarbamol in hospitalised patients. It can be exceedingly difficult to perform a reliable neurological examination in an anxious patient with muscle spasm, with or without true radicular pain. It has been the author's frequent experience that many of the original 'objective neurological findings' will disappear once the patient relaxes and cooperates with the examination.

Within a few days, most instances of radicular pain due to mild disc protrusion or facet arthrosis will begin to relent. It is common practice to require a period of strict bedrest in these cases, but the duration of rest is a subject of some controversy. One randomized clinical trial (Deyo et al 1986) showed that 2 days of bedrest was as effective as a longer period in patients with acute low back pain, even when minor sensory and motor deficits were present. Patients with more obvious root damage may require a longer period of rest. If there is adequate relief after this trial of rest, and resolution of neurological deficits, there may be no need for further restriction of activities or for diagnostic tests. If pain and deficits do not improve, CT or MRI studies of the appropriate level of the spine should be obtained. If the diagnosis remains in doubt, electromyography, spinal fluid analysis or other tests may be indicated.

Recurrence of lumbosacral root compression can sometimes be prevented by a course of supervised exercises to strengthen the abdominal muscles and gently stretch the taut spine extensors. In one series of 100 patients with signs of acute lumbosacral radiculopathy, conservative management and occasional short-term use of oral corticosteroids produced satisfactory relief in 95% (Johnson & Fletcher 1981). Another series of 100 patients with radicular pain due to myelographically-proven herniated lumbar discs were treated with an initially high but tapering dose of intramuscular dexamethasone for 7 days. All had relief of pain in 24–48 hours and only nine subsequently required surgery (Green 1975). Oral steroids do have serious potential adverse effects, most of which can be prevented by a brief duration of use. Randomized controlled trials of oral steroids with CT or MRI correlation are needed to establish their role in treating early root lesions.

Epidural steroid injection is widely advocated for pain associated with nerve root compression due to disc protrusion and spondylosis. Unfortunately, most of the available literature at present suffers from inadequate methodological design. Only a few randomized, controlled trials are available, and none of these is substantiated by electromyography, CT or MRI to document objectively the presence of nerve root damage. Indeed, it appears that when frank root damage is already present, the chances of benefit from epidural steroids are greatly diminished. The best chance of success with this treatment is within the first month of a mild disc protrusion. Even then, reported success rates in better-controlled studies range from 0–70% using rather lenient criteria, such as the disappearance of pain on straight-leg-raising and the patient's subjective improvement early after the procedure (Dilke et al 1973; Snoek et al 1977; Breivik et al 1976; Cuckler et al 1985). Even enthusiasts admit that patients with chronic sciatica do not fare as well, and those with previous surgery, entrapment of roots by bone or scar tissue, or demonstrable behavioural disturbances are even less likely to respond (White et al 1980). In successful cases, as many as three injections may be needed, and beneficial effects are often delayed for 2–6 days (Green et al 1980). There is some evidence that intrathecal steroids can lead to arachnoiditis, probably due to the vehicle polyethylene glycol (Nelson et al 1973). Intrathecal steroid injection can aggravate radicular pain acutely and administration by this route is inadvisable. Epidural injections of the steroid triamcinolone in cats failed to produce any histological signs of damage in lumbar roots (Delaney et al 1980). At present there is no evidence that epidural steroid use in humans causes further root damage. Steroids given in this way are absorbed systemically and can suppress adrenal function for 3 weeks (Gorski et al 1982).

Long-term management of both cervical and lumbar radiculopathy due to mechanical spine problems should not neglect dietetic referral for weight loss in obese patients. In most cases, this goal will only be achieved by a 1- or 2-year period of supervised diet and physical activity. If surgery is undertaken, the operation should not be treated as a substitute for these other measures which are still needed to counteract progressive postural deterioration and spondylosis.

Surgical decompression of a compromised nerve root is warranted by progression of the neurological deficit or by intractable pain. Signs of compression of the cord or cauda equina are urgent indications for surgery regardless of the amount of pain. Disc surgery is reviewed elsewhere in this volume. Here, a few generalities will serve to indicate typical current practice. At levels between C3 and T1, root compression at one or two levels is best treated by anterior cervical discectomy with removal of osteophytes and wide lateral exposure of the affected roots. Dowel bone grafts are inserted to fuse the adjoining vertebrae at those levels. More than two levels of involvement are usually treated by cervical laminectomies. All sites of root compression are relieved by foramenotomy, creating a 5 × 8 mm slot behind each. Failure to explore and decompress roots adequately by either the anterior or posterior approach is a common reason for persistent radicular pain.

Lumbar root compression is usually treated by a posterior surgical approach. Again, thorough removal of any disc, bone, or thickened ligament distorting the involved root is the goal. Some surgeons advocate wide exposure, while others practise 'microsurgical discectomy'. Several series of lumbar 'microdiscectomies' have been reported in which over 90% of patients were relieved of their symptoms and returned to their previous activities (Wilson & Kenning 1979; Goald 1980; Williams 1983; Maroon & Abla 1985). Wilson & Harbaugh (1981) reported a 50% earlier return to work with microdiscectomy than with standard laminectomy, but Kahanovitz et al (1989) found that the only significant advantage of microdiscectomy was that the patients left the hospital earlier. Bertrand (1975) and Fager (1986) have criticized the use of microdiscectomy technique on the grounds that bony ridges, thickened ligament material, and freely extruded disc fragments may be inaccessible through a 'micro' approach. Moreover, limited exposure during discectomy may make it necessary to use greater retraction pressure on the neighboring nerve root, and this may damage the root. With careful preoperative radiological studies, it is currently possible, and indeed essential, to document all of the relevant anatomical factors causing root distortion before embarking on surgery. An experienced surgeon can probably deal with unilateral facet hypertrophy and free herniated disc fragments as well as disc protrusion per se through a small incision, provided that the preoperative radiological studies make the structural abnormalities quite clear and they are unilateral. Sadly, the large population of patients with persistent radiculopathy following inadequate disc surgery suggests that there must be few truly 'experienced' surgeons. The author continues to practise a rather wide surgical exposure.

Postoperative epidural scar encasement of the root may be a cause for failure of disc surgery. This tissue can be distinguished from disc material by means of intravenous contrast-enhanced CT, which shows uptake of contrast by vascular scar tissue but not by disc (Teplick & Haskin 1984). If postoperative radiological studies document persistent root distortion due to osteophytes, thick or calcified annulus fibrosus, or disc material, reoperation and completion of the root decompression should be considered. Pain of chronically damaged roots does not respond to these basic measures, though. Repeated exploration and decompression of traumatised roots is usually futile. Rhizotomy at the time of reexploration is not apt to be beneficial (Bertrand 1975) and may lead to a very unpleasant deafferentation pain syndrome. Dorsal root ganglionectomy has been advocated for pain traced to a single damaged root, but this procedure has not been convincingly shown to be more effective (or less likely to cause deafferentation dysaesthesia) than rhizotomy at lumbar levels.

Symptomatic lumbar spinal stenosis, particularly if neurogenic claudication is present, is an indication for surgical decompression of the involved levels. Rarely, a single level of stenosis can be relieved by limited surgery, but far more often laminectomies and foramenotomies are required at multiple levels between L2 and sacrum.

Chymopapain or collagenase injected into the centre of a degenerated disc digests and shrinks the nucleus pulposus. In North America, following earlier decades of moderate enthusiasm, chemonucleolysis of discs has largely ceased to be used. This is so because its success rate is less than that of open discectomy and because its complications are not insignificant. As early as 1978, questions were raised about the effectiveness of the procedure, which was said to be similar to that of a placebo in one randomized, double-blind study (Martins et al 1978). Further studies since then have documented a 60–70% rate of neurological improvement and pain relief after chemonucleolysis when an appropriate clinical deficit, mechanical signs of root compression, and objective radiological evidence of root compression by the disc are present. Postchemonucleolysis CT scans may show impressive changes. Unfortunately, they do not always reflect the clinical outcome. About 25% of patients undergoing chymopapain discolysis experience severe back muscle spasm after the procedure. The degree of muscle spasm is sometimes incapacitating and often worse than that seen after open surgery. The reasons for this are still unknown. Other reported complications include anaphylaxis and discitis (Watts 1977), and neural toxicity. Shields (1985) found 35 documented cases of paraplegia due to cauda equina syndrome or acute transverse myelitis in patients undergoing lumbar chemonucleolysis. Experimental demyelination and disruption of the vasa nervorum in rabbit tibial nerves has been reported as a toxic effect of chymopapain (Rydevik et al 1976).

The complications associated with chemonucleolysis led to further efforts to treat lumbar discs percutaneously, including the mechanical nucleotome, an automated suction/cutting probe (Onik & Maroon 1988). This device was subjected to a multiinstitutional study (Onik et al 1990) with about 75% of patients obtaining relief from sciatica in a carefully selected group of cases. Workmen's compensation patients were excluded, as were those with significant facet joint disease, spinal stenosis, extruded disc fragments and other degenerative changes contributing to radiculopathy. While the complication rate of the procedure was only about 1% overall, the results still did not equal those of open discectomy. Moreover, patients with spondylotic joint enlargement, osteophytes and thickened ligaments will not likely be helped by this or any other percutaneous method.

TREATMENT OF CHRONIC RADICULOPATHIES AND ARACHNOIDITIS

The most treatable of the severe chronic radicular pain syndromes are undoubtedly the paroxysmal lower cranial neuralgias. Though unresponsive to ordinary analgesics, glossopharyngeal and geniculate neuralgia can frequently be managed with anticonvulsants (carbamazepine and phenytoin). These can sometimes be used in combination, with better results than when used singly. Monitoring of serum drug levels and periodic blood counts is advisable. Failures of drug therapy may be considered for surgical rhizotomy which is likely to be curative, but with significant risks.

Chronic radicular pain of postherpetic neuralgia, diabetic neuropathy, and failed disc surgery sometimes respond to anticonvulsants, but this group of patients is liable to failure of all conservative measures. Some cases of postherpetic neuralgia benefit from transcutaneous electrical nerve stimulation (Nathan & Wall 1974), epidural steroid injections (Forrest 1980), or psychotropic drugs (amitriptyline and fluphenazine; Taub & Collins 1974). Of the various neurosurgical options, dorsal root entry zone lesions currently offer the best chance of long-term relief, about 60% in cases of postherpetic neuralgia (Friedman & Nashold 1984). The same procedure gives 62–82% chance of long-term relief in pain due to brachial plexus root avulsion (Nashold & Ostdahl 1979; Thomas & Jones 1984; Samii & Moringlane 1984).

The management of pain in chronic arachnoiditis continues to be a discouraging problem. Initially, cultures of cerebrospinal fluid should be done to eliminate the possibility of a chronic low-grade infection. The presence of fibrosis in the spinal canal may make it dangerous to attempt administration of epidural drugs for pain management in these cases (O'Connor et al 1990). Steroids have been advocated; there is no objective proof of their effectiveness, and as noted above, their use intrathecally may even contribute to arachnoiditis. The rationale of steroid therapy has its basis in animal studies showing diminution of the aseptic meningeal inflammatory reaction to blood and radiographic contrast agents (Howland & Curry 1966). This may not be analogous to the severe chronic adhesive process seen in humans. Lumbar air insufflation and radiation therapy have not been shown to have any value in this condition (Whisler 1978). In occasional cases, the inflammatory process is focal enough that dorsal rhizotomics or dorsal root ganglionectomies help (Jain 1974), but the risks of postoperative dysaesthesias and deafferentation pain are unattractive ones. Lysis of intradural adhesions by tedious microsurgery has its proponents, but the results are equivocal. Microscopic lysis in 28 patients did not produce better results than conservative treatment, according to Johnston & Matheny (1978). Myelography showed reaccumulation of arachnoid loculations in all cases examined. Wilkinson & Schuman (1979) reported initial pain relief in 76% of cases after extensive dissection of adhesions under the operating microscope, and 50% were still relieved after 1 year. Gourie-Devi & Satish (1984) described intrathecal use of the proteolytic enzyme hyaluronidase in chronic spinal arachnoiditis. Early improvement of neurological status was seen in 11 of 15 patients, with no serious toxic effects. Of 66 patients with spinal arachnoiditis secondary to tuberculous meningitis, 39 were given intrathecal hyaluronidase in addition to the usual antituberculous drugs. These patients appeared to have reduced mortality and improved functional deficit scores in comparison with the group not receiving hyaluronidase (Gourie-Devi & Satishchandra 1991). Hyaluronidase therapy has not received widespread usage outside India, so far, and its potential role in the treatment of arachnoiditis after failed back surgery remains to be determined.

More commonly used is electrical spinal cord stimulation (Meilman et al 1990; North et al 1991), which carries very little risk. After failed surgery, arachnoiditis typically affects roots in the lumbar spine, but the segmental anatomy of the spinal cord dictates electrode placement in the lower thoracic region. Therefore patients wary of further spinal surgery are usually relieved to learn that the implantation procedure will not require a reexploration of the original laminectomy site. Cord stimulation for failed back surgery syndrome carries approximately a 50% long-term improvement rate (North et al 1991). When arachnoiditis is present, the outcome of stimulation appears primarily related to the number of roots involved (Meilman et al 1990). As might be expected, patients with injury to a single root respond more favorably than do those with multiple nerve root damage. Technical failures such as difficulty finding an effective stimulation target, or electrode migration, may impede the success of deep brain and cord electrical stimulation. However, when stimulation is effective, it can provide a welcome respite for these patients.

REFERENCES

Adams J H 1976 Virus diseases of the nervous system. In: Blackwood W, Corsellis J A N (eds) Greenfield's neuropathology. Edward Arnold, London, p 292–326

Aminoff M J, Goodin D S, Barbaro N M, Weinstein P R, Rosenblum M L 1985 Dermatomal somatosensory evoked potentials in unilateral lumbosacral radiculopathy. Annals of Neurology 17: 171–176

Auld A W 1978 Chronic spinal arachnoiditis. A postoperative syndrome that may signal its onset. Spine 3: 88–91

Baker A S, Ojemann R G, Swartz M N, Richardson E P 1975 Spinal epidural abscess. New England Journal of Medicine 293: 463–468

Barron K D, Rowland L P, Zimmerman H M 1960 Neuropathy with malignant tumor metastases. Journal of Nervous and Mental Diseases 131: 10–31

Bertrand G 1975 The 'battered' root problem. Orthopedic Clinics of North America 6: 305–309

Bohm E, Franksson C 1959 Coccygodynia and sacral rhizotomy. Acta Chirurgica Scandinavica 116: 268–274

Boulton A M J, Angus E, Ayyar D R, Weiss R 1984 Diabetic thoracic polyradiculopathy presenting as abdominal swelling. British Medical Journal 289: 798–799

Breivik H, Hesla P E, Molnar I, Lind B 1976 Treatment of chronic low back pain and sciatica: comparison of caudal epidural steroid injections of bupivacaine and methylprednisolone with bupivacaine followed by saline. In: Bonica J J, Albe-Fessard D (eds) Advances in pain research and therapy, vol 1. Raven Press, New York, p 927–932

Burton C V 1978 Lumbosacral arachnoiditis. Spine 3: 24–30

Calvin W H, Loeser J D, Howe J F 1977 A neurophysiological theory for the pain mechanism of tic douloureux. Pain 3: 147–154

Caplan L R, Norohna A B, Amico L L 1990 Syringomyelia and arachnoiditis. Journal of Neurology, Neurosurgery and Psychiatry 53: 106–113

Chapman E M, Shaw R S, Kubik C S 1964 Sciatic pain from arteriosclerotic aneurysm of pelvic arteries. New England Journal of Medicine 271: 1410–1411

Christensen E 1942 Chronic adhesive spinal arachnoiditis. Acta Psychiatrica Scandinavica 17: 23–38

Chung J M, Lee K H, Coggeshall R E 1984 Nociceptive role of ventral root afferents. In: Fields H L, Dubner R, Cervero F (eds) Advances in pain research and therapy, vol 9. Raven Press, New York, p 103–109

Coggeshall R E, Applebaum M L, Fazen M, Stubbs T B, Sykes M T 1975 Unmyelinated axons in human ventral roots, a possible explanation for the failure of dorsal rhizotomy to relieve pain. Brain 98: 157–166

Cuckler J M, Bernini P A, Wiesel S W, Booth R E, Rothman R H, Pickens G T 1985 The use of epidural steroids in the treatment of lumbar radicular pain: a prospective, randomized, double-blind study. Journal of Bone and Joint Surgery 67A: 63–66

Davis C H 1982 Extradural spinal cord and nerve root compression from benign lesions of the lumbar area. In: Youmans J R (ed) Neurological surgery. W B Saunders, Philadelphia, p 2535–2561

Davis D 1957 Radicular syndromes. Year Book, Chicago

Delamarter R B, Ross J S, Masaryk T J, Modic M T, Bohlman H H 1990 Diagnosis of lumbar arachnoiditis by magnetic resonance imaging. Spine 15: 304–310

Delaney T J, Rowlingson J C, Carron H C, Butler A 1980 Epidural steroid effects on nerves and meninges. Anesthesia and Analgesia 59: 610–614

Denny-Brown D, Kirk E J, Yanagisawa N 1973 The tract of Lissauer in relation to sensory transmission in the dorsal horn of the spinal cord in the macaque monkey. Journal of Comparative Neurology 151: 175–200

Deparis M 1968 Glossopharyngeal neuralgia. In: Vinken P J, Bruyn G W (eds) Handbook of clinical neurology, vol 5. Headaches and cranial neuralgias. North-Holland, Amsterdam, p 350–361

Deyo R A, Diehl A K, Rosenthal M 1986 How many days of bed rest for acute low back pain? A randomized clinical trial. New England Journal of Medicine 315: 1064–1070

Dilke T F W, Burry H C, Grahame R 1973 Extradural corticosteroid injection in management of lumbar nerve root compression. British Medical Journal 2: 635–637

Dubuisson D 1980 Time course of descending excitation of single units recorded in laminae 1, 2 and 3 of cat spinal cord. Journal of Physiology 307: 56–57 P

Dubuisson D, Melzack R 1976 Classification of clinical pain descriptions by multiple group discriminant analysis. Experimental Neurology 51: 480–487

Dubuisson D, Wall P D 1980 Descending influences on receptive fields and activity of single units recorded in laminae 1, 2 and 3 of cat spinal cord. Brain Research 199: 283–298

Dubuisson D, Fitzgerald M, Wall P D 1979 Ameboid receptive fields of cells in laminae 1, 2 and 3. Brain Research 177: 376–378

Dugan M C, Locke S, Gallagher J R 1962 Occipital neuralgia in adolescents and young adults. New England Journal of Medicine 267: 1166–1172

Dujovny M, Barrionuevo P J, Kossovsky N, Laha R K, Rosenbaum A E 1978 Effects of contrast media on the canine subarachnoid space. Spine 3: 31–35

Dullerud R, Morland T J 1976 Adhesive arachnoiditis after lumbar radiculography with Dimer-X and Depo-Medrol. Radiology 119: 153–155

Dyck P 1976 The femoral nerve traction test with lumbar disc protrusions. Surgical Neurology 6: 163–166

Dykes R W, Terzis J K 1981 Spinal nerve distributions in the upper limb; the organization of the dermatome and afferent myotome. Philosophical Transactions of the Royal Society of London (Biology) 293: 509–554

Ehni G, Benner B 1984 Occipital neuralgia and the C1-2 arthrosis syndrome. Journal of Neurosurgery 61: 961–965

Eisen A 1981 Identifying a spinal nerve lesion. American Academy of Neurology, Special Courses 22: 81–92

Eisen A, Elleker G 1980 Sensory nerve stimulation and evoked cerebral potentials. Neurology 30: 1097–1105

Elkington J St C 1951 Arachnoiditis. In: Feiling A (ed) Modern trends in neurology. Hoeber, New York, p 149–161

Epstein J A, Epstein B S, Rosenthal A D, Carras R, Lavine L S 1972 Sciatica caused by nerve root entrapment in the lateral recess: the superior facet syndrome. Journal of Neurosurgery 36: 584–589

Esses S I, Morley T P 1983 Spinal arachnoiditis. Canadian Journal of Neurological Sciences 10: 2–10

Fager C A 1986 Lumbar microdiscectomy: a contrary opinion. Clinical Neurosurgery 33: 419–456

Feder B H, Smith J L 1962 Roentgen therapy in chronic spinal arachnoiditis. Radiology 78: 192–198

Fincham R W, Cape C A 1968 Sensory nerve conduction in syringomyelia. Neurology 18: 200–201

Fisher M A, Shivde A J, Teixera C, Grainer L S 1978 Clinical and electrophysiological appraisal of the significance of radicular injury in back pain. Journal of Neurology, Neurosurgery and Psychiatry 41: 303–306

Foerster O 1933 The dermatomes in man. Brain 56: 1–39

Forrest J R 1980 The response to epidural steroid injections in chronic dorsal root pain. Canadian Anesthetists Society Journal 27: 40–46

French J D 1946 Clinical manifestations of lumbar spinal arachnoiditis. Surgery 20: 718–729

Friedman A II, Nashold B S 1984 Dorsal root entry zone lesions for the treatment of postherpetic neuralgia. Neurosurgery 15: 969–970

Frykholm R 1951 Cervical root compression resulting from disc degeneration and root sleeve fibrosis. Acta Chirurgica Scandinavica (suppl) 160: 1–149

Gilroy J, Meyer J S 1975 Medical neurology, Macmillan, New York

Goald H 1980 Microlumbar discectomy: followup of 477 patients. Journal of Microsurgery 2: 95–100

Gorski D W, Rao T L K, Glisson S N, Chintagada M, El-Etr A 1982 Epidural triamcinolone and adrenal response to hypoglycemic stress in dogs. Anesthesiology 57: 364–366

Gourie-Devi M, Satish P 1984 Intrathecal hyaluronidase treatment of chronic spinal arachnoiditis of noninfective etiology. Surgical Neurology 22: 231–234

Gourie-Devi M, Satishchandra P 1991 Hyaluronidase as an adjuvant in the management of tuberculous spinal arachnoiditis. Journal of the Neurological Sciences 102: 105–111

Green L N 1975 Dexamethasone in the management of symptoms due to herniated lumbar disc. Journal of Neurology, Neurosurgery and Psychiatry 38: 1211–1217

Green P W B, Burke A J, Weiss C A, Langan P 1980 The role of epidural cortisone injection in the treatment of discogenic low back pain. Clinical Orthopedics 153: 121–125

Guyer D W, Wiltse L L, Eskay M L, Guyer B H 1989 The long-range prognosis of arachnoiditis. Spine 14: 1332–1341

Haughton V M, Ho K C 1982 Effect of blood on arachnoiditis from aqueous myelographic contrast media. American Journal of Roentgenology 139: 569–570

Haughton V M, Ho K C, Larson S J, Unger G F, Correa-Paz F 1977 Experimental production of arachnoiditis with water-soluble myelographic media. Rudiology 123: 681–685

Head H, Campbell A W 1900 The pathology of herpes zoster and its bearing on sensory localization. Brain 23: 353–523

Hitselberger W E, Witten R M 1968 Abnormal myelograms in asymptomatic patients. Journal of Neurosurgery 28: 204–206

Horwich M S, Cho L, Porro R S, Posner J B 1977 Subacute sensory neuropathy: a remote effect of carcinoma. Annals of Neurology 2: 7–19

Hosobuchi Y 1980 The majority of unmyelinated afferent axons in human ventral roots probably conduct pain. Pain 8: 167–180

Howe J F, Loeser J D, Calvin W H 1977 Mechanosensitivity of dorsal root ganglia and chronically injured axons: a physiological basis for the radicular pain of nerve root compression. Pain 3: 25–41

Howland W J, Curry J L 1966 Pantopaque arachnoiditis. Experimental study of blood as a potentiating agent and corticosteroids as an ameliorating agent. Acta Radiologica 5: 1032–1041

Hoyland J A, Freemont A J, Denton J, Thomas A M, McMillan J J, Jayson M I 1988 Retained surgical swab debris in post-laminectomy arachnoiditis and peridural fibrosis. Journal of Bone and Joint Surgery 70: 659–662

Hunt J R 1915 The sensory field of the facial nerve: a further contribution to the symptomatology of the geniculate ganglion. Brain 38: 418–446

Hunter C R, Mayfield F H 1949 Role of the upper cervical roots in the production of pain in the head. American Journal of Surgery 78: 743–751

Inman V T, Saunders J B DeC M 1944 Referred pain from skeletal structures. Journal of Nervous and Mental Diseases 99: 660–667

Jain K K 1974 Nerve root scarring and arachnoiditis as a complication of lumbar intervertebral disc surgery. Surgical treatment. Neurochirurgia 17: 185–192

Johnson C E, Sze G 1990 Benign lumbar arachnoiditis: MR imaging with gadopentetate dimeglumine. American Journal of Neuroradiology 11: 763–770

Johnson E W, Fletcher E R 1981 Lumbosacral radiculopathy: review of 100 consecutive cases. Archives of Physical Medicine and Rehabilitation 62: 321–323

Johnston J D H, Matheny J B 1978 Microscopic lysis of lumbar adhesive arachnoiditis. Spine 3: 36–39

Junck L, Marshall W H 1983 Neurotoxicity of radiological contrast agents. Annals of Neurology 13: 469–484

Kahanovitz N, Viola K, McCulloch J 1989 Limited surgical discectomy and microdiscectomy. A clinical comparison. Spine 14: 79–81

Keegan J J, Garrett F D 1948 The segmental distribution of the cutaneous nerves in the limbs of man. Anatomical Record 102: 409–437

Kellgren J H 1939 On the distribution of pain arising from deep somatic structures with charts of segmental pain areas. Clinical Science 4: 35–46

Kelly M 1956 Is pain due to pressure on nerves? Neurology 6: 32–36

Kendall H O, Kendall F P, Wadsworth G E 1971 Muscles: testing and function. Williams & Wilkins, Baltimore

Kerr F W L 1961 A mechanism to account for frontal headache in cases of posterior fossa tumors. Journal of Neurosurgery 18: 605–609

Kibler R F, Nathan P W 1960 Relief of pain and paresthesiae by nerve block distal to the lesion. Journal of Neurology, Neurosurgery and Psychiatry 23: 91–98

King R B 1980 Pain and tryptophan. Journal of Neurosurgery 53: 44–52

Kirk E J, Denny-Brown D 1970 Functional variation in dermatomes in the macaque monkey following dorsal root lesions. Journal of Comparative Neurology 139: 307–320

Kunc Z 1965 Treatment of essential neuralgia of the ninth nerve by selective tractotomy. Journal of Neurosurgery 23: 494–500

Laha R K, Jannetta P J 1977 Glossopharyngeal neuralgia. Journal of Neurosurgery 47: 316–320

Lance J W, Anthony M 1980 Neck-tongue syndrome on sudden turning of the head. Journal of Neurology, Neurosurgery and Psychiatry 43: 97–101

Lindahl O, Rexed B 1951 Histologic changes in spinal nerve roots of operated cases of sciatica. Acta Orthopaedica Scandinavica 20: 215–225

Lindblom K, Rexed B 1948 Spinal nerve injury in dorsolateral protrusions of lumbar discs. Journal of Neurosurgery 5: 413–432

Lipton S 1979 Relief of pain in clinical practice. Blackwell, Oxford, p 231–248

Little J R, Dale A J D, Okazaki H 1974 Meningeal carcinomatosis: clinical manifestations. Archives of Neurology 30: 138–143

Loeser J D, Ward A A, White L E 1968 Chronic deafferentation of human spinal cord neurons. Journal of Neurosurgery 29: 48–50

Long D M 1982 Pain of spinal origin. In: Youmans J R (ed) Neurological surgery. W B Saunders, Philadelphia, p 3613–3626
MacNab I 1971 Negative disc exploration. An analysis of the causes of nerve root involvement in 68 patients. Journal of Bone and Joint Surgery 53A: 891–903
Maigne J-Y, Rime B, Deligne B 1992 Computed tomographic follow-up study of forty-eight cases of nonoperatively treated lumbar intervertebral disc herniation. Spine 17: 1071–1074
Maroon J C, Abla A A 1986 Microlumbar discectomy. Clinical Neurosurgery 33: 407–417
Maroon J C, Onik G 1987 Percutaneous automated discectomy: a new method for lumbar disc removal. Technical note. Journal of Neurosurgery 66: 143–146
Martin G 1980 Recurrent pain of a pseudotabetic variety after laminectomy for lumbar disc lesion. Journal of Neurology, Neurosurgery and Psychiatry 43: 283–284
Martins A N, Ramirez A, Johnston J, Schwetschenau P R 1978 Double-blind evaluation of chemonucleolysis for herniated lumbar discs. Journal of Neurosurgery 49: 816–827
Meilman P W, Leibrock L G, Leong F T 1989 Outcome of implanted spinal cord stimulation in the treatment of chronic pain: arachnoiditis versus single nerve root injury and mononeuropathy. Clinical Journal of Pain 5: 189–193
Murphey F 1968 Sources and patterns of pain in disc disease. Clinical Neurosurgery 15: 343–350
Murphey F, Simmons J C H, Brunson B 1973 Ruptured cervical discs, 1939 to 1972. Clinical Neurosurgery 20: 9–17
Murphy F, Hartung W, Kirklin J W 1947 Myelographic demonstration of avulsion injury of the brachial plexus. American Journal of Roentgenology 58: 102–105
Nachemson A L 1977 Pathophysiology and treatment of back pain: a critical look at the different types of treatment. In: Buerger A A, Tobis J S (eds) Approaches to the validation of manipulation therapy. C C Thomas, Springfield, Illinois, p 769–779
Nagashima C, Sakaguchi A, Kamisasa A, Kawanuma S 1976 Cardiovascular complications on upper vagal rootlet section for glossopharyngeal neuralgia. Journal of Neurosurgery 44: 248–253
Nashold B S, Ostdahl R H 1979 Dorsal root entry zone lesions for pain relief. Journal of Neurosurgery 51: 59–69
Nashold B S, Ostdahl R H, Bullitt E, Friedman A, Brophy B 1983 Dorsal root entry zone lesions. A new neurosurgical therapy for deafferentation pain. In: Bonica J J, Lindblom U, Iggo A (eds) Advances in pain research and therapy, vol 5. Raven Press, New York, p 739–750
Nathan P, Wall P D 1974 Treatment of postherpetic neuralgia by prolonged electric stimulation. British Medical Journal 14: 645–647
Neiri R L, Burgert E O, Groover R V 1968 Central nervous system leukemia: a review. Mayo Clinic Proceedings 43: 70–79
Nelson D A, Vates T S, Thomas R B 1973 Complications from intrathecal steroid therapy in patients with multiple sclerosis, Acta Neurologica Scandinavica 49: 176–188
North R B, Ewend M G, Lawton M T, Kidd D H, Piantadosi S 1991 Failed back surgery syndrome: 5-year followup after spinal cord stimulator implantation. Neurosurgery 78: 692–699
O'Connor M, Brighouse D, Glynn C J 1990 Unusual complications in the treatment of chronic spinal arachnoiditis. Clinical Journal of Pain 6: 240–242
Olson M E, Chernik N L, Posner J B 1974 Infiltration of the leptomeninges by systemic cancer. A clinical and pathologic study. Archives of Neurology 30: 122–137
Onik G, Mooney V, Maroon J C et al 1990 Automated percutaneous discectomy: a prospective multi-institutional study. Neurosurgery 26: 228–232
Pedersen H E, Blunck C F J, Gardner E 1956 The anatomy of the lumbosacral posterior rami and meningeal branches of spinal nerves (sinu-vertebral nerves), with an experimental study of their functions. Journal of Bone and Joint Surgery 38A: 377–391
Poletti C E 1983 Proposed operation for occipital neuralgia: C2 and C3 root decompression. Neurosurgery 12: 221–224
Quiles M, Marchisello P J, Tsairis P 1978 Lumbar adhesive arachnoiditis. Etiologic and pathologic aspects. Spine 3: 45–50
Rasminsky M 1980 Ephaptic transmission between single nerve fibres in the spinal nerve roots of dystrophic mice. Journal of Physiology 305: 151–169
Ray C G 1980 Chickenpox (varicella) and herpes zoster. In: Isselbacher K J et al (eds) Harrison's principles of internal medicine. McGraw-Hill, New York, p 801–804
Robson J T, Bonica J J 1950 The vagus nerve in surgical consideration of glossopharyngeal neuralgia. Journal of Neurosurgery 7: 482–484
Rocovich P M 1947 Adhesive spinal arachnoiditis. Bulletin of the Los Angeles Neurological Society 12: 69–77
Rothman S L G, Glenn W V, Kerber C W 1985 Postoperative fractures of lumbar articular facets: occult cause of radiculopathy. American Journal of Neuroradiology 145: 779–784
Rushton J G, Stevens J C, Miller R H 1981 Glossopharyngeal (vagoglossopharyngeal) neuralgia. Archives of Neurology 38: 201–205
Rydevik B, Branemark P I, Nordborg C et al 1976 Effects of chymopapain on nerve tissue. Spine 1: 137–139
Samii M, Moringlane J R 1984 Thermocoagulation of the dorsal root entry zone for the treatment of intractable pain. Neurosurgery 15: 953–955
Schutz H, Lougheed W M, Wortzman G, Awerbuck B G 1973 Intervertebral nerve root in the investigation of chronic lumbar disc disease. Canadian Journal of Surgery 16: 217–221
Seaman W B, Marder S N, Rosenbaum H E 1953 The myelographic appearance of adhesive spinal arachnoiditis. Journal of Neurosurgery 10: 145–153
See D H, Kraft G H 1975 Electromyography in paraspinal muscles following surgery for root compression. Archives of Physical Medicine and Rehabilitation 56: 80–83
Shaw M D M, Russell J A, Grossart K W 1978 The changing pattern of spinal arachnoiditis. Journal of Neurology, Neurosurgery and Psychiatry 41: 97–107
Sherrington C S 1898 Experiments in the examination of the peripheral distribution of the fibres of the posterior roots of some spinal nerves. Part II. Philosophical Transactions B 190: 45–186
Shields C B 1985 In defense of chemonucleolysis. Clinical Neurosurgery 33: 397–405
Skalpe I O 1976 Adhesive arachnoiditis following lumbar radiculography with water-soluble agents. A clinical report with special reference to metrizamide. Radiology 121: 647–651
Smith R W, Loeser J D 1972 A myelographic variant in lumbar arachnoiditis. Journal of Neurosurgery 36: 441–446
Smyth M J, Wright V 1958 Sciatica and the intervertebral disc. Journal of Bone and Joint Surgery 40A: 1401–1418
Snoek W, Weber H, Jorgensen B 1977 Double blind evaluation of extradural methylprednisolone for herniated lumbar discs. Acta Orthopaedica Scandinavica 48: 635–641
Spangfort E V 1972 The lumbar disc herniation. Acta Orthopaedica Scandinavica (suppl) 142: 1–95
Stewart J D 1987 Focal peripheral neuropathies. Elsevier, New York
Storm-Mathisen A 1978 Syphilis. In: Vinken P J, Bruyn G W (eds) Handbook of clinical neurology. North-Holland, Amsterdam, p 337–394
Tarlov I M 1970 Spinal perineurial and meningeal cysts. Journal of Neurology, Neurosurgery and Psychiatry 33: 833–843
Taub A, Collins W F 1974 Observations on the treatment of denervation dysesthesia with psychotropic drugs: postherpetic neuralgia, anesthesia dolorosa, peripheral neuropathy. Advances in Neurology 4: 309–315
Teplick J G, Haskin M E 1984 Intravenous contrast-enhanced CT of the postoperative lumbar spine: improved identification of recurrent disk herniation, scar, arachnoiditis, and diskitis. American Journal of Roentgenology 143: 845–855
Thomas D G T, Jones S J 1984 Dorsal root entry zone lesions (Nashold's procedure) in brachial plexus avulsion. Neurosurgery 15: 966–968
Turnbull I M, Shulman R, Woodhurst W B 1980 Thalamic stimulation for neuropathic pain. Journal of Neurosurgery 52: 486–493
Upton A R M, McComas A J 1973 The double crush in nerve entrapment syndromes. Lancet 2: 359–360
Verbiest H 1954 A radicular syndrome from developmental narrowing of the lumbar vertebral canal. Journal of Bone and Joint Surgery 36B: 230–237
Wall P D 1977 The presence of ineffective synapses and the circumstances which unmask them. Philosophical Transactions of the Royal Society of London 278: 361–372

Wall P D 1980 The role of substantia gelatinosa as a gate control. In: Bonica J J (ed) Pain. Raven Press, New York, p 205–231

Wall P D, Devor M 1983 Sensory afferent impulses originate from dorsal root ganglia as well as from the periphery in normal and nerve-injured rats. Pain 17: 321–339

Wall P D, Waxman S, Basbaum A I 1974 Ongoing activity in peripheral nerve: injury discharge. Experimental Neurology 45: 576–589

Warren J, Guttman L, Figueroa A P, Bloor B M 1969 Electromyographic changes of brachial plexus root avulsions. Journal of Neurosurgery 31: 137–140

Wasserstrom W R, Glass J P, Posner J B 1982 Diagnosis and treatment of leptomeningeal metastases from solid tumors. Cancer 49: 759–772

Watts C 1977 Complications of chemonucleolysis for lumbar disc disease. Neurosurgery 1: 2–4

Weinstein P R, Ehni G, Wilsou C B 1977 Lumbar spondylosis. Year Book, Chicago

Whisler W W 1978 Chronic spinal arachnoiditis. In: Vinken P J, Bruyn G W (eds) Handbook of clinical neurology, vol 33. North-Holland, New York, p 263–274

White A A, Derby R, Wynne G 1980 Epidural injections for the diagnosis and treatment of low back pain. Spine 5: 78–86

White J C, Sweet W H 1969 Pain and the neurosurgeon. C C Thomas, Springfield, Illinois

Wiesel S W, Tsoumas N, Feffer H L, Citrin C M, Patronas N 1984 A study of computer-assisted tomography. The incidence of positive CAT scans in an asymptomatic group of patients. Spine 9: 549–551

Wilkinson H A 1992 Intrathecal Depo-Medrol: a literature review. Clinical Journal of Pain 8: 49–52

Wilkinson H A, Schuman N 1979 Results of surgical lysis of lumbar adhesive arachnoiditis. Neurosurgery 4: 401–409

Wilkinson M 1971 Cervical spondylosis. Heinemann, London

Williams R W 1983 Microsurgical discectomy: a surgical alternative for initial disc herniation. In: Cauthen J (ed) Lumbar spine surgery. Williams & Wilkins, Baltimore, p 85–98

Wilson D H, Harbaugh R 1981 Microsurgical and standard removal of the protruded lumbar disc: a comparative study. Neurosurgery 8: 422–425

Wilson D H, Kenning J 1979 Microsurgical lumbar discectomy: preliminary report of 83 corrective cases. Neurosurgery 4: 137–140

Wynn Parry C B 1980 Pain in avulsion lesions of the brachial plexus. Pain 9: 41–53

Children

41. Pain experience in children: developmental and clinical characteristics

Ronald G. Barr

PAIN IN CHILDREN

An essential dilemma for paediatric clinicians is the ability to gain access to the child's *experience* of pain. This is difficult enough in adults, with whom we have a shared language. In children, we are not as certain that they have the same vocabulary, use it in the same way, or are as articulate in describing their pain sensations (e.g. Harbeck & Peterson 1992). As a result, we often depend on parents' descriptions of their children's pain, sometimes to the exclusion of their child's description (Barr 1989a).

This dilemma is exacerbated further with children in whom verbal descriptions are not available, most notably prematures, newborns, and preverbal infants, but also older nonverbal children with cognitive and language delays. For such children, we must rely on other behavioural channels of communication, such as posture, motor response, and facial expression (e.g. Craig 1992). However, in many clinical situations, these behaviours too are unavailable when children are under anaesthesia or otherwise constrained.

In part, this dilemma is a direct consequence of the nature of pain experience. For the clinician, access to the patient's pain experience is limited to overt behaviour (Turk & Flor 1987). However, for the patient, pain behaviour is only the public expression of pain experience, which is virtually universal but essentially private. Furthermore, pain is the outcome of sensory, emotional and situational factors which contribute to the experience. It is communicated by a verbal, facial and motoric behavioural 'language' reflecting universal features modulated by learned responses. The behavioural signal is a powerful elicitor of reactions from the community, thereby assuring that the experience is not simply an isolated, private event (Craig 1978). Consequently, the overt behaviour acts as a signal which integrates a multitude of inputs and influences, but only indirectly reflects the experiences which it represents.

A second component of the dilemma is the fact it is often not clear whether children, especially preverbal infants, are experiencing or expressing pain or generalized distress in their verbal, behavioural and physiological reactions to a noxious stimulus. However, one can say that infants and children manifest nociceptive responses, that is, responses to stimuli or tissue injury or insults which are 'known' to be painful in adults. Indeed, the terms 'pain' and nociception' are often used interchangeably. This permits the description of responses to noxious stimuli in infants at a variety of levels (except the verbal subjective one), as is done in adults. What is measured, however, is not the pain experience, but the behavioural and physiological response to the stressful, and presumably painful, stimulus. This means that evidence concerning pain experience in children is indirect and inferential. Thus, the term 'pain stress' will be used to refer to the presumed pain experience which accompanies the general stress of noxious stimuli or tissue injury.

Thirdly, the characteristics and interrelationships of all these levels (the experience, its representation, and the community response) are constrained by the developmental evolution of the child. Thus, the crying behaviour of a 3-month-old child is likely to reflect a different experience, carry a different message, and evoke a different response than the crying of a school-aged child. In principle, a description of pain in children should include the developmental changes in each of the factors contributing to the pain experience as well as their interactions. Pain behaviour in children is not the pain behaviour of 'little adults'. It is not just an adult experience in a smaller person, or a smaller amount of otherwise adult experience.

Because of the indirectness and developmental complexity of the evidence of pain experience in children, the importance of interpreting that evidence correctly is heightened for both diagnosis and treatment. For example, one would probably accept an adult's assertion that he is not moving to avoid exacerbating pain postoperatively and not withold analgesic medication, whereas the nonverbal infant or child who did not move to avoid pain exacerbation might not receive medication because he did not 'look uncomfortable'. Even in older verbal children, pain may be expressed differently. LeBaron & Zeltzer (1984) make the important observation that, in response to bone marrow aspiration procedures, younger children cry, scream, express verbal anxiety, and need restraint more often than adolescents. However, groaning and flinching are significantly more frequent in adolescents, and minimal in children. If groaning and flinching are not included in the pain assessment, younger children would be interpreted as experiencing more pain than adolescents; if they are included, no difference in pain intensity would be found (LeBaron & Zeltzer 1984).

In the light of these dilemmas, this chapter focuses on two aspects of pain experience in children. The first section provides a summary of developmental characteristics of pain experience. The second section describes clinical pain syndromes. Particular emphasis will be placed on those syndromes which are specific to the pediatric age group and, in particular, their clinical presentations and diagnostic considerations.

DEVELOPMENTAL CHANGES

Pain perception is usually conceived of as including a sensory component referring to the sensory qualities (such as intensity, temporal features, location) associated with noxious stimuli, and a motivational-affective component referring to the emotional and aversive aspect (such as the 'hurting' quality) of the perception leading to behaviour that will avoid or reduce the stimulus (Melzack & Wall 1970). It is reasonable to expect that underlying changes in sensory maturation and cognitive–affective development contribute to changes in pain perception. However, inferences about these conceptually distinguishable underlying processes on the basis of observed pain reactivity are indirect and difficult to substantiate. Significant recent developments have been the inclusion of both behavioural and physiological measures in developmental studies (e.g. Lewis & Thomas 1990; Gunnar et al 1992), and the use of these measures in studies of pain stress reactivity in prematures (e.g. Anand et al 1987; Fitzgerald et al 1988, 1989; Anand et al 1992).

Perhaps the most significant change is the shift away from the interpretation that pain reactivity reflects a gradient starting with pain insensitivity at birth to increased sensitivity in older children. In its place, developmental changes are interpreted as reflecting a sensitivity (or even hypersensitivity) to pain at birth, with a developmental gradient to increasing ability to *modulate* pain reactivity as the child grows older. These interpretations are important because the same *behaviours* characteristic of a response to a noxious stimulus have been interpreted as evidence both against and for the presence of a functional pain system. In the former interpretation, the behavioural reaction is taken to reflect a developmentally 'decorticate' response due to an immature nervous system with the absence of the ability to localize the stimulus; in the latter interpretation, the reaction is taken to reflect an immature but intact response (Barr 1983a; Shulman et al 1983; Barr 1989a; Fitzgerald et al 1989), with the possibility that there is early hypersensitivity to the stimulus (Shulman et al 1983; Fitzgerald et al 1989).

Recent studies demonstrate that an organized response for pain stress is evident at an early age: 2- to 3-day-old infants exhibit a distinct set of facial changes accompanying the cry response to a heel lance compared to the reaction to the preliminary heel rub required for the procedure (Grunau & Craig 1987; Grunau et at 1990). Even at this age, the facial reaction pattern is subject to modification by the state of the infant at the time of stimulus onset, although the cry (fundamental frequency) is not (Grunau & Craig 1987). There is some evidence that this sophisticated response system would include directed defensive motor activity (swiping movements) if the infant were not constrainted (Frank 1986). Furthermore, facial reactivity is sensitive to variations in handling during the post-stimulus manipulations suggesting some degree of specificity to the response (Grunau & Craig 1987). In response to immunizations, there is a substantial difference in reactivity manifested by infants older than 1 year compared to younger infants, primarily apparent in reduction of torso rigidity, duration of crying post-stimulus, and orientation to the site of injection (Craig et al 1984). Even within the first 6 months, there is an age-related decrease in the time taken to become quiet following a diphtheria–pertussis–tetanus (DPT) immunization, but not in the intensity of crying and facial reaction to the initial stimulus (Lewis & Thomas 1990). Using a predefined coding system for facial motor patterns, Izard and his colleagues argue that, in response to heel lance, all infants manifest a pain reaction consisting of a specific facies and crying, but that the pain expression decreases and an anger expression increases with age in response to inoculations (Izard et al 1983, 1987). In addition, the duration of negative emotion displayed poststimulus diminishes with increasing age. Within an episode, progressively less of the displayed negative emotion is pain and more is anger as the infant grows older. While the specificity of the predefined 'pain' facies may be questioned, these observations are nevertheless consistent with the developmental trend towards an increasing ability to modulate the behavioural response to a noxious stimulus.

In an elegant series of studies, Fitzgerald and colleagues have extended the developmental observations 'downwards' into the premature age range using the cutaneous flexor reflex (Fitzgerald et al 1988, 1989). The reflex consists of withdrawal of the leg in response to application of standard calibrated stimuli (von Frey hairs) to the sole of the foot. This reflex is of particular interest because it accesses a pathway for somatosensory input and, in adults, correlates strongly with subjective pain sensation (Willer 1977; Willer & Bussel 1980; Chan & Dallaire 1989). Furthermore, in premature infants, the reflex threshold is lowered following tissue injury (repeated heelsticks), and the lowered threshold is blocked by the application of anaesthetic cream to the injury site (Fitzgerald et al 1989). The post-injury hypersensitivity to cutaneous stimulation closely parallels post-injury hyperalgesia in adults, suggesting that the reflex measures an aspect of the pain response in infants (Fitzgerald 1991b).

Of particular interest are the findings in normal premature infants. Between 27 and 40 weeks postmenstrual age (PMA), flexor reflex thresholds increase gradually, and this increase is strictly a function of postmenstrual age, not time since birth (Fitzgerald et al 1988). However, even for infants born at term, flexor reflex thresholds remain very low (2 g) relative to those that are perceived as noxious by adults (30–75 g). Furthermore, prior to about 32 weeks postconceptual age, infants are likely to manifest sensitization to repeated stimulation (increased intensity of withdrawal, rhythmic movements, mass body movement), whereas after 32 weeks they are more likely to demonstrate habituation (absence of response after repeated stimulation). These characteristics hold across species, since analogous responses can be elicited in rat pups at developmentally analogous ages (Fitzgerald et al 1988; Fitzgerald 1991b).

Fitzgerald et al interpret these changes in reflex threshold and early sensitization as reflecting properties of the cutaneous interneurons within the spinal cord because they are more excitable and/or lack the degree of inhibitory control characteristic of the adult (Fitzgerald et al 1988). The low threshold and lack of inhibitory control may contribute at a physiological level to the difficulty in defining responses which are specific to pain in infants. Furthermore, these findings may mean that there is less endogenous 'gate control' of noxious inputs to both pain and repeated handling, making the premature infant 'hyperalgesic' (Fitzgerald, 1991b).

In summary, the behavioural data from prematures through to early infancy consistently support a developmental gradient beginning initially with relatively diffuse reactions to low threshold stimuli, more organized reactions to higher threshold stimuli later, and some evidence that the reaction is brought under control more quickly as the infant matures. Whether these behaviours represent early pain insensitivity or early pain sensitivity (or even hypersensitivity) being brought under control depends in part on whether an intact functional system for pain perception is present and underlies these responses.

Evidence from preclinical and human studies increasingly supports the presence of such a system, and this evidence has been thoroughly and articulately reviewed (e.g. Anand & Hickey 1987; Anand & Carr, 1989; Zeltzer et al 1990; Fitzgerald 1991a, 1991b). These findings include anatomical evidence that:

1. Cutaneous nociceptive nerve endings are present in all cutaneous and mucous surfaces by the 20th week of gestation; furthermore, the density of these nerve endings may equal or exceed that found in adult skin.
2. Myelination to the thalamus is complete by 30 weeks.
3. Dendritic arborization of cortical neurons, and synaptogenesis between thalamic afferents and cortical neurons begin to be established between 20 and 24 weeks of gestation.
4. Myelination of thalamocortical fibres is complete by 37 weeks.

Evidence for the functional operation of these pathways includes:

1. Cortical components of visual, auditory and somatosensory evoked potentials are present by 30 weeks' gestation.
2. EEG patterns and behavioural evidence of well-defined periods of sleep and wakefulness.
3. In vivo measures of maximal rates of cerebral glucose utilization in the essential sensory areas of the neonatal brain (Anand & Carr 1989).

Although an intact, functional pain transmission system appears to be in place, it continues to develop and to produce subsystems that modulate and/or inhibit the afferent signal, including reorganization of connections between neurons, the development of neurotransmitters and their receptors, and the establishment of local and descending control circuits (Fitzgerald 1991a, 1991b). In the rat, for example, axons of descending brainstem projection neurons are present in the cord from early fetal life, but their influence on dorsal horn cells is delayed pending the extension of collaterals into the dorsal horn and the development of neurotransmitters and receptors. As a result, electrophysiological evidence of inhibition from the dorsolateral funiculus is not detectable until the postnatal period (Fitzgerald 1991a). To the extent that similar processes take place in the development of the human nervous system, such evidence implies that the early diffuse reaction to noxious stimuli represents experienced but relatively unorganized and unmodulated perceptions, while the later development of endogenous control systems could contribute to the better organized, higher threshold, and shorter recovery reactions seen in the postnatal period.

Recent psychobiological studies contribute to our understanding of the developmental changes in infants' experience of noxious stimuli. The ability to measure cortisol noninvasively in saliva has permitted the direct comparison of behavioural and cortisol responses to the same noxious stimuli. These two levels of description are often dissociated. For example, Gunnar et al (1989a) reported significant, similar increases in cortisol to discharge examinations and a heelstick procedure, but more crying to the heelstick. Cortisol levels were elevated to the first physical examination but habituated to the second, while crying remained elevated for both (Gunnar et al 1989a, 1992). In addition, the habituation of cortisol levels was stimulus specific, occuring only in response to the repeated physical examination, but not to the repeated heelstick procedure. There was no habituation reflected in crying levels (Gunnar et al 1992). Finally, infants who had experienced mild obstetric and peripartum risk ('non-optimal' infants) did not show the cortisol habituation to repeated physical examination. It is apparent that different measures at different levels of description may be necessary to track developmental changes in pain stress responses.

In a cross-sectional study of 2-, 4-, and 6-month-old infants' responses to inoculations, Lewis & Thomas (1990) reported an age-related trend to blunted cortisol responses in older infants. Interestingly, parallel behavioural changes were seen in the latency to calm following the inoculation, but not in the intensity of the initial behavioural response. These observations may reflect developmental processes by which the pituitary–adrenocortical axis becomes buffered in responses to commonly occuring stressors (Gunnar et al 1989b; Lewis & Thomas 1990) or a decrease in the intensity of the pain stress due to continuing development of endogenous control systems. Furthermore, some features of the behavioural responses may parallel cortisol responses but not others.

Developmental changes may also be tracked by observing how responses are modified by simple interventions. Blass & Hoffmeyer (1991) reported approximately 50% reductions in crying following heelstick and circumcision when newborn infants were first provided with a sucrose taste. In parallel studies in rat pups, similar sucrose effects on distress vocalizations and pain thresholds were shown to be naloxone-reversible, implicating mediation by an endogenous opioid system (Blass et al 1987, 1990). In the newborn period, sucrose does not affect the immediate response to heelstick, but does reduce crying during the recovery phase (Barr et al 1993a). However, similar or even increasing doses of sucrose are not as effective at reducing crying at 6 weeks of age, nor at affecting the behavioural reaction to inoculation at 2 and 4 months of age (Barr et al 1933b, 1993c). However, in preadolescents, sucrose in the mouth increased 'pain threshold' in response to a cold pressor experience by about 30% (Miller et al 1993). Such relatively substantial changes in a short period of time postnatally imply considerable reorganization underlying central processing of noxious stimuli in the post-newborn period. The detection of a sucrose effect in preadolescents raises the possibility that the role of this central system may vary in salience at different periods of development.

There are fewer systematic studies of developmental changes in pain reactivity of children following infancy. In a study of 'pain threshold' to anterior tibial pressure with 5–18-year-olds, Haslam (1969) reported generally increasing stimulus thresholds in older children. Similar findings were reported by Tucker et al (1989) using threshold responses (prickling pain sensation) to transcutaneous neuronal electrical stimulation. Threshold values continued to rise between the ages of 5 and 25 years, after which they plateaued until after 80 years of age. Consistent with these results, two studies of self-reported and behavioural distress reactions to routine venipunctures (one in inpatients who had previously experienced 20 or more venipunctures) reported a generally linear decline in distress response to the procedure (Fradet et al 1990; Humphrey et al 1992). Importantly, the absence of gender differences has been a consistent finding in pain stress responses to venipuncture in this age range (Fradet et al 1990; Lander et al 1992; Humphrey et al 1992).

In certain clinical conditions, some suggestions of age-related trends have been noted. For example, in recurrent abdominal pain syndrome, the pain is more often nonspecific and diffuse in younger children, but becomes increasingly localized and less likely to be limited to the periumbilical region in older children (Heinild et al 1959; Barr 1983b). Older children aged 4–19 rate the intensity of pain as depicted in pictures as being less than do younger children, and children whose previous pain experience was considerable rate the intensity of the pictured pains as being less (Lollar et al 1982). Studies of children of preschool through adolescent ages undergoing bone marrow aspirations provide evidence of age-related changes in distress associated with the procedure. As might be expected, younger children's distress tends to be characterized by resistance to the procedure and diffuse vocal protest, while older children react with more specific verbal expressions, muscle rigidity, flinching and groaning, and self control with fewer emotional outbursts (Katz et al 1980; Jay et al 1983; Lebaron & Zeltzer 1984; Lavigne et al 1986; van Aken et al 1989). Similar age-related trends for uncooperative behaviour and anxiety are found in relation to dental treatment (Zachary et al 1985). These behaviours are associated with predictable rather than unanticipated pain in clinical rather than normal children, and therefore the extent to which these changes represent differences with age in pain reactivity rather than distress in acute pain situations is questionable. However, the findings are consistent with a trend toward increasing pain threshold and greater ability to modulate the pain experience.

The developmental changes in overt pain response are also subject to developmental contraints on factors which contribute to the subject's assessment and modulation of the sensation, including changes in cognitive strategies, available pain 'language', and community responses to the pain behaviour. Virtually all studies of coping with medical procedures in children refer to coping dimensions of passive or avoidant on the one hand or active and information-seeking on the other (Peterson 1989). Moreover, most studies indicate that children who tend to utilize active coping strategies demonstrate more beneficial responses to procedural pain. Active coping also tends to be more likely with increasing age. Thus, for example, the number of children between the ages of 8 and 18 who can describe the use of positive cognitive coping strategies ('copers') as compared to those who focus on the negative aspects of pain and stress experiences ('catastrophizers') increases with age, and the total number of types of strategies available to them does as well (Brown et al 1986; Branson et al 1990). The most common types of coping strategies for an imagined dental visit were positive self-talk and diverting attention. Similarly, descriptions of active coping increase with age in children approaching surgery (Peterson & Toler 1986).

The pain 'language' available to children changes and probably performs different functions as development progresses. In preverbal children, it is thought that crying in the first few months of life reflect more 'physiological' stimuli, whereas later in the first year it has a more 'instrumental' function (Bell & Ainsworth 1972; Barr 1990). At both of these developmental stages, the power of crying to attract caregiver attention and support is functionally appropriate. However, crying in a school-aged child may not be the most competent or functional behaviour. The onset of language permits a considerable increase both in the ability to specify sensory and motivational-affective characteristics and to describe what the pain experience signifies. In fact, the ability of even very young children to describe pain experiences is striking (Ross & Ross 1984a; Harbeck & Peterson 1992). Whether there is a developmental progression in the language available to describe pain in the preadolescent child is uncertain. While no age-related trends were noted for pain concepts or descriptors in one study (Ross & Ross 1984a), others have shown a clear trend for increasing number and types of themes and descriptors being incorporated into children's pain descriptions (Jeans 1983; Gaffney & Dunne 1986). The differences that exist in the few available studies (see also Schultz 1971; Scott 1978; Savedra et al 1982, 1988) may be related more to differences in methods, measures, and age ranges studied than to irreconcilable disagreement in the findings (Ross & Ross 1984b; Savedra et al 1982). Harbeck & Peterson (1992) have shown that, in response to three vignettes representing an injury (skinned knee), a medical intervention (injection), and an illness (headache), there were age-related differences in children's descriptions of the pains, why they hurt, and what the value of the pain was. The developmental differences were not based on the number or types of words used, but rather on the complexity and precision of the descriptions. Interestingly, these developmental differences were to some extent pain-specific. Thus, for example, third graders' most precise description was of a shot, while sixth graders' most precise description was of a headache. This implies that there may not be a unitary concept of 'pain', but rather that different aspects of pain are better understood at different developmental levels (Harbeck & Peterson 1992). Importantly for clinical assessment, there also appears to be an age-related trend in the consistency with which children rate the intensity of remembered painful events, with satisfactory consistency (>80%) being achieved only at about 8 years of age (Lehmann et al 1990).

Because of the powerful influence of behavioural pain expression on the response of the community (Melzack 1973; Weisenberg 1977), and because pain expressions are influenced by the social context in which the child develops (Craig 1983), a third developmental influence on pain responses is the reactions of observers in the presence of whom the pain behaviour occurs. As might be expected, these reactions differ as a function of the age, sex, and culture of the respondent. A well-studied example is the almost obligatory response to infant crying which can elicit responses ranging from positive, nurturant and empathetic to egoistic, avoiding and abusive (Murray 1979). While mothers, fathers and adolescent boys and girls all show a similar physiological arousal to infant cries, fathers and adolescent boys are more likely than mothers and adolescent girls respectively to ignore the infant's behaviour or report less extreme emotional responses to it (Frodi & Lamb 1978; Frodi et al 1978). In the !Kung hunter–gatherers, even minimal crying elicits a positive caretaker response within 15 seconds in over 90% of observations (Barr et al 1987) compared to the lower response rate (about 40%) typical in North American societies (Lozoff & Brittenham 1979). Furthermore, the same behaviour is responded to differently depending on real or perceived characteristics (e.g. age, temperament, 'normality') of the infant (Frodi et al 1978; Frodi & Senchak 1990). The cry of a normal infant described as 'premature' elicits greater physiological arousal in both men and women (Frodi et al 1978). Over the first 2 years, the profile of caregiving to infant crying changes in the !Kung, with increasing likelihood of social verbal responses, and decreasing likelihood of behavioural responses (Barr et al 1987). Similarly, maternal verbal responses to distress behaviour associated with inoculations change from being more soothing in younger infants to more verbal distraction in older infants (Craig et al 1984). In short, while pain expression is a powerful eliciting stimulus at all ages, the likely responses are subject to age-related and developmental changes in the character and perceptions of the respondents.

Our increasing understanding of developmental changes in pain perception is of more than theoretical interest. For clinicians, beliefs in the presence of pain and the extent to which one appropriately reads the patient's pain 'language' is likely to affect one's use of medications and techniques for pain relief. That this has been a problem for pediatric clinicians is indicated by the well documented 'undertreatment' of pain in children. In general, adults tend to be prescribed and to receive full analgesic doses for various conditions or procedures, while for the same painful conditions, children tend to be prescribed only partial analgesic doses, and often do not receive them (Eland & Anderson 1977; Perry & Heidrich 1982; Beyer et al 1983; Mather & Mackie 1983; Schechter et al 1986; Franck 1987). The reduction in actual delivery of prescribed doses is particularly noticeable for infants less than 5 years of age (Schechter et al 1986). There is a striking decrease in the likelihood that analgesia will be provided for the same invasive procedure in neonatal intensive care units (NICU) compared to a pediatric intensive care unit (PICU). For example, 66% of PICU patients, but only 26% of NICU patients, are likely to receive analgesia for an arterial line placement (Bauchner et al 1992).

While there are many contributing factors, one is the beliefs of physicians concerning the pain experiences of infants and children. In a study by Schechter & Allen (1986), physicians believed that the pain experience of children was 'similar to adults' only by 12 years of age. Only 50% felt that the pain was similar in infants under 1 year of age. Of the three groups of physicians surveyed (family practitioners, pediatricians, pediatric surgeons), surgeons were the least convinced, with only 30% believing that infants under 1 month felt pain similar to adults.

The weight of the developmental evidence now supports the concept that infants can experience pain stress, that pain threshold probably increases with age, and that children are increasingly competent in modulating their pain response. However, treatment decisions remain difficult, in part because of inadequate understanding of developmental changes in pain perception.

One of the difficulties is that the apparently simple question of whether infants experience pain (and therefore whether they should be treated) is actually a complicated one (Barr 1992a). In one sense in which the question is asked, the emphasis is on the word 'experience' (i.e. do infants *experience* pain?). The evidence (reviewed above) reveals a functional cortical neural substrate for perception of a noxious stimulus and argues that infants do have these experiences. The question of whether this perception represents 'consciousness' is theoretical and the answer depends on philosophical and semantic considerations (see e.g. Merskey 1970; Craig 1980; Lewis & Michalson 1983; Owens 1984; Grunau & Craig 1987; Izard et al 1987).

In a second sense in which the question is asked, the emphasis is on the word 'pain' (i.e. do infants experience *pain*?). In this case, the challenge is to understand whether infants experience the particular sensation of pain or just generalized distress. As previously discussed, to the extent that our understanding of pain depends on verbal report, this question may never be answered for infants. Furthermore, the developmental of the neural substrate for pain sensation may not provide a behavioural or physiological response specific to pain experience (Fitzgerald et al 1988; Fitzgerald 1991b). However, it is increasingly clear that *treatment* for 'pain stress' is beneficial to the infant whether or not the specific experience of the infant is that of pain.

Such treatment is often absent in a wide range of common procedures (heel lance, venipunture, innoculations, and lumbar puncture) and even in more invasive surgical procedures such as circumcision. Even in major surgery such as ligation of a patent ductus arteriosus in prematures, anaesthesia is usually limited to the use of muscle relaxants with or without intermittent nitrous oxide (Anand et al 1985). It is well documented that, in response to tissue damage, almost all infants have, or are capable of having, a stress response which includes a constellation of behaviours (crying, facial patterning, motoric activity; Izard et al 1980, 1983; Owen & Todt 1984; Johnston & Strada 1986; Franck 1986; Grunau & Craig 1987; Izard et al 1987) and physiological changes (adrenocortical, heart rate, transcutaneous oxygen pressure and respiratory rate, palmar water loss, vagal tone; Anders et al 1972; Talbert et al 1976; Rawlings et al 1980; Harpin & Rutter 1982; Owens & Todt 1984; Gunnar et al 1984, 1985, 1989a, 1992; Porter 1989). Furthermore, the stress response is modifiable by behavioural techniques (Field & Goldson 1984; Campos 1989), procedural techniques (Harpin & Rutter 1982) and analgesic techniques (Halperin et al 1989; Kapelushnik et al 1990; Robieux et al 1991), and even taste stimuli (Blass & Hoffmeyer 1991; Barr et al 1993a). The behavioural and physiological changes during and after circumcision are clearly improved by the use of regional anaesthesia (penile dorsal nerve block; Kirya & Werthmann 1978; Williamson & Williamson 1983; Holve et al 1983; Dixon et al 1984).

Perhaps the most important demonstration of the role of pain stress in the response to surgery was a randomzied controlled trial in preterms undergoing ligation of a patent ductus arteriosus (Anand et al 1987). In the group that received the opioid fentanyl as well as curare and nitrous oxide, there were significantly reduced hormonal responses during surgery and fewer metabolic and circulatory complications following surgery, with some of these changes (particularly protein breakdown) persisting until the third postoperative day. The conclusion was that the reduced stress response was due to the more effective dampening of pain perception by the addition of fentanyl to the anaesthetic regimen (Anand et al 1987). Similar findings were reported in a more recent study, in which newborn infants undergoing surgery for complex congenital heart defects were randomly assigned to receive 'deep' intraoperative anaesthesia (high-dose sufentanil) and postoperative opiate infusion or 'light' anaesthesia (halothane plus morphine) and postoperative intermittent morphine and diazepam (Anand et al 1992). In addition to significantly reduced endogenous opioid, catecholamine, and adrenocortical responses, the deep anaesthesia group had a decreased incidence of sepsis, metabolic acidosis, disseminated intravascular coagulation, and fewer postoperative deaths. Such findings demonstrate that the treatment of pain stress has significant health benefits to the infant, even if the specificity of the stress experience cannot be determined with certainty.

The third sense in which the question 'Do infants experience pain?' is asked relates to whether infants have *memory* for pain. Withholding analgesia for this reason provides a 'weaker' rationale, since infants may be neurologically capable of experiencing pain even if they do not remember it. The fact that infants may show anticipatory fear reactions only at 7–12 months (McGraw 1941) is consistent with evidence for increasing cognitive capacity and memory at this age (Kagan et al 1978; Kagan 1984). However, there is clear evidence of much earlier memory in infants and even in fetuses for stimuli that are probably less salient than the nociceptive stimuli of most medical procedures. For example, DeCaspar & Fifer (1980) reported that infants who had been read passages from 'The cat in the hat' repeatedly by their mothers before birth responded with a higher rate of sucking (indicating attention and recognition of the stimulus) when hearing the same story after birth. Zelazo and colleagues reported the ability of newborns to remember the difference between hearing words such as 'tinder' and 'beagle' 24 hours later using an information processing paradigm (Swain et al 1993). Furthermore, there is increasing evidence that early experiences are remembered in later life. For example, Clifton and her colleagues demonstrated that 2.5-year-old children showed evidence of having remembered a single experience to which they were exposed beginning at 6 months of age (Perris et al 1990). These and other studies demonstrate that infants have the capacity to create memories of incoming sensory information, and to attend to that information. If this ability extends to the more salient experiences of noxious stimuli, it suggests that pain may be remembered, whether or not infants are able to use it as a 'learned experience' in later behaviour.

The understanding of developmental changes also raises questions concerning appropriate treatment approaches in older children. For example, the fact that active coping responses become more prevalent as children grow older and that they tend to be associated with better outcomes suggests that active coping strategies should be encouraged. However, it remains unclear whether measures to facilitate active coping should be encouraged in all children, especially in those who have an avoidant coping style (Peterson 1989). Zeltzer and her colleagues reported that encouraging specific coping procedures may be of benefit only to some children and only when the facilitation method matches the subject's style (Fanurik et al 1993). Some of the children who were 'distractors' (as compared to 'attenders') were taught to use imagery (a distraction technique *matched* to distraction coping preference) and some were taught to focus on the sensations of the cold pressor task (a sensory monitoring attention technique *mismatched* to distraction coping preference). The greatest *increase* in pain tolerance was found for the distractors who were taught imagery (the matched intervention) and the greatest *decrease* in tolerance (and *increase* in pain ratings) was found for the distractors provided with sensory monitoring (the mismatched intervention). The attenders did not significantly change their pain responsivity with either intervention strategy, whether matched or mismatched.

Finally, a still unanswered but important question concerning the development of pain perception is whether early pain experience modifies later pain experience. While there is no direct evidence for this in children, the results of some preclinical studies suggest mechanisms by which 'pain vulnerability' might develop. In response to peripheral nerve section in newborn rats, dorsal root ganglion cells die, nearby intact nerves develop sprouting with functional connections in areas outside their normal termination area, and areas surrounding the denervated skin contribute inputs via this permanently changed neural architecture (Himes & Tessler 1989; Fitzgerald et al 1990; Shortland & Fitzgerald 1993). Furthermore, the effects of nerve injury may spread centrally to the cortex (Fitzgerald 1991a). In addition, opioid peptides are implicated not only in the neural transmission of the pain stress response, but also in the regulation of neural growth (Stiene-Martin & Hauser 1991; Stiene-Martin et al 1991; Zagon & McLaughlin 1991).

In summary, early nociceptive experiences may be experienced and remembered, and there are biologically plausible reasons why they may also affect the development of the 'hard wiring' of the neural architecture. To the extent that descending and local 'gating' mechanisms in the spinal cord are still developing, these early nociceptive experiences may be less well modulated and make more significant contributions to pain vulnerability than later pain experiences. Consequently, an appropriate understanding of the development of pain perception is important as a guide to appropriate assessment and treatment of concurrent pain, and because it elucidates mechanisms which prevent subsequent pain experience.

CLINICAL PAIN SYNDROMES IN CHILDREN

Although pain is a common experience of childhood, most of what we know concerns pain behaviours transformed into complaints which are taken to the physician, and behaviours related to medical and dental procedures. In general, the behaviour attributed to the perception of pain in the narrow sense can rarely be distinguished from the behaviour representing the distress of pain in the broader sense, especially in infants (Owens 1984; McGrath 1987). There is increasing retrospective information about some pain syndromes obtained in nonclinical settings (reviewed by Goodman & McGrath 1991), although there are as yet no prospective epidemiological studies of pain in children. We know virtually nothing of incidental pain experiences in normal childen who are never brought to the physician but which are so important to our understanding of pain behaviour (Craig 1983). As a result, our understanding of pain in children tends to be based on selective samples, biased towards assuming a pathological process underlying the complaint, and confounded by factors which might be as much determinants of the act of seeking care as they are determinants of the pain experience itself (Barr & Feuerstein 1983). Despite these difficulties, the patterns of clinical pain in children are becoming increasingly subject to better controlled and more systematic study (McGrath & Unruh 1987; McGrath 1990; 1991, 1993; Goodman & McGrath 1991).

For most purposes, the presentation of clinical pain can be usefully described as syndromes or episodes, as acute, recurrent, or chronic, and as predictable or unpredictable. These dimensions overlap and may be important for both diagnosis and management. For example, recurrent abdominal pain syndrome consists of recurrent episodes of paroxysmal (unpredictable) abdominal pain. In contrast, procedure-associated pain is usually acute and predictable, at least to the extent that it is known when it is going to occur. In the syndrome, diagnosis tends to be a major problem, in part because of the relative lack of organic pathology (Apley 1975). In procedures, however, the pain stimulus is clear, and the primary concern is management of the accompanying pain and distress. However, these distinctions are often blurred in the clinical setting, and should not be considered analogous to their use in adults. For example, the child with recurrent abdominal pain may first present with an acute episode or may experience an intercurrent episode of acute organic pain in addition to his recurrent pain syndrome. While the pain stimulus may be apparent in procedures with infants, the painfulness of the stimulus may not, especially when the procedure is chronic or does not involve a needle. Finally, truly chronic pain continuing for days or weeks, as occurs in adults with low-back pain, is relatively rare in children. Although the *syndromes* of recurrent pain are sometimes considered chronic, the pattern of pain experience is recurrent with completely pain-free intervals. In most cases, chronic pain in children is associated with chronic diagnosed disease, of which pain is a part.

COLIC

In pediatrics, the term 'colic' is usually reserved for a syndrome of recurrent crying which occurs during the first 3 months of life. Typically, the crying occurs in a pattern characterized by an increase in overall duration per 24 hours until about 6 weeks of age, followed by a decline and resolution at 4 months. Each day, the crying clusters during the evening hours. There is considerable variation in both the amount and pattern of crying, both within and between individuals. While the term 'colic' implies that this behaviour pattern represents a distinct clinical syndrome, identical crying characteristics are described in normal (nonclinical) children (Brazelton 1962; Hunziker & Barr 1986), making the diagnostic differential of clinical from nonclinical infants difficult (Barr 1989b). As a result, many definitions of colic specify the amount of crying necessary to fulfill the criteria as well as additional features such as presence of gas and abdominal distention, motoric behaviour patterns (pulled up legs, body writhing, 'pain' facies), or lack of response to parental intervention (Illingworth 1954; Paradise 1966; Lothe et al 1982; Barr 1991). The commonest criterion defining crying behaviour is Wessel's (1954) 'rule of threes' (i.e. greater than 3 hours/day for greater than 3 days/week for 3 weeks). In a study of characteristics of crying in infants whose crying was considered a problem by their parents, approximately two-thirds had durations, bout lengths, perceived temperament profiles, and patterns of crying facies after meals similar to those of nonreferred infants (Barr et al 1992). However, the one-third who met Wessel's criterion differed from both the nonreferred and the referred infants who did not meet the criterion, implying that there may be subgroups of infants whose crying is seen as a problem.

The classification of colic as a pain syndrome highlights the difficulty of defining the pain experience in this age group in the absence of a clear precipitating stimulus (Barr & Geertsma 1993). Unless one assumes that all crying behaviour is due to pain, there is little direct convergent evidence that colic is, in fact, a pain syndrome. Infants meeting Wessel's criterion have longer, but not more frequent, crying bouts (Barr et al 1992). Their crying post-feeding is also more likely to have a characteristic 'pain facies' (brow bulge, eye squeeze, nasolabial furrow, and open lips) but this does not occur only in infants with colic and is prevalent when noncolic infants cry as well (Barr et al 1992). Other than this, there is almost no detailed description of the crying, facial, or motoric behaviour of the colicky infant to compare with the characteristic 'pain' behaviour of normal infants in response to a known stimulus. Furthermore, the biobehavioural determinants of this crying pattern remain largely unknown, in both colicky and noncolicky infants.

Most hypotheses concerning aetiology, including parental anxiety, birth order, breast versus bottle feeding, intestinal gas, and allergic reactivity, have found support only in methodologically weak studies, have not been replicated, or have not been supported by controlled studies (Illingworth 1954; Paradise 1966; Evans et al 1981; Lothe et al 1982; Forsyth 1983; Thomas et al 1987). The only clearly demonstrated effective therapy is the use of the 'antispasmodic' medication dicyclomine hydrochloride (Illingworth 1959; Grunseit 1977; Weissbluth et al 1984), although it is no longer available for clinical use because of presumed side-effects. While these findings may implicate gastrointestinal tone and/or motility in the pathogenesis of colic, the specific aetiology remains unknown. Increased carrying of the infant beyond the duration typical in our society reduces crying and fussing duration in nonclinical infants by about 40% at 6 weeks of age (Hunziker & Barr 1986) but is not effective as a treatment once colic has been established (Barr et al 1991b). However, mixed intensive behavioural interventions may reduce crying in clinical infants (Taubman 1984; 1988). While these findings may implicate nonorganic mechanisms, the same difficulty of arguing from therapy to aetiology remains for both the behavioural and medication strategies (Miller & Barr 1991).

One of the few mechanisms most clearly implicated in crying behaviour is hunger. In infants with gastrostomies, it can be experimentally demonstrated that gastric filling and not sucking (two elements of feeding usually confounded with one another in normal infants) is a sufficient condition for arresting crying (Wolff 1969). This may help explain the positive relationship between short interfeed intervals and reduced crying and fretting in nonclinical infants (Barr & Elias 1988). Consistent with these findings, crying is less in newborns fed on a 3- versus 4-hour schedule, and awake and alert behaviour clusters in the immediate postfeed period, regardless of nutrient composition (Oberlander et al 1992). Furthermore, crying duration (but not frequency) is reduced in societies where caretaking includes short interfeed intervals, more carrying, and increased responsivity to infant distress (Barr et al 1991a). However, the extent to which these mechanisms might account for or prevent 'colic' remains unclear.

In short, both the behavioural descriptions and experimental evidence are insufficient to determine whether the behaviour of the infant with colic represents an infant in pain. The clinical problem of colic illustrates the difficulty of attempting to determine the presence of pain in infants in the absence of a clear noxious stimulus.

EAR PAIN

Ear pain typically presents as an unpredictable episode of acute pain. It is a common experience of early childhood primarily because of its strong association with acute otitis media which is most prevalent in the first 6 years of life (Bluestone 1982). However, not all otitis media is associated with pain, nor is all ear pain due to otitis media (Ingvarsson 1982; Pukander 1983; Hayden & Schwartz 1985).

In the nonclinical setting, predictable ear pain can be experienced at all ages in response to a rapid change in altitude, unless relatively simple measures such as activation of the tensor veli palatini by yawning or swallowing are taken. However, infants are particularly predisposed to such episodes, not only because they are neither aware of the association nor know how to equalize atmospheric and middle ear pressure, but also because the eustachian tubes of infants are more compliant and therefore susceptible to collapse (Bluestone 1983). This has been demonstrated in infants during aircraft descent (Byers 1986). Crying which did not respond to mothers' soothing strategies was significantly increased during descent, typically began after adults had voluntarily sensed the need to clear their ears, was less likely to occur if the infant was bottle-feeding at the time, and was more likely if the infant had a cold – all features consistent with the predicted mechanism of inability to voluntarily open the eustachian tube and equalize middle ear pressure during descent (Patterson & Pettyjohn 1983; Byers 1986).

In the clinical setting, ear pain is usually seen because of inflammation of the external canal or the middle-ear. The pain of external otitis is diagnostically notable for being easily exacerbated by movement of the pinna or tragus of the ear which does not occur with middle-ear disease, and because it may appear out of proportion to the degree of inflammation (Bluestone 1983). Middle-ear disease is thought to be primarily due to dysfunction of the eustachian tube with secondary inflammation of the mucosa (Bluestone 1982). When the tube is closed, the pressure of exudate on inflamed mucosa can produce severe pain (Shambaugh & Girgis 1980) which is often dramatically relieved when the tube opens or spontaneous rupture of the tympanic membrane occurs. The pain seldom persists for more than 24 hours before being seen by a clinician (Ingvarsson 1982; Pukander 1983).

Despite its commonness, we know very little more about the pain of otitis media, illustrating the previously mentioned problems of studying pain in children. For example, Hayden & Schwartz (1985) graded clinically the severity of otalgia associated with acute otitis media with effusion by questioning the parent and/or child. They reported that pain was 'severe' in 42%, more likely to be present in association with redness, and more likely to be absent in children less than two years of age (25% versus 7%). However, as the authors noted, it is not possible to determine whether the age difference in pain is related to bacterial aetiology, pain perception, pain tolerance, or difficulty in communicating pain in this age group.

RECURRENT ABDOMINAL PAIN

The syndrome of recurrent abdominal pain (RAP) in

children typically consists of recurrent episodes of unpredictable acute pain in the abdomen. Although it is sometimes considered as a form of 'chronic' pain, this can only be meaningfully applied to the duration of the syndrome, since each pain episode in quite distinct, and the child is perfectly well between episodes. Since the recurrent nature of the pain is the cardinal symptom and probably most important for understanding the functional and emotional consequences, it is better understood as a form of recurrent rather than chronic pain.

Virtually all authors follow Apley (1975) in defining the syndrome as abdominal pain which is paroxysmal in nature, occurs frequently over an extended time period (at least three episodes over a period of 3 months), and is severe enough to result in a change of activity. The pain is often difficult to describe, other than its location which is typically but not consistently periumbilical. Nonperiumbilical pain has been taken to be a sign that the pain is more likely due to organic disease (Apley 1975) although this distinction may be less helpful in adolescents who often describe pain in other locations even in the absence of disease (Heinild et al 1959; Barr 1983b). The pain usually lasts less than 1 hour but is often associated with a number of additional complaints, such as nausea, vomiting, pallor, perspiration, headache and limb pains (Stone & Barbero 1970; Apley 1975; Liebman 1978). The frequency of these 'functional' symptoms is in sharp contrast to the low likelihood of symptoms implicating organic disease such as fever, jaundice, bloody stools and weight loss. In unreferred school children, the complaint has a prevalence of 10–15% (Oster 1972b; Apley 1975; Parcel et al 1977) although estimates as high as 25% have been reported in 6 year olds (Faull & Nicol 1986). The data for prevalence in the adolescent age group are less solid than that for preadolescents. The few follow-up studies suggest that the complaint persists for many years in about one-third of the patients seen clinically (Apley & Hale 1973; Christensen & Mortensen 1975; Stickler & Murphy 1979). The clinical similarities with the adult irritable bowel syndrome are suggestive of a causal connection, but this has not been demonstrated.

The classification of recurrent abdominal pain syndrome is described in terms of demonstrated or, more often, presumed aetiology. In developed Western countries, organic diseases are found to account for less than 10% of cases (Apley 1975; Liebman 1978), although the variety of diseases which may present with this syndrome is many (Bain 1974; Apley 1975; Barr 1983b). The common clinical assumption that the remainder represent manifestations of 'psychogenic', stress-related, or specific personality-related factors is not clearly supported by controlled studies using objective measures (e.g. McGrath et al 1983; Raymer et al 1984; Ernst et al 1984; Greene et al 1985; Sawyer et al 1987; Walker & Greene 1989; Osborne et al 1989; Sharrer & Ryan-Wenger 1991). Neither is it clear that stomach aches are characteristic symptoms in children with diagnosed anxiety disorders (Beidel et al 1991). The evidence that the parents of children with the syndrome may differ psychologically from the parents of children without it is somewhat more consistent (Routh & Ernst 1984; Hodges et al 1985a, 1985b, Zuckerman et al 1987; Walker & Greene 1989; Garber et al 1990), although whether this is aetiological or facilitates the complaint being seen clinically is unclear (Walker & Greene 1989). In addition, there is some evidence that parents and other significant adults may provide models for pain behaviour of children presenting with abdominal or chest pain (Osborne et al 1989). Earlier evidence based on a single laboratory measure (pupillary response) of a difference in autonomic reactivity to a cold pressor stress (Rubin et al 1967; Apley et al 1971) could not be replicated using phenylephrine instillation (Battistella et al 1992) or different autonomic measures and better matched controls (Feuerstein et al 1982). The possibility of an intestine-specific sensitivity to parasympathetic stimulation has been suggested (Kopel et al 1967) and deserves replication. Furthermore, the belief that children with RAP react differently to a pain stimulus was not confirmed in a laboratory situation with regard to facial reactivity, verbal report of pain or distress, or forearm EMG activity (Feuerstein et al 1982). In short, the clinical impression and many anecdotal reports suggesting that all 'nonorganic' recurrent abdominal pain should be considered as 'psychogenic' has not received substantial support in controlled systematic studies.

Given the nonspecific definition of the syndrome, the probable multifactorial nature of the predisposing influences, and the recognized difficulties of studying pain phenomena in children, the relative ignorance concerning the biobehavioural influences and mechanisms underlying the syndrome is not surprising. In part, this may be a function of the tendency to classify all children with the syndrome into 'organic' or 'psychogenic', and proceed on the assumption that there is something abnormal to be corrected (Barr & Feuerstein 1983). Usually, however, the role of psychosocial factors is ill-defined. It is often unclear, for example, whether 'stress' should be understood to predispose to, exacerbate, or maintain the complaint. Furthermore, it is difficult to know whether the stress is related directly to the pain complaint, or whether it acts to bring the complaint to medical attention (Roghmann & Haggerty 1973).

The pain episodes in many children may not represent symptoms of organic, psychological, or interactional 'disease', but may simply be due to normal physiological and environmental influences (Barr & Feuerstein 1983). For example, abdominal pain may be a manifestation of intolerance to incompletely absorbed lactose or other carbohydrates in disease-free children, although the extent to which the syndrome can be explained in this way is unclear (Barr et al 1979; Lebenthal et al 1981; Wald et al 1982; Hyams 1983; Barr et al 1985; Ceriani et al 1988). In the light of these uncertainties, it has been suggested that a third 'dysfunctional' category be included in the clinical classification to encompass those in whom neither organic disease nor psychosocial factors can reasonably be considered causal, and in whom the complaint represents a symptom of disease in an otherwise well child (Barr & Feuerstein 1983). Whether this or other subclassifications prove to be more accurate and helpful descriptions of this pain behaviour remains to be determined.

To date, little attention has been given to developmental changes potentially relevant to the complaint. Although it is commonly considered a complaint of school-aged children, the syndrome arguably might include the few well-documented cases in 1 year olds, as well as preschoolers and adults with irritable bowel syndrome (Hayden & Grossman 1959; Zuckerman et al 1987). Furthermore, there are limited data on adolescents and little direct comparison with the syndrome in preadolescents despite changes which might be important for understanding the pain behaviour (Barr 1992b). Among these changes is the fact that the history is more often taken from the patient directly, the same disease may manifest differently at different ages, and new disease aetiologies enter the differential, especially those referable to the genitourinary tract in females (Barr 1983b). The 'typical' lifestyle changes of adolescents may also contribute to difficulties in diagnosis (e.g. deliberate weight loss), and may be difficult to differentiate from pain as a conversion symptom (Friedman 1973; Barr 1992b).

Recent work in children and adults raises the possibility that clinically distinct presentations of children presenting with recurrent pain syndromes may be usefully delineated, including the syndrome of primary periumbilical pain as classically described, lower abdominal pain syndromes with altered bowel habits analogous to the 'spastic colon' subgroup of adult irritable bowel syndrome, and 'non ulcer dyspepsia' characterized by upper abdominal location of the pain. 'Spastic colon' in adults is similar to RAP and is typically associated with symptoms of distension, pain relief with a bowel movement, looser and more frequent stools, mucus, and a feeling of incomplete evacuation, and lower abdominal tenderness on examination. Nonulcer dyspepsia, although ill-defined, is usually characterized by upper abdominal pain and variably associated with nausea, postprandial fullness, distention, gas symptoms (belching, hiccups), and early satiety. Interest in this latter symptom complex has been heightened by the more common use of endoscopy for the identification of ulcers, and derives its name from the presence of ulcer-like symptoms in the absence of ulcer pathology. In addition, a new organism (*Helicobactor pylori*) has been identified as an aetiological agent in antral gastritis (Drumm et al 1987; Czinn & Speck 1989; Oderda et al 1989) which can also present with the same symptom complex. Symptomatic differentiation of ulcer from nonulcer patients has always been difficult in children (Tomomasa et al 1986), thereby increasing the use of endoscopy and other diagnostic techniques to identify these conditions (Vandenplas et al 1992). The mechanisms underlying the symptoms of nonulcer dyspepsia when these or other organic diseases are not identified remain obscure. However, there is some evidence that upper gastrointestinal motility changes are associated with the syndrome (Malagelada & Stanghellini 1985; Pineiro-Carrero et al 1988; Talley & Phillips 1988), and possibly duodenal inflammation (van der Meer et al 1990). There is reason to expect that further systematic attention to these clinical patterns in clinical and nonclinical settings will be required to understand the nature and significance of recurrent abdominal pain syndrome.

HEADACHE

While RAP is usually considered a syndrome, recurrent headaches in children are typically understood as a cluster of syndromes. By extrapolation from adults, most clinicians think of headache syndromes as tension headaches, migraine and its variants, and cluster headaches. Depending on how specifically the label 'tension headache' is used, another group of children with functional, chronic, or nonspecific headache may be distinguished (Rothner 1983). Cluster headaches, although recognized, are rare in children (Curless 1982). In addition to these 'primary' headache syndromes, the symptom can be secondary to a wide variety of important and often life-threatening organic diseases. These aetiologies are most important in acute, severe, often localized, isolated symptom presentations or chronic progressive presentations involving increased intracranial pressure.

The characteristics of the migraine syndrome have been described in more detail than nonmigraine headaches, despite the greater prevalence of the latter (Bille 1962; Sillanpaa 1983a, 1983b; Linet et al 1989; Mortimer et al 1992). The prevalence of both tends to increase almost linearly during childhood, with migraine affecting somewhat less than 3% at 7 years of age to 5–10% at 15 years (Bille 1962; Sillanpaa 1983a; Linet et al 1989; Mortimer et al 1992). Preadolescent boys and adolescent girls are preferentially affected in their respective age groups (Sillanpaa 1983a; Linet et al 1989) and girls tend to be headache-free during pregnancy (Bille 1981), characteristics which may reflet a relationship to oestrogenic hormones as a predisposing factor. Cases considered to be migraine are notable for an increased likelihood of unilateral pulsatile headache, positive family histories, the presence of aura (especially visual), abdominal discomfort, and sensory disturbances, although none of these criteria are 'necessary'. In general, aura in children with migraine ('classical migraine') occurs in approximately one-third of the cases, and increases with age in the preadolescent years (Mortimer et al 1992). The sensory disturbances can be quite striking, as in the Alice in Wonderland variant (Golden 1979). The association with motion sickness seen in adults also appears to hold in children, occuring in 45% of migraine cases compared to less than 7% in other headache and clinical groups (Barabas et al 1983), although this association is not confirmed in all studies (Deubner 1977). The prognosis of childhood migraine has not been adequately studied, but Bille's follow-up of children with 'pronounced' migraine until 30 years of age suggests persistence of the syndrome in 60%, with permanent remission in 40% during adolescence, and a hiatus in symptomatology during this time for the remainder (Bille 1981).

Despite the similarities, some features of migraine are thought to differ in children. These include shorter duration of attacks (usually 2–6 hours), lack of unilaterality (about 50%), and an association with concurrent or alternating abdominal pain attacks. This association does not, however, persist into adulthood (Bille 1981; Rothner 1983). Some variants, such as basilar migraine and paroxysmal vertigo, appear to be more common in children (Fenichel 1968; Rothner 1983). Many of these observations are based on the assumption of distinct headache syndromes presumed to have different pathogeneses. The epidemiological identification of migraine with aura (as compared to migraine without aura) is stable using various sets of criteria, suggesting that this subgroup may be a distinct syndrome (Mortimer et al 1992). Interestingly, the interval between the aura and the onset of headache tends to be shorter in males (15 min) than in females (25 min) (Linet et al 1992). Furthermore, visual aura headaches with associated tension-type symptoms (pain in the back of the head, neck and shoulders, and/or a feeling of a 'tight band' around the head) compared to visual aura headaches without tension symptoms tend to increase with age in females but not males, and tend to be more painful (Linet et al 1992). However, in a clinical study of 'problem headaches' using children's own descriptions over a 3-week period, typical 'muscle contraction' or 'migraine' symptoms were more likely to correlate with each other or with measures of headache severity (e.g. number of headache hours, number of locations affected) than with features typical of the respective syndromes (Joffe et al 1982). At the clinical level, these preliminary findings are consistent with a construct of continuing severity of headaches rather than headache types, but what they reflect is uncertain. They may reflect substantial differences between child and adult headache experience or simply that, contrary to most studies, the children themselves were the respondents. In this case, the childrens' reports may have been describing the motivational–emotional aspects of their subjective experience of pain intensity, whereas parent reports would be more likely to refer to objective occurences. Even in adults, self-report of the headache experience may not be distinguishable between adult migraine and tension headache patients (Hunter & Philips 1981). The almost complete lack of direct comparisons of migraine and headache phenomena between children and adults leaves the significance of these apparent differences uncertain.

The role of stress or psychosocial factors in the pathogenesis of headache syndromes not due to organic disease is commonly assumed and seems apparent clinically, but systematic demonstration of the relationship remains problematic (Cunningham et al 1988; Kowal & Pritchard 1990). In migraine, it is typically of interest as a precipitant or 'trigger factor', whereas in functional or tension headache it is usually considered aetiological. In addition, considerable clinical experience but no systematic study suggests that relatively well-defined behavioural and psychiatric syndromes (depression, conversion hysteria, malingering, school phobia) may present with headache as the primary complaint (Ling et al 1970; Schmitt 1971; Friedman 1973; Rothner 1983), but headache complaints are not characteristic of diagnosed anxiety syndromes (Beidel et al 1991), nor do they appear to be related to anxiety or depression in well-controlled studies using standardized instruments (Cunningham et al 1988; Kowal & Pritchard 1990). However, these important clinical assumptions have rarely been tested in appropriately controlled studies, and the available results are conflicting. In some studies using questionnaires and retrospective histories, 'emotional upsets', fear of failure, school problems, an especially hard day, and anxiety and depression were associated with headache symptomatology (Maratos & Wilkinson 1982; Leviton et al 1984; Passchier & Orlebeke 1985). However, in the best controlled study of children presenting with migraine to a referral centre using objective instruments, there were no differences in anxiety, behavioural–emotional problems, or life events changes between the patients and controls, nor between their respective parents (Cooper et al 1987). Nevertheless, although all the patients scored within the normal range for anxiety, those with the highest rating had more frequent and severe headaches during follow-up.

Another clinical entity which presents an instructive variant on the theme of head pain in children is the problem of temporomandibular joint (TMJ) dysfunction or myofascial pain-dysfunction (MPD), the former implicating the joint and the latter the masticatory muscles, but usually considered to be aspects of one syndrome. In the majority of cases, the pain is thought to be related to muscle fatigue, most often created by chronic bruxism (Guralnick et al 1978). The cardinal symptoms are dull, aching pain in the ear or periauricular area, tenderness of the masticatory muscles, clicking on movement of the temporomandibular joint, and limitation of movement on jaw opening. In children, as in adults, the syndrome may be a secondary manifestation of organic disease processes, but most often is not (Simon & Marbach 1976; Guralnick et al 1978; Belfer & Kaban 1982). In children, the primarily adolescent syndrome appears to differ from that in adults in not showing any gender preference compared to the 20:1 likelihood of the adult patient being female, and in being more likely to present in association with a reactive depression in adolescents (35%) than in adults (6.3%) (Belfer & Kaban 1982). A tripartite classification of the syndrome has been proposed for children and adolescents based on presence of organic pathology, interaction of physiological and psychological vulnerabilities, and absence of organic or anatomic dysfunction (Pillemer et al 1987).

The syndrome is also notable, however, because it represents an exception to two common generalizations often used to diagnose 'nonorganic' pain syndromes in children. The first is that the pain may be truly chronic, being present daily for weeks and months at a time – a feature which helps distinguish it clinically from childhood headaches (Holmes & Zimmerman 1983). Second, rather than being nonspecific or bilateral, the pain is most often unilateral, a characteristic which is often considered a cardinal sign of 'organicity' in other recurrent pain syndromes. Furthermore, diagnosis of the disorder can be difficult, since most of the cardinal symptoms and signs are common in unreferred populations (Nilner & Lassing 1981; Nilner 1981). For example, the presence of clicking sounds from the joint, which may be produced factitiously, is reported in about 17% of adolescents (Nilner 1981; Belfer & Kaban 1982). The syndrome underlines the implications for diagnosis of nonorganic pain syndromes when symptoms defining the syndrome are at variance with diagnostic generalizations thought to distinguish disease-related conditions, and when the symptoms are common outside of the clinical setting.

LEG PAIN

Leg pains in childhood that are not secondary to disease processes have also been considered as a recurrent pain syndrome. Historically, they generated most interest as a possible subacute form of rheumatic carditis, until important clinical differences (muscular versus joint location, nighttime versus daytime predominance respectively), absence of other signs of organic disease, and long-term follow-up studies established the lack of relationship between the two (Shapiro 1939; Hawksley 1939). Subsequently, it has usually been labelled and discussed as the syndrome of 'growing pain', despite its lack of relationship to growth parameters of childen (Oster 1972b; Oster & Neilsen 1972; British Medical Journal Editorial 1972).

Although clinical descriptions vary in details, there is considerable consensus about the primary clinical symptomatology (Hawksley 1939; Oster 1972a; Peterson 1977; Ansell 1980; Bowyer & Hollister 1984). The pain (or ache) is intermittent, deep, bilateral, most often localized in the muscles of thighs and calves but not in joint regions, and completely resolved in the morning. Naish & Apley (1951) stress differences between a diurnal and nocturnal form, the former including upper and lower limb pain with possible exacerbation by fatigue and heavy exercise. Usually, the criteria include the requirement that the pain be severe enough to wake the child from sleep or otherwise interfere with normal activity. The prevalence will vary depending on the restrictiveness of the definitions used (Peterson 1977). In the largest community sample of school-aged children and adolescents, the overall prevalence was 15.5%, with a predominance of the complaint in girls (18.4 versus 12.5%) mostly due to their persistently high rate of complaint throughout adolescence (Oster & Neilsen 1972).

Even in comparison to other childhood recurrent pain, there is relatively little understanding of this syndrome other than the objective clinical description. Descriptions of severity have ranged from minimal to 45% of children being 'reduced to crying with the pain' (Hawksley 1939). The validity of the observation that the pains are most pronounced at 3–5 years has been understandably questioned (Brenning 1960; Oster 1972a). This may reflect the occurrence in younger children of pains ascribed to hypermobility of the joints which is thought to predispose to leg pains often more prominent in the evening and after prolonged activity (Gedalia et al 1985; Sherry 1990). Growing pains have been compared to the adult syndrome of leg cramps or 'restless legs' (Oster 1972a; Ekbom 1975), and have also been thought of as a manifestation of fibrositis in children, a syndrome of unknown origin which in adults is characterized by multiple tender points at the site of tendon insertions (Calabro et al 1976; Campbell et al 1983; Malleson 1992). Some authors have stressed the cooccurrence of complaints of leg pains, recurrent abdominal pain and headache, because more than a third of the children may report more than type of pain at the time of questioning (Oster 1972b; Oster & Neilsen 1972). This has been interpreted as evidence for pain-proneness in the families of these children, suggesting a role for social modelling in the genesis of the complaint. However, evidence for the assumption that stress, emotional upset, or personality differences are differentially associated with the complaint is suggestive at best and often absent.

An interesting and increasingly recognized variant is the syndrome of reflex sympathetic (or neurovascular) dystrophy. In the classical description, this syndrome differs in being chronic, with paroxysmal exacerbations in pain severity, and a tendency to increase prior to treatment (Bernstein et al 1978; Silber & Majd 1989; Wilder et al

1992). The cardinal symptom is pain, but it typically has a qualitatively unusual character (burning, dyaesthesia, or paraesthesia), or is associated with extreme sensitivity to light touch (allodynia) or cold. The second major criterion includes the presence of autonomic signs, such as cyanosis, skin mottling, hyperhidrosis, oedema, and extremity coolness in the absence of other evidence of organic disease. In all series, it is present most commonly but not exclusively (about 80%) in lower extremities (Bernstein et al 1978; Silber & Majd 1989; Wilder et al 1992). Although originally considered more benign in children than in adults (Berstein et al 1978), secondary muscle atrophy and skin deterioration can occur when the condition is longstanding and severe (Silber & Majd 1989; Wilder et al 1992). The most frequently elicited historical stimulus is some form of antecedent injury, often related to sports activities, although identifiable lesions are rare (Silber & Majd 1989; Wilder et al 1992). Younger patients appear to have a milder course than older ones, with less functional disability, and there tends to be a predominance of females (Silber & Majd 1989; Wilder et al 1992). As with other recurrent and chronic pain syndromes, both the importance and the specific role, if any, of psychological factors in aetiology remain obscure, subject to conflicting findings, and deserving of better controlled evaluation (Sherry & Weisman 1988; Wilder et al 1992). In those children in whom it has been tried, sympathetic blocks can be helpful but they are not universally so, and physical therapy and remobilization remain the mainstay of therapy (Malleson 1992; Wilder et al 1992). Although uniformly good outcomes have been reported by some (Bernstein et al 1978; Sherry & Weisman 1988; Silber & Majd 1989), persistent dysfunction has been reported after a median 3-year follow-up of multidisciplinary therapy in a tertiary-care referral clinic (Wilder et al 1992). Because of its chronic character in the absence of clearly identifiable organic disease, this syndrome provides a particularly interesting contrast to the more typical recurrent pain syndromes of otherwise well children and adolescents.

As a possible third group of well children with leg pains, Sherry and colleagues (1991) described 100 children presenting to a tertiary-care referral centre with complaints of musculoskeletal pain, typically at multiple sites (66%), with hyperaesthesia in 45%, and a notable prevalence of a cheerful affect. In contrast to reflex sympathetic dystrophy, these children did not have objective signs of sympathetic hyperactivity, and the pain was constant in about two-thirds, but recurrent in one-third. The authors also eliminated children with 'growing pains' from the sample (Sherry 1990). There was a clear predilection to female patients (76%) with a mean age of 13 (range 3–20). No evidence of organic disease conditions was detected in any of them. The authors present evidence for a strong association with 'cohesive' (44%) and chaotic (40%) family clusters, enmeshment (76%) in parent-child relationships, a low prevalence (11%) of depression in the patients, and dramatic response to physical and occupational therapy (78%), which they interpret as evidence for a nonorganic and psychogenic aetiology, and label the syndrome as 'psychosomatic musculoskeletal pain'. Whether this label is appropriate in the absence of control groups, particularly in view of the difficulty of distinguuishing cause and effect when psychosocial and medical assessments are made concurrently, remain problematic as with other chronic and recurrent pain syndromes. Nevertheless, these children represent a group whose symptoms and associated findings tend to 'bridge' the phenomena typically described as 'growing pain' and those that are now recognized as reflex sympathetic dystrophy.

CHEST PAIN

Chest pain may present as an isolated episode or as a syndrome of recurrent episodes. It is not typically considered as part of a broader complex of recurrent pain complaints with headache, abdominal and leg pains. Although headache is less commonly reported as an associated complaint for chest rather than abdominal pain, it is more commonly reported in children with chest pain than in a clinical control group (Goodman & Pantell 1984). The epidemiology of chest pain is almost completely unknown (Goodman & MacGrath 1991), except for a study of urban black adolescents. In this study, chest pain occured in 12.8% of the adolescents, of whom only 32% had seen a physician for the complaint (Brunswick et al 1979).

In most of those who present clinically, the symptom presentation is that of a stable pattern of recurrent intermittent episodes (Pantell & Goodman 1983; Rowe et al 1990). It is usually substernal or left praecordial in location, thought of as sharp, and seldom radiates. Half of the episodes last less than 5 minutes; only 20% last an hour. Almost 70% of adolescents report restricting their physical activity as a result of the pain (Pantell & Goodman 1983) but that is more likely a reflection of anxiety about presumed underlying heart disease than an index of pain severity. In another clinical population presenting to the emergency room, 31% reported being awakened from sleep by the pain (Selbst et al 1987). Metaphorical descriptions (e.g. 'sharp like a knife') were offered by 97% of patients during a psychiatric interview, but by only 38% of the same patients during the medical interview (Driscoll et al 1976), strikingly illustrating the effect of context on pain description in children.

Compared with other recurrent pain syndromes, organic disease accounts for a greater proportion but still less than 25% of clinical complaints (Driscoll et al 1976; Pantell & Goodman 1983; Selbst et al 1987, 1988; Rowe et al 1990). These are usually cardiorespiratory and rarely gastrointestinal. In contrast to other recurrent pain syndromes, about 40% can be attributed to recognizable benign clinical syndromes, the most common of which are musculoskeletal, particularly costochondritis and chest wall syndrome, and the unique and easily indentifiable 'pericordial catch syndrome' (Reynolds 1989). In another 20–40%, there is no recognizable mechanism, and these are usually referred to as 'idiopathic'. There is a striking lack of relationship between any symptom patterns and the likelihood of a particular underlying aetiology, and lack of difference between organic and idiopathic (Driscoll et al 1976; Pantell & Goodman 1983; Rowe et al 1990). However, an aetiology is more likely to be recognizable in syndromes being evaluated within 6 months of onset (Driscoll et al 1976; Selbst et al 1987). In the emergency room setting, pain that occurs in younger children, presents within 48 hours of onset of the first episode, and wakes the patient from sleep is less likely to be idiopathic (Selbst et al 1987, 1988).

The fact that chest pain not attributed to a recognizable cause is typically referred to as idiopathic (rather than functional or psychogenic) may reflect the relative lack of clinical evidence for psychosocial stresses in these patients. Children with chest pain are notably similar to their non-complaining peers in not reporting family problems, insomnia, or fatigue. Life stresses are similar to those of other populations, and similar between aetiological categories (Pantell & Goodman 1983). School absence or difficulties with social activities may or may not be characteristic of children with chest pain, depending on the population, but is more often thought of as a consequence of the pain symptom (Driscoll et al 1976; Pantell & Goodman 1983; Selbst et al 1988). The relative infrequency of headache complaints compared to abdominal pain controls argues against the likelihood that they are 'pain prone' patients (Goodman & Pantell 1984). While the pain clearly produces anxiety concerning its aetiology, psychiatric interviews do not reveal evidence that anxiety predisposes to the pain (Driscoll et al 1976). The complaint can be the presenting symptom of childhood depression, but this is not common, and children are no more likely than healthy adolescents to report symptoms characteristic of depression (Kashani et al 1982; Goodman & Pantell 1984; Rowe et al 1990).

There has been no direct comparison between the description of chest pain in adults and children. However, the aetiological significance of the symptom is clearly different. Nevertheless, the *belief* that the aetiology is similar appears to have distinct functional consequences related to physical activity, self-concept, and possibly school function, even in an age group of the population who consider themselves to be, and are, relatively invulnerable (Pantell & Goodman 1983). The disjunction between the belief and the reality is all the more striking in the light of the fact that knowledge about the relationship between chest pain and self-perception of health is the same in adolescents who have or have not complained of chest pain themselves (Kaden et al 1991), and that, subjectively, none of the adolescents who attributed their pain to heart disease had ever known of someone their age who had suffered a heart attack (Pantell & Goodman 1983). Objectively, the pain of only one of 242 subjects in three studies was clinically attributable to a cardiac origin (mitral valve prolapse) on the basis of a mid-systolic click, murmur, and prolapse by echocardiography (Driscoll et al 1976; Pantell & Goodman 1983; Brenner et al 1984). In a recent study of all cases presenting to tertiary-care pediatric referral emergency rooms in a 1 year period, five of 325 cases (1.5%) were found to have cardiac diseases (myocarditis, atrial septal defect, idiopathic hypertrophic subaortic stenosis, Wolff-Parkinson-White syndrome, and congenital heart block) but none had myocardial infarction (Polly & Mason 1991). Nine of 407 patients (4%) had cardiac disease in another study (Selbst et al 1988). These data are consistent with previous demonstrations of the morbidity of cardiac nondisease in the pediatric population (Bergman & Stamm 1967). However, myocardial infarction and cardiac-related chest pain have been reported in adolescents using cocaine (Woodward & Selbst 1987; Choi & Pearl 1989).

In a follow-up study of the available 37% of the latter cohort (Selbst et al 1990), recurrent pain persisted in 43% of the children for 6 months or more. More of the children were assessed as idiopathic at follow-up (34%) than at initial presentation (13%) and a few more as psychogenic (11% versus 9% respectively). One patient was subsequently determined to have mitral valve prolapse which may have been related to the pain (Selbst et al 1990).

While the pain pattern is considered crucial to clinical assessment and diagnosis in adults, it is less helpful in diagnosing underlying causes in children (Selbst et al 1988; Rowe et al 1990). Furthermore, the finding of objective evidence of mitral valve prolapse does not assure that the pain is 'cardiac' in origin. Chest pain is a less frequent finding in community samples of children with mitral valve prolapse than those without it (Arfken et al 1990). Woolf et al (1991) presented evidence of gastroenterological abnormalities and response to therapy in 13 of 17 preadolescents and adolescents with mitral valve prolapse and chest pain as the presenting symptom. Similarly, systematic laboratory evaluation of exercise-induced reactive airways of otherwise typical children and adolescents with exertional chest pain suggests that pulmonary aetiologies may be more common than predicted on the basis of standard clinical assessments (Wiens et al 1992). Whether more multidimensional descriptions of the pain experience would be more discriminating is untested. Compared to other recurrent pain syndromes in children, it clearly produces recognizable anxiety in the patient, and is less likely to be considered psychogenic in aetiology. It provides one of the best examples of the importance of determining the patient's understanding of the significance of the pain symptom in order to comprehensively treat the complaint and prevent morbidity.

PAIN SECONDARY TO DISEASE

While the pain complaints of these recurrent syndromes are usually primary, they may also present as symptoms secondary to underlying organic or psychiatric diseases. In some cases, the syndrome of recurrent pain may itself be the manifestation of the disease process; in others, the symptom of acute pain may present as an isolated episode secondary to an intercurrent disease process. Across all studies of the syndromes discussed, two generalizations have been repeatedly confirmed in industrialized Western clinical populations. The first is that organic disease entities account for somewhat less than 10% of the presenting cases, with the possible exception of higher percentages in children with chest pain. The second is that the number of possible organic processes presenting as pain is very extensive. Almost any disease entity of the relevant organ system which includes pain as a symptom may present in this manner. For RAP syndrome, for example, it has been estimated that well over 100 conditions may present in this way (Bain 1974). The complaint of back pain appears to represent an important exception to these generalizations, however. Back pain in children is always considered significant and most clinical classifications do not even include a category of 'idiopathic' or 'functional' back pain (Bunnell 1982; King 1984; Harvey & Tanner 1991). The dramatic differences in prevalence (Olsen et al 1992) and relationship to organic aetiology both from other childhood pain complaints and from the highly prevalent adult syndrome may provide an interesting model for studying the role of pain proneness and complaint modelling in the generation of pain complaints. A third generalization may also hold true, at least in the clinical setting: namely, that single acute presentations are more likely to be due to organic disease processes than recurrent presentations.

Whether these generalizations also hold for the likelihood that the symptoms represent psychiatric diseases is considerably less clear. In part this is due to the relatively more difficult tasks of objectively establishing psychiatric diagnoses and of defining the appropriate borders of the construct of 'disease' in psychosocial and behavioural terms (Large 1986; Dworkin 1992; Pilowsky 1992; Tunks 1992). It is complicated further by the still prevalent clinical practice of considering all nonorganic disease as 'psychogenic' or as being a manifestation of abnormal psychosocial processes (e.g. Sherry et al 1991). It has been argued that such a practice inappropriately assumes that a symptom of disease entails the presence of disease itself, assumes that aetiologies must be reduced to organic or psychological, goes beyond what we know on the available evidence, and makes no provision for the possibility that pain complaints may be due to normal, nondisease mechanisms (Barr & Feuerstein 1983). If the construct of 'psychiatric disease' is limited to well-established clinical entities and the clinical decision is based on positive criteria for diagnosis, then the relative prevalence of attributable 'psychogenic' pain may be similarly low (Apley 1975; Barr 1983b, Barr & Feuerstein 1983; Goodman & Pantell 1984). Psychiatric syndromes most likely to manifest with pain syndromes appear to be conversion/hysteria reactions, depression, acute anxiety, and school phobia (Ling et al 1970; Schmitt 1971; Smith & Eastham 1973; Friedman 1973; Asnes et al 1981; Astrada et al 1981; Kashani et al 1982; Moffatt 1982; Ernst et al 1984; Hughes 1984; Routh & Ernst 1984; Friedman 1985). In addition, the extent to which these complaints may be reflections of complex psychosocial trauma such as child abuse and sexual assault remains unknown, but deserves systematic study. Unfortunately, with few exceptions (Osborne et al 1989), studies of the relationship between psychosocial factors and recurrent pain syndromes are simply concurrent and correlational, and rarely specify clearly which of the many proposed mechanisms by which the two might be related is being tested.

The organic diseases entering the differential of these syndromes have been well reviewed recently (*general*: McGrath & Unruh 1987; *recurrent abdominal pain*: Bain 1974; Barr 1983b; Levine & Rappaport 1984; *headache*: Rothner 1983; *limb pains*: Peterson 1977; Bowyer & Hollister 1984; Sherry 1990; Malleson 1992; *chest pain*: Coleman 1984; Selbst 1990; *back pain*: Dyment 1991). Of the extensive list which may manifest as pain syndromes, many have characteristics typical of that seen in adults. However, they often have characteristics specific to children which help define the clinical approach.

First, it is an important clinical principle that the same disease does not necessarily present similarly in all age groups. Within the pediatric age group, for example, urinary tract infection is more likely to present as vomiting in infants and children but as abdominal pain in adolescents (Carvajal 1978). Gallstones present predominantly as right upper quadrant pain in older children, but not in children under 6 years of age (Reif et all 1991). With the exception of pregnant adolescents, the female predominance seen in adults is not present in children with gallstones (Reif et al 1991). Ulcer disease tends to present as blood loss in younger children (even though abdominal pain is present historically), but as abdominal pain in older children and adolescents (Drumm et al 1988; Gold et al 1990). In adults, the pain of ulcer disease is characteristically improved with food intake, but it is typically unchanged or made worse in adolescents (Deckelbaum et al 1974; Gold et al 1990). Secondly, there are some diseases which have particular prominence in children, either because they are limited to a certain age group ('developmental' conditions), or because they are present at all ages but become more prevalent in particular age groups. Notable examples of 'developmental' diseases are Legg-Calve-Perthe's disease under age 10 and slipped capital femoral epiphyses over age 10 as causes of hip pain (Bowyer & Hollister 1984), inflammatory bowel diseases, appendicitis, and dysmenorrhoea as causes of abdominal pain (Barr 1983b), and infections and tumours as causes of back pain up to 10 years of age (King 1984). The pain manifestations of other diseases may be age-related because of changes in life-style and environmental exposure. For example, abdominal pain may be due to acute intermittent porphyria interacting with barbiturates, or dysmenorrhoea secondary to the use of intrauterine devices (Tschudy et al 1975; Barr 1983b). Similarly, chest pain may present in adolescents due to smoking, cocaine, or contraceptive use (Friedman et al 1975; Bernstein et al 1986; Luque et al 1987; Selbst 1990). Thirdly, diseases may enter the differential not so much because they are causal of the pain, but rather because anxiety concerning these diseases is causal of the pain being presented as a clinical complaint. The prototypical example of this is fear of atherosclerotic heart disease as a cause of chest pain, as previously discussed (Pantell & Goodman 1983). However, fear of cancer is a prominent aetiological concern in all childhood pain syndromes. With the possible exception of chest pain, these fears are more often those of the parent than the patient.

Despite the presence of recognized pathogeneses in many disease-related pains, there is relatively little additional understanding of childhood pain which has been gained through systematic study of these disease entities. Reports directly comparing the pain experience of children and adults with the same disease are extremely rare. Generally, comparisons of children with organic and nonorganic pain syndromes, while differing with regard to the presence of associated symptoms and laboratory findings, have not been strikingly so in their descriptions of the pain. In some cases, the time course of the pain, both at the level of episodes and syndrome description, may be useful, but this has not been systematically evaluated (Driscoll et al 1976; Rothner 1983; Selbst et al 1987). Even in sickle-cell disease, a disease in which severe pain episodes are due to acute vasoocclusive crises, there has been little detailed description of the pain characteristics. Prior to understanding its pathogenesis, the predominance of the pain manifestations was such that it was apprently identified and recognized in Africa by tribal onomatopoeic names stressing the relentless, repetitive gnawing nature of the pains in the bones during crisis (Konotey-Ahulu 1974). Although painful crises may be the cause of death (Parfrey et al 1985), and the frequency of painful crises has typically been used to index disease severity, only recently has it been determined what the natural history of crisis frequency is (Greenberg et al 1983). Nevertheless, the potential benefit of studying pain descriptions was illustrated by the reports of children with sickle-cell disease (Walco & Dampier 1990) using the Pediatric Pain Questionnaire (Varni et al 1987). These children reported a broad range of pain intensities but higher mean intensities for episodes than reported by children with juvenile rheumatoid arthritis, and longer duration of episodes than the equally high intensity pains reported with procedures. Importantly, parent- and children-reported pain intensity did not correlate well for average pain, worst pain in the past week, worst pain ever managed at home, and worst pain managed in the hospital, underlining the importance of 'asking the child'. The intensity rating did not correlate with the number of painful sites reported, suggesting that any 'objective' scale based on number of pain sites would be misleading, at least for this condition. Finally, although not specific, the choice of sensory descriptors was different for these children than for patients with juvenile rheumatoid arthritis, with the former more often endorsing 'aching', and the latter more often endorsing 'sore' as descriptors. This is of interest since the mechanisms underlying the pains is different in these two diseases. Since sickle-cell pain is recurrent, variable and unpredictable, these findings may provide interesting comparisons for other recurrent pain syndromes as well. However, such instructive disease-specific comparisons are rare in children. Whether this is a reflection of the rather inclusive and nonspecific definitions of nonorganic pain syndromes, the commonality of pain pathogenesis, difficulties in measurement, lack of interest in pediatric pain phenomena, or other factors is unclear.

Juvenile rheumatoid arthritis is one of the few diseases in which comparisons with adult descriptions have been studied. In two comparisons of adult and child joint pain using globally defined pain severity or visual analogue scales, the number of painful joints and the severity of pain was considered less in children (Laaksonen & Laine 1961; Scott et al 1977). Interestingly, the number of patients with severe pain was similar and there was no difference in pain report when inflamed joints were subject to passive movement in the former study (Laaksonen & Laine 1961). Consequently, the results leave the question open as to whether the child patients actually experience less pain or underreport it. In the latter study, the pain severity ratings correlated poorly with disease severity indices in children, this being in contrast to what occurs in adults (Scott et al 1977). Recent evidence confirms that disease severity has little relation to child patient-reported pain, with joint inflammation accounting for only 10% of the variance in perceived pain severity (Ilowite et al 1992). Some children with the disease may not report any pain at all (Sherry et al

1990). These results raise the question as to whether disease severity and pain are related in analogous ways in adults and children.

Other studies limited to children have explored aspects of the pain description other than intensity. When presented with a list of descriptors of possible joint sensations, all children were able to report some sensations from their affected joints (Beales et al 1983). In contrast to the previous study (Varni et al 1987), 'aching' was reported by all children (100%), perhaps because of the limited descriptor list provided, followed by words describing a sharp sensation, and then burning sensations. In another study of similar patients using pain descriptor lists, a similar ranking of descriptors was picked (sore, aching, sharp, burning), but this distribution was not markedly different from comparison groups of hospitalized and nonhospitalized children (Savedra et al 1982; Varni et al 1987). When asked to interpret the meanings of these sensations, however, there were striking differences in the attributed meanings, with adolescents most often indicating that it implied continuing disability and preadolescents rarely reporting any particular attribution (Beales et al 1983). Older children also reported more unpleasantness and more severe pain using visual analogue scales (Beales et al 1983). In sum, while the sensations reported were similar across age groups, the cognitive and emotional meaning of the experiences were different. The authors plausibly argue that the increased severity ratings in the older childen were influenced by their attributions of the significance of the pain for them.

PAIN SECONDARY TO PROCEDURES

Pain secondary to procedures, broadly speaking, is commonly acute (as in venipuncture) and sometimes chronic (as in chemotherapy-related side effects). Procedural pain is recurrent only in the sense that the procedures themselves may be repeated. The cardinal feature differentiating procedural pain is its predictability, at least with regard to time of occurrence. This attribute means that interpretation of the behaviour elicited with painful procedures is likely to be confounded with anticipatory and concurrent anxiety, usually considered together as procedure-related 'distress'. Whether the difficulty of distinguishing these two aspects of the experience is due to their mutual interdependence or the inability to cognitively differentiate them remains a problem for measurement, especially in children (e.g. Sacham & Daut 1981; Katz et al 1981; Winer 1982; Lebaron & Zeltzer 1984). However, the predictability provides the opportunity to use contextual, behavioural and analgesic techniques to modify the pain and/or anxiety.

Procedural pain has provided a model for the study and evaluation of pain in children. In part this is due to its predictability, and in part due to the ethical constraints on inducing pain which has no clear benefit to the child. While procedures are performed for preventive, diagnostic, or therapeutic purposes other than our understanding of pain phenomena, the fact that their performance entails potential suffering permits, indeed mandates, their study.

Procedures may range from relatively acute, mild acts (venipuncture, inoculations, lumbar puncture, dressing changes, especially in burn patients) to longer, more severe insults (operations: Marshall 1993). Often overlooked is the potential discomfort associated with prolonged monitoring or therapeutic manoeuvres such as indwelling catheters and feeding tubes, procedures that are common in infants and prematures. Since any particular procedure is usually performed in a relatively standard way, one is presented with the possibility of observing distress behaviours in response to a standard stimulus across a variety of individual, group, and situational variables. For example, there is a clinically striking difference between the reaction of children with leukaemia and children with haemophilia when receiving intravenous lines for therapeutic purposes. While the act is similar, it is usually occasioned by disease recurrence and associated with unpleasant side-effects of medication in the former compared to imminent relief from a painful bleed in the latter. Indeed, for some children with cancer, the treatments are more salient stresses than the disease itself (Zeltzer et al 1980). Such differences are consistent with observations that, in comparison to other children with chronic diseases, even 6- to 10-year-old children with leukaemia tell stories expressing more anxiety, concern for body integrity and distancing from important adults, and that this increases with subsequent hospitalizations (Spinetta et al 1973; 1974). Anxiety and concern for bodily integrity are similar for clinic patients in remission as well as hospitalized children under treatment, while the distancing from adults is not apparent in the clinic (Spinetta & Maloney 1975). The comparisons further suggest that children with other chronic illnesses accommodate to the 'procedure' of the clinic visit, while the children with leukaemia do not (Spinetta & Maloney 1975).

Others have used these standard pain experiences to advantage to delineate some of the influences which may modulate the pain response. For example, Schechter et al (1991) exploited the opportunity of examining the range of self-report and behavioral 'pain' responses of normal 5-year-old children to diphtheria–pertussis–tetanus (DPT) immunization. On both measures, a considerable range of response was reported (from no response in 26% to extreme responses in 11%) despite the absence of illness and standardization of setting and procedure (Schechter et al 1991). Children previously rated by their parents as less 'adaptable' and as more 'difficult' temperamentally were more likely to have higher distress scores.

Interestingly, parental attitudes towards medical procedures or attitudes which might emphasize or denigrate pain expression had little effect (Schechter et al 1991). These kinds of studies underline the importance of individual differences in pain response, and support the notion that information and preparation for procedures may need to be individualized to have optimum benefit (Peterson 1989; Fanurik et al 1993). Similarly, Fowler-Kerry & Lander (1991) used the venipuncture procedure to report the most systematic assessment of the role of gender in pain response. Importantly, in the age range of 5–12 years, females were no different on their self-reported sensory and affective pain ratings, nor did they report different state anxiety or amount of pain expected from the procedure. On a measure of pain estimation (actual sensory pain minus expected pain on a visual analogue scale), females were more likely to overestimate, and males to underestimate, the pain experienced (Lander et al 1992). These results suggest that while management of pain expectations may need to be gender-specific, management of sensory and affective pain should not be (see also Fradet et al 1990; Humphrey et al 1992).

Bone marrow aspirations are performed only in children with diseases, and therefore the reactions may be modulated by disease severity, manifestations of anxiety, different perceptions of the meaning of the procedure and associated contextual differences (e.g. sedation, physician, subsequent procedures, parent presence or absence). In an investigation of behavioural distress in response to bone marrow aspirations in children with cancer across the pediatric age range and in two cultures (United States and Holland), differences in response were noted for age, sex and culture, with the largest differences due to age (van Aken et al 1989). Studies such as these emphasize the importance of developmental changes as significant determinants despite the many influences contributing to the pain stress response. In addition, direct observations of interactions involved in bone marrow aspirations suggest that what the adult and child participants actually do makes a difference (Blount et al 1991). Coping or distress responses of children are contingent upon whether the adults' behaviours tend to facilitate coping (e.g. humour, coaching to breathe) or distress (e.g. reassurance, apologies, criticism) respectively. Adults interacting with children who are 'high coping' engage in more coping-promoting behaviours, and these children respond with coping behaviours (e.g. deep breathing, humour), indicating that the types of behaviour that constitute the contingent interactions can modify the distress response.

While anticipation of a procedure may contribute to the distress, it also provides the opportunity to structure the context to optimize the patient's ability to cope with the event. Consequently, procedural pain in children has been used to evaluate psychological coping strategies thought to be helpful in adults, including previous instruction, influencing the sense of control of the patient, the presence of observers-models, attention-distraction, increasing predictability, and the presence of suggestion or expectation of relief (e.g. Weisenberg 1977; Zeltzer & LeBaron 1982; Katz et al 1987; Fowler-Kerry & Lander 1987; Gonzalez et al 1989; Manne et al 1990; Blount et al 1991). Interestingly, 5-year-old children overwhelmingly (86%) express the preference to have a parent present, even though more distress is displayed in that context (Gonzalez et al 1989). Zeltzer & LeBaron (1982) reported a controlled comparison of hypnotic (active facilitation of pleasant fantasies or images) and nonhypnotic (distraction, deep breathing, practised self-control) behavioural techniques to control pain and anxiety in lumbar puncture and bone marrow aspiration procedures. The results suggested that both techniques helped, but that hypnosis was more helpful in reducing pain and anxiety during both procedures (Zeltzer & LeBaron 1982). In more recent work, they have found evidence that behavioural techniques might be more successful if tailored to the particular coping style of the individual patient (Fanurik et al 1993).

In an attempt to reduce the psychopathology associated with chronic burn patients, the predictability of the procedure of burn debridement was increased by focusing the child on the procedure, describing sensations to be expected, and signalling that this nursing interaction was for debridement by wearing a red tape on the nurse's apron (Kavanaugh 1983). Patient control was increased by encouraging the patient to aid actively in the removal of dressings, debridement and application of silver nitrate. Compared to children receiving standard practice characterized by verbal support, distraction and staff control of the procedure, the children in the experimental group demonstrated fewer maladaptive responses, particularly lower hostility, less 'stress analgesia' withdrawal episodes, and less depression at discharge (Kavanaugh 1983). Of the two, the element of controllability was thought to contribute the most. Although the groups were small, the results were impressive in illustrating the importance of attention to how the process of the procedure is structured and the potential power of the patient's involvement in the process (Beales 1979).

Other notable research applications which have capitalized on the standardization of the procedural stimulus include the study of measurement and assessment techniques related to bone marrow aspiration and dental visits (e.g. Katz et al 1980; Winer 1982; Jay et al 1983; LeBaron & Zeltzer 1984) and developmental differences in pain reactivity to immunizations in infants (see Developmental changes above).

Interestingly, the studies on predictable, anticipated pain related to immunization and dental visits provide almost all of the information available on pain and pain-related distress in normal 'non-clinical' infants and children. The extent to which these findings can be generalized to unanticipated pain occurring in nonclinical settings has not been assessed.

SUMMARY

There has been a remarkable increase in our understanding of children's pain, and there remains a remarkable amount that is unknown. Since the last edition of this text, the literature on pain in children has grown exponentially. In addition, there is a considerable body of literature concerning diagnosis and treatment in children which has been implicitly though not specifically addressed in this chapter, but which has recently been well reviewed elsewhere (Schechter 1985; McGrath & Unruh 1987; Ross & Ross 1988; McGrath 1990, 1991, 1993) and in Chapters 80 and 81 of this volume. Throughout this literature, it is clear that the increasing recognition of the sensory and motivational–affective aspects of the pain experience, how they are affected by biological, behavioural and situational variables, and the importance of developmental changes have stimulated attempts to find more appropriate and more effective modalities for assessment and intervention.

Despite this effort, our knowledge of pain in children has significant gaps which often put us at risk of biasing our understanding and our practice. While a number of these gaps have been illustrated in the descriptions of specific pain syndromes, a few of the limitations which cross most of the pain syndromes deserve explicit mention.

There is a remarkable asymmetry in the amount we know about pain depending on the setting in which it is studied. Our knowledge of the pain representing disease far surpasses that which we have of 'nonorganic' pain. Some implications of this asymmetry are that we still have considerable difficulty diagnostically distinguishing the two, and probably overestimate the extent to which nonorganic pain is attributable to 'psychogenic' aetiologies. Our concentration on pattern recognition of pain syndromes derived primarily from organic disease tends to entail a thoroughgoing, expensive medical investigation for all pain complaints.

Even more striking, however, is the difference between what we know about pain (organic or nonorganic) which presents in clinical settings compared to what is not brought to the physician. The absence of information about pain that is not referred clinically, its associated symptomatology, and especially its relationship to psychosocial stresses leaves us without a baseline for comparison in order to designate appropriately non-organic pain complexes as syndromes. As a result, the attempt to understand the appropriate role of personality, family factors, and psychosocial stress has been confounded by the difficulty of parsing out the extent to which these factors predispose to *pain* as opposed to predisposing to *pain being seen as a clinical complaint* (Barr & Feuerstein 1983). Arguably, the relative lack of substantial evidence implicating these factors as causal in the better-designed, controlled studies implies that their role as referral-generating rather than pain-generating is larger than previously considered.

The second major asymmetry concerns the extent to which we have accumulated semiquantitative 'sensory' descriptions of pain severity, frequency and location characteristics, but lack descriptions of other qualities of the pain experience. Two other qualities in particular probably deserve more attention: namely, the time course of the pain (both intraepisode and intrasyndrome), and the motivational–affective qualities of the pain perception. With the possible exception of headache pain (Rothner 1983), there has been little attention to the value of the time course in distinguishing disease-related and nondisease-related pain, or in subdividing nonorganic pain presentations. It has also meant that virtually all of our epidemiological data have been limited to point prevalence estimates, leaving questions of duration and stability of pain complexes unanswered (Goodman & McGrath 1991). Despite the fact that attention to other, more subjective qualities of the pain experience has been limited to a few studies, the findings have already raised interesting questions concerning the clinical appropriateness of the migraine–tension headache distinction, prior assumptions about lack of pain in juvenile rheumatoid arthritis patients, and putative differences in the pain experience of children with juvenile rheumatoid arthritis and sickle-cell disease. Similar systematic studies in other pain syndromes are likely to raise similar challenges to prior assumptions.

Moving from more objective sensory descriptions to more subjective qualitative descriptions has required a significant change of focus from 'asking the parent' to 'asking the child'. Indeed, the use of the parent as primary information source both in epidemiological and clinical studies might possibly prove to have been the single most important systematic bias in our past conceptualization of children's pain. However, the increasing willingness to 'ask the child' will only prove fruitful if appropriate attention is paid to questions of validity and reliability of measures, an effort which has certainly begun and is now being pursued more vigorously (see Ch. 16). As a corollary, this shift of focus should permit better understanding of the meaning of the pain complaint to the child patient, as well as the functional consequences. The apparent value of these aspects of the pain experience in childen with chest pain may only be the most salient example of a largely neglected aspect of childhood pain experience.

The final asymmetry is the relative lack of attention to the importance of developmental changes in understanding, assessing and treating the child in pain. While the most striking clinical illustrations of this point are apparent in the way analgesic techniques have been used (or, rather, not used), the most difficult methodological questions relate to the problems posed for pain measurement. The adoption of multidimensional verbal approaches and parallel verbal, behavioural, and physiological descriptions of pain reactivity have substantially changed our perception of the pain experience of infants and across age groups of children. However, the clinical, as opposed to research, application of these approaches still faces the considerable challenge of finding measures which are *specific* as well as sensitive to the pain experience (Craig 1992; Barr 1992c). As illustrated by the question of whether colic is really a pain syndrome at all, the issue of measure specificity is particularly salient for infants in situations where the noxious stimulus may be chronic and not as apparent as during an injection (Barr & Geertsma 1993). It is also to be expected that, with the advent of valid multidimensional measures appropriate for use with children, more direct adult-child comparisons in disease- and nondisease-related pain syndromes will contribute to our understanding of the developmental changes in pain experiences across the life span.

Acknowledgements

The author's research is supported by the Medical Research Council of Canada (MA-11083) and the McGill University–Montreal Children's Hospital Research Institute Telethon Fund.

REFERENCES

Anand K J S, Carr D B 1989 The neuroanatomy, neurophysiology, and neurochemistry of pain, stress, and analgesia in newborns and children. Pediatric Clinics of North America 36: 795–822

Anand K J S, Hickey P R 1987 Pain and its effects in the human neonate and fetus. New England Journal of Medicine 317: 1321–1347

Anand K J S, Brown R C, Causon R et al 1985 Can the human neonate mount an endocrine and metabolic response to surgery? Journal of Pediatric Surgery 20: 41–48

Anand K J S, Sippell W G, Aynsley-Green A 1987 A randomised trial of fentanyl anesthesia undergoing surgery: effect on the stress response. Lancet 1: 243–248

Anand K J S, Phil D, Hickey P R 1992 Halothane-morphine compared with high dose sufentanil for anesthesia and postoperative analgesia in neonatal cardiac surgery. New England Journal of Medicine 326: 1–9

Anders T F, Sachar E J, Kream J, Roffwarg H, Hellman L 1972 Behavioural state and plasma cortisol response in the human newborn. Pediatrics 49: 250–259

Ansell B M 1980 Aches and pains. In: Ansell B M (ed) Rheumatic disorders of childhood. Butterworth, Boston 6–7

Apley J 1975 The child with abdominal pain, 2nd edn. Blackwell, Oxford

Apley J, Hale B 1973 Children with abdominal pain. How do they grow up? British Medical Journal 3: 7–9

Apley J, Haslam D R, Tulloch G 1971 Pupillary reactions in children with recurrent pain. Archives of Disease in Childhood 46: 337–340

Arfken C L, Lachman A S, McLaren M J et al 1990 Mitral valve prolapse: associations with symptoms and anxiety. Pediatrics 85: 311–315

Asnes R S, Santulli R, Bemporad J R 1981 Psychogenic chest pain in children. Clinical Pediatrics 20: 788–791

Astrada C A, Licamele W L, Walsh T L, Kessler E S 1981 Recurrent abdominal pain in children and associated DSM-III diagnoses. American Journal of Psychiatry 138: 687–688

Bain H W 1974 Chronic vague abdominal pain in children. Pediatric Clinics of North America 21: 991–1000

Barabas G, Matthews W S, Ferrari M 1983 Childhood migraine and motion sickness. Pediatrics 72: 188–190

Barr R G 1983a Pain tolerance and developmental change in pain perception. In: Levine M D, Carey W B, Crocker A C, Gross R T (eds) Developmental-behavioural pediatrics. W B Saunders, Philadelphia, p 505–512

Barr R G 1983b Abdominal pain in the female adolescent. Pediatrics in Review 4: 281–289

Barr R G 1989a Pain in children. In: Wall P D Melzack R (eds) Textbook of pain, 2nd edn. Churchill Livingstone, Edinburgh, p 568–588

Barr R G 1989b Recasting a clinical enigma: the problem of early infant crying. In: Zelazo P H, Barr R G (eds) Challenges to developmental paradigms. Lawrence Erlbaum, New York, p 43–64

Barr R G 1990 The normal crying curve: what do we really know? Developmental Medicine and Child Neurology 32: 356–362

Barr R G 1991 Colic and gas. In: Walker W A, Durie P R, Hamilton J R, Walker-Smith J A, Watking J G (eds) Pediatrics gastrointestinal disease: pathophysiology, diagnosis and management. Decker, Burlington VT, p 55-61

Barr R G 1992a Les nourissons ressentent-ils la douleur? Trois reponses possibles. Psychiatrie, Recherche et Intervention en Sante Mentale de l'Enfant 2: 484–495

Barr R G 1992b Recurrent abdominal pain. In: Friedman S B, Fisher M, Schonberg S K (eds) Comprehensive adolescent health care. Quality Medical Publishing, St Lois, p 755–760

Barr R G 1992c Is this infant in pain? Caveats from the clinical setting. American Pain Society Journal 1: 187–190

Barr R G, Elias M F 1988 Nursing interval and maternal responsivity: effect on early infant crying. Pediatrics 81: 529–536

Barr R G Feuerstein M 1983 Recurrent abdominal pain in children: How appropriate are our usual clinical assumptions? In: Firestone P, McGrath P (eds) Pediatric and adolescent behavioral medicine. Springer-Verlag, New York, p 13–27

Barr R G, Geertsma M A 1993 Colic: the pain perplex. In: Schechter N L, Berde C B, Yaster M (eds), pain in infants, children and adolescents. Williams & Wilkins, Philadephia p 587–596

Barr R G, Watkins J B, Levine M D 1979 Recurrent abdominal pain (RAP) of childhood due to lactose intolerance: a prospective study. New England Journal of Medicine 300: 1449–1452

Barr R G, Francoeur T E, Westwood M, Walsh S 1985 Recurrent abdominal pain and lactose intolerance revisited. American Journal of Diseases of Children 140: 320

Barr R G, Bakemen R, Konner M, Adamson L 1987 Crying in !Kung infants: distress signals in a responsive context. American Journal of Diseases of Children 141: 386

Barr R G, Bakeman R, Konner M, Adamson L 1991a Crying in !Kung infants: a test of the cultural specificity hypothesis. Developmental Medicine and Child Neurology 33: 601–610

Barr R G, McMullan S J, Spiess H et al 1991b Carrying as colic 'therapy': a randomized controlled trial. Pediatrics 87: 623–630

Barr R G, Rotman A, Yaremko J, Leduc D, Francoeur T E 1992 The crying of infants with colic: a controlled empirical description. Pediatrics 90: 14–21

Barr R G, Oberlander T F, Quek V S H et al 1993a Dose-response analgesic effect of intraoral sucrose in newborns. Society for Research in Child Development Program Abstracts

Barr R G, Quek V, Cousineau D, Oberlander T F, Brian J A, Young S N 1993b Effects of intraoral sucrose on crying, mouthing and hand-mouth contact in newborn and six-week old infants. (Submitted)

Barr R G, Young S N, Wright J H, et al 1993c "Sucrose analgesia" and DTP immunizations at two and four months: clinical effects and developmental changes. (submitted)

Battistella P A, Carra S, Zaninotto M, Ruffilli R, Da Dalt L 1992 Pupillary reactivity in children with recurrent abdominal pain. Headache 32: 105–107

Bauchner H, May A, Coates E 1992 Use of analgesic agents for invasive medical procedures in pediatric and neonatal intensive care units. Journal of Pediatrics 121: 647–650

Beales J G 1979 Pain in children with cancer. In: Bonica J J, Ventafridda V (eds) Advances in pain research and therapy. Raven Press, New York, p 89–98

Beales J G, Keen J H, Holt P J L 1983 The child's perception of the disease and the experience of pain in juvenile chronic arthritis. Journal of Rheumatology 10: 61–65

Beidel D C, Christ M A G, Long P J 1991 Somatic complaints in anxious children. Journal of Abnormal Child Psychology 19: 659–670

Belfer M L, Kaban L B 1982 Temporomandibular joint dysfunction with facial pain in children. Pediatrics 69: 564–567

Bell S M, Ainsworth D S 1972 Infant crying and maternal responsiveness. Child Development 43: 1171–1190

Bergman A B, Stamm S J 1967 The morbidity of cardiac nondisease in schoolchildren. New England Journal of Medicine 276: 1008–1013

Bernstein B H, Singsen B H, Kebt J T et al 1978 Reflex neurovascular dystrophy in childhood. Journal of Pediatrics 93: 211–215

Berstein D, Coupey S, Schonberg S K 1986 Pulmonary embolism in adolescents. American Journal of Diseases of Children 140: 667–671

Beyer J, DeGood D, Ashely L , Russell G 1983 Patterns of post-operative analgesic use with adults and children following cardiac surgery. Pain 17: 71–81

Bille B S 1962 Migraine in school children. Acta Paediatrica Scandinavica 51 (suppl 136): 1–151

Bille B 1981 Migraine in childhood and its prognosis. Cephalalgia1: 71–75

Blass E M, Hoffmeyer L B 1991 Sucrose as an analgesic for newborn infants. Pediatrics 87: 215–218

Blass E M, Fitzgerald E, Kehoe P 1987 Interactions between sucrose, pain and isolation distress. Pharmacology Biochemistry and Behavior 26: 438–489

Blass E M, Fillion T J, Weller A 1990 Separation of opioid from nonopioid mediation of affect in neonatal rates: nonopioid mechanisms mediate maternal contact influences. Behavioral Neuroscience 104: 625–636

Blount R L, Landolf-Fritsche B, Powers S W, Sturges J W 1991 Differences between high and low coping children and between parent and staff behaviors during painful medical procedures. Journal of Pediatric Psychology 16: 795–809

Bluestone C D 1982 Otitis media in children: to treat or not to treat? New England Journal of Medicine 306: 1399–1404

Bluestone C D 1983 The ear. In: Nelson W E, Behrman R E, Vaughan C V (eds) Nelson's textbook of pediatrics, 12th edn. Saunders, Philadelphia, p 1022–1031

Bowyer S L, Hollister J R 1984 Limb pain in childhood. Pediatric Clinics of North America 31: 1053–1081

Branson S, McGrath P J, Craig K D, Rubin S W, Vair C 1990 Spontaneous coping strategies for coping with pain and their origins in adolescents who undergo surgery. In: Tyler D, Krane E (eds) Pediatric pain. Pain research and therapy, Raven Press, vol 15. New York, p 237–245

Brazelton T B 1962 Crying in infancy. Pediatrics 29: 579–588

Brenner J I, Ringel R E, Berman M A 1984 Cardiologic perspectives of chest pain in childhood: a referral problem? to whom? Pediatric Clinics of North America 31: 1241–1258

Brenning R 1960 Growing pains. Acta Societatis Medicorum Upsaliensis 65: 185–201

British Medical Journal Editorial 1972 Growing pain. British Medical Journal 2: 365–366

Brown J M, O'Keeffe J, Sanders S H, Baker B 1986 Developmental changes in children's cognition of stress and painful situations. Journal of Pediatric Psychology 11: 343–357

Brunswick A F, Boyle J M, Tarica C 1979 Who sees the doctor? A study of urban black adolescents. Social Science and Medicine 13A: 45–56

Bunnell W P 1982 Back pain in children. Orthopedic Clinics of North America 12: 587–604

Byers P H 1986 Infant crying during aircraft descent. Nursing Research 35: 260–262

Calabro J J, Wachtel A I, Holgerson W B et al 1976 Growing pains. Postgraduate Medicine 59: 66–72

Campbell S M, Clark S, Tindall C A, Forehand M E, Bennett R M 1983 Clinical characteristics of fibrositis I: A clinical controlled study of symptoms and tender points. Arthritis and Rheumatism 26: 817–824

Campos R G 1989 Soothing pain-elicited distress in infants with swaddling and pacifiers. Child Development 60: 781–792

Carvajal H F 1978 Kidney and bladder infections. Advances in Pediatrics 25: 383–413

Ceriani R, Zuccato E, Fontana M et al 1988 Lactose malabsorption and recurrent abdominal pain in Italian children. Journal of Pediatric Gastroenterology and Nutrition 7: 852–857

Chan C W Y, Dallaire M 1989 Subjective pain sensation is linearly correlated with the flexion reflex in man. Brain Research 479: 149–150

Choi Y S, Pearl W R 1989 Cardiovascular effects of adolescent drug abuse. Journal of Adolescent Health Care 10: 332–337

Christensen M F, Mortensen O 1975 Long-term prognosis in children with recurrent abdominal pain. Archives of Disease in Childhood 50: 110–114

Coleman W L 1984 Recurrent chest pain in children. Pediatric Clinics of North America 31: 1007–1026

Cooper P J, Bawden H N, Camfield P R, Camfield C S 1987 Anxiety and life events in childhood migraine. Pediatrics 79: 999–1004

Craig K D 1978 Social modelling influences on pain. In: Sternbach R A (ed) The psychology of pain. Raven Press, New York, p 73–109

Craig K D 1980 Ontogenetic and cultural influences on the expression of pain in man. In: Kosterlitz H W, Terenius L Y (eds) Pain and society. Verlag Chemie, Weinheim, p 37–52

Craig K D 1983 Modeling and social learning factors in chronic pain. In: Bonica J J, Lindblom U, Iggo A (eds) Advances in pain research and therapy, vol 5. Raven Press, New York, p 813–827

Craig K D 1992 The facial expression of pain: better than a thousand words? American Pain Society Journal 1: 153–162

Craig K D, McMahon R J, Morison J D, Zaskow C 1984 Developmental changes in infant pain expression during immunization injections. Social Science and Medicine 19: 1331–1337

Cunningham S J, McGrath P J, Fergusson H B et al 1988 Personality and behavioral characteristics in pediatric migraine. Headache 28: 16–20

Curless R G 1982 Cluster headaches in childhood. Journal of Pediatrics 101: 393–395

Czinn S J, Speck W T 1989 *Campylobacter pylori*: a new pathogen. Journal of Pediatrics 114: 670–671

DeCaspar A J, Fiter W P 1980 Of human bonding: newborns prefer their mothers' voices. Science 208: 1174–1176

Deckelbaum R J, Roy C C, Lussier-Lazaroff J et al 1974 Peptic ulcer disease: a clinical study in 73 children. Canadian Medical Association Journal 111: 225–228

Deubner D C 1977 An epidemiologic study of migraine and headache in 10–20 year olds. Headache 17: 173–180

Dixon S, Snyder J, Holve R, Bromberger P 1984 Behavioral effects of circumcision with and without anesthesia. Journal of Development Behavior and Pediatrics 5: 246–250

Driscoll D J, Glicklich L B, Gallen W J 1976 Chest pain in children. a prospective study. Pediatrics 57: 648–651

Drumm B, Sherman P, Cutz E, Karmali M 1987 Association of *Camplylobacter pylori* on the gastric mucosa with antral gastritis in children. New England Journal of Medicine 316: 1557–1561

Drumm B, Rhoads J M, Stringer D A et al 1988 Peptic ulcer disease in children: etiology, clinical findings, and clinical course. Pediatrics 82: 410–414

Dworkin S F 1992 Perspectives on psychogenic versus biogenic factors in orofacial and other pain states. American Pain Society Journal 1: 172–180
Dyment P G 1991 Low back pain in adolescents. Pediatric Annals 20: 170–178
Ekbom K A 1975 Growing pains and restless legs. Acta Paediatrica Scandinavica 64: 264–266
Eland J M, Anderson J E 1977 The experience of pain in children. In Jacox A (ed) Pain: a source book for nurses and other health professionals. Little, Brown, Boston, p 453–473
Ernst A R, Routh D K, Harper D C 1984 Abdominal pain in children and symptoms of somatization disorder. Journal of Pediatrics and Psychology 9: 77–86
Evans R W, Fergusson D M, Allardyce R A, Taylor B 1981 Maternal diet and infantile colic in breast-fed infants. Lancet 1: 1340–1342
Fanurik D, Zeltzer L, Roberts M C, Blount R L 1993 The relationship between children's coping style and psychological interventions for cold pressor pain. Pain (in press)
Faull C, Nicol A 1986 Abdominal pain in six-year-olds: an epidemiologic study in a new forum. Journal Child Psychology and Psychiatry 27: 251–260
Fenichel G M 1968 Migraine as a cause of benign paroxysmal vertigo of childhood. Journal of Pediatrics 71: 114–115
Feuerstein M, Barr R G, Francoeur T E, Houle M M, Rafman S 1982 Potential biobehavioural mechanisms of recurrent abdominal pain in children. Pain 13: 287–298
Field T, Goldson E 1984 Pacifying effects of nonnutritive sucking on term and preterm neonates during heelstick procedures. Pediatrics 74: 1012–1025
Fitzgerald M 1991a Development of pain mechanisms. British Medical Bulletin 47: 667–675
Fitzgerald M 1991b The developmental neurobiology of pain. In: Bond M R, Charlton J E, Woolf C J (eds) Proceedings of the VIth World Congress on Pain. Elsevier, Amsterdam, p 253–261
Fitzgerald M, Shaw A, MacIntosh N 1988 Postnatal development of the cutaneous flexor reflex: comparative study of preterm infants and newborn rat pups. Developmental Medicine and Child Neurology 30: 520–526
Fitzgerald M, Millard C, MacIntosh N 1989 Cutaneous hypersensitivity following peripheral tissue damage in newborn infants and its reversal with topical anaesthesia. pain 39: 31–36
Fitzgerald M, Woolf C J, Shortland P 1990 Collateral sprouting of the central terminals of cutaneous primary afferent neurons in the rat spinal cord: pattern, morphology, and influence of targets. Journal of Comparative Neurology 300: 370–385
Forsyth B W C 1983 A partially blind study. Pediatrics 771: 667
Fowler-Kerry S, Lander J R 1987 Management of injection pain in children. Pain 30: 169–175
Fradet C, McGrath P J, Kay J, Adams S, Luke B 1990 A prospective survey of reactions to blood tests by children and adolescents. Pain 40: 53–60
Franck L S 1986 A new method to quantitatively describe behavior in infants. Nursing Research 35: 28–31
Franck L S 1987 A national survey of the assessment and treatment of pain and agitation in the neonatal intensive care unit. Journal of Obstetric, Gynecologic and Neonatal Nursing 16: 387–393
Friedman S 1973 Conversion symptoms in adolescents. Pediatric Clinics of North America 20: 873–882
Friedman S 1985 Psychosocial factors in the somatic symptoms of children and adolescents. In: Green M (ed) Psychosocial aspects of the family: the new pediatrics. Lexington Books, Lexington
Friedman G D, Siegelaub A B, Dales L G 1975 Cigarette smoking and chest pain. Annals of Internal Medicine 83: 1–7
Frodi A M, Lamb M E 1978 Sex differences in responsiveness to infants: a developmental study of psychophysiological and behavioral responses. Child Development 49: 1182–1188
Frodi A, Senchak M 1990 Verbal and behavioral responsiveness to the cries of atypical infants. Child Development 61: 76–84
Frodi A M, Lamb M E, Leavitt L A, Donovan W L 1978 Fathers' and mothers' responses to infant smiles and cries. Infant Behavior and Development 1: 187–198
Gaffney A, Dunne E A 1986 Developmental aspects of children's definitions of pain. Pain 26: 105–117
Garber J, Zeman J, Walker L S 1990 Recurrent abdominal pain in children: psychiatric diagnoses and parental psychopathology. Journal of the American Academy of Child and Adolescent Psychiatry 29: 648–656
Gedalia A, Person D A, Brewer E J, Giannini E H 1985 Hypermobility of the joints in juvenile episodic arthritis/arthralgia. Journal of Pediatrics 107: 873–876
Gold M S, Hill I D, Bowie M D 1990 Primary peptic ulcer disease in childhood. South African Medical Journal 77: 183–185
Golden G S 1979 The Alice in Wonderland syndrome in juvenile migraine. Pediatrics 63: 517–519
Gonzalez J C, Routh D K, Saab P G et al 1989 Effects of parent presence on children's reactions to injections: behavioral, physiological, and subjective aspects. Journal of Pediatric Psychology 14: 449–462
Goodman J E, McGrath P J 1991 The epidemiology of pain in children and adolescents: A review. Pain 46: 247–264
Goodman B W, Pantell R H 1984 Chest pain in adolescents – functional consequences. Western Journal of Medicine 141: 342–346
Greenberg J, Ohene-Frempong K, Halus J, Way C, Schwartz E 1983 Trial of low doses of aspirin as prophylaxis in sickle cell disease. Journal of Pediatrics 102: 781–784
Greene J W, Walker L S, Hickson G, Thompson J 1985 Stressful life events and somatic complaints in adolescents. Pediatrics 75: 19–22
Grunau R V E, Craig K D 1987 Pain expression in neonates: facial action and cry. Pain 28: 295–410
Grunau R V E, Johnston C C, Craig K D 1990 Neonatal facial and cry responses to invasive and non-invasive procedures. Pain 42: 295–305
Grunseit F 1977 Evaluation of the efficacy of dicyclomine hydrochloride ('Merbentyl') syrup in the treatment of infantile colic. Current Medical Research and Opinion 5: 258–261
Gunnar M R, Fisch R O, Malone S 1984 The effects of a pacifying stimulus on behavioural and adrenocorticol responses to circumcision. Journal of the American Academy of Child Psychiatry 23: 34–38
Gunnar M R, Malone S, Vance G, Fisch R O 1985 Coping with aversive stimulation in the neonatal period: quiet sleep and plasma cortisol levels during recovery from circumcision. Child Development 56: 824–834
Gunnar M, Connors J, Isensee J 1989a Lack of stability in neonatal adrenocortical reactivity because of rapid habituation of the adrenocortical response. Developmental Psychobiology 22: 221–233
Gunnart M R, Mangelsdorf S, Larson M, Hertsgaard L 1989b Attachment, temperament, and adrenocortical activity in infancy: a study of psychoendocrine regulation. Developmental Psychology 25: 355–363
Gunnar M R, Hertsgaard L, Larson M, Rigatuso J 1992 Cortisol and behavioral responses to repeated stressors in the human newborn. Developmental Psychobiology 24: 487–505
Guralnick W, Kaban L B, Merrill R G 1978 Temporomandibular-joint afflictions. New England Journal of Medicine 299: 123–129
Halperin D L, Koren G, Attias D, Pellegrini E, Greenberg M L, Wyss M 1989 Topical skin anesthesia for venous, subcutaneous drug reservoir and lumbar punctures in children. Pediatrics 84: 281–284
Harbeck C, Peterson L 1992 Elephants dancing in my head: a developmental approach to children's concepts of specific pains. Child Development 63: 138–149
Harpin V A, Rutter N 1982 Making heel pricks less painful. Archives of Disease in Childhood 71: 226–228
Harvey J, Tanner S 1991 Low back pain in young athletes: a practical approach. Sports Medicine 12: 394–406
Haslam D 1969 Age and the perception of pain. Psychonomic Science 15: 86–87
Hawksley J C 1939 The nature of growing pains and their relation to rheumatism in children and adolescents. British Medical Journal 1: 155–157
Hayden R, Grossman M 1959 Rectal, ocular, and submaxillary pain. A familial autonomic disorder related to proctalgia fugax: Report of a family. American Medical Association Journal of Diseases of Childhood 97: 479–482
Hayden G F, Schwartz R H 1985 Characteristics of earache among children with acute otitis media. American Journal of Diseases of Children 139: 721–723

Heinild S V, Malner E, Roelsgaard G, Worning B 1959 A psychosomatic approach to RAP pain in childhood with particular reference to the X-ray appearances of the stomach. Acta Paediatrica Scandinavica 48: 361–370
Himes B T, Tessler A 1989 Death of some DRG neurons and plasticity of others following sciatic nerve section in adult and neonatal rats. Journal of Comprehensive Neurology 204: 215–230
Hodges K, Kline J J, Barbero G, Flanery R 1985a Depressive symptoms in children with recurrent abdominal pain and in their families. Journal of Pediatrics 107: 622–626
Hodges K, Kline J J, Barbero G, Woodruff C 1985b Anxiety in children with recurrent abdominal pain and their parents. Psychosomatics 26: 859–866
Holmes G L, Zimmerman A W 1983 Temporomandibular joint pain – dysfunction syndrome: a rare cause of headaches in adolescents. Developmental Medicine and Child Neurology 25: 601–605
Holve R L, Bromberger P J, Groveman H D et al 1983 Regional anesthesia during newborn circumcision. Clinics in Pediatrics 22: 813–818
Hughes M C 1984 Recurrent abdominal pain and childhood depression: clinical observation of 23 children and their families. Amerian Journal of Orthopsychiatry 54: 146–155
Humphrey G B, Boon C M J, Chiquit van Linden van den Heuvell G F E, van de Wiel H B M 1992 The occurrence of high levels of acute behavioral distress in children and adolescents undergoing routine venipunctures. Pediatrics 90: 87–91
Hunter M, Philips C 1981 The experience of headache – assessment of the qualities of tension headache pain. Pain 10: 209–219
Hunziker U A, Barr R G 1986 Increased carrying reduces infant crying: a randomized controlled trial. Pediatrics 77: 641–648
Hyams J 1983 Chronic abdominal pain caused by sorbitol malabsorption. Journal of Pediatrics 100: 772–773
Illingworth R S 1954 'Three months' colic'. Archives of Disease in Childhood 29: 165–174
Illingworth R S 1959 Evening colic in infants: a double blind trial of dicyclomine hydrochloride. Lancet ii: 1119–1120
Ilowite N T, Walco G A, Pochaczevsky R 1992 Assessment of pain in patients with juvenile rheumatoid arthritis: relation between pain intensity and degree of joint inflammation. Annals of Rheumatic Diseases 51: 343–346
Ingvarsson L 1982 Acute otalgia in children – findings and diagnosis. Acta Paediatrica Scandinavica 71: 705–710
Izard C E, Huebner R R, Risser D, McGinnes G C, Dougherty L M 1980 The young infant's ability to produce discrete emotion expressions. Developmental Psychology 16: 132–140
Izard C E, Hembree E A, Dougherty L M, Spizzirri C C 1983 Changes in facial expressions of 2–19 month old infants following acute pain. Developmental Psychology 19: 418–426
Izard C E, Hembree E A, Hembree R R 1987 Infants' emotional expressions to acute pain: developmental changes and stability of individual differences. Developmental Psychology 23: 105–113
Jay S M, Ozolins M, Elliott C H 1983 Assessment of children's distress during painful medical procedures. Heath Psychology 2: 133–147
Jeans M E 1983 Pain in children: a neglected area. In: Firestone P, McGrath P J, Feldman W (eds) Advances in behavioral medicine for children and adolescents. Lawrence Elbaum, Hillsdale NJ, p 23–37
Joffe R, Bakal D A, Kaganov J 1982 A self-observation study of headache symptoms in children. Headache 23: 20–25
Johnston C C, Strada M E 1986 Acute pain response in infants: a multidimensional description. Pain 24: 373–382
Kaden G G, Shenker I R, Gootman N 1991 Chest pain in adolescents. Journal of Adolescent Health 12: 251–255
Kagan J 1984 The nature of the child. Basic Books, New York
Kagan J, Kearsley R B, Zelazo P R 1978 Infancy: its place in human development. Harvard University Press, Cambrige
Kapelushnik J, Koren G, Sohl H, Greenberg M, DeVeber L 1990 Evaluating the efficacy of EMLA in alleviating pain associated with lumbar puncture: comparison to open and double-blinded protocols in children. Pain 42: 31–34
Kashani J H, Lababidi Z, Jones R S 1982 Depression in children and adolescents with cardiovascular symptomatology: the significance of chest pain. Journal of the American Academy of Child Psychiatry 21: 187–189
Katz E R, Kellerman J, Siegel S E 1980 Behavioral distress in children with cancer undergoing medical procedures: developmental considerations. Journal of Consulting and Clinical Psychology
Katz E R, Kellerman J, Siegel S E 1981 Anxiety as an effective focus in the clinical study of acute behavioral distress: a reply to Sacham and Daut. Journal of Consulting and Clinical Psychology 49: 470–471
Katz E R, Kellerman J, Ellenberg L 1987 Hypnosis in the reduction of acute pain and distress in children with cancer. Journal of Pediatric Psychology 12: 379–394
Kavanaugh C 1983 Psychological intervention with the severely burned child: report of an experimental comparison of two approaches and their effects on psychological sequelae. Journal of the American Academy of Child Psychiatry 22: 145–156
King H A 1984 Back pain in children. Pediatric Clinics of North America 31: 1083–1095
Kirya C, Werthmann M W 1978 Neonatal circumcision and penile dorsal nerve block – a painless procedure. Journal of Pediatrics 92: 998–1000
Konotey-Ahulu F I D 1974 The sickle cell diseases: clinical manifestations including the 'sickle crisis'. Archives of Internal Medicine 133: 611–619
Kopel F B, Kim I C, Barbero G J 1967 Comparison of rectosigmoid motility in normal children, children with recurrent abdominal pain, and children with ulcerative colitis. Pediatrics 39: 539–545
Kowal A, Prichard D 1990 Psychological characterictics of children who suffer from headache: a research note. Journal of Child Psychology and Psychiatry 31: 637–649
Laaksonen A-L, Laine V 1961 A comparative study of joint pain in adult and juvenile rheumatoid arthritis. Annals of Rheumatic Diseases 20: 386–387
Lander J, Hodgins M, Fowler-Kerry S 1992 Children's pain predictions and memories. Behavior Research and Therapy 30: 117–124
Large R G 1986 DSM-III diagnosis in chronic pain: confusion or clarity. Journal of Nervous and Mental Disease 174: 295–303
Lavigne J V, Schulein M J, Hahn Y S 1986 Psychological aspects of painful medical conditions in children I. Developmental aspects and assessment. Pain 27: 133–146
LeBaron S, Zeltzer L 1984 Assessment of acute pain and anxiety in children and adolescents by self-reports, observer reports, and a behaviour checklist. Journal of Consulting and Clinical and Psychology 55: 729–738
Lebenthal E, Rossi T M, Nord K S, Branski D 1981 Recurrent abdominal pain and lactose absorption in children. Pediatrics 67: 828–832
Lehmann H P, Bendebba M, DeAngelis C 1990 The consistency of young children's assessment of remembered painful events. Journal of Developmental and Behavioral Pediatrics 11: 128–134
Levine M D, Rappaport L A 1984 Recurrent abdominal pain in school children: the loneliness of the long distance physician. Pediatric Clinics of North America 31: 969–991
Leviton A, Slack W V, Masek B, Bana D, Graham J R 1984 A computerized behavioral assessment for children with headaches. Headache 24: 182–185
Lewis M, Michalson L 1983 Children's emotions and moods: developmental theory and measurement, Plenum, New York
Lewis M, Thomas D 1990 Cortisol release in infants in response to inoculation. Child Development 61: 50–59
Liebman W 1978 Recurrent abdominal pain in children. Pediatrics 17: 149–153
Linet M S, Stewart W F, Celentano D D, Ziegler D, Sprecher M 1989 An epidemiologic study of headache among adolescents and young adults. Journal of the American Medical Association 261: 2211–2216
Linet M S, Ziegler D K, Stewart W F 1992 Headaches preceded by visual aura among adolescents and young adults: a population-based survey. Archives of Neurology 49: 512–516
Ling W, Oftedal G, Weinberg W 1970 Depressive illness in childhood presenting as severe headache. American Journal of Diseases of Children 120: 122–124
Lollar D J, Smits S J, Patterson D L 1982 Assessment of pediatric pain: an empirical perspective. Journal of Pediatric Psychology 7: 267–277
Lothe L, Lindberg T, Jakobsson I 1982 Cow's milk formula as a cause of infantile colic: a double-blind study. Pediatrics 70: 7–10

Lozoff B, Brittenham G 1979 Infant care: cache or carry. Journal of Pediatrics 95: 478–483
Luque M A 3rd, Cavallaro D L, Torres M, Emmanuel P, Hillman J V 1987 Pneumomediastinum, pneumothorax, and subcutaneous emphysema after cocaine inhalation and marijuana smoking. Pediatric Emergency Care 3: 107–109
McGrath P A 1987 An assessment of children's pain: a review of behavioral, physiological and direct scaling techniques. Pain 31: 147–176
McGrath P A 1990 Pain in children: nature, assessment and treatment. Guilford Press, New York
McGrath P A 1991 Children in pain. Clinical research issues from a developmental perspective. Springer Verlag, New York
McGrath P A 1993 Psychological aspects of pain perception. In: Schechter N L, Berde C B, Yaster M (eds) Pain in infants, children and adolescents. Williams & Wilkins, Baltimore, p 39–63
McGrath P J, Unruh A M 1987 Pain in children and adolescents. Elsevier, Amsterdam
McGrath P J, Goodman J J, Firestone P, Shipman P, Peters S 1983 Recurrent abdominal pain: a psychogenic disorder: Archives of Disease in Childhood 58: 888–890
McGraw M B 1941 Neural maturation as exemplified in the changing reactions of the infant to pin prick. Child Development 12: 31–42
Malagelada J-R, Stanghellini V 1985 Manometric evaluation of functional upper gut symptoms. Gastroenterology 88: 1223–1231
Malleson P N 1992 Pain syndromes, disability, and chronic disease in childhood. Current Opinion in Rheumatology (in press)
Manne S L, Redd W H, Jacobsen P B, Gorfinkle K, Schorr O, Rapkin B 1990 Behavioral intervention to reduce child and parent distress during venipuncture. Journal of Consulting and Clinical Psychology 58: 565–572
Maratos J, Wilkinson M 1982 Migraine in children: a medical and psychiatric study. Cephalalgia 2: 179–187
Marshall R E 1993 Neonatal pain associated with caregiving procedures. Pediatric Clinics of North America 36: 885–903
Mather L, Mackie J 1983 The incidence of postoperative pain in children. Pain 15: 271–282
Melzack R 1973 The puzzle of pain. Basic Books, New York
Melzack R, Wall P D 1970 Psychophysiology of pain. Internal Anesthesiology Clinics 8: 3–34
Merskey H 1970 On the development of pain. Headache 10: 116–123
Miller A R, Barr R G 1991 Infantile colic: Is it a gut issue? Pediatric Clinics of North America 38: 1407–1423
Miller A, Barr R G, Young S N 1993 The cold pressor test in children: methodological aspects and the analgesic effect of intraoral sucrose. Pain (in press)
Moffatt M E K 1982 Epidemic hysteria in a Montreal train station. Pediatrics 70: 308–310
Mortimer M J, Kay J, Jaron A 1992 Epidemiology of headache and childhood migraine in an urban general practice using ad hoc, Valquist and IHS criteria. Development Medicine and Child Neurology 34: 1095–1101
Murray A D 1979 Infant crying as an elicitor of parental behavior: an examination of two models. Psychology Bulletin 86: 191–215
Naish J M, Apley J 1951 'Growing pains': a clinical study of non-arthritic limb pains in children. Archives of Disease in Childhood 26: 134–140
Nilner M 1981 Prevalence of functional disturbances and diseases of stomatognathic system in 15–18 year olds. Swedish Dental Journal 5: 189–197
Nilner M, Lassing S A 1981 Prevalence of functional disturbances and diseases of the stomatognathic system in 7–14 year olds. Swedish Dental Journal 5: 173–187
Oberlander T F, Barr R G, Young S N, Brian J A 1992 Short-term effects of feed composition on sleeping and crying in newborn infants. Pediatrics 90: 733–740
Oderda G, Vaira D, Holton J, Dowsett J F, Ansaldi N 1989 Serum pepsinogen I and IgG antibody to *Campylobacter pylori* in non-specific abdominal pain in children. Gut 30: 912–916
Olsen T L, Anderson R L, Dearwater S R et al 1992 The epidemiology of low back pain in an adolescent population. American Journal of Public Health 82: 606–608
Osborne R B, Hatcher J W, Richtsmeier A J 1989 The role of social modeling in unexplained pediatric pain. Journal of Pediatric Psychology 14: 43–61
Oster J 1972a Growing pains: a symptom and its significance. Danish Medical Bulletin 19: 72–79
Oster J 1972b Recurrent abdominal pain, headache, and limb pains in children and adolescents. Pediatrics 50: 429–436
Oster J, Neilsen A 1972 Growing pains: a clinical investigation of a school population. Acta Paediatrica Scandinavica 61: 329–334
Owens M E 1984 Pain in infancy: conceptual and methodological issues. Pain 20: 213–230
Owens M E, Todt E H 1984 Pain in infancy: neonatal reaction to heel lance. Pain 20: 77–86
Pantell R H, Goodman B W 1983 Adolescent chest pain: a prospective study. Pediatrics 71: 881–887
Paradise J L 1966 Maternal and other factors in the etiology of infantile colic. Journal of the American Medical Association 197: 123–131
Parcel G S, Nader P R, Meyer M P 1977 Adolescent health concerns, problems, and patterns of utilization in a triethnic urban population. Pediatrics 60: 157–164
Parfrey N A, Moore G W, Hutchins G M 1985 Is pain crisis a cause of death in sickle cell disease? American Journal of Clinical Pathology 84: 209–212
Passchier J, Orlebeke J F 1985 Headaches and stress in schoolchildren: an epidemiological study. Cephalalgia 5: 167–176
Patterson H S, Pettyjohn F S 1983 Otalgia in infants travelling in airplanes. New England Journal of Medicine 308: 781–782
Perris E E, Myers N A, Clifton R K 1990 Long-term memory for a single infancy experience. Child Development 61: 1796–1807
Perry S, Heidrich G 1982 Management of pain during debridement: A survey of US burn units. Pain 13: 267–280
Peterson HA 1977 Leg aches. Pediatric Clinics of North America 24: 731–736
Peterson L 1989 Coping by children undergoing stressful medical procedures: some conceptual, methodological, and therapeutic issues. Journal of Consulting and Clinical Psychology 57: 380–387
Peterson L, Toler S M 1986 An information seeking disposition in child surgery patients. Health Psychology 5: 343–358
Pillemer F G, Masek B J, Kaban L B 1987 Temporomandibular joint dysfunction and facial pain in children: an approach to diagnosis and treatment. Pediatrics 80: 565–570
Pilowsky I 1992 The problem of 'psychogenic' pain. American Pain Society Journal 1: 181–184
Pineiro-Carrero V M, Andres J M, Davis R H, Mathias J R 1988 Abnormal gastroduodenal motility in children and adolescents with recurrent functional abdominal pain. Journal of Pediatrics 113: 820–825
Polly D W, Mason D E 1991 Congenital absence of a lumbar pedicle presenting as back pain in children. Journal of Pediatric Orthopedics 11: 214–219
Porter F 1989 Pain in the newborn. Clinics in Perinatology 16: 549–564
Pukander J 1983 Clinical features of acute otitis media among children. Acta Otolaryngologia 95: 117–122
Rawlings D J, Miller P A, Engel R R 1980 The effect of circumcision on transcutaneous PO_2 in term infants. American Journal of Diseases of Children 134: 676–678
Raymer D, Weinberger O, Hamilton J R 1984 Psychological problems in children with abdominal pain. Lancet I: 439–440
Reif S, Sloven D G, Lebenthal E 1991 Gallstones in children: characterization by age, etiology, and outcome. American Journal of Diseases of Children 145: 105–108
Reynolds J L 1989 Precordial catch syndrome in children. Southern Medical Journal 82: 1228–1230
Robieux I, Kumar R, Radhakrishnan S, Koren G 1991 Assessing pain and analgesia with a lidocaine-prilocaine emulsion in infants and toddlers during venipuncture. Journal of Pediatrics 118: 971–973
Roghmann K J, Haggerty R J 1973 Daily stress, illness, and use of health services in young families. Pediatric Research 7: 520–526
Ross D M, Ross S A 1984a Childhood pain: the school-aged child's viewpoint. Pain 20: 179–191
Ross D M, Ross S A 1984b The importance of type of question, psychological climate and subject set in interviewing children about pain. Pain 19: 71–79

Ross D M, Ross S A 1988 Childhood pain: current issues, research and management. Urban & Schwarzenberg, Baltimore

Rothner A D 1983 Diagnosis and management of headache in children and adolescents. Neurologic Clinics 1: 511–526

Routh D K, Ernst A R 1984 Somatization disorder in relatives of children and adolescents with functional abdominal pain. Journal of Pediatric Psychology 9: 427–437

Rowe B H, Dulberg C S, Peterson R G, Vlad P, Li M M 1990 Characteristics of children presenting with chest pain to a pediatric emergency department. Canadian Medical Association Journal 143: 388–394

Rubin L S, Barbero G J, Sibinga M S 1967 Pupillary reactivity in children with recurrent abdominal pain. Psychosomatic Medicine 29: 111–120

Sacham S, Daut R 1981 Anxiety or pain: what does the scale measure? Journal of Consulting and Clinical Psychology 49: 486–489

Savedra M, Gibbons P, Tesler M, Ward J, Wegner C 1982 How do children describe pain? A tentative assessment. Pain 14: 95–104

Savedra M C, Tesler M D, Ward J D, Wegner C 1988 How adolescents describe pain. Journal of Adolescent Health Care 9: 315–320

Sawyer M G, Davidson G P, Goodwin D, Crettenden A D 1987 Recurrent abdominal pain in childhood. Relationship to psychological adjustment of children and families: a preliminary study. Australian Pediatric Journal 23: 121–124

Schechter N L 1985 Pain and pain control. In: Lockhart J D (ed) Current problems in pediatrics, vol 15. Yearbook Medical Publishers, Chicago, p 1–63

Schechter N L, Allen D A 1986 Physicians' attitudes toward pain in children. Journal of Developmental and Behavioural Pediatrics 7: 350–354

Schechter N L, Allen D A, Hanson K 1986 Status of pediatric pain control: a comparison of hospital analgesic usage in children and adults. Pediatrics 77: 11–15

Schechter N L, Bernstein B A, Beck A, Haret L, Scherzer L 1991 Individual differences in children's response to pain: role of temperament and parental characteristics. Pediatrics 87: 171–177

Schmitt B D 1971 School phobia – the great imitator. Pediatrics 48: 433–441

Schultz N V 1971 How children perceive pain. Nursing Outlook 19: 670–673

Scott R 1978 'It hurts red': a preliminary study of children's perception of pain. Perceptual and Motor Skills 47: 787–791

Scott P J, Ansell B M, Huskisson E C 1977 Measurement of pain in juvenile chronic polyarthritis. Annals of Rheumatic Diseases 36: 186–187

Selbst S M 1990 Chest pain in children. American Family Physician 41: 179–186

Selbst S, Ruddy R, Clark B J, Henretig F, Santulli T 1987 Prospective study of chest pain in children. American Journal of Diseases of Children

Selbst S M, Ruddy R M, Clark B J, Henretig F M, Santulli T 1988 Pediatric chest pain: a prospective study. Pediatrics 82: 319–323

Selbst S M, Ruddy R, Clark B J 1990 Chest pain in children: Follow-up of patients previously reported. Clinical Pediatrics (Philadephia) 29: 271–276

Shambaugh G E, Girgis T F 1980 Acute otitis media and mastoiditis. In: Paparella MM, Shumrick D A (eds) Otolaryngology, vol 2. Saunders, Philadelphia, 1445–1451

Shapiro M J 1939 Differential diagnosis of non-rheumatic 'growing pain' and subacute rheumatic fever. Journal of Pediatrics 14: 315–322

Sharrer V W, Ryan-Wenger N M 1991 Measurements of stress and coping among school-aged children with and without recurrent abdominal pain. Journal of School Health 61: 86–91

Sherry D D Limb pain in childhood. Pediatric Reviews 12: 39–46

Sherry D D, Weisman R 1988 Psychologic aspects of childhood reflex neurovascular dystrophy. Pediatrics 81: 572–578

Sherry D D, Bohnsack J, Salmonson K, Wallace C A, Mellins E 1990 Painless juvenile rheumatoid arthritis. Journal of Pediatrics 116: 921–924

Sherry D D, McGuire T, Mellins E, Salmonson K, Wallace C A, Nepom B 1991 Psychosomatic musculoskeletal pain in childhood: clinical and psychological analyses of 100 children. Pediatrics 88: 1093–1099

Shortland P, Fitzgerald M 1993 Functional connections formed by saphenous nerve terminal sprouts in the dorsal horn following neonatal sciatic nerve section. European Journal of Neuroscience (in press)

Shulman R J, Wong W W, Irving C S, Nichols B L, Klein P D 1983 Utilization of dietary cereal by young infants. Journal of Pediatrics 103: 23–28

Silber T J, Majd M 1989 Reflex sympathetic dystrophy syndrome in children and adolescents: report of 18 cases and review of the literature. American Journal of Diseases of Children 142: 1325–1330

Sillanpaa M 1983a Changes in the prevalence of migraine and other headaches during the first 7 school years. Headache 23: 15–19

Sillanpaa M 1983 Prevalence of headache in puberty. Headache 23: 10–14

Simon G, Marbach J J 1976 Familial Mediterranean fever with temporomandibular joint arthritis. Pediatrics 57: 810–812

Smith H C T, Eastham E J 1973 Outbreak of abdominal pain. Lancet 2: 956–958

Spinetta J J, Maloney L J 1975 Death anxiety in the outpatient leukemic child. Pediatrics 56: 1034–1037

Spinetta J J, Rigler D, Karon M 1973 Anxiety in the dying child. Pediatrics 52: 841–845

Spinetta J J, Rigler D, Karon M 1974 Personal space as a measure of a dying child's sense of isolation. Journal of Consulting and Clinical Psychology 42: 751–756

Stickler G, Murphy D B 1979 Recurrent abdominal pain. American Journal of Diseases of children 133: 486–489

Stiene-Martin A, Hauser K F 1991 Glial growth is regulated by agonists selective for multiple opioid receptor types in vitro. Journal of Neuroscience Research 29: 538–548

Stiene-Martin A, Gurwell J A, Hanser K F 1991 Morphine alters astrocyte growth in primary cultures of mouse glial cells: Evidence for a direct effect of opiates on neural maturation. Developmental Brain Research 60: 1–7

Stone R T, Barbero G J 1970 Recurrent abdominal pain in childhood. Pediatrics 45: 732–738

Swain I U, Zelazo P R, Clifton R K 1993 Newborn memory for speech sounds retained over 24 hours. Developmental Psychology (in press)

Talbert L M, Kraybill E N, Potter H D 1976 Adrenal cortical response to circumcision in the neonate. Obstetrics and Gynecology 48: 208–210

Talley N J, Philips S F 1988 Non-ulcer dyspepsia: potential causes and pathophysiology. Annals of Internal Medicine 108: 865–879

Taubman B 1984 Clinical trial of the treatment of colic by modification of parent–infant interaction. Pediatrics 74: 998–1003

Taubman B 1988 Parental counselling compared with elimination of cow's milk or soy milk protein for treatment of infant colic syndrome: a randomized trial. Pediatrics 81: 756–761

Thomas D W, McGilligan K, Eisenberg L D, Lieberman H M, Rissman E M 1987 Infantile colic and type of milk feeding. American Journal of Diseases in Children 141: 451–453

Tomomasa T, Hsu J Y, Shigeta M et al 1986 Statistical analysis of symptoms and signs in pediatric patients with peptic ulcer. Journal of Pediatric Gastroenterology and Nutrition 5: 711–715

Tschudy D P, Valsamis M, Magnussen C R 1975 Acute intermittent porphyria: clinical and selected research aspects. Annals of Internal Medicine 83: 851–864

Tucker M A, Andrew M F, Ogle S J, Davison J G 1989 Age-associated change in pain threshold measured by transcutaneous neuronal electrical stimulation. Age and Ageing 18: 241–246

Tunks E 1992 'Psychogenic pain': the validity of the concept. American Pain Society Journal 1: 163–166

Turk D C, Flor H 1987 Pain > pain behaviours: the utility and limitations of the pain behavior construct. Pain 31: 277–295

van Aken M A, van Lieshout C F, Katz E R, Heezen T J 1989 Developmental of behavioral distress in reaction to acute pain in two cultures. Journal of Pediatrics Psychology 14: 421–432

van der Meer S B, Forget P P, Arends J W 1990 Abnormal small bowel permeability and duodenitis in recurrent abdominal pain. Archives of Disease in Childhood 65: 1311–1314

Vandenplas Y, Blecker U, Devreker T et al 1992 Contribution of the C-Urea breath test to the detection of *Helicobacter pylori* gastritis in children. Pediatrics 90: 608–611

Varni J W, Thompson K L, Hanson V 1987 The Varni/Thompson Pediatric Pain Questionnaire. I. Chronic musculoskeletal pain in juvenile rheumatoid arthritis. Pain 28: 27–38

Walco G A, Dampier C D 1990 Pain in children and adolescents with sickle cell disease: a descriptive study. Journal of Pediatric Psychology 15: 643–658

Wald A, Chaudra R, Fisher S E, Gartner J C, Zitelli B 1982 Lactose malabsortion in recurrent abdominal pain of childhood. Journal of Pediatrics 100: 65–68

Walker L S, Greene J W 1989 Children with recurrent abdominal pain and their parents: more somatic complaints, anxiety, and depression than other patient families? Journal of Pediatric Psychology 14: 231–243

Weisenberg M 1977 Pain and pain control. Psychological Bulletin 84: 1008–1041

Weissbluth M, Christoffel K K, Davis T 1984 Treatment of infantile colic with dicyclomine hydrochloride. Journal of Pediatrics 104: 951–955

Wessel M A, Cobb J C, Jackson E B, Harris G S, Detwiler A C 1954 Paroxysmal fussing in infancy, sometimes called 'colic'. Pediatrics 14: 421–434

Wiens L, Sabath R, Ewing L, Gowdamarajan R, Portnoy J, Scagliotti D 1992 Chest pain in otherwise healthy children and adolescents in frequently caused by exercise-induced asthma. Pediatrics 90: 350–353

Wilder R T, Berde C B, Wolohan M, Vieyra M A, Masek B J, Micheli L J 1992 Reflex sympathetic dystrophy in children: clinical characteristics and follow-up in seventy patients. Journal of Bone and Joint Surgery 74A: 910–919

Willer J C 1977 Comparative study of perceived pain and the nociceptive flexion reflex in man. Pain 3: 69–80

Willer J C, Bussel B 1980 Evidence for a direct spinal mechanism in morphine-induced inhibition of nociceptive reflexes in humans. Brain Research 187: 212–215

Williamson P S, Williamson M L 1983 Physiologic stress reduction by a local anesthetic during newborn circumcision. Pediatrics 71: 36–40

Winer G A 1982 A review and analysis of children's fearful behavior in dental settings. Child Development 53: 111–1133

Wolff P H 1969 The natural history of crying and other vocalizations in early infancy. In: Foss B M (ed) Determinants of infant behavior. Methuen, London, pp 81–108

Woodward G A, Selbst S M 1987 Chest pain secondary to cocaine use. Pediatric Emergency Care 3: 153–154

Woolf P K, Gewitz M H, Berezin S et al 1991 Noncardiac chest pain in adolescents and children with mitral valve prolapse. Journal of Adolescent Health 12: 247–250

Zachary R A, Friedlander S, Huang L N, Silverstein S, Leggott P 1985 Effects of stress-relevant and -irrelevant filmed modeling on children's responses to dental treatment. Journal of Pediatrics and Psychology 10: 383–401

Zagon I S, McLaughlin P J 1991 Identification of opioid peptides regulating proliferation of neurons and glia in the developing nervous system. Brain Research 542: 318–323

Zeltzer L K, Lebaron S 1982 Hypnosis and nonhypnotic techniques for reduction of pain and anxiety during painful procedures in children and adolescents with cancer. Journal of Pediatrics 101: 1032–1035

Zeltzer L, Kellerman J, Ellenberg L, Dash J, Rigler D 1980 Psychological effects of illness in adolescence II. Impact of illness in adolescents – crucial issues and coping styles. Journal of Pediatrics 97: 132–138

Zeltzer L K, Anderson C T M, Schechter N L 1990 Pediatric pain: current status and new directions. Current Problems in Pediatrics 20: 411–430

Zuckerman B, Stevenson J, Bailey V 1987 Stomachaches and headaches in a community sample of preschool children. Pediatrics 79: 677–682

Geriatrics

42. Geriatric pain

Stephen W. Harkins, Donald D. Price, Francis M. Bush and Ralph E. Small

INTRODUCTION

This review considers the effects of chronological age on pain in the later years of adult life. In contrast to fairly well defined age changes in most sensory systems (Fozard 1990), it is unclear whether age, in the adult years of life, influences sensory processes involved in pain perception. Yet many clinicians and many elderly people themselves assume that aging is associated with both a loss in ability to perceive and report accurately pain and an increase in nonspecific pain-related suffering and pain complaints (Harkins 1988). Such assumptions are derived from scant findings and inadequate research (Melding 1991).

EFFECTS OF AGE ON PAIN PERCEPTION

BACKGROUND

Psychophysical evaluation of the effects of age on pain has a history differing considerably from that of other sensory modalities. While the physical, psychological and physiological attributes of the major and most 'minor' sensory modalities have been characterized, those defining pain are less well documented.

At least four reasons account for this comparative lag in understanding the effects of age on pain. First is the precision to which stimuli that activate the various sensory modalities can be controlled and quantified. For example, in auditory psychophysics, the case of quantification and control of sound has facilitated the study of age changes in hearing (presbycusis) (Olsho et al 1985). In contrast, quantification and control of stimuli that produce pain have been far less precise, largely because many such stimuli, by their very nature, are potentially damaging and difficult to present repeatedly with the same effect. Others, like electrical stimuli, while more easily controlled, lack a natural physical counterpart.

A second reason relates to attitudes about pain. Confusion exists whether pain operates more as a motivational system or as a sensory modality (Wall 1979; Mayer & Price 1982; Price 1988), and/or whether the pain system is limited to dealing with crude discriminative information only (Mountcastle 1974; Wall 1979). In the extreme, some consider pain a private experience that does not lend itself readily to experimental examination. This logic has led to the position that pain is not measurable. Such attitudes belied the fact that pain can be analysed in the same way as other sensory modalities and dissuaded many from attempting to do so.

A third reason is the magnitude of the effort directed toward the study of different sensory modalities. Perhaps because of the first two factors, the number of researchers exploring the psychophysics of other sensory modalities and the effects of age on these senses has been far greater than that devoted to the study of adult age differences in pain.

A final reason is that it has been assumed by many that age results in loss of pain perception. In the clinical setting, particularly multidisciplinary pain clinics, it has also been inappropriately assumed that the older adult with a chronic pain complaint is not a good candidate for treatment (Harkins 1988; Harkins & Price 1992). This logic is compounded by atypical presentation of acute pain as a symptom in the elderly, which may be more a result of pathophysiology than as a direct result of developmental changes due to aging (Harkins et al 1990).

Thus, ageist attitudes, the view that pain is not measurable, and the perceived difficulty in stimulus presentation and control have limited advances in our understanding of adult developmental factors influencing pain perception.

EXPERIMENTAL STUDIES OF AGE AND PAIN

Although some efforts have been made to document the effects of adult age on pain perception, findings of experimental studies are contradictory. Studies of adult age differences in pain are limited almost exclusively to evaluation of the sensory/discriminative dimension (Harkins & Warner 1980; Harkins 1988; Harkins et al 1990; Ferrell 1991; Harkins & Price 1992). These studies are summarized in Table 42.1.

Table 42.1 Laboratory studies on the effect of age on psychophysical indices of pain sensitivity (updated from Harkins & Price 1992 as modified from Harkins & Warner 1980)

Stimulus	Source (reference)	Psychophysical end points and findings
1. Thermal		
A. Radiant heat	Schumacher et al (1940)	Sensory thresholds: no age effects
	Hardy et al (1943)	Sensory thresholds: no age effects Sensory thresholds: higher in elderly
	Chapman & Jones (1944)	Reaction thresholds: higher in elderly
	Birren et al (1950)	Pain, sensory thresholds: no age effects Pain, reaction thresholds: no age effects
	Sherman & Robillard (1960, 1964a, 1964b)	Sensory thresholds: higher in elderly Reaction thresholds: higher in elderly
	Procacci et al (1970)	Sensory thresholds: higher in elderly*
	Clark & Mehl (1971)	Sensory thresholds: higher in 55 year olds compared to younger adults
B. Contact heat	Kenshalo (1986)	Sensory thresholds: no age effects
	Harkins et al (1986)	Magnitude matching: slight age effects (see text and Fig. 42.1)
C. Cold pressor	Walsh et al (1989)	Tolerance (time) Males: lower with increasing age Females: minimal increase with increasing age
2. Electrical shock		
A. Cutaneous	Collins & Stone (1966)	Sensory threshold: lower in elderly Tolerance: lower in elderly
	Tucker et al (1989)	Sensory threshold: higher in elderly
	Evans et al (1992)	Sensory thresholds: no age effect in non-diabetics; older diabetics higher thresholds than younger diabetics
B. Tooth	Mumford (1965)	Sensory threshold: no age effects
	Mumford (1968)	Sensory threshold: no age effects
	Harkins & Chapman (1976)	Sensory threshold: no age effects Discrimination accuracy: lower in elderly Response bias (criteria): age effects variable
	Harkins & Chapman (1977b)	Sensory threshold: no age effects Discrimination accuracy: lower in elderly Response bias (criteria): age effects variable
3. Pressure		
Achilles tendon	Woodrow et al (1972)	Tolerance: lower in elderly
	Jensen et al (1992)	Muscle tenderness and pressure: pain to age 65 Sensory thresholds: higher in elderly

*Noted that the elevated sensory thresholds in elderly volunteers were due, in part, to increased thermal dispersion of radiant heat by senescent skin.

As shown in Table 42.1, stimuli used in the laboratory have included electrical shock (both cutaneous and tooth electrical shock), thermal (radiant heat, contact heat and cold pressor), and mechanical (pressure) stimuli. Psychophysical endpoints included pain threshold, pain tolerance, reaction thresholds (i.e. wincing), pain discrimination, pain response criteria and magnitude matching.

The studies shown in Table 42.1 are not easily interpreted as a whole, partly because of the differences in the methods of pain induction and the psychophysical procedures employed. Variability in findings also reflects a lack of standards in definition of age as a variable, differences between studies in training, practice, instructions and subject selection criteria.

Psychophysical procedures using traditional end points, such as thresholds or more complex procedures, such as signal detection theory tasks in the study of pain, have been increasingly replaced by magnitude matching and estimation procedures (Marks 1974; Stevens 1975; Stevens & Marks 1980; Price 1988). These procedures have proved powerful in the study of age differences in the chemical senses (Bartoshuck et al 1986; Cain & Stevens 1989) and pain (Harkins et al 1986; Kenshalo 1986).

Within the last decade there has been increasing interest in psychophysical studies of pain in the elderly.

Methodological changes, for example, have led to experimental paradigms that directly relate suprathreshold contact thermal stimuli to neural responses and pain-related behaviour (Price 1988; Price & Harkins 1992). Conceptual changes relate to the recognition of the importance of the distinction between 'nociception', the manner in which the nervous system signals the presence of potentially tissue-damaging stimuli, and 'pain', the sensory and affective reactions based on these neural processes (see Zimmermann 1976; Price & Harkins 1992). This approach has potential for a refined analysis of the effects of chronological age on understanding how components of pain are synthesized under normal conditions (Price & Harkins 1992).

Figure 42.1 presents results employing contact heat stimuli in the study of age differences in pain perception. Stimuli were heat pulses of 5-second duration delivered to the inside of the forearm from an adapting temperature of 34°C. While some older individuals tended to rate lower-level cutaneous heat pulses as less intense compared to younger individuals, the magnitude of this effect was slight and was considered unlikely to be clinically relevant (Harkins et al 1986).

Since there are no longitudinal studies of pain in the elderly, data on pain sensitivity related to adult age are confounded by birth cohort effects, providing information on group differences only and not within-individual changes across time. This confound of birth cohort with biological effects of aging is important since cultural history and life-experience differences between age groups may influence willingness to report a sensation as painful. Age differences in response bias can result in false elevations in sensory thresholds in old compared to young individuals. Age-group differences in life history of clinical, procedural and illness-related pains create the potential for differences in what constitutes significant nociceptive events and suffering. Cross-sectional studies are also subject to the limitation that individuals surviving into their seventh and eighth decades of life constitute a group selected by survivorship. Survivors may well be biologically different from their birth cohort peers.

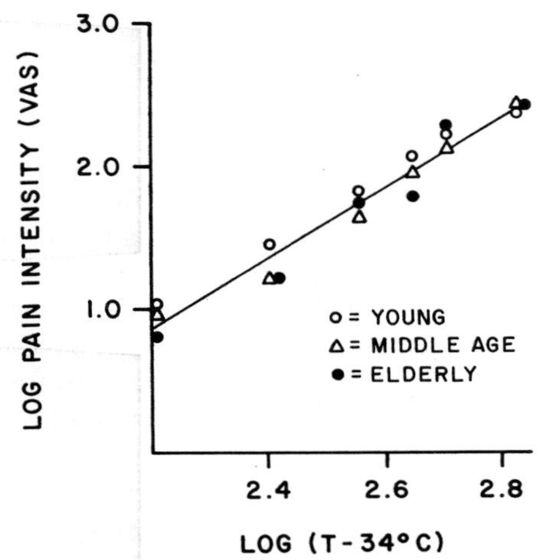

Fig. 42.1 Combined visual analogue scale (VAS) pain intensity and pain unpleasantness ratings of contact thermal stimuli applied to the volar surface of the forearm in young (mean age of 25.3 years, sd = 4.2; n = 21), middle-aged (53.4 years, sd = 5.7; n = 10) and elderly (72.5 years, sd = 4.6; n = 13) healthy volunteers. Stimuli were 5-second duration heat pulses from an adapting temperature of 34°C to 43, 45, 47, 48, 49 or 51°C. Note that data are well fit by a single psychophysical function. No significant overall age effect was observed, though there was a significant age groups effect over the temperature range of 48–51°C. Combined intensity and unpleasantness ratings were suggestive of an 'intensity recruitment' effect in the elderly group. (From Harkins et al (1986) with permission.)

SUMMARY

Based on the literature presented in Table 42.1 and the preceding review, we conclude that age does not significantly influence the sensory–discriminative dimension of the human pain experience in healthy, well-instructed elderly when psychophysical tasks are used which do not present a performance challenge to the subject. This does not mean, however, that the elderly, particularly the frail–old with chronic health problems, do not experience atypical pain as a symptom. Experimental pain studies in the laboratory involve presentation of brief noxious stimuli which do not have any necessary relation to emotions and suffering due to acute, recurrent or chronic pain. Thus, it is inappropriate to conclude from the literature summarized in Table 42.1 that age does or does not affect discomfort and suffering associated with clinical, recurrent or chronic pains.

GERIATRIC PAIN

This section discusses (i) prevalence of pain in community-dwelling populations; (ii) acute pain as a symptom in the old; and (iii) chronic pain in the elderly.

PREVALENCE OF GERIATRIC PAIN

Most illnesses of old age are chronic. A study of new-pain visits to physicians in over 70 million individuals found *first time* pain complaints occurred most frequently in individuals between 15 and 44 years. First-time pain visits to office-based physicians were at their lowest in the elderly. In the old, pains related to degenerative conditions lose their newness quickly (Knapp & Koch 1984; Harkins 1988; Harkins et al 1990). Unlike new pain visits, persistent pain was found to occur more frequently in older than younger individuals in a community-dwelling sample (Crook et al 1984). Age-specific morbidity rates of persistent pain were 76 cases per 1000 in individuals aged 18–30 years and 400 per 1000 in those above 81 years of age (Crook et al 1984).

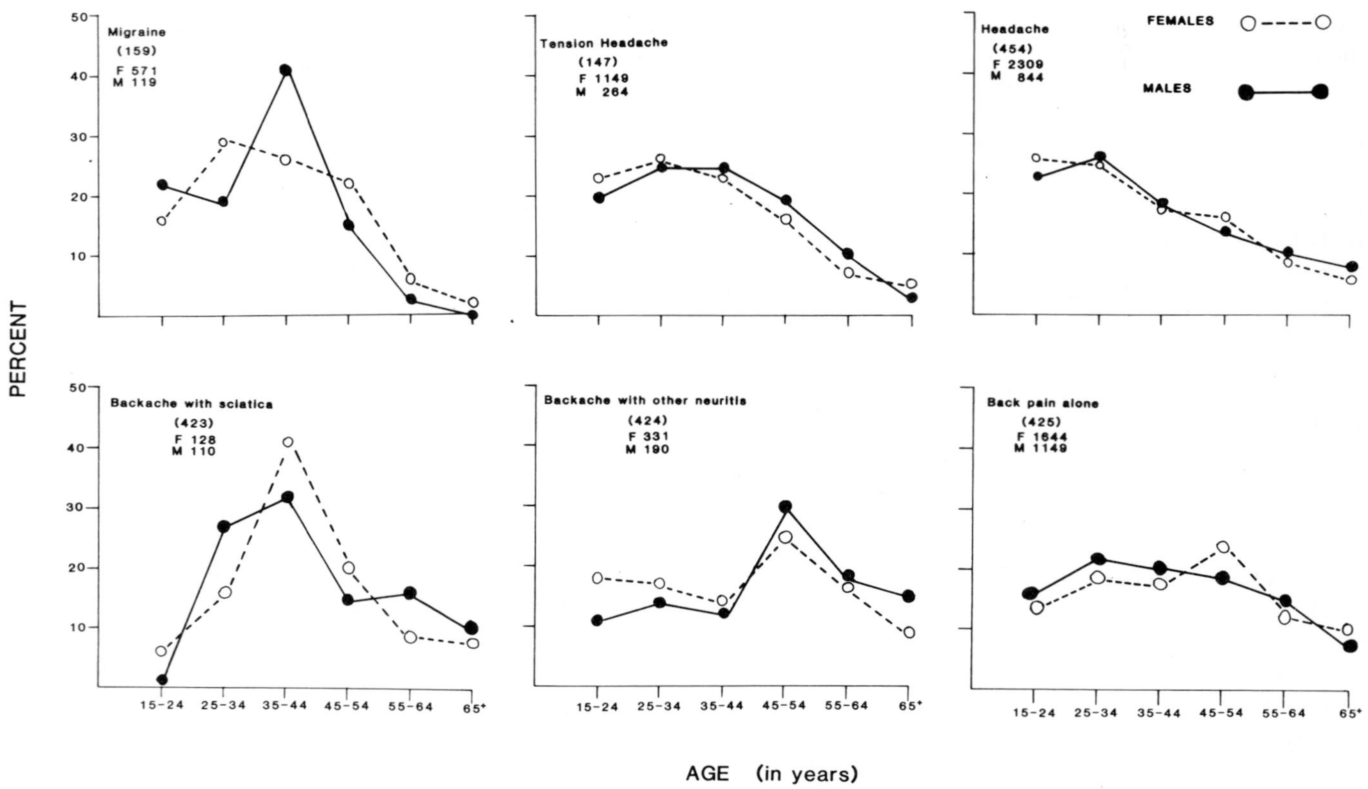

Fig. 42.2 **A–D** Frequency (%) of over 86 000 primary care patients making over half a million patient visits for selected reasons for visits. Patient visits over a 2-year period to Medical College of Virginia, Virginia Commonwealth University's family practice clinical centres. **A** Frequency of headache and backache in men and women of different ages. Note the peak in migraine and backaches in the middle years of life. **B** Other reasons for visit that are likely to be accompanied by pain as a presenting symptom. Note the increase in Herpes zoster with increasing age in both men and women; this is likely to reflect age-related change in immune function. **C** Conditions which typically show increased incidence with age and that have pain as a primary presenting symptom. **D** Age-related prevalence of selected fractures in the primary care setting. Numbers in parentheses are diagnoses that were classified according to the problem-oriented disease classification of the Royal College of General Practitioners. Substantially modified from Marsland et al (1976). (Figures from Harkins et al (1990) with permission.)

The elderly as a group are at considerable risk of conditions which predispose to chronic pain. Estimates are that 80–85% of individuals above 65 years have at least one significant health problem that predisposes to pain (Harkins 1988). Valkenburg (1988) noted that 30% of men and 53% of women over the age of 55 years have peripheral joint pain complaints. His findings are important because they are based on a community-dwelling and randomly sampled population.

Based on a review of findings from a family practice centre (Marsland et al 1976), Harkins et al (1984, 1990) summarized reasons for visits by the physician that were likely to be pain-related in over 86 000 patients, making approximately half a million patient visits over a 2-year period. A summary of selected reasons for primary care physician visits for different age and sex groups is presented in Figure 42.2A-D. The pattern of occurrence of the pain problems frequently encountered in the pain clinic (headaches and backaches) decreased with increasing age in the family practice patients (Fig. 42.2A), while chronic health problems associated with pain-related degenerative problems increased with age (Fig. 42.2C).

Not surprisingly, there is an increase with age in fractures (Fig. 42.2D). Fractures are a major source of morbidity and mortality in the aged. The specific relation of pain and pain-associated disability due to fractures and resulting fracture-pain-related mortality and morbidity in the aged is not known. It is likely to be considerable. Similarly, the interactions of age and pain with the health problems (reasons for visits) shown in Figure 42.2A–D have not been systematically studied in relation to psychological well-being, activities of daily living, dependency and quality of life.

Sternbach (1986) also reported age-related differences in pain report. This study, the Nuprin pain survey, involved a cross-sectional sample of individuals aged 18 and older in the continental United States. The results showed that the frequencies of headaches, backaches, muscle pains, stomach pain and dental pain were lower in older (aged 65 and above) compared to younger individ-

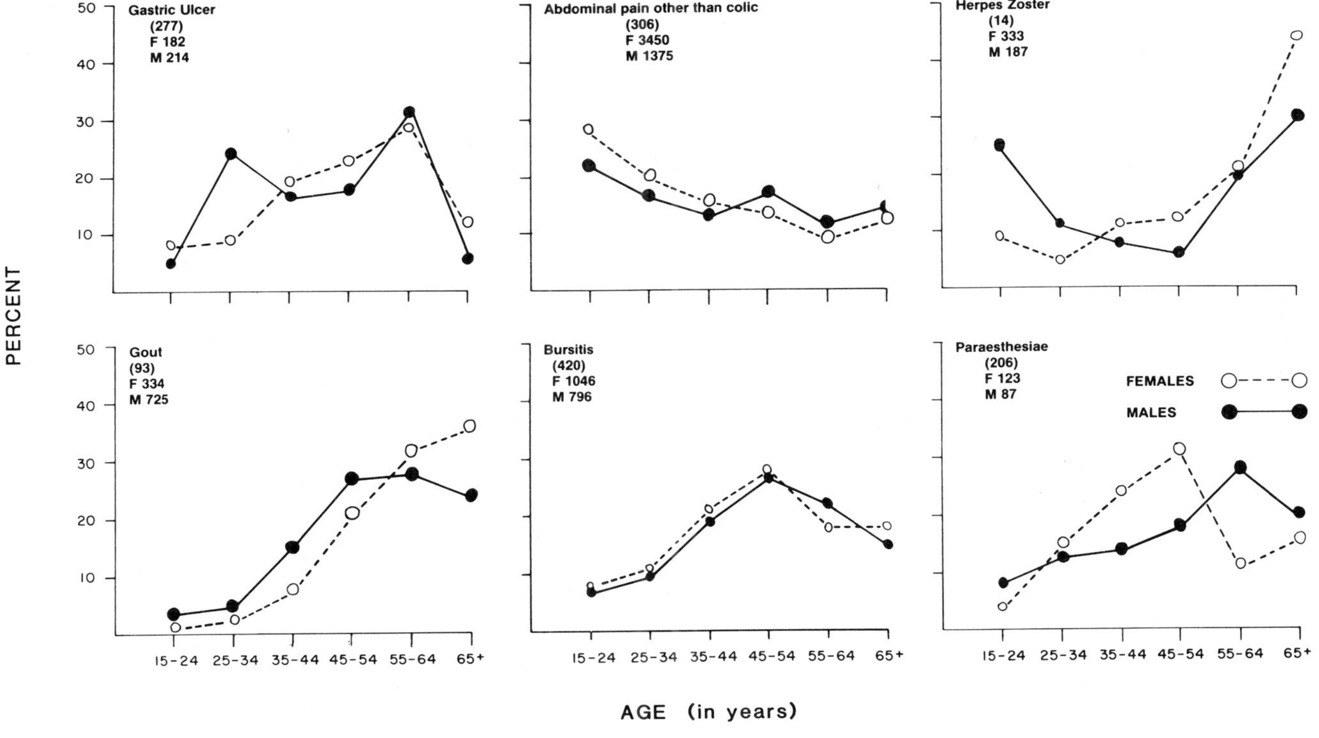

Fig. 42.2 *Contd*

uals (18–24 years of age). Joint pains were more frequent in the older compared to the younger individuals.

Lavsky-Shulan et al (1985) evaluated the prevalence of low-back pain in people over 65 years of age in a geographically defined, community-dwelling sample. Low-back pain caused much discomfort, dysfunction and medical service utilization. While back pain may well decrease with age (see Fig. 42.2A and Sternbach 1986), it represents an important source of morbidity in the elderly. Yet, as noted above, the impact of such pains in the elderly have not been systematically evaluated, even though they are likely to be a major, causal factor in depression and suffering in the elderly.

Another survey which contains information on pain in the general population is the National Health and Nutrition Survey I Epidemiological Follow-up Study (NHANES 1987), conducted between 1982 and 1984, which contained questions concerning musculoskeletal pain lasting at least 1 month and which was present during the week previous to the interview. Questions concerned the presence and intensity of neck, back, hip, knee and joint pain, and stiffness of painful joints upon wakening. The study population was a representative sample of individuals between the ages of 32 and 86 living in the United States who were not institutionalized. In this regard, it is similar to the sample population evaluated in the Nuprin study (Sternbach 1986).

Table 42.2 shows the frequency of each of six musculoskeletal pains, lasting 1 month or longer, that was present during the week prior to the interview for younger individuals (mean age = 39.6; SD= 3.3; n = 2796) and older individuals (mean age = 74.7; SD = 5.5; n = 2863) participating in the NHANES follow-up survey. Five of the six pains were more frequent in the old. Only neck pain did not occur more frequently in the older group. These data contrast with those shown in Figure 42.2A from the family practice sample (Marsland et al 1976; Harkins 1988; Harkins et al 1990), and the findings of the Nuprin study (Sternbach 1986). In the case of the family practice data, this is likely to be due to age differences in self-referral for clinical care for these types of pain problem. As noted earlier, the chronic nature of these pains means that the older individual has probably developed coping skills, is knowledgeable about the source of the pain, has experienced it before and is therefore aware of the pain's implications for activities of daily living, and either has maintenance prescriptions for analgesics or knows which nonprescription medications are most effective for pain control. The reason the Nuprin survey showed an age decrease in certain pains may be due to choice of age groups. In the Nuprin study, younger subjects were those in their late teens and early 20s, and this highlights the need to specify carefully the definition of age as a variable.

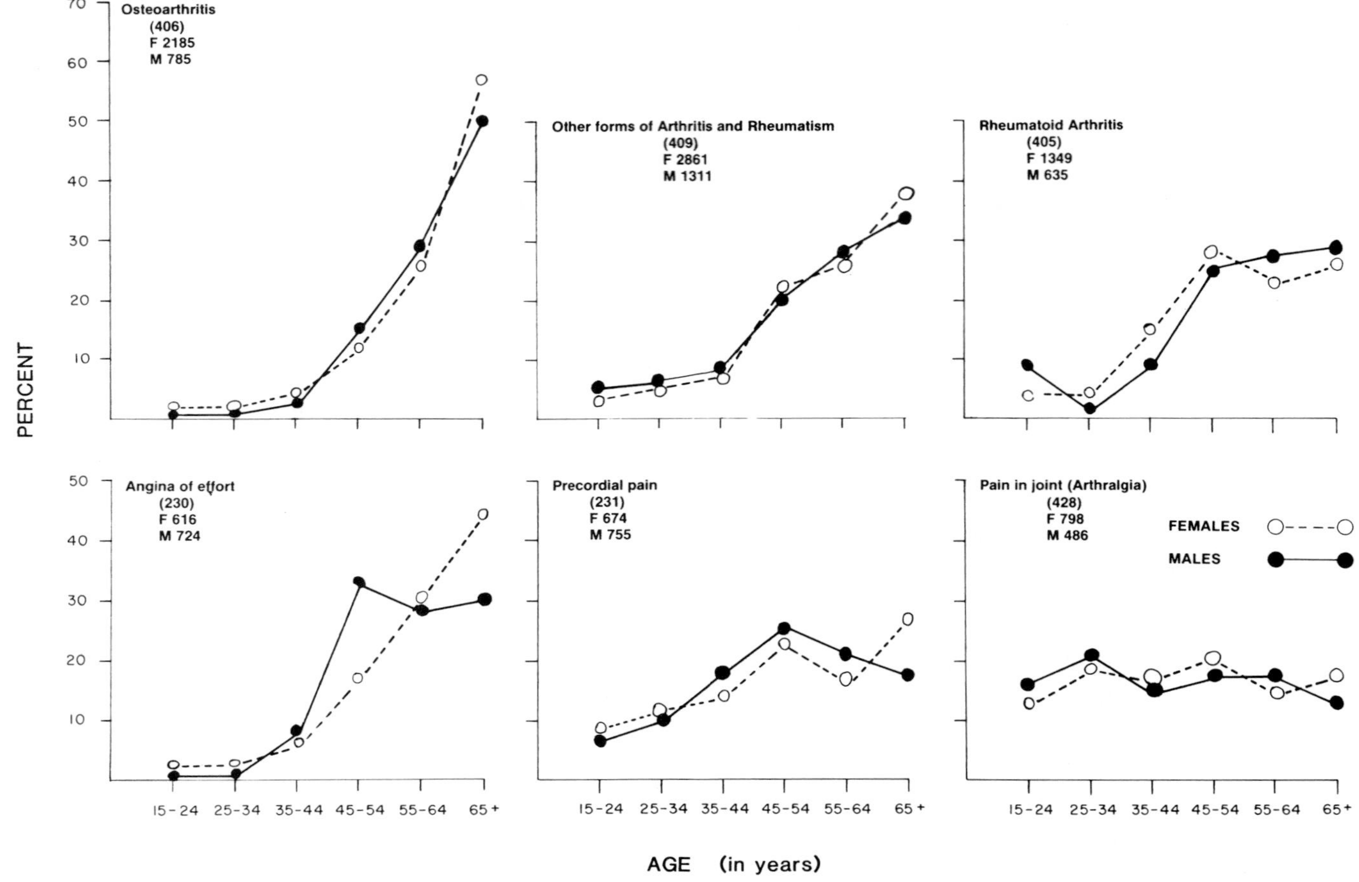

Fig. 42.2 *Contd*

The NHANES follow-up survey also includes information on pain intensity, depression and activities of daily living. The lower section of Table 42.2 presents information on these measures for each age group and type of pain. For example, the 239 individuals of 2796 in the younger group who had neck pain reported a mean pain intensity of 35.2 (out of 100 on the VAS), had a score on the Centre for Epidemiology Studies–Depression (CESD) inventory (Radloff 1977) of 10.8 (SD = 10.6), and an Activities of Daily Living (ADL) (Lawton & Brody 1969) score of 28.2 (SD = 8.7).

Furthermore, pain intensity, depression, and impairment in ADL were consistently greater in the older compared to the younger pain patients. These results indicate that older age in the general population is associated with increased risk for: (i) musculoskeletal pain; (ii) greater pain intensity; (iii) depression; and (iv) limitations in ADL. Causal relations cannot be determined from such cross-sectional data. Longitudinal research with appropriate causal modelling is necessary to address the relationship of pain, depression and limitation of activities of daily living in the elderly.

ACUTE GERIATRIC PAIN

Different forms of acute pain and referred pain have not been systematically evaluated in the elderly. Acute pain is primarily a symptom of disease or injury, whereas chronic pain represents a disease in itself (Sternbach 1981). Acute pain arising from superficial structures and that arising from deeper structures are likely to represent different types of pain (Lewis 1942; Bonica 1990). In contrast, acute pains associated with cutaneous structures, most fractures, and muscle, joint and tendon strain probably *do not change in a clinically significant manner with age in otherwise healthy, elderly people.*

Acute pain as a symptom has signal value, warning of actual or pending tissue damage. If it changes significantly with age, this would delay and confuse diagnosis and treatment. Whether changes in acute pain presentation are due to age-related developmental (ontogenetic) changes in physiology or anatomy, or are due to currently unrecognized disease processes, is a question for research. The answer, however, is one that has little immediate relevance in diagnosis and treatment of the elderly emergency-room

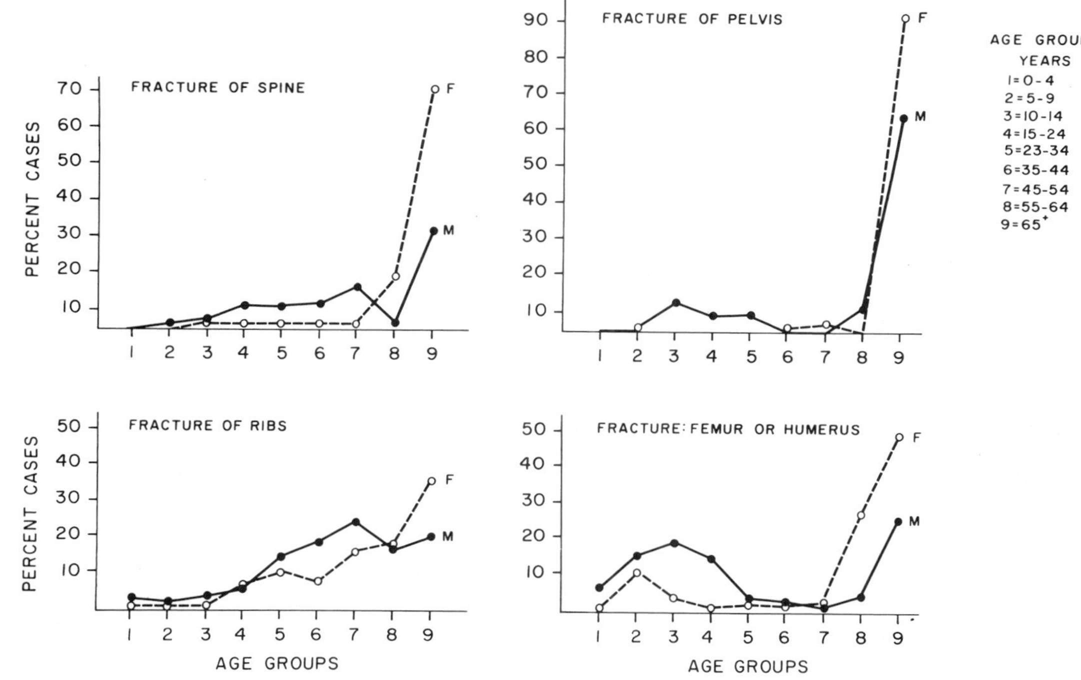

Fig. 42.2 *Contd*

patient with painless acute myocardial infarct (MI), mesenteric infarct, or appendicitis.

Acute pain may not be a primary presenting symptom in the elderly in several conditions in which pain is a key diagnostic symptom in younger individuals. For example, age is an independent risk factor for decreased ischaemic cardiac pain (MacDonald et al 1983; Applegate et al 1984; Miller et al 1990; Montague 1990; Murry et al 1990). Silent, acute MI occurs more frequently in the old than the young. Estimates of painless MI in the elderly range widely from approximately 30%–80% of patients over 65 years of age (Pathy 1967; Montague et al 1990).

Pain consequent to MI develops when sufficient levels of afferent impulses are reached and when an appropriate activation of central ascending pathways has been established. In silent MI, such levels are apparently not reached because of insufficient stimulation of the myocardium, decreased capacity for cephalad transmission or for other unknown pathophysiological reasons (Harkins et al 1990). This should not be taken as evidence that age dulls pain sensibilities in some general sense, since silent ischaemia and atypical chest pain also occur in acute MI with significant frequency in younger individuals, though to a lesser extent than observed in the elderly (Montague et al 1990; Glaxier et al 1991).

At any age, the absence of pain in acute MI is associated with increased morbidity (Montague et al 1990). The fact that the old are more at risk for atypical symptom presentation requires knowledge, vigilance and care. This presents a difficult challenge in the provision of medical care to these individuals, requiring a considerable range of knowledge across disciplines (Calkins et al 1986).

There is no 'catalogue' of acute, potentially catastrophic conditions usually characterized by pain which frequently present without pain in the elderly. Because of the differences in acute pain associated with superficial and deep structures, as well as referred pain, and the pattern of pain-symptom presentation in the elderly, future research should actively strive to define the patterns of 'atypical' pain presentation in the young–old, the old–old and in the frail-old. A better understanding of the mechanisms of deep and referred pain will aid this effort.

GERIATRIC CHRONIC PAIN

Chronic pain is defined here as pain that persists at least 1 month beyond the usual course of an acute disease or beyond a reasonable time for an injury to heal or pain *'that is associated with a chronic pathologic process that causes continuous pain or the pain recurs at intervals for months or years'* (Bonica 1990, p 19; emphasis added). This definition has quite important implications for the elderly. It differs from some definitions in that the time-course is set at 1 month, emphasizing the importance of intervention in cases at risk of developing conditions requiring

Table 42.2 Summary of original tabulations of prevalence of pain lasting at least 1 month and present during the week immediately prior to interview in 5659 community-dwelling individuals. Prevalence of six selected pains, and pain intensity, depression and activities of daily living. Previously unpublished data, compiled from The National Health and Nutrition Follow-Up Survey (NHANES 1987)

	Age		Neck	Back	Hip	Knee	Other joint pain	Stiff joints
(N)	Mean	SD	% (N)	% (N)	% (N)	% (N)	% (N)	% (N)
2796	39.6	3.3	8.55(239)	19.17(536)	9.33(261)	10.26(287)	11.48(321)	14.5(406)
2863	74.7	5.5	9.71(278)	21.34(611)	14.98(429)	21.31(610)	13.66(391)	26.1(748)
χ^2			NS	4.13*	42.2***	123.7****	6.09**	117.4****
VAS[1] pain intensity	Young		35.18(30.2)	31.6(30.8)	35.7(32.3)	32.0(31.0)	34.7(31.9)	37.9(28.9)
	Old		44.39(30.6)	40.2(32.0)	43.6(32.0)	45.2(31.3)	42.7(30.5)	44.7(29.6)
	F		11.7**	21.2****	9.8**	34.3****	11.4***	14.0***
	(df)		(1, 513)	(1, 1129)	(1, 683)	(1, 878)	(1, 702)	(1, 1137)
CESD[2]	Young		10.8(10.6)	10.6(11.0)	10.2(11.1)	10.9(11.5)	10.67(10.5)	12.3(11.5)
	Old		12.9(10.8)	11.9(9.9)	12.2(10.1)	12.2(10.1)	11.7(9.4)	12.9(10.2)
	F		4.9*	4.2*	5.7*	2.62	1.85	0.74
	(df)		(1, 515)	(1, 1145)	(1, 688)	(1, 895)	(1, 712)	(1, 1152)
ADL score[3]	Young		28.2(8.7)	27.4(7.3)	28.0(8.2)	28.0(8.1)	27.5(7.7)	28.1(7.5)
	Old		35.7(15.3)	34.6(14.2)	36.8(15.2)	36.0(14.9)	35.5(14.7)	36.3(15.0)
	F		44.1****	112.8****	75.6****	72.6***	77.6***	107.0****
	(df)		(1, 515)	(1, 1145)	(1, 688)	(1, 895)	(1, 710)	(1, 1152)
Age	Young		40.2(3.1)	39.8(3.31)	40.0(3.1)	39.5(3.5)	40.1(3.45)	40.0(3.2)
	Old		75.0(5.8)	74.6(5.8)	75.7(5.7)	75.1(5.8)	74.8(5.7)	74.7(5.7)

*<0.05; **<0.01; ***<0.001; ****<0.0001.
[1]VAS = visual analogue scale.
[2]CESD = Center for Epidemology Studies–Depression inventory (Radloff 1977).
[3]ADL = activities of daily living inventory (Lawton & Brody 1969).
NS = not significant.

immediate intervention to avoid irreversible chronic pain (i.e. reflex sympathetic dystrophy). It also stresses that degenerative musculoskeletal conditions, such as osteoarthritis, be included in the definition of chronic pain. Pain of osteoarthritis serves no warning of impending or actual tissue damage, has no survival value and is a malefic force that is deleterious to the patient, the family and to society (Bonica 1990, p 20).

Chronic pain intensity and unpleasantness in the elderly

It is possible that chronic pain intensity and unpleasantness differ with chronological age and this might explain, in part, the low frequency of old chronic-pain patients attending chronic pain clinics (Harkins et al 1986, 1990). A first step in addressing this question is the development of pain assessment tools appropriate for the elderly. Magnitude-matching procedures have not been systematically applied to age differences in intensity and unpleasantness of chronic pain.

Visual analogue scales (VASs) have been shown to be reliable and easily administered tools for the study of intensity and negative affect (unpleasantness) of experimental pain (Harkins et al 1986, 1989; Price 1988), labour pain (Price et al 1987), and chronic pain (Price & Harkins 1987). The validity of appropriately formulated VASs in well-instructed patients for the assessment of sensory intensity and unpleasantness of pain has been established (Price et al 1983; Price et al 1986; Price 1988; Price & Harkins 1992).

In a pilot study, we evaluated intensity and unpleasantness of chronic pain in young and old patients. Figure 42.3 shows pain intensity and unpleasantness ratings in 81 younger (mean age 35.6 years) and in 19 older (mean age 71.3 years) consecutive patients at a multidisciplinary chronic pain clinic. Pain ratings were made for pain sensory intensity at its lowest, usual, and highest over the past week on a 150 mm VAS. Similar VAS pain unpleasantness ratings were made (see Harkins & Price 1992).

No significant age differences in pain intensity or unpleasantness ratings were observed in these patients (see Fig. 42.3). These results, while consistent with those employing magnitude-matching procedures in the study of experimental pain (Harkins et al 1986; Kenshalo 1986), are based on a select sample of older individuals who were accepted for evaluation and treatment at a multidisciplinary pain clinic and may not be representative of elderly people with chronic pain in the general population (see Table 42.2). Nevertheless, the data in Figure 42.3 suggest

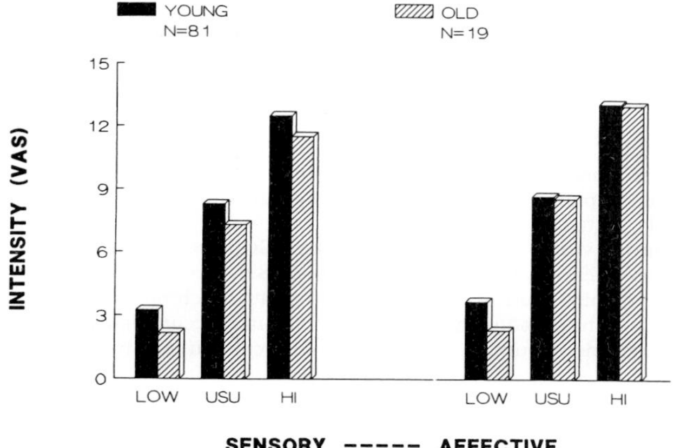

Fig. 42.3 Visual analogue scale (VAS) ratings of the sensory intensity (SENSORY) and unpleasantness (AFFECTIVE response ratings) of chronic pain over the past week at its lowest (LOW), usual (USU) and its highest (HI) levels. Data from patients attending a chronic pain clinic at evaluation visit. The young group had a mean age of 35.6 years. The old group had a mean age of 71.3 years. (Unpublished data collected with the Virginia Commonwealth University Pain Assessment Scales (VCU-PASs).

that chronic pain intensity and unpleasantness are quite similar in patients of quite different ages attending a chronic-pain centre.

Similar results have been reported by Sorkin et al (1990). In two studies these investigators evaluated physical and psychological characteristics of elderly and young chronic-pain patients. Though elderly patients had more abnormal physical findings, the age groups did not differ on self-reported activity, pain severity, pain interference with life events, or emotional or worry reactions in response to pain. Importantly, Sorkin et al (1990) concluded that age should not be a factor in offering either psychological or physical treatments to elderly chronic-pain patients by multidisciplinary pain clinics. Similar results were also reported by Puder (1988), who observed no age differences in outcome in response to 10-week cognitive-behavioural group therapy (a stress inoculation training intervention for chronic pain) in 69 outpatients between the ages of 27 and 80. Age appears not to be a contraindication for standard chronic pain interventions.

Frequency and prevalence of pain as well as depression increase with closeness to death (Moss et al 1991) and pain is an under-recognized source of morbidity in the nursing homes (Ferrell et al 1990; Parmelee et al 1991). Nevertheless, age does not appear to affect success of traditional interventions for the treatment of chronic pain (Middaugh et al 1988; Puder 1988; Sorkin et al 1990).

Unfortunately, a view that is currently expressed is that there is a decrease in perception of pain in the elderly (Enck 1991; Egbert 1991). The findings summarized here concerning experimental pain, pain prevalence, chronic pain and pain-treatment outcome suggest that age does not decrease pain perception in the elderly, though there is evidence that emotional suffering specifically related to pain may be less in older than in younger chronic-pain patients (Harkins & Price 1992). Assessment and intervention for pain in the elderly should begin with the assumption that all neurophysiological processes subserving nociception are intact.

SPECIAL CONSIDERATIONS IN ASSESSMENT AND TREATMENT OF GERIATRIC PAIN

It must be recognized there are no universally accepted methods for pain assessment, though we have been impressed with the utility and ease of administration of VASs in the evaluation of geriatric pain. Each special group requires special considerations. For example, pain assessment procedures change with developmental stage in children (McGrath 1990; Bush & Harkins 1991). Similarly, assessment tools which are valid and efficacious in the general population of the elderly may not be useful in assessment of pain in individuals with cognitive impairment. Noncognitively impaired elderly people with significant physical limitations require special considerations to assure compliance with treatment. Treatment of cognitively impaired pain patients, who make up more than 50% of the nursing-home population, requires other special considerations. Considerations that are important in the assessment and treatment of older pain patients are presented in Tables 42.3 and 42.4.

SENSITIVITY TO NOCICEPTIVE INPUT

The position that age dulls the sense of pain is untenable. Assertions that the elderly tolerate tooth extractions and minor surgical procedures with little or no discomfort (Critchley 1931) cannot be accepted. Also, no evidence exists that qualitative properties of pain (location, extent or quality) are different in older compared to younger pain patients. Older patients, who have come to accept pain as a 'normal' part of their daily lives, should be encouraged to discuss their pain. Discussion should centre on expectations, evaluation if the patient views pain as a 'natural' fact of aging, and most importantly the impact of pain on activities of daily living.

COMORBIDITY

Interpretation of symptoms and signs in the elderly are a challenge. Chronic degenerative conditions occur with high frequency in the old and these include the dementias and stroke. Among the frail old it is not surprising to find multiple overlapping sources contributing to chronic pain.

Table 42.3 Selected drugs useful in the management of pain in the elderly

Drug	Indication	Adverse effects	Special considerations
Narcotic analgesics Morphine Meperidine (Demerol®)* Codeine Oxycodone (Percodan®) Hydrocodone (Vicodin®) Hydromorphone (Dilaudid®) Levorphanol (Levo-Dromoran®) Fentanyl (Sublimaze®, Duragesic®) Propoxyphene (Darvon®)	Relief of moderate to severe pain or when nonnarcotic analgesics are ineffective	Respiratory depression, apnoea, respiratory arrest. Dizziness, sedation, nausea, vomiting, sweating. Euphoria, dysphoria, delirium, insomnia, agitation, anxiety, hallucinations, blurred vision, tremor, depression. Urinary retention, hesitancy, reduced libido or potency. Pruritus, urticaria, other skin rashes. Abdominal pain, taste alterations, dry mouth, anorexia, constipation	Addiction, physical dependence. Acute abstinence syndrome (withdrawal). Exercise caution in elderly or debilitated patients, and in those with hypoxia or hypercapnia, patients taking CNS depressants. Meperidine inappropriate for chronic pain, metabolite may accumulate and lead to CNS excitation (e.g. tremors, twitches, seizures)
Narcotic agonist–antagonist analgesics Buprenorphine (Buprenex®) Butorphanol (Stadol®) Dezocine (Dalgan®) Nalbuphine (Nubain®) Pentazocine (Talwin®)	Relief of moderate to severe pain	Respiratory depression, hypotension, hypertension, chest pain, sedation, nausea, vertigo, dyspepsia, bitter taste, confusion, psychosis, slurred speech, constipation, dry mouth	Use with caution in elderly and debilitated, renal or hepatic dysfunction.Lower abuse potential than narcotic analgesics. CNS side-effects are most common for group
Analgesic Acetaminophen	Relief of mild to moderate pain	Hepatotoxicity	Avoid excessive use
Nonsteroidal antiinflammatory drugs Aspirin Ibuprofen (Motrin®, Rufen®) Fenoprofen (Nalfon®) Naproxen (Naprosyn®) Tolmetin (Tolectin®) Diclofenac (Voltaren®) Ketorolac (Toradol®) Diflunisal (Dolobid®) Piroxicam (Feldene®) Etodolac (Lodine®) Flurbiprofen (Ansaid®) Nabumetone (Relafen®) Ketoprofen (Orudis®) Indomethacin (Indocin®) Sulindac (Clinoril®) Meclofenamate (Meclomen®) Mefenamic Acid (Ponstel®) Oxaprozin (Dzypro®)	Rheumatoid arthritis, osteoarthritis, ankylosing spondylitis, mild to moderate pain, tendinitis, bursitis, acute gout, migraine and cluster headache	Gastrointestinal toxicity such as bleeding, ulceration and perforation. May aggravate depression or other psychiatric disturbances. Headache. Hypersensitivity. Acute renal insufficiency, nephritis, hyperkalaemia, hyponatraemia, renal papillary necrosis. Inhibition of platelet aggregation (bleeding time prolonged). Decreased haemoglobin. Blurred vision. Increased liver function tests. Nausea, vomiting, diarrhoea, constipation, dyspepsia	Assess renal function before and during therapy.Caution in patients with impaired hepatic function. Gastrointestinal toxicity increases with age.May cause fluid retention and peripheral oedema. Avoid aspirin, ibuprofen and alcoholic beverages. May take with food or antacids. Decrease dose of ketoprofen and naproxen in the elderly. Alter doses of diflunisal, ibuprofen, ketoprofen, naproxen, diclofenac, etodolac, indomethacin, ketorolac and sulindac in chronic renal insufficiency. Nonacetylated salicylates and fenoprofen may alter thyroid function tests
Non-acetylated salicylates Sodium salicylate Magnesium salicylate Choline salicylate Choline magnesium trisalicylate Trolamine salicylate Salsalate (Disalcid®) Diflunisal (Dolobid®)			
Benzodiazepines Alprazolam (Xanax®) Chlordiazepoxide (Librium®) Clonazepam (Klonopin®) Diazepam (Valium®) Halazepam (Paxipam®) Lorazepam (Ativan®) Oxazepam (Serax®) Prazepam (Centrax®) Clorazepate (Tranxene®) Midazolam (Versed®)	Management of anxiety and panic attacks. Muscle relaxant	Drowsiness, ataxia and confusion. Sedation, depression, lethargy, apathy, memory impairment, delirium, slurred speech, nervousness, inability to perform complex mental functions. Constipation, diarrhoea, dry mouth, incontinence, urinary retention. Bradycardia, tachycardia, hypertension, hypotension, palpitations. Visual disturbances, auditory disturbances	Avoid alcohol or other CNS depressants. Long-term or high-dose therapy may cause withdrawal symptoms upon abrupt cessation. Observe caution in patients with renal or hepatic dysfunction. Small initial dose with gradual increases in elderly.
Temazepam (Restoril®) Flurazepam (Dalmane®) Triazolam (Halcion®)	Insomnia		

Table 42.3 *(contd)*

Drug	Indication	Adverse effects	Special consideration
Tricyclic antidepressants Amitriptyline (Elavil®) Amoxapine (Asendin®) Desipramine (Norpramine®) Doxepin (Sinequan®) Imipramine (Tofranil®) Nortriptyline (Aventyl®, Pamelor®) Protriptyline (Vivactil®) Trimipramine (Surmontil®)	Relief of symptoms of depression. Chronic pain (migraine, chronic tension headache, diabetic neuropathy, tic douloureux, cancer pain, postherpetic neuralgia, arthritic pain)	Sedation and anticholinergic effects. Orthostatic hypotension, syncope, tachycardia, palpitations, heart block. Nausea, vomiting. Confusion, hallucinations, delusions, agitation, insomnia, hypertonia, paraesthesia, akathisia, ataxia, tardive dyskinesia, EEG alterations.Bone marrow depression	Avoid alcohol and/or other CNS depressants. Lowered seizure threshold. Monitor ECG, Photosensitivity may occur
Tetracyclic antidepressants Maprotiline (Ludiomil®)	Same as above		Seizure risk in overdose
Other antidepressants Trazodone (Desyrel®)	Treatment of depression	Skin rash, hypertension, hypotension, tachycardia, arrhythmias. Hostility, confusion, drowsiness, insomnia, blurred vision, tinnitus. Anaemia	Increased risk in patients with preexisting cardiac disease
Fluoxetine (Prozac®) Sertraline (Zoloft®)	Treatment of major depressive disorders	Most commonly observed: anxiety, nervousness, insomnia, fatigue, tremor, dizziness, anorexia, nausea, diarrhoea, headache, dry mouth, sweating, constipation	Inhibition of serotonin uptake. Alteration of appetite and weight may occur. Activation of mania/hypomania may occur. *Very long* elimination half-life for fluoxetin (e.g. 7–9 days)
Bupropion (Wellbutrin®)	Treatment of depression	Seizures. Constipation, weight loss, nausea, vomiting, dry mouth, headache, tremor, sedation, dizziness, rash, agitation, confusion, blurred vision	Increased seizure risk. Avoid alcohol
Phenothiazine Methotrimeprazine (Levoprome®)	Depression of thalamus, hypothalamus, reticular and limbic systems. Sedative and analgesic for moderate to severe pain.	Drowsiness, sedation, amnesia, respiratory depression, nausea, vomiting, jaundice, blood dyscrasias. Constipation. Urinary retention, extrapyramidal symptoms	Marked hypotension may develop. For intramuscular use only. Tardive dyskinesia
Anticonvulsants Phenytoin (Dilantin ®)	Control of grand mal and psychomotor seizures. Antiarrhythmic. Treatment of trigeminal neuralgia (tic douloureux)	CNS reaction such as nystagmus, ataxia, slurred speech, confusion, insomnia, diplopia, drowsiness, tremor and headache most common. Nausea, vomiting, constipation, gingival hyperplasia, toxic hepatitis, liver damage. Dermatologic reactions such as morbilliform, maculopapular, urticarial and nonspecific rashes. Stevens–Johnson syndrome and toxic epidermal necrolysis. Thrombocytopenia, leucopenia, granulocytopenia and pancytopenia	Blood counts and urinalysis should be done before and during therapy. Discontinue if skin rash develops. Saturable metabolism 87–93% plasma protein bound. Monitor closely with total and free serum levels if low albumin
Carbamazepine (Tegretol®)	Partial seizures with complex symptoms. Trigeminal neuralgia, glossopharyngeal neuralgia. *Not* for relief of minor aches or pains	Dizziness, drowsiness, nausea, vomiting are most common. Aplastic anaemia, leucopenia, agranulocytopenia, eosinophilia, bone marrow depression. Fever. Abnormal liver function tests, hepatitis. Urinary frequency, urinary retention, pulmonary hypersensitivity, dermatologic reactions including Stevens–Johnson syndrome. Cardiovascular reactions such as hypertension or hypotension and syncope	Baseline liver function tests and periodic monitoring recommended. Pretreatment haematological testing then every 2 months advised (CBC, white cell differential and platelet counts)

Table 42.3 *(contd)*

Drug	Indication	Adverse effects	Special consideration
Agents for migraine headache			
Methysergide (Sansert®)	Prevention or reduction of intensity of severe vascular headaches, such as migraine and cluster headache	Retroperitoneal fibrosis, pleuropulmonary fibrosis and may involve aorta, inferior vena cava. Nausea, vomiting, diarrhoea, insomnia, dizziness, ataxia, weakness. Facial flush, nonspecific rashes, peripheral oedema. Cold extremities. Neutropenia, eosinophilia, insomnia, dizziness, ataxia, weakness.	Adverse reactions occur in up to 30–50% of patients. Fibrosis more common with prolonged, uninterrupted therapy
Ergotamine tartrate (Ergostat®) Dihydroergotamine mesylate (D.H.E.45®)	To abort or prevent vascular headaches	Nausea, vomiting in up to 10%. Numbness and tingling of toes, weakness, tachycardia, bradycardia, local oedema, itching	Initiate therapy at first sign of attack. Avoid prolonged administration to avoid dependence and tolerance
Propranolol (Inderal®)	Prophylaxis of common migraine headache	Bradycardia, hypotension, fluid retention. Lightheadedness, ataxia, visual disturbances, vivid dreams, hallucinations, insomnia, depression, nausea, vomiting, diarrhoea, increased BUN and serum creatinine	Use with caution in patients with heart failure. Gradually reduce doses over 2 weeks. May mask hyperthyroidism and inhibit bronchodilation
Steroids			
Dexamethasone (Decadron®) Prednisone (Deltasone®) Prednisolone (Prelone®)	Antiinflammatory agent. Tumour involvement in nervous system or compression by tumour. Cancer pain	Adrenocortical insufficiency, muscle wasting, weakness, increased susceptibility, sodium retention, potassium loss, exophthalmos, decreased glucose tolerance, nausea, vomiting, increased appetite, gastric irritation, mental disturbances, impaired wound healing. Osteoporosis	Patients should be instructed to notify physician if any infection or signs of infection. Evaluation of HPA-axis function recommended
Skeletal muscle relaxants			
Baclofen (Lioresal®) Carisoprodol (Soma®) Methocarbamol (Robaxin®) Cyclobenzaprine (Flexeril®)	Relief of discomfort associated with acute, painful musculoskeletal conditions. Management of spasticity	Drowsiness, dry mouth, dizziness, headache, blurred vision, nervousness, confusion, nausea, vomiting, postural hypotension, facial flushing	Additive CNS toxicity if given with other CNS depressants. Slow dosage increase recommended in the elderly. Cautious use in renal or hepatic insufficiency
Topical ointments			
Capsaicin (Zostrix®)	Postherpetic neuralgia, pain, diabetic neuropathy. Investigational use for cutaneous disorders such as psoriasis, vitiligo, and intractable pruritus	Burning sensation, erythema, stinging	Avoid getting in eyes or on broken or irritated skin
Local anaesthetics			
Short acting Lidocaine (Xylocaine®) Mepivacaine (Carbocaine®) *Long acting* Bupivacaine (Marcaine®)	Infiltration anaesthesia, nerve block. Palliation of acute pain	CNS stimulatory effects such as anxiety, nervousness, confusion, blurred vision, tremors, then followed by CNS depression. Bradycardia, cardiac arrhythmias, hypotension. Hypersensitivity or allergic reactions. Burning at site of injection,swelling, neuritis, tissue necrosis and sloughing. Allergic reactions with cutaneous lesions such as urticaria, oedema, contact dermatitis and anaphylactoid reactions with use of topical agents	Local anaesthetics should be used only by experienced clinicians. Patients with cardiac disease, hyperthyroidism or other endocrine disease may be more susceptible to toxic effects. Caution in patients with liver disease.
Topical Ethyl chloride Benzocaine Cocaine Fluori-Methane® Fluro-Ethyl® Dyclonine (Dyclone®)	Topical vapocoolant to control pain associated with minor surgical procedures, athletic injuries, myofascial pain, restricted motion and muscle spasm		Some topicals can be used for anaesthetizing mucous membranes in nose and throat. Use minimal doses in the elderly

*Less desirable than others because of more side-effects.

Table 42.4 Psychosocial management of pain in the elderly (from Harkins et al (1990) with permission)

Factors enhancing painful experiences	Assessment	Intervention
Loneliness and social isolation	Family interview	Increase family interaction
Learned helplessness	Family interview	Increase social interaction
Acute stress and anxiety	Patient catharsis	Time-limited psychotherapy, occasional benzodiazepines
Maladaptive environment	Family interview, staff interview	Behaviour modification through family and staff
Autonomous depression	Vegetative signs, biological markers	Antidepressant therapy
Personality disorder	Past history of interpersonal relationships, particularly with professionals	Limit setting, good communication from treating physicians
Organic syndrome	Status, drug history	Determine cause, limit dose of analgesic, provide educational support to the family
Hypochondriasis	Review of previous medical history	Long-term, personalized physician–patient relationship, occasional anxiolytic

MENTAL STATUS

Many elderly people complain of memory impairment. Benign senescent forgetfulness is likely to be associated with complaints of memory loss without impairment of daily functioning, self-care or social functioning. These individuals are likely to be as accurate in reports of pain symptoms as are younger patients, and pain-treatment outcome is likely to be very good.

Dementia in late life presents special challenges. Patients with significant cognitive impairment are not likely to be able to schedule themselves or attend an outpatient pain clinic alone. Currently, little is known of the neurophysiological relationships between pain and age-related degenerative brain diseases.

ACTIVITIES OF DAILY LIVING (ADL)

Increasing frailty in the elderly results in a decrease in ability to perform the activities of daily living, together with significant emotional distress (Moss et al 1991). In ambulatory individuals, the ADL scale developed by Lawton & Brody (1969) is recommended. For individuals with significant functional impairments, the observational scale of Katz et al (1969) is useful. No validated instrument exists for the determination of the impact of pain on ADL in older adults. This is unfortunate, since pain contributes to significant social, psychological and physical activity limitations in the old (Ferrell et al 1990; Moss et al 1990; Williamson & Schulz 1992).

MEDICATIONS

Table 42.3 presents some recommendations concerning drug therapy for pain in the elderly. The patient should bring all the medications they are taking or are 'storing' in the house to their first visit to the clinic. This 'brown bag of pills' will likely contain some surprises. The potential for drug–drug interactions needs to be assessed prior to pain treatment.

A rule for pharmacological intervention in the elderly is 'start low and go slow'. However, this rule of thumb may also lead to overly conservative pharmacological therapy resulting in unnecessary suffering and expense (Melzack et al 1987). Clinical experience indicates that the elderly without renal or hepatic dysfunctions tolerate analgesics well. Problems develop when physiological integrity is compromised, resulting in changes in pharmacokinetics. Appropriate screening and clinical examination are therefore crucial for effective use of analgesics with minimal complications. Age-related increased fat deposition and decreased lean body mass and water may influence drug effects but, in general, response to analgesics is not greatly affected by normal aging.

The use of a combined approach of medication and rehabilitative therapy (counselling, physical therapy, biofeedback) is likely to be more beneficial than a single therapeutic approach. Guidelines for medications are: know the risks; use correctly according to indications; start low and go slow; achieve adequate dose; anticipate side-effects; reassess response frequently; be ready to modify as needed.

In general, pharmacodynamics are unaffected in the normal aging process. Since centrally active drugs may interact with a preexisting disease state, care must be taken in individuals with central nervous system disease (e.g. Parkinsonism, Alzheimer's dementia, stroke). Age is not a contraindication for patient-controlled analgesia (PCA). PCA is effective with noncognitively impaired elderly people and should be used. Nurse-assisted 'patient-controlled' analgesia should be considered when patient conditions limit PCA.

The last months of life are associated with significant psychological morbidity and limitations in activities due to pain (Moss et al 1991). This is an area, like those of pain assessment in the nursing home and in the older postsurgical patient, that is in need of systematic research and improvement in standards for intervention.

FAMILY AND SOCIAL SUPPORT SYSTEMS

Involvement of family and friends in the treatment of the older pain patient can be beneficial not only for psychosocial management (see Table 42.4), but also in aiding with compliance during treatment. Family assistance becomes important if cognitive impairment or nonpain related limitations in activities of daily living are present.

SUMMARY

The literature reviewed in this chapter suggests that the intensity of experimental and chronic pain do not appear to differ appreciably across healthy adult age groups. This may reflect sample biases, since recurrent and chronic pain intensity and prevalence increase with age in the general population (Table 42.2). Further, pain in the dying (Moss & Lawton 1990) and the nursing-home resident (Ferrell et al 1990; Parmelee et al 1991) is associated with significant pain-related psychological morbidity.

Pain lasting for more than 1 month in the aged should be considered for evaluation and treatment in multidisciplinary pain clinics. Treatment of these individuals can be expected to be as positive as that in the younger patient. Pain assessment and treatment, particularly in the frail –old represents a particular challenge. This challenge has not been met. Elderly people and young children are often perceived by the health-care delivery system as being insensitive to pain. This is a mistaken perception resulting in systematic undertreatment of pain in these individuals (Melzack et al 1987). It is unfortunate that those who are most dependent are most likely to receive the least optimal care for pain (Wall 1979; Butler & Gastel 1980).

REFERENCES

Applegate W B, Graves S, Collins T, Zwaag R V, Akins D (1984) Acute myocardial infarction in elderly patients. Southern Medical Journal 77: 1127–1129

Birren J E, Shapiro H B, Miller J H (1950) The effect of salicylate upon pain sensitivity. Journal of Pharmacology and Experimental Therapy 100: 67–71

Bonica J J (1990) The management of pain, 2nd edn. Lea & Febiger Philadelphia

Bush J, Harkins S W (1991) Children in pain: clinical and research issues from a developmental perspective. Springer-Verlag, New York

Butler R N, Gastel B (1980) Care of the aged: perspectives on pain and discomfort. In: Ng L K Y, Bonica J J (eds) Pain and discomfort. Elsevier/North Holland, Amsterdam

Calkins E, Davis P J, Ford A B (1986) The practice of geriatrics. W B Saunders, Philadelphia, p 617

Cassel E J (1982) The nature of suffering and the goals of medicine. New England Journal of Medicine 306: 639–645

Chapman W P, Jones C M (1944) Variations in cutaneous and visceral pain sensitivity in normal subjects. Journal of Clinical Investigation 23: 81–91

Clark W C, Mehl L (1971) Thermal pain: a sensory decision theory analysis of the effect of age and sex on d', various response criteria, and 50 percent pain threshold. Journal of Abnormal Psychology 78: 202–212

Clinch D, Banerjee A K, Ostick G (1984) Absence of abdominal pain in elderly patients with peptic ulcer. Age and Ageing 13: 120–123

Coleman J A, Denham M J (1980) Perforation of peptic ulceration in the elderly. Age and Ageing 9: 257–261

Collins G, Stone L A (1966) Pain sensitivity, age and activity level in chronic schizophrenics and in normals. British Journal Psychiatry 112: 33–35

Critchley M (1931) The neurology of old age. Lancet 225: 1221–1230

Crook J, Rideout E, Browne G (1984) The prevalence of pain complaints in a general population. Pain 18: 299–314

Egbert A M (1991) Help for the hurting elderly. Safe use of drugs to relieve pain. Postgraduate Medicine 89: 217–228

Enck R E (1991) Pain control in the ambulatory elderly. Geriatrics 46: 49–60

Evans E R, Rendell M S, Bartek J P et al 1992 Current perception thresholds in ageing. Age and Ageing 21: 273–279

Ferrell B A (1991) Pain management in elderly people. Journal of the American Geriatrics Society 39: 64–73

Ferrell B A, Ferrell B R, Osterweil D (1990) Pain in the nursing home. Journal of the American Geriatrics Society 38: 409–414

Fozard J (1990) Vision and hearing in aging. In: Birren J E, Schaie K W (eds) Handbook of the psychology of aging, 3rd edn. Academic Press, San Diego, p 150–170

Glazier J J, Vrolix M, Kesteloot H, Piessens J (1991). Silent ischaemia: an update on current concepts. Acta Cardiologica 46: 461–469

Hardy J D, Wolff H G, Goodell H (1943) The pain threshold in man. American Journal of Psychiatry 99: 744–751

Hardy J D, Wolff H G, Goodell H, (1952) Pain sensation and reactions. Williams & Wilkins, Baltimore

Harkins S W (1988) Pain in the elderly. In: Dubner R, Gebhart F G, Bond M R (eds) Proceedings of the Vth World Congress on Pain. Elsevier, Amsterdam, p 355–357

Harkins S W, Chapman C R (1976) Detection and decision factors in pain perception in young and elderly men. Pain 2: 253–264

Harkins S W, Chapman C R (1977a) The perception of induced dental pain in young and elderly women. Journal of Gerontology 32: 428–435

Harkins S W, Chapman C R (1977b) Age and sex differences in pain perception. In: Anderson B, Matthews B (eds) Pain in the trigeminal region. Elsevier/North Holland, Amsterdam, p 435–441

Harkins S W, Price D D (1992) Assessment of pain in the elderly. In: Turk D, Melzack R (eds) Handbook of pain measurement and assessment. Guilford Press, New York, p 315–351

Harkins S W, Warner M H (1980) Age and pain. In: Eisdorfer C (ed) Annual review of gerontology and geriatrics, vol 1. Springer, New York, p 121–131

Harkins S W, Kwentus J, Price D D (1984) Pain and the elderly. In: Benedetti C et al Advances in pain research and therapy, vol 7. Raven Press, New York, p 103–212

Harkins S W, Price D D, Martelli M (1986) Effects of age on pain perception: thermonociception. Journal of Gerontology 41: 58–63

Harkins S W, Price D D, Braith J (1989) Effects of extraversion and neuroticism on experimental pain, clinical pain, and illness behavior. Pain 36: 209–218

Harkins S W, Kwentus J, Price D D (1990) Pain and suffering in the

elderly. In: Bonica J J (ed) Management of pain, 2nd edn. Lea & Febiger, Philadelphia, p 552–559
Helme R D, Katz B, Neufeld S, Lachal J, Corron H T (1989) The establishment of a geriatric pain clinic: a preliminary report of the first 100 patients. Australian Journal on Ageing 8: 27–30
Jensen R, Rasmussen B K, Pedersen B, Lous I, Olesen J (1992) Pain 48: 197–203
Katz S, Downs T D, Cash H R, Grotz R C (1970) Progress in development of the index of ADL. Gerontologist 1: 20–30
Keefe F J, Williams D A (1990) A comparison of coping strategies in chronic pain patients in different age groups. Journal of Gerontology 45: 161–165
Kenshalo D R Snr 1986 Somesthetic sensitivity in young and elderly humans. Journal of Gerontology 41: 732–742
Knapp D A, Koch H (1984) The management of new pain in office-based ambulatory care: National Ambulatory Medical Care Survey, 1980 and 1981. Advance data from Vital and Health Statistics, No. 97, DHHS Pub. No (PHS) 84–1250. Public Health Service, Hyattsville, Maryland
Lawton M P, Brody E M (1969) Assessment of older people; self-maintaining and instrumental activities of daily living. Gerontologist 9: 179–186
Lavsky-Shulan M, Wallace R B, Kohout F J, Lemke J H, Morris M C, Smith I M (1985) Prevalence and functional correlates of low back pain in the elderly: the Iowa 65+ Rural Health Study. Journal of the American Geriatrics Society 33: 23–28
Lewis T (1942) Pain. MacMillan, New York
MacDonald J B, Baillie J, Williams B O, Ballantyne D (1983) Coronary care in the elderly. Age and Ageing 12: 17–20
Marks L E 1974 Sensory processes: the new psychophysics. Academic Press, New York
Marsland D W, Wood M, Mayo F (1976) Content of family practice: a statewide study in Virginia with its clinical educational, and research implications. Appleton–Century–Crofts, New York
Mayer D J, Price D D (1982) A physiological and psychological analysis of pain: a potential model of motivation. In: Pfaff D W (ed) The physiological mechanisms of motivation. Springer-Verlag, New York, p 433–471
McGrath P A (1990) Pain in children: nature assessment and treatment. Guilford New York
McKhann G, Drachman D, Folstein M, Katzman R, Price D, Stadlan E M (1984) Clinical diagnosis of Alzheimer's disease: report of the NINCDS-ADRDA Work Group under the auspices of the Department of Health and Human Services Task force on Alzheimer's Disease. Neurology 34: 939–944
Melding P S (1991) Is there such a thing as geriatric pain? Pain 46: 119–121
Melzack R (1973) The puzzle of pain. Basic Books, New York
Melzack R, Casey K L (1968) Sensory, motivational, and central control determinants of pain. In: Kenshalo D R (ed) The skin senses. Charles C. Thomas, Springfield, pp 423–443
Melzack R, Wall P O (1965) Pain mechanisms: a new theory. Science 150: 971–979
Melzack R, Abbott F V, Zackon W, Mulder D S, Davis M W L (1987) Pain on a surgical ward: a survey of the duration and intensity of pain and the effectiveness of medication. Pain 29: 67–72
Middaugh S J, Levin R B, Lee W G, Barchie S I, Roberts J M (1988) Chronic pain: its treatment in geriatric patients. Archives of Physical Medicine and Rehabilitation 69: 1021–1026
Miller P F, Sheps D S, Bragdon E E et al (1990) Aging and pain perception in ischaemic heart disease. American Heart Journal 120: 22–30
Montague T, Wong R, Crowell R et al (1990) Acute myocardial infarction: contemporary risk and management in older versus younger patients. Canadian Journal of Cardiology 6: 241–246
Mountcastle V B (1974) Pain and temperature sensibilities. In: Mountcastle V B (ed) Medical Physiology 13th edn. Mosby C V, St Louis, vol 1, p 348–381
Moss M S, Lawton M P, Glicksman A (1991) The role of pain in the last year of life of older persons. Journal of Gerontology 46: 51–57
Mumford J M (1965) Pain perception threshold and adaptation of normal human teeth. Archives of Oral Biology 10: 957–968
Mumford J M (1968) Pain perception in man on electrically stimulating the teeth. In: Soulairac A, Cahn J, Charpentier J (eds) Pain. Academic Press, London, p 224–229
NHANES I Epidemiological Follow-up Study (1982–1984) 1987 Plan and operation of the National Health and Nutrition Survey. I Epidemiological follow-up study, 1982–1984 Vital and health statistics, Series I, No. 22, DHHS Pub. No. (PHS) 87–1324
Olsho L W, Harkins S W, Lenhardt M L (1985) Aging and the auditory system. In: Birren J E, Schaie K W (eds) Handbook of the psychology of aging 2nd edn. Van Nostrand Reinhold, New York, p 332–277
Parmelee P A, Katz I R, Lawton M P (1991) The relation of pain to depression among institutionalized aged. Journal of Gerontology 46: 15–21
Pathy M S (1967) Clinical presentation of myocardial infarction in the elderly. British Heart Journal 29: 190–199
Price D D (1988) Psychological and neural mechanisms of pain. Raven Press, New York
Price D D, Harkins S W (1987) Combined use of experimental pain and visual analogue scales in providing standardized measurement of clinical pain. Clinical Journal of Pain 3: 1–8
Price D D, Harkins S W (1992) The affective-motivational dimension of pain: a two-stage model. American Pain Society Journal 1: (in press)
Price D D, McGrath P A, Rafii A, Buckingham B (1983) The validation of visual analogue scales as ratio scale measures for chronic and experimental pain. Pain 17: 45–56
Price D D, Harkins S W, Rafii A, Price C (1986) A simultaneous comparison of fentanyl's analgesic effects on experimental and clinical pain. Pain 24: 197–203
Price D D, Harkins S W, and Baker F (1987) Sensory-affective relationships among different types of clinical and experimental pain. Pain 28: 297–307
Procacci P, Bozza G, Buzzelli G, Della Corte M (1970) The cutaneous pricking pain threshold in old age. Gerontologic Clinics 12: 213–218
Procacci P, Della Corte M, Zoppi M, Romano S, Maresca M, Voegelin M (1974) Pain threshold measurement in man. In: Bonica J J, Procacci P, Pagoni C (eds) Recent advances on pain: pathophysiology and clinical aspects. C C Thomas, Springfield, p 105–147
Puder R S (1988) Age analysis of cognitive–behavioral group therapy for chronic pain outpatients. Psychology of Aging 3: 204–207
Radloff L S (1977) The CES-D scale: a self-report depression scale for research in the general population. Applied Psychological Measurement 1: 385–401
Ready B L, Edwards W T (1992) Management of acute pain: a practical guide. IASP Publications, Seattle
Scapa E, Horowitz M, Avtalion J, Waron M, Eshchar J (1992) Appreciation of pain in the elderly. Israel Journal Medical Science, 28: 94–96
Schluderman E, Zubek J P (1952). Effect of age on pain sensitivity. Perceptual and Motor Skills 14: 295–301
Schumacher G A, Goodell H, Hardy J D, Wolff H G (1940) Uniformity of the pain threshold in man. Science 92: 110–112
Sherman E D, Robillard E (1960) Sensitivity to pain in the aged. Canadian Medical Association Journal 83: 944–947
Sherman E D, Robillard E (1964a) Sensitivity to pain in relationship to age. In: Hansen P F (ed) Age with a future: proceedings of the sixth international congress of gerontology, Copenhagen 1963. F A Davis, Philadelphia, p 325–333
Sherman E D, Robillard E (1964b) Sensitivity to pain in relationship to age. Journal of the American Geriatric Society 12: 1037–1044
Sorkin B S A, Rudy T E, Hanlon R B, Turk D C, Stieg R L (1990) Chronic pain in old and young patients: differences appear less important than similarities. Journal of Gerontology: Psychological Sciences 45: 64–68
Sternbach R A (1981) Chronic pain as a disease entity. Triangle 20: 27
Sternbach R A (1986) Survey of pain in the United States: the Nuprin Pain Report. Clinical Journal of Pain 2: 49–53
Stevens S S 1975 Psychophysics: introduction to its perceptual, neural and social prospects. Wiley, New York
Stevens S S, Marks L E 1980 Cross-modality matching function generated by magnitude estimation. Perception and Psychophysics 27: 379–389
Tait R C, Chibnall J T, Margolis R B (1990) Pain extent: relations with

psychological state, pain severity, pain history, and disability, Pain 41: 295–301

Tucker M A, Andrew M F, Ogle S J et al (1989) Age associated change in pain threshold measured by transcutaneous neuronal electrical stimulation. Age and Aging 18: 241–246

Valkenburg H A (1988) Epidemiological considerations of the geriatric populations. Gerontology 34: 2–10

Wall P D (1979) On the relation of injury to pain. (The first John J Bonica lecture). Pain 6: 253–264

Walsh N E, Schoenfeld L, Ramamurthy S, Hoffman J (1989) Normative model for cold pressor test. American Journal of Physical Medicine and Rehabilitation 68: 6–11

Whiteside L A (1991) The effect of patient age, gender, and tibial component fixation on pain relief after cementless total knee arthroplasty. Clinical Orthopedics 271: 21–27

Williams A K, Schulz R (1988) Association of pain and physical dependency with depression in physically ill middle-aged and elderly persons. Physical Therapy 68: 1226–1230

Williamson G M, Schulz R (1992) Pain, activity restriction, and symptoms of depression among community-residing elderly adults. Journal of Gerontology 47: 367–372

Woodrow K M, Friedman G D, Siegelaub A B, Collen M F (1972) Pain tolerance: differences according to age, sex, and race. Psychosomatic Medicine 34: 548–556

Ysia R, Rosonoff R S, Rosomoff H L (1986) Functional improvement in geriatric chronic pain patients. Archives of Physical Medicine Rehabilitation 67: 685 (abstract)

Zimmerman M (1976) Neurophysiology of nociception. In: Porter R (ed) International review of physiology II, vol 10. University Park Press, Baltimore p 179–221

Carcinoma

43. Cancer pain: principles of assessment and sydromes

Nathan I. Cherny and Russell K. Portenoy

INTRODUCTION

The prevalence of acute and chronic cancer pain (Bonica 1989), and the profound psychological and physical burdens engendered by this symptom, oblige all treating clinicians to be skilled in pain management (Edwards 1989; Martin 1989; Wanzer et al 1989). Relief of pain in cancer patients is an ethical imperative and it is incumbent upon clinicians to maximize the knowledge, skill and diligence needed to attend to this task (Edwards 1989; Martin 1989; Wanzer et al 1989). Unfortunately, undertreatment continues to be common (Bonica 1985; Stjernsward & Teoh 1990) despite the availability of established therapeutic strategies that could benefit most patients (Jorgensen et al 1990). Undertreatment has many causes, among the most important of which is inadequate assessment (Grossman et al 1991; Von Roenn et al 1993). Assessment is an ongoing and dynamic process that includes evaluation of presenting problems, elucidation of pain syndromes and pathophysiology, and formulation of a comprehensive plan for continuing care (Coyle 1987; Ventafridda 1989; Shegda & McCorkle 1990; Levy 1991). In this process, pain treatment must be incorporated within a broader therapeutic agenda, so that needs for tumour control, symptom palliation (physical and psychological) and functional rehabilitation are concurrently addressed (Ventafridda 1989; World Health Organization 1990).

PAIN ASSESSMENT – GENERAL PRINCIPLES

NOCICEPTION, PAIN AND SUFFERING

Pain assessment in the cancer population begins with an appreciation of the relationships among pain, nociception and suffering.

Pain and nociception

Nociception can be defined as the activity produced in the nervous system by potentially tissue-damaging stimuli. Although nociception cannot be directly observed in the clinical setting, it is imputed to occur whenever a potentially tissue-damaging stimulus impinges on a pain-sensitive structure. Nociception is not equivalent to pain. There may be no report of pain despite overt tissue injury, and should pain occur, it may or may not be perceived by the clinician to be commensurate with the degree of the injury. This complex relationship between tissue injury and pain is emphasized in the definition of pain promulgated by the International Association for the Study of Pain: 'an unpleasant sensory and emotional experience associated with actual or potential tissue damage or described in terms of such damage' (International Association for the Study of Pain: Subcommittee on taxonomy 1980).

Pain can be conceptualized as the perception of nociception. Like other perceptions, pain is determined by an interaction between activity in sensorineural pathways and other factors. These other factors presumably comprise two broad categories of pathophysiological mechanisms, specifically neuropathic processes and psychological disturbances (Fig. 43.1). Although psychological processes can strongly influence the expression and impact of pain (Derogatis et al 1983; Breitbart 1989), nociceptive and neuropathic factors predominate in the cancer population (Gonzales et al 1991). Elucidation of the lesions that induce these processes is an essential element in the assessment, and may alter prognosis, provide an opportunity for primary therapy, or suggest application of a specific analgesic modality.

Pain, psychological distress and suffering

The assessment of cancer pain requires a careful evaluation of the complex relationship between pain and psychological well-being. The complexity of this relationship is illustrated by numerous studies that have explored the link between pain and psychological distress in the cancer population. Mood disturbance and beliefs about the meaning of pain in relation to illness have been shown to

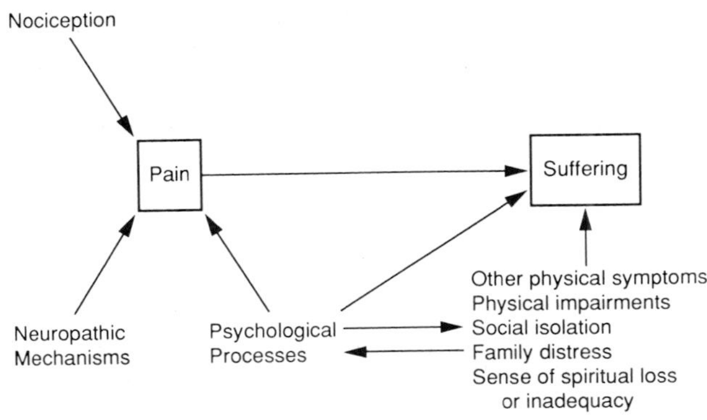

Fig. 43.1 Factors contributing to pain and the relationship between pain and suffering (see text). (From Portenoy 1992 with permission.)

be significant predictors of perceived pain intensity (Bond & Pearson 1969) and the perceived meaning of the pain is a major determinant of function and mood (Daut & Cleeland 1982). In one large prospective study (Derogatis et al 1983), the prevalence of cancer-related pain was 39% in those who had a psychiatric diagnosis and only 19% in those without such a diagnosis; the most important psychiatric diagnoses among those with pain were adjustment disorder with depressed mood, or mixed depression and anxiety, and major depression. It has been observed that uncontrolled pain is a major factor in cancer-related suicide (Cleeland 1984; Bolund 1985; Breitbart 1987) and that psychiatric symptoms commonly disappear with adequate pain relief (Breitbart 1990).

The presence of cancer pain can disturb normal processes of coping and adjustment, which are fundamental to the patient's reactions to the stresses imposed by the cancer and its treatment (Lazarus & Folkman 1984; Fishman 1990). Pain may augment a sense of vulnerability, contributing to a preoccupation with the potential for catastrophic outcomes (Fishman 1990). In some cases unrealistic or distorted attitudes towards the pain problem (e.g. assumptions, beliefs, expectations) can undermine the ability to cope so that the patient becomes utterly helpless and desperate (Fishman 1990). This situation can be reflected in the development of pain behaviours characterized by increasing passivity and dependency, or the uncontrolled expression of negative attitudes and feelings. These behaviours can, in turn, exacerbate social isolation (Fishman 1990).

Suffering can be defined as the global perception of distress engendered by adverse factors that together undermine quality of life (Cassel 1982). Pain may contribute profoundly to suffering, but numerous other factors, such as the experience of other symptoms, progressive physical impairment or psychosocial disturbances, may be equally or more important (Saunders 1984; Ventafridda et al 1990a) (Fig. 43.1). Analgesia alone may not lessen suffering, and consequently, pain therapy is not the sole objective in the supportive care of the cancer patient. Rather, pain therapy must be a critical component of a more comprehensive therapeutic plan designed to address the diverse factors that impair quality of life (Ventafridda 1989; World Health Organization 1990).

CANCER PAIN PATHOPHYSIOLOGY

As suggested previously, three broad categories of pain mechanisms may be posited: ongoing nociception, neuropathic processes and psychological influences. These putative mechanisms are used to label pains according to the predominant pathophysiologies that are inferred to exist from the information acquired through the assessment process. The clinical lexicon now commonly refers to 'nociceptive pain' and 'neuropathic pain' (Arner & Meyerson 1988; Ventafridda & Caraceni 1991). A third category, which is sometimes termed 'idiopathic pain' (Arner & Meyerson 1988), includes both those pains that are presumed to have an organic aetiology that has not yet been identified and those that are perceived to have a psychological cause (American Psychiatric Association 1987).

It should be appreciated that the labelling of a pain according to its inferred pathophysiology is a simplification of very complex processes that can involve multiple interacting mechanisms that can evolve over time (Wall 1989; Dubner 1991b; Ventafridda & Caraceni 1991). These constructs have not been validated and cannot be proven to exist in any individual case. Indeed, the basic validity of the distinction between nociceptive and neuropathic pains has been questioned by some researchers, who note the similarities between experimental models that evaluate injury to nonneural tissue (the substrate for nociceptive pain) and peripheral nerve injury (a substrate for neuropathic pain) (Besson & Chaouch 1987; Devor et al 1991). Nonetheless, this terminology has clinical utility, and is now generally accepted by practitioners.

Nociceptive pain

The term, nociceptive pain, is applied when pain is perceived to be commensurate with tissue damage associated with an identifiable somatic or visceral lesion. The persistence of pain is presumed to be related to ongoing activation of primary afferent neurons responsive to noxious stimuli (nociceptors), which have been identified in skin, muscle, connective tissues, and viscera (Mense & Stahnke 1983; Ness & Gebhart 1990; Willis 1985; Besson & Chaouch 1987; Wall 1989). Nociceptive pain that originates from somatic structures (also known as somatic pain) is typically well localized and described as sharp, aching, throbbing or pressure-like. Pain originating from viscera (visceral pain) is often more diffuse, and is usually described as gnawing or cramping when due to obstruction of a hollow viscus, and aching, sharp or throbbing when due to involvement of organ capsules or other mesentery. From the clinical perspective, nociceptive pains (particularly somatic pains) often respond to opioid drugs (Arner & Meyerson 1988; Cherny et al 1992) or to interventions that ameliorate or denervate the peripheral lesion.

Neuropathic pain

The term 'neuropathic pain' is applied to a pain that is believed to be sustained by a site of aberrant somatosensory processing in the peripheral or central nervous system (Devor et al 1991; Portenoy 1991). Neuropathic pain is most strongly suggested when a dysaesthesia (abnormal, unfamiliar pain) occurs in a region of motor, sensory or autonomic dysfunction that is attributable to a discrete neurological lesion (Portenoy 1991). The diagnosis can be challenging, however, since neuropathic pain may not be dysaesthetic, and the associated neurological deficit may be minimal or absent. In many cases, the diagnosis is inferred from the distribution of the pain and identification of a lesion in neural structures that innervate this region.

Although neuropathic pain can be described in terms of pain characteristics or site of injury, it is useful to distinguish these syndromes according to the presumed site of the aberrant neural activity ('generator') that sustains the pain (Fig. 43.2) (Portenoy 1991). Peripheral neuropathic pain is caused by injury to a peripheral nerve or nerve root and is presumably sustained by aberrant processes originating in the nerve root, plexus or nerve. Neuropathic pains believed to be sustained by a central 'generator' include sympathetically-maintained pain and a group of syndromes traditionally known as the deafferentation pains. The latter pains comprise a subgroup caused by injury to the central nervous system (also known as central pains, the prototype of which is thalamic pain) and a group precipitated by a peripheral nerve injury (e.g. phantom pain). Sympathetically-maintained pain (also known as reflex sympathetic dystrophy or causalgia) may occur following injury to soft tissue, peripheral nerve, viscera or central nervous system, and is characterized by focal autonomic dysregulation in a painful region (e.g. vasomotor or pilomotor changes, swelling, or sweating abnormalities) or trophic changes (Janig et al 1991). Sympathetically-maintained pain is presumably induced or sustained by a process that involves efferent activity in the sympathetic nervous system.

The diagnosis of neuropathic pain has important clinical implications. Neuropathic pains are widely believed to respond relatively less well to opioid drugs than nociceptive pains (Arner & Meyerson 1988; Portenoy et al 1990; Dubner 1991a). Optimal treatment may depend on the use of so-called adjuvant analgesics

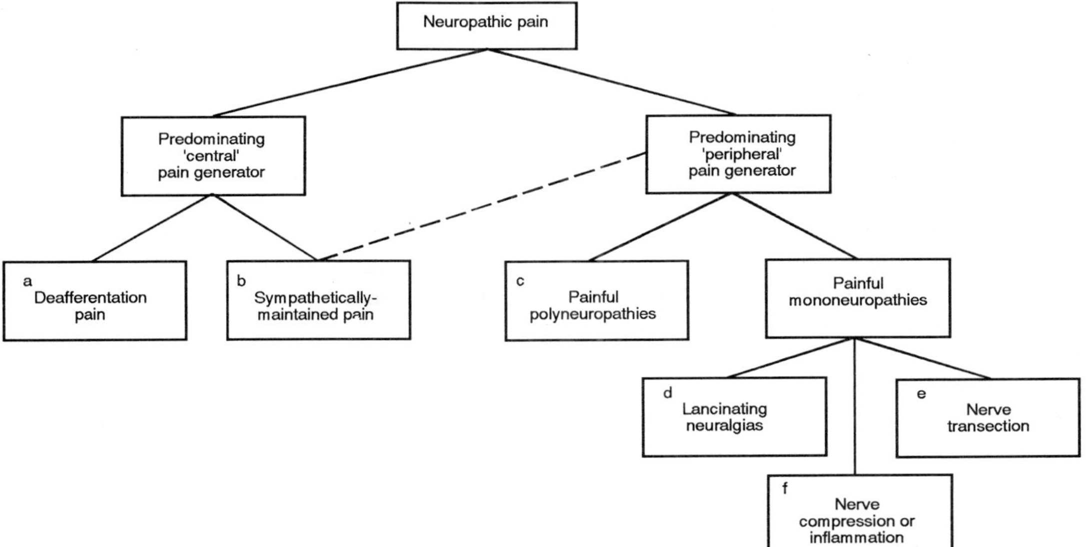

Fig. 43.2 Taxonomy of neuropathic pain by a putative predominating mechanism. (From Portenoy 1992 with permission.) (a) Response to either peripheral or central nervous system injury. (b) Associated with focal autonomic dysregulation (e.g. oedema, vasomotor disturbances), involuntary motor responses and/or trophic changes that may improve with sympathetic nerve blocks. (c) Multiple mechanisms probably involved. (d) The patterns of peripheral activity, or peripheral and central interaction, that yield the lancinating quality of these pains are unknown. (e) Injury to axons may be followed by neuroma formation, a source of aberrant activity likely to be involved in pain. (f) If nociceptive nervi nervorum (small afferents that innervate larger nerves) are confirmed, they may account for neuropathic pain accompanying nerve compression or inflammation.

(Portenoy 1991, 1993a) or other specific approaches, such as sympathetic nerve block. A central neuropathic mechanism also may augur poorly for the response to some neurolytic procedures (Tasker 1990).

Idiopathic pain

Pain that is perceived to be excessive for the extent of organic pathology can be termed idiopathic. Some patients with idiopathic pain present with affective and behavioral disturbances sufficient to infer a predominating psychological pathogenesis, in which case a specific psychiatric diagnosis can be applied (American Psychiatric Association 1987). When this inference cannot be made, however, the label 'idiopathic' should be retained, and assessments should be repeated at appropriate intervals. Idiopathic pain in general, and pain related to a psychiatric disorder specifically, are distinctly rare in the cancer population, notwithstanding the importance of psychological factors in the quality of life.

PAIN CHARACTERISTICS AND SYNDROME IDENTIFICATION

A syndrome is a temporal and qualitative convergence of symptoms and signs, which conforms to a recognized pattern. Specific syndromes may be associated with distinct aetiologies, pathophysiologies, and prognostic and therapeutic implications. In the context of cancer pain, syndromes are defined by the association of particular pain characteristics and physical signs with specific complications of the underlying disease or its treatment.

Pain characteristics

Pain intensity

In the cancer population, evaluation of pain intensity is pivotal to therapeutic decision-making. The selection of an analgesic drug, route of administration and rate of dose titration may all be influenced by reported pain intensity. Furthermore, intensity may also help characterize the pain mechanism and underlying syndrome. For example, clinical observation strongly suggests that the pain associated with radiation-induced nerve injury is rarely severe; the occurrence of severe pain in a previously irradiated region, therefore, suggests the existence of occult neoplasm.

Pain quality

The quality of the pain often suggests its pathophysiology. As noted previously, somatic nociceptive pains are usually well localized and described as sharp, aching, throbbing or pressure-like. Visceral nociceptive pains are generally diffuse and may be gnawing or crampy when due to obstruction of a hollow viscus, or aching, sharp or throbbing when due to involvement of organ capsules or mesentery. Neuropathic pains are often described as burning, tingling or shock-like (Boureau et al 1990).

Pain distribution

Patients with cancer pain commonly experience pain at more than one site (Twycross & Lack 1984; Coyle et al 1990; Banning et al 1991; Portenoy et al 1992). In ambulatory cancer patients the number of pain sites has been identified as a salient determinant of the impact of pain on mood and function (Portenoy et al 1992), and should be queried during the pain assessment. The topographic distribution of a specific pain also may have implications for diagnosis and treatment. For example, the distinction between focal, multifocal and generalized pain may be important in the selection of therapy, such as nerve blocks, radiotherapy or surgical approaches.

The distribution of the pain often clarifies its relationship to the underlying organic lesion. The term 'focal pain', which is used to denote one site of pain, is also used to depict pain that is experienced in the region of the underlying lesion. The term 'referred pain' is applied when pain is experienced in a distribution remote to the lesion. Pain referral patterns, which have been characterized for both nociceptive (somatic and visceral) pain and neuropathic pain (Kellgren 1939; Torebjörk et al 1984; Ness & Gebhart 1990), must be recognized to evaluate the underlying organic aetiology. For example, neuropathic pain is associated with several characteristic patterns, including : (i) pain referred anywhere in the distribution of a peripheral nerve from a lesion involving the nerve itself or the plexus from which it arises, (ii) pain referred anywhere in the dermatome innervated by a damaged nerve root (radicular pain), (iii) pain referred anywhere in the region of the body innervated by a damaged central pathway, and (iv) symmetrical extremity pain from a generalized axonopathy (painful peripheral neuropathy). Similarly, somatic and visceral nociceptive stimuli are associated with characteristic pain referral patterns. For example, neck and arm pain is associated with cardiac pathology, shoulder pain can be caused by diaphragmatic irritation, and knee pain can result from hip pathology.

Temporal relationships

Cancer-related pain may be acute or chronic. Acute pain is defined by a recent onset and a natural history characterized by transience. Most often, acute pain is associated with a well-defined onset and a readily identifiable cause, such as chemotherapy-induced stomatitis or a postlumbar puncture headache. The pain may or may not be associated with overt pain behaviours (such as moaning, grimacing and splinting), anxiety, or signs of generalized sympathetic hyperactivity, including diaphoresis, hypertension and tachycardia.

Chronic pain has been defined by persistence for 1 month or more beyond the usual course of an acute illness or injury, a pattern of recurrence at intervals over months or years, or by association with a chronic pathological process (Bonica et al 1990). Chronic tumour-related pain is usually insidious in onset and has a course that is characterized by fluctuations in intensity. Pain often increases progressively with tumour growth, and may regress as the tumour shrinks in response to anticancer therapy. Chronic pain due to cancer may be associated with affective disturbances (anxiety and/or depression) and vegetative symptoms, such as asthenia, anorexia and sleep disturbance; overt pain behaviours and sympathetic hyperactivity are often absent (McCaffery & Thorpe 1989). Vegetative symptoms, particularly asthenia and anorexia, are also commonly experienced by patients with advanced cancer who report no pain (Reuben et al 1988; Coyle et al 1990; Ventafridda et al 1990c).

Transitory exacerbations of severe pain over a baseline of moderate pain or less may be described as breakthrough pain (Portenoy & Hagen 1990). Breakthrough pains can occur in either acute or chronic pain states. In a survey of patients with chronic cancer pain, almost two-thirds of patients experienced severe or excruciating breakthrough pains (Portenoy & Hagen 1990). These exacerbations may be precipitated by volitional actions of the patient (incident pains), such as movement, micturition, cough or defaecation, or nonvolitional events such as bowel distension. Spontaneous fluctuations in pain intensity can also occur without an identifiable precipitant.

Pain aetiology

Whereas acute cancer-related pains are usually caused by diagnostic or therapeutic interventions, chronic pains are most commonly due to direct effects of the tumour. Adverse consequences of cancer therapy, including surgery, chemotherapy and radiation therapy, account for 15–25% of chronic cancer pain problems, and an even smaller proportion (5–15%) is caused by pathology unrelated to either the cancer or its treatment (Foley 1982; Twycross & Fairfield 1982; Twycross & Lack 1984; Banning et al 1991).

APPROACH TO CANCER PAIN ASSESSMENT

Cancer pain assessment has two major objectives: (i) the accurate characterization of the pain, including the pain syndrome and inferred pathophysiology, and (ii) the evaluation of the impact of the pain and the role it plays in the overall suffering of the patient. This assessment is predicated on the establishment of a trusting relationship with the patient. Even with such a relationship, however, the clinician should not be cavalier about the potential for symptom underreporting. Symptoms are frequently described as complaints, and there is a common perception that the 'good patient' refrains from complaining (Cleeland 1989). The clinician must maintain a clinical posture that affirms relief of pain and suffering as central goals of therapy, and encourages open and effective communication about symptoms. If the patient is either unable or unwilling to describe the pain, a family member may need to be questioned to assess the distress or disability of the patient. The prevalence of pain is so great that an open-ended question about the presence of pain should be included at each patient visit in routine oncological practice.

A practical approach to cancer pain assessment incorporates a stepwise approach that begins with data collection and ends with a clinically relevant formulation (Table 43.1).

DATA COLLECTION

History

A careful review of past medical history and the chronology of the cancer is important to place the pain complaint in context. The pain-related history must elucidate the relevant pain characteristics, as well as the responses of the patient to previous disease-modifying and analgesic therapies. The presence of multiple pain problems is common, and if more than one is reported, each must be assessed independently. The use of validated pain assessment instruments can provide a format for communication between the patient and health care professionals, and can also be used to monitor the adequacy of therapy (Melzack 1975; Daut & Cleeland 1982; Fishman et al 1987; Foley 1989).

The consequences of the pain must also be assessed. These may include, for example, impairment in activities of daily living; psychological, familial and professional dysfunction; disturbed sleep, appetite and vitality; and financial concerns. The patient's psychological status, including current level of anxiety or depression, suicidal ideation, and the perceived meaning of the pain, is similarly relevant. Pervasive dysfunctional attitudes, such as pessimism, idiosyncratic interpretation of pain, self-blame, catastrophizing, and perceived loss of personal control, can usually be detected through careful questioning. It is important to assess the patient-family interaction, and to note both the kind and frequency of pain behaviours and the nature of the family response.

Most patients with cancer pain have multiple other symptoms (Reuben et al 1988; Coyle et al 1990; Ventafridda et al 1990c). The clinician must evaluate the

Table 43.1 Stepwise assessment of the patient with cancer patient

Step 1: Data collection			
Pain related history	*Other relevant history*	*Available laboratory and imaging data*	*Physical examination*
Chronology Characteristics Impact on function Prior treatment Other pain history	Disease-related Other symptoms Psychiatric history Social resources		
Step 2: Provisional assessment			
Provisional pain diagnosis (1) Syndrome identification (2) Inferred pathophysiology	*Global assessment* (1) Extent of disease (2) Goals of care Prolongation of survival Augmentation of function Provision of comfort	*Concurrent concerns* (1) Other symptoms (2) Untreated concurrent diseases (3) Psychosical needs (4) Rehabilitative needs (5) Financial needs	
Step 3 Diagnostic investigations and other assessments			
	Diagnostic investigations (1) Symptom-specific (2) Extent of disease	*Other assessments* (1) Psychological (2) Social (3) Financial (4) Functional	
Step 4: Initial formulation and problem list			
	(1) Pain syndromes and pathophysiology (2) Extent of disease (3) Concurrent concerns (4) Anticipated contingencies		
Step 5 Patient review and formulation of prioritized problem list			
	Current problems (1) .... (2) .... (3) .... (4)	*Anticipated contigencies* (1) .... (2) .... (3) .... (4)	
Step 6 Multimodality therapeutic plan			
	(1) Primary anticancer treatment: Chemotherapy Radiotherapy Surgery Immunotherapy Other (2) Treatment of concurrent disease processes (3) Symptom-directed pharmacotherapy (4) Rehabilitative approaches (5) Psychological approaches (6) Anaesthetic approaches (7) Neurostimulatory approaches		

severity and distress caused by each of these symptoms. Symptom checklists and quality of life measures may contribute to this comprehensive evaluation (Moinpour et al 1989; Moinpour et al 1991).

Examination

A physical examination, including a neurological evaluation, is a necessary part of the initial pain assessment. The need for a thorough neurological assessment is justified by the high prevalence of painful neurological conditions in this population (Gonzales et al 1991; Clouston et al 1992). The physical examination should attempt to identify the underlying aetiology of the pain problem, clarify the extent of the underlying disease, and discern the relationship of the pain complaint to the disease.

Review of previous investigations

Careful review of previous laboratory and imaging studies can provide important information about the cause of the pain and the extent of the underlying disease.

PROVISIONAL ASSESSMENT

The information derived from these data provides the basis for a provisional pain diagnosis, an understanding of the disease status, and the identification of other concurrent concerns. This provisional diagnosis includes inferences about the pathophysiology of the pain and an assessment of the pain syndrome. An understanding of disease status requires an evaluation of the extent of the disease, prognosis, and the anticipated goals of therapy (Haines et al 1990). Evaluation of concurrent concerns includes other symptoms and related psychosocial problems.

DIAGNOSTIC INVESTIGATIONS

Additional investigations are often required to clarify areas of uncertainty in the provisional assessment (Gonzales et al 1991). The extent of diagnostic investigation must be appropriate to the patient's general status and the overall goals of care. For some patients, comprehensive evaluation may require numerous investigations, some targeted at the specific pain problem and others needed to clarify extent of disease or concurrent symptoms. In specific situations, algorithms have been developed to facilitate an efficient evaluation. This is well illustrated by established algorithms for the investigation of back pain in the cancer patient (Portenoy et al 1987; Posner 1987) which provide a straightforward approach for those patients at highest risk for epidural cord (see p. 803).

The lack of a definitive finding on an investigation should not be used to override a compelling clinical diagnosis. In the assessment of bone pain, for example, plain radiographs provide only crude assessment of bony lesions and further investigation with bone scintigrams, computerized tomography (CT) or magnetic resonance imaging (MRI) may be indicated. To minimize the risk of error, the physician ordering the diagnostic procedures should personally review them with the radiologist to correlate pathological changes with the clinical findings.

Pain should be managed during the diagnostic evaluation. Comfort will improve compliance and reduce the distress associated with procedures. No patient should be inadequately evaluated because of poorly controlled pain.

Additional assessments

The comprehensive assessment may also require additional evaluation of other physical or psychosocial problems identified during the initial assessment. Expert assistance from other physicians, nurses, social workers or others may be essential.

FORMULATION AND THERAPEUTIC PLANNING

The evaluation should enable the clinician to appreciate the nature of the pain, its impact and the concurrent concerns that further undermine quality of life. The findings of this evaluation should be reviewed with the patient and other appropriate people. Through candid discussion, current problems can be prioritized to reflect their importance to the patient.

This evaluation may also identify potential outcomes that would benefit from contingency planning. Examples include evaluation of resources for home care, prebereavement interventions with the family, and the provision of assistive devices in anticipation of compromized ambulation.

ACUTE PAIN SYNDROMES

Although acute cancer pain syndromes often pose little diagnostic difficulty, a comprehensive pain assessment in such patients is usually valuable, potentially yielding important information about the extent of disease or concurrent issues relevant to therapy. Cancer-related acute pain syndromes are most commonly due to diagnostic or therapeutic interventions (Table 43.2) Pains due to the neoplasm tend to be either chronic or recurrent. Although some tumour-related pains have an acute onset (such as pain from a pathological fracture), most of these will persist unless effective treatment for the underlying lesion is provided.

ACUTE PAIN ASSOCIATED WITH DIAGNOSTIC AND THERAPEUTIC INTERVENTIONS

Many investigations and treatments are associated with predictable, transient pain. For those patients with a preexisting pain syndrome, otherwise innocuous manipulations can also precipitate an incident pain.

Acute pain associated with diagnostic interventions

Lumbar puncture headache

The best characterized acute pain syndrome associated with a diagnostic intervention is lumbar puncture (LP) headache. LP can be followed by the delayed development of a positional headache, which is precipitated or markedly exacerbated by upright posture. The pain is believed to be related to reduction in cerebrospinal fluid volume, which is perhaps due to ongoing leakage through the defect in the dural sheath (Raskin 1990; Grant et al 1991a). The incidence of headache is related to the calibre of the LP needle (0.5–3% with 25–26 gauge, 5–8% with 22-gauge, 10–15% with 20-gauge and 20–30% with 18-gauge needles) (Bonica 1953). The overall incidence can be reduced by the use of small-gauge needle and by longitudinal insertion of the needle bevel, which presumably induces less trauma to the longitudinal elastic fibres in the dura (Fink & Walker 1989). There is no evidence that recumbency after LP reduces the incidence of this syndrome (Cook et al 1989; De Boer 1989).

Table 43.2 Cancer-related acute pain syndromes

Acute pain associated with diagnostic and therapeutic interventions
Acute pain associated with diagnostic interventions
Lumbar puncture headache
Arterial or venous blood sampling
Bone marrow biopsy
Lumbar puncture
Colonoscopy
Myelography
Percutaneous biopsy
Thoracocentesis
Acute postoperative pain
Acute pain caused by other therapeutic interventions
Pleurodesis
Tumour embolization
Suprapubic catheterization
Intercostal catheter
Nephrostomy insertion
Acute pain associated with analgesic techniques
Injection pain
Opioid headache
Spinal opioid hyperalgesia syndrome
Epidural injection pain
Acute pain associated with anticancer therapies
Acute pain associated with chemotherapy infusion techniques
Intravenous infusion pain
Venous spasm
Chemical phlebitis
Vesicant extravasation
Anthracycline-associated flare reaction
Hepatic artery infusion pain
Intraperitoneal chemotherapy abdominal pain
Acute pain associated with chemotherapy toxicity
Mucositis
Corticosteroid-induced perineal discomfort
Steroid pseudorheumatism
Painful peripheral neuropathy
Headache
Intrathecal methotrexate meningitic syndrome
L-asparaginase associated dural sinus thrombosis
Transretinoic acid headache
Diffuse bone pain
Transretinoic acid
Colony stimulating factors
5-Flurouracil-induced anginal chest pain
Postchemotherapy gynaecomastia
Acute pain associated with hormonal therapy
Luteinizing hormone releasing factor tumour flare in prostate cancer
Hormone-induced pain flare in breast cancer
Acute pain associated with immunotherapy
Interferon-induced acute pain
Acute pain associated with radiotherapy
Incident pains associated with positioning
Oropharyngeal mucositis
Acute radiation enteritis and proctocolitis
Early onset brachial plexopathy
Subacute radiation myelopathy
Acute pain associated with infection
Acute herpetic neuralgia

LP headache, which usually develops hours to several days after the procedure, is typically described as a dull occipital discomfort that may radiate to the frontal region or to the shoulders (Bonica 1953; Raskin 1990). When severe, the pain may be associated with diaphoresis and nausea (Raskin 1990). The duration of the headache is usually brief, hours to days, and routine management relies on bedrest, hydration and analgesics. Persistent headache may necessitate application of an epidural blood patch (Olsen 1987). Although a recent controlled study suggested that prophylactic administration of a blood patch may reduce this complication (Heide & Diener 1990), the incidence and severity of the syndrome do not warrant this treatment. Severe headache has also been reported to respond to treatment with intravenous caffeine (Ford et al 1989).

Acute pain associated with invasive therapeutic interventions

Postoperative pain

Acute postoperative pain is universal unless adequately treated. Unfortunately, undertreatment is endemic despite the availability of adequate analgesic and anaesthetic techniques (Agency for Health Care Policy and Research: Marks & Sachar 1973; Edwards 1990; Acute Pain Management Panel 1992). Guidelines for management have recently been reviewed (Ready 1991; Agency for Health Care Policy and Research: Acute Pain Management Panel 1992). Postoperative pain that exceeds the normal duration or severity should prompt a careful evaluation for the possibility of infection or other complications.

Invasive interventions other than surgery are commonly used in cancer therapy and may also result in predictable acute pain syndromes. Examples include the pains associated with tumour embolization techniques and chemical pleurodesis.

Acute pain associated with analgesic techniques

Injection pain

Intramuscular (IM) and subcutaneous (SC) injections are painful. When repetitive dosing is required, the IM route of administration is not recommended (Agency for Health Care Policy and Research: Acute Pain Management Panel 1992). If the volume of analgesic is small, repetitive SC boluses can be administered through a 27 gauge 'butterfly' that is maintained in situ (Payne 1989a; Mather 1991). Alternatively, continuous infusion techniques should be considered.

Opioid headache

Rare patients develop a reproducible generalized headache after opioid administration. It can be speculated that this may be caused by opioid-induced histamine release.

Spinal opioid hyperalgesia syndrome

Intrathecal and epidural injection of high opioid doses is

occasionally complicated by a paradoxical response characterized by pain (typically perineal, buttock or leg), hyperalgesia and associated manifestations, including segmental myoclonus, piloerection and priapism. This is an uncommon phenomenon that remits after discontinuation of the drug (Stillman et al 1987; De Castro et al 1991; De Conno et al 1991).

Epidural injection pain

Back, pelvic or leg pain may be precipitated by epidural injection or infusion. The incidence of this problem has been estimated at approximately 20% (De Castro et al 1991). It is speculated that it may be caused by the compression of an adjacent nerve root by the injected fluid (De Castro et al 1991).

ACUTE PAIN ASSOCIATED WITH ANTICANCER THERAPIES

Acute pain associated with chemotherapy infusion techniques

Intravenous infusion pain

Infusion site pain is a common problem in patients receiving cancer chemotherapy. Four intravenous infusion-related pain syndromes are recognized: venous spasm, chemical phlebitis, vesicant extravasation and anthracycline-associated flare (Molloy et al 1989; Curran et al 1990). Venous spasm, which produces pain without inflammation, may be modified by application of a warm compress or reduction of the rate of infusion (Molloy et al 1989). Chemical phlebitis causes pain and linear erythema and may be produced by the infusion of cytotoxic drugs (including amasarcine, decarbazine and carmustine), potassium chloride or hyperosmolar solutions (Hundrieser 1988; Mrozek et al 1991). Phlebitis must be distinguished from the more serious complication of a vesicant cytotoxic extravasation which may cause intense pain followed by desquamation and ulceration (Table 43.3) (Schneider & Distelhorst 1989). Finally, transient pain may be associated with local urticaria in the so-called venous flare reaction often caused by intravenous administration of the anthracycline, doxorubicin (Curran et al 1990).

Table 43.3 Commonly used tissue vesicant cytotoxic drugs

Amasarcine
BCNU
Cis-platinum
Decarbazine
Daunorubicin
Doxorubicin
Etoposide
Mitomycin C
Mitoxantrone
Streptozotocin
Teniposide
Vinblastine
Vincristine
Vindesine

Hepatic artery infusion pain

Chemotherapy infusions into the hepatic artery for patients with hepatic metastases are often associated with the development of a diffuse abdominal pain (Kemeny et al 1990). Continuous infusions can lead to persistent pain. In some patients , the pain is due to the development of gastric ulceration or erosions, or cholangitis (Botet et al 1985). If the latter complications do not occur, the pain usually resolves with discontinuation of the infusion. A dose relationship is suggested by the observation that some patients will comfortably tolerate reinitiation of the infusion at a lower dose (Kemeny et al 1990).

Intraperitoneal chemotherapy pain

Abdominal pain is a common complication of intraperitoneal chemotherapy (IPC). A transient mild abdominal pain, associated with sensations of fullness or bloating , is reported by approximately 25% of patients receiving IPC (Almadrones & Yerys 1990). A further 25% of patients report moderate or severe pain necessitating opioid analgesia or discontinuation of therapy (Almadrones & Yerys 1990). Moderate or severe pain is usually caused by chemical serositis or infection (Markman 1986). Drug selection may be a factor in the incidence of chemical serositis; it is a common complication of intraperitoneal anthracycline agents, such as mitoxantrone (Gitsch et al 1990; Dufour et al 1991) and doxorubicin (Markman et al 1984; Deppe et al 1991), but it is relatively infrequent with 5-fluorouracil (Schilsky et al 1990). Abdominal pain associated with fever and leucocytosis in blood and peritoneal fluid is suggestive of infectious peritonitis (Kaplan et al 1985).

Acute pain associated with chemotherapy toxicity

Mucositis

Severe mucositis is an almost invariable consequence of the myeloablative chemotherapy and radiotherapy that precede bone marrow transplantation (Chapko et al 1990). It is less common with standard intensity therapy. Although the clinical syndrome usually involves the oral cavity and pharynx, the underlying pathology commonly extends to other gastrointestinal mucosal surfaces, and symptoms may occur as a result of involvement of the oesophagus, stomach or intestine (e.g. odynophagia, dyspepsia or diarrhoea). Damaged mucosal surfaces may become superinfected with microorganisms, such as

Candida albicans or herpes simplex. The latter complication is most likely in neutropenic patients, who are also predisposed to systemic sepsis arising from local invasion by aerobic and anaerobic oral flora. Numerous therapies have been developed to reduce the risk of mucositis, including the use of cryotherapy (Mahood et al 1991), surface coating agents (Pfeiffer et al 1990; Barker et al 1991), antibiotics (Spijkervet et al 1991), antiviral agents (Redding 1990) and disinfectant mouthwashes (Ferretti et al 1990). Severe mucositis usually requires both local and systemic analgesic therapies Studies in bone marrow transplant patients have demonstrated the efficacy of patient-controlled analgesic techniques in this setting (Hill et al 1990, 1991).

Corticosteroid-induced perineal discomfort

A transient burning sensation in the perineum is described by some patients following rapid infusion of large doses (20–100 mg) of dexamethasone (Elliott & Foley 1989). Patients need to be warned that such symptoms may occur. Clinical experience suggests that this syndrome is prevented by slow infusion.

Steroid pseudorheumatism

A second acute pain syndrome associated with the use of corticosteroids manifests as diffuse myalgias, arthralgias, and tenderness of muscles and joints following dose reduction. These symptoms occur with rapid or slow withdrawal and may occur in patients taking these drugs for long or short periods of time. The pathogenesis of this syndrome is poorly understood, but it has been speculated that steroid withdrawal may sensitize joint and muscle mechanoreceptors and nociceptors (Rotstein & Good 1957). Treatment consists of reinstituting steroid therapy and tapering the drug more slowly (Rotstein & Good 1957).

Painful peripheral neuropathy

Chemotherapy-induced painful peripheral neuropathy, which is usually associated with vinca alkaloids and cisplatinum, can have an acute course. The vinca alkaloids (particularly vincristine) are also associated with other, presumably neuropathic, acute pain syndromes, including pain in the jaw, legs, arms or abdomen that may last from hours to days (Holland et al 1973; McDonald 1991).

Headache

Intrathecal methotrexate therapy produces an acute meningitic syndrome in 5–50% of patients treated for leukaemia or leptomeningeal metastases (Weiss et al 1974). Headache is the prominent symptom and may be associated with vomiting, nuchal rigidity, fever, irritability and lethargy. Symptoms usually begin hours after intrathecal treatment and persist for several days. Cerebrospinal fluid (CSF) examination reveals a pleocytosis that may mimic bacterial meningitis. Patients at increased risk for the development of this syndrome include those who have received multiple intrathecal injections and those patients undergoing treatment for proven leptomeningeal metastases (Weiss et al 1974). The syndrome tends not to recur with subsequent injections.

Systemic administration of L-asparaginase for the treatment of acute lymphoblastic leukaemia is associated with thrombosis of cerebral veins or dural sinuses in 1-2% of patients (Feinberg & Swenson 1988). This complication occurs as a result of depletion of asparagene, which, in turn, leads to the reduction of plasma proteins involved in coagulation and fibrinolysis. Headache is the most common initial symptom, and seizures, hemiparesis, delirium, vomiting or cranial nerve palsies may also occur. This complication typically occurs after a few weeks of therapy, but its onset may be delayed until after the completion of treatment. The diagnosis may be established by angiography or by gradient echo sequences on MRI scan (Moots et al 1987).

Transretinoic acid therapy, which may be used in the treatment of acute promyelocytic leukaemia (APML), can cause a transient severe headache (Huang et al 1988). The mechanism may be related to pseudotumour cerebri induced by hypervitaminosis A.

Diffuse bone pain

Acute bone pain is another common adverse effect of transretinoic acid therapy in patients with APML (Castaigne et al 1990). The pain is generalized, variable in intensity, and closely associated with a transient neutrophilia. The latter observation suggests that the pain may be due to marrow expansion, a phenomenon that may underlie a similar pain syndrome that occurs following the administration of colony stimulating factors (Balmer 1991; Hollingshead & Goa 1991).

5-Fluorouracil-induced anginal chest pain

Patients receiving continuous infusions of 5-fluorouracil (5-FU) may develop ischaemic chest pain (Freeman & Costanza 1988; Eskilsson & Albertsson 1990). Continuous ambulatory electrocardiographic (ECG) monitoring of patients undergoing 5-FU infusion demonstrated a near three-fold increase in ischaemic episodes over pretreatment recordings (Rezkalla et al 1989); these ECG changes were more common among patients with known coronary artery disease. It is widely speculated that coronary vasospasm may be the underlying mechanism

(Freeman & Costanza 1988; Rezkalla et al 1989; Eskilsson & Albertsson 1990).

Postchemotherapy gynaecomastia

Painful gynaecomastia can occur as a delayed complication of chemotherapy. Testis cancer is the most common underlying disorder (Trump et al 1982; Saeter et al 1987) but other cancers may also be associated (Schorer et al 1978; Sherins et al 1978; Trump et al 1982). Gynaecomastia typically develops after a latency of 2–9 months and resolves spontaneously within a few months. Persistent gynaecomastia is occasionally observed (Trump et al 1982). Cytotoxic-induced disturbance of androgen secretion is the probable cause of this syndrome (Trump et al 1982; Saeter et al 1987 ; Hands & Greenall 1991). In patients with testicular cancer, this treatment-related syndrome must be differentiated from tumour-related gynaecomastia, which may herald early recurrence (see p. 813) (Trump & Anderson 1983; Tseng et al 1985; Saeter et al 1987).

Acute pain associated with hormonal therapy

Luteinizing hormone releasing factor (LHRF) tumour flare in prostate cancer

Initiation of LHRF hormonal therapy for prostate cancer produces a transient symptom flare in 5–25% of patients (Thompson et al 1990; Chrisp & Sorkin 1991). The flare is presumably caused by an initial stimulation of luteinizing hormone release before suppression is achieved (Chrisp & Sorkin 1991; Goldspiel & Kohler 1991). The syndrome typically presents as an exacerbation of bone pain or urinary retention; spinal cord compression and sudden death have also been reported (Ahmann et al 1987; Thompson et al 1990). Symptom flare is usually observed within the first week of therapy and lasts 1–3 weeks in the absence of androgen antagonist therapy. Coadministration of an androgen antagonist at the start of LHRF agonist therapy can prevent this phenomenon (Labrie et al 1987; Lunglmayr 1989; Crawford & Nabors 1991).

Hormone-induced pain flare in breast cancer

Any hormonal therapy for metastatic breast cancer can also precipitate a sudden onset of diffuse musculoskeletal pain that usually commences within hours to weeks of the initiation of therapy. Other manifestations of this syndrome include erythema around cutaneous lesions, changes in liver function studies mechanism and hypercalcaemia. Although the underlying is not understood, there is little evidence that the flare is caused by tumour stimulation, and it is speculated that it may reflect normal tissue response (Henderson & Harris 1991).

Acute pain associated with immunotherapy

Interferon (IFN)-induced acute pain

Virtually all patients treated with IFN experience an acute syndrome consisting of fever, chills, myalgias, arthralgias and headache (Quesada et al 1986). The syndrome usually begins shortly after initial dosing and frequently improves with continued administration of the drug (Jones & Itri 1986; Quesada et al 1986). The severity of symptoms is related to type of IFN, route of administration, schedule and dose. Doses of 1–9 million units of alpha-interferon are usually well tolerated, but doses greater than or equal to 18 million units usually produce moderate to severe toxicity (Quesada et al 1986). Acetaminophen pretreatment is often useful in ameliorating these symptoms (Jones & Itri 1986).

Acute pain associated with radiotherapy

Incident pains can be precipitated by transport and positioning of the patient for radiotherapy. Other pains can be caused by acute radiation toxicity, which is most commonly associated with inflammation and ulceration of mucous membranes within the radiation port. The syndrome produced is dependent upon the involved field: head and neck irradiation can cause a stomatitis or pharyngitis (Rider 1990), treatment of the chest and oesophagus can cause an oesophagitis, and pelvic therapy can cause a proctitis, cystitis-urethritis or vaginal ulceration. Rare syndromes involve skin or neural tissues.

Oropharyngeal mucositis

Radiotherapy-induced mucositis is invariable with doses above 1000 cGy, and ulceration is common at doses above 4000 cGy. Although the severity of the associated pain is variable, it is often severe enough to interfere with oral alimentation. Painful mucositis can persist for several weeks after the completion of the treatment (Epstein et al 1991).

Acute radiation enteritis and proctocolitis

Abdominal or pelvic radiotherapy causes acute radiation enteritis in as many as 50% of patients. Involvement of the small intestine can present with cramping abdominal pain associated with nausea and diarrhoea (Earnest & Trier 1989; Buchi 1991). Proctocolitis produces rectal pain, tenesmus, diarrhoea, mucous discharge and bleeding (Earnest & Trier 1989). These complications typically resolve shortly after completion of therapy, but may have a slow resolution over 2–6 months (Earnest & Trier 1989; Buchi 1991). Acute enteritis is associated with an increased risk of late-onset radiation enteritis (see p. 816) (Earnest & Trier 1989).

Early-onset brachial plexopathy

A transient brachial plexopathy has been described in breast cancer patients immediately following radiotherapy to the chest wall and adjacent nodal areas. In retrospective studies, the incidence of this phenomenon has been variably estimated as 1.4–20% (Salner et al 1981; Fulton 1987); clinical experience suggests that lower estimates are more accurate. The median latency to the development of symptoms was 4.5 months (range 3–14 months) in one survey (Salner et al 1981). Paraesthesias are the most common presenting symptom, and pain and weakness occur less frequently. The syndrome is self-limiting and does not predispose to the subsequent development of delayed onset, progressive plexopathy (see p. 808).

Subacute radiation myelopathy

Subacute radiation myelopathy can occur following radiotherapy of extraspinal tumours (Cascino 1991). It is most frequently observed involving the cervical cord after radiation treatment of head and neck cancers and Hodgkin's disease. In the latter case, patients develop painful, shock-like pains in the neck that are precipitated by neck flexion (Lhermitte's sign); these pains may radiate down the spine and into the one or more extremities. The syndrome usually begins weeks to months after the completion of radiotherapy, and typically resolves over a period of 3–6 months (Cascino 1991).

ACUTE PAIN ASSOCIATED WITH INFECTION

Acute herpetic neuralgia

Cancer patients, especially those with haematological or lymphoproliferative malignancies and those receiving immunosuppressive therapies, have a significantly increased incidence of acute herpetic neuralgia (Portenoy et al 1986; Rusthoven et al 1988b). Pain or itch usually precedes the development of a dermatomal rash by several days and may occasionally occur without the development of skin eruption. The pain, which may be continuous or lancinating, usually resolves within 2 months (Portenoy et al 1986). Pain persisting beyond this interval is referred to as postherpetic neuralgia (see p. 807). Patients with active tumour are also more likely to disseminate the infection (Rusthoven et al 1988a). In those predisposed by chemotherapy, zoster usually develops less than 1 month after the completion of treatment. The location of the infection is associated with the site of the malignancy (Rusthoven et al 1988a): Patients with primary tumours of gynaecological and genitourinary origin have a predilection to lumbar and sacral involvement, and those with breast or lung carcinomas tend to present with thoracic involvement; patients with haematologic tumours appear to be predisposed to cervical lesions. The infection also occurs twice as frequently in previously irradiated dermatomes as nonradiated areas.

CHRONIC PAIN SYNDROMES

Most chronic cancer-related pains are caused directly by the tumour (Table 43.4) (Twycross & Fairfield 1982; Daut & Cleeland 1982; Foley 1985, 1987; Banning et al 1991). Bone pain and compression of neural structures are the most prevalent conditions (Daut & Cleeland 1982; Twycross & Fairfield 1982; Foley 1985, 1987; Banning et al 1991; Portenoy et al 1992).

Table 43.4 Cancer-related chronic pain syndromes

Tumour-related pain syndromes
Bone pain
Multifocal or generalized bone pain
Multiple bony metastases
Marrow expansion
Vertebral syndromes
Atlantoaxial destruction and odontoid fractures
C7–T1 syndrome
T12–L1 syndrome
Sacral syndrome
Back pain and epidural compression
Pain syndromes of the bony pelvis and hip
Hip joint syndrome
Headache and facial pain
Intracerebral tumour
Leptomeningeal metastases
Base of skull metastases
Orbital syndrome
Parasellar syndrome
Middle cranial fossa syndrome
Jugular foramen syndrome
Clivus syndrome
Sphenoid sinus syndrome
Painful cranial neuralgias
Glossopharyngeal neuralgia
Trigeminal neuralgia
Tumour involvement of the peripheral nervous system
Tumour-related radiculopathy
Postherpetic neuralgia
Cervical plexopathy
Brachial plexopathy
Malignant brachial plexopathy
Idiopathic brachial plexopathy associated with Hodgkin's disease
Malignant lumbosacral plexopathy
Tumour-related mononeuropathy
Paraneoplastic painful peripheral neuropathy
Subacute sensory neuropathy
Sensorimotor peripheral neuropathy
Pain syndromes of the viscera and miscellaneous tumour-related syndromes
Hepatic distension syndrome
Midline retroperitoneal syndrome
Chronic intestinal obstruction
Peritoneal carcinomatosis
Malignant perineal pain
Malignant pelvic floor myalgia
Ureteric obstruction
Paraneoplastic nociceptive pain syndromes
Tumour-related gynaecomastia

Table 43.4 *(contd)*

Chronic pain syndromes associated with cancer therapy
Postchemotherapy pain syndromes
Chronic painful peripheral neuropathy
Avascular necrosis of femoral or humeral head
Plexopathy associated with intraarterial infusion
Chronic pain associated with hormonal therapy
Gynaecomastia with hormonal therapy for prostate cancer
Chronic postsurgical pain syndromes
Postmastectomy pain syndrome
Postradical neck dissection pain
Postthoracotomy pain
Postoperative frozen shoulder
Phantom pain syndromes
Phantom limb pain
Phantom breast pain
Phantom anus pain
Phantom bladder pain
Stump pain
Postsurgical pelvic floor myalgia
Chronic postradiation pain syndromes
Plexopathies
Radiation-induced brachial and lumbosacral plexopathies
Radiation-induced peripheral nerve tumour
Chronic radiation myelopathy
Chronic radiation enteritis and proctitis
Burning perineum syndrome
Osteoradionecrosis

BONE PAIN

Bone metastases are the most common cause of chronic pain in the cancer population (Twycross & Lack 1984; Foley 1985; Payne 1989b; Banning et al 1991; Nielsen et al 1991). Cancers of the lung, breast and prostate most often metastasize to bone, but any tumour type may be complicated by painful bony lesions. Although bone pain is usually associated with direct tumour invasion of bony structures, more than 25% of patients with bony metastases are pain-free (Wagner 1984) and patients with multiple bony metastases typically report pain in only a few sites (Fig. 43.3). The factors that convert a painless lesion to a painful one are unknown. Bone metastases could potentially cause pain by any of multiple mechanisms, including endosteal or periosteal nociceptor activation (by mechanical distortion or release of chemical mediators) or tumour growth into adjacent soft tissues and nerves (Nielsen et al 1991).

Bone pain due to metastatic tumour needs to be differentiated from less common causes of chronic bone pain in cancer patients. Nonneoplastic causes in this population include osteoporotic fractures (including those associated with multiple myeloma) and focal osteonecrosis, which may be idiopathic or related to corticosteroids or radiotherapy (see p. 814, 817).

Multifocal or generalized bone pain

Bone pain may be focal, multifocal or generalized. A generalized pain syndrome, which is well recognized in patients with multiple bony metastases, is also rarely produced by replacement of bone marrow (Jonsson et al 1991). This bone marrow replacement syndrome has been observed in both haematogenous malignancies and, less commonly, solid tumours (Jonsson et al 1991). This syndrome can occur in the absence of abnormalities on bone scintigraphy or radiography, increasing the difficulty of diagnosis.

Vertebral syndromes

The vertebrae are the most common sites of bony metastases. More than two-thirds of vertebral metastases are located in the thoracic spine; lumbosacral and cervical metastases account for approximately 20% and 10% respectively (Gilbert et al 1978; Sorensen et al 1990). Multiple level involvement is common, occurring in greater than 85% of patients (Constans et al 1983). The early recognition of pain syndromes due to neoplastic invasion of vertebral bodies is essential, since pain usually precedes compression of adjacent neural structures and prompt treatment of the lesion may prevent the subsequent development of neurological deficits. Clinical recognition often requires substantial acumen; referral of pain is common and the associated symptoms and signs can mimic a variety of other disorders, both malignant (e.g. paraspinal masses) and nonmalignant.

Atlantoaxial destruction and odontoid fracture

Destruction of the atlas or fracture of the odontoid process typically presents with nuchal or occipital pain. Pain often radiates over the posterior aspect of the skull to the vertex and is exacerbated by movement of the neck, particularly flexion (Phillips & Levine 1989). Pathological fracture may result in secondary subluxation with compression of the spinal cord at the cervicomedullary junction. Compression is usually insidious and may begin with symptoms or signs in one or more extremity. There may be early involvement of the upper extremities and the occasional appearance of so-called ‘pseudolevels' suggestive of more caudal spinal lesions; these deficits can slowly progress to involve sensory, motor and autonomic function in the extremities (Sundaresan et al 1981). MRI is probably the best method for imaging this region of the spine (Bosley et al 1985), but clinical experience suggests that CT is also sensitive. Plain radiography, tomography and bone scintigraphy should be viewed as ancillary procedures.

C7–T1 syndrome

Invasion of the C7 or T1 vertebra can result in pain referred to the interscapular region. These lesions may be missed if radiographic evaluation is mistakenly targeted to the painful area caudal to the site of damage. Additionally,

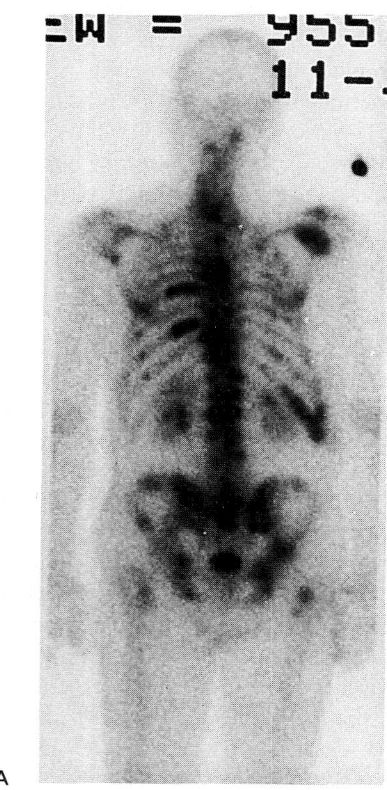

A

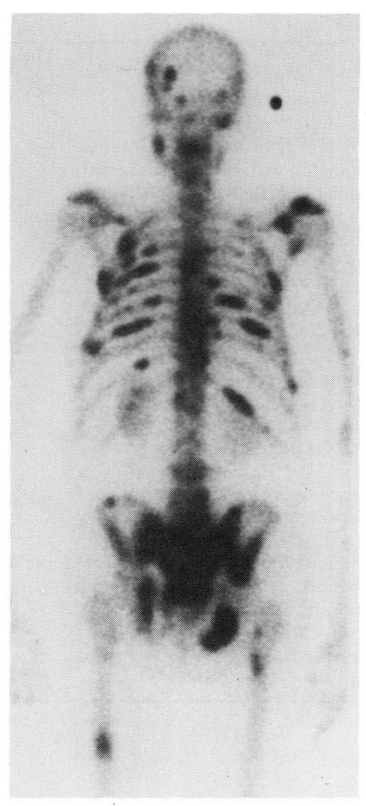

B

Fig. 43.3 Bone scans of two patients with prostate cancer – one with and one without bone pain. Scan A is that of a 64-year-old man with diffuse multifocal bone pain involving ribs, back and pelvis. Scan B was performed as a staging investigation in an asymptomatic 70 year old.

visualization of the appropriate region on routine radiographs may be inadequate due to obscuration by overlying bone and mediastinal shadows. Patients with interscapular pain should therefore undergo radiography of both the cervical and the thoracic spine. Bone scintigraphy may assist in targeting additional diagnostic imaging procedures, particularly CT or MRI. The latter procedures can also be useful in assessing the possibility that pain is referred from an extraspinal site, such as the paraspinal gutter.

T12–L1 syndrome

A T12 or L1 vertebral lesion can refer pain to the ipsilateral iliac crest or the sacroiliac joint. Imaging procedures directed at pelvic bones can miss the source of the pain.

Sacral syndrome

Severe focal pain radiating to buttocks, perineum or posterior thighs may accompany destruction of the sacrum. The pain is often exacerbated by sitting or lying and is relieved by standing or walking. The neoplasm can spread laterally to involve muscles that rotate the hip (e.g. the pyriformis muscle).This may produce severe incident pain induced by motion of the hip, or a malignant 'pyriformis syndrome', characterized by buttock or posterior leg pain that is exacerbated by internal rotation of the hip. Local extension of the tumour mass may also involve the sacral plexus (see p. 809).

Back pain and epidural compression

Epidural compression (EC) of the spinal cord or cauda equina is the second most common neurological complication of cancer, occurring in up to 10% of patients (Posner 1987). In the community setting, EC is often the first recognized manifestation of malignancy (Stark et al 1982); at a cancer hospital it is the presenting syndrome in only 8% of cases (Posner 1987). Most EC is caused by posterior extension of vertebral body metastasis to the epidural space. Occasionally, EC is caused by tumour extension from the posterior arch of the vertebra or infiltration of a paravertebral tumour through the intervertebral foramen.

Untreated, EC leads inevitably to neurological compromise, ultimately including paraplegia or quadriplegia.

Effective treatment can potentially prevent these complications. The efficacy of treatment is determined by numerous factors, the most salient of which is the degree of neurological impairment at the time therapy is initiated. Of patients who begin treatment while ambulatory, 75% remain so; the efficacy of treatment declines to 30–50% for those who begin treatment while markedly paretic and is less than 10% for those who are plegic (Gilbert et al 1978; Barcena et al 1984; Posner 1987; Portenoy et al 1989; Ruff & Lanska 1989). Treatment generally involves the administration of corticosteroids (see p. 803) and radiotherapy. Surgical decompression is considered for some patients with radioresistant tumours, those who have previously received maximal radiotherapy to the involved field, those with spinal instability, and those for whom no other tissue is available for histological diagnosis (Posner 1987; Grant et al 1991b). Decompressive laminectomy for posteriorly located lesions and anterior vertebrectomy with spinal stabilization for lesions arising from the vertebral body are the currently recommended procedures (Harrington 1984; Sundaresan et al 1984, 1985). Decompressive laminectomy in the setting of vertebral body collapse is not recommended because of the risk of neurological deterioration or spinal instability (22–25%) induced by the procedure (Brice & McKissock 1965; Findlay 1987).

Back pain is the initial symptom in almost all patients with EC (Posner 1987) and in 10% it is the only symptom at the time of diagnosis (Greenberg et al 1980). Since pain usually precedes neurological signs by a prolonged period, it should be viewed as a potential indicator of EC, which could lead to treatment at a time that a favourable response is most likely. Back pain, however, is a nonspecific symptom that can result from bony or paraspinal metastases without epidural encroachment, from retroperitoneal or leptomeningeal tumour, or from a large variety of benign conditions. Since it is infeasible to pursue an extensive evaluation in every cancer patient who develops back pain, the complaint should impel a systematic evaluation that determines the likelihood of EC and thereby selects patients appropriate for definitive imaging of the epidural space. This selection process is based on symptoms and signs and the results of simple and inexpensive imaging techniques.

Clinical features of epidural extension

Some pain characterisitics are particularly suggestive of epidural extension (Obbens & Posner 1987). Rapid progression of back pain in a crescendo pattern is a particularly ominous occurrence. Radicular pain, which can be constant or lancinating, has similar implications. Radicular pain is usually unilateral in the cervical and lumbosacral regions and bilateral in the thorax, where it is often experienced as a tight, belt-like band across the chest or abdomen. The likelihood of EC is greater when back or radicular pain is exacerbated by recumbency, cough, sneeze or strain (Obbens & Posner 1987; Ruff & Lanska 1989). Other types of referred pain are also suggestive, including Lhermitte's sign (Stillman & Foley 1991) and central pain from spinal cord compression, which is usually perceived some distance below the site of the compression and is typically a poorly localized, nondermatomal dysaesthesia.

Weakness, sensory loss, autonomic dysfunction and reflex abnormalities usually occur after a period of progressive pain. Weakness may begin in a segmental distribution if related to nerve root damage or in a multisegmental or pyramidal distribution if the cauda equina or spinal cord, respectively, is injured. The rate of progression of weakness is variable; in the absence of treatment paralysis will follow the onset of weakness within 7 days in one-third of patients (Barron et al 1959). Patients whose weakness progresses slowly have a better prognosis for neurological recovery with treatment than those who progress rapidly (Helweg et al 1990). Without effective treatment, sensory abnormalities, which may also begin segmentally, may ultimately evolve to a sensory level, with complete loss of all sensory modalities below the site of injury. The upper level of sensory findings may correspond to the location of the epidural tumour or be below it by many segments. Ataxia without pain is the initial presentation of epidural compression in only 1% of patients; this finding is presumably due to early involvement of the spinocerebellar tracts (Gilbert et al 1978). Bladder and bowel dysfunction occur late, except in patients with a conus medullaris lesion who may present with acute urinary retention and constipation without preceding motor or sensory symptoms (Stillman & Foley 1991).

Other features that may be evident on examination of patients with EC include scoliosis, asymmetrical wasting of paravertebral musculature and a gibbus (palpable step in the spinous processes). Spinal tenderness to percussion, which may be severe, often accompanies the pain.

Imaging modalities

Definitive imaging of the epidural space confirms the existence of EC (and thereby indicates the necessity and urgency of treatment), defines the appropriate radiation portals and determines the extent of epidural encroachment (which influences prognosis and may alter the therapeutic approach) (Portenoy et al 1987). The options for definitive imaging include MRI, myelography, and CT-myelography (Figs 43.4 and 43.5). MRI, which is noninvasive and offers accurate soft-tissue imaging and multiplanar views, is generally preferred. It should be recognized, however, that there are no studies comparing state-of-the-art MRI techniques with myelog-

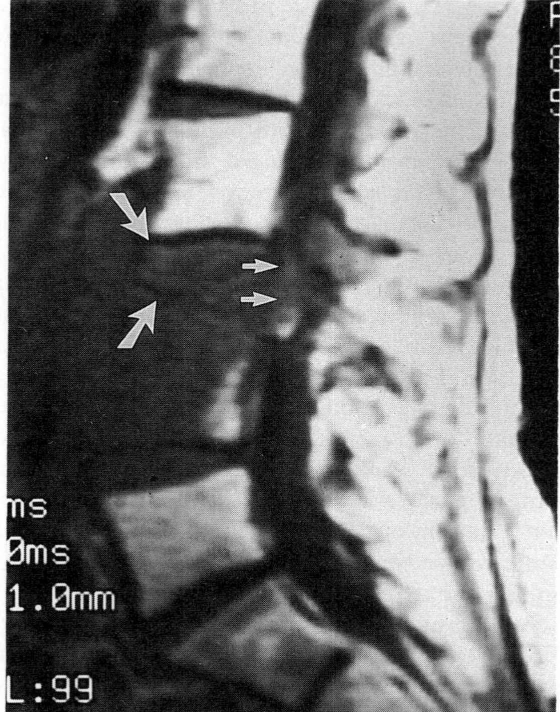

A

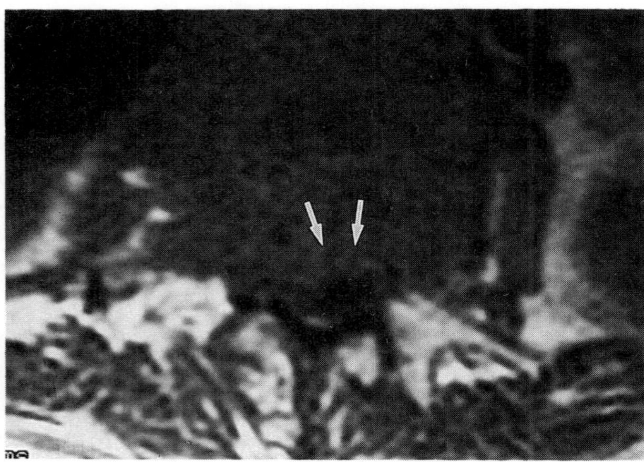

B

Fig. 43.4 Sagittal (A) and axial (B) MRI scans of the lumbar spine in a 56-year-old woman with carcinoma of the colon who presented with back pain and L3 radicular pain in the right leg. The sagittal scan demonstrates extensive destruction of both L3 and L4 vertebral bodies (vertical arrows). There is posterior extension of the tumour into the epidural space, which compress the spinal cord (horizontal arrows). The axial scan performed through L3 demonstrates complete obliteration of the epidural space (arrows) and severe compression of the thecal sac.

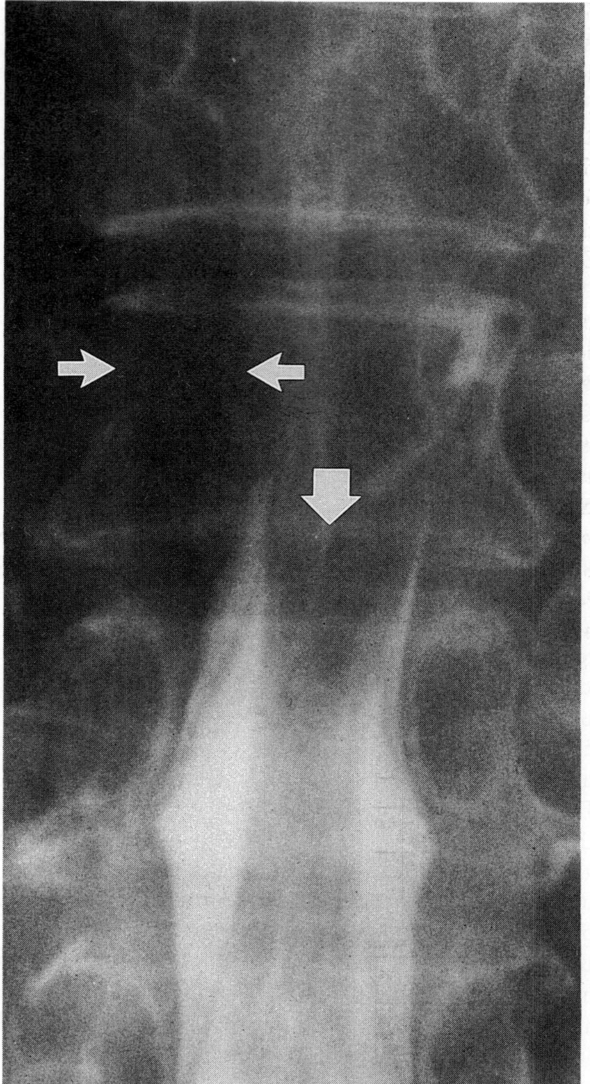

Fig. 43.5 Segment of thoracic myelogram (T8, 9, 10 and 11) performed on a 54-year-old woman with severe mid-back pain. There is a complete block to the flow of contrast at the T9 level (large arrow) The left pedicle of the T9 vertebra is absent due to metastatic erosion (small arrows).

raphy in the evaluation of EC, and some data suggest that some techniques, such as a 'scanning' mid-sagittal MRI, are clearly inadequate (Hagen et al 1989). Myelography remains the investigation of choice for patients who lack access to MRI and those unable to undergo the procedure. MRI is relatively contraindicated in patients with severe claustrophobia and absolutely contraindicated for patients with metallic implants, cardiac pacemakers or aneurysm clips. Myelography may be the only feasible procedure in some who would benefit from total spinal imaging (such as those with multifocal pain or multiple spinal metastases who have a 10% chance of EC remote from the symptomatic site (Stark et al 1982) and others with severe kyphosis or scoliosis. Myelography should also be considered following a MRI scan that is suboptimal or nondiagnostic, particularly in the setting of neurological deterioration.

Algorithm for the investigation of cancer patients with back pain

Given the prevalence and the potentially dire consequences of EC, and the recognition that back pain is a marker of early (and therefore treatable) EC, algorithms have been developed to guide the evaluation of back pain in the cancer patient. The objective of these algorithms is to select a subgroup who should undergo definitive imaging of the epidural space from amongst the large number of patients who develop back pain. Effective treatment of EC before irreversible neurological compromise occurs is the overriding goal of these approaches.

One such algorithm defines both the urgency and course of the evaluation (Fig. 43.6) (Portenoy et al 1987). Patients with emerging symptoms and signs indicative of spinal cord or cauda equina dysfunction are designated Group 1. The evaluation (and if appropriate, treatment) of these patients should proceed on an emergency basis. In most cases, these patients should receive an intravenous dose of corticosteroid before epidural imaging is performed. Dexamethasone is used customarily. High doses have been advocated on the basis of animal studies (Delattre et al 1989), analgesic efficacy (Greenberg et al 1980) and the dose–response relationship that has been observed during treatment of intracranial hypertension from mass lesions. One regimen advocates an initial IV bolus of 100 mg followed by 96 mg per day in divided doses, which is tapered over 3–4 weeks. Although a randomized trial failed to identify any difference in neurological outcome between a high (100 mg) and low (10 mg) initial dose (Vecht et al 1989a), these findings need to be replicated on a larger sample, and high doses can still be recommended on the basis of a favourable clinical experience.

Patients with symptoms and signs of radiculopathy or stable or mild signs of spinal cord or cauda equina dysfunction are designated Group 2. These patients are also usually treated presumptively with a corticosteroid (typically with a more moderate dose) and are scheduled for definitive imaging of the epidural space as soon as possible.

Group 3 patients have back pain and no symptoms or signs suggesting EC. These patients should be evaluated in routine fashion. The first step consists of plain spine radiographs. The presence at the appropriate level of any abnormality consistent with neoplasm indicates a high probability (60%) of EC (Rodichok et al 1981). This likelihood varies, however, with the type of radiological abnormality; for example, one study noted that EC

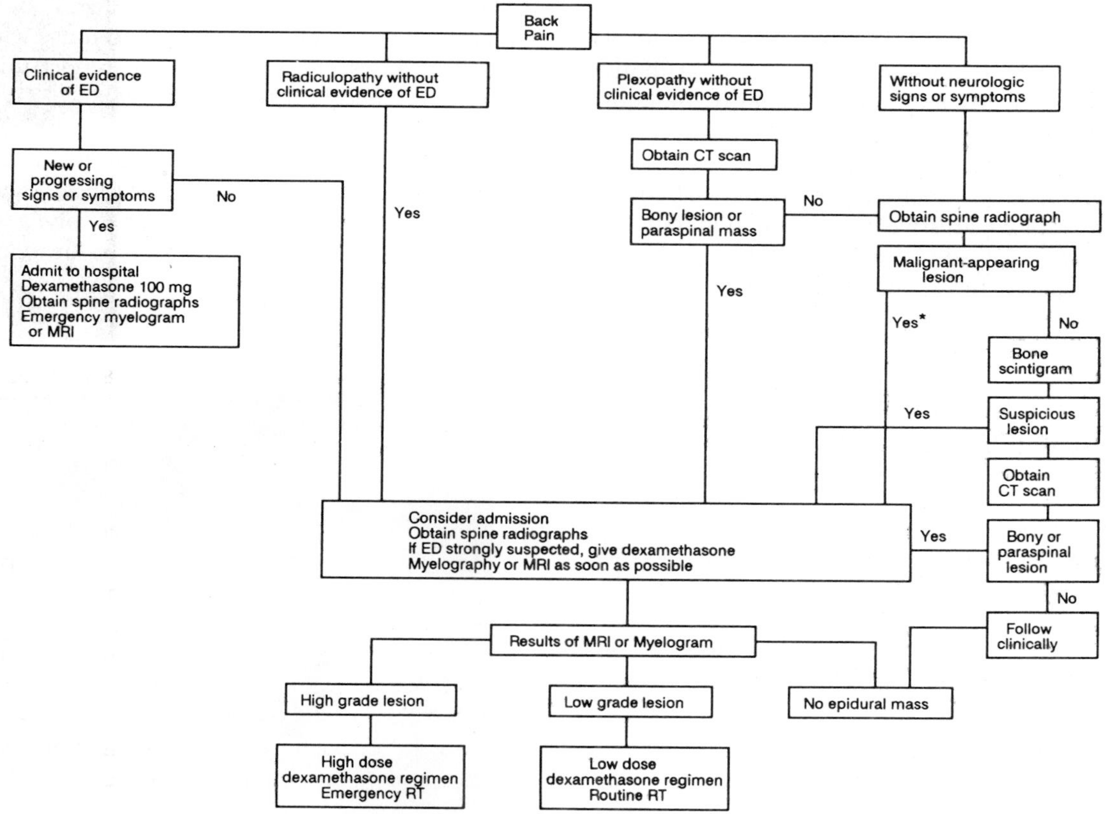

Fig. 43.6 Algorithm for the mangement of back pain in the cancer patient. (From Portenoy 1993b with permission.)
ED = epidural disease; CT = computerized tomogram; MRI = magnetic resonance imaging; RT = radiation therapy.
* Definitive imaging is strongly recommended if vertebral collapse is present. The clinician may consider foregoing definitive imaging if lesion is limited to the body of the vertebra. A CT scan may be needed to define the limits of the lesion; definitive imaging should be done if the bony cortex adjacent to the spinal canal is comprised.

occurred in 87% patients with greater than 50% vertebral body collapse, 31% with pedicle erosion, and only 7% with tumour limited to the body of the vertebra without collapse (Graus et al 1986b). Definitive imaging of the epidural space is thus strongly indicated in patients who have >50% vertebral body collapse, and is generally recommended for patients with pedicle erosion. Some patients with neoplasm limited to the vertebral body can be followed expectantly; imaging should be performed if pain progresses or changes (e.g. become radicular), or if radiographic evidence of progression is obtained.

Normal spine radiographs alone are not adequate to ensure a low likelihood of epidural tumour in patients with back pain. The bone may not be sufficiently damaged to change the radiograph or the tumour may involve the epidural space with little or no involvement of the adjacent bone (such as may occur when paraspinal tumour grows through the intervertebral foramen). The latter phenomenon has been most strikingly demonstrated in patients with lymphoma, in whom EC presents with normal radiography more than 60% of the time (Haddad et al 1976). Damage to the vertebra that is not seen on the plain radiograph may potentially be demonstrated by bone scintigraphy. In patients with back pain and normal bone radiography, a positive scintigram at the site of pain is associated with a 12–17% likelihood of epidural disease (O'Rourke et al 1986; Portenoy et al 1989). Although such patients can also be followed expectantly, definitive imaging of the epidural space should be considered, particularly if the pain is progressive.

If both radiographs and scintigraphy are normal but the patient has severe or progressive pain, evaluation with CT, or preferably MRI, may still be warranted. If the CT scan demonstrates either a bony lesion abutting the spinal canal or a paraspinal mass, imaging of the epidural space is still justified (Portenoy et al 1989).

Pain syndromes of the bony pelvis and hip

The pelvis and hip are common sites of metastatic involvement. Lesions may involve any of the three anatomic regions of the pelvis, (ischiopubic, illiosacral or periacetabular), the hip joint itself or the proximal femur (Sim 1988). The weight-bearing function of these structures, essential for normal ambulation, contributes to the propensity of disease at these sites to cause incident pain with ambulation.

Hip joint syndrome

Tumour involvement of the acetabulum or head of femur typically produces localized hip pain that is aggravated by weight bearing and movement of the hip. The pain may radiate to the knee or medial thigh and, occasionally, pain is limited to these structures (Sim 1988). Medial extension of an acetabular tumour can involve the lumbosacral plexus as it traverses the pelvic sidewall (Fig. 43.7). Evaluation of this region is best accomplished with CT or MRI, both of which can demonstrate the extent of bony destruction and adjacent soft tissue involvement more sensitively than other imaging techniques (Beatrous et al 1990).

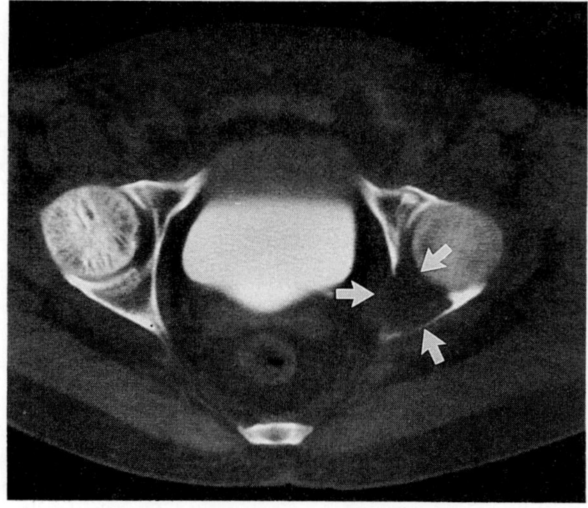

Fig. 43.7 CT scan demonstrating lytic lesion of the right acetabulum (arrows) with tumour extension into the pelvis.

HEADACHE AND FACIAL PAIN

Headache in the cancer patient results from traction, inflammation or infiltration of pain-sensitive structures in the head or neck (Posner 1992). Early evaluation with appropriate imaging techniques may identify the lesion and allow prompt treatment, which may reduce pain and prevent the development of neurological deficits.

Intracerebral tumour

The prevalence of headache in patients with brain metastases or primary brain tumours is 60–90% (Forsyth & Posner 1993). The headache is presumably produced by traction of pain-sensitive vascular and dural tissues. Patients with multiple metastases and those with posterior fossa metastases are more likely to report this symptom (Posner & Chernik 1978; Fadul et al 1987; Forsyth & Posner 1993). The pain may be focal, overlying the site of the lesion, or generalized. Posterior fossa lesions often cause a bifrontal headache (Posner 1992). The quality of the headache is usually throbbing or steady, and the intensity is usually mild to moderate. The headache is often worse in the morning and is exacerbated by stooping, sudden head movement or valsalva manoeuvres (cough, sneeze or strain). In patients with increased intracranial pressure, these manoeuvres can also precipitate transient elevations in intracranial pressure called 'plateau waves.' These plateau waves, which may also be spontaneous, can be associated with short periods of severe headache, nausea, vomiting, photophobia, lethargy and transient neurological deficits (Vick & Rottenberg 1992). Occasionally these plateau waves produce life-threatening herniation syndromes (Vick & Rottenberg 1992).

Leptomeningeal metastases

Leptomeningeal metastases are characterized by diffuse or multifocal involvement of the subarachnoid space by metastatic tumour. Autopsy studies demonstrate an incidence of 1–8% in patients with systemic cancer (Posner & Chernik 1978). Non-Hodgkin's lymphoma and acute lymphocytic leukaemia both demonstrate predilection for meningeal metastases; the incidence is lower for solid tumours alone. Of solid tumours, adenocarcinomas of the breast and lung predominate.

Leptomeningeal metastases present with focal or multifocal neurological symptoms or signs that may involve any level of the neuraxis (Henson & Urich 1982; Wasserstrom et al 1982). More than one-third of patients presents with evidence of cranial nerve damage, including double vision, hearing loss, facial numbness, or decreased vision (Wasserstrom et al 1982). Less common features include seizures, papilloedema, hemiparesis and ataxic gait.

Generalized headache, and radicular pain in the low back and buttocks are the most common pains associated with leptomeningeal metastases (Wasserstrom et al 1982; Kaplan et al 1990). The headache is variable and may be associated with changes in mental status (e.g. lethargy, confusion or loss of memory), nausea, vomiting, tinnitus or nuchal rigidity. Pains that resemble cluster headache (DeAngelis & Payne 1987), or glossopharyngeal neuralgia with syncope (Sozzi et al 1987) have also been reported.

The diagnosis of leptomeningeal metastases is confirmed through analysis of the CSF. The CSF may reveal elevated pressure, elevated protein, depressed glucose, and/or lymphocytic pleocytosis. Some 90% of patients ultimately show positive cytology, but multiple analyses may be required. After a single LP, the false negative rate may be as high as 55%; this declines to only 10% after three LPs (Olsen et al 1974; Wasserstrom et al 1982; Kaplan et al 1990). Tumour markers, such as lactic dehydrogenase (LDH) isoenzymes (Fleisher et al 1981), carcinoembryonic antigen (Twijnstra et al 1986b) and beta-2-microglobulin (Twijnstra et al 1986a) may help establish the diagnosis. Flow cytometry for detection of abnormal DNA content may be a useful adjunct to cytologic examination (Cibas et al 1987). Imaging studies may also be of value. MRI of the cranium and spinal cord with gadolinium enhancement is the most sensitive imaging modality (Fig. 43.8) (Dillon 1991; Manelfe 1991), but cost and availability may limit its utility at present. Myelography is abnormal in up to 30% of patients and CT or MRI of the head may demonstrate enhancement of the dural membranes or ventricular enlargement (Lee et al 1984; Krol et al 1988).

Untreated leptomeningeal metastases cause progressive neurological dysfunction at multiple sites, followed by death in 4–6 weeks. Treatment, which includes radiation therapy to the area of symptomatic involvement, corticosteroids, and intraventricular or intrathecal chemotherapy, can be salutary; for example, patients with breast carcinoma have a median survival of 7 months following therapy (Glass & Foley 1991).

Base of skull metastases

Base of skull metastases are associated with well-described clinical syndromes (Greenberg et al 1981) metastatic which are named according to the site of involvement: orbital, parasellar, middle fossa, jugular foramen, occipital condyle, clivus and sphenoid sinus. Cancers of the breast, lung and prostate are most commonly associated with this complication (Greenberg et al 1981), but any tumour type that metastasizes to bone may be responsible (Bingas 1974). When base of skull metastases are suspected, axial imaging with CT (including bone window settings) is the usual initial procedure (Fig. 43.9) (Greenberg et al 1981). MRI is

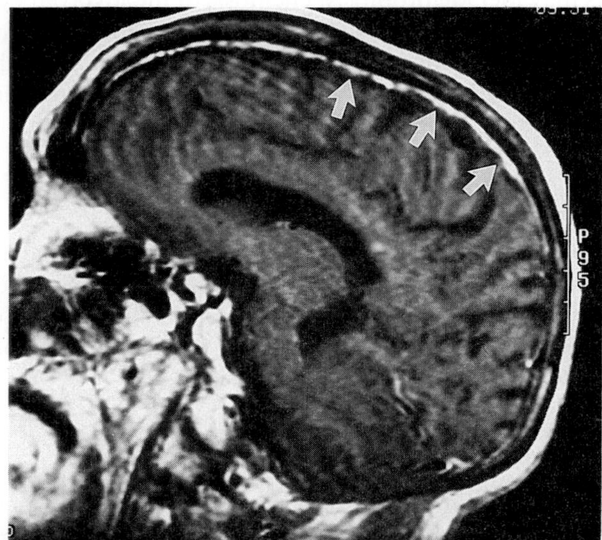

Fig. 43.8 Gadolium-enhanced MRI scan of the cranium in a 37-year-old woman with non-Hodgkin's lymphoma demonstrating meningeal enhancement (arrows) consistent with leptomeningeal metastases.

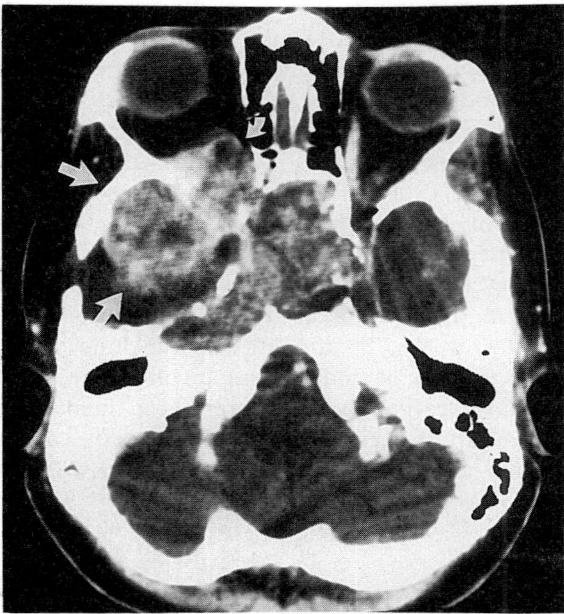

Fig. 43.9 CT scan of the base of skull of a woman with proptosis and right-sided facial pain. There is extensive tumour erosion of the orbital wall, clivus and the floor of the middle cranial fossa (arrows).

more sensitive for assessing soft-tissue extension, and CSF analysis may be needed to exclude leptomeningeal metastases.

Orbital syndrome

Orbital metastases usually present with progressive pain in the retroorbital and supraorbital area of the affected eye. Blurred vision and diplopia may be associated complaints. Signs may include proptosis, chemosis of the involved eye, external ophthalmoparesis, ipsilateral papilloedema and decreased sensation in the ophthalmic division of the trigeminal nerve. Imaging with MRI or CT scan can delineate the extent of bony damage and orbital infiltration.

Parasellar syndrome

The parasellar syndrome typically presents as unilateral supraorbital and frontal headache, which may be associated with diplopia. There may be ophthalmoparesis or papilloedema, and formal visual field testing may demonstrate hemianopsia or quadrantinopsia.

Middle cranial fossa syndrome

The middle cranial fossa syndrome presents with facial numbness, paraesthesias or pain, which is usually referred to the cheek or jaw (in the distribution of second or third divisions of the trigeminal nerve). The pain is typically described as a dull continual ache, but may also be paroxysmal or lancinating. On examination, patients may have hypaesthesia in the trigeminal nerve distribution and signs of weakness in the ipsilateral muscles of mastication. Occasional patients have other neurological signs, such as abducens palsy (Greenberg et al 1981; Bullitt et al 1986).

Jugular foramen syndrome

The jugular foramen syndrome usually presents with hoarseness or dysphagia. Pain is usually referred to the ipsilateral ear or mastoid region and may occasionally present as glossopharyngeal neuralgia, with or without syncope (Greenberg et al 1981). Pain may also be referred to the ipsilateral neck or shoulder. Neurological signs include ipsilateral Horner's syndrome and paresis of the palate, vocal cord, sternocleidomastoid or trapezius. Ipsilateral paresis of the tongue may also occur if the tumour extends to the region of the hypoglossal canal.

Occipital condyle syndrome

The occipital condyle syndrome presents with unilateral occipital pain that is worsened with neck flexion. The patient may complain of neck stiffness. Pain intensity is variable, but can be severe. Examination may reveal a head tilt, limited movement of the neck, and tenderness to palpation over the occipitonuchal junction. Neurological findings may include ipsilateral hypoglossal nerve paralysis and sternocleidomastoid weakness.

Clivus syndrome

The clivus syndrome is characterised by vertex headache, which is often exacerbated by neck flexion. Lower cranial nerve (VI–XII) dysfunction follows and may become bilateral.

Sphenoid sinus syndrome

A sphenoid sinus metastasis often presents with bifrontal and/or retroorbital pain, which may radiate to the temporal regions. There may be associated features of nasal congestion and diplopia. Physical examination is often unremarkable, although unilateral or bilateral sixth nerve paresis can be present.

Painful cranial neuralgias

As noted, specific cranial neuralgias can occur from metastases in the base of skull or leptomeninges. Invasion of the soft tissues of the head or neck, or involvement of sinuses can also eventuate in such lesions. Each of these syndromes has a characteristic presentation. Early diagnosis may allow effective treatment of the underlying lesion before progressive neurological injury occurs.

Glossopharyngeal neuralgia

Glossopharyngeal neuralgia has been reported in patients with leptomeningeal metastases (Sozzi et al 1987), the jugular foramen syndrome (Greenberg et al 1981) or head and neck malignancies (MacDonald et al 1983; Weinstein et al 1986; Dalessio 1991). This syndrome presents as severe pain in the throat or neck, which may radiate to the ear or mastoid region. Pain may be induced by swallowing. In some patients, pain is associated with sudden orthostasis and syncope.

Trigeminal neuralgia

Trigeminal pains may be continual, paroxysmal or lancinating. Pain that mimics classical trigeminal neuralgia can be induced by tumours in the middle or posterior fossa (Bullitt et al 1986) or leptomeningeal metastases (DeAngelis & Payne 1987). All cancer patients who develop trigeminal neuralgia should be evaluated for the existence of an underlying neoplasm.

Uncommon causes of headache and facial pain

Headache and facial pain in cancer patients may have many other causes. Unilateral facial pain can be the initial symptom of an ipsilateral lung tumour (Bindoff & Heseltine 1988). Presumably this referred pain is mediated by vagal afferents. Patients with Hodgkin's disease may have transient episodes of neurological dysfunction that has been likened to migraine (Feldmann & Posner 1986; Dulli et al 1987). Headache may occur with cerebral infarction or haemorrhage, which may be due to nonbacterial thrombotic endocarditis, disseminated intravascular coagulation or other cancer-related phenomena. Headache is also the usual presentation of sagittal sinus occlusion, which may be due to tumour infiltration, hypercoagulable state or treatment with L-asparaginase therapy (Feinberg & Swenson 1988). Headache due to pseudotumour cerebri has also been reported to be the presentation of superior vena canal obstruction in a patient with lung cancer (Portenoy et al 1983).

NEUROPATHIC PAINS INVOLVING THE PERIPHERAL NERVOUS SYSTEM

Neuropathic pains involving the peripheral nervous system are common and clinically challenging problems in the cancer population. The syndromes include painful radiculopathy, plexopathy, mononeuropathy or peripheral neuropathy.

Painful radiculopathy

Radiculopathy or polyradiculopathy may be caused by any process that compresses, distorts or inflames nerve roots.

Tumour-related radiculopathy

Painful radiculopathy is an important presentation of epidural tumour and leptomeningeal metastases (see p. 801, 805).

Postherpetic neuralgia

Postherpetic neuralgia is defined solely by the persistence of pain in the region of a zoster infection. Although some authors apply this term if pain continues beyond lesion healing, most require a period of weeks to months before this label is used; a criterion of pain persisting beyond 2 months after lesion healing is recommended (Portenoy et al 1986). One study suggests that postherpetic neuralgia is two to three times more frequent in the cancer population than in the general population (Rusthoven et al 1988a). In patients with postherpetic neuralgia and cancer, changes in the intensity or pattern of pain, or the development of new neurological deficits, may indicate the possibility of local neoplasm and should be investigated.

Cervical plexopathy

The ventral rami of the upper four cervical spinal nerves join to form the cervical plexus between the deep anterior and lateral muscles of the neck. Cutaneous branches emerge from the posterior border of the sternocleidomastoid. In the cancer population, plexus injury is frequently due to tumour infiltration or treatment (including surgery or radiotherapy) of neoplasms in this region (Hollinshead 1982; Jaeckle 1991).

Malignant cervical plexopathy

Tumour invasion or compression of the cervical plexus can be caused by direct extension of a primary head and neck malignancy or neoplastic (metastatic or lymphomatous) involvement of the cervical lymph nodes (Hollinshead 1982; Jaeckle 1991). Pain may be experienced in the preauricular (greater auricular nerve) or postauricular (lesser and greater occipital nerves) regions, or the anterior neck (transverse cutaneous and supraclavicular nerves). Pain may refer to the lateral aspect of the face or head, or to the ipsilateral shoulder. The overlap in the pain referral patterns from the face and neck may relate to the close anatomic relationship between the central connections of cervical afferents and the afferents carried in the fifth, seventh, ninth and tenth cranial nerves in the upper cervical spinal cord (Brodal 1981). The pain may be aching, burning or lancinating, and is often exacerbated by neck movement or swallowing. Associated features can include ipsilateral Horner's syndrome or hemidiaphragmatic paralysis. The diagnosis must be distinguished from epidural compression of the cervical spinal cord and leptomeningeal metastases. MRI or CT imaging of the neck and cervical spine is usually required to evaluate the aetiology of the pain.

Brachial plexopathy

The two most common causes of brachial plexopathy in cancer patients are tumour infiltration and radiation injury. Less common causes of painful brachial plexopathy include trauma during surgery or anaesthesia, radiation-induced second neoplasms, acute brachial plexus ischaemia and paraneoplastic brachial neuritis.

Malignant brachial plexopathy

Plexus infiltration by tumour is the most prevalent cause of brachial plexopathy. Malignant brachial plexopathy is most common in patients with lymphoma, lung cancer or breast cancer. The invading tumour usually arises from adjacent axillary, cervical and supraclavicular lymph nodes (lymphoma and breast cancer) or from the lung (superior sulcus tumours or so-called Pancoast tumours) (Kori et al 1981). Pain is nearly universal, occurring in 85% of patients, and often precedes neurological signs or symptoms by months (Tsairis et al 1972; Foley 1991). Lower plexus involvement (C7, C8, T1 distribution) is typical, and is reflected in the pain distribution which usually involves the elbow, medial forearm and fourth and fifth fingers. Pain may sometimes localize to the posterior arm or elbow. Severe aching is usually reported, but patients may also experience constant or lancinating dysaesthesias along the ulnar aspect of the forearm or hand.

Tumour infiltration of the upper plexus (C5–C6 distribution) is less common. This lesion is characterized by pain in the shoulder girdle, lateral arm and hand. Of patients presenting with upper plexopathy, 75% subsequently develop a panplexopathy and 25% of patients present with panplexopathy (Kori et al 1981).

Cross-sectional imaging is essential in all patients with symptoms or signs compatible with plexopathy (Fig. 43.10). In one study, CT scanning had 80–90% sensitivity in detecting tumour infiltration (Cascino et al 1983); others have demonstrated improved diagnostic yield with a multiplanar imaging technique (Fishman et al 1991). Although there are no comparative data on the sensitivity and specificity of CT and MRI in this setting, MRI does have some theoretical advantages; changes in soft-tissue signal intensity on T2-weighted images may help distinguish between tumour and radiation fibrosis, and MRI

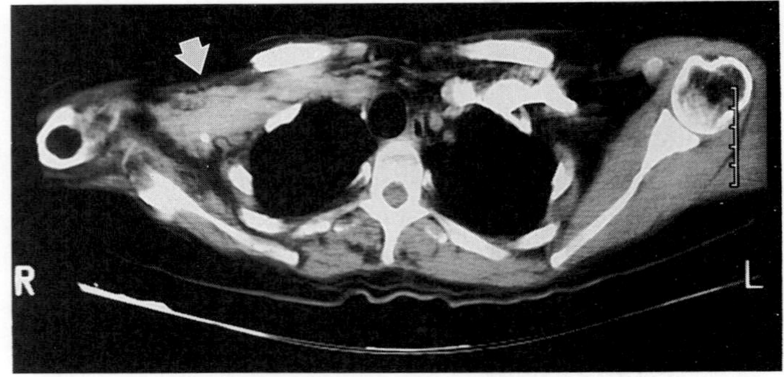

Fig. 43.10 Contrast-enhanced CT scan of the brachial plexus in a 57-year-old woman who has a past history of breast cancer and presented with right arm and hand pain. There is a mass in the right brachial plexus (arrow).

can reliably assess the integrity of the adjacent epidural space (Hagen et al 1989).

Electrodiagnostic studies may be helpful in patients with suspected plexopathy, particularly when neurological examination and imaging studies are normal (Synek 1986; Foley 1991). Although not specific for tumour, abnormalities in electromyography (EMG) or somatosensory evoked potentials may establish the diagnosis of plexopathy, and thereby confirm the need for additional evaluation (which may potentially include exploratory surgery) (Foley 1991).

Patients with malignant brachial plexopathy are at high risk for epidural extension of the tumour (Portenoy et al 1989; Jaeckle 1991). Epidural disease can occur as the neoplasm grows medially and invades vertebrae or tracks along nerve roots through the intervertebral foramina (Fig. 43.11). In the latter case, there may be no evidence of bony erosion on imaging studies. The development of Horner's syndrome, evidence of panplexopathy, or finding of paraspinal tumour or vertebral damage on CT or MRI are highly associated with epidural extension and should lead to definitive imaging of the epidural space (Portenoy et al 1989; Jaeckle 1991).

Radiation-induced brachial plexopathy

Two distinct syndromes of radiation-induced brachial plexopathy have been described: (i) early-onset transient plexopathy (see above) and (ii) delayed-onset progressive plexopathy. Delayed-onset progressive plexopathy can occur 6 months to 20 years after a course of radiotherapy that included the plexus in the radiation portal. In contrast to tumour infiltration, pain is a relatively uncommon presenting symptom (18%) and, when present, is usually less severe (Kori et al 1981). Weakness and sensory changes predominate in the distribution of the upper plexus (C5, C6 distribution) (Kori et al 1981; Mondrup et al 1990; Vecht 1990). Radiation changes in the skin and lymphoedema are commonly associated. The CT

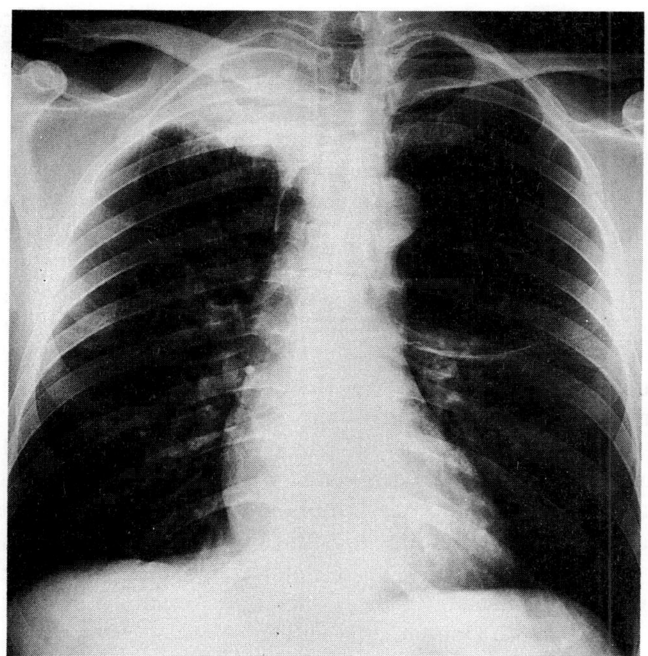

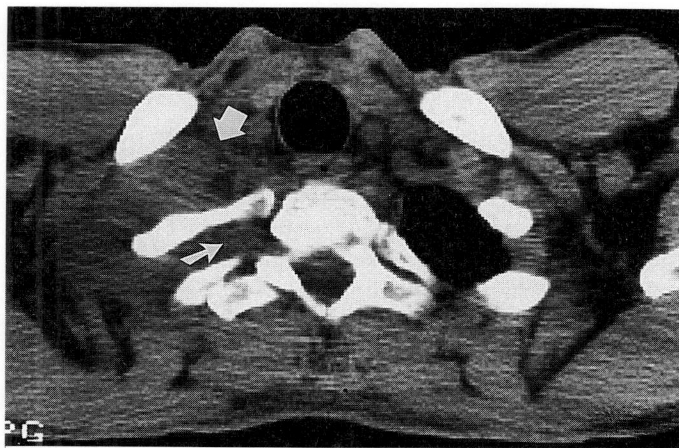

Fig. 43.11 Chest radiograph (A) and CT scan (B) of a 63-year-old man with an apical tumour of the right lung involving the brachial plexus (Pancoast tumour). The CT scan demonstrates the apical tumour (large arrow) with extension of the lesion into the intervertebral foramina (small arrow).

scan usually demonstrates diffuse infiltration that cannot be distinguished from tumour infiltration. Electromyography may demonstrate myokymia (Lederman & Wilbourn 1984; Harper et al 1989; Foley 1991). Although a careful history, combined with these neurological findings and the results of CT scanning and electrodiagnostic studies can strongly suggest the diagnosis of radiation-induced injury, repeated assessments over time are needed to confirm the diagnosis. Rare patients require surgical exploration of the plexus to exclude neoplasm and establish the aetiology. When due to radiation, plexopathy is usually progressive (Killer & Hess 1990; Jaeckle 1991), although some patients plateau for a variable period of time.

Uncommon causes of brachial plexopathy

Malignant peripheral nerve tumour or a second primary tumour in a previously irradiated site can account for pain recurring late in the patient's course (Foley et al 1980; Aho & Sainio 1983). Pain has been reported to occur as a result of brachial plexus entrapment in a lymphoedematous shoulder (Vecht 1990) and as a consequence of acute ischaemia many years after axillary radiotherapy (Mumenthaler et al 1987; Gerard et al 1989). An idiopathic brachial plexopathy has also been described in patients with Hodgkin's disease (Lachance et al 1991).

Lumbosacral plexopathy

The lumbar plexus, which lies in the paravertebral psoas muscle, is formed primarily by the ventral rami of L1–4. The sacral plexus forms in the sacroiliac notch from the ventral rami of S1–3 and the lumbosacral trunk (L4–5), which courses caudally over the sacral ala to join the plexus (Chad & Bradley 1987). Lumbosacral plexopathy may be associated with pain in the lower abdomen, inguinal region, buttock or leg (Jaeckle et al 1985). In the cancer population, lumbosacral plexopathy is usually caused by neoplastic infiltration or compression. Radiation-induced plexopathy also occurs and occasional patients develop the lesion as a result of surgical trauma, infarction, cytotoxic damage, infection in the pelvis or psoas muscle, abdominal aneurysm or idiopathic lumbosacral neuritis. Polyradiculopathy from leptomeningeal metastases or epidural metastases can mimic lumbosacral plexopathy and the evaluation of the patient must consider these lesions as well.

Malignant lumbosacral plexopathy

The primary tumours most frequently associated with malignant lumbosacral plexopathy include colorectal, cervical, breast, sarcoma and lymphoma (Jaeckle et al 1985; Jaeckle 1991). Most tumours involve the plexus by direct extension from intrapelvic neoplasm; metastases account for only one-fourth of cases. In one study, two-thirds of patients developed plexopathy within 3 years of their primary diagnosis and one-third presented within 1 year (Jaeckle et al 1985).

Pain is the first symptom reported by most patients with malignant lumbosacral plexopathy. Pain is experienced by almost all patients during the course of the disease and it is the only symptom in almost 20% of patients The quality is usually aching, pressure-like or stabbing; dysaesthesias appear to be relatively uncommon. Most patients develop numbness, paraesthesias or weakness weeks to months after the pain begins. Common signs include leg weakness that involves multiple myotomes, sensory loss that crosses dermatomes, reflex asymmetry, focal tenderness, leg oedema and positive direct or reverse straight leg-raising signs.

An upper plexopathy occurs in almost one-third of patients with lumbosacral plexopathy (Jaeckle et al 1985). This lesion is usually due to direct extension from a low abdominal tumour, most frequently colorectal. Pain may be experienced in the back, lower abdomen, flank or iliac crest, or the anterolateral thigh. Examination may reveal sensory, motor and reflex changes in a L1–4 distribution. A subgroup of these patients presents with a syndrome characterized by pain and paraesthesias limited to the lower abdomen or inguinal region, variable sensory loss and no motor findings. CT scan may show tumour adjacent to the L1 vertebra (the L1 syndrome) (Jaeckle et al 1985) or along the pelvic sidewall, where it presumably damages the ilioinguinal, iliohypogastric or genitofemoral nerves. Another subgroup has neoplastic involvement of the psoas muscle and presents with a syndrome characterized by upper lumbosacral plexopathy, painful flexion of the ipsilateral hip and positive psoas muscle stretch test. This has been termed the malignant psoas syndrome (Stevens & Gonet 1990).

A lower plexopathy occurs in just over 50% of patients with lumbosacral plexopathy (Jaeckle et al 1985). This lesion is usually due to direct extension from a pelvic tumour, most frequently rectal cancer, gynaecological tumours or pelvic sarcoma. Pain may be localized in the buttocks and perineum, or referred to the posterolateral thigh and leg. Associated symptoms and signs conform to an L4–S1 distribution. Examination may reveal weakness or sensory changes in the L5 and S1 dermatomes and a depressed ankle jerk. Other findings include leg oedema, bladder or bowel dysfunction, sacral or sciatic notch tenderness and a positive straight leg-raising test. A pelvic mass may be palpable.

Sacral plexopathy may occur from direct extension of a sacral lesion or a presacral mass. This may present with predominant involvement of the lumbosacral trunk, characterized by numbness over the dorsal medial foot and sole, weakness of knee flexion, ankle dorsiflexion and inversion. Other patients demonstrate particular involvement of the coccygeal plexus, with prominent sphincter dysfunction and perineal sensory loss. The latter syndrome occurs with low pelvic tumours, such as those arising from the rectum or prostate.

A panplexopathy with involvement in a L1–S3 distribution occurs in almost one-fifth of patients with lumbosacral plexopathy (Jaeckle et al 1985). Local pain may occur in the lower abdomen, back, buttocks or perineum. Referred pain can be experienced anywhere in the distribution of the plexus. Leg oedema is extremely common. Neurological deficits may be confluent or patchy within the L1–S3 distribution and a positive straight leg-raising test is usually present.

Autonomic dysfunction, particularly anhydrosis and vasodilation, has been associated with plexus and peripheral nerve injuries. Focal autonomic neuropathy, which may suggest the anatomic localization of the lesion (Evans & Watson 1985), has been reported as the presenting symptom of metastatic lumbosacral plexopathy (Gilchrist & Moore 1985; Dalmau et al 1989).

Cross-sectional imaging, with either CT or MRI, is the usual diagnostic procedure to evaluate lumbosacral plexopathy (Fig. 43.12). Scanning should be done from the level of the L1 vertebral body, through the sciatic notch. When using CT scanning techniques, images should include bone and soft-tissue windows. Definitive imaging of the epidural space adjacent to the plexus should be considered in the patient who has features indicative of a relatively high risk of epidural extension including bilateral symptoms or signs, unexplained incontinence or a prominent paraspinal mass (Jaeckle et al 1985; Portenoy et al 1989).

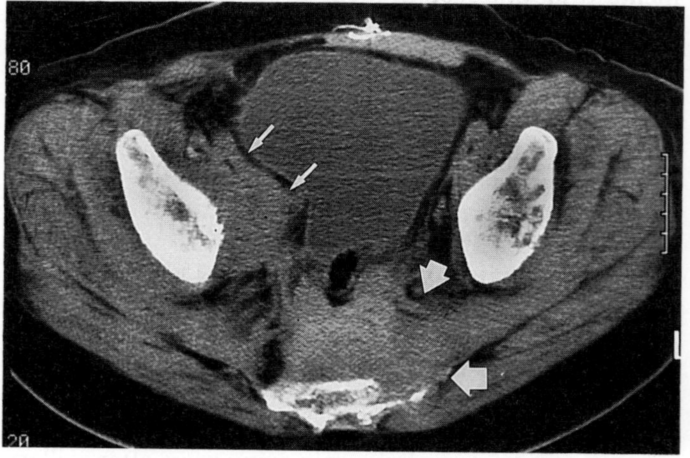

Fig. 43.12 Pelvic CT scan of a 60-year-old man with unresectable carcinoma of the bladder who presented with severe pain radiating down the posterior aspect of both legs. There is a presacral mass that erodes the sacrum (large arrows) and extends to the right pelvic side-wall (small arrows).

Radiation-induced lumbosacral plexopathy

Radiation fibrosis of the lumbosacral plexus is a rare complication that may occur from 1 to over 30 years following radiation treatment. The use of intracavitary radium implants for carcinoma of the cervix may be an additional risk factor (Glass et al 1985; Stryker et al 1990). Radiation-induced plexopathy typically presents with progressive weakness and leg swelling; pain is not usually a prominent feature (Thomas et al 1985; Stryker et al 1990). Weakness typically begins distally in the L5–S1 segments and is slowly progressive. The symptoms and signs may be bilateral (Thomas et al 1985). If CT scanning demonstrates a lesion, it is usually a nonspecific diffuse infiltration of the tissues. Electromyography may show myokymic discharges (Thomas et al 1985).

Uncommon causes of lumbosacral plexopathy

Lumbosacral plexopathy may occur following intraarterial cis-platinum infusion (see below) and embolization techniques. This syndrome has been observed following attempted embolization of a bleeding rectal lesion. Benign conditions that may produce similar findings include haemorrhage or abscess in the iliopsoas muscle (Chad & Bradley 1987), abdominal aortic aneurysms (Garcia-Diaz et al 1988) and diabetic radiculoplexopathy (Brown & Asbury 1984; Chad & Bradley 1987). Vasculitis may also result in lumbosacral plexopathy (Chad & Bradley 1987) and an idiopathic lumbosacral plexitis analogous to acute brachial neuritis has been described (Evans 1981). A subgroup of patients with the latter syndrome have an elevated erythrocyte sedimentation rate and respond to immunosuppressive therapy (Bradley et al 1984).

Painful mononeuropathy

Tumour-related mononeuropathy

Tumour-related mononeuropathy usually results from compression or infiltration of a nerve from tumour arising in an adjacent bony structure. The most common example of this phenomenon is intercostal nerve injury in a patient with rib metastases. Constant burning pain and other dysaesthesias in the area of sensory loss are the typical clinical presentation. Other examples include the cranial neuralgias previously described, sciatica associated with tumour invasion of the sciatic notch and common peroneal nerve palsy associated with primary bone tumours of the proximal fibula.

Other causes of mononeuropathy

Cancer patients also develop mononeuropathies from many other causes. Postsurgical syndromes are well described (see below) and radiation injury of a peripheral nerve occurs occasionally. Rarely, cancer patients develop nerve entrapment syndromes (such as carpal tunnel syndrome) related to oedema.

Painful peripheral neuropathies

Painful peripheral neuropathies have multiple causes, including nutritional deficiencies, other metabolic derangements (e.g. diabetes and renal dysfunction), neurotoxic effects of chemotherapy and, rarely, paraneoplastic syndromes (Henson & Urich 1982).

Toxic peripheral neuropathy

Chemotherapy-induced peripheral neuropathy is a common problem, which is typically manifested by painful paraesthesias in the hands and/or feet and signs consistent with an axonopathy, including 'stocking–glove' sensory loss, weakness, hyporeflexia and autonomic dysfunction (Delattre & Posner 1989; McDonald 1991). The pain is usually characterized by continuous burning or lancinating pains, either of which may be increased by contact. The drugs most commonly associated with a peripheral neuropathy are the vinca alkaloids (especially vincristine) (Casey et al 1973) and cis-platinum (Mollman et al 1988a, 1988b). Procarbazine, carboplatinum, misonidazole and hexamethylmelamine have also been implicated as causes of this syndrome (Weiss et al 1974; Delattre & Posner 1989). One small study has suggested that the neuropathy associated with cis-platinum can be prevented by the coadministration of the radioprotective agent S-2-(3-aminopropylamino)-ethylphosphorothioic acid (WR-2721) (Mollman et al 1988a).

Paraneoplastic painful peripheral neuropathy

Paraneoplastic painful peripheral neuropathy can be related to injury to the dorsal root ganglion (also known as subacute sensory neuronopathy or ganglionopathy) or injury to peripheral nerves. These syndromes may be the initial manifestation of an underlying malignancy. Except for the neuropathy associated with myeloma (Davis 1972; Bardwick et al 1980), their course is usually independent of the primary tumour (Anderson et al 1987).

Subacute sensory neuronopathy is characterized by pain (usually dysaesthetic), paraesthesias, sensory loss in the extremities and severe sensory ataxia (Henson & Urich 1982; Anderson et al 1987; Posner 1991). Although it is usually associated with small-cell carcinoma of the lung, other tumour types, including Hodgkin's disease and varied solid tumours, are rarely associated (Henson & Urich 1982; Anderson et al 1987; Posner 1991). Both constant and lancinating dysaesthesias occur and typically predate other symptoms. The pain usually develops before the tumour is evident and its course is typically independent. The syndrome, which results from an inflammatory process involving the dorsal root ganglia, may be part of a more diffuse autoimmune disorder that can affect the limbic region, brainstem and spinal cord (Henson & Urich 1982). An antineuronal IgG antibody ('anti-Hu'), which recognizes a low-molecular-weight protein present in most small cell lung carcinomas, has been associated with the condition (Graus et al 1986a; Anderson et al 1988; Posner 1991).

A sensorimotor peripheral neuropathy, which may be painful, has been observed in association with diverse neoplasms, particularly Hodgkin's disease and paraproteinaemias (Henson & Urich 1982; Chad & Recht 1991). The peripheral neuropathies associated with multiple myeloma, Waldenstrom's macroglobulinaemia, small-fibre amyloid neuropathy and osteosclerotic myeloma (McLeod et al 1984; Chad & Recht 1991) are thought to be due to antibodies that cross-react with constituents of peripheral nerves (Davis 1972; Bardwick et al 1980; McLeod et al 1984). Clinically evident peripheral neuropathy occurs in approximately 15% of patients with multiple myeloma and electrophysiological evidence of this lesion can be found in 40% (Walsh 1971).

PAIN SYNDROMES OF THE VISCERA AND MISCELLANEOUS TUMOUR-RELATED SYNDROMES

Pain may be caused by pathology involving the luminal organs of the gastrointestinal or genitourinary tracts, the parenchymal organs, the peritoneum or the retroperitoneal soft tissues. Obstruction of hollow viscus, including intestine, biliary tract and ureter, produces visceral nociceptive syndromes that are well described in the surgical literature (Silen 1983). Pain arising from retroperitoneal and pelvic lesions may involve mixed nociceptive and neuropathic mechanisms if both somatic structures and nerves are involved.

Hepatic distension syndrome

Pain-sensitive structures in the region of the liver include the liver capsule, vessels and biliary tract (Coombs 1990; Mulholland et al 1990). Nociceptive afferents that innervate these structures travel via the coeliac plexus, the phrenic nerve and the lower right intercostal nerves. Extensive intrahepatic metastases, or gross hepatomegaly associated with cholestasis, may produce discomfort in the right subcostal region, and less commonly in the right mid-back or flank (Coombs 1990; Mulholland et al 1990). Referred pain may be experienced in the right neck or shoulder or in the region of the right scapula (Mulholland et al 1990). The pain, which is usually described as dull and aching, may be exacerbated by movement, pressure in the abdomen and deep inspiration. Pain is commonly accompanied by symptoms of anorexia and nausea. Physical examination may reveal a hard, irregular subcostal mass that descends with respiration and is dull to percussion. Other features of hepatic failure may be present. Imaging of the hepatic parenchyma by either ultrasound or CT will usually identify the presence of space-occupying lesions or cholestasis.

Occasional patients who experience chronic pain due to hepatic distension develop an acute intercurrent subcostal pain that may be exacerbated by respiration. Physical examination may demonstrate a palpable or audible rub. These findings suggest the development of an overlying peritonitis, which can develop in response to some acute event, such as a haemorrhage into a metastasis.

Midline retroperitoneal syndrome

Retroperitoneal pathology involving the upper abdomen may produce pain by injury to deep somatic stuctures of the posterior abdominal wall, distortion of pain-sensitive connective tissue and vascular structures, local inflammation and direct infiltration of the coeliac plexus. The pain is experienced in the epigastrium, in the low thoracic region of the back or in both locations. It is usually dull and boring in character, exacerbated with recumbency and improved by sitting. The lesion can usually be demonstrated by CT or MRI scanning of the upper abdomen (Fig. 43.13). If tumour is identified in the paravertebral space, or vertebral body destruction is

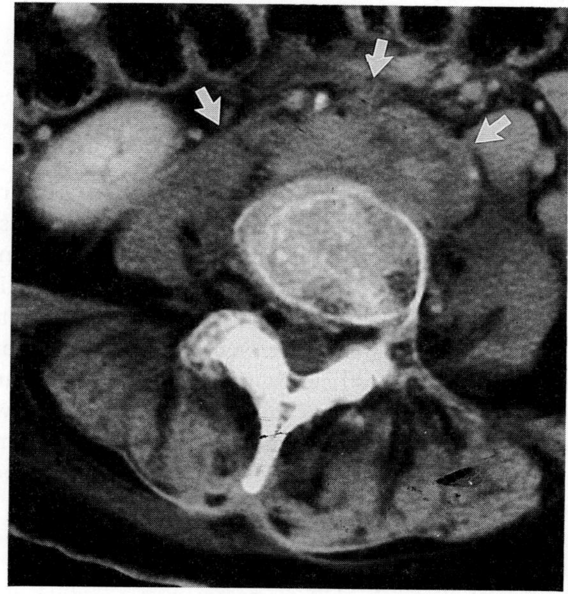

Fig. 43.13 Abdominal CT scan of a 52-year-old woman with metastatic cancer of the colon who presented with upper abdominal and mid-back pain. There is lymphadenopathy in the retroperitoneal space immediately anterior to the vertebral body (arrows).

identified, consideration should be given to careful evaluation of the epidural space.

Chronic intestinal obstruction

Abdominal pain is an almost invariable manifestation of chronic intestinal obstruction, which may occur in patients with abdominal or pelvic cancers (Baines 1990; Ventafridda et al 1990b). The factors that contribute to this pain include smooth muscle contractions, mesenteric tension and mural ischaemia. Obstructive symptoms may be due primarily to the tumour or, more likely, to a combination of mechanical obstruction and other processes, such as autonomic neuropathy and ileus from metabolic derangements or drugs. Both continuous and colicky pains occur (Baines 1990; Ventafridda et al 1990b), and are referred to the dermatomes represented by the spinal segments supplying the affected viscera. Vomiting, anorexia and constipation are important associated symptoms. Abdominal radiographs taken in both supine and erect positions may demonstrate the presence of air-fluid levels and intestinal distension. CT or MRI scanning of the abdomen can assess the extent and distribution of intraabdominal neoplasm, which has implications for subsequent treatment options.

Peritoneal carcinomatosis

Peritoneal carcinomatosis occurs most often by transcoelomic spread of abdominal or pelvic tumour; haematogenous spread of an extraabdominal neoplasm in this pattern is rare (Walsch & Williams 1971; Bender 1989). Carcinomatosis can cause peritoneal inflammation, mesenteric tethering, malignant adhesions and ascites (Bender 1989), all of which can cause pain. Mesenteric tethering and tension appear to cause a diffuse abdominal or low-back pain. Tense malignant ascites can produce diffuse abdominal discomfort and a distinct stretching pain in the anterior abdominal wall. Adhesions can also cause obstruction of hollow viscus, with intermittent colicky pain (Lynch et al 1988). CT scanning may demonstrate evidence of ascites, omental infiltration and peritoneal nodules.

Malignant perineal pain

Tumours of the colon or rectum, female reproductive tract and distal genitourinary system are most commonly responsible for perineal pain (Stillman 1990). Severe perineal pain following antineoplastic therapy may precede evidence of detectable disease and should be viewed as a potential harbinger of progressive or recurrent cancer (Stillman 1990). There is evidence to suggest that this phenomenon is caused by microscopic perineural invasion by recurrent disease (Seefeld & Bargen 1943). The pain, which is typically described as constant and aching, is often aggravated by sitting or standing and may be associated with tenesmus or bladder spasms (Stillman 1990).

Tumour invasion of the musculature of the deep pelvis can also result in a syndrome that appears similar to the so-called tension myalgia of the pelvic floor (Sinaki et al 1977). The pain is typically described as a constant ache or heaviness that exacerbates with upright posture. When due to tumour, the pain may be concurrent with other types of perineal pain. Digital examination of the pelvic floor may reveal local tenderness or palpable tumour.

Ureteric obstruction

Ureteric obstruction is most frequently caused by tumour compression or infiltration within the true pelvis (Fair 1989; Greenfield & Resnick 1989; Talner 1990). Less commonly, obstruction can be more proximal, associated with retroperitoneal lymphadenopathy, an isolated retroperitoneal metastasis, mural metastases or intraluminal metastases. Cancers of the cervix, ovary, prostate and rectum are most commonly associated with this complication. Nonmalignant causes, including retroperitoneal fibrosis resulting from radiotherapy or graft-versus-host disease, occur rarely (Fair 1989).

Pain may or may not accompany ureteric obstruction. When present, it is typically a dull chronic discomfort in the flank, which may radiate into the inguinal region or genitalia. If pain does not occur, ureteric obstruction may be discovered when hydronephrosis is discerned on abdominal imaging procedures or renal failure develops. Ureteric obstruction can be complicated by pyelonephritis or pyonephrosis, which often present with features of sepsis, loin pain and dysuria. Diagnosis of ureteric obstruction can be confirmed by the demonstration of hydronephrosis on renal sonography (Fair 1989; Frohlich et al 1991). The level of obstruction can be identified by pyelography and CT scanning techniques will usually demonstrate the cause (Fig. 43.14) (Fair 1989; Greenfield & Resnick 1989).

PARANEOPLASTIC NOCICEPTIVE PAIN SYNDROMES

Tumour-related gynaecomastia

Tumours that secrete chorionic gonadotrophin (HCG), including malignant and benign tumours of the testis (Tseng et al 1985; Haas et al 1989; Mellor & McCutchan 1989; Cantwell et al 1991) and rarely cancers from other sites (Sapone & Reyes 1985; Wurzel et al 1987; McCloskey et al 1988; Herr et al 1990; Hands & Greenall 1991), may be associated with chronic breast tenderness or gynaecomastia. Approximately 10% of patients with

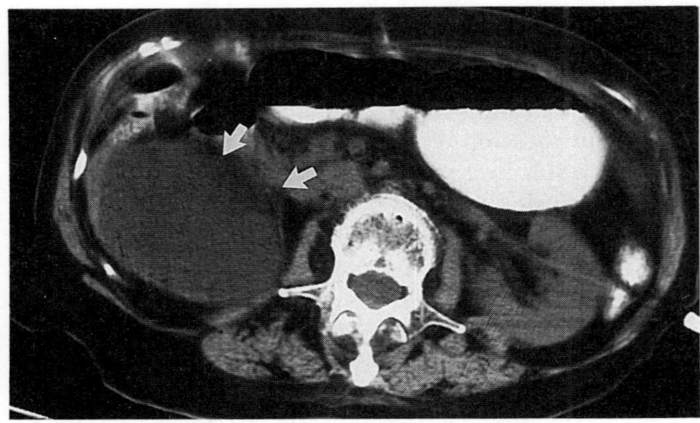

Fig. 43.14 Abdominal CT scan of a 70-year-old woman with carcinoma of the cervix who developed right-flank discomfort. There is massive right-sided hydronephrosis with marked cortical thinning (arrows).

testis cancer have gynaecomastia or breast tenderness at presentation and the likelihood of gynaecomastia is greater with increasing HCG level (Tseng et al 1985). Breast pain can be the first presentation of an occult tumour (Haas et al 1989; Mellor & McCutchan 1989; Cantwell et al 1991).

CHRONIC PAIN SYNDROMES ASSOCIATED WITH CANCER THERAPY

Most treatment-related pains are caused by tissue-damaging procedures. These pains are acute, predictable and self-limited. Chronic treatment-related pain syndromes are associated with either a persistent nociceptive complication of an invasive treatment (such as a postsurgical abscess) or, more commonly, neural injury. In some cases, these syndromes occur long after the therapy is completed, resulting in a difficult differential diagnosis between recurrent disease and a complication of therapy.

Postchemotherapy pain syndromes

Chronic painful peripheral neuropathy

Although most patients who develop painful peripheral neuropathy due to cytotoxic therapy gradually improve, some develop a persistent pain. The characteristics of this pain syndrome were described previously (p. 811).

Avascular (aseptic) necrosis of femoral or humeral head

Avascular necrosis of the femoral or humeral head may occur either spontaneously or as a complication of intermittent or continuous corticosteroid therapy. Osteonecrosis may be unilateral or bilateral. Involvement of the femoral head is most common and typically causes pain in the hip, thigh or knee. Involvement of the humeral head usually presents as pain in the shoulder, upper arm or elbow. Pain is exacerbated by movement and relieved by rest (Foley 1987). There may be local tenderness over the joint, but this is not universal. Pain usually precedes radiological changes by weeks to months; bone scintigraphy and MRI are sensitive and complementary diagnostic procedures. Early treatment consists of analgesics, decrease or discontinuation of steroids and sometimes surgery. With progressive bone destruction, joint replacement may be necessary.

Plexopathy

Lumbosacral or brachial plexopathy may follow cisplatinum infusion into the iliac artery (Castellanos et al 1987) or axillary artery (Kahn et al 1989), respectively. Affected patients develop pain, weakness and paresthaesias within 48 hours of the infusion. The mechanism for this syndrome is thought to be due to small vessel damage and infarction of the plexus or nerve. The prognosis for neurological recovery is not known.

Chronic pain associated with hormonal therapy

Gynaecomastia with hormonal therapy for prostate cancer

Chronic gynaecomastia and breast tenderness are common complications of antiandrogen therapies for prostate cancer (Chrisp & Sorkin 1991). The incidence of this syndrome varies between drugs; it is frequently associated with diethyl stilboestrol (Eberlein 1991), is less common with flutamide and cyproterone (Delaere & Van Thillo 1991; Goldenberg & Burchovsky 1991; Neumann & Kalmus 1991) and is uncommon among patients receiving LHRF agonist therapy (Chrisp & Sorkin 1991). Gynaecomastia in the elderly must be distinguished from primary breast cancer or a secondary cancer in the breast (Olsson et al 1984; Ramamurthy & Cooper 1991).

Chronic postsurgical pain syndromes

Surgical incision at virtually any location may result in chronic pain. Although persistent pain is occasionally encountered after nephrectomy, sternotomy, craniotomy, inguinal dissection and other procedures, these pain syndromes are not well described in the cancer population. In contrast, several syndromes are now clearly recognized as sequelae of specific surgical procedures. The predominant underlying pain mechanism in these syndromes is neuropathic, resulting from injury to peripheral nerves or plexuses.

Postmastectomy pain syndrome

Postmastectomy pain is a chronic and distressing outcome that affects 4–10% of women who undergo breast surgery (Foley 1979; Granek et al 1983). Although it has been reported to occur after almost any surgical procedure on the breast (from lumpectomy to radical mastectomy) (Foley 1979), it is most common after procedures involving axillary dissection (Vecht et al 1989b; Watson et al 1989; Vecht 1990). Pain may begin immediately or as late as many months following surgery. The natural history of this condition appears to be variable, and both subacute and chronic courses are possible (International Association for the Study of Pain: Subcommittee on taxonomy 1986). The onset of pain later than 18 months following surgery is unusual and a careful evaluation to exclude recurrent chest wall disease is recommended in this setting.

Postmastectomy pain is usually characterized as a constricting and burning discomfort that is localized to the medial arm, axilla and anterior chest wall (Wood 1978; Granek et al 1983; Vecht et al 1989b; Paredes et al 1990). On examination, there is often an area of sensory loss within the region of the pain. In some cases a trigger point can be palpated in the axilla or chest wall. The patient may restrict movement of the arm, leading to frozen shoulder as a secondary complication.

The aetiology of postmastectomy pain is believed to be related to damage to the intercostobrachial nerve, a cutaneous sensory branch of T1,2,3 (Vecht et al 1989b). There is marked anatomic variation in the size and distribution of the intercostobrachial nerve and this may account for some of the variability in the distribution of pain observed in patients with this condition (Assa 1974).

Postradical neck dissection pain

Several types of postradical neck dissection pain are recognized. A persistent neuropathic pain can develop weeks to months after surgical injury to the cervical plexus. Tightness, along with burning or lancinating dysaesthesias in the area of the sensory loss, are the characteristic symptoms.

A second type of chronic pain can result from musculoskeletal imbalance in the shoulder girdle following surgical removal of neck muscles. Similar to the droopy shoulder syndrome (Swift & Nichols 1984), this syndrome can be complicated by development of a thoracic outlet syndrome or suprascapular nerve entrapment, with selective weakness and wasting of the supraspinatus and infraspinatus muscles (Stewart 1987).

Escalating pain in patients who have undergone radical neck dissection may signify recurrent tumour or soft-tissue infection. These lesion may be difficult to diagnose in tissues damaged by radiation and surgery. Repeated CT or MRI scanning may be needed to exclude tumour recurrence. Empiric treatment with antibiotics should be considered (Bruera & McDonald 1986).

Postthoracotomy pain

In the largest study of postthoracotomy pain (Kanner et al 1982), three groups were identified. The largest (63%) had prolonged postoperative pain that abated within 2 months after surgery; recurrent pain following resolution of the postoperative pain was usually due to neoplasm. A second group (16%) experienced pain that persisted following the thoracotomy, then increased in intensity during the follow-up period; local recurrence of disease and infection were the most common causes of the increasing pain. A final group had a prolonged period of stable or decreasing pain that gradually resolved over a maximum 8 month period; this pain was not associated with tumour recurrence. Overall, the development of late or increasing postthoracotomy pain was due to recurrent or persistent tumour in greater than 95% of patients.

Patients with recurrent or increasing postthoracotomy pain should be carefully evaluated, preferably with a CT scan through the chest (Fig. 43.15). MRI presumably offers a sensitive alternative. Chest radiographs are insufficient to evaluate recurrent chest disease.

Postoperative frozen shoulder

Patients with postthoracotomy pain, like those with postmastectomy pain, are at risk for the development of a frozen shoulder. This lesion may become an independent focus of pain, particularly if complicated by reflex sympathetic dystrophy. Adequate postoperative analgesia and active mobilization of the joint soon after surgery are necessary to prevent these problems.

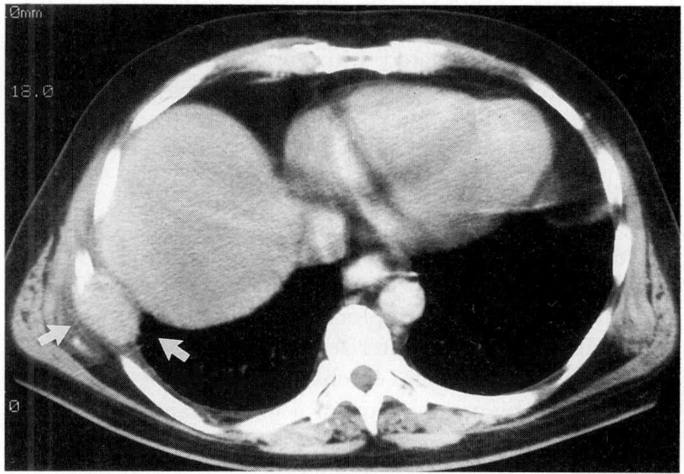

Fig. 43.15 Chest CT scan of a 50-year-old man who had recurrent right-sided chest wall pain 9 months after right lower lobectomy for squamous-cell carcinoma of the lung. There is a chest wall recurrence associated with rib destruction and soft tissue mass (arrows).

Phantom pain syndromes

Phantom limb pain is perceived to arise from an amputated limb, as if the limb were still contiguous with the body. The incidence of phantom pain is significantly higher in patients with a long duration of preamputation pain and those with pain on the day before amputation (Katz & Melzack 1990). Patients who had pain prior to the amputation may experience phantom pain that replicates the earlier one (Katz & Melzack 1990). The pain may be continuous or paroxysmal and is often associated with bothersome paraesthesias. The phantom limb may assume painful and unusual postures and may gradually telescope and approach the stump. Phantom pain may initially magnify and then slowly fade over time. Two small studies suggested that preoperative or postoperative neural blockade reduces the incidence of phantom limb pain during the first year after amputation (Bach et al 1988; Fisher & Meller 1991).

Some patients have spontaneous partial remission of the pain. The recurrence of pain after such a remission, or the late onset of pain in a previously painless phantom limb, suggests the appearance of a more proximal lesion, including recurrent neoplasm (Elliott & Foley 1989).

Phantom pain syndromes have also been described after other surgical procedures. Phantom breast pain after mastectomy, which occurs in 15–30% of patients, also appears to be related to the presence of preoperative pain (Bressler et al 1955; Kroner et al 1989). The pain tends to start in the region of the nipple and then spread to the entire breast (Kroner et al 1989). The character of the pain is variable and may be lancinating, continuous or intermittent (Kroner et al 1989). A phantom anus pain syndrome occurs in approximately 15% of patients who undergo abdominoperineal resection of the rectum (Boas 1983; Ovesen et al 1991). Phantom anus pain may develop either in the early postoperative period or after a latency of months to years (Boas 1983 1990). Late-onset pain is almost always associated with tumour recurrence (Boas 1990). Rare cases of phantom bladder pain after cystectomy have also been reported (Brena & Sammons 1979).

Stump pain

Stump pain occurs at the site of the surgical scar several months to years following amputation. It is usually the result of neuroma development at a site of nerve transection. This pain is characterized by burning or lancinating dysaesthesias, which are often exacerbated by movement and blocked by an injection of a local anaesthetic (Foley 1987).

Postsurgical pelvic floor myalgia

Surgical trauma to the pelvic floor can cause a residual pelvic floor myalgia which, like the neoplastic syndrome described previously, mimics so-called tension myalgia (Sinaki et al 1977). The risk of disease recurrence associated with this condition is not known and its natural history has not been defined. In patients who have undergone anorectal resection, this condition must be differentiated from the phantom anus syndrome (see above).

Chronic postradiation pain syndromes

Chronic pain complicating radiation therapy tends to occur late in the course of a patient's illness. These syndromes must always be differentiated from recurrent tumour.

Radiation-induced brachial and lumbosacral plexopathies

Radiation-induced brachial and lumbosacral plexopathies were described previously (see p. 808, 809).

Chronic radiation myelopathy

Chronic radiation myelopathy is a late complication of spinal cord irradiation. The latency is highly variable but is most commonly 12–14 months. The most common presentation is a partial transverse myelopathy at the cervicothoracic level, sometimes in a Brown–Sèquard pattern (Jellinger & Strum 1971). Sensory symptoms, including pain, typically precede the development of progressive motor and autonomic dysfunction (Cascino 1991). The pain is usually characterized as a burning dysaesthesia and is localized to the area of spinal cord damage or below. Imaging studies, particularly MRI, are important to exclude an epidural lesion and demonstrate the nature and extent of intrinsic cord pathology, which may include atrophy, swelling or syrinx (Cascino 1991). The course of chronic radiation myelopathy is usually characterized by steady progression over months, followed by a subsequent phase of slow progression or stabilization.

Chronic radiation enteritis and proctitis

Chronic enteritis and proctocolitis occur as a delayed complication in 2–10% of patients who undergo abdominal or pelvic radiation therapy (Earnest & Trier 1989; Buchi 1991). The rectum and rectosigmoid are more commonly involved than the small bowel (Earnest & Trier 1989), a pattern that may relate to the retroperitoneal fixation of the former structures. The latency is variable (3 months–30 years) (Earnest & Trier 1989; Buchi 1991). Chronic radiation injury to the rectum can present as proctitis (with bloody diarrhoea, tenesmus and cramping pain), obstruction due to stricture formation or fistulae to the bladder or vagina. Small-bowel radiation damage typically causes colicky abdominal pain, which can be associated with chronic nausea or malabsorption (Earnest & Trier 1989; Buchi 1991). Barium studies may demonstrate a narrow tubular bowel segment resembling Crohn's disease or ischaemic colitis. Endoscopy and biopsy may be necessary to distinguish suspicious lesions from recurrent cancer (Earnest & Trier 1989).

Burning perineum syndrome

Persistent perineal discomfort is an uncommon delayed complication of pelvic radiotherapy. After a latency of 6–18 months, burning pain can develop in the perianal region, the pain may extend anteriorly to involve the vagina or scrotum (Minsky & Cohen 1988). In patients who have had abdominoperineal resection, phantom anus pain and recurrent tumour are major differential diagnoses.

Osteoradionecrosis

Osteoradionecrosis is another late complication of radiotherapy. Bone necrosis, which occurs as a result of endarteritis obliterans, may produce focal pain. Overlying tissue breakdown can occur spontaneously or as a result of trauma, such as dental extraction or denture trauma (Epstein et al 1987, 1991). Delayed development of a painful ulcer must be differentiated from tumour recurrence.

CONCLUSION

Adequate assessment is a necessary precondition for effective pain management. In the cancer population, assessment must recognize the dynamic relationship between the symptom, the illness and larger concerns related to quality of life. Syndrome identification and inferences about pain pathophysiology are useful elements that may simplify this complex undertaking.

REFERENCES

Agency for Health Care Policy and Research: Acute Pain Management Panel 1992 Acute pain management: operative or medical procedures and trauma. Clinical Practice Guideline. US Dept. of Health and Human Services.

Ahmann F R, Citrin D L, deHaan H A et al 1987 Zoladex: a sustained-release, monthly luteinizing hormone-releasing hormone analogue for the treatment of advanced prostate cancer. Journal of Clinical Oncology 5: 912–917

Aho K A, Saino K 1983 Late irradiation-induced lesions of the lumbosacral plexus. Neurology 33: 953–955

Almadrones L, Yerys C 1990 Problems associated with the administration of intraperitoneal therapy using the Port-A-Cath system. Oncology Nursing Forum 17: 75–80

American Psychiatric Association 1987 Somatoform disorders. In: Spitzer R L (ed) Diagnostic and statistical manual of mental disorders, 3rd edn. American Psychiatric Association, Washington, p 255–267

Anderson N E, Cunningham J M, Posner J B 1987 Autoimmune pathogenesis of paraneoplastic neurological syndromes. Critical Review of Neurobiology 3: 245–299

Anderson N E, Rosenblum M K, Graus F, Wiley R G, Posner J B 1988 Autoantibodies in paraneoplastic syndromes associated with small cell carcinoma. Neurology 38: 1391–1398

Arner S, Meyerson B A 1988 Lack of analgesic effect of opioids on neuropathic and idiopathic forms of pain. Pain 33: 11–23

Assa J 1974 The intercostobrachial nerve in radical mastectomy. Journal of Surgical Oncology 6: 123–126

Bach S, Noreng M F, Tjellden N U 1988 Phantom limb pain in amputees during the first 12 months following limb amputation, after preoperative lumbar epidural blockade. Pain 33: 297–301

Baines M J 1990 Management of malignant intestinal obstruction in patients with advanced cancer. In: Foley K M, Bonica J J, Ventafridda V (eds) Second International Congress on Cancer Pain. Advances in pain research and therapy, vol 16. Raven Press, New York, p 327–336

Balmer C M 1991 Clinical use of biologic response modifiers in cancer treatment: an overview. Part II. Colony-stimulating factors and interleukin-2. DICP 25: 490–498

Banning A, Sjogren P, Henriksen H 1991 Pain causes in 200 patients referred to a multidisciplinary cancer pain clinic. Pain 45: 45–48

Barcena A, Lobato R D, Rivas J J et al 1984 Spinal metastatic disease: analysis of factors determining functional prognosis and choice of treatment. Neurosurgery 15: 820–827

Bardwick B A, Zvaifler N J, Gill N et al 1980 Plasma cell dyscrasia with polyneuropathy organomegaly, endocrinopathy, M protein , and skin changes. Medicine 59: 311–322

Barker G, Loftus L, Cuddy P, Barker B 1991 The effects of sucralfate suspension and diphenhydramine syrup plus kaolin–pectin on radiotherapy-induced mucositis. Oral Surgery, Oral Medicine, Oral Pathology 71: 288–293

Barron K D, Hirano A, Araki S et al 1959 Experience with metastatic neoplasms involving the spinal cord. Neurology 9: 91–100

Beatrous T E, Choyke P L, Frank J A 1990 Diagnostic evaluation of cancer patients with pelvic pain: comparison of scintigraphy, CT and MRI imaging. American Journal of Roentgenology 155: 85–88

Bender M D 1989 Diseases of the peritoneum, mesentery and diaphragm. In: Sleisenger M H, Fordtran J S (eds) Gastrointestinal disease: pathophysiology diagnosis management, 4th edn. Saunders, Philadelphia, p 1932–1967

Besson J M, Chaouch A 1987 Peripheral and spinal mechanisms of nociception. Physiological Reviews 67: 67–186

Bindoff L A, Heseltine D 1988 Unilateral facial pain in patients with lung cancer: a referred pain via the vagus? Lancet 1: 812–815

Bingas B 1974 Tumors of the base of the skull. In: Vinken P J, Bruyn G W (eds) Handbook of clinical neurology, vol 17 Elsevier, Amsterdam, p 136–233

Boas R A 1983 Phantom anus syndrome. In: Bonica J J, Lindblom U, Iggo A (eds) Proceedings of the Third World Congress on Pain. Advances in pain research and therapy, vol 5. Raven Press, New York, p 947–951

Boas R A 1990 Post-surgical perineal pain in cancer: a 5 year follow-up. Pain (suppl 5): 376

Bolund C 1985 Medical and care factors in suicides by cancer patients in Sweden. Journal of Psychosocial Oncology 3: 31–52

Bond M R, Pearson I B 1969 Psychosocial aspects of pain in women with advanced cancer of the cervix. Journal of Psychosomatic Research 13: 13–21

Bonica J J 1953 Headache and other visceral disorders of the head and neck. In: Bonica J J (ed) The management of pain, 1st edn. Lea & Febiger, Philadelphia, p 1263–1309

Bonica J J 1985 Treatment of cancer pain: current status and future needs. In: Fields H L, Dubner R, Cervero F (eds) Advances in pain research and therapy, vol 9. Raven Press, New York, p 589–616

Bonica J J, Ventafridda V, Twycross R G 1990 Cancer pain. In: Bonica J J (ed) The management of pain, 2nd edn. Lea & Febiger, Philadelphia, p 400–460

Bosley T M, Cohen D A, Schatz N J et al 1985 Comparison of metrimazole computed tomography with magnetic resonance imaging in the evaluation of lesions at the cervicomedullary junction. Neurology 35: 485–492

Botet J F, Watson R C, Kemeny N, Daly J M, Yeh S 1985 Cholangitis complicating intraarterial chemotherapy in liver metastasis. Radiology 156: 335–337

Boureau F, Doubrere J F, Luu M 1990 Study of verbal description in neuropathic pain. Pain 42: 145–152

Bradley W G, Chad D, Verghese J P et al 1984 Painful lumbosacral plexopathy with elevated erythrocyte sedimentation rate: a treatable inflammatory syndrome. Annals of Neurology 15: 457–464

Breitbart W 1987 Suicide in the cancer patient. Oncology 1: 49–54

Breitbart W 1989 Psychiatric management of cancer pain. Cancer 63: 2336–2342

Breitbart W 1990 Cancer pain and suicide. In: Foley K M, Bonica J J, Ventafridda V (eds) Second International Congress on Cancer Pain. Advances in pain research and therapy, vol 16. Raven Press, New York, p 399–412

Brena S F, Sammons E E 1979 Phantom urinary bladder pain – case report. Pain 7: 197–200

Bressler B, Cohen S I, Magnussen S 1955 The problem of phantom breast and phantom pain. Journal of Nervous and Mental disorders 123: 181–187

Brice J, McKissock W 1965 Surgical treatment of malignant extradural tumors. British Journal of Medicine 1: 1341–1346

Brodal A 1981 Neurological anatomy. Oxford University Press, Oxford

Brown M J, Asbury A K 1984 Diabetic neuropathy. Annals of Neurology 15: 2–12

Bruera E, McDonald N 1986 Intractable pain in patients with advanced head and necks tumors: possible role of local infection. Cancer Treatment Reports 70: 691–692

Buchi K 1991 Radiation proctitis: therapy and prognosis. Journal of the American Medical Association 265: 1180

Bullitt E, Tew J M, Boyd J 1986 Intracranial tumors in patients with facial pain. Journal of Neurosurgery 64: 865–(871

Cantwell B M, Richardson P G, Campbell S J 1991 Gynaecomastia and extragonadal symptoms leading to diagnosis delay of germ cell tumours in young men. Postgraduate Medical Journal 67: 675–677

Cascino T L 1991 Radiation myelopathy. In: Rottenberg D A (ed). Neurological complications of cancer treatment. Butterworth-Heinemann, Boston, p 69–78

Cascino T L, Kori S, Krol G, Foley K M 1983 CT scan of brachial plexus in patients with cancer. Neurology 33: 1553–1557

Cassel E B, Jellife A M, LaQuesne P M et al 1973 Vincristine neuropathy: clinical and electrophysiological observations. Brain 96: 69–86

Cassel E J 1982 The nature of suffering and the goals of medicine. New England Journal of Medicine 306: 639–645

Castaigne S, Chomienne C, Daniel M T et al 1990 All-trans retinoic acid as a differentiation therapy for acute promyelocytic leukemia. I. Clinical results. Blood 76: 1704–1709

Castellanos A M, Glass J P, Yung W K 1987 Regional nerve injury after intraarterial chemotherapy. Neurology 37: 834–837

Chad D A, Bradley W G 1987 Lumbosacral plexopathy. Seminars in Neurology 7: 97–104

Chad D A, Recht L D 1991 Paraneoplastic syndromes. Neurologic Clinics 9: 901–918

Chapko M K, Syrjala K L, Schilter L, Cummings C, Sullivan K M 1990 Chemoradiotherapy toxicity during bone marrow transplantation: time course and variation in pain and nausea. Bone Marrow Transplantation 4: 181–186

Cherny N I, Thaler H T, Friedlander-Klar H, Lapin J, Portenoy R K 1992 Opioid responsiveness of neuropathic cancer pain: combined analysis of single-dose analgesic trials. Proceedings of the American Society of Clinical Oncology 11: abstract 1330

Chrisp P, Sorkin E M 1991 Leuprorelin. A review of its pharmacology and therapeutic use in prostatic disorders. Drugs and Aging 1: 487–509

Cibas E S, Malkin M G, Posner J B et al 1987 Detection of DNA abnormalities by flow cytometry in cells from cerebrospinal fluid. American Journal of Clinical Pathology 88: 570–577

Cleeland C S 1984 The impact of pain on the patient with cancer. Cancer 54: 2635–2641

Cleeland C S 1989 Pain control : public and physicians' attitudes. In: Hill C S, Fields W S (eds) Drug treatment of cancer pain in a drug-oriented society, vol 11. Raven Press, New York, p 81–89

Clouston P, De Angelis L, Posner J B 1992 The spectrum of neurologic disease in patients with systemic cancer. Annals of Neurology 31: 268–273

Constans J P, DeVitis E, Donzelli R et al 1983 Spinal metastases with neurological manifestations: review of 600 cases. Journal of Neurosurgery 59: 111–118

Cook P T, Davies M J, Beavis M J 1989 Bed rest and post lumbar puncture headache. Anaesthesia 44: 389–391

Coombs D W 1990 Pain due to liver capsular distention. In: Ferrer-Brechner T (ed) Common problems in pain management. Common problems in anesthesia . Year Book Medical Publishers, Chicago, p 247–253

Coyle N 1987 A model of continuity of care for cancer patients with chronic pain. Medical Clinics of North America 71: 259–270

Coyle N, Adelhardt J, Foley K M, Portenoy R K 1990 Character of terminal illness in the advanced cancer patient: pain and other symptoms during last four weeks of life. Journal of Pain and Symptom Management 5: 83–89

Crawford E D, Nabors W 1991 Hormone therapy of advanced prostate cancer: where we stand today. Oncology 5: 21–30

Curran C F, Luce J K, Page J A 1990 Doxorubicin-associated flare reactions. Oncology Nurses Forum 17: 387–389

Dalessio D J 1991 Diagnosis and treatment of cranial neuralgias. Medical Clinics of North America 75: 605–615

Dalmau J, Graus F, Marco M 1989 'Hot and dry foot' as initial manifestation of neoplastic lumbosacral plexopathy. Neurology 39: 871–872

Daut R L, Cleeland C S 1982 The prevalence and severity of pain in cancer. Cancer 50: 1913–1918

Davis D 1972 Myeloma neuropathy. Archives of Neurology 27: 507–511

De Boer W 1989 Bed rest after lumbar puncture is obsolete. Anaesthesia 44: 934

De Castro M D, Meynadier M D, Zenz M D 1991 Regional opioid analgesia. Developments in critical care medicine and anesthesiology, vol 20. Kluwer Academic Publishers, Dordrecht

De Conno F, Caracenti A, Martini C, Spoldi E, Salvetti M, Ventafridda V 1991. Hyperalgesia and myoclonus with intrathecal infusion of high-dose morphine. Pain 47: 337–339

DeAngelis L M, Payne R 1987 Lymphomatous meningitis presenting as atypical cluster headache. Pain 30: 211–216

Delaere K P, Van Thillo E 1991 Flutamide monotherapy as primary treatment in advanced prostatic carcinoma. Seminars in Oncology 5: 13–18

Delattre J Y, Posner J B 1989 Neurological complications of chemotherapy and radiation therapy. In: Aminoff M J (ed). Neurology and general medicine. Churchill Livingstone, New York, p 365–387

Delattre J Y, Arbit E, Thaler H T, Rosenbaum M K, Posner J B 1989 A dose response study of dexamethasone in a model of spinal cord compression caused by epidural tumor. Journal of Neurosurgery 70: 920–925

Deppe G, Malviya V K, Boike G, Young J 1991 Intraperitoneal doxorubicin in combination with systemic cisplatinum and cyclophosphamide in the treatment of stage III ovarian cancer. European Journal of Gynaecological Oncology 12: 93–97

Derogatis L R, Morrow G R, Fetting J, Penman D, Piasetsky S, Schmale A M 1983 The prevalence of psychiatric disorders among cancer patients. Journal of the American Medical Association 249: 751–757

Devor M, Basbaum A I, Bennett G et al 1991 Group Report: mechanisms of neuropathic pain following peripheral injury. In: Basbaum A, Besson J-M (eds) Towards a new pharmacotherapy of pain. John Wiley, New York, p 417–440

Dillon W P 1991 Imaging of central nervous system tumors. Current Opinion in Radiology 3: 46–50
Dubner R 1991a A call for more science, not more rhetoric, regarding opioids and neuropathic pain. Pain 47: 1–2
Dubner R 1991b Neuronal plasticity and pain following peripheral tissue inflammation or nerve injury. In: Bond M R, Charlton J E, Woolf C J (eds) Proceedings of the VIth World Congress on Pain. Elsevier, Amsterdam, p 263–276
Dufour P, Maloisel F, Bergerat J P et al 1991 Intraperitoneal mitoxantrone as consolidation treatment for stage III ovarian carcinoma: a pilot study. Bulletin du Cancer (Paris) 78: 273–280
Dulli D A, Levine R L, Chun R W et al 1987 Migrainous neurological dysfunction in Hodgkin's disease. Archives of Neurology 44: 689–693
Earnest D L, Trier J S 1989 Radiation enteritis and colitis. In: Sleisenger M H, Fordtran J S (eds). Gastrointestinal disease: pathophysiology diagnosis management, vol 2. Saunders, Philadelphia, p 1369–1382
Eberlein T J 1991 Gynecomastia. In: Harris J R, Hellman S, Henderson I C, Kinne D (eds) Breast diseases, 2nd end. Lippincott, Philadephia, p 46–50
Edwards R B 1989 Pain management and the values of health care providers. In: Hill C S, Fields W S (eds). Drug treatment of cancer pain in a drug oriented society. Advances in pain research and therapy, vol 11. Raven Press, New York, p 101–112
Edwards W T 1990 Optimizing opioid treatment of postoperative pain. Journal of Pain and Symptom Management 5 (suppl 1) : 24–36
Elliott K, Foley K M 1989 Neurologic pain syndromes in patients with cancer. Neurologic Clinics 7: 333–360
Epstein J B, Wong F L W, Stephenson-Moore P 1987 Osteoradionecrosis: clinical experience and a proposal for classification. Journal of Oral and Maxillofacial Surgery 45: 104–110
Epstein J B, Schubert M M, Scully C 1991 Evaluation and treatment of pain in patients with orofacial cancer. Pain Clinic 4: 3–20
Eskilsson J, Albertsson M 1990 Failure of preventing 5-fluorouracil cardiotoxicity by prophylactic treatment with verapamil. Acta Oncologica 29: 1001–1003
Evans B A 1981 Lumbosacral plexus neuropathy. Neurology 31: 1327–1330
Evans R J, Watson C P N 1985 Lumbosacral plexopathy in cancer patients. Neurology 35: 1392–1393
Fadul C, Misulis K E, Wiley R G 1987 Cerebellar metastases: diagnostic and management considerations. Journal of Clinical Oncology 5: 1110–1115
Fair W R 1989 Urologic emergencies. In: DeVita V T, Hellman S, Rosengerg S A (eds). Cancer principles and practice of oncology, 3rd edn. Lippincott, Philadelphia, p 2016–2028
Feinberg W M, Swenson M R 1988 Cerebrovascular complications of L-asparaginase therapy. Neurology 38: 127–133
Feldmann E, Posner J B 1986 Episodic neurologic dysfunction in patients with Hodgkin's disease. Archives of Neurology 43: 1227–1233
Ferretti G A, Raybould T P, Brown A T et al 1990 Chlorhexidine prophylaxis for chemotherapy- and radiotherapy-induced stomatitis: a randomized double-blind trial. Oral Surgery, Oral Medicine, Oral Pathology 69: 331–338
Findlay G F 1987 The role of vertebral body collapse in the management of malignant spinal cord compression. Journal of Neurology, Neurosurgery and Psychiatry 50: 151–154
Fink B R, Walker S 1989 Orientation of fibres in human dorsal lumbar dura mater in relation to lumbar puncture. Anesthesia and Analgesia 69: 768–772
Fisher A, Meller Y 1991 Continuous postoperative regional analgesia by nerve sheath block for amputation surgery - a pilot study. Anesthesia and Analgesia 72: 300–303
Fishman B 1990 The treatment of suffering in patients with cancer pain: cognitive behavioral approaches. In: Foley K M, Bonica J J, Ventafridda V (eds) Second International Congress on Cancer Pain. Advances in pain research and therapy, vol 16. Raven Press, New York, p 301–316
Fishman B, Pasternak S, Wallenstein S L, Houde R W, Holland J C, Foley K M 1987 The memorial pain assessment card: a valid instrument for the evaluation of cancer pain. Cancer 60: 1151–1158
Fishman E K, Campbell J N, Kuhlman J E, Kawashima A, Ney D R, Friedman N B 1991 Multiplanar CT evaluation of brachial plexopathy in breast cancer. Journal of Computer Assisted Tomography 15: 790–795
Fleisher M, Wasserstrom W R, Schold S C, Schwartz M K, Melamed M R, Posner J B 1981 Lactic dehydrogenase isoenzymes in cerebrospinal fluid in patients with systemic cancer. Cancer 47: 2654–2659
Foley K M 1979 Pain syndromes in patients with cancer. In: Bonica J J, Ventafridda V (eds) Advances in pain research and therapy, vol 2. Raven Press, New York, p 59–75
Foley K M 1982 Clinical assessment of pain. Acta Anaesthiologica Scandinavica 74 suppl: 91–96
Foley K M 1985 The treatment of cancer pain. New England Journal of Medicine 313: 84–95
Foley K M 1987 Pain syndromes in patients with cancer. Medical Clinics of North America 71: 169–184
Foley K M 1989 Controversies in cancer pain: medical perspective. Cancer 63: 2257–2265
Foley K M 1991 Brachial plexopathy in patients with breast cancer. In: Harris J R, Hellman S, Henderson I C, Kinne D (eds) Breast diseases, 2nd edn. Lippincott, Philadelphia, p 722–729
Foley K M, Woodruff J M, Ellis F T 1980 Radiation-induced malignant and atypical peripheral nerve sheath tumors. Archives of Neurology 7: 311–318
Ford C D, Ford D C, Koenigsberg M D 1989 A simple treatment of post-lumbar-puncture headache. Journal of Emergency Medicine 7: 29–31
Forsyth P A, Posner J B 1993 Headache associated with intracranial neoplasms. In: Olesen J, Tfelt-Hansen P, Welch K M A (eds) The headaches. Raven Press, New York (in press)
Freeman N J, Costanza M E 1988 5-Fluorouracil-associated cardiotoxicity. Cancer 61: 36–45
Frohlich E P, Bex P, Nissenbaum M M, Epstein B M, Sonnondecker E W 1991 Comparison between renal ultrasonography and excetory urography in cervical cancer. International Journal of Gynecology and Obstetrics 34: 49–54
Fulton D S 1987 Brachial plexopathy in patients with breast cancer. Developmental Oncology 51: 249–257
Garcia-Diaz J, Balseiro J, Calandre L, Bermejo F 1988 Aortic dissection presenting with neurologic signs. New England Journal of Medicine 318: 1070
Gerard J M, Franck N, Moussa Z, Hilderbrand J 1989 Acute ischemic brachial plexus neuropathy following radiation therapy. Neurology 39: 450–451
Gilbert R W, Kim J H, Posner J B 1978 Epidural spinal cord compression from metastatic tumor: diagnosis and treatment. Annals of Neurology 3: 40–51
Gilchrist J M, Moore M 1985 Lumbosacral plexopathy in cancer patients. Neurology 35: 1392
Gitsch E, Sevelda P, Schmidl S, Salzer H 1990 First experiences with intraperitoneal chemotherapy in ovarian cancer. European Journal of Gynaecological Oncology 11: 19–22
Glass P J, Foley K M 1991 Carcinomatous meningitis. In: Harris J R, Hellman S, Henderson I C, Kinne D (eds) Breast diseases, 2nd edn. Lippincott, Philadelphia, p 700–710
Glass J P, Pettigrew L C, Maor M 1985 Plexopathy induced by radiation therapy. Neurology 35: 1261
Goldenberg S L, Bruchovsky N 1991 Use of cyproterone acetate in prostate cancer. Urologic Clinics of North America 18: 111–122
Goldspiel B R, Kohler D R 1991 Goserelin acetate implant: a depot luteinizing hormone-releasing hormone analog for advanced prostate cancer. DICP 25: 796–804
Gonzales G R, Elliot K J, Portenoy R K, Foley K M 1991 The impact of a comprehensive evaluation in the management of cancer pain. Pain 47: 141–144
Granek I, Ashikari R, Foley K M 1983 Postmastectomy pain syndrome: clinical and anatomic correlates. Proceedings of the American Society of Clinical Oncology 3: abstract 122
Grant R, Condon B, Hart I, Teasdale G M 1991a Changes in intracranial CSF volume after lumbar puncture and their relationship to post-LP headache. Journal of Neurology, Neurosurgery and Psychiatry 54: 440–442

Grant R, Papadopoulos S M, Greenberg H S 1991b Metastatic epidural spinal cord compression. Neurologic Clinics 9: 825–841

Graus F, Elkon K B, Cordon-Cardo C, Posner J B 1986a Sensory neuropathy and small cell lung cancer. Antineuronal antibody that also reacts with the tumor. American Journal of Medicine 80: 45–52

Graus F, Krol G, Foley K M 1986b Early diagnosis of spinal epidural metastasis: correlation with clinical and radiological findings. Proceedings of the American Society of Clinical Oncology 5: abstract 1047

Greenberg H S, Kim J, Posner J B 1980 Epidural spinal cord compression from metastatic tumor: results with a new treatment protocol. Annals of Neurology 8: 361–366

Greenberg H S, Deck M D F, Vikram B et al 1981 Metastasis to the base of the skull: clinical findings in 43 patients. Neurology 31: 530–537

Greenfield A, Resnick M I 1989 Genitourinary emergencies. Seminars in Oncology 16: 516–520

Grossman S A, Sheidler V R, Swedeen K, Mucenski J, Piantadosi S 1991 Correlation of patient and caregiver ratings of cancer pain. Journal of Pain and Symptom Management 6: 53–57

Haas G P, Pittaluga S, Gomella L et al 1989 Clinically occult Leydig cell tumor presenting with gynecomastia. Journal of Urology 142: 1325–1327

Haddad P, Thaell J F, Kiely J M, Harrison E G, Miller R H 1976 Lymphoma of the spinal epidural space. Cancer 38: 1862–1866

Hagen N, Stulman J, Krol G, Foley K M, Portenoy R K 1989 The role of myelography and magnetic resonance imaging in cancer patients with symptomatic and asymptomatic epidural disease. Neurology 39: 309

Haines I E, Zalcberg J, Buchanan J D 1990 Not-for-resuscitation orders in cancer patients: principles of decision making. Medical Journal of Australia 153: 225–229

Hands L J, Greenall M J 1991 Gynaecomastia. British Journal of Surgery 78: 907–911

Harper C M, Thomas J E, Cascino T L, Litchy W J 1989 Distinction between neoplastic and radiation-induced brachial plexopathy, with emphasis on EMG. Neurology 39: 502–506

Harrington K D 1984 Anterior cord decompression and spinal stabilization for patients with metastatic lesions of the spine. Journal of Neurosurgery 61: 107–117

Heide W, Diener H C 1990 Epidural blood patch reduces the incidence of post lumbar puncture headache. Headache 30: 280–281

Helweg L S, Rasmusson B, Sorensen P S 1990 Recovery of gait after radiotherapy in paralytic patients with metastatic epidural spinal cord compression. Neurology 40: 1234–1236

Henderson I C, Harris J R 1991 Principles in the management of metastatic disease. In: Harris J R, Hellman S, Henderson I C, Kinne D (eds) Breast diseases, 2nd edn. Lippincott, Philadelphia, p 547–678

Henson R A, Urich H (eds) 1982 Cancer and the nervous system. Blackwell, Boston, p 100–119, 368–405

Herr H W, Hennessy W T, Kantor A 1990 Pelvic sarcoma causing gynecomastia. Journal of Urology 143: 1008–1009

Hill H F, Chapman C R, Kornell J, Sullivan K, Saeger L, Benedetti C 1990 Self-administration of morphine in bone marrow transplant patients reduces drug requirement. Pain 40: 121–129

Hill H F, Mackie A M, Coda B A, Iverson K, Chapman C R 1991 Patient-controlled analgesic administration. A comparison of steady-state morphine infusions with bolus doses. Cancer 67: 873–882

Holland J F, Scharlau C, Gailani S et al 1973 Vincristine treatment of advanced cancer: a cooperative study of 392 cases. Cancer Research 33: 1258–1264

Hollingshead L M, Goa K L 1991 Recombinant granulocyte colony-stimulating factor (rG-CSF). A review of its pharmacological properties and prospective role in neutropenic conditions. Drugs 42: 300–330

Hollinshead W H 1982 Anatomy for surgeons: the head and neck. Harper & Row, Philadelphia, p 472–476

Huang M E, Ye Y C, Chen S R et al 1988 Use of all-trans retinoic acid in the treatment of acute promyelocytic leukemia. Blood 72: 567–572

Hundrieser J 1988 A non-invasive approach to minimizing vessel pain with DTIC or BCNU. Oncology Nurses Forum 15: 199

International Association for the Study of Pain: Subcommittee on taxonomy 1980 Pain terms: a list with definitions and notes on usage. Pain: 8: 249–252

International Association for the Study of Pain: Subcommittee on taxonomy 1986 Classification of chronic pain. Pain (Suppl 3) 135–138

Jaeckle K A 1991 Nerve plexus metastases. Neurologic Clinics 9: 857–866

Jaeckle K A, Young D F, Foley K M 1985 The natural history of lumbosacral plexopathy in cancer. Neurology 35: 8–15

Janig W, Blumberg H, Boas R A, Campbell J N 1991 The reflex sympathetic dystrophy syndrome: consensus statement and general recommendations for diagnosis and clinical research. In: Bond M R, Charlton J E, Woolf C J (eds) Proceedings of the VIth World Congress on Pain. Pain research and clinical management, vol 4. Elsevier, Amsterdam, p 373–382

Jellinger K, Strum K W 1971 Delayed radiation in myelopathy in man. Journal of the Neurological Sciences 14: 389–408

Jones G J, Itri L M 1986 Safety and tolerance of recombinant interferon alfa-2a (Roferon-A) in cancer patients. Cancer 8: 1709–1715

Jonsson O G, Sartain P, Ducore J M, Buchanan G R 1991 Bone pain as an initial symptom of childhood acute lymphoblastic leukemia: association with nearly normal hematologic indexes. Journal of Pediatrics 117: 233–237

Jorgensen L, Mortensen M B, Jensen N H, Eriksen J 1990 Treatment of cancer pain patients in a multidisciplinary pain clinic. Pain Clinic 3: 83–89

Kahn C E, Messersmith R N, Samuels B L 1989 1989 Brachial plexopathy as a complication of intraarterial cisplatin. Cardiovascular and Interventional Radiology 12: 47–49

Kanner R, Martini N, Foley K M 1982 Nature and incidence of postthoracotomy pain. Proceedings of the American Society of Clinical Oncology 1: abstract 590

Kaplan R A, Markman M, Lucas W E, Pfeifle C, Howell S B 1985 Infectious peritonitis in patients receiving intraperitoneal chemotherapy. American Journal of Medicine 78: 49–53

Kaplan J G, DeSouza T G, Farkash A et al 1990 Leptomeningeal metastases: comparison of clinical features and laboratory data of solid tumors, lymphomas and leukemias. Journal of Neuro-oncology 9: 225–229

Katz J, Melzack R 1990 Pain 'memories' in phantom limbs: review and clinical observations. Pain 43: 319–336

Kellgren J G 1939 On distribution of pain arising from deep somatic structures with charts of segmental pain areas. Clinical Science 4: 35–46

Kemeny N, Cohen A, Bertino J, Sigurson E R, Botet J, Oderman P 1990 Continuous intrahepatic infusion of floxuridine and leucovorin through an implantable pump for the treatment of hepatic metastases from colorectal carcinoma. Cancer 65: 2446–2450

Killer H E, Hess K 1990 Natural history of radiation-induced brachial plexopathy compared to surgically treated patients. Journal of Neurology 237: 247–250

Kori S H, Foley K M, Posner J B et al 1981 Brachial plexus lesions in patients with cancer: 100 cases. Neurology 31: 45–50

Krol G, Sze G, Malkin M, Walker R 1988 MR of cranial and spinal meningeal carcinomatosis. American Journal of Neuroradiology 9: 709–714

Kroner K, Krebs B, Skov J, Jorgensen H S 1989 Immediate and long-term phantom breast syndrome after mastectomy: incidence, clinical characteristic relationship to pre-mastectomy breast pain. Pain 36: 327–335

Labrie F, Dupont A, Belanger A, Lachance R 1987 Flutamide eliminates the risk of disease flare in prostatic cancer patients treated with a luteinizing hormone-releasing hormone agonist. Journal of Urology 138: 804–806

Lachance D H, O'Neil B P, Harper C J, Banks P M, Cascino T L 1991 Paraneoplastic brachial plexopathy in a patient with Hodgkin's disease. Mayo Clinic Proceedings 66: 97–101

Lazarus R S, Folkman C 1984 Stress, appraisal and coping. Springer, New York.

Lederman R J, Wilbourn A J 1984 Brachial plexopathy: recurrent cancer or radiation? Neurology 34: 1331–1335

Lee Y Y, Glass J P, Geoffray A et al 1984 Cranial computed tomographic abnormalities in leptomeningeal metastasis. American Journal of Neuroradiology 5: 559–563

Levy M H 1991 Effective integration of pain management into comprehensive cancer care. Postgraduate Medical Journal 67 (suppl 2) 35–43

Lunglmayr G 1989 'Zoladex' versus 'Zoladex' plus flutamide in the treatment of advanced prostate cancer. First interim analysis of an international trial. International Prostate Cancer Study Group. Progress in Clinical and Biological Research 303: 145–151

Lynch M A, Cho K C, Jeffrey R J, Alterman D D, Federle M P 1988 CT of peritoneal lymphomatosis. American Journal of Roentgenology 151: 713–715

McCaffery M, Thorpe D M 1989 Differences in perception of pain and the development of adversarial relationships among health care providers In: Hill C S, Fields W S (eds) Drug treatment of cancer pain in a drug oriented society. Advances in pain research and therapy, vol 11. Raven Press, New York, p 19–26

McCloskey J J, Germain L E, Perman J A, Plotnick L P, Janoski A H 1988 Gynecomastia as a presenting sign of fibrolamellar carcinoma of the liver. Pediatrics 82: 379–382

McDonald D R 1991 Neurological complications of chemotherapy. Neurologic Clinics 9: 955–967

MacDonald D R, Strong E, Nielson S et al 1983 Syncope from head and neck cancer. Journal of Neurological Oncology 1: 257–267

McLeod J G, Walsh J C, Pollard I D et al 1984 Neuropathies associated with paraproteinemias and dysproteinemias. In: Dyck P J Thomas P K, Lambert E H, Bunge R (eds) Peripheral neuropathy, vol 2. Saunders, Philadelphia, p 1847–1865

Mahood D J, Dose A M, Loprinzi C L et al 1991 Inhibition of fluorouracil-induced stomatitis by oral cryotherapy. Journal of Clinical Oncology 9: 449–452

Manelfe C 1991 Imaging of the spine and spinal cord. Current Opinion in Radiology 3: 5–15

Markman M 1986 Cytotoxic intracavitary chemotherapy. American Journal of Medical Science 291: 175–179

Markman M, Howell S B, Lucas W E, Pfeifle C E, Green M R 1984 Combination intraperitoneal chemotherapy with cisplatin, cytarabine, and doxorubicin for refractory ovarian carcinoma and other malignancies principally confined to the peritoneal cavity. Journal of Clinical Oncology 2: 1321–1326

Marks RM, Sachar EJ 1973 Undertreatment of medical inpatients with narcotic analgesics.Annals of Internal Medicine 78: 173–181

Martin R S 1989 Mortal values: healing, pain and suffering. In: Hill C S, Fields W S (eds) Drug treatment of cancer pain in a drug oriented society. Advances in pain research and therapy vol 11. Raven Press, New York, p 19–26

Mather L E 1991 Novel methods of analgesic drug delivery. In: Bond M R, Charlton J E and Woolf C J (eds) Proceedings of the VIth World Congress on Pain. Pain research and clinical management, vol 4. Elsevier, Amsterdam, p 159–174

Mellor S G, McCutchan J D 1989 Gynaecomastia and occult Leydig cell tumour of the testis. British Journal of Urology 63: 420–422

Melzaçk R 1975 The McGill pain questionnaire: major properties and scoring methods. Pain 1: 277–299

Mense S, Stahnke M 1983 Responses in muscle afferent fibers of slow conduction velocity to contractions and ischaemia in the cat. Journal of Physiology (London) 342: 343–348

Minsky B, Cohen A 1988 Minimizing the toxicity of radiation therapy in rectal cancer. Oncology 2: 21–25

Moinpour C M, Feigi P, Metch B et al 1989 Quality of life endpoints in cancer clinical trials. Journal of the National Cancer Institute 81: 485–495

Moinpour C M, Hayden K A, Thomson I M, Feigi P, Metch B 1991 Quality of life assessment in Southwest Oncology Group trials. In: Tchekmedyian N S, Cella D (eds) Quality of life in oncology practice and research. Dominus Publishing, Williston Park, p 43–50

Mollman J E, Glover D J, Hogan W M, Furman R E 1988a Cisplatin neuropathy: risk factors. prognosis and protection by WR-2721. Cancer 61: 2192–2195

Mollman J E, Hogan W M, Glover D I, McCluskey L F 1988b Unusual presentation of cis-platinum neuropathy. Neurology 38: 488–490

Molloy H S, Seipp C A, Duffey P 1989 Administration of cancer treatments: practical guide for physicians and oncology nurses. In: De Vita V T, Hellman S , Rosenberg S A (eds) Cancer: principles and practice of oncology, 3rd edn. Lippincott, Philadelphia, p 2369–2402

Mondrup K, Olsen N K, Pfeiffer P, Rose C 1990 Clinical and electrodiagnostic findings in breast cancer patients with radiation-induced brachial plexus neuropathy. Acta Neurologica Scandinavica 81: 153–158

Moots P L, Walker R W, Sze G, Mast J 1987 Diagnosis of dural venous sinus thrombosis by magnetic resonance imaging. Annals of Neurology 2: 431–432

Mrozek-Orlowski M, Christie J, Flamme C, Novak J 1991 Pain associated with peripheral infusion of carmustine. Oncology Nurses Forum 18: 942

Mulholland M W, Debas H, Bonica J J 1990 Diseases of the liver, biliary system and pancreas. In: Bonica J J (ed) The management of pain, vol 2. Lea & Febiger, Philadelphia, p 1214–1231

Mumenthaler M, Narakas A, Billiat R W 1987 Brachial plexus disorders. In: Dyck J P, Thomas P K, Lambert E H, Bunge R (eds) Peripheral neuropathy, vol 2. Saunders, Philadelphia, p 1384–1424

Ness T J, Gebhart G E 1990 Visceral pain: a review of experimental studies. Pain 41: 167–234

Neumann F, Kalmus J 1991 Cyproterone acetate in the treatment of sexual disorders: pharmacological base and clinical experience. Experimental and Clinical Endocrinology 98: 71–80

Nielsen O S, Munro A J, Tannock I F 1991 Bone metastases: pathophysiology and management policy. Journal of Clinical Oncology 9: 509–524

Obbens E A M T, Posner J B 1987 Systemic cancer involving the spinal cord. In: Davidoff R A (ed) Handbook of the spinal cord. Marcel Dekker, New York, p 451–489

Olsen K S 1987 Epidural blood patch in the treatment of post-lumbar puncture headache. Pain 30: 293–301

Olsen M E, Chernik N L, Posner J B 1974 Infiltration of the leptomeninges by systemic cancer. Archives of Neurology 30: 122–137

Olsson H, Alm P, Kristoffersson U, Landin O M 1984 Hypophyseal tumor and gynecomastia preceding bilateral breast cancer development in a man. Cancer 53: 1974–1977

O'Rourke T, George C B, Redmond J 1986 Spinal computed tomography and computer tomographic metrimazide myelography in the early diagnosis of spinal metastatic disease. Journal of Clinical Oncology 4: 576–581

Ovesen P, Kroner K, Ornsholt J, Bach K 1991 Phantom-related phenomena after rectal amputation: prevalence and characteristics. Pain 44: 289–291

Paredes J P, Puente J L, Potel J 1990 Variations in sensitivity after sectioning the intercostobrachial nerve. American Journal of Surgery 160: 525–528

Payne R 1989a Novel routes of opioid administration. In: Hill C S, Fields W S (eds) Drug treatment of cancer pain in a drug oriented society, vol 11. Raven Press, New York, p 319–338

Payne R 1989b Pharmacological management of bone pain in the cancer patient. Clinical Journal of Pain 5 (suppl 2): S43–50

Pfeiffer P, Madsen E L, Hansen O, May O 1990 Effect of prophylactic sucralfate suspension on stomatitis induced by cancer chemotherapy. A randomized, double-blind cross-over study. Acta Oncologica 29: 171–173

Phillips E, Levine A M 1989 Metastatic lesions of the upper cervical spine. Spine 14: 1071–1077

Portenoy R K 1991 Issues in the management of neuropathic pain. In: Basbaum A, Besson J-M (eds) Towards a new pharmacotherapy of pain. Wiley, New York, p 393–416

Portenoy R K 1992 Cancer pain: pathophysiology and syndromes. Lancet 339: 1026–1031

Portenoy R K 1993a Adjuvant analgesics. In: Doyle D, Hanks G W, MacDonald N (eds) Oxford textbook of palliative medicine. Oxford University Press, Oxford, p 187–203

Portenoy R K 1993b Evaluation of back pain in the patient with cancer. Journal of Back Pain and Musculoskeletal Rehabilitation 3: 44–52

Portenoy R K, Hagen N A 1990 Breakthrough pain: definition, prevalence and characteristics. Pain 41: 273–281

Portenoy R K, Abissi C J, Robbins et al 1983 Increased intracranial pressure with normal ventricular size due to superior vena cava obstruction. Archives of Neurology 40: 598

Portenoy R K, Duma C, Foley K M 1986 Acute herpetic and postherpetic neuralgia: clinical review and current management. Annals of Neurology 20: 651–664

Portenoy R K, Lipton R B, Foley K M 1987 Back pain in the cancer patient: an algorithm for evaluation and management. Neurology 37: 134–138

Portenoy R K, Galer B S, Salamon O et al 1989 Identification of epidural neoplasm. Radiography and bone scintigraphy in the symptomatic and asymptomatic spine. Cancer 64: 2207–2213

Portenoy R K, Foley K M, Inturrisi C E 1990 The nature of opioid responsiveness and its implications for neuropathic pain: new hypotheses derived from studies of opioid infusions. Pain 43: 273–286

Portenoy R K, Miransky J, Thaler H T et al 1992 Pain in ambulatory patients with lung or colon cancer: prevalence, characteristics and impact. Cancer 7: 1616–1624

Posner J B 1987 Back pain and epidural spinal cord compression. Medical Clinics of North America 71: 185–206

Posner J B 1991 Paraneoplastic syndromes. Neurologic Clinics 9: 919–936

Posner J B 1992 Headache and other head pain. In: Wyngaarden J B, Smith L H, Claude Bennett J (eds) Cecil's textbook of medicine, 19th edn. W B Saunders, Philadelphia, p 2117–2123

Posner J B, Chernik N L 1978 Intracranial metastases from systemic cancer. Advances in Neurology 19: 575–587

Quesada J R, Talpaz`M, Rios A, Kurzrock R, Gutterman J U 1986 Clinical toxicity of interferons in cancer patients: a review. Journal of Clinical Oncology 4: 234–243

Ramamurthy L, Cooper R A 1991 Metastatic carcinoma to the male breast. British Journal of Radiology 64: 277–278

Raskin N H 1990 Lumbar puncture headache: a review. Headache 30: 197–200

Ready L B 1991 The treatment of post operative pain. In: Bond M R, Charlton J E, Woolf C J, (eds) Proceedings of the VIth World Congress on Pain. Pain research and clinical management, vol 4. Elsevier, Amsterdam, p 53–58

Redding S W 1990 Role of herpes simplex virus reactivation in chemotherapy-induced oral mucositis. NCI Monograph 9: 103–105

Reuben D B, Mor V, Hiris J 1988 Clinical symptoms and length of survival in patients with terminal cancer. Archives of Internal Medicine 148: 1586–1591

Rezkalla S, Kloner R A, Ensley J et al 1989 Continuous ambulatory ECG monitoring during fluorouracil therapy: a prospective study. Journal of Clinical Oncology 7: 509–514

Rider C A 1990 Oral mucositis. A complication of radiotherapy. New York State Dental Journal 56: 37–39

Rodichok L D, Harper G R, Ruckdeschel J C et al 1981 Early diagnosis of spinal epidural metastases. American Journal of Medicine 70: 1181–1188

Rotstein J, Good R A 1957 Steroid pseudorheumatism. Archives of Internal Medicine 99: 545–555

Ruff R L, Lanska D J 1989 Epidural metastases in prospectively evaluated veterans with cancer and back pain. Cancer 63: 2234–2241

Rusthoven J J, Ahlgren P, Elhakim T et al 1988a Risk factors for varicella zoster disseminated infection among adult cancer patients with localized zoster. Cancer 62: 1641–1646

Rusthoven J J, Ahlgren P. Elhakim T et al 1988b Varicella-zoster infection in adult cancer patients: a population study. Archives of Internal Medicine 148: 1561–1566

Saeter G, Fossa S D, Norman N 1987 Gynecomastia following cytotoxic therapy for testicular cancer. British Journal of Urology 59: 348–352

Salner A L, Botnick L, Hertzog A G et al 1981 Reversible transient plexopathy following primary radiation therapy for breast cancer. Cancer Treatment Reports 65: 797–801

Sapone F M, Reyes C V 1985 Unusual faces of lung cancer. Journal of Surgical Oncology 30: 1–5

Saunders C 1984 The philosophy of terminal care. In: Saunders C (ed) The management of terminal malignant disease, 2nd edn Arnold, Baltimore, p 232–241

Schilsky R L, Choi K E, Grayhack J, Grimmer D, Guarnieri C, Fullem L 1990 Phase I clinical and pharmacologic study of intraperitoneal cisplatin and fluorouracil in patients with advanced intraabdominal cancer. Journal of Clinical Oncology 8: 2054–2061

Schneider S M, Distelhorst C W 1989 Chemotherapy-induced emergencies. Seminars in Oncology 16: 572–578

Schorer A E, Oken M M, Johnson G J 1978 Gynecomastia with nitrosurea therapy. Cancer Treatment Reports 62: 574–576

Seefeld P H, Bargen J A 1943 The spread of carcinoma of the rectum: invasion of lymphatics, veins and nerves. Annals of Surgery 118: 76–90

Shegda L M, McCorkle R 1990 Continuing care in the community. Journal of Pain and Symptom Management 5: 279–286

Sherins R J, Olweny C L M, Ziegler J L 1978 Gynecomastia and gonadal dysfunction in adolescent boys treated with combination chemotherapy for Hodgkin's disease. New England Journal of Medicine 299: 12–16

Silen W 1983 Cope's early diagnosis of the acute abdomen, 16th edn. Oxford, New York

Sim F H 1988 Metastatic bone disease: lesions of the pelvis and hip. In: Sim F H (ed) Diagnosis and management bone disease. A Multidisciplinary approach. Raven Press, New York, p 183–198

Sinaki M, Merritt J L, Stilwell G K 1977 Tension myalgia of the pelvic floor. Mayo Clinic Proceedings 52: 717–722

Sorensen S, Borgesen S E, Rohde K et al 1990 Metastatic epidural spinal cord compression. Results of treatment and survival. Cancer 65: 1502–1508

Sozzi C, Marotta P, Piatti L 987 Vagoglossopharyngeal neuralgia with syncope in the course of carcinomatous meningitis. Italian Journal of Neurological Science 8: 271–276

Spijkervet F K, Van S H, Van S J et al 1991 Effect of selective elimination of the oral flora on mucositis in irradiated head and neck cancer patients. Journal of Surgical Oncology 46: 167–173

Stark R J, Hensin R A, Evans S J W 1982 Spinal metastases: a retrospective survey from a general hospital. Brain 105: 189–197

Stevens M J, Gonet Y M 1990 Malignant psoas syndrome: recognition of an oncologic entity. Australasian Radiology 34: 150–154

Stewart J D 1987 Focal peripheral neuropathies. Elsevier, New York.

Stillman M 1990 Perineal pain: diagnosis and management, with particular attention to perineal pain of cancer. In: Foley K M, Bonica J J, Ventafridda V (eds) Second International Congress in Cancer Pain. Advances in pain research and therapy, vol 16. Raven Press, New York, p 359–377

Stillman M, Foley K M 1991 Breast cancer and epidural spinal cord compression: diagnostic and therapeutic strategies. In: Harris J R, Hellman S, Henderson I C, Kinne D (eds) Breast diseases, 2nd edn. Lippincott, Philadelphia, p 688–700

Stillman M J, Moulin D E, Foley K M 1987 Paradoxical pain following high-dose spinal morphine. Pain (suppl 4): 389

Stjernsward J, Teoh N 1990 The scope of the cancer pain problem. In: Foley K M, Bonica J J, Ventafridda V (eds) Second International Congress on Cancer Pain, vol 16 Raven Press, New York, p 7–12

Stryker J A, Sommerville K, Perez R, Velkley D E 1990 Sacral plexus injury after radiotherapy for carcinoma of cervix. Cancer 66: 1488–1492

Sundaresan N, Galicich J H, Lane J M et al 1981 Treatment of odontoid fractures in cancer patients . Journal of Neurosurgery 54: 187–192

Sundaresan N, Galicich J H, Bains M S, Martini N, Beattie E 1984 Vertebral body resection in the treatment of cancer involving the spine. Cancer 53: 1393–1396

Sundaresan N, Galicich J H, Lane J M, Bains M S, McCormack P| 1985 Treatment of neoplastic epidural cord compression by vertebral resection and stabilization . Journal of Neurosurgery 63: 676–684

Swift T R, Nichols F T 1984 The droopy shoulder syndrome. Neurology 34: 212–215

Synek V M 1986 Validity of median nerve somatosensory evoked potentials in the diagnosis of supraclavicular brachial plexus lesions. Electroencephalography and Clinical Neurophysiology 65: 27–35

Talner L B 1990 Specific causes of obstruction. In: Pollack H M (ed) Clinical urography, vol 2. Saunders, Philadelphia, p 1629–1751

Tasker R 1990 Management of nociceptive, deafferentation, and central pain by surgical intervention. In: Fields H L (ed). Pain syndromes in neurology. Butterworths International Medical Reviews: Neurology, vol 10. Butterworths, London, p 143–200

Thomas J E, Cascino T L, Earl J D 1985 Differential diagnosis between radiation and tumor plexopathy of the pelvis. Neurology 35: 1–7

Thompson I M, Zeidman E J, Rodriguez`F R 1990 Sudden death due to disease flare with luteinizing hormone-releasing hormone agonist therapy for carcinoma of the prostate. Journal of Urology 144: 1479–1480

Torebjörk H E, Ochoa J L, Schady W 1984 Referred pain from intraneural stimulation of muscle fascicles in the median nerve. Pain 18: 145–156

Trump D L, Anderson S A 1983 Painful gynecomastia following cytotoxic therapy for testis cancer: a potentially favorable prognostic sign? Journal of Clinical Oncology 1: 416–420

Trump A R, Pavy M D, Staal S 1982 Gynecomastia in men following antineoplastic therapy. Archives of Internal Medicine. 142: 511–513

Tsairis P, Dyck P J, Mulder D et al 1972 Natural history of brachial plexus neuropathy. Archives of Neurology 27: 109–117

Tseng A J, Horning S J, Freiha F S, Resser K J, Hannigan J J, Torti F M 1985 Gynecomastia in testicular cancer patients. Prognostic and therapeutic implications. Cancer 56: 2534–2538

Twijnstra A, van Zanten A P, Nooyen W J, Hart A A M, Ongerboer de Visser B W 1986a Cerebrospinal fluid beta-2-microglobulin: a study in controls and patients with metastatic and non-metastatic neurological disease. European Journal of Cancer and Clinical Oncology 22: 387–391

Twijnstra A, van Zanten A P, Nooyen W J, Hart A A M, Ongerboer de Visser B W 1986b Cerebrospinal fluid carcinoembryonic antigen in patients with metastatic and non-metastatic neurological disease. Archives of Neurology 43: 269–272

Twycross R G, Fairfield S 1982 Pain in far-advanced cancer. Pain 14: 303–310

Twycross R G, Lack S A 1984 Symptom control in far-advanced cancer: pain relief. Pitman, London

Vecht C J 1990 Arm pain in the patient with breast cancer. Journal of Pain and Symptom Management 5: 109–117

Vecht C J, Haaxma-Reiche H, van Putten W L J, de Visser M, Vries E P, Twijnstra A 1989a Initial bolus of conventional versus high-dose dexamethasone in metastatic spinal cord compression. Neurology 39: 1255–1257

Vecht C J, Van de Brand H J, Wajer O J 1989b Post-axillary dissection pain in breast cancer due to a lesion of the intercostobrachial nerve. Pain 38: 171–176

Ventafridda V 1989 Continuing care: a major issue in cancer pain management. Pain 36: 137–143

Ventafridda V, Caraceni A 1991 Cancer pain classification: a controversial issue. Pain 46: 1–2

Ventafridda V, DeConno F, Ripamonti C, Gamba A, Tamburini M 1990a Quality of life assessment during a palliative care program. Annals of Oncology 1: 415–420

Ventafridda V, Ripamonti C, Caraceni A, Spoldi E, Messina L, De Conno F 1990b The management of inoperable gastrointestinal obstruction in terminal cancer patients. Tumori 76: 389–393

Ventafridda V, Ripamonti C, De Conno F, Tamburini M, Cassileth B R 1990c Symptom prevalence and control during cancer patients' last days of life. Journal of Palliative Care 6: 7–11

Vick N A, Rottenberg D A 1992 Disorders of intracranial pressure. In: Wyngaaden J B, Smith L H, Claude Bennett J (ed). Cecil's textbook of medicine, 19th edn. Saunders, Philadelphia, p 2221–2224

Von Roenn J H, Cleeland C S, Gonin R, Hatfield A, Pandya K J 1993 Physicians' attitudes and practice in cancer pain management. A survey from the Eastern Cooperative Oncology Group. Annals of Internal Medicine 119: 121–126

Wagner G 1984 Frequency of pain in patients with cancer. Recent Results in Cancer Research 89: 64–71

Wall P D 1989 Introduction. In: Wall P D, Melzack R (eds) Textbook of pain, 2nd edn. Churchill Livingstone, Edinburgh, p 1–18

Walsch D, Williams G 1971 Surgical biopsy studies of omental and peritoneal nodules. British Journal of Surgery 58: 428–432

Walsh I C 1971 The neuropathy of multiple myeloma: An electrophysiological and histological study. Archives of Neurology 25: 404–414

Wanzer S H, Federman D D, Adelstein S H et al 1989 The physician's responsibility toward hopelessly ill patients – a second look. New England Journal of Medicine 120: 844–849

Wasserstrom W R, Glass J P, Posner J B 1982 Diagnosis and treatment of leptomeningeal metastasis from solid tumors: Experience with 90 patients. Cancer 49: 579–772

Watson C P N, Evans R J, Watt V R 1989 The post-mastectomy pain syndrome and the effect of topical capsaicin. Pain 38: 177–186

Weinstein R E, Herec D, Friedman J H 1986 Hypotension due to glossopharyngeal neuralgia. Archives of Neurology 40: 90–92

Weiss H D, Walker M D, Wiernik P H et al 1974 Neurotoxicity of commonly used antineoplastic agents. New England Journal of Medicine 291: 75–81

Willis W D 1985 The pain system: the neural basis of nociceptive transmission in the mammalian nervous system. Karger, Basel

Wood I M 1978 Intercostobrachial nerve entrapment syndrome. Southern Medical Journal 76: 662–663

World Health Organization 1990 Cancer pain relief and palliative care. World Health Organization, Geneva

Wurzel R S, Yamase H T, Nieh P T 1987 Ectopic production of human chorionic gonadotropin by poorly differentiated transitional cell tumors of the urinary tract. Journal of Urology 137: 502–504

44. Psychiatric and psychosocial aspects of cancer pain

William Breitbart, Steven D. Passik and Barry D. Rosenfeld

INTRODUCTION

The cancer patient faces a wide range of psychological and physical stressors throughout the course of illness. These stressors include fears of a painful death, physical disability, disfigurement and growing dependency on others. Although such fears exist in most if not all cancer patients, the degree of psychological distress experienced varies greatly between individuals and depends in part on the patient's personality style, coping abilities, available social supports and medical factors (Holland & Rowland 1989). One of the most feared consequences of cancer, however, is the potential for pain. Pain has a profound impact on a patient's level of emotional distress and psychological factors such as mood, anxiety and the meaning attributed to pain can intensify a patient's experience of cancer pain (Ahles et al 1983). Because of the relationship between psychological factors and pain experience, clinicians who treat patients with cancer pain face complex diagnostic and therapeutic challenges. Appropriate management of cancer pain therefore requires a multidisciplinary approach, recognizing the importance of accurate diagnosis and treatment of concurrent psychological symptoms and psychiatric syndromes (Breitbart 1989a). This chapter reviews the common psychological issues and psychiatric complications (e.g. anxiety, depression, delirium) seen in cancer pain patients and provides guidelines for their assessment and management. In addition, psychiatric and psychological interventions in cancer pain management are reviewed. Finally, the problem of pain in AIDS is addressed with special focus on psychiatric issues in pain assessment and management.

PSYCHOLOGICAL IMPACT OF CANCER AND THE ROLE OF PAIN

Patients diagnosed with cancer often demonstrate a consistent pattern of emotional responses that have been described by Holland, Massie and others (Massie & Holland 1987; Breitbart & Holland 1988; Breitbart 1989a). These responses usually consist of an initial period of shock, denial and disbelief, followed by a period of anxiety and/or depression. Disturbed sleep, diminished appetite and concentration, irritability, pervasive thoughts about cancer and fears about the future often interfere with normal daily activities. These 'stress responses' generally occur at specific points in the course of cancer and its treatment: after diagnosis, with relapse, prior to diagnostic tests, surgery, radiation and chemotherapy, as well as after treatment has concluded and patients enter the phase of survivorship. Distress usually resolves slowly over a period of several weeks and patients gradually return to their prior level of homeostasis once a treatment plan has been agreed upon and emotional supports arise. Psychiatric intervention is not typically necessary for most cancer patients, although anxiolytic or sedative medications and relaxation techniques may be helpful in restoring sleep patterns and minimizing emotional distress in many cancer patients and/or their family members. The support of family and friends, social workers, clergy and hospital staff are usually sufficient to help patients cope with these brief crisis periods.

The degree of psychological distress observed in cancer patients also varies considerably between individuals. Some patients experience persistently high levels of anxiety and depression for weeks or months which significantly hinder their ability to function independently or even comply with cancer treatment. Others experience only mild or transient symptoms which remit rapidly without intervention. This variability is influenced by a number of different factors, most notably medical variables (the presence and degree of pain, stage of disease), and psychological issues (preexisting psychiatric disorders, coping abilities, level of emotional development). Such significant levels of distress generally require psychiatric intervention and are often the result of psychiatric disorders that have developed as a complication of cancer. For the most part, however, physicians treating cancer patients are confronted with psychologically healthy individuals who are reacting to the stresses imposed by cancer and its treatment. Nearly 90% of the psychiatric disorders observed in cancer patients are reactions to or manifestations of the disease or treatments (Derogatis et al 1983; Massie & Holland 1987). Along with an expectation of psychological distress associated with cancer, the public perceives cancer as an extremely painful disease, and pain is one of the most feared consequences of the disease process (Levin et al 1985). Approximately 15% of all cancer patients without metastatic disease report significant pain (Kanner & Foley 1981; Daut & Cleeland 1982). In patients with advanced disease, between 60 and 90% of all patients report debilitating pain and as many as 25% of all cancer patients die while still experiencing considerable pain (Foley 1975, 1985; Twycross & Lack 1983; Cleeland 1984). These findings highlight the importance of understanding the factors which influence the experience of pain for effective management of cancer pain.

Not only does pain have a profound impact on psychological distress in cancer patients, but psychological factors appear to influence the experience and intensity of cancer pain. Psychological variables such as perceived control, meaning attributed to the pain experience, fear of death, hopelessness and anxious or depressed mood all appear to contribute to the experience of cancer pain and suffering (Bond 1979; Spiegel & Bloom 1983a; Ahles et al 1983). These interrelationships have been supported by considerable psychosocial research exploring the relationship between psychological variables and cancer pain. In a study of women with metastatic breast cancer, Spiegel & Bloom (1983a) found that although the site of metastasis did not predict intensity of pain report, greater depression and the belief that pain represented the spread of disease (e.g. the meaning attributed to the pain) did significantly predict a greater degree of pain experienced. Daut & Cleeland (1982) also found that cancer patients who believed that their pain represented disease progression reported significantly more interference with their ability to function and enjoy daily activities that did patients who attributed their pain to a benign cause. Other research has demonstrated that patients with advanced disease who report high levels of emotional disturbance also report more pain (McKegney et al 1981), as do patients with more anxiety and depression (Bond & Pearson 1969; Bond 1973).

Current conceptual models of cancer pain emphasize the multidimensional nature of the pain experience, incorporating the contribution of cognitive, motivational, behavioural and affective components, as well as sensory (nociceptive) phenomena. This multidimensional formulation of cancer pain has opened the door to psychiatric and psychological participation in pain research, assessment and treatment (Melzack & Wall 1983; Lindblom et al 1986). Pain is no longer considered simply as a nociceptive event, but is widely recognized and accepted as a psychological process involving nociception, perception and expression. Because of the important role played by psychological variables in the experience and intensity of cancer pain, appropriate and effective management of cancer pain requires a multidisciplinary approach that incorporates neurology, neurosurgery, anaesthesiology and rehabilitative medicine in addition to a considerable reliance on the input of psychiatrists or psychologists (Foley 1975, 1985; Breitbart 1989a). The challenge of untangling and addressing both the physical and psychological issues involved in cancer pain is essential to developing a rational and effective management strategy. Psychosocial therapies directed primarily at psychological variables have a profound impact on nociception, while somatic therapies directed at nociception have beneficial effects on psychological sequelae of cancer pain. Ideally such somatic and psychosocial therapies are used simultaneously in a multidisciplinary approach to cancer pain management (Breitbart 1989a, Breitbart & Holland 1990; Ahles & Martin 1992).

Unfortunately, psychological variables are too often proposed as the sole explanation for continued pain or lack of response to conventional therapies when in fact medical factors have not been adequately appreciated or examined. The psychiatrist or psychologist is often the last member of the treatment team to be asked to consult on a cancer patient with unrelieved pain and, in that role, must be vigilant that an accurate pain diagnosis is made. They also must be capable of assessing the adequacy of the medical analgesic management provided. Psychological distress in patients with cancer pain should be initially assumed to be the consequence of uncontrolled pain. Personality factors may appear distorted or exaggerated by the presence of pain and the relief of pain often results in the disappearance of a perceived psychiatric disorder (Marks & Sachar 1973; Cleeland 1984).

PSYCHIATRIC DISORDERS IN CANCER PAIN PATIENTS: ASSESSMENT AND MANAGEMENT

While recognizing the potential for psychological disturbance as the result of uncontrolled cancer pain, research has suggested an increased frequency of psychiatric disorders in cancer patients with pain. The Psychosocial Collaborative Oncology Group, which described the prevalence of psychiatric disorders in cancer patients (see Table 44.1), noted that 39% of patients with a psychiatric diagnosis also reported experiencing significant pain, while only 19% of patients without a psychiatric diagnosis reported significant pain (Derogatis et al 1983). The most frequent psychiatric diagnoses seen in cancer patients with pain include adjustment disorder with depressed or anxious mood and major depression. In a specific cancer-related painful condition, epidural spinal cord compres-

Table 44.1 Rates of DSM-III psychiatric disorders and prevalence of pain observed in 215 cancer patients from three cancer centres*

Diagnostic category	Number diagnostic class	Psychiatric diagnoses (%)	Number with significant pain**
Adjustment disorders	69 (32%)	68	
Major affective disorders	13 (6%)	13	
Organic mental disorders	8 (4%)	8	
Personality disorders	7 (3%)	7	
Anxiety disorders	4 (2%)	4	
Total with DSM III psychiatric disorder diagnosis	101 (47%)		39 (39%)
Total without DSM III psychiatric disorder diagnosis	114 (53%)		21 (19%)
Total patient population	215(100%)		60 (28%)

* Adapted from Derogatis et al 1983.
**Score greater than 50 mm on a 100 mm VAS for pain severity.

sion (ESCC), the prevalence of psychiatric disorders is as high as 52% (Breitbart et al 1993). ESCC is a common neurological complication of cancer that occurs in 5–10% of cancer patients and often presents initially as severe pain. These patients are typically treated with a combination of high-dose dexamethasone and radiotherapy, receiving as much as 96 mg/day of dexamethasone for up to a week with gradually tapering doses for up to 3–4 weeks. Such treatments for ESCC are reported to be complicated by significantly high rates of both depression and delirium (Stiefel et al 1989; Breitbart et al 1993). A diagnosis of a major depressive episode was warranted in 22% of all patients undergoing this treatment regimen compared with only 4% so diagnosed in a control sample of cancer patients. Delirium was diagnosed during the course of treatment in 24% of the ESCC patients compared to 10% of a comparison sample. These findings of increased frequency of psychiatric disturbances in cancer patients with pain have been supported by a number of other researchers (e.g. Woodforde & Fielding 1970; Ahles et al 1983).

Because of the confounding influence of pain on a patient's psychological condition, it is imperative that the patient's mental state be reassessed after pain has been adequately controlled in order to determine whether a psychiatric disorder is indeed present. Psychiatric complications of cancer pain can result in increased morbidity and mortality. Management of psychiatric complications of cancer pain is essential for patients to maintain an optimal quality of life. For cancer pain patients, interventions that help decrease mood disturbance also help to reduce pain. A multidisciplinary approach, incorporating psychotherapeutic, behavioural and psychopharmacological interventions is the optimal method for treating psychiatric complications in cancer pain patients. Treatment decisions, however, are predicated on the assumption that a thorough medical and psychiatric assessment has led to an accurate diagnosis, thus allowing specific and effective intervention. The management of specific psychiatric disorders such as depression, delirium and anxiety in cancer patients (including those with pain) has been reviewed in detail in the *Handbook of Psychooncology* edited by Holland & Rowland (1989) as well as in other sources (Massie & Holland 1987; Breitbart & Holland 1988; Holland 1989b; Massie & Holland 1990). A brief guide to the diagnosis and management of these disorders is presented below.

DEPRESSION IN CANCER PAIN PATIENTS

Depression occurs in roughly 20–25% of all cancer patients and the prevalence increases with higher levels of disability, advanced illness and pain (Plumb & Holland 1977; Massie & Holland 1990; Bukberg et al 1984). The somatic symptoms of depression (e.g. anorexia, insomnia, fatigue and weight loss) are unreliable and lack specificity in the cancer patient (Endicott 1983). Thus, the psychological symptoms of depression take on greater diagnostic value and include the following: dysphoric mood, hopelessness, worthlessness, guilt and suicidal ideation (Plumb & Holland 1977; Endicott 1983; Bukberg et al 1984; Massie & Holland 1990). A family history of depression and a history of previous depressive episodes further support the reliability of a diagnosis. A number of specific types of cancer are also associated with higher rates of depression; for example, patients with pancreatic cancer are more likely to develop depression than patients with other types of intraabdominal malignancy (Holland et al 1986). Once the presence of depressive symptomatology has been established, evaluation of potential organic aetiologies such as corticosteroids (Stiefel et al 1989), chemotherapeutic agents (vincristine, vinblastine, asparaginase, intrathecal methotrexate, interferon, interleukin) (Holland et al 1974; Young 1982; Adams et al 1984; Denicoff et al 1987), amphotericin (Weddington 1982), whole-brain radiation (DeAngelis et al 1989), central nervous system metabolic–endocrine complications (Breitbart 1989b) and paraneoplastic syndromes (Posner 1988; Patchell & Posner 1989) that can present as depression must precede initiation of treatment.

TREATMENT OF DEPRESSION

Depressed cancer-pain patients are usually treated with a combination of antidepressant medications, supportive psychotherapy and cognitive-behavioural techniques (Massie & Holland 1990). Many of these techniques are useful in the management of psychological distress in cancer patients and have been applied to the treatment of depressive and anxious symptoms related to cancer and cancer pain. Psychotherapeutic interventions, either in the form of individual or group therapy, have been shown to effectively reduce psychological distress and depressive symptoms in cancer-pain patients (Spiegel et al 1981; Spiegel & Bloom 1983a; 1983b; Massie et al 1989). Cognitive-behavioural interventions, such as relaxation, distraction with pleasant imagery, and cognitive restructuring also appear to be effective in reducing symptomatology in patients with mild to moderate levels of depression (Holland et al 1991).

Psychopharmacological interventions (i.e. antidepressant medications), however, are the mainstay of symptom management in cancer patients with severe depressive symptoms (Massie & Holland 1990). The efficacy of antidepressants in the treatment of depression in cancer patients, including those with or without pain, has been well established in case observations and clinical trials (Purohit et al 1978; Costa et al 1985; Popkin et al 1985; Rifkin et al 1985; Massie & Holland 1987, 1990; Breitbart & Holland 1988; Breitbart 1989a). Antidepressant medications used in cancer-pain patients are listed in Table 44.2.

Table 44.2 Antidepressant medications used in cancer-pain patients*

Drug	Therapeutic daily dosage (mg, p.o.)
Tricyclic antidepressants	
Amitriptyline	25–125
Doxepin	25–125
Imipramine	25–125
Desipramine	25–125
Nortriptyline	25–125
Clomipramine	25–125
Second generation antidepressants	
Buproprion	200–450
Trazodone	150–300
Serotonin specific re-uptake inhibitors	
Fluoxetine	20–60
Sertraline	50–200
Paroxetine	10–40
Heterocyclic antidepressants	
Maprotiline	50–75
Amoxapine	100–150
Monoamine oxidase inhibitors	
Isocarboxazid	20–40
Phenelzine	30–60
Tranylcypromine	20–40
Psychostimulants	
Dextroamphetamine	5–30
Methylphenidate	5–30
Pemoline	37.5–150
Benzodiazepines	
Alprazolam	0.75–6.00
Lithium carbonate	600–1200

*Adapted from Massie & Holland 1990.

Tricyclic Antidepressants

Among the multitude of available antidepressant medications, tricyclic antidepressants (TCAs) are the most frequently used in the cancer setting. Treatment is initiated at low dose (10–25 mg at bedtime), particularly with debilitated patients, and slowly increased by 10–25 mg every 1–2 days until a therapeutic effect has been achieved. Depressed cancer patients often respond to doses considerably lower (25–125 mg orally) than those typically required by the physically healthy (150–300 mg o.d.) (Massie & Holland 1990). The choice of TCA depends on the side-effects profile, existing medical problems, the nature of depressive symptoms and past response to specific antidepressants. Sedating TCAs like amitriptyline or doxepin are prescribed for the agitated, depressed patient with insomnia. Doxepin is highly antihistaminic and as such is useful in improving appetite. Desipramine and nortriptyline are relatively nonanticholinergic and are therefore used when concerns about urinary retention, decreased intestinal motility or stomatitis exist. Patients receiving multiple drugs with anticholinergic properties (e.g. meperidine, atropine, diphenhydramine, phenothiazines) are at risk for developing an anticholinergic delirium, and so TCAs with potent anticholinergic properties should be avoided or used with caution. Amitriptyline, imipramine and doxepin can be given intramuscularly in patients unable to use an oral route. Rectal suppositories containing amitriptyline or other TCAs can also be used. Although not approved for use in the United States, TCAs such as amitriptyline have been used safely by the intravenous route as a slow infusion (Breitbart & Holland 1988; Massie & Holland 1990).

Second generation antidepressants

If a patient does not respond to a TCA, or cannot tolerate its side-effects, a second generation (buproprion, trazodone), heterocyclic (maprotiline, amoxapine) or serotonin-specific reuptake-inhibiting (fluoxetine, sertraline, paroxetine) antidepressants can be used. The second generation antidepressants are generally considered to be less cardiotoxic than the TCAs (Glassman 1984). Trazodone is highly sedating and, in low doses (100 mg at bedtime), is particularly helpful for treating depressed cancer patients with insomnia. Trazodone has been associated with priapism and should, therefore, be used with caution in male patients (Sher et al 1983). Buproprion is a relatively new drug in the United States and its efficacy in cancer patients is unclear. At present, it is not the first drug of choice for depressed patients with cancer; however, buproprion may be considered if patients have a poor response to a reasonable trial of other antidepressants. Buproprion may be somewhat activating in medically-ill patients. It should be avoided in patients with seizure disorders and brain tumours and in those who are malnourished (Peck et al 1983).

Serotonin specific reuptake inhibitors

Fluoxetine, a selective inhibitor of neuronal serotonin uptake, has fewer sedative and autonomic effects than the TCAs (Cooper 1988). The most common side-effects are mild nausea and a brief period of increased anxiety. Fluoxetine can cause appetite suppression, usually lasting for a period of several weeks and, although some patients experience transient weight loss, weight usually returns to baseline level. The anorectic properties of fluoxetine have not been a limiting factor in our use of this drug in cancer patients at Memorial Hospital. Although the side-effect profile of fluoxetine makes it a favourable treatment for depressed medically ill patients, the relatively long half-lives of fluoxetine and its active metabolite norfluoxetine (1–3 and 7–9 days, respectively) can be problematic. Medically-ill patients may take even longer to clear this drug than healthy depressives. In addition, coadministration of fluoxetine and TCAs has resulted in increased blood tricyclic concentration (von Ammon Cavanaugh 1990). Fluoxetine can also increase blood levels of a variety of commonly used medications that are typically metabolized by the cytochrome P3450 enzyme system of the liver (Fuller et al 1976). Two new selective reuptake inhibitors, paroxetine and sertraline, have recently become available in the United States, have shorter half-lives and inactive metabolites and may therefore prove to be useful additions to our armamentarium of antidepressants.

Heterocyclic antidepressants

The heterocyclic antidepressants have side-effect profiles similar to those of the TCAs. Maprotiline should be avoided in patients with brain tumours and in those with seizures since the incidence of seizures is increased by this medication (Lloyd 1977). Amoxapine has mild dopamine blocking activity. Hence, patients who are taking other dopamine blockers (e.g. antiemetics) have an increased risk of developing extrapyramidal symptoms and dyskinesias (Ayd 1979). Mianserin (not available in the USA) is a serotonergic antidepressant with adjuvant analgesic properties that is used widely in Europe and Latin America. Costa and colleagues (1985) found mianserin to be a safe and effective drug for the treatment of depression in cancer patients.

Psychostimulants

The psychostimulants (dextroamphetamine, methylphenidate and pemoline) have been shown to be effective antidepressants in cancer patients with and without pain as well as other medically-ill populations (Katon & Raskind 1980; Kaufmann et al 1982; Fisch 1985; Chiarillo & Cole 1987; Fernandez et al 1987b). They are most helpful in the treatment of depression in cancer patients with pain and advanced disease and in those cases where dysphoric mood is associated with psychomotor retardation, aesthenia, and mild cognitive impairment. Psychostimulants have been shown to improve attention, concentration and overall performance on neuropsychological testing in the medically ill (Fernandez et al 1988). In relatively low dose, psychostimulants can increase appetite, promote a sense of well being and decrease weakness and fatigue in cancer pain patients. Treatment with dextroamphetamine or methylphenidate is usually initiated with a dose of 2.5 mg at 8.00 a.m. and at noon, and gradually increased over several days until a desired effect is achieved or side-effects (overstimulation, anxiety, insomnia, paranoia, confusion) intervene. Most patients respond to doses of 30 mg or less per day, although occasionally patients require up to 60 mg per day. Patients are usually maintained on psychostimulants for 1–2 months, and approximately two-thirds will be able to be withdrawn from this medication without a recurrence of depressive symptoms. Patients whose symptoms reemerge after treatment has been withdrawn can be maintained on a psychostimulant for up to 1 year without significant abuse problems (although tolerance will develop and dose adjustments may be necessary). An additional benefit of such stimulants as methylphenidate and dextroamphetamine is that they have been shown to reduce sedation secondary to opioid analgesics and provide adjuvant analgesia in cancer pain patients (Bruera et al 1987). See section on psychotropic adjuvant analgesics later in this chapter.

Pemoline is a unique psychostimulant chemically unrelated to amphetamine. It is a less potent stimulant with little abuse potential (Chiarillo & Cole 1987). Advantages of pemoline as a psychostimulant in cancer pain patients include the lack of abuse potential, the lack of governmental regulation (in the USA) through special triplicate prescriptions, milder sympathomimetic effects as compared to other psychostimulants and, most importantly, availability in chewable tablet form that can be absorbed through the buccal mucosa and can therefore be used by cancer patients who have difficulty swallowing or have intestinal obstruction. In our clinical experience, pemoline is as effective as methylphenidate or dextroamphetamine in the treatment of depressive symptoms in cancer-pain patients (Breitbart & Mermelstein 1992). Pemoline is usually started at a dose of 18.75 mg at 8.00 a.m. and noon, and increased gradually over the next several days. Typically, patients require 75 mg a day or less. Pemoline should be used with caution in patients with liver impairment and liver function tests should be monitored periodically with longer term treatment (Nehra et al 1990).

Monamine oxidase inhibitors

In the cancer-pain patient, use of a monamine oxidase inhibitor (MAOI) must be accompanied by caution. Dietary restrictions, such as the avoidance of tyramine-containing foods while on an MAOI, are often unpopular among cancer patients who may already have dietary and nutritional restrictions. Narcotic analgesics may also be problematic or even dangerous in patients taking MAOIs, since myoclonus and delirium have been reported (Breitbart & Holland 1988), thus limiting the utility of these agents in cancer patients with pain. The use of meperidine in patients taking an MAOI is absolutely contraindicated and can lead to hyperpyrexia and cardiovascular collapse.

Sympathomimetic drugs and other less obvious monoamine oxidase inhibitors such as the chemotherapeutic agent procarbazine can cause a hypertensive crisis in patients taking an MAOI. If a patient has responded well to an MAOI for depression in the past, its continued use is warranted, but again with extreme caution.

Lithium carbonate

Patients who have been treated with lithium carbonate prior to a cancer illness can be maintained on it throughout cancer treatment, although close monitoring is necessary, especially in preoperative and postoperative periods when fluids and salt may be restricted and fluid balance shifts can occur. Maintenance doses of lithium may need reduction in seriously-ill patients. Lithium carbonate is primarily eliminated through renal excretion and so should be prescribed with caution in patients receiving cisplatinum and other nephrotoxic agents. Several authors have reported possible beneficial effects from the use of lithium in neutropenic cancer patients; however, the functional capabilities of these leucocytes have not been determined. This leucocyte stimulation effect appears to be transient (Stein et al 1980).

Benzodiazepines

The triazolobenzodiazepine alprazolam has been shown to be a mildly effective antidepressant as well as an anxiolytic. Alprazolam is particularly useful in cancer patients who have mixed symptoms of anxiety and depression (i.e. adjustment disorder with anxious and depressed mood). Alprazolam alone is probably not adequate in the treatment of major depressive syndromes. The starting dose is 0.25 mg three times a day, although therapeutic effects may require 4–6 mg daily (Holland et al 1991).

Electroconvulsive therapy

Occasionally, it is necessary to consider electroconvulsive therapy (ECT) for severely depressed cancer-pain patients such as those whose depression includes psychotic features or patients for whom treatment with antidepressants pose unacceptable side-effects. The safe, effective use of ECT in depressed cancer patients has been reviewed by others (Massie & Holland 1990) and will not be elaborated here, although this alternative may yield secondary analgesic benefits for the depressed patient with otherwise unrelieved pain.

ANXIETY IN CANCER PAIN PATIENTS

A number of different types of anxiety syndrome commonly appear in cancer patients with and without pain, including: (i) reactive anxiety related to the stresses of cancer and its treatment; (ii) anxiety that is a manifestation of a medical or physiological problem related to cancer, such as uncontrolled pain (organic anxiety disorder), and (iii) phobias, panic and chronic anxiety disorders that predate the cancer diagnosis but are exacerbated during illness (Massie & Holland 1987; Holland 1989b).

REACTIVE ANXIETY

Although many, if not all, patients experience some anxiety at critical moments during the evaluation and treatment of cancer (i.e. while waiting to hear of diagnosis or possible recurrence, before procedures, diagnostic tests, surgery or while awaiting test results), such anxiety may disrupt a patient's ability to function normally, interfere with interpersonal relationships and even impact upon the ability to understand or comply with cancer treatments. In such cases, anxiety can be effectively treated pharmacologically with benzodiazepines such as alprazolam, oxazepam or lorazepam. In patients whose level of anxiety is relatively mild, and when sufficient time exists for the patient to learn a behavioral technique, relaxation and imagery exercises or cognitive restructuring can be useful in reducing levels of distress (Holland et al 1991). Optimal treatment of anxiety generally incorporates both a benzodiazepine and relaxation exercises or other behavioural interventions.

ORGANIC ANXIETY

The diagnosis of organic anxiety disorder assumes that a medical factor is the aetiological agent in the production of anxious symptoms. Cancer patients with pain are exposed to multiple potential organic causes of anxiety, including medications, uncontrolled pain, infection, metabolic derangements, etc. Patients in acute pain and those with acute or chronic respiratory distress often appear anxious.

The anxiety that accompanies acute pain is best treated with analgesics; the anxiety that accompanies severe respiratory distress is usually relieved by oxygen and the judicious use of morphine and/or antihistamines. Many patients receiving corticosteroids experience insomnia and anxiety symptoms which vary from mild to severe. Since steroids prescribed as part of cancer therapy usually cannot be discontinued, anxiety symptoms are often relieved with benzodiazepines or low-dose antipsychotics (Stiefel et al 1989). Patients developing an encephalopathy (delirium) or who are in early stages of dementia can also appear restless or anxious. Symptoms of anxiety are also frequent sequelae of a withdrawal from narcotics, alcohol, benzodiazepines and barbiturates. Since patients who abuse alcohol often inaccurately report alcohol intake prior to admission, the physician needs to consider alcohol withdrawal in all patients who develop otherwise unexplained anxiety symptoms during early days of admission to the hospital. Other medical conditions that may have anxiety as a prominent or presenting symptom include hyperthyroidism, phaeochromocytoma, carcinoid, primary and metastatic brain tumour and mitral valve prolapse (Holland 1989b; Breitbart 1989b).

PHOBIAS AND PANIC

Occasionally, patients have their first episode of panic or phobia while in the cancer setting. Approximately 20% of Memorial Hospital patients scheduled to have an MRI scan examination developed anxiety (typically claustrophobia) of such intensity that they were unable to complete the procedure (Brennan et al 1988). A number of variants of anxiety disorders (e.g. panic attack, needle phobia or claustrophobia) can complicate treatment and thus a prompt psychiatric consultation is recommended. The techniques available to treat these disorders include both behavioural interventions (such as relaxation training, systematic desensitization and in vivo or imaginative exposure for specific phobias) and more rapid pharmacological approaches for both phobias and panic. If there is the luxury of time (days to weeks) and the patient will have to face the stress (venipunctures, bone marrow aspirations) repeatedly, behavioural interventions may be advisable in order to enable the patient to gain some control over such fear. Often, however, the need for anxiety relief is immediate because of the urgency of many medical procedures and benzodiazepines (e.g. alprazolam 0.25–1.0 mg p.o.), in addition to providing emotional support, are used to help the phobic patient undergo necessary procedures.

PHARMACOLOGICAL TREATMENT OF ANXIETY SYMPTOMS AND DISORDERS

The most commonly used drugs for the treatment of anxiety are the benzodiazepines (Massie & Holland 1987; Holland 1989b). Other medications used to alleviate anxiety include buspirone, antipsychotics, antihistamines, beta-blockers and antidepressants (Table 44.3).

Benzodiazepines

For cancer pain patients, the preferred benzodiazepines are those with shorter half-lives (i.e. alprazolam, lorazepam and oxazepam). These medications are better tolerated and are complicated less frequently by toxic accumulation of active metabolites when combined with other sedating medications (e.g. analgesics, diphenhydramine). Determining the optimal starting dose depends on a number of factors, including the severity of the anxiety, the patient's physical state (respiratory and hepatic impairment), estimated tolerance to benzodiazepines and the concurrent use of other medications (antidepressants, analgesics, antiemetics). The dose schedule also depends on the half-life of the drug; shorter-acting benzodiazepines must be given three to four times a day, while longer acting diazepam can be used on a twice-daily schedule. Anxiolytic medications are often

Table 44.3 Anxiolytic medications used in cancer-pain patients

Generic name	Approximate daily dosage range (mg)	Route*
Benzodiazepines		
Very short acting		
Midazolam	10–60 per 24h	i.v., s.c.
Short acting		
Alprazolam	0.25–2.0 t.i.d–q.i.d	p.o., s.l.
Oxazepam	10–15 t.i.d–q.i.d	p.o
Lorazepam	0.5–2.0 t.i.d–q.i.d	p.o., s.l., i.v., i.m.
Intermediate acting		
Chlordiazepoxide	10–50 t.i.d–q.i.d	p.o., i.m.
Long acting		
Diazepam	5–10 b.i.d–q.i.d	p.o., i.m., i.v., p.r.
Clorazepate	7.5–15 b.i.d–q.i.d	p.o.
Clonazepam	0.5–2 b.i.d–q.i.d	p.o.
Nonbenzodiazepines		
Buspirone	5–20 t.i.d	p.o.
Neuroleptics		
Haloperidol	0.5–5 q 2–12 h	p.o., i.v., s.c., i.m.
Methotrimeprazine	10–20 q 4–8 h	p.o., i.v., s.c.
Thioridazine	10–75 t.i.d–q.i.d	p.o.
Chlorpromazine	12.5–50 q 4–12 h	p.o., i.m., i.v.
Antihistamine		
Hydroxyzine	25–50 q 4–6 h	p.o., i.v., s.c.
Tricyclic antidepressants		
Imipramine	12.5–150 h	p.o., i.m.
Clomipramine	10–150 h	p.o.

*p.o., per oral; i.m., intramuscular; p.r., per rectum; i.v., intravenous; s.c., subcutaneous; s.l., sublingual; b.i.d, two times a day; t.i.d, three times a day; q.i.d, four times a day; q (2–12) h, every (2–12) hours. Parenteral doses are generally twice as potent as oral doses; intravenous bolus injections or infusions should be administered slowly.

prescribed only on an 'as needed' basis for patients whose anxiety is limited to specific events such as medical procedures or chemotherapy treatments. However, patients with chronic anxiety should be treated with anxiolytics on an around-the-clock schedule as with analgesics for chronic pain. The most common side-effects of the benzodiazepines are drowsiness and motor incoordination. Physicians must be aware of synergistic effects when they are used with other CNS depressants and the possibility of resulting confusional states. If these occur, the dose should be lowered. If side-effects persist, the anxiolytic should be discontinued and another class of medication used. In patients taking benzodiazepines chronically (for periods of several weeks), abrupt discontinuation can lead to a serious withdrawal syndrome similar to alcohol withdrawal.

Midazolam (Versed) is a very short-acting benzodiazepine that is administered, usually as an intravenous infusion, in critical care settings where sedation is the goal in an agitated or anxious patient on a respirator. Clonazepam, a long-acting benzodiazepine, has been found to be extremely useful in cancer patients for a multitude of symptoms and treatment needs. Symptoms of anxiety and depersonalization or derealization, particularly in the presence of seizure disorders, brain tumours and mild organic mental disorders, are often successfully treated with clonazepam. Patients who experience end-of-dose failure with breakthrough anxiety on shorter-acting drugs also find clonazepam helpful, as do patients with organic mood disorders who have symptoms of mania and as an adjuvant analgesic in patients with neuropathic pain (Chouinard et al 1983; Walsh 1990). Clonazepam is also frequently used when attempting to taper off a shorter-acting benzodiazepine such as alprazolam and in the treatment of panic disorder.

Nonbenzodiazepine anxiolytics

Buspirone is a nonbenzodiazepine anxiolytic that is useful, along with psychotherapy, in patients with chronic anxiety or anxiety related to adjustment disorders. The onset of anxiolytic action is delayed relative to a benzodiazepine, taking 5–10 days for relief of anxiety to begin. Since buspirone is not a benzodiazepine, it is not useful in preventing benzodiazepine withdrawal, and so one must be cautious when switching from a benzodiazepine to buspirone. The effective dose of buspirone is 10–20 mg p.o. t.i.d (Robinson et al 1988).

Antipsychotics such as thioridazine are useful in treating severe anxiety unresponsive to high doses of benzodiazepines and in treating anxiety in patients with cognitive impairment (e.g. encephalopathy or dementia) in whom benzodiazepines may worsen an organic mental syndrome. Thioridazine can be started at a low dose (10–20 mg p.o. two to three times per day) and increased, if necessary up to 100 mg three times per day. Antihistamines are infrequently prescribed for anxiety because of their low efficacy; hydroxyzine can be useful for anxious patients with respiratory impairment in whom benzodiazepines are relatively contraindicated. Acute panic is best treated with alprazolam or clonazepam. For maintenance treatment of panic disorder, the tricyclic antidepressant imipramine (used in doses comparable to those for the treatment of depression), alprazolam, clonazepam and the monamine oxidase inhibitors (e.g. phenalzine) all have demonstrated antipanic effects. Propranolol can be a helpful adjunct in blocking the physiologic manifestations of anxiety in patients with panic disorders (Holland 1989b).

DELIRIUM (ORGANIC MENTAL DISORDERS)

Delirium and other organic mental disorders occur in roughly 15–20% of hospitalized cancer patients (Levine et al 1978; Posner 1979) and are the second most common group of psychiatric diagnoses ascribed to cancer patients. Delirium and other organic mental disorders are an even more common occurrence in patients with advanced illness. Massie et al (1983) found delirium in more than 75% of terminally ill cancer patients they studied. The *Diagnostic and Statistical Manual of Mental Disorders*, 3rd edn (revised) (DSM-III-R) (American Psychiatric Association, 1987) divides organic mental disorders and syndromes into the subcategories of delirium, dementia, amnestic disorder, organic delusional disorder, organic hallucinosis, organic mood disorder, organic anxiety disorder, organic personality disorder, intoxications and withdrawal states. Lipowski (1987) has grouped these different disorders into those characterized by general cognitive impairment, (i.e. delirium and dementia), and those in which cognitive impairment is selective, limited or nonexistent (i.e. amnestic disorder, organic hallucinosis, organic mood disorder, etc.). In organic mental disorders where cognitive impairment is selective, limited or not observable, prominent symptoms tend to consist of anxiety, mood disturbance, delusions, hallucinations or personality change.

Delirium has been described as an aetiologically non-specific, global cerebral dysfunction characterized by concurrent disturbances in any of a number of different functions, including level of consciousness, attention, thinking, perception, emotion, memory, psychomotor behaviour and sleep–wake cycle. Disorientation, fluctuation, or waxing and waning of the above symptoms, as well as acute or abrupt onset of such disturbances are critical features of a delirium. Delirium is also conceptualized as a reversible process (e.g. as compared to dementia), even in patients with advanced illness. Delirium, however, may not be reversible in the last 24–48 hours of life. This is most likely to be due to the influence of irreversible processes such as multiple organ failure occurring in the final hours of life. Delirium in these last days of life is often referred to as 'terminal restlessness' or 'terminal agitation' in the palliative care literature.

Early symptoms of delirium or other organic syndromes are often misdiagnosed as anxiety, anger, depression or psychosis. Because of the potential for diagnostic error, the diagnosis of an organic mental disorder should be considered in *any* medically-ill patient demonstrating an acute onset of agitation or uncooperative behaviour, impaired cognitive function, altered attention span, a fluctuating level of consciousness or intense, uncharacteristic anxiety or depression (Lipowski 1987). A common error among medical and nursing staff is to conclude that a new psychological symptom represents a functional psychiatric disorder without adequately considering, evaluating and/or eliminating possible organic aetiologies. For example, the patient with mood disturbance meeting DSM-III-R criteria for major depression, who is severely hypothyroid or on high-dose corticosteroids may be more accurately diagnosed as having an organic mood disorder, depressed type (if organic factors are judged to be the primary aetiology related to the mood disturbance). Similarly, the patient with hyponatraemia, or the patient on acyclovir for CNS herpes, who is experiencing visual hallucinations but has an intact sensorium with minimal cognitive deficits, is more accurately diagnosed as having an organic hallucinosis rather than a psychotic disorder.

In many cases, differentiating between delirium and dementia can be extremely difficult, since they frequently share clinical features such as impaired memory, thinking, judgment and disorientation. Dementia, however, typically appears in relatively alert individuals with little or no clouding of consciousness. The temporal onset of symptoms in dementia is also less acute (i.e. chronically progressive) and the sleep–wake cycle appears less impaired. Most prominent in dementia are difficulties in short- and long-term memory, impaired judgment and abstract thinking as well as disturbed higher cortical functions (e.g. aphasia, apraxia). Occasionally one will encounter delirium superimposed on an underlying dementia, particularly in elderly patients or patients with AIDS or a paraneoplastic syndrome. A number of different clinical scales or instruments have also been developed to facilitate the diagnosis of delirium, dementia or other cognitive impairments. The delirium rating scale (DRS) developed by Trzepacz et al (1988) is a 10-item clinician-rated symptom measure assessing delirium. The scale is based on DSM-III-R diagnostic criteria for delirium and is designed to be used by the clinician to identify delirium and reliably distinguish it from dementia or other neuropsychiatric disorders. Each item consists of a series of descriptive statements or behaviours, each weighted with a numerical value reflecting the similarity of that feature with the phenomenology of delirium. The scale is completed by clinicians and the weighted statements are summed to generate a DRS score. A cut-off score of 12 or greater differentiates delirious from non-delirious patients. The mini-mental-state examination (MMSE) (Folstein et al 1975) is also a useful tool for the screening of cognitive deficits, but does not distinguish between delirium and dementia. The MMSE is a series of questions and tasks which assess five general cognitive areas including orientation, registration, attention and calculation, recall and language. The MMSE quantifies the patient's level of cognitive impairment and is more sensitive to cortical dementias such as Alzheimer's disease than it is in detecting subcortical deficits such as those found in AIDS dementia.

Organic mental disorders can be due either to the direct effects of cancer on the central nervous system (CNS), or to indirect CNS effects of the disease or treatments (medications, electrolyte imbalance, failure of a vital organ or system, infection, vascular complications and preexisting cognitive impairment or dementia). Given the large numbers of medications cancer-pain patients require, and their fragile physiological state, even routinely ordered hypnotics may engender an episode of delirium. Perhaps most relevant to cancer pain management is the role that narcotic analgesics play in the development of delirium. Certainly opioid analgesics such as meperidine, morphine sulfate, hydromorphone and levorphanel have been reported to cause confusional states, particularly in the elderly cancer patient and in the terminally ill patient (Bruera et al 1989b, 1990b). The toxic accumulation of meperidine's metabolite, normeperidine, is associated with florid delirium accompanied by myoclonus and possible seizures. The routine use of stable regimens of oral narcotic analgesics for the control of cancer pain is rarely complicated by overt delirium or confusional states (Liepzig et al 1987); in fact, most patients have minimal functional or cognitive impairment. There have been reports of organic hallucinosis, complicating standard regimens of oral opioids (Jellema 1987). Significant cognitive impairment as well as delirium can, however, occur during periods of rapid opioid dosage escalation, especially in older patients receiving intravenous infusions of opioids (Portenoy 1987; Bruera et al 1989b; Eller et al 1992). Eller et al (1992) recently studied the incidence of acute confusional states in 94 adult cancer patients receiving continuous intravenous morphine infusion for pain control. In this retrospective review, 68% exhibited some alteration in mental status and 53% had symptoms suggestive of delirium. Factors that increased risk of developing delirium included opioid dosage (higher dosage) age (over 65) and impaired renal function (creatinine >1.5 mg/100 ml).

Chemotherapeutic agents known to cause delirium (Table 44.4) include methotrexate, fluorouracil, vincristine, vinblastine, bleomycin, BCNU, cis-platinum,

Table 44.4 Neuropsychiatric side-effects of chemotherapeutic drugs

Drug	Neuropsychiatric symptoms
Methotrexate (intrathecal)	Delirium, dementia, lethargy, personality change
Vincristine, vinblastine	Delirium, hallucinations lethargy, depression
Asparaginase	Delirium, hallucinations, lethargy, cognitive dysfunction
BCNU	Delirium, dementia
Bleomycin	Delirium
Fluorouracil	Delirium
Cis-platinum	Delirium
Hydroxyurea	Hallucinations
Procarbazine	Depression, mania, delirium, dementia
Cytosine arabinoside	Delirium, lethargy cognitive dysfunction
Hexylmethylamine	Hallucinations
Isophosphamide	Delirium, lethargy, hallucinations
Prednisone	Depression, mania, delirium, psychoses
Interferon	Flu-like syndrome, delirium, hallucinations, depression
Interleukin	Cognitive dysfunction, hallucinations

asparaginase, procarbazine and the glucocorticosteroids (Holland et al 1974; Weddington 1982; Young 1982; Adams et al 1984; Denicoff et al 1987; Stiefel et al 1989). With the exception of steroids, however, most patients receiving chemotherapeutic agents do not develop prominent CNS effects. The spectrum of mental disturbances caused by corticosteroids ranges from minor mood lability to mania or depression, cognitive impairment (reversible dementia) to delirium (steroid psychosis). The incidence of these disorders varies greatly, with 3–57% of noncancer patients developing an organic mental disorder. Although these disturbances are most common with higher doses and usually develop within the first 2 weeks of steroid use, they can occur at any time, on any dose, even during the tapering phase (Stiefel et al 1989). Prior psychiatric illness or prior mental disturbance due to steroid use does not predict susceptibility to, or the nature of, subsequent mental disturbance with steroids. These disorders often reverse rapidly upon dose reduction or discontinuation (Stiefel et al 1989).

MANAGEMENT OF DELIRIUM

The appropriate approach in the management of delirium in the cancer-pain patient includes interventions that are directed both at the underlying causes and symptoms of delirium. Identification and correction of the underlying cause(s) for delirium must take place while symptomatic and supportive therapies are initiated (Lipowski 1987; Fleishman & Lesko 1989). In the case of the cancer patient in pain who develops delirium while on a high dose opioid infusion, often the mere reduction of dose or infusion rate (if pain is controlled) will begin to resolve symptoms of delirium within hours. Other strategies include switching from one opioid (e.g. morphine) to another (e.g. hydromorphone). Often, delirium will occur or persist even after such manoeuvres or pain may require continued high-dose infusion. The use of a concomitant neuroleptic drug (e.g. haloperidol) is indicated. Symptomatic treatment measures include support for and communication with the patient and family, reassurance, manipulation of the environment to provide a reorienting, safe millieu and then appropriate use of pharmacotherapies. Measures to help reduce anxiety and disorientation (i.e. increased structure and familiarity) may include a quiet, well-lit room with familiar objects, a visible clock or calendar and the presence of family. Judicious use of physical restraints, along with one-to-one nursing observation, may also be necessary and useful. Often, these supportive techniques alone are not effective and symptomatic treatment with neuroleptic or sedative medications is necessary (Table 44.5).

Table 44.5 Medications useful in managing delirium in cancer-pain patients

Generic name	Approximate daily dosage range (mg)	Route*
Neuroleptics		
Haloperidol	0.5–q 2–12 h	p.o., i.v., s.c., i.m.
Thioridazine	10–75 q 4–8 h	p.o.
Chlorpromazine	12.5–50 q 4–12 h	p.o., i.v., i.m.
Methotrimeprazine	12.5–50 q 4–8 h	p.o., i.v., s.c.
Benzodiazepines		
Lorazepam	0.5–2.0 q 1–4 h	p.o., i.v., i.m.
Midazolam	30–100 per 24 h	i.v., s.c.

*Parenteral doses are generally twice as potent as oral doses; i.v., intravenous infusions or bolus injections should be administered slowly; i.m., intramuscular injections should be avoided if repeated use becomes necessary; p.o., oral forms of medication are preferred, or s.c., subcutaneous infusions are generally accepted modes of drug administration in the terminally ill, q (2–12)h, every (2–12) hours.

Neuroleptic medications in the management of delirium

Neuroleptic medications vary in their sedating properties and in their potential for producing orthostatic hypotension, neurological side-effects (acute dystonia, extrapyramidal symptoms) and anticholinergic effects. The acutely agitated cancer patient requires a sedating medication; the patient with hypotension requires a drug with the least effect on blood pressure; the delirious postoperative patient who has an ileus or urinary retention should receive an antipsychotic with the least anticholinergic effects.

Haloperidol, a neuroleptic agent that is a potent dopamine blocker, is the drug of choice for the treatment of delirium in the cancer-pain patient because of its useful sedating effects and low incidence of cardiovascular and anticholinergic effects (Adams et al 1986; Lipowski 1987; Murray 1987). Relatively low doses of haloperidol (1–3 mg/day) are usually effective in targeting agitation, paranoia and fear. Typically 0.5–1.0 mg haloperidol (p.o., i.v., i.m., s.c.) is administered initially, with repeat doses every 45–60 minutes titrated against symptoms (Massie et al 1983; Fleishman & Lesko 1989). Peak plasma concentrations are achieved in 2–4 hours after an oral dose and measureable plasma concentrations occur 15–30 minutes after intramuscular administrations. Although not yet approved by the Food and Drug Administration for intravenous use, haloperidol is commonly and safely administered by this route. The intravenous route is preferable in agitated or paranoid patients as it facilitates rapid onset of medication effects (Lipowski 1987; Adams 1988; Fleischman & Lesko 1989). If intravenous access is unavailable, we suggest starting with intramuscular or subcutaneous administration and switching to the oral route when possible. The majority of delirious patients can be managed with oral haloperidol. Parenteral doses are roughly twice as potent as oral doses. Delivery of haloperidol by the subcutaneous route is utilized by many palliative care practitioners (Fainsinger & Bruera 1992). Although our experience has been that most patients respond to doses of less than 20 mg of haloperidol in a 24 hour period, others advocate high doses (up to 250 mg/24 hour of i.v. haloperidol) in selected cases (Adams et al 1986; Murray 1987; Fernandez et al 1989).

A drawback to the use of haloperidol is the potential for causing extrapyramidal side-effects and movement disorders. Acute dystonias and extrapyramidal side-effects can generally be controlled by use of antiparkinsonian medications (e.g. diphenhydramine, benztropine, trihexyphenidyl); akathisia responds either to low doses of propranolol (e.g. 5 mg two to three times per day), lorazepam (0.5–1.0 mg two to three times per day) or benztropine (1–2 mg once to twice per day). A rare but at times fatal complication of antipsychotics is the neuroleptic malignant syndrome (NMS). NMS usually occurs after prolonged, high dose administration of neuroleptics and is characterized by hyperthermia, increased mental confusion, leucocytosis, muscular rigidity, myoglobinuria and high serum creatine phosphokinase (CPK). Treatment consists of discontinuing the neuroleptic and use of dantrolene sodium (0.8–10 mg per kilogram per day) or bromocriptine mesylate (2.5–10 mg three times per day) (Fleishman & Lesko 1989).

Benzodiazepines in the management of delirium

A common strategy in the management of agitated delirium is to add parenteral lorazepam to a regimen of haloperidol (Adams et al 1986; Murray 1987; Fernandez et al 1989). Lorazepam (0.5–1.0 mg every 1–2 h p.o. or i.v.) along with haloperidol, may be more effective in rapidly sedating the agitated delirious patient. Despite these clinical observations suggesting lorazepam as an effective adjunct to antipsychotic medications, benzodiazepines alone have limited benefit in the treatment of delirium. In a double-blind, randomized comparison trial of haloperidol versus chlorpromazine versus lorazepam, we demonstrated that lorazepam alone, in doses up to 8 mg in a 12 hour period, was ineffective in the treatment of delirium and in fact contributed to worsening delirium and cognitive impairment (Breitbart et al 1991b). Both neuroleptic drugs, however, in low doses (approximately 2 mg of haloperidol equivalent/per 24 hours), were highly effective in controlling the symptoms of delirium (dramatic improvement in DRS scores) and improving cognitive function (dramatic improvement in MMSE scores). Perhaps the only setting in which benzodiazepines alone have an established role is in the management of delirium in the dying patient.

Management of delirium in the dying cancer-pain patient

The treatment of delirium in the dying cancer-pain patient is unique for the following reasons. (i) Most often, the aetiology of terminal delirium is multifactorial or may not be found; Bruera et al (190b) reported that an aetiology was discovered in less than 50% of terminally-ill patients with cognitive dysfunction. (ii) When a distinct cause is found, it is often irreversible (such as hepatic failure or brain metastases). (iii) Work-up may be limited by the setting (home, hospice). (iv) The consultant's focus is usually on the patient's comfort and ordinarily helpful diagnostic procedures that are unpleasant or painful (i.e. CT scan, lumbar puncture) may be avoided. When confronted with a delirium in the terminally ill or dying cancer patient, a differential diagnosis should always be formulated; however, studies should be pursued only when a suspected factor can be identified easily and treated effectively.

The use of medications in the management of delirium in the dying patient remains controversial in some circles. Some have argued that pharmacological interventions with neuroleptics or benzodiazepines are inappropriate in the dying patient. Delirium is viewed as a natural part of the dying process that should not be altered. Another rationale that is often raised is that these patients are so close to death that aggressive treatment is unnecessary. Parenteral neuroleptics or sedatives may be mistakenly avoided because of exaggerated fears that they might hasten death through hypotension or respiratory depression. Many clinicians are unnecessarily pessimistic about the possible results of neuroleptic treatment for delirium. They argue that since the underlying pathophysiological process often continues unabated (such as hepatic or renal failure), no improvement can be expected in the patient's mental status. There is concern that neuroleptics or sedatives may worsen a delirium by making the patient more confused or sedated. Clinical experience in managing delirium in dying cancer patients suggests that the use of neuroleptics in the management of agitation, paranoia, hallucinations and altered sensorium is safe, effective and quite appropriate. Management of delirium on a case-by-case basis is always the most logical course of action. The agitated, delirious dying patient should probably be given neuroleptics to help restore calm. A 'wait and see' approach, prior to using neuroleptics, may be most appropriate with patients who have a lethargic or somnolent presentation of delirium. The consultant must educate staff and patients and weigh each of these issues in making the decision as to whether or not to use pharmacological interventions for the dying patient who presents with delirium.

Methotrimeprazine (i.v. or s.c.) is often utilized to control confusion and agitation in terminal delirium (Oliver 1985). Dosages range from 12.5–50 mg every 4–8 hours up to 300 mg per 24 hours for most patients. Hypotension and excessive sedation are problematic limitations of this drug. Midazolam, given by subcutaneous or intravenous infusion in doses ranging from 30–100 mg/24 hours are also used to control agitation related to delirium in the terminal stages (De Sousa & Jepson 1988; Bottomley & Hanks 1990). The goal of treatment with midazolam, and to some extent with methotrimeprazine, is quiet sedation only. As opposed to neuroleptic drugs such as haloperidol, a midazolam infusion does not clear a delirious patient's sensorium or improve cognition. These clinical differences may be due to the underlying pathophysiology of delirium. One hypothesis postulates that an imbalance of central cholinergic and adrenergic mechanisms underlies delirium and so a dopamine blocking drug may initiate a rebalancing of these systems (Itil & Fink 1966). While neuroleptic drugs such as haloperidol are most effective in achieving the goals of diminishing agitation, clearing the sensorium and improving cognition in the delirious patient, this is not always possible in the last days of life. Processes causing delirium may be ongoing and irreversible during the active dying phase. Ventafridda et al (1990a) and Fainsinger et al (1991) have reported that a significant group (10–20%) of terminally-ill patients experience delirium that can be controlled only by sedation to the point of a significantly decreased level of consciousness.

CANCER PAIN AND SUICIDE, PHYSICIAN-ASSISTED SUICIDE, EUTHANASIA

Uncontrolled pain is a major factor in cancer suicide (Breitbart 1987, 1990b). Cancer is perceived by the public as an extremely painful disease compared to other medical conditions. In Wisconsin, a study revealed that 69% of the public agreed that cancer pain could cause a person to consider suicide (Levin et al 1985). The majority of suicides observed among patients with cancer had severe pain, which was often inadequately controlled or tolerated poorly (Bolund 1985). Although relatively few cancer patients commit suicide, they are at increased risk (Farberow et al 1963; Breitbart 1987). Factors associated with increased risk of suicide in cancer patients are listed in Table 44.6. Patients with advanced illness are at highest risk and are the most likely to have the complications of pain, depression, delirium and deficit symptoms. Psychiatric disorders are frequently present in hospitalized cancer patients who attempt suicide. A review of the psychiatric consultation data at Memorial Sloan-Kettering Cancer Center (MSKCC) showed that one-third of cancer patients who were seen for evaluation of suicide risk received a diagnosis of major depression; approximately 20% met criteria for delirium and more than 50% were diagnosed with an adjustment disorder (Breitbart 1987).

Thoughts of suicide probably occur quite frequently, particularly in the setting of advanced cancer and, seem to act as a steam valve for feelings often expressed by patients as 'If it gets too bad, I always have a way out'. It has been our experience in working with cancer pain patients that once a trusting and safe relationship develops, patients almost universally reveal that they have occasionally had persistent thoughts of suicide as a means of escaping the threat of being overwhelmed by pain. Recent published reports, however, suggest that suicidal ideation is relatively infrequent in cancer and is limited to those who are significantly depressed. Silberfarb et al (1980) found that only 3 of 146 breast cancer patients had suicidal thoughts, whereas none of the 100 cancer patients interviewed in a Finnish study expressed suicidal thoughts (Achte & Vanhkouen 1971). A study conducted at St Boniface Hospice in Winnipeg, Canada, demonstrated that only 10 of 44 terminally-ill cancer patients were suicidal or desired an early death and all 10 were suffering from clinical depression (Brown et al 1986). At the MSKCC, suicide

Table 44.6 Cancer pain suicide vulnerability factors

Pain; suffering aspects
Multiple physical symptoms
Advanced illness; poor prognosis
Depression; hopelessness
Delirium; disinhibition
Control; helplessness
Preexisting psychopathology
Suicide history; family history
Inadequate social support

risk evaluation accounted for 8.6% of psychiatric consultations, usually requested by staff in response to patients verbalizing suicidal wishes (Breitbart 1987). In the 71 cancer patients who had suicidal ideation with serious intent, significant pain was a factor in only 30% of cases. In striking contrast, virtually all 71 suicidal cancer patients had a psychiatric disorder (mood disturbance or organic mental disorder) at the time of evaluation (Breitbart 1987).

We recently examined the role of cancer pain in suicidal ideation by assessing 185 cancer pain patients involved in ongoing research protocols of the MSKCC Pain and Psychiatry Services (Saltzburg et al 1989). Suicidal ideation occurred in 17% of the study population with the majority reporting suicidal ideation without intent to act. Interestingly, in this population of cancer patients who all had significant pain, suicidal ideation was not directly related to pain intensity but was strongly related to degree of depression and mood disturbance. Pain was related to suicidal ideation indirectly in that patients' perception of poor pain relief was associated with suicidal ideation. Our group at Memorial (Breitbart et al 1991b) examined these same issues in an AIDS population and found similar relationships between pain, mood and suicidal ideation. Perceptions of pain relief may have more to do with aspects of hopelessness than pain itself. Pain plays an important role in vulnerability to suicide; however, associated psychological distress and mood disturbance seem to be essential cofactors in raising the risk of suicide in cancer patients. Pain has adverse effects on patients' quality of life and sense of control and impairs the family's ability to provide support. Factors other than pain, such as mood disturbance, delirium, loss of control and hopelessness, contribute to cancer suicide risk (Breitbart 1990b).

In a 1988 survey of Californian physicians, 57% of those responding reported that they had been asked by terminally-ill patients to hasten death. Persistent pain and terminal illness were the primary reasons for those requests for physician-assisted suicide (Helig 1988). What is the appropriate response to such a request? The clinician in the oncology setting faces a dilemma when confronting the issue of assisted suicide or euthanasia in the cancer patient. From the medical perspective, professional training reinforces the view of suicide as a manifestation of psychiatric disturbance to be prevented at all costs. However, from the philosophical perspective, many in our society view suicide in those who face the distress of an often fatal and painful disease like cancer as 'rational' and a means to regain control and maintain a 'dignified death'. An internal debate thus often takes place within the cancer care professional that is not dissimilar to the public debate that surrounds celebrated cases in which the rights of patients to terminate life-sustaining measures or receive active euthanasia are at issue.

The term 'euthanasia' encompasses a number of concepts, all of which have become controversial but important issues in the care of terminally-ill patients. Active euthanasia refers to the intentional termination of a patient's life by a physician. Physician-assisted suicide is the provision by a physician of the means by which patients can end their own lives. Passive euthanasia refers to the withholding or withdrawal of life-sustaining measures and is viewed as acceptable in many societies (Pellegrino 1991). Active euthanasia and physician-assisted suicide, however, are perhaps the most intensely and bitterly debated issues in medical ethics today.

Active euthanasia has been taking place in the Netherlands for a decade (deWachter 1989; van der Maas et al 1991). While still illegal, the active termination of a patient's life by a physician is tolerated under the condition that: (i) the patient's consent is free, conscious, explicit and persistent; (ii) the patient and physician agree that the suffering is intolerable; (iii) other measures for relief have been exhausted; (iv) a second physician must concur; and (v) these facts must be documented. A best estimate is that 1.8% of deaths in the Netherlands are the result of euthanasia with physician involvement (van der Maas et al 1991). Common reasons for requesting euthanasia included: loss of dignity (57%), pain (46%), unworthy dying (sic) (46%), being dependent on others (33%) and tiredness of life (sic) (23%) (van der Maas 1991). Recently, the states of California and Washington have considered initiatives that would allow active euthanasia along the Netherlands model. Physician opponents of Washington State's recent referendum on euthanasia (Initiative 119) agreed that the vote was as much about pain control as it was about dying, and proposed that the state require physicians to take pain management courses in order to maintain licenses. Many supporters of Initiative 1991 voted for the measure because of fear that their death would be painful (American Medical News 1992). The case of 'Debbie', published in the Journal of the American Medical Association in 1988, forced a debate on active euthanasia in the USA that is ongoing (Gaylin et al 1988; Wanzer et al 1989; Singer 1990).

Physician-assisted suicide has also become a topic of public debate, following the dramatic case in 1990 of a woman with Alzheimer's disease who utilized Dr Kevorkian's 'suicide machine'. Dr Kevorkian was acquitted by a Michigan Court of any wrongdoing. Dr Timothy E. Quill, a physician who assisted a leukaemia patient in committing suicide, was not indicted by a Rochester grand jury in July 1991. Dr Quill's account of his participation in his patient's suicide was published in the March 7, 1991 issue of the New England Journal of Medicine (Quill 1991) and sparked a continuing debate regarding the physician's role in aiding dying patients. In interviews after he published this article, Dr Quill said he had decided to go public in order to present an alternative to Dr Kevorkian's approach, using a machine in the death of a patient whom Dr Kevorkian did not know well. In contrast to the Kervorkian case, Dr Quill had been treating the patient with leukaemia for 8 years and knew her quite well. In his article, Dr Quill described the process which he and the patient undertook, exploring her choice actively to take her life. He also described recommending that the patient contact the Hemlock Society and prescribing barbiturates for sleep 1 week later at the patient's request. While Dr Quill's patient was not suffering with uncontrolled pain, many physicians who care for cancer-pain patients report interactions with patients where requests for assistance in suicide are expressed. Foley (1991) reports that, in a large cancer centre pain clinic, patients not uncommonly consider suicide or request hastened death or physician-assistance, but change their minds once adequate pain control has been provided.

'The Humane and Dignified Death Act', a proposed law that would free doctors from criminal and civil liability if they participated in voluntary active euthanasia, did not appear on the 1988 California ballot because the sponsoring group (Americans Against Human Suffering) failed to get the required number of signatures. That group, an affiliate organization of the National Hemlock Society, did however undertake a survey of Californian physicians, as part of their efforts to build up support for the act, that was quite revealing (Helig 1988). Of the physicians who responded, 70% agreed that patients should have the option of active euthanasia in terminal illness. More than half of the physicians said that they would practise active voluntary euthanasia if it were legal. Some 23% revealed that they had already practised active euthanasia at least once in their careers. Of the 60% of physicians who indicated that they had been asked by patients with terminal illness to hasten death, nearly all agreed that such requests from patients can be described as 'rational'. Public support for the 'right to die' has been growing as well. Of the general population, 65–85% support a change in the law to permit physicians to help patients die and there is greater acceptance by the public of suicide when pain and suffering coexist with terminal illness.

Those of us who provide clinical care for cancer patients with pain and advanced illness are sympathetic to the goals of symptom control and relief of suffering, but are also obviously influenced by those who view suicide or active voluntary euthanasia as rational alternatives for those already dying and in distress. Ironically, while inadequate pain control seems to be a factor in driving patients towards suicide or assisted suicide/euthanasia, an obstacle to adequate pain control is the concern by many that aggressive pain control (e.g. opioid infusions) is a form of euthanasia. Many have argued that adequate pain control is not physician-assisted suicide or euthanasia (Wanzer et al 1989; Foley 1991; Pellegrino 1991). Danger lies in the premature assumption that suicidal ideation or a request to hasten death in the cancer patient represents a 'rational act' that is unencumbered by psychiatric disturbance. Accepted criteria for 'rational suicide' (Siegel 1982; Siegel & Tuckel 1984) include the following. (i) The person must have clear mental processes that are unimpaired by psychological illness or severe emotional distress, such as depression. (ii) The person must have a realistic assessment of the situation. (iii) The motives for the decision of suicide are understandable to most uninvolved observers. Clearly there are suicides that occur in the cancer setting that meet these criteria for rationality; however, a significant percentage, possibly the majority, do not, by virtue of the fact that significant psychiatric comorbidity exists. By reviewing the current research data on cancer suicide and the role of such factors as pain, depression and delirium, we hope to provide a factual framework on which to base guidelines for management of this vulnerable group of patients.

ASSESSMENT ISSUES IN THE TREATMENT OF CANCER PAIN: OBSTACLES TO ADEQUATE PAIN CONTROL

Cancer pain is often inadequately managed. Recently, a survey of 1177 oncologists who participate in the Eastern Cooperative Oncology Group (ECOG) was undertaken to assess cancer pain management (von Roenn et al 1993). Over 85% reported that they felt the majority of cancer patients are undermedicated for pain. Only 51.4% believed that pain control in their own setting was good or very good. Barriers to adequate pain management described by this survey of oncologists included: (i) patient reluctance to report pain (62%); (ii) patient reluctance to take medications (62%); (iii) physician reluctance to prescribe pain medication (61%); and, most importantly; (iv) poor pain assessment knowledge and skills (61%). Inadequate management of cancer pain is often due to a lack of ability to properly assess pain in all its dimensions (Marks & Sachar 1973; Foley 1985; Breitbart 1989a). All too frequently, psychological variables are proposed to explain continued pain or lack of response to therapy, when in fact medical factors have not been adequately appreciated. Other causes of inadequate cancer pain management include: (i) lack of knowledge of current therapeutic approaches; (ii) focus on prolonging life and cure versus alleviating suffering; (iii) inadequate physician-patient relationship; (iv) limited expectations of patients; (v) unavailability of narcotics; (vi) fear of respiratory depression, and, most important, (vii) fear of addiction.

Fear of addiction affects both patient compliance and physician management of narcotic analgesics leading to undermedication of cancer pain (Marks & Sachar 1973);

Macaluso et al 1988). Studies of the patterns of chronic narcotic analgesic use in patients with cancer have demonstrated that, although tolerance and physical dependence commonly occur, addiction (psychological dependence) is rare and almost never occurs in an individual without a history of drug abuse prior to cancer illness (Kanner & Foley 1981). Passik (1992) reviewed the requests for psychiatric consultation at Memorial Sloan-Kettering Cancer Centre for a 1 year period. In only 36 of 1200 (3%) requests for psychiatric consultation was substance abuse cited as the primary reason for the request. Interestingly, in one-third of these cases the psychiatry service consultant did not go on to concur with the labelling of the patient as a substance abuser (usually citing uncontrolled pain as the reason for the supposedly aberrant behaviour on the part of the patient). Fears of iatrogenic addiction result largely from the erroneous assumption the the opioids are highly addictive drugs and that the problem of addiction resides in the drugs themselves. Cancer patients allowed to self-administer morphine for several weeks during an episode of painful mucositis do not demonstrate escalating use (Chapman 1989). Of 11 882 inpatients surveyed in the Boston Collaborative Drug Surveillance Project, who had no prior history of addiction and were administered opioids, only 4 cases of psychological dependence could be documented (Porter & Jick 1980). A survey of burn centers identified no cases of iatrogenic addiction in a sample of over 10 000 patients without prior drug abuse history, who were administered opioids for pain (Perry & Heidrich 1982). A study of opioid use in headache patients identified opioid abuse in only three of 2369 patients prescribed opioids (Medina & Diamond 1977). These data suggest that patients without a prior history of substance abuse are highly unlikely to become addicted following the administration of opioid drugs as part of their medical treatment.

Escalation of narcotic analgesic use by cancer-pain patients is usually due to progression of cancer or the development of tolerance. Tolerance means that a larger dose of narcotic analgesic is required to maintain an original analgesic effect. Physical dependence is characterized by the onset of signs and symptoms of withdrawal if the narcotic is suddenly stopped or a narcotic antagonist is administered. Tolerance usually occurs in association with physical dependence but does not imply psychological dependence or addiction, is not equivalent to physical dependence or tolerance and is a behavioural pattern of compulsive drug abuse characterized by a craving for the drug and overwhelming involvement in obtaining and using it for effects other than pain relief. The cancer-pain patient with a history of intravenous opioid abuse presents an often unnecessarily difficult management problem. Macaluso et al (1988) reported on their experience in managing cancer pain in such a population. Of 468 inpatient cancer pain consultations, only eight (1.7%) had a history of intravenous drug abuse, but none had been actively abusing drugs in the previous year. All eight of these patients had inadequate pain control and more than half were intentionally undermedicated because of concern by staff that drug abuse was active or would recur. Adequate pain control was ultimately achieved in these patients by using appropriate analgesic dosages and intensive staff education. The reader is referred to the section below on Psychotherapy and Cancer Pain for more extensive review of the management of substance abuse problems in cancer pain patients.

The risk of inducing respiratory depression is too often overestimated and can limit appropriate use of narcotic analgesics for pain and symptom control. Bruera et al (1990a) demonstrated that, in a population of terminally-ill cancer patients with respiratory failure and dyspnoea, administration of subcutaneous morphine actually improved dyspnoea without causing a significant deterioration in respiratory function. The adequacy of cancer-pain management can be influenced by the lack of concordance between patient ratings or complaints of their pain and those made by caregivers. Persistent cancer pain is often ascribed to a psychological cause when it does not respond to treatment attempts. In our clinical experience we have noted that patients who report their pain as ‘severe’ are quite likely to be viewed as having a psychological contribution to their complaints. Staff members’ ability to empathize with a patient’s pain complaint may be limited by the intensity of the pain complaint. Grossman et al (1991) found that while there is a high degree of concordance between patient and caregiver ratings of patient pain intensity at the low and moderate levels, this concordance breaks down at high levels. Thus, a clinician’s ability to assess a patient’s level of pain becomes unreliable once a patient’s report of pain intensity rises above 7 on a visual analogue rating scale of 0 to 10. Physicians must be educated as to the limitations of their ability objectively to assess the severity of a subjective pain experience. Additionally, patient education is often a useful intervention in such cases. Patients are more likely to be believed and adequately treated if they are taught to request pain relief in a nonhysterical, business-like fashion.

Optimal treatment of cancer pain is multimodal and includes pharmacological, psychotherapeutic, cognitive-behavioural, anaesthetic, stimulatory and rehabilitative approaches. Psychiatric participation in cancer pain management involves the use of psychotherapeutic, cognitive-behavioural, and psychopharmacological interventions which are described below.

PSYCHOTHERAPY AND CANCER PAIN

The goals of psychotherapy with cancer pain patients are to provide support, knowledge and skills (Table 44.2).

Utilizing short-term supportive psychotherapy based on a crisis intervention model, the therapist provides emotional support, continuity, information and assists in adaptation to the crisis. The therapist has a role in emphasizing past strengths, supporting previously successful coping strategies, and teaching new coping skills such as relaxation, cognitive restructuring, use of analgesics, self-observation, assertiveness and communication skills. Communication skills are of paramount importance for both patient and family, particularly around pain and analgesic issues. The patient and family are the unit of concern, and often require a more general, long-term, supportive relationship within the health care system in addition to specific psychological approaches dealing with pain that a psychiatrist, psychologist, social worker or nurse can provide.

Group interventions with individual patients, spouses, couples and families are a powerful means of sharing experiences and identifying successful coping strategies. Utilizing psychotherapy to decrease symptoms of anxiety and depression, factors that can intensify pain, has been empirically demonstrated to have beneficial effects on cancer pain and overall quality of life. Spiegel & Bloom (1983b) demonstrated, in a controlled randomized prospective study, the effect of both supportive group therapy for metastatic breast cancer patients in general and, in particular, the effect of hypnotic pain control exercises. Patients were divided into either a support group focused on the practical and existential problems of living with cancer, a self-hypnosis exercise group or a control group. Results indicated that the patients receiving treatment experienced significantly less pain that the control patients. Passik et al (1991) described the efficacy of a psychoeducational group for the spouses of brain tumour patients. They have demonstrated the importance of addressing bereavement issues at an early stage in the patient's illness. The group members reported considerable benefit from one another's emotional support into widowhood and described improved quality of patient care (including pain management and all forms of nursing care) as a result of the support group.

While psychotherapy in the cancer pain setting typically focuses on more current issues around illness and treatment (rather than psychoanalytic or insight-oriented approaches), exploration of reactions to cancer often facilitates insight into more pervasive life issues. Some patients opt to continue with exploratory psychotherapy during extended illness-free periods or survivorship. Theoretical constructs derived from psychotherapy with chronic noncancer-pain patients can be helpful in guiding psychotherapy with the cancer-pain patient. Alexithymia and pain-induced dissociative symptoms (remnants of early life trauma) have proven to be useful adjuncts to the psychotherapeutic treatment of many cancer-pain patients and are discussed in detail below. Psychiatric observations of chronic noncancer-pain patients may have relevance to a subset of cancer-pain patients, although the degree of overlap between these two populations has received little empirical investigation.

Alexithymia, or the inability to express and articulate emotional experiences, is considered a personality trait associated with chronic pain and somatization. Recent research has demonstrated the utility of this construct in understanding the cancer-pain patient as well. Dalton & Feuerstein (1989), for example, demonstrated that patients who reported more prolonged and severe pain also scored higher on a measure designed to assess alexithymia when compared to patients experiencing sporadic or less intense pain. The cancer setting is characterized by highly emotionally charged issues revolving around loss, disability, disfigurement and death (Massie & Holland 1987). Patients are faced with intense emotions that can be threatening or difficult to articulate. Therapists can be quite helpful to alexithymic patients by acknowledging such feelings and allowing for their verbalization. In many instances, the therapist must actually provide the patient with a lexicon for their expression (Passik & Wilson 1987). Analogously, the meaning patients attribute to their pain can influence the amount of pain they report. Therapists can help to correct misperceptions about pain when appropriate and allow for the open discussion of issues and fears that might prolong or intensify a pain experience.

Increased awareness of the impact of traumatic events on psychological functioning and, in particular, on the development of dissociative states and disorders (psychogenic amnesia, fugue states, multiple personality disorder, conversion, posttraumatic stress disorder), has led to a growing acknowledgment of the traumatic impact of pain. Patients with dissociative disorders suffer from a wide variety of transient physical problems such as dysaesthesias, anaesthesias and pain (Terr 1991). In the chronic nonmalignant pain population there has also been growing empirical support for the existence of such sequelae of chronic pain. Patients with chronic pelvic pain and premenstrual syndrome, for example (Walker et al 1988; Paddison et al 1990), were found to have an unusually high prevalence of early sexual abuse. The prevalence of such phenomena in the cancer pain population is unknown. However, the cancer setting, with its life-threatening backdrop, toxic and disfiguring treatments and invasive procedures, can reawaken long-dormant traumata in even high-functioning patients with abuse histories. Inquiry into such issues can be essential to the evaluation and treatment of such patients. Although not generally a part of a routine psychiatric assessment in the medical setting, the recognition of the need to inquire into these areas requires attentive listening with the 'third ear' (Reik 1948).

THE SUBSTANCE-ABUSING PATIENT

Substance abuse is increasingly prevalent in the population at large and so will be encountered in the care of cancer-pain patients. The management of cancer pain in the active abuser and in the patient with a history of substance abuse is a particularly difficult and challenging problem (Payne 1989; McCaffery & Vourakis 1992). Portenoy & Payne (1992) have outlined a range of aberrant drug-taking behaviours that help to identify the substance-abusing cancer-pain patient. When patients obtain and use street drugs, purchase opioids from nonmedical sources or engage in illegal behaviours such as forging prescriptions or selling their prescription medications, a diagnosis of substance abuse is clear. More subtle and difficult to interpret are behaviours such as dose escalation without contact with the physician, contacting multiple physicians to obtain opioids, making frequent visits to emergency rooms, hoarding medications and using medications to relieve symptoms other than pain. What renders these behaviours difficult to interpret (though many physicians might feel that they are uniformly aberrant regardless of mitigating circumstances) is that such behaviours usually arise in the setting of an evolving pain complaint with fluctuating intensity and degree of relief. Many behaviours that are used to define addiction in the physically healthy have limited utility when assessing the cancer-pain patient. Relapse after withdrawal from a substance is a common feature in definitions of addiction (Jaffe 1985). However, relapse of pain complaints after decrease or withdrawal from a particular medication in a cancer-pain patient may simply signal the return to the baseline level of the underlying pain and may reflect the need for continued treatment with opioids. Furthermore, the need for chronic use of an opioid presupposes that the patient will become tolerant and physiologically dependent. The fact that the patient develops an abstinence syndrome upon abrupt discontinuation of the drug or requires higher doses for continued pain control has little bearing upon the diagnosis of drug abuse.

Psychological dependence is generally accepted as central to the definition of addiction and can be inferred from such behaviors as loss of control over the drug, compulsive use or use despite harm. Patients may directly state that they have lost control over their pain medicines or have become overly concerned with acquisition of these drugs. They may even be aware that their behaviour in seeking pain medicines has alienated their health care team and jeopardized their cancer treatment. Pain, psychological distress, the adequacy and duration of pain relief and the patient's prior cancer-pain experience must be taken into account when assessing the 'drug-seeking' patient. What appears to be highly aberrant drug seeking behaviour (obsessive preoccupation with the availability of opioids) may simply be a reflection of inadequate pain control. The term 'pseudoaddiction' (Weissman & Haddox 1989) has been coined to describe the phenomenon in which the highly preoccupied and apparently out-of-control patient ceases to act in an aberrant fashion upon the provision of adequate pain control. Drug-taking behaviours that are unsanctioned by the physician and that fall in the less severe end of the range of these behaviours should be given the benefit of the doubt and seen as reflections of inadequate pain control, especially if the physician's expectations about the patient's responsibility for communication about dose escalation has not been made explicit. Some patients, such as those with a prior history of drug abuse (but not actively abusing), may require more explicit discussions of the rules for treatment than that given to other patients being started on opioid therapy. Paradoxically, such an explicit outline of the parameters of opioid therapy will provide structure as well as comfort to patients who are concerned about relapsing into active abuse.

The psychiatrist or psychologist in the oncology setting who consults in the care of the active substance-abusing patient is faced with many obstacles. Foremost among them is the limited access patients with serious medical illnesses have to traditional modes of treatment for drug and alcohol problems. The demands of cancer treatment are not generally accommodated by inpatient drug treatment centers. Twelve-step and methadone maintenance programmes can be rigid in their approach to the cancer patient's use of opioids and psychiatric medications for symptom control. Hospital staff members are often resentful and frightened of the substance-abusing patient and this can detract from the psychiatrist's or psychologist's ability to create a caretaking environment and alliance with the patient. The addict, frightened and regressed in the face of potentially life-threatening illness, can be tremendously distrustful of the staff and may attempt to cope through drug use, guile and manipulation rather than trusting in the staff's competence and goodwill. At Memorial Hospital we have established several guidelines for the inpatient treatment of the active substance-abusing cancer-pain patient (in concert with hospital administration and security) that have allowed us to provide surveillance of illicit drug use and control over manipulation. The structured treatment guidelines set clear limits, help avoid medications appropriately used for pain and symptom control from becoming a focus of conflict and communicate knowledge about pain and substance-abuse management. In return for compliance, the patient, through the collaborative efforts of staff, is afforded a consistent and caring approach to pain and symptom control. In extreme cases, patients are informed that they will receive cancer treatment at our facility only if they comply with the recommendations of the pain/psychiatry team.

The active substance abuser is, when possible, admitted to the hospital with forewarning of the type of management he will receive. The patient admitted for a surgical procedure is brought into the hospital earlier to allow for stabilization of drug regimens and to avoid the development of withdrawal syndromes. The patient is admitted to a private room as close to the nursing station as possible to allow for monitoring and is informed that a search of his possessions will be conducted. Drugs, alcohol and previously prescribed medications are removed from the patient's possession. The patient is restricted to his room or floor until the danger of withdrawal or illicit drug use has been judged to be diminished. The patient is required to wear hospital pyjamas in an effort to render less likely his leaving the hospital to buy drugs. The patient's visitors are restricted to family and friends that are known to be drug-free (the psychiatry service consultant interviews those whom the patient would like to have visit). Packages brought to the hospital by family members and friends are searched by members of hospital security to ensure that they do not contain contraband. The patient is instructed to produce a urine specimen daily and more frequently if deemed necessary because of unconventional behaviour. Most laboratories in general hospitals are like our own in that they cannot return results of urine toxicology screens in a timely fashion. Thus, we collect daily specimens (for surveillance) and have them sent to the laboratory when clinically indicated.

Once these parameters are established, the patient is assessed several times daily for the adequacy of pain and other physical and psychological symptom control. Medications are prescribed in a manner that takes the patient's tolerance into account. Furthermore, medications are given on an around-the-clock basis so as to avoid frequent encounters with floor staff that center upon obtaining medications. Through the use of these guidelines, we have assisted in the management of patients who might otherwise have difficulty in rendering themselves 'treatable'. The plan also helps to contain staff sentiments such as anger and mistrust that might otherwise become a self-fulfilling prophecy in which the undertreated substance-abusing cancer-pain patient acts in an aberrant fashion that compromises treatment.

THE DYING CANCER-PAIN PATIENT

Psychotherapy with the dying patient in pain consists of active listening with supportive verbal interventions and the occasional interpretation (Cassem 1987). Despite the seriousness of the patient's plight, it is not necessary for the psychiatrist or psychologist to appear overly solemn or emotionally restrained. Often, it is only the psychotherapist, of all the patient's caregivers, who is comfortable enough to converse lightheartedly and allow the patient to talk about his life and experiences, rather than focus solely on impending death. The dying patient who wishes to talk or ask questions about death and pain and suffering should be allowed to do so freely, with the therapist maintaining an interested, interactive stance. It is not uncommon for the dying patient to benefit from pastoral counselling. If a chaplaincy service is available, it should be offered to the patient and family. As the dying process progresses, psychotherapy with the individual patient may become limited by cognitive and speech deficits. It is at this point that the focus of supportive psychotherapeutic interventions shifts primarily to the family. In our experience, a very common issue for family members at this point is the level of alertness of the patient. Attempts to control pain are often accompanied by sedation that can limit communication between patient and family. This can sometimes become a source of conflict, with some family members disagreeing amongst themselves or with the patient about what constitutes an appropriate balance between comfort and alertness. It can be helpful for the physician to clarify the patient's preferences as they relate to these issues early so that conflict can be avoided and work related to bereavement can begin.

CANCER PAIN AND THE FAMILY

The many stressors faced by the families of cancer patients have prompted mental health professionals who work with such patients to refer to them as 'second order patients' (Rait & Lederberg 1990). Family members face a difficult and ongoing process of adjustment throughout the stages of the cancer patient's illness. They are called upon to perform the sometimes onerous tasks of providing emotional support, meeting basic caretaking needs, sharing responsibility for medical decision-making, weathering financial and social costs and maintaining stability in the midst of the changes caused by cancer. Cancer pain can impact upon the performance of each of these tasks and the presence of pain has been found to be associated with increased emotional and financial burden in the family (Mor et al 1987). Pain is viewed as a major concern by family members of cancer patients and, perhaps more than other physical symptoms, it is perceived as a powerful threat to the ongoing ability to manage the disease (Ferrell 1991). Many studies have documented the concern family members have about cancer pain and the priority families place upon patient comfort (Hinds 1985; Rowat 1985; Kristjanson 1986; Blank et al 1989; Hull 1989). The management of cancer pain should provide for the inclusion of family members. A programme for family members should include education in pain management issues (i.e. the assessment of pain, proper administration and scheduling of medications, addiction), emotional support and stress management skills and structured opportunities for respite from caregiving responsibilities (Warner 1992).

As was noted above, cancer patients with pain are more likely to develop psychiatric disorders than are patients without pain. The presence of serious depression or organic mental syndromes can seriously disrupt family–

patient relationships and render the provision of ongoing emotional support for the patient difficult if not impossible. Family members themselves are vulnerable to developing stress-related emotional disorders which can further break down the support they can afford the patient. Ferrell et al (1991) examined patients with pain and its effects upon caregivers. Caregivers consistently described the patient's pain as highly distressing to themselves. They rated the patient's pain as more intense than did the patient and viewed the patient as extremely distressed by the pain. Thus pain heightened the burden of caregiving, especially in the areas of sleep disturbance, physical strain and emotional adjustment. In the advanced cancer patient, whose pain may be difficult to relieve without some sacrifice of mental clarity, family members may come into conflict with the patient or amongst one another if there is disagreement about the goals of pain treatment (mental clarity with residual pain versus greater comfort even if accompanied by sedation). Discussions of the patient's and family members' goals for treatment should be held early in the disease course, so that the patient and family can resolve conflicts with the full participation of the patient. Another issue which can lead to difficulty in the provision of emotional support are misconceptions harboured by family members about drug tolerance, dependence and addiction. Family members often become alarmed at the patient's increasing need for opioids and can withold treatment or their advocacy for the patient for fear that the patient will become addicted or 'use up' the drug's ability to relieve pain. Education about addiction, tolerance and the meaning of physiological dependence is crucial in the avoidance of such unnecessary conflicts. As described earlier in this chapter, some family members may view aggressive pain control as a form of euthanasia, and so may become quite distressed and act to prevent adequate pain control in a dying patient.

The family's tasks of providing basic caregiving and weathering the financial and social strains are also complicated by the presence of cancer pain. New technologies in pain treatment necessitate that family members become skilled in increasingly complex pain regimens, including the administration of medications and the coordination of multiple drug regimens. Learning how to assess pain and the side-effects of pain treatment can vastly complicate the caregiver's burden. These advances can also dramatically increase the financial and social costs of cancer care for the family. The prescription of various modalities for pain control needs to take into account family resources so as to avoid overburdening the family emotionally and financially.

Finally, the family's ability to provide the patient with continuity in the midst of change can be seriously threatened by the development of or changes in cancer pain. To provide for such continuity, family members need to feel as if they are able to predict or exert some control over the disease course. Cancer pain is often viewed as a harbinger of disease progression and as such can be a signal for the patient and family that they are about to enter a new phase of the disease. When cancer pain is continually unrelieved, it can confuse such signals and sacrifice family members' sense of control. The ability to maintain stability and provide the patient with a safe and supportive family environment can thus be disrupted.

CANCER PAIN AND STAFF STRESS

Those of us who work intensively with cancer patients have chosen a rewarding but stressful occupation. The painful nature of cancer and cancer treatment, difficult ethical dilemmas in treatment decision making, emotional reactions of patients and staff to cancer pain, and poor staff communication or conflict all contribute to the stressful cancer work environment.

Vachon (1987) described the stressors that are regularly encountered by oncologists and oncology nurses. These include caring for the patient who is extremely ill, dealing with the deaths of patients of all ages, poor staff communications, being intensely involved with patients and their families, conflicts between research and clinical care goals and the work load imposed by the complicated and taxing work of palliative care.

A survey conducted by Schmale and colleagues (1987) of 147 physicians who were members of the American Society of Clinical Oncology indicated that oncologists felt challenged by oncology but, nevertheless, they felt pressured, suffering from the negative responses and emotional problems of patients and families, the burden of dealing with dying patients, the frustration of ineffective treatments and the impact of negative personal life events. They identified a need for more emotional support for themselves as well as their patients. In a study done at Dana-Farber Cancer Institute (Peteet et al 1989), the greatest source of stress for physicians was their inability to help patients. Nurses felt that ethical issues, particularly as they revolve around 'do not resuscitate' (DNR) status, and competing research and clinical goals were the most stressful. von Roenn and colleagues (1993) found that the majority of oncologists felt they were inadequately trained in pain assessment and management. Thus, dealing with cancer patients who have difficult pain problems can increase this sense of inability to help and can intensify physician and nurse stress.

Intense medical involvement with cancer pain patients tends to elicit common reactions which are well known to health care workers in the field. The first is the need to try to 'save' patients from their cancer illness or death. The health care worker may wish to rescue patients from their dreadful plight. Unfortunately, disease often progresses, and failure to save or rescue patients provokes feelings of helplessness, impotence and a sense of futility. Low self-esteem and depression may result and sometimes lead to a sense of resentment towards the patient. In an attempt to deal with these feelings of helplessness and futility, the physician or nurse may become over-involved in the patient's medical care, encouraging or demanding inappropriately aggressive or unrealistic interventions. Staff members often find the transition from active treatment to palliative care difficult. Accepting altered treatment goals and relinquishing the hope of survival for a special patient can be very painful (Spikes & Holland 1975). Inability to recognize that such a transition in care is necessary can lead to a delay in dealing with issues such as DNR orders or other practical issues. Unaware of such reactions, a nurse or physician with a cancer patient may develop an adversarial relationship with other health professionals involved in that individual's care. A grandiose or self-serving attitude may develop in which the nurse or physician feels that only he or she understands the patient and knows how best to care for him medically. Unchecked, such attitudes can lead to staff conflict. More commonly, such an attitude reflects an overinflated sense of responsibility for the patient's fate, which can result in enormous guilt once the patient's condition ultimately worsens. An alternative response to feelings of helplessness and futility involve avoidance of or premature withdrawal from the patient. Such avoidance or withdrawal is often based on unrecognized angry feelings that reflect the impotence felt in dealing with a patient whose condition progresses and deteriorates despite all efforts (Massie et al 1989).

A second common reaction is the need to 'protect' the patient. This often takes the form of an avoidance to confront or bring up for discussion, even when appropriate, topics that may be painful or emotionally distressing to the patient. Consequently, important issues may go unaddressed such as the patient's feelings about pain, suffering and death, practical issues such as a will, DNR status and tying up financial loose ends. It is also important for the health professional to confront extreme denial and other maladaptive defenses on the part of the patient, especially when they interfere with treatment compliance. Recognition of our human limitations and personal vulnerabilities to loss are as important as being aware of these common countertransference reactions. Hopefully such awareness can benefit our patients, colleagues and ourselves.

A third common reaction is the tendency to blame the patient for his continued complaints of pain and discomfort. Ignoring the fact that cancer pain management is complex, this reaction takes the form of interpreting the patient's failure to respond to efforts at pain and symptom control as a desire on his part to perpetuate his symptomatology. Patients who have failed to respond to efforts at pain control are seen as 'needing their pain', 'communicating through pain' or drug-seeking. In an effort to protect oneself from feelings of inadequacy, the health care worker can displace his anger upon the patient and withold appropriate diagnostic tests or interventions.

The consequences of stress in the cancer work environment include the development of physical symptoms, psychological symptoms, 'burnout', or even more serious psychiatric impairment (e.g. alcoholism, drug abuse or depression). The most frequent physical symptoms of chronic stress include tension headache, exhaustion, fatigue, insomnia, gastrointestinal disturbances (with increase or decrease in appetite) when no medical explanation can be found and minor aches and pains (often questioned as signs of leukaemia or cancer). Psychological symptoms of stress in cancer staff include loss of enthusiasm for work, depression, irritability and frustration and a cynical view of medicine and colleagues (Hall et al 1979; Maslach 1979; Holland & Holland 1985; Mount 1986). Physicians and nurses can become overinvolved in their work, with excessive dedication and commitment, spend longer hours with less productivity and show decreased sensitivity to the emotional needs of patients and others; conversely, they may become detached and disinterested in medical practice. These two presentations of 'burnout' in oncologists and oncology nurses have been described as the 'I must do everything' syndrome and the 'I hate medicine' syndrome. Potential outcomes of both of these syndromes, if allowed to progress, include alcoholism, substance abuse, depression and even suicide (Hall et al 1979; Holland & Holland, 1985; Mount 1986).

The 'burnout' syndrome, described by Maslach (1979), is characterized by emotional exhaustion, depersonalization and lack of a sense of personal accomplishment. Emotional exhaustion is experienced as being emotionally overextended and exhausted by work. Depersonalization is a poor term to describe the sense of distance and reduced empathy that the person usually feels toward patients. Lack of personal accomplishment is expressed by such comments as 'What do I ever accomplish anyway?' Staff begin to feel that all treatment is futile in cancer, so why bother at all. Millerd (1977) conceptualized these problems as a form of survivor syndrome, as posttraumatic stress disorder, in health caregivers who have dealt repeatedly with losses from death; some of the adverse symptoms are the same as those seen in survivors of natural disasters.

A variety of coping methods can be introduced at both the personal and organizational levels and can be useful in the prevention and management of 'burnout' (Hartl 1979; Koocher 1979; Mount 1986). One of the most important strategies is to be able to recognize the physical and psychological symptoms of stress in oneself. If is additionally important to identify them in colleagues and point out that such symptoms are common, transient and reversible when dealt with early. Discomfort in pointing out emotional distress in a colleague should not be any greater than suggesting a consultation for a medical symptom. In the cancer centre, having the support of one's peers helps to decrease feelings of demoralization (Kash & Holland 1990). Providing ongoing education in pain management can help reduce stress and feelings of inadequancy for staff members.

Mental health professionals can perform several staff support roles in the oncology setting. Lederberg (1989) categorizes these roles into two: (i) support and backup to unit leaders, and (ii) facilitator of communications. Fulfilling such roles can be accomplished with activities that range from providing support to colleagues or helping identify and deal with troubled staff, to leading groups and conferences or participating in daily rounds. Ideally, an active role on the unit makes the liaison psychiatrist most familiar with the problems of the unit. The mental health consultant can be an outsider, but this usually limits one's effectiveness.

COGNITIVE-BEHAVIOURAL INTERVENTIONS IN CANCER PAIN

Cognitive-behavioural interventions are effective in the management of acute procedure-related cancer pain and as an adjunct in the management of chronic cancer pain (Table 44.7). Hypnosis, biofeedback and multicomponent cognitive behavioural interventions have been used to provide comfort and minimize pain in adults, children and adolescents undergoing bone marrow aspirations, spinal taps and other painful procedures (Hilgard & LeBaron 1982; Zeltser & LeBaron 1982; Redd et al 1982; Kellerman et al 1983; Jay et al 1986). In chronic cancer pain, cognitive behavioural techniques are most effective when they are employed as part of a multimodal, multidisciplinary approach that has assured adequate medical assessment and management, including appropriate use of opioid and nonopioid analgesics (Breitbart & Holland 1990). Cognitive behavioural intervention in chronic cancer pain has included such techniques as biofeedback, group therapy and self-hypnosis, music therapy, relaxation, imagery–distraction, behavioural rehearsal and positive reinforcement (occasionally as part of a multicomponent study) (Fotopoulos et al 1979; Turk & Rennert 1981; Spiegel & Bloom 1983b; Graffam & Johnson 1987; Zimmerman et al 1989; Beck 1991). Syrjala and colleagues (1992) tested the efficacy of psychological techniques for reducing pain related to oral mucositis in patients receiving bone marrow transplantation. This controlled clinical trial compared four interventions: (i) hypnosis training – combined relaxation and imagery; (ii) cognitive behavioural coping skills training – relaxation, cognitive restructuring, information, short-term goal-setting, exploration of meaning of pain; (iii) therapist contact control, and (iv) treatment as usual.

Table 44.7 Selected studies demonstrating efficacy of cognitive-behavioural interventions in cancer pain

Study	Type of pain	Intervention	Outcome
Hilgard & LeBaron (1982)	Bone marrow aspiration in children	Hypnosis	↓pain
Kellerman et al (1983)	Bone marrow aspiration; lumbar puncture in adolescents	Hypnosis	↓pain
Zeltzer & LeBaron (1982)	Bone marrow aspiration; lumbar puncture in adolescents	Hypnosis	↓pain
Redd et al (1982)	Hyperthermia adults	Hypnosis	↓pain
Jay et al (1986)	Bone marrow aspiration; lumbar puncture	Cognitive[b]-behavioural multicomponent programme	↓pain
Spiegel and Bloom (1983b)[a]	Chronic pain breast cancer	Group therapy and self-hypnosis	↓pain
Fotopoulos et al (1979)	Chronic cancer pain	EMG, EEG, biofeedback	↓pain
Turk & Rennert (1981)	Chronic cancer pain; terminally ill	Cognitive-behavioural multicomponent programme	↓pain
Syrjala et al (1992)[a]	Oral mucositis in BMT patients	Hypnosis versus cognitive behavioural training versus control	↓pain with hypnosis

[a] Controlled study.
[b] Filmed modelling, breathing training, imagery/distraction, behavioural rehearsal, positive reinforcement.
BMT = bone marrow transplant.

Patients in these groups met the psychologist twice pretransplant and then had 10 in-hospital sessions during the course of transplantation. All patients received opioids for their pain and opioid use was monitored. Interestingly, hypnosis was the most effective technique in reducing reported oral pain, even more effective than cognitive behavioural training.

Cognitive-behavioural techniques useful in cancer pain (Table 44.8) include passive relaxation with mental imagery, cognitive distraction or focusing, cognitive restructuring, progressive muscle relaxation, biofeedback, hypnosis, systematic desensitization and music therapy (Cleeland & Tearnan 1986; Cleeland 1987; Fishman & Loscalzo 1987). Some techniques are primarily cognitive in nature, focusing on perceptual and thought processes and others are directed at modifying patterns of behaviour that help cancer patients cope with pain. Behavioural techniques include methods of modifying physiological pain reactions, respondent pain behaviours and operant pain behaviours. The most fundamental technique is self-monitoring. The development of the ability to monitor one's behaviours allows a person to notice dysfunctional

Table 44.8 Cognitive-behavioural techniques used by cancer-pain patients

Psychoeducation
Preparatory information
Relaxation
Passive breathing
Progressive muscle relaxation
Distraction
Focusing
Controlled mental imagery
Cognitive distraction
Behavioural distraction
Combined relaxation and distraction techniques
Passive relaxation with mental imagery
Progressive muscle relaxation with imagery
Systematic desensitization
Meditation
Hypnosis
Biofeedback
Music therapy
Cognitive therapies
Cognitive restructuring
Behavioural therapies
Self-monitoring
Modelling
Behavioural rehearsal
Graded task management
Contingency management

reactions and learn to control them. Systematic desensitization is useful in extinguishing anticipatory anxiety that leads to avoidant behaviours and in remobilizing inactive patients. Graded task assignment is analogous to in vivo systematic desensitization, in which patients are encouraged to delineate and then execute a series of small steps towards an ultimate goal. Contingency management, a behavioural intervention in which healthy or adaptive behaviours are reinforced, has also been applied to the management of chronic pain as a method for modifying dysfunctionl operant pain behaviours associated with secondary gain (Cleeland 1987; Loscalzo & Jacobsen 1990). Primarily cognitive techniques for coping with pain are aimed at increasing relaxation and reducing the intensity and emotional distress that accompany the pain experience. Cognitive restructuring, a technique often used in the treatment of depression or anxiety, is an effective method of altering a patient's interpretation of events and bodily sensations. Because many patients are plagued by disturbing and maladaptive thoughts or beliefs, identifying and modifying these beliefs can allow for more accurate assessment of the situation and thereby decrease subjective distress (Fishman & Loscalzo 1987).

Most cancer patients with pain are appropriate candidates for useful application of cognitive and behavioural techniques; the clinician, however, should take into account the intensity of pain and the mental clarity of the patient. Ideal candidates have mild to moderate pain and can benefit from these interventions, whereas patients with severe pain can expect limited benefit from psychological interventions unless somatic therapies can lower the level of pain to some degree. Confusional states also interfere dramatically with a patient's ability to focus attention and thus limit the usefulness of these techniques (Loscalzo & Jacobsen 1990). Occasionally these techniques can be modified to enable patients with mild cognitive impairments to benefit. This often involves the therapist taking a more active role by orienting the patient, creating a safe and secure environment and evoking a conditioned response to the therapist's voice or presence.

Cancer patients are usually highly motivated to learn and practise cognitive-behavioural techniques because they are often effective not only in symptoms control, but in restoring a sense of self-control, personal efficacy and active participation in their care. It is important to note that these techniques must not be used as a substitute for apropriate analgesic management of cancer pain but rather as part of a comprehensive multimodal approach. The lack of side-effects associated with psychological interventions makes them particularly attractive in the oncology setting as a supplement to already complicated medication regimens. The successful use of these techniques should never lead to the erroneous conclusion that the pain was of psychogenic origin and therefore not 'real'. Although the specific mechanisms by which these cognitive and behavioural techniques relieve pain vary, most share the elements of relaxation and distraction. Distraction or redirection of attention helps reduce awareness of pain and relaxation reduces muscle tension and sympathetic arousal (Cleeland 1987).

RELAXATION TECHNIQUES

Several techniques are used to achieve a mental and physical state of relaxation. Muscular tension, autonomic arousal and mental distress exacerbate pain (Cleeland 1987; Loscalzo & Jacobsen 1990). Some specific relaxation techniques include (i) passive relaxation, (ii) progressive muscle relaxation, and (iii) meditation. Other methods that employ both relaxation and cognitive techniques include hypnosis, biofeedback, and music therapy and are discussed later in this chapter. Passive relaxation, focused breathing and passive muscle relaxation exercises involve the focusing of attention systematically on one's breathing, on sensations of warmth and relaxation or on release of muscular tension in various body parts. Verbal suggestions and imagery are used to help promote relaxation. Muscle relaxation is an important component of the relaxation response and can augment the benefits of simple focused breathing exercises, leading to a deeper experience of relaxation and self-control. Progressive or active muscle relaxation involves the active tensing and relaxing of various muscle groups in the body, focusing attention on the sensations of tension and relaxation. Clinically, in the hospital setting, relaxation is most commonly achieved through the use of a combination of focused breathing and progressive muscle relaxation exercises. Once patients are in a relaxed state, imagery techniques can then be used to induce deeper relaxation and facilitate distraction from or manipulation of a variety of cancer-related symptoms. Scripts that can be utilized by therapists to aid in teaching patients passive and/or active relaxation techniques are available in the literature (McCaffery & Beebe 1989; Loscalzo & Jacobsen 1990; Horowitz & Breitbart 1993).

IMAGERY/DISTRACTION TECHNIQUES

Clinically, relaxation techniques are most helpful in managing pain when combined with some distracting or pleasant imagery. The use of distraction or focusing involves control over the focus of attention. Imagery refers to the use of one's imagination, usually during a relaxed state or hypnotic trance, to manipulate some aspect of the pain experience or enhance distraction. Once in a relaxed state, the cancer patient with pain can use a variety of imagery techniques including: (i) pleasant distracting imagery; (ii) transformational imagery, and (iii) dissociative imagery (Breitbart 1987; Fishman & Loscalzo 1987; Breitbart & Holland 1990; Loscalzo & Jacobsen 1990). Transformational imagery involves the imaginative transformation of either the painful sensation itself, or the context of pain, or both. Patients can imaginatively transform a sensation of pain in their arm, for instance, into a sensation of warmth or cold. They can use such imagery as 'dipping their arm into a bucket of cold spring water', or into a 'vat of warm honey'. Such techniques can also be used to alter the context of the pain. Dissociative imagery or dissociated somatization refers to the use of one's imagination to disconnect or dissociate from the pain experience. Specifically, patients can sometimes imagine that they leave their pain-racked body in bed and walk about for 5 or 10 minutes pain-free. Patients can also imagine that a particularly painful part of their body becomes disconnected or dissociated from the rest of them, resulting in a period of freedom from pain. These techniques can provide much-needed respite from pain. Even short periods of relief from pain can break the vicious pain cycle that entraps many cancer patients. Again, scripts for imagery exercises are available in the literature (McCaffery & Beebe 1989; Loscalzo & Jacobsen 1990; Horowitz & Breitbart 1993).

HYPNOSIS

Hypnosis is efficacious in the treatment of some cancer pain (Barber & Gitelson 1980; Redd et al 1982; Spiegel & Bloom 1983b; Spiegel 1985). The hypnotic trance is essentially a state of heightened and focused concentration and thus it can be used to manipulate the perception of pain. The depth of hypnotizability may determine the effectiveness as well as the strategies employed during hypnosis. One-third of cancer patients are not hypnotizable and it is recommended that other techniques be employed for them. Of the two-thirds of patients who are identified as being less, moderately, and highly hypnotizable, three principles underlie the use of hypnosis in controlling pain (Spiegel 1985): (i) use self-hypnosis; (ii) relax, do not fight the pain, and (iii) use a mental filter to ease the hurt in pain. Patients who are moderately or highly hypnotizable can often alter sensations in a painful area by changing temperature sensation or experiencing tingling. Patients who are hypnotizable to a lesser degree can still utilize techniques that distract attention, such as concentrating on a mental image of a pleasant scene.

BIOFEEDBACK

Fotopoulos et al (1979) noted significant pain relief in a group of cancer patients who were taught electromyographic (EMG) and electroencephalographic (EEG) biofeedback-assisted relaxation. Only two of 17 were able to maintain analgesia after the treatment ended. A lack of generalization of effect can be a problem with biofeedback techniques. Although physical condition may make a prolonged training period impossible, especially for the terminally ill, most cancer patients can utilize EMG and temperature biofeedback techniques for learning relaxation-assisted pain control (Cleeland 1987).

MUSIC THERAPY

Munro & Mount (1978) have written extensively on the use of music therapy with cancer patients, documenting clinical examples and suggesting mechanisms of action. Music can often capture the focus of attention like no other stimulus and helps patients distract their attention away from pain, while expressing themselves in meaningful ways. Several studies have demonstrated beneficial effects of pain experience through the use of patient-selected instrumental audiotapes, and by listening to music or humming sounds (Zimmerman et al 1989; Beck 1991).

AROMA THERAPY

Aromas have been shown to have innate relaxing and stimulating qualities. Our colleagues at Memorial Hospital have recently begun to explore the use of aroma therapy for the treatment of procedure-related anxiety (i.e. anxiety related to MRI scans). Utilizing the scent of heliotropin, Manne et al (1991) reported that two-thirds of the patients found the scent especially pleasant and reported much less anxiety than those who were not exposed to the scent during MRI. As a general relaxation technique, aroma therapy may have an application for pain management, but this is as yet unstudied.

PSYCHOTROPIC ADJUVANT ANALGESICS FOR CANCER PAIN

While the mainstay of pharmacological management of cancer pain is the aggressive use of narcotic analgesics, there is a growing appreciation for the role of adjuvant analgesic drugs in providing maximal comfort (Breitbart 1989a; Breitbart & Holland 1990; Walsh 1990). Psychotropic drugs, particularly antidepressants, psychostimulants, neuroleptics and anxiolytics, are useful as adjuvant analgesics in the pharmacologic management of cancer pain. Psychiatrists are often the most experienced in the clinical use of these drugs and so can play an important role in assisting pain control. Table 44.9 lists the various psychotropic medications with their analgesic properties, routes of administration and approximate daily doses. These medications have been shown earlier (see Tables 44.2 and 44.3) to be effective in managing symptoms of depression, anxiety or delirium that commonly complicate the course of cancer patients with pain. They also potentiate the analgesic effects of opioid drugs and often have analgesic properties of their own.

Table 44.9 Psychotropic adjuvant analgesic drugs for cancer pain

Generic name	Trade name	Approximate daily dosage range (mg)	Route
Tricyclic antidepressants			
Amitriptyline	Elavil	10–150	p.o., i.m., p.r.
Nortriptyline	Pamelor, Aventyl	10–150	p.o.
Imipramine	Tofranil	12.5–150	p.o., i.m.
Desipramine	Norpramin	10–150	p.o.
Clomipramine	Anafranil	10–150	p.o.
Doxepin	Sinequan	12.5–150	p.o., i.m.
Heterocyclic and noncyclic antidepressants			
Trazodone	Desyrel	25–300	p.o.
Maprotiline	Ludiomil	50–300	p.o.
Serotonin specific reuptake inhibitors			
Fluoxetine	Prozac	20–60	p.o.
Paroxetine	Paxil	10–40	p.o.
Amine precursors			
L-Tryptophan		500–3000	p.o.
Psychostimulants			
Methylphenidate	Ritalin	2.5–20 b.i.d	p.o.
Dextroamphetamine	Dexedrine	2.5–20 b.i.d.	p.o.
Phenothiazines			
Fluphenazine	Prolixin	1–3	p.o., i.m.
Methotrimeprazine	Levoprome	10–20 q 6 h	i.m., i.v.
Butyrophenones			
Haloperidol	Haldol	1–3	p.o., i.m., i.v.
Pimozide	Orap	2–6 b.i.d.	p.o.
Antihistamines			
Hydroxyzine	Vistaril	50 q 4–6 h	p.o., i.m., i.v.
Steroids			
Dexamethasone	Decadron	4–16	p.o., i.v.
Benzodiazepines			
Alprazolam	Xanax	0.25–2.0 t.i.d.	p.o.
Clonazepam	Klonopin	0.5–4 b.i.d.	p.o.

p.o., per oral; i.m., intramuscular; p.r., parenteral; i.v., intravenous; q 6 h, every 6 hours, b.d., two times a day; t.i.d., three times a day.

ANTIDEPRESSANTS

The current literature supports the use of antidepressants as adjuvant analgesic agents in the management of a wide variety of chronic pain syndromes, including cancer pain (Walsh 1983, 1990; Butler 1986; France 1987; Getto et al 1987; Magni et al 1987; Ventafridda et al 1987). There is substantial evidence (see Ch. 50) that the tricyclic antidepressants, in particular, are analgesic and useful in the management of such chronic pain syndromes as postherpetic neuralgia, diabetic neuropathy, fibromyalgia, headache and low-back pain. Amitriptyline is the tricyclic antidepressant most studied, and proven effective as an analgesic, in a large number of clinical trials, addressing a wide variety of chronic pain syndromes (Pilowsky et al 1982; Watson et al 1982; Max et al 1987, 1988; Sharav et al 1987). Other tricyclic antidepressants that have been shown to have efficacy as analgesics include imipramine (Kvindesal et al 1984; Young & Clarke 1985; Sindrup et al 1989), desipramine (Kishore-Kumar et al 1990; Max et al 1991), nortriptyline (Gomez-Perez et al 1985), clomipramine (Langohr et al 1982; Tiengo et al 1987) and doxepin (Hammeroff et al 1982).

The heterocyclic and noncyclic antidepressant drugs such as trazodone, mianserin, maprotiline and the newer serotinin-specific reuptake inhibitors (SSRIs) fluoxetine and paroxetine may also be useful as adjuvant analgesics for chronic pain syndromes, including cancer pain; however, clinical trials of their efficacy as analgesics have been equivocal. Trazodone has been found to be analgesic in a cancer pain population; however, a trial for dysaesthetic pain in patients with traumatic myelopathy failed to show efficacy (Davidoff et al 1987; Magni et al 1987; Ventafridda et al 1987). Mianserin is a potent serotonin reuptake blocker with few adverse side-effects, thus making it an attractive choice as an antidepressant or adjuvant analgesic in the cancer-pain patient (Costa et al 1985). Maprotiline, a norepinephrine reuptake blocker, demonstrated moderate analgesic properties in a controlled comparison study against clomipramine (Eberhard et al 1988). In a double-blind crossover trial, maprotiline relieved pain related to postherpetic neuralgia, but was not as effective as amitriptyline (Watson et al 1992). Fluoxetine, a potent antidepressant with specific serotonin reuptake inhibition activity (Feighner 1985), has been shown to have analgesic properties in experimental animal pain models (Hynes et al 1985). There are no well-controlled studies of fluoxetine as an analgesic for chronic pain; however, several case reports suggest that fluoxetine may be a useful adjuvant analgesic in the management of headache (Diamond & Frietag 1989), fibrositis (Geller 1989) and diabetic neuropathy (Theesen & Marsh 1989). Paroxetine is the first SSRI shown to be a highly effective analgesic in the treatment of neuropathic pain (Sindrup et al 1990) and may be a useful addition to our armamentarium of adjuvant analgesics for cancer pain.

Tryptophan, a serotonin precursor, has been used for chronic pain (King 1980; Seltzer et al 1983) in doses of 2–4 g; however, nausea is a common side-effect with higher doses, thus limiting usefulness in debilitated cancer patients. Monoamine oxidase inhibitors (MAOIs) are also less useful in the cancer setting because of dietary restriction and potentially dangerous interactions between MAOIs and narcotics such as meperidine. Among the MAOI drugs available, phenelzine has been shown to have adjuvant analgesic properties in patients with atypical facial pain and migraine (Lascelles 1966; Anthony & Lance 1969).

Table 44.10 is a compilation of the studies, both controlled and uncontrolled, that demonstrate adjuvant analgesic efficacy of antidepressants for cancer pain. The antidepressants most commonly used in clinical studies on the management of cancer pain include amitriptyline, imipramine, clomipramine, trazodone and doxepin (Walsh 1986; Magni et al 1987; Ventafridda et al 1987). In a placebo-controlled double-blind study of imipramine in chronic cancer pain, Walsh (1986) demonstrated that imipramine had analgesic effects independent of its mood effects and was a potent coanalgesic when used along with morphine. In general, the antidepressants are utilized in cancer pain as adjuvant analgesics, potentiating the effects of opioid analgesics and are rarely used as the primary analgesic (Botney & Fields 1983; Walsh 1986; Ventafridda et al 1987). Ventafridda et al (1987) reviewed a multicentre clinical study with antidepressant agents (trazodone and amitriptyline) in the treatment of chronic cancer pain that included a deafferentation or neuropathic component. Almost all of these patients were already receiving weak or strong opioids and experienced improved pain control. A subsequent randomized double-blind study showed both amitriptyline and trazodone (a triazolo pyridine) to have similar therapeutic analgesic efficacy (Ventafridda et al 1987). Magni et al (1987) reviewed the use of antidepressants in Italian cancer centres and found that a wide range of antidepressants were used for a variety of cancer pain syndromes, with amitriptyline being the most commonly prescribed, for a variety of cancer pains. In nearly all cases, antidepressants were used in association with opioids. Good or fair analgesic results were reported in 51% of patients and the inclusion of all worthwhile responses (improved sleep, etc.) raised the proportion with benefit to 98%.

Table 44.10 Studies of antidepressants for cancer pain

Study	Drug	Efficacy of pain relief (%)
Gebhardt et al (1969)	Clomipramine	67
Adjan (1970)	Clomipramine	90
Bernard & Scheuer (1972)	Clomipramine + neuroleptic	87
Adjan (1970)	Imipramine	80
Monkemeier & Steffen (1970)	Imipramine	75
Barjou (1971)	Imipramine	70–80
Deutschmann (1971)	Imipramine	80
Hughes et al (1963)	Imipramine	70
Fiorentino (1969)	Imipramine[a]	p
Walsh (1986)	Imipramine[a]	p
Ventafridda et al (1987)	Amitriptyline[a]	p
	vs trazodone	p
Magni et al (1987)	Amitriptyline Imipramine Clomipramine Trazodone Doxepin	51–98
Breivik & Rennemo (1982)	Amitriptyline	67
Bourhis et al (1978)	Amitriptyline	0
	Trimipramine	0
Carton et al (1976)	Amitriptyline	70–80
Fernandez et al (1987a)	Alprazolam	75
Bruera et al (1989a)	Methylphenidate[a]	p

[a] Controlled study.
p = Drug more effective than placebo.

MECHANISMS OF ANTIDEPRESSANT ANALGESIA

The antidepressants are effective as adjuvants in cancer pain through a number of mechanisms that include: (i) antidepressant activity (France 1987), (ii) potentiation or enhancement of opioid analgesia (Malseed & Goldstein 1979; Botney & Fields 1983; Ventafridda et al 1990b), and (iii) direct analgesic effects (Spiegel et al 1983). Relief of depression in patients with chronic pain has been demonstrated to result in reported pain relief (Bradley 1963); thus, the antidepressant effects of the tricyclics and other antidepressants probably make an important contribution to the analgesic properties of this class of drugs. Antidepressants, however, also potentiate the analgesic effects of the opioid drugs. This occurs through direct action of the antidepressants on the central nervous system (CNS) that is likely mediated through serotonergic, catecholaminergic and anticholinergic effects (Botney & Fields 1983). Manipulation of CNS serotonin can dramatically influence the degree of analgesia produced by an opioid analgesic such as morphine. Increasing levels of CNS serotonin result in greater degrees of analgesia produced by an opioid drug, while depletion of CNS serotonin results in decreased opioid analgesia (Botney & Fields 1983). Serotonin is an important neurotransmitter mediator of opioid analgesia. Modulation of the noradrenergic and cholinergic systems in the brain also have profound effects on opioid analgesia (Basbaum & Fields 1978; Botney & Fields 1983; Gram 1983). Additionally, antidepressants can potentiate the analgesic effects of opioids through pharmacokinetic mechanisms. Imipramine, orally administered, can increase the bioavailability of morphine by reducing its rate of elimination (Feinman 1985). Desipramine can elevate methadone levels in serum (Liu & Wang 1975).

Antidepressants have direct analgesic properties of their own, independent of their effects on mood or potentiation of opioid analgesia (Gram 1983; Fields & Basbaum 1984). A leading hypothesis is that mechanisms involving serotonin and norepinephrine mediate clinical analgesia via descending systems originating in the brainstem and influencing the dorsal horn of the spinal cord (Basbaum & Fields 1978; Watson et al 1992; Fields & Basbaum 1984). The various tricyclic, heterocyclic and noncyclic antidepressants have effects on a number of neurotransmitters and their receptors (Charney et al 1981). A drug like amitriptyline acts to elevate levels of serotonin and noradrenaline in the nervous system by blocking the synaptic reuptake of both catecholamines (Basbaum & Fields 1978; Dubner & Bennett 1983). Other antidepressants have been demonstrated to have more specific serotonergic or noradrenergic properties. Many antidepressants with mixed or predominantly serotonergic properties such as amitriptyline, imipramine, nortriptyline, clomipramine, doxepin and trazadone have been shown to have direct analgesic effects. However, newer, more selective serotonin reuptake inhibitors such as zimelidine and fluoxetine as well as serotonin antagonists such as buspirone have proven disappointing in clinical studies of neuropathic pain (Watson & Evans 1985; Kishore-Kumar et al 1989). Maprotiline and desipramine, both rather selective noradrenergic agents, have now been demonstrated to have direct analgesic properties (Kishore-Kumar et al 1990; Watson et al 1992). Given these findings, the mechanisms of analgesia shared universally by all antidepressants are still not agreed upon. Variation among individuals in pain (as to the status of their own neurotransmitter systems) is an important variable (Watson et al 1992). Other possible mechanisms of antidepressant analgesic activity have been proposed (see Ch. 50).

RECOMMENDATIONS FOR CLINICAL USE

At this point, it is clear that many antidepressants have analgesic properties. There is no definite indication that any one drug is more effective than the others, although the most experience has been accrued with amitriptyline which remains the drug of first choice. What is the appropriate dose of tricyclic antidepressant when the drug is utilized as an analgesic and not as an antidepressant? Sharav et al (1987) argued that a low dose (10–30 mg) of amitriptyline is as analgesic as a high dose (75–150 mg). Zitman et al (1990), however, demonstrated only modest analgesic results from low-dose amitriptyline. More recently, Max et al (1987, 1988) presented compelling evidence that the therapeutic analgesic effects of amitriptyline are correlated with serum levels just as the antidepressant effects are, and analgesic treatment failure is due to low serum levels. A high-dose regimen of up to 150 mg of amitriptyline or higher is suggested (Kvindesal 1984; Watson & Evans 1985). The time course of onset of analgesia appears to be a biphasic process. There are immediate or early analgesic effects occurring within hours or days that are probably mediated by inhibition of synaptic reuptake of catecholamines (Botney & Fields 1983; Spiegel et al 1983; Tiengo et al 1987). Additionally, there are later, longer analgesic effects that peak over a 4–6 week period that are likely to be due to receptor effects of the antidepressants (Max et al 1987, 1988; Pilowsky et al 1982).

Treatment should be initiated with a small dose of amitriptyline (i.e. 10–25 mg at bedtime), especially in debilitated patients and increased slowly by 10–25 mg every 2–4 days towards 150 mg with frequent assessment of pain and side-effects until a beneficial effect is achieved. Maximal effect as an adjuvant analgesic may require continuation of the drug for 2–6 weeks. Serum levels of antidepressant drug, when available, may also help in management to assure that therapeutic levels are being achieved. Both pain and depression in cancer patients often respond to lower doses (25–100 mg) of antidepressant than are usually required in the physically healthy (100–300 mg), most likely because of impaired metabolism of these drugs. The choice of drug often depends on the side-effect profile, existing medical problems, the nature of depressive symptoms if present and past response to specific antidepressants. Sedating drugs like amitriptyline are helpful when insomnia complicates the presence of pain and depression in a cancer patient. Anticholinergic properties of some of these drugs should also be kept in mind. Occasionally, in patients who have limited analgesic response to a tricyclic, potentiation of analgesia can be accomplished with the addition of lithium augmentation (Tyler 1974).

PSYCHOSTIMULANTS

The psychostimulants, dextroamphetamine and methylphenidate, are useful agents prescribed selectively for medically-ill cancer patients with depression (Kaufmann et al 1982; Fernandez et al 1987b). Psychostimulants are also useful in diminishing excessive sedation secondary to narcotic analgesics and are potent adjuvant analgesics. Bruera et al (1987, 1989a) demonstrated that a regimen of 10 mg methylphenidate with breakfast and 5 mg with lunch significantly decreased sedation and potentiated the analgesic effect of narcotics in patients with cancer pain. Methylphenidate has also been demonstrated to improve functioning on a number of neuropsychological tests, including tests of memory, mental speed and concentration, in patients receiving continuous infusions of opioids for cancer pain (Bruera et al 1992).

Dextroamphetamine has also been reported to have additive analgesic effects when used with morphine in postoperative pain (Forrest et al 1977). In relatively low dose, psychostimulants stimulate appetite, promote a sense of well being, and improve feelings of weakness and fatigue in cancer patients. Treatment with dextroamphetamine or methylphenidate usually begins with doses of 2.5 mg at 8.00 a.m. and at noon. The dosage is slowly increased over several days until a desired effect is achieved or side-effects (overstimulation, anxiety, insomnia, paranoia, confusion) intervene. Typically, a dose greater than 30 mg per day is not necessary, although occasionally patients require up to 60 mg per day. Patients usually are maintained on methylphenidate for 1–2 months and approximately two-thirds will be able to be withdrawn from the drug without a recurrence of depressive symptoms. If symptoms recur, patients can be maintained on a psychostimulant for up to 1 year without significant abuse problems. Tolerance can develop and adjustment of dose may be necessary.

NEUROLEPTICS

Methotrimeprazine is a phenothiazine that is equianalgesic to morphine, has none of the opioid effects on gut motility and probably produces analgesia through alpha-adrenergic blockade (Beaver et al 1966). In patients who are opioid tolerant, it provides an alternative approach to providing analgesia by a nonopioid mechanism. It is a dopamine blocker and so has antiemetic as well as anxiolytic effects. Methotrimeprazine can produce sedation, anticholinergic symptoms and hypotension, and should be given cautiously by slow intravenous infusion, or subcutaneous infusion. Dosages for methotrimeprazine range from 12.5–50 mg every 4–8 hours up to 300 mg per 24 hours for most patients. In addition to its analgesic effects, methotrimeprazine is used as an anxiolytic and in the management of agitation and confusion in the terminally ill (Oliver 1985). Other phenothiazines such as chlorpromazine and prochlorperazine (Compazine) are useful as antiemetics in cancer patients, but probably have limited use as analgesics (Houde & Wallenstein 1966). Fluphenazine in combination with TCAs has been shown to be helpful for neuropathic pains (Gomez-Perez et al 1985). Haloperidol is the drug of choice in the management of delirium or psychoses in cancer patients and has clinical usefulness as a coanalgesic for cancer pain (Maltbie et al 1979). Both fluphenazine and haloperidol are most commonly used in low doses (2–8 mg per day) for neuropathic pain. The benefits of prolonged use of neuroleptics for analgesia must be weighed against the risk of developing tardive dyskinesia, particularly in the young patient with good long-term prognosis. Pimozide (Orap), a butyrophenone, has been shown to be effective as an analgesic in the management of trigeminal neuralgia at doses of 4–12 mg per day (Lechin et al 1989).

ANXIOLYTICS

Hydroxyzine is a mild anxiolytic with sedating and analgesic properties that are useful in the anxious cancer patient with pain (Beaver & Feise 1976). This antihistamine has antiemetic activity as well. 100 mg of parenteral hydroxyzine has analgesic activity approaching 8 mg of morphine and has additive analgesic effects when combined with morphine. Adding 25 mg to 50 mg of hydroxyzine every 4–6 hours orally, intravenously or subcutaneously to a regimen of opioids often helps relieve anxiety as well as providing adjuvant analgesia. Benzodiazepines have not been felt to have specific analgesic properties, although they are potent anxiolytics and anticonvulsants. Some authors have suggested that their anticonvulsant properties make certain benzodiazepine drugs useful in the management of neuropathic pain. Recently, Fernandez et al (1987b) showed that alprazolam, a unique benzodiazepine with mild antidepressant properties, was a helpful adjuvant analgesic in cancer patients with phantom limb pain or deafferentation (neuropathic) pain. Clonazepam (Klonopin) may also be useful in the management of lancinating neuropathic pains in the cancer setting, and has been reported to be an effective analgesic for patients with trigeminal neuralgia, headache and posttraumatic neuralgia (Caccia 1975; Swerdlow & Cundill 1981).

PSYCHIATRIC ASPECTS OF PAIN IN AIDS

According to several preliminary clinical studies (Lebovits et al 1989; Newshan et al 1989; Breitbart et al 1991a), pain is a significant problem for patients with HIV infection, and is associated with significant psychological and functional morbidity. Clinicians have neglected pain management in AIDS patients, focusing instead on treating life-threatening opportunistic infections, cancers and neuropsychiatric syndromes such as AIDS dementia complex. Health care professionals working with HIV-infected patients must be aware of the prevalence and types of pain encountered and of pain's potential role in initiating and sustaining psychological distress.

PREVALENCE OF PAIN IN HIV DISEASE

There are few systematic studies that examine the prevalence of pain, describe specific pain syndromes or examine the relationship of pain experience and psychological factors in the AIDS population (Breitbart 1990a). A recent retrospective chart review of hospitalized patients with AIDS revealed that over 50% of patients required treatment for pain; pain was the presenting complaint in 30% (second only to fever) (Lebovits et al 1989). In this study, chest pain occurred in 22%, headache in 13%, oral cavity pain in 11%, abdominal pain in 9% and peripheral neuropathy in 6%. A second retrospective review of pain in an AIDS population reported abdominal pain, peripheral neuropathy and Kaposi's sarcoma as the three most frequent pain problems, affecting 15% of hospitalized AIDS patients (Newshan et al 1989). Schofferman & Brody (1990) described pain in patients with far advanced AIDS. Of patients surveyed, 53% had pain, most commonly peripheral neuropathy, abdominal pain, headaches and Kaposi's sarcoma. At Memorial Hospital (Breitbart et al 1991a), we examined the prevalence and characteristics of pain in a population of HIV infected persons receiving medical care in an ambulatory setting. Of ambulatory HIV-infected patients, 38% reported significant pain. Patients had an average of two or more pains at any given time. Painful sensory neuropathy made up 50% of pain diagnoses. Kaposi's sarcoma resulted in lower extremity pain in an additional 45% of patients. Those with pain are more likely to have advanced HIV disease (i.e. CDC Class IV–AIDS), with low T4 cell counts, history of multiple opportunistic infections and lower Karnofsky performance scores (less able to function independently). HIV-related peripheral neuropathy is an often painful condition, affecting up to 30% of people with AIDS (Snider et al 1983; Levy et al 1985; Cornblath & McArthur 1988; Parry 1988), and characterized by a sensation of burning, numbness or pins and needles. It is important to note, however, that several antiviral drugs like ddI and ddC, chemotherapy agents used to treat Kaposi's sarcoma (vincristine), as well as Dilantin and isoniazid (INH) can cause painful peripheral neuropathy. Colony stimulating factor (GM-CSF) can cause transient bone pain. Barone et al (1986) observed abdominal pain in 12% of AIDS patients. Rabeneck et al (1990) reported 16 cases of painful swallowing due to oesophageal ulcers in HIV-infected men. Reiter's syndrome, reactive arthritis and polymyositis are other painful conditions reported to occur in early HIV infection (Kaye 1989).

IMPACT OF PAIN: PSYCHOLOGICAL DISTRESS

The patient with HIV disease faces many stessors during the course of illness, including dependency, disability and fear of pain and painful death. Such concerns are universal; the level of psychological distress, however, is variable and depends on social support, individual coping capacities, personality and medical factors, such as extent or stage of illness. It is important to remember that pain has a profound impact on levels of emotional distress and that psychological factors, such as anxiety and depression, can intensify pain.

In a study of the impact of pain on ambulatory HIV-infected patients (Breitbart et al 1991a), depression was significantly correlated with the presence of pain. In addition to being significantly more distressed and depressed, those with pain were twice as likely to have suicidal ideation (40%) as those without pain (20%). HIV-infected patients with pain were more functionally impaired and this was highly correlated with levels of pain intensity and depression. Those who felt that pain represented a threat to their health reported more intense pain than those who did not see pain as a threat. Patients with pain were more likely to be unemployed or disabled and reported less social support.

The effective treatment of pain often decreases psychiatric morbidity and occasionally eliminates a perceived psychiatric disorder. Conversely, interventions that diminish anxiety and mood disturbances also can reduce pain. When treating uncontrolled pain, clinicians should consider that psychological distress may be the consequence of the pain itself and not of other factors, such as an adjustment reaction to life-threatening illness, since personality factors may be distorted by the presence of pain.

CONCERNS ABOUT NARCOTIC ABUSE AMONG AIDS PATIENTS

Fears of addiction and concerns regarding drug abuse affect both patient compliance and physician management of narcotic analgesics and often lead to the undermedication of HIV-infected patients with pain. Studies of patterns of chronic narcotic analgesic use in patients with cancer, however, have demonstrated that although tolerance and physical dependence commonly occur, addiction (psychological dependence) and drug abuse are rare and almost never occur in individuals who do not have histories of drug abuse.

More problematic, however, is managing pain in the growing segment of HIV-infected people who are actively using i.v. drugs. Such use, specifically of i.v. opiates, raises several pain treatment questions including: how to treat pain in people who have a high tolerance to narcotic analgesics; how to mitigate this population's drug-seeking and potentially manipulative behaviour; how to deal with patients who may offer unreliable medical histories or who may not comply with treatment recommendations; and how to counter the risk of patients spreading HIV while high and disinhibited. In addition, clinicians must rely on a patient's subjective report, which is often the best or only indication of the presence and intensity of pain, as well as the degree of pain relief achieved by an intervention. Physicians who believe they are being manipulated by drug-seeking patients often hesitate to use appropriately high doses of narcotic analgesics to control pain.

Most clinicians experienced in working with this population of patients recommend that practitioners set clear and direct limits. While this is an important aspect of the care of i.v. drug-using people with HIV disease, it is by no means the whole answer. As much as possible, clinicians should attempt to eliminate the issue of drug abuse as an obstacle to pain management by dealing directly with the problems of opiate withdrawal and drug treatment. Clinicians should err on the side of believing patients when they complain of pain and should utilize knowledge of specific HIV-related pain syndromes to corroborate the report of a patient perceived as being unreliable.

PSYCHIATRIC MANAGEMENT OF PAIN IN AIDS

The psychiatric management of HIV-related pain involves the use of psychotherapeutic, cognitive-behavioural, and psychopharmacological techniques. Psychotherapists can offer short-term, supportive psychotherapy, based on a crisis–intervention model, and provide emotional support, continuity of care, information about pain management, and assistance to patients in adapting to their crises. This often involves working with 'families' that are not typical and that may consist of gay lovers, estranged spouses or parents, and fragmented or extended families. People with HIV disease may also require treatment for substance abuse.

Cognitive-behavioural techniques for pain-control, such as relaxation, imagery, hypnosis and biofeedback, are effective as part of a comprehensive multimodal approach, particularly among patients with HIV disease who may have an increased sensitivity to the side-effects of medications. Nonpharmacological interventions, however, must never be used as a substitute for appropriate analgesic management of pain. The mechanisms by which these nonpharmacological techniques work are not known; however, they all seem to share the elements of relaxation and distraction. Additionally, patients often feel a sense of increased control over their pain and their bodies. Ideal candidates for the application of these techniques are mentally alert and have mild to moderate pain. Confusion interferes significantly with a patient's ability to focus attention and so limits the usefulness of cognitive-behavioural interventions.

Psychiatric disorders, particularly organic mental disorders such as AIDS dementia complex, can occasionally interfere with adequate pain management in patients with HIV disease. Opiate analgesics, the mainstay of treatment for moderate to severe pain, may worsen dementia or cause treatment-limiting sedation, confusion or hallucinations in patients with neurological complications of AIDS. The judicious use of psychostimulants to diminish sedation and neuroleptics to clear confusion can be quite helpful.

Psychotropic drugs, particularly the tricyclic antidepressants and the psychostimulants, are useful in enhancing the painblocking properties of analgesics in pharmacological management of HIV-related pain. The tricyclic antidepressants (amitriptyline, nortriptyline, imipramine, desipramine, doxepin) and some of the newer noncyclic antidepressants (trazodone and fluoxetine) have potent analgesic properties and are widely used to treat a variety of chronic pain syndromes. They may have their most beneficial effect in the treatment of neuropathic pain, that is, pain due to nerve damage, such as the peripheral neuropathies seen commonly in people with HIV infection. Antidepressants have direct analgesic effects and the capacity to enhance the analgesic effects of morphine.

Psychostimulants such as dextroamphetamine or methylphenidate are useful antidepressants in people with HIV disease who are cognitive impaired and are also helpful in diminishing sedation secondary to narcotic analgesics. Psychostimulants also enhance the analgesic effects of opiate analgesics.

Inadequate management of pain is often due to the inability to properly assess pain in all its dimensions. All too frequently, physicians presume that psychological variables are the cause of continued pain or lack of response to medical treatment, when in fact they have not adequately appreciated the role of medical factors. Other causes of inadequate pain management include: lack of knowledge of current pharmaco- or psychotherapeutic approaches; a focus on prolonging life rather than alleviating suffering; lack of communication or unsuccessful communication between doctors and patients; limited expectations of patients to achieve pain relief; limited capacity of patients impaired by organic mental disorders to communicate; unavailability of narcotics; doctors' fear of causing respiratory depression; and, most importantly, doctors' fear of amplifying addiction and drug abuse.

SUMMARY

Unfortunately, cancer patients with pain are most vulnerable to such psychiatric complications of cancer as depression, anxiety and delirium. The clinician who wants to provide comprehensive management of cancer pain must be familiar with or have available expertise in psychiatric assessment and intervention in the cancer patient. Knowledge of the indications and usefulness of psychotropic drugs in the cancer pain population will be most rewarding, particularly since these drugs are useful not only in the treatment of psychiatric complications of cancer, but also as adjuvant analgesic agents in the management of cancer pain. Psychotherapy and cognitive-behavioural techniques have also been shown to decrease psychological distress in cancer-pain patients and provide useful tools for regaining a sense of control and reducing cancer pain. Psychopharmacological, psychotherapeutic and cognitive-behavioural interventions are all powerful psychiatric contributions to a multidisciplinary approach to the management of cancer pain. The mainstay of pharmacological interventions for cancer pain continues to be the appropriate use of narcotic analgesics. There is, however, growing awareness and acceptance of the benefits for cancer-pain patients derived from psychiatric contributions to pain control. These same principles may be applied to patients with HIV infection and pain with beneficial results.

REFERENCES

Achte K A, Vanhkouen M L 1971 Cancer and the psyche. Omega 2: 46–56

Adams F 1988 Neuropsychiatric evaluation and treatment of delirium in cancer patients. Advances in Psychosomatic Medicine 18: 26–36

Adams F, Quesada J R, Gutterman J U 1984 Neuropsychiatric manifestations of human leukocyte interferon therapy in patients with cancer. JAMA 252: 938–941

Adams F, Fernandez F, Andersson B S 1986 Emergency pharmacotherapy of delirium in the critically ill cancer patient. Psychosomatics 27: 33–37

Adjan M 1970 Uber therapeutischen beeinflussung des schmerzsmptoms bei unheilboren tumorkranken. Therapie der Hergenwart 10: 1620–1627

Ahles T A, Martin J B 1992 Cancer pain: a mutidimensional perspective Hospice Journal 8: 25–48

Ahles T A, Blanchard E B, Ruckdeschel J C 1983 The multidimensional nature of cancer related pain. Pain 17: 277–288

American Medical News, January 20, 1992, p 9

American Psychiatric Association Diagnostic and Statistical Manual of Mental Disorders, 3rd edn (revised) 1987 Spitzer R L, Williams J B W(eds) American Psychiatric Association, Washington, DC

Anthony M, Lance J W 1969 MAO inhibition in the treatment of migraine. Archives of Neurology 21: 263

Ayd F 1979 Amoxapine: a new tricyclic antidepressant. International Drug Therapy Newsletter 14: 33–40

Barber J, Gitelson J 1980 Cancer pain: psychological management using hypnosis. CA: a Cancer Journal for Clinicians 3: 130–136

Barjou B 1971 Etude du Tofranil sules douleurs en chirugie. Revue de Medecine de Tours 6: 473–482

Barone S E, Gunold B S, Nealson T F et al 1986 Abdominal pain in patients with acquired immune deficiency syndrome. Annals of Surgey 204: 619–623

Basbaum A I, Fields H L 1978 Endogenous pain control mechanisms: review and hypothesis. Annals of Neurology 4: 451–462

Beaver W T, Feise G 1976 Comparison of the analgesic effects of morphine, hydroxyzine and their combination in patients with post-operative pain. In: Advances in pain research and therapy. Bonica J J, Albe-Fessard D. (eds) Raven Press, New York, p 533–557

Beaver W T, Wallenstein S L, Houde R W et al 1966 A comparison of the analgesic effect of methotrimeprazine and morphine in patients with cancer. Clinical Pharmacology and Therapeutics 7: 436–446

Beck E 1967 Depression: clinical experimental and theoretical aspects. Harper & Row, New York

Beck S L 1991 The therapeutic use of music for cancer-related pain. Oncology Nursing Forum 18: 1527–1537

Bernard A, Scheuer H 1972 Action de la clomipramine (Anafranil) sur la douleur des cancers en pathologie cervico-faciale. Journal Francais d'Oto-Rhino-Laryngologie 21: 723–728

Blank S S, Clark L, Longman A J, Atwood J R 1989 Perceived home care needs of cancer patients and their caregivers. Cancer Nursing 12: 78–84

Bolund C 1985 Suicide and cancer: II. Medical and care factors in suicide by cancer patients in Sweden. 1973–1976. Journal of Psychosocial Oncology 3: 17–30

Bond M R 1973 Personality studies in patients with pain secondary to organic disease. Journal of Psychosomatic Research 17: 257–263

Bond M R 1979 Psychological and emotional aspects of cancer pain. In: Bonica J J, Ventafridaa V (eds) Advances in pain research and therapy, vol 2. Raven Press, New York, p 81–88

Bond M R, Pearson I B 1969 Psychological aspects of pain in women with advanced cancer of the cervix. Journal of Psychosomatic Research 13: 13–19

Botney M, Fields H C 1983 Amitriptyline potentiates morphine analgesia by direct action on the central nervous system. Annals of Neurology 13: 160–164

Bottomley D M, Hanks G W 1990 Subcutaneous midazolam infusion in palliative care. Journal of Pain Symptom Management 5: 259–261

Bourhis A, Boudouresue G, Pellet W, Fondarai J, Ponzio J, Spitalier J M 1978 Pain, infirmity and psychotropic drugs in oncology. Pain 5: 263–274

Bradley J J 1963 Severe localized pain associated with the depressive syndrome. British Journal of Psychiatry 109: 741–745

Breitbart W 1987 Suicide in cancer patients. Oncology 1: 49–53

Breitbart W 1989a Psychiatric management of cancer pain. Cancer 63: 2336–2342

Breitbart W B 1989b Endocrine-related psychiatric disorder. In: Holland J, Rowland J (eds) The handbook of psychooncology: the psychological care of the cancer patient. Oxford University Press, New York, p 356–366

Breitbart W 1990a Psychiatric aspects of pain and HIV disease. Focus, a Guide to AIDS Research and Counselling 5: 1–3

Breitbart W 1990b Cancer pain and suicide. In: Foley K M et al (eds) Advances in pain research and therapy, vol 16. Raven Press, New York, p 399–412

Breitbart W, Holland, J C 1988 Psychiatric complications of cancer. In: Brain M C, Carbone P P (eds) Current therapy in hematology oncology—3. B C Decker, Toronto, p 268–274

Breitbart W, Holland J 1990 Psychiatric aspects of cancer pain. In: Foley K M et al (eds) Advances in pain research and therapy, vol 16. Raven Press, New York, p 73–87

Breitbart W, Mermelstein H 1992 Pemoline: an alternative psychostimulation in the management of depressive disorders in cancer patients. Psychosomatics 33: 352–356

Breitbart W, Passik S, Bronaugh T et al 1991a Pain in the ambulatory AIDS patient: prevalence and psychosocial correlates (abstract). 38th Annual Meeting, Academy of Psychosomatic Medicine, October 17–20, Atlanta

Breitbart, Platt M, Marotta R et al 1991b Low-dose neuroleptic treatment for AIDS delirium (abstract). 144th Annual Meeting, American Psychiatric Association, New Orleans, May 11–16

Breitbart W, Stiefel F, Pannulo S, Kornblith A, Holland J C 1993 Neuropsychiatric cancer patients with epidural spinal cord compression receiving high dose corticosteroids: a prospective comparison study. Psycho-oncology (in press)

Breivik H, Rennemo F 1982 Clinical evaluation of combined treatment with methadone and psychotropic drugs in cancer patients. Acta Anaesthesiologica Scandinavica (Suppl) 74: 135–140

Brennan S C, Redd W H, Jacobsen P B et al 1988 Anxiety and panic during magnetic resonance scans. Lancet 2: 512

Brown J H, Henteleff P, Barakat S, Rowe J R 1986 Is it normal for terminally ill patients to desire death. American Journal of Psychiatry 143: 208–211

Bruera E, Chadwick S, Brennels C, Hanson J, MacDonald R N 1987 Methylphenidate associated with narcotics for the treatment of cancer pain. Cancer Treatment Reports 71: 67–70

Bruera E, Brenneis C, Paterson A H, MacDonald R N 1989a Use of methylphenidate as an adjuvant to narcotic analgesics in patients with advanced cancer: Journal of Pain Symptom Management 4: 3–6

Bruera E, MacMillan K, Kuehn N et al 1989b The cognitive effects of the administration of narcotics. Pain 39: 13–16

Bruera E, MacMillan K, Pither J, MacDonald R N 1990a Effects of morphine on the dyspnea of terminal cancer patients. Journal of Pain Symptom Management 5: 341–344

Bruera E, Miller L, McCalion S 1990b Cognitive failure in patients with terminal cancer: a prospective longitudinal study. Psychosocial Aspects of Cancer 9: 308–310

Bruera E, Miller M J, MacMillan K, Kuehn N 1992 Neuropsychological effects of methylphenidate in patients receiving a continuous infusion of narcotics for cancer pain. Pain 48: 163–166

Bukberg J, Penman D, Holland J 1984 Depression in hospitalized cancer patients. Psychosomatic Medicine 43: 199–122

Butler S 1986 Present status of tricyclic antidepressants in chronic pain therapy. In: Benedetti C et al (eds) Advances in pain research and therapy, vol 7. Raven Press, New York, p 173–196

Caccia M R 1975 Clonazepam in facial neuralgia and cluster headache: clinical and electrophysiological study. European Neurology 13: 560–563

Carton M, Cabarrot E, Lafforque C 1976 Interest de l'amitriptyline utilisee comme antalgique en cancerologie. Gazette Medicale de France 83: 2375–2378

Cassem N H 1987 The dying patient. In: Hacket T P, Cassem N H (eds) Massachusetts General Hospital handbook of general hospital psychiatry, 2nd edn. PSG Publishing, Littleton, MA, p 332–352

Chapman C R 1989 Giving the patient control of opioid analgesic administration. In: Hill C S, Fields W S (eds) Advances in pain research and therapy, vol 11. Raven Press, New York, p 339–352

Charney D S, Meukes D B, Heniuger P R 1981 Receptor sensitivity and the mechanism of action of antidepressant treatment: Archives of General Psychiatry 38: 1160–1180

Chiarillo R J, Cole J O 1987 The use of psychostimulants in general psychiatry. A reconsideration. Archives of General Psychiatry 44: 286–295

Chouinard G, Young S N, Annable L 1983 Antimanic effect of clonazepam. Biological Psychiatry 18: 451–466

Cleeland C S 1984 The impact of pain on the patient with cancer. Cancer 54: 2635–2641

Cleeland C S 1987 Nonpharmacologic management of cancer pain. Journal of Pain and Symptom Control 2: 523–528

Cleeland C S, Tearnan B H 1986 Behavioral control of cancer pain. In: Holzman D, Turk DC (eds) Pain management. Pergamon Press, New York: p 193–212

Clifford D B, Rutherford J L, Hicks F G, Zorumski C F 1985 Acute effects of antidepressants on hippocampal seizures. Annals of Neurology 18: 692–697

Cooper G 1988 The safety of fluoxetine – an update. British Journal of Psychiatry 153: 77–86

Cornblath D R, McArthur I C 1988 Predominantly sensory neuropathy in patients with AIDS and AIDS-related complex. Neurology 38: 794–796

Costa D, Mogos I, Toma T 1985 Efficacy and safety of mianserin in the treatment of depression of women with cancer. Acta Psychiatrica Scandinavica 72: 85–92

Dalton J A, Feuerstein M 1989 Fear, alexithymia and cancer pain. Pain 38: 159–170

Daut R L, Cleeland C S 1982 The prevalence and severity of pain in cancer. Cancer 50: 1913–1918

Davidoff G, Guarracini M, Roth E et al 1987 Trazodone hydrochloride in the treatment of dysesthetic pain in traumatic myelopathy: a randomized, double-blind, placebo-controlled study. Pain 29: 151–161

de Sousa E, Jepson A 1988 Midazolam in terminal care. Lancet 1: 67–68

de Wachter M A H 1989 Active euthanasia in the Netherlands. JAMA 262: 3316–3319

DeAngelis L M, Delattre J, Posner J B 1989 Radiation-induced dementia in patients cured of brain metastases. Neruology 39: 789–796

Denicoff K D, Rubinow D R, Papa M Z et al 1987 The neuropsychiatric effects of treatment with interleukin-w and lymphokine-activated killer cells. Annals of Internal Medicine 107: 293–300

Derogatis L R, Morrow G R, Fetting J et al 1983 The prevalence of psychiatric disorders amonǵ cancer patients. JAMA 249: 751–757

Deutschmann W 1971 Tofranil ider schmerzbehandlung de krebskranken. Medizinische Welt 22: 1346–1347

Devor M 1983 Nerve pathophysiology and mechanisms of pain in causalgia. Journal of the Autonomic Nervous System 7: 371–384

Diamond S, Frietag F G 1989 The use of fluoxetine in the treatment of headache. Clinical Journal of Pain 5: 200–201

Dubner R, Bennett G J 1983 Spinal and trigeminal mechanisms of nociception Annual Review of the Neurosciences 6: 381–418

Eberhard G et al 1988 A double-blind randomized study of clomipramine versus maprotiline in patients with idiopathic pain syndromes. Neuropsychobiology 19: 25–32

Eller K C, Sison A C, Breitbart W, Passik S 1992 Morphine-induced acute confusional states: a retrospective analysis (abstract). Academy of Psychosomatic Medicine 39th Annual Meeting, San Diego, CA

Endicott J 1983 Measurement of depression in patients with cancer. Cancer 53: 2243–2248

Fainsinger R, Bruera E 1992 Treatment of delirium in a terminally ill patient. Journal of Pain Symptom Management 7: 54–56

Fainsinger R, MacEachern T, Hanson J et al 1991 Symptom control during the last week of life in a Palliative Care Unit. Journal of Palliative Care 7: 5–11

Farberow N L, Schneidman E S, Leonard C V 1963 Suicide among general medical and surgical hospital patients with malignant neoplasms. Medical Bulletin 9, Washington DC, US Veterans Administration

Feighner J P 1985 A comparative trial of fluoxetine and amitriptyline in patients with major depressive disorder. Journal of Clinical Psychiatry 46: 369–372

Feinman C 1985 Pain relief by antidepressants: possible modes of actions. Pain 23: 1–8

Fernandez F, Adams F, Holmes V F 1987a Analgesic effect of alprazolam in patients with chronic, organic pain of malignant origin. Journal of Clinical Psychopharmacology 3: 167–169

Fernandez F, Adams F, Holmes V F et al 1987b Methylphenidate for depressive disorders in cancer patients. Psychosomatics 28: 455–461

Fernandez F, Adams F, Levy J et al 1988 Cognitive impairment due to AIDS related complex and its response to psychostimulants. Psychosomatics 29: 38–46

Fernandez F, Levy J K, Mansell PWA 1989 Management of delirium in terminally ill AIDS patients. International Journal of Psychiatry in Medicine 19: 165–172

Ferrell B 1991 Pain as a metaphor for illness: impact of cancer pain on family caregiver. Oncology Nursing Forum 18: 1303–1308

Ferrell B R, Ferrell B A, Rhiner M, Grant M 1991 Family factors influencing cancer. Pain Management Postgraduate Medical Journal 67: 564–569

Fields H L, Basbaum A I 1984 Endogenous pain control mechanisms. In: Wall P D, Melzack R (eds) Textbook of pain. Churchill Livingstone, Edinburgh, p 142–152

Fiorentino M 1969 Sperimentazione controllata dell' Imipramina come analgesico maggiore in oncologia. Revista Medica de Trentina 5: 387–396

Fisch R 1985–1986 Methylphenidate for medical inpatients. International Journal of Psychiatry in Medicine 15: 75–79

Fishman B, Loscalzo M 1987 Cognitive-behavioral interventions in the management of cancer pain: principles and applications. Medical Clinics of North America 71: 271–287

Fleishman S B, Lesko L M 1989 Delirium and dementia. In: Holland J, Rowland J (eds) The handbook of psychooncology: psychological care of the cancer patient. Oxford University Press, New York, p 342–355

Foley K M 1975 Pain syndromes in patients with cancer. In: Bonica J J, Ventafridda V, Fink R B, Jones L E, Loeser J D (eds) Advances in pain research and therapy, vol 2. Raven Press, New York, p 59–75

Foley K M 1985 The treatment of cancer pain. New England Journal of Medicine 313: 845

Foley K M 1991 The relationship of pain and symptom management to patient requests for physician-assisted suicide. Journal of Pain and Symptom Management 6: 289–295

Folstein M F, Folstein S E, McHugh P R 1975 Mini-mental state. Journal of Psychiatric Research 12: 189–198

Forrest W H, Brown B W, Brown C R et al 1977 Dextroamphetamine with morphine for the treatment of post-operative pain. New England Journal of Medicine 296: 712–715

Fotopoulos S S, Graham C, Cook M R 1979 Psychophysiologic control of cancer pain. In: Bonica J J, Ventafridda, V (eds) Advances in pain research and therapy, vol 2. Raven Press, New York, p 231–244

France R D 1987 The future for antidepressants: treatment of pain. Psychopathology 20: 99–113

Fuller R W, Rathbun R C, Parli C J 1976 Inhibition of drug metabolism by fluoxetine. Research Communications in Chemical Pathology and Pharmacology 13: 353–356

Gaylin W, Kass L R, Pellegrino E D, Siegler M 1988 'Doctors must not kill.' JAMA 259: 2139–2140

Gebhardt K H, Beller J, Nischk R 1969 Behandlung des karzinomschmerzes mit chlorimipramin (Anafrani). Mediziniche Klinik 64: 751–756

Geller S A 1989 Treatment of fibrositis with fluoxetine hydrochloride (Prozac). American Journal of Medicine 87: 594–595

Getto C J, Sorkness C A, Howell T 1987 Antidepressants and chronic nonmalignant pain: a review. Journal of Pain Symptom Control 2: 9–18

Glassman A H 1984 The newer antidepressant drugs and their cardiovascular effects. Psychopharmacology Bulletin 20: 272–279

Goldsmith L, Warsh J 1982 Amitriptyline versus placebo in postherpetic neuralgia. Neurology 32: 671–673

Gomez-Perez F J, Rull J A, Dies H et al 1985 Nortriptyline and fluphenazine in the symptomatic treatment of diabetic neuropathy. A double-blind cross-over study. Pain 23: 395–400

Graffam S, Johnson A 1987 A comparison of two relaxation strategies for the relief of pain and its distress. Journal of Pain and Symptom Management 2: 229–231

Gram L F 1983 Antidepressants: receptors, pharmacokinetics and clinical effects. In: Burrows G D et al (eds) Antidepressants. Elsevier, Amsterdam, p 81–95

Grossman S A, Sheidler V R, Swedeon K et al 1991 Correlations of patient and caregiver ratings of cancer pain. Journal of Pain and Symptom Management 6: 53–57

Hall R C W, Gardner E R, Perl M, Stickney S K, Pfefferbaum B 1979 The professional burnout syndrome. Psychiatric Opinion 16: 12–17

Hammeroff S R, Cork R C, Scherer K et al 1982 Doxepin effects on chronic pain, depression and plasma opioids. Journal of Clinical Psychiatry 2: 22–26

Hartl D E 1979 Stress management and the nurse. In: Sutterley D C, Donnelly G F (eds) Stress management. Aspen, Germantown MD, p 163–172

Helig S 1988 The San Francisco Medical Society euthanasia survey. Results and analysis. San Francisco Medicine 61: 24–34

Hilgard E, LeBaron S 1982 Relief of anxiety and pain in children with cancer: quantitative measures and clinical observations. International Journal of Clinical and Experimental Hypnosis 30: 417–422

Hinds C 1985 The needs of families who care for patients with cancer at home: are we meeting them? Journal of Advanced Nursing 10: 575–585

Holland J C 1989a Stresses on the mental health professionals. In: Holland J C, Rowland J (eds) Handbook of psychooncology: psychological care of the patient with cancer. Oxford University Press, New York, p 678–682

Holland J C 1989b Anxiety and cancer: the patient and family. Journal of Clinical Psychiatry 50: 20–25

Holland J C, Holland J F 1985 A neglected problem: the stresses of cancer care on physicians. Primary Care and Cancer 5: 16–22

Holland J C, Rowland J (eds) 1989 Handbook of Psychooncology. Psychological care of the patient with cancer. Oxford University Press, New York

Holland J C, Fassanellos, Ohnuma T 1974 Psychiatric symptoms associated with L-asparaginase administration. Journal of Psychiatric Research 10: 165

Holland J C, Hughes Korzun A, Tross S et al 1986 Comparative psychological disturbance in pancreatic and gastric cancer. American Journal of Psychiatry 143: 982–986

Holland J C, Morrow G, Schmale A et al 1991 A randomized clinical trial of alprazolam versus progressive muscle relaxation in cancer patients with anxiety and depressive symptoms. Journal of Clinical Oncology 9: 1004–1011

Horowitz S A, Breitbart W 1993 Relaxation and imagery for symptom control in cancer patients. In: Breibart W, Holland J C (eds) Psychiatric aspects of symptom management in cancer patients. American Psychiatric Press, Washington DC, p 147–172

Houde R W, Wallenstein S L 1966 Analgesic power of chlorpromazine alone and in combination with morphine (abstract). Federation Proceedings 14: 353

Hughes A, Chauverghe J, Lissilour T, Lagarde C 1963 L'imipramine utilisee comme antalgique majeur en carcinologie: Etude de 118 cas. Presse Medicale 71: 1073–1074

Hull, M M 1989 Family needs and supportive nursing behaviors during terminal cancer: a review. Oncology Nursing Forum 16: 787–792

Hynes M D, Lochner M A, Bemis K et al 1985 Fluoxetine, a selective inhibitor of serotonin uptake, potentiates morphine analgesia without altering its discriminative stimulus properties or affinity for opioid receptors. Life Sciences 36: 2317–2323

IASP Subcommittee on Taxonomy Pain Terms 1979 A list with definitions and notes on usage. Pain 6: 249–252

Itil T, Fink M 1966 Anticholinergic drug-induced delirium: experimental modifaction, quantitative EEG and behavioral correlations. Journal of Nervous and Mental Disease 143: 492–507

Jaffe J H 1985 Drug addition and drug abuse. In: Gilman A G, Goodman L S, Rall T W, Murad F (eds) The pharmacological basis of therapeutics, 7th edn. Macmillan, New York, p 532–581

Jay S, Elliott C, Varnis J 1986 Acute and chronic pain in adults and children with cancer. Journal of Consulting and Clinical Psychology 54: 601–607

Jellema J C 1987 Hallucinations during sustained-release opioid and methadone administration. Lancet 2: 392

Kanner R M, Foley K M 1981 Patterns of narcotic use in a cancer pain clinic. Annals of the New York Academy of Sciences 362: 161–172

Kash K M, Holland J C 1990 Reducing stress in medical oncology house officers: a preliminary report of a prospective intervention study. In: Hendrie H C, Lloyd C (eds) Educating competent and humane physicians. Indiana University Press, Bloomington, p 183–195

Katon W, Raskind M 1980 Treatment of depression in the medically ill elderly with methylphenidate. American Journal of Psychiatry 137: 963–965

Kaufmann M W, Murray G B, Cassem N H 1982 Use of psychostimulants in medically ill depressive patients. Psychosomatics 23: 817–819

Kaye B R 1989 Rheumatologic manifestations of infection with human immunodeficiency virus. Annals of Internal Medicine 111: 158–167

Kellerman J, Zetter L, Ellenberg L et al 1983 Adolescents with cancer: hypnosis for the reduction of acute pain and anxiety associated with medical procedures. Journal of Adolescent Health Care 4: 85–90

King R B 1980 Pain and tryptophan. Journal of Neurosurgery 53: 44–52

Kishore-Kumar R, Schafer S C, Lawlow B A, Murphy D L, Max M B 1989 Single doses of the serotonin agonists buspirone and chlorophenylpiperazine do not relieve neuropathic pain. Pain 37: 233–227

Kishore-Kumar R, Max M B, Schafer S C et al 1990 Desipramine relieves postherpetic neuralgia. Clinical Pharmacology and Therapeutics 47: 305–312

Koocher G P 1979 Adjustment and coping strategies among the caretakers of cancer patients. Social Work in Health Care 5: 145–150

Kristjanson L J 1986 Indications of quality of palliative care from a family perspective. Journal of Palliative Care 1: 8–17
Kvindesal B, Molin J, Froland A, Gram L F 1984 Imipramine treatment of painful diabetic neuropathy. JAMA 251: 1727–1730
Langohr H D, Stohr M, Petruch F 1982 An open and double-blind crossover study on the efficacy of clomipramine (anafranil) in patients with painful mono- and polyneuropathies. European Neurology 21: 309–315
Lascelles R G 1966 Atypical facial pain and depression. British Journal of Psychology 122: 651
Lebovits A K, Lefkowitz M, McCarthy D et al 1989 The prevalence and management of pain in patients with AIDS. A review of 134 cases. Clinical Journal of Pain 5: 245–248
Lechin F et al 1989 Pimozide therapy for trigeminal neuralgia. Archives of Neurology 9: 960–964
Lederberg M 1989 Psychological problems of staff and their management. In: Holland J C, Rowland J (eds) Handbook of psychooncology: psychological care of the patient with cancer. Oxford University Press, New York, p 678–682
Levin D N, Cleeland C S, Dan R 1985 Public attitudes toward cancer pain. Cancer 56: 2337–2339
Levine P M, Silverfarb P M, Lipowski Z J 1978 Mental disorders in cancer patients: a study of 100 psychiatric referrals. Cancer 42: 1385–1391
Levy R M, Bredesen D E, Rosenblum M L 1985 Neurological manifestations of the AIDS experience at UCSF and review of the literature. Journal of Neurosurgery 62: 475–495
Liepzig R M, Goodman H, Gray P et al 1987 Reversible narcotic-associated mental status impairment in patients with metastatic cancer. Pharmacology 53: 47–57
Lindblom U, Merskey H, Mumford J M et al 1986 Pain terms: a current list with definitions and notes on usage. Pain 3: 5215–5221
Lipowski Z J 1987 Delirium (acute confusional states) JAMA 285: 1789–1792
Liu S F, Wang R I H 1975 Increased analgesia and alterations in distribution and metabolism of methadone by desipramine in the rat. Journal of Pharmacology and Experimental Therapeutics 195: 94–104
Lloyd A H 1977 Practical consideration in the use of maprotiline (ludiomil) in general practice. Journal of International Medical Research 5: 122–125
Loscalzo M, Jacobsen P B 1990 Practical behavioral approaches to the effective management of pain and distress. Journal of Psychosocial Oncology 8: 139–169
Macaluso C, Weinberg D, Foley K M 1988 Opiod abuse and misuse in a cancer pain population (abstract). Second International Congress on Cancer Pain, July 14–17, Rye, New York
McCaffrey M, Beebe A 1989 Pain: clinical manual for nursing practice. C V Mosby, Philadelphia, p 353–360
McCaffrey M, Vourakis C 1992 Assessment and relief of pain in chemically dependent patients. Orthopaedic Nursing 11: 13–27
McKegney F P, Bailey C R, Yates J W 1981 Prediction and management of pain in patients with advanced cancer. General Hospital Psychiatry 3: 95–101
Magni G, Arsie D, DeLeo D 1987 Antidepressants in the treatment of cancer pain. A survey in Italy. Pain 29: 347–353
Malseed R T, Goldstein F J 1979 Enhancement of morphine analgesics by tricyclic antidepressants. Neuropharmacology 18: 827–829
Maltbie A A, Cavenar J O, Sullivan J L et al 1979 Analgesia and haloperidol: a hypothesis. Journal of Clinical Psychiatry 40: 323–326
Manne S, Redd W, Jacobsen P, Georgiades I 1991 Aroma for treatment of anxiety during MRI scan. American Psychiatric Association Annual Meeting, 7–12 May, New Orleans (abstract)
Marks R M, Sachar E J 1973 Undertreatment of medical inpatients with narcotic analgesics. Annals of Internal Medicine 78: 173–181
Maslach C 1979 The burnout syndrome and patient care. In: Garfield C A (ed) Stress and survival, the emotional realities of life-threatening illness. Mosby St Louis, p 89–96
Massie M J, Holland J C 1987 The cancer patient with pain: psychiatric complications and their management. Medical Clinics of North America 71: 243–258
Massie M J, Holland J C 1990 Depression and the cancer patient. Journal of Clinical Psychiatry 51: 12–17
Massie M J, Holland J C, Glass E 1983 Delirium in terminally ill cancer patients. American Journal of Psychiatry 140: 1048–1050
Massie M J, Holland J C, Straker N 1989 Psychotherapeutic interventions. In: Holland J C, Rowland J (eds) Handbook of psychooncology: psychological care of the patient with cancer. Oxford University Press, New York, p 455–469
Max M B, Culnane M, Schafer S C, Gracely R H, Walther D J, Smoller B, Dubner R 1987 Amitriptyline relieves diabetic-neuropathy pain in patients with normal and depressed mood. Neurology 37: 589–596
Max M B, Schafer S C, Culnane M, Smollen B, Dubner R, Gracely R H 1988 Amitriptyline, but not lorazepam, relieves postherpetic neuralgia. Neurology 38: 1427–1432
Max M B, Kishore-Kumar R, Schafer S C et al 1991 Efficacy of desipramine in painful diabetic neuropathy: a placebo-controlled trial. Pain 45: 3–10
Melzack R, Wall P D 1983 The challenge of pain. Basic Books, New York
Merskey H, Hamilton J T 1989 An open trial of possible analgesic effects of dipyridamole. Journal of Pain and Symptom Management 4: 34–37
Millerd E J 1977 Health professionals as survivors. Journal of Psychiatric Nursing and Mental Health Services 15: 33–36
Monkemeir D, Steffen U 1970 Zur schmerzbehandlung mit Imipramin bei krebserkrankungen. Medizinische Klinik 65: 213–215
Mor V, Guadagnoli E, Wool M 1987 An examination of the concrete service needs of advanced cancer patients. Journal of Psychosocial Oncology 5: 1–17
Mount B M 1986 Dealing with our losses. Journal of Clinical Oncology 4: 1127–1134
Munro S M, Mount B 1978 Music therapy in palliative care. Canadian Medical Association Journal 119: 1029–1034
Murray G B 1987 Confusion, delirium, and dementia. In: Hackett T P, Cassem N H (eds) Massachusetts General Hospital handbook of general hospital psychiatry, 2nd. PSG Publishing, Littleton, MA, p 84–115
Nehra A, Mullick F, Ishak K G, Zimmerman A J 1990 Pemoline associated hepatic injury. Gastroenterology 99: 1517–1519
Newshan G, Wainapel S, Schmitz D 1989 Pain related syndromes and their treatment in persons with AIDS (abstract). Eighth Annual Scientific Meeting of the American Pain Society, Phoenix, Arizona
Oliver O J 1985 The use of methotrimeprazine in terminal care. British Journal of Clinical Practice 39: 339–340
Paddison P L, Gise L H, Lebovits A et al 1990 Sexual abuse and premenstrual syndrome: comparison between a lower and higher socioeconomic group. Psychosomatics 31: 265–272
Parry G J 1988 Peripheral neuropathies associated with human immunodeficiency virus infection. Annals of Neurology 23 (suppl): 349–553
Passik S 1992 Psychotherapy of the substance abusing cancer patient. American Psychiatric Association Annual Meeting, May 4–10, Washington, DC (abstract)
Passik S, Wilson A 1987 Technical considerations of the frontier of supportive and expressive modes in psychotherapy. Dynamic Psychotherapy 5: 51–62
Passik S, Horowitz S, Malkin M, Gargan R 1991 A psychoeducational support group for spouses of brain tumor patients. American Psychiatric Association Annual Meeting, 7–12 May, New Orleans (abstract)
Patchell R A, Posner J B 1989 Cancer and the nervous system. In: Holland J, Rowland J (eds) The handbook of psychooncology: the psychological care of the cancer patient. Oxford University Press, New York p 327–341
Payne R M 1989 Pain in the drug abuser. In: Foley K M, Payne R M (eds) Current therapy of pain. B C Decker, Philadelphia, p 46–54
Peck A W, Stern W C, Watkinson C 1983 Incidence of seizures during treatment with tricyclic antidepressant drugs and buproprion. Journal of Clinical Psychiatry 44: 197–201
Pellegrino E D 1991 Ethics. JAMA 265: 3188
Perry S, Heidrich G 1982 Management of pain during debridement: a survey of US burn units. Pain 13: 267–280
Peteet J R, Murrary-Ross D, Medeiros C et al 1989 Job stress and satisfaction among the staff members at a cancer center. Cancer 64: 975–982

Pilowsky I, Hallett E C, Bassett D L, Thomas P G, Penhall R K 1982 A controlled study of amitriptyline in the treatment of chronic pain. Pain 14: 169–179

Plumb M M, Holland J C 1977 Comparative studies of psychological function in patients with advanced cancer. Psychosomatic Medicine 39: 264–276

Popkin M K, Callies A L, Mackenzie T B 1985 The outcome of antidepressant use in the medically ill. Archives of General Psychiatry 42: 1160–1163

Portenoy R K 1987 Continuous intravenous infusion of opioid drugs. Medical Clinics of North America 71: 233–241

Portenoy R K, Hagen N A 1990 Breakthrough pain: definition, prevalence and characteristics. Pain 41: 273–282

Portenoy R K, Payne R 1992 Acute and chronic pain. In: Lowinson J H, Ruiz P, Millman R B (eds) Comprehensive textbook of substance abuse. Williams & Wilkins, Baltimore, p 691–721

Porter J, Jick H 1980 Addiction rate in patients treated with narcotics. New England Journal of Medicine 302: 123

Posner J B 1979 Delirium and exogenous metabolic brain disease. In: Beeson P B et al (eds) Cecil's textbook of medicine. W B Saunders, Philadelphia, p 644–651

Posner J B 1988 Nonmetastatic effects of cancer on the nervous system. In: Wyngaarden J B et al (eds) Cecil's textbook of medicine. W B Saunders, Philadelphia, p 1104–1107

Purohit D R, Navlakha P L, Modi R S et al 1978 The role of antidepressants in hospitalized cancer patients. Journal of the Association of Physicians of India 26: 245–248

Quill T E 1991 Sounding board: death and dignity: a case of individualized decision making. New England Journal of Medicine 324: 691–694

Rabeneck L, Popovic M, Gartner S et al 1990 Acute HIV infection presenting with painful swallowing and esophageal ulcers. JAMA 263: 2318–2322

Rait D, Lederberg M 1990 The family of the cancer patient. In: Holland J, Rowland J (eds) The handbook of psychooncology. Oxford University Press New York, p 585–598

Redd W B, Reeves J L, Storm F K, Minagawa R Y 1982 Hypnosis in the control of pain during hyperthermia treatment of cancer. In: Bonica J J et al (eds) Advances in pain research and theory, vol 5. Raven Press, New York, p 857–861

Reik T 1948 Listening with a third ear. Farrar Straus, New York

Rifkin A, Reardon G, Siris S et al 1985 Trimipramine in physical illness with depression. Journal of Clinical Psychiatry 46: 4–8

Robinson D, Napoliello M J, Schenk J 1988 The safety and usefulness of buspirone as an anxiolytic drug in elderly versus young patients. Clinical Therapeutics 10: 740–746

Rowat K 1985 Chronic pain: a family affair. In: King K (ed) Recent advances in nursing long term care. Churchill Livingstone, Edinburgh

Salter M H, Henry J L 1987 Evidence that adenosine moderates the depression of spinal dorsal horn neurones induced by peripheral vibration in the rat. Neuroscience 22: 631–650

Saltzburg D, Breitbart W, Fishman B et al 1989 The relationship of pain and depression to suicidal ideation in cancer patients (abstract). ASCO Annual Meeting, May 21–23, San Francisco

Schmale J, Weinberg N, Pieper S 1987 Satisfactions, stresses, and coping mechanisms of oncologists in clinical practice (abstract). Proceedings of the American Society of Clinical Oncology 6: 255

Schofferman J, Brody R 1990 Pain in far advanced AIDS. In: Foley K M et al (eds) Advances in pain research and therapy, vol 16. Raven Press, New York, p 379–386

Seltzer S, Dewart D, Pollack R L, Jackson E 1983 The effects of dietary tryptophan on chronic maxillofacial pain and experimental pain tolerance. Journal of Psychiatric Research 17: 181–186

Sher M, Krieger J N, Juergen S 1983 Trazodone and priapism. American Journal of Psychiatry 140: 1362–1364

Sharav Y, Singer E, Schmidt E, Dione R A, Dubner R 1987 The analgesic effect of amitriptyline on chronic facial pain. Pain 31: 199–209

Siegel K 1982 Rational suicide: considerations for the clinician. Psychiatric Quarterly 54: 77–83

Siegel K, Tuckel P 1984 Rational suicide and the terminally ill cancer patient. Omega 15: 263–269

Silberfarb P M, Manrer L H, Cronthamel C S 1980 Psychological aspects of neoplastic disease. I: Functional status of breast cancer patients during different treatment regimens. American Journal of Psychiatry 137: 450–455

Sindrup S H, Ejlertsen B, Froland A et al 1989 Imipramine treatment in diabetic neuropathy: relief of subjective symptoms without changes in peripheral and autonomic nerve function. European Journal of Clinical Pharmacology 37: 151–153

Sindrup S H, Gram L F, Brosen K, Eshoj O, Mogenson E F 1990 The selective serotonin reuptake inhibitor paroxetine is effective in the treatment of diabetic neuropathy symptoms. Pain 42: 135–144

Singer P A 1990 Euthanasia: a critique. New England Journal of Medicine 322: 1881–1883

Snider W D, Simpson D M, Nielsen S et al 1983 Neurological complications of AIDS: analysis of 50 patients. Annals of Neurology 14: 403–418

Spiegel D 1985 The use of hypnosis in controlling cancer pain. CA: A Cancer Journal for Clinicians 4: 221–231

Spiegel D, Bloom J R 1983a Pain in metastatic breast cancer. Cancer 52: 341–345

Spiegel D, Bloom J R 1983b Group therapy and hypnosis reduce metastatic breast carcinoma pain. Psychosomatic Medicine 4: 333–339

Spiegel D, Bloom J R, Yalom I D 1981 Group support for patients with metastatic cancer: a randomized prospective outcome study. Archives of General Psychiatry 38: 527–533

Spiegel K, Kalb R, Pasternak G W 1983 Analgesic activity of tricyclic antidepressants. Annals of Neurology 13: 462–465

Spikes J, Holland J 1975 The physician's response to the dying patient. In: Strain J J, Grossman S (eds) Psychological care of the medically ill. Appleton–Century–Crofts, New York p 138–148

Stein R S, Flexner J H, Graber S E 1980 Lithium and granulocytopenia during induction therapy of acute myelogenous leukemia: update of an ongoing trial. Advances in Experimental Medicine and Biology 127: 187–198

Stiefel F C, Breitbart W, Holland J C 1989 Corticosteroids in cancer: neuropsychiatric complications. Cancer Investigation 7: 479–491

Swerdlow M, Cundill J G 1981 Anticonvulsant drugs used in the treatment of lancinating pains: a comparison. Anesthesia 36: 1129–1134

Syrjala K L, Cummings C, Donald G W 1992 Hypnosis or cognitive behavioral training for the reduction of pain and nausea during cancer treatment: a controlled clinical trial. Pain 48: 137–146

Terr L 1991 Childhood traumas: an outline and overview. American Journal of Psychiatry 148: 10–20

Theesen K, Marsh W 1989 Relief of diabetic neuropathy with fluoxetine. DICP (Annals of Pharmacotherapy) 3: 572–574

Tiengo M, Pagnoni B, Calmi A, Rigoli M, Braga P C, Panerai A E 1987 Chlorimipramine compared to pentazocine as a unique treatment in post-operative pain. International Journal of Clinical Pharmacology Research 7: 141–143

Trzepacz P T, Baker R W, Greenhouse J 1988 A symptom rating scale for delirium. Psychiatric Research 23: 89–97

Turk D, Rennert K 1981 Pain and the terminally ill cancer patient: a cognitive–social learning perspective. In: Sobel H (ed) Behavior therapy in terminal care. Ballinger, Cambridge

Twycross R G, Lack S A 1983 Symptom control in far advanced cancer: pain relief. Pitman Books, London

Tyler M A 1974 Treatment of the painful shoulder syndrome with amitriptyline and lithium carbonate. Canadian Medical Association Journal 111: 137–140

Vachon M L S 1987 Occupational stress in the care of the critically ill, the dying, and the bereaved. Hemisphere, Washington DC

van der Maas P J, van Delden J J M, Piznenborg L, Looman C W N 1991 Euthanasia and other medical decisions concerning the end of life. Lancet 338: 669–674

Ventafridda V, Bonezzi C, Caraceni A et al 1987 Antidepressants for cancer pain and other painful syndromes with deafferentation component: comparison of amitriptyline and trazodone. Italian Journal of Neurological Sciences 8: 579–587

Ventafridda V, Ripamonti C, DeConno F et al 1990a Symptom prevalence and control during cancer patients' last days of life. Journal of Palliative Care 6: 7–11

Ventafridda V, Bianchi M, Ripamonti C et al 1990b Studies on the effects of antidepressant drugs on the antinociceptive action of morphine and on plasma morphine in rat and man. Pain 43: 155–162

von Ammon Cavanaugh S 1990 Drug-drug interactions of fluoxetine with tricyclics. Psychosomatics 31: 273–276

von Roenn J H, Cleeland C S, Gonin R et al 1993 Physicians' attitudes toward cancer pain management survey: results of the Eastern Cooperative Oncology Group survey. Annals of Internal Medicine (in press)

Walker E, Katon W, Griffins J H et al 1988 Relationship of chronic pelvic pain to psychiatric diagnosis and childhood sexual abuse. American Journal of Psychiatry 145: 75–80

Walsh T D 1983 Antidepressants and chronic pain. Clinical Neuropharmacology 6: 271–295

Walsh T D 1986 Controlled study of imipramine and morphine in chronic pain due to advanced cancer (abstract). ASCO, May 4–6, Los Angeles

Walsh T D 1990 Adjuvant analgesic therapy in cancer pain. In: Foley K M et al (eds) Advances in pain research and therapy, vol 16. Second International Congress on Cancer Pain. Raven Press, New York, p 155–166

Wanzer S H, Federman D D, Edelstein S T et al 1989 The physician's responsibility toward hopelessly ill patients: a second look. New England Journal of Medicine 320: 844–849

Warner M M 1992 Involvement of families in pain control of terminally ill patients. Hospice Journal 8: 155–170

Watson C P, Evans R J 1985 A comparative trial of amitriptyline and zimelidine in postherpetic neuralgia. Pain 23: 387–394

Watson C P, Evans R J, Reed K, Merskey H, Goldsmith L, Warsh J 1982 Amitriptyline versus placebo in postherpetic neuralgia. Neurology 32: 671–673

Watson C P, Evans R J, Reed K, Merskey H, Watson C P N 1984 'Therapeutic window' for amitriptyline analgesia. Canadian Medicial Association Journal 130: 105

Watson C P, Chipman M, Reed K, Evans R J, Birkett N 1992 Amitriptyline versus maprotiline in postherpetic neuralgia: a randomized, double-blind, cross over trial. Pain 48: 29–36

Weddington W W 1982 Delirium and depression associated with amphotericin B. Psychosomatics 23: 1076–1078

Weissman D E, Haddox J D 1989 Opioid pseudoaddiction – an iatrogenic syndrome. Pain 36: 363–366

Woodforde J M, Fielding J R 1970 Pain and cancer. Journal of Psychosomatic Research 4: 365–370

Young D F 1982 Neurological complications of cancer chemotherapy. In: Silverstein A (ed) Neurological complications of therapy: selected topics. Futura Publishing, New York, p 57–113

Young R J, Clarke B F 1985 Pain relief in diabetic neuropathy: the effectiveness of imipramine and related drugs. Diabetic Medicine 2: 363–366

Zeltzer L, LeBaron S 1982 Hypnosis and non-hypnotic techniques for reduction of pain and anxiety in painful procedures in children and adolescents with cancer. Journal of Pediatrics 101: 1032–1035

Zimmerman L, Porzehl B, Duncan K, Schmitz R 1989 Effects of music in patients who had chronic cancer pain. Western Journal of Nursing Research 11: 298–309

Zitman F G, Linssen A C G, Edelbroek P M, Stijnen T 1990 Low dose amitriptyline in chronic pain: the gain is modest. Pain 42: 35–42

45. Pain and impending death

Dame Cicely Saunders

Evidence from various sources (Hinton 1963; Parkes 1978; Keane et al 1983; Wilkes 1984) shows that while the majority of patients may find dying peaceful at the end, sufficient attention and skill is not always given to what has by then become a multisystem disease or deterioration. Among more recent studies, quoted below, concerning patients with advanced cancer, only Coyle et al (1990) review this important area of management and show what can be done by an experienced team incorporated into standard medical care. *How* people die remains in the memories of those who live on, and for them (as for the patient) we need to be aware of the nature and management of terminal pain and distress. What happens in the last hours may heal some earlier memories or remain as disturbing recollections that hinder the resolution of bereavement.

STUDIES OF DYING

The first clinical study of the way patients die was reported by Sir William Osler in his lecture 'Science and immortality' (1906). He states:

> In our modern life the educated man dies . . . generally unconscious and unconcerned. I have careful records of about 500 deathbeds, studies particularly with reference to the modes of death and the sensations of the dying. The latter alone concerns us here. 90 suffered bodily pain or distress of one sort or another, 11 showed mental apprehension, 2 positive terror, 1 expressed spiritual exaltation, 1 bitter remorse. The great majority gave no signs one way or the other; like their birth, their death was a sleep and a forgetting.

Exton-Smith (1961) studied 220 patients (80 men and 140 women) in a geriatric unit. The mean age was 80 years. Pain was recorded as 'moderate' or 'severe' when it did not respond to aspirin or related compounds and occurred at some time in 30 patients (13.6%). A further 17 patients (7.7%) complained of other distressing symptoms such as persistent nausea and vomiting, dysphagia, severe dyspnoea and suffocation. Less than a quarter of those dying of malignant disease had pain and this was well controlled with opioid drugs given regularly. Those patients with locomotor disorders, especially rheumatoid arthritis, had severe pain of longer duration (months to several years). The suffering of this group was greater 'because they were alert and recognized their helplessness. By contrast, more than 40% of patients were confused, usually persistently and were unaware of the extent of their disabilities and their progressive physical decline'.

Most of the patients were peaceful during their terminal hours. 88 (40%) were unconscious for 3 hours or more before death and only seven 'showed considerable anxiety and feared to be left alone . . . The *angor animi* of one patient with severe substernal pain due to coronary thrombosis was striking'. At least a quarter of the patients were aware that they were dying and the approach of death was met by most with calmness and without fear or misgiving.

Witzel (1975) reported clinical observations of 360 dying patients in a brief paper which is evidently a summary of a survey more fully reported in German (Witzel 1971, 1973). Of the 360, 110 were observed continuously on hospital wards during their final 24 hours and 250 were seen during the last days and weeks before their death. The mean age of the first group was 72.4 years. About 28% suffered from diseases of the cardiovascular system, 19% from cancer, 18% from diseases of the gastrointestinal tract, 10% from pulmonary disease, 7% from renal failure, 6% from metabolic diseases and 11% from other diseases. Nine died suddenly, 16 were in a comatose state and 12 were mentally disturbed. The other 73 patients were aware of time and place 24 hours before death, and 29 had such awareness up to 15 minutes before death. Nine patients of the whole group were treated with analgesics for pain relief. There was often a brief improvement in condition with reduced need for analgesics shortly before death. The conversations reported showed that while 27 said spontaneously that they were dying, and 29 believed death was near when asked, only two wanted 'information about their health'. Only two were afraid of death.

The second group of 250 patients, whose mean age was 73.97 years, included 30% with cancer, 19% with diseases of the cardiovascular system, 16% of the gastrointestinal tract, 10% of the kidney, 8% of the pulmonary system, 3% with metabolic diseases and 12% with other diseases. This group all had some physical symptoms, including pain, dyspnoea, nausea, vomiting, cough, hiccups, dysphagia and anorexia. These physical symptoms and the various 'neuropsychiatric' symptoms, such as fear, depression, weakness, uncoordinated thinking, hallucinations and irritability, influenced one another. The patients were more afraid of pain, physical distress or chronic debility than of death itself.

Witzel emphasizes that an understanding of the interdependence of physical and neuropsychiatric symptoms is essential for good management, listing the relationship between fear and dyspnoea. We would agree, linking also nausea, incontinence and fungating, smelly tumours with depression, but would hesitate to label these normal reactions to adversity as 'psychiatric'. This may, of course, be merely a matter of semantics.

Hinton (1963), in a uniquely detailed study, compared the physical discomfort and mental state of 102 dying patients with 102 patients in the same wards who were suffering from diseases in the same systems that were serious but not fatal. He found that the physical discomfort among the dying patients was 'disturbingly greater' than among the control patients. Pain was adequately relieved in 82% of 82 patients with malignant disease, but vomiting and nausea were relieved in 63% and dyspnoea in only 18%. These symptoms were more common in patients dying of renal and cardiac failure, a total of 14 patients in all. The physical symptoms increased in the last week; 16% had almost continuous distress and a further 27% had physical distress for some of the time.

Hinton's patients were less alert than Witzel's as death approached. Of the 71 of his 102 patients who died in hospital, 11% were unrousable for most of the last week of life; 34% were unconscious for at least 24 hours, and 60% for 6 or 9 hours before death; only 6% were conscious just before they died. Many of these patients were receiving drugs likely to impair consciousness. The act of dying was rarely distressful. Hinton noted a significant degree of depression in 46%, with a rise in the last week or two of life. The nursing staff reported obvious grief in about a quarter of the patients before death. The incidence of anxiety was 38% and this was frequently associated with unrelieved dyspnoea. Hinton comments that whereas methods of controlling dyspnoea, vomiting and severe malaise were not always adequate, pain 'against which we have powerful weapons [was] not always controlled, owning to various delays'.

RETROSPECTIVE STUDY OF PATIENTS IN ST CHRISTOPHER'S HOSPICE

Data were collected from the medical and nursing records of 200 consecutive patients dying at St Christopher's Hospice, London, in 1978–79. The aim was to examine the incidence of clinical problems noted in the last 24 hours of life and to look at the use of oral morphine and parenteral diamorphine in these patients. It must be noted that this is not a random selection of patients but a group who were admitted to the hospice for the control of symptoms found difficult elsewhere, with pain predominant (about 75% of 657 patients admitted in 1978). The most common clinical problems recorded in the last 24 hours were 'chestiness' and 'drowsiness'. Other problems included agitation, dyspnoea, pain, confusion, twitching and vomiting. Only 47 of the 200 had pain the last 24 hours and about a third of these patients had pain recorded only on movement.

Most patients received intramuscular (i.m.) diamorphine in the last 24 hours and younger patients seemed to get i.m. diamorphine prior to the last 24 hours more frequently than older patients. This was not statistically significant, nor were any of the other differences found in the survey. Oral morphine was the opioid of choice for most patients until the last 48 or 24 hours; 20 mg oral morphine given 4-hourly was the highest dose for the majority. Many patients were given chlorpromazine in the last 72 hours, particularly elderly males (Walsh et al 1982).

A further examination of the nursing notes of the first 100 of these patients was made to assess the effectiveness of this treatment during the last 48 hours before death and showed that most of these symptoms caused only intermittent distress or were controlled as the medical and nursing staff continually reviewed each patient's condition and titrated the drugs according to need.

Patients in the first 100 who did not die peacefully

One died in acute dyspnoea while an injection was being prepared. He was in the hospice 1 day only. One died suddenly on the commode. The clinical diagnosis of pulmonary embolism was not confirmed by autopsy.

Patients in the first 100 who died peacefully

Of the 100 patients, 98 were recorded as dying peacefully. The following observations were made: peaceful for 24 hours or longer – 60, distress recorded between 4 and 24 hours – 27; distress recorded within 4 hours or less – 13. Of the latter 13 patients, six were agitated or restless, four had dyspnoea, one was confused, one had pain on movement and one vomited with distress.

It was observed in this group that six patients were alone when they died, six patients had family with them, 28 patients had family and nurse(s), 60 patients had nurse(s) with them.

An interesting change has taken place since then. Of 100 patients in 1992, 21% died alone (often at night),

26% with family, 25% with family and nurse and 28% with nurse(s) only. Family involvement and support has obviously developed considerably.

State of consciousness

Observations were made at various times during the 24 hours before death: 10 patients were recorded as 'alert', 23 were recorded as 'unrousable', 'unresponsive' or 'unconscious', and the remaining 67 were recorded as 'drowsy', 'rousable' or 'semiconscious'; that is, still responding to those with them.

OBSERVATIONS FROM THE HOSPICE TEAM

The first signs of impending death were discussed with two staff groups consisting mainly of nurses. In patients already mortally ill with advanced malignant or motor neuron disease, staff observed a deepening of feelings of profound illness and weakness and an increasing irritability of mood and sensitivity to minor discomforts during their last few days. Night nurses reported that patients became difficult to settle, while day nurses found previously equable patients more demanding or moody. They noted that the patients became more easily upset by their own disabilities and were sometimes obsessional about their belongings. Comfort and reassurance were usually accepted but had to be repeated continually. Most patients in a hospice sleep well, but as these patients neared the end of their lives they sometimes had recurrent nightmares, reliving traumatic experiences of past life such as war and internment or dreaming of bizarre situations of peril.

This tendency to 'irritation' would seem to match with the 63 of 200 patients recorded as 'agitated' in the last 24 hours. Terminal restlessness may be caused by various factors, such as pain, dyspnoea, metabolic disturbances leading to confusion, retention or the inability to move without assistance any longer, but in many it may be that the 'irritability' escapes self-control. Families are understandably disturbed if these symptoms are not controlled, and many need an explanation that this is not a new mental illness but a common part of severe illness. Hospice nurses (and others) are anxious that their patients should not be sedated to the point where they cannot recognize or speak to their families and a careful balance must be kept between an individual's need and the drugs and the dosages used.

The pain of the last few days which most concerned the nurses was the pain on movement that causes a patient to moan or cry out, disturbing everyone around (family, other patients and staff) even though the patient might appear to be unconscious. The nurses believed that as the patients were no longer able to move in periods between turning, washing or changing, this was sometimes due to stiffness; but it also seems to have much in common with the 'disturbance reaction' in the geriatric unit described below. It can be alleviated by careful announcement of what is to be done and by whom, by gentle, slow manoeuvres and by reducing disturbance to the minimum. Such activities should be carried out at a time related to the maximum action of the medication being given. Even if a patient seems to be deeply unconscious, such reaction needs to be anticipated. Experienced nurses note that these patients frequently do not wince when given injections or when a hand is gently taken.

'Chesty' symptoms have been differentiated from dyspnoea in the survey of these 200 patients. The former are rarely of great anxiety for the patient, while the latter can be very distressing. Both are relieved by the use of opioids. The fact that laboured breathing is rarely a cause for complaint in the alert patient is probably due to the concurrent use of these drugs for pain control.

The anxiety of dyspnoea is seen frequently in patients dying of motor neuron disease, and these patients, like those with terminal malignancy, respond well to the use of opioids, accompanied if necessary by diazepam or chlorpromazine or related drugs (O'Brien et al 1992). Experience and a study on opioids and respiratory depression (Walsh 1984) both suggest that these drugs, properly titrated to a patient's need, are not only indicated but are unlikely to hasten death. Prospective studies are in progress. Even if respiratory depression should be considered a risk in these patients, effective control of very distressing symptoms should not be withheld at a stage when there is nothing else to offer. Oxygen has been found to be of little help and may only serve to keep the family at a distance. It too is being investigated.

These terminal symptoms can be relieved but call for constant vigilance by the nursing staff and prompt action by the medical staff. The group surveyed in the study of 200 were sent to the hospice because of problems in symptom control. The median length of stay during that year was 11 days with 12.5% dying within 48 hours and 39.75% within a week. Often there was little time to know the patient or his family, although, as at all moments of crisis, a surprising amount of progress of all kinds may be made in a short time.

The change from oral medication to injections occurs for most hospice patients only during the last 48 hours. A balance has to be struck between giving extra responsibility for this decision to a nurse or leaving a patient in distress until a doctor is available. Sometimes heroic efforts are made to help a patient to swallow in order to avoid the change to injections, since such responsibility can be given only to the experienced person. Setting up a syringe driver may solve this problem, especially in home care (Hawkett & Nicholson 1987). The family also needs an explanation if this necessary changeover is not to become threatening or misunderstood. Even then, difficulty in distinguishing between post hoc and propter hoc may cause distress. Every time a patient dies within a short time of an injection, many families (and indeed many nurses) need reassurance that this was not the cause of death, and that 'the proper medical treatment that is administered and that has an incidental effect on determining the exact moment of death is not the cause of death in any sensible use of the term' (Devlin 1985).

Fear is occasionally an overwhelming symptom of impending death and calls for physical contact and adequate medication. All the common fears of the dying (see below) may be exacerbated as death finally approaches, but more commonly patients show the transformation reported by Brain (1934) of Dr Johnson: 'Having struggled with the fear of death all his life, he finally capitulated and, having ceased to struggle, ceased to fear and died in peace'.

Hospice nurses and volunteers endeavour when possible to ensure that no patient dies alone and sit to hold a hand if there is no relative or friend to keep this vigil. The same concern has been reported from general hospitals, in spite of all the other demands. It is a comfort to other patients and their visitors, as well as to the one concerned. This touch appears to be comforting even to the unrousable patient. Furthermore, the person who is physically present will also observe the first, treatable signs of the 'death rattle', which is profoundly disturbing to the family and other patients, though rarely to the patient himself. Since nurses need to explain any manoeuvre to the patient at this stage, the family should be encouraged to talk gently or to sit in a last companionable silence. The 'lightening before death', or the unexpected lucid interval, is still occasionally seen, though no doubt less often now that we are so concerned with relieving terminal distress with suitable medication.

The wife of a patient who was in the hospice for 10 weeks in 1977 wrote:

> One thought I would like to pass on to you. I think one of the greatest aids I personally received from St Christophers's was being able to watch other patients die peacefully and easily without being shuffled off behind curtains and so on. I think those experiences have been of great therapeutic value to me so that when the time came for Eric to die, I felt no panic or even great distress and consequently was able just to concentrate on sharing his last moments.

This lady had time to learn this confidence for herself, but the process of dying often needs explaining to the watching family. They face many fears if the patient remains at home, and they need to voice and discuss them. Their fears are often macabre and unrealistic but, given support, many will give excellent care to the end and gain a sense of great achievement in so doing. This will often be the patient's choice and can greatly ease the long pain of bereavement. Whenever care is given, it is important to emphasize that the dying, unconscious patient is not suffering but rather that any suffering is now being borne by those who watch. Noisy breathing or even moaning can be explained by telling the family: 'He is no more conscious of this than he was of his snoring when he was well', which has often brought the response: 'He was always a noisy sleeper'.

SOME MORE RECENT STUDIES

Coyle et al (1990) reported on their experience with a subgroup of patients with advanced cancer who experienced difficulties in the last 4 weeks of life that led to their referral to this very experienced team. In a detailed report they concluded that ongoing monitoring and adjustments of treatment were essential. Setbacks and limited successes may be frequent but they showed how recognition of carer and professional fatigue, coupled with flexibility in managing multiple problems, can provide ongoing support for the patient and family and expert symptom control.

Several other recent studies have looked at the end stages of cancer. Lombard & Oliver (1989) showed that 66% of 236 patients were able to take oral medication in the last day of life. They found that the need for parenteral medication over long periods is small and that this in itself should not preclude home care. The use of a syringe driver will also reduce these specific demands on the professional team, although the family may need other support.

Lichter & Hunt (1990) followed 200 consecutive patients in an integrated hospice inpatient and home care programme. Some 40% died in their own homes but, in identifying and treating the same common symptoms found in the Walsh study, they found that with a ready awareness of the problems that may arise in the last 48 hours of life it was possible to keep their patients comfortable to the end. They concluded that those who have had good control at an earlier stage may expect final relief. Although 36% of their group experienced difficulties in the last 48 hours, these were controlled.

One study, carried out among home care patients (Ventafridda et al 1990) gives a different picture. A prospective study of 120 patients found that more than 50% of them had suffering which they considered unendurable in their last days. These were controlled only by means of sedation. Pain was the problem for 31 patients, dyspnoea 33, delirium 11 and vomiting 5. In a guest editorial, Mount (1990) asks whether this may be a different patient population and points out that many patients, such as the St Christopher's group, are admitted to hospice units when control at home breaks down (often coupled with carer exhaustion). He considers that, while it may be that cancer patients experience pain with increasing frequency and severity as death approaches, it does not indicate that the pain becomes more difficult to treat. He points out that less than a quarter of St

Christopher's patients died in a comatose state, including those unconscious due to tumour, metabolic state and all other causes combined, while more than half the Milan patients died in iatrogenic coma (Mount 1990).

A study from the Edmonton team of the last week of 100 patients with details recorded from Visual Analogue Scales showed that 2–7% of the patients had poor symptom control and 16% appeared to have symptoms controllable only by sedation (Faisinger et al 1991). None of us can cease from our efforts at accurate assessment and treatment with ever-developing skills.

Mount believes that Ventafridda's study should stimulate others and looks for better ways of comparing populations, such as the Edmonton system, for staging pain proposed by Bruera et al (1989).

OBSERVATIONS FROM THE INTENSIVE CARE UNIT (ICU) (Dr R Baxter)

The problems involved in coping with death in the ICU are really the problems of staff and relatives. The patients themselves are (hopefully) virtually unaware of the ICU and are usually on ventilators and other life-support systems.

Acute episodes (sudden coronaries, trauma, acute infection) requiring ICU admission almost invariably need rapid ventilation and full technological back-up. The patient is usually unconscious, either from disease or sedatives, so is not in distress. The relatives need gentle, considerate reassurance, and as much optimism as the facts will allow; however, it is essential that they are given an honest opinion, even if shaded a little toward reassurance. The patient nowadays is likely to be unsedated and not ventilated only during the recovery period. It is clear that our sedation techniques are not fully adequate, since 30–50% of former ICU patients show some detectable, although not overt, signs of psychological disturbance. Relatives are overawed by the unit, and although they are intimidated by the technology, they also find it reassuring in that they feel everything possible is being done.

Deaths from nonmalignant disease fall broadly into two groups. The acute group is usually fought for determinedly in ICU or the resuscitation room and the patient is generally totally unaware. The relatives normally feel that everyone has tried very hard and the most common reaction is a kind of stunned gratitude. Anger, resentment, bitterness and aggression all occur and are best met with gentleness and compassion. Just allowing the aggression an outlet is usually enough to produce a complete change of attitude.

The more chronic cases are usually well prepared for the end. The relatives are resigned and symptom control is generally fairly good. Respiratory and cardiac deaths are often accompanied by dyspnoea, but this usually responds well to morphine in these patients, who have had little previous exposure to the drug. The presumptive mechanism is mild vasodilation and cardiac stimulation. Hypercarbic dyspnoea is quite rare, the patients tend to stabilize quite rapidly (over 24–28 hours) to the changes induced by hypercarbia and the dypsnoea resolves.

On the whole, ICU cases have few symptom problems, as death usually occurs on a ventilator, where the patient is effectively anaesthetized. Symptom control in nonmalignant disease is fairly good, with the exception of dysphagia and spastic spasms, although there is a great tendency to compensate for therapeutic failure by oversedating at the end.

DEATH FROM RESPIRATORY FAILURE (Dr G Spencer)

Death from acute respiratory failure may be dreaded even more than death in pain. However, Dr Spencer reports that the stubborn 'responauts', many of whom have experienced near-death from respirator disconnections or a similar mishap, are not really as afraid of this as might be expected. The most difficult problem when they are dying is dyspnoea, for which oral morphine is given, with cocaine added during the day. Staff may be reluctant to give this mixture for the treatment of dyspnoea and terminal dyspnoea can thus be more difficult to manage than terminal pain.

DEATH FROM RENAL FAILURE (Dr A Wing)

Death from uncomplicated renal failure does not present particular pain problems. Successful dialysis may eventually present more difficult challenges, involving much distress for these patients. They may become so incapacitated from intercurrent problems that the clinical team is faced with the necessity of withdrawing dialysis support from an alert patient and concentrating on symptom control. Pope Pius XII's distinction (1957) between ordinary and extraordinary treatment, and his pronouncement concerning the patient's freedom to refuse the latter, has been helpful to some in enabling them to ask to stop dialysis without regarding this as tantamount to suicide.

When treatment itself is a cause of pain, as with recurrent peritonitis in a patient on continuous ambulatory peritoneal dialysis, a decision may finally be taken not to treat an episode with anything other than what is necessary to relieve the pain.

DEATH IN A GERIATRIC UNIT (Professor B Livesley)

Professor Livesley points out that lower doses of drugs are often adequate for the 'elderly' patient compared with younger patients. This demands that we pay attention to the overall physical and mental state of a patient rather than the chronological age, and to a number of disease-associated conditions common to this age group, such as poor myocardial performance, impairment of renal function and the masked presence of hypothyroidism.

Professor Livesley draws attention to the pain on movement suffered by a proportion of his patients, and comments:

> Since rest on its own can relieve pain, movement of patients to reposition them in bed can aggravate severe pain, and analgesics may need adjusting to anticipate this problem. In fact, I have wondered if tranquilisers aid pain relief by reducing the patient's restlessness. It can be difficult to differentiate this severe pain-response to positional change from the sometimes considerable discomfort that patients can experience when they are moved from a settled position. Rightly or wrongly, I have accepted that if a patient's symptoms are immediately relieved once they have been repositioned this 'disturbance reaction' does not require further analgesics but simply an increased awareness by medical and nursing staff of the need for particularly gentle handling of affected patients.
>
> When adequate pain control has been obtained, the observer can sometimes be misled into recommending the dosage be increased. This is most likely to occur in those patients who have an 'alarm response' to being disturbed – when they are blind, deaf, confused, or have been asleep. Sometimes these patients may call out when they are unattended not because they are in obvious pain but because they need to be reassured they are not alone. I have had these observations confirmed by two of my most senior nurses (Livesley 1985).

PAIN AND SUDDEN DEATH

Death from injury in an accident is remembered by several witnesses as apparently painless. Worcester (1935) pointed out that those who have been rescued from death by drowning, even after apparently hopeless hours of artificial respiration, always say that before losing consciousness they experienced no suffering whatever. Melzack & Wall (1982) reported that, of patients admitted to an emergency room, 37% had no pain in the initial phase of injury, although they point out that 40% reported very severe pain.

Sudden death from coronary occlusion may also be painless, although some of those who survive for long enough to speak may refer to most severe pain. An elderly nurse died recently after a series of myocardial infarcts. Talking with a friend, she suddenly interrupted her to say, quite calmly, 'I need one of my pills', and died without another breath or sign of distress. The same evidently happens after some cerebrovascular accidents

Many would choose this way of dying, although research on bereavement suggests that it is more difficult for the survivors to come to terms with than the slower, expected death when there has been opportunity to bid farewell and resolve outstanding difficulties.

Lewis Thomas (1980) discussed the apparent painlessness of some traumatic deaths in his essay, 'On natural death'. He writes:

> Pain is useful for avoidance, for getting away when there's time to get away, but when it is endgame, and no way back, pain is likely to be turned off, and the mechanisms for this are wonderfully precise and quick. If I had to design an ecosystem in which creatures had to live off each other and in which dying was an indispensable part of living, I could not think of a better way to manage.

FEAR AND IMPENDING DEATH

Dying is not a mental illness and most patients will not require referral to a psychiatrist during the last days or weeks of life. Psychiatrists have recorded that they are needed more for support for the staff than for interviewing their patients. However, Parkes (1973), who has performed both kinds of activity in hospice wards over a number of years, saw 61 patients dying of cancer in the course of a typical year. Some 47 (77%) discussed their fears spontaneously with him and he classified them in the following categories:

1. Fear of separation from loved people, homes or jobs (38%).
2. Fear of being unable to complete some unfinished task or responsibility (10%) – 'There's so much left to be done'.
3. Fear of the consequences of the patient's death for his dependants (20%) – 'What will become of them?'
4. Fear of becoming dependent on others, of losing control of physical faculties, of being a nuisance (23%).
5. Fear of pain or mutilation (7%).
6. In addition, there were nine patients (15%) who were fearful but who never specified what it was they were afraid of . Several seemed anxious to be reassured of their own worth and one might conclude that, as religious persons, they were afraid of the judgement of God. More often, however, they seemed afraid of other unknown things that they must face at the time of, or after, death and of their incapacity to cope with these. It is this last fear, fear of the unknown, which comes closest to what most people mean by the fear of death (Parkes 1973).

As Parkes suggests, although one cannot deal effectively with everyone's fear, 'there are no cases for whom nothing can be done'. Fears of separation and loss are proper causes of grief, but if expressions of appropriate sorrow are encouraged, the patient can often move on to a deeper enjoyment of the life left to him. Fear of failure may lead to what has been termed (Butler 1963) 'the life review', in which problems of long standing are sometimes worked through at surprising speed. Crises of all kinds can lead to different forms of acceleration. Fears for dependants are frequently realistic and instituting or planning practical arrangements can bring comfort to all who are involved. Fears of losing physical function 'seem to derive mainly from fantasies of the effects of this loss of control on those around'. This is an obvious component of the widespread fear of incontinence. Parkes also found that patients who had been in pain were often more afraid of disgracing themselves by crying aloud than they were of the pain itself. This fear of physical pain is often unrealistic, or should be made so by effective treatment both for the patient and others around him. Such fear should be listened to and the possibilities of relief explained and given.

Fear of mutilation or physical deterioration may be helped by the attitude of the staff towards the weakening body. This attitude is reflected in verbal reassurances that the essence of this person still remains and is recognized and respected. Fear of the unknown is helped when the known, as seen by the patient, is rendered attentive and reassuring. Trust and faith in life and death are interwoven and both are enhanced by the attitude of those around.

It is most important that the staff should be at ease, with some confidence that both life and death are meaningful and that death is a necessary and fitting end to the accomplishment of living. A supportive atmosphere is best created with few if any words.

THE NEED FOR RESEARCH INTO SYMPTOM CONTROL OF THE DYING

Hinton (1964) suggested that if comparisons of the distress of dying after different treatments were available, it would add another factor to decisions made at an earlier stage. Such assessments have been made in combined pathological (clinical and therapeutic) studies. Of 18 patients with head-and-neck cancer submitted to salvage surgery and 26 with no salvage surgery, there were no significant differences in terminal pain or in difficulty of speech and swallowing. These symptoms were all common but success was achieved in terms of pain relief and a 'quiet' death in the special units in which these patients died. The results in this study suggest that a decision not to operate on older patients with advanced tumours would not condemn them to a more unpleasant death and would avoid the added trauma of unsuccessful major surgery (Pittam 1982).

A clinical and pathological study was made of 40 patients with intestinal obstruction due to far advanced abdominal and/or pelvic malignant disease. Surgical intervention was feasible in only two cases. The remaining 38 patients were managed medically without intravenous fluids and nasogastric suction. Obstructive symptoms such as intestinal colic, vomiting, and diarrhoea were effectively controlled by drugs (Baines et al 1985).

Recent discussion on 'necessary sustenance' when a patient is dying tends to ignore the fact that patients gradually lose their urge to eat and that feelings of thirst are better helped by the slow giving of normal fluids and of ice to suck, and by scrupulous mouth care, than by intravenous fluids.

Intravenous infusions are often continued until death in seriously ill patients because it is thought that electrolyte imbalance and dehydration may cause distress. However, the infusion may cause discomfort and distress to the patient, act as a barrier to relatives and divert the attending medical and nursing personnel from the care of the patient to that of the electrolyte and fluid balance.

We await definitive studies in this area.

EXPERIENCES OF 'DEATH'

Books have been written about patients who, in accident or illness, have 'died' and returned to life with clear memories of 'out-of-body experiences'. The fact that fear and pain seem to have been entirely absent, and that these experiences have been full of peace and light, has evidently comforted many people. Whether these are in fact experiences of 'death' rather than of some form of altered consciousness appears unproven, indeed unprovable.

Among many thousands of patients I have known as they faced their death, only one, a former nurse in her mid-40s with multiple sclerosis, had told me such a story. These stories, as they stand, have helped some patients to lose their fear of death. In no way are they proof of immortality; that seems to remain a matter of faith.

THERAPY

The limited number of studies and the series of contributions from different settings present the challenge of pain and impending death. The demand, for most patients, is for skilled symptom control. When this is won, as it commonly appears to be, at the cost of some diminution of consciousness, it would seem for most patients and, above all, their families, to be the preferred choice. An agitated and restless patient can do little to prepare himself or his family for the final parting; death in 'a sleep and a forgetting' can bring comfort and peace. For some this will be achieved by nature but others may demand constant vigilance and skill.

When specific treatments are no longer possible and death is likely within a few days, the major weapon for the control of pain, dyspnoea and other distress is the opioids. It may still be possible to give these drugs orally but the change to subcutaneous or intramuscular injections either regularly or by syringe driver must be planned and made with due regard to comparative potencies (orally, 15 mg morphine = 10 mg diamorphine; parenterally, 20 mg morphine = 10 mg diamorphine; oral morphine is approximately half as powerful as the same dose by injection). Many hospices in the United Kingdom use diamorphine rather than morphine in this way because of its greater solubility and therefore smaller volume. Hydromorphone may take this place elsewhere. Morphine would be entirely satisfactory for many patients, but, although only a few are likely to require large doses and therefore a large volume, this is important for the often emaciated patients.

Slow-release morphine or suppositories such as oxycodone (Proladone) may help maintain constant analgesia for the patient at home and a syringe driver containing either an opioid alone or a combination of drugs has enabled many families to care for a patient to the end. Haloperidol and midazolam can be used in this way with hyoscine added to dry up terminal lung secretions. Methotrimeprazine is a useful drug for a very restless patient but may occasionally produce a skin reaction (Hanks 1987).

Various combinations of these drugs with doses titrated to need may be required to ease a patient through his dying, whether at home or as an inpatient. There are of course other drugs in these groups but St Christopher's Hospice has kept to a rather limited pharmacopoeia as it is better to use a drug whose doses, effects and side-effects are well known than constantly to be making changes (Baines 1990). It has been suggested that, for some patients, pain decreases as death approaches (Witzel 1975). Studies since then have shown that there is a substantial number for whom this is not so and some for whom pain may become more severe. Because increased pain may be accompanied by a decreased ability to communicate, it seems important that drugs found necessary at an earlier stage should be continued and increased if there is any reason to believe that pain is present, even intermittently.

The selection of these drugs and others, such as phenobarbitone for seizures, needs to be individualized. A blanket ordering of what may be an overdose for a particular patient would hardly seem to be the way to end a long-term commitment to a patient's care on the part of his doctors and nurses. Drugs are used as fine instruments, and to turn to their use as a blunderbuss at the end would intimate a final attitude tantamount to 'writing off the patient. Clinical assessment and response to the needs of the patient cease only at death and support for the family afterwards depends on the doctor's presence and interest throughout the illness he has committed himself to manage.

Acknowledgements

Dr R Baxter (Intensive Care Unit), Professor B Livesley (Geriatric Unit), Dr G Spenser (Respiratory Unit), and Dr A Wing (Renal Unit) very kindly contributed to sections of this paper and Dr T D Walsh and his team carried out the survey of 200 patients in St Christopher's Hospice. To all these my grateful thanks.

REFERENCES

Baines M B 1990 Drug control of common symptoms. St Christopher's Hospice, London
Baines M B, Oliver D J, Carter R L 1985 Medical management of intestinal obstruction in patients with advanced malignant disease. Lancet ii: 990–993
Brain W R 1934 A post mortem on Dr Johnson. London Hospital Gazette 37: 225–230
Bruera E, Macmillan K, Hanson J, MacDonald R N 1989 The Edmonton staging system for cancer pain: preliminary report. Pain 37: 203–209
Butler R N 1963 The life review. An interpretation of reminiscence in the aged. Psychiatry 26: 65
Coyle N, Adelhardt J, Foley K M, Portenoy R K 1990 Character of terminal illness in the advanced cancer patient: pain and other symptoms during the last four weeks of life. Journal of Pain and Symptom Management 5: 83–93
Devlin P 1985 Easing the passing. Bodley Head, London, p 171
Exton-Smith A N 1961 Terminal illness in the aged. Lancet ii: 305–308
Faisinger R, MacEachern T, Hanson J, Miller M, Bruera E 1991 Symptom control during the last week of life in a palliative care unit. Journal of Palliative Care 7: 1
Hanks G W 1987 Opioid analgesics in the management of pain in patients with cancer. A review. Palliative Medicine 1: 1–25
Hawkett S, Nicholson R 1987 Syringe drivers. Journal of District Nursing 1: 4–6
Hinton J M 1963 The physical and mental distress of the dying. Quarterly Journal of Medicine 32: 1–21
Hinton J M 1964 Editorial: problems in the care of the dying. Journal of Chronic Diseases 17: 201–205
Keane W G, Gould J H, Millard P H 1983 Death in practice. Journal of the Royal College of General Practitioners 1: 347–351
Lichter I, Hunt E 1990 The last 48 hours of life. Journal of Palliative Care 6: 7–15
Livesley B 1985 The management of the dying patient. In: Pathy M S J (ed) Principles and practice of geriatric medicine. John Wiley, London, p 1287–1295
Lombard D J, Oliver D J 1989 The use of opioid analgesics in the last 24 hours of life of patients with advanced cancer. Palliative Medicine 3: 27–29
Melzack R, Wall P D 1982 Acute pain in an emergency clinic: latency of onset and description patterns related to different injuries. Pain 14: 33–43
Mount B 1990 Editorial: a final crescendo of pain? Journal of Palliative Care 6: 5–6
O'Brien T, Kelly M, Saunders C 1992 Motor neurone disease: a hospice perspective. British Medical Journal 304: 471–473
Osler W 1906 Science and immortality. Constable, London, p 36
Parkes C M 1973 Attachment and autonomy at the end of life. In: Gosling R (ed) Support, innovation and autonomy. Tavistock, London, p 151–166
Parkes C M 1978 Home or hospital? Terminal care as seen by surviving spouses. Journal of the Royal College of General Practitioners 28: 19–30
Pittam M R 1982 Does unsuccessful salvage surgery modify the terminal course of patients with squamous carcinomas of head and neck? Clinical Oncology: 195–200
Pius XII Pope 1957 Acta apostolicae sedia 49: 1027–1033
Thomas L 1980 On natural death. In Thomas L (ed) The medusa and the snail – more notes of a biology watcher. Allen Lane, London, p 102
Ventafridda V, Ripamonti C, De Conno F, Tamburini M 1990 Symptom prevalence and control during cancer patients' last days of life. Journal of Palliative Care 6: 7–11
Walsh T D 1984 Opiates and respiratory function in advanced cancer. Recent Results in Cancer Research 89: 115–117
Walsh T D, Bowman K B, Leber B, Daly E 1982 Unpublished data.
Wilkes E 1984 Occasional survey: dying now. Lancet i: 950–952
Witzel L 1971 Das Verhalten von sterbenden Patienten. Medizinische Klinik 66: 557
Witzel L 1973 Der Sterbende als Patient. Medizinische Klinik 68: 1378
Witzel L 1975 Behaviour of the dying patient. British Medical Journal ii: 81–82
Worcester A 1935 The care of the aged, the dying and the dead. C C Thomas, Springfield, Illinois

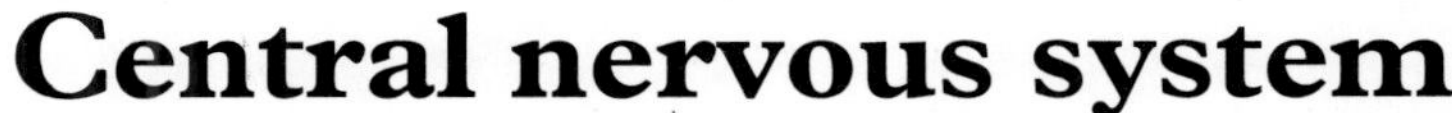

46. Central pain

Jörgen Boivie

DEFINITIONS

The International Association for the Study of Pain (IASP) has defined central pain as pain caused by a lesion or dysfunction in the central nervous system (CNS) (Merskey et al 1986). Note that the cause shall be a primary process in the CNS. Thus, peripherally induced pain with central mechanisms is not central pain, even if the central mechanisms are prominent. As with all definitions, there are conditions which may or may not be included. In the present context, pain due to brachial plexus evulsion and phantom pain are such examples. They will not be discussed in this chapter. Painful epileptic seizures are evoked by primary processes in the CNS and may thus be considered central pain.

The term *thalamic pain* is often used in a general sense for all central pain and the expression *pseudothalamic pain* is sometimes used for central pain caused by extrathalamic lesions. The term *dysaesthetic pain* is also sometimes used for central pain in general, probably due to the belief that all or almost all central pain has a predominantly dysaesthetic character, which is incorrect. Dysaesthetic pain can have either central or peripheral causes. It is recommended that the general term 'central pain' be used in most instances, and that only central pain caused by lesions in the thalamus should be labelled thalamic pain.

The term *anaesthesia dolorosa* has been used chiefly for head and face pain, and in particular for the neurogenic pain that sometimes develops after neurosurgical lesions of the trigeminal nerve or ganglion, or after destructive nerve blocks carried out to treat trigeminal neuralgia (see Ch. 39). It has also been used for central pain in an anaesthetic region caused by neurosurgical brain lesions created in the treatment of severe pain.

The term *deafferentation pain* is used for similar conditions, but it is more commonly used in patients with lesions of spinal nerves.

INTRODUCTION AND HISTORICAL PERSPECTIVE

Central pain is commonly thought of as being excruciating pain with a bizarre character and covering large areas of the body. This is only part of the truth, however, because central pain can appear in many guises. It can have a trivial character and be restricted to a relatively small area, such as distal pain in one arm, or in the face. It is true, though, that central pain is mostly severe in the sense that it causes the patient much suffering, even though its intensity may be relatively low. This is due to the fact that central pain is commonly very irritating and is largely constant.

Central pain has often been overlooked as a possibility in patients with CNS diseases because of poor knowledge of its characteristics. This may cause puzzling symptoms when several coexisting pains of an unusual nature exist. Not infrequently has central pain been thought to be of psychogenic origin. One reason for the lack of knowledge concerning central pain is the fact that relatively little systematic research has been done on the clinical aspects of central pain. Publications in the literature consist largely of case reports, reviews and studies on particular aspects, rather than more general studies characterizing central pain occurring after various kinds of lesions and diseases in the CNS. The lack of experimental models for central pain until recently has also contributed to the situation, since this has hampered research into its mechanisms.

Historically, central pain appears to have first been knowingly described as early as 1883 by Greiff in a patient who, following cerebrovascular lesions developed lasting pain ('reissende Schmertzen' – tearing pain; Greiff 1883). The lesion included the thalamus. Some 8 years later Edinger (1891) presented arguments for the existence of central pain. By then it was known that sensory pathways project to the thalamus, which was therefore at an early stage thought to play a crucial role in central pain. Throughout the years thalamic pain, i.e. pain caused by thalamic lesions, has remained the best-known form of central pain. It is for this reason that all kinds of central pain are often called thalamic pain, although only a minority are related to thalamic lesions.

The most cited early description of central pain is Dejerine & Roussy's classic report from 1906 (Dejerine & Roussy 1906). They studied six patients with thalamic syndromes, including central pain. According to them, the syndrome is characterized by: (i) slight hemiplegia, (ii) disturbances of superficial and deep sensibility, (iii) hemiataxia and hemiastereognosia, (iv) intolerable, persistent and paroxysmal pain, and (v) choreoathetoid movements. The cause of the syndrome is usually a thalamic infarction or haemorrhage (Garcin 1968). However, in the three patients in which Dejerine & Roussy did postmortem microscopy the lesions extended lateral to the thalamus to include the posterior part of the internal capsule where the thalamocortical fibres from the ventroposterior thalamic region pass to the cerebral cortex. This has been a common feature also in other patients with thalamic lesions reported in the literature. Few patients have had complete thalamic syndromes, which are evidently very rare, but thalamic pain, i.e. pain caused by a thalamic lesion, is less rare (Riddoch 1938; Schott et al 1986; Leijon et al 1989; Bogousslavsky et al 1988).

Although interest in central pain was focused mainly on thalamic pain for many years, Edinger had already in 1891 introduced the idea that cortical lesions might also cause pain (Edinger 1891). He also mentioned that the aura of epileptic seizures can include the experience of pain, which has since been reported by several authors. It has now also been demonstrated beyond doubt that lesions above the thalamus can cause central pain (Davidson & Schick 1935; Schuster 1936; Ajuraguerra 1937; Biemond 1956; Garcin 1968; Fields & Adams 1974; Leijon et al 1989; Michel et al 1990; Schmahmann & Leifer 1992; cases 29 and 32), but it is still uncertain whether a lesion strictly limited to the cortex can lead to central pain because in all cases published the lesions have also included some subcortical white matter (Breuer et al 1981; Sandyk 1985; Michel et al 1990).

Evidence showing that lesions in the brainstem can evoke central pain has also been accumulating (Riddoch 1938; Garcin 1968; Cassinari & Pagni 1969; Tasker 1990). The most common site of these lesions has been the medulla oblongata, whereas few cases of pontine and midbrain lesions with central pain have been reported. Only rare cases of midbrain lesions are known, mainly after mesencephalic tractotomies (Drake & Mckenzie 1953). Pontobulbar lesions have been dominated by infarctions in the territory of the posterior inferior cerebellar artery (PICA), but also syringobulbia, multiple sclerosis and tumours can give rise to central pain.

An early description of central pain after traumatic spinal cord injuries (SCI) was published by Holmes, who had noticed this form of pain in soldiers from the First World War (Holmes 1919). In the report he did not use the term 'central pain', but remarked that the pain and hypersensitivity resembled that found in thalamic syndromes. This pain started shortly after the injury and subsided spontaneously after about 1 month. It has since been shown that long-lasting central pain is common after SCI and is actually one of the major problems in patients with traumatic SCI. Central pain is also common in several other forms of myelopathy, for instance, in multiple sclerosis, syringomyelia and vascular malformations.

Many descriptions of central pain syndromes were published during the first three decades of this century, showing that the character of this pain can vary considerably from patient to patient and that central pain can be excruciating. Since these case reports vividly illustrate this kind of pain some of the descriptions given by Head & Holmes will be cited: crushed feeling; scalding sensation, as if boiling water was being poured down the arm; cramping; aching; soreness, as if the leg was bursting; something crawling under the skin; pain pumping up and down the side; as if the painful region was covered with ulcers; as if pulling a dressing from a wound; as if a log of wood was hanging down from the shoulder; as if little pins were sticking into the fingers; like a wheel running over the arm; cold stinging feeling (Head & Holmes 1911); as if knives heated in Hell's hottest corner were tearing me to pieces (Holmes 1919). In a more recent report of a patient with central poststroke pain with unknown location, the following pain components were described: boiling hot; deep as though in the bones; showers of pain like electric shocks or red-hot needles evoked by touch; as though the arm and leg were being twisted; continuous sensation of pins and needles; a strange sensation of the limbs being abnormally full (Loh et al 1981).

AETIOLOGY AND EPIDEMIOLOGY

LESIONS CAUSING CENTRAL PAIN

Structure and location of the lesion

It appears that all kinds of lesion in the brain and spinal cord can cause central pain (Table 46.1). These lesions and dysfunctions are due to many different disease processes. The macrostructure of the lesion is probably less important than its location as regards the probability that it will induce central pain. This does not mean that the structure of the lesion has no significance, because it is conceivable that the microstructure of the lesion in some instances is critical, but there is to date no information from research on this matter.

Pain in Parkinson's disease has previously not been considered central pain. Recent surveys show that pain is common in this disease, but it is at present not clear to

Table 46.1 Causes of central pain

Vascular lesions in the brain and spinal cord
infarct
haemorrhage
vascular malformation
Multiple sclerosis
Traumatic spinal cord injury; cordotomy
Traumatic brain injury
Syringomyelia and syringobulbia
Tumours
Abscesses
Inflammatory diseases other than MS; myelitis caused by viruses, syphilis
Epilepsy
Parkinson's disease

what extent this pain is caused directly by the brain pathology. It is possible, though, that much of the pain is of central origin and thus central pain.

The lesions that lead to central pain include rapidly and slowly developing lesions. There appears to be no difference in the tendency to cause central pain between rapidly developing haemorrhages, infarcts (Leijon et al 1989) and traumatic spinal cord lesions, and slowly developing demyelination or arteriovenous malformations. Syringomyelia very often leads to central pain, but it is unlikely that this has anything to do with the fact that the lesion develops extremely slowly. Since the prevalence of central pain is very low in patients with intracranial tumours and spinal tumours it is difficult to know whether or not they differ in this respect and if there is any difference between intra- and extraparenchymal tumours. Besides the common kind of constant central pain, tumours may also cause painful epileptic seizures.

It is now clear that lesions at any level along the neuraxis can cause central pain. Thus, lesions at the first synapse in the dorsal horn of the spinal cord or trigeminal nuclei, along the ascending pathways through the spinal cord and brainstem, in the thalamus, in the subcortical white matter and probably in the cerebral cortex have all been reported to cause central pain (Riddoch 1938; Garcin 1968; Cassinari & Pagni 1969; Leijon et al 1989; Tasker 1990). The highest prevalences have been noticed after lesions in the spinal cord, lower brainstem and ventroposterior part of the thalamus (Tasker 1990; Bonica 1991; Boivie 1992).

The location of lesions that produce central pain has been best studied in central poststroke pain (CPSP). The role of thalamic lesions is one of the recurrent questions in this context. In one study it was found that nine of 27 patients had lesions involving the thalamus, but the lesions were restricted to the thalamus in only two of these (Leijon et al 1989). These results were based on X-ray computerized tomography (CT) scans. A later study using magnetic resonance imaging (MRI) indicated that about 50% of all CPSP patients have lesions engaging the thalamus (Lewis-Jones et al 1990).

The importance of the location of the thalamic lesion within the thalamus was elucidated in a study of the clinical consequences of thalamic infarcts. The results showed that only patients with lesions including the ventroposterior thalamic region developed central pain (Bogousslavsky et al 1988). Three of 18 patients with such infarcts had central pain at follow-up, whereas none of the 22 patients with other locations, including a medially located one, had central pain. In the other cited study, all nine thalamic lesions included part of the ventroposterior thalamic region (Leijon et al 1989). This is in accordance with Hassler's idea that the posterior inferior part of the ventroposterior region, i.e. his V.c.p.c or VPI in recent terminology, is the crucial location for thalamic lesions causing central pain (Hassler 1960). This region receives a particularly dense spinothalamic projection in primates (Boivie 1979).

It was recognized at an early stage that subcortical lesions can induce central pain, but there has been continuing argument whether superficial lesions in the cerebral cortex can also have that effect. This question can still not be given a definite answer because lesions restricted to the cortex are rare. Usually the lesions damage more or less of the subcortical white matter, too. Several central pain patients with such combined lesions, and lesions located just deep to the cortex, have been described, particularly with lesions in the insular region, i.e. in the second somatosensory region (Michelson 1943; Biemond 1956; Bender & Jaffe 1958; McNamara et al 1990; Michel et al 1990; Schmahmann & Leifer 1992). These lesions have included infarcts, haematomas, meningiomas and traumatic lesions. Some of the patients with superficial lesions have had painful partial epileptic seizures. This is a strong argument for the idea that cortical lesions can lead to central pain, because epileptic seizures are cortical phenomena.

Lesions affect somatic sensibility

The first requisite for a disease process to produce central pain seems to be that it affects structures involved in somatic sensibility, which is not surprising, since pain is part of somaesthesia. This notion is based on previous reviews, case reports and recent studies in patients with central pain caused by stroke, multiple sclerosis and syringomyelia, which indicate that central pain is independent of nonsensory symptoms and signs (Leijon et al 1989; Tasker 1990; Boivie & Rollsjö, unpublished observations). This excludes many lesion sites as possible causes of central pain. Fortunately, however, only a minority of the patients with lesions that carry a risk will develop central pain. The risk differs very much between diseases and locations of the lesion (see below; Bonica 1991).

Most patients with central pain reported in the literature have had sensory abnormalities and the dominating features have been abnormal sensibility to temperature and pain and hyperaesthesia (Riddoch 1938; Pagni 1989; Tasker 1990). Depending on the location of the lesion the sensibility profiles differ, often in a predictable way. For instance, after ventroposterior thalamic lesions there is usually a general profound loss of all modalities. After low brainstem infarcts of the Wallenberg type there is a crossed dissociated sensory loss and after complete spinal cord injuries all sensibility is lost. However, if one looks for a common denominator among these patients, abnormal pain and temperature sensibility, together with hyperaesthesia, stands out.

These observations, and results from studies on patients with central pain due to cerebrovascular lesions, multiple sclerosis, traumatic spinal cord injuries and syringomyelia employing quantitative methods to assess the sensory abnormalities, form the basis for the hypothesis that central pain occurs only after lesions that affect the spinothalamic pathways, i.e. the pathways that are most important for temperature and pain sensibility (Berić et al 1988; Boivie et al 1989; Pagni 1989; Boivie & Leijon 1991; Boivie 1992). If this hypothesis turns out to be correct it means that lesions of the dorsal column–medial lemniscal pathways are not a requisite for the occurrence of central pain. Such lesions were for many years thought to be essential in the mechanism of central pain (see below). This hypothesis states that central pain is the result of lesions of the lemniscal system which remove the inhibition normally exerted on the spinothalamic projections. Undoubtedly the lemniscal projections are affected in many central pain patients, but the question is whether or not this part of the lesion is of importance for the pain. It certainly affects sensibility. No reports of patients with central pain and lesions unequivocally restricted to the lemniscal pathways appear to have been published, whereas many cases of lesions strictly limited to the spinothalamic pathways have been reported, for instance in the Wallenberg syndrome and after cordotomy.

EPIDEMIOLOGY

There are large differences in the prevalence of central pain among the disorders that may lead to such pain (Table 46.2; Bonica 1991). No true epidemiological studies have been done, so the figures are estimates. Such estimates are difficult to make, because it is sometimes difficult to distinguish central pain from other possible causes of the pain. This, for instance, is the case in many patients with pain after spinal injury and multiple sclerosis. Nevertheless, the figures given in Table 46.2 are probably in the right range, which means that, even if pain in epilepsy and Parkinson's disease are excluded, in the order of about 130 000 Americans have central pain, i.e. a prevalence of about 54 per 100 000 individuals. The reader is referred to Bonica's article for details.

Table 46.2 Estimated prevalence in 1989 of major disorders with central pain (CP) in the USA (population about 250 million)[1]

Disease	Total number of patients	Patients with CP	Patients with CP(%)
Spinal cord injury	225 000	68 000	30
Multiple sclerosis	150 000	35 000	23
Stroke	2 000 000	30 000	1.5
Epilepsy	1 600 000	45 000	2.8
Parkinson's disease	500 000	50 000	10

[1]From Bonica (1991).

The highest prevalence is found with traumatic spinal cord injuries, multiple sclerosis and syringomyelia. The latter is a rare disease with a very high incidence of central pain, probably the highest of any disease. In a recent survey of 22 patients it was found that most had central pain at some stage of the disease (Boivie & Rollsjö, unpublished observations).

PATHOPHYSIOLOGY

HYPOTHESES CONCERNING THE MECHANISMS INVOLVED

The lesions that cause central pain vary enormously in location, size and structure. There is no study indicating that a small lesion in the dorsal horn of the spinal cord carries less risk for central pain than a huge infarct involving much of the thalamus and large parts of the white matter lateral and superior to the thalamus. This raises the question as to whether or not the same pathophysiology underlies all central pain. The fact that the character of the pain also differs widely between patients with the same kind of lesion, and between groups, points in the same direction. However, this does not exclude the possibility that some common pathophysiological factors may be involved in all central pain.

For many reasons, knowledge about the pathophysiology of central pain is incomplete. This has stimulated several investigators to propose hypotheses concerning the mechanisms involved. The most important are briefly summarized below.

Irritable focus

One of the first hypotheses was that the pain is the result of activity produced by an irritable focus created at the site of injury. This was the explanation of Dejerine & Roussy (1906) for thalamic pain.

Disinhibition by lesions in the medial lemniscal pathways

The notion that central pain is caused by lesions in the dorsal column-medial lemniscal pathway has been one of the most favoured hypotheses. The crucial physiological consequence of the lesions is thought to be a disinhibition of neurons in the pain-signalling system, i.e. in the spinothalamic pathways (when this term is used in this chapter it also includes the thalamocortical projections activated via the spinothalamic and spinoreticulothalamic pathways and the cortical projections via the spinomesencephalic tract). Head & Holmes (1911) were among the first to embrace this notion. They mainly discussed it with regard to corticothalamic connections. Later Foerster (1927) formulated the hypothesis slightly differently when he argued that the epicritic sensibility normally exerts control over the protopathic sensibility. The term epicritic sensibility includes the sensory modalities thought to depend on activity through the lemniscal pathways, i.e. touch, pressure, vibration and kinaesthesia, whereas protopathic sensibility includes pain and temperature. According to this hypothesis, central pain can occur only when there is a loss of epicritic sensibility, i.e. a lesion in the lemniscal system.

Lesion in the spinothalamic pathway

In recent years most investigators have found indications that the spinothalamic system is affected in the majority of central pain patients (Boivie et al 1989; Pagni 1989; Tasker 1990). These indications include, for instance, the finding that central pain patients have abnormal temperature and pain sensibility, but they may have normal threshold to touch, vibration and joint movements (Berić et al 1988; Boivie et al 1989), and that low brainstem infarcts (= Wallenberg syndrome) and cordotomies, in which the spinothalamic but not the lemniscal pathways are injured, cause central pain. This is the basis for the hypothesis that central pain occurs only after lesions affecting the spinothalamic system (Boivie et al 1989). In many patients the lemniscal pathways are also affected by the lesion, but this does not appear to be necessary for the occurrence of central pain. It even appears possible that the involvement of the lemniscal pathway in no way affects the character of the pain, but it does of course affect the character of the sensory abnormalities. Further elaboration has been made on this hypothesis and it has been proposed that the crucial lesion is one that affects the neospinothalamic projections, by which is meant the projections to the ventroposterior thalamic region (Bowsher 1959; Garcin 1968; Pagni 1989). This kind of lesion is thought to leave the more medially and inferiorly terminating paleospinothalamic projections anatomically intact. This idea is somewhat related to the hypothesis proposing that a lemniscal lesion is crucial, because it is based on the idea that the neospinothalamic projections carry the sensory-discriminative aspects of pain and temperature sensibility (location, intensity, sensory character). There is some support in the literature for this notion, but it cannot be considered proven.

Removal of inhibition exerted by the reticular thalamic nucleus

A recent hypothesis focuses on the role of the reticular thalamic nucleus, and the medial and intralaminar thalamic regions receiving spinothalamic projections. According to this hypothesis the lesion removes the suppressing activity exerted by the reticular thalamic nucleus on medial and intralaminar thalamic nuclei, thereby releasing abnormal activity in this region, which, in turn, leads to pain and hypersensitivity (Schott et al 1986; Mauguière & Desmedt 1988; Cesaro et al 1991).

Experimental studies have shown that the reticular thalamic nucleus receives collateral input from the thalamocortical projections, and that it in turn projects to the medially located spinothalamic projection zones. In an investigation aimed at showing whether there was neuronal hyperactivity in the brain of four patients with central pain caused by cerebrovascular lesions in the thalamus (one patient) and in the thalamocortical projection path (three patients), using the SPECT-technique (= single photon emission computerized tomography), Cesaro et al (1991) found signs of hyperactivity in the thalamus, possibly in its medial part, in two patients with hyperpathia, but not in the other two patients without hyperpathia. It is interesting to note that, in one of the patients, hyperactivity was not found during successful treatment with amitriptyline, but reappeared when the treatment had to be stopped and the pain had returned. The technique, however, has a very poor spatial resolution, so it could not be determined in which part of the thalamus the hyperactivity was located. In accordance with this hypothesis it appears from the literature that most thalamic lesions that cause central pain might involve part of the reticular nucleus, as well as parts of the ventroposterior nuclei.

Cellular pain

A theory of 'cellular pain' was proposed 70 years ago (Foix et al 1922). The hypothesis proposes that central pain is the result of 'disorganization of integration at the level of cellular relays' (cited from Garcin 1968). This is a modern idea that fits well with current knowledge about the neurophysiological correlates of pain (see below).

Sympathetic mechanisms

Sympathetic dysfunction has long been suspected of playing a role in central pain because signs of abnormal sympathetic activity – including oedema, decreased sweating, lowered skin temperature, change in skin colour and trophic skin changes – have been observed in many patients (Riddoch 1938). It is difficult to evaluate the significance of these abnormalities, however, because they may be secondary to the change in mobility. Many patients with central pain avoid using the painful arm or foot because of the hypersensitivity to skin contact and the aggravating effect of movements or because of paresis. This total or partial immobilization could, itself, lead to changes in the sympathetic outflow and in the microcirculation of the region. Attempts have been made to study these relationships, but it has been difficult to determine if the abnormalities are causal or coincidental with regard to central pain, or caused by the central pain. The results of sympathetic blockade might give some clue about these relationships, but the case reports show contradictory results with only some patients reporting pain relief (Loh et al 1981; Leijon et al, unpublished observations).

THALAMIC AND CELLULAR MECHANISMS

In most hypotheses the thalamus is believed to play a major role in the mechanism of central pain. Three of its regions are in focus, namely the ventroposterior part including also the posteriorly and inferiorly located nuclei bordering on this region, the medial-intralaminar region and the reticular nucleus (see above). All three regions receive spinothalamic projections, directly or indirectly. The role of the ventroposterior region in central pain was recently analysed in a series of articles in the *APS Journal* (Boivie 1992; Jones 1992; Lenz 1992; Salt 1992). Lenz proposed that the ventroposterior thalamic region is heavily involved in the mechanism of central pain and summarized data showing that, in primates, large parts of the ventroposterior nuclei (VP) receive nociceptive inputs, although these may be restricted to the so-called shell zones in the outer part of the complex. Many of these thalamic neurons appear to be wide dynamic range neurons, receiving inputs via the lemniscal pathways as well, but there are also nociceptive-specific neurons in the nuclei.

Neurophysiological studies in the human ventroposterior thalamus

Burst activity and neurochemistry of sensory projections

Recordings from the thalamus in patients with central pain following spinal cord injuries have demonstrated increased spontaneous activity characterized by bursts of action potentials in the portions of the ventroposterior nuclei representing the anaesthetic or painful area of the body. This activity has similarities to calcium spikes shown in animal studies, i.e. activity related to the function of calcium channels, and it has been proposed that excitatory amino acids acting through N-methyl-D-aspartate (NMDA) receptors are involved (Lenz 1992). In this context it is of interest to note that such receptors are crucial in the relaying of inputs from nociceptors in the thalamus (Eaton & Salt 1990) and that the spinothalamic and lemniscal systems differ neurochemically, for instance with regard to the calcium-binding proteins. Thus, parvalbumin immunoreactivity has been found in the lemniscal projections, whereas calbindin is present in the spinothalamic system. Jones (1992) concluded that current evidence suggests that the calbindin cells in the posterior, anterior pulvinar, caudal intralaminar, ventral posterior inferior, VPL, VPM, and parts of the ventral lateral and ventral medial nuclei form a small-celled spinothalamic- and caudal trigeminothalamic-recipient matrix that projects diffusely to widespread areas of the cerebral cortex. In monkeys with long-term deafferentation after cervical rhizotomy there was an increase in calbindin in this small-celled matrix (Rausell et al 1991). It was speculated that this might underlie the signs of deafferentation pain that were observed.

Pain memory – possible long-term potentiation

Lenz, Tasker, Dostrovsky and collaborators showed that electrical stimulation in a ventroposterior zone deprived of its peripheral input due to a spinal cord lesion or amputation might evoke pain in the deafferented, but painful region (Lenz et al, 1988). Stimulation at these thalamic sites in patients without pain did not evoke pain. The fact that the stimulation evoked pain in deafferented regions indicates that there remains a representation in the CNS of the somatic sensibility for the deafferented region, a kind of long-term memory, which need not necessarily be located in the thalamus. Hypothetically it is possible that such a memory could be activated long after the lesion appeared, which may explain the long delay in the onset of central pain in some patients. Long-term potentiation is thought to be an important aspect in the memory processes. It seems probable that some kind of long-term potentiation is involved in chronic central pain, which is really a long-term process. NMDA receptors and associated calcium conduction have been implicated in long-term potentiation, thus representing another possible connection with excitatory amino acids (Collingridge & Singer 1990).

Lesions in the ventroposterior thalamus and central pain

An important question regarding Lenz's hypothesis is whether the observed abnormal activity observed in the ventroposterior thalamus is the primary event, or whether it is mainly a reflection of primary events occurring somewhere else in the CNS, for instance in the spinal cord, the brainstem, some other part of the thalamus or in the cerebral cortex. This question cannot be answered at present.

The observations reviewed above have been made in patients with spinal cord injuries. It is reasonable to suspect some common mechanisms in all central pain conditions, but it is also conceivable that there are differences depending on where the primary lesion is located. It would thus be surprising if the physiological abnormalities are identical in a patient with a large supratentorial cerebrovascular lesion affecting much of the thalamus, including the ventroposterior region, and one with a small spinal cord lesion mainly affecting the dorsal horn. As regards the hypothesis postulating a crucial role for abnormal neuronal activity in the ventroposterior thalamic region in central pain, the mere location of the lesion sometimes makes this impossible, because, in some patients with central pain, this region is completely silent, namely, in many patients with central pain due to thalamic infarct or haemorrhage. In fact, it appears that this is where the thalamic lesions that cause central pain have to be located (see above in section on lesions).

In a study of the clinical consequences of thalamic infarct it was found that only patients with thalamic lesions including the ventroposterior thalamic region developed central pain (Bogousslavsky et al 1988). Three of 18 patients with such infarcts had central pain at follow-up, whereas none of the 22 patients with other locations had central pain. In our own material with central post-stroke pain (CPSP), all nine thalamic lesions included part of the ventroposterior thalamic region (Leijon et al 1989). This is in accordance with Hassler's idea that the posterior inferior part of the ventroposterior region, i.e. his V.c.p.c or ventroposterior inferior nucleus (VPI) in recent terminology, is the crucial target for thalamic lesions causing central pain (Hassler 1960).

Submedius nucleus

The medially located submedius nucleus has been proposed to play a role in the pathophysiology of central pain (Craig 1991). The experimental results that form the basis for this hypothesis were recently reviewed by Craig (1991). Nociceptive projections have been shown to the submedius nucleus (Sm), which projects to the ventral lateral orbital cortex (VLO). This cortical zone is reciprocally connected with area 3a, the caudal aspect of the second somatosensory region (SII), area 5a and the anterior cingulate region. It has descending projections to the ventrolateral periaqueductal grey (PAG). These connections support a sensory role of the submedius nucleus, possibly in affective aspects of pain. 'A lesion of lateral spinothalamic terminations in the ventral caudal part of the VP nuclei that produced a contralateral hypalgesia could result in release of corticocortical control by the ventral VP projection areas on the Sm projection area in VLO' (Craig 1991). This would lead to 'dysfunctional activity' in the Sm and VLO, which could possibly be part of the mechanism causing central pain.

A POSSIBLE EXPERIMENTAL MODEL FOR CENTRAL PAIN

Experience from many fields of medical research has shown that experimental models are most valuable in the search for mechanisms and treatments. Early experience from a recently developed technique for producing experimental lesions in the spinal cord gives hope that the use of the model will lead to new insights into central pain. In this model ischaemic lesions are produced by a photochemical process involving the injection of erythrosin B parenterally followed by irradiation with an argon laser (Watson et al 1986). The size of the lesions depends on the energy transferred to the spinal cord by the laser, but it has so far not been possible to predetermine the exact location and size of the lesions. In a series of studies Wiesenfeld-Hallin and collaborators have tested the model on rats and reported interesting results (Hao et al 1991a, 1991b, 1991c, 1991d). It has been shown for instance that the lesion strikes both white and grey matter, that the rats almost immediately, after induction of the lesion, develop tactile allodynia, which is morphine-resistant but responds to the gamma amino butyric acid (GABA)-B-agonist baclofen given systemically and that the allodynia is prevented by pretreatment with the NMDA-antagonist MK-801 in rats with short irradiation times, that pretreatment with guanethidine or the opioid antagonist naltrexone does not prevent the development of allodynia, and that the sensitivity of wide-dynamic-range neurons in Rexed's lamina I-V to mechanical pressure is greatly increased with lowered threshold and more vigorous response. This is, no doubt, a promising experimental model of central pain, but further studies are needed to establish its similarity to chronic central pain in humans.

SUMMARY OF PATHOPHYSIOLOGY

1. The disease process, here called the lesion, involves the spinothalamic pathways, including the indirect spinoreticulothalamic and spinomesencephalic projections, as indicated by abnormalities in the sensibility to pain and temperature.
2. The lesion probably does not have to involve the dorsal column–medial lemniscal pathways to invoke central pain.
3. The lesion can be located at any level of the neuraxis, from the dorsal horn to the cerebral cortex.
4. It is probable that all kinds of disease process may cause central pain, but the probability of central pain occurring varies greatly between these diseases, from being rare to occurring in the majority of patients.

5. As yet, no single region has been shown to be crucial in the processes underlying central pain, but three thalamic regions have been focused upon, namely, the ventroposterior, the reticular and the medial/intralaminar regions. The role of the cerebral cortex in central pain is unclear, but this issue has not been specifically studied.

6. The pain and hypersensitivity experienced by central pain patients are compatible with the increased burst activity that has been found in the ventroposterior thalamic region in spinal cord injury patients with central pain. It is conceivable that this kind of cellular activity is also present at other levels of the sensory pathways, including the cerebral cortex.

7. The cellular processes underlying central pain are still unknown, but processes involving excitatory amino acids, and, in particular glutaminergic NMDA-receptors have been implicated.

CLINICAL CHARACTERISTICS

DIAGNOSIS OF A CNS PROCESS

The definition of central pain states that it is caused by a lesion or dysfunction in the CNS. The first step in the diagnostic procedure is therefore to ensure that the patient has a CNS disorder. This is often obvious, as in many patients with stroke or multiple sclerosis, but it is sometimes not clear that there is a CNS lesion, as in some patients with moderate spinal trauma or suspected minor stroke. A detailed history of the neurological symptoms and a neurological examination are important parts of the diagnostic procedure, but laboratory examinations are often necessary. These include computerized tomography with X-ray or magnetic resonance, i.e. a CT scan or MRI, assays of the cerebrospinal fluid (CSF), neurophysiological examinations, and other tests.

In addition to confirming the presence of a CNS process, one must also consider whether or not the patient has pain due to peripheral neuropathy. Polyneuropathy is not uncommon in, for instance, stroke patients, a group with a high incidence of diabetes. Neurography and electromyography are therefore indicated in some patients. Quantitative sensory tests are also valuable in the diagnosis of neuropathy. They include examination of sensibility to temperature and pain, as well as to vibration and touch (Lindblom & Ochoa 1986). Whereas neurography can demonstrate abnormalities only in large fibres, these tests can show dysfunction in both large and small sensory fibres.

DIFFERENTIAL DIAGNOSIS OF CENTRAL VERSUS NOCICEPTIVE AND PSYCHOGENIC PAIN

Central pain can usually be distinguished from other forms of pain provided that one is familiar with the characteristics of central pain, but in some patients it is difficult to determine whether the pain is central, peripheral neurogenic, nociceptive or psychogenic. Some patients have more than one kind of pain. A hemiplegic stroke patient, for instance, can have a nociceptive shoulder pain in addition to central pain. The examination of patients suspected of having central pain has to be individually tailored in order to identify possible noncentral causes of the pain. Diagnostic problems are particularly difficult in some patients with MS and spinal cord injury (SCI), because of the complex clinical picture, with a mixture of motor and sensory symptoms, and pain. Paresis and dyscoordination may lead to abnormal strain in musculoskeletal structures and development of nociceptive pain. The diagnostic procedure often calls for consultations by specialists, particularly orthopaedics.

Psychogenic factors are important in central pain, as in all pain, but with increasing knowledge of the characteristics of central pain it rarely turns out that pain suspected of being central is truly psychogenic. Psychiatric and psychological consultations may be indicated in some patients, even if there is definite certain central pain, because the patient may also be depressed, although patients with central pain do not appear to be more depressed than other pain patients.

PAIN CHARACTERISTICS

The next step is to analyse the characteristics of the pain, i.e. its location, quality, intensity, onset and development after onset, variation with time and influence by external and internal events.

Pain location

It is usually stated with considerable emphasis that central pain is diffusely located. This notion appears to be largely derived from the fact that central pain often extends over large areas of the body, for instance the whole right or left side, or the lower half of the body. However, central pain can also involve one hand only, or just the ulnar or radial side of the hand, or one side of the face. Even patients with extensive central pain find it relatively easy to describe the extent of the painful regions, as shown in studies of patients with central pain after stroke and MS (Leijon et al 1989; Österberg, Boivie & Henriksson, unpublished observations). It is therefore more correct to state that most central pain is extensive, than to describe it as diffuse.

The location of the lesion determines the location of the pain (Table 46.3). Thus, large lesions in the ventroposterior thalamic region or the posterior limb of the internal capsule tend to cause hemibody pain, whereas large spinal cord lesions cause bilateral pain involving the body regions innervated by the segments caudal to the

Table 46.3 Common locations of central pain

Stroke
All of one side
All of one side, except the face
Arm and/or leg on one side
Face on one side, extremities on the other side
The face
Multiple sclerosis
Lower half of the body
One or both legs
Arm and leg on one side
Trigeminal neuralgia
SCI
Whole body below the neck
Lower half of the body
One leg
Syringomyelia
Arm and thorax on one side
One arm
Thorax on one side
One leg in addition to one of the above

lesion. Even lesions that cause extensive loss of somatic sensibility may lead to central pain restricted to a small portion of the deafferented region. Examples of central pain engaging small regions were recently shown in patients with superficial cortical/subcortical vascular lesions (Michel et al 1990).

Cerebrovascular lesions in the medulla oblongata, i.e. mainly lesions caused by thrombosis in the posterior inferior cerebellar artery leading to Wallenberg syndromes, can induce central pain on both sides, the face and head being involved on the lesion side, and the rest of the body on the contralateral side (Riddoch 1938; Leijon et al 1989). This pattern is due to injury to the ipsilateral spinal trigeminal nucleus and the crossed spinothalamic tract. Lesions affecting the spinothalamic tract in the spinal cord will lead to pain on the contralateral side, after cordotomy for example. In syringomyelia central pain may be restricted to part of one side of the thorax, but it may also be more extensive, including the arm and even the lower body regions.

Central pain is experienced as superficial or deep pain, or with both superficial and deep components, but the high incidence of cutaneous hyperaesthesias contributes to the impression that superficial pain dominates, although deep pain is also common. Among 27 central poststroke pain (CPSP) patients, eight described the pain as superficial, eight as deep and the remaining 11 as both superficial and deep (Leijon et al 1989).

Quality of pain

No pain quality is pathognomonic for central pain. Central pain is thus not always burning or 'dysaesthetic', as one might believe from reading some of the literature on the subject. In fact, central pain can have any quality,

Table 46.4 Qualities of pain reported by patients with central pain*

*Burning	Shooting	Stabbing
*Aching	Squeezing	Cramping
*Lancinating	Throbbing	Smarting
*Pricking	Cutting	Pulling
*Lacerating	Crushing	Sore
*Pressing	Splitting	Icy feeling
	Stinging	

*Indicates the most common qualities.

and the variation between patients is great, although some qualities are more common than others (Table 46.4).

Another basic feature is the presence of more than one pain quality in many patients. The different pains can coexist in a body region, or may be present in different parts of the body. A patient with CPSP, for instance, may have burning and aching pain in the leg and arm, and burning and stinging pain in the face. Other patients have a less complex pain condition, with aching pain in the arm or leg. Some patients have pain with bizarre character, as was illustrated by citations from the early literature in the Introduction.

One would expect the location of the lesion to be a deciding factor with regard to the quality of pain. This appears to be partly true, but it is also apparent that similar lesions can lead to different pain qualities, as illustrated by central pain caused by cerebrovascular lesions in the thalamus. Nine patients with such pain reported more than eight types of pain and none of these qualities was experienced by all patients (Leijon et al 1989). All of the lesions involved the ventroposterior thalamic region, but in seven of the patients the lesions extended lateral to the thalamus. It was not possible to correlate a particular pain character to the site of the lesion.

The description of the various central pain conditions given later in this chapter shows that, just as with central pain in general, no pathognomonic pain character has been found in any of these conditions. Perhaps the most homogeneous group consists of patients with central pain after spinal cordotomy, in whom the pain has mostly been described as dysaesthetic (see below), but the incidence is low, so that only small numbers of patients have been reported from each centre (Cassinari & Pagni 1969; White & Sweet 1969; Tasker 1990). When comparing central pain conditions one gets the impression that the variation in pain qualities may be largest among stroke patients (Table 46.10). This is not surprising since the variation in the structure and location of the lesion is largest in this group.

The most common central pain quality is probably burning pain, which has been found to be frequent in most central pain conditions (Cassinari & Pagni 1969; Schott et al 1986; Berić et al 1988; Moulin et al 1988; Leijon et al 1989; Tasker 1990). However, it was recently reported that burning pain is rare in patients with cortical/subcortical lesions (Michel et al 1990). As mentioned above, dysaesthetic pain has been reported to be common in some conditions, for instance, in MS and incomplete SCI, and after cordotomy, which also is a form of incomplete SCI. However, the term has not been well defined and evidently it has often been used to indicate a combination of dysaesthesias and spontaneous pain of differing qualities. This is indicated in a recent article by Davidoff & Roth (1991) in which 19 SCI patients with 'dysesthetic pain syndrome' were reported. They experienced the following pain qualities: cutting (63%), burning (58%), piercing (47%), radiating (47%), tight (37%). The descriptions 'cruel' and 'nagging' were each used by 37%. Since dysaesthesias are common in most central pain conditions, this results in high figures for 'dysaesthetic' pain. It would seem logical to reserve this term for painful dysaesthesias which occur spontaneously or which are evoked by cutaneous stimuli, and also to specify any other forms of pain that the patient experiences.

Central pain caused by spinal cord processes commonly includes a pressing belt-like pain (= a girdle pain) at the level of the upper border of the lesion, in addition to other pains. This pain occurs in patients with MS and traumatic SCI and is similar to pain caused by lesions or inflammation affecting the spinal dorsal roots, which may present a diagnostic problem in SCI patients. For instance, an MS patient with a complete transverse lesion at T9 experienced a girdle pain with the character of tight armour at the level of the umbilicus, in addition to a constant burning pain in both legs and feet (Österberg, Boivie & Henriksson, unpublished observations).

Intensity of pain

From much of the early literature one gets the impression that central pain is always excruciating. This is incorrect, because the intensity of central pain ranges from low to extremely high. However, even if the pain is of low or moderate intensity the patients assess the pain as severe because it causes much suffering due to its irritating character and constant presence. Thus, a patient may indicate a pain intensity of 28 on a visual analogue scale (VAS; 0–100) and yet explain that the pain is a great burden, making life very miserable. Interviews with patients show that many patients with central pain and severe motor handicap following strokes, MS or SCI, often rate the pain as their worst handicap (Britell & Mariano 1991; Leijon, Boivie & Österberg, unpublished observations). SCI patients with minor motor handicap have stated that they would prefer to trade their pain for a severe paresis if it were possible (Nepomuceno et al 1979). The results of such surveys differ, though, as shown by Davidoff et al (1987b), who reported that many SCI patients did not consider their pain to be a great problem.

Table 46.5 Pain intensity in patients with central poststroke pain; assessment with VAS 0–100[1]

Lesion site	N	Mean	Range
Brainstem	8	61	39–94
Thalamus	9	79	68–98
Extrathalamic	6	50	30–91

[1]From Leijon et al (1989).

In a study of patients with central poststroke pain with different lesion sites, it was found that the pain intensity was highest in the groups with lesions in the thalamus and low brainstem lesions, with mean VAS values of 79 and 61, respectively, compared to patients with suprathalamic lesions, who scored 50 (Table 46.5; Leijon et al 1989). The ranges were large, and the number of patients in each group was small, so no definite conclusions can be drawn from these data, but a picture emerges that the pain intensity is higher with some lesion sites than with others. Thalamic lesions probably tend to cause more intense pain than nonthalamic lesions, since all patients with such lesions scored high.

Central pain may have a constant intensity or the intensity may vary. These variations seem to occur spontaneously or under the influence of external somatic or psychological stimuli or they may be due to internal events. In patients with more than one central pain quality, the variation in intensity may differ between pain forms.

Onset and other temporal aspects

Central pain may start almost immediately after occurrence of the lesion or it may be delayed for up to several years. Delays are well known in poststroke central pain. This delay may be as long as 2–3 years, but in most patients the pain starts within a couple of weeks of the stroke (Mauguière & Desmedt 1988; Michel et al 1990; Boivie & Leijon 1991; Fig. 46.1). In some patients the pain starts immediately after the stroke. When the onset is delayed it frequently coincides with changes in the subjective sensory abnormalities. For example, a patient with dense sensory loss may start to experience paraesthesias or dysaesthesias and soon afterwards the pain starts. With successively developing lesions, such as the lesions of patients with spinal vascular malformations, MS and syringomyelia, it is difficult to know the temporal relationship between the lesion and onset of pain. In such diseases the pain can be the first symptom, or it may start later at any stage of the disease. In MS the prevalence of central pain is higher after the fifth year than earlier in the disease (Moulin et al 1988). The situation is complex in SCI because these patients frequently have multiple injuries with a mixture of different kinds of pain during the initial

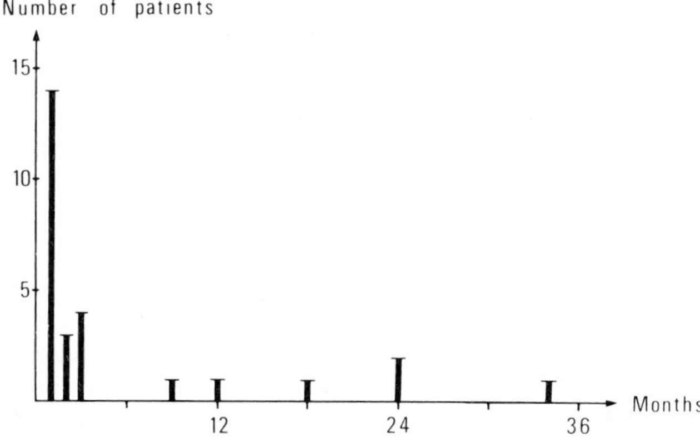

Fig. 46.1 Interval between onset of stroke and onset of central poststroke pain in 27 patients. (From Boivie & Leijon 1991.)

period following injury, which makes it more difficult to distinguish central pain in the early stages.

Most spontaneous central pain is constantly present, with no pain-free intervals. In central poststroke pain 23 of 27 patients reported constant pain, whereas the other four patients had some pain-free intervals lasting, at most, a few hours each day (Leijon et al 1989). In addition to the spontaneous pain, many patients experience intermittent pain evoked by external and internal stimuli. Intermittent pain is well known in MS as part of tonic painful seizures and as trigeminal neuralgia. MS patients may also develop intermittent aching pain during physical activity, for instance during walking. This pain often seems to be central, but it is also conceivable that it can be nociceptive.

Unfortunately, central pain is commonly permanent, but it may remit completely. This occurs spontaneously or as a result of new lesions or other changes in the underlying disease. A small fraction of CPSPs successively cease completely, but most CPSP continues throughout life, (Leijon & Boivie, unpublished observations). A few cases have been reported in which a new supratentorial stroke abolished the pain (Soria & Fine 1991). In SCI the central pain can be temporary, lasting a few months only, but more commonly it is permanent (Berić et al 1988; Britell & Mariano 1991), which is similar to central pain in MS. A few patients with syringomyelia have described temporary pain with features characteristic of central pain during the early phase of the disease, but no central pain later (Boivie & Rollsjö, unpublished observations).

Stimuli affecting central pain

Many internal and external events influence central pain, such as cutaneous stimuli, body movements, visceral stimuli, emotions and changes in mood. Allodynia, i.e. pain evoked by a stimulus that is normally not painful, e.g. touch, light pressure or moderate heat or cold, is common in patients with central pain (Riddoch 1938; Berić et al 1988; Boivie 1992; Boivie et al 1989; Pagni 1989; Tasker 1990; Hansson & Lindblom 1992). Such stimuli often give prolonged after-effects, and they may increase ongoing pain. Patients with central pain frequently experience an increase in pain associated with body movement, such as changes in body posture, nonstrenuous walking or movement of the extremities (Leijon et al 1989; Österberg, Boivie & Henriksson, unpublished observations). Visceral stimuli, particularly from a full bladder or rectum, have long been thought to influence central pain (Riddoch 1938). Several case reports in the early literature and current experience from SCI patients support this notion.

It is also common that patients with central pain experience an immediate increase in pain after sudden fear, joy, loud noise or bright light (Riddoch, 1938; Leijon et al 1989; Tasker, 1990). Experience from clinical practice indicates that central pain is as affected by psychological factors as other pain conditions, i.e. anxiety and depression aggravate central pain. This has not been well documented, however, although studies from SCI patients point in this direction (Britell & Mariano 1991). On the other hand, there is no reason to believe that psychological factors per se are important in the development of central pain, which is clearly somatic organic pain caused by lesions in the CNS. This concept is supported by studies of 22 CPSP patients, none of whom had major depression or other psychiatric disease (Leijon and Boivie, unpublished observations).

NEUROLOGICAL SYMPTOMS AND SIGNS

Since central pain is a neurological symptom emanating from processes in the CNS it is of interest to know whether central pain is accompanied by any other particular neurological symptoms and signs, which should then be included in the criteria for the diagnosis. All investigators agree that central pain is caused by perturbations of the somatosensory systems, usually a lesion. It is thus a somatosensory symptom and it is therefore natural that abnormalities in somatic sensibility are the only symptoms and signs besides pain that are present in all patients with central pain. Several studies have shown that central pain is independent of abnormalities in muscle function, coordination, vision, hearing, vestibular functions and higher cortical functions (Riddoch 1938; Berić et al 1988; Leijon et al 1989; Pagni 1989; Tasker 1990). In a study on CPSP all 27 patients had sensory abnormalities, whereas only 48% had paresis and 58% ataxia (Leijon et al 1989). Other neurological symptoms were present in a few patients.

This statement is not contradicted by the fact that symptoms of the aforementioned kind are common in patients with central pain, because these nonsensory symptoms are a natural consequence of the lesion, which is seldom restricted to somatosensory structures. The important point is that the nonsensory symptoms are not necessary for the development of central pain. This is supported by the fact that many patients with central pain lack nonsensory symptoms. This has been shown in CPSP (Riddoch 1938; Leijon et al 1989) and MS (Österberg, Boivie & Henriksson, unpublished observations) and syringomyelia (Boivie & Rollsjö, unpublished observations).

SOMATOSENSORY ABNORMALITIES

Abnormalities in somatic sensibility are important in patients with central pain, both as criteria for diagnosis and as symptoms contributing to the patient's handicap. All central pain is probably accompanied by such symptoms and signs, although they may be subtle and may elude detection with clinical test methods which only provide a rough qualitative estimate. To be able to demonstrate small changes in sensibility one needs to use quantitative sensory tests (QST). Devices for such tests are now available for clinical use. They include calibrated vibrameters, sets of von Frey filaments for the analysis of touch, devices for quantitative testing of temperature and temperature pain sensibility with Peltier element stimulators and devices for measuring mechanical pain (Lindblom & Ochoa 1986; Boivie et al 1989). To date few systematic studies have been done with QST to analyse the sensory abnormalities in central pain conditions. Much is uncertain regarding these abnormalities. It is postulated that central pain is always accompanied by sensory abnormalities, but we have examined a few patients in whom the clinical criteria have strongly indicated central pain and yet not even quantitative sensibility tests have shown abnormal sensibility (Boivie & Leijon, unpublished observations).

There is a large variation in the spectrum of sensory abnormalities among patients with central pain. It ranges from a slightly raised threshold for one of the submodalities, to complete loss of all somatic sensibility in the painful region. Hyperaesthesia often occurs as well as abnormal sensations. The most important sensory abnormalities are listed in Table 46.6. They include changes in detection thresholds and in stimulus–response function, spontaneous or evoked abnormal sensations, radiation of sensations from the stimulus site, prolonged response latency and spatial and temporal summation. They represent both quantitative and qualitative abnormalities. The occurrence of these abnormalities in patients with central pain will be briefly summarized.

Table 46.6 Somatosensory abnormalities

Threshold (detection) hypo-, hyper-	Numbness
Intensity functions hypo-, hyper-	Allodynia
Abnormal sensations paraesthesias dysaesthesias	Radiation of sensation Prolonged response latency Prolonged aftersensations Spatial and temporal summation Hyperpathia

Hypoaesthesia

This term is usually used to denote a raised threshold, but can also mean that the sensation evoked by a stimulus is weaker than normal. Raised thresholds or total loss of sensibility is common in central pain. It can affect some or all submodalities. In a study in CPSP it was found that all patients had hypoaesthesia to temperature, whereas only about half of the patients had hypoaesthesia to touch, vibration and kinaesthesia (Boivie et al 1989). Similar results, but less pronounced, were found in another CPSP study (Leijon & Bowsher 1990). Hypoaesthesia to noxious thermal and mechanical stimuli (heat, cold, pinprick or pinching), i.e. hypoalgesia, was also found. In other studies using QST, similar observations were made in patients with MS (Österberg et al 1993) and SCI with central pain (Berić et al 1988), and in syringomyelia (Boivie & Rollsjö, unpublished observations). This is the basis for the hypothesis that central pain occurs only in patients who have dysfunctions in the spinothalamic systems, i.e. in the pathways that are most important for temperature and pain sensibility (Boivie et al 1989; Boivie & Leijon 1991).

Hyperaesthesia

This denotes increased sensation to a stimulus, i.e. a steeper than normal stimulus–response curve. If this hypersensitivity occurs to noxious stimuli it is termed *hyperalgesia*. *Allodynia* is the name for pain evoked by stimuli that under normal conditions do not evoke pain, e.g. touch, vibration, moderate joint movements or moderate heat or cold. It often occurs as touch-evoked painful dysaesthesia. Hyperaesthesia to touch, moderate cold and heat, allodynia to touch and cold, and hyperalgesia to cold, heat or pin-prick are common in many central pain conditions (Riddoch 1938; Garcin 1968; Boivie et al 1989; Pagni 1989; Tasker 1990; Hansson & Lindblom 1992). Combinations of hypoaesthesia and allodynia to touch or cold are not uncommon. For instance, some CPSP patients with severely decreased touch sensibility, even with total loss, have allodynia to touch (Boivie et al 1989). Head and Holmes, as early as 1911, claimed that over-reaction to somatic stimuli was the most typical sign of central pain.

Paraesthesias and dysaesthesias

These are common in central pain (Riddoch 1938; Garcin 1968; Pagni 1989; Tasker 1990). In a study of CPSP,

85% and 41%, respectively, of the patients reported spontaneous and evoked dysaesthesia, whereas 41% experienced paraesthesia (Boivie et al 1989). Dysaesthesia is often evoked by touch and cold and is sometimes painful. It is possible that painless dysaesthesia together with nondysaesthetic central pain may result in the pain being classified as dysaesthetic (see section on quality of pain). This could partly explain the claim expressed in some articles that dysaesthetic pain dominates in central pain, since dysaesthesia is one of the most frequent symptoms in central pain patients. This kind of pain has been reported to be common in MS (Moulin et al 1988) and after incomplete SCI (Berić et al 1988; Davidoff et al 1987b).

Numbness

Many central pain patients experience numbness, but it is not clear what underlies the perception of numbness. Is it primarily related to loss of tactile sensibility? Undoubtedly total sensory loss leads to numbness, but evidently it can also occur with normal threshold to touch, as shown in CPSP (Boivie et al 1989). Patients will sometimes use the term numbness when they experience paraesthesias or dysaesthesias.

Radiation, prolonged response latency, after-sensations, summation

These features are indicative of neurogenic pain and seem to be more common in central pain than in peripheral neurogenic pain. The term 'radiation' means that the sensation spreads outside the site of stimulation, such as when touch with cotton wool or pin-prick on the dorsum of the foot evokes a sensation in both the leg and foot. Radiation was demonstrated in 12 of 24 patients with CPSP (Boivie et al 1989), and is also found in other central pain conditions (Riddoch 1938; Garcin 1968; Tasker et al 1991).

Prolonged latency between the stimulus and perception of the sensation can in some patients be demonstrated with tactile and pin-prick stimulation. This appears to occur only when there is a hyperaesthetic/hyperalgesic response, which includes spatial and temporal summation. It is then that the delay in sensation is mostly prolonged and it may also be of an explosive, hyperpathic kind. Hyperalgesia is found in many, but not all central pain patients.

Neurophysiological examinations

The central somatosensory pathways can be examined with neurophysiological techniques, which offer objective information regarding the function of the pathways. The most commonly employed method is to study somatosensory evoked potentials (SEP) evoked by electrical stimulations of the median and tibial/sural nerves. This method tests the function of the dorsal column–medial lemniscal pathways, because the stimulation activates large primary afferent fibres innervating low threshold mechanoreceptors. Studies have shown that abnormalities in SEP evoked with this technique correlate well with abnormalities in the sensibility to touch and vibration (Schott et al 1986; Mauguière & Desmedt 1988; Holmgren et al 1990).

As the sensory disturbances in central pain indicate that the lesions affect the spinothalamic pathways, it is of interest to study SEP evoked by peripheral stimulation of afferents that activate the spinothalamic pathways. This can be done by using lasers to stimulate cutaneous heat receptors (Bromm & Treede 1987; Pertovaara et al 1988; Treede et al 1988). A study with this technique on patients with central poststroke pain showed that abnormalities in the laser evoked cortical potentials, which have a long latency, correlate well with abnormalities in the sensibility to temperature and pain, but not to touch and vibration (Casey et al 1990).

Willer and collaborators have extensively studied the flexion reflex in patients with central pain and found that the latency of this reflex is prolonged in these patients. This reflex, the R III reflex, is dependent on activation of nociceptor afferents. Lesions in the CNS leading to decreased pain sensibility have been found to result in a delay of this reflex following electrical stimulation of the sural nerve (Dehen et al 1983).

PSYCHOLOGICAL FACTORS

Central pain patients have CNS disease that is mostly chronic and in many cases causes severe handicap. It is therefore natural that these diseases per se can lead to depression, for example poststroke depression, and depression in SCI patients. Since many investigations have shown that there is mutual correlation between pain and depression (see Ch. 47), one would expect to find a high incidence of depression in central pain patients. This has not been well studied and available data are incomplete and somewhat conflicting. In a group of SCI patients depression, anxiety, loneliness and several other psychosocial factors correlated significantly with the degree of pain, but this study also included nociceptive pain (Umlauf et al 1992), whereas a study of 24 CPSP patients could not identify any signs of depression (Leijon & Boivie, unpublished observations). Neither were these CPSP patients different from a control group with regard to social situation or major life events.

There has previously been a tendency among those not familiar with central pain to consider it as psychogenic pain. It is now absolutely clear that central pain is somatic organic pain and that it is not caused by psychological factors, but, like all other pains, the experience of central pain is influenced by such factors and central pain may of course also affect the afflicted both psychologically and socially.

TREATMENT

GENERAL ASPECTS

Treating central pain is no easy task because there is no universally effective treatment. This means that one often has to try various treatment modalities to get the best results (Table 46.7). Combination of treatments sometimes gives the best results. With each treatment it is important that the patient is well informed about possible adverse side-effects, and how these should be regarded and when they should contact the doctor responsible. Treatment usually reduces the pain, rather than giving complete relief, and patients should be aware of this, so that they have realistic expectations. In this context it is interesting to note that relatively small decreases in pain intensity are often highly valued by the patients, with the result that they want to continue treatment even if the clinican responsible is doubtful.

Most treatment regimes for central pain are empirical and based on clinical experience. Many treatments in the literature have been claimed to be effective, mostly based on experience with small groups of patients. Few treatments have been tested in well-designed clinical trials. There is thus a great need for such trials on homogeneous patient groups. Furthermore, since it is conceivable that treatment affects some aspects of central pain but not others, it would be desirable to assess the effect of treatment on each pain modality separately. The practical problems in performing such studies are obvious. One has therefore to compromise, which often results in a global assessment of the effect on the spontaneous pain, whereas the effect on the painful hyperaesthesia is not assessed.

Table 46.7 Treatment modalities for central pain, including methods with unproven effect

Pharmacological
Antidepressant drugs (AD)
Antiepileptic drugs (AED)
Antiarrhythmic drugs, local anaesthetics
Analgesics
Other drugs
adrenergic drugs
cholinergic drugs
naloxone
neuroleptic drugs
Sensory stimulation
Transcutaneous electrical stimulation (TENS)
Dorsal-column stimulation (DCS)
Deep-brain stimulation (DBS)
Neurosurgery
Cordotomy
Dorsal root entry zone (DREZ) lesions
Cordectomy
Mesencephalic tractotomy
Thalamotomy
Cortical and subcortical ablation
Sympathetic blockade

An important, but still largely unanswered question concerning treatment is whether or not the different central pain conditions respond differently to one particular treatment. This has not been systematically studied, but such differences appear to exist. From a study of the literature and from clinical experience one gets the impression that CPSP responds better to antidepressants than the central pain in SCI and MS. Conversely paroxysmal pain in MS seems to respond much better to antiepileptic drugs than do other kinds of central pain.

One of the similarities between central pain and peripheral neurogenic pain is treatment. In both pain categories antidepressants and antiepileptic drugs are the most frequently used drugs. These are also the ones with the best documented effects and virtually the only ones tested in well-conducted clinical trials. They are the first-line treatments, together with transcutaneous electrical nerve stimulation (TENS), which can only have a chance of giving relief, however, if the dorsal column–medial lemniscal pathways are not totally damaged. The other treatments listed in Table 46.6 are more of an experimental character, although some of them are used quite frequently by some pain specialists.

The ideal would be to use only treatments with well-documented effects and this is the goal for the future. This goal can only be reached through carefully planned and well-designed evaluation of the results of treatment. This can be included in everyday practice, by choosing methods that are manageable in clinical practice. Scientific studies require more rigid and elaborate regimes. Treatments may affect spontaneous and/or painful hyperaesthesia, or both. It is desirable that both effects are evaluated. It has also been strongly recommended that the effects are analysed separately with regard to pain intensity (sensory aspect) and unpleasantness (affective aspect) of the pain (Gracely 1991) (see Ch. 19). Further features to consider are the effects on anxiety, depression and other psychological factors. There is thus a risk for overload in evaluation and this should be taken into account when studies are planned.

ANTIDEPRESSANTS (AD)

Documentation of effects, clinical aspects

These are the firstline drugs for central pain (Table 46.8). Controlled trials have been done only on CPSP and the central pain in SCI, with conflicting results. The CPSP study was a crossover study on 15 patients (mean age 66 years) in which the effects of amitriptyline (25 plus 50 mg), carbamazepine (400 mg b.i.d.) and placebo, given

Table 46.8 Antidepressant drugs used in central pain

Relatively unselective with regard to 5-HT and NA
Amitriptyline
Doxepin
Nortriptyline
Some selectivity for 5-HT
Clomipramine
Imipramine
High selectivity for 5-HT
Fluvoxamine
Paroxetine
Trazodone
Zimelidine
Some selectivity for NA
Desipramine
Maprotiline
Mianserin

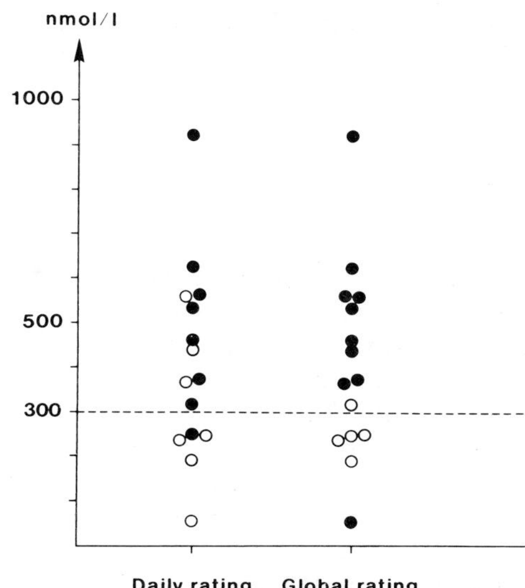

Fig. 46.3 The relationship between plasma concentration of amitriptyline and nortriptyline and the response in 15 patients with central poststroke pain. ● = responder (median 497); ○ = nonresponder (median 247). (From Leijon & Boivie 1989c.)

in randomized order, were assessed during three treatment periods, each 4 weeks long (Fig. 46.2; Leijon & Boivie 1989c). Assessment was done by daily ratings of pain intensity with a 10-step verbal scale (morning and evening), posttreatment global ratings of pain relief and depression scores (comprehensive psychopathological rating scale = CPRS) on days 0 and 28. The cut-off for responders was 20% pain reduction, as compared to the placebo period. Of the 15 patients, 10 were responders to amitriptyline with both assessment modes and there was a statistically significant reduction in pain as compared to placebo. No difference was noted between patients with thalamic (five patients) and nonthalamic lesions, but the groups were small. The order in which the drugs were given did not affect the outcome. There appeared to be a correlation between pain relief and the plasma concentrations of amitriptyline and its active metabolite nortriptyline (Fig. 46.3), the responders having a mean concentration of 497 nmol/l, whereas the corresponding value was 247 nmol/l, for the nonresponders. The results also indicated that the pain-relieving effect could not depend on an improvement of depression, because none of the patients were depressed according to assessment and their depression scores did not decrease during treatment.

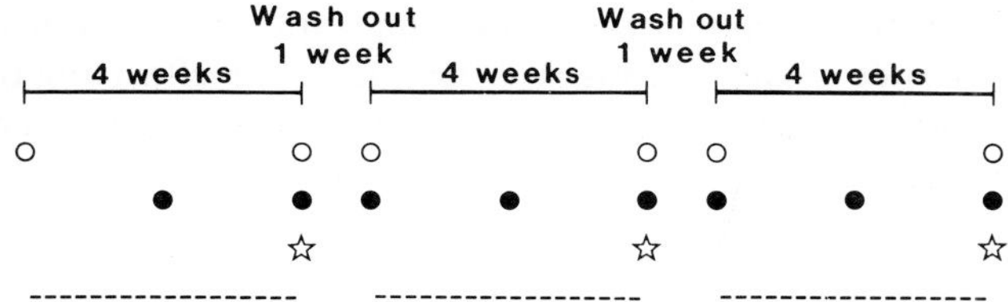

Fig. 46.2 Design of a study of the treatment with amitriptyline, carbamazepine and placebo in patients with central poststroke pain (CPSP). CPRS = comprehensive psychopathological rating scale. (From Leijon & Boivie 1989c.)

These results contrast with those from a controlled study of the effect of trazodone (a tricyclic AD with specific action on serotonin reuptake) on central pain in 18 patients with SCI (Davidoff et al 1987a). No significant effects were found, compared to placebo. The trial was done with parallel groups, so that only nine patients tried each treatment, but there was not even a tendency towards an effect of the active drug.

One possible explanation for the differences in effect on the two pain conditions is a difference in pharmacodynamics, i.e. specific serotonin reuptake inhibitors may be less effective than drugs also acting on the noradrenergic systems (see below). Another possible explanation is differences in susceptibility to treatment with AD in the two central pain conditions. The idea that central pain conditions may respond differently to AD therapy is supported by clinical experience from the use of AD in an open way. However, such conclusions may be affected by strong bias. It is our impression that CPSP may be more amenable to relief by AD than the central pain in MS and SCI (Boivie & Leijon, unpublished observations). The favourable responsiveness in CPSP has also been found by Bowsher et al (unpublished observations) in a retrospective review of 31 CPSP patients and by Tourian (1987) in 10 patients treated with a combination of doxepin and propranolol. About 50% of these patients had long-lasting pain relief with AD.

Mechanisms of action, adverse side-effects

The mechanisms underlying the pain-relieving effect of AD are unclear. For a long time it has been believed that they depend on inhibition of the reuptake of serotonin, but this idea has been contested over recent years. Instead it has been argued that they depend on their effects on the noradrenergic systems (Lenz 1992). This conclusion is based on observations that AD having major effects on noradrenaline function and minor or no effects on serotonin (e.g. desipramine, maprotiline, mianserin) appear to be more effective in relieving neurogenic pain that the specific serotonin uptake inhibitors (= SSRIs, including, amongst others, fluvoxamine, paroxetine, trazodone, zimelidine). However, this issue has not been finally clarified yet, because results have been obtained indicating an effect of SSRIs on peripheral neurogenic pain (Sindrup et al 1990). No controlled studies have been done using these drugs on central pain.

Amitriptyline and doxepin have effects on both noradrenergic and serotoninergic systems, in addition to rather strong anticholinergic, and even some dopaminergic effects. It is possible that it is an advantage to use drugs with mixed effects, since several of the transmitter systems that they affect are involved in pain and pain inhibition. However, there are undoubtedly problems in managing treatment with the first-generation tricyclics because of their side effects, mainly the anticholinergic ones. Thorough pretreatment information, slow dose increases, the whole dose at bedtime and close monitoring with frequent contacts are important steps to minimize the problems of treatment. In this way most patients can tolerate the drugs and test the effect. The new ADs also have adverse effects that prevent their use in some patients, which is not surprising considering that they are very potent drugs. It is too early to recommend general use of the new ADs in the treatment of central pain, because there are still uncertainties regarding their effects in clinical use.

Several studies on AD and neurogenic pain have shown that their pain-relieving effect is independent of their effect on depression (see Ch. 50). In addition to relieving the pain the ADs may thus decrease depression and may also allow the patient to sleep better. The temporal relationship between the onset and full development of the analgesic and antidepressive effects is unclear, as with many other questions regarding the place of the AD in the treatment of central pain. One such aspect is the dose–response relationship.

Dose–response relationships

In the CPSP study of amitriptyline the results indicated a correlation between the plasma concentration and the degree of pain relief (Leijon & Boivie 1989c; 1991) and some other studies have yielded similar results (Watson et al 1982; Max et al 1988; Sindrup et al 1990) but results to the contrary have also been obtained. Usually doses of 50–100 mg/day are used, but it has also been claimed that small doses of the order of 10–20 mg of tricyclics are sufficient for some patients. No controlled studies have provided support for this. In one of the studies on postherpetic neuralgia the results indicated that there might be a therapeutic window for the tricyclics (Watson et al 1982), but the study on CPSP was not in accordance with that idea, since good responses were found only in some patients with high plasma concentrations.

The large inter-individual differences in plasma concentration between patients on the same dose are probably due to a large extent to genetically determined differences in the rate of drug metabolism (Gram 1990). A fixed dose regime will thus lead to underdosage in some patients and toxic levels in others. This is well illustrated by investigations on imipramine showing that to obtain similar plasma concentrations the dose may vary between 25 and 350 mg/day. It is therefore recommended that the dose be titrated individually. If insufficient effect is obtained with doses of 50–100 mg/day one should either check the plasma concentration or try a higher dose, provided that side-effects do not prevent dose increase.

ANTIEPILEPTIC DRUGS (AED)

Documentation of effects, clinical aspects

These drugs are widely used for central and peripheral neurogenic pain. However, an effect has not been demonstrated in well-designed clinical trials, except in idiopathic tic douloureux (Tomson 1980). In the only two controlled studies on the effect of an AED (carbamazepine) on central pain, an effect significantly better than placebo could not be demonstrated in one (Leijon & Boivie 1989) and in the other only three MS patients were studied, all of whom obtained good pain relief (Espir & Millac 1970). Their use in central pain is thus largely based on tradition, rather than on results from systematic research. This does not mean that they have no effect on central pain. Clinical experience speaks strongly in favour of an effect on tic douloureux and painful tonic seizures in MS (Osterman & Westerberg 1975). Based on experience, it has been suggested that AEDs can only be expected to relieve paroxysmal central pain. Although this may be the most suitable condition to treat with AEDs, it is thus conceivable that other kinds of central pain may also respond. This conclusion is supported by the results from the CPSP study mentioned above, in which the responders did not have paroxysmal pain (Leijon & Boivie 1989c). It is recommended that an AED be included in the list of treatments for central pain.

In the study on the effect of carbamazepine on CPSP, 800 mg/day for 4 weeks was compared with amitriptyline and placebo in 14 patients (Leijon & Boivie 1989c). Five patients responded, but the effect did not reach statistical significance. In the other study, all three MS patients with pain responded to carbamazepine (Espir & Millac 1970). From two open label studies on paroxysmal central pain it was reported that all six MS patients and all seven patients with tabetic lightning pain had excellent results with carbamazepine (Ekbom 1966; Shibasaki & Kuroiwa 1974). A few cases have also been reported in which phenytoin was found beneficial in CPSP and MS (Leijon & Boivie 1991). Clonazepam was likewise reported to be better than other AEDs in 7/9 central pain patients (Swerdlow 1986).

Mechanism of action

The commonly used AEDs are listed in Table 46.9. Carbamazepine is probably the most widely used drug, but in recent years clonazepam has gained popularity (Swerdlow 1986). The rationale underlying the use of AEDs for central pain is their ability to suppress discharge in pathologically altered neurons, an effect that is also the basis for their use in epilepsy. Carbamazepine and phenytoin probably exert their effect by inactivation of sodium channels (McLean & Macdonald 1986). Clonazepam, like other benzodiazepines, binds to a receptor associated with the GABA–chloride iontophoric complex, thus facilitating GABA-mediated inhibition, which is also thought to be the mechanism for sodium valproate (Budd 1989).

Dose–response relationships, adverse side-effects

In trigeminal neuralgia it is clear that the pain-relieving effect of carbamazepine is strongly correlated with the plasma concentration, as in epilepsy (Tomson 1980). It is not known whether or not this is also the case with AEDs in central pain. No such correlation was found in the study on CPSP (Leijon & Boivie 1989c).

Like the antidepressants, the AEDs have a tendency to cause troublesome side-effects and must therefore be managed with caution. It is possible that some groups of central pain patients are more amenable to the side-effects than other patients with neurological diseases, because many neurologists have the impression that carbamazepine, and possibly also other AEDs, causes more problems in MS patients than in patients with idiopathic trigeminal neuralgia or epilepsy. This could be explained by the fact that carbamazepine has effects on cerebellar centres for the coordination of movements which are frequently affected by the disease process in MS.

Table 46.9 Antiepileptic drugs used in central pain

Carbamazepine
Phenytoin
Barbiturates
Clonazepam
Sodium valproate
Vigabatrin

LOCAL ANAESTHETICS, ANTIARRHYTHMIC DRUGS

These substances have structural similarities and are thought to act on the same kind of pathophysiology as the antiepileptic drugs, i.e. to reduce pathological neuronal activity to a more normal level, mainly by acting on ion channels in the peripheral and central nervous systems (Wiesenfeld-Hallin & Lindblom 1985; Woolf & Wiesenfeld-Hallin 1985; Chabal et al 1989). In controlled clinical trials, intravenous lidocaine (= lignocaine) and oral mexiletine have been shown to have a pain-relieving effect in painful diabetic neuropathy (Dejgard et al 1988) and oral tocainide in trigeminal neuralgia (Lindström & Lindblom 1987). The duration of effect of an intravenous infusion of lidocaine is short, lasting 3–21 days in diabetics (Kastrup et al 1987). Tocainide was probably about as effective as carbamazepine in trigeminal neuralgia, but it had to be withdrawn from the market because of serious adverse effects.

No controlled clinical trials have been published on the use of these substances in central pain, but according to preliminary results from a placebo-controlled study of intravenous lidocaine in 10 CPSP patients, four of the patients responded with short-term relief, two on placebo and two on lidocaine (Coe et al, unpublished observations). A few patients with central pain have responded well in open-label treatment studies using lidocaine (Boas et al 1982; Edwards et al 1985). Similar experiences were made with oral mexiletine in seven CPSP patients, of whom five responded well (Awerbuch 1990). Controlled clinical trials are evidently needed to establish the role of these substances in the treatment of central pain.

ANALGESICS

The question as to whether or not neurogenic pain responds to analgesics is controversial. Some claim that their material indicates that neuropathic pain in general responds poorly or not at all. Others report experience to the contrary. Apparently most clinicians agree that neurogenic pain in general responds less well to analgesics than does most nociceptive pain and that many patients do not respond at all to opioids. Portenoy, Foley and collaborators reason that neurogenic pain may respond to some but not to all opioids, in other words, that differences in pharmacological properties may be important, and that it is partly a matter of dosage (Portenoy & Foley 1986; Portenoy et al 1990). There may also be differences between different neurogenic pains in this respect, presumably because of differences in the pathophysiology involved. The positive effects of morphine on postherpetic neuralgia shown recently in a well-designed trial might be an illustration of this (Rowbotham et al 1991).

Most of the patients referred to specialists because of central pain have tried analgesics, often in relatively high doses, without experiencing relief, but a few have obtained some pain reduction, mostly with weak opioids such as codeine and dextropropoxyphene. The results from acute, single-blind tests of opioids on central pain also provide strong evidence for a low sensitivity to opioids (Arnér & Meyerson 1991; Kupers et al 1991; Kalman et al 1993). We tried doses of the order of 30–50 mg morphine over 2 hours, i.e. close to doses causing the patient to sleep or develop confusion and found no analgesic effects on CPSP and central pain in MS. It is also common that patients with central pain who undergo operations and receive opioids postoperatively report that they have a good effect on the pain related to the operation, but no effect on the central pain. Portenoy et al however have reported good effects of long-term treatment with moderate doses of opioids in central pain (Portenoy & Foley 1986; Portenoy et al 1990).

A reasonable conclusion from the evidence available seems to be that a few central-pain patients may benefit from analgesics and that it is important to evaluate these effects carefully in each individual before prescribing them for long-term use. If the patient reports that the opioid clearly reduces the pain, and thereby the suffering significantly, then he should not be denied this relief.

ADRENERGIC AND CHOLINERGIC DRUGS; NALOXONE

Adrenergic synapses play a role in the mechanisms of pain (see Chs 9 and 12). It has therefore been postulated that adrenergic drugs may contribute to pain relief (Scadding et al 1982; Glynn et al 1986). For some years the interest has focused on the α_2-agonist clonidine, which has been shown to block the release of transmitters and peptides in primary afferent terminals by presynaptic action. In a double-blind study, patients with pain induced by arachnoiditis responded equally well to 150 μg clonidine as to morphine, both given epidurally (Glynn et al 1988), as well as in an open trial in patients with MS/SCI and painful spasms (Glynn et al 1986). Clonidine gave fewer side-effects and longer lasting relief. Agents acting on beta adrenergic receptors have also been tried in neurogenic pain.

The β_2-antagonist propranolol was found to relieve trigeminal neuralgia, phantom pain and diabetic neuropathy pain, but none of eight patients with post-traumatic neuralgia responded to 240 mg/day (Scadding et al 1982). Tourian (1987) reported that propranolol enhances the effectiveness of doxepin, a tricyclic antidepressant, in open-label treatment of CPSP.

Cholinergic systems are involved in pain and analgesia (Hartvig et al 1989). Acetylcholinesterase inhibitors and muscarinic receptor agonists increase pain thresholds after both systemic and spinal administration. In an open study, 2/5 patients reported long-term relief of CPSP during treatment with physostigmine and pyridostigmine (Schott & Loh 1984). One group has extensively tried the combination of distigmine and tricyclic antidepressants in an open-label trial and has found this to be beneficial in CPSP patients, but it is unclear whether this is obtained by suppression of the anticholinergic side-effects of the tricyclic or by more effective analgesia, or both (Hampf et al 1989). However, data from well-designed clinical trials are needed before this combination can be recommended for general use.

The μ-receptor opioid antagonist naloxone has been given to CPSP patients in high doses to alleviate pain, but the results are conflicting (Budd 1985; Bainton et al 1992). Budd, who introduced the therapy, claims that one injection of huge doses of about 20–50 mg gives good, long-lasting relief in many patients, whereas Bainton et al (1992) found in a controlled study that 10 mg did not differ from placebo. Budd reported that X-ray CT scans showed signs of increased blood flow in the thalamus on the injured side after naloxone injections, but the methods employed did not have sufficiently high sensitivity to show this.

NEUROLEPTIC DRUGS

There is a long clinical tradition for the use of phenothiazines and other neuroleptic drugs in pain treatment. They are believed to increase the effect of analgesics and to have analgesic properties of their own. In neurogenic pain they are particularly used for dysaesthesia and hyperaesthesia. However, such effects have not been shown in controlled studies on any pain condition, or in any form of convincing study. Their potentially severe and partially irreversible adverse effects and the lack of documented effects are strong enough reasons to caution against the use of these drugs in the treatment of central pain. This is particularly so as many of these patients have brain lesions which increases the risk for the occurrence of irreversible tardive dyskinaesia, which is the most serious side-effect of neuroleptics.

SENSORY STIMULATION

Transcutaneous nerve stimulation (TENS)

This form of treatment provides relief for some central pains and has the advantage of few and mild adverse effects, apart from possible effects on cardiac pacemakers (Sjölund 1991). It is applied in one of two modes: high-frequency stimulation (80–100 Hz, called conventional

TENS by Sjölund) aiming at activation of myelinated cutaneous sensory fibres, or low-frequency stimulation (short trains of impulses with 1–4 Hz repetition rate, called acupuncture-like TENS) aiming at activation of muscle efferents or muscle cells, thereby evoking muscle afferent inputs to the CNS. The mechanisms are believed to be mainly segmental, but suprasegmental mechanisms also exist (see Ch. 12). It is unclear how the effect of TENS in central pain is explained, but it appears that TENS can reduce central pain only if the dorsal column–medial lemniscal pathways are uninjured or only mildly injured. This hypothesis is based on a study of TENS in CPSP. Three of 15 CPSP patients obtained long-term relief (Leijon & Boivie 1989b). All three had normal or almost normal thresholds to touch and vibration, indicating good function in the lemniscal pathways. Two of the three suffered from brainstem infarction, but in the third the location of the lesion could not be identified. One of the Wallenberg patients had facial pain on one side and extremity pain on the other. He used high-frequency TENS for the facial pain, but this had no effect on the arm or leg. High- and low-frequency stimulation had approximately equal effect in the other two. Our continued use of TENS in CPSP follows these results, but a better yield had been reported in an earlier study (Eriksson et al 1979). In this study good results were also reported in SCI patients, with seven of 11 patients responding well to TENS. These patients probably had incomplete lesions because it would be surprising if one could obtain relief with stimulation that cannot affect the structures located rostral to the lesion, which would be the case with a complete SCI.

Spinal cord and deep-brain stimulation

From a review of the literature, and of his own patients, Tasker concluded that spinal cord stimulation is not effective enough in central pain to be recommended, a view shared by Gybels & Sweet, Nashold, and Pagni (Gybels & Sweet 1989; Pagni 1989; Tasker 1990; Tasker et al 1991), though he and others have had patients with successful results from spinal cord stimulation in central pain due to SCI. Instead, he favours deep-brain stimulation (DBS). Richardsson et al observed good results at 1-year follow-up in six of 19 paraplegics, and Siegfried reported good to excellent relief at 1- to 4-year follow-up in about 70% of 84 patients with 'deafferentation' pain caused by various central and peripheral lesions (Richardsson et al 1980; Siegfried 1983).

DBS is an exclusive mode of treatment that should be reserved for particularly severe and treatment-resistant pain conditions. The severe pain suffered by many central-pain patients fulfils these criteria. The periaqueductal and periventricular grey regions (PAG, PVG) are the primary targets for stimulation in the treatment of nociceptive pain, whereas stimulation for neurogenic pain is usually done along the lemniscal pathways in the ventroposterior thalamic region or the posterior limb of the internal capsule. Tasker reported successful results in 5/12 patients following thalamic stimulation, similar to the results of Siegfried & Demierre, whereas only 3/19 gained relief from stimulation of the PVG (Siegfried & Demierre 1984; Tasker et al 1991). Excellent results were recently reported following surface stimulation of the motor cortex in central pain (Tsubokawa et al 1990).

NEUROSURGICAL ABLATIVE PROCEDURES

Many different surgical lesions have been tried to find relief for central pain, but no particular lesion has been found that reliably results in successful outcome (Tasker 1990; Sjölund 1991; Tasker et al 1991). Lesions have been made at almost all levels of the neuraxis from the spinal cord to the cerebral cortex. Even lesions of peripheral nerves, mainly rhizotomy, have been tried. It is interesting to note that such lesions have not had an effect on steady ongoing pain, but in some cases there has been improvement of hyperaesthesia (Tasker 1990). According to Tasker et al (1991) ablative procedures in the spinal cord and the brain have also given better results with the intermittent and evoked components of central pain.

Three main kinds of spinal cord lesion have been performed for the treatment of central pain, namely, anterolateral cordotomy, dorsal root entry zone (DREZ) lesion and cordectomy. The underlying lesion has usually been a traumatic cord lesion. A fair proportion of patients with sacrococcygeal lesions have been found to obtain relief from cordotomy, but there has been a tendency for the pain to recur, as after cordotomy for nociceptive pain (Tasker 1990). The more rostral the lesion, the lesser the chance that cordotomy will do anything for the patient.

DREZ lesions have gained interest over recent years for the treatment of central SCI pain (Nashold & Bullitt 1981; Edgar et al 1993). The procedure aims at destroying the Lissauer tract and the superficial part of the dorsal horn. One would thus expect the DREZ lesion to affect pain emanating from the segment where the original lesion is located, i.e. in the transitional zone of partially injured cord tissue. So far results have not been consistent, but some centres have reported a success-rate of about 50% (Nashold & Bullitt 1981; Gybels & Sweet 1989; Tasker 1990; Sjölund 1991). Cordectomy is a more robust method to achieve a similar goal as the DREZ lesion, namely to interfere with the local pain-generating process. As with cordotomy, and probably also DREZ lesions, it appears that cordectomy rarely affects steady ongoing pain, but rather intermittent pain and hyperaesthesia, but has a low success rate (Gybels & Sweet 1989; Tasker 1990).

Among the many intracranial ablative procedures that have been tried for central pain can be mentioned mesencephalic tractotomy, medial and lateral thalamotomies, cingulotomy and cortical ablation. None of these have turned out to produce successful long-term outcomes. Some operations have resulted in postoperative pain relief in some patients, but the overall results have not been good because of unacceptably high complication rates or return to preoperative pain levels after some time. From a review of the literature, and of his own material, Tasker concluded that the only procedures that can be recommended in selected cases are stereotactic mesencephalic tractotomy and/or medial thalamotomy (Tasker 1990). Of his own nine patients with central pain caused by brain lesions in whom such operations were performed, only three had 'modest' relief of steady pain and another four had some effect on intermittent pain. Three had transient complications. It has been suggested that the pain-relieving effect of the mesencephalic lesion is obtained by interfering with the spinoreticulothalamic projections. Medial thalamotomy appears to affect the intralaminar–submedius region and the spinal and trigeminal projections to this.

SYMPATHETIC BLOCKADE

In the section on pathophysiology the idea that sympathetic dysfunction may be part of the mechanism underlying central pain was discussed. Oedema, decreased sweating, lowered skin temperature, change in skin colour and trophic skin changes occur in regions affected by central pain. Based on these observations, sympathetic blockade has been tried in the treatment of central pain. Loh et al (1981) gave a detailed report of the results of sympathetic blockade in three patients with CPSP, one with a traumatic brainstem lesion, two with MS, one with a spinal cord tumour, and one with traumatic SCI. The short-term effects were remarkable. All patients experienced at least 50% pain reduction in pain and disappearance or improvement of hyperaesthesia, but the effects usually lasted only 1–24 hours, apart from the patient with a traumatic brainstem lesion who experienced long-term relief. In some cases symptom reduction was noticed outside the region involved by the sympathetic block, for instance in the leg after a stellate ganglion block. These results are interesting and raise important questions that ought to be explored further. Firstly, these clinical effects need to be studied in larger patient groups because experience with sympathetic blockade in clinical practice has shown this procedure not to give consistent results. Secondly, what can be the explanation for the dramatic effects of a distal regional block in the arm on symptoms caused by a lesion in the brain? Could this indicate that there is a peripheral component affecting the central pain generator, or that the spinal grey matter also plays a role in the central pain caused by brain lesions and that altered peripheral input affects this mechanism? Furthermore, can similar effects be obtained by the blockade of somatic nerves?

INDIVIDUAL CENTRAL PAIN CONDITIONS

In this section some features of particular interest regarding individual central pain conditions will be summarized. Many of the features of individual central pain conditions have been discussed in the section on the general aspects of central pain. Much of this information will not be repeated in this section.

CENTRAL POSTSTROKE PAIN (CPSP)

The lesions

All kinds of cerebrovascular lesion (CVL) can cause central poststroke pain (CPSP). There appears to be no difference between haemorrhages and infarcts as regards the tendency to induce central pain (Leijon et al 1989; Boivie & Leijon 1991). The consequence of this is that there are many more patients with CPSP caused by infarct than haemorrhages since approximately 85% of all strokes are caused by infarct.

Different principles can be used to classify CVL. One principle is according to the artery involved, giving two major groups, namely, carotid and vertebrobasilar strokes. About 80% of all infarcts occur in the carotid territories. Infarcts in the territories of the thalamostriate and the posterior inferior cerebellar arteries (PICA) are particularly interesting because they engage the ventroposterior part of the thalamus and the lower brainstem, respectively. These infarcts are probably among the most frequent causes of central pain.

Haemorrhages can induce central pain only when they damage the brain parenchyma. It is thus unusual that subarachnoid haemorrhage causes central pain, but it occurs when severe vasospasm develops and leads to an infarct (Bowsher et al 1989).

As regards central pain caused by vascular malformation, this mainly concerns arteriovenous malformations (AVM) and the result is similar to CVL. They can cause central pain in two ways, namely, through rupture and haemorrhage, or if they increase in size and cause parenchymal damage. Patients with CPSP due to both these forms of lesion have been reported. The lesions were located cortically and subcortically in the parietal region and in the thalamus (Silver 1957; Waltz & Ehni 1966).

The location of the CVL, and not its size, is crucial as regards the probability that it will produce central pain (see section on pathophysiology). The following major locations have been shown to be associated with central pain: lateral medulla oblongata (PICA), thalamus, posterior limb of the internal capsule, subcortical and cortical zones in the postcentral gyrus (i.e. in the regions of the first somatosensory area, SI), and the insular regions (second somatosensory area, SII). A crude picture of the relative prevalence of CPSP according to the different lesion locations was obtained in a study of 27 patients of whom eight had low brainstem lesions, nine thalamic lesions, and six supratentorial, extrathalamic lesions (Leijon et al 1989). Only two of the thalamic lesions were restricted to the thalamus, the other seven extended laterally and superior to the thalamus. The location could not be determined in the four remaining patients.

Current available information is not sufficient to enable definite conclusions concerning the incidence of central pain following stroke in general to be made, or as regards the various locations of the CVL. A rough estimate would be that around 1–2 % of all stroke patients develop central pain (Boivie, Leijon & Bowsher, unpublished results; estimation not based on epidemiological studies). It appears that CVL in the lower brainstem and thalamus more often results in central pain than CVL in other locations, since these are not the most frequent locations of CVL and yet these locations are common in CPSP studies (Riddoch 1938; Garcin 1968; Leijon et al 1989). In the study by Leijon et al (1989) 33% of the patients with CPSP had CVL involving the thalamus. This conclusion was based on X-ray CT scans. A later study using MRI indicated that about 50% of all CPSP patients have lesions engaging the thalamus (Lewis-Jones et al 1990) but that study included few patients with low brainstem lesions. It thus appears probable that, at the most, 50% of all CPSP patients have lesions that involve the thalamus.

CPSP associated with thalamic lesions has attracted much attention over the years, probably because Dejerine & Roussy's early description of cases of thalamic pain provided the archetypal characteristics of central pain (Dejerine & Roussy 1906). (The reader is referred to the section on pathophysiology for a discussion of the role of thalamic lesions in central pain.) In brief, recent and old data indicate that lesions in the ventroposterior thalamic region relatively often cause central pain. In one study, three of 18 patients with such lesions developed central pain (Bogousslavsky et al 1988). It has also been shown that a small, but strategically located thalamic lesion may result in central pain.

Pain characteristics

The major problem in the diagnosis of CPSP is to distinguish central pain from nociceptive pains of various kinds, particularly hemiplegic shoulder pain, which is common in hemiplegic stroke patients. The development of shoulder pain can to a large extent be prevented by physiotherapy and information to everyone involved in the care of the patient.

The onset of CPSP is delayed in many patients. In one study, about half of the patients noticed the pain within a few days or during the first month, but in half of the patients the onset was delayed by more than 1 month (Fig. 46.1; Leijon et al 1989). The longest delay was 34 months.

CPSP is commonly experienced in a large part of the right or left side. This was the case in 20 of 27 patients in our study, but the face was involved in only six of them (Leijon et al 1989). However, some patients have pain in only a small region, such as the distal part of the arm and hand, or in the face. Two of the eight patients with brainstem infarcts had pain in the face on one side and in the rest of the body on the other side. In this study two-thirds of the patients had left-sided pain, which was in accord with the material of Schott et al (1986), but dominance of one side did not appear in a larger series (Bowsher & Leijon, unpublished observations).

Patients with CPSP report a large variety of pain qualities. Most patients experience two to four qualities. A burning sensation is the most frequent quality reported by about 60% of patients, with aching, pricking and lacerating sensations being next in frequency (Table 46.10). In a recent study of CPSP patients with superficial cortical lesions, burning pain was not common; instead, lacerating and cutting pain were more often experienced (Michel et al 1990). Bizarre pain qualities do occur, as mentioned in the first part of this chapter, but they are the exception rather than the rule.

Assessment of the intensity of CPSP reveals large individual variations (Table 46.11). In a global sense most patients consider the pain to be severe, though some of them rate the pain intensity rather low on scales such as the VAS, but a few patients have a mild form of CPSP. There are also patients in whom it is difficult to determine whether the sensation experienced should be classified as pain or not. This, for instance, is true for some dysaesthesias, because there is no sharp transition from nonpainful to painful dysaesthesias.

In many patients the pain is affected by internal and external stimuli. Such stimuli usually increase the pain

Table 46.10 Quality of central post-stroke pain (CPSP): proportion of patients (%)[1]

	BS ($n = 8$)	TH ($n = 9$)	SE ($n = 6$)	UI ($n = 4$)	All ($n = 27$)
Burning	75	22	83	75	59
Aching	38	22	33	25	30
Pricking	25	22	33	50	30
Lacerating	0	44	33	25	26
Shooting	13	22	0	0	11
Squeezing	13	22	0	0	11
Throbbing	0	22	17	0	11
Other	13	22	17	25	19

[1] From Leijon et al (1989).
BS = CVL in brainstem. TH = CVL involving thalamus. SE = supratentorial, extrathalamic CVL. UI = location of CVL not identified.

Table 46.11 Factors increasing central poststroke pain: proportion of patients (%)[1]

	BS ($n = 8$)	TH ($n = 9$)	SE ($n = 6$)	UI ($n = 4$)	All ($n = 27$)
Movements	38	89	83	75	70
Cold	63	33	33	75	48
Warmth	20	11	33	35	22
Touch	63	4	17	50	44
Emotions	25	33	0	0	19

[1] From Leijon et al (1989).
For explanation of BS, TH etc. please see footnote to Table 46.10.

(Leijon et al 1989). Table 46.11 provides some information on this. It can be seen that many patients report that body movement increases the pain. CPSP patients are also sensitive to cold (see also Michel 1990). In the cited study, relatively few patients had observed that strong emotions affected the pain, but this has been common in previous case reports.

Neurological symptoms and signs

Since pain is a somatosensory symptom it is not surprising that somatosensory symptoms and signs regularly accompany CPSP, whereas other symptoms may or may not be present in patients with CPSP (Table 46.12). Among 27 CPSP patients more than half had no paresis (Leijon et al 1989) and other nonsensory symptoms were much more uncommon. In a subgroup of nine patients with thalamic lesions only one had choreoathetosis, a symptom that others have found to be more common.

Some of the sensory abnormalities are subtle and are not noticed by the patients or revealed in the clinical sensory examination, but can be demonstrated by QST. However, we have had a few patients with CPSP, and other forms of central pain, in whom it has not been possible even with quantitative methods to show any sensory disturbances.

Some of the sensory abnormalities are of a quantitative nature; others are more qualitative (Table 46.6). The spectrum of quantitative and qualitative abnormalities is shown in Tables 46.13 and 46.14 for CPSP patients with different lesion locations (results from Boivie et al 1989).

Table 46.12 Neurological signs in 27 patients with central poststroke pain: proportion of patients (%)[1]

Sensory abnormality	100
Paresis (moderate/severe)	37/11
Ataxia	62
Choreoathetosis	4
Agnosia	17
Apraxia	17
Dysphasia (light)	7
Hemianopia	22

[1] From Leijon et al (1989).

Table 46.13 Sensory abnormalities in 27 patients with central poststroke pain as revealed with quantiative (Q) and clinical (CL) tests: proportion of patients (%)[1]

	BS ($n = 8$)	TH ($n = 9$)	SE ($n = 6$)	UI ($n = 4$)	All ($n = 27$)
Vibration (Q)					
Moderate	0	22	0	0	7
Severe	12	56	50	0	33
Touch (Q)					
Moderate	0	22	33	50	23
Severe	25	67	0	0	29
Innocuous temperature (Q)					
Moderate	25	11	17	25	19
Severe	75	89	83	75	81
Temperature pain (Q)					
Moderate	12	0	33	25	15
Severe	75	100	50	75	78
Touch (CL)					
Hypo-	50	33	50	75	48
Hyper-	38	56	33	0	37
Pinprick (CL)					
Hypo-	63	11	33	50	37
Hyper-	38	89	50	50	59
Kinaesthesia (CL)					
Hypo-	0	78	25	33	37

[1] From Boivie et al (1989).
For explanation of BS, TH etc. please see footnote to Table 46.10

Table 46.14 Quantitative sensory abnormalities in 27 patients with central poststroke pain: proportion of patients.[1]

	BS	TH	SE	UI	All
Numbness	3/8	5/9	6/8	4/4	18/22 (67%)
Paraesthesia	3/8	1/9	5/6	2/4	11/27 (41%)
Dysaesthesia	7/8	7/9	5/6	4/4	23/27 (85%)
Hyperaesthesia	7/7	8/9	3/5	4/4	22/25 (88%)
Allodynia	2/7	3/8	0/4	0/3	5/22 (23%)
Radiation	2/7	4/8	3/4	3/3	12/22 (55%)
Aftersensations	4/7	4/8	2/4	0/3	10/22 (45%)

[1] From Boivie et al (1989).
For explanation of BS, TH etc. please see footnote to Table 46.10.

The dominating features are abnormal temperature and pain sensibility, which were found in all of the patients examined, and hyperaesthesias and dysaesthesias, which were found in about 85% of the patients. The abnormalities in temperature sensibility were pronounced. Of the 81% who could not identify temperatures between zero and 50°C, about half had normal thresholds to touch and vibration. These results indicate that all CPSP patients have lesions affecting the spinothalamic pathways, which are those most important for the sensibility of temperature and pain, whereas only some of the patients have lesions that affect the dorsal column–medial lemniscal pathways. A similar, but less pronounced tendency has been found in a larger study (Leijon & Bowsher 1990). These results are the basis for the hypothesis that CPSP occurs only in patients who have lesions affecting the spinothalamic pathways (see above).

Treatment

The reader is referred to the general section on treatment of central pain for details. In this section only a few comments will be made. It is recommended that transcutaneous electrical stimulation (TENS) is tried as the primary treatment in patients who have not lost touch and vibration sensibility in the painful region because this relatively inexpensive treatment with almost no adverse side-effects will give some patients long-lasting relief.

Antidepressants have undoubtedly been most useful among the drugs. About 50–70% of CPSP patients have been found to benefit from these drugs. Next in order are antiepileptic drugs, which should not be restricted to patients with tic-like pain. Other drugs are not well documented, but may nevertheless be tried. The same is true for sympathetic blockade.

MULTIPLE SCLEROSIS (MS)

Epidemiology and pain characteristics

Multiple sclerosis is a severe chronic neurological disease that, in many patients, causes serious handicap and suffering. The disease process is of neuroinflammatory nature and results in destruction of myelin, and eventually of the axons and cell bodies, in the CNS. The characteristic lesion is the plaque, which is a zone of demyelination. Such plaques may occur anywhere in the CNS and in the optic nerves, but are most frequently found in the spinal cord, particularly in the dorsal columns, in the brainstem, and periventricularly in the forebrain. The two major clinical forms are the slowly progressive and relapsing forms. The cause of the inflammatory process is as yet unknown, but much is known about the various stages in the process in which different lymphatic T-cell populations play a crucial role.

In a fairly recent comprehensive review on MS it was stated that pain is uncommon in this disorder (Tourtellotte & Baumhefner 1983). This reflects the common view of MS, which is believed to be dominated by problems concerning mobility, incoordination of movements, balance control and vision, when in fact pain is a major problem for many MS patients. Ironically, trigeminal neuralgia, which is one of the most infrequent pain types associated with MS, has been the MS-related pain usually quoted.

As soon as investigations were made on the prevalence of pain in MS it became evident that the majority of MS patients experience pain. Four of five recent studies obtained prevalence figures indicating that 54–65% of all MS patients have clinically significant pain (Table 46.15). These results were based on interviews and examination of 614 patients. The figures include almost all forms of pain except headache. In one of the studies it was found that 45% had pain at the time of the investigation, and that 32% considered the pain to be one of their worst symptoms (Stenager et al 1991).

Not all MS pain is central. It is to be expected that MS patients with paresis, spasticity and incoordination of movements will develop nociceptive musculoskeletal pain. This is also the case. Vermote et al (1986) found that about 20% had such pain, including back pain, which is comparable to the 14% with back pain reported by Moulin et al (1988). It is also conceivable that peripheral neurogenic pain will be found in some MS patients. Primary psychogenic pain, i.e. pain as part of a major psychiatric disease, appears to be rare in MS. Vermote et al (1986) found only two such cases in their material of 83 patients.

It is important to analyse carefully the characteristics of the various pains experienced by MS patients to form a basis for the optimal management of the pain. According to the prevalence studies cited in Table 46.15 such an analysis will show that the majority of MS patients with pain have central pain caused by the disease itself. The figures for central pain in Table 46.15 are estimates made from the descriptions of the pain, and were not made by the authors themselves. They are thus somewhat uncertain and may be an overestimation. The figures include

Table 46.15 Results from prevalence studies of pain in multiple sclerosis

Study	Clifford & Trotter (1984)	Vermote et al (1986)	Moulin et al (1988)	Stenager et al (1991)	Österberg et al (1993)
Number of patients	317	83	159	117	255
Patients with pain (%)	29	54	55	65	58
Patients with central pain (%)	17	31	34	52	22
Trigeminal neuralgia (%)	1.6	4	4.4	1	5
Paroxysmal pain (%)	6	4	5	6	?
Pain quality/ number of patients( )	Burning (18) Toothache (15)	Burning (12) Pricking (10) Stabbing (9) Dull (5)	Burning (46)		Burning (21) Aching (20) Pricking (13) Stabbing (9) Squeezing (8)

Table 46.16 Prevalence of central pains in multiple sclerosis.[1]

	Number of patients	Percentage of all patients
Paroxysmal pain		
Trigeminal neuralgia	7	4.4
Painful Lhermitte sign	4	
Tic-like extremity pain	2	
Painful tonic seizures	2	
Chronic pain		
Dysaesthetic extremity pain	46	29
Painful leg spasms	21	13

[1] Figures obtained by Moulin et al (1988) in a study of 159 MS patients.

both paroxysmal/acute and chronic pain. Table 46.16 lists most types of pain classified as central pain and gives the prevalences found by Moulin et al (1988). These relative prevalences of the various forms of central pain are in accordance with most other studies.

Idiopathic trigeminal neuralgia is usually considered to be peripherally induced, but it appears likely that in MS this pain is caused by demyelination in the brainstem and it is therefore classified as central pain in this context. Its prevalence is probably higher than the previous estimate of about 2% of all MS patients. Recent studies indicate that its prevalence is about 4–5% (Moulin et al 1988; Österberg et al 1993).

In a retrospective study it was concluded that pain increases with age in MS (Clifford & Trotter 1984). A similar trend was found by Moulin et al (1988). No such trend was found regarding the age at onset of MS or disease duration, apart from the fact that pain was less common during the first 5 years of the disease, than later (Clifford & Trotter 1984; Moulin et al 1988; Stenager et al 1991). These relationships were not analysed specifically for central pain, however.

Pain characteristics and neurological symptoms

The characteristics of trigeminal neuralgia are described in Chapter 39. Its character is similar in MS and idiopathic tic douloureux.

The Lhermitte sign is classical of MS. It consists of rapidly spreading paraesthesias or dysaesthesias, sometimes like an electric current, down the back and radiating to the extremities. It is mostly bilateral and sometimes painful. It is usually evoked by bending the head forward and it has been proposed that it is produced when the cervical part of the inflamed dorsal columns are stretched.

Painful tonic seizures constitute another kind of paroxysmal pain in MS. A detailed description of these attacks is found in Shibasaki & Kuroiwa's report (1974). They found 11 such cases among 64 patients with MS, which is higher than in other studies. The attacks consist of spreading paraesthesias, pain and muscle spasm in the spinal segments involved. They are evoked by light touch or movement. No correlation was found between the pain and the degree of paresis or spasticity, but with sensory signs. The attacks usually occurred during exacerbation of spinal cord symptoms, i.e. during bouts of increased myelopathy. Painful paroxysms without muscle engagement also occur, but very infrequently (Osterman & Westerberg 1975).

The most common form of central pain in MS is nonparoxysmal extremity pain, usually termed dysaesthetic pain. The quality of this pain shows a large interindividual variation, and most patients experience more than one pain quality. In a group of 40 patients with this pain it was found that burning and aching pains were most frequent, occurring in about half, with pricking, stabbing and squeezing being next in frequency (Österberg et al 1993). In this group, 30 patients had pain in the lower extremity/ies, whereas only 10 had engagement of the arms. A few had trunk pain and one had hemipain. Multiple locations were common.

The combination of different pain locations and qualities can be illustrated by one of our patients. He is a 53-year-old clerk with central pain of 4 years' duration. The pain started about 2 months after he rapidly developed signs of a transverse myelitis at T9, with total loss of voluntary motor and bladder control, and total sensory loss below the waist. He now has steady pain of three distinctly different kinds. The first is a burning pain from the waist down. The second is a tight belt-like pain just above the waist; it feels like tight armour. The third pain is described as if he is sitting heavily on a tennis ball. It is interesting to know that the first symptom this patient noticed was hyperaesthesia to heat, i.e. an indication of dysfunction in the spinothalamic pathways.

Most investigators have found that MS patients with nonparoxysmal central pain have disturbed somatic sensibility. It has usually been found that the patients have sensory abnormalities indicating posterior column involvement, whereas not all patients have shown signs of dysfunction in the spinothalamic pathways (Moulin et al 1988). These results have been based on clinical examinations of sensibility. In a study of 29 patients using both clinical and quantitative sensory tests only one patient was found to have completely normal sensibility (Österberg et al 1993). The abnormalities found were dominated by abnormal temperature and pain sensibility, only two patients having normal pain and temperature sensibility, whereas more than one-third of the patients had normal threshold to touch. The vibration sense was also severely affected, but not to the same degree as temperature and pain. These results are in accordance with the results from patients with CPSP (see above).

As regards nonsensory symptoms and signs, it appears that, at the most, half of MS patients with nonparoxysmal central pain have paresis, ataxia or bladder dysfunction (Österberg et al 1993). Only four of 33 patients had severe paresis, and only one-third of them had ataxia. This conforms with the results of other studies failing to find any covariation between central pain and disability (Vermote et al 1986; Moulin et al 1988; Stenager et al 1991). This also seems to be true for central pain and depression in MS (Stenager et al 1991; Österberg et al 1993). Stenager et al (1991) found no differences between MS patients with and without pain with respect to depressive symptoms.

Treatment

Antiepileptic drugs (AEDs) are the treatment of choice for trigeminal neuralgia and other paroxysmal pains in MS (Shibasaki & Kuroiwa 1974). These treatments are generally very successful. Carbamazepine is the first-line drug, but most other AEDs have a good effect too (see section on these drugs in this chapter). The effects of treatment are dependent on the plasma concentration. It appears that many MS patients have difficulty in tolerating sufficiently high doses of AED, probably more so than other patient groups. One possible way around such problems is to try a combination of baclofen and an AED.

The AEDs generally have not been found effective against steady extremity pain (Clifford & Trotter 1984; Moulin et al 1988), but this has not been tested in controlled studies, which is true for all forms of treatment of central pain or other kinds of pain in MS. Antidepressants are recommended for nonparoxysmal central pain, but the outcome of such treatment is debated. Thus Clifford & Trotter (1984) reported excellent results, while Moulin et al (1988) had a poor outcome, with only nine of 46 patients responding well to amitriptyline and imipramine.

TENS can be tried in patients with at least some preservation of dorsal column function. Electrical stimulation of the spinal cord (DCS) has been tried quite extensively, but the outcome has been poor (Rosen & Barsoum 1979; Young & Goodman 1979; Tasker 1990) and the method is not recommended. Intrathecal baclofen has been used successfully to treat severe spasticity, but its direct effect on central pain in MS is not known.

SPINAL CORD INJURY (SCI)

Differential diagnosis of pain categories and epidemiology

Spinal trauma affects the individual in many ways. Besides pain, many of the patients have severe physical handicaps with severe effects on their social life, and they are also afflicted by psychological stress in their new life situation. In addition to this, many of them have intense pain. It is therefore important to apply a holistic view when analysing and treating pain in SCI patients. The various pains experienced by SCI patients need to be thoroughly analysed to find out what is nociceptive and what is neurogenic pain, and to what extent the pain is dependent on psychological factors. Most pain in SCI patients is undoubtedly organic.

The pain is particularly difficult to analyse during the early posttrauma period, because many patients are immobilized and have nociceptive musculoskeletal pain, which makes it difficult to determine when the central pain started.

Five studies from the last 13 years show that many SCI patients have chronic pain, with a moderate to severe pain prevalence of 42–77% of all SCI patients (Britell & Mariano 1991). Bonica estimated that about 30% of these patients have central pain (Bonica 1991). This calculation is difficult because many of the patients have more than one kind of neurogenic pain, for instance, pain due to lesions of the nerve roots and peripheral nerves. Some of the pain emanating from all three kinds of lesion has been described as dysaesthetic, although most of the dysaesthetic pain after SCI is considered to be central. Dysaesthetic pain is said to be more common after high spinal lesion than after low lesions, which, on the other hand, often result in lesions of the cauda equina, i.e. root lesions, and such lesions are known to cause severe pain.

Many SCI patients suffer from visceral pain. This is sometimes related to disturbed function in the intestines, bowel or bladder, but it is conceivable that some of this pain is central.

The practical consequence of chronic pain in SCI patients was illustrated in a study in which 36% of 885 out-patients who were unemployed stated that the severity of the pain, rather than their paralyses prevented them from working (Nepomuceno et al 1979). In this survey, 37% of lower-level SCI patients with chronic pain would rather have pain relief than recovery of motor function.

The lesions are classified as complete or incomplete, depending on whether they result in total loss of voluntary motor control, i.e. complete paralysis, and total loss of sensibility below the lesion, or in partial loss of these functions, which reflects the extent of the damage to the white and grey matter in the cord.

Cordotomies performed to relieve intractable pain are rare causes of 'dysaesthetic' central pain. This happens after 3–5% of all cordotomies (Tasker 1990).

Characteristics of central pain in SCI

Currently available information about the characteristics of central pain in SCI patients is incomplete. It is thus uncertain whether or not the character of central pain is different in patients with complete and incomplete lesions. In studies from recent years the term 'dysaesthetic' has been used for all SCI pain (Davidoff et al 1987b; Berić et al 1988; Britell & Mariano 1991), although one might get the impression from one of the studies that dysaesthetic pain occurs mainly after incomplete lesions (Berić et al 1988). By analysing pain in 19 patients, Davidoff et al (1987b) showed that the term 'dysaesthetic pain' corresponds to many pain qualities. When these SCI patients described their central pain according to the McGill Pain Questionnaire (MPQ) it was found that 58% experienced cutting pain, 47% burning pain, 47% radiating pain, and 37% tight pain. Some 37% chose the word 'cruel' and 37% the word 'nagging'. In most of the patients the pain was deep (83%), whereas it was both deep and superficial in the others. All 13 patients of Lenz et al (1988) had burning pain. Most patients have constant pain, but paroxysmal pain is not uncommon.

The onset of central pain in SCI is sometimes immediate; in other patients there is a considerable delay (Berić et al 1988). It is evident that its location depends on the segmental level of the lesion and one can predict that the extension of the lesion in the cord also influences the regional extension of the pain. A complete transverse lesion carries the risk of inducing central pain in all of the regions innervated by the segments below the lesion. This is in accordance with most reported material, in which pain in the legs dominates, because low-level lesions are more frequent than high lesions. All three quadriplegic patients of Davidoff et al (1987b) had pain from the upper extremities down. It seems probable that in some patients one part of the central pain complex is caused by damage to the grey matter at the level of the lesion. This pain can be expected to engage the dermatomes of the injured segments and to be similar to the pain in syringomyelia. Another part is caused by injury to the ascending pathways. The extension of this pain is determined by the extent of the lesion in the pathways, and can engage all of the body caudal to the lesion. In some patients there is a pain-free zone from the segment of the lesion to the upper level of the pain (Berić et al 1988).

The profile of the sensory abnormalities was investigated by QST in 13 patients with 'dysaesthetic' burning central pain following SCI (Berić et al 1988). All but one had incomplete lesions. The sensibility to temperature and pain were more severely affected than vibration and touch. These results are in accordance with the results from patients with central poststroke pain, i.e. they may indicate that spinothalamic tract lesions are more important for central pain than lesions in the dorsal column–medial lemniscal pathways.

Painful hyperaesthesias, for instance touch and cold allodynia, occur in some SCI patients. Their spontaneous central pain is sometimes also influenced by body movement, external stimuli and emotions.

Treatment

The reader is referred to the general section on treatment of central pain for details. TENS can be expected to produce relief only in patients with some preserved dorsal column function but, in general, TENS has not been found effective in SCI. The same appears to be true for dorsal-column stimulation. Among drugs, antidepressants and antiepileptic drugs are most used (Farkash & Portenoy 1986). Only one controlled study has been published. In this study, trazodone, a serotonin reuptake blocker, was not more effective than placebo (Davidoff et al 1987a). However, it is conceivable that antidepressants with effects also on the noradrenergic systems are more effective, for instance amitriptyline, doxepin and desipramine. A recent report of a single case points to the possibility that a combination of an antidepressant and an antiepileptic drug may sometimes be effective (Sandfjord et al 1992). DREZ lesions have been tried for many years as a treatment for central pain in SCI patients, with varying success (Nashold & Bullitt 1981; Friedman & Nashold 1986). This treatment has recently gained new interest in a modified form, but the effectiveness of this modification has not yet been well evaluated (Edgar et al 1993).

SYRINGOMYELIA AND SYRINGOBULBIA

Syringomyelia (in the spinal cord) and syringobulbia (in the lower brainstem) are rare diseases with a very high incidence of central pain. From a scientific point of view they are of particular interest for the understanding of the mechanisms that underly central pain and sensory disturbances because they illustrate the possible consequences of internal lesions in the spinal cord and brainstem. The lesion is a cystic cavity filled with a fluid that is similar to normal cerebrospinal fluid. The size and extension of the cavity, i.e. the syrinx (from the Greek word for 'flute'), varies enormously between patients, from a small lesion in the dorsal part of the spinal cord over a couple of segments to huge cavities extending from the most caudal part of the cord into the medulla oblongata, as illustrated by findings at autopsy, and in recent years by examination with MRI (Foster & Hudgson 1973; Schliep 1978). The largest cavities leave only a thin layer of spinal cord tissue undamaged at the maximally cavitated regions.

Much is still unknown about how the cavities develop and particularly about the cause of the disease. According to the most-embraced theory, hydromechanical forces are important for the expansion of the cavity. This theory states that the cavity develops as an enlargement of the central canal. Waves of increased pressure are thought to descend from the fourth ventricle in moments of increased intracranial pressure. Incomplete closure of the upper part of the central canal may enhance such a process. This means that the cavity starts in the centre of the spinal cord, which is where the spinothalamic fibres cross the midline to reach their position in the ventrolaterally located spinothalamic tract. A lesion with this location will affect the sensibility to temperature and pain, i.e. a dissociated sensory loss will appear. Studies have shown that this in fact happens, because this sensory abnormality was found in 248 of 250 patients with syringomyelia and syringobulbia (Foster & Hudgson 1973; Schliep 1978). Syringomyelia can also be posttraumatic and can be caused by spinal cord haematomas.

Pain is common in syringomyelia (when this term is used in this chapter it also includes syringobulbia). In a recent survey of 22 patients it was found that all had pain, and that 16 (73%) had central pain (Boivie & Rollsjö, unpublished results). In most patients this pain was located in one of the upper extremities, seldom in both. The thorax was another rather common location and a few patients had pain in the lower extremities. Burning, aching and pressing were the most common pain qualities. Pain, often central pain, was a frequent initial symptom in this disease, which usually progresses slowly over decades.

The results from our study cast doubt over the notion that the somatosensory symptoms of syringomyelia, including central pain, are mainly caused by damage to the spinothalamic fibres as they cross the midline because it has been found that the symptoms and signs are strictly unilateral in several patients who are probably in an early stage of the disease. Thus, some patients have central pain and dissociated sensory loss in one arm and hand. This could be explained by either a lesion affecting the dorsal horn or one affecting the spinothalamic fibres on that side, before they cross. Unfortunately, no MRI verification is available for these patients. It can be speculated that the syrinx expands from the central canal into the dorsal horn grey matter because the mechanical resistance is lower there than in the white matter. This would fit the clinical features. However, there is as yet no support for this idea from MRI or postmortem examinations, which usually show that the cavities are very extensive both longitudinally and across the cord.

Quantitative sensory tests show that all patients with syringomyelia have abnormal temperature and pain sensibility (Boivie 1984; Boivie & Rollsjö, unpublished results). These abnormalities are mostly pronounced, with total loss of temperature sensibility. Patients in advanced stages of the disease have abnormal touch, vibration and kinaesthesia too, indicating that either the dorsal root fibres or the dorsal columns are affected by the syrinx. Some, but not all, patients with central pain have hyperaesthesias of the hyperpathic kind, or allodynia.

The treatment of central pain in syringomyelia is similar to that of central pain after traumatic SCI. In our clinical experience tricyclic antidepressants have been moderately successful.

PARKINSON'S DISEASE

Parkinson's disease (PD) is rightfully considered to be a movement disorder. The dominating symptoms are rigidity, bradykinesia, tremor and defective postural control. However, it is now becoming increasingly clear that many patients with PD have pain and sensory symptoms (Snider et al 1976; Koller 1984; Goetz et al 1985; Schott 1985; Quinn et al 1986). In some patients these symptoms precede the onset of the motor symptoms. The mechanisms behind these symptoms are unknown. It is thus unclear to what extent the pain in PD should be classified as central pain, but it appears likely that at least part of it is of primarily central origin, i.e. central pain. A brief summary of published reports on this pain will be made.

In an investigation of 105 ambulatory PD patients it was found that 43% had sensory symptoms (pain, tingling, numbness; Snider et al 1976). Pain was the most common complaint, reported by 29%. 'It was usually described as an intermittent, poorly localized, cramp-like or aching sensation, not associated with increased muscle contraction and not affected by movement or pressure. It was often proximal and in the limb of greatest motor deficit.' (Snider et al 1976). Some 11% had burning sensations and 12% had painful muscle spasm or cramps. In 7% the pain preceded the motor symptoms. In a similar study of 94 patients, 46% were found to have pain (Goetz et al 1985). The major pains were 'muscle cramps or tightness' (34% of all patients) and painful dystonias (13% of all patients).

A classification for the pain directly related to PD was proposed by Quinn et al (1986):

A. Pain preceding the diagnosis of PD
B. Off-period pain (without dystonia) in patients with fluctuating response to levodopa (four subgroups)
C. Painful dystonic spasms (four subgroups)
D. Peak-dose pain.

Quinn et al (1986) did not give any prevalence figures for the four groups. They concluded that most of the pain is related to fluctuations in motor symptoms, which, in turn, are related to the response to the drug treatment. This idea was supported by observations in two patients in which the fluctuations in motor symptoms and pain were recorded (Nutt & Carter 1984). These observations are compatible with a modulatory influence of the basal ganglia on somatic sensibility, including pain. In all of the studies cited no significant abnormalities in the sensibility to cutaneous stimuli were found.

From the case reports of Quinn et al (1986) it appears that much of the pain in PD can be relieved by careful adjustment of the antiparkinson medication, but they also show that this is sometimes a difficult task.

EPILEPSY, BRAIN TUMOURS AND ABSCESSES

Only a brief comment will be given on central pain in these disease states. In a survey of 858 patients with epilepsy it was found that 2.8% (24) had pain as part of epileptic seizures (Young & Blume 1983). In several of the patients the cause of the epilepsy was unknown. Many were children. No patients with cerebrovascular lesions were included. The pain was either a symptom during the major part of the seizure or part of the aura.

Three groups were recognized. (i) Unilateral pain in the face, arm, leg or trunk (10 patients). Various pain qualities were experienced, including, for instance, burning, tingling, cramp-like, aching, throbbing, stinging, like a sharp knife or like an electric shock. These seizures were thought to emanate from activity in the first somatosensory cortical region in the postcentral gyrus. (ii) Head pain, mainly headache (11 patients). These attacks included pain described as throbbing, pricking or diffuse headache. The cortical focus of these attacks could not be determined. (iii) Abdominal pain (three patients). These attacks were different from the epigastric rising sensations that are sometimes part of the aura of temporal lobe seizures, but the attacks were still considered to be a feature of temporal lobe epilepsy. Since then the same investigators have described a patient with bilateral extremity pain during epileptic seizures, which they proposed to originate in the second somatosensory cortical region (Young et al 1988).

Patients with cerebrovascular lesions that engage the cerebral cortex may develop epilepsy. Fine reported five such patients with epileptic seizures that included severe pain (Fine 1967). This pain had qualities similar to central poststroke pain, but it occurred spontaneously in short attacks, and disappeared completely when antiepileptic drugs were given.

In general, brain tumours rarely induce central pain, but several patients with meningiomas and central pain have been reported (Bender & Jaffe 1958). Surprisingly, not even thalamic tumours have a tendency to cause central pain. In a retrospective study only one of 49 patients with thalamic tumours had central pain (Tovi et al 1961).

Finally, a late 20th century illustration of the fact that all kinds of lesion can result in central pain. Recently, two patients with brain abscesses in the thalamus and internal capsule were reported to have central pain (Gonzales et al 1992). The cause of the abscesses was *Toxoplasma* infection – the patients had AIDS!

CONCLUDING COMMENTS

For the patient it is important to identify central pain when present because this is the basis for its rational management. An ad hoc committee in the Special Interest Group on Central Pain of the IASP has worked out an examination protocol for the diagnosis of central pain. This protocol can be recommended for clinical use. It has the components listed below.

Historical information

1. Is pain the major or primary complaint? If not, indicate the alternative
2. Nature of primary neurological disability:
   (a) Primary diagnosis (e.g. stroke, tumour, etc.)
   (b) Location of disability (e.g. left hemiparesis)
3. Date of onset of neurological signs/symptoms
4. Date of onset of pain
5. Description of pain:
   (a) Location:
   Body area – preferably use pain drawing
   Superficial (skin) and/or deep (muscle, viscera)
   Radiation or referral
   (b) Intensity (1–10 or VAS or categorical scaling); most common intensity at maximum, at minimum
   (c) Temporal features:
   Steady, unchanging; intermittent
   Fluctuates over minutes, hours, days, weeks
   Paroxysmal features (shooting pain, tic-like)
   (d) Quality:
   Thermal (burning, freezing, etc.)
   Mechanical (pressure, cramping, etc.)
   Chemical (stinging etc.)
   Other (aching, etc.)
   (e) Factors increasing the pain (cold, emotions, etc.)
   (f) Factors decreasing the pain (rest, drugs, etc.)
6. Neurologial symptoms besides pain:
   (a) Motor (paresis, ataxia, involuntary movements)
   (b) Sensory (hypo-, hyperaesthesia, paraesthesia, dysaesthesia, numbness, overreaction)
   (c) Others (speech, visual, cognitive, mood, etc.).

Examination

1. Neurological disease; results of CT, MRI, SPECT, PET, CSF assays, neurophysiological examinations, etc.
2. Major neurological findings (e.g. spastic paraparesis)
3. Sensory examination; preferably use sensory chart with the dermatomes. Indicate whether modalities listed have normal, increased or decreased threshold, and paraesthesias or dysaesthesias are evoked:
   (a) Vibratory sense (tuning fork, biothesiometer or vibrameter)
   (b) Tactile (cotton wool, hair movement)
   (c) Skin direction sense, graphaesthesis
   (d) Kinaesthesia
   (e) Temperature (specify how tested; cold and warm, noxious and innocuous)

(f) Pinprick
(g) Deep pain (specify how tested)
(h) Allodynia to mechanical stimuli, cold, heat
(i) Hyperpathia (specify how tested)
(j) Other abnormalities such as radiation, summation, prolonged aftersensation.

Criteria for the diagnosis of central pain

In most patients the examination protocol will lead to information that will enable the examiner to determine whether central pain is at hand. For this decision the following criteria for central pain may be used:

1. The presence of CNS disease. The lesion/dysfunction can be located at any level of the neuraxis from the dorsal horn grey matter of the spinal cord, and the trigeminal spinal nucleus, to the cerebral cortex, i.e. either engaging the ascending pathways and/or their brainstem or cortical relays.
2. Pain that started after the onset of this disease. The pain can be steady, intermittent or paroxysmal or can be present in the form of painful hyperaesthesias such as allodynia or hyperpathia. Its onset can be immediate or delayed up to several years.
3. The pain can have virtually any quality, including trivial aching pain. More than one pain quality is often experienced in the same region or in different regions.
4. The pain can engage large parts of the body (hemipain, one quarter, lower body half, etc.) or can be restricted to a small region such as one arm or the face.
5. The pain can be of high or low intensity. It is often increased, or evoked, by various internal or external stimuli, such as touch, cold and sudden emotions.
6. The presence of abnormalities in somatic sensibility. The abnormalities can be subtle and in some patients it takes quantitative sensory tests to demonstrate their presence. However, in rare cases not even the quantitative methods can show such abnormalities. They are dominated by abnormal sensibility to temperature and pain, indicating involvement of the spinothalamic pathways. Abnormalities are common in touch, vibration and kinaesthesia too, but their presence is not mandatory in central pain, and many patients with central pain have normal thresholds for these submodalities. Hyperaesthesias such as allodynia, hyperalgesia and hyperpathia are common, but not demonstrable in all patients with central pain. Most patients with central pain experience paraesthesias or dysaesthesias that sometimes are painful and thus themselves are a kind of central pain.
7. Nonsensory neurological symptoms and signs may or may not be present. There is thus no correlation between central pain and motor disturbances.
8. Psychological or psychiatric disturbances may or may not be present. A large majority of central pain patients are normal in these respects.
9. The pain should not appear to be of psychic origin.
10. The diagnosis of certain central pain should be ascertained on clinical grounds/criteria or with the help of laboratory examinations that show that the pain is not of nociceptive or peripheral neurogenic origin.

Treatment

Since no universally effective treatment is available for central pain it is important to try available modalities in a systematic way to find the best treatment for the individual patient. In this endeavour it is important to keep the patient well-informed and to monitor treatment closely because of potential side-effects. When drugs are used, increases in dosage should be gradual. It is also wise to inform the patient that the treatment may not relieve the pain completely, which it seldom does.

Central pain is truly chronic pain, often lasting for the rest of the patient's life, and it mostly causes the patient much suffering. It is therefore important that the patient has a reliable, long-lasting relationship with the physician so that he/she knows whom to contact when the pain brings him/her into despair. Support by a psychotherapist may then be indicated. Furthermore, there is reason to include physiotherapy in the treatment programme aiming at increased activity and rehabilitation.

The first-line specific treatments are TENS, antidepressants and antiepileptic drugs. The reader is referred to the sections on these treatments or on the individual pain conditions for detailed information. In some patients the treatment of the central pain needs to be combined with other forms of treatment, because other pains may also be present.

REFERENCES

Ajuraguerra D J 1937 La douleur dans les affections du système nerveux central. Doin, Paris

Arnér S, Meyerson B A 1991 Genuine resistance to opioids – fact or fiction? Pain 47: 116–118

Awerbuch G 1990 Treatment of thalamic pain syndrome with Mexiletone. Annals of Neurology 28: 233

Bainton T, Fox M, Bowsher D, Wells C 1992 A double-blind trial of naloxone in central post-stroke pain. Pain 48: 159–162

Bender M B, Jaffe R 1958 Pain of central origin. Medical Clinics of North America 42: 691–700

Berić A, Dimitrijević M R, Lindblom U 1988 Central dysesthesia syndrome in spinal cord injury patients. Pain 34: 109–116

Biemond A 1956 The conduction of pain above the level of the thalamus opticus. Archives of Neurology and Psychiatry 75: 231–244

Boas R A, Covino B G, Shahnarian A 1982 Analgesic responses to i.v. lignocaine. British Journal of Anaesthesiology 54: 501–505

Bogousslavsky J, Regli F, Uske A 1988 Thalamic infarcts: clinical syndromes, etiology, and prognosis. Neurology 38: 837–848

Boivie J 1979 An anatomic reinvestigation of the termination of the spinothalamic tract in the monkey. Journal of Comparative Neurology 168: 343– 370

Boivie J 1984 Disturbances in cutaneous sensibility in patients with central pain caused by spinal cord lesions of syringomyelia. Pain (suppl 2): 82

Boivie J 1992 Hyperalgesia and allodynia in patients with CNS lesions. In: Willis W D J (ed) Hyperalgesia and allodynia. Raven Press, New York, p 363–373

Boivie J, Leijon G 1991 Clinical findings in patients with central post-stroke pain. In: Casey K L (ed) Pain and central nervous system disease: the central pain syndromes. Raven Press, New York, p 65–75

Boivie J, Leijon G, Johansson I 1989 Central post-stroke pain – a study of the mechanisms through analyses of the sensory abnormalities. Pain 37: 173–185

Bonica J J 1991 Introduction: sematic, epidemiologic, and educational issues. In: Casey K L (ed) Pain and central nervous disease: the central pain syndromes: Raven Press, New York, p 13–29

Bowsher D 1959 The anatomy of thalamic pain. Journal of Neurology, Neurosurgery and Psychiatry 22: 81–82

Bowsher D, Foy P M, Shaw M D M 1989 Central pain complicating infarction following subarachnoid haemorrhage. British Journal of Neurosurgery 3: 435–442

Breuer A C, Cuervo H, Selkoe D J 1981 Hyperpathia and sensory level due to parietal lobe arteriovenous malformation. Archives of Neurology 38: 722–724

Britell C W, Mariano A J 1991 Chronic pain in spinal cord injury. Physical Medicine and Rehabilitation: State of Art Reviews 5: 71–82

Bromm B, Treede R D 1987 Human cerebral potentials evoked by CO_2 laser stimuli causing pain. Experimental Brain Research 67: 153–162

Budd K 1985 The use of the opiate antagonist naloxone, in the treatment of inreactable pain. Neuropeptides 5: 419–422

Budd K 1989 Sodium valproate in the treatment of pain. In: Chadwick D (ed) Fourth international symposium on sodium valproate and epilepsy. Royal Society of Medicine, London, p 213–216

Casey K L, Boivie J, Leijon G, Morrow T J, Sjölund B I R 1990 Laser-evoked cerebral potentials and sensory function in patients with central pain. Pain (suppl 5): 204

Cassinari V, Pagni C A 1969 Central pain. A neurosurgical survey. Harvard University Press, Cambridge, Massachusetts

Cesaro P, Mann M W, Moretti J L 1991 Central pain and thalamic hyperactivity: a single photon emission computerized tomographic study. Pain 47: 329–336

Chabal C, Russel L C, Burchiel K J 1989 The effect of intravenous lidocaine, tocainide, and mexiletine on spontaneous active fibres originating in rat sciatic neuromas. Pain 38: 333–338

Clifford D B, Trotter J L 1984 Pain in multiple sclerosis. Archives of Neurology 41: 1270–1272

Collingridge G L, Singer W 1990 Excitatory amino acid receptors and synaptic plasticity. Trends in Pharmacological Science 11: 290–296

Craig A D 1991 Supraspinal pathways and mechanisms relevant to central pain. In: Casey K L (ed) Pain and central nervous disease: the central pain syndromes. Raven Press, New York, p 157–170

Davidoff G, Roth J E 1991 Clinical characteristics of central (dysesthetic) pain in spinal cord injury patients. In: Casey K L (ed) Pain and central nervous diseases: the central pain syndromes. Raven Press, New York, p 77–83

Davidoff G, Guarrachini M, Roth E, Sliwa J, Yarkony G 1987a Trazodone hydrochloride in the treatment of dysesthetic pain in traumatic myelopathy: a randomized, double-blind, placebo-controlled study. Pain 29:151–161

Davidoff G, Roth E, Guarracini M, Sliwa J, Yarkony G 1987b Function-limiting dysesthetic pain syndrome among traumatic spinal cord injury patients: a cross-sectional study. Pain 29: 39–48

Davidson C, Schick W 1935 Spontaneous pain and other subjective sensory disturbances: a clinicopathological study. Neurology 34: 1204–1237

Dehen H, Willer J C, Cambier J 1983 Pain in thalamic syndrome: electrophysiological findings in man. Advances in Pain Research and Therapy 5: 936–940

Dejerine J, Roussy G 1906 Le syndrome thalamique. Revue Neurologique (Paris) 14: 521–532

Dejgard A, Petersen P, Kastrup J 1988 Mexiletine for treatment of chronic painful diabetic neuropathy. Lancet 1: 9–11

Drake C G, McKenzie K G 1953 Mesencephalic tractotomy for pain. Journal of Neurosurgery 10: 457–462

Eaton S A, Salt T E 1990 Thalamic NMDA receptors and nociceptive sensory synaptic transmission. Neuroscience Letters 110: 297–302

Edgar R E, Best L G, Quail P A, Obert A D 1993 Computer-assisted DREZ microcoagulation: posttraumatic spinal deafferentation pain. Journal of Spinal Diseases 6: 48–56

Edinger L 1891 Giebt es central antstehender Schmerzen. Deutche Zeitschrift für Nervenheilkunde 1: 262–282

Edwards W T, Habib F, Burney R G, Begin G 1985 Intravenous lidocaine in the management of various chronic pain states. Regional Anaesthesie 10: 1–6

Ekbom K 1966 Tegretol, a new therapy of tabetic lightning pains. Acta Medica Scandinavica 179: 251–252

Eriksson M B E, Sjölund B H, Nielzén S 1979 Long term results of peripheral conditioning stimulation as an analgesic measure in chronic pain. Pain 6: 335–347

Espir M L E, Millac P 1970 Treatment of paroxysmal disorders in multiple sclerosis with carbamazepine (Tegretol). Journal of Neurology, Neurosurgery and Psychiatry 33: 528–531

Farkash A E, Portenoy R K 1986 The pharmacological management of chronic pain in the paraplegic patient. Journal of American Paraplegia Society 4: 41–50

Fields H L, Adams J E 1974 Pain after cortical injury relieved by electrical stimulation of the internal capsule. Brain 97: 169–178

Fine W 1967 Post-hemiplegic epilepsy in the elderly. British Medical Journal 1: 199–201

Foerster O 1927 Die Laitungsbahnen des Schmerzgefuhls und die chirurgische Behandlung der Schmerzzustande. Urban & Schwarzenberg, Berlin, p 77–80

Foix C, Thévenard A, Nicolesco 1922 Revue Neurologique (Paris) 29: 990

Foster J B, Hudgson P 1973 Clinical features of syringomyelia. In: Barnett H J, Foster J B, Hudgson P (eds) Syringomyelia. Saunders, London, p 1–123

Friedman A H, Nashold B S 1986 DREZ lesions for relief of pain related to spinal cord injury. Journal of Neurosurgery 65: 465–469

Garcin R 1968 Thalamic syndrome and pain of central origin. In: Soulairac A, Cahn J, Charpentier J (eds) Pain. Academic Press, London, p 521–541

Glynn C J, Jamous M A, Teddy P J, Moorem R A, Lloyd J W 1986 Role of spinal noradrenergic system in transmission of pain in patients with spinal cord injury. Lancet 2: 1249–1250

Glynn, C, Dawson D, Sanders R A 1988 A double-blind comparison between epidural morphine and epidural clonidine in patients with chronic non-cancer pain. Pain 34: 123–128

Goetz, C G, Tanner C M, Levy M, Wilson R S, Garron D G 1985 Pain in idiopathic Parkinson's disease. Neurology 35: 200

Gonzales G R, Herskovitz S, Rosenblum M et al, 1992 Central pain from cerebral abscess: thalamic syndrome in AIDS patients with toxoplasmosis. Neurology 42: 1107–1109

Gracely R H 1991 Theoretical and practical issues in pain assessment in central pain syndromes. In: Casey K (ed) Pain and central nervous system disease: the central pain syndromes. Raven Press, New York, p 85–101

Gram L 1990 Inadequate dosing and pharmacokinetic variability as confounding factors in assessment of efficacy of antidepressants. Clinical Neuropharmacology 13 (suppl 1): 35–44

Greiff 1883 Zur Localisation der Hemichorea. Archiv fur Psychologie und Nervenkrankheiten 14: 598

Gybels J M, Sweet W H 1989 Neurosurgical treatment of persistent pain. Karger, Basel

Hampf G, Bowsher D, Nurmikko T 1989 Distigmine and amitriptyline in the treatment of chronic pain. Anesthesia Progress 36: 58–62

Hansson P, Lindblom U 1992 Hyperalgesia assessed with quantitative sensory testing in patients with neurogenic pain. In: Willis W D J (ed) Hyperalgesia and allodynia. Raven Press, New York, p 335–343

Hao J X, Xu X J, Aldskogius H, Sieger Å, Wiesenfeld-Hallin Z 1991a The excitatory amino acid receptor antagonist MK-801 prevents the hypersensitivity induced by spinal cord ischemia in the rat. Experimental Neurology 113: 182–191

Hao J X, Xu X J, Aldskogius H, Sieger Å, Wiesenfeld-Hallin Z 1991b Beneficial effect of opioid receptor antagonist naltrexone on hypersensitivity induced by spinal cord ischemia in rats: dissociation with MK-801. Restorative Neurology and Neuroscience 3: 357–366

Hao J X, Xu X J, Aldskogius H, Sieger Å, Wiesenfeld-Hallin Z 1991c Allodynia-like effects in rat after ischaemic spinal cord injury photochemically induced by laser irradiation. Pain 45: 175–185

Hao J X, Xu X J, Yu Y X, Sieger Å, Wiesenfeld-Hallin Z 1991d Hypersensitivity of dorsal horn wide dynamic range neurons to cutaneous mechanical stimuli after transient spinal cord ischemia in the rat. Neuroscience Letters 128: 105–108

Hartvig P, Gillberg P G, Gordh T, Post C 1989 Cholinergic mechanisms in pain and analgesia. TIPS(December 1989 suppl): 76–79

Hassler R 1960 Die zentrale Systeme des Schmerzes. Acta Neurochirurgica 8: 353–423

Head H, Holmes G 1911 Sensory disturbances from cerebral lesions. Brain 34: 102–254

Holmes G 1919 Pain of central origin. In: Osler W (ed) Contributions to medical and biological research. Paul B Hoeber, New York, p 235–246

Holmgren H, Leijon G, Boivie J, Johansson I, Ilievska L 1990 Central post-stroke pain – somatosensory evoked potentials in relation to location of the lesion and sensory signs. Pain 40: 43–52

Jones E G 1992 Thalamus and pain. ASP Journal 1: 58–61

Kalman S, Sörensen J, Österberg A, Boivie J, Bertler Å 1993 Is central pain in multiple sclerosis opioid sensitive? Pain (in press)

Kastrup J, Petersen P, Dejgård A, Angelo H R, Hilsted J 1987 Intravenous lidocaine infusion – a new treatment of chronic painful diabetic neuropathy? Pain 28: 69–75

Koller W C 1984 Sensory symptoms in Parkinson's disease. Neurology 34: 957–959

Kupers R C, Konings H, Adriasen H, Gybels J M 1991 Morphine differentially affects the sensory and affective ratings in neurogenic and ideopathic forms of pain. Pain 47: 5–12

Leijon G, Boivie J 1989a Treatment of neurogenic pain with antidepressants. Nordisk Psykiatrisk Tidsskrift 43 (suppl 20): 83–87

Leijon G, Boivie J 1989b Central post-stroke pain – the effect of high and low frequency TENS. Pain 38: 187–191

Leijon G, Boivie J 1989c Central post-stroke pain – a controlled trial of amitriptyline and carbamazepine. Pain 36: 27–36

Leijon G, Boivie J 1991 Pharmacological treatment of central pain. In: Casey K L (ed) Pain and central nervous disease: the central pain syndromes. Raven Press, New York, p 257–266

Leijon G, Bowsher D 1990 Somatosensory findings in central post-stroke pain (CPSP) and controls. Pain (suppl 5): S468

Leijon G, Boivie J, Johansson I 1989 Central post-stroke pain – neurological symptoms and pain characteristics. Pain 36: 13–25

Lenz F A 1992 Ascending modulation of thalamic function and pain; experimental and clinical data. In: Sicuteri F (ed) Advances in pain research and therapy. Raven Press, New York, p 177–196

Lenz A F, Tasker R R, Dostrovsky J O et al 1988 Abnormal single-unit activity and response to stimulation in the presumed ventrocaudal nucleus of patients with central pain. In: Dubner R, Gebhart G F, Bond M R (eds) Pain research and clinical management. Elsevier, Amsterdam, p 157–164

Lewis-Jones H, Smith T, Bowsher D, Leijon G 1990 Magnetic resonance imaging in 36 cases of central post-stroke pain (CPSP). Pain (suppl 5): 278

Lindblom U, Ochoa J 1986 Somatosensory function and dysfunction. In: Asbury A K, McKhann G M, McDonald I W (eds) Diseases in the nervous system, clinical neurobiology. W B Saunders, Philadelphia, p 283–298

Lindström P, Lindblom U 1987 The analgesic effect of tocainide in trigeminal neuralgia. Pain 28: 45–50

Loh L, Nathan P W, Schott G D 1981 Pain due to lesions of central nervous system removed by sympathetic block. British Medical Journal 282: 1026–1028

McLean M J, Macdonald R L 1986 Carbamazepine and 10,11-epoxycarbamazepine produce use- and voltage-dependent limitation of rapidly firing action potentials of mouse central neurons in cell culture. Journal of Pharmacology and Experimental Therapeutics 238: 727–738

McNamara P J, Albert M L, Tanaka Y, Miyazaki M 1990 Pain associated with cerebral lesions. Pain (suppl 5): 434

Mauguière F, Desmedt J E 1988 Thalamic pain syndrome of Dejérine-Roussy. Differentation of four subtypes assisted by somatosensory evoked potentials data. Archives of Neurology 45: 1312–1320

Max M B, Schafer S C, Culnane M, Smoller B, Dubner R, Gracely R H 1988 Amitriptyline, but not lorazepam, relieves postherpetic neuralgia. Neurology 38: 1427–1432

Merskey H, Lindblom U, Mumford J M, Nathan P W, Noordenbos W, Sunderland S 1986 Pain terms. A current list with definitions and notes on usage. Pain (suppl 3): 217–221

Michel D, Laurent B, Convers P et al 1990 Douleurs corticales. Étude clinique, électrophysiologique et topographie de 12 cas. Revue Neurologique (Paris) 146: 405–414

Michelson J J 1943 Subjective disturbances of the sense of pain from lesions of the cerebral cortex. Research Publications–Association for Research in Nervous and Mental Disease 23: 86–99

Moulin D E, Foley K M, Ebers G C 1988 Pain syndromes in multiple sclerosis. Neurology 38: 1830–1834

Nashold B S, Bullitt E 1981 Dorsal root entry zone lesions to control central pain in paraplegics. Journal of Neurosurgery 55: 414–419

Nepomuceno C, Fine P R, Richards S et al 1979 Pain in patients with spinal cord injury. Archives of Physical Medicine and Rahabilitation 60: 605–609

Nutt J G, Carter J H 1984 Sensory symptoms in parkinsonism related to central dopaminergic function. Lancet 2: 456–457

Österberg A, Boivie J, Henriksson A, Holmgren H, Johansson I 1993 Central pain in multiple sclerosis. Pain (suppl) (in press)

Osterman P O, Westerberg C-E 1975 Paroxysmal attacks in multiple sclerosis. Brain 98: 189–202

Pagni C A 1989 Central pain due to spinal cord and brainstem damage. In: Wall P D, Malzack R (eds) Textbook of pain, 2nd edn. Churchill Livingstone, Edinburgh, p 634–655

Pertovaara A, Morrow T J, Casey K L 1988 Cutaneous pain and detection thresholds to short CO_2 laser pulses in humans: evidence on afferent mechanisms and the influence of varying stimulus conditions. Pain 34: 261–269

Portenoy R K, Foley K M 1986 Chronic use of opioid analgesics in non-malignant pain: report of 38 cases. Pain 25: 171–186

Portenoy R K, Foley K M, Inturrisi C E 1990 The nature of opioid responsiveness and its implications for neuropathic pain: new hypothesis derived from studies of opioid infusions. Pain 43: 273–286

Quinn N P, Koller W C, Lang A E, Marsden C D 1986 Painful Parkinson's disease. Lancet 1: 1366–1369

Rausell E, Cusick C G, Taub E, Jones E G 1991 Chronic deafferentation in monkeys differentially affects nociceptive and non-nociceptive pathways distinguished by specific calcium binding proteins and down regulates GABA-A receptors at thalamic levels. Proceedings of the National Academy of Sciences USA 89: 2571–2575

Richardsson R R, Meyer P R, Cerullo L 1980 Neurostimulation in the modulation of intractable paraplegic and traumatic neuroma pains. Pain 8: 75–84

Riddoch G 1938 The clinical features of central pain. Lancet 234: 1093–1098, 1150–1156, 1205–1209

Rosen J A, Barsoum A H 1979 Failure of chronic dorsal column stimulation in multiple sclerosis. Annals of Neurology 6: 66–67

Rowbotham M C, Reisner-Keller L A, Fields H L 1991 Both intravenous lidocaine and morphine reduce the pain of postherpetic neuralgia. Neurology 41: 1024–1028

Salt T E 1992 The possible involvement of excitatory amino acids and NMDA receptors in thalamic pain mechanisms and central pain syndromes. APS Journal 1: 52–54

Sandfjord P R, Lindblom L B, Haddox J D 1992 Amitriptyline and carbamazepine in the treatment of dysesthetic pain in spinal cord injury. Archives of Physical Medicine and Rehabilitation 73: 300–301

Sandyk R 1985 Spontaneous pain, hyperpathia and wastings of the hand due to parietal lobe haemorrhage. European Neurology 24: 1–3

Scadding J W, Wall P D, Parry C B W, Brooks D M 1982 Clinical trial of propranolol in post-traumatic neuralgia. Pain 14: 283–292
Schliep G 1978 Syringomyelia and syringobulbia. In: Vinken G, Bruyn G (eds) Handbook of neurology. North-Holland, Amsterdam, p 255–327
Schmahmann J D, Leifer D 1992 Parietal pseudothalamic pain syndrome. Clinical features and anatomic correlates. Archives of Neurology 49: 1032–1037
Schott B, Laurent B, Mauguière F 1986 Les douleurs thalamiques: étude critique de 43 cas. Revue Neurologique (Paris) 142: 308–315
Schott G D 1985 Pain in Parkinson's disease. Pain 22: 407–411
Schott G D, Loh L 1984 Anticholinesterase drugs in the treatment of chronic pain. Pain 20: 201–206
Schuster P 1936 Beiträge zur patologie des Thalamus opticus. Archiv fur Psychiatrie und Nervenkrankheiten 105: 550–622
Shibasaki H, Kuroiwa Y 1974 Painful tonic seizure in multiple sclerosis. Archives of Neurology 30: 47–51
Siegfried J 1983 Long term results of electrical stimulation in the treatment of pain by means of implanted electrodes. In: Rizzi C, Visentin T A (eds) Pain therapy. Elsevier, Amsterdam, p 463–475
Siegfried J, Demierre B 1984 Thalamic electrostimulation in the treatment of thalamic pain syndrome. Pain (suppl 2): 116
Silver M L 1957 'Central pain' from cerebral arteriovenous aneurysm. Journal of Neurosurgery 14: 92–97
Sindrup S H, Gram L F, Brosen K, Eshöj O, Mogensen E F 1990 The selective serotonin reuptake inhibitor paroxetine is effective in treatment of diabetic neuropathy symptoms. Pain 42: 135–144
Sjölund B H 1991 Role of transcutaneous electrical nerve stimulation, central nervous system stimulation, and ablative procedures in central pain syndromes. In: Casey K L (ed) Pain and central nervous disease: the central pain syndromes. Raven Press, New York, p 267–274
Snider S R, Fahn S, Isgreen W P, Cote L J 1976 Primary sensory symptoms in parkinsonism. Neurology 26: 423–429
Soria E D, Fine E J 1991 Disappearance of thalamic pain after parietal subcortical stroke. Pain 44: 285–288
Stenager E, Knudsen L, Jensen K 1991 Acute and chronic pain syndromes in multiple sclerosis. Acta Neurologica Scandinavica 84: 197–200
Swerdlow M 1986 Anticonvulsants in the therapy of neuralgic pain. Pain Clinic 1: 9–19
Tasker R 1990 Pain resulting from nervous system pathology (central pain). In: Bonica J J (ed) The management of pain. Lea & Febiger, Philadelphia, p 264–280
Tasker R R, de Carvalho G, Dostrovsky J O 1991 The history of central pain syndromes, with observations concerning pathophysiology and treatment. In: Casey K L (ed) Pain and central nervous disease: the central pain syndromes. Raven Press, New York, p 31–58
Tomson T 1980 Carbamazepine therapy in trigeminal neuralgia. Archives of Neurology 37: 699–703
Tourian A Y 1987 Narcotic responsive 'thalamic' pain treatment with propranolol and tricyclic antidepressants. Pain (suppl 4): 411
Tourtellotte W W, Baumhefner W W 1983 Comprehensive management of multiple sclerosis. In: Hallpike J F, Adams C W M, Tourtellotte W W (eds) Multiple sclerosis. Williams & Wilkins, Baltimore, p 513–578
Tovi D, Schisano G, Liljequist B 1961 Primary tumours of the region of the thalamus. Journal of Neurosurgery 18: 730–740
Treede R D, Kief S, Bromm B 1988 Late somatosensory evoked cerebrals in response to cutaneous heat stimuli. Electroencephalography and Clinical Neurophysiology 70: 429–441
Tsubokawa T, Katayama T, Hirayama T, Koyama S 1990 Motor cortex stimulation for control of thalamic pain. Pain (suppl 5): 491
Umlauf R L, Moore J E, Britell C W 1992 Relevance and nature of the pain experience in spinal cord injured. Journal of Behavioural Medicine (in press)
Vermote R, Ketelaer P, Carton H 1986 Pain in multiple sclerosis patients. Clinical Neurology and Neurosurgery 88: 87–93
Waltz T A, Ehni G 1966 The thalamic syndrome and its mechanism. Journal of Neurosurgery 24: 735–742
Watson C P, Evans R J, Reed K, Merskey H, Goldsmith L, Warsh J 1982 Amitriptyline versus placebo in postherpetic neuralgia. Neurology 32: 671–673
Watson B D, Prado R, Diedrich W D 1986 Photochemically induced spinal cord injury in the rat. Brain Research 367: 296–300
White J C, Sweet W H 1969 Pain and the neurosurgeon. A forty-year experience. C C Thomas, Springfield Illinois
Wiesenfeld-Hallin Z, Lindblom U 1985 The effect of systemic tocaimide, lidocaine and bupivacaine on nociception in the rat. Pain 23: 357–360
Woolf C J, Wiesenfeld-Hallin Z 1985 The systematic administration of local anesthetics produces a selective depression of C-afferent fibre evoked activity in the spinal cord. Pain 23: 361–374
Young B G, Blume W T 1983 Painful epileptic seizures. Brain 106: 537–554
Young G B, Barr H W K, Blume W T 1988 Painful epileptic seizures involving the second sensory area. Neurology 19: 412
Young R F, Goodman S J 1979 Dorsal spinal cord stimulation in the treatment of multiple sclerosis. Neurosurgery 5: 225–230

47. Pain and psychological medicine

H. Merskey

INTRODUCTION

Although psychological medicine is still used in the title of a fairly young journal, the words have a slightly old-fashioned tone. Nevertheless they are an apt description for a topic of much current importance. Pain may be a result of emotional factors and is well-established as a consequence of psychological illness. It is often a cause of emotional change. In Britain these topics are part of psychological medicine, or general hospital psychiatry. In the United States they are known as liaison psychiatry.

The phenomena are wider than questions of illness alone. That this is so can be seen in Chapters 13 and 14, among others. In this chapter, I will consider a more limited field and I will describe, firstly, the ways in which psychological illness is believed to be responsible for pain, and, secondly, the way in which sustained noxious input which is experienced as severe pain may itself affect the emotional state. Common features of the pain in psychiatric patients and in pain-clinic patients with psychiatric problems will then be described. This approach reverses the order of proceeding from symptom and pattern of illness to aetiology and treatment. It does so mainly because the patterns of pain in psychological illness are not so distinct that they form neat and convenient groupings for diagnostic purposes. It is true that they have some idiosyncrasies and special features which enable them to be distinguished at times, but these are perhaps less important than the general understanding of the relationship between emotion and pain.

PSYCHOLOGICAL CAUSES OF PAIN

Pain is frequent in psychiatric patients. Klee et al (1959) found it occurred in 61% of a Veterans Administration outpatient population. Spear (1967) found it in 65.6% of psychiatric inpatients and outpatients. It was a spontaneous complaint in more than 50% of them. Delaplaine et al (1978) examined patients in a psychiatric hospital on admission and found, as anticipated, the lowest rate, namely 38%, with 22% of the patients having no physical cause to account for their symptoms. It was anticipated that these figures would be relatively low in a psychiatric hospital because the association of pain with neurosis is, in fact, much more prominent than that of pain with psychosis or many types of personality disorder (Merskey 1965a). In any case, the view generally goes without challenge that there is an important minority of psychiatric patients in whom pain results from their mental state. In many instances the pain is not a major complaint; it is incidental and is mentioned only after rather full enquiries have been made. Even so, severe or moderately severe pain affects a minimum of 25% of psychiatric patients (Delaplaine et al 1978). In other settings (e.g. clinics for headache and low-back pain and in pain clinics generally) the importance of emotional disorders as a cause of pain, or as an agent in increasing it, is usually recognised as a matter of course (see, for example, Chs 27 and 57).

The sample of patients which is seen by any practitioner – whether family practitioner, psychiatrist, neurologist, neurosurgeon or anaesthetist – is almost always influenced by psychological and social selection factors. People who are concerned about their bodies, hypochondriacal or tenacious will seek medical help more often than those who do not have these characteristics. It is easy to see this, for example, with migraine. Studies which rely on clinic patients find them to have marked psychological disturbance (Klee 1968). When migraine-clinic patients are compared with migraine patients who did not attend a special clinic, the former are the more emotionally disturbed (Henryk-Gutt & Rees 1973). When a more complete epidemiological study was done (Crisp et al 1977), it was found that there was a little excess anxiety in patients with migraine but that that was the main difference between them and others, and overall they much resemble the general population, as might be expected. There is probably a relationship between episodes of depression and an increased frequency of migraine, as any clinician will observe. However, the overall link between migraine and the emotional state is much less strong than is sometimes suggested (Merskey 1982).

Hospital clinics inevitably acquire patients who do not rest content with symptoms that are not completely removed by their doctors. Indeed one can say that even general practitioners see a selected sample of the population. In one study, patients were asked to keep a sickness diary of the number of episodes of illness which they underwent (Banks et al 1975). Only 3% of such complaints as headache, vomiting, diarrhoea, etc. were reported to the general practitioners. The scope for self-selection in this context is enormous. Even a general practitioner can be expected to see patients whose personal and psychological characteristics differ from those of the general population. Accordingly, no medical practitioner can expect to find that all the patients whom he sees with chronic pain will be free from emotional disorder. In fact, the more specialized and highly regarded his practice, the more this will happen. Thus it must always be recognized that the clinical material on which we form our opinion about pain is biased by these selection problems. General conclusions about the psychology of pain which would apply to all groups of pain must be made very cautiously. On the other hand, the role of psychiatry in accounting for pain in psychiatric patients is quite well-developed, since psychiatric patients with pain have been studied by a number of authors. It is merely necessary to recognize that the psychiatry of patients with pain, seen by a psychiatrist, or seen in pain clinics, only allows qualified generalizations about pain overall.

DEFINITION OF PAIN

Before proceeding to discuss the psychiatry of pain it is important to emphasize that the pain which psychiatric patients have, often without lesions, is as 'real' as that of those people whose pain is due to lesions or pathophysiological states. This observation is embodied in the definition of the International Association for the Study of Pain (IASP), which is as follows: 'an unpleasant sensory and emotional experience associated with actual or potential tissue damage or described in terms of such damage' (IASP 1979).

PAIN IN PSYCHIATRIC PATIENTS

Walters (1961) was the first to describe a large series of psychiatric patients with pain and demonstrate their main diagnostic and personal characteristics. In 430 patients whom he had seen in consultation concerning pain, 185 had a pain in the head and neck, 133 in the chest and upper limbs, 112 in the low back and the lower limbs, 61 in the trunk and back, 50 in the genitals or pelvis and seven had pain all over. Others had pain in the abdomen, all four limbs or both limbs on one side. Sometimes but not invariably, the pain was described dramatically. Only 26 patients had conversion hysteria and only 68 had psychoses (including 45 with depression). The majority (336) had 'other neuroses and situational states'. Walters emphasized, besides, that many patients had minor physical lesions which gave rise to much more pain in the presence of emotional disturbance than would otherwise have been expected. Merskey & Spear (1967) found, like Walters, that pain was more often located in the head than in any other region of the body in psychiatric patients. Merskey (1965a), examining a group of psychiatric patients with pain as a major complaint and no physical lesions, found that 57 out of 76 had a diagnosis of neurosis, six out of 76 had a diagnosis of reactive depression and nine had a diagnosis of endogenous depression. There were four with other diagnoses. When compared with a control group of psychiatric patients who did not have pain, the proportions with neurosis were very much higher and the proportions with endogenous depression, schizophrenia and other diagnoses were lower. Thus Merskey found the primary association of pain in psychological illness to be with neurotic illnesses.

The frequency of the diagnosis of hysteria either on the basis of a history of conversion symptoms or personality disorder was relatively high. Spear (1967), whose patients were less chronic, found lower percentages of hysteria but still showed the same predominance of neurotic conditions relating to psychiatric illness in those who had pain compared with those who did not have pain. The above work was some of the earliest to provide controlled comparisons of psychiatric patients with pain and without pain and the diagnosis of hysteria today requires much stricter criteria than were acceptable at that time.

Large (1980), examining patients referred to a psychiatrist in a pain clinic, found the following distributions: among 110 diagnoses of psychiatric illness, reactive depression and neurotic conditions accounted for 69 patients and endogenous depression for 33, while others numbered eight; 50 patients had personality disorders. Thus, the psychiatric findings in these cases are quite consistent and indicate that those patients who have pain with psychological illness appear to be suffering for the most part from neurotic or depressive disorders.

Pilowsky & Spence (1976) used an illness behaviour questionnaire (IBQ) to characterize pain-clinic patients and observed six taxonomic clusters which have much in common with the traditional results described above. Demjen & Bakal (1981) found very similar results with headache sufferers, but observed more general hypochondriasis and greater unwillingness to see their trouble in psychological terms. Large & Mullins (1981) reported findings which were essentially confirmatory of those of Pilowsky & Spence, but from a different clinic.

Psychological test studies yield comparable results. Pilling et al (1967) showed the occurrence of the conversion V triad pattern in the Minnesota Multiphasic Personality Inventory (MMPI) in patients who had pain as a presenting symptom with psychological illness. In this pattern, the scale for hypochondriasis is elevated, that for depression is elevated but less than that for hypochondriasis, and the scale for hysteria is also elevated more than for depression. These findings were attributed early on to low-back pain (Hanvik 1956) and have been found in a wide range of studies of patients with chronic pain (Merskey 1980). It is noteworthy however that, as Fordyce (1976) recognizes, this pattern is common to pain patients whether or not they have physical lesions. Watson (1982) showed that chronic pain patients obtained elevated hysteria and hypochondriasis scores on the MMPI because they endorsed items that were relevant to their problem and not because they were hypochondriacal. Smythe (1984) and Merskey et al (1985) have emphasized that the use of these scales in the MMPI can be seriously misleading. They rely to a considerable extent upon symptoms like pain in different locations, fatigue, other bodily complaints and insomnia as evidence for hypochondriasis depression (HsD) and hysteria (Hy). In the presence of physical illness this will often be invalid. Love & Peck (1987) reviewed 56 studies and concluded that the MMPI should not be used in the attempt to distinguish psychological causes of pain. Some use remains for the MMPI as a measure of severity or for the analysis of different profiles (Bradley et al 1978).

Sternbach (1974) who demonstrated the conversion V pattern in many pain clinic patients, also showed that it was especially associated with chronicity and could improve with treatment (Sternbach et al 1973). Naliboff et al (1988) confirmed that reductions appear in MMPI scores with successful treatment. This may be as much because physical symptoms abate as because psychological improvement occurs.

It is worth mentioning that the term 'hysterical pain' which the writer sometimes considers to be justified, is often best avoided. There are a number of practical reasons for this, especially the difficulty in conveying the concept directly to patients. Another term used for patients who seem to have pain for psychological reasons is 'operant pain'. The writer has reservations about this term, about its applications to the theory of pain and psychological illness, and about the validity of many of the claims which have been made for treatments based upon the notion of operant pain. Those grouped under it probably include patients whose pain is related to anxiety, depression and many psychiatric characteristics. It is of practical importance to distinguish these phenomena in order to apply appropriate treatment, whether antidepressants, psychotherapy or rehabilitative measures.

The literature on pain patients has frequently commented upon a number of characteristics which are said to be typical of them (Hart 1947; Engel 1959). In fact, more than 30 authors who mention such characteristics have been listed (Merskey & Spear 1967). The traits noted particularly include guilt, resentment, hostility, multiple somatic complaints, excessive consultations and numerous operations. Most of these features have been confirmed and reconfirmed in subsequent literature. Many of the reports are anecdotal but the systematic ones have shown an increased frequency of operations (Spear 1967) in psychiatric patients with pain and an increased frequency of resentment in the same group compared with those without pain (Merskey 1965b). The marital relationships of the patients have been noted to be disturbed (Merskey 1965b) and this was systematically investigated and confirmed by Mohamed et al (1978) and by many subsequent workers (e.g. Rowat & Knafl 1985; Payne & Norfleet 1986). Several investigators, including Rowat & Knafl (1985), have found the spouses of patients with pain suffer in addition (Flor et al 1987, 1989; Watson et al 1988; Romano et al 1989; Thomas & Roy 1989). On the whole, among these reports the tendency is greater for the wives of male patients to be affected by their partner's pain rather than for the husbands to be affected by their wives' pain. However, Dura & Beck (1988) did show that a wife's chronic pain also had an effect on the husband. Labbe (1988) concluded that the literature suggests that about two-thirds of all back pain patients report sexual problems after the onset of pain, the frequency and quality of activity both being affected. There are increasing reports of sexual abuse in childhood among patients with chronic pain, but the material is not yet sufficient to evaluate satisfactorily. The problems of sampling and comparisons with the base rate for sexual abuse in the population have yet to be dealt with adequately.

PSYCHOLOGICAL ILLNESS IN PAIN CLINICS

Engel (1959) advanced the view, which has been supported also by Blumer (1975), that many patients could adapt themselves to life only by reason of having a traumatic social or personal relationship, such as a bad marriage in which they played a masochistic role, or by suffering from chronic pain.

Engel's hypothesis has been quite influential but only partly confirmed. It suffers from the serious weakness of lack of controlled evidence and the possibility that the cases reported were very highly selected. Merskey (1965b) did find that psychiatric patients with chronic pain were more resentful than psychiatric patients without pain, and irritability in pain patients is a common observation which probably has a biological basis. If pain reflects damage to the body which can, on occasion, result from the actions of an aggressor, it may be expected that it will not only promote rest or retreat but also a more active defence by aggression. However while resentment was shown to be a feature of some chronic pain, Spear (1967) was quite unable to demonstrate that psychiatric patients with pain were more hostile either covertly or overtly than those without. Adler et al (1989) in a small scale but intensive controlled study found that female pain patients experienced more brutality, sexual abuse, punishment and guilt feelings in childhood than three other types of patient. They saw more illness and pain in their parents as well. This evidence is not strong, and could be related to social class differences and differences in employment, but it matches a popular view in support of Violon-Jurfest (1980) who argued that, because of their past experiences, patients could only relate to other individuals through the experience of pain and could not have an affectionate or loving relationship except if they suffered in that way. In other words, one would suppose that although they did not necessarily seek masochistic patterns of relationship, pain offered the same function for them, enabling them to feel that they could be loved. These views tend to be speculative and are not well supported by controlled evidence, but they almost certainly apply to some patients whether or not they have lesions to promote their pain.

Several reports from pain clinics have been discussed already. They represent only some samples from the earlier papers in the very large literature on the psychological aspects of patients in pain clinics. In particular, the number of reports of MMPI findings and of other psychological test results is very great. Perhaps the most important observation in regard to all these reports is that they inevitably reflect the variety of types of clinics, the pattern of selection (which is also called referral bias), and the different tests employed. Many of the findings include reports on the frequency of depression which will be considered further below. They also provide information on the diagnosis of neurotic conditions such as anxiety or hysteria, or characteristics which are held to be typical of anxiety or hysterical personality patterns.

Except where the results are defined by sets of criteria on psychological test scores, these findings may be hard to replicate and criteria are not uniform. However, even where the criteria are uniform, it is not clear that they are reliable or always meaningful. For example, criteria for hypochondriasis which are invariably linked with the MMPI depend upon the proof of the absence of physical illness, which is almost never provided in these populations. The problems of relying upon such test data have been considered by a number of authors.

Where psychiatric techniques are used for the diagnosis of neurotic illness, the criteria are also often somewhat variable and it is only lately that the same criteria have been used, even in a semistandardised form, by different investigators. The principal agent for this purpose has been the Diagnostic and Statistical Manual of the American Psychiatric Association in its third edition (DSM-III 1980 and DSM-III[R] 1987). This manual gives precise criteria, sometimes criticized as a checklist approach, for the diagnosis of psychiatric illnesses. The trouble with those particular illnesses in which we are most interested, namely the so-called 'somatoform disorders', is that the criteria are mostly rather loose and still unsatisfactory. Suggestions for drastic official revisions have been put forward in a current document the 'DSM IV Options Book' (American Psychiatric Association 1991). These suggestions effectively change the title of the condition to 'pain disorder' and require much more substantial evidence of psychiatric problems in order to make an attribution of psychological illness in this diagnosis. The manual as a whole, however, is an unquestionable step forward which will lead to considerable improvement in the reliability of reports on psychiatric illness in various circumstances. Meanwhile, the information which is available is based, for the most part, on the individual diagnostic judgements of psychiatrists, sometimes corroborated by reliability studies or concomitant psychological tests.

One of the first DSM-III studies was by Reich et al (1983). The authors reviewed the psychiatric diagnoses of 43 patients with chronic pain who had not responded well to conventional treatment and found that 98% of the patients had an axis I disorder, i.e. a diagnosis of an illness rather than a personality disorder. Sixteen patients, or 37%, had an axis II disorder, i.e. a personality disorder.

Another paper (Fishbain et al 1986), also using DSM-III criteria, presented data on 283 patients seen consecutively in a comprehensive pain centre. Of these patients, 85% had a 'myofascial syndrome' and all the rest also had an organic diagnosis. Most of the patients appear to have had at least two and sometimes three physical diagnoses, including the myofascial syndrome diagnosis. The commonest secondary diagnosis was degenerative spinal disease, affecting 35%. Only 5.7% of the males and 4.7% of the females did not have at least one diagnosis from DSM-III on axis I.

More than 95% of the patients were seen to have a formal psychiatric condition. Anxiety and adjustment disorders affected 62.5% of all patients, while 56% had an affective disorder; 38% had a conversion disorder and 10% a problem with substance abuse. A number of other diagnoses related to the above were also present, as were a few organic cerebral conditions. Thus, the picture is largely one of anxiety and affective illness, found in almost all patients who also have physical problems.

Personality disorders (axis II) were found in 59%, including dependent personality disorder in 17.4%, passive–aggressive personality in 14.9% and histrionic personality in 11.7%.

The authors wisely note weaknesses in the DSM-III system for diagnosing conversion disorder and for so-called 'psychogenic pain'. They recognize that there is physiological evidence, summarized in the first edition of this book (Wall 1984), which casts grave doubt on the common view that nonanatomical sensory loss implies a hysterical symptom.

The profusion of both physical and psychiatric diagnoses in this report suggests that the patients were a relatively selected sample. Even so, the paper shows much psychiatric disorder in the presence of physical disorder, and anxiety and depression as the principal psychiatric phenomena.

As one might expect psychiatric illness is most often found in those patients where no lesion is evident and it is found less often in patients who do have a lesion. Chaturvedi et al (1984) made a psychiatric diagnosis in 50% only of patients who had lesions with chronic pain, and in 86% of patients who had no lesions. Magni & Merskey (1987) recorded psychiatric diagnoses in 61% of patients with lesions and in 97% of patients without lesions.

Another approach to the examination of psychiatric illness in pain clinics is to undertake screening tests, not measuring the severity of psychiatric illness but its frequency. This does not necessarily give a diagnostic breakdown but will indicate the extent to which a population is thought to suffer from psychiatric illness. A recent survey by Merskey et al (1987) used the General Health Questionnaire 28-item version (GHQ-28). This questionnaire has some advantages over the usual psychiatric questionnaires when employed in nonpsychiatric populations, since it tends to be based on items concerning physical function in the first instance, and then only secondarily does it ask about psychological status. One disadvantage is that it requires adjustment for the presence of physical illness, but this can be made. It has been standardized in numerous studies in the past. When several different types of clinic were compared it was found that an anaesthetist's pain clinic serving a mixed urban and rural population had 37% of patients positive for psychiatric illness. An oral medicine facial pain clinic had 30% positive for psychiatric illness and a rural hospital pain clinic had 37% positive for psychiatric illness. The writer's own personal series of patients, using the same test, had 51% positive for psychiatric illness. This demonstrates the effects of selection on the psychiatric characteristics of different pain populations. However it should be noted that current psychiatric illness was never present in more than approximately half of the population. This is a much lower rate than that found either by Reich et al (1983) or by Fishbain et al (1986). It is certainly possible that some of the difference relates to a lack of sensitivity on the part of the screening test, although this seems somewhat unlikely considering that it is usually more than 80% sensitive and specific in comparison with psychiatric interview. Some part of the difference between the screening test paper by Merskey et al and these two papers may be due to a superior technique of case-finding in the other papers.

Retrospective examination of the writer's own practice by chart review showed that a much higher proportion of the patients than 50% had a psychological problem at some time. Some 47% were positive for definite psychiatric illness using DSM-III criteria and a further 37% had atypical or minor forms of psychological disturbance making 84% affected altogether. Perhaps the most important observation here is that psychological illness in the presence of chronic pain with lesions tends to fluctuate and that it will be present at one time and not at another. This may well depend upon the severity of the pain and the process through which the patient is going. For example, after injury many patients suffer difficulties in employment and marital relationships, as well as continuing insomnia from pain, and become depressed. After a while treatment may take the edge off the worst of their pain, and some of their social difficulties may be resolved, so that although the pain persists, depression and other psychological problems subside. This observation would indicate that much of the depression found with chronic pain with lesions is secondary rather than primary in causing the pain.

Fibromyalgia provides another group of patients in whom psychological changes are evident without accounting for all the cases. It appears from a review of several sources that between 35 and 72% of patients with fibromyalgia have current or past psychiatric disturbance (Merskey 1989). Such a finding leads to the conclusion that while psychiatric factors might promote some cases of fibromyalgia, they are very unlikely to be a principal cause of the illness and the same conclusion probably applies to most cases with chronic pain in medical practice.

Overall, there is no doubt that there is an increased frequency of psychological illness in pain-clinic patients, although it does not necessarily rise to 100%. The most characteristic findings in the psychiatric population within a pain clinic are that depression was found in a significant minority of the patients as well as other anxiety symptoms and social dysfunction; irritability is also a marked feature of the depression seen in pain clinics, especially in comparison with depression seen in other settings. Epidemiological evidence supports this position. Crook et al (1984), in a community survey, found chronic pain in 11% of the adult population and acute pain in a further 5%. Crook et al (1989) have since shown that, compared with the community sample, patients in a pain clinic were more likely to have been injured, reported a greater intensity and constancy of pain and had more difficulties with the activities of daily living. They were more depressed and withdrawn socially and showed more long-term consequences due to unemployment, litigation and alcohol and drug abuse.

Magni et al (1990) reported the relationship between pain and depression in a very carefully chosen epidemiological sample. We obtained data from the United States National Center for Health Statistics based on a survey of a stratified sample of 3023 subjects, aged 25–74 years, 1319 males and 1704 females. Of these, 416 (14.4%) definitely suffered from pain in the musculoskeletal system which had been present on most days for at least 1 month in the 12 months preceding the interview. A total of 219 patients (7.4%) were 'uncertain' cases in the sense that they had some pain, but it was not possible to determine that the duration of their symptoms was at least 1 month, or that they had been present during the previous 12 months. The remaining 2388 (78.1%) had no chronic pain. All these subjects were also given the Depression Scale of the Center for Epidemiologic Studies (CESD). The chronic pain subjects scored significantly higher than normals, and those with pain of uncertain duration scored similar to the definite chronic pain population. In a conservative (i.e. high) cut-off score for depression, 18% of the population with chronic pain were found to have depression compared with 8% of the population who did not have chronic pain. To date these are the most definitive data we have on the relationship in the population between chronic pain and depression, indicating that depression occurs twice as frequently in those with chronic pain as in a controlled sample. There are two questions in the CESD which relate to somatic items that could be due to physical effects (e.g. insomnia), but the use of the high cut-off score effectively cancels their possible influence. In the pain group there were also significantly more females and older people and people with a lower income.

Incidentally, it is worth noting that Merskey et al (1987) obtained a measure of the personality features of the pain population with the hysteroid–obsessoid questionnaire of Caine & Hope (1967) and the mean score for the pain population was slightly towards the obsessional side of the hysteroid–obsessoid continuum. A significant difference was found by clinic, with the psychiatric clinic population being somewhat more obsessoid than the populations of the other three clinics. Premorbid personality did not appear to contribute to the pain complaints themselves nor to social dysfunction. Tauschke et al (1990) also obtained evidence that adult defence mechanisms in patients with pain were related to the presence or absence of psychiatric illness and immature defence mechanisms were greater in patients who had psychiatric illness with or without pain than in those who did not have psychological illness.

A number of the studies in pain clinics have reported upon the frequency of depression in the patients there. Studies of pain in psychiatric patients have also produced data about the frequency of depression. This is an important topic which has been much discussed lately. Before considering it, it is desirable to examine the accepted mechanisms by which psychological illness may produce pain, and also the question of hysteria.

STRESS FACTORS AND CHRONIC PAIN

The influence of psychological factors in causing pain is often thought to be mediated through stress. Vulnerable individuals faced with difficult circumstances may develop pain in response. Three principal phenomena should be associated with this hypothesis. First, there should be evidence of stress sufficient to cause emotional change. Second, there should be evidence of emotional change. Third, the people affected should be at greater risk than average.

Although it is often recognized that stress occurs in conjunction with chronic pain, particularly the sort of chronic pain for which patients are referred to hospital, there is little satisfactory evidence on the topic. Good evidence is hard to obtain because the task is very time-consuming. The popular checklists for stress are not efficient or satisfactory and an adequate measure usually requires a lengthy interview to determine prior life events. The methodology is difficult (Brown et al 1973). Jensen (1988) compared patients with low-back pain, with and without nerve-root compression, and two groups of headache patients. Comparison of the frequency of single life events within the previous 12 months revealed no statistically significant differences among the diagnostic groups. The same applied to the total number of life events and the number of life events with transient distress or enduring distress. A number of life events with transient distress were found to show a significant negative association with the persistence of pain in patients with headache but not in other groups. However, even this finding does not appear to be significant after correction for multiple tests.

Atkinson et al (1988) hypothesized that low-back pain patients with depressed mood would report significantly more untoward life events and ongoing life difficulties than chronic low-back pain patients without depressed mood and controls. Their prediction was confirmed. However, the increased stress reported by the depressed group appeared to be a direct consequence of life events related to back pain rather than from other life problems. This supports a model of pain causing disability or disadvantage rather than the latter causing the pain. Kukull et al (1986) showed similarly that, among outpatients in a general medical clinic, depression appeared to result most often from physical illness. Those who were not depressed initially but became depressed had more new physical illness.

Marbach et al (1988) undertook a thorough study of life events in patients with temporomandibular pain and dysfunction syndrome. They found no preponderance of life events in the patients with facial pain compared with controls except after the onset of the symptom. The occurrence of other physical illness was more common in these patients. This may suggest an association of types of musculoskeletal change but it does not suggest an effect of stress in producing the illnesses originally. Speculand et al (1984) found some evidence with a similar syndrome which they felt favoured the occurrence of life events as a precipitating factor.

In none of this work does it appear that life events reflect even a large subordinate portion of the variance in explaining the appearance of pain. The NUPRIN Study (Sternbach 1986) showed that individuals approached by telephone in the community reported a strong association between stress and pain in that minor ongoing stresses and strains of daily living – 'hassles' – were related to pain in different locations, including headache and backache. It would fly in the face of ordinary experience to suggest that stress does not cause chronic pain but it seems equally clear that the contribution is not large. Most studies have not shown either that stressful life events will precipitate or increase headache or low-back pain and life events have not been used for predicting the results of treatment (Jensen 1988).

Another perspective is suggested by the Boeing study in Seattle, Washington (Bigos et al 1991). This study has been widely taken as indicating that one of the most important factors in back pain is the satisfaction of the employee with his or her job. This was a prospective study of workers in an aircraft factory of whom 279 out of 3020 reported back problems when followed longitudinally. The subjects who stated they 'hardly ever' enjoyed their job tasks were 2.5 times more likely to report a back injury ($P = 0.0001$) than subjects who 'almost always' enjoyed their job tasks. There are some limitations to this study. Only 75% of those who were solicited to take part in the study actually participated, and only 54% of these respondents, i.e. only 40.5% of the total, were studied. Some 279 out of 1569 reported back pain but only 89 of them (32%) actually did not enjoy their job. After deducting from this figure the 40% who presumably had other reasons for sickness, although they were also discontented, we are left with 53 workers (19%) who are likely to have been off work because they were discontented. In any case, this is a short-term study, dealing with relatively acute pain and does not demonstrate the factors involved in chronic pain. There is reason to believe that many people who dislike work and have adequate insurance will take extra time off, or take some time off, when they have a modest illness, but not that they will prolong this into chronic pain which requires much more substantial treatment and is much more disruptive to the working life. In a substantial study of large numbers of patients with chronic pain in different centres, Gamsa (1990) provided evidence that psychological changes were more related to the occurrence of pain than to premorbid characteristics. The same implication appears from several studies in which we have undertaken screening procedures for psychological illness in relation to chronic pain (Salter et al 1983; Merskey et al 1985, 1987; Zilli et al 1989). As we have already noticed, less than 50% of patients receiving treatment for chronic pain show significant evidence of psychiatric illness. This means that even if all such cases had pain because of their emotional state the hypothesis of psychogenesis of pain could fit only a minority. There is also only a small relationship at most between previous personality and current symptoms of anxiety and depression in patients with pain (Merskey et al 1987). The foregoing indicates that although there may be a relationship between stress and the production of pain, the relationship is not a strong one and in the absence of psychological illness has not been shown to account for pain syndromes which appear to have a pathophysiological or organic basis.

MECHANISMS OF PAIN

There are five ways in which psychological illness may be causally related to the appearance or increase of pain. The first is perhaps one of the most common and has to do with the increase of pain which occurs when patients who have a lesion are worried about it. The precise psychological mechanism of this effect is unknown. Nevertheless, it is frequently observed that patients who have a state of anxiety experience much greater pain from lesions than would otherwise be expected. A reduction of their anxiety leads to a considerable reduction in their pain. Perhaps this is the situation where gate-theory-type explanations are most relevant to pain due to psychological causes. It is plausible to suppose that pain which is related to some existing activity in peripheral nerve pathways may be greatly increased as a result of heightened arousal in the patient, so that an effect is transmitted through descending pathways to the spinal cord, thus increasing the abnormal activity which itself is ultimately the basis for the experience of pain in consciousness. This explanation remains speculative but pain in clinical practice is frequently much relieved by measures which relieve the patient's anxiety about the provocative lesion.

Pain may also at times, but very rarely, be due to psychotic hallucinations. The most clear-cut and most rare example of this is in schizophrenia. Typical schizophrenic hallucinations are almost never concerned with pain. Schizophrenic patients do have some pains, for example, dull headache, which may be hallucinatory but which are not readily recognizable as such. They have frequent bodily experiences of other people doing things to them, such as hypnotising them, influencing them with rays and so forth, but it is astonishing how rarely they indicate that these bodily changes are painful. In a series of

78 patients with schizophrenia only one was found whose pain might be attributed to her delusion (Watson et al 1981) and, as it happens, that patient was suffering from an atypical or schizoaffective illness. Perhaps slightly more often, depressive patients may have delusions which appear to give rise to hallucinations – for example, a patient who felt that she was being punished and who was experiencing stabbing pains in her buttocks and genitals. Usually it is reasonable to suppose that the pain associated with depression is like that found with anxiety or with hysterical conditions to be discussed below.

The third mechanism of the production of pain which may be considered is the well-known tension pain mechanism. There is no doubt that, if muscles are exercised in the absence of adequate circulation, they will give rise to discomfort and even very severe pain. This was demonstrated over 60 years ago (Lewis et al 1931). The common hypothesis holds that inadequate removal of waste products from the tissues provides noxious stimulation.

Unaccustomed exercise of almost any bodily part, especially under conditions of emotional tension, may hence give rise to pain which is attributable to muscle contraction. The very term 'muscle contraction headache', which is a popular diagnostic category, implies this aetiological theory. Anyone who has driven a new car (or one with which he was not very familiar) in difficult driving conditions over long distances may have experienced comparable aching and discomfort in muscles which were used in an unaccustomed fashion. Thus the notion of muscle tension pain is easily understood and widely popular. It is a perfectly acceptable explanation for many cases in ordinary life and also for many people who have anxiety and who have increased muscle tension. The limitation to this theory is that it is probably excessively applied to all types of pain from psychological causes. Thus there are many patients who have chronic pain who do not show the increase in muscular tension which might be expected (Sainsbury & Gibson 1954). This has been particularly well-known in studies where patients with so-called muscle contraction headache had less frontal muscle tension than patients with migraine (Pozniak-Patewicz 1976; Bakal & Kaganov 1977). Muscle tension in patients with chronic headache only accounts for a very small proportion of the pain, as little as 5% of the variance (Epstein et al 1978; Martin & Mathews 1978). The pain is more related to personality disorder and measures thereof (Harper & Steger 1978). Moreover, traditional methods of relieving anxiety and muscle tension (relaxation, psychotherapy, anxiolytic-medication) are largely ineffective in these chronic cases. It is therefore felt that there is a group of patients for whom another explanation must be provided.

The fourth explanation, and one which presumably applies to many of the patients with chronic headache and other chronic pains without clear evidence of physical illness, is the production of pain by hysterical mechanisms. The idea that pain can be a hysterical symptom has been recognised since antiquity and has been popular since the Middle Ages at least. Perhaps it has been too popular and some pains which were not due to hysteria were too readily explained in that way. However, there are several anecdotal and observational instances which give an indication of how such a pain may appear. The best example of pain due to the patient's thoughts or due to a hysterical process may be that of the couvade syndrome where husbands have the pains which their wives would normally experience in labour. This has been well studied by Reik (1914), Bardhan (1965a, 1965b), Curtis (1965), Trethowan & Conlon (1965) and Trethowan (1968).

Another striking example of pain due to hysterical mechanisms is probably to be found in the report by Rawnsley & Loudon (1964) who were able to show that many patients in a group whom they studied and who had a history of headache had a previous history of gross hysterical fits. Anecdotal instances which have some theoretical significance have been described in several places by the present writer. An important study by Kudrow & Sutkus (1979) showed that, the longer patients were in a headache clinic, the more evidence they had of hysterical patterns, i.e. of the conversion V triad in MMPI test results. Thus it is reasonable to suppose that the psychological mechanisms of chronic pain in psychiatric and other patients include hysterical conversion. Also, the more intractable the pain the more it appears that hysterical patterns of behaviour will be found.

While this may not be a mechanism of pain in exactly the same way as the other factors just discussed, hypochondriasis is liable to promote pain and may transform a minor physical complaint into a substantial psychological and medical problem. Occasionally too, the hypochondriacal nature of the pain symptom is more marked than any other pattern and represents the principal diagnosis and explanation. Mild hypochondriasis amounts to excessive concern with bodily symptoms and is often dispelled by reassurance when that can be given appropriately. It is then a form of expression of anxiety, very well considered recently by Kellner (1986) and Barsky & Klerman (1983). Barsky & Wyshak (1990) provided evidence of a tendency of hypochondriacal patients to amplify bodily sensations in response to a questionnaire. This extends the earlier fundamental work of Pilowsky (1967) in which it was well demonstrated that the other principal phenomena of hypochondriasis are fear of disease combined with a conviction that disease is present, as well as bodily preoccupation. Such tendencies are common among patients who have chronic pain, but the recognition should not, as with hypochondriasis in general, overshadow the need to appreciate the existence of a physical mechanism in many instances.

PROBLEMS OF HYSTERIA

Some comments were made on hysteria earlier. However, no discussion of hysteria as a cause of pain is sufficient without a warning. The mere absence of physical evidence for a cause of pain does not justify a diagnosis of hysteria. This diagnosis must always be made on positive evidence. In cases of paralysis and some other types of loss of function, it can be shown by neurological examination that there is positive evidence that the patient is able to do things which he or she thinks are not feasible. In the case of pain itself, that opportunity does not exist. On the contrary, there are probably certain signs which are traditionally taken to be evidence of hysteria which are misleading in that respect in patients with pain. The first of these signs is the so-called 'give-way' weakness. Many patients in a state of pain who frankly are able to use their limbs in different ways will refuse to do so, knowing that to comply with the examiner's request would hurt them. Either consciously or unconsciously they are affected by 'pain inhibition'. That should not be taken to suggest that they have hysteria or even that they are 'hysterical'. Further, the occurrence of non-anatomical sensory loss is not necessarily hysterical either. Wall (1984) summarized evidence which indicates that at least some cells in the dorsal horn may have receptive fields from the whole of a limb. Thus, as Fishbain et al (1986) point out, the issue of nondermatomal sensory abnormalities and their significance may need more research. These findings are extremely frequent and may well reflect an aspect of pain physiology which has not been properly understood. Particularly in view of the findings by Wall and his colleagues that receptive fields of cells in the spinal cord can change enormously in response to pain in a limb, it becomes evident that regional nondermatomal changes cannot be relied upon as signs of hysteria. This view is reinforced from another direction by the work of Gould et al (1986) who examined 30 patients with acute organic disease of the nervous system and demonstrated that they showed a high frequency of signs which are supposed to be characteristic of hysteria. Seven traditional signs were examined; namely, a history suggestive of hypochondriasis, potential secondary gain, belle indifference, nonanatomical or patchy sensory loss, changing boundaries of hypoalgesia, sensory loss (to pinprick or vibratory stimulation) that splits at the midline and give-way weakness. All the patients demonstrated at least one of the above. Of these 30 patients, 29 showed at least one feature of a supposedly nonphysiological sensory examination. The mean number of these items per patient was 3.4. The authors infer that hysteria is easily misdiagnosed if the above signs or items of history are accepted as pathognomonic, and many tests which are said to provide good evidence of hysteria lack validity.

There are several conditions which are basically physical and have been mistaken for hysteria or even for malingering. The writer has known some of them to be diagnosed as psychiatric, e.g. pain from ectopia cerebelli, facial pain with dyskinetic movements, and even the thoracic outlet syndrome in the presence of physical signs. In recent years the fibrosis or diffuse myofascial pain syndrome (IASP category 1.9, code X33.X8a) has been well-characterized as a physical disorder (Smythe 1985; Wolfe et al 1990). Localized myofascial syndromes have also been increasingly recognized (Littlejohn, 1986; IASP 1986). Such relatively subtle syndromes which depend for their recognition on advances or improvement in clinical method may have often been misdiagnosed as hysteria in the past and the possibility still exists of such a misdiagnosis.

If the diagnosis of hysteria is to be made on psychiatric grounds, there must be evidence for this from psychological examination, to an extent which shows that psychological problems and causes are present in proportion to the symptom. Moreover, they should ideally be accepted by the patient as the principal causes of his complaint. This situation is rarely achieved.

It is relevant at this point to comment on the relationship between psychiatry and pain in routine practice. Most psychiatric patients are seen in outpatient departments, and pain is a major problem in only a minority. Even when they do present with pain, particularly headache, which is the commonest type of pain in psychiatric patients (Merskey 1965b; Spear 1967), the pain is frequently relegated to a secondary place whilst the psychiatrist concentrates on the psychiatric disorders and causes of illness which he is able to find. More often, patients who have pain about which they are particularly concerned tend to appear in headache clinics or in pain clinics, and the psychiatrist there has the extra task of adding his advice on the care of individuals who are generally disinclined to think of their illness in psychological terms and are more prone to think of it in physical terms. This is perhaps even more often a problem for nonpsychiatrists who seek to refer the patient to the psychiatrist. The management of this objection is difficult for all physicians and surgeons, and it is normally handled in several different ways depending on the individual case. Some patients who are able to accept the advice that they need psychological help – or who even volunteer for it themselves – are readily referred. Others are persuaded to see psychiatrists because they are told that the individual doctor has experience or an interest in the treatment of pain which goes beyond his particular specialty, and this is to some extent a justifiable approach. Still others are seen in psychiatric practice because the patients are told that automatically everybody entering a pain clinic or centre is assessed in both physical and psychological respects. This is perhaps one of the easiest and most effective ways of providing a psychological assessment and is one of the particular advantages of pain clinics.

PHYSICAL SIGNS AND PSYCHOLOGICAL ILLNESS

The detection of psychological illness, or a psychological problem, by means of supposedly 'nonorganic' physical signs has long been popular, and it was noted above that this can be a useful method for demonstrating the presence of psychological problems. Difficulties were recognized in applying some of these approaches to patients with pain. Nevertheless, an impressive sustained effort has been made to do this, particularly by Waddell and his colleagues (1980, 1984, 1987, 1989). The fundamental initial study in this series demonstrated the use of five types of physical sign to indicate the occurrence of psychological problems. They were tenderness (superficial or nonanatomic), simulated physical stresses leading to a report of pain (either from axial loading or rotation), distraction (in straight leg raising), regional alterations (weakness or sensory change) and overreaction. Patients without back pain had none of these. British patients with previously untreated back pain referred to a routine hospital orthopaedic clinic had one or more of these signs in about 10% of cases. This figure compares with one-third of cases in both Canadian and British patients with more persistent problems (failed surgery, chronic disability, etc.). These signs had a strong relationship to the judgement by a surgeon that the condition was 'nonorganic' or that the patient was unsuitable for surgery. They also had a strong relationship to general somatic and neurotic symptoms, so-called disability behaviour and 'inappropriate symptoms'. There was a low but consistent correlation in one study in which the neurotic triad of scores of the MMPI was used but no relationship with the Eysenck Personality Questionnaire (EPQ) in British patients.

Subsequent work demonstrated a great deal of consistency and reliability in the measurements of these signs (Waddell & Main 1984) and that both objective physical impairment and psychological distress accounted for significant proportions of the disability observed. Thus, physical impairment was thought to account for about 40% of the disability observed, depression and increased bodily awareness for 22.5% between them and 'magnified illness behaviour' for 8.4% of the variance (Waddell et al 1984b). Four patients with partial cord lesions, three with cauda equina lesions and two with lumbosacral injuries did not show these signs. The authors concluded very reasonably that 'Disability in low back pain can be understood in terms of physical impairment, psychological distress and illness behaviour, each of which can be defined, observed and measured'. Those patients who had more evidence of inappropriate illness behaviour received more treatment (Waddell et al 1984a). The implications of these findings and further studies were explored by Waddell et al (1989) with the use of the Illness Behaviour Questionnaire of Pilowsky & Spence (1976). Disease affirmation or disease conviction were observed to be prominent in patients with chronic low-back pain.

This series of studies is unmatched in methodology, numbers and attention to detail. The result might be thought to imply that much disability from back pain is due to the mental state of the patients rather than the physical illness. The authors themselves are cautious about such a conclusion. They suggested that these signs should not be sought to indicate psychological problems in patients who are over the age of 55–69 or who have acute causes of pain. Waddell et al (1980) also point out that it is wise to assume that there is a physical basis in most cases of back pain. Further, the figures quoted show that 40% of the variance with disability is related to demonstrable physical illness and 31% to the psychological state. The contributions of the two types of factor appear to be fairly similar.

Two more qualifications should be expressed concerning this phenomenon. The first qualification is that some of the so-called nonorganic physical signs are less nonorganic than was thought. I discussed earlier the difficulty of proving that signs of 'hysteria' were free from organic influence as shown by Gould et al (1986). It is true that the work of Waddell does not utilize the same signs as that of Gould except for give-way weakness which only appeared in one of Gould's cases. Nevertheless as with regional weakness it is not accurate to interpret superficial tenderness or regional pain syndromes as due to psychological factors. Among the other signs on which reliance has been placed, simulation and overreaction place a burden (which may be legitimate) on the judgement of the examiner. One also has to note that in the instructions connected with the measurement of responses to simulated stresses, the stress of pressure on the neck giving rise to pain is found to be common and should be discounted, whereas the same effect lower down the vertebral column is not common and is taken into account as psychological. Further, if the more severe cases of pain have more of these findings is it because they are a nonspecific accompaniment of the more intense physical disorder or because they are due primarily to a psychological cause? This is a substantial problem which has not been resolved.

In order to show that the 'nonorganic' signs are attributable to something other than the severity of the painful disorder, and are due to an independent variable, such as a wish for compensation or a state of depression due to bereavement and not connected with the physical disorder, it is necessary to establish the occurrence of stressful events or other psychological causes more often in those individuals who show significant amounts of 'nonorganic' signs compared with those who have a comparable physical state but do not show those signs. This does not appear to have been done. As noted above it is not an easy task. It certainly must apply at times. However, in so far as investigations of stress factors in relation to chronic pain have been successful they have mostly shown that the worst stresses appear to arise in relation to consequences of pain and the disability associated with it.

Some other correlates of the 'nonorganic' signs are also misleading. A modest relationship with the MMPI is not meaningful in terms of a psychological aetiology since, as mentioned earlier, that test merely counts symptoms, many of which on the most relevant scales relate to complaints about the physical state of the body.

Lastly, and most importantly, even if pain is due to a physical cause it will in that case, as in any other case, be experienced as a subjective condition. This is inherent in all accepted definitions of pain. The final statement about pain is subjective. The associated experience of the patient is subjective. Subjective psychological measures, whether they reflect independent psychological causes, or the mental state of an individual suffering from significant physical problems will always show the closest relationships between pain and subjective measures. Pain cannot be expressed otherwise than through reports of distress and subjective experience. Measures of distress will always be powerfully influenced by it. It follows that the patient's subjective awareness may well give a better estimate of the actual physical state than the physician's external measurements.

BEHAVIOURAL THEORIES OF PAIN – BEHAVIOURAL MEASURES

Fordyce et al (1981) have shown systematically that exercise helps to reduce pain or the behaviour related to it. It has long been recognized that exercise can be beneficial in some cases of pain. Stiffness produced by overactivity may be abated by further activity (a day or two later). In clinical practice however it remains very difficult at times to know which patients will benefit from exercise and which will be made worse. Hilton (1863) argued that rest is also beneficial for pain and despite some qualifications this remains true for many cases. Pain which is related to disuse and inactivity of muscles may be the sort which will respond best to behavioural measures. Pain which is related to current tenderness and spasm is much less likely to benefit. Hence exercise programmes which are increasingly common in North America appear to have great success with relatively easy cases but give rise to a good deal of discontent on the part of patients when the effort is made to apply exercise in the more protracted cases with continuing indications of some sort of musculoskeletal dysfunction, and no improvement after continuing effort.

The question of exercise is a subordinate topic within the larger issue of behavioural treatment of patients with chronic pain. Indeed, it can be separated from it since it also has a physiological rationale. Efforts to treat patients by behavioural means which discourage so called 'pain behaviour' and encourage activity have continued through the 1980s. Current books or articles on pain frequently indicate a behavioural element in programmes for the treatment of pain (Sternbach 1987; Aronoff 1988; Loeser & Egan 1989; Bonica 1990). The theory of this treatment has been advanced (Fordyce et al 1985, 1988; Rachlin 1985) and criticized (Atkinson & Kremer 1985; Merskey 1985; Schmidt 1987, 1988). Critics of the theoretical position of the operant school of treatment are extremely wary of Fordyce's view that '... *behavioural methods* in pain treatment programs *are intended to treat excess disability and expressions of suffering*'. They wonder if the clinician is going to be as skilful as is necessary in defining 'excess disability and expressions of suffering'. Anyone who gets this wrong is going to be pushing patients repeatedly to do things which are increasingly difficult and painful for them. We have seen this often and it is not a pretty matter. This is a lesser point, though a grievous one in practice, than the fundamental issue which Fordyce (1976) previously stated, namely, that the subjective state of the patient is not a matter of concern to him, provided behaviour can change. Rachlin (1985) complained that Fordyce makes it harder to defend his valid position by this particular notion. Schmidt (1988), however, demonstrated that the operant approach by Fordyce and colleagues has confused pain, ratings of pain by the sufferer and pain behaviours, although Fordyce (1990) disputes this. No matter how much argument there is around this topic it seems that the notion of treating pain behaviour involves some denial of the patient's experience.

Although I have not seen this discussed it appears that there is a significant potential problem of conflict of interest in programmes which aim to treat patients behaviourally. Of course all practitioners who follow such a policy are likely to establish a contract with the patient and obtain the patient's agreement and informed consent. If the therapist has a special interest, he makes it clear to the patient. In many countries such as Great Britain or Canada the problem of conflict of interest in this connection will not often arise because medical care is often wholly funded from public sources or directly by the patient. A different situation obtains in many jurisdictions, particularly in the United States where a considerable proportion of the patients in pain clinics have their treatment funded by insurance carriers. The best interest of an insurance company lies in getting the insured person back to health and strength, but also in establishing that the insured person will receive treatment directed to his employability. That, too, is in the interest of the insured. Nevertheless it appears that patients are more interested than insurance companies in relieving pain but in order to satisfy the companies, clinics have to provide programmes which offer to remove *disability* rather than necessarily remove *pain*. In fact one aim may be sacrificed for the sake of another. The considerable popularity of behavioural programmes in the United States may have something to do with the need to talk to insurance companies in terms which encourage them to provide funds for treatment of the affected individuals. The style of treatment adopted in consequence is not necessarily one which would otherwise be favoured.

As an alternative, many psychologists have adopted cognitive approaches which are dealt with elsewhere in this volume. It is worthwhile pointing out here that Flor & Turk (1989) have shown that cognitive variables in rheumatoid arthritis explain between 32 and 60% of the variance in pain and disability and did so more effectively than physical measures. There is increasing recognition that the patient's awareness of disability and distress predicts outcome better than the physician's estimate of the physical status in a number of instances. Perhaps this is because the patient's awareness effectively takes into account both his physical state and his feelings.

Anderson et al (1988) showed that psychological variables did not independently predict pain behaviour in rheumatoid arthritis. This particular study was accompanied by a thorough rating of pain behaviours such as guarding, bracing, grimacing, sighing, rigidity, passive rubbing and active rubbing. One of the most striking findings was that pain behaviour was most closely related to physical illness. This ought to be in accordance with expectation since the model of pain behaviour was developed out of the model of physical disease. Pain behaviour is thought to be anomalous only when it is not matched by physical disease to a considerable extent. Thoughts on this have been confused at times by the fact that some physical measures are not very satisfactory, e.g. X-ray measurements are a poor organic index for the pain of patients with osteoarthritis. Anderson et al, like Keefe et al (1990) demonstrate effectively that the strongest relationship of pain behaviour is found to be with physical illness. As Anderson et al state 'in our prior investigations . . . rigidity and guarding were the behaviours that were the most highly associated with disease activity variables and self report of functional disability . . . the results of multiple studies support the validity of guarding and rigidity as measures of RA pain . . . '.

Meanwhile, the studies of Keefe and his colleagues do identify a subgroup of patients with low-back pain who have some evidence of pain behaviour and only moderate complaints of pain. This group remains a focus of attention and amounted to 19% of the sample of Keefe et al taken from patients referred to a pain management programme who were participating in structured inpatient treatment. Whether or not this group had its pain from mainly psychological or behavioural reasons is not clear. The findings are somewhat reminiscent of the conclusions of Leavitt et al (1982) on another occasion that perhaps 10% of patients with chronic back pain are not adequately diagnosed psychiatrically or physically. Keefe's subgroup may also only have had less severe pain than others. In summary the work of this group suggests that pain behaviour can be measured quite effectively but that it should not be misinterpreted as merely a sign of operant pain. This type of pain behaviour is more marked with movement and cannot easily be measured without inducing movement.

Psychological studies of coping and behaviour bear obvious links with other issues that we have been considering. Thus, the way in which individuals cope may be influenced by or may influence the relationships within the family, the frequency of pain or its severity and the extent of the emergence of depression. Watt-Watson et al (1988) have demonstrated relationships between depression and coping responses, pain intensity and family function. Coping responses also had a significant relationship with pain intensity and family functioning. This is but one of numerous papers which indicate the importance of a comprehensive appraisal of the situation of individuals with chronic pain.

DEPRESSION IN PATIENTS WITH PAIN

In the discussion of psychiatric illness in patients with pain and also in examining the frequency of psychiatric illness in patients attending pain clinics, it was observed that depression is often found in both such populations. Some workers have reported that a particularly high proportion of pain-clinic patients have depression. For example, Lindsay & Wyckoff (1981), from the University of Washington Pain Clinic in Seattle, indicated that, out of 150 consecutive referrals to the clinic of patients with nonmalignant pain, at least 85% had depression according to the research diagnostic criteria of Feighner et al (1972). Perhaps those criteria were easier to satisfy than some others. In contrast, Large (1980), as described above, found 46 diagnoses of one type of depression or another among 172 pain-clinic patients. Using quite stringent psychological screening tests, Pilowsky et al (1977) demonstrated that depression affected only 10% of their series of patients. Pelz & Merskey (1982) observed that 83 pain-clinic patients, all with lesions, had a mean score on the Levine–Pilowsky depression questionnaire of 7.13, which placed them in the 'nondepressed group'. Even 12 patients who were receiving tricyclic antidepressants were also in this category. Thus, although occasional cases of depressive illness were recognized in pain-clinic patients, they were only a minority. On the other hand, a far larger number of patients may express some complaint of dysphoric mood or depression as a symptom, such as 'feeling blue'. Thus, 26.5% of patients confessed to 'feeling blue' compared with the very small number who admitted to depression in that study.

A specific study by Kramlinger et al (1983), using Research Diagnostic Criteria (Spitzer et al 1978) found that 25 were definitely depressed, 39 were probably depressed and 36 were not depressed. In the author's own chart review of patients seen in psychiatric consultation for painful conditions, nine out of 32 patients had major affective disorder and 12 had atypical affective disorder (Merskey et al 1987). Thus, the proportion with a well-defined affective illness was limited to 28%. Only with the inclusion of atypical affective disorder does the figure for depression reach 66%. However, atypical affective disorder is so easily diagnosed as to be commonplace in innumerable medical settings, and perhaps in the general population. The importance to be given to depression when it is found frequently in pain-clinic patients may thus be very much diminished if the finding of high frequency is based on a very mild state.

The numerous reports of pain in relation to depression have been reviewed by Roy et al (1984), Romano & Turner (1985), and Gupta (1986). All these reviews point to the inconsistency of the data available in the literature and the limitations of the different studies and their methodological differences. There are few controlled studies and the diagnostic criteria in relation to both depression and pain are often not rigorous enough. The populations are extremely heterogeneous, different instruments are used, some patients come from one source and some from another, as already considered, and some have organic lesions and some not. Overall, while there is probably an increased frequency of depression in pain-clinic patients and of pain in patients with depression, the frequency will vary with the sample and with the method used for measuring depression, and in most pain-clinic populations, other than specialized centres, the writer estimates that the frequency of sustained depression will be of the order of about 10–30%. The frequency of depression in patients with chronic musculoskeletal pain is 14.4% compared with a population incidence of depression of 8%. However, we cannot tell from that finding alone whether the pain causes depression or the depression is due to pain. Other data which suggest that the depression is often due to pain were discussed above, particularly the appearance of depression in patients whose burdens from pain become sufficiently high, and whose depression reduces when the severity of the pain and burden decrease. Some direct, albeit retrospective evidence, comes from the work of Atkinson et al (1991) who showed that patients with chronic pain from industrial injuries had depression twice as often after their injury as prior to it. The same patients also showed more evidence of alcoholism prior to their injuries compared with controls which tends to suggest that the recording of illness before and after the injury was objective.

Another condition which provides increasing evidence to suggest organic effects in causing depression or psychological change is the cervical sprain ('whiplash') syndrome. Macnab (1964) has long established that this is a condition with an important physical basis in terms of torn muscles, ligaments and even disks. Taylor (1991) has shown from postmortem examinations that many patients with relatively 'minor' cervical injury suffer splitting of their cervical disks. Radanov et al (1991) found that the only variable which they could discover to predict cognitive function at 6 months was the severity of the pain at the time of the initial injury. Patients with this problem frequently become depressed in the course of the illness when they were not depressed previously.

One aspect of the relationship between pain and depression which has often been considered deserves further comment. There are some patients who appear to have no explanation for their pain physically and who also do not seem to be depressed. Moreover, no other psychiatric diagnosis seems to be feasible. No doubt in some of these cases further inquiry and time will reveal an unknown physical cause or a psychiatric one. Recently, Magni et al (1987a) collected a group of patients who had such a pattern of pain and examined them systematically for phenomena associated with depression such as a family history of depressive disorders and related phenomena. They found that this group of patients had an increased family history of so-called 'depressive spectrum disorders' compared with a normal group. Further they found that imipramine binding was reduced in patients with this pattern of illness in the same direction as patients with depression but not to the same extent. These authors then went on to show (Magni et al 1987b) that the pain responded to antidepressant treatment, particularly in those patients who had a reduced number of imipramine binding sites and also a family history of depression. This leads to the conclusion that there are sometimes patients whose cerebral pathophysiology is such that they will respond to antidepressants in the same way as patients with depression, but who lack the evidence of a depressed mood.

Patients who have this condition, or this state, have previously been diagnosed as having 'depressive equivalents'. Such a diagnosis, however, lacks clinical criteria and ought to be avoided. The best term for those patients for whom no physical or organic cause can be shown is probably 'indeterminate pain'. Magni (1987) has recently reviewed the evidence for the explanation of indeterminate pain as being related to depression at times.

PAIN PROMOTING PSYCHOLOGICAL ILLNESS

Most authors who have worked with patients with chronic pain due to lesions have come to the conclusion that changes are liable to occur in the emotional state of people who are otherwise normal as a result of their experience of prolonged pain. Weir Mitchell (1872) observed the condition of a man with causalgia who, from being 'one of gay and kindly temper', became morose and apparently furious. Patients with pain, and especially with chronic pain from physical lesions, may be expected to be worn down and generally made miserable by their experience. Taub (personal communication 1972) observed that patients in a neurological clinic with such conditions tended to present a picture initially of anxiety and depression. This contrasts with the expectation that patients with pain of psychological origin will have slightly more hypochondriacal or hysterical aspects to their emotional disorder. Comparing patients with physical lesions and those without Woodforde & Merskey (1972) found that those who had their pain from lesions actually became more anxious, more depressed and more subject to signs of neuroticism than patients whose pain had no physical cause and who were known to have psychiatric illness. Patients with physical causes for their pain did, however, tend to see themselves as being persons who in the past were well-adjusted, stable, successful and well-controlled. This gave them high scores on the L-scale of the Eysenck Personality Inventory. That scale was at first thought to indicate a tendency to falsify the account of the individual's previous personality by 'faking good'. Evidence from other studies such as Morgenstern (1967) and Bond (1971) indicates that higher scores are also associated with physical disability, and it appears that, in patients with pain of organic origin, high L scores accompanied by raised neuroticism scores may have the following explanation (Woodforde & Merskey 1972); they represent the response of individuals struggling to keep themselves stable in the face of damage done to their personalities who nevertheless feel that they were once fit, well and effective people. Despite increasing anxiety and depression, the patient looks back to a time when perhaps, in fact, he was indeed free from those psychological troubles because he was not beset by intractable pain. Evidence from another direction supports this, in that Sternbach et al (1973) showed that chronic-pain patients had increased hysteria, depression and hypochondriasis scores on the MMPI compared with patients with acute back pain, while Sternbach & Timmermans (1975) showed a reduction of neuroticism in patients whose pain was relieved by back surgery. Crown & Crown (1973) showed that patients with late rheumatoid arthritis had more personality change than those with early arthritis (who resembled normals). In the case of animals, experimental pain gives rise to aggressive responses – biting the bars of the cage or the neighbour (O'Kelly & Steckley 1939). Aggression in response to pain is presumably part of the fight or flight mechanism, the alternative being retreat. Thus it seems that we should also expect emotional change to appear quite consistently in patients who have chronic lesions.

Fordyce (1976) has noted that the degree of neuroticism shown in the MMPI studies is related more to the chronicity of the pain than to its basis in physical lesions. This particularly applies to the conversion V pattern. Nevertheless, the predominance of obsessional anxiety and depressive symptoms in patients with physical lesions studied by Woodforde & Merskey (1972) does support Taub's idea, mentioned above, that anxiety and depression are more characteristic of patients with troublesome lesions.

Studies which enable us to discriminate between patients with lesions and those without lesions on the basis of MMPI scores or other psychological techniques are rather few or slight. Other studies using the MMPI have, however, been used to predict successfully which patients would respond to organic treatment (chemonucleolysis), to surgery (Wiltse & Rocchio 1975; Smith & Duerksen 1980; Oostdam et al 1981), or to conservative treatment (McCreary et al 1979). Not all studies have agreed that it is possible to discriminate in this way (Waring et al 1976). Another approach to the separation of patients by psychological techniques on the basis of their psychiatric characteristics has been made by Bradley et al (1978) who have tried to discern MMPI groupings which would signify different types of pain patients. Sternbach did so earlier (1974) and the effort should be continued. Meanwhile, one approach which has helped in the discrimination, by psychological means, of groups of patients with lesions and without lesions is the use of the McGill Pain Questionnaire (MPQ). Although it has been argued by the present writer that in general the descriptions of pain by patients with lesions and without lesions are remarkably similar (Devine & Merskey 1965), it appears that there are times and occasions when a distinction can be made between the two groups of patients on the basis of their response to the adjectival check lists of the MPQ. Leavitt & Garron (1979a, 1979b) have indeed reported substantial success in this respect. They were also able to show that patients who did not have a detectable lesion, but who did not have psychiatric illness either, used language which suggested that they fell in the group of patients with organic lesions which had not yet been discovered.

PATTERNS OF ILLNESS

Overall, the patterns of psychological illness which are associated with pain are essentially those of the particular psychological conditions with which the pain is occurring. Pain has not so far been shown to differ significantly in patients according to psychiatric diagnosis. Nevertheless, there are some patterns of pain which may be recognized in patients whose pain is primarily of psychological origin. The pain may be expected to occur more often in women than in men, but if it occurs in men it will be more often in association with a disability which has occurred at work and provides some compensatory benefits, at least financially. In chronic pain of psychological origin, the pain is usually severe. The commonest sites nowadays in the United States and Britain are first of all the head, and secondly the low back. The genitals may be affected in as many as 10% of patients but special enquiry may be needed to show this. Frequently the patient has pain in more than one part of the body and indeed, unless a well-recognized organic diagnosis is evident, pain in more than two sites of the body is suggestive of pain of psychological origin. The pain is bilateral or symmetrical in approximately half the patients and there is a tendency in some studies for it to be commoner on the left side (Merskey & Watson 1979). It has been disputed whether this is true for all pain, and it has been suggested that it applied only to pain of psychological origin and especially to pain where there are hysterical features (Hall et al 1981). At the present time, the only safe conclusion on this point is that pain on the left side has only been shown to be commoner in patients where there is evidence of hysterical patterns. Pain of psychological origin usually appears with the illness and is coexistent with it. If pain has been present before the onset of the psychological illness, it may be presumed to be due to another cause. It will usually get worse with the illness and improve afterwards.

Pain from psychological illness is usually continuously present with rather irregular fluctuations. It rarely, if ever, keeps the patient awake at night and it rarely, if ever, wakens the patient from sleep. If pain actually wakes the individual (and he is not merely conscious of pain after waking for some other reason) it gives very strong reason to think that the diagnosis is not wholly psychiatric. In studies of the actual words used by patients to describe their pains, it has been found that approximately 50% do not use unusual descriptions (Gittleson 1961; Devine & Merskey 1965). Physical factors sometimes relieve pain even though it is of psychological origin – mild analgesics, heat or cold may help. The response never appears to be great, at least not for long. Many patients with pain of psychological origin may recognize the relationship between it and worry or emotional difficulties.

The psychiatric conditions associated with pain of psychological origin are primarily those of neurosis, as already indicated. No description will be given of neurosis in general, since one chapter cannot be a textbook on psychiatry. It is worth emphasizing that the common associations of hysterical patterns, anxiety and neurotic or reactive depression will be found more often in that order in patients with chronic pain, whereas with acute pain anxiety may well be the most frequent phenomenon. Endogenous depressive illnesses represent a small but significant group which if recognized responds very well to treatment. Schizophrenia is a very rare cause indeed of chronic pain. The causes of the pain are implicit in the diagnoses and discussions of mechanisms which have been provided already.

The primary treatment of these pain problems is that of the underlying psychiatric condition. Perhaps the most important distinction from ordinary psychiatric work is a careful study of the pain. This itself is therapeutic for those patients in whom it is a very prominent and troublesome aspect of their symptoms. So many of them feel that physicians and others have neglected to consider their pain while diagnosing them as having something wrong with their minds. Thus the writer's practice of taking a careful direct history from the patient about this pain, before even beginning to look at psychological aspects, is frequently helpful in forming a relationship with the patient. One does not have to accept that pain has an organic basis when it is largely of psychological origin. One must accept the need to take seriously the patient's description of his symptoms and to treat this as a priority at the initial part of the relationship. Once that is done, it is usually possible to take an ordinary or conventional psychiatric history and establish at least some information about the psychological disorder which may be promoting the illness. In patients with chronic pain and psychiatric illness, and where the clinician is not initially acquainted with the individual, the interview normally takes more than 1 hour. If only 1 hour has been booked, it is best to say that more time is needed and allow for a second hour before coming to a moderately definitive opinion. This works well enough with many patients who have had the experience of seeing other doctors either for short periods which proved unsatisfactory or for longer periods which were demonstrably necessary in order to review the total history of the individual's experience.

If a diagnosis has been made and the clinician is satisfied that he has appropriate guidelines for treatment of the individual, psychiatric treatment may then proceed in conventional fashion whether by marital guidance, psychotherapy, drug treatment or whatever is most appropriate. Many of these different forms of treatment are considered in other chapters and so their special application to pain will not be described here. It should be noted, however, that it is occasionally worth giving minor analgesics if only to establish that they do not work. Patients for whom other forms of treatment are more appropriate will perhaps accept them somewhat more readily if it has been shown that the physician has a sincere interest in attempting to use the sort of medication and the sort of approach which, on common-sense grounds, the patient favours. A 1-week trial of a nonnarcotic antiinflammatory drug, whether it is acetylsalicylic acid or indomethacin or ketorolac, is frequently useful in demonstrating the open-mindedness of the clinician and the effectiveness, or lack of effectiveness, of the medication.

REFERENCES

Anderson K O, Keefe F R, Bradley L A et al 1988 Prediction of pain behavior and functional status of rheumatoid arthritis patients using medical status and psychological variables. Pain 3: 25–32

Aronoff G M 1988 Pain centers: a revolution in health care. Raven Press, New York

Atkinson J H, Kremer E F 1985 Behavioral definition of pain: necessary but not sufficient. Behavioral and Brain Sciences 8: 54–55

Atkinson J H, Slater M A, Grant I, Patterson T L, Garfin S R 1988 Depressed mood in chronic low back pain: relationship with stressful life events. Pain 35: 47–55

Atkinson J H, Slater M A, Patterson T L, Grant I, Garfin S R 1991 Prevalence, onset, and risk of psychiatric disorders in men with chronic low back pain: a controlled study. Pain 45: 111–121

Bakal D A, Kaganov J A 1977 Muscle contraction and migraine headache: psychophysiologic comparison. Headache 17: 208–215

Banks M H, Beresford S H A, Morrell D C, Waller J J, Watkins C J 1975 Factors influencing demand for primary medical care in women aged 20–40 years; a preliminary report. International Journal of Epidemiology 4: 189–255

Bardhan P N 1965a The fathering syndrome. US Armed Forces Medical Journal 20: 200–208

Bardhan P N 1965b The couvade syndrome. British Journal of Psychiatry 111: 908–909

Barsky A J, Klerman G L 1983 Overview: hypochondriasis, bodily complaints, and somatic styles. American Journal of Psychiatry 140: 273–283

Barsky A J, Wyshak G 1990 Hypochondriasis and somatosensory amplification. British Journal of Psychiatry 157: 404–409

Bartels E M, Danneskiold-Samsoe B 1986 Histological abnormalities in muscle from patients with certain types of fibrositis. Lancet i: 755–757

Bigos S J, Battie M C, Spengler D M et al 1991 A prospective study of work perceptions and psychosocial factors affecting the report of back injury. Spine 16: 1–6

Blumer D 1975 Psychiatric considerations in pain. In: Rothman R H, Simeone F A (ed) The spine. W B Saunders, Philadelphia

Bond M R 1971 The relation of pain to the Eysenck personality inventory, Cornell medical index and Whiteley index of hypochondriasis. British Journal of Psychiatry 119: 671–678

Bonica J J 1990 The management of pain, 2nd edn. Lea & Febiger, Philadelphia

Bradley L A, Prokop C K, Margolis R, Gentry W D 1978 Multivariate analysis of the MMPI profiles of low back pain patients. Journal of Behavioral Medicine 1: 253–272

Brown G W, Sklair F, Harris T O, Birley J L T 1973 Life events and psychiatric disorders. Part I: Some methodological issues. Psychological Medicine 3: 74–87

Caine T H, Hope K 1967 Manual of the hysteroid-obsessed questionnaire. University of London Press, London

Chaturvedi S K, Michael A 1986 Chronic pain in a psychiatric clinic. Journal of Psychosomatic Research 30: 347–354

Chaturvedi S K, Varma V K, Malhotra A 1984 Non-organic intractable pain: a comparative study. Pain 19: 87–94

Crisp A H, Kalucy R S, McGuinness B, Ralph P C, Harris G 1977 Some clinical, social and psychological characteristics of migraine subjects in the general population. Postgraduate Medical Journal 53: 691–697

Crook J, Tunks E 1985 Defining the 'chronic pain syndrome': an epidemiological method. In: Fields H L, Dubner R, Cervero F (eds) Advances in pain research and therapy, vol 9. Raven Press, New York, p 871–877

Crook J, Rideout E, Browne G 1984 The prevalence of pain complaints in a general population. Pain 18: 299–314

Crook J, Weir R, Tunks E 1989 An epidemiological follow-up survey of persistent pain sufferers in a group family practice and specialty pain clinic. Pain 36: 49–61

Crown S, Crown J M 1973 Personality in early rheumatic disease. Journal of Psychosomatic Research 17: 189–196

Curtis J L 1965 A psychiatric study of 55 expectant fathers. US Armed Forces Medical Journal 6: 937–950

Delaplaine R, Ifabumuyi O I, Merskey H, Zarfas J 1978 Significance of pain in psychiatric hospital patients. Pain 4: 361–366

Demjen S, Bakal D A 1981 Illness behavior and chronic headache. Pain 10: 221–229

Devine R, Merskey H 1965 The description of pain in psychiatric and general medical patients. Journal of Psychosomatic Research 9: 311–316

Diagnostic and Statistical Manual 1980, 3rd edn. American Psychiatric Association, Washington, DC

Diagnostic and statistical manual (revised) 1987 3rd edn. American Psychiatric Association, Washington, DC

Dura J R, Beck S J 1988 A comparison of family functioning when mothers have chronic pain. Pain 35: 79–89

Engel G L 1959 'Psychogenic' pain and the pain prone patient. American Journal of Medicine 26: 899–918

Epstein L H, Abel G G, Collin F, Parker L, Cinciripini P M 1978 The relationship between frontalis muscle activity and self-reports of headache pain. Behaviour Research and Therapy 16: 153–160

Eysenck H J, Eysenck S B G 1964 Manual of the Eysenck personality inventory. University of London Press, London

Fam A G, Smythe H A 1985 Musculoskeletal chest wall pain. Canadian Medical Association Journal 133: 379–389

Feighner P, Robins E, Guze S B et al 1972 Diagnostic criteria for use in psychiatric research. Archives of General Psychiatry 26: 56–63

Fishbain D A, Goldberg M, Meagher B R et al 1986 Male and female chronic pain patients categorized by DSM-III psychiatric diagnostic criteria. Pain 26: 181–197

Flor H, Kerns R D, Turk D C 1987 The role of the spouse in the maintenance of chronic pain. Journal of Psychosomatic Research 31: 251–260

Flor H, Turk D C, Rudy T E 1989 Relationship of pain impact and significant other reinforcement of pain behaviors: the mediating role of gender, marital status and marital satisfaction. Pain 38: 45–50

Fordyce W E 1976 Behavioural methods in chronic pain and illness. C V Mosby, St Louis, p 236

Fordyce W E 1990 A response to Schmidt et al (1989 Pain 38: 137–140). Pain 43: 133–134

France R D, Krishnan K R R 1985 The dexamethasone suppression test as a biologic marker of depression in chronic pain. Pain 21: 49–55

Fordyce W E, McMahon R, Rainwater G et al 1981 Pain complaint–exercise performance relationship in chronic pain. Pain 10: 311–321

Fordyce W E, Roberts A H, Sternbach R A 1985 The behavioral management of chronic pain: a response to critics. Pain 22: 113–125

Fordyce W E, Roberts A H, Sternbach R A 1988 The behavioral management of pain: a critique of a critique (letter to the editor). Pain 33: 385–387

Gamsa A 1990 Is emotional status a precipitator or a consequence of pain? Pain 42: 183–195

Gittleson N L 1961 Psychiatric headache: a clinical study. Journal of Mental Science 107: 403–416

Gould R, Miller B L, Goldberg M A, Benson D F 1986 The validity of hysterical signs and symptoms. Journal of Nervous and Mental Diseases 174: 593–598

Gupta M A 1986 Is chronic pain a variant of depressive illness? A critical review. Canadian Journal of Psychiatry 31: 241–248

Hall W, Hayward L, Chapman C R 1981 On 'the lateralization of pain'. Pain 10: 337–351

Hanvik L H 1956 MMPI profiles in patients with low-back pain. Journal of Consulting and Clinical Psychology 15: 350–353

Harper R C, Steger J C 1978 Psychological correlates of frontalis EMG and pain in tension headache. Headache 18: 215–218

Hart H 1947 Displacement, guilt and pain. Psychoanalysis Review 34: 259–273

Henryk-Gutt R, Rees W L 1973 Psychological aspects of migraine. Journal of Psychosomatic Research 17: 141–153

Hilton J 1863 Rest and pain. London

International Association for the Study of Pain (Subcommittee on Taxonomy) 1979 Pain terms: a list with definitions and notes on usage. Pain 6: 249–252

International Association for the Study of Pain (Subcommittee on Taxonomy) 1986 Classification of chronic pain: descriptions of chronic pain syndromes and definitions of pain terms. Pain (suppl 3). Elsevier, Amsterdam

Jensen J 1988 Life events in neurological patients with headache and low back pain (in relation to diagnosis and persistence of pain). Pain 27: 203–210

Keefe F J, Bradley L A, Crisson J E 1990 Behavioral assessment of low back pain: identification of pain behavior subgroups. Pain 40: 153–160

Kellner R 1986 Somatization and hypochondriasis. Prager, New York

Klee A 1968 A clinical study of migraine with particular reference to the most severe cases. Munksgaard, Copenhagen

Klee G D, Ozelis S, Greenberg I, Gallant L J 1959 Pain and other somatic complaints in a psychiatric clinic. Maryland State Medical Journal 8: 188–191

Kramlinger K G, Swanson D W, Maruta T 1983 Are patients with chronic pain depressed? American Journal of Psychiatry 140: 6

Kudrow L, Sutkus B J 1979 MMPI pattern specificity in primary headache disorders. Headache 19: 18–24

Kukull W A, Koepsell T D, Inui T S et al 1986 Depression and physical illness among elderly general medical clinic patients. Journal of Affective Disorders 10: 153–162

Labbe E E 1988 Sexual dysfunction in chronic back pain patients. Clinical Journal of Pain 4: 143–149

Large R G 1980 The psychiatrist and the chronic pain patient: 172 anecdotes. Pain 9: 253–263

Large R G, Mullins P R 1981 Illness behaviour profiles in chronic pain: the Auckland experience. Pain 10: 231–239

Leavitt F, Garron D C 1979a Validity of a back pain classification scale among patients with low back pain not associated with demonstrable organic disease. Journal of Psychosomatic Research 23: 301–306

Leavitt F, Garron D C 1979b Psychological disturbance and pain report differences in both organic and non-organic low back pain patients. Pain 7: 187–195

Leavitt F, Garron D C, McNeill T W et al 1982 Organic status, psychological disturbance, and pain report characteristics in low-back pain patients on compensation. Spine 7: 398–402

Lewis T, Pickering G W, Rothschild P 1931 Observations upon muscular pain in intermittent claudication. Heart 15: 359–383

Lindsay P G, Wyckoff M 1981 The depression–pain syndrome and its response to antidepressants. Psychosomatics 22: 571–577

Littlejohn G O 1986 Repetitive strain syndrome: an Australian experience (editorial). Journal of Rheumatology 13: 1004–1006

Loeser J, Egan K J 1989 Managing the chronic pain patient. Raven Press, New York

Love A W, Peck D L 1987 The MMPI and psychological factors in chronic low back pain: a review. Pain 28: 1–12

McCreary R P, Turner J, Dawson E 1979 The MMPI as a predictor of response to conservative treatment for low back pain. Journal of Clinical Psychology 35: 278–284

Macnab I 1964 Acceleration injuries of the cervical spine. Journal of Bone and Joint Surgery 46A: 1797–1799

Magni G 1987 On the relationship between chronic pain and depression when there is no organic lesion. Pain 31: 1–21

Magni G, Merskey H 1987 A simple examination of the relationships between pain, organic lesions and psychiatric illness. Pain 29: 295–300

Magni G, Andreoli F, Arduino C et al 1987a 3H imipramine binding sites are decreased in platelets of chronic pain patients. Acta Psychiatrica Scandinavica 75: 108–110

Magni G, Andreoli F, Arduino C et al 1987b Modifications of ^{3}H-imipramine binding sites in platelets of chronic pain patients treated with mianserin. Pain 30: 311–320

Magni G, Caldieron C, Rigatti-Luchini S, Merskey H 1990 Chronic musculoskeletal pain and depressive symptoms in the general population. An analysis of the 1st National Health and Nutrition Examination survey data. Pain 43: 299–307

Marbach J J, Lennon M C, Dohrenwend B P 1988 Candidate risk factors for temporomandibular pain and dysfunction syndrome: psychosocial, health behaviour, physical illness and injury. Pain 34: 139–151

Martin P R, Mathews A M 1978 Tension headaches: psychophysiological investigation and treatment. Journal of Psychosomatic Research 22: 389–399

Merskey H 1965a The characteristics of persistent pain in psychological illness. Journal of Psychosomatic Research 9: 291–298

Merskey H 1965b Psychiatric patients with persistent pain. Journal of Psychosomatic Research 9: 299–309

Merskey H 1980 The role of psychiatrist in the investigation and treatment of pain. In: Bonica J J (ed) Pain. Raven Press, New York, p 249–260

Merskey H 1982 Pain and emotion: their correlation in headache. In: Critchley M et al (eds) Advances in neurology, 3rd edn. Raven Press, New York, p 135–143

Merskey H 1985 A mentalistic view of 'Pain and behaviour'. Commentary on Rachlin. Behavioral and Brain Sciences 8: 68

Merskey H, Spear F G 1967 Pain: psychological and psychiatric aspects. Baillière, Tindall & Cassell, London

Merskey H, Watson G D 1979 The lateralization of pain. Pain 7: 271–280

Merskey H, Brown A, Brown J, Malhotra L, Morrison D, Ripley C 1985 Psychological normality and abnormality in persistent headache patients. Pain 23: 35–47

Merskey H, Lau C L, Russell E S et al 1987 Screening for psychiatric morbidity: the pattern of psychological illness and premorbid characteristics in four chronic pain populations. Pain 30: 141–147

Mitchell S W 1872 Injuries of nerves and their consequences. Reprinted 1965 Dover Publications, New York

Mohamed S N, Weisz G M, Waring E M 1978 The relationship of chronic pain to depression, marital adjustment and family dynamics. Pain 5: 285–292

Morgenstern F S 1967 Chronic pain. D M Thesis, Oxford

Naliboff B D, McCreary C P, McArthur D L, Cohen M J, Gottlieb H J 1988 MMPI changes following behavioral treatment of chronic low back pain. Pain 35: 271–277

O'Kelly L E, Steckley L C 1939 A note on long enduring emotional responses in the rat. Journal of Psychology 8: 125 (cited by Ulrich R E, Hutchinson P R, Azrin N H 1965 Pain-elicited aggression. Psychological Research 15: 11)

Oostdam E M M, Duivenvoorden H J, Pondaag W 1981 Predictive value of some psychological tests on the outcome of surgical intervention in low back pain patients. Journal of Psychosomatic Research 3: 227–235

Payne B, Norfleet M A 1986 Chronic pain and the family: a review. Pain 26: 1–22

Pelz M, Merskey H 1982 A description of the psychological effects of chronic painful lesions. Pain 14: 293–301

Pilling L F, Brannick T L, Swenson W M 1967 Psychological characteristics of patients having pain as a presenting symptom. Canadian Medical Association Journal 97: 387–394

Pilowsky I 1967 Dimensions of hypochondriasis. British Journal of Psychiatry 113: 89

Pilowsky I, Spence D N 1976 Pain and illness behaviour: a comparative study. Journal of Psychosomatic Research 20: 131–134

Pilowsky I, Chapman C R, Bonica J J 1977 Pain, depression and illness behaviour in a pain clinic population. Pain 4: 183–192

Pozniak-Patewicz E 1976 'Cephalgic' spasm of head and neck muscles. Headache 15: 261–266

Rachlin H 1985 Pain and behavior. Behavioral and Brain Sciences 8: 43–83

Radanov B P, Stefano G D, Schnidrig A, Ballinari P 1991 Role of psychosocial stress in recovery from common whiplash. Lancet 338: 712–715

Rawnsley K, Loudon J B 1964 Epidemiology of mental disorders in a closed community. British Journal of Psychiatry 110: 830–839

Reich J, Tupin J P, Abramowitz S I 1983 Psychiatric diagnosis of chronic pain patients. American Journal of Psychiatry 140: 1495–1498

Reik T 1914 Ritual: psychoanalytical studies. Hogarth, London

Romano J M, Turner J A 1985 Chronic pain and depression: does the evidence support a relationship? Psychological Bulletin 97: 18–34

Romano J M, Turner J A, Clancy S L 1989 Sex differences in the relationship of pain patient dysfunction to spouse adjustment. Pain 39: 289–295

Rowat K M, Knafl K A 1985 Living with chronic pain: the spouse's perspective. Pain 23: 259–271
Roy R, Thomas M, Matas M 1984 Chronic pain and depression. Comprehensive Psychiatry 25: 96–105
Sainsbury P, Gibson J G 1954 Symptoms of anxiety and tension and the accompanying physiological changes in the muscular system. Psychosomatic Medicine 17: 216–224
Salter M, Brooke R I, Merskey H, Fichter G F, Kapusianyk D H 1983 Is the temporomandibular pain and dysfunction syndrome a disorder of the mind? Pain 17: 151–166
Schmidt A J M 1987 The behavioral management of pain: a criticism of a response. Pain 30: 285–291
Schmidt A J M 1988 Reply to letter from Fordyce, Roberts and Sternbach (letter to the editor). Pain 33: 388–389
Smith W L, Duerksen D L 1980 Personality in the relief of chronic pain: predicting surgical outcome. In: Smith W L, Merskey H, Gross S C (eds) Pain: meaning and management. Spectrum, New York
Smythe H A 1985 Fibrositis and other diffuse musculoskeletal syndromes. In: Kelley W N, Harris E D Jr, Ruddy S et al (eds) Textbook of rheumatology. W B Saunders, Philadelphia p 481–489
Spear F G 1967 Pain in psychiatric patients. Journal of Psychosomatic Research 11: 187–193
Speculand B, Hughes A O, Goss A N 1984 Role of recent stressful life event experiences in the onset of TMJ dysfunction pain. Community Dental and Oral Epidemiology 12: 197–202
Spitzer R L, Endicott Robins E 1978 Research diagnostic criteria: rationale and reliability. Archives of General Psychiatry 35: 773–782
Sternbach R A 1974 Pain patients. Traits and treatment. Academic Press, New York
Sternbach R A, Timmermans G 1975 Personality changes associated with reduction of pain. Pain 1: 177–181
Sternbach R A 1986 Survey of pain in the United States: the NUPRIN Pain Report. Clinical Journal of Pain 2: 49–53
Sternbach R A 1987 Mastering pain. G P Putnam's Sons, New York
Sternbach R A, Wolf S R, Murphy R W, Akeson W H 1973 Traits of pain patients: the low-back 'loser'. Psychosomatics 14: 226–229
Taub A 1972 Personal communication
Tauschke E, Merskey H, Helmes E 1990 A systematic inquiry into recollections of childhood experience and their relationship to adult defence mechanisms. British Journal of Psychiatry 157: 392–398
Thomas M, Roy R 1989 Pain patients and marital relations. Clinical Journal of Pain 5: 255–259
Trethowan W H 1968 The couvade syndrome – some further observations. Journal of Psychosomatic Research 12: 107–115
Trethowan W H, Conlon M F 1965 The couvade syndrome. British Journal of Psychiatry 3: 57–76
Violon-Jurfest A 1980 The onset of facial pain: a psychological study, Psychotherapy and Psychosomatics 34: 11–16
Waddell G 1987 A new clinical model for the treatment of low-back pain. Spine 12: 632–644
Waddell G, Main C J 1984 Assessment of severity in low-back disorders. Spine 9: 204–208
Waddell G, McCulloch J A, Kummel E G, Venner R M 1980 Non-organic physical signs in low back pain. Spine 5: 117–125
Waddell G, Gircher M, Finlayson D, Main C J 1984a Contemporary themes: symptoms and signs: physical disease or illness behaviour? British Medical Journal 289: 739–741
Waddell G, Main C J, Morris E W, Di Paola M, Gray I C M 1984b Chronic low-back pain, psychologic distress, and illness behavior. Spine 9: 209–213
Waddell G, Pilowsky I, Bond M R 1989 Clinical assessment and interpretation of abnormal illness behaviour in low back pain. Pain 39: 41–53
Wall P D 1984 The dorsal horn. In: Wall P D, Melzack R (eds) Textbook of pain, 1st edn. Churchill Livingstone, Edinburgh, p 80–87
Walters A 1961 Psychogenic regional pain alias hysterical pain. Brain 84: 1–18
Waring E M, Weisz G M, Bailey S I 1976 Predictive factors in the treatment of low back pain by surgical intervention. In: Bonica J J, Albe-Fessard D (eds) Advances in pain research and therapy. Raven Press, New York, p 939–942
Watson D 1982 Neurotic tendencies among chronic pain patients: an MMPI item analysis. Pain 14: 365–385
Watson G D, Chandarana P C, Merskey H 1981 Relationships between pain and schizophrenia. British Journal of Psychiatry 138: 33–36
Watt-Watson J H, Evans R J, Watson C P N 1988 Relationships among coping responses and perceptions of pain intensity, depression, and family functioning. Clinical Journal of Pain 4: 101–106
Wiltse L L, Rocchio P D 1975 Preoperative psychological tests as predictors of success of chemonucleolysis in the treatment of low-back syndrome. Journal of Bone and Joint Surgery 57AI: 478–483
Wolfe F, Smythe H A, Yunus M B et al 1990 The American College of Rheumatology 1990 criteria for the classification of fibromyalgia. Report of the Multicenter Criteria Committee. Arthritis and Rheumatism 33: 160–172
Woodforde J M, Merskey H 1972 Personality traits of patients with chronic pain. Journal of Psychosomatic Research 16: 167–172
Zilli C, Brooke R I, Merskey H, Lau C L 1989 Screening for psychiatric illness in patients with oral dysaesthesia using the GHQ-28 and the IDA. Oral Surgery, Oral Medicine, Oral Pathology 67: 384–389

Pharmacology

48. Nonnarcotic analgesics

Abraham Sunshine and Nancy Z. Olson

INTRODUCTION

The objective of this chapter is to provide a review of currently available, generally accepted worldwide, nonnarcotic analgesics as well as certain analgesic adjuvants. We have not discussed therapies for specific clinical pain conditions, such as migraine, discussed elsewhere in this book.

The nonnarcotic analgesics, such as aspirin, acetaminophen and dipyrone, and the nonsteroidal antiinflammatory drugs (NSAIDs) constitute a heterogeneous group of compounds differing in chemical structure and sharing certain pharmacological and therapeutic actions. Nonnarcotic analgesics have their main pharmacological action in the periphery where the pain originates; however, they do have some activity in the central nervous system as well (Malmberg & Yaksh 1992). They are distinct from narcotic analgesics in that they do not bind to the narcotic receptor sites. Nonnarcotic analgesics are used alone or in combination with narcotic analgesics or analgesic adjuvants for an enhanced effect. As a group, these drugs are commonly administered orally, although some are available for parenteral administration as well as for topical and rectal administration. Unlike narcotic analgesics, tolerance or physical dependence does not develop with the use of these drugs. Nonnarcotic analgesics have a ceiling effect in that increasing the dose beyond a certain level does not produce additional analgesic effects, although it may increase the duration of effect. Since many of the peripherally acting analgesics act as potent prostaglandin synthetase inhibitors, they possess analgesic, antipyretic, antiplatelet and antiinflammatory properties.

Well designed clinical trials with internal standards to measure assay sensitivity are not always available to compare the analgesic efficacy of the NSAIDs relative to each other or to some of the older nonnarcotic analgesics. Nonetheless, the available data suggest that the NSAIDs have varying efficacy and side-effect profiles. The variability in adverse effects is clear from the reactions seen with NSAIDs such as benoxaprofen, fenbufen, indoprofen, isoxicam, suprofen and zomepirac which have been withdrawn from the market or are restricted in their use because of side-effects. Some NSAIDs have been shown to be equivalent to aspirin, others are clearly more efficacious than aspirin and are equivalent to drugs used for more severe pain, such as aspirin with codeine, oxycodone and morphine. This variability in efficacy among the NSAIDs may be a result of differences in their pharmacological effects on the prostaglandin cascade (Day & Brooks 1987). There are also interpatient variations in response. This may be a result of genetic differences in the mediating pathways by which an inflammatory response is controlled or differences in the mediators utilized in pain transmission and modulation (Kantor 1984). NSAID blood levels achieved from a specific dose may vary from patient to patient as a result of differences in the rate of absorption, metabolism and elimination and differences in the ratio of bound to unbound drug (Birkett 1985; Brune 1985). This variability in blood level concentrations can account for differences in response. Laska et al (1986) showed that there was a correlation between serum blood levels of an NSAID and clinical efficacy. In addition, many of the propionic acid NSAIDs (i.e. ibuprofen, naproxen, fenoprofen, ketoprofen and flurbiprofen) are chiral and, with the exception of naproxen, are administered as their racemates, although their activity resides primarily in one isomer (Williams & Day 1985). For those compounds which undergo chiral conversion, individual variability in the rate of inversion of the inactive to active isomer may be another factor contributing to the difference in clinical response.

ACETAMINOPHEN (PARACETAMOL)

Acetaminophen is an effective oral analgesic and antipyretic. It is equipotent to aspirin as an analgesic and antipyretic. It is the active metabolite of phenacetin and has less overall toxicity than phenacetin. Unlike aspirin and NSAIDs, its antiinflammatory activity is weak and it has practically no antiplatelet effect. The mechanism of action of acetaminophen is poorly defined, although it has been speculated that it may selectively inhibit brain prostaglandin synthetase. This has been proposed to account for its antipyretic action and possibly for its analgesic effect as well (Flower & Vane 1972; Flower et al 1985). The lack of any significant influence on peripheral cyclo-oxygenase would explain the absence of its antiinflammatory activity.

Pharmacokinetics and metabolism

Acetaminophen is rapidly absorbed from the gastrointestinal tract and reaches peak plasma concentrations in 30–60 minutes. It is metabolized in the liver and excreted in the urine. The plasma half-life for acetaminophen is about 2–3 hours in the usual dose range. Its plasma-protein binding is negligible, approximately 10% (Levy 1981).

Safety

At the recommended therapeutic dosage, acetaminophen is well tolerated and side-effects are mild. Acetaminophen does not attack the gastric mucosa nor does it affect platelet function. However, patients with chronic alcoholism and liver disease can develop severe hepatotoxicity, including jaundice, from acetaminophen even when taken in usual therapeutic doses (Seeff et al 1986). Acetaminophen should be considered as a possible cause of progressive liver disease in patients with chronic alcoholism. Blood levels of acetaminophen should be evaluated in these patients. The most serious potentially fatal adverse effect of acute overdosage of acetaminophen is hepatic necrosis; the ingestion of a single dose of 25 g or more can be fatal (Flower et al 1985).

Drug interactions

Acetaminophen is absorbed in the small intestine and drugs delaying gastric emptying delay absorption. Pectin which is found in foods high in carbohydrates, decreases the rate of acetaminophen absorption (Hayes 1981).

Dosage and clinical efficacy

The conventional adult oral or rectal dose of acetaminophen is 500–1000 mg every 4–6 hours. Increasing the dose above 1000 mg will result in little added analgesia because of the shallow dose–response curve (Laska et al 1984). The total daily dose should not exceed 4000 mg. For children, the dose is dependent on age and weight.

SALICYLATES

ACETYLATED (ASPIRIN) AND NON-ACETYLATED SALICYLATES

Acetylsalicylic acid (aspirin) is one of the oldest nonnarcotic oral analgesics used for over 100 years for the treatment of a variety of painful illnesses. One of its principal mechanisms of action is believed to be inhibition of the biosynthesis and release of prostaglandins from cells by acetylating the active site of cyclo-oxygenase, thereby destroying its enzyme function. It does not antagonize the action of prostaglandins which have been released. The inhibitory effects of aspirin on cyclo-oxygenase in platelets are irreversible. In other tissues this inhibition is transient, and prostaglandin production recovers, due to new enzyme synthesis (Higgs et al 1987). In vitro nonacetylated salicylate has no acetylating capacity and does not inhibit prostaglandin synthesis. In man, the nonacetylated salicylates are devoid of significant adverse effects associated with prostaglandin inhibition such as gastric ulceration, inhibition of platelet function and bronchospasm (Abramson 1991), yet they are effective analgesics (Sunshine et al 1992). In vivo, both aspirin and nonacetylated salicylate may have a variety of nonprostaglandin mechanisms that result in analgesia (Abramson 1991). Thus, aspirin may have two mechanisms of action; one related to the effects of the acetyl radical on prostaglandin and the other to the effects of the metabolite salicylate on nonprostaglandin mechanisms.

Pharmacokinetics and metabolism

Aspirin is absorbed passively from the stomach and upper small intestine. Appreciable concentrations are found in the plasma in less than 30 minutes. Aspirin is hydrolysed in the body to salicylic acid; the plasma half-life of aspirin is about 15 minutes, and that of salicylic acid is 2–3 hours (Levy 1981). The rate of absorption of aspirin is determined by the disintegration and dissolution rate of the tablet or capsule, the pH of the gastric contents, presence of food in the stomach and the rate of gastric emptying. Nonionized lipid-soluble aspirin is the only form capable of crossing the mucosal membrane. If the pH is increased, aspirin is more ionized and this tends to decrease the rate of absorption. However, a rise in pH increases the solubility of aspirin which enhances its absorption and also promotes gastric emptying (Clissold 1986). The net effect of this is a shorter time to peak effect.

Aspirin must penetrate the mucosal cells to cause damage. When the nonionized aspirin enters the mucosal cells it dissociates to the ionized form and produces mucosal damage. The gastric mucosal damage caused by aspirin can be assessed endoscopically, or indirectly by measuring gastrointestinal blood loss. The occurrence is related to the dose administered and the presence of acid in the stomach. These gastric mucosal haemorrhages and small erosions do not predict onset of massive gastrointestinal bleeding or gastric ulcer (Graham & Smith 1986). Chronic aspirin administration results in gastric adaptation or lessening injury with continuing treatment. The development of a chronic ulcer probably reflects either a failure of adaptation or a locally susceptible patch of mucosa or both. The absence of symptoms has no predictive value in identifying gross gastric damage. Patients taking aspirin may experience heartburn or burning upper abdominal discomfort. This can occur in over 5–25% of all aspirin users. Importantly, dyspepsia does not relate to intestinal blood loss or endoscopic appearance of the gastric mucosa.

Safety

Occasional use of usual dosages of aspirin for analgesia or antipyretic purposes generally causes few adverse effects. However, the use of larger doses for a sustained period of time results in an increase in the incidence of side-effects. The most common adverse effects occurring with therapeutic doses of aspirin are gastrointestinal disturbances such as nausea, dyspepsia and vomiting. Irritation of the gastric mucosa may occur; slight blood loss may occur in about 70% of patients with most aspirin preparations, whether buffered, soluble, or plain, and often this is not accompanied by dyspepsia. Slight blood loss is not usually of clinical significance but may cause iron deficiency anaemia during long-term salicylate therapy (Reynolds 1989). Generally, renal function is not adversely affected by intermittent use of aspirin and related salicylates. However aspirin should be used with caution in patients with impaired renal function and those likely to have increased dependence on renal prostaglandins for maintenance of renal blood flow.

Aspirin affects platelet function. Single oral doses of aspirin above 40 mg inhibit platelet aggregation and prolong bleeding time by blocking synthesis of thromboxane A_2 (Flower et al 1985). The effect on platelets is irreversible. Only new platelets are not inhibited. The effect of aspirin on platelet aggregation does not normally result in any morbidity in healthy subjects. However, it may be a problem in patients at risk of bleeding such as those with haemophilia, thrombocytopenia, patients on anticoagulants or patients about to undergo certain types of surgery.

Aspirin has been reported to cause tinnitus, deafness, headache and dizziness. Symptoms rapidly disappear after the dosage is reduced.

Acute overdoses can lead to gastrointestinal disturbances, tinnitus, deafness, hyperventilation, disturbed acid-base balance, convulsions, cyanosis, coma, respiratory or cardiovascular failure and death.

Aspirin hypersensitivity

Aspirin hypersensitivity usually occurs in middle-aged adults and is more common in females (Reynolds 1989). The exact mechanism underlying aspirin hypersensitivity is not known and it therefore cannot be classified as an allergic reaction. Two subgroups of aspirin-sensitive patients have been reported. One subtype develops a respiratory reaction with rhinitis, asthma or nasal polyps. Another subtype develops urticaria, wheals, angioneurotic oedema, hypotension, shock and syncope (Clissold 1986; Szczeklik 1986). The response to aspirin usually occurs within minutes of ingestion and almost always within an hour. Patients who are sensitive to aspirin may also develop cross-sensitivity to NSAIDs. Aspirin-induced asthma can be precipitated by aspirin as well as other NSAIDs that inhibit cyclo-oxygenase, but not by the nonacetylated salicylate salts (Hoigne & Szczeklik 1992).

Drug interactions

Aspirin interacts with oral anticoagulants and methotrexate, enhancing their activity. It also interacts with probenecid and sulfopyrazones, diminishing the action of these drugs. Aspirin can compete for protein-binding sites with other NSAIDs.

Dosage and clinical efficacy

The usual dosage is 500–1000 mg every 4–6 hours. The higher dose results in increased analgesia and a longer duration of effect; however the dose–response curve for aspirin is shallow, and doses above 1000 mg should not be used. The total daily dose should be kept under 4000 mg/day.

DIFLUNISAL

Pharmacokinetics and metabolism

Diflunisal is a long-acting salicylic acid derivative analgesic which is effective with twice-a-day dosing. Diflunisal is an inhibitor of prostaglandin synthesis (Tempero et al 1977). It is rapidly and completely absorbed following oral administration with peak plasma concentrations usually attained in 2 hours. Unlike other salicylates, diflunisal is not metabolized to salicylic acid and its elimination is almost entirely dependent on glucuronidation. The drug is excreted in the urine; little or no diflunisal is excreted in the faeces. At the usual analgesic dose of 500–750 mg/day, the plasma half-life ranges between 8 and 12 hours (Flower et al 1985). Several days are required for diflunisal plasma levels to reach steady-state following multiple doses. For this reason an initial loading dose is necessary to shorten the time to reach steady-state levels. Forbes et al (1982) conducted a series of 12-hour studies in patients with oral surgery pain and found onset of mean analgesic effect for the usual 500 mg dose of diflunisal significantly slower than that of aspirin. Doubling the dose to 1000 mg shortened the mean time to onset; patients treated with diflunisal continued to have a good analgesic effect 8–12 hours after dosing.

Safety

The most common side-effects occurring with diflunisal are gastrointestinal disturbances, although the incidence is reportedly slightly less than that seen with aspirin. Peptic ulceration and gastrointestinal bleeding have been reported. Diflunisal increases the clearance of uric acid at therapeutic doses. Skin rash, pruritus, dizziness, drowsiness, headache and tinnitus may also occur. Patients who are hypersensitive to aspirin or other NSAIDs should not take diflunisal. See section on general considerations, below.

Drug interactions

Diflunisal prolongs the prothrombin time in patients who are on oral anticoagulants by competitively displacing Coumadin from protein-binding sites. The concomitant administration of diflunisal and indomethacin decreases the renal clearance and significantly increases the plasma levels of indomethacin. In some patients the combined use of indomethacin and diflunisal has been associated with fatal gastrointestinal haemorrhage. Diflunisal also interacts with hydrochlorthyazide, acetaminophen, aspirin, indomethacin, sulindac and naproxen and increases plasma levels of these drugs. Concomitant administration of antacids may reduce plasma levels of diflunisal.

Dosage and clinical efficacy

Diflunisal (Dolobid) is indicated for mild to moderate pain. An initial dosage of 1000 mg followed by 500 mg every 12 hours is recommended. Following the initial dose, some patients may require 500 mg every 8 hours. A lower dosage may be appropriate depending upon pain severity, patient's response and age. Clinical trials indicate that diflunisal 500 mg, after 2 hours, is more effective than aspirin 650 mg and has a longer duration of effect.

PYRAZOLONE DERIVATIVES

DIPYRONE

The pyrazolone derivatives are widely used analgesics in many countries. Dipyrone, the sodium sulphonate of amidopyrine, is the most widely used pyrazolone and has analgesic antiinflammatory and antipyretic activity. The analgesic activity of dipyrone is attributed to inhibition of prostaglandin biosynthesis (Brogden 1986b). Studies indicate that dipyrone is a prodrug which undergoes extensive biotransformation and is hydrolysed to biologically active metabolites (Levy 1986; Roth 1986). It is excreted in the urine. Although dipyrone is extensively used both orally and parenterally, few studies exist that would meet current standards of evaluating analgesics. Two studies in episiotomy pain reported dipyrone 500 mg to be more effective than the same amount of aspirin or acetaminophen. No studies were found comparing dipyrone to the NSAIDs. The risk of agranulocytosis is small but a real concern and has resulted in dipyrone being removed from the market in the United States and other countries. In some countries, it has been removed from over-the-counter self-care prescription use only. The risk of fatal toxic effects which appear silently, and the failure to demonstrate any significant therapeutic analgesic advantage, makes this drug one which should not be recommended as an analgesic.

Safety

The most frequently reported side-effects of the pyrazolone derivatives are skin rashes. Skin reactions to dipyrone usually appear within the first 7 days of drug administration and may be severe. Toxic epidermal necrolysis, exfoliative dermatitis and acute anaphylactic shock have all been reported with the pyrazolone derivatives. Agranulocytosis has been reported.

Dosage and clinical efficacy

The usual oral dose of dipyrone (Novalgina, Metamizol) is 500–1000 mg given up to three times daily. It is also given by subcutaneous, intramuscular or intravenous injection in doses of 500–1000 mg.

GENERAL CONSIDERATIONS OF NSAIDs OTHER THAN SALICYLATES

General considerations of the NSAIDs are presented below. As far as possible the NSAIDs will be discussed by chemical class. These compounds can be classified as shown in Figure 48.1. An effort will be made to emphasize clinical aspects associated with the use of these agents as analgesics.

PHARMACOLOGICAL PROPERTIES

Mechanism of analgesic action

Tissue damage initiates a complex set of events leading to activation of primary afferent nociceptors (Fields 1987). Prostaglandins sensitize and activate nociceptors in peripheral nerves to the pain producing effects of

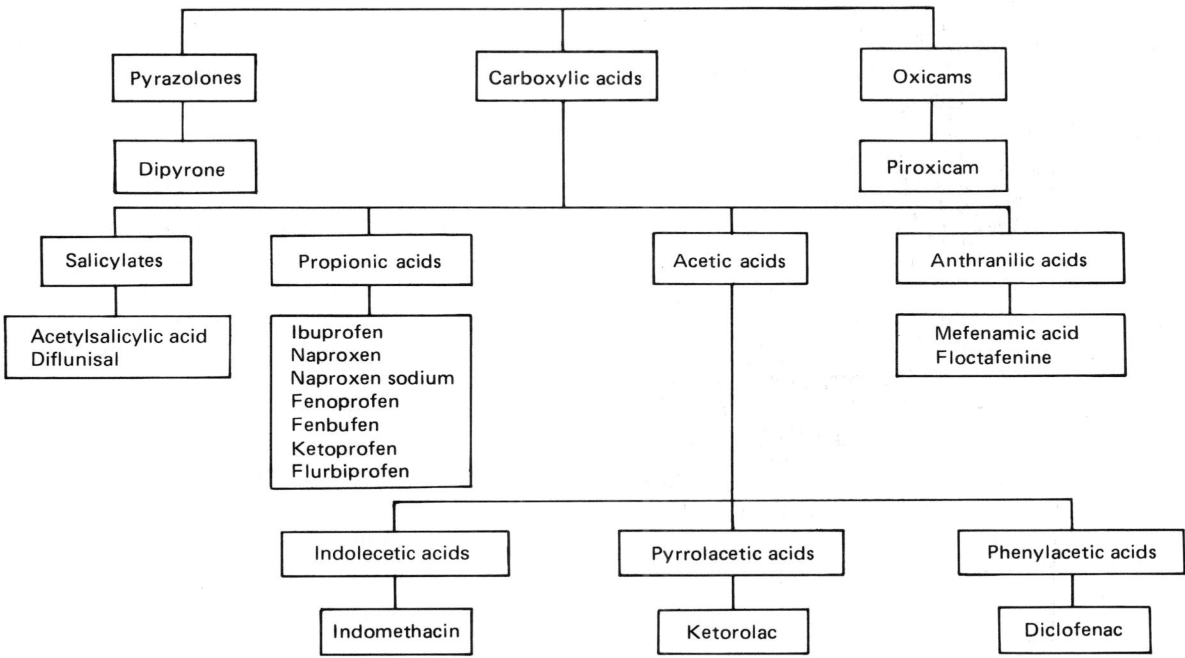

Fig. 48.1 Selected nonsteroidal antiinflammatory drugs.

substances such as bradykinin. NSAIDs are thought to exert their analgesic antiinflammatory effect in part by inhibiting prostaglandin biosynthesis through inhibition of the enzyme cyclo-oxygenase (Vane 1973). Most of the available NSAIDs inhibit cyclo-oxygenase which catalyses the conversion of arachidonic acid to prostaglandins F, D and E as well as prostacyclin and thromboxane. NSAIDs have recently been shown in the rat to exert a direct spinal action most likely by inhibiting spinal cyclo-oxygenase and blocking hyperalgesia (Malmberg & Yaksh 1992). In addition, unrelated to prostaglandins, they inhibit the release of mediators of inflammation from neutrophils and macrophages (Abramson 1991).

Haematological effects

The NSAIDs inhibit platelet aggregation by affecting prostaglandin synthetase through a reversible mechanism. This is in contrast to aspirin which has an irreversible effect on platelets. Thus the inhibition of platelet aggregation by NSAIDs only lasts as long as there is an effective drug concentration. All NSAIDs by inhibiting platelets can render the patient more susceptible to bleeding. Patients who are receiving anticoagulants should be carefully evaluated before using NSAIDs. In addition to the above haematological effect resulting from the pharmacological properties of the drug, there is a category of drug-dependent immune mechanisms that result in blood dyscrasias such as anaemia, agranulocytosis and thrombocytopenia (Rybak 1992).

Gastrointestinal effects

Serious gastrointestinal toxicity, such as bleeding, ulceration and perforation, can occur at any time with or without warning symptoms in patients treated with NSAIDs. Factors increasing the risk of gastrointestinal adverse effects include: a prior history of serious gastrointestinal events; age over 60 years; smoking; alcoholism; the concomitant use of anticoagulants and/or corticosteroids, and the use of high doses of NSAIDs; in addition, women appear to be at a greater risk than men (Borda 1992).

Several factors should be considered in addition to the above in preventing gastrointestinal adverse effects. NSAIDs should be taken with sufficient water to facilitate dissolution. Misoprostol has been shown effective in both short- and long-term double blind placebo-controlled trials for the prevention of NSAID gastropathy. The recommended adult oral dose of misoprostol for the prevention of NSAID-induced gastric ulcers is 200 μg four times daily with food. If this dose cannot be tolerated, a dose of 100 μg can be used (Physicians' Desk Reference 1992). The use of H_2 receptor antagonists has been shown to be especially effective in the presence of duodenal ulcers. If NSAIDs are taken with or immediately after meals, the adverse effects may be lessened but the pharmacokinetic parameters may be altered as well. Antacids when administered with NSAIDs can reduce the absorption of the NSAID and therefore its effectiveness. The concomitant use of antacids or H_2 blockers with enteric-coated NSAIDs or enteric-coated aspirin results in an alkaline pH which promotes release of the drug in the stomach and is counterproductive (Roth et al 1992).

Renal effects

NSAIDs can cause drug-induced renal insufficiency and significant nephrotoxicity. The mechanisms by which NSAIDs can affect renal function include: decreased synthesis of renal vasodilatory prostaglandins; interstitial nephritis; impaired renin secretion, and enhanced tubular water and sodium reabsorption.

The NSAIDs vary in their ability to inhibit renal prostaglandins. Renal adverse effects are more frequently reported with indomethacin than with ibuprofen or naproxen and this is explained by the fact that indomethacin is a more potent renal prostaglandin inhibitor than ibuprofen or naproxen. Aspirin has the least effect on the kidney.

The acute reversible renal insufficiency induced by NSAIDs is most likely a result of the blockade of intrarenal vasodilatory prostaglandins. Patients who are at risk for developing acute renal failure when treated with NSAIDs are those with congestive heart failure, chronic renal insufficiency, cirrhosis with ascites, systemic lupus erythematosus, intravascular volume depletion, elderly patients with significant atherosclerotic disease and patients being treated with diuretics. These patients may have a decrease in renal perfusion and activation of the renin angiotensin pathway. The blockade of prostaglandin synthesis results in acute decline in renal blood flow and glomerular filtration rate (Cooper & Bennett 1987). With the availability of parenteral NSAIDs for use in the perioperative and immediate postoperative period, the clinician should be alerted to the potential renal failure which may occur in surgical patients receiving parenteral NSAIDs. Signs of NSAID-induced acute renal failure include abrupt onset of oliguria, sodium and water retention and these are rapidly reversed after discontinuing the NSAID. Most NSAIDs have been implicated as a cause of acute renal failure.

NSAIDs are a known cause of allergic interstitial nephritis and nephrotic syndrome. Interstitial nephritis has been reported with several NSAIDs, most commonly with fenoprofen (Cooper & Bennett 1987). Patients present with the nephrotic syndrome, including oedema, proteinuria, and hypoalbuminaemia. Renal insufficiency may or may not be present. There is usually no associated fever, rash or eosinophilia. The syndrome is rapidly reversible after discontinuation of the NSAID.

NSAIDs may also affect tubular function, including renal handling of potassium, sodium and water. Prostaglandins stimulate the production of renin which leads to increased secretion of aldosterone. The decrease in renal prostaglandins can result in hyperkalaemia in patients who develop hyporeninaemic hypoaldosteronism. This reaction has been reported with indomethacin but can occur with all NSAIDs. High-risk patients include patients with preexistent renal insufficiency, vascular disease, diabetes and mild hyperkalaemia.

Prostaglandins also antagonize the effects of the antidiuretic hormones. Consequently, NSAIDs by blocking prostaglandins can enhance ADH action, resulting in a decrease in water excretion leading to hyponatraemia.

Acute renal failure has been reported in patients with multiple myeloma who have been treated with naproxen (Wu et al 1987). In the two reported cases it was not apparent that the patients had myeloma until after they were treated with naproxen. Therefore, patients who develop acute renal failure on NSAIDs should be screened for possible myeloma.

The key to the diagnosis and treatment of NSAID-related renal syndromes requires the physician to be alert to the possibility and ready to discontinue the NSAID.

Central nervous system dysfunction

Central nervous system dysfunction has long been recognized as a manifestation of salicylate toxicity and a side-effect reported with indomethacin. Cognitive dysfunction (comprising decreased attention span, loss of short-term memory and difficulty with calculations) has been noted in the elderly with naproxen and ibuprofen. The NSAID doses in these patients with cognitive dysfunction were within the accepted range and not excessive (Goodwin & Regan 1982). Patients are unaware of these symptoms of cognitive dysfunction and mood alteration and are reluctant to volunteer this information. Thus the physician must be alert to make this diagnosis. These cognitive effects probably occur with other NSAIDs as well.

PHARMACOKINETIC PROPERTIES

Selected pharmacokinetic data, such as time to peak, median half-life, and percentage protein-bound, for each NSAID, are presented in Table 48.1

Absorption

Absorption of orally ingested drugs is believed to occur primarily from the upper small intestine with its greater surface area, and to a lesser extent from the stomach. There are several factors affecting the rate of absorption. Absorption is promoted by rapid gastric emptying time as would occur with the patient in the fasted state and with the patient upright or lying on his right side. The presence of food in the stomach usually delays absorption and may diminish the peak plasma effect and onset of analgesia, although the total amount of drug absorbed remains the same. Gastric emptying times have been shown to be

Table 48.1 Pharmacokinetic properties of selected nonnarcotic analgesics following oral administration

Drug	Plasma half-life $t^{1}/_{2}$ (h)	Plasma peak effect (h)[1]	Percentage protein binding	Main route of excretion of drug and metabolites
Acetaminophen	2–3	0.5–1.0	10	Renal
Salicylates				
Aspirin	0.25	2.0[2]	80–90[2]	Renal
Diflunisal	8–12	2.0	>99	Renal (90%)
Choline magnesium trisalicylate	9–17	1–2	NA	Renal
Magnesium salicylate	2	1.5[2]	50–90[2]	Renal
Pyrazolones				
Dipyrone	7	1–1.5	Minimal	Renal (65%)
Propionic acids				
Ibuprofen	2–2.5	0.5–1.5	99	Renal
Naproxen	12–15	2.0	99.6	Renal (95%)
Fenoprofen	2–3	1.0–2.0	>99	Renal (90%)
Ketoprofen	1.5	1.0	98.7	Renal
Flurbiprofen	3–4	1.5–3.0	99	Renal
Oxybutyric acids				
Fenbufen	10	1.0–2.0	>98	Renal, active metabolite
Acetic acids				
Indoleacetic acids				
Indomethacin	6	2	>90	Renal (60%)
Pyrrolacetic acids				
Ketorolac tromethamine	6	0.5–1.0	>99	Renal (91%)
Phenylacetic acid				
Diclofenac sodium	1	2	99.7	Renal (61%), faecal (30%)
Anthranilic acids				
Meclofenamate sodium	0.8–2.1	0.5–2.0	>99	Renal (70%), Faecal and biliary (30%)
Mefenamic acid	2	2–4	48	Renal (67%), faecal (25%)
Floctafenine	1	1–2	NA	Faecal and biliary (60%), Renal (40%)
Glafenine	1.25	1–2	NA	Renal and faecal
Pyranocarboxylic acid				
Etodolac	7	1–2	>99	Renal (72%), faecal (16%)
Oxicams				
Piroxicam	36–45	2–3	>99	Renal and faecal

NA = not available.
[1]Peak effect refers to peak plasma concentrations,
[2]For active metabolite, salicylic acid.

significantly longer when an NSAID was administered in the fed versus fasted state (Dressman et al 1992). Different formulations can influence the rate of absorption. Certain salts, such as the aluminum salt of ibuprofen, are poorly absorbed (Laska et al 1986), whereas the lysine salt of ibuprofen is reported to enhance its absorption (Merckle 1986).

Elimination

Elimination of NSAIDs depends largely on hepatic biotransformation and the metabolites are then excreted by the kidney. As a rule, only a small proportion of the dose is excreted unchanged. Some of the drugs undergo enterohepatic circulation and 30–40% of the dose is excreted in bile.

Protein binding

Once the NSAID is absorbed from the gastrointestinal tract, over 90% of the dose is bound to serum albumin. Only the unbound fraction which is in equilibrium with the bound fraction exerts pharmacological activity. Other protein-bound drugs administered concomitantly may compete for binding sites, resulting in increased serum concentrations of the free drug. When a patient's condition requires administration of two or more drugs that are albumin-bound, such as anticoagulants, oral hypoglycaemics, sulphonamides or anticonvulsants, potentiation of the pharmacological action of the drug displaced from its binding sites usually occurs. A reduction in dosage of such drugs and careful clinical monitoring therefore is advisable. Generally, the potentiation of pharmacological action of the displaced drug is temporary and is not a factor in chronic coadministration.

Drug interactions

The NSAIDs as a group decrease lithium clearance and result in clinically relevant elevation of plasma lithium levels.

The concomitant administration of aspirin and an NSAID results in a significant decrease in the plasma concentration of the NSAID. However, the clinical significance of this interaction is uncertain.

Chronic administration of phenobarbital, a known enzyme inducer, may be associated with a decrease in the plasma half-life of fenoprofen and other NSAIDs.

Reduced clearance of methotrexate has been associated with aspirin, indomethacin, ketoprofen and diclofenac administration (Kantor 1984).

Probenecid decreases renal excretion of NSAIDs. It also appears to interfere with NSAID conjugation in the liver (Harth 1992). Probenecid increases the plasma concentrations of many NSAIDs, including carprofen, diflunisal, indomethacin, ketoprofen and naproxen. Probenecid has been shown to increase the naproxen steady-state concentration by 50%.

NSAIDs in lactating women

Because of the possible adverse effect of prostaglandin-inhibiting drugs on neonates, NSAIDs are generally not recommended for use in nursing mothers. However, if NSAIDs are used in lactating women for pain relief and for the treatment of arthritis they should provide minimum drug exposure for the child (Brooks & Needs 1992). Therefore, the drug should be taken just before breast-feeding as plasma drug levels are just then beginning to rise. Drugs most appropriate in this situation are those that have short half-lives and whose metabolites are inert and rapidly excreted. NSAIDs in this category are ibuprofen and flurbiprofen (Brooks & Needs 1992).

PROPIONIC ACID DERIVATIVES

The propionic acid derivatives are a class of compounds which includes ibuprofen, naproxen, fenoprofen, ketoprofen and flurbiprofen. They are a rather homogeneous group of compounds. Selected propionic acid derivatives are generally thought to be safer than aspirin and are better tolerated by most patients.

Gastrointestinal irritation is the most common side-effect seen with these compounds, but it is less severe than with aspirin at equianalgesic doses. All of these agents alter platelet function and prolong bleeding time. However, the inhibition of cyclo-oxygenase produced by the propionic acid derivatives is reversible. Most of these compounds are available commercially as a racemic mixture of R(–) and S(+) isomers, except for naproxen which is available as the S(+) isomer (Williams & Day 1985). In man, the S(+) isomer has been found to be the active portion of the racemic mixture. For ibuprofen and fenoprofen the R(–) is converted to the S(+) isomer while for ketoprofen and flurbiprofen little, if any, conversion occurs in man (Jamali 1989).

IBUPROFEN

Pharmacokinetics and metabolism

Ibuprofen is rapidly absorbed following oral administration. Peak effect is usually attained in 1–2 hours. Ibuprofen is extensively metabolized in the liver and the metabolites are excreted in the urine, primarily as the S(+) isomer. The renal excretion of ibuprofen metabolites is virtually complete 24 hours after the last dose. The plasma half-life is approximately 2 hours. Ibuprofen is more than 99% albumin-bound.

Safety

Gastrointestinal side-effects are experienced by 5–15% of patients taking ibuprofen; however this incidence is less with ibuprofen than with aspirin or indomethacin at equianalgesic doses. Data from endoscopic studies of gastric injury indicate that dosage levels of ibuprofen at 1600 or 2400 mg daily, given for 3 days or less, produced little or no injury to the gastric mucosa. In contrast, aspirin 600 mg every 4 hours in the same study model produced gastric injury (Lanza 1984).

Aseptic meningitis has been observed in patients taking ibuprofen, particularly in patients with systemic lupus erythematosus (Rainsford 1987).

Renal toxicity in the form of interstitial nephritis has been reported for ibuprofen but it is rare. Renal effects of the NSAIDs are discussed under the section on general considerations, above.

For discussion of the use of ibuprofen in lactating females, see section on general considerations, above.

Drug interactions

The possibility of interaction with albumin-bound drugs must be considered and is discussed in the section on general considerations, above. Data regarding warfarin-ibuprofen interaction are conflicting. Clinicians should be aware that warfarin anticoagulant effects may be potentiated in rare instances.

Dosage and clinical efficacy

Ibuprofen (Motrin, Rufen) is available as 200, 300, 400

and 600 mg tablets. An ibuprofen suspension of 100 mg/5 ml is also available. For mild to moderate pain, the usual adult dose is between 200 and 400 mg every 4–6 hours as needed, not exceeding 3200 mg/day.

In several clinical trials, 200 mg ibuprofen has been shown to be more effective than acetaminophen 650 mg; ibuprofen 400 mg has been shown to be more effective than aspirin 650 mg, acetaminophen 600 mg, and both aspirin and acetaminophen when combined with codeine 60 mg (Cooper 1984).

NAPROXEN

Pharmacology and pharmacokinetics

Naproxen is a long-acting drug with analgesic activity requiring only twice-a-day dosage. It is the only drug marketed as the S(+) isomer rather than the racemic mixture. It is rapidly and completely absorbed, especially when administered as the sodium salt. Onset of analgesia may be accelerated by the use of the sodium salt of naproxen. Peak plasma levels of naproxen-anion are attained in 2–4 hours. The mean plasma half-life is approximately 13 hours and it is greater than 99% albumin-bound. Naproxen and its metabolites are almost entirely excreted in the urine. The administration of only the active d-isomer of naproxen instead of the racemic mixture is said to reduce side-effects (Allison et al 1985).

Safety

Most of the gastrointestinal side-effects seen in patients taking naproxen have been mild. Occasional cases of interstitial nephritis, reversible acute renal failure and nephrotic syndrome have been reported (Allison et al 1985). Patients with myeloma have been reported developing renal failure after short-term administration (Wu et al 1987). Pseudoporphyria from naproxen therapy has been reported as a rare complication (Physicians' Drug Alert 1986).

Drug interactions

Absorption may be accelerated by the concurrent administration of sodium bicarbonate or reduced by magnesium oxide or aluminum hydroxide. Probenecid decreases clearance of naproxen (Brogden 1986a).

Dosage and clinical efficacy

Naproxen (Naprosyn) is available as 250, 375 or 500 mg tablets for oral administration. Naproxen sodium (Anaprox) is available in tablets of 275 and 550 mg of the salt (equivalent to 250 and 500 mg of naproxen respectively). A suspension for oral administration containing 125 mg/5ml of naproxen is also available. The recommended starting dose of naproxen is 500 mg followed by 250 mg every 6–8 hours as required. There is a need for a priming dose because the 250 mg dose generally has slower onset of effect than standard aspirin. The total daily dose should not exceed 1250 mg for adults.

The efficacy of naproxen as an analgesic has been shown in several clinical studies. The 550 mg dose of naproxen sodium has provided significantly greater pain relief than standard doses of aspirin (650 mg), and a longer duration. Based on hourly analgesic scores and time to remedication, it appears to have an 8-hour duration of analgesic effect in most patients (Forbes et al 1986).

FENOPROFEN CALCIUM

Pharmacokinetics and metabolism

Fenoprofen has a half-life of approximately 3 hours. It is rapidly absorbed with peak plasma levels achieved within 2 hours after oral administration. The drug is extensively (90%) metabolized and excreted almost entirely in the urine.

Safety

Gastrointestinal side-effects are the most frequently reported. These side-effects are almost always less than with equipotent doses of aspirin. Interstitial nephritis has also been reported. See section on general considerations, above.

Drug interactions

The coadministration of aspirin with fenoprofen decreases the half-life of fenoprofen because of an increase in metabolic clearance.

Dosage and clinical efficacy

Fenoprofen calcium (Nalfon) is available in capsules and tablets containing 200–600 mg of active drug for oral administration. For the treatment of mild to moderate pain, the recommended dosage is 200 mg every 4–6 hours as needed.

Analgesic clinical trials (Sunshine et al 1978) have shown a dose-response between 50 and 200 mg of fenoprofen in postoperative pain; however a shallow dose-response was reported from 200–600 mg with very little enhancement of analgesic effect above 200 mg. Fenoprofen 200 mg was shown to be comparable to codeine 60 mg and also to aspirin 650 mg (Sunshine et al 1981).

KETOPROFEN

Pharmacokinetics and metabolism

Ketoprofen is rapidly absorbed after oral administration with peak plasma levels reached in 1–2 hours. The plasma half-life is about 1.5–2 hours. Ketoprofen is largely eliminated in the urine (60%) within 24 hours. Enterohepatic recirculation of the drug has been thought to account for the remaining 40% of the drug. There are no active metabolites (Harris & Vavra 1985).

Safety

The most common side-effects of ketoprofen involve the gastrointestinal system. However, comparative studies with aspirin show that the incidence of adverse gastrointestinal reaction is significantly lower with ketoprofen (Rahbeck 1976).

Drug interactions

Concurrent administration of aspirin reduced ketoprofen protein binding and accelerated plasma clearance. Protein binding and clearance of ketoprofen were reduced by probenecid, which appeared to inhibit ketoprofen glucuronidation. Cross-sensitivity between ketoprofen and aspirin does exist and one case of death attributable to this cause has been reported in the literature (Harris & Vavra 1985). Therefore, combined treatment with these agents should be avoided. See section on general considerations, above.

Dosage and clinical efficacy

Ketoprofen (Orudis) is available for oral use in 25, 50, 75 and 100 mg capsules, 50 mg injectable preparation, 100 mg suppositories and a topical gel. The usual recommended dose for mild-to-moderate pain is 25–50 mg every 6–8 hours as necessary. A larger dose may be tried if the patient's response to a previous dose was unsatisfactory. The recommended total daily dose ranges from 200–300 mg.

Oral analgesic studies suggest that ketoprofen at 25 mg is equal to or more effective than aspirin 650 mg (Cooper et al 1984; Sunshine et al 1986a) or codeine 90 mg (Mehlisch et al 1984). Ketoprofen 50 mg has been shown to be significantly more effective than aspirin 650 mg, while the 100 mg dose provided no added analgesia above that achieved with 50 mg ketoprofen (Sunshine et al 1986). More recent work (Sunshine et al 1992) demonstrates that ketoprofen 100 mg is significantly more effective than ketoprofen 50 mg; equivalent to acetaminophen 650 mg in combination with oxycodone 10 mg and of longer duration of effect in the treatment of postoperative pain.

FLURBIPROFEN

Pharmacokinetics and metabolism

Flurbiprofen is well absorbed after oral administration with peak mean plasma levels occurring within 1.5–3 hours after a dose. The half-life is approximately 3–4 hours. Oxidation and conjugation are the major pathways of metabolism. A total of 20–25% of the drug is excreted unchanged in urine; the remainder is primarily excreted as metabolites. Flurbiprofen is more than 99% albumin-bound.

Safety

Premarketing studies of 4123 patients treated with flurbiprofen revealed that 9.4% of the patients dropped out of the studies because of an adverse reaction, principally involving the gastrointestinal tract (5.8%), central nervous system and special senses (1.4%), skin (0.6%) and genitourinary tract (0.5%). Dyspepsia, diarrhoea, abdominal pain and nausea were the predominant gastrointestinal effects and headache was the more frequently reported central nervous system effect (Physicians' Desk Reference 1992).

For discussion of the use of flurbiprofen in lactating females, see section on general considerations, above.

Drug interactions

Drug interactions with the benzodiazepines may occur due to displacement from albumin binding sites. See section on general considerations, above.

Dosage and clinical efficacy

Flurbiprofen (Ansaid) is available as tablets of 50 and 100 mg. The analgesic dose ranges from 25–50 mg every 4–6 hours, with 50 mg being the preferred dose. Maximum daily dose is 300 mg/day.

Oral analgesic studies suggest that 50 mg of flurbiprofen is more effective than 650 mg of acetaminophen alone or in combination with 60 mg of codeine (Sunshine et al 1986b). Cooper et al (1988) demonstrated a linear dose effect from 50–150 mg of flurbiprofen.

OXYBUTYRIC ACIDS

FENBUFEN

Pharmacokinetics and metabolism

Fenbufen is classified as an oxybutyric acid (Humber 1992). It is a prodrug and is inactive until it is metabolized. It is converted to the active metabolites biphenylacetic acid and hydroxy-biphenylbutanoic acid (Greenberg & Bernstein 1985). Following oral administration, fenbufen is rapidly and essentially completely absorbed and converted to the active metabolites. Fenbufen and its metabolites are more than 98% bound to plasma proteins. Peak serum concentrations of fenbufen are reached by 1–2 hours. Half-lives range from 9–12 hours for all of the metabolites.

Safety

Skin rashes are more frequently reported with fenbufen than with aspirin or indomethacin and occur predominantly in women during the second or third week of therapy. In its mild form, the rash occurs on the trunk, extremities and face and may be characterized as morbilliform. In its severe form, erythroderma, facial and periorbital oedema, mucous membrane erythema and fever occur. Rarely, Stevens–Johnson syndrome or toxic epidermal necrolysis has been reported (Sloboda et al 1987).

Drug interactions

Fenbufen interacts with Coumadin-like drugs. Concomitant administration of fenbufen and aspirin may result in decreased serum concentration of fenbufen and its metabolites. See section on general considerations, above.

Dosage and clinical efficacy

Fenbufen (Cinopal, Bufemid) is available as 300 mg capsules and tablets of 300 or 450 mg. Effervescent tablets of 450 mg are also available. The exact analgesic dose is not specified. The daily dose for rheumatoid arthritis is 600–900 mg.

Studies on the analgesic efficacy of fenbufen are limited. Fenbufen was assessed in a double-blind postoperative clinical trial; fenbufen at a dose of 500 mg was similar in efficacy to aspirin 600 mg and at 900 mg it was significantly more effective than both the lower dose of fenbufen and aspirin 600 mg (Sunshine 1975). In another study, a single dose of fenbufen 800 mg was as effective as aspirin 600 mg for the relief of postoperative pain (Coutinho et al 1976). Fenbufen 500 mg was superior to aspirin 750 mg and placebo for the treatment of pain following the surgical removal of an impacted lower wisdom tooth (Henrikson et al 1979). Because of its poor efficacy and safety profiles, the use of this drug is questionable.

ACETIC ACIDS

This section discusses selected acetic acid derivatives from the indoleacetic, pyrrolacetic and phenylacetic groups. These include indomethacin, ketorolac and diclofenac sodium respectively (Fig. 48.1).

INDOMETHACIN

Pharmacokinetics and metabolism

Indomethacin is an indoleacetic with antiinflammatory and analgesic-antipyretic properties. It is readily absorbed from the gastrointestinal tract following oral ingestion; peak plasma concentrations are reached within 2 hours. Peak plasma concentrations are generally achieved sooner following rectal administration than with oral administration, but are lower (Verbeck et al 1983). Marked inter- and intraindividual differences in plasma concentrations following oral administration have been reported. The half-life of indomethacin is estimated to be about 4.5 hours. Indomethacin undergoes appreciable enterohepatic circulation. It is largely converted to inactive metabolites in the liver and kidneys and is excreted in the urine (60%) and to a much lesser extent (about 33%) in the faeces.

Safety

A very high percentage (35–50%) of patients receiving usual therapeutic doses of indomethacin experience adverse effects and about 20% must discontinue its use. The adverse effects are dose-related. Gastrointestinal complaints and complications consist of anorexia, nausea and abdominal pain in high incidence. Rectal administration of indomethacin is used in an attempt to minimize the gastrointestinal side-effects of orally administered indomethacin. A common side-effect is severe frontal headache, occurring in 25–50% of patients who take the drug chronically. Indomethacin may aggravate depression or other psychiatric disturbances, epilepsy and parkinsonism and should be used with caution in these conditions. Dizziness, drowsiness and lightheadedness have also been reported. If severe central nervous system reactions develop, indomethacin should be discontinued. Indomethacin is a potent inhibitor of renal prostaglandin and can lead to renal insufficiency in certain clinical states. See section on general considerations, above.

Drug interactions

The concurrent administration of probenecid increases the total plasma concentration of indomethacin plus its inactive metabolites, therefore a lower total daily dosage of indomethacin may be called for. Indomethacin antagonizes the natriuretic and antihypertensive effects of furosemide; the antihypertensive effects of thiazide diuretics may also be reduced. Acute renal failure has been associated with the concomitant administration of indomethacin and triamterene.

Dosage and clinical uses

The usual dose of indomethacin (Indocin) is 25–50 mg

three times a day. Few patients tolerate more than 100 mg/day without severe side-effects. The analgesic properties of indomethacin 50 mg are generally believed to be in the range of aspirin 650 mg (Sunshine et al 1964). Because of the high incidence and severity of side-effects associated with chronic administration, and the fact that its efficacy is equivalent to aspirin 650 mg, indomethacin is not routinely used as an analgesic or antipyretic.

KETOROLAC TROMETHAMINE

Pharmacokinetics and metabolism

Ketorolac tromethamine is a nonsteroidal analgesic agent approved for oral and intramuscular administration. The drug is a pyrrolo-pyrrole derivative chemically related to tolmetin and indomethacin. It is metabolized in the liver with some of the drug excreted unchanged in the urine. When given intramuscularly or orally, ketorolac is rapidly absorbed, achieving peak plasma concentration in 30–50 minutes. It has a plasma half-life of 5–6 hours and this is similar whether given orally or intramuscularly. Ketorolac is more than 99% albumin-bound. Ketorolac administered orally is bioequivalent to ketorolac administered intramuscularly.

Safety

The most serious risks associated with ketorolac are gastrointestinal, renal, haemorrhage and hypersensitivity reactions. The use of ketorolac at recommended doses for more than 5 days is associated with increased frequency and severity of adverse effects. The use of ketorolac^{oral} 10 mg on a long-term basis is associated with more gastrointestinal tract adverse effects than aspirin 650 mg four times a day. The gain in efficacy with the higher intramuscular dose regimen is achieved without a significant increase in adverse events for short term use (4–5 days). In general, ketorolac should not be administered for longer than 5 days. Renal adverse effects for ketorolac are similar to other NSAIDs. However, since ketorolac is available intramuscularly for use in the perioperative and postoperative period, patients with reduced blood volume and/or reduced renal blood flow may be exposed to this drug which can result in progressive renal failure.

Drug interactions

Concurrent administration of salicylate may increase unbound ketorolac plasma levels.

Dosage and clinical efficacy

Ketorolac tromethamine (Toradol^{im}) is available in 15, 30 or 60 mg syringe or cartridge needle units and is indicated for the short-term management of pain (not over 5 days). The recommended initial dose is 30 or 60 mg intramuscularly, as a loading dose, followed by half of the loading dose (i.e. 15 or 30 mg, every 6 hours). The maximum daily dose is 150 mg for the first day and 120 mg/day thereafter. Toradol^{oral} is available in 10 mg tablets. The recommended oral dose is 10 mg as needed every 4–6 hours for limited duration. Oral dosage should not exceed the recommended daily maximum of 40 mg for 5 days.

The clinical efficacy of ketorolac was investigated in general postoperative and oral surgery pain models. Ketorolac 30 or 90 mg intramuscularly was equivalent and was comparable in pain relief to meperidine 100 mg or morphine 12 mg (Yee et al 1986; O'Hara et al 1987) and ketorolac 10 mg intramuscularly was comparable to 50 mg of meperidine or 6 mg of morphine. In dental surgery, ketorolac 10 or 20 mg orally gave comparable pain relief to ibuprofen 400 mg, and superior relief to aspirin 650 mg, acetaminophen 600 mg and acetaminophen 600 mg in combination with codeine 60 mg (Forbes et al 1990a, 1990b).

DICLOFENAC SODIUM

Pharmacokinetics and metabolism

Diclofenac sodium is a phenylacetic acid derivative available for oral and parenteral use. Orally administered diclofenac undergoes first-pass metabolism with about 60% of the drug reaching the systemic circulation in unchanged form. After oral administration of enteric-coated tablets, the onset of absorption is delayed and peak plasma concentrations are attained within 2 hours. The mean half-life of orally administered diclofenac is 1.2–1.8 hours. Following intramuscular injection the maximum plasma concentration is found after approximately 15 minutes and the area under the curve is approximately twice that seen with oral or rectal formulations. This is due to hepatic first-pass effect.

Diclofenac and its metabolites are excreted mainly in the urine (61%) and faeces (30%). About 90% of an oral or intravenous dose of diclofenac is excreted in the first 96 hours. Enterohepatic recirculation of the unchanged active substance is minimal. Renal excretion of diclofenac has been found to correlate with creatinine clearance.

Safety

Gastrointestinal side-effects are the most frequently reported adverse effects of diclofenac and occur in about 5–25% of patients. Isolated cases have been reported of anaphylactoid reactions, skin rash and oedema. Elevations of transaminases have been reported in about 15% of patients treated with diclofenac sodium. If abnormal liver tests persist or worsen, or clinical signs or symptoms consistent with liver disease develop or if systemic manifestations occur, diclofenac should be discontinued. The optimum time for making the first transaminase measurements is not known; however the first measurement should be made no later than 8 weeks after the start of treatment. To minimize the possibility that hepatic injury will become severe between transaminase measurements, physicians should inform patients of the warning signs or symptoms of hepatotoxicity (e.g. nausea, fatigue, lethargy, pruritus, jaundice, right upper quadrant tenderness and 'flu-like' symptoms) and take the appropriate actions if these symptoms should occur (Physicians' Desk Reference 1992).

Drug interactions

Diclofenac increases steady-state plasma levels of digoxin (Sengupta et al 1985). Diclofenac decreases lithium renal clearance and increases lithium plasma levels. In patients taking diclofenac and lithium concomitantly, lithium toxicity may occur.

Dosage and clinical efficacy

Diclofenac sodium (Voltaren, Voltarol) is available in enteric-coated tablets of 25 and 50 mg, sustained release tablets of 100 mg and ampules of 75 mg in 3 ml. The oral adult dosage is 50 mg every 6–8 hours. For children aged 1 year or over the daily analgesic dose is 0.25–3 mg per kg body weight. The parenteral form has been used in a variety of painful conditions in a dose up to 75 mg intramuscularly every 12 hours for up to 1 week.

The available studies comparing diclofenac sodium with indomethacin suggest that the two drugs are comparable in analgesic efficacy. Preliminary studies suggest that the parenteral form may be very effective in renal colic. The analgesic efficacy of the potassium salt of diclofenac was compared to aspirin 650 mg in a double-blind study; diclofenac potassium 50 and 100 mg was found to be statistically superior to aspirin 650 mg in the treatment of postepisiotomy pain (Sunshine et al 1990).

ANTHRANILIC ACIDS (FENAMATES)

The fenamates are derivatives of N-phenylanthranilic acid. Select members of this group discussed here are meclofenamate sodium, mefenamic acid, floctafenine and glafenine. Pharmacologically the fenamates are cyclo-oxygenase inhibitors. While these substances have been reported to inhibit prostaglandin synthesis and antagonize the effects of prostaglandins at the myometrium, they are only as effective as other NSAIDs (Scherrer 1985). The absence of well-controlled clinical analgesic studies plus frequent adverse effects, including allergic diarrhoea, central nervous system effects and the scarcity of chronic safety data, have limited their application (Corbin & Upton 1987).

MECLOFENAMATE SODIUM

Pharmacokinetics and metabolism

Meclofenamate sodium is rapidly absorbed in man following single and multiple oral doses with peak plasma concentrations occurring in 0.5–2 hours. The half-life ranges from 0.8–2.1 hours with no evidence of accumulation of meclofenamic acid in plasma. Meclofenamic acid is extensively metabolized to an active metabolite (metabolite I) and to at least six other minor metabolites. Approximately 70% of the administered dose is excreted by the kidney and the remaining 30% is eliminated through biliary excretion (in the faeces). Meclofenamic acid is greater than 99% bound to plasma proteins. Meclofenamic acid has a decrease in both the rate and extent of absorption when taken with food.

Safety

The most frequently reported adverse reactions associated with meclofenamate sodium involve the gastrointestinal system. In controlled studies of up to 6 months these disturbances occurred in the following order of decreasing frequencies: diarrhoea (10–33%), nausea with or without vomiting (11%), other gastrointestinal disorders (10%) and abdominal pain. The occurrence of the diarrhoea is dose related, generally subsides with dose reduction and clears with termination of therapy.

Drug interactions

Meclofenamate sodium enhances the effect of warfarin. Concurrent administration of aspirin may lower meclofenamate sodium plasma levels.

Dosage and clinical efficacy

Meclofenamate sodium (Meclomen) is available in 50 or 100 mg capsules. For mild to moderate pain, the recommended dose is 50 mg every 4–6 hours. Doses of 100 mg may be needed in some patients for optimal relief. The daily dose should not exceed 400 mg.

In controlled clinical trials of patients with episiotomy or dental pain, meclofenamate sodium 100 mg provided benefit in some patients. The onset of analgesic effect was generally within 1 hour with a duration of 4–6 hours. In controlled trials of patients with dysmenorrhoea, meclofenamate sodium 100 mg three times a day provided significant reduction in the symptoms associated with dysmenorrhoea.

MEFENAMIC ACID

Pharmacokinetics and metabolism

Mefenamic acid is absorbed from the gastrointestinal tract. Peak concentrations in plasma are reached in 2 hours after a single oral dose. The plasma half-life is 2–3 hours. In man, approximately 67% of a dose of mefenamic acid is excreted in the urine, and 20–25% of the dose is accounted for in the faeces.

Safety

The most common side-effects involve the gastrointestinal tract. Diarrhoea in particular may be severe. Peptic ulceration and gastrointestinal bleeding have also been reported, as well as headache, drowsiness, dizziness and nervousness. Skin rashes may also occur. If diarrhoea or skin rash appears the drug should be stopped at once. Mefenamic acid has been shown to increase blood urea nitrogen. It is occasionally associated with serious bone marrow toxicity and hepatic toxicity.

Dose and clinical efficacy

Mefenamic acid (Ponstel, Ponstan) is indicated for acute pain. The initial dose for adults and children over 14 years of age is 500 mg; thereafter 250 mg every 6 hours with food. It is available over the counter in Japan. In the USA its use is restricted to intervals of 7 days.

Clinical trials suggest that mefenamic acid is approximately equivalent to aspirin.

FLOCTAFENINE

Pharmacokinetics and metabolism

Floctafenine is an anthranilic acid derivative. Floctafenine is well absorbed after oral administration and peak plasma levels are attained 1–2 hours after administration. Floctafenine has a half-life of approximately 1 hour. Floctafenine is rapidly hydrolysed in the liver to floctafenic acid, which becomes the main circulating metabolite. Elimination of floctafenine and its metabolites is virtually complete 24 hours after administration (Reynolds 1989).

Safety

The most commonly reported side-effects include drowsiness, dizziness, headache, insomnia, nausea, diarrhoea, abdominal pain or discomfort, heartburn and gastrointestinal bleeding. In clinical trials dysuria without apparent changes in renal function was reported.

Dosage and clinical use

Floctafenine (Idarac) is indicated for short-term use in acute pain of mild to moderate severity. The usual adult dosage is 200–400 mg every 6–8 hours as required. The maximum recommended daily dose is 1200 mg.

In postoperative pain, floctafenine 200 mg was not significantly different from aspirin 600 mg (Reynolds 1989).

GLAFENINE

Pharmacokinetics and metabolism

Glafenine is an anthranilic acid derivative. It is absorbed from the gastrointestinal tract with peak plasma concentrations occurring about 1–2 hours after ingestion. The half-life is about 75 minutes. It is metabolized to glafenic acid and is excreted in the urine and bile.

Safety

Side-effects reported with glafenine include gastrointestinal disturbances, headache, drowsiness, fever and renal failure. Allergic reactions may occur.

Dosage and clinical use

Glafenine (Exidol, Glifan) is indicated for acute and chronic pain. The usual adult dosage is 200–400 mg every 5–6 hours as required. For acute pain, 400 mg by mouth followed by 200 mg as required up to a total of 1000–1200 mg daily. For less severe pain the initial dose is 200–400 mg followed by 200 mg doses up to a total of 600–800 mg daily. It is also available as the hydrochloride, in 500 mg suppositories (Reynolds 1989).

PYRANOCARBOXYLIC ACID

ETODOLAC

Pharmacokinetics and metabolism

Etodolac is a pyranocarboxylic acid. It is well absorbed with a peak effect occurring in 1–2 hours. The mean plasma half-life is about 7 hours and it is more than 99% albumin-bound. Etodolac is extensively metabolized in the liver, with renal elimination of etodolac and its metabolites being the primary route of excretion.

Safety

Reported side-effects with etodolac include gastrointestinal disturbances, headache, drowsiness, dizziness, tinnitus and skin rashes. The presence of metabolites in the urine may give rise to a false-positive reaction for bilirubin.

Drug interactions

Coadministration of etodolac with an antacid decreases the peak concentration. Food intake reduces the peak concentration by one-half and increases the time-to-peak concentration by 1.4–3.8 hours.

Dosage and clinical efficacy

Etodolac (Lodine) is available as 200 or 300 mg capsules for oral administration. The recommended dose for acute pain is 200–400 mg every 6–8 hours as needed, not to exceed a total daily dose of 1200 mg.

The efficacy of etodolac as an analgesic has been shown in clinical studies (Mizraji 1990). Onset of analgesia occurred approximately 30 minutes after oral administration and was comparable for etodolac (200–400 mg), aspirin (650 mg), and acetaminophen with codeine (600 mg + 60 mg). Duration of relief averaged 4–5 hours for 200 mg of etodolac and 5–6 hours for 400 mg of etodolac as measured by when approximately half the patients required remedication. Etodolac 50, 100 and 200 mg was compared to aspirin 650 mg and placebo in the treatment of pain after oral surgery and was found comparable to aspirin (Nelson et al 1985).

OXICAMS

Pharmacologically the oxicams share the properties of other NSAIDs. Clinically, they have shown antirheumatic, antiinflammatory and analgesic activity. Oxicams are structurally distinct from other classes of NSAIDs and they have extended plasma half-lives (Wiseman 1982). This enables the oxicams to maintain therapeutic plasma drug concentrations throughout the day from a single daily dose.

PIROXICAM

Pharmacokinetics and metabolism

Piroxicam is completely absorbed after oral administration. The mean peak plasma concentrations are reached within 2–3 hours after oral administration and 5–6 hours after rectal administration. The plasma half-life ranges

Table 48.2A Average analgesic dosage of selected nonnarcotic analgesics and comparative efficacy to aspirin[1]

Drug	Proprietary name (not all-inclusive)	Average analgesic dose (mg)	Dose interval (h)	Maximal daily dose (mg)	Analgesic efficacy compared to aspirin 650 mg (oral formulation only)	Comments
Acetaminophen	Numerous	p.o. 500–1000	4–6	4000	Comparable	No antiplatelet effect; hepatotoxicity seen with sustained high doses
Salicylates						
Acetylsalicylic acid	Numerous; Aspegic (lysine aspirin)	p.o. 500–1000 i.v. 900–1800	4–6 prn	4000 7200	900 mg of lysine aspirin contains 500 mg of aspirin	Irreversible antiplatelet effect
Diflunisal	Dolobid	p.o. 1000 p.o. 500	initial dose 8–12 h thereafter	 1500	500 mg superior in efficacy to aspirin with slower onset and longer duration; an initial dose of 1000 mg significantly shortens time to onset of effect	No antiplatelet effect at lower doses
Magnesium salicylate	Doan's, Magan	p.o. 1000	4–6	4000		No antiplatelet effect; less GI effect than aspirin
Choline magnesium trisalicylate	Trilisate	p.o. 1000–1500	12	4000		No antiplatelet effect; less GI effect than aspirin
Pyrazolones						
Dipyrone	Novalgina, Metamizol	p.o. 500–1000 i.m., i.v., 500–1000	t.i.d t.i.d	3000 3000	Superior (based on limited data)	Reversible antiplatelet effect; withdrawn in some countries because of toxicity

[1]Not all drugs and formulations are available in all countries.
prn = as needed for pain

Table 48.2B Average analgesic dosage of selected nonnarcotic analgesics and comparative efficacy to aspirin[1]

Drug	Proprietary name (not all-inclusive)	Average analgesic dose (mg)	Dose interval (h)	Maximal daily dose (mg)	Analgesic efficacy compared to aspirin 650 mg (oral formulation only)	Comments
Propionic acids						
Ibuprofen	Motrin, Rufen Nuprin, Advil	p.o. 200–400	4–6	3200	Superior at both doses	
Naproxen	Naprosyn	p.o. 500 p.o. 250	Initial dose 6–8 h thereafter	1250		
Naproxen sodium	Anaprox	p.o. 550 p.o. 275	Initial dose 6–8 h thereafter	1375	275 mg is comparable in efficacy to aspirin with slower onset and longer duration. 550 mg is superior to aspirin	
Fenoprofen	Nalfon	p.o. 200	4–6	800	Comparable	
Ketoprofen	Orudis	p.o. 25–50–75 i.m., i.v. 100	6–8	300 100	25 mg is comparable in efficacy to aspirin (based on limited data); 50 mg is superior to aspirin	Data on parenteral ketoprofen are limited; it is recommended that only one dose be given i.m., followed by p.o. dosage
Flurbiprofen	Ansaid	p.o. 50	4–6	300	Superior	
Oxybutyric acids						
Fenbufen	Cinopal, Bufemid	p.o. 300	b.i.d	900	Inferior (based on limited data)	Frequent severe skin rashes can occur

[1]Not all drugs and formulations are available in all countries.

from 36–45 hours. Piroxicam is more than 99% albumin-bound. There is enterohepatic recycling of piroxicam. Metabolic transformation in man accounts for about 60% of the drug being excreted in the urine and faeces (Flower et al 1985).

Safety

Gastrointestinal reactions are the most common side-effects reported with the use of piroxicam. Peptic ulceration, perforation and gastrointestinal bleeding, in some instances fatal, have been reported with patients treated with piroxicam. Other than the gastrointestinal symptoms, oedema, dizziness, headache, changes in haematological parameters and rash have also been reported.

Drug interactions

Piroxicam has been reported to potentiate the anticoagulant effect of acenocoumarol (Wiseman 1985). Plasma levels of piroxicam are decreased approximately 80% when administered in conjunction with aspirin. See section on general considerations, above.

Dosage and clinical efficacy

Piroxicam (Feldene) is available in 10 and 20 mg capsules for oral administration. The usual single daily dose is 20 mg. The analgesic dose and antiinflammatory doses are the same. Recent clinical studies suggest that a priming dose of 40 mg enhances the analgesic response on first administration.

Piroxicam 20 mg exerted analgesic activity comparable to that of aspirin 648 mg in subjects with postoperative, postfracture, postepisiotomy, postpartum and dental pain, but of longer duration of effect. Piroxicam 20 mg daily also provided effective management for symptoms of dysmenorrhoea (Wiseman 1985). In general, as with all the longer acting NSAIDs, the onset of action and the mean effects in the first 2 hours are usually less than that of aspirin.

ANALGESIC ADJUVANTS

Analgesic adjuvants are drugs that enhance the response of known analgesics. The drugs in this category which have been shown to have proven effect are caffeine, amphetamines, antihistamines and tricyclic antidepressants. The antidepressants are discussed elsewhere in this text.

CAFFEINE

Clinical studies have indicated that caffeine significantly enhances the analgesic effect of aspirin, acetaminophen

Table 48.2C Average analgesic dosage of selected nonnarcotic analgesics and comparative efficacy to aspirin[1]

Drug	Proprietary name (not all-inclusive)	Average analgesic dose (mg)	Dose interval (h)	Maximal daily dose (mg)	Analgesic efficacy compared to aspirin 650 mg (oral formulation only)	Comments
Acetic acids						
Indoleacetic acids						
Indomethacin	Indocin	p.o. 25–50	b.i.d. or t.i.d. 8–12	100	Comparable	Not routinely used as an analgesic because of high incidence of side-effects
Pyrrolacetic acids						
Ketorolac tromethamine	Toradol	p.o. 10 i.m. 30–60 i.m. 15–30	4–6 Initial dose 6 h thereafter	40 150 first day, 120 thereafter	Superior	Ketorolac should be limited to short-term therapy (not over 5 days); when oral ketorolac is used as follow-on therapy to i.m. ketorolac, the total combined dose should not exceed 120 mg on day of transition with a maximum of 40 mg orally
Phenylacetic acids						
Diclofenac sodium	Voltaren, Voltarol	p.o. 25–50 i.m. 25–75	6–8 12	150 150	Diclofenac potassium at 50 mg and 100 mg has been reported to be superior to aspirin	i.m. diclofenac has been reported to be efficacious in renal colic. Monitor for abnormal liver chemistries (see text)

[1]Not all drugs and formulations are available in all countries.

and ibuprofen and shortens the time to onset of effect (Laska et al 1984; Forbes et al 1990c; Schachtel et al 1991). The suggested oral dose for caffeine is 65 to 130 mg in combination with an analgesic.

AMPHETAMINES

Forrest et al (1977) showed that dextroamphetamine 10 mg in combination with morphine markedly enhanced the analgesic response and overcame the sedating effect of morphine. The clinical application of amphetamines is in situations where it is important to have the patient alert and to minimize the amount of morphine or other narcotics necessary for analgesia.

ANTIHISTAMINES

Antihistamines have been shown to be analgesic adjuvants in both animal and human studies. Hydroxyzine is widely used as an adjuvant in preoperative analgesia as well as in postoperative and cancer pain. Hydroxyzine in a dose of 100 mg intramuscularly enhances the analgesic response of morphine. Hydroxyzine itself has some analgesic effect (Beaver & Freise 1976). Clinically, hydroxyzine decreases the amount of narcotic that is necessary and in addition provides sedating and other antihistaminic effects that are helpful in certain clinical situations. Phenyltoloxamine has also been shown to be an orally effective analgesic adjuvant (Sunshine et al 1987b).

COMBINATIONS

The nonnarcotic analgesics have a ceiling effect. To achieve a greater analgesic response, the use of these drugs in combination with the narcotic analgesics has proven to be clinically useful. These combinations provide enhanced efficacy through the additive effect of two drugs producing analgesia by different mechanisms. These combinations can also result in reduced adverse reactions because each of the analgesic components can be used at a reduced dose. Some representative oral narcotics that are used in combination with NSAIDs are codeine, hydrocodone, oxycodone and propoxyphene.

There are no well-controlled clinical trials demonstrating that the combination of an NSAID with another NSAID provides analgesic effect superior to either one of the drugs alone. The addition of acetaminophen to aspirin has raised the questions of enhanced renal toxicity and the

Table 48.2D Average analgesic dosage of selected nonnarcotic analgesics and comparative efficacy to aspirin[1]

Drug	Proprietary name (not all-inclusive)	Average analgesic dose (mg)	Dose interval (h)	Maximal daily dose (mg)	Analgesic efficacy compared to aspirin 650 mg (oral formulation only)	Comments
Anthranilic acids						
Meclofenamate sodium	Meclomen	p.o. 50 p.o. 100	4–6 prn	400	NA	Indicated for mild to moderate pain, and for excessive menstrual blood loss and primary dysmenorrhoea
Mefenamic acid	Ponstel	p.o. 500 p.o. 250	Initial dose 6 h thereafter	1500	Comparable	In the USA its use is restricted to intervals of 1 week
Floctafenine	Idarac	p.o. 200–400	6–8	1200	Comparable	
Glafenine	Exidol, Glifan	p.o. 400 p.o. 200	Initial dose prn	1200	NA	500 mg suppository of the hydrochloride is available
Pyranocarboxylic acid						
Etodolac	Lodine	p.o. 200–400	6–8	1200	Comparable	Food markedly decreases absorption
Oxicams						
Piroxicam	Feldene	p.o. 20	24	20	Comparable in efficacy to aspirin with slower onset and much longer duration	A 40 mg loading dose which hastens onset is approved in some countries

[1]Not all drugs and formulations are available in all countries.
NA = not available.
prn = as needed for pain.

use of acetaminophen in combination with an NSAID is therefore also questionable.

GUIDELINES IN THE SELECTION OF NSAIDs AS ANALGESICS

Selecting and using the most appropriate nonnarcotic analgesic for a patient requires a knowledge of the unique properties of that analgesic. Table 48.2 provides the usual recommended dosages, dosing intervals and a statement of the drug's relative efficacy in comparison to aspirin. Unique features of the particular compounds are presented as well. Where platelet function is of particular concern, drugs such as acetaminophen or one of the nonacetylated salicylates could be considered. Particular attention should be paid to gastrointestinal and renal adverse effects and their prevention discussed above.

NSAIDs vary in time to onset and duration of analgesic effect. Generally, the longer the half-life of a drug, the slower the onset of effect. In treating patients with acute pain there appears to be an advantage in starting with the highest approved dose of a short half-life drug and then adjusting the dose downward. With many NSAIDs the higher dose has a faster onset rate, higher peak effect and a longer duration. Most NSAIDs have a dose-response relationship and a ceiling effect. In chronic pain conditions, the use of once-a-day or twice-a-day administration of a long half-life drug is a clear advantage. The longer acting once-a-day or twice-a-day drugs usually require a priming dose to achieve increased blood levels and shortened onset of effect. Factors of patient compliance, drug interaction and conditions influencing drug absorption, as well as any underlying disease processes should be considered if there is treatment failure. If a patient fails to respond to a particular NSAID, it is advisable to select another, perhaps of another class. Careful adjustment of the dose of the analgesic to the individual patient is important. For chronic use, the lowest dose that provides satisfactory results should be maintained. Particular attention should be paid to the elderly because of the increase in incidence of adverse effects, such as gastrointestinal bleeding, which may be dose-related. As data accumulate from pharmacodynamic studies, therapeutic ranges will hopefully become available to assist clinicians in determining the appropriate dosage regimen for the management of more difficult cases.

Acknowledgement

The authors thank J Rodriguez for her help in the preparation of this manuscript.

REFERENCES

Abramson S 1991 Therapy with and mechanisms of nonsteroidal anti-inflammatory drugs. Current Opinion in Rheumatology 3: 336–340

Allison A C, Rooks W H, Segre E J 1985 Naproxen. In: Rainsford K D (ed) Anti-inflammatory and anti-rheumatic drugs, vol 2. Newer anti-inflammatory drugs. CRC Press, Boca Raton, Florida, p 171–188

Beaver W J, Freise G 1976 Comparison of the analgesic effect of morphine, hydroxyzine and their combination in patients with postoperative pain. Advances in Pain Research Therapy 1: 553–557

Birkett D J 1985 The importance of unbound drug. In: Agents and Actions Supplement 17 (Proceedings of a Symposium on non-steroidal anti-inflammatory drugs – basis for variability in response). Birkhauser Verlag, Basel, p 79–84

Borda I T 1992 The spectrum of adverse gastrointestinal effects associated with nonsteroidal anti-inflammatory drugs. In: Borda I T, Koff R S (eds) NSAIDs: a profile of adverse effects. Hanley & Belfus, Philadelphia and Mosby-Yearbook, St Louis, p 25–80

Brogden R N 1986a Non-steroidal anti-inflammatory analgesics other than salicylates. In: Lasagna L, Prescott L F (eds) Non-narcotic analgesics today: benefits and risks. Drugs 32 (suppl 4): 27–45

Brogden R N 1986b Pyrazolone derivatives. In: Lasagna L, Prescott L F (eds) Non-narcotic analgesics today: benefits and risks. Drugs 32 (suppl 4): 60–70

Brooks P M, Needs C J 1992 NSAIDs in lactating women. In: Famaey J P, Paulus H E (eds) Therapeutic applications of NSAIDs subpopulations and new formulations. Marcel Dekker, New York, p 157–162

Brune K 1985 Pharmacokinetic factors as causes of variability in response to non-steroidal anti-inflammatory drugs. In: Agents and Actions Supplement 17 (Proceedings of a symposium on non-steroidal anti-inflammatory drugs: basis for variability in response). Birkhauser Verlag, Basel, p 59–63

Clissold S P 1986 Aspirin and related derivatives of salicylic acid. In: Lasagna L, Prescott L F (eds) Non-narcotic analgesics today: benefits and risks. Drugs 32 (suppl 4): 8–26

Cooper S 1984 Five studies on ibuprofen for postsurgical dental pain. In: Proceedings of a symposium – Motrin (ibuprofen) past, present and future. American Journal of Medicine 77: 70–77

Cooper K, Bennett W 1987 Nephrotoxicity of common drugs used in clinical practice. Archives of Internal Medicine 147: 1213–1218

Cooper S A, Gelbs, Goldman E H et al 1984 An analgesic relative potency assay comparing ketoprofen and aspirin in postoperative dental pain. Advances in Therapy 1: 410

Corbin A, Upton G V 1987 Nonsteroidal anti-inflammatory drugs in dysmenorrhea. In: Lewis A J, Furst D E (eds) Nonsteroidal anti-inflammatory drugs: mechanisms and clinical use. Marcel Dekker, New York, p 89–105

Coutinho A, Bonelli J, De Carvalho P 1976 A double-blind comparative study of the analgesic effects of fenbufen, codeine, aspirin, propoxyphene and placebo. Current Therapeutic Research 19: 58–65

Day R O, Brooks P M 1987 Variations in response to non-steroidal anti-inflammatory drugs. British Journal of Clinical Pharmacology 23: 655–658

Dressman J B, Berardi R R, Elta G H et al 1992 Absorption of flurbiprofen in the fed and fasted states. Pharmaceutical Research 9: 901–907

Fields H 1987 Pain. McGraw-Hill, New York, p 13–40

Flower R J, Vane J R 1972 Inhibition of prostaglandin synthetase in brain explains the anti-pyretic activity of paracetamol (4-Acetamidophenol). Nature 240: 410–411

Flower R J, Moncada S, Vane J R 1985 Analgesic-antipyretics and the anti-inflammatory agents: drugs employed in the treatment of gout. In: Gilman A G et al (eds) The pharmacological basis of therapeutics, 7th edn. MacMillan, New York, p 674–715

Forbes J A, Beaver W T, White E H et al 1982 A new oral analgesic with an unusually long duration of action. Journal of the American Medical Association 248: 2139–2142

Forbes J A, Keller C K, Smith J W et al 1986 Analgesic effect of naproxen sodium, codeine, a naproxen–codeine combination and aspirin on the postoperative pain of oral surgery. Pharmacotherapy 6: 211–218

Forbes J A, Butterworth G A, Burchfield W H et al 1990a Evaluation of ketorolac, aspirin, and an acetaminophen–codeine combination in postoperative oral surgery pain. Pharmacotherapy 10: 77S–93S

Forbes J A, Kehm C J, Grodin C D et al 1990b Evaluation of ketorolac, ibuprofen, acetaminophen, and an acetaminophen–codeine combination in postoperative oral surgery pain. Pharmacotherapy 10: 94S–105S

Forbes J A, Jones K F, Kehm C J et al 1990c Evaluation of aspirin, caffeine, and their combination in postoperative oral surgery pain. Pharmacotherapy 10: 387–393

Forrest W H, Brown B W, Brown C R et al 1977 Dextroamphetamine with morphine for treatment of postoperative pain. New England Journal of Medicine 296: 712–715

Goodwin J S, Regan M 1982 Cognitive dysfunction association with naproxen and ibuprofen in the elderly. Arthritis and Rheumatism 25: 1013–1015

Graham S, Smith J L 1986 Aspirin and the stomach. Annals of Internal Medicine 104: 390–398

Greenberg B P, Bernstein J 1985 Fenbun. In: Rainsford K D (ed) Anti-inflammatory and anti-rheumatic drugs, vol 2. Newer anti-inflammatory drugs. CRC Press, Boca Raton, Florida, p 87–104

Harris R H, Vavra I 1985 Ketoprofen. In: Rainsford K D (ed) Anti-inflammatory and anti-rheumatic drugs, vol 2. Newer anti-inflammatory drugs. CRC Press, Boca Raton, Florida, p 151–170

Harth M 1992 Rare miscellaneous adverse drug reactions and interactions of NSAIDs. In: Borda I T, Koff R S (eds) NSAIDs: a profile of adverse effects. Hanley & Belfus, Philadelphia and Mosby-Yearbook, St Louis, p 219–231

Hayes A H 1981 Therapeutic implications of drug interactions with acetaminophen and aspirin. Archives of Internal Medicine 141: 301–304

Henrikson P A, Tiernberg A, Ahlstrom U, Petersen L E 1979 Analgesic efficacy and safety of fenbufen following surgical removal of a lower wisdom tooth: a comparison with acetyl salicylic acid and placebo. Journal of International Medical Research 7: 107–116

Higgs G A, Salmon J A, Henderson B, Vane J R 1987 Pharmacokinetics of aspirin and salicylate in relation to inhibition of arachidonate cyclo-oxygenase and anti-inflammatory activity. Proceedings of the National Academy of Sciences USA 84: 1417–1420

Hoigne R V, Szczeklik A 1992 Allergic and pseudoallergic reactions associated with nonsteroidal anti-inflammatory drugs. In: Borda I T, Koff R S (eds) NSAIDs: a profile of adverse effects. Hanley & Belfus, Philadelphia and Mosby-Yearbook, St Louis, p 57–184

Humber L G 1992 On the Classification of NSAIDs. Drug News and Perspectives 5: 102–103

Jamali F, Mehvar R, Pasutto R M 1989 Eantioselective aspects of drug action and disposition: therapeutic pitfalls. Journal of Pharmaceutical Sciences 78: 695–715

Kantor T G 1984 Peripherally acting analgesics. In: Kuhar M, Pasternak G (eds) Analgesics: neurochemical, behavioral and clinical perspectives. Raven Press, New York, p 289–312

Lanza F L 1984 Endoscopic studies of gastric and duodenal injury after the use of ibuprofen, aspirin and other nonsteroidal anti-inflammatory agents. Proceedings of a symposium – Motrin (ibuprofen) past, present, and future. American Journal of Medicine 77: 19–24

Laska E M, Sunshine A, Mueller F et al 1984 Caffeine as an analgesic adjuvant. Journal of the American Medical Association 251: 1711–1718

Laska E M, Sunshine A, Marrero I et al 1986 The correlation between blood levels of ibuprofen and clinical analgesic response. Clinical Pharmacology and Therapeutics 40: 1–7

Levy G 1981 Comparative pharmacokinetics of aspirin and acetaminophen. Archives of Internal Medicine 141: 279–281

Levy M 1986 Pharmacokinetics of metamizol metabolites. In: Brune K (ed) 100 years of pyrazolone drugs. Agents and actions, vol 19. Birkhauser Verlag, Basel, p 199–204

Malmberg A B, Yaksh T L 1992 Hyperalgesia mediated by spinal glutamate or substance receptor blocked by spinal cyclo-oxygenase inhibition. Science 257: 1277–1280

Mehlisch D, Frakes L, Cavaliere M B et al 1984 Double-blind parallel comparison of single oral doses of ketoprofen, codeine, and placebo in patients with moderate to severe dental pain. Journal of Clinical Pharmacology 24: 486

Merckle 1986 Imbun 400/500 Rheuma-analgetikum Mit der wirksubstanz ibuprofen–lysinat-auf der basis von ibuprofen. Jahre Merckle Arznelmittel, Blaubeuren

Mizraji M 1990 Clinical response to etodolac in the management of pain. European Journal of Rheumatology and Inflammation 10: 35–43

Nelson S L, Bergman S A 1985 Relief of dental surgery pain: a controlled 12-hour comparison of etodolac, aspirin, and placebo. Anesthesia Progress 32: 151–156

O'Hara D A, Fragen R J, Kinzer M, Pemberton D 1987 Ketorolac tromethamine as compared with morphine sulfate for treatment of postoperative pain. Clinical Pharmacology and Therapeutics 41: 556–561

PEM News, Drug Surveillance Research Unit, University of Southampton, no 3, December 1985

Physicians' Desk Reference 1992 46th Edition, Medical Economics Data, Montvale, New Jersey, p 1043

Physicians' Drug Alert 1986 Pseudoporphyria from the naproxen therapy, vol VII, no 10, October 1986, p 73–74

Rahbek I 1976 Gastroscopic evaluation of the effect of a new anti-rheumatic compound, Ketoprofen (19, 583 RP) on the human gastric mucosa. Scandinavian Journal of Rheumatology 5 (suppl 14): 63

Rainsford K D 1987 Toxicity of currently used anti-inflammatory and anti-rheumatic drugs. In: Lewis A J, Furst D E (eds) Nonsteroidal anti-inflammatory drugs – mechanism and clinical use. Marcel Dekker, New York, p 215–244

Reynolds J E F (ed) 1989 Martindale: the extra pharmacopoeia, 29th edn. Analgesic and anti-inflammatory agents. Pharmaceutical Press, London, p 1–49

Roth H J 1986 Pharmacokinetics and biotransformation of pyrazolinones. In: Brune K (ed) 100 years of pyrazolone drugs. Agents and actions, vol 19. Birkhauser Verlag, Basel, p 205–221

Roth S H, Bennett R E 1992 NSAIDs, peptic ulcer, esophageal disease, and gastropathy. In: Famaey J P, Paulus H E (eds) Therapeutic applications of NSAIDs – subpopulations and new formulations. Marcel Dekker, New York, p 279–298

Rybak M E M 1992 Hematologic effects of nonsteroidal anti-inflammatory drugs. In: Borda I T, Koff R S (eds) NSAIDs: a profile of adverse effects. Hanley & Belfus, Philadelphia and Mosby-Yearbook, St Louis, p 113–132

Schactel B P, Fillingim J M, Lane A L et al 1991 Caffeine as an analgesic adjuvant. A double-blind study comparing aspirin with caffeine to aspirin and placebo in patients with sore throat. Archives of Internal Medicine 151: 733–737

Scherrer R A 1985 Fenamic acids. In: Rainsford K D (ed) Anti-inflammatory and anti-rheumatic drugs, vol 2. Newer anti-inflammatory drugs. CRC Press, Boca Raton, Florida, p 65–87

Seeff L B, Cuccherini B A, Zimmerman H J et al 1986 Acetaminophen hepatotoxicity in alcoholics. Annals of Internal Medicine 104: 399–404

Sengupta C, Afeche P, Meyer-Brunot H G et al 1985 Diclofenac sodium. In: Rainsford K D (ed) Anti-inflammatory and anti-rheumatic drugs, vol 2. Newer anti-inflammatory drugs. CRC Press, Boca Raton, Florida, p 49–64

Sloboda A E, Oronsky A L, Kerwar S S 1987 Fenbufen. In: Lewis A J, Furst D E (eds) Nonsteroidal anti-inflammatory drugs – mechanism and clinical use. Marcel Dekker, New York, p 371–392

Sunshine A 1975 Analgesic value of fenbufen in postoperative patients. A comparative oral analgesic study of fenbufen, aspirin, and placebo. Journal of Clinical Pharmacology 15: 591–597

Sunshine A, Laska E, Meisner M, Morgan S 1964 Analgesic studies of indomethacin as analyzed by computer techniques. Clinical Pharmacology and Therapeutics 5: 699–707

Sunshine A, Slafta J, Gruber C 1978 A comparative analgesic study of propoxyphene, fenoprofen, the combination of propoxyphene and fenoprofen, aspirin and placebo. Journal of Clinical Pharmacology 18: 556–563

Sunshine A, Laska E, Zighelboim I et al 1981 A comparison of the analgesic responses of fenoprofen, codeine, and placebo in postpartum and postoperative pain. Current Therapeutic Research 29: 771–777

Sunshine A, Zighelboim I, Laska E et al 1986a Double-blind parallel comparison of ketoprofen, aspirin, and placebo in patients with postpartum pain. Journal of Clinical Pharmacology 26: 706–711

Sunshine A, Marrero I, Olson N et al 1986b Comparative study of flurbiprofen, zomepirac sodium, acetaminophen plus codeine and acetaminophen for the relief of postsurgical pain. American Journal of Medicine 80 (suppl 3A): 50–54

Sunshine A, Zighelboim I, Sorrentino J V, Bartizek R D 1989 Augmentation of acetaminophen analgesia by phenyltoloxamine. Journal of Clinical Pharmacology 29: 660–664

Sunshine A, Laska E, Siegel C et al 1990 Duration of analgesic efficacy of diclofenac potassium in postepisiotomy pain. Clinical Pharmacology and Therapeutics 47: 164

Sunshine A, Marrero I, Olson N Z et al 1992a Analgesic efficacy of choline magnesium trisalicylate alone and in combination with controlled-release codeine for the treatment of postsurgical pain assessed with a new method for duration (submitted for publication)

Sunshine A, Olson N Z, Zighelboim I et al 1992b Duration of analgesic efficacy of ketoprofen, acetaminophen alone, acetaminophen plus oxycodone and placebo in postoperative pain. Clinical Pharmacology and Therapeutics 51: 123

Szczeklik A 1986 Analgesics, allergy and asthma. In: Lasagna L, Prescott L F (eds) Non-narcotic analgesics today: benefits and risks. Drugs 32 (suppl 4): 148–163

Tempero K F, Cirillo V J, Steelman S L 1977 The clinical pharmacology of diflunisal. In: Miehlke K (ed) Diflunisal in clinical practice (proceedings of a special symposium held at the XIV Congress of Rheumatology). Futura Publishing, Mt Kisco, New York

Vane J R 1973 Inhibition of prostaglandin synthesis as a mechanism of action for aspirin-like drugs. Nature 231: 232–235

Verbeck R K, Blackburn J L, Loewen G R 1983 Clinical pharmacokinetics of non-steroidal anti-inflammatory drugs. Clinical Pharmacokinetics 8: 297–331

Williams K M, Day R O 1985 Stereoselective disposition – basis for variability in response to NSAIDs. In: Agents and actions, vol 17. (Proceedings of a symposium on non-steroidal anti-inflammatory drugs – basis for variability in response). Birhauser Verlag, Basel, p 119–126

Wiseman E H 1982 Pharmacologic studies with a new class of nonsteroidal anti-inflammatory agents – the oxicams – with special reference to piroxicam (Feldene). In: Piroxicam Symposium. American Journal of Medicine (Feb 16): 2–8

Wiseman E H 1985 Piroxicam and related oxicams. In: Rainsford K D (ed) Anti-inflammatory and anti-rheumatic drugs, vol 2. Newer anti-inflammatory drugs. CRC Press, Boca Raton, Florida, p 209–248

Wu M J, Kumar K S, Kulkarni G, Kaiser H 1987 Multiple myeloma in naproxen-induced acute renal failure. New England Journal of Medicine 317: 170–171

Yee J T, Brown C R, Allbon C et al 1986 Analgesia from intramuscular ketorolac tromethamine compared to morphine in severe pain following major surgery. Pharmacotherapy 6: 253–261

49. Opioids

Robert G. Twycross

INTRODUCTION

The following is highly selective. The emphasis is on the use of strong opioids for the relief of cancer pain. Although opioids have been described as 'the mainstay of cancer pain management' (World Health Organization 1986), in many countries morphine and codeine are not available for this purpose or, if available, are underused (World Health Organization 1990). As a result, many cancer patients suffer pain needlessly. The World Health Organization is attempting to correct this by promoting wider knowledge among health-care workers about orally administered opioids in the management of cancer pain and by encouraging drug regulatory authorities to make sufficient quantities of these drugs available (Stjernsward 1991).

Although there is consensus among specialists internationally about the use of codeine and morphine for cancer pain (World Health Organization 1986, 1990), conflicting views are still expressed about a number of issues (Portenoy & Coyle 1990):

1. responsiveness of neuropathic pain to opioids
2. respiratory depression
3. tolerance
4. addiction
5. route of administration
6. timing of administration
7. morphine versus diamorphine
8. metabolism of morphine
9. oral-to-parenteral potency ratio of morphine
10. alternatives to morphine.

The key to the resolution of several of these areas of controversy lies in a realization that there are significant differences in man between opioid *clinical* pharmacology (i.e. patients) and opioid *laboratory* pharmacology (i.e. volunteers). These differences appear to relate to the presence or absence of pain. For example, in the absence of pain, respiratory depression and tolerance may well occur. In patients being treated for opioid responsive pain, however, these phenomena are rarely of clinical importance.

Many of the controversial issues apply to both cancer pain management and postoperative care. It is important to recognize that the pharmacological differences between oral and parenteral administration of any given opioid may be greater than those between different opioids given by the same route. As the goal of treatment is pain relief with the minimum of adverse effects, a rational approach requires an understanding of the clinical pharmacology of both oral and parenteral use.

OPIOID CLASSIFICATION AND RECEPTOR SITES

Clinically, opioids can be conveniently classified as weak (e.g. codeine) and strong (e.g. morphine). These terms are necessarily imprecise but refer principally to *relative efficacy* rather than potency (Hanks & Hoskin 1987). Weak opioids exhibit a ceiling to their analgesic effect because of an increased incidence of adverse effects. Thus, it is rarely possible to increase the dose of codeine above 200 mg every 4 hours. In contrast, strong opioids have a much wider range of efficacy and can relieve more severe pain.

Opioids may also be classified in terms of receptor site affinities. There is general agreement on the relevance to pain modulation of three subtypes of opioid receptor, namely, mu, delta and kappa (Fig. 49.1). Most clinically used opioids are predominantly mu agonists. Of the more recently introduced opioids, buprenorphine, profadol and propiram are partial mu agonists, whereas butorphanol and nalbuphine are partial kappa agonists. Because the latter two are antagonists at the mu receptor, they are commonly called *mixed agonist–antagonists* (Table 49.1). Nalophine and pentazocine also come into this category. Mixed agonist–antagonists should not be used in conjunction with mu agonists.

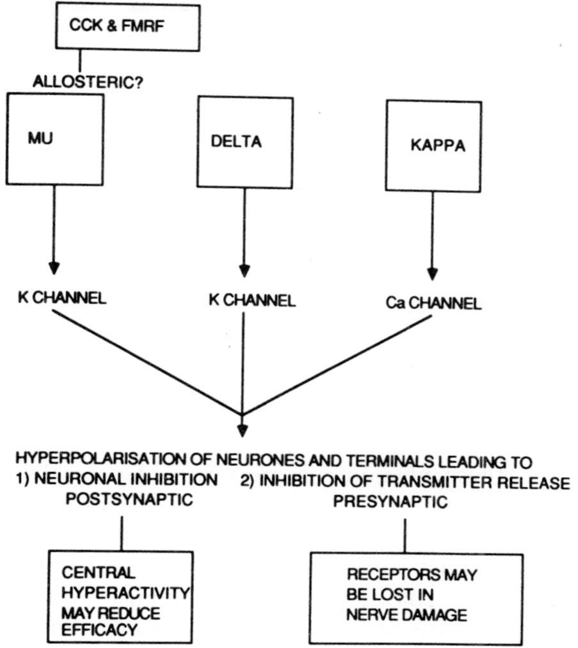

Fig. 49.1 The three main opioid receptor subtypes and their effector mechanisms together with the interactions between the opioid and other systems which may interfere with analgesia. (From Dickenson 1991 with permission.)

Evidence for the differential roles of the opioid receptor subtypes has accumulated since the identification of relatively selective agonists and antagonists for the three receptors (Table 49.2). The actions of opioids in the spinal cord are reasonably well understood and there is increasing knowledge of supraspinal sites of action, peripheral analgesic effects in inflammatory states (Hargreaves et al 1988) and interactions between opioid and nonopioid systems at spinal levels (Dickenson 1991).

OPIOID-RESISTANT PAIN

All pain is not equally responsive to opioid analgesics (Schulze et al 1988; Hanks 1991a). It is useful therefore to have a working classification of pain based on anticipated response to opioids (Table 49.3). There is much debate about whether neuropathic pain is intrinsically resistant (Arner & Meyerson 1988; Wall 1990; Portenoy et al 1990). Three questions need to be addressed:

1. Does opioid-resistant pain exist?
2. If so, is it relative rather than absolute?
3. Can it be predicted on the basis of whether the pain is nociceptive or neuropathic?

In practice, a pain may be said to be opioid-resistant if:

1. there is little or no relief despite a progressive increase in opioid dose
2. there are intolerable adverse effects despite the use of standard measures to control them.

The concept of opioid resistance stems from clinical observation and is supported by animal studies (Woolf & Wall 1986; McQuay & Dickenson 1990). Studying the phenomenon under controlled conditions, however, is not easy. If opioid resistance is a relative rather than an absolute phenomenon, imposition of dose limits in a study might produce false negative results, particularly if the subject has been previously exposed to opioid administration and in whom there may be a shift to the right in the dose–response curve because of tolerance. One group has used intravenous patient-controlled analgesia (PCA) to circumvent this problem (Jadad et al 1992).

Table 49.1 Alternative classification of opioids

Class	Definition	Example
Agonist	A drug which, when bound to the receptor, stimulates the receptor to the maximum level; by definition, the intrinsic activity of a full agonist is unity	Morphine
Antagonist	A drug which, when bound to the receptor, fails completely to produce any stimulation of that receptor; by definition, the intrinsic activity of a pure antagonist is zero	Naloxone
Partial agonist	A drug which, when bound to the receptor, stimulates the receptor to a level below the maximum level; by definition, the intrinsic activity of a partial agonist lies between zero and unity	Buprenorphine (partial mu agonist)
Mixed agonist–antagonist	A drug which acts simultaneously on different subtypes, with the potential for agonist action on one or more subtypes and antagonist action on one or more subtypes	Pentazocine (partial mu agonist, kappa agonist, delta antagonist)

Table 49.2 Opioid receptors and their ligands[1]

Receptor	Mu	Delta	Kappa
Endogenous ligands	β-Endorphin Dermorphin Metorphamide	Met-enkephalin Leu-enkephalin	Dynorphins
Exogenous ligands	Morphine[2] Fentanyl Methadone DAGOL[3]	DPDPE[3] DTLET DSTBULET	U50488H[4] U69893 PD117302 Pentazocine
Antagonists	Naloxone (low dose) β-FNA[5]	Naloxone (medium dose) ICI174864	Naloxone (high dose) nor-BNI[6]

1 From Dickenson (1991) with permission.
2 Most clinically used opioids are predominantly mu agonists.
3 DAGOL, DPDPE, DTLET and DSTBULET are all peptide analogues based on enkephalin.
4 U50488H, U69893 and PD117302 are nonpeptide kappa agonists.
5 β-FNA is β-funaltrexamine, an irreversible antagonist.
6 nor-BNI is nor-binaltorphimine.

Perhaps the most striking study is that of intravenous lignocaine and morphine in postherpetic neuralgia (Rowbotham et al 1991). This demonstrated clear and equal response to both drugs (Fig. 49.2). Others also have shown response to morphine with neuropathic pain under double-blind conditions (Jadad et al 1992). On the other hand, there are those who claim that morphine has only a differential effect on neuropathic pain. In other words, the sensory dimension of the pain is unchanged but the patient's affective response to it alters (Kupers et al 1991).

Such a view would fit with the results of an open study in which 16 patients with neuropathic pain were given IV morphine 3–4 mg every 10 minutes up to a total of 18–20 mg (Tasker et al 1983). Relief was graded as follows: complete 2; partial 7; none 7. In eight of these IV naloxone 0.4 mg was subsequently given, including five who had obtained pain relief. The naloxone did not reverse the analgesia, suggesting that the relief obtained was mediated by nonopioid receptor pathways (Tasker et al 1983).

The concept of opioid resistance is still important. The message from recent studies, however, is to stress that the situation in relation to neuropathic pain is more complex and less clear-cut than previously thought.

Table 49.3 Opioid-resistant cancer pain: clinical classification

Pseudoresistant
Underdosing
Poor alimentary absorption (*rare*)
Poor alimentary intake because of vomiting
Ignoring psychological aspects of care

Semiresistant
Bone metastasis
Neuropathic (some)
Raised intracranial pressure
Activity-related

Resistant
Neuropathic (some)
Muscle spasm

RESPIRATORY DEPRESSION

The respiratory depressant effect of opioid agonists can be demonstrated easily in volunteer studies. When the dose of morphine is titrated against a patient's pain, however, clinically important respiratory depression does not occur. This is because *pain acts as a physiological antagonist to the central depressant effects of morphine*. As a double dose of morphine at bedtime causes no excess night-time mortality (Regnard & Badger 1987), there is presumably a relatively broad margin of safety. In 20 cancer patients, of median age 59 years, who were taking more than 100 mg of morphine sulphate by mouth per 24 hours, all had respiratory rates of 12 or more breaths per minute at rest (Walsh 1984). Twelve of the patients had a history of chronic bronchitis and eight had carcinoma of the

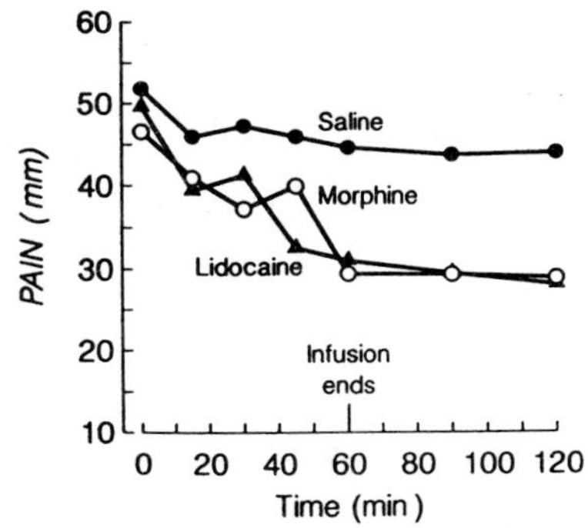

Fig. 49.2 Mean pain intensity visual analogue scale scores during the 60-minute infusion and 60-minute postinfusion observation period. (From Rowbotham et al 1991 with permission.)

bronchus. All $Paco_2$ values except one were within the normal range (i.e. < 45 mmHg); 12 were hypoxic but only one severely so (Po_2 = 48 mmHg). If $Paco_2$ is used as the index of ventilatory failure, this appears to be neither common nor severe in advanced cancer patients in pain treated with oral morphine. Given the frequency of respiratory tract disease in this group of patients, some degree of hypoxia would be expected.

Respiratory depression does occur, however, if the pain is removed suddenly and the dose of morphine is not reduced. A 76-year-old man with a pleural mesothelioma required oral morphine 90 mg every 4 hours to control severe chest pain (Hanks et al 1981). After a successful thoracic intrathecal nerve block with chlorocresol, respiratory depression was produced by doses of morphine which had been used without trouble before the block, and also by substantially smaller doses (Fig. 49.3). This indicates the need for caution, particularly in those with limited respiratory reserve if the level of pain is suddenly altered as a result of nondrug measures.

Thus, if a patient's pain is treated successfully by neurolytic or neuroablative techniques, life-threatening respiratory depression can be avoided if the dose of morphine is reduced immediately to, say, 25% of the previous analgesic dose. If the nerve block is totally successful, it will be possible to curtail the morphine completely in stages over the next 1–2 weeks. However, if only partly successful, it may be necessary to increase the dose again to 50–60% of the original dose, or more.

Respiratory depression may also occur with spinal opioids. This is more likely in opioid-naive patients (Writer et al 1985). In advanced cancer, patients will invariably have been exposed previously to oral and/or parenteral opioids. In this circumstance, respiratory depression is a rare complication. Guidance about appropriate monitoring over the first 24 hours is available (Etches et al 1989).

Differences between postoperative and cancer patients should be noted. Unlike the former, the cancer pain patient:

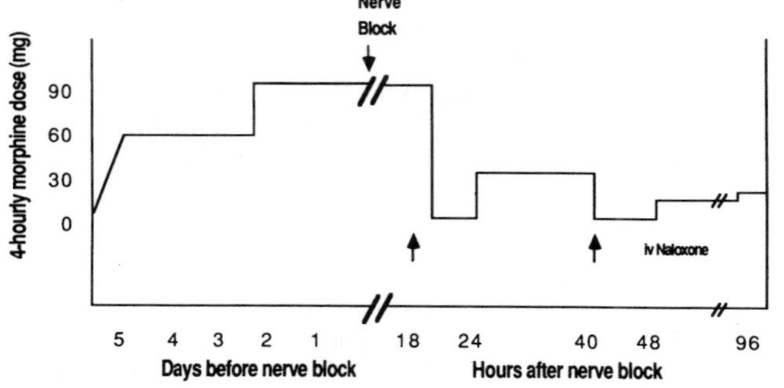

Fig. 49.3 Morphine requirements in a 76-year-old man with a pleural mesothelioma before and after intrathecal chlorocresol nerve block.

1. has usually been receiving a weak opioid for some time (i.e. is not opioid naive)
2. takes medication by mouth (slower absorption, lower peak concentration)
3. titrates the dose upwards step by step (less likelihood of an excessive dose being given).

Postoperative respiratory depression is caused by both pulmonary (atelectasis) and drug-related factors (Brismar et al 1985; Heneghan & Jones 1985; Jones & Jordan 1987). Opioid doses larger than those required for pain relief will increase the depression. The risk of this occurring is greater with continuous opioid infusions than with on demand bolus administration.

In conclusion, morphine is a safe drug for the relief of cancer pain, provided the patient is not dying from exhaustion as a result of weeks or months of intolerable pain associated with insomnia and poor nutrition. In this circumstance, almost anything that eases the patient's mental or physical distress is likely to 'tip the scales' further in the direction of death. Circumstantial evidence suggests, however, that the correct use of morphine *prolongs* the life of a cancer patient because he is free of pain, better able to rest, sleep and eat, and is more physically active.

TOLERANCE

In the past, predictions about dose 'escalation' were made on the basis of animal and volunteer studies. The subjects were not in pain and the emphasis was on inducing tolerance and physical dependence as rapidly as possible by using maximum tolerated doses rather than by administering the drugs in doses and at intervals comparable to a clinical regimen. Although such studies may be useful in predicting abuse liability, they are irrelevant to clinical practice. Several published studies review the long-term opioid requirements of patients with advanced cancer (Twycross 1974; Twycross & Wald 1976; Twycross & Lack 1983). They demonstrate that the longer the duration of treatment:

1. the slower the rate of rise in dose
2. the longer the periods without a dose increase
3. the greater the likelihood of a dose reduction
4. the greater the likelihood of stopping medication altogether.

Of nearly 1000 advanced cancer patients who received opioids, only 5% of patients required an average daily increase of more than 10% of the previous dose; 81% were said to have a stable dose pattern, and 14% discontinued opioids (Brescia et al 1992). Thus, when used within the context of comprehensive biopsychosocial and continuing care, morphine may be used for long periods in cancer patients without concern about tolerance. Further, although physical dependence may develop after several weeks of continuous treatment, this does not prevent a downward adjustment of dose should the pain be relieved by nondrug measures (e.g. radiation therapy or neurolytic block).

With the exception of constipation and miosis, tolerance to the adverse effects of morphine develops more readily than tolerance to analgesia (Bruera et al 1989). Should tolerance develop, an upward adjustment of dose is all that is necessary to regain pain control. The main reason for increasing the dose is not tolerance, however, but progression of the disease (Twycross 1974; Kanner & Foley 1981; Brescia et al 1992).

Tolerance does occur in other contexts. Street addicts develop tolerance and may need increasing doses to obtain the same effect. They use opioids in the absence of pain. Acute tolerance in the absence of pain has also been shown in animals (Colpaert et al 1980).

ADDICTION

The term 'drug addiction' has been replaced by 'drug dependence' and is defined as:

> A state, psychic and sometimes also physical, resulting from the interactions between a living organism and a drug, characterized by behavioural and other responses that always include a compulsion to take the drug on a continuous or periodic basis in order to experience its psychic effects, and sometimes to avoid the discomfort of its absence. Tolerance may or may not be present. (World Health Organization 1969.)

This definition approximates closely to the popular conception of addiction as a compulsion or overpowering drive to take the drug in order to experience psychological effects.

The fear of causing psychological dependence is still a potent cause of under-prescription and under-use of strong opioid analgesics (Hill 1987). Published data indicate that this fear is unfounded and unnecessary. Among nearly 12 000 hospital patients who received strong opioids, there were only four reasonably well-documented cases of addiction in patients who had no history of drug abuse (Porter & Jick 1980). The dependence was considered major in only one instance, which suggests that the medical use of strong opioids rarely leads to addiction.

The diversion of strong opioids for illicit use by non-patients is a parallel concern, particularly of governments and law-enforcement agencies. The experience in Sweden allays this fear. There, the medicinal use of morphine and methadone increased 17 times between 1975 and 1982 because of an increasing use of oral strong opioids to control cancer pain (Agenas et al 1982). There was, however, no associated increase in illicit drug use or diversion of strong opioids to established addicts.

Studies of chronically ill patients have shown that abuse of nonopioid analgesics or combinations of weak opioids and nonopioids is more common than abuse of strong opioids (Maruta et al 1979; Tennant & Rawson 1982; Tennant & Uelman 1983). In patients with pain of nonmalignant origin, studies indicate that long-term opioid use is not associated with psychological dependence (Taub 1982; Portenoy & Foley 1986). These studies suggest that drug use alone is not the major factor in the development of psychological dependence and that other factors are more important. Support for this view comes from studies of USA military personnel addicted to strong opioids in Viet Nam (Robins et al 1974). In this group, drug abuse was strongly dependent on factors such as underlying personality, social environment and availability of money.

From time to time, a patient is encountered who appears to be addicted, demanding 'an injection' every 2 or 3 hours (Weissman & Haddox 1989). Typically, such a patient has a long history of poor pain control and for several weeks will have been receiving fairly regular ('4-hourly as needed') but inadequate injections of one or more opioid analgesics. Given time, it is usually possible to control the pain, prevent clock-watching and demanding behaviour and transfer the patient to an oral preparation. Even here, however, it cannot be said that the patient is addicted because he is not demanding an opioid in order to experience its psychological effects but to be relieved from pain for at least an hour or two.

More difficult to deal with is the rare patient, usually young, who was a 'street addict' before becoming ill. Usually one of two errors will be made. On the one hand his pain is discounted by the professional staff and requests for strong opioids resisted: 'After all, he is an addict'. At the other extreme the patient is treated as a nonaddict patient and allowed to escalate his opioid intake far beyond reasonable estimates of what is needed to control his pain. This is one situation in which the patient's statements about what hurts must be carefully balanced by the judgement of an experienced and compassionate physician (Twycross & Lack 1983).

OPIOIDS AND PAIN MANAGEMENT

The use of analgesics and pain management are not synonymous. The use of analgesics should be regarded as one part of a multimodality approach to treatment. From a therapeutic point of view, pain in cancer falls into three categories:

1. opioid responsive pains, i.e. pain that is relieved by opioidan alone
2. opioid semi-responsive pains, i.e. pain that is relieved by the concurrent use of an opioid, an adjuvant drug and/or nondrug measures
3. opioid resistant pains, i.e. pain that is not relieved by

opioids but is relieved by other drugs and/or nondrug measures.

This classification is important because it reminds doctors that opioids are sometimes of limited value. The classification holds true, however, only for opioids given by mouth or by conventional parenteral routes. Anecdotal evidence suggests that by a spinal route (epidural or intrathecal) 'opioid resistant' pains may well be more opioid responsive (Ottesen et al 1990).

OPIOID RESPONSIVE PAINS

Visceral pains generally come into this category, and so do many deep soft-tissue pains. Five important concepts govern the use of analgesics in the management of opioid responsive pains:

1. 'by the mouth'
2. 'by the clock'
3. 'by the ladder'
4. 'for the individual'
5. 'use adjuvant medication'.

'By the mouth'

Morphine is effective by mouth (Hanks 1991b). Thus, apart from the last few hours or days of life, few patients require injections to control their pain. Because of reduced bioavailability, the oral dose needs to be two to three times larger than the parenteral one (see p. 953). Patients with intractable vomiting as well as pain will need parenteral medication – both antiemetic and analgesic. Once the vomiting has been controlled it is generally possible to revert to the oral route. Suppositories are a useful alternative, particularly in the home. The dose of morphine by mouth and per rectum is the same (Pannuti et al 1982; Kaiko et al 1989).

'By the clock'

To allow pain to reemerge before administering the next dose causes unnecessary suffering and encourages tolerance. 'As needed' medication has no place in the treatment of persistent pain (Fig. 49.4). Whatever the cause, continuous pain requires regular prophylactic therapy. The next dose is given before the effect of the previous one has worn off and, therefore, before the patient may think it necessary.

For codeine and morphine 'every 4 hours' is usually optimal. If a strong analgesic other than morphine is used, the doctor must be familiar with its pharmacology. Pethidine is generally effective for only 2–3 hours, though is commonly given every 4–6 hours. On the other hand, levorphanol and phenazocine are satisfactory when given every 6 hours; and buprenorphine and methadone every 8 hours. With methadone, which has a plasma half-life of over 2 days when taken regularly by mouth (Inturrisi & Verebely 1972), there is a likelihood of cumulation leading to worsening adverse effects, particularly in the elderly and debilitated (Twycross 1977).

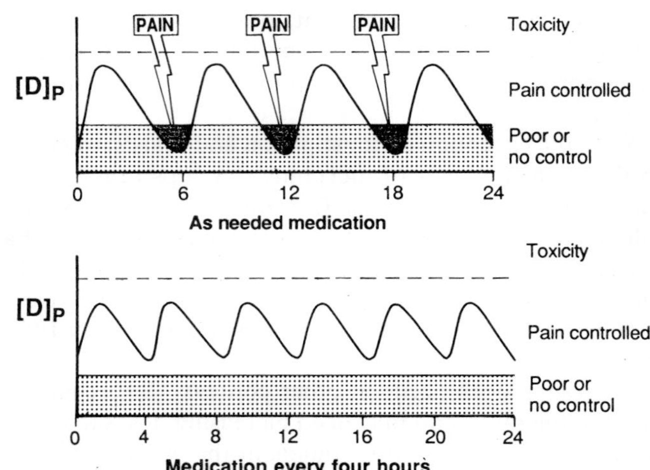

Fig. 49.4 Diagram to illustrate the results of 'as needed' compared with regular 'every 4 hours' morphine [D]p = plasma concentration of drug. (From Twycross & Lack 1983.)

'By the ladder'

The three standard analgesics are aspirin, codeine and morphine (Fig. 49.5). Other analgesics should be considered as alternatives of fashion or convenience. Appreciating this helps prevent 'kangarooing' from one analgesic to another in a desperate search for some drug that will suit the patient better. If a preparation containing a nonopioid and a weak opioid, such as aspirin–codeine or paracetamol–dextropropoxyphene, fails to relieve, it is usually best to move directly to a small dose of oral morphine sulphate than, for example, to prescribe dihydrocodeine.

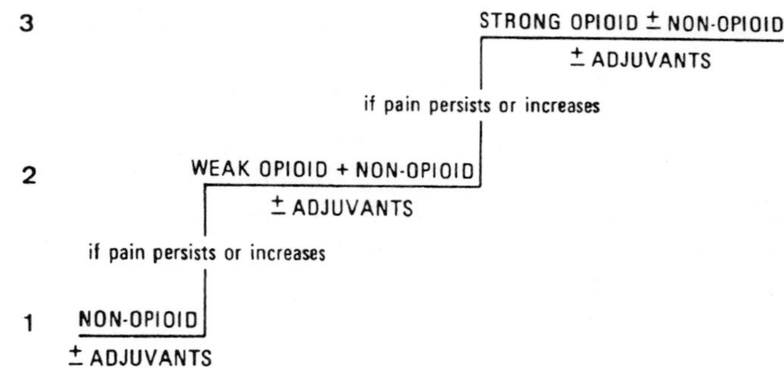

Fig. 49.5 The analgesic ladder for cancer pain management. (From World Health Organization 1986.)

It is necessary to be familiar with one or two alternatives for patients who cannot tolerate the standard preparations (Table 49.4). Aspirin has two alternatives: paracetamol which has no antiinflammatory effect, and the non-steroidal antiinflammatory drugs (NSAIDs). For step 2, the author uses dextropropoxyphene in preference to codeine. It is less constipating and, in the UK, the compound tablet with paracetamol (co-proxamol) has a considerably greater 'codeine-equivalent' content than most other weak opioid compound tablets.

Oral codeine is about one-twelfth as potent as oral morphine (Lasagna & Beecher 1954) and dihydrocodeine about one-tenth. Although dextropropoxyphene is less potent than codeine in single doses, it has a prolonged plasma half-life and can, in practice, be regarded as equipotent with codeine when given regularly (Beaver 1984; Twycross 1984). Tramadol is one-tenth as potent as morphine.

The use of morphine is determined by analgesic need and not, for example, by the doctor's estimate of life expectancy – which is often wrong. The right dose of morphine is the one which gives adequate relief for 4 hours without unacceptable adverse effects. 'Maximum' or 'recommended' doses, derived mainly from postoperative parenteral single dose studies, are not applicable for cancer pain (Brescia et al 1992; McCormack et al 1992). The following points should be noted:

Table 49.4 A basic list of opioids for cancer pain relief[1]

Category	Basic drugs	Alternatives
Weak opioids[2]	Codeine[3]	Dextropropoxyphene Dihydrocodeine Tramadol
Strong opioids[2]	Morphine	Standardized opium[4] Pethidine Oxycodone Methadone Levorphanol Hydromorphone Buprenorphine[5]
Opioid antagonist	Naloxone	

Modified from the revised method for relief of cancer pain (World Health Organization 1994).

[1] All the drugs listed except tramadol are contained in the WHO *Model List of Essential Drugs*.

[2] The opioids are divided into those for mild to moderate pain ('weak opioids') and those for moderate to severe pain ('strong opioids') principally on the grounds of common patterns of use. There is, however, no pharmacological difference between a high dose of codeine and an equianalgesic low dose of morphine.

[3] Codeine and some other weak opioids are *not* scheduled drugs in most countries. This may make them more readily available.

[4] Standardized opium is equivalent to 10% morphine (13% morphine sulphate) on a weight-for-weight basis.

[5] Buprenorphine is a partial agonist (i.e. has a pharmacological ceiling). At doses of 0.4–1 mg every 8 hours, it can substitute for up to 30 mg of oral morphine every 4 hours.

1. It is pharmacological nonsense to prescribe simultaneously two weak opioids or two strong opioids.
2. It is sometimes justifiable for a patient on a strong opioid to be given another weak or strong opioid as a second 'as needed' analgesic for breakthrough pain. Generally, with troublesome breakthrough pain, patients should be advised to take an extra dose of their regular medication.
3. Avoid short-acting preparations like pentazocine, pethidine, and dextromoramide.
4. Do not prescribe a mixed agonist–antagonist (e.g. pentazocine) with a strong opioid agonist (e.g. morphine). It is unnecessary and may well lead to antagonism.

'For the individual'

Morphine can be given either as an aqueous solution of morphine sulphate, as ordinary tablets or as slow-release tablets (Hanks et al 1987). The latter are available in many countries as 10, 30, 60, 100 and 200 mg strengths. Most patients changing from a weak opioid commence with 60 mg a day, i.e. morphine sulphate 10 mg every 4 hours or slow-release morphine 30 mg every 12 hours (Levy 1990). As the effective dose of oral morphine ranges from as little as 5 mg to more than 1 g every 4 hours (Fig. 49.6), the top of the ladder is not reached simply by prescribing morphine. Most patients, however, never need more than 100 mg every 4 hours. The majority continue to be well-controlled on doses as small as 10–30 mg (or slow-release morphine 30–100 mg twice a day). Older patients on average require less morphine than young patients (Kaiko 1980; Rees 1990). The use of morphine by mouth has been described fully elsewhere (Twycross & Lack 1990). The salient points are summarized in Table 49.5.

Adjuvant medication

Laxatives are almost always necessary when a patient is prescribed morphine, unless there is a definite reason for not doing so, e.g. steatorrhoea or an ileostomy (Twycross & Harcourt 1991). Experience at many centres strongly suggests that a combination of a contact laxative (peristaltic stimulant) and a surface-wetting agent (faecal softener) achieves the best results, for example, standardized senna (up to 75 mg a day) and docusate (up to 600 mg a day). Combination preparations reduce the number of tablets/capsules the patient has to swallow (e.g. co-danthrusate (UK) and casanthranol-docusate (USA)). More than one-third of inpatients with terminal cancer continue to need rectal measures (suppositories, enemas or manual evacuations) in addition to oral laxatives (Twycross & Lack 1986).

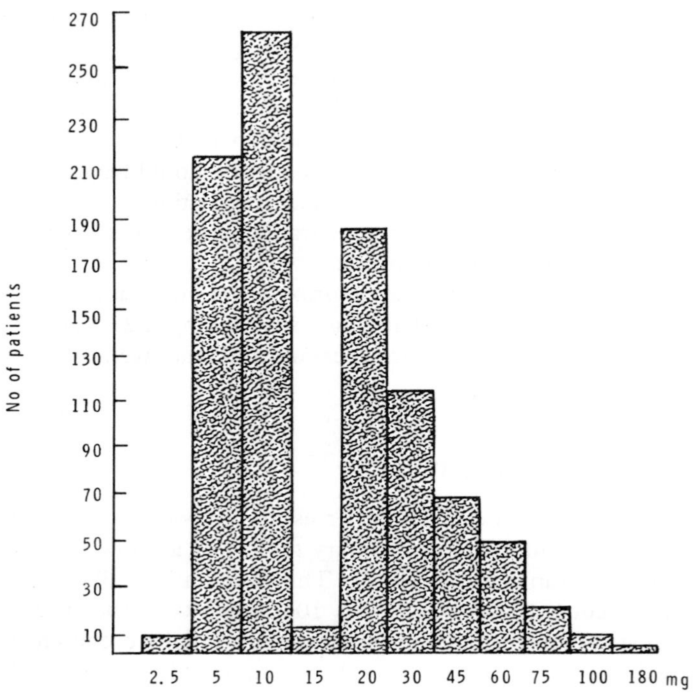

Fig. 49.6 Histogram of maximum dose of morphine sulphate administered orally every 4 hours to 955 patients at St Christopher's Hospice (1978–79). Median dose = 10 mg. Note: 75 includes 80 and 90 mg; 100 includes 110 and 120 mg.

Table 49.5 Use of oral morphine

1. Morphine by mouth is the strong opioid of choice for cancer patients
2. Available as aqueous solution and tablet; also as slow release (SR) tablet
3. If previously receiving a weak opioid, begin with aqueous morphine 10 mg every 4 hours (SR morphine 30 mg every 12 hours)
4. With frail elderly patients, consider starting on a smaller dose to reduce the likelihood of initial drowsiness and unsteadiness; initially, back-up with 'rescue' doses of previously used weak opioid
5. If changing from alternative strong opioid (e.g. buprenorphine, levorphanol, methadone), a much higher dose of morphine may be needed
6. If using aqueous solution or standard tablets, give advice about 'rescue' doses for breakthrough pain (e.g. an extra dose if pain returns in less than 2 hours or half a dose if more than 2 hours)
7. If using SR tablets, prescribe aqueous solution or standard tablets for 'rescue' doses
8. After 24 hours, if pain not 90% controlled, increase dose by 50%
9. Two-thirds of patients are pain-controlled on a dose of 30 mg every 4 hours or less (SR morphine 100 mg every 12 hours). The rest need higher doses, up to 200 mg every 4 hours and occasionally more (SR morphine 600 mg every 12 hours)
10. With aqueous morphine and standard tablets, a double dose at bedtime usually enables a patient to go through the night without waking in pain
11. Use adjuvants for bone pain (NSAID) and nerve compression pain (corticosteroid)
12. Supply an antiemetic for regular use should nausea or vomiting develop, e.g. haloperidol 1.5 mg stat and nocte or 1 mg stat and twice daily
13. Prescribe a laxative, e.g. co-danthrusate, casanthranol-docusate (Peri-Colace); adjust dose according to response. Suppositories often also necessary
14. Write out regimen with times and amount to be taken; arrange for close liaison and follow-up
15. If swallowing becomes difficult or vomiting persists, morphine sulphate may be administered by suppository
16. Alternatively, give one-third of previously satisfactory dose of morphine as diamorphine hydrochloride (UK) or one-half of previous dose as morphine (elsewhere) by subcutaneous injection

About two-thirds of patients prescribed morphine need an antiemetic. Haloperidol 1–1.5 mg stat and at bedtime is the antiemetic of choice if nausea or vomiting is opioid-induced. In some patients haloperidol is ineffectual because of morphine-induced delayed gastric emptying. Thus, if a patient does not respond to haloperidol and the pattern of vomiting is suggestive of gastric stasis, a prokinetic agent (e.g. metoclopramide, cisapride) should be substituted (Rowbotham et al 1988).

If the patient is very anxious, an anxiolytic should be prescribed (e.g. diazepam 5–10 mg at bedtime). If a patient remains depressed after 1–2 weeks of much improved pain relief, an antidepressant should be considered. Discomfort is worse at night when the patient is alone with his pain and his fears. The cumulative effect of many sleepless, pain-filled nights is a substantial lowering of the patient's pain threshold with a concomitant increase in pain intensity. Many patients benefit by the use of a night sedative (e.g. temazepam or chloral hydrate).

Sometimes, it is necessary to use morphine at night in patients well-controlled by a weak opioid during the day or to use a considerably larger dose of morphine at bedtime to relieve pains which are particularly troublesome when lying down for a prolonged period.

At some centres, aqueous morphine is prescribed for cancer pain with a second drug, either cocaine (a stimulant) or a phenothiazine (an anxiolytic–sedative). Sometimes both are given – which is pharmacological nonsense. Increasing the dose of morphine can be hazardous in these circumstances because, by increasing the volume of the mixture to be taken, the dose of the second drug is increased automatically. Depending on what the second drug is, this could lead either to agitation or to somnolence. It is better to give psychotropic drugs separately so that the dose of each drug can be adjusted individually according to need. Cocaine is no longer recommended (Melzack et al 1979; Twycross 1979). Patients on high doses may sometimes benefit from a morning dose of dexamphetamine or methylphenidate (Bruera et al 1992).

The central depressant effects of morphine tend to be potentiated by psychotropic drugs and alcohol. It is generally wise, therefore, to prescribe relatively small doses of psychotropic drugs initially. The effect of hypotensive drugs, phenothiazines and benzodiazepines on blood pressure is potentiated, and the cardiac slowing effect of adrenergic beta-blockers may be enhanced.

OPIOID SEMIRESPONSIVE PAINS

Bone pain

Pain caused by bone metastases is often not wholly responsive to opioids. The same is true for some soft-tissue pains. Best results are obtained with a combination of an NSAID and morphine. Many osseous metastases produce a prostaglandin (PG) which causes osteolysis (Galasko 1981). The PG also lowers the 'peripheral pain threshold' by sensitizing the nerve endings (Ferreira 1972). NSAIDs inhibit the synthesis of PGs and thereby alleviate pain. Response to PG inhibitors, however, is variable.

Neuropathic pain

Pain caused by nerve compression is often not controlled with morphine alone. In this situation a corticosteroid should be prescribed (e.g. dexamethasone 4–8 mg daily). Commonly a marked improvement is seen within 48 hours. If the nerve compression relates to an identifiable bone metastasis or soft-tissue mass, radiotherapy should be considered. It is normally possible to reduce the dose of morphine and dexamethasone after radiotherapy.

Patients with neural injury pain often do not respond to morphine and dexamethasone. With these patients other drugs will be needed, either alone or in combination (see Chs 50 and 51). The need for neurolytic and neuroablative procedures has decreased dramatically as a result of the better use of drug combinations. In 158 patients admitted to a Palliative Care Unit in the United Kingdom, neurolysis (coeliac axis plexus block) was used only once (Walker et al 1988). At the Palliative Care Service, National Cancer Institute, Milan, fewer than 10% of pain patients now need such procedures (Ventafridda 1989). The use of spinal morphine and bupivacaine has almost totally replaced the use of neurolytic and neuroablative procedures at many centres (Hogan et al 1991; Sjoberg et al 1991). Preliminary results with subcutaneous morphine and ketamine (an anaesthetic induction agent and NMDA (N-methyl D-aspartate) receptor antagonist) are equally promising (Luczak et al 1992).

EXPECTATIONS

All cancer patients receiving analgesics need close supervision to achieve maximum relief with minimal adverse effects. A number of studies indicate the degree of success that may be anticipated (Table 49.6). Relief is obtained within 2 or 3 days in some patients, but in others (particularly those whose pain is made worse by movement and in the very anxious and depressed) it may take up to 4 weeks of inpatient treatment to obtain a satisfactory result. Even so, it should be possible to achieve significant improvement within 24–48 hours in all patients, particularly at night or at rest.

MORPHINE VERSUS DIAMORPHINE

Diamorphine is a classical prodrug. It does not bind to opioid receptors (Inturrisi et al 1983) and is devoid of analgesic activity itself. It is metabolized into analgesically active 6-monoacetylmorphine, morphine and M6G (Fig. 49.7). In terms of both analgesic efficacy and effect on mood, diamorphine has no clinical advantage over morphine by oral or intramuscular routes (Twycross 1977; Inturrisi et al 1984).

Intramuscularly, diamorphine has a slightly earlier onset of action than morphine, whereas intravenously morphine acts more quickly (Morrison et al 1991). This probably relates to differences in lipid-solubility (diamorphine > morphine), plasma protein binding (diamorphine 40%, morphine 20%) and the need for diamorphine to be converted into an active metabolite.

The use of diamorphine in some centres in the UK as the *parenteral* strong opioid of choice has caused a number of doctors elsewhere to believe that diamorphine is better than morphine (Tattersall 1981, Katz et al 1984, Levine et al 1986, Sellers 1986). This is not so. There is no pharma-

Table 49.6 Evaluation of WHO method for relief of cancer pain[1]

Study	Year	Country	Number of patients	Pain control (%)
Rappaz et al	1985	Switzerland	63	90
Takeda	1986	Japan	156	87
Ventafridda et al	1987b	Italy	1229	71
Walker et al	1988	UK	20	100
Vijayaram et al	1989	India	88	86
Schug et al	1990	Germany	174	92
Zech et al	1990	Germany	1070	70
WHO Collaborating		25 countries	261[2]	75
Centre in Milan			100[3]	50

[1] From Stjernsward (1991) with permission.
[2] Centres familiar with WHO method.
[3] Centres not familiar with WHO method.

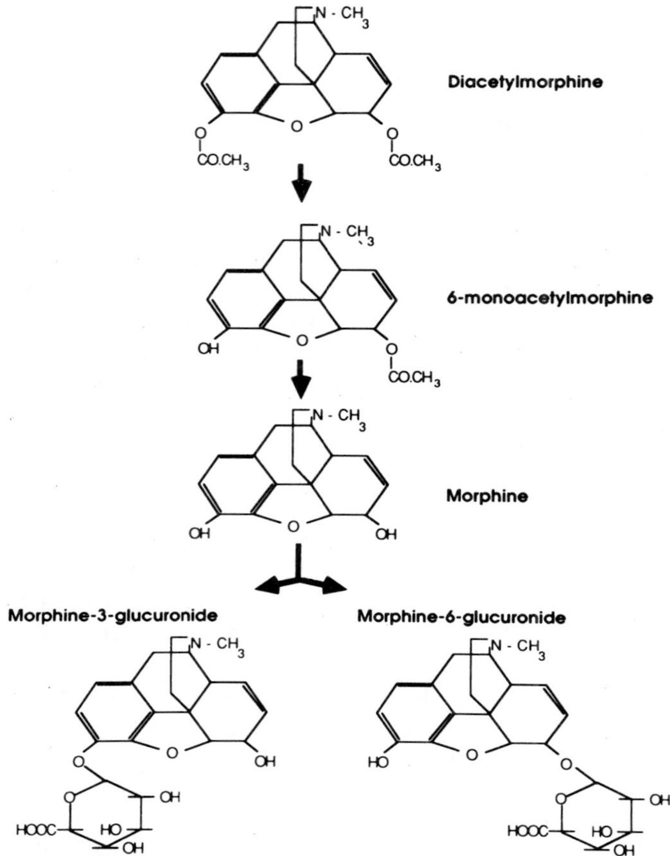

Fig. 49.7 Metabolic pathway of diamorphine and morphine. 6-monoacetylmorphine, morphine and morphine-6-glucuronide bind to opioid receptors; diacetylmorphine and morphine-3-glucuronide do not.

cological justification for seeking to introduce diamorphine for medicinal use on the grounds that it is better than morphine. It is not. If a pain is opioid responsive it will respond equally well to both morphine and diamorphine. If the pain is opioid nonresponsive it will respond equally badly. The major advantage of diamorphine over morphine is that, when injections are necessary, the high solubility of diamorphine means that large doses can be given in a small volume (Hanks & Hoskin 1987). This advantage is irrelevant if hydromorphone is available, as in the USA and Canada. Hydromorphone is more potent than diamorphine and almost as soluble.

METABOLISM OF MORPHINE

PHARMACOLOGY

Recent reports about the metabolism of morphine have focused attention on the metabolites (Fig. 49.7), the site of metabolism and the method of excretion. Diamorphine (diacetylmorphine) and morphine-3-glucuronide (M3G) do not bind to opioid receptors; 6-monoacetylmorphine, morphine and morphine-6-glucuronide (M6G) all do. It is the analgesic activity of M6G which has captured recent interest. M3G and M6G are the major metabolites of morphine in man (Sawe et al 1981; McQuay et al 1990). In rats, M6G is 45 times more potent than morphine intracerebrally and nearly four times more potent subcutaneously (Shimomura et al 1971). Prolonged respiratory depression has been reported in man in association with negligible plasma concentrations of morphine but with very high concentrations of M3G and M6G (Osborne et al 1986). M6G may contribute substantially to the analgesic effect of morphine, in both single and repeated doses.

A recent report demonstrates that M6G and M3G are far more lipophilic than expected (Carrupt et al 1991). Glucuronides are normally highly polar hydrophilic compounds which are unable to cross the blood–brain barrier. M6G and M3G, however, exist in equilibrium between extended and folded forms. Whereas the extended form is highly hydrophilic, the folded form is almost as lipophilic as morphine itself. This form may well predominate in biological membranes, thereby facilitating movement into the central nervous system.

INFLUENCE OF RENAL FUNCTION

> Of all the lessons which were hammered into me during my hospital career, none was more persistently driven home than the fact that it is extremely dangerous to administer morphia in kidney disease or derangement. (Toogood 1898)

In patients with severely impaired renal function, morphine and its active congeners have an increased and prolonged effect (McQuay & Moore 1984; Barnes et al 1985). A series of case reports confirm this observation (Mostert et al 1971; Don et al 1975; Barnes & Goodwin 1983; Redfern 1983). Cumulation of the active metabolite M6G is the probable explanation of this phenomenon, as elimination of morphine itself is unimpaired in renal failure, even in anephric patients (Aitkenhead et al 1984; Sawe et al 1985b; Woolner et al 1986).

HEPATIC FUNCTION

Evidence favours the liver as the principal site of morphine metabolism in man (Sawe et al 1985a; Hasselstrom et al 1986). The arguments that, as in other species, metabolism also occurs in other organs are summarized elsewhere (McQuay 1986). Glucuronidation is rarely impaired in hepatic failure (Patwardhan et al 1981; Hasselstrom et al 1986). This reflects clinical experience; morphine is well tolerated in patients up to the point of hepatic precoma (Laidlaw et al 1961; Regnard & Twycross 1984).

MORPHINE-INDUCED PAIN

Occasionally, at very high doses, additional morphine exacerbates rather than relieves pain. In a patient with metastatic pelvic and back pain, this occurred with a daily dose of 60 mg *intrathecal* morphine (Morley et al 1992). Cerebrospinal fluid (CSF) analysis showed a very high concentration of M3G but no M6G. When the patient was given intrathecal injections of M6G 1 mg, there was complete pain relief for 7 hours on each occasion.

It has been suggested that morphine-induced pain may be the result of abnormal morphine metabolism, i.e. production of only M3G and no M6G. It has also been suggested that M3G antagonizes the effects of both morphine and M6G (Smith et al 1990; Gong et al 1992). Normally, however, M3G does not bind to opioid receptors. However, perhaps in the absence of M6G and at very high concentrations, receptor-binding might occur. M3G may also be a nonspecific cerebral stimulant.

ORAL-TO-PARENTERAL POTENCY RATIO OF MORPHINE

In the USA, it is often stated that the oral-to-parenteral potency ratio of morphine is 1:6. This view is based on the results of a single-dose study in postoperative cancer patients (Houde et al 1965). The bioavailability of orally administered morphine varies, however, between 15 and 64%, with a mean of 38% (Sawe et al 1981). Using intravenous PCA, it has been shown that approximately three times as much oral morphine is needed to match the previously satisfactory parenteral dose, i.e. the *oral-to-intravenous* potency ratio is 1:3 (Kalso & Vainio 1990), reflecting the earlier bioavailability study. Bioavailability by subcutaneous injection, however, is only about 80% (Hanna et al 1993). This means that the *oral-to-subcutaneous* potency ratio should be regarded as 1:2 (Consensus Statement 1994).

The discrepancy between a ratio of 1:6 with single doses for acute pain and 1:3 or 1:2 with repeated doses for chronic pain has led to much confusion (Kaiko 1986). The reason for the discrepancy may relate to a greater contribution by M6G to the analgesic effect of repeatedly administered morphine (Hanks 1991; Portenoy et al 1992). Enterohepatic recirculation of morphine – a possible alternative explanation – has been shown in rodents (Walsh & Levine 1975, Dahlstrom & Paalzow 1978) but not in man. The phenomenon of greater efficacy with repeat oral doses is seen with codeine in acute pain (McQuay et al 1988).

ALTERNATIVE STRONG OPIOIDS

Of the other strong opioids, none has any clear advantage over morphine. Tramadol, however, has a unique mode of action (see p. 955). It is necessary to have an alternative strong opioid available for the small minority of patients who cannot tolerate morphine. The only common form of intolerance is vomiting caused by morphine-induced delayed gastric emptying. Those patients who fail to respond to the prescription of a prokinetic agent (e.g. metoclopramide, cisapride; Rowbotham et al 1988) should be changed to an alternative strong opioid. Those few patients who remain psychologically averse to taking morphine in any form also require an alternative opioid. When changing from one strong opioid to another it is important to give an adequate dose (Table 49.7). The following factors may also need to be taken into account:

Table 49.7 Opioids by mouth: approximate equivalence to oral morphine sulphate[1]

Analgesic	Proprietary name	Potency ratio with morphine sulphate	Duration of action (hours)[2]
Codeine[3]		1/12	3–5
Tramadol[3]	Tramal	1/10	4–5
Pethidine/meperidine[4]	Demerol (USA)	1/8	2–3
Papaveretum[5]	Omnopon (UK), Pantopon (USA)	2/3	3–5
Oxydodone[6]	in Percodan, Percocet, Tylox (USA)	1	5–6
Methadone[7]	Physeptone (UK), Dolophine (USA)	(3–4)	6–12
Levorphanol[3]	Dromoran (UK), Levo-dromoran (USA)	5	6–8
Phenazocine[8]	Narphen (UK)	5	6–8
Hydromorphone[3]	Dilaudid (USA)	6	3–5
Buprenorphine[9]	Temgesic	60	6–8

[1] Multiply dose of opioid by its potency ratio to determine the equivalent dose of morphine sulphate.
[2] Dependent in part on severity of pain and on dose; often longer lasting in very elderly and those with renal dysfunction.
[3] Vickers et al (1992).
[4] Extrapolation from parenteral ratio and relative bioavailability, supported by clinical experience.
[5] Papaveretum (strong opium) is standardized to contain 50% morphine base. Potency ratio expressed in relation to morphine sulphate.
[6] Kalso & Vainio (1990).
[7] Methadone single 5 mg dose is equivalent to morphine 7.5 mg. Has a long plasma half-life which leads to cumulation when given repeatedly; overall potency ratio adjusted accordingly; Verebely & Inturrisi (1972).
[8] Unpublished observations, Twycross (1973).
[9] Must be taken *sublingually*; potency diminished if swallowed; Zenz et al (1985).

1. prescriber preference
2. speed of onset and duration of action
3. adverse effects
4. drug interactions
5. whether agonist or mixed agonist–antagonist.

PRESCRIBER PREFERENCE

In the USA, *hydromorphone* is widely used. It is available as 1, 2, 3 and 4 mg tablets, as a 3 mg rectal suppository and in ampoules containing 1, 2 and 4 mg/ml. A dose of 1.5 mg is equivalent to 10 mg of morphine; adverse effects are comparable. The analgesic effect lasts 3–5 hours. A concentrated injection is also available (Dilaudid-HP). This contains hydromorphone hydrochloride 10 mg/ml, and is equivalent to 60 mg of morphine sulphate or 25–30 mg of diamorphine hydrochloride. Dilaudid-HP is useful when a large dose of 'morphine equivalent' has to be administered parenterally.

In Britain, *phenazocine* is commonly used in cancer patients who are intolerant of morphine. It is available as a 5 mg tablet, equivalent to 20–25 mg of morphine sulphate by mouth (Twycross 1973, unpublished observations). One tablet every 4 hours may therefore be excessive. The tablets can, however, be halved and need not be taken as often as morphine. For example, 2.5 mg four times a day is approximately equivalent to 10 mg of morphine sulphate every 4 hours. Although not manufactured specifically for sublingual use, the tablets dissolve readily in the mouth. Phenazocine appears to be equipotent whether taken sublingually or swallowed.

Levorphanol, available in both Britain and the USA, can also be used for morphine intolerant patients. In animal receptor-binding studies, levorphanol demonstrated high affinity for mu, kappa and delta receptors, whereas morphine was relatively selective for mu receptors (Moulin et al 1988). Levorphanol infusions resulted in tolerance to both morphine and levorphanol whereas morphine infusions selectively produced tolerance to morphine. Thus, in terms of receptor subtype affinity, levorphanol is more broad-spectrum than morphine. It is not known whether this observation is of clinical importance.

Oxycodone is widely used in the USA. For many years its use was largely limited to several popular compound tablet or capsule formulations with either aspirin (Percodan) or paracetamol/acetaminophen (Perocet, Tylox). The potential toxicity of the nonopioid component restricted the amount of oxycodone which could be taken. This situation is now changing and the usefulness of oxycodone alone as an alternative strong opioid is increasingly recognized (Poyhia et al 1993). It has a plasma half-life of about 5 hours (Poyhia et al 1992), compared with 2.5 hours for morphine. Parenterally it is three-quarters as potent as morphine (Kalso & Vainio 1990). Oral bioavailability is about two-thirds, compared with one-third for morphine. This means that by mouth, oxycodone and morphine are more or less equipotent.

Buprenorphine is used at some centres as an alternative to morphine in the lower part of morphine's dose range (Table 49.8; Atkinson et al 1990). As a partial agonist it can never be a total substitute for morphine. Opinions differ as to the presence or the height of a therapeutic ceiling. It has been suggested that it may be effective only in doses up to about 5 mg in 24 hours (Zenz et al 1985). This view has been vigorously challenged (Budd 1990).

SPEED OF ONSET AND DURATION OF ACTION

There is little to choose between the various opioids in terms of speed of onset of action. Most begin to take effect about 20–30 minutes after oral administration. If a rapid onset of action is desirable, the intravenous route should be used. Speed of absorption after intramuscular injection varies according to the vascularity of the muscle. Uptake from the gluteal muscles is slower in females than in males and uptake from deltoid is faster than from the gluteal muscles (Kaiko 1986). Rapid onset is not a critical factor, however, for patients receiving medication by the clock.

A longer duration of action means that fewer doses are needed each day. The advent of slow-release formulations of morphine means, however, that there is now less reason for choosing an opioid other than morphine on the grounds of longer duration of effect. Opioids that last

Table 49.8 Guide to the use of sublingual buprenorphine

1. A semisynthetic thebaine derivative with potent partial mu-agonist properties
2. An alternative to oral morphine in the low–middle part of morphine's dose range
3. In low doses, buprenorphine and morphine are additive in their effects; at high doses, antagonism by buprenorphine may occur
4. Buprenorphine is available as a sublingual tablet; ingestion reduces bioavailability
5. Needs to be given only every 8 hours; to give more often is to make life unnecessarily harder for a hard-pressed patient
6. With daily doses of over 3 mg, patients may prefer to take fewer tablets more often, i.e. every 6 hours
7. Analgesic ceiling at a daily dose of 3–5 mg; this is equivalent to 180–300 mg of morphine
8. Buprenorphine is *not* an alternative to codeine or dextropropoxyphene; like morphine, it should be used when a weak opioid has failed
9. Assuming previous regular use of codeine or dextropropoxyphene, patients should commence on 0.2 mg every 8 hours with the advice that: 'If it is not more effective than your previous tablets take a further 0.2 mg after 1 hour, and 0.4 mg every 8 hours after that'
10. When changing to morphine, multiply total daily dose of buprenorphine by 60; if pain previously poorly controlled, multiply by 100
11. Adverse effects need to be monitored as with morphine: nausea, vomiting, constipation, drowsiness
12. There is never need to prescribe both buprenorphine and morphine; use one or the other, then unintended antagonism cannot occur

longer than morphine include methadone, buprenorphine, levorphanol, phenazocine and possibly oxycodone.

With chronic use, the plasma half-life of *methadone* increases from 17–24 hours to 2–3 days (Inturrisi & Verebely 1972) compared with 2.5 hours for oral morphine (Brunk & Delle 1974). As a result, methadone requires a different approach from morphine to dose titration (Ventafridda et al 1986). Central depressant effects may well become a limiting factor as a result of cumulation (Ettinger et al 1979). Although methadone has been used successfully twice a day at some centres (Jakobsson et al 1980, Breivik & Rennemo 1982), the duration of analgesic effect frequently does not extend beyond 6–8 hours.

Levorphanol also has a long plasma half-life, about 12–16 hours. It, too, can be taken 6–8-hourly. The potential impact of hepatic and renal dysfunction on the metabolism of opioids should not be forgotten (Table 49.9).

ADVERSE EFFECTS

For the clinically important adverse effects of constipation and nausea there are no comparative data from chronic studies to suggest that any of the alternatives are consistently preferable to morphine. In a postoperative study, a higher incidence of nausea and vomiting has been demonstrated for pethidine (Morrison et al 1968). In another postoperative study, oxycodone was shown to have significantly fewer adverse effects than morphine (Kantor et al 1981).

A study of cancer patients suggested that oxycodone may have a greater propensity to cause sweating (Kalso & Vainio 1990). On the other hand, patients who experienced hallucinations with morphine did not with oxycodone. This may indicate a different pattern of receptor subtype affinity.

Dysphoria

The use of opioids which produce a higher incidence of dysphoria than codeine or morphine without any specific advantage is clearly inadvisable. The mixed agonist–antagonists *butorphanol*, *nalbuphine* and *pentazocine* all have this potential (Houde 1986; Wallenstein et al 1986). In patients with acute pain, the incidence of dysphoria with pentazocine is about 10% (Woods et al 1974). This is much higher than the 1–2% seen with opioid agonists. Pentazocine has no place in the management of cancer pain.

Toxic metabolite

This is a potential problem with *pethidine*. Its chief metabolite, norpethidine, causes central nervous system excitation, tremor, twitching, agitation and convulsions (Szeto et al 1977). The incidence of these problems increases considerably at oral doses above 200 mg and at lower doses in patients with impaired renal function (Szeto et al 1977). Phenobarbitone and chlorpromazine enhance the production of norpethidine (Stambaugh et al 1977; Stambaugh & Wainer 1981). As its duration of action is only some 2–3 hours, pethidine is clearly a poor choice in the management of cancer pain.

DRUG INTERACTIONS

There is general need for caution when using strong opioids and psychotropic drugs concurrently. There are reports of important interactions between opioids and a number of drugs (Table 49.10). For example, cimetidine inhibits the metabolism of methadone, which may lead to increasing drowsiness or even coma (Sorkin & Ugawa 1983). Rifampicin, which speeds up methadone metabolism, has on occasion precipitated opioid withdrawal symptoms (Kreek et al 1976).

TRAMADOL

Tramadol is a synthetic centrally-acting analgesic with a unique mode of action, displaying both weak opioid and

Table 49.9 Disease induced alterations in opioid pharmacokinetics[1]

Opioid		References
	Cirrhosis	
Pethidine	Increased bioavailability and decreased clearance = accumulation	Klotz et al (1974) Pond et al (1981)
Pentazocine	Increased bioavailability and decreased clearance = accumulation	Neal et al (1979)
Dextropropoxyphene	Increased bioavailability and decreased clearance = accumulation	Giacomini et al (1980)
	Renal failure	
Pethidine	Increased norpethidine, a toxic metabolite = accumulation	Szeto et al (1977)
Dextropropoxyphene	Increased norpropoxyphene, a toxic metabolite = accumulation	Gibson et al (1980)
Morphine	Increased morphine-6-glucuronide, an active metabolite = accumulation	Inturrisi (1990) Osborne et al (1986) Sawe et al (1985b)
Dihydrocodeine	Decreased clearance = accumulation	Barnes et al (1985)

[1]From Inturrisi (1989) with permission.

Table 49.10 Drug-induced alterations in opioid pharmacokinetics and/or pharmacodynamics[1]

Opioid	Interaction	Result	Reference
Morphine	Clomipramine	Increased bioavailability	Ventafridda et al (1987a)
Morphine	Amitriptyline	Increased bioavailability	Ventafridda et al (1987a)
Pethidine	Phenobarbitone	Increased biotransformation = accumulation of norpethidine	Stambaugh et al (1977)
Pethidine	Phenytoin	Increased biotransformation = accumulation of norpethidine	Pond and Kretachzmar (1981)
Methadone	Phenytoin	Increased biotransformation = faster elimination	Tong et al (1981)
Methadone	Rifampicin	Increased biotransformation = faster elimination	Kreck et al (1976)
Pethidine	Monoamine oxidase inhibitors	Excitation, hyperpyrexia and convulsions	Inturrisi (1990)
Any opioid	Alcohol or other CNS depressants	Enhanced depressant effects	Inturrisi (1990)

[1]From Inturrisi (1989) with permission.

nonopioid properties (Raffa et al 1992). The opioid properties relate to mu, delta and kappa opioid receptor agonism, with a 20-fold preference for the mu receptor ((+)enantiomer). The nonopioid properties result from stimulation of serotonin release ((+)enantiomer) and inhibition of presynaptic re-uptake of noradrenaline and serotonin ((–)enantiomer). Noradrenaline and serotonin are neurotransmitters involved in the activation of descending inhibitory pathways which modulate nociception. (see Chs 9 and 12)

The principal metabolite of tramadol, mono-O-desmethyl tramadol, is also pharmacologically active. It has a higher affinity for opioid receptors than tramadol itself. The quantity produced in man is small, however, and its contribution to analgesia is probably small. Parenterally, tramadol and pethidine are equipotent, and one-tenth as potent as morphine (Vickers et al 1992). Although tramadol has a higher oral bioavailability than morphine, the same potency ratio should be used when converting from tramadol to morphine, whether oral to oral or injection to injection (Zech, personal communication). Oral tramadol is therefore a step 2 analgesic, i.e. an alternative to codeine.

Tramadol is usually administered in doses of 50–100 mg 4–6-hourly; experience with higher doses is limited. A typical *daily* dose for moderately severe pain is 200 mg. Tramadol causes much less constipation and respiratory depression than equianalgesic doses of other opioids (Houmes et al 1992; Vickers et al 1992). Its dependence liability is also considerably less (Preston et al 1991). On the other hand, it is as effective as codeine when used as a cough suppressant (Szekely & Vickers 1992).

ALTERNATIVE ROUTES OF ADMINISTRATION

PER RECTUM

Morphine sulphate suppositories offer an alternative mode of administration (Ripamonti & Bruera 1991). In Britain 15 mg and 30 mg suppositories are commercially available. Plasma morphine concentration after oral and rectal routes suggests that the oral to rectal potency ratio for morphine sulphate is 1:1 (Hanning et al 1985). Thus, the same dose is given per rectum as by mouth. Slow-release morphine tablets can be given per rectum in patients no longer able to swallow tablets (Kaiko et al 1989; Maloney et al 1989).

Oxycodone pectinate suppositories (30 mg) are available in the UK and Canada. These need be given only every 8 hours. Oxycodone pectinate 30 mg 8-hourly is equivalent to morphine 15 mg 4-hourly.

CONTINUOUS SUBCUTANEOUS INFUSION

Terminally ill cancer patients with, for example, inoperable bowel obstruction may need parenteral medication for several days or weeks. Portable battery-driven syringe drivers are increasingly used to deliver a continuous subcutaneous infusion of morphine or diamorphine together with an antiemetic (Walsh et al 1992). Other drugs may also be included provided they are miscible and stable in combined solution (Table 49.11). Tissue irritability must also be considered; a factor which precludes, for example, the use of chlorpromazine by this route.

INTRAVENOUS

An increasing number of cancer patients have a permanent indwelling silicone central venous catheter to facilitate chemotherapy and repeated blood sampling. Catheters have been kept in situ for periods of up to 3 years, with a median duration of 40 days (McCredie & Lawson 1984). These catheters can be used for morphine (and other symptom-control drugs) by either continuous infusion or intermittent bolus (Portenoy et al 1986).

As intravenous administration limits the mobility of the patient, it is generally not preferable to the oral, rectal or subcutaneous routes. Acute tolerance to the analgesic effect of repeat intravenous bolus injections of diamorphine hydrochloride has been reported (Hanks & Thomas

Table 49.11 Drugs given in various combinations by continuous subcutaneous infusion by more than 10% of 97 UK hospices[1]

	Percentage of respondents using drug (n = 97)	Range of maximum 24 h doses (mg)	Median of range (mg)
Diamorphine[2]	99	300–10 000	2200
Haloperidol	95	5–100	12.5
Methotrimeprazine	93	25–400	150
Cyclizine	85	50–150	150
Midazolam	64	10–160	40
Metoclopramide	64	10–200	30
Dexamethasone	39	4–30	15.5
Hyoscine hydrobromide	39	0.4–4	1.2
Hyaluronidase	16	1500 IU	1500 IU

[1]From Johnson & Patterson (1992) with permission.
[2]Used in place of morphine in the UK.

1985). On the other hand, continuous intravenous infusions of morphine have been used successfully in children for long periods (Miser et al 1980).

NEW ROUTES OF ADMINISTRATION

A number of new routes have been explored in recent years, notably the sublingual/buccal and spinal, and also the transdermal, nasal and inhalational (nebulized). Two issues tend to become confused. The first is clinical necessity; some patients cannot take oral medication for physical reasons, e.g. intractable vomiting. The second is the potential of new routes to provide better pain relief and/or fewer adverse effects.

SUBLINGUAL/BUCCAL ROUTE

The kinetic logic behind the sublingual/buccal route is that the drug is absorbed systemically without a hepatic 'first-pass' effect. Compared to ingested oral medication, the relative systemic bioavailability is potentially increased.

Sublingual buprenorphine provides the best example of kinetic gain in bioavailability. Postoperatively 0.4 mg sublingually produces analgesia equivalent to 0.3 mg intramuscularly. Relative systemic availability was 55% (range 16–94%). The systemic availability of oral buprenorphine, in contrast, is about 15% (McQuay et al 1986a). Substantial gains in onset time for analgesic effect, however, have not been achieved; 30 minutes is the accepted time for chronic dosing. Phenazocine has also been used clinically by the sublingual route but as yet there are no controlled data (Blane & Robbie 1972).

Opioids with a high oral bioavailability (e.g. methadone) do not demonstrate significant kinetic gain when taken sublingually (McQuay et al 1986b). The same is true for morphine (Pannuti et al 1982; McQuay et al 1986b). Sublingual preparations are particularly useful when strong opioids are necessary but cannot be taken by mouth and injections are problematic (e.g. in children, haemophiliacs and home care).

SPINAL OPIOIDS

The presence of opioid receptors in high density in the dorsal horn of the spinal cord (Pert & Snyder 1973) provides the logical basis for spinal opioid use (Sabbe & Yaksh 1990). Compared with conventional routes, extradural and intrathecal administration carry a potentially higher morbidity. The use of the spinal route can be justified only if it results in equal or greater pain relief than conventional routes with less troublesome or fewer adverse effects (Hogan et al 1991; Sjoberg et al 1991).

Duration of analgesic effect after spinal opioids is considerably longer than after intramuscular injection. In patients having cardiac surgery, analgesia of about 36 hours' duration was achieved by lumbar intrathecal injection of 2–4 mg of morphine (Mathews & Abrams 1980). In patients having total hip replacement, lower doses gave 24–48 hours' analgesia (Kalso 1983; Paterson et al 1984). Diamorphine gives an equivalent duration of analgesia to morphine at the same dose.

The advantage of the epidural route is the potentially lower morbidity, notably headache and infection. On the other hand, in chronic use the catheter tip may occlude (it is not bathed in CSF) or migrate intrathecally. Further, spinal opioid availability is less certain than with the intrathecal route. Systemic absorption adds another dimension to both pharmacokinetic and pharmacodynamic considerations. Only 10–20% of an epidural dose of morphine (low lipid-solubility) crosses the dura into the CSF. This is reflected in the higher doses used by this route. Extradural morphine (5 mg) twice daily is equivalent to 1 mg of intrathecal morphine once a day (Watson et al 1984). In a postoperative study of lumbar epidural analgesia, 5 mg of morphine gave a median duration of relief of 10 hours (Watson et al 1984). A second study gave comparable results (Nordberg 1984). Doses used with infusions, however, have been as low as 0.3 mg/h (Cullen et al 1985). This suggests that the dose–response for morphine differs with bolus and infusion.

Adverse effects

Adverse effects vary according to dose, whether the opioid is given intrathecally or epidurally, and whether usage is acute or chronic. Troublesome adverse effects are generally less with chronic compared with acute use. The incidence of adverse effects and complications after postoperative epidural morphine are summarized in Table 49.12. Intramuscular naloxone reverses most of the adverse effects associated with epidural morphine notably respiratory depression, urinary retention and pruritus, without reducing analgesia, (Korbon et al 1985; Ueyama et al 1992). However, rectovaginal muscle spasms seen in one patient receiving intrathecal morphine necessitated the ongoing use of midazolam by PCA (Littrell et al 1992).

Tolerance to spinal opioids may occur with chronic use; it is a predictable consequence of the very high local concentrations of opioid in the cerebrospinal fluid. Tolerance develops more rapidly with infusions than with on demand bolus injections (Erickson et al 1984). It is not an insuperable problem, as increasing the dose corrects the reduced response. Abstention for about a week leads to a reversal of tolerance.

Spinal opioids have a definite place in the relief of pain after major surgery and after injuries such as multiple rib fractures (Ullman et al 1989). In these situations the use is self-limiting and is unlikely to exceed 14 days. With chronic pain, until the promise of higher quality pain relief is realized, the spinal route should be used only after systemically administered opioids have been shown to be ineffective or associated with intolerable adverse effects (Sjostrand & Rawal 1986).

Before instituting long-term treatment, it is important to determine whether the pain is responsive to opioids. It has been recommended that a test injection of an appropriate dose of morphine should be given epidurally and compared with the effect of normal saline (Erickson et al 1984). Increasingly, however, a combination of morphine and bupivacaine is being used for pains which are not wholly responsive to morphine (Hogan et al 1991; Sjoberg et al 1991).

A safe method of converting from conventional parenteral routes to intrathecal administration is to use 1% of the former total daily dose (Coombs 1986); some centres, however, use 2%. In Oxford, the following guidelines are followed:

1. oral to epidural morphine, *divide 24-hour dose by 10*
2. subcutaneous to epidural, *divide 24-hour dose by 5*
3. intrathecal doses are *10 times smaller* than epidural ones.

Table 49.12 Incidence of complications in opioid-naive patients after 5 mg epidural morphine (n = 128)[1]

Complications	Incidence (%)
Nausea	48
Vomiting	30
Pruritus	41
Urinary retention	34
Hypotension	4
Respiratory depression	4

[1] From Writer et al (1985) Canadian Anaesthesiological Society Journal 32: 330–338, with permission.

Table 49.13 Strong opioids in the management of chronic pain of nonmalignant origin[1]

1. There must be a clear understanding that opioids are to be used for a limited term in the first instance
2. Their use is contingent upon certain obligations or goals being met by the patient, e.g. increased mobilization, return to work, no unauthorized demands for emergency injectable opioids from locum services, and changes in unacceptable or nonproductive behaviours, i.e. a contractual arrangement (which can be in the form of a written document) that opioids will be supplied for a limited term in exchange for agreed goals
3. Extension of the initial term can be contemplated only upon agreed improvements being met by patients
4. The patient understands that there will be regular and random blood samples collected to ensure compliance with dosing schedule and that other opioid drugs are not being consumed

[1] From Gourlay & Cherry (1991).

OPIOIDS AND CHRONIC PAIN OF NONMALIGNANT ORIGIN

While there is a clear consensus about the use of morphine and other strong opioids for severe pain in cancer, its use for chronic pain of nonmalignant origin is still controversial (Coniam 1989; Brena & Sanders 1991; Glynn et al 1991; Gourlay & Cherry 1991). An absolute embargo on their use is, however, unsustainable. Clinical experience demonstrates that some chronic pain patients derive considerable benefit from opioids (Knight 1989; Portenoy 1990; Zenz et al 1992). Controlled data confirm this (Rowbotham et al 1991; Jadad et al 1992). The situation is comparable to cancer pain in that it is important to recognize that not all chronic pains respond equally to opioids. On the other hand, the situation differs in as much as the chronic use of opioids in nonterminal conditions could well mean 10–50 years, compared with weeks or months.

The use of intravenous PCA comparing morphine with placebo may well become a standard test for opioid-responsiveness in chronic pain patients (Jadad et al 1992). The guidelines suggested by the Pain Management Unit at Flinders Medical Centre should be noted (Table 49.13).

REFERENCES

Agenas I, Gustafsson L, Rane A, Sawe J 1982 Analgetikaterapi for cancerpatienter. Lakartidningen 79: 287–289

Aitkenhead A R, Vater M, Achola K, Cooper C M S, Smith G 1984 Pharmacokinetics of single dose IV morphine in normal volunteers and patients with end-stage renal failure. British Journal of Anaesthesia 56: 813–819

Arner S, Meyerson B A 1988 Lack of analgesic effect of opioids on neuropathic and idiopathic forms of pain. Pain 33: 11–23

Atkinson R E, Schofield P, Mellor P 1990 The efficacy in sequential use of buprenorphine and morphine in advanced cancer pain. In: Doyle D (ed) Opioids in the treatment of cancer pain. Royal Society of Medicine Services, London, p 81–87

Barnes J N, Goodwin F J 1983 Dihydrocodeine narcosis in renal failure. British Medical Journal 286: 438–439

Barnes J N, Williams A J, Tomson M J, Toseland P A, Goodwin F J 1985 Dihydrocodeine in renal failure: further evidence for an important role in the kidney in the handling of opioid drugs. British Medical Journal 290: 740–742

Beaver W T 1984 Analgesic efficacy of dextropropoxyphene and dextropropoxyphene-containing combinations: a review. Human Toxicology 3: 191S–220S

Blane G F, Robbie D S 1972 Agonist and antagonist actions of narcotic analgesic drugs. In: Kosterlitz H W, Collier A O J, Villareal J E (eds) Proceedings of the Symposium of the British Pharmaceutical Society. Macmillan, London, p 120–127

Breivik K, Rennemo F 1982 Clinical evaluation of combined treatment with methadone and psychotropic drugs in cancer patients. Acta Anaesthesiologica Scandinavica 26: 135–140

Brena S F, Sanders S H 1991 Opioids in nonmalignant pain: questions in search of answers. Clinical Journal of Pain 7: 342–345

Brescia F J, Portenoy R K, Ryan M, Krasnoff L, Gray G 1992 Pain, opioid use, and survival in hospitalized patients with advanced cancer. Journal of Clinical Oncology 10: 149–155

Brismar B, Hedenstierna G, Lundquist H, Strandberg A, Svensson L, Tokics L 1985 Pulmonary densities during anesthesia with muscular relaxation: a proposal of atelectasis. Anesthesiology 62: 422–428

Bruera E, Macmillan K, Hanson J, MacDonald R N 1989 The cognitive effects of the administration of narcotic analgesics in patients with cancer pain. Pain 39: 13–16

Bruera E, Miller M J, Macmillan K, Kuehn N 1992 Neuropsychological effects of methylphenidate in patients receiving a continuous infusion of narcotics for cancer pain. Pain 48: 163–166

Brunk S F, Delle M 1974 Morphine metabolism in man. Clinical Pharmacology and Therapeutics 16: 51–57

Budd K 1990 Experience with partial agonists in the treatment of cancer pain. In: Doyle D (ed) Opioids in the treatment of cancer pain. Royal Society of Medicine Services, London, p 51–55

Carrupt P-A, Testa B, Bechalany A, El Tayar N, Descas P, Perrissoud D 1991 Morphine 6-glucuronide and morphine 3-glucuronide as molecular chameleons with unexpected lipophilicity. Journal of Medicinal Chemistry 34: 1272–1275

Colpaert F C, Niemegeers C J E, Janssen P A J, Maroli A N 1980 The effects of prior fentanyl administration and of pain on fentanyl analgesia: tolerance to and enhancement of narcotic analgesia. Journal of Pharmacology and Experimental Therapeutics 213: 418–426

Coniam S W 1989 Prescribing opioids for chronic pain in nonmalignant disease. In: Twycross R G (ed) The Edinburgh symposium on pain control and medical education. Royal Society of Medicine Services, London, p 205–210

Consensus Statement 1994 Use of morphine for cancer pain. European Association for Palliative Care (In press)

Coombs D W 1986 Management of chronic pain by epidural and intrathecal opioids: newer drugs and delivery systems. In: Sjostrand U H, Rawal N (eds) International anesthesiology clinics 24(2): regional opioids in anesthesiology and pain management. Little Brown, Boston, p 59–74

Cullen M L, Staren E D, El-Ganzouri A, Logas W G, Ivkanovich A D, Economou S G 1985 Continuous epidural infusion for analgesia after major abdominal operations: a randomised prospective double-blind study. Surgery 98: 718–726

Dahlstrom B E, Paalzow L K 1978 Pharmacokinetic interpretation of the enterohepatic recirculation and first-pass elimination of morphine in the rat. Journal of Pharmacokinetics and Biopharmaceutics 6: 505–519

Dickenson A H 1991 Mechanisms of the analgesic actions of opiates and opioids. British Medical Bulletin 47: 690–702

Don H F, Dieppa R A, Taylor P 1975 Narcotic analgesics in anuric patients. Anesthesiology 42: 745–747

Eddy N B, Friebel H, Hahn K-J, Halbach H 1968 Codeine and its alternatives for pain and cough relief. Bulletin of the World Health Organization 38: 637–741

Erickson D L, Lo J, Michaelson M 1984 Intrathecal morphine for treatment of pain due to malignancy. Pain (suppl) 2: S19

Etches R C, Sandler A N, Daley M D 1989 Respiratory depression and spinal opioids. Canadian Journal of Anaesthesiology 36: 165–185

Ettinger D S, Vitale P J, Trump D L 1979 Important clinical pharmacological considerations in the use of methadone in cancer patients. Cancer Treatment Reports 63: 457–459

Ferreira S H 1972 Prostaglandins, aspirin-like drugs and analgesics. Nature New Biology 240: 200–203

Galasko C S B 1981 The development of skeletal metastases. In: Weiss L, Gilbert H A (eds) Bone metastasis. G K Hall, Boston, p 83–113

Giacomini K M, Giacomini J C, Gibson T P, Levy G 1980 Propoxyphene and norpropoxyphene plasma concentrations after oral propoxyphene in cirrhotic patients with and without surgically constructed portacaval shunt. Clinical Pharmacology and Therapeutics 30: 183–188

Gibson T P, Giacomini K M, Briggs W A, Whitman W, Levy G 1980 Propoxyphene and norpropoxyphene plasma concentrations in the anephric patient. Clinical Pharmacology and Therapeutics 27: 665–670

Glynn C J, McQuay H, Jadad A R, Carroll D 1991 Response to controversy corner: 'Opioids in nonmalignant pain: questions in search of answers'. Clinical Journal of Pain 7: 346

Gong Q-L, Hedner J, Bjorkman R, Hedner T 1992 Morphine 3-glucuronide may functionally antagonize morphine-6-glucuronide induced antinociception and ventilatory depression in the rat. Pain 48: 249–255

Gourlay G K, Cherry D A 1991 Response to controversy corner: 'Can opioids be successfully used to treat severe pain in nonmalignant conditions?' Clinical Journal of Pain 7: 347–349

Hanks G W 1991a Opioid responsive and opioid non-responsive pain in cancer. British Medical Bulletin 47: 718–731

Hanks G W 1991b Morphine pharmocokinetics and analgesia after oral administration. Postgraduate Medical Journal 67: (suppl 2) S60–S63

Hanks G W, Hoskin P J 1987 Opioid analgesics in the management of pain in patients with cancer: a review. Palliative Medicine 1: 1–25

Hanks G W, Thomas E A 1985 Intravenous opioids in chronic cancer pain. British Medical Journal 291: 1124–1125

Hanks G W, Twycross R G, Lloyd J W 1981 Unexpected complication of successful nerve block. Anaesthesia 36: 37–39

Hanks G W, Twycross R G, Bliss J M 1987 Controlled-release morphine tablets: a double-blind trial in patients with advanced cancer. Anaesthesia 42: 840–844

Hanna M 1993 British Journal of Anaesthesia (in press)

Hanning C D, Smith G, McNeill M, Graham N B 1985 Rectal administration of morphine from a sustained release hydrogel suppository. British Journal of Anaesthesia 236p–237p

Hargreaves K M, Dubner R, Joris J 1988 Peripheral actions of opiates in the blockade of carrageenan-induced inflammation. In: Dubner R, Gebhart G F, Bond M R (eds) Proceedings of the Vth World Congress on Pain. Elsevier, Amsterdam, p 55–60

Hasselstrom J, Eriksson L S, Persson A, Rane A, Svensson J, Sawe J 1986 Morphine metabolism in patients with liver cirrhosis. Acta Pharmacologica et Toxicologica (suppl V): abstract 101

Heneghan C P H, Jones J G 1985 Pulmonary gas exchange and diaphragmatic position. British Journal of Anaesthetics 57: 1161–1166

Hill S C 1987 Painful prescriptions. Journal of the American Medical Association 257: 2081

Hogan Q, Haddox J D, Abram S, Weissman D, Taylor M L, Janjan N 1991 Epidural opiates and local anesthetics for the management of cancer pain. Pain 46: 271–279
Houde R W 1986 Discussion. In: Bonica J J (ed) Advances in pain research and therapy, vol 8. Raven Press, New York p 261–263
Houde R W, Wallenstein S L, Beaver W T 1965 Clinical measurement of pain. In: de Stevens G (ed) Analgetics. Academic Press, New York, p 75–122
Houmes R J M, Voets M A, Verkaaik A, Erdmann W, Lachmann B 1992 Efficacy and safety of tramadol versus morphine for moderate and severe postoperative pain with special regard to respiratory depression. Anesthesia and Analgesia 74: 510–514
Inturrisi C E 1989 Management of cancer pain: pharmacology and principles of management. Cancer 63: 2308–2320
Inturrisi C E 1990 Effects of other drugs and pathologic states on opioid disposition and response. In: Benedetti C, Giron G, Chapman C R (eds) Advances in pain research and therapy, vol 14. Raven Press, New York, p 171–180
Inturrisi C E, Verebely K 1972 The levels of methadone in the plasma in methadone maintenance. Clinical Pharmacology and Therapeutics 13: 633–637
Inturrisi C E, Schultz M, Shin S, Umans J G, Angel L, Simon E J 1983 Evidence from opiate binding studies that heroin acts through its metabolites. Life Sciences 33: 773–776
Inturrisi C E, Max M B, Foley K M, Schultz M, Shin S U, Houde R W 1984 The pharmacokinetics of heroin in patients with chronic pain. New England Journal of Medicine 310: 1213–1217
Jadad A R, Carroll D, Glynn C J, Moore R A, McQuay H J 1992 Morphine sensitivity of chronic pain: a double-blind randomised crossover study using patient-controlled analgesia. Lancet i: 1367–1371
Jakobsson P A, Ginman C, Hanson J et al 1980 Clinical evaluation of methadone treatment in cancer pain. Presented at symposium on narcotic analgesics, Stockholm
Johnson I, Patterson S 1992 Drugs used in combination in the syringe driver: a survey of hospice practice. Palliative Medicine 6: 125–130
Jones J G, Jordan C 1987 Postoperative analgesia and respiratory complications. Hospital Update 13: 115–124
Kaiko R F 1980 Age and morphine analgesia in cancer patients with postoperative pain. Clinical Pharmacology and Therapeutics 28: 823–826
Kaiko R F 1986 Discussion. In: Foley K, Inturrisi C E (eds) Advances in pain research and therapy. Vol 8. Raven Press, New York, p 235–237
Kaiko R F 1989 The pre- and post-operative use of controlled release morphine (MS contin) tablets. In: Twycross R G (ed) The Edinburgh symposium on pain control and medical education. Royal Society of Medicine Services, London, p 147–160
Kaiko R F, Healy N, Pav J, Thomas G B, Goldenheim P D 1989 The comparative bioavailability of MS Contin tablets (controlled release oral morphine) following rectal and oral administration. In: Twycross R G (ed) 1989 The Edinburgh symposium on pain control and medical education. Royal Society of Medicine Services, London, p 235–241
Kalso E 1983 Effects of intrathecal morphine injected with bupivacaine on pain after orthopaedic surgery. British Journal of Anaesthesia 55: 415–422
Kalso E, Vainio A 1990 Morphine and oxycodone in the management of cancer pain. Clinical Pharmacology and Therapeutics 47: 639–646
Kanner R M, Foley K M 1981 Patterns of narcotic drug use in cancer pain clinic. Annals of the New York Academy of Sciences 362: 162–172
Kantor T G, Hopper M, Laska E 1981 Adverse effects of commonly ordered oral narcotics. Journal of Clinical Pharmacology 21: 1–8
Katz M D, Fritz W L, Lor E 1984 Heroin: should it be legalized for the treatment of cancer pain? Arizona Medicine 51: 602–603
Klotz U, McHorse T S, Wilkinson G R, Schenker S 1974 The effect of cirrhosis on the disposition and elimination of meperidine in man. Clinical Pharmacology and Therapeutics 16: 667–675
Knight C L 1989 The use of opioids in chronic low back pain. In: Twycross R G (ed) 1989 The Edinburgh symposium on pain control and medical education. Royal Society of Medicine Services, London, p 201–204
Korbon G A, James D J, Verlander J M et al 1985 Intramuscular naloxone reverses the side effects of epidural morphine while preserving analgesia. Regional Anaesthesia 10: 16–20
Kreek M J, Garfield J W, Gutjahr C L, Giusti L M 1976 Rifampin-induced methadone withdrawal. New England Journal of Medicine 294: 1104–1106
Kupers R C, Konings H, Adriaensen H, Gybels J M 1991 Morphine differentially affects the sensory and affective pain ratings in neurogenic and idiopathic forms of pain. Pain 47: 5–12
Lasagna L, Beecher K H 1954 The analgesic effectiveness of codeine and meperidine (Demerol). Journal of Pharmacology and Experimental Therapeutics 112: 306–311
Levine M N, Sackett D L, Bush H 1986 Heroin versus morphine for cancer pain? Archives of Internal Medicine 146: 353–356
Levy M 1990 Oral controlled release morphine: guidelines for clinical use. In: Benedetti C, Chapman C, Giron G (eds) Advances in pain research and therapy, vol 14. Raven Press, New York, p 285–295
Littrell R A, Kennedy L D, Birmingham W E, Leak W D 1992 Muscle spasms associated with intrathecal morphine therapy: treatment with midazolam. Clinical Pharmacy 11: 57–59
Luczak J, Okupny M, Sopata M 1992 The use of ketamine in the palliative care. Paper presented at the Advanced Palliative Care Course, Lad, Poland, June 1992
McCormack A, Hunter-Smith D, Piotrowski Z H, Grant M, Kubik S, Kessel K 1992 Analgesic use in home hospice cancer patients. Journal of Family Practice 34: 160–164
McCredie K B, Lawson M 1984 Percutaneous insertion of silicone central venous catheters for long term intravenous access in cancer patients. Internal Medicine 5: 100–105
McQuay H J 1986 Opiate metabolism and excretion. In: Levy J, Budd K (eds) Opioids: use and abuse. Royal Society of Medicine Services, London, p 27–34
McQuay H J, Dickenson A H 1990 Implications of nervous system plasticity for pain management. Anaesthesia 45: 101–102
McQuay H J, Moore R A 1984 Be aware of renal function when prescribing morphine. Lancet ii: 284–285
McQuay H J, Moore R A, Bullingham R E S 1986a Buprenorphine kinetics. In: Foley K M, Inturrisi C E (eds) Opioid analgesics in the management of cancer pain. Raven Press, New York, p 271–278
McQuay H J, Moore R A, Bullingham R E S 1986b Sublingual heroin morphine methadone and buprenorphine. In: Foley K M, Inturrisi C E (eds) Advances in pain research and therapy opioid analgesics in the management of cancer pain, vol 8. Raven Press, New York, p 407–412
McQuay H J, Carroll D, Watts P G, Juniper R P, Moore R A 1988 Codeine increases pain relief from ibuprofen after third molar surgery. Pain 37: 7–13
McQuay H J, Carroll D, Faura C C, Gavaghan D J, Hand C W, Moore R A 1990 Oral morphine in cancer pain: influences on morphine and metabolite concentration. Clinical Pharmacology and Therapeutics 48: 236–244
Maloney C M, Kesner R K, Klein G, Bockenstette J 1989 The rectal administration of MS Contin: clinical implications of use in end stage cancer. American Journal of Hospice Care 6: 34–35
Maruta T, Swanson D W, Finlayson R E 1979 Drug abuse and dependency in patients with chronic pain. Mayo Clinic Proceedings 54: 241–244
Mathews E T, Abrams L D 1980 Intrathecal morphine in open heart surgery Lancet i: 543
Melzack R, Mount B M, Gordon J M 1979 The Brompton mixture versus morphine solution given orally: effects on pain. Canadian Medical Association Journal 120: 435–439
Miser A W, Miser J S, Clark B S 1980 Continuous intravenous infusion of morphine sulphate for control of severe pain in children with terminal malignancy. Journal of Paediatrics 96: 930–932
Morley J S, Miles J B, Wells J C, Bowsher D 1992 Paradoxical pain. Lancet 340: 1045
Morrison J D, Hill G B, Dundee J W 1968 Studies of drugs given before anaesthesia XV: evaluation of the method of study after 10,000 observations. British Journal of Anaesthesia 40: 890–900
Morrison L M, Payne M, Drummond G B 1991 Comparison of speed of onset of analgesic effect of diamorphine and morphine. British Journal of Anaesthesia 66: 656–659

Mostert J W, Evers J L, Hobika G H, Moore R H, Ambrus J L 1971 Cardiorespiratory effects of anaesthesia with morphine or fentanyl in chronic renal failure and cerebral toxicity after morphine. British Journal of Anaesthesia 43: 1053–1060
Moulin D E, Ling G S F, Pasternak G W 1988 Unidirectional analgesic cross-tolerance between morphine and levorphanol in the rat. Pain 33: 233–239
Neal E A, Meffin P J, Gregory P B, Blaschke T F 1979 Enhanced bioavailability and decreased clearance of analgesics in patients with cirrhosis. Gastroenterology 77: 96–102
Nordberg G, Hedner T, Mellstrand T, Dahlstrom B 1984 Pharmacokinetic aspects of intrathecal morphine analgesia. Anesthesiology 60: 448–454
Osborne R J, Joel S P, Slevin M L 1986 Morphine intoxication in renal failure: the role of morphine-6-glucuronide. British Medical Journal 292: 1548–1549
Ottesen S, Minton M, Twycross R G 1990 The use of epidural morphine at a palliative care centre. Palliative Medicine 4: 117–122
Pannuti F, Rossi A P, Iafelice G et al 1982 Control of chronic pain in very advanced cancer patients with morphine hydrochloride administered by oral, rectal and sublingual route. Clinical report and preliminary results on morphine pharmacokinetics. Pharmacological Research Communications 14: 369–380
Paterson G M C, McQuay H J, Bullingham R E S, Moore R A 1984 Intradural morphine and diamorphine dose-response studies. Anaesthesia 39: 113–117
Patwardhan R V, Johnson R F, Hoyumpa A et al 1981 Normal metabolism of morphine in cirrhosis. Gastroenterology 81: 1006–1011
Pert C B, Snyder S H 1973 Opiate receptor: demonstration in nervous tissue. Science 179: 1011–1014
Pond S M, Kretschzmar K M 1981 Effect of phenytoin on meperidine clearance and normeperidine formation. Clinical Pharmacology and Therapeutics 30: 680–686
Pond S M, Tong T, Benowitz N L, Jacob P, Rigod J 1981 Presystemic metabolism of meperidine to normeperidine in normal and cirrhotic subjects. Clinical Pharmacology and Therapeutics 30: 183–188
Portenoy R K 1990 Chronic opioid therapy in nonmalignant pain. Journal of Pain and Symptom Management 5 (suppl): S46–S62
Portenoy R K, Coyle N 1990 Controversies in the long-term management of analgesic therapy in patients with advanced cancer. Journal of Pain and Symptom Management 5: 307–319
Portenoy R K, Foley K M 1986 Chronic use of opioid analgesics in non-malignant pain: report of 38 cases. Pain 25: 171–186
Portenoy R K, Foley K M, Inturrisi C E 1990 The nature of opioid responsiveness and its implications for neuropathic pain: new hypotheses derived from studies of opioid infusions. Pain 43: 273–286
Portenoy R K, Moulin D E, Rogers A, Inturrisi C E, Foley K M 1986 Intravenous infusion of opioids for cancer pain: clinical review and guidelines for use. Cancer Treatment Reports 70: 575–581
Portenoy R K, Thaler H T, Inturrisi C E et al 1992 The metabolite morphine-6-glucuronide contributes to the analgesia produced by morphine infusion in patients with pain and normal renal function. Clinical Pharmacology and Therapeutics 51: 422–431
Porter J, Jick J 1980 Addiction rare in patients treated with narcotics. New England Journal of Medicine 302: 123
Poyhia R, Seppala T, Olkkola K T, Kalso E 1992 The pharmacokinetics and metabolism of oxycodone after intramuscular and oral administration to healthy subjects. British Journal of Clinical Pharmacology 33: 617–621
Poyhia R, Vainio A, Kalso E 1993 Oxycodone: an alternative to morphine for cancer pain. A review. Journal of Pain and Symptom Management (in press)
Preston K L, Jasinski D R, Testa M 1991 Abuse potential and pharmacological comparison of tramadol and morphine. Drug and Alcohol Dependency 27: 7–18
Raffa R B, Friderichs E, Reimann W, Shank R P, Codd E E, Vaught J L 1992 Opioid and nonopioid components independently contribute to the mechanism of action of tramdol, an 'atypical' opioid analgesic. Journal of Pharmacology and Therapeutics 260: 275–285
Rappaz O, Tripiana J, Rapin C-H, Stjernsward J, Junod J O 1985 Soins palliatifs et traitement de la douleur cancéreuse en gériatrie. Therpeutische Umschau/Revue Therapeutique 42: 843–848
Redfern N 1983 Dihydrocodeine overdose treated with naloxone infusion. British Medical Journal 287: 751–752
Rees W D 1990 Opioid needs of terminal care patients: variation with age and primary site. Clinical Oncology 2: 79–83
Regnard C F B, Badger C 1987 Opioids, sleep and the time of death. Palliative Medicine 1: 107–110
Regnard C F B, Twycross R G 1984 Metabolism of narcotics (letter). British Medical Journal 288: 860
Ripamonti C, Bruera E 1991 Rectal, buccal, and sublingual narcotics for the management of cancer pain. Journal of Palliative Care 7: 30–35
Robins L N, Davis D H, Nurco D N 1974 How permanent was Viet Nam drug addiction? American Journal of Public Health 64: 38–43
Rowbotham D J, Bamber P A, Nimmo W S 1988 Comparison of the effect of cisapride and metoclopramide on morphine-induced delay in gastric emptying. British Journal of Clinical Pharmacology 26: 741–746
Rowbotham M C, Reisner-Keller L A, Fields H L 1991 Both intravenous lidocaine and morphine reduce the pain of postherpetic neuralgia. Neurology 41: 1024–1028
Sabbe M B, Yaksh T L 1990 Pharmacology of spinal opioids. Journal of Pain and Symptom Management 5: 191–203
Sawe J, Dahlstrom B, Paalzow L, Rane A 1981 Morphine kinetics in cancer patients. Clinical Pharmacology and Therapeutics 30: 629–635
Sawe J, Kager L, Svensson J O, Rane A 1985a Oral morphine in cancer patients: in vivo kinetics and in vitro hepatic glucuronidation. British Journal of Clinical Pharmacology 19: 495–501
Sawe J, Svensson J O, Odar-Cederlof I 1985b Kinetics of morphine in patients with renal failure. Lancet ii: 211
Schug S A, Zech K, Dorr U 1990 Cancer pain management according to WHO analgesic guidelines. Journal of Pain and Symptom Management 5: 27–32
Schulze S, Roikjaer O, Hasselstrom L, Jensen N H, Kehlet H 1988 Epidural bupivacaine and morphine plus systemic indomethacin eliminates pain but not systemic response and convalescence after cholecystectomy. Surgery 103: 321–327
Sellers E M 1986 Therapeutic use of heroin: the scientist's role in social policy development. Clinical and Investigative Medicine 9: 139–140
Shimomura K, Kamata O, Ueki S, Ida S, Oguri K, Yoshimura H, Tsukamoto H 1971 Analgesic effect of morphine glucuronides. Tohoku Journal of Experimental Medicine 105: 45–52
Sjoberg M, Appelgren L, Einarsson S, Hultman E, Linder L E, Nitescu P, Curelaru I 1991 Long-term intrathecal morphine and bupivacaine in 'refractory' cancer pain. Results from the first series of 52 patients. Acta Anaesthesiologica Scandinavica 35: 30–43
Sjostrand U H, Rawal N (eds) 1986 Regional opioids in anaesthesiology and pain management. International Anesthesiology Clinics 24(2). Little, Brown, Boston, p 135
Smith M T, Watt J A, Cramond T 1992 Morphine-3-glucuronide: a potent antagonist of morphine analgesia. Life Sciences 47: 579–585
Sorkin E M, Ugawa C S 1983 Cimetidine potentiation of narcotic action. Drug Intelligence and Clinical Pharmacy 17: 60–61
Stambaugh J E, Wainer I W 1981 Drug interaction: meperidine and chlorpromazine, a toxic combination. Journal of Clinical Pharmacology 21: 140–146
Stambaugh J E, Wainer I W, Hemhill D M, Schwartz I 1977 A Potentially toxic drug interaction between pethidine (meperidine) and phenobarbitone. Lancet i: 398–399
Stjernsward J 1991 WHO cancer pain relief programme and future challenges. In: Takeda F (ed) Cancer pain relief and quality of life. WHO Collaborative Center for Cancer Pain Relief and Quality of Life, Saitama, p 5–9
Szekely S M, Vickers M D 1992 A comparison of the effects of codeine and tramadol on laryngeal reactivity. European Journal of Anaesthesiology 9: 111–120
Szeto H H, Inturrisi C E, Houde R et al 1977 Accumulation of normeperidine, an active metabolite of meperidine, in patients with renal failure or cancer. Annals of Internal Medicine 86: 738–741
Takeda F 1986 Results of field-testing in Japan of the WHO draft interim guidelines on relief of cancer pain. Pain Clinic 1: 83–89

Tasker R R, Tsuda T, Hawrylyshyn P 1983 Clinical neurophysiological investigation of deafferentation pain. In: Bonica J J, Lindblom U, Iggo A (eds) Advances in pain research and therapy, vol 5. Raven Press, New York, p 713–738

Tattersall M H N 1981 Pain: heroin versus morphine. Medical Journal of Australia 1: 492

Taub A 1982 Opioid analgesics in the treatment of chronic intractable pain of non-neoplastic origin. In: Kitahata L M, Collins J D (eds) Narcotic analgesics in anaesthesiology. Williams & Wilkins, Baltimore, p 199–208

Tennant F S, Rawson R A 1982 Outpatient treatment of prescription opioid dependence. Archives of Internal Medicine 142: 1845–1847

Tennant F S, Uelman G F 1983 Narcotic maintenance for chronic pain: medical and legal guidelines. Postgraduate Medicine 73: 81–94

Tong T G, Pond S M, Kreek M J, Jaffery N F, Benowitz N L 1981 Phenytoin-induced methadone withdrawal. Annals of Internal Medicine 94: 349–351

Toogood F S 1898 The use of morphia in cardiac disease. Lancet ii: 1393–1394

Twycross R G 1974 Clinical experience with diamorphine in advanced malignant disease. International Journal of Clinical Pharmacology Therapy and Toxicology 9: 184–198

Twycross R G 1977 A comparison of diamorphine with cocaine and methadone. British Journal of Clinical Pharmacology 4: 691–692

Twycross R G 1979 Effect of cocaine in the Brompton Cocktail. In: Bonica J J, Liebeskind J C, Albe-Fessard D G (eds) Advances in pain research and therapy, vol 3. Raven Press, New York, p 927–932

Twycross R G 1984 Plasma concentrations of dextropropoxyphene and norpropoxyphene. Human Toxicology 3: 58S–59S

Twycross R G, Harcourt J M V 1991 Use of laxatives at a palliative care centre. Palliative Medicine 5: 27–33

Twycross R G, Lack S A 1983 Symptom control in far advanced cancer: pain relief. Pitman, London, p 334

Twycross R G, Lack S A 1986 Control of alimentary symptoms in far-advanced cancer. Churchill Livingstone, Edinburgh, p 368

Twycross R G, Lack S A 1990 Therapeutics in terminal cancer, 2nd edn. Churchill Livingstone, Edinburgh, p 175–206

Twycross R G, Wald S J 1976 Longterm use of diamorphine in advanced cancer. In: Bonica J J, Albe-Fessard D G (eds) Advances in pain research and therapy, vol 1. Raven Press, New York, p 653–661

Ueyama H, Nishimura M, Tashiro C 1992 Naloxone reversal of nystagmus associated with intrathecal morphine administration (letter). Anesthesiology 76: 153

Ullman D A, Fortune J B, Greenhouse B B, Wimpy R E, Kennedy T M 1989 The treatment of patients with multiple rib fractures using continuous thoracic epidural narcotic infusion. Regional Anesthesia 14: 43–47

Ventafridda V 1989 Continuing care: a major issue in cancer pain management. Pain 36: 137–143

Ventafridda V, Ripamonti C, Bianchi M, Sbanotto A, De Conno F 1986 A randomized study on oral administration of morphine and methadone in the treatment of cancer pain. Journal of Pain and Symptom Management 1: 203–207

Ventafridda V, Ripamonti C, De Conno F, Bianchi M, Pazzuconi F, Panerai A E 1987a Antidepressants increase bioavailability of morphine in cancer patients (letter). Lancet i: 1204

Ventafridda V, Tamburini M, Caraceni A, De Conno F, Naldi F 1987b A validation study of the WHO method for cancer pain relief. Cancer 59: 851–856

Vickers M D, O'Flaherty D, Szekely S M, Read M, Yoshizumi J 1992 Tramadol: pain relief by an opioid without depression of respiration. Anaesthesia 47: 291–296

Vijayaram S, Bhargava M K, Ramamani P V et al 1989 Experience with oral morphine for cancer pain relief. Journal of Pain and Symptom Management 4: 130–134

Walker V A, Hoskin P J, Hanks G W, White I D 1988 Evaluation of WHO analgesic guidelines for cancer pain in a hospital based palliative care unit. Journal of Pain and Symptom Management 3: 145–149

Wall P D 1990 Neuropathic pain. Pain 43: 267–268

Wallenstein S L, Rogers A G, Kaiko R F, Houde R W 1986 Nalbuphine: clinical analgesic studies. In: Foley K M, Inturrisi C E (eds) Advances in pain research and therapy, vol 8. Raven Press, New York, p 247–252

Walsh T D 1984 Opiates and respiratory function in advanced cancer. Recent Results in Cancer Research 89: 115–117

Walsh C T, Levine R R 1975 Studies of the enterohepatic circulation of morphine in the rat. Journal of Pharmacology and Experimental Therapeutics 195: 303–310

Walsh T D, Smyth E M S, Currie K, Glare P A, Schneider J 1992 A pilot study, review of the literature, and dosing guidelines for patient-controlled analgesia using subcutaneous morphine sulphate for chronic cancer pain. Palliative Medicine 6: 217–226

Watson P J Q, Moore R A, McQuay H J, Teddy P, Baldwin D, Allen M C, Bullingham R E S 1984 Plasma morphine concentrations and analgesic effects of lumbar extradural morphine and heroin. Anesthesia and Analgesia 63: 629–634

Weissman D E, Haddox J D 1989 Opioid pseudoaddiction: an iatrogenic syndrome. Pain 36: 363–366

Woods A J J, Moir D C, Campbell C et al 1974 Medicines evaluation and monitoring group: central nervous system effects of pentazocine. British Medical Journal 1: 305–307

Woolf C J, Wall P D 1986 Morphine-sensitive and morphine-insensitive actions of C-fibre input on the rat spinal cord. Neuroscience Letters 64: 221–225

Woolner D F, Winter D, Frendin T J, Begg E J, Lynn K L, Wright G J 1986 Renal failure does not impair the metabolism of morphine. British Journal of Clinical Pharmacology 22: 55–59

World Health Organization 1969 Expert committee on drug dependence, 16th report. Technical report series 407. World Health Organization, Geneva

World Health Organization 1986 Cancer pain relief. World Health Organization, Geneva

World Health Organization 1990 Report of a WHO expert committee: cancer pain relief and palliative care. Technical report series 804. World Health Organization, Geneva

World Health Organization 1994 Revised method for relief of cancer pain. (in press)

Writer W D R, Hurtig J B, Evans D 1985 Epidural morphine prophylaxis of postoperative pain: report of a double-blind multicentre study. Canadian Anaesthesiological Society Journal 32: 330–338

Zech D 1990 Pain control according to WHO guidelines in 1140 cancer patients. Abstract presented at the First European Congress on Palliative Care, Paris

Zenz M, Piepenbrock S, Tryba M, Glocke M, Everlien M, Klauke W 1985 Kontrollierte studie mit buprenorphine. Deutsche Medizinische Wochenschrift 110: 448–453

Zenz M, Strumpf M, Tryba M 1992 Long-term opioid therapy in patients with chronic non-malignant pain. Journal of Royal Society of Medicine 7: 69–77

50. Psychotropic drugs

Richard Monks

INTRODUCTION

The aim of this chapter is to describe the clinical use of various psychotropic drugs in the treatment of pain states, especially those of chronic duration. Because human pain is an experience with an affective element, it is not surprising that these substances have been used as part of the therapeutic approach to this complex problem. However, there is also reason to believe that some of them have analgesic properties which are independent of their psychological effects. In the following pages, the rationale and indications for use, effectiveness and adverse effects of antidepressants, neuroleptics, lithium carbonate and the antianxiety–sedative drugs will be discussed.

RATIONALE FOR TREATMENT

ANTIDEPRESSANTS

Tricyclic–type antidepressant and monoamine oxidase inhibitors

A number of different but related mechanisms have been suggested to explain the presumed efficacy of tricyclic and heterocyclic antidepressants (TCAD) and monoamine oxidase inhibitors (MAOI) in various pain conditions.

Antidepressant action

Analgesic effects of these drugs may result from their antidepressant action. Paoli et al (1960) were the first to report TCAD therapy of chronic pain states, noting that they had intended to improve the 'reactive' depression which was often present. Others speculated that various pain states were masked depressions (Lopez Ibor 1972) or variants of depression (Blumer & Heilbronn 1982).

Various studies have shown that a substantial minority of chronic pain patients are clinically depressed and, compared with nondepressed pain controls, show an increased incidence of familial affective disorders, biological markers of depression and response to TCAD (Blumer & Heilbronn 1982; Blumer et al 1982; Krishnan et al 1985; Atkinson et al 1986, France et al 1986; Magni et al 1987; Mellerup et al 1988).

In clinical trials with adequate data, the vast majority of patients with coexisting chronic pain and depression obtained relief from both disorders when responding to MAOI or TCAD therapy (Okasha et al 1973; Couch et al 1976; Jenkins et al 1976; MacNeill & Dick 1976; Ward et al 1979; Turkington 1980; Lindsay & Wyckoff 1981; Watson et al 1982; Hameroff et al 1984; Magni et al 1986; Puttini et al 1988; Saran 1988; Loldrup et al 1989; Nappi et al 1990). Also, the onset of a depressive disorder preceding or coinciding with the onset of a chronic atypical pain complaint predicted a much better response to TCAD or MAOI than if the depression followed the pain onset (Bradley 1963).

Separate analgesic effect

There is evidence to suggest the existence of an analgesic action of TCAD and MAOI which is not mediated by any measurable antidepressant action. The onset of analgesia with TCAD in chronic pain states is more rapid than the usual onset of an antidepressant effect in some clinically depressed patients (3–7 days versus 14–21days) (Monks 1981; Langohr et al 1982; Mitas et al 1983; Hameroff et al 1984; Smoller 1984; Montastruc et al 1985; Gourlay et al 1986; Levine et al 1986).

Also, chronic pain relief with TCAD and MAOI has been reported despite a lack of antidepressant response (Lascelles 1966; Couch & Hassanein 1976; Alcoff et al 1982; Watson et al 1982; Ward et al 1984; Fogelholm & Murros 1985; Gourlay et al 1986; Macfarlane et al 1986). Similar improvements were obtained in patients without detectable depression (Lance & Curran 1964; Couch et al 1976; Jenkins et al 1976; Watson et al 1982; Feinmann et al 1984; Kvinesdal et al 1984; Montastruc et al 1985;

Watson & Evans 1985; Zeigler et al 1987; Puttini et al 1988).

Neurotransmitter alteration

It has been suggested that both the analgesic and antidepressant action of TCAD and MAOI are caused by their action on central neurotransmitter functions, particularly those mediated by the catecholamine and indolamine systems (Sternbach et al 1976; Lee & Spencer 1977; Messing & Lytle 1977; Basbaum & Fields 1978; Murphy et al 1978; Schildkraut 1978). Also, increased synaptic monoamines may inhibit nociception at thalamic (Andersen & Dafny 1983), brainstem (Roberts 1984) and spinal cord levels (Dubner & Bennet 1983; Hammond 1985; Hwang & Wilcox 1987; Proudfit 1988). Given acutely (minutes to hours), TCAD and MAOI increase synaptic levels of dopamine, noradrenaline or serotonin. Chronic administration (days to weeks) probably stabilises acute changes by regulating central and peripheral monoamine receptors or altering the activities of cerebral and spinal cord monoamine comodulators, such as substance P, thyrotropin-releasing hormone-like peptides and gamma amino-butyric acid GABA (Fuxe et al 1983; Sugrue 1983; Lloyd & Pile 1984; Willner 1985; Young & Clarke 1985).

Animal experiments on acute pain suggest the existence of both serotonin and noradrenaline bulbospinal antinociceptive pathways which interact in a complex way (Basbaum & Fields 1978; Soja & Sinclair 1983; Butler 1984; Barber et al 1989). The analgesic effects observed with TCAD alone in such studies seem to depend on monoamine neurotransmission and, to a lesser extent, opiate neurotransmission (Biegon & Samuel 1980; Eschalier et al 1981; Spiegal et al 1983).

Similar findings in some human acute and chronic pain studies suggest that analgesic properties of TCAD depend on interrelated central serotonergic and opiate mechanisms (Sternbach et al 1976; Johansson & Von Knorring 1979; Willer et al 1984). Human acute pain studies with the newer antidepressants fluoxetine (selective serotonergic reuptake blocker) and ritanserin (a 5-HT_2 antagonist) reveal antinociceptive properties that likely occur centrally and are not blocked by naloxone (Messing et al 1975; Sandrini et al 1986). Drug trials comparing various TCAD used for patients with chronic pain tend to favour more serotonergic drugs (Sternbach et al 1976; Carasso 1979; Ward et al 1984; Eberhard et al 1988; Loldrup et al 1989; Sindrup et al 1990a). However, there is evidence that noradrenergic mechanisms may also be involved, at least where pain and depression coexist (Ward et al 1983). Also, antidepressants with predominantly noradrenergic effects have been shown to be effective in adequate, controlled trials (Fogelholm & Murros 1985; Loldrup et al 1989; Kishore–Kumar et al 1990; Sindrup et al 1990a; Max et al 1991).

Further, most controlled clinical trials with antidepressants, such as fluoxetine, paroxetine, trazodone and zimelidine, that are selectively serotonergic in their effects have shown results that are no better than those of a placebo (Johansson & Von Knorring 1975; Gourlay et al 1986; Lynch et al 1990) or are inferior to those of a less selective antidepressant (Watson & Evans 1985; Frank et al 1988; Sindrup et al 1990b). Trazodone and ritanserin provided pain relief equal to that of low-dose amitriptyline in two nonplacebo-controlled trials which were the exception (Ventafridda et al 1987; Nappi et al 1990). In keeping with these findings, a recent meta-analysis of 39 placebo-controlled studies of antidepressant analgesia in chronic pain found that antidepressants with mixed serotonergic and noradrenergic properties had a larger effect size than that of drugs with more specific properties when other patient disorders and study variables were eliminated (Onghena & Van Houdenhove 1992).

Opiate effects

The analgesic effect of the opiates, like TCAD and MAOI, appears to be modulated by central biogenic amines, at least in animal acute pain trials (Lee & Spencer 1977). TCAD and MAOI effect opiate analgesia and tolerance in animal experiments (Contreras et al 1977; Fuentes et al 1977, Lee & Spencer 1977; Tofanetti et al 1977; Gonzales et al 1980; Botney & Fields 1983). These effects may be mediated by changes in serotonin and catecholamine neurotransmitters but TCAD may also bind directly to opiate receptors (Biegon & Samuel 1980).

Endogenous morphine-like substances (endorphins) seem to have a role in acute and chronic pain in animals and man (Terenius 1978, 1979). Preliminary work with a selective serotonergic TCAD, zimelidine, found therapeutic efficacy to be correlated with changes in cerebrospinal fluid (CSF) endorphin and indolamine activity in human chronic pain (Johansson et al 1980). However, more recent clinical trials did not show a correlation of TCAD-induced improvement with changes in CSF beta endorphin (Ward et al 1984; France & Urban 1991) or with plasma beta endorphin and enkephalin-like activity (Hameroff et al 1984).

Miscellaneous effects

Analgesic properties of antidepressants also have been attributed to nonspecific physiological effects such as sedation, diminished anxiety, muscle relaxation and restored sleep cycles. These effects alone do not seem adequate to explain the superiority of TCAD to more powerful anxiolytics such as the benzodiazepines in relieving chronic pain. Also, changes in anxiety, depression and chronic pain with TCAD treatment were not significantly correlated with each other in one double-blind controlled trial (Ward et al 1984).

Other specific TCAD effects which have been invoked to explain their analgesic effects include: central or peripheral histamine receptor blockade (Rumore & Schlichting 1986), inhibition of prostaglandin synthetase (Krupp & Wesp 1975) and a calcium channel blocking effect (Peroutko et al 1984). Antiinflammatory effects of TCAD have been demonstrated in two recent chronic pain experiments using arthritic rats (Butler et al 1985; Godefroy et al 1986).

NEUROLEPTICS

Commonly used neuroleptics include the phenothiazines, thioxanthenes and butyrophenones. Mechanisms of action responsible for any analgesic effects of these drugs are unknown. However, various possibilities have been considered.

Antipsychotic action

The vast majority of clinical pain syndromes relieved by neuroleptics are not delusional in nature and do not occur in the presence of a psychotic disorder.

Neurotransmitter alteration

Neuroleptic drugs show a wide range of actions on neurotransmitter systems centrally and peripherally. Based on results from acute animal pain studies, it has been suggested that neuroleptic analgesia might be mediated by inhibition of dopamine, noradrenaline, serotonin or histamine neurotransmission (Malec & Langwinski 1981; Tricklebank et al 1984; Rumore & Schlichting 1986). The limited data from human clinical trials do not suggest a correlation of analgesic effectiveness and adrenergic or muscarine blocking effects of specific neuroleptics.

Opiate effects

Haloperidol shows isomorphic similarity to meperidine and morphine (Maltbie et al 1979). Various neuroleptics inhibit naloxone or met-enkephalin binding to opiate receptors (Creese et al 1976; Somoza 1978). These observations have been cited to explain neuroleptic analgesia effects, synergistic action with narcotics and amelioration of narcotic withdrawal.

Miscellaneous effects

Potentiation of analgesia and anaesthesia in animals has been reported for different phenothiazines (Courvoisier et al 1957). The analgesic properties of phenothiazines and morphine were comparable for acute pain in mice (Maxwell et al 1961). Dundee et al (1963) found a weak analgesic action with some phenothiazines used preoperatively and tested by a pressure–pain threshold technique. Other phenothiazines had a more marked antianalgesic effect. A biphasic phenomenon was noted in these acute investigations with the analgesic effect succeeding the antianalgesic one.

Sedation may explain single-dose analgesic effects of more sedating neuroleptics, although sedation alone does not guarantee pain relief (Petts & Pleuvry 1983). Additionally, high-potency alerting neuroleptics diminish chronic pain. Anxiolytic properties of neuroleptics in chronic pain patients have been reported (Hackett et al 1987) but are insufficient to explain their analgesic effects in patients who have not responded to benzodiazepines. Local anaesthetic and skeletal muscle relaxant effect of neuroleptics only occur at higher concentrations of these drugs than are obtained at usual clinical doses.

Combined neuroleptic–antidepressant regimens might provide superior analgesic effectiveness because neuroleptics inhibit TCAD degradation and enhance TCAD plasma levels (Hirschowitz et al 1983). Similarly, carbamazepine may augment TCAD levels in combined antidepressant anticonvulsant regimens (Gerson et al 1977).

LITHIUM CARBONATE

Ekbom's initial use of lithium in cluster headache was based on the observation that this disorder, like bipolar affective disorders, is cyclic in nature (Ekbom 1974). However, analgesic effects of lithium in cluster headache occur in the absence of depression or antidepressant effect and at lower serum levels than in bipolar affective disorders (Kudrow 1977; Mathew 1978; Pearce 1980). Lithium has complex acute and chronic effects on neurotransmission which may influence pain. It enhances serotonin availability in the brain, diminishes catecholamine neurone activity, alters central adrenergic, dopaminergic, GABA and opiate receptor binding and inhibits various central and peripheral adenylate cyclase–mediated cyclic adenosine monophosphate production, including that induced by prostaglandin E (Gold & Byck 1978; Bunney & Garland 1984).

ANTIANXIETY AND SEDATIVE DRUGS

Benzodiazepines are usually given to pain sufferers in an attempt to diminish the anxiety, excessive muscle tension and insomnia felt to contribute adversely to acute and chronic pain states (Lasagna 1977; Shimm et al 1979; Hollister et al 1981). One benzodiazepine, alprazolam, also has demonstrable antidepressant properties (Feighner et al 1983; Fernandez et al 1987). Another, clonazepam, may achieve analgesic effects by its anticonvulsant properties (Swerdlow & Cundill 1981).

Stimulation of BDZ receptors effects noradrenaline,

serotonin, dopamine and GABA neurotransmission (Hamlin & Gold 1984). While benzodiazepine failed to produce antinociceptive activity in some animal studies (Bodnar et al 1980), diazepam analgesic effects were partially antagonised by naloxone in other trials with animals and humans (Wüster et al 1980; Haas et al 1982). However, more prolonged benzodiazepine use may decrease serotonin turnover and induce benzodiazepine receptor subsensitivity (Snyder et al 1977; Hamlin & Gold 1984), potentially reversing the analgesic effects of benzodiazepines and other drugs.

INDICATIONS FOR USE

It is important to recognize that the use of psychotropic drugs is only one of the adjunctive measures available in the comprehensive approach required for many pain problems, especially those of more chronic duration. A careful evaluation of some of the psychological and social factors contributing to the pain complaint is necessary to prescribe these drugs rationally (Bonica 1977).

The TCAD, neuroleptics and benzodiazepines are often used for initial control of target symptoms such as depression, anxiety, abnormal muscle tension, insomnia and fatigue (Merskey 1974). The TCAD and occasionally the neuroleptics are also used for withdrawal/detoxication from narcotics, other analgesics, minor tranquillizers and alcohol (Sternbach et al 1973; Khatami et al 1979; Halpern 1982). TCAD/narcotic regimens are used for some pain disorders refractory to either alone (Urban et al 1986).

TREATMENT INDICATIONS FOR EACH PSYCHOTROPIC GROUP

A review of the pain literature was used to delineate specific treatment indications for each psychotropic drug group.

ANTIDEPRESSANTS (TCAD AND MAOI)

Depression

A trial of antidepressants (TCAD or in some cases MAOI) is usually indicated if the patient with acute or chronic pain is clinically depressed (Bradley 1963; Lascelles 1966; Merskey & Hester 1972; Ward et al 1979; 1983, 1984; Lindsay & Wyckoff 1981; Hameroff et al 1984; Smoller 1984; Magni et al 1987; Max et al 1991). This is particularly so if the onset of depression preceded or coincided with the onset of pain (Bradley 1963), if there is a past history of favourable response of depression or pain to antidepressants or if the current episode of depression is 'endogenous' in nature (anorexia, early morning awakening, psychomotor changes or anhedonia).

Biological markers of depression such as dexamethasone nonsuppression, shortened rapid eye movement sleep latency and level of urinary 3-methoxy-4-hydroxyphenethylene glycol (MHPG) have been noted to predict pain relief with TCAD in depressed patients (Blumer et al 1982; Ward et al 1983; Smoller 1984). A newer marker, [^{3}H] imipramine platelet-binding site density, was found to be diminished in chronic idiopathic pain patients without major depression. Binding site density, pain scores and depression ratings were all improved after TCAD treatment with a family history of depressive spectrum disorder (Magni et al 1987).

Tricyclic-type antidepressants

Acute pain

Only one paper was found in which TCAD were used to treat acute clinical pain (Levine et al 1986). Neither amitriptyline nor desipramine given for 7 days was found to be superior to placebo in alleviating postoperative dental pain. However, desipramine significantly enhanced morphine analgesia in these patients. Although TCAD have been found effective in treating migraine headache, the papers listed in Table 50.1 reported on patients suffering chronic high-frequency attacks of this disorder. In short, there is no well substantiated indication for TCAD use for acute pain alone.

Chronic pain

A total of 99 papers described 119 trials of TCAD alone given for chronic pain. Success was reported for those disorders listed in Table 50.1. Pain of 'psychological origin' refers to disorders in which structural damage was not found and in which anxiety and depression were obvious and antedated or coincided with the onset of atypical pain. 'Mixed' pain refers to various nonneoplastic chronic pain disorders grouped together to compare treatment groups in those papers reviewed.

Unfortunately, most of the trials reviewed suffered from inadequacies of various sorts. However, Table 50.2 details the results of adequately controlled trials using TCAD for chronic pain. In 40 out of 46 trials, TCAD produced pain relief which was statistically and clinically superior to that obtained with placebo ('positive'). In two low-back pain studies and two rheumatoid arthritis studies, the TCAD and comparison placebo both produced clinically important pain relief which did not differ statistically in the two groups ('tie'). In one low-back pain and one 'mixed' pain study, neither TCAD nor placebo were found to change pain or depression ratings ('negative').

Clinical use of imipramine for chronic osteoarthritis and rheumatoid arthritis, amitriptyline and imipramine for diabetic neuropathy, amitriptyline for migraine, amitripty-

Table 50.1 Disorders treated with antidepressants

Disorder	Total trials	References/(number of trials)
Tricyclic-type drugs		
Arthritis	11	Kuipers 1962(3); McDonald Scott 1969; Thorpe & Marchant-Williams 1974; Gingras 1976; MacNeill & Dick 1976; Ganvir et al 1980; Macfarlane et al 1986; Frank et al 1988; Puttini et al 1988
Central post-stroke	1	Leijon & Boivie 1989
Fibromyalgia	4	Bibolotti et al 1988; Carette et al 1986; Goldenberg et al 1986; Caruso et al 1987
Low-back pain	6	Kuipers 1962; Jenkins et al 1976; Sternbach et al 1976; Alcoff et al 1982; Ward et al 1984(2)
Migraine	8	Gomersall & Stuart 1973; Couch & Hassanein 1976; Couch et al 1976; Noone 1977; Mørland et al 1979; Langohr et al 1985; Martucci et al 1985; Zeigler et al 1987
Mixed	17	Rafinesque 1963; Adjan 1970; Desproges-Gotteron et al 1970; Radebold 1971; Evans et al 1973; Kocher 1976; Duthie 1977; Johansson & Von Knorring 1979; Pilowsky et al 1982; Hameroff et al 1984; Zitman et al 1984; Edelbeck et al 1986; Gourlay et al 1986; Sharav et al 1987(2); Nappi et al 1990(2)
Mixed neurological	7	Paoli et al 1960; Laine et al 1962; Merskey & Hester 1972; Castaigne et al 1979; Montastruc et al 1985; Ventafridda et al 1987(2)
Myofascial dysfunction	2	Gessel 1975; Smoller 1984
Neoplastic	7	Hugues et al 1963; Parolin 1966; Fiorentino 1967; Gebhardt et al 1969; Adjan 1970; Bernard & Scheuer 1972; Bourhis et al 1978
Neuralgia postherpetic	10	Woodforde et al 1965; Taub 1973; Hatangdi et al 1976; Carasso 1979(2); Watson et al 1982; Watson & Evans 1985(2); Max et al 1988; Kishore-Kumar et al 1990
Neuralgia trigeminal	2	Carasso 1979(2)
Neurological perineal	1	Magni et al 1982
Neuropathy		
diabetic	16	Davis et al 1977; Gade et al 1980; Turkington 1980(2); Khurana 1983; Mitas et al 1983; Kvinesdal et al 1984; Max et al 1987; Sindrup et al 1989; Lynch et al 1990(2); Sindrup et al 1990a(2), 1990b(2); Max et al 1991
mononeuropathy	1	Langohr et al 1982
Painful shoulder syndrome	1	Tyber 1974
Phantom limb	1	Urban et al 1986
Psychological origin	13	Bradley 1963; Singh 1971(2); Okasha et al 1973(2); Ward et al 1979; Lindsay & Wyckoff 1981; Feinmann et al 1984; Magni et al 1987; Eberhard et al 1988(2); Saran 1988; Valdes et al 1989
Tension headache	11	Lance & Curran 1964(2); Diamond & Baltes 1971; Carasso 1979(2); Kudrow 1980; Sjaastad 1983; Fogelholm & Morros 1985; Martucci et al 1985; Loldrup et al 1989(2).
MAOI-type drug		
Facial pain of psychological origin	2	Lascelles 1966(2)
Migraine	1	Anthony & Lance 1969
Psychological origin	3	Bradley 1963; Lindsay & Wyckoff 1981; Raskin 1982

line for postherpetic neuralgia and amitripyline for chronic tension headaches is supported by at least two adequately controlled studies each.

Monoamine oxidase inhibitors

Chronic pain

As noted in Table 50.1 and 50.2 phenelzine has been reported to be efficacious in treating facial pain of psychological origin in one uncontrolled and one adequately controlled trial (Lascelles 1966). A few case reports support the use of phenelzine or tranylcypromine for patients suffering from depression and pain of psychological origin (Bradley 1963; Lindsay & Wyckoff 1981; Raskin 1982). One uncontrolled trial showed marked analgesic effects of phenelzine in chronic high-frequency migraine headache (Anthony & Lance 1969).

NEUROLEPTICS

Psychosis

Neuroleptics are indicated for those psychiatric disorders which are associated with delusional or hallucinatory pain such as schizophrenia, delusional depressions and monosymptomatic hypochondriacal psychosis (Munro & Chmara 1982).

Table 50.2 Antidepressants: adequately controlled trials

Disorder	Drug	Positive	Tie	Negative	References
Arthritic	Amitriptyline	1	–	–	Frank et al 1988
	Desipramine	–	1	–	Frank et al 1988
	Dibenzepin	1	–	–	Thorpe & Marchant-Williams 1974
	Dothiepin	1	–	–	Puttini et al 1988
	Imipramine	2	–	–	Gingras 1976; McDonald Scott 1969
	Trazodone	–	1	–	Frank et al 1988
	Trimipramine	1	–	–	Macfarlane et al 1986
Central poststroke	Amitriptyline	1	–	–	Leijon & Boivie 1989
Fibromyalgia	Amitriptyline	1	–	–	Goldenberg et al 1986
	Dothiepin	1	–	–	Caruso et al 1987
Low-back	Amitriptyline	–	1	–	Sternbach et al 1976
pain	Clomipramine	1	–	–	Sternbach et al 1976
	Imipramine	1	1–		Alcoff et al 1982; Jenkins et al 1976
	Trazodone	–	–	1	Goodkin et al 1990
Migraine	Amitriptyline	3	–	–	Gomersall & Stuart 1973
					Couch et al 1976; Zeigler et al 1987
Mixed	Amitriptyline	2	–	1	Pilowsky et al 1982; Sharav et al 1987(2)
	Doxepin	1	–	–	Hameroff et al 1984
	Zimelidine	1	–	–	Gourlay et al 1986
Neoplastic	Imipramine	1	–	–	Fiorentino 1967
Neuropathy					
diabetic	Amitriptyline	2	–	–	Turkington 1980; Max et al 1987
	Clomipramine	1	–	–	Sindrup et al 1990a
	Desipramine	1	–	–	Max et al 1991
	Imipramine	4	–	–	Turkington 1980; Kvinesdal et al 1984; Sindrup et al 1989, 1990b
	Paroxetine	1	–	–	Sindrup et al 1990b
mono	Clomipramine	1	–	–	Langohr et al 1982
Neuralgia	Amitriptyline	2	–	–	Watson et al 1982; Max et al 1988
post herpetic	Desipramine	1	–	–	Kishore-Kumar 1990
Psychological	Amitriptyline	1	–	–	Okasha et al 1973
origin	Dothiepin	1	–	–	Feinmann et al 1984
	Doxepin	1	–	–	Okasha et al 1973
	Phenelzine	1	–	–	Lascelles 1966
Tension	Amitriptyline	2	–	–	Lance & Curran 1964; Diamond & Baltes 1971
headache	Clomipramine	1	–	–	Loldrup et al 1989
(chronic	Maprotyline	1	–	–	Fogelholm & Murros 1985
form)	Mianserin	1	–	–	Loldrup et al 1989

Pain-associated problems

Overwhelming pain characterised by anxiety, psychomotor agitation and insomnia which does not respond to benzodiazepines in acute pain or TCAD in chronic pain may be treated, at least on a short-term basis, by neuroleptics. In patients with neoplastic pain, neuroleptics are useful in managing nausea, vomiting, bladder or rectal tenesmus and ureteral spasm (Twycross 1979).

Acute pain

In 13 papers describing 20 trials in which neuroleptics alone were given for acute pain (Table 50.3), the most common indication for use in the mixed and postoperative group was abdominal, dental or postpartum pain.

Only four of these trials were judged to be adequate. In two studies of acute postoperative pain (Taylor & Doku 1967; Fazio 1970) and one of acute myocardial infarction (Davidson et al 1979), methotrimeprazine 10–20 mg intramuscularly gave analgesic results equivalent to meperidine 50 mg intramuscularly. In the remaining trial, premedication with haloperidol 5 or 10 mg orally was no better than placebo in diminishing analgesic requirements or providing pain relief. However, a potent antiemetic effect of haloperidol was demonstrated (Judkins & Harmer 1982).

Chronic pain

In 26 papers describing 31 trials of neuroleptics alone administered for chronic pain (Table 50.3), the main indication for the use of neuroleptics in chronic pain is for patients with recognizable organic lesions which are not treatable by more conservative means. Because of their adverse effects, neuroleptics should only be given after transcutaneous electrical nerve stimulation; other benign local measures and regular nonnarcotic analgesics at fixed times have been tried. Neuroleptics may be strongly

Table 50.3 Disorders treated with neuroleptics

Disorder	Total trials	References
Acute pain		
Mixed	1	Montilla et al 1963
Herpes zoster	3	Sigwald et al 1959(2); Farber & Burks 1974
Postoperative	14	Jackson & Smith 1956(3); Lasagna & DeKornfeld 1961(3); Bronwell et al 1966; Stirman 1967; Taylor & Doku 1967; Fazio 1970; Minuck 1972(2); Judkins & Harmer 1982(2)
Migraine	1	Iserson 1983
Myocardial infarction	1	Davidson et al 1979
Chronic pain		
Arthritis	1	Breivik & Slørdahl 1984
Migraine	1	Polliack 1979
Mixed	6	Sadove et al 1955; Bloomfield et al 1964; Kast 1966; Cavenar & Maltbie 1976; Kocher 1976; Langohr et al 1982
Mixed neurological	1	Merskey & Hester 1972
Myofascial dysfunction	1	Raft et al 1979
Neoplastic	10	Beaver et al 1966(2); Maltbie & Cavenar 1977; Bourhis et al 1978; Schick et al 1979(2); Breivik & Rennemo 1982; Hanks et al 1983(2); Landa et al 1984
Neuralgia (Postherpetic)	5	Sigwald et al 1959(2); Nathan 1978(2); Duke 1983
Neuropathy (diabetic)	2	Davis et al 1977; Mitas et al 1983
Radiation fibrosis	1	Daw & Cohen-Cole 1981
Tension headache (chronic)	2	Hakkarainen 1977; Hackett et al 1987
Thalamic pain	1	Margolis & Gianascol 1956

indicated in the management of pain which wakes patients from sleep (e.g. cluster headache or persistent early-morning migraine). They are most commonly employed with a variety of neurological disorders which are notoriously resistant to other forms of intervention. They may be used for thalamic or similar central pain which does not respond to antidepressants, carbamazepine or clonazepam. They are often helpful in nerve lesions including causalgias, neuralgias, neuropathies, traumatic avulsion of the brachial plexus and some instances of back pain, particularly if there is clear evidence of associated damage to nerves or nerve roots. Often they are of value as an adjunct in the treatment of painful neoplasms, allowing decreased doses or discontinuation of narcotics in some patients (Parolin 1966; Cavenar & Maltbie 1976; Schick et al 1979; Breivik & Rennemo 1982).

Only five adequate controlled trials of neuroleptic therapy for chronic pain were found. Single doses of methotrimeprazine 15 mg were found to have analgesic properties equal to 8–15 mg of morphine in patients with mixed sources of chronic pain (Bloomfield et al 1964; Kast 1966) and in patients with chronic pain of neoplastic origin (Beaver et al 1966). Fluphenazine and flupenthixol each at 1 mg orally per day were both clinically and statistically superior to placebo in the treatment of chronic tension headache in trials of 2 months and 6 weeks respectively (Hakkarainen 1977; Hackett et al 1987). Preliminary reports of two placebo-controlled crossover trials of flupenthizol for severe cancer pain (Landa et al 1984) and for chronic osteoarthritic hip pain (Breivik & Slørdahl 1984) suggest that this neuroleptic may exhibit significant analgesic and antidepressant properties.

COMBINED THERAPHY

Antidepressant and anticonvulsant

A combination of TCAD and an anticonvulsant may be useful for neuralgias which are resistant to either drug alone. Three clinical trials were found describing the successful treatment of chronic postherpetic neuralgia with combinations of TCAD with carbamazepine or with diphenylhydantoin (Hatangdi et al 1976; Gerson et al 1977) or with valproic acid (Raferty 1979).

Antidepressant and neuroleptics

No evidence was found to support the use of TCAD–neuroleptic combined therapy for acute pain but such therapy was used for chronic pain in the 17 trials listed in Table 50.4. Combined therapy is usually indicated when either drug group alone is indicated but has not proven efficacious and adverse effects are not a contraindication. The best results seem to occur with arthritic pain, treatment-resistant headaches, neoplastic pain and a variety of neurological pain disorders such as causalgias, de-afferentation syndromes, neuralgias and neuropathies.

Only one adequately controlled trial of TCAD–neuroleptic was found. Nortriptyline and fluphenazine were found to be clearly superior to placebo in decreasing pain and paraesthesias in patients with diabetic polyneuropathy (Gomez–Perez et al 1985).

Table 50.4 Disorders treated with antidepressant and neuroleptics combination

Disorder	Total trials	References
Head pain of psychological origin	1	Sherwin 1979
Mixed	3	Kocher 1976(2); Duthie 1977
Mixed neurological	2	Merskey & Hester 1972; Langohr et al 1982
Neoplastic	3	Bernard & Scheuer 1972; Bourhis et al 1978; Breivik & Rennemo 1982
Neuralgia (postherpetic)	3	Taub 1973; Langohr et al 1982; Weis et al 1982
Neuropathy (diabetic)	5	Davis et al 1979; Gade 1980; Khurana 1983; Mitas et al 1983; Gomez-Perez et al 1985

Lithium

As already noted, lithium alone has been reported to be useful in episodic and chronic cluster headaches (Ekbom 1974, 1981; Kudrow 1977, 1978; Mathew 1978; Bussone et al 1979; Pearce 1980) and, when combined with amitriptyline, in the treatment of painful shoulder syndrome (Tyber 1974). Lithium alone or combined with TCAD or with neuroleptics may be useful for pain syndromes which are associated with bipolar affective disorders and some recurrent unipolar depressions. No controlled adequate trials of lithium therapy for acute or chronic pain were found.

ANTIANXIETY–SEDATIVE DRUGS

Anxiety

The benzodiazepines may be useful in the short-term (4 weeks or less) management of anxiety, muscle spasm and insomnia which are frequently associated with acute pain and which may occur during acute exacerbations of chronic pain disorders. Nondrug psychological management techniques for these pain-related problems should be tried first where time and resource availability permit.

Acute pain

There is suggestive evidence that short-term benzodiazepine use may diminish the acute pain associated with myocardial infarction (Wheatley 1979; Dixon et al 1980; Monks 1981), anxiety-related gastrointestinal disorders (Lasagna 1977) and acute and chronic intervertebral disc problems with skeletal muscle spasm (Greenblatt & Shader 1974; Lasagna 1977; Hollister et al 1981).

Chronic pain

In general, reservations must be expressed about the use of benzodiazepines for chronic pain. Benzodiazepines cause dependency and cognitive impairment, thus promoting the complaint of chronic pain (see section on adverse effects). Although it may be necessary to continue established use of benzodiazepines for certain patients, initiation of their use in chronic pain is seldom indicated.

In one uncontrolled study of chronic neoplastic pain, alprazolam was found to be very effective in relieving causalgic but not other types of pain (Fernandez et al 1987).

A small number of controlled studies have reported on the treatment of chronic pain with benzodiazepines. While some analgesic effect was observed in the treatment of pain of psychological origin (Okasha et al 1973) and chronic tension headache (Lance & Curran 1964), the results are definitely inferior to those obtained with the TCAD with which the benzodiazepine was being compared.

However, a benzodiazepine (diazepam) and a neuroleptic (flupenthixol) were equally superior to placebo in diminishing pain and analgesic use in persons with chronic tension headache in one adequately controlled study (Hackett et al 1987).

A benzodiazepine was without effect on pain of diabetic neuropathy, despite excellent response to two TCAD for which it was the control treatment (Turkington 1980).

Similarly, a TCAD was clearly superior to lorazepam and placebo, neither of which were effective for postherpetic neuralgia pain (Max et al 1988).

Clonazepam, a newer benzodiazepine with sedative and anticonvulsant properties, has shown some promise in the treatment of neuralgias (Swerdlow & Cundill 1981) and deserves further investigation in view of its relative freedom from adverse effects as compared with other anticonvulsants.

EFFECTIVENESS

ANTIDEPRESSANTS

Tricyclic antidepressants

Chronic pain

The outcome of the 119 TCAD trials for chronic pain listed in Table 50.1 may be summarized. Although none of these directly compared TCAD with nondrug therapies, nearly one-half of the trials reported failure of previous analgesic and/or nondrug therapy. Only four of the 119 trials failed to show clinically important analgesic effects of TCAD. In the first trial zimelidine failed to alleviate postherpetic neuralgia, whereas subsequent treatment with amitriptyline provided good or excellent relief in nine out of 15 of the same patients (Watson & Evans 1985). In the second trial, amitriptyline showed no analgesic effects in nondepressed patients with mixed chronic nonneoplastic pain. A rather high percentage of patients had compensation or litigation problems and there was a high drop-out rate (19%) for both amitriptyline and placebo groups (Pilowsky et al 1982). In the third trial, neither trazodone nor placebo had an effect on chronic back pain in patients with organic findings. However, the pain was of very long duration (average 20 years), patients with depressive disorders excluded; doses and plasma levels of trazodone were rather modest and litigation issues and narcotic use quite common (Goodkin et al 1990). In the last of the four trials, amitriptyline and subsequently phenelzine (a MAOI) were without analgesic effect despite a mild antidepressant action in a short (4 weeks each drug) uncontrolled study in a small (n=10) number of persons suffering from depression and chronic headache associated with minor closed head injury (Saran 1988).

In another three controlled trials, TCAD were compared with nonplacebo control drugs commonly used in the disorder under study. Amitriptyline and propranolol proved equally effective and clearly superior to placebo in decreasing the pain associated with high-frequency chronic migraine (Zeigler et al 1987). Low-dose amitriptyline was superior to naproxen and to placebo in alleviating pain and fatigue associated with fibromyalgia (Goldenberg et al 1986). Amitriptyline provided greater pain relief than carbamazepine and placebo and was better tolerated than carbamazepine in the treatment of persons with central post-stroke pain (Leijon & Boivie 1989).

The outcome of adequately controlled trials has been presented (see section on indications).

In 61 of the 78 trials giving details, ≥50% of patients obtained moderate to total pain relief. Analgesic use was significantly diminished in those studies giving this information. A variety of measures indicated acceptable patient compliance with TCAD regimens. In the vast majority of trials, drop-out rates were less than 10%, no different from the rates for comparison placebos. TCAD blood levels, where measured, were in the expected range for doses employed. When asked, patients and physicians preferred TCAD to placebo.

Unfortunately, the length of follow-up on TCAD was rather limited in the trials (80% ≤3 months). However, two recent papers have reported on longer-term treatment. One questionnaire follow-up study reported on 104 patients with chronic nonneoplastic pain who were treated with a variety of TCAD (Blumer & Heilbronn 1981). At 9–16 months, 57% were significantly improved but still on TCAD and 31% had dropped out. At 21–28 months, about one-quarter of the 104 patients were improved or free of pain and still on TCAD while an additional one-tenth were able to discontinue TCAD with sustained relief. It was noted that some patients only began to improve after months of TCAD therapy. The other study concerned 93 patients with chronic facial pain of psychological origin treated with dothiepin (Feinmann et al 1984). At 12 months, 73% were painfree; 38% of the painfree group were still obliged to take dothiepin to prevent relapse of pain. An additional 8% continued to take dothiepin with partial relief and 9% were lost to follow-up.

A number of clinical and laboratory factors may predict increased TCAD analgesic effect in chronic pain disorders. The presence of clinically important depression (Bradley 1963; Rafinesque 1963; Lascelles 1966; Radebold 1971; Gessel 1975; Loldrup et al 1989), a family history of depressive spectrum disorders (Magni et al 1987), an absence of previous analgesic use (Bourhis et al 1978; Kudrow 1980), dexamethasone nonsuppression (Smoller 1984) and increased MHPG levels in CSF associated with increased anxiety scores (Ward et al 1983) have all been noted to correlate with TCAD-induced pain relief.

Newer studies have reported conflicting evidence on the value of the dexamethasone suppression test (DST) results (Valdes et al 1989; Nappi et al 1990).

Head pain, except that from closed head injury, is more likely to be associated with good outcome than that with other body sites (Lodrup et al 1989; Ohghena & Van Houdenhove 1992). Blood levels of TCAD and their metabolites have been positively correlated with analgesic response in some studies (Johansson & Von Knorring 1979; Lindsay & Wyckoff 1981; Watson et al 1982; Hameroff et al 1984; Kvinesdal et al 1984; Zitman et al 1984; Montastruc et al 1985; Max et al 1987; Max et al 1988; Leijon & Boivie 1989) but not in others (Loldrup et al 1989; Kishore-Kumar et al 1990; Sindrup et al 1990a; Max et al 1991). Specific therapeutic blood levels for analgesic response to amitriptyline (Watson et al 1982; Max et al 1987), imipramine (Sindrup et al 1990b) and clomipramine (Montastruc et al 1985) have been suggested.

Poorer outcomes with TCAD for chronic pain have been reported with certain Minnesota Multiphasic Personality Inventory (MMPI) profiles (Pheasant et al 1983), DST nonsuppression (Nappi et al 1990), increased analgesic use (Nappi et al 1990), a family history of pain disorders (Valdes et al 1989) and increased levels of E-10-hydroxy nortriptyline, an inactive metabolite of amitriptyline (Edelbrock et al 1986).

Evidence for specific predictors which are clinically useful is still sparse and most of the work cited above requires replication.

Monoamine oxidase inhibitors

Chronic pain

A majority of patients experienced ≥50% pain relief in

those MAOI trials listed in Table 50.1. In most instances, depression and pain were alleviated at the same time. Substantial previous therapies had not been helpful for a majority of patients. Patient compliance was acceptable; drop-out rates were from 0–12%. The length of follow-up was 7 months and 12 months in the two studies with details. Decreased pretreatment plasma 5-hydroxytryptamine during an attack was correlated with successful treatment of migraine headaches using phenelzine (Anthony & Lance 1969).

The efficacy of MAOI for chronic pain remains unestablished in view of the small number of patient studies. Unfortunately, no trials are available to compare directly the analgesic effects of MAOI with other drug or nondrug forms of therapy, save the one adequate placebo-controlled trial already mentioned.

Neuroleptics

Acute pain

Of the 20 trials listed in Table 50.3, 19 reported clinically important analgesic effects of neuroleptics in patients with acute pain. In 15 of these trials, a single dose of methotrimeprazine was found to compare favourable with a narcotic control and/or to be superior to placebo in postoperative pain (see section on indications). In one other paper the authors found no significant difference in postoperative pain scores or narcotic use among patients premedicated with haloperidol 5 or 10 mg or placebo (Judkins & Harmer 1982). One additional single group outcome study reported 96% of patients experienced total relief from acute migraine attacks following a single intramuscular dose of chlorpromazine (Iserson 1983).

The remaining three trials were concerned with ongoing regimens of neuroleptic therapy for acute herpes zoster neuralgia. Treatment with chlorpromazine, chlorprothixene or methotrimeprazine (one trial each) produced total relief in 92–100% of patients within 1–5 days if the therapy was started within 3 months of the onset of the disorder (Sigwald et al 1959; Farber & Burks 1974). These trials were uncontrolled and did not detail previous failed therapies.

Chronic pain

Of the 31 trials listed in Table 50.3, 29 reported clinically important analgesic effects of neuroleptics given for chronic pain. In one retrospective study, haloperidol 5 and 10 mg did not decrease narcotic use in patients with neoplastic pain (Hanks et al 1983) but in an adequate, controlled trial, minor analgesic use was significantly more diminished with flupenthixol than with placebo in patients with chronic tension headache (Hackett et al 1987). Four of the 31 trials were single-dose experiments or therapy. Methotrimeprazine compared favourably with narcotic controls in mixed or neoplastic chronic pain in three trials (see section on indications). One uncontrolled trial reported 'success' in treating chronic recurrent headaches with one dose of trifluoperazine combined with a nonsteroidal antiinflammatory agent (Polliack 1979). In the remaining 27 trials, longer-term continuous neuroleptics regimens were used to manage various chronic pain disorders. In 16 of the 20 trials with relevant data, the majority of patients experienced moderate to total pain relief with neuroleptics.

Unfortunately, the majority of trials lasted less than 3 months. The importance of this limitation is demonstrated in the case of chronic postherpetic neuralgia, where two trials lasting more than 6 months reported almost total failure after initial impressive relief (Nathan 1978). On the other hand, in another trial, 75% of patients with this disorder maintained their initial painfree state for 10–20 months following inception of neuroleptic therapy (Duke 1983).

The duration of the disorder may be of importance. In herpes zoster neuralgia, if neuroleptic therapy was started within 3 months of onset, more than 90% of patients experienced total pain relief, whereas less than 20% of patients obtained good or total pain relief if the condition had been of longer duration (Sigwald et al 1959).

In addition to the controlled trials already mentioned (see section on indications), the evidence for neuroleptic-induced pain relief is supported by a series of anecdotal, single-patient experiments and uncontrolled group reports of patients with diabetic neuropathy, neoplastic pain, post-herpetic neuralgia and thalamic pain (Margolis & Gianascol 1956; Sigwald et al 1959; Cavenar & Maltbie 1976; Davis et al 1977; Maltbie & Cavenar 1977; Daw & Cohen-Cole 1981; Duke 1983). Patients with very chronic, stable baseline pain disorders, refractory to many interventions, responded rapidly (≤4 days), frequently had total pain relief and suffered relapse rapidly with placebo substitution or stopping the neuroleptic.

Treatment acceptability in all but one trial was good (≤10% drop-out). In the remaining study, a moderate-dose chlorprothixene (50–100 mg/day orally) regimen was associated with a 35% patient refusal to take the drug for more than 2 weeks despite significant analgesic effects.

In one other trial, the addition of haloperidol to relaxation training led to important pain relief in a group of patients with chronic myofascial dysfunction who were previously unresponsive to this and other forms of behaviour therapy (Raft et al 1979).

Combined therapy

TCAD and anticonvulsant

In three trials 72–89% of patients with chronic post

herpetic neuralgia experienced moderate to complete relief. Follow-up ranged from 1–18 months with a mean of 3 months. In two of the three trials drop-out rates were similar to those noted for TCAD alone, i.e. with nortriptyline plus diphenylhydantoin or carbamazepine, the rate was 12% (Hatangdi et al 1976) and with amitriptyline plus valproic acid 8% (Raferty 1979). In the third trial, patients were entered into a limited cross-over nonblind study in which a regimen of clomipramine plus carbamazepine was compared with transcutaneous nerve stimulation, with each being given for 8 weeks. The drop-out rate for the drug group was 50% while that for transcutaneous nerve stimulation was 70%. Clearly superior analgesic results were reported for the drug group (Gerson et al 1977).

TCAD and neuroleptic

All 16 of the 17 combined TCAD and neuroleptic trials for chronic pain listed in Table 50.4 reported good to total pain relief in the majority of patients. Follow-up was ≤3 months in five trials and 6–36 months in five further trials. The average drop-out rate in 13 trials with information was 12%. Most patients had received extensive previous therapy and those disorders treated tended to be resistant to other forms of therapy.

There is evidence to suggest that combined therapy may be more efficacious than TCAD or neuroleptic therapies alone for a significant group of patients. In three trials with flexible drug schedules, about one-third of patients responded to the combined regimen but not TCAD or neuroleptics alone (Davis et al 1977; Khurana 1983; Mitas et al 1983). One controlled trial, comparing clomipramine plus neuroleptic to neuroleptic therapy alone for mixed neurological chronic pain, found 67% compared with 47% good to total relief in the combined and neuroleptic groups respectively with the drop-out rate being lower in the combined therapy group (Langohr et al 1982).

Lithium

Most evidence for the use of lithium in the management of pain is derived from studies with cluster headache. Combining the results of six trials, about one-third of the 69 patients treated with lithium for episodic cluster headache experienced good to total control of pain during a 1-month treatment period (Mathew 1978; Ekbom 1981). In 10 trials of lithium given for chronic cluster headache, more than two-thirds of 118 patients obtained good to total pain relief for periods of up to 6 months or longer (Ekbom 1974, 1981; Kudrow 1977; Mathew 1978; Bussone et al 1979; Pearce 1980). Although no adequate controlled trials were found, the evidence that lithium helps to relieve chronic cluster headache is compelling, given the natural history of the disorder and its non-response to other treatments. Also, one open controlled trial reported lithium to be strikingly superior to methysergide and to prednisone in the treatment of this disorder (Kudrow 1978).

In one uncontrolled trial of lithium and amitriptyline for painful shoulder syndrome, 40% of patients experienced complete pain relief and increased range-of-motion of the joint, while 20% showed resolution of radiographic abnormalities (Tyber 1974).

Lithium therapy was well tolerated in all but one trial with drop-out rates being ≤3%.

ADVERSE EFFECTS

Extensive reviews of the adverse effects of psychotropic drugs are available elsewhere (Greenblatt & Shader 1974; Hollister 1978; Klein et al 1980; Baldessarini 1990). In this section, discussion is directed towards those problems more specifically encountered in treatment of patients with pain disorders.

ANTIDEPRESSANTS

Tricyclic-type antidepressants

Adverse effects with TCAD include anticholinergic autonomic effects, allergic and hypersensitivity reactions, cardiovascular and central nervous system problems, drug interactions, overdoses, drug withdrawal effects and weight gain. The safety of TCAD during pregnancy and lactation has not been established.

Anticholinergic autonomic effects are usually transient and irritating at worst (dry mouth, palpitations, decreased visual accommodation, constipation and oedema) but may occasionally be more serious (postural hypotension, loss of consciousness, aggravation of narrow-angle glaucoma, urinary retention and paralytic ileus). There is more risk in the elderly or those on other anticholinergic drugs (e.g. neuroleptics, antiparkinsonian drugs). Slowing initial administration, lowering TCAD doses, discontinuing other drugs or using a less anticholinergic drug (see Table 50.5) may be necessary. TCAD may cause sexual dysfunctions such as loss of libido, impotence and ejaculatory problems. Trazodone may cause priapism and permanent impotence.

Allergic/hypersensitivity reactions such as cholestatic jaundice, skin reactions and agranulocytosis are quite uncommon but require giving the patient adequate precautions. Zimelidine has been withdrawn from use because of hepatotoxicity and haemolytic anaemia associated with its use.

Anticholinergic and quinidine-like cardiac effects of tricyclic antidepressants are relative contraindications to their use in patients with preexisting conduction defects (Glassman & Bigger 1981). Of the tricyclic antidepressants with demonstrated analgesic properties, desipramine,

Table 50.5 Antidepressant drugs used in management of chronic pain

Drug	Oral dosage range (mg/day)	Anticholinergic potency	Orthostatic hypotension	Sedation
Tricyclic-type antidepressants				
Amitriptyline	10–300	High	Moderate	High
Clomipramine	20–300	Moderate	Moderate	Moderate
Desipramine	25–300	Low	Low	Low
Doxepin	30–300	Moderate	Moderate	High
Fluoxetine	5–40	Nil	Nil	Nil
Imipramine	20–300	High	High	Moderate
Maprotiline	50–300	Low	Low	High
Nortriptyline	50–150	Moderate	Low	Moderate
Paroxetine	40	Nil	Nil	Nil
Ritanserin	10	Nil	Nil	Nil
Trazodone	50–600	Low	Moderate	High
Trimipramine	50–300	Moderate	? Moderate	High
Monoamine oxidase inhibitors				
Phenelzine	30–90	Low	High	None
Tranylcypromine	10–40	Low	? Moderate	None

nortriptyline or low-dose doxepin may be the available drugs of choice with vulnerable patients (Monks 1981).

Orthostatic hypotension is common with TCAD which block adrenergic receptors (see Table 50.5) Imipramine is more hazardous for the elderly and others vulnerable to falls or hypotension. Those at risk require safer drugs and measurement of orthostatic change before and after an initial test dose. Possible interventions include patient education, use of a bedside commode and night light, surgical support stockings and in severe cases, 9-alpha-fluorhydrocortisone 0.025–0.05 mg orally twice a day.

Various central nervous system (CNS) adverse effects have been reported (sedation, tremor, seizures, insomnia, exacerbation of schizophrenia or mania and atropine-like delirium). The elderly are at particular risk, especially if there is previous brain damage or when combinations of drugs with anticholinergic properties are used.

TCAD potentiate CNS depressants (alcohol, anxiolytics, narcotics) potentiate other anticholinergics, antagonize certain antihypertensives (alpha methyldopa, guanethidine) and may produce lethal hypertensive episodes with MAOI.

Acute overdoses of TCAD in excess of 2000 mg can be fatal. Initial prescriptions of greater than 1 week's supply are unwise for the depressed patient.

Mild withdrawal reactions have been observed after abrupt cessation of imipramine 300 mg/day given for 2 months. Gradual termination of TCAD seems prudent.

Although the selective serotonin reuptake blockers such as paroxetine and fluoxetine require further study to demonstrate any analgesic properties in human chronic pain, they appear to have adverse effect profiles which may make them attractive in persons at risk of adverse effect from tricyclic antidepressants. They are free of anticholinergic, adrenergic and histaminergic receptor action and thus are relatively unlikely to produce anticholinergic autonomic, cardiac, orthostatic hypotension, sedation or weight gain problems. Overdosage with these drugs would appear to be less dangerous than those with tricyclic antidepressants.

On the other hand, their use may be associated with increased insomnia, diarrhoea, nausea, agitation, anxiety, headache and tremor. Akasthaesia, other extrapyramidal effects, anorgasmia and a serum sickness-like illness have been reported with fluoxetine. A central hyperserotonergic syndrome, including autonomic instability, hyperthermia, rigidity, myoclonus and delirium may occur when these drugs are prescribed with other serotonergic drugs like lithium and/or monoamine oxidase inhibitors (Sternbach 1991). Also, fluoxetine may increase serum concentration of tricyclic antidepressants and neuroleptics (Medical Letter on Drugs and Therapeutics 1990).

In considering TCAD trials listed in Table 50.1, severe adverse effects were rare. Delirium (8–13% of patients in papers with data) and drowsiness (3–28%) were the most common reasons for discontinuing therapy and were usually noted with high doses and drug combinations (TCAD with neuroleptics or with anticonvulsants), especially in the elderly. Delirium (2%) and dissociative reactions (5%) were noted with TCAD-lithium combined therapy (Tyber 1974). One case of myocardial infarction and one case of suicide occurred in trials of TCAD alone; both patients were suffering from advanced neoplastic conditions. One other death occurred in an 80-year-old male with preexisting 'severe cardiac decompensation' within 1 month of starting amitriptyline and valproic acid for postherpetic neuralgia (Raferty 1974).

Adverse effects and drop-out rates were correlated with higher plasma levels of TCAD and their metabolites in at least two studies (Gerson et al 1977; Kvinesdal et al 1984).

Although little is known about adverse effects of long-term TCAD administrations, one study reported on 46 depressed patients treated with doxepin for 2–10 years (Ayd 1979). No patients were noted to have any serious side-effects or any drug-caused impairment of intellectual, social or other functions.

Monoamine oxidase inhibitors

Although relatively free of anticholinergic side-effects, MAOI may cause urinary retention, orthostatic hypotension, severe parenchymal hepatotoxic reactions, central nervous system effects (insomnia, agitation, exacerbation of mania or schizophrenia), hypertensive crises and drug interactions.

Fortunately, serious adverse effects are rare if medications, foods and beverages with sympathomimetic activities are avoided (Hartshorn 1974; Tyrer 1976; Baldessarini 1990). In pain patients, narcotics, especially meperidine, should be avoided and anaesthetics used with great caution (Janowski & Janowski 1985). Hypertensive crises resulting from enhanced sympathomimetic action are best treated with immediate but slow intravenous injection of phentolamine 5 mg or, in an emergency, chlorpromazine 50–100 mg intramuscularly.

In those trials in which MAOI were used to treat pain disorders, phenelzine was discontinued because of jaundice in 4%, impotence in 4% and insomnia in 16% of patients in one study (Anthony & Lance 1969), while orthostatic hypotension was found in 6% and headache in 3% of patients in another (Lascelles 1966).

Long-term MAOI use in chronic pain is unreported, but efficacious and acceptably safe use has been described for up to several years in patients with anxiety disorders (Tyrer 1976).

A new class of compounds, the reversible inhibitors of MAO type A (RIMA), such as moclobemide, brofaromine and toloxatone appear to be effective antidepressants and are reported to be virtually free of the hepatotoxicity, hypertensive crises and orthostatic hypotension encountered with the older irreversible mixed MAO-A and MAO-B inhibitors reported on in this chapter (Da Prada et al 1990). Unfortunately, it is not known whether RIMA have any analgesic properties.

Neuroleptics

Neuroleptics may also cause anticholinergic effects, orthostatic hypotension, quinidine-like cardiac effects and sedation (see Table 50.6). These side-effects are more prominent with the low-potency phenothiazines and thiothixenes, particularly when they are combined with TCAD or carbamazepine.

CNS effects are a frequent source of patient noncompliance. Patients may note malaise, dysphoria (boring, 'unpleasant' or 'wretched' feelings) or even overt depression. Acute extrapyramidal syndromes (parkinsonism, akasthaesia and dystonia) usually occur early in treatment, especially with high-potency drugs (see Table 50.6).

Other neurological syndromes include neuroleptic malignant syndrome, perioral tremor (relatively benign and responsive to anticholinergic drugs) and tardive dyskinesia. Tardive dyskinesia may occur in up to 40% of those who have taken neuroleptics regularly over periods of 12 months or more. The likelihood of developing tardive dyskinesia seems to be proportional to the total quantity of neuroleptic taken over time but occasionally may occur even with low doses taken over several months (Monks 1980). It is more likely to occur in elderly females and in those with previous brain damage and may be more frequent in those who have also received antiparkinsonian drugs. Tardive dyskinesia is best managed by prevention (adequate indication for use, alterative regimen if possible), informed consent (patient and family adequately informed and vigilant regarding the emergence of tardive dyskinesia), regular examination for tardive dyskinesia by the

Table 50.6 Neuroleptic drugs used in the management of chronic pain

Drug	Oral dosage range (mg/day)	Anti cholinergic potency	Orthostatic hypotension	Sedative potency	Extra pyramidal effects
Phenothiazines					
Chlorpromazine	25–500	High	High	High	Low
Fluphenazine	1–10	Low	Low	Low	High
Methotrimeprazine	15–100	High	High	High	Moderate
Pericyazine	5–200	High	High	High	Low
Perphenazine	8–64	Moderate	Moderate	Moderate	Moderate
Thioridazine	10–200	High	High	High	Low
Trifluoperazine	3–20	Low	Low	Low	High
Thioxanthenes					
Chlorprothixene	50–200	High	High	High	Low
Flupenthixol	0.5–2	Low	? None	Absent	High
Miscellaneous					
Haloperidol	0.5–30	Low	Low	Moderate	High

physician at follow-up visits and the use of low-dose, short-term therapy with regular attempts to decrease or discontinue the neuroleptic should it no longer be necessary (American Psychiatric Association 1980). If neuroleptics are stopped at the first sign of tardive dyskinesia, the symptoms become worse but gradually fade over a period of 2 or 3 months in most cases. Once tardive dyskinesia has developed, the continued use of neuroleptics is inadvisable.

Other adverse effects of neuroleptics include weight gain, sexual dysfunction, endocrine disorders, exacerbation of epileptic disorders, photosensitivity, blood dyscrasias (agranulocytosis, leucopenia), cholestatic jaundice and ocular and skin pigmentation. The neuroleptics also increase the effects of central nervous system depressants and block the action of guanethidine.

In the trials of neuroleptics alone or in combination with TCAD, the commonest problems were somnolence and delirium with a higher incidence of these problems occuring with high-dose chlorprothixene or methotrimeprazine therapy. Myoclonus and tardive dyskinesia were both noted in a single patient in these predominantly short-term trials (Sigwald et al 1959).

Lithium

Reported hazards of lithium administration include intoxication and the development of renal, thyroid, cardiac, neuromuscular, neurotoxic, dermatological and birth abnormalities (Klein et al 1980; Bendz 1983; Baldessarini 1990). With careful monitoring of clinical symptoms and blood levels of the drug, short-term lithium use is reasonably safe. The issue of renal morphological changes (interstitial fibrosis and nephron atrophy) with longer-term use is still a cause of concern and preventive measures should include using the lowest dose of lithium for the least time possible and monitoring renal function (Amdisen & Grof 1980; Bendz 1983). Lithium-induced goitre and hypothyroidism usually respond to thyroid hormone.

In studies of lithium use for cluster headaches, the drug had to be discontinued because of lithium headaches (3%), severe nausea and vomiting (6%), lethargy and general weakness (6%) severe tremor (1%). The most common minor symptom was tremor, which was treatable by propranolol (Kudrow 1977; Mathew 1978; Pearce 1980). Long-term lithium use in pain patients has yet to be reported in detail.

Antianxiety sedative drugs

Although physical dependency and withdrawal may occur with prolonged (≥6 weeks) moderate to high dosage use of benzodiazepines, such problems are rarely encountered at therapeutic doses (Marks 1980; Medical Letter on Drugs and Therapeutics 1981).

Daytime sedation, impaired coordination and judgement and other forms of cognitive impairment have been reported to be common with prolonged steady use of these drugs for chronic pain (Hendler et al 1980; McNairy et al 1984). These adverse effects are more likely if the patient is elderly or brain-damaged, if longer-acting benzodiazepines are used or if other central-depressant drugs are drugs are given at the same time (Committee on the Review of Medicine 1980; Marks 1980; Medical Letter on Drugs and Therapeutics 1981). Other reported adverse effects include depression, suicidal thoughts, impulsivity and rebound insomnia.

Studies of patients treated in pain centres suggest that global and specific neuropsychological test impairments and electroencephalogram abnormalities occur more often in patients on benzodiazepines than in comparable controls (Hendler et al 1980; McNairy et al 1984). However, in the general population, 15% of all benzodiazepine users continue these drugs on a daily long-term basis. Most claim continued benefit without tolerance to the drugs developing. A similar result was reported in one study of long-term diazepam use (1 month–16 years) in a neurosurgical clinic for patients with chronic pain and muscle spasm (Hollister et al 1981). Despite daily use, an older population and concomitant use of other drugs, 77% of patients felt that diazepam benefited them. Only a small number (10 out of 108) reported any side-effects (usually oversedation). Side-effects could not be correlated with plasma levels of diazepam or nordiazepam and the values did not suggest abuse of the drug. Unfortunately, neuropsychological testing of these patients was not reported.

DESCRIPTION OF TREATMENT

GENERAL CONSIDERATIONS

Certain principles of psychotropic drug use are worth mentioning (Klein et al 1980):

1. There must be adequate indications for the use of these drugs. Moreover, this symptomatic management must not delay discovery of treatable causes of pain.
2. Every effort must be made to establish a working alliance with the patient and his or her support system (family, other health professionals). A clear explanation of indications, goals, methods, alternative management and risk of intervention and nonintervention is helpful in this regard.
3. Management should begin with the most benign efficacious intervention and a more hazardous regimen used only if treatment fails and informed consent is given (e.g. transcutaneous nerve stimulation → TCAD → TCAD and neuroleptic therapy). Figures 50.1 and 50.2 depict one possible protocol based on this approach.
4. The therapeutic trial must be at an adequate dose for a sufficient length of time.

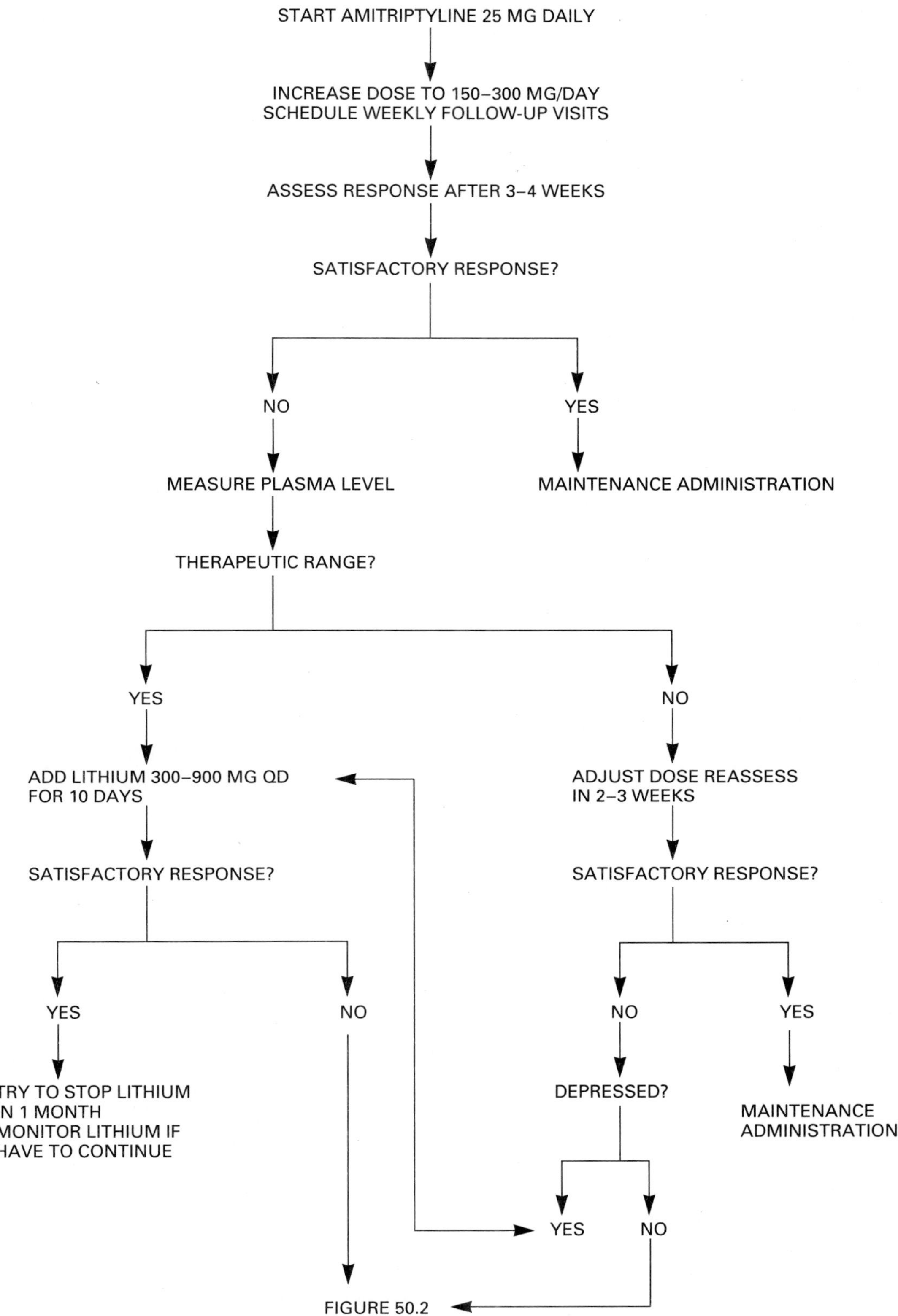

Fig. 50.1 Suggested sequence of psychotropic drug use in chronic pain disorders listed in Table 50.1. (Continued in Fig. 50.2.)

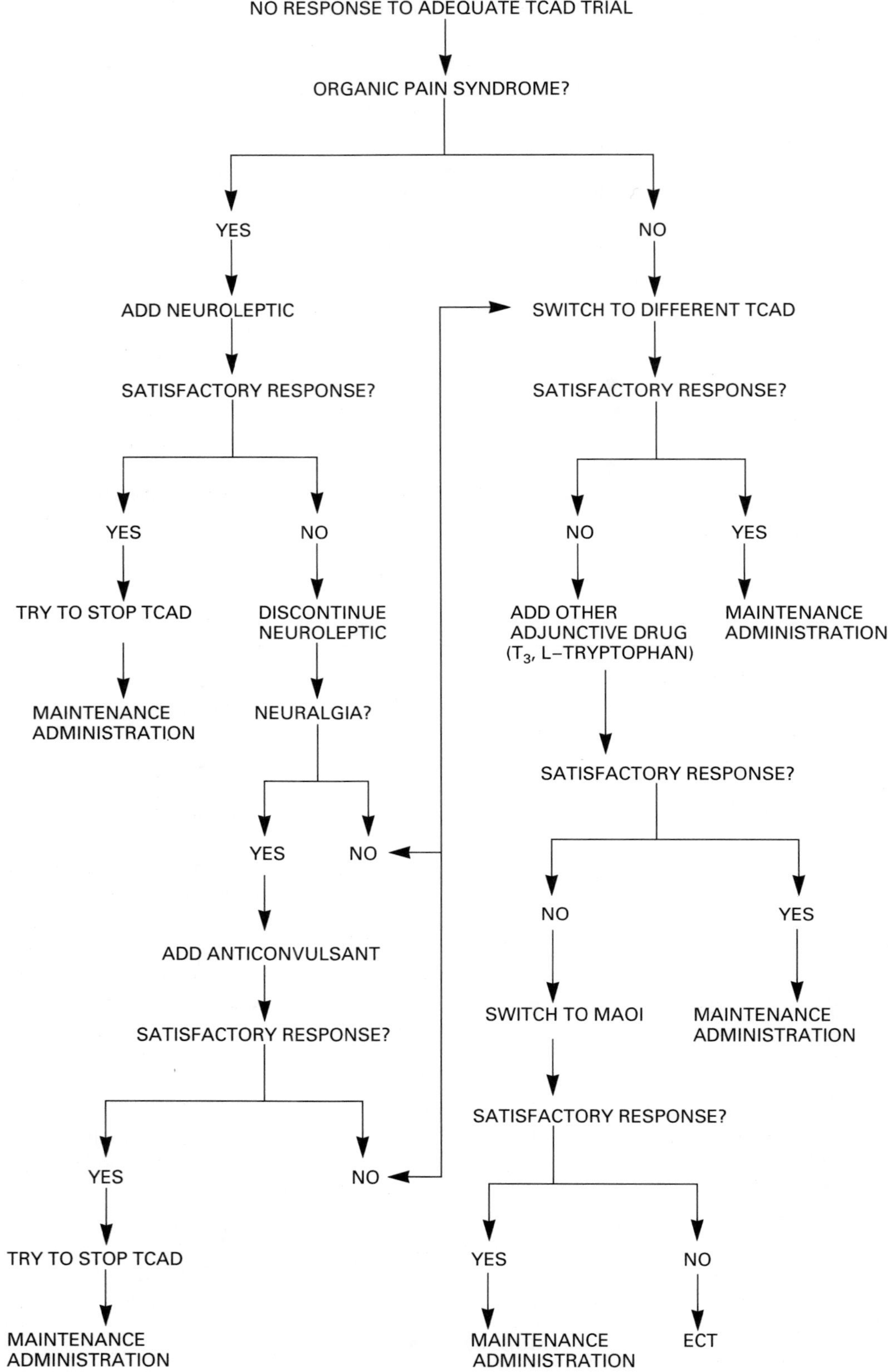

Fig. 50.2 Suggested sequence of psychotropic drug use in chronic pain disorders listed in Table 50.1. (Continued from Fig. 50.1.)

5. Other drugs should be reduced or eliminated, if at all feasible, as soon as possible. Detoxification from narcotics, alcohol, hypnotics and antianxiety drugs is often necessary to obtain a therapeutic response (Halpern 1982; Buckley et al 1986).

6. The physician must be available during the initiation of therapy and during changes in regimen.

7. Elderly patients usually require only one-third to one-half of the usual adult daily doses. Cumulative increases in psychotropics and their metabolics occur over a much longer period and maximum adverse effects may not be seen for weeks.

ANTIDEPRESSANTS

Tricyclic antidepressant

The generic names and approximate dosage ranges of some of the tricyclic-type antidepressants (bicyclic, tricyclic, tetracyclic and similar drugs) are indicated in Table 50.5. Figures 50.1 and 50.2 illustrate the approach to antidepressant use outlined below.

Precautions

Baseline blood studies (liver function, haemoglobin measurement and blood count) are performed. An electrocardiogram is obtained in all elderly patients and those with cardiovascular problems. Patients at risk from possible hypotension may have lying and sitting blood pressure determination before and 1–2 hours following an initial oral 10–50 mg test dose.

Choice of drugs

There is little evidence to support the use of one TCAD over any other. However, a past positive response of pain or depression in the patient or his blood relatives to a particular TCAD would favour its use. A history of therapeutic failure or adverse effects with a TCAD requires further information. These difficulties are usually due to inadequate trials, noncompliance or avoidable adverse effects. If the drug history is not helpful, patients with disorders listed in Table 50.2 should start one of the drugs proven effective in these adequately controlled trials. Evidence from studies directly comparing one TCAD with another provides slight support for the superiority of doxepin to amitriptyline in head pain of psychological origin (Okasha et al 1973), of clomipramine to amitriptyline in trigeminal neuralgia (Carasso 1979), of doxepin to desipramine in low back pain and depression (Ward et al 1984), of amitriptyline to desipramine or trazodone in rheumatoid arthritis (Frank et al 1988), of clomipramine to maprotyline in fibromyalgia (Bibolotti et al 1986) and in psychogenic pain (Eberhard et al 1988) and of clomipramine or imipramine to desipramine or paroxetine in diabetic neuropathy (Sindrup et al 1988, 1990b). As already discussed in the rationale section of this chapter, for most chronic pain disorders there appears to be an advantage to initiating therapy with a tricyclic antidepressant with mixed neurotransmitter properties (e.g. amitriptyline, imipramine, clomipramine or doxepin) unless the potential side-effects of these drugs dictate otherwise.

Drug side-effects may be exploited (e.g. by the use of a more sedating TCAD such as amitriptyline, doxepin or trimipramine for patients with marked sleep disturbance or high daytime arousal). For example, a single dose of 50–75 mg of one of these TCAD at bedtime is often used in substitution–detoxification programmes during the initial 1–2 months of treatment to obtain rapid symptomatic relief, prevent exacerbation of anxiety and depression and to facilitate optimal levels of function (Halpern 1982).

TCAD may be taken to minimize adverse effects. For example, there are fewer anticholinergic effects with desipramine, trazodone or fluoxetine as discussed in the section on adverse effects (see Table 50.5).

Initial administration

In dealing with chronic pain, schedules and doses of TCAD are best arranged to increase compliance and decrease adverse effects. Using amitriptyline or imipramine as examples, the patient is instructed to start with 25 mg orally 1–2 hours before bedtime. The dose is then increased to 25 mg each day, using a divided dosage schedule with the greater part taken in the evening. This is continued until a therapeutic response is obtained or a total daily dose of 150 mg/day is reached. If undue side-effects supervene, a lower dose should be employed than the one at which these effects appeared. If there is no response after 150 mg/day for 1 week and there are no medical contraindications or serious adverse effects, the dose may be increased by 25 mg/day to the maximum dose indicated in Table 50.5. If there is no therapeutic effect after a further 3 weeks, a TCAD blood level should be performed (see Fig. 50.1). If plasma levels are lower than usual antidepressant levels i.e. amitriptyline plus nortriptyline metabolite >120 ng/ml, imipramine >225 ng/ml or nortriptyline between 50 and 150 ng/ml (Perry et al 1987), check for noncompliance and attempt to achieve these plasma levels for at least 3–4 weeks. If there is no direct response in spite of adequate levels or if it is not possible to achieve these levels through discussion and regimen alterations to improve side-effects and compliance, either discontinue the drug by 25 mg/day decrements or move to one of the alternative strategies outlined for nonresponse below.

In the majority of reported clinical trials and in clinical practice, the therapeutic dose of TCAD like amitriptyline, even in the initial phase, is between 50 and 150 mg/day orally (average 75 mg). There is some evidence that head pain (migraine, psychogenic head and face pain and chronic tension headache) may respond at lower dose (25–75 mg/day) (Lance & Curran 1964; Diamond and Baltes 1971; Okasha et al 1973; Gessel 1975; Carasso 1979; Kudrow 1980; Sharav et al 1987).

Lower doses and slower rates of administration of the TCAD are necessary in patients over 60 years old (Nies et al 1977). Treatment is usually initiated at 20–30 mg/day and increased by 10 mg with total daily doses of 50–150 mg/day usually being adequate.

Initial parenteral TCAD administration for pain patients has been advocated by some authors (Fiorentino 1967; Gebhardt et al 1969; Adjan 1970; Desproges-Gotteron et al 1970; Radebold 1971; Bernard & Scheuer 1972; Monstastruc et al 1985). A typical regimen would be clomipramine 25–50 mg/day intravenously for 3–5 days in hospital, then switching to usual oral doses.

Maintenance administration

There are several clinical reports of TCAD pain therapy lasting more than 3 months (Kuipers 1962; Gade et al 1980; Blumer & Heilbronn 1981; Feinmann et al 1984; Urban et al 1986; Theesen & Marsh 1989; Valdes et al 1989). Despite the lack of detail in many of these reports, certain patients require maintenance TCAD for months to years, and in most instances the daily dose approximated the initial dose (20–75 mg). In usual clinical practice, especially with higher initial doses, some slow reduction to lower maintenance levels is possible 1 month after maximum therapeutic response has been obtained. After a further 3–6 months of remission, slow discontinuation of the drug may be tried as the patients are closely watched for relapse of pain and for depressive symptoms.

During maintenance therapy, a single daily evening dose of the more sedating TCAD may be used to improve compliance, decrease daytime adverse effects and provide hypnotic effect. Patients vulnerable to nocturnal disorientation or postural hypotensive episodes may require continued divided doses.

Nonresponse or relapse

Many instances of nonresponse are due to poor compliance or an inadequate regimen. Careful preparation of patients, close initial follow-up, simplified, typed drug schedules and the support of the family and of the primary physician are all important in increasing compliance.

In the case of nonresponse to an adequate trial of TCAD and where an alternative drug or nondrug therapy is unhelpful or unavailable, other strategies may be used:

1. *Lithium potentiation.* If depression and chronic pain are present, lithium carbonate 300–900 mg/day may be added to the TCAD (see Fig. 50.1). If an antidepressant response is not seen within 10 days lithium should be stopped and further alternatives considered (Fig. 50.2). If there is a satisfactory response, lithium may be discontinued after another month of therapy in a majority of persons (De Montigny et al 1981). Where there is an antidepressant but no analgesic response, additional therapy may be attempted (Fig. 50.2).

2. *Alternate TCAD.* In the obviously depressed patient, especially when depression is felt to be the primary disorder, a second therapeutic trial with a TCAD with different monoamine properties is initiated after tapering off the first TCAD over a period of 7–10 days. For example, if a more serotonergic drug was used first and failed, a drug with stronger noradrenergic effects (desipramine, imipramine, nortriptyline or maprotyline) would be substituted and a second adequate trial instituted. If adverse effects prevent the use of the less selective TCAD, a trial of a selective serotonin re-uptake inhibitor (fluoxetine, paroxetine) may be tried.

3. *TCAD–neuroleptic combination.* For the patient with milder or no depressive symptoms or where an organic pain generator is present, an alternative approach would be to add a neuroleptic to the first TCAD regimen instead of switching to a second TCAD (see Fig. 50.2 and Table 50.4). In order to decrease adverse effects (Table 50.6), oral doses of haloperidol 0.5–5 mg/day (Bernard & Scheuer 1972; Kocher 1976), fluphenazine 1–3 mg/day (Hatangdi et al 1983; Gomez-Perez et al 1985) or perphenazine 4–16 mg/day (Taub 1973; Duthie 1977; Weis et al 1982) are used. If one of these drugs is ineffective, if extrapyramidal adverse effects are a problem or if more sedation is required, a low-potency neuroleptic such as methotrimeprazine 15–100 mg/day, chlorpromazine 25–100 mg/day or pericyazine 5–100 mg/day may be used (Sigwald et al 1959; Merskey & Hester 1972).

The neuroleptic is started at the lowest dose listed above and stepped up by increments of this dose daily until a clear therapeutic effect or the maximum recommended dose is reached. If no therapeutic response is obvious by 2 weeks, the neuroleptic and then the TCAD are tapered off over 7–10 days each and discontinued. A different TCAD may then be tried (Fig. 50.2).

If the combination is effective, an attempt should be made to taper off the TCAD as the neuroleptic alone may be adequate. If both drugs are necessary, it is worth trying to taper off the neuroleptic after 3 months of stable response as it may no longer be necessary (Khurana 1983). Otherwise, maintenance administration guidelines are those described for each drug group used alone.

4. *TCAD–anticonvulsant combination.* Patients with neuralgias that are resistant to TCAD or a TCAD–neuroleptic combination may be aided by the addition of clonazepam 1.5–10 mg/day (Swerdlow & Cundhill 1981),

carbamazepine 150–1000 mg/day (Hatangdi et al 1976; Gerson et al 1977) or valproic acid 25–75 mg/day (Raferty 1979) to an adequate TCAD regimen. Because of frequent adverse effects, especially with TCAD–carbamazapine combinations, blood level monitoring of both drugs is advisable. Hospitalization of frail elderly patients during the initiation of therapy is advisable. If the combination is effective, attempt to taper off the TCAD after 3 months of stable response. Further maintenance administration guidelines are those for each drug group used alone. If there is no response, a different TCAD may be tried (Fig. 50.2).

5. *Other alternatives*. The addition of an adjunctive drug, such as triiodothyronine (25–50 μg/day) to an adequate TCAD regimen may produce an antidepressant response in a minority of depressives not responding to TCAD alone (Goodwin et al 1982). L-tryptophan (2–4 g/day) may have some analgesic properties when used alone or with TCAD but further studies are needed (France & Krishnan 1986).

For a patient with pain of psychological origin, especially in the presence of depressive symptoms, a trial with MAOI would be warranted following failed treatment with adequate trials of two different TCADs. Also, atypical depressive symptoms such as hypersomnia, increased appetite and weight, panics, phobias and depersonalization may respond preferentially to MAOI (Liebowitz et al 1988). A wash-out period of 2 weeks between TCAD and MAOI trials is essential.

Finally, electroconvulsive therapy has been used successfully in a small number of drug-refractory pain patients with or without TCAD therapy (Lascelles 1966; Mandel 1975). It is likely this treatment is not indicated unless warranted by the clinical depression alone.

Monamine oxidase inhibitors

The characteristics of the irreversible mixed type MAO-A and MAO-B inhibitors, phenelzine and tranylcypromine, are listed in Table 50.5. The newer RIMA drugs are not described here as their analgesic properties are unknown.

Precautions

Because of potential adverse reactions and a narrower spectrum of antidepressant action, MAOI are usually reserved for TCAD-resistant chronic pain disorders. The MAOI should only be used with patients capable of following stringent restrictions of foods, beverages and other medications and not suffering from a variety of medical ailments (see section on adverse effects: Hartshorn 1974; Baldessarini 1977, 1990). The patient should be given a list of potentially dangerous items and a card to carry which details the drug and specific countermeasures for medical emergencies.

Initial administration

Phenelzine is started at 15 mg/day orally and an additional 15 mg/day is added each day to a total dose of 45 mg/day. Because insomnia is a common side-effect, the drug is given in two divided doses in the morning. If there is no response within 1 week, the total daily dose is increased by 15 mg every 3 days to a total of 60–90 mg. If no response occurs within a further 2 weeks, the total daily dose is diminished by 15 mg each day until discontinued.

Maintenance administration

Despite the absence of published data concerning MAOI and chronic pain, clinical experience suggests that the initial therapeutic and maintenance doses are of the same magnitude.

Nonresponse or relapse

Measures of platelet MAOI may be used to determine adequate dosage and patient compliance (Baldessarini 1990). Although only anecdotal evidence exists, it is possible that the compliance and therapeutic outcome may be enhanced by the addition of minor tranquillizers or small-dose neuroleptics to the MAOI (Bradley 1963; Lascelles 1966).

L-Tryptophan 0.5–1.0 g three times a day may be added to phenelzine in order to obtain improvement in patients with depression who have not responded sufficiently to the MAOI. There is evidence that this combination has a very potent antidepressant effect (Coppen 1972). Once improvement appears, some side-effects such as sluggish behaviour, slurred speech and ataxia may also develop. These are easily dealt with by reduction of the dose of each drug (usually by about one-third). This combination does not seem to be particularly analgesic.

NEUROLEPTICS

Dosages for neuroleptics used in the treatment of chronic pain are listed in Table 50.6.

Precautions

As indicated, neuroleptics are best employed for pain associated with organic lesions. In general, antidepressants should be considered before neuroleptics since, for the most part, they are better tolerated by patients and are much less prone to be associated with long-term complications such as tardive dyskinesia. Baseline laboratory tests are identical to those for TCAD. A written informed consent is advisable, especially regarding the risk of tardive dyskinesia.

Initial administration

The physician should familiarize himself with one or two of the neuroleptics and use them preferentially. There is no convincing evidence that one neuroleptic is more effective than another.

Among the low-potency neuroleptics, methotrimeprazine is a reasonable choice. This drug is started at 5–10 mg about 2–3 hours before bedtime. This often enables a reduction to be made in the use of other night sedatives. If the medication is taken too near bedtime, the hypnotic effect will not occur for several hours and there may be morning drowsiness. If proven acceptable in the evening, enabling good sleep without waking from pain, the use of the medication may be extended to daytime with 2.5 mg taken three times a day. In general, it is not advisable to exceed 75–100 mg/day of methotrimeprazine. Most depressive adverse effects seem to occur above the 50 mg daily level. The same pattern of use may be applied with any of the other sedative phenothiazines, such as chlorpromazine or pericyazine, varying the dose with the potency of the individual medication.

High-potency neuroleptics are utilized for patients at risk from autonomic, anticholinergic or sedative adverse effects, especially those on TCAD–neuroleptic combinations. Neuroleptics such as haloperidol or fluphenazine are started with a 1 mg oral test dose (0.25–0.5 in elderly) and, if tolerated, increased by 1 mg/day to the usual effective dose of 3–5 mg/day (0.5–2 mg/day in the elderly). If there is no response after 1 week, the drug is further increased by 1 mg/day, as tolerated, to effective or maximum dosage.

With either high- or low-potency neuroleptics, a therapeutic response should be seen within 2 weeks of maximum tolerable dosage; if not, the drug is tapered off and discontinued.

Maintenance administration

It is important to emphasize that the dose of any psychotropic drug must be tailored to the individual's response and his or her needs. As with TCAD – neuroleptic combinations, intermittent (3-monthly) attempts should be made to lower and discontinue the neuroleptic in view of the risk of tardive dyskinesia.

A careful clinical examination and chart notation regarding involuntary movements should be made at each follow–up visit.

LITHIUM CARBONATE

Lithium salts are given orally, usually in the form of lithium carbonate.

Precautions

Lithium use for pain is contraindicated in the presence of certain medical conditions (renal tubular disease, myocardial infarction, myasthenia gravis and cardiac conduction defects) and in early pregnancy (Klein et al 1980). Patients must cooperate with regular blood tests and be capable of recognizing early signs of intoxication. Baseline investigations include serum creatinine and electrolytes, thyroid tests, haemogram, pregnancy test, urinalysis, 24-hour urine volume and creatinine clearance. Close monitoring of lithium blood levels is necessary for patients who are also taking drugs that may increase lithium levels, such as diuretics, carbamazepine and various nonsteroidal antiinflammatory agents.

Initial administration

In studies reporting on the treatment of cluster headaches, lithium carbonate 300 mg was given orally on the first day and increased to 300 mg two or three times per day by the end of the first week (Ekbom 1974; Kudrow 1977; Mathew 1978). The dosage was adjusted according to clinical response, severity of side-effects and in order to keep weekly serum lithium levels between 0.5 and 1.2 mmol/l.

Maintenance therapy

Little data are available for episodic cluster headache beyond 2 weeks' administration (Mathew 1978). In the chronic cluster group, maintenance periods of 16–32 weeks are reported with continuing improvement despite lowered lithium dosages and mean serum levels (0.3–0.4 mmol/l; Kudrow 1977; Mathew 1978). In another report even lower lithium levels were possible (0.3–0.4 mmol/l; Pearce 1980).

Once maintenance dosage is achieved, lithium determinations may be performed less frequently (monthly, then 3-monthly). Serum creatinine and thyroid-stimulating hormone levels are repeated 6-monthly. Creatinine clearance and 24-hour urine volume are repeated each year. Other tests are undertaken if clinically indicated. After a 3–6 month symptom-free interval, lithium dosage may be tapered off and, and if possible, discontinued.

Nonresponse or relapse

Most treatment failures were due to intolerable adverse effects despite serum lithium levels less than 1.2 mmol/l. Some patients were able to continue with lower doses of lithium (Kudrow 1977) and others with incapacitating tremor were helped by propranolol (Mathew 1978).

Table 50.7 Benzodiazepines used in the management of pain

Drug	Oral dosage range (mg/day)	Main indications
Alprazolam	0.75–8.0	Panics, anxiety-depression
Chlordiazepoxide	10–100	Generalized anticipatory anxiety
Clonazepam	1.5–10	Panics, seizures, neuralgias
Clorazepate	7.5–60	Generalized anticipatory anxiety
Diazepam	4–40	Generalized anticipatory anxiety, muscle spasm
Lorazepam	1–6	Generalized anticipatory anxiety
Oxazepam	30–120	Generalized anticipatory anxiety

ANTIANXIETY – SEDATIVE DRUGS

Benzodiazepine preparations used in the management of anxiety and pain are listed in Table 50.7.

Precautions

Patients should be educated to expect only short-term benzodiazepine use. Alternative therapies for anxiety and muscle tension, such as behavioral–cognitive techniques, should be started as soon as possible. Benzodiazepines should not be used for those subjects who are dependent on alcohol or other drugs. Baseline tests are only performed if clinically indicated, except for clonazepam, where a complete haemogram should be done.

Initial administration

Benzodiazepine choice, dose and administration schedules are those used in the treatment of anxiety and are well described elsewhere (Lasagna 1977; Hollister et al 1981; Monks 1981; Greenblatt et al 1983; Baldessarini 1986). Doses of benzodiazepines in excess of diazepam 10–15 mg/day orally or its equivalent are seldom indicated.

After 3–4 weeks of therapy, benzodiazepines are tapered off and withdrawn over 1–2 weeks. A longer period of withdrawal may be necessary for alprazolam, i.e. decrease by 0.125–0.25 mg each 4–7 days. Further brief, intermittent courses of benzodiazepines may be used for exacerbations of the pain disorder.

CONCLUSIONS

Additional adequate clinical trials are required to establish psychotropic efficacy in most pain disorders. There is a particular need for psychotropic regimens to be compared or combined with other somatic therapies (TENS, nerve blocks) and various nondrug interventions. One relevant study in persons with psychogenic pain disorder found that the combination of amitriptyline and psychotherapy was superior to either treatment alone (Pilowsky & Barrow 1990).

Antidepressants are indicated in most pain patients with clinically detectable depression. They may be useful in relieving pain-related problems such as anxiety, panics and insomnia. They may help in the early stages of detoxification from narcotics and antianxiety–sedative drugs. They probably have an analgesic effect in specific chronic pain states such as chronic osteo- and rheumatoid arthritis, diabetic neuropathy, migraine, head and face pain of psychological origin, postherpetic neuralgia and chronic tension headaches.

Neuroleptics are the treatment of choice for delusional pain. They may be efficacious alone or in combination with TCAD for some types of chronic pain which are often resistant to other forms of therapy, i.e. arthritic pain, causalgias, neuralgias, neuropathies, phantom pain and thalamic pain.

Lithium carbonate is effective in relieving chronic cluster headache and may prevent episodic cluster headache.

The benzodiazepines may be useful in short-term management of acute or chronic pain which is closely related to anxiety. Continuous benzodiazepine use for chronic pain is not recommended.

In general, with reasonable precautions, psychotropic regimens are well tolerated and acceptably free from important adverse effects.

Acknowledgements

The author wishes to express his gratitude to Ms Andrée Curtis for her patience and skill, and to Dr H. Merskey for his contributions to earlier editions of this chapter and for his continued support.

REFERENCES

Adjan M 1970 Uber therapeutischen Beeinflussung des Schmerzsumptoms bei unheilbaren Tumorkranken. Therapie der Gegenwart 10: 1620–1627

Alcoff J, Jones E, Rust P, Newman R 1982 Controlled trial of imipramine for chronic low back pain. Journal of Family Practice 14: 841–846

Amdisen A, Grof P 1980 Lithium and the kidneys. International Drug Therapy News 15: 3–4

American Psychiatric Association 1980 Task force on late neurological effects of antipsychotic drugs. Tardive dyskinesia. American Journal of Psychiatry 137: 1163–1172

Andersen E, Dafny N 1983 An ascending serotonergic pain modulation pathway from the dorsal raphe nucleus to the parafascicularis nucleus of the thalamus. Brain Research 269: 57–67

Anthony M, Lance J W 1969 Monoamine oxidase inhibitors in the treatment of migraine. Archives of Neurology 21: 263–268

Atkinson J H, Kremer E F, Risch S C, Jankowsky D S 1986 Basal and post-dexamethasone cortisol and prolactin concentrations in depressed and non-depressed patients with chronic pain syndromes. Pain 25: 23–24

Ayd F J 1979 Continuation and maintenance doxepin therapy: 10 years' experience. International Drug Therapy News 14: 9–16

Baldessarini R J 1977 Chemotherapy in psychiatry. Harvard University Press, Cambridge, Massachusetts, p 101–121

Baldessarini R J 1990 Drugs and the treatment of psychiatric disorders In: Goodman Gilman A, Rall T T W, Nies A S, Taylor P (eds) The pharmacological basis of therapeutics, vol 8. Pergamon Press, New York, p 383–435

Barber A, Harting S, Wolf H P 1989 Antinociceptive effects of the $5HT_2$ antagonist ritanserin in rats: evidence for an activation of descending monoaminergic pathways in the spinal cord. Neuroscience Letters 99: 234–238

Basbaum A I, Fields H L 1978 Endogenous pain control mechanisms: review and hypothesis. Annals of Neurology 4: 451–462

Beaver W T, Wallenstein S L, Houde R W et al 1966 A comparison of the analgesic effect of methotrimeprazine and morphine in patients with cancer. Clinical Pharmacology and Therapeutics 7: 436–446

Bendz H 1983 Kidney function in lithium-treated patients. A literature survey. Acta Psychiatrica Scandinavica 68: 303–324

Bernard A, Scheuer H 1972 Action de la clomipramine (Anafranil) sur la douleur des cancers en pathologie cervico-faciale. Journal Français d'Oto-rhino-laryngologie 21: 723–728

Bibolotti E, Borghi C, Pasculli E et al 1986 The management of fibrositis: a double blind comparison of maprotyline (Ludiomil®, chlorimipramine and placebo. Clinical Trials Journal 23: 269–280

Biegon A, Samuel D 1980 Interaction of tricyclic antidepressants with opiate receptors. Biochemical Pharmacology 29: 460–462

Bloomfield S, Simard-Savoie S, Bernier J, Tétreault L 1964 Comparative analgesic activity of levomepromazine and morphine in patients with chronic pain. Canadian Medical Association Journal 90: 1156–1159

Blumer D, Heilbronn M 1981 Second-year follow-up study on systematic treatment of chronic pain with antidepressants. Henry Ford Hospital Medical Journal 29: 67–68

Blumer D, Heilbronn M 1982 Chronic pain as a variant of depressive disease. The pain-prone disorder. Journal of Nervous and Mental Disease 170: 381–394

Blumer D, Zorick F, Heilbronn M, Roth T 1982 Biological markers for depression in chronic pain. Journal of Nervous and Mental Disease 170: 425–428

Bodnar R J, Kelly D D, Thomas L W, Mansour A, Brutas M, Glusman M 1980 Chlordiazepoxide antinociception: cross tolerance with opiates and stress. Psychopharmacology 69: 107–110

Bonica J J 1977 Basic principles in managing chronic pain. Archives of Surgery 112: 783–788

Botney M, Fields H L 1983 Amitriptyline potentiates morphine analgesia in a direct action on the central nervous system. Annals of Neurology 13: 160–164

Bourhis A, Boudouresque G, Pellet W, Fondarai J, Ponzio J, Spitalier J M 1978 Pain infirmity and psychotropic drugs in oncology. Pain 5: 263–274

Bradley J J 1963 Severe localized pain associated with the depressive syndrome. British Journal of Psychiatry 109: 741–745

Breivik H, Rennemo F 1982 Clinical evaluation of combined treatment with methadone and psychotropic drugs in cancer patients. Acta Anaesthetica Scandinavica 74: 135–140

Breivik H, Slørdahl J 1984 Beneficial effects of flupenthixol for osteoarthritic pain of the hip: a double blind cross-over comparison with placebo. Pain 2 (suppl): 5254

Bronwell A W, Rutledge R, Dalton M L 1966 Analgesic effect of methotrimeprazine and morphine. Archives of Internal Medicine 111: 725–728

Buckley F P, Sizemore W A, Charlton J E 1986 Medication management in patients with chronic non-malignant pain: a review of the use of a drug withdrawal protocol. Pain 26: 153–165

Bunney W E, Garland M A 1984 Lithium and its possible modes of action. In: Post R M, Ballenger J C (eds) Neurobiology of mood disorders. Williams & Wilkins, London, p 731–743

Bussone G, Boiardi A, Merati B, Crenna P, Picco A 1979 Chronic cluster headache: response to lithium treatment. Journal of Neurology 221: 181–185

Butler S 1984 Present status of tricyclic antidepressants in chronic pain therapy. In: Benedetti C, Chapman C R, Moricca G (eds) Advances in pain research and therapy , vol 7. Raven Press, New York, p 173–197

Butler S H, Weil-Fugazza J, Godefroy F, Besson J M 1985 Reduction of arthritis and pain behavior following chronic administration of amitriptyline or imipramine in rats with adjuvant-induced arthritis. Pain 23: 159–175

Carasso R L 1979 Clomipramine and amitriptyline in the treatment of severe pain. International Journal of Neuroscience 9: 191–194

Carette S, McCain G A, Bell D A, Fam A G 1986 Evaluation of amitriptyline in primary fibrositis: a double blind, placebo controlled trial. Arthritis and Rheumatism 29: 655–659

Caruso I, Sarzi Puttini P C, Boccassini L et al 1987 Double blind study of dothiepin versus placebo in the treatment of primary fibromyalgia syndrome. Journal of International Medical Research 15: 154–159

Castaigne P, Laplane D, Morales R 1979 Traitement par la clomipramine des douleurs des neuropathies périphériques. Nouvelle Presse Médicale 8: 843–845

Cavenar J O, Maltbie A A 1976 Another indication for haloperidol. Psychosomatics 17: 128–130

Committee on the Review of Medicine 1980 Systematic review of the benzodiazepines. Guidelines for data sheets on diazepam, chlordiazepoxide, medazepam, clorazepate, lorazepam, oxazepam, temazepam, trazolam, nitrazepam and flurazepam. British Medical Journal 280: 910–912

Contreras E, Tamayo L, Quijada L 1977 Effects of tricyclic compounds and other drugs having a membrane stabilising action on analgesia, tolerance to and dependence on morphine. Archives of Internal Psychodynamics 228: 293–299

Coppen A 1972 Indoleamines and affective disorders. Journal of Psychiatric Research 9: 163–171

Couch J R, Hassanein R S 1976 Migraine and depression: effect of amitriptyline prophylaxis. Transactions of the American Neurological Association 101: 1–4

Couch J R, Ziegler D K, Hassanein R 1976 Amitriptyline in the prophylaxis of migraine. Effectiveness and relationship of antimigraine and anti-depressant effects. Neurology 26: 121–127

Courvoisier S, Ducrot R, Fournel J, Julou L 1957 Propriétés pharmacodynamiques générales de la levomepromazine. Comptes Rendus des Séances de la Société de Biologie et de ses Filiales 151: 1378

Creese I, Feinberg A P, Snyder S H 1976 Butyrophenone influences on the opiate receptor. European Journal of Pharmacology 36: 231–235

Da Prada M, Kettler R, Burkard W P, Lorez H P, Haefely W 1990 Some basic aspects of reversible inhibitors of monoamine oxidase-A. Acta Psychiatrica Scandinavia (suppl 360): 7–12

Davidoff G, Guarracini M, Roth E, Sliwa J, Yarkony G 1987 Trazodone hydrochloride in the treatment of dysesthetic pain in traumatic myelopathy: a randomized double-blind placebo controlled study. Pain 29: 151–161

Davidson O, Lindeneg O, Walsh M 1979 Analgesic treatment with levomepromazine in acute myocardial infarction. Acta Medica Scandinavica 205: 191–194

Davis J L, Lewis S B, Gerich J E, Kaplan R A, Schultz T A, Wallin J D 1977 Peripheral diabetic neuropathy treated with amitriptyline and fluphenazine. Journal of the American Medical Association 238: 2291–2292

Daw J L, Cohen-Cole S A 1981 Haloperidol analgesia. Southern Medical Journal 74: 364–365

De Montigny C, Grunberg F, Mayer A, Deschenes J P 1981 Lithium induces rapid relief of depression in tricyclic antidepressant drug non-responders. British Journal of Psychiatry 138: 252–256

Desproges-Gotteron R, Abramon J Y, Borderie J, Lathelize H 1970 Possibilités thérapeutiques actuelles dans les lombalgies d'origine névrotique. Rheumatologie 22: 45–48

Diamond S, Baltes B J 1971 Chronic tension headache–treatment with amitriptyline–double blind study. Headache 11: 110–116

Dixon R A, Edwards R I, Pilcher J 1980 Diazepam in immediate post myocardial infarct period. A double blind trial. British Heart Journal 43: 535–540

Dubner R, Bennett G J 1983 Spinal and trigeminal mechanisms of nociception. Annual Review of Neuroscience 6: 381–418

Duke E E 1983 Clinical experience with pimozide: emphasis on its use in post herpetic neuralgia. Journal of the American Academy of Dermatology 8: 845–850

Dundee J W, Love W J, Moore J 1963 Alterations in response to somatic pain associated with anaesthesia. XV. Further studies with phenothiazine derivatives and similar drugs. British Journal of Anaesthesia 35: 597–609

Duthie A M 1977 The use of phenothiazines and tricyclic antidepressants in the treatment of intractable pain. South African Medical Journal 51: 246–247

Eberhard G, Von Knorring L, Nilsson H L et al 1988 A double-blind randomized study of clomipramine versus maprotyline in patients with idiopathic pain syndromes. Neuropsychobiology 19: 25–34

Ekbom K 1974 Lithium vid kroniska symptom av cluster headache. Preliminart Meddelande Opuscula Medica (Stockholm) 19: 148–158

Ekbom K 1981 Lithium for cluster headache: review of the literature and preliminary results of long-term treatment. Headache 21: 132–139

Eschalier A, Montastruc J L, Devoice J L, Rigal F, Gaillard-Plaza G, Pechadre J C 1981 Influence of naloxone and methylsergide on the analgesic effect of clomipramine in rats. European Journal of Pharmacology 74: 1–7

Evans W, Gensler F, Blackwell B, Galbrecht C 1973 The effects of anti-depressant drugs on pain relief and mood in the chronically ill. Psychosomatics 14: 214–219

Farber G A, Burks J W 1974 Chlorprothixene therapy for herpes zoster neuralgia. Southern Medical Journal 67: 808–812

Fazio A N 1970 Control of postoperative pain: a comparison of the efficacy and safety of pentazocine, methotrimeprazine, meperidine and placebo. Current Therapeutic Research and Clinical Experimentation 12: 73–77

Feighner J P, Aden G C, Fabre L F, Rickels K, Smith W T 1983 Comparison of alprazolam, imipramine, and placebo in the treatment of depression. Journal of the American Medical Association 249: 3057–3064

Feinmann C, Harris M, Cawley R 1984 Psychogenic facial pain: presentation and treatment. British Medical Journal 288: 436–438

Fernandez F, Frank A, Holmes V F 1987 Analgesic effect of alprazolam in patients with chronic organic pain of malignant origin. Journal of Clinical Psychopharmacology 7: 167–169

Fiorentino M 1967 Sperimentazione controllata dell'imipramina come analgesico maggiore in oncologia. Rivista Medica Trentina 5: 387–396

Fogelholm R, Murros K, 1985 Maprotyline in chronic tension headaches: a double blind crossover study. Headache 25: 273–275

France R M, Krishnan K R R 1988 Psychotropic drugs in chronic pain. In: France R D, Krishnan K R R (eds) Chronic pain. American Psychiatric Press, Washington DC, p 343–346

France R D, Urban B J 1991 Cerebrospinal fluid concentrations of beta-endorphin in chronic low back pain patients. Influence of depression and treatment. Psychosomatics 32: 72–77

France R D, Krishnan K R R, Trainor M 1986 Chronic pain and depression. III. Family history studies of depression and alcoholism in chronic low back pain patients. Pain 24: 185–190

Frank R G, Kashani J H, Parker J C et al 1988 Antidepressant analgesia in rheumatoid arthritis. Journal of Rheumatology 15: 1632–1638

Fuentes J A, Garzon J, Del Rio J 1977 Potentiation of morphine analgesia in mice after inhibition of brain type B monoamine oxidase. Neuropharmacology 16: 857–862

Fuxe K, Ogren S O, Agnati L F et al 1983 Chronic antidepressant treatment and central 5-HT synapses. Neuropharmacology 22: 389–400

Gade G N, Hofeldt F D, Treece G L 1980 Diabetic neuropathic cachexia. Journal of the American Medical Association 243: 1160–1161

Ganvir P, Beaumont G, Seldrup J 1980 A comparative trial of clomipramine and placebo as adjunctive therapy in arthralgia. Journal of International Medical Research 8 (suppl 3): 60–66

Gebhardt K H, Beller J, Nischik R 1969 Behandlung des Karzinomschmerzes mit Chlorimipramin (Anafranil). Medizinische Klinik 64: 751–756

Gerson G R, Jones R B, Luscombe D K 1977 Studies on the concomitant use of carbamazepine and clomipramine for the relief of post-herpetic neuralgia. Postgraduate Medical Journal 53 (suppl 4): 104–109

Gessel A H 1975 Electromyographic biofeedback and tricyclic anti-depressant in myofascial pain–dysfunction syndrome: Psychological predictors of outcome. Journal of the American Dental Association 91: 1048–1052

Gingras M 1976 A clinical trial of Tofranil in rheumatic pain in general practice. Journal of International Medical Research 4 (suppl 2): 41–49

Glassman A H, Bigger J T 1981 Cardiovascular effects of therapeutic doses of tricyclic antidepressants. Archives of General Psychiatry 36: 815–819

Godefroy F, Butler S H, Weil-Fugazza J, Besson J M 1986 Do acute or chronic tricyclic antidepressants modify morphine antinociception in arthritic rats? Pain 25: 233–244

Gold M S, Byck R 1978 Endorphins, lithium and naloxone: their relationship to pathological and drug induced manic euphoric states. In: Petersen R C (ed) The international challenge of drug abuse. National Institute on Drug Abuse, Rockville, p 192

Goldenberg D L, Felson D T, Dinerman H 1986 A randomized controlled trial of amitriptyline and naproxen in the treatment of patients with fibromyalgia. Arthritis and Rheumatism 29: 1371–1377

Gomersall J D, Stuart A 1973 Amitriptyline in migraine prophylaxis. Changes in pattern of attacks during a controlled clinical trial. Journal of Neurology, Neurosurgery and Psychiatry 36: 684–690

Gomez-Perez F J, Riell J A, Dies H, Rodriguez-Rivera J G, Gonzalez-Barranco J, Lozano-Castaneda O 1985 Nortriptyline and fluphenazine in the symptomatic treatment of diabetic neuropathy. A double-blind cross-over study. Pain 23: 395–400

Gonzalez J P, Sewell R D E, Spencer P S 1980 Antinociceptive activity of opiates in the presence of the antidepressant agent nomifensine. Neuropharmacology 19: 613–618

Goodkin K, Gullion C M, Agras W S 1990 A randomized double-blind placebo controlled trial of trazodone hydrochloride in chronic low back pain syndrome. Journal of Clinical Psychopharmacology 10: 269–278

Goodwin R K, Prange A J, Post R M, Muscettola G, Lipton M A 1982 Potentiation of antidepressant effect by L-Triiodothyronine in tricyclic nonresponders. American Journal of Psychiatry 139: 34–38

Gourlay G K, Cherry D A, Cousins M F, Love B L, Graham J R, McLachlan M O 1986 A controlled study of a serotonin reuptake blocker, zimelidine, in the treatment of chronic pain. Pain 25: 35–52

Greenblatt D J, Shader R I 1974 Benzodiazepines. Parts I and II. New England Journal of Medicine 291: 1011–1015, 1239–1243

Greenblatt D J, Shader R I, Abernathy D R 1983 Current status of benzodiazepines, Parts I and II. New England Journal of Medicine 309: 354–358, 410–416

Haas S, Emrich H M, Beckmann H 1982 Analgesic and euphoric effects of high dose diazepam in schizophrenia. Neuropsychobiology 8: 123–128

Hackett G, Boddie H G, Harrison P 1987 Chronic muscle contraction headache: the importance of depression and anxiety. Journal of the Royal Society of Medicine 80: 689–691

Hakkarainen H 1977 Brief report, fluphenazine for tension headache; double blind study. Headache 17: 216–218

Halpern L 1982 Substitution-detoxification and the role in the management of chronic benign pain. Journal of Clinical Psychiatry 43: 10–14

Hameroff S R, Weiss J L, Lerman J C et al 1984 Doxepin effects on chronic pain and depression: a controlled study. Journal of Clinical Psychiatry 45: 45–52

Hamlin C, Gold M S 1984 Anxiolytics: predicting response/maximizing efficacy. In: Gold M S, Lydiard R B, Carman J S (eds) Advances in psychopharmacology: predicting and improving treatment response. CRC Press, Boca Raton, p 238–244

Hammond D L 1985 Pharmacology of central pain-modulating networks (biogenic amines and nonopioid analgesics). In: Field H L, Dubner R, Cervero F (eds) Advances in pain research and therapy. Raven Press, New York, p 499–511

Hanks G W, Thomas P J, Trueman T, Weeks E 1983 The myth of haloperidol potentiation. Lancet ii: 523–524

Hartshorn E A 1974 Interaction of CNS drugs, psychotherapeutic agents–antidepressants. Drug Intelligence and Clinical Pharmacy 8: 591–606

Hatangdi V S, Boa R A, Richards E G 1976 Post herpetic neuralgia: management with antiepileptic and tricyclic drugs. In: Bonica J J, Albe Fessard D (eds) Advances in pain research and therapy, vol 1. Raven Press, New York, p 583–587

Hendler N, Cimini A, Terence M A, Long D 1980 A comparison of cognitive impairment due to benzodiazepines and to narcotics. American Journal of Psychiatry 137: 828–830

Hirschowitz J, Bennett J A, Zemlan F P, Garrer D L 1983 Thioridazine effect on desipramine plasma levels. Journal of Clinical Psychopharmacology 3: 376–379

Hollister L E 1978 Drug therapy, tricyclic antidepressants. Parts I and II. New England Journal of Medicine 229: 1106–1109, 1168–1171

Hollister L E, Conley F K, Britt R H, Shuer L 1981 Long-term use of diazepam. Journal of the American Medical Association 246: 1568–1570

Hugues A, Chauvergne J, Lissilour T, Lagarde C 1963 L'imipramine utilisée comme antalgique majeur en carcinologie. Etude de 118 cas. Presse Médicale 71: 1073–1074

Hwang S A, Wilcox G L 1987 Analgesic properties of intrathecally administered heterocyclic antidepressants. Pain 28: 343–355

Iserson K V 1983 Parenteral chlorpromazine treatment of migraine. Annals of Emergency Medicine 12: 756–758

Jackson G L, Smith D A 1956 Analgesic properties of mixtures of chlorpromazine with morphine and meperidine. Annals of Internal Medicine 45: 640–652

Janowski E C, Janowski D S 1985 What precautions should be taken if a patient on an MAOI is scheduled to undergo anaesthesia? Journal of Clinical Psychopharmacology 5: 128–129

Jenkins D G, Ebbutt A F, Evans C D 1976 Imipramine in treatment of low back pain. Journal of International Medical Research 4 (suppl 2): 28–40

Johansson F, Von Knorring L 1979 A double-blind controlled study of a serotonin uptake inhibitor (zimelidine) versus placebo in chronic pain patients. Pain 7: 69–78

Johansson F, Von Knorring L, Sedvall G, Terenius L 1980 Changes in endorphins and 5-hydroxyindoleacetic acid in cerebrospinal fluid as a result of treatment with a serotonin reuptake inhibitor (zimelidine) in chronic pain patients. Psychiatry Research 2: 167–172

Judkins K C, Harmer M 1982 Haloperidol as an adjunct analgesic in the management of postoperative pain. Anaesthesia 37: 1118–1120

Kast E C 1966 An understanding of pain and its measurement. Medical Times 94: 1501–1513

Khatami M, Woody G, O'Brien C 1979 Chronic pain and narcotic addiction: a multitherapeutic approach – a pilot study. Comprehensive Psychiatry 20: 55–60

Khurana R C 1983 Treatment of painful diabetic neuropathy with trazodone. Journal of the American Medical Association 250: 1392

Kishore-Kumar R, Max M B, Schafer S C et al 1990 Desipramine relieves posherpetic neuralgia. Clinical Pharmacology and Therapeutics 47: 305–312

Klein D F, Gittlemann R, Quitkin F, Rifkin A 1980 Diagnosis and drug treatment of psychiatric disorders: adults and children. Williams & Wilkins, Baltimore, p 470–486

Kocher R 1976 Use of psychotropic drugs for treatment of chronic severe pain. In: Bonica J J, Albe Fessard D (eds) Advances in pain research and therapy, vol 1. Raven Press, New York, p 579–582

Krishnan K R R, France R D, Pelton S, McCann U D, Davidson J, Urban B J 1985 Chronic pain and depression. I. Classification of depression in chronic low back pain patients. Pain 22: 279–287

Krupp P, Wesp M 1975 Inhibition of prostaglandin synthetase by psychotropic drugs. Experientia 31: 330–331

Kudrow L 1977 Lithium prophylaxis for chronic cluster headache. Headache 17: 15–18

Kudrow L 1978 Comparative results of prednisone, methylsergide and lithium therapy in cluster headache. In: Greene R (ed) Current concepts in migraine research. Raven Press, New York, p 159–163

Kudrow L 1980 Analgesics and headache. In: The use of analgesics in the management of mild to moderate pain. Postgraduate Medical Communications: Riker Laboratories, Northridge, California, p 60–62

Kuipers R K W 1962 Imipramine in the treatment of rheumatic patients. Acta Rheumatologica Scandinavica 8: 45–51

Kvinesdal B, Molin J, Frøland A, Gram L F 1984 Imipramine treatment of painful diabetic neuropathy. Journal of the American Medical Association 251: 1727–1730

Laine E, Linguette M, Fossati P 1962 Action de l'imipramine injectable dans les symptômes douloureux. Lille Médicale 7: 711–716

Lance J W, Curran D A 1964 Treatment of chronic tension headache. Lancet 1: 1236–1239

Landa L, Breivik H, Husebo S, Elgen A, Rennemo F 1984 Beneficial effects of flupenthixol on cancer pain patients. Pain 2 (suppl): S253

Langohr H D, Stöhr M, Petruch F 1982 An open and double-blind cross-over study on the efficacy of clomipramine (Anafranil) in patients with painful mono- and polyneuropathies. European Neurology 2: 309–317

Langohr H D, Gerber W D, Koletzki E, Mayer K, Schroth G 1985 Clomipramine and metoprolol in migraine prophylaxis: a double blind crossover study. Headache 25: 107–113

Lasagna L 1977 The role of benzodiazepines in nonpsychiatric medical practice. American Journal of Psychiatry 134: 656–658

Lasagna R G, DeKornfeld T J 1961 Methotrimeprazine. A new phenothiazine derivative with analgesic properties. Journal of the American Medical Association 178: 887–890

Lascelles R G 1966 Atypical facial pain and depression. British Journal of Psychiatry 122: 651–659

Lee R, Spencer P S J 1977 Antidepressants and pain: a review of the pharmacological data supporting the use of certain tricyclics in chronic pain. Journal of International Medical Research 5 (suppl 1): 146–156

Leijon G, Boivie J 1989 Control post-stroke pain: a controlled trial of amitriptyline and carbamazepine. Pain 36: 27–36

Levine J D, Gordon N C, Smith R, McBryde R 1986 Desipramine enhances opiate postoperative analgesia. Pain 27: 45–49

Liebowitz M R, Quitkin F M, Stewart J W et al 1988 Antidepressant specificity in atypical depression. Archives of General Psychiatry 45: 129–137

Lindsay P G, Wyckoff M 1981 The depression–pain syndrome and its response to antidepressants. Psychosomatics 22: 571–577

Lloyd K G, Pile A 1984 Chronic antidepressants and GABA synapses. Neuropharmacology 23: 841–842

Loldrup D, Langemark M, Hansen H J, Olesen J, Bech P 1989 Clomipramine and mianserin in chronic idiopathic pain syndrome. Psychopharmacology 99: 1–7

Lopez Ibor J J 1972 Masked depressions. British Journal of Psychiatry 120: 245–257

Lynch S A, Max M B, Muir J, Smoller B, Dubner R 1990 Efficacy of antidepressants in relieving diabetic neuropathy pain: amitriptyline vs desipramine, and fluoxetine vs placebo. Neurology 40 (suppl 1): 437

McDonald Scott W A 1969 The relief of pain with an antidepressant in arthritis. Practitioner 202: 802–807

Macfarlane J G, Jalali S, Grace E M 1986 Trimipramine in rheumatoid arthritis: a randomized double-blind trial in relieving pain and joint tenderness. Current Medical Research and Opinion 10: 89–93

McNairy S L, Maruta T, Ivnik R J, Swanson D W, Ilstrup D M 1984 Prescription medication dependence and neuropsychologic function. Pain 18: 169–178

Macneill A L, Dick W C 1976 Imipramine and rheumatoid factor. Journal of Internal Medicine Research 4 (suppl 2): 23–27

Magni G, Bertolini C, Dodi G 1982 Treatment of perineal neuralgia with antidepressants. Journal of the Royal Society of Medicine 75: 214–215

Magni G, Andreoli F, Arduino C et al 1987 Modifications of [^{3}H] imipramine binding sites in platelets of chronic pain patients treated with mianserin. Pain 30: 311–320

Malec D, Langwinski R 1981 Central action of narcotic analgesics. VIII. The effect of dopaminergic stimulants on the action of analgesics in rats. Polish Journal of Pharmacologic Pharmacology 33: 243–282

Maltbie A A, Cavenar J O 1977 Haloperidol and analgesia: case reports. Military Medicine 142: 946–948

Maltbie A A, Cavenar J O, Sullivan J L, Hammett X X, Zung W W K 1979 Analgesia and haloperidol: a hypothesis. Journal of Clinical Psychiatry 40: 323–326

Mandel M R 1975 Electroconvulsive therapy for chronic pain associated with depression. American Journal of Psychiatry 132: 632–636

Margolis L H, Gianascol A J 1956 Chlorpromazine in thalamic pain syndrome. Neurology 6: 302–304

Marks J 1980 The benzodiazepines – use and abuse. Arzneimittel Forschung/Drug Research 30(I)(5a): 889–891

Martucci N, Manna V, Porto C, Agnoli A 1985 Migraine and the noradrenergic control of vasomotricity: a study with alpha-2 stimulated and alpha-2 blocker drugs. Headache 25: 95–100

Mathew N T 1978 Clinical subtypes of cluster headache and response to lithium therapy. Headache 18: 26–30

Max M B, Culnane M, Schafer S C et al 1987 Amitriptyline relieves diabetic neuropathy pain in patients with normal or depressed mood. Neurology 37: 589–596

Max M B, Schafer S C, Culnane M, Smoller B, Dubner R, Gracely R H 1988 Amitriptyline, but not lorazepam, relieves postherpetic neuralgia. Neurology 38: 1427–1432

Max M B, Kishore-Kumar R, Schafer S C et al 1991 Efficacy of desipramine in painful diabetic neuropathy: a placebo-controlled trial. Pain 45: 3–9

Maxwell D R, Palmer H T, Ryall R W 1961 A comparison of the analgesic and some other central properties of methotrimeprazine and morphine. Archives Internationaux de Pharmacodynamie 132: 60–73

Medical Letter on Drugs and Therapeutics 1981 Choice of benzodiazepines 23: 41–42

Medical Letter on Drugs and Therapeutics 1990 Fluoxetine (Prozac) revisited. 32: 83–85

Mellerup E T, Bech P, Hansen H J, Langemark M, Loldrup D, Plenge P 1988 Platelet 3H–imipramine binding in psychogenic pain disorders. Psychiatry Research 29: 149–156

Merskey H 1974 Psychological aspects of pain relief: hypnotherapy; psychotropic drugs. In: Swerdlow M (ed) Relief of intractable pain. Elsevier, Amsterdam, p 90–115

Merskey H, Hester R N 1972 The treatment of chronic pain with psychotropic drugs. Postgraduate Medical Journal 48: 594–598

Messing R B, Lytle L D 1977 Serotonin-containing neurons: their possible role in pain and analgesia. Pain 4: 1–21

Messing R B, Phebus L, Fisher L A, Lytle L D 1975 Analgesic effect of fluoxetine hydrochloride (Lilly 110140), a specific inhibitor of serotonin uptake. Psychopharmacology Communications 1: 511–521

Minuck R 1972 Postoperative analgesia – combination of methotrimeprazine and meperidine as postoperative analgesic agents. Canadian Medical Association Journal 90: 1156–1159

Mitas J A, Mosley C A, Drager A M 1983 Diabetic neuropathic pain: control by amitriptyline and fluphenazine in renal insufficiency. Southern Medical Journal 76: 462–467

Monks R C 1980 Tardive dyskinesia with low dose neuroleptic therapy. Modern Medicine 519

Monks R C 1981 Psychopharmacological management of post myocardial depression and anxiety. Canadian Family Physician 27: 1117–1121

Montastruc J L, Tran M A, Blanc M et al 1985 Measurement of plasma levels of clomipramine in the treatment of chronic pain. Clinical Neuropharmacology 8: 78–82

Montilla E, Fredrik W S, Cass L J 1963 Analgesic effect of methotrimeprazine and morphine. Archives of Internal Medicine 111: 91–94

Mørland T J, Storli O V, Mogstead T E 1979 Doxepin in the prophylactic treatment of mixed 'vascular' and tension headache. Headache 19: 382–383

Munro A, Chmara J 1982 Monosymptomatic hypochondriacal psychoses. A diagnostic checklist based on 50 cases of the disorder. Canadian Journal of Psychiatry 27: 374–376

Murphy D L, Campbell I, Costa J L 1978 Current status of the indoleamine hypothesis of the effective disorders. In: Lipton M A, Mascio A D, Killam K F (eds) Psychopharmacology: a generation of progress. Raven Press, New York, p 1235–1247

Nappi G, Sandrini G, Granella F et al 1990 A new 5-HT_2 antagonist (ritanserin) in the treatment of chronic headache with depression. A double-blind study vs amitriptyline. Headache 30: 439–444

Nathan P W 1978 Chlorprothixene (Taractan) in post herpetic neuralgia and other severe chronic pain. Pain 5: 367–371

Nies A, Robinson D S, Friedman M J et al 1977 Relationship between age and tricyclic antidepressant levels. American Journal of Psychiatry 134: 790–793

Noone J F 1977 Psychotropic drugs and migraine. Journal of International Medical Research 5 (suppl 1): 66–71

Okasha A, Ghaleb H A, Sadek A 1973 A double-blind trial for the clinical management of psychogenic headache. British Journal of Psychiatry 122: 181–183

Onghena P, van Houdenhove B 1992 Antidepressant-induced analgesia in chronic non-malignant pain: a meta-analysis of 39 placebo controlled studies. Pain 49: 205–219

Paoli F, Darcourt G, Cossa P 1960 Note préliminaire sur l'action de l'imipramine dans les états douloureux. Revue Neurologique 102: 503–504

Parolin A R 1966 El tratamiento del dolor y la ansiedad en el carcinoma avanzado. El Medico Practico 21: 3–4

Pearce J M S 1980 Chronic migraneous neuralgia, a variant of cluster headache. Brain 103: 149–159

Peroutko S J, Banghart S B, Allen G S 1984 Relative potency and selectivity of calcium antagonists used in the treatment of migraine. Headache 24: 55–58

Perry P J, Pfohl B M, Holstad G 1987 The relationship between antidepressant response and tricyclic antidepressant plasma concentration. A retrospective analysis of the literature using logistic regression analysis. Clinical Pharmacokinetics 13: 381–392

Petts H V, Pleuvry B J 1983 Interactions of morphine and methotrimeprazine in mouse and man with respect to analgesia, respiration and sedation. British Journal of Anaesthesia 55: 437–441

Pheasant H, Bursk A, Goldfarb J et al 1983 Amitriptyline and chronic low back pain: a randomized double blind cross over study. Spine 8: 552–557

Pilowsky I, Barrow C G 1990 A controlled study of psychotherapy and amitriptyline individually and in combination in the treatment of chronic intractable 'psychogenic' pain. Pain 40: 3–19

Pilowsky I, Hallett E C, Bassett D L, Thomas P G, Penhall R K 1982 A controlled study of amitriptyline in the treatment of chronic pain. Pain 14: 169–179

Polliack J 1979 Chronic recurrent headaches. South African Medical Journal 56: 980

Proudfit H K 1988 Pharmacological evidence for the modulation of nociception by noradrenergic neurons. In: Field H L, Besson J M (eds) Pain modulation. Progress in brain research. Elsevier, Amsterdam, p 357–370

Puttini P S, Cazzola M, Boccasini L et al 1988 A comparison of dothiepin versus placebo in the treatment of pain in rheumatoid arthritis and the association of pain with depression. Journal of International Medical Research 16: 331–337

Radebold H 1971 Behandlung chronischer Schmerzzustande mit Anafranil. Medizinische Welt 22: 337–339

Rafinesque J 1963 Emploi du Tofranil à titre antalgique dans les syndromes douloureux de diverses origines. Gazette Médicale de France 1: 2075–2077

Raferty H 1979 The management of post herpetic pain using sodium valproate and amitriptyline. Journal of the Irish Medical Association 72: 399–401

Raft D, Toomey T, Gregg J M 1979 Behavior modification and haloperidol in chronic facial pain. Southern Medical Journal 72: 155–159

Raskin D E 1982 MAO inhibitors in chronic pain and depression. Journal of Clinical Psychiatry 43: 122

Roberts M H T 1984 5-Hydroxytryptamine and antinociception. Neuropharmacology 23: 1529–1536

Rumore M M, Schlichting D A 1986 Clinical efficacy of antihistamines as analgesics. Pain 25: 7–22

Sadove M S, Rose R F, Balagot R C, Reyes R 1955 Chlorpromazine in the management of pain. Modern Medicine 23: 117–120

Sandrini G, Alfonsi E, DeRysky C, Marini S, Facchinetti F, Nappi G 1986 Evidence for serotonin-S_2 receptor involvement in analgesia in human. European Journal of Pharmacology 130: 311–314

Saran A, 1988 Antidepressants not effective in headache associated with minor closed head injury. International Journal of Psychiatry in Medicine 18: 75–83

Schick E, Wolpert E, Reichert A, Queisser W 1979 Neuroleptanalgesie mit einen hechpotenten Depotneuroleptikum zur Schmerztherapie bei metastasierenden Malignomen. Verhandlungen der Deutschen Gesellschaft fur Innere Medizin 85: 1113–1114

Schildkraut J N 1978 Current status of the catecholamine hypotheses of affective disorders. In: Lipton M A, Mascio A D, Killam K F (eds) Psychopharmacology: a generation of progress. Raven Press, New York, p 1223–1234

Sharav Y, Singer E, Schmidt E, Dionne R A, Dubner R 1987 The analgesic effect of amitriptyline on chronic facial pain. Pain 31: 199–209

Sherwin D 1979 A new method for treating 'headaches'. American Journal of Psychiatry 136: 1181–1183

Shimm D S, Logue G L, Maltbie A A, Dugan S 1979 Medical management of chronic cancer pain. Journal of the American Medical Association 241: 2411

Sigwald J, Bouttier D, Caille F 1959 Le traitement du zona et des algies zostériennes. Etude des résultats obtenus avec la levomepromazine. Thérapie 14: 818–824

Sindrup S H, Ejlertsen B, Frøland A, Sindrup E H, Brøsen K, Gram L F 1989 Imipramine treatment in diabetic neuropathy: relief of subjective symptoms without changes in peripheral and autonomic nerve function. European Journal of Clinical Pharmacology 37: 151–153

Sindrup S H, Gram C F, Skjold T et al 1990a Clomipramine vs desipramine vs placebo in the treatment of diabetic neuropathy symptoms: a double-blind crossover study. British Journal of Clinical Pharmacology 30: 683–691

Sindrup S H, Gram L F, Brosen K, Eshoj O, Mogensen E F 1990b. The selective serotonin reuptake inhibitor paroxetine is effective in the treatment of diabetic neuropathy symptoms. Pain 42: 135–144

Singh G 1971 Drug treatment of chronic intractable pain in patients referred to a psychiatry clinic. Journal of the Indian Medical Association 56: 341–345

Sjaastad O 1983 So-called 'tension headache' – the response to a 5-HT uptake inhibitor: femoxetine. Cephalgia 3: 53–60

Smoller B 1984 The use of dexamethasone suppression test as a marker of efficacy in the treatment of a myofascial syndrome with amitriptyline. Pain (suppl) 2: S250

Snyder S, Enna J J, Young A B 1977 Brain mechanisms associated with the therapeutic actions of benzodiazepines: focus on neuro-transmitters. American Journal of Psychiatry 134: 662–664

Soja P F, Sinclair J G 1983 Evidence that noradrenaline reduces tonic descending inhibition of cat spinal cord nociceptor-driven neurones. Pain 15: 71–81

Somoza E 1978 Influence of neuroleptics on the binding of metenkephalin, morphine and dihydromorphine to synaptosome-enriched fractions of rat brain. Neuropharmacology 17: 577–581

Spiegel K, Kalb R, Pasternak G W 1983 Analgesic activity of tricyclic antidepressants. Annals of Neurology 13: 462–465

Sternbach R A, Murphy R W, Akeson W H, Wolf S R 1973 Chronic low back pain, the 'low back loser'. Postgraduate Medical Journal 53: 135–138

Sternbach R A, Janowsky D S, Huey I Y, Segal D S 1976 Effects of altering brain serotonin activity on human chronic pain. In: Bonica J J, Albe Fessard D (eds) Advances in pain research and therapy, vol 1. Raven Press, New York, p 601–606

Sternback H 1991 The serotonin syndrome. American Journal of Psychiatry 148: 705–713

Stirman J 1967 A comparison of methotrimeprazine and meperidine as analgesic agents. Anesthesia and Analgesia 46: 176–180

Sugrue M F 1983 Chronic antidepressant therapy and associated changes in central monoaminergic receptor functioning. Pharmacology and Therapeutics 21: 1–33

Swerdlow M, Cundill J G 1981 Anticonvulsant drugs used in the treatment of lancinating pain. A comparison. Anaesthesia 36: 1129–1132

Taub A 1973 Relief of post herpetic neuralgia with psychotropic drugs. Journal of Neurosurgery 39: 235–239

Taylor R G, Doku H C 1967 Methotrimeprazine: evaluated as an analgesic following oral surgery. Journal of Oral Medicine 22: 141–144

Terenius L 1978 Endogenous peptides and analgesia. Annual Review of Pharmacology 18: 189

Terenius L 1979 Endorphins in chronic pain. In: Bonica J J, Liebeskind J C, Albe Fessard D (eds) Advances in pain research and therapy, vol 3. Raven Press, New York, p 458–471

Theesen K A, Marsh W R 1989 Relief of diabetic neuropathy with fluoxetine. DICP, The Annals of Pharmacotherapy 23: 572–574

Thorpe P, Marchant-Williams R 1974 The role of an antidepressant, dibenzepin (Noveril), in the relief of pain in chronic arthritic states. Medical Journal of Australia 1: 264–266

Tofanetti O, Albiero L, Galatulas I, Genovese E 1977 Enhancement of propoxyphene-induced analgesia by doxepin. Psychopharmacology 51: 213–215

Tricklebank M D, Huston P H, Curzon G 1984 Involvement of dopamine in the antinociceptive response to footshock. Psychopharmacology 82: 185–188

Turkington R W 1980 Depression masquerading as diabetic neuropathy. Journal of the American Medical Association 243: 1147–1150

Twycross R G 1979 Non-narcotic, corticosteroid and psychotropic drugs. In: Twycross R G, Ventafridda V (eds) The continuing care of terminal cancer patients. Pergamon Press, Oxford, p 126–128

Tyber M A 1974 Treatment of the painful shoulder syndrome with amitriptyline and lithium carbonate. Canadian Medical Association Journal 111: 137–140

Tyrer P 1976 Towards rational therapy with monoamine oxidase inhibitors. British Journal of Psychiatry 128: 354–360

Urban B J, France R D, Steinberger E K, Scott D L, Maltbie A A 1986 Long term use of narcotic/antidepressant medication in the management of phantom limb pain. Pain 24: 191–196

Valdes M, Garcia L, Treserra J, De Pablo J, De Flores T 1989 Psychogenic pain and depressive disorders: an empirical study. Journal of Affective Disorders 16: 21–25

Ventafridda V, Bonezzi C, Caraceni A et al 1987 Antidepressants for cancer pain and other painful syndromes with deafferentation component: comparison of amitriptyline and trazodone. Italian Journal of Neurological Sciences 8: 579–587

Ward N G, Bloom V L, Friedel R O 1979 The effectiveness of tricyclic antidepressants in the treatment of coexisting pain and depression. Pain 7: 331–341

Ward N G, Bloom V L, Fawcett J, Friedel R P 1983 Urinary 3-methoxy-4-hydroxyphenethylene glycol in the prediction of pain and depression relief with doxepin: preliminary findings. Journal of Nervous and Mental Disease 171: 55–58

Ward N, Bokan J A, Phillips M, Benedetti C, Butler S, Spengler D 1984 Antidepressants in concomitant chronic back pain and depression: doxepin and desipramine compared. Journal of Clinical Psychiatry 45: 54–59

Watson C P N, Evans R J 1985 A comparative trial of amitriptyline and zimelidine in post-herpetic neuralgia. Pain 23: 387–394
Watson C P N, Evans R J, Reed K, Merskey H, Goldsmith L, Warsh J 1982 Amitriptyline versus placebo in postherpetic neuralgia. Neurology 32: 671–673
Weis O, Sriwatanakul K, Weintraub M 1982 Treatment of post-herpetic neuralgia and acute herpetic pain with amitriptyline and perphenazine. South African Medical Journal 62: 274–275
Wheatley D 1979 Clorazepate in the management of coronary disease. Psychosomatics 20: 195–205
Willer J C, Roby A, Maulet C, Gerard A 1984 Possible tryptaminergic involvement of pain and of endogenous opiate activity in man. Pain 2 (suppl): 251
Willner P 1985 Antidepressants and serotonergic neurotransmission: an integrative review. Psychopharmacology 85: 387–404
Woodforde J M, Dwyer B, McEwen B W et al 1965 Treatment of post-herpetic neuralgia. Medical Journal of Australia 2: 869–872
Wüster M, Duka T, Herz A 1980 Diazepam effects on striatal metenkephalin levels following long-term pharmacological manipulation. Neuropharmacology 19: 501–505
Young R J, Clarke B F 1985 Pain relief in diabetic neuropathy: the effectiveness of imipramine and related drugs. Diabetic Medicine 2: 363–366
Zeigler D K, Hurwitz A, Hassanein R S, Kodanaz H A, Preskorn S H, Mason J 1987 Migraine prophylaxis. A comparison of popranolol and amitriptyline. Archives of Neurology 44: 486–489
Zitman F G, Linssen A C G, Edelbroek P M 1984 Amitriptyline versus placebo in chronic benign pain: a double blind study. Pain 2 (suppl): S250

51. Peripheral neuropathic pain: an approach to management

Howard L. Fields

INTRODUCTION

There are two broad classes of peripheral nerve injury: mononeuropathies (e.g. traumatic, or ischaemic) and polyneuropathies (e.g. toxic, hereditary, inflammatory or 'metabolic'). Most peripheral neuropathies are associated with a loss of function, either sensory, motor, or both, and are typically nonpainful. Pain is, however, characteristic of some neuropathic diseases (e.g. diabetic and alcohol-deficiency neuropathies and herpes zoster). Although very little is known about the pathophysiology of human neuropathic pain, animal models of focal traumatic neuropathies have contributed significantly to our knowledge about the factors that could contribute to this type of pain and have provided clues about potentially useful treatments. In this chapter I will outline a systematic approach to management that is based on emerging knowledge of the pathophysiology of neuropathic pain and of treatment efficacy based on data from controlled clinical trials.

Clinical features of neuropathic pain

Pain associated with peripheral nerve injury has several clinical characteristics, including localization of the pain in an area of sensory deficit (the deficit is usually to noxious and thermal stimuli which indicates damage to small-diameter afferent fibres); the pain commonly has a burning and/or shooting quality with unusual tingling, crawling or electrical sensations (dysaesthesiae); there is often a delay between the causative nerve injury and the onset of pain; gentle mechanical stimuli such as bending of hairs may evoke severe pain (allodynia). Although these characteristics are neither universally present in, nor diagnostic of neuropathic pain, when they are present the diagnosis of neuropathic pain is not difficult.

MECHANISMS THAT MAY CONTRIBUTE TO NEUROPATHIC PAIN

CENTRAL MECHANISMS

Loss of large-fibre afferent inhibition

The clinical paradox that injury to peripheral nerves often produces an association of increased pain with loss of sensory function was cited by Melzack & Wall (1965) as a major impetus to their Gate Control hypothesis which presented a detailed explanation for neuropathic pain. Because selective blockade of large-diameter myelinated sensory axons increases pain, they proposed that these large-diameter fibres normally inhibit pain-transmitting spinal-cord neurons. They further proposed that the pain of nerve injury was due to selective damage to these pain-inhibiting large-diameter myelinated sensory axons. They predicted that selective activation of myelinated axons, for example by electrical stimulation of a peripheral nerve, would decrease pain. In fact, there are cases of dramatic pain relief produced by transcutaneous electrical nerve stimulation (TENS) (Meyer & Fields 1972). Thus it seems likely that release of dorsal horn pain transmission cells from inhibition by myelinated axons does contribute to the pain that occurs in some cases of focal nerve injury.

Deafferentation hyperactivity

Deafferentation has been shown to produce hyperactivity in dorsal horn cells. Following dorsal rhizotomy, many dorsal horn cells begin to fire spontaneously at high frequencies (Lombard & Larabi 1983). Such a mechanism may underlie the pain that occurs following extensive denervating injuries. For example, pain is a characteristic sequela of the deafferentation produced by brachial plexus avulsion (Wynn-Parry 1980) and this pain seems to respond to surgical procedures which destroy nociceptive dorsal horn neurons (Nashold et al 1979).

PERIPHERAL MECHANISMS OF NEUROPATHIC PAIN

Ectopic impulse generation

Although release phenomena may account for some of the features observed in patients with neuropathic pains, there are some features that remain obscure. Relative loss of large fibres is not always seen in painful generalized neuropathies. Thomas (1974) reviewed this topic and pointed out that when fibre counts are actually done on biopsies, some painful neuropathies are associated with a specific loss of *small*-diameter fibres (e.g. Fabry's disease, amyloid neuropathy and dominantly inherited sensory neuropathy) (Kocen & Thomas 1970). In addition, Friedreich's ataxia and uraemic neuropathy, which are characterized by selective *large*-fibre loss, are characteristically *not* painful. Another observation that is not accounted for by putative mechanisms which depend on the partial or complete deafferentation of spinal pain-transmission neurons is that sympathetic nerve block can often completely relieve neuropathic pain. Major progress in understanding these clinical observations has come from studies of experimental neuromas.

When the sciatic nerve is cut and allowed to regenerate and form a neuroma, spontaneous activity and exquisite mechanical sensitivity develops in the afferent axons innervating the neuroma (Wall & Gutnick 1974; Scadding 1981). Some of these primary afferents are of small diameter (A-delta and C-fibres), contain substance P (Fried et al 1989) and thus may have originally been nociceptors (Welk et al 1990). Similarly, within hours of damaging the small-diameter nociceptive axons innervating the cornea, these axons become spontaneously active (Tanelian & MacIver 1991).

Ectopic impulses may be generated at sites other than the damaged and regenerating distal axon terminals. For example, when a peripheral nerve is damaged, a region near the dorsal root ganglion (which is distant from the site of injury) becomes capable of generating 'spontaneous' impulses (Devor & Rappaport 1990). In addition, small patches of demyelination on, for example, the axon of an A-delta nociceptor, can become a source of ectopic impulses.

Sympathetically maintained pain

Causalgia is the classic example of a sympathetically maintained pain. It is characterized by a burning sensation which is exacerbated by cold, loud noises, and slight mechanical stimulation (Mitchell 1965). It is dramatically and virtually completely relieved by sympathetic block (Richards 1967). Animal studies have shown that, in addition to the development of spontaneous ectopic impulse activity, damaged nociceptive afferents that have regenerated into a neuroma can be excited by i.v. adrenaline or by stimulation of sympathetic efferents (Devor & Janig 1981). Furthermore, Sato & Perl (1991) have shown that sympathetic activity can sensitize identified nociceptors following damage to the nerve in which they run. These animal studies are supported by human research demonstrating that adrenaline applied directly to a neuroma produces severe burning pain (Chabal et al 1992). Thus, damage to a peripheral nerve seems to induce in primary afferent nociceptors a state of sensitivity to sympathetic activity. Ultrastructural studies have demonstrated that regenerating axonal sprouts come into close apposition with each other during posttraumatic regeneration (Aguayo & Bray 1975). There is immunocytochemical evidence that some of these regenerating sprouts are derived from small-diameter primary afferents and others from sympathetic postganglionic axons (Fried et al 1989); this feature may provide an anatomical substrate for sympathosensory activation.

Antidromic release of sensitizing neuromediators

Many unmyelinated primary afferent nociceptors contain neuropeptides (e.g. substance P and calcitonin-gene-related peptide) that can produce a local inflammatory process (vasodilatation, plasma extravasation, accumulation of white blood cells and hyperalgesia). These peptides can be released during stimulation induced activation of primary afferent nociceptors and they undoubtedly contribute to the neurally mediated cutaneous wheal and flare produced by noxious stimuli (Levine et al 1993).

Ochoa and his colleagues have presented data on a small number of patients with chronic pain which document that C-fibre nociceptors innervating a painful region can become chronically sensitized. Recordings of C-fibres in these patients suggests that the sensitization is maintained in part by antidromic release of some neuromediator (e.g. substance P) from the peripheral terminals of C-nociceptors (Cline et al 1989). If damaged or sensitized unmyelinated afferents generate spontaneous ectopic impulses this will lead to chronic neuropeptide release and contribute to inflammation and pain.

What all these observations suggest is that, as part of the regenerative reaction to local injury of nerve, a peripheral irritative focus develops which can be maintained by some combination of mechanical stimulation, ectopic impulse generation, neurogenic inflammation and sympathetic efferent outflow to the region of damage. This notion is supported by the clinical observations that local anaesthetics, at levels which block ectopic impulse generation, topical cyclo-oxygenase inhibitors and the C-fibre neurotoxin (capsaicin) may all relieve the pain (see below). It may also explain why sympathetic or alpha-adrenergic blockade frequently gives dramatic relief of causalgia and posttraumatic neuralgias (e.g. Hannington-Kiff 1974; Loh & Nathan 1978).

Inflammation of the nerve trunk

It is important to point out that the connective tissue sheath surrounding a peripheral nerve is innervated, presumably by nociceptive primary afferents. These *nervi nervorum* may enter the nerve trunk with a neurovascular bundle (Hromada 1963; Appenzeller et al 1984). Because of these nervi nervorum, peripheral nerve can be a source of pain in a manner similar to joints, muscles and ligamentous structures. The acute pain of a herniated inflamed disc, or that seen with an infection of nerve such as acute leprous neuropathy, are probably mediated by the physiological activation of the nervi nervorum (Asbury & Fields 1984).

THE TREATMENT OF NEUROPATHIC PAIN

Except for trigeminal neuralgia, which responds reliably and specifically to anticonvulsant medications, the treatment of neuropathic pain has until recently been largely hit or miss, mostly miss. Fortunately, over the past few years, clinical research has led to significant improvements in therapy of neuropathic pain.

Tricylic antidepressants

Tricyclics are clearly valuable in the treatment of a variety of painful conditions, including cancer, low-back pain, different types of headache and, obviously, pain accompanied by significant affective disorder (Fields 1987). Amitriptyline is currently the most widely prescribed of the antidepressants used for the treatment of chronic pain. However, it has significant side-effects (Richelson 1990). Amitriptyline produces orthostatic hypotension, due largely to an alpha-adrenergic blocking action. Other serious problems include urinary retention, memory loss and cardiac conduction abnormalities (largely due to the muscarinic anticholinergic actions of the drug). In addition, most patients find amitriptyline to be very sedating and this is probably due to its antihistamine action. Patients who are to be treated with this drug should be started at a very low dose, even as low as 10 mg, and built up slowly at about 25 mg every fourth day until the empirically determined therapeutic range is reached. Desipramine, another tricyclic, appears to be as effective as amitriptyline in most of the conditions studied (Kishore-Kumar et al 1990; Max et al 1992). Patients respond to desipramine at doses comparable to those of amitriptyline but with fewer anticholinergic side-effects and significantly less sedation. All patients undergoing treatment with any tricyclic should have a cardiogram at the onset of treatment. Cardiac conduction defects are a contraindication to their use. Blood levels and repeated cardiograms should be taken if the dose is pushed above 100 mg/24 h.

There are very few studies of nontricyclic antidepressants for pain management. The much heralded fluoxetine (Prosac), which is almost a pure 5HT reuptake inhibitor, has virtually none of the serious side-effects common with desipramine or amitriptyline. It is nonsedating, and side-effects such as heart block, memory loss and orthostatic hypotension are rare. Although a very closely related drug (paroxetine) has been reported to help the pain of diabetic neuropathy (Sindrup et al 1990), results with fluoxetine for neuropathic pain have been disappointing (e.g. Max et al 1992). It is important to point out that although fluoxetine may not be helpful for neuropathic pain per se, it is an effective antidepressant and some patients report an improvement in pain as their depression clears. This point should be kept in mind with the use of all antidepressants. In the absence of a response at low doses, and especially in patients with clinically significant depression, the drugs should be pushed until limiting side-effects ensue or the maximum recommended plasma concentration is achieved.

Although touted in early papers as a useful adjunct to tricyclics in the treatment of neuropathic pain, phenothiazines have not been shown to be helpful for any pain problem (McGee & Alexander 1979). Furthermore, the side-effect profile of phenothiazines demands that they be used with great caution.

Membrane-stabilizing agents

This group includes the anticonvulsants and the lidocaine-like cardiac antiarrhythmics.

In contrast to the consistently good results obtained with antidepressants in the treatment of neuropathic pain, anticonvulsants such as Dilantin and Tegretol are helpful for a more restricted patient population. However, if a patient reports pain with a sharp shooting or electric shock-like component, anticonvulsants are much more likely to be helpful and should be tried. Drugs such as baclofen, clonazepam, and valproate may be used as alternatives to carbamazepine and phenytoin.

Lidocaine by intravenous infusion produces significant relief for patients with postherpetic neuralgia (Rowbotham et al 1991) and a variety of other neuropathic pain syndromes (Glazer & Portenoy 1991). Although the site of action of membrane-stabilizing drugs for relief of pain has not been proven, in vitro studies have shown that ectopic impulses generated by damaged primary afferent nociceptors are abolished by concentrations of local anaesthetics much lower than that required for blocking normal axonal conduction (Chabal et al 1989; Tanelian & MacIver 1991). This principle has been used in the treatment of certain cardiac arrhythmias and has led to the marketing of oral drugs that, like lidocaine, produce a use-dependent block of voltage-dependent sodium channels. Tocainide and mexiletine are two drugs of this class that are currently available. Mexiletine is less toxic and has been shown to be effective for pain in diabetic neuropathy (Dejgard et al 1988) and other peripheral neuropathic pains (Chabal et al 1992). We are currently using it as a second-line drug after tricyclics for a variety of neuropathic pains.

Opioid analgesics in neuropathic pain

The use of narcotic analgesics for patients with chronic neuropathic pain is highly controversial, even among experts in the field of pain management. Unfortunately, the data available on this question are mostly anecdotal. Some controlled trials have indicated that narcotics have no analgesic effect in patients with neuropathic pain (Arner & Meyerson 1988; Max et al 1988). In contrast, our double-blind placebo controlled study demonstrated that infusions of morphine give significant relief to patients with postherpetic neuralgia (Rowbotham et al 1991). This result is supported by a study using patient-controlled analgesia (Jadad et al 1992). My (anecdotal) experience and that of others (Portenoy & Foley 1986) is that many patients with pain due to central and peripheral nerve injury can be successfully treated on a chronic basis with stable doses of narcotic analgesics. I recommend the use of a long-acting narcotic analgesic (methadone, levorphanol or a sustained release morphine preparation) when alternative approaches to treatment have failed. The danger of addiction in patients with no prior history of drug abuse is miniscule. Clearly, long-term prospective trials of this approach need to be carried out.

Topical medications

Many patients with neuropathic pain suffer from a condition, termed allodynia, in which light mechanical stimulation of the skin produces pain (allodynia). Allodynia is very common in postherpetic neuralgia, causalgia and traumatic mononeuropathies, such as accompany surgical scars. One approach to the treatment of such conditions is the use of capsaicin extracts. Capsaicin is a neurotoxin that targets unmyelinated sensory axons, predominantly nociceptors (Lynn 1990). Capsaicin extracts are commercially available in a 0.025% and a 0.075% preparation. The 0.075% preparation has been reported to reduce the pain of postherpetic neuralgia (Bernstein et al 1989) and postmastectomy pain (Watson & Evans 1992). The 0.075% preparation has also been advocated for pain in diabetic neuropathy, however, without convincing data supporting this indication. These capsaicin preparations often produce intolerable burning so that many patients discontinue their use (Watson et al 1988). My own experience with these capsaicin preparations has been disappointing.

Topical application of aspirin in either a chloroform or ethyl ether suspension has been reported to produce profound pain relief for some patients with postherpetic neuralgia (King 1988; DeBenedittis et al 1992).

A third promising topical medication for neuropathic pain is local anaesthetics. The rationale is similar to that discussed above in the section on membrane-stabilizing drugs. There are several uncontrolled studies that report pain relief with topically applied special formulations of local anaesthetic (e.g. Rowbotham & Fields 1989; Stow et al 1989).

The use of clonidine patches to relieve cutaneous hypersensitivity in patients with sympathetically maintained pain has recently been reported (Davis et al 1991). My experience with this modality is positive but limited.

In summary, the medical management of neuropathic pain consists of three main classes of oral medication (opioids, tricyclics, membrane-stabilizing agents) and several categories of topical medications for patients with cutaneous hyperalgesia (cyclo-oxygenase inhibitors, capsaicin in either 0.025% or 0.075% preparations, local anaesthetics and adrenergic antagonists).

NEUROPATHIC PAIN MANAGEMENT
Phase I

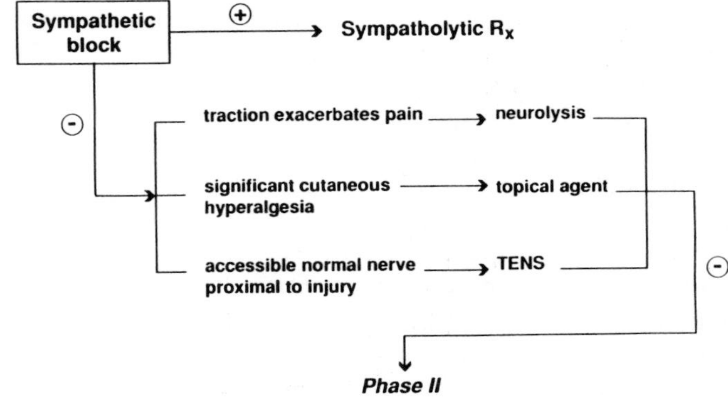

NEUROPATHIC PAIN MANAGEMENT
Phase II

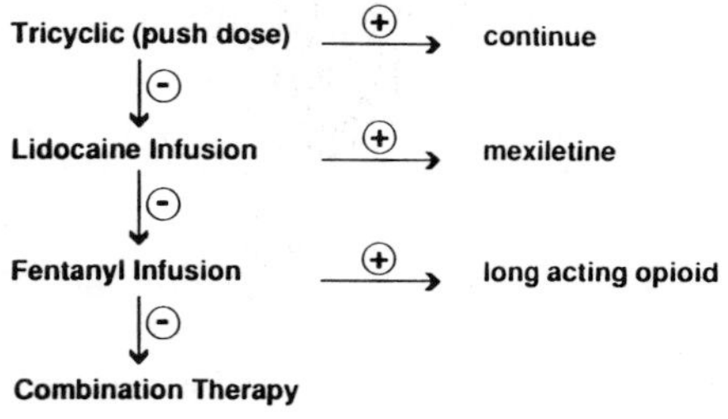

Fig. 51.1 Algorithm for approaching pain associated with peripheral nerve damage. Phase I outlines the steps to be taken prior to instituting long term medical management. Phase II illustrates one systematic approach to long term pharmacological treatment of neuropathic pain.

A systematic approach to patients with neuropathic pain

The ideal in medicine is to treat the cause of the disease rather than the symptom. For patients with painful nerve injuries this is often not possible. Entrapment neuropathies can be treated by neurolysis, transposition or decompression (Dawson et al 1983). If scar-induced mechanical traction is a factor, this approach is particularly worthwhile. Transcutaneous electrical stimulation of nerves (TENS) is a viable option for some patients with focal nerve injury, particularly if the nerve trunk can be stimulated proximal to the site of injury. The majority of patients, however, require medical management. When cutaneous hyperalgesia and/or allodynia are present we usually initiate therapy with a topical agent, either local anaesthetic, cyclo-oxygenase inhibitor or capsaicin.

Once the decision is made to pursue medical management we currently use the algorithm illustrated in Figure 50.1. The most useful diagnostic procedure, particularly in patients with focal neuropathies, is a sympathetic block. Because it is less invasive and technically simpler, we begin with intravenous phentolamine (e.g. Arner 1991). If that does not produce striking relief we proceed to a standard sympathetic chain local anaesthetic block. Patients with sympathetically maintained pain may be cured by a series of sympathetic blocks combined with vigorous physical therapy. Although the results are rarely dramatic, oral sympatholytics such as phenoxybenzamine (Ghostine et al 1984), reserpine or guanethidine may be helpful for some patients who obtain only transient relief with sympathetic blockade.

If the sympatholytic intervention does not provide adequate relief, the next line of therapy is tricyclics. With tricyclics it is best to initiate therapy with a very low dose (e.g. 10 mg) and gradually increase it to optimize pain relief. It is often necessary to raise the dose into the antidepressant range (over 200 mg). It is important to check plasma levels of antidepressant medications before concluding that they are of no value. If patients obtain inadequate relief from tricyclics and plasma levels are at the top of the therapeutic range, or if they do not tolerate the side-effects, we then pursue membrane-stabilizing drugs. We begin with a lidocaine infusion. If the patient does get a good response with the lidocaine we will begin treatment with either mexiletine or one of the anticonvulsants. If the patient does not obtain relief with a lidocaine infusion our experience is that the pain is much less likely to respond to drugs of this class and we give the patient a fentanyl infusion to determine the opioid sensitivity of their pain. With a good response to fentanyl we initiate opioid therapy. At the present time, levorphanol is our first line drug but MS-Contin (sustained release morphine) and methadone are probably just as good. There is evidence for an additive effect of opioids with tricyclics and cyclo-oxygenase inhibitors so we usually try these combinations before abandoning this approach. The majority of our patients require a combination of therapies for optimal results.

Although this approach does not help all patients it does cast a broad net across potential sources of pain and it is gratifying for those patients who obtain significant relief.

REFERENCES

Aguayo A J, Bray G M 1975 Pathology and pathophysiology of unmyelinated nerve fibers. In: Dyck P J, Thomas P K, Lambert E H (eds) Peripheral neuropathy. Saunders, Philadelphia, p 363–378

Appenzeller O, Dhital K K, Cowen T, Burnstock G 1984 The nerves to blood vessels supplying blood to nerves: the innervation of vasa nervorum. Brain Research 304: 383–386

Arner S 1991 Intravenous phentolamine test: diagnostic and prognostic use in reflex sympathetic dystrophy. Pain 46: 17–22

Arner S, Meyerson B 1988 Lack of analgesic effect of opioids on neuropathic and idiopathic forms of pain. Pain 33: 11–23

Asbury A K, Fields H L 1984 Pain due to peripheral nerve damage: an hypothesis. Neurology 34: 1587–1590

Bernstein J E, Korman N J, Bickers D R et al 1989 Topical capsaicin treatment of chronic postherpetic neuralgia. Journal of the American Academy of Dermatology 21: 265–270

Chabal C, Russell L C, Burchiel K J 1989 The effect of intravenous lidocaine, tocainide, and mexiletine on spontaneously active fibers originating in rat sciatic neuromas. Pain 38: 333–338

Chabal C, Jacobson L, Mariano A, Chaney E, Britell C W 1992 The use of oral mexiletine for the treatment of pain after peripheral nerve injury. Anesthesiology 76: 513–717

Chabal C, Jacobson L, Russell L C, Burchiel K J 1992b Pain response to perineuromal injection of normal saline, epinepherine, and lidocaine in humans. Pain 49: 9–12

Cline M A, Ochoa J, Torebjork H E 1989 Chronic hyperalgesia and skin warming caused by sensitized C nociceptors. Brain 112: 621–647

Davis K D, Treede R D, Raja S N, Meyer R A, Campbell J N 1991 Topical application of clonidine relieves hyperalgesia in patients with sympathetically maintained pain. Pain 47: 309–317

Dawson D M, Hallet M, Millender L H 1983 Entrapment neuropathies. Little, Brown, Boston

DeBenedittis G, Besana F, Lorenzetti A 1992 A new topical treatment for acute herpetic neruralgia and post-herpetic neuralgia: the aspirin/diethyl ether mixture. An open-label study plus a double-blind controlled clinical trial. Pain 48: 383–390

Dejgard A, Petersen P, Kastrup J 1988 Mexiletine for the treatment of chronic painful diabetic neuropathy. Lancet 1: 9–11

Devor M, Janig W 1981 Activation of myelinated afferents ending in neuroma by stimulation of the sympathetic supply in the rat. Neuroscience Letters 24: 43–47

Devor M, Rappaport Z H 1990 Pain and the pathophysiology of damaged nerve. In: Fields H L (ed) Pain syndromes in neurology. Butterworths, London, p 47–84

Fields H L 1987 Pain McGraw-Hill, New York, p 133–170

Fried K, Brodin E and Theodorsson E 1989 Substance P-, CGRP- and NPY-immunoreactive nerve fibers in rat sciatic nerve-end neuromas. Regulatory Peptides 25: 11–24

Ghostine S Y, Comair Y G, Turner D M, Kassell N F, Azar C G 1984 Phenoxybenzamine in the treatment of causalgia. Journal of Neurosurgery 60: 1263–1268

Glazer S, Portenoy R K 1991 Systemic local anaesthetics in pain control. Journal of Pain Symptom Management 6: 30–39

Hannington-Kiff J G 1974 Intravenous regional sympathetic block with guanethidine. Lancet 1: 1019–1020

Hromada J 1963 On the nerve supply of the connective tissue of some peripheral nervous system components. Acta Anatomica 55: 343–351

Jadad A R, Carroll D, Glynn C J, Moore R A, McQuay H J 1992 Morphine responsiveness of chronic pain: double-blind randomized crossover study with patient-controlled analgesia. Lancet 339: 1367–1371

King R B 1988 Concerning the management of pain associated with herpes zoster and of postherpetic neuralgia. Pain 33: 73–78

Kishore-Kumar R, Max M B, Schafer S C et al 1990 Desipramine relieves post-herpetic neuralgia. Clinical Pharmacology and Therapeutics 47: 305–312

Kocen R S, Thomas P K 1970 Peripheral nerve involvement in Fabry's disease. Archives of Neurology 22: 81–88

Levine J D, Fields H L, Basbaum A I 1993 Peptides and primary afferent nociceptors. Journal of the Neuroscience 13: 2273–2286

Loh L, Nathan P W 1978 Painful peripheral states and sympathetic blocks. Journal of Neurology, Neurosurgery and Psychiatry 41: 664–671

Lombard M C, Larabi Y 1983 Electrophysiological study of cervical dorsal horn cells in partially deafferented rats. In: Bonica J J et al (eds) Advances in pain research and therapy. Raven Press, New York, p 147–154

Lynn B 1990 Capsaicin: actions on nociceptive C-fibers and therapeutic potential. Pain 41: 61–69

McGee J L, Alexander M R 1979 Phenothiazine analgesia – fact or fantasy? American Journal of Hospital Pharmacy 1: 39–49

Max M B, Schafer S C, Culnane M et al 1988 Association of pain relief with drug side effects in postherpetic neuralgia: a single dose study of clonidine codeine, ibuprofen and placebo. Clinical Pharmacology and Therapeutics 43: 363–371

Max M B, Lynch S A, Muir J, Shoaf S E, Smoller B, Dubner R 1992 Effects of desipramine, amitriptyline, and fluoxetine on pain in diabetic neuropathy. New England Journal of Medicine 326: 1250–1256

Melzack R, Wall P D 1965 Pain mechanisms: a new theory. Science 150: 971–978

Meyer G A, Fields H L 1972 Causalgia treated by selective large fibre stimulation of peripheral nerve. Brain 95: 163–168

Mitchell S W 1965 Injuries of nerves and their consequences. Dover Publications, New York

Nashold B S Jr, Ostdahl R H 1979 Dorsal root entry zone lesions for pain relief. Journal of Neurosurgery 51: 59–69

Portenoy R, Foley K 1986 Chronic use of opioid analgesics in non-malignant pain: report of 38 cases. Pain 25: 171–186

Richards R L 1967 Causalgia. Archives of Neurology 16: 339–350

Richelson E, 1990 Antidepressants and brain neurochemistry. Mayo Clinic Proceedings 65: 1227–1236

Rowbotham M C, Fields H L 1989 Topical lidocaine reduces pain in post-herpetic neuralgia. Pain 38: 297–302

Rowbotham M C, Reisner L M, Fields H, L, 1991 Both intravenous lidocaine and morphine reduce the pain of post-herpetic neuralgia. Neurology 41: 1024–1028

Sato J, Perl E R 1991 Adrenergic excitation of cutaneous pain receptors induced by peripheral nerve injury. Science 251: 1608–1610

Scadding J W 1981 Development of ongoing activity, mechanosensitivity, and adrenaline sensitivity in severed peripheral nerve axons. Experimental Neurology 73: 345–364

Sindrup S H, Gram L F, Brosen K et al (1990) The selective serotonin reuptake inhibitor paroxetine is effective in the treatment of diabetic neuropathy symptoms. Pain 42: 135–144

Stow P J, Glynn C J, Minor B 1989 EMLA cream in the treatment of post-herpetic neuralgia. Efficacy and pharmacokinetic profile. Pain 39: 301–305

Tanelian D L, MacIver M B 1991 Analgesic concentrations of lidocaine suppress tonic A-delta and C fibre discharges produced by acute injury. Anesthesiology 74: 934–936

Thomas P K 1974 The anatomical substratum of pain. Canadian Journal of Neurological Sciences 1: 92–97

Wall P D, Gutnick M 1974 Ongoing activity in peripheral nerves: The physiology and pharmacology of impulses originating from a neuroma. Experimental Neurology 43: 580–593

Watson C P N, Evans R J 1992 The postmastectomy pain syndrome and topical capsaicin: a randomized trial. Pain 51: 375–375

Watson C P N, Evans R J, Watt V R 1988 Post-herpetic neuralgia and topical capsaicin. Pain 33: 333–340

Welk E, Leah J D, Zimmerman M 1990 Characteristics of A- and C-fibers ending in a sensory nerve neuroma in the rat. Journal of Neurophysiology 63: 759–766

Wynn-Parry C B 1980 Pain in avulsion lesions of the brachial plexus. Pain 9: 41–53

52. Local anaesthesia and regional blocks

J. J. Bonica and S. H. Butler

INTRODUCTION

Local and regional analgesia, achieved by injecting a local anaesthetic into tissues, or in proximity to certain parts of the peripheral nervous system, to relieve pain has been used for nearly a century (Bonica 1953). For many years these various techniques were used in an empirical and often haphazard fashion resulting not infrequently in failures and, at times, complications. Fortunately, during the past 30 years a number of factors have helped to clarify their proper role as diagnostic and therapeutic tools in managing patients with acute and chronic pain. During this period, much new scientific knowledge has been acquired about pain and a variety of new therapeutic modalities have been developed which have altered the role of nerve blocks in pain therapy. Nevertheless, while nerve blocks no longer have the preeminent role of three to four decades ago, when properly applied they remain a useful tool in managing patients with acute, chronic and cancer pain.

The purpose of this chapter is to present an updated version of the material presented in the last (second) edition of this textbook. A significant portion of the text is taken from the second edition of *The Management of Pain* and is reproduced with permission of the publishers. This includes a brief discussion of the indications, efficacy, side-effects, complications and techniques, of local analgesia and regional nerve blocks. There have been few changes in the book since the second edition but rather the important areas are application with an increasing interest in their use for acute pain states (US Department of Health 1992). This is well detailed in other chapters, notably by Cousins in Chapter 19. Because the painful conditions for which these procedures are used are described in detail elsewhere in this book, only brief mention is made of them here. The material will be presented in the following order:

1. fundamental considerations, including basic, general indications and basic principles of application
2. block of spinal nerves distal to their exit from the spinal canal and their distal branches
3. block of cranial nerves.

The technical aspects of local and regional analgesia are presented very briefly and consist of illustrations and concise discussion of technique in the figure legend. This is not intended to provide instructions to readers who wish to learn to apply these procedures, because this requires much more information available in books devoted to regional anaesthesia and, most importantly, requires personal instruction by experienced teachers. This is to conform with Bonica's long-held conviction that anyone managing patients with pain should be acquainted with *all* therapeutic modalities currently available (Bonica 1953, 1955, 1958, 1959, 1974, 1990). Only with such knowledge and broad perspective is a physician able to inform and guide the patient. Rather, the objective of including the techniques in this chapter is to give readers who do not practise regional anaesthesia an idea of what the procedure entails, as well as discussing the indications, advantages, disadvantages and complications. Detailed description of these techniques can be found in textbooks on the subject (Bonica 1953, 1990; Moore 1979; Winnie 1983; Cousins & Bridenbaugh 1988).

With renewed interest in acute pain therapy, especially perioperative pain, more research is proving the benefits of regional anaesthesia used pre-, intra- and postoperatively. Those beneficial effects have been documented in many areas, including the surgical stress response, blood loss, postoperative thromboembolism, intraoperative and postoperative cardiovascular problems, pulmonary complications, gastrointestinal function, not to mention marked improvement in pain relief and a decrease in narcotic consumption. This information is detailed in Chapter 19.

FUNDAMENTAL CONSIDERATIONS

BASIS FOR USE

The basis for the efficacy and utility of local analgesia and somatic nerve blocks in patients with acute or chronic pain is the interruption of nociceptive input at its very source or the blocking of nociceptive impulses coursing in peripheral nerve fibres. In addition, blockade may interrupt the afferent and efferent limbs of abnormal reflex mechanisms which contribute to the pathophysiology of some pain syndromes. Moreover, since sympathetic fibres destined for somatic structures, particularly the limbs, course through somatic spinal nerves, the blocking of these nerves may be used to eliminate sympathetic hyperactivity which often contributes to the pathophysiology of certain pain syndromes.

Low concentrations of local anaesthetics block the unmyelinated C- and B- fibres and small myelinated A-delta fibres with only minor or no interruption of somatic motor function. On the other hand, in certain conditions it may be useful to block somatomotor nerves to relieve severe muscle spasm. By producing one or more of these effects, there is often prompt relief of pain which may last for varying periods of time, depending on the concentration and characteristics of the local anaesthetic used. Moreover, in certain conditions, the pain relief outlasts by hours, and sometimes days and weeks, the transient pharmacological action of the local anaesthetics. It has been suggested that the blocking of sensory input for several hours stops the self-sustaining activity of the neuron pools in the neuraxis which may be responsible for some chronic pain states (Bonica 1953, 1990, Melzack 1971). In recent years animal experiments and clinical studies have shown that infiltration of the site of operation with a local anaesthetic or block of the nerves that supply the site carried out before the initiation of the operation prevents or markedly reduces the incidence and intensity of pain and the delay of normal functional activity that invariably follow some surgical procedures. This beneficial action which some have called 'preemptive analgesia' is achieved by block of the nociceptive input to the spinal cord that occurs from stimulation of afferents particularly of C-fibres that supply periosteum, A-delta innervated joints, muscles and structures around them. Even with general anaesthesia, this massive afferent barrage produces sensitization decreasing the threshold of not only peripheral nociceptive receptors but also dorsal horn neurons, intraneurons and anterior motor neurons (see Bonica 1990 for detailed description of the pathophysiological process). Therefore, these procedures can be used as diagnostic, prognostic, prophylactic and/or therapeutic measures as summarized in Table 52.1.

Table 52.1 Indications for nerve blocks with local anaesthetics

1. *Diagnostic blocks*
   a. Ascertain specific nociceptive pathways
   b. Help determine mechanism of chronic pain syndromes
   c. Aid differential diagnosis of the site and cause of pain
   d. Determine patient's reaction to pain relief
2. *Prognostic blocks*
   a. Predict the effects of neurolytic blocks or neurosurgery
   b. Afford the patient an opportunity to experience the numbness and other side-effects that follow destructive procedures and thus help patient decide whether or not to have it done
3. *Therapeutic blocks*
   a. Control severe acute postoperative, posttraumatic pain and pain from self-limiting diseases
   b. Breaking of 'vicious circle' involved in some pain syndromes may provide prolonged relief
   c. Provide temporary relief to permit other therapies, or used in combination with other therapies

DIAGNOSTIC BLOCKS

Neural blockade can be used as part of an integrated diagnostic process and specific nerve block procedures can be useful in helping the physician to obtain information and attain the goals listed above and presented here.

Determination of source of pain and nociceptive pathways

Local infiltration and block of small or large nerves or plexuses can provide information about the source of the pain and the pathways that mediate the nociceptive impulses. Thus, prompt and complete relief of pain following two or three direct injections of a dilute solution of local anaesthetic into a trigger point, painful scar, neuroma, joint (e.g. a facet or temporomandibular joint) or spasmodic muscle helps to determine the source of pain and helps in making the diagnosis. Similarly, prompt relief of pain following injection of 2–3 ml of a local anaesthetic on a spinal nerve as it exits from its intervertebral foramen provides information about the nociceptive pathway(s) involved in the projected pain caused by a herniated intervertebral disc, osteophytes, fracture of the vertebra or other vertebral pathology.

Visceral versus somatic pain

In most patients a complete history and physical examination are sufficient to differentiate pain in the chest, abdomen or pelvis caused by visceral disease from pain in the chest wall, abdominal wall or somatic structures of the pelvis caused by pathology. In patients who present confusing symptoms and signs, however, blockade of the thoracic intercostal nerves at the posterior axillary line relieves pain caused by pathological processes in the ribs or anterior chest wall but does not relieve pain caused by disease of the thoracic viscera, the nociceptive pathways of which pass through the sympathetic nerves close to the vertebral column. Because pain in the epigastrium can be caused by disease of the thoracic viscera or of the upper abdominal viscera or by pathology in the ribs, cartilages, or soft tissue or nerves that supply the abdominal wall, blocks can be used to differentiate among these three sources of pain. Thus, blockade of the T6–T9 nerves at the posterior axillary line relieves pain arising in the abdominal wall but does not relieve pain caused by visceral disease. If such a procedure does not relieve the pain, the visceral source of the pain can be ascertained by blocking the upper thoracic sympathetic chain (T1 to T5 or T6), a technique that relieves pain arising from the thoracic viscera. This procedure, however, does not relievie pain arising from the abdominal viscera because these are supplied by afferent fibres contained in the thoracic splanchnic nerves (T6–T12), which can be interrupted by a coeliac plexus or splanchnic nerve block. The various pathophysiological conditions for which these procedures can be used as diagnostic tools are dicussed in more detail below.

Local versus referred somatic pain

In addition to differentiating referred pain arising from visceral disease from pain caused by somatic pathology, nerve blocks can also be used to differentiate referred pain in somatic structures that is caused by a distant somatic pathological process from pain arising locally. Thus, pain referred to the knee is frequently caused by a pathological process in the head and neck of the femur. Such pain can be relieved by injection of an anaesthetic into the hip joint or by blockade of the nerves that supply the joint. Similarly, pathology in a facet joint in the lumbar region can cause pain referred to the low back, thigh or even the leg and this can be relieved by injection of the facet joint or of the medial branches of the posterior primary division that supply the joint. This procedure does not relieve pain caused by pathology at the site of referred pain, but this can be relieved by infiltration into the area of the pain.

Sympathetic versus somatic origin of peripheral pain

Sympathetic hyperactivity can cause or contribute to pain by the following mechanisms:

1. Sensitization of peripheral nociceptors
2. Production of vasoconstriction with subsequent local ischaemia, which causes direct nociceptor stimulation
3. Reflex changes involving afferent and efferent fibres
4. Coupling between noradrenergic postganglionic fibres and afferent fibres at the site of the lesion in tissue or a nerve trunk
5. Liberation of norepinephrine by postganglionic axon terminals, possibly leading to the release of prostaglandins that in turn decrease the threshold of nociceptive afferents (Janig 1988)
6. Sensitization of wide dynamic range neurons in the dorsal horn and other parts of the neuraxis
7. Other mechanisms.

Recent evidence (Bengtsson & Bengtsson 1988) also indicates that sympathetic hyperactivity contributes to the development and maintenance of trigger points of myofascial pain syndromes. Moreover, sympathetic hyperactivity can cause inhibition of the gastrointestinal and genitourinary tracts with consequent ileus and a decrease in urinary output, both of which can be a source of abdominal or suprapubic pain.

The role of sympathetic hyperactivity in causing these changes can be ascertained by blocking the regional sympathetic supply to various structures at anatomical sites that are separate from somatic nerve fibres. Thus, paravertebral block of the T2 and T3 sympathetic ganglia relieves pain in the upper limb as a result of reflex sympathetic dystrophy without involving roots of the branchial plexus. Similarly, blockade of the lumbar sympathetic chain relieves sympathetically maintained pain in the foot or leg without involving the roots of somatic nerves. Injection of neuromata, painful scars, trigger points or other sites of localized disease usually results in a pure somatic block. Blockade of the lateral femoral cutaneous nerve to help establish the diagnosis of meralgia paraesthetica or blockade of the saphenous nerve at the ankle also results in a purely somatic block.

Peripheral versus central pain

Various techniques can be used to differentiate peripheral pain from central pain that is caused by pathology in the neuraxis. As already mentioned, evidence now shows that blockade of afferent and efferent nerves or intravenous injection of local anaesthetics can be helpful in providing transient partial relief of central pain (Boas et al 1982). Another technique is the use of 'differential' subarachnoid or epidural blockade extended to the T1 thoracic spinal segment, which should eliminate pain of peripheral origin. This procedure is unlikely to eliminate pain caused by disease of the spinal cord or brainstem completely, however, and the efficacy of such methods has been questioned. A recently introduced technique is a diagnostic epidural opioid block that might prove useful in differentiating peripheral from central pain and pain primarily of psychological origin from pain arising from other sources.

Reaction to pain relief

Most patients, especially those with severe pain, are grateful when pain is relieved following neural blockade. Some patients with mild or moderate pain that is being used for secondary or tertiary gains, however, might become alarmed by the realization that the pain could be permanently eliminated. Although such instances are rare they do occur and require that the physician, with the help of nurses and others, evaluates the effects of the pain relief on patients' behaviour and attitudes. At the other end of the spectrum are patients whose severe pain is caused by a musculoskeletal injury and who, on relief of pain, might disgregard the physician's advice and resume strenuous activity prematurely before healing at the injury site has occured.

Prognostic blocks

The primary purpose of prognostic nerve blocks is to afford patients an opportunity to experience the sensory changes and other effects that follow neuro-ablative surgical procedures or neurolytic blocks, thus helping patients to decide whether or not to undergo such a procedure. It was previously believed that a single block with a local anaesthetic could predict the pain-relieving effects of a neurosurgical section or neurolytic block. Ample clinical evidence now shows, however, that one such block does not predict the *long-term* effects of neurosurgical section, such as spinal posterior rhizotomy (Loeser 1972). Loeser (1972) noted that, whereas the pain relief obtained immediately after a spinal posterior rhizotomy was similar to that obtained after a prior prognostic paravertebral block of certain spinal segments, many of the patients had a return of their pain in the months following the operation. It is not known whether the return of pain was the result of an incomplete operation (i.e. the nociceptive fibres in the anterior root were not divided), regeneration of the nerve or the development of other new nociceptive pathways or other mechanisms. In many patients the decision to carry out the surgical rhizotomy was done on the basis of the results of one prognostic block, an error that Bonica considers to be a 'cardinal sin' in this field. In any case, we believe that prognostic blocks continued for 2–3 days (by continuous techniques) are still useful, not only in providing patients with the experience of sensory change but also in predicting the effects of neurolytic blockade in patients with cancer pain whose life expectancy is limited.

Prophylactic blocks

Various nerve blocks are used to prevent pain and thus prevent or minimize the delay of return to normal functional activity that often follows trauma, infections or operations. In some centres nerve block procedures are considered to be one of the most efficient methods for controlling postoperative or posttraumatic pain and result in earlier functional rehabilitation, prevention of complications and shorter hospitalization (Pflug et al 1974; see Ch. 19). Blockade of nociceptive afferent and efferent pathways in patients with acute pancreatitis, ileus or other visceral disorders relieves pain, decreases morbidity and possibly decreases mortality. In addition, evidence has shown that analgesia achieved with regional block for several days prior to the operation can decrease the incidence of phantom limb pain following amputation, reflex sympathetic dystrophy and other chronic pain syndromes (Bach et al 1988). As previously mentioned, there is now evidence that infiltration of the proposed site of the operation for blockade of the nerves supplying the site prevents or reduces the incidence and intensity of pain and the delay of normal functional activity that follows posttraumatically, postoperatively and postinfection. In the last several years, a number of reports have suggested that, during back operation or other major procedures carried out with general anaesthesia, a massive nociceptive input into the spinal cord occurs from noxious stimulation of afferents, particularly of the L5 roots that supply periosteum, richly innervate joints, muscles and structures around them. Moreover, this operation entails severance of or injury to small peripheral nerves which generate a brief maximal injury discharge that triggers prolonged spinal cord hyperexcitability. This sensitizies spinal cord nociceptive specific cells as well as cells that respond to both light and intense stimulation–wide-dynamic-range (WDR) neurons. All of this facilitation is triggered by the arrival of impulses at the L5 level of the dorsal horn. It is sustained by an intrinsic spinal cord process. Consequently, tactile and nociceptor afferent activity by nonnoxious stimulation causes intense activation of the anterior horn cells that produce muscle spasm. This, together with activation of dorsal horn, causes the excruciating pain. A number of studies have shown that carrying out local infiltration or nerve block before starting the operation is much more effective than the procedures used postoperatively. Studies have shown that this preemptive analgesia not only provides pain relief but results in earlier functional rehabilitation, prevention or reduction of complications and shorter hospitalization.

Therapeutic blocks

A recent study by Levine and colleagues showed that pain can contribute to morbidity in a disease model of experimental arthritis in rats which typically lost weight and were considerably less active than normal rats. To test the hypothesis that pain contributed to the general morbidity of the rats with experimental arthritis, the major ascending nociceptive transmission pathways in the ventrolateral funiculus of the spinal cord were interrupted and the effect on weight loss and decrease in activity were noted. It was found that following the relief of pain, the treated rats had significantly less weight loss and decrease in activity as compared to those in the control group. These data provide strong evidence that the pain that accompanies various disease states makes an important contribution to morbidity and should therefore be eliminated promptly.

BASIS FOR USE OF NEURAL BLOCKADE

The primary reason for the effectiveness and usefulness of neural blockade in patients with acute or chronic pain is the interruption of nociceptive input at its source or the blocking of nociceptive fibres coursing in peripheral nerves. Blockade also interrupts the afferent limb of abnormal reflex mechanisms that may contribute to the pathogenesis of some chronic pain syndromes. Moreover, sympathetic blockade may be used to eliminate sympathetic hyperactivity that often contributes to the pathophysiology of postoperative and posttraumatic pain and plays an important role in chronic pain syndromes. In addition, through changes in peripheral blood flow, sympathetic blocks may decrease tissue damage and re-establish tissue homeostasis. By using low concentrations of the local anaesthetic, blockade of the unmyelinated C- and B-preganglionic fibres and of the small myelinated A-delta nociceptive fibres is achieved, with only minimal effect on somatic motor function. On the other hand, in certain conditions it may be useful to block somatomotor nerves to relieve severe skeletal muscle spasm.

By producing one or more of these effects, there is often prompt relief of pain that may last for varying periods of time, depending on the characteristic of the local anaesthetic used. Moreover, in certain conditions, the pain relief outlasts by hours, and sometimes days and weeks, the transient pharmacological action of the local anaesthetic. Melzack has suggested that the blockade of sensory input for several hours stops the self-sustaining activity of the neuron pools in the neuraxis that may be responsible for some chronic pain states. Based on the concept of 'hyperstimulation analgesia' first described by Melzack et al (1977), it has been suggested that neural blockade may alter or 'jam' a pattern of central neural activities.

There are two other points on which agreement has been reached regarding the role of neural blockade in patients with multiple physical and emotional impairments:

1. because such patients usually have difficulty in accepting the idea that their discomfort is related to psychological/emotional factors, targeting of a medical intervention at the pain location may facilitate the patient's willingness to undertake psychophysiological rehabilitation
2. when structured as part of the behavioural modification programme, nerve blocking enhances the patient–physician relationship and strengthens the physician's role as an educator who reinforces the global roles of rehabilitation.

INDICATIONS FOR CLINICAL APPLICATION

Neural blockade may be used as a diagnostic, prognostic, prophylactic or therapeutic tool.

Diagnostic blocks

Certain nerve blocks are useful in ascertaining specific nociceptive pathways, differentiating referred from local pain, and determining the possible mechanisms of chronic pain states. Nerve block is also useful in the differential diagnosis of the site and cause of the pain and in determining the reaction if the pain is eliminated. Blockade of the appropriate nerves helps to differentiate trigeminal neuralgia from atypical facial neuralgia, neuralgia involving the third division of trigeminal nerve from glossopharyngeal or vagal neuralgia, and pain due to visceral disease from pain of somatic origin. For example, complete relief of chest or epigastric pain following intercostal nerve block at the midaxillary line suggests that the pain is of somatic origin in the chest or abdominal wall, whereas lack of relief suggests that it is a pain referred from viscera.

Prognostic blocks

Properly applied, certain nerve blocks may be used prior to prolonged interruption either by injection of neurolytic agents or by neurosurgical section. Moreover, prognostic blocks may give patients an opportunity to experience the numbness and other side-effects following surgery or neurolytic block and help them to decide whether to have the procedure. Although clinical evidence suggests that this tool has certain limitations in predicting the long-term effects of spinal rhizotomy, it is still useful, especially when prolonged interruption is to be carried out in patients with cancer pain.

Prophylactic blocks

A variety of nerve blocks are used to prevent pain and the delay of normal functional activity that follows trauma, infections or operations. In some centres, nerve block procedures are considered some of the most efficient methods for controlling postoperative or posttraumatic pain, thus effecting earlier functional rehabilitation and preventing complications. Moreover, there is evidence that analgesia achieved with regional blockade for several days decreases the incidence of reflex sympathetic dystrophy and other chronic pain syndromes.

Therapeutic blocks

Local anaesthesia and nerve blocks using local anaesthetics are effective in treating self-limiting disease accompanied by severe pain and in breaking up the so-called 'vicious circle' in patients with causalgia and reflex sympathetic dystrophy, myofascial syndromes and reflex muscle spasm. It provides symptomatic relief to permit other therapeutic measures or to use as an adjunct to other therapeutic modalities. Therapeutic blocks with neurolytic agents are usually limited to patients with cancer pain, although they may be indicated in selected patients with trigeminal neuralgia, causalgia, chronic pancreatitis, severe angina pectoris or other chronic disorders in patients who cannot tolerate a neurosurgical operation. Neurolytic blocks are especially useful in patients with chronic peripheral vascular disease.

BASIC PRINCIPLES OF APPLICATION

The aforementioned failures and complications of the past resulted from a number of deficiencies in the application of this method by anaesthetists and other physicians (Bonica 1953: Cousins & Bridenbaugh 1990). These included:

1. Inadequate knowledge of pain syndromes
2. Inadequate evaluation of patients
3. Lack of knowledge of other therapeutic modalities that might be used in each patient
4. Inadequate management of the patient before, during and after the block
5. Lack of appreciation of the specific indications, limitations and possible complications of these procedures

Requisite for optimal results

The realization that many practitioners are unfamiliar with these problems prompted Bonica, as soon as he began to use these tools, to develop certain basic principles which he first stated in 1953 and which have been repeatedly confirmed with greater conviction with the results of increasing experience (Bonica 1955, 1958, 1959, 1974, 1990). These are listed in Table 52.2

Table 52.2 Basic principles of application of nerve block

1. Physicians using this method must have ample knowledge of pain syndromes and of all diagnostic and therapeutic measures that can be applied to each patient; knowledge of advantages, disadvantages, limitations and complications of each modality provides the broad perspective essential to decide the best therapy or combination of therapies
2. Physicians must be willing and able to devote necessary time and effort to evaluate patient through history, general physical and neurological examination and other studies, even when patient referred by respected colleagues
3. Physicians must be highly skilled in the technique and have thorough knowledge of:
   a. Anatomical basis of the procedure
   b. Pharmacology of the local anaesthetics
   c. Side-effects and possible complications of each procedure and how to prevent and treat them *promptly*
4. Patients must be fully informed of what, how and why the block is being done:
   a. Unless patients realise that the procedure is done only to gain information rather than to cure, he/she may be disappointed prematurely and may not return for futher care
   b. Patients must be assured that all will be done to minimize discomfort

Diagnostic/prognostic blocks require:
   a. Precise localization of nerve blocks with X-ray or image intensifier with or without prior injection of contrast medium
   b. Injection of small (2–4 ml) volumes of local anaesthetic to avoid spillage to adjacent nerves which may give misleading information
   c. No decisions should be made until two or three blocks produce consistent results
   d. Use local anaesthetics of different duration and correlate duration of block with duration of subjective pain relief (placebo block may be included)

Careful assessment of patients and results by physician, nurses and others:
   a. Reaction of the patient to needle insertion and other manipulation to help evaluate 'pain threshold'
   b. Ascertain if intended nerves have been blocked
   c. Evaluate efficacy of block in relieving pain and pathophysiology, and duration of the relief
   d. Record results in detail in patient's chart

Consider the results of diagnostic/prognostic block within the framework of all other information acquired; to make final decision on basis of the results of only one or two blocks is conducive to error and to performing useless, destructive procedures

General principles concerning agents and techniques

A thorough knowledge of pharmacology and optimal concentration of local anaesthetic agents is required for their proper use. Table 52.3 lists the most common local anaesthetics in current use, together with the clinical characteristics and optimal concentrations for various procedures as well as the maximum therapeutic dose. It deserves emphasis that the practice of many physicians in using higher concentrations, such as 1% procaine or 1% lidocaine or 0.25% bupivacaine, for local infiltration is unnecessary because the local anaesthetic promptly comes into contact with bare nerve endings which are easily and rapidly blocked with much lower concentrations. The lower concentration for nerve block is sufficient for blockade of A-delta and C-fibres, while the high concentration will produce blockade of many somatomotor fibres (Bonica 1959; Covino & Vassallo 1976).

For diagnostic and prognostic purposes short-acting agents may be used, but, for therapeutic action, long-lasting agents such as bupivacaine are best.

In regard to technique, it is essential to have high-quality equipment, including sharp needles of proper length, well-fitting syringes, high-quality local anaesthetics in the proper concentrations and other drugs and equipment necessary for the procedure (Fig. 52.1) and for prompt treatment of complications (Fig. 52.2). Just

Table 52.3 Clinical characteristics and dosage of local anaesthetics

	Procaine (Novocaine)	2-Chloroprocaine (Nesacaine)	Lidocaine (Xylocaine)	Mepivacaine (Carbocaine)	Prilocaine (Citanest)	Tetracaine (Pontocaine)	Bupivacaine (Marcaine)	Etidocaine (Duranest)
Latency (speed of onset)	Moderate	Fast	Fast	Moderate	Moderate	Very slow	Fast	Very fast
Penetration (diffusibility)	Moderate	Marked	Marked	Moderate	Moderate	Poor	Moderate	Moderate
Duration	Short	Very short	Moderate	Moderate	Moderate	Long	Long	Long
Optimal concentrations (%)								
Infiltration	0.5	0.5	0.25	0.25	0.25	0.05	0.05	0.1
Spinal nerve and plexus block	1.5–2	1.0–2	0.5–1.0	0.5–1.0	0.5–1.0	0.1–0.2	0.25–0.5	0.5–1.0
Maximum amount (mg/kg)	12	15	6	6	6	2	2	2

prior to the blockade, details of the procedure should be repeated to the patient, written consent for the procedure obtained and vital signs measured and recorded. If the neurological examination has not been done, it should be carried out to determine sensory, motor or reflex dysfunctions. The patient should be placed in the position which best facilitates execution of the block and allows the greatest amount of comfort possible. Obviously, these invasive procedures require that sterile techniques be used, including application of appropriate antiseptic to the skin and proper draping. Prior to the insertion of large needles, the skin should be anaesthetized by injecting a small amount of dilute local anaesthetic with a thin (26- or 30-gauge) needle into the skin to produce what is usually called a 'skin wheal'.

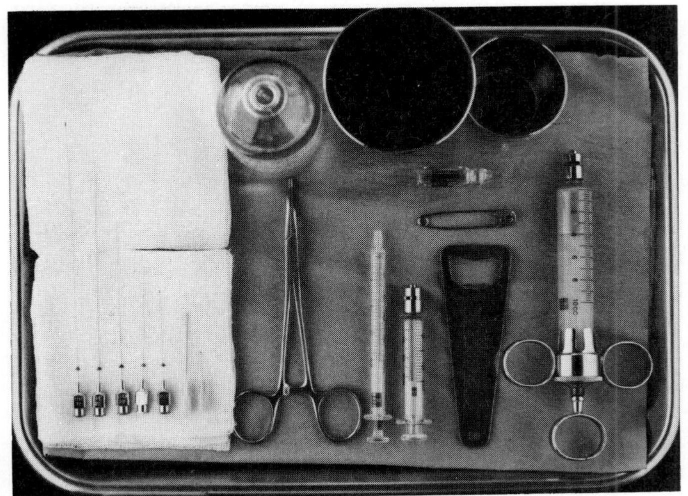

Fig. 52.1 Equipment for local anaesthesia and nerve blocks. From left to right: 22-gauge 15-cm, 12-cm, 8-cm and 5-cm needles; 25-gauge 4-cm needle, 3-cm, 0.5-cm disposable needles; ring forceps, to grasp sponges to apply antiseptic solution to the skin; 1 ml tuberculin syringe to measure accurately adrenalin solution; 2-ml Luer-Lok syringe for injection of small volumes and, if preferable, to carry out aspiration tests; bottle opener to use in opening sterile bottles of saline shown above or bottles of local anaesthetics which are sterilized as separate units to provide flexibility of selecting the optimal local anaesthetic agent; Luer-Lok control syringe best used for any regional anaesthetic block because it facilitates aspiration and other manoeuvres with one hand; above the bottle opener is a safety-pin used for skin testing and above that an ampoule of adrenalin 1:1000(1 mg). The containers in the uppermost part of the figure include (left to right) one for the antiseptic, the middle one for saline to dilute the local anaesthetic to any desired concentration and the one on the right is for the local anaesthetic.

SIDE-EFFECTS AND COMPLICATIONS OF LOCAL AND REGIONAL ANALGESIA

A number of the procedures that will be described have side-effects and some are associated with complications of varying severity. To avoid repetition with each procedure the following complications will be briefly considered:

1. Systemic toxic reactions
2. Other systemic reactions
3. Very high or total spinal anaesthesia
4. Pneumothorax
5. Neurological complications.

It deserves reemphasis that none of these procedures should be done by staff unable to diagnose promptly and treat these complications. Moreover, other than infiltration of 3–5 ml of dilute solution into superficial structures, *no block should be done without:*

1. having an intravenous infusion running for prompt injection of therapeutic drugs
2. having an assistant present to help with the therapy
3. *having resuscitative drugs and equipment for immediate use.*

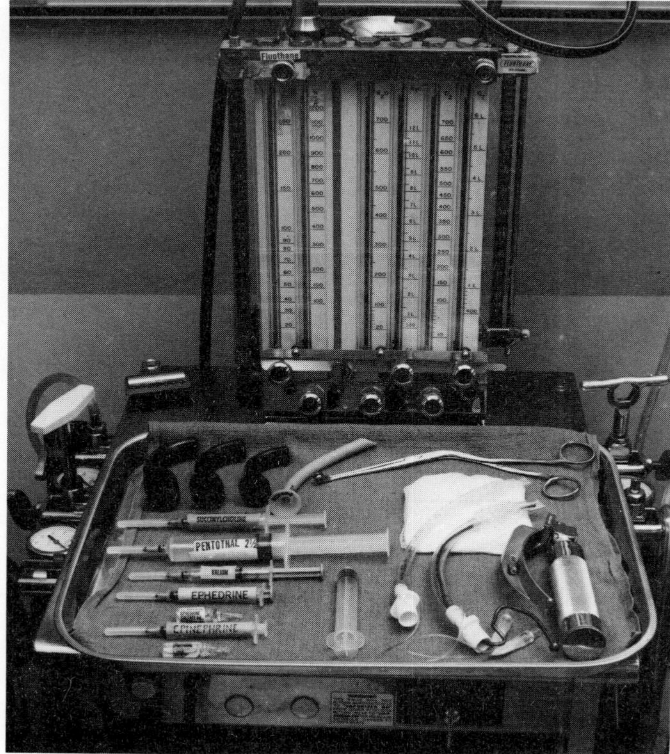

Fig. 52.2 Equipment and drugs needed to treat complications of nerve blocks. A tray placed on top of the anaesthetic machine contains ampoules and syringes to administer adrenalin (epinephrine), ephedrine, diazepam (Valium), thiopental (Pentothal) or succinylcholine. Behind these are different sizes of oropharyngeal and nasopharyngeal airways. On the right, the tray contains a Macintosh laryngoscope, two endotracheal tubes, a Macintosh forceps to guide tubes into the trachea and a syringe to inflate the cuff of the endotracheal tube. The anaesthetic machine is equipped with tubes and mask to permit immediate administration of oxygen.

Systemic toxic reactions to local anaesthetic

Systemic toxic reactions to local anaesthetic result from:

1. injection of an excessive dose
2. accidental intravenous injection of a therapeutic dose
3. abnormal rates of absorption and biotransformation.

Toxic reactions to the local anaesthetic may be arbitrarily classified as mild, moderate and severe. *Mild* reactions occur when the blood level of the drug is just above therapeutic limits and are manifested by palpitation, a metallic taste, dryness of the mouth and throat, tinnitus, vertigo, dysarthria and confusion. *Moderate* reactions are manifested by severe confusion and muscular twitchings that progress to convulsions. *Severe* reactions result from massive overdosage of the drug and are manifested by severe hypotension, bradycardia and respiratory depression which may progress to cardiovascular standstill and respiratory arrest.

Preventive measures include:

1. using the lowest concentration and volume of local anaesthetic that assures good results (Table 52.3)
2. use of adrenaline 1:200 000 in the solution to retard the rate of local anaesthetic absorption
3. repeated aspiration to ascertain that the needle point is not in a blood vessel prior to each injection
4. prior to injecting large amounts, inject 3 ml of solution as a test dose; if injection is intravenous the 15 μg of adrenaline in the solution will cause transient (30–90 s) tachycardia and hypertension (Bonica et al 1971; Moore & Batra 1981).

Treatment

Treatment of mild reactions includes encouragement of the patient and administration of oxygen. Convulsions must be treated *immediately* so that the patient does not suffer asphyxia, because as long as the patient is convulsing he/she is not ventilating adequately. Oxygen is administered promptly under positive pressure and muscular hyperactivity is controlled by intravenous injection of 40–80 mg succinylcholine. If any difficulty is encountered in keeping the airway patent, tracheal intubation is promptly carried out. In addition, 5–10 mg diazepam or 50–100 mg thiopental should be given intravenously to control seizure activity of the cerebral cortex and additional increments of these drugs given as needed. Severe reactions require support of the circulation with fluids, vasopressors and artificial ventilation.

Other systemic reactions

Undesirable systemic reactions to local and regional analgesia frequently occur from causes other than systemic toxicity produced by the local anaesthetic. These include psychogenic reactions, epinephrine reactions, allergic reactions and idiosyncratic reactions.

Psychogenic reactions

Psychogenic reactions constitute the most frequent undesirable response to local and regional analgesia. Such reactions are usually caused by fear and apprehension regarding the block procedure and frequently occur in the dentist's office, especially in a patient who is in a sitting position. They are usually manifested by dizziness, faintness, occasionally ringing in the ears, marked perspiration, tachycardia, paleness of the skin, and marked arterial hypotension, which can cause loss of consciousness. A characteristic of this type of reaction is that it occurs as soon as the procedure is initiated, even before any needle is inserted into the skin or any solution is injected, sometimes causing the reaction to be labelled by the misinformed as a sensitivity or 'allergic' reaction. Treatment consists of placing the patient in the recumbent position, administering oxygen and, if the hypotension is moderate to severe, giving small i.v. increments of ephedrine.

Adrenaline (epinephrine) reactions

Another common cause of reactions, especially those that occur in the dentist's chair, is overdosage of adrenaline or of some other vasoconstrictor. The patient can experinece an extreme degree of palpitation, tachycardia, dizziness, perspiration and paleness of the skin. Treatment consists of the administration of a small dose of a fast-acting barbiturate to allay apprehension and to reduce the blood pressure to normal limits. If the hypertension is severe it might be necessary to administer a vasodilator such as nitroglycerine, amyl nitrite or sodium nitrate, or to use a more potent ganglionic blocking agent.

Allergic reactions

Allergic reactions to local anaesthetics occur rarely following repeated exposure, as occurs in dentistry, and with the use of procaine or other paraaminobenzoic acid esters. They rarely, if ever, are caused by amide compounds, such as lidocaine. The patient can experience generalized urticaria, joint pains and oedema, particularly of the eyelids, hands, joints and larynx. Treatment consists of the administration of antihistamines or adrenaline. The patient should then be observed closely for severe laryngeal oedema; if this occurs it might be necessary to carry out a tracheostomy.

Idiosyncratic (anaphylaxis hypersensitivity) reactions

On extremely rare occasions the administration of small amounts of a local anaesthetic, properly given, can result in sudden cardiovascular and respiratory collapse, possibly followed rapidly by death. Although such a phenomenon could presumably occur with the use of local anaesthetics, the incidence must be extremely rare; Bonica, with 45 years of experience, has never seen or heard of one. Such a reaction must be classified as idiosyncratic because it occurs rarely and bears no relation to dosage. Treatment is the same as that described for severe toxic reactions and includes prompt artificial ventilation with oxygen, administration of vasopressors and, if necessary, cardiac massage.

Very high or total spinal anaesthesia

Very high or total spinal anaesthesia, and consequent respiratory paralysis and hypotension, may develop from accidental subarachnoid injections during attempts at paravertebral block. Within a few minutes of such an accident, there is a rapid development of bilateral analgesia and, if more than 3–4 ml of solution has been used, it will ascend rapidly to involve the cervical and cranial nerves, especially if the injection is in the upper thoracic or cervical region. The patient usually becomes restless, drowsy, dyspnoeic, is unable to speak, develops apnoea and may lose consciousness.

Preventive measures include aspiration before injection and observing the needle for passive cerebrospinal fluid flow after the syringe has been detached.

Treatment consists of:

1. prompt artificial ventilation through an endotracheal tube
2. support of blood pressure with fluids and intravenous ephedrine administered in increments of 5–10 mg
3. prompt removal of 5–15 ml of cerebrospinal fluid, depending on the amount of drug injected, in order to remove as much drug as possible before it becomes fixed to spinal nerve roots.

If these measures are carried out, there is rapid regression of the spinal anaesthetic and no residual morbidity.

Pneumothorax

Pneumothorax may occur as a complication of thoracic paravertebral, intercostal or supraclavicular brachial plexus block if the needle is advanced too deeply and the lung is punctured. This will produce a bronchopleural fistula through which air is aspirated into the pleural cavity during inspiration. Using the techniques described in the pages that follow, and exercising proper precautions, the incidence of pneumothorax should be less than 1% (Bonica 1953; Moore 1955, 1971, 1975). Signs and symptoms are usually apparent within a short interval of lung puncture, but they may not appear until as late as 12 hours after the puncture. A patient with less than 15–20% pneumothorax may have only mild pain in the chest accentuated by deep breathing and occasional cough, but with a larger amount of lung collapse, the pain is more severe and the patient becomes dyspnoeic and hypoxic. An upright X-ray of the chest should be taken to confirm the diagnosis and, if negative, it should be repeated in several hours. Treatment of mild pneumothorax consists of sedation, reassurance and bedrest. Moderate or severe cases require systemic analgesics, aspiration of air from the pleura, underwater negative pressure drainage and the administration of 100% oxygen under slight pressure to assist reexpansion of the lung.

Hypotension

This complication is usually due to extensive vasomotor blockade consequent to extensive subarachnoid or epidural block. It occurs rarely with local infiltration or peripheral nerve block and only when excessive doses of local anaesthetics are used.

Neurological complications

Gentle contact with a nerve or plexus by the point of a needle to elicit paraesthesia is very unlikely to cause neurological sequelae, and if such complications do occur after nerve block with local anaesthetic other causes should be considered (Dhuner 1950; Bonica 1953; Swerdlow 1988). The incidence of such nerve dysfunction has been reported to be 0.35% or less (Bonica 1953; Moore 1955, 1971; Winchell & Wolfe 1985; Swerdlow 1988). On the other hand, if there are repeated insertions of needles with long bevels or hooks into the nerve, or a rapid intraneural injection, transient nerve dysfunction may develop. In such cases signs of neuropathy may appear 1 week or more after the block, become maximal in about 3 weeks, and begin to diminish after 2–3 months; complete recovery of nerve function usually occurs (Lofstrom et al 1966). To minimize the occurrence of such complication following peripheral nerve block, it is recommended that short-bevelled (45°) needles be used, that location of the nerve be achieved by very gentle paraesthesiae or by use of a nerve stimulator and that the concentration of the local anaesthetic listed in Table 52.3 not be exceeded.

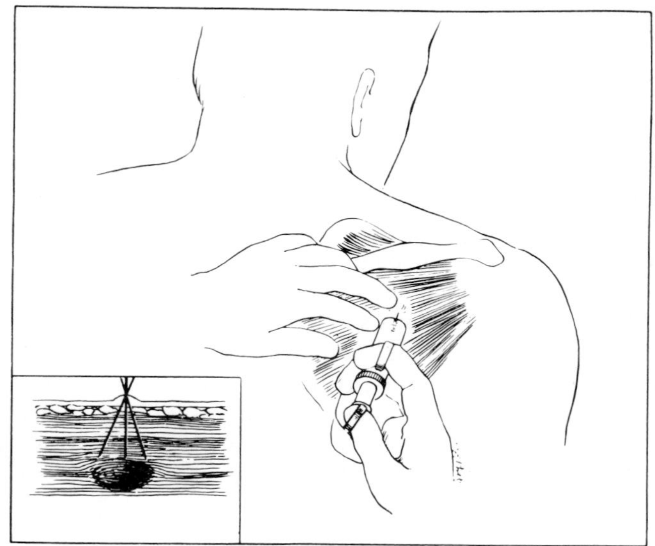

Fig. 52.3 Technique of injecting a trigger point located in the infraspinous muscle. After indentifying the trigger point and disinfecting the skin, a 25-gauge 5-cm needle attached to a 10-ml syringe containing local anaesthetic solution is advanced slowly toward the trigger point. As the needle approaches the trigger area the patient experiences more local and referred pain and tenderness and this is further aggravated during the injection of the local anaesthetic solution. It is best to carry out a fan-like injection by repeatedly withdrawing the needle and redirecting it as shown in the insert. (From Bonica 1953).

LOCAL BLOCKS

Infiltration and topical application of local anaesthetics are frequently used techniques of analgesic blocks in the treatment of pain. Simplicity, facility and apparent innocuousness make local block the method of choice among many physicians working in their office. By producing physicochemical blockade of nervous pathways almost at the very source of the nociceptive process, it effectively relieves the pain and other symptomatology of many disorders, including myofascial pain syndromes, sprains and strains, tendinitis, epicondylitis, periarthritis, severe muscle spasm, scalenus anticus syndrome and some simple fractures.

MYOFASCIAL PAIN SYNDROMES

One of the most productive clinical applications of local block therapy is in the management of myofascial pain syndromes with trigger points (Bonica 1957, 1990, Kraus 1970; Simon 1975, 1976; Travell 1976; Sola 1981; Travell & Simons 1983; Gunn 1989). Trigger points can be found in virtually every muscle of the body, in tendons and in ligaments. The injection of the trigger point is accomplished with a 25-gauge, 5-cm needle, as depicted in Figure 52.3. Usually 5 ml of dilute solution of long-lasting anaesthetic suffices, e.g. 0.05% bupivacaine (see Table 52.3). It deserves reemphasis that the practice of some anaesthetists and other clinicians of using 1% lidocaine or 0.25% bupivacaine or equivalent concentration of other drugs is unnecessary for local infiltration. As the point of the needle nears or actually touches the trigger point, the patient experiences exaggeration of the local and referred pain and tenderness and these are further aggravated during the injection. If complete relief of pain is not achieved in 3–5 minutes it is likely that the trigger point was not injected and may require another trial. A fan-like approach is made by inserting the needle at different angles until the most sensitive region is contacted. Since many patients have more than one trigger point, it is essential to block all of them to obtain optimal results. Some clinicians have found saline injections or simply needle-point stimulation of trigger points (many of which are located in areas in which acupuncture points are found) almost as effective as the injection of the local anaesthetic (Melzack et al 1977).

Another approach to the treatment of myofascial pain, as proposed by Gunn, is the use of acupunture needles to penetrate trigger points to provide short- and long-term muscle relaxation. This ‘intramuscular stimulation’ has, for many, supplanted trigger point injections (Gunn 1989).

The relief of pain, tenderness and muscle spasm persists for several hours and sometimes for days and weeks or even months, especially if the condition is treated early. In acute cases, one or two treatments are sometimes sufficient, whereas in chronic cases a series of treatments is usually necessary. Injections are repeated every second, third and fourth day, depending on the severity and acuteness of the condition. After the trigger points have been injected, adjunctive therapy, including physical therapy, massage, application of ice or spraying of coolant should be used. Some clinicians use the spraying of a coolant on the skin as another method of therapy. More detailed discussion of the subject is presented in Chapter 67.

Muscle spasms

Another effective application of infiltration of dilute solutions of local anaesthetics is relief of severe pain caused by skeletal muscle spasm following accidental or surgical trauma or that associated with certain visceral diseases. This technique is also effective in relieving severe low-back pain (lumbago) due to sudden lumbosacral muscle strain or caused by poor posture or deformity of the spine (Bonica 1953, 1959; Finneson 1973). In all such cases local anaesthetic infiltration should be used as an adjunct to heat, massage and corrective exercises. Local anaesthetic muscle infiltration may be used as a diagnostic/therapeutic procedure in the rare cases of pyriformis syndrome and scalenus anticus syndrome (Bonica 1953, 1990; Wyant 1979).

Pain due to disorders of joints and periarticular structures

Acute bursitis is another important indication for infiltration of local anaesthetics and long-lasting steroids. Usually 10–15 ml of dilute solution of a long-acting agent, such as 0.25% bupivacaine, with 40 mg methylprednisolone (Depo Medrone) or other long-acting steroid will suffice. Pain relief occurs in 10–15 minutes and is likely to last 4–8 hours, after which pain returns and is often more intense. Therefore, the patient should be given systemic analgesics to manage the postblock pain. Frequently, several injections are necessary. Although this procedure is best known for the treatment of subacromial (subdeltoid) bursitis, it is also effective in the management of subscapular, prepatellar and other painful bursae. If the effusion of the joint is pronounced, frequent aspiration of the bursa is indicated.

Tendonitis is another very painful condition for which infiltration of local anaesthetic and steroid compounds is effective in relieving the associated pain. Lateral humeral epicondylitis (tennis elbow), medial humeral epicondylitis (golfer's elbow) and supraspinatus tendinitis associated with subacromial bursitis are frequent indications for this form of therapy (Bonica 1959; Littler 1980). This is supplemented with systemic analgesic for postblock pain and these procedures are repeated several times until permanent relief is achieved.

Ligamentous sprains are another indication for local anaesthetic infiltration therapy. This condition may affect ligaments of any major joint, including the lumbosacral, sacroiliac, sacrococcygeal (coccydynia) interspinous and lateral or medial patellar ligaments. Injections of 5–10 ml of local anaesthetic and steroid into the tender areas usually produces effective relief for many hours and this is repeated until prolonged relief is achieved.

Intraarticular injection of local anaesthetic along or in combination with steroids is also indicated as a diagnostic/prognostic procedure in patients with severe pain or chronic arthritis involving major joints in the limbs or spine or the temporomandibular joint. It is also useful as a prognostic procedure in facet syndrome, involving the thoracic or lumbar spine and in which facet rhizotomy is indicated (Finneson 1973; Sedzimir 1980).

In many of the foregoing conditions, patients are likely to have pain after the effects of the local anaesthetic dissipate. Therefore, it is essential to provide the patient with a prescription of systemic analgesic to be taken by mouth at fixed intervals until the pain subsides. The application of ice to the region may also relieve the pain by reducing oedema and pressure within the bursa or joint.

Postoperative pain

Infiltration of a dilute solution of long-acting local anaesthetic (e.g. 0.05% bupivacaine) in the region of the surgical incision will produce effective relief of postoperative pain for up to 16 hours and results in a decrease in the total dosage of narcotic medication required (Owen et al 1985; Porter & Davies 1985). Infiltration of such solution through catheters placed in the wound at the end of the operation provides even longer pain relief.

'Preemptive' or preincision infiltration of the wound has been shown to provide superior postoperative pain relief when compared to all other methods, including post-surgery infiltration (Tverskoy et al 1990). Such prophylactic use of local infiltration, or peripheral nerve block, has been shown to be effective in preventing the hyperexcitability of the spinal cord caused by massive nociceptive barrage and thus prevents or delays the onset of pain and the neuroendocrine response. (Kehlet 1989; McQuay 1992)

Other painful disorders

Painful scars are not an infrequent cause of chronic postoperative or posttraumatic pain. Infiltration of the scar with local anaesthetics is a useful diagnostic and therapeutic procedure. A series of six to eight injection with 0.125% bupivacaine given at intervals of 3–5 days frequently produces persistent relief (Bonica 1953, 1990; Hannington-Kiff 1974).

Infiltration of neuroma is a useful diagnostic/prognostic procedure in patients with postamputation pain in the stump or phantom limb (Bonica 1953, 1990; Churcher 1978) and also in neuroma that develops after mastectomy or radical neck dissection.

TOPICAL APPLICATION

Topical application of local anaesthetic drugs, either in solution or as a paste, is used to relieve temporarily severe excruciating pain of the mucous membrane in the mouth, throat and frequently the bladder. The most frequently used agents are 2–4% lidocaine, 4–6% cocaine, 1–2% tetracaine or 0.25% dibucaine solution to produce topical analgesia for 30–60 minutes, or 0.5–1% tetracaine or dibucaine or 2.5–5% lidocaine or 30% benzocaine as constituents of an ointment, jelly or cream to produce longer topical analgesia, with benzocaine producing the longest duration. Since topical anaesthetic solutions are absorbed very rapidly from the vascular mucous membrane, the amount applied must be carefully measured and limited to a total dose of one-third to one-half of the total dose shown in Table 52.3. Ointments are used to relieve the excruciating pain of mucositis in cancer patients receiving chemotherapy or as rectal suppositories in patients with anal/rectal pain, while jellies and creams may be applied to the urethra and into the urinary bladder.

BLOCKS OF SPINAL NERVES

Outside the spinal canal the spinal nerves may be blocked in the paravertebral region or at certain points along their course. These procedures are usually employed primarily to interrupt nociceptive pathways in the management of severe acute or chronic pain but some may be used to block somatomotor nerves to relieve pain of muscle spasm or to block sympathetic fibres to the limbs.

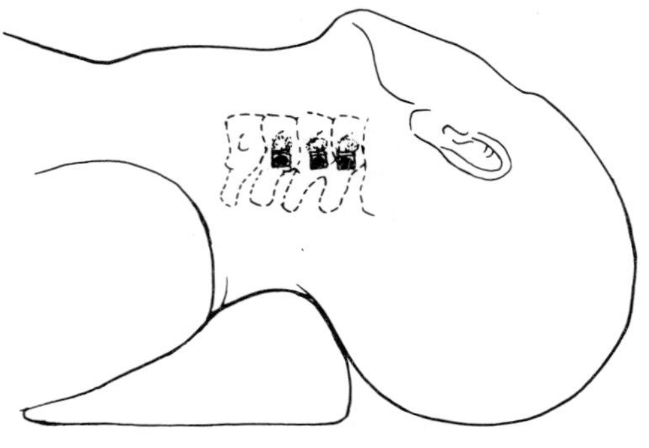

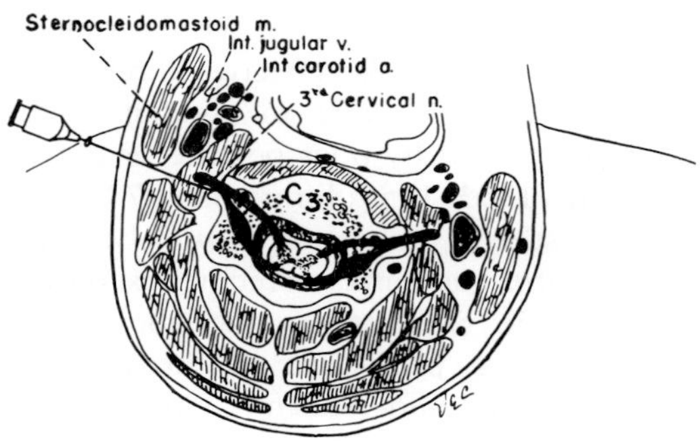

Fig. 52.4 Technique of paravertebral cervical nerve block. Upper figure illustrates the position of the patient while the lower shows a cross-section with the needle in place. Note that the patients's head is turned to the opposite side and a small pillow is placed under the upper portion of the thoracic spine and neck in order to make the transverse processes of the cervical vertebrae more prominent. The tips of the transverse processes are palpated and identified with the tips of the last four fingers, a line is drawn on the skin over them extending from Chassaignac's (C6) tubercle to the mastoid process, and a second line is made parallel and 1 cm posterior to the first. After preparing the skin with an antiseptic solution, three skin wheals are made on the second line with the first wheal made 1.5 cm caudad to the tip of the mastoid process and the other two wheals produced at similar intervals caudally on the same line. A 22-gauge 5-cm needle is directed medially and slightly caudad to avoid unintentional insertion of the needle into the intervertebral foramen. The nerve or the transverse process should be contacted at a depth of about 2.5–3 cm. (From Bonica 1959).

CERVICAL SPINAL NERVES

Paravertebral block

Technique

The lateral approach is the most frequently used technique for blocking the cervical spinal nerves. The techniques of blocking the upper cervical nerves is shown in Figure 52.4. Blockade of the other cervical nerves, except the eighth, is achieved in the same manner. To block the eighth nerve, a wheal is made in the skin overlying the transverse process of the seventh cervical vertebra and the needle is directed caudad and slightly mesiad and advanced until contact with the nerve is made.

Indications

Paravertebral block of the cervical nerves can be used as a diagnostic procedure to identify the specific nerve segment in patients with segmental neuralgia due to intervertebral disc, root–sleeve fibrosis or osteophytes. Since these patients already have a mechanical neuropathy, extreme care must be exercised to avoid further damage to the nerve with the needle point. The procedure may also be used as a prognostic measure in patients with cancer pain and to relieve temporarily severe pain due to musculoskeletal pathology.

Complications

Complications include accidental injection into the subarachnoid space, with consequent total spinal anaesthesia, or injection into the vertebral artery, which immediately brings the bolus of drug to the brainstem and brain with consequent seizures and/or transient paralysis of vital centres and often unconsciousness. Both of these complications must be treated *promptly* with artificial ventilation and support of the circulation until the local anaesthetic drug is redistributed and biotransformed. Possible side-effects include concomitant block of the cervical sympathetic chain, with development of Horner's syndrome, or involvement of the superior aspect of recurrent laryngeal nerves and perhaps even the trunk of vagus. All of these can be avoided by using proper techniques and small amounts of solutions.

Occipital nerve block

Blockade of the greater and third occipital nerve may be used as a diagnostic, prognostic or therapeutic measure for managing patients with occipital headache, neuralgia and other painful conditions in the posterior portion of the head (Bonica 1953).

Technique

The greater occipital nerve is usually blocked just above the superior nuchal line about 2.5–3 cm lateral to the external occipital protuberance. The occipital artery, which serves as the most reliable landmark, is palpated, an antiseptic solution is applied, and a 25-gauge needle, attached to a 5-ml syringe filled with local anaesthetic, is introduced perpendicular to the scalp just medial to the artery. It is advanced until paraesthesia along the course of the nerve until paraesthesia along the course of the nerve is obtained, whereupon 2–3 ml of solution is injected. Anaesthesia of the scalp in the distribution of the nerve develops within 5–10 minutes. The third occipital nerve is just medial to the greater nerve and is often involved in the block.

Side-effects

There are no side-effects other than accidental intra-arterial injection, which is usually of no consequence because of the small volume of the drug.

BRACHIAL PLEXUS BLOCK

Block of the brachial plexus may be used as a diagnostic or prognostic measure in patients with causalgia and other sympathetically mediated pain, phantom limb pain and other types of postamputation pain, and to differentiate pain of peripheral neuralgia from that caused by disorders of the central nervous system. Since all of the sympathetic fibres destined for the hand, forearm and lower two-thirds of the arm are carried by the nerves derived from the brachial plexus, block of this structure is a most effective measure to confirm the results of cervicothoracic sympathetic block in the management of patients with causalgia or other sympathetically mediated pains or those with painful peripheral vascular disorders. It is also useful for providing temporary relief of severe acute pain that follows trauma or operation or in patients with severe spasm caused by accidental intraarterial injection of agents such as thiopental and in patients with severe pain consequent to an embolus. Continuous brachial plexus block is especially useful in patients who have undergone re-implantation of a severed limb or digits and in patients who have other problems in which the blood supply to the extremities is compromised. In such circumstances, prolonged sympathetic block and analgesia enhance the survival of the limb and concomitantly provide pain relief (DeKrey et al 1969; Menriques & Pallers 1978; Rosenblatt et al 1979; Vatashsky & Aronson 1980; Rosenblatt & Cress 1981).

Technique

Although many techniques to block the brachial plexus have been described, the most commonly used are the supraclavicular, interscalene and axillary approaches (Bonica et al 1949; Accardo & Adriani 1949; Bonica 1953; Eather 1958; Winnie 1970). These techniques are depicted in Figures 52.5–52.7. For diagnostic/prognostic purposes, 1% lidocaine produces a block for 2–4 hours, whereas for therapeutic blocks 0.25% bupivacaine with adrenaline will produce analgesia and sympathetic block for 8–12 hours or longer. The 'continuous' technique is achieved by introducing an intravenous plastic catheter until its tip is near the target nerves, as determined by eliciting paraesthesia, or with a nerve stimulator and then removing the stylet and taping the catheter in place. Sustained analgesia is produced by injection of 20–25 ml of 0.25% bupivacaine every 6 hours or, alternatively, by continuous infusion of 0.25% bupivacaine at a rate of 6–10 ml/h (DeKrey et al 1969; Selander 1977; Menriques & Pallares 1978; Rosenblatt et al 1979; Vatashsky & Aronson 1980; Ang et al 1984).

Complications

The most serious complication of supraclavicular brachial plexus block is pneumothorax, which is reported to occur in between 0.5 and 6% of blocks (Moore 1955), but in the hands of the skilled operator it occurs in less than 0.4% (Bonica et al 1949; Bonica 1953; Moore 1955, 1971; Swerdlow 1980; Winchell & Wolfe 1985). Other complications with large volumes of drug include ipsilateral block of the phrenic nerve, which causes no symptomatology except in patients with severe chronic lung disease, and/or block of the cervicothoracic sympa-

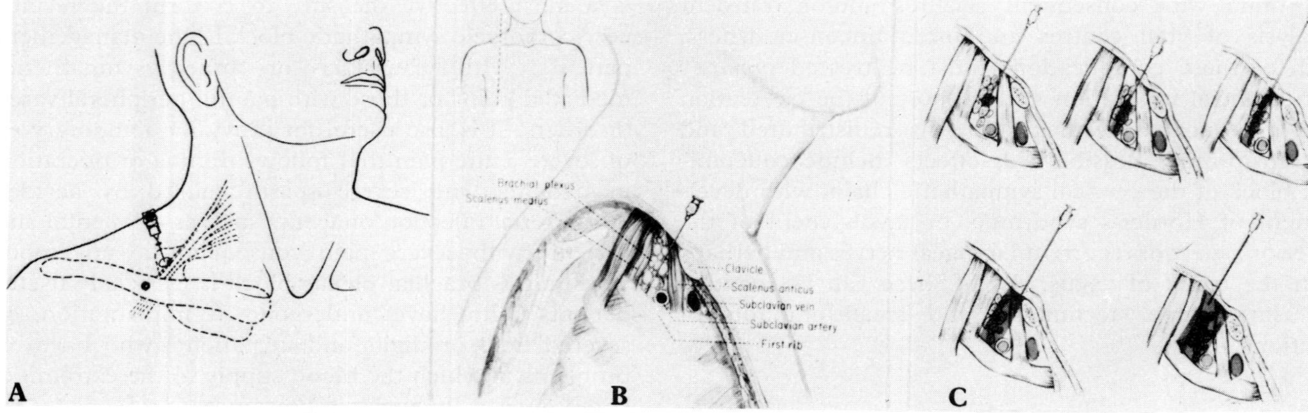

Fig. 52.5 Brachial plexus block by the supraclavicular technique. **A** Anterior schematic view depicting the position of the plexus and direction of the needle. **B** Parasagittal section to show the relationship of the subclavian artery and brachial plexus between the anterior and middle scalenus muscles and the direction of the first needle insertion. **C** Deposition of the solution (dark) with each of three insertions. After thoroughly informing the patient about the procedure and giving the instruction to signal promptly any feeling of paraesthesia, the two ends of the clavicle are identified and the subclavian artery is palpated. After disinfecting the skin, towels are placed along the inferior and posterior edge of the triangle of the neck and the skin wheal is formed about 1 cm above the midpoint of the clavicle and just posterior to the palpable artery. A 22-gauge 5- or 8-cm needle (depending on the size of the patient) attached to a 10-ml Luer-Lok control syringe filled with local anaesthetic solution is inserted in a caudad and slightly dorsad and mesiad direction (**A** and **B**) until paraesthesia is elicited, whereupon the needle is arrested, aspiration in two places is carried out and, if negative, 3–4 ml of solution is injected (**C** upper left). The needle is then carefully advanced until the upper surface of the first rib just posterior to the artery is contacted. After injecting 2–3 ml on the rib, the remainder of the solution is injected as the needle is withdrawn between the first rib and superficial fascia. To avoid accidental intravenous injection, the needle should be withdrawn in stepwise fashion and aspiration made prior to the injection of 1–2 ml of solution. The needle is then introduced 0.5 cm posterior and parallel to the first insertion and the same procedure repeated, after which a third insertion is made 0.5 cm posterior to the second and the same steps repeated. By injecting 10 ml of solution through each of these three insertions, a wall of anaesthesia is created between the first rib and the skin and within the sheath encasing the neurovascular bundle through which the plexus must pass (**C** lower right).

thetic chain with consequent Horner's syndrome. Accidental intravenous injection with consequent systemic toxicity can occur if repeated aspiration tests are not used. As already mentioned, transient or prolonged nerve dysfunction due to trauma by the needle point is rare.

The possible complications of interscalene block are accidental epidural or subarachnoid injection or injection into the vertebral artery, all of which can be obviated with proper technique. Phrenic nerve block occurs more frequently with this technique than with the supraclavicular approach. Possible complications of axillary brachial block include accidental intravenous injection with systemic reaction, haematoma or nerve damage if poor equipment and poor techniques are used.

Suprascapular nerve block

Block of the suprascapular nerve, a branch of the brachial plexus and the major sensory nerve supply to the shoulder joint, is useful for the management of severe pain due to bursitis, periarthritis or arthritis if these conditions are not amenable to intraarticular and periarticular injection of local anaesthetic and steroids (Bonica 1953).

Technique

Suprascapular nerve block is accomplished at the suprascapular notch, as depicted in Figure 52.8. Although in most instances this block is relatively simple, occasionally it is difficult to contact the nerve and the solution is injected within the muscle mass, resulting in failure. X-rays may be used to aid the placement of the needle.

Side-effects

Side-effects include:

1. paralysis of the supraspinatus and infraspinatus muscles which results in transient disability
2. (rarely) pneumothorax if the needle misses the upper border of the scapula and is advanced too far inferiorly and anteriorly into the lung.

BLOCK OF THORACIC SPINAL NERVES

Paravertebral block

Paravertebral block of the thoracic spinal nerves is a useful procedure in managing painful disorders involving the thoracic spine, the thoracic cage and the abdominal wall. Since this procedure includes block of the recurrent nerve and posterior division and its branches which supply the vertebra, the facet joint, the meninges, and the paraverte-

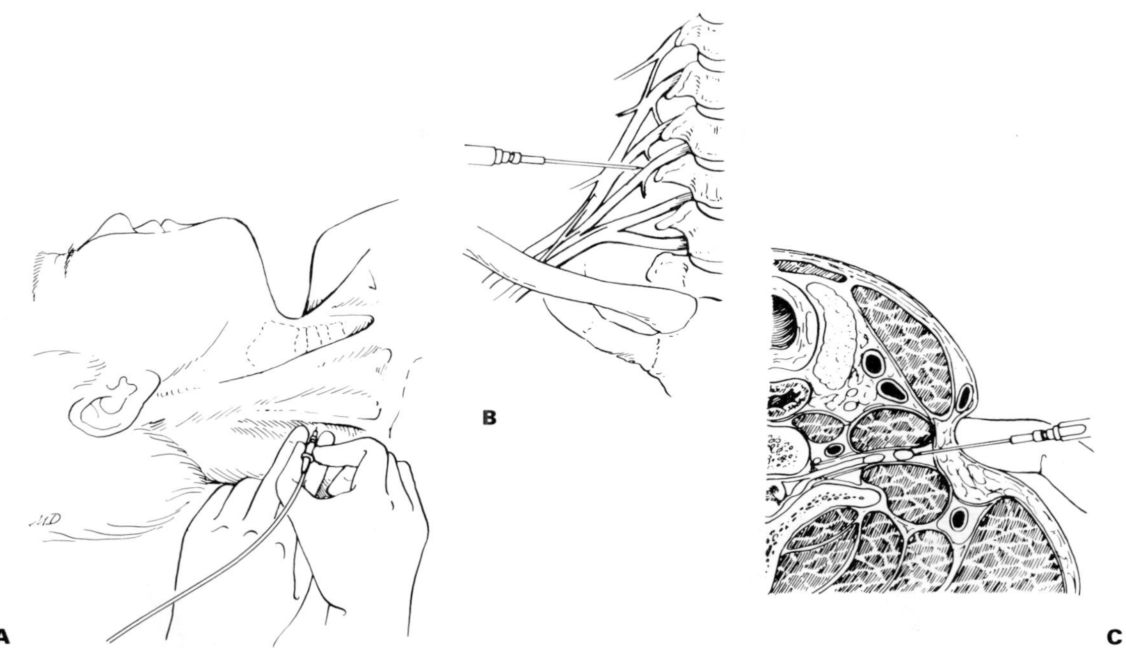

Fig. 52.6 Technique of interscalene block of the brachial plexus. **A**. The patient lies supine with the head on a pillow and rotated to the opposite side. The interscalene groove is identified by asking the patient to lift the head, which places the scaleni muscles in tension. The insertion point is determined by drawing a line that extends laterally from the cricoid cartilage to intersect the interscalene groove; a 3- or 5-cm 23- or 25-gauge short-bevelled needle is inserted in a medial and slightly caudad direction toward the sulcus of the C6 transverse process. **B**. The needle is advanced slowly for 1.5–2 cm until paraesthesia is elicited; this indicates contact with a nerve, which is usually the C7 root of the plexus. **C**. Cross-section at level of C6 vertebra showing the bevel of the needle approaching the nerve, which is located between the anterior and middle scalenus muscles. The 30–40 ml of local anaesthetic solution injected diffuses cephalad, caudad and laterally to block the roots, trunks and divisions of the brachial plexus and often the roots of the cervical plexus. Although this volume of solution can be injected by adapting a 10-ml Luer-Lok syringe directly to the hub of the needle, it is best to attach a length of tubing to the needle hub with its proximal end adapted to a 50-ml syringe containing the local anaesthetic (as shown in **A**). To avoid unintentional intravenous or subarachnoid injection, attempts at aspiration are made before and after injection of 1–2 ml of solution and repeated frequently as the entire volume of the solution is injected. For a continuous technique, an 18- or 20-gauge intravenous catheter is similarly introduced, the stylet is removed and the catheter taped into place with its hub connected to a 10- to 15-cm length of tubing attached to the syringe containing the local anaesthetic. Repeated injections of 20–30 ml of 0.25–0.357% bupivacaine every 6 hours, or an infusion of 0.25% bupivacaine at a rate 6–12 ml/h, produces continuous blockade.

bral muscles, skin and tissues, it is useful to help determine the nociceptive pathways in patients with segmental neuralgia due to vertebral pathology, such as osteoporosis and metastatic fracture, narrowing of the intervertebral foramen due to osteophytes or scoliosis or herniated intervertebral disc which, though rare in this part of the spine, are sometimes the cause of severe pain. Paravertebral block with 0.25%–0.5% bupivacaine–adrenaline solution is also useful for the relief of severe pain of rib fractures, acute herpes zoster and pleurisy (Bonica 1953, 1959; Hannington-Kiff 1974). There is evidence that repeated or continuous paravertebral somatic block (which also involves the sympathetic supply to the segment) decreases the incidence of postherpetic neuralgia (Findley & Patzer 1945; Colding 1969; Dan et al 1979).

Thoracic paravertebral block with a long-acting anaesthetic (e.g. 0.5% bupivacaine–adrenaline) may also be used to control severe acute postthoracotomy pain if the chest incision extends to the paravertebral region. This procedure is also being used to manage patients with chronic post thoracotomy, posttraumatic pain or postinfectious neuralgia. In a significant percentage of patients, a series of paravertebral local anaesthetic blocks produces lasting benefits (Bonica 1953, 1959; Hannington-Kiff 1971, 1974; Miller et al 1975, 1988). In more than two dozen patients with segmental neuralgia due to osteoporosis, a series of paravertebral blocks, and in two patients a single block, produced prolonged relief of pain. A possible explanation for the prolonged relief is interruption of a 'vicious circle' that involved severe skeletal muscle spasm which had caused decrease of the interspace and thus contributed to the chronic irritation of the nerve root (Howe 1979). Prolonged relief for up to 21 days following block with 0.25% bupivacaine, 1:400 000 adrenaline in patients with cancer pain, postherpetic

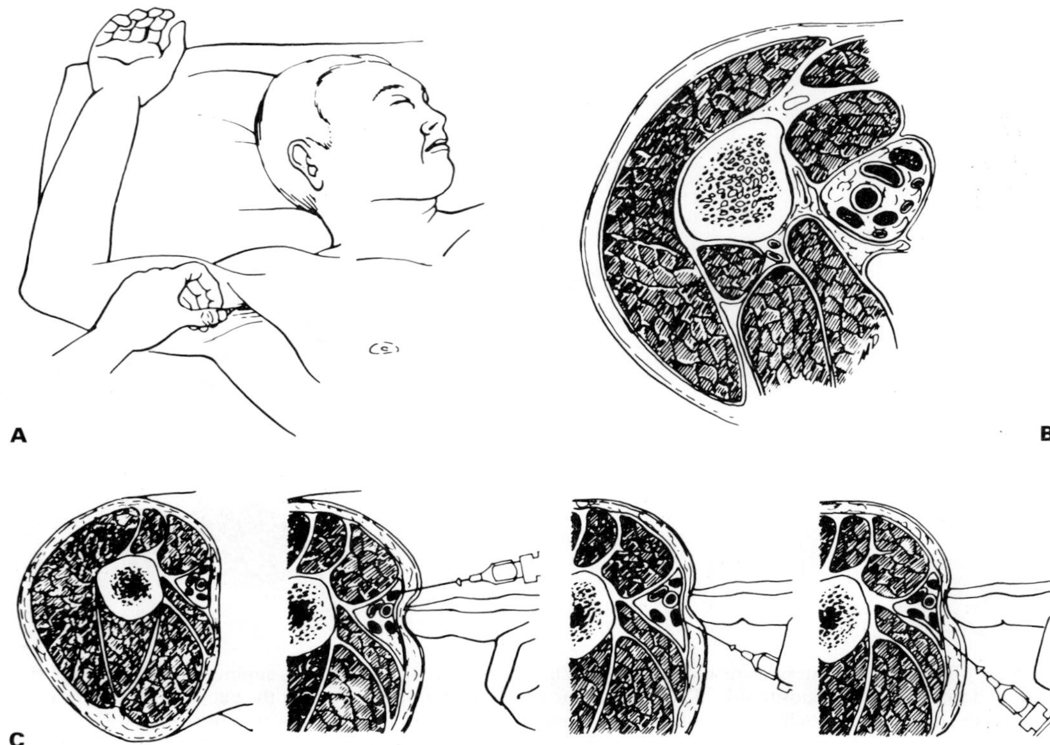

Fig. 52.7 Technique of axillary block of the brachial plexus. **A.** The patient is supine with the arm abducted to 90° and rotated externally. **B**. Cross-section of the upper part of the axilla showing the relationship of the nerves to the axillary arteries. The axillary artery is palpated and traced as far as possible proximally within the axilla, ideally to the pectoralis major muscle. After appropriate preparation of the skin a skin wheal is formed over the artery and a 3- or 5-cm or 25-gauge short-bevelled needle (attached to tubing connected to an anaesthetic-filled syringe; not shown) is inserted through a wheal. The shaft of the needle should be at a 45° angle with the medial aspect of the arm (**A**), directing its point cephalad toward the apex of the axilla and advancing it slowly. A short-bevelled needle can be felt to penetrate the sheath, within which lie the lower portion of the axillary artery and the four major nerves of the plexus. Penetration of the fascial sheath is felt as 'click', after which the needle is advanced 1–2 mm to ensure that the bevel is within the fascial sheath. Elicitation of paraesthesia obviously indicates contact with one of the major nerves. Injection to 30–40 ml of solution while pressure is placed firmly on the neurovascular bundle and its surrounding sheath below the needle enhances diffusion of the solution proximally so as to involve all the branches of the brachial plexus, except those that leave it above the 1st rib. **C**. Some physicians prefer to elicit paraesthesia and inject each of the three major nerves at the uppermost part of the arm at the beginning of the brachial artery. (1) After identifying the artery, an intracutaneous wheal is formed just medial to the artery. A 5-cm 25-gauge short-bevelled needle attached to a 10-ml Luer-Lok control syringe containing the local anaesthetic solution is inserted through the wheal and the skin is moved anteriorly about 0.5 cm. While palpating the artery with the second and third fingers of one hand, with the other hand the needle is advanced laterally through the fascial sheath, which can be felt. The needle is advanced another 2 or 3 mm until contact with the median nerve produces paraesthesia in its distribution. (2) Injection of 2–3 ml of solution is sufficient to anaesthetize the nerve. For blockade of the ulnar nerve, the manoeuvre is repeated except, after inserting the needle through the wheal, the skin is moved posteriorly 0.5 cm and advanced until contact with the ulnar nerve elicits paraesthesia in its distribution. (3) To reach the radial nerve, which is posterolateral to the artery, the needle must be inserted 0.5 cm posterior to the plane of injection of the ulnar nerve, with the needle passing posterior to the ulnar nerve in a lateral and slightly anterior direction. (4) At this level the musculocutaneous nerve has passed laterally and is in the substance of the coracobrachialis muscle. To block this nerve it is necessary to insert the needle 0.5 cm anteriorly to where the median nerve is located and to advance the needle laterally into the substance of the muscle, in which 5 ml of solution is usually sufficient to diffuse and block the nerve. For a continuous technique, a 5-cm 18-gauge intravenous catheter is introduced through an opening in the anaesthetized skin that has been made with a larger sharp needle. The catheter is directed at an angle of 30° with the skin in a central direction toward the apex of the axilla. Once the tip of the catheter pierces the sheath containing the neurovascular bundle, it is advanced about 2 cm along the side of the artery, the stylet is removed, the solution is injected and the catheter is fixed firmly in place. Subsequent injections are repeated as necessary.

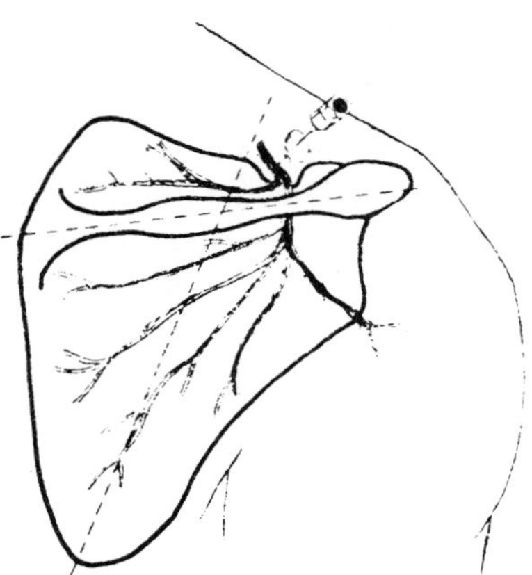

Fig. 52.8 Technique of suprascapular nerve block. After identifying the spine of the scapula a line is drawn on the skin overlying it and another one bisecting the inferior angle of the scapula. The outer triangle formed by the two intersecting lines is bisected and a wheal is formed on this bisector about 1.5 cm from the angle. Through this wheal a 22-gauge 8-cm needle is introduced so that its shaft is directed anteriorly, slightly caudad and mesiad to make contact with the supraspinatus fossa just lateral to the suprascapular notch. The needle is then withdrawn and reintroduced medially until the point enters the notch, makes contact with the nerve and elicits paraesthesia. In the event that the first insertion fails to produce paraesthesia, a second and third insertion are made in search of paraesthesia. Usually 5 ml of local anaesthetic solution will produce blockade of the nerve.

neuralgia and compression of nerve roots for vertebral pathology has been reported by Hannington-Kiff (1971), who believes that the block interrupts self-perpetuating activity in the central nervous system.

Technique

The classical technique of blocking the thoracic paravertebral nerve entails the insertion of the needle 4–5 cm lateral to the spinous process and advancing it anteriorly and slightly medially so that the shaft of the needle makes an angle of 45° with the midsaggital plane. This will frequently cause the needle to traverse the deep concavity on either side of the vertebral column which contains the posterior border of the lung, with the inherent risk of pneumothorax or passage of the needle point into an intravertebral foramen, possibly causing accidental epidural or subarachnoid injection. To obviate these serious problems, many years ago Bonica developed the paralaminar technique depicted in Figure 52.9 (Bonica 1959). For diagnostic or prognostic purposes, 2–3 ml of a local anaesthetic solution is used and the position of the needle is verified with X-ray. For therapy of severe acute pain, 5 ml of 0.5% bupivacaine with adrenaline will produce analgesia for 5–8 hours or longer. To achieve a 'continuous' technique, a catheter is placed with its tip in the paravertebral space to permit injection of 10–15 ml of 0.25–0.5% bupivacaine, producing a block of 2–3 segment.

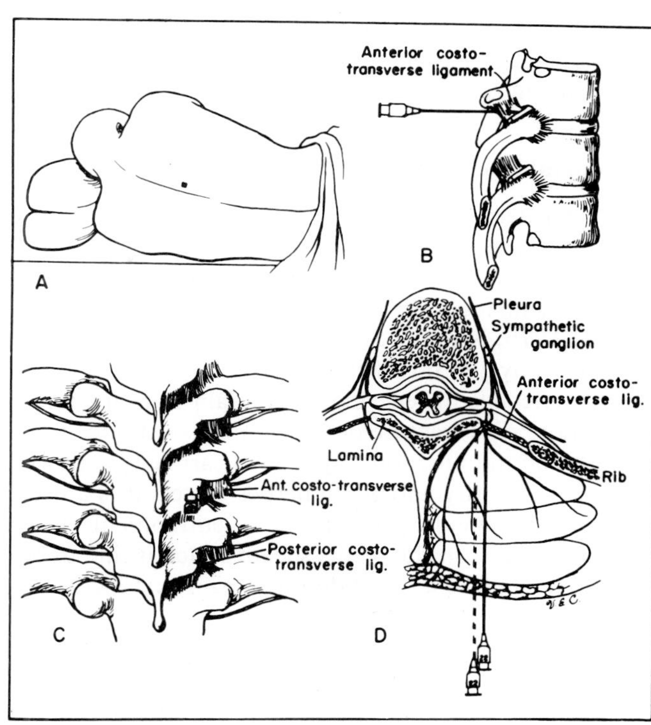

Fig. 52.9 Technique of thoracic paravertebral somatic nerve block. **A** Position of the patient for block on the right side. After identifying the appropriate spinous process and disinfecting the skin, a skin wheal is formed 1.5 cm lateral to the tip of the spinous process of the vertebrae above, as shown in **C**. A 22-gauge 5- or 8-cm needle with a short bevel is inserted through the skin wheal perpendicular to the skin and advanced until the lateral edge of the lamina is contacted as depicted in **C**. The needle is then withdrawn until its point is in subcutaneous tissue, the skin moved laterally about 0.5 cm and the needle readvanced until it slips just lateral to the lateral edge of the lamina and its point engages the anterior (superior) costotransverse ligament. Once the point of the needle is in the ligament, a syringe filled with saline is attached to the needle and attempt is made to inject. As long as the tip of the needle is within the ligament, there is some resistance to the injection. By exerting constant pressure on the plunger of the syringe with the right hand and advancing the needle *very slowly* with the left hand, a lack of resistance is felt as soon as the bevel of the needle passes through the ligament and is in the paravertebral region in the immediate vicinity of the nerve (**B**). If paraesthesia is not elicited, a nerve stimulator is used to ascertain that the bevel of the needle is near the target. For diagnostic/prognostic block 3–4 ml of solution is injected. Note in **D** that the needle is directed in true sagittal plane rather than at an angle, as is the case with the traditional approach. (From Bonica 1959.)

Complications

Possible complications with the paralaminar technique include accidental subarachnoid injection (in patients with a very prolonged dural cuff that extends to the paravertebral region), accidental intravenous injection and pneumothorax if the needle is advanced too far anteriorly. All of these can be obviated by using patience, caution and skill in carrying out the procedures. If many segments are blocked, there may be sufficient interruption of the sympathetic chain to produce orthostatic arterial hypotension for the duration of the block. If the patient needs to be ambulant, the hypotension can be minimized or prevented by using tight stockings and an abdominal binder to decrease pooling of blood in the lower limbs and abdomen and by giving intravenous fluids.

Intercostal block

Intercostal nerve block is one of the most useful procedures for the relief of severe acute posttraumatic, postoperative or postinfectious pain in the thoracic or abdominal wall (Bridenbaugh et al 1973; Delilkan et al 1973; Engberg 1975; Nunn & Slavin 1980; Crawford & Skinner 1982; Murphy 1983; Restelli et al 1984; Buckley 1985). It is highly effective in relieving severe pain from fracture of one or more ribs, fracture of the sternum or dislocation of the costocondral junction, slipped rib cartilage, contusion chest pain, pleurisy and acute herpes zoster. It is a useful diagnostic/therapeutic procedure in entrapment of the intercostal nerves in the rectus sheath which is said to be a not infrequent cause of abdominal pain and occasional chest pain (Applegate 1972).

Perhaps the most frequent use of intercostal block is to relieve severe pain following cholecystectomy, gastrectomy, mastectomy, thoracotomy and sternotomy. In such cases it not only relieves pain but also reduces or eliminates reflex muscle spasm and other reflex phenomena initiated by the nociceptive input. A number of studies have shown the superiority of intercostal nerve block over conventional narcotics in managing postoperative pain (Bergh et al 1966; Bridenbaugh et al 1973; Delilkan et al 1973; Engberg 1975; Buckley & Simpson 1980).

The peak expiratory flow (PEF), forced vital capacity (FVC), forced expiratory volume in one second (FEV_1) and partial pressure of oxygen in arterial blood (Pa_{O_2}), which are usually reduced by 50% or more by postoperative pain in the abdomen or thorax, are improved after intercostal block. Postthoracotomy patients managed with intercostal block show less impairment on effort-dependent tests of respiratory function such as FVC, PEF (Galway et al 1975; Faust & Nauss 1976; Toledo-Peraya & DeMeester 1978; Murphy 1983) and Pa_{O_2} (Delilkan et al 1973). When compared with narcotic analgesia for the relief of postoperative pain following upper abdominal surgery, patients who receive intercostal blocks have a better and earlier global recovery and discharge from the hospital (Bridenbaugh et al 1973), better effort-dependent tests of respiratory function, better Pa_{O_2} and a reduced incidence of respiratory complications (FVC and PEF) (Engberg 1975). For postthoracotomy pain, fractured ribs on one side or subcostal abdominal incisions which do not extend beyond the midline, a unilateral block is sufficient, whereas for sternotomy and for many upper abdominal operations, where incisions are in the midline or transverse, a bilateral block is necessary.

Although segmental epidural block is commonly used for post operative or posttraumatic pain relief, intercostal block has the significant advantage of producing analgesia two to four times the duration of that achieved with the same drug dose injected into the epidural space. Moore et al (1978) reported that following intercostal block with 4 ml of 0.25% bupivacaine with adrenaline, analgesia lasted 10–12 hours. This makes it practical to induce intercostal block in the morning and have the patient ambulate, cough and be as active as possible during the analgesic stage for the remainder of the day. If necessary, the block can be repeated in the evening or at least each morning. Disadvantages of intercostal block compared with epidural block are the need to make multiple injections once or twice a day and that it carries the risk of pneumothorax.

Technique

Although the intercostal nerves may be blocked at any point along their course, the angle of the rib offers the best site because:

1. it is the most superficial and therefore the most easily palpable point
2. the rib is thickest and the intercostal groove broadest and deepest
3. the collateral branch is in the same triangular space and therefore more accessible to the local anaesthetic solution (Moore et al 1980; Nunn & Slavin 1980).

The technique of posterior intercostal block is shown in Figure 52.10. The injection of 3–4 ml of solution at the angle of the rib will spread proximally to involve the sympathetic chain as well as distally for several centimetres (Moore et al 1980). While some believe that blockade of the sympathetic chain has the advantage of also interrupting visceral nociceptive pathways (Nunn & Slavin 1980), it has the disadvantage of producing orthostatic hypotension if a large number of segments are blocked.

Lateral intercostal block

This entails blockade of the intercostal nerve along the posterior axillary line, which is several centimetres posterior to the midaxillary line, the point at which the lateral cutaneous nerves pierce the intercostal muscles and fascia to divide into the anterior and posterior branches. The anterior branch supplies the skin and subcutaneous tissues of the chest and abdominal wall, as far as 7 cm from the anterior midline, while the posterior branch supplies these tissues as far as 7–10 cm from the spine. Although Moore et al (1980) suggest that, with this technique, there is a risk of producing inadequate analgesia, this has not been my experience or that of my colleagues using the techniques shown in Figure 52.11. Blockade at this site is

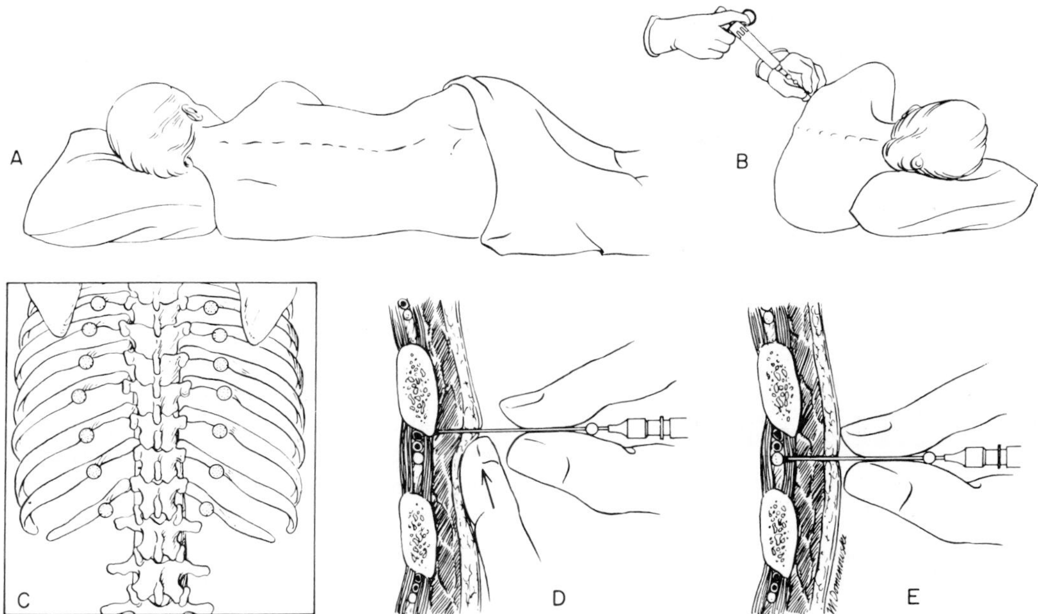

Fig. 52.10 Technique of posterior intercostal block. The injections are done at the angles of the ribs. **A** and **B** Patient in comfortable position for unilateral and bilateral block. **C** The dots indicate sites of injection. **D** and **E** Details of injection. The second finger of the left hand is placed over the intercostal space and pushes the skin cephalad slightly so that the lower edge of the rib above can be palpated and at the same time immobilise the skin over the rib. This finger also protects the intercostal space and thus decreases the risk of passing the needle too far into the lung. A 25-gauge short bevel needle 1–2 cm in length (depending on the thickness of the subcutaneous tissue) attached to a 10 ml Luer-Lok control syringe filled with local anaesthetic solution held in the right hand is inserted perpendicular to the skin and advanced until the lowermost part of the lateral aspect of the rib is contacted. After the rib is impinged upon, the needle is grasped between the thumb and index finger of the left hand about 0.5 cm from the skin; the skin is moved caudad to allow the needle to slip below the lower border of the rib. It is then advanced until the fingertips grasping the needle are flush with the skin. This is a simple manoeuvre which minimises the chance of advancing the needle too deeply and entering the lung. With the needle held firmly and steadily between the second and third fingers of the left hand an attempt at aspiration is made and, if negative, 3–4 ml of solution is injected. (From Bonica 1967.)

particularly useful in differentiating thoracic or abdominal visceral pain from somatic pain caused by disorders of the chest or abdominal wall. For example, in patients complaining of anterior chest pain, the use of intercostal nerve block of the appropriate segments will relieve the pain of somatic origin but will not relieve pain arising in thoracic viscera which, of course, are supplied by nociceptive fibres that follow sympathetic pathways. Similarly, intercostal block will relieve abdominal wall pain but not pain arising in the abdominal viscera.

Anterior intercostal block

This is done along the midclavicular line, which is proximal to the take-off of the anterior cutaneous branch and thus very useful to relieve severe pain of sternotomy and/or fracture of the sternum or of the costal cartilages (Fig. 52.12).

Continuous intercostal block

This may be accomplished by inserting a catheter percutaneously into each of several intercostal spaces (Ablondi et al 1966) or by inserting one catheter and injecting large volumes (15–20 ml) of the local anaesthetic solution. With the latter technique, good unilateral analgesia involving several segments is obtained (Murphy 1983; Restelli et al 1984; Lyles et al 1986), but this technique carries the risk of extensive paravertebral or epidural block involving many vasomotor segments with consequent hypotension (Moore et al 1980).

Complications

The most important complication of intercostal block is pneumothorax, which has been reported to occur in an incidence of 0.09–19% (Moore et al 1980), but, skilfully done, the incidence should be less than 1% (Bonica 1953; Moore et al 1980). Because the absorption of local anaesthetic from the intercostal space is faster and greater than it is after injection in other sites (Tucker & Mather 1988), systemic toxic reactions may occur after the injection of large therapeutic doses. This problem

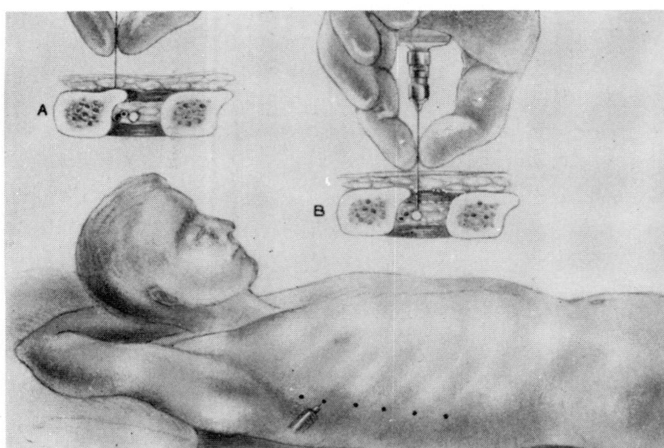

Fig. 52.11 Lateral intercostal block. Dots indicate sites of injection along the posterior axillary line about 7 cm posterior to the point where the lateral cutaneous branch emerges at the midaxillary line. The technique of introducing the needles is similar to that described in Figure 52.10. (From Bonica 1959.)

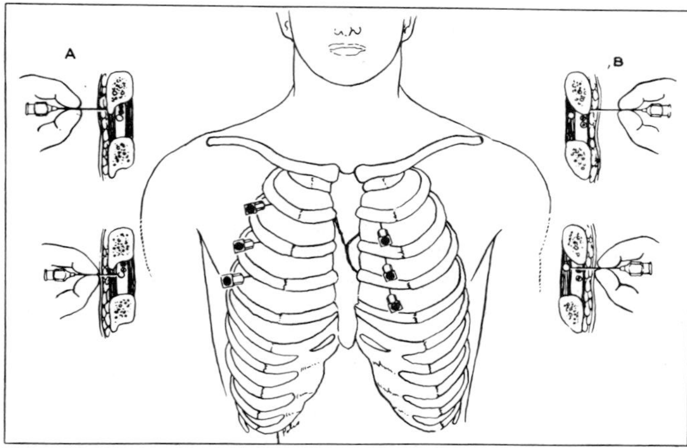

Fig. 52.12 Anterior intercostal block. **A** Block done along the midclavicular line to relieve pain in distal portion of the rib or cartilages. **B** Intercostal block in the parasternal region to relieve pain in the sternum. The technique of introducing the needle is similar to that in Figure 52.10. (From Bonica 1953.)

can be obviated or at least minimized by adding adrenaline to the solution to retard absorption and by using optimal concentrations and reasonable volumes of the drug.

BLOCKADE OF THE LUMBAR AND SACRAL NERVES

The lumbar and sacral nerves are here considered together because they have a common function (nerve supply of the pelvis and lower extremity) and consequently are frequently involved together in conditions which indicate nerve blocks. Since these nerves, like those to the upper extremity, contain somatic sensory, motor and sympathetic fibres, blockade may be employed in the management of the same disorders discussed in connection with the upper extremity.

Paravertebral block

Lumbar paravertebral block is very useful for determining the specific nociceptive pathway or pathways associated with herniated intervertebral disc or other vertebral pathology. For this purpose, the nerve must be identified either by eliciting paraesthesia or by the use of a nerve stimulator and then carrying out X-ray verification. Lumbar paravertebral block is also useful in providing relief of severe postnephrectomy pain and severe pain produced by fracture of one of the lumbar vertebrae. Block of S1 is often used to ascertain the specific nociceptive pathways in patients with herniated intervertebral disc of this root. Transsacral block may also be used to evaluate the effects of individual nerve block on pain and pelvic structures (Goffen 1982; Simon et al 1982; Robertson 1983) and is a valuable prognostic procedure prior to injection of neurolytic agents to relieve severe bladder pain (Goffen 1982; Simon et al 1982) or perineal pain of cancer (Robertson 1983).

Technique

The technique of lumbar paravertebral block of spinal nerves is similar to that of blocking the thoracic nerves (Fig. 52.13). For diagnostic or prognostic purposes, only 3–4 ml of solution should be injected *after* X-ray verification of the position of the bevel of the needle in the correct segment. The technique of transsacral block is depicted in Figure 52.14.

Complications

Complications of lumbar paravertebral block are similar to those of thoracic block, except that pneumothorax does not occur. Complications associated with transsacral block are limited to accidental intravenous injection or transient nerve dysfunction from damage by the needle, both of which can be obviated with proper technique.

Sciatic nerve block

Since the sciatic nerve contains the majority of the sensory and sympathetic fibres for the lower extremity, sciatic nerve block may be used to control severe acute pain temporarily and to produce complete sympathetic interruption of the foot and leg. The technique of the block is depicted in Figure 52.15. Continuous sciatic nerve block

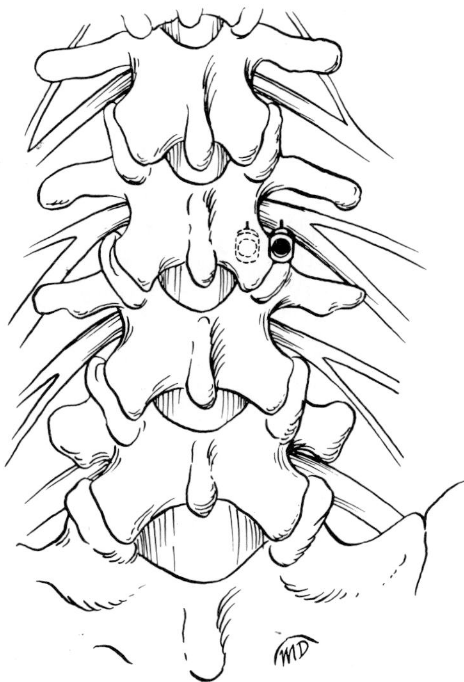

Fig. 52. 13 The technique of lumbar paravertebral block. After identification of the spinous process and preparation of the skin, a wheal is produced 1.5 cm lateral to the midpoint of the quadrilaterally shaped spinous process. By using a 25-gauge 3- or 5-cm needle, one can anaesthetize the skin, subcutaneous tissue, fascia and deeper painsensitive structures and thus make the insertion of the 22-gauge 8-cm needle painless. The 22-gauge needle is then inserted perpendicular to the skin and advanced until it makes contact with the lateral part of the ipsilateral lamina of the vertebra. Once the lamina is contacted, a rubber marker is placed on the needle shaft 1.5 cm from the skin, the needle withdrawn and moved laterally about 0.5 cm and advanced until either the lateral edge of the lamina is contacted or the needle passes 1.5 cm deeper than the lamina. It may be necessary to carry out two or three insertions before the needle passes just lateral to the edge of the lamina. Because of the large size of the lumbar nerves, contact is easily made and paraesthesia elicited, but if this is difficult a nerve stimulator is used.

may be achieved by introducing a catheter close to the sciatic nerve via the posterior approach (Smith 1984). Complications are rare and are limited to accidental intravenous injection or transient nerve dysfunction due to trauma during the procedure.

Femoral and lateral cutaneous nerve

Block of the femoral nerve is rarely used as a therapeutic measure but may be useful as a diagnostic procedure in the management of neuralgia and other severe pain in the anterior thigh, or it can be used concomitantly with sciatic block to effect sympathetic interruption of the entire lower limb. Blockade of the lateral femoral cutaneous nerve is indicated in unusual circumstances where there is severe pain in the anterolateral aspect of the thigh and in managing meralgia paraesthetica. The latter condition is due to a variety of factors, most of which can be eliminated by conservative treatment. Blockade of nerve is used to confirm the diagnosis.

Technique

The femoral nerve is blocked just below the inguinal ligament in its position lateral to the femoral artery, as shown in Figure 52.16. The technique of lateral femoral cutaneous nerve block is shown in Figure 52.17. Winnie et al (1973) have described a perivascular technique of blocking the lumbar plexus which includes the femoral, lateral femoral cutaneous and obturator nerves. This technique entails insertion of a short bevel needle into the fascial compartment or 'sheath' which contains the femoral nerve, eliciting paraesthesia, then changing direction of the needle so that its shaft is parallel to the nerve and advancing it cephalad 1 cm. A total of 30 ml of local anaesthetic is injected while placing firm pressure distal to the point of needle insertion to enhance diffusion of the drug centrally to reach the roots of the lumbar plexus. Side-effects of these procedures include transient paralysis of the anterior thigh muscles and complications may include injury to the femoral nerve.

Obturator nerve block

Obturator nerve block may be used in the management of adductor muscle spasm and in the differential diagnosis in patients with a painful hip. Since this nerve contributes the major portion of the nerve supply to the hip joint, it was formerly used as a diagnostic or prognostic procedure prior to obturator neurectomy in patients with severe intractable pain in the hips due to osteoarthritis. However, the advent of arthroplasty has virtually eliminated this application. Although this procedure is rarely used, the technique is depicted in Figure 52.18 for the sake of completeness.

Pudendal nerve block

Pudendal nerve block may be used as a diagnostic or prognostic procedure in patients with perineal pain. The optimal site for injection of the nerve is just posterior to the attachment of the sacrospinous ligament to the ischial spine. In the female this can be done transvaginally using the technique shown in Figure 34.15. In males the transperineal approach is used. A 22-gauge 10-cm needle is inserted through a skin wheal made 2.5 cm posteromedial to the ischial tuberosity and, with the index finger in the rectum to guide the needle, it is advanced through the ischiorectal fossa toward the ischial spine (Bonica 1967). As the needle approaches the spine, it is pushed posterior to it by the guiding finger. Once the point of the needle is just posterior to the ligament near its attachment to the

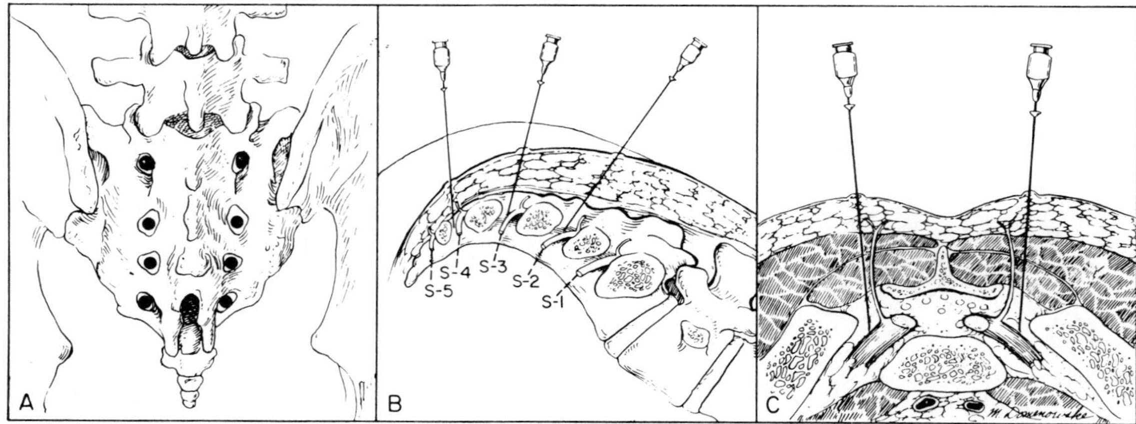

Fig. 52.14 Transsacral nerve block. **A** Posterior view of the sacrum showing location of points of insertion **B** Sagittal view showing directions of needles. **C** Cross-section showing needles in position for block of the second sacral nerves. After identifying the posterior superior iliac spine and the sacral cornu on the ipsilateral side, a line is drawn 1.5 cm medial to the spine and 1.5 cm lateral and cephalad to the ipsilateral cornu. For block of S1 a wheal is made 1.5 cm cephalad to the level of the iliac spine. For S2 the wheal is made 1.5 cm below the level of the iliac spine. Since there is some variation in the location of the foramina, it is necessary to make a systematic search until the needle is felt to go through the posterior foramen to the transsacral canal. Contact with the nerve will produce paraesthesia. (From Bonica 1967.)

spine, 10 ml of solution is injected. Side-effects include unintentional involvement of the sciatic nerve and accidental intravenous injection.

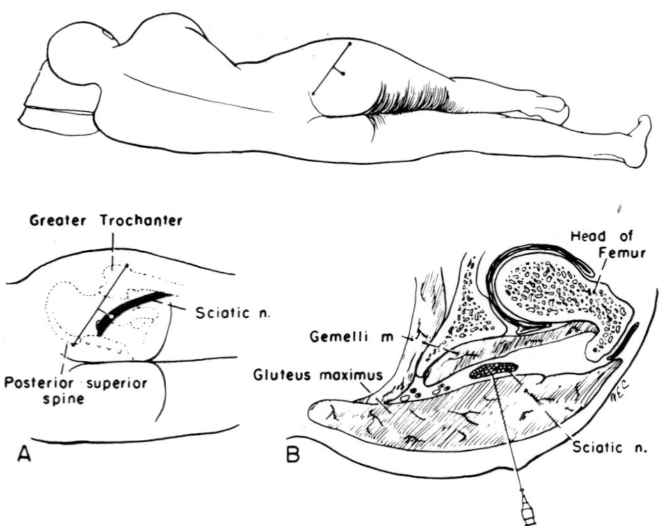

Fig. 52.15 Technique of sciatic nerve block. The top figure shows the patient in Sims' position and the landmarks marked on the skin. **A** Relationship of the nerves to the bones and the method of locating the nerve. The line extending from the upper portion of the greater trochanter to the posterior superior iliac spine is bisected and a perpendicular line is drawn from the point of bisection in an inferior and medial direction for a distance of 3 cm. This is the site of the puncture. After formation of the skin wheal a 22-gauge 10-cm needle is introduced perpendicular to the skin and advanced until paraesthesia is obtained or bone is contacted. If paraesthesia is not obtained, the skin wheal is moved 0.5 cm cephalad and the needle reintroduced until paraesthesia is elicited or bone contacted. Several insertions made along the bisector permit the exact location of the nerve. As soon as paraesthesia is elicited 15–20 ml of solution is injected. **B** Cross-section showing point of the needle on the nerve.

Penile nerve block

Penile nerve block is very useful as a diagnostic procedure but its most important application is to provide post-operative analgesia subsequent to penile operations, particularly in children. The most effective technique is to insert a 25-gauge 2-cm needle through the skin at the 2 o'clock position and another at the 10 o'clock position at the base of the penis and advance them slowly until the deep (Buck's) fascia is pierced, which is often perceived as a 'pop' or 'click'. An attempt is made to aspirate and, if negative, 0.2% bupivacaine *without* adrenaline is injected. The volumes used vary from 1 ml for a child less than 1 year old to 5–7 ml for a patient who is 13 years or older. Complications include puncture of the corpus cavernosum or the dorsal vessel of the penis, but these can be avoided with proper technique.

BLOCKADE OF CRANIAL NERVES: TRIGEMINAL NERVE OR ITS BRANCHES

Since the trigeminal nerve supplies the sensory fibres to the entire face and the anterior two-thirds of the head, it is often involved in painful conditions. Consequently, block of the gasserian ganglion or one of the main branches of the fifth nerve with local anaesthetics is a useful diagnostic/prognostic aid. Although the advent of anticonvulsant drugs, reintroduction of the thermocoagulation of the gasserian ganglion and other operations specific for trigeminal neuralgia have markedly decreased the use of alcohol block, in skilled hands this technique still has a place in controlling severe trigeminal neuralgia or severe cancer pain in situations where neurosurgical procedures

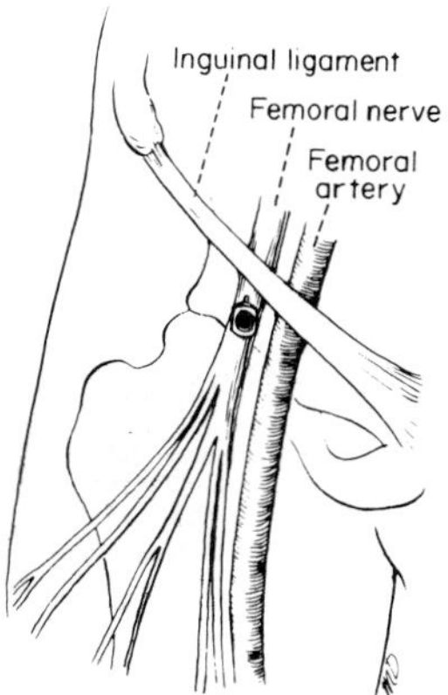

Fig. 52.16 Technique of femoral nerve block. After preparation of the skin an anaesthetic wheal is made 1 cm lateral to the femoral artery and a 22-gauge 5-cm needle is introduced perpendicular to the skin and advanced until paraesthesia is elicited in the distribution to the cutaneous branches of the femoral nerve. Since the nerve often branches above the inguinal ligament, paraesthesia is more difficult to elicit than is the case with sciatic block. To search for paraesthesia several insertions of the needle may be necessary, beginning with the first insertion made just lateral to the artery and making repeated insertions 0.5 cm lateral to each preceding one. If several trials do not elicit paraesthesia a nerve stimulator should be used. Injection of 10–15 ml of solution in the region of the nerve is usually effective in blocking it.

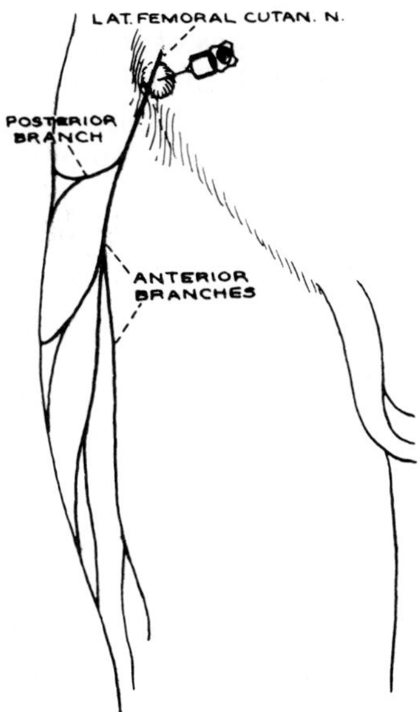

Fig. 52.17 Technique of lateral cutaneous nerve block. After identifying the anterior superior iliac spine and the inguinal ligament, the skin is disinfected and a skin wheal made 1.5 cm medial to the spine immediately below the inguinal ligament. Then a 22- or 25-gauge 5-cm needle is introduced through the skin wheal perpendicular to the skin and slowly advanced until paraesthesia is obtained or the bone is contacted. In the latter case, the needle is withdrawn until its point is subcutaneous, the skin wheal is moved 0.5 cm lateral and superior and the needle advanced until paraesthesia is elicited or the bone contacted. By making several insertions through this same wheal in a line parallel to the inguinal ligament, the nerve is usually located and paraesthesia elicited. Injection of 5 ml of local anaesthetic suffices. (From Bonica 1953.)

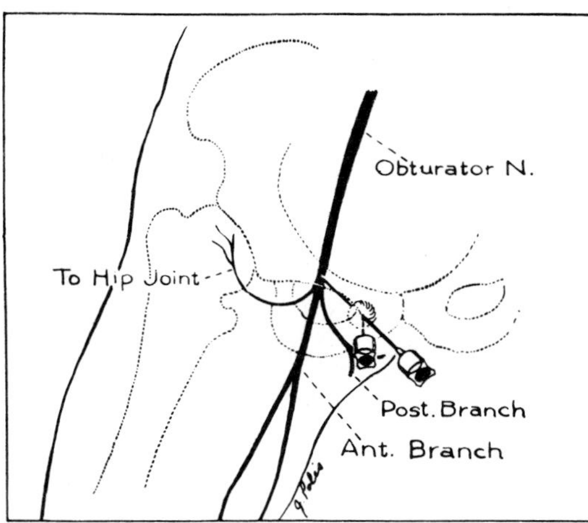

Fig. 52.18 Technique of obturator nerve block. With the patient lying supine and thighs separated, the pubic tubercle of the affected side is palpated and the skin wheal raised 1 cm lateral and inferior to it. A 22-gauge 8-cm needle is introduced through the wheal perpendicular to the skin and slowly advanced until the upper part of the inferior ramus of the pubis is contacted. A needle recorder is placed 2.5 cm from the skin and the point of the needle is redirected in a lateral and slightly superior and posterior direction so that the shaft is parallel with the superior ramus of the pubis and the point of the needle directed laterally and slightly superiorly. The needle is then slowly advanced while its point is kept in constant contact with the inferomedial surface of the superior ramus of the pubis until the recorder is flush with the skin or contact with the bone is lost. Since paraesthesia is rather difficult to elicit, a nerve stimulator is used to position the point of the needle near the nerve. After negative aspiration 10 ml of solution is injected. A successful block is evidenced by the loss of power in the abductor muscles within 15–20 minutes of the injection. (From Bonica 1953.)

are not available (Bonica 1953, 1959; Hannington-Kiff 1974). More recently, the technique of injection of glycerol into the trigeminal cistern for the treatment of trigeminal neuralgia has been reported (Hakansson 1981). I believe that no neurolytic or ablative procedure should be done without prior diagnostic/prognostic blocks with local anaesthetics.

Gasserian ganglion block

Gasserian ganglion block with a local anaesthetic is indicated as a diagnostic/prognostic procedure *only* in patients with severe intractable cancer pain and in cases of patients with trigeminal neuralgia involving the three divisions and in whom trigeminal rhizotomy is contemplated. The technique of gasserian ganglion block is depicted in Figure 52.19.

Complications

Complications will occur unless precautions are taken and skill is used. The most serious complication is accidental subarachnoid injection which invariably produces unconsciousness and palsy of other cranial nerves. When this complication occurs with a local anaesthetic, proper resus-

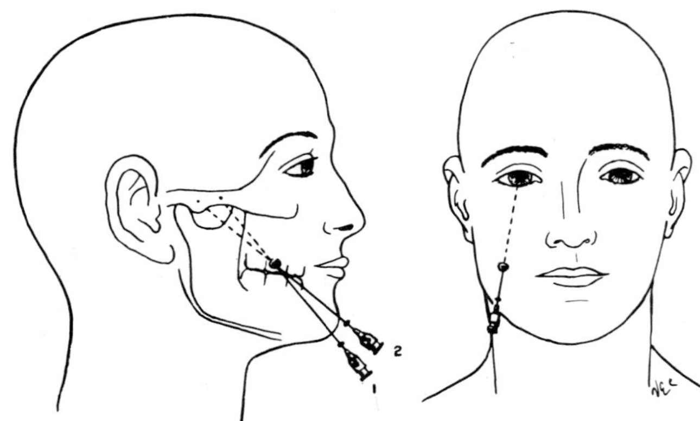

Fig. 52.19 Technique of block in the gasserian ganglion or the mandibular nerve by the anterolateral (Hartel) approach. The needle is inserted through a skin wheal which is on the skin overlying the second upper molar tooth. It is advanced in a direction so that viewed from the side its point is directed to the midpoint of the zygomatic arch and viewed from the front it is directed to the pupil of the ipsilateral eye. It is advanced in this direction until it contacts the infratemporal plate lateral to the base of the pterygoid process just anterior to the foramen ovale. The depth mark is then set 1.5 cm from the skin surface and the needle withdrawn until its point is in the subcutaneous tissue, then reinserted so that its point will go through the foramen ovale which is about 1 cm from the point of contact of the infratemporal plate. Passage of the needle through the foramen ovale often elicits paraesthesia in the distribution of the mandibular nerve. Once the point of the needle is 1.5 cm deeper than the bone, it is considered to be in the gasserian ganglion. An attempt at aspiration is made in several planes and the syringe is then detached to watch for cerebrospinal fluid. If no evidence of fluid or blood is noted, 1–1.5 ml of solution is injected. Analgesia will develop within 5–8 minutes of the injection. (From Bonica 1959.)

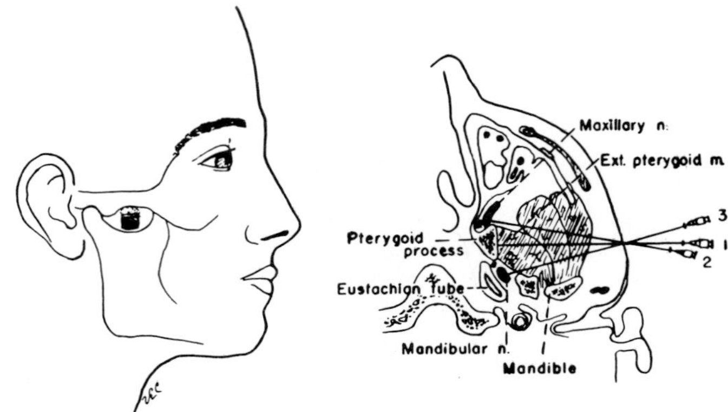

Fig. 52.20 Technique of maxillary and mandibular nerve block by the lateral extraoral route. Figure on the left indicates point of entrance into the skin just below the midpoint of the zygomatic arch. Figure on the right shows a schematic cross-section. The point of the needle (1) is impinging on the lateral pterygoid plate. To carry out maxillary nerve block, the needle is withdrawn until its point is in the subcutaneous region and then reinserted so that it will pass slightly anterior and superior, and advanced until its point enters the pterygopalatine fossa and contacts the maxillary nerve therein (2). In carrying out mandibular nerve block, needle 1 is withdrawn and reinserted in a direction slightly posterior. It is advanced until its point contacts the mandibular nerve just below the foramen ovale (3). After contacting each nerve eliciting paraesthesia, 2–3 ml of solution is injected. (From Bonica 1959.)

citative measures will avoid morbidity, but when it occurs with alcohol, it may cause permanent neurological sequelae. Haematoma of the face is likely to occur with repeated punctures using dull needles with hooks.

Blockade of the maxillary and mandibular nerves

Blockade of one or both of these nerves may be indicated as diagnostic/prognostic procedures in patients with trigeminal neuralgia, cancer pain or atypical facial pain. Blockade of the mandibular nerve is useful to help in the differential diagnosis of mandibular neuralgia from glossopharyngeal neuralgia in a patient in whom the lancinating pain is localized in the angle of the jaw (Bonica 1953, 1959). In patients with cancer pain in the lower jaw and upper neck it is necessary to combine mandibular nerve blocks with blockade of C2 and C3. The technique of blocking each of these nerves is depicted in Figure 52.20.

Complications

Blockade of the maxillary nerve may result in diffusion of the drug to adjacent nerves which supply eye muscles and laceration of vessels caused by needles with hooks or repeated haphazard insertions of the needle. Side-effects of mandibular nerve block include involvement of the motor fibres with paresis or paralysis of the ipsilateral muscles of mastication and deviation of the lower jaw to the affected side. Injection of large amounts of local anaesthetics or intraneural injection of the therapeutic

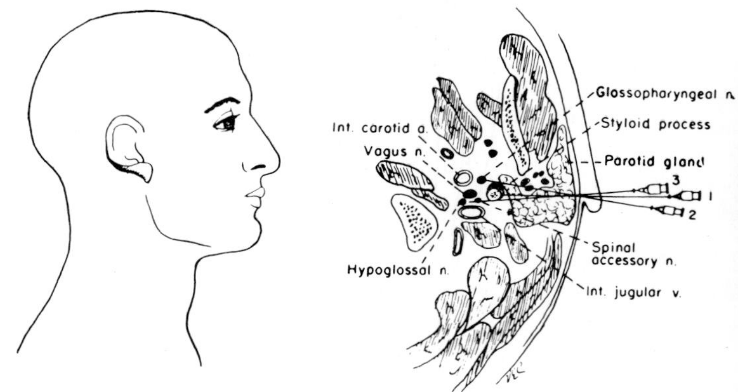

Fig. 52.21 Technique of blocking the glossopharyngeal and vagus nerves. Figure on the left shows the site where the skin wheal is formed, approximately midway between the posterior border of the mandible and tip of the mastoid process. The needle is inserted perpendicular to the skin and advanced until its point impinges on the styloid process, as depicted by needle 1 in the cross-sectional diagram on the right. The needle is then withdrawn and redirected so that it will pass anterior to the styloid process and slightly deeper until its point is in contact with the glossopharyngeal nerve (2). The vagus nerve is blocked by passing the needle posterior to the styloid process and advancing it about 1 cm deeper than the bone (3). Injection of 3–5 ml of solution is sufficient. (From Bonica 1959.)

dose may cause diffusion centrally to involve the gasserian ganglion.

Blockade of the glossopharyngeal and vagus nerves

Blockade of the glossopharyngeal nerve alone or in combination with blockade of the vagus nerve is useful as a diagnostic/prognostic procedure in patients with glossopharyngeal neuralgia, severe cancer pain of the throat or other severe painful conditions in the region innervated by the glossopharyngeal nerve. For the diagnosis of pure glossopharyngeal neuralgia, topical anaesthesia of the throat usually relieves the patient completely; this may be confirmed by blocking the glossopharyngeal nerve. In some atypical cases, the vagus nerve is also involved and it then becomes necessary to do diagnostic/prognostic blocks of both nerves at the base of the skull just below the jugular foramen (Robson & Bonica 1950; Bonica 1953). The technique of blocking the glossopharyngeal and vagus nerves is depicted in Figure 52.21.

Complications

Since this procedure produces paralysis of the pharyngeal muscles, a bilateral block is contraindicated. Moreover, blockade of the vagus nerve is likely to affect all of its branches ipsilaterally. If a large volume of drug is injected, the accessory and hypoglossal nerves become involved with consequent paralysis of the trapezius muscles and half of the tongue on the same side. Horner's syndrome is a frequent side-effect because of the proximity of the site of injection to the upper cervical sympathetic ganglion. A preventable complication of these procedures is accidental injection of the local anaesthetic into the internal jugular vein with consequent rapid onset of systemic toxic reaction.

REFERENCES

Ablondi M A, Ryan J F, O'Connell C T, Haley R W 1966 Continuous intercostal blocks for postoperative pain relief. Anesthesia and Analgesia 45: 185–189

Accardo N J, Adriani J A 1949 Brachial plexus block–a simplified technique using the axillary route. Southern Medical Journal 42: 920–923

Ang E T, Lassale B, Goldfarb G 1984 Continuous axillary brachial plexus block–a clinical and anatomical study. Anesthesia and Analgesia 63: 680–684

Applegate W V 1972 Abdominal cutaneous nerve entrapment syndrome. Surgery 71: 118–124

Bach S, Noreng M F Tjellden N U 1988 Phantom limb pain in amputees during the first 12 months following limb amputation after preoperative lumbar epidural blockade. Pain 33: 297

Bengtsson A, Bengtsson M 1988 Regional sympathetic blockade in primary fibromyalgia. Pain 33: 161

Bergh W P, Dottori O, Axisonhof B, Simonsson B G, Ygge H 1966 Effect of intercostal block of lung function after thoracotomy. Acta Anaesthesiologica Scandinavica 24 (suppl): 85–95

Berry F R, Bridenbaugh L D 1988 Upper extremity somatic blockade. In: Cousins M J, Bridenbaugh P O (eds) Neural blockade in clinical anesthesia and management of pain, 2nd edn. J B Lippincott, Philadelphia

Boas R A, Covino B G, Shahwarina A 1982 Analgesic response to IV lignocaine. British Journal of Anaesthesia 54: 501

Bogduk N 1988 Back pain: zygapophysial blocks and epidural steroids. In: Cousins M J, Bridenbaugh P O (eds) Neural blockade in clinical anaesthesia and management of pain, 2nd edn. Lippincott, Philadelphia

Bonica J J 1953 management of pain, 1st edn. Lea & Febiger, Philadelphia

Bonica J J 1955 Teaching residents diagnostic and therapeutic nerve blocks. Anesthesia and Analgesia 34: 202–213

Bonica J J 1957 Management of myofascial pain syndromes in general practice. Journal of the American Medical Association 165: 732–738

Bonica J J 1958 Diagnostic and therapeutic blocks. A reappraisal based on 15 years' experience. Anesthesia and Analgesia 37: 58–68

Bonica J J 1959 Clinical applications of diagnostic and therapeutic nerve blocks. C Thomas, Springfield, Illinois

Bonica J J 1967 Principles and practice of obstetric analgesia and anesthesia, vol 1. F A Davis, Philadelphia

Bonica J J 1974 Organization and function of a pain clinic. In: Bonica J J (ed) International symposium on pain. Raven Press, New York

Bonica J J 1990 Management of pain, 2nd edn. Lea & Febiger, Philadelphia

Bonica J J, Moore D C, Orlov M 1949 Brachial plexus block anesthesia. American Journal of Surgery 78: 65–79

Bonica J J, Akamatsu T J, Berges P U, Morikawa K, Kennedy W F Jr 1971 Circulatory effects of peridural block. II. Effects of epinephrine. Anesthesiology 34: 514–522

Bridenbaugh P O (ed) 1988 Neural blockade in clinical anesthesia and management of pain, 2nd edn. J B Lippincott, Philadelphia

Bridenbaugh P O, DuPen S L, Moore D C Bridenbaugh I D, Thompson G E 1973 Postoperative intercostal nerve block analgesia versus narcotic analgesia. Anesthesia and Analgesia 52: 85–85

Buckley F P 1985 Somatic nerve block for postoperative analgesia. In: Smith G, Covino B A (eds) Acute pain. Butterworth, London

Buckley F P, Simpson B R 1988 Acute traumatic and postoperative pain management. In: Cousins M J, Bridenbaugh P O (eds) Neural blockade in clinical anesthesia and management of pain, 2nd edn. J B Lippincott, Philadelphia

Churcher M 1978 Peripheral nerve blocks in relief of intractable pain. In: Swerdlow M (ed) Relief of intractable pain. Excerpta Medica, Amsterdam

Colding A 1969 The effect of regional sympathetic blocks in the treatment of herpes zoster. Acta Anaesthesiologica Scandinavica 13: 133–141

Cousins M J, Bridenbaugh P O 1988 Neural blockade in clinical anesthesia and management of pain, 2nd edn. J B Lippincott, Philadelphia

Covino B G, Vassallo H G 1976 Local anesthetics: mechanisms of action and clinical use. Grune & Stratton, New York

Crawford E D, Skinner D B 1982 Intercostal nerve block with thoracoabdominal and flank incisions. Urology 19: 25–28

Dan K, Tanaka H, Kamihara Y 1979 Herpetic pain and T-cell subpopulation. In: Bonica J J, Liebeskind J C, Albe-Fessard D (eds) Advances in pain research and therapy, vol 3. Raven Press, New York

DeJong R H 1977 Local anesthetics, 2nd edn. C C Thomas, Springfield, Illinois

DeKrey J A, Schroeder D F, Buechel D R 1969 Continuous brachial plexus block. Anesthesiology 30: 332

Delilkan A E, Lee C K, Young W K, Ong S C, Gannendran A I 1973 Post-operative local analgesia for thoracotomy with direct bupivacaine intercostal blocks. Anaesthesia 28: 561–567

Dhuner K G 1950 Nerve injuries following operations. A survey of

cases occurring during a six year period. Anesthesiology 11: 289–293
Eason M J, Wyatt R 1979 Paraurethral thoracic block – a reappraisal. Anaesthesia 34(7) 827–836
Eather K F 1958 Axillary brachial plexus block. Anesthesiology 19: 683–685
Engberg G 1975 Single dose intercostal nerve block for pain relief after upper abdominal surgery. Acta Anaesthesiologica Scandinavica 60 (suppl): 43–49
Faust R J, Nauss L A 1976 Post-thoracotomy intercostal block: comparison of its effects on pulmonary function with those of intramuscular meperidine. Anesthesia and Analgesia 55: 542–546
Findley T, Patzer R 1945 The treatment of herpes zoster by paravertebral procaine block. Journal of the American Medical Association 128: 1217–1221
Finneson B E 1973 Low back pain. J B Lippincott, Philadelphia
Galway J E, Caves P K, Dundee J W 1975 Effect of intercostal nerve block during operation of lung function and the relief of pain following thoracotomy. British Journal of Anaesthesia 47: 730–735
Goffen B S 1982 Transsacral block. Anesthesia and Analgesia 61: 623–624
Gunn C C 1989 Treating myofascial pain. Health Sciences Center for Educational Resources, University of Washington, Seattle
Hakansson S 1981 Trigeminal neuralgia treated by injection of glycerol into the trigeminal cistern. Neurosurgery 9: 638–666
Hannington-Kiff J G 1971 Treatment of intractable pain by bupivacaine nerve block. Lancet ii: 1392–1394
Hannington-Kiff J G 1974 Pain relief. Heinemann, London
Howe J F 1979 A neurophysiological basis for the radicular pain of nerve root compression. In: Bonica J J, Liebeskind J C, Albe-Fessard D G (eds) Advances in pain research and therapy, vol 3. Raven Press, New York
Janig W 1988 The pathophysiology of nerve following mechanical injury. In Dubner R, Gebhart G F, Bond M R (eds). Pain research and clinical management, vol 3. Proceedings of the Fifth World Congress on Pain. Elsevier, Amsterdam
Kehlet H 1989 Surgical stress: the role of pain and analgesia. British Journal of Anaesthesia 63(2) 189–195
Kraus H 1970 Clinical treatment of back and neck pain. McGraw-Hill, New York
Levine J D, Dardick S J, Roizen M F et al 1986 Contribution of sensory afferents and sympathetic efferents to joint injury in eperimental arthritis. Journal of Neuroscience 6(12) 3423–3429
Littler T R 1980 Pain relief in rheumatic conditions, part I. In: Lipton S (ed) Persistent pain: modern methods of treatment, vol 2. Academic Press, London
Loeser J D 1972 Dorsal rhizotomy for the relief of chronic pain Journal of Neurosurgery 36: 745
Lofstrom B, Wennberg A, Widen L 1966 Late disturbances in nerve function after block with local anaesthetic agents. Acta Anaesthesiologica Scandinavica 10: 111–122
Lyles R, Skurdal P, Stene J, Jaberi M 1986 Continuous intercostal catheter techniques for treatment of post-traumatic thoracic pain. Anesthesiology 65: A205
McQuay H J 1992 Pre-emptive analgesia (editorial). British Journal of Anaesthesia 69(1): 1–3
Melzack R 1971 Phantom limb pain: implication for treatment of pathologic pain. Anesthesiology 35: 409–419
Melzack R, Stillwell D M, Fox E J 1977 Trigger points and acupuncture points for pain: correlations and implications. Pain 3: 2–23
Menriques R G, Pallares V 1978 Continuous brachial plexus block for prolonged sympathectomy in control of pain. Anesthesia and Analgesia 57: 128–130
Miller R D, Johnston R R, Hosobuchi Y 1975 Treatment of intercostal neuralgia with 10% ammonium sulfate. Journal of Thoracic and Cardiovascular Surgery 69: 476–478
Miller R D, Munger W L, Powell P E 1988 Chronic pain and local anesthetic neural blockade. In: Cousins M J, Bridenbaugh P O (eds) Neural blockade in clinical anesthesia and management of pain, 2nd edn. J B Lippincott, Philadelphia
Moore D C 1955 Complications of regional anesthesia. C C Thomas, Springfield, Illinois
Moore D C 1971 Complications of regional anesthesia. In: Bonica J J (ed) Regional anesthesia. F A Davis, Philadelphia
Moore D C 1975 Intercostal nerve block for postoperative somatic pain following surgery of thorax and upper abdomen. British Journal of Anaesthesia 47: 284–286
Moore D C 1979 Regional nerve block, 4th edn. C C Thomas, Springfield, Illinois
Moore D C, Batra M S 1981 The components of an effective test dose prior to epidural block. Anesthesiology 55: 393–396
Moore D C, Bridenbaugh L D, Thompson G E et al 1978 Bupivacaine: a review of 11 080 cases. Anesthesia and Analgesia 57: 42–53
Moore D C, Bush W H, Scurlock J E 1980 Intercostal nerve block: a roentgenographic anatomic study of technique and absorption in humans. Anesthesia and Analgesia 59: 815–825
Murphy D F 1983 Intercostal nerve blockade for fractured ribs and postoperative analgesia. Description of new technique. Regional Anaesthesia 10: 151–153
Nunn J F, Slavin G 1980 Posterior intercostal nerve block for pain relief after cholecystectomy: anatomical basis and efficacy. British Journal of Anaesthesia 52: 253–260
Owen M, Galloway D J, Mitchell K G 1985 Analgesia by wound infiltration after surgical excision of benign breast lumps. Annals of the Royal College of Surgeons of England 67: 130–131
Pflug E A, Murphy, T M, Butler S H 1974 The effects of postoperative peridural analgesia on pulmonary therapy and pulmonary complications Anesthesiology 41: 8
Porter K M, Davies J 1985 The control of pain after Keller's procedure–a controlled double blind prospective trial with local anaesthetic and placebo. Annals of the Royal College of Surgeons of England 67: 293–294
Restelli L, Movilia P, Bossi L 1984 Management of pain after thoracotomy and technique of multiple intercostal blocks. Anesthesiology 61: 353–354
Robertson D M 1983 Transsacral neurolytic blocks. An alternative approach to intractable perineal pain. British Journal of Anaesthesia 55: 873–874
Robson J T, Bonica J J 1950 The vagus nerve in surgical consideration of glossopharyngeal neuralgia. Journal of Neurosurgery 7: 482–486
Rosenblatt R M, Cress J C 1981 Modified Seldinger technique for continuous interscalene brachial plexus block. Regional Anesthesia 6: 82–84
Rosenblatt R M, Pepitone-Rockwell F, McKillop, M J 1979 Continuous axillary analgesia for traumatic hand surgery. Anesthesiology 51: 565–566
Scott D B, Cousins M J 1988 Clinical pharmacology of local anesthetic agents. In: Cousins M J, Bridenbaugh P O (eds) Neural blockade in clinical anesthesia and management of pain, 2nd edn. J B Lippincott, Philadelphia
Sedzimir C B 1980 Lumbo-sacral root pain. In: Lipton S (ed) Persistent pain: modern methods of treatment, vol 2. Academic Press, London
Selander D 1977 Catheter technique in axillary brachial plexus block. Acta Anaesthesiologica Scandinavica 21: 324–329
Simons D L, Carron H, Rowlingson J C 1982 Treatment of bladder pain with transsacral nerve blocks. Anesthesia and Analgesia 61: 46–48
Simons D G 1975 Muscle pain syndromes: part I. American Journal of Physical Medicine 54: 289–311
Simon D G 1976 Muscle pain syndromes: part II. American Journal of Physical Medicine 55: 15–42
Smith B E 1984 Continuous sciatic nerve block. Anaesthesia 39: 155–157
Sola A E 1981 Myofascial trigger point therapy. Resident and Staff Physician 27: 38–45
Swerdlow M 1988 Complications of local anesthetic neural blockade. In: Cousins M J, Bridenbaugh P O (eds) Neural blockade in clinical anesthesia and management of pain, 2nd edn. J B Lippincott, Philadelphia
Toledo-Peraya L M, DeMeester T R 1978 Prospective randomized evaluation of intrathoracic block with bupivacaine in postoperative ventilatory function. Annals of Thoracic Surgery 19: 355–363

Travell J 1976 Myofascial trigger points. In: Bonica J J, Albe-Fessard D G (eds) Advances in pain research and therapy, vol 1. Raven Press, New York

Travell J G, Simons D G 1983 Myofascial pain and dysfunction. The trigger point manual. Williams & Williams, Baltimore

Tucker G T, Mather L E 1988 Absorption and disposition of local anesthetic agents. In: Cousins M J, Bridenbaugh, P O (eds) Neural blockade, 2nd edn. J B Lippincott, Philadelphia

Tverskoy M et al 1990 Postoperative pain after inguinal herniorrhaphy with different types of anaesthesia. Anaesthesia and Analgesia 70: 29–35

U S Department of Health and Human Services Agency for Health Care Policy and Research 1992 Acute pain management: operative or medical procedures and trauma. Clinical Practice Guidelines, AHCPR Publication No 91–0046, Rockville

Vatashsky E, Aronson H B 1980 Continuous interscalene brachial plexus block for surgical operation on the hand. Anesthesiology 53: 356

Wall P D 1988 The prevention of postoperative pain. Pain 33(3): 289–290

Winchell S W, Wolfe R 1985 The incidence of neuropathology following upper extremity blocks. Regional Anaesthesiology 10: 12–15

Winnie A P 1970 Interscalene brachial plexus block. Anesthesia and Analgesia 49: 455–466

Winnie A P 1983 Plexus anesthesia, vol I. W B Saunders, Philadelphia

Winnie A P, Ramamurthy S, Durrani Z 1973 The inguinal paravascular technic of lumbar plexus anesthesia. The 3-in-1 block. Anesthesia and Analgesia 52: 989–996

Woolf C J 1984 Long term alterations in the excitability of the flexion reflex produced by peripheral tissue injury in the chronic decerebrate rat. Pain 18(4): 325–343

Woolf C J 1986 Morphine-sensitive and morphine insensitive actions of C-fibre in the rat spinal cord. Neuroscience Letters 64(2) 221–225

Wyant G M 1979 Chronic pain syndromes and their treatment: III. The pyriformis syndrome. Canadian Anaesthetists Society Journal 26: 305–308

53. Epidural analgesics

Henry J. McQuay

INTRODUCTION

For nearly 20 years we have known that opioids applied to the spinal cord have analgesic effect. It has proved surprisingly difficult to define a clinical role for spinal (epidural and intrathecal) opioids, maximizing the analgesic benefit while minimizing the risk. The original question addressed was the advantage of spinal opioids over spinal local anaesthetics. The next question was the advantage of spinal opioids over intramuscular, oral or subcutaneous opioids. Now we have come full circle because it is the use of spinal combinations of local anaesthetic and opioid which promises the greatest clinical benefit.

It is ironic that these questions are being addressed for spinal opioids while our ignoranace about the conventional routes of administration for opioids, whether oral, subcutaneous, intramuscular or intravenous, remains profound. The single most important point is to distinguish between the phenomenon 'it can be done' and the clinical questions 'should it be done?' and 'if so, when and to whom?' New routes often have a high profile so that it may be very difficult to determine their real clinical role. The ultimate arbiter of the clinical role is the risk:benefit ratio. The aim is better analgesia with fewer adverse effects and with no increase in morbidity. For instance, in chronic pain oral opioids can provide good relief with manageable adverse effects for the majority of patients. New routes must be considered as replacements, adjuncts or alternatives to the oral route.

Well-designed randomized controlled trials which compared the new route with the established routes would give us the answers. Very few such trials are available. A good example of just how few such trials are done is the fact that 'Although millions of women have been offered epidural block for pain relief in labour over the past 20 years or so, fewer than 600 women have participated in reasonably well controlled comparisons with other forms of pain relief' (Howell & Chalmers 1991).

The underlying issues for new routes are kinetic and clinical logic. The spinal routes have the kinetic logic of applying the opioid directly to opioid receptors in the cord. The clinical advantage sought is better analgesia without the problems of systemic opioid use, or even the same analgesia with fewer adverse effects. Proposed alternatives must provide an improved risk:benefit ratio and be logistically feasible.

UNDERLYING ISSUES

THE EPIDURAL SPACE

The spinal epidural space extends from the sacral hiatus to the base of the skull. Drugs injected into the epidural space can then block or modulate afferent impulses and cord processing of those impulses. The way in which they block and modulate impulses and processing is probably the same as the mechanism which operates when the same drugs are injected intrathecally. There are some important differences between the epidural and intrathecal spaces, however, which affect clinical practice. It is the fact that the epidural space is a relatively indirect method of access compared with intrathecal that provides potential clinical advantage compared with the intrathecal route, and it is this which complicates matters.

The advantage is the fact that the meninges are not physically breached, so that headache from cerebrospinal fluid (CSF) leakage does not occur and the danger of meningitis is also reduced. Chronic administration through catheters should therefore be safer by the epidural route than by the subarachnoid route. The first disadvantage is that the epidural space is vascular and contains fat. A large proportion of the epidural dose is taken up by extradural fat and by vascular absorption and so less drug is immediately available for neural blocking action. The second disadvantage is that the epidural tissues react to foreign bodies more than the sheltered subarachnoid space. Epidural catheters often become walled off by fibrous tissue within days to weeks, whereas intrathecal catheters are much less prone to blockage (Durant &

Yaksh 1986); this problem is in part overcome by using continuous infusion rather than intermittent bolus.

The epidural space provides access for drugs to the neuraxis. When percutaneous catheters are used to provide continuous drug delivery the epidural route has advantages over the intrathecal route.

REACHING THE SITE OF ACTION

It used to be thought that the dura mater was impermeable to local anaesthetics and that epidural block with local anaesthetic occurred at the mixed nerve and dorsal root ganglia beyond the dural sleeves surrounding each pair of anterior and posterior spinal roots. Radioactive tracer studies have shown that the dura mater is not impermeable and that subarachnoid and epidural local anaesthetics act at precisely the same sites, namely, the spinal roots, mixed spinal nerves and the surface of the spinal cord to a depth of 1 mm or more, depending on the lipid solubility of the anaesthetic (Bromage et al 1963). With both epidural and subarachnoid injection the local anaesthetic drug entered the CSF and remained there until taken up by the lipids of the cord and spinal roots or until 'washed out' by vascular uptake into the blood vessels of the region.

Opioids have to reach the opioid receptors in the substantia gelatinosa of the cord in order to have spinal effect. Some of the opioid injected into the epidural space will reach the CSF and then the cord. Some will be absorbed into the blood stream and some will be bound by fatty tissue in the epidural space. The proportion of the dose injected which goes in each of these directions depends on lipid solubility and on molecular weight (Moore et al 1982). Lipid-soluble opioids will be subject to greater vascular uptake from the epidural space than lipid-insoluble opioids. High-molecular-weight drugs diffuse across the dura with less ease than drugs of low molecular weight. Once across the dura, drugs which have low lipid solubility may maintain high concentrations in the CSF for long periods of time and so can spread rostrally. Sampling at cisternal level after lumbar intrathecal injection of morphine has confirmed that high concentrations are found within an hour (Moulin et al 1986). Drugs with high lipid-solubility will be bound much faster in the cord, leaving lower concentrations of drug in the CSF available to spread rostrally.

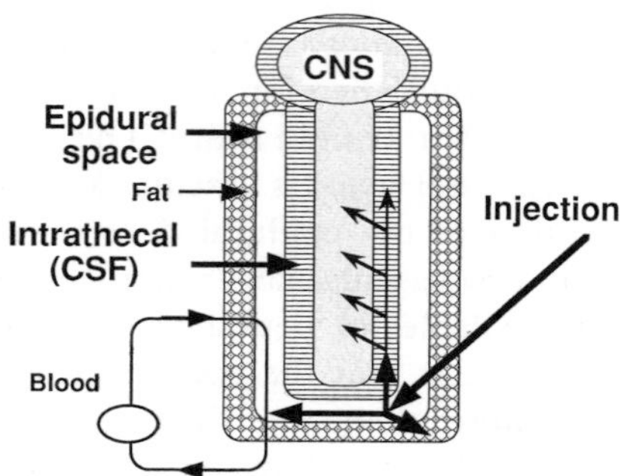

Fig. 53.1 Diagram of epidural space and fate of injected drugs, which may go into fat, into blood or into CSF and then into the spinal cord.

There is a similar range of lipophilicity and molecular size for the two drug classes, local anaesthetics and opioids, so that the journey from the place of injection to the target sites is likely to be accomplished in roughly the same time span for both classes of drug and proportional losses by vascular absorption and uptake into neighbouring fat depots are also likely to be similar. With both local anaesthetics (Burm et al 1986) and opioids (Jamous et al 1986), vascular uptake is slowed and neural blockade increased by adding a dilute concentration of adrenaline (3–5 μg/ml) to the injected agent.

LIPOPHILICITY AND POTENCY

Within each class of drug, however, there is a wide range of lipophilicity and this may have considerable influence on the relative potencies of the drugs within a class. Using an electrophysiological model, single unit recordings were made in the lumbar dorsal horn in the intact anaesthetized rat from convergent, multireceptive neurons. Activity was evoked by Aβ and C-fibre transcutaneous electrical stimulation of hindpaw receptive fields. With intrathecal application of opioids the effect of lipid solubility in determining relative intrathecal potency was measured. Initially, four μ opioid receptor agonists were used – morphine, pethidine, methadone and normorphine – because all four drugs had relatively high affinity for μ and little for δ and κ, precluding receptor affinity to other receptor subtypes as a complicating factor. The ED_{50} values from the dose–response curves were expressed against the partition coefficients. A significant correlation ($P = 0.002$) was found between the log ED_{50} and lipophilicity, but this was an inverse relationship, so that the least-lipid-soluble agonists, morphine and normorphine, were the most potent and the highly lipid-soluble methadone was considerably the least potent.

The same approximate order of potency, morphine = normorphine > pethidine > methadone, was seen in behavioural hot-plate and tail-flick tests, although the cut-off maxima necessary in those tests made it difficult to determine an ED_{50} for the more lipophilic and hence less potent compounds (Yaksh & Noueihed 1985). In a second study (Dickenson et al 1990) three opioids, fentanyl, etorphine and buprenorphine, all highly potent by the systemic route in man and animals, were applied either intrathecally or intravenously. Figure 53.2 shows the relationship between intrathecal potency and lipophilicity for the seven opioids tested. For fentanyl and buprenorphine potency correlated well with lipophilicity.

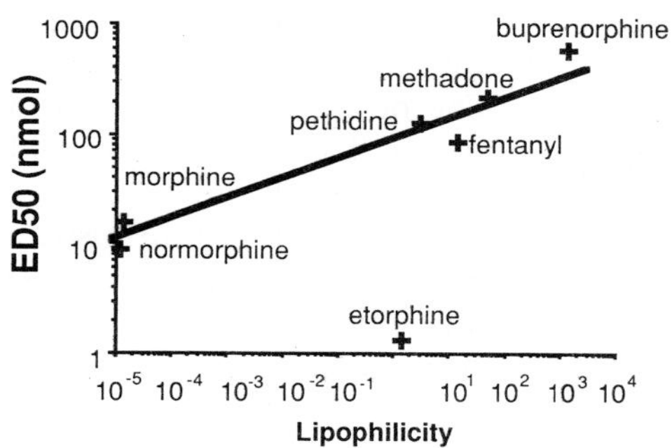

Fig. 53.2 The relationship between lipophilicity (heptane/water partition coefficient) and potency (ED_{50} nmol) for morphine, normorphine, pethidine, methadone buprenorphine, etorphine and fentanyl. Equation to the line (y = 94.4*x^0.19, r^2 = 0.93). (Redrawn from Dickenson et al 1990.)

The potency of etorphine, however, was considerably greater than would be expected if lipophilicity was the only determinant.

Nonspecific binding is the probable explanation of the inverse correlation between intrathecal potency and lipid solubility. When radiolabelled opioid distribution was visualized by autoradiography (Herz & Teschemacher 1971) the highly lipid-soluble opioids were found to be restricted largely to fibre tracts and penetrated the grey matter poorly. The thickly myelinated large A-fibres cap the spinal cord grey matter; they pass medially over the dorsal horn before penetrating the grey matter. This means that the lipid-rich A-fibres come between the injection site and the opioid receptors in the grey matter. Lipid-soluble opioids will be taken up rapidly but preferentially in this lipid-rich tissue. Drug bound in this nonspecific way cannot then go on to bind to the receptors.

Systemic potency ratios in man are thus unlikely to be accurate guides to spinal effectiveness, which makes it difficult to choose the dose of intrathecal (or extradural) opioid necessary to produce the same analgesia as a given dose of morphine. Many of the epidural opioid studies which used opioids other than morphine have used the systemic potency ratio to morphine as the guide for spinal potency. Extrapolation from the animal data suggests that, for drugs with high lipophilicity, the intrathecal dose required to give analgesia equivalent to that produced by a 0.5 mg bolus dose of intrathecal morphine is likely to be of the order of 5 mg for pethidine and close to 8.5 mg for methadone.

Clinical studies support this argument. Systemically, methadone is equipotent to morphine. From the animal work intrathecal methadone was approximately 18-fold less potent than intrathecal morphine (McQuay et al 1989). An intrathecal dose of 0.5 mg of morphine provided analgesia significantly superior to 20 mg of methadone (Jacobson et al 1990).

For extradural use, life is even less straightforward. Previous calculations showed that the proportion of an extradural dose transferred across the dura could vary from up to 20% for morphine (low lipid-solubility) to 0.2% for buprenorphine (high lipid-solubility) (Moore et al 1982). Because of the significant inverse correlation between lipid solubility and potency shown for the drug once in the CSF, the extradural dose of highly lipid-soluble drugs may have to be surprisingly high to give an effect equianalgesic to that of 5 mg of extradural morphine. Again, there are clinical data to support the theory. No clinical advantage was seen with extradural fentanyl compared with i.v. either in postoperative orthopaedic pain (Loper et al 1990) or after caesarean section (Ellis et al 1990). This finding is disputed (Salomäki et al 1991); these authors found epidural fentanyl to provide superior analgesia compared with intravenous fentanyl after thoracotomy, although the study design made this an inevitable result. These papers emphasize the necessity of systemic controls in extradural studies, because the vascular uptake of a lipophilic drug from the epidural space will, in itself, result in analgesia and is similar in its time course and extent to the uptake seen after the same dose given parenterally.

The theory then is that lipophilic opioids on their own (not combined with local anaesthetic) may be a poor choice for epidural use; nonspecific binding means that they have low spinal potency and substantial systemic analgesic effect makes it difficult to determine any spinal action. In practice, bolus injection of epidural opioid is often given with, or soon after, injection of epidural local anaesthetic. Clinical impressions of good analgesia after epidural injection of lipophilic opioid may reflect synergism between the opioid and the local anaesthetic and systemic effect of the opioid.

COMBINATIONS OF LOCAL ANAESTHETIC AND OPIOID

Epidural opioids on their own did not provide reliable analgesia in several pain contexts (Husemeyer et al 1980; Hogan et al 1991). Empirically combinations of local anaesthetic and opioid were found to work well and extradural infusions of these combinations are used widely for postoperative pain. The benefit is analgesia with minimal motor block and hypotension.

Two experimental studies have confirmed synergism between local anaesthetic and opioid (Fig. 53.3). Using visceral as well as conventional behavioural tests, Maves & Gebhart did an isobolographic analysis for morphine and lignocaine (Maves & Gebhart 1992). They showed that the analgesic effect of the intrathecal combination was greater than would be expected for a simply additive relationship. Using an electrophysiological model Fraser et al compared the dose–response curve for lignocaine combined with a dose of morphine with the dose–response

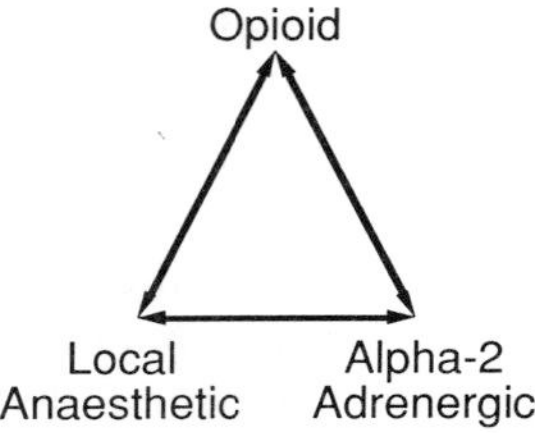

Fig. 53.3 Diagram of interactions between epidural local anaesthetic, opioid and alpha-2 adrenergic agonists. The relationships with midazolam are not clear.

curve for lignocaine alone; adding morphine, at a dose well below the ED_{50}, produced a 10-fold leftward shift in the lignocaine dose–response curve (Fraser et al 1992).

These studies support what has been observed clinically, that doses of local anaesthetic and opioid, doses which might be regarded as homeopathic for either drug independently, can produce good analgesia. Neither study was designed to answer the important question of the minimal effective doses of the combination components. While the minimum effective doses will vary with pain context, studies answering the question for one type of pain may tell us which component is the prime mover. The mechanism of the synergism is not known. It may be that the local anaesthetic, by reducing the afferent input, is moving the opioid dose–response to the right. Such explanations, however, account for only one direction of synergism and the evidence suggests that the synergism is bidirectional (Fig. 53.3). Clinical observations suggest that chronic infusion of the combination can produce selective blockade, blocking pain fibres while leaving other sensory input (and motor function) intact. These contradict the observation that blockade of pain by epidural opioid alone is associated with blunting of sensitivity to cold and pin-scratch sufficient for a segmental effect on cutaneous sensation to be detectable (Bromage et al 1982a). Such selectivity may of course be dose-dependent.

OTHER DRUGS

Many drugs have been given as analgesics via the epidural route. Steroids given for the management of back pain may in fact block C-fibre transmission (Johannson et al 1990). Other contenders have less logic behind their use, and caveats about toxicity are necessary. Two classes of drug are discussed below because both have had high profiles recently.

Alpha-2 adrenergic agonists

In both electrophysiological (Sullivan et al 1987) and behavioural studies, alpha-2 adrenergic agonists have antinociceptive effect. Much of the early work was with clonidine and this may have been misleading in terms of the properties of purer alpha-2 adrenergic agonists. Intrathecal clonidine showed a plateau at 50% of maximum effect. The newer drug, dexmedetomidine, is considerably more potent than clonidine and did not show such a ceiling to antinociception (Sullivan et al 1992a).

Alpha-2 adrenergic agonists have synergistic effect with both spinal opioid anaesthetic (Ossipov et al 1989; Sullivan et al 1987; 1992b) and spinal local anaesthetic (Fig. 53.3). The evidence for the local anaesthetic interaction comes mainly from clinical studies (Racle et al 1988; Bonnet et al 1989b, 1990; Huntoon et al 1992; Carabine et al 1992).

Midazolam

Midazolam on its own has very limited antinociceptive effect in standard behavioural or electrophysiological models (Clavier et al 1992), although effects have been found in other models (Niv et al 1983; Goodchild & Serrao 1987). Midazolam may have effects on Aδ fibres (Clavier et al 1992). There may well be interaction when combined with opioid (Moreau & Pieri 1988).

THERAPEUTIC ASPECTS

Both epidural local anaesthetics and epidural opioids can produce analgesia. The adverse effects of the two classes of drug are different. Epidural local anaesthetics can produce hypotension because of sympathetic blockade and carry the risks of local anaesthetic toxicity for which there is no specific antagonist. Epidural local anaesthetics produce motor block in a dose-dependent way. Epidural opioids can produce delayed respiratory depression, urinary retention, pruritus and nausea and vomiting, particularly in the opioid-naive patient. Naloxone is a specific antagonist. Epidural opioids do not produce a motor block. The combination of epidural local anaesthetic and opioid can also produce pain relief and the synergism between the drug classes offers the potential of effective analgesia at low doses of the components, minimizing the adverse effects of both. These features are summarized in Table 53.1.

The analgesic effect of epidural analgesics can be measured by a number of techiques; directly by measuring decrease in intensity or increase in pain relief, or indirectly via decreased need for other (parenteral) analgesics. Comparison with other, nonepidural methods of pain relief has also involved indirect measures, such as the relative effects on respiration, time for patients to recover and effects on stress hormones. The ultimate arbiter has to be analgesic effect, because indirect measures, such as reduction of the expected rise of stress hormones, do not have a direct relationship with analgesia.

For many years randomized controlled trials which compared the analgesia and adverse effects of oral or parenteral analgesics used the rule that sensible compar-

Table 53.1 Effects of local epidural anaesthetics, epidural opioids and of the combination

	Local anaesthetics	Opioids	Combination
Quality of blockade			
Sensory block	All modalities, dose-dependent	Mainly pain	Mainly pain LA dose-dependent
Sympathetic block	Yes, dose-dependent	None	LA dose-dependent
Motor block	Slight to complete, dose-dependent	None	LA dose-dependent
Vascular uptake	Dose-dependent and reduced by adrenaline	Reduced by adrenaline 1:200 000	
Possible to limit segmental blockade	Yes	Yes, but may spread rostrally	
Duration of action	Short	Variable, drug-dependent	Infusion
Adverse effects			
Central respiratory depression	No	Yes, dose-dependent	Minimal (low doses)
Urinary retention	Yes, relatively short	Yes, may be very prolonged	Minimal (low doses)
Pruritus	No	Yes	Minimal (low doses)
Nausea and vomiting	No	Yes	Minimal (low doses)

LA = local anaesthetic

isons of adverse effect incidence can be made only when the study drugs are compared at equianalgesic dosage. Very few randomized controlled trials which compare the adverse effects of different epidural opioids (or indeed epidural opioids with other techniques) have made equianalgesia the criterion which it should have been. Pronouncements about relative incidence of adverse effects can carry little weight unless the disparity in incidence or severity is measured at doses which produce equivalent analgesic effect.

The clinical decision to use epidural analgesia for pain relief is just that: a clinical decision. It presupposes that the analgesia is as good or better than analgesia from lower technology methods, that the potentially higher risk of adverse effects is worthwhile and that the facilities exist to deliver the epidural analgesia effectively and safely. Combination techniques are superseding the use of epidural opioids on their own and the randomized controlled trials to define the clinical role are still emerging.

ACUTE PAIN

ANALGESIA

Although both epidural local anaesthetics and epidural opioids can produce analgesia, there is some doubt about the ability of epidural opioids to produce analgesia as good (Husemeyer et al 1980) as epidural local anaesthetics in severe pain states. In childbirth the degree of analgesia was inadequate to relieve the pain of second stage labour (Husemeyer et al 1980; Hughes et al 1984), although satisfactory relief of first-stage pain could be achieved. No such doubt is seen with the epidural combination of local anaesthetics and opioids. The difference between the pain severity of different pain states should be emphasized, because it also means that categoric prescriptions for the doses to be used in combination infusions are likely to be valid only for a particular pain state or set of circumstances. Indeed, the dynamic nature of postoperative pain means that the dosage required on the day of surgery may be much higher than the dosage required on subsequent days.

A clear demonstration of the advantage of the combination of local anaesthetic and opioid was seen in a comparison of 0.125% bupivacaine in saline, diamorphine 0.5 mg in 15 ml and diamorphine mixed with 0.125% bupivacaine (0.5 mg in 15 ml) infused at a rate of 15ml/h for pain after major gynaecological surgery. The combination produced significantly superior analgesia to either of its components alone, without major adverse effects (Lee et al 1988). Giving the diamorphine intravenously with epidural bupivacaine was significantly less effective than giving the same dose epidurally in combination with epidural bupivacaine (Lee et al 1991).

Many important questions are still to be answered. A practical issue is the ability of combination infusions to control pain remote from the catheter site, as with thoracic pain and a lumbar catheter.

Combination dosage

Three strategies in dosage are discernible, the low (Cullen et al 1985; Logas et al 1987; Lee et al 1988), the intermediate (Bigler et al 1989; Seeling et al 1990) and the high (Hjortso et al 1985; Schulze et al 1988; Scott et al 1989). High doses (bupivacaine 0.5% 25 mg/h and morphine 0.5 mg/h) were used to produce analgesia immediately after upper abdominal surgery, but at some risk (Scott et al 1989). The stress response was not blocked. Lower doses (bupivacaine 0.1% 4 mg/h and morphine 0.4 mg/h) did not provide total pain relief after thoracotomy (Logas et al 1987). The issue of the minimum effective dose is of great importance and unfortunately may have to be defined for particular circumstances. It is too early (and too circumstance-dependent) for consensus to emerge, but an intermediate dose, 0.25% bupivacaine 10 mg/h with morphine 0.2 mg/h, has its advocates for use in pain after major surgery.

Other analgesics

Many other drugs have been used by the epidural route to provide analgesia, often with little underlying logic. The two major current contenders are alpha-2 adrenergic agonists and benzodiazepines (see Underlying Issues, above). The use of drugs by the epidural route which have not had adequate neurotoxicology must be discouraged.

Alpha-2 adrenergic agonists

The rôle of these drugs as analgesics on their own remains unclear. It is very difficult to preserve the double-blinding in studies of alpha-2 adrenergic agonists because of the hypotensive and sedative effects of the drugs. Comparisons of epidural clonidine with epidural placebo for postoperative pain relief are all marred by this fault because significant hypotension was a feature (Gordh 1988; Bonnet et al 1989a; Bernard et al 1991). No analgesic dose–response curve could be defined for clonidine (Mendez et al, 1990).

There is clear evidence, however, for both enhancement of the effect of local anaesthetics (Racle et al 1988; Bonnet et al 1989b, 1990; Huntoon et al 1992; Carabine et al 1992) and enhancement of the effect of opioids. With fentanyl (Rostaing et al 1991) and sufentanil (Vercauteren et al 1990) duration of effect was extended; with morphine Motsch et al (1990) found that adding clonidine produced significantly better pain scores. There may thus be an adjuvant rôle for alpha-2 adrenergic agonists.

Midazolam

Midazolam is reported to have analgesic effect in postoperative pain (Serrao et al 1992) but further studies are necessary to establish the benefits and risks compared with other techniques and other epidural analgesics.

ADVERSE EFFECTS

Toxicity

Epidural delivery necessarily places drugs at the neuraxis. Toxicity is therefore a real risk. Standard epidural analgesics, specifically local anaesthetics and opioids, have not produced toxicity to date, and clonidine was tested before it was used. Perhaps the major worry is if new analgesics without toxicology are introduced.

Motor block

Techniques of epidural local anaesthesia have been refined to a point where the neural pathways conducting pain can be blocked with a high degree of anatomical selectivity, but motor block is an inevitable accompaniment if large doses of local anaesthetic are needed to stop the pain. In labour pain, the motor block results in a higher incidence of instrumental delivery compared with nonepidural pain relief (Howell & Chalmers 1991). This block is not seen with epidural opioids or with the low doses used when local anaesthetic is combined with opioid.

Vasodilatation and hypotension

Vasodilatation in the lower parts of the body from blockade of sympathetic vasomotor nerves in the segments involved is another inevitable accompaniment of epidural local anaesthetic. In labour this requires prophylaxis. Hypotension also occurs with alpha-2 adrenergic agonists, and their use in combination with local anaesthetics could accentuate the risk. Again, the risk is minimized with epidural opioids alone or with the low doses of local anaesthetic used when combined with opioid.

Respiratory depression

Epidural block with local anaesthetics of intercostal and abdominal muscles is unlikely to cause significant impairment of respiratory function unless the phrenic segments (C3, C4 and C5) are also blocked. Respiratory depression after epidural opioids in opioid-naive subjects is much more subtle, more delayed in onset and longer lasting. The epidural opioids all reach the CSF by diffusion through the meninges and variable degrees of cephalad spread occur within the CSF. Morphine, being relatively lipid-soluble, will maintain substantial CSF concentrations to a greater extent than more lipid-soluble drugs, increasing the chance of drug reaching opioid receptors in the brain and so increasing the chance of respiratory depression. In volunteers, 10 mg of epidural morphine produced a depression of the CO_2-response curve far greater than that seen after intravenous administration, with the nadir of depression between the 6th and 12th hours after administration (Camporesi et al 1983).

Profound respiratory depression may be precipitated if other opioids are given parenterally during this danger period. Precautions must be taken to see that this mixed type of medication is avoided, and that patients are under appropriate surveillance, so that any case of delayed respiratory depression can be treated promptly (Ready et al 1988). Life-threatening apnoeic intervals can also arise abruptly after small doses of epidural opioids alone, with little warning. Theoretically, highly lipid-soluble opioids such as fentanyl and sufentanil should be less prone to rostral spread in the CSF. In practice, volunteer studies suggest that, although apnoeic intervals after epidural sufentanil were less frequent and less prolonged than after morphine (Klepper et al 1987), at equianalgesic doses of the drugs the CO_2-response curve was depressed and displaced equally severely.

Epidural opioids given on their own for relief of acute pain in opioid-naive subjects are only as safe as the quality of surveillance that is given. Whether the lower doses used in combination with local anaesthetics reduce the risk has still to be established.

Systemic effects

With epidural opioids, systemic effects of the opioid are to be expected. Vascular uptake from the epidural space is appreciable, with blood concentration curves of opioid which are almost indistinguishable from those after intramuscular or intravenous administration (for morphine, see Bromage et al 1982a; Chauvin et al 1982; Nordberg et al 1983). All the adverse effects of systemic opioids should therefore be expected. Placental transfer of opioid to the fetus and subsequent neonatal respiratory depression are thus not prevented by changing from parenteral opioid to epidural opioid.

Bladder function

Urinary retention is a common complication of epidural analgesic techniques after either local anaesthetics or opioids. The incidence appears to be dose-related and, in the case of local anaesthetics, retention is probably due to bladder deafferentation because the distended bladder does not give rise to discomfort. With epidural opioids the mechanism seems to be more complicated because retention and bladder distension to volumes above 800 ml in volunteers gave rise to marked discomfort and distress (Bromage et al 1982b).

Urodynamic and electromyographic studies in male volunteers indicated that the cause was detrusor muscle relaxation and not increased motor activity in the pelvic floor muscles (Rawal et al 1983). The origin of this detrusor relaxation is unclear, but the time sequence mirrors that of antinociception, beginning within 15 minutes but taking about 60 minutes to reach peak effect, and then lasting 14–16 hours. The overall intensity and duration of bladder relaxation appears to be independent of dose within the range of 2–10 mg. Retention with epidural opioids, like all the other adverse effects of epidural opioids, can be relieved by naloxone, although repeated doses may be needed to ensure complete evacuation of the bladder (Bromage et al 1982b).

The high incidence of retention from either local anaesthetic or opioid blockade is a factor in the clinical decision to use epidural analgesia.

Pruritus

Pruritus is not seen after epidural local anaesthetics, but it is a frequent adverse effect of epidural opioids in the opioid-naive patient. The itching is usually generalized but can be in the analgesic segments. The cause of the pruritus is unclear. The onset is often hours after analgesic effect is established, perhaps suggesting modulation of cutaneous sensation in the cord. Pruritus can be a major problem in acute pain management with epidural opioids, severe enough to cause distress. It can be reversed by naloxone, but then the analgesia is likely to be reversed.

Long-term risks

The spectre of a link between epidural local anaesthetics in childbirth and chronic backache has emerged (MacArthur et al 1990). These survey data do not prove causation, but prospective studies are needed to clarify the issue; difficult labours are more likely to need epidural block and may be associated with a higher risk of backache. If it is indeed motor block with local anaesthetic which is the cause, rather than the delivery or the epidural procedure per se, then the use of opioids or combinations should be preferred.

CHRONIC PAIN

Epidural analgesics have roles in both chronic nonmalignant pain and cancer pain.

CHRONIC NONMALIGNANT PAIN

In chronic nonmalignant pain the primary role for epidural local anaesthetics is their injection combined with steroid for the management of back pain with the object of reducing local oedema and nerve-root compression, although block of C-fibre transmission (Johannson et al 1990) may be the mechanism of the analgesia claimed. There are surprisingly few randomized controlled trials to support the use of epidural steroids for back pain management. Of the randomized controlled trials which compared epidural steroids with epidural local anaesthetic (Beliveau 1971; Breivik et al 1976; Yates 1978; Cuckler et al 1985; Rogers et al 1992), two showed significant difference between the two treatments. Each of the studies has some methodological problems, such as blinding technique, assessment methods, timing of subsequent treatments or use of concurrent treatments during the assessment period.

Epidural opioids have little place in the long-term management of ongoing nonmalignant pain (but see Plummer et al 1991), although acute exacerbations may be handled on a one-off basis.

The rôle of epidural clonidine is contentious. Apart

from its ability to extend the duration of local anaesthetics it may have the ability to relieve some forms of neuropathic or deafferentation pain. Glynn et al (1988) found epidural clonidine to be as effective as epidural morphine in 20 chronic pain patients using a cross-over design. As in earlier studies, there was a suggestion that clonidine was more effective than morphine for neuropathic pain and it may be that alpha-2 adrenergic drugs find a place as adjuvants in local anaesthetic and opioid combinations for resistant neuropathic pain.

Epidural midazolam was found in one randomized controlled trial to be as effective as epidural steroid in the management of chronic back pain (Serrao et al 1992). Experience is limited, so that more studies are needed to clarify whether there is a clinical rôle.

CANCER PAIN

Epidural opioids are used in chronic cancer pain as an alternative to other (oral or subcutaneous) routes (Plummer et al 1991). There has been little evidence from randomized controlled trials to support the argument that better analgesia is provided at lower incidence of adverse effects. Long-term administration, either as intermittent bolus or by infusion, has shown that this is technically feasible. The choice of delivery system lies between percutaneous exterior epidural catheter and micropore filter, tunnelled subcutaneous catheter with external injection port and micropore filter, totally implanted system with small subcutaneous reservoir and injection port, totally implanted system with large internal reservoir and automatic metered or manually controlled dosing device. Implanted systems are more likely to maintain hygiene and convenience, in theory protecting from infection and mechanical displacement. Implanted devices have high initial costs compared with simple percutaneous approaches, but over a period of months this may even out because of the higher costs of maintaining or replacing percutaneous catheters.

These technical approaches for administering small metered doses of spinal morphine over periods of weeks or months have proved to be well suited to home management and highly appreciated by the patients and their families. The problems include blockage, infection, pain on injection and leaks (Plummer et al 1991). It is important to be sure that the patient's pain cannot be controlled by simpler routes and that it can indeed be controlled by this method before embarking on what is a substantial undertaking (Jadad et al 1991). Preliminary trials with a percutaneous catheter to assess the effectiveness and the acceptability of adverse effects are necessary.

The main argument against the use of the epidural route as (merely) an alternative way to deliver opioid is that the opioid, whether given orally or spinally, must in the end be working at the opioid receptor. Failed management with oral opioid, failed because the pain was not responsive (Arner & Meyerson 1988; Jadad et al 1992) rather than because the opioid was not absorbed, is thus a questionable indication for epidural opioid. The protagonists can point to many thousands of patients treated. Epidural opiates alone, however, are not a universal panacea in cancer pain (Hogan et al 1991); if conventional routes for opioids do not relieve the pain, combinations of local anaesthetic and opioid appear to have a higher success rate than opioid alone.

Combination of local anaesthetic and opioid

The situation is changing with the advent of epidural infusion of a combination of local anaesthetics and opioid. Intrathecal use of such combinations in cancer pain is described by Sjöberg et al (1991). Most cancer pain, some 80%, responds to simple management with oral opioid and other analgesics. The two kinds of pain which respond badly to simple management are movement-related pain and neuropathic pain.

Movement-related pain can theoretically be controlled with oral opioid. In practice the dose of opioid required to control the patient's pain on movement is such that the patient is soundly sedated when not moving (not in pain). Conventional wisdom is that nonsteroidal antiinflammatory drugs should be added if they have been omitted. In practice this often has little impact. Some such pains, for instance due to vertebral metastases, can be helped by extradural steroid. The final resort is to use continuous epidural infusion of a combination of local anaesthetic and opioid. The synergism between the local anaesthetic and the opioid means that low doses can provide analgesia with little loss of mobility. There are few randomized controlled trials of this usage. The need for greater volume means that few of the devices available for implanted infusion of opioid alone are suitable, so that percutaneous catheters and external syringe drivers may be necessary. This method appears to produce analgesia for pains poorly responsive to opioids alone. The logic then is that pains poorly responsive to opioid orally are unlikely to improve simply by changing the route by which the opioid is given. Epidural use of local anaesthetic and opioid can produce the necessary analgesia.

The management of neuropathic cancer pain is often not straightforward. If such pain cannot be controlled by opioid, antidepressant or anticonvulsant, and steroids are inappropriate, then the same technique, epidural infusion of a combination of local anaesthetic and opioid, should be considered.

CONCLUSION

Epidural local anaesthetics have been used for many years in the management of acute pain in trauma, surgery and obstetrics, as well as in chronic pain, and their limitations and capabilities are well understood in these clinical areas. Opioids by this route are a new departure and our short experience in human subjects dates from as recently as 1979. Early enthusiasm in this field has been tempered by randomized controlled trials, and the field remains dynamic, with a switch from the use of either local anaesthetics or opioids on their own to the combination of the two. The alpha-2 adrenergic agonists in existing forms may also have a limited role on their own but may interact with local anaesthetics and opioids to provide a clinical advantage. Their importance is that they suggest that other beneficial interactions may emerge.

The fact that the field is dynamic, with a recent switch to the combination of local anaesthetics and opioids, means that we do not yet have the necessary information as to minimal effective dose. Randomized controlled trials are then required to define the clinical role of epidural combinations versus nonepidural pain relief in all the various pain contexts. There is still major concern that these powerful analgesic tools should be used effectively, safely and economically. The dream of attaining prolonged and powerful analgesia without adverse effects has not yet been realized and, as far as these epidural techniques are concerned, pain relief must still be bought at the cost of some risk. In some areas of pain management, however, these techniques are radically changing the quality of the service we deliver.

REFERENCES

Arner S, Meyerson B A 1988 Lack of analgesic effect of opioids on neuropathic and idiopathic forms of pain. Pain 33: 11–23

Beliveau P 1971 A comparison between epidural anaesthesia with and without corticosteroid in the treatment of sciatica. Rheumatology and Physical Medicine 11: 40–43

Bernard J-M, Hommeril J-L, Passuti N, Pinaud M 1991 Postoperative analgesia by intravenous clonidine. Anesthesiology 75: 577–582

Bigler D, Dirkes W, Hansen R, Rosenberg J, Kehlet H 1989 Effects of thoracic paravertebral block with bupivacaine versus combined thoracic epidural block with bupivacaine and morphine on pain and pulmonary function after cholecystectomy. Acta Anaesthesiologica Scandinavica 33: 561–564

Bonnet F, Boico O, Rostaing S et al 1989a postoperative analgesia with extradural clonidine. British Journal of Anaesthesia 63: 465–469

Bonnet F, Diallo A, Saada M, Belon M, Guilbaud M, Boico O 1989b Prevention of tourniquet pain by spinal isobaric bupivacaine with clonidine. British Journal of Anaesthesia 63: 93–96

Bonnet F, Buisson V B, Francois Y, Catoire P, Saada M 1990 Effects of oral and subarachnoid clonidine on spinal anesthesia with bupivacaine. Regional Anesthesia 15: 211–214

Broivik H, Hesla P E, Molnar I, Lind B 1976 In: Bonica J J, Albe-Fessard D (eds) Advances in pain research and therapy, vol 1. Raven Press, New York, p 927–932

Bromage P R, Joyal A C, Binney J C 1963 Local anaesthetic drugs: penetration from the spinal extradural space into the neuraxis. Science 140: 392–393

Bromage P R, Camporesi E M, Durant P A C, Nielson C H 1982a Rostral spread of epidural morphine, Anesthesiology 56: 431–436

Bromage P R, Camporesi E M, Durant P A C, Nielson C H 1982b Nonrespiratory side effects of epidural morphine. Anesthesia and Analgesia 61: 490–495

Burm A G L, van Kleef J W, Gladines M P R R, Olthof G, Spierdijk J 1986 Epidural anesthesia with lidocaine and bupivacaine: effects of epinephrine on the plasma concentration profiles. Anesthesia and Analgesia 65: 1281–1284

Camporesi E M, Nielson C H, Bromage P R, Durant P A C 1983 Ventilatory CO_2 sensitivity following intravenous and epidural morphine in volunteers. Anesthesia and Analgesia 62: 633–640

Carabine U A, Milligan K R, Moore J 1992 Extradural clonidine and bupivacaine for postoperative analgesia. British Journal of Anaesthesia 68: 132–135

Chauvin M, Samii K, Schermann J M, Sandouk P, Bourdon R, Viars P 1982 Plasma pharmacokinetics of morphine after i.m. extradural and intrathecal administration. British Journal of Anaesthesia 54: 843–847

Clavier N, Lombard M-C, Besson J-M 1992 Benzodiazepines and pain: effects of midazolam on the activities of nociceptive non-specific dorsal horn neurons in the rat spinal cord. Pain 48: 61–71

Cohen K L, Lucibello F E, Chomiak M 1990 Lack of effect of clonidine and pentoxifylline in short term therapy of diabetic peripheral neuropathy. Diabetes Care 13: 1074–1077

Cuckler J M, Bernini P A, Wiesel S W, Booth R E, Rothman R H, Pickens G T 1985. The use of epidural steroids in the treatment of lumbar radicular pain. Journal of Bone anad Joint Surgery 67A: 63–66

Cullen M L, Staren E D, El-Ganzouri A, Logas W G, Ivankovich D, Economou S G 1985 Continuous epidural infusion for analgesia after major abdominal operations: a randomised, prospective, double-blind study. Surgery 10: 718–728

Dickenson A H, Sullivan A F, McQuay H J 1990 Intrathecal etorphine, fentanyl and buprenorphine on spinal nociceptive neurones in the rat. Pain 42: 227–234

Durant P A C, Yaksh T L 1986 Distribution in cerebrospinal fluid, blood, and lymph of epidurally injected morphine and insulin in dogs. Anesthesia and Analgesia 65: 583–592

Ellis D J, Millar W L, Reisner L S 1990 A randomised double-blind comparison of epidural versus intravenous fentanyl infusion for analgesia after cesarian section. Anesthesiology 72: 981–986

Fraser H M, Chapman V, Dickenson A H 1992 Spinal local anaesthetic actions on afferent evoked responses and wind-up of nociceptive neurones in the rat spinal cord: combination with morphine produces marked potentiation of nociception. Pain 49: 33–41

Glynn C, Dawson D, Sanders R 1988 A double blind comparison between epidural morphine and epidural clonidine in patients with chronic non cancer pain. Pain 34: 123–128

Goodchild C S, Serrao J M 1987 Intrathecal midazolam in the rat: evidence for spinally-mediated analgesia. British Journal of Anaesthesia 59: 1563–1570

Gordh T Jr 1988 Epidural clonidine for treatment of postoperative pain after thoracotomy. A double blind placebo controlled study. Acta Anaesthesiologica Scandinavica 32: 702–709

Herz A, Teschemacher H J 1971 Activities and sites of antinociceptive action of morphine like analgesics. Advances in Drug Research 6: 79–119

Hjortso N C, Neumann P, Frosig F et al 1985 A controlled study on the effect of epidural analgesia with local anaesthetics and morphine on morbidity after abdominal surgery. Acta Anaesthesiologia Scandinavica 29: 790–796

Hogan Q, Haddox J D, Abram S, Weissman D, Taylor M L, Janjan N 1991 Epidural opiates and local anaesthetics for the management of cancer pain. Pain 46: 271–279

Howell C J, Chalmers I 1991 A review of prospectively controlled comparisons of epidural forms of pain relief during labour. International Journal of Obstetric Anesthesia 2: 1–17

Hughes S C Rosen M A, Shnider S M, Abboud T K, Stefani S J, Norton M 1984 Maternal and neonatal effects of epidural morphine for labor and delivery. Anesthesia and Analgesia 63: 319–324

Huntoon M, Eisenach J C, Boese P 1992 Epidural clonidine after cesarian section. Anesthesiology 76: 187–193

Husemeyer R P, O'Connor M C, Davenport H T 1980 Failure of epidural morphine to relieve pain in labour. Anaesthesia 35: 161–163

Jacobson L, Chabal C, Brody M C, Ward R J, Wasse L 1990 Intrathecal methadone: a dose–response study and comparison with intrathecal morphine 0.5 mg. Pain 43: 141–148

Jadad A R, Popat M T, Glynn C J, McQuay H J 1991 Double-blind testing fails to confirm analgesic response to extradural morphine. Anaesthesia 46: 935–937

Jadad A R, Carroll D, Glynn C J, Moore R A, McQuay H J 1992 Morphine responsiveness of chronic pain: double-blind randomised crossover study with patient-controlled analgesia method. Lancet 339: 1367–1371

Jamous M A, Hand C W, Moore R A, Teddy P J, McQuay H J 1986 Epinephrine reduces systemic absorption of extradural heroin. Anesthesia and Analgesia 65: 1290–1294

Johannson A, Hao J, Sjölund B 1990 Local corticosteroid application blocks transmission in normal nociceptive C-fibers. Acta Anaesthesiologica Scandinavica 34: 335–338

Klepper I D, Sherrill D L, Boetger C L, Bromage P R 1987 The analgesic and respiratory effects of epidural sufentanil and the influence of adrenaline as an adjuvant. Anesthesiology 59: 1147–1159

Lee A, Simpson D, Whitfield A, Scott D B 1988 Postoperative analgesia by continuous extradural infusion of bupivacaine and diamorphine. British Journal of Anaesthesia 60: 845–850

Lee A, McKeown D, Brockway M, Bannister J, Wildsmith J A W 1991 Comparison of extradural and intravenous diamorphine as a supplement to extradural bupivacaine. Anaesthesia 46: 447–450

Logas W G, El Baz N, El Ganzouri A et al 1987 Continuous thoracic epidural analgesia for postoperative pain relief following thoracotomy: a randomized prospective study. Anesthesiology 67: 787–791

Loper K A, Ready B L, Downey M et al 1990 Epidural and intravenous fentanyl infusions are clinically equivalent after knee surgery. Anesthesia and Analgesia 70: 72–75

MacArthur C, Lewis M, Knox E G, Crawford J S 1990 Epidural analgesia and long term backache after childbirth. British Medical Journal 301: 9–12

McQuay H J, Sullivan A F, Smallwood K, Dickenson A H 1989 Intrathecal opioids, potency and lipophilicity. Pain 36: 111–115

Maves T J, Gebhart G F 1992 Antinociceptive synergy between intrathecal morphine and lidocaine during visceral and somatic nociception in the rat. Anesthesiology 76: 91–99

Mendez R, Eisenach J C, Kashtan K 1990 Epidural clonidine analgesia after cesarean section. Anesthesiology 73: 848–852

Moore R A, Bullingham R E S, McQuay H J et al 1982 Dural permeability to narcotics: in vitro determination and application to extradural administration. British Journal of Anaesthesia 54: 1117–1128

Moreau J-L, Pieri L 1988 Effects of an intrathecally administered benzodiazepine receptor agonist, antagonist and inverse agonist on morphine-induced inhibition of a spinal nociceptive reflex. British Journal of Pharmacology 93: 964–968

Motsch J, Graber E, Ludwig K 1990 Addition of clonidine enhances postoperative analgesia from epidural morphine: a double blind study. Anesthesiology 73: 1067–1073

Moulin D E, Inturrisi C E, Foley K M 1986 Epidural and intrathecal opioids: cerebrospinal fluid and plasma pharmacokinetics in cancer pain patients. In: Foley K M, Inturrisi C E (eds) Opioid analgesics in the management of cancer pain. Advances in pain research and therapy, vol 8. Raven Press, New York, p 369–383

Niv D, Whitwam J G, Loh L 1983 Depression of nociceptive sympathetic reflexes by the intrathecal administration of midazolam. British Journal of Anaesthesia 55: 541–547

Nordberg G, Hedner T, Mellstrand T, Dahlstrom B 1983 Pharmacokinetic aspects of epidural morphine analgesia. Anesthesiology 58: 545–551

Ossipov M H, Suarez L J, Spaulding T C 1989 Antinociceptive interactions between alpha2-adrenergic and opiate agonists at the spinal level in rodents. Anesthesia and Analgesia 68: 194–200

Plummer J L, Cherry D A, Cousins M J, Gourlay G K, Onley M M, Evans H K A 1991 Long term spinal administration of morphine in cancer and non-cancer pain: a retrospective study. Pain 44: 215–220

Racle J P, Poy J Y, Benkhadra A, Jourdren L, Fockenier F 1988 Prolongation of spinal anesthesia with hyperbaric bupivacaine by adrenaline and clonidine in the elderly. Annales Francaises d'Anesthesie et de Reanimation 7: 139–144

Rawal N, Möllefors K, Axelsson K, Lingårdh G, Widman B 1983 An experimental study of urodynamic effects of epidural morphine and naloxone reversal. Anesthesia and Analgesia 62: 641–647

Ready L B, Oden R, Chadwick H S et al 1988 Development of an anesthesiology based postoperative pain management service. Anesthesiology 68: 100–106

Rogers P, Nash T, Schiller D, Norman J 1992 Epidural steroids for sciatica. Pain Clinic 5: 67–72

Rostaing S, Bonnet F, Levron J C, Vodinh J, Pluskwa F, Saada M 1991 Effect of epidural clonidine on analgesia and pharmacokinetics of epidural fentanyl in postoperative patients. Anesthesiology 75: 420–425

Salomäki T E, Laitinen J O, Nuutinen L S 1991 A randomised double-blind comparison of epidural versus intravenous fentanyl infusion for analgesia after thoracotomy. Anesthesiology 75: 790–795

Schulze S, Roikjaer O, Hasselstrom L, Jensen N H, Kehlet H 1988 Epidural bupivacaine and morphine plus systemic indomethacin eliminates pain but not systemic response and convalescence after cholecystectomy. Surgery 103: 321–327

Scott N B, Mogensen T, Bigler D, Lund C, Kehlet H 1989 Continuous thoracic extradural 0.5% bupivacaine with or without morphine: effect on quality of blockade, lung function and the surgical stress response. British Journal of Anaesthesiology 62: 253–257

Seeling W, Bruckmooser K P, Hufner C, Kneitinger E, Rigg C, Rockemann M 1990 No reduction in postoperative complications by the use of catheterized epidural analgesia following major abdominal surgery. Anaesthesist 39: 33–40

Serrao J M, Marks R L, Morley S J, Goodchild C S 1992 Intrathecal midazolam for the treatment of chronic mechanical low back pain: a controlled comparison with epidural steroid in a pilot study. Pain 48: 5–12

Sjöberg M, Applegren L, Einarsson S et al 1991 Long-term intrathecal morphine and bupivacaine in 'refractory' cancer pain. I. Results from the first series of 52 patients. Acta Anaesthesiologica Scandinavica 35: 30–43

Sullivan A F, Dashwood M R, Dickenson A H 1987 Alpha adrenoceptor modulation of nociception in rat spinal cord: location, effects and interactions with morphine. European Journal of Pharmacology 138: 169–177

Sullivan A F, Kalso E, McQuay H J, Dickenson A H 1992a The antinociceptive actions of dexmedetomidine on dorsal horn neuronal responses in the anaesthetised rat. European Journal of Pharmacology 215: 127–133

Sullivan A F, Kalso E, McQuay H J, Dickenson A H 1992b Evidence for the involvement of the μ but not the δ opioid receptor subtype in the synergistic interaction between opioid and alpha-2 adrenergic antinociception in the rat spinal cord. Neuroscience Letters 139: 65–68

Vercauteren M, Lauwers E, Meert T, De Hert S, Adriaensen H 1990 Comparison of epidural sufentanil plus clonidine with sufentanil alone for postoperative pain relief. Anaesthesia 45: 531–534

Yaksh T L, Noueihed R 1985 The physiology and pharmacology of spinal opiates. Annual Review of Pharmacology and Toxicology 25: 433–462

Yates D W 1978 A comparison of the types of epidural injection commonly used in the treatment of low back pain and sciatica. Rheumatology and Rehabilitation 17: 181–186

54. Sympathetic nerve blocks in painful limb disorders

J. G. Hannington-Kiff

INTRODUCTION

The idea of sympathy between various organs and regions of the body has been around at least since the time of Galen in the early 16th century. The anatomical ease of demonstrating the wide distribution of the vagus and the connections of the thoracolumbar outflow throughout the body presented an obvious mechanism for the functional concept of sympathy, serving to explain the link between the activity of visceral and somatic structures. The time has undoubtedly come for a revaluation of the sympathetic nervous system to incorporate modern views about the functional diversity of the sympathetic nervous system and its currently recognized capability of interacting with peripheral somatic nerves following injury and in the presence of inflammation.

The sympathetic nervous system should be considered as efferent with the ability to alter cutaneous and possibly muscle sensory mechanisms at a peripheral level and to contribute to the sensitization of neuron pools in the spinal cord as well as the classical effects on the viscera and the cardiovascular system. Unless the clinician becomes aware of these new possibilities, it is difficult to get away from the traditional view that sympathetic block affects only blood flow in the limb and that any other benefits, for instance pain relief, must stem from the effects of increased blood flow in washing away accumulated noxious metabolic products. A glimpse of the complexity of the interacting neurotransmitters and the neuromodulators in the postganglionic sympathetic nerve endings is provided by Burnstock (1986) so that considering the sympathetic nervous system as purely efferent need not mean that there is a poverty of interactive possibilities between the postganglionic nerve endings and the target receptors wherever they are located.

Though the sympathetic nerve endings are efferent, they may be considered as having an indirect afferent effect by virtue of changing the nature of the afferent receptors upon which they impinge. Consequently, regional blockade of the sympathetic nervous system, especially in the presence of disease, may be expected to produce more changes than simply those due to altered blood flow in the affected part. Clearly, we need to revise our views about the sympathetic nervous system (Hannington-Kiff 1992).

The purpose of this chapter is to outline the methods by which the regional sympathetic nerves to limbs can be blocked and to provide a clinical guide to assist the clinician in selecting the most appropriate kind of block to suit the condition requiring treatment. The emphasis will be on the integration of sympathetic blocks into the programme of the general management and the rehabilitation of the patient with the objective of promoting the best possible functional outcome for the affected limb.

The various methods of blocking the paravertebral ganglia have been dealt with in copious detail in the various sumptuously illustrated atlases and manuals that are currently available. Accordingly, the only comment that will be made in relation to paravertebral ganglion blocks will be by way of practical hints and cautions.

The intravenous regional technique of blocking the sympathetic nervous system will be considered in more detail because such accounts do not appear elsewhere and the subject lends itself well to introducing the use of a spectrum of blocking agents which exploit the burgeoning information about the galaxy of neurotransmitters and neuromodulators known to be present in the postganglionic nerve endings.

BLOCKS OF THE SYMPATHETIC NERVOUS SYSTEM

These blocks may be classified as follows with regard to limbs:

Component of any local anaesthetic regional block
Paravertebral ganglion block
Interpleural anaesthesia (upper limb)
Transdermal (topical) block
Intravenous regional block

Systemic intravenous infusion of alpha adrenoreceptor blocking agent

LOCAL ANAESTHETIC REGIONAL BLOCK

Any regional block with local anaesthesia, whether intrathecal, epidural, plexus or peripheral, will produce some degree of regional sympathetic block, the extent depending upon the proximity to the spinal cord or to a major neurovascular bundle. It should not be forgotten, for example, that local anaesthetic solution introduced in substantial volume in the various approaches to the brachial plexus not infrequently reaches the stellate ganglion. Moreover, systemically absorbed local anaesthetic agents can have a generalized effect on the sympathetic nervous system and on the perception of pain.

PARAVERTEBRAL GANGLION BLOCK

Stellate ganglion block

It should be recalled that the left and right stellate ganglia have different controlling functions on the heart; for instance blocking the right stellate ganglion can prolong the electrocardiographic Q–T interval and render the patient more prone to dysrhythmia (Yanagida et al 1976; Kettler & Stene 1987). I prefer to perform stellate ganglion block with the patient sitting from the beginning (rather than lying down at first) and to use a volume of about 12 ml of 0.5% bupivacaine plain with 5 ml of a suitable water-soluble contrast medium to enable the progress of the injected material to be followed down over the heads of the first two ribs with the aid of the X-ray image intensifier. Blockade of the sympathetic nervous supply to the arm requires a fair volume of local anaesthetic solution; the appearance of Horner's syndrome is not testimony to sympathetic block in the arm; indeed, good blockade in the arm can be achieved with careful attention to technique with only minor, evanescent eye signs.

It should be recalled that the cervicothoracic sympathetic chain can be blocked by appropriate posturing of the patient and by the use of a long catheter during interpleural local anaesthesia. This will also block the brachial plexus but the wide extent of the block can be most useful if pain and sympathetic dystrophy involve much of the upper quadrant and shoulder as well as the arm.

LUMBAR PARAVERTEBRAL BLOCK

This block should always be targeted with X-ray image intensification, the use of which is mandatory when neurolytic agents are employed. The target should be identified with a small volume of full-strength water-soluble contrast medium; about 0.3–0.5 ml is enough to produce the linear, slightly curved 'thumb-nail impression' at the edge of the vertebral body when the needle tip is in the correct position. It is naive and unhelpful to drench the edge of the psoas muscle with contrast medium as is so often depicted in the textbooks.

Though the one-needle technique has become popular, it is wiser when using a neurolytic agent to introduce a small volume of the agent at 2–3 levels rather than to inject a substantial volume at one level with the attendant risk of spreading the agent laterally to affect the genitofemoral nerve and posteriorly to affect the spinal nerve roots.

During the targeting with contrast medium the image intensifier should be in 'real time' to ensure that the material is not being injected into a blood vessel or ureter (when the image of the injected material will shoot off the screen). Care should be taken thereafter not to move the needle point. If the neurolytic agent is labelled with some of the contrast medium, this, too, can be monitored in real time with the image intensifier, adding an extra dimension of safety.

PHARMACOLOGICAL TARGET BLOCKS

When a variety of drugs, including local anaesthetic agents, can be delivered to a discrete part of the body to remain there in high concentration for a period of time, it seems appropriate to identify the procedure in general terms as a pharmacological block.

The principle of the target block is to deliver a drug or prodrug in high concentration directly to a selected tissue or area of the body (Hannington-Kiff 1984). The objective is to affect profoundly a defined geographical area without as far as possible producing a significant plasma level and unwanted systemic effects. Moreover, there is a high degree of assurance that most of the agent will reach the target tissue compared with the vagaries of oral administration and patient compliance. The dimension of time can be added to these spatial considerations by using drugs with a high affinity for selected tissues or by using slow-release preparations of drugs in appropriate locations.

The limbs uniquely provide a simple clinical method of confining drugs in high local concentration as it is possible to isolate the regional circulation with an arterial tourniquet and aim the drug at the tissues by back-perfusion through the veins. It is astonishing that back-perfusion to the tissues from the veins is so effective. The use of guanethidine in this way has become an established method of procuring peripheral sympathetic block in limbs. Not only has this technique stood the test of time but it has offered a method of selective noradrenergic block, whereas the classical method of sympathetic ganglion block also blocks cholinergic sympathetic fibres. The regional use of guanethidine has not only transformed the management of certain types of disabled limbs but has helped to generate new ideas about the peripheral sympathetic nervous system. Consequently, a major part of this chapter will be devoted to the technique of intravenous regional noradrenergic neuron block with guanethidine (guanethidine block, for simplicity) with particular reference to the treatment of reflex sympathetic dystrophy syndromes (RSDS, codes 203.91b and 603.91b; Merskey 1986). Other methods of aiming or confining drugs to specific targets must perforce be considered in outline only, but in sufficient detail to illustrate the principle and effects of strategically applying agents to selected tissues in high concentration. Agents applied in a pharmacological magnitude of concentration can produce different effects from those normally encountered when they are given in their usual therapeutic systemic dilution. The targeting of drugs on a cellular scale through the circulation (for example in macrophages) and by intraarterial injection will not be discussed.

CLINICAL AIMING METHODS

There are basically three methods of targeting drugs readily available to clinicians: transdermal inunction, percutaneous injection and intravenous regional injection.

TRANSDERMAL INUNCTION

The simple inunction of substances is possibly the oldest type of medication known to man. Proprietary rubefacient and counterirritant creams abound in domestic medicine cabinets but few drugs penetrate the skin to any appreciable depth, except in infants. The interesting effect of capsaicin on C-afferents, most of which are nociceptive, suggests that further consideration should be given to the possibility of developing a more effective modern equivalent of traditional liniments, many of which contain this substance.

Attempts have been made to aid the passive transdermal absorption of drugs by the use of penetrating vehicles such as the evil-smelling dimethyl sulphoxide (DMSO) but they have not been very successful. Lately, the serendipitous finding that a mixture of equal parts of lignocaine and prilocaine crystals forms an eutectic compound which is liquid at room temperature has made it possible to formulate a highly effective transdermal local anaesthetic cream (Brodin et al 1984). This cream, called EMLA (eutectic mixture of local anaesthetics) contains droplets of the eutectic liquid; those droplets which penetrate the superficial layers of the dermis produce a profound effect on nerve endings equivalent to applying 80% local anaesthetic agent. Clinically useful local anaesthesia takes 60–90 minutes to develop but this relatively minor disadvantage can be overcome by planning. EMLA has proved of great help in my clinic as an aid to the rehabilitation of painful hands and as a means of providing cutaneous anaesthesia prior to nerve blocks. A particular advantage of using EMLA prior to performing a delicate nerve block with an injected agent or with a lesion-producing probe is that the contours of the tissues overlying the target are not distorted, as they can be after an intracutaneous or subcutaneous injection of local anaesthetic solution. Consequently, the chances of successful location of the target are increased.

Simple inunction is a passive process and I have attempted to power-assist the process by applying direct current (iontophoresis) or ultrasound (phonophoresis). The guanethidine molecule bears two strong positive charges and should consequently be a good prospect for use with iontophoresis. Guanethidine has been applied with iontophoresis to relieve causalgia (Hannington-Kiff 1984) and with phonophoresis to promote the healing of ischaemic leg ulcers (unpublished). A note of caution is that informed care is required to avoid burning the patient during iontophoresis. Phonophoresis would appear to be the safer technique but controlled studies are required to establish whether either technique regularly increases the transdermal penetration of selected drugs.

It is to be hoped that a drug which has negotiated the dermal barrier will be selectively taken up by the target tissue. In the case of guanethidine the target (the sympathetic nerve endings) selectively and actively takes up the drug. One explanation of the way guanethidine can destroy sympathetic neurons in certain laboratory animals is that guanethidine blocks the retrograde axon transport of nerve growth factor to the cell body from the periphery (Johnson 1978). Csillick et al (1982) proffered a similar explanation for the method of action on sensory nerves of vinca alkaloids applied transdermally by iontophoresis for the clinical relief of various types of neuralgia.

A special case of the topical application of guanethidine to produce pain relief is the successful use of this solution in the alleviation of dentinal hypersensitivity when painted with a cotton pledget on to acutely exposed dentine (Hannington-Kiff & Dunne 1993; Dunne & Hannington-Kiff 1993.) Guanethidine applied in this way removes the typical hypersensitivity of exposed dentine to cold within a couple of minutes. This analgesic effect of guanethidine is seemingly not the result of local anaesthetic action as there is no loss of sensibility in the adjacent gum margin. Since there is no initial exacerbation of pain, the effect is unlikely to involve noradrenergic mechanisms. Guanethidine has proved to be a useful and superior alternative to local anaesthesia in certain areas of conservative dentistry when dentine is exposed: indeed it has proved to be a rescue technique when local anaesthetic block has failed. The efficacy of guanethidine in relieving dentinal pain has important theoretical implications as well as providing a useful new technique in dental practice.

PERCUTANEOUS INJECTION

By injecting solutions into the fascial sheaths and potential spaces between tissue planes it is possible to guide drugs blindly to relatively distant targets: for instance, the cervical sympathetic chain can be reached by local anaesthetic solution injected through the usual anterior route in the neck, through the posterior paravertebral route in the upper thoracic region and through the subclavian route when a large volume is injected into the axillary sheath. Apart from the targeting principle, there are other advantages to confining volumes of solution containing an active agent within fascial sheaths or potential spaces between tissue planes. For instance, the deposited solution can act as a pool or depot from which the active principle may slowly leach on to the target. It may be possible, as in the case of a local anaesthetic, to choose different concentrations of active agent which will selectively or differentially affect different classes of nerve fibre.

The following case report illustrates how natural fascial sheaths and tissue planes can be used to guide a drug to a relatively distant target.

Case report

An elderly lady had severe intercostal neuralgia associated with a malignant secondary deposit in the seventh left rib in the anterior axillary line. The patient was receiving a variety of analgesics, including opiates. It was decided to provide regional pain relief prior to performing a cryosurgical intercostal nerve block on the routine surgical session later in the week. A fine catheter was directed towards the vertebral column in the subcostal groove of the affected rib through a Tuohy needle introduced near the edge of the rib. About 17 ml of a solution containing 2.5 mg diamorphine and a trace of a radionuclide dissolved in 20 ml normal saline was injected and followed with a gamma camera (much as described by Middaugh et al 1985). Pain relief occurred when the leading edge of the radioactive puddle had traversed the paravertebral space and had just reached the epidural region. An interesting theoretical implication is that the opiate did not produce analgesia whilst in contact with the intercostal nerve, as there is some controversy about whether opiates can affect peripheral nerve fibres along their length. Good regional pain relief lasted 8 hours from the one injected dose of diamorphine.

The aiming and arrival on target of a needle-cannula, a cryoprobe and a radiofrequency heated probe can be monitored with image-intensified X-ray control or computerized axial tomography. These aids are now widely available and there is little justification for taking risks with blind neurolytic injections. For example, biplanar image-intensified X-ray control should be considered mandatory in lumbar sympathectomy using phenol solution or other neurolytic agents.

INTRAVENOUS REGIONAL INJECTION

After arterial occlusion with a tourniquet, the veins provide a fast and effective method of transporting drugs in high concentration to the tissues of the isolated segment of a limb. Unwanted systemic effects are unusual if careful attention is given to the application of a pneumatic tourniquet by experienced personnel. Premature release or accidental failure of the pneumatic tourniquet poses the greatest unforeseen hazards to the patient. Otherwise the most unpredictable stage of intravenous regional (IVR) techniques is associated with the release of the tourniquet at the end of the procedure. Systemic effects at this time should be minimal if the tourniquet is kept inflated for at least 20 minutes to allow fixation of the injected drug in the tissues. The affinity of the drug for the tissues and other factors, such as the degree of plasma-binding, must be taken into consideration, as well as the nature of the drug. I overcome the relative hazard associated with the period of tourniquet release in IVR anaesthesia for surgical procedures by the application of an extra distal tourniquet (Hannington-Kiff 1980, 1984, 1990a). In this technique the local anaesthetic is injected into the confined veins in the compartment of the limbs between the tourniquets. This produces local anaesthesia in the terminal part of the limb because nerves traversing the intertourniquet compartment undergo a conduction block as local anaesthetic diffuses on to them from the venous reservoir in the isolated compartment. Because the local anaesthetic is contained in a well-demarcated venous reservoir, it is feasible to wash out the dregs of the unfixed drug with saline before releasing the tourniquets. There are surgical advantages associated with the use of IVR compartment blocks which are especially important in delicate reconstructive operations on the hand: the surgical field is not suffused with local anaesthetic solution oozing from the distended veins and the extra tourniquet reduces the bleeding in general. For these reasons I often refer to this type of block as bloodless intravenous regional anaesthesia, or BIVRA (Hannington-Kiff 1984).

ANTISYMPATHETIC IVR BLOCKS

The injection of local anaesthetic solution into the vicinity of the stellate ganglion and the lumbar ganglion chain is the usual clinical method of temporarily blocking the sympathetic nerve supply to the upper and lower limbs respectively. The stellate ganglion block is disliked by patients who are generally fearful of injections into the neck and the effects of sympathetic block in the face and occasional hoarseness are unwelcome. If the posterior paravertebral approach is used there is an increased risk of pneumothorax. In the case of lumbar sympathetic block, the target of the needle should preferably be identified with the aid of an X-ray image-intensifier. On the whole, sympathetic ganglion blocks require skill beyond the experience of most doctors and the logistical difficulty of procuring sympathetic blocks in our community has undoubtedly been a considerable handicap in the rational management of pain and disability in dystrophic limb conditions.

Sympathetic ganglion blocks with local anaesthetic, even with the relatively long-acting bupivacaine, last only several hours and most clinical conditions will require a series of blocks. In selected patients, lumbar sympathetic blocks can justifiably be performed with neurolytic agents such as phenol to give more prolonged effects, lasting several days or weeks. In these circumstances control of the injection with an X-ray image-intensifier is mandatory to minimise complications and ensure the most effective block with a small volume of neurolytic agent. Neurolytic block of the stellate ganglion has only limited application because of the unwanted effects in the face and the possibility of complications.

Sympathetic ganglion blocks are contraindicated in patients on continued anticoagulant therapy because of the risks of serious haemorrhage associated with the deep penetration of tissues required in these procedures. Lumbar sympathetic ganglion blocks are not uncommonly requested in patients who are on long-term anticoagulant therapy. Considerable haemorrhage can occur into the psoas fascia in these circumstances.

It is quite common for sympathetic tone to return to a limb within a year or two of adequate surgical sympathectomy. In this case the usual anatomy has been altered and there is no concentration of sympathetic ganglion cells to inject. It is likely that the return of sympathetic activity after a delay of at least months is the result of regeneration of sympathetic nerves, possibly in relation to the major arteries, rather than to the appearance of denervation supersensitivity in peripheral small blood vessels. I have found the galvanic skin response to be present in patients who have developed clinical evidence of returning sympathetic tone: this suggests that the sympathetic nerves have become reestablished.

Faced with these problems, I wondered if there was an easier way of blocking the sympathetic nerves to the limbs and decided to try blocking the postganglionic sympathetic terminals in the periphery; in other words, attacking the nerve fibres from the other end. It seemed possible that a specific sympathetic nerve terminal blocker, such as guanethidine, might diffuse from the venous system into the autonomic nerves in a kind of Bier block. I had first to find a clinical method of determining whether I had produced a local sympathetic (noradrenergic) block. Knowing that causalgia is regularly relieved by sympathetic block, I performed the first guanethidine block on an elderly lady with severe causalgia in the hand associated with irradiation of the axillary region after radical mastectomy. The irradiation had presumably caused scarring of the axillary plexus and the kind of partial nerve damage that gives rise to causalgia. With the informed consent of the patient and the family doctor, I applied a venous tourniquet to the forearm and injected 0.1 ml (1 mg) undiluted guanethidine solution into the dorsal vein located in the interspace between the fourth and fifth metacarpals. Within 2 minutes the burning pain had been relieved in the little finger and most of the ring finger. The relief lasted 3 days and the patient was insistent that I treat the whole hand. This was done by diluting 10 mg guanethidine (the contents of one ampoule) to 25 ml with saline and injecting into a dorsal hand vein after isolation of the limb with an arterial tourniquet on the upper arm. The tourniquet was kept on for 10 minutes. Following a brief period of exacerbation of pain for about 2 minutes, the burning pain was relieved whilst the tourniquet was still in place. After the tourniquet was released the patient was delighted to be free of pain in the hand for the first time in 2 years. Relief lasted for several weeks.

Further studies in other patients confirmed that a simple and effective way of blocking the sympathetic nervous system in a limb was now possible. Its performance required care rather than exceptional expertise and it was hopeful that sympathetic blocks would become more readily available in pain clinics and rehabilitation centres. There was the unexpected bonus that guanethidine blocks, which were in any case easily repeated, were found to last several days. In fact they become more effective and longer-lasting upon repetition. Moreover, guanethidine blocks solved the problem of providing sympathetic block in the limbs of patients who were either on anticoagulants or had been sympathectomized without lasting result. Subsequently, other drugs were used in the isolated limb technique and their use will be touched upon later.

One of the main objectives of this chapter is to discuss the use of guanethidine, which has proven to be a reliable and effective noradrenergic blocking agent in the IVR technique. The subject will be considered under the following headings: principle, technique, effectiveness, unwanted effects, indications, phentolamine test and clinical syndromes.

PRINCIPLE

The principle of the IVR technique is to limit the effect of a potent drug to the tissues of the treated limb. By the use of selected agents, a specific target in the tissues can be attacked and, since a high concentration of the drug can be used, effects may be obtained more akin to the realms of pharmacology than therapeutics. Such a 'pharmacological target block' with guanethidine, which is selectively taken up by noradrenergic nerve endings, has a persistence of activity rarely encountered in therapeutics. Guanethidine has a strong affinity for its target and it can take 21 days for its clearance from the tissues. Clinically, the effects of guanethidine are obvious for a lesser period of 3–5 days but careful testing of the extremity reveals that its effects are still detectable beyond this period.

When guanethidine first enters the endings of the postganglionic neurons it releases noradrenaline from the storage sites. The concentration of guanethidine builds up at these sites and the continued presence of guanethidine prevents the reuptake of noradrenaline from the synaptic cleft. The postganglionic neurons depend upon the recapture of much of the released noradrenaline to maintain normal sympathetic tone. Another effect of intraneural guanethidine is to inhibit the release of any remaining noradrenaline. The overall effect is a profound sympathetic block. It is important to note that the effect of guanethidine is biphasic, first releasing noradrenaline and then causing noradrenergic block. Furthermore, the clinical results of a guanethidine block can take time to develop and are dose-dependent. In sufficient concentration guanethidine can cause permanent damage to the noradrenaline reuptake 'pump'. This concentration can be reached progressively in repeated blocks because the guanethidine accumulates in the nerves for a prolonged period. In animal studies guanethidine doses of the order of 30 mg/kg can cause the remarkable phenomenon of axon retraction (Burnstock & Costa 1975) which causes sympathetic nerve endings to withdraw from their effector sites. This kind of 'microsurgical' sympathectomy is probably attainable with the doses used in the IVR technique with guanethidine. The effect would very likely be produced by repeated blocks.

TECHNIQUE

BASIC REQUIREMENTS

Skin marker to identify treated limb
Ampoules of drugs, saline and water
Syringes, including 50-ml size
Butterfly needles, preferably size 23
Skin-cleaning swabs and dry gauze swabs
Firm quality 'dental' rolls to be strapped over sites of venepuncture after removal of butterfly needles
Reliable pneumatic tourniquet, preferably automatic
Soft material, e.g. Velband, to pad area under tourniquet
Operating table, tilting trolley or tilting bed
Resuscitation equipment, preferably anaesthetic machine
Trough for warm water to aid vasodilatation in extremity

MONITORING EQUIPMENT

Stopwatch
Blood pressure machine
Pulse monitor
Thermistor thermometer to measure skin temperature at selected points
Thermographic system to visualize temperature differences over whole area – liquid crystal thermography is particularly convenient
Sensory testing equipment
Apparatus to record galvanic skin response – an ECG machine can be used
Sweat tests
Ice response test
Grip strength–the patient can be asked to squeeze the rubber bulb of a standard mercury-in-glass blood pressure machine kept inflated at about 40 mmHg
Protractor to measure range of joint movement
Calipers or bands to assess swelling at selected points, e.g. Vernon finger joint comparator
Camera

The above lists are given to emphasize safety and the wealth of clinical information which can be recorded to assess *objectively* the progress of the patient. It is possible to manage with basic equipment but the blocks give so much rewarding clinical and theoretical information that the opportunity should not be lost of recording relevant information with the untreated extremity as control. Such information is invaluable during prolonged therapy in limb rehabilitation when both doctor and patient can find it difficult to remember exactly what a limb was like a few months previously. Detailed records are particularly useful in medicolegal work.

EVOLUTION OF THE BASIC TECHNIQUE

As originally described (Hannington-Kiff 1974a, 1974b) the dose of guanethidine was 10–20 mg in the upper limb and 20 mg in the lower limb. These doses do not need to be exceeded for diagnostic tests and should not be exceeded when an early vasolidatation is required, especially in vasospastic disorders. I now often use a larger dose of 30 mg (Hannington-Kiff 1980), especially in repeat blocks, for reasons which will become clear, but it is important to realise that larger doses of guanethidine may not be followed by early vasodilatation after release of the tourniquet and the block may be considered mistakenly to have failed. Vasodilatation may be delayed for several hours in sensitive patients with a history of Raynaud's phenomenon. Guanethidine releases some noradrenaline at first and this may delay the vasodilating effect of the drug. A sign to look for in these circumstances is the piloerection which mirrors the effect of this noradrenaline: this sign can be quite dramatic in patients with obvious Raynaud's phenomenon. I find that a high proportion of patients with Sudeck's atrophy and other types of sympathetic dystrophy have a history of Raynaud's phenomenon and I warn these patients that the limb will be warmest on the day after the block, which should not be confused with the effects of infection.

The addition of an alpha adrenoceptor blocker (AAB), such as phentolamine 5–10 mg, will prevent this effect of the released noradrenaline and allow an early vasodilatation. A similar but less specific effect in allowing early vasodilatation after the higher dose regimen with guanethidine is achieved by the addition of a local anaesthetic, for example 5 ml 0.5% lignocaine, to the solution of guanethidine. Local anaesthetic is added when a guanethidine block is administered to patients with conditions such as causalgia, in which the initial release of noradrenaline can cause a considerable exacerbation of pain. This exacerbation lasts only a minute or so but is unbearable in causalgic patients.

A useful long-acting AAB is phenoxybenzamine, but I usually limit its use to inpatients because its long duration of action causes prolonged sedation. This drug is indicated when vasodilatation is of paramount importance, for example in conditions which threaten the viability of the limb. The dose is about 25 mg.

In repeated guanethidine blocks, especially when only a few days have passed since the last block, there is no need for an AAB because the residual guanethidine will abolish the noradrenaline-releasing phase of subsequent doses of guanethidine.

TECHNICAL DETAILS

The steps of the IVR procedure are basically as follows:

1. The solution for injection is prepared by diluting guanethidine in the syringe by drawing up saline and any additional agents to make a volume of about 30 ml for the upper limb and 50 ml for the lower limb. The dose of guanethidine is up to 30 mg, the precise dose depending upon the objective of the block, the mass of the limb beyond the tourniquet and the robustness of the patient. On the whole, repeated blocks are performed with the higher dosages of guanethidine.

It has already been mentioned that the initial block with guanethidine (especially in Raynaud's phenomenon, causalgia and high dosage of guanethidine) should include an AAB. Agents may be given mixed or it may be preferred to administer the drugs separately in some convenient dilution, bearing in mind that the total volume injected should approach the target volume usually employed in this kind of Bier block. I usually administer the diluted AAB about 2 minutes before the diluted guanethidine. When lignocaine is used, I normally mix it with the guanethidine solution in the syringe. The dose of lignocaine is about 5–7 ml of 0.5% solution (the preparation of lignocaine containing adrenaline must, of course, never be used).

2. A 23-gauge butterfly needle is introduced into a vein on the dorsal surface of the hand or foot of the treated limb. (Another butterfly needle is introduced into a free hand to facilitate the injection of a sedative and to provide access to a vein for safety's sake should a reaction occur to the drugs used in the block.) If the veins are thready, the extremity should be held well below heart level in a container of warm water until the veins fill. In 'stubborn' cases I have found that the application of a smear of glyceryl trinitrate 2% w/w ointment (Percutol) over a limited area on the back of the treated extremity will bring up a vein. This is a spin-off of my work with this agent in patients who have persistently cold dystrophic extremities with venospasm. After introduction, the butterfly needles should be filled with saline to prevent blockage by blood clot in the period before the agents are introduced through them.

3. A thin layer of padding (e.g. Velband) is wrapped around the limb and the correct size of tourniquet cuff is carefully applied and secured. The limb is raised well above heart level for about 60 seconds to drain the venous blood, and the tourniquet is inflated to at least 50 mm and 100 mmHg above systolic pressure, in the case of the arm and leg respectively. In the sedated patient, higher pressures can be used in the tourniquet. It is worth noting that a tourniquet which is slightly lower in pressure than fully desirable to save the patient the initial discomfort of considerable tightness may be associated with more discomfort later in the procedure if arterial blood creeps in to swell the limb.

In the upper extremity the site of the tourniquet is usually the upper arm, though the forearm can be used. When less tissue is isolated, the dose of drugs can be reduced without loss of effect. Digits can be isolated and their veins cannulated if causalgia is limited to a distal phalanx, for instance. If guanethidine is used in a digit, an AAB should definitely be used in the initial block to avoid the effect of noradrenaline release. In the lower limb it is unwise to apply the tourniquet to the calf because of the risks of deep vein thrombosis and pulmonary embolus.

4. The limb is returned to the horizontal position and the solution is injected at the rate it will conveniently pass from a 50-ml syringe through a 23-gauge butterfly needle. The treated limb will soon show patchy areas of pallor caused by arteriolar constriction. This is probably the result of the noradrenaline released by guanethidine and it is at this time that burning pain may occur. By about 6 minutes the limb becomes uniformly pale and I believe that it is relatively safe to let the tourniquet down at this stage if needed. It may seem paradoxical at first but the main complication likely to occur after the accidental deflation of the tourniquet early in the procedure is a precipitous rise in blood pressure owing to the general release of noradrenaline when unfixed guanethidine enters the general circulation. Of course, this complication would be countered by the inclusion of an AAB in the technique.

5. The distribution of the guanethidine solution in the limb can be hastened by brief periods of active or passive movements of the extremity.

6. The tourniquet is released in one step but it is kept in place ready to be reinflated for about 3–4 minutes. I have

never had to reinflate the tourniquet. Patients are confined to bed for 2 hours after the block; they lie horizontal on the side for the first half-hour, especially if they have had any form of anaesthesia. These are arbitrary precautions. Most of my patients are treated as day-cases and receive their blocks in the earlier part of the morning. As soon as they are sufficiently rested, they begin physiotherapy and occupational therapy if indicated. Patients with disabled limbs should be 'attacked' by their therapists soon after the block, which usually produces an early and dramatic relief of pain and stiffness.

7. Blocks may need to be repeated at 3-day intervals at first, in severe cases, and then less often. In some cases only one block, or two blocks about 3 weeks apart, may suffice. The most common requirement is for two or three blocks.

8. If parenteral guanethidine is unavailable, reserpine (2–5 mg) and bretylium (100–200 mg) are possible substitutes. The use of reserpine in the IVR technique has been reported by Gorsky (1977) and McKain et al (1983).

Rocco et al (1989) have shown that there is no significant difference between guanethidine and reserpine when used in the intravenous regional technique to treat reflex sympathetic dystrophy in a double-blind, cross-over study. It is, however, noteworthy that repeated treatments with intravenous regional reserpine could cause depression and excessive sedation because reserpine is a tertiary amine capable of crossing the blood–brain barrier whereas guanethidine is a quarternary ammonium compound which does not pass across into the brain.

Bretylium, like guanethidine, is a quarternary ammonium compound and therefore probably does not cross the blood–brain barrier. I have found bretylium to be useful diagnostically rather than therapeutically because its effects last only a few hours, unlike the prolonged effects of guanethidine. Hanowell et al (1989) found that bretylium provided 2–7 hours of pain relief after intravenous regional block. Ford et al (1988) have reported good results with bretylium blocks in four cases of reflex sympathetic dystrophy but this was not the experience of Manchikanti (1990) who repeated the study in another four cases. Ford (see Johnson & Ford 1990) subsequently suggested that Manchikanti's results were different because the patients were diagnostically different. The cost of an ampoule of bretylium in the United Kingdom is £23.00 (US$35 in May, 1993) compared with 27 pence (£0.27) for an ampoule of guanethidine. When a drug is as cheap as guanethidine there is a risk that it will be taken off the market, which would be a great loss. Moreover, parenteral guanethidine is an orphan drug in the United States.

EFFECTIVENESS

In the IVR technique it is possible to use concentrations of drugs at the target organ which are beyond the usual therapeutic range. Consequently, it is helpful to summarize the possible advantages and disadvantages of what may conveniently be called pharmacological target blocks.

ADVANTAGES

The advantages of depositing high doses of drugs in the extremities may be summarized as follows:

1. The general systemic effects of the drugs are eliminated, reduced or rendered predictable by limiting their activity to the tissues requiring treatment.

2. Large doses can be applied to the tissues in the affected limb only, which would otherwise be impossible because of adverse general systemic effects. Moreover, the effect can be limited to the actual tissues desired; for example, guanethidine is 6800 times more effective in blocking the sympathetic nerve fibres than procaine. Guanethidine could thus be called the local anaesthetic of the sympathetic nervous system.

3. Drugs can have different effects on tissues in high concentration; for example, guanethidine in doses (especially repeated doses) of 30–60 mg/kg can cause axon retraction in the sympathetic nervous system – a sort of sympathectomy in the surgical sense as well as in the chemical sense. This sort of high-dose pharmacology is usually only possible in animal work.

4. In high doses drugs can be used to block enzymes; for example, lysine acetylsalicylate probably acetylates and destroys all the prostaglandin synthetase present in the limb for a time after an IVR block.

5. The effects of the drug are fully monitored at the time by the doctor in attendance, unlike a continuous intravenous infusion which is given over a period of hours. This has the potential to make the IVR techniques safer than an infusion: naftidrofuryl is an example of a drug that could be more safely used in a regional technique and its high local concentration can have an unexpectedly longer duration of action (Hannington-Kiff 1980). The IVR technique with the alpha adrenoreceptor blocking agent phentolamine has proved useful for diagnostic purposes. The effect lasts only an hour or so and does not cause an exacerbation of pain. The use of a tourniquet confuses the test because it is unclear whether the short period of pain relief achieved by this method is really the effect of tourniquet ischaemia rather than that produced by the phentolamine. For this reason it has become popular to use phentolamine in a systemic intravenous infusion as discussed later in this chapter.

6. The slow leaching of drug into the systemic circulation could be a useful side-effect. In a way it is a type of depot injection, with the advantage that it is not going to cause toxic, mechanical and necrotic effects in tissues with a limited blood supply, which are risks after deep injections of slow-release preparations. These depot prepara-

tions are usually expensive; the IVR technique could be a cheaper way of matching their effects, although there may be a lesser period of activity. Some drugs, like guanethidine, take up to 21 days to be eliminated completely. Even atropine takes up to 20 minutes to produce tachycardia after using it in an IVR technique and then it releases slowly and not in a flush, in my experience.

7. A good proportion of any drug, however it is administered, is rendered inactive by plasma-binding. The high dose of drug applied to the tissues in an IVR block may be proportionately more effective because it is only exposed to the plasma pool remaining in the limb before it is taken up by the tissues.

8. Any drug given by mouth has to be absorbed and then passed through the liver before it can get to the target tissues. The first pass through the liver can remove or inactivate a great part of the drug. Consequently, the big dose given in an IVR block can in effect be very much larger than first considered.

9. After oral administration many factors influence the availability of the drug where it is needed. Not the least problem is patient compliance – many patients fail to take their drugs. The effect of a drug in an IVR block is predictable at the time, except in cases of hypersensitivity, and later the rate of release can usually be relied upon to be slow. The incidence of systemic hypersensitivity to the low circulating level of drug should be no higher than after oral administration.

10. Since the drug is given well-diluted in the IVR technique, there is a low incidence of irritation of the veins, except with drugs known to be very active in this respect.

11. The opposite limb is available as a control, an exceptional luxury in medicine. The treated limb can also be used as its own control in sequential studies.

12. The IVR technique is safe in patients on anticoagulants in whom deep injections are contraindicated. The technique has solved the problem of how to provide sympathetic blocks for the symptomatic relief of ischaemic limbs in such patients. A strategy that is sometimes used in patients on warfarin or dicoumarol anticoagulants is to transfer them to heparin for 48 hours. Heparin can then be stopped a few hours before the sympathetic ganglion block, the theory being that heparin has a shorter action and therefore provides more controllable anticoagulation. This changing about can prejudice the continuity of the patient's treatment and is perhaps not really effective in any case. All can be avoided by the guanethidine technique.

13. The guanethidine technique has solved the problem of what to do for patients who have the symptoms and signs of regeneration of the regional sympathetic nerve supply despite initially adequate surgical sympathectomy.

14. IVR blocks are simple to perform. They are within the capabilities of all doctors who will require none of the special skills necessary for the competent performance of stellate ganglion blocks, lumbar paravertebral blocks, lumbar epidural blocks, etc.

15. IVR blocks are easily repeated at regular intervals provided a vein can be found. They cause little discomfort and the risks are very small. The technique can be performed on painful limbs if consideration is given to providing sedation/analgesia. Entonox inhalation is helpful in these cases: it not only provides analgesia but gives extra oxygen, which is a useful safety precaution.

16. IVR blocks can be used to deliver drugs to extremities in which there is no major arterial supply, because the drug is introduced to the tissues in a retrograde fashion.

17. IVR blocks are valuable in diagnosis, prophylaxis and therapy. They have already thrown new light on the aetiology of certain enigmatic conditions affecting limbs and have been instrumental in formulating new ideas.

18. Since there is no prolonged sensory deficit in IVR sympathetic blocks with noradrenergic neuron blockers or alpha adrenoreceptor blockers, the limb pain in causalgia, Sudeck's atrophy and ischaemia can be relieved for quite lengthy periods without the risk of untoward damage, such as pressure sores or accidental burns.

19. An interesting corollary of the IVR technique of depositing drugs in the limb is that the isolation of the circulation to the limb by a tourniquet can be used to keep drugs out of that limb. This strategy has been used to keep muscle-relaxant drugs out of one limb in an experimental study of the depth of unconsciousness during general anaesthesia with muscle relaxation (Tunstall 1977). It is not unknown for patients to be paralysed yet conscious during modern light anaesthesia.

DISADVANTAGES

The disadvantages are largely technical and may be summarized as follows:

1. The tightness of the tourniquet is uncomfortable. This is usually bearable with reassurance but occasionally the inhalation of Entonox or the intravenous injection of diazepam may be required.

2. Some drugs cause an initial burning after injection even when diluted. Diagnostic use of this burning has been made in the case of guanethidine. The burning can be overcome by the use of a little local anaesthetic agent in the IVR block. When the burning is believed to be the effect of noradrenaline release, as in the case of guanethidine injection, the prior use of an AAB can reduce the discomfort and increase the vasodilatation.

3. In the ischaemic limb isolation of the circulation with a tourniquet could cause further deterioration. In practice this does not seem to happen.

4. A tight tourniquet could conceivably cause

neurapraxia, especially if it is applied where the nerve crosses bone. I have never encountered this complication.

5. Occlusion of the circulation could cause intravascular coagulation, especially when the veins have been relatively empty for a period. In risky lower extremities heparin 500–1000 units could be added to the solution used in the IVR block. Heparin is a reactive substance and could interact with the active principle needed for the block. I rarely find it necessary to use heparin.

6. Not all drugs are available in parenteral form and not all of these are suitable for intravenous administration.

7. Not all drugs have the high affinity for tissue which is an advantage in the IVR technique. Local anaesthetics soon escape into the general circulation when the tourniquet is released after a Bier block. It is surprising how tenacious most drugs are for the tissues after an IVR block.

8. There is a possibility of unwanted effects when the blocking drug enters the systemic circulation on release of the tourniquet. These have proved rare in practice.

UNWANTED EFFECTS

No serious unwanted effects have been encountered in over 14 years' experience with the IVR technique using guanethidine and a variety of other drugs. The only reaction I have seen in the skin of the isolated limb is the occasional appearance of a few livid itchy patches which disappear in a few hours at most. This reaction has followed the use of guanethidine, lysine acetylsalicylate and naftidrofuryl and bupivacaine, and is clearly nonspecific. I have not encountered venous thrombosis at the injection sites and there have been no complications in relation to the use of the tourniquets.

General reactions just after the release of the tourniquet are uncommon and never serious. When the shorter tourniquet time of 10 minutes was used in guanethidine blocks it was not unusual for the patient to report an evanescent slight burning sensation in the throat and later there might be pinkness of the conjunctivae and slight drooping of the eyelids for an hour or so. These effects are uncommon with a tourniquet time of 20 minutes. The blood pressure is not significantly affected at the time of tourniquet release in supine patients.

In the first day or two after a guanethidine block the patient may feel slightly tired and weak. These effects could simply be due to the successful abatement of intense stimulation in patients who have long suffered from severe pain. If the patient has received intravenous sedation with diazepam, then recurring periods of tiredness and weakness would be expected from the enterohepatic recirculation of this type of drug. The reporting of mild muscle weakness after guanethidine may be genuine rather than imagined because I have found guanethidine relieves muscle spasticity in the extremities in a variety of conditions. I believe this is the result of reducing the sympathetic tone in the muscle spindles (Hannington-Kiff 1980). It is important to note that none of the patients has ever felt depressed after guanethidine blocks, whereas this is a possible complication if reserpine is used as a substitute for guanethidine.

INDICATIONS FOR ANTISYMPATHETIC IVR BLOCKS

Regional sympathetic blockade by whatever means may relieve a variety of limb pains and disabilities whether or not there are overt clinical signs of autonomic hyperactivity in the extremity. In recognition of this finding, clinicians often perform a trial sympathetic block in unexplained limb disabilities involving pain, altered sensation or impaired mobility. Classical views and definitions of the sympathetic nervous system do not serve well in explaining clinical experience. There are few procedures in medicine which are as dramatic as the instant relief of pain and disability (without sensory loss) which can follow successful sympathetic block.

In the management of a patient with unexplained limb pain, it is important to consider the possibility of underlying sympathetic hyperactivity. If overt clinical signs of sympathetic hyperactivity are not present, clues suggesting that a sympathetic component subserves the pain may nevertheless be gathered from the nature of the pain itself.

OVERT SIGNS OF REGIONAL SYMPATHETIC HYPERACTIVITY

Altered skin colour

There may be inappropriate regional pallor or lividity, particularly in the distal parts of the extremity where the cutaneous vessels are normally most strongly under the control of the sympathetic nervous system. The colour of the affected parts may alter rapidly in response to environmental temperature owing to a combination of colour changes in stagnant blood and hyperactive vascular reflexes altering blood flow.

Hyperhydrosis

Sweating may be generally increased in the affected extremity or limited to the territory adjacent to a painful scar. Of course, sweating can only occur in those areas of skin which bear sweat glands.

Temperature

The affected limb may feel warm or cold depending on the blood flow. Changes in the environmental temperature usually trigger the vascular responses which determine the skin temperature but there is sometimes a diurnal variation.

Sympathetic nervous activity is highest in the evening (at about 2100h) and the patient may well report that vascular changes and pain are most pronounced at this time.

Piloerection

This important finding is frequently missed or ignored, which is a pity because I find that pilomotor activity confined to the affected limb is arguably the earliest incontrovertible physical sign of impending reflex sympathetic dystrophy syndrome. Strong contraction of the arrectores pili causes gooseflesh as well as piloerection. Since pilomotor activity is specifically noradrenergic, both piloerection and gooseflesh may appear in the treated portion of a limb during the initial stage of a guanethidine block, especially in a patient who has a history of Raynaud-type circulatory reactivity.

Swelling

This may be confined to the digits or more widely spread in the extremity. It is an unpitting kind of oedema which can rapidly fluctuate in size during the early stages when swelling is caused directly by altered vascular mechanisms. If the limb is not used, the 'muscle-pump' in the hand or foot, as the case may be, fails to assist the venous return and further extravasation occurs to add to the swelling. Pain, swelling and stiffness are the main components of the vicious circle that must be broken in the management of sympathetic dystrophy. Treatment must be aimed at promoting reuse of the limb: unfortunately, the relief of pain associated with immobilisation is often irresistible but this short-term solution can be disastrous for the rehabilitation of the limb.

PAIN AND ASSOCIATED CHANGES IN SYMPATHETIC HYPERACTIVITY

The nature of pain as described by the patient and the associated findings on sensory testing are often bizarre and may lead to unfair aspersions about the patient's emotional state. The pain is usually described as burning in the skin with a deeper ache inside the limb. A more complete description of the pain will emerge during the physical examination: at this juncture the patient will be hard put to find words to describe his feelings and the general physician will not fare much better in choosing apt words to record the findings. This is the sort of occasion when the 'Classification of Chronic Pain' (Merskey 1986) can be most helpful. Pain subserved by sympathetic hyperactivity is often associated with the following findings, which will be listed under technical headings with supporting brief definitions from the 'Classification of Chronic Pain'. In each case the associated finding can be removed by sympathetic block.

Allodynia

Pain due to a stimulus which does not normally provoke pain. This term implies that the threshold is lowered. Patients with sympathetic dystrophy often have allodynia to light moving touch, especially if there is a degree of peripheral nerve damage, whereas moderate stationary pressure/touch is unremarkable. Cold allodynia is not uncommon after hand surgery.

Hyperpathia

A painful syndrome, characterized by increased reaction to a stimulus, especially a repetitive stimulus, as well as an increased threshold. This is probably the most constant feature of sympathetic hyperactivity. The patient feels that sensation is generally blunted in the limb but experiences an agonizing response, after a delay, to any prolonged cutaneous stimulus.

Hyperaesthesia

Increased sensitivity to stimulation, excluding the special senses. Light touch, temperature (cold rather than warmth) and tickle all cause discomfort, if not frank pain.

Dysaesthesia

An unpleasant abnormal sensation, whether spontaneous or evoked. Perhaps the emphasis should be on the spontaneous nature of the condition. For example, in postherpetic neuralgia, dysaesthesia is a most apt term. Though postherpetic neuralgia is not considered a sympathetic dystrophy, dysaesthesia in this condition can usually be temporarily abated by sympathetic block.

Hyperalgesia

An increased response to a stimulus which is normally painful. This is usually a feature of inflamed tissues and might be encountered in the moderately early florid stage of sympathetic dystrophy. The term hyperalgesia does not contribute much to the description of chronic clinical pain, as it seems to involve mainly the judgement of the observer. In the circumstances it is not profitable to speculate whether sympathetic block will alleviate hyperalgesia.

OTHER CLINICAL FEATURES OF REGIONAL SYMPATHETIC HYPERACTIVITY

Reflex nature

The description *reflex* preceding sympathetic dystrophy is apt in the sense that sympathetic block instantly alleviates pain and altered sensation in the affected limb.

Subsequently, these features can arise again as soon as the block has worn off.

Quadrant radiation

The features of sympathetic dystrophy often spread beyond a limb to engage a quadrant of the body. For example, pain and stiffness in the hand with a sympathetic trigger are commonly followed by pain and stiffness in the shoulder; these events may themselves be sequential to myocardial ischaemia. Seemingly, the sympathetic nervous system is divided into quadrants based upon the main conglomerations of sympathetic postganglionic cell bodies – the stellate and lumbar ganglia.

Dermatomal radiation

Isosegmental referral of pain from a viscus to the corresponding dermatome and sclerotome is well-recognized. Referred pain in a strip down the inner aspect of the left (occasionally the right) arm is a common complication of myocardial ischaemia, owing to the shared thoracic segmental levels: paravertebral sympathetic block at TI–T2 will relieve the referred pain.

Crossed lateral radiation

When one extremity is affected by sympathetic dystrophy and a sympathetic block is performed, it is not unusual for the patient to report that the relief of pain and stiffness in the affected extremity is associated with similar improvements in the opposite, seemingly normal, extremity. This is particularly noticeable in the case of the hands. Moreover, radionuclide scans, which provide a sensitive way of revealing early changes in the bone of the affected extremity in sympathetic dystrophy, often show a slight degree of change in the opposite extremity. Repeat bone scans 12–14 days after guanethidine block in the affected limb will usually show considerable improvement in the scan on the treated side. Occasionally, successful treatment of sympathetic dystrophy in one extremity will be followed after an interval of about 12 weeks by a flare-up of similar changes in the opposite limb.

Longitudinal and oblique radiation

Evidence of the spread of influence vertically within the sympathetic nervous system is given by the clinical finding that a sympathetic block which relieves pain in a hemiplegic upper extremity may also relieve pain in the hemiplegic lower limb. Very occasionally pain in an upper limb may be associated with pain in the obliquely opposite lower limb. Clearly all these features emphasise the widely linked reflexogenic nature of the sympathetic nervous system.

Postsympathectomy pain

It is curious that surgical sympathectomy can give rise to neuralgia in the sympathectomized limb. The neuralgia usually begins abruptly after an interval of about 1–6 weeks. Pain is described as deep and aching and there is tenderness, particularly over neurovascular bundles. After a few weeks the pain usually disappears as abruptly as it started. Sometimes sweating occurs in association with the pain in the sympathectomised limb. The reasons for these perverse effects of sympathectomy are unclear.

SYSTEMIC IV INFUSION OF ALPHA ADRENORECEPTOR BLOCKING AGENT (PHENTOLAMINE TEST)

To overcome the possibility that the period of ischaemia associated with the use of an arterial tourniquet contributes significantly to the efficacy of the IVR guanethidine blocking technique, Arner (1991) and Raja et al (1991) have recommended the systemic intravenous infusion of phentolamine to predict whether a particular pain has a sympathetic component and whether IVR guanethidine and other sympatholytic blocks are likely to be successful in relieving pain in a given patient. The method is also, of course, not limited in application to a limb when it is necessary to test whether a particular pain has a sympathetic component.

Since the infusion can be started with saline and switched to phentolamine solution it is possible to eliminate any placebo response. A disadvantage of the method is that phentolamine administered in this way can cause tachycardia and other unwanted effects so that it should not be used in patients with cardiac disease. The phentolamine test should only be carried out in locations where full resuscitation equipment is readily available whether or not the patient is robust.

One of the characteristic features of sympathetically maintained pain is that the pain can vary throughout the day or over a period of days, probably in accord with the amount of underlying sympathetic activity. The phentolamine test depends upon blocking adrenergic activity and I have found that some patients tested with a systemic intravenous infusion of phentolamine can be judged to have responded positively one day and negatively the next. In such doubtful cases of sympathetically maintained pain (SMP) in a limb, I have administered edrophonium (Tensilon, Roche) through an intravenous infusion of physiological saline established in the unaffected extremity, first in a test dose of 2 mg, then followed by 6–8 mg if there are no adverse effects. It is known that the cholinergic activity of edrophonium can release noradrenaline from postganglionic sympathetic nerve endings (Leveston et al 1979), which will conceivably be able to challenge and trigger any existing SMP in the affected area. If the result of this edrophonium challenge (or Tensilon Test) is positive, I administer phentolamine through the infusion to assess whether the pain is switched off or not (Hannington-Kiff 1980). In this way the positive and negative aspects of the presumed noradrenergic trigger of the pain are tested.

The inhalation of tobacco smoke by virtue of its nicotine content can release noradrenaline. This is probably the reason for my clinical impression that reflex sympathetic dystrophy in habitual smokers is often refractory to treatment with sympathetic blocks. In a retrospective epidemiological study reflex sympathetic dystrophy was proved statistically to be associated with cigarette smoking (An et al 1988).

CLINICAL SYNDROMES

The effects of IVR sympathetic blocks will be illustrated in a selection of pain syndromes involving the extremities.

CAUSALGIA

Burning pain, allodynia and hyperpathia, usually in the hand or foot after partial injury of a nerve or one of its major branches. Fully developed causalgia is an extremely distressing condition. It usually accompanies incomplete severance of a limb nerve, most commonly the median, the brachial plexus and the sciatic nerve but in my experience the ulnar nerve has increasingly suffered from this complication following the rise in popularity of surgical transposition of this nerve at the elbow (Hannington-Kiff 1982). Causalgia may be an immediate complication of nerve damage but this is rare and it is more common for the onset to be delayed for a few weeks. The severely affected patient will go to considerable lengths to protect the painful limb from environmental stimuli and the limb quickly becomes atrophic through disuse.

Sympathetic blocks, by whatever means, are the only consistently effective treatment of causalgia. Repeated IVR guanethidine blocks are useful, especially if begun at an early stage, and early recognition, preferably *anticipation*, of this dreadful complication is vital (Hannington-Kiff 1979, 1982). The patient will require general anaesthesia for the block in the presence of severe causalgia. If prilocaine (currently favoured for Bier's blocks) is used to provide local anaesthesia it must be preservative-free (Hannington-Kiff 1983). Physiotherapy should be instituted during the pain-free period after each guanethidine block in an effort to rehabilitate the limb and reduce the severity of the discomforts associated with the complications of disuse, such as swelling and stiffness. Sympathetic blocks are less effective in the late stages of the disease and many patients will end up having a surgical sympathectomy. After a couple of years the severe pain may spontaneously resolve but the ravages of the dystrophy and the disuse will have permanently disabled the limb.

REFLEX SYMPATHETIC DYSTROPHY

Continuous pain in a portion of an extremity after trauma which may include fracture but does not involve a major nerve, associated with sympathetic hyperactivity. Mild forms of this condition are probably commoner than acknowledged because they remit before the signs become obvious enough to make the diagnosis. Moreover, there is often reluctance to label the condition 'reflex sympathetic dystrophy' (RSD) until the signs are florid and X-ray films show osteoporosis. At this stage the condition is called Sudeck's atrophy and certainly most letters of referral to pain clinics in the UK must mention this name. Usually 2–3 months or longer pass before patients with RSD appear in the pain clinic, whereas the relatively subtle signs of sympathetic hyperactivity are to be seen within days. Perhaps earlier awareness of RSD changes would be promoted if the condition were given the acronym SOS, standing for *sympathetic overdrive syndrome.*

The inclusion of dystrophy in the diagnostic label is probably part of the problem. Other factors which mitigate against early diagnosis are: the patient who is developing RSD is often agitated and, therefore, suspected of being neurotic; there may be an existing tendency to Raynaud-type reactivity of peripheral blood vessels which leads to misinterpretation of the early signs, and there is often a period of 4–6 weeks during which the patient is not seen, especially when a plaster cast has been applied. Not infrequently it is only when the plaster cast is removed that the signs of RSD are noted. Then a period of observation will follow before treatment is contemplated. During this period there is a natural tendency to give the patient further splintage, albeit with lighter materials, because the patient is relieved of pain by immobilisation.

Instead the patient should be encouraged to use the extremity, otherwise the lack of a muscle-pump will greatly add to the dystrophic complications of RSD. Use of the extremity will be promoted by the early institution of some kind of sympathetic block and there are clear advantages for the IVR guanethidine technique (Hannington-Kiff 1977; McKay et al 1977; Glynn et al 1981; Bonelli et al 1983; Driessen et al 1983).

The most useful investigation is a radionuclide scan of both extremities for comparison, paying particular attention to the delayed findings 3 hours after radionuclide injection (which shows the uptake in bone). An increased radionuclide uptake in the bone in the affected extremity (reflecting high-turnover osteoporosis) will be seen at an early stage of RSD long before signs of osteoporosis are evident on an X-ray film. Increased uptake in the bone associated with the original injury will need to be differentiated if the scan is carried out at a very early stage. (Simple disuse osteoporosis is not associated with increased uptake.)

On the whole, treatment rests upon two pillars: sympathetic block and vigorous rehabilitation with physical methods and occupational therapy. Fully trained occupational therapists have a great deal of expertise to offer in the assessment, rehabilitation and reeducation of painful and disabled hands.

The use of a short, high-dose course of an oral corticosteroid is occasionally advocated as an alternative to sympathetic block but the possibility of unwanted effects should be borne in mind, especially in these patients who are very likely to be already taking an oral antiinflammatory agent so that gastric ulceration and perforation are distinct possibilities.

CENTRAL PAIN (INCLUDING THALAMIC AND PSEUDOTHALAMIC PAIN)

Diffuse unilateral pain, often burning with allodynia, hypoaesthesia, hyperalgesia, hyperpathia, dysaesthesia and neurological signs of damage to structures which supply the affected region. Intractable pain in the hemiparetic limbs of six patients, diagnosed as thalamic pain by the referring physicians, was found to respond very well to IVR guanethidine block (Hannington-Kiff 1980). Though there were no overt signs of RSD the quality of pain was very similar to that found in RSD. A curious and rewarding feature was that in each case there was a varying degree of improvement in memory, which lasted from 2–4 days. In two patients the improvement in mental processes and articulation was spectacular. Guanethidine does not cross the normal blood–brain barrier but it is interesting to speculate that somehow the treatment favoured an alteration of adrenergic/cholinergic balance in the brain in favour of the cholinergic mechanisms. This would fit in with current ideas about memory (Annotation 1987). Otherwise, is it outrageous to ask whether a painful hemiparetic limb can control the damaged brain in the sense that noxious input engages brain areas and brain mechanisms, which can be ill-afforded? This would certainly be a novel concept. Loh et al (1981) reported the benefits of IVR guanethidine blocks and local anaesthetic sympathetic ganglion blocks in relieving pain in the limbs of three patients with the thalamic syndrome but made no mention of changes in the mental faculties of the patients. Subsequently, these workers (Schott & Loh 1984) found that limb pain in two patients with the thalamic syndrome was relieved for a few hours after the administration of physostigmine by various routes. These patients had previously had pain relief following IVR guanethidine blocks and hence there is some suggestion that the promotion of cholinergic mechanisms in the brain (or peripherally) may account for the pain relief. Schott & Loh (1984) do not state whether their patients became more mentally alert during the few hours of pain relief after the administration of physostigmine. The preoccupation of these two patients with the muscarinic side-effects of the physostigmine would no doubt have masked any improvement in their mental faculties.

TRAUMA

The relatively prolonged increased local blood supply produced by guanethidine block could just make the difference to the survival of threatened tissues after degloving injuries, plastic surgery with extensive skin flaps and the replantation of digits. In serious cases the increased regional blood flow after IVR sympathetic block could be combined with the effects of hyperbaric oxygen to promote the survival of damaged tissues. The successful replantation of a thumb with the aid of a guanethidine block has been described by Davies (1976). The use of guanethidine combined with an AAB may be helpful in vascular anastomoses, which can if necessary be bathed with the solution during surgery. This treatment may make the difference when a narrow artery with a powerful muscular wall has to be grafted on to a larger more elastic artery.

The profound peripheral vascular dilatation after IVR guanethidine can facilitate angiography. For example, adequate angiographic views of the arterial system of the hand prior to thumb reconstruction by toe transplantation are crucial, and the use of IVR guanethidine, shortly before arterial cannulation and injection of contrast medium, will ensure the best possible chance of demonstrating the whole vascular bed (Vaughan et al 1985; Hannington-Kiff 1986a).

Before treating a painful peripheral nerve lesion (pseudoneuroma) in the extremity with cryosurgery (Wang 1985) it is necessary to look for associated signs of RSD and treat these first with IVR guanethidine or another kind of sympathetic block (Hannington-Kiff 1986b). This anti-sympathetic–cryoanalgesia sequential regimen may successfully remove cold-intolerance and persistent vasospasm which not infrequently complicate otherwise successful microsurgical replantation of digits. (Hannington-Kiff 1986b).

VASCULAR INSUFFICIENCY

Occasionally, sympathetic blocks improve the circulation in the lower extremity in arteriopathy but the main indication for sympathetic blockade in this instance is the relief of rest pain. Guanethidine block can be used instead of the usual lumbar ganglion block for this purpose. Lumbar ganglion block is contraindicated in the patient taking anticoagulants and a guanethidine block offers a solution to providing sympathetic block in these circumstances. The occlusion of the circulation for 10 – 20 minutes has not been found to cause obvious deterioration in the chronically ischaemic limb in my experience. Patients certainly appreciate the relief of pain, even if it lasts only for a matter of days.

In patients who have been treated by lumbar sympathectomy yet show a return of sympathetic tone with deterioration of the peripheral circulation, a single guanethidine block can cause an increase in blood flow lasting several weeks longer than usual (Hannington-Kiff 1974a, 1974b, 1980). During this period ischaemic ulcers may heal and guanethidine blocks have undoubtedly saved a number of patients from amputation in these circumstances.

RAYNAUD'S DISEASE

Episodic attacks of aching, burning pain associated with vasoconstriction of the arteries of the extremities in response to cold or emotional stimuli. Patients with severe Raynaud's disease can be tided over the coldest winter months by repeated guanethidine blocks (Hannington-Kiff 1974a, 1974b, 1980) as an alternative to surgical excision of the regional sympathetic ganglia. This is more rational therapy than surgery in the patient who is only troubled during the cold spells. In any event, the results of surgery are not usually permanent and the signs of returning sympathetic tone may be encountered as early as 6 months after surgery.

Eriksen (1981) has confirmed the superiority of guanethidine blocks compared with injections of bupivacaine into the stellate ganglion in the relief of Raynaud's phenomenon in the hands because of the longer duration of the effect of guanethidine and the absence of the complications associated with stellate ganglion block. Eriksen used my original technique and did not include an AAB in the injected solution. It is interesting that he reports a slight vasoconstriction at first in the initial guanethidine block which did not occur after the second block 3 days later. The reasons for this finding have been explained above. Patients with Raynaud's phenomenon are very sensitive to noradrenaline and should be protected from the initial release of this substance in the guanethidine block by the prior use of an AAB such as thymoxamine, phentolamine or phenoxybenzamine. If guanethidine blocks are repeated at intervals of less than a week or so, the AAB is probably unnecessary because the residual guanethidine prevents or reduces the release of noradrenaline.

Guanethidine block may be the only sensible recourse in some patients with severe Raynaud's disease in whom sympathetic tone has returned after adequate sympathectomy and in whom there has been no response to medication. Work is required to establish whether the return of excessive tone after sympathectomy is the result of regeneration, or rerouting of sympathetic nerves, or the appearance of vascular supersensitivity to circulating noradrenaline. Since guanethidine has some direct relaxing effect on vascular smooth muscle, this agent should also be effective in supersensitivity.

RHEUMATOID ARTHRITIS

Aching, burning joint pain due to systemic inflammatory disease affecting all synovial joints, muscle, ligaments and tendons in accordance with diagnostic criteria below. The invitation to read on in this definition from the 'Classification of Chronic Pain' gives some indication of the semantic difficulties posed by the wide array of conditions which are lumped together as rheumatoid arthritis.

Autonomic neuropathy can be demonstrated in some patients with rheumatoid arthritis by comparative assessment of cardiovascular reflexes (Edmonds et al 1979). Some of the symptoms and signs of rheumatoid arthritis, certainly in the early stages, are reminiscent of RSD and it is possible that peripheral sympathetic hyperactivity might be a contributory factor in the initiation and progression of rheumatoid arthritis in genetically predisposed patients. The nature of the pain and its exacerbation by changes in the weather (such as damp-cold, humid-warmth and low barometric pressure) suggest some contribution from the sympathetic nervous system. The symmetrical involvement of the joints on the two sides of the body could be a reflection of the symmetry of the sympathetic nervous system.

Is there any evidence of peripheral sympathetic involvement? I have successfully used IVR guanethidine blocks to provide symptomatic relief in patients with rheumatoid arthritis who are experiencing exacerbations of their disease as seasons change or whose nonsteroidal antiinflammatory drug (NSAID) is beginning to lose its effect (Hannington-Kiff 1990b). The following case report illustrates the use of IVR guanethidine to alleviate rheumatoid arthritis.

Case report

A woman of 47 with active painful rheumatoid arthritis, mainly in the hands and elbows, was referred to the pain clinic because her current NSAID was beginning to fail to control her disease. This was a matter for concern, as she had experienced side-effects from the previous NSAID. She felt it was the damp-cold (it was late November) that had made her arthritis worse. An IVR block (with 10 mg guanethidine in 25 ml normal saline, tourniquet time 20 minutes) relieved some pain and muscle stiffness within a few minutes and within a few hours the treated hand was warm and rewardingly comfortable. She noted that the treated limb remained warmer than the opposite limb for 6 days, even outside in the cold. As the raised temperature in the treated limb waned she noted that morning stiffness began to reappear in the hand. For about 8 days she was relieved of pain in the treated limb and was able to move her fingers, wrist and elbow more easily, grip and twist bottle-tops better and firmly hold her front door key. She was also able to resume driving for a few days. During this 8-day period the weather grew colder and wetter and she noticed that the arthritic pain in the untreated limbs had grown worse, as she would normally have expected for the whole body. She was most impressed by the protective effect of the IVR guanethidine and wondered if she could be tided over 'bad patches' in this way. She had not stopped taking her current NSAID.

The above patient was a relatively typical example of rheumatoid arthritis and there was no sign of peripheral neuritis (which can complicate this disease) to explain the pain relief achieved with the IVR guanethidine block. It must be concluded that the pain relieved by the guanethidine is none other than the 'rheumatoid' pain. The use of antisympathetic drugs for the symptomatic relief of rheumatoid arthritis merits further study.

Since the early stages of rheumatoid arthritis and RSD have features in common, it would be interesting to know whether IVR guanethidine blocks are capable of arresting the progression of early rheumatoid arthritis with the same efficacy as they relieve RSD. Immunocompetent cells possess adrenoceptors of high affinity and specificity and lymphoid tissue has an ample sympathetic nerve supply (Sanders & Munson 1985). It is conceivable, therefore, that sympathetic hyperactivity is a correlate of immune responsiveness and could play a part in the genesis of rheumatoid arthritis. I have found that the use of IVR blocks can abort and cut short episodes of palindromic rheumatism (Hannington-Kiff 1984). It is interesting to speculate whether treatment aimed at modulating the sympathetic nervous system could be an early line of defence in members of families with a predisposition to rheumatoid arthritis. First, new families of antisympathetic drugs are needed.

NEW HYPOTHESIS ABOUT THE CAUSE OF REFLEX SYMPATHETIC DYSTROPHY (RSD)

One of the most puzzling features of RSD is that it characteristically complicates a minor injury. For instance, a patient may have had major limb fractures in the past without RSD supervening but a subsequent minor injury such as a sprain might be followed by months of painful disability in the affected extremity. This disproportional relationship between the injury and the outcome has prompted me to suggest that a minor injury may fail to trigger or maintain some kind of opioid modulation within the regional sympathetic paravertebral ganglia which otherwise naturally accompanies an injury to a limb (Hannington-Kiff 1991).

Some support for this contention is provided by the beneficial effects observed in a limb affected by RSD when a small dose of an opioid is injected in the close vicinity of the adjacent regional sympathetic ganglia. For instance, a stellate ganglion block with morphine 3–4 mg diluted in about 12–16 ml physiological saline may relieve pain and muscle spasm in minutes and somewhat later may reduce swelling – all without the usual local accompaniments of increased arterial blood flow, raised skin temperature and anhydrosis. The alleviation of muscle spasm may be the result of pain relief, but may be a more direct effect, and the reduction in swelling may be the result of the venous dilatation that occurs because patients with swelling usually have constricted veins.

It is possible that lack of opioid modulation in the regional sympathetic ganglia in RSD permits the release of more noradrenaline (and other factors) from the sympathetic postganglionic nerve endings, hence precipitating the chain of events leading to RSD.

The pain of RSD usually becomes clinically manifest about 3–6 weeks after injury, perhaps testimony to the failure or waning of natural opioid modulation in the regional sympathetic ganglia which is conceivably normally raised after injury. It is interesting that autotomy in rats (the biting of claws after peripheral nerve damage which probably resembles RSD in man) also supervenes after this kind of interval (Wall et al 1980).

When the severe pain of RSD appears from the beginning and remains unabated, it is possible that opioid modulation in the regional sympathetic ganglia fails to rise in conjunction with the injury from the start.

The common clinical expedient of immobilizing even minor injuries may serve to favour the waning of opioid modulation in the regional sympathetic ganglia. Many patients need no encouragement to stop moving a painful limb; indeed in RSD the degree of suppression of the part from the body image (neglect) can occasionally approach that seen after a stroke. The overriding anxiety of the typical RSD patient may also be testimony to opioid withdrawal generally. Finally, the observation that RSD can be particularly intractable in habitual smokers may reflect their general need to seek stimulation to bolster their precarious supply of natural opioids.

It is possible that systemic absorption of the injected material is responsible for the beneficial effects of opioid regional ganglionic block but this is unlikely for the following reasons: the dose of opioid is small, a similar dose injected elsewhere does not produce improvements in the affected extremity, and measurements of the near point of visual accommodation shows the relief of pain and muscle spasm in the affected extremity precede the ocular changes (unpublished).

The practical message arising from the theory of failed opioid modulation in the regional sympathetic ganglia is that supervised 'aggressive' physiotherapy should be introduced to promote and preserve an appropriate opioid bias in the regional sympathetic ganglia in any patient who is considered to be at risk of developing RSD. The incidence and severity of RSD could conceivably be limited by early efforts to promote movement, despite the associated discomforts, in all patients following minor injuries rather than recommending conventional immobilisation and analgesia.

It should not be forgotten that surgery is 'planned

trauma' and the opportunity might be taken with advantage to preempt the complication of RSD, especially in patients considered to be at risk by performing a prophylactic regional sympathetic block just before surgery begins under general anaesthesia. Otherwise it might be wise to prevent the ingress of noxious input into the spinal cord by carrying out all limb surgery under local anaesthetic regional block even when the patient is rendered unconscious by general anaesthesia. Crile made a plea in 1913 for local anaesthetic solution to be injected at the site of operation in all patients under general anaesthesia to prevent shock of the central nervous system. We are all children of our age and today such a concept would be described in terms of the need to avoid sensitization of the wide-dynamic-range (WDR) neurons in the spinal dorsal horn. Add subsequently the reinforcing efferent effects of the sympathetic postganglionic nerves on the sensitized mechanoreceptors in the periphery and the scene is set for sympathetically maintained pain as described by Roberts (1986).

REFERENCES

An H S, Hawthorne K B, Jackson W T 1988 Reflex sympathetic dystrophy and cigarette smoking. Journal of Hand Surgery 13A: 470–472

Annotation 1987 Cholinergic treatment in Alzheimer's disease: encouraging results. Lancet i: 139–141

Arner S 1991 Intravenous phentolamine test: diagnostic and prognostic use in reflex sympathetic dystrophy. Pain 46: 17–22

Bonelli S, Conoscente F, Movilia P G, Restelli L, Francucci B, Grossi E 1983 Regional intravenous guanethidine vs. stellate ganglion block in reflex sympathetic dystrophies: a randomised trial. Pain 16: 297–307

Brodin A, Nyqvist-Mayer A, Wadsten T, Forslund B, Broberg F 1984 Phase diagram and aqueous solubility of the lidocaine-prilocaine binary system. Journal of Pharmaceutical Sciences 73: 481–484

Burnstock G 1986 The changing face of autonomic neurotransmission. Acta Physiologica Scandinavica 126: 67–91

Burnstock G, Costa M 1975 Adrenergic neurons. Chapman & Hall, London

Crile G 1913 The kinetic theory of shock and its prevention through anoci-association (shockless operation). Lancet ii: 7–16 (see also subsequent correspondence ibid 557 and 721–722)

Csillick B, Knyihar-Csillick E, Szucs A 1982 Treatment of chronic pain syndromes with iontophoresis of vinca alkaloids to the skin of patients. Neuroscience Letters 31: 87–90

Davies K H 1976 Guanethidine sympathetic blockade: its value in reimplantation surgery. British Medical Journal i: 876–877

Driessen J J, van der Werken C, Nicolai J P A, Crul J F 1983 Clinical effects of regional intravenous guanethidine (Ismelin) in reflex sympathetic dystrophy. Acta Anaesthesiologica Scandinavica 27: 505–509

Dunne S M, Hannington-Kiff J G 1993 The use of topical guanethidine in the relief of dentine hypersensitivity: a controlled study. Pain 165–168

Edmonds M E, Jones T C, Saunders W A, Sturrock R D 1979 Autonomic neuropathy in rheumatoid arthritis. British Medical Journal ii: 173–175

Eriksen S 1981 Duration of sympathetic blockade. Stellate ganglion versus intravenous regional guanethidine block. Anaesthesia 36: 768–771

Ford S R, Forrest W H, Eltherington L 1988 The treatment of reflex sympathetic dystrophy with intravenous regional bretylium. Anesthesiology 68: 137–140

Glynn C J, Basedow R W, Walsh J A 1981 Pain relief following postganglionic sympathetic blockade with i.v. guanethidine. British Journal of Anaesthesia 53: 1297–1301

Gorsky B H 1977 Intravenous perfusion with reserpine for Raynaud's phenomenon. Regional Anaesthesia 2: 5

Hannington-Kiff J G 1974a Intravenous regional sympathetic block with guanethidine. Lancet i: 1019–1020

Hannington-Kiff J G 1974b Pain relief. Heinemann, London

Hannington-Kiff J G 1977 Relief of Sudeck's atrophy by regional intravenous guanethidine. Lancet i: 1132–1133

Hannington-Kiff J G 1979 Relief of causalgia in limbs by regional intravenous guanethidine. British Medical Journal ii: 367

Hannington-Kiff J G 1980 In limbo. Jacksonian Prize Dissertation, *in libris* Royal College of Surgeons of England, London

Hannington-Kiff J G 1982 Hyperadrenergic-effected limb causalgia: relief by i.v. pharmacologic norepinephrine blockade. American Heart Journal 103: 152–153

Hannington-Kiff J G 1983 Prilocaine for Bier's block needs methylene-blue but not preservative. Lancet ii: 1085

Hannington-Kiff J G 1984 Pharmacological target blocks in hand surgery and rehabilitation. Journal of Hand Surgery 9B: 29–36

Hannington-Kiff J G 1986a Intravenous regional sympathetic block in upper limb angiography. Annals of the Royal College of Surgeons of England 68: 58–59

Hannington-Kiff J G 1986b Local cold block and guanethidine. Pain 26: 130–131

Hannington-Kiff J G 1990a Bier's block revisited: intercuff block. Journal of the Royal Society of Medicine 83: 155–158

Hannington-Kiff J G 1990b Rheumatoid arthritis – interventional treatment with regionally applied drugs and the use of sympathetic modulation: discussion paper. Journal of the Royal Society of Medicine 83: 373–376

Hannington-Kiff J G 1991 Does failed natural opioid modulation in regional sympathetic ganglia cause reflex sympathetic dystrophy? Lancet 338: 1125–1127

Hannington-Kiff J G 1992 Pain: sympathetic maintenance and central nervous sensitization. In: Kaufman L (ed) Anaesthesia review 9. Churchill Livingstone, Edinburgh p 112–126

Hannington-Kiff J G, Dunne S M 1993 Topical guanethidine relieves dentinal hypersensitivity and pain. Journal of the Royal Society of Medicine 86: 514–515

Hanowell L H, Kanefield J K, Soriano S G 1989 A recommendation for reduced lidocaine dosage during intravenous regional bretylium treatment of reflex sympathetic dystrophy. Anesthesiology 71: 811–812

Johnson E M 1978 Destruction of the sympathetic nervous system in neonatal rats and hamsters by vinblastine: prevention by concomitant administration of nerve growth factor. Brain Research 141: 105–118

Johnson R V, Ford S R 1990 Correspondence. Anesthesiology 73: 586

Kettler R E, Stene E 1987 Reflex sympathetic dystrophy in a patient with pre-existing torsade de pointes. Pain 28: 197–200

Leveston S A, Shah S D, Cryer P E 1979 Cholinergic stimulation of norepinephrine release in man. Journal of Clinical Investigation 64: 374–380

Loh L, Nathan P W, Schott G D 1981 Pain due to lesions of the central nervous system removed by sympathetic block. British Medical Journal i: 1026–1028

Manchikanti L 1990 Role of intravenous bretylium in reflex sympathetic dystrophy. Anesthesiology 73: 585–586

McKain C W, Urban B J, Goldner J L 1983 The effects of intravenous regional guanethidine and reserpine. Journal of Bone and Joint Surgery 65A: 808–811

McKay N N S, Woodhouse N J Y, Clarke A K 1977 Post-traumatic reflex sympathetic dystrophy syndrome (Sudeck's atrophy): effects of regional guanethidine infusion and salmon calcitonin. British Medical Journal ii: 1575–1576

Merskey H 1986 (ed) Classification of chronic pain. International Association for the Study of Pain Subcommittee on Taxonomy. Pain Supplement 3

Middaugh R E, Menk E J, Reynolds W J, Bauman J M, Cawthon M A, Hartshorne M F 1985 Epidural block using large volumes of local anaesthetic solution for intercostal nerve block. Anesthesiology 63: 214–216

Raja S N, Treede R-D, Davies K D, Campbell J N 1991 Systemic alpha-adrenergic blockade with phentolamine: a diagnostic test for sympathetically maintained pain. Anesthesiology 74: 691–698

Roberts W J 1986 A hypothesis on the physiological basis for causalgia and related pains. Pain 24: 297–311

Rocco A G, Kaul A F, Reisman R M, Gallo J P, Lief P A 1989 A comparison of regional intravenous guanethidine and reserpine in reflex sympathetic dystrophy. A controlled, randomized, double-blind crossover study. Clinical Journal of Pain 5: 205–209

Sanders V M, Munson A E 1985 Norepinephrine and the antibody response. Pharmacological Reviews 37: 229–248

Schott G D, Loh L 1984 Anticholinesterase drugs in the treatment of chronic pain. Pain 20: 201–206

Tunstall M E 1977 Detecting wakefulness during general anaesthesia for Caesarian section. British Medical Journal i: 1321

Vaughan R S, Lawrie B W, Sykes P J 1985 Use of intravenous regional sympathetic block in upper limb angiography. Annals of the Royal College of Surgeons of England 67: 309 – 312

Wall P D Devor M, Inbal F R et al 1980 Autotomy following peripheral nerve lesions: experimental anaesthesia dolorosa. Pain 7: 103–113

Wang J K 1985 Cryoanalgesia for painful peripheral nerve lesions. Pain 22: 191–194

Yanagida H, Kemi C, Suwa K 1976 The effects of stellate ganglion block on the idiopathic prolongation of the Q–T interval with cardiac arrhythmia (the Romano–Ward syndrome). Anesthesia and Analgesia 55: 782–787

Lesions

55. Root surgery

David Dubuisson

INTRODUCTION

This chapter gives the uses and consequences of root section and some of its variants (Fig. 55.1). When spinal dorsal root section was introduced by Bennett (1889) and Abbe (1889), the risk of the procedure was considerable, but anatomical principles suggested that it would relieve many types of pain. Today, the risks of general anaesthesia and surgery to carry out spinal root section are much less, although they are not negligible. Of greater concern is the frequent failure of spinal root surgery to provide permanent relief, and the possibility of causing anaesthesia dolorosa in the denervated area. Sectioning of lower cranial nerve roots carries a slighly larger operative risk, but its reliability in appropriately chosen cases seems well established. The topics of dorsal root ganglionectomy and dorsal entry zone lesions are dicussed in Chapter 59.

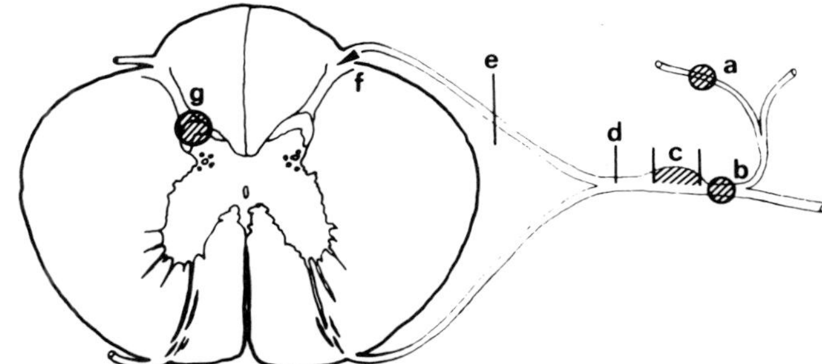

Fig. 55.1 Targets of root surgery. **a** Coagulation of medial branch of posterior primary ramus; **b** coagulation of spinal nerve trunk; **c** excision of dorsal root ganglion; **d** extradural section of dorsal root; **e** intradural section of dorsal root; **f** selective dorsal rhizidiotomy (partial section of rootlets); **g** coagulation of dorsal root entry zone.

DESCRIPTION

SECTION OF LOWER CRANIAL NERVES

Since the time of Dandy (1927), the usual approach to cranial neves VII, IX and X has been posterior fossa craniectomy. White & Kjellberg (1973) described the use of 'wake-up anaesthesia' to observe the patient's response to electrical stimulation of individual lower cranial nerve rootlets. However, this type pf surgery is more commonly done under general anaesthesia. Cranial nerves VII through X are all visible through a single small opening in the skull. In cases of glossopharyngeal neuralgia or other throat pain, the ninth and tenth nerves are identified at the jugular foramen, where they are separated by a dural septum. In most cases of this type, all of the glossopharyngeal nerve rootlets and one to three rostral filaments of the vagus nerve are sectioned. In an effort to reduce the risk of dysphonia, White & Sweet (1969) stimulated individual vagus filaments to reproduce the patient's pain, avoiding filaments that did not contribute. Robson & Bonica (1950) recommended a preoperative trial of cocainisation of the tonsillar fossa; persisting pain in the ear relieved by nerve block at the jugular foramen was felt to be evidence of a vagal contribution. Cardiovascular instability at the time of root section may be damped to some extent by applying a small cotton pledget soaked in Xylocaine before cutting the nerves. In some cases, microvascular decompression without section of the nerves may be sufficient (Laha & Jannetta 1977). When a tortuous vertebral or posterior inferior cerebellar artery is found to be causing focal pressure on the ninth or tenth nerve, the vessel can be dissected away from the nerve under high magnification. A small piece of polyvinyl chloride or silicone sponge or muscle is left between nerve and vessel.

If it is necessary to section the intermedius component of the seventh nerve, attention is directed instead to the internal auditory meatus. The nervus intermedius (Fig. 55.2) is hidden from view by the eighth nerve which must be separated from it by microdissection. In an awake patient, mechanical or electrical stimulation of the nervus intermedius may reproduce the patient's pain and thus confirm that section is necessary (White & Sweet 1969). The patient must be warned before stimulation because there is risk of destroying the facial nerve if he moves suddenly. The anatomy of the nervus intermedius is highly variable and the sensory component of the seventh nerve may consist of numerous tiny filaments which join the rest

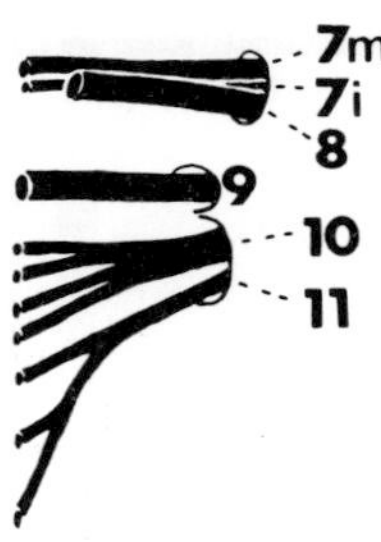

Fig. 55.2 Relationships of the lower cranial nerves. **7m** Motor division of facial nerve; **7i** sensory division of facial nerve (nervus intermedius); **8** vestibulocochlear nerve; **9** glossopharyngeal nerve; **10** vagus nerve; **11** accessory nerve. Note that nervus intermedius is largely hidden from view by the eighth nerve as it approaches the internal auditory canal. The ninth nerve is separated from the tenth in the jugular foramen by a dural septum.

of the nerve. White & Sweet (1969) sectioned the vestibular component of the eight nerve when a distinct nervus intermedius could not be identified.

PERCUTANEOUS THERMOCOAGULATION OF THE NINTH AND TENTH NERVES

Radio frequency thermocoagulation of the petrous ganglion in the jugular foramen has been used to treat pain due to oropharyngeal cancer (Lazorthes & Verdie 1979; Tew 1982; Giorgi & Broggi 1984) and idiopathic glossopharyngeal neuralgia (Lazorthes & Verdie 1979; Isamat et al 1981; Tew 1982; Giorgi & Broggi 1984). After local anaesthesia, an electrode is introduced through the cheek and guided, with appropriate radiological confirmation, into the neural portion of the jugular foramen. Low-intensity electrical stimulation through the correctly positioned electrode should provoke pain or dysaesthesia in the ear and throat without substantial alterations of blood pressure or electrocardiogram. During the thermocoagulation, the patient is heavily sedated and a lesion is made by heating the tip of the probe with a radiofrequency current generator. The size of the lesion is limited by careful timing of the heating phase and by monitoring of probe temperature.

INTRADURAL SPINAL ROOT SECTION

Root section in subarachnoid space is convenient at cervical and thoracic levels where the cord segments are near the corresponding intervertebral foramina. In the lumbosacral region, the nerve roots exit far caudal to the cord, which usually ends behind the first lumbar vertebra. Intradural section near the conus medullaris is feasible if stimulation is used to identity the involved roots, but since it is rarely desirable to section completely more than one or two lumbosacral roots, a smaller extradural exposure of the root sheaths near the intervertebral foramina is usually preferred. For intradural root section, the correct vertebral level must first be identified by suitable radiological technique. The operation is usually performed under general anaesthesia, but White & Kjellberg (1973) thought it advantageous to wake the patient during the procedure in order to choose roots for sectioning.

To treat truncal pain, posterior rootlets in the cord segment corresponding to the painful area are sectioned along with one or two roots below and above that level. For intradural root section, this requires a series of laminectomies or hemilaminectomies. The posterior rootlets leave their parent root to enter the cord as a fan-shaped array (Fig. 55.3). The appropriate rootlets are freed of accompanying blood vessels by microdissection before dividing them. It is sometimes necessary to divide anastomotic connections with rootlets of adjacent cord segments (Schwartz 1956).

Six or more consecutive thoracic dorsal roots can be sectioned without important loss of function. In the cervical and lumbosacral regions, the number of roots which can safely be sectioned is limited by loss of function in the limb. White & Kjellberg (1973) found minimal hypoaesthesia and no proprioceptive deficit after section of a single dorsal root of the brachial or lumbosacral plexus. Section of two major plexus roots did not result in serious loss of function provided the second and third sacral roots were spared. These authors also recommended preserving at least C6 or C7 or else both C5 and C8 to protect proprioception in the upper limb in cases of extensive brachial rhizotomy, and at least one root of the L2–L3–L4 group in cases of extensive lumbosacral rhizotomy. Section of both L5 and S1 may be done at some risk of interfering with proprioception in the foot. Combined cranial and upper cervical rhizotomies are occasionally undertaken in cases of head and neck cancer.

EXTRADURAL ROOT SECTION

In the lumbosacral region where roots do not exit at the level of the corresponding cord segments, it is preferable to identify the dorsal roots near the intervertebral foramina. This can be done by opening the subarachnoid space, but most surgeons (e.g. Scoville 1966; White &

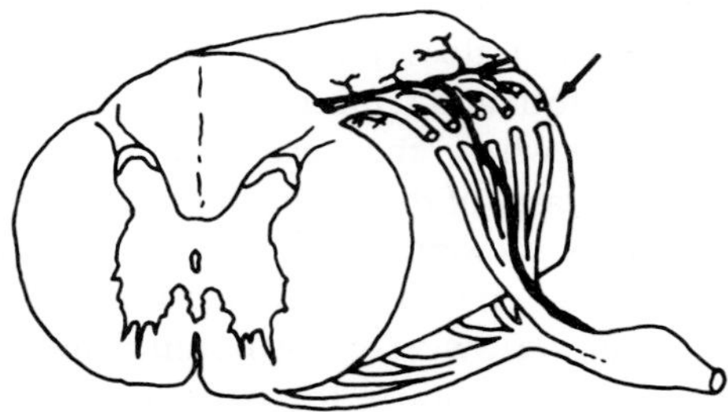

Fig. 55.3 Intradural dorsal rhizotomy. Individual rootlets fan apart to enter the cord. Note sparing of the radicular artery. Arrow marks point at which rootlets have been sectioned.

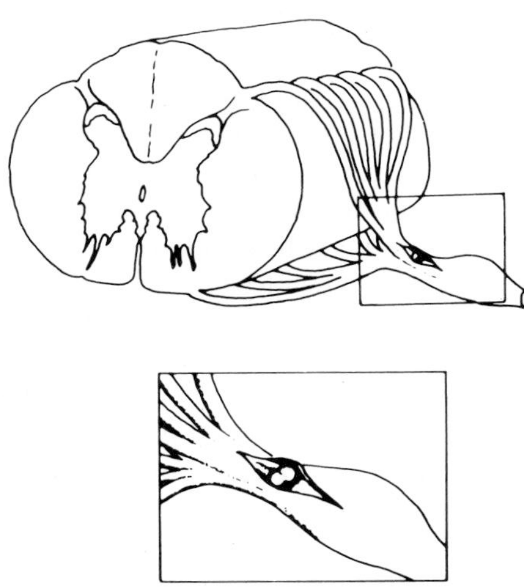

Fig. 55.4 Extradural dorsal rhizotomy. The root sheath is opened proximal to the ganglion and the root, frequently bifid at that point, is sectioned.

Kjellberg 1973; Bertrand 1975; Strait & Hunter 1981) prefer an intraspinal extradural approach (Fig. 55.4). If previous discectomy or other spinal surgery has been done, the presence of thick epidural scar tissue may obscure the root, making it necessary to remove additional bone from the laminae and from the medial aspect of the articular facets for adequate exposure. Two distinct dorsal root fascicles are usually present, posterior to a ventral root bundle (Osgood et al 1976). Electrical stimulation can be used to distinguish ventral root filaments but in chronically damaged roots the threshold for excitation of motor responses is higher than usual and in some cases it is impossible to produce muscle contractions (Bertrand 1975). Stimulation of dorsal roots may be used in an awake patient to confirm the contribution of individual roots to the patient's pain. When the appropriate fascicles have been identified, they are dissected free of blood vessels and sectioned. Leakage of cerebrospinal fluid (CSF) is seldom a problem if section is carried out close to the dorsal root ganglion. Scoville (1966) described a similar approach for extradural section of cervical dorsal roots but he recommended a slightly different technique for extradural section of thoracic roots. He exposed the dorsal root ganglion laterally by removing a small amount of bone from the outer edge of the lamina just caudal to the transverse process.

For the treatment of certain cases of intractable perineal and perianal pain due to advanced malignancy, a simplified extradural method of sectioning the lower sacral roots has been advocated (Crue & Todd 1964; Felsööry & Crue 1976). The dural tube is exposed by a laminectomy of the upper sacrum. The entire theca and its contents are ligated and divided caudal to the S1 root sheaths when bladder function is no longer important. In occasional patients whose pain extends to the leg, the S1 root is included on the painful side. In patients with residual bladder function, the S2 root on the least painful side is excluded from section.

In general, the limitations of extradural root section are the same as those outlined above for intradural section.

SELECTIVE POSTERIOR RHIZIDIOTOMY

The term 'selective posterior rhizidiotomy' refers to partial section of individual posterior rootlets at their junction with the spinal cord. This technique, developed by Sindou (Sindou et al 1974a, 1974b, 1974c, 1976, 1981), postulates an anatomical separation of large and small primary afferent axons within each rootlet at the dorsal root entry zone. It is suggested that small-diameter afferents cluster in the lateral aspect of each rootlet and penetrate the Lissauer tract where they can be divided by a microsurgical incision (Fig. 55.5).

The approach is similar to that used for intradural dorsal root section but the rootlets are not completely divided. Near the cord, the individual rootlets are dissected free of blood vessels and arachnoid strands under an operating microscope. Each rootlet is then lifted medially with a blunt microsurgical hook. Underlying pial vessels are dissected away or lightly coagulated with a bipolar forceps. A microsurgical blade is used to make an incision 1 – 2 mm deep in the ventrolateral aspect of the rootlet – cord junction at an angle of 45° from the sagittal plane (Fig. 55.6). A similar incision is made along each rootlet of the involved segments. There are no strict limitations of the number and levels of rootlets treated. Since the points of entry of the lumbosacral rootlets are nearly continuous, it may be easier in this region to retract all of the selected rootlets medially and, after moving or

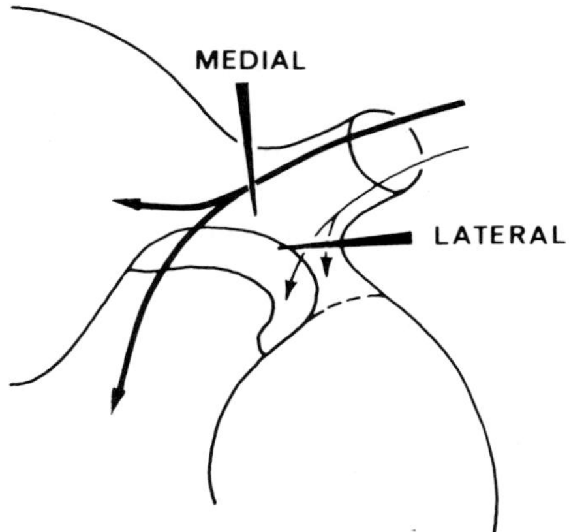

Fig. 55.5 The parcellation of primary afferent fibres postulated by Sindou et al (1976). Small-diameter primary afferent are preferentially destroyed by a lesion placed in the Lissauer tract at the lateral side of the entering dorsal rootlet. Large-diameter primary afferent fibres from muscle spindles and proprioceptive elements would be disrupted by a lesion at the medial side of the dorsal rootlet, where the large fibres merge with the dorsal column.

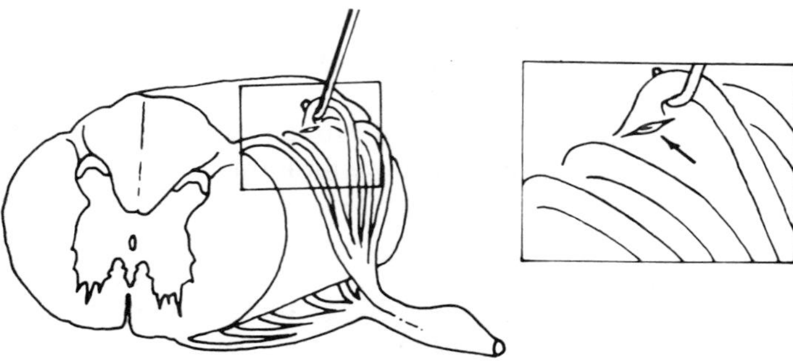

Fig. 55.6 Selective dorsal rhizidiotomy (after Sindou et al 1976). Each dorsal rootlet is lifted medially with a small nerve hook to permit section of the lateralmost fibres. An incision 1–2 mm deep is made in the ventrolateral aspect of the cord–rootlet junction (inset).

coagulating pial vessels, to make a continuous 1–2 mm incision along the posterolateral sulcus of the cord (Sindou et al 1976). Identification of lumbar and sacral rootlets is aided by electrical stimulation of corresponding ventral rootlets looking for muscle contractions, and by measurements. The dorsal rootlets of S2 and S3 spread rostrally 20–35 mm from the coccygeal root entry zone (Sindou et al 1976). Stimulation of ventral rootlets arising from the second, third and fourth sacral segments may produce contractions of the urinary bladder (Rockswold et al 1974).

PERCUTANEOUS SPINAL ROOT LESIONS

Radio-frequency lesions of the spinal nerve roots and ganglia can be performed by a percutaneous technique under local anaesthesia (Uematsu et al 1974; Lazorthes et al 1976; Nash 1986; van Kleef et al 1993). To reach spinal roots at cervical, thoracic or lumbosacral levels, a guide needle is introduced through the skin and paraspinal muscles. Needle position is confirmed radiologically, usually by intermittent fluoroscopy. When the root is contacted, an electrode is inserted through the guide needle and low-intensity electrical stimulation is used to verify that the root innervates the painful region. Further confirmation of root level can sometimes be provided by the pattern of muscle contractions induced by stimulation. The patient is then sedated and the root is lesioned with a radio-frequency current generator. The use of a temperature-monitoring electrode and timer helps to limit the size of the lesion. With careful technique, motor function can usually be preserved along with some cutaneous sensation.

PERCUTANEOUS MEDIAL BRANCH NEUROTOMY

Several techniques attempt to denervate the lumbar articular facets as a treatment of back pain. Rees (1976) described a 'facet rhizolysis' in which he claimed to sever the articular branches of posterior primary rami using a long scaplel blade. A percutaneous radio-frequency technique was later devised by Shealy (1975). With local anaesthesia, a hollow guide needle is introduced under fluoroscopic control, to contact the facet joint. Then a temperature monitoring probe is inserted through the guide needle and the tip is heated with a radio-frequency current generator to create a lesion. This is repeated at all of the levels which are thought to be involved. Other authors recommend slightly different electrode placements (Bogduk & Long 1979). The target (Fig. 55.1) is the medial branch of the posterior primary ramus of the spinal nerve so that the procedure is actually a medial branch neurotomy. It may also be performed at cervical or thoracic levels. Some technical aspects of this procedure have been called into question, as discussed later in this chapter.

RATIONALE

The basic purpose of spinal dorsal root section and of cranial sensory root section is to denervate the area in which pain is felt, without compromising the spinal cord or brainstem. It is often assumed that root section is of greatest benefit in pain due to intrinsic lesions of the sensory ganglion or root itself where the underlying disturbance is thought to be disordered or excessive activity of primary afferent fibres. It is also commonly assumed that root section should effectively relieve pain which is peripheral and circumscribed since the afferent territory of a few adjacent spinal nerves might completely encompass the painful region. Judging from the long-term results of root section, however, neither of these assumptions seems entirely accurate.

Some of the reasons for failure are already known. For instance, herpes zoster produces segmental pain with prominent lesions of individual sensory ganglia, yet root section usually fails to provide relief (White & Sweet 1969; Onofrio & Campa 1972). This might be due to additional herpetic lesions of adjacent ganglia or of the spinal cord. The result of dorsal root section for pain associated with chronic mechanical damage and scarring of roots are also poor in the long term. We know from the work of Howe et al (1977) that chronic nerve and ganglion compression in animals leads to the development of mechanosensitivity of primary afferents. In man, dorsal root section for postlaminectomy radicular pain might reasonably be expected to interrupt abnormal trains of nerve impulses from the damaged sites, yet the late success rate is poor (Loeser 1972; Onofrio & Campa 1972; Bertrand 1975). This might be explained by spontaneous activity of chronically deafferented transmission neurons in the cord (Loeser & Ward 1967; Loeser et al 1968) which would not be helped by rhizotomy. Indeed there are reasons to suspect that further deafferentation might even aggravate the problem. Ovelmen-Levitt et al (1984) reported that receptive fields of deep dorsal horn neurons expanded to the flank and thoracic dermatomes after lumbar dorsal rhizotomies or root avulsions. Receptive fields after avulsion were smaller and required more intense stimuli. Histological analysis showed damage to Lissauer tract and gliosis in the substantia gelatinosa after avulsion, but not after simple rhizotomy.

Some peripheral sources of pain fail to respond to root section but it can often be argued that too few roots were divided. It has been known since the time of Sherrington that each cutaneous region is innervated by at least three consecutive roots (Sherrington 1898; Foerster 1933). Recent studies in primates (Dykes & Terzis 1981) make it clear that the full extent of dermatomal overlap is more extensive than this. Moreover the extent of the dermatomes supplied by peripheral processes of A delta and C primary afferents has never been mapped specifically in any species, even though it is obviously relevant to root section for pain in humans.

Anatomical and physiological studies stress the presence of long-ranging primary afferent fibres which, in some species, may travel six or more segments to contact distant cord neurons (Imai & Kusuma 1969; Wall & Werman 1976). We know that some dorsal horn neurons deprived of their most direct primary afferent contacts by multiple root section begin to respond to these long-ranging afferents, taking on new and 'distant' receptive fields (Wall 1977). These facts may partly explain the recurrence of some types of pain after section of a limited number of dorsal roots. Also, root section may provide initial relief of pain from a small region of infection or malignancy yet a recurrence of pain might result from spread of the disease to involve intact neighbouring afferent dermatomes and sclerotomes.

The rationale of conserving some important dorsal roots of the brachial or lumbosacral plexus is that a completely deafferented limb is useless. Obviously this could limit the success of multiple rhizotomy for process such as lung apex tumours or tumours in the pelvis since some of the afferent fibres which serve the painful area are not sectioned. Sindou's technique of selective dorsal rhizidiotomy may largely circumvent this problem since it leaves intact at least some of the large proprioceptive and low-threshold mechanoreceptive axons in the medial portion of the root entry zone. Sindou et al (1986) have used a similar lesion to relieve pain in the arm associated with severe spasticity in hemiplegic patients. Certainly prolonged muscle contraction must contribute to other types of pain. We do not know which population of primary afferent fibres are excessively active in such conditions as chronic low back pain, painful surgical scars or amputation.

The lesion described by Sindou et al (1976) involves the lateral division of the Lissauer tract. However, the term 'Lissauer tractotomy' refers to an older procedure devised by Hyndman (1942) in which transverse sections were made in the tract. It should be noted that some disruption of pial arteries and veins occurs in these procedures, particularly if coagulation is used. Vascular compromise of the dorsal horn might create a functionally more extensive lesion than the one visible to the surgeon. Wall (1962) carried out physiological and anatomical studies of the dorsal horn and ascending sensory tracts following tiny lesions of the ventrolateral cord–rootlet junction in cats. Using a dye perfusion technique, he detected a massive decrease in perfusion of the entire dorsal horn after seemingly minor interference with the pial vessels. A variety of physiological recordings suggested that the only remaining dorsal horn activity was transmission through the large group Ia proprioceptive afferents.

Not all authors find a distinct lateral separation of small afferent at the cord–rootlet junction. Wall (1962) felt that the longitudinally directed fibres of the Lissauer tract might be deflected by entering rootlets so as to create a false impression of large numbers of fine primary afferents entering laterally. Snyder (1977) failed to find a lateral subdivision of the dorsal rootlet in the cat, but he agreed that such a parcellation of small and large afferents was present in the monkey. Kerr (1975) studied thin sections of rootlets cut tangential to the root entry zone of monkey and cat cord and concluded that the distribution of large and small fibres within the rootlet was random until they were within 1 mm of the cord. Then fine afferents tended laterally. While such an arrangement appears to exist in man, Sindou et al (1976) admit that other patterns may sometimes be present. The ultrastructural anatomy of this region of human cord deserves further study. Certainly the lack of fibre subdivisions within rootlets could be a cause for failure in some cases of selective rhizidiotomy.

Radiofrequency thermocoagulation of roots and root branches is based on the assumption that heat lesions preferentially destroy small myelinated and unmyelinated fibres, including the bulk of known nociceptive afferents, but leave intact the majority of innocuous mechanoreceptors and proprioceptors (Letcher & Goldring 1968). This concept is questioned by authors who find that large and small fibres are destroyed indiscriminately (Uematsu 1977; Smith et al 1981). Widespread experience with thermocoagulation of the trigeminal ganglion supports the view that sparing of at least some innocuous mechanoreceptive afferents can be achieved by careful control of temperature. This is not necessarily true of spinal dorsal root thermocoagulations which may or may not involve the dorsal root ganglia. One obvious difference is that the trigeminal ganglion is actually a cistern filled with CSF. Nevertheless, percutaneous spinal dorsal root ganglion lesions have been accomplished safely at mid-cervical levels, without loss of motor function in the arms or long-term signs of de-afferentation syndrome (van Kleef et al 1993).

It is not unreasonable to think that some of the success

of thermocoagulation is due to destruction of large-diameter afferents which might contribute importantly to pain in many of the cases treated. The pain of cranial neuralgias is known to be triggered by innocuous stimuli. In many cases of pain associated with cancer, herpes zoster and other causes of deafferentation, light touch or brushing of hairs may provoke intense burning pain. Since the altered synaptic relationships and physiology of partially deafferented cord and brainstem neurons are not yet understood, it seems premature to interpret the results of root or ganglion thermacoagulations solely in terms of large and small afferent fibre spectra.

There is some controversy in the use of selective nerve root blocks with local anaesthetics to predict the result of root section. Many surgeons rely on preliminary root blocks to determine the segmental level involved, to decide whether a permanent root lesion might relieve the patient's pain and to give the patient some warning of what to expect should section be carried out. Some patients cannot tolerate numbness and should not be subjected to rhizotomy. Some reports (Loeser 1972; Onofrio & Campa 1972) indicate that an effective root block does not reliably predict a good response to subsequent root section. We do not know how reliably such blocks, if ineffective, can identify the patients who should not have root surgery. It is difficult to eliminate the possibility that spread of the anaesthetic agent reaches adjacent roots. There is the additional possibility that many instances of apparent monoradicular pain actually involve afferents from several dorsal roots. Blocking one root may reduce the total afferent drive of transmission neurons of neighbouring cord segments. Bonica (1974) argues that three or more selective root blocks of differing duration may be needed to predict the result of root section with any accuracy. Johnson et al (1974) used intercostal nerve conduction studies to investigate levels of involvement prior to thoracic root section. These studies were felt to increase the likelihood of pain relief in patients chosen to have surgery.

There are additional reasons to question the rationale of root surgery. In the monkey, dorsal rhizotomy depletes the substantia gelatinosa of opiate receptors which are associated with terminals of primary afferent axons (Lamotte et al 1976). If this is also the case in man, root surgery could conceivably cause a decrease of the effectiveness of narcotic analgesic drugs. Such a decrease has been difficult to demonstrate convincingly, perhaps because the underlying conditions are so often refractory to narcotics prior to surgery. Subtance P, somatostatin and other neuroactive peptides are depleted from the dorsal horn by dorsal rhizotomy. The physiological consequences of this are not known.

Strictly speaking, 'facet denervation' is not root surgery and it does not have the same rationale as nerve root and ganglion lesions. Its practitioners hold that back pain, neck pain and radicular pain are often referred from sites of degeneration of inflammation of the spinal zygapophyseal joints (Rees 1976). This is largely a matter of speculation. Because the procedure is done percutaneously with no confirmation of the lesions, there is considerable scepticism concerning its rationale. King (1976) reported that in an average patient the lumbosacral facet joints could not in fact be denervated by the Rees procedure, since the blade which is used is not long enough to reach them. Bogduk & Long (1979), noting several anatomical innaccuracies in descriptions of 'facet rhizotomy', studied the anatomy of the posterior primary rami and their articular branches. The articular branches lie rostral and caudal to the zygapophyseal joint, yet most of the reported techniques describe electrode placements lateral to the joint. Bogduk & Long (1979) concluded that is probably not possible to denervate the zygapophyseal joints selectively by a percutaneous approach.

Despite its many irrational aspects, root surgery is still useful in carefully selected cases to reduce noxious inputs from a circumscribed part of the body. With careful attention to technique, it is possible to spare motor fibres and, to some extent, proprioceptive afferent fibres. There are some adverse consequences of extensive denervation (see Complications and Side-Effects, below), but in general the zone of sensory loss produced by rhizotomy is more permanent than that produced by cordotomy (Loeser 1982).

INDICATIONS

The indications for section of lower cranial nerves are clearer than those for spinal root surgery. A long history of glossopharyngeal neuralgia or intermedius neuralgia refractory to medical management is a suitable indication for root section, microsurgical decompression or thermocoagulation provided the patient is in good enough general health to undergo surgery. Cancer of the head and neck associated with intractable pain in the throat or ear may require section of some combination of the fifth, seventh (intermedius), ninth and upper tenth nerves in addition to section of the upper cervical nerves. Of course such extensive surgery is only warranted in a patient whose life expectancy is subtantially greater than the time required for hospitalisation, operation and recovery. This applies to multiple root section for malignancy elsewhere in the body, especially when another treatment might be equally effective. In some of these cases it seems preferable to choose percutaneous root coagulation or cordotomy, which may require a day or two in the hospital, than to choose an open surgical procedure which may demand weeks in hospital for an already debilitated patient.

Spinal root surgery is often useful for pain associated with tumours of the lung apex and brachial plexus region. Here, selective rhizidiotomy can be used to prevent total denervation of the arm. For pain due to malignant perineal and pelvic tumours, bilateral section of the third, fourth and fifth sacral and of the coccygeal roots can be effective. Crue's method is probably the simplest way to achieve this but concern for remaining bladder function may demand a more restricted approach with intraoperative stimulation of individual roots. Pain limited to the superficial anococcygeal region may require section of only S4, S5 and the coccygeal roots. Deeper perineal and pelvic pain is not as easily managed by root section and may require additional division of S3 and even unilateral section of S2. Pelvic pain extending to the leg might require additional section of S1 or of lumbar roots. Selective rhizidiotomy is the procedure of choice to preserve some useful afferent function in the lower limb in these cases (Sindou et al 1981). Obviously, when previous colostomy and urinary diversion have been done, bilateral section of sacral roots can be done with impunity. Pain associated with chest wall malignancies may also respond well to multiple root section or ganglionectomy. Ordinarily, at least two roots above and two below the painful segments should be sectioned in addition to the roots of the involved dermatomes.

Root surgery for pain associated with benign conditions has widely varying success rates that appear to depend mainly on the underlying disease process and location of pain. Occipital neuralgia can usually be relieved by section of the first, second and third cervical roots if the patient is willing to accept a zone of anaesthesia in the scalp. The author has treated refractory occipital neuralgia by selective posterior rhizidiotomy at C1–C3, sparing scalp sensation in all cases. Results in nine cases have been similar to those obtained with complete rhizotomies. Good initial results of rhizotomy for occipital neuralgia tend to be permanent, especially in posttraumatic cases (Hunter & Mayfield 1949). The author has noted that patients with demonstrable radiological abnormalities, such as fractures and arthritis, tend to fare better than do patients with idiopathic occipital pain.

Postherpetic neuralgia is seldom adequately relieved by dorsal rhizotomy alone (White & Sweet 1969). Multiple thoracic ganglionectomies have been used, but the number of reported cases is small (Smith 1970). Postthoracotomy incisional pain, idiopathic intercostal neuralgia and chest-wall pain associated with irradiated tumours can often be effectively managed by multilevel ganglionectomies. This procedure has the advantage that laminectomies are not required, although there may still be considerable incisional discomfort due to disruption of the paraspinal muscles. Also, multiple rhizotomies or ganglionectomies at truncal level can be followed at least transiently by dysaesthesias in neighbouring dermatomes, as discussed later in this chapter.

'Facet denervation' seems to be used mainly for refractory low back pain. There is no indisputable indication for the procedure. We do not know if the technique is more suitable for cases in which there is definite radiological evidence of articular damage. If the procedure is to be used at all, the radiofrequency thermocoagulation method with strict X-ray control of electrode placements is clearly preferable to a blind approach. Familiarity with the anatomy of the articular nerve branches is required (Bogduk & Long 1979).

RESULTS

The success of standard dorsal rhizotomy and of dorsal root ganglionectomy seems to depend less on the exact technique employed than on the problem treated. Long-term results sampled at least three months after the procedure are invariably worse than immediate results. Table 55.1 shows the percentages of patients who reported either substantial relief or complete relief of their pain after root surgery for various conditions. These percentages were derived by adding patients from several series of intradural or extradural rhizotomies or ganglionectomies for which some useful data were given concerning follow-up. Admittedly, careful descriptions of both immediate and long-term results are seldom given in these series and, in most, the criteria for good results are either not specified by the authors or, if specified, not always objective. There is a need for further studies of root surgery using objective pain-rating scales and measures of the descriptions of pain before and after surgery. These should preferably be administered by someone other than the surgeon and his team.

It can be seen from Table 55.1 that the most consistent results are reported for idiopathic cranial neuralgias, although section of the ninth and upper tenth cranial nerve roots via suboccipital craniectomy carries a mortality rate of around 5%. The results of microvascular decompression alone (Laha & Jannetta 1977) are not better than the results of root section. Deaths following section of the nervus intermedius are not described in the modern literature. This may be partly because, in contrast to section of the ninth and tenth cranial nerves, section of the sensory component of the seventh does not case cardiovascular instability. However, there are too few cases of intermedius section in the recent literature to conclude reliably on the surgical mortality rate of the procedure. In cases of glossopharyngeal neuralgia, section of only the ninth nerve is not as consistently effective as section of the ninth plus upper rootlets of the tenth (White & Sweet 1969).

Root surgery has not been conspicuously successful in the treatment of widespread arachnoiditis, although occasional cases of localized intradural scarring may benefit (Jain 1974). Dorsal rhizotomy for cases of 'battered root' syndrome following lumbar disc surgery or spinal fusion has a very poor success rate with essentially all patients reporting eventual failure, and most describing dysaesthesias as a complication (Bertrand 1975). Ganglionectomy

Table 55.1 Results of standard rhizotomy or ganglionectomy

Condition	Levels	Immediate relief	Relief after 3 monthss	Mortality	No. of cases	Authors
Intermedius neuralgia	VII	100%	86%	(? nil)	7	cited in White & Sweet 1969
Glossopharygeal neuralgia	IX (±X)	83%	77%	5%	166	Robson & Bonica 1950; Bohm & Strang 1962; Walker 1966; White & Sweet 1969; Laha & Jannetta 1977; Rushton et al 1981
Occipital neuralgia	C1–C3	76%	69%	(? nil)	54	Hunter & Mayfield 1949;Chambers 1954; Cusson & King 1960; Scoville1966;White & Sweet 1969; Echols 1970; Onofrio & Campa 1972
Postherpetic neuralgia	Multiple spinal roots	36%	29%	(? nil)	11	White & Sweet 1969; Smith 1970; Loeser 1972; Onofrio & Campa 1972
Truncal pain: postsurgical posttraumatic idiopathic	Multiple spinal roots	81%	65%	(? nil)	106	Scoville1966; Echols1970; Smith 1970; Loeser 1972; Onofrio & Campa 1972; White & Kjellberg 1973; Osgood et al 1976; Hosobuchi 1980; Dubuisson (this chapter)
Failed lumbar disc surgery	L4, L5, S1	74%	33%	(? nil)	168	Loeser 1972; Onofrio & Campa 1972; White & Kjellberg 1973; Jain 1974; Bertrand 1975; Osgood et al 1976; Strait & Hunter 1981
Coccygodynia	S3–Col	79%	58%	nil	52	Echols 1970; Bohm 1962; Albrektsson 1981; Saris et al 1986
Cancer	Multiple spinal ± cranial	59%	47%	5%	585	cited in Sindou et al 1976 (153 cases with long follow-up)

appears to have no advantage in this patient group. North (1991) reported that no patients in a group of 13 were satisfied with the results of dorsal root ganglionectomy for failed back surgery after 5.5 years of follow-up. The author has carried out selective posterior rhizidiotomy in two cases of persistent sciatica and failed disc surgery. Both patients experienced proprioceptive difficulties in the leg, and neither reported adequate pain relief. Pain associated with failed disc surgery and nerve root damage would therefore appear to be a poor indication for any type of dorsal root surgery because of its high failure rate and the likelihood of dysaesthesias or frank anaesthesia dolorosa. It seems likely that the underlying root damage in these cases has already led to disordered afferent impulse generation and perhaps irreversible patterns of function within the central nervous system, so that further de-afferentation by rhizotomy will often be futile or even detrimental.

Rhizotomy for posthherpetic neuralgia cannot be strongly endorsed, as it carries only a 29% long-term success rate. Root surgery for cancer pain has a slightly better overall success rate (47% late pain relief), but the results are still discouraging. Patient selection in cancer cases is a critical issue. Some of the best published results pertain to selective posterior rhizidiotomy for tumours of the brachial and lumbosacral plexus regions, where initial relief can be as high as 87–100% of cases (Vlahovitch & Fuentes 1975; Sindou et al 1981). Relief is generally sustained over the survival period of the patient. Unfortunately, not all cancer patients with tumours in suitable locations can submit to selective rhizidiotomy, because of the high anaesthetic risk associated with systemic malignancy. It has been the author's experience that root surgery for chest wall and brachial plexus invasion is best carried out rather early in the course of the disease while the patient's general health permits a safer peri-operative course. Inclusion of additional roots above and below the segmental levels of obvious involvement gives some insurance against pain recurrence due to spread of the tumour.

As noted earlier, selective posterior rhizidiotomy can also provide relief in cases of severe spasticity (Vlahovitch & Fuentes 1975; Sindou et al 1986). Late results of selective rhizidiotomy for pain associated with amputation, nerve injury or herpes zoster infection are said not to be satisfactory unless there is a prominent degree of cutaneous hyperaesthesia (Sindou et al 1981).

Percutaneous electrocoagulation of spinal and lower cranial roots or ganglia provides respectable early relief of pain due to malignancy or glossopharyngeal neuralgia (Table 55.2). Late results of spinal root coagulation are hard to judge since this technique is used primarily to treat pain of terminal malignancy. Long-term results would be expected to be less satisfactory because the root lesions created in this way are not as complete as those achieved by open surgery and, unless the dorsal root ganglion is

Table 55.2 Results of percutaneous thermocoagulation of spinal and cranial roots (selected series)

Authors	Levels treated	Initial relief	Late relief	Mortality	No. of cases
Uematsu et al (1974)	Spinal roots	39%	?	0	13
Lazorthes et al (1976)	Spinal roots	65%	?	0	20
Nash (1986)	Spinal ganglia	58%	50%	0	26
van Kleef et al (1993)	Spinal ganglia	75%	39%	0	20
Lazorthes & Verdie (1979)	Ninth/tenth cranial (cancer)	?	73%	0	11
	(glossopharyngeal neuralgia)	?	100%	0	1
Isamat et al (1980)	Ninth/tenth cranial (glossopharyngeal neuralgia)	100%	75%	0	4
Tew (1982)	Ninth/tenth cranial (cancer)	56%	?	0	9
	(glossopharyngeal neuralgia)	100%	?	0	2
Giorgi & Broggi (1984)	Ninth\tenth cranial (cancer)	100%	100%	0	5
	(glossopharyngeal neuralgia)	100%	60%	0	5

destroyed, some fibre regeneration is possible after thermocoagulation. Late results of ninth and tenth cranial root coagulation are good, but late recurrences are noted and some patients experience serious difficulties with swallowing postoperatively.

Shealy (1975) reported that percutaenous radiofrequency 'facet denervation' for chronic back pain and sciatica was effective for more than six months in 79% of previously unoperated patients, in 41% of those with a previous laminectomy and in 27% of patients with a previous spinal fusion. In a series of 149 patients treated by Long (1982), excellent relief of chronic low back pain was described after 'facet denervation' in 61% of cases with no prior surgery, in 27% of those with one previous operation and in no case with two or more previous spinal fusion. Deaths and serious complications of the procedure were not encountered by these authors.

Results of several series of radio-frequency root or ganglion coagulation procedures are given in Table 55.2.

COMPLICATIONS AND SIDE-EFFECTS

Some of the risks root surgery were mentioned in the preceding discussion and in Table 55.1 – namely, the frequent failure to achieve pain relief; the risk of loss of proprioception in arm or leg after multiple root section; the possible loss of control of anal and urethral sphincters, weakness of the bladder or impotence after sacral root section; and the relatively small risk of death due to complications of open surgery.

Possible complications of suboccipital craniectomy for glossopharyngeal and upper vagal root section include severe cardiovascular instability with sudden pronounced arterial hypotension or hypertension, cardiac arrhythmias or cardiac arrest, or intracranial bleeding. Cerebellar haemorrhage can occur postoperatively due to a sudden surge of blood pressure and to the changes which may follow prolonged retraction of the cerebellar hemisphere at the time of surgery. These patients require zealous postoperative monitoring and observation in a neurosurgical intensive care unit. Cerebellar dysfunction per se after surgery of the lower cranial nerves is almost always mild and transient.

Denervation of the larynx and pharynx has the obvious risk of interfering with swallowing and coughing, which sometimes leads to pneumonitis due to inadvertent aspiration of vomitus or secretions. Dysphonia due to vocal cord paralysis is sometimes permanent. This complication can best be avoided by stimulation of the upper vagal filaments before sectioning them in an awake patient (White & Sweet 1969) or by careful testing with stimulation delivered through the thermocouple electrode prior to coagulation lesion. Temporary facial weakness after section of the nervus intermedius is not unexpected since the motor portion of the seventh nerve is manipulated to some degree. There is of course the uncommon risk of permanent facial paralysis should accidental section or vascular compromise of the facial nerve occur. This has nor been reported in the available surgical series however.

Following spinal root surgery, there is the unfortunate possibility of failure to achieve relief because the wrong roots were sectioned. This requires reoperation. Numbness is seldom a major problem after rhizotomy but an occasional patient who has not been exposed to this feeling by prior anaesthetic root block may find it more disturbing than his original pain. Distressing numbness in the genitalia may follow sacral root surgery and cause impotence or limitation of sexual function.

Some patients will experience severe pain in the deafferented dermatomes (anaesthesia dolorosa) following rhizotomy or ganglionectomy. It might be thought that the number of roots sectioned would be an important factor, but the condition is frequent after limited rhizotomy for damaged roots after failed disc surgery (Bertrand 1975). Sweet (1984) estimated a 4% incidence of lasting dysaesthesias after rhizotomy, but this figure is probably too low. Sweet noted that the unpleasant sensations are often referred to the margins of the denervated zone. This is also the author's experience, at least in patients undergoing multilevel thoracic ganglionectomies. Hosobuchi (1980) described the same phenomenon after ganglionectomies. van Kleef et al (1993) reported transient burning sensations, lasting 6 weeks or less, in 12 of 20 patients who underwent percutaneous radio-frequency lesions of the cervical dorsal root ganglia for neck pain of benign aetiology. They felt that permanent complications could be minimized by the use of a small-diameter electrode.

Paraplegia can occur after spinal root surgery due either to vascular compromise of the cord or to the formation of a blood clot in the epidural or subarachnoid space. The former can be avoided by meticulous attention to all of the vessels around the ganglion, rootlets and root entry zone. Prompt recognition of a postoperative clot requires frequent examination of the patient. Certainly this complication is less likely after extradural rhizotomy or ganglionectomy. Another advantage of these extradural procedures is the reduced risk of CSF leakage since there is no entry of the subarachnoid space. The risk of postoperative meningitis and arachnoiditis is also less. Moderate incisional pain and paraspinous muscle spasm are expected after either an intradural or an extradural approach and this may continue for weeks while wound healing progresses.

Spinal thermocoagulation procedures are generally free of side-effects other than local bruising and swelling at the needle sites. Undetected breaks in cable insulation can cause superficial burns (Shealy 1975). A more serious complication of percutaneous medial branch neurotomy is a neuralgia-like pain syndrome ('lumbar lateral branch neuralgia') resulting from inadvertent transection of lateral branches of the lumbar posterior primary rami (Bogduk 1981). Burning pain and hyperaesthesia to pinprick are said to occur in the buttock above the iliac crest. The frequency of this complication is not yet known.

REFERENCES

Abbe R 1889 A contribution to the surgery of the spine. Medical Record 35: 149–152

Albrektsson B 1981 Sacral rhizotomy in cases of anococcygeal pain. Acta Orthopaedica Scandinavica 52: 187–190

Bennett W H 1889 A case in which acute spasmodic pain in the left lower extremity was completely relieved by subdural division of the posterior roots of certain spinal nerves. Medico-Chirurgical Transactions 72: 329–348

Bertrand G 1975 The 'battered' root problem. Orthopedic Clinics of North America 6: 305–310

Bogduk N 1981 Lumbar lateral branch neuralgia: a complication of rhizolysis. Medical Journal of Australia 1: 242–243

Bogduk N, Long D M 1979 The anatomy of the so-called 'articular nerves' and their relationship to facet denervation in the treatment of low back pain. Journal of Neurosurgery 51: 172–177

Bohm E 1962 Late results of sacral rhizotomy in coccygodynia. Acta Chirurgica Scandinavica 123: 6–8

Bohm E, Strang R R 1962 Glossopharyngeal neuralgia. Brain 85: 371–388

Bonica J J 1974 Floor discussion: dorsal rhizotomy. In: Bonica J J (ed) Pain. Advances in neurology, vol 4. Raven Press, New York, p 626

Chambers W R 1954 Posterior rhizotomy of the second and third cervical nerves for occipital pain. Journal of the American Medical Association 155: 431–432

Crue B L, Todd E M 1964 A simplified technique of sacral rhizotomy for pelvic pain. Journal of Neurosurgery 21: 835

Cusson D L, King A B 1960 Cervical rhizotomy in the management of some cases of occipital neuralgia. Guthrie Clinic Bulletin 29: 198–208

Dandy W E 1927 Glossopharyngeal neuralgia (tic douloureux): its diagnosis and treatment. Archives of Surgery 15: 198–214

Dykes R W, Terzis J K 1981 Spinal nerve distributions in the upper limb: the organization of the dermatome and afferent myotome. Philosophical Transactions of the Royal Society of London Series B: Biological Sciences 293: 509–554

Echols D H 1970 The effectiveness of thoracic rhizotomy for chronic pain. Neurochirurgia 13: 69–74

Felsööry A, Crue B L 1976 Results of 19 years' experience with sacral rhizotomy for perineal and perianal cancer pain. Pain 2: 431–433

Foerster O 1933 The dermatomes in man. Brain 56: 1–39

Giorgi C, Broggi G 1984 Surgical treatment of glossopharyngeal neuralgia and pain from cancer of the nasopharynx. A 20 year experience. Journal of Neurosurgery 61: 952–955

Hosobuchi Y 1980 The majority of unmyelinated afferent axons in human ventral roots probably conduct pain. Pain 8: 167–180

Howe J F, Loeser J D, Calvin W H 1977 Mechanosensitivity of dorsal root ganglia and chronically injured axons: a physiological basis for the radicular pain of nerve root compression. Pain 3: 25–41

Hunter C R, Mayfield F H 1949 Role of the upper cervical roots in the production of pain in the head. American Journal of Surgery 78: 743–751

Hyndman O R 1942 Lissauer's tract section. Journal of the International College of Surgeons 5: 394–400

Imai Y, Kusama T 1969 Distribution of the dorsal root fibres in the cat. Brain Research 13: 338–359

Isamat F, Ferran E, Acebes J J 1981 Selective percutaneous thermocoagulation rhizotomy in essential glossopharyngeal neuralgia. Journal of Neurosurgery 55: 575–580

Jain K K 1974 Nerve root scarring and arachnoiditis as a complication of lumbar intervertebral disc surgery: surgical treatment. Neurochirurgia 17: 185–192

Johnson E R, Powell J, Caldwell J, Crane C 1974 Intercostal nerve conduction and posterior rhizotomy in the diagnosis and treatment of thoracic radiculopathy. Journal of Neurology, Neurosurgery and Psychiatry 37: 330–332

Kerr F W L 1975 Neuroanatomical substrates of nociception in the spinal cord. Pain 1: 325–356

King J S 1976 Randomized trial of the Rees and Shealy methods for the treatment of low back pain. In: Morley T P (ed) Current controversies in neurosurgery. W B Saunders, Philadelphia p 89–94

Laha R K, Jannetta P J 1977 Glossopharyngeal neuralgia. Journal of Neurosurgery 47: 316–320

Lamotte C, Pert C B, Snyder S H 1976 Opiate receptor binding in primate spinal cord: distribution and changes after dorsal root section. Brain Research 112: 407–412

Lazorthes Y, Verdie J C 1979 Radiofrequency coagulation of the petrous ganglion in glossopharyngeal neuralgia. Neurosurgery 4: 512–516

Lazorthes Y, Verdie J C, Lagarrigue J 1976 Thermocoagulation percutanée des nerfs rachidiens à visée analgésique. Neurochirurgie 22: 445–453

Letcher F S, Goldring S 1968 The effect of radiofrequency current and heat on peripheral nerve action potential in the cat. Journal of Neurosurgery 29: 42–47

Loeser J D 1972 Dorsal rhizotomy for the relief of chronic pain. Journal of Neurosurgery 36: 745–750

Loeser J D 1982 Dorsal rhizotomy. In: Youmans J R (ed) Neurological surgery, vol 6. W B Saunders, Philadelphia, p 3664–3671

Loeser J D, Ward A A 1967 Some effects of deafferentation on neurons of the cat spinal cord. Archives of Neurology 17: 629–636

Loeser J D, Ward A A, White L E 1968 Chronic deafferentation of human spinal cord neurons. Journal of Neurosurgery 29: 48–50

Long D M 1982 Pain of spinal origin. In: Youmans J R (ed) Neurological Surgery, vol 6. W B Saunders, Philadelphia, p 3613–3626
Nash T P 1986 Percutaneous radiofrequency lesioning of dorsal root ganglia for intractable pain. Pain 24: 67–73
North R B, Kidd D H, Campbell J N, Long D M 1991 Dorsal root ganglionectomy for failed back surgery syndrome: a 5-year follow-up study. Journal of Neurosurgery 74: 236–242
Onofrio B M, Campa H K 1972 Evaluation of rhizotomy. Review of 12 years' experience. Journal of Neurosurgery 36: 751–755
Osgood C P, Dujovny M, Faille R, Abassy M 1976 Microsurgical ganglionectomy for chronic pain syndromes. Journal of Neurosurgery 45: 113–115
Ovelmen-Levitt J, Johnson B, Bedenbaugh P, Nashold B S 1984 Dorsal root rhizotomy and avulsion in the cat: a comparision of long term effects on dorsal horn neuronal activity. Neurosurgery 15: 921–927
Rees S 1976 Disconnective neurosurgery: multiple bilateral percutaneous rhizolysis (facet rhizotomy). In: Morley T P (ed) Current controversies in neurosurgery. W B Saunders, Philadelphia, p 80–88
Robson J T, Bonica J 1950 The vagus nerve in surgical consideration of glossopharyngeal neuralgia. Journal of Neurosurgery 7: 482–484
Rockswold G L, Bradley W E, Chou S N 1974 Effect of sacral nerve blocks on the function of the urinary bladder in humans. Journal of Neurosurgery 40: 83–89
Rushton J G, Stevens J C, Miller R H 1981 Glossopharyngeal (vagoglossopharyngeal) neuralgia. Archives of Neurology 38: 201–205
Saris S C, Silver J M, Vieira J F S, Nashold B S 1986 Sacrococcygeal rhizotomy for perineal pain. Neurosurgery 19: 789–793
Schwartz H G 1956 Anastomoses between cervical nerve roots. Journal of Neurosurgery 13: 190–194
Scoville W B 1966 Extradural spinal sensory rhizotomy. Journal of Neurosurgery 25: 94–95
Shealy C N 1975 Percutaneous radiofrequency denervation of spinal facets. Journal of Neurosurgery 43: 448–451
Sherrington C S 1898 Experiments in the examination of the peripheral distribution of the fibres of the posterior roots of some spinal nerves. Part II. Philosophical Transactions of the Royal Society of London Series B: Biological Sciences 190: 45–186
Sindou M, Fischer G, Goutelle A, Mansuy L 1974a La radicellotomie postérieure sélective. Premiers résultats dans la chirurgie de la douleur. Neurochirurgie 20: 391–408
Sindou M, Fischer G, Goutelle A, Schott B, Mansuy L 1974b La radicellotomie postérieure sélective dans le traitement les spasticités. Revue Neurologique 130: 201–215
Sindou M, Quoex C, Baleydier C 1974c Fiber organization at the posterior spinal cord–rootlet junction in man. Journal of Comparative Neurology 153: 15–26
Sindou M, Fischer G, Mansuy L 1976 Posterior spinal rhizotomy and selective posterior rhizidiotomy. Progress in Neurological Surgery 7: 201–250
Sindou M, Fischer G, Goutelle A, Allegré G E 1981 Microsurgical selective posterior rhizotomy. Pain (suppl) 1: 354
Sindou M, Mifsud J J, Boisson D, Goutelle A 1986 Selective posterior rhizotomy in the dorsal root entry zone for treatment of hyperspasticity and pain in the hemiplegic upper limb. Neuurosurgery 18: 587–595
Smith F P 1970 Trans-spinal ganglionectomy for relief of intercostal pain. Journal of Neurosurgery 32: 574–577
Smith H P, McWhorter J M, Challa V R 1981 Radiofrequency neurolysis in a clinical model. Neuropathological correlation. Journal of Neurosurgery 55: 246–253
Snyder R 1977 The organization of the dorsal root entry zone in cats and monkeys. Journal of Comparative Neurology 174: 47–70
Strait T A, Hunter S E 1981 Intraspinal extradural sensory rhizotomy in patients with failure of lumbar disc surgery. Journal of Neurosurgery 54: 193–196
Sweet W H 1984 Deafferentation pain after posterior rhizotomy, trauma to a limb, and herpes zoster. Neurosurgery 15: 928–932
Tew J M 1982 Treatment of pain of glossopharyngeal and vagus nerve by percutaneous rhizotomy. In: Youmans J R (ed) Neurological Surgery, vol 6. Saunders, Philadelphia, p 3609–3612
Uematsu S 1977 Percutaneous electrothermocoagulation of spinal nerve trunk, ganglion and rootlets. In: Schmidek H H, Sweet W S (eds) Current techniques in operative neurosurgery. Grune & Stratton, New York, p 469–490
Uematsu S, Udvarhelyi G B, Benson D W, Siebens A A 1974 Percutaneus radiofrequency rhizotomy. Surgical neurology 2: 319–325
van Kleef M, Spaans F, Dingemans A, Barendse G A M, Floor E, Sluijter M E 1993 Effects and side effects of a percutaneous thermal lesion of the dorsal root ganglion in patients with cervical pain syndrome. Pain 52: 49–53
Vlahovitch B, Fuentes J M 1975 Résultats de la radicellotomie sélective postérieure à l'étage lombaire et cervicale. Neurochirurgie 21: 29–42
Walker A E 1966 Neuralgias of the glossopharyngeal, vagus and intermedius nerves. In: Knighton R S, Dumke P R (eds) Pain. Little, Brown, Boston, p 421–429
Wall P D 1962 The origin of a spinal cord slow potential. Journal of Physiology 164: 508–526
Wall P D 1977 The presence of ineffective synapses and the circumstances which unmask them. Philosophical Transactions of the Royal Society of London 278: 361–372
Wall P D, Werman R 1976 The physiology and anatomy of long-ranging afferent fibres within the spinal cord. Journal of Physiology 255: 321–334
White J C, Kjellberg R N 1973 Posterior spinal rhizotomy: a subsitute for cordotomy in the relief of localized pain in patients with normal life expectancy. Neurochirurgia 16: 141–170
White J C, Sweet W H 1969 Pain and the neurosurgeon. C C Thomas, Springfield, Illinois

56. Disc surgery

Erik Spangfort

THE DEVELOPMENT OF DISC SURGERY

Although ruptured intervertebral discs had been described and operated on previously, the era of disc surgery unquestionably began in September 1933, when Mixter & Barr presented a series of successful operations for disc herniation, or ruptured discs as they preferred to call it, to the New England Surgical Society in Boston (Mixter & Barr 1934).

The original series presented by Mixter & Barr included disc ruptures in the cervical and thoracic spine. Surgical treatment of disc herniations in the cervical and especially the thoracic spine is, however, rare compared with herniations of the lower lumbar discs and is not discussed in detail in this presentation.

The simplistic concept that low back pain with or without sciatica was usually caused by a disc herniation and cured by a fairly simple operation was readily and rapidly accepted all over the world, and maintained an overwhelming dominance over lay and medical minds for the next 40 years.

Throughout these years a vast number of papers dealing with all aspects of the disc problem were published, and when the results of disc surgery were compiled, it became obvious that discectomy was not always a successful procedure.

The reported rate of surgical failures was usually 5–10%, but there were large variations among the reports, and some claimed more than 50% failures. A growing number of unfortunate, severely disabled patients with 'failed back-surgery syndrome' became a highly complex challenge, and a heavy burden to the medical profession. Distrust of discectomy was spreading widely (Wilson 1967). Evidently, some pertinent questions concerning disc surgery had to be answered.

Studies to identify the causes of surgical failures revealed that inaccuracy of diagnosis and a poor selection of patients for initial lumbar disc operation were more important factors than technical errors during the operation itself (Macnab 1971; Nachemson 1976; Finneson 1978; Spengler & Freeman 1979). The operation, discectomy, was used inappropriately on loose and wide indications.

It was shown that the single most important factor for prediction of a successful discectomy is the degree of herniation found by the operation (Spangfort 1972). In patients with complete herniations, i.e. rupture of the annulus and extrusion of fragments of disc tissue into the spinal canal, complete relief of sciatic pain was achieved immediately in more than 90% of the patients, independent of age, sex, level of herniation and other variables (Fig. 56.1). As the degree of herniation decreases, the rate of failure increases significantly, and the majority of patients with a 'negative exploration' do not benefit from the operation.

Obviously, improvement of surgical results was crucially dependent on accurate preoperative diagnosis and a strict selection of patients with high-grade herniations for discectomy.

In the last 15 years, the development in this field has been intensive and interesting. The complete explanation for this is complex, but a basic feature is, no doubt, a

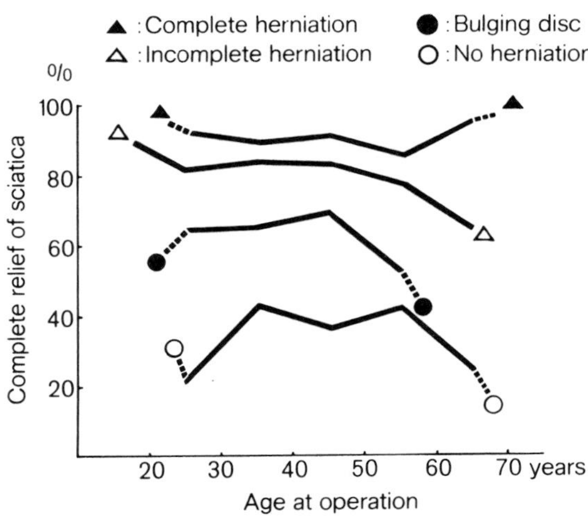

Fig. 56.1 The rate of complete relief of sciatica by age at operation and degree of herniation in 2503 operations. (From Spangfort 1972.)

growing awareness among low back specialists of the fact that the damage caused by a disc herniation depends not only on the volume of disc tissue protruding or extruding into the spinal canal, but also on the space available for herniated disc tissue in the individual spinal canal.

In this broader context, disc herniation is only one of several pathomechanisms causing mechanical compression syndromes and nerve entrapments in the lumbar spine.

Reduction of the space available for the neural elements, generally called spinal stenosis of developmental, posttraumatic or degenerative type, is recognized as a nosological entity, which, alone or in combination with disc herniation, may produce disabling symptoms of the spine. It is also recognized that when stenosis is involved in a disc syndrome, the results of surgical treatment with traditional discectomy are usually unsatisfactory or frankly disastrous. Spinal stenosis requires a radical change in surgical technique.

As well as growing awareness of clinical problems attributed to spinal stenosis, several other changes have recently influenced the surgical treatment of spinal disorders.

Diagnostic methods necessary to analyse the complicated pathological anatomy of the diseased spine have been highly amplified by the advent of computerized tomography (CT), ultrasonography, epidural venography, safer water-soluble contrast agents, epidural contrast CT-technique (Hårdstedt & Vucetic 1986) and magnetic resonance imaging (MRI).

In spite of this impressive development of technological investigative methods, it may still be an extremely difficult task to supply the necessary diagnostic foundation for decisions about proper surgical treatment in individual cases of lumbar pain syndromes. Surgical management of these conditions cannot be satisfactorily improved without a better clinical analysis and interpretation of the main symptom, i.e. pain.

DISC OPERATION

SURGICAL TECHNIQUE

The earliest cases of disc herniation were classified as tumours, and removed by a neurosurgical approach with complete laminectomy on at least two vertebrae and transdural extirpation of the herniated disc tissue.

In 1939, Love described the unilateral interlaminar approach, which is still the routine technique in most quarters. The laminae of the two vertebrae between which the herniation has occurred are exposed by subperiosteal dissection, and the strong ligamentum flavum is resected – if necessary together with some part of the adjacent lamina. In most cases this exposure allows identification of the underlying nerve root, inspection of the surface of the intervertebral disc after medial retraction of the root and removal of the possible herniation. Occasionally more bone has to be removed, and in some cases a hemilaminectomy and/or a partial resection of the posterior facet joint is performed to obtain an adequate exposure of the suspected area.

Bilateral exposure is usually not necessary in typical cases of disc herniation.

EXTENT OF EXPOSURE

It is, of course, desirable to minimize surgical damage to the anatomical structures as much as possible, even if it is still unproven that the extent of exposure has any major effect on the results of disc operation (Busch et al 1950; Eyre-Brook 1952; Naylor 1974; Fager & Freidberg 1980; Weber 1983). Inadequate exposure, on the other hand, greatly increases the risk of surgical injuries to the nerve roots, the dura and the vessels, and also the risk of failure to locate displaced and migrating fragments extruded from a ruptured disc.

We do not share the opinion that the lower two or three disc spaces should always be explored during a disc operation. With modern diagnostic methods applied in a meticulous preoperative investigation, the extent and type of appropriate exposure should be clearly defined before the operation. When the preoperative diagnosis is found to be wrong, which is still unavoidable in some cases, it is wise to abstain from unplanned exploration.

In recent years the development of microsurgical technique has reduced the risks associated with a limited exposure.

Percutaneous discectomy is still at an experimental stage, but the results do not seem to be as predictable or successful as the results after surgical discectomy (Kahanovitz et al 1990).

VOLUME OF TISSUE REMOVED

Free fragments and disc tissue protruding into the spinal canal must be removed for a good operative result. There is, however, no general agreement about the need to remove as much tissue as possible from the interior of the disc space. It has been presumed by many that a radical excision of the disc improves surgical results and reduces the rate of recurrence, but so far there is no evidence in support of this assumption. Hirsch & Nachemson (1963) reported that the results were not improved by extensive removal of disc tissue. We have followed the principle expressed by Busch et al (1950), that the disc space should be evacuated 'but without fanaticism'.

In several reports the specimens of disc tissue removed by operation are measured by weight, and the reported mean values range from 0.79 g (Boemke 1951) to 9.88 g (Hanraets 1959). O'Connell (1951) found a mean weight of 1.95 g; he also reported that the mean weight of lumbar discs excised at autopsy was 24.6 g. He concluded that only exceptionally does the specimen removed at operation represent more than 20% of the average normal intervertebral disc by weight.

Capanna et al (1981), applying a technique of intraoperative discography, estimated the percentage of disc volume removed by disc surgery. The average volume removed was found to equal only 6% of the total disc volume. There was little difference in the percentage of disc removal when different operative approaches were used or when more or less 'extensive' disc extirpation was performed.

In my study of the lumbar disc operation (Spangfort 1972) the volume of disc tissue removed was analysed in 645 cases (unpublished). The volume was measured by replacement of water in a graded tube immediately after removal, and the total mean in this series was 2.14 (s.d. 1.04) ml, with no single specimen larger than 7 ml. The mean volume was correlated with the degree of herniation, and increased from 1.25 ml in negative explorations to 1.52 ml in 'bulging discs', 2.01 ml in incomplete herniations and 2.36 ml in ruptured discs. In 90 reoperations, where a disc herniation was found, the mean volume was almost the same (2.09 ml).

These studies all indicate that the average volume of disc tissue removed by discectomy represents only 6–8% of the total disc volume and apparently it is not easy to excise disc tissue with the instruments usually applied for this purpose (rongeur and curette) unless the disc is already in a certain condition of degeneration and fragmentation.

THE 'COMBINED OPERATION'

Since 1940 it has become increasingly common to advocate concomitant discectomy and some type of fusion operation as a standard procedure in an attempt to improve the results of disc surgery. Arthrodesis of the spine (or fusion) was already an established and approved operation, based on the principles of Albee and Hibbs, in the treatment of an unstable spine. Compared with simple discectomy, fusion is a surgical procedure of considerable magnitude with prolonged convalescence and more serious postoperative complications.

Most studies comparing discectomy with and without concomitant fusion indicate that the results after the 'combination operation' are 5–10% better than after simple discectomy (Nachlas 1952; van Hoytema & Oostrom 1961; White 1966). The issue is still controversial, but the dominating conclusion has been that the advantage of the 'combined operation' is too small to warrant the use of this method as a routine in patients with typical lumbar disc herniations. The surgical indications for discectomy and spine fusion are different and the decision to recommend a fusion depends on many factors. The special indications for this procedure should be considered separately in each individual case when disc surgery is planned (Symposium 1981).

REOPERATION AFTER DISCECTOMY

The rate of reoperations after a first disc operation is usually reported at 10–15% and the risk of acquiring a new disc herniation is probably considerably increased in patients with a verified herniation in their medical history.

Recurrences occur both on the same side and level and at other locations, but rarely within the first year after a discectomy. The mean interval between the first and second operation for true disc herniation is 5–6 years in our experience, but a true recurrence from the same disc may occur more than 20 years after the first operation.

The pathological process, which in some patients results in a true disc herniation, tends to begin at the lumbosacral level and proceed in the cranial direction with age. The mean age at operation for verified ruptures at the level L5–S1 was found to be 38 years, at the level L4–L5 42 years, and in the unusual herniations at the three higher levels (L1–L4) 47 years (Spangfort 1972). Simultaneous complete ruptures of two different discs were never found during the same operation in this series and seem to be rare.

Thus, symptoms of a recurrent disc herniation may be expected with a certain degree of probability approximately 5 years after a first operation, although not necessarily severe enough to motivate a reoperation. In this situation there is no reason to classify the first operation as a failure.

In patients without relief of pain for at least 6 months after a first operation, the operation has usually been an outright failure, in some cases caused by techincal errors during the operation (e.g. failure to locate an offending fragment or exposure at a wrong level), but in the majority caused by an incomplete or wrong preoperative diagnosis: another type of operation should have been performed or the patient should not have been exposed to surgical treatment at all. In the latter group the probability of a successful reoperation with the same technique is low. If the first operation was a negative exploration, the risk of a second negative exploration is about 50%.

The results of reoperations are generally less favourable than those of first operations. This is partly due to a higher rate of surgical complications at reoperation, but the main reason is diagnostic difficulties in patients assessed for repeat surgery, which results in high rates of negative explorations in this group. When the degree of herniation found by reoperation is considered, the results are, however, almost as good.

In my study of disc operations, the rate of excellent results (i.e. complete relief of both low back pain and sciatica) decreased from 62.0% after first operations to

43.1% after second operations and 28.6% after third operations. If a disc herniation was found by reoperation (161 cases) the rate of excellent results was still 53.4%, but if the reoperation was a negative exploration (69 cases) the rate was as low as 14.5%. Again, preoperative diagnosis is crucial for the result of operation. Proper selection of patients for reoperation is, however, often a difficult task even for the experienced low back specialist.

The multioperated low back patient with a 'failed back surgery syndrome', who seldom achieves satisfactory relief of pain by any combination of measures, should be carefully examined by a qualified investigation, preferably in a centre specialising in assessing these highly complicated patients, before further 'salvage surgery' is attempted: 'no matter how severe or how intractable the pain, it can always be made worse by surgery' (Finneson 1978).

EPIDURAL SCAR FORMATION

The prevalent pathological condition found in reoperations for recurrent pain after disc surgery is often a dense fibrous scar formation strangling the dura and nerve roots. This scar formation is considered a major cause of recurrent symptoms after discectomy; it also complicates correct diagnosis and reoperation of a true recurrent disc herniation. Excision of the scar tissue (neurolysis) is difficult and the results are usually poor.

LaRocca & Macnab (1974) called this excessive fibrosis 'the laminectomy membrane' and showed that the main source is fibrous tissue from traumatized surrounding muscles. Langenskiöld & Kiviluoto (1976) reported efficient prevention of epidural scar formation by the use of free grafts of subcutaneous fat tissue placed outside the spinal canal.

It has been confirmed that covering raw bone, muscles and nerve roots with free fat grafts effectively prevents epidural scar formation (Yong-Hing et al 1980).

URGENT DISC SURGERY

The only indication for immediate disc surgery is acute compression of the cauda equina by a large herniation causing a sacral syndrome with neurological signs from the second and lower sacral roots, i.e. dysfunction of the bladder and bowel with loss of sphincter control, impairment of sexual function and saddle-shaped loss of sensation in the sacral dermatomes. In most cases the herniation is large, situated in the midline and ruptured. The condition is rare, probably less than one case per year in a population of 200 000.

In patients with symptoms of acute cauda equina compression a qualified examination, including cystometry and myelography, CT or MRI, is urgent. Bladder dysfunction is, however, a common symptom in patients with severe low back pain and not necessarily caused by a large disc herniation. Immediate surgical decompression is generally considered mandatory when an acute disc herniation is identified as the cause of the syndrome. Severe impairment of bladder function, bilateral saddle anaesthesia and a preoperative duration of more than 2 days appear to imply a poor prognosis for satisfactory neurological recovery after surgical decompression (Aho et al 1969).

SURGICAL INDICATIONS AND SELECTION OF PATIENTS

Except for the rare cases of acute cauda equina syndrome, the purpose of discectomy is relief of pain, in particular severe sciatic pain, caused by a disc herniation, i.e. by dislocated (protruding or extruding) disc tissue. The disc herniation is a special lesion occurring sometimes in the course of disc degeneration. However, disc degeneration in itself is not an indication for discectomy.

Complete relief of sciatic pain after discectomy is correlated almost exclusively and completely with the degree of herniation (Fig. 56.2). The rate of complete relief is excellent in patients with high-grade herniations, and the ideal indications for discectomy are recently ruptured herniations and large incomplete herniations in the process of rupturing or dissecting beneath the posterior longitudinal ligament. Only by meticulous selection of patients with high-grade herniations is it possible to improve the results of discectomy and avoid a growing number of disastrous failures.

Disc surgery is pain surgery: the first condition for considering the possibility of discectomy is that the pain is severe enough to motivate surgical treatment. The next

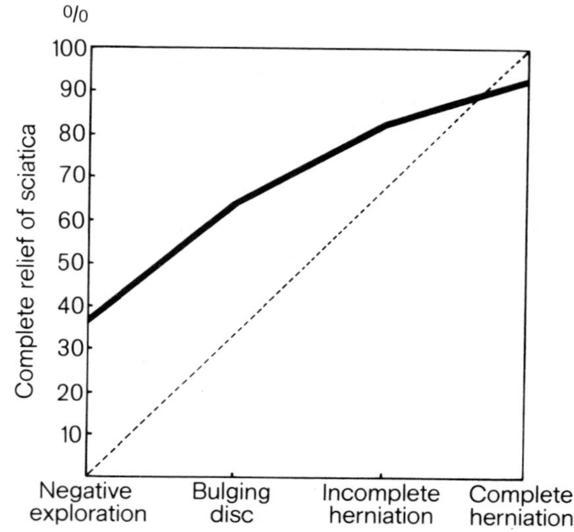

Fig. 56.2 The correlation between complete relief of sciatica and the degree of herniation in 2503 operations. (From Spangfort 1972.)

condition is that the pain is caused predominantly by a high-grade herniation. These conditions must be strictly respected. The point is to establish the presence and location of an offending disc herniation and, unfortunately, surgical exposure is still the only way to do so with complete certainty.

The decision to advise discectomy must, therefore, be based on a systematic and comprehensive diagnostic investigation, comprising a detailed history and an adequate analysis of the pain syndrome, disentangling in each case debut and duration of pain, temporal pattern, activities and circumstances affecting the pain, anatomical and topographical patterns, sensory modalities and an assessment of the intensity of the pain. Furthermore, a complete physical examination is necessary, including the recording of posture and gait, degree of lordosis, range and pattern of spinal motion, pattern of pain by rest, motion and weight-bearing and a neurological examination, as well as psychological assessment, routine laboratory tests and plain radiographs of the spine and pelvis.

In detailed analyses of the pain syndrome–particularly of the topographical pattern and sensory modalities, which are of fundamental importance in diagnosing a disc herniation–we have found diagnostic thermography of little value. To achieve this information, in our experience, a pain-drawing method is definitely superior, as well as being cheap and convenient. Our present pain-drawing system (Fig. 56.3) was developed from the model published by Ransford et al (1976), and has become indispensable in our preoperative investigation.

We use myelography and CT as routine examinations to support the clinical diagnosis and localize the herniation accurately, but we do not consider a positive myelogram, in itself, to be a sufficient indication for surgical treatment. Occasionally we advise discectomy in spite of a negative myelography, if the clinical diagnosis is clear. In such cases CT is now reducing the diagnostic confusion caused by a 'false negative' myelography.

We do not consider a discogram helpful in deciding whether or not to recommend a discectomy.

Electrodiagnostic examination may add information to the diagnosis, but there is no single test that measures all aspects of nerve root function and there is no test measuring sciatic pain, which may be present in the absence of nerve root pathology.

Progressive neurological deficits are usually listed as an indication for disc surgery. Strictly speaking, we do not agree with this. We consider neurological deficits important diagnostic signs, but not an independent indication for discectomy, as surgical treatment has not been shown to improve the average prognosis of peripheral neurological deficits. If surgical treatment of a disc herniation cures neurological deficits (which is most likely in some cases) we still cannot identify the subgroup of patients who will benefit from discectomy in this respect.

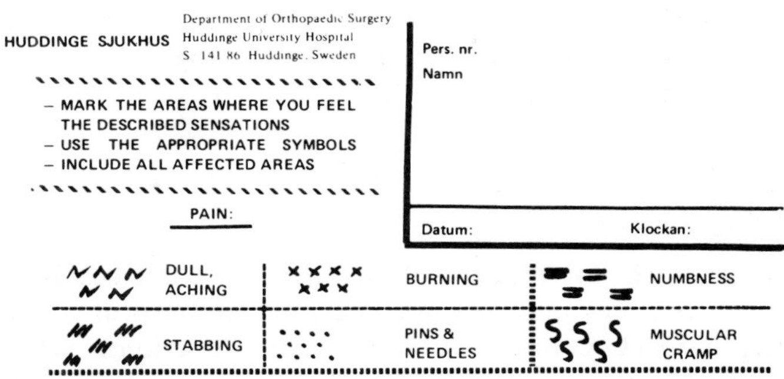
HUDDINGE SJUKHUS Department of Orthopaedic Surgery Huddinge University Hospital S 141 86 Huddinge, Sweden

Pers. nr.
Namn

– MARK THE AREAS WHERE YOU FEEL THE DESCRIBED SENSATIONS
– USE THE APPROPRIATE SYMBOLS
– INCLUDE ALL AFFECTED AREAS

PAIN:

Datum: Klockan:

DULL, ACHING | BURNING | NUMBNESS
STABBING | PINS & NEEDLES | MUSCULAR CRAMP

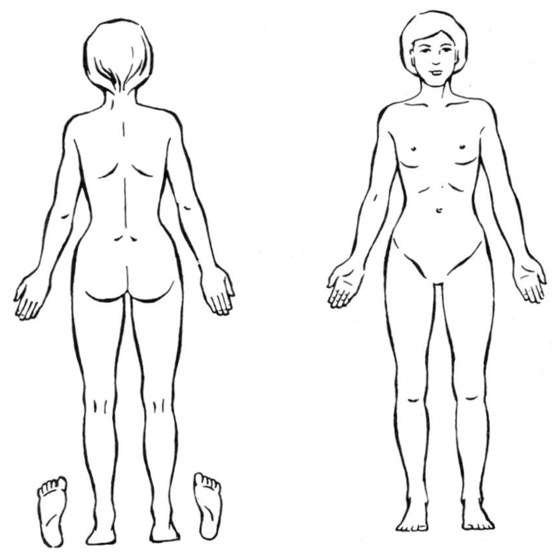

Fig. 56.3 Main form for pain-drawing used for patients with low-back pain. (Modified from Ransford et al 1976.)

The rupture of a disc herniation into the spinal canal is an anatomical disaster and surgical measures against it are widely independent of the patient's general psychological status. Certainly, individual psychological experience of pain and suffering is the main indication for discectomy, and inappropriate or incomprehensible description of the symptoms and unusual or pathological pain behaviour may seriously complicate the objective diagnostic interpretation and assessment, but in the case of an unequivocal diagnosis of disabling disc herniation we do not deny the patient surgical relief for psychological reasons. The emotionally unstable patient may, indeed, be in greater need of immediate pain relief than the stable one.

The situation is somewhat different in other types of low back surgery, especially 'salvage surgery', in which the psychological variables apparently play a more dominating role in surgical treatment.

It is generally recognized that, with the exceptions already mentioned, surgical treatment of a disc herniation should be advised only if nonsurgical treatment fails. A reasonable trial period is 2–3 months in many cases, but we hesitate to accept rigid rules, as a wide variety of circumstances necessitates individual evaluation and decision in every case.

NONSURGICAL VERSUS SURGICAL TREATMENT

So far, it has not been possible to design a clinical trial of the differences between nonsurgical and surgical treatment, which completely fulfils scientific criteria. One problem is that a disc herniation can be definitely confirmed and classified only by surgical exposure. Another obstacle is the fact that, when patients with a convincing clinical diagnosis of disc herniation are allocated at random to comparable groups for one of the two treatment modalities, there are always some patients, allocated to nonsurgical treatment, in whom the pain becomes so excruciating that they cannot reasonably be denied surgical relief. This important group is therefore lost for comparison.

A few studies from which it is possible to draw tentative conclusions (e.g. Hakelius 1970; Nashold & Hrubec 1971; Hasue & Fujiwara 1979) do, however, indicate that surgical treatment does not necessarily improve the prognosis in the long term, either as regards pain or the risk of persistent neurological deficits.

Weber (1983), in his controlled prospective study, allocated 126 patients with questionable indications for discectomy to either operation or physiotherapy, and then compared the groups for 10 years. After 1 year the results were significantly better after surgical treatment than after nonsurgical treatment. After 4 years the operated patients still showed better results, but the difference was no longer significant. Only minor changes occurred throughout the last 6 years of observation. After 10 years no patients in the two groups complained of sciatic pain, and the rates of persistent low-back pain were equal in the groups. The severity of low-back pain decreased over the last 6 years in both groups.

If the clinical situation allows a choice between nonsurgical and surgical treatment, the patient should be informed that the benefit expected from the operation is immediate relief of sciatic pain and not necessarily an improvement of the long-range prognosis, which is fairly good anyway.

CHEMONUCLEOLYSIS

Chemonucleolysis was introduced as a nonsurgical treatment, a last alternative to surgical treatment, and randomized studies comparing chemonucleolysis and saline injections indicate some beneficial effect of chemonucleolysis (Fraser 1984).

Considering the invasive procedure and the complications, chemonucleolysis should, however, be classified as surgery and the results of chemonucleolysis have been found inferior to those of traditional surgical discectomy (Ejeskar et al 1983; Crawshaw et al 1984).

COMPLICATIONS OF DISC SURGERY

MORTALITY RATE

The mortality rate associated with disc surgery is low. In a survey of 54 reports from the period 1937–72 with a total of 25 392 operations the mean rate was 0.3% (72 cases), constantly decreasing over the last 35 years. Pulmonary embolism and postoperative infections were the most frequent causes of death (Spangfort 1972).

INJURY TO VESSELS AND VISCERA

Injury to abdominal vessels is an uncommon but extremely dangerous complication in disc surgery. Not all cases are reported in the literature, but an estimated incidence of this complication is less than 1 case in 2000 operations (DeSaussure 1959; Birkeland & Taylor 1969).

The disaster usually occurs when the instrument used for evacuating tissue from the interior of the disc space accidentally and without the surgeon being aware of it passes through a fissure in the anterior wall of the disc. The major vessels (the abdominal aorta, the inferior vena cava and the common iliac vessels) are in close proximity to the anterior surface of the lumbar discs and easily within range of the biting rongeur (Nilsonne & Hakelius 1965). Laceration of these vessels may cause a dramatic retroperitoneal haemorrhage, which is detectable in the surgical field in only half of the cases: the first warning of a vascular catastrophe may be symptoms of severe hypovolaemic shock during or after surgery. Immediate laparotomy and repair of the injured vessel is imperative.

Arteriovenous fistula is another type of vascular injury, which may produce complex circulatory impairment and cardiac failure. The diagnosis is often delayed for months or years, but the mortality rate is lower.

Injuries to the bowel, the ureter and the sympathetic trunk may occur by the same mechanism, but are less commonly reported in the literature.

In 95% of all disc operations the total loss of blood is less than 500 ml. Damage to the epidural veins is the usual cause of more extensive bleeding and, although this type of haemorrhage is almost always well within safe limits, the bleeding may cause troublesome difficulties, at least in the narrow field exposed by the interlaminar approach.

INJURIES TO NEURAL STRUCTURES

Injuries to the nerve roots, and even to the cauda equina, may occur during the operation in spite of careful surgical technique. Surgical damage to nerve roots is reported by surgeons in 0.5–3% of all operations; in reoperations the rate is two or three times higher. Verified damage to a nerve root is not always followed by significant clinical symptoms. Motor weakness in the leg, obviously caused by the operation, occurs in at least 5% of all operations, but in the majority the paresis is partial and recovers satisfactorily with time.

DURA LESIONS

Minor surgical lesions to the dura are not uncommon and are often revealed by leakage of cerebrospinal fluid during the operation. If the lesion is located and closed with fine sutures, the complication is usually harmless. In rare cases a dura lesion results in the formation of an extradural pseudocyst or a fistula leaking cerebrospinal fluid, which requires secondary surgery.

THROMBOEMBOLISM

Postoperative thromboembolism is reported to average 2% in the literature. The complication is usually diagnosed between the fourth and 12th day after the operation, and is rare in patients below 40 years. A period of immobilization before surgery is probably a pathogenetic factor.

POSTOPERATIVE INFECTIONS

With modern surgical technique and facilities, the mean rate of postoperative wound infections after discectomy should not exceed a total of 2–3%, with severe infections accounting for less than 0.5%.

Septic meningitis, epidural abscess and frank pyogenic spondylitis are rare and major complications.

POSTOPERATIVE DISCITIS

This condition is now recognized as a complication to disc surgery. Most cases are caused by a low-grade infection of the disc space, but an aseptic or 'mechanical' type of postoperative discitis also seems to occur (Fouquet et al 1992). The true incidence is unknown, but probably does not exceed 1–2%.

The most typical symptom, almost pathognomonic, is violent, spasmodic pain in the back precipitated by the slightest movement and in most cases appearing during the second week, after an otherwise uneventful postoperative course. The pain is referred to the lower abdomen, the groins, hips or upper thighs. True root pain is unusual, and the patient often describes the pain as a new and terrible experience.

Systemic reactions are scarce. Some patients have a moderate fever and/or infection of the surgical wound. The sedimentation rate (ESR) is usually elevated, and a second rise of the postoperative ESR, which normally reaches its peak 3–4 days after the operation, is a significant warning. Needle aspiration results in a positive culture in less than 50%.

Early radiological changes may appear 3–4 weeks after the onset of pain and the main features are fuzzines and irregular defects of the end-plates, cavitations into one or both of the adjacent vertebrae, marked narrowing of the intervertebral disc space and vertebral sclerosis. Later, there is abundant new bone formation, which often results in solid bony fusion. MRI is now considered the best method for diagnosing the condition.

The acute pain syndrome lasts between 6 and 12 weeks in most cases and complete immobilization is the most effective management. Adequate treatment with antibiotics until the ESR is normal is recommended. There is no indication for surgical intervention when the clinical picture is typical. The course is always prolonged and the pain may be a frightening experience to the patient. The complication seems to increase the risk of chronic low-back pain and vocational disability, but otherwise most studies indicate a fairly good long-term prognosis (Iversen et al 1992).

SPINAL ARACHNOIDITIS

An association between lumbar disc disease and arachnoiditis (a progressive inflammatory reaction of the pia arachnoid) was suspected long ago (French 1946), but the condition is difficult to diagnose, the more so because intradural exploration is seldom performed during a disc operation and the complication has been considered rare. Recent studies indicate, however, that some degree of arachnoiditis is common, at least in patients with severe pain and disability secondary to disc surgery. Arachnoiditis may be clinically silent and the correlation between the pathology and pain is still poorly defined (Symposium 1978).

Many aetiological factors are apparently involved in the development of arachnoiditis: injection of contrast media, anaesthetics and other agents into the subarachnoid space, infection, the presence of blood, trauma, disc lesions and spinal stenosis, surgical injuries and unknown individual factors (Ransford & Harries 1972).

Symptoms vary considerably and mild cases are probably often overlooked. In severe cases, the condition is extremely distressing. The pain is constant in the back and radiates to one or both legs, often in a well-defined distribution of more than one root. The pain is described as burning or cramping – painful muscle cramps and violent spasms of the legs are usual. The cauda equina may be involved. Pain is unrelieved by rest and poorly correlated to weight-bearing and motion.

Treatment of this neuralgic pain syndrome is extremely difficult, but the condition is not inevitably progressive – a slow recovery over the years occurs in some patients. Severe psychological complications in response to the constant torturing pain are, however, the rule.

STRUCTURAL IMPAIRMENT

It has not been established that simple discectomy, without removal of the articular facets or the pedicles, is associated with an increased risk of disc degeneration, recurrent herniations, segmental instability or arthrosis of the intervertebral joints.

REFERENCES

Aho A J, Auranen A, Pesonen K 1969 Analysis of cauda equina symptoms in patients with lumbar disc prolapse. Acta Chirurgica Scandinavica 135: 413–420

Birkeland I W Jr, Taylor T K F 1969 Major vascular injuries in lumbar disc surgery. Journal of Bone and Joint Surgery 51B: 4–19

Boemke F 1951 Feingewebliche Befunde beim Bandscheibenvorfall. Langenbecks Archiv 267: 484–492

Busch E, Andersen A, Broager B et al 1950 Le prolapsus discal lombaire. Acta Psychiatrica et Neurologica 25: 443–500

Capanna A H, Williams R W, Austin D C, Darmody W R, Thomas L M 1981 Lumbar discectomy – percentage of disc removal and detection of anterior annulus perforation. Spine 6: 610–614

Crawshaw C, Frazer A M, Merriam W F, Mulholland R C, Webb J K 1984 A comparison of surgery and chemonucleolysis in the treatment of sciatica. A prospective randomized trial. Spine 9: 195–198

DeSaussure R L 1959 Vascular injury coincident to disc surgery. Journal of Neurosurgery 16: 222–229

Ejeskar A, Nachemson A, Herberts P 1983 Surgery versus chemonucleolysis for herniated lumbar discs. A prospective study with random assignment. Clinical Orthopaedics and Related Research 174: 236–242

Eyre-Brook A L 1952 A study of late results from disc operations. British Journal of Surgery 39: 289–296

Fager C A, Freidberg S R 1980 Analysis of failures and poor results of lumbar spine surgery. Spine 5: 87–94

Finneson B E 1978 A lumbar disc surgery predictive score card. Spine 3: 186–188

Fouquet B, Goupille P, Jattiot F et al 1992 Discitis after lumbar disc surgery. Features of 'aseptic' and 'septic' forms. Spine 17: 356–358

Fraser R D 1984 Chymopapain for the treatment of intervertebral disc herniation. The final report of a double-blind study. Spine 9: 815–818

French J D 1946 Clinical manifestations of lumbar spinal arachnoiditis. Surgery 20: 718–729

Hakelius A 1970 Prognosis in sciatica. Acta Orthopaedica Scandinavica Supplementum 129: 1–76

Hanraets P R M J 1959 The degenerative back and its differential diagnosis. Elsevier, Amsterdam

Hårdstedt C, Vucetic N 1986 Lumbosacral epidurography and computed tomography. Acta Radiologica 27: 173–178

Hasue M, Fujiwara M 1979 Epidemiologic and clinical studies of long-term prognosis of low-back pain and sciatica. Spine 4: 150–155

Hirsch C, Nachemson A 1963 The reliability of lumbar disk surgery. Clinical Orthopaedics an Related Research 29: 189 –195

Iversen E, Herss Nielsen V A, Gadegaard Hansen L 1992 Prognosis in postoperative discitis. A retrospective study of 111 cases. Acta Orthopaedica Scandinavica 63: 305–309

Kahanovitz N, Viola K, Goldstein T, Dawson E 1990 A multicenter analysis of percutaneous discectomy. Spine 15: 713–715

Langenskiöld A, Kiviluoto O 1976 Prevention of epidural scar formation after operations on the lumbar spine by means of free fat transplants. Clinical Orthopaedics and Related Research 115: 92–95

LaRocca H, Macnab I 1974 The laminectomy membrane. Journal of Bone and Joint Surgery 56B: 545–550

Love J G 1939 Removal of protruded intervertebral disks without laminectomy. Proceedings of the Staff Meetings of the Mayo Clinic 14: 800 (1940 15: 4)

Macnab I 1971 Negative disc exploration. Journal of Bone and Joint Surgery 53A: 891–903

Mixter W J, Barr J S 1934 Rupture of the intervertebral disc with involvement of the spinal canal. New England Journal of Medicine 211: 210–215

Nachemson A L 1976 The lumbar spine – an orthopaedic challenge. Spine 1: 59–71

Nachlas W 1952 End-result study of the treatment of herniated nucleus pulposus by excision with fusion and without fusion. Journal of Bone and Joint Surgery 34A: 981–988

Nashold B S, Hrubec Z 1971 Lumbar disc disease. A 20-year clinical follow-up study. C V Mosby, St Louis

Naylor A 1974 The late results of laminectomy for lumbar disc prolapse. Journal of Bone and Joint Surgery 56B: 17–29

Nilsonne U, Hakelius A 1965 On vascular injury in lumbar disc surgery. Acta Orthopaedica Scandinavica 35: 329–337

O'Connell J E A 1951 Protrusions of the lumbar intervertebral discs. Journal of Bone and Joint Surgery 33B: 8–30

Ransford A O, Harries B J 1972 Localised arachnoiditis complicating lumbar disc lesions. Journal of Bone and Joint Surgery 54B: 656–665

Ransford A O, Cairns D, Mooney V 1976 The pain drawing as an aid to the psychologic evaluation of patients with low back pain. Spine 1: 127–134

Spangfort E V 1972 The lumbar disc herniation – a computer-aided analysis of 2504 operations. Acta Orthopaedica Scandinavica Supplementum 142: 1–95

Spengler D M, Freeman C W 1979 Patient selection for lumbar discectomy – an objective approach. Spine 4: 129–134

Symposium 1978 Lumbar arachnoiditis: nomenclature, etiology, and pathology. Spine 3: 21–92

Symposium 1981 The role of spine fusion for low-back pain. Spine 6: 277–314

van Hoytema G, Oostrom J 1961 The operation for herniation of the nucleus pulposus with intervertebral body fusion. Archivum Chirurgicum Neerlandicum 13: 71–80

Weber H 1983 Lumbar disc herniation – a controlled, pros pective study with 10 years of observation. Spine 8: 131–140

White J C 1966 Results in surgical treatment of herniated lumbar intervertebral discs. Clinical Neurosurgery 13: 42–51

Wilson J C Jr 1967 Low back pain and sciatica – a plea for better care of the patient. Journal of the American Medical Association 200: 705–712

Yong-Hing K, Reilly J, de Korompay V, Kirkaldy-Willis W H 1980 Prevention of nerve root adhesions after laminectomy. Spine 5: 59–64

57. The failed back

C. B. Wynn Parry

Since the last edition of the book there have been major advances in the multidisciplinary team management of chronic intractable pain. These include refinement of pain-relieving modalities as well as the psychological approach with cognitive behavioural therapy. These advances are considered in this chapter. The natural history and clinical profiles of the common causes of the 'failed back' remain unaltered and this material in the chapter of the 2nd edition has been retained.

One of the major problems confronting the rheumatologist and orthopaedic surgeon is the patient suffering from intractable backache and sciatica. Such patients have frequently had symptoms for many years and many have been subjected to multiple operations without relief of symptoms. There is a general belief amongst specialists in this field that surgery for low-back pain has been overprescribed in the past. A study of the natural history of acute back pain and sciatica reveals that the vast majority of patients lose their symptoms in time. Nachemson (1982) has shown that in several thousand patients who were off work with back pain, 90% were back to work in 6 weeks, 60% being back to work within 1 week. The same author has also shown that there is little evidence that any of the standard physiotherapy measures demonstrate any significant effect on the natural history of low-back pain or on return to work.

Hakelius (1970) compared 517 patients with sciatica who were treated conservatively with 66 patients who had been treated surgically. At 6 months the results were almost identical. He concluded that acute sciatica with neurological symptoms is a transient condition which, with a few exceptions, subsides after a relatively brief period. Green (1975) showed that after an attack of acute pain has subsided, a large majority of patients would either have no further recurrence or only mild residual pain. Only 7–12% of patients ultimately required surgery. Friedenberg & Shoemaker (1954) also showed that with conservative management a substantial number of patients with back pain and radiculopathy secondary to ruptured disc had complete remission of symptoms and returned to full-time employment. Shannon & Paul in 1979 reported on 323 operations for backache and sciatica. At follow-up, 86% of males and 70% of females were symptom-free, 9% of males and 15% of females had persistent low-back pain and only 2% of males and 6% of females had severe permanent symptoms. Weber (1983) showed in a prospective study comparing surgery with conservative treatment that the surgical group did significantly better at 1 and 4 years, but at 10 years there was no difference between the groups.

Saal & Saal (1989) studied 64 patients with classical clinical prolapsed intervertebral discs who were submitted to an intensive and aggressive physical rehabilitation programme in order to see whether such a programme could obviate the necessity for surgery. Their inclusion criteria were complaints of leg pain primarily, positive straight-leg raising less than 60°, computerized tomography (CT) scan demonstrating a herniated nucleus pulposus without significant stenosis and positive electromyogram (EMG) demonstrating radiculopathy. A subgroup was identified with actual neurological signs. At an average of 31 months follow-up, the results showed that 90% had good or excellent outcome with a 92% return-to-work rate. Only six patients required surgery for removal of disc and decompression of nerve roots. This important study thus shows that it is possible to relieve symptoms and return patients back to work with classical disc lesions by a nonoperative, intensive rehabilitation programme.

The importance of understanding the natural history of back pain is further emphasized when studying the long-term results of repeated surgery for intractable back pain. Nachemson (1976) has pointed out that the success rate drops in a dramatic fashion after the first operation and second or subsequent operations for back pain have only a 5% chance of success. Selecki et al (1975) reported that only 8% of patients undergoing multiple back operations had a good result. Finnegan et al (1979) reported that in 67 of 80 patients who had more than one operation on the back followed for more than 1 year, only eight had good results with no pain, 13 had continued disabling pain, and 46 had fair results necessitating periodic bed rest and analgesics. No patient with scarring had a good result.

Kircaldy-Willis et al (1974, 1982) reviewed the causes of failure of disc surgery; in their experience, the commonest causes were wrong operations, operations at the wrong level or the existence of arachnoiditis. Kirwan (personal communication) found in 196 operations that 13 had been at the wrong level and six on the wrong side.

Burton (1983) carried out an extensive review of the causes of the failed back surgery syndrome, as he calls it. The most important surgical causes were failure to diagnose lateral spinal stenosis in 58%; the development of central stenosis, including fusion overgrowth, 7%; the development of adhesive arachnoiditis in 16%; recurrent or persistent disc herniation, 12%; epidural fibrosis, 8%; the so-called 'transitional syndrome', 5%, where increased stress had enhanced degenerative disease of the facet joints at the segments above the fusion, producing a localized low-back pain syndrome. He stresses, as do many other authors, that overlooking psychological and emotional factors is an extremely important cause of failure after surgery. We are constantly surprised at the failure by many surgeons to institute an intensive rehabilitation programme after spinal surgery, particularly after spinal fusion, for such patients are certain to have had pain for months, or even years, and be not only unfit generally but also have poor spinal muscles and very stiff joints, muscles and ligaments. As will be seen later, the results of intensive rehabilitation in patients with the failed back syndrome can be extremely rewarding.

Graham Smith (1990) emphasizes the importance of patient selection for surgery, particularly if there has been previous surgery. If he is in any doubt he admits patients for 5 days' in-depth assessment and we also subscribe to this view. This gives a chance for the rehabilitation team to assesss the patient's physical, emotional, psychological and social status in depth. It allows full investigation to make sure that no surgically remediable lesion remains and it allows one to assess whether the patient is likely to respond to the intensive rehabilitation programme necessary after further surgery. It is possible also to make a detailed assessment of the patient's expectations from surgery and his likely lifestyle as a result. The role of the psychologist in exploring patients' attitude to disease and their ability to cope with disability is of paramount importance in this respect. At the same time a psychotherapist can reinforce the psychologist's approach, exploring any emotional problems that may underline the chronic pain syndrome.

It may then become apparent that the cause of pain is not predominantly a surgical problem and an intensive progressive rehabilitation programme with appropriate counselling by the various members of the team may be the most appropriate approach.

Hsu et al (1988) reviewed 68 patients with breakdowns after lumbar fusions. Of these patients, 30 had good or excellent results lasting more than 16 months from the time of their fusions, but they eventually developed severe clinical deterioration due to herniated disc, degenerative stenosis, segmental instability, spondylolisthesis or retrolisthesis at the motion segment adjacent to the fused levels. Clinical symptoms developed from 16 months to 28 years after fusion. They noted that the rate of deterioration was most rapid when rigid internal fixation was used and slowest when there had been no fixation.

Graham Smith (1990) has summarized the surgical causes of failed back syndrome. Like other authors, he notes that immediate failure is likely to be due to an unrecognized diagnosis such as:

1. an internal disc derangement in the segment above an extruded disc fragment
2. operation at the wrong intervertebral space
3. immediate recurrent disc herniation
4. infection
5. a technical error resulting in neural damage or a cerebrospinal fluid (CSF) fistula.

The commonest causes of late failure were nonunion of spinal fusion, late segmental instability and lateral spinal stenosis, recurrent disc herniation, epidural fibrosis, segmental failure above the spinal fusion, infection and meningocele.

Mooney (1989b) has argued that there is a good case for using external pulsed electromagnetic field stimulation in all spinal fusions, as these have been shown to improve incorporation of the bone graft.

DIAGNOSIS

The last 10 years have seen marked advances in the diagnostic facilities for the condition of the disc and the root canals, and a combination of magnetic resonance imaging (MRI) discography and CT scan, with or without enhancement with contrast medium, has greatly increased the possibility of diagnosing the cause of surgical failures. When there is doubt about the actual root involved or if multiple root involvement is suspected, then selective nerve root block combined with EMG studies can be most helpful in deciding which nerve roots are at fault.

Leyshon et al (1981) showed that careful electromyography could be most helpful in delineating those patients with root stenotic lesions by the detection of denervation in one or more nerve roots. Young & Wynn Parry (1988) studied 146 patients with lateral root stenotic lesions and showed that straight-leg raising was diminished in only 32%, sensory impairment was very variable and tender points in the muscles were only present in 25%. Pain in the foot was common, as was nocturnal pain. One-third of their patients had normal physical findings despite clear evidence of nerve damage on electromyography.

Dooley and his colleagues (1988) have reviewed the value of nerve root infiltration in the diagnosis of radicular pain. They classified their patients' responses into four groups: in group 1 the patient felt typical leg pain on introducing the needle into the epiradicular sheath and the pain was completely relieved by the local anaesthetic during its time of action; in group 2 the patient felt typical leg pain on needle insertion but was not completely relieved by the local anaesthetic; in group 3 the typical pain was not reproduced on needle insertion but the patient was completely relieved by the local anaesthetic, and in group 4 the pain was not reproduced on introduction of the needle or relieved by the local anaesthetic. In the 46 patients in group 1, in which all but one patient had surgical confirmation of root pathology, eight had a herniated nucleus pulposus, 17 had bony entrapment as the cause of the radicular symptoms, and 12 had lumboradicular arachnoiditis. In group 2, three patients were found to have multiple root involvement and one had a peripheral neuropathy. Patients in groups 3 or 4 were seldom relieved of radicular pain by surgery. They therefore recommend nerve root infiltration as a useful diagnostic aid in patients with radicular symptoms in whom other investigations are either normal or show multiple level involvement or are difficult to interpret because of previous surgery. They were also able to show that it was only necessary to decompress the root in which the nerve infiltration test had been positive. This obviates the need for multiple level surgery when radiographic signs may suggest multiple disorders.

Dooley et al (1988) also comment on two patients who presented with the hip/spine syndrome where it was unclear whether the pain was predominantly coming from the hip or the spine. In both patients nerve root infiltration relieved the majority of pain, indicating a spinal pathology. We too have found this a useful diagnostic aid. In addition, we would carry out local anaesthetic injection of the hip joint under an image intensifier to ascertain whether hip disease was the cause of the symptoms if nerve root block had been unsuccessful.

If patients have clear clinical and radiological evidence of nerve root damage, they are referred for consideration of further surgery. There may well be a variety of reasons that makes surgery inadvisable, e. g. obesity, multiple operations, abnormal psychological reaction and predominance of back pain over sciatica, or the patient's natural reluctance to undergo further surgery. Unfortunately, a significant proportion of patients in whom the correct operation has been carried out by an experienced surgeon, decompressing an obviously compressed nerve root in the lateral canal, do not lose their symptoms. We now appreciate that surgery has failed because nerve damage has been so pronounced for so long that permanent peripheral and central changes have taken place. Clearly in such patients further surgery is doomed to failure and a conservative approach must therefore be adopted.

Recent advances in the basic sciences have given us a much clearer understanding of the probable causes of intractable backache and sciatica, despite operations designed to relieve the cause of symptoms, in particular by decompressing nerve roots. In 1974 Wall & Gutnik showed that experimental neuromas were the seat of spontaneous electrical discharges which were mechanosensitive, highly sensitive to circulating noradrenaline, but whose discharges could be substantially modified or even abolished by antidromic electrical stimulation. Occasionally one sees patients with nerve root compression syndrome with allodynia and hyperpathia in the leg. Wall & Gutnik (1974) also showed that sprouts from neuromas, whether from compression or section, could course far proximally. Subsequently it was shown that abnormally myelinated fibres resulting from chronic compression are the seat of ectopic discharges. Wall & Devor (1981) have shown that the normal resting spontaneous discharges in dorsal root ganglia are markedly increased as a result of peripheral neuroma formation. In the intact dorsal root ganglion some 4–5% of units are discharging spontaneously. After nerve section distally this increases to 10%. There is a spontaneous low rate of discharge of some three to four impulses per second and this frequency rises dramatically to up to 50 per second after peripheral damage. Thus, individual axons may contain many loci of generation of abnormal afferent impulses and this can be a major cause of pain in chronic root compression.

Howe et al in 1977 created a chronic lesion by tying a ligature round the dorsal root ganglion in cats, causing chronic demyelination. An increased rate of spontaneous firing in the dorsal root ganglion was produced – a slight increase in mechanical stimulation producing very prolonged firing at high frequencies. The authors imitated both the Lasègue sign and forward flexion by attaching a small thread to the dorsal root ganglion leading it out externally. Slight tension on this thread produced prolonged firing in the damaged dorsal root ganglion for minutes or hours on end. They suggested that the scarring excites mechanosensitivity of the nerve root on movement.

Wall & Devor (1978) have drawn our attention to the central effects that occur after peripheral deafferentation. Even mild damage to peripheral nerve can, within 1 week, cause remarkable changes in the spinal cord at that level. These include hypersensitivity of deafferented neurons, sprouting causing abnormal networks and response of deafferented cells to neuronal circuits to which they are normally not responsive. There is thus a marked change in the activities of the spinal cord both at the level of the lesion and further centrally as a result of peripheral damage.

Albe Fessard & Lombard (1983) caused deafferentation of the brachial plexus in rats by cutting the roots of the brachial plexus. Spontaneous discharges could be detected within a week in the dorsal horn at the level of the cervical enlargement and some weeks later spontaneous firing could be detected as far cephalad as the thalamus. There are thus profound peripheral and central effects of nerve damage which become permanent within a comparatively short time and may well explain the failure of decompression operations to relieve pain. We thus have the paradoxical situation whereby surgeons are loath to operate because of the poor results of recurrent procedures for intractable back pain and yet with this new knowledge of the effects of nerve damage there must be a strong case for early surgery before the nerve changes become permanent and irreversible. Clearly a very fine clinical judgement backed up by all the modern means of investigation needs to be mobilised to choose the right time for surgery in a particular patient. Some surgeons are fond of saying that patients must earn their disc operation. This may in fact be misguided for, by waiting, chronic irreversible nerve root damage may result. Certainly these recent experimental findings make it much clearer as to why patients who have seemingly had the correct operation for decompression of a compressed nerve root are not relieved of their pain, for if the peripheral and central damage has persisted for long enough, surgery clearly cannot reverse the situation. Surgery, in fact, can only make things worse by adding more nerve damage, with its effects of ectopic discharges and central deafferentation to an already abnormal peripheral and central nervous system.

The major syndromes causing intractable back pain due to spinal mechanical disorders have characteristic clinical pictures.

SPINAL STENOSIS

This condition has only relatively recently been recognized, partly because of the somewhat bizarre clinical picture and the frequent absence of any obvious neurological changes. Symptoms can be episodic and variable and can be explained by the somewhat random ischaemia created by vascular blocking along the spinal nerves and a patchy distribution of complaints is common. Clinicians are frequently confronted with a differential diagnostic problem and it may be necessary to carry out extensive investigations to exclude peripheral neuropathy. Both central and lateral canal stenosis can coexist, thus giving a complex clinical picture. Pain is felt in the buttocks, legs and low back. It can be extremely severe with a feeling of heaviness and uselessness in the legs. Sometimes there is a burning quality and the legs may feel as if they are gripped in a vice. Back pain may be less troublesome than the symptoms in the legs. Standing and walking are particularly painful. Characteristically, walking uphill is much worse than on the flat due to the hyperextension which narrows the canal. Pain is dramatically relieved by forward flexion; such patients can cycle long distances but only walk a short way. The walking distance progressively diminishes with time.

It can be very difficult to distinguish this from vascular disease and indeed the two may coexist. Demonstration of normal peripheral pulses is helpful, as are the characteristic X-ray appearances of diffuse degenerative disease with facet joint abnormalities and a narrowing of the anteroposterior diameter of the canal. EMG studies are helpful in demonstrating denervation and localizing the root or affected roots. Myelography and CT scan are valuable in central stenosis but myelograms are unhelpful in lateral canal stenosis as the canal is in the hidden zone where the contrast medium is obscured by the lamina.

In lateral canal stenosis, severe pain is felt in the back radiating down the particular nerve root encroached on by the facetal joint arthritis and ligament hypertrophy. Compressions of L5 and S1 roots account for the overwhelming majority of cases. Pain is felt down the side of the leg and into the big toe in L5 lesions and along the back of the calf and into the little toe in S1 lesions. However, the clinical picture is often confusing with bizarre sensory symptoms and normal straight-leg raising. It is only comparatively recently that the syndrome of lateral canal stenosis has been clearly defined and many cases have been, and still are missed.

> 'Bony entrapment of a single nerve root is a clearly recognizable entity which deserves much greater diagnostic attention' (Waddell 1982).

Macnab et al (1987) studied 635 patients with surgically-confirmed spinal stenosis. Some 382 had presented with unilateral leg pain and clinical evidence of single nerve root symptoms. These were treated by unilateral single nerve root decompression. Of these patients, 337 were reviewed at an average of 5.6 years postoperatively (45 having been lost to follow-up) and nerve root infiltration as a diagnostic aid was carried out. Decompression was carried out at L3 in 12, L4 in 98, L5 in 215 and S1 in 12. Some 92% of patients achieved significant and sustained relief. Bilateral or multilevel involvement was demonstrated on the myelogram in 60% of patients and on CT in 67%. Macnab et al also emphasize, that the mere radiographic demonstration of spinal stenosis does not indicate that the abnormality is necessarily a source of root compression causing pain. Equally and additionally the presence of stenosis at other levels does not influence the results of single root decompression and at follow-up rarely becomes a source of symptoms.

Porter et al (1984), in England, studied the natural history of lateral canal stenosis in 2360 patients who attended a back pain clinic. Some 6.5% of these patients had spinal stenosis and 10.5% had nerve root entrapment. They confirmed that lack of extension was the most notable physical sign. Despite obvious sensory symptoms, 85% had normal reflexes and 95% normal muscle power. In their series 81% of the patients required no specific treatment other than advice regarding home care and natural history of the process. In 14% they carried out epidural injections and only in 9.6% of patients was decompression undertaken. They state that the problem seems gradually to resolve with time and only 6% of those patients with clinical nerve root entrapment were over 65 years of age. They conclude that the degenerative process is gradually progressive with varying degrees of severity, inconsistently related to the passage of time and tends to be self-limiting in many cases. They therefore encourage alternating rest and physical activity with occasional epidural blocks.

FACET JOINT SYNDROME

There has been increasing recognition over the last few years of the importance of this syndrome. The facet joints are, of course, synovial joints and can become inflamed like any other such joint. Thus an acute inflammatory flare-up in chronic degenerative joint disease is to be expected. Furthermore it is recognized that extension and rotation injuries at any age can cause sudden acute facet joint derangement. In the younger person these are the acute backs that are so often helped by the osteopath or chiropractor and, when allowed to, by the physiotherapists who are now fully trained in manipulation techniques. The pathophysiology of the facet joints has been carefully studied by a number of authors and it is well-recognized that injection of the facet joint with hypertonic saline can produce pain not only locally but radiating with increasing strength of solution into the buttocks, thigh, knee and often into the calf. It is now known that chronic disc degeneration results in disturbance of the facet joints with loss of height, increased bone formation, synovial changes with chronic capsular thickening and contraction causing the full-blown facet joint syndrome. Later, with continued deterioration, there may be increasing facet joint deterioration with massive bony outgrowths causing the classical lateral stenotic lesion. This can, as previously described, coexist with central stenosis. These changes can often be seen clearly on plain X-rays, of which the anterior/posterior view is the most useful. CT scanning is the most reliable means of demonstrating the degree of involvement. Several authors have described the value of local anaesthetic injection into the facet joint to determine whether this is the source of pain. Dooley et al in 1988, as previously described.(p 1077) showed how valuable the reponse to local injection could be. Clinically the classical facet joint derangement causes pain in the back radiating to the buttocks, worse on extension and rotation and relieved by flexion. There may be marked morning stiffness.

Straight-leg raising is usually normal. Pressure over the facet joint may reproduce the pain. The patient usually points to the facet joint as the source of the pain and, in our experience, the patient's description of the site and radiation is very accurate. Marks et al (1992) were disappointed in the use of facet joint anaesthetic injections or blocks. They compared facet joint injection or facet nerve block, in which the medial articular branch of the posterior primary ramus was blocked. They found no difference in the two groups and a disappointing number of patients who had prolonged relief. They found that patients who had complained of pain for more than 7 years were more likely to have good or excellent pain relief. However, they emphasized that their patients were not subjected to a rehabilitation programme thereafter and suggested that such patients should be offered a rehabilitation programme during the time of pain relief, as they say, to take advantage of the brief window in their pain. Helbig & Lee in 1988 designed a points system to determine whether patients were likely to respond to a facet joint injection. They gave 30 points to the presence of back pain and radiation to the groin or thigh, 20 to well-localized paraspinal tenderness, 30 to reproduction of pain with extension and rotation, 20 to X-ray changes and 10 to pain below the knee. If the patient scored more than 60 points he was likely to respond to injection. Marks (1989) showed that stimulation of the posterior primary ramus electrically was more likely to produce distally-referred pain and respond to intraarticular facet joint injection. He indicates that absence of referred pain should not be regarded as excluding the facet joint as the source of pain since 76% of patients complained only of local pain when the joints were directly stimulated electrically. It was reasonable to infer a low lumbar origin for pain radiating to the buttock or trochanteric region since this pattern did not occur when stimulating the nerves at a higher level. Pain in the groin could equally be experienced from L2 to L5. Pain felt in the midline was unlikely to arise at a different level and coccygeal pain was unlikely to arise from a facet joint.

Silvers in 1990 reported on 223 patients who underwent lumbar percutaneous facet rhizotomy for chronic low-back pain or back pain and leg pain. The overall success rate was 69%. Their follow-up period was a mean of 6.2 years and all patients had had pain for at least 6 months and most for more than 1 year. The rhizotomy was only carried out on patients who had successfully undergone two successive facet nerve blocks at monthly intervals which had produced complete relief of symptoms. There was no correlation between the length of time of symptoms and the success of the injection. They noted, as have others, that the success rate was significantly higher in patients who had not had previous operations on the back although there was a 50% success rate in operated patients. However, they were very disappointed in the results in those patients who had had previous lumbar posterior fusion.

Mehta & Wynn Parry (1992) have routinely carried out facet joint injections with local anaesthetic and steroid in all patients presenting with a classical facet joint syndrome irrespective of previous surgery or not. In our series the injection is simply a prelude to an intensive rehabilitation programme, for all these patients have the characteristics of the chronic back syndrome with stiff joints, weak muscles and poor general fitness. The injections are always carried out under careful radiological control with an image intensifier. Our patients are admitted for two nights and re-assessed the morning following injection. Some days later the patients are admitted to an intensive progressive rehabilitation programme as described later. We found that it was undesirable to follow the injections immediately with a rehabilitation programme as this would often cause recrudescence of pain. Some 83 patients who had failed to respond to long-term conservative measures, such as long periods of rest, analgesia, transcutaneous electrical nerve stimulation (TENS) and antiinflammatory preparations, were treated. In 16 patients transient relief only was noted, but in 63 significant relief was achieved with little or no pain at 2-year follow-up. All members of our rehabilitation team are impressed with the necessity of offering the patient complete or substantial pain relief before they can be expected to undertake rehabilitation as we regard the rehabilitation programme as the single most important factor in the management of chronic back pain.

CHRONIC MECHANICAL LOW-BACK PAIN

The classical clinical picture in this condition is of a middle-aged person complaining of virtually chronic low-back pain with or without referral to the buttock, thigh or occasionally below the knee. In the most florid cases there may be generalized degenerative changes in the spine with disc degeneration and facet joint arthritis. There may, of course, be concomitant osteoporosis, particularly in women. However, the radiological changes may not necessarily be relevant to the symptoms for it is well recognized that marked X-ray changes can be present despite minimal or absent symptoms. Mooney (1989a) has also drawn our attention to the fact that the incidence of back pain peaks in middle years and diminishes in the aged and therefore degenerative arthritis of the spine cannot be regarded always as a determinant of back pain. The typical natural history starts with an acute attack of pain in adolescence or youth following some sporting activity, heavy lifting or in the later stages of pregnancy. There follows periodic attacks of back pain lasting a few days once every year or two. The patient may require to take a few days off from work or sport and may occasionally seek help from osteopathy or physiotherapy. Gradually, over the years, he or she becomes aware of 'having a back'. Eventually a severe episode occurs which may last several weeks and may even require admission to hospital or a prolonged period of rest at home. This is followed by the patient giving up sport and curtailing their do-it-yourself activities, including gardening and jobs around the house and regular help is sought from osteopath, chiropractor, acupuncturist and other fringe practitioners. Finally the patient appears in the back specialist's clinic with chronic low-back pain with restriction in most activities of daily life, having to take great care with driving, not being able to garden or play any sport. Some of such patients, on careful examination, may present with the facet joint syndrome. Some may have developed a classical nerve root compression syndrome which rarely may be a prolapsed disc, this being far commoner in the younger age group, but is much more likely to be a lateral canal stenotic lesion. Most patients complain predominantly of back pain with occasional reference to the sacroiliac area and the buttock. The likely cause of this condition is that over the years, with recurrent attacks of back pain and reducing physical activity, the small joints of the spine have become stiff, the ligaments have become tight and inflexible and the muscles of the lower back and abdomen have become progressively weaker. Thus on examination the patient may have a very stiff lumbar spine, particularly in forward flexion and extension but relative freedom laterally. There may be tenderness over the interspinous areas indicating chronic strain of the interspinous ligaments. There may be multiple trigger spots which can cause pain radiating into areas of which the patient complains and there will be very weak lower spinal and abdominal muscles. Sometimes one may find preexisting conditions that have rendered the spine more vulnerable, in particular Scheurmann's disease, scoliosis, old infections of the spine (particularly tuberculosis), inequality of leg length or osteoarthritis of the hips and knees producing secondary problems in the back. An unsuspected spondylolisthesis may be demonstrated for the first time. In some cases there may be radiation of pain into the groin, the abdomen and occasionally into the perineum and in such cases full investigations to exclude intraabdominal causes of pain are necessary. It is, of course, essential to distinguish the pain of chronic hip disease from chronic back pain and occasionally injection of local anaesthetic into the hip joint as a diagnostic aid can be most helpful. Some patients, such as nurses, dentists and doctors, may have classical postural backache through prolonged stooping causing stiffness of the lower spine and weakness of muscles. Many sedentary workers who do not take regular exercise can be martyrs to this condition. Patients presenting in this manner seek help not only for the immediate acute attack of pain, superimposed on a chronic condition, but are also seeking guidance for their lifestyle and whether they have to live with this condition. It is most important to emphasize that such patients do *not* need to 'live with' this condition; a very great deal can be done to minimize their symptoms and prevent further trouble. Clearly, a specific condition that is amenable to a specific treatment must be diagnosed, in particular, nerve root compression syndromes, lateral and central canal stenosis, spondylolisthesis or, rarely, a prolapsed intervertebral disc (PID). An acute or chronic facet joint problem without root impingement must be treated, but the patient with generalized chronic back pain without particular localizing features such as just described can be greatly helped by a change of lifestyle. This will involve taking off weight, following an intensive progressive programme to restore movement in the stiff spine and regain spinal and abdominal muscle power, and achieving a general higher standard of cardiovascular and musculoskeletal fitness. Many of such patients have become demoralized through increasing amounts of back pain and a short spell of intensive inpatient therapy can be most helpful. This allows the patient to learn the lessons of back discipline and back care.

It is often very difficult for patients to achieve the necessary speedy improvement with an outpatient programme, often travelling long distances for their physiotherapy and continuing to run their jobs and/or home at the same time. Often the patient's spouse suffers from the increasing disability suffered by the patient as social activities are cut to the minimum, holidays have to be abandoned and the family becomes consumed by the patient's chronic pain. Drug abuse is not uncommon and one of the most valuable means of treatment in somebody with chronic back pain is to remove all analgesics and antiinflammatory drugs; this, of course, is best done on an inpatient basis.

FUNCTIONAL BACK PAIN

Much has been written about the so-called functional or inorganic signs in patients with chronic back pain. Here the clinical situation suggests that the patient's signs and symptoms are inconsistent with known organic clinical syndromes. Waddell et al (1980) have contributed significantly in this field and described a number of inappropriate symptoms and signs which indicate that whereas there may be an organic basis to the patient's symptoms, there is a good deal of overreaction, which may be significant in the total management of the patient's problems. The inappropriate symptoms described are as follows: whole leg pain, whole leg numbness, whole leg giving way, pain at the tip of the tailbone, complete lack of pain-free intervals, intolerance of any treatment and emergency admissions to hospital. Inappropriate signs are: superficial nonanatomic tenderness, simulation of pain by axial loading (pressing on the head) or rotation. Distraction allows painless flexion of the spine in sitting from lying, yet straight-leg raising is grossly restricted by pain. Cogwheel weakness, stocking sensory disorder, overreacting with verbalization and facial expressions, muscle tension, tremor, collapse and sweating. It has been shown that these symptoms and signs correlate well with general somatic and neurotic symptoms, disability behaviour, exaggerated pain drawings and the surgeon's view of unsuitability for surgery.

Leavitt et al (1979) point out that it is possible to distinguish patients without organic disease using a standard nine-point assessment scale. Pain in nonorganic disease is invariably diffuse, variable and more intense. Many more words are used to describe the pain than in those with known organic disease. Keefe & Hill (1985) described a 10-minute video tape-recording session in which five pain-related behaviours were studied: these were guarded movements, bracing, rubbing the painful area, grimacing and sighing, and were much more frequent in the group with nonorganic disease. These patients were more demonstrative, less active, they took more medication and made considerable demands on their families.

Leavitt & Sweet (1986) circulated a questionnaire to 105 orthopaedic surgeons asking their opinion on nonorganic back pain. Some 70% or more physicians were in agreement on six findings:

1. weakness to manual testing not seen in other activities, e.g. heel to toe walking
2. disablement disproportionate to objective findings
3. pain not following an organic pattern
4. endorsement of false symptom suggestions
5. cogwheel weakness
6. reaction during examination.

Such patients tend to describe their symptoms in melodramatic form, like: 'a spear going through my back', or 'tight vices being compressed round my spine and down my leg'. Some of the patients exert the most extraordinary amount of energy in their attempts to walk (or not to walk!) or to turn over in bed and may go into chronic spasms affecting the whole of the body except the limb that they are being asked to move. Patients may present with frank paralysis. This usually is global and involves all muscles below the knee or all muscles in one leg. The simplest and most effective way of demonstrating the functional nature of such paralysis is by stimulating the nerves at the knee and demonstrating normal strong contraction in all the relevant muscles. The demonstration of normal function is then accompanied by praise from the examiner who is delighted to reassure the patient that the muscles and nerves are working normally but that there is some block to transmission of the message from the brain down to the leg. Treatment, it is then suggested, will be addressed to releasing this block. Patients usually accept this explanation and, provided that they are allowed time to regain function, supportive treatment with positive enforcement is often highly successful (Withrington & Wynn Parry 1985).

Leavitt & Sweet (1986) point out that malingering is extremely rare and that the vast majority of patients are not simulating weakness or symptoms but are genuinely disturbed. We feel that it is important to emphasize that the presence of inappropriate signs and inappropriate behaviour, excessive overreaction and the rest, should not debar a patient either from possible curative surgery nor from admission to a pain management programme. The patient is in fact desperate to seek attention and does not believe that the physician or surgeon will believe him unless he overreacts. We stress that this is an entirely unconscious performance and the patient must not be regarded as not 'genuine'. We have had some of the most gratifying results both from surgery and from rehabilitation in such patients.

A number of surgeons use the Minnesota Multiphasic Personality Inventory (MMPI) index test as a means of determining which patients will be suitable for surgery or rehabilitation. If the MMPI shows a strong conversion hysterical reaction, the surgeons will refuse the patient treatment. This seems a pity because it may well be that the patients are reacting in this way because they have failed to convince surgeons of the reality of their symptoms. Roberts & Reinhardt (1980) showed that as a result of successful operant conditioning for intractable back pain, the MMPI might change to normal, since the abnormal result was originally due to disability, use of drugs or frustrations through living an abnormal life rather than the cause of the pain. This seems to us an important observation and we deplore the decision to accept or reject a patient simply on the MMPI alone. A full psychological assessment is of vital importance in all patients coming to a pain management programme. Watkins et al (1986), in studying 42 patients with spinal fusion, showed that the MMPI was no predictor of the functional results.

REHABILITATION PROGRAMME

The value of a multidisciplinary rehabilitation programme for patients with chronic back pain is becoming increasingly accepted. The underlying rationale is to restore the patient to maximum physical and psychological fitness by a progressive programme of exercises to restore locomotor and cardiovascular fitness and to help the patient to gain control over his symptoms.

In our view successful back rehabilitation programmes incorporate both physical reconditioning and pain management strategies. This requires the integrated efforts of a team of physiotherapists, occupational therapists, nurses, psychologist, psychotherapist and social worker, coordinated by a specialist conversant with relevant clinical and managerial skills.

Many authors have reported on their specific programmes. The following account can be taken as representative of most such programmes. Most of our experience was obtained at the Royal National Orthopaedic Hospital, the rehabilitation unit of a National Health Service hospital and, latterly, at the Alexandra Rehabilitation Centre at King Edward VII Hospital in Midhurst a private hospital where all patients have their own rooms. The principles underlying the programmes are identical. Exercise is the fundamental basis of the rehabilitation programme.

EXERCISE

In the last 5 years there has been a considerable interest shown in the value of an intensive progressive exercise programme for patients with chronic back pain. Manniche et al (1991) have given an extensive review of the evidence indicating the value of such an exercise programme. They quote work by Holm & Nachemson (1983) on the positive influence exercise has on the nutrition of disc and refer to the work of Cady et al (1979) showing a physical conditioning programme reduces the risk of recurrence of low back pain in firefighters. Several reports show that a combination of weak spinal muscles and back-straining work increases the risk of development of back trouble. Manniche and colleagues studied 105 patients with chronic low-back pain, dividing them into three groups. The first group had an intensive progressive treatment programme; the second had one-fifth of the exercise programme per session, whilst in the third group the treatment consisted of heat, massage and very mild exercise. Patients had to have had chronic low-back pain for at least 6 months and an acute attack of back pain within the last half-year. At 1-year follow-up only those patients who continued the back training at least once a week achieved significant progress. They concluded that intensive back training can effect a lasting improvement of pain but continued training is essential to avoid relapse. They were surprised, as indeed we were when we began this work with patients with very severe disabling back pain, to find how many patients were able to perform the exercises without difficulty. Linton et al (1989) looked at the value of intensive exercises as a preventive measure for recurrences of back pain. They had noted that only 35–45% of patients with chronic low-back pain were able to manage a job a year after treatment and that persons who had been off work for more than three consecutive months with low-back pain had little chance of recovery. The goals in their study were to reduce current pain problems and increase levels of functioning, teach patients skills to prevent reinjury and to prevent minor benign bouts of pain developing into chronic pain. Some 66 nurses were admitted to the trial, all of whom were suffering pain at the time they entered the programme. A very detailed assessment was carried out which included daily ratings of pain, pain behaviour (which was observed by video recording), activities of daily living, depression, helplessness, marital satisfaction assessed on the appropriate inventories, absenteeism and the level of medication. The controls were those on a waiting-list who did not have active treatment. An intensive inpatient programme was carried out with activities for at least 8 hours a day during a 5-week period. The programme was varied, including walking, swimming, jogging, cycling, ergonomic education, teaching of self-care methods and behavioural therapy techniques. Significant differences were found between the groups on all the variables that were evaluated, ratings of pain intensity, fatigue, anxiety, sleep, depression, helplessness and marital satisfaction. The improvement in pain behaviour was especially dramatic. They concluded that a secondary prevention programme was an effective method for dealing with musculoskeletal pain problems and was particularly helpful in preventing recurrences. Deardorff et al (1991) came to similar conclusions when treating 42 chronic pain patients with a multidisciplinary programme compared with 15 not so treated. As well as counselling, relaxation and reduction in medication, a very intensive progressive exercise programme was introduced for 3 weeks as an inpatient, followed by a 10-week outpatient continuation programme. There was no change in the nontreatment group, but in the treated group a high percentage continued their exercises and a year later 64% were medication-free and 76% had returned to work or were in training for work. They felt that the improvement was likely to be due to modification of beliefs rather than a change in the physical status, i.e. the orthopaedic condition, and it was improved physical function with more appropriate perceptions of such improvement that was responsible. They feel that determinants of return to work are more psychosocially based than physically and organically based. They emphasize that when there is a cognitive shift early in the phase of treatment there is an excellent chance of a successful result. We have certainly found this in our patients, both at the Royal National Orthopaedic Hospital and at the Alexandra Rehabilitation Centre at King Edward VII Hospital, Midhurst. This shift is shown by a much more positive and cheerful approach with patients volunteering that they now understand the point of the regime and are delighted to see improvements in their functioning and ability to take charge of their own health.

There are many reasons why exercises are helpful for patients with back pain. The vast majority, of course, will have poor spinal musculature through years of disuse. It is only to be expected that prolonged sitting, standing or walking or sudden movements will cause pain because there is not the muscle power to stabilize the spine or the reflex action to protect it with sudden changes of movement. The small joints of the spine almost inevitably become stiff and it is rare in somebody with chronic back pain not to find a very stiff spine, particularly in forward flexion and extension. Exercises, therefore, to improve strength and stamina in the spine and to increase mobility are of obvious benefit. Furthermore they must be continued on an indefinite basis, on a daily basis, to be effective. In addition, patient's general health has suffered and a generalized exercise programme to develop cardiovascular fitness as well as improvement in locomotor function is of great benefit. The effect of exercise is to improve mood and instil a sense of wellbeing which in itself leads to a positive optimistic attitude and a better ability to cope with pain and return to a normal life. Indeed, the benefits of general exercise have been well-publicized and are well-known, but what is important is to reassure patients that they cannot possibly do themselves harm by an exercise programme under careful supervision and that inactivity and lack of exercise are positively dangerous and will lead to morbidity and mortality. Unfortunately, many patients will have been advised not to exercise and to 'look after their backs' and have not been given a conditioning or back discipline programme; it is thus up to the team to instil the correct attitudes and explain the scientific basis and evidence for this approach. Most middle-aged patients can return to their chosen sport, provided they have become fit for it and obey the basic rules; for example, many patients are surprised to be told that they can return to playing golf and that the better the golfer the less likely they are to do themselves harm. We encourage patients, if necessary, to have one or two sessions from a professional to learn correct techniques and the correct presport conditioning programme. Obviously, a careful choice of equipment and pacing themselves throughout their sport is important. Similarly, advice on how to cope with daily living activities and sensible gardening techniques will reassure patients that they can get back to meaningful and enjoyable activities which in themselves promote wellbeing and improve fitness. All patients are given an intensive session of back discipline by the combined teaching of physiotherapists and occupational therapists, stressing an exercise regime, correct sitting and posture at work, choice of bed and chair, correct lifting techniques and all the factors that prevent problems to the back in daily living. This may require ergonomic assessment of the workplace, even a change of motor car or bed. Attention to such detail, examining all aspects of the patient's daily life at home, at work and at play, make all the difference to a successful result. The aim of the rehabilitation programme is to improve patients' general function and hopefully to reduce pain, to help them to cope with their disability, to give them a more positive approach to life, to educate themselves and their families in the effect of their back problem and to take control of their own symptoms. The most successful pain management programmes incorporate the skills of a variety of different professions, each having their own particular contribution and these will be described in some detail. The patients are enormously cheered to find themselves the subject of attention of a team of highly-skilled and knowledgeable professionals who all really understand the problem and have a positive and optimistic attitude. Despite the tendency to develop more and more outpatient programmes, mainly because of the cost and reimbursement by insurance companies, an inpatient programme is without doubt the most effective in somebody who has had pain for a long time, who is despondent and depressed and pessimistic about the outcome. We tell patients that they will be working hard for 6–7 hours a day and at the end of the day they will be exhausted. The one thing they do not want to do is to go home to cook meals or run the house, or try and organize their business from home. They are strongly encouraged to eat meals together and spend the evening in social pursuits. This brings them out of themselves and re-introduces them to social life. They return home at the weekends but are made to promise that they will not indulge in any physical activities that would obviate the improvement that has occurred during the week.

Throughout the rehabilitation programme careful objective measurements are made by all the therapists so that the patients, the doctor and the team can see tangible results. At the outset appropriate, realistic goals are set and a time set for their achievement. Thus at the end of the first week it may be that the patient will only be expected to be sitting for 1 hour and walking 100 yards and these objectives are increased in difficulty as the programme progresses. Throughout the programme achievements are praised and as little notice as possible taken of negative responses. All members of the team must be fully conversant with the aims, particularly that of reinforcing positive achievements and disregarding negative reponses. If patients complain of pain then a careful assessment will reveal whether this is because the exercise programme is beginning to be effective and muscles that have not been used for years are beginning to respond or whether there is an exacerbation of the underlying pathology, when some form of pain relief such as TENS or acupuncture may be introduced, but solely with the purpose of allowing the patient to continue with the rehabilitation programme.

REHABILITATION PROGRAMME AT THE ROYAL NATIONAL ORTHOPAEDIC HOSPITAL

All patients are admitted to the minicare wards at the Royal National Orthopaedic Hospital at Stanmore. Patients are up and dressed having treatment throughout the day in the departments and simply use the wards for sleeping and evening activities. Patients have their own dining room, games room and television room. There is also an interview room where quiet discussions can be held with the patient and his or her family. A special rehabilitation sister and nurses are in charge of the ward. Their role is to help the patients to learn to be independent, encourage them to do as much for themselves as they can, to chart their progress objectively and to study their reactions to their disease. They are particularly skilled in observing inappropriate behaviour and whether the patients are cooperating with the programme or resisting attempts to help. Nurses, in turn, attend the treatment departments and cooperate with the therapists in the assessment and management of the patient's programme. Each nurse on the staff is encouraged to take a specific interest in two or three patients, together with the patient's therapists. The information the nurses glean and the observations they make throughout the week can be of great help on the weekly ward rounds and team conferences. Patients arrive on Monday morning and throughout Monday and Tuesday morning are assessed in detail by all members of the rehabilitation team.

Before entering any pain programme a full reassessment is made irrespective of the distinction of the referring surgeon or physician. This of course is particularly important when patients have not been through a specialist unit before. Particular attention is paid to the exclusion of any underlying malignancy, metabolic disorder (particularly in the Asian population), endocrine disease or general rheumatic disorder. An excellent account of screening procedures in patients with chronic back pain to exclude nonmechanical causes is given by Waddell (1982). In 5.5% of referrals of back pain to his service, underlying spinal pathology was found – malignancy, infection or metabolic bone disease.

All X-rays and blood tests are reviewed and a definitive diagnosis made where possible. This may well be modified as a result of the detailed assessment made by the therapists; thus, for example, the proportion of symptoms due to mechanical problems as opposed to neural damage may become clearer after these assessments.

On the Tuesday afternoon the ward round or case conference is held. Before the patient attends the meeting the doctor presents the history and relevant clinical examination and each member of the team in turn presents his or her findings. The patient is then invited to attend and the various aspects of the problems are discussed. At the end of the meeting specific goals are agreed and the timing of the treatment programme is negotiated. Most patients stay for 2 or 3 weeks but we indicate to all patients that most of the first week will be devoted to detailed assessment and the treatment programme is unlikely to start until the latter end of the first week. Thus at least 2 weeks are required to achieve any significant progress and the majority of patients will be encouraged to stay at least 3 weeks. As at least 60% of our referrals are from distant parts of the country, it is thus not possible to involve the patient's family or general practitioner except on rare occasions, but when this is possible, it is strongly encouraged. Each therapist has a specific area of interest, as follows.

PHYSIOTHERAPY

The physiotherapist takes a detailed history of past treatment. It is vital to have a clear knowledge of past treatment in order to decide whether further physiotherapy is likely to be beneficial and, if so, what type of modality. This is particularly relevant when considering TENS. The patient may already have tried this modality with no benefit but it is most important to establish that the patient has had a thorough trial of the technique supervised by someone fully versed in it. A high proportion of patients who claim to have tried TENS without success are found on detailed discussion not to have been given instruction in correct use of the machine or to have been told to use it for only half an hour three times a week for 10 minutes at a time. Our physiotherapist will invariably give TENS another proper trial if there is any doubt about the efficacy of previous attempts. She will also assess what other therapeutic modalities have been tried and whether they have been given effectively and for long enough. Patients easily lose heart if they feel in their first 2 days that they are merely going to be given the same treatments they have already tried, probably on a number of different occasions in the past.

The physiotherapist in her examination pays particular attention to the patient's posture, range-of-movement, affected joints, factors limiting movement (such as pain, stiffness and muscle spasm), muscle power, undue tenderness, abnormal muscle tone and localized joint movements reproducing the patient's pain. She will then assess activities such as walking, sitting, standing, squatting and mounting stairs. She will look for inconsistent signs and symptoms; for example, inability to dorsiflex the foot with a functional foot drop, yet able to contract the tibialis anterior when rocking back on the heels or walking. She will assess how easily symptoms are aroused or exacerbated and how long they take to settle. It is important to determine this to make an assessment of how vigorous a treatment can be introduced. Video recordings are taken of the patient's gait and movements; for example, the way he gets off a couch on to a chair or from a chair to standing position. Keefe & Hill in 1985 described the use of a transducer in the patient's shoes to measure walking parameters at the same time as video recordings. They noticed that patients with severe back pain walked more slowly with shorter steps with an asymmetrical pattern and showed a higher level of pain behaviour than normal controls and these observations were very useful to judge progress on a serial basis.

Assessment is of course a continuing process and patients will be reassessed two or three times a week. The physiotherapist will then be able to suggest a plan of treatment with a scale of priorities and an indication of how long it is expected before they can be achieved.

Treatment plans are always made in conjunction with the occupational therapist particularly, and with other members of the team, so that an integrated progressive programme is constructed. Hydrotherapy is an essential part of treatment, all patients with back problems going into the pool twice a day. At the start this is used for gentle mobilization and relaxation to relieve pain and to start exercising the muscles and improving range of movement in the joints. As progress is made the water can be used for resistance rather than assistance and eventually swimming several lengths and even water games can be introduced. If pain is interfering with the rehabilitation programme and if the patient cannot accept TENS or it is ineffective, then interferential has been found to be a very useful pain-relieving modality. Acupuncture is more successful for neck pain than for back pain in our experience although if there are clear trigger points which are either too numerous or inappropriate to be treated with local injections of local anaesthetic and steroid, these are treated with acupressure or acupuncture. There was some suggestion in our work at the Royal National Orthopaedic Hospital that electroacupuncture was more effective than conventional acupuncture and the brief, almost painful, mode was more effective than the prolonged TENS with trigger-point pains. Stretching is an important part of treatment and patients with long-standing chronic back pain have shortening of their spinal muscles and ligaments and, in addition, can have tight hamstrings, calf and hip muscles. This will obviate proper lifting procedures to protect the back. Therefore all these muscles are progressively stretched, mobilized and a specific exercise programme for these lower-limb muscles is introduced. Throughout, there is a close liaison with the psychologist and psychotherapist so that appropriate attitudes in treatment are adopted and the psychological strategies are reinforced. Every patient is given a structured, detailed, written home programme and all patients are followed up at 4–6 weeks to make sure that the programme is understood and being followed. Objective measurements are recorded regularly and serve to reassure patients that progress is being made. This will include standard ranges of movement, muscle power, strength and stamina, walking distance and time taken, up time, sitting time and pain ratings.

All patients attend relaxation classes at the end of each day and are given a tape to use at home after discharge.

OCCUPATIONAL THERAPY

The occupational therapist's assessment is particularly concerned with functional activities and thus careful objective records are made of daily living, tolerance of sitting and standing, walking distances and time taken to effect these. She will obtain full details of the social history and lifestyle and, in particular, a detailed day's activity, indicating what household activities can be achieved, how long they take, and how they are organized throughout the week. She will be particularly concerned with the type of living accommodation, work situation, methods of transport, role in the family and the expectations of other family members.

Either the physiotherapist or the occupational therapist will supervise the keeping of a careful pain diary by the patient and both these therapists will record the effect of treatment on pain ratings.

Our occupational therapist recognises four distinct areas in which she is concerned; these are as follows.

1. Organization of the environment

This is to ensure the efficient function of the patients at home or within their working environment. This means careful attention to height of work surfaces, position of equipment and articles in the kitchen, introduction of grab rails in the toilet and supporting rails along the stairs. Indeed, a work study of the whole of the patient's home, in the case of a housewife, is well worthwhile undertaking and will of course necessitate a home visit. Our resettlement officer and occupational therapist will together visit the patient's work in special circumstances.

2. Coping strategies

Patients are encouraged to find hobbies and activities as a means of distraction for pain relief and to counteract the feeling of depression. Whenever possible they are encouraged to get out of the house and if necessary to develop activities in a day centre. The proper use of relaxation techniques between functional activities is stressed.

3. Organization of self

This is attempted by trial and error in the department to appreciate and understand patients' tolerance to pain and activity. It is important to plan the day and the week so that activities are evenly spaced and to encourage a structured approach to their lives.

Patients are encouraged not to dwell on their pain but to indulge in meaningful activities. Goals are drawn up by the patient and therapist together and these are broken down in parts; for example, if the patients decide that their goal is to go shopping then the component parts can be split up as follows: walking, measuring the distance to the car from the home, sitting in the car for a specific period, walking to and around the shops, standing in a checkout queue, returning to the car and then going home. These individual targets can be achieved one by one through simulation in the occupational therapy department. The activities are then put together until the whole activity can be achieved in one session.

Case history

Mr W, aged 66, came to the unit in 1986 with a 12-year history of low-back pain and sciatica. In 1980 a lumbar decompression was carried out with no relief of pain. Eight epidural injections were unhelpful. In 1982 decompression of both S1 nerve roots and spinal fusion were carried out. He continued to suffer severe back pain and sciatica and had not responded significantly to TENS, physiotherapy, drugs or acupuncture. He was able to sit or stand for only a few minutes and walking was restricted to 20 metres. Realistic goals were discussed and are listed in Table 57.1, as are targets for the first week in the programme, and the activities introduced into the occupational therapy programme to prepare him for these targets. Table 57.2 shows his progress at 3-month follow-up. The patient reported that pain was now more under his control. He was less anxious, spent more time with his wife, had more shared interests and was a happier man.

CLINICAL PSYCHOLOGY IN THE MANAGEMENT OF CHRONIC PAIN

The role of psychological factors in the personal and subjective experience of medical conditions has gained greater recognition in the scientific literature in recent years. This has been particularly so in those conditions which are accompanied by pain and where there is currently a limit in the efficacy of purely medical interventions. Thus, in a study with sufferers of rheumatoid arthritis (Flor & Turk 1988), attitudes and beliefs appeared to be better predictors of pain disability than the disease variables themselves. Such very subjective factors of personal meaning and understanding will greatly influence the reaction to the objective reality of any pathological agent.

Pain has been associated with what has been described as 'illness behaviours'. The event of pain can produce reactions and adaptations in the manner in which people think, feel and behave. Rather than being transitory phenomena these can become habitual parts of a person's behavioural repertoire that serve no real functional purpose except in attenuating the experience. Clinical psychologists, therefore, utilizing theories from cognitive psychology and learning theory, have sought to tease out the salient features in perception and thinking and then to modify them with the purpose of altering the subjective experience of pain. This approach is called cognitive – behaviour therapy. This has gained attention and yielded some positive results in the management of chronic pain.

Table 57.1 Royal National Orthopaedic Hospital Occupational Therapy Department treatment plan for Mr W

Goals	Targets	Activities	M	T	W	T	F	S	S
	Week 1								
1. Help in domestic activities to take the strain off my wife	Standing 15 minutes Sitting 15 minutes	Woodwork							
2. Extend ability to go for walks	Walking – easy route to Occupational Therapy Department	Walking							
3. Find a hobby	Get fit								
4. Cut myself off from my business or increase ratio of satisfaction to worry, or replace by other brain activity	Cycling	Cycling Alexander relaxation tape							
5. Take up do-it-yourself activities									
6. Take up gardening		Washing-up							
7. Take up some mild social activity such as touring									
8. Lose a little weight									
	Weekend arrangements								
	Alexander technique on floor (20 min) Walk 20 min first day Walk 30 min second day	Shopping							
	Tape relaxation Find better position for watching television Work in garden – 30 min Saturday, 30 min Sunday Washing-up each day	In garden							

Table 57.2 Mr W: progress in achieving goals after 3 months

Goals	Action and outcome
1. Domestic activities	Washing-up Cleaning Make beds Learning to cook
2. Walking	Maintains 30 min
3. Hobby	Very interested in do-it-yourself activities Completed electrical jobs Completed woodwork jobs Completed plastering jobs
4. Business	Wound up business affairs in a satisfactory manner Now acts in consultancy capacity
5. Do-it-yourself	Very interested in do-it-yourself activities (see above)
6. Gardening	Spending time planning and landscaping garden
7. Social activity	Joined Rotary Club with his wife
8. Weight	Maintained weight

Cognition, which refers inter alia to styles of thinking, attitudes, expectations and beliefs, interacts with an experience to produce a certain reaction or mood.

In the assessment phase, cognitive – behavioural techniques focus on establishing the individual's personal and idiosyncratic cognitions. Then, during the treatment phase, these are subjected to systematic challenge and scrutiny with alternative strategies being both proposed and instigated. The behaviours targetted for modification include activity levels, the use of analgesics and the utterance of negative comments, each of which can be quantified. Goals can be set, within certain time limits, and thereby attained, allowing the patient to recapture the experience of success which repeated treatment failures may well have submerged.

To maintain progress in this approach it is important for there to be a genuinely consistent therapeutic environment in which everyone involved collaborates. While the clinical psychologist may possess the knowledge and skills to elicit awareness of the individual cognitions, others in the multidisciplinary clinical team, and in the patient's life, will need to share the reinforcing of the positive behaviour while they concentrate upon their own unique contribution to the patient's life.

THE SOCIAL WORKER

The social worker will pay particular attention to the patient's problems at home. She will make a detailed inventory of the various financial ingoings and outgoings and whether the patient is receiving all the allowances to which he or she is entitled. She will make a detailed study of the family situation and pay particular attention to any interfamily problems and the role that the patient takes in the family setting. She will attempt to gain an idea of the patient's motivation, expectations and general mood. Patients will often speak more freely to social workers because they do not have the medical image to the same extent.

PSYCHOTHERAPY

The rehabilitation centre at King Edward VII Hospital has been greatly strengthened by the addition of a psychotherapist to the team. Her major input is in the elucidation of emotional problems that are preventing satisfactory rehabilitation. She will help the patient to face the traumas of childhood, marriage, relationships with relatives, friends and colleagues at work that lead to insecurity, fear of failure and inappropriate attitudes. Often a few sessions are sufficient to help the patient appreciate the emotional background to symptoms and may lead to a dramatic improvement in acceptance of life and readiness to cooperate with the rehabilitation strategies.

Sometimes this is only the beginning of long-term therapy, for many patients have deep-seated fears and irrational beliefs that need time to bring out.

The psychotherapist advises the team on the significance of these problems in the patient's behaviour and this can lead to an alteration in the team's attitude and strategies.

We would not now be without a psychotherapist's contribution.

PHYSICAL MODALITIES

TRANSCUTANEOUS ELECTRICAL NERVE STIMULATION (TENS)

The one modality that we find most helpful is TENS. Most patients will have tried this before but it is surprising in how many the technique has been poorly used. So often patients are handed a stimulator at a pain clinic or by their general practitioner with scant or no instructions on how to use it. Many of our patients have been told to try it for half an hour a day twice a week, and have abandoned it because not surprisingly it has proved useless. We insist that patients who are considered for TENS for chronic pain admitted as inpatients to our pain service and our physiotherapists who are specially trained in the application of TENS will assess the effect of stimulation for at least 2 weeks. They will experiment with electrodes in different positions with different settings of pulse rate, amplitude and repetition rate and for varying lengths of time. It is well known that TENS has a cumulative effect and that the longer the treatment is used the more likely it is to be beneficial (Melzack 1975). All our patients try TENS for at least 8 hours a day for 2 weeks. If there is a significant response the patient will be allowed to take the stimulator away and no further attempts to relieve his back pain are considered until a proper and intensive trial of this technique has been given for at least 3 months. Many of our patients are able to return to work or to activities in the home using their stimulator regularly, and in our view this is one of the most important modern advances in the management of chronic pain.

ACUPUNCTURE

The literature is full of reports of acupuncture being singularly unsuccessful in severe chronic pain; this is well reviewed by Richardson & Vincent (1986). Most studies show initial good response, only to relapse later. However, Coan et al (1980) found a 58% improvement at 10-month follow-up when traditional acupuncturists were given full rein in choice of technique. The whole field is bedevilled by poorly controlled studies and the difficulty of providing satisfactory controlled ineffective acupuncture. Lehman et al (1986) compared pain estimates and disability in three treatment groups – conventional TENS, placebo TENS and electroacupuncture. Electroacupuncture constantly demonstrated the greatest improvement on outcome measures. We have had one or two spectacular successes with electroacupuncture and, as this is a noninvasive technique, it is worth trying.

The enthusiasm for biofeedback techniques to teach relaxation and thus hopefully relief of pain has waned considerably and the general consensus is that biofeedback has little or no place in the control of symptoms.

DRUGS

Some patients are on a veritable pharmacopoeia of drugs and we have seen a number of patients who are almost zombie-like as a result of the large number of different drugs they are taking.

A careful drug history is essential, particularly concerning the effect of a drug on the patient's symptoms and performance. Surprisingly, dramatic relief of pain can result from rapid detoxification of such patients. Pain is often worsened by these drugs and we explain to the patient that it is quite impossible for him to mobilize his own pain-inhibiting pathways, nor can he expect such pain-relieving modalities as TENS to be effective if he is damping down the responses of his pain factory.

Turk & Flor (1984) in their excellent review article on physical methods of treatment in back pain suggest that medication is no solution to chronic back pain and its only use is in the acute exacerbations. However, the centrally acting pain-relieving compounds which are also antidepressants are worth trying because of occasional spectacular results – we have found Triptafen to be the most successful. If patients suffer from severe paroxysmal shooting pains down the leg, suggesting a highly irritable focus of spontaneously firing cells in the spinal cord, it is worth trying carbamazepine and its analogues, but it is rather rare to find a significant effect. Obviously, if a patient is clinically depressed, appropriate antidepressants are prescribed.

DORSAL COLUMN STIMULATION

The vogue for this modality has waned as a long-term follow-up showed a dramatic fall in the numbers gaining permanent relief (Leibrock et al 1984). Leibrock et al (1984) reported on 14 patients with organic findings relating to their low-back pain who received dorsal column stimulation. Two were unable to obtain stimulation over the distribution of the pain, in one the pain became intolerable, three had less than 70% relief, four had a good result, with two returning to work. Two had some relief still requiring analgesia. Thomas (personal communication) finds that some 50% of patients with arachnoiditis respond to dorsal column stimulation. We have three patients (in his series) who have had dramatic relief. The treatment is complex and expensive but is clearly worth serious consideration in well motivated patients who have responded to TENS but who can no longer tolerate the electrode jelly and who have failed to respond to a comprehensive pain management programme. The subject is well reviewed by Krainick & Thoden (1984).

RESULTS

In 1988 we reported a prospective study on 101 patients who were admitted to a comprehensive rehabilitation programme as described, with a minimum, 2-year follow-up. A total of 72 patients had received surgery which had failed to relieve their symptoms – often two or more procedures. Some 58% gained complete or substantial relief of pain and were living useful and fulfilling lives. There was no relation to length of symptoms and number of operations between those who improved and those who did not. The average duration of symptoms was 10 years. Of those who improved, 13% were able to return to work, but a further 20% were past retirement age. Of those who did not improve, 6% returned to work, and a futher 19% were past retirement age. In total, 60% of those who improved with rehabilitation and had had surgery found TENS the single most successful modality and 19% of those who did not improve found some benefit. An exercise programme was found to be the second most beneficial item in the programme, helping 40% of those who had had surgery.

Some 29 patients did not have surgery, mostly because back pain predominated over leg pain and because our surgical team believe that surgery rarely helps backache, being specifically designed to abolish leg pain by relieving nerve root compression. Of these, 61% found that TENS was the most effective modality and 28% found that an exercise programme was most effective.

Overall, 58% of all patients benefited significantly from the rehabilitation programme.

RETURN TO WORK

A distressingly small percentage of patients with chronic back pain are able to return to work. Most men do not return to work (Watkins et al 1986). Beals & Hickman (1972) studied 180 industrially injured men admitted to a rehabilitation programme. Only 29% were employed 6 months after discharge. The longer the interval between injury and assessment the less likely was their return to work, and the percentage fell as physical and psychological handicaps increased and in proportion to the number of surgical procedures. Gottlieb et al (1982) found that 45% of chronic low back patients were in employment at 6 months after a comprehensive rehabilitation programme.

Guck et al (1985) found that 64% of a treated group (20 patients) returned to work, while none of the control group were able so to do. Malec et al (1981) found 36% (32 patients) were employed at 6-month to 3-year follow-up. Rosomoff et al (1981) studied 128 patients with an intensive rehabilitation programme concentrating on activities and disregarding pain. A total of 29% were able to work, but 16% were unemployable owing to their history of back pain. Trief (1983), in a series of 132 patients admitted to a 6-week rehabilitation programme reinforcing well behaviour and extinguishing illness behaviour, found that although 75% felt better for the programme, only 37% were able to return to work. Gottlieb et al (1982) studied 78 subjects, of whom 72 were unemployed on admission to a back pain rehabilitation programme. At 12 months, 35 were working.

There is no doubt that a comprehensive inpatient back programme incorporating physical and behavioural techniques can help some patients to return to work but, although this is a desirable outcome, organizers must not be disappointed if the number of patients who return to work is small. Considerable gains in lifestyle, activities in the home, reduction in medication, improved social life and reduced complaining can be expected. Sometimes men will accept role reversal and this can be a most satisfactory answer.

Even if there is a strong suspicion that the patient is motivated towards obtaining compensation this should not necessarily debar him from admission to the programme. It is important however to establish quite clearly what the legal issues are, how long it is likely to be before the case will be heard and to reassure the patient that acceptance into a programme and possible return to work will not militate against his settlement. If necessary, the positive rehabilitation programme should be discussed with the legal advisers and these issues clarified at an early stage. The disastrous results of inactivity and accepting a chronic illness role must be stressed.

A number of authors have studied criteria that will predict the likely success in a pain management programme. Guck et al (1985) showed that prognosis was worse with increasing age, the existence of compensational problems, poor education, use of psychotrophic medication and number of operations for relief of back pain. Maruta et al (1979) applied a seven-item rating scale to 69 patients; 34 did well on a pain-management programme whilst 35 failed. Those in whom pain had lasted for less than 3 years and who had been off work for less than a year did well. Those who had had three or more operations, were dependent on drugs and those who had a low educational standard did badly. Such poor prognostic signs should not debar a patient from a pain-management programme but should alert the team to the fact that considerably more problems are likely to be encountered than with those patients in whom the prognostic signs are better.

However, a more optimistic report is given by Deardorff et al (1991) who described a comprehensive multidisciplinary treatment of chronic pain with a follow-up study of treated and nontreated groups. They pointed out that there are relatively few outcome studies of such pain programmes which have utilised no-treatment comparison groups. Some 42 patients were in the treated group and 15 were in the untreated group. They assessed the following parameters: subjective ratings of pain, physical functioning, reduction of pain medication, health care utilization, return to work. The treated group followed a programme of progressive conditioning with stretching and strengthening activities with occasional use of pain-relieving modalities such as spray and TENS. Occupational therapists emphasized body mechanics training, increased sitting and standing tolerance, muscle strengthening, work simulation and retraining in the activities of daily living. Psychological interventions involved individual pain management, group activities, biofeedback, family counselling and relaxation training. Finally, medication management was arranged with the pain cocktail procedure. The number of inpatient days was 20.32. Following the inpatient programme, outpatient treatment was offered for 5 days a week for 2–3 weeks and then gradually reduced to 1 day a week. In the treated group the return to work rate or vocational training was 76%, whereas none of the untreated group returned to work or training. All patients in the treated group increased their physical functioning, decreased their medication use and achieved considerable improvement in wellbeing.

Gallagher et al (1989) studied 150 subjects with severe back pain in an attempt to pick predictors of successful rehabilitation involving locomotor, psychological and emotional assessments. They studied illness behaviour, the patient's attitude to their disease, their hypochondriasis index, effective inhibition and somatising tendencies. They found that the physical examination was not predictive of the patient's likelihood to return to work. If patients perceived that their job change was difficult they were unlikely to return to work. The hysteria scale was highly relevant and their ability to do daily living tasks was also relevant. If they were convinced that their disease was serious, this was very relevant. They found in their rehabilitation programme that the most significant factors were helping patients develop a sense of control over their pain and noted that small changes in several areas of functioning had a greater impact on the probability of return to work than large change in one area.

As in all rehabilitation programmes for chronic intractable pain, one cannot expect 100% results and one should not be deterred from accepting patients on the grounds that they are likely to be failures. One cannot tell in an individual case who will succeed and who will not, and statistics are of no interest to the individual.

One thread that is common throughout all these studies, and which we have continued at both our units, is that the patient must be given permission to exercise and become fit. So much of the medical advice given to them previously has been to rest, to take things easy and to beware of reinjuring the back. They therefore come to the rehabilitation programme convinced that any effort is likely to damage their back. Time spent explaining the nature and pathology of the disease and the extreme unlikelihood that anything they do under a supervised exercise programme can cause reinjury is most important. Careful explanation of the danger of inactivity and the pathophysiological changes that occur with disuse will convince patients that they are safe to exercise. This is where the inpatient structured programme is so valuable where patients are supervised and observed throughout the day and, indeed, throughout the 24 hours, and are given a promise that nothing that they will be encouraged to do can possibly cause them injury or exacerbation of their problem. The increase in symptoms after a few days of intensive exercise is due, of course, to the effect on muscles and joints that have not been used for a very long time. Such symptoms are expected and are welcomed. We tell patients that by the end of the first week they will feel worse, by the middle of the second week they will begin to feel the improvement and by the third week they will feel a different person. It is rare that we are proved wrong.

Cairns et al (1984) described a spinal pain rehabilitation programme and compared the results of inpatient and outpatient treatment. They emphasized that chronic spinal pain does not respond to one modality only. Their outpatient programme consisted of graded walking, sitting, standing, muscle strengthening exercise, attention to posture, relief of stress and use of biofeedback and relaxation for 3 hours daily, 5 days a week for 4 weeks. At 1-year follow-up, the results were considerably better in the outpatients, presumably because much more severe cases were selected for inpatient treatment. They showed that half the inpatients maintained decrease in pain at 1-

year follow-up, 68% had maintained an increase in activity, and 50% a decrease in medication. Only two of 20 patients who could have returned to work, did so. Decrease in pain did not mean a return to work. These authors therefore showed that an intensive inpatient programme does significantly reduce disability and that this reduction is maintained at 1-year follow-up.

A new dimension was achieved when Fordyce et al (1968) introduced the technique of operant conditioning. The rationale of this pain management programme was quite different from previous programmes in that it was not concerned with reducing pain but in achieving physical activity and reducing medication. To quote Fordyce: 'behaviour is all that can be observed and measured as representative of the other's unknowable experience'. Original tissue damage may cause persistence of pain, for this is reinforced by contingencies in the patient's environment. Thus the encouragement of the spouse in learned illness behaviour is a potent factor in the maintenance of symptoms. A fear of return to work or involvement in activities which might increase the pain leads the patient to become progressively more dependent. The end result is a patient with a set of learned behaviours – inactivity at home and much display of suffering. Eventually the patient unconsciously (or rarely consciously) manipulates his family and environment to such an extent that he is the centre of attraction.

Fordyce et al (1981) showed that pain behaviour may be little if at all related to inferences about underlying noxious stimulation. In a study of 150 patients with chronic back pain who were asked to record a pain diary and to assess their pain on a 0–10 scale, it was found that there were few relationships to consumption of medication or utilization of health care. The diary recorded levels of activity or frequency of engaging in commonplace activities that were not related to recording of pain. In chronic pain a questionable relationship exists between what people say about their pain and what they actually do and therefore any assessment of pain must include analysis of the patient's behaviour.

Fordyce's revolutionary approach involves the aim of treating the behaviour consequent on pain, not the pain itself. Behavioural methods, he has pointed out repeatedly, do not have as their principal objective a modification of nociception or direct modification of experiences of pain. The aim is to improve the patient's lifestyle by increasing his activity and reducing his dependence on medication (Fordyce et al 1985). A vital component is the involvement of the family so that they understand the rationale of the programme, disregarding complaints of suffering but praising and rewarding achievements such as increased activity or reduced medication (Fordyce et al 1973, 1974, 1985, 1986). Anderson (1977) has summarized the objectives of a behavioural modification programme as follows:

> to increase physical activity to normal levels appropriate to the age and sex, to reduce or eliminate medication, to return the patient to a satisfying lifestyle with his family, to change family interactions so that these is less need to use pain to control the relationships, to eliminate the dependency on the medical profession, to change attitudes to health care and thus decrease pain complaints.

The classical method involves an inpatient programme with gradually decreasing medication using a pain cocktail in which the active ingredients are successfully reduced on a time-related and not on a demand basis. The patient is aware that medication is being reduced but does not know the rate or when the active ingredient has been entirely removed. A number of authors have reported results showing that this system certainly works with long-term effects (Cinciripini & Floreen 1982). Of 130 patients screened for the programme in Anderson's group, 60 were accepted but only 37 chose to enter and 34 were studied. At 2-year follow-up 70% were living normal lives without medication. This was assessed by the level of activity, cessation of medication and decreased use of health care. It must be remembered that patients in these groups are very severe chronic sufferers and successful rehabilitation in all cases cannot be expected. To achieve these results in even a small number of patients represents a considerable advance. Fordyce himself reported that 31 out of 36 patients has less pain, more increased activity, more time up, less medication, increased walking time and increased activity as assessed by occupational therapists and physiotherapists.

Linton (1982, 1986) reviewed the current state of the art of operant conditioning therapy and concluded that operant procedures are to be recommended for the objectives of increasing activity levels and decreasing medicine consumption and that there are now at least 30 studies reported in the literature indicating that these techniques can be successful. Linton proposes that clinicians should match treatment methods to patient needs based on a thorough analysis of the problem. The goals to be achieved should be considered after a thorough behavioural analysis and then methods selected that are known to help and are appropriate for that particular patient.

In organizing such a pain management programme the constitution of the group is all important. Results may be significantly affected by one individual with negative attitudes to treatment who may adversely affect the rest of the group. Conversely, an enthusiastic individual can often 'carry' some less motivated members of the group. Regular and careful assessment by all members of the team, particularly the nurses, is vital to spot this problem and take appropriate action. One must not forget that patients exist who want to 'beat the system', prove the doctors incapable, or prove to the team that they are incurable and deserve their life on their back at the state's expense.

Moore et al (1984) emphasize the effect of other group members in their study.

An important feature of all these operant conditioning programmes is that they are organized by the psychologists and not by the physician. Once it has been established that there is no further surgery and no further medical treatment appropriate, then the patient is urged to accept that it is his responsibility to change his lifestyle and to try to cope with the pain without having recourse to continual visits to the doctor in the vain hope of finding a new drug that will solve all his problems or a new operation which will cure his pain. It is therefore important to withdraw physician involvement and the patient must understand that he is learning to be the master of his own destiny. If the doctor continues to see the patient regularly there will always be the feeling on both sides that some form of medical intervention is still expected. Latterly a compromise has been reached in many centres in that both approaches, physical rehabilitation and behavioural modification, act concurrently.

Whilst all these inpatient programmes are expensive and labour-intensive they do hold out hope for some return of function for a significant proportion of people who have suffered severe symptoms for many years. Patient selection is all-important and the patient must be absolutely clear at the outset what his expectations are and what the goals are that he wishes to achieve. The family must be prepared to enter wholeheartedly into the regime, otherwise the programme is doomed to failure.

One of the most depressing situations for the patient with chronic back pain is to be told by his surgeon that 'there is nothing more I can do for you'. Strictly speaking this may well be true – in that there is no further surgical procedure that can help. However, the patient quite rightly interprets this to mean that nothing more can be done.

It is hoped that this chapter has indicated that there is, indeed, a great deal that can be done for such unfortunate people. At the very least they can be helped with pain-coping strategies and an exercise programme to achieve control over their life. At the best they can be restored to an active, fulfilling life – and even return to work.

It is certain that with a comprehensive, structured rehabilitation programme, using the skills of a multidisciplinary team, the lot of the chronic-back-pain sufferer needs no longer to be one of despair.

The following three case histories illustrate three typical problems encountered in rehabilitation of the failed back:

- a patient with multiple operations and no subsequent rehabilitation
- a patient with severe osteoporosis and crush fractures
- a young girl with back pain and 'functional paralysis'.

Case history: Miss S.P. (aged 52)

This lady had a very long history of intractable back pain, having had multiple operations. She had diastematomyelia of the thoracic lumbar spine. She had had six operations in all, including decompressions, discectomies, two fusions and further fusion following collapse of a T5 vertebra. When we saw her in April 1991 she was in constant pain, could walk only a few yards, could not sit for any length of time and spent her whole time at home either on the bed or in the chair. It was clear that she had totally lost confidence in herself and this was not surprising because she had never had any rehabilitation following any of the surgical procedures and she had been told by several surgeons that she should be careful, not exercise and not indulge in any vigorous activities. She was admitted to the intensive inpatient rehabilitation programme but it took 3 weeks before she was prepared to accept the advice given which was that she must undertake a progressive, structured exercise programme to build up the power of her muscles, mobilize her joints and get her generally fit. She was still convinced that this was dangerous and that her back would break if she indulged in any physical activity. We were gradually able to persuade her that the reverse was in fact the case and that it was dangerous to be inactive. We relieved some of her pain temporarily with pain-relieving injections so that it would allow her to be active in the pool and later on dry land. There were several long sessions with the consultant and with the psychologist and psychotherapist. Eventually she accepted that further surgery would be contraindicated and that the programme we had outlined was the only way that she was going to get increased function and some quality to her life. By the time she left after 8 weeks, she was walking from the ward to the gym, was up all day complaining of very little pain and had a very positive attitude. Some months later she wrote to us saying how grateful she was for the opportunity to improve her function, that she was driving her car again, she was swimming, doing her exercises regularly, going for short walks and doing all the activities in the house, including ironing. Hopefully, in these days the lessons of inactivity and lack of rehabilitation after surgery have been learned and patients will be offered a progressive structured programme to get them back to full activities as soos as possible.

Case history: Mrs M.A.B.

This lady had long-standing osteoporosis of the spine with multiple crush fractures in lower thoracic and mid-lumbar vertebrae. She developed very severe chronic mid-thoracic and upper lumbar back pain and was unable to undertake any activities around the house. She could only sleep sitting in a chair propped up with pillows and cushions and was quite unable to lie flat in bed. The situation was complicated by the fact that her husband was an amputee who was deteriorating and she found that she was having to cope with him as well as herself. We were able to persuade her to come in for an intensive structured programme and her husband was admitted at the same time for rehabilitation to see whether he could be made more mobile and change his attitude. She started with a very limited programme of gentle exercises in the pool twice a day, gradually building up to dry land exercises, increased sitting and standing time and a more intensive programme to build up the spinal muscles. On review 3 months later she was now able to lie flat and could sleep throughout the night, she was up and about, active and looking after her husband, and had virtually completely lost her pain. Such a result could not be achieved on an outpatient basis, partly for social reasons and partly because the fatigue of getting to and from the hospital department obviated the value of the treatment. In addition, an intensive progressive programme was essential in her case for she had virtually lost complete muscle activity in the whole of the thoracic and lumbar spine and, of course, had totally lost her confidence.

Case history: Miss F.M. (aged 13)

This young girl of 13 years went over the handlebars of her bicycle in June 1991. She cut her knee but seemed to recover quickly. However, she began to get pain in the knee when she returned to school and then developed severe back pain. Eventually she ended up with complete paralysis below the waist of a functional type and spent her days at home lying motionless in bed. There was generalized tenderness of the back and she was unable to get any contraction of her lower limb muscles. She was eventually transferred to the rehabilitation unit where this physical condition of total paralysis was confirmed. There was no wasting. Electrical stimulation of the femoral, lateral and medial popliteal nerves all showed strong contraction in all muscles, so a confident diagnosis of functional paralysis was made.

She complained bitterly of pain in her knee and was unable to move any of her joints. Our orthopaedic colleague carried out an examination of the knee under anaesthetic – a complete free range of movement was found. The knee was irrigated and examined with an arthroscope. The patient could then be assured that the knee was now 'clean', a full range of movement had been noted and there was now no impediment to a full functional recovery.

Gradually, with a great deal of persuasion, she was mobilized and regained full range of movement of her hips, knees and ankles and excellent muscle power. However, she remained very stiff in the back with no appreciable movement and still continuing pain.

It was decided that this was an inhibitory phenomenon and she was given a general anaesthetic and an epidural. Subsequent to this she regained full range of movement and, on last follow-up, she was living a full, active life.

Apart from the progressive, structured rehabilitation programme, the most useful contribution came from the psychotherapist who was able to unravel a lot of emotional problems within the family and ongoing family therapy was instituted with good effect.

This case, which is not at all unique, illustrates the fundamental importance of combining a progressive, structured rehabilitation programme with an attention to psychological and emotional underlying factors and treating them accordingly.

The multidisciplinary team approach is vital to the success in such cases. The total overall treatment time was 3 months.

REFERENCES

Albe Fessard D, Lombard M C 1983 Use of an animal model to evaluate the origin of and protection against deafferentation pain. Advances in pain research and therapy, vol 5. Raven Press, New York, p 691–700

Anderson T P 1977 Behavioural modification of chronic Pain. Clinical Orthopaedics and Related Research 129: 96–101

Beals R K, Hickman N W 1972 Industrial injuries of the back and extremity. Journal of Bone and Joint Surgery 54A: 1593–1611

Burton C V 1983 Aetiology of the failed back syndrome. In: Carthen J C (ed) Lumbar spine surgery - indications, techniques, failures and alternatives. Williams & Wilkins, Baltimore, p 190–203

Cairns D, Mooney V, Crane P 1984 Spinal pain rehabilitation: in-patient and out-patient treatment results and development of predictors for outcome. Spine 9: 91–95

Cady L D, Bischoff D P, O'Connell E R, Thomas P C, Allen J H 1979 Strength and fitness and subsequent back injuries in fire fighters. Journal of Occupational Medicine 21: 269–272

Chaffin D B 1974 Human strength capability and low back pain. Journal of Occupational Medicine 16: 248–254

Cinciripini P M, Floreen A 1982 An evaluation of a behavioural programme for chronic pain. Journal of Behavioural Medicine 5: 375–389

Coan R M, Wong G, Su Lianaku et al 1980 The acupuncture treatment of low back pain. A randomised control study. American Journal of Clinical Medicine 8: 181–189

Deardorff W W, Rubin M S, Scott D W 1991 Comprehensive multidisciplinary treatment of chronic pain – a follow up study of treated and non-treated groups. Pain 45: 35–43

Donovan W H, Dwyer A P, White B W S et al A multidisciplinary approach to chronic low back pain in Western Australia. Spine 6: 591–597

Dooley J F, McBroom J, Taquchi T, MacNab I 1988 Nerve root infiltration in the diagnosis of muscular pain. Spine 13: 79–83

Finnegan W J, Fenlin J M, Marvel J P, Nardini R D, Rothman R H 1979 Results of surgical intervention in the symptomatic multiplyoperated back patient. Journal of Bone and Joint Surgery 61A: 1077–1082

Flor H, Turk D C 1988 Chronic back pain and rheumatoid arthritis predicting pain and disability from cognitive variables. Journal of Behavioral Medicine 11: 251–265

Fordyce W E 1974 Treating chronic pain by contingency management. Advances in Neurology 4: 583–589

Fordyce W E 1986 Behavioural methods for chronic pain and illness. C V Mosby, St Louis

Fordyce W E, Fowler R S, DeLateur B 1968 An application of behaviour modification technique to a problem of chronic pain. Behaviour Research and Therapy 6: 105–106

Fordyce W E, Fowler R S, Lehmann J F, DeLateur B J, Sand P L, Trieschmann R B 1973 Operant conditioning in the treatment of chronic pain. Archives of Physical Medicine and Rehabilitation 54: 399–408

Fordyce W E, McMahon G, Rainwater S et al 1981 Pain complaint – exercise performance relationship in chronic pain. Pain 10: 311–321

Fordyce W E, Roberts A H, Sternbach R A 1985 The behavioural management of chronic pain. A response to critics. Pain 22: 113–125

Friedenberg Z B, Shoemaker R C 1954 The results of non-operative treatment of ruptured lumbar discs. American Journal of Surgery 86: 933–935

Gallagher R M, Rauh V, Haugh L D et al 1989 Determinants of return to work among old back patients. Pain 39: 55–67

Getty C J M 1980 Lumbar spinal stenosis. The clinical spectrum and the results of operations. Journal of Bone and Joint Surgery 62B: 481–485

Getty C J M, Johnson J R, Kirwan E O'G, Sullivan M F 1981 Partial undercutting facetectomy for bony entrapment of the lumbar nerve root. Journal of Bone and Joint Surgery 63B: 330–335

Gottlieb H J, Koller R, Alperson B L 1982 Low back pain comprehensive rehabilitation program: a follow-up study. Archives of Physical Medicine and Rehabilitation 63: 458–461

Graham Smith A 1990 'Failed back surgery syndrome.' Florida Orthopedic Journal (in press)

Green L N 1975 Dexamethasone in management of symptoms due to herniated lumbar disc. Journal of Neurology, Neurosurgery and Psychiatry 38: 1211–1221

Guck T P, Skultety F M, Meilman P W, Dowd E T 1985 Multidisciplinary pain center follow-up study: evaluation with a no-treatment control group. Pain 21: 295–306

Hakelius A 1970 Prognosis in sciatica. Acta Orthopaedia Scandinavica (suppl) 129: 1076

Helbig I T, Lee C K 1988 The lumbar facet syndrome. Spine 13: 61–64

Holm S, Nachemson A 1983 Variations in the nutrition of the canine intervertebral disc induced by motion. Spine 8: 866–874

Howe J F, Loeser J D, Calvin W H, 1977 Mechano-sensibility of dorsal root ganglia and from focal nerve injuries. Brain Research 116: 139

Hsu K Y, Zucherman J, White A, Reynolds J, Goldthwaite N 1988 Deterioration of motion segments adjacent to lumbar spine fusions (abstracts). International Society for the Study of the Lumbar Spine, Miami, Florida

Keefe F J, Hill R W 1985 An objective approach to quantifying pain behaviour and gait patterns in low back pain patients and controls. Pain 21: 153–161

Kircaldy-Willis W H, Pain K W E, Canchoix J, McIvor G 1974 Lumbar spinal stenosis. Clinical Orthopaedics 99: 30–50

Kircaldy-Willis W H, Wedge J H, Yong Hing A 1982 Lumbar spine nerve lateral entrapment. Clinical Orthopaedics 169: 171–178

Krainick J V, Thoden V 1984 Dorsal column stimulation. In: Wall P D, Melzack R (eds) Textbook of pain, 1st edn. Churchill Livingstone, Edinburgh, p 701–715

Leavitt F, Sweet J Z 1986 Characteristics and frequency of malignancy among patients with low back pain. Pain 25: 357–364

Leavitt F, Garron D C, D'Angelo C M, McNeill T W 1979 Low back pain in patients with and without demonstrable organic disease. Pain 6: 191–200

Lehman T R, Russell D W, Spralt K F et al 1986 Efficacy of electroacupuncture and TENS in the rehabilitation of chronic low back pain patients. Pain 26: 277–290

Leibrock L G, Mellman P, Cuka D 1984 Spinal cord stimulation in the treatment of chronic back pain and lower extremity pain syndromes. Nebraska Medical Journal 69: 180–183

Leyshon A, Kirwan E O, Wynn Parry C B 1981 Electrical studies in the diagnosis of compression of the lumbar root. Journal of Bone and Joint Surgery 63B: 51–75

Linton S J 1982 A critical review of behavioural treatments for chronic benign pain other than headache. British Journal of Clinical Psychology 21: 321–337

Linton S J 1986 Behavioural remediation of chronic pain. A status report. Pain 24: 125–141

Linton S J, Bradley L A, Jenson I, Sprangfort E, Sundell L 1989 The secondary prevention of low back pain - a controlled study with follow up. Pain 36: 197–207

Lora J, Long D 1976 Facet denervation in the management of intractable back pain. Spine 1: 121

Macnab I, McBroom R J, Parrott T 1987 Unilateral root decompression in lumbar spinal stenosis (abstract). International Society for the Study of the Lumbar Spine, Rome, Italy

Malec J, Cayner J J, Harvey R F 1981 Pain management: long-term follow up of an inpatient program. Archives of Physical Medicine and Rehabilitation 62: 362–372

Manniche C, Lundberg E, Christensen I, Bentzen L, Hasselsoe G 1991 Intensive dynamic back exercises for chronic low back pain. A clinical trial. Pain 47: 53–63

Marks R 1989 Distribution of pain provoked from lumbar facet joints and related structures during diagnostic spinal infiltration. Pain 39: 37–40

Marks R C, Houston T, Thulbourne T 1992 Facet joint injection and facet nerve block. A randomised comparison in 86 patients with chronic low back pain. Pain 49: 325–328

Maruta T, Swanson D W, Swenson W M 1979 Chronic pain. What patients may pain management programmes help. Pain 7: 321–329

Mayer T G, Gatchel J, Kishiono N et al 1985 Objective assessment of spine function following industrial injury. A prospective study with comparison group and one year follow up. Spine 10: 482–493

Mehta M, Wynn Parry C B 1992 Mechanical back pain and the facet joint syndrome. International Disability Studies (in press)

Melzack R 1975 Prolonged relief of pain by brief intense transcutaneous somatic stimulation. Pain 1: 357–374

Melzack R, Wall P D 1965 Pain mechanisms – a new theory. Science 150: 971–979

Mooney V 1989a Where is the lumbar pain coming from? Annals of Medicine 21: 373–379

Mooney V 1989b A randomised double blind prospective study of the efficacy of electromagnetic fields for interbody fusion. Fourth Annual Meeting North American Spinal Society

Moore M E, Berk S N, Nyparer A 1984 Chronic pain in-patient treatment with small group effects. Archives of Physical Medicine and Rehabilitation 65: 516

Nachemson A 1976 A critical look at conservative treatment for low back pain. In: Jayson M (ed) The lumbar spine and back pain. Sector Publishing, London

Nachemson A 1982 The natural course of low back pain. In: White A A, Gordon S L (eds) Symposium on idiopathic low back pain. C V Mosby, St Louis, p 46–51

Porter R W, Hibbert C, Evans C 1984 The natural history of root entrapment syndrome. Spine 7: 374–389

Redmond J 1989 Functional restoration with behavioural support. A one year prospective study of patients with low back pain. Part 1. Scandinavian Journal of Rehabilitation Medicine 26: 81–89

Richardson P H, Vincent C A 1986 Acupuncture for the treatment of pain. A review of evaluative research. Pain 24: 15–40

Roberts A H, Reinhardt L 1980 The behavioural management of chronic pain. Long-term follow up with comparison groups. Pain 8: 151–162

Rosomoff H L, Green C, Silbert M, Steele R 1981 Pain and low back rehabilitation program at the University of Miami School of Medicine. In: Ng L K Y (ed) New approaches to treatment of chronic pain: a review of multidisciplinary pain clinics and centers. National Institute of Drug Abuse, New York, p 92–111

Saal J A, Saal J S 1989 Non operative treatment of herniated lumbar intervertebral disc with radiculopathy. An outcome study. Spine 14: 431–437

Selecki B P, Ness T D, Limbers P, Blum P W, Stening W A 1975 The surgical management of low back and sciatic syndrome in disc disease or injury: results of a joint neurosurgical and orthopaedic project. Australian and New Zealand Journal of Surgery 45: 183–191

Shannon N, Paul E A 1979 L4/5 and L5/S1 disc protrusion – analysis of 323 cases operated on over 12 years. Journal of Neurology, Neurosurgery and Psychiatry 42: 804–809

Silvers H R 1990 Lumbar pencutaneous facet rhizotomy. Spine 15: 36–40

Sjolund B 1988 'TENS for low back problems.' Report of the Intractable Pain Society of Great Britain and Ireland, Basingstoke, April 1988

Trief P M 1983 Chronic back pain. A tripartite model of outcome. Archives of Physical Medicine and Rehabilitation 64: 53–56

Turk D C, Flor H 1984 Etiological theories and treatments for chronic back pain. Psychological models and interventions. Pain 19: 209–234

Waddell G 1982 An approach to backache. British Journal of Hospital Medicine 28: 187–219

Waddell G, McCulloch J A, Kummel E G, Venner R M 1980 Non organic signs in low back pain. Spine 5: 117–125

Waddell G, Pilowsky I, Bond M R 1989 Clinical assessment and interpretation of abnormal illness behaviour in low back pain. Pain 39: 41–54

Wall P D, Devor M 1978 Physiology of sensation after peripheral nerve injury regeneration and neuroma formation. In: Waxman S G (ed) Physiology and pathology of axons. Raven Press, New York

Wall P D, Devor M 1981 The effect of peripheral nerve injury on dorsal root potentials and on transmission of afferent signals into the spinal cord. Brain Research 209: 95–111

Wall P D, Gutnik M 1974 Properties of afferent nerve impulses originating from a neuroma. Nature (London) 248: 740–743

Watkins R G, O'Brien J P, Dyangelis R, Jones D 1986 Comparison of preoperative and postoperative MMPI data in chronic back patients. Spine 11: 385–390

Weber J 1983 Lumbar disc herniation. A controlled prospective study with 10 years of observation. Spine 8: 131–140

Withrington R W, Wynn Parry C B 1985 Rehabilitation of conversion paralysis. Journal of Bone and Joint Surgery 67B: 635–637

Wynn Parry C B, Girgis F 1988 The assessment and management of the failed back, Part II. International Disability Studies 10: 25–28

Young A, Wynn Parry C B 1988 The assessment and management of the failed back. International Disability Studies 10: 21–23

58. Orthopaedic surgery

Robert F. McLain and James N. Weinstein

INTRODUCTION

The orthopaedist is called on to treat a wide variety of musculoskeletal disorders, among which pain is often the common denominator. These disorders are exceptionally diverse in nature, arising out of neoplastic, inflammatory, developmental, metabolic or traumatic conditions, and so are the mechanisms by which they produce pain. Pain is the symptom that most often drives the patient to seek treatment; it is, however, a nonspecific symptom and provides little insight, by itself, as to the serious or benign nature of the underlying malady. Whether the pain source is a life-threatening tumour or an ankle sprain, one of the patient's key concerns is the alleviation of pain; it is, therefore, the physician's responsibility to formulate a plan that offers the best treatment of the underlying disease while effectively limiting or eliminating the symptom of pain.

When the physician encounters the patient complaining of musculoskeletal pain, his initial task is to identify the true nature of the patient's problem: is the pain severe and debilitating in and of itself or does it simply trigger the patient's fear of a possible malignant cause? Is it a manifestation of underlying psychological turmoil or is it physiologically normal pain interfering with an active, functional patient? The next task is to seek out the source and cause of the pain, if possible, and to exclude the possibility of an underlying systemic or malignant process that may threaten the patient's life. Finally, the orthopaedic surgeon reviews the treatment options and formulates a treatment plan suited to the individual patient and the specific disorder. The physician's objectives in treating the orthopaedic patient are to reduce the patient's pain, to correct the underlying musculoskeletal disorder and to improve overall function, and he or she may take advantage of a wide variety of modalities to accomplish these goals.

MECHANISMS OF MUSCULOSKELETAL PAIN

The musculoskeletal system consists of the bones and articulations of the skeleton and the ligaments, muscles and tendons that connect and mobilize them. The system is made up of diverse tissues with radically different characteristics. Injuries or disorders of the musculoskeletal system may directly affect muscle, bone, tendon, ligament, articular cartilage, periosteum, synovium or articular capsule and may directly or indirectly affect the overlying integument, the indwelling haematopoietic tissues or neural elements associated with or contained within the skeletal framework. These tissues are richly innervated by a variety of neural receptors (transducers) that inform, modulate and coordinate their individual and collective musculoskeletal functions.

JOINT PAIN

The articulations of the appendicular skeleton are specialized to bear loads and allow motion through specific, proscribed arcs of excursion. In the extremities, and in the posterior elements of the spine, these are synovial joints. The components of these joints are specialized to meet specific demands of function: articular cartilage absorbs and distributes loads; subchondral bone resists deformation and supports and nourishes the cartilage; ligaments maintain alignment and constrain joint excursion; musculotendinous units flex, extend and stabilize the joint. Derangement of the joint may result in destruction of the articular cartilage, fracture of the subchondral bone, attenuation or disruption of the ligaments and excessive strains and inflammation of the muscles. Nerve endings in these or other tissues may signal the presence of ongoing or incipient tissue damage, producing the sensation of pain.

Synovial joints enjoy a dual pattern of innervation: *primary articular nerves* are independent branches from larger peripheral nerves, which specifically supply the joint capsule and ligaments; *accessory articular nerves* reach the joint after passing through muscular or cutaneous tissues to which they provide primary innervation (Wyke 1972). These muscular tissues may overlie or run adjacent to the joint in question and the musculotendinous insertion often ramifies with connective tissues of the joint capsule, allowing intramuscular nerves embedded in the intrafascicular connective tissue to extend branches that reach the joint (Gardner 1944, 1948). Both primary and accessory articular nerves are mixed afferent nerves, containing proprioceptive and nociceptive fibres. These fibres supply innervation to virtually all of the periarticular soft tissues, though some structures are more heavily innervated than others.

Freeman & Wyke have described four basic types of afferent nerve endings in articular tissues and have documented the presence of those endings in a wide variety of joints (Freeman & Wyke 1967). While the type 4 receptors (free nerve endings) are the only ones thought to be exclusively nociceptive, it is known that the proprioceptive endings of groups 1–3 are capable of responding to excessive joint excursion as a noxious stimulus and that they play an important role in mediating protective muscular reflexes that maintain joint stability (Palmer 1958; Eckholm et al 1960). Deandrade and Kennedy have both demonstrated that the presence of a joint effusion, a common finding in patients with inflammatory, traumatic or degenerative joint disease, can produce significant reflex inhibition of the quadriceps mechanism (Deandrade et al 1965; Kennedy et al 1982). Histological studies have demonstrated receptors in ligaments (Gardner 1948; O'Connor & Gonzales 1979; DeAvila et al 1989, capsule (Freeman & Wyke 1967; Grigg et al 1982) and meniscal tissues (O'Connor & McConnaughey 1978), as well as periarticular fat and muscle (Freeman & Wyke 1967; Dee 1978). Giles & Harvey have demonstrated nociceptive free nerve endings in capsular tissue from human facets and reported similar endings in the apophyseal synovium (Giles & Harvey 1987). These nociceptive endings are supplied by small myelinated type 3 nerve fibres and small unmyelinated type 4 fibres.

While capsule, fat and muscle are richly supplied with nociceptive free nerve endings, investigators have previously reported a relative paucity of these receptors in the synovium, ligaments and menisci. In most situations the neural impulses that signal joint pain have been thought to be generated by receptors in surrounding the joint and not by the tissues directly exposed to mechanical stresses or trauma. The stimuli that these periarticular receptors respond to may be either mechanical (capsular distension, ligamentous instability, direct trauma) or chemical (Wyke 1981).

The role of the synovium in producing and releasing kinins, prostaglandins and other chemical irritants has been suggested to explain why joints with synovitis are frequently painful, even though the synovium has long been thought to have few receptors. However, it now appears that the synovial tissues may produce joint pain by both direct and indirect mechanisms. Using antisera against specific neuronal markers, investigators reexamining synovial innervation have found vastly greater numbers of small-diameter nerve fibres than were previously reported using standard histological methods (Gronblad et al 1988, 1991; Weinstein et al 1988a; Kidd et al 1990). Nearly all of these fibres have been immunoreactive for vasoactive and pain-related neuropeptides. Substance P (sP) has been shown to accumulate in articular fluid following capsaicin injection and is known to produce plasma extravasation and vasodilatation (Yaksh 1988; Lam & Ferrell 1989, 1991). Levels of sP are higher in joints with more severe arthritis and infusion of the neuropeptide into joints with mild disease has been shown to accelerate the degenerative process (Levine et al 1984). Calcitonin-gene-related peptide (CGRP) has also been implicated as a mediator in the early stages of arthritis (Konttinen et al 1990). Whether sP plays a direct role in the stimulation or sensitization of intraarticular pain receptors is not established, but sensitization is important and several mechanisms have been confirmed experimentally. Grigg et al have shown that the induction of experimental arthritis results in sensitization of free nerve endings in the joint capsule (Grigg et al 1986). When acute inflammation is induced, afferent receptors which are normally silent during joint motion become responsive to previously innocuous stimuli, including motion in the normal range. A similar sensitizing effect is produced by intraarticular infusion of prostaglandins or bradykinin (Schaible et al 1987; Neugebauer et al 1989), providing further evidence that local sensitization is at least partly responsible for the pain felt in arthritic or inflamed joints. There is also strong evidence of a central nervous system component in sensitizing spinal cord neurons that receive input from these joint afferents, a means of further amplifying the nociceptive discharges from the joint (Neugebauer & Schaible 1990).

BONE AND PERIOSTEUM

Bone is a dynamic composite tissue involved in a variety of physiological processes and capable of a number of biological responses to injury or stress. It is the one tissue in the body able to repair itself after injury without forming scar. It responds to minute pizo-electric currents generated by stresses by increasing its mass in areas of increased load and by removing support from areas seeing little load. It is sensitive to pressure internally and to direct injury externally.

The external covering of the bone is the periosteum. This tough fibrous sheath adheres to the outer cortex of the bone and contains the pluripotent mesenchymal cells necessary for bone growth and fracture healing. The periosteum is highly vascular and copiously supplied with both free nerve endings and encapsulated endings; the complex free nerve endings are thought to generate painful discharges, while the encapsulated endings are thought to be sensitive to pressure (Ralston et al 1960; Cooper 1968). In periosteal tissue, Hill and others have documented the presence of nerves immunoreactive to a wide variety of pain-related and vasoactive neuropeptides (Hill & Elde 1991). Gronblad et al have demonstrated an extensive ramification of sP-reactive nerve fibres in both the superficial and deep layers of the periosteal sheath (Gronblad et al 1984). They also reported the presence of sP immunoreactivity in some encapsulated, glomerular-type receptors from the same tissue. Encapsulated sP-reactive nerve endings have previously been reported in the posterior longitudinal ligament of the spine, implicating that structure as a source of low back pain (Liesi et al 1983).

Bjurholm et al have demonstrated both sP- and CGRP-containing nerves in the marrow, periosteum and cortex of long bones, as well as the associated muscles and ligaments (Bjurholm et al 1988a). They noted a higher density of sP- and CGRP-immunoreactive fibres in epiphyseal rather than diaphyseal marrow and saw that some fibres from the abundantly innervated periosteum penetrated the cortex and entered the marrow space by way of the Volkmann's canals. These two neuropeptides, sP and CGRP, have been associated with nociceptor transmission (Skofitsch & Jacobowitz 1985; Badalamente et al 1987) as well as an acceleration of experimental arthritis and an increase in its severity following local infusion (Colpaert et al 1983; Levine et al 1984).

Vasoactive intestinal peptide (VIP), and a number of other vasoactive neuropeptides, have also been localized to fine nerve fibres predominantly found in cancellous bone of the epiphysis and in the periosteum (Bjurholm et al 1988b). The vasodilatory effect of VIP has been clearly demonstrated (Said & Mutt 1970), while neuropeptide Y (NPY) has been shown to be a powerful vasoconstrictor (Lundberg et al 1982). Fibres containing these neuropeptides tend to congregate at the osteochondral junction of the epiphyseal plate, with VIP fibres running in the marrow spaces while NPY fibres follow the small vessels nourishing the epiphysis. Although the primary role of these peptides is likely to be related to the regulation of growth, it is possible that these or similar peptides might also play a role in the production or prevention of intraosseous hypertension, a proposed cause of bone and joint pain.

As a result, bone is a tissue capable of responding to both internal and external pressure changes, physical distortion, inflammation and periosteal injury by transmitting pain signals proximally. Bone pain may be produced by microfracture and subsidence in osteoarthritis, by periosteal elevation and disortion in infection or tumour, by vascular congestion and infarction in sickle-cell crisis and by mechanical disruption in fractures and other traumatic conditions.

MUSCULOTENDINOUS PAIN

The nociceptive innervation of muscle has been discussed previously (Ch. 1). The primary nociceptive endings in muscle are unencapsulated free nerve endings similar to those seen in periarticular tissues, which transmit their impulses centrally by way of type III and IV afferent fibres. Intramuscular mechanoreceptors may also produce pain impulses when exposed to noxious stimuli. Muscular pain receptors may be either chemonociceptive or mechanonociceptive and may respond to stimuli as either specific or poly-modal receptors. Chemonociceptive endings may respond to metabolites that accumulate during anaerobic metabolism, to products of cell injury produced by trauma or ischaemia or to chemical irritants such as bradykinin, serotonin or potassium. Mechanonociceptive units may respond to stretch, pressure or disruption. Some receptors may also respond to thermal stimuli (Kumazawa & Mitzumura 1977; Mense & Schmidt 1977). Recent studies have demonstrated that intramuscular injection of CGRP in combination with either sP or neurokinin A elicits a significant pain sensation though, when injected alone, none of the neuropeptides produces muscular pain (Pedersen-Bjergaard et al 1989, 1991). It is thought that the neurogenic inflammatory response produced by CGRP, which results in persistent vasodilatation, erythema and oedema formation, may also serve to sensitize nociceptors to the presence of other pain-related neuropeptides (Piotrowski & Foreman 1986; Fuller et al 1987). This receptor sensitization, as well as the increase in intramuscular blood flow and interstitial oedema, may represent a primary mechanism of muscular pain.

Muscular pain may be the result of a direct injury, such as a blow or puncture, which disrupts or damages the muscle tissue and its intrafascicular nerve fibres, or the distension and pressure produced by the ensuing haematoma and oedema. Pain also results from indirect trauma, such as athletic injuries, where the muscle is torn or ruptured as it strains against an excessive resistance force. Inflammation and oedema, components of the normal healing process, play a role in the mediation of pain symptoms. In major musculoskeletal injuries persistent spasm may occur, resulting in severe muscle pain as well as further trauma to the muscle and other tissues of the soft-tissue envelope.

A more ominous type of muscle pain occurs when excessive pressure in or around the muscle results in ischaemia. Compartment syndromes occur in patients with bleeding disorders, vascular injuries, musculoskeletal trauma, systemic infections and can result from constrictive dressings or casts. They are also a common finding in patients with stroke, intoxication, metabolic disorders or head injuries; patients with these conditions are often 'found down' and have lain in one position for so long that the blood supply to an extremity has been compromized. Pain in compartment syndrome is severe and unremitting and out of proportion to the injury sustained. The clinical condition mimics the symptoms produced by experimental tourniquet pain and it is likely that the pathophysiology of the two conditions is the same (Smith et al 1968; Sternbach et al 1974). Like tourniquet pain, compartment syndrome pain is progressive in intensity and rapidly resolves if pressure is released in a timely fashion, either by removing the constricting dressing or by performing a surgical release of the compartmental fascia (Matsen 1975; Mubarak & Owen 1977).

NEURAL ELEMENTS

Nerves are subject to injury and irritation as they pass through the muscular compartments and around the bony articulations of the extremities. Several recent studies have shown that environmental stimuli can produce histological changes in dorsal root ganglion neurons similar to those seen following injury and can induce marked changes in the levels of pain-related neuropeptides contained within the ganglion (Weinstein 1986; Weinstein et al 1988; McLain & Weinstein 1991, 1992). Compression and injury to the spinal nerves and dorsal root ganglion are discussed in detail in Chapters, 40 and 55.

TREATMENT MODALITIES – PRINCIPLES AND APPLICATION

The goals of orthopaedic treatment are to reduce pain, correct deformity and to improve function. To accomplish these goals the surgeon may employ any of a number of different treatment modalities, both surgical and nonsurgical. These modalities can be roughly segregated into four different levels:

1. Immobilization
2. Fusion
3. Resection
4. Reconstruction.

In addition, the orthopaedist routinely uses a number of tools available to the primary care physician – injections, physical therapy, nonsteroidal antiinflammatory medications and oral analgesics – to supplement or augment the pain relief provided by these modalities.

IMMOBILIZATION

The immobilization of injured extremities and joints is among the oldest and most effective means of controlling musculoskeletal pain. Archaic splints have been discovered among the burial trappings of Egyptian mummies and are described throughout medieval writings (Colton 1992). In modern orthopaedic care the splint is only the simplest of the many forms of immobilization available to the patient.

Immobilization of an injured extremity can be accomplished by either direct or indirect means, using internal splints, external splints or traction. Splinting effectively reduces pain in both soft-tissue and bony trauma, inflammatory conditions, infections of the soft tissues or joints, joint instability, intraarticular derangements and a variety of other musculoskeletal conditions. By preventing joint excursion, muscle contraction and displacement of bony fractures, splinting insures appropriate immobilization and enforces rest on the injured tissues, eliminating many of the stimuli that trigger local nociceptors.

In the fractured limb, pain is initially produced by the distortion or disruption of intramedullary nerve fibres and receptors in the broken bone, by stretched or disrupted receptors in the torn periosteum and by injury or pressure on receptors in the muscle and soft tissue overlying the fracture (Fig. 58.1). A haematoma rapidly accumulates and expands until the pressure within the compartment is significantly elevated; distension of the fascia and soft tissue triggers further pain receptors. Damaged tissues release bradykinin, histamine, potassium and neurotransmitters which sensitize local nociceptors, alter vascular permeability and mediate the influx of inflammatory cells. The result is oedema, inflammation and irritation of the injured muscle, triggering muscle spasms and involuntary contractions. This produces further tissue damage and increasing deformity, as well as uncontrolled pain. In a patient with multiple fractures this may lead to life-

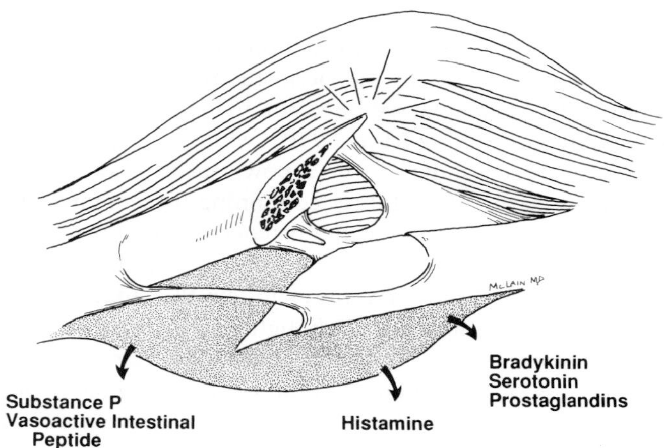

Fig. 58.1 Pain in musculoskeletal trauma. Fractures, dislocations and sprains elicit pain through a variety of interrelated and independent mechanisms which act locally and systemically to generate and mediate the pain sensation: fine nerve endings in the cancellous bone and periosteal lining are triggered by the physical disruption of the bone and the tearing and stretching of the periosteum; nerve endings in the surrounding muscle and soft tissue may be damaged directly or subjected to pressure or stretch by the displaced fracture fragments or the expanding haematoma; inflamed muscle may be triggered to spasm, producing pain and further distortion of tissues; damaged cells, nerve endings and inflammatory cells elaborate a variety of neurochemical mediators, including neuropeptides, algesic chemicals and inflammatory components.

threatening haemorrhage and systemic shock (Chapman 1989). A variety of splinting techniques may be needed to manage such a patient through the course from initial resuscitation to definitive fixation (Fig. 58.2). External splints are the simplest of orthopaedic interventions, yet provide satisfactory treatment for injuries ranging from ligamentous sprains to long-bone fractures. By preventing motion, the splint reduces the stimulation of nociceptors in injured tissues and reduces tension on irritated muscles, reducing spasm and promoting rest.

In conditions of joint inflammation, haemarthrosis or pyarthrosis, pain is produced by the distension of the joint capsule. Chemical pain mediators which sensitize receptors in the fat pads and joint capsule directly stimulate chemonociceptors (Heppelmann et al 1985, 1986). Irritation of the synovium results in secondary oedema, synovial hypertrophy and an effusion, which stretch and distort the capsule. Any motion of the joint serves to increase the tension on the capsule and mechanically distorts the inflamed tissues, resulting in increased pain. What is ordinarily benign movement is now extremely painful. Joint motion in this inflammed state causes further release of noxious neuropeptides, kinins and inflammatory agents which act to stimulate receptors in the capsule and surrounding periosteum. Inflammation results in the appearance or increase in spontaneous activity in fine joint afferents and an increase in sensitivity to movement (Schaible & Schmidt 1985). By immobilizing the joint in a splint, these mechanisms can be attenuated. An appropriately applied splint will control joint motion while healing occurs and, by immobilizing the irritated tissues, can be instrumental in treating soft tissue inflammation such as occurs in tendonitis. The period of immobilization depends not only on pain and swelling, but also on the aetiology of the problem as well as the specific tissues involved. Bony injuries heal well with rigid immobilization, while ligamentous injuries often heal better with early motion despite pain.

Traction has long been recognized as an effective means of obtaining and maintaining a reduction in fractures of long bones (Charnley 1961a). By applying persistent longitudinal traction, muscle spasm can often be overcome and bony alignment restored. This prevents further tissue damage and reduces pain caused by distortion of soft-

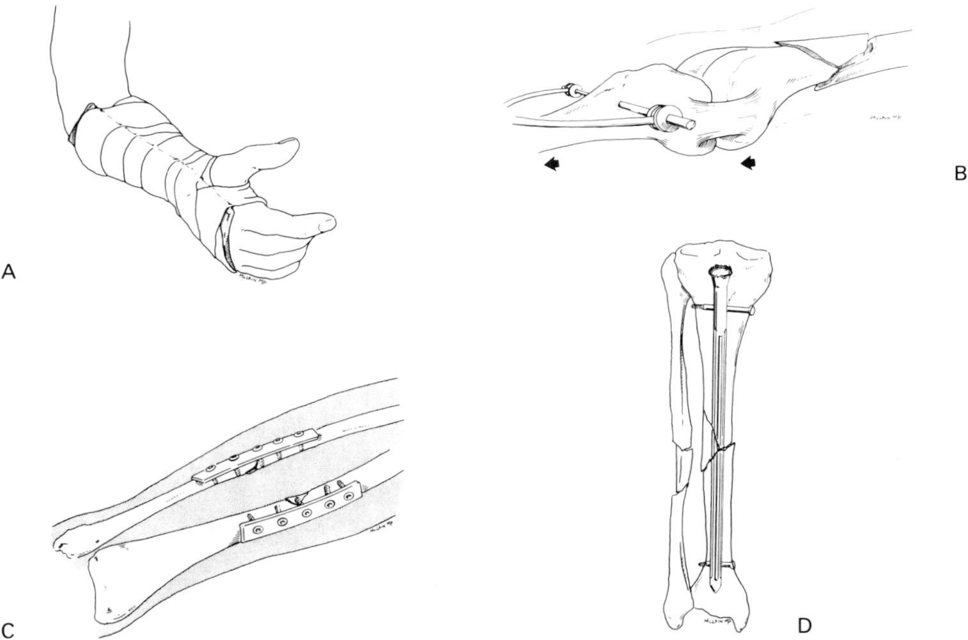

Fig. 58.2 Immobilization of musculoskeletal injuries: methods of immobilizing injured limbs range from passive, noninvasive techniques to sophisticated methods of internal fixation. **A**. Splint immobilization can be applied to any extremity. The external splint is easy to apply, prevents excessive motion of joints and stabilizes soft tissues and allows the patient to return to limited function. **B**. Skeletal traction is applied primarily in fractures of the femur, but can be used in any long-bone fracture. The longitudinal traction overcomes powerful muscle spasm and controls alignment in injuries which cannot be splinted. **C**. Internal fixation, using plates and screws, allows the surgeon to reduce anatomically the fracture fragments and rigidly fix the fracture. This assures the best possible result in terms of alignment, joint congruency and anatomical relationships and also permits the patient to start range of motion exercises before the fracture has healed. **D**. Intramedullary fixation restores alignment without exposing the fractures site, thereby reducing the risk of infection. By sharing the load applied to the limb, the intramedullary device minimizes the risk of nonunion and allows early mobilization.

tissues and movement of the ends of the fractured bone. Once the muscle fatigues and the spasm is overcome, muscle pain quickly subsides. Traction is typically used by emergency personnel for the transport of injured patients or as temporary treatment prior to casting or internal fixation. In patients who cannot tolerate surgery, skeletal traction remains a viable method of treating fractures. The complications of traction and prolonged immobilization (deep venous thrombosis, pulmonary embolus, pneumonia, infection) must be weighed against the risk of operative treatment or the disability associated with a poorly aligned fracture should neither traction nor surgery be employed.

Internal fixation or 'internal splintage' provides all the benefits of fracture reduction, tissue immobilization and protection from additional injury, but offers the additional benefit of early functional return. Because the bone is fixed internally, the adjacent joints can be left free for early range of motion. This reduces the complications of joint stiffness, muscular adhesions and atrophy which commonly accompany treatment with external casts, splints or traction. Rigid fixation of fractures eliminates motion at the injured bone ends and hence the pain caused by the abrading fracture surfaces. Immobilization limits the extent of subsequent muscle and periosteal damage, reducing the quantity of noxious metabolites, kinins and debris produced at the site of injury.

Depending on the location and the comminution of a fracture the surgeon may elect to stabilize it using either plates and screws or an intramedullary device. In applying a plate to the fracture the surgeon opens the fracture site and reduces the fragments under direct vision. The plate is then applied so that it compresses the fracture fragments and promotes healing. Additional screws may be used to reduce and fix additional fragments which have broken off from the main segments of bone (Fig. 58.2). In this way complex fractures may be fixed rigidly enough to allow beneficial early motion of the adjacent joints and active movement of the muscles and tendons overlying the injury. This is particularly important in fractures of the upper extremity where malalignments are poorly tolerated and joint and muscle contractures result in persistent pain and permanent disability. In fractures of the forearm, for instance, cast treatment requires prolonged immobilization of the elbow, the wrist and the hand; this form of treatment is rarely adequate to control the position of the broken bones. The result is stiffness and pain in the joints, adhesions of the finger flexor muscles and loss of forearm rotation because of bony malalignment. Rehabilitation may be prolonged and painful and the patient's final function is often compromized. Open reduction and internal fixation of this injury is universally recommended; the patient is able to begin elbow motion the day after surgery and begins active finger motion and grip within a few days. Range of motion is restored to nearly normal and pain is a rare complication.

Intramedullary fixation of long bone fractures has become the standard of care in most trauma centres around the world. The technique involves opening a portal into the medullary canal at a site remote to the actual fracture. A rod is then passed down the medullary canal, across the fracture, and into the canal of the far fragment. Locking screws can be placed proximally and distally to control shortening and rotation (Küntscher 1968; Winquist & Hanson 1978). The use of intramedullary rods has two advantages over plate fixation. First, the surgeon does not have to open the fracture site to fix the fracture, thus reducing the risk of infection. Second, the device allows the natural forces of gravity and muscle contraction to compress the fracture, stimulating the healing process. Intramedullary fixation is most commonly used in femur fractures, but can be applied to injuries of the tibia, humerus and ulna as well (Fig. 58.3).

Specialized fixation devices have been developed for fractures which have proven to be particularly difficult to treat by conservative means. Hip fractures, for example, are common injuries among elderly patients. In 1931 Smith-Peterson demonstrated a reduction in mortality from 75 to 25% and an increase in union rate from 30–70% when femoral neck fractures were internally fixed (Smith-Peterson et al 1931). Intertrochanteric hip fractures are particularly serious injuries, and even as late as 1966, Horowitz reported a 35% mortality rate in patients treated nonoperatively (Horowitz 1966). In more than half of the patients that survive, the residual pain, deformity, prolonged recumbency and high rate of nonunion result in a significant loss of independence. For this reason, open treatment of intertrochanteric fractures is the treatment of choice for most patients. Although a number of devices have been developed to address the unique anatomy of the proximal femur, since the mid 1970s the sliding hip screw and side plate have been the gold standard for internal fixation (Fig. 58.4). The biomechanical principles of this fixation system allow the patient to bear weight on the injured limb immediately postoperatively, permitting rehabilitation of muscles and avoiding recumbency and contractures. Failure rates have been reduced to around 4% (Rao et al 1983) and 70% will regain good to excellent function (Miller 1978). Most patients are able to ambulate with a walker or crutches, using only oral analgesics for pain, within the first week after their operation.

FUSION

Joint fusion represents a permanent form of musculoskeletal immobilization. Fusions are carried out in patients with pain secondary to joint infections, severe degenerative disease, severe articular trauma or disabling ligament instability, with the goal of restoring maximum function while eliminating pain. Although fusion is

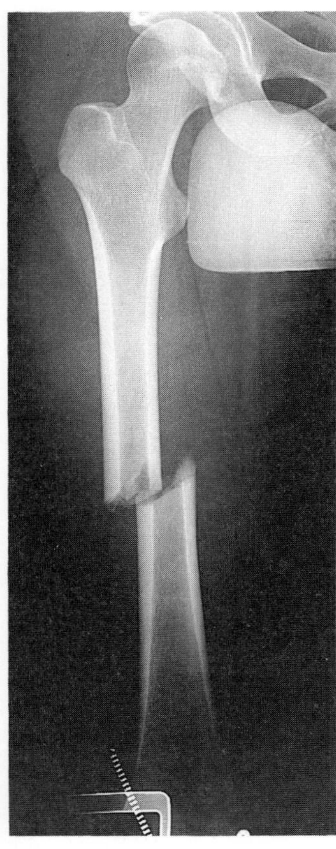

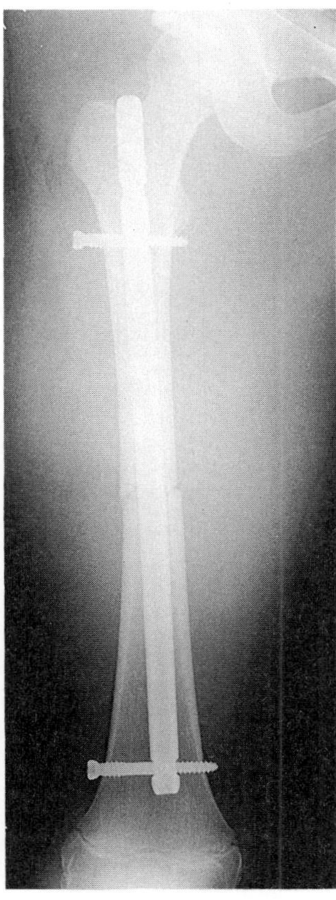

A B

Fig. 58.3 Intramedullary fixation of a femur fracture. Intramedullary rodding allows the surgeon to restore length and axial alignment of this long-bone fracture without opening the fracture site or damaging the massive muscular sheath that surrounds the femur. **A**. AP radiograph of transverse femur fracture sustained in an auto accident; alignment and length are being maintained by longitudinal skeletal traction. **B**. Same extremity after intramedullary fixation. Locking screws have been placed proximally and distally to prevent rotational or angular displacement. This patient was able to walk with crutches within 48 hours of surgery, and was full weight-bearing at 3 weeks.

unglamorous, and modern technology has provided us with so many options as to make fusion seem like a last resort for most patients, joint arthrodesis is still a highly successful operation for young patients with rugged functional demands. Patients who are younger than 40 years, weigh in excess of 200 lbs and/or have excessive activity requirements, are at high risk for failure when treated with a conventional total joint prosthesis. In these patients a hip or knee fusion may be the right choice.

Callaghan et al (1985) reviewed 28 patients with hip fusions, followed-up for an average of 35 years. Although most patients eventually developed some degree of pain in the ipsilateral knee or low back, these patients had enjoyed years to decades of physical activity before developing symptoms. Over half these patients had returned to manual labour occupations, which would have been discouraged even with modern arthroplasty techniques. Approximately one-fourth of the patients underwent a late conversion to a total hip arthroplasty, with subsequent relief of their pain. Arthrodesis has been shown in this study and others reliably to relieve hip pain and improve function in selected, physically active patients (Sponseller et al 1984).

Another area in which fusion is often the best choice for pain relief and improved function is the wrist. Wrist arthrodesis has long enjoyed a reputation for reliable and satisfactory reconstruction in patients suffering severe trauma, infection, inflammatory disease or tumour. Steindler recommended the procedure for patients with polio or spastic hemiparesis (Steindler 1918) and later for tuberculosis (Steindler 1921), and others have described the procedures and outcomes for rheumatoid arthritis, posttraumatic arthritis and infections (Abbott et al 1942; Haddad & Riordan 1967; Millender & Nalebuff 1973). In these patients, end-stage joint destruction results in chronic resting pain, severe pain with activity, wrist deformity and loss of grip strength. Arthrodesis removes the painful joint tissues, eliminates motion and restores alignment and power grip. For patients with limited areas of joint disease within the wrist a variety of intercarpal fusions have been described which maintain some joint motion while relieving pain and instability (Watson & Hempton 1980).

Arthrodesis is performed by removing the articular cartilage and preparing the bone ends so that broad areas of bleeding, cancellous bone can be approximated and held firmly in place. Either internal or external fixation may be applied to ensure compression of the surfaces until fusion occurs. The surgical technique used is designed to maximize both the potential for fusion and the function of the limb after fusion. This means that the positioning of the limb at the time of surgery is critical to the patient's ability to use the extremity productively and painlessly. Optimal positions of function have been described for the wrist, hip, knee, shoulder, elbow and ankle, as well as the digits of both feet and hands. A patient with a solid arthrodesis in a position of function will consistently demonstrate greater function and satisfaction than a patient with a mobile but painful joint.

RESECTION

The ability surgically to remove the pathological tissue, segment or limb from a patient provides the orthopaedist with a variety of options in palliating painful musculoskeletal conditions. The simplest resections may require only the removal of a small piece of tissue, as in the patient with a torn meniscal cartilage, while the most complex of procedures may result in the internal resection of an entire long bone and its muscular envelope, for the patient with a primary bone tumour. Modern techniques allow us to consider limb-salvaging operations where terminal

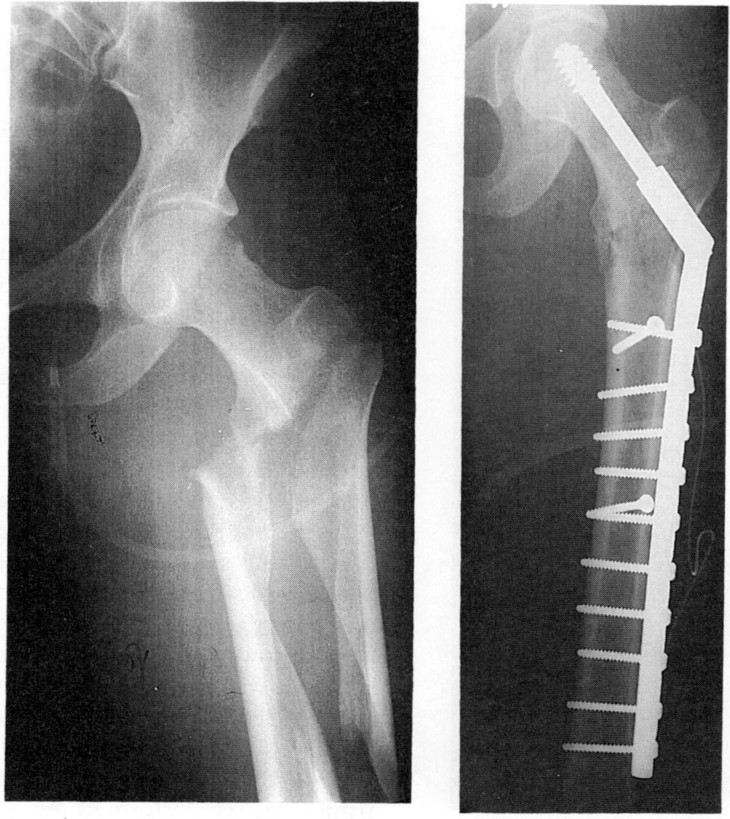

Fig. 58.4 Hip screw and side-plate. **A**. Severely comminuted fracture of the proximal femur in a middle-aged patient. Nonoperative management is likely to result in nonunion, deformity and pain. **B**. Specially designed hip screw provides fixation of long spiral fracture of the femoral shaft while maintaining alignment of the femoral head and neck. The screw placed in the femoral head is designed to slide through the barrel of the side-plate, allowing this fragment to collapse down on the shaft fragments during weight-bearing while maintaining an appropriate angle between the neck and the shaft.

amputations are a viable but less satisfactory option. Modern prosthetics provide superior function and cosmesis where amputation is the logical and preferred choice.

Removal of pathological tissue from within a joint is a commonly performed procedure in patients with post-traumatic or inflammatory problems involving the articular cartilage, menisci or synovium. Arthroscopic surgery now allows surgeons to perform many of these procedures without opening the joint and, although most commonly performed in the knee, arthroscopy can be used in the shoulder, hip, wrist or ankle. In some situations, as with meniscal tears, arthroscopy actually provides better visualization and easier access to the damaged tissue than can be obtained through open methods.

Osteochondral loose bodies can occur in any joint, but are most common within the knee. These fragments usually result from previous cartilage injuries and may produce pain by impinging between the joint surfaces, compressing the synovial lining or irritating the capsular tissues (O'Connor & Shahriaree 1984). Simply removing the loose bodies and lavaging the joint can result in significant pain relief, particularly if there is a component of crystal-induced synovitis (O'Connor 1973). Meniscal tears are very common problems, resulting in pain and dysfunction in the most active and productive segment of our population. Depending on the size and pattern of a tear, the patient may present with persistent, nagging pain, occasional, severe pain or an acutely 'locked' knee, in which the torn meniscal tissue is found incarcerated within the joint, preventing flexion or extension. Through the arthroscope the orthopaedist is able to diagnose and access the injury and, as indicated, partially or completely resect the torn meniscus, or repair it when possible. Since total meniscectomy has been shown to precipitate degenerative changes in the knee, partial meniscectomy or repair is widely recommended (Dandy & Jackson 1975; Jackson & Rouse 1982).

Synovial inflammation and hypertrophy may occur with any chronic inflammatory process, but are particularly prominent in rheumatoid and tuberculous arthritis, haemophilic arthritis and in pigmented villonodular synovitis (Wilkinson 1969; Montane et al 1986). It has previously been reported that the synovium is a relatively insensitive tissue (Kellgren & Samuel 1950) and that the pain of synovitis was produced by distortion of the capsule and the elaboration of inflammatory factors. As noted above, more recent techniques have demonstrated free nerve endings and neuropeptide-containing nerve fibres within the synovium which suggest a much greater role in pain sensation and mediation than previously thought (Kidd et al 1990; Konttinen et al 1990).

Synovectomy, either open or arthroscopic, has been shown to be effective in reducing pain and disability in patients with persistent synovitis due to haemophilia. Montane et al (1986) demonstrated that open synovectomy was able to eliminate recurrent haemarthroses, reduce pain and arrest the progressive arthrosis in 12 of 13 patients with haemophilic synovitis. Although some studies have questioned the efficacy of synovectomy in treating clinical symptoms of rheumatoid arthritis (Arthritis Foundation 1977), others have shown significant benefit to function and pain relief when carried out in early stages of the disease (Ishikawa et al 1986).

Resection of tumours of bone or soft tissue, and of destructive infections of bone, are often necessary for patient welfare as well as pain relief. Tumours produce pain as they displace normal tissues during growth. Expansile lesions, whether tumour or infection, may elevate the periosteum away from the bone, producing local pressure and disrupting nerve endings. Destructive lesions may weaken bone to the point of fracture or impending fracture and pathological fractures may prove very reluctant to heal. Compression of vascular structures may produce ischaemia or venous congestion, and of nerves, paralysis, paresthesias or pain. Some neoplastic lesions, such as osteoid osteomas and osteoblastomas, may elaborate factors which produce pain directly (Sherman & McFarland 1965; Marsh et al 1975). Pain relief can be obtained by any means that reduces the distension of the soft tissues or compression of neurovascular structures. In cases of soft-tissue infection, simple drainage of the abscess provides prompt and dramatic pain relief. Antibiotic therapy also provides rapid pain relief as the infection subsides and swelling is reduced. Pain due to expanding tumour mass can be reduced or eliminated by radiotherapy or chemotherapy; necrosis and shrinkage of the tumour relieves pressure on surrounding structures. While medical management is often able to control pain or slow the progress of disease, in many cases surgery is needed to ensure the best chance of curing the patient. In infections, debridement or resection of infected bone is necessary to prevent recurrence and in tumours, removal of the tumour, the surrounding soft tissues and sometimes all of the associated musculature may be necessary to provide local tumour control, depending on the tumour type. In any case, the type of resection chosen is determined on the basis of the location and nature of the lesion involved and the health and prognosis of the patient. Quality of life issues must always be considered – in some cases surgical resection may be the safest and most efficacious treatment available to the patient, while in others it may provide little benefit despite an extensive, debilitating operation.

The oldest and most straightforward form of resection is amputation, until this century the only rational treatment of tumours, infections, open fractures or other severely painful or potentially lethal lesions of the extremities. Although modern antibiotics, chemotherapeutic agents and surgical techniques have made it possible to salvage the vast majority of infected and injured limbs, and many of those affected by tumour, amputation is still indicated in a number of clinical situations. Diabetic patients, with poor sensation, poor circulation and impaired healing potential, often require amputation to eliminate chronic and recurrent infections, nonhealing wounds and neuropathic pain (Ecker & Jacobs 1970; Wagner 1986). Vascular insufficiency, whether associated with atherosclerosis or diabetes mellitus, accounts for nearly 80% of all lower extremity amputations (Glatty 1964; Mazet 1968). Tumours requiring a wide resection distal to the mid-tibia are still best treated by amputation, as reconstruction of this area is very difficult and the results somewhat unreliable.

Amputation remains an appropriate alternative in the care of some traumatic injuries. Advances in surgical technique, microvascular repair and soft tissue transfers have made it possible to 'save' almost any extremity; the decision to do so may be a disservice to some patients, however (Lange et al 1985). Patients with severe injuries to the lower leg, with open fractures and significant muscle and soft-tissue damage, often require extensive reconstruction and multiple surgeries to repair the damage. These patients who, in the past, would have lost their legs, can now retain their limb and obtain a good outcome in terms of pain and long-term disability (Chapman & Mahoney 1979; Cierny et al 1983). However, patients with prolonged ischaemia of the limb, disruption of major nerves or mangling injuries of hand or foot have a poor prognosis; the patient is often left with a viable but functionless extremity, prone to infection and often painful. In these patients primary amputation offers the best likelihood of rapid return to painless activity and function (Hanson 1987; Caudle & Stern 1987).

Limb-salvage surgery has made tremendous advances in the past decade. Limb-salvage resections amount to 'internal amputations', and their success depends on the surgeon's ability to replace adequately the resected tissue elements with something that will function in an acceptably similar way. Likewise, the segment of the limb being salvaged has to be of enough importance to warrant a highly technical and demanding operation and extensive rehabilitation. Below-knee prostheses provide excellent, pain-free function with few problems in terms of fit, cosmesis or activity restrictions. Reconstructions of the foot and ankle often function poorly; stiffness and pain are frequent complications which may severely limit the patient. Hence, salvage of the foot and ankle is rarely warranted. On the other hand, patients with above-knee amputations expend significantly more energy in walking than do those with below-knee amputations. The fitting of above knee prostheses can be more difficult and, when the amputation is performed high up on the thigh, the fit becomes more difficult and the function poorer; these patients have a greater tendency to become wheelchair-bound than patients with below-knee amputations (Volpicelli et al 1983). For this reason, a tumour of the femur or knee in a young, active individual is one of the most common indications for limb-salvage surgery (Fig. 58.5).

RECONSTRUCTION

Of all procedures performed by the orthopaedic surgeon, joint reconstruction can have the most dramatic impact on the patients' function and satisfaction with life.

Regardless of the initial insult (trauma, rheumatic disease, osteoarthritis, ligamentous instability, metabolic disorders, neoplasia or infection) the fundamental problem in end-stage joint disease is the erosion or destruction of the articular surfaces. Operative treatment seeks to remedy this problem by accomplishing one or more of the following:

A

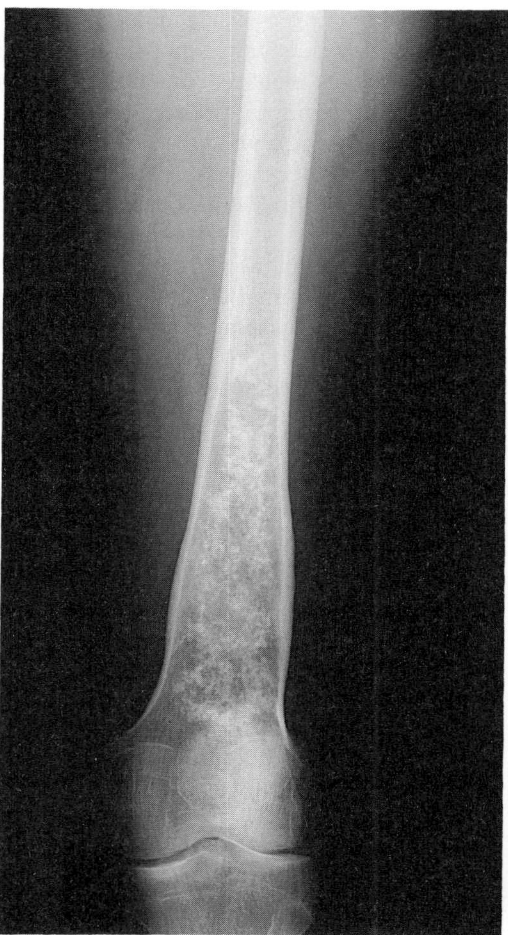

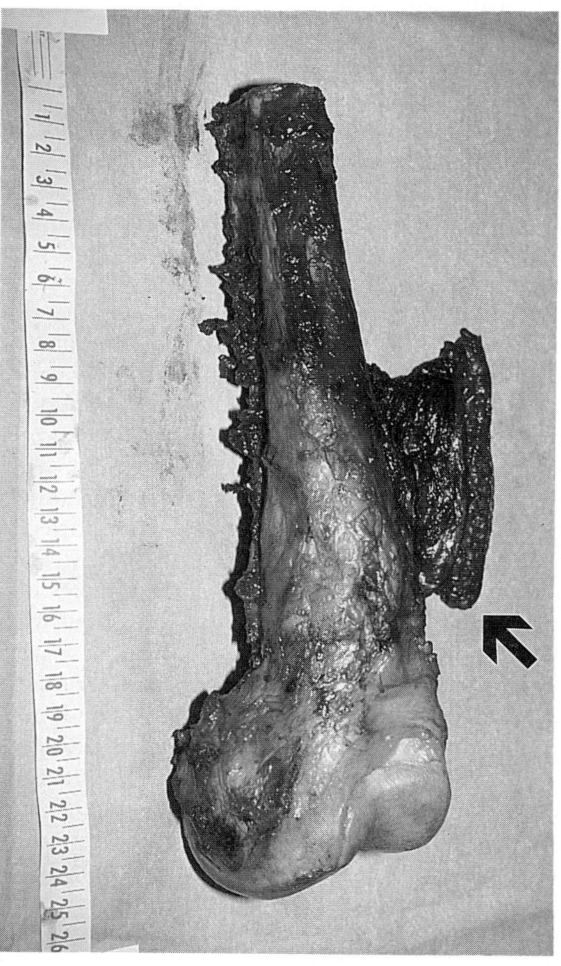

B

Fig. 58.5 Limb salvage surgery. **A**. Grade I chondrosarcoma of the distal femur in a 40-year-old man; the tumour is confined to the medullary canal but has extended well up the shaft. The prognosis for this lesion, which has a tendency to recur locally, is good if local control can be obtained. Traditional treatment would have been a high thigh amputation. **B**. Resection of the tumor involves removal of the entire distal femur, with a suitable margin of normal bone at the proximal end. The biopsy tract has also been excised enbloc with the specimen to limit the chances of local recurrence (arrow). **C**. A custom endoprosthesis was implanted to salvage the limb. This prosthesis has a long proximal stem which is cemented into the amputated end of the femur and an artificial knee joint which replaces both the femoral and tibial side of the articulation. Pain relief is excellent with this implant and the patient has near-normal function despite the wide resection of this tumour.

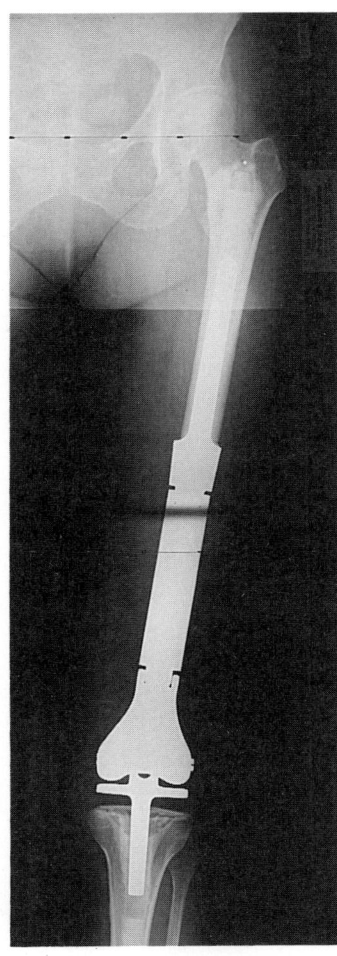

Fig. 58.5C *Contd*

1. Eliminating the contact between the two damaged joint surfaces. Excisional arthroplasty and interposition arthroplasty are techniques used to either remove the damaged joint surfaces or place tissue between them to reduce contact.

2. Transferring contact from the damaged articular surface to areas of healthy cartilage. Osteotomies alter joint contact by changing the alignment of the limb or the orientation of the joint surfaces.

3. Replacing the joint surfaces. Total joint arthroplasty can be performed in virtually any joint of the appendicular skeleton, but has had its most profound effect on the treatment of disorders of the hip, knee and shoulder.

Excisional arthroplasty

One of the earliest forms of joint reconstruction was the excisional arthroplasty, performed by excising the joint surfaces and surrounding bone and allowing a pseudarthrosis to form which might allow reasonable motion and function with tolerable pain. This procedure is still used, primarily in patients who cannot tolerate a total joint arthroplasty, or in joints unsuitable for that procedure.

The Girdlestone excision of the hip remains a viable option for the treatment of hip fractures or infections in elderly or feeble patients whose primary goal is to be able to sit or transfer comfortably (Girdlestone 1943). It may be the only option in patients with infections of the hip joint or those who have failed previous total joint arthroplasty. The cost to the patient is significant shortening of the limb and instability; patients are able to walk on a Girdlestone hip, but usually have a significant limp and require some assistive device. The quality of the outcome depends on the formation of a tough scar around the proximal end of the femur. Prolonged traction and bracing may be required to allow that scar to mature between the femur and acetabulum, providing enough stability to walk on. Girdlestone patients treated for infection appear to have somewhat better results than those treated for fracture or degenerative disease and it is thought that the presence of infection, by producing a more intense scarring response, may actually lead to a stronger pseudarthrosis (Parr et al 1971). Nonetheless, few patients are very satisfied with the long-term results of resection arthroplasty (Petty & Goldsmith 1980).

Interpositional arthroplasty

Soft-tissue arthroplasties are performed by interposing adjoining soft tissues between the joint's ends to provide a resilient, biologically active gliding surface where the original articular surface has been worn away. Interposition of deep fascia has been tried in large weight-bearing joints, such as the hip, with limited success and has largely been abandoned in favour of fusion or joint replacement. In smaller joints, however, fascial interposition remains a successful operation, providing excellent symptomatic relief and good function in the joints of the elbow, wrist and thumb (Smith-Peterson et al 1943; Froimson 1970; Beckenbaugh & Linscheid 1982).

Osteotomy

Osteotomy is a commonly applied procedure in orthopaedics and is primarily used in one of two scenarios: cases in which deformity or malalignment result in poor function and predispose to early joint degeneration, and cases in which degenerative disease has damaged one area of weight-bearing cartilage while sparing the rest. Congenital and acquired deformities of the lower extremity (Blount's disease, congenital coxa vara, rickets) may sufficiently derange the weight-bearing axis of the limb so as to assure progressive deformity and early joint destruction (Langenskiold & Riska 1964; Schoeneker et al 1985). In these patients, corrective osteotomies, performed at the

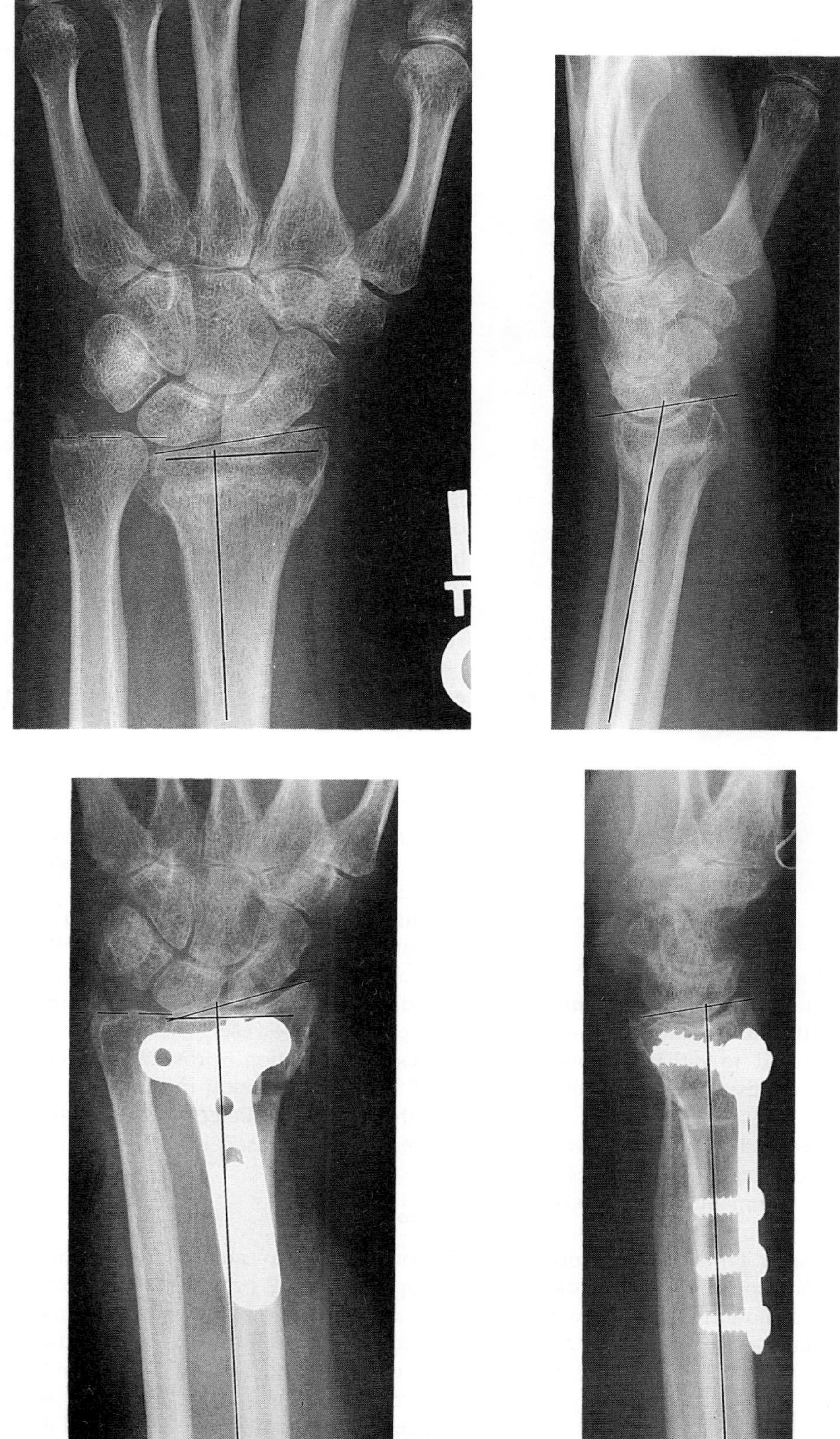

Fig. 58.6 Distal radial osteotomy. **A**. AP and lateral views show mal-union of wrist. Note on the AP view that radial inclination is reduced to 5°, (normal, 20–25°) and that the radius is considerably shortened relative to the ulna. On the lateral view, the wrist is *dorsally* angulated 18°, compared to a normal *palmar* tilt of 10–25°, resulting in derangement of the radiocarpal articulation. This patient has chronic pain, weakness and a predisposition to severe degenerative disease. **B**. A distal radial osteotomy was performed using an iliac crest bone graft to restore the normal orientation of the radiocarpal joint. Following the corrective osteotomy the radial inclination is improved and length restored. The normal volar tilt has also been restored.

right age, may restore alignment, height and function, with relatively little risk (Deitz & Weinstein 1988). In children with congenital dislocation of the hip, osteotomy may be necessary to correct the rotational deformity of the proximal femur and to allow reduction of the coxa-femoral joint without applying excessive pressure to the femoral head.

Osteotomies are sometimes needed for posttraumatic malunion, particularly when the deformity is in a plane other than that of the joint's motion. Injuries resulting in a varus or valgus deformity of the lower extremity force the weight-bearing joints to be loaded eccentrically, causing pain and early joint destruction. Corrective osteotomies are designed to return the limb to its natural alignment and restore normal joint mechanics. For instance, malunion of a distal radius fracture (Colles' fracture) can be satisfactorily corrected with a distal radius osteotomy to restore joint alignment and stability, grip strength and pain-free function (Fernandez 1988) (Fig. 58.6).

Proximal tibial osteotomy (Fig. 58.7) remains the most successful operation for osteoarthritis of the knee, short of joint replacement (Jackson & Waugh 1961). In younger patients with greater functional demands this procedure is the treatment of choice, allowing the patient unrestricted activity without lifting limits, or restrictions of sports or recreation. By transferring contact forces from the side of the joint with advanced degenerative disease to the side with residual healthy cartilage, tibial osteotomy may provide the patient with years of unrestricted function before replacement arthroplasty is necessary, which, for many patients, translates to additional years of gainful employment, recreation and fitness (Holden et al 1988). Although results do deteriorate over time, 40% of patients with a high tibial osteotomy remain pain-free more than 9 years after their operation (Insall et al 1984). A variety of osteotomies have been described for treatment of disorders of the hip joint, but are no longer commonly used. With consistently excellent results, total hip arthroplasty has largely displaced hip osteotomies as a treatment of osteoarthritis. A proximal femoral osteotomy requires a longer convalescence than a total hip arthroplasty and greater patient compliance is required for success. Also, since the range of motion of the hip is not improved by osteotomy, patients with contractures or limited motion are poor candidates. Nonetheless, in young, active patients at risk for early total joint failure, osteotomies of the hip provide a valuable treatment alternative and may provide definitive correction in 15–20% of cases (Fortune 1990).

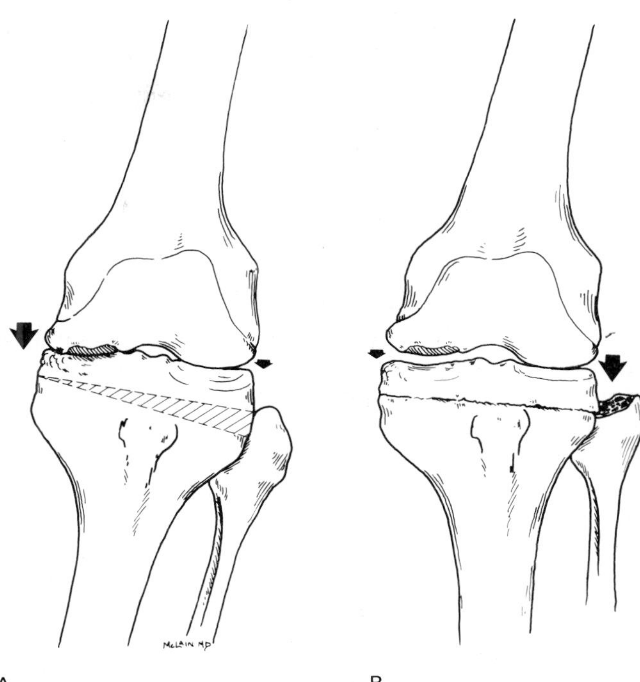

Fig. 58.7 Proximal tibial osteotomy. Osteotomy to correct deformity of the knee and reduce stress on a joint compartment with severe arthritis is an effective and commonly used operation. **A**. Patients with severe medial compartment osteoarthritis develop genu valgum, which result is a progressive shift of loads onto the injured side (large arrow). As weight is shifted to the diseased compartment, the healthy cartilage in the lateral compartment sees less load and remains intact. A corrective osteotomy performed through the cancellous bone of the proximal tibia (cross-hatched area) corrects the valgus deformity, shifting weight away from the damaged medial cartilage and on to the healthy lateral cartilage. **B**. By restoring the normal alignment of the knee, ligament and muscle stresses are normalized. An osteotomy performed through the vascular cancellous bone of the tibial metaphysis heals reliably.

Total joint arthroplasty

There are few, if any, operations as successful for managing pain and restoring function as joint replacement arthroplasty. In the 30 years since Charnley first reported his hip replacement procedure (Charnley 1961b), total joint arthroplasty has become the most frequently performed reconstructive procedure in orthopaedic surgery. Replacement joints are now available for most joints of the extremities and are routinely applied in the treatment of arthrosis of the hip, knee and shoulder. Technical advances now allow the surgeon to chose between cemented and bone-ingrowth methods of fixation and modular implants allow the surgeon to customize implants to fit the needs of individual patients.

Total hip arthroplasty can provide dramatic and long-lasting pain relief in patients with osteoarthritis , rheumatoid arthritis, avascular necrosis of the femoral head, nonunions of the femoral neck, post posttraumatic degenerative disease and a number of other congenital or acquired maladies of the hip joint. Total hip arthroplasty can also be performed in patients with previous fusions or osteotomies and in patients with previous arthroplasties which have loosened. Relative contraindications to arthroplasty include obesity, youth, high functional demands and active or chronic infection in the joint (Chandler 1981; Salvati et al 1991). The use of bone in-growth (cementless) prostheses promises improved success even in these difficult patients.

Although modern implants are the product of significant technological evolution, the basic concept behind the original plastic and metal prosthesis of Charnley still pertains: a small-diameter, polished metal head mounted on a femoral stem, articulates with a metal-backed high-density polyethylene socket embedded in the acetabulum, with both components fixed so as to restore anatomical alignment and range of motion (Fig. 58.8). Because the longevity of the device is determined, in part, by the positioning and fixation of the components, attention to surgical technique is critical to the survival of the implant and the duration of symptomatic relief. Failure of the arthroplasty usually occurs because of loosening or infection, or a combination of the two. The earliest symptom of failure is recurrence of groin or thigh pain, usually worse with weight-bearing, which may appear before any radiographic evidence of loosening can be detected.

In performing a total hip arthroplasty, the hip joint may be exposed through one of several surgical approaches. The capsule of the joint is excised and the femoral head dislocated from the acetabulum. The femoral neck is transected and the femoral head discarded. The acetabulum is prepared by removing the remaining articular cartilage and any medial osteophytes with a domed reamer, and the femoral shaft by the insertion of a broach contoured to match the femoral implant being used. The implant is then inserted and either fixed in place with polymethylmethacrylate (PMMA) cement or press-fit in the case of bone in-growth components. The patient is usually out of bed on the first postoperative day and ambulating independently within the week. In patients with severe degenerative disease pain relief is often immediate and range of motion improved. Although long-term results are not yet available for cementless prostheses, cemented prostheses have provided good to excellent results in the majority of patients in long-term follow-up studies (Charnley 1973). A review of Charnley low-friction arthroplasties at 15 – 21 year follow-up showed that less than 4% had become painful, 11% produced occasional discomfort and 85% were still functioning painlessly (Wroblewski 1986). McCoy et al (1988) reported good to excellent results in 88% of Charnley hips followed for 15 years or more.

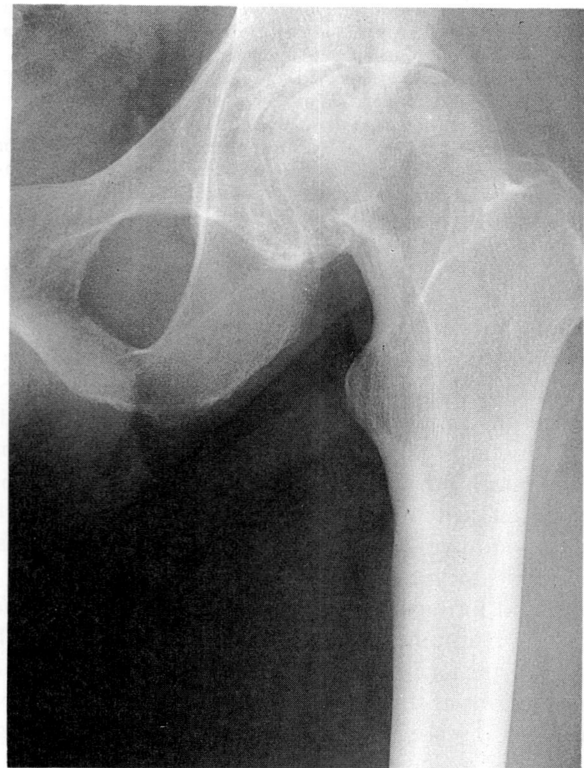

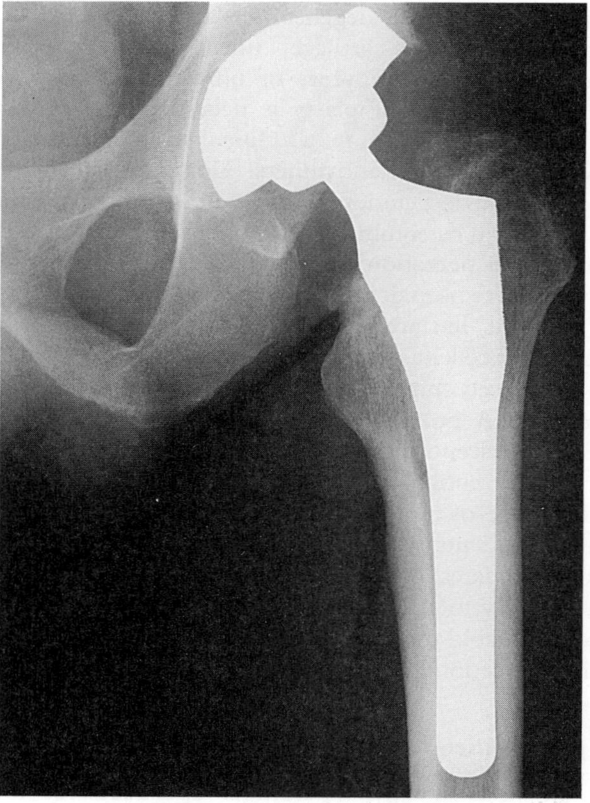

Fig. 58.8 Total hip arthroplasty. **A**. AP view of the pelvis, showing severe, unilateral degenerative disease of the hip. Loss of the joint space is apparent, while several signs of DJD (sclerosis of the subchondral bone, formation of subchondral cysts, osteophyte formation) are also seen. **B**. A total hip arthroplasty, with a metal-backed acetabular cup and an uncemented femoral component. Pain relief is reliably excellent.

Improvements in cement technique promise even greater longevity for the hips currently being implanted (Harris & McGann 1986; Russotti et al 1988).

Total knee arthroplasty has enjoyed a similar rise in popularity as component design has evolved and implant technology has been refined; the clinical success of knee arthroplasty now equals or exceeds that of total hip arthroplasty with respect to pain relief, functional restoration and survival of the implant at 10 years (Insall et al 1983; Ewald et al 1984). Modern implant designs simulate the geometry of the normal knee, providing eccentric femoral condylar surfaces, broad, nonconforming tibial surfaces of high density polyethylene and a replacement surface for the patella. Failure to replace the patellar surface was a source of clinical failure in the past, while attempts to increase implant stability by constraining the femoral and tibial components led to loosening and mechanical failure. Currently, most knee implants are cemented in place with PMMA, as bone in-growth implants have proven less reliable in knee surgery than in the hip.

SUMMARY

The orthopaedic surgeon has a wide variety of techniques and a vast array of technology available for the treatment of musculoskeletal disorders. The rational treatment of musculoskeletal problems requires that the surgeon match the treatment to the disease and that options be tried in the order of their invasiveness and potential risk. Likewise, the natural history of the disorder must be considered in order to weigh the risks of intervention against those of observation and supportive therapy. As many interventions provide only transient pain relief, the patient may require a series of procedures over the course of his or her lifetime and the physician must use good judgement early on to avoid 'burning bridges' with respect to later procedures. The majority of patients will be well cared for with a judicious combination of medical management and an occasional surgical intervention, well-timed and tailored to the patient's needs. The injudicious application of technology to orthopaedic problems can lead to unmanageable problems in later life; cementing a total hip implant into a young, noncompliant patient is bound to lead to early failure, repeated revisions and, in the end, an excisional arthroplasty before the patient reaches middle-age. On the other hand, a patient with a traumatic injury to the knee might undergo an acute ligament or meniscal repair as a young man, arthroscopic debridement or synovectomy to control symptoms in middle age, a high tibial osteotomy for unicompartmental degenerative disease at 50, a hemiarthroplasty at 60 and a total condylar knee replacement at the age of 70, at which time that arthroplasty could be expected to provide excellent function for another 15–20 years. The goal of such a treatment hierarchy, as aggressive as it may appear, is to keep the patient functioning at the highest possible level throughout his life, with a minimal or acceptable level of pain; such a patient is pleased with his care and an asset to his family and community rather than a burden. Regardless of the nature of the disorder, the orthopaedist's challenge is to maintain the patient as an independent, productive member of society, capable of enjoying and participating in life; if this can be accomplished both the physician and the patient will be well satisfied.

Despite the great advances made over past decades in the diagnosis and treatment of most common orthopaedic disorders, the source of musculoskeletal pain is often an enigma to the treating physician. With proper education, appropriate expectations and a comprehensive approach to orthopaedic disease and pain management, the majority of our patients can expect successful outcomes. Still, in many cases, residual pain must be expected and dealt with. It is only through a better understanding of pain itself – the pathophysiology, neurochemistry, anatomy and psychology of pain – that we as treating physicians can continue to offer our patients more efficacious and responsible therapy. We hope this chapter has effectively touched on many of the common orthopaedic disorders that produce musculoskeletal pain and has provided some insight into the current principles of orthopaedic management.

REFERENCES

Abbott L C, Saunders J B de C M, Bost F C 1942 Arthrodesis of the wrist with the use of grafts of cancellous bone. Journal of Bone and Joint Surgery 24: 883–898

Arthritis Foundation Committee on Evaluation of Synovectomy 1977 Multicenter evaluation of synovectomy in the treatment of rheumatoid arthritis. Report of results at the end of three years. Arthritis and Rheumatology 20: 765–771

Badalamente M A, Dee R, Ghillani R, Chien P F, Daniels K 1987 Mechanical stimulation of dorsal root ganglia induces increased production of Substance P: a mechanism of pain following nerve root compromise? Spine 12: 552–555

Beckenbaugh R D, Linscheid R L 1982 Arthroplasty in the hand and wrist. In: Green D P (ed) Operative hand surgery. Churchill Livingstone, New York, p 141–184

Bjurholm A, Kreicbergs A, Brodin E, Schultzberg M 1988a Substance P and CGRP immunoreactive nerves in bone. Peptides 9: 165–171

Bjurholm A, Kreicbergs A, Terenius L, Goldstein M, Schultzberg M 1988b Neuropeptide Y-, tyrosine hydroxylase-, and vasoactive intestinal peptide-immunoreactive nerves in bone and surrounding tissues. Journal of the Autonomic Nervous System 25: 119–125

Callaghan J J, Brand R A, Petersen D R 1985 Hip arthrodesis. Journal of Bone and Joint Surgury 67A: 1328–1325

Caudle R J, Stern P J 1987 Severe open fractures of the tibia. Journal of Bone and Joint Surgury 69A: 801–807

Chapman M W, Mahoney M 1979 The role of early internal fixation in the management of open fractures. Clinical Orthopaedics and Related Research 138: 120–131

Chapman M W 1989 Orthopaedic management of the multiply injured patient. In: Evarts C M (ed) Surgery of the musculoskeletal system, 2nd edn. Churchill Livingstone, New York, p 19–35

Charnley J 1961a The closed treatment of common fractures. Churchill Livingstone, Edinburgh, p 1–67

Charnley J 1961b Arthroplasty of the hip. Lancet 1: 1129–1132

Charnley J, Cupic Z 1973 The nine and ten year results of the low-friction arthroplasty of the hip. Clinical Orthopaedics and Related Research 95: 9–25

Cierny G, Byrd H S, Jones R E 1983 Primary versus delayed soft tissue coverage for severe open tibial fractures. A comparison of results. Clinical Orthopaedics and Related Research 178: 54–63

Colpaert F C, Donnerer J, Lembeck F 1983 Effects of capsaicin on inflammation and on the Substance P content of nervous tissues in rats with adjuvant arthritis. Life Sciences 32: 1827–1834

Colton C L 1992 The history of fracture treatment. In: Browner B D, Jupiter J B, Levine A M, Trafton P G (eds) Skeletal trauma. W B Saunders, Philadelphia, p 3–30

Cooper R R 1968 Nerves in cortical bone. Science 160: 327–328

Dandy D J, Jackson R W 1975 The diagnosis of problems after meniscectomy. Journal of Bone and Joint Surgery 57B: 349–352

Deandrade J R, Grant C, Dixon A 1965 Joint distension and reflex muscle inhibition in the knee. Journal of Bone and Joint Surgery 47A: 313–332

DeAvila G A, O'Connor B L, Visco D M, Sisk T D 1989 The mechanoreceptor innervation of the human fibular collateral ligament. Journal of Anatomy 162: 1–7

Dee R M 1978 The innervation of joints. In: Sokoloff L (ed) Joints and synovial fluid. Academic Press, New York

Dietz F R, Weinstein S L 1988 Spike osteotomy for angular deformities of the long bones Journal of Bone and Joint Surgery 70A: 848–852

Ecker M D, Jacobs B S 1970 Lower extremity amputations in diabetic patients. Diabetes 19: 189–195

Eckholm J, Eklund G, Skoglund S 1960 On the reflex effects from the knee joint of the cat. Acta Physiologica Scandinavica 50: 167–174

Ewald F C, Jacobs M A, Miegel R E, Walker P S, Poss R, Sledge C B 1984 Kinematic total knee replacement. Journal of Bone and Joint Surgery 66A: 1032–1040

Fernandez D L 1988 Radial osteotomy and Bowers arthroplasty for malunited fractures of the distal end of the radius. Journal of Bone and Joint Surgery 70A: 1538–1551

Fortune W P 1990 Hip osteotomies. In: Evarts C M (ed) Surgery of the musculoskeletal system, vol 3. Churchill Livingstone, New York, p 2795–2832

Freeman M A R, Wyke B D 1967 The innervation of the knee joint. An anatomical and histological study in the cat. Journal of Anatomy 101: 505–532

Froimson A I 1970 Tendon arthroplasty of the trapeziometacarpal joint. Clinical Orthopaedics and Related Research 70: 191–199

Fuller R W, Conradson T B, Dixon C M S, Crossman D C, Barnes P J 1987 Sensory neuropeptide effects in human skin. British Journal of Pharmacology 92: 781–788

Gardner E 1944 The distribution and termination of nerves in the knee joint of the cat. Journal of Comparative Neurology 80: 11–32

Gardner E 1948 The innervation of the knee joint. Anatomical Record 101: 109–130

Giles L G F, Harvey A R 1987 Immunohistochemical demonstration of nociceptors in the capsule and synovial folds of human zygapophyseal joints. British Journal of Rheumatology 26: 362–364

Girdlestone G R 1943 Acute pyogenic arthritis of the hip. An operation giving free access and effective drainage. Lancet 1: 419–421

Glatty H 1964 A statistical study of 12 000 new amputees. Southern Medical Journal 57: 1373–1378

Grigg P, Hoffman A H, Fogarty K E 1982 Properties of Golgi–Mazzoni afferents in cat knee joint capsule as revealed by mechanical studies in isolated joint capsule. Journal of Neurophysiology 47: 31–40

Grigg P, Schaible H G, Schmidt R F 1986 Mechanical sensitivity of group III and IV afferents from posterior articular nerve in normal and inflammed cat knee. Journal of Neurophysiology 55: 635–643

Gronblad M, Liesi P, Korkala O, Karaharju E, Polak J 1984 Innervation of human bone periosteum by peptidergic nerves. Anatomical Record 209: 297–299

Gronblad M, Konttinen Y, Korkala O, Liesi P, Hukkanen M, Polak J 1988 Neuropeptides in synovium of patients with rheumatoid arthritis and osteoarthritis. Journal of Rheumatology 15: 1807–1810

Gronblad M, Weinstein J N, Santavirta S 1991 Immunohistochemical observations on spinal tissue innervation. Acta Orthopaedica Scandinavica 62: 614

Haddad R J, Riordan D C 1967 Arthrodesis of the wrist. A surgical technique. Journal of Bone and Joint Surgery 49A: 950–954

Hansen S T 1987 The type-IIIC tibial fracture. Salvage or amputation. Journal of Bone and Joint Surgery 69A: 799–800

Harris W H, McGann W A 1986 Loosening of the femoral component after use of the medullary plug cementing technique. Journal of Bone and Joint Surgery 68A: 1064–1066

Heppelmann B, Schaible H-G, Schmidt R F 1985 Effects of prostaglandin E1 and E2 on the mechanosensitivity of group III afferents from normal and inflammed cat knee joints. In: Fields H L, Dubner R, Cervero F (eds) Advances in pain research and therapy. Raven Press, New York, p 91–101

Heppelmann B, Pfeffer A, Schaible H-G, Schmidt R F 1986 Effects of acetylsalicylic acid and indomethocine on single group III and IV sensory units from acutely inflammed joints. Pain 26: 337–351

Hill E L, Elde R 1991 Distribution of CGRP-, VIP-, DβH-, SP-, and NPY-immunoreactive nerves in the periosteum of the rat. Cell and Tissue Research 264: 469–480

Holden D L, Stanley L J, Larson R L, Slocum D B 1988 Proximal tibial osteotomy in patients who are fifty years old or less. Journal of Bone and Joint Surgery 70A: 977–982

Horowitz B G 1966 Retrospective analysis of hip fractures. Surgery, Gynecology and Obstetrics 123: 565–570

Insall J N, Hood R W, Flawn L B, Sullivan D J 1983 The total condylar knee prosthesis in gonarthrosis. A five to nine year follow-up of the first one hundred consecutive replacements. Journal of Bone and Joint Surgery 65A: 619–628

Insall J N, Joseph D M, Msika C 1984 High tibial osteotomy for varus gonarthrosis. Journal of Bone and Joint Surgery 66A: 1040–1048

Ishikawa H, Ohno O, Hirohata K 1986 Long-term results of synovectomy in rheumatoid patients. Journal of Bone and Joint Surgery 68A: 198–205

Jackson R W, Rouse D W 1982 The results of partial arthroscopic meniscectomy in patients over 40 years of age. Journal of Bone and Joint Surgery 64B: 481–486

Jackson J P, Waugh W 1961 Tibial osteotomy for osteoarthritis of the knee. Journal of Bone and Joint Surgery 43B: 746–751

Kellgren J H, Samuel E P 1950 Sensitivity and innervation of the articular cartilage. Journal of Bone and Joint Surgery 32B: 84–92

Kennedy J C, Alexander I J, Hayes K C 1982 Nerve supply of the human knee and its functional importance. American Journal of Sports Medicine 10: 329–335

Kidd B L, Mapp P I, Blake D R, Gibson S J, Polak J M 1990 Neurogenic influences in arthritis. Annals of the Rheumatic Diseases 49: 649–652

Konttinen Y, Rees R, Hukkanen M et al 1990 Nerves in inflammatory synovium: immunohistochemical observations on the adjuvant arthritic rat model. Journal of Rheumatology 17: 1586–1591

Kumazawa T, Mizumura K 1977 Thin fiber receptors responding to mechanical, chemical and thermal stimulation in the skeletal muscle of the dog. Journal of Physiology 273: 179–194

Küntscher G 1968 The intramedullary nailing of fractures. Clinical Orthopaedics and Related Research 60: 5–12

Lam F Y, Ferrell W R 1989 Inhibition of carrageenan-induced inflammation in the rat knee joint. Annals of the Rheumatic Diseases 48: 928–932

Lam F Y, Ferrell W R 1991 Neurogenic component of different models of acute inflammation in the rat knee model. Annals of the Rheumatic Diseases 50: 747–751

Lange R H, Bach A W, Hansen S T, Johansen K H 1985 Open tibial fractures with associated vascular injuries. Prognosis for limb salvage. Journal of Trauma 25: 203–208

Langenskiold A, Riska E B 1964 Tibia vara (osteochondrosis deformans tibia). A survey of seventy-one cases. Journal of Bone and Joint Surgery 46A: 1405–1420

Levine J D, Clark R, Devor M, Helms C, Moskowitz M, Basbaum A I 1984 Interneuronal Substance P contributes to the severity of experimental arthritis. Science 226: 547–549

Liesi P, Gronblad M, Korkala O, Karaharju E, Rusanen M 1983 Substance P. A neuropeptide involved in low back pain? Lancet 1: 1328–1329

Lundberg J M, Terenius L, Hokfelt T et al 1982 Neuropeptide Y (NPY)-like immunoreactivity in peripheral noradrenergic neurons and effects of NPY on sympathetic function. Acta Physiologica Scandanavica 116: 477–480

McCoy T H, Salvati E A, Ranawat C S 1988 A fifteen year follow-up study of one hundred Charnley low-friction arthroplasties. Orthopedic Clinics of North America 19: 467–476

McLain R F, Weinstein J N 1991 Ultrastructural changes in the dorsal root ganglion associated with whole body vibration. Journal of Spinal Disorders 4: 142–148

McLain R F, Weinstein J N 1992 Nuclear clefting in dorsal root ganglion neurons. A response to whole body vibration. Journal of Comparative Neurology (in press)

Marsh B W, Bonfiglio M, Brady L P, Enneking W F 1975 Benign osteoblastoma: range of manifestations. Journal of Bone and Joint Surgery 57A: 1–9

Matsen F A 1975 Compartmental syndrome: a unifying concept. Clinical Orthopaedics and Related Research 113: 8–14

Mazet R 1968 Syme's amputation. A follow-up study of fifty-one adults and thirty-two children. Journal of Bone and Joint Surgery 50A: 1549–1563

Mense S, Schmidt R F 1977 Muscle pain. Which receptors are responsible for the transmission of noxious stimuli? In: Clifford Rose (ed) Physiological aspects of clinical neurology. Blackwell, Oxford, p 265–278

Millender L H, Nalebuff E A 1973 Arthrodesis of the rheumatoid wrist. An evaluation of sixty patients and a description of a different surgical technique. Journal of Bone and Joint Surgery 55A: 1026–1034

Miller C W 1978 Survival and ambulation following hip fracture. Journal of Bone and Joint Surgery 60A: 930–934

Montane I, McCollough N C, Lian E C-Y 1986 Synovectomy of the knee for hemophilic arthropathy. Journal of Bone and Joint Surgery 68A: 210–216

Mubarak S J, Owen C A 1977 Double incision fasciotomy of the leg for decompression of compartment syndromes. Journal of Bone and Joint Surgery 59A: 184–187

Neugebauer V, Schaible H G 1990 Evidence for a central component in the sensitization of spinal neurons with joint input during development of acute arthritis in cat's knee. Journal of Neurophysiology 64: 299–311

Neugebauer V, Schaible H G, Schmidt R F 1989 Sensitization of articular afferents to mechanical stimuli by bradykinin. Pflügers Archiv 415: 330–335

O'Connor B L, Gonzales J 1979 Mechanoreceptors of the medial collateral ligament of the cat knee joint. Journal of Anatomy 129: 719–729

O'Connor B L, McConnaughey J S 1978 The structure and innervation of the cat knee menisci and their relation to a 'sensory hypothesis' of meniscal function. American Journal of Anatomy 153: 431–442

O'Connor R L 1973 The arthroscope in the management of crystal-induced synovitis of the knee. Journal of Bone and Joint Surgery 55A: 1443–1449

O'Connor R L, Shahriaree H 1984 Arthroscopic technique and normal anatomy of the knee. In: Shahriaree H, O'Connor R L (eds) O'Connor's textbook of arthroscopic surgery. J B Lippincott, Philadelphia

Palmer I 1958 Pathophysiology of the medial ligament of the knee joint. Acta Chirurgica Scandinavica 115: 312–318

Parr P L, Croft C, Enneking W F 1971 Resection of the head and neck of the femur with and without angular osteotomy. Journal of Bone and Joint Surgery 53A: 935–944

Pedersen-Bjergaard U, Nielsen L B, Jensen K, Edvinsson L, Jansen I, Olesen J 1989 Algesia and local responses induced by neurokinin A and substance P in human skin and temporal muscle. Peptides 10: 1147–1152

Pedersen-Bjergaard U, Nielsen L B, Jensen K, Edvinsson L, Jansen I, Olesen J 1991 Calcitonin gene-related peptide, neurokinin A, and substance P. Effects on nociception and neurogenic inflammation in human skin and temporal muscle. Peptides 12: 333–337

Petty W, Goldsmith S 1980 Resection arthroplasty following infected total hip arthoplasty. Journal of Bone and Joint Surgery 62A: 889–896

Piotrowski W, Foreman J C 1986 Some effects of calcitonin gene-related peptide in human skin and on histamine release. British Journal of Dermatology 114: 37–46

Ralston H J, Miller M R, Kasahara M 1960 Nerve endings in human fasciae, tendons, ligaments, periosteum, and joint synovial membrane. Anatomical Record 136: 137–148

Rao J P, Banzon M T, Weiss A B, Raychack J 1983 Treatment of unstable intertrochanteric fractures with anatomic reduction and compression hip screw fixation. Clinical Orthopaedics and Related Research 175: 65–71

Russoti G M, Coventry M B, Stauffer R N 1988 Cemented total hip arthroplasty with contemporary techniques. A five-year minimum follow-up study. Clinical Orthopaedics and Related Research 235: 141–147

Said S I, Mutt V 1970 Polypeptide with broad biological activity isolation from small intestine. Science 169: 1217–1218

Salvati E A, Huo M H, Buly R L 1991 Cemented total hip replacement long-term results and future outlook. In: Tullos H S (ed) Instructional course lectures, vol XL. AAOS, p 121–134

Schaible H G, Schmidt R F 1985 Effects of an experimental arthritis on the sensory properties of fine articular afferent nerves. Journal of Physiology 54: 1109–1122

Schaible H G, Schmidt R F, Willis W D 1987 Spinal mechanisms in arthritis pain. In: Schaible H G, Schmidt R F, Vahle-Hinz C (eds) Fine afferent nerve fibers and pain. VCH Publishers, Weinheim, p 399–409

Sherman M S, McFarland G 1965 Mechanism of pain in osteoid osteomas. Southern Medical Journal 58: 163

Shoenecker P L, Meade W C, Pierron R L, Sheridan J J, Capelli A M 1985 Blount's disease. A retrospective review and recommendations for treatment. Journal of Pediatric Orthopedics 5: 181–186

Skofitsch G, Jacobowitz D M 1985 Calcionin gene-related peptide co-exists with Substance P in capsaicin sensitive neurons and sensory ganglia of the rat. Peptides 6: 747–754

Smith G M, Egbert L D, Markowitz R A, Mosteller F, Beecher H K 1966 An experimental pain method sensitive to morphine in man. The submaximal effort tourniquet technique. Journal of Pharmacology and Experimental Therapeutics 154: 324–332

Smith-Peterson M N, Cave E F, Vangorder G W 1931 Intracapsular fractures of the femoral neck – treatment by internal fixation. Archives of Surgery 23: 715–759

Smith-Peterson M N, Aufranc O E, Larson C B 1943 Useful surgical procedures for rheumatoid arthritis involving joints of the upper extremity. Archives of Surgery 46: 764–770

Sponseller P D, McBeath A A, Perpich M 1984 Hip arthrodesis in young patients. A long-term follow-up study. Journal of Bone and Joint Surgery 66A: 853–859

Steindler A 1918 Orthopaedic operations on the hand. Journal of the American Medical Association 71: 1288–1291

Steindler A 1921 Operative methods and end-results of disabilities of the shoulder and arm. Journal of Orthopaedic Surgery 3: 652–658

Sternbach R A, Murphy R W, Zimmermans G, Greenhoot J H, Akeson W H 1974 Measuring the severity of clinical pain. In: Bonica J J (ed) Advances in neurology, vol 4. Raven Press, New York

Volpicelli L J, Chambers R B, Wagner F W 1983 Ambulation levels of bilateral lower extremity amputees. Journal of Bone and Joint Surgery 65A: 599–604

Wagner F W Jr 1986 Amputations of the foot. In: Chapman M W (ed) Operative orthopaedics. J B Lippincott, Philadelphia, p 1777–1797

Watson H K, Hempton R F 1980 Limited wrist arthrodeses I: the triscaphoid joint. Journal of Hand Surgery 5: 320–327

Weinstein J N 1986 Mechanisms of spinal pain. The dorsal root ganglion and its role as a mediator of low-back pain. Spine 11: 999–1001

Weinstein J N 1988 New perspectives on low back pain. Workshop, Airlie, Virginia. Supported by the AAOS/NIH/NASS. American Academy of Orthopaedic Surgeons, p 35–130

Weinstein J N 1991 Anatomy and neurophysiologic mechanisms of spinal pain. In: Frymoyer J W (ed) The adult spine: principles and practice. Raven Press, New York, Ch 30

Weinstein J N 1992 The role of neurogenic and non neurogenic mediators as they relate to pain and the development of osteoarthritis. A clinical review Spine 17: S356–S361
Weinstein J N, Claverie J, Gibson S 1988a The pain of discography. Spine 13: 1444–1448
Weinstein J N, Pope M, Schmidt R, Serroussi R 1988b Neuropharmacological effects of vibration on the dorsal root ganglion. An animal model. Spine 13: 521–525
Wilkinson M C 1969 Tuberculosis of the hip and knee treated by chemotherapy, synovectomy, and debridement. Journal of Bone and Joint Surgery 51A: 1343–1359
Winquist R A, Hanson S T 1978 Segmental fractures of the femur treated by closed intramedullary nailing. Journal of Bone and Joint Surgery 60A: 934–993
Wroblewski B M 1986 15–21 year results of the Charnley low-friction arthroplasty. Clinical Orthopaedics and Related Research 211: 30–35
Wyke B 1972 Articular neurology – a review. Physiotherapy 58: 94–99
Wyke B 1981 The neurology of joints. A review of general principles. Clinics in Rheumatology disease 7: 233–239
Yaksh T L 1988 Substance P release from knee joint afferent terminals: modulation by opioids. Brain Research 458: 319–324
Yamashita T, Cavanaugh J M, El-Bohy A, Getchell T V, King A I 1990 Mechanosensitive afferent units in the lumbar facet joint. Journal of Bone and Joint Surgery 72A: 865–870

59. Operations in the brainstem and spinal canal, with an appendix on the relationship of open to percutaneous cordotomy

William H. Sweet, Charles E. Poletti and Jan M. Gybels

SPINAL GANGLIONECTOMY

In an effort to improve the success rate of cutting thoracic spinal posterior roots, Smith (1970) added avulsion of the sympathetic rami communicantes and removal of the dorsal root ganglion. His rationale was that 'afferent fibers might convey pain from the spinal ganglion to the sympathetic chain and then enter the spinal cord at higher or lower levels.' His seven patients with post-thoracotomy pain and two with thoracic postherpetic pain could stop their narcotics after this procedure. He has not supplemented this brief report.

However, the concept that spinal ganglionectomy might improve the results of posterior rhizotomy received tremendous impetus from a series of careful studies showing that afferents exist in the ventral roots. Prior to these studies, many other investigators had adduced evidence for and against conduction of impulses of pain via ventral roots. This was reviewed by White & Sweet (1955). However until 1980 there was still no report of altered response to objective sensory tests after anterior rhizotomy in man, no published report of relief by this procedure of pain unassociated with muscle spasm, and no case of relief after anterior rhizotomy of pain persisting after posterior rhizotomy. The first clearcut evidence that the ventral roots in man may contain unmyelinated afferent axons related to pain was provided by Hosobuchi (1980). In three patients he removed thoracic dorsal root ganglia, after dorsal rhizotomy at the same levels had either failed to relieve the original pain or had been followed by disabling hyperaesthesias and dysaesthesias. All three patients had postthoracotomy or posttraumatic chest pain. The first and third patients had maintained relief for over 5 years after the last operation. There remains a possibility that uncut posterior root fibres were the crucial structures removed at the ganglionectomies.

The first systematic effort to add only ganglionectomy to posterior rhizotomy in man was that of Osgood and colleagues (1976) who reported on 18 patients with a 2–20-month follow-up. However, in 1982 Osgood reported (personal communication) that recurrence of pain occurred in enough of the patients for him to conclude that pain relief was about the same as after posterior rhizotomy alone. Based on his earlier good results, Hosobuchi (personal communication, 1982) went on to do thoracic spinal ganglionectomies on 17 patients; five failed.

Our own experience has been limited to five cases because four failed to obtain more than transitory relief, even though repeated nerve blocks at the relevant levels had given temporary relief before operation. In the sole patient to retain 2-year relief of his pain (disabling dysaesthesias in the first $3\frac{1}{2}$ fingers) only the C5 ganglion had been removed. At the C4 and C6 levels an intradural posterior rhizotomy was done because of the difficulty even under the microscope of finding the plane of cleavage between ventral root and posterior root ganglion. No such difficulty was encountered at the T2–T5, and T11–T12, L1–L3 and S1 levels. These were the levels of ganglionectomy in the four failures. There was no motor disability in them, as had occurred related to the C5 ventral root in the first case. The patients were awakened on the operating table after dorsal and ventral roots had been separated from each other extradurally but leaving the ventral root still attached to the ventral surface of the ganglion. In three of six extradurally exposed ventral roots, pain in the distribution of the root was elicited by electrical stimulation. About twice the voltage was required as compared with the threshold for pain at the corresponding posterior root. In our first patient, who was operated on in 1973, leg movements which had consistently evoked pain no longer did so after the nerve was blocked before operation or following local block into the S1 ganglion at operation. Yet the pain recurred a few weeks after operation. The fourth patient was not relieved of left lateral 'deep' crural pain by radio-frequency lesions in the first three left lumbar spinal ganglia which produced crural analgesia without anaesthesia of all but the posterior thigh. Ganglionectomy at these levels which added anaesthesia to the analgesia also failed to stop the pain. Scratching the periosteum over the lower third of the anterior femur was still painful, as was squeezing of the left quadriceps. Even the ganglionectomy has not rendered the deep structures analgesic. Perhaps more careful selection of our patients would yield results approaching those of Hosobuchi, Taub and Pawl.

A happier picture emerges from the work of Pawl and Taub. The former (personal communication, 1982) carried out lower lumbar or S1 ganglionectomies at one or more levels in 30 patients whose unilateral sciatica was associated with arachnoiditis. The patients were carefully studied at a comprehensive pain treatment centre. Selection of patients for surgery and levels for excision were based finally on responses to stimulation via an electrode inserted into the ganglia. Of the 30 similar patients with 'failure of lumbar disc surgery', 63% were able to return to their premorbid activities, all having been followed for more than 1 year. As in Taub's cases, those with only a single ganglion implicated had the best results. These series contrast with Strait & Hunter's (1981) report on 47 similar patients, only 30% of whom had improvement in activity after spinal extradural rhizotomy of one or two roots, sparing the ganglia. The degree of improvement was not specified.

Taub (personal communication, 1985, 1986) has the largest series; it is a relatively homogeneous group, well studied originally, critically selected and carefully followed. From about 1500 patients with persistent back and sciatic pain related to disc disease and an average of three previous operations, he selected 55 (two-thirds of whom were on workmen's compensation). The clinical criteria included elimination of any directly treatable residual herniation of disc, stenosis or infection and adequate outcome of psychological assessment. Final selection in every case was by inducing via local analgesia of a single spinal root a totally painfree state in that limb. Electrically induced paraesthesias in some were used to identify the appropriate spinal root, and the expected neural deficits corresponding to a proper block were confirmed, as was absence of significant pain relief with verified analgesia of the roots above and below. All but two of the ganglia were at L5 and/or S1; 14 of the patients had two ganglia resected – usually at two separate procedures. The sciatica was markedly reduced or eliminated in 56% of the 55 patients, only 34 of whom were thought likely before operation to be able to return to their previous activity should the pain be relieved. In fact, 21 or 68% of the surgically successful group – 38% of the total – did go back to work. The remainder were disabled by age, persistent back pain and/or other unrelated illness. Relief of the sciatica, if it occurred, was nearly always on the first postoperative day, and if present, was lasting. Follow-up was for 4.8 years in 48 of the 55.

The principal postoperative complication, critically analysed by Taub for the first time after this procedure, is a spontaneous and evoked dysaesthesia confined to the dermatome of the resected ganglion, and appearing in the domains of only 51% of the resected ganglia. It usually did not appear until 10–14 days after operation, often beginning as pain in the calf and hence confused with thrombophlebitis, but then spreading both proximally and distally. The pain gradually rose to a peak in 7–10 days. In 68% of those affected it was graded as 1–2+ on a scale of 0 to 4 lasting 2–3 weeks. In 27% it was graded 3 and lasted 3–6 weeks; finally, a rare chronic form has persisted for months or years with occasional brief, distal dysaesthetic spontaneous bursts, and tactile evoked dysaesthesia, often nocturnal. Recently Taub (1986; personal communication) has found that the five patients with this dysaesthesia, in whom he injected subcutaneously 150 mg of 2% lidocaine, had total relief for 3.5–6 hours. Four of them continued a self-injection regime at 150 mg about every 4 hours with no decrease in the relief obtained and no side-effects for respectively 1 week, 1 month, 3 months and in one patient continuing at 18 months. Osgood et al (1976) mention in their table lasting dysaesthesias in four of their 18 cases. Three had had two and one had had three ganglia removed ipsilaterally. The dysaesthesia was increased on urination in two and during bowel movement in one. In two patients the dysaesthesia was mild; in two others it persisted at 8 and 14 months In the rigorously selected cases of Taub and Pawl among the great pool of patients with failed surgery on the low back, useful results have clearly been secured.

LESIONS IN DORSAL ROOT ENTRY ZONE (DREZ) FOR PAIN AFTER AVULSION OF BRACHIAL PLEXUS

Nashold & Ostdahl (1979) have proposed the operation of coagulation of the substantia gelatinosa of Rolando and the overlying structures dorsal to the posterior horns of the spinal cord for the treatment of pains which may be due to abnormal impulses arising in this area of the cord. The pain in their first group of patients had developed following avulsion from the cord of some or all of the roots of the brachial plexus. This mechanism of injury seemed especially likely to set up some type of irritative phenomenon in the tract of Lissauer and more dorsal layers of the posterior horns of the grey matter. Nashold operated on his first patient in March 1975, making a series of focal radiofrequency heat lesions 2–3 mm apart along the line of the posterolateral fissure at the site of the avulsion of the rootlets. The lesions usually extended for several centimetres to the first normal rootlets above and below the injury, so that 10–20 lesions were made (see Fig. 59.1). Originally he extended his lesion for 3 mm deep to the pia. In his first 21 patients this led to some persistent new postoperative weakness in 11 of them, which was 'barely detectable in some cases'. Some new sensory deficit was also present in 15 of the 21, the most severe and consistent

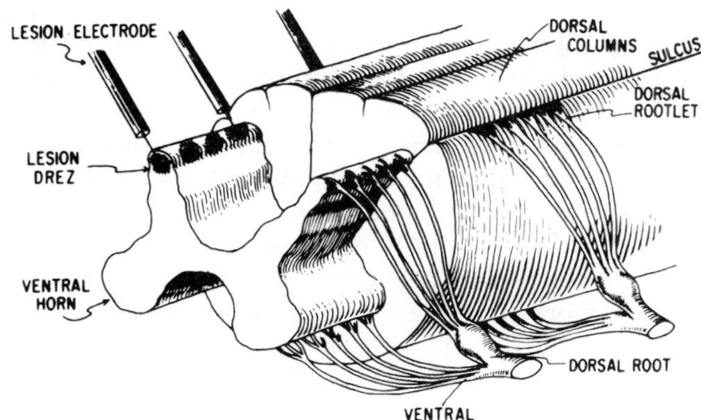

Fig. 59.1 Nashold's diagram of location of his lesions in dorsal root entry zone (from Nashold & Ostdahl 1979).

change being a proprioceptive deficit in the ipsilateral lower limb.

Cosman et al (1984) reduced the complication rate by completely redesigning the electrode to include near the pointed tip of a cylinder a thermocouple only 0.25 mm in diameter (rather than 0.45 mm) with a 1 mm teflon sleeve providing an insulated shoulder above the 2 mm uninsulated portion manufactured by Radionics (Massachusetts). Nashold has been using this electrode since 1982. The reports by nine other centres of 109 cases include four deaths. All of the eight centres which use the less precise method of monitoring by milliamperage of a larger, deeper electrode, as originally proposed by Nashold, describe few neurological complications. In our personal experience with radiofrequency heat lesions in the trigeminal rootlets, the actual temperature is a far more reliable indicator of lesion size than the voltage and milliamperage used.

At present, the temperature-controlled radiofrequency method competes with the argon laser as the tactic for making the lesions. Levy et al (1985) and Powers et al (1984), studying the histology of such lesions in cats, noted smaller lesions with the laser than with the original Nashold technique. Three postmortem analyses of the RF cord lesions in man are also available (Richter & Sietz 1984; Barcia Salorio et al 1985; Iacono et al 1988). In the case of Barcia Salvorio et al (1985), the lesions were made at 40 mA for 15 s and extended deeply to include Rexed's lamina IV of the posterior horn as well as some of the column of Burdach medially and the lateral corticospinal tract laterally. In the case of Richter & Seitz (1984) the lesions were made at 45–50 mA for 5–10 s and included Rexed's laminae I–IV and parts of Clarke's column of cells but the adjoining posterior and posterolateral white columns were less involved. The lesions in the third patient, who died on the 28th postoperative day, were made with temperature control at the appropriate 75–80°C for 15 s. Although there were 48 lesions on one side and 35 on the other in the lumbar cord which extended halfway into lamina VI, there was minimal impingement on the white matter – indicating that the current technique is accomplishing its objective. The groups of Makachinas et al (1988), Campbell & Miles (1984) and Powers (Powers et al 1984) are all exploring the evoked potential techniques during operation as an aid to control of lesion size.

Nashold's original method and his subsequent improvements have enabled him and his colleagues to operate on over 400 cases without mortality. Classifying as 'good' only those meeting the rigorous criteria of being off all analgesics with no limitation of activity by pain, Nashold (Friedman & Bullitt 1988) had 54% such results in 39 cases of brachial plexus avulsion followed for 1–8 years. A further 13% were 'fair', i.e., off all narcotics with no limitation of activity by pain – or a total of 67% reasonably satisfactory long-term results. These were obtained at the price, in 60% of the patients postoperatively, of subjective change in sensation and/or weakness in the ipsilateral leg with preservation of independent ambulation. It is important that the present lesion technique used since 1982 has yielded 82% in the good category.

This injury in motocycle riders appears to be a British specialty. Wynn Parry's series of brachial plexus lesions stood at 540 by September 1981. He states that in that one year in Britain there were 497 total avulsions of C5–T1. In a series of 122 avulsions he studied, 44 were still in severe pain 3 or more years later. Thomas & Sheehy (1982) at the National Hospital for Nervous Diseases have reported on 34 patients treated by the Nashold procedure after personal tutelage from Nashold himself. In a follow-up at 4–44 months, 60% had a good result, i.e. 20 patients had 75–100% pain relief, nine had 20–70% relief and only five had less than 20% relief. Thomas comments that he too reduced the undesirable spread of lesions to the posterior and posterolateral columns by carrying out Nashold's technical improvements. However, 12% have persisting new neurological deficits although all his patients are ambulant.

From nine other services come accounts of 91 cases. Although different grading systems were used for the results, 61 (67%) may be classed as having had roughly 70% or more relief at the last follow-up, which was relatively short in many of the patients.

CENTRAL PAIN OF PARAPLEGICS

Nashold (1988) has expanded the use of the technique to treat paraplegics with central pain, i.e. pain referred to an anaesthetic, analgesic area below the level of the lesion in the cord or cauda equina. In 5–10% of severe injuries of cord or cauda equina, such pain remains a major problem, tending to persist if it lasts over 6–8 months. Friedman & Bullitt (1988) note that the results of their DREZ lesions vary markedly depending on the locus and type of pain.

Those patients with 'end zone' pain, i.e. beginning at the dermatomal level of the cord injury and extending a variable distance caudally, tend to have both a constant aching and burning together with paroxysms of another pain, often cramping in character, lasting from 1 to several minutes. Of the 31 of their patients in this category, 80% had good or fair relief by their stringent criteria (see above).

In a second group are patients with diffuse pain which often involves the entire body and limbs below the level of the cord lesion. It tends to be worst in the saddle region and may be confined solely to the sacral segments. Of their 25 patients in this group only eight (32%) had good or fair relief. Having found that electrical signals from the posterior columns do not become normal up to two to three segments above the level of the obvious injury, the authors usually made their DREZ lesions from a few segments above to a few below this level. Extending the DREZ lesions down through the sacral dermatomes improved the pain in only one of the patients in whom it was diffuse or sacral. Most of the affected patients had bilateral leg pain, but in the subgroup of 10 with only unilateral pain, nine had good relief.

In another favourable group were those found to have nerve root avulsions at the DREZ operation. Those whose pain was worsened by distension of bowel or bladder were also improved. Complications included three patients with new postoperative weakness and three with other neurological change but no loss of useful function. New dysaesthesias appeared in only two patients referred above or below the level of the old pain, as one may see after posterior rhizotomy.

In those 18 cases with an intramedullary cyst, this was identified by a combination of myelogram, computed tomography and magnetic resonance scanning plus ultrasound at operation (Vieira 1987). In seven patients there were two independent cysts, one above and one below the horizontal lesion. Drainage of the cyst alone did not suffice, whereas in the 18 in whom this was combined with DREZ lesions, 12 good and two fair results were achieved.

In the most extensive trial elsewhere of the operation in these patients, Wiegand & Winkelmüller (1985) followed 20 patients from 5–34 months. They described nine as maintaining 100% relief and one with 80% relief. In agreement with Nashold's results, they found at follow-up that 10 had maintained their early postoperative relief; in fact, one moved from 80 to 100% relief. Only one of the 20 developed a new paresis.

In another series of seven cases with lesser lesions followed for 5–19 months, Powers et al (1984) controlled the 'end zone' pain at a level of 80–100% relief in six of the seven. However, in two patients with 90–100% relief of this pain, low back and coccygeal pain were not helped at all, confirming the experience of Nashold's group. Samii & Moringlane (1984) achieved 70–100% relief in two of five patients, but three other groups (Dieckmen & Veras 1984; Richter & Seitz 1984; Thomas & Jones 1984) had no benefit in any of their total of patients and did not use the procedure further in this group.

We venture to describe our results in detail in one patient with a traumatic total transverse lesion at T5 in whom pain was both of upper thoracic 'end zone' location, as well as coccygeal and in one foot. Since such patients are much less subject to further serious deficits and may also have more extensive lesions of deeper lying nociceptive neurons in Rexed's layer V we have elected to make deeper more extensive lesions. We describe these as a *posterior poliotomy* rather than a root entry zone lesion. In this case, 48 lesions were made, half on each side, each at 85°C for 15 s, extending for 40 mm from the lower T3–T5 levels down into abnormal cord. There was a striking difference in the electrical parameters required; the voltage varied (from site to site) from 12–20 V and the milliamperage from 20 – 50 mA to maintain 85°C. Complete relief lasted only 3 months; at 13 months the patient said his worst pains were two-thirds as bad as those he had suffered preoperatively, with an average of 40% of the original. Despite this discouraging aspect of his appraisal he stopped all of his preoperative narcotics and alcohol, and reports that his 'personality is now 10 times better'. His neurological deficits are unchanged despite the lesions in the presumed normal cord. In another patient with an arteriovenous malformation and a massive infarct at T12, extensive lesions were fruitless to deal with diffuse bilateral pain from the lower abdomen down.

POSTHERPETIC NEURALGIA

Another probable group of candidates for the operation seemed to Nashold (Friedman & Bullitt 1988) to be those with intractable postherpetic pain. This is a third group of difficult patients, once such pain becomes well established for a year or more after the acute attack. Nashold's series of 32 spinal cases includes only two less than 60 years of age, with some over 80 years old. The subjects were followed for 6 months to 6 years. Although in 90% there was early relief, the pain recurred by 6 months in 50%, with a present recurrence rate of 66%. Only three remain relieved at 25, 36 and 48 months, with only 25% continuing with excellent pain relief. This contrasts with the low recurrence rate in root avulsions and spinal cord injuries. In 10 of the 24 recurrences a new type of pain has appeared, which is not as severe and has been rated as 20 – 60% of the original pain, called aching in six, indescribable in three and cold in one case. These 10 cases were all limited in activity by pain and required analgesics. The original hyperpathia usually does not reappear. One-quarter of this older group of patients must walk with a cane and 44% have mild unsteadiness, along with increased deep tendon reflexes. In three patients the surgical lesion had failed to denervate a 1-cm strip along one margin of the painful area. Accordingly, the technique was changed so that the DREZ lesions are made from half a spinal segment above to half a segment below the area of pain. About 25 lesions were made at each spinal segment. No other group has used the operation extensively for the spinal postherpetics. Thomas & Jones (1984) record one failure.

PAIN IN AMPUTATION STUMP AND PHANTOM LIMB PAIN

Saris et al (1988), reporting their experience with 22 patients, note a difference in the results correlated with the site of the pain. Grading as a good result an overall improvement of three points on a scale of 1–10, they saw six of nine 'good' outcomes if the pain was confined to the phantom limb, whereas there were only two good results in the seven whose pain was in both stump and phantom, and no good results in those with pain only in the stump. No other report appraises outcomes according to site of pain. However, of six patients in whom a traumatic amputation was associated with root avulsion, five had good results, In the five other reports (Dieckmann & Veras 1984; Powers et al 1984; Samii and Moringlane 1984; Thomas & Jones 1984; Wiegand & Winkelmüller 1985) totalling 17 patients, six were described as totally relieved and two as having greater than 50% relief. The rest had little or no sustained relief. Although all five of Wiegand & Winkelmüller's lower-limb amputees lost any original DREZ relief, two of Powers et al's three amputees below the knee were still fully relieved at 1 year. In the Duke series (Saris et al 1988) there was no difference in the results of lower versus upper limb amputation. In two of the cases of Powers et al, new persistent dysaesthesias occurred; the operation in one was for amputation stump and phantom pain and in the other for dysaesthesias after posterior rhizotomy.

LUMBAR ARACHNOIDITIS AND FAILED BACK OPERATIONS

Hopes that DREZ lesions may be of help in this vexing group of patients have not been realised. In a thorough trial Powers et al (1984, 1988) have recorded an uninterrupted succession of early or late failures in 20 cases; two operations were done in two of these cases. Other neurosurgeons (Dieckmann & Veras 1984; Wiegand & Winkelmüller 1985), both groups with one case of arachnoiditis, describe no relief.

CONCLUSION

Those neurosurgeons who consider adding the DREZ procedure to their repertoire would do well to study carefully the full accounts of its brilliant pioneer, Nashold, and his industrious colleagues.

BULBAR TRIGEMINAL NUCLEOTOMY AND TRIGEMINAL DREZ LESIONS

The making of radiofrequency heat lesions in the secondary afferent neurons of the descending cephalic pain pathway in nucleus caudalis was first described by Hitchcock & Schvarcz (1972) and used by them for postherpetic facial pain. Further cases were reported by Schvarcz (1975) under the rubric of trigeminal nucleotomy and by 1979 he could give us the results on 115 such operations. Of these, 53 were carried out on 52 patients with syndromes of central pain. Via stereotactic instrumentation he sought, by enlarging a lesion at one site toward the rostral pole of nucleus caudalis, to induce hypalgesia rather than dense analgesia in those with preoperative preserved sensation. At times, contralateral lumbosacral hypalgesia was produced, but as expected, facial touch was preserved. No new facial or contralateral dysaesthesias ensued. Elimination of hyperpathia when present and marked reduction or abolition of deep burning pain were achieved in nine of 16 (56%) with anaesthesia dolorosa and 20 of 27 (74%) of those with dysaesthesia: 'mostly sequelae of Gasserian ganglion alcohol injections performed elsewhere, with additional superimposed tic pain'. Follow-ups were from 0.55–6.5 years. In his 1985 report on 21 patients with postherpetic neuralgia, this involved VI in 19 cases, VIII in 1, VII, IX and X in 4 and C2–3 in 5. In 16 (76%) hyperpathia and constant pain were significantly reduced or gone. One patient who had recurrent pain at 5 years was reoperated on and relieved until death 3 years later. Schvarcz was encouraged to perform his operations on nucleus caudalis by Black's demonstration that deafferentation by retrogasserian rhizotomy was gradually followed by grossly abnormal spontaneous activity in nucleus caudalis. Satisfactory relief was attained in 84% who were followed from 2–30 months.

The extensive overlap between V, VII, IX, X and upper cervical afferents in nucleus caudalis described by Kerr (1970) and the origin from it of an important ascending polysynaptic intranucleus pathway demonstrated by Stewart et al (1964) have been shown by Schvarcz (1979, 1985) to represent a fruitful zone for attack.

MULTIPLE LESIONS OF DESCENDING CEPHALIC PAIN TRACT AND NUCLEUS CAUDALIS

Extending his concept of making a row of lesions in the long axis of the spinal grey column and Lissauer's tract receiving afferent input, Nashold and his group made a line of such spinobulbar lesions 2 mm deep and about 1 mm apart from the uppermost C2 dorsal root 'along the dorsolateral sulcus' up to or slightly above the level of the obex (Bernard et al 1987, 1988). Thermocouple-controlled temperatures of a 0.2 mm-diameter electrode were kept at 75–80°C for 15 s. In the largest group, those with postherpetic pain, six of the nine maintained good to excellent relief at 4–39 months. The remaining 18 patients fell into seven diagnostic categories. There were five patients whose tic douloureux became atypical after treatment, four with pain due to neoplasm and three to anaesthesia dolorosa. The pain in four was due to neoplasm and in three it was provoked by a dental procedure. There was one good result in each of these three groups. Although the mean age of the patients was 58 years, only two had major complications and there were no deaths from this extensive procedure. Hypalgesia of all three trigeminal divisions was produced in the patients. A mild transient dysmetria was the only neurological impairment and none developed secondary dysaesthesias. Prognostic factors favourable for relief included a lesser preoperative sensory deficit, restriction of the pain to the trigeminal zone and a burning, lancinating or penetrating quality to the pain in contrast to a dull pain. If only one trigeminal division was involved, 75% had a good result; if two were involved, only 50% were in this category and this dropped to 38% if all three divisions were affected.

Ishijima et al (1988), using an even shorter electrode only 1.2 mm long and extending the lesions up to only 5 mm below the obex, have carried out an otherwise similar procedure in four patients. The two with postherpetic neuralgia have had 100% relief; of the two with anaesthesia dolorosa one was a complete failure and the other had residual medial pain. Complications were a slight truncal ataxia in two and a slight paresis of an upper limb in one. These radiofreqency lesions were monitored only with milliamperage measurement, which is perhaps the explanation for the complications which had not been experienced by Nashold.

We doubt that bulbar lesions only a little more than 1.5 or 2 mm deep are as much nucleotomies as they are tractotomies, but the results in the usually intractable trigeminal postherpetic pain are indeed encouraging.

COMMISSURAL MYELOTOMY

OPEN OPERATION

Rationale: early French experience

Greenfield suggested and Armour (1927) first carried out the division of the decussating fibres in the midline commissures of the spinal cord with the objective of severing at one operation the fibres for pain and temperature from both sides of the body. Since these are the principal fibres presumed to be in the commissures, the hope was that all other functions would be less disturbed than after bilateral anterolateral cordotomy. For the next quarter-century the French neurosurgeons were the principal pioneers. Even though Wertheimer & Lecuire (1953) conceded that pain fibres might be running in the anterior as well as the posterior commissures they made their incisions only 3–4 mm deep, intending them for the posterior commissure only. Although pain from cancer in the lower torso and legs led to the operation in 87% of their 107 cases they made their cord incision opposite the fourth to sixth thoracic vertebral levels in 80% of them. Of 80 patients followed more than 1 month, 33% had complete disappearance of all preoperative pain, 32% needed only small doses of analgesics and 35% still had significant pain. After operation one-third of the patients had radicular pain at the level of the cord lesion and another third had dysaesthesias in the legs. Except for one patient in each group these symptoms were transitory. Hyper- or hyper-aesthesia to touch occurred in 22 cases, proprioceptive loss in six. Decreased appreciation of pain and temperature was seen in 26, none of whom was in the group of failures. Leg weakness in 18% was always temporary and bladder complications exceptional.

Guillaume took the view that a much more precise placement of the cord incision was necessary, based on the assumption that all of the pain fibres crossed to the opposite side within two segments of the level at which the corresponding posterior root entered the cord, e.g. for postherpetic pain at C6–C7 one should, he said, divide the commissures of C5–C6. He even contended that one need cut only one cord segment if the postherpetic pain involved only one segment (Guillaume et al 1945). The relationship of the cord segments to the vertebral bodies is well described by Guillaume et al (1949). They recommended local anaesthetic for the procedure. This permitted use of the patient's responses to mechanical stimulation of the posterior roots to confirm that the proper level had been selected. The surgeon could also lengthen the myelotomy in the proper direction until the patient's pain was all gone. These surgeons urged total division of the commissures – a tactic which has been followed by all other reporting surgeons since then. They recommended confining the incision to three segments of the cord and advised against this operation in the cervical region, having had two deaths from 'late respiratory troubles' (Guillaume et al 1949). They give us no comprehensive account of their results.

Later experiences

Table 59.1 summarizes many of the results of those authors who have given us detailed accounts.

The next surgeon with a significant series, Lembcke (1964), describes the most drastic technique at the most dangerous level with the most spectacular results. In the cervical cord in 12 patients he made 'one smooth even cut' from the surface of the posterior median sulcus through the middle of the cord until he felt the bone in the anterior

Table 59.1 Results of commissural myelotomy

	Wertheimer & LeCuire 1953	Lembcke 1964	Sourek 1969, 1977	Grunert et al 1970	Broager 1974	Lippert et al 1974	Adams et al 1977	Cook 1977	King 1977	Sweet & Poletti 1984
Number of cases	107	12	39	24	34	16	30	24	9	9
Early complete relief of original pain (%)	–	92	96	92	90	Saddle area (68) Limbs (14)	91	70	100	67
Levels incised and length of incision	Usually 3 cord segments	Usually 5 cervical segments	2 segments (19) 3 segments (13) > 3 segments (6) 25–40 mm	Usually 3–5 segments	40 mm or slightly more	25–40 mm	25–40 mm	40–110 mm	35–100 mm	40–80 mm
Mortality (%)	14	0	3	8	3	0	0	0	0	0
Leg weakness (%)	18 transient	0 or transient	0	16	17 mild	13	7	0	20 mild	44 mild 22 severe
Bowel and/or bladder dysfunction	Unusual	0 or transient	0	8	0	0 or transient	10	0	0	11 incontinent
Initial analgesia			Bilateral girdle-shaped zone in most	Band of analgesia only in a minority; hypalgesia in most	Not mentioned	0 analgesia; small zone hypalgesia only (55%)	Minimal	Small zone early; gone later	Erratic; no band-like analgesia	Varies from extensive to minimal; soon fades
Dysaesthesias or radicular pain (%)										
Up to 1 month	68	–	Most	–	Almost all	55	In most	50	Never severe	Never severe
> 1 month	2	–	10	–	6	–	27	0	0	0
Cord level of operation		Usually C4–C5 to C8–T1	D10 or below in 26	T9–L2 area in 21 cases	D11 or below	T10–S5 in 13 cases	95% T10 Column	Various; C5–C5	Various all below T7 and down to S1 in 7	From mid-canus upward
Cause of pain (%)										
Cancer	87	42	76	91	90	75	91	67	67	100
Multiple sclerosis	–	–	4	–	–	6	3	–	–	–
Other	–	58	20	9	10	19	6	33	33	–
Proprioceptive loss (%)	5	–	Slight	–	–	–	Persisted 13	Early in $\frac{1}{2}$ cases; mild later	Many early, usually gone soon	Early in 44; remained severe in 11

wall of the spinal canal. He used an ultra-thin blade tipped with a tiny ball which 'pushed the anterior spinal artery to one side'. He usually carried this smooth cut from C4 or C5 cord segment down through C8 or T1. The first operations were done under local anaesthesia and on two occasions, based on the patient's first statement of persistent pain, he lengthened the incision. There was no operative mortality. In only one of the 12 was the pain relief inadequate and in only one was there a lasting neurological deficit, a severe ataxia, present only when the patient walked in the dark. At follow-up of more than 10 years in six of the patients, all remained painfree. These six had unilateral pain related to an amputation stump, phantom limb, brachial plexus injury or avulsion thereof. No mention was made of zones of.decreased appreciation of joint position, pin or touch. Cook & Kawakami (1977) also had one dramatic success in a patient with invasion of both brachial plexuses from bilateral breast carcinoma. Her constant pain in both arms was relieved by a 110 mm incision from C4–T1 at a small price of transitory hypernoia for 4 days. At the present time Nashold's procedure (Nashold et al 1976), or posterior-column stimulation, seems preferable for the unilateral cervical lesions which comprised the six long-time cases of Lembcke.

Sourek (1969) also divided the cord into two halves (Fig. 59.2), usually over two to three segments. He describes early analgesia involving two to six dermatomal segments in all of his 25 patients, but four in whom only one segment showed this deficit. A girdle-shaped area of bilateral analgesia in one patient had disappeared in 6 months. The three patients followed over 6 months had no recurrence of pain; one of these with 'arachnoiditis' rather than cancer was still painfree at 36 months.

Grunert et al (1970) tried only one myelotomy in the cervical region – a C3–T1 section which was followed by death on the fourth post-operative day. Follow-up in 11 of

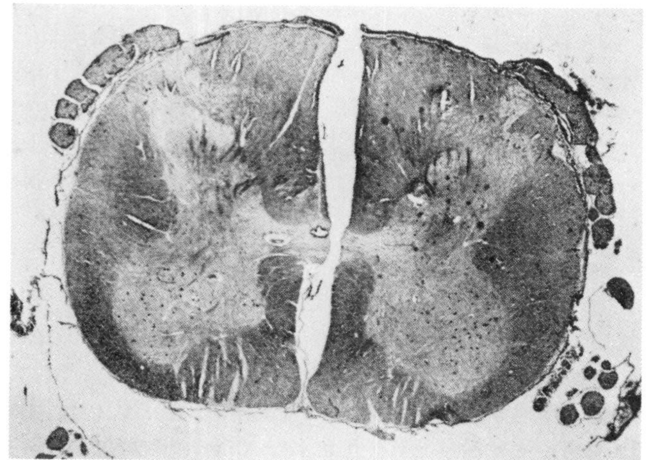

Fig. 59.2 Commissural myelotomy: postmortem section of Sourek's (1969) patient illustrating relatively atraumatic division of cord into two halves.

their cancer patients revealed that three had pains later above or below the original level at which they had become painfree. A recurrence of the original pain had taken place in three other patients. Hence these authors recommended longer incisions. Five of the 11 remained painfree.

Broager (1974) used a technique similar to Sourek's. He noted that diffuse tingling in the lower torso and legs, even painful dysaesthesias, were likely to be present for days or weeks after operation and in two of his cases persisted until death at 3 and 6 months. Two-thirds of his patients were at first freed of their pre-operative pains with no major side-effects. However, the pain recurred in one-third of these early excellent results. Almost all had such poor position sense that difficulty in walking lasted for days or weeks.

Lippert et al (1974) have used a more drastic technique. They coagulated the midline dorsal median vein and any tiny arteries crossing the posterior median sulcus for the full length of the proposed incision. Then they divided the cord either with a knife or a blunt microdissector for 6–8 mm down to the anterior median fissure. Their illustration suggests that this yields a more extensive injury of posterior and posterolateral column than Sourek's method. They made a short incision in the cord, only 25–40 mm long, which is probably correlated with the fact that leg pains were relieved, even initially, in only 14% of their patients.

The operating microscope has facilitated a more precise separation of the medial aspects of the two posterior columns with reduction of the diffuse dysaesthesias in the legs. Thus Adams et al (1977) noted their persistence in only four of 24 patients (who also maintained a proprioceptive loss). They appeared in only half of Cook & Kawakami's cases and had disappeared by 10–14 days after operation. They attributed this prompt subsidence to large doses of corticosteroids initially after operation with rapid tapering of the dose. Their patients with bilateral carcinomatous metastases were the ones showing the most dramatic relief, which was unusually maintained until they died. They gave the procedure a thorough trial for arachnoiditis of the cauda equina and lumbar radiculopathy in eight cases, classifying the late results as a total failure after months to 5 years in every case. Likewise in King's (1977) two similar patients the pain recurred after about 1 year.

Robert King (1977) has brought his customary perspicacity and thoroughness to bear on this problem. He emphasizes the extreme variability in the sensory loss to pain. His diagrams of this early postoperative loss reveal two patients with bilateral total analgesia from the costal margins downwards on both sides. One of these two patients had only a 41-mm incision from T8–T10. At the other extreme was a third patient with a 35-mm incision who did not even have hypalgesia anywhere, although the pain was relieved for 12 months. The rest had loss intermediate in degree and extent. Despite the erratic sensory loss, pain in legs as well as the lower torso was satisfactorily relieved in six of the cancer patients until they died in

4–6 months, and in the seventh such patient for 5 months – at the price of relatively inconsequential sequelae, i.e. two minor monopareses in all seven.

Our own experience and biases concerning technique in nine patients agree with those of King. We operated only on patients with pelvic cancers and devastating bilateral pain. We too used generous magnification with the microscope, sought to ease aside the midline vein at the posterior fissure, gently dissected apart the dorsal columns and spared small vessels crossing the midline in the septum. We usually used a delicate 7-mm wire with a ball tip (a Jacobson dissector) to complete the myelotomy down to the anterior median fissure, encountering virtually no bleeding. Dysaesthesias related to the separation of the posterior columns usually subsided promptly. Even initial major zones of analgesia did not persist. Thus one patient with an 80-mm long myelotomy had on his third postoperative day bilateral analgesia from L1–S5 except for sparing of S2–S5 on one side. This loss had disappeared in all but the feet by 6 weeks; nevertheless total pain relief persisted until death at 11 weeks. The typical early relief in these patients lasted less than 2 months in two of them and for about 1 year in a third. However one lady remains active and pain-free at 7.5 years, complaining only of tingling in the legs at night. In the hope of maintaining longer periods of relief we have lengthened our incision to 80 mm. Even though a paraparesis, severe in one leg, ensued in one such patient, he was grateful for the total relief of pain which had previously been inadequate even with epidural morphine and dilaudid.

Guesses concerning the mechanisms of relief

Sourek (1969, 1977) and Broager (1974) have both explained the common finding of relief of pain in areas not rendered analgesic to pinprick by hypothesising the presence of slowly conducting fibres related to pain in the medial parts of the dorsal horns. Guillaume et al (1945) described flashes of pain evoked by spreading the posterior columns in patients under local anaesthesia. Sourek (1969, 1977) confirmed work of Forster and of White & Sweet (1969) that mechanical stimulation of the dorsal columns with the patient awake causes somatotopically organized reference of pain. King (1977) points out that explanations for the relief remain speculative; he concludes that a combination of lesions in the commissures, the nonlemniscal systems in the grey matter along with some medial posterior column deficit may perhaps be responsible for the good clinical results.

Conclusion

The place of this operation is challenged by the much lower-risk use of epidural morphine or other pain suppressors. However pains in the saddle area, especially in the male, may be controlled only with such large narcotic doses that rapidly developing tolerance may lead to the need for a midline myelotomy.

STEREOTACTIC UPPER CERVICAL C1 MIDLINE MYELOTOMY

Hitchcock (1969), having developed an apparatus for stereotactic spinal surgery, used it to introduce an electrode and make relatively midline electrical heat lesions near the cervicobulbar junction. With the patient seated so as to keep the cord's midline close to the skeletal midline and with the head flexed to keep the cord taut he carries his electrode through the atlanto-occipital ligament into the cord. Subsequent refinements include impedance monitoring to determine when the 1-mm bare electrode has penetrated the cord. The patient is tested for distribution and depth of analgesia immediately after the lesion is made. The early extent and severity of the loss to pinprick often seen can only be described as astounding. Figure 59.3 displays the loss 24 days after operation, 2 days before the patient died. Early after operation there was complete analgesia to pin in the cross-hatched areas on both sides. The patient remained completely free of the pain in the neck and both arms related to his metastatic cancer in the lower cervical vertebrae. The postmortem

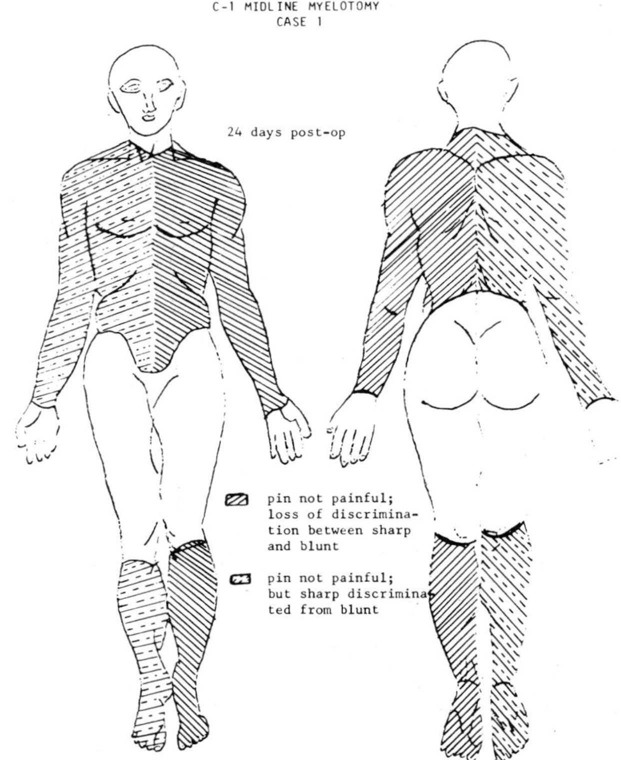

Fig. 59.3 Stereotactic C1 mid-line myelotomy (Hitchcock's case 1). Early after operation there was symmetrical loss of discrimination between sharp and blunt – the same on the right side as that persisting 24 days later only on the left.

study revealed an electrode track the full dorsoventral height of the cord 1–2 mm to one side of the midline. The unexpected analgesia in both legs led Hitchcock logically to try the method for lower midline pain. In his case 2 this was perineal from spreading cancer and was stopped for the 4 months of follow-up by a lesion which preserved the patient's ability to distinguish sharp from blunt but rendered pinprick painless literally everywhere except the medial parts of the face. Even though completely normal sensation was recovered in the saddle area by 6 weeks, pain relief persisted. In 1974 Hitchcock reported these C1 operations at the near the midline in 26 patients, mainly with cancer pain. There was no operative mortality, although the procedure was not completed in five patients due to technical problems. Of 19 patients who were followed until death or for up to 4 years, eight remained completely relieved without analgesics and five did not require strong analgesics. In these two groups there was well marked sensory loss in 75 and 80% respectively. Poor or no relief occurred in six patients who had but little sensory loss.

Hitchcock's pupil Schvarcz has an even larger experience, reporting on 17 patients by 1974 and 45 by 1976. His target was in the midline 5 mm from the dorsal surface of the cord. The lesion was usually made at the sites at which threshold stimulation – usually 0.5–1.0 V at 50–75 Hz evoked a tingling or electrical feeling in one or both distal lower limbs.The lesions averaged 2.5–3 mm in diameter. In 35 of the patients the pain was related to tumour; four had causalgia; three had postherpetic neuralgia; three had other painful central lesions in the cord. In the tumour group 22 had lower torso midline and/or bilateral pain; 13 had unilateral upper body pain. Satisfactorily relief ensued in 30; there was early partial recurrence of pain in the remaining five. Of the group with a nonmalignant cause of pain, one postherpetic patient had no relief and one with dysaesthesia after a Brown-Séquard syndrome had a recurrence in 6 months. The other eight were still painfree at the relatively short follow-up times of 9–24 months.

The only neurological deficit in most of Schvarcz's cases was the description of a pinprick as sharp but not painful. In only a few was there inability to distinguish sharp from blunt stimuli, i.e. conventional analgesia. This might be in one or both arms or the face; more rarely it occurred below the waist. These deficits could not be correlated with the responses to stimulation induced at operation. There were no lasting neurological disturbances of any kind, including no postoperative dysaesthesias.

A lesion of decussating spinothalamic fibres is an even less likely explanation for the sensory losses and relief of pain in these patients than in those after the much larger open commissural myelotomies lower in the cord. Hitchcock (1970, 1974) considers the possibility of 'an entirely separate purely pain pathway ascending in the spinal cord, possibly multisynaptically, close to the midline'.

Papo & Luongo (1976) have tried the operation in 10 patients. Relief until death at 5 weeks–3 months occurred in four. Initial complete surcease from pain in five of the remaining six was followed by relapse in 2 weeks–2 months. Only three patients showed a mild hypalgesia from C2–T10; this lasted only 3–4 weeks. The only side-effect was a transient ataxia either in the lower or in all four limbs, noted in seven patients. The period of relief was too brief even in these short-lived patients to encourage these surgeons to pursue the procedure.

The results of the operation do emphasise our bewilderment as to the mechanism of chronic pain.

CORDECTOMY

The first operation of this type carried out for the treatment of pain appears to have been that of Armour (1927). He did this in 1916 on a posttraumatic paraplegic in whom he excised totally from above the lesion downwards a mass of scar tissue including cord and cauda equina from the upper border of T12 to the L2 vertebral levels. The patient's intense pain in lower abdomen, legs and especially the thighs was totally relieved. In the same article Armour cites an operation late in 1916 by Cushing, who transected the entire cord rostral to spinal metastases; the excruciating pain these were causing was handled 'with an entirely satisfactory result'.

The pain in patients with total transverse lesions of the cord has been considered to be of at least three types:

1. root, segmental or girdle; these loci are related to the dermatomal level of the lesion
2. pains usually referred to lower bowel or bladder or general visceral
3. either diffuse or more focal pains referred lower to one or more insentient areas below the level of sensory loss.

As mentioned in the section on DREZ lesions, the more rostral of these three types of pain is more likely to be relieved by neurosurgical measures than those in the other two categories.

STUDIES OF A. JEFFERSON

The most encouraging presentation on both the value and the limitations of cordectomy for pain has been provided by A. Jefferson (1983). His operations on 19 cases – about as many as have been done by the rest of the neurosurgical world put together – were all carefully analysed at the Sheffield Spinal Injuries Unit. Jefferson states: 'The low overall incidence of intractable pain is a tribute to the quality of pain management by the staff of the unit'. Major pain did not develop in many of the patients until years later; the mean elapsed time after injury was 5.8 years. Those who did develop severe pain did so despite excellent care. An open mind as to the need for surgery was constantly maintained; e.g. one patient who was considered a candidate for cordectomy has his pain controlled by clonazepam and carbamazepine, remaining free of pain for the subsequent 4 years of follow-up. The mean time of conservative management following the onset of severe pain and before operation was 3.4 years. No operated patients had any useful function below the hips.

An especially encouraging feature of Jefferson's series is the fact that such good results were obtained in the pain of diffuse or caudal type in all 15 of the patients whose cordectomy (at and below the level of injury) was at or below D11 vertebra. Relief to the extent of 70–100% was obtained in 14 of the 15 patients whose pain was in thighs, knees or legs; in half of the 14 the relief was in fact 100%. In the 15th patient the leg pain disappeared but the patient graded himself as having only 50% relief due to continuing pain in buttocks, genitals and lower abdomen. There was a puzzling and striking contrast in those results with the outcome in three patients whose cordectomies were one level higher, opposite T10 or T10–T11. Two of these patients had pains in the tops of the thighs, lower abdomen, buttocks and rectum and derived no benefit; only 25% relief occurred in the third patient whose pain was throughout the legs. Likewise there was no relief given to a fourth patient with a higher lesion and a cordectomy from the body of D3 to the upper border of D7. Episodic pains were most likely to respond to operation.

Touch to the abdomen triggered the pain in the legs in four other patients. The effort to deal with this by section of one or two posterior roots at and above the level of the cord section despite being carried out bilaterally relieved none of them. Several of us have sought to extend the excision rostrally into normal cord; Jefferson did not find this necessary. In some of his patients who were cured of their pains 'there was still severe widespread cord damage at the level of the upper incision into it'. In a subsequent letter, Jefferson (1987) informs us that in his Sheffield Unit severe pain was present in almost none of the patients whose lesion was above D10 vertebra. Others have not commented on this preponderance of pain at the lower levels of the cord.

REPORTS OF OTHERS

The paper of Durward et al (1982) emphasizes the findings associated with posttraumatic syringomyelia, present in five of his six patients in addition to their severe pain. There were three whose progressive syringomyelic deficit included the production of new pain in the upper limb. This syndrome had appeared 2, 2 and 15 years respectively after the injury. A further substantial interval of 4, 4 and 1 year respectively was devoted to conservative therapy before cordectomy was done. In all three cases the upper level of surgical transection, although placed somewhat above the area of trauma at T6, T7 and T8 respectively, was well below the upper level of the syrinx. Accordingly, the upper ends of the specimens of removed cord were pathological in all three patients. Nevertheless they were all relieved of their arm pain. These three outcomes suggest that the pathological changes accompanying a syrinx may not be a generator of pain. In three other patients whose buttock and leg pain came on 13, 1 and 5 years respectively after injury, the cordectomies at T10–T12, T2 and T4–T5 gave rise to no relief at all. The excision at T2 was for a C6 lesion; the one at T10–T12 was for an injury at that level and the one at T4–T5 was well above the major injury at T7. However, in this last case there was a rostral syrinx lined by gliosis through the level of the upper end of the operative specimen. Hence the rostral incision was not into histologically normal cord in any of these three cases. A posttraumatic syringomyelia in two of them had been initially treated by drainage of the cyst which had improved other aspects of the syndrome, but the pain continued. All three of these lesions were at levels at which Jefferson's cordectomies had also failed to give relief.

In all of six earlier reports, each describing one or two cases, further successes have been described (Botterell et al 1954; Smolik et al 1960; Druckman & Lende 1965; White & Sweet 1969; Melzack & Loeser 1978; Tasker 1984). Botterell et al, in addition to excising into grossly normal cord at T5, also carried out a bilateral posterior rhizotomy at both T4 and T5. The operation relieved the root pain and burning pain in the feet was less severe. At late follow-up the authors graded the result as 'good'. This is the only case report in which additional posterior rhizotomy appears to have contributed to a useful result.When Druckman & Lende (1965) carried the upper transection of the removed cord through gliotic tough tissue at the junction of the T10–T11 vertebral bodies they did not relieve the patient's pain. Shortly after they carried out a second transection 3 cm higher through histologically normal cord, following which the original bilateral lower abdominal and groin pain was completely relieved, remaining so at 40-month follow-up. In a second patient studied by these authors a cordectomy through normal cord at the upper end again yielded relief persisting at over 12 months. White & Sweet (1969) also failed to relieve pain when their resection at T2–T3 was through a gliotic area; the opposite was true for a second patient whose resection was though normal cord at the T11 vertebral level. He had lasting relief of severe burning pain in both legs at 4-year follow-up. This good result ensued despite gliosis at the rostral end of the removed cord. Another resection at the T10–T11 level carried out by Collin MacCarty (Melzack & Loeser's case 3) had 11.5 years of complete relief of pain in the low back, hips, posterior thighs and calves. This relieved pain was of unusually episodic type in that there were attacks of spontaneous shooting pains each lasting only 3–4 seconds but occurring up to 60 times an hour. In the late recurrence the pain was of exactly the same type. In case 5 of Melzack & Loeser (1978) the pain was unusually high in relation to the site of cord injury. A T10–T11 total tranverse traumatic lesion was accompanied by pain around the right lower chest and abdomen. In this patient cordectomy at T8–T9 achieved partial success with initial disappearance of the pain; however it gradually returned to its original severity by 5 years.

Although failures dominate the accounts of the 11 patients described in this paragraph, Tasker (1984) noted in one of his six cases the cure of another case of episodic, severe sharp pain with ability of the patient to return to work. However, in this and in five other cases of his, pain in the anaesthetic lower limbs was not relieved. Such diffuse burning pain also persisted in the case of Davis & Martin (1947). Likewise, Freeman & Heimburger (1947) after removal of a 2.3 cm segment of cord at the T3–T4 level failed to relieve pain in a leg. The entire operative specimen was abnormal on microscopy. Cases 1, 2 and 4 of Melzack & Loeser (1978) were not helped. The T6 cordectomy in their case 1 was of no benefit for the principal pain in the abdomen and legs. In their case 2, a T11 cordectomy likewise failed to alter burning pain in distal legs, perirectal or buttock regions. This is the only reported case of total failure of a cordectomy at this low level. Even more difficult to handle are those patients with intrinsic cord disease, as illustrated by their case 4. Extensive unilateral operations preceded two cordectomies, one from T9–T12 and a second one at T4–T5. Although the first cordectomy stopped the pain completely for 2 years with only gradual worsening during a third year, the second cordectomy did nothing for pain extending from the right chest to the right toes. Melzack & Loeser had determined by appropriate sympathetic blocks that autonomic routes were not being used by the impulses causing the pain in their patients. This leaves essentially no other source of the generation of the pain impulses than the CNS somewhere above the cord transection.

CORDECTOMY FOR SPASTICITY PLUS PAIN

MacCarthy (1954), a pioneer in the field, has done the most extensive total cordectomies either for spasticity or for intramedullary tumour. He treated pain at the T5–T6 segments and the severely spastic legs of a patient with a traumatic T7 total transverse lesion by removing the lower 21 cm of the cord from T5 down. Although annoying girdle sensations and occasional root pain at the T5 segment persisted, the patient could stop narcotics and begin effective rehabilitation with a good result continuing at follow-up 6 months later. Smolik et al (1960) have also treated spastic paraplegia by cordectomy in four cases, in three of whom the spasms were very painful. The cord was removed from the T10 level down through the conus and upper cauda equina in all of four cases with the anticipated flaccid paralysis of the legs ensuing. When the muscle spasms stopped, the pain stopped in two of the patients but it continued diffusely in both legs in the third patient despite complete flaccidity throughout them. The diagnosis in this last case of thrombosis of the anterior spinal artery suggests again, as in case 5 of Melzack & Loeser, that intrinsic disease of the cord is less likely to be giving rise to pain treatable by cordectomy than sharply localised trauma. Latash et al (1990) have described gratifying effects of intrathecal baclofen on voluntary motor control in spastic paresis.

SUMMARY AND CONCLUSIONS

We are all encouraged to take a more optimistic look at cordectomy for the control of persistent pain after total transverse lesions of the cord by the outstanding success of Jefferson (1983), whose cord resections were at the level of the T11 vertebra and below. The mystifying abrupt decline of good results when the lesions are above this remains to be explained. Clearly the three successes of Durward et al (1982) in dealing with a painful upper limb associated with a posttraumatic syringomyelic syndrome by much higher cord resections make it clear that at least in certain situations higher cord resections also have something to offer.

BULBAR TRIGEMINAL TRACTOTOMY

Operations in these areas have for the most part been superseded by less hazardous procedures. However there remain special problem patients in whom such operations continue currently to be tried. The following list of further reading will aid an exploration of this subject.

BULBAR TRIGEMINAL TRACTOTOMY

Crue B L, Todd E M, Carregal E J 1970 Percutaneous radiofrequency stereotactic trigeminal tractotomy. In: Crue B L (ed) Pain and suffering. C C Thomas, Springfield, Illinois, p 69

Falconer M A 1949 Intramedullary trigeminal tractotomy and its place in the treatment of facial pain. Journal of Neurology, Neurosurgery and Psychiatry 12: 297–311

Hitchcock E R 1970 Stereotactic trigeminal tractotomy. Annals of Clinical Research 2: 131–135

Hosobuchi Y, Rutkin B 1971 Descending trigeminal tractotomy. Neurophysiological approach. Archives of Neurology 25: 115–126

Kunc Z 1970 Significant factors pertaining to the results of trigeminal tractotomy. I. In: Hassler R, Walker A E (eds) Trigeminal neuralgia. Georg Thieme, Stuttgart, p 90

Sjoqvist O P 1938 Studies on pain conduction in the trigeminal nerve: a contribution to the surgical treatment of facial pain. Acta Psychiatrica et Neurologica (suppl) 17: 1–139

BULBAR AND PONTINE SPINOTHALAMIC TRACTOTOMY

Hitchcock E R 1973 Stereotaxic pontine spinothalamic tractotomy. Journal of Neurosurgery 39: 746–752
Schwartz H G, O'Leary J L 1941 Section of the spinothalamic tract in the medulla with observations on the pathway for pain. Surgery 9: 183–193
White J C 1941 Spinothalamic tractotomy in the medulla oblongata. An operation for the relief of intractable neurolysis of the occiput, neck and shoulder. Archives of Surgery 43: 113–127
White J C, Sweet W H (eds) 1969 Spinothalamic tractotomy at the medullary, pontine and mesencephalic levels. In: Pain and the neurosurgeon. A 40 year experience. C C Thomas, Springfield, Illinois, p 712

MESENCEPHALIC TRACTOTOMY

Amano K, Kitamura K, Sano K, Sekino H 1976 Relief of intractable pain from neurosurgical point of view with reference to present limits and clinical indications – a review of 100 consecutive cases. Neurologica Medico-Chirurgica 16: 141–153
Liberson W T, Voris H C, Uematsu S 1970 Recording of somatosensory evoked potentials during mesencephalotomy for intractable pain. Confinia Neurologica 34: 382
Nashold B S Jr 1972 Extensive cephalic and oral pain relieved by midbrain tractotomy. Confinia Neurologica 34: 382
Nashold B S Jr, Slaughter D G, Wilson W P, Zorub D 1977 Stereotactic mesencephalotomy. In: Krayenbühl H, Maspes P, Sweet W H (eds) Progress in neurological surgery, vol 8. Karger, Basel, p 35
Walker A E 1942 Relief of pain by mesencephalic tractotomy. Archives of Neurology and Psychiatry 48: 865–883

Open cervical and thoracic cordotomy

INTRODUCTION

Division at open operation of the anterolateral quadrants of the spinal cord to cut the pain and temperature pathways concentrated therein was first carried out by Spiller & Martin (1912) in January 1911. Förster's independently conceived operation was reported the following year (1913). For decades this operation, unilateral or bilateral, remained one of the most successful for pain control in the neurosurgical repertoire. The perfection of methods to achieve the same result by the less stressful tactic of introducing an electrode through the intact skin into the relevant part of the cervical cord in the middle 1960s led in the most practised hands to excellent results with fewer complications (Tasker 1982; see also Ch. 60). For a decade it seemed as though open cordotomy might be superseded by the percutaneous approach. In the past few years, however, a number of factors have decreased the trend in this direction:

1. New therapy for many cancers has reduced the number of patients in this group with intractable pain.

2. Nondestructive neurosurgical alternatives, such as electrical stimulation of the posterior columns of the cord and chronic administration by catheter of epidural narcotics, are controlling the pain in many patients (see Ch. 53).

3. The percutaneous tactic requires a technical skill many of us never succeeded in bringing up to the level of the above-cited reports; the decreasing need for the operation means we shall not acquire this skill.

4. The secondary afferent fibres in the cord related to pain may be so diffusely distributed that lasting relief is more likely to be achieved by section of essentially the entire anterior quadrant on one or both sides. This is more certainly accomplished by open operation.

5. Physiological location of the pain pathway by the patient's sensation upon electrical stimulation within the cord's fibre tracts is nowhere near as reliable as this method for locating an electrode in the primary afferent pathways (Sweet 1976). Mazars (1976) and Rosomoff et al (1965), for example, have abandoned entirely the use of stimulation to localise the electrode.

Consequently we regard open cordotomy as an operation of immediate as well as historic interest.

INDICATIONS

The pain of cancer referred to one or both sides of torso and/or lower limbs remains the principal disorder calling for the procedure. Cancer pain referred only to one upper limb is a slightly less clear-cut basis for the operation, since it is a bit more difficult to secure sustained analgesia to pinprick in the upper limb by a C1–C2 cordotomy, whether open or closed.

Opinions diverge concerning the place of cordotomy for many of the types of severe chronic pain unrelated to malignant tumour. We have firm long-term data on relatively few of these syndromes (see Table 59.2).

LOCATION IN THE CORD OF THE PATHWAYS FOR PAIN

Although the pain tract was depicted in the earlier texts of neuroanatomy as a small compact bundle, it early became apparent that these fibres often extend throughout much of the anterior quadrant. Consequently Olivecrona (1947), Kahn & Peet (1948), White et al (1950), Nathan & Smith (1979), among many others, have recommended transection of virtually the entire anterior quadrant of the cord. Happily the inclusion in such a cut of vestibulo-, rubro-, tecto- and ventral corticospinal tracts as well as the ascending ventral spinocerebellar tract usually carries with it no consequential deficit from a unilateral incision at the mid and lower cervical and upper thoracic levels.

Table 59.2 Mortality and results with regard to pain early or until death from cancer

Authors	*n*	Mortality	Number with cancer	Number without cancer	Level of incision	Unilateral	Bilateral	Results
Cowie & Hitchcock 1982	56	3.5%	43	13	C1–C2 T2–T3	44 5	5 2	Of 43 with cancer grades I, II in 97% early relief, 55% at 12 months 0% at 18 months
Diemath et al 1961	126	5%	88	33	Upper C Upper T	23 38 11 secondary not described	6 43	Cancer 67% complete relief early; noncancer 67% complete relief early
Ehni unpublished observations	35	0%	19	16	C2	29	6	69% 'satisfied with pain relief'
Frankel & Prokop 1961	75	11% (all cancer)	59	16	C2–C3 Upper T		5 70	Cancer 67% complete relief noncancer 71% early relief; 30% later relief
French 1974	200	7.5% When bilateral 1 stage operations were stopped, dropped to 4%	177	23	C2			Grade I–II in 96% early
Grant & Wood 1958	129 86 66 31	5% 8% 18% 10%	244	72	Upper T, low C C2–C5 Upper T, low C C2–C5	129 86	66 Cancer 31	Grade I 51% of 92 Grade I 44% of 68 Grade I 40% of 50 Grade I 53% of 30 Grade I 44% of 72 with nonmalignant disease all early
Guzmán-Ramos et al 1979	257	5.3%	257			71%	14% 1 stage 15% 2 stage	Grades I, II 87.5% early relief
Mansuy et al 1976	124	3%	124		C8–C6 C7 C2	 43 18	1 stage 59	Grades I, II 85% to 64% at death Grades I, II 54% to 40% at death Grades I, II 88% to 72% at death
O'Connell 1969	56	4%	56		Upper T	2	54	63% complete relief till death or loss to follow-up
Perneczky & Sunder-Plassmann 1975	14	0%	14 all phantom limb pain		C2 Upper T	1 13		Grades I, II relief in all but 1 early postop
Piscol 1975	103	5%	80	23				Grades I, II 80% Grades I, II 61%
Porter et al 1966	34	0%	all cauda equina injury	34	T2 T1, T3	3	31	Grades I, II 87% 1–3 months postop
Raskind 1969	237	2.5% (all cancer)	207	30	T in 242 C in 32	28 with cancer 16 without cancer	1 stage 66 with cancer 9 without cancer 2 stage 105 with cancer 5 without cancer	Grades I, II 78% early postop Grades I, II 44% early postop Grades I, II 82% early postop Grades I, II 67% early postop Gardes I, II 90% early postop Grades I, II 100% early postop
Schwartz 1960	120	20% 1.5%	106	14	C1–2 C1–2	 64	56	Grades I, II 78% of 45 Grades I, II 69% of 62

Table 59.2 *(contd)*

Authors	*n*	Mortality	Number with cancer	Number without cancer	Level of incision	Unilateral	Bilateral	Results
White & Sweet 1969	21%				C1–2	28 with cancer		Grades I, II 54% early
	3%				C1–2	30 without cancer		Grades I, II 70% early
	6%				T2–3	138 with cancer		Grades I, II 73% early
	12%				T2–3		1 stage 86 with cancer	Grades I, II 81% early
	2%				T2–3		2 stage 47 with cancer	Grades I, II 85% early
	0%				T2–3	70 without cancer		Grades I, II 86% early

The safety of a transection of the entire quadrant at T1–T2 has been increased by the technique of Poletti (1982), who divides the fibres using an instrument with an insulated small round shaft having a tiny, smooth, uninsulated sphere at its tip. This is carried to the pia of the anterior median fissure and ventral surface of the cord without the risk of injury to the anterior spinal artery. Lateral and ventral corticospinal motor fibres are stimulated by the current from the ball tip and the incision is kept free of such responses.

Marked variations may occur in the number of cord segments above the level of entry required for crossover of the pain fibres to the opposite side. Förster & Gagel (1932) recorded numerous patients in whom the crossover was prompt, with analgesia extending up to within one or two segments of the level of incision in the cord. However, the crossover may be delayed for many segments. White & Sweet (1955) described a patient whose entire anterior quadrant was divided at T3, but who had analgesia only to T10. Hence, there is general agreement that the incision in the cord should be made no lower than T2 or T3.

Several authorities prefer the high cervical level for all unilateral incisions, both because complete crossover is more likely to have occurred, and because some think the pain tract is more accessible, having become more compact and more dorsal at this level (Grant & Wood 1958; Schwartz 1960; French 1974). Sweet et al (1950) found during electrical stimulation within the anterior quadrant that 12% of the responses were ipsilateral and 6% simultaneously bilateral. The ipsilateral responses tended to lie deeper in the quadrant. Persistent ipsilateral conduction may make necessary a second operation on the side ipsilateral to the pain (Voris 1951; White & Sweet 1955; Grant & Wood 1958). French (1974) points out that some patients after initial cordotomy even show analgesia to tests for both superficial and deep pain in an area of continuing pain, yet are relieved by a second cordotomy ipsilateral to that area. There are three reported patients in whom upper thoracic cordotomies yielded only an *ipsilateral* loss of pain and temperature sensation (French & Peyton 1948; Voris 1951; von Brenner & Pendl 1966). In Voris' patient the first left-sided cordotomy at T6 produced ipsilateral analgesia to T10, but a complete section of the right anterior quadrant yielded finally only hypalgesia from T10–L3 on the right, indicating an aberrant placement of these left-sided pain tracts, presumably into the posterolateral quadrant. Diemath et al (1961) described similar evidence for a grossly asymmetrical disposition of the pain tracts. Their patient with two ostensibly symmetrical 3-mm incisions at C1 on the right and C3 on the left had analgesia below T3 on the right but almost no sensory loss on the left.

Another major anatomical variation has been demonstrated by Moossy & Rosomoff (cited by Sweet 1976). They reported postmortem examinations after percutaneous cordotomies on three patients who had an analgesic level to pin, relief of pain and no hemiparesis following lesions confined to *the posterolateral column of white matter at the C1–C2 level.*

The topographic representation within the pain tracts usually places the sacral segments most posterolaterally with the segments lying more and more ventromedially as one ascends the cord – as though the crossing fibres at each higher level push more dorsolaterally those which have already crossed. This however is not invariable and Schwartz (1960) found three cases and Voris (1951) one case with reversal of the usual disposition such that the sacral dermatomes lay far ventrally. In general there is a sufficient mixing and dispersal of the pain fibres to make it inadvisable to try for a selective analgesia of only part of the area below the lesion (White & Sweet 1969; French 1974).

There are a few reports of a small lesion in the anterolateral quadrant producing a dense extensive contralateral lesion (Sweet 1976). Unfortunately there is as yet no reliable, feasible, systematic way to explore the interior of the human cord to seek out the fortunate and unfortunate anatomical variations.

RESULTS

These can be most succinctly presented in tabular form. Patients with the pain of cancer comprise by far the largest group, as is clear from the citations in Table 59.2. We classify the good results as grade I: no pain; grade II: pain relieved by nonnarcotics analgesics. The results recorded in the table represent our best guess at interpreting the authors' phraseology on this score. Cowie & Hitchcock (1982) classify in grade II only those in whom 'weak' nonnarcotics are effective for infrequent and/or mild pain and place in grade III those requiring 'strong' nonnarcotics for frequent and/or moderate pain. A disadvantage of the operation, as is indeed the case for virtually all other medical and surgical treatments for severe chronic pain, is the marked tendency for recurrence. The pain often comes back within months to a year or so. During this interval most of the cancer patients will have died so that the severity of their suffering and their short life expectancies make them the prime candidates for this procedure. When it is successful it has the priceless advantage of enabling many patients to derive some pleasure from the remainder of their lives and frees them from the incessant need to determine whether they can hold out for another hour or two until their next pain medication is due. Table 59.3 illustrates a quantification of this problem which we owe to the distinguished clinical pharmacologist Dr Raymond Houde (Houde et al 1965).

The operation has found less favour for those with nonlethal causes of disabling pain. Only the papers giving long-term follow-up results help us with this evaluation. Our own appraisal is that the results we and some others have had over the long term deserve a cautiously favourable bias when the less risky newer procedures have failed. Table 59.4 summarizes the evidence in support of this statement. In all but the publication of French (1974) we cite only the results in those without cancer. His experience of 64 patients with 84% good or excellent relief of pain at 1 year following C1–C2 cordotomy, including those with cancer, is so outstanding as to warrant special mention.

The data with regard to relief of the individual types of noncancerous pain are too sparse to warrant comment by type, with the exception of pain in two general categories: those related to amputation stumps and phantom limbs.

In the first group Porter et al (1966) carried out cordotomies in 34 patients, bilateral in all but three; all had shooting, stabbing or electric shock-like pains related to cauda equina injuries with a complete neural deficit below the level of injury in 21. After their exceptionally long follow-ups, from 8–20 years, 62% continued with either no significant pain at any time or relief by nonnarcotic agents. These results become the more impressive in view of the continuation of pain throughout the follow-up period in every one of the 13 patients who failed to get relief after operation. The authors point out that cordotomies were not done for the much less troublesome burning pain in the legs and did not affect such pains when present in these patients. Botterell et al (1954) with persistent failure after three unilateral cordotomies in one patient advise the bilateral operation. Unlike Porter et al (1966), they also used the procedure in five complete cord injuries low in the thoracic canal, achieving long-lasting relief in three. Burning pain in the saddle area was eliminated in one of them. White & Sweet (1969) gave lasting relief to six of 10 patients with cord injuries and four of seven with cauda equina damage.

In the second group, mainly with painful phantom limbs, Falconer (1966) and Perneczky & Sunder-Plassmann (1975) each have lasting encouraging results in 67% in their series of 12 cases each. White & Sweet (1969) had 12 early or late failures and 11 well relieved patients followed from 2.25–15 years, with an average of 6.4 years. It is worth noting that neither the patients with phantom pain nor those with major cord or caudia injuries can be tested objectively for analgesia in absent or insentient areas. Hence in them open operation with direct visualization of the extent of the lesion is especially indicated in preference to percutaneous cordotomy.

The series of White & Sweet (1969) remains the largest in the general group without cancer. We have had much less satisfactory early results after high cervical cordotomy than French (1974) and wonder if our incisions at this level were inadequate. We focus on the fact that over half of the patients have long relief after a thoracic cordotomy, but only those willing to face the thought that they may be

Table 59.3 Control of cancer pain by medication: double-blind study of Dr Raymond Houde and colleagues (1965)

Saline versus morphine Hypodermic injection	Percentage of patients with 50% pain relief	
Saline	40%	at 1 hour
Morphine 10 mg	65%	at 1 hour
Saline	8%	at 4 hours
Morphine 10 mg	30%	at 4 hours
Chlorpromazine alone Same effect as saline		
Chlorpromazine plus morphine Same pain relief as with morphine alone Drowsier than with morphine alone		

Table 59.4 Open cordotomy: long-term results, usually in patients without cancer

Authors	n	Disorder	Level of incision	Results	
Cowie & Hitchcock 1982	13	Noncancer pain		Grades I, II 46% at 12 months 38% at 18 months 23% at 3 years	
Diemath et al 1961	2 1 1	Gastric crises Tabes thoracic lightning pain Lumbar spondylosis No other long-term results given in 29 patients without cancer	T C	2 relieved at 5.5 and 7.5 years Relief at 5 years Relief complete at 6.5 years	
French 1974	104	Usually cancer	All C1–2	86% satisfactory sensory level without hypalgesic islands at 6 months	
	64	Usually cancer		84% (54) satisfactory sensory level without hypalgesic islands at 12 months Of these 10 with recovery of some algesia, recurrence of pain in only 4 – no recurrence of pain 94%	
McKissock 1961	8	Noncancer pain		Recurrence in few weeks in 2 Recurrence at 2 and 9 years in 2 4 painfree at 1.5, 5, 5, 10 years	
White & Sweet 1969	30	Noncaner pain (includes 39 cases below)	Upper C	Early postop grades I, II 1–12-year follow-up grades I, II	70% 33%
	70		Upper T	Early postop grades I, II 1–32-year follow-up grades I, II	86% 56%
Pain after injuries in spinal canal					
Botterell et al 1954	7	2 partial injuries cauda equina 5 complete injuries low throacic cord	1 bilateral high T; 1 unilateral T3 5 bilateral high T	Grade 1 at 8 years Failure after 3 operations 1 early failure 1 failure at 6 years 3 grades I-II at 2, 3 and 8 years	
Porter et al 1966	34	All cauda equina injury; operations only for sharp, stabbing pains not for burning pains	All but 3 bilateral T1–T3	1–3 months postop grades I, II 8–20-year follow-up grades I, II	87% 62%
				Early success / Late success	
White & Sweet 1969	4 6 7	Lower cord Lower cord Cauda equina	Mid-thoracic T8–T12 L1 or lower	2 / 2 5 / 4 6 / 4 } Follow-up 13 months–8 years	
Pain in phantom limb and/or amputation stump					
Falconer 1966	12	All phantom limb	6 upper C 6 upper T	4 grade I relief 2–15 years postop 4 grade I, II relief for years – 1 at 15 and 1 at 16 years	
Perneczky & Sunder-Plassmann	12	All phantom limb	1 upper C 11 upper T	Followed 1–9 years, average 5.5 years 8 grade I, II; 3 late failures; 1 immediate failure: analgesia only ipsilateral to incision in cord	
White & Sweet 1969	22	Mainly phantom limb	1 bulbar 3 upper C 18 C7–T3	Relief till recurrence at 5 years 1 recurrence at 3 months 1 recurrence at 9 months 1 relief at 15 years 4 early failures 5 recurrences at 1, 1, 2, 2, 8 years 9 continued relief at last follow-up – average 4 years	

in the unfortunate half as regards recurrence should elect this route.

The problem of selection for cordotomy of patients who do not have cancer is highlighted by the comment of Cowie & Hitchcock (1982) that seven of their 13 such patients cordotomized subsequently came under psychiatric care with the diagnosis of functional disorder. Of the 33 patients of Diemath et al (1961) with pain unrelated to cancer, nine were operated on despite an associated diagnosis of neurosis; five of the nine had recurrence of pain in a few weeks. Frankel & Prokop's (1961) series included five patients thought preoperatively to have an excessive reaction to pain; in four of these 'return of pain was explained solely by psychological factors, including hysteria'. Schwartz (1960) mentions 'four patients in whom emotional factors played a role so great that I should not have expected any significant degree of success'. We have encountered this problem infrequently since we have adhered to the policy of routinely consulting a psychiatric colleague especially versed in appraising patients with chronic pain. That the psychiatrists do not enjoy much more infallibility than we do is emphasized by the account of Porter et al (1966). After close protracted psychological evaluations the advice was that nine of their patients should not have cordotomy. This operation was nevertheless performed, giving grade I or II relief to four of the nine. (All but one of 16 for whom the operation was recommended after psychological evaluation had such relief after operation.)

COMPLICATIONS

LIMB WEAKNESS, AND BLADDER, BOWEL AND SEXUAL DYSFUNCTION

The mortality and lasting morbidity of unilateral cordotomy is uniformly and gratifyingly low. However, the bilateral operation carry a much higher morbidity rate for the two major problems of ipsilateral weakness or paralysis of limbs and urinary tract dysfunction. With the latter there is often faecal incontinence and, in the male, inability to develop erections or to ejaculate. There are major variations in the incidence of these problems in different hands, apparent on inspection of Table 59.5. As shown by Nathan & Smith (1958), the fibres for autonomic control of bowel and bladder lie in the white matter at the equator of the cord. Hence they are likely to be interspersed among the nociceptive fibres from the sacral segments. These autonomic fibres on at least one side of the cord usually need to be intact to maintain sexual, bowel and bladder function.

DYSAESTHESIAS

New types of very disagreeable sensations, which may be in new locations, may appear early or late after operation. They may even be of terrible severity with such intense hyperpathia that the patient cannot tolerate touch even of clothing to the affected skin. Tasker et al (1980) emphasize the difficulty in distinguising bizarre types of pain pre and postoperatively from such dysaesthesias, all of which may be related to intrinsic disorder in the central nervous system. Happily these are uncommon problems, as attested in Table 59.5. The complaints usually appear only after analgesia has given way to hypalgesia and are hence more likely in patients who live longer. However, Grant & Wood (1958) saw this symptom in 10 patients whose burning sensations were referred below their level of good analgesia; in only four were hypalgesic zones involved. Most of their cases improved spontaneously but the pain persisted for over 10 years in one person. In Falconer's (1966) series of 12 patients with phantom limb pain, new painful paraesthesias appeared following one high thoracic cordotomy after the initial analgesia receded. Extensive cordotomy at a higher level did not stop the pain in our experience (White & Sweet 1969) or that of Schwartz (1960). However relief has been achieved by several of the newer forms of antalgic neurosurgery. We do not regard the possibility of intense dysaesthesias as a flat contraindication to cordotomy for noncancerous pain.

HYPOTENSION

The descending vasoconstrictor pathway terminating in the intermediolateral cell column of the cord's grey matter may be cut sufficiently at the second side of a bilateral operation to produce a hypotension at what would ordinarily be a 'shock level'. However these patients typically remain normally alert and show no sign of vasomotor collapse. Later, orthostatic hypotension may appear even though the blood pressure in the horizontal position has returned to normal. In the experience of White & Sweet (1969) this symptom never persisted. Mansuy et al (1976) state that it was 'always gone in 10 days'. French (1974) found it to be 'temporary after bilateral C1–C2 incisions in 22% and permanent in 5%'. Diemath et al (1961) describe the worst experiences, i.e. a 'shock' level of blood pressure, after three of 49 bilateral operations. In one patient this lasted for over 5 years; in another patient it resulted in death on the eighth postoperative day despite massive supportive pharmacotherapy. There are other isolated nonfatal single case reports of this as a rare long-lasting complication.

RESPIRATORY FAILURE

The production of extensive analgesia up to the C4–C5 range bilaterally is dangerous to voluntary respiratory pathways which lie just lateral to the ventral horns of grey matter and are likely to be interspersed with deeper nociceptive fibres. Even if the patient has useful respiration when awake he may stop breathing when asleep (nocturnal respiratory paralysis). Although this dangerous state tends not to persist, the severity of the complication has led most of us to abandon bilateral high cervical incisions. In fact a unilateral incision may also lead to serious or even fatal respiratory failure if preexisting diaphragmatic paralysis or major pulmonary pathology on the painful side is added to injured ventilatory motor power on the operated side. Such patients have been reported by Grant & Wood (1958), White & Sweet (1969), Mansuy et al (1976), Tasker (1977) and Cowie & Hitchcock (1982).

POSTOPERATIVE RADICULAR PAIN AT LEVEL OF INCISION

This usually disappears in a few weeks. It persisted in only three of the 126 patients of Diemath et al (1961) after

Table 59.5 Open cordotomy complications

Authors	Level of incision	Weakness	Urinary dysfunction	Dysaesthesias
Cowie & Hitchcock 1982	88% C1–C2 incisions	Temporary in 2% of 49 unilateral and 14% of 7 bilateral	10% of 49 unilateral 14% of 7 bilateral	3 of 49 unilateral 1 of 7 bilateral
Diemath et al 1961	67% upper T incisions; 33% upper C 40% of ops bilateral	2 of 121 weakness on discharge but soon able to walk	Permanent in 13% of 126	1 of 148 cordotomies in 121 patients
Ehni 1974 unpublished observations	All C2 incisions	8 of 39 transient paresis only	Permanent in 7% unilateral Permanent in 18% bilateral	
Frankel & Prokop 1961	93% of 75 upper T	5% of 67 paralysis permanent in 3%; temporary early weakness in 41%	Permanent in 4.5%	
French 1974	200–all C2 incisions	5% paresis or paralysis after unilateral; 12% paresis of paralysis after bilateral	30% persistent if preop deficit (unilateral) 6% persistent if no preop deficit (unilateral) 92% persistent (bilateral)	
Grant & Wood 1958	C7–D3 unilateral C7–D3 bilateral C2–C5 unilateral C2–C5 bilateral	Moderate 4% of 98 to severe 18% of 33 10% of 86 20% of 30	7% moderate to severe 70% moderate to severe 9% moderate to severe 76% moderate to severe	8 of 105 C7–D3 incisions 4 of 98 C2–C5 incisions
Guzmán-Ramos et al 1979	90% of 300 ops upper T	3.6% permanent weakness or paralysis	6% in unilateral 93% in bilateral	
Mansuy et al 1976	C2 18 cases C7 unilateral 43 cases C6–C8 bilateral 59 cases	Paraplegia 0.8% of 124 4% moderate paresis of the leg but able to walk	'Frequent after bilateral'	None – all cancer patients Average life 6 months postop
Nathan & Smith 1972	23 C2 unilateral	Both limbs weak in 16%; transient in 8%; severe lasting in 8%; slight weakness lower limb in 22%	Only temporary after unilateral; persistent in 80% after bilateral	1 of 41 bilateral 3 of 79 unilateral
	45 upper T unilateral	Weakness of the leg: slight in 13%, marked in 13%		
	41 upper T bilateral	24% severe weakness lower limbs		
O'Connell 1969	56 upper T Bilateral in 96%	Paresis lower limb 11%– permanent but slight in half of these	Persistent in 13% after bilateral	
Perneczky & Sunder-Plassmann 1975	14; in 13 upper T	0 with permanent weakness	Persistent in 2 after unilateral	
Piotrowski & Panitz 1975	11 upper T bilateral 2 upper T unilateral 2 upper C unilateral	1 case		
Porter et al 1966	44 ops in 31 patients upper T bilateral 3 ops in 3 patients upper T unilateral	Transitory early new weakness in 1 of 13 with incomplete caude equina injury	All severely impaired preop	
Raskind 1969	46 unilateral 76 bilateral 1 stage 115 bilateral 2 stage	0 weakness 2 transient on 1 side 2 transient on 1 side	0 Persistent in 55% Persistent in 18%	
Schwartz 1960	62 C1–C2 unilateral	Weakness temporary 9; permanent 1	Persistent in 8%	In 2 of 120 patients
	45 C1–C2 bilateral	Weakness temporary 6; permanent 1 in 2 limbs	Persistent in 31%	
Tasker 1977	51 unilateral 62 bilateral	'Significant paresis' 15% 'Significant paresis' 39%	Nearly all in patients with pelvic cancer 2% increased impairment 25% increased impairment	
White & Sweet 1969	58 C1–C2 unilateral	Weakness temporary 8; permanent 1 in 1 limb	0	3 severe; 9 mild of 276 for cancer
	194 upper T unilateral	Permanent weakness 0.5%	Persistent in 1.5%	3 severe; 6 mild of 50 upper T for noncancer
	111 upper T bilateral	Permanent weakness 13%	Persistent in 23%	1 severe; 3 mild of 30 C1–2 for noncancer

discharge from the hospital. We have had one patient in whom it continued for 3 years before the annoyance stopped. Care in rotating the cord so as to place minimal tension on the posterior roots is the principal prophylactic manoeuvre.

CAUSES OF FAILURE

The principal reason of inadequate relief of pain is *an inadequate incision in the anterior quadrant of the cord.* Although many of us have adduced evidence to support this statement, the most extensive documentation is provided by Nathan & Smith (1979) who have postmortem studies on 80 cordotomized patients with cancer. They say that after the 27 cordotomy incisions which 'divided all the ascending sensory fibres of the anterolateral column', 'the original pain is no longer felt and it does not return; there is lasting sensory loss with dense analgesia'. These statements apply to their cancer group, in which their longest survival was for 2 years. They illustrate 14 erratically placed or inadequate cuts from their necroscopies with corresponding poor analgesia and relief. However, as already described in the section on location of the pain pathways, it is these which may at times be aberrant rather than the surgeon. A detailed sensory examination may be helpful. Thus White & Sweet (1969) found in four patients islands of hypalgesia in which multiple rapid pinpricks were sharp; at a second operation a deeper incision in the anterior quadrant stopped the pain in all of them. The sacral dermatomes are more likely to escape total section partly because of their usual proximity to the lateral corticospinal tract. Thus O'Connell (1969) recorded recurrences of pain in 17 of 56 cancer patients associated with patchy return of pain sensibility in the previously analgesic sacral segments.

When cancer pain is near the midline or slight on the second side, opinions are divided as to the advisability of doing at once a bilateral one-stage operation. All are agreed though that major pain on the second side is likely to occur soon in this situation.

Infrequently, pain persists well within the upper and lower levels of a zone of complete cutaneous analgesia to pin jabs. At times a pressure algometer induces deep pain in such an area. Nathan & Smith (1979) regard analgesia to such a device as correlating best with clinical relief from cancer pain. We agree with Diemath et al (1961) and Porter et al (1966) that the degree of relief does not always parallel the degree and extent of sensory loss.

LATE RECURRENCES

Late recurrences, as described in Table 59.4, may be due to redevelopment of some form of nociception via the anterior quadrant. Thus the recrudescence of pain in the patient H H (White & Sweet 1969) took place 15 years after a bilateral cordotomy. Another incision in the anterior quadrant contralateral to the pain restored objective analgesia and pain relief. Graf (1960) describes two similar cases. Late recurrences after fading of long-sustained analgesia are however more likely to be due to reestablishment of nociceptive pathways at other sites, since the uniform experience is that secondary cordotomies in this situation have a lesser chance of providing relief. White & Sweet (1969) illustrate the postmortem confirmation of a virtually complete incision of the anterior quadrant 5.5 years earlier; yet the clinical pain and that on pricking any part of the leg had returned after 8 months.

DRUG ADDICTION

It is certainly preferable to move to cordotomy before drug addiction becomes likely. Thus 22% of Diemath's addicted patients (Diemath et al 1961) failed to get relief, whereas failure occured in only 4% of the nonaddicted. Kanner et al (1981) noted two patients in whom major withdrawal symptoms complicated the result of otherwise successful cordotomy. However, Frankel & Prokop's (1961) series of 75 includes 32 with narcotic addiction; their success rate was the same in the addicted and nonaddicted groups. White & Sweet (1969) agree with six others whom they cite that addiction rarely remains a problem once the pain had been relieved.

CONCLUSION

It is the tremendous gratitude of the patient with sustained relief of pain that leads us to continue to recommend this operation to those willing to face its complications and risks of failure.

Acknowledgement

The authors wish to express their thanks to the Neuro-Research Foundation for its help in the preparation of this manuscript.

REFERENCES

Adams J E, Lippert R, Hosobuchi Y 1977 Commissural myelotomy. In: Schmidek H H, Sweet W H (eds) Current techniques in operative neurosurgery. Grune & Stratton, New York, p 427–434

Armour D 1927 Surgery of spinal cord and its membranes. Lancet i: 691–697

Barcia Salorio J L, Broseta J et al 1985 Lesion de la zona de entrada de las racies posteriores (DREZ) en el dolor por afectacion traumatica o neoplasia del plexo braquial. In: Arjuna V (ed) Combined Meeting/ Reunion Conjunta, Society of British Neurological Surgeons, Society of Neurosurgeons of South Africa, Sociedad Luso-Espanola de

Neurocirugia, 29 y 30 Abril, 1 Mayo 1985, Granada, Graficos Arte, Granada, p 149–159

Bernard E J, Nashold B S, Caputi F 1988 Clinical review of nucleus caudalis dorsal root entry zone lesions for facial pain. Applied Neurophysiology 51: 218–224

Bernard E J, Nashold B S Jr, Caputi F, Moossy J J 1987 Nucleus caudalis DREZ lesions for facial pain. British Journal of Neurosurgery 1: 81–92

Botterell E H, Callaghan C, Jousse A T 1954 Pain in paraplegia: Clinical management and surgical treatment. Proceedings of the Royal Society of Medicine 47: 281–288

Broager B 1974 Commissural myelotomy. Surgical Neurology 2: 71–74

Campbell J A, Miles J M 1984 Evoked potentials as an aid to lesion making in the dorsal root entry zone. Neurosurgery 15: 951–952

Cook A W, Kawakami Y 1977 Commissural myelotomy. Journal of Neurosurgery 47: 1–6

Cosman E R, Nashold B S, Ovelman-Levitt J 1984 Theoretical aspects of radiofrequency lesions in the dorsal root entry zone. Neurosurgery 15: 945–950

Cowie R A, Hitchcock E R 1982 The late results of antero-lateral cordotomy for pain relief. Acta Neurochirurgica 64: 39–50

Davis L, Martin J 1947 Studies upon pain of spinal cord injuries. II. The nature and treatment of pain. Journal of Neurosurgery 4: 483–491

Dieckmann G, Veras G 1984 II. Plexus avulsion pain (neurogenic pain). High frequency coagulation of dorsal root entry zone in patients with deafferentation pain. Acta Neurochirurgica (suppl) 33: 445–450

Diemath E E, Heppner F, Walker A E 1961 Anterolateral cordotomy for relief of pain. Postgraduate Medicine 29: 485–495

Druckman R, Lende R 1965 Central pain of spinal cord origin. Pathogenesis and surgical relief in one patient. Neurology 15: 518–522

Durward Q J, Rice J P, Ball M J, Gilbert J J, Kaufman J C 1982 Selective spinal cordectomy: clinicopathological correlation. Journal of Neurosurgery 56: 359–367

Falconer M A 1966 Relief of phantom pain by cordotomy. In: Knighton R S, Dumke R P (eds) Pain. Little, Brown, Boston, p 273

Förster I, Gagel O 1932 Die Vordenseitenstrang Durchschneidung beim Menschen. Zeitschrift für die Gesamte Neurologie und Psychiatrie 138: 1–92

Förster O 1913 Vorderseitenstrangdurchschneidung im Rückenmark zur Beseitigung von Schmerzen. Berliner Klinische Wochenschrift 50: 1499

Frankel S A, Prokop J D 1961 Value of cordotomy for the relief of pain. New England Journal of Medicine 264: 971–974

Freeman L W, Heimburger R F 1947 Surgical relief of pain in paraplegic patients. Archives of Surgery 55: 433–440

Friedman A H, Bullitt E 1988 Dorsal root entry zone lesions in the treatment of pain following brachial plexus avulsion, spinal cord injury and herpes zoster. Applied Neurophysiology 51: 164–169

French L A, 1974 High cervical tractotomy: technique and results. Clinical Neurosurgery 21: 239–245

French L A, Peyton W T 1948 Ipsilateral sensory loss following cordotomy. Journal of Neurosurgery 5: 403–404

Graf C 1960 Consideration in loss of sensory level after bilateral cervical cordotomy. Archives of Neurology 3: 410–415

Grant F C, Wood F A 1958 Experiences with cordotomy. Clinical Neurosurgery 5: 38–65

Grunert V, Kraus H, Sunder-Plassman M, Gestring G F 1970 Commissural myelotomy: indications and results. Wiener Klinische Wochenschrift 82: 865–868

Guillaume J, Mazars G, de Monillac V 1945 La myelotomie commissurale. Presse Medicale 53: 666–667

Guillaume J, de Seze S, Mazars G 1949 Chirurgie cerebrospinale de la douleur. Presses Universitaires de France, Paris

Guzmán-Ramos J, Anda-Ponce de León S, Mateos-Gómez J H 1979 Control del dolor incoercible por medio de cordotomia. Revision de trescientas intervenciones quirurgicas. Gaceta Medica de Mexico 115: 113–117

Hitchcock E 1969 An apparatus for stereotactic spinal surgery. Lancet i: 705–706

Hitchcock E 1970 Stereotactic cervical myelotomy. Journal of Neurology, Neurosurgery and Psychiatry 33: 224–230

Hitchcock E 1974 Stereotactic myelotomy. Proceedings of the Royal Society of Medicine 67: 771–772

Hitchcock E R, Schvarcz J R 1972 Stereotaxic trigeminal tractotomy for post-herpetic facial pain. Journal of Neurosurgery 37: 412–417

Hosobuchi Y 1980 The majority of unmyelinated afferent axons in human ventral roots probably conduct pain. Pain 8: 167–180

Houde R, Wallenstein S L, Beaver W T 1965 Clinical measurement of pain. In: deStevens G (ed) Analgetics. Academic Press, New York, p 75

Iacono R P, Aguirre M L, Nashold B S 1988 Anatomic examination of human dorsal root entry zone lesions. Applied Neurophysiology 51: 225–229

Ishijima B, Shimoji K, Shimizu H, Takahashi H, Suzuki I 1988 Lesions of spinal and trigeminal dorsal root entry zone for deafferentation pain. Experience of 35 cases. Applied Neurophysiology 51: 175–187

Jefferson A 1982 Cordectomy for the pain of paraplegics referred below the level of the lesion. Personal communication

Jefferson A 1983 Cordectomy for intractable pain in paraplegia. In: Lipton S, Miles Y (eds) Persistent pain, vol 4. Grune & Stratton, Orlando, p 115–132

Kahn E A, Peet M M 1984 The technique of antero-lateral cordotomy. Journal of Neurosurgery 5: 276–283

Kanner R M, Foley K M, Galicich 1981 Patient selection for cordotomy in cancer pain. Third World Congress on Pain of the International Association for the Study of Pain, Edinburgh, September (abstract) 4–11

Kerr F W L 1970 The fine structure of the subnucleus caudalis of the trigeminal nerve. Brain Research 23: 129–145

King R B 1977 Anterior commissurotomy for intractable pain. Journal of Neurosurgery 47: 7–11

Latash M L, Penn R O, Corescos D M, Gottlieb G L 1990 Journal of Neurosurgery 72: 388–393

Lembcke W 1964 Uber die mediolongitudinale Chordotomie im Halsmarkbereich. Zentralblatt für Chirurgie 89: 439–443

Levy W J, Gallo C, Watts C 1985 Comparison of laser and radiofrequency dorsal root entry zone lesions in cats. Neurosurgery 16: 327–330

Lippert R G, Hosobuchi T, Nielsen S L 1974 Spinal commissurotomy. Surgical Neurology 2: 373–377

Loeser J D, Ward A A Jr, White L E Jr 1968 Chronic deafferentation of human spinal cord neurons. Journal of Neurosurgery 29: 48–50

McKissock W 1961 Spinothalamic chordotomy. Second International Congress of Neurological Surgery, Washington D C (abstract no S17): D31–D34

Makachinas T, Ovelmen-Levitt J, Nashold B S 1988 Intraoperative somatosensory evoked potentials. A localizing technique in the DREZ operation. Applied Neurophysiology 51: 146–153

Mansuy L, Sindou M, Fischer G, Brunon J 1976 Spinothalamic cordotomy in cancerous pain. Results of a series of 124 patients operated on by the direct posterior approach. Neurochirurgie 22: 437–444

Mazars G 1976 Etat actuel de la chirurgie de la douleur. Neurochirurgie (suppl 1) 22: 1

Melzack R, Loeser J D 1978 Phantom body pain in paraplegics: Evidence for a central 'pattern generating mechanism' for pain. Pain 4: 195–210

Nashold B S Jr 1988 Neurosurgical technique of the dorsal root entry zone operation. Applied Neurophysiology 51: 136–145

Nashold B S Jr, Ostdahl R H 1979 Dorsal root entry zone lesions for pain relief. Journal of Neurosurgery 51: 59–69

Nashold B S Jr, Urban B, Zorub D S 1976 Phantom relief by focal destruction of substantia gelatinosa of Rolando. In: Bonica J J, Albe-Fessard D (eds) Advances in pain research and therapy, vol 1. Raven Press, New York, p 959

Nathan P W, Smith M C 1958 The centrifugal pathway for micturition within the spinal cord. Journal of Neurology, Neurosurgery and Psychiatry 21: 177–189

Nathan P W, Smith M C 1972 Pain in cancer: comparison of results of cordotomy and chemical rhizotomy. In: Fusek I, Kunc Z (eds) Present limits of neurosurgery. Excerpta Medica, Amsterdam, p 513–519

Nathan P W, Smith M C 1979 Clinico-anatomical correlation in anterolateral cordotomy. In: Bonica J J, Liebeskind J C,

Albe-Fessard D G (eds) Advances in pain research and therapy, vol 3. Raven Press, New York, p 921
O'Connell J E A 1969 Anterolateral chordotomy for intractable pain in carcinoma of the rectum. Proceedings of the Royal Society of Medicine 62: 1223–1225
Olivercrona H 1947 The surgery of pain. Acta Psychiatrica Scandinavica (suppl) 46: 268–280
Osgood C P 1982 Personal communication
Osgood C P, Dujovny M, Faille R, Abassy M 1976 Microsurgical lumbar ganglionectomy, anatomic rationale and surgical results. Acta Neurochirurgica 35: 197–204
Papo I, Luongo A 1976 High cervical commissural myelotomy in the treatment of pain. Journal of Neurology, Neurosurgery and Psychiatry 39: 705–710
Pawl R P 1982 Microsurgical ganglionectomy for treatment of arachnoiditis-related unilateral sciatica. In: Program and Abstracts, The American Pain Society, Third General Meeting, Miami Beach, No. 44
Perneczky A, Sunder-Plassmann M 1975 Anterolateral cordotomy in cases of phantom limb pain. In: Penzholz H, Brock M, Hamer J, Klinger M, Spoerri I (eds) Advances in neurosurgery, vol 3, Springer Verlag, New York, p 170–173
Piotrowski W, Panitz C 1975 Results after open cordotomy. In: Penzholz H, Brock M, Hamer J, Klinger M, Spoerri I (eds) Advances in neurosurgery, vol 3. Springer Verlag, New York, p 174
Piscol K 1975 Open spinal surgery for (intractable) pain. In: Penzholz H, Brock M, Hamer J, Klinger M, Spoerri I (eds) Advances in neurosurgery, vol 3. Springer Verlag, New York, p 157–169
Poletti C E 1982 Open cordotomy – new techniques. In: Schmidek H H, Sweet W H (eds) Operative neurosurgical techniques. Grune & Stratton, New York, p 1155–1168
Porter R W, Hohmann G W, Bors E, French J D 1966 Cordotomy for pain following cauda equina injury. Archives of Surgery 92: 765–770
Powers S K, Adams J E, Edwards M S B, Boggan J E, Hosobuchi Y 1984 Pain relief from dorsal root entry zone lesions made with argon and carbon dioxide microsurgical lasers. Journal of Neurosurgery 61: 841–847
Powers S K, Barbaro N M, Levy R M 1988 Pain control with laser-produced dorsal root entry zone lesions. Applied Neurophysiology 51: 243–254
Raskind R 1969 Analytical review of open cordotomy. International Surgery 51: 226–231
Richter H P, Seitz H 1984 Dorsal root entry zone lesions for the control of deafferentation pain: experiences in 10 patients. Neurosurgery 15: 956–959
Rosomoff H L, Carroll F, Brown J, Sheptak P 1965 Cordotomy: technique. Journal of Neurosurgery 23: 639–644
Samii M, Moringlane J R 1984 Thermocoagulation of the dorsal root entry zone for the treatment of intractable pain. Neurosurgery 15: 953–955
Saris S C, Iacono R P, Nashold B S 1984 DREZ for postamputation pain. Neurosurgery 15: 269–270
Saris S C, Iacono R P, Nashold B S 1988 Successful treatment of phantom pain with dorsal root entry zone coagulation. Applied Neurophysiology 51: 188–197
Schvarcz J R 1974 Spinal cord stereotactic surgery. In: Sano K, Ishii S (eds) Recent progress in neurological surgery. Excerpta Medica, Amsterdam, p 234–241
Schvarcz J R 1975 Stereotactic trigeminal tractotomy. Cofinia Neurologica 37: 73–77
Schvarcz J R 1976 Stereotactic extralemniscal myelotomy. Journal of Neurology, Neurosurgery and Psychiatry 39: 53–57
Schvarcz J R 1979 Stereotactic spinal trigeminal nucleotomy for dysesthetic facial pain. In: Bonica J J et al (eds) Advances in pain research and therapy, vol 3. Raven Press, New York, p 331–336
Schvarcz J R 1985 Trigeminal, glosso-vagal and high cervical post-herpetic neuralgia treated by stereotactic spinal trigeminal nucleotomy. Presented at the VIIIth International Congress of Neurological Surgery, Toronto, Ontario
Schwartz H G 1960 High cervical tractotomy – technique and results. Clinical Neurosurgery 8: 282–293
Smith F P 1970 Trans-spinal ganglionectomy for relief of intercostal pain. Journal of Neurosurgery 32: 574–577
Sourek K 1969 Commissural myelotomy. Journal of Neurosurgery 31: 524–527
Sourek K 1977 Mediolongitudinal myelotomy. In: Krayenbühl H, Maspes P, Sweet W H (eds) Progress in neurological surgery, vol 8. Karger, Basel, p 15–34
Spiller W G, Martin E 1912 The treatment of persistent pain of organic origin in the lower part of the body by division of the anterolateral column of the spinal cord. Journal of the American Medical Association 58: 1489–1490
Stewart W A, Stoops W L, Pillone P R, King R B 1974 An electrophysiologic study of ascending pathways from nucleus caudalis of the spinal trigeminal nuclear complex. Journal of Neurosurgery 21: 35–48
Strait T A, Hunter S E 1981 Intraspinal extradural sensory rhizotomy in a patient with failure of lumbar disc surgery. Journal of Neurosurgery 54: 193–196
Sweet W H 1976 Recent observations pertinent to improving anterolateral cordotomy. Clinical Neurosurgery 23: 80–95
Sweet W H, Poletti C E 1984 Operations in the brain stem and spinal canal, with an appendix on open cordotomy. In: Wall P D, Melzack R (eds) Textbook of pain, 1st edn. Churchill Livingstone, Edinburgh, p 615–631
Sweet W H, White J C, Selverstone B, Nilges R 1950 Sensory responses from anterior roots and from surface and interior of spinal cord in man. Transactions of the American Neurological Association 74: 165–169
Tasker R R 1977 Open cordotomy. In: Krayenbühl H H, Maspes P E, Sweet W H (eds) Progress in neurological surgery, vol 8. Karger, Basel, p 1–14
Tasker R R 1982 Percutaneous cordotomy – the lateral high cervical technique. In: Schmidek H H, Sweet W H (eds) Operative neurosurgical techniques. Grune & Stratton, New York, p 1137
Tasker R R, Organ L W, Hawrylshyn P 1980 In: Bonica J J (ed) Pain, vol 58. Association for Research in Nervous and Mental Diseases. Raven Press, New York, p 305–329
Taub A 1982 Relief of chronic intractable sciatica by dorsal root ganglionectomy. In: Program and Abstracts, The American Pain Society, Third General Meeting, Miami Beach, No. 45
Thomas D G T, Sheehy J 1982 Dorsal root entry zone coagulation. (Nashold's procedure) for pain due to brachial plexus avulsion Journal of Neurology, Neurosurgery and Psychiatry 45: 949
Thomas D G T, Jones S J 1984 Dorsal root entry zone lesions (Nashold's procedure) in brachial plexus avulsion. Neurosurgery 15: 966–968
Thomas J H, MacArthur R I, Pierce G E, Hermreck A S 1980 Hickman-Broviac catheters. Indications and results. American Journal of Surgery 140: 791–796
Vieira J F S 1987 DREZ lesions in post-traumatic intramedullary cysts. Presented to the DREZ Symposium, Duke, Duke University, Durham, North Carolina, April 23–25
von Brenner H, Pendl G 1966 Ipsilateraler Chordotomieeffekt – ein seltener Fall einer ungekruezten Schmerzbhan. Wiener Medizinsche Wochenschrift 116: 1041–1042
Voris H C 1951 Ipsilateral sensory loss following chordotomy. Archives of Neurology and Psychiatry 65: 95–96
Wertheimer P, LeCuire J 1953 La myelotomie commissurale postérieure. A propos de 107 observations. Acta Chirurgica Belgica 52: 568–574
White J C, Sweet W H 1955 Pain: its mechanisms and neurosurgical control. C C Thomas, Springfield, Illinois
White J C, Sweet W H 1969 Pain and the neurosurgeon. A 40 year experience. C C Thomas, Springfield, Illinois
White J C, Sweet W H, Hawkins R, Nigles R G 1950 Anterolateral cordotomy: results, complications and causes of failure. Brain 73: 346–367
Wiegand H, Winkelmuller W 1985 Behandlung des Deafferentierungsschemerzes durch Hochfrequenzläsion der Hinterwurzeleintrittszone. Deutsche Medizinische Wochenschrift 110: 216–220
Wynn Parry C B 1981 Therapies of pain due to spinal root avulsion. Pain (suppl) 1: S84

Addendum on the relationship of open to percutaneous cordotomy

Jan. M. Gybels

In 1963 Mullan et al introduced a percutaneous method for performing an anterolateral cordotomy. The different techniques available for this procedure have been described in detail by a number of authors (Mullan et al 1963, 1965; Rosomoff et al 1965; Lin et al 1966; Rosomoff 1968; Gildenberg et al 1968; Crue et al 1968; Hekmatpanah 1968; Taren et al 1969; Lorenz 1976; Tasker 1976/77; Gildenberg 1976/77, 1982; Ganz & Mullan 1977; Lipton & McLennan 1980; Tasker 1982; Ischia et al 1983). It is not an easy procedure and, since indications for destructive interventions designed to interrupt nociceptive pathways have become exceptional, not many individuals acquire the necessary skills to perform the procedure safely and successfully. There is no basic difference in the indication for percutaneous versus open anterolateral cordotomy (Gybels & Sweet 1989). I now see as an indication for both procedures the situation in which nociceptive pain is due to cancer, preferably in the trunk and lower limb on one side, when survival time is estimated to be more than, say, 5 months and other more conservative treatment modalities have failed. Due to the marked tendency – as time passes – for recurrence of the original pain, or the appearance of a new type of pain, I do not think that anterolateral cordotomy is, at present, indicated for pain of non-cancerous origin. Not everybody will agree with this statement and reasons not to agree can be found in the data collected by Sweet & Poletti in this chapter, particularly the data in Table 59.4

REFERENCES

Crue B L, Todd E M, Carregal J A 1968 Posterior approach for high cervical percutaneous radiofrequency cordotomy. Confinia Neurologica 30: 41–52

Ganz E, Mullan S 1977 Percutaneous cordotomy. In: Lipton S (ed) Persistent pain: modern methods of treatment, vol 1. Academic Press, London/Grune & Stratton, New York, p 21–33

Gildenberg P L 1976/77 Percutaneous cervical cordotomy. Applied Neurophysiology 39: 97–113

Gildenberg P L 1982 Spinal stereotaxic procedures. In: Schaltenbrand G, Walker A E (eds) Stereotaxy of the human brain, 2nd edn. Thieme, Stuttgart, p 469–474

Gildenberg P L, Lin P M, Polakoff P P, Flitter M A 1968 Anterior percutaneous cervical cordotomy: determination of target point and calculation of angle of insertion. Journal of Neurosurgery 28: 173–177

Gybels J, Sweet W H 1989 Neurosurgical treatment of persistent pain. Karger, Basel

Hekmatpanah J 1968 Techniques and results of percutaneous cordotomy. Medical Clinics of North America 52: 189–201

Ischia S, Luzzani A, Maffezzoli G F, Pacini L, Nicolini F 1983 Percutaneous cervical cordotomy: technical considerations and results in 400 treated cases. In: Rizzi R, Visentin M (eds) Pain therapy. Elsevier, Amsterdam, p 367–379

Lin P M, Gildenberg P L, Polakogg P P 1966 An anterior approach to percutaneous lower cervical cordotomy. Journal of Neurosurgery 25: 553–560

Lipton S, McLennan J E 1980 Percutaneous spinothalamic tractotomy: the prototype of neurosurgical pain control. In: Cousins M J, Bridenbaugh P O (eds) Neural blockade. Lippincott, Philadelphia, p 679–690

Lorenz R 1976 Methods of percutaneous spinothalamic tract section. In: Krayenbühl H (ed) Advances and technical standards in neurosurgery, vol 3. Springer, Wien, p 123–145

Mullan S, Harper P V, Hekmatpanah J, Torres H, Dobben G 1963 Percutaneous interruption of spinal-pain tracts by means of a strontium needle. Journal of Neurosurgery 20: 931–939

Mullan S, Hekmatpanah J, Dobben G, Beckman F 1965 Percutaneous intramedullary cordotomy utilizing the unipolar anodal electrolytic lesion. Journal of Neurosurgery 22: 548–553

Rosomoff H L 1968 Cordotomy: 1967. Lancet ii: 23–27

Rosomoff H L, Carroll F, Brown J, Sheptak P 1965 Percutaneous radiofrequency cervical cordotomy technique. Journal of Neurosurgery 23: 639–644

Taren J A, Davis R, Crosby E C 1969 Target physiologic corroboration in stereotaxic cervical cordotomy. Journal of Neurosurgery 30: 569–584

Tasker R R 1976/77 Percutanous cervical cordotomy. Applied Neurophysiology 39: 114–121

Tasker R R 1982 Percutaneous cordotomy – the lateral high cervical technique. In: Schmidek H H, Sweet W H (eds) Operative neurosurgical techniques: indications, methods and results. Grune & Stratton, New York, vol 2, p 1137–1153

Addendum on the relationship of open to percutaneous cordotomy

60. Sterotactic surgery

R. R. Tasker

INTRODUCTION

The management of chronic pain must have tested the ingenuity of man from earliest times. Even now, so desperate can the problem be that surgeons have felt justified in destroying parts of the nervous system in the hope of lessening the suffering. Pain surgery can be said to have 'come of age' with the demonstration by Spiller & Martin (1912) that pathways apparently responsible for the perception of pain could be selectively severed in the spinal cord with preservation of essential sensory and motor function, a concept that soon became well established at the level of the spinal cord and which was then extended to the brain. Open procedures for severing sensory cranial nerves and brainstem pain pathways were developed, particularly medullary and mesencephalic tractotomy – rostral extensions of Spiller & Martin's cordotomy – to cope with pain located in parts of the body not amenable to control by making lesions in the spinal cord or spinal nerves. Unfortunately the impact of such major procedures on the patient already ill with a chronic pain syndrome detracted from their cost-effectiveness.

The dream of guiding a probe through a small opening in the skull towards an unseen target located anywhere within the brain and of manipulating that target with minimal impact on the patient caught the imagination of surgeons at an early age, being apparently first put to practical use in 1889 by Zernov in Moscow (Kandel 1989). By 1908 Horsley & Clarke had devised a sophisticated apparatus for the accomplishment of just such manoeuvres in the animal laboratory. However, these techniques depended for guidance on surface skull landmarks, a strategy not sufficiently reliable for localizing a probe at any depth within the human brain. The problem was solved by Spiegel & Wycis (1949) who showed that depth explorations could be done accurately in man if structures were localized with reference to deep landmarks identified by contrast studies of the ventricular system. This made it possible to introduce brain probes with various capabilities (EEG recording, stimulation, single unit recording, chemical injection, lesion-making) to any site within the brain through a small opening in the skull using only local anaesthesia.

Stereotaxic, or stereotactic surgery as it was called, rapidly became a neurosurgical subspecialty. Because its early popularity in the 1950s and 1960s was mainly in the treatment of Parkinson's disease, with the advent of L-dopa in 1967 its utilization declined, although small numbers of stereotactic procedures continued to be done. With the introduction of modern imaging in the 1980s however, computerized tomography (CT) and magnetic resonance imaging (MRI) guidance have generated a renaissance of stereotactic surgery to a level of utilization far beyond that of the early years, including its applications in pain.

Controversy over the term used to describe the surgery was largely settled in 1973 when the International Society for Research in Stereoencephalotomy pointed out that the term 'stereotactic', derived from Greek and Latin words implying touching a target in three-dimensional space, was more appropriate than 'stereotaxic' derived from Greek words implying a system for displaying structures in three dimensions (Gildenberg 1988).

SELECTION OF PATIENTS

The decision to treat chronic pain by surgical means is a major and sometimes difficult one quite apart from whether the surgery should be directed at the brain or not or effected by stereotactic means. Before considering any form of surgical therapy, the surgeon must be assured that the pain is truly intractable and treatment of the primary cause is not possible. Next, all appropriate nonsurgical measures should have been exhausted. Once a surgical approach is appropriate there must be assurance that the patient's chief disability for which relief is sought is the result of pain and not of other accompanying factors, including psychological ones. Moreover, the procedure being considered should have a reasonable chance of significantly lessening the particular patient's pain and the balance between likely rates of success and complications should be acceptable to surgeon and patient alike. Finally, the simplest procedure capable of doing the job should be chosen, whether directed towards the brain, spinal cord or peripheral nervous system. It is this author's opinion that cranial pain surgery should be accomplished by stereotactic means whenever possible to take advantage of its precision, accompanying imaging, ready incorporation of physiological control, minimal impact on the patient and the capability of using local anaesthesia. Only a few operations for pain performed on the brain cannot be accomplished stereotactically.

MECHANISMS OF CHRONIC PAIN

Formal education regarding mechanisms of chronic pain still tends to dwell on the same simple Cartesian concepts that guided the pioneering neurosurgeon to attempt to treat all chronic pain syndromes by separating nociceptors from consciousness. As our understanding of various pain syndromes (discussed elsewhere in this textbook) has grown, this limited approach has been seen to lead frequently to failure or, even worse, aggravation of the pain for which relief was sought (Livingston 1976). The ideal in the best of possible worlds where the pathophysiology of every pain syndrome was fully understood would be to tailor therapy precisely, including surgical therapy, to correct the specific defects of function responsible for the pain. Unfortunately, knowledge falls far short of this goal and even consensus about pain taxonomy is lacking.

In an attempt to begin to deal with this void, a conceptualization of pain mechanisms is cautiously and humbly offered in Table 60.1 as a first step in trying to rationalize surgical approaches to pain. In this table, the entries A1cii, A1d (Lhermitte's sign), A3 (tic douloureux), A4 (sympathetic involvement; Roberts 1986) and B1 (psychogenic pain) will not be further considered as they are dealt with elsewhere in this textbook. Entries A1a, A1ci (common pain mechanisms) constitute what is usually considered as nociceptive pain, treated by interrupting or modulating transmission in pain pathways. Entry B2 is the commonest type of pain seen after injuries to the peripheral or central nervous system for which a number of possible mechanisms are possible (Zimmermann 1979) and which is seldom relieved by interrupting or modulating pain pathways but which may respond to chronic stimulation of sensory pathways (Tasker & Dostrovsky 1988). Entry B3 is included on the basis of a traditional explanation for central pain – imbalanced input – particularly Bowsher's (1980) suggestion that it results from selective damage to spinothalamic sparing reticulospinal tracts and the observation that a small number of patients with constant pain respond to destructive surgery. Entry A1b follows Lindblom's (1985) concept of evoked pain supported by much subsequent work summarized by Woolf (1992a, 1992b) and by our own experience with its surgical relief in patients with cord (Tasker et al 1992) and brain lesions (Tasker & de Carvalho 1990; Parrent et al 1992a). Woolf concluded that, for evoked pain

Table 60.1 Suggested classification of pain mechanisms

- A. Dependent upon transmission in sensory paths
  1. Dependent upon receptors
     a. *Peripheral nociceptors, normal transmission and central reception*
        Acute pain, cancer in bone, osteoarthritis, etc.
     b. *peripheral nociceptors, other receptors, normal transmission, abnormal central reception*
        Allodynia, hyperpathia, hyperaesthesia in neural injury pain.
     c. *Direct stimulation of nerve trunks ?Via nervi nervorum, nervi arteriorum*
        (i) sciatica from ruptured disc, cancerous involvement of lumbosacral plexus
        (ii) direct stimulation of neuroma, direct stimulation of abnormal nerve trunks – (Tinel's sign)
     d. *Ditto, spinal cord*
        Lhermitte's sign
  2. Not dependent on receptors but dependent on transmission
     ?Spontaneous ectopic impulses generated from, or proximal to, a neural injury site
     Intermittent lancinating pain in neural injury pain
  3. Tic douloureux
     ? Dependent on antidromic impulses
  4. Dependent on sympathetic function
     a. *Sympathetic dystrophy accompanying neural injury, other conditions*
        Swelling, colour, sweat changes, osteoporosis, not pain
     b. *Sympathetic drive to pain perception*
        Sympathetically maintained pain
- B. Not dependent on receptors or transmission in sensory pathways
  1. Cortically generated in an otherwise normally functioning nervous system. Psychogenic pain
  2. Cortically generated in damaged nervous system? from a focus generated by the neural damage
     Constant causalgic, dysaesthetic pain of neural injury responding to chronic stimulation
  3. ? Cortically generated from imbalance of spinothalamic and reticulothalamic input
     Constant causalgic dysaesthetic pain of neural injury responding to destructive surgery

caused by peripheral lesions, C-fibre activity modifies central neuronal excitability at the cord level so that A-fibre input is perceived as pain whether ectopically or naturally stimulated. In addition, A-fibre input activates a structurally reorganized dorsal horn, the result of deafferentation, so as to induce pain by reorganization of synaptic input into lamina I. For evoked pain caused by lesions of the central nervous system the mechanism has still not yet been worked out (Boivie 1992). Entry A2 is based on a traditional explanation for the pain of neural injury (Tasker & Dostrovsky 1988), our own experience with surgical treatment of central pain of cord origin (Tasker et al 1992) and observations such as those of Nashold & Wilson (1966) who reported six patients with neural injury pain with a mesencephalic EEG focus firing in time with pain paroxysms at which site stimulation aggravated and lesioning relieved the patient's pain. Entries A1b, A2, B2 and B3 constitute what is often referred to as neuropathic or neural injury pain.

Thus, our as yet limited understanding of the elements of chronic pain suggests a variety of components distinguished by the words patients use to describe their pain experience as suggested by the work of Boureau et al (1990), each with different mechanisms requiring specifically tailored treatment strategies. For example, if a patient described sharp pain in a leg aggravated by weight-bearing and associated with an intractable cancerous lesion of bone or lumbosacral plexus, an example of nociceptive pain, treatment such as cordotomy that interrupts spinothalamic function or that modulates it, such as morphine instillation, might be considered. If he described constant burning in an area of partial denervation of the trigeminal nerve, chronic stimulation of the nerve might be the procedure of choice. Our experience, along with that of various authors, suggests that the intermittent neuralgia-like lancinating pain associated with neural injury, particularly damage to the conus-cauda equina, responds to the same strategies as nociceptive pain, as does our limited experience with allodynia and hyperpathia in central pain.

A special note is necessary with respect to cancer pain. Fortunately the days have passed when pain was classified as 'benign' or 'malignant'. However, not all cancer pain is the result of nociceptor stimulation and transmission in pain pathways and not all nociceptive pain is the result of cancer. For the nociceptive pain of intractable cancer, a warning that tissue destruction is imminent, unfortunately progresses till actual tissue destruction takes place. Moreover when, as is commonly the case, that warning pain results from compression of lumbosacral or brachial plexus, the destruction that follows sets the stage for two common examples of deafferentation pain (Tasker 1987). Moreover, arthritis is a common cause of nociceptive pain.

CHOICE OF SURGICAL PROCEDURES

The review of stereotactic approaches to the treatment of chronic pain will be organized as indicated in Table 60.2. Although procedures performed on cord are not usually done stereotactically, but rather percutaneously freehand, Crue et al (1968) and Hitchcock (1969) have developed stereotactic techniques for high cervical dorsal cordotomy, trigeminal tractotomy and commissurotomy at the high cervical level so that cord procedures will be included in this discussion for completeness.

Of the procedures listed in Table 60.2, those intended to sever pain pathways are self-evident rostal extensions of cordotomy (Willis 1984, 1985). The spinoreticulothalamic tract ascends first in spinal cord and then the brainstem to separate at the level of the upper midbrain into a medial nonsomatotopographically organized portion, thought to be the continuation of the spinoreticulothalamic tract, that passes medially to end in medial thalamic nuclei. The somatotopographically organized lateral portion passes first to Hassler's (1972) parvicellular ventrocaudal (VCpc) and then the main ventrocaudal nucleus (VC) of thalamus on its way to sensory cortex (Bowsher 1957, 1961). Decussation in the pain pathway, apart from that of spinothalamic tract in the spinal cord, is thought to occur throughout the spinal cord and brainstem within the nonsomatotopographically organized reticulothalamic tract (Noordenbos 1959). Although it is well known that pain perception and its somatotopic local-

Table 60.2 Stereotactic procedures for the relief of chronic pain

I.	Procedures that interrupt transmission in pain pathways	
	Cord	Percutaneous cordotomy, dorsal high cervical approach
		Percutaneous commissurotomy, high cervical approach
		Percutaneous trigeminal tractotomy
	Brain	Pontine tractotomy
		Mesencephalic tractotomy
		Medial thalamotomy
		Thalamotomy in Hassler's parvicellular ventrocaudal nucleus
		Ventrocaudal thalamotomy
		Lesions in thalamic radiations
		Pulvinarotomy
		Hypothalamotomy
		?Cingulotomy
II.	Procedures that modulate transmission in pain pathways	
	Intraventricular morphine infusion	
	Chronic stimulation of periventricular grey (PVG)	
	? Hypophyseal ablation	
	Chronic stimulation of hypothalamus	
III.	Procedures that modulate pain generation at a central focus generated by neural injury	
	Chronic stimulation of medial lemniscus, ventrocaudal nucleus or sensory internal capsule	
	Chronic stimulation of sensorimotor cortex	
IV.	Procedures that modulate suffering	
	? Cingulotomy	

ization persist in man after hemispherectomy and hemithalamotomy (Gardner et al 1955; Ralston 1962) and there is evidence that central pain after stroke may be ipsilaterally processed (Parrent et al 1992b), it is uncertain how such ipsilateral somatotopographic processing can take place. The corpus callosum is inactivated after hemispherectomy or massive supratentorial stroke leaving decussation in the region of the posterior commissure (Chang & Ruch 1947), ipsilaterally distributed spinothalamic fibres or fibres travelling and decussating with the dorsal columns (Willis 1985) as possibilities (Tasker et al 1982).

Commissurotomy at the high cervical level is thought to interrupt a separate unknown pain-generating system (Cook et al 1984) relieving pain nonsomatotopically with respect to the anatomical site of the lesion made in the cord or to the sensory loss induced.

Trigeminal tractotomy is thought to sever the caudal portion of the trigeminal nucleus and/or tracts serving it, structures believed involved with facial pain perception.

The function of the pulvinar (Richardson & Zorub 1970) and hypothalamus (Spiegel et al 1954b) in pain perception is poorly understood, as is the role of destructive surgery aimed at the pituitary gland and now usually carried out with alcohol (Moricca 1974) sometimes stereotactically (Levin 1988).

Modulatory procedures such as morphine infusion, usually not requiring the stereotactic approach, and chronic stimulation of the periventricular grey (PVG) that does, (Richardson & Akil 1977a, 1977b) are thought to activate the brain's own pain suppressing circuitry involving nucleus raphe magnus and a descending serotoninergic pathway that blocks impulse access to spinothalamic tract (Mayer & Price 1976).

Chronic stimulation of the lemniscal pathway so as to produce paraesthesiae in the area of the patient's pain (Adams et al 1974; Mazars et al 1974; Mazars 1975) is thought to function similarly to peripheral nerve stimulation (Wall & Sweet 1967) and dorsal column stimulation (Shealey et al 1970), suppressing in an unknown way a central generator for pain that has been caused by neural injury.

The role of cingulotomy not always performed stereotactically but for which the stereotactic technique affords superb control, (see Ch. 62), appears to be receiving increasing attention. Whether the relief cingulotomy affords is related to interruption of pain pathways or effects on suffering is uncertain (Bouckoms 1988; Talbot et al 1991).

It is difficult to know the current extent of stereotactic surgery for the relief of pain. Probably chronic stimulation of PVG and the lemniscal pathway are the most frequently employed with medial thalamotomy, mesencephalic tractotomy and hypophyseal alcohol injection also being popular.

TECHNIQUE OF CRANIAL STEREOTACTIC SURGERY

Except for spinal cord procedures which will be briefly separately mentioned, most stereotactic procedures depend on the following components:

1. suitable frame
2. brain atlas
3. imaging – usually CT or MRI
4. computer facilities
5. suitable set of probes and back-up for physiological corroboration of target site
6. suitable set of probes with back-up for manipulating the chosen target.

Probably most readers will be familiar with the technique of stereotactic biopsy where the stereotactic coordinates of the lesion to be biopsied are determined directly from the scan and the biopsy probe introduced towards it. Most functional stereotactic targets except for cingulum bundle are not directly visible in CT or MRI scans so that their locations must be extrapolated from identifiable 'landmarks', usually anterior (AC) and posterior (PC) commissures.

Our practice is to apply the frame to the head (in our case the Leksell CT or MRI compatible frame) under local anaesthetic and to complete stereotactic imaging the day prior to surgery. (The frame is available from Elekta Instruments Inc, Tucker, Georgia, USA.) Usually a series of 1.5 mm axial cuts are made with CT traversing the thalamus from which the stereotactic coordinates of AC and PC are determined using the computer software in the scanner in the same mannner as for stereotactic biopsy (Tasker et al 1988). PC is usually 1.5 mm cut above the last slice displaying the collicular plate and AC (which may be poorly visualized in CT scans), 3 mm below the foramen of Monro. Alternatively MRI may be used, taking advantage of its better demonstration of AC when it is probably best to identify AC and PC in a single mid-sagittal slice and then determine actual coordinates by coronal or axial cuts 'bracketing' their locations as determined from the sagittal scans. We have satisfied ourselves that CT and MRI are thoroughly accurate for stereotactic localization (Kondziolka et al 1992; Tasker et al 1993), in keeping with many published observations. For functional targets whose coordinates cannot be read directly from the scan, coordinates are determined by extrapolotion with reference to a suitable brain atlas calibrated with respect to the AC/PC line such as that by Schaltenbrand & Bailey (1959) or Schaltenbrand & Wahren (1977). This anatomical localization is facilitated by a simple computer program (Hawrylyshyn et al 1976; Tasker & Dostrovsky 1992) available for use with a PC computer and laser printer, in which the digitized atlas diagrams are redrawn, stretched or compressed as need be, until their AC/PC line coincides with that of the individual patient determined from the imaging and ruled in millimetres corresponding to the scales on the frame as positioned on the particular patient's head.

On the day of surgey (the frame can be either left in situ or replaced in the morning if skull fixation pin lengths and positions are matched) the target is selected from the computer diagram and its stereotactic coordinates read off. If a target structure can be identified directly from the scan, physiological corroboration is optional but enhances accuracy; otherwise it is mandatory since anatomical variation between patients of the relationship of targets to the AC/PC line can be large enough to result in failure of the surgery or complications (Tasker et al 1982). Under local anaesthetic a suitable probe is introduced through a twist drill hole in the same sagittal plane as the target and advanced towards the target. This facilitates plotting of physiological data collected to corroborate probe localization on a single sagittal brain diagram.

The technique of physiological localization depends upon the target and the surgeon's preferences. Two techniques are in common use – microelectrode recording with microstimulation (Lenz et al 1988) or macrostimulation (Tasker et al 1982). Recording is useful in nuclear structures where single-cell activity can be studied, while microstimulation is universally applicable. Use of a microelectrode on the one hand enchances precision since structures recorded and current spread of microstimulation are restricted to the immediate vicinity of the electrode but demands more complex equipment and technical skill than macrostimulation. Macrostimulation, though simple, is diminished in usefulness by the degree of current spread over several millimetres. The latter, however, results in a greater variety of stimulation-induced responses than that seen with microstimulation and makes it more likely that responses will be obtained on any given trajectory, albeit at high thresholds; microstimulation may not 'see' very far so that a poorly placed trajectory may yield no useful information.

With microelectrode recording we have been able to identify neurons that respond to contralateral superficial and deep tactile stimuli, muscle squeezing, passive joint movement, deep tissue deformation, voluntary movement and auditory stimuli, and, occasionally as others have reported, responses to noxious stimuli (Sano et al 1970, 1977; Sano 1977; Amano et al 1978, 1979, 1986).

With either micro- or macrostimulation, a limited number of usually contralateral effects are induced (Table 60.3) (Tasker et al 1982), the only differences between the two modalities being threshold: as low as 2 μA with microstimulation, about 300 μA with macrostimulation; and size of projected field: as small as a tactile neuron's receptive field with microstimulation, large with macrostimulation. In some patients with neural injury pain, stimulation of the spinothalamic path can be unpleasent or painful, usually in patients with allodynia or hyperpathia. Or else nonsomatotopically organized burning or painful effects may be elicited widely in the brainstem, in the general area of the reticulothalamic path and medial thalamus, usually referred to the painful part of the patient's body (Tasker et al 1982; Tasker 1982a).

Table 60.3 Effects elicited by simulation of the brain

Structure	Threshold effect in somatotopically appropriate location
Motor cranial nerve nuclei or fibres	Tetanization
Corticospinal tract,	Tetanization
Certain correlating tracts in brainstem	Tetanization
Dentatothalamic tract	Unsustained motor contraction at onset of stimulus train
Kinaesthetic including ? spindle pathway	Paraesthesiae, sometimes sense of movement though none occurred
Tactile pathway	Paraesthesiae
Spinothalamic tract	Warm or cold paraesthesiae
Auditory paths	Buzzing
Primary visual paths	Coloured phosphenes
Secondary visual paths	White phosphenes Other effects
Reticulothalamic pathway including medial thalamus	No response
PVG	No response or general feeling of satiety, warmth, various bizarre effects
Periaqueductal grey (PAG)	No response or unpleasant feelings or bizarre effects

On the basis of recordings and/or stimulation-induced effects in an appropriate number of electrode trajectories, the desired target is selected and the chosen manipulation carried out – usually the introduction of a chronic stimulating electrode or the making of radiofrequency (RF) lesion. The latter is accomplished in our practice with a temperature-monitored electrode with a 1.1 × 3 mm bare tip, the latter serially heated for 60 seconds at progressively higher current flows and temperatures until a lesion of the desired size has made. (This is available from Diros Technology Inc, 965 Pape Ave, Toronto, Canada.) A minimal lesion occurs in the brain at about 25 mA and at temperatures below 70°C, the lesion size steadily increasing to maximum at 65 mA and 90°C.

STEREOTACTIC PROCEDURES FOR THE RELIEF OF PAIN

The remainder of this chapter will briefly review the indications, technique and published experience with stereotactic procedures with added personal comments.

PRODECURES PERFORMED ON THE CORD

Though percutaneous cordotomy is a common procedure, it is not often performed by a truly stereotactic method, though Hitchcock has described a special frame and myelographic technique for a high cervical dorsal approach to cordotomy (Hitchock 1969) as well as commissurotomy. (Schvarcz 1978) and Crue et al (1968) have used a Todd Wells frame for the purpose.

PERCUTANEOUS CORDOTOMY

Hitchcock (1988) has recently reviewed the status of stereotactic procedures on the spinal cord. Hitchcock (1969) and Crue et al (1968) independently developed dorsal high cervical stereotactically aimed approaches for percutaneous cordotomy, at the C1–C2 and at the occipital–C1 space respectively. Hitchcock preferred the seated, head-flexed position in order to stabilize the cord as much as possible. A cordotomy electrode was then advanced dorsoventrally to the appropriate site in the spinothalamic tract for the location of the patient's pain, guided by myelography, confirming location by stimulation, and making an RF lesion as in other cordotomy techniques. Hitchcock (1977) reported that 90% of his patients, mostly suffering from cancer, were initially relieved of their pain, 79% after 6 months, 72% after 9 months, and 57.6% at latest follow-up or death. Transient paresis affected 10%, more persistent paresis 3%, while disturbance of bladder function occurred in 5%. It would be interesting to complement stereotactic cordotomy with CT-guidance as performed by Kanpolat et al (1989, 1990).

While cordotomy is perhaps the most useful, precise and successful surgical procedure for the relief of chronic pain in properly selected patients, it is discussed elsewhere in this textbook. Suffice it to say that, in this author's opinion, percutaneous cordotomy, particularly using the lateral high cervical approach (Tasker 1990), is the treatment of choice for cancer-induced nociceptive pain below the level of the C4–C5 dermatomal junction, particularly if not midline, in a patient with a normally functioning lung and phrenic nerve on the opposite side to the cordotomy lesion. It is also very useful in patients with neuralgic-like pain in the lower limb(s) caused by lesions of the conus and cauda equina (Tasker et al 1992a).

The application of cordotomy in the treatment of cancer-induced nociceptive pain has declined radically in recent years because of the increased use of various techniques for morphine infusion. This is unfortunate for those carefully selected patients for whom cordotomy is well suited. For cordotomy offers a once-only encounter rather than a treatment modality that requires continuous patient care, continual attendance at treatment facilities, using expensive equipment which exposes the patient to the effects of escalating dosages of morphine and complications that are at least as great as those of cordotomy performed by an experienced surgeon.

COMMISSUROTOMY

Armour (1927) originally introduced the notion of dorsoventral midline commissurotomy by open means, suggesting that it would relieve pain by interrupting decussating spinothalamic fibres, which it apparently does do. In contemporary neurosurgery it is usually done percutaneously in the high cervical region but with a different concept. As reviewed by Cook et al (1984), there is evidence to suggest that commissurotomy interrupts an extralemniscal pain pathway, there being no relationship between the known somatotopographic location of the lesion in the cord, the location of the pain or of any sensory loss induced.

Using myelographic control and a suitable stereotactic frame (Hitchcock 1970a), a fine needle is introduced dorsoventrally in the midline of the cord, in the occipital–C1 interspace, using macrostimulation for control, to a point 5 mm beneath the dorsal pia where a radiofrequency lesion is made. Hitchcock (1970a) reported 10 excellent and two good results in 14 patients with nociceptive pain without inducing sensory loss. Hitchcock (1988) reported 42.1% of 19 cancer patients pain-free, 26.3% significantly relieved over a 4-year follow-up or until the patient's death. Some 80% of patients with pain relief showed analgesia, while those with poor pain control showed little sensory loss. Eiras et al (1980) reported excellent early pain relief, but later recurrence at the expense of transient dysmetria and ataxic gait. Schvarcz (1984) described 78% satisfactory results in 79 patients with nociceptive pain, transient ataxia being frequently encountered. Papo (1979), however, found the procedure less than satisfactory because of pain recurrence. Kanpolat et al (1990) reported total pain control in two out of six, and 50% reduction in three patients with unspecified pain operated upon with CT-guidance.

The only experience in patients with pain caused by neural injury is that of Hitchcock (1970a), reporting relief in all three patients treated.

In summary, the limited published experience makes it impossible to judge the effectiveness of commissurotomy in deafferentation pain. It would seem preferable to choose percutaneous cordotomy in cancer pain wherever applicable and to consider commissurotomy in patients unsuited to cordotomy on the basis of the balance between possible risks and effectiveness.

LESIONS OF THE DESCENDING TRACT AND CAUDAL NUCLEUS OF THE TRIGEMINAL NERVE

Hitchcock (1969, 1970b), Schvarcz (1978, 1979) and Hitchcock & Schvarcz (1972) have developed stereotactic-guided percutaneous techniques for lesioning the caudal nucleus and descending tract of the trigeminal nerve.

Kanpolat et al (1990) have developed CT-guidance for the procedure. Crue et al (1967, 1970), Todd et al (1969) and Fox (1972, 1974) have developed techniques for medullary tractotomy.

With the medullary technique, with the patient prone, the floor of fourth ventricle, obex and dorsal brainstem are visualized myelographically, allowing the introduction of a cordotomy-type electrode through an 18-gauge thin-walled lumbar puncture needle towards the target whose position is extrapolated with reference to the above structures. Stimulation (50 Hz) producing facial paraesthesiae confirms correct positioning when an RF lesion is made, as in cordotomy.

In the cervical approach, with the patient seated and head flexed, myelographic demonstration of the antero-posterior extent of the cord and cisterna magna is done and a cordotomy-type electrode advanced at C1 towards the expected target site of the 'caudal trigeminal dematome' about 6 mm lateral to midline and 3 mm anterior to the posterior aspect of the cord. Representation of central segments is said to lie further laterally, anteriorly and rostral. Lower cranial nerves are represented more posteriorly and medially. Impedance and stimulation monitoring are used as in cordotomy followed by RF lesioning.

Fox (1972) reported satisfactory pain relief with facial analgesia but ipsilateral ataxia, postoperative pyrexia and contralateral body analgesia. Schvarcz (1978, 1979) reported 84% relief over 2–30 months in 30 cancer patients, ipsilateral ataxia and contralateral body analgesia being complications. Kanpolat et al (1990) reported good results in three of five patients with unspecified pain. Hitchcock (1988) reported good to excellent pain relief till death in 47% of an early series of 21 patients, most apparently suffering from cancer, with no operative mortality, 40% transient mild, 4.8% severe paresis or ataxia; 4.8% had transient severe dysaesthesiae, and 4% minor pain recurrence. The procedure relieved the pain of cancer better (60% good to excellent long-term relief) than it did the pain of other conditions. Out of Schvarcz's series of 104 which he quoted, nearly 87% of cancer patients were relieved.

Subsequently, Hitchcock (1970b) and Hitchcock & Schvarcz (1972) explored the usefulness of nucleotomy specifically in the treatment of deafferentation pain syndromes. They induced dissociated sensory loss in the face with some degree of dysaesthesia and hypoaesthesia in three patients with postherpetic neuralgia, relieving their pain in each case, but with recurrence after a few months in two. Schvarcz (1978, 1979) reported 88% relief in eight patients with postherpetic neuralgia, 57% in 14 cases of anaesthesia dolorosa, 72% of 25 unspecified cases of dysaesthetic pain over a 0.5–5.5-year follow-up. Hitchcock (1988) reviewed the role of nucleotomy as opposed to tractotomy to treat deafferentation syndromes, particularly postherpetic neuralgia, citing Schvarcz's experience with 104 nucleotomies relieving 57% of patients with anaesthesia dolorosa, 72% with 'dysaesthesia' and 87% of those with postherpetic neuralgia. Hitchcock concluded: 'In general, however, the procedure should be limited to patients with oropharyngeal head malignancy and selected cases of atypical facial pain or facial deafferentation pain'. However, Schvarcz's growing experience with the procedure in deafferentation pain warrants particular attention.

In summary, though percutaneous trigeminal nucleotomy–tractotomy appears to be effective for the relief of cancerous nociceptive pain in trigeminal territory, if it is technically feasible it would appear to be easier and safer to make percutaneous RF lesions in Meckel's cave. The operation would seem most valuable when cancer prevents access to Meckel's cave or when cancer pain extends into the territories of the lower cranial nerves when, through the posterior nucleotomy approach, the lesion can be extended dorsomedially into their territory (Kanpolat et al 1990). The use of the procedure in facial deafferentation syndromes is interesting in view of the later introduction by Nashold et al (1986) of the open 'trigeminal DREZ' procedure which, in their hands, has also proven very successful in the treatment of deafferentation pain syndromes, especially trigeminal postherpetic neuralgia (Bernard et al 1988). It would seem most useful to make a direct comparison of the successes and risks of the two procedures in treating the different facial deafferentation pain syndromes.

PONTINE TRACTOTOMY

Hitchcock (1973) and Hitchcock et al (1985a, 1985b, 1988) described a technique for severing the spinothalamic tract at the pontine level using his special frame designed for spinal and posterior fossa surgery. Localization was based on ventriculographic demonstration of the aqueduct and floor and fastigium of fourth ventricle. In eight patients with cancer, pain was completely relieved in three until their deaths 6 days to 1.5 months later and partially relieved in the remainder. One more patient was relieved of deafferentation pain over a 2.5 year follow-up. Four suffered complications, and analgesic levels tended to fall with time. Barbéra et al (1979) reported relief of pain till death in five patients with cancer pain, at least two of whom had a deafferentation component from brachial plexus destruction.

Clearly, pontine tractotomy has a role in treating nociceptive cancer pain when cordotomy is not indicated. It would appear to fill a similar niche, and to offer the same advantages and disadvantages, as the more well-known mesencephalic tractotomy. A comparison study would be most useful to determine the relative merits and disadvantages of the two operations.

MESENCEPHALIC TRACTOTOMY

The history of mesencephalic tractotomy is a long one, beginning with open techniques but revolutionized by the introduction of the stereotactic method by Spiegel & Wycis (1949) and its application to mesencephalic tractotomy (Spiegel & Wycis 1962; Wycis & Spiegel 1962). Stereotactic mesencephalotomy has remained popular ever since because of its diminished morbidity, including, strangely, a far lower incidence of postoperative iatrogenic dysaesthetic pain and mortality compared with the open operation in, usually, mortally ill patients.

The current strategy is to make RF lesions stereotactically in both the somatotopographically organized spinothalamic and, especially, the more medially located nonsomatotopographically organized reticulothalamic tract as outlined in various reviews (Pagni 1974; Nashold et al 1974, 1977; Nashold 1982). The location of the spinoreticulothalamic pathway in upper midbrain is first determined anatomically with reference to the AC-PC line and then physiologically using stimulation. Medial and somewhat dorsal to the medial lemniscus, which is located 10–12 mm from midline, and whose stimulation induces contralateral paraesthesiae, lies the spinothalamic tract, 7–9 mm laterally. Stimulation of the latter induces contralateral warm or cold somatotopographically organized sensations, sometimes pain in patients with allodynia or hyperpathia (Tasker 1982a; Tasker et al 1982), while lesions here produce dissociated sensory loss. Medially again in, presumably reticulothalamic tract, 5–7mm from the midline, stimulation usually induces no specific effect, except in some patients with neural injury pain (Tasker 1982a; Tasker et al 1982), but effects from volume conduction (often paraesthesiae) or from PVG–PAG grey stimulation (a variety of bizarre responses) (Richardson & Akil 1977a, 1977b; Tasker et al 1986) may also be seen; lesions made in the reticulothalamic tract produce no clinically detectable effects. Figure 60.1 indicates the types of responses obtained in mesencephalic exploration with microstimulation; Figure 60.2 illustrates a typical lesion demonstated with MRI.

Experience with mesencephalic tractotomy is usually different in patients with nociceptive pain than in those with neural injury pain. Spiegel & Wycis (1962) and Wycis & Spiegel (1962) reported their experience in 54 patients, 42 apparently suffering from neural injury pain, 12 from cancer pain. Significant long-term relief occurred in 31% at the expense of a 7.4% mortality, 15% contralateral dysaesthesia, 50% hearing loss (at least in earlier cases), 7.4% facial or limb paresis, 16.7% oculomotor palsies, 3.7% ataxia, 3.7% tremor or tremor and ataxia. Many of these defects were transient. Mazars et al (1960a) obtained good results in six cancer patients and unspecified results in four with deafferentation pain. A further report (Mazars et al 1960a, 1960b) on 86 procedures, 27 for unspecified facial pain, documented total relief in 25 with one postoperative death. Helfant et al (1965) achieved total relief in three, partial relief in three, out of eight patients with cancer pain and in 11 with various other pain syndromes. Some 63.6% suffered oculomotor complications, 45.5% from paresis, 27.3% from dysaesthesiae and 9.1% from ataxia. In 27.3% some loss of lemniscal function occurred. Gioia et al (1967) reported 66.7% relief in 15 cancer patients with 6.7% mortality. The contributions of Nashold and his group to our understanding of stereotactic mesencephalic tractotomy is enormous and cannot be given due attention in a review such as this, working out the locations and somatotopographic organization of the spinothalamic tract and nearby structures (Nashold 1970; Nashold & Wilson 1966; Nashold et al 1969a, 1969b). Turnbull (1972) recommended combining cingulotomy with mesencephalic tractotomy, reporting relief of pain in nine of 10 cancer patients. Voris & Whisler (1975) reported relief of upper body cancer pain in 26 of 27 patients with complications in 37%, dysaesthesiae in 12%, ocular palsies in 17%. A further report (Whisler & Voris 1978) recorded 92% pain relief in 38 cancer patients. Frank et al (1982) reported significant relief of upper body cancer pain in all 14 of their patients over a follow-up of up to 4.9 months at the expense of ocular palsies in 78.6%, permanent in 21.4%. Some 14.3% suffered from dysaesthesiae and 7.1% from cognitive disorders. In three patients the procedure was done bilaterally and in two it was repeated. De Montreuil et al (1983) reported striking short-term relief in 90.9% of 11 cancer patients but with recurrence in 3 months at the expense of 18.2% oculomotor disturbances. Amano et al (1986) reported 83% good results in six cancer patients followed 1–70 months, 26% developing Parinaud's syndrome. Frank et al (1987), in a combined study by the Bologna and Freiburg groups of 109 cancer patients followed 2–7 months, reported 83.5% pain relief, 1.8% mortality, 13% oculomotor disturbances, 6.5% dysaesthesiae and 15.4% recurrence of pain. Bosch (1991) reported 87.9% initial, 59.3% long-term good results in 33 cancer patients, especially those with pain in the extremities. There was a 6.1% incidence of dysaesthesiae, 3% of lemniscal damage, 3% myoclonus and all had initial, 1% persistent, diplopia. Frank et al (1989), in their most recent publication reviewing 202 personal patients, concluded that mesencephalotomy is to be preferred to cordotomy in patients with upper body pain, for their mortality was 0.5%, early (less than 1 month) pain recurrence was 15%, late, 4%. Complications included 9% early, 3% late gaze palsy, 6% permanent dysaesthetic problems. Our own experience consists of 34 procedures with a mortality of 8.8%, serious complications in 5.9%,

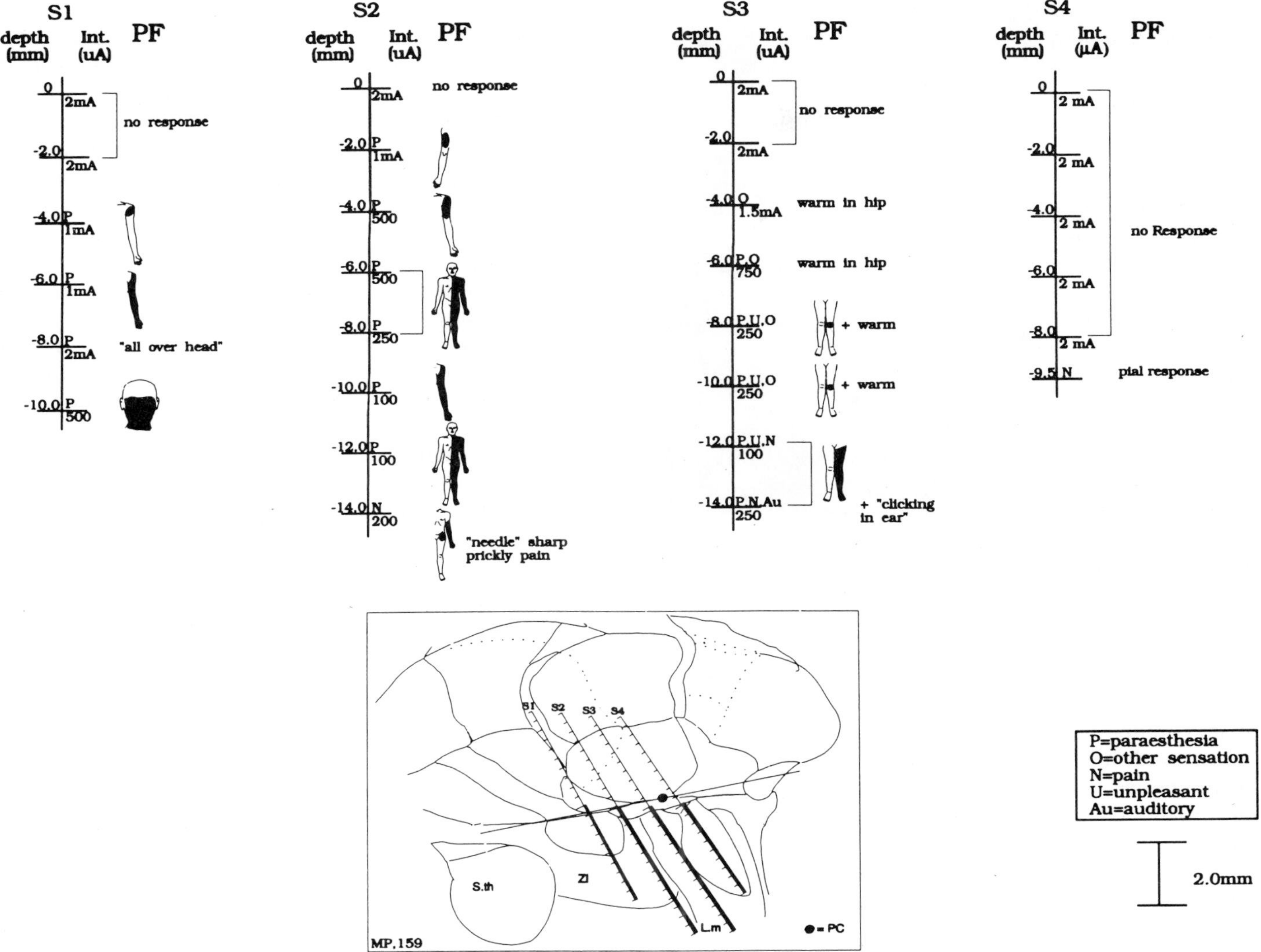

Fig. 60.1 Inset. A 9 mm left sagittal brain diagram showing four electrode trajectories (S1, S2, S3, S4). Sth = subthalamic nucleus; Z1 = zona incerta; Lm = medial lemniscus; PC = posterior commissure. **Above**. Figurine maps depicting PFs (responses to stimulation) in the four trajectories in the portions shaded in black. Numbers on left indicate sites stimulated in mm below the top of the shaded portions. Numbers to right indicate threshold in µA unless stated in mA. Note that most responses are described as paraesthetic in the two rostal trajectories in keeping with stimulation of medial lemniscus while the deepest response in S2 is painful, those in S3 warm, in keeping with stimulation of spinothalamic tract. The auditory response in S3 probably arose in lateral lemniscus, the pial response in S4 from mechanical stimulation of the dorsum of the midbrain.

transient in 20.6%; 41.7% of the 24 cancer patients had nearly complete relief till they died, 29.2% significant but incomplete relief. Clinical results were compared with lesion sites at autopsy in three cases (Tasker et al 1982).

Pagni (1974), Nashold (1982), ourselves and Gybels & Sweet (1989) have reviewed published results. Pagni (1974) concluded that, for pain caused by cancer, thalamotomy or mesencephalotomy was often the only surgical method of relieving pain. He suggests the thalamic lesion 'should encompass the specific neospinothalamic (VPL-VPM, VCpc) and nonspecific palaeospinothalamic (CM, Pf, intralaminar, limitans) pathways' while the mesencephalic lesion should interrupt the spinothalamic tract with the lesion 'widely impinging on the adjacent spinoreticulothalamic systems'. Yet even extensive tractotomy plus thalamotomy resulted in pain relief in only 30% of his patients. Nashold concluded: 'At this time mesencephalotomy including a portion of the dorsomedian midbrain and adjacent periaqueductal grey is the treatment of choice for either intractable unilateral or bilateral pain caused by extensive carcinoma involving the head, neck and/or arm. Significant relief of pain and suffering can be expected for the lifetime of these patients.' He concluded that the mortality ranged from 3–5%, morbidity was 37%, chiefly from oculomotor disturbances, with usually transient dysaesthesiae in 5%.

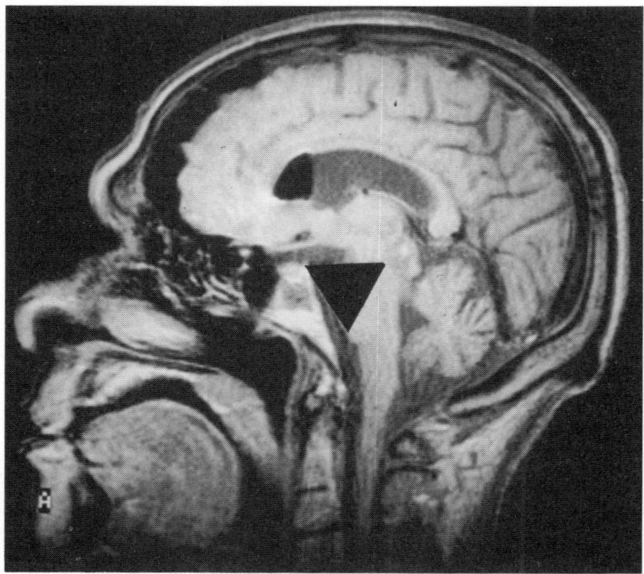

Fig. 60.2 Sagittal MRI image of patient with pain from head and neck cancer 2 days after stereotactic mesencephalic tractotomy showing lesion (arrowhead) and postoperative ventricular air.

Our review (Tasker 1984) of 92 published protocols allowing separation of results between nociceptive and neural injury pain suggested 80% good results in the former with a 5–10% mortality, a 15–20% incidence of dysaesthesiae and a similar incidence of oculomotor disturbances. Gybels & Sweet (1989) reviewed 270 published cases in cancer pain and concluded that 85% of patients experienced significant pain relief till they died from their disease. Frank et al (1987) carried out an informative comparison of the results in mesencephalic tractotomy and medial thalamotomy in cancer pain in collaboration with the Freiburg group with a 2–7 month follow-up. Only 51.9% enjoyed persisting relief after medial thalamotomy while 83.5% did so after mesencephalic tractotomy. However, the risk of thalamotomy was less: 0 versus 1.8% mortality, 70% transient confusion and 1.9% aphasia for thalamotomy versus 13% oculomotor, 6.5% dysaesthetic disturbances after mesencephalotomy. Laitinen (1988), however, concluded that mesencephalic tractotomy had no place in the treatment of chronic pain since it was no more successful than the much less risky medial thalamotomy or pulvinarotomy–26% (best in cancer pain) long-term relief in a mixed group of patients with cancer and neural injury pain with a 42.1% incidence of dysaesthesiae, 15.8% of lemniscal damage, 21.1% of ocular disturbance.

Pain relief with mesencephalic tractotomy in neural injury pain is considerably less than that in cancer pain. Wycis & Spiegel (1962) achieved 29% permanent relief in 42 patients. Von Roeder & Orthner (1961) and Orthner & von Roeder (1964) reported complete relief in three, partial relief in two out of 12 patients after mesencephalotomy combined with lesions at additional sites; 17% suffered from dysaesthesiae. Helfant et al (1965) reported relief in one out of three patients, Gioia et al (1967) 0 out of two. Although Voris & Whisler (1975) noted 80% immediate relief, only 28% continued to do well after 1 year, 12% suffering from dysaesthesiae, 17% oculomotor palsies. Amano et al (1979) reported 84.6% relief in 13 patients, all but two of whom suffered from neural injury pain. Turnbull (1972) relieved three patients of 16 with neural injury pain by combining mesencephalic tractotomy with cingulotomy. Amano et al (1986) obtained good relief in 64% of 28 patients over a 1–70 month follow-up, 20% of whom developed Parinaud's syndrome. Shieff & Nashold (1987, 1988, 1990) have published their remarkable experience of achieving 66.7% relief in 27 patients with central pain caused by stroke over follow-up of up to 5 years; three patients could not be followed and mortality was 7.4%. Results were better (75% long-term relief) when lesions were made at the level of the posterior commissure where usually transient oculomotor disturbances affected all patients rather than at the level of the superior colliculus where they occurred in only 23–54%. Usually transient complications affected half the others. Bosch (1991) obtained only brief relief in 57.1% of patients with neural injury pain, with a 57.1% incidence of dysaesthesiae. Half of our 10 patients with central pain had significant relief from mesencephalic tractotomy, nine with transient, but none with serious complications (Tasker et al 1982; Tasker 1984), lesions in spinothalamic tract appearing more successful than those in reticulospinal tract.

For the most part, then, mesencephalic tractotomy carries a lower chance of relief of neural injury pain than of nociceptive pain like destructive lesions elsewhere in the nervous system. Reviews by Cassinari & Pagni (1969) and Davis & Stokes (1966) suggest that the chance of relieving central pain by destructive surgery was about 50%, while Nashold (1982) conluded: 'central pains, such as the "thalamic syndrome" the "lateral medullary plate syndrome", postcordotomy dysaesthesia, phantom pain following avulsion of the brachial plexus, or postherpetic pain, can be relieved 50% of the time by stereotactic mesencephalotomy'. A personal review of 92 published protocols in which nociceptive and neural injury syndromes could be differentiated suggested that 27% of patients with the latter were relieved by mesencephalotomy (Tasker 1984). Nevertheless, Pagni (1974) stated that stereotactic surgery in cases of nonmalignant origin: 'is still the unique way to relieve, at least temporarily, the atrocious suffering of pain due to central nervous system lesions . . . after every other . . . procedure has failed'. Gybels & Sweet (1988) reviewed published data in 150 cases of neural injury pain, finding 44% of patients enjoying long-term relief, 39% short-term relief.

The general failure of destructive lesions to relieve neural injury pain has become widely known during the 1980s (Tasker & Dostrovsky 1988) and has become associated with the notion that such pain is centrally generated by such mechanisms as denervation neuronal hypersensitivity, somatotopographic reorganization, loss of or rearrangement of input which arise in response to deafferentation. However, such pain appears to respond a little better, by some unknown mechanism, to chronic stimulation producing paraesthesiae in the area of pain. Yet chronic stimulation remains an acceptable strategy for two reasons: lack of surgical alternatives and the fact that stimulation is a reversible procedure with a much lower risk than destructive surgery. Our differential experience (Tasker et al 1992) with stimulation and destructive lesions in central pain caused by cord lesions is clearcut: stimulation, despite its relatively low yield, is superior to destructive surgery in treating the commonest feature of such central pain, the steady causalgic, dysaesthetic or aching component, while destructive surgery is much superior for the less frequent intermittent neuralgia-like pain and for allodynia and hyperpathia. This observation suggests that these components of neural injury pain may depend on transmission in spinoreticulothalamic tracts, unlike the steady component. Our much less extensive experience with central pain caused by brain lesions points in the same direction as shown in Table 60.4. Thus it is possible that reported outcomes in treating neural injury pain may differ from one patient or one series to the next depending upon relative incidence of these three basic components in the syndrome: steady, intermittent lancinating and evoked pain.

Yet a small percentage (in our case 30%) of patients with steady pain still appear to derive relief from destructive lesions. Bowsher (1980) has offered a possible explanation – that steady pain in such patients, though centrally generated, is the result of differential damage to spinothalamic tract sparing reticulothalamic tract destructive surgery reestablishing equilibrium. Yet it is well-known that apparent damage to both pathways can also result in central pain.

It is difficult to summarize the role of mesencephalic tractotomy. For nociceptive pain, usually caused by cancer, affecting head and neck, proximal upper limbs or elsewhere where percutaneous cordotomy is not indicated, it is the most familiar and best studied procedure for interrupting pain pathways along with medial thalamotomy to which it is superior, though at the expense of a greater morbidity and mortality. It constitutes, if you will, the cranial counterpart of percutaneous cordotomy. There is insufficient experience to assess pontine tractotomy or thalamotomy in Hassler's VCpc, though both procedures appear promising. Intraventricular morphine infusion is an alternative, easier to carry out and probably safer, though experience with it is limited, particularly in North America. Yet this latter procedure, along with spinal infusion of morphine, has a retinue of disadvantages mentioned earlier.

For neural injury pain, successful outcome after mesencephalic tractotomy is usually much less frequent, though the results reported by Nashold's group are encouraging in stroke-induced central pain. It seems prudent to this author, however, to reserve the technique for carefully selected patients with neural injury pain who have failed trials of less risky procedures such as chronic nerve, cord, or brain stimulation, and particularly for those with a major component of neuralgia-type pain, allodynia or hyperpathia.

PROCEDURES ON THE THALAMUS

The first stereotactic pain operation (in 1947) appears to have been a dorsomedian thalamotomy (Spiegel & Wycis 1962). In the intervening years attention has been addressed to various thalamic sites with varying degrees of success. Attention was first directed to the VC, but soon turned to the medial thalamus instead where results appeared better and complications fewer. Over recent years, as the number of cancer patients referred for surgery has diminished and awareness of neural injury pain has increased, attention has turned away from lesion-making

Table 60.4 Surgical treatment: 73 cases of brain central pain

	Stimulation				Destructive	
	Trigeminal		Stereotactic lemniscal pathway*		Mesencephalic tractotomy and/or medial thalamotomy	
	Relief	Fail	Relief	Fail	Relief	Fail
Steady	4	2	5**	7***	3	7****
Intermittent	0	1	0	0	1	0
Evoked	1	2	2	7	3	2

* 1 Case with PVG, 11 lemniscal relay.
** 3 with evoked pain, 2 relieved
*** 6 with evoked pain, stimulation painful in 3.
**** 2 temporary relief.

towards chronic stimulation of the brain instead (discussed elsewhere in this textbook), either in VC, to produce paraesthesiae in the patient's area of pain, or PVG, supposedly activating the descending serotoninergic pathway through nucleus raphe magnus to inhibit activation of spinothalamic tract in the cord. This latter strategy, though seemingly best suited for the treatment of nociceptive pain, has also been reported useful in other pain syndromes though it appears to have been used most frequently in patients with chronic nociceptive pain associated with degenerative disc disease (Young et al 1985; Young & Brechner 1986; Levy et al 1987). We have now studied four patients, however, with stroke-induced central pain with allodynia and/or hyperpathia relieved by PVG stimulation, suggesting that these pain phenomena are dependent upon spinothalamic transmission and capable of treatment by the same strategies as nociceptive pain (Parrent et al 1992a).

Be that as it may, this author sees little current application for destructive thalamic procedures. For nociceptive pain not amenable to cordotomy, mesencephalic tractotomy is more effective, though at a cost. If that cost is not acceptable, medial thalamotomy can be considered, accepting its lower success rate. In cases of neural injury pain, chronic stimulation should be tried first because of its low risk and reversibility and destructive surgery – either in medial thalamus or mesencephalic tract, considered only as a last resort, particularly if neuralgic or evoked pain is prominent. However, not all authors will share these views.

THE VENTROCAUDAL NUCLEUS

It was only natural when stereotactic surgery first became available that attention would be focused on the VC – the major thalamic relay for somatotopographically organized sensory input, including that of the spinothalamic tract. Hécaen et al (1949) and Monnier & Fischer (1951) pioneered stereotactic thalamotomy both in VC and medial nuclei. There then followed a series of papers by Mark and his group (Ervin & Mark 1960; Mark et al 1960, 1961, 1963; Mark & Ervin 1965) comparing the two procedures and concluding that lesions in centre median were not only more effective but also avoided sensory loss and dysaesthesiae. Bettag & Yoshida (1960) reported only transient relief of cancer pain in four patients, one of whom developed postoperative paresis after VC thalamotomy. Uematsu et al (1974) reported relief of cancer pain in 53.8% of 13 patients. Tasker (1982b) carried out a review of world literature concerning VC thalamotomy in nociceptive pain, finding 82% relief in 22 patients with complications in 32%, usually dysaesthesiae.

As with other destructive operations, thalamotomy has been less successful in neural injury pain. In 31 cases of neural injury pain Bettag & Yoshida (1960) reported 6.5% mortality, 35.5% paresis and 19.4% persisting pain relief after VC thalamotomy. Kandel (1990) arrested both the pain and disease process in three children with erythromelagia with VC plus medial thalamotomy. In a review (Tasker 1982b) of VC thalamotomies reported in the literature in neural injury pain, 36% of 56 patients enjoyed good relief and 34% complications, mostly dysaesthesiae. Our own experience is limited to three cases of VC thalamotomy, all for cancer pain, two undergoing thalamotomy alone. The third who had a simultaneous medial thalamotomy had had a previous unsuccessful mesencephalic tractotomy. All three were significantly relieved of pain till their deaths at the expense of dysaesthesiae.

VC thalamotomy is probably of historical interest today, partly because of the associated high incidence of dysaesthesiae and the danger of loss of position sense.

PARVICELLULAR VENTROCAUDAL THALAMOTOMY

Despite declining interest in VC thalamotomy, there has been increasing interest in making destructive lesions in the posteroinferior margin of VC, 14–17 mm from midline probably in VCpc (Hassler & Riechert 1959; Hassler 1972) which is probably a way-station for the spinothalamic tract. It is identified in man (Tasker et al 1982) as a site where somatotopographic arrangement of stimulation-induced responses in VC (e.g. in hand) shift dramatically, within 1– 2 mm to responses often in leg, frequently accompanied by a change in quality from paraesthesiae to warm or cold sensations (Fig. 60.3). Lesions here produce dissociated sensory loss.

Hassler & Riechert (1959) achieved short-term relief in five patients with neural pain, while Siegfried & Krayenbühl (1972) obtained pain relief in only one of nine patients with pain of unspecified type. Halliday & Logue (1972) also published experience with the operation. Hitchcock & Teixeira (1981) relieved two of three patients with stroke-induced pain, four of six with postherpetic neuralgia, all five with postcordotomy or posttractotomy dysaesthesiae and all three with multiple sclerosis for an overall success rate of 82.4% with a 48% complication rate, 18% permanent. Some 36% showed cognitive and 52% oculomotor disturbances, 16% of the latter being permanent.

MEDIAL THALAMOTOMY

Mention has been made of the pioneering work of Hécaen et al (1949) Monnier & Fischer (1951) and Mark and his colleagues. There has been a lack of consensus as to which site in medial thalamus should be the target for interruption of the reticulothalamic tract, various authors suggesting centre median, parafascicular or centrolateral

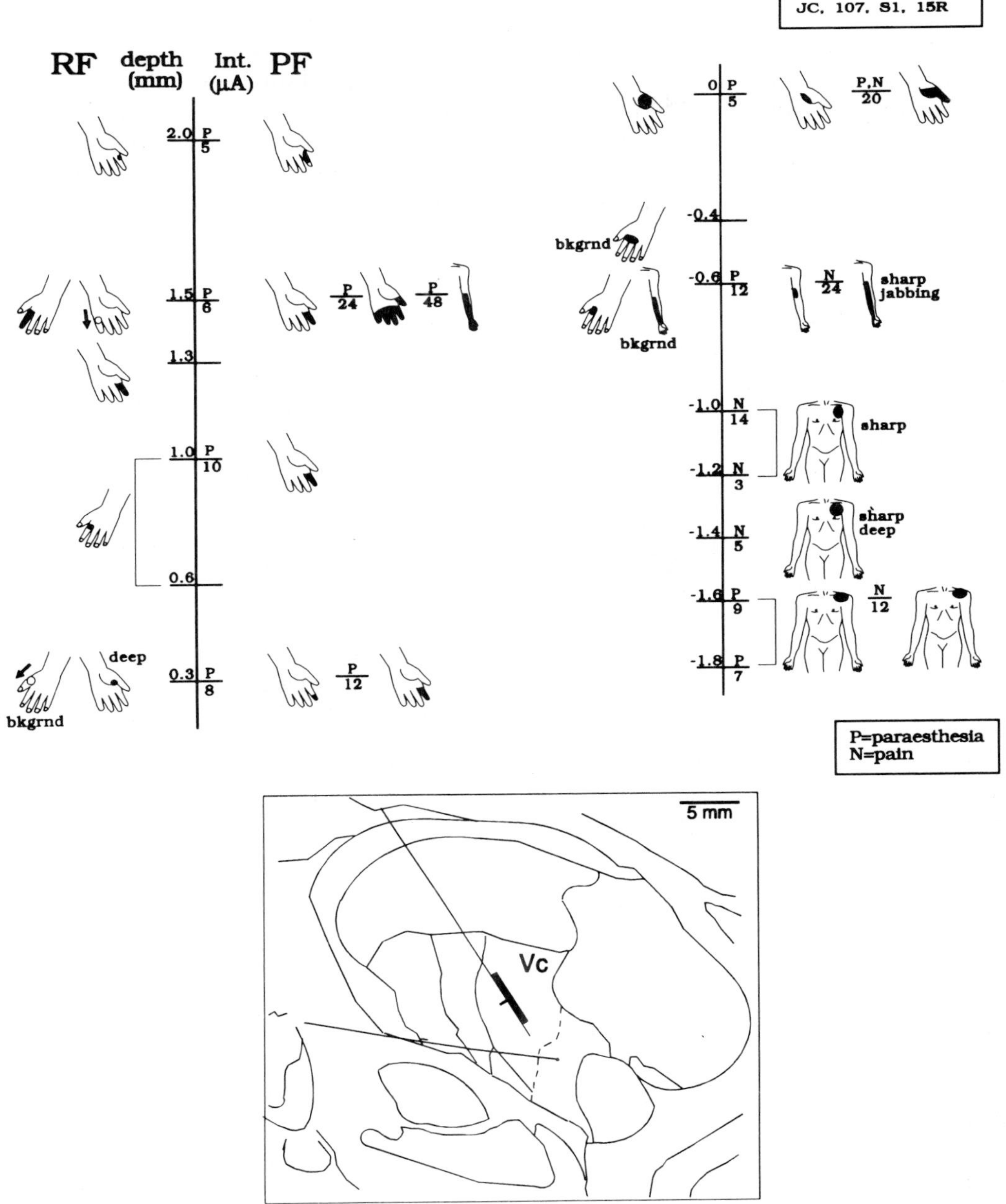

Fig. 60.3 A 15 mm lateral sagittal atlas diagram showing location of a single electrode trajectory with a partial figurine map showing receptive fields (RF), determined with a microelectrode, to the left of the trajectory, projected fields (PF) to microstimulation with the same microelectrode to the right. Low threshold mechanoreceptor multiunit responses with paraesthetic (P) PFs are recorded for upper extremity throughout most of the trajectory. At the base of VC where RFs cease the PFs suddenly shift in somatotopy to trunk and the stimulation-induced responses change from P to noxious (N). There is a small anatomical–physiological mismatch in that the position of VC as determined by CT from the locations of the anterior and posterior commissures lies more anterior and lower than would have been expected from the physiological responses. Numbers to the left indicate distance along trajectory in mm with respect to the tick in the atlas diagram, and numbers to the right indicate threshold in microamperes for response elicited neurons responding to passive digital movements (not shown) extended from +4.3 to +3.3 and to tactile stimuli of index from +2.9 to +2.0 (not shown). 'Bkgrnd' indicates sites where increase in background (baseline noise) was elicited. (From Dostrovsky et al 1992 with permission.)

nucleus, internal thalamic lamina and nucleus submedius (Willis 1985).

The technique of medial thalamotomy is similar to that of mesencephalic tractotomy except that the location of VC is determined anatomically and confirmed physiologically as shown in Figure 60.3. The location of the appropriate target in medial thalamus is then extrapolated from that of VC as physiologically confirmed. Physiological studies in medial thalamus are not diagnostic, as shown in Figure 60.4, and RF lesions here produce no clinically detectable neurological change (Fig. 60.5).

Urabe & Tsubokawa (1965) performed unilateral centre median lesions in seven patients with, probably, cancer pain relieving two (28.6%); bilateral procedures in seven were all successful. Postoperative confusion affected three (21.4%) and dysaesthesiae two (14.3%), but

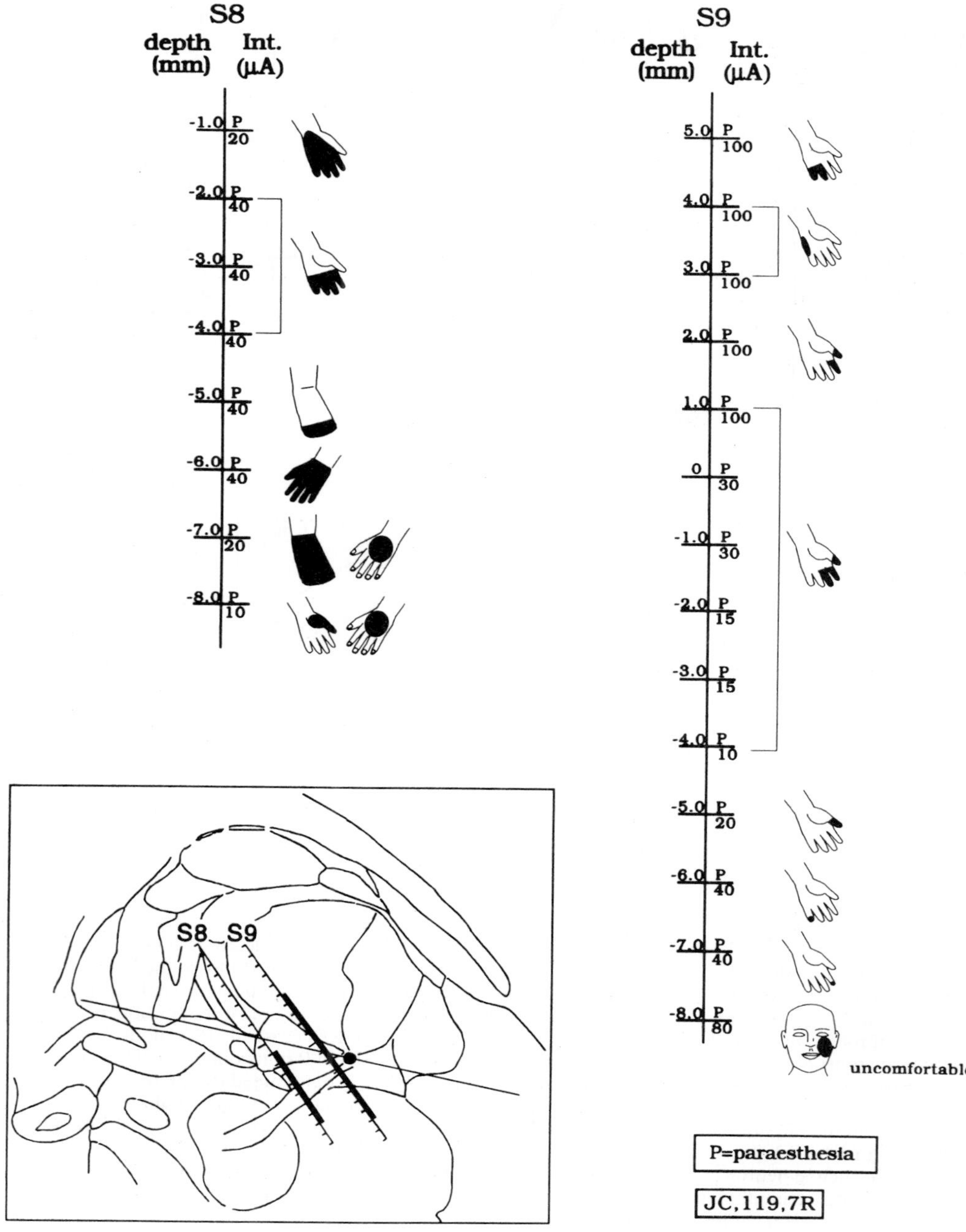

Fig. 60.4 A 7 mm right sagittal atlas diagram showing the locations of two microelectrode trajectories (S8, S9) through the medial thalamus. Data displayed as in Figure 60.3. No indentifiable units were recorded and PFs with paraesthetic responses referred mostly to contralateral upper extremity and with relatively high thresholds presumably arise from volume conduction to VC.

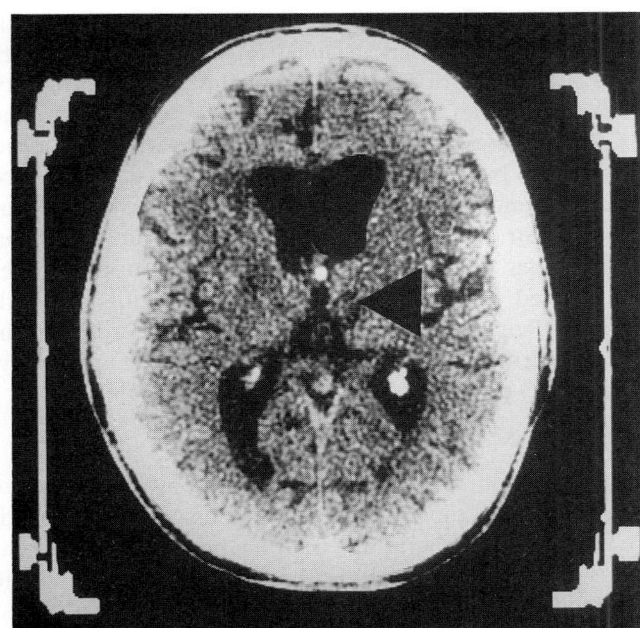

Fig. 60.5 CT scan of a patient who has undergone a medial thalamotomy 6 days before, showing lesion (arrowhead) and postoperative ventricular air. He is fitted with a Leksell stereotactic frame in order to undergo a mesencephalic tractotomy since the thalamotomy did not relieve his pain, induced by cancer of the head and neck.

Tsubokawa & Mariyasu (1975) noted an eventual recurrence of pain in 45% of 25 cases. Sugita et al (1972) reported relief of cancer pain in 81% of 47 patients, 15% suffering from confusion. Siegfried & Krayenbühl (1972) noted pain recurrence after medial thalamotomy in 60% of 19 patients with various pain syndromes in 6 months, 70% in a year and 75% in 3 years – an event less likely in cancer patients. They reported no complications. Sano (1977) and Sano et al (1966, 1970) concluded that the results of medial thalamic lesions were best in the posterior portion of the intralaminar complex and published detailed physiological criteria for target identification while autopsy studies (Yoshimasu 1982) pointed to the thalamic lamina or centrolateral nucleus as the preferred target. Sano (1979) reported that 31% of patients with cancer pain were relieved by lesions of the internal thalamic lamina and 20% by lesions in the centre median-parafascicular area. Leksell et al (1972) reported 40% relief of cancer pain in 25 patients treated by 'gamma knife' lesions in centre median-parafascicular complex with no complications, while Steiner et al (1980) found useful relief in 46% of cancer patients with the same operation. Hitchcock & Teixeira (1981) relieved all eight patients operated on for cancer pain by medial thalamotomy.

Our own experience with 80 lesions made in medial thalamus is that no responses are elicited by its stimulation, except in some patients with neural injury pain, and no detectable neurological effects follow lesions made there (Tasker et al 1982). Some 55% of our 22 patients with cancer pain derived useful pain amelioration, sometimes in conjunction with lesions in dorsomedian nucleus or mesencephalic tract. Use of multiple lesion sites precludes reliable data on complications or comparison with the results of others. A literature review (Tasker 1982b) of 175 patients apparently suffering nociceptive pain from cancer suggested a 46% relief rate after medial thalamotomy, not including the large series of 521 patients presented in very limited detail by Fairman (1967, 1972) and Fairman & Llavallol (1973) in which 70% were relieved with 10% morbidity. Pagni (1974) concluded that medial thalamotomy resulted in only a transient 'leucotomic' effect; bilateral lesions only increased the risk of cognitive problems. As mentioned previously, Frank et al (1987) compared medial thalamotomy with mesencephalic tractotomy in the treatment of cancer pain, recording 83.5% pain relief, a mortality of 1.8% and a morbidity of 10.1% after mesencephalic tractotomy, with 57.9% pain relief and a tendency for recurrence, no mortality and a low morbidity from cognitive problems after medial thalamotomy.

Turning to the more intractable problem of neural injury pain, in their pioneering work Hécaen et al (1949) relieved three of six patients with neural injury pain, Bettag & Yoshida (1960) one of four; dorsomedian lesions were sometimes included in the latter's hands. Voris & Whisler (1975) relieved 30.4% of 23 cases but the lesions were variously located throughout upper brainstem. Sano (1979) induced 50% significant relief with thalamolaminotomy, 60% after centre median-parafascicular lesions. Niizuma et al (1980) found their 56% improvement tended to be transient. Laitinen (1988) noted long-term relief in five patients without complications. Only 18% of our 17 patients with neural injury pain treated with medial thalamotomy (some with additional lesions elsewhere) were relieved, a considerably less successful outcome than mesencephalic tractotomy achieved in our hands for this difficult type of pain (Tasker 1982b updated). Summarizing published data in patients with neural injury pain, Tasker (1982b) found 29% satisfactory, 38% fair relief in 47 patients, with lesions often made at multiple sites with a 4–21% complication rate.

Thus, medial thalamotomy, like other destructive lesions, is more effective for the relief of cancer than for neural injury pain. However, if the quality of the pain caused by neural injury is taken into account, there may be a differential effect, destructive lesions in the pain processing paths being much more effective for evoked (allodynia, hyperpathia) and intermittent shooting pain than for steady pain while the reverse is true for chronic stimulation procedures. This effect is statistically significant in central pain from cord injury (Tasker & de Carvalho 1990), while the same trend applies in the smaller numbers of patients with central pain induced by brain lesions (see Table 60.4).

PULVINAR LESIONS

Virtually nothing is known about the physiology of the pulvinar and its relationship to pain perception; Willis (1985) doesn't mention it. Richardson & Zorub (1970) considered it an extension of the medial thalamic group just discussed and a target for lesions made for the relief of cancer pain (Richardson 1967). Fraioli & Guidetti (1975) reported early recurrence of neural injury pain after pulvinotomy. Mayanagi & Bouchard (1976/77) felt that medial thalamic lesions were more effective for cancer pain if they encroached on pulvinar, producing 89% longer-term relief, compared with 60%. Only 33% of their patients with neural injury pain were relieved. Siegfried (1977) reported experience with the operation in 13 patients with neural injury pain, eight with cancer, two of whom died. Despite early relief in 77%, pain tended to recur and mortality was 9% with 14% sensory complications. Laitinen (1977) reported experience with 41 patients with difficult pain syndromes noting that relief tended to be transient; 15% suffered transient complications. Yoshii et al (1980) reported that both of his patients with cancer pain surviving over a year continued to be relieved. Laitinen (1988) concluded that results were best with cancer pain and postherpetic neuralgia, four of six recent cases with neural injury pain enjoying good early relief. He concluded that pulvinotomy 'may be as good as CM thalamotomy' and that lesions in nonspecific thalamic lesions were sufficiently useful in neural injury pain that they should be kept equally in mind with chronic neurostimulation, having the advantage of being a once-only procedure not requiring ongoing management of expensive and, for the patient, technically complex equipment. Yoshii et al (1990) did postmortem studies of cancer patients whose pain had been relieved by pulvinotomy, concluding that the supranucleus pulvinaris was the target of choice. Tasker's literature review (1982b) found 81% of 76 patients with nociceptive pain relieved by pulvinotomy, 21% suffering complications, though recurrence was a problem; 22% of patients with neural injury pain were relieved.

THE HYPOTHALAMUS

As early as 1954 Spiegel et al (1954a, 1954b) suggested that the hypothalamus had a role in pain processing. Fairman (1973, 1976) reported 70% relief in 54 patients after hypothalamotomy. Sano (1977, 1979) and Mayanagi et al (1978) have reported a considerable experience with posteromedial hypothalamotomy in cancer pain, finding 60–69% relief. They also found it useful in neural injury pain. A literature review (Tasker 1982b) suggests a two-thirds chance of relief in cancer pain with 10% complications. Mayanagi & Sano (1988) reported 28 procedures up to 1977 (18 for cancer, 10 for neural injury pain) with 71.4% pain relief after unilateral operation, relief in the rest after bilateral surgery. The cancer patients enjoyed better relief but there was a tendency for postoperative pain recurrence. They observed however that the stimulation used for physiological localization also induced pain relief so that nine patients with various pain syndromes were treated with chronic hypothalamic stimulation with four excellent results and two good results, especially in cancer. Fairman (1976) also used this treatment modality.

HYPOPHYSECTOMY

In contradistinction to hypothalamotomy, destructive lesions of the pituitary gland have long been employed, usually by open operation, to treat hormone-dependent cancer and its pain. Various percutaneous and stereotactic approaches to hypophysectomy have been considered (Zervas 1969; Moser et al 1980) and tried over the years, but Moricca's (1974) technique of alcohol injection introduced in 1963 was instantly accepted and popularized. The suprising observation was made that the pain not only of hormone-dependent but also of other cancer was relieved by the simple procedure – applicable even in the very ill – of injecting alcohol percutaneously with a transnasal approach. This procedure, the mechanism of which is unknown, has been reviewed by Levin (1988) who, with Katz (Levin & Katz 1977), introduced a stereotactic approach in an attempt to reduce cerebrospinal fluid (CSF) rhinorrhoea and increase the volume of alcohol delivered to the pituitary through a single needle insertion. His review of the published experience of others suggested 75–94% relief of cancer pain. His own experience with 110 patients gave equally favourable results – 73–97% relief in different types of cancer over a mean 5-month survival; 16–30%, depending on cancer type, experienced transient pain exacerbations postoperatively and there was a tendency to pain recurrence. In his series only one patient had a CSF leak; six suffered oculomotor palsies, some with visual field defects. His excellent results contrast with earlier experience in the literature reviewed by this author (Tasker 1993) with the technique performed freehand in which reported pain relief was 41–95% in hormonally-dependent cancer, 69% in other types, with a tendency for pain recurrence within 3–4months, mortality 2–6.5%, rhinorrhoea 3–20%, meningitis 0.3–1%, visual and oculomotor effects 2–10%, diabetes insipidus 5–60%, hypothalamic disturbance and headache being frequent.

OTHER TARGET SITES

Talairach et al (1960) treated neural injury pain in eight patients with lesions in the thalamic radiations to the second somatosensory cortex, little or no clinically detectable sensory loss being induced. Martinez et al (1975) reported 65% relief of a mixed group of pain syndromes with the same operation. Andy (1973) performed successful anterior thalamotomy in a patient with hysterical pain. Dorsomedian thalamotomy has usually been combined with lesions elsewhere so that its effects on pain cannot be evaluated Tasker (1982b). Spiegel et al (1966) found lesions in Forel's fields questionable. Psychosurgery and stereotactic brain stimulation are discussed in Chapters 62 and 60.

SUMMARY AND CONCLUSIONS

This chapter cannot be summarized in isolation. The stereotactic approach is just one of those available, should surgical treatment of chronic pain be considered, and must be put in perspective according to its complexity, risk and likelihood for success.

NOCICEPTIVE PAIN

Patients with nociceptive pain referred to the neurosurgeon often suffer from cancer, though low-back pain is probably the commonest cause. For cancer pain, percutaneous radiofrequency neurectomy or rhizotomy are the obvious solution in those very few patients for whom the procedures are applicable. Otherwise percutaneous cordotomy is the treatment of choice and the best surgical procedure available to control pain in appropriately selected patients. If the patient cannot cooperate, the procedure can be done very effectively under general anaesthesia without muscle paralysis (Tasker 1990). However, for pain above the C5 dermatome, or in patients with respiratory contraindications, cordotomy is contraindicated and there is no substitute that is nearly as satisfactory. Intraspinal morphine infusion is not ideal in these situations. Third ventricle morphine infusion (Dennis & DeWitty 1990) can be considered but experience with the technique is still limited. Mesencephalic tractotomy requires the stereotactic approach and has a significant mortality and morbidity. Medial thalamotomy is attractive because of its simplicity and low risk, but it often fails. Pontine tractotomy and VCpc thalamotomy appear promising but experience with them is limited. For truncal, especially midline pelvic, pain caused by cancer where cordotomy is less successful, spinal morphine infusions would appear preferable (Meyerson et al 1984). Chronic stimulation of PVG would seldom seem cost-effective in cancer patients with a short life expectancy because of the cost of the equipment but can be used long-term transcutaneously (Meyerson et al 1978). Gybels (1991) recommended that, for cancer patients with a 1–2-month life expectancy, only percutaneous neurolytic or morphine infusion procedures be used. For patients expected to survive 2–5 months, ablative procedures could also be considered. For patients with longer survival, ablative procedures and PVG stimulation should be considered. Neurostimulation is Gybels' treatment of choice in neural injury pain.

Chronic low-back pain is perhaps the commonest pain syndrome referred for surgical treatment. It is a complex entity, considered in detail in Chapter 24, consisting of a variety of interrelated pain syndromes, often complicated by psychogenic magnification and seldom managed adequately by any one procedure. In rare cases, so-called facet rhizotomy – really percutaneous RF section of posterior rami – may be useful; in the occasional, carefully investigated patient, selective dorsal rhizotomy, or else, if a root deafferentation syndrome is prominent, dorsal column stimulation. This author would caution against the use of cordotomy or stereotactic destructive procedures because of their risks and low yield. Of the various stereotactic procedures available, only chronic stimulation of PVG would appear appropriate in those patients with severe nociceptive back pain who have consistently failed to respond to other simpler approaches. Other types of noncancerous nociceptive pain are sufficiently uncommon to require case-by-case assessment.

NEURAL INJURY PAIN

Neural injury pain, whether caused by peripheral or central lesions, nearly always has a constant burning, dysaesthetic or aching element. No matter whether this is the result of an infraorbital nerve lesion caused by a fracture or of stroke, this constant pain usually responds poorly to destructive surgery but has a 50% chance of amelioration by chronic stimulation. This should be accomplished by the simplest possible means – percutaneous trigeminal or dorsal cord stimulation if possible, otherwise stereotactic stimulation of the lemniscal pathway. Except for the percutaneous trigeminal technique, peripheral nerve stimulation has the disadvantage of being an open operation on an already damaged nerve in which it may be difficult to find the appropriate sensory fascicles, leaving dorsal column stimulation as the procedure of choice. When the latter fails or is technically impossible, stereotactic brain stimulation is indicated, a practical alternative despite its 50% success rate because of its low risk and reversibility.

Stereotactic destructive surgery in neural injury pain should be restricted to patients in whom stimulation has failed, particularly patients with prominent intermittent neuralgic pain or allodynia and hyperpathia. The commonest cause of neuralgic pain is thoracolumbar cord injury in which condition it is very effectively relieved by cordotomy, cordectomy or the dorsal root entry zone procedure (Nashold & Ostdahl 1979). In other neural injury pain syndromes in which these cord lesions are inappropriate, neuralgic pain, if not relieved by stimulation, may respond to destructive surgery such as medial thalamotomy. For allodynia or hyperpathia that is still a problem after stimulation has been used, destructive lesions can be considered, such as rhizotomy in the quadriplegic with allodynia in root distribution at the level of the lesion. Otherwise destructive cord or stereotactic lesions can be considered – always trying the simplest and safest technique first. Or else, particularly after stroke when it is common, allodynia or hyperpathia may be relieved by PVG stimulation.

The use of morphine infusion techniques in pain of nonmalignant origin deserves mention. There would be nothing surprising about the control by opiates of nociceptive pain caused by noncancerous disease. It would seem likely to this author that morphine would also relieve the intermittent neuralgic or evoked elements of neural injury pain but not the constant causalgic, dysaesthetic component.

Thus, stereotactic procedures occupy a very limited but specific niche in the treatment of chronic pain; less sophisticated procedures should be considered first and, in neural injury pain, stimulation techniques should take preference over destructive ones.

REFERENCES

Adams J E, Hosobuchi Y, Fields H L 1974 Stimulation of internal capsule for relief of chronic pain. Journal of Neurosurgery 41: 740–744

Amano K, Tanikawa T, Iseki H et al 1978 Single neuron analysis of the human midbrain tegmentum. Rostral mesencephalic reticulotomy for pain relief. Applied Neurophysiology 41: 66–78

Amano K, Iseki H, Notani M et al 1979 Rostral mesencephalic reticulotomy for pain relief with reference to electrode trajectory and clinical results. Applied Neurophysiology 42: 316

Amano K, Kawamura H, Tanikawa T et al 1986 Long-term followup study of rostral mesencephalic reticulotomy for pain relief – report of 34 cases. Applied Neurophysiology 49: 105–111

Andy O J 1973 Successful treatment of long-standing hysterical pain and visceral disturbances by unilateral anterior thalamotomy. Journal of Neurosurgery 39: 252–254

Armour D 1927 Surgery of the spinal cord and its membranes. Lancet ii: 691–697

Barbéra J, Barcia-Salorio J L, Broseta J 1979 Stereotaxic pontine spinothalamic tractotomy. Surgical Neurology 11: 111–114

Bernard E J Jr, Nashold B S Jr, Caputi F 1988 Clinical review of nucleus caudalis dorsal root entry zone lesions for facial pain. Applied Neurophysiology 51: 218–224

Bettag W, Yoshida T 1960 Uber stereotaktische Schmerzoperationen. Acta Neurochirurgica 8: 299–317

Boivie J 1992 Hyperalgesia and allodynia in patients with CNS lesions. In: Willis W (ed) Hyperalgesia and allodynia. Raven Press, New York, p 363–373

Bosch D A 1991 Stereotactic rostral mesencephalotomy in cancer pain and deafferentation pain. A series of 40 cases with follow-up results. Journal of Neurosurgery 75: 747–751

Bouckoms A J 1988 Psychosurgery for pain. In: Wall P D, Melzack R (eds) Textbook of pain, 2nd edn. Churchill Livingstone, Edinburgh p 868–881

Boureau F, Doubrère J F, Luu M 1990 Study of verbal description in neuropathic pain. Pain (suppl) 42: 145–152

Bowsher D 1957 Termination of the central pain pathway in man: the conscious appreciation of pain. Brain 80: 606–622

Bowsher D 1961 The termination of secondary somatosensory neurons within the thalamus of Macaca mulatta: an experimental degeneration study. Journal of Comparative Neurology 116: 213–277

Bowsher D 1980 The problem of central pain. Verhandlungen der Deutschen Gesellschaft für innere Medizin 86: 1525–1527

Cassinari V, Pagni C A 1969 Central pain: a neurosurgical survey. Harvard, Cambridge.

Chang H T, Ruch T C 1947 Topographical distribution of spinothalamic fibers in the thalamus of the spider monkey. Journal of Anatomy 81: 150–164

Cook A W, Nathan P W, Smith M C 1984 Sensory consequences of commissural myelotomy. A challenge to traditional anatomical concepts. Brain 107: 547–568

Crue B L Jr, Todd E M, Carregal E J A, Kilham O 1967 Percutaneous trigeminal tractotomy. Case report utilizing stereotactic radiofrequency lesion. Bulletin of the Los Angeles Neurological Society 32: 86–92

Crue B L, Todd E M, Carregal E J A 1968 Posterior approach for high cervical percutaneous radiofrequency cordotomy. Confinia Neurologica 30: 41–52

Crue B L, Todd E M, Carregal E J 1970 Percutaneous radiofrequency stereotactic trigeminal tractotomy. In: Crue B L (ed) Pain and suffering. Thomas, Springfield, p 69–79

Davis R A, Stokes J W 1966 Neurosurgical attempts to relieve thalamic pain. Surgery, Gynecology and Obstetrics 123: 371–384

DeMontreuil C B, Lajat Y, Resche F, Boutet J J, Legent F 1983 Apport de la neuro-chirurgie stéréotaxique dans le traitement des algies des cancers cervico-faciaux. Annales Oto-Laryngologie (Paris) 100: 181–186

Dennis G C, DeWitty R L 1990 Long-term intraventricular infusion of morphine for intractable pain in cancer of the head and neck. Neurosurgery 26: 404–408

Dostrovsky J O, Wells F E B, Tasker R R 1992 Pain evoked by stimulation in human thalamus. In: Inoki R, Shigenaga Y, Tohyama M (eds) Processing and inhibition of nociceptive information. International Congress Series 989. Excerpta Medica, Amsterdam, p 115–120

Eiras J, Garcia J, Gomes J, Carcavalla L I, Ucar J 1980 First results with extralemniscal myelotomy. Acta Neurochirurgica (suppl) 30: 377–381

Ervin F R, Mark V H 1960 Stereotactic thalamotomy in the human. II. Physiologic observations on the human thalamus. Archives of Neurology 3: 368–380

Fairman D 1967 Unilateral thalamic tractotomy for the relief of bilateral pain in malignant tumours. Confinia Neurologica 29: 146–158

Fairman D 1972 Hypothalamotomy as a new perspective for alleviation of intractable pain and regression of metastatic malignant tumours. In: Fusek I, Kunc Z (eds) Present limits of neurosurgery. Avicenum, Prague p 525–528

Fairman D 1973 Stereotactic hypothalamotomy for the alleviation of pain in malignant disease. Journal of Surgical Oncology 5: 79–84

Fairman D 1976 Neurophysiological bases for the hypothalamic lesion and stimulation by chronic implanted electrodes for the relief of intractable pain in cancer. In: Bonica J J, Albe-Fessard D (eds) Advances in pain research and therapy, vol 1. Raven Press, New York, p 843–847

Fairman D, Llavallol M A 1973 Thalamic tractotomy for the alleviation of intractable pain in cancer. Cancer 31: 700–707

Fox J L 1972 Delineation of the obex by contrast radiography during percutaneous trigeminal tractotomy. Technical note. Journal of Neurosurgery 36: 107–112

Fox J L 1974 Percutaneous trigeminal tractotomy. Variations in delineation of the obex using emulsified pantopaque. Confinia Neurologica 36: 97–100

Fraioli B, Guidetti B 1975 Effect of stereotactic lesions of the pulvinar and lateralis posterior nucleus on intractable pain and dyskinetic syndromes of man. Applied Neurophysiology 38: 23–30

Frank F, Tognetti F, Gaist G, Frank G, Galassi E, Sturiale C 1982 Stereotaxic rostral mesencephalotomy in treatment of malignant facial thoracobrachial pain syndromes. Journal of Neurosurgery 56: 807–811

Frank F, Fabrizi A P, Gaist G, Weigel K, Mundinger F 1987 Stereotactic lesions in the treatment of chronic cancer pain syndromes: mesencephalotomy or multiple thalamotomies. Applied Neurophysiology 50: 314–318

Frank F, Fabrizi A P, Gaist G 1989 Stereotactic mesencephalic tractotomy in the treatment of chronic cancer pain. Acta Neurochirurgica 99: 38–40

Gardner W J, Karnosh L J, McClure C C Jr, Gardiner A K 1955 Residual function following hemispherectomy for tumour and for infantile hemiplegia. Brain 78: 487–502

Gildenberg P L 1988 General concepts of stereotactic surgery. In: Lunsford L D (ed) Modern stereotactic neurosurgery. Martinus Nijhoff, Boston p 3–11

Gioia D F, Wallace P B, Fuste F J, Greene M 1967 A stereotaxic method of surgery for the relief of intractable pain. International Surgery 48: 409–416

Gybels J M 1991 Indications for the use of neurosurgical techniques in pain control In: Bond M R, Charlton J E, Woolf C J (eds) Proceedings of the VIth World Congress on Pain. Pain research and clinical management, vol 4. Elsevier, Amsterdam, p 475–482

Gybels J M, Sweet W H 1989 Stereotactic mesencephalotomy. In: Gybels J M, Sweet W H (eds) Neurosurgical treatment of persistent pain. Karger, Basel, p 210–219

Halliday A M, Logue V 1972 Painful sensations evoked by electrical stimulation in the thalamus. In: Somjen G G (ed) Neurophysiology studied in man. Excerpta Medica, Amsterdam, p 221–230

Hassler R 1972 The division of pain conduction into systems of pain and pain awareness. In: Janzen R, Keidel W D, Herz A, Steichele C (eds) Pain: basic principles – pharmacology – therapy. Thieme, Stuttgart, p 98–112

Hassler R, Riechert T 1959 Klinische und anatomische Befunde bei stereotaktischen schmerzoperationen im Thalamus. Archiv für Psychiatric und Nervenkrankheiten 200: 93–122

Hawrylyshyn P, Rowe I H, Tasker R R, Organ LW 1976 A computer system for stereotaxic surgery. Computers in Biology and Medicine 6: 87–97

Hécaen H, Talairach J, David M, Dell M B 1949 Coagulations limitées du thalamus dans les algies du syndrome thalamique. Révue Neurologique (Paris) 81: 917–931

Helfant M H, Leksell L, Strang R R 1965 Experiences with intractable pain treated by stereotaxic mesencephalotomy. Acta Chirurgica Scandinavica 129: 573–580

Hitchcock E R 1969 Stereotactic spinal surgery. A preliminary report. Journal of Neurosurgery 31: 386–399

Hitchcock E R 1970a Stereotactic cervical myelotomy. Journal of Neurology, Neurosurgery Psychiatry 33: 224–230

Hitchcock E R 1970b Stereotactic trigeminal tractotomy. Annals of Clinical Research 2: 131–135

Hitchcock E R 1973 Stereotaxic pontine spinothalamic tractotomy. Journal of Neurosurgery 39: 746–752

Hitchcock E R 1977 Stereotactic spinal surgery. In: Proceedings of the VIth International Congress of Surgery. Garrea R, LeVay D (eds) Neurological Surgery International Congress Series 433. Excerpta Medica, Amsterdam, p 271–280

Hitchcock E R 1988 Spinal and pontine tractotomies and nucleotomies. In: Lunsford L D (ed) Modern stereotactic neurosurgery. Martinus Nijhoff, Boston, p 279–295

Hitchcock E R, Schvarcz J R 1972 Stereotaxic trigeminal tractotomy for post-herpetic facial pain. Journal of Neurosurgery 37: 412–417

Hitchcock E R, Teixeira M J A 1981 A comparison of results from center-median and basal thalamotomies for pain. Surgical Neurology 15: 341–351

Hitchcock E R, Kim M C, Sotelo M 1985a Further experience in stereotactic pontine tractotomy. Applied Neurophysiology 48: 242–246

Hitchcock E, Sotelo M G, Kim M Ch 1985b Analgesic levels and technical method in stereotactic pontine spinothalamic tractotomy. Acta Neurochirurgica 77: 29–36

Horsley V, Clarke R H 1908 The structure and functions of the cerebellum examined by a new method. Brain 31: 45–124

Kandel E I 1989 Functional and stereotactic neurosurgery. Plenum, New York, p 67–72

Kandel E I 1990 Stereotactic surgery of erythromelalgia. Stereotactic and Functional Neurosurgery 54, 55: 96–100

Kanpolat Y, Deda H, Akyar S, Bilgi C S 1989 CT-guided percutaneous cordotomy. Acta Neurochirurgica (suppl) 46: 67–68

Kanpolat Y, Deda H, Akyar S, Caglar S 1990 CT-guided pain procedures. Neurochirurgie 36: 394–398

Kondziolka D, Dempsey P K, Lunsford L D et al 1992 A comparison between magnetic resonance imaging and computed tomography for stereotactic coordinate determination. Neurosurgery 30: 402–407

Laitinen L 1977 Anterior pulvinotomy in the treatment of intractable pain. Acta Neurochirurgica (suppl) 24: 223–225

Laitinenn L V 1988 Mesencephalotomy and thalamotomy for chronic pain. In: Lunsford L D (ed) Modern stereotactic neurosurgery. Martinus Nijhoff, Boston p 269–277

Leksell L, Meyerson B A, Forster D M C 1972 Radiosurgical thalamotomy for intractable pain. Confinia Neurologica 34: 264

Lenz F A, Dostrovsky J O, Kwan H C, Tasker R R, Yamashiro K, Murphy J T 1988 Methods for microstimulation and recording of single neurons and evoked potentials in the human central nervous system. Journal of Neurosurgery 68: 630–634

Levin A B 1988 Stereotactic chemical hypophysectomy. In: Lunsford L D (ed) Modern stereotactic neurosurgery. Martinus Nijhoff, Boston, p 365–375

Levin A B, Katz J 1977 Treatment of diffuse cancer pain by instillation of alcohol into the sella turcica. Anesthesiology 46: 115–121

Levy R M, Lamb S, Adams J E 1987 Treatment of chronic pain by deep brain stimulation: long term follow-up and review of the literature Neurosurgery 21: 885–893

Lindblom U 1985 Assessment of abnormal evoked pain in neurological pain patients and its relation to spontaneous pain: a descriptive and conceptual model with some analytical results in: Fields H L, Dubner R, Cervero F (eds) Advances in pain research and therapy , vol 9. Raven Press, New York, p 409–423

Livingston W K 1976 Pain mechanisms: a physiologic interpretation of causalgia and its related causes, 2nd edn. Plenum, New York

Mark V H, Ervin F R 1965 Role of thalamotomy in treatment of chronic severe pain. Postgraduate Medicine 37: 563–571

Mark V H, Ervin F R, Hackett T P 1960 Clinical aspects of stereotactic thalamotomy in the human. I. The treatment of chronic severe pain. Archives of Neurology 3: 351–367

Mark V H, Ervin F R, Yakovlev P I 1961 Correlation of pain relief sensory loss, and anatomical lesion sites in pain patients treated by stereotactic thalamotomy. Transactions of the American Neurological Association 86: 86–90

Mark V H, Ervin F R, Yakovlev P 1963 Stereotactic thalamotomy. III. The verification of anatomical lesion sites in the human thalamus. Archives of Neurology 8: 78–88

Martinez S N, Bertrand C, Molina Negro P, Perez-Calvo J M 1975 Alterations of pain perception by stereotactic lesions of frontothalamic pathways. Confinia Neurologica 37: 113–118

Mayanagi Y, Bouchard G 1976/77 Evaluation of stereotactic thalamotomies for pain relief with reference to pulvinar intervention. Applied Neurophysiology 39: 154–157

Mayanagi Y, Sano K 1988 Posteromedial hypothalamotomy for behavioural disturbances and intractable pain. In: Lunsford L D (ed) Modern stereotactic neurosurgery. Martinus Nijhoff, Boston, p 377–388

Mayangi Y, Hori T, Sano K 1978 The posteromedial hypothalamus and pain behaviour with special reference to endocrinological findings. Applied Neurophysiology 41: 223–231

Mayer D J, Price D D 1976 Central nervous system mechanisms of analgesia. Pain 2: 379–404

Mazars G L 1975 Intermittent stimulation of nucleus ventralis posterolateralis for intractable pain. Surgical Neurology 4: 493–495

Mazars G, Pansini A, Chiarelli J 1960a Coagulation du faisceau spinothalamique et du faisceau quinto-thalamique par stéréotaxie. Indications-résultats. Acta Neurochirurgica 8: 324–326

Mazars G, Roge R, Pansini A 1960b Stereotactic coagulation of the spinothalamic tract for intractable trigeminal pain. Journal of Neurology, Neurosurgery and Psychiatry 23: 352

Mazars G L, Merienne L, Ciolocca C 1974 Treatment of certain types of pain by implantable thalamic stimulators. Neurochirurgie 29: 117–124

Meyerson B A, Boethius J, Carlson A M 1978 Percutaneous central gray stimulation for cancer pain. Applied Neurophysiology 41: 57–65
Meyerson B A, Arner S, Linderoth B 1984 Pros and cons of different approaches to the management of pelvic cancer pain. Acta Neurochirurgica (suppl) 33: 407–419
Monnier M, Fischer R 1951 Localisation, stimulation et coagulation du thalamus chez l'homme. Journal de Physiologie 43: 818
Moricca G 1974 Chemical hypophysectomy for cancer pain In: Bonica J J (ed) Advances in neurology, vol 4. Raven Press, New York, p 707–714
Moser R P, Yap J C, Fraley E E 1980 Stereotactic hypophysectomy for intractable pain secondary to metastatic prostate carcinoma. Applied Neurophysiology 43: 145–149
Nashold B S Jr 1970 Ocular reactions from brain stimulation in conscious man. Neuroophthalmology 5: 92–103
Nashold B S Jr 1982 Brainstem stereotaxic procedures. In: Schaltenbrand G, Walker A E (eds) Stereotaxy of the human brain. Anatomical, physiological and clinical applications. Thieme, Stuttgart, p 475–483
Nashold B S Jr, Ostdahl R H 1979 Dorsal root entry zone lesions for pain relief. Journal of Neurosurgery 51: 59–69
Nashold B S Jr, Wilson W P 1966 Central pain. Observations in man with chronic implanted electrodes in the midbrain tegmentum. Confinia Neurologica 27: 30–44
Nashold B S Jr, Wilson W P, Slaughter D G 1969a Sensations evoked by stimulation in the midbrain of man. Journal of Neurosurgery 30: 14–24
Nashold B S, Wilson W P, Slaughter D G 1969b Stereotaxic midbrain lesions for central dysesthesia and phantom pain. Journal of Neurosurgery 30: 116–126
Nashold B S Jr, Wilson W P, Slaughter G 1974 The midbrain and pain. In: Bonica J J (ed) Advances in neurology, vol 4. Raven Press, New York, 191–196
Nashold B S, Slaughter D G, Wilson W P, Zorub D 1977 Stereotactic mesencephalotomy. In: Krayenbühl H, Maspes P E, Sweet W H (eds) Progress in neurological surgery, vol 8. Karger, Basel, p 35–49
Nashold B S, Lopes H, Chodakiewitz J, Bronec P 1986 Trigeminal DREZ for craniofacial pain. In: Samii M (ed) Surgery in and around the brain stem and the third ventricle. Springer-Verlag, Berlin, p 54–59
Niizuma H, Kwak R, Saso S et al 1980 Follow-up results of center median thalamotomy for central pain. Applied Neurophysiology 43: 336
Noordenbos W 1959 Pain. Elsevier, Amsterdam
Orthner H, von Roeder F 1966 Further clinical and anatomical experiences with stereotactic operations for relief of pain. Confinia Neurologica 27: 418–430
Pagni C A 1974 Place of stereotactic technique in surgery for pain. Advances in neurology, vol 4. Raven Press, New York, p 699–706
Papo I 1979 Spinal posterior rhizotomy and commissural myelotomy in the treatment of cancer pain. In: Bonica J J, Ventafridda V (eds) Advances in pain research and therapy vol 2. Raven Press, New York, p 439–447
Parrent A, Lozano A, Tasker R R, Dostrovsky J 1992a Periventricular gray stimulation suppresses allodynia and hyperpathia in man. Stereotactic and Functional Neurosurgery 59: 82
Parrent A G, Lozano A M, Dostrovsky J O, Tasker R R 1992b Central pain in the absence of functional sensory thalamus . Stereotactic and Functional Neurosurgery 59: 9–14
Ralston B L 1962 Hemispherectomy and hemithalamectomy in man. Journal of Neurosurgery 19: 909–912
Richardson D E 1976 Recent advances in the neurosurgical control of pain. Southern Medical Journal 60: 1082–1086
Richardson D E, Akil H 1977a Pain reduction by electrical brain stimulation in man. I. Acute administration in periaqueductal and periventricular sites. Journal of Neurosurgery 47: 178–183
Richardson D E, Akil H 1977b Pain reduction by electrical brain stimulation in man. II. Chronic self-administration in the periventricular grey matter. Journal of Neurosurgery 47: 184–194.
Richardson D E, Zorub D S 1970 Sensory function of the pulvinar. Confinia Neurologica 32: 154–173
Roberts W J 1986 A hypothesis on the physiological basis for causalgia and related pain. Pain 24: 297–311
Sano K 1977 Intralaminar thalamotomy (thalamolaminotomy) and posterior hypothalamotomy in the treatment of intractable pain. In: Krayenbühl H, Maspes P E, Sweet W H (eds) Progress in neurological surgery, vol 8, Karger, Basel, p 50–103
Sano K 1979 Stereotaxic thalamolaminotomy and posteromedial hypothalamotomy for the relief of intractable pain. In: Bonica J J, Ventrafridda V (eds) Advances in pain research and therapy , vol 2. Raven Press, New York, p 475–485
Sano K, Yoshioka M, Ogashiwa M, Ishijima B, Ohye C 1966 Thalamolaminotomy: a new operation for relief of intractable pain. Confinia Neurologica 27: 63–66
Sano K, Yoshioka M, Sekino H, Mayanagi Y, Yoshimasu Y, Tsukamoto Y 1970 Functional organization of the internal medullary lamina in man. Confinia Neurologica 32: 374–380
Schaltenbrand G, Bailey P 1959 Introduction to stereotaxis with an atlas of the human brain. Thieme, Stuttgart
Schaltenbrand G, Wahren W 1977 Atlas for stereotaxy of the human brain, 2nd edn. Thieme, Stuttgart
Schvarcz J R 1978 Spinal cord techniques re trigeminal nucleotomy and extralemniscal myelotomy. Applied Neurophysiology 41: 99–112
Schvarcz J R 1979 Stereotactic spinal trigeminal nucleotomy for facial pain. In: Bonica J J, Liebeskind J C, Albe-Fessard D G (eds) Advances in pain research and therapy, vol 3. Raven Press, New York, p 331–336
Schvarcz J R 1984 Stereotactic high cervical extralemniscal myelotomy for pelvic cancer pain. Acta Neurochirurgica (suppl) 33: 431–435
Shealy C N, Mortimer J T, Hagfors N R 1970 Dorsal column electroanalgesia. Journal of Neurosurgery 32: 560–564
Shieff C, Nashold B S 1987 Mesencephalotomy for thalamic pain. Neurological Research 9: 101–104
Shieff C, Nashold B S Jr 1988 Thalamic pain and stereotactic mesencephalotomy. Acta Neurochirurgica (suppl) 42: 239–242
Shieff C, Nashold B S Jr 1990 Stereotactic mesencephalotomy. In: Friedman W A (ed) Neurosurgery clinics of North America . Saunders, Philadelphia, p 825–859
Siegfried J 1977 Stereotactic pulvinarotomy in the treatment of intractable pain. In: Krayenbühl H, Maspes P E, Sweet W H (eds) Progress in neurological surgery, vol 8, Karger, Basel, p 104–113
Siegfried J, Krayenbühl H 1972 Clinical experience with the treatment of intractable pain In: Janzen R, Keidel W D, Herz A, Steichele C (eds) Pain: basic principles – pharmacology – therapy. Thieme, Stuttgart, p 202–204
Spiegel E A, Wycis H T 1949 Pallidothalamotomy in chorea. Presented at Philadelphia Neurological Society, April 22
Spiegel E A, Wycis H T 1962 Stereoencephalotomy. II. Clinical and physiological applications. Grune & Stratton, New York
Spiegel E A, Kletzkin M, Szekely E G, Wycis H T 1954a Pain reactions upon stimulation of the tectum mesencephali. Journal of Neuropathology and Experimental Neurology 13: 212–220
Spiegel E A, Kletzkin M, Szekely E G ,Wycis H T 1954b Role of hypothalamic mechanisms in thalamic pain. Neurology 4: 739–751
Spiegel E A, Wycis H T, Szekely E G, Gildenberg P L 1966 Medial and basal thalamotomy in so-called intractable pain. In: Knighton R S, Dumke P R (eds) Henry Ford Hospital International Symposium on Pain. Little, Brown, Boston, p 503–517
Spiller W G, Martin E 1912 The treatment of persistent pain of organic origin in the lower part of the body by division of the anterolateral column of the spinal cord. Journal of the American Medical Association 58: 1489–1490
Steiner L, Forster D, Leksell L, Meyerson B A, Boethius J 1980 Gammathalamotomy in intractable pain. Acta Neurochirurgica 52: 173–184.
Sugita K, Mutsuga N, Takaoka Y, Doi T 1972 Results of stereotaxic thalamotomy for pain. Confinia Neurologica 34: 265–274
Talairach J, Tournoux P, Bancaud J 1960 Chirurgie pariétale de la douleur. Acta Neurochirurgica 8: 153–250
Talbot J D, Marrett S, Evans A C, Meyer E, Bushnell C, Duncan G H 1991 Multiple representations of pain in human cerebral cortex. Science 251: 1355–1358
Tasker R R 1982a Identification of pain processing systems by electrical stimulation of the brain. Human Neurobiology 1: 261–272
Tasker R R 1982b Thalamic stereotaxic procedures. In: Schaltenbrand

G, Walker A E (eds) Stereotaxy of the human brain. Anatomical, physiological and clinical applications. Thieme, Stuttgart, p 484–497

Tasker R R 1984 Stereotaxic surgery. In: Wall P D, Melzack R (eds) Textbook of pain, 1st edn. Churchill Livingstone, Edinburgh, p 639–655

Tasker R R 1987 The problem of deafferentation pain in the management of the patient with cancer. Journal of Palliative Care 2: 8–12

Tasker R R 1990 Percutaneous cordotomy In: Youmans J R (ed) Neurological surgery, 3rd edn. A comprehensive reference guide to the diagnosis and management of neurosurgical problems. Saunders, Philadelphia, p 4045–4058

Tasker R R 1993 Neurosurgical and neuroaugmentative intervention In: Patt R B (ed) Cancer pain. Lippincott, Philadelphia, p 471–500

Tasker R R, de Carvalho G 1990 Pain in thalamic stroke. Proceedings of the 13th Annual Meeting of the Inter-Urban Stroke Academic Association, Toronto, Queen Elizabeth Hospital, p 1–25

Tasker R R, Dostrovsky J O 1988 Deafferentation and central pain. In: Wall P D, Melzack R (eds) Textbook of pain, 2nd edn. Churchill Livingstone, Edinburgh p 154–180

Tasker R R, Dostrovsky J O 1992 Computers in functional stereotactic surgery In: Kelly P J, Kall B A (eds) Computers in stereotactic neurosurgery: contemporary issues in neurological surgery. Blackwell, Boston, p 155–164

Tasker R R, Organ L W, Hawrylyshyn P A 1982 The thalamus and midbrain of man. A physiological atlas using electrical stimulation. In: Wilkins R H (ed) The Bannerstone division of American lectures in neurosurgery. C C Thomas, Springfield, Illinois

Tasker R R, Yoshida M, Sima A A F, Deck J 1986 Stimulation mapping of the periventricular-periaqueductal gray (PVG-PAG) in man: an autopsy study In: Samii M (ed) Surgery in and around the brain stem and the third ventricle. Springer-Verlag, Berlin, p 161–167

Tasker R R, Yamashiro K, Lenz F, Dostrovsky J O 1988 Thalamotomy for Parkinson's disease: microelectrode technique In: Lunsford L D (ed) Modern stereotactic surgery. Martinus Nijhoff, Boston, p 297–314

Tasker R R DeCarvalho G T C, Dolan E J 1992 Intractable pain of spinal cord origin: clinical features and implications for surgery. Journal of Neurosurgery 77: 373–378

Tasker R R, Dostrovsky J O, Dolan E J 1993 Computerized tomography (CT) is just as accurate as ventriculography for functional stereotactic thalamotomy. Stereotactic and Functional Neurosurgery 57: 157–166

Todd E M, Crue B L, Carregal E J A 1969 Posterior percutaneous tractotomy and cordotomy. Confinia Neurologica 31: 106–115

Tsubokawa T, Moriyasu N 1975 Follow-up results of centre median thalamotomy for relief of intractable pain. Confinia Neurologica 37: 280–284

Turnbull I M 1972 Bilateral cingulumotomy combined with thalamotomy or mesencephalic tractotomy for pain. Surgery, Gynecology and Obstetrics 134: 958–962

Uematsu S, Konigsmark B, Walker A E 1974 Thalamotomy for alleviation of intractable pain. Confinia Neurologica 38: 88–96

Urabe M, Tsubokawa T 1965 Stereotaxic thalamotomy for the relief of intractable pain. Tohoku Journal of Experimental Medicine 85: 286–300

von Roeder F, Orthner H 1961 Erfabrungen mit stereotaktischen Eingriffen. III. Mitteilung. Confinia Neurologica 21: 51–97

Voris H C, Whisler W W 1975 Results of stereotaxic surgery for faciothoracobrachial pain syndromes. Journal of Neurosurgery 56: 807–811

Wall P D, Sweet W H 1967 Temporary abolition of pain in man. Science 155: 108–109

Whisler W W, Voris H C 1978 Mesencephalotomy for intractable pain due to malignant disease. Applied Neurophysiology 47: 52–56

Willis W D 1984 The origin and destination of pathways involved in pain transmission. In: Wall P D, Melzack R (eds) Textbook of pain, 2nd edn. Churchill Livingstone, Edinburgh, p 112–127

Willis W D 1985 The pain system. The neural basis of nociceptive transmission in the mammalian nervous system. Karger, Basel

Woolf C J 1992a Excitability changes in central neurons following peripheral damage: role of central sensitization in the pathogenesis of pain In: Willis W (ed) Hyperalgesia and allodynia. Raven Press, New York, p 221–243

Woolf C J 1992b Current understanding of the mechanisms of neuropathic pain. Acta Neurochirurgica 117: 86

Wycis H T, Spiegel E A 1962 Long-range results in the treatment of intractable pain by stereotaxic midbrain surgery. Journal of Neurosurgery 19: 101–107

Yoshii N, Mizokami T, Ushikubo T, Kuramtsu T, Fukuda S 1980 Long-term follow-up study after pulvinotomy for intractable pain. Applied Neurophysiology 43: 128–132

Yoshii N, Mizokami T, Usikubo Y, Samejima H, Adachi K 1990 Postmortem study of stereotactic pulvinarotomy for relief of intractable pain. Stereotactic and Functional Neurosurgery 54, 55: 103

Yoshimasu N, Ishijima B, Sano K 1982 Pain and the internal medullary lamina. Applied Neurophysiology 45: 498–499

Young R F, Brechner T 1986 Electrical stimulation of the brain for relief of intractable pain due to cancer. Cancer 57: 1266–1272

Young R F, Kroening R, Fulton W, Feldman R A, Chambi I 1985 Electrical stimulation of the brain in the treatment of chronic pain: experience over 5 years. Journal of Neurosurgery 62: 389–396

Zervas N T 1969 Stereotaxic radiofrequency surgery of the normal and the abnormal pituitary gland. New England Journal of Medicine 280: 429–437

Zimmermann M 1979 Peripheral and central nervous mechanisms of nociception pain, and pain therapy: facts and hypotheses. In: Bonica J J, Liebeskind J C, Albe-Fessard D G (eds) Advances in pain research and therapy, vol 3. Raven Press, New York, p 3–32

61. Pituitary destruction

John Miles

HISTORY AND EVOLUTION OF TECHNIQUES

The function of the pituitary gland, tucked away as it is in its own compartment in the base of the skull, was not immediately clear and is still ill-understood. Galen is reputed to have named the gland on the presumption that it produced pituita, the phlegmonous secretion from the mucous membranes of the nose. However, this great anatomist was somewhat limited by the contemporary restriction of his morbid studies to the animal rather than to the human. The association of acromegaly with a tumour of the pituitary was made by Marie in 1886, but the major advances in endocrinology and its orchestration from the pituitary gland have been made in this century. Houssay pursued his interest in pituitary function from an initiation as a medical student in the first decade of this century through continuous study involving many separate hormones to a Nobel prize in 1947 (Asimov 1972). The controlling influence of the hypothalamus on pituitary endocrinological function was an important development and the integration has now extended beyond the field of pure hormones into the semantically ill-defined area of neuromodulators and neurotransmitters.

A historic correlation between endocrine hormones and cancer was made in 1896 by Beatson. His studies in histology showed the striking similarity between the cellular proliferation in the mammary ducts of farm animals in the prelactation stage of oestrus and carcinoma of the human breast. This temporary proliferation in the sheep clears quickly on lactation with breakdown of the cells by fatty degeneration. On learning that in some countries oophorectomy was practised on cows in order to prolong lactation, he made the major extrapolation to the human with advanced carcinoma of the breast and proposed oophorectomy for such patients. Being something of a scientist he first undertook an experimental study on lactating rabbits. Being human, when oophorectomy failed to prolong lactation in the rabbit, he rationalized that the generalized adiposity that had followed castration was, in fact, a form of occult lactation, and proceeded to perform oophorectomy in three patients with inoperable cancer of the breast. The results were strikingly successful, with carefully recorded tumour regression. Oophorectomy has been extensively practised for advanced carcinomatosis from the breast since that time.

In 1941 Huggins & Hodges reported histological changes in the prostate as a result of castration and likewise this was then applied to the human with advanced carcinoma of the prostate. In 1952 Huggins & Bergenstahl extended the surgical manipulations to include adrenalectomy for carcinoma of both the breast and the prostate. In 1953 Luft & Olivercrona performed hypophysectomy, on a similar rationale, for advanced carcinoma of the breast and prostate. With each of the surgical ablative techniques already mentioned only a proportion of cases appeared to respond. Following hypophysectomy there was not only a similar proportionate regression of tumour but also a striking amount of pain relief. Pain relief had been recorded following oophorectomy and adrenalectomy but appeared to have been associated with tumour regression (Beatson 1896; I have found no mention of immediate relief). Pain relief following hypophysectomy was noted to correlate only in part with tumour regression and also, on occasion, to appear with striking speed, even within hours of recovery from anaesthetic. Over the next 20 years extensive endocrine manipulation was practised by various surgical techniques, but oophorectomy and adrenalectomy were much more common than hypophysectomy. On the rationale that improvement presumably related to depression of gonadatrophin hormones, oophorectomy was considered to be particularly appropriate for premenopausal patients with advanced carcinoma of the breast and was indicated by some even immediately after recognition of the primary tumour.

In general, adrenalectomy was the next choice. It is probable that it was preferred to hypophysectomy primarily because it could be performed by the same surgeon who had undertaken the primary breast surgery. To a lesser extent, hypophysectomy, by craniotomy, may also have suggested a greater risk to the patient than adrenalectomy.

In 1971 Hardy advocated increased use of hypophysectomy by virtue of the reduced morbidity of the transsphenoidal surgical approach he advocated. Cushing (1914) had extensively used this approach to the pituitary fossa earlier in the century, after it had been first proposed by Schloffer in 1907.

Alternatives were proposed in order to overcome the resistance to formal craniotomy and pituitary resection, such as that of pituitary stalk section by Ehni & Eckles in 1959. Zervas in 1969 used a stereotactically guided radiofrequency system for achieving pituitary ablation. Again a proportion of patients obtained amelioration of their cancer and, as particularly emphasised by Zervas, a separate proportion experienced pain relief, commonly immediate, even when objective remission in tumour growth did not occur.

In 1974 Morrica presented a massive experience of nearly 1000 cases of advanced cancer in whom there was virtual total relief of pain by the use of a technique of injecting alcohol into the pituitary gland. This technique he described as new and having first been used in 1963. It is of some interest to note that Greco et al first described the technique in 1957 and by 1973 had published at least 13 papers describing it and its use for advanced carcinoma of the breast, prostate and even a whole range of carcinomatoses not usually considered to be hormonally influenced. Regression of the tumour process and its effect on relieving pain were also described in detail. The consistency of pain relief as described by Morrica was almost unbelievable. However, when practised by others–Katz & Levin (1977); Lipton et al (1978); Takeda et al (1978) and Madrid (1979)–it clearly did have an important part in the management of persistent malignant pain.

The general experience is that persistent malignant pain can undoubtedly be relieved and that while it may be long-lasting, that is, more than 1 year, it is more common for it to be temporary, lasting weeks or months.

There may be associated tumour regression, but this does not necessarily correlate with the pain relief. Hormonal monitoring has tended to show varying degrees of pituitary functional impairment, but again this does not necessarily correlate with pain relief. Morbidity can attend this technique and therefore, in the main, it is reserved for cases of persistent malignant pain.

TECHNIQUES FOR PITUITARY DESTRUCTION

TRANSCRANIAL SURGICAL RESECTION (Fig. 61.1)

Ray (1960) had extensive experience of this technique and achieved effective ablation with low morbidity. Modern microsurgical technique, and the reintroduction of the transsphenoidal route, has rendered it obsolete.

TRANSCRANIAL PITUITARY STALK SECTION

This technique was advocated by Ehni & Eckles (1959) with the theoretical advantage of reducing morbidity, but most would consider that such a modification has little significance. The degree of hypopituitarism resulting from such a section is undoubtedly more erratic. Pain relief still occurs.

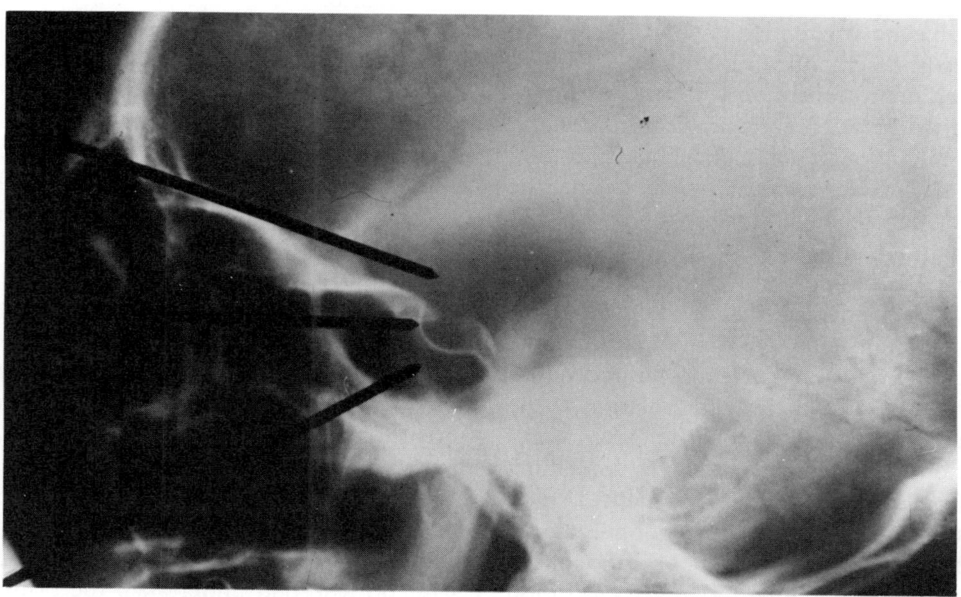

Fig. 61.1 Routes to sella for pituitary destruction: transcranial, transethmoidal–transsphenoidal.

TRANSSPHENOID HYPOPHYSECTOMY

This technique was proposed by Schloffer (1907) and used extensively by Cushing (1914) and then repopularized by Hardy in 1971 with the major advantage of microsurgical technique. This procedure involves the introduction of a speculum through a nasal passage or, as advocated by Hardy, through the position of the resected nasal septum, or through a medial orbital incision via the ethmoidal sinuses. The end result is the same, namely, that the sphenoidal sinus is entered and the anterior wall of the pituitary fossa is resected. After removal of the whole gland or its anterior lobe the sella is packed with muscle and further reinforced by a graft of dural substitute of some kind. Hardy used further support in the form of a transplanted piece of nasal septum. The procedure carries low morbidity and the main risk is cerebrospinal fluid (CSF) rhinorrhoea and/or meningitis. The use of interoperative radiographic screening is recommended in order to avoid inadvertent exploration beyond the sella.

RADIOFREQUENCY PITUITARY DESTRUCTION

This is achieved percutaneously by the transsphenoidal route, originally employing some form of stereotactic guidance system. A cannula is introduced through a nasal passage and, with radiographic screening, is directed through the sphenoidal sinus and through the anterior wall of the pituitary fossa. Through it is passed an electrode with a retractable side tip so that a wide area of the pituitary gland can be explored and coagulated. This technique, designed by Zervas (1969), carries even less morbidity, but also less certainty of achieving total pituitary ablation.

A modification of this method, with the electrode being introduced through a cannula of the Greco/Morrica type and using intermittent screening, but without stereotactic equipment, I have found to be equally effective and simple.

CRYOGENIC PITUITARY DESTRUCTION

This is also achieved percutaneously by the transsphenoidal route and has been extensively used (Bleasel 1965; Wilson & Frewer 1971). It is similar to the technique described above for radiofrequency coagulation, with less potential for lateral gland destruction.

RADIATIONAL PITUITARY DESTRUCTION

External irradiation is said to demand dosages above the safety limits for the surrounding structures, such as the optic nerves. Proton irradiation is probably safer by virtue of the focusing used (Donegan 1967).

Interstitial radiation using radon seeds, radioactive gold and yttrium have all been used. Yttrium appears to be the choice for destruction of the normal pituitary (Forrest et al 1959). There is a significant risk of meningitis and also irradiation injury to the adjacent cranial nerves and this, together with the special facilities required for using radioisotopes, has tended to limit its use.

Stereotactic radiosurgical destruction of pituitary tumours has been proven to be both accurate and free from most of the complications of the more invasive techniques and therefore, in centres that have the facilities, it should provide for pituitary destruction as a continuing option in the treatment of pain due to malignancy.

ULTRASONIC PITUITARY DESTRUCTION

This can be achieved but the gland, or at least the intrasellar dura, needs to be exposed. Having done so, and with the posssibly greater risk of unwanted spread of effect beyond the gland, this technique would appear to offer little advantage.

CHEMICAL PITUITARY DESTRUCTION

Greco et al described the technique in 1957 and it was applied to various carcinomatoses. Carbonin (1978) reminded us of the reports of tumour regression and pain relief that emanated from Greco's group.

Morrica described in 1974 his use of this technique and its almost total efficiency in relieving pain. Since then it has been used by many groups throughout the world with only minor modifications in technique and varying, though lesser, degrees of success.

The patient is slightly anaesthetised such that the pupils still react to light. A strong cannula is passed through a nasal passage and often enters the sphenoidal sinus, with ease, through the ostium. With radiographic screening it is directed to the anterior wall of the pituitary fossa. The obturator of the cannula is sharp and the cannula plus obturator are tapped through the anterior pituitary wall. When the obturator is removed the cannula tip is either in the subarachnoid space surrounding the gland or in the gland itself. The exact site can be determined by injecting a little fluid along the cannula. If it is in the subarachnoid space there is no resistance to injection, while if it is in the pituitary gland there is a very definite and immediate resistance that can, however, be overcome with further injection. If a radiocontrast fluid is injected this clearly shows up the subarachnoid space within the sella and the flow from there into the general subarachnoid space (Fig. 61.2). If the tip is in the gland the initial picture is of a gradually extending bolus within the gland. In the latter circumstances in more than one-quarter of the patients, further injection will clearly show spread of the radiocontrast up the pituitary stalk into the region of the hypothalamus and

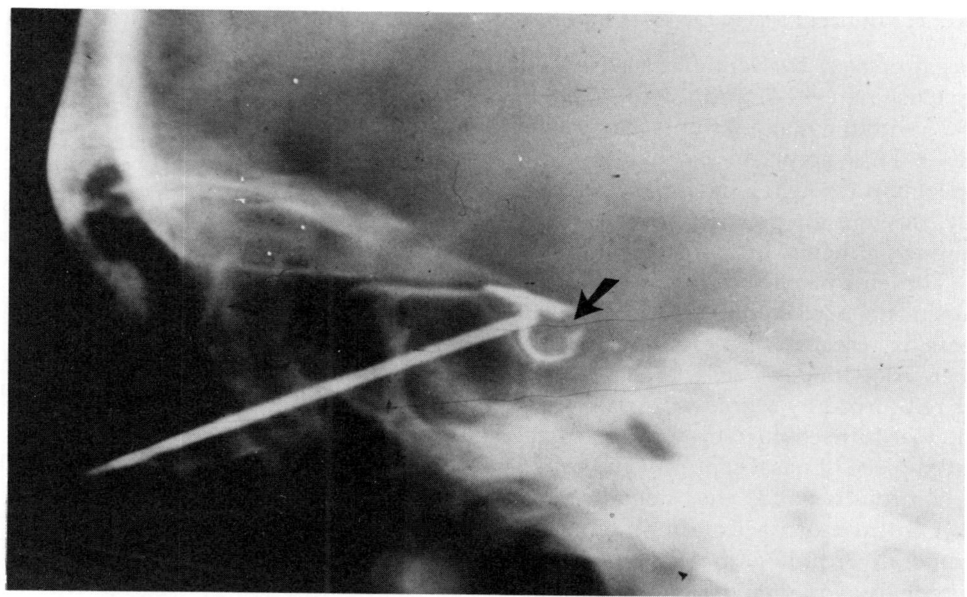

Fig. 61.2 Iodophylate (Myodil) injected through cannula into subarachnoid space within the sella with some escaping out. Pituitary gland and stalk (arrowed) outlined.

even into the third ventricle (Fig. 61.3). After the first contrast has gone in this direction there is little resistance to injection and, unless the position of the cannula is changed, subsequent material tends to follow that route. Between 1 and 6 ml of alcohol is then injected in increments of around 0.1 ml. The pupillary reaction to light is tested between each injection. If the pupillary reaction fails, the injection of alcohol is terminated and 25 mg prednisolone is quickly instilled into the spinal subarachnoid space. This is most expeditiously achieved by a lateral high cervical puncture at the same position as is used for entry in percutaneous cordotomy.

RESULTS OF PITUITARY DESTRUCTION

There is probably little difference in the results obtained by using the various techniques. Surgical hypophysectomy by the transcranial or the transsphenoidal approach almost certainly more completely ablates anterior pituitary function. On theoretical grounds, when the aim was to suppress carcinoma, total anterior pituitary ablation was considered desirable, and therefore these surgical techniques were preferred. However, there has been considerable disagreement as to the absolute necessity of achieving total suppression or destruction. Tindall et al (1979), Edelstyn et al (1965), Brodkey et al (1978) and, regarding alcohol injection, Takeda et al (1978) have argued for the correlation between effective pituitary ablation and the pain relief achieved. La Rossa et al (1978) and Zervas (1969), with regard to breast cancer, and Norrell et al (1970), Thompson et al (1974) and West et al (1979), regarding prostatic cancer, have emphasised the disparity between the degree of pain relief and the objective hypopituitarism with the obvious conclusion that the latter is not necessary to achieve the former.

The percentage relief of pain by the various strictly surgical techniques has varied little, being around 80% for carcinoma of the breast and as high as 90% with carcinoma of the prostate. It has been as good for other carcinomatoses though the experience is less (Tindall et al 1977). The duration of relief has varied widely, with the majority being months, but all series have included patients who have gone more than 1 year with total relief of pain.

Using chemical pituitary destruction, as described by Morrica (1974), no one has been able to match his results (Table 61.1). The nearest was the study reported by Katz & Levin (1977) using larger volumes of alcohol (up to 6 ml). Madrid (1979) described in 329 patients total relief of pain in 67%, partial relief in 27% and no relief in 6%. Our series (Lipton et al 1978) of 155 injections in 106 patients gave total relief in 41%, partial relief in 30% and no relief in 28%. The majority of our patients experienced relief for less than 3 months, with only 21% achieving relief lasting more than 3 months. We have always used less alcohol and rarely injected more than 2 ml.

Edelstyn et al (1965), Tindall et al (1977) and Schwarz et al (1981) have emphasized the apparent preferential relief of pain due to bony metastases rather than to soft tissue deposits. This opinion is propagated in many publications, but it is only in these two reports that the conclusions appear justified. Even then there is no doubt that there is disparity between the ease with which delineation of bony metastases could be achieved compared with soft

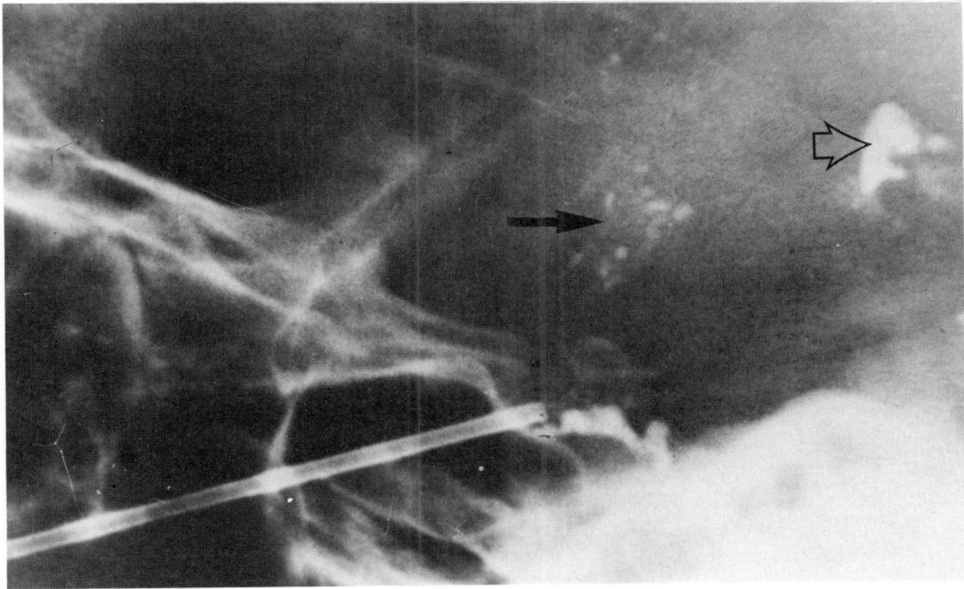

Fig. 61.3 Iodophylate in subarachnoid space and within hypothalamic tissue (solid arrow) and within the third ventricle (outlined arrow).

Table 61.1 Comparative efficiency of alcohol injection into the pituitary gland in relieving pain

	Patients	Injections	Excellent	Some	None
Morrica 1977	822	1906	809	12	1
Katz & Levin 1977	13	15	6	7	0
Lipton 1978	106	155	38	28	26
Madrid 1979	329		220	89	20

tissue masses and this might well make direct comparison invalid. Using the alcohol injection technique, we have certainly had excellent pain relief from soft tissue masses, not only those from breast or prostatic cancers. Persistent malignant pain in the head and neck region has proved equally amenable to alcohol injections into the pituitary gland and this has been particularly satisfying in view of the paucity of effective alternative treatments.

COMPLICATIONS

There is no doubt that injection of alcohol into pituitary fossa can be associated with significant complications. We have now performed this procedure for more than 250 patients and seen six cases in whom death appeared to be directly related to the technique. One of these was meningitis and two certainly involved hypothalamic injury. We have had two permanent visual field losses, one being bitemporal hemianopia. CSF rhinorrhoea only proved refractory to natural healing in one instance and in this case we satisfactorily plugged the hole by recannulation and packing with absorbable haemostatic tissue (Fig. 61.4).

SELECTION OF PATIENTS FOR PITUITARY DESTRUCTION

It will be clear from the foregoing that pituitary destruction is probably better reserved for persistent pain associated with malignancies. It would now seem utterly reasonable to include all carcinomatoses. We would still preferentially use cordotomy if the pain is suitably lateralized, reserving pituitary destruction for bilateral pains or pain in the head or neck region.

If one is also seeking tumour regression, as with carcinoma from the breast or prostate, then there is a wealth of opinion to encourage pituitary destruction if there has already been a response to hormonal manipulation, either medical or surgical (Thompson et al 1974; Tindall et al 1977, 1979).

Oestrogen receptor estimation, in the case of carcinoma of the breast, is said to have proved useful in predicting a response from endocrine manipulation other than by hypophysectomy (Leung et al 1973). McGuire (1978) considers oestrogen receptor assessment as of uncertain value in the prediction of response to pituitary destruction.

McCalister et al (1961) attempted a careful assessment of factors influencing the response of advanced cancer to hypophysectomy and included pain relief as evidence of objective remission, but unfortunately it is not possible to extract from the report how much remission was that of pain relief and how much was that of tumour mass shrinkage. The conclusions were that slightly more evidence of remission occured when there were bony mestastases; that premenopausal patients did better than postmenopausal patients, and that early hypophysectomy

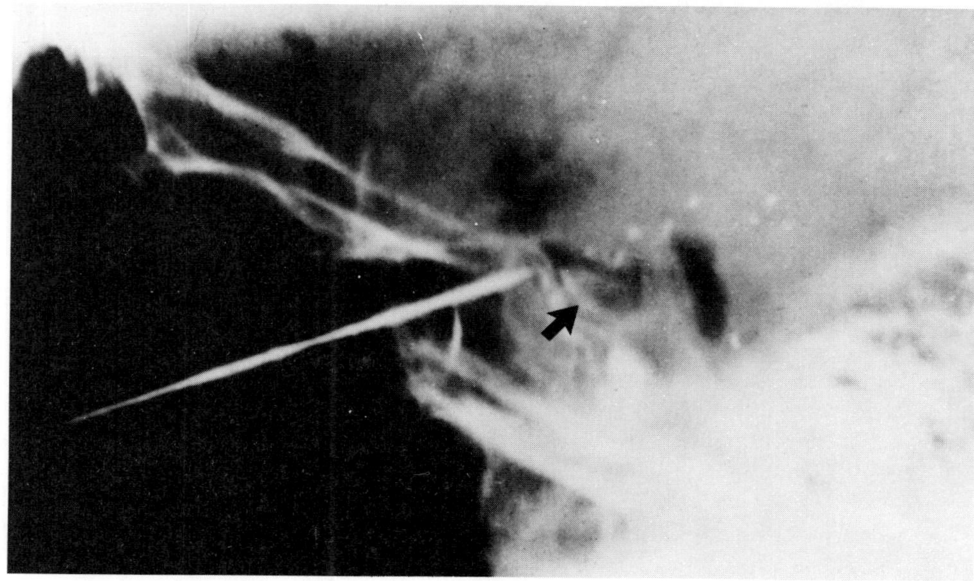

Fig. 61.4 Haemostatic tissue soaked in iodophylate and packed into pituitary fossa with successfully stopped cerebrospinal fluid rhinorrhoea.

appeared to be associated with a better response than late hypophysectomy. Their series did not appear to confirm the predictive value of previous endocrine manipulation, but in 1961 the potential for medical manipulation would have been rather limited.

The freer and more rational use of morphia, particularly in its long-acting form, and also its more direct application to the spinal subarachnoid space or the ventricle by the use of delivery pumps, has radically reduced the need to resort to pituitary destruction.

THE MODE OF ACTION

ENDOCRINE EFFECT

When pituitary destruction was used to suppress tumour, it was naturally expected that the relief of pain would result from reduction in tumour tissue. Such pain relief undoubtedly occurs and was described with endocrine ablative techniques other than those applied to the pituitary (Beatson 1896).

However, it is with pituitary destruction that the disparity between the occurrence and the degree of pain relief and tumour regression was clearly seen and mentioned (Schwartz et al 1981). This led to quite a hot debate concerning the certainty with which total anterior pituitary suppression should be sought (Edelstyn et al 1965; Norrell et al 1970; Brodkey et al 1978; La Rossa et al 1979). This debate concerns not only the discrepancy between pain relief and subsequent hypopituitarism, but also tumour regression and hypopituitarism. Attempts have been made to associate pain relief with particular forms of anterior hypopituitarism, but such claims have not been substantiated. Using the less certain techniques, such as alcohol injection, there has understandably been even greater doubt as to these correlations. Takeda et al (1978) considered that it was necessary to aim for major anterior pituitary dysfunction in order to get lasting pain relief, while we did not (Williams et al 1980). Deshpandi et al (1981) studied cases who had all obtained long-lasting pain relief, and they found normal adrenocorticotrophin function and only relatively minor reductions in the basal levels of thyroid-stimulating hormone and responsiveness to thyrotrophin-releasing hormone.

Takeda et al (1978) considered that diabetes insipidus, as indicated by polyuria, seemed to be associated with more than twice the amount of persisting relief from pain that was found in those without polyuria. All groups have shown at least relative preservation of adrenocorticotrophic hormone (ACTH) function following alcohol injection.

Since the discovery that beta endorphin occured in high concentration in the anterior pituitary gland, attempts have been made to correlate the pain relief resulting from destruction of the pituitary with the endorphin concentration in body fluids. Deshpandi et al (1981) found elevation in serum beta endorphin, beta lipotrophin and ACTH approximately 2 weeks after alcohol injection in four patients, but the levels were still within the normal range. Takeda et al (1978) found an abrupt increase in alpha endorphin in both CSF and serum 1 hour after injection in a single patient with a CSF shunt system in situ. The elevation of this substance and that of ACTH, which had also occured, returned to zero within 24 hours. In four other cases delayed postinjection estimations of alpha endorphin and ACTH in serum and CSF showed no significant change.

Our own studies on cervical CSF immediately after pituitary destruction (using radiofrequency coagulation) have shown a slight but extremely erratic increase in beta endorphin when pain relief has occurred. The increases ranged from minimal to more than 1000 fmol/ml, while the baseline levels ranged from below detection (less than 10) to 385 fmol/ml.

Takeda et al (1978) reported that naloxone had no pain-precipitating effect when given after alcohol injection. A minority (three out of nine) of our cases subjected to naloxone testing after alcohol injection into the pituitary fossa suffered recurrence of this pain (Bowsher 1978). In one case this recurrence occurred after 20 minutes, in an apparently agonizing form and in the same region as the original pain, and required morphine to suppress it. It had cleared 40 minutes after the original naloxone injection and 15 minutes after the morphine injection and did not return again for the remaining 3 months of the patient's life. A small amount of experimental animal work continues correlating the pituitary gland and neuropeptide with pain and analgesia (Przewlocki et al 1982).

Millan et al (1986) suggest a positive correlation between anterior pituitary concentrations of various neuropeptides and painful arthropathy in rats. Hargreaves et al (1990) describe an increase in the threshold of the paw-lick test when b-endorphin release from the pituitary was stimulated by corticotrophin-release factor.

Extrapolation to the human circumstance should be made cautiously, but Hargreaves et al (1987) also reported that suppressing b-endorphin release by intravenous dexamethazone was associated with an increase in pain in dental patients. The finding that the significant increase in pain appeared only with the lowest dose of dexamethazone (0.1 mg), although 0.32 mg and 1 mg also suppressed bendophin, is disquieting.

NEUROGENIC EFFECT

When hypophysectomy by the transcranial approach was occasionally noted to give rise to pain relief immediately on recovery of the patient from the anaesthetic, it was suggested that injury to the pituitary stalk or hypothalamus might have resulted from the brain retraction necessary to gain exposure and that this was responsible for the immediate effect. When the same phenomenon was noted after transsphenoidal hypophysectomy, the original explanation was clearly untenable.

Injection of alcohol into the pituitary fossa was initially carried out without general anaesthetic and this phenomenon of early relief of pain, again occurring in a minority of cases, was noted within minutes of the injections. Although the majority of pain relief tended to develop gradually, over perhaps 48 hours, this immediatė phenomenon suggested the possibility of a neurogenic mediation. This hypothesis was further supported by observations emanating from the practice of injecting radiocontrast along the cannula immediately before the alcohol. We noted that, in more than 20% of patients, radiocontrast could be seen rapidly ascending the pituitary stalk into the

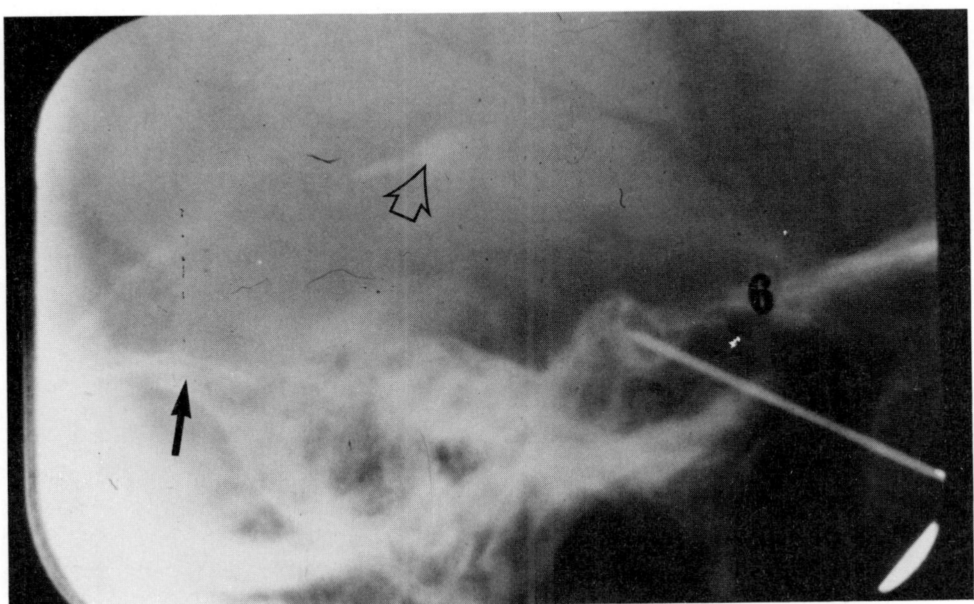

Fig. 61.5 Water-soluble radiocontrast within the pituitary fossa and third ventricle (outlined arrow) and also in the venous sinuses (solid arrow).

hypothalamic region and breaking through into the third ventricle (Fig. 61.3). We were initially uncertain as to why this should occur, but now realise that it is a tendency that relates to injecting into the anterior lobe, rather than into the subarachnoid space surrounding the gland. It therefore seemed logical to assume that hypothalamic injury was occurring. It is well known that the hypothalamus is involved in the suffering of pain states and that ablative procedures on the hypothalamus have proved useful in relieving pain in humans (Sano et al 1966) and in animals (Millan et al 1980a). A study was therefore undertaken in an attempt to correlate the radiographic and histological evidence of spread of the injected fluid from the pituitary fossa (Miles & Lipton 1976).

In 15 cadavers a technique of injecting into the pituitary fossa was undertaken which was identical to that used in clinical practice. The injecting fluid however consisted of equal parts of radiocontrast, of either the water-soluble or the insoluble type, together with a suspension of Indian ink. Under radiographic control the puncture was made before the head was opened. The injection was made at the same rate as in patients, using increments of 0.1 ml. Radiographic screening and still radiography revealed a higher incidence of spread to the hypothalamus, but also revealed that there was extensive spread outward from the pituitary gland into the draining basal venous sinuses (Fig. 61.5). This was recognised in the cadaver, presumably because of the absence of flow in the veins, while in the clinical situation the radiocontrast would have been quickly dispersed in the active venous flow.

After completing the injection the skull was opened and the brain removed with the pituitary gland attached and intact. The brain was immediately suspended in and fixed by formalin solution. After 2 weeks an accurate sagittal section was made and a careful note made of the macroscopic evidence of the Indian ink staining. A routine pattern of sectioning was undertaken involving the pituitary gland, the stalk and the hypothalamus (Fig. 61.6).

In all cases the anterior lobe of the pituitary gland was heavily impregnated with Indian ink particles. Towards the posterior part of the anterior lobe the particles were concentrated within the draining sinusoids.

In the pituitary stalk the particles were almost entirely within the portal venous system (Fig. 61.7) and the same could be recognised in the hypothalamus adjacent to the pituitary stalk. Indian ink-impregnated clefts were recognised in the hypothalamus posterior to the pituitary stalk as far back as the mammillary bodies (Fig. 61.8) and Indian ink particles were frequently seen on the ependymal epithelium. As a result of this study, it seemed likely that hypothalamic injury was occurring as a result of injection of alcohol into the pituitary gland.

We had autopsy evidence that this was happening in the clinical experience (Fig. 61.9). This evidence was naturally positively weighted, in that our autopsy material came from those patients succumbing quickly after pituitary alcohol injection, that is, while still in hospital with us.

Takeda et al (1978) also described hypothalamic injury in some 6% of their cases, but tended to deny its significance. The next important correlation necessary was that between clinical pain relief and clinical evidence of spread of radiocontrast during injection. Woo et al (unpublished observations) have now collected 75 cases in

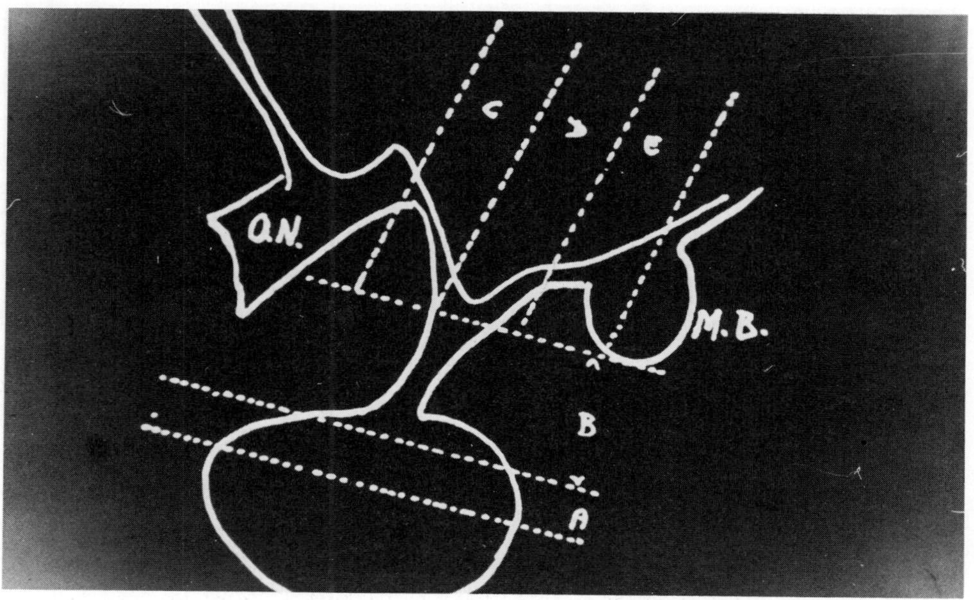

Fig. 61.6 Diagrammatic pattern of sectioning pituitary gland and hypothalamus after injection of radiocontrast and Indian ink mixture.

which there is unequivocal record of the spread of radiocontrast and for which we have accurate details as to the degree of pain relief and its duration, the patient's age and sex and diagnosis of malignancy. The spread of contrast has been recorded within the sella subarachnoid space, within the pituitary gland, in the pituitary stalk, in the hypothalamus and in the ventricular system. No correlation has been observed between any single position of radiocontrast or combination of positions with the quality of pain relief. Neither has there been any correlation between the tumour diagnosis and the occurrence of pain relief. Age and sex, similarly, do not seem to influence the prognosis.

Takeda et al (1978) appear not to have seen any spread of radiocontrast into the stalk or into the hypothalamus. Likewise Katz & Levin (1977) do not consider this to be frequent. Madrid (1979) sees this spread as commonly as we do and Morrica (1977) noted the same phenomenon.

We remain convinced that alcohol is likely to spread up into the hypothalamus and to give rise to injury there. We

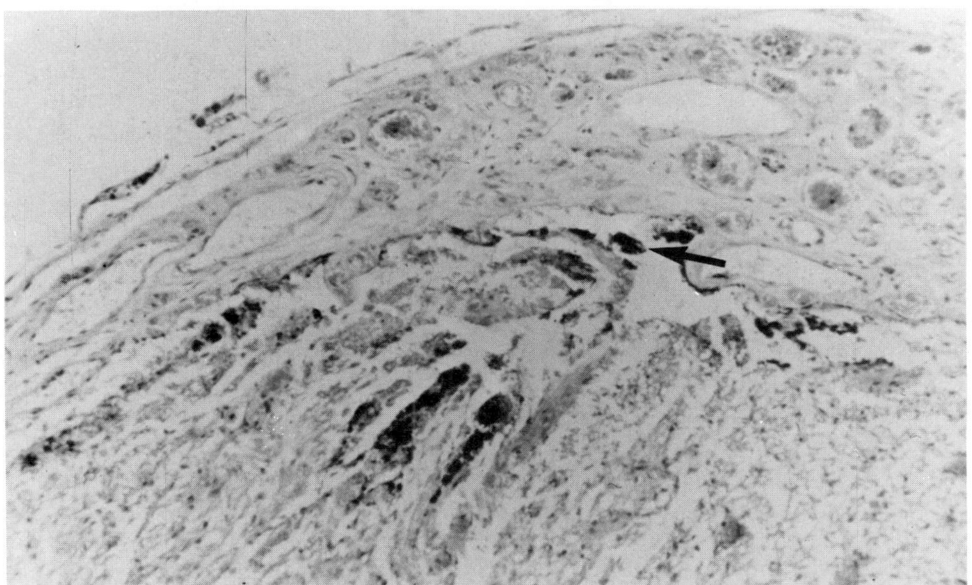

Fig. 61.7 Transverse section of pituitary stalk showing Indian ink particles in portal veins (arrow). Pars tuberalis in the upper part of the picture.

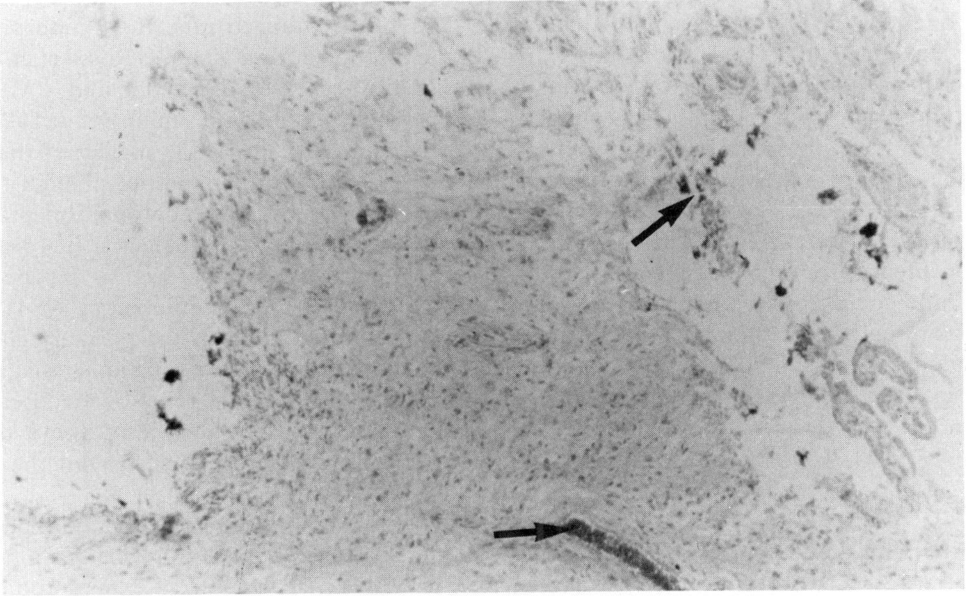

Fig. 61.8 Section of hypothalamus disrupted by clefts containing Indian ink particles (arrows).

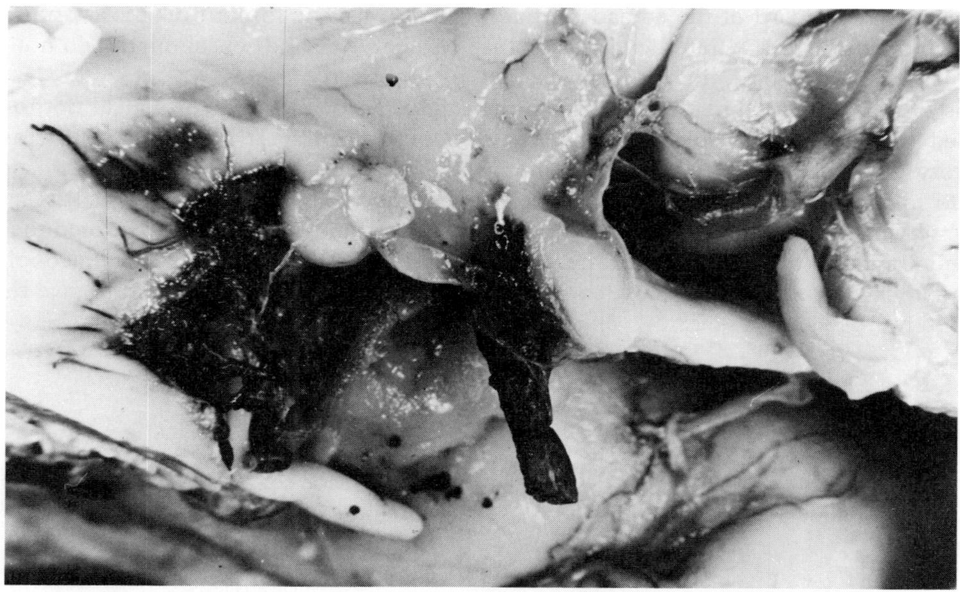

Fig. 61.9 Sagittal screening through hypothalamus of patient dying 36 hours after alcohol injection, showing massive infarction of pituitary stalk extending up into the anterior hypothalamus.

believe that we have autopsy evidence of the same and also experimental evidence in the cadaver. We can find no correlation between apparent spread and quality or incidence of pain relief.

PSYCHOSURGICAL EFFECT

As an extrapolation of the former impression of hypothalamic injury it seemed possible that some kind of frontothalamic leucotomy might be occurring and that a resulting change in the affect or behaviour of the patient might be responsible for the relief from pain. Most groups have noticed infrequent evidence of behavioural change towards euphoria (Takeda et al 1978). In our series this occurred in only around 1% of cases; even then the degree of inappropriate humour was only mild (Lipton et al 1978). In the group under consideration, namely those with advanced malignancy, the more usual psychometric methods involving questionnaires tend to be rather inap propriate. It seems likely that, in order to establish a change in mood or affect, pre- and postinjection studies would have to include social management in the home. Again this is an extremely difficult area to investigate, given the group under study. It would seem likely that in a small minority of cases there is evidence of a minor degree of modification of affect.

STRESS ANALGESIC EFFECT

Stories of apparently painfree heroism in people severely injured during warfare or catastrophe are well known. Observations of animals in similar states are readily recognized. Study of experimental stress on animals reveals unequivocal analgesia (Amir & Amit 1978) which is suppressed by hypophysectomy (Gispen et al 1970; Haybach et al 1978; Millan et al 1980). It is partially reversed by naloxone (Chester et al 1977; Bodnar et al 1978) but not affected by dexamethasone or Metapyrone (Millan et al 1980), though ACTH and beta endorphin are secreted concomitantly by the pituitary gland (Guillemin et al 1977). Contrary findings have been reported during swimming-stress analgesia (Liu 1987) and pregnancy-stress analgesia (Baron & Gintzler 1987), recording no significant difference between intact and hypophysectomized rats. Beta endorphin is released into the blood during stress (Rossier et al 1977) and its significance has been debated (Millan et al 1980; Przewlocki et al 1980; Kulling et al 1988).

Millan et al, in 1983, suggested that something other than beta endorphin is responsible for the stress analgesia, but evidence for specific neuropeptide release during pituitary destructive analgesia (in part discussed previously in this chapter) has so far been found wanting (Capper et al 1984; Conlon et al 1984).

On the logic that, if the pituitary gland were involved, through stress, in producing analgesia, attempts have been made to achieve pain relief by electrically stimulating the gland and in the short term (days or weeks) this has proved as satisfactory as destroying the gland (Yanagida et al 1984).

With present techniques it is difficult to justify stimulating the pituitary gland when a long-term application method is not available. We have studied CSF concentrations of beta endorphin, beta lipotrophin, Met and Leu enkephalin, somatostatin and substance P in the CSF of three anaesthetised patients during electrical stimulation of the gland prior to coagulation and observed no significant changes. Again this does not imply that there are not profound tissue changes of these neuropeptides.

If stress analgesia is the explanation for pain relief after interference of the pituitary gland, it is difficult to explain a system that allows it to occur in the intact animal under stress and yet sees it effective for varying periods after destruction of the pituitary gland, and again sees it operative for brief periods after pituitary stimulation. It does offer continuing prospect, perhaps through telemetric destruction or stimulation, and it is scientifically rather disappointing that there has been little recent progress or even apparent research interest.

SUMMARY AND CONCLUSIONS

Destruction of the pituitary gland by any of the methods described, in patients with pain due to malignancy, is associated with relief of that pain in more than 70% of cases (Table 61.1). When the malignancy is from the breast or prostate, pain relief can be associated with evidence of regression of the tumour. Pain relief can occur immediately on pituitary destruction. The duration of pain relief varies greatly and while, in the majority of cases, the pain returns within 3 months, it is possible for the relief to last for more than 1 year.

Pituitary destruction also relieves pain associated with carcinomatosis other than that from the breast and prostate. In the series quoted the incidence of relief is equal to that found with carcinoma of the breast and prostate. There is no substantial evidence of regression of these tumours. There is still debate as to whether major suppression of pituitary hormonal function (as currently determined) correlates with better or more persistent pain relief.

Although hypothalamic injury would appear to occur in association with alcohol injection into the pituitary fossa, it is very unlikely to occur with some of the other techniques and does not seem to correlate with the degree of pain relief.

There is little evidence for correlating pain relief with neuropeptides released into the CSF following destruction or electrical stimulation of the pituitary gland; however, it is probably simplistic to assume that such changes would be found. Changes in neuropeptide concentration within the tissue may still be occurring.

Destruction of the pituitary has proved a useful method of relieving the otherwise persisting pain associated with malignancy, with stereoradiosurgery and radiofrequency coagulation carrying the lowest risk. There would appear to be every justification for continuing studies of electrical stimulation of the gland or of its neural connections, and of the telemetric equipment that would be necessary chronically to achieve this.

REFERENCES

Amir S, Amit Z 1978 Endogenous opiate ligands may mediate stress-induced changes in the affects of pain related behaviour in rats. Life Sciences 18: 1143–1152

Asimov I 1972 In: Biographical encyclopaedia of science and technology. Pan Books, London

Baron S A, Gintzler A R 1987 Effects of hypophysectomy and dexamethasone treatment on plasma b-endorphin and pain threshold in pregnancy. Brain Research 418: 138–145

Beatson G T 1896 On the treatment of inoperable cases of cancer of the mamma. Suggestions for a new method of treatment with illustrative cases. Lancet ii: 104–106, 162–165

Bleasel K 1965 Cryogenic hypophysectomy. Medical Journal of Australia 2: 148–156

Bodnar R J, Kelly D D, Spaggia A, Errenberg C, Glusman M 1978 Dose dependent reduction by naloxone induced by cold water stress. Pharmacology, Biochemistry and Behaviour 8: 667–672

Bowsher D 1978 Naloxone after surgical procedures to relieve pain. Unpublished material presented at the Second World Congress of the International Association for the Study of Pain, Montreal, Canada, August 27–September 1

Brodkey J S, Pearson O H, Mann A 1978 Hypophysectomy for relief of bone pain in breast cancer (letters). New England Journal of Medicine 299: 1016

Capper S, Morley J B, Miles J B 1984 New methodology in raising antibodies to small peptides leading to highly specific radio immunoassay for encephalus. Neuropeptide 4: 447–482

Carbonin G 1978 Hypophysectomy and pain relief in cancer (letter). Journal of Neurosurgery 48: 666

Chester G B, Chan B 1977 Footshock induced analgesia; its reversal by naloxone and cross tolerance with morphine. Life Sciences 21: 1569–1574

Conlon J M, Laherta J, Lipton S, Miles J B 1984 Changes in the concentration of somatostatin and substance P in the CSF following injection of alcohol into the pituitary gland. Neuropeptides 4: 227–236

Cushing H 1914 Surgical experiences with pituitary disorders. Journal of the American Medical Association 63: 1515–1525

Deshpandi N, Morrica G, Saullo F, Di Martino L, Kwa G 1981 Some aspects of pituitary function after neuroadenolysis in patients with metastatic cancer. Tumori 67: 355–359

Donegan W L 1967 Endocrine ablation, hormone therapy and chemotherapy. In: Spratt, Donegan W L (eds) Cancer of the breast. W B Saunders, Philadelphia, p 201–244

Edelstyn G, Gleadhill C, Lyons A 1965 A rational approach to hypophysectomy. British Journal of Surgery 52: 953–957

Ehni G, Eckles N E 1959 Interruption of the pituitary stalk in the patients with mammary cancer. Journal of Neurosurgery 16: 628–652

Forrest A P M, Blair D W, Pebles Brown A D et al 1959 Radioactive implantation of the pituitary. British Journal of Surgery 47: 61–70

Gispen W H, Van Wimersima-Greidanus T B, de Weid D 1970 Effects of hypophysectomy and ACTH and responsiveness to electric shock in rats. Physiological Behaviour 5: 143–146

Greco T, Sbaragli F, Cammili L 1957 L'alcoolizazione della ipofisi per via transfenoidale nella terapia di particolari tumori maligni. Settimana Medicale 45: 355–356

Guillemin R T, Vargo T, Rossier J et al Beta endorphin and adrenocorticotrophin are secreted concomitantly by the pituitary gland. Science 197: 1367–1369

Hardy J 1971 Transphenoidal hypophysectomy. Journal of Neurosurgery 34: 582–594

Hargreaves K M, Schmidt E A, Mueller G P, Dionne R A 1987 Dexamethasone alters plasma levels of b-endorphin and postoperative pain. Clinical Pharmacological Therapy 42: 601–607
Hargreaves K M, Flores C M, Dionne R A, Mueller G P 1990 The role of pituitary b-endorphin in mediating corticotrophin-releasing factor-induced antinociception. American Journal of Physiology 258: 235–242
Haybach J P, Vernikos J, Danielli S 1978 The effect of pituitary–adrenal function in the modulation of pain sensitivity in the rat. Journal of Physiology 283: 331–340
Huggins C, Bergenstahl D M 1952 Inhibition of mammary and prostatic cancers by adenalectomy. Cancer Research 12: 131–141
Huggins C, Hodges C V 1941 Studies on prostatic cancer. Cancer Research 1: 293–297
Katz J, Levin A B 1977 Treatment of diffuse metastatic cancer pain by instillation of alcohol into the sella turcica. Anesthesiology 46: 115–121
Kulling P, Frishknecht H R, Pasi A, Waser P G, Siegfried B 1988 Social conflict-induced changes in nociception and b-endorphin-like immunoreactivity in pituitary and discrete brain areas of C57BL/6 and DBA/2 mice. Brain Research 450: 237–246
La Rossa J T, Strong M S, Melby J C 1978 Endocrinologically incomplete transethmoidal transphenoidal hypophysectomy with relief of bone pain in breast cancer. New England Journal of Medicine 298: 1332–1335
Leung B S, Fletcher W S, Krippaehne W 1973 Oestrogen receptor, a valid test for selection of breast cancer patients for endocrine ablation. Surgical Forum 24: 125–127
Lipton S, Miles J B, Williams N, Bark-Jones N 1978 Pituitary injections of alcohol for widespread cancer pain. Pain 5: 73–81
Lui H M 1986 The effect of swimming stress on tail-flick latency of normal and hypophysectomised rats. Clinical Journal of Physiology 29: 65–69
Luft R, Olivercrona H 1953 Experiences with hypophysectomy. Journal of Neurosurgery 10: 301–316
McCalister A, Wellbourn R B, Edelstyn G J A et al 1961 Factors influencing response to hypophysectomy for advanced cancer of the breast. British Medical Journal i: 613–617
McGuire W L 1978 Hormone receptors: their role in predicting progress and response to endocrine therapy. Seminars in Oncology 5: 428–433
Madrid J 1979 Chemical hypophysectomy. In: Bonica J J, Ventafridda V (eds) Advances in pain research and therapy, vol 2. Raven Press, New York, p 381–391
Miles J B, Lipton S 1976 Mode of action by which pituitary alcohol injection relieves pain. In: Bonica J J, Albe-Fessard D (eds) Advances in pain research and therapy, vol 1. Raven Press, New York, p 867–869
Millan M J Gramsch C, Przewlocki R, Hollt V, Herz A 1980a Lesions of the hypothalamic arcuate nucleus produce a temporary hyperalgesia and attenuate stress evoked analgesia. Life Sciences 27: 1513–1523
Millan M J, Przewlocki R, Herz A 1980b A non beta-endorphinergic adenohypophyseal mechanism is essential for an analgetic response to stress. Pain 8: 343–353
Millan M J, Przewlocki R, Millan M H, Herz A 1983 Evidence for ventral–medial posterior hypothalamus in nociceptive processes in rat. Pharmacology, Biochemistry and Behaviour 18: 901–907
Millan M J, Millan M H, Czlonkowshi A et al 1986 A model of chronic pain in the rat: response of multiple opioid systems to adjuvant induced arthritis. Journal of Neurosciences 6: 899–906
Morrica G 1974 Chemical hypophysectomy for cancer pain. In: Bonica J J (ed) Advances in neurology, vol 4. Raven Press, New York, p 707–714
Morrica G 1977 Pituitary neuroadenolysis. In: Lipton S (ed) Persistent pain, vol 1. Academic Press, London
Norrell H, Alvars A M, Winternitz W W 1970 A clinicopathologic analysis in cryohypophysectomy in patients with advanced cancer. Cancer 25: 1050–1060
Przsewlocki R, Millan M J, Herz A 1980 Is beta-endorphin involved in the analgesia generated by stress? In: Way E L (ed) Endogenous and exogenous opiate agonists and antagonists. Pergamon Press, New York, p 391–394
Przsewlocki R, Millan M J, Gramsch C H, Millan M H, Herz A 1982 The influence of selective adeno- and neuro–intermedio hypophysectomy upon plasma and brain levels of β-endorphin and their response to stress in rats. Brain Research 242: 1–11
Ray B S 1960 Neurosurgeons' interest in pituitary. Journal of Neurosurgery 17: 1–21
Rossier J, French E D, Rivier C, Ling N, Guillemin R, Bloom F E 1977 Footshock induced stress increases beta-endorphin levels in blood but not brain. Nature 270: 618–620
Sano K, Yoshioka M, Ogashiwa M, Ishijima B, Ohye C 1966 Thalamolaminectomy. A new operation for relief of intractable pain. Confinia Neurologica 27: 63–66
Schloffer H 1907 Erfolgreiche Operation eines Hypophysentumours auf nasalem Wege. Wiener Klinischer Wochenschrift 20: 621–624
Schwartz M, Tindall G T, Nixon D W 1981 Transphenoidal hypophysectomy in disseminated breast cancer. Southern Medical Journal 73: 315–317
Takeda F, Fuji T, Tozawa R, Kitani Y, Fujita T 1978 Endocrinological aspect of transphenoidal adenohypophyseal neurolysis for cancer pain. In: Abstracts, Second World Congress of the International Association for the Study of Pain, Montreal, Canada, August 27-September 1, p 145
Thompson J B, Greenberg L S, Pazianos A, Pearson O H 1974 Hypophysectomy in metastatic prostate cancer. New York State Journal of Medicine 74: 1006–1008
Tindall G T, Nixon D W, Christy J H, Neil J D 1977 Pain relief in metastatic cancer other than breast and prostate gland following transphenoidal hypophysectomy. Journal of Neurosurgery 50: 275–282
Tindall G T, Nixon D W, Christy J H, Neill J D 1979 Transphenoidal hypophysectomy. Journal of Neurosurgery 47: 659–662
West C R, Avellanosa A M, Bremer A M, Yamado K 1979 Hypophysectomy for disseminated carcinoma of the prostate. In: Bonica J J, Ventafridda V (eds) Advances in pain research and therapy, vol 2. Raven Press, New York, p 393–400
Williams N E, Miles J B, Lipton S, Hipkin L, Davis J C 1980 Pain relief and pituitary function following injection of alcohol into the pituitary fossa. Annals of the Royal College of Surgeons of England 62: 203–207
Wilson C B, Frewer D 1971 The role of neurosurgery in the management of patients with cancer of the breast. Cancer 28: 1681–1685
Yanagida H, Corssen G, Trouwborst A, Erdmann 1984 Relief of cancer pain in man; alcohol induced neuroadenolysis vs. electrical stimulation of the pituitary gland. Pain 19: 133–142
Zervas N 1969 Stereotactic, radiofrequency surgery of the normal and the abnormal pituitary gland. New England Journal of Medicine 280: 429–437

62. Limbic surgery for pain

A. J. Bouckoms

INTRODUCTION

This chapter reviews ablative limbic and frontal neurosurgery for the relief of chronic intractable pain. This kind of surgery has been called psychosurgery, in order to distinguish it from surgical interruption of the afferent spinothalamic tracts, brain stem neurosurgery, and pituitary ablation. Limbic surgery is the more appropriate term, since limbic-frontal structures are the targets, not the mind. Cingulotomy and anterior capsulotomy are the two currently reported operations that lesion limbic-frontal structures for the relief of pain, depression and anxiety. Cingulotomy has been studied specifically for pain treatment. In 1977, when the US National Commission for the Protection of Human Subjects of Biomedical and Behavioral Research published the results of a 10-year study of psychosurgery, their definition was:

> Psychosurgery means brain surgery on normal or diseased brain tissue of an individual, if the sole object of the perfomance of such surgery is to control, change, or effect any behavioral or emotional disturbance of such individual. Psychosurgery includes the implantation of electrodes, destruction or direct stimulation of brain tissue by any means (e.g. ultrasound, laser beams), and the direct application of substances to the brain, when the primary purpose of such intervention is to change or control behavior or emotions.

Limbic surgery directed at pain, not 'change of behaviour or emotions' is not psychosurgery by the definition of the National Commission. Accordingly, the Cingulotomy report of the US Department of Health and Human Services mentioned pain only briefly (Carter & Marshall 1985). The Commission's specification, that surgery or other invasions of the brain that interrupt the transmission of pain signals along sensory pathways should not be considered to be psychosurgery, is not pure sophistry. Indeed, this distinction between pain and behaviour begs two questions that will determine the future of frontal-limbic neurosurgery for pain.

Can chronic pain be shown to have a central nervous system pathophysiology that might be treated with brain surgery? Gybels & Sweet (1989) answer this question with an encyclopaedic update of the neurosurgery and clinical pathophysiology of persistent pain as they review bulbar and pontine tractotomy, mesencephalotomy, thalamotomy, hypothalamotomy, gyrectomy, pituitary and telencephalic surgery for pain. This erudite treatise describes the critical problems of pain as a disease unto itself, with a central nervous system pathophysiology.

Are there psychiatric diseases associated with suffering and pain that are treatable by frontal-limbic neurosurgery? The fact that primary psychiatric illnesses, namely, depression and obsessive anxiety disorders, have become the major indications for limbic psychosurgery in the United States and Europe in the last 5 years answers this question affirmatively (Mindus 1991). This 3rd edition of the Textbook of Pain will describe the advances that have been made in the last 5 years concerning the limbic-frontal dysfunction that justify modern selective neuroablative procedures on the brain for pain and suffering.

HISTORY

Neurological surgery developed rapidly at the turn of the 20th century because of the serendipitous confluence of new theoretical knowledge and technical advances. Between 1885 and 1927, Walter Dandy discovered the technique of ventriculography, Egas Moniz discovered cerebral angiography and Wagner Juaregg won the Nobel prize for his biological treatment of psychiatric illness – namely, the use of malaria to treat neurosyphilis. Walter Freeman, the father of psychosurgery, was born in 1885 (Shutts 1982).

During the 1930s the central nervous system was still being functionally defined, and Adolph Meyer, the father of psychobiological psychiatry, founded the American Psychiatric Association in an attempt to bridge the gap between psychotherapy-performing psychiatrists and anatomically oriented neurologists. One such bridge was the Second International Neurological Congress in London in 1935, which was attended by Moniz, Freeman, Penfield, Fulton and Jacobsen. At the Congress, Fulton and Jacobsen reported on the resistance of two monkeys with frontal lobe lesions to 'experimental neurosis'. This was a form of behavioural distress induced by failure to reach a desired object in a laboratory test. Egas Moniz coupled these findings with his knowledge of angiographic anatomy and his belief that Pavlov's 'conditioning' was produced by aberrant neuronal connections, and hypothesized that sectioning connections between the cortex of the frontal lobe and thalamic nuclei might relieve psychic distress. Returning to Lisbon, he operated on 20 severely disturbed mental patients with 'good results ... a decreased intensity of emotional reaction to delusions or hallucinations' (Shutts 1982).

At about the same time, Freeman enlisted the help of neurosurgeon Watts, and on 14 September 1936 performed the first of many of his standard prefrontal leucotomy operations. Freeman noted that several patients who complained of unbearable pain as well as nervous symptoms stopped complaining of pain after leucotomy. As the patients returned for follow-up examination and were questioned about their previous symptoms, it was found that they admitted having had pain only when questioned. Their fearful attitude was gone, as if the residual pain were an emotionless sensation rather than a threat. In response to this finding, Freeman changed the title of the second edition of his textbook from 'Psychosurgery' to 'Psychosurgery in the treatment of mental disorders and intractable pain' (Freeman et al 1950).

In 1936, Dogliotti & Fiamberti performed the first transorbital approach to the frontal area in their search for improved approaches to ventriculography. In 1937, Papez proposed that the thalamus was not simply a rudimentary element located at the top of the brain stem, but formed part of the neuronal circuit involving the mamillary bodies, anterior thalamic nuclei, gyrus cingulatus and hippocampus. He stated that this circuit constituted a harmonious mechanism which may elaborate functions of the central emotion as well as participate in emotional expression. MacLean (1952) was to call this the limbic system. Freeman combined Moniz's earlier theory about frontal thalamic connections with Papez's notion of the limbic circuit and explained the indifference to pain of his postleucotomy patients as due to their inability to elaborate on emotional distress. This work laid the basis for the current thinking that recruitment of the limbic system is the key to the suffering of pain, which is what defines chronic intractable pain.

The indications, benefits and risks of psychosurgery needed more definition. An influx of emotionally disabled World War II veterans provided a large population for frontal ablative procedures. It was estimated, at the end of the 1940s, that approximately 5000 frontal ablative procedures per year were done in the United States. Vindication for such surgery seemed to be provided by Egas Moniz winning the Nobel prize in 1949 for 'his discovery of the therapeutic value of prefrontal leucotomy in certain psychoses'. However, the reckless and sometimes indiscriminant manner of performing frontal lobotomy raised a certain amount of ire. Freeman had performed lobotomies in his office, in a motel room, and often with the disapproval of his neurosurgical colleague Watts. It is estimated that Freeman personally performed over 3500 cases during his peak years of the late 1940s to early 1950s.

The ethics of medicine and behavioural change were further examined under the US Nuremberg code of medical ethics, a reaction to the indiscriminant experimentation on human subjects during World War II. In 1949 the first US research project on lobotomy patients, Columbia Greystone Project, found that although many of the chronic institutionalized 'schizophrenic' patients had clinically improved and been discharged from hospital, their relief of anxious suffering was proportional to the severity of their frontal lobe syndrome. There was a tenuous balance between the benefits of the surgery and further deterioration of the patient. It was not until 1952 when the Columbia Greystone Associates produced their second publication on psychosurgery that Poole endorsed psychosurgery and was the first prominent neurosurgeon to do so. Transorbital lesions with an ice-pick were the common procedure of the time. Meanwhile, despite his successes, Freeman was noting an 85% failure rate of lobotomy in patients who had auditory hallucinations and a 20% incidence of seizures. Concomitant with the discovery of chlorpromazine in 1954, there was a decline in lobotomies from approximately 5000 per year in the early 1950s to 300 per year in the early 1970s. As psychotropic drugs decreased the need for ablative procedures in the psychiatric population, interest increased in the use of central neurosurgery for the treatment of epilepsy, movement disorders, episodic violence and pain.

Pain complaints were common, but were never assiduously studied in leucotomy patients. Freeman spoke of pain relief, but never focused on pain in his frontal lobotomies. Other surgeons who continued selective pain ablative procedures such as Schwartz's medullary spinothalamic tractotomy (Schwartz & O'Leary 1941), were hampered by the technical difficulty of the operation and the high risk of complications and mortality. These specific 'pain' operations appeared to be significantly more dangerous and less effective than Freeman's ice-pick transorbital leucotomy. Modified procedures followed (Retif 1966). The results of 40 years' experience with modified leucotomy were reviewed by White & Sweet (1969) with the conclusion:

> Resort to frontal leucotomy should be recommended only for the hopeless victims of malignant disease and other non-fatal neuralgias when mental suffering, anxiety and depression are predominant factors. In this situation excellent results can be obtained and the patient remain a useful and acceptable

member of society. If pain alone is the predominant problem, relief is unlikely short of carrying the leucotomy to the state of severe dementia.

Modern stereotactic psychosurgery for pain began in 1947 when Spiegel & Wycis made a lesion in the dorsomedial nucleus of the thalamus and the midbrain spinothalamic tract. Successful results with low morbidity and mortality showed these techniques to be a major advance for temporary pain relief and decreased suffering. Theoretical interest in stereotactic approaches to the limbic system continued, and in 1948 Fulton performed the first cingulate lesion in the monkey. The first human cingulotomy followed in 1952. Spiegel & Wycis (1962) added stereotactically placed lesions of the reticular formation to their previous spinothalamic lesions, and noted considerable efficacy for the control of pain. They routinely stimulated the brain before making a lesion, could make a more accurate lesion than with the ice-pick leucotomy and noticed a very low incidence of painful dysaesthesias.

The new era of modern ablative procedures began in the 1960s with a 50% good or excellent relief rate from stereotactic thalamotomy for the relief of cancer pain (Sweet 1980). Since then lesions have been successfully placed in the cingulum, inferoposteromedial or subcaudate (preinnominate) frontal white matter, medial thalamus, internal medullary lamina of the thalamus, pulvinar, amygdala, frontothalamic tracts, pituitary, hypothalamus and its periventricular nuclei (Gybels 1989). Lesions of these sites appear effective in controlling chronic pain, yet are ineffective for acute pain. The immediate results are reduction in narcotic requirements, a more placid appearance and less preoccupation with pain (Sweet 1980).

INDICATIONS

A decision to treat pain and suffering with frontal-limbic surgery requires specific indications for the surgery and information about alternative treatments. Consideration of a frontal-limbic procedure for pain control often occurs in the context of failed deafferentation, ongoing neuropathic pain, tolerance/addiction to narcotics and upper body pain that limits spinal options. Frontal leucotomy is no answer; although it is not a deafferenting procedure, it does not relieve deafferentation pain. The propensity for pain to 'run in front of the knife' with peripheral ablative procedures suggests the use of more selective central nervous system interventions, such as cingulotomy, before other extensive neurolytic procedures have been tried, depression has supervened, or the person has become addicted to narcotics.

Consideration of a cingulotomy for pain should weigh the following six alternatives. First, that spinal deafferentation surgery such as percutaneous cordotomy or midline myelotomy can carry a significant risk of dyaesthesias that are very difficult to treat. Second, pain in the upper body, head, neck or face cannot be safely treated with spinal procedures because of respiratory and motor compromise. Third, high level lesions such as mesencephalotomy or pontine tractotomy have brief efficacy (a few weeks), significant mortality (10–15%) and produce dysaesthesias, oculomotor disorders (80%) and reticular dysfunction leading to confusion. Deafferentation pain may even be exacerbated (Siegfried 1984). Fourth, intrathecal or intraventricular morphine is more suitable for terminal patients given the problems of tolerance, monitoring and follow-up. Fifth, patients who have already had deafferentation procedures or narcotics may benefit from cingulotomy, where nothing else is known to work. Sixth, chronic stimulation of deep brain structures is complex, expensive and unavailable.

If these six issues are considered to exclude spinal, brain stem, stimulation and narcotic therapies then specific indications for cingulotomy should then be considered.

Severe anxiety has been the prime indication for psychosurgery (Scoville 1949; Lehmann & Ostrow 1973; Martin-Rodriguez 1977; Jenike 1991). Depression is also especially amenable to psychosurgery; it was the symptom with the greatest change in those with a favourable outcome (Mirsky & Orzack 1976). The Health Care Technology Assessment Report (1985) quotes Teuber et al (1977a, 1977b), stating that the results of limbic surgery have been generally optimistic, with highest rates of favourable results among subjects with chronic pain or depression. The American Association of Neurological Surgeons in a joint statement with the Congress of Neurological Surgeons has endorsed the performance of lesions in the inferior frontal or cingulate regions, with particular reference to chronic pain where there has been drug failure and the patient remains totally disabled. Lehmann notes that persons should have had a 2-year plus history of chronic anxiety, depression and a good premorbid personality. Psychological tests have proven 'very disappointing' as indicators of good response (Lehmann & Ostrow 1973). Denial of affect carries a worse prognosis, in that high deniers require more extensive leucotomies for relief of their pain and hence have more psychological deterioration (White & Sweet 1969). A literature survey was conducted by Valenstein (1977) at the request of the National Commission for the Protection of Human Subjects of Biomedical and Behavioural Research. He found that the patients most likely to improve with psychosurgery were those with 'severe disturbances of mood and emotion, e.g. the severely depressed, anxious and the obsessive–compulsive neurotic'. Pain specifically was not mentioned. Although there is unanimity that the symptoms of anxiety and depression predict good response to psychosurgery, the definitions of terms are not clear. State symptoms, traits, primary anxiety disorders, primary mood disorders, personality disorder and psychotic illness are not distinguished. Typical is

Hirose's (1977) study on 523 orbitoventromedial undercutting operations. He states that the premorbid personality is the most important prognostic indicator but then discusses psychotic and neurotic diagnoses. One infers he is really talking about anxious or depressive symptoms, not personality traits or diagnoses. Until Bouckoms' 1985 report on cingulotomy for pain, and then Ballantine's 1987 publication on the treatment of psychiatric illness by cingulotomy, there were no studies of psychosurgery where DSM-III or similar standard psychiatric diagnostic systems had been used. There were no studies differentiating indications for relief of pain versus the relief of psychiatric illness, and no prognostic indicators for the relief of various pain types such as somatic or deafferentation pain.

In response to these questions, this reviewer examined 22 patients with a primary psychiatric diagnosis, age-matched with 22 patients with a primary pain diagnosis, all of whom were treated with bilateral anterior cingulotomy (Bouckoms et al 1985). The purpose was to determine which pain types, psychiatric diagnoses and follow-up psychotropic medicines correlated with the best outcome. DSM-III (American Psychiatric Association 1980) diagnoses were used for the psychiatric diagnosis.

Pain types were divided into somatic and neuropathic, and the painful physical diagnosis defined. Of the 22 pain patients, 13 could be completely evaluated for an average follow-up of 11 months. The physical diagnoses were seven failed low-back syndromes, one spinal cord tumour, two stump amputation pain, one intractable abdominal pain and two deafferentation dysaesthesia. The concurrent primary psychiatric diagnoses were four major depression, four mixed personality disorders and five psychological factors affecting physical condition. In the primary psychiatric group, the psychiatric diagnoses were 20 with major affective disorder, seven with personality disorder and two with depressive symptoms. Pain patients had a different spectrum of affective disorders from the psychiatric patients. The main difference is that in the pain group, eight of the 22 people met DSM-III criteria for major affective disorder. In the psychiatric group, 20 of the 22 people had major affective disorder. The average status on a 1 (very sick) to 5 (very well) categorical scale of overall functioning was 2.1 at follow-up compared with 1 at the time of the initial evaluation. Typically, this degree of improvement meant that these patients did not complain of pain unless specifically asked, used nonnarcotic analgesics in moderation, pursued some normal activities of daily living and enjoyed an improved family life. There was no statistically significant correlation between the psychiatric diagnosis and status at follow-up. However, there was a trend for those with major depression without personality disorder to do better than those with personality disorders. Somatic and neuropathic pain types both responded well to cingulotomy. In particular, the two patients with amputation pain and two with deafferentation dysaesthesia had significant improvement.

Follow-up treatment after cingulotomy played an important part in the outcome. Five of the 13 pain patients had temporary relapses in their condition after they had stopped taking the antidepressant medication which is standard treatment after cingulotomy. When the medicine was reinstituted, the patients again resumed their improved mental status. Eight patients who maintained their antidepressant drug regimen over the course of the follow-up had no recurrence of their condition. Clonazepam was used in three patients as an anticonvulsant where it was required either for deafferentation pain or because of a previous history of seizures. These patients did well and tolerated the medicine well. The indications are that allodynia may be the indication for the use of clonazepam in this setting. The results of follow-up on these 13 patients suggest the following indications for optimal outcome from cingulotomy:

1. Patients with a primary pain diagnosis do as well after cingulotomy as those with a primary psychiatric diagnosis.
2. Personality disorder is a relative contraindication to cingulotomy.
3. The benefits from cingulotomy are sustained as long as antidepressant and/or anticonvulsant medicines are maintained.
4. Intractable somatic and neuropathic pain types respond equally well to cingulotomy.
5. The reports of electrical stimulation of the periaqueductal or periventricular areas producing poor results in deafferentation pain (Young et al 1984) suggest that cingulotomy may be the surgical treatment of choice for intractable deafferentation pain patients (Bouckoms et al 1985).

These general observations about what constitutes appropriate indications for limbic surgery can be summarized in Sweet's (1973) principal indication for limbic surgery as 'stereotypy of an excessive and futile emotional response to pain'. This succinct statement has now been operationalized into a detailed, precise list of particular indications and contraindications for the intractable pain patient.

SELECTION CRITERIA FOR LIMBIC SURGERY FOR INTRACTABLE PAIN

The following selection criteria have been used at Massachusetts General Hospital since 1987. They constitute the minimum criteria each patient must meet to be considered for limbic surgery for pain. The judgement of the referring physician, the treating neurosurgeon and consultant psychiatrist must agree on these points.

1. DIAGNOSIS

a. Pain. The patient has intractable severe pain with associated suffering. The patient rates the pain as greater than 4 over 10 at least half of the time. The duration of pain must be at least 12 weeks and the life expectancy of the patient at least 8 weeks.
b. Psychiatric diagnosis. The majority of patients will have a major psychiatric diagnosis of either major affective disorder or anxiety disorder (DSM-III/III-R criteria must be met). The absence of these two major categories of psychiatric diagnoses does not exclude the patient from limbic surgery for pain. Certain psychiatric diagnoses are exclusion criteria, as described in Section 6.
c. Disability. 'The patient must show significant disability during the 12 weeks or more that he or she has been in pain. Significant disability is defined on DSM-III Axis V as the highest level of adaptive functioning. Poor (5) to grossly impaired (7) constitutes significant disability.

2. INTRACTABILITY

The disorder must have been unsuccessfully treated by all of the following, with reasonable level of intensity or dosage and reasonable duration, pertinent to the patient's disorder.

a. Pharmacotherapy. Medications to treat the pain and suffering have either resulted in a lack of response, intolerance precluding a therapeutic treatment trial or severe side-effects that limit the quality of life. Medicine trials would typically have included oral/parenteral narcotics and psychotropic adjuvants such as antidepressants, stimulants, neuroleptics, antihistamines and nonsteroidal antiinflammatory drugs. Typically other medicines would also have been used either orally or parenterally or both. These medicines would include membrane-stabilizing drugs (xylocaine-like agents, neuroleptics, antidepressants), anticonvulsants (Klonopin, Tegretol, Dilantin) and GABA-agonist-like agents (benzodiazepines, baclofen).
b. Electrical stimulation with transcutaneous nerve stimulators or dorsal column stimulation has either not worked or is contraindicated.
c. The patient has not responded to or it is impractical to use focal deafferentation interventions (e.g. nerve blocks, intraspinal blocks, neurectomy, rhizotomy or cordotomy).
d. Psychotherapy, hypnosis, behavioural treatment, inpatient pain unit therapy and physical therapy are all potentially available to the patient, and are either not indicated or have been tried and failed.

3. INFORMED CONSENT

The patient must be informed as to the nature of the surgery and its risks and benefits, as well as of alternative treatments. The patient should consent to the procedure. The family should be involved in consent discussions but need not necessarily agree with the patient. However, the patient may not exclude the family from discussion of the procedure.

4. TREATING PROFESSIONALS

a. Limbic surgery is done at a tertiary care centre in which chiefs of neurosurgery, psychiatry and neurology have approved the evaluating clinicians from each service.
b. The evaluation consists of a multidisciplinary team of physicians who can evaluate the pain and psychiatric diagnosis. It is recommended that screening of applicants and their records should occur well in advance of the initial visit of the patient to the treatment centre.

5. EVIDENCE

Past records of treatment and hospitalization from each significant hospital and physician. Family history, corroborated by family members if living and available.

6. EXCLUSION CRITERIA

a. Delusional psychosis.
b. Somatoform disorders.
c. Principal psychopathology of a personality disorder, Axis II in DSM-III R (e.g. borderline personality disorder, antisocial personality disorder or mixed personality disorder).
d. Primary substance abuse.
e. A history of criminality or other evidence of lack of reliability with regard to conscientious cooperation with medical treatment and the exercise of good judgement.
f. Factitious disorders or malingering.
g. Lack of willingness of the person to be maintained on a postsurgical drug regimen, and/or confer regularly with a psychiatrist and another primary physician.

TYPES OF PSYCHOSURGERY AND THEIR SEQUELAE: EFFICACY, RISKS, SIDE-EFFECTS

Nineteen different types of neurosurgery have been described for the relief of intractable pain. These are listed in Table 62.1 as early nonselective ablative procedures,

Table 62.1 Central surgical procedures for pain

Early procedures
Prefrontal leucotomy*(Moniz 1936)
Orbital undercutting*(Scoville 1949)
Transorbital lobotomy*(Freeman & Watts 1937)
Topectomy (Lebeau 1950)
Postcentral gyrectomy (Gutierrez-Mahoney 1944)
Bimedial leucotomy (Greenblatt & Solomon 1952)
Modified procedures
Unilateral frontal leucotomy (Koskoff et al 1948)
Bilateral prefrontal modified leucotomy
Frontothalamic tractotomy*(Sertrand et al 1966)
Posteromedial hypothalamotomy*(Sano et al 1975)
Thalamotomy – medial, ventral posterior (Mark 1960)
thalamolaminotomy (Sano 1966)
posterior (pulvinotomy) (Kudo 1966)
Amygdalotomy*(Jelasic 1966)
Multitarget lesions: cingulum, subcaudate, amygdala (Brown 1973)
Bilateral anterior capsulotomy*(Bingley 1973)
Hypothalamotomy – periventricular nuclei*(Fairman 1976)
Modern stereotactic procedures
Bilateral frontal medial subcaudate tractotomy (Knight 1969; Sweet 1982)
Cingulotomy (Foltz & While 1962)

*Procedures with insufficient data for their utility in pain.

modified procedures and modern, limited stereotactic procedures. Only those operations with efficacy reported by multiple authors will be discussed: thalamotomy, leucotomy and cingulotomy.

THALAMOTOMY

The first reports of medial thalamic nuclei lesions were described in 1960 by Mark et al. Sweet (1980) reviewed the literature of 1052 patients, primarily with cancer pain, who had undergone medial or intralaminar thalamotomies. In these 18 studies, an average of 83% of subjects received excellent early pain relief from the surgery, often with the ability to stop taking narcotics. Of the total group, 62% experienced protracted relief for many months or to the point of death from their malignancy. Review of three additional reports of thalamotomy on 155 patients (Bouchard et al 1977; Martin-Rodriguez et al 1977; Mundinger & Becker 1977) showed that an average of 62% of their patients had prolonged pain relief from the operation, similar to the more extensive review by Sweet. Shieff (1987) reports his best results in poststroke thalamic pain, where 16/27 had long-term pain relief. There were visual problems in 20%, and a mortality of 7.4%.

Studies by Hécaen et al (1949), Bouchard et al (1977), Mundinger & Becker (1977) and Laitinen (1977) describe impressive results with nonmalignant pain. Laitinen describes 50% of his 41 patients with deafferentation pain as sustaining some lasting benefit. Mundinger & Becker describe 40% with good to permanent absence of pain in their deafferentation pain patients, followed for up to 14.5 years. Bouchard et al note that phantom pain patients within their group of 68 were among those who did not respond. Steiner (1980) and Niizuma (1982) found similarly poor results, 8/52 incurring good relief from ventromedial thalamotomy, and minimal efficacy for deafferentation syndromes. Tasker (1982) reported only 36% of 56 patients with neurogenic pain had good relief. Clearly, the variability of response to thalamotomy is very much greater for patients with neurogenic or deafferentation pain, and hence detracts from the value of thalamic lesions.

One limitation of the thalamic procedures reported is that most involve lesions in the inferoposteromedial thalamus, especially the centrum medianum and parafascicular nuclei. However, it is the intralaminar nuclei of the thalamus that receive many projections from pain receptors, and their projections are more to the striatum, including the limbic striatum or nucleus accumbens, rather than the cortex. Perhaps this potential pathway into the limbic system could be much more pertinent to chronic pain with limbic/effective components (Jones 1985). We do not know whether neuropathic pain, or pain with depression and anxiety might respond differentially well to intralaminar thalamic lesions.

Side-effects of thalamic surgery are another limitation. There is a 10–50% chance of recurrence of severe pain, which is directly associated with the length of survival. Paraesthesias, severe dysaesthesias, hypoaesthesias, sensory ataxia, coma, disorientation and confusion also occur. The mortality rate is up to 7%, larger than in other stereotactic procedures, but lower than in comparable open operations. There have been no formal studies of the more subtle cognitive sequelae of thalamic lesions, because most of the patients so treated have had widespread cancer in the head or neck. Choppy et al (1977) did review the effects of primarily subthalamic lesions on IQ, finding an increase in verbal performance (P = 0.05) and no change in performance score.

In summary, thalamic lesions of the medial, intralaminar, anterior and posterior areas have proven efficacy in cancer pain. Pain will be relieved in at least 60% of such patients; however, the chance of recurrence, operative mortality, dysphasia and dysaesthesias make this operation uncommon today.

LEUCOTOMY

Leucotomy may be divided into those procedures that ablate matter superoanterior to the tips of the lateral ventricles and those that ablate limited amounts of white matter inferoposteromedial to the tips of the lateral ventricles. The former group subsumes lobotomy and its modifications; orbital undercutting, topectomy, gyrectomy and bimedial, unilateral and staged modifications of leucotomy. The latter (inferoposteromedial) procedures include medial-frontal leucotomy, preinnominate tractotomy, anterior capsulotomy, subcaudate tractotomy and some of the multitarget limbic procedures.

The first known leucotomy for pain was performed by Freeman & Watts in 1936. A woman who had been confined to bed for 2 years with severe back pain and conversion neurosis received a radical frontal leucotomy with the result that she was out of bed within a few days and was known to be still working some 15 years later. In 1943 Watts performed his first leucotomy with the sole purpose of relieving pain. In 1948, Freeman & Watts published their first article recommending the procedure for relief of painful suffering connected with nonpsychiatric disease. They found that when the postleucotomy patient is asked about pain, he almost always reports a sensation of pain, but does not react with the same suffering as before the surgery. Leucotomy was noted to be much more effective when fear, agitation and depression were associated problems than when pain alone was the presenting symptom (Elithorn et al 1958; Barber 1959). Peraita et al (1977) report a series of 424 leucotomy patients, some with intractable metastatic pain. They found that only those patients with functional neurotic manifestations of pain were susceptible to improvement. The poorest results were in those with pain alone, who had the largest incidence of psychological deterioration. Despite success in relieving suffering and drug addiction, psychological deterioration following large ablations of white matter was a major problem. Excessive masturbation, disorientation, incontinence and unruly behaviour were the norm (White & Sweet 1969). Falconer (1948) and Rylander (1948) believed that extensive frontal lobe lesions were a treatment of therapeutic desperation because of the mental deterioration that followed. Subsequent modifications included orbital undercutting, topectomy, gyrectomy and bimedial, unilateral and staged radiofrequency medial-frontal modifications of leucotomy. These limited the amount of white matter destroyed. Greenblatt & Solomon (1952) reported that modified leucotomy reduced the destruction of white fibres by one-third. Smith (1977) estimated that two-thirds of patients with affective psychoses achieved excellent or satisfactory results. Nevertheless, when these modified procedures were performed for the primary complaint of pain, mental changes appeared which were as severe as in the unmodified procedure. White's report of nine subjects undergoing modified frontal leucotomy showed that the only long-term survivor after 3 years remained so indolent that he was a severe burden to his family. Relief of pain and suffering was satisfactory, but the loss of initiative and interest in their surroundings negated the utility of the operation. Deficits in problem-solving and conceptual thinking resulted in such a profound apathy that the side-effects outweighed the benefits (Walsh 1977).

The main advantage of these first modified procedures was reduction in mortality and epilepsy, not improved efficacy for the relief of pain. Sykes & Tredgold (1964), reporting on orbital undercutting in 177 patients, found a 1.5% mortality, 16% epilepsy and only 5% with adverse behavioural effects. Scoville (1949) stated that there was no personality change in 90% of his orbital undercutting cases after 6 months. He found that only close relatives noticed subtle changes of either improvement or diminution of creative thinking and 75% of his patients returned to their premorbid occupation. These positive notes were generally impressionistic or depended on Wechsler intelligence scales to assess intellectual deterioration. These studies involved subjects not in optimal condition to perform well on tests prior to surgery, probably lowering initial scores and confounding the effects of surgery on subsequent scores. Scoville's last follow-up report on orbital undercutting in 1977 described only transient lethargy, hostility and garrulousness, but 4% mortality and 13% seizures. Smith (1964) has noted that some of the adverse effects as judged by psychological testing may not become evident until 10–12 years after surgery. Thus early reports of the absence of adverse effects from these modified procedures were misleading, particularly in pain patients, who suffered more adverse psychological sequelae than psychosurgery patients with affective illness (White & Sweet 1969).

Further restriction to staged and unilateral medial-frontal leucotomy did not avoid psychological deterioration. Nine of 27 patients who underwent unilateral frontal leucotomy suffered serious, depressed affect postoperatively, and four of 23 patients suffered a return or persistence of pain at a 3-month follow-up. They spoke more slowly, less often and with a slower response time. There was a recovery towards normal, but the pain benefits lasted only as long as the psychological alterations persisted (White & Sweet 1969). Hackett's analysis (in White & Sweet 1969) of staged medial-frontal leucotomy found psychological sequelae from mild transient disorientation to profound apathy and inappropriate behaviour. Limited ablations initially had less adverse sequelae, but the need for repeated procedures because of recurrence of pain ultimately resulted in the same apathetic state as occured after the unmodified procedures.

In summary, frontal leucotomy is efficacious for the relief of the suffering of intractable pain, for a short duration, and with a significant chance of marked mental deterioration. Hence, even when the surgery was the only type available, it was marginally indicated for those with an advanced malignant aetiology for their pain and a limited life expectancy. As a result of the evolution of limited inferoposteromedial procedures and cingulotomy, these earlier frontal leucotomies have been relegated to historical importance only.

Psychosurgical lesions of the ventromedial quadrants of the frontal lobes were found to have optimal results and less chance of side-effects (Fulton 1951; Greenblatt & Solomon 1952; Knight 1969, Sweet 1973, 1980; Bartlett et al 1981). Knight (1969) developed a technique of small radiofrequency lesions in the inferoposteromedial frontal lobes, treating over 200 psychiatric patients with this procedure. Strom-Olsen & Carlisle (1971) and Goktepe et al (1975) reported on Knight's patients with the finding that two-thirds had less depression and one-third to two-thirds had significant improvement in anxiety. Mortality was less than 1%, epilepsy less than 2% and behavioural problems occurred in 3%. Of patients treated with these subcaudate lesions, 93% suffered no undesirable side-effects (Shevitz 1976).

This procedure of subcaudate tractotomy, alone or in combination with other limbic surgery, has become the psychosurgical treatment of choice in intractable affective disease (Bartlett et al 1981). There are limited data on its utility in pain. Corkin & Hebben (1981) have reported on five of Sweet's subcaudate leucotomy patients who were operated on for nonneoplastic pain. Comparison of pre- and post-treatment ratings indicated a significant decrease in pain for cingulotomy patients, but not for leucotomy or pain behaviour unit-treated groups. It appeared that the subcaudate leucotomy or pain behaviour unit-treated groups did not maintain their decreased level of pain for a sustained period postoperatively, in contrast to the cingulotomy patients. Sweet (1982) has reported on 35 cancer pain patients, treated with subcaudate lesions, with the goal of allaying psychological distress and pain associated with the relentless advance of the disease: 22 of 31 patients whose status could be assessed had excellent relief that persisted until death in 17 of the 22. Abrupt cessation of narcotic intake was the rule. Even those patients who lived for a few more weeks were grateful for the relief of both organic pain and psychological suffering. One patient, who lived for a further 15.5 months, had excellent relief for 1 year but then required oral narcotics for her final 14 weeks. As with cingulotomy, half the subcaudate patients required more than one operation. No gross adverse psychological effects could be clinically observed, with detailed neuropsychological testing precluded because of the terminal disease state of the patients. Two patients who required a third pair of lesions had mild abulia, but no other adverse mental changes were noted. Two sisters of one patient concurred that their brother's postoperative willingness to speak to them without his dentures was not a terribly unfavourable personality change. Gybels (1988) has reported on the use of radiofrequency subcaudate tractotomy with extensive medial orbital white matter destruction for atypical facial neuralgia – results pending. Multitarget limbic lesions in the subcaudate area, cingulum and amygdala were reported in 43 patients with intractable pain, psychogenic fixation and drug dependence (Brown 1977). All patients had cingulum lesions, with nine of 43 having amygdala lesions and two of 43 subcaudate lesions in addition. Follow-up of 1–20 years showed 90% of these patients were significantly better, in that their psychiatric distress was decreased.

Thus, while subcaudate lesions are effective and safe in psychiatric conditions, their role for the relief of pain is still being established. The evidence so far is that they have one of the highest benefit–risk ratios for all intracerebral neurosurgery (Sweet 1982). In summary, inferoposteromedial frontal lesions have low morbidity, low mortality and some efficacy in reducing the suffering of intractable pain. The specific efficacy of these lesions in long-term reduction of nonmalignant pain is unproven. The relief of suffering that these operations can produce is remarkable in some cases, and hence further study is indicated. The efficacy of subcaudate tractotomy and anterior capsulotomy in the treatment of malignant and nonmalignant pain is of major interest, and rests on the continuation of studies such as those of Corkin (1981) and Mindus (1991).

CINGULOTOMY

Cairns & LeBeau in 1947 introduced human cingulate lesions following Fulton's lesioning of the cingulum in monkeys. Foltz & White (1962), using evoked potentials, demonstrated that the cingulum was a multisynaptic pathway connecting the medial-frontal cortex, anterior thalamic nuclei, rostral midline and intralaminar nuclei with the hippocampal formation. They postulated that transection of the cingulum might modify the patient's emotional response as well as relieve intractable pain. In 1962 they reported their first results, where five out of six patients with malignant disease and severe anxiety-depression achieved good relief, and four out of five patients with depression and nonmalignant pain (causalgia, paraplegia, angina) achieved good to excellent results. The best results from cingulotomy occurred when anxiety–depressive states coexisted with pain.

Bilateral but not unilateral lesions produced lasting benefit in nonmalignant pain. Bilateral severance of the cingulum deep to the anterior cingulate gyrus resulted in less apathy, due to minimal involvement of thalamic projections, and more lasting relief of suffering, due to maximal involvement of the association tracts of the outer limbic ring.

Later reviews of cingulotomy for chronic pain showed its efficacy. Gutierrez-Lara (1973) reported on 14 patients with severe causalgic pain refractory to neurolysis, sympathetic blocks or cordotomy. Abolition of pain was achieved in all patients, although four had to use simple analgesics occasionally. Six patients who were drug addicts did not exhibit withdrawal symptoms, a unanimous finding with other researchers. They found no evidence of psychological deficit. Wilson & Chang (1974) reported on 23 patients who underwent bilateral anterior cingulotomy for intractable pain: 19 suffered from metastatic disease, three had pain from arachnoiditis, and one had phantom limb pain. Ten of 19 metastatic pain patients obtained significant relief; one of the three arachnoiditis patients obtained pain relief. The single case of phantom limb syndrome also obtained good relief. Wilson & Chang conclude that significant relief of pain symptoms was achieved in 12 out of 23 patients. Of their patients, 57% had flattened affect postsurgery which remained at the time of discharge. Three patients had seizures postoperatively which were easily controlled with anticonvulsant medication.

Teuber et al (1977a) reported on 11 patients with a 10-year history of persistent pain. Nine of the 11 had complete or near complete relief of pain for many years to decades. None required a repeat procedure, unlike many of the primary psychiatric cases. Those who had a primary complaint of depression as well as pain did not do as well. Narcotic drug withdrawal was again noted to be a marked benefit to the surgery. Hurt & Ballantine (1974) reported on 32 cancer pain patients and nine other patients with persistent pain who had cingulotomies for pain. He found that while 12 patients had complete or marked relief of pain for 3 months or less, only one of the 41 had marked relief of pain for over 3 months. Overall, 60% of patients obtained some relief, but many required narcotics a few months later.

A total of 557 cingulotomies on 390 patients were performed by Ballantine as of July 1982 (1982). He noted that 34% of his total series complained of pain preoperatively which was reduced to 15% postoperatively. Nervousness and anxiety were most relieved with a decrease from 80 to 38% and 60 to 20% respectively. A total of 112 patients underwent cingulotomy primarily for chronic pain. This number subsumes the series of Teuber et al (1977b). Of the 112, 35 suffered from terminal cancer pain and 77 from nonmalignant conditions. The 77 include 43 with back pain, seven with abdominal and flank pain and a remaining 27 of miscellaneous origin. Of the 35 patients with pain from terminal cancer, 25 lived 3 months or less. During that period of time, 20 of them were felt to have obtained moderate to complete relief. Of the 10 who survived more than 3 months, pain relief was sustained in only two. The 77 patients with chronic pain of nonmalignant origin have been evaluated over a period from 3 months to 18 years, with an average follow-up of 7 years. Of the 43 patients with 'failed back syndrome', a significant postoperative improvement occurred in 34; eight were completely relieved and 18 had marked relief, with eight having moderate improvement. Four of the seven abdominal and flank pain patients had complete to marked relief. Five of seven patients with pain of undetermined aetiology had marked pain relief. Five of the 20 miscellaneous pain patients had significant relief. Ballantine's rating of outcome involved an assessment of pain relief per se, subjective assessment of percentage of normal functioning and the amount and type of medication taken. By 1 January 1986, Ballantine had performed 696 separate bilateral cingulate lesions on 465 patients, of which 33% were for intractable pain.

A detailed on-going analysis of these patients is being undertaken by Corkin & Hebben. They have reported on 22 bilateral anterior cingulotomy pain patients compared with five bilateral medial-frontal leucotomy patients and three patients treated in a comprehensive pain unit. These patients complained mainly of back or leg pain. It was found that cingulotomy decreases pain postoperatively and that the decrement is maintained over a follow-up period ranging from 1–12 years. Comparison of pre- and post-treatment ratings indicated a significant decline in pain for cingulotomy patients but not for pain unit or leucotomy patients. Unlike the two other groups, the cingulotomy patients had a significant decrease in thermal pain equivalent. All of these patients had nonmalignant pain. Corkin & Hebben (1981) tentatively concluded that cingulotomy was more effective than either leucotomy or noninvasive therapy in chronic nonmalignant pain. The decrement in pain magnitude estimation, and in the number and severity of adjectives applied to that pain, suggest that the benefit of cingulotomy is reflected in both the sensory and affective components of the patient's pain. A summary of the neuropsychological sequelae of cingulotomy is provided by Teuber et al (1977a). They concluded that:

1. There is currently no evidence of lasting neurological behavioural deficits after surgery.
2. A comparison of preoperative and postoperative scores reveals significant gains in the Wechsler IQ ratings.
3. When the total group of patients was subdivided according to diagnosis the incidence of improvement was high in patients with persistent pain and also in those with depression but low in those with a diagnosis of schizophrenia or obsessive-compulsive neurosis.

The only decrement is an irreversible decrease in performance of the Rey-Taylor complex figure test (Corkin & Hebben 1981).

A coincidental finding by Corkin (1979) concerned age related variance in post cingulotomy perceptual performance. Younger patients (less than 30 years) showed a statistically significant increase in the hidden figures test ability after surgery in contrast to a significant decrease in test performance among older postoperative cases. This is consistent with the improvement in cognition found by Teuber et al, but suggests that cognitively there is a smaller margin of safety in older patients undergoing cingulotomy.

There have been two major complications in Ballantine's series of 696 cingulotomies. They were caused by laceration of cortical arteries during introduction of ventricular needles. These acute subdural haematomas resulted in one transient hemiparesis and one persistent hemiparesis. A 1972 symposium where seven surgeons reported on 683 cingulotomies showed a total complication rate of one death and two hemiplegias. The consensus was that these 683 cingulotomies produced good results, with no worsening of behaviour or cognition in 70–90% of their patients. Smith (1977) and Long et al (1978) concur on the safety of the procedure. Riddle & Roberts' study (1978) of Porteus maze scores in various cingulate lesions concluded that, although there was initial postoperative decrement in performance after the surgery, it was not clear if there was complete recovery or complete loss. Teuber notes that, even though such patients performed less well than preoperatively on these conceptual tests, this was in sharp contrast to the fact that they were clinically improved, coping with their occupations at the preoperative level.

In summary, cingulotomy provides significant pain relief in half to three-quarters of all patients. The short-term benefits are clear. The long-term benefits, particularly in cancer pain patients, are equivocal. The reported mortality is 0.1%, physical morbidity 0.3% and psychological morbidity between 10 and 30%.

MECHANISMS OF ACTION OF PSYCHOSURGERY

The one consistent finding is that the mechanism of action of limbic surgery does not involve the abolition of nociception (Sweet 1980). Pinprick, temperature, pressure and acute pain are perceived as before. In contrast, lesions in the specific thalamic sensory relay nuclei, nuclei ventralis posteromedialis and posterolateralis do not relieve the suffering of chronic pain; sensation may be lost, dysaesthesias occur and the pain continues.

We shall consider the mechanisms of action of psychosurgery from the perspectives of anatomy, physiology, neuropsychology, anxiety, personality change and neurochemistry.

ANATOMY

Anatomical evaluation of frontal lobotomy, cingulotomy or thalamotomy reveals a common involvement of the outer limbic ring and its projections from the anterior thalamus. The cingulum is connected with the striatum, anterior thalamus, septal region, fornix, supralimbic cortex and hippocampus. One of these circuits is a cingulum-caudate-pallidum-thalamic circuit that links limbic, sensory, motor and affective elements (Willner 1991). Cingulotomy interrupts supracallosal, frontohippocampal, frontal-cingulate, thalamic-cingulate, thalamic-parahippocampal and limbic-temporal connections (Pandya et al 1981). That is, cingulotomy lesions certain mesocortical and mesolimbic circuits. Sweet's metaphorical description of a 'stereotypy of an excessive and futile emotional response' in chronic pain prophetically leads to the analogue of stereotypy as a symptom of a dysfunctional mesolimbic system, from the dopaminergic ventral tegmentum ascending to the limbic-frontal projections. The hypothesis of uncontrolled feedback between the frontal and limbic system, with the cingulum playing a major role, first proposed by Livingston in 1969, is even more apropos with the neurophysiological knowledge of the present day. The studies of Knight (1969) and Strom-Olsen & Carlisle (1977), using anatomicoclinical correlations in psychiatric patients, found that goods results followed when thalamofrontal radiations had been cut. Lesions largely above the cingulum were less effective compared with those involving the superior fibres of the corpus callosum (Ballantine et al 1977). When failed patients with more superficial cingulate lesions had superior fibres of the corpus callosum interrupted, the percentage of useful improvement increased from 53–80% (Ballantine et al 1977). Picaza & Hunter (1982) studied 50 rostral limbotomy patients and concluded that interruption of the cingulum, not its projections, was responsible for the behaviour modification that is seen. These studies were not double-blind and were primarily in patients with intractable affective disorders. It remains to be proven whether it is the same inferomedial thalamofrontal radiations that are critical for the relief of suffering in chronic pain.

PHYSIOLOGY

The last 10 years have seen physiological evidence that chronic pain involves the midbrain from the periaqueductal grey into the tegmentum and limbic system plus ascending projections (Bonica 1980). Poletti & Sandrew (1984) were the first to demonstrate in a squirrel monkey single unit study that there were extensive anatomical and physiological connections between the limbic system and the pain centres in the periaqueductal grey. The neurophysiological significance of the cingulum-thalamic-forebrain circuit in pain has been best demonstrated in central pain syndromes and in the neuropsychological processing of information necessary for task performance. Neuronal hyperactivity (spontaneous + evoked) has been found in the sensory thalamic nucleus (ventralis posterolateralis) (Gorecki 1989; Hirayama 1989) and in the intralaminar and medial thalamic nuclei of patients with central pain. This burst activity has been previously shown with sleep, alerting responses and now with pain. Rinaldi (1991) showed that these 'non-sensory' intralaminar nuclei (connected to the cingulum) are spontaneously hyperactive in patients with chronic pain. The clinical results of stimulating these neurons is to provoke 'a sensation of movement, throbbing or pulling'. These neurons have large receptive fields and have spatial and modality convergence responses to stimuli. In this way these forebrain circuits connecting the thalamus–basal ganglia–cingulum may explain the role of the cingulotomy in abating pathological convergence of sensory, affective, motor and behavioural aspects of pain. This widespread multifocal hyperactivity in chronic pain may explain why peripheral, spinal or purely opioid interventions do not work consistently. The susceptibility of thalamic, hippocampal and septal areas to kindling suggests that there may be permanent changes in neuronal excitability in the limbic system or cortex via this mechanism (Sramka et al 1977). Wycis & Spiegel (1961) have shown that after ablation of the ventroposterior nuclei of the thalamus, stimulation of afferent nerves evokes potentials in the hypothalamus that have a higher amplitude than preablation, and Bouchard (1977) found that evoked potentials were decreased in thalamic structures contralateral to the side of pain. Evoked potentials have been studied as physiological correlates of certain pain types, but not in relation to resolution of pain in psychosurgery. Kullberg & Risberg (1978) found a localised decrease in frontal blood flow following capsulotomy. Deafferentation pain treated with cingulotomy may be time-sensitive regarding outcome (Caputi 1984). In rats, cingulate lesions made prior to the denervation injury delayed the onset and decreased the severity of pain behaviour by one-third to one-half respectively. Controls with craniotomies or lesions made after the denervation showed no such reduction in pain-related behaviour.

NEUROPSYCHOLOGY

Psychological function of the anterior cingulate cortex has been shown to be important for mediating selection responses necessary for task selection. Pardo (1990) showed that it is the anterior cingulate cortex that is responsible for responding to conflicting or incongruent information. The cingulum is a conflict resolver, whereby competing behaviours are processed for a decision about task execution. The inability to adapt flexibly to chronic pain and suffering may reflect cingulate dysfunction and hence a mechanism of action of cingulotomy.

ANXIETY

Anxiolysis is one mechanism of improvement following psychosurgery. Anxiety reduction of 60–90% following psychosurgery is one of the most common findings (Smith 1964; Bailey 1977; Ballantine 1977; Hirose 1977; Ibor 1977; Martin-Rodriguez 1977; Vilkky 1977). The same anxiolytic effect has been noted in cingulotomy, capsulotomy, orbital undercutting and prefrontal leucotomy (Smith 1964; Bailey et al 1977; Ballantine et al 1977; Kullberg & Risberg 1978). Following the immediate postoperative reduction of anxiety, there is a euphoric phase in the first few weeks, irrespective of any preexisting psychiatric diagnosis. The alleviation of anxiety does not prove it is the change in this symptom which is responsible for the efficacy of the operation. Schumacher & Velden (1981) have demonstrated that, in experimental pain, induced anxiety can either increase discrimination between stimuli when the pain is strong or decrease discrimination when it is weak. Reduction in anxiety may increase or decrease both general suffering and pain complaints depending on the strength of the pain. Patients' subjective comments about decreased pain may mean a decreased discrimination between different stimuli secondary to a reduction in anxiety. Furthermore, lesions in the orbital undersurface of the frontal lobes usually result in disinhibition of emotional response. Bailey (1977) found similar decreased inhibition of cortical functioning in cingulate lesions. The evidence does not favour an interpretation of diminished emotionality or stimulus receptivity in psychosurgical operations (Adams et al 1977). Anxiety may be decreased, but there is no generalised diminished emotionality. Stimulus receptivity is unchanged. The disinhibition of some cortical functions may explain the measured increased cognitive skills, euphoric affect and perception of new pain as distinctly as before.

PERSONALITY CHANGE

Personality change as a result of the surgery is the most commonly offered rationale for its effectiveness (Koskoff et al 1948; Ward 1948a; Elithorn et al 1958; Foltz & White 1962; White & Sweet 1969; Walsh 1977). A reduction of tortured self-concern, decreased rumination and worrying, impairment of the ability to form appropriate worried emotional responses and a decreased social conscience have been offered as generalized personality changes that lie behind the mechanism of psychosurgery. The question is whether these are real trait changes in the personality or rather state changes associated with pain and suffering. Personality change is more than simply a theoretical question of mechanism, because its status as the sine qua non of pain relief becomes critical in the overall assessment of benefits versus risks. 'Personality' profiles of anxiety and depression as described on Minnesota Multiphasic Personality Inventory (MMPI) scores are generally found to have been significantly lowered in successful cases (Mirsky & Orzack 1976; Walsh 1977). Koskoff et al (1948) and Freeman (1971) have stated that the beneficial effect of psychosurgery on pain remains only as long as the mental alterations can be demonstrated.

Without these changes in personality, pain relief does not occur. This perspective comes from the earlier large frontal ablative procedures performed by Freeman, but is also supported by the work of Foltz & White (1973) with more limited cingulate lesions. There is evidence that personality change is not the sine qua non for efficacy. An analogy would be with anterior–temporal lobectomy for epilepsy which, although effective for the epilepsy, does not alter the personality disorder that often goes with it. Likewise, a change in the limbic suffering of pain need not be associated with a change in personality traits, defined as those lifelong patterns of interaction with people and emotions. Hackett's analysis (in White & Sweet 1969) of 22 patients who had undergone staged medial leucotomy found that the severity of adverse personality change was not related to relief of pain. Walsh (1977) found that although self-concern, introversion and depression decreased overall, particularly in the more improved cases, the items unchanged after surgery were the basic personality structure as reflected in the person's attitude to morality, sex, religion and family. This suggests that true personality traits are not changed but state variables related to depressed affect are.

The Canadian Psychiatric Association and Bridges & Bartlett (1977) reject the notion of primary behavioural change in the personality of the individual as the purpose of psychosurgery. Indeed, if one examines those proponents of personality change as the mechanism, the word 'personality' is used quite loosely, not distinguishing between state and trait affective attributes. For example, 'personality profiles of anxiety and depression on an MMPI' (mentioned above) are highly susceptible to acute painful distress, and are more likely to be reflections of pain than personality. Ibor (1977) and Walsh (1977), both proponents of the 'change in personality' theory, state that previous personality or psychiatric illness does not correlate with outcome Teuber et al (1977a), after their independent study of cingulotomy for pain and affective dysfunction, commented on the lack of overall change in the person following surgery. It was originally very difficult for these investigators to find any test capable of demonstrating a change in personality or cognition. The changes found were in subtle cognitive skills, not in the overall personality.

NEUROCHEMISTRY

Neurochemical knowledge about mechanisms of action had been sparse and inchoate. Monoamines had been implicated in psychosurgery with limited correlative findings. Fowler et al (1981) showed that monoamine oxidase B (MAOB) was no different at postmortem in psychotic lobotomized compared with nonlobotomized cases. MAOB is typically increased in the brains of psychotics and cases of degenerative brain processes resulting in loss of neuronal activity. Endorphins from periventricular nuclei stimulation can also lessen pain, but endorphin changes after cingulotomy are unknown (Connolly 1982). However, dopamine blockers enhance endorphin release in vivo (Head 1979). Carter (1978) showed in clinically improved cases of depression 1 year postleucotomy that a relative decrease in conjugated and free tyramine output after an oral tyramine load remained unchanged and abnormal. While a direct deficit in intestinal tyramine and conjugating ability still needs to be ruled out, it suggests that there is a deficit in membrane transport intrinsic to depressive illness which is not affected by psychosurgery.

The last decade has established that the neurochemistry of the cingulum involves catecholamines (e.g. dopamine and serotonin), acetylcholine, benzodiazepine receptors, glutamate, neuropeptides (P, CCK, neurotensin) and opiates. The cingulum is unique among limbic structures in that there is relatively increased cingulate glucose metabolism in depressed patients (Wu 1992), focusing attention on cingulate neurochemistry per se, in our efforts to try and understand the mechanisms of pain and suffering. Cholinergic and dopaminergic dysfunction are the two most interesting new developments in the field. Cholinergic input from the forebrain innervates the cingulum (Borst 1987) and depressed patients can have an overactive cholinergic system. The cingulate gyrus is unique among cortical structures in that it has a higher metabolic rate during rapid eye movement (REM) sleep than during normal waking, REM sleep being associated with relatively more cholinergic activity and less aminergic activity. This cholinergic cingulate overactivity model is consistent with our knowledge of pain and affective disease and may link the sleep abnormalities, hypervigilance/superattentiveness to physical complaints, monoaminergic dysfunction and mood disturbance that often accompany chronic pain that responds to cingulotomy. This overactivity focused in the cingulum may provide a clue to the unique potential of a cingulate lesion in the depressed patient. Dopaminergic (DA) modulation in the mesolimbic pathways has been shown to be important for pain. Opiate receptors comodulate dopamine. Stress, shock, conditioned fear and anxiogenic beta-carbolines can activate mesocortical DA. Antidepressant drugs, both tricyclics and serotonin selective reuptake inhibitors, upregulate mesolimbic dopamine. These particular mesolimbic/cortex dopaminergic cells lack autoreceptors and have very fast basal firing and burst activity, compared to nigrostriatal cells (Chiodo 1984). We know dopamine and pain cohabitate and share many of the same comodulating factors. Precision about any of the neurochemical mechanisms is still lacking.

In summary, disruption of the frontal limbic connections is an important mechanism of effective psychosurgery. Decreased anxiety is the most consistently altered state variable. Change in personality trait variables does not explain the mechanism of modern selective limbic procedures. Kindling, dopaminergic and cholinergic neurochemical changes or changes in mesolimbic physiology are likely candidates for the mechanism of action of psychosurgery.

CONTROVERSY

Controversy in the use of psychosurgery involves lack of defined terminology, the personalities of the surgeons involved, the question of how far to go in treating the intractably suffering and the historical ethos when psychosurgery was born. The lack of clear definition of psychosurgery was epitomized by the National Commission's exclusion of pain from their definition of psychosurgery. Such a stand-off presumably rests with a lack of appreciation that the complaint of chronic intractable pain involves 'suffering' as well as the sensory (or nociceptive) dimension of pain. The limbic system appears to be intimately involved in the 'suffering' that defines the distress of chronic pain. The relief of perseverative anquish related to pain is no different from the relief of perseverative tremor in parkinsonism. Both involve relief of symptoms by effecting changes in the central nervous system, which sometimes modify the affective state of the individual. The use of psychosurgery for pain should rest on the benefits versus risks of the particular procedure, not on an emotional response to the prefix 'psycho', implying something unusual, sacred or inviolate.

The International Association for the Study of Pain's taxonomy system (1979, 1982), and Loeser's (1981) definitions of pain, nociception, suffering and pain behaviour, have been critical first steps in defining what is meant by pain. Lack of definition of terms has fuelled not only controversy, but also ambiguous research and criticism about lack of controlled data. For example, controls consist of occasional patients who have not had the procedure completed, comparison of ineffective superficial cingulate lesions with effective deep cingulate lesions (Ballantine et al 1977) and the finding (Bouchard et al 1977) of thalamic pain responding to the homolateral operation after an ineffective operation contralateral to the pain. The main problem with study design is that ethically controlled studies cannot be done if limbic surgery is a lesioning treatment of last resort. It would be unethical to subject a patient to the risks of neurosurgery with no expectation of improvement.

The social persona of Walter Freeman was another factor in the controversy surrounding psychosurgery. He embodied both some of the best and most maladroit physicianly traits, placing him in an ambiguous position within medical society (Shutts 1982). His knowledge of anatomy, dedication to his work and patients, surgical skill, innovation and humanitarian concern made him one of the pioneers of his time. At other times he was viewed as a nonsurgeon performing operations which were sometimes inappropriate, reckless and of an experimental nature. Intense need breeds intense feelings. Psychosurgery treats the sickest, most disabled patients one can find anywhere. Severe illness carries with it intensely ambivalent feelings about the extent to which treatment should go. Often the ambivalence at a human level is projected on the procedure itself. Thus the wish to deal somehow with the severe illness results in strong protagonists and antagonists of particular procedures.

The third element that has fuelled controversy over psychosurgery lies in the need for effective biological treatments of affective illness and pain. Some patients did benefit from modified lobotomy, and this seemed better than leaving these people in permanent anguish (Sweet 1973). Martin-Rodriguez et al (1977) report better results with additional somatic therapy following psychosurgery. Psychosurgery has a good record of efficacy compared with other pain-relieving procedures. The benefits of anterior quadrant cordotomy outweigh the side-effects only with lower limb unilateral malignant pain (Connolly 1982). After cordotomy, there is a 15–50% incidence of painful dysaesthesias over several years of follow-up.

Rhizotomy frequently carries the risks of more painful denervation dysaesthesia and trophic sores. Peripheral nerve blocks have a 40% incidence of painful dysaesthesias and are often not effective, either because peripheral causes of pain are too diffuse or because anxiety or suffering have become paramount (White & Sweet 1969). Modern psychopharmacology can be of benefit in 80% of severe chronic pain patients, but in 20% the severity of the pain and psychological variables make all pharmacological treatment useless (Brown 1977).

Electroconvulsive therapy is usually not helpful in treating pain patients. Mandel (1975) has shown that intractable pain, unless associated with a major depression, correlates with nonresponse to electroconvulsive therapy ($P < 0.01$). Overall, psychosurgery has an efficacy at least comparable to other procedures for the relief of intractable pain.

The fourth element in the controversy was the historical ethos at the time when the treatment became possible. The same technological advances that allowed stereotactic neurosurgical procedures produced a reaction wherein it was thought that the technology of science might intrude on a person's rights. This reaction was fuelled by the atrocities against humans during World War II and then by the civil unrest during the 1960s. Psychosurgery attracted vehement criticism as a culprit in the inappropriate use of medical technology on human beings. Critics picked on a comment made by Mark & Ervin (1970) regarding the possible control of violence in society with stereotactic brain lesions, an ironic and unfortunate emphasis. The work that Mark & Ervin had actually done was on a limited number of patients with clearly defined electrical abnormality in the brain recorded by in-depth electrodes. Strictly speaking, according to the National Commission Report, surgery on such patients does not even fall under the rubric of 'psychosurgery' because it involves lesions of abnormal tissue.

Thus, the controversy over psychosurgery at this time was fuelled by one of the most uncommon reasons for psychosurgery – documented focal brain disease in an atypical group of patients. It focused on a comment made by a surgeon out of context with what was actually going on in clinical practice. Thus, psychosurgery became a convenient scapegoat for other social concerns. Ethical issues in psychosurgery have been reviewed in a very scholarly manner by Kleinig (1985). His critical thinking about past problems leads us to advance a set of ethical standards for psychosurgery in the future. First, psychosurgery is indicated only when the patient is competent and personally wants the procedure without any other contingency attached. Second, the patient should meet the selection criteria previously described, pain being one of them. Finally, the procedures of cingulotomy or subcaudate tractotomy are the only two procedures currently justifiable for intractable pain (Lange 1973; Kleinig 1985; Lowinger 1987; Ostow 1987).

There are problems in the accurate assessment of psychosurgical patients, particularly pain patients. There have been few prospective studies which have followed these patients with any kind of sophisticated psychiatric assessment. Corkin & Hebben's follow-up on cingulotomy pain patients is the notable exception. We really do not know if particular types of pain or suffering respond differentially to psychosurgery, what type of depression or depressive symptoms respond to surgery or even if depressive illness is a sine qua non for good response to psychosurgery for pain. In sum, controversy has centred on the psychosocial aspects of psychosurgery. The progress of psychosurgery has been defined more by the milieu in which it operates than by objective data.

CONCLUSIONS

The last decade has shown that chronic pain is an illness in its own right. It has a central nervous system pathophysiology characterized by limbic system dysfunction and neuronal plasticity. These dual features confer a relentless morbidity and mortality in some cases. The failures of neurostimulation, deafferentation and narcotics draw attention back to the central nervous system and hence the search for selective brain therapies. Despite scientific clarifications of the limbic substrate of suffering compared with the spinothalamic substrate of the sensory dimension of pain, this distinction is rarely made and seldom appreciated. It underlies the definition, indications, and mechanism of action of limbic surgery for 'pain'.

The challenges of the future in the use of limbic surgery for intractable pain are immediate and compelling. First, accurately diagnosed patients, using DSM-IIIR and International Association for the Study of Pain diagnostic criteria and studied prospectively, would provide invaluable data on the exact kind of affective disorder and pain syndrome that is most amenable to psychosurgical treatment. Secondly, confirmation of the value of cingulotomy for neuropathic pain and somatic pain types should be instituted. Cingulotomy may be the only surgical treatment with any efficacy in the treatment of central pain syndromes, unlike the poor results seen with periaqueductal grey stimulation or other ablative procedures of afferent tracks. Third, the role of anterior capsulotomy for anxiety and affective disorders in pain patients requires definition, because of its known efficacy for anxiety disorder. Fourth, the maintenance of antidepressants and/or anticonvulsants seems to be extremely important in good outcome in these patients. This tenet needs confirmation so that the initially good postsurgical results are maintained. Finally, the human suffering alleviated by cingulotomy needs to be made more public, at least among the medical profession. The fact that intractably ill patients feel well again is simply not appreciated by most laymen or physicians.

Just as the history of psychosurgery was defined by serendipitous personal and social factors of the time, its future may be similarly defined. Currently, psychosurgery has been restricted to very few centres and has been performed by few surgeons. Bilateral anterior cingulotomy, anterior capsulotomy, and medial frontal leucotomy of the subcaudate fibres are the three operations of primary interest. These three operations have demonstrated efficacy for general suffering in psychiatric patients, with cingulotomy appearing to be the most promising for the relief of suffering from chronic pain. This is partly because of the paucity of data on subcaudate tractotomy and anterior capsulotomy for pain. Paradoxically, it is the failure of the decade's exciting new knowledge about central pain and therapeutic technologies to deliver consistent pain relief that reinvigorates psychosurgery. The difficulty involved in treating severely ill patients, the costs and uncertain remuneration of multiphysician teams and limitations of psychopharmacology and analgesic delivery systems redirect attention to the brain as the home of pain. Frontal–limbic pain surgery may be the only hope for effective treatment for a few patients.

REFERENCES

Adams P M, Barratt E S, O'Neal J T 1977 Behavioral effects of bilateral cingulum bundle lesions in the squirrel monkey. In: Sweet W H, Obrador S, Martin-Rodriguez J G (eds) Neurosurgical treatment in psychiatry, pain, and epilepsy. University Park Press, Baltimore, p 709

American Psychiatric Association 1980 Diagnostic and statistical manual for mental disorders, 3rd edn (DSM-III). American Psychiatric Association, Washington, DC

Bailey H R 1977 Cingulotractotomy and related procedures for severe depressive illness. In: Sweet W H, Obrador S, Martin-Rodriguez J G (eds) Neurosurgical treatment in psychiatry, pain, and epilepsy. University Park Press, Baltimore, p 229

Ballantine H T 1982 Cingulotomy for chronic pain. Unpublished manuscript

Ballantine H T, Levy B S, Dagi T F, Giriunas I E 1977 Cingulotomy for psychiatric illness: reports of 13 years' experience. In: Sweet W H, Obrador S, Martin-Rodriguez J G (eds) Neurosurgical treatment in psychiatry, pain, and epilepsy. University Park Press, Baltimore, p 333

Ballantine H T, Bouckoms A J, Thomas E K, Giriunas I E 1987 Treatment of Psychiatric illness by stereotactic cingulotomy. Biological Psychiatry 22: 807–819

Barber T X 1959 Toward a theory of pain: relief of chronic pain by prefrontal leukotomy, opiates, placebos, and hypnosis. Psychological Bulletin 56: 430–460

Bartlett J, Bridges P, Kelly D 1981 Contemporary indications for psychosurgery. British Journal of Psychiatry 138: 507–511

Bertrand C, Martinez N, Hardy J 1966 Frontothalamic section for intractable pain. In: Knighton R S, Dumke P R (eds) Pain. Little, Brown, Boston, p 531–535

Bingley T, Leksell L, Meyerson B A, Rylander G 1973 Stereotactic anterior capsulotomy in anxiety and obsessive-compulsive states. In: Laitinen L, Livingston K E (eds) Surgical approaches in psychiatry. University Park Press, Baltimore, p 159–164

Bonica J (ed) 1980 Pain. Association for Research in Nervous and Mental Disease, vol 58. Raven Press, New York

Borst J G G, Leung W S, MacFabe D F (1987) Electrical activity of the cingulate cortex. II. Cholinergic modulation. Brain Research 407: 81–93

Bouchard G, Mayanagi Y, Martins L F 1977 Advantages and limits of intracerebral stereotactic operations for pain. In: Sweet W H, Obrador S, Martin-Rodriguez J G (eds) Neurosurgical treatment in psychiatry, pain, and epilepsy. University Park Press, Baltimore, p 693

Bouckoms A J, Ballantine H T, Thomas E J 1985 Cingulotomy for pain. Proceedings of the IVth World Congress of Biological Psychiatry. Elsevier, Amsterdam

Bridges P K, Bartlett J R 1977 Psychosurgery: yesterday and today. British Journal of Psychiatry 131: 249–260

Brown M H 1973 Further experiences with multiple limbic lesions for schizophrenia and aggression. In: Laitinen L V, Livingston K E (eds) Surgical approaches in psychiatry. University Park Press, Baltimore, p 189–195

Brown M H 1977 Limbic target surgery in the treatment of intractable pain with drug addition. In: Sweet W H, Obrador S, Martin-Rodriguez J G (eds) Neurosurgical treatment in psychiatry, pain, and epilepsy. University Park Press, Baltimore, p 699

Caputi F, Ovelmen-Levitt J, Makachinas T, Nashold B S 1984 Neuroscience Abstracts 87: 330

Carter E O, Marshall J E (eds) 1985 Stereotactic cingulotomy as a means of psychosurgery. US Department of Health and Human Services. Health Technology Assessment Reports 9

Carter S B, Sandler M, Goodwin B L, Sepping P, Bridges P K 1978 Decreased urinary output of tyramine and its metabolites in depression. British Journal of Psychiatry 132: 125–132

Chido L A, Bannon M J, Grace A A (1984) Evidence for the absence of impulse-regulating somatodendritic and synthesis-dopamine neurons. Neuroscience 12: 1–16

Choppy M, Demaria C, LeBeau J 1977 Psychological assessment of personality following peripheral and central surgery of pain. In: Sweet W H, Obrador S, Martin-Rodriguez J G (eds) Neurosurgical treatment in psychiatry, pain, and epilepsy. University Park Press, Baltimore, p 657

Columbia Greystone Associates Second Group (eds) 1952 Psychosurgical problems. Blakiston, New York

Connolly R C 1982 Pain as a problem to the neurosurgeon. Journal of the Royal Society of Medicine 75: 160–165

Corkin S 1979 Hidden figures test performance: lasting unilateral penetrating head injury and transient effects of bilateral cingulotomy. Neuropsychologia 17: 585–605

Corkin S, Hebben N 1981 Subjective estimates of chronic pain before and after psychosurgery or treatment in a pain unit. Paper presented at the Third World Congress on Pain of the International Association for the Study of Pain, Edinburgh, Scotland

Elithorn A, Glithero E, Slater E 1958 Leucotomy for pain. Journal of Neurology, Neurosurgery and Psychiatry 21: 249–260

Fairman D 1976 Neurophysiological basis for the hypothalamic lesions and stimulation by chronic implanted electrodes for the relief of intractable pain in cancer. Advances in Pain Research and Therapy 1: 842–847

Falconer M A 1948 Relief of intractable pain of organic origin by frontal lobotomy. Research Publications, Association for Research in Nervous and Mental Disease 27: 706–714

Foltz E L, White L E 1962 Pain 'relief' by frontal cingulotomy. Journal of Neurosurgery 19: 89–100

Foltz E L, White L E 1973 Affective disorders involving pain. In: Youmans J (ed) Neurological surgery: a comprehensive reference guide to diagnosis and management of neurosurgical problems I. W B Saunders, Philadelphia, p 1772

Fowler C J, Carlsson A, Winblad B 1981 Monoamine oxidase A and B activities in the brain stem of schizophrenics and nonschizophrenic psychotics. Journal of Neural Transmission 52: 23–32

Freeman W 1971 Frontal lobotomy in early schizophrenia: long follow-up in 415 cases. British Journal of Psychiatry 119: 621–624

Freeman W J, Watts J 1937 Prefrontal lobotomy in the treatment of mental disorders. Southern Medical Journal 30: 23–31

Freeman W, Watts J W 1948 Pain mechanisms and the frontal lobes: a study of prefrontal lobotomy for intractable pain. Annals of Internal Medicine 28: 747–754

Freeman W, Watts J W, Robinson M F 1950 Psychosurgery in the treatment of mental disorders and intractable pain. C C Thomas, Springfield, Illinois

Fulton J F 1951 Frontal lobotomy and affective behavior. A neurophysiological analysis. Norton, New York

Goktepe E O, Young L B, Bridges P K 1975 A further review of the results of stereotactic subcaudate tractotomy. British Journal of Psychiatry 126: 270–280

Gorecki J, Hirayama T, Dostrovsky J O (1989) Thalamic stimulation and recording in patients with deafferentation and central pain. Stereotactic and Functional Neurosurgery 52: 219–226

Greenblatt M, Solomon H C 1952 Survey of nine years of lobotomy investigations. American Journal of Psychiatry 109: 262–265

Gutierrez-Lara F 1973 Stereotactic cingulotomy, a rational and effective approach for causalgia (report 14 cases). Excerpta Medica, Amsterdam, p 233–238

Gutierrez-Mahoney C G 1944 The treatment of painful phantom limb by removal of post-central cortex. Journal of Neurosurgery 1: 156–162

Gybels J M, Sweet W H (1989) Neurosurgical treatment of persistent pain. Karger, Houston, Texas

Head M, Lal H, Puri S, Mantione C, Valentine D 1979 Enhancement of morphine analgesia after acute and chronic haloperidol. Life Sciences 24: 2037–2044

Hécaen H, Talairach J, David M, Dell M D 1949 Coagulations limitées du thalamus dans les algies du syndrome thalamique. Résultats thérapeutiques et physiologiques. Revue Neurologique 81: 917–931

Hirayama T, Dostrovsky J O, Gorecki J (1989) Recordings of abnormal activity in patients with deafferentation and central pain. Stereotactic Functional Neurosurgery 52: 120–126

Hirose S 1977 Psychiatric evaluation of psychosurgery. In: Sweet W H, Obrador S, Martin-Rodriguez J G (eds) Neurosurgical treatment in psychiatry, pain, and epilepsy. University Park Press, Baltimore, p 203

Hurt R W, Ballantine H T 1974 Stereotactic anterior cingulate lesions for persistent pain: a report on 68 cases. Clinical Neurosurgery 21: 334–351

Ibor J J 1977 Selection criteria for patients who should undergo psychiatric surgery. In: Sweet W H, Obrador S, Martin-Rodriguez J G (eds) Neurosurgical treatment in psychiatry, pain, and epilepsy. University Park Press, Baltimore, p 151

International Association for the Study of Pain 1979 Pain terms: a list with definitions and notes on usage. Pain 6: 249–252

International Association for the Study of Pain 1982 Pain terms: a supplementary note. Pain 14: 204–206

Jelasic F 1966 Relation of the lateral part of the amygdala to pain. Confinia Neurologica 27: 53–55

Jenike M A, Baer L, Ballantine H T et al (1991) Cingulotomy for refractory obsessive-compulsive disorder. Archives of General Psychiatry 48: 548–554

Jones E G (1985) The thalmus Plenum Press, New York Mindus P, Nyman H (1991) The role of capsulotomy in the treatment of chronic, severe, and otherwise intractable anxiety disorder. Acta Psychiatrica Scandinavica 83: 283–291

Journal of the American Medical Association 1980 Treating the brain by cingulotomy. Medical News 244: 2161

Kleinig J 1985 Ethical issues in psychosurgery. Allen & Unwin, London

Knight G C 1969 Bifrontal stereotactic tractotomy: an atraumatic operation of value in the treatment of intractable psychoneurosis. British Journal of Psychiatry 115: 257–266

Koskoff Y D, Dennis W, Lazovik D, Wheeler E T 1948 E T 1948 The psychological effects of frontal lobotomy performed for the alleviation of pain. Association for Research in Nervous and Mental Disease Proceedings 27: 723–753

Kudo T, Yoshii N, Shimizu S, Akawa S, Nakahama H 1966 Effects of stereotactic thalamotomy to (sic) intractable pain and numbness. Keio Journal of Medicine 15: 191–194

Kullberg G, Risberg J 1978 Changes in regional cerebral blood flow: following stereotactic psychosurgery. Applied Neurophysiology 41: 79–85

Laitinen L V 1977 Anterior pulvinotomy in the treatment of intractable pain. In: Sweet W H, Obrador S, Martin-Rodriguez J G (eds) Neurosurgical treatment in psychiatry, pain, and epilepsy. University Park Press, Baltimore, p 669–672

Lange S A 1973 Ethical implications of psychosurgery. Psychiatrie, Neurologie und Neurochirurgie 76: 383–389

LeBeau J 1950 Experience with topectomy for the relief of intractable pain. Journal of Neurosurgery 7: 79–91

Lehmann H E, Ostrow D E 1973 Quizzing the expert: clinical criteria for psychosurgery. Hospital Medicine, Feb: 24–31

Livingston K E 1969 Anatomical bias of the limbic system concept. Archives of Neurology 20: 90–95

Loeser J 1981 Concepts of pain. Presentation at Low Back Pain Seminar, Harvard Medical School

Long C J, Pueschel K, Hunter S E 1978 Assessment of the effects of cingulate gyrus lesions by neuropsychological techniques. Journal of Neurosurgery 49: 264–271

Lowinger P 1987 Two comments on psychosurgery. New England Journal of Medicine 316: 114

Mandel M R 1975 Electroconvulsive therapy for chronic pain associated with depression. American Journal of Psychiatry 132: 632–636, plus personal communication data

Mark V H, Ervin F R 1970 Violence and the brain. Harper & Row, New York

Mark V H, Ervin F R, Hackett T P 1960 Clinical aspects of stereotactic thalamotomy in the human. I The treatment of chronic pain. Archives of Neurology 3: 351–367

Martin-Rodriguez J G, Delgado J M R, Obrador S, Santo-Domingo J, Alonso A 1977 Intractable pain: dynamics of its psychoneurosurgical approach and brain stimulation. In: Sweet W H, Obrador S, Martin-Rodriguez J G (eds) Neurosurgical treatment in psychiatry, pain, and epilepsy. University Park Press, Baltimore, p 639

Mirsky A F, Orzack M H 1976 Final report on psychosurgery pilot study. In: Psychosurgery appendix of the National Commission for the Protection of Human Subjects of Biomedical and Behavioral Research II-2-168. US Government Printing, Washington, DC

Moniz E 1936 Tentatives operataires operataires dans le traitement de certaines psychoses. Masson, Paris

Mundinger F, Becker P 1977 Long-term results of central stereotactic interventions for pain. In: Sweet W H, Obrador S, Martin-Rodriguez J G (eds) Neurosurgical treatment in psychiatry, pain, and epilepsy. University Park Press, Baltimore, p 685

Niizuma H, Kwak R, Ikeda S, Ohyama H, Suzuki J, Saso S (1982) Follow-up results of centromedian thalamotomy for central pain. Applied Neurophysiology 45: 324–325

Ostow M 1987 Two comments on psychosurgery. New England Journal of Medicine 316: 114–115

Pandya D N 1981 The connections of the cingulate gyrus. Experimental Brain Research 42: 319–330

Pardo J V, Pardo P J, Janer K W, Raichele M E (1990) The anterior cingulate cortex mediates processing selection in the stroop attentional conflict paradigm. Neurobiology 87: 256–259

Peraita P, Lopez de Lerma J 1977 Frontal psychosurgery: a review of 424 cases. In: Sweet W H, Obrador W, Martin-Rodriguez J G (eds) Neurosurgical treatment in psychiatry, pain, and epilepsy. University Park Press, Baltimore, p 211

Picaza J A, Hunter S E 1982 Selective limbotomy. Applied Neurophysiology 45: 528–537

Retif J, Crahay S, Brihaye J (1966) Minimum frontal leucotomy with selective interruption of the cingulate gyrus, uni- or bilateral in the surgical treatment of pain. Acta Neurologica et Psychiatrica Belgica 66: 499–513

Riddle M, Roberts A H 1978 Psychosurgery and the porteus maze tests: review and reanalysis of data. Archives of General Psychiatry 35: 493–497

Rinaldi P C, Young R F, Albe-Fessard D, Chodakiewitz J (1991) Spontaneous neuronal hyperactivity in the medial and intralaminar thalamic nuclei of patients with deafferentation pain. Journal of Neurosurgery 74: 415–421

Rylander G 1948 Personality analysis before and after frontal lobotomy. Research Publications – Association for Research in Nervous and Mental Disease 27: 691–705

Sandrew B B, Poletti C E (1984) Limbic influence on the periaqueductal grey: a single unit study in the awake squirrel monkey. Brain Research 303: 77–86

Sano K, Yoshioka M, Ogashiwa M, Ishijima B, Ohye C 1966 Thalamolaminotomy. A new operation for relief of intractable pain. Confinia Neurologica 27: 63–66

Sano K, Sekina H, Hashimoto I, Amano K, Sugiyama H 1975 Posteromedial hypothalamatomy in the treatment of intractable pain. Confinia Neurologica 37: 285–290

Schumacher R, Velden M 1981 Effects of anxiety on experimental pain using SDT. Pain (suppl 1): 1–319

Schwartz H G, O'Leary J L 1941 Section of the spinothalamic tract in the medulla with observations on the pathway for pain. Surgery 9: 183–193

Scoville W 1949 Selective cortical undercutting. Journal of Neurosurgery 6: 65–73

Scoville W B, Bettis D B (1977) Result of orbital undercutting today: a personal series. In: Sweet W H, Obrador S, Martin-Rodriguez J G (eds) Neurosurgical treatment in psychiatry, pain and epilepsy. University Park Press, Baltimore, p 189–202

Shevitz S A 1976 Psychosurgery: some current observations. American Journal of Psychiatry 133: 266–270

Shieff C, Nashold B S (1987) Stereotactic mesencephalic tractotomy for thalamic pain. Neurological Research 9: 101–104

Shutts D 1982 Lobotomy: resort to the knife. Van Nostrand Reinhold, New York

Smith A 1964 Changing effects of frontal lesions in man. Journal of Neurology, Neurosurgery and Psychiatry 27: 511–515

Smith J S 1977 Prospective evaluation of prefrontal leucotomy. In: Sweet W H, Obrador S, Martin-Rodriguez J G (eds) Neurosurgical treatment in psychiatry, pain, and epilepsy. University Park Press, Baltimore, p 217

Spiegel E A, Wycis H T 1962 Stereoencephalotomy. Part II: Clinical and physiological applications. Grune & Stratton, New York, p 504

Šramka M, Sedlák P, Nádvornik P 1977 Observation of kindling phenomenon in treatment of pain by stimulation in thalamus. In: Sweet W H, Obrador S, Martin-Rodriguez J G (eds) Neurosurgical treatment in psychiatry, pain, and epilepsy. University Park Press, Baltimore, p 651

Steiner L, Forster D, Leksell L (1980) Gammathalamotomy in intractable pain. Acta Neurochirurgica 52: 173–184

Ström-Olsen R, Carlisle S 1971 Bi-frontal stereotactic tractotomy: a follow-up of its effects on 210 patients. British Journal of Psychiatry 118: 141–154

Sweet W H 1973 Treatment of medically intractable mental disease by limited frontal leucotomy – justifiable? New England Journal of Medicine 289: 1117–1125

Sweet W H 1980 Central mechanisms of chronic pain (neuralgias and certain other neurogenic pain). In: Bonica J (ed) Pain. Raven Press, New York

Sweet W H 1982 Neurosurgical aspects of primary affective disorders. In: Youmans J (ed) Neurological surgery: a comprehensive reference guide to diagnosis and management of neurosurgical problems II. W B Saunders, Philadelphia

Sweet W H (1988) Deafferentation pain in man. Applied Neurophysiology 51: 117–127

Sykes M K, Tredgold R F 1964 Restricted orbital undercutting: a study of its effects on 350 patients over the 10 years 1951–1960. British Journal of Psychiatry 110: 609–640

Tasker R R (1982) Stereotaxy of the human brain , 2nd edn. Thieme-Stratton, Stuttgart

Teuber H L, Corkin S, Twitchell T E 1977a A study of cingulotomy in man. Appendix to Psychosurgery. Reports prepared for the National Commission for the Protection of Human Subjects of Biomedical and Behavioral Research. US Department of Health, Education and Welfare, publication no (OS) 77–0002, 3, p 1–115

Teuber H L et al 1977b Study of cingulotomoy in man. In: Sweet W H, Obrador S, Martin-Rodriguez J G (eds) Neurosurgical treatment in psychiatry, pain, and epilepsy. University Park Press, Baltimore, p 355

US Department of Health and Welfare 1977 Protection of human subjects. Federal Register 42(99): 26318–26332

US Department of Health, Education and Welfare 1978 Determination of the Secretary regarding the recommendation on psychosurgery of the National Commission for the Protection of Human Subjects of Biomedical and Behavioral Research. Federal Register 43: 221: 53244M

US National Commission for the Protection of Human Subjects of Biomedical and Behavioural Research 1977 Report and recommendations: psychosurgery. Department of Health, Education and Welfare publication no (OS) 77–0001. US Government Printing Office, Washington, DC

Valenstein E S 1977 The practice of psychosurgery. A survey of the literature (1971–1976). In: Appendix to psychosurgery. US Department of Health, Education and Welfare publication no (OS) 77–00002, New York, p 11–183

Vilkky J 1977 Effects of pulvinotomy and ventrolateral thalamotomy on some cognitive functions. In: Sweet W H, Obrador S, Martin-Rodriguez J G (eds) Neurosurgical treatment in pyschiatry, pain, and epilepsy. University Park Press, Baltimore, p 672

Walsh K W 1977 Neuropsychological aspects of modified leucotomy. In: Sweet W H, Obrador S, Martin-Rodriguez J G (eds) Neurosurgical treatment in psychiatry, pain, and epilepsy. University Park Press, Baltimore, p 163

White J C, Sweet W H 1969 Pain and the neurosurgeon. C C Thomas, Springfield, Illinois

Willner P, Scheel-Kruger J (1991) The mesolimbic dopamine system: from motivation to action. John Wiley, Chichester

Wilson D H, Chang A E 1974 Bilateral anterior cingulectomy for the relief of intractable pain. Report of 23 patients. Confinia Neurologica 36: 61–68

Wu J C, Gillin J C, Buchsbaum M D, Hershey T, Johnson J C, Bunney W E (1992) Effect of sleep deprivation on brain metabolism of depressed patients. American Journal of Psychiatry 149: 538–543

Wycis H T, Spiegel E A 1961 Long-range results in the treatment of intractable pain by stereotaxic midbrain surgery. Journal of Neurosurgery 19: 101–107

Young R F, Feldman R A, Kroening R, Fulton W, Morris J 1984 Electrical stimulation of the brain in the treatment of chronic pain in man. In: Kruger L, Liebeskind J C (eds) Advances in pain research and therapy. Raven Press, New York

Stimulation

63. Stimulation-induced analgesia: transcutaneous electrical nerve stimulation (TENS) and vibration

Clifford J. Woolf and John W. Thompson

The ability of a clinician to reduce pain in a patient by exploiting the patient's own in-built neurobiological control mechanisms must surely rank as one of the great achievements of contemporary medical science. Acute pain can be diminished in over 60% of all patients, and chronic intractable pain, refractory to all conventional treatments, can be controlled for prolonged periods in up to 30% of patients, by the selective stimulation of particular subtypes of primary afferent nerve fibres. Afferent fibres can be activated by transcutaneous electrical nerve stimulation (TENS), by implanted electrodes or by natural stimuli such as vibration.

This modern therapeutic success has a historical antecedent in the Socratic era. The first reported use of electricity in medicine was the exploitation of the electrogenic torpedo fish (Scribonius longus) to treat the pain of arthritis and headache. Much later electrostatic generators combined with Leyden jar condensers resulted in the reintroduction of electrotherapy in the late Middle Ages. With the discovery of the electric battery in the 19th century a large number of charlatans and possibly a few genuine researchers continued to investigate electroanalgesia, but the phenomenon remained largely ignored by the mainstream of clinical practice (see Kane & Taub 1975 for historical review). The current use of peripheral stimulation of afferent fibres to control pain owes itself directly to the publication in 1965 of Melzack & Wall's spinal gate control theory. This theory directed attention to the active role of the dorsal horn of the spinal cord in modulating sensory transmission. One of the predictions of the theory was that activity generated by myelinated primary afferent fibres (the A fibres) would, acting via inhibitory circuits in the superficial laminae of the dorsal horn, inhibit the transmission of activity in the small unmyelinated primary afferent fibres (the C fibres). Several aspects of the original theory have since been shown to be untenable (Nathan 1976), but this key aspect, the inhibitory effect of A afferent fibre input on C fibre-evoked activity, has been amply confirmed electrophysiologically, behaviourally and clinically.

The first clinical test of the spinal gate control theory was performed on eight patients with chronic cutaneous pain by Wall & Sweet in 1967. They also demonstrated that prolonged stimulation of peripheral nerves with percutaneous needle electrodes modified the reaction of healthy human volunteers to acute noxious stimuli, without any ill-effects. Since then there has been enormous progress both in the clinical application of TENS and vibration to treat pain and in the understanding of the neurophysiological mechanisms involved. This chapter will discuss the techniques used for transcutaneous and direct peripheral nerve stimulation and for mechanical stimulation, the indications for these forms of therapy, their efficacy and associated complications. To complete the chapter a brief review will be made of our current understanding of the mechanism of the antinociceptive/analgesic action of primary afferent fibre stimulation.

THE RATIONALE OF PERIPHERAL NERVE OR MECHANICAL STIMULATION

The primary intention, in choosing peripheral nerve stimulation or vibration to relieve pain, clearly is to utilise myelinated afferent nerve fibres to activate local inhibitory circuits within the dorsal horn of the spinal cord. The arrangement of the inhibitions mediated by A beta fibres is largely segmental. Polysegmental inhibitory circuits also exist, but they tend to require higher intensity stimuli to activate them, since these inhibitory mechanism are largely induced by A delta and C afferent fibre inputs.

Therefore, in order to relieve pain using segmental afferent fibre stimulation, either low-threshold electrical stimulation should be used or, alternatively, the afferents can be activated by mechanical stimulation of their peripheral receptors with vibratory stimuli. Such treatment requires the generation of non-painful paraesthesia in the region of the body where the pain is located. This is in marked contrast to acupuncture and other counterirritant techniques which are extrasegmental and use painful stimuli, and which will not be discussed in this chapter.

TECHNIQUES

Non-painful paraesthesia can be produced by five different techniques – four electrical and one natural:

1. TENS, using surface electrodes applied to the skin
2. Peripheral nerve stimulation through subcutaneously implanted electrodes
3. Peripheral nerve stimulation using electrodes implanted directly on the nerve
4. Antidromic activation of primary afferent collaterals by the stimulation of the dorsal columns either directly or through the dura
5. Activation of rapidly adapting low-threshold afferents by the cutaneous application of a vibrator.

Electrical stimulation of the nervous system requires a pulse generator, an amplifier and a system of electrodes.

Electrical stimulation

The pulse generator and amplifier

The pulses produced by a pulse generator may be of different configurations (Fig. 63.1), pulse-widths and frequencies. The train of pulses need not be continuous but can consist of short trains of high frequency pulses delivered at fairly low frequency (Fig. 63.2). The output from the pulse generator is fed into an amplifier which amplifies the signal to a level where sufficient current is delivered to the electrodes. The amount of current required will depend on the impedance of the electrodes and the impedance of the body tissue that separates the electrodes and the peripheral nerve (see section on electrodes). Since the total impedance can change (for example, by drying of the gel interface between the electrodes and the skin), it is best to use a constant current amplifier, where the delivered current will not change with changes in the impedance of the system. A constant voltage amplifier, on the other hand, can cause sudden uncontrolled surges of current if the impedance drops.

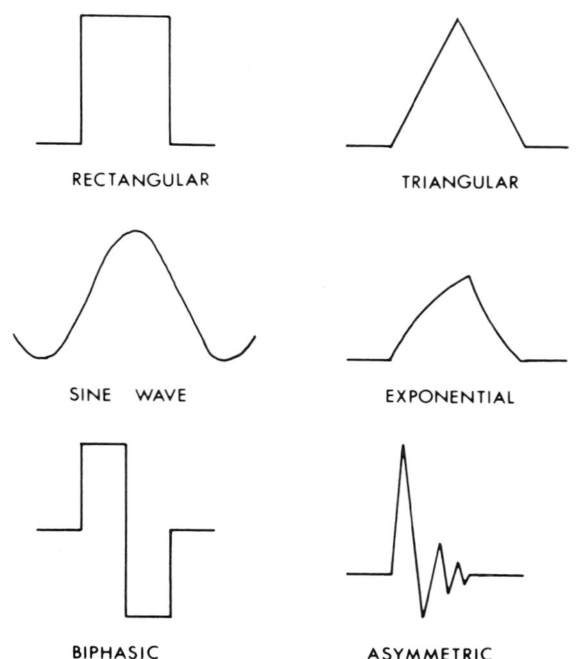

Fig. 63.1 The different configurations of pulses that can be generated by electrical pulse generators.

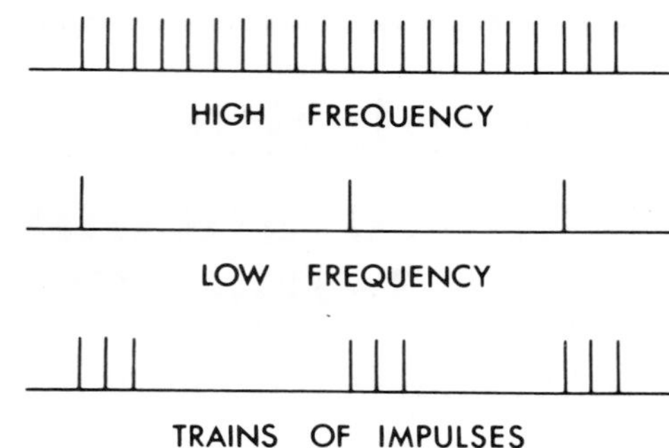

Fig. 63.2 The different patterns of pulse output used in TENS.

The typical range of controls for a stimulator suitable for TENS would be: current 0–50 mA, frequency 0–100 Hz, pulse width 0.1–0.5 ms. Although there are theoretical advantages in using biphasic pulses (see section on electrodes), in practice rectangular pulses are simplest to generate and are satisfactory for delivering a controlled charge to the skin (Bütikofer & Laurence 1979). Unlike sine waves, rectangular waves do not show a change in the charge/pulse at different frequencies.

With modern solid-state electronic technology, such stimulators are simple and inexpensive to build. The ideal stimulator should be small, but not so small as to make it difficult for the elderly to operate and read the controls; it should have rechargeable batteries, and in certain cases it should have the facility to drive more than one pair of electrodes. In the case of implanted electrodes for direct stimulation of nerves, the stimulator must have, in addition, a radiofrequency transmitter which can signal to a coil-receiver located subcutaneously.

The electrodes

Transcutaneous electrodes. The aim of TENS is to deliver sufficient charge to a pair of electrodes so that the current density produced by the resultant electric field is able to excite the afferent fibres in an adjacent nerve in a controllable manner. The stimulation must in addition be performed without damaging the skin. A variety of different electrodes have been used for this purpose, e.g. electrolyte gel-impregnated sponges, silver/silver chloride electrodes and silver-impregnated tapes. The most widely used electrodes are silicone rubber impregnated with carbon particles (Brennan 1976). These electrodes have the advantage of being strong, flexible and inert and are able to follow the shape of the body's contours. Their main disadvantage is that they require adhesive tape to attach them to the skin. Recently, disposable and reusable electrodes which are self-adhesive have become available.

Figure 63.3 illustrates the arrangement of an electrode on the skin. Electrically this arrangement can be represented by the circuit diagram in Figure 63.3, with R_e representing the resistance of the electrode, R_i the resistance of the electrode-skin interface and C_i the capacitance of the interface and tissue elements. The typical resistivity of silicone rubber/carbon electrodes is in the order of 10 Ω/cm. The current density distributed along the surface of the electrode falls off exponentially from the contact point with the stimulator, as indicated in Figure 63.3. This fall depends on the length of the electrode, its resistivity, its thickness and the complex impedance of the contact gel, skin and underlying tissue (Brennan 1976). The current density required for TENS typically is 1–5 mA/cm^2 and electrodes should be at least 4 cm^2 in size to prevent skin irritation from too high a current density in too small an electrode. Very large electrodes would, however, deliver insufficient current to stimulate peripheral nerves because of the fall-off in current density with length.

The electrode/skin impedance can be reduced by applying electrolyte gel. Without such gel, stimulation at an intensity that produces a pleasant vibration or tingling sensation can change to a sudden pricking pain due to thermal damage to the corneal layer of the skin. The high energy densities required to produce such damage occur because of localised areas of low impedance produced by

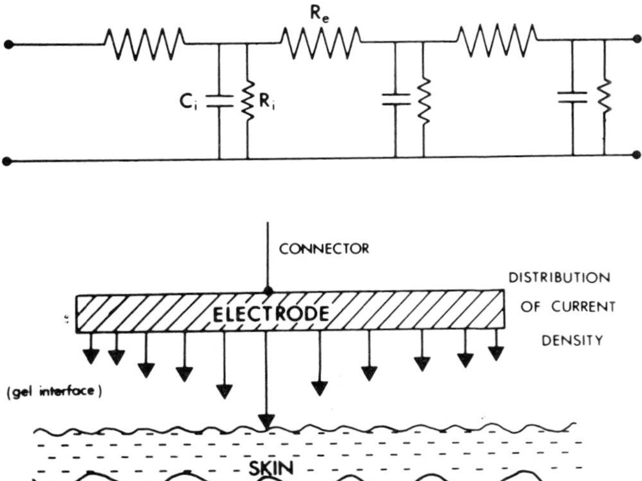

Fig. 63.3 Top A circuit diagram of the electrode/skin interface. R_e = resistance of the electrode; R_i = resistance of the skin interface; C_i = the capacitance of the skin interface. **Bottom A** diagrammatic representation of the current density distributed along an electrode used for TENS (after Brennan 1976).

perspiration (Mason & Mackay 1976). Consequently, electrolyte gel should always be used between the skin and the electrode.

The impedance of the skin and underlying tissues is very complex and non-homogeneous. Different skin thicknesses can produce significant changes in the impedance. The electrode performance also depends on the frequency of stimulation because of the capacitance of the tissue elements, with a decrease in impedance at higher frequencies.

Complex electrochemical changes can occur at the electrode-skin interface. The most important of these is the formation of an ionic bilayer which increases the electrode impedances, thereby diminishing the current density. This can be minimised by having zero charge flow using biphasic stimuli. In practice, the commonly used cathodal rectangular pulses are not accompanied by significant electrochemical problems because the amplitude of the anodal charge recovery during the period between the pulses is much less than that which causes damage at either the electrodes or the skin (Seligman 1982).

Electrodes which are used for postoperative pain control must be of such a design that they can be satisfactorily sterilised and positioned adjacent to surgical incisions.

Implanted electrodes Two types of implanted electrodes have been used. Ledergerber (1978) has used fine steel wire electrodes, placed subdermally adjacent to a surgical incision, to provide postoperative electroanalgesia. The second type of implanted electrodes are those designed to stimulate peripheral nerves directly in order to treat chronic pain. The early experience with this approach largely involved cuff electrodes placed around the appropriate nerve. However, because of problems with compression and movement (Nielson et al 1976), a new generation of electrodes has been developed (Nashold et al 1979). These electrodes consist of 2 × 1 mm platinum-iridium buttons attached to small sheets of Dacron impregnated with Silastic, with a connector to a lead. Typically, four of these button electrodes are then sutured to the epineurium in a manner that produces a maximal stimulation of the sensory afferents in the nerve. Although implanted electrodes will require much less current to stimulate nerves than surface electrodes, there is a risk of damage to tissues by electrochemical changes at the metal-tissue interface of the electrode (Dymond 1976). The implanted electrodes are attached via leads to a sealed and encapsulated receiver which is positioned subdermally. The coil of the receiver is driven by a pulse-modulated radiofrequency transmitter which is positioned externally on the surface of the skin at the site of the receiver. A more detailed discussion of the electrical stimulation of peripheral nerves is given in Swett & Bourassa (1981).

Mechanical stimulation

Rapidly adapting low-threshold mechanoreceptive primary afferents from skin and deeper tissue can be activated by applying the probe (approximately 3 cm diameter) of an electromechanical vibration to the skin. The vibrator should generate a sinusoidal mechanical oscillation of between 300 and 1000 μm when applied to the skin, over a frequency range of 50–250 Hz (Ottoson et al 1981; Lundeberg 1984a, 1984b).

THE USE OF PERIPHERAL ELECTRICAL STIMULATION TO TREAT PAIN

THEORETICAL CONSIDERATIONS

It is possible to produce complex theoretical analyses of the factors that affect stimulation of peripheral nerves by electric pulses. If one assumes that a peripheral nerve is a passive conducting cable, contained within a volume conductor formed by the body's tissues, then one can theoretically predict the current densities required to activate the nerve from electrodes of a particular size and electrical property (Long & Hagfors 1975). However, because the local conditions in the environment of the electrode are difficult to measure, and because of the heterogeneity of the body's impedance and the non-passive properties of peripheral nerves, such an analysis is of little practical help. It is useful, though, to appreciate the factors that affect the threshold for stimulating peripheral nerves. The larger the individual nerve fibres, the lower their threshold. Fibres on the surface of a nerve will be activated before deep ones. In isolated nerves, the excitability of the nerve by electrical stimulation can be expressed as a strength-duration curve. The greater the pulse-width, the lower the current required to excite the nerve, until a stable maximum is activated. There are also pulse-widths which are so short that, no matter how high the current, the nerve will not be excited. In addition to the pulse-width, increasing the frequency of stimulation can also reduce the threshold of the nerve. Figure 63.4 illustrates the theoretical relationship between pulse-width, frequency and the amplitude required to stimulate a peripheral nerve.

PRACTICAL CONSIDERATIONS

For practical purposes, the aim of all peripheral stimulating techniques is to activate sensory myelinated fibres without producing muscle contraction or dysaesthesia. Of great importance is the positioning of the electrodes. Usually these are aligned over the course of a peripheral nerve innervating the site of the pain. The optimal site of stimulation should be proximal to the pain but this is not absolutely essential and TENS can be used successfully to

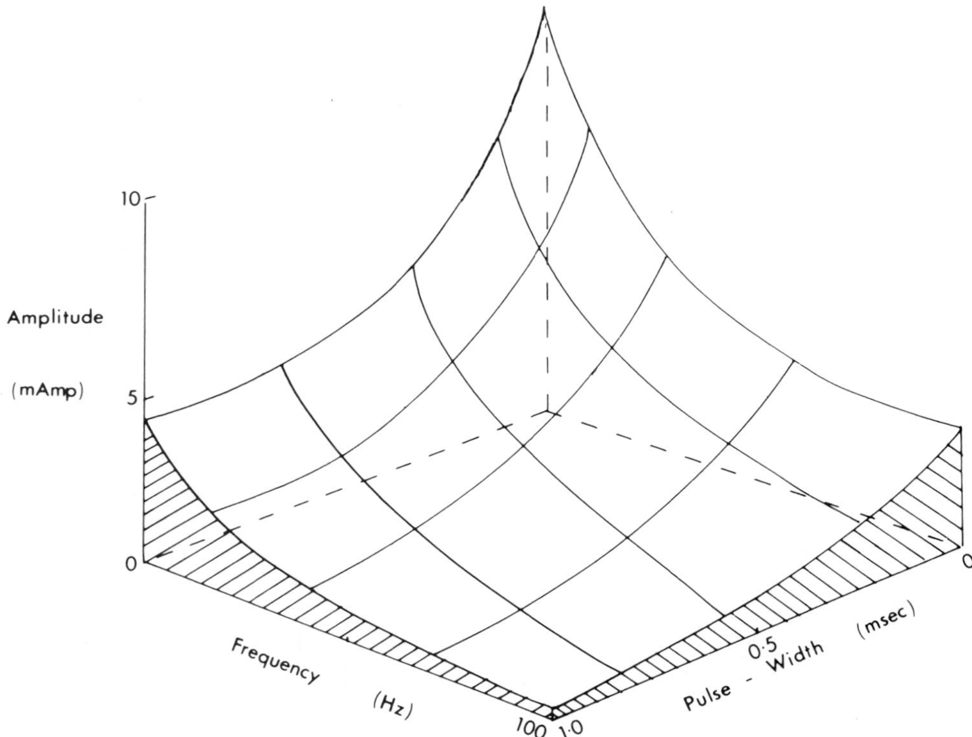

Fig. 63.4 A three-dimensional surface indicating the theoretical relationship between pulse-width and frequency in determining the amplitude of a pulse necessary to activate a nerve.

treat spinal root pain, the pain of brachial avulsion injury, etc. The site of stimulation should however be chosen to produce a maximal input in the same segment as the pain. Extrasegmental stimulation is only as effective as placebo stimulation (Cottingham et al 1985; Ekblom & Hansson 1985). The closer the electrodes are to a nerve, the lower the current required, although this will also depend on the thickness of the skin. When the stimulation of a large peripheral nerve, such as the sciatic nerve, is not practical, the electrodes can be positioned so that they stimulate the afferent nerve endings in their immediate vicinity rather than a nerve trunk. This will obviously produce a more localised area of paraesthesia.

It is often not possible to predict the most effective site for the stimulating electrodes, and some time should be spent by the patient and his medical assistants in optimising the stimulating conditions. In the case of TENS, although the stimulating apparatus is fairly straightforward, many patients are somewhat overawed or frightened by electronic devices. Therefore it is often useful for the clinician to use trained, experienced, paramedical personnel to explain to the patient in simple, non-technical terms the aim and methods of the treatment, and to perform an adequate trial of the stimulation at an appropriate strength for an appropriate time and with the electrodes at appropriate positions. Many of the treatment failures of TENS are likely to be due to the technique not being applied adequately.

Some clinicians find that admitting patients to a rehabilitation unit for a week or more is the only way to ensure an adequate trial of TENS (Wynn Parry 1980). Unless the patient feels adequate paraesthesia at the site of the pain it is unlikely that the pain will be satisfactorily reduced. As far as the appropriate frequency, pulse-width and amplitude are concerned, the aim once again is to generate the maximal comfortable paraesthesia; thus, the patient might be given the freedom to find empirically the appropriate stimulation parameters that are comfortable and reduce the pain. Although there may be an argument for attempting to activate the small myelinated A delta fibres in addition to the large A beta afferents to maximise inhibition in the spinal cord (see below), in practice patients find prolonged continuous stimulation at very high intensities intolerable. Experimental evidence does however indicate that maximal comfortable stimulation produces a greater reduction in pain than stimulation at an intensity just above detectable levels (Woolf 1979; Roche et al 1984). The vast majority of patients prefer frequencies between 40 and 70 Hz with pulse-widths of 0.1–0.5 ms. Stimulation at low frequencies requires a higher intensity and tends to produce painful muscle contraction. By using short trains of high-frequency bursts repeated at low frequency (see Fig. 63.3), it is possible to use a fairly high intensity of stimulation (Eriksson et al 1979).

The induction time for TENS to produce analgesia ranges from immediate to several hours, the average time being about 20 minutes. In the case of patients with chronic pain, there is often a cumulative effect of TENS in that the degree of pain relief produced by continuous stimulation slowly builds up over several weeks (Wynn Parry 1980). Some reports of treatment failure, when only 30 minutes of stimulation were attempted (Wolf et al 1981), indicate the need to persevere if maximal benefits are to be obtained. The duration of the stimulation also varies considerably from patient to patient, some requiring continuous, others intermittent, stimulation. Some patients find that TENS only produces analgesia during the stimulation, while others find considerable periods of poststimulation relief (Meyer & Fields 1972; Andersson et al 1976; Johnson et al 1991a). Unfortunately, the reasons for these differences in different patients are not clear but most probably reflect the nature of their pain and the degree of peripheral stimulation achieved.

Before electrodes are implanted to stimulate peripheral nerves it is necessary that a rigorous selection be performed. This should include a trial of TENS, a diagnostic local anaesthetic block, and percutaneous stimulation with needle electrodes. Since different nerves have different distributions of sensory fascicles, the implanted electrodes should be sutured in a manner such that maximal paraesthesia is achieved with minimal muscle contraction. The optimal positioning of the electrodes can be achieved only if the electrodes are implanted under local anaesthesia (Nashold 1980).

PRACTICAL USE OF THE EQUIPMENT

Equipment for TENS

Equipment for TENS consists of three parts: stimulator, leads and electrodes.

Stimulator

This is a transistorized, battery-operated pulse generator, usually controlled by:

1. combined on/off switch/amplitude (intensity) control
2. frequency control (low (c.2–5 Hz) to high (c.100–250 Hz)
3. mode selector switch for continuous/pulsed (burst) ± ramped ± random
4. width control (c.40–500 μsec) (when provided)
5. on multi channel instruments an amplitude (intensity) control is provided for each channel.

Leads

A pair of insulated wires that connect the stimulator to the electrodes. On one end of the lead is mounted a miniature jack (double pole) plug for connection to the stimulator. On the opposite end of the lead there are two individual plugs, each of which is connected either directly to a socket moulded into the electrode, or indirectly via a socket mounted on the end of a short single lead fixed to the electrode.

Important: The leads are the weakest component in TENS equipment, especially at the junction between the lead and the plugs mounted on each end. Wherever possible, the most supple leads should be used, because the wires inside the cable are less likely to fracture and also because supple leads are much more comfortable for the patient, especially when worn under clothing.

Electrodes

These are of two main types:

1. carbon-rubber (rubber impregnated with carbon to make it conduct)
2. self-adhesive (often each one has its own short lead and socket).

Use of the equipment

The following procedure should be employed.

Positioning the electrodes. First, decide where the electrodes should be positioned. Stimulating electrodes are used in pairs and are positioned so that their edges are never less than 1 cm apart so as to avoid direct conduction (i.e. short circuiting between the electrodes). In general, electrodes should be positioned so that they lie along the main direction of the nerves in the part of the body to be treated. For example, with the limbs, the electrodes should be placed longitudinally (rather than transversely). On the trunk the electrodes should be placed along the main axis of the nerves or dermatomes.

Applying the electrodes. Apply the electrodes to the selected site. Note that it is easier and more convenient if the leads are connected to the electrodes *before* the latter are applied to the skin.

Carbon-rubber. These are applied to the skin using conductive saline jelly and tape for fixation. The use of saline jelly is essential in order to achieve adequate electrical contact between the electrode and the skin. For this reason *the jelly must be applied evenly over the whole of the surface* of the electrode. Use only jelly designed for use with TENS; this normally contains 2% sodium chloride (and a bactericide). It is important to note that *ECG jelly is not recommended* because it often contains much higher concentrations of sodium chloride which will irritate the skin. The most satisfactory tape is Micropore because it is thin, flexible, easy to cut or tear into strips and does not usually irritate the skin. Alternatively, specially shaped pieces of tape designed to fit over an electrode can be obtained but are more expensive.

Self-adhesive. When not in use, these must be stored in contact with waxed paper to prevent drying. To use, peel the electrode off the wax backing and apply to the selected area of skin. Ensure that the whole surface of the electrode is applied evenly to the skin. To remove from the skin, pick up one corner of the electrode and peel it off. Immediately reapply the electrode to the waxed paper.

Important: Before applying electrodes always ensure that the skin is clean and dry and is also free from grease and powder. If this is not done, conduction between the electrode and the skin will be impaired; self-adhesive electrodes will become clogged with these substances and rapidly lose their ability to stick to the skin.

Connecting the electrodes. Connect the electrodes to the stimulator by means of the leads (having first checked that the stimulator is switched OFF).

Switching on the stimulator. Switch on and adjust the stimulator according to the procedure set out below (see later under TENS trial).

Important: Electrodes of all types must be removed from the skin at least once every 24 hours in order to allow it to recover its normal state.

Types of equipment

Three types of TENS may be used (Thompson & Filshie 1993):

1. Continuous (conventional): high-frequency (40–150Hz)/low-intensity (10–30 mA)
2. Pulsed (burst): low frequency (bursts of 100 Hz at 1–2 Hz)/low intensity (10–30 mA)
3. Acupuncture-like (Acu-TENS): low-frequency (bursts of 100 Hz at 1–2 Hz)/high intensity (15–50 mA).

Select which one of the three types of TENS is to be used, bearing in mind the following points:

a. On some stimulators, the pulsed forms of TENS referred to above (2 and 3) are available in a ramped or amplitude-modulated form so that each burst of shocks forms a rising staircase of increasing intensity. This pattern of pulsing produces a stroking sensation which is more comfortable for the patient. Stimulators with frequency-modulated pulses are also now available.

b. On some stimulators a randomized continuous output is available. The purpose of this is to reduce the development of tolerance to TENS; this may occur less readily than with a regular pattern of stimulation, which is more likely to encourage habituation of the nervous system.

c. Stimulators are now available which produce complex wave forms designed to (a) achieve deeper stimulation of the tissues with a single pair of electrodes (LIKON) or (b) further reduce the risk of tolerance by utilising multiple electrodes activated randomly (CODETRON). The possible advantages of these new stimulators remain to be fully assessed.

General points

1. The stimulus sensation should be directed into the painful area
2. The sensation produced by TENS should be strong but comfortable (not just tolerable)
3. Neither continuous (conventional) TENS nor pulsed (burst) TENS should be permitted to produce muscle twitching or spasm
4. By contrast, acupuncture-like TENS (Acu-TENS) is deliberately adjusted to a strength that evokes muscle twitching
5. To treat large areas of pain, dual (or multiple) pairs of electrodes may be needed. In order to achieve this, a double adaptor lead with a single-channel stimulator OR a dual-channel stimulator with two leads are required).

TENS TRIAL

The purpose of this is threefold:

1. To ensure that the pain condition is not aggravated by TENS
2. To familiarize the patient with the use of TENS
3. It may also indicate whether the patient obtains pain relief within the trial period. But if pain relief is not achieved within this time, the patient may well achieve pain relief with longer periods of stimulation.

Important: *It is essential that in a TENS trial, stimulation should be carried out for a minimum of 1 hour.* If this is not done then a patient who fails to respond to TENS in less than 1 hour may be wrongly assumed to be non-responsive to TENS (see later section on Relationship between patient variables, stimulator variables and outcome variables, p 1201).

Trial session-setting of controls

CONTINUOUS (conventional) stimulation

1. Set all controls to *zero* (or minimal setting), and set mode switch to continuous position
2. Increase pulse *amplitude* slowly to maximum comfortable level i.e. 'strong but comfortable'. N.B. This is usually a distinct end-point
3. Increase pulse *frequency* to maximum comfortable level. N.B. This is usually a distinct end-point
4. Where available, increase pulse *width* to comfortable level.

PULSED (burst) stimulation

Set all controls to zero (or minimal setting) and set mode switch to pulsed position. Then proceed with steps 2–4 as for continuous stimulation (see above).

ACUPUNCTURE-LIKE TENS (Acu-TENS)

Proceed as for pulsed TENS, but in step 2 adjust pulse amplitude so that muscles underlying the electrodes twitch visibly but not painfully.

After the initial TENS trial it is extremely important to ensure that the patient is given a trial period of TENS *over a period of at least 14 days.*

Which type of TENS should be used?

The form of TENS that is optimum for a particular pain *must be discovered by trial and error.* Both continuous and pulsed TENS should always be tried for every new pain treated.

TREATMENT PLAN (Thompson 1986; Thompson & Filshie 1993)

As for all other forms of treatment, it is important that the diagnosis should be established first. Even when a precise diagnosis cannot be made it is essential to establish that TENS is an appropriate treatment for a particular pain, i.e. that other, possibly more radical treatment, for example surgery, is not required. Once the decision to use TENS has been made, the following procedure is adopted:

1. Trial session (see above under Trial session – setting of controls)
2. Instruct patient in the use of equipment
3. Directions to patient:
   a. begin with a minimum of 1 hour, three times a day
   b. adjust according to need
   c. use as much as you like
   d. try comparing the pain-relieving effect of continuous and burst TENS and then use whichever is best for you; both forms if necessary
   e. you may get a bonus of a period of poststimulation pain relief (postTENS analgesia)
   f. if you have any problems with the use of TENS, please contact the clinic immediately
4. Review:
   1 month
   3 months
   6 months
   12 months

Thereafter according to need.

THE USE OF PERIPHERAL MECHANICAL STIMULI TO TREAT PAIN

Electrical stimulation of peripheral nerves is indiscriminate. All afferents with a particular threshold will be activated by a given stimulus if it exceeds that threshold. Therefore the paraesthesia resulting from TENS will be due to the activation of both rapidly and slowly adapting afferents because they have similar electrical thresholds. A more selective input can be generated by using natural stimuli that are adequate for only certain functional classes of afferents. Vibratory stimuli at frequencies of greater than 50 Hz will predominantly activate rapidly adapting low-threshold afferents. By varying the contact pressure, activation of only cutaneous or cutaneous and deep afferents (from muscle, bone, joints, etc.) can be selected (Lundeberg 1984a). Maximal efficacy is achieved by applying the vibration to the painful area, with the greatest reduction in pain at 25–45 minutes after stimulation (Lundeberg et al 1984). Optimum frequencies vary between 100 and 200 Hz, with no effect below 50 Hz.

INDICATIONS FOR THE USE OF AFFERENT FIBRE STIMULATION TO TREAT PAIN

The indication for an optimal form of pain therapy should be that it is effective with minimal or no side-effects. It is convenient for this reason to separate the indications for using TENS and vibration from those of using implanted electrodes, since the former two are non-invasive forms of therapy while the latter is associated with a variety of unique problems.

TENS

Essentially, TENS can be used to treat any localised pain of somatic or neurogenic origin, provided paraesthesia can be generated in the region of the pain or within the same or a closely related dermatome. TENS can also be effective in the treatment of pain of visceral origin, for example, angina pectoris (Mannheimer et al 1986). In this instance, stimulation is applied to a dermatome of which the cutaneous afferent nerve fibres enter the spinal cord at the same or a closely related level to that of the visceral afferents which are signalling the particular visceral pain. Because acute and chronic pain studies have different aetiologies and natural histories, they will be dealt with separately.

Acute pain

Acute pain is generally of sudden onset and can usually be attributed to an easily identifiable site of tissue injury or inflammation. The pain tends to diminish as the lesion heals, although in some cases a chronic unremitting pain can occur following acute injury. Most minor trauma produces pain of such short duration that TENS is not indicated. Sports injuries, such as torn ligaments, pulled muscles, back strain etc. can usefully be treated by TENS. Major trauma associated with multiple injuries is likely initially to produce pain of such a severity and distribution that TENS will be ineffective and a systemic analgesic is more appropriate. One situation where TENS is highly effective in treating traumatic pain is the case of fractured ribs (Myers et al 1977). A good example of inflammatory pain that is amenable to TENS is acute orofacial pain due to periodontal infections and pulpal inflammations (Hansson & Ekblom 1983; Black 1986) and the pain associated with acute arthritis, acute myalgia and the myofascial syndrome is also responsive to TENS therapy.

Labour pain has successfully been reduced by TENS, although two sets of electrodes are optimally required, one pair at T10–L1 to treat the pain associated with the first stage of labour and a pair at S2–S4 for the second stage (Augustinsson et al 1977; Nesheim 1981; Polden 1984; Davies 1989). The pain in primary dysmenorrhoea is also sensitive to TENS therapy (Lundeberg et al 1985).

Postoperative pain was the first form of acute pain successfully treated with TENS (Hymes et al 1974). Since then the treatment of postoperative pain by TENS has increased dramatically. The technique is simple and sterilised electrodes can be placed adjacent to the incision by the surgeon at the end of an operation. TENS has been used for abdominal surgery and thoracic surgery (Cooperman et al 1977; Ali et al 1981), total hip replacements (Pike 1978), lumbar spine operations (Solomon et al 1980), hand operations (Bourke et al 1984) and post-Caesarean pain (Smith et al 1986). The main advantages of TENS over opioid (narcotic) therapy is that the pain relief is continuous, there is no respiratory depression or sedation and there are no deleterious effects on bowel motility.

Chronic pain

The satisfactory management of chronic pain remains a major problem for the clinician. Initially, TENS was tried on these patients when all other forms of conventional therapy had failed. Now that more is known about how to use TENS and its efficacy, it is often appropriate to use TENS as a first-line form of therapy.

TENS is particularly suited to the treatment of pain of neurogenic origin, including peripheral nerve injury, causalgia, postherpetic neuralgia and intercostal neuritis (Wall & Sweet 1967; Meyer & Fields 1972; Nathan & Wall 1974; Loeser et al 1975; Ersek 1977; Győry & Caine 1977; Miles & Lipton 1978; Magora et al 1978; Bates & Nathan 1980). Chronic back pain, radiculopathies, compression syndromes etc. are also suitable for treatment by TENS (Cauthen & Renner 1975; Hachen 1978;

Eriksson et al 1979) as are chronic facial pains (atypical facial pain and trigeminal neuralgia; Eriksson et al 1984). Central pain states, such as brachial avulsion injury (Wynn Parry 1980) and the pain of spinal injury (Bannerjee 1974; Richardson et al 1980), can also be treated by TENS, although success can only be expected if sufficient paraesthesia can be generated. One novel use of TENS is that for treating angina pectoris. Not only is pain reduced but there is an increase in working capacity, diminished ST segment depression and an increased tolerance to pacing (Mannheimer et al 1986).

Chronic pain states that are less likely to be suitable for treatment by TENS are those that are widespread and poorly localized, including visceral pain and psychogenic pain (Johansson et al 1980; Nielzen et al 1982; Sylvester 1986). TENS has also been used to control itch (Augustinsson et al 1976).

VIBRATION

Vibration has been successfully used to treat both acute and chronic pain states. Acute orofacial pain due to pulpal inflammation, apical periodontitis and postoperative pain are reduced by this form of therapy (Ottoson et al 1981). Acute and chronic musculoskeletal pain is also diminished by vibration, with an associated increase in social activity (Lundeberg et al 1984).

INDICATIONS FOR IMPLANTED ELECTRODES

Relatively few patients have been treated by this technique because of the complexity of the apparatus, the skill required by the surgeon, possible complications, apparatus failure and resistance by patients. The criteria for selecting patients for this technique must be rigorous and include the existence of severe, unremitting, intractable pain and the fact that the pain is relieved by TENS and by nerve block. The most suitable patients tend to be those with peripheral nerve injury (Long 1973; Picaza et al 1975b; Campbell & Long 1976; Law et al 1980; Nashold 1980).

In general, TENS should be attempted in all patients with chronic pain before more invasive treatment is attempted, such as dorsal column stimulation, brain stimulation or neurosurgical lesions. It must be stressed that an adequate and supervised trial of TENS must be attempted before the treatment is judged as being ineffective.

THE EFFICACY OF TENS IN RELIEVING PAIN

CLINICAL TRIALS

In common with all other forms of pain therapy, peripheral stimulation has a significant placebo component. Early trials reporting the success of TENS or implanted devices failed to take the placebo element into account by not performing adequate controls. The problem of measuring pain is one that also makes assessment of TENS very difficult. Nevertheless, recent double-blind, randomized controlled trials and the use of techniques other than the patient's verbal report of pain have confirmed the impression of the earlier uncontrolled trials and of anecdotal reports that electrical stimulation of peripheral nerve is an effective technique in controlling pain.

ACUTE VERSUS CHRONIC PAIN

The bulk of controlled trials on the efficacy of TENS have been performed on patients with postoperative pain, since in these cases it is easier to compare the pain suffered in experimental groups and those given sham stimulation only. Vander Ark & McGrath, in 1975, showed in patients with abdominal and thoracic operations that only 7 out of 39 sham-stimulated patients reported pain relief as opposed to 47 of 61 patients with real stimulation. In a trial on 50 patients, Cooperman et al (1977) found a 33% placebo effect and a 77% TENS relief of postoperative pain. These results have been confirmed by other trials (Solomon et al 1980; Ali et al 1981). In a trial on the effect of TENS on acute orofacial pain, Hansson & Ekblom (1984) found that the stimulation was more effective than both sham stimulation and aspirin.

TENS was also more effective than placebo in reducing cutaneous pain associated with an incision for Caesarean section, but did not influence deep pain (Smith et al 1986). Several double-blind trials on the use of TENS on postoperative pain have failed to find an effect exceeding sham stimulation (Conn et al 1986; Gilbert et al 1986) and a similar report has been made for labour pain (Cushieri et al 1985; Harrison et al 1986). Why TENS failed in these particular trials is not clear. An interesting feature of the trial by Harrison et al is that while the patients commented very favourably on TENS they did not report a reduction in peak pain. TENS may act therefore in certain circumstances to make pain less disturbing without affecting its intensity.

One study that strongly counters these negative reports is that of Bourke et al (1984) who found that patients given TENS required reduced amounts of halothane to maintain adequate anaesthesia during hand surgery. This study shows that in a situation devoid of any psychological component (because the patients are unconscious) TENS is still effective. Another example of acute pain where TENS has been found to be more effective than placebo is that following intra-articular haemorrhage in haemophiliacs. A total of 71% patients receiving TENS reported pain relief, exceeding 50% compared with 21% in the sham TENS group (Roche et al 1985).

In the case of chronic pain, Thorsteinsson et al (1977) reported that stimulation was three times more effective than placebo in treating chronic neuropathies. Long et al (1979) found that the placebo effect is highest on day 1 of treatment and falls close to zero by 1 month, while the electrically treated patients with chronic pain show a considerably higher pain relief. A long-term, double-blind, controlled trial using TENS to treat the pain of osteoarthritis confirms that the analgesia produced by the electrical stimulation is significantly greater than placebo even when used over 1 year (Taylor et al 1981).

Recently, the efficacy of TENS has been questioned by Deyo et al (1990) who were unable to detect any statistically significant effect when it was compared under controlled conditions with sham TENS in 145 patients with chronic back pain. However, several factors may have contributed to this negative result. The use of strong suggestion during sham TENS may have markedly increased the placebo response. In addition, recruitment of the patients by newspaper advertisements probably attracted an atypical sample into this trial which was biased towards non-responders (Leading article, Lancet 1991).

In addition to reducing the patients' subjective complaints of pain, TENS has been found to diminish significantly the narcotic requirements of patients postoperatively (Pike 1978; Rosenberg et al 1978; Schuster & Infante 1980; Solomon et al 1980; Ali et al 1981). In a trial comparing TENS and vibration with aspirin the patients judged the former to be more effective than the latter in reducing myofascial or musculoskeletal pain (Lundeberg 1984a). However, the pain relief produced by afferent stimulation was found to be insufficient to permit dental and oral surgery (Hansson & Ekblom 1984). The pattern then is one of a reduction in pain, making it more bearable but not necessarily eliminating it.

Ali et al (1981) found that the postoperative PO_2, vital capacity and functional residual capacity of patients treated with TENS for upper abdominal surgery are much less depressed than in sham-stimulated patients. They conclude that TENS minimizes the tendency towards postoperative alterations in respiratory mechanics and thereby decreases pulmonary complications. These changes can all be attributed to an alleviation of the incisional pain.

Most clinical trials agree that maximum pain relief is obtained when the stimulation is performed in the same region as the pain. Ebershold et al (1975) found no relief of chronic intractabale pain when TENS was applied to an unrelated nerve trunk. Similar findings have been reported by Thorsteinsson et al (1977), Eriksson et al (1979), and Cottingham et al (1985).

MODE OF STIMULATION

The frequency of stimulation used by different clinicians to treat pain has varied from very low frequencies, 1–5 Hz, to frequencies of 100–150 Hz. When the patients are given the choice of frequency, most select frequencies in the range of 40–70 Hz (Linzer & Long 1976; Ledergerber 1978). Mannheimer & Carlsson (1979) have compared the effect of stimulating at 70 Hz and at 3 Hz on the pain of rheumatoid arthritis. Only 5 of 20 patients obtained relief at 3 Hz, while 18 of 20 had a reduction of pain at 70 Hz. When 70 Hz brief trains were applied three times a second, the pain relief was better than that at 3 Hz but less than that with continuous 70 Hz stimulation. Andersson et al (1976) found very similar results, with low-frequency stimulation only reducing chronic pain in 1 of 12 patients as opposed to 7 or 12 who were successfully treated at a frequency of 50–100 Hz. In a trial comparing stimulation at 2 and 100 Hz for acute orofacial pain, Hansson & Ekblom (1983) reported significant pain relief at both frequencies but a greater patient preference for the high-frequency stimulation. Low-frequency stimulation requires a higher intensity of stimulation to produce pain relief equivalent to that found at higher frequencies since, in contrast to TENS where cutaneous afferents are being stimulated, the low-frequency stimulation aims to stimulate muscle afferents (Andersson 1979).

High-intensity, low-frequency stimulation, while effective in controlling pain, can cause unpleasant muscle contraction (Melzack 1975; Andersson et al 1976). An attempt to solve this problem has been to use trains of high-frequency stimuli repeated at a low frequency. Eriksson et al (1979) reported that in patients who do not respond to conventional TENS the trains of high-intensity pulses are often effective.

Of great interest is the phenomenon of poststimulation analgesia. Meyer & Fields (1972), while treating patients with causalgia, found that the poststimulation effect lasted from 5 minutes to 10 hours in different patients. Andersson et al (1976) found a poststimulation effect of 30–60 minutes, while Augustinsson et al (1976) reported pain relief up to 18 hours after the stimulation. Bates & Nathan (1980) found that 30% of patients with postherpetic neuralgia have a permanent reduction in pain after long-term TENS (see also pp 1201–1202).

TOLERANCE

A major problem that has emerged from the use of TENS in the treatment of chronic pain is that the efficacy of the treatment tends to fall with time. The rate of attrition varies considerably from trial to trial. Loeser et al (1975) found that while 68% of 198 patients obtained short-term relief with TENS, this fell to only $12\frac{1}{2}$% over the long term. In a carefully monitored and supervised 2-year follow-up trial, Eriksson et al (1979) reported that at 2 months 55% of patients had effective relief but that at 2 years this had fallen to 30%, with a 41% relief rate at 1 year. The relief obtained over this 2-year period was estimated by the successfully treated patients to be substantial and was associated with a reduced analgesic drug requirement. Long et al (1979) found a more rapid fall-off in effective pain control, with only 35% of patients reporting satisfactory relief at 1 month, but this group of patients continued to get relief for over a year. In a controlled trial using TENS to treat the pain of osteoarthritis, Taylor et al (1981) reported a 50% reduction in pain initially falling to only 20% at 1 year. A 7-year follow-up by Bates & Nathan (1980), while affirming the success of TENS in treating a wide variety of chronic intractable painful conditions, also reported a gradual fall-off in the efficacy of the treatment over time until only 25% of patients continued to think it useful to use TENS over several years.

Figure 63.5 summarises the time-course of the efficacy of TENS reported by several authors who made long-term studies. In the early stages, TENS produces a 60–80% relief of chronic pain, figures which are similar to those found for the treatment of acute pain. A proportion of this early success can be ascribed to the placebo phenomenon, shown in Figure 63.5. The placebo effect falls off very rapidly, while the therapeutic efficacy of TENS tends to decrease more slowly until a stable long-term success rate of 20–30% is achieved.

PREDICTIVE FACTORS

It would obviously be extremely valuable if one could predict whether a particular patient is going to achieve long-term pain relief. Several attempts have been made to do this. Johansson et al (1980) found that age and sex were not useful as predictors of the outcome of therapy but that pain on the extremities responded better than axial pain. Mental illness and pathological personality traits were found by Nielzen et al (1982) to be negative factors, as was the absence of a relevant physical cause of their pain. Bates & Nathan (1980) were unable, however, to find any suitable criteria to select patients who would respond to long-term TENS. Widerström et al (1992) have demonstrated the existence of relationships between changes in experimentally induced tooth pain threshold, psychometric tests and clinical pain relief with TENS in patients suffering from chronic musculoskeletal pain of the neck and shoulders. They found that these relationships differ between responders and non-responders to TENS and if this is shown to be a general phenomenon, might clearly have predictive value. Elucidating the mechanism for this fall-off in the efficacy of TENS is the great challenge of this form of therapy. On the positive side, though, it must be recognised that the successful treatment of 20–30% of patients with chronic pain refractory to other non-invasive forms of treatment is still a major achievement.

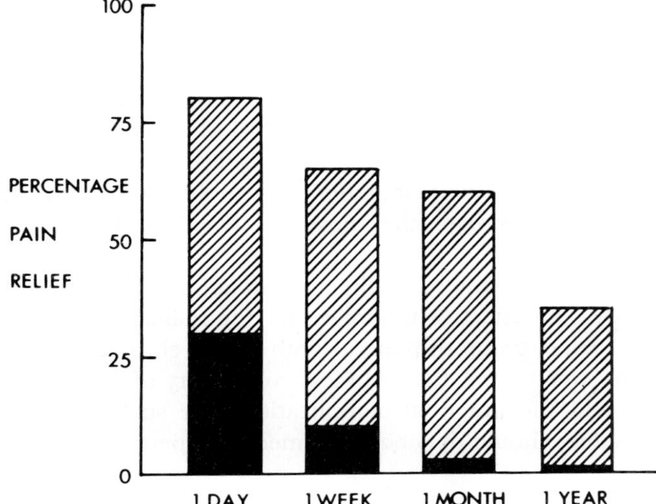

Fig. 63.5 A histogram indicating the time course of the effectiveness of TENS in controlling chronic pain. The solid area represents the contribution of the placebo effect while the cross-hatched areas represent the contribution made by TENS.

While most published clinical studies on the efficacy of TENS tend to emphasise the success of this form of treatment in managing a variety of pain conditions, it is clear that certain patients do not benefit from the treatment. Some of these treatment failures can be ascribed to technical problems with insufficient paraesthesia being generated to relieve the pain, but this is clearly not the reason in all cases. Unfortunately the types of pain which fail to respond to TENS in one trial are often reported to be satisfactorily controlled in others, and it is difficult to label TENS as being inappropriate to manage a certain condition when some patients with that condition get good long-term relief. In general, though, the types of pain least suitable for treatment with TENS are axial, diffuse, psychogenic and central pain states.

RELATIONSHIP BETWEEN PATIENT VARIABLES, STIMULATOR VARIABLES AND OUTCOME VARIABLES

When TENS is used for the treatment of a patient's pain, there are three sets of important variables that may influence the final outcome namely, *patient variables* (age, sex, cause and site of pain, personality and use of drugs); *stimulator variables* (model of stimulator, site of electrodes, pulse waveform and pulse frequency (Hz), pulse pattern, pulse intensity (mA) and pulse width (μSec) and *outcome variables* (analgesic efficacy, onset of analgesia, postTENS analgesia and adverse effects).

In two recent studies, Johnson et al (1991a, 1991b) examined these variables in nearly 200 patients who were known to respond to TENS. A number of important conclusions were drawn as follows:

1. No significant relationships were observed between the region, cause or diagnosis of pain with any patient, stimulator or outcome variable.
2. Patients applied stimulation so as to produce a strong but comfortable paraesthesia within the painful area
3. In 47% of patients, TENS reduced the intensity of their pain by more than half
4. The onset of analgesia occurred within 0.5 hour in over 75% of patients and within 1 hour in over 95% of patients
5. PostTENS analgesia lasted for less than 30 minutes in 51% of patients, for more than 1 hour in 30% of patients and for more than 2 hours in only 20%
6. 75% of patients used TENS on a daily basis and 30% used it for more than 49 hours each week, i.e. more than 7 hours daily
7. 44% of the patients benefited from the use of pulsed (burst) mode stimulation
8. Patients show individual preferences for particular pulse frequencies and patterns and consistently adjust their stimulators to these settings on subsequent treatment sessions
9. Skin irritation occurred in one-third of the patients, probably due, at least in part, to drying out of the electrode jelly.

These findings have a number of clinical implications of which the two most important are that clinicians must never assume that any particular pain will not respond to TENS, and that initially, at least, TENS should be tried for a *minimum* of 1 hour in order to establish (a) whether the patient will respond to TENS, (b) that the pain condition is not aggravated by TENS and (c) that no immediate adverse skin reaction develops. In the majority of patients analgesia only occurs during stimulation. Some patients will need to use TENS for at least 9 hours daily in order to control their pain. Other patterns of stimulation, for example burst (pulse) mode, should always be available on all stimulators because some patients fail to respond to continuous stimulation. Patients need to be instructed on the use and care of TENS equipment with particular respect to the electrodes.

In general, TENS can be considered to be useful in reducing pain for a wide variety of acute and chronic conditions. The fact that the placebo effect contributes to the pain relief should be regarded as a bonus, but there is little doubt that there is in addition, a genuine alteration in sensibility produced by TENS. TENS has, however, limited efficacy in the sense that while it can reduce or eliminate moderate or mild pain, it is less effective against severe pain. In these cirucmustances TENS should be regarded as an adjunct, permitting the reduction of other pain therapies such as the opioids (narcotics), but unable by itself to produce complete pain relief.

THE EFFICACY OF IMPLANTED ELECTRODE STIMULATION IN TREATING PAIN

Considerably fewer patients have been treated with the direct stimulation of peripheral nerves than with TENS. The first use of this technique was reported by Sweet & Wepsic in 1968. Picaza et al (1975a) reported that 20 of 23 patients with implanted stimulators obtained between 50 and 100% pain relief using cuff electrodes to stimulate the sciatic, ulnar, peroneal, occipital, obturator and pudendal nerves. A variety of pain conditions were treated in this trial, most of which were postspinal surgery but also included compression neuropathy, causalgia, syringomyelia, atypical facial pain and phantom limb pain. Long (1973) reported relief in 6 of 10 patients with pain from chronic nerve injury to the ulnar and sciatic nerves and to the brachial plexus. A subsequent trial by Campbell & Long (1976) showed excellent results in only 8 of 33 patients, 7 patients having an intermediate degree of relief. They found the best results in patients with nerve injury, while sciatica responded poorly.

These early trials used wrap-around cuff electrodes which had a risk of compressing the nerve and of movement. Picaza et al (1975a) reported a high rate of complications, including infection, equipment malfunction and postoperative tenderness. Ten of their 23 patients suffered some complication, which in six required reoperation, and left permanent nerve damage in two patients. Complications from the cuff electrodes have also been reported by Nielson et al (1976). Because of these problems, Nashold (1980) has adopted a new form of electrode, the button electrode (see section on electrodes). In a 10-year follow-up of 35 patients, he found that the stimulation of the median, ulnar and radial nerves respond much more satisfactorily than the sciatic; he ascribes this to the greater size of the sciatic nerve, with its deep sensory fascicles. Law et al (1980) used the button electrodes, although in a somewhat different manner to that of Nashold, and reported that 13 of 22 patients with posttraumatic neuropathy were successfully treated. However, 50% of their patients required reoperation in order to improve the position of the stimulating electrodes.

Therefore, while the direct stimulation of peripheral nerves is an effective treatment for the management of a small select group of patients with severe chronic pain of neurogenic origin, the technical complexity of the operation and the potential complications are such that the procedure should only be performed by experts.

COMPLICATIONS

Unlike implanted stimulating electrodes, the use of TENS is remarkably free from side-effects.

Skin irritation

A mild erythema can occur at the site of stimulation. This is not uncommon, is usually symptomless and fades after stimulation has been stopped. However, if insufficient electrolyte gel is used, a burning or pricking sensation can occur under the electrodes due to concentration of the stimulating current through a limited number of contact points. The commonest cause of skin irritation is failure to clean the skin and the carbon-rubber electrodes after use. Both must always be washed with soap, well rinsed and dried after use so as to remove dried jelly, tape adhesive and skin debris. Electrodes of all types must be removed from the skin at least once every 24 hours. Electrodes should not be applied to the same piece of skin every day but instead to an adjacent piece of 'fresh' skin which has not been used for TENS during the preceding 24 hours.

In a recent survey of long-term users of TENS (Johnson et al 1991a) the only common problem encountered was skin irritation, which occurred in one-third of the patients. It was found that to avoid inconvenience, some of the patients used TENS for 7 hours without replenishing the electrode jelly. The irritation was probably due either to drying out of the electrode jelly (Mason & Mackay 1976; Yamamoto el al 1986) or to irritation (not allergy) by the tape. It is essential to impress upon users of TENS the great importance of proper care of the skin and electrodes.

Allergic reaction

This is very uncommon, but when it occurs it may be due to some constituent of (a) the electrodes, (b) the electrode jelly or (c) the fixative, e.g. tape or adhesive, the latter being responsible in less than 1.6% (Fisher, 1978). When this problem arises, the culprit (a), (b) or (c) must be identified and changed appropriately. Thus, carbon-rubber electrodes can be replaced by self-adhesive electrodes; TENS saline jelly can be replaced by KY jelly; the tape can be replaced by another which is not antigenic.

Electrical skin burn

As indicated above, a mild and symptomless erythema can occur at the site of stimulation. By contrast, excessive electrical current applied to denervated or poorly innervated areas of skin can result in an electrical burn. Therefore, before TENS is even contemplated for a patient, *it is mandatory to test that there is normal sensation in the skin to which the electrodes are to be applied.*

Equipment failure

This is uncommon with equipment that has been well designed and constructed and marketed by reputable suppliers. Nevertheless, the stimulator, battery, leads, charger (when rechargeable batteries are used) and the electrodes can all fail and may need to be repaired or replaced. The most vulnerable part of the system is the pair of leads of which the wires are most likely to fracture where these are connected to the plugs. When equipment failure occurs, first check the battery and if in doubt, replace with a new one. Then check the continuity of the leads ensuring that the plugs connected to the electrodes (and also the mini-jack connected to the stimulator) are neither dirty, corroded nor heavily oxidized. Finally, check the continuity of the electrodes. For clinic use, a simple test rig should be constructed which can be used to test quickly any stimulator that is thought to have developed a fault. In addition, the rig can be used to carry out routine checks on all stimulators, new and old, before these are issued to new patients.

Development of tolerance to the analgesic effect (see also under Tolerance)

First check that the stimulator is working normally and that it is being used correctly. Apparent tolerance may be due to worsening of the pain problem. Nevertheless in about 30% of patients tolerance develops slowly with the passage of time (Johnson et al 1991b) and when this occurs the following courses of action should be considered:

1. Change the pulse pattern, e.g. from continuous to pulsed or to random (if available)
2. Temporarily withdraw treatment with TENS to permit reversal of tolerance
3. Use an alternative method of analgesia.

CONTRAINDICATIONS

There are few contraindications for using TENS and these can be summarised as follows:

1. Do not stimulate over the anterior part of the neck because of the risk of stimulating the nerves to the laryngeal muscles and so causing laryngeal spasm. There is also a remote risk of stimulating the carotid sinus which could result in an acute hypotensive response through the activation of the vasovagal reflex.

2. Do not stimulate over a pregnant uterus because of the possibility of producing unwanted, but as yet unknown, effects on pregnancy, and also the remote possibility of inducing labour. This raises the general question as to whether TENS should be used at all during pregnancy. Although the authors are unaware of any unwanted effects produced by TENS during pregnancy, it seems prudent to avoid using it, particularly during the first trimester. From a medico-legal point of view, if TENS were to have been used during a pregnancy that was subsequently abnormal, it might be difficult to exclude TENS as a possible cause

of the problems that ensued. On the other hand, the use of TENS for the control of pain *during labour* is well established (Augustinsson et al, 1976; Nesheim 1981; Polden 1984; Davies 1989).

3. Do not use TENS in the presence of a cardiac pacemaker or other implanted electrical device because of the risk of inducing dangerous malfunction in these devices due to the field generated by TENS equipment. Whenever the need arises to consider the use of TENS in a patient fitted with any pacemaker, the first step must be *to discuss the problem with the patient's cardiologist.* In practice, as reported by Eriksson et al (1978), this contraindication applies particularly to demand pacemakers; TENS can usually be operated without risk in the presence of fixed-rate pacemakers, but this should never be assumed.

4. Do not use TENS for the non-adaptable or non-compliant patient because this will result inevitably in therapeutic failure. In a pain relief clinic, the occasional patient is encountered who is unable or unwilling to manage the use of TENS. This may be the result of ineptitude, a deeply rooted fear of electrical devices or frank non-compliance. The first two types of patient can usually be spotted at the time of carrying out a TENS trial, but the third may only become apparent during follow-up.

THE MECHANISM OF ACTION OF PERIPHERAL NERVE STIMULATION IN CONTROLLING PAIN

Electrophysiological studies in the primate, cat and rat have clearly demonstrated that segmental cutaneous A fibre stimulation selectively inhibits C fibre and noxious-evoked activity in dorsal horn neurones of spinalized animals (Wagman & Price 1969; Handwerker et al 1975; Woolf & Wall 1982; Chung et al 1984). Prolonged A-conditioning stimuli have also been shown to diminish C fibre-evoked ventral root reflexes in spinalized cats (Cervero et al 1981) and rats (Sjölund 1985) and the reflex withdrawal response to noxious thermal stimuli in both intact and spinalized rats (Woolf et al 1980). In man such stimulation reduces noxious or A delta-evoked flexion reflexes (Willer et al 1982; Chan & Tsang 1987). These results confirm the clinical finding that the activation of myelinated primary afferents segmentally modifies the response of the spinal cord to noxious stimuli and show that analgesic effects of afferent stimulation operate by genuine neural mechanisms in situations where placebo stimulation is not relevant.

The precise way in which A fibre input generates activity in local inhibitory circuits within the spinal cord, which can then act to diminsh C fibre-evoked activity in dorsal horn neurones, is not known. Pre- and postsynaptic inhibitory mechanisms are likely to contribute. Stimulation of A fibres has been found, for example, to produce a depolarization of C fibre terminals (Fitzgerald & Woolf 1981). Such a primary afferent depolarization (PAD) is thought to be an indication of the release of a presynaptic inhibitory transmitter from an axoaxonic synapse which diminishes the afferent terminals' synaptic effectiveness. Stimulation of A fibres also produces an excitatory postsynaptic potential/inhibitory postsynaptic potential complex (EPSP/IPSP complex) in many dorsal horn neurones (Hongo et al 1968; Woolf & King 1987). The duration of the EPSP is about 10–20 ms, while that of the following IPSP is 30–60 ms. Therefore, if A fibres are stimulated at a frequency such that the interspike interval is 40 ms or less (>25 Hz), each stimulus will be associated with a short-latency, short-lasting EPSP sitting on top of a fused IPSP. This hyperpolarization may be sufficient to diminish C afferent-evoked responses in dorsal horn neurones. Which interneurones are responsible for producing the pre-and postsynaptic inhibitions is not known.

Both the A on C inhibitions of dorsal horn neurones and the PAD of C terminals occur in spinalized animals. There is evidence, though, that the A fibre stimulation, in addition to activating local inhibitory circuits, also activates some descending inhibitory pathways from the brain stem. In the rat and mouse at least, depletion of 5-hydroxytryptamine, the transmitter contained in raphe-spinal pathways, diminishes the effectiveness of the antinociceptive effect of peripheral A fibre stimulation in intact but not in spinal animals (Woolf et al 1980; Shimizu et al 1981). It is likely though that descending inhibitory mechanisms contribute more to extrasegmental stimulation-produced analgesia (Le Bars et al 1979) than to segmental analgesia.

Of great interest is the possible role of endogenous opioids in primary afferent-mediated inhibitions. Opioid receptors are present on C fibre terminals in the dorsal horn (Fields et al 1980), and enkephalin and dynorphin-containing neurones are concentrated in the substantia gelatinosa adjacent to C terminals (Aronin et al 1981). Because of this it seemed probable that these compounds would contribute to segmental analgesic mechanisms. Naloxone, an opioid receptor antagonist, fails however to reverse the analgesic effect of high-frequency TENS in patients with acute and chronic pain (Woolf et al 1978; Abrams et al 1981; Hansson et al 1986). It is quite conceivable that the dose of naloxone used in these clinical trials, although sufficient to antagonise the effect of morphine on mu receptors, is insufficient to antagonise the action of the enkephalins on kappa or delta receptors, and that it is these receptors that are responsible for producing inhibition in the spinal cord. Until specific antagonists for all three receptors become available the role of the enkephalins, dynorphins or β-endorphin in segmental afferent-induced analgesia remains unproven. Interestingly, it has been possible to produce evidence for a role for these endogenous morphine-like compounds in afferent-mediated inhibitions in laboratory animals (Woolf et al 1980; Chung et al 1983).

Whatever the role opioid peptides may ultimately turn out to have, non-opioid mechanisms are likely to be as important, and in particular ones involving the inhibitory transmitter gamma amino butyric acid (GABA); Duggan & Foong 1985).

In animals, the reflex response to a thermal noxious stimulus is attenuated by A fibre stimulation (Woolf et al 1980) but in human subjects the threshold and tolerance levels for thermal stimuli are unchanged by low-intensity conditioning stimuli (Woolf 1979). Such low-intensity stimuli do however reduce the pain produced by experimental ischaemic pain (Woolf 1979) and by electric shock-induced pain (Janko & Trontelj 1980). This finding is of some interest because morphine does not modify human thermal pain thresholds (Beecher 1959) but does reduce experimental ischaemic pain ratings (Smith et al 1966) and indicates a possible differential sensitivity of different types of pain to afferent conditioning stimuli.

Conditioning stimuli at a very high intensity, which themselves produce pain, and presumably recruit A delta afferents, do reduce thermal pain in man (Woolf 1979). The fibres activated by TENS in clinical practice are almost certainly A beta afferents (because of patients' intolerance to high-intensity stimulation), while those activated by vibration are definitely A beta. It is not clear whether A beta and A delta afferents have an identical action on the spinal cord or whether they operate on different inhibitory mechanisms. In animal experiments A delta stimulation produces a more powerful inhibition than A beta afferents (Chung et al 1984; Sjölund 1985).

Peripheral blockade of afferents has been introduced as one explanation for the mechanism of action of TENS (Campbell & Taub 1973); Ignelzi & Nyquist 1976). This is most unlikely, however, because careful experimental studies have shown that the afferent barrage evoked by painful stimuli remains intact during conditioning stimuli (Janko & Trontelj 1980). An alternative possibility is that conditioning stimuli could activate the release of pituitary and hypothalamic opioid peptides into the systemic circulation or into the cerebrospinal fluid (Facchinetti et al 1984). However, the most likely mechanism remains the activation of segmental inhibitory circuits in the spinal cord supplemented by descending inhibitory pathways. These inhibitory mechanisms operate on spinothalamic tract cells (Chung et al 1984) and on the flexion reflex pathway (Woolf et al 1980). One other pathway that may be sensitive to afferent conditioning stimuli is that mediating sympathetic reflexes. Interruption or inhibition of these reflexes would have two peripheral effects. First it could diminish the sensitizing action that noradrenaline is presumed to have on injured axons and on axon terminals in inflamed tissue (Levine et al 1986) interrupting the reflex sympathetic circuit. Second, it could increase bloodflow, aiding wound healing.

The parameters required to affect the sympathetic outflow may be different from those that interrupt the somatosensory pathways, and clinical and laboratory trials are urgently required on this subject. The beneficial effect of TENS on angina pectoris (Mannheimer et al 1986) is certainly an example of how activation of somatosensory afferents can modulate the autonomic system.

REFERENCES

Abrams S E, Reynolds A C, Cusick J F 1981 Failure of naloxone to reverse analgesia from transcutaneous electrical stimulation in patients with chronic pain. Anesthesia and Analgesia 60: 81–84

Ali J A, Yaffee C S, Serretti C 1981 The effect of transcutaneous electric nerve stimulation on postoperative pain and pulmonary function. Surgery 89: 507–512

Andersson S A 1979 Pain control by sensory stimulation. In: Bonica J J, Liebeskind J C (eds) Pain research and therapy 3. Raven Press, New York, p 569–585

Andersson S A, Hahsson G, Holmgren E 1976 Evaluation of the pain suppressant effect of different frequencies of peripheral electrical stimulation in chronic pain conditions. Acta Orthopaedica Scandinavica 47: 149–157

Aronin N, Difiglid M, Liotta A S, Martin J B 1981 Ultrastructural localisation and biochemical features of immunoreactive leuenkephalin in monkey dorsal horn. Journal of Neuroscience 1: 561–577

Augustinsson L E, Carlsson C A, Pellettieri L 1976 Transcutaneous electrical stimulation for pain and itch control. Acta Neurochirurgica 33: 342

Augustinsson L E, Bohlin P, Bundsen P et al 1977 Pain relief during delivery by transcutaneous nerve stimulation. Pain 4: 59–65

Bannerjee T 1974 Transcutaneous nerve stimulation for pain after spinal injury. New England Journal of Medicine 291: 796

Bates J A V, Nathan P W 1980 Transcutaneous electrical nerve stimulation for chronic pain. Anaesthesia 35: 817–822

Beecher H K 1959 Measurement of subjective responses. Oxford University Press, New York

Black R R 1986 Use of transcutaneous electrical nerve stimulation in dentistry. Journal of the American Dental Association 113: 649–652

Bourke D L, Smith B A C, Erickson J, Gwartz B, Lessard L 1984 TENS reduces halothane requirement during hand surgery. Anesthesiology 61: 769–722

Brennan K R 1976 The characterisation of transcutaneous stimulating electrodes. IEEE Transactions on Biomedical Engineering 23: 337–340

Bütikofer R, Laurence P D 1979 Electrocutaneous nerve stimulation. II Stimulus waveform selection. IEEE Transactions on Biomedical Engineering 26: 69–74

Campbell J N, Long D M 1976 Peripheral nerve stimulation in the treatment of intractable pain. Journal of Neurosurgery 45: 692–699

Campbell J N, Taub A 1973 Local analgesia from percutaneous electrical stimulation. Archives of Neurology 28: 347–350

Cauthen J C, Renner E J 1975 Transcutaneous and peripheral nerve stimulation for chronic pain states. Surgical Neurology 4: 102–104

Cervero F, Schounberg J, Sjölund B H 1981 Effects of conditioning stimulation of somatic and visceral afferent fibres on viscerosomatic and somatosomatic reflexes. Journal of Physiology 317: 84P

Chan C W Y, Tsang H 1987 Inhibition of the human flexion reflex by low intensity high frequency transcutaneous electrical nerve stimulation (TENS) has a gradual onset and offset. Pain 28: 239–254

Chung J M, Fang Z R, Cargill C L, Willis W D 1983 Prolonged naloxone reversible inhibition of the flexion reflex in the cat. Pain 15: 35–53

Chung J M, Lee K H, Hari Y, Endo K, Willis W D 1984 Factors influencing peripheral nerve stimulation produced inhibition of primate spinothalamic tract cells. Pain 19: 277–293

Conn I G, Marshall A H, Yadav S N, Daly J C, Jalfer M 1986 Transcutaneous electrical nerve stimulation following appendectomy: the placebo effect. Annals of the Royal College of Surgeons of England 68: 191–192

Cooperman A M, Hall B, Mikalacki K, Hardy R, Sadar E 1977 Use of transcutaneous electrical stimulation in control of postoperative pain-results of a prospective, randomized, controlled study. American Journal of Surgery 133; 185–187

Cottingham B, Philips P D, Davis G K, Getty C J M 1985 The effect of subcutaneous nerve stimulation (SCNS) on pain associated with osteoarthritis of the hip. Pain 22: 243–248

Cushieri R J, Morran C G, McArdle C S 1985 Transcutaneous electrical stimulation for postoperative pain. Annals of the Royal College of Surgeons of England 67: 127–129

Davies P 1989 An evaluation of transcutaneous nerve stimulation for the relief of pain in labour. Journal of the Association of Chartered Physiotherapists in Obstetrics and Gynaecology 65: 2–7

Deyo R A, Walsh N E, Martin D G, Schoenfeld L S, Ramamurthy S 1990 A controlled trial of transcutaneous electrical nerve stimulation (TENS) and exercise for chronic low back pain. New England Journal of Medicine 322: 1627–1634

Duggan A W, Foong F W 1985 Bicuculline and spinal inhibition produced by dorsal column stimulation in the cat. Pain 22: 249–259

Dymond A M 1976 Characteristics of the metal-tissue interface of stimulation electrodes. IEEE Transactions on Biomedical Engineering 23: 274–286

Ebershold M J, Laws E K, Stonnington H, Stillwell G K 1975 Transcutaneous electrical stimulation for treatment of chronic pain: a preliminary report. Surgical Neurology 4: 96–99

Ekblom A, Hansson P 1985 Extrasegmental transcutaneous electrical nerve stimulation and mechanical vibrating stimulation as compared to placebo for the relief of acute oro-facial pain. Pain 23: 223–229

Eriksson M B E, Schuller H S, Sjölund B H 1978 Letter: Hazard from transcutaneous stimulators in patients with pacemakers. Lancet i: 1319

Eriksson M B E, Sjölund B H, Nielzen S 1979 Long term results of peripheral conditioning stimulation as an analgesia measure in chronic pain. Pain 6: 335–347

Eriksson M, Sjölund B H, Sundberg G 1984 Pain relief from peripheral conditioning stimulation in patients with chronic facial pain. Journal of Neurosurgery 61: 149–155

Ersek R A 1977 Transcutaneous electrical neuro-stimulation – new therapeutic modality for controlling pain. Clinical Orthopedics and Related Research 1977: 314–324

Facchinetti F, Sandrini G, Petraglia F, Alfonsi E, Nappi G, Genazzani A R 1984 Concomitant increase in nociceptive flexion reflex threshold and plasma opioids following transcutaneous nerve stimulation. Pain 19: 295–307

Fields H L, Emson P C, Leigh B K, Gilbert R F T, Iversen L L 1980 Multiple opiate receptor sites on primary afferent fibres. Nature 184: 351–353

Fisher A A 1978 Dermatitis associated with transcutaneous electrical nerve stimulation. Current Contact News 21: 24

Fitzgerald M, Woolf C J 1981 Effects of cutaneous nerve and intraspinal conditioning on C-fibre afferent terminal excitability in decerebrate spinal rats. Journal of Physiology 318: 25–39

Gilbert J M, Gledhill D, Law N, George C 1986 Controlled trial of transcutaneous electrical nerve stimulation (TENS) for postoperative pain relief following inguinal herniorrhaphy. British Journal of Surgery 73: 749–751

Györy A N, Caine D C 1977 Electric pain control of a painful forearm amputation stump. Medical Journal of Australia 2: 156–158

Hachen H J 1978 Psychological, neurophysiological and therapeutic aspects of chronic pain – preliminary results with transcutaneous electrical stimulation. Paraplegia 25: 353–367

Handwerker H O, Iggo A, Zimmermann M 1975 Segmental and supraspinal actions on dorsal horn neurons responding to noxious and non-noxious skin stimuli. Pain 1: 147–165

Hansson P, Ekblom A 1983 Transcutaneous electrical nerve stimulation (TENS) as compared to placebo-TENS for the relief of acute orofacial pain. Pain 15: 157–165

Hansson P, Ekblom A 1984 Afferent stimulation induced pain relief in acute orofacial pain and its failure to induce sufficient pain reduction in dental and oral surgery. Pain 20: 273–278

Hansson P, Ekblom A, Thornsson H, Fjellner B 1986 Influence of naloxone on relief of acute oro-facial pain by transcutaneous nerve stimulation (TENS) or vibration. Pain 24: 323–329

Harrison R F, Woods T, Shore M, Mathews G, Unwin A 1986 Pain relief in labour using transcutaneous electrical nerve stimulation (TENS). A TENS/TENS placebo controlled study in two parity groups. British Journal of Obstetrics and Gynaecology 93: 739–746

Hongo T, Jankowska E, Lundberg A 1968 Postsynaptic excitation and inhibition for primary afferents in neurons of the spinocervical tracts. Journal of Physiology 199: 569–592

Hymes A C, Raab D E, Yonchiro E G, Nelson G D, Drintz A L 1974 Acute pain control by electrostimulation: a preliminary report. In: Bonica J J (ed) Advances in neurology 4. Raven Press, New York, p 761–773

Ignelzi R J, Nyquist J K 1976 Direct effect of electrical stimulation on peripheral nerve evoked activity: implications in pain relief. Journal of Neurosurgery 45: 159–165

Janko M, Trontelj J V 1980 Transcutaneous electrical nerve stimulation: a neurographic and perceptual study. Pain 9: 219–230

Johansson F, Almay B G L, Von Knorring L, Terenius L 1980 Predictors for the outcome of treatment with high frequency transcutaneous electrical nerve stimulation in patients with chronic pain. Pain 9: 55–61

Johnson M I, Ashton C H, Thompson J W 1991a An in-depth study of long-term users of transcutaneous electrical nerve stimulation (TENS). Implications for clinical use of TENS. Pain 44: 221–229

Johnson M I, Ashton C H, Thompson J W 1991b The consistency of pulse frequencies and pulse patterns of transcutaneous electrical nerve stimulation (TENS) used by chronic pain patients. Pain 44: 231–234

Kane K, Taub A 1975 A history of local electrical analgesia. Pain 1: 125–138

Law J D, Swett J, Kirsch W M 1980 Retrospective analysis of 22 patients with chronic pain treated by peripheral nerve stimulation. Journal of Neurosurgery 52: 482–485

Leading article 1991 TENS for chronic low-back pain. Lancet 337: 462–463

Le Bars D, Dickinson A H, Besson J M 1979 Diffuse noxious inhibitory controls (DNIC). I Effects on dorsal horn convergent neurones in the rat. Pain 6: 283–304

Ledergerber C P 1978 Postoperative electro-analgesia. Obstetrics and Gynaecology 151: 334–338

Levine J D, Taiwo Y O, Collins S D, Tam J K 1986 Noradrenaline hyperalgesia is mediated through interaction with sympathetic postganglionic neurone terminals rather than activation of primary afferent nociceptors. Nature 323: 158–160

Linzer M, Long D M 1976 Transcutaneous neural stimulation for relief of pain. IEEE Transactions on Biomedical Engineering 23: 341–345

Loeser J D, Black R G, Christman R M 1975 Relief of pain by transcutaneous stimulation. Journal of Neurosurgery 42: 308–314

Long D M 1973 Electrical stimulation for relief of pain from chronic nerve injury. Journal of Neurosurgery 39: 718–722

Long D M, Hagfors N 1975 Electrical stimulation in the nervous system: the current status of electrical stimulation of the nervous system for relief of pain. Pain 1: 109–123

Long D M, Campbell J N, Gurer G 1979 Transcutaneous electrical stimulation for relief of chronic pain. In: Bonica J J, Liebeskind J C, Albe-Fessard D G (eds) Advances in pain research and therapy 3. Raven Press, New York, p 593–599

Lundeberg T 1984a Long-term results of vibratory stimulation as a pain relieving measure for chronic pain. Pain 20: 25–44
Lundeberg T C M 1984b The pain suppressive effect of vibratory stimulation and transcutaneous electrical nerve stimulation (TENS) as compared to aspirin. Brain Research 294: 201–209
Lundeberg T, Nordener R, Ottoson D 1984 Pain alleviation by vibratory stimulation. Pain 20: 25–44
Lundeberg T, Bondesson C, Lindström V 1985 Relief of primary dysmenorrhea by transcutaneous electrical nerve stimulation. Acta Obstetricia et Gynecologica Scandinavica 64: 491–497
Magora F, Aladjemoff L, Tannenbaum J, Magora A 1978 Treatment of pain by transcutaneous electrical stimulation. Acta Anaesthesiologica Scandinavica 22: 587–592
Mannheimer C, Carlsson C A 1979 The analgesic effect of transcutaneous electrical nerve stimulation in patients with rheumatoid arthritis. A comparative study of different pulse patterns. Pain 6: 329–334
Mannheimer C, Carlsson C A, Vedin A, Wilhemssen C 1986 Transcutaneous electrical nerve stimulation (TENS) in angina pectoris. Pain 26: 291–300
Mason J L, Mackay N A M 1976 Pain sensations associated with electrocutaneous stimulation. IEEE Transactions on Biomedical Engineering 23: 405–409
Melzack R 1975 Prolonged relief of pain by brief transcutaneous somatic stimulation. Pain 1: 357–373
Melzack R, Wall P D 1965 Pain mechanisms: a new theory. Science 150: 971–979
Meyer G A, Fields H L 1972 Causalgia treated by selective large fibre stimulation of peripheral nerves. Brain 95: 163–167
Miles J, Lipton S 1978 Phantom limb pain treated by electrical stimulation. Pain 5: 373–382
Myers R A, Woolf C J, Mitchell D 1977 Management of acute traumatic pain by peripheral transcutaneous electrical stimulation. South African Medical Journal 52: 309–312
Nashold B S 1980 Peripheral nerve stimulation for pain. Journal of Neurosurgery 53: 132–133
Nashold B S, Muller J B, Avery R 1979 Peripheral nerve stimulation for pain relief using a multicontact electrode system. Journal of Neurosurgery 51: 872–873
Nathan P W 1976 The gate control theory of pain. A critical review. Brain 99: 123–158
Nathan P W, Wall P D 1974 Treatment of post-herpetic neuralgia by prolonged electrical stimulation. British Medical Journal iii: 645–647
Nesheim B I 1981 The use of transcutaneous nerve stimulation for pain relief during labour. Acta Obstetricia et Gynecologica Scandinavica 60: 13–16
Nielson D, Watts C, Clark W K 1976 Peripheral nerve injury from implantation of chronic stimulating electrodes for pain control. Surgical Neurology 5: 51–53
Nielzen S, Sjölund B H, Eriksson B E 1982 Psychiatric factors influencing the treatment of pain with peripheral conditioning stimulation. Pain 13: 365–371
Ottoson D, Ekblom A, Hanssen P 1981 Vibratory stimulation for the relief of pain of dental origin. Pain 10: 37–45
Picaza J A, Cannon B W, Hunter S E, Boyd A S, Guma J, Maurer D 1975a Pain suppression by peripheral nerve stimulation. Part I. Observations with transcutaneous stimuli. Surgical Neurology 4: 105–114
Picaza J A, Cannon B W, Hunter S E, Boyd A S, Guma J, Maurer D 1975b Pain suppression by peripheral nerve stimulation. Part II. Observations with implanted devices. Surgical Neurology 4: 115–126
Pike P M 1978 Transcutaneous electrical stimulation: its use in management of postoperative pain. Anaesthesia 33: 165–171
Polden M 1984 Transcutaneous nerve stimulation used in labour. Journal of the Association of Chartered Physiotherapists in Obstetrics and Gynaecology 54: 13–16
Richardson R R, Meyer P R, Cerullo L J 1980 Neurostimulation in the modulation of intractable paraplegic and traumatic neuroma pains. Pain 8: 75–84
Roche P A, Gijsbers K, Belch J J F, Forbes C D 1984 Modification of induced ischaemic pain by transcutaneous electrical nerve stimulation. Pain 20: 45–52
Roche P A, Gijsbers K, Belch J J F, Forbes C D 1985 Modification of haemophilic haemorrhage pain by transcutaneous electrical nerve stimulation. Pain 21: 43–48
Rosenberg M, Curtis L, Bourke D L 1978 Transcutaneous electrical nerve stimulation for the relief of postoperative pain. Pain 5: 129–135
Schuster G D, Infante M C 1980 Pain relief after low back surgery : the efficacy of transcutaneous electrical nerve stimulation. Pain 8: 299–302
Seligman L J 1982 Physiological stimulators: from electric fish to programmable implants. IEEE Transactions on Biomedical Engineering 29: 270–284
Shimizu T, Koja T, Fujisaki T, Fukuda T 1981 Effects of methysergide and naloxone on analgesia induced by the peripheral electric stimulation in mice. Brain Research 208: 463–467
Sjölund B H 1985 Peripheral nerve stimulation suppression of C-fibre evoked flexion reflex in rats. Journal of Neurosurgery 63: 612–616
Smith C M, Guralnick M S, Gelfund M M, Jeans M E 1986 The effects of transcutaneous nerve stimulation on post-Cesarian pain. Pain 27: 181–194
Solomon R A, Viernstein M C, Long D M 1980 Reduction of postoperative pain and narcotic use by transcutaneous electrical nerve stimulation. Surgery 87: 142–146
Sweet W H, Wepsic J G 1968 Treatment of chronic pain by stimulation of fibres of primary afferent neurons. Transactions of the American Neurological Association 93: 103–105
Swett J E, Bourassa C M 1981 Electrical stimulation of peripheral nerve. In: Patterson M M, Kerner R P (eds) Electrical stimulation research techniques. Academic Press, New York, p 243–295
Sylvester K, Kendall G P N, Lennard-Jones J E 1986 Treatment of functional abdominal pain by transcutaneous electrical nerve stimulation. British Medical Journal 293: 481–482
Taylor P, Hallett M, Flaherty L 1981 Treatment of osteoarthritis of the knee with transcutaneous electrical nerve stimulation. Pain 11: 233–246
Thompson J W 1986 The role of transcutaneous electrical nerve stimulation (TENS) for the control of pain. In: Doyle D (ed) International Symposium on Pain Control. Royal Society of Medicine Services International Congress and Symposium Series 123. Royal Society of Medicine Services Limited, London p 27–47
Thompson J W, Filshie J 1993 Transcutaneous electrical nerve stimulation (TENS) and acupuncture. In: Doyle D, Hanks G, MacDonald N (eds) Oxford textbook of palliative medicine. Oxford University Press. Oxford, p 229–244
Thorsteinsson G, Stonnington H H, Stillwell G K, Elveback L R 1977 Transcutaneous electrical stimulation: a double-blind trial of its efficacy for pain. Archives of Physical and Medical Rehabilitation 58: 8–13
Vander Ark G D, McGrath K A 1975 Transcutaneous electrical stimulation in treatment of postoperative pain. American Journal of Surgery 130: 338–340
Wagman I H, Price D D 1969 Responses of dorsal horn cells of *M. mulatta* to cutaneous and sural nerve A and C fibre stimulation. Journal of Neurophysiology 32: 803–817
Wall P D, Sweet W H 1967 Temporary abolition of pain in man. Science 155: 108–109
Widerström E G, Åslund, P G, Gustafsson LE, Mannheimer C, Carlsson S G, Andersson S A 1992 Relations between experimentally induced tooth pain threshold changes, psychometrics and clinical pain relief following TENS. A retrospective study in patients with long-lasting pain. Pain 51: 281–287
Willer J C, Roby A, Boulu P, Boureau F 1982 Comparative effects of electroacupuncture and transcutaneous electrical nerve stimulation on the human blink reflex. Pain 14: 267–278
Wolf S L, Gersh M R, Rao V K 1981 Examination of electrode placements and stimulating parameters in treating chronic pain with conventional transcutaneous electrical nerve stimulation (TENS). Pain 11: 37–47
Woolf C J 1979 Transcutaneous electrical nerve stimulation and the reaction to experimental pain in human subjects. Pain 7: 115–127

Woolf C J, King A E 1987 The physiology and morphology of multireceptive neurons with C-afferent fibre inputs in the deep dorsal horn of the rat lumbar spinal cord. Journal of Neurophysiology 58: 460–479

Woolf C J, Wall P D 1982 Chronic peripheral nerve section diminishes the primary afferent A-fibre mediated inhibition of rat dorsal horn neurones. Brain Research 242: 77–85

Woolf C J, Mitchell D, Myers R A, Barrett G D 1978 Failure of naloxone to reverse peripheral transcutaneous electro-analgesia in patients suffering from acute trauma. South African Medical Journal 53: 179–180

Woolf C J, Mitchell D, Barrett G D 1980 Antinociceptive effect of peripheral segmental electrical stimulation in the rat. Pain 8: 237–252

Wynn Parry C B 1980 Pain in avulsion lesions of the brachial plexus. Pain 9: 41–53

Yamamoto T, Yamamoto Y, Akiharu Y 1986 Formative mechanisms of current concentration and breakdown phenomena dependent on direct current flow through the skin by a dry electrode. Institute of Electrical and Electronic Engineers Transactions of Biomedical Engineering 33: 396–404

64. Folk medicine and the sensory modulation of pain

Ronald Melzack

INTRODUCTION

The study of folk medicine by anthropologists and medical historians has revealed an astonishing array of ingenious methods to relieve pain (Brockbank 1954; Wand-Tetley 1956). In addition to the use of herbs, poultices, chants and prayers, every culture appears to have learned to fight pain with pain – in general, to produce brief, moderate pain in the attempt to abolish severe, prolonged pain.

ANCIENT FORMS OF PAIN TREATMENT

One of the oldest methods of treating pain is cupping, in which a glass cup is heated up (by hot coals or flaming alcohol) and then inverted over the painful area and held against it. As the air in the cup cools and contracts, it creates a partial vacuum so that the skin is sucked up into the cup. The procedure produces bruising of the skin with concomitant pain and tenderness. Cupping was practised in ancient Greece and Rome as early as the 4th century BC, and was also practised in ancient India and China. Over the centuries, the method spread to virtually all parts of the world, and cups of various sizes, shapes and materials have evolved. Cupping has been used – and is still widely practised – for a large variety of ailments, including headaches, backaches and arthritic pains.

Scarification is another ancient practice in which the skin was cut by a sharp knife or by awesome devices with lever-driven multiple blades. Scarification has been widely practised and, sometimes, was part of 'wet cupping', in which a hot cup was placed over the cut skin and sucked out blood. Wet cupping and scarification, like leech-induced bleeding, were used for a variety of diseases ranging from heart failure to hallucinations. In addition, they were used to produce pain as well as local irritation and inflammation to combat disease and severe, chronic pain. Old medical texts describe the methods in great detail, and it is evident that they were used for common diseases as well as for the treatment of headache, backache and sciatica, and other forms of chronic pain.

Cauterisation is yet another ancient method. Generally, the end of an iron rod was heated until it was red-hot, and was then placed on the painful area, such as the foot in the case of gout, or on the buttock, back or leg in patients with low-back pain. Often, however, the cautery was applied to specifically prescribed sites distant from the painful area. The procedure, of course, produced pain and subsequent blistering of the area that was touched by the cautery. The same effect was achieved by two other procedures: rubbing blistering fluids into the skin, or applying a cone of moxa (made from the leaves of the mugwort plant) to a site on the body, setting the tip of the cone aflame, and allowing it to burn slowly until it approached or reached the skin ('moxibustion'). Again, the procedure produced pain and, while used for all kinds of diseases, was often prescribed specifically for painful conditions.

There are countless related methods, such as scraping the skull ('trepanation') to relieve headache (Meschig & Schadewaldt 1982) and producing severe skin abrasions of the neck (*cao gio*) for toothache (Primosch & Young 1980). It is evident that the one factor common to all of them is that they produce pain to abolish pain. The pain was usually brief and moderate but the desired effect was to relieve or abolish a much more severe, chronic pain. These methods, of course, did not always work, but they obviously worked well enough to have survived throughout the world for thousands of years. Do these procedures work better than a placebo? There are no experimental studies, but the evidence from studies of acupuncture – a related procedure – suggests that they do.

The methods just described are generally known as 'counterirritation', and some are still frequently used although there has not been, until recently, any theoretical or physiological explanation for their effectiveness. Suggestion and distraction of attention are the usual mechanisms invoked, but neither seems capable of explaining the power of the methods or the long duration of the relief they may afford. Because they involve painful, or near-painful levels of stimulation to relieve pain, these methods have also been labelled 'hyperstimulation analgesia' (Melzack 1973).

The multitude of procedures produced by folk medicine, which includes the use of heat, cold, electric shock in a variety of forms, vigorous massage and manipulation, have evolved into the modalities of contemporary physical therapy. These are described and evaluated in the chapters in this textbook on electrical stimulation (Ch. 63), heat and cold (Ch. 67) and manipulation and massage (Ch. 68). This chapter provides a brief examination of physical therapies and physiological concepts to explain the effects of such varied sensory inputs. Most of the procedures are ancient. Even electric shocks produced by eels were used about 2000 years ago to relieve headaches. Some procedures have vanished, but many are still used because they are effective.

ACUPUNCTURE ANALGESIA

Interest in folk medicine gained enormous impetus in recent years by the rediscovery of the ancient Chinese practice of acupuncture, which has been in continuous practice for at least 2000 years. Basically, the procedure involves the insertion of fine needles (made of steel, gold or other metals) through specific points at the skin and then twirling them for some time at a slow rate. The needles may also be left in place for varying periods of time. Acupuncture charts are extremely complex and consist, traditionally, of 361 points which lie on 14 meridians, most of which are named after internal organs, such as the large intestine, the heart or the bladder (Kao 1973). Traditional acupuncture is still more complicated: the points chosen for treatment of a given malady are held to be influenced by the time of day, the weather and a multitude of other variables. Despite its apparent complexity, however, acupuncture analgesia may be explained by one or more basic physiological principles. Even acupuncture points, when displayed according to syndrome, appear to present a coherent picture. Most points are at or near the site of pain and a few are distant from it (Melzack et al 1977) (Figs 64.1 and 64.2).

Acupuncture was first described in the western world by the Dutch physician Willem ten Rhyne in 1683. After great initial enthusiasm, interest in acupuncture soon diminished. Since that time, acupuncture has been 'rediscovered' in the west about two or three times a century. Presently, acupuncture is used for various aches and pains, often with impressive results in cases of low-back pain, myofascial pain and some of the neuralgias (Macdonald 1982). The discovery by physiologists in China that peripheral nerves (rather than meridians) are essential for effective pain relief by acupuncture placed the practice on a firm scientific basis (Nathan 1978; Han & Terenius 1982; Takagi 1982). The importance of afferent transmission to achieve analgesia was demonstrated by observations that the analgesic effect is blocked by procaine infiltration of acupuncture points and that analgesia of rostral body areas cannot be induced by applying acupuncture to distant caudal sites in paraplegic or hemiplegic patients. The involvement of specific neurotransmitters in acupuncture analgesia was also indicated in early studies carried out in China, in which cerebrospinal fluid from donor rabbits after acupuncture raised pain thresholds in recipient rabbits, and by a large number of subsequent neuropharmacological studies reviewed by Han & Terenius (1982) and Takagi (1982).

Several kinds of evidence, obtained in western countries as well as in China, reveal the nature of acupuncture's action on pain. The first is the demonstration, in carefully controlled studies, that acupuncture has significantly greater effects on pain than placebo stimulation. An excellent review paper by Reichmanis & Becker (1977) examined 24 controlled studies on acupuncture analgesia for the relief of pain produced experimentally by radiant heat, electrical stimulation of tooth pulp, ischaemic pain and other procedures. Of the 24, three reported unequivocally negative results, four contained equivocal results and 17 demonstrated significant analgesic effects during electrical or manual stimulation at acupuncture loci. Most studies utilised manual stimulation, d.c. electrical stimulation, or very low frequency a.c. stimulation (usually 2 Hz). An induction time of about 20 minutes for full analgesia was reported in some of these studies. Several investigators (Anderson & Holmgren 1975; Jeans 1979; Chapman et al 1980) have also compared the relative effectiveness of near and distant acupuncture points and concluded that stimulation at sites close to the painful area is more effective than distant sites. The latter, however, frequently produces analgesic effects greater than a placebo. In general, the evidence acquired in controlled laboratory conditions has shown that acupuncture produces significantly greater analgesia than appropriate placebos, and that stimulation close to the site of pain is more effective than distant sites.

An impressive number of studies show that acupuncture stimulation need not be applied at the precise points indicated on acupuncture charts. It is possible, for example, to achieve as much control over dental pain by stimulating an area between the fourth and fifth fingers, which is not designated on acupuncture charts as related to facial pain, as by stimulating the Hoku point between the thumb and index finger which is so designated (Taub et al 1977). The decreases in pain obtained by stimulation at either site are so large and occur in so many patients that it is unlikely that the pain relief is due to placebo effects. Rather, the results suggest that the site that can be effectively stimulated is not a discrete point but a large area, possibly the whole hand.

The same conclusion can be drawn from another study – a double-blind experiment on the efficacy of acupuncture on osteoarthritic pain – in which the control patients received 'placebo' acupuncture stimulation at sites just

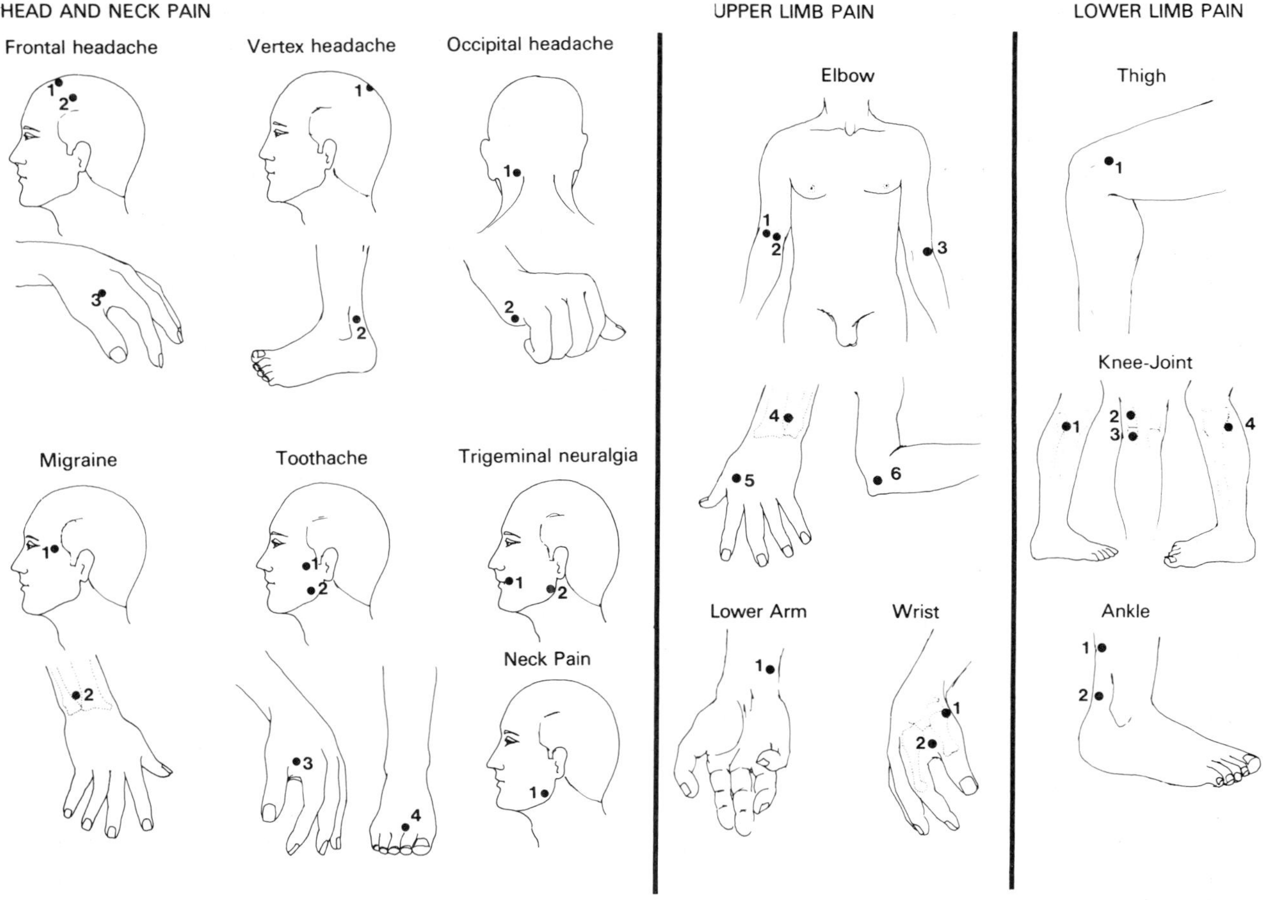

Fig. 64.1 Acupuncture points associated with head and neck pain, upper limb pain and lower limb pain (reprinted, with modifications, from Kao 1973). The acupuncture points for each syndrome are: *Head and neck pain*: frontal headache 1–Gv23, 2–S8, 3–Li4; vertex headache 1–Gv20, 2–B60; occipital headache 1–G20, 2–Si3; migraine 1–*t'ai yang*, 2–T5; toothache 1–S7, 2–S6, 3–Li4, 4–S44; trigeminal neuralgia 1–S4, 2–S6; neck pain 1–S6. *Upper limb pain*: elbow 1–L5, 2–B3, 3–Li11, 4–T4, 5–Li4, 6–T10; lower arm 1–H5; wrist 1–Li5, 2–Li4. *Lower limb pain*: thigh 1–Sp10; knee joint 1–G34, 2–S34, 3–S35, 4–Sp9; ankle 1–Sp6, 2–B60. Abbreviations of the acupuncture points: B = bladder; Cv = conception vessel; G = gall bladder; Gv = governing vessel; H = heart; K = kidney; L = lung; Li = large intestine; Liv = liver; P = pericardium; S = stomach; Si = small intestine; Sp = spleen; T = triple warmer; XH = nonmeridial point.

adjacent to the 'real' acupuncture points (Gaw et al 1975). Patients in both groups showed significant improvement in tenderness and subjective report of pain as evaluated by two independent observers, as well as in activity of the joint. Because there was no difference between the two groups, the improvement was attributed to a placebo effect. It is more likely, however, that it is stimulation within a large area and not merely at a particular point that has an effect. Similar conclusions can be drawn from an excellent study of acupuncture control over pain in patients with sickle cell anaemia (Co et al 1979). In fact, intense stimulation at many sites of the body may be effective. It is the intense stimulation rather than the precise site that appears to be the crucial factor. This is exactly the conclusion drawn by several writers (Ghia et al 1976; Lewit 1979), who showed that acupuncture stimulation of the painful area is as effective as stimulation at designated distant points. From all this it may be concluded that intense stimulation is the necessary factor, and the precise site of stimulation is less important than the intensity of the input.

That the pain relief produced by acupuncture cannot be attributed simply to a placebo effect is also indicated by the fact that partial analgesia can be produced in animals such as monkeys and mice (Vierck et al 1974; Pomeranz et al 1977; Sandrew et al 1978), and that acupuncture stimulation inhibits or otherwise changes the transmission of pain-evoked nerve impulses at several levels of the central nervous system (Kerr et al 1978). However, acupuncture needles are not essential to produce these effects. They are also produced by intense electrical stimulation, heat and a variety of intense sensory inputs (Le Bars et al 1983). The effectiveness of all of these forms of stimulation indicates that acupuncture is not a magical

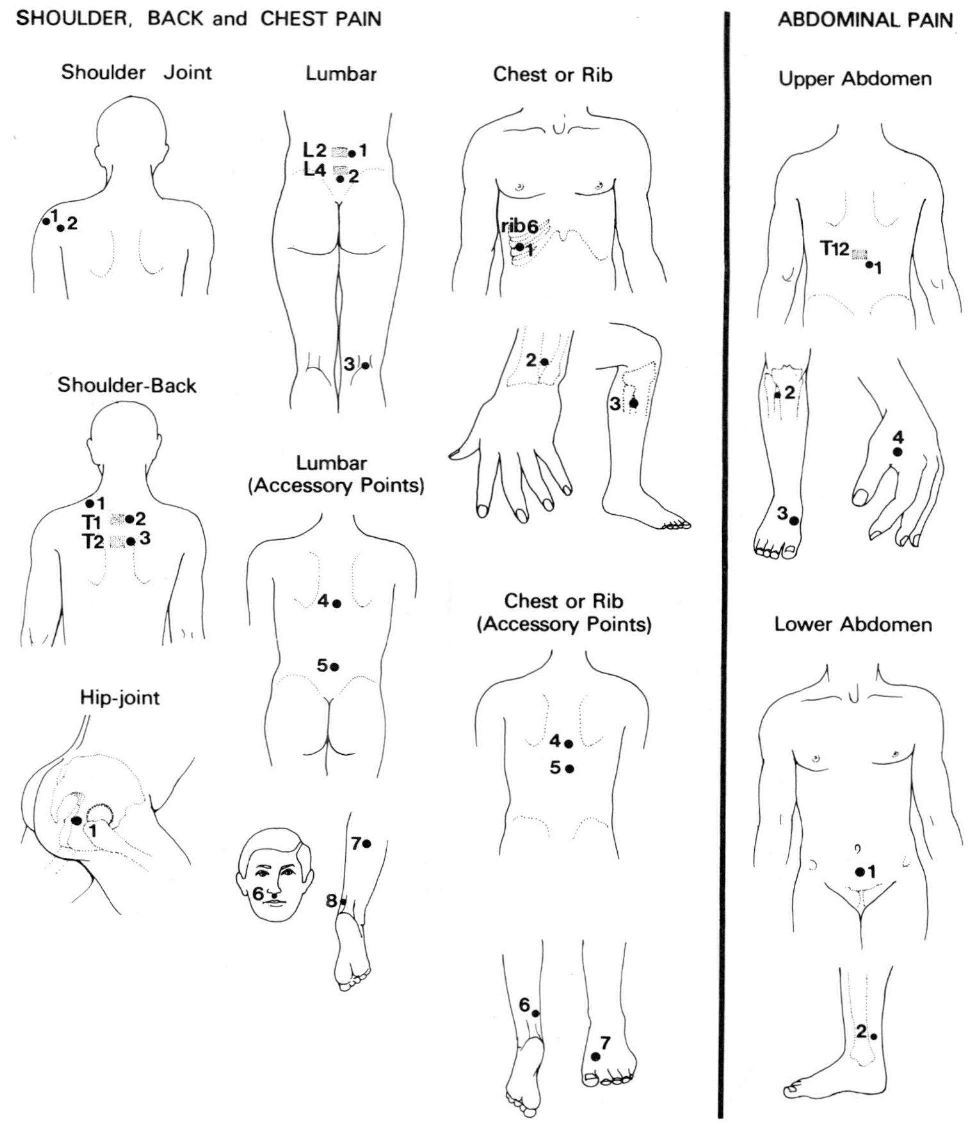

Fig. 64.2 Acupuncture points associated with shoulder, back and chest pain and abdominal pain (reprinted, with modifications, from Kao 1973). The acupuncture points for each syndrome are: *Shoulder, back and chest pain*: shoulder joint 1–Li15, 2–T14; shoulder-back 1–G21, 2–B12, 3–B43; hip joint 1–G30; lumbar 1–B23, 2–Gv3, 3–B54 (accessory points), 4–Gv9, 5–Gv4, 6–Gv26, 7–B57, 8–K3; chest or rib 1–Liv14, 2–T5, 3–G34, 4–B17, 5–B18, 6–Sp6, 7–Liv3. *Abdominal pain*: upper abdomen 1–B21, 2–S36, 3–Li4, 4–Sp4; pain around navel 1–S25; lower abdomen 1–Cv4, 2–Sp6. Abbreviations as in Fig. 64.1.

procedure, but only one of many ways to produce analgesia by an intense sensory input which may be labelled generally as 'hyperstimulation analgesia'.

HYPERSTIMULATION ANALGESIA

INTENSE TRANSCUTANEOUS ELECTRICAL NERVE STIMULATION

The concept that acupuncture is only one of many ways to deliver intense stimulation led Melzack (1975) to examine the effects of brief, intense transcutaneous electrical nerve stimulation (TENS) at trigger points or acupuncture points on severe clinical pain. The data indicated that the procedure produced significant relief of several forms of pathological pain. The duration of relief frequently outlasted the 20-minute period of stimulation by several hours, occasionally for days or weeks. Different patterns of the amount and duration of pain relief were observed. Daily stimulation carried out at home by the patient sometimes provided gradually increasing relief over periods of weeks or months. That these effects were not due to placebo phenomena was demonstrated in double-blind studies (Melzack 1975; Jeans 1979). Having established the effectiveness of brief periods of intense TENS, a study was then carried out by Fox & Melzack (1976) to compare the relative effectiveness of TENS and acupuncture on low-back pain. The results showed that both forms of stimulation at the same points produce substantial decreases in pain intensity but neither procedure is statistically more effective than the other. Most patients were relieved of pain for several hours, and some for 1 or more days. Statistical analysis also failed to reveal any differences in the duration of pain relief between the two procedures. Interestingly, an almost identical study was carried out independently in Finland at the same time (Laitinen 1976), in which it was also found that the two procedures are equally effective in relieving low-back pain. In a study of experimentally evoked tooth pain, Andersson & Holmgren (1975) similarly found that TENS and electroacupuncture through needles were equally effective.

These findings have important practical implications. The chief advantage of acupuncture is that the procedure is of short duration – at intense levels, stimulation may sometimes last only a few minutes. The method, however, is invasive and requires licensed practioners with specialised training. TENS, on the other hand, is non-invasive; once the appropriate points are located, it can be administered by paramedical personnel. Furthermore, once the procedure is found to be effective for a given patient, it can be self-administered by the patient with supervision by the physician.

Our understanding of hyperstimulation analgesia is further enhanced by studies which show that the distribution of acupuncture points is similar to that of trigger points (Travell & Rinzler 1952) and motor points (the points which produce maximal contraction of muscles and which have been shown to lie above the area of highest density of innervating motor neurons on the muscle). When acupuncture needles are inserted into sites that reduce pain, they produce a deep, aching feeling when twirled manually or electrically stimulated. This is reminiscent of the deep, aching feeling reported by patients when a trigger point is stimulated by the pressure of a finger pushing on it. This similarity led Melzack et al (1977) to examine the correlation between trigger points and acupuncture points for pain. The results of their analysis showed that every trigger point reported in the western medical literature has a corresponding acupuncture point. Furthermore, there is a close correspondence – 71% – between the pain syndromes associated with the two kinds of points. This close correlation suggests that trigger points and acupuncture points for pain, though discovered independently and labelled differently, represent the same phenomenon and can be explained in terms of similar underlying neural mechanisms.

A comparable study (Liu et al 1975) investigated the relationship between motor points and acupuncture loci and also found a remarkably high correspondence. This shows that there are sensitive sites on the body which produce a deep, aching feeling when they are palpated or needled, that they are intimately related to many common forms of chronic myofascial pains, and that many of these sites are related to the most densely innervated and most sensitive areas of muscles.

ICE MASSAGE

Ice massage is another way to produce intense sensory input. At first, ice massage of an area makes it feel numb. If ice massage is maintained, however, it produces aching, burning pain, and therefore may act like acupuncture or intense TENS. Melzack et al (1980a) treated patients suffering from acute dental pain with ice massage of the back of the hand (at the hoku area between the thumb and index finger) on the same side as the pain. The ice massage decreased the intensity of the dental pain by 50% or more in the majority of patients. Furthermore, ice massage of the hand on the side opposite to the pain also produced significant pain relief (Melzack & Bentley 1983).

Another study (Melzack et al 1980b) examined the relative effectiveness of ice massage and TENS for the relief of low-back pain. Patients suffering chronic low-back pain were treated with both ice massage and TENS. The results showed that both methods are equally effective: about 65% of patients obtained pain relief greater than 33% with each method. The results also revealed that ice massage is more effective than TENS for some patients, while TENS is more effective for others. Ice massage, then, may serve as an additional sensory-modulation method to alternate with TENS to overcome adaptation effects. Taken together, the results of both studies point to neural mechanisms that are similar to those of acupuncture and intense TENS.

The fact that stimulation of the hand persistently diminishes dental pain is one of the most dramatic examples of stimulation diminishing distant pain. It is known (Rossi & Brodal 1956; Torvik 1956) that there are direct projections from the spinal cord to the trigeminal nucleus which could mediate inhibitory effects of inputs from the limbs on trigeminal neurons. However, there is no information about the somatotopic organisation of these projections. In the light of recent evidence, a more likely mechanism to explain the effects of distant stimulation on dental pain is the loop involving afferent fibres from the upper limbs to the brainstem inhibitory control structures, and descending control fibres which go to the trigeminal subnucleus caudalis. This hypothesis receives strong support from the observation by Sessle et al (1981) that direct stimulation of the periaqueductal grey and related structures has a marked inhibitory effect on responses evoked in neurons in subnucleus caudalis by stimulation of the tooth pulp in the cat. Furthermore, responses evoked in individual neurons in the subnucleus caudalis by stimulating the tooth pulp are markedly inhibited by stimulation of the forepaws.

THE 'NEEDLE EFFECT'

The striking effectiveness of methods to relieve chronic pain by brief, intense sensory inputs has led several investigators to question whether their anaesthetic blocks relieve myofascial and back pains because of the anaesthetic agents or because of the insertion of the hypodermic needle. Astonishingly, the results are in favour of needling. Lewit (1979) has called this phenomenon the 'needle effect'.

In the 1950s several investigators discovered, independently of one another, that the insertion of a hypodermic needle through the skin, without injecting an anaesthetic or injecting only normal saline, often produces a dramatic relief of myofascial pains associated with the musculoskeletal system. Travell & Rinzler, in a classic paper published in 1952, summarised the work they carried out over a period of years demonstrating that 'dry needling' of trigger points – simply moving a needle in and out of the area without injecting any substance – produced striking relief of myofascial pain. Similarly, Sola & Williams (1956) discovered that injecting normal saline was highly effective. In fact, Kibler (1958) reported that different kinds of anaesthetics have virtually identical effects which are barely influenced by the amount and concentration of the anaesthetic injected.

These observations led Frost et al (1980) to carry out a double-blind comparison of a local anaesthetic (mepivacaine) and saline injected into trigger points for myofascial pain. To their astonishment, the group that received saline tended to have significantly more relief of pain: 80% of patients with saline reported pain relief compared with 52% with mepivacaine. Furthermore, the average duration of relief was 3 hours for saline and 30 minutes for mepivacaine. Clearly, the pain relief could not be due to the anaesthetic but was more likely to be due to the insertion of the needle into the trigger point. The saline was more effective, the authors proposed, because it irritated tissues, which is the essential ingredient of the treatment, while the mepivacaine actually blocked the irritating effect of the needle.

These results are in agreement with Lewit's observations that the 'needle effect' is the crucial factor in relieving myofascial pain. The effectiveness of the treatment, he observes, bears little relationship to the agent injected, but is 'related to the intensity of pain produced at the trigger zone, and to the precision with which the site of maximal tenderness was located by the needle' (Lewit 1979). The needle, in short, must penetrate at the point of maximum pain. While this sounds like torture, the brief shot of pain produced by the needle resulted in striking relief of pain in 86.8% of cases and persistent relief for months or even permanently in about 50% of the cases.

AURICULOTHERAPY

The claim by the French physician Nogier (1972) that electrical stimulation at points of the outer ear abolishes pain has led to widespread use of 'auriculotherapy'. Nogier argued, moreover, that the body is represented at the ear in the shape of an inverted homunculus. These claims are so remarkable that several serious investigators have set out to examine them. Bossy et al (1977) have observed a highly complex neural and vascular organisation of the auricle which they believe provides the basis for Nogier's proposed somatotopic map. Far more remarkable is a clinical demonstration (Oleson et al 1980), in a well-designed double-blind trial, of a somatotopic organisation at the ear. A physiological basis of auriculotherapy has also been reported. Pert et al (1981) found that auricular electrostimulation produced naloxone-reversible analgesia in the rat accompanied by increased endorphin levels in the cerebrospinal fluid and evidence of depletion of endorphin in the periaqueductal grey matter.

Despite these positive data, Melzack & Katz (1983) were unable to confirm Nogier's claims with subjects suffering a variety of pain problems. The first part of a double-blind study was undertaken to see whether pain is relieved more effectively by stimulation at designated 'Nogier' points on the ear than at 'control' spots elsewhere on the ear. The experiment failed to show any difference. A second study was therefore carried out in which stimulation at 'Nogier' points was compared with a placebo control which provided no stimulation. Again, there was no greater relief of pain after stimulation of the 'Nogier' points. However, about a third of the patients reported that they felt warmth, 'glowing feelings' and other sensations in distant parts of the body when the ear was stimulated (Katz & Melzack 1987). These referred sensations indicate that inputs from the ear project to central integrating structures which may play a role in the important clinical phenomenon of referred sensation. In their most recent study, using only patients with phantom limb pain, Katz & Melzack (1991) found that auricular stimulation produced modest though statistically significant relief of pain compared to a no-stimulation control group. Clearly, further studies are needed (see Johnson et al 1991).

PHYSIOLOGICAL MECHANISMS

The evidence examined so far indicates that there are three major properties of acupuncture and other forms of hyperstimulation analgesia:

1. a moderate-to-intense sensory input is applied to the body to alleviate pain
2. the sensory input is sometimes applied to a site distant from the site of pain, and
3. the sensory input, which is usually of brief duration (ranging from a few seconds to 20 or 30 minutes) may relieve chronic pain for days, weeks, sometimes permanently.

Recent physiological research allows speculation about the first and second properties, while the third property remains as elusive as the physiological basis of learning and memory.

CONTROL OF PAIN BY INTENSE STIMULATION

It is widely held (Melzack 1971, 1973; Mayer & Price 1976; Basbaum & Fields 1978; Watkins & Mayer 1982) that this property is best explained in terms of brainstem mechanisms that exert a descending inhibitory control over transmission through the dorsal horns as well as at higher levels in the somatic projection system. Intense somatic stimuli of almost any kind would produce pain but would also activate the brainstem mechanisms which could exert an inhibitory effect on transmission through the dorsal horns (Le Bars et al 1983). Basically, the concept holds that intense inputs activate small-diameter

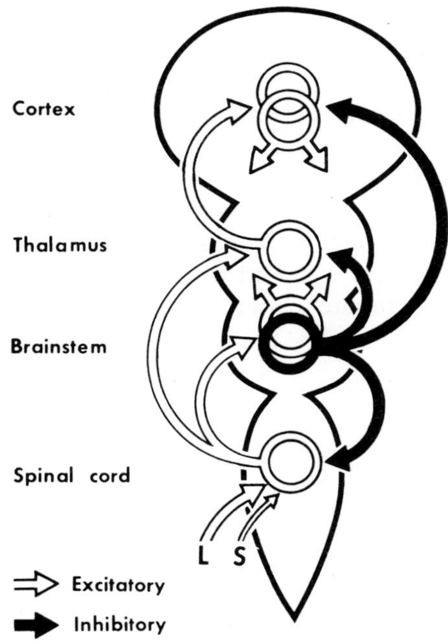

Fig. 64.3 Schematic diagram of the central biasing mechanism. Large (L) and small (S) fibres from a limb activate a neuron pool in the spinal cord, which excites neuron pools at successively higher levels. The central biasing mechanism, represented by the inhibitory projection system that originates in the brainstem reticular formation, modulates activity at all levels. Loss of inputs to the system would weaken the inhibition. Increased sensory input or direct electrical stimulation would increase the inhibition.

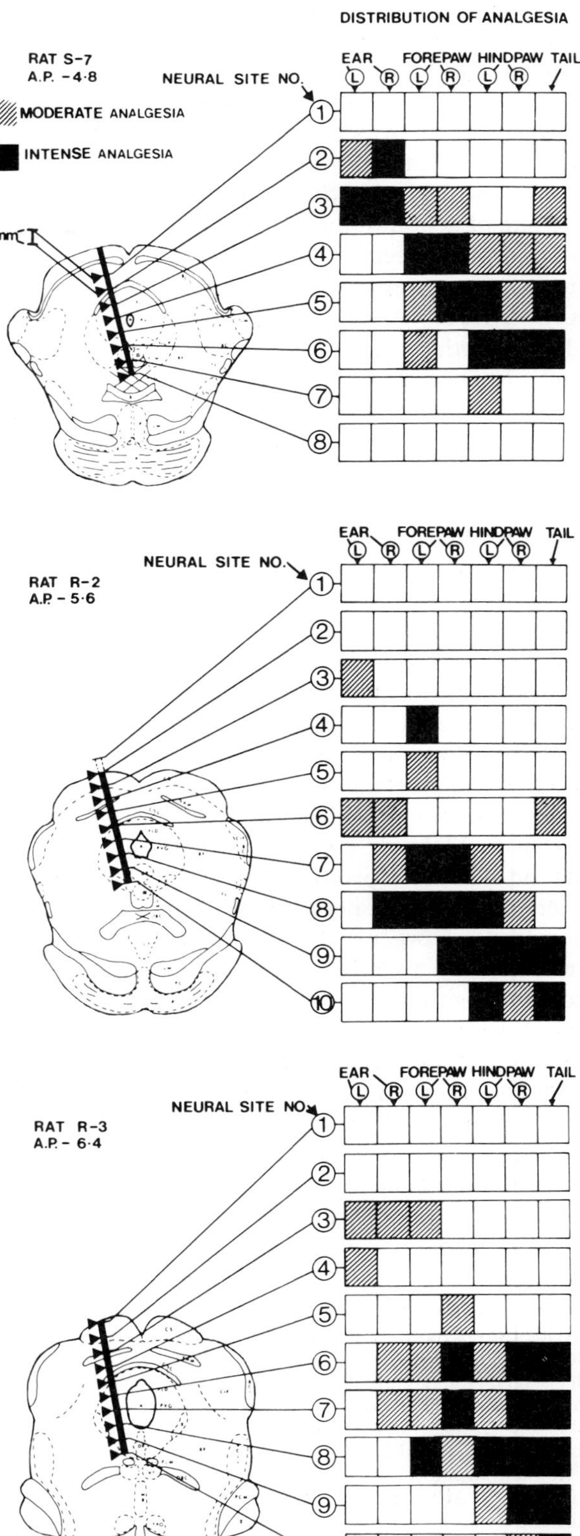

Fig. 64.4 Histological reconstruction of the series of stimulation sites in three subjects and the corresponding distribution of cutaneous analgesic fields. Moderate analgesia is denoted by the hatched squares and intense analgesia by the solid black squares.

fibres which project to cells in the periaqueductal grey. These in turn activate a serotonergic system that ultimately modulates transmission through the dorsal horns. The entire system, then, comprises a complex feedback loop in which small-fibre inputs comprise the feedforward segment while the descending inhibitory system is the feedback. Since the periaqueductal grey is a major site of action of morphine and contains endorphins and endorphin receptors (Snyder 1980), the observation that naloxone reverses needle-acupuncture analgesia totally (Mayer et al 1977) and electroacupuncture analgesia partially (Sjolund & Eriksson 1979) is cited as strong evidence that acupuncture and related forms of treatment are mediated by means of this neural loop through the brainstem. However, the failure to demonstrate a reversal by naloxone of the effects of acupuncture applied at near or distant sites on evoked responses and subjective pain report (Chapman et al 1980) suggests that additional mechanisms may be operating.

DISTANT BODY SITES

The brainstem mechanisms can also explain the second property – relief of pain by intense stimulation at a distant site. These brainstem areas may be conceptualised as a `central biasing mechanism' (Melzack 1971, 1973) which acts as an inhibitory feedback system (Fig. 64.3).

Soper & Melzack (1982) systematically mapped the analgesic skin areas produced by electrical stimulation of discrete points of the periaqueductal grey. They observed a dorsoventral organisation in which the face is represented dorsally and the more caudal parts of the body become analgesic as the electrode tip is moved ventrally (Fig. 64.4). This organisation was maintained throughout the rostrocaudal extent of the midbrain. However, rostral stimulation sites tended to produce analgesia in smaller, more discrete fields than those produced by caudal stimulation sites. Further studies showed that the relationship between stimulation-produced analgesia and stimulation site is influenced by the electrical stimulation current level. Each site had an optimum current level, so that current intensities higher or lower than the optimum produced decreased analgesia. These results reveal a possible neural mechanism for somatotopic organisation in hyperstimulation analgesia in which an intense somatic input at a body site produces analgesia in the same or distant segments. Particular body areas project especially strongly to discrete regions of the periaqueductal grey (Groves et al 1973). These regions, in turn, exert an inhibitory control over pain signals from particular parts of the body. However, it is important to keep in mind that cells in the periaqueductal grey at adjacent areas project rostrally as well as caudally, and the effects of localised brain stimulation may also be exerted on structures in the forebrain (Abbott & Melzack 1982).

PAIN RELIEF OUTLASTS STIMULATION

The final property – prolonged relief of pain by brief stimulation – may be explained by assuming that the physiological processes which subserve pain may persist as a result of abnormal, memory-like activity produced by injury (Katz & Melzack 1990; Katz et al 1991). Intense stimulation could block this activity by direct spinal inhibition or by means of inhibition through the structures that comprise the central biasing mechanism. The increased physical activity permitted by the relief of pain, which would produce normally patterned sensory inputs, would tend to prevent the recurrence of the abnormal neural activity and the pain it produces. Repeated periods of pain relief followed by increased physical activity and normal inputs might be the basis of the gradually increasing effectiveness of intense TENS which is sometimes observed (Melzack 1975). The duration and degree of relief sometimes become progressively greater over a period of weeks or months. In the occasional fortunate patient, the pain may disappear altogether.

REFERENCES

Abbott F V, Melzack, R 1982 Brainstem lesions dissociate neural mechanisms of morphine analgesia in different kinds of pain. Brain Research 251: 149–156

Andersson A, Holmgren E 1975 On acupuncture analgesia and the mechanism of pain. American Journal of Chinese Medicine 3: 311–334

Basbaum A E, Fields H L 1978 Endogenous pain control mechanisms: review and hypothesis. Annals of Neurology 4: 451–462

Bonica J J 1974 Anesthesiology in the People's Republic of China. Anesthesiology 40: 175–186

Bossy J, Golewski G, Maurel J C, Seoane M 1977 Innervation and vascularization of the auricula correlated with the loci of auriculotherapy. Acupuncture and Electrotherapeutics Research, the International Journal 2: 247–257

Brockbank W 1954 Ancient therapeutic arts. Heinemann, London

Chapman C R, Colpitts Y M, Benedetti C, Kitaeff R, Gehrig J D 1980 Evoked potential assessment of acupunctural analgesia: attempted reversal with naloxone. Pain 9: 183–197

Co L L, Schmitz T H, Havdala H, Reyes A, Westerman M P 1979 Acupuncture: an evaluation in the painful crises of sickle cell anaemia. Pain 7: 181–185

Fox E J, Melzack R 1976 Transcutaneous electrical stimulation and acupuncture: comparison of treatment for low-back pain. Pain 2: 141–148

Frost F A, Jessen B, Siggaard-Andersen J 1980 A control, double-blind comparison of mepivacaine injection versus saline injection for myofascial pain. Lancet 8 March: 499–501

Gaw A C, Chang L W, Shaw L C 1975 Efficacy of acupuncture on osteoarthritic pain. New England Journal of Medicine 293: 375–378

Ghia J N, Mao W, Toomey T C, Gregg J M 1976 Acupuncture and chronic pain mechanisms Pain 2: 285–299

Groves P M, Miller S W, Parker M V, Rebec G V 1973 Organization by

sensory modality in the reticular formation of the rat. Brain Research 54: 207–212
Han J S, Terenius L 1982 Neurochemical basis of acupuncture analgesia. Annual Review of Pharmacology and Toxicology 22: 193–220
Jeans M E 1979 Relief of chronic pain by brief, intense transcutaneous electrical stimulation – a double-blind study. In: Bonica J J, Liebeskind J C, Albe-Fessard D G (eds) Advances in pain research and therapy 3. Raven Press, New York, p 601–606
Johnson M I, Hajela V K, Ashton C H, Thompson J W 1991 The effects of auricular transcutaneous electrical nerve stimulation (TENS) on experimental pain threshold and autonomic function in healthy subjects. Pain 46: 337–342
Kao F F 1973 Acupuncture therapeutics. Eastern Press, New Haven, Conn.
Katz J, Melzack R 1987 Referred sensations in chronic pain patients. Pain 28: 51–59
Katz J, Melzack R 1990 Pain 'memories' in phantom limbs; review and clinical observations. Pain 43: 319–336
Katz J, Melzack R 1991 Auricular transcutaneous electrical nerve stimulation (TENS) reduces phantom limb pain. Journal of Pain and Symptom Management 6: 73–83
Katz J, Vaccarino A L, Coderre T J, Melzack R 1991 Injury prior to neurectomy alters the pattern of autotomy in rats. Anesthesiology 75: 876–883
Kerr F W L, Wilson P R, Nijensohn D E 1978 Acupuncture reduces the trigeminal evoked response in decerebrate cats. Experimental Neurology 61: 84–95
Kibler M 1958 Das Storungsfeld bei Gelenkserkrankungen und inneren Krankheiten. Hippokrates, Stuttgart
Laitinen J 1976 Acupuncture and transcutaneous electric stimulation in the treatment of chronic sacrolumbalgia and ischialgia. American Journal of Chinese Medicine 4: 169–175
Le Bars D, Dickenson A H, Besson J M 1983 Opiate analgesia and descending control systems. In: Bonica J J, Lindblom U, Iggo A (eds) Advances in pain research and therapy. Raven Press, New York, p 341–372
Lewit K 1979 The needle effect in the relief of myofascial pain. Pain 6: 83–90
Liu Y K, Varela M, Oswald R 1975 The correspondence between some motor points and acupuncture loci. American Journal of Chinese Medicine 3: 347–358
Macdonald A J R 1982 Acupuncture from ancient art to modern medicine. Allen & Unwin, London
Mayer D J, Price D D 1976 Central nervous system mechanisms of analgesia. Pain 2: 379–404
Mayer D J, Price D D, Rafii A 1977 Antagonism of acupuncture analgesia in man by the narcotic antagonist naloxone. Brain Research 121: 368–372
Melzack R 1971 Phantom limb pain: implications for treatment of pathological pain. Anesthesiology 35: 409–419
Melzack R 1973 The puzzle of pain. Basic Books, New York
Melzack R 1975 Prolonged relief of pain by brief, intense transcutaneous somatic stimulation. Pain 1: 357–373
Melzack R, Bentley K C 1983 Relief of dental pain by ice massage of either hand or the contralateral arm. Journal of the Canadian Dental Association 106: 257–260
Melzack R, Katz J 1984 Auriculotherapy fails to relieve chronic pain. Journal of the American Medical Association 251: 1041–1043
Melzack R, Stillwell D M, Fox E J 1977 Trigger points and acupuncture points for pain: correlations and implications. Pain 3: 3–23
Melzack R, Guité S, Gonshor A 1980a Relief of dental pain by ice massage of the hand. Canadian Medical Association Journal 122: 189–191
Melzack R, Jeans M E, Stratford J G, Monks R C 1980b Ice massage and transcutaneous electrical stimulation: comparison of treatment for low-back pain. Pain 9: 209–217
Meschig R, Schadewaldt H 1982 Skull trepanation in Eastern Africa. Hexagon <Roche> 9: 17–24
Nathan P W 1978 Acupuncture analgesia. Trends in Neurosciences July: 21–23
Nogier P F M 1972 Treatise of auriculotherapy. Maisonneuve, Moulin-les-Metz
Oleson T D, Kroening R J, Bressler D E 1980 An experimental evaluation of auricular diagnosis: the somatotopic mapping of musculo-skeletal pain at ear acupuncture points. Pain 8: 217–229
Pert A, Dionne R, Ng L et al 1981 Alterations in rat central nervous system endorphins following transauricular electroacupuncture. Brain Research 224: 83–93
Pomeranz B, Cheng R, Law P 1977 Acupuncture reduces electrophysiological and behavioural responses to noxious stimuli: pituitary is implicated. Experimental Neurology 54: 172–178
Primosch R E, Young S K 1980 Pseudobattering of Vietnamese children (*cao gio*). Journal of the American Dental Association 101: 47–48
Reichmanis M, Becker R O 1977 Relief of experimentally induced pain by stimulation at acupuncture loci. Comparative Medicine East and West 5: 281–288
Rossi G F, Brodal A 1956 Spinal afferents to the trigeminal sensory nuclei and to the nucleus of the solitary tract. Confinia Neurologica 16: 321–332
Sandrew B B, Yang R C C, Wang S C 1978 Electro-acupuncture analgesia in monkeys: a behavioural and neurophysiological assessment. Archives Internationales de Pharmacodynamie et de Thérapie 231: 274–284
Sessle B J, Hu J W, Dubner R, Lucier G E 1981 Functional properties of neurons in cat trigeminal subnucleus caudalis (medullary dorsal horn). II. Modulation of responses to noxious and non-noxious stimuli by periaqueductal grey, nucleus raphe magnus, cerebral cortex, and afferent influences, and effect of naloxone. Journal of Neurophysiology 45: 211–255
Sjolund B H, Eriksson M B E 1979 Endorphins and analgesia produced by peripheral conditioning stimulation. In: Bonica J J, Albe-Fessard D, Liebeskind J C (eds) Advances in pain research and therapy 3. Raven Press, New York, p 587–599
Snyder S 1980 Brain peptides as neurotransmitters. Science 209: 976–983
Sola A E, Williams R L 1956 Myofascial pain syndromes. Neurology 6: 91–95
Soper W Y, Melzack R 1982 Stimulation-produced analgesia: evidence for somatotopic organisation in the midbrain. Brain Research 251: 301–311
Takagi H 1982 Critical review of pain relieving procedures including acupuncture. Advances in pharmacology and therapeutics II. CNS pharmacology. Neuropeptides 1: 79–92
Taub H A, Beard M C, Eisenberg L, McCormack R K 1977 Studies of acupuncture for operative dentistry. Journal of the American Dental Association 95: 555–561
Torvik A 1956 Afferent connections to the sensory trigeminal nuclei, the nucleus of the solitary tract and adjacent structures. Journal of Comparative Neurology 106: 51–132
Travell J, Rinzler S H 1952 The myofascial genesis of pain. Postgraduate Medicine 11: 425–434
Vierck C J, Lineberry C G, Lee P K, Calderwood H W 1974 Prolonged hypalgesia following 'acupuncture' in monkeys. Life Sciences 15: 1277–1289
Wand-Tetley J I 1956 Historical methods of counter-irritation. Annals of Physical Medicine 3: 90–98
Watkins L R, Mayer D J 1982 Organization of endogenous opiate and nonopiate pain control systems. Science 216: 1185–1192

65. Spinal cord stimulation

J. -U. Krainick and U. Thoden

DESCRIPTION OF THE TREATMENT

The argument for the development of dorsal column stimulation (DCS) for pain relief has been the gate control theory of Melzack & Wall (1965) and the therapeutic success in stimulating peripheral nerves and dorsal roots (Wall & Sweet 1967). In 1967 Shealy et al described relief of chronic intractable pain by a radiofrequency-induced electrical stimulation of the spinal cord using implanted electrodes over the dorsal columns. Since that time many reports have been published on DCS, not only for pain relief (Nashold & Friedman 1972; Hunt et al 1975; Krainick et al 1975, 1980; Nielson et al 1975; Pineda 1975; Burton 1977; Lazorthes et al 1978; Krainick & Thoden 1981a, 1981b) but also for movement disorders (Cook 1974; Illis et al 1976; Krainick et al 1977; Siegfried et al 1978; Tallis et al 1983; Barolat-Romana et al 1985) and peripheral vascular diseases (Cook et al 1976; Meglio et al 1981; Tallis et al 1983; Augustinsson et al 1985; Broseta et al 1986; Linderoth 1992).

Although the initial concept involved stimulation of the dorsal columns, it became obvious from ventral electrode placements (Larsen et al 1975) that the actual neural tissues stimulated by the electrodes were unknown and that stimulation applied to the ventral surface, or from dorsal to ventral surfaces, could also be effective in relieving pain. The actual current pathways are difficult to determine and the physiological basis of pain relief from spinal cord stimulation (SCS) is still uncertain. Whether the effect of electrical stimulation is to activate certain axons which inhibit pain, or to block transmission in axons subserving pain sensation, is unknown.

In recent studies it was supposed that central neurohumoral systems may be activated by the electrical stimulation. Originally stimulation was achieved by the surgical implantation of electrodes close to the dorsal columns after laminectomy. Electrodes (unipolar or bipolar) were fixed at the dura in the subarachnoidal space (Nashold & Friedman 1972; Shealy et al 1967). However, the spinal cord may also be stimulated by electrodes inserted percutaneously into the epidural space. It thus seems more appropriate to use the term 'spinal cord stimulation' (SCS) instead of 'dorsal column stimulation' (DCS).

Two important facts should be mentioned, as they were the reasons for further development of new techniques. First, in some patients the induced paraesthesias are more unpleasant than the pain itself. Second, the pain is only alleviated when the electrically-induced paraesthesias cover the painful area; this means that the induced input to the fast-fibre system should be identical to the chronic-pain input (Krainick et al 1975). This may explain why, in cases of cervical root avulsion, the patient reports no paraesthesia in the painful area during stimulation and no pain relief, depending on degeneration of afferent fibres and their connections (Wall 1984).

For both reasons in the beginning of this method a preoperative test stimulation was done either by direct puncture of the spinal cord or by intrathecal electrodes. These methods for testing could not guarantee the final projection of the paraesthesias induced by stimulation of the surgically-implanted electrodes. These problems nowadays are solved by electrode placements in local anaesthesia with continuous verbal contact with the patient during surgery.

METHOD AND DEVICES

SURGICAL PROCEDURE

The implantation of a spinal cord stimulation system is a surgical procedure which requires the highest level of asepsis. The rate of infection ranges from 80% under worst conditions to below 1% under optimal conditions. The implantation is carried out under local anaesthesia, the patient places in a prone position on an X-ray table. One spinal interspace is selected for puncture of the epidural space from a paramedian lateral approach using Thouhy-type needles.

It is important that the path of the electrode through the muscle has to be as short as possible, because the displacement is almost always caused by contractions of paraspinal muscles. The tips of the needle should be positioned in the midline, in order to avoid lateral or ventral drifting of the electrode. The electrode is inserted through the needle and advanced in cranial direction. The final position of the tip of the electrode is determined by electrical stimulation. The electrode is brought into that position in which the patient reports electrically-induced paraesthesias exactly in the painful area. It is also possible to stimulate the root selectively with a lateral position of the electrode, e.g. in patients with pain after lesion of peripheral nerves of the upper extremities.

The distance between the insertion and the tip of the electrode should be as long as possible to avoid dislocation. The best level of electrode position in pain of lower extremities is the middle and lower thoracic region and for upper extremities the higher thoracic or lower cervical region. Positioning the tip in the middle or higher cervical level should be avoided, because of the alteration in the intensity of stimulation during head movements. This phenomenon is also observed in the lumbar and thoracic region, but to a lesser degree. If stimulation fails to produce paraesthesias in the painful areas, the electrode is removed.

If the test stimulation alleviates the pain, a receiver is internalised in a second surgical step, connecting the electrode. The patient is able to stimulate the implanted system either inductively by an external transmitter and to vary the combinations of the active polesor using a fully-implantable system in which the battery-powered stimulator is subcutaneous.

PATIENT SELECTION

It was clear very soon that a twofold selective process was indicated, psychological and technical.

Trial stimulation that is performed during surgery must have as an objective to cover the painful area with tingling induced by electric stimulation. Most authors stress the congruence of satisfactory pain relief and a complete covering of pain area and induced paraesthesias. A good covering yields successful results in 64% and failures in only 9%. Long & Erickson (1975) found that in 33% of their failures this covering could not be obtained. However, even a good covering cannot guarantee complete pain relief.

The second step of the selective process (the psychological investigation of the patient) is much more complicated. There are various psychological aspects that have to be taken into consideration. Patients with major psychological problems should not be operated on, but it is not always easy to detect these problems and the help of a psychiatrist is indicated. The stimulation procedures seem to be much more effective in subjects without severe psychological overlay, and the majority of the failures consisted of patients with serious psychological or psychiatric problems (Long et al 1981; Ray 1988). The presence of drug addiction is not an absolute contraindication for the operation, but it should be treated separately after pain relief has been obtained. Naturally a search should be made for the aetiology of the pain, because it is preferable, whenever possible, to treat the underlying cause specifically, rather than symptomatically.

In order to obtain good results implantation of a spinal cord stimulation system should be performed only on patients whose pain is well defined in localisation and origin. Patients with neurogenic pain are the best qualified to undergo this implantation. Neurogenic pain occurs when a nerve or a nerve root is damaged and ectopic receptors develop. These ectopic receptors appear in patients with epidural fibrosis after disc surgery and after damage of peripheral nerves. The localisation and origin of this type of pain are evident and can be verified by performing anaesthetic blocks. Moreover it must be proven by nuclear magnetic resonance imaging or computed tomography that this pain is caused by epidural fibrosis. If lateral or central stenosis or instability of the lumbar spine is the source of pain in patients with failed-back-surgery syndrome, it stands to reason a decompression or fusion is to be preferred.

RESULTS OF SPINAL CORD STIMULATION

PERCUTANEOUS TEST STIMULATION

Two surgical steps are needed when an implantation of a spinal cord stimulator is performed. These steps should not be carried out at the same time because prior trial stimulation has great prognostic value for the success of the method of final implantation of a neurostimulation system. Prospective studies led to the conclusion that the efficacy of the selective process doubles the success rate of the late outcome.

After a positive stimulation test the patient has a 70% chance to benefit from the operation while a negative result of the stimulation test reduces the chance to 25%. The value of test stimulation was also confirmed by Burton (1975) and North et al (1977/78). Since the transcutaneous electric nerve stimulation (TENS) has no prognostic value for the late outcome of spinal cord stimulation, as recently stated by Spiegelmann & Friedman (1991), it is only logical and absolutely essential to perform the trial stimulation under exactly the same conditions as the final implantation. The trial electrode which has been implanted can remain as the final electrode or it can be replaced by a plate electrode but must be kept at exactly the same localisation (Table 65.1).

INITIAL AND LONG-TERM RESULTS

Table 65.2 shows the overall results of early and late observation periods for SCS with implanted electrodes via

Table 65.1 Test stimulation versus operative results

Pain relief during test stimulation	Pain relief after operation					
	n	0	0–25%	25–50%	50–75%	75–100%
Excellent pain relief	46	10	6	7	11	12
Marked reduction of pain	12	5	2	4	0	1
Painfree interval	8	1	4	1	1	1
No statement of value	7	3	1	1	1	1
Total	73	19	13	13	13	15

Table 65.2 Early results of 726 patients: European study group (1977) 168; Nashold 30; Sweet 97; Burton 63; Pineda 79; Hunt 10; Nielson 130; Shealy 80; Long 69. Late results of 468 patients: Nashold 25; Shealy 80; Nielson 130; Long 55; Sheldon 27; Krainick 73; Sweet 68.

	Pain relief				
	0	0–25%	25–50%	50–75%	75–100%
Early results	241	81	129	71	204
(n = 726)	33%	11%	18%	10%	28%
Late (n = 468)	232	72	54	17	83
	50.5%	15.5%	11.5%	3.5%	19%

laminectomy. Our own results of a long-term follow-up over 5 years are shown in Table 65.3

Winkelmüller (1981) reported results on percutaneous test stimulation. Out of 94 patients tested 71 were finally implanted. For a group of 56 patients with low-back pain, a success rate of 87% short-term follow-up and 69% long-term follow-up was reported.

De la Porte & van de Kelft (1992) reviewed their experience in SCS in treating 64 patients with failed-back surgery syndromes for a mean follow-up period of 4 years: 35 patients (55%) continued to experience at least 50% of pain relief, 58 patients (90%) could reduce their medication, 39 patients (61%) reported that their ability to perform daily activities had improved significantly and 53 patients (83%) continued to use their device at the latest follow-up.

Pain after damage of peripheral nerves is a reasonable indication for spinal cord stimulation. Amputees who have massive damage to their peripheral nerves represent a homogeneous group of candidates for this method. In their case the localisation and origin of pain are also obvious. With careful screening early results of 60% of pain relief and 40% for long-term results can be realised (Krainick et al 1980).

DISCUSSION

METHODS, SIDE-EFFECTS, COMPLICATIONS AND MODIFICATIONS

For chronic implantation via laminectomy nowadays multipolar electrodes are preferred. Monopolar electrodes, especially those placed below the dura, lose their efficacy rapidly and are responsible for more side-effects, i.e. radicular dysaesthesias (Sedan & Lazorthes 1978). Pineda (1975) has observed that bipolar electrodes produce more direct failures at the outset, whereas unipolar electrodes produce more delayed failures. He found 25.5% of late failures with bipolar electrodes, and in monopolar implantation 45.5%. This may be due to the smaller size of the unipolar electrode and the associated higher current density. The larger bipolar electrode allows electrical stimulation to leak through the developing thickening of the surrounding tissue. This may account for the intermittent or irregular stimulation sometimes seen.

Today these problems are historical, because percutaneous multipolar electrodes in the epidural space are now in use. Implantations via laminectomy are only performed when puncture of the epidural space is not possible.

Due to technical problems, dislocations of the percutaneously inserted electrodes has often been seen. This dislocation results from a coiling of the electrode, which develops between the epidural space and the external fascia of the contracting muscle resulting in an ineffective stimulation. If this happens twice, we perform a small laminectomy in general or spinal anaesthesia and implant a multipolar-plated electrode at the same level.

The possible side-effects of the stimulating electrodes in the epidural space include radicular dyaesthesias if the electrodes are more than about 2 mm paramedian. Infections are relatively rare (4 out of 126). In these instances the system has to be removed immediately.

Location and level of implantation

At first all authors reported implantation of the electrodes below the dura (extra of subarachnoidal). Later, in order to avoid arachnoidal reactions and cerebrospinal fluid leakage, endodural implantations were preferred (Burton 1975; Krainick et al 1975). Some authors preferred stimulation of the anterior part of the spinal cord, since it seems to be more efficient in obtaining pain relief without the disturbing paraesthesias (Hoppenstein 1975; Larson et al 1975; Lazorthes et al 1978). However, in clinical efficacy no difference was evident. In our series we saw uncomfortable motor side-effects.

Stimulation should take place in the segments above the painful dermatomes (4–5 segments according to Shealy (1975), 1–2 segments according to Sweet & Wepsic 1975). For practical use, Nashold (1975) recommended implantation at C2–C4 for pain in the upper extremities and trunk and implantation at T2–T7 for pain states below. We observed in some patients that stimulation at the level of T4 was able to induce paraesthesia and pain relief in the upper extremities as well.

Table 65.3 Pain relief in patients with spinal cord stimulation

Diagnosis	No. of cases	Pain relief				
		0	0–25%	25–50%	50–75%	75–100%
Initial results (evaluated 1974 to 1975)						
Arm amputated	13	4	0	0	6	3
Leg amputated	51	14	10	7	10	10
Total amputees	64		43.7%		56.3%	
Spinal, radicular peripheral nerve lesions	12	6	2	2	1	1
Other pain syndromes	8	4	0	2	1	1
Total	84		47.6%		52.4%	
Long-term results (evaluated 1977)						
Arm amputated	13	5	1	2	4	1
Leg amputated	48	23	6	10	9	0
Total amputees	61		57.4%		42.6%	
Spinal, radicular peripheral nerve lesions	12	8	–	4	–	–
Other pain syndromes	4	4	–	–	–	–
Total	77	61%			39%	

Superposition of painful segments and induced paraesthesias

Most authors stress the congruence of good pain relief and a complete superposition of pain and induced paraesthesias. A good superposition yields good results in 64% and failures in only 9.5% (Krainick et al 1975, 1980). In addition, Long & Erikson (1975) found that in 33% of their failures this superposition could not be obtained. But even a good superposition cannot guarantee a complete pain relief (see also Nielson & Hunt (1975)).

INDICATIONS FOR SPINAL CORD STIMULATION

The German Society for Neurosurgery (Arbeitsgruppe Schmerztherapie) gives the following guidelines for indications, possible indications and no indications for implantation of spinal cord stimulation systems for pain control.

Main indications

1. Failed-back surgery syndromes
2. Postamputation pain
3. Incomplete plexus lesions (cervical, brachial, lumbar)
4. Peripheral nerve lesions
5. Sympathetic reflex dystrophy
6. Rest pain in peripheral vascular disease.

Possible indications

1. Peripheral vascular disease, angina pectoris
2. Incomplete transverse lesion of the spinal cord.

No indication

1. Complete transverse lesions of the spinal cord
2. Cancer pain
3. Deafferentation pain in spinal-root avulsion
4. Postherpetic neuralgia.

In summary the best results will be obtained:

1. with multipolar electrodes
2. with epidural placement
3. when electrodes are localised above the pain segments
4. if stimulation paraesthesias and pain segments superimpose without radicular irritation
5. when the patient has no secondary gain from his pain
6. when the pain is localised rather than diffuse.

REFERENCES

Augustinsson L E, Holm J, Jivegard L, Carlsson C A 1985 Epidural electrical stimulation in severe limb ischaemia. Evidences of pain relief, increased blood flow and a possible limb-saving effect. Annals of Surgery 202: 104–111

Barolat-Romana G, Myklebust J B, Hemmy D C, Myklebust B, Wenninger W 1985 Immediate effects of spinal cord stimulation in spinal spasticity. Journal of Neurosurgery 62: 558–562

Broseta J, Barbera J, De Vera J A et al 1986 Spinal cord stimulation in peripheral arterial disease. Journal of Neurosurgery 64: 71–80

Burton C 1975 Dorsal column stimulation: optimization of application. Surgical Neurology 4: 171–176

Burton C 1977 Safety and clinical efficacy of spinal cord stimulation. Neurosurgery 1: 214–215

Cook A W 1974 Stimulation of the spinal cord in motor neurone disease. Lancet ii: 230–231

Cook A W, Oygar A, Baggenstos P, Pacheco S, Kleriga E 1976 Vascular disease of extremities. Journal of Medicine 3: 46–48

De la Porte Ch, van de Kelft E 1992 Spinal cord stimulation in failed back surgery syndrome. Pain (in press)

Hoppenstein R 1975 Percutaneous implantation of chronic spinal cord electrodes for control of intractable pain: preliminary report. Surgical Neurology 4: 195–198

Hosobuchi Y, Adams J E, Weinstein P R 1972 Preliminary percutaneous dorsal column stimulation prior to permanent implantation. Technical note. Journal of Neurosurgery 37: 242–245

Hunt W E, Goodman J H, Bingham W G 1975 Stimulation of the dorsal spinal cord for treatment of intractable pain: a preliminary report. Surgical Neurology 4: 153–156

Illis L S, Oygar A E, Segwick E M, Awadalla M S A S (1976) Dorsal column stimulation in the rehabilitation of patients with multiple sclerosis. Lancet i: 1383–1386

Krainick J-U, Thoden U 1981a Experience with spinal cord stimulation for the control of postamputation pain. In: Hosobuchi Y, Corbin T (eds) Indications for spinal cord stimulation. Excerpta Medica, Amsterdam, p 42–45

Krainick J-U, Thoden U 1981b Spinal cord stimulation in postamputation pain. In: Siegried J, Zimmerman M (eds) Phantom and stump pain. Springer Verlag, Berlin, pp 163–166

Krainick J-U, Thoden U, Riechert T 1975 Spinal cord stimulation in postamputation pain. Surgical Neurology 4: 167–170

Krainick J U, Thoden U, Strassburg H M, Wenzel D 1977 The effects of electrical spinal cord stimulation on spastic movement disorders. Advances in Neurosurgery 4: 257–260

Krainick J, Thoden U, Riechert T 1980 Pain reduction in amputees by long-term spinal cord stimulation. Journal of Neurosurgery 52: 346–350

Larson S J, Sances A Jr, Cusick J F, Meyer G A, Swiontek T 1975 A comparison between anterior and posterior spinal implant systems. Surgical Neurology 4: 180–186

Lazorthes Y, Verdie J C, Arbus L 1978 Stimulation analgésique médullaire antérieure et postérieur par technique d'implantation percutanée. Acta Neurochirurgica 40: 253–276

Linderoth B 1992 Dorsal column stimulation and pain. Experimental studies of putative neurochemical and neurophysiological mechanisms. Stockholm Kongl Carolinska Medico chirurgiska institutet

Long D M, Erickson D E 1975 Stimulation of the posterior columns of the spinal cord for relief of intractable pain. Surgical Neurology 4: 134–141

Long D M, Erickson D, Campbell J, North R 1981 Electrical stimulation of the spinal cord and peripheral nerves for pain control – 10 years' experience. Applied Neurophysiology 44: 207–217

Meglio M, Cioni B, Dal Lago A et al 1981 Pain control and improvement of peripheral blood flow following epidural spinal cord stimulation. Journal of Neurosurgery 54: 821–823

Melzack R, Wall P D 1965 Pain mechanisms: a new theory. Science 150: 971–979

Nashold B S Jr 1975 Dorsal column stimulation for control of pain: a three-year follow-up. Surgical Neurology 4: 146–147

Nashold B S, Friedman H 1972 Dorsal column stimulation for control of pain: a preliminary report on 30 patients. Journal of Neurosurgery 36: 590

Nielson K D, Adams J E, Hosobuchi Y 1975 Experience with dorsal column stimulation for relief of chronic intractable pain. Surgical Neurology 4: 148–152

North R S, Fischell T A, Long D M 1977/78 Chronic dorsal column stimulation via percutaneously inserted epidural electrodes. Applied Neurophysiology 40: 181–191

Pineda A 1975 Dorsal column stimulation and its prospects. Surgical Neurology 4: 157–163

Sedan R, Lazorthes Y 1978 La neurostimulation électrique thérapeutique. Neurochirurgie 24 (suppl 1): 53–57

Ray Ch D 1988 Implantation of spinal cord stimulators for relief of chronic and severe pain. In: Cauthen J C (ed) Lumbar spine surgery. Indications, techniques, failures, and alternatives, 2nd edn. Williams & Wilkins, Baltimore

Shealy C N 1975 Dorsal column stimulation: optimization of application. Surgical Neurology 4: 142–145

Shealy C N, Mortimer J T, Reswick J 1967 Electrical inhibition of pain by stimulation of the dorsal column: preliminary clinical reports. Anesthesia and Analgesia 46: 489–491

Siegfried J, Krainick J-U, Haas H, Adorjani C, Meyer M, Thoden U 1978 Electrical spinal cord stimulation for spastic movement disorders. Applied Neurophysiology 41: 134–141

Spiegelmann R, Friedman W 1991 Spinal cord stimulation: a contemporary series. Neurosurgery 28: 65–77

Sweet W H, Wepsic J G 1975a Stimulation of the posterior columns of the spinal cord for pain control. Indications – techniques and results. Clinical Neurosurgery. 21: 278–310

Sweet W H, Wepsic J G 1975b Stimulation of the posterior columns of the spinal cord for pain control. Surgical Neurology 4: 133

Tallis R C, Illis L S, Sedgwick E M, Hardwidge C, Garfield J S 1983 Spinal cord stimulation in peripheral vascular disease. Journal of Neurology, Neurosurgery and Psychiatry 46: 478–484

Tallis R C, Illis L S, Sedgwick E M 1983 The quantitative assessment of the influence of spinal cord stimulation on motor function in patients with multiple sclerosis. International Rehabilitation Medicine 5: 10–16

Wall P, Melzack R 1984 Introduction. Textbook of pain. Churchill Livingstone, Edinburgh, p 1–16

Wall P D, Sweet W H 1967 Temporary abolition of pain in man. Science 155: 108–109

Winkelmüller W 1981 Experience with control of low-back pain by the dorsal column stimulation (DCS) system and by the peridural electrode system (PISCES). In: Hosobuchi Y, Corbin T (eds) Indications for spinal cord stimulation. Excerpta Medica, Amsterdam, p 34–40

66. Brain stimulation for relief of chronic pain

Ronald F. Young and Patricia C. Rinaldi

INTRODUCTION

Electrical stimulation of the human brain for the treatment of chronic pain began in the 1950s with reports by Heath (1954) and Pool et al (1956) that successful pain relief was produced by stimulation in the septal region anterior and lateral to the anterior columns of the fornix in patients with significant psychopathology. In 1960 Heath & Mickle reported relief from pain during septal stimulation in nonpsychiatric patients. Ervin et al (1966) reported pain relief in a single patient with stimulation of the caudate nucleus. At about the same time Gol (1967) described limited success in attempts to stimulate both the septal region and the caudate nucleus for the treatment of pain.

The phenomenon of stimulation-produced analgesia (SPA) following electrical stimulation of the periaqueductal grey (PAG) region of the rat mesencephalon was described by Reynolds in 1969. Subsequent studies, also in animals, showed that SPA was at least partially reversed by the narcotic antagonist naloxone and that cross-tolerance could be demonstrated between repeated PAG stimulation and analgesia from exogenous opioids (Mayer & Hayes 1975; Basbaum & Fields 1978; Sherman & Liebeskind 1980). These findings led to the hypothesis that in animals SPA depended upon release of naturally occurring opioid compounds, most notably β-endorphin and metenkephalin.

Effective pain relief from acute and chronic electrical stimulation in the periventricular grey (PVG) region of the posterior third ventricle in humans was reported in 1977 by Richardson & Akil (1977a, 1977b). Adams (1976) and later others (Hosobuchi et al 1977, 1979, 1980a, 1980b; Akil et al 1978) suggested that, in humans, release of naturally occurring opioid compounds accounted for pain relief elicited by such stimulation. Subsequently, many groups have reported successful attempts to relieve pain in humans by chronic electrical stimulation in either the PAG or PVG (Meyerson et al 1979; Thoden et al 1979; Amano et al 1980; Gybels 1980; Ray & Burton 1980; Dieckmann & Witzmann 1982; Plotkin 1982; Richardson 1982: Young et al 1984, 1985; Hosobuchi 1986). The role of opiates as it relates to stimulation-induced pain relief in humans is less clear. Elevation in endogenous opiate levels and related compounds in cerebrospinal fluid sampled from the third ventricle following PAG or PVG stimulation was observed by both the Richardson and Hosobuchi groups (Akil et al 1978; Hosobuchi et al 1979, 1980b). However, our own studies indicate that the relationship between SPA and opioid compounds is not simple (Young & Chambi 1987); previous observations of elevations in endogenous opiate levels may have been, at least in part, a function of cross-reaction of materials used in ventriculography for contrast with the radioimmunoassays for opioid compound identification (Dionne et al 1984; Fessler et al 1984).

The relationship of SPA to opioid mediation and the possibility of other mediators has been, and continues to be, a controversial subject. It appears likely that other neuromodulatory systems, possibly acting through collateral and other descending pathways, may be involved in chronic pain relief via PVG/PAG stimulation (Bonica et al 1990; Young 1990; Duncan et al 1991; Bartolini et al 1992). More medial structures (i.e. centre median–CM, parafascicularis–Pf, centralis lateralis–CL) may also contribute to modulating the classical pain relays and centres (Bushnell & Duncan 1989; Guilbaud et al 1989). Recently, in our patients, it has been observed that electrical stimulation of PVG has a profound inhibitory effect on spontaneous activity of both nociceptive and nonnociceptive neurons in the thalamic somatosensory nuclei, the ventroposterolateral and the ventroposteromedial (VPL and VPM, also called the ventrocaudalis, Vc of Hassler). The length of inhibition appears to vary with the intensity or length of stimulation and the inhibition outlasts the stimulation by 20 – 30 minutes in some patients (Rinaldi et al 1991b). This modification of somatosensory thalamic activity may well play a role in pain relief elicited by PVG stimulation.

Early attempts to stimulate the somatosensory pathways for treatment of chronic pain, particularly the neospinothalamic tract at its termination in the thalamic relay nucleus VPL, were reported by Mazars et al in 1960. Hosobuchi et al (1973) and Adams et al (1974) also reported early experience with chronic stimulation in the sensory thalamic relay nuclei and internal capsule for treatment of neuropathic or deafferentation pain. All three groups produced subtantial pain relief.

A number of reports have subsequently appeared which describe the clinical results of somatosensory thalamic stimulation for treatment of chronic pain in humans (Mazars et al 1974; Mazars 1975; Schvarcz 1980; Turnbull et al 1980; Siegfried 1982; Tsubokawa et al 1982; Young et al 1984, 1985). The mechanisms for pain relief from somatosensory thalamic stimulation are less understood than those of PVG/PAG stimulation. Studies with monkeys suggest that VPL stimulation-produced inhibition of spinothalamic tract neurons located in the dorsal horn of the spinal cord may play a role in VPL stimulation pain relief (Gerhart et al 1981, 1983). Abnormal activity of somatosensory thalamic neurons in patients with pain of deafferentation origin has been studied by Tasker's group (Lenz et al 1987; Hirayama et al 1989). Lenz has proposed that the abnormal bursting of thalamic cells may be mediated by NMDA regulated calcium-binding protein changes and may be involved in the development of central pain syndromes (Lenz 1992). This apparently abnormal hyperactivity and bursting recorded in VPM/VPL may be more widespread in the thalamus than previously thought, since we have recently recorded similar bursting in the medial and intralaminar thalamic nuclei (Rinaldi et al 1991a). The importance of medial thalamic nuclei and supraspinal structures, including cortex, in modulating pain and participating in pain relief have recently received renewed interest (Bushnell & Duncan 1989; Guilbaud et al 1989; Casey 1991; Talbot et al 1991).

Electrical stimulation of several other brain targets has been shown to inhibit nociceptive-induced activation of dorsal horn neurons. Katayama and colleagues described electrical stimulation of the parabrachial region of the mesencephalon in cats (Katayama et al 1984a, 1984b) and in two patients (Katayama et al 1985) with chronic pain due to cancer. In cats, the inhibitory effect of parabrachial stimulation was antagonised by anticholinergic agents, which suggested a cholinergic mechanism. We are not aware of any other attempts to stimulate this target for treatment of chronic pain in humans.

Associated with the parabrachial area is the so-called Kolliker-Fuse nucleus. Hodge and colleagues demonstrated that electrical stimulation of this nucleus in cat inhibited dorsal horn neuronal activity and that pretreatment with reserpine antagonised the inhibitory effects of stimulation, which suggested a catecholamine mechanism (Hodge et al 1986). Recently, Young and colleagues described successful relief of intractable pain in three of six patients treated by electrical stimulation in the Kolliker-Fuse region. This region lies just medial to the ventral end of the superior cerebellar peduncle and is considered part of the pedunculopontine nucleus by some (Olszewski & Baxter 1982). The actual target area employed by Young and colleagues was just lateral to the locus coeruleus and included the pedunculopontine nucleus rostrally and the lateral parabrachial region caudally (Young et al 1992).

PATIENT SELECTION

Stimulation of the brain by chronically implanted electrodes for treatment of chronic pain is usually employed solely in patients who are incapacitated by their pain and in whom other more conventional methods of pain treatment have been unsuccessful. A minimum of approximately 6 months should elapse from the onset of the pain before brain stimulation is considered, in order to allow sufficient time for spontaneous resolution of the pain and for a thorough trial of treatment alternatives. Indeed, most patients who undergo stimulation have had pain for many years.

Treatment prior to brain stimulation may include pharmacological agents, physical therapy, nerve blocks, acupuncture, biofeedback and psychotherapy. In our experience, treatment in a multidisciplinary pain-management clinic is very helpful, and nearly all of our patients have had such treatment before electrode implantation.

Psychological assessment is also essential prior to consideration of electrode placement. The Minnesota Multiphasic Personality Inventory (MMPI), together with a psychological interview, has been our choice of phychological evaluation techniques useful for screening candidates for electrode implantation (Long 1981). Patients with psychoses are immediately excluded from further consideration. Patients with a strong psychological component to their pain are encouraged to undergo further psychological treatment prior to consideration of brain stimulation. Such patients often show marked elevations of the hysteria and hypochondriasis scales of the MMPI, and low scores in the depression scale producing the so-called 'conversion-V' pattern (Wiltse & Rocchio 1975). Patients with excessive neurotic concern with bodily functions and disease processes and a prior history of frequent surgical procedures for equivocal indications are also considered relatively poor candidates for stimulation. Likewise, patients with complaints of chronic pain in the genital, rectal or pelvic region, in whom the pain aetiology is unclear, are excluded from treatment by brain stimulation based on our lack of long-term success in treating such patients. In general, any patients with longstanding pain complaints without a clearly defined aetiology are not candidates for treatment by brain stimulation.

Brain stimulation has the potential to diminish chronic pain of any aetiology and in any location. It has not, however, been applied to the treatment of certain chronic pain problems such as headache, nor to intermittent acute pain such as trigeminal neuralgia. It has been used to treat virtually every other kind of chronic pain of both nociceptive and neuropathic origin. These include chronic pain due to spinal disorders (e.g. disc disease, arachnoiditis, epidural fibrosis), cancer, postherpetic neuralgia, thalamic syndrome, anaesthesia dolorosa, pain due to spinal cord injury and a variety of other causes. More important than the aetiology of the patient's pain or its location is the psychological state of the patient. Brain stimulation cannot relieve the suffering of life's tribulations which come to be expressed in the word 'pain'. Unfortunately even with the most sophisticated psychological assessment available, errors in patient selection probably account for many failures.

Several authors have recommended that patients should discontinue all narcotics usage prior to electrode placement in the PAG or PVG regions, based on the idea that pain relief from stimulation in such sites depends on activation of an endogenous opioid system and that cross tolerance between exogenous opioids and stimulation may prevent effective pain relief (Adams 1976; Hosobuchi et al 1977, 1979, 1980a, 1980b; Hosobuchi 1978; Richardson 1982). We originally employed such a requirement but currently do not do so. Patients are encouraged to discontinue opiate use if possible, but successful pain relief has, in fact, been obtained in patients who were taking large doses of narcotics at the time of electrode implantation. In addition, we no longer routinely screen patients with intravenous narcotics prior to PAG or PVG electrode placement. Hosobuchi (1986) recommended the morphine saturation test, in which increasing doses of morphine sulphate are given intravenously until pain relief occurs or respiratory depression is noted (Plotkin 1982), as a means of selecting patients for PAG or PVG electrode implantation. Relief of pain by intravenous opiates and reversal by naloxone was thought to predict successful pain relief by PAG-PVG stimulation but, as previously mentioned, this has not been our experience (Young & Chambi 1987).

TARGET SELECTION AND LOCALISATION

The general recommendation of many authors has been to employ PAG–PVG stimulation for treatment of so-called nociceptive, peripheral or nondeafferentation pain, based on the hypothesis that pain elicited by such stimulation depends on an endogenous opioid mechanism and that opiates are generally effective for relief of nociceptive pain. Stimulation of other targets, notably the thalamic sensory relay nuclei ventralis posterolateralis (VPL) or ventralis posteromedialis (VPM) or the internal capsule, has been recommended for treatment of central pain related to deafferentation or neuropathic pain. Examples of the latter include anaesthesia dolorosa, postcordotomy dysaesthesias, the thalamic syndrome, brachial plexus avulsion, postherpetic neuralgia and spinal cord and peripheral nerve injuries.

We find that rigid adherance to a 'rule' such as VPM/VPL stimulation for neuropathic pain and PAG/PVG for nociceptive pain does not hold and is not clinically valid. In addition, many chronic-pain patients present with combinations of nociceptive and neuropathic pain. Indeed, the largest number of patients with combined pain are those with the 'failed-back' syndrome. Such patients often complain of low-back pain of a nociceptive origin and neuropathic leg pain associated with paraesthesias and sensory loss due to deafferentation at the root level. Results of stimulation in such patients are unpredictable, with some patients achieving relief of both the back and leg pain with PAG/PVG stimulation, while others require stimulation in both PAG–PVG and somatosensory thalamus (Hosobuchi 1983). Occasionally such patients derive no relief from PAG/PVG stimulation, but nearly complete pain relief from somatosensory thalamic stimulation alone. We have also noted unpredictable results with neuropathic pain due to postherpetic neuralgia and spinal cord injury.

Another aspect of target selection concerns whether pain is unilateral or bilateral. In animal models, analgesia from PVG stimulation is generally bilateral, but Soper & Melzack (1982) have shown a somatotopic relationship between stimulation sites in the PAG and analgesia. Our general approach has been to place PAG or PVG electrodes contralateral to the side of unilateral pain and to employ an electrode placed in the non-dominant hemisphere for bilateral pain. However, in at least one patient (a right-handed woman), a right-sided PAG electrode relieved only back and leg pain but not neck pain, whereas the placement of a second left-sided PAG electrode relieved both neck and back pain. During an earlier period, we employed bilateral PAG/PVG electrodes for bilateral pain but concerns about potential morbidity from insertion of electrodes in both hemispheres have resulted in our present infrequent use of bilateral electrodes.

Somatosensory thalamic or internal capsular stimulation produces effective relief of pain only contralateral to electrode placement. Interestingly, in monkeys, VPL stimulation results in suppression of activity generated in spinothalamic tract neurons by noxious stimuli, both contralateral and ipsilateral to VPL stimulation (Gerhart et al 1981, 1983).

Considerable differences exist among the sensations evoked by stimulation in various target sites. In the PAG, patients often note pleasant sensations of warmth, floating, dizziness, and well-being at threshold stimulation amplitudes. At higher amplitudes PVG stimulation may

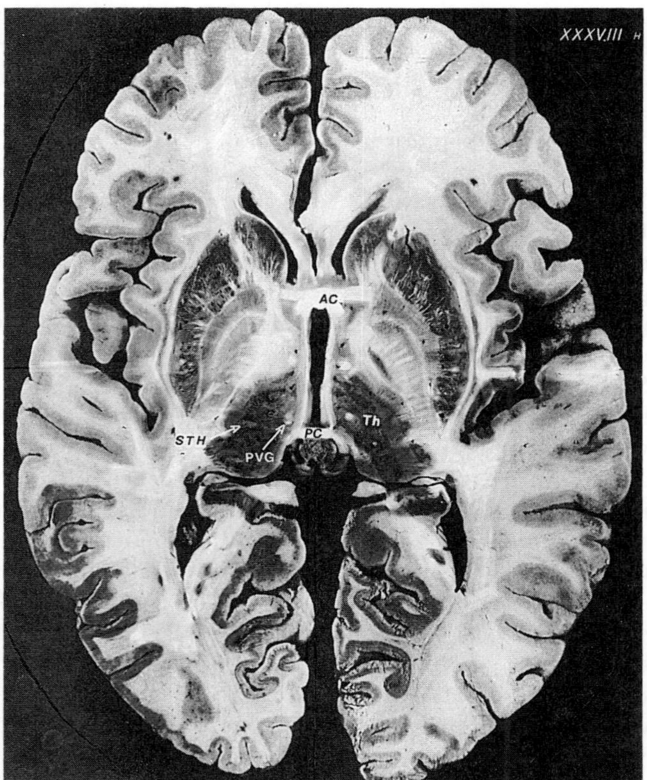

Fig. 66.1 Anatomical section of the brain at the level of the anterior (AC) and posterior (PC) commissures. The typical targets for electrode implantation in periventricular grey (PVG) and the somatosensory thalamus (STH right side and Th on left side) are shown. (Adapted from Schaltenbrand & Wahren 1977.)

evoke feelings of nervousness, anxiety and diffuse burning. Similar sensations, but less noticeable burning, nervousness and anxiety are produced by ventral PAG stimulation. Dorsal PAG stimulation usually evokes unpleasant sensations of fear, doom, severe anxiety and agitation. High-amplitude stimulation in both the dorsal and ventral PAG, as well as PVG, produces limitation in vertical gaze, occasionally complete gaze paralysis, and sometimes conjugate eye deviation or oscillopsia.

Stimulation in the somatosensory thalamus typically evokes a sensation of paraesthesia in the contralateral face or body which is somatotopically related to the site of stimulation. Occasionally, VPL or VPM stimulation evokes contralateral tonic muscular contractions of the face and/or limbs at stimulus frequencies of 50 –60 Hz. Generally such motor signs occur at stimulus amplitudes greater than those which evoke paraesthesias, presumably from current spread into the adjacent internal capsule or thalamic nucleus ventralis intermedius.

Stimulation of the postrior limb of the internal capsule also evokes paraesthesias in contralateral regions of the body, but thresholds for contralateral muscular contractions are often nearly identical to those for paraesthesias. For this reason, we rarely employ this stimulation site in our patients. Capsular stimulation is also occasionally perceived as painful, a sensation rarely evoked by VPL or VPM stimulation except at very high stimulus amplitudes. The anatomical locations of the two targets which we commonly employ, namely PVG and somatosensory thalamus (VPL and VPM) are demonstrated in Fig 66.1 and Fig. 66.2.

SURGICAL TECHNIQUE

Electrodes are implanted stereotactically under local anaesthesia via a 15-mm burr hole centred anterior to the coronal suture and 15 –20 mm lateral to the midline. In the past, stereotactic calculations of the various targets were based on contrast ventriculography and reference to standard atlases of stereotactic anatomy. Target coordinates employed by the author for the common stimulation targets are shown in Table 66.1.

For a period of time from 1986 –88 we employed computerised tomographic (CT) scanning for target localisation, but since 1988 we have used magnetic resonance (MR) imaging. Our technique is to obtain a mid-sagittal T-1 weighted MR image to locate the anterior (AC) and posterior (PC) commissures. An Axial T-1 weighted

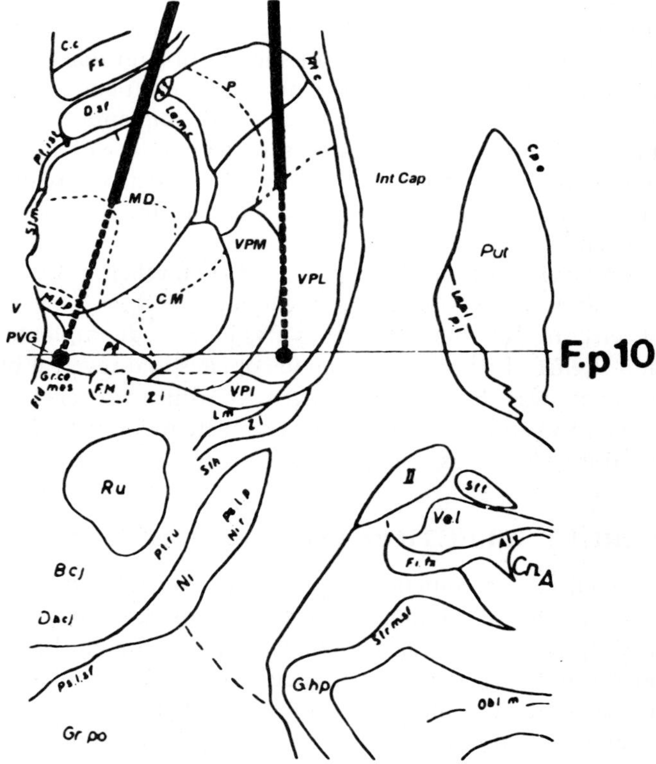

Fig. 66.2 Diagrammatic coronal representation of the brain which demonstrates electrode trajectories into PVG and VPL. The section is 10 mm posterior to the midpoint of the AC–PC plane (F.p 10). (Adapted from Schaltenbrand & Wahren 1977.)

Table 66.1 Stereotactic coordinates for stimulation targets

	X	Y	Z
Periventricular grey	3–4	10	0
Ventral periaqueductal grey	2–3	12–14	-6 to -10
Somatosensory thalamus			
VPL	14–18	10–13	+2 to -5
VPM	8–14	8–12	+2 to -5
Internal capsule	25	12–14	+4 to -4

VPL = ventral posterolateral nucleus ; VPM = ventral posteromedial nucleus.
All coordinates (in mm) are referred to the line connecting the anterior (AC) and posterior (PC) commissures, the AC–PC plane. X = distance right or left of midline; Y=distance posterior to midpoint of AC–PC plane; Z=distance superior (+) or inferior (-) to AC–PC horizontal plane.

image at the level of the AC–PC plane is then obtained (Fig. 66.3). We have made a careful comparison of target selection by standard ventriculography, by CT and by MR techniques and we believe that MR is the best method available. If implanted metallic hardware makes MR imaging impossible, CT localisation is employed.

Intraoperative physiological target localisation is essential since the stereotactic coordinates represent only starting points for localisation of the physiological targets. We employ microelectrode recording, microstimulation and finally macrostimulation to identify accurately our intended targets. The electrode used is custom-designed, bipolar and concentric, consisting of an inner fine tungsten rod microelectrode and an outer stainless steel tube insulated except for 0.5 mm around the end nearest the tip of the microelectrode. Microstimulation is accomplished through the fine recording electrode tip while macrostimulation is accomplished through the uninsulated portion of the outer tube. The latter closely approximates the stimulation delivered by the permanent electrode implanted for chronic stimulation purposes. Stimulation can be monopolar or bipolar as required. Assessment of the target location by stimulation has been our most successful tool, but cellular activity recorded by the microelectrode has also begun to prove useful. We are often able to recognise neurophysiologic activity patterns of single cells peculiar to the medial dorsal, endymalis and parafascicularis nuclei through which the microelectrode passes on its way to the PVG target (Rinaldi et al 1991a).

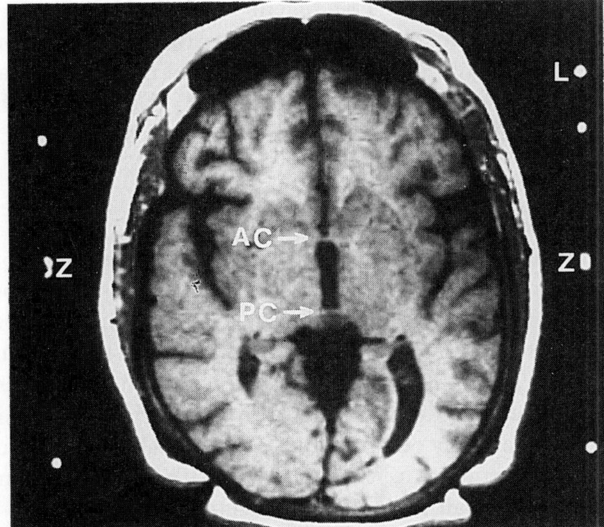

Fig. 66.3 MRI scan at the level of the anterior (AC) and posterior (PC) commissures. Dots at the sides of the figure represent fiducials of stereotactic frame used to calculate the depth or Z coordinate.

Single-unit recording in the VPL and VPM thalamic targets allows identification of the somatotopic organisation of the thalamus by plotting of receptive fields of neurons in patients in a manner similar to that accomplished for many years in animal research (Lenz et al 1988). Microstimulation and macrostimulation elicit contralateral paraesthesias in a distribution similar, but not necessarily identical, to the location of receptive fields recorded from the same locus in the somatosensory thalamus. The correct target in the somatosensory thalamus is one from which stimulation-induced paraesthesias encompass the body region where the patient's pain is located. Unless this correspondence between pain location and stimulation-induced paraesthesias is accomplished, pain relief is unlikely to result from somatosensory thalamic stimulation.

The purpose of intraoperative physiological studies is to locate correctly the intended target. We do not attempt to assess the effect of stimulation on the patient's pain during the electrode implantation. The stress and distraction of the operating-room environment do not lend themselves to the patient's accurate assessment of pain relief.

When the stereotactic coodinates of the desired targets have been physiologically indentified, permanent stimulating electrodes are introduced into the brain at these sites and the connecting electrode leads are brought out of the scalp through small wounds. Typically a postoperative CT scan (Fig. 66.4) or MRI scan is obtained to confirm correct electrode placement and to assess possible intracerebral haemorrhage. About 24–48 hours postoperatively, trial stimulation is begun to evaluate the effectiveness of stimulation for pain relief. We have employed exclusively the four contact Medtronic platinum wire electrode, which allows flexibility in final stimulation site as well as a variety of bipolar and monopolar stimulation combinations. All possible stimulation combinations are explored during the trial stimulation period which lasts from about 3 days to 3 weeks, but is generally 5–7 days in length.

If pain relief ensues, the electrodes are connected either to a radiofrequency receiver or to a fully implanted pulse generator for chronic stimulation. If pain relief does not occur during trial stimulation, the electrodes are removed.

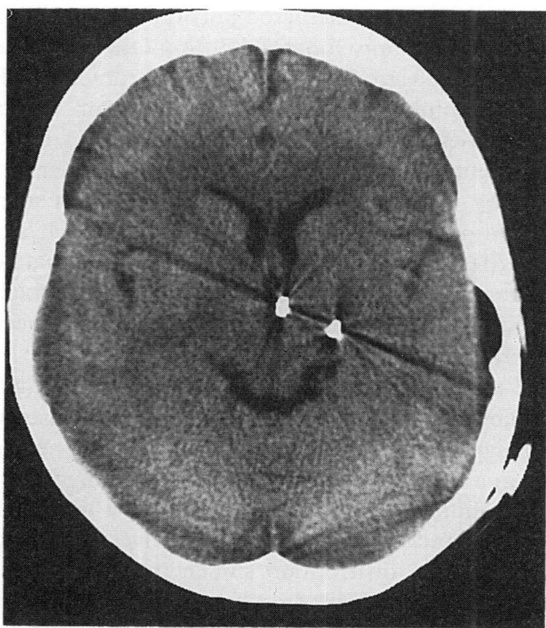

Fig. 66.4 Postimplant CT scan which demonstrates electrodes in both left PVG and somatosensory thalamus.

RESULTS

Our own experience includes 178 patients implanted between 1978 and 1992. The aetiology of pain in these patients is shown in Table 66.2. The largest single group of patients suffered chronic pain related to spinal disorders, mainly in the lumbar spine. Patients with cancer pain constituted the second largest group. A total of 383 electrodes were implanted in a variety of targets as described in Table 66.3. Our most common combinations of electrodes and targets were two electrodes, one in PVG and one in VPL, located contralateral to the side of the patient's pain, which was used in 143 patients. Some 23 patients had unilateral PAG or PVG electrodes and 15 had bilateral PAG or PVG electrodes; 151 patients had electrodes implanted on a single occasion while 27 others had a second (21 patients), third (five patients) or fourth (one patient) operation, either to implant additional electrodes or to replace broken or displaced electrodes.

Overall, 80.3% of our patients (143/176) experienced pain relief during the trial stimulation period and went on to have a permanent stimulator implanted. Of those patients with a permanent implant 62.2% (89/143) experienced long-term relief of their pain. Our criteria for pain relief include at least 50% reduction in pain intensity measured on the Visual Analogue Scale, cessation of chronic narcotic analgesic usage and improvement in functional capacities as measured by the Functional Capacity Questionnaire. The latter is designed to assess in a quantifiable manner the patient's ability to function in physical, personal care, social and interpersonal spheres of life. It also provides information on medications which may be required by the patients. These data are obtained prior to surgery and at follow-up interviews.

Table 66.2 Pain Aetiology

Failed back	61
Failed neck	8
Cancer	30
Brain infarct or injury	14
Postherpetic neuralgia	13
Spinal-cord injury	12
Anaesthesia dolorosa	5
Miscellaneous	35
Total	178

Table 66.3 Electrode locations

PAG/PVG	205
Sensory thalamus	171
K-F	6
Internal capsule	1
Total	383

Patients with nociceptive pain have fared considerably better than those with pain of neuropathic origin. In the former group, 70% of those who underwent permanent implants achieved long-term relief of their pain whereas in the group with neuropathic pain, only 50% experienced long-term relief.

We have previously reviewed the world literature regarding electrical stimulation of the brain for treatment of chronic pain. A total of 916 patients were available for analysis (Amano et al 1980; Gybels 1980; Schvarcz 1980; Boivie & Meyerson 1982; Dieckmann & Witzmann 1982; Groth et al 1982; Siegfried 1982; Young 1985; Hosobuchi 1986). Of these 916 patients, 542 (59%) experienced satisfactory relief of pain. The recent study by Kumar et al (1990) on 48 patients from 6 months to 10 years reports similar success (63%). Our conclusion that nociceptive pain responds better (70% of patients relieved) than neuropathic pain (50% relieved) has also been confirmed by others.

COMPLICATIONS

Complications experienced by the 178 patients in our series are shown in Table 66.4. Permanent complications occurred in 7 patients (3.9%). One death which occurred in the postoperative period was unrelated to the implant itself. The permanent complications included hemiparesis and disorders of extraocular movements, primarily persistent diplopia. Only one patient remains disabled as a result of a permanent complication. Two of the seven patients experienced small intrathalamic haemorrhages. In one of the former, neglect of the left side of the body was noted after a right-sided haemorrhage which relieved the patient of her pain (brain stimulation was unnecessary)

Table 66.4 Complications

	Temporary	Permanent
Neurological deficit	13	5
Infection	12	
Thalamic haemorrhage	2	2
Hardware	9	
Subdural haematoma	2	
Spinal accessory palsy	1	
Aqueduct obstruction	1	
Respirator dependant	1	
Totals	41*	7 (3.9%)

* 37 patients (20.7%)

until her death from cancer. In the other patient, a haemorrhage at the junction of the lateral sensory thalamus and the internal capsule caused a contralateral hemiparesis which has nearly completely resolved.

Only five other patients have experienced permanent complications. Of these, two patients have persistent diplopia and gaze paresis following placement of electrodes in the PAG. One of the latter patients, in whom the electrode was left in place, has experienced excellent pain relief for 9 years and has remained gainfully employed. In the other patient, sudden forced tonic downward eye deviations and adduction occurred as an electrode was advanced into the PAG and the electrode was immediately removed. Marked improvement occurred within hours, but the patients continues to experience diplopia. A third patient developed compulsive stimulation behaviour from an electrode placed in the right (nondominant) VPL nucleus. Stimulation at maximal amplitude apparently produced a diffuse pleasant sensation. The patient's compulsion to self-stimulation caused her to isolate herself and interfered with most normal activities. Upon removal of the electrode the patient's behaviour returned to normal. Portenoy et al (1986) reported a similar patient with compulsive self-stimulation of an electrode in the right somatosensory thalamus (VPL). Stimulation in this patient was accompanied by erotic sensation, pupillary dilatation, left hemiparesis and left hemisensory loss. We are not aware of any other reports of patients with compulsive stimulation involving electrodes in PAG, PVG, thalamus or internal capsule for treatment of pain.

The fourth and fifth patients with permanent complications developed hemiparesis following placement of a right VPL electrode. One patient is now ambulating with a cane and one requires a wheelchair. In neither of these was a lesion demonstrated with follow-up scanning which might account for their hemiparesis.

In the group of 178 patients 12 infections (6.7%) occurred and of these, four were superficial and were resolved with antibiotics. Eight deep infections occurred which required electrode removal in six cases. In two patients the infections resolved with antibiotics and the electrode implants remained. Nine patients experienced either electromechanical problems or local pain related to the implanted stimulating hardware but these problems were all eventually resolved.

One death occurred following electrode implantation but it did not relate directly to the implant. Injection of morphine via a ventricular reservoir resulted in ventriculitis which was treated successfully from a bacteriological standpoint with antibiotics. The patient, who suffered from pain due to metastatic lung cancer to the brachial plexus, remained comatose and after further aggressive treatment was declined by the family, the patient died.

In total, 37 patients (20.7%) experienced a total of 42 complications, whereas the other 141 patients were complication free. Hosobuchi (1986) reported complication in only 14 of his 122 patients (11.5%), a rate considerably lower than that noted in our group. However, two other patients described by Hosobuchi experienced electrode migration requiring electrode replacement, and two others had skin erosion overlying the implant hardware. If these four patients are included as complications, then the complication rate in Hosobuchi's patients increases to 14.7%. Complications reported by other authors, including the recent study by Kumar et al (1990) are similar to those described for ours and Hosobuchi's patient groups. Thus, complications occur relatively frequently related to implanted electrodes for pain relief, but most are relatively minor and can be resolved. Permanent complications are uncommon and death is rare.

CONCLUSIONS

Electrical stimulation of the brain is a valuable tool for the treatment of chronic pain which has failed to respond to other treatment techniques. This is probably the most invasive technique available but offers hope to a group of patients who are otherwise hopelessly incapacitated and condemned to a life of despair and suffering. The technique is expensive. In our hospital the total cost for implantation of two electrodes, our most common scenario, is about $60 000. Although expensive, the cost pales in comparison to the cost of continuing medical treatment of pain, lost wages, disability payments and the incalculable toll on the psychological health of not only the patients but their families and friends as well. About 70% of patients with pain of nociceptive origin and 50% of patients with neuropathic pain obtain substantial reductions in pain with brain stimulation. About 20% of patients experience complications of the procedure but only about 4% are permanent and less than 1% of patients experience either permanent disability or death.

REFERENCES

Adams J E 1976 Naloxone reversal of analgesia produced by brain stimulation in the human. Pain 2: 161–166

Adams J E, Hosobushi Y, fields H L 1974 Stimulation of internal capsule for relief of chronic pain. Journal of Neurosurgery 41: 740–744

Akil H, Richardson D E, Hughes J et al 1978 Enkephalin-like material elevated in ventricular cerebrospinal fluid of pain patients after analgetic focal stimulation. Science 201: 463–465

Amano K, Kitamura K, Kawamura H et al 1980 Alterations of immunoreactive beta-endorphin in the third ventricular fluid in responses to electrical stimulation of the human periaqueductal gray matter. Applied Neurophysiology 43: 150–158

Bartolini A, Ghelardini C, Malcangio M et al 1992 Physiological analgesia is obtainable by potentiating presynaptic mechanisms involved in central control. In Sicuteri F, Terenius L, Vecchiet L, Maggi C, Advances in pain research and therapy 20: 81–92

Basbaum A I, Fields H L 1978 Endogenous pain control mechanism: review and hypothesis. Annals of Neurology 4: 451–462

Boivie J, Meyerson B A 1982 Correlative anatomical and clinical study of pain suppression by deep brain stimulation. Pain 13: 113–126

Bonica JJ, Yaksh T, Liebeskind J C, Pechnick R N, Depaulis A 1990 Biochemistry and modulation of nociception and pain. In J J Bonica (eds) The management of pain. Lea & Febiger, Pennsylvania, p 95–121

Bushnell M C, Duncan G H 1989 Sensory and affective aspects of pain perception: is medial thalamus restricted to emotional issues? Experimental Brain Research 78: 415–418

Casey K L 1991 Pain and the central nervous system. Raven Press, New York

Dieckmann G J, Witzmann A 1982 Initial and long-term results of deep brain stimulation for chronic intractable pain. Applied Neurophysiology 45: 167–172

Dionne R A, Muller G P, Young R F et al 1984 Contrast medium causes the apparent increase in β-endorphin levels in human cerebrospinal fluid following brain stimulation. Pain 20: 313–321

Duncan G H, Bushell M C, Marchand S 1991 Deep brain stimulation: a review of basic research and clinical studies. Pain 45: 49–59

Ervin F R, Brown C E, Mark V H 1966 Striatal influence on facial pain. Confinia Neurologia 27: 75–86

Fessler R G, Brown F D, Rachlin J R et al 1984 Elevated β-endrophin in cerebrospinal fluid after electrical brain stimulation: artifact of contrast infusion? Science 224: 1017–1019

Gerhart K D, Yezierski R P, Wilcox T K, Grossman A E, Willis W D 1981 Inhibition of primate spinothalamic tract neurons by stimulation in ipsilateral or contralateral ventral posterior lateral (VPL) thalamic nucleus. Brain Research 229: 514–519

Gerhart K D, Yezierski R P, Fang Z R, Willis W D 1983 Inhibition of primate tract neurons by stimulation in ventral posterior lateral (VPL) thalamic nucleus: possible mechanisms. Journal of Neurophysiology 49: 406–423

Gol A 1967 Relief of pain by electrical stimulation of the septal area. Journal of Neurological Science 5: 115–120

Groth K, Adams J, Richardson D et al 1982 Deep brain stimulation for chronic intractable pain. Medtronic, Minneapolis In: Wall P D, Melzack R (eds) Textbook of Pain, 2nd edn.

Guilbaud G, Peschanski M, Besson J M 1989 Experimental data related to pain at the supraspinal level. In: Wall: P D Melzack R (eds) Textbook of pain. 2nd edn. Churchill Livingstone, Edinburgh, p 141–153

Gybels J 1980 Electrical stimulation of the brain for pain control in human. Verhandlungen der Deutschen Gesellschaft für Innere Medizin 86: 1553–1559

Heath R G 1954 Studies in schizophrenia. Harvard University Press, Cambridge, Massachusetts

Heath R G, Mickle W A 1960 Evaluation of 7 years' experience with depth electrode studies in human patients. In: Ramey E R, O'Doherty D S (eds) Electrical studies in the anesthetized brain. Harper & Row, New York, p 214–247

Hirayama T, Dostrovsky J O, Gorecki J, Tasker R R, Lenz F A 1989 Recordings of abnormal activity in patients with deafferentation and central pain. Proceedings of the Microelectrode Meeting, Stereotactic Functional Neurosurgery 52: 120–126

Hodge C J Jr, Apkarian A V, Stevens R T 1986 Inhibition of dorsal-horn cell responses by stimulation of the Kolliker-Fuse nucleus. Journal of Neurosurgery 65: 825–833

Hosobuchi Y 1978 Trytophan reversal of tolerance to analgesia induced by central grey stimulation. Lancet 2: 47

Hosobuchi Y 1983 Combined electrical stimulation of the periaqueductal grey matter and sensory thalamus. Applied Neurophysiology 46: 112–115

Hosobuchi Y 1986 Subcortical electrical stimulation for control of intractable pain in humans. Journal of Neurosurgery 64: 543–553

Hosobuchi Y, Adams J E, Rutkin B 1973 Chronic thalamic stimulation for the control of facial anesthesia dolorosa. Archives of Neurology 29: 158–161

Hosobuchi Y, Adams J E, Linchitz R 1977 Pain relief by electrical stimulation of the central gray matter in humans and its reversal by naloxone. Science 197: 183–186

Hosobuchi Y, Adams J E, Bloom F E, Guilleum R 1979 Stimulation of human periaqueductal grey for pain relief increases immunoreactive β-endorphin in ventricular fluid. Science 203: 279–281

Hosobuchi Y, Lamb S, Bascim D 1980a Trytophan loading may reverse tolerance to opiate analgesics in humans: a preliminary report. Pain 9: 161–169

Hosobuchi Y, Rossier J, Bloom F E 1980b Oral loading with L-trytophan may augment the simultaneous release of ACTH and beta-endorphin that accompanies periaqueductal stimulation in humans. Advances in Biochemical Psychopharmacology 22: 563–570

Katayama Y, Dewitt D S, Becker D P 1984a Behavioral evidence for a cholinoceptive pontine inhibitory area: descending control of spinal motor output and sensory input. Brain Research 296: 241–262

Katayama Y, Watkins L R , Becker D P 1984b Evidence for involvement of cholinoceptive cells of the parabrachial region in environmentally induced nociceptive suppression in the cat. Brain Research 299: 348–353

Katayama Y, Tsubokawa T, Hirayama T 1985 Pain relief following stimulation of the pontomesencephalic parabrachial region in humans: brain sites for nonopiate-mediated pain control. Applied Neurophysiology 48: 195–200

Kumar K, Wyant G M, Nath R 1990 Deep brain stimulation for control of intractable pain in humans, present and future: a ten-year follow-up. Neurosurgery 26: 774–782

Lenz F A 1992 The ventral posterior nucleus of thalamus is involved in the generation of central pain syndromes. American Pain Society Journal 1: 42–51

Lenz F A, Tasker R R, Dostrovsky J O et al 1987 Abnormal single-unit activity recorded in the somatosensory thalamus of a quadriplegic patient with central pain. Pain 31: 225–236

Lenz F A, Dostrovsky J O, Tasker R R et al 1988 Single-unit analysis of human ventral thalamic nuclear group: somatosensory responses. Journal of Neurophysiology 59: 299–316

Long C J 1981 The relationship between surgical outcome and MMPI profiles in chronic pain patients. Journal of Clinical Psychology 37: 744–749

Mayer D H, Hayes R L 1975 Stimulation produced analgesia: development of tolerance and cross tolerance to morphine. Science 188: 941–943

Mazars G 1975 Intermittent stimulation of nucleus ventralis posterolateralis for intractable pain. Surgical Neurology 4: 93–95

Mazars G, Roge R, Mazars Y 1960 Stimulation of the spinothalamic fasciculus and their bearing on the physiopathology of pain (in French). Revue Neurologique 103: 136–138

Mazars G, Merienne L, Cioloca C 1974 Treatment of certain types of pain by implantable thalamic stimulators (in French). Neurochirurgie 20: 117–124

Meyerson B A, Boethius J, Carlsson A M 1979 Alleviation of malignant pain by electrical stimulation in the periventricular–periaqueductal region: pain relief as related to stimulation sites. Advances in Pain Research Therapy 3: 525–533

Olsxewski J, Baxter D 1982 Cytoarchitecture of the human brain stem, 2nd edn. S Karger, Basel.

Plotkin R 1982 Results in 60 cases of deep brain stimulation for chronic intractable pain. Applied Neurophysiology 45: 173–178

Pool J L, Clark W D, Hudson P, Lombardo M 1956 Hypothalamic-hypophyseal interrelationships. C Thomas, Springfield, Illinois
Portenoy R K, Jarden J O, Sidtis J J et al 1986 Compulsive thalamic self-stimulation: a case with metabolic, electrophysiologic and behavioural correlates. Pain 27: 277–290
Ray C D, Bruton C V 1980 Deep brain stimulation for severe, chronic pain. Acta Neurochirurgica (Wien) (suppl) 3: 289–293
Reynolds D V 1969 Surgery in the rat during electrical analgesia induced by focal brain stimulation. Science 164: 444–445
Richardson D E 1982 Analgesia produced by stimulation of various sites in the human beta-endorphin system. Applied Neurophysiology 45: 116–122
Richardson D E, Akil H 1977a Pain reduction by electrical brain stimulation in man, Part I. Acute administration in periaqueductal and periventricular sites. Journal of Neurosurgery 47: 178–183
Richardson D E, Akil H 1977b Pain reduction by electrical brain stimulation, Part II. Chronic self-administration in the periventricular gray matter. Journal of Neurosurgery 47: 184–194
Rinaldi P C, Young R F, Albe-Fessard D, Chodakiewitz J 1991a Spontaneous neuronal hyperactivity in the medial and intralaminar thalamic nuclei of patients with deafferentation pain. Journal of Neurosurgery 74: 415–421
Rinaldi P C, Young R F, Tronnier V M 1991b Bursting activity of thalamic neurons recorded from chronic pain patients is modified by electrical stimulation in PVG. Society for Neuroscience Abstracts 17, Part II, 1560
Schaltenbrand G, Wahren W 1977 Atlas for stereotaxy of the human brain. George Thieme Verlag, New York
Schvarcz J R 1980 Chronic self-stimulation of the medial posterior inferior thalamus for alleviation of deafferentation pain. Acta Neurochirurgica (Suppl) 30: 295–301
Sherman J E, Liebeskind J C 1980 An endorphinergic centrifugal substrate of pain modulation: recent findings, current concepts and complexities. In: Bonica J J (ed) Pain research publications of the Association for Research in Nervous and Mental Disease, vol 58. Raven Press, New York, p 190–204
Siegfried J 1982 Monopolar electrical stimulation of nucleus ventroposteromedialis thalami for postherpetic facial pain. Applied Neurophysiology 45: 179–184
Soper W Y, Melzack R 1982 Stimulation-produced analgesia: evidence for somatotopic organization in the midbrain. Brain Research 251: 301–312
Talbot J D, Marrett S, Evans A C, Meyer E, Bushnell M C, Duncan G H 1991 Multiple representations of pain in human cerebral cortex. Science 251: 1355–1358
Thoden U, Doerr M, Dieckmann G, Krainick J U 1979 Medial thalamic permanent electrodes for pain control in man: an electrophysiological and clinical study. Electroencephalography and Clinical Neurophysiological 47: 582–591
Tsubokawa T, Ramamoto T, Katayama Y, Moriyasu N 1982 Clinical results and physiological basis of thalamic relay nucleus stimulation for relief of intractable pain with morphine tolerance. Applied Neurophysiology 45: 143–155
Turnbull I M, Shulman R, Woodhurst W B 1980 Thalamic stimulation for neuropathic pain. Journal of Neurosurgery 52: 486–493
Wiltse L L, Rocchio P D 1975 Preoperative psychological tests as predictors of success of chemonucleolysis in the treatment of the low-back syndrome. Journal of Bone and Joint Surgery 57A: 478–483
Young R F 1990 Brain stimulation. Neurosurgery Clinics of North America 1: 865–879
Young R F, Chambi V I 1987 Pain relief by electrical stimulation of the periaqueductal and periventricular gray matter. Journal of Neurosurgery 66: 364–371
Young R F, Feldman R A, Kroening R, Fulton W, Morris J 1984 Electrical stimulation of the brain in the treatment of chronic pain in man. In: Druger L, Liebeskind J C (eds) Advances in pain research and therapy vol 6 Raven Press, New York, p 289–303
Young R F, Kroening R, Fulton W, Feldman R A, Chambi I 1985 Electrical stimulation of the brain in treatment of chronic pain. Journal of Neurosurgery 62: 389–396
Young R F, Tronnier V M, Rinaldi PC 1992 Chronic stimulation of the Kolliker-Fuse nucleus region for relief of intractable pain in humans. Journal of Neurosurgery 76: 979–985

Physiotherapy

67. Ultrasound, shortwave, microwave, laser, superficial heat and cold in the treatment of pain

Justus F. Lehmann and Barbara J. de Lateur

INTRODUCTION

Heat and cold applications are commonly used as adjuncts to other therapy in order to relieve painful conditions which often involve the musculoskeletal system. Both modalities may relieve pain through a 'counterirritant' effect. The application of heat and cold may also reduce pain by direct effects on peripheral nerve and free nerve endings.

REDUCTION OF PAIN BY RELIEVING PAINFUL CONDITIONS

Both heat and cold are commonly used to reduce painful muscle spasms secondary to underlying skeletal or neurological pathology. This painful muscle spasm is associated with low-back pain of various causes such as degenerative joint disease or intervertebral disc disease, with or without resultant nerve root irritation. The physiological basis for the relief of the muscle spasm is incompletely understood. Mense (1978), who studied temperature effects on muscle spindles, found that in a prestretched preparation the rate of firing of the group Ia afferents was increased by warming and decreased by cooling. The secondary afferents with a high background discharge responded in a similar manner whereas those with a low initial discharge rate showed a cessation of firing. One could speculate, assuming that a secondary muscle spasm is to large degree a tonic phenomenon, that the selective cessation of firing from the secondary endings may reduce the muscle tone, an effect which may be supplemented by the increased firing from the Golgi tendon organs which in turn increase the inhibitory impulses. The temperatures that produced these effects were within the lower therapeutic range. At higher temperatures it could be shown that the spindle sensitivity dropped (Ottoson 1965).

When cold is applied to the spindle, it has been shown that the spindle response is reduced (Ottoson 1965). Eldred and associates (1960) cooled single spindles and found that the rate of discharge from the spindle followed the temperature curve precisely. He felt that this represented a direct effect on the sensory terminal while all the other neural elements within the muscle, such as the alpha motor neuron fibres, the gamma fibres, the Ia afferents and the secondary afferents, the neuromuscular junction and the muscle fibre itself, require lower temperatures to be significantly affected by cooling than does the spindle itself (Lehmann & de Lateur 1990a, 1990b). Consistent with these findings, Miglietta (1973) found, in stroke patients, that the spasticity and clonus disappeared only when the muscle itself was significantly cooled.

There is also evidence that skin heating may produce muscle relaxation. Stimulation of the skin in the neck region decreases gamma fibre activity resulting in a decreased spindle excitability (Fischer & Solomon 1965). This may explain why superficial heating devices that primarily raise the skin temperature may also decrease muscle spasms.

Knutsson & Mattsson (1969) found a reduction of amplitude of the Achilles tendon reflex with local cold application. In some cases, they found an immediate temporary increase of the reflex muscle tone after cold application. The Hoffmann (H) response seemed to be enhanced in some, and in other cases the increase was minimal and insignificant. They concluded that the initial increase in tone and H response may be the result of an increased excitability of the alpha motor neuron through stimulation of the exteroceptors of the skin. All cases ultimately showed a decline of the tendon jerk and reflex muscle tone, which they attributed to an effect of cold on the muscle and the peripheral nerve.

Hartviksen (1962) found a decrease of foot clonus in all of his patients. At the moment the ice packs were applied, the spasticity increased temporarily. After 15–30 seconds, it decreased. The reduction of the clonus lasted 60–90 minutes. Hartviksen felt that spasticity disappeared while intramuscular temperature was still normal. The long-lasting effect was attributed by him to the lower intramuscular temperature, which probably affected the spindles.

Miglietta (1973) also found a decrease in clonus. He

found an almost immediate decrease in the mechanically induced stretch response. However, clonus was unchanged in the majority of patients (80%) after 10 minutes of exposure, and it was evident that clonus started to decrease and became absent only after the intramuscular temperature started to drop. He suggested that the relief of clonus in spasticity following local cold application is not related to changes in the mechanical contraction of the muscle, but to direct effect of cold on muscle spindle excitability.

Trnavsky (1983) found decreased muscle tone after cold application. Here, again, this occurred only when the local muscle temperature was reduced. It should be noted that both Knutsson & Mattsson and Hartviksen spot-measured the temperature only at one place in the musculature, and had no data available as to whether, at the time of the earliest decreased reflex activity, another part of the muscle was already cooled.

Knuttsson & Mattsson found an increased H response during the first minutes of cold application in most of the subjects, indicating a facilitation of the alpha motor neuron discharge. Urbscheit & Bishop (1970) also found an increase in the H response without a significant change of the Achilles tendon tap. Lightfoot et al (1975) applied cooling for 45 minutes, and found no significant change in the H to M (direct muscle response) ratio. They concluded that, in addition to an effect on the spindle reducing the muscle tone, other factors were involved, including slowing of conduction in muscle or motor nerve fibres and prolonging of twitch contraction and half-relaxation time.

Bell & Lehmann (1987) measured skin and muscle temperature during cold application. The location of the temperature probe in the muscle was determined by soft-tissue X-ray. They found an average decrease in skin temperature of 18.4°C and in muscle temperature of 12.1°C. Before, during and after cold application, they examined the H response by a series of recruitment curves and related the maximal H response to the M response with supramaximal stimulation. They found that in all 16 cases the amplitude of the maximal M response decreased significantly in response to cooling. These changes in the recording of the compound action potentials should be considered when cooling experiments result in alterations in H or electromyogram (EMG) response to tendon tap, since the changes in recording may affect all three potentials, the H response, the M response and the tendon tap EMG. When using the M response as a covariant in this analysis, there were no significant changes in the H reflex amplitude. However, the tendon tap amplitude decreased significantly.

Thus, these findings do not support the claims that simple cooling facilitates the alpha motor neuron discharge measured by the H reflex. However, rubbing with ice may stimulate the mechanoreceptors. Hagbarth (1952) has clearly shown that this may lead to facilitation of muscle tone. The study of Bell & Lehmann (1987) does confirm that the tendon tap reflex is decreased by muscle cooling.

The clinically effective use of ice application to the skin and some of the references cited suggest that, as long as the exteroceptors of the skin are stimulated, a facilitation of the alpha motor neuron discharge may occur. One may conclude that, to decrease muscle tone, i.e. spasticity, cooling should be applied in such a way that the muscle temperature is lowered. All authors agree that under those circumstances, reflex activity is diminished and the therapeutic effect of spasticity is achieved and maintained for an adequate period of time.

Another condition that creates a great deal of discomfort to the patient is joint or 'morning' stiffness as it is encountered in collagen diseases, most commonly in rheumatoid arthritis. Wright & Johns (1960) and Bäcklund & Tiselius (1967) showed that the complaint correlated closely with physical measurements of the viscoelastic properties of the joints. Specifically they measured maximal elasticity in extension and flexion, as well as resistance to motion due to viscous properties and to friction. There was a 20% decrease in stiffness at 45°C as compared with 33°C when a superficial joint was treated with infrared radiation (Wright & Johns 1961).

A well-documented physiological response to heat application is the increase in blood flow with a corresponding decrease when cold is applied. In an active organ, local temperature elevation will lead to a marked increase in blood flow (Guy et al 1974; Lehmann et al 1979; Sekins et al 1980, 1982; Lehmann & de Lateur 1990b). Reflexly induced changes usually consist of an increase of blood flow to the skin and superficial tissues and of a decrease of the blood flow to an inactive organ. Thus, when heat is applied to the skin, blood flow to the underlying musculature will be reduced. When the skin is heated, blood flow to the skin is increased not only in the area heated but also in other areas of the skin which are not heated (consensual reaction; Fischer & Solomon 1965). On the other hand, cooling produces vasoconstriction. Vasodilatation in response to cold – the 'hunting reaction' – occurs only if the temperatures are low enough to be potentially destructive to the tissues. The increase in vascularity and blood flow due to heating may play a role in obtaining relief from painful conditions such as myofibrositis or fibrositis, a poorly defined syndrome which responds to heating the tender muscular nodes. In the same fashion a resolution of painful inflammatory reactions may be achieved.

Pain in trauma, as it is commonly encountered in sports injuries, can be alleviated and to a degree prevented by early cold application, often in combination with application of pressure, for instance via an elastic bandage. In these cases cold not only reduces pain perception but also reduces bleeding and oedema formation as a result of vasoconstriction (Nilsson 1983; Derscheid & Brown 1985; Kay 1985). At a later date, heat application with vasodilatation may help with the healing and haematoma resolution (Perkins et al 1948, Clarke et al 1958; Schmidt et al 1979; Lehmann et al 1983; Lehmann & de Lateur 1990b).

Heat and cold application to the skin of the abdominal wall has a profound effect on pain resulting from spasm of the smooth musculature in the gastrointestinal tract or in the uterus. This pain is commonly associated with gastrointestinal upset resulting from viral enteritis, dietary indiscretion or with menstrual cramps. It has been shown (Bisgard & Nye 1940; Molander 1941; Fischer & Solomon 1965) that there is a marked reduction of peristalsis of the gastrointestinal tract with heat application and an increase of the peristalsis with cold application. This is associated with a decrease in acid production of the stomach and blanching of the mucous membrane when heat is applied. Acid production and blood flow to the mucous membrane are increased with cold application.

'COUNTERIRRITANT' EFFECTS

Parsons & Goetzl (1945) showed that cold applied with ethyl chloride spray for 20 seconds to the skin covering the tibia increased the pain threshold of the tooth pulp as measured by electrical stimulation. Similarly Melzack et al (1980a) reduced dental pain by ice massage applied to the web of the thumb and index finger of the hand on the same side as the painful region. Melzack et al (1980b) also showed that ice massage and transcutaneous electrical stimulation are equally effective in relieving low-back pain. Murray & Weaver (1975) showed that counterirritation (consisting of 10-second immersion of the finger into a 2°C water bath) reduced itching significantly more than a control procedure. Melzack et al (1980a) suggested that the observations could be explained on the basis of the gate theory (Melzack & Wall 1965). Studies of morphine receptors in the central nervous system and of the role of enkephalins and endorphins (Fields & Basbaum 1978) suggested that this mechanism could play a role in explaining the counterirritant effect, especially when the stimulus is applied distant from the site of the pain-producing process (Kerr & Casey 1976). Gammon & Starr (1941) also showed that heat producing a significant temperature elevation resulted in the same analgesic effect as cold application. The effects produced by this mechanism seem to be of the same order of magnitude as those obtained by transcutaneous electrical nerve stimulation (Melzack et al 1980b).

Benson & Copp (1974) found that heat and cold both raised the normal pain threshold significantly. Ice therapy was more effective than heat, but following either form of treatment the effect declined within 30 minutes.

EFFECTS ON NERVE AND NERVE ENDINGS

Douglas & Malcolm (1955), in experiments with cats, studied the differential effect of cold on fibres of various diameters. Small medullated fibres were affected first, then the large medullated fibres and finally the unmedullated fibres. In man (Ganong 1979), pain impulses are carried in part by the small medullated A delta fibres. Unfortunately, data like these are somewhat species-dependent and generalisation can only be tentative. However, it has been shown by Goodgold & Eberstein (1977) and de Jong et al (1966) that, in general, nerve conduction drops with decreasing temperature and that finally (Li 1958) nerve fibres cease conducting. Therefore it can be assumed that pain sensation may be markedly reduced by significant local cooling through an indirect effect on nerve fibres and free endings. There is also evidence that heat applied to the peripheral nerve or free nerve endings reduces pain sensation (Lehmann et al 1964). The pain threshold was measured with the Hardy-Wolff-Goodell method (Hardy et al 1940) before and after heat application to the ulnar nerve and to the pad of the little finger. However, a counterirritant effect could not absolutely be ruled out in these experiments.

In a study by Barker et al (1991), administration of cold saline prior to injection of propofol (2,6-diisopropylphenol) anaesthetic increased the amount of pain relief obtained as compared with propofol injection alone. Recently, it has been shown (Hong 1991) that ultrasound therapy with therapeutic dosage may cause a reversible nerve conduction block and pain relief in patients with polyneuropathy.

LASERS

While lasers have many characteristics in common with diffuse light, the main difference between laser and diffuse light is that the laser is a columnated beam of photons of the same frequency with the wavelength in phase. In therapy, except for surgical purposes, lower level intensities are used. Unfortunately, most studies on the use of laser for the relief of pain in various conditions do not have suitable controls. Therefore the results are equivocal and the effectiveness of lasers in treatment of painful syndromes is not well documented. Attempts have been made to show benefits in various arthritides, myofascial pain syndromes, back pain, epicondylitis (tennis elbow), and others. Where well-controlled studies have been done, they have usually failed to show benefit.

Goldman et al (1980) treated 30 patients with rheumatoid arthritis with the neodymium laser. It operated at a wavelength of 1060 nanometres (nm) with output of 15 joules per square centimetre, and a pulse duration of 30 nanoseconds. The duration of the laser exposure was not stated. One hand was treated at the proximal interphalangeal and metacarpophalangeal joints, whereas the other hand received a sham exposure. They found improvement in both hands. However, the hand that had laser treatment had a greater improvement in erythema and pain. On the other hand, laboratory data which included the titre of rheumatoid arthritis, antinuclear antibody or polyethylene glycol precipitates showed no change. No controls were used. On physical examination the lateral pinch was the same for treated and untreated hands as well as range of motion of the joints. However, over time a difference was found in both treated and untreated hands with regard to grasp strength. The increase was greater on the treated side.

In a study by Bliddal et al (1987) nine treatments with helium-neon laser, 6 joules per square centimetre, were given in a double-blind study to the hands of patients with rheumatoid arthritis. One hand was irradiated with laser, the other with a sham exposure. The laser therapy gave some pain relief, but no difference in morning stiffness or joint performance was obtained.

Basford et al (1987) carried out a randomised controlled and double-blind study of the effects of low-energy 0.9 milliwatt helium-neon laser treatment of osteoarthritis of the thumb. 81 subjects were studied; 47 were treated and 34 served as controls. Subjectively, a slight but significant decrease in tenderness in the laser-treated group was noted. However, all objective measures such as grip strength and range of motion showed no significant difference between the control group and the treated group. The authors concluded that this treatment was safe but ineffective for osteoarthritis of the thumb.

Waylonis et al (1988) treated chronic myofascial pain with low output helium-neon laser. They found no statistical difference between treatment and placebo groups. They treated 62 patients by using acupuncture points. Clinical response was assessed using a portion of the McGill Pain Questionnaire.

Ceccherelli et al (1989) used laser for the treatment of 37 women with muscular neck pain. Differences between the treated and the control group were statistically significant.

Hansen & Thorøe (1990) treated chronic orofacial pain in 40 patients in a controlled study. They did not find any statistically significant difference in the analgesic effect between the groups treated with laser and with placebo, although they found a substantial placebo response in both groups.

Walker (1983) used a low-power, one milliwatt helium-neon laser over various peripheral nerves, such as the radial, median and saphenous nerves, in the treatment of pain syndromes. Pain relief occurred only when the appropriate peripheral nerve was treated. When patients with trigeminal neuralgia, postherpetic pain, sciatica, and osteoarthritis were treated, 19 of 26 had relief of pain without medication, whereas those who received sham stimulation reported no improvement of pain. Similarly, Iijima et al (1989), in an uncontrolled study, reported that laser treatment produced relief of postherpetic pain.

Walker et al (1988) also used the helium-neon laser (1 milliwatt, 20 Hz) to treat trigeminal neuralgia. Control subjects received placebo treatment. The experimental group contained 18 patients and the control group 17. Assignment to the experimental or control group was on a random basis. Pain was assessed subjectively on a scale from 0 to 100. The results suggested improvement with the laser therapy.

Laser also has been used in the treatment of epicondylitis (tennis elbow). Lundeberg et al (1987a) compared the pain-relieving effect of laser treatment versus placebo in tennis elbow. The results showed that laser treatment is not significantly better than placebo.

In a study by Siebert et al (1987) the efficacy of helium-neon laser and gallium-aluminum-arsenic lasers in treatment of tendinopathies was compared with placebo in a double-blind controlled study. No therapeutic effect was found.

Lundeberg et al (1987b) also compared the pain-relieving effect of laser treatment and acupuncture. They found that neither neon-helium nor gallium-arsenide low-power irradiation produced any change in response. The study was performed in 36 male white rats; 12 of them served as a control group. An antinociceptive effect was assessed using the tail-flick test and compared with the mean prolongation of the response time in intact rats, compared with the responses of rats who had acupuncture, one of the two lasers or morphine. Lasers did not produce any changes compared to the control group, whereas acupuncture and morphine did.

Haker et al (1990) applied laser treatment, in a double-blind study, to acupuncture points in lateral humeral epicondylalgia. No significant differences were observed between laser and the placebo groups in relation to the subjective and objective outcome after 10 treatments. These authors used a wavelength of 904 nanometres, a mean power output of 12 milliwatts with a peak value of 8.3 watts, and a pulse frequency of 70 Hz.

In a study on the effect of laser in lateral epicondylalgia, Haker & Lundeberg (1991a) used a wavelength of 904 nanometres, output of 12 milliwatts with a frequency of 70 Hz and a pulse train of 8000 Hz. They assigned 49 patients consecutively to a control group or to a laser treatment group; they concluded that laser may be a valuable therapy, but that further studies will be necessary.

Haker & Lundeberg (1991b) compared the effectiveness of application of laser, using specific stimulation parameters, to acupuncture points in the treatment of lateral epicondylalgia. They used a gallium-arsenide and helium-neon laser. The combined application was compared with red-light application in a control group of patients. 58 patients were consecutively assigned to the laser and placebo groups. There was no statistical difference in the outcome between the two treatments using objective and subjective measures.

Klein & Eek (1990) studied the effects of low-energy laser treatment and exercise for low-back pain in a controlled trial. They found that exercises had an effect, whereas there was no significant difference between the two groups, one receiving laser and exercise and the other receiving exercise only.

Finally, helium-neon laser has been used in dentistry to prevent pain and swelling after tooth extraction. Taube et al (1990) found no difference in postoperative swelling and pain relief between the test and the control groups. Carrillo et al (1990) on the other hand found in a controlled study of patients treated with helium-neon laser, ibuprofen or placebo, that trismus was significantly reduced in the helium-neon laser and the ibuprofen treated groups compared with the placebo group. Pain, however, was significantly less only with the ibuprofen group. Swelling was the same in the laser, ibuprofen, and control groups.

In summary, laser may be useful for pain relief, but more controlled studies which give the specific parameters of the laser application will be necessary to assess the efficacy of this new modality. Further studies are also required to understand the mechanism of interaction with biological tissues under therapeutic conditions.

DIFFERENCES IN THE EFFECTS OF HEAT AND COLD APPLICATION

From the review of the literature it is apparent that the effect of heat and cold may be similar in many cases. In others cold produces effects in the opposite direction of heat. Both heat and cold reduce muscle spasm secondary to underlying joint and skeletal pathology and nerve-root irritation, as in low-back syndromes, and therefore relieve the associated pain. A vicious cycle consisting of muscle spasm, ischaemia, pain and more muscle spasm is interrupted. In case of upper motor neuron lesions with painful spasticity the effect of heat is short-lived because the temperature in the muscle is rapidly restored to its pretreatment level as a result of the increase in blood flow. If the reduction in spasticity with reduction in pain relief is produced by muscle cooling, this effect lasts much longer. Rewarming from the outside is slow because of the insulating subcutaneous fat layer, and rewarming from the inside is retarded because of the vasoconstriction in the muscle. However, neither heat nor cold has a permanent effect on spasticity.

In the presence of an acute deep-seated inflammatory reaction, vigorous heat application is contraindicated. It usually increases hyperaemia and oedema with pain and acceleration of abscess formation. This does not contradict the fact that such heat application is used in superficial boils to bring the abscess to a head with subsequent easy evacuation. Mild-heat application is used in superficial thrombophlebitis. In contrast to the effects of heat, in an inflammatory reaction it is generally agreed that cold may reduce oedema, hyperaemia and pain.

In acute rheumatoid arthritis, vigorous deep-heat application is likely to aggravate the pain and discomfort. On the other hand, painful joint stiffness is measurably improved by heat and aggravated by cold application (Wright & Johns 1960, 1961; Bäcklund & Tiselius 1967). However, an intensive cooling may numb pain in spite of the increase in stiffness.

In acute trauma with aggravation of pain resulting from oedema and bleeding, cold application will reduce both because of vasoconstriction. Heat will increase both oedema and bleeding tendency.

THE USE OF HEAT FOR PAIN RELIEF

DOSIMETRY AND TECHNIQUE OF HEAT APPLICATION

The physiological effects which produce pain relief when heat is applied may be achieved by direct effects of the temperature elevation on the tissue and cellular functions. They may also be achieved through local reflexes with the reaction occurring at the site of the tissue temperature elevation. However, the type and extent of the reaction may depend largely on whether the site of the pain-producing pathology is heated or whether one relies on distant heating and on effects produced by reflex or other neuromechanisms.

Local heating

Local temperature elevation at the site of the pathology can produce a large number of different responses, including changes in neuromuscular activity, blood flow, capillary permeability, enzymatic activity and pain threshold. These reactions can be produced to varying degrees depending on the condition of heating. Thus vigorous local responses may be produced.

Distant heating

If the site of temperature elevation is distant from the painful pathology to be treated, only a limited number of physiological responses, reflexogenic in nature, can be obtained at the site of the pathology. These reactions are always milder than those produced locally at the site of the temperature elevation. These distant reactions include blood-flow changes in skin and in the mucous membranes of the gastrointestinal tract. They include reflexogenic changes in muscle activity, both relaxation of voluntary striated muscle and of smooth muscle of the gastrointestinal tract and uterus. They also include reflex reduction of gastric acidity.

In conclusion, when vigorous responses are desired, local heat is strongly preferred. The factors which determine the intensity of the physiological reaction locally are, first, the level of tissue temperature elevation (approximately 40–50°C) and, second, the duration of tissue temperature elevation (5–30 min).

Mild versus vigorous effects

In order to obtain vigorous responses to heat therapy, it is necessary to attain the highest temperature at the site of the tissue pathology to be treated and to elevate this temperature close to the maximally tolerated level. Dosimetry and proper technique of application of the modalities are essential, since the therapeutic range for a given effect extends only over a few degrees.

If a mild limited response is desired one can select a modality which produces the highest temperature at the site of the pathology, but then limit the output of the modality so that only a moderate temperature rise occurs; this, in turn, produces a mild effect. The alternative to this procedure is to heat the superficial tissues and rely on mild limited reflexogenic responses at the site of the pathology in the depth of the tissues.

Selection of modality according to temperature distribution

From this it becomes apparent that if vigorous heating is indicated, one must select that type of heating modality which produces the highest temperature in the distribution at the site of the treatable pathology. Since the temperature at this site is brought to tolerance level, this method avoids burns elsewhere. This represents the rationale for having the various deep-heating devices: shortwave diathermy, a high-frequency elecromagnetic current operating at the frequency of 27.12 Megahertz (MHz) microwaves, an electromagnetic radiation of the frequency of 2456 and 915 MHz, and ultrasound, a high-frequency acoustic vibration at a frequency of 0.8–1 MHz. The approach to using these modalities primarily as deep-heating agents is justified in the light of overwhelming experimental evidence that most of the therapeutically desirable effects are due to heating, and not due to non-thermal reactions (Lehmann & de Lateur 1982, 1990a, 1990b; Kramer 1985). It is conceivable that some non-thermal effects may play a role in the outcome. It has been documented, however, that some undesirable side-effects are clearly due to non-thermal mechanisms and should be avoided (Lehmann & de Lateur 1982, 1990a, 1990b). The superficial heating agents such as hot packs, paraffin bath, Fluidotherapy, hydrotherapy and radiant heat will produce temperature distributions similar to one another, with the highest temperature in the most superficial tissues. Some of these modalities have non-thermal effects of therapeutic advantage; for instance, hydrotherapy allows exercise of painful joints with reduced stress because the buoyancy of the water reduces the gravitational forces. Also, the cleansing action of a whirlpool bath can be beneficial in wound treatments and the drying action of radiant heat may be desirable in weeping lesions.

In order to select the appropriate modality for a given site of a treatable pathology, one must take into account the propagation and absorption characteristics of the tissues for each form of energy used for heating. In general one can state that skin and superficial subcutaneous tissues are selectively heated by infrared, visible light, hot packs, paraffin bath, Fluidotherapy and hydrotherapy. Subcutaneous tissues and superficial musculature are selectively heated by shortwave diathermy with condenser application and by microwaves at a frequency of 2456 MHz. Superficial musculature is heated preferentially by shortwave diathermy using induction coil applicators. Deep-seated joints and fibrous scars within soft tissues are selectively heated by ultrasound as are myofascial interfaces, tendon and tendon sheath and nerve trunks. Pelvic organs are selectively heated by shortwave diathermy using internal vaginal or rectal electrodes.

In addition it is most important to realise that the desirable temperature distribution can be achieved only if proper technique of application and proper dosimetry are used. Several of these modalities are very powerful and if inappropriately used can do severe tissue damage in a short period of time. Details of the techniques of application are beyond the scope of this chapter. The reader is referred to Lehmann & de Lateur (1990b).

Nonthermal effects of the diathermy modalities, i.e. shortwave, microwave and ultrasound, have been well documented (Lehmann & de Lateur 1990a, 1990b, 1990c). However, none of them has been proven to be essential for therapeutic effectiveness. Some nonthermal effects may represent potential hazards; however, few of them have been documented to be destructive. These can be avoided by use of proper equipment and proper technique of application. In shortwave diathermy, among others, pearl-chain formation of blood corpuscles has been documented without any relation to physiological effects (Herrick et al 1950; Herrick & Krusen 1953; Texeira-Pinto et al 1960). Possible nonthermal changes of macromolecules were reported by Bach (1965), Bach et al (1960) and Heller (1960), who exposed human gamma globulin to radiofrequency and microwave energy. However, such changes were not observed at therapeutic frequencies. Pearl-chain formation can also be produced by microwave application (Saito & Schwan 1961; Lehmann & de Lateur 1990c). In microwaves, the controversy ranges primarily around safety standards and inadvertent exposure of sensitive organs. Physiological and hazardous responses claimed at low intensities below 10 mW/cm^2 are not well documented (Michaelson 1972,

1990; Lehmann 1990b), whereas thermal damage at intensities above 100 mW/cm^2 is clearly established. Specifically sensitive areas include the eye, the lens, the testicles and the brain. With ultrasound it is important to avoid the occurrence of gaseous cavitation, which occurs more readily in media with low-volume percentage of cells and low viscosity. Such media are found in the eye and also include amniotic fluid, cerebrospinal fluid and joint effusions. Under therapeutic conditions the occurrence is avoided by using adequate equipment with adequate uniformity in the spatial and temporal distribution of the intensity of the beam. Aggregation of platelets and accumulation of red cells in wave nodes can be avoided by using a stroking technique of application. While some other-than-thermal mechanism, such as acceleration of diffusion processes, may be produced by ultrasound and may be therapeutically helpful, the importance of this has not been clearly documented.

TECHNIQUES OF COLD APPLICATION

Melting ice together with water is commonly used for cryotherapy, since it assures a steady temperature of 0°C. Most commonly a rubber bag containing ice cubes with water is applied as a compress. A layer of terry cloth between the ice bag and the skin may slow down cooling. Other methods use terry cloth dipped into a mixture of ice shavings with water. The cloth is wrung out and then applied to the body part. This application has to be repeated frequently. Finally a part may be treated by immersion in ice water; this, however, is a potentially more dangerous method because of the possibility of development of necrosis of fingers or toes. If it is the objective to cool musculature to relieve muscle spasm or spasticity, it is necessary to apply the ice for a significant period of time. Even in a relatively slender individual with a subcutaneous fat layer of less than 1 cm, more than 10 minutes of ice application is necessary to get significant cooling of the underlying musculature. In many cases 20–30 minutes may be necessary to achieve the desired result, which can be gauged by clinical observation of the resolution of the muscle spasm, the reduction of spasticity, clonus and the spindle reflexes (Bierman & Friedlander 1940; Hartviksen 1962).

Ice massage, in which a block of ice is rubbed over the skin surface, is also used for the same purpose. However, it must be remembered that short-term ice massage is more likely just to cool the skin and therefore facilitate alpha motor neuron discharge with subsequent increase in muscle tone, as documented by Hartviksen (1962).

Evaporative cooling with ethyl chloride spray is done by spraying the skin from a distance of about 1 metre with stroking motion. Bierman (1955) suggested a movement of the spray of 4 inches/second. Each area should be exposed only for a few seconds, followed by a pause. More recently, chlorofluoromethanes have been used since they are less flammable than ethyl chloride (Traherne 1962). This method is more frequently used as a 'counterirritant'. It is doubtful that it is suitable for cooling a large muscle covered by a significant fat layer.

COMMON THERAPEUTIC APPLICATIONS OF HEAT AND COLD FOR PAIN RELIEF

It is essential for successful therapeutic application of heat and cold that the correct diagnosis be made first. The local condition to be treated is assessed and a judgement is made as to whether or not it is treatable with heat or cold. The location of the pathological process is clearly identified and correspondingly the proper modality is selected. It is equally important that the application should be done with appropriate technique. Painful skeletal muscle spasms, which frequently occur in the back as a result of nerve root irritation or spinal pathology, may be successfully treated with heat or cold to achieve muscle relaxation and thus abolishment of pain. Shortwave diathermy may be applied with either induction coil applicators or condenser pads. Treatment should occur once or twice daily for 20–30 minutes. Relaxation may be achieved by direct muscle heating and an effect on the spindle mechanism as well as reflexly by surface heating. Microwave direct contact applicators can be used for this purpose. Also helpful are superficial heating agents, including hot packs such as Hydrocollator packs or radiant heat with heat lamp or cradle. Treatment should be for 20–30 minutes. In this case reflexogenic relaxation is achieved.

As an alternative mode of treatment ice pack or ice massage may be applied so as to cool the muscle and thus reduce spindle sensitivity. Therefore applications for a minimum of 10 minutes (although 20 min would be better) would be required. Landen (1967) showed in 117 patients with back pain that heat and cold applications were equally effective. In acute conditions heat was found to reduce hospital stay more effectively than ice applications, while in chronic conditions ice was more effective than heat application. All of these treatments are for symptomatic relief and produce their effects by reduction of the painful muscle spasm.

In myofibrositis in the presence of so-called trigger points, both cold application, often with ethyl chloride spray, and local application of heat have been used successfully. Ultrasound in low or medium dose applied to the painful area has also been found to be effective. In this condition heat application is often followed by deep-seated sedative massage. In cases of mild fibrositis more vigorous friction massage may also be used.

In tension states with increased EMG activity, discomfort can be relieved by heat application; commonly shortwave or superficial heat are used. These forms of heat application are often followed by deep sedative massage. This treatment is usually combined with relaxation training with biofeedback to reduce the muscle tension. In any one of these conditions, but specifically in myofibrositis, there is also evidence that these modalities represent a 'counterirritant' and reduce pain as explained on the basis of the gate theory (Parsons & Goetzl 1945; Melzack & Wall 1965).

In gastrointestinal upset, cramping of the smooth musculature of the tract produces pain. The peristalsis and discomfort can be reduced by superficial heat application to the abdomen in the form of hot packs (Bisgard & Nye 1940; Molander 1941; Fischer & Solomon 1965). This reduction of cramps is associated with reduction of blood flow to the mucous membranes and hydrochloric acid secretion in the stomach. Cold application aggravates the discomfort. Menstrual cramps seem to respond in the same fashion.

In persons with Raynaud's phenomenon, Delp & Newton (1986) assessed hand function after cold stress. Both two-point discrimination and finger dexterity were assessed. The results showed a decreased performance on the Purdue Pegboard test and decreased two-point discrimination after cold application. Similar findings were observed in a normal control group.

The common complaint of joint stiffness and pain in rheumatic diseases such as rheumatoid arthritis is alleviated measurably by heat application (Wright & Johns 1960, 1961; Johns & Wright 1962; Bäcklund & Tiselius 1967). Cold application aggravates the objective signs. Clinically, superficial heat such as radiant heat and hot tub bath is commonly used for this purpose. Also, the secondary muscle spasms can be treated in this fashion. Modalities, such as ultrasound, which selectively heat the joints, are not used in this condition because the vigorous heating of the inflamed synovium may produce exacerbation. The whirlpool bath or the dip method of paraffin may be used for mild heating of hands and feet. If the Hubbard tank is used, exercise of the joints can occur at the same time with elimination of the force of gravity by buoyancy. Futhermore, contrast baths, according to Martin et al (1946), may be used to relieve stiffness.

Contrast baths are often recommended for the treatment of stiffness associated with Heberden's nodes. If many joints of the upper and lower extremity are involved in the rheumatic process, radiant heat applied with a double baker is a method of heat application. It has been suggested that ice should be used to numb the pain of the joint and this application has been advocated on the basis that Harris & McCroskery (1974) found that the activity of destructive enzymes such as collagenase is reduced at lower temperatures. These same experiments have been quoted to indicate that heating of the joint itself is contraindicated. This conclusion exceeds the parameters of the experiment which investigated the effects on the collagenase of temperatures only up to 36°C whereas therapeutic temperatures reach or exceed 43°C. At these therapeutic temperatures other enzyme systems have shown a markedly reduced activity (Harris & Krane 1973; Harris & McCroskery 1974).

Joint contractures due to capsular tightness or synovial scarring are frequently painful when mobilised by range of motion exercises and stretch. The effectiveness of the treatment can be increased and the associated pain can be markedly reduced by using ultrasound in high dosage which has been shown selectively to raise the temperature in the tight structures, which in turn show an increase in extensibility rendering the treatment programme less painful and more effective (DePreux 1952; Friedland 1975). Depending on the soft tissue covering of the joint, ultrasound applied with the multiple field method is used at intensities between 2 and 4 W/cm^2 with a total output between 20 and 40 W. The application is with a stroking technique.

In acute calcific bursitis of the subdeltoid and subacromial bursae the acute pain is due to swelling and pressure within the content of the bursa resulting in an inflammatory reaction. Ice application may alleviate the acute pain especially if used in conjunction with removal of bursal content and hydrocortisone injection combined with local anaesthetic. At the later stage the limitation of the range of motion of the shoulder joint, which is frequently associated with calcific tendinitis, should be appropriately treated with ultrasound in combination with range of motion exercises and stretch (Lehmann & de Lateur 1990b).

In the shoulder-hand syndrome or reflex sympathetic dystrophy, superficial heat and ultrasound treatment in combination with a programme to increase range of motion may be used as an adjunct to other therapy, including stellate ganglion blocks.

In painful lateral epicondylitis or 'tennis elbow' the primary treatment should consist of rest, splinting, ice application and possibly also an injection of hydrocortisone and local anaesthetic. During the later stage of resolution superficial heat may be used. Also, ultrasound in low dosage to produce mild effects could be used at this stage since ultrasound selectively raises the temperature at the common tendon of origin and the extensor aponeurosis. The dosage should be approximately 0.5 W/cm^2. Recently Binder et al (1985) treated 76 patients with lateral epicondylitis. The patients were randomly allocated to groups such that 38 received ultrasound and 38 received placebo treatment. A total of 63% of the patients treated with ultrasound were improved, compared with 29% of those given placebo treatment.

Steinberg & Callies (1992) treated epicondylitis with ultrasound and with ultrasound in combination with prednisolone ointment (phonophoresis). They found that ultrasound significantly reduced the pain. However, there was no difference between ultrasound application alone or with phonophoresis; Haker & Lundeberg (1991c) did not find pulsed application of ultrasound effective in this condition.

In a retrospective analysis of medical records of acute surgical trauma patients, Schaubel (1946) found that cold application reduced the need for recasting due to swelling from 42.3 to only 5.3% of the cases. Also he found a marked reduction in the requirement for narcotics for pain relief. Cohn et al (1989) found that cooling after surgical repair of the anterior cruciate ligament reduced the need for pain medication. Seino et al (1985) used intercostal nerve blocks to produce cryoanalgesia. They used a freezing technique to control pain after thoracotomy. The cryoanalgesia group had lower postoperative pain scores and required less than half the analgesia compared with the control group. Moore & Cardea (1977) found that the combination of intermittent pressure and ice application promptly reduced the compartmental pressures in the calf which were markedly increased as a result of tibial and fibular fractures. Only Matsen et al (1975) found in animal experiments that swelling after fracture was not reduced, perhaps even increased when cold was applied. In case of minor sports injuries, cryotherapy in combination with compression, for instance using an elastic bandage, is usually used (Basur et al 1976). Also elevation of the limb and immobilisation are recommended. It must be remembered, however, that this application of ice should be extended only over a period long enough to prevent swelling and bleeding since prolonged ice application may unnecessarily retard healing (Vinger & Hoerner 1982). At a later date resolution can be assisted by heat application.

In superficial thrombophlebitis, one adjunct of therapy may be application of moist hot packs or the heat cradle with reduction of discomfort.

Painful amputation neuromas can be treated successfully with ultrasound, provided that the origin of pain is local, for instance due to adhesions and irritation of the neuroma and not phantom limb pain of other origin. Ultrasound selectively raises the temperature of the neuroma and is given in high dosage which is probably destructive to the nerve fibres. The alternative to conservative treatment is the surgical revision of the stump. It is clinically suggested that postherpetic pain can be treated on the same basis. This indication is based purely on clinical (that is, empirical) evidence.

In other conditions, Balogun & Okonofua (1988) reported successful use of shortwave diathermy applied to the pelvic organs in chronic pelvic inflammatory disease which was not responsive to antibiotic therapy.

CONTRAINDICATIONS OR PRECAUTIONS

In general there are conditions when heat should be used with special precautions. These include heat application to anaesthetic areas or to an obtunded patient. Dosimetry, especially in the deep-heating modalities, is not developed to the point that the tissue temperatures can be safely controlled and that destructive temperatures can be reliably avoided. Therefore pain is an essential signal that safe temperature limits are exceeded and it has been documented that if the signal is heeded tissue destruction does not occur. Also, tissues with inadequate vascular supply should not be heated since the temperature elevation increases metabolic demand without associated vascular adaptations. As a result ischaemic necrosis may occur. Heat should not be applied if there is a haemorrhagic diathesis, since the increase in blood flow and vascularity will produce more bleeding. Heat should not be applied to malignancies without exact tissue temperature monitoring since otherwise therapeutic temperatures may accelerate tumour growth. Heat should not be applied to the gonads or the developing fetus because of the possibility of development of congenital malformations (Mussa 1955; Edwards 1967, 1972; Dietzel & Kern 1971a, 1971b; Moayer 1971; Dietzel et al 1972; Edwards et al 1974; Menser 1978; Smith et al 1978; Hendrickx et al 1979; Harvey et al 1981).

Some specific contraindications also exist for specific diathermy modalities. Shortwave diathermy is contraindicated if an appreciable amount of energy can reach the site of a metal implant (Lehmann et al 1979). The dangers involved are caused by shunting of current through the metal implant or by increasing the current density surrounding the implant. In either case excessively high temperatures are produced. This contraindication includes intrauterine devices containing copper or other metals until proven otherwise. However, these devices would be reached by significant amounts of current only with application with internal vaginal or rectal electrodes (Sandler 1973). Also, electronic implants such as cardiac pacemakers and electrophysiological orthoses represent contraindications. Contact lenses may lead to excessive heating of the eye (Scott 1956). Some clinicians have suggested that shortwave diathermy applied to the low back may result in increased menstrual flow (Lehmann & de Lateur 1990c). The use of pelvic diathermy in the pregnant woman is contraindicated for the reasons given under general contraindications. Safe levels of stray radiation have not been worked out for shortwave diathermy.

Sensitive organs which should not be exposed to any significant amount of microwave radiation include the eyes, since in experimental animals (Carpenter & Van Ummerson 1968; Guy et al 1975) cataracts were produced due to a selective heating effect. The testicles should not be exposed because of the great sensitivity of these reproductive organs to temperature elevation. Exposure of the skull and the brain could lead to focusing of the intensity inside the skull and produce higher levels of exposure than anticipated from measurement outside the body (Johnson & Guy 1972). In the USA, safety standards proposed by the Food and Drug Administration for therapeutic application specify a level of 5 mW/cm^2 at a distance of 5 cm from the applicator. Damage under therapeutic exposure, however, has not been observed under 100–150 mW/cm^2 (Michaelson 1990) and is clearly related to the heating effect. Precautions should be used when microwaves are applied over bony prominences, since the reflection of the wave at the bone interface may produce increased absorption in the tissues superficial to the bone. Burns have been observed under these circumstances.

In the case of ultrasound, as mentioned previously, proper equipment and technique of application must be used to avoid the occurrence and destructive effects of gaseous cavitation. Also, exposure of the fluid media of the eye, of the cerebrospinal fluid and of effusions should be avoided because in these media with low cellular content and low viscosity, gaseous cavitation can occur even at therapeutic intensities. For the same reason the amniotic fluid of the pregnant uterus should not be exposed and the heating effect of ultrasound would represent a contraindication when ultrasound is applied to the fetus. However, due to the excellent beaming properties of ultrasound, exposure of the pregnant uterus can easily be avoided. Thus ultrasound can be used for other indications. Also, ultrasound can be applied to the intervertebral joints without significant exposure of cerebrospinal fluid and spinal cord because of the intervening tissues such as bone, ligaments and muscles and because the beam can be aimed at the joint facets.

If superficial heat is applied by means of a Hubbard tank or hot tub and the entire body is submerged, the body temperature should be monitored. In this situation, the heat regulatory mechanisms are disabled and therefore an artificial fever is easily produced. Oral temperatures should be taken at water temperatures over 100°F (37.8°C).

There are also contraindications to the use of cold. Severe adverse effects to local cold application are rare and are usually due to hypersensitivity to cold. Four groups of hypersensitivity may be distinguished (Juhlin & Shelley 1961). The first group of hypersensitivity syndromes is a result of release of histamine or histamine-like substances. It presents itself frequently as classical cold urticaria. The pathogenesis is primarily due to an effect of histamine on capillary vessels and smooth musculature with skin manifestations of urticaria, erythema, itching and sweating. There may be facial flush, puffiness of the eyelids and laryngeal oedema with respiratory impairment. In severe cases there is shock or so-called anaphylaxis with syncope, hypotension and tachycardia. Gastrointestinal symptoms are associated with gastric hyperacidity and include dysphagia, abdominal pain, diarrhoea and vomiting. Horton et al (1936) demonstrated that this type of sensitivity is treatable by a programme of careful desensitisation.

The second group of hypersensitivity is due to the presence of cold haemolysins and agglutinins. Renal haemoglobinuria and skin manifestations of urticaria and Raynaud's phenomenon are part of the symptomatology.

The third group of syndromes is due to the presence of cryoglobulins. There are severe manifestations such as reduced vision, impairment of hearing, conjunctival haemorrhages, epistaxis, cold urticaria, Raynaud's phenomenon and ulceration and necrosis. Also, gastrointestinal upset with melaena and gingival bleeding have been observed.

Finally, a marked cold pressor response may be observed in some patients with submersion of limbs in ice water (Wolf & Hardy 1941; Wolff 1951; Boyer et al 1960; Larson 1961; Shelley & Caro 1962).

Some of these responses are severe. Prominent vasospasm can produce a necrosis of fingers and toes in submersion of the limbs. Therefore careful medical evaluation of the patients is essential and also a trial of localised ice application over a small area – for instance, on the thigh – may produce skin manifestations of sensitivity as a warning sign.

REFERENCES

Bach S A 1965 Biological sensitivity to radio-frequency and microwave energy. Federation Proceedings 24 (suppl 14): S22–S26

Bach S A, Luzzio A J, Brownell A S 1960 Effects of radio-frequency energy on human gamma globulin. Proceedings of the Fourth Annual TriService Conference on the Biological Effects of Microwave Radiation 1: 117–133

Bäcklund L, Tiselius P 1967 Objective measurement of joint stiffness in rheumatoid arthritis. Acta Rheumatologica Scandinavica 13: 275–288

Balogun J A, Okonofua F E 1988 Management of chronic pelvic inflammatory disease with shortwave diathermy. Physical Therapy 68: 1541–1545

Barker P, Langton J A, Murphy P, Rowbotham D J 1991 Effect of prior administration of cold saline on pain during propofol injection. Anaesthesia 46: 1069–1070

Basford J R, Sheffield C G, Mair S D, Ilstrup D M 1987 Low-energy helium-neon laser treatment of thumb osteoarthritis. Archives of Physical Medicine and Rehabilitation 68: 794–797

Basur R L, Shephard E, Mouzas G L 1976 A cooling method in the treatment of ankle sprains. Practitioner 216: 708–711

Bell K R, Lehmann J F 1987 Effect of cooling on H- and T-reflexes in normal subjects. Archives of Physical Medicine and Rehabilitation 68: 490–493

Benson T B, Copp E P 1974 The effects of therapeutic forms of heat and ice on the pain threshold of the normal shoulder. Rheumatology and Rehabilitation 13: 101–104

Bierman W 1955 Therapeutic use of cold. Journal of the American Medical Association 157: 1189–1192

Bierman W, Friedlander M 1940 The penetrative effect of cold. Archives of Physical Therapy 21: 585–591

Binder A, Hodge G, Greenwood A M, Hazleman B L, Page Thomas D P 1985 Is therapeutic ultrasound effective in treating soft tissue lesions? British Medical Journal 290: 512–514

Bisgard J D, Nye D 1940 The influence of hot and cold application upon gastric and intestinal motor activity. Surgery, Gynecology and Obstetrics 71: 172–180

Bliddal H, Hellesen C, Ditlevsen P, Asselberghs J, Lyager L 1987 Soft-laser therapy of rheumatoid arthritis. Scandinavian Journal of Rheumatology 16: 225–228

Boyer J T, Fraser J R E, Doyle A E 1960 The haemodynamic effects of cold immersion. Clinical Science 19: 539–550

Carpenter R L, Van Ummerson C A 1968 The action of microwave power on the eye. Journal of Microwave Power 3: 3–19

Carrillo J S, Calatayud J, Manso F J et al 1990 A randomized double-blind clinical trial on the effectiveness of helium-neon laser in the prevention of pain, swelling and trismus after removal of impacted third molars. International Dental Journal 40: 31–36

Ceccherelli F, Altafini L, Lo Castro G et al 1989 Diode laser in cervical myofascial pain: a double-blind study versus placebo. The Clinical Journal of Pain 5: 301–304

Clarke R S J, Hellon R F, Lind A R 1958 Vascular reactions of the human forearm to cold. Clinical Science 17: 165–179

Cohn B T, Draeger R I, Jackson D W 1989 The effects of cold therapy in the postoperative management of pain in patients undergoing anterior cruciate ligament reconstruction. American Journal of Sports Medicine 17: 344–349

de Jong R H, Hershey W N, Wagman I H 1966 Nerve conduction velocity during hypothermia in man. Anesthesiology 27: 805–810

Delp H L, Newton R A 1986 Effects of brief cold exposure on finger dexterity and sensibility in subjects with Raynaud's phenomenon. Physical Therapy 66: 503–507

DePreux T 1952 Ultrasonic wave therapy of osteoarthritis of the hip joint. British Journal of Physical Medicine 15: 14

Derscheid G L, Brown W C 1985 Rehabilitation of the ankle. Clinics in Sports Medicine 4: 527–544

Dietzel F, Kern W 1971a Kann hohes mütterliches Fieber beim Kind auslösen? Originalmitteilungen ist ausschliesslich der Verfasser verantwortlich. Naturwissenschaften 2: 24–26

Dietzel F, Kern W 1971b Kann hohes mütterliches Fieber Missbildungen beim Kind auslösen? Geburtshilfe und Frauenheilkunde 31: 1074–1079

Dietzel F, Kern W, Steckenmesser R 1972 Missbildungen und intrauterines Absterben nach Kurzwellenbehandlung in der Frühschwangerschaft. Münchener medizinische Wochenschrift 114: 228–230

Douglas W W, Malcolm J L 1955 The effect of localized cooling on conduction in cat nerves. Journal of Physiology 130: 53–71

Edwards M J 1976 Congenital defects in guinea pigs. Archives of Pathology 84: 42–48

Edwards M J 1972 Influenza, hyperthermia, and congenital malformation. Lancet i: 320–321

Edwards M J, Mulley R, Ring S, Wanner R A 1974 Mitotic cell death and delay of mitotic activity in guinea-pig embryos following brief maternal hyperthermia. Journal of Embryology and Experimental Morphology 32: 593–602

Eldred E, Lindsley D F, Buchwald J S 1960 The effect of cooling on mammalian muscle spindles. Experimental Neurology 2: 144–157

Fields H L, Basbaum A I 1978 Brainstem control of spinal pain-transmission neurons. Annual Review of Physiology 40: 217–248

Fischer E, Solomon S 1965 Physiological responses to heat and cold. In: Licht S (ed) Therapeutic heat and cold, 2nd edn. Waverly Press, p 126–169

Friedland F 1975 Ultrasonic therapy in rheumatic diseases. Journal of the American Medical Association 163: 799

Gammon G D, Starr I 1941 Studies on the relief of pain by counter-irritation. Journal of Clinical Investigation 20: 13–20

Ganong W F 1979 The nervous system, 2nd edn. Lange Medical Publications, Los Altos, California

Goldman J A, Chiapella J, Casey H et al 1980 Laser therapy for rheumatoid arthritis. Lasers in Surgery and Medicine 1: 93–101

Goodgold J, Eberstein A 1977 Electrodiagnosis of neuromuscular diseases, 2nd edn. Williams & Wilkins, Baltimore

Guy A W, Lehmann J F, Stonebridge J B 1974 Therapeutic applications of electromagnetic power. Proceedings of the Institute of Electrical and Electronic Engineers 62: 55–75

Guy A W, Lin J C, Kramar P O, Emery A F 1975 Effect of 2450-MHz radiation on the rabbit eye. Institute of Electrical and Electronic Engineers, Transactions on Microwave Theory and Techniques MTT 23: 492–498

Hagbarth K-E 1952 Excitatory and inhibitory skin areas for flexor and extensor motoneurons. Acta Physiologica Scandinavica 26 (suppl 94): 1–58

Haker E, Lundeberg T 1990 Laser treatment applied to acupuncture points in lateral humeral epicondylalgia. A double-blind study. Pain 43: 243–247

Haker E, Lundeberg T, 1991a Is low-energy laser treatment effective in lateral epicondylalgia? Journal of Pain and Symptom Management 6: 241–245

Haker E H K, Lundeberg T C M 1991b Lateral epicondylalgia: report of non-effective midlaser treatment. Archives of Physical Medicine and Rehabilitation 72: 984–988

Haker E, Lundeberg T 1991c Pulsed ultrasound treatment in lateral epicondylalgia. Scandinavian Journal of Rehabilitation Medicine 23: 115–118

Hansen H J, Thorøe U 1990 Low-power laser biostimulation of chronic orofacial pain. A double-blind placebo controlled cross-over study in 40 patients. Pain 43: 169–179

Hardy J D, Wolff H G, Goodell H 1940 Studies on pain. A new method for measuring pain threshold: observations on spatial summation of pain. Journal of Clinical Investigation 19: 649–657

Harris E D Jr, Krane S M 1973 Cartilage collagen: substrate in soluble and fibrillar form for rheumatoid collagenase. Transactions of the Association of American Physicians 86: 82–94

Harris E D Jr, McCroskery P A 1974 The influence of temperature and fibril stability on degradation of cartilage collagen by rheumatoid synovial collagenase. New England Journal of Medicine 290: 1–6

Hartviksen K 1962 Ice therapy in spasticity. Acta Neurologica Scandinavica 38 (suppl 3): 79–84

Harvey M A S, McRorie M M, Smith D W 1981 Suggested limits of exposure in the hot tub and sauna for the pregnant woman. Canadian Medical Association Journal 125: 50–53

Heller J H 1960 Reticuloendothelial structure and function. Roland Press, New York

Hendrickx A G, Stone G W, Henrickson R V, Matayoshi K 1979 Teratogenic effects of hyperthermia on the bonnet monkey (Macaca *radiata*). Teratology 19: 177–182

Herrick J F, Krusen F H 1953 Certain physiologic and pathologic effects of microwaves. Electrical Engineering 72: 239–244

Herrick J F, Jelatis D G, Lee G M 1950 Dielectric properties of tissues important in microwave diathermy. Federation Proceedings 9: 60

Hong C-Z 1991 Reversible nerve conduction block in patients with polyneuropathy after ultrasound thermotherapy at therapeutic dosage. Archives of Physical Medicine and Rehabilitation 72: 132–137

Horton B T, Browne G E, Roth G M 1936 Hypersensitiveness to cold. Journal of the American Medical Association 107: 1263–1268

Iijima K, Shimoyama N, Shimoyama M et al 1989 Effect of repeated irradiation of low-power He-Ne laser in pain relief from postherpetic neuralgia. The Clinical Journal of Pain 5: 271–274

Johns R J, Wright V 1962 Relative importance of various tissues in joint stiffness. Journal of Applied Physiology 17: 824–828

Johnson C C, Guy A W 1972 Nonionizing electromagnetic wave-effects in biological materials and systems. Proceedings of the Institute of Electrical and Electronic Engineers 66: 692–718

Juhlin L, Shelley W B 1961 Role of mast cell and basophil in cold urticaria with associated systemic reactions. Journal of the American Medical Association 117: 371–377

Kay D B 1985 The sprained ankle: current therapy. Foot and Ankle 6: 22–28

Kerr F W L, Casey K L 1976 Pain. Neurosciences Research Program Bulletin 16: 1–207

Klein R G, Eek B C 1990 Low-energy laser treatment and exercise for chronic low-back pain: double-blind controlled trial. Archives of Physical Medicine and Rehabilitation 71: 34–37

Knutsson E, Mattsson E 1969 Effects of local cooling monosynaptic reflexes in man. Scandinavian Journal of Rehabilitation Medicine 1: 126–132

Kramer J F 1985 Effect of therapeutic ultrasound intensity on subcutaneous tissue temperature and ulnar nerve conduction velocity. American Journal of Physical Medicine 64: 1–9

Landen B R 1967 Heat or cold for the relief of low back pain? Physical Therapy 47: 1126–1128

Larson D L 1961 Systemic lupus erythematosus. Little, Brown, Boston

Lehmann J F, de Lateur B J 1990a Cryotherapy. In: Lehmann J F (ed) Therapeutic heat and cold, 4th edn. Williams & Wilkins, Baltimore

Lehmann J F, de Lateur B J 1990b Therapeutic heat. In: Lehmann J F (ed), Therapeutic heat and cold, 4th edn. Williams & Wilkins, Baltimore

Lehmann J F, de Lateur B J 1990c Diathermy, superficial heat, laser and cold therapy. In: Kottke F J, Lehmann J F (eds), Handbook of physical medicine and rehabilitation, 4th edn. W B Saunders, Philadelphia

Lehmann J F, Brunner G D, McMillan J A, Silverman D R, Johnson V C 1964 Modification of heating patterns produced by microwaves at the frequencies of 2456 and 900 mc by physiologic factors in the human. Archives of Physical Medicine and Rehabilitation 45: 555–563

Lehmann J F, Stonebridge J B, Guy A W 1979 A comparison of patterns of stray radiation from therapeutic microwave applicators measured near tissue-substitute models and human subjects. Radio Science 14: 271–283

Lehmann J F, Dundore D E, Esselman P C, Nelp W B 1983 Microwave diathermy: effects on experimental muscle hematoma resolution. Archives of Physical Medicine and Rehabilitation 64: 127–129

Li C-L 1958 Effect of cooling on neuromuscular transmission in the rat. American Journal of Physiology 194: 200 –206

Lightfoot E, Verrier M, Ashby P 1975 Neurological effects of prolonged cooling of the calf in patients with complete spinal transection. Physical Therapy 55: 251–258

Lundeberg T, Haker E, Thomas M 1987a Effect of laser versus placebo in tennis elbow. Scandinavian Journal of Rehabilitation Medicine 19: 135–138

Lundeberg T, Hode L, Zhou J 1987b A comparative study of the pain-relieving effect of laser trearment and acupuncture. Acta Physiologica Scandinavica 13: 161–162

Martin G M, Roth G M, Elkins E C, Krusen F H 1946 Cutaneous temperature of the extremities of normal subjects and of patients with rheumatoid arthritis. Archives of Physical Medicine 27: 665–682

Matsen F A III, Questad K, Matsen A L 1975 The effect of local cooling on post fracture swelling. Clinical Orthopedics and Related Research 109: 201–206

Melzack R, Wall P D 1965 Pain mechanisms: a new theory. Science 150: 971–979

Melzack R, Guite S, Gonshor A 1980a Relief of dental pain by ice massage of the hand. Canadian Medical Association Journal 122: 189–191

Melzack R, Jeans M E, Stratford J G, Monks R C 1980b Ice massage and transcutaneous electrical stimulation: comparison of treatment for low-back pain. Pain 9: 209–217

Mense S 1978 Effects of temperature on the discharges of muscle spindles and tendon organs. Pflügers Archiv 374: 159–166

Menser M 1978 Does hyperthermia affect the human fetus? Medical Journal of Australia 2: 550

Michaelson S M 1972 Human exposure to nonionizing radiant energy – potential hazards and safety standards. Proceedings of the Institute of Electrical and Electronic Engineers 60: 389–421

Michaelson S M 1990 Bioeffects of high frequency currents and electromagnetic radiation. In: Lehmann J F (ed) Therapeutic heat and cold, 4th edn. Williams & Wilkins, Baltimore

Miglietta O 1973 Action of cold on spasticity. American Journal of Physical Medicine 52: 198–205

Moayer M 1971 Die morphologischen Veränderugen der Plazenta unter dem Einfluss der Kurzwellendurchflutung. Tierexperimentelle Untersuchungen. Strahlentherapie 142: 609–614

Molander C O 1941 Physiologic basis of heat. Archives of Physical Therapy 22: 335–340

Moore C D, Cardea J A 1977 Vascular changes in leg trauma. Southern Medical Journal 70: 1285–1286

Murray F S, Weaver M M 1975 Effects of ipsilateral and contralateral counter-irritation on experimentally produced itch in human beings. Journal of Comparative and Physiological Psychology 89: 819–826

Mussa B 1955 Embriopatie da cause fisiche. Minerva Nipiologica 5: 69–72

Nilsson S 1983 Sprains of the lateral ankle ligaments, an epidemiological and clinical study with special reference to different forms of conservative treatment. Part II, a controlled trial of different forms of conservative treatment. Journal of the Oslo City Hospitals 33: 13–36

Ottoson D 1965 The effects of temperature on the isolated muscle spindle. Journal of Physiology 180: 636–648

Parsons C M, Goetzl F R 1945 Effect of induced pain on pain threshold. Proceedings of the Society for Experimental Biology and Medicine 60: 327–329

Perkins J F, Li M-C, Hoffman F, Hoffmann E 1948 Sudden vasoconstriction in denervated or sympathectomized paws exposed to cold. American Journal of Physiology 155: 165–178

Saito M, Schwan H P 1961 The time constants of pearl-chain formation. Biological effects of microwave radiation. Proceedings of the Fourth Annual Tri-Service Conference on the Biological Effects of Microwave Radiation 1: 85–91

Sandler B 1973 Heat and the IUCD. British Medical Journal 25: 458

Schaubel H J 1946 The local use of ice after orthopedic procedures. American Journal of Surgery 72: 711–714

Schmidt K L, Ott V R, Röcher G, Schaller H 1979 Heat, cold and inflammation. Rheumatology 38: 391–404

Scott B O 1956 Effect of contact lenses on short wave field distribution. British Journal of Ophthalmology 40: 696–697

Seino H, Watanabe S, Tanaka J et al 1985 Cryoanalgesia for postthoracotomy pain. Masui 34: 842–845

Sekins K M, Dundore D, Emery A F, Lehmann J F, McGrath P W, Nelp W B 1980 Muscle blood flow changes in response to 915 MHz diathermy with surface cooling as measured by Xe^{133} clearance. Archives of Physical Medicine and Rehabilitation 61: 105–113

Sekins K M, Lehmann J F, Esselman P et al 1984 Local muscle blood flow and temperature responses to 915 MHz diathermy as simultaneously measured and numerically predicted. Archives of Physical Medicine and Rehabilitation 65: 1–7

Shelley W B, Caro W B 1962 Cold erythema. Journal of the American Medical Association 180: 639–642

Siebert W, Seichert N, Siebert B, Wirth C J 1987 What is the efficacy of 'soft' and 'mid' lasers in therapy of tendinopathies? Archives of Orthopaedic and Trauma Sugery 106: 358–363

Smith D W, Clarren S K, Harvey M A S 1978 Hyperthermia as a possible teratogenic agent. Journal of Pediatrics 92: 878–883

Steinberg R, Callies R 1992 Vergleichsstudie Ultraschall und Prednisolonphonophorese bei Patienten mit Epicondylopathia humeri. Physikalische Medizin Rehabilitationsmedizin Kurortmedizin 2: 84–87

Taube S, Piironen J, Ylipaavalniemi P 1990 Helium-neon laser therapy in the prevention of postoperative swelling and pain after wisdom tooth extraction. Proceedings of the Finnish Dental Society 86: 23–27

Texeira-Pinto A A, Nejelski L L, Cutler J L, Heller J H 1960 The behavior of unicellular organisms in an electromagnetic field. Experimental Cell Research 20: 548–564

Traherne J B 1962 Evaluation of the cold spray technique in the treatment of muscle pain in general practice. Practitioner 189: 210–212

Trnavsky G 1983 Die Beeinflussing des Hoffmann-Reflexes durch Kryolangzeittherapie. Wiener Medizinische Wochenschrift 11: 287–289

Urbscheit N, Bishop B 1970 Effects of cooling on the ankle jerk and H-response. Physical Therapy 50: 1041–1049

Vinger P F, Hoerner E F (eds) 1981 Sports injuries, the unthwarted epidemic. PSG Publishing, Littleton, Massachusetts

Walker J 1983 Relief from chronic pain by lower power laser irradiation. Neuroscience Letters 43: 339–344

Walker J B, Akhanjee L K, Cooney M M et al 1988 Laser therapy for pain of trigeminal neuralgia. The Clinical Journal of Pain 3: 183–187
Waylonis G W, Wilke S, O'Toole D, Waylonis D A, Waylonis D B 1988 Chronic myofascial pain: management by low-output helium-neon laser therapy. Archives of Physical Medicine and Rehabilitation 69: 1017–1020
Wolf S, Hardy J D 1941 Studies on pain. Observations on pain due to local cooling and on factors involved in the 'cold pressor' effect. Journal of Clinical Investigation 20: 521–533
Wolff H H 1951 The mechanism and significance of the cold pressor response. Quarterly Journal of Medicine 20: 261–273
Wright V, Johns R J 1960 Physical factors concerned with the stiffness of normal and diseased joints. Bulletin of the Johns Hopkins Hospital 106: 215–231
Wright V, Johns R J 1961 Quantitative and qualitative analysis of joint stiffness in normal subjects and in patients with connective tissue diseases. Annals of the Rheumatic Diseases 20: 36–46

68. Manipulation and massage for the relief of back pain

Scott Haldeman

INTRODUCTION

The laying on of hands is questionably the oldest, most universally utilised and probably the most appreciated means of relieving pain and suffering. Touching, massaging or manipulating areas that are painful, tense or tight is used in every household and much of the animal kingdom. Parents learn very early that rubbing or kissing a child's bruise or scratch may be all that is necessary to change a scream of pain to a smile of contentment. Tension headaches and neck pain are probably relieved more often by a spouse's massage than by a physician. Animals lick, scratch or rub wounds or areas of irritation both on themselves and on their offspring or mates. Horses, cats and dogs, amongst other animals, are commonly noted to stretch, roll on their backs or scratch against objects, presumably because it feels good.

Manipulation and massage in their various forms have also been offered as methods of relieving pain by physicians throughout history. The history of manipulation and massage as treatment modalities is extensive and has been reviewed by a number of authors in detail (Schiotz 1958; Lomax 1975, 1976; Gibbons 1980; Tappan 1984; Kamenetz 1985). The debate on the etymology of the words 'manipulation and massage' is an indication of their wide usage. Many ancient languages have similar sounding words. Manipulation is commonly thought to originate from the Latin word 'manus', hand or 'manipulare', to use the hands. Massage, however, has been variously attributed to the Arab verb 'mass', to touch, the Greek work 'massein', to knead, the Hebrew 'mashesh', to feel, touch or grope, or the Sanskrit term 'makeh', to stroke, press or condense (Kamenetz 1985). Writings, diagrams, paintings and sculpture showing or describing various methods of massage and manipulation can be found in virtually all recorded civilisations, including Babylon, Assyria, ancient China as far back as 1000 BC, India, Greece, Rome and Egypt. The formalised use of manipulation of the spine is commonly attributed to Hippocrates and Galen, both of whom recommended manipulating the spine in certain cases. Similarly, a number of cultures, without written history, including the Eskimos, South American Indians and African tribal natives, have been noted to utilise massage and manipulation techniques as part of their healing rituals. This author has personally witnessed a Bushman ceremony to drive out evil spirits where the healer repeatedly massaged and thrust on the spine of the person whose affliction was to be relieved. It was not possible, however, even with a competent translator, to determine what was wrong with the patient beyond the explanation that there was an evil spirit preventing the patient from running and that such spirits were most likely to be expelled through this ritual.

Until recently, the history of manipulation and massage has been dominated by a love–hate relationship between the medical establishment and the numerous groups which practise these techniques. In the 19th and early 20th centuries, many well-respected physicians, such as Paget (1867) and Percivall Pott (1936) recommended that physicians should study the techniques of bone-setting. During this period an occasional textbook on the topic was published (Hoffa 1897; Graham 1902). The introduction of manipulation and massage into mainline medical practice is often attributed to James Mennell (1917, 1934) and E F Cyriax (1904), both of whom were followed by sons, John Mennell and James Cyriax, who became advocates, authors and teachers of manipulation. There was, however, considerable scepticism, and ostracism of practitioners of manipulation by mainstream medical physicians was common.

This reluctance by medical physicians to incorporate manipulation into their practice led in part to the development of other groups of practitioners, including osteopaths, naturopaths and chiropractors, who began to fill the public demand for this treatment modality. Gibbons (1980) feels that the development of chiropractic was part of a social protest in the early 20th century against medical treatments which were often ineffective and either dangerous or unpleasant.

One of the most remarkable events in the recent history of musculoskeletal pain management is the transformation of massage and manipulation from fringe or marginal procedures into primary, first-line therapies for certain types of spinal pain. This transformation is one of the best examples of scientific research supplanting ignorance and dogma. The acceptance of manipulation has been fuelled by an international search for a low-technology, low-cost, low-risk, effective method of dealing with the worldwide epidemic of back pain and its related disability.

This acceptance has led to the rapid growth in the number of professionals who practise manipulation. Chiropractors, in particular, have been responsible for the bulk of the research and have benefited from the resultant prestige. In North America, chiropractic care is now covered by almost all private, governmental and workers' compensation health benefits. It is not uncommon for chiropractors to practise in hospitals, health maintenance organizations and group practices with medical physicians and specialists. Osteopathic physicians and colleges have begun to increase their research efforts and teaching of manipulation. At the same time, physical therapists have increasingly been incorporating massage and manipulation techniques into their practices. In Europe, in particular, the medical community has developed associations, courses and certification to serve those physicians who practise manipulation. Previously ostracised medical practitioners who have developed their manipulation skills are finding themselves in demand by patients and by research and teaching institutions. Chiropractic, which at one time was primarily a North American profession, is spreading throughout the world with colleges in Europe, Australia and South Africa. Even the World Health Organization is acknowledging this reality by co-sponsoring meetings and texts with the World Federation of Chiropractic.

The primary impetus for the recognition of manipulation is the change of emphasis by its practitioners from territorial protection and dogmatic theoretical beliefs to scientific investigation. The past decade has seen the publication of more clinical trials, scientific conferences and experimental research papers on the topic than the previous 2000 years. There are now more prospective controlled clinical trials on manipulation published in peer-reviewed journals than any other treatment for low-back pain. It is still not clear exactly why massage and manipulation cause relief of pain, and the type of patient and clinical entities most likely to respond to manipulation are only now being defined. These questions, however, are being subjected to scientific investigation and debate. The traditional methods of discussion of this topic, based on dogmatic acceptance or rejection of its clinical value and blind belief in a particular theory based on the teachings of charismatic individuals, has been placed in the annals of history.

MASSAGE AND MANIPULATION TECHNIQUES

Massage and manipulation fall into the larger field referred to as manual medicine, manual therapy or manipulative therapy. All techniques, where the hands are used to touch, feel, massage or manipulate tissue therapeutically in order to directly benefit a patient, can be included under these headings. The number of methods and techniques of massage and manipulation is too great to include in a short chapter on the topic. Clinicians who use manual therapy to treat patients begin to modify methods they have been taught very early in their career and adapt their approach to the particular patient and tissue they are treating. Techniques are also adapted to suit a clinician's level of strength, dexterity, training and confidence. There are, however, a number of principles which allow for a classification of the various manual therapeutic approaches. The most common classification of manual techniques is based on a differentiation between massage, passive movement, mobilisation and the manipulative or adjusting techniques. These techniques are applied at different positions within a specific range of motion of a joint, as shown in Figure 68.1.

MASSAGE

Massage is the application of touch or force to soft tissues, usually muscles, tendons or ligaments, without causing movement or change in position of a joint. Each massage technique is performed with a specific goal in mind. The most commonly applied techniques are as follows:

Stroking or effleurage

This is the light movement of the hands over the skin in a slow, rhythmic fashion. The hands mould to the contour of the area being massaged and are in constant contact with the skin. The hands may gently stroke the skin or

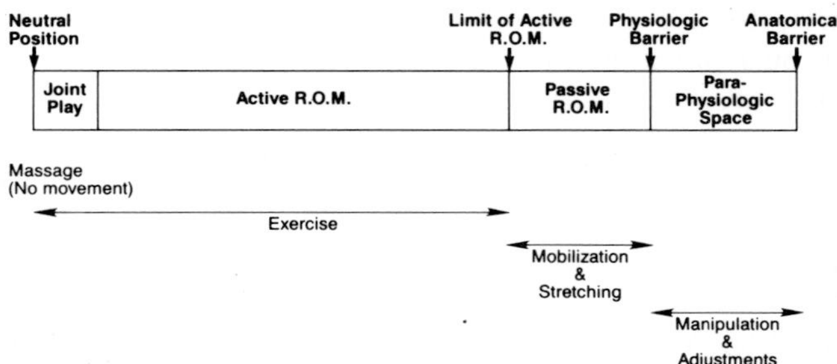

Fig. 68.1 The presumed barriers to motion in a joint and the position or range of motion where the various forms of manual therapy are performed.

influence deeper tissues depending on the amount of pressure exerted. Light stroking tends to be non-painful and soothing and can be either centripetal or centrifugal. Deeper pressure techniques can be slightly uncomfortable and are always taught to be in the direction of venous or lymph flow with the stated goal of reducing oedema.

Connective tissue massage

This technique uses deeper stroking motions and is presumed to free subcutaneous connective tissue adhesions. The technique initially described by Elizabeth Dicke (1953) was popularised by Marie Ebner (1960). This deep stroking in specifically defined patterns results in a sensation of warmth and hyperaemia of the skin.

Kneading and pétrissage

These techniques require the clinician to grasp, lift, squeeze or push the tissues being massaged. The skin moves with the hands over the underlying tissues. This differs from stroking, where the hands move over the skin. Commonly these techniques are applied to muscles which can be gripped and alternately compressed and then released before moving on to another area.

Friction and deep massage

The theoretical goal of these techniques is the loosening of scars or adhesions between deeper structures such as ligaments, tendons and muscles (Cyriax 1971; Wood 1974). These procedures are presumed to aid in the absorption of local effusion within these tissues. The direction of movement of the fingers over the tissues being massaged is described by Wood as circular, whereas Cyriax insists that the movement should be transverse across the fibres of the structure being massaged. The massage is continued until a muscle is mobilised from its surrounding tissues or any palpated effusions or thickening in a ligamentous structure is dispersed. It may require several sessions to achieve this result and the massage should be followed by exercise to maintain mobility.

Tapotement, percussion or clapping

These techniques consist of a series of gentle taps or blows applied to the patient (Hofkosh 1985). These techniques have been described as hacking (using the ulnar border of the hand), clapping or cupping (using the palm either flat or concave), tapping (using the tips of the fingers) or beating (using the fists if closed). These percussive movements have been used primarily in postural drainage of the lungs, to obtain muscle contraction and relaxation or to increase circulation. They are generally not recommended for the treatment of pathological tissues (Wood 1974) and are commonly used on athletes to tone and relax muscles.

Shaking and vibration

These massage methods require the clinician to take hold of a portion of the patient's body and apply either a coarse shaking or a fine vibration motion. They are not widely used except in postural drainage of the lungs.

PASSIVE MOVEMENT

The use of the hands to maintain passive motion in a joint falls into the category of manual therapy although these procedures are often performed by nurses, aides and patients' families. They are briefly mentioned here to demonstrate the wide spectrum of manual therapeutic techniques. The techniques are relatively simple to teach and perform. They require an understanding of the different directions of movement a joint may traverse. The clinician takes hold of the peripheral arm of the joint and systematically moves the joint through each of its normal motions, from the neutral point to the point of resistance or pain. No attempt is made to force the joint but the entire length of the range of motion must be traversed and each direction of potential motion must be included. The procedure is repeated and performed several times a day. The goal is to prevent stiffening or shortening of the ligamentous structures as well as to maintain motion and lubrication in the joint and surrounding tissues.

The natural progression from passive motion is to active motion or exercise. Exercise is performed within the same boundaries of joint motion as is passive motion, although not all directions of motion which can be achieved passively can be reproduced by exercise. Exercise has the additional advantage of including muscle activity and developing strength and coordination. Passive movement, except in paralysis or severe muscle injury requiring a period of healing, is usually discontinued, where possible, in favor of active exercise assuming the therapeutic goal is maintenance of range of motion.

MOBILISATION AND STRETCHING

Mobilisation includes those manual procedures which attempt to increase the range of motion beyond the resistance barrier which limits passive range of motion or exercise (Fig. 68.1). Certain mobilisation methods include stretching of muscles and ligaments while others include movement of joints in non-physiologic directions of motion. Mobilisation differs from manipulation or adjustments by the absence of a forceful thrust or jerking motion.

Graded oscillation or mobilisation

These techniques were popularised by Maitland (1973) who proposed four levels or grades of mobilisation. Grade I mobilisation is a fine oscillation with very little force or depth. Grade II is a mobilisation with greater depth but within the first half of the range of motion. Grade III is a deeper mobilisation at the limits of the motion, whereas Grade IV is a deep, fine oscillation at the limits of potential motion. The clinician tends to start at Grade I and increase to Grade IV as greater motion becomes possible. The ranges of motion of each of these grades are illustrated in Figure 68.2B.

Progressive stretch mobilisation

These techniques require the application of successive short-amplitude stretching movements to the joint. The depth of the stretching into the resisted range of motion is increased as permitted by the joint. Again four grades or depths are described (Nyberg 1985) but in this situation the grades refer to each quarter of the potential motion of the joint as illustrated in Figure 68.2C. These techniques are used primarily to overcome soft tissue restriction to joint motion.

Sustained progressive stretch

This is a sustained stretching motion with progressively increasing pressure. This sustained force technique is recommended to stretch shortened periarticular soft tissues and is performed slowly and carefully to avoid tearing of tissues (Fig. 68.2D).

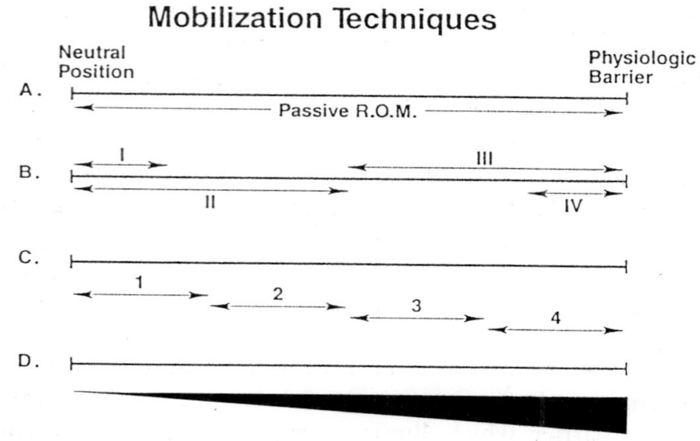

Fig. 68.2 The different forms of mobilisation. Active and passive ranges of motion are included under 'passive range of motion' as all of these mobilisations are performed passively. **A** Continuous passive range of motion; **B** graded oscillations; **C** progressive stretch mobilisation; **D** sustained progressive stretching.

Spray and stretch

These techniques have been taught widely by Janet Travell (1976) and John Mennell (1960) for the treatment of painful muscular trigger points. The muscle being treated is placed in a light stretch and a fluoromethane spray is applied to the muscle in a specific pattern. This results in a cooling of the skin as the fluoromethane evaporates. The muscle can then be stretched further, allowing increased range of motion and, theoretically, the elimination of the trigger point.

Muscle energy

These methods require the use of muscle activity and subsequent relaxation to set the stage for increasing range of motion. In peripheral joint mobilisation it has been called the 'hold–relaxation' technique. The clinician places the muscle in light stretch. The patient then contracts the muscle against resistance applied by the clinician. The contraction is held for a brief period and the patient then relaxes. The clinician can then increase the stretch of the muscle and joint. Certain osteopathic physicians (Kimberly 1979; Goodridge 1981) have modified these techniques with sophisticated positioning of the patient to allow for specific directional mobilisation or manipulation of vertebrae.

MANIPULATION OR ADJUSTIVE THRUSTS

The difference between mobilisation and manipulation or adjustment is the application of a high velocity, low amplitude thrust to the joint. Many chiropractors feel that there is a difference between non-specific manipulation and the classical adjustment which has specific direction, force and presumed physiologic effects. Other clinicians include mobilisation techniques and muscle-energy techniques under the heading of manipulation. There is, however, fairly clear differentiation between the previously described non-thrust techniques and the thrusting techniques described under this heading. These techniques force the joint beyond the physiologic range of motion, through the paraphysiological space, to the anatomical limits of motion (Fig. 68.1). The thrust is commonly followed by a 'click' or 'pop' which is audible and is felt to be related to release of gases within the joint space.

Non-specific long-lever manipulations

These techniques are becoming less popular because of the potential to exert large forces which could damage bones, ligaments or discs. Force is applied via a long bone as a lever. Commonly a shoulder or leg is used to exert force into the spine (Cyriax 1971; Coplans 1978).

These techniques, in the past, were commonly used under anaesthesia, allowing for the exertion of strenuous forces to a joint. In large patients treated by small clinicians, the utilisation of long levers with directed force may be the only way in which a joint can be manipulated.

Specific spinal adjustment

The application of high velocity, small amplitude thrusting techniques to short levers of the spine such as a spinous or transverse process has been the mainstay of traditional chiropractic practice. The goal has been variously described as correcting misalignments or subluxations, eliminating fixations in intersegmental motion and bringing about a variety of neural and muscular reflex changes. There are numerous techniques which have been described in textbooks (Logan 1950; Greco 1953; States 1968; Haldeman 1980, 1992). Each vertebra can be adjusted in a number of different directions and the patient can be placed in very specific positions prior to the administration of an adjustment to allow for control of the depth and direction of the force to be applied. It has yet to be established, however, that such precise application of force does in fact bring about specific vertebral movements as claimed. A number of chiropractic techniques require specialised tables which allow for the positioning of the patient.

Toggle-recoil

Certain chiropractic techniques (Thompson 1973) require the patient to be placed on a table which is constructed so that one vertebral segment is locked or blocked while a rapidly controlled force is applied to the adjacent vertebra. The portion of the table supporting the vertebra being adjusted then drops approximately 1 cm, allowing for a concussion or recoil effect. Properly performed, high velocity forces can be applied very specifically to a vertebra without the clinician exerting much force or effort.

Joint play

John Mennell (1960) has been instrumental in teaching techniques of moving joints in directions not commonly moved during exercise. Most joints have some degree of play at rest because of ligamentous elasticity. When joints cease to have this play due to tightening of the ligaments and especially if the joint is locked in a slightly abnormal position, Mennell recommends that the joint be manipulated in specific directions to increase the play. A number of manipulation techniques for increasing joint play in both vertebral and peripheral joints have been described.

Traction and distraction

Manual traction and the combination of mechanical traction or distraction with manipulation techniques are perhaps not properly included in this section. They are, however, commonly accompanied by pulling or thrusting methods while the patient is in traction (Cox 1980) and are widely used by chiropractors under the term 'adjustments'. Manual traction without thrusting is also used as a standard physiotherapeutic technique and could be included under mobilisation methods.

THE EFFECTIVENESS OF MASSAGE AND MANIPULATION

By far the majority of people who request massage or manipulation do so for relief of pain, muscle spasm, tension or stiffness. Surveys reviewing the reason why patients seek chiropractic treatment reveal that 80–90% of them do so for the relief of spinal pain or headaches (Vear 1972; Breen 1977; Nyiendo et al 1987). The anecdotal surveys and descriptive studies on patients who attend both chiropractors and other practitioners of manipulation demonstrate a very high success or satisfaction rate. The success rates reported for manipulation in uncontrolled trials and in various comparative trials are between 60 and 100% (Haldeman 1978; Brunarski 1984; Bronfort 1992). This type of study with its lack of controls ignores the well-recognised problems of spontaneous recovery, placebo effect, difficulty in quantitating pain and natural prejudice of practitioners reporting on the success of their own treatment. In the case of spinal pain, the problem of different populations of patients and pathological causes of pain also makes it difficult to compare studies and determine the success of treatment. The fact that the majority of patients visiting a practitioner of manipulation feel better while undergoing treatment is the primary reason for its popularity.

For the entire field of massage, despite its universal usage, there have not been many serious controlled trials. There are, however, few clinicians or patients who would deny that rubbing or massaging sore muscles or stiff joints produces a soothing feeling and pain relief. It can be argued that even if the relief described after massage and manipulation is due to placebo or psychological effects, such treatments should not be discarded. The goal of any treatment is to make people feel and function better and any treatment that has this effect should be considered beneficial. Pope et al (1992) found that satisfaction rates in patients who were receiving massage were significantly higher than in those patients being treated with corsets or transcutaneous muscle stimulation (TMS). These rates increased with repeated treatments, thus demonstrating the high acceptance of this procedure by patients.

Manipulation, on the other hand, has been the subject

of increasing clinical research. A growing number of prospective, randomised controlled trials have studied the effectiveness of manipulation compared to placebo and other conservative treatments. As is often the case in the early trials of any treatment, the results of such research can be confusing and difficult to interpret. In the case of manipulation, the problem is greater than usual because there are few standards with regard to technique used, the skill of the manipulator, the number and frequency of manipulations, patient selection or outcomes which have to be adhered to.

The number of published controlled clinical trials has grown rapidly during the past few years. Shekelle et al (1992) lists 29 controlled clinical trials on low-back pain, and Bronfort has reviewed 47 randomised, comparative trials on the treatment of back pain, neck pain and headaches using manipulation. These authors and others (Oltenbacher & DiFabio 1985) have found sufficient numbers of well-designed trials to perform meta-analyses and to sort the trials into different subgroups of patients. This has made it possible to discuss the effectiveness of manipulation in more specific forms, such as condition or diagnosis, and expected outcome measures.

ACUTE UNCOMPLICATED LOW-BACK PAIN:

The majority of the controlled clinical trials on manipulation was performed on patients with recent onset of symptoms (within 2–4 weeks). These studies tended to exclude patients with complicating factors such as systemic or metabolic diseases, sciatica or disc herniation, workers' compensation or other psychosocial factors. There are many difficulties in reviewing these papers. The paper by Jayson (1986), for example, found that manipulation was superior in controls when given in an outpatient clinic, but was ineffective in hospitalised patients with back pain who presumably had more severe pathology. The paper by Bergquist-Ullman & Larsson (1997) found manipulation to be more effective than placebo but no better than a comprehensive education programme. Glover et al (1974, 1977) found that manipulation had a significant positive effect in patients with acute pain when assessed immediately after treatment but not in more chronic cases. Doran & Newell (1975), Coxhead et al (1981) and Sloop et al (1982) each showed non-statistically significant trends towards improvement in their manipulation groups when compared to controls. Greenland et al (1979) suggest that a different statistical analysis of Doran Newell's data would find manipulation significantly more effective than the controls.

Even in the trials where manipulation was reported as clearly more successful than controls, the picture is not clear. The studies by Coyer & Curwen (1955) and by Lewith & Turner (1982) were not blinded nor statistically analysed. The studies by Sims-Williams et al (1978, 1979), Buerger (1978, 1979) and Hoehler et al (1981) were well controlled but showed only short-term changes with no long-lasting results from manipulation. However, one point is clear: the multiple comparative trials have shown that no other conservative treatment is superior to manipulation. Of particular interest is the observation that none of the trials reported any complications from the application of manipulation.

In order to assess the results of manipulation on acute low-back pain better, it is useful to look at the meta-analyses and critical reviews of these papers. The most recent and comprehensive review is by Shekelle et al (1992). They analysed all the controlled trials on manipulation and assigned quality scores on the published research designs. They then selected seven papers which had used single outcome measures or assessed outcome measures independently. Table 68.1 lists these papers and the number of patients who recovered. They then developed differences in probability of recovery from back pain

Table 68.1 Outcome measures combined in meta-analysis of acute low-back pain studies

Author (reference)	Outcome measure	When assessed	Number of patients recovered	
			Manipulated group	Comparison group
Coyer & Curwen 1955	'Well' (relief of symptoms)	3 wk	58 of 76	36 of 60
Bergquist-Ullman & Larsson 1977	Return to work	3 wk	30 of 61	25 of 56
Farrell et al 1982	'Symptom-free', very low pain score, can do all functional activity without difficulty, and objective lumbar movements are without pain	3 wk	22 of 24	15 of 24
Godfrey et al 1984	1–5-point scale of 'general symptomatology' dichotomised by the original authors into 'marked improvement' or not	Mean, 2 wk	14 of 39	7 of 33
Rasmussen 1979	'Fully restored', no pain, normal function, no sign of disease, fit to work	2 wk	11 of 12	3 of 12
Matthews et al 1987	6-point pain scale divided into 'recovered' and 'not recovered'	2 wk	116 of 152	73 of 108
Waterworth & Hunder 1985	'Excellent overall improvement' by patient self-report	12 d	23 of 38	15 of 36

(From Shekelle et al 1992.)

for each of the seven studies (Fig. 68.3). The results show that manipulation increased the probability of recovery at 2 or 3 weeks after start of treatment by 0.17 (95% probability limits, 0.07–0.28), indicating that manipulation hastens recovery from acute uncomplicated low-back pain.

The meta-analyses to date have not been able to detect a long-term effect of manipulation in patients. This, in part, is due to the fact that most of the studies have not included long-term follow-up. There are two studies which have recently attempted to look at long-term effects. The paper by Meade (1990) compared the effects of hospital-based, outpatient, physical-therapy department treatment to office-based chiropractic treatment, and noted a small but detectable (7%) long-term effect on Oswestry scores over a 2-year period. Waagen et al (1990) also demonstrated a long-term (2-year) higher satisfaction rate with chiropractic care compared to care received from a family physician's office. The significance of these studies, however, is not clear but at least raises the possibility that manipulation is of greater benefit than simple acute pain relief.

CHRONIC LOW-BACK PAIN

There are only a few studies on the effect of manipulation in patients with chronic low-back pain and these are more difficult to interpret. Waagen et al (1986), for example, showed a statistical benefit from manipulation in patients with recurrent or chronic low-back pain at 2 weeks, whereas Gibson (1985) failed to show such an effect in patients undergoing osteopathic manipulation. Evans (1978), using patients as their own controls in a crossover-designed clinical trial, showed diminished codeine use in patients undergoing manipulation, and a trial by Ongley (1987) demonstrated that a group that received both rotational manipulation and proliferent injections showed significant improvement. It may be that, in patients with chronic back pain, the support of a physician and the relief, even if temporary, following manipulation serves to make the patients tolerate their pain and thereby reduce pain scores.

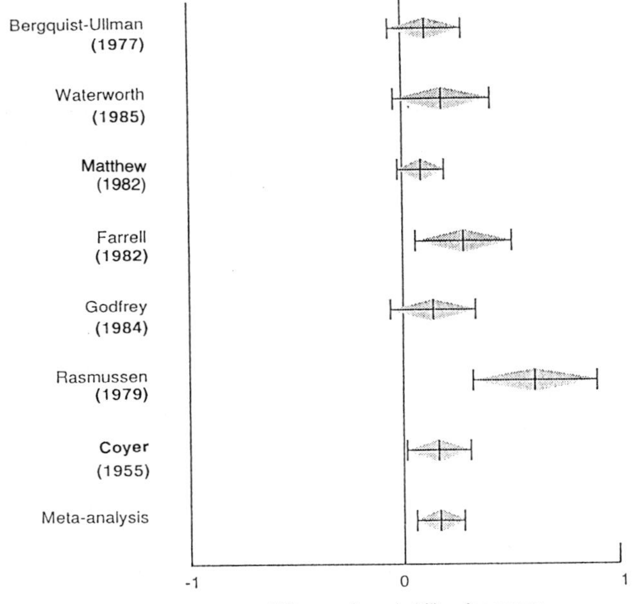

Fig. 68.3 Difference in probability of recovery in seven trials of manipulation. A difference in probability of greater than zero represents a beneficial effect of manipulation. For individual studies, 95% confidence intervals are shown; for the meta-analysis, the 95% probability limits are shown. (From Shekelle et al 1992.)

SCIATICA

Only three studies have looked specifically at patients with sciatica. Although Nwuga (1982), Coxhead et al (1981) and Edwards (1969) all report improvement in certain outcome measures following manipulation in patients with sciatica, the significance of these studies is not clear. It appears from uncontrolled studies by Chrisman et al (1964) and Cassidy & Kirkaldy-Willis (1985) that patients with demonstrated disc herniation and sciatica do less well following manipulation than patients with back pain alone.

NECK PAIN AND HEADACHES

After low-back pain, neck pain and headaches are the most common complaints for which manipulation has been recommended. This has primarily been based on descriptive clinical studies and large case series (see Bronfort 1992). These case series cover an extremely broad and often poorly defined group of patients with cervical and thoracic pain, and cervicogenic and migraine headaches. These reports have been universally enthusiastic but without controls or even proper research protocols.

The few prospective controlled clinical trials that have been performed have covered such a wide variety of conditions and outcome parameters that it is difficult to reach specific conclusions. Parker et al (1978) and Hoyt (1979) reported significant improvement in headache severity and frequency when compared to controls but not in all parameters which were measured. Brodin (1982) and Howe et al (1983) reported decreased neck pain following manipulation when compared with analgesics or no treatment. In addition, Howe et al (1983) described increased cervical rotation following manipulation on goniometric examination. Bitterli et al (1977), on the other hand, did not show a change in headache following mobilisation in a small sampling of patients and Sloop et al (1982) failed to show improvement in neck pain following a single manipulation.

MECHANISMS OF PAIN RELIEF BY MASSAGE AND MANIPULATION

The exact mechanism by which massage and manipulation relieves pain has been the subject of a great deal of debate but relatively little experimentation. It has been the topic of two conferences sponsored by the National Institutes of Health (Goldstein 1975; Korr 1978) and has been the topic of discussion in multiple other conferences and articles. The problem, in part, has been the difficulty of isolating the primary cause of low-back pain. For virtually every theory as to the cause of spinal pain there has been a corresponding theory as to how manipulation might reverse the pain-producing process. The following are the more prominent theories under debate.

CHANGE IN PAIN THRESHOLD

Since many of the effects of manipulation are immediate (Glover et al 1974; Hoehler et al 1981), the possibility that a manipulation may somehow increase the pain threshold has been raised. Terrett & Vernon (1984) attempted to investigate this phenomenon by measuring tolerance to electrically induced pain in paraspinal tissues before and after spinal manipulation, and before and after joint play. Both groups showed increases in pain tolerance but in the manipulation group the increase was significantly higher than in the group undergoing joint play. In order to investigate possible mechanisms for this phenomenon, Vernon et al (1985) analysed serum β-endorphin levels before and after chiropractic adjustments. They report a small but significant increase in serum β-endorphin levels in subjects undergoing spinal manipulation. Christian et al (1988) and Sanders et al (1990), however, were not able to confirm these results.

RELIEF OF MUSCLE PAIN OR SPASM

One of the primary goals of many massage techniques is the relief of muscle spasm and the assumption that such spasm is painful. Anyone who has had a muscle massage will recognise that a good practitioner can find sore spots in muscles and the soothing effect of massage makes it a luxury much in demand. There has not, however, been much study as to what actually occurs. Cyriax (1971) has stated that deep friction separates adhesions and restores movement between individual muscle fibres. Wakim (1980) describes the effects of massage as relieving muscle fatigue from overexertion by improving circulation and removing waste products.

Spinal manipulation has similarly been considered to reduce muscle spasm. In this case it has been proposed that the sharp thrust of a manipulation results in stretch of the muscle and subsequently reflex relaxation of the muscle. A number of studies (Diebert & England 1972; Grice 1974; Grice & Tschumi 1985; Shambaugh 1987) report decreased muscle activity in patients after manipulation using surface muscle electrical activity measurement techniques. These studies all suffer from small sample size and methodologic problems and are not conclusive. A recent study by Zhu et al (1992) reports normalisation of magnetically induced muscle contraction cortical-evoked responses following manipulation and suggests that this may reflect changes in muscle spindle activity.

IMPROVED CIRCULATION

The theory that the effect of massage and manipulation is primarily on circulation has many supporters. The erythema that follows massage is presumed to be due to an increase in blood flow. A number of individuals have reported measuring increased circulation from various massage techniques (Skull 1945; Wakim et al 1949). This phenomenon in turn has been extrapolated to suggest that massage removes waste products and promotes healing.

The early research of Starling (1894), in which the role of muscle contraction on lymph flow was demonstrated, is often quoted to suggest that massage, passive motion and exercise may have its primary effect on lymphatic drainage. A few researchers (Elkins et al 1953; Wakim et al 1955) have demonstrated that massage and compression of an oedematous extremity can increase lymph flow and reduce oedema. Extrapolation of these theories to the massage of areas of tenderness in muscles and ligaments, however, has yet to be demonstrated.

REDUCTION IN DISC PROTRUSION

This theory proposed by Cyriax (1971) was based partially on the observations of Matthews & Yates (1969) using epidural venography before and after manipulation. Many of the traction-distraction techniques have also been proposed on the basis of a presumed effect on the intervertebral disc (Cox 1980). There remains, however, considerable scepticism concerning this theory since the clinical studies by Chrisman et al (1964) and Cassidy & Kirkaldy-Willis (1985) have demonstrated that patients with demonstrated disc herniation respond relatively poorly to manipulation.

CHANGES IN POSTERIOR JOINT FUNCTION

Pathology of the posterior facets and its relationship to posture and leg length has been studied intensively by Giles & Taylor (1982, 1984, 1985). The discovery of intraarticular synovial protrusions with nerve endings containing substance P has led to the suggestion that these protrusions may become entrapped within the joint, resulting in pain. Giles (1986) has suggested that manipulation may relieve this entrapment and any muscle spasm which results from it. This is by no means a new theory and has previously been postulated by a number of practitioners of manipulation, but without the anatomical studies of Giles & Taylor. Other anatomists (Bogduk & Jell 1985), however, are not as yet convinced that the anatomy is consistent with the ability of the posterior facets to entrap the synovial folds.

INCREASED RANGE OF MOTION

By far the most popular theory regarding the effect of manipulation is that it increases range of motion. This concept has been incorporated into the theories of chiropractic, medical, osteopathic and physical therapy practitioners of manipulation. Variations of Figure 68.1 can be seen in the literature of all practitioners of manipulative therapy. According to this theory, spinal or peripheral joint motion can become restricted, and such restrictions can be detected by palpation and other examination techniques. This restricted motion has been referred to as a 'fixation' or 'blockage'.

The restricted motion theory is based on the assumption that there are barriers which normally restrict range of motion. Figure 68.4 illustrates these presumed barriers and the proposed mechanisms through which they can be shifted under different pathological situations resulting in restricted joint motion. For example, the active range of motion can be restricted by muscle spasm or any other pathology which results in shortening of the muscle (Fig. 68.4, second line). The goal of treatment in this situation is therefore to relax or stretch the muscle. The passive range of motion may be normal and there may be little or no bony pathology.

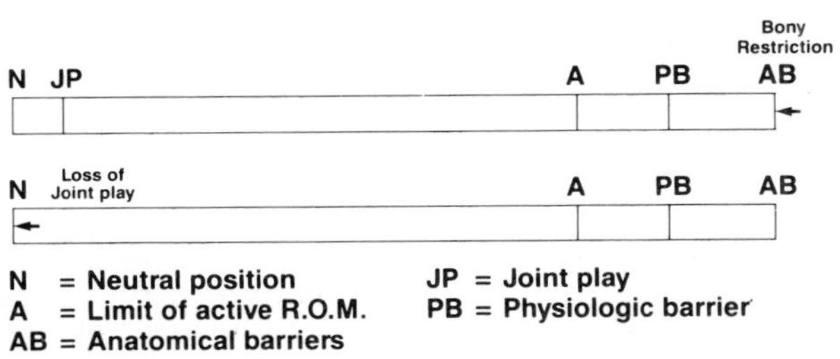

Methods of Restricting Joint Motion

N JP Normal A PB AB

Muscle Spasms
N JP A PB AB

Ligamentous Shortening
N JP A PB AB

Bony Restriction
N JP A PB AB

Loss of Joint play
N A PB AB

N = Neutral position
A = Limit of active R.O.M.
AB = Anatomical barriers
JP = Joint play
PB = Physiologic barrier

Fig. 68.4 The mechanisms by which a joint can become restricted (see text).

The second method by which joint motion can be restricted is the shortening of ligamentous or capsular structures (Fig. 68.4, third line). The bony elements of the joint may be normal but the joint cannot be passively moved through its normal range. The goal of treatment in this situation is the stretching of ligamentous structures to increase range of motion. The third mechanism by which joints can be restricted is through pathology in the bony elements themselves, primarily through degenerative spondylosis (Fig. 68.4, fourth line). It is generally assumed that manipulation will not result in any change in this form of restriction but instead is aimed at any concomitant ligamentous or muscular changes. The fourth mechanism by which motion is restricted is by limitation of joint play in the neutral position or at some point in the normal range of motion (Fig. 68.4, fifth line). Such joint play is usually for accessory movements and may be in planes other than the direction in which a joint usually moves. Such accessory movements are felt to be essential for the full smooth motion of a joint. Treatment is directed at restoring the joint play. Combinations of these various methods of restricting range of motion of a joint are also thought to occur.

The exact mechanism through which restricted motion can cause pain is not clear and is probably multifactoral. A totally fused joint is not generally painful, but spinal joints where manipulation is being considered are not completely fused. There is still movement in the joint which can stretch strained ligaments or pull on inflamed or contracted muscles, resulting in pain. Restricted motion may also reduce nutrition to the intervertebral disc or joint cartilage, resulting in breakdown of these tissues and resulting inflammation. The latter changes have been noted in peripheral joints which have been restricted in animals (Akeson et al 1980). Holm & Nachemson (1982) have demonstrated the importance of motion in intervertebral disc nutrition.

There is a growing body of evidence that manipulation can increase spinal range of motion. Many of the research trials used range of motion as one of the measures of successful treatment. Evans et al (1978), Rasmussen (1979), Nwuga (1982) and Waagen et al (1986) all demonstrated increases in the gross range of motion following manipulation of the lumbar spine. Howe et al (1983) demonstrated increased rotation and lateral flexion of the neck when compared to controls, It appears, however, from these studies that only certain directions of movement show increased range after manipulation. Jirout (1972a, 1972b) reported changes in range of motion on X-rays before and after manipulation. Of particular interest in this regard is the paper by Fisk (1979), where straight-leg raising was noted to increase in patients with low-back pain following manipulation, but not when manipulation was applied to asymptomatic patients. Buerger (1978, 1979) also demonstrated increased straight-leg raising after manipulation but only when pelvic rotation was used as an end-point.

PSYCHOLOGICAL EFFECTS OF MANIPULATION

The growing recognition of the close relationship between psychosocial and psychological factors and back pain with its related disability has resulted in a closer look at the psychological effects of manipulation. This method has many advantages over other pain-relief procedures. Most patients and their physicians who offer this modality have a strong, enthusiastic belief in the effectiveness of manipulation. Furthermore, there is confidence in a physician who uses his or her hands to 'find' the pain and then apply a treatment directly to the painful area, especially when other physicians have looked at the pain from a distance. In addition, there is the soothing effect of laying on of hands and the natural empathy and concern which is commonly found in practitioners of manipulation.

There are now some data which actually document these changes. Kane et al (1974) were the first to demonstrate that patients were more satisfied when chiropractors took time to explain their opinions and make patients feel welcome. Pope et al (1992) have furthermore shown that not only are patients' confidence levels for massage and manipulation higher than for TMS and corsets, but also that the confidence levels increase with ongoing treatment.

SUMMARY AND CONCLUSION

Massage and manipulation, the so-called manual therapies, remain amongst the most universally applied techniques for relieving pain and discomfort. There is great variation in techniques which have been described and taught over the centuries. It is possible to group these techniques according to the position within the range of motion of a joint where the treatment is being applied, the depth and direction and nature of the tissue being massaged and mobilised, and whether stretching or thrusting motions are applied to a joint. It cannot be assumed that all forms of massage or manipulation are equivalent or have similar effects because there are marked differences between these techniques. Clinical research is now available to substantiate a role for manipulation in the treatment of acute, uncomplicated low-back pain. Lesser evidence is available for justifying the use of manipulation in the management of chronic back pain, sciatica, neck pain and headaches.

The most commonly accepted theory on manipulation is based on the concept of restricted barriers in joint range of motion. Manipulation is assumed to improve range of motion with subsequent positive effects on the intervertebral disc, joints, muscles and ligaments. Massage and manipulation are also felt to increase thresholds for pain, relax muscles, increase circulation and reduce oedema, and in this way result in relief of pain. There is also growing objective evidence that patients have high satisfaction and confidence in manipulation which may also explain the growing use of this procedure around the world.

REFERENCES

Akeson W H, Amiel D, Woo S 1980 Immobility effects on synovial joints. The pathomechanics of joint contracture. Biorheology 17: 95–110

Bergquist-Ullman M, Larsson U 1977 Acute low back pain in industry. Acta Orthopaedica Scandinavica (Suppl.) 170: 11–117

Bitterli J 1977 Zur Objektivierung der manual therapeutischen Beeinflussbarkeit des spondylogenen Kopfschmerzes. Nervenarzt 48: 259–262

Bogduk N, Jell G 1985 The theoretical pathology of acute locked back: a basis for manipulation. Manual Medicine 1: 78–82

Breen A C 1977 Chiropractors and the treatment of back pain. Rheumatology and Rehabilitation 16: 46–53

Brodin H 1982 Cervical pain and mobilization. Manual Medicine 20: 90–94

Bronfort G 1992 Effectiveness of spinal manipulation and adjustment. In: Haldeman S (ed) Principles and practice of chiropractic. Appleton & Lange, Norwalk, Connecticut, p 415–441

Brunarski D J 1984 Clinical trials of spinal manipulation: a critical appraisal and review of the literature. Journal of Manipulative and Physiological Therapeutics 7: 243–249

Buerger A A 1978 A clinical trial of rotational manipulation. International Association for the Study of Pain. Second World Congress on Pain, Montreal, Canada. Pain Abstracts 1: 248

Buerger A A 1979 A clinical trial of spinal manipulation. Federation Proceedings 38: 1250

Cassidy J D, Kirkaldy-Willis W H, McGregor M 1985 Spinal manipulation for the treatment of chronic low back and leg pain: An observational study. In: Buerger A A, Greenman P E (eds) Empirical approaches to the validation of spinal manipulation, C C Thomas, Springfield, Illinois, p 119–148

Chrisman O D, Mittnacht A, Snook G A 1964 A study of the results following rotatory manipulation in the lumbar intervertebral disc syndrome. Journal of Bone and Joint Surgery 46A: 517–524

Christian G F, Stanton G J, Sissons D, How H Y, Jamison J, Alder B, Fullerton M and Funder J W 1988 Immunoreactive ACTH, beta-endorphin and cortisol levels in plasma following spinal manipulative therapy. Spine 13: 1411–1417

Coplans C W 1978 The conservative treatment of low back pain. In: Helfet A J, Gruebel Lee D M (eds) Disorders of the lumbar spine. J B Lippincott Co., Philadelphia, p 145–183

Cox J M 1980 Low back pain, 3rd edn. Self-published, Fort Wayne, Indiana

Coxhead C E, Inskip H, Meade T W, North W R S, Troup J D G 1981 Multicentre trial of physiotherapy in the management of sciatic symptoms. Lancet 1: 1065–1068

Coyer A B, Curwen I H M 1955 Low back pain treated by manipulation: a controlled series. British Medical Journal March 19: 705–707

Cyriax E F 1904 The elements of Kellgren's manual treatment. London 1903, New York 1904

Cyriax J 1971 Textbook of orthopaedic medicine, diagnosis of soft tissue lesions, vol 1, 6th edn. Baillière Tindall, London

Dicke E 1953 Meine Bindegewebs Massage. Stuttgart

Diebert P, England R 1972 Electromyographic studies. Part 1: Consideration in the evaluation of osteopathic therapy. Journal of the American Osteopathic Association 72: 162–169

Doran D M L, Newell D J 1975 Manipulation in treatment of low back pain: a multicentre study. British Medical Journal 2: 161–164

Ebner M 1960 Connective tissue massage, therapy and therapeutic application. Williams & Wilkins, Baltimore

Edwards B C 1969 Low back pain resulting from lumbar spine conditions. A comparison of treatment results. Australian Journal of Physiotherapy 15: 104–110

Elkins E C, Herrick J F, Grindlay J H, Mann F C, DeForrest R E 1953 Effect of various procedures on the flow of lymph. Archives of Physical Medicine 34: 31

Evans D P, Burke M S, Lloyd K N, Roberts E E, Roberts G M 1978 Lumbar spinal manipulation on trial. Part 1: Clinical assessment. Rheumatology and Rehabilitation 17: 46–53

Farrell J P, Twomey L T 1982 Acute low back pain. Comparison of two conservative treatment approaches. Medical Journal of Australia 1: 160–164

Fisk J W 1979 A controlled trial of manipulation in a selected group of patients with low back pain favouring one side. New Zealand Medical Journal 645: 288–291

Gibbons R W 1980 The evolution of chiropractic: medical and social protest in America. In: Haldeman S (ed), Modern developments in the principles and practice of chiropractic. Appleton-Century-Croft, New York, pp 3–24

Gibson T, Grahame R, Harkness J et al 1985 Controlled comparison of short wave diathermy treatment with osteopathic treatment in non-specific low back pain. Lancet 1: 1258–1260

Giles L G F 1986 Lumbosacral and cervical zygapophyseal joint inclusions. Manual Medicine 2: 89–92

Giles L G F, Taylor J R 1982 Intra-articular synovial protrusions in the lower lumbar apophyseal joints. Bulletin of the Hospital for Joint Diseases Orthopaedic Institute 42: 248–254

Giles L G F, Taylor J R 1984 The effect of postural scoliosis on lumbar apophyseal joints. Scandinavian Journal of Rheumatology 13: 209–220

Giles L G F, Taylor J R 1985 Osteoarthritis in human cadaveric lumbo-sacral zygapophyseal joints. Journal of Manipulative and Physiological Therapeutics 8: 239–243

Glover J R, Morris J G, Khosla T 1974 Back pain: a randomized clinical trial of rotational manipulation of the trunk. British Journal of Industrial Medicine 31: 59–64

Glover J R, Morris J G, Khosla T 1977 A randomized clinical trial of rotational manipulation of the trunk. In: Buerger A A, Tobis J S (eds) Approaches to the validation of manipulation therapy, C C Thomas, Springfield, Illinois, p 271–283

Godfrey C M, Morgan P P, Schatzker J 1984 A randomized trial of manipulation for low back pain in a medical setting. Spine 9: 301–304

Goldstein M (ed) 1975 The research status of spinal manipulative therapy. NINCDS Monograph no. 15, DHEW Publication no. (NIH) 76–998, Bethesda, Maryland

Goodridge J P 1981 Muscle energy technique: definition, explanation, methods of procedure. Journal of the American Osteopathic Association 81: 249

Graham D A 1902 Treatise on massage, 3rd edn. New York 1884, Philadelphia

Greco M A 1953 Chiropractic technique illustrated. Jarl Publishing Co., New York

Greenland S, Reisbord L, Haldeman S, Buerger A A 1979 Controlled clinical trials of manipulation: a review and proposal. Journal of Occupational Medicine 22: 670–676

Grice A A 1974 Muscle tonus changes following manipulation. Journal of the Canadian Chiropractic Association, 19 no. 4: 29–31

Grice A S, Tschumi P C 1985 Pre- and post-manipulation lateral bending radiographic study and relation to muscle function of the low back. Annals of the Swiss Chiropractic Association 8: 149–165

Haldeman S 1978 The clinical basis for discussion of mechanisms of manipulative therapy. In: Korr I (ed) The neurobiologic mechanisms in manipulative therapy. Plenum, New York, p 53–75

Haldeman S 1980 Modern developments in the principles and practice of chiropractic. Appleton-Century-Croft, New York

Haldeman S 1992 Principles and practice of chiropractic. Appleton & Lange, Norwalk, Connecticut

Hoehler F K, Tobis J S, Buerger A A 1981 Spinal manipulation for low back pain. Journal of the American Medical Association 245: 1835–1838

Hoffa A 1897 Technik des Massage, 13th edn. Hoffa-Gocht-Starck, Stuttgart (Quoted by Kamenetz 1980)

Hofkosh J M 1985 Classical massage. In: Basmajian J V (ed), Manipulation, traction and massage, 3rd edn, Williams & Wilkins, Baltimore

Holm S, Nachemson A 1982 Variations in the nutrition of canine intervertebral disc induced by motion. Orthopaedic Transactions 6: 48

Howe D H, Newcombe R G, Wade M T 1983 Manipulation of the cervical spine – a pilot study. Journal of the Royal College of General Practitioners 33: 574–579

Hoyt W H, Schafter F, Bard D A et al 1979 Osteopathic manipulation in the treatment of muscle contraction headache. Journal of the American Osteopathic Association 78: 332–325

Jayson M I V 1986 A limited role for manipulation. British Medical Journal 293: 1454–1455

Jirout J 1972a The effect of mobilization of the segmental blockade on the sagittal component of the reaction on lateral flexion of the cervical spine. Neuroradiology 3: 210–215

Jirout J 1972b Changes in the sagittal component of the reaction of the cervical spine to lateroflexion after manipulation of blockade. Ceskoslovenska Neurologie a Neurochirurgie 35: 175–180

Kane R, Olsen D, Leymaster C 1974 Manipulating the patient: a comparison of the effectiveness of physician and chiropractor care. Lancet 1: 1333

Kamenetz H L 1985 History of massage. In: Basmajian J V (ed), Manipulation, traction and massage, 3rd edn. Williams & Wilkins, Baltimore

Kimberly P E 1979 Outline of osteopathic manipulative procedures. Kirksville College of Osteopathic Medicine, Kirksville

Kirkaldy-Willis W H, Cassidy J D 1985 Spinal manipulation in the treatment of low back pain. Canadian Family Physician 31: 535–540

Korr I M (ed) 1978 The neurobiologic mechanisms in Manipulative Therapy. Plenum Press, New York

Lewith G T, Turner G M T 1982 Retrospective analysis of the management of acute low back pain. The Practitioner 226: 1614–1618

Logan H B 1950 Textbook of Logan basic methods. L B M, St Louis

Lomax E 1975 Manipulative therapy: a historical perspective from ancient times to the modern era. In: Goldstein M (ed) The research status of spinal manipulative therapy. NINCDS monograph no. 15. DHEW Publication no. (NIH) 76–998

Lomax E 1976 Manipulative therapy: a historical perspective. In: Buerger A A, Tobis J S (eds) Approaches to the validation of manipulative therapy. C C Thomas, Springfield, Illinois, p 205–216

Maitland G D 1973 Vertebral manipulation, 3rd edn. Butterworth, London

Matthews J A, Yates D A H 1969 Reduction of lumbar disc prolapse by manipulation. British Medical Journal Sept 20: 696–699

Matthews J A, Mills S B, Jenkins V M et al 1987 Back pain and sciatica: controlled trials of manipulation, traction, sclerosal and epidural injections. British Journal of Rheumatology 26: 416–423

Meade T W, Dyer S, Browne W, Townsend J, Frank A O 1990 Low back pain of mechanical origin: randomized comparison of chiropractic and hospital outpatient treatment. British Medical Journal 300: 1431–1437

Mennell J B 1917 Massage: its principles and practice. London

Mennell J B 1934 Physical treatment by movement, manipulation and massage. Philadelphia

Mennell J McM 1960 Back pain – diagnosis and treatment using manipulative therapy. Little, Brown, Boston

Nyiendo J, Haldeman S 1987 A prospective study of 2000 patients attending a chiropractic college teaching unit. Medical Care 25: 516–527

Nwuga V C B 1982 Relative therapeutic efficacy of vertebral manipulation and conventional treatment in back pain management.

American Journal of Physical Medicine and Rehabilitation 61: 273–278

Nyberg R 1985 The role of physical therapists in spinal manipulation. In: Basmajian J V (ed) Manipulation, traction and massage, 3rd edn. Williams Wilkins, Baltimore

Oltenbacher K, DiFabio R P 1985 Efficiency of spinal manipulation/mobilization therapy. A meta-analysis. Spine 10: 833–837

Ongley M J, Klein R G, Droman T A, Eck B C, Hubert L J 1987 A new approach to the treatment of chronic low back pain. Lancet 2: 143–146

Paget J 1867 Cases that bone-setters cure. British Medical Journal 1: 1–4

Parker G B, Tupling H, Pryor D S 1978 A controlled trial of cervical manipulation for migraine. Australian and New Zealand Journal of Medicine 8: 589–593

Pope M H, Phillips R B, Haugh L D, MacDonald L, Haldeman S 1992 A prospective randomized three week trial of spinal manipulation, transcutaneous muscle stimulation, massage and corset in the treatment of subacute low back pain. (Submitted)

Pott P 1936 Remarks on that kind of palsy of the lower links which is frequently found to accompany a curvature of the spine, is supposed to be caused by it, together with its method of cure. Medical Classics 1: 281–322

Rasmussen G G 1979 Manipulation in low back pain: a randomized clinical trial. Manuelle Medizin 1: 8–10

Sanders G E, Reinert O, Tepe R, Maloney P 1990 Chiropractic adjustive manipulation on subjects with acute low back pain: Visual analog pain scores and plasma beta-endorphin levels. Journal of Manipulative and Physiological Therapeutics 13: 391–395

Schiotz E H 1958 Manipulation treatment of the spinal column from the medical–historical viewpoint. Tidsshr Nor Laegeform (NIH Library translation) 78: 359–372

Shambaugh P 1987 Changes in electrical activity in muscles resulting from chiropractic adjustment: a pilot study. Journal of Manipulative and Physiological Therapeutics 10: 300–303

Shekelle P G, Adams A H, Chassin M R, Hurwitz E C, Brook R H 1992 Spinal manipulation for low back pain. Annals of Internal Medicine 117: 590–598

Sims-Williams H, Jayson M I D C, Young S M S, Baddeley H, Collins E 1978 Controlled trial of mobilization and manipulation for patients with low back pain in general practice. British Medical Journal 2: 1338–1340

Sims-Williams H, Jayson M I C, Young S M S, Baddeley H, Collins E 1979 Controlled trial of mobilization and manipulation for patients with low back pain: hospital patients British Medical Journal 2: 1318–1320

Skull C W 1945 Massage – physiologic basis. Archives of Physical Medicine 261: 159

Sloop P R, Smith D S, Boldenberg S R N, Dore C 1982 Manipulation for chronic neck pain. A double-blind controlled study. Spine 7: 532–535

Starling E H 1984 The influence of mechanical factors on lymph production. Journal of Physiology 16: 224

States A Z 1968 Spinal and pelvic technics. Atlas of chiropractic technic, 2nd edn. National College of Chiropractic, Lombard, Illinois

Tappan F 1984 Massage. In: Wall P D, Melzack R (eds) Textbook of pain, 1st edn. Churchill Livingstone, Edinburgh

Terrett A C J, Vernon H 1984 Manipulation and pain tolerance. A controlled study of the effects of spinal manipulation on paraspinal cutaneous pain tolerance levels. American Journal of Physical Medicine 63: 217–225

Thompson J C 1973 Thompson technique. J C Thompson, Davenport

Travell J 1976 Myofascial trigger points: clinical view. advances in pain research and therapy 1: 919–926

Vear H J 1972 A study into the complaints of patients seeking chiropractic care. Journal of the Canadian Chiropractic Association Oct 9–13

Vernon H T, Dhami M S I, Annett R 1985 Abstract, Canadian Foundation for Spinal Research. Symposium of low back pain, Vancouver B C, March 15–16

Waagen G N, Haldeman S, Cook G, Lopez D, DeBoer K F 1986 Short term trial of chiropractice adjustments for the relief of chronic low back pain. Manual Medicine 2: 63–67

Waagen G N, DeBoer K, Hansen J, McGhee D, Haldeman S 1990 A prospective comparative trial of general practice medical care, chiropractic manipulative therapy and sham manipulation in the management of patients with chronic or repetitive low back pain. Abstract, International Society for the Study of the Lumbar Spine, Boston

Wakim K G, Martin G M, Terrier J C, Elkins E C, Krusen E H 1949 The effects of massage on the circulation in normal and paralyzed extremities. Archives of Physical Medicine 30: 135

Wakim K G, Martin G M, Krusen E H 1955 Influence of centripetal rhythmic compression on localized edema of an extremity. Archives of Physical Medicine 36: 98

Wakim K G 1980 Physiologic effects of massage. In: Rogoff J B (ed) Manipulation, massage and traction, 2nd edn. Williams & Wilkins, Baltimore Ch. 2

Waterworth R F, Hunder I A 1985 An open study of diflunisal, conservative and manipulative therapy in the management of acute mechanical low back pain. New Zealand Medical Journal 98: 327–328

Wood E C 1974 Beard's massage principles and techniques. W B Saunders, Philadelphia

Zhu Y, Starr A, Haldeman S, Seffinger M A, Su S H 1992 Paraspinal muscle evoked cerebral potentials in patients with unilateral low back pain. (Submitted)

69. Movement education and limitation of movement

Patricia Wells and Eva Lessard

INTRODUCTION

Humans are dependent upon the integrity of their locomotor system: muscles, ligaments, joints, bones and nerves. If this integrity is lost through disease or trauma, the resulting limitation of movement may be regained in whole or in part through movement education, i.e. therapeutic exercises. Rehabilitation involves a complex interaction between patient and therapist. Treatment of each patient requires the therapist to design a unique programme which addresses identified needs. To develop a sound therapeutic programme the physiotherapist must identify the patient's problem(s) through assessment, establish functional outcome goals and determine the appropriate treatment.

A purposeful treatment using movement should improve function and relieve pain. The physiotherapist's role is to assist the patient at each stage of recovery by recognising the ability to function at a higher level and instituting the appropriate therapeutic measures to achieve the next level. An additional role of the physiotherapist in rehabilitation is to educate patients to prevent recurrence of pain by teaching proper body mechanics in their activities of daily living.

HISTORY

The therapeutic value of exercises for the human body was recognised in ancient times. MacAuliffe (1904) reported that in ancient China therapeutic exercises were prescribed for the relief of pain and other symptoms. In the 19th century the famous British surgeon John Hunter had an extensive appreciation of the value of early mobilisation following injury or disease to relieve pain and enhance return of function. Hunter (1841) demonstrated not only knowledge in the area of surgery but also an appreciation of kinesiology. He felt that voluntary movements were superior to passive movements in helping the patient to regain function. Licht (1978), in a historical review of exercises, reported on the work of Lucas-Championnière, a 19th-century French physician, who discovered the value of mobilisation following a fracture of the radius. He noted that a patient who was not immobilised following a fracture of the radius regained function quickly. Moreover, the pain associated with the fracture appeared to lessen more quickly than in persons with similar fractures who were immobilised (without exercise), the accepted form of treatment for fractures at the end of the 19th century.

In Britain at the beginning of the 20th century, the emphasis of the newly formed Chartered Society of Physiotherapy was on massage and medical electricity (Wicksteed 1948). Physiotherapists perfected their skills in these techniques while the orthopaedists, neurologists and physicians at the spas continued to develop and prescribe therapeutic exercises. Davies (1976) reported that following an outbreak of poliomyelitis in 1914 in the United States, care-givers other than physicians (physiotherapists) were trained in the use of therapeutic exercises, massage and electricity. It became increasingly evident, especially with poliomyelitis, that movement re-education was of greater value than either massage or electrotherapy.

The 20th century has been one of advancement of knowledge and technology in all areas of medicine. During the past 50 years, physiotherapy has evolved and became an important component of the health-care team. Advances in the areas of biomechanics, neurophysiology, motor control, motor learning, motor development and cognitive training have provided new and more effective methods to treat patients with movement disorders. Recently, research activities in both the basic and clinical areas has increased significantly. For example, Tipton et al (1986) in an experimental study on the influences of physical activity on ligaments, tendons and joints concluded that immobilisation of a limb will markedly reduce muscle strength and the functioning of ligaments and tendons. Prescribed exercises which increase the forces being transmitted to ligaments, tendons and bones will maintain and generally increase the strength and functional capacity of these structures. Other researchers

(Murray 1988; Godges et al 1989; Feine et al 1990; Mitchell & Carmen 1990; Donelson et al 1991; Kakigi & Shebasoki 1992) whose studies have focused on pain and movement have shown that sound therapeutic exercise programmes can be instrumental in the relief of pain. Farrell (1985) suggests that exercise activiates the endogenous opiate system, which may also decrease pain.

THERAPEUTIC MOVEMENTS

When there is a disruption of the integrity and functioning of the locomotor system, the individual experiences difficulty with activities of daily living. The degree to which this difficulty is experienced depends upon the severity of the trauma and/or disease process which affects normal functioning of the system. Frequently, the method of choice to restore lost function and decrease pain is through the use of therapeutic exercises. An extensive survey of physiotherapy students' clinical experiences (Wells & Lessard 1983) indicated that 45% of the patients are referred from orthopaedics, 32% from medicine, 19% from neurology and that therapeutic exercises are the most frequently used method in the rehabilitation of patients with disorders affecting the locomotor system.

The goals of therapeutic exercises are determined following assessment and identification of the patient's problem(s) (Fig. 69.1). Once the problem has been identified, the goals and treatment programme are planned and treatment commences. It is usual for a therapist to reassess the condition at least every 10–14 days following the beginning of treatment, assuming that the usual smooth course in the rehabilitation programme is seen. The therapist may at an earlier time or with greater frequency reassess the situation if events warrant such a course of action. These events may include:

1. further deterioration of the locomotor system
2. improvement greater than usual for the problem assessed initially, or
3. complications, such as venous thrombosis, which require changes in programme (including its cessation) until the problem is removed.

PASSIVE MOVEMENTS

In a passive movement, there is no active force generated by the muscles of the body part receiving therapy. The force to move the joint or limb may be provided manually by the therapist, by the patient (autoassisted) or by a continuous passive motion machine (Walker et al 1991). Passive movement is slightly greater than active movement as each joint has a small amount of available motion that is not under voluntary control. Passive motion is used in assessing and evaluating patient problems as it provides information about the integrity of the articular surfaces, extensibility of the joint capsule and associated ligaments and muscles (Montgomery & Connelly 1991). In treatment, the therapist supports the weight of the limb throughout the movement in such a way that the joint being moved has both proximal and distal support. The direction of the movement is guided by placing the hands on the appropriate surface, e.g. in passive flexion of the elbow, the hand is placed on the anterior surface of the forearm. As well as maintaining joint range, passive movements are thought to be useful in providing appropriate tactile and proprioceptive stimulation. The range of motion achieved depends on the normal degrees of freedom of the particular joint being moved, the subjective sensation of pain, the stretchability of muscles and ligaments and other macro and micro changes in the joint.

Harris & Lundgren (1991) hypothesis that articular nerve supply has provided some understanding of the effect of passive movement on modulating pain. Passive movement stimulates Type I, II and III mechanoreceptors in joint capsules and ligaments. End-of-range passive movement may reduce peripheral input and therefore decrease pain by decreasing intraarticular pressure. End-range passive movement also reduces peripheral input to the central nervous system through the adaptation of the encapsulated joint nerves.

Salter (1980) states that passive movement may trigger pain as a result of reflex inhibition of muscle action at each end of the range of motion. Therefore, passive movement has to be administered very carefully as it is potentially

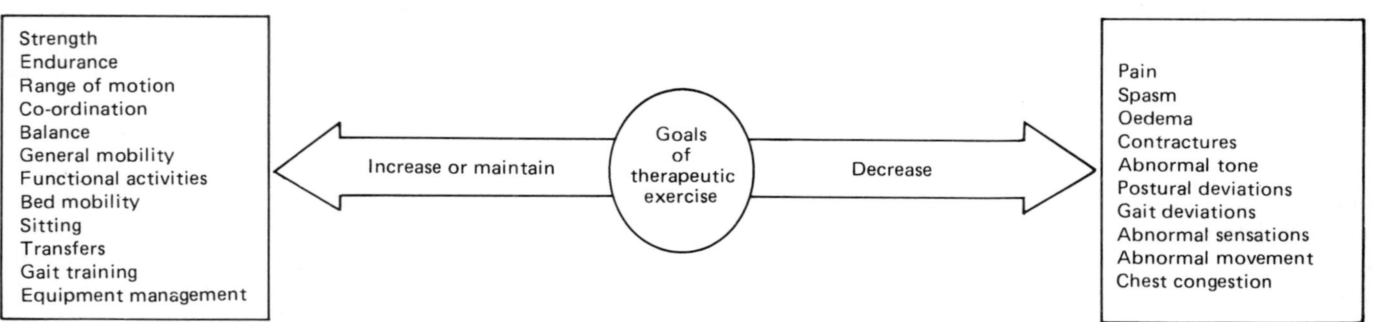

Fig. 69.1 Goals of therapeutic exercises.

dangerous and may produce further irritation to the abnormal synovial membrane and joint capsule resulting in increasing stiffness and pain. Salter considers passive movements to be of greatest value in paralysis and in the gradual stretching of existing muscle contractures. Wilson (1984) cautions that if passive movement is chosen as the method for beginning rehabilitation of arthritic joints, this should be done only to the degree that pain and spasm will permit.

Passive movements which provide a form of mobilisation may be effective in preventing the occurrence of advanced changes seen in joints following periods of immobilisation. Ebel (1978), in discussing the rationale for passive movements, noted that passive movements increased blood flow and thereby nutrition to the body part in disorders of the lymphatic circulation. In oedematous conditions, the same author states that venous return may be augmented and venous congestion possibly prevented by passive movements.

Strickland & Glogovac (1980), in reporting on digital function following flexor tendon repair, give some support to early passive mobilisation. In a controlled study, they demonstrated that early mobilisation of flexor tendon repairs has better effects than immobilisation methods, and they concluded that passive movement has an adhesion-limiting effect which substantially improves the results of flexor-tendon repair in finger joints and reduces pain.

Saunders (1989) claims that passive range of motion assists articular cartilage healing, and reduces swelling and stiffness in a hand fracture. She encourages the use of passive range of motion as a primary modality before active range of motion can be obtained. Evans (1989) gives a rationale for early passive motion technique in the treatment of extension tendon injury of the hand based on research studies in biomechanics, physiological studies on the healing extensor tendons and their reaction to controlled stress, and clinical results. Philips (1989), in her discussion on rehabilitation of the patient with a rheumatoid hand, suggests that in cases of acute synovitis associated with pain and muscle spasm, gentle passive range of motion may be less stressful to the joints than other movement therapy.

Swenson (1984) feels that daily range-of-motion exercises will prevent contractures in cases of upper motor neuron lesions which result in paralysis of the limbs. Bromley (1976) concurs with this opinion and advocates daily passive movement of the paralysed limbs in the early management of spinal-cord injuries. An exception to the effectiveness of passive movement of paralysed limbs is in cases of hysterical paralysis. Dodgson (1977) feels that movement therapy in hysterical paralysis is contraindicated as it focuses further attention on the paralysed limbs. Knapp (1984) reports that having therapists perform passive motion of the strong muscles while the patient performs active motion of the weak muscles helps restore muscle balance in lower motor neuron lesions. This specific use of passive movements is referred to as localised differential exercise. If muscle balance is restored, contractures are prevented. While this is an interesting theory on the use of passive movement, further study must be done to validate the effectiveness of this procedure. For the moment, until further scientific research is carried out, most writers agree that frequent motion through an adequate range is the only way to prevent contractures.

Currently, passive movement therapy is accepted as a starting modality in the rehabilitation of an extremity which has lost the voluntary control to move the joints. Neurological conditions such as spinal-cord lesions, head trauma, peripheral nerve lesions, poliomyelitis, polyneuropathies or unconscious states from varying causes may result in loss of voluntary control of the extremities. If complete loss is present, passive movement is the only choice of therapeutic movement available to the therapist. Carr & Shepherd (1980), in discussing passive range-of-motion activities in an unconscious patient, feel that administering passive movements gives necessary proprioceptive feedback. Renfrew (1977) states that in the treatment of head-injured patients isolated passive joint movements are not recommended. He suggests that total patterns of passive movement should be carried out. However, if there is any voluntary activity, a quasipassive movement will be performed with the therapist encouraging active participation during the phases of movement in which there is contraction of the muscles responsible for the movement. The therapist must be extremely sensitive to returning function and should encourage active movement where possible. Passive movements have been criticised recently from proponents of neurorehabilitation who advocate the multisensory approach (Farber 1982). The multisensory approach – which includes vestibular input, quick stretch, joint compression, tapping, vibration, facilitation of phasic flexor patterns and normalisation of touch – is considered to be more effective in developing patterns of movement. The multisensory approach has a strong theoretical base, supported by recent findings by neurologists who have shown that the central nervous system is capable of structural repair after injury (Harris 1984). Given this new information regarding the plasticity of the central nervous system, an even more critical look will be taken at traditional passive movements.

Griffin & Reddin (1981) feel that improperly administered passive movement, especially when abducting the shoulder, may contribute to the pain factor by causing compression trauma. They are adamantly against passive abduction by the patients themselves using pulley systems prescribed by physiotherapists. They are supported by Voss (1969) who concurs with this view, since passive abduction may contribute to shoulder pain. Griffin &

Reddin, in their review of the literature pertaining to shoulder pain in patients with hemiplegia, warn against unskilled forced passive movements of the shoulder in the abducted position, as bursa and rotator-cuff damage may occur. Moreover, improper exercise techniques are considered to be a possible cause of subluxation, rotator-cuff lesion and pain. They encourage an understanding of the biomechanics of the shoulder before undertaking a treatment programme. Overall, the authors conclude that early treatment helps to prevent pain. On the whole, therapists employ traditional passive movements reluctantly in the rehabilitation of patients with orthopaedic conditions. Further research is warranted on this type of therapeutic intervention. It appears that judicious use of passive movements has a place in today's movement education.

ACTIVE ASSISTED EXERCISES

In active assisted exercises, a force is applied which is equal to but not greater than the absent force of the muscle. The aim of this movement therapy is to augment, but never substitute for, the active muscle forces; otherwise it becomes passive movement therapy. Assistive forces may be provided manually by the therapist, by mechanical means such as slings and springs, by gravity, by the individual (autoassisted) or by the use of hydrotherapy.

Three important points should be considered in administering this type of exercise:

1. The correction or prevention of factors limiting range of motion, such as pain, spasm and joint stiffness.
2. Utilisation of the afferent side of the motor pattern by tactile, visual, auditory and proprioceptive stimuli. Knapp (1984) states that Sister Kenny, well known for her rehabilitation programme for poliomyelitis, calls stimulation of the afferent side of the motor pattern 'restoration of mental awareness'. The modern concept of this restoration process is seen in the electromyographic biofeedback method of treatment.
3. Re-education of the efferent side of the motor pattern by active participation on the part of the patient until function improves to the level where the entire treatment programme is an active one. Sister Kenny referred to this process as the 'restoration of muscle function'.

The transition from assisted to active free movements may be achieved by giving exercises with progressive loading, with gravity eliminated or counterbalanced. Carr & Shepherd (1980), in discussing treatment for lower motor neuron lesions, especially Guillain-Barré, suggest that active assisted movement should be used once the patient stabilises and the recovery stage begins. Active assisted exercises are followed by active mobilising and resisted active exercises. Shestack (1977) also encourages the use of assistive exercises in the treatment of polyneuropathies. Active assisted exercises serve as a transition state, the patient going on to active exercises when muscle function returns.

ACTIVE EXERCISES

Active exercise, as indicated, is one where the entire movement is carried out under the voluntary control of the individual. During the past 20 years efforts have been made to merge the physical and life sciences in the study of human motion. Increasing utilisation of engineering skills has occurred in rehabilitation medicine. The principles of mechanics have been incorporated in courses of study in the training of physiotherapists.

The principles of mechanics include such concepts as statics (where bodies are in static or dynamic equilibrium with no great acceleration) and dynamics (study of motion where bodies are in motion but not in equilibrium). Dynamics are further divided into the area of kinematics (study of the characteristics of motion – displacement, velocity, acceleration and time) and kinetics (study of the relationship existing among forces acting on the mass of the body). Kinetics is used to predict the motion caused by given forces, such as gravity, friction, water, air resistance, resistance of muscle contraction and the elastic components of tissue. Montgomery & Connelly (1991) state that the study of dynamics is invaluable in the field of medicine as indicated by the role that biomechanical investigations have played in analysis of walking patterns, development of orthotics and prosthetics, analysis of the role that muscles play in functional activities, tendon transfers, sport injuries, etc. It is not within the scope of this chapter to deal with these concepts in detail; we wish, however, to give a brief description of the neuromusculoskeletal system's contribution to active exercises.

In active exercises there is an orchestrated integration of effort from several systems to produce the desired movement. The causes of movement in the human body are internal forces, such as those produced by muscles, ligaments and joints, and external forces such as gravity and other mechanical forces. The passive elements (bone, tendons and ligaments) provide a framework for the active elements, i.e. muscles. Movement control is a highly interactive process of the central and peripheral nervous systems and the musculoskeletal system. Before an active movement occurs, the brain interprets a stimulus and then it chooses the appropriate action; integration, sequencing, coordination and timing of the motor output take place. In addition, the memory system is also involved and must be intact to assist in carrying out the activity. Changes in any of the above will result in inappropriate and/or altered movement response.

A joint is a junction between two bones and unites the various body segments. We speak of body segments when describing body links and kinematic chain concepts.

When a number of links are united they form what are called a kinematic or joint chain. A kinematic chain is a combination of several successively arranged joints constituting a complex motor system (Galley & Forster 1991). Joints exhibit either one, two or three degrees of freedom of motion which means that they have the capacity to provide movement in one, two or three planes and axes. The kinematic chain system allows the degrees of freedom of several joints in the chain to be pooled, giving the segments greater opportunity to achieve variety of movement than any one joint acting alone. An analysis of the apparently simple task of taking a glass off a shelf, filling it with a liquid and drinking it demonstrates that the pooling of several joints in the kinematic chain with their degrees of freedom of motion are necessary to provide the versatility of movement which no one joint could provide by acting alone. Should a joint in the chain become restricted due to pain, the pooling becomes impossible and deficiency of active movement occurs. Muscles make up the largest mass of the human body. Muscles convert energy into mechanical work. They allow us to play the piano or swim the English Channel. The elements of skeletal muscle are protein and they are the responsive elements. Muscle proteins can be divided into three broad categories: the contractile proteins which make up approximately 60% of the total protein content, the soluble proteins which encompass most of the energy-producing enzymes and the stromal or connective tissue proteins. A decrease of the contractile proteins is evident in muscles that are immobilised in a shortened state. The quantity of this protein affects the ability of the muscle to develop tension.

The smallest active part of the muscle is called the motor unit, which consists of motor neurons located in the spinal cord, axons that conduct the impulse to the neuromuscular junction and the motor end-plate. Muscles are elongated cells containing nuclei, intricate cytoplasmic systems, mitochondria in large numbers that provide adenosine triphosphate and myofibrils (Boyd & Sheldon 1980). A muscle is made up of two types of fibre: red (a slow fibre) and white (a fast-twitch fibre). Physical training causes adaptation in muscle cells. For example, a weight-lifter shows an increase in the number of myofibrils of the fast-twitch fibres in the trained muscles; a marathon runner demonstrates adaptation of muscles by an increase in the number and size of mitochondria of the slow-twitch fibres. The enzyme system also changes with respect to the content of enzymes. It appears that training enables the muscle to use this substrate more efficiently. Transport of glycogen and calcium is also improved. According to Boyd & Sheldon (1980), there is considerable evidence that increased training creates a microvascular bed that enhances oxygenation of the muscle. Therapeutic training, according to some evidence, may affect the following factors in muscle metabolism: the glycolytic and anaerobic enzymes may increase or remain unchanged, the Krebs cycle and respiratory chain enzymes show a similar pattern, carbohydrate metabolism is likely to increase, fat metabolism increases, mitochondrial changes occur and oxygen consumption capacity may increase (St-Pierre & Gardiner 1987).

Atrophy occurs in muscles that are not used. Edington & Edgerton (1976) state that changes in the contractile machinery of muscle that are atrophied from disuse occur. In slow-twitch red muscle fibres absolute maximum tension is lowered in the atrophied muscle because of the loss of muscle mass. The loss in muscle mass results from the loss of myofibrils within existing fibres. In fast-twitch, white-muscle fibres the same loss occurs more slowly. Atrophied muscles are known to be more susceptible to fatigue.

Recent evidence suggests the following changes with respect to immobilisation and atrophy (Table 69.1).

There are four different levels at which muscles may be affected by disease:

1. motor neuron loss that leads to denervation atrophy, e.g. poliomyelitis
2. interference with conduction or disease that leads to atrophy, e.g. peripheral nerve injury
3. interference with the neuromuscular junction, e.g. myasthenia gravis
4. primary disease of the muscle cells, e.g. muscular dystrophy.

A muscle rarely acts alone to produce movement. In order that the desired movement may be achieved, an orchestrated action of the muscles must occur. This is accomplished by muscles playing various roles in movement. They can be prime movers or agonists where

Table 69.1 Summary of references on the effect of immobilisation on muscle metabolism

1. Glycolytic and other anaerobic enzymes: no change and/or decreased	4. Free fatty acid metabolism oxidation of free fatty acids: maintained or decreased
2. Krebs cycle and respiratory chain enzymes: no change and/or decreased	5. Mitochondrial changes: ADP: O is maintained or decreased
3. Carbohydrate metabolism: uptake of 2-deoxyglucose in the absence of insulin is decreased	state III respiration is decreased only in subsarcolemma mitochondria
uptake of 2-deoxyglucose in the presence of insulin is decreased	state IV respiration of subsarcolemma and intermyofibrillar mitochondria is maintained
oxidation of carbohydrates is either maintained or decreased	respiration control index is decreased
activation of glycogen synthesis by insulin is decreased	6. Oxygen consumption capacity: decreased
glycogen concentration is decreased	

the muscle(s) initiate, carry out and maintain a particular movement. Smaller muscles that contribute are referred to as assistant movers. The muscle(s) may take the role of antagonist by reciprocal relaxation during the contraction of the prime mover. Muscle can play the role of stabiliser or fixator by contracting to position a bone to provide a stable base from which the prime mover can act. Another role is one of synergist where the muscle teams up with others to enhance the action of the prime mover. A good example of this orchestration is in doing a sit-up from a knees-bent, feet-flat-on-floor lying position. In this action, rectus abdominis and the obliques act as the prime mover, and the obliques are also helping synergists by counter-acting each other's rotational and lateral flexion action. Upon the return from the sit-up position, the flexor component of the external obliques and the rectus abdominis act as antagonists to gravity to provide a controlled descent to the starting position.

Contraction of muscles may be classified as isometric or dynamic. The isometric contraction is one in which the internal force developed by the muscle is such that the total muscle neither shortens nor lengthens. No motion is produced because the internal and external forces are in equilibrium. Dynamic muscle work is divided into concentric, eccentric and isokinetic. Concentric contraction is one where the internal force generated is greater than the external force applied, the muscle actively shortens and movement of the body part occurs. The eccentric or lengthening type of contraction is one where the internal force is less than the external force applied; the muscle lengthens while maintaining tension. Isokinetic contraction occurs when the rate of shortening and lengthening of the muscle is constant. The subject contracts the muscle group being exercised; an electromechanical device controls the speed of movement without permitting acceleration to occur. During isokinetic exercise the resistance accommodates the external force at the skeletal lever so that the muscle maintains maximum output throughout the full range of motion. Before development of this device, a skilled therapist could apply similar accommodating resistance throughout the range of motion by manually resisting the motion. The therapist could continually adjust the amount of resistance being offered so that the motion produced is approximately constant throughout the range, thereby approaching an isokinetic condition (Brunnstrom 1983). The manual resistance of the therapist cannot be precisely measured.

Active exercises are classified as free or resisted. The active, free movements are a progression from the assistive stage. Active exercises are used to improve strength, endurance and flexibility, maintain and improve joint mobility, improve skill in performance, break down adhesions, prevent contractures and decrease pain.

Pain may be thought of as a sensation calling attention to possible tissue damage or disease and has affective, motivational and cognitive dimensions. Levenson (1971), in discussing the shoulder–hand dystrophy frequently seen in hemiplegia, advocates mobilisation of the shoulder joint to relieve deep pain. Deep pain may originate in muscles, tendons and joints. This type of pain is difficult to locate at times since it tends to radiate. He further states that the pain can be prevented by early mobilisation using active assisted and active exercises. Bobath (1979) claims that mobilising the shoulder is necessary to prevent pain. Todd & Davies (1977) reported that, after spasticity around the scapula and trunk is released, careful mobilisation will free the shoulder and relieve pain. Swenson (1984), in discussing the hemiplegic patient, feels that positioning and active exercises are necessary to prevent contractures which cause pain.

Andrews (1980), Paulos et al (1980), Walsh (1980), in discussing rehabilitation of the postsurgical knee, put forward the suggestion that isometric exercises minimise pain and hasten return of function. St-Pierre & Gardiner (1987), in a review of the literature on the effect of immobilisation and exercise on muscle function, state that the benefit of isometric exercise in preventing muscle atrophy is controversial. Bennett & Stauber (1986), in a study on the evaluation and treatment of anterior knee pain using eccentric exercises, demonstrated that those subjects who fit the criteria for anterior knee pain syndrome demonstrated remarkable improvement after training. In some cases, the pain was relieved after 2 weeks of training while others required up to 4 weeks before significant change was experienced. Nordemar (1981) and Nordemar et al (1981), in a controlled long-term study on physical training in rheumatoid arthritis, concluded that extreme loading of tendons, muscles, collateral ligaments and joints is contraindicated but that physical exercises in rheumatoid arthritis as a therapy helped patients in all respects, including improvement in articular cartilage and nutrition, strengthening ligaments and tendons and decreasing pain.

Wilson (1984), in discussing movement therapy for arthritic joints, noted that opinion is divided on the type of exercise to be given in the acute phase where pain and spasm are present. While some advocate passive movement he feels the most effective method is active assisted exercise. He further cautions that whatever method is used an increase in pain or spasm for more than 1 hour after exercise indicates excessive motion and so the method must be modified in future therapy sessions.

A common condition treated in physiotherapy departments is low-back pain. Raskin (1981) reports that the most widely known disorder of the low back is herniated nucleus pulposus; other disorders, such as degenerative changes in the posterior elements of the spine, changes occurring in the normal ageing process, abnormal stress due to congenital defects, trauma, etc. may have greater clinical significance. According to Macnab (1978), the common problem encountered in the clinical picture of back pain is the emotional overtone. This factor is not to be confused with purely psychogenically induced back pain, which is relatively infrequent.

Physiotherapists may select isometric abdominal exercises, flexion/extension exercises, manipulation, transcutaneous electrical nerve stimulation (TENS), ice or biofeedback in conjunction with back exercises and back-care education routine in the treatment of low-back pain. Currey et al (1979), in reporting the early management of low-back problems, indicated that, with regard to primary treatment, 66% of 188 cases received physical treatment (exercises), 34% received analgesic drugs, 31% surgical corset, 12% bed rest at home, 3% observation, and 1% were admitted to hospital. Wells & Lessard (1983) in a survey of students' clinical experiences, found that flexion exercises prevailed as the method of choice in the management of back pain. Davies et al (1979), in reviewing back-pain management, reported that exercises are used more frequently than any other method of treatment. A study conducted by Zylbergold & Piper (1981) comparing three approaches to treatment of low-back pain found no statistically significant differences in the pain measurements. However, the authors suggest that manual therapy may have provided somewhat more relief of pain than the other methods. In the 1930s Dr Paul Williams developed a set of exercises of the lumbar flexion type which he felt would provide stability of the lower trunk, passively stretch the extensor muscles and reduce pain. Blackburn & Portney (1981) studied the electromyographic activity of back musculature during Williams's flexion exercises. They reported that to minimise the electromyographic activity of the paraspinal muscles the optimum position would be supine, lying with knees bent and posterior pelvic tilt. This position and the posterior pelvic tilt movement tended to minimise clinical symptoms as compared with posterior pelvic tilt in the standing position. Kvien et al (1984) report that two groups of patients they studied benefited from satisfactory information regarding back-care education and that this approach was more beneficial to patients than the traditional physiotherapeutical methods practised in the hospital. Relevant education which emphasised exercises and the correct use of the back enhanced the patients' self-care.

Jensen (1980), in a study of lumbar interdiscal pressures, reported that the largest pressure increases were recorded during hyperextension and sit-up exercises. The author advocates, in the treatment of low-back pain, that one should focus on resisted knee extension exercises and resisted isometric abdominal exercises to increase intraabdominal pressure which, in his opinion, reduces intradistal pressure and pain. Sarno (1984), in discussing therapeutic exercises and back pain, feels that the deeply ingrained concept that low-back and neck pain must be accounted for by structural disorders of the lumbosacral and neck regions is not supported by objective data. He suggests that the majority of cases of low-back pain are from benign, reversible, psychosomatic processes involving the musculature of the back: 'tension myositis syndrome' (TMS). While admitting that no hard data on this syndrome exist, he feels that clinical studies support it. In a retrospective study of patients treated by physical exercise for TMS, 84% derived benefit, 76% were essentially cured, while 16% failed to improve. Sarno concludes that a proper understanding of the course of back pain in combination with intelligently applied therapeutic exercise can eliminate pain and restore physical competence.

Beekman & Axtell (1985) investigated ambulation distance, activity level, medical care sought and perceived pain in 49 patients with chronic spinal pain who completed an inpatient 4-week rehabilitation programme. The patients were followed for 6 months. The postintervention test (at 6 months) of the factors studied revealed significant increases in distance walked, cardiovascular efficiency and in reports of participation in exercise activities. There was also a significant decrease in self-rated pain and a decrease in medical care sought. The finding on pain is consistent with results of other investigators (Seres & Newman 1976; Gottlieb et al 1977; Roberts & Reinhardt 1980; Keefe et al 1981; Cinciripini & Floreen 1982).

Saal (1990) completed a 3 year study on patients with herniated nucleus pulposus and leg pain where straight leg raising of 60° or less reproduced radiculopathy. All patients underwent an aggressive physical therapy programme. Successful outcomes were achieved in 50 of 52 non-operatively treated patients (96%).

Exercises also have a role in the postoperative management of patients with low-back pain. Mooney (1979) reports that early mobilisation and gentle movements help to prevent complications seen following discoidectomy. Among these complications are urinary tract infections, thrombophlebitis, gastrointestinal disturbances and muscle atrophy. Mitchell et al (1990) conducted a multicentre study on effective treatment of acute soft tissue and back injuries using a specific exercise regimen. The authors reported that movement therapy appears to overcome muscle spasm and reduce pain. Active exercises produce a release of endorphins and this was thought to be a factor in the diminution of pain. Kellett et al (1991) in their study of the effects of exercise on low-back pain found that 81% of the patients reported a subjective improvement in low-back pain following exercises. Elnaggar et al (1991) in their study on the effect of flexion and extension exercises on low-back pain concluded that both types of exercises provided significant reduction in the severity of low-back pain but no significant difference in pain reduction was perceived by either type of exercise group. Mannicke et al (1991) in a clinical trial using 105 patients tested the effect of intensive dynamic back exercises for chronic low-back pain. The outcome revealed a statistically significant improvement in the group receiving the exercise regimen compared to the control group.

Donelson (1990), in a review paper on the McKenzie approach to evaluating and treating low-back pain states that patients treated by this method were able to decrease the recurrence of low-back pain and that groups treated by alternate approaches were unable to do so. He suggests that no other treatment for acute back pain has shown such long-term benefit. Lindström et al (1992) conducted a study on patients who had non-specific mechanical low-back pain. There were two randomly assigned groups: activity group (N=51) and control group (N=53). The study found that the subjects in the activity group returned to work significantly earlier than the control group. Deyo et al (1990) examined the effectiveness of TENS, a programme of stretching exercises and a combination of both on patients with chronic low-back pain. It was found that, after 1 month, subjects in the exercise group had significant improvement in self-rated pain scores, reduction in the frequency of pain and greater levels of activity as compared with subjects who did not exercise. The authors feel that 1 month of intervention may be insufficient to observe the full effect. Donchin et al (1990), using 142 subjects, randomly assigned the subjects to a flexion exercise programme for 3 months, a back school programme and a control group. The two intervention programmes were evaluated over a 1 year period. The results show that the exercise group had a mean of 4.5 painful months as compared to 7.3 and 7.4 painful months for the back school and control groups respectively.

Feine et al (1990) state that there is now considerable evidence that movement reduces the transmission of somatosensory information within the dorsal column-medial lemniscal system in both humans and animals. It seems most likely that shaking a painful body part suppresses pain by the high frequency stimulation of muscle afferents. Kakigi & Shibasaki (1992) applied vibratory stimuli to the fingers concurrently with active movement and found that they significantly reduced pain.

Mullins (1989) states that early mobilisation following trauma increases large-diameter nerve-fibre stimulation, which aids in decreasing pain. She also says that the reflex sympathetic dystrophies (well described by Lankford & Thompson 1977) are helped by active exercises in conjunction with TENS for pain relief.

Resisted exercises require the patient to work beyond those limits which are easily met. Progressive resisted exercises for the quadriceps developed by Delorme – brief maximal exercises (BME), weight-lifting, underwater-resisted and isometric-resisted exercises, manual and springs resistance, and isokinetic exercises–are commonly used by physiotherapists. Ideally a progressive increase of repetition and/or an increase in load are the most efficient approaches. Hettinger & Muller (1953) report that isometric-resisted exercise is the most rapid method of increasing muscle strength (force production). These authors believe that regardless of how much the muscles are used they will not grow in mass or strength unless they are overloaded. Paulos et al (1980), in discussing a treatment rationale for patellar malalignment state, suggest that, at the intermediate stage of rehabilitation, the progressive resistance exercise approach should be used to increase muscle strength, but these exercises must not increase pain or effusion. Rasch & Burke (1978) claim that if the resistance is greater than that to which the muscle is accustomed, even a single daily contraction stimulates a significant strength increase. With weight-training equipment, the amount of resistance, the number of repetitions and the number of sets of exercises can be regulated precisely to bring about efficient strength adaptation. Lateur & Lehmann (1990) in discussing isokinetic motion, which is a resisted exercise, state that the Cybex system has the advantage that it automatically accommodates to any torque the muscle can produce at any rate of contraction. The device provides accommodating resistance that matches anything that the muscle can produce throughout the range. If pain is present, it affects the muscle contraction and the machine will adjust to this factor. A disadvantage is that the patient is dependent on equipment.

In discussing patients with central nervous system damage, such as spastic hemiplegia, Carr & Shepherd (1988) claim that there is no evidence that activation of an increasing number of motor units (resisted exercise) will alone produce improvement in function. Norton & Sahrmann (1978) proposed that unnecessary voluntary effort may be a major contribution to dysfunction of the spastic hemiplegia because the muscles may be exercised to the exclusion of their antagonists, reinforcing the muscular imbalance so typical after a stroke. Often the intact limb is treated by resistive techniques which result in muscle activity in the affected limb. Given this information one must be cautious in using resistive techniques.

In rehabilitation programmes using exercises as a therapeutic modality, the idiom 'do no harm' must prevail. Grabois (1979) infers that 15–20% of patients must discontinue or decrease exercise programmes because of injuries sustained while undergoing therapeutic treatment. On the other hand, he states that therapeutic exercise programmes are an indispensable part of the treatment of subacute and chronic pain syndromes. Salter (1980) states that when pain is experienced by the patient while doing an exercise, the therapist must reassess the situation and modify the exercise because further synovial membrane or joint capsule damage may occur. Amundsen (1979) feels that strengthening and endurance exercises should not cause pain. Exercise should be stopped if chest, joint or upper extremity pain occurs, since it may be a symptom of angina pectoris and myocardial ischaemia. McClellan (1951) states that overdoing or incorrect performance of an exercise following fracture may delay union, and may result in trauma and ankylosis. Exercises that are too vigorous in the aged may result in cardiac insufficiency and an acute cardiac situation with fatal results. Wolf (1984) reports that few clinical studies on quantitative and qualitative changes in muscle during therapeutic exercises have been carried out, but suggests that muscle strength is increased by both concentric and eccentric contractions. Eccentric contractions appear to be more beneficial for patients with painful limitation of joint range. For instance, eccentric abdominal contraction with low-back pain is less painful than concentric muscle work.

There is some significant evidence that active exercises increase endorphin levels. Endorphins are morphine-like substances produced in the central nervous system. They are endogenous-signalling molecules that regulate pain perception and affective states (Alberts et al 1983). Grossman & Sutton (1985) report that endorphins and enkephalins are measurable in the circulation and their concentration increases with exercise. Farrell (1985) also reports that an increase in the peripheral plasma levels of beta-endorphins in humans after exercise has been noted by all investigators to date. However, these findings cannot be extrapolated to pain relief following therapeutic exercise. To date, the role of therapeutic exercises in the relief of pain seems to lie in the restoration of function through the reduction of oedema, circulatory improvement, increase in muscle strength, flexibility, improvement in joint range and functional ability.

Galley & Forster (1990), in discussing the use of movement for an injured body part, suggest that early movement therapy may not be permitted until healing has occurred. Often during this period, when pain is experienced at the traumatised area, the patient keeps the whole limb tense, causing secondary pain. In order to prevent this occurring, early movement therapy to all unaffected joints should encouraged. As knowledge of muscle cell physiology, biomechanics and kinesiology unravels the effect of exercise on pain, improved application of therapeutic exercise may result.

STRETCHING EXERCISES

Stretching exercises were utilised by athletes and dancers who had an appreciation of their value long before scientific investigators attempted to understand the physiological mechanisms involved. According to Stanish (1982), stretching techniques affect the elastic component of the muscle in such a way that the stretching will maximise the elastic recoil properties of the muscle tendon units. Bowling & Rockar (1985) define contractures as a lesion of non-contractile and contractile elements, a macro- or microscopic tear of the connective tissue and/or the substance of the muscolotendinous unit. Both passive and active stretching exercises are used by therapists today to relieve contractures. Jacobs (1976) does not promote passive stretching, preferring slow active stretching. Salter (1980) concurs with this point of view. Jacobs believes that passive stretching may cause damage to muscles. The technique of slow active stretching is explained and described by Stanish (1982) after the method of Holt. He explains that, with an isometric contraction of a previously passively stretched muscle, a firing of the Golgi tendon organ takes place within the stretched muscle, thus facilitating relaxation of the muscle. If a particular muscle is to be stretched it should be passively stretched to minimal discomfort and then exposed to an isometric contraction which facilitates relaxation of the muscle; further relaxation of the stretched muscle will occur if the agonist contracts. This technique exploits the reciprocal innervation and contraction inhibition theory. He further states that the entire process must be totally painfree. A study by Wallin et al (1985) on 47 male subjects revealed that passive stretching of a muscle after a short (7–8 seconds) isometric contraction of the muscle allows a greater lengthening of the muscle and an increased range of motion of the corresponding joint than the classic ballistic swing method.

Sady et al (1982) reported in a study that proprioceptive neuromuscular facilitation techniques elicited a greater acute stretch from a muscle group during exercise than either the ballistic or static method, even though the duration of stretch was the same for all three methods. This study appears to support Holt's claim that stretch of the muscle followed by isometric contraction, then relaxation, increases further stretchability of the muscle; however, the effect is temporary.

Godges et al (1989) compared two commonly used stretching techniques (static stretching and soft-tissue mobilisation with proprioceptive neuromuscular facilitation) and found that static stretching was the treatment of choice for improving hip range of motion as well as for reducing the metabolic cost of submaximal walking and running. Khalil et al (1992) studied 28 chronic low-back pain patients in whom the effect of stretching manoeuvres was evaluated. Their findings demonstrated that immediate as well as cumulative gains in reduction of pain level was obtained. They concluded that a scheduled stretching protocol can be useful in restoring functional abilities as well as pain reduction. Some contraindications to stretching include myositis ossificans, inflamed joints after a period of prolonged disuse, certain neurological disorders and osteoporosis.

RELAXATION EXERCISES

In this movement therapy, the patient is taught to recognise unnecessary tension and methods to avoid it. Tension is primarily caused by stress and pain. Farber (1982), in discussing Seyle's stress studies, defines stress as the body's non-specific over-reaction to any demand. Seyle defined the general adaptation syndrome as an entity with three components:

1. alarm reaction component to harmful stimuli
2. stage of resistance by increasing general bodily defence reactions
3. exhaustion.

According to Rosch (1979), stress has been characterised as the most prevalent health problem in America. Kottke (1990) states that anxiety produces a state of tension that causes increased activity in the central nervous system and affects many other systems. Tension causes pain in the muscles, joints, neck and head.

Physiotherapists have long recognised the need for relaxation prior to initiation of and during treatment programmes. Tension states often interfere with the therapeutic effect of exercise. If, during a treatment, unnecessary or excessive muscle contraction is noted or altered breathing rate is observed, the therapist brings this to the patient's attention. Galley & Forster (1990) suggest that localised relaxation leads to a lessening of pain and increased movement potential. The techniques employed by physiotherapists include the methods of Jacobson, Fair & Basmajian, Fink & Mitchell, yoga and meditation (if qualified to use) and biofeedback. Breathing exercises are usually incorporated into most of these techniques.

Pregnant women comprise one of the largest groups who undergo structured relaxation training. Marshall (1981) reports that selective or differential relaxation is important during the second stage of labour, when relaxation of the pelvic floor is of utmost importance to facilitate expulsion of the baby. A tense pelvic floor acts as a counterforce to the downward pressure created by the contraction of the abdomen, the uterus and the descending baby.

Relaxation techniques are also useful in asthmatic and emphysematous patients. It is believed that reduction in wasteful associated movements will result in energy conservation. Sorbi & Tellegen (1986), studying the differential effects of relaxation training and stress-coping training in 29 patients with migraine headaches, found significantly beneficial effects of relaxation training on migraine headaches. Blanchard et al (1986) also found significant reduction of headache distress using relaxation therapy.

MOVEMENT THERAPY BASED ON HIERARCHIAL AND DISTRIBUTED CONTROL MODELS

Movement therapy in the rehabilitation of patients with neurological deficits prior to the 1980s was largely based on the work of Bobath, Knott, Voss, Brunnstrom & Rood who developed therapeutic programmes. These programmes were developed using the theoretical concepts available to them at the time as well as their own knowledge derived from practice in the clinical setting. During the 1980s there was a tremendous increase in research in neuroscience, biomechanics and psychology which provided physiotherapists with information to modify their approach in the treatment of neurological disorders.

The approaches to treatment developed in the past were primarily based on the *hierarchial model of motor control*. This model views the cortex as the highest functioning component and the spinal level reflexes as the lowest. Using this model the physiotherapist assessed reflexive behaviour, i.e. righting and equilibrium reactions, tonic neck reflex or tonic labyrinthine reflexes, etc. and used their findings to develop a treatment programme.

Keshner (1981) describes the conceptual framework of neurodevelopmental theory, as presented in the writing of Bobath, which was based on Jackson's theoretical approach. Jackson described the central nervous system (CNS) as a hierarchically functioning structure in which the normal, more complex patterns of behaviour, such as righting and equilibrium reactions, are at a higher level of organisation than, for example, tonic neck or tonic labyrinthine reflexes. We suggest that the CNS does not function as a strictly descending hierarchy but as a network of independent systems that support desired movement through their interactions (systems theory). It must be remembered that the neurodevelopmental and systems theories are only suggestions about the structure of the CNS. Keshner feels that research is necessary to substantiate both theories.

Montgomery & Connelly (1991) describe the Bobath method of treatment as one where an attempt was made to normalize muscle tone (flaccidity, spasticity and rigidity), inhibit or integrate primitive postural patterns and facilitate normal postural reactions. The main thrust of Bobath's approach was on altered reflex mechanisms. During the same time period Margaret Jonstone, a Scottish physiotherapist, based her treatment approach on reflex inhibition with special attention to tonic neck reflexes through use of air splints and positioning. Harris (1984) sees a deficiency in the Bobath approach and states that the symptoms of cerebral palsy are not solely determined by altered reflex mechanisms. Postmortem neuropathological studies of central nervous system specimens of cerebral palsy patients showed diffuse anoxic destruction of somatosensory and motor neurons of the cerebral cortex. Moreover, damage of the subcortical relay nuclei for sensory pathways was seen.

Brunnstrom, in her treatment, uses a combination of central facilitation, proprioceptive and peripheral stimulation to take the patient from the initial stage of mass synergic reaction to an intermediate stage of voluntary motion dominated by synergy. Finally, she breaks away from synergies to approach a stage of refined functional voluntary control of limbs (Harris 1984). According to Harris, Brunnstrom feels that mass synergist reactions are dominated by spinal reflex mechanisms but, it is believed, most likely involve intra- and interhemispheric cortical interconnections as well. Hughes (1972), in her comparison of two methods of treatment of left hemiplegia, expresses the view that treatments which employ abnormal patterns cannot be nearly as beneficial as one which takes a patient through many varied sensory and motor experiences. Hughes feels that Bobath, by putting patients in reflex-inhibiting patterns, enables the patient to relearn the prestroke patterns. Brunnstrom, on the other hand, attempts to return the central integration to normal by using abnormal patterns to facilitate function. Once the patient is able to move voluntarily through the synergies, only then is the patient encouraged to peform normalised movement functions.

The proprioceptive neuromuscular facilitation (PNF) technique of Kabat, Knott & Voss makes explicit use of proprioceptive stimulation. The therapist facilitates the contraction of muscle groups. The patient executes diagonal spiral movements which start with placing the muscle to be facilitated under maximal stretch (by the therapist) and end with the muscles at the maximally shortened part of their range. Graded resistance is applied throughout the range in order to facilitate weak muscle contraction through overflow from strong muscles during maximal effort. Auditory stimulation is also a part of this exercise routine. In addition to muscle joint compression, the therapist uses other forms of peripheral stimulation as an adjunct to the method, e.g. cold in the form of compresses is used to relax muscle spasm and eliminate pain. Surburg (1979), in comparing interactive effects of resistance and facilitation patterning upon reaction and response times, found no significant difference between PNF with resistance, PNF without resistance and weight-training.

Semans (1965), in comparing PNF with the Bobath technique, says that although both were based on Sherrington's theory, different aspects were applied to clinical problems and as a result took different directions in developing a treatment programme. Bobath, in describing the difference between PNF and the Bobath method, stated that Kabat & Knott made use of spinal, cerebellar and cortical mechanisms and emphasised facilitation through the contribution of these mechanisms. Bobath, on the other hand, placed the emphasis on utilising reflex-inhibiting patterns. Semans finds many similarities in the two systems, such as the need to focus attention on movement patterns rather than movement of individual parts and the necessity for skilled use of hands.

Dickstein et al (1986) conducted a study on 131 hemiplegic patients, comparing conventional exercise, PNF (Knott & Voss 1956) and Bobath approaches to treatment. Despite the differences in theory and practice, no treatment-related variances in the outcomes of patients after 6 weeks of treatment were found. Carr & Shepherd (1980) state that, in their opinion, PNF techniques used to facilitate relaxation of spastic muscles are contraindicated since the technique may actually increase hypertonus.

Sady et al (1982), in a flexibility training programme, compared ballistic, static and PNF routines and found that PNF elicited greater muscle stretch from a muscle group than the other two techniques. There is some evidence from the study by Pink (1981) that electromyographic activity is prevalent in the non-exercised limb during the administration of a resisted PNF pattern to the other limb. Pink suggests that patients with burns, fractures and arthritis who are unable to exercise the involved limb due to pain and other factors could benefit from the indirect approach of exercising the non-involved limb. The positive results of this study may aid in setting up treatment programmes when difficulty is encountered in exercising the affected limb.

Rood's technique (1956) is based on the theory that cutaneous stimulation modifies tone and promotes muscular contraction and that the two are inseparable. Her treatment techniques are also based on the neurodevelopmental sequence, i.e. withdrawal–spine, rolling over, pivot prone, co-contraction neck, leaning on elbow in prone, four-foot kneel, standing and walking. Montgomery & Connelly (1991) state that the purpose of her treatment is to restore that component in the sequence in the manner in which it is normally acquired. The sensory stimulation is applied through mechanical and thermal modalities, i.e. mechanical (stroking pressure and stretch) and thermal (icing).

The sensory motor integrative theory advanced by Farber (1982) proposes the knowledgeable use of sensory stimuli to bring about improvement in maladaptive behavioural manifestations caused by the inability of the CNS to filter properly, and to organise and process incoming sensory information. Although the general theories presented so far do not seem to be in conflict with Farber's approach, the research studies Farber cites do not provide enough support for acceptance of the sensory motor integrative therapy approach. The specific therapeutic modalities Farber uses include touch, vestibular, olfactory, gustatory, temperature, stretch, traction, resistance, vibration, auditory and visual input.

In addition to multiple-stimulation therapeutic treatment approaches, the use of a monostimulation treatment approach is also practised. Fiebert & Brown (1979), in a pilot study of vestibular stimulation to improve ambulation in 20 hemiplegic patients, demonstrated that patients who received the vestibular stimulation showed greater improvement in functional ambulation than did the patients who did not receive the stimulation. Farber (1982) warns of the common misuse of the vestibular stimulation modality. Inadequate monitoring during and following stimulation, and improper rotating patterns and velocities, may be dangerous. Poor application of vestibular stimulation may have a deleterious effect since the system has many interconnections within the central nervous system.

Two Australian physiotherapists, Carr & Shepherd (1988), developed a treatment for stroke patients called motor relearning programme. The major assumptions about motor control underlying this model is relearning life activities: those which have meaning for the patient and non facilitation or the practice of non-specific exercises. The assumptions made to support this model are:

1. learning needs are the same for both disabled and able-bodied people, i.e. they need to practise, get feedback, understand the goals, etc.
2. specific motor tasks can be learned by practice of the same task, i.e. getting up from lying to sitting to standing
3. sensory input is important in accomplishing the task. Emphasis is on normal movement and how it is used in daily living, how it is learned and relearned. Carr & Shepherd feel that the developmental sequence approach should not be adhered to in the treatment of adults.

The *distributed control model* (closed system) is based on a neural organisation different from the hierarchial model (open system). In this model the control element of movement varies depending on the task to be accomplished. The model embraces the closed system which has multiple feedback loops and supports the concept of distributed control. The theory attempts to explain motor control, motor learning and motor development. Additionally, in the closed system, the CNS is viewed as an active agent with structures that enable the initiation and generation of movement not merely as an agent that reacts to incoming stimuli. (The open system model is characterised by a single transfer of information without feedback loops.) Diagnosis and treatment approaches using this model relate to functional goals, functional objectives, functional assessments, functional problems and functional outcomes (Montgomery & Connelly 1991).

We are aware that in discussing neurorehabilitation approaches the pain factor was not emphasised. Little if any concrete research on the effect of these techniques on the relief of pain was evident in a search of the literature.

CONCLUSIONS

In recent years there has been an increase in the number of well-designed clinical studies which investigate movement therapy and its effect on the pain factor; however, many of the therapeutic exercise programmes are still based on empirical evidence. Current writings indicate that movement therapy has value for the relief of pain; the concept of pain is neither simple nor linear in relation to the physiological and psychological functioning in humans. Further studies on how therapeutic exercise affects the cell, tissue, organs and systems will no doubt enhance the development of movement therapy and its effects on the reduction of pain.

REFERENCES

Alberts B, Bray D, Lewis J, Raff M, Robert K, Watson J D 1983 Molecular biology of the cell. Garland, New York

Amundsen L R 1979 Assessing exercise tolerance: a review. Physical Therapy 59: 534–537

Andrews J R 1980 Posterolateral rotary instability of the knee; surgery for acute and chronic problems. Physical Therapy 60: 1637–1639

Beekman C E, Axtell L 1985 Ambulation, activity level, and pain. Physical Therapy 65: 1649–1655

Bennett J G, Stauber W T 1986 Evaluation and treatment of anterior knee pain using eccentric exercise. Medicine and Science in Sports and Exercise 18: 526–530

Blackburn S E, Portney L G 1981 Electromyographic activity of back musculature during Williams' flexion exercises. Physical Therapy 61: 878–885

Blanchard E B, Andrasik F, Appelbaum B A, Evans D D, Myers P, Barron K D 1986 Three studies of the psychologic changes in chronic headache patients associated with biofeedback and relaxation therapies. Psychomatic Medicine 48: 73–83

Bobath B 1979 Adult hemiplegia: evaluation and treatment, 2nd edn. Heinemann, London

Bobath K, Bobath B 1952 Treatment of cerebral palsy based on analysis of patient's motor behaviour. British Journal of Physical Medicine 15: 107–117

Bowling R W, Rockar P A 1985 The elbow complex. In: Gould J A, Davies G J (eds) Orthopaedics and sports physical therapy, vol 2. Mosby, St Louis, Missouri

Boyd W, Sheldon H 1980 Introduction to the study of disease, 8th edn. Lea & Febiger, Philadelphia

Bromley I 1976 Tetraplegia and paraplegia. Churchill Livingstone, Edinburgh

Brunnstrom S 1970 Movement therapy in hemiplegia. Harper & Row, New York

Brunnstrom S 1983 Clinical kinesiology, 4th edn. F A Davis, Philadelphia

Carr J H, Shepherd R B 1988 A motor relearning programme for stroke. Aspen Publishers, Rockville, Maryland

Carr J H, Shepherd R 1980 Physiotherapy in disorders of the brain. Heinemann, London

Cinciripini P M, Floreen A 1982 An evaluation of a behavioral program for chronic pain. Journal of Behavioral Medicine 5: 375–389

Currey H L F, Greenwood R M, Lloyd G G, Murray R S 1979 A prospective study of low back pain. Rheumatology and Rehabilitation 18: 94–104

Davies E J 1976 The emergence of our profession. Physical Therapy 56: 11–12

Davies J E, Gibson T, Tester L 1979 The value of exercises in the treatment of low back pain. Rheumatology and Rehabilitation 18: 243–247
Deyo R A, Walsh N E, Martin D C, Schoenfeld L S, Ramamurthy S 1990 A controlled trial of transcutaneous electrical nerve stimulation (TENS) and exercise for chronic low back pain. New England Journal of Medicine 322: 1627–1634
Dickstein R, Hocherman S, Pillar T, Shaham R 1986 Stroke rehabilitation: three exercise therapy approaches. Physical Therapy 66: 1233–1238
Dodgson J M 1977 Physiotherapy in some psychiatric conditions. In: Cash J (ed) Neurology for physiotherapists, 2nd edn. Faber & Faber, London
Donchin M, Woolf O, Kaplan L, Floman Y 1990 Secondary prevention of low-back pain: a clinical trial. Spine 15: 1317–1320
Donelson R, Grant W, Kamps C, Medcalf R 1991 Pain response to sagittal end-range spinal motion. Spine 72: 210–211
Ebel A 1978 Exercise in peripheral vascular diseases. In: Basmajian J V (ed) Therapeutic exercise, 3rd edn. Williams & Wilkins, Baltimore
Edington D W, Edgerton V R 1976 The biology of physical activity. Houghton Mifflin, Boston
Elnaggar I M, Nordin M, Sheikhzadeh A, Parnianpour M, Kahanovitz N 1991 Effects of spinal flexion and extension exercises on low-back pain and spinal mobility in chronic mechanical low-back pain patients. Spine 16: 967–971
Evans R B 1989 Clinical application of controlled stress to the healing extensor tendon: a review of 112 cases. Physical Therapy 69: 1041–1049
Farber S D 1982 Neurorehabilitation. W B Saunders, Philadelphia
Farrell P A 1985 Exercise and endorphins–male response. Medicine and Science in Sports and Exercise 17: 89–93
Feine J S, Chapman C E, Lund J P, Duncan G H, Bushnell M C 1990 The perception of painful and nonpainful stimuli during voluntary motor activity in man. Somatosensory and Motor Research 7: 113–124
Fiebert I M, Brown E 1979 Vestibular stimulation to improve ambulation after a cerebral vascular accident. Physical Therapy 59: 423–426
Galley P M, Forster A L 1990 Human movement: an introductory text for physiotherapy students. Churchill Livingstone, London
Godges J J, Holden M R, Longdon C, Tinberg C, MacRae P 1989 The effects of two stretching procedures on hip range of motion and gait economy. Journal of Orthopaedic and Sports Physical Therapy 10: 350–357
Gottlieb H, Strite L C, Koller R et al 1977 Comprehensive rehabilitation of patients having chronic low back pain. Archives of Physical Medicine and Rehabilitation 58: 101–108
Grabois M 1979 Treatment of pain syndromes through exercise. In: Lowenthal D T, Bharadwaja K, Oaks W W (eds) Therapeutics through exercise. Grune & Stratton, New York
Griffin J, Reddin G 1981 Shoulder pain in patients with hemiplegia: a literature review. Physical Therapy 61: 1041–1045
Grossman A, Sutton J R 1985 Endorphins: what are they? How are they measured? What is their role in exercise? Medicine and Science in Sports and Exercise 17: 74–81
Harris F A 1984 Facilitation techniques in therapeutic exercise. In: Basmajian J V (ed) Therapeutic exercise, 4th edn. Williams & Wilkins, Baltimore
Harris S R, Lundgren B D 1991 Joint mobilization for children with central nervous system disorders: indications and precautions. Physical Therapy 71: 890–896
Hettinger T, Muller E A 1953 Muskelleistung und Muskel Training. Arbeitsphysiologie 15: 111–114
Hugues E 1972 Bobath and Brunnstrom: comparison of two methods of treatment of a left hemiplegia. Physiotherapy (Canada) 24: 262–266
Hunter J 1841 The complete works. Haswell, Barrington & Haswell, Philadelphia
Jacobs M 1976 Neurophysiological implications of the slow act of stretching. Correlative Technique Journal 30: 151–154
Jensen G M 1980 Biomechanics of the lumbar intervertebral disk; a review. Physical Therapy 60: 765–773
Jones D A, Newham D J, Torgan C 1989 Mechanical influences on long-lasting human muscle fatigue and delayed-onset pain. Journal of Physiology 412: 415–427
Kakigi R, Shibasaki H 1992 Mechanisms of pain relief by vibration and movement. Journal Neurology, Neurosurgery and Psychiatry 55: 282–286
Keefe F J, Block A R, Williams R B, Surwit P S 1981 Behavioral treatment of chronic low back pain: clinical outcome and individual differences in pain relief. Pain 11: 221–231
Kellett K M, Kellett D A, Nordholm L A 1991 Effects of an exercise program on sick leave due to back pain. Physical Therapy 71: 283–291
Keshner E A 1981 Reevaluating the theoretical model underlying the neurodevelopmental theory: a literature review. Physical Therapy 61: 1035–1040
Khalil T M, Asfour S S, Martinez L M et al 1992 Stretching in the rehabilitation of low-back pain patients. Spine 17: 311–317
Knapp M K 1984 Exercises for lower motor neuron lesions. In: Basmajian J V (ed) Therapeutic exercise, 4th edn. Williams & Wilkins, Baltimore
Knott M, Voss D E 1956 Proprioceptive neuromuscular facilitation: patterns and techniques. Paul B Hoeber, New York
Kottke F J 1990 Therapeutic exercise to maintain mobility. In: Krusen F M (ed) Handbook of physical medicine and rehabilitation, 4th edn. W B Saunders, Philadelphia
Kvien T K, Nilsen H, Vik P 1984 Education and self-care of patients with low back pain. Scandinavian Journal of Rheumatology 10: 318–320
Lankford L L, Thompson J E 1977 Reflex sympathetic dystrophy, upper and lower extremity: diagnosis and management. In: American academy of orthopaedic surgeons: instructional course lectures, vol 26. Mosby, St Louis, Missouri
Lateur B J, Lehmann J F 1990 Therapeutic exercise to develop strength and endurance. In: Krusen F M (ed) Handbook of physical medicine and rehabilitation, 4th edn. W B Saunders, Philadelphia
Levenson C 1971 Rehabilitation of the stroke hemiplegia patient. In: Krusen F M (ed) Handbook of physical medicine and rehabilitation, 2nd edn. W B Saunders, Philadelphia
Licht S 1978 History. In: Basmajian J V (ed) Therapeutic exercise, 4th edn. Williams & Wilkins, Baltimore
Lindström I, Öhlund C, Eek C et al 1992 The effect of graded activity on patients with subacute low back pain: a randomized prospective clinical study with an operant-conditioning behavioral approach. Physical Therapy 72: 279–290
Lund J P, Donga R, Widmer C G, Stohler C S 1991 The pain-adaptation model: a discussion of the relationship between chronic musculoskeletal pain and motor activity. Canadian Journal of Physiology and Pharmacology 69: 683–694
MacAuliffe L 1904 La thérapeutique physique d'autrefois. Masson, Paris
McClellan W S 1951 Physical medicine and rehabilitation for the aged. C C Thomas, Springfield, Illinois
Macnab I 1978 Backache. Williams & Wilkins, Baltimore
Manniche C, Lundberg E, Christensen I, Bentzen L, Hesselsoe G 1991 Intensive dynamic back exercises for chronic low back pain: a clinical trial. Pain 47: 53–63
Marshall K 1981 Pain relief in labour. Physiotherapy 67: 8–11
Mitchell R I, Carmen G M 1990 Results of a multicenter trial using an intensive active exercise program for the treatment of acute soft tissue and back injuries. Spine 15: 514–521
Mooney V 1979 Surgery and post surgical management of the patient with low back pain. Physical Therapy 59: 1000–1006
Montgomery P C, Connolly B H 1991 Motor control and physical therapy: theoretical framework and practical applications. Chattanooga Group Inc., Hixson, TN
Mullins P A T 1989 Management of common chronic pain problems in the hand. Physical Therapy 69: 1050–1057
Murray P B 1988 Case study: rehabilitation of a collegiate football placekicker with patellofemoral arthritis. Journal of Orthopaedics and Sports Physical Therapy 10: 224–227
Nordemar R 1981 Physical training in rheumatoid arthritis: a controlled long term study. Scandinavian Journal of Rheumatology 10: 25–30
Nordemar R, Ekblom B, Zachrisson L, Lundquist K 1981 Physical training in rheumatoid arthritis: a controlled long term study. Scandinavian Journal of Rheumatology 10: 17–23

Norton B J, Sahrmann S A 1978 Reflex and voluntary electromyographic activity in patients with hemiparesis. Physical Therapy 58: 951–955
Paulos L, Rusche K, Johnson C, Noyes F 1980 Patellar malalignment: a treatment rationale. Physical Therapy 60: 1624–1632
Philips C A 1989 Rehabilitation of the patient with rheumatoid hand involvement. Physical Therapy 69: 1091–1098
Pink M 1981 Contralateral effects of upper extremity proprioceptive neuromuscular facilitation patterns. Physical Therapy 61: 1158–1162
Rasch P J, Burke R K 1978 Kinesiology and applied anatomy, 6th edn. Lea & Febiger, Philadelphia
Raskin S P 1981 Degenerative changes of the lumbar spine: assessment by computed tomography. Orthopedics 4: 186–195
Renfrew E L 1977 Head injuries. In: Cash J (ed) Neurology for physiotherapists, 2nd edn. Faber & Faber, London
Roberts A H, Reinhardt L 1980 The behavioral management of chronic pain: long term follow-up with comparison groups. Pain 8: 151–162
Rood M S 1956 Neuromuscular mechanisms utilized in the treatment of neuromuscular dysfunction. American Journal of Occupational Therapy 10: 220–225
Rosch P J 1979 Stress and illness. Journal of the American Medical Association 242: 427–428
Ruch T C, Patton H D, Woodbury J W, Towe A L 1965 Neurophysiology, 2nd edn. W B Saunders, Philadelphia
Saal J A 1990 Dynamic muscular stabilization in the nonoperative treatment of lumbar pain syndromes. Orthopaedic Review 19: 691–699
Sady S P, Wortman M, Blanke D 1982 Flexibility training: ballistic, static or proprioceptive neuromuscular facilitation. Archives of Physical Medicine and Rehabilitation 63: 261–263
St-Pierre D, Gardiner P F 1987 The effect of immobilization and exercise on muscle function: a review. Physiotherapy (Canada) 39: 24–36
Salter R B 1980 Textbook of disorders and injuries of the musculoskeletal system. Williams & Wilkins, Baltimore
Sarno J E 1984 Therapeutic exercise for back pain. In: Basmajian J V (ed) Therapeutic exercise, 4th edn. Williams & Wilkins, Baltimore
Saunders S R 1989 Physical therapy management of hand fractures. Physical Therapy 69: 1065–1076
Semans S 1985 Treatment of neurological disorders. Physical Therapy 45: 11–16
Seres J L, Newman R I 1976 Results of treatment of chronic low back pain at the Portland Pain Center. Journal of Neurosurgery 45: 32–36
Shestack R 1977 Handbook of physical therapy. Springer Verlag, New York
Sorbi M A, Tellegen B 1986 Differential effects of training in relaxation and stress-coping in patients with migraine. Headache 26: 473–481
Stanish W D 1982 Neurophysiology of stretching. In: D'Ambrosia D D, Drez D (eds) Prevention and treatment of running injuries. Slack, New Jersey
Stichbury J 1981 Physiotherapy: assessment and treatment of disordered motor function. In: Evans C D (ed) Rehabilitation after severe head injury. Churchill Livingstone, Edinburgh
Strickland J W, Glogovac S V 1980 Digital function following flexor tendon repair in zone II: a comparison of immobilization and controlled passive motion techniques. Journal of Hand Surgery 5: 537–543
Surburg P D 1979 Interactive effects of resistance and facilitation patterning upon reaction and response times. Physical Therapy 59: 1513–1517
Swenson J R 1984 Therapeutic exercise in hemiplegia. In: Basmajian J V (ed) Therapeutic exercise, 4th edn. Williams & Wilkins, Baltimore
Tipton C M, Vailas A C, Matthes R D 1986 Experimental studies on the influences of physical activity on ligaments, tendons and joints: a brief review. Acta Medica Scandanavica (Suppl) 711: 157–168
Todd J H, Davies P M 1977 Hemiplegia II. In: Cash J (ed) Neurology for physiotherapists, 2nd edn. Faber & Faber, London
Voss D 1969 Should patients with hemiplegia wear a sling? Physical Therapy 49: 1030–1033
Walker R H, Morris B A, Angulo D L, Schneider J, Colwell C W J 1991 Postoperative use of continuous cooling pad following total knee arthroplasty. Journal of Arthroplasty 6: 151–156
Wallin D, Ekblom B, Grahn R, Nordenborg T 1985 Improvement of muscle flexibility. A comparison between two techniques. American Journal of Sports Medicine 13: 263–268
Walsh W M 1980 Anteromedial rotatory instability of the knee: present state of the art of surgery. Physical Therapy 60: 1633–1635
Wells P A, Lessard E 1983 Analysis of clinical experiences of physical therapy students in a Canadian university. Physiotherapy (Canada) 35: 92–99
Wicksteed J 1948 Growth of a profession. Edward Arnold, London
Wilson C H 1984 Exercises for arthritis. In: Basmajian J V (ed) Therapeutic exercise, 4th edn. Williams & Wilkins, Baltimore
Wolf S L 1984 The morphological and functional basis of therapeutic exercise. In: Basmajian J V (ed) Therapeutic exercise, 4th edn. Williams & Wilkins, Baltimore
Zylbergold R S, Piper M C 1981 Lumbar disc disease: comparative analysis of physical therapy treatments. Archives of Physical Medicine and Rehabilitation 62: 176–179

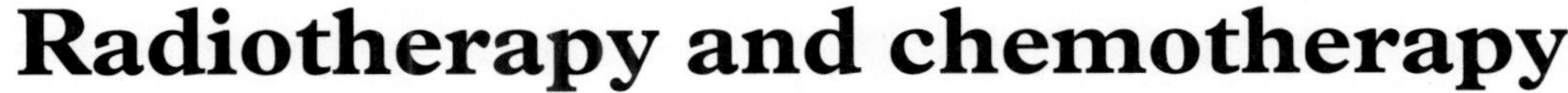

Radiotherapy and chemotherapy

70. Radiotherapy, chemotherapy and hormone therapy: treatment for pain

A. M. Hoy and C. F. Lucas

INTRODUCTION

Radiotherapy, chemotherapy and hormone therapy are mainly used as antitumour treatment in the relief of pain. The rational use of any of these types of treatment demands knowledge both of tumour biology and also of the mechanisms of action of these specific oncological techniques. The therapeutic aim should be clearly understood prior to starting treatment. Radical treatment should be given if the disease is potentially curable, but the intent should be symptomatic or palliative if the tumour is advanced or widely disseminated.

Pain may be a feature of both early and advanced cancer. In early cases it may be a presenting symptom, have clinical usefulness and therefore be understandable (and at least partly acceptable) to the patient. In advanced disease it no longer has a specific meaning diagnostically but only serves to underline the patient's illness (Saunders 1984).

The overall incidence of chronic pain in cancer patients is about 30%, but as patients enter the terminal phase of their illness this figure rises to 70–90% (Twycross & Lack 1983). This is higher than an earlier estimate that 50% of patients dying from cancer experienced pain (Aitken-Swan 1959). The incidence of pain in advanced cancer patients admitted to St Christopher's Hospice is 75%; this higher figure probably reflects the selection of such cases for admission (Haram 1984).

Pain may be directly attributable to tumour growth in three main categories which include tumour infiltration of bone, nerve or a hollow viscus. Rarely, pain may occur as a nonmetastatic manifestation such as in hypertrophic pulmonary osteoarthropathy (Coombes 1982). Pain may also be caused by factors unrelated to cancer. One survey showed that pain was directly due to cancer, related to cancer treatment or unrelated to either in 77%, 19% and 3% of patients respectively (Foley 1979).

The percentage of patients with cancer pain varies according to the primary site of the tumour. Cancers involving bone or the oral cavity are often painful, whereas lymphomas and leukaemias tend to be less so (Foley 1979; Bonica 1980).

Surgery, radiotherapy, chemotherapy or hormone therapy are used separately or in combination in the treatment of cancer. The choice of treatment will depend on whether the therapeutic aim is curative or palliative, which in turn will be decided by a number of factors, including tumour site, histology, stage and the patient's clinical condition (both physical and emotional). Although therapies are developing which will target tumour cells specifically, most commonly used techniques will continue to result in a degree of damage to normal tissues with consequent side-effects.

This chapter briefly describes the development and delivery of radiotherapy, chemotherapy and hormone therapy. The mechanism of action, rationale for use and the painful conditions for which they may be effective are discussed with reference to possible side-effects.

RADIOTHERAPY

DEVELOPMENT

X-rays were discovered by Wilhelm Roentgen on 8 November 1895 at the University of Würzburg, and amazingly the first recorded use of ionising radiation for cancer took place on 29 January 1896. A Chicago instrument maker named Emil Grubbé used it to treat a patient referred to him with a breast cancer (Grubbé 1933).

The discovery of naturally occurring radioactivity was made on 1 March 1896 by Antoine-Henri Becquerel in Paris, who observed the effects of radiation emitted from uranium. It was two years later that Pierre and Marie Curie, together with M G Bemont, announced the discovery of the new element radium which was to become such an important radionuclide for cancer treatment (Curie et al 1898).

Radiotherapy has developed over the past century from these early beginnings. Initially, localised skin lesions could be readily treated with X-rays from a single conventional X-ray beam, but because of the physical limitations of the equipment it was difficult to achieve high doses to deep-seated tumours. Various 'cross-fire' techniques were employed, but the limiting factor was always that the highest dose from the beam of radiation fell on the skin and thereafter the dose decreased rapidly the greater the depth from the surface. The effect of this was relative overtreatment of the skin surface with subsequent and often serious side-effects and undertreatment of deep-seated tumours with inadequate arrest of tumour growth.

Before the 1940s so-called 'deep X-ray treatment' (DXT) represented the most powerful conventional X-rays from machines the most sophisticated of which operated at a maximum energy of 300 kV. External radiotherapy always produced dose-limiting DXT skin reactions until the introduction of the more powerful X-ray equipment in the 1940s which evolved into the linear accelerators of today. Almost simultaneously improvements in apparatus such as the radium bomb took place and external beam cobalt machines became available. These technical advances led to the megavoltage era which saw not only much higher radiation doses achieved at depth in the body, but also sparing of the skin from the previously limiting severe reactions. This 'skin-sparing' effect is a physical characteristic of high-voltage radiation (Lederman 1981).

The discovery of new radioisotopes also allowed the development of sealed sources for use in interstitial and intracavity localised treatments (^{192}Ir and ^{60}Co), and unsealed sources for the administration of radioactive material for systemic use (^{131}I, ^{32}P and ^{89}Sr).

When a high absorbed dose of radiation is required at the skin surface, but the underlying tissues must be spared, then a beam of electrons is more useful than superficial X-rays. Such electron beams can be readily produced by linear accelerators, and the sharp cut-off in dose at depth can be varied with the generating energy. Other forms of radiotherapy employing particles such as neutrons or protons are still experimental.

Finally, the use of total-body or hemibody external beam radiotherapy has been used both for radical and palliative treatments.

PRINCIPLES OF RADIOBIOLOGY

The biological effects of artificially produced X-rays or electrons are identical to those of naturally occurring γ-rays, provided that the variables of quality (penetrating power) and absorbed dose are taken into account.

The desired therapeutic aim of radiotherapy is achieved by tumour cell destruction with minimal destruction of normal tissues. Radiation may be considered as quanta or packets of energy which are deposited in tissue. The absorbed dose will depend on the type of tissue and the energy of the radiation. This absorbed energy causes a series of complex radiochemical events ending in 'free radical' formation. The free radicals are highly reactive abnormal ions that disrupt the nucleic acids of the cell nucleus. This disruption prevents or delays mitosis so that the cell is unable to repair itself.

In general, radiation damage to any cell becomes evident when it enters mitosis, and it follows that the response of a cell to radiotherapy will vary as a function of the speed of cell turnover or cell cycle time. Very rapidly dividing cells will show response quicker than slowly dividing cells. Furthermore, both normal tissues and tumours vary widely in their intrinsic response to radiation. For example, gut and central nervous tissue are radiosensitive (although they have very different cell cycle times) whereas uterus, bladder and retina are far more radioresistant (Strickland 1980). It is often the normal tissue radiosensitivity of adjacent organs that limits the dose of radiation which can be delivered to a tumour.

RADIOTHERAPY AS TREATMENT FOR PAIN

External beam radiotherapy, like surgery, is a localised or regional form of treatment and cannot be curative for disseminated disease. The choice of radical radiotherapy is determined by tumour operability, accessibility, clinical stage, histology, likely morbidity from the particular mode of treatment, intrinsic radiosensitivity, the tolerance of adjacent tissues and patient fitness. Radiotherapy may be used alone or in combination with surgery and/or chemotherapy.

Localised pain may be a presenting symptom of primary cancer and will usually be relieved by successful radical treatment. The overall role of radiotherapy in cancer treatment is beyond the scope of this chapter. It is discussed in detail in various standard texts (del Regato et al 1985; Souhami & Tobias 1986; DeVita et al 1989; Sikora & Halnan 1990) and review articles (Paine 1980; Drug and Therapeutics Bulletin 1981).

Pain due to bone infiltration

This is the most common form of cancer pain, usually due to metastatic involvement (discussed in detail in Ch. 43). The role of radiotherapy in the management of pain due to bone metastases is unquestioned, and this indication constitutes approximately 15% of the total number of patients referred to an average radiotherapy department (Bates 1987). The commonest primary tumours associated with bone metastases are those of breast, lung, prostate, thyroid, kidney and multiple myeloma (Allen et al 1976; Gilbert et al 1977).

Radiotherapy techniques vary widely – from a large dose given as a single treatment to as many as 20 smaller treatments given over 4 weeks. It must be borne in mind that the biological effect of the radiation depends not only on the total dose delivered but also on the number of separate treatments and the total time over which the course is given (dose–time factors). Standard palliative treatment has been 20 Gy in 5 fractions over 5 days for a small volume, but for larger volumes (such as a hemipelvic field, where there is closely related bowel) 30 Gy in 10 fractions over 12 days has been used (Ford & Yarnold 1983).

Some authors have advocated single palliative doses of 8–15 Gy (Vargha et al 1969; Jensen & Roesdahl 1976; Penn 1976) for speed of effect and to avoid repeated tiring attendances or the need for hospitalisation. Retrospective comparisons found single and multiple fraction courses of treatment to be equally effective (Ford & Yarnold 1983). A prospective randomised trial of a single 8 Gy fraction compared with 10 fractions of 3 Gy each showed equally effective palliation, even if the original bone pain had been severe. There was no advantage for multiple fractionation in terms of pain relief, speed of onset or limitation of gut toxicity (Price et al 1986). A further randomised trial indicated good palliation of pain when comparing 24 Gy in 6 fractions with a single dose of 8 Gy. 25% of patients in the single-fraction group required retreatment at some stage, but all subsequently responded (Cole 1989).

If the bone to be treated is superficial (e.g. ribs, scapula) then a single field using orthovoltage (300 kV) or ^{137}Cs gives a sufficient tumour dose without irradiating underlying tissues too heavily. However, more homogeneous treatment, irradiating for example a hip joint, can be achieved with a parallel opposed pair of megavoltage fields. Field size is a compromise. It should be generous, bearing in mind that a palliative dose (that is, less than maximum tolerance dose) will be given, and also that radiological evidence of a lytic deposit may considerably underestimate the extent of disease. However, it is also important to avoid treating larger volumes than necessary in order to minimise morbidity.

Administration of high dosage has been regarded as important by some radiotherapists. Patients with renal, breast and thyroid tumours may be expected to have a longer life expectancy than those with lung tumours, and the deposits may also be less radiosensitive. Higher total doses in such cases have therefore been advised. However, no dose–response relationship has so far been shown using single low- and high-dose fractions in comparative surveys (Vargha et al 1969; Jensen & Roesdahl 1976; Hoskin 1988). Earlier studies have not suggested that dose is important in determining the duration of pain relief (Allen et al 1976; Penn 1976; Hoskin 1988). Recently, however, a prospective study comparing single fractions of 4 Gy and 8 Gy has shown that the higher dose gives increased probability of pain relief (Hoskin et al 1992). It is also possible that where the tumour is amenable to systemic therapy as well as local measures, such as myeloma, the total dose may positively influence length of relief (Adamietz et al 1991). Apart from this study, there has been no demonstrable effect of histology of the primary on the effectiveness of pain relief.

In summary, conventional radiotherapy for metastatic bone pain is beneficial in the majority of patients, and this effect does not appear to be significantly influenced by dose–time relationships or histology. The proportion of patients achieving complete pain relief approaches 80% (Ford & Yarnold 1983; Bates 1989).

Special techniques

It is common for patients with widespread metastatic disease to present with multiple painful areas, usually due to bony but also visceral deposits. Wide-field or hemibody irradiation (HBI) was proposed in such patients who had received previous heavy conventional palliation (Saenger et al 1973), since low-dose, total-body irradiation had already been shown to be effective for haematological malignancies (Medinger & Craver 1942).

The main indications have been for widespread disease such as advanced-stage multiple myeloma, prostatic or breast carcinoma. There is also considerable interest in HBI as a systemic treatment for widespread non-Hodgkin's lymphoma or small-cell lung cancer which has failed to respond to chemotherapy.

Several authors reported prompt pain relief in up to 80% of patients with a variety of tumours, using HBI with 8 Gy in a single fraction (Rowland 1979; Qasim 1981; Salazar et al 1981). However, the cost in terms of acute radiation sickness (Danjoux et al 1979) and radiation pneumonitis (Fryer et al 1978) was high. If doses as high as 10 Gy to the upper hemibody were given, there was a 70% mortality from acute radiation pneumonitis by 100 days after irradiation.

When the upper hemibody dose was reduced to 6 Gy, this toxicity was avoided while maintaining a response rate in terms of pain relief as high as 82% (Wilkins & Keen 1987). A report from the Royal Marsden Hospital on 50 patients with metastatic myeloma or prostatic cancer replicated these findings with an overall response rate of 83%, but a complete response rate of only 5%. Pain relief was apparent within 24 hours in 25% of patients and lasted until death in 74% (Hoskin et al 1989). However, significant gastrointestinal or marrow toxicity occurred in 60% of patients.

Sequential upper and lower HBI, using doses of no more than 6 and 8 Gy respectively, is now becoming standard palliative treatment in many radiotherapy departments.

Widespread axial skeletal involvement in prostate cancer has been successfully treated with systemically administered radioactive ^{32}P. It was shown that testosterone increased the uptake of ^{32}P in normal bone by a factor of 2–3, and in tumour deposits by a factor of 20–30 (Hertz 1950). These early findings encouraged the use of

^{32}P with androgen priming. A recent report on 53 treatments shows a worthwhile response in terms of pain reduction and improved mobility in 87% of patients (Burnet et al 1990).

An alternative bone-seeking isotope is ^{89}Sr. A large series assessing the efficacy of strontium showed a response rate of 75% in patients with prostatic cancer (Robinson 1986). Strontium follows the biochemical pathways of calcium and is taken up preferentially by osteoblastic metastases compared with normal bone. It is less marrow depressant in therapeutic doses than ^{32}P. A recent multicentre study of 83 patients indicated benefit in 75% of patients with 27% becoming painfree at 6 weeks following a dose of 1.5 MBq/kg. This treatment may be repeated at not less than 3-monthly intervals (Laing et al 1991).

A retrospective comparison was undertaken between patients receiving HBI or ^{89}Sr (Dearnaley et al 1992). Pain control was assessed at 3 months and found to be similar for matched HBI and ^{89}Sr patients with 63% and 52% respectively showing benefit. Clinically significant falls in white blood cell and platelet counts were similar in both groups. Strontium had an advantage in its ease of administration and lack of gastrointestinal toxicity, but was more expensive.

The use of other bone-seeking isotopes has been investigated. Initial trials with $^{185}Re(Sn)HEDP$ (hydroxyethylidene diphosphonate) indicate prompt and significant improvements in quality of life in 80% of patients treated with a single intravenous injection. The speed and overall rate of response were similar to those reported after HBI. Minimal marrow toxicity was seen compared with ^{32}P and HBI, and tumour/marrow dose ratios were twice those for ^{89}Sr (Maxon 1991).

Differentiated carcinomas of the thyroid (both papillary and follicular) often spread to bone but may retain the ability of the parent tissue to take up iodine. These patients may experience bone pain, and they can be treated after surgical thyroid ablation by both external beam radiation and systemic ^{131}I. This treatment is given with curative intent, and bone pain is relieved as long as there is uptake. Usually 5.5 GBq ^{131}I is given by mouth every 6 months until no further uptake is detected. Side-effects are minimal (Beierwaltes 1986).

Pathological fracture through a bony metastasis may be both painful and disabling and, when possible, weight-bearing bones should be internally fixed (British Medical Journal Editorial 1981). This should be followed by postoperative radiotherapy because there is a real danger of continued tumour growth and further structural weakness is spite of fixation if radiation is withheld (Galasko 1980). If the patient is considered unsuitable for internal fixation because of a short prognosis, the advisability of radiotherapy should also be questioned. If more than 50% of the thickness of the cortex of a long bone is eroded by metastasis, prophylactic fixation rather than radiotherapy alone should be considered. With or without fixation, radiotherapy should not be withheld for fear of inhibiting bone healing and regrowth. There is good evidence that palliative doses of radiotherapy are associated with recalcification (Ford & Yarnold 1983).

Pain due to nerve infiltration and compression

Head and neck

Tumours of the head and neck frequently cause pain by nerve compression. The more common pain syndromes have been described by Foley (1979), Molinari (1979) and Portenoy (1992).

Nasopharyngeal cancer may cause the jugular foramen syndrome where there is occipital pain radiating to the vertex of the head and 9th–12th cranial nerve palsies, or the petrosphenoidal syndrome with frontal, supraorbital and maxillary pain associated with 2nd–4th cranial nerve dysfunction. Cancers of the tongue, tonsil and oropharynx may cause pain involving the 5th–10th cranial nerves and this often includes painful trismus. Cancers of the floor of the mouth cause lingual nerve infiltration and neuralgic pain, while cancers of the maxillary antrum cause pain due to maxillary nerve compression.

In addition to these presenting pain syndromes, head and neck cancers have a tendency to cause severe pain due to local mucosal involvement, bone necrosis and infection.

Radiotherapy (alone or in combination with surgery or chemotherapy) is the mainstay of radical treatment for head and neck cancers (Wang 1975). Even in relatively advanced disease, a case for 'radical palliation' with high-dose radiation can be made, as the pain from uncontrolled local tumour is likely to be far more distressing than the transient acute reaction associated with higher dose radiotherapy. Large total doses of the order of 55–65 Gy are required for growth control in squamous head and neck cancers.

Once a radical course of radiation has been given, it is rare that retreatment will be helpful because of the danger of pain from radionecrosis.

Intracranial tumour

This may be due to primary or secondary tumour. The site of involvement will determine the presenting symptoms and signs. Bulky supratentorial tumours or small deposits adjacent to the ventricles may obstruct the flow of cerebrospinal fluid (CSF), leading to symptoms and signs of raised intracranial pressure such as vomiting and headache.

Craniotomy and excision of tumour where accessible may relieve symptoms temporarily. Radiotherapy is often used where surgery is impossible, inappropriate or as an adjunct to surgery. Metastases are likely to be multiple and therefore palliative radiotherapy should normally include the whole brain. It is more likely to be successful if there has been an initial symptomatic response to high-dose dexamethasone (Ashby 1991).

A large collaborative study (Borgelt et al 1980) showed that 52% of patients with headache due to metastases obtained complete relief from radiotherapy. If partial relief was included, then the response rate rose to 82%. This study compared dose–time–fraction schedules and could find no difference in response between 20 Gy in five daily fractions and longer schedules such as 40 Gy in 20 daily fractions over 4 weeks. A shorter course provided quicker relief, was more convenient and cheaper. The results are awaited of a multicentre trial of 12 Gy in two fractions versus 30 Gy in 10 fractions (Royal College of Radiologists). Kramer et al (1977) showed that in up to 40% of patients irradiated, death was due not to brain metastases but to other manifestations of systemic malignancy. Whole-brain radiotherapy is usually well tolerated but always causes temporary epilation. It is advisable to continue corticosteroids (dexamethasone 12–16 mg/day) until after the end of radiotherapy.

It has been demonstrated that prophylactic cranial irradiation for small-cell lung cancer, may reduce the occurrence of cerebral metastases from 22% to 8%, although there is no survival advantage (Bleehan 1986).

Leptomeningeal infiltration by tumour may occur, particularly in breast cancer. Such 'carcinomatous meningitis' may be associated with severe pain in the head, back and limbs. The diagnosis is made by CSF examination, and treatment is with neuroaxis radiotherapy and intrathecal chemotherapy.

Spinal cord compression

Spinal cord compression may be due to collapse of a vertebral body or to pressure from extradural tumour within the spinal canal and prodromal pain is a feature in 96% of these patients (Gilbert et al 1978). In adults, spinal cord compression occurs most commonly with tumours arising from lung, breast, unknown primary site, lymphoma, multiple myeloma, sarcoma, prostate and kidney, in descending order of frequency (Bruckman & Bloomer 1978). The overall incidence in cancer patients is 3–5%, although the figure rises to 10% and 15% for prostatic cancer and multiple myeloma respectively. Thoracic cord compression is the commonest area (70%) and the incidence of multiple extradural sites may be as high as 18% (Kramer 1992).

The treatment of spinal cord compression remains controversial. Corticosteroids are used empirically, based on the assumption of oedema of the cord. Traditionally dexamethasone 16 mg daily is used, although doses as high as 100 mg daily have been advocated in some centres (Posner 1987). The response is short-lived and probably dose-dependent. Definitive treatment with surgery or radiotherapy should therefore be considered.

Gilbert et al (1978) advocated the use of primary radiotherapy and high-dose dexamethasone following localisation of the level of compression by myelography, irrespective of the histology of the tumour. However, others believe that emergency surgical decompression followed by postoperative radiation offers the best chance of reversing incipient paraplegia in all but the most radiosensitive tumours (Benson et al 1979). When myelography demonstrates a complete block in CSF flow, radiotherapy alone is unlikely to result in neurological improvement (Tomita et al 1983). No comparative trials have been conducted between surgical decompression and radiotherapy versus radiotherapy alone. However, the advent of techniques of anterior decompression with spinal stabilisation would seem to favour the surgical approach, provided that the patient is fit enough initially (Kornblith & Cassady 1985; Closs & Bates 1987). Radicular pain associated with spinal cord compression may not necessarily be relieved by definitive oncological treatment as irritation may persist where the nerve root exits from the intervertebral foramen. Sometimes the symptom of local back pain disappears despite increasing motor deficit. This is due to the evolving sensory component of the paraplegia.

Nerve plexus compression

Brachial, lumbar and sacral nerve plexus compression give rise to characteristic pain syndromes. The compression may be due to a variety of primary tumours including breast, head and neck, gastrointestinal, genitourinary, soft-tissue sarcomas and lymphomas. If radiotherapy can induce tumour shrinkage, the pain will be relieved, but not all these tumours are radiosensitive, and palliative radiation particularly of lumbar nerve roots may involve irradiating gut.

A further problem arises if radiation has been used before, e.g. prophylactic cervicoaxillary treatment in breast cancer. It may then be difficult to differentiate radiation-induced peripheral neuropathy (Stoll & Andrews 1966) from recurrent tumour. Some patients may be helped by pelvic radiation for the pain of recurrent colorectal cancer but this will not be as rewarding as relieving bony pain, and patient selection is more difficult (Bates 1984).

Pain due to soft-tissue and hollow-viscus invasion

Pain from tumour invasion of soft tissues may occur in various ways. Skin is an effective barrier to infection, and if this is broken by tumour, then pain may be produced by consequent ulceration or fungation. A classic example of this is a locally advanced breast cancer eroding the chest wall. As well as being painful, this may be both psychologically distressing and malodorous.

Successful palliative treatment must be individualised and may include radiotherapy, chemotherapy, hormone therapy and even limited toilet surgery, alone or in combination. Unless the prognosis is very poor, local disease control should always be a priority. Opposed radiation fields applied tangentially across the breast will control the tumour and allow reepithelialisation in most cases. The dose and fractionation will depend on the presence or absence of distant disease and fitness of the patient. If the patient has only a few months to live, 35 Gy in six fractions over 18 days is a well-tolerated regimen (Bates 1984), and Stoll (1964) has sucessfully used 10 Gy on each of 2 consecutive days.

Hepatic invasion by secondary tumour is a common cause of right hypochondrial pain, often radiating to the back and shoulder tip. The mechanism may be stretching of nerve endings in the liver capsule, diaphragmatic irritation or haemorrhage into a necrotic area of tumour. Liver pain can often be controlled by conventional titration of appropriate analgesics against the pain or with corticosteroids.

Whole liver palliative radiotherapy can also be useful in carefully selected patients with refractory pain, with far fewer side-effects than the alternatives of intraarterial chemotherapy or hepatic artery embolisation. In a series reported by Borgelt et al (1981), abdominal pain was improved by hepatic irradiation in over half the patients with little toxicity. Doses should not exceed 30 Gy in 15 daily fractions or its equivalent if radiation hepatitis is to be avoided.

Malignant mesothelioma arising from the pleura frequently causes severe chest-wall pain. Although mesothelioma is usually considered to be radioresistant, short-lived pain relief can be obtained with doses of 30 Gy in 10 fractions to the hemithorax involved with minimal toxicity (Bissett et al 1991).

Invasion and compression of major blood vessels by tumour may cause pain. Superior vena caval obstruction (SVCO) is often caused by bronchial tumours producing the distressing syndrome of upper limb and head oedema, associated with pain and dyspnoea. If SVCO is rapid, radiation should be given as a matter of urgency, together with high doses of corticosteroids.

Advanced tumours of the cervix, bladder, bowel or bronchus may invade neighbouring hollow viscera. Under these circumstances, palliative radiotherapy should be used with caution as there is a significant risk of precipitating fistula formation between two hollow viscera (e.g. rectovaginal, vesicovaginal or bronchooesophageal fistulae). Rather than palliating existing symptoms, a fistula thus formed will cause further problems.

Radiotherapy for benign painful conditions

As ionising radiation has been implicated in leukaemogenesis and carcinogenesis (Duncan & Nias 1977), radiotherapy for benign conditions is strictly limited. However, there are still a few rare clinical indications for its use.

For many years, pain due to ankylosing spondylitis was relieved by low-dose X-rays in a variable number of patients, depending on whether their disease was in limb joints or spine. However, since the classical study of Court-Brown & Doll (1965) showing a greatly increased risk of leukaemia in irradiated ankylosing spondylitic patients, radiotherapy is now restricted to severe inflammation refractory to any other treatment (Hickling & Wright 1982).

Intraarticular injection of the β-emitter ^{90}Y has been used for the relief of pain in rheumatoid arthritis, and it is also effective in reducing joint swelling and increasing mobility (Bridgman et al 1973). However, a clinical trial comparing the effectiveness of ^{90}Y with that of intraarticular triamcinalone hexacetamide was inconclusive.

The use of total lymphoid irradiation (TLI) for active rheumatoid arthritis has been investigated and the results are encouraging. The variables of dose and technique have been studied by groups at Stanford and Harvard, USA. At present, TLI seems safe and effective in reducing disease activity, morning stiffness and joint tenderness and in improving global well-being. However, further long-term prospective studies are required before it becomes standard treatment (Calin 1985).

Primary proliferative polycythaemia may be present with headache and epigastic pain due to the associated peptic ulceration. Treatment of choice is with the β-emitter ^{32}P. A dose of 180 MBq intravenously will produce complete clinical and haematological remission in 85% of patients (Szur et al 1959) and a partial response in a further 12% of cases.

Aneurysmal bone cysts usually present with pain and swelling (Ruiter et al 1977). They often occur in the second and third decades and may be confused with giant-cell tumour pathologically. Treatment is generally surgical, but recurrence depends on how radical the curettage has been (Ruiter et al 1977). Recurrence rates of approximately 30% can be reduced by postoperative radiotherapy (Nobler et al 1968).

Giant-cell tumour of bone (formerly called osteoclastoma) commonly presents with a painful swelling of a long bone in a young adult. Females are affected more often than males (Dahlin et al 1970). These tumours recur locally in 40–75% of cases after incomplete surgical excision (Dahlin et al 1970; Goldenberg et al 1970) and up to one-quarter of all giant-cell tumours will behave in a frankly malignant fashion not easily predicted from the histological features (Ashley 1978). Radiotherapy is effective as a local treatment (Bradshaw 1964) and is the treatment of choice if surgery would be incomplete or produce dysfunction (del Regato et al 1985).

Langerhans' cell histiocytosis includes a spectrum of disorders of children of the mononuclear phagocytic system which may range from localised eosinophilic granuloma to the generalised Letterer-Siwe disease (Nesbit 1986). A painful bony lesion is a common feature, particularly of the more benign members of this group of diseases. Some of these lesions will resolve spontaneously, some can be effectively curetted, but others may recur or be inaccessible. Low-dose radiotherapy (1–6 Gy) is successful in controlling these painful areas in 95% of cases (Smith et al 1973; Greenberger et al 1979). In the systemic disease, chemotherapy will also be indicated.

SIDE-EFFECTS OF RADIOTHERAPY

Side-effects of radiotherapy are due to unavoidable irradiation of normal tissues. Radiation side-effects are all dose-dependent and therefore assume most importance in relation to radical treatment. When palliative doses are used toxicity should be minimal.

The cell kinetic characteristics of tissues determine whether the effects are immediate or delayed. Thus, normal gut has a rapid cell turnover and toxicity appears immediately, as nausea, vomiting, abdominal colic, diarrhoea or tenesmus. Irradiation of the mouth or throat will cause a similar acute mucositis. These acute radiation reactions are self-limiting, lasting from 1–2 days to 2 weeks. Other sites that will show an acute reaction are the bladder and the skin, particularly moist skin creases.

Bone marrow is very radiosensitive but this is only of significance if the fields employed include a large volume of red marrow or the patient has little marrow reserve, perhaps because of replacement by tumour or suppression by previous chemotherapy. Sequential HBI can usually be tolerated from a haematological point of view, provided that at least a 6-week gap is allowed between treatments to the two halves of the body.

Lung toxicity is a problem if doses in excess of 20 Gy in 10 fractions are given to the whole of both lungs, when a potentially fatal radiation pneumonitis may result. This lung toxicity is rarely seen with palliative treatments for bronchial and mediastinal tumours as normal lung can always be spared by selection of suitable radiation fields. However, if the fields are very large or the dose applied is high, then a self-limiting pneumonitis occurs. Symptoms of cough present a few weeks following radiation and symptomatic relief may be obtained with a short course of corticosteroids.

Radiation nephritis is a possibility if doses of 20 Gy in 10 fractions to the kidneys are exceeded. Both ovary and testis are relatively radiosensitive and even stray dosage to the gonads may cause sterility. Dosage of 10 Gy to the whole pelvis in two fractions is an adequate method of inducing amenorrhoea in women approaching the menopause but this dose may be tolerated by the cells of younger ovaries. Testicular irradiation to moderate dosage does not affect secondary sexual characteristics or potency even though spermatogenesis is abolished. Radiation hepatitis is seen when doses exceed 30 Gy to the whole liver in 3 weeks.

Delayed toxicity can be seen if brain or spinal cord are irradiated to doses above 40 and 50 Gy respectively, given in daily 2 Gy fractions. The clinical effects in the brain of high-dosage irradiation may mimic recurrent tumour and the true cause may only be found at autopsy. Radiation myelopathy causes the clinical syndrome of cord transection. As mentioned above, peripheral nerves may be damaged following high-dose radiation producing, for example, a brachial plexus syndrome (Stoll & Andrews 1966). The lens of the eye may become opaque 12 months or more after doses as low as 2 Gy. Complications of radiotherapy are more fully reviewed by Strickland (1980).

In summary, radiotherapy may cause considerable toxicity, some of which will be permanent if high doses are used and normal-tissue tolerance is not respected. However, if radiotherapy is prescribed skilfully, palliative treatment for pain should almost never cause lasting significant side-effects.

CHEMOTHERAPY

Cytotoxic chemotherapy drugs are conventionally divided into five classes depending on their biochemical characteristics: alkylating agents, antimetabolites, plant alkaloids, antimitotic antibiotics and miscellaneous other compounds. A variety of hormones have cytotoxic or cytostatic activity. The use of hormonal manipulation as an antitumour technique for pain control will be considered separately.

DEVELOPMENT

It had been noted during the First World War that survivors from mustard-gas poisoning had low white-cell counts (Stewart 1918), but it was not until the early 1940s that any medical application for this leucopaenic effect was realised. The beginning of cancer chemotherapy was the use of the alkylating agent mustine hydrochloride for leukaemias and lymphomas (Goodman et al 1946; Rhoads 1946). A variety of other alkylating agents were discovered to have clinical usefulness during the 1950s, including cyclophosphamide, melphalan, chlorambucil, busulphan and thiotepa (Shay et al 1953).

The discovery of the importance of nucleic acid synthesis in cell division stimulated the investigation of antimetabolites. The folate antagonist methotrexate (Farber et al 1948) was the first antimetabolite found to be useful clinically. The development of the purine and pyrimidine antagonists (6-mercaptopurine and 5-fluorouracil) paralleled the elucidation of the structure of DNA. Both methotrexate and some of the later alkylating agents were found to have activity against solid tumours as well as in haematological malignancies.

In 1963 plant extracts from the periwinkle (*Vinca rosea*) were found to have antimitotic activity (Johnson et al 1963). All three members of this group, the vinca alkaloids, have neurotoxic effects, but nevertheless have a wide spectrum of clinical usefulness. More recently, derivatives of podophyllin, extracted from the mandrake or May apple plant, have been found to be active. This group includes etoposide (VP16–213) (Arnold 1979).

As in antimicrobial chemotherapy, antibiotics produced by micro-organisms were found to be clinically useful for cancer. Various *Streptomyces* species produce such cytotoxics as actinomycin (Pinkel 1959), mitomycin and doxorubicin (Bonadonna et al 1969). These drugs have increased the treatment options in various sarcomas, germ-cell tumours, and gastrointestinal and breast cancers.

Various other agents have been discovered over the past 35 years which do not fit into any particular chemical classification. These include dacarbazine, mitozantrone, the platinum complexes, cisplatin and carboplatin, and the monoamine-oxidase inhibitor procarbazine. By 1970 nearly 100 000 new compounds had been investigated but less than 30 had proved useful (Bodley Scott 1970). This was usually because of widespread toxicity.

MECHANISM OF ACTION

All cytotoxic drugs interfere with cell division, some by disturbing mitotic spindle formation, some by cross-linkage of DNA or RNA, some by specific enzyme inhibition and some by several actions simultaneously at different sites in the cell. The exact mode of action varies with each drug and for some it is not yet fully elucidated. This variation is reflected in different patterns of normal tissue toxicity. The effects of chemotherapy, like radiotherapy, are not specific to tumour cells so that all cytotoxic drugs have some dose-limiting normal-tissue toxicity. A list of commonly used drugs, classification and limiting toxicities is given in Table 70.1.

Most cytotoxic drugs are administered directly into the circulation, although some are absorbed well enough by the gut to be taken orally. Anticancer chemotherapy is therefore systemic treatment. However, only a few agents (e.g. lomustine, carmustine and vincristine) cross the blood–brain barrier in sufficient quantities to be useful.

Table 70.1 Commonly used cytotoxic drugs and limiting toxicities

Class	Drug	Toxicity
Alkylating agents	Mustine	Marrow, gut
	Cyclophosphamide	Marrow, gut, bladder, alopecia
	Ifosfamide	Marrow, gut, bladder, alopecia
	Melphalan	Marrow, gut
	Chlorambucil	Marrow, skin
	Busulphan	Marrow, lung fibrosis
	Lomustine	Marrow, gut
	Carmustine	Marrow, gut
	Treosulfan	Marrow
	Thiotepa	Marrow
Antimetabolites	Methotrexate	Marrow, gut
	Fluorouracil	Marrow, gut
	Cytarabine	Marrow
Plant alkaloids	Vincristine	Neuropathy
	Vinblastine	Neuropathy, marrow
	Vindesine	Neuropathy, marrow
	Etoposide	Marrow, gut, alopecia
Antimitotic antibiotics	Actinomycin	Marrow, gut, alopecia
	Mitomycin	Marrow, gut, kidney, lung
	Doxorubicin (Adriamycin)	Marrow, gut, heart, alopecia
	Bleomycin	Gut, skin, lung fibrosis
	Mithramycin	Marrow, gut, kidney, liver
Miscellaneous	Procarbazine	Marrow, gut
	Cisplatin	Marrow, gut, kidney, neuropathy
	Carboplatin	Marrow
	Dacarbazine	Gut, photosensitivity, marrow
	Mitozantrone	Marrow, heart

Because of this effect, late 'sanctuary site' relapse can occur in the central nervous system. In acute lymphoblastic leukaemia of childhood this can be reduced by a combination of intrathecal methotrexate and cranial irradiation (Medical Research Council 1973).

CHEMOTHERAPY AS TREATMENT FOR PAIN

Different tumour types vary in their response rates to chemotherapy. Conventionally, a complete response represents total disappearance of all observable disease for a variable length of time (usually 1–3 months depending on the trial criteria). A partial response represents a decrease in measurable tumour size of 50% or more. It would seem likely that a drug showing a good objective response rate for any given tumour would be useful for pain relief. Table 70.2 lists approximate response rates to various drug combinations in advanced solid tumours.

However, a patient may experience pain relief (and therefore good palliation) without showing objective tumour response. Pain relief has always been notoriously difficult to quantify, although two notable attempts have been made to standardise improvements in a patient's quality of life. These are changes in performance status or Karnofsky index (Karnofsky & Burchenal 1949), and

Table 70.2 Approximate response rates of some solid tumours to various combined cytotoxic drugs

Tumour	% CR	% CR + PR
Hodgkin's disease	70–80	85–95
Non-Hodgkin's lymphoma	50–70	60–90
Testis	70–80	85–95
Ovary	20–30	50–70
Breast	10–20	50–80
Lung (small cell)	30–60	60–85
(non-small cell)	15–20	30–50
Head and neck squamous carcinoma	25–60	60–95
Gastrointestinal	10–40	40–70
Uterine corpus	10	10–20
Uterine cervix	10–15	50–70
Oesophagus	10	20
Malignant melanoma	10–20	30–40

CR = complete response; PR = partial response

more recently the application of linear analogue techniques to chemotherapy assessment by Priestman & Baum (1976). While quality of life is now rightly regarded as an important parameter in cancer therapy assessment (Fallowfield 1990), Brewin (1986) has emphasised the complexity of its measurement.

Although pain relief may be one of the most important aspects of response to treatment as far as the patient is concerned, most investigators have sought to use other criteria of response such as measurable regression of soft-tissue masses or recalcification of lytic bone deposits. Comparison of results is complicated by the lack of standardisation of even the objective criteria of response.

The mechanism of pain production has already been discussed. If there are multiple painful areas of tumour, systemic treatment is theoretically more promising than local palliative radiotherapy. However, only some tumours show consistent chemosensitivity and, as Table 70.2 indicates, many of the common cancers show very limited response. The concept of treatment being radical/curative, as opposed to palliative, is as important with chemotherapy as with radiotherapy. A reasonable expectation of cure with chemotherapy is at present only found in a few tumours such as some leukaemias, lymphomas, choriocarcinoma, testicular cancers and some childhood tumours. In most other tumours the results of chemotherapy are purely palliative, and this implies that symptomatic benefit must be balanced against toxicity. Curative chemotherapy is beyond the scope of this chapter and the reader is directed to standard texts for further information (DeVita et al 1985; Priestman 1989; Sikora & Halnan 1990).

Breast cancer

This is a common disease that shows some degree of chemoresponsiveness. Single-agent studies suggest that cyclophosphamide, fluorouracil and doxorubicin give objective response rates of 12–50% (Nemoto & Dao 1971; Hoogstraten 1975; Rubens et al 1975). Objective response in bone metastases is less than in soft-tissue disease, but the only report which specifically noted bone-pain relief (Hoogstraten 1975) did so in as many as 50% of patients. This would suggest that response in bone may be as likely as in other tissues but is harder to measure objectively (e.g. by radiological recalcification) (Russell 1983). Newer cytotoxics have been developed, such as epirubicin and mitozantrone, which are less cardiotoxic than doxorubicin, and cause less alopecia.

Combination chemotherapy will produce objective remission rates (50–80%) that are usually better than those obtained with single agents. Pain relief is reported in a similar proportion of patients (40–94%) (Smalley et al 1977; Muss et al 1978; Salmon & Jones 1979). No particular combination of agents emerges as the best, and the median duration of response is between 8 and 10 months (Henderson & Canellos 1980). Although a patient may respond to palliative chemotherapy, it is doubtful whether survival is increased (Powles et al 1980). This would imply that at present routine chemotherapy should only be given to palliate symptoms.

Multiple myeloma

This disease can be one of the most painful of all malignancies because of frequent widespread bone involvement. Standard chemotherapy with melphalan and prednisolone will give a 60% response rate, but complete clearance of myeloma to the point at which it is undetectable by bone-marrow examination or serum protein electrophoresis is uncommon, occurring in less than 10% of patients (Scarffe 1982). Recent treatment using vincristine, doxorubicin and methylprenisolone (VAMP), followed by high-dose melphalan with autologous bone-marrow rescue, has given an overall response rate of 74% with 50% achieving complete haematological and biochemical remission (Gore et al 1989). Although these results are impressive, this regime is potentially very toxic.

Radiotherapy given to local painful areas is often useful. HBI is effective but may be contraindicated if there is insufficient marrow reserve.

Lymphomas

When high-grade lymphoma is disseminated, chemotherapy is usually indicated as radical treatment. Not all patients will be cured, however, and recurrent disease may well produce pain. In such cases, useful palliation, or even a limited complete response, may be obtained with second-line chemotherapy. However, this is usually more toxic than standard chemotherapy and the patient may have only limited bone-marrow reserve. Palliative treatment has therefore to be selected on an individual basis, and because of previous toxic chemotherapy or radiotherapy it may be better to rely on nononcological methods of analgesia. Palliative single-agent chemotherapy (such as chlorambucil) may be useful in symptom control for disseminated low-grade non-Hodgkin lymphoma.

Lung cancer

In the last few years considerable changes have taken place in the treatment of small-cell lung cancer. Combination chemotherapy has produced complete response rates in limited and extensive disease of 70 and 25% respectively (Arnold & Williams 1979). Similar results have been obtained with various combinations of drugs giving up to 90% overall response rates (Souhami & Tobias 1986). Although pain relief is not assessed, it is a common experience of oncologists treating these patients that while they are in complete remission, they have complete symptomatic relief. Drugs used include cyclophosphamide, vincristine, methotrexate, doxorubicin, etoposide, cisplatin, procarbazine and lomustine. Although many patients relapse, a few have maintained disease-free survival which is much longer than the median survival of untreated patients. Chemotherapy would therefore appear to be, at the least, good palliative treatment, and when combined with other modalities it may even be curative.

Chemotherapy for non-small-cell lung cancer is disappointing. Few complete responses are obtained even with highly toxic combinations, and median survival is not improved. Palliative chemotherapy for pain in these patients is not successful.

Testicular tumours

Over the past 20 years the prognosis of disseminated testicular teratoma has improved considerably due to the use of effective combination chemotherapy. One of the most active combinations was proposed by Einhorn & Donohue (1977). This regimen of cisplatin, vinblastine and bleomycin gives complete response rates of over 70%, of which two-thirds will be cures. Toxicity is considerable; indeed most series include a small percentage of deaths due to treatment complications rather than disease. There is no information available as to pain relief from this regime.

Ovarian tumours

These tumours will respond to a variety of drugs but single agents or combinations often cause toxicity. Recent reports give response rates of 50–60% for combination regimes with cisplatin and carboplatin, toxicity being less with carboplatin (Cancer Topics 1992). A frequent symptom in advanced disease is abdominal distension and pain due to ascites. This may be controlled for a time by chemotherapy. Although single agents such as chlorambucil, thiotepa or melphalan will result in lower response rates than combinations, they may, nevertheless, be more appropriate for elderly and frail patients.

Special techniques

Intraarterial chemotherapy has been claimed to give good pain relief in certain situations; fluorouracil and methotrexate have mainly been used. One report quotes 60% symptomatic improvement following intraarterial fluorouracil for hepatocellular carcinoma (Cady & Oberfield 1974). Intraarterial methotrexate has also been claimed to be effective for pain due to advanced head and neck tumours (Bonadonna & Molinari 1979). However, this technique is complicated to perform, and morbidity (usually thrombosis) is high. It has not been widely adopted.

Isolated limb perfusion by cytotoxic agents with or without heating of the perfusate is reported to give good palliation without systemic toxicity in the case of melanomas of the extremities (del Regato et al 1985).

Hyperthermia applied both locally and as whole-body therapy has been investigated, as it has a cytotoxic effect which differs in mechanism from that of radiotherapy or chemotherapy. In theory, pain due to widespread metastases could be palliated usefully by whole-body hyperthermia combined with chemotherapy. In practice, the procedure requires lengthy general anaesthesia and is hazardous. Further development and evaluation are required before it can be recommended (Stewart 1985).

SIDE-EFFECTS OF CHEMOTHERAPY

Like radiotherapy, chemotherapy affects normal tissue as well as tumour cells. Toxicity may be negligible or considerable depending on drug type, regime and dosage. Immediate effects include anaphylaxis (rarely) and cardiac arrhythmias. If there is extravasation of drug during intravenous injection, this may produce local pain which may develop into tissue necrosis.

Early toxic effects occur a few hours after administration, and include nausea, vomiting, diarrhoea, fever, 'flu-like syndrome and hypersensitivity skin reactions. Intermediate effects occurring after a few days include marrow depression, stomatitis, alopecia, constipation (due to ileus), renal failure and immunosuppression. Late effects occur after some months and may only become apparent years afterwards if the patient survives. These include congestive cardiomyopathy, lung fibrosis, renal and hepatic impairment, amenorrhoea and sterility, carcinogenesis, depression and other psychological effects of prolonged chemotherapy.

The use of chemotherapy is still a comparatively young discipline. The potential toxicity is great and the palliative benefits in many instances are uncertain. New drugs, combinations and schedules being developed must be explored for the benefit of all, but this must be balanced against the possible toxicity for the individual patient. This toxicity may be difficult to evaluate for the doctor giving the treatment, as the patient may fail to communicate and the doctor fail to appreciate reported problems. This is especially the case with nonphysical symptoms (Coates 1986). Some oncologists have found patient self-assessment linear analogue scales useful in balancing this cost–benefit equation.

HORMONE THERAPY

DESCRIPTION AND RATIONALE

Beatson (1896) first suggested hormone therapy in the form of oophorectomy for patients with advanced breast cancer, while Huggins & Hodges (1941) first noted the effect of exogenous oestrogen administration on prostatic carcinoma. Since then, several other tumours have been shown to respond to changes in the hormonal environment of the individual. These changes or manipulations may be achieved either by ablating endocrine glands or by the administration of exogenous hormones or hormone antagonists. Table 70.3 lists various tumours which may respond to hormone therapy.

Hormone ablation may be surgical, as with oophorectomy, adrenalectomy and hypophysectomy, but artificial menopause may also be induced by irradiating the ovaries, while high doses of radioactive ^{90}Y have been used to ablate the pituitary. 'Medical adrenalectomy' is possible by using aromatase inhibitors, such as aminoglutethimide, which block corticosteroid synthesis.

Table 70.3 Tumours which may respond to hormone therapy

Primary tumour	Hormone manipulation
Breast carcinoma	Oestrogens
	Androgens
	Antioestrogens
	Progestogens
	Aromatase inhibitors
	GnRH analogues
	Corticosteroids
	Oophorectomy
	Adrenalectomy
	Hypophysectomy
Prostatic carcinoma	Orchidectomy
	GnRH analogues
	Oestrogens
	Antiandrogens
	Hypophysectomy
	Aminoglutethimide
	Corticosteroids
Endometrial carcinoma	Progestogens
Renal carcinoma	Progestogens
Ovarian carcinoma	GnRH analogues
	Progestogens
Thyroid carcinoma	Thyroxine
Lymphomas and leukaemias	Corticosteroids

Hormone additive therapy is mainly by the administration of oestrogens, progestogens, androgens, antioestrogens, corticosteroids and thyroid hormone. The doses used (excepting antioestrogens) generally produce plasma levels that are substantially higher than physiological levels, and such hormone changes may cause complex endocrine effects, such as pituitary inhibition of luteinising hormone (LH), follicle-stimulating hormone (FSH) and prolactin, as well as changes in endogenous corticosteroid hormone production (Powles et al 1982).

The rationale for hormone therapy in cancer is mainly empirical. Many normal cells are under hormonal control, particularly those of the breast, prostate and endometrium. Steroid hormones exert their influence largely by combining to nuclear receptors. The resulting hormone receptor complex interacts with specific target genes. This association with 'promotor enhancer' regions in the genome results in activation of transcription and altered mRNA production. Some tumour tissues, particularly the better differentiated ones, retain these hormone receptors and it is our ability to measure concentrations of these oestrogen and progestogen receptors in tumour tissue that has greatly improved the prediction of hormone response (Leake 1981).

HORMONE THERAPY AS TREATMENT FOR PAIN

As with radiotherapy and chemotherapy, assessment of pain relief as a measure of response to hormone therapy has usually been avoided and most investigators have sought to use objective criteria for response. Those writers who have assessed pain relief by hormone therapy have rarely attempted to quantify that relief.

Breast cancer

The objective response rate to any hormone manipulation in advanced breast cancer rarely exceeds 30–40% in unselected series (Stoll 1969). In the past, high doses of oestrogen were given to postmenopausal patients, and oestrogen deprivation by means of oophorectomy or ovarian irradiation was used for premenopausal women. Objective response rates for bone metastases to hormone therapy tend to be lower than for soft-tissue disease, although pain relief may be very prompt after bilateral oophorectomy (Stoll 1983). Similarly, bilateral adrenalectomy may give relief from bone pain within 1–2 days of operation, being most useful in patients who have relapsed after remission with oophorectomy (Kiang 1981). However, pain relief may occur in the absence of subsequent bone recalcification and it is possible that the subjective benefit may be due to replacement corticosteroid therapy used after adrenalectomy.

If pain is due predominantly to bone metastases, androgen therapy with intramuscular testosterone or oral fluoxymesterone will give relief in up to 80% of patients, although objective response is seen in only about 20% (Stoll 1969). Patients generally have an improved sense of well-being with androgens which is not seen with oestrogens, but there is usually some degree of androgenic virilisation.

The antioestrogen tamoxifen has fewer side-effects than other additive hormone manipulations, and it has been shown to be as effective. It is therefore the drug of first choice. It acts by competition with oestrogen for oestrogen receptors (ER), but may occasionallv show intrinsic oestrogenic activity resulting in transient tumour stimulation. The overall objective response rate is 25–30% in unselected patients but up to 60% in ER-positive patients. Following relapse after an initial response, a withdrawal response may be seen in 20% of patients (Canney et al 1987). Tamoxifen can be used in premenopausal patients as an alternative to surgical ablation. Other methods of additive hormone therapy (androgens, corticosteroids, progestogens, aminoglutethimide plus hydrocortisone) may give better bone-pain relief because they have additional mechanisms of action over and above oestrogen receptor depletion (Stoll 1983).

Progestogen therapy was initially given in the form of high-dose injectable medroxyprogesterone acetate (MPA). Pannuti et al (1979) reported pain relief in over 90% of patients with predominantly bone metastases, although only 50% had objective evidence of tumour response. In view of the corticosteroid side-effects reported from these large doses of MPA, it seems possible that much of the subjective response is due to nonspecific steroid action. Recently lower oral doses of MPA (500 mg/day) or megestrol acetate (160 mg/day) have been just as effective with much less toxicity (Gallagher et al 1987).

Aminoglutethimide acts as a competitive inhibitor of aromatase in the steroid synthetic pathway. It is as effective as adrenalectomy as second-line therapy but without the need for major surgery. Hydrocortisone replacement is usually needed unless doses are reduced to 250 mg daily, when aromatase inhibition is confined to peripheral tissues and not the adrenals. This low-dose regime may, however, be as effective as conventional higher doses and be particularly useful when additional steroids are undesirable (Stuart-Harris et al 1984).

4-Hydroxy-androstenedione is a synthetic analogue of the oestrogen precursor androstenedione, acting as a competitive substrate for the aromatase enzyme. Hydrocortisone replacement is not required and it appears to be as effective as aminoglutethimide and less toxic (Brodie et al 1988).

A recent medical alternative to oophorectomy or hypophysectomy is the use of the gonadotrophin-releasing hormone (GnRH) analogues, such as goserelin. This is given as a monthly subcutaneous depot injection, and it may be useful after tamoxifen has failed.

Corticosteroid therapy gives a rather low objective response rate of 14% (Minton et al 1981) when doses of prednisolone 15 mg/day are given. However, patients also experience a sense of well-being, increase in appetite and strength and subjective pain relief. Massive-dose parenteral methylprednisolone has been claimed to give rapid pain relief in over 60% of advanced cancer patients (Cappelaere & Adenis 1977).

Prostatic carcinoma

Widespread bony metastases causing multifocal pain are often seen in patients with advanced prostatic carcinoma. A variety of additive or ablative hormone manipulations have been employed, including oestrogen, antiandrogen (cyproterone, flutamide), oestrogen-mustine complex (estramustine), progestogens, aminoglutethimide, GnRH analogues, orchidectomy, adrenalectomy and hypophysectomy.

Pain relief in collected series has been estimated as between 35% (Stoll 1981) and 70% (Pannuti et al 1979). The differences may be due to selection of patients and problems in pain measurement. Well-differentiated prostatic carcinoma is more likely to respond to hormones than is poorly differentiated carcinoma. Manipulations that include replacement corticosteroid therapy or have additional corticoid effects (high-dose MPA) seem to give higher response rates.

Endometrial carcinoma

Progestogens were initially introduced for the treatment of endometrial cancer because of experimental evidence that they opposed the tumour-promoting effect of oestrogens. MPA 100 mg tds. orally will yield approximately a 30% objective response rate (Ehrlich & Young 1981), while subjective improvement is seen in up to 70% of patients (Pannuti et al 1979). Well-differentiated tumours are most likely to show objective evidence of response.

Renal carcinoma

Androgens and progestogens in various doses have been used for the treatment of disseminated renal carcinoma. Objective response is said to be seen in over 20% of patients, more often in men than in women (Bloom 1971), but most authors find objective response to be rare. Subjective response including pain relief has been reported, mainly with progestogen therapy, in up to 50% of patients (van der Werf-Messing & van Gilse 1971; Pannuti et al 1979).

Ovarian carcinoma

In spite of the presence of steroid receptors in ovarian carcinoma, little objective response to hormones has been demonstrated, apart from a recent report on the use of the GnRH analogue, Decapeptyl. Parmar et al (1988) have shown a 26% response rate occurring more reliably in the elderly. Subjective response is obtained in some patients with progestogen therapy but no information is available concerning pain relief (Kohorn 1981).

Thyroid carcinoma

Well-differentiated papillary thyroid carcinomas (found typically in women below the age of 40) are likely to be dependent on thyroid-stimulating hormone (TSH). Pituitary TSH secretion can be suppressed by thyroxine administration. Over 50% of this subgroup of thyroid cancers will respond objectively (Crile 1981).

Corticosteroids

As well as having nonspecific euphoric, appetite-stimulating and antiinflammatory effects, corticosteroids have direct antitumour activity in lymphomas and leukaemias (Lister & Malpas 1981). This has been exploited in the many successful chemotherapy regimes for this group of cancers. Corticosteroids are also used for the palliation of pain, particularly that due to bone deposits.

SIDE-EFFECTS OF HORMONE THERAPY

Compared with chemotherapy, hormone therapy is generally much better tolerated. In particular marrow suppression does not occur, and indeed peripheral blood counts tend to improve on hormone therapy. Corticosteroids and high-dose MPA, if given for long periods, are associated with classical Cushingoid side-effects, including peptic ulceration, osteoporosis, neuropathy and myopathy (Fischer 1984). Parenteral MPA is also associated with various local complications, such as gluteal abscess, in 18% of patients (Pannuti et al 1979).

Tamoxifen is remarkably free of side-effects although, like other hormone manipulations, it may precipitate hypercalcaemia in patients with widespread bony metastases. There may also be a 'flare' or temporary exacerbation of pain, which is generally a predictor of subsequent response (Stoll 1983). Aminoglutethimide is less well tolerated, being associated with transient rashes, lethargy and ataxia in about 50% of cases. Flutamide commonly causes gynaecomastia if used alone, but this is not seen when it is given in combination with GnRH analogues.

Sex hormones, in particular oestrogens, may cause intermittent uterine bleeding, which can be upsetting, especially for postmenopausal women. Androgens cause variable virilisation and increased libido in some women. Oestrogens given to men cause loss of body hair, testicular atrophy, gynaecomastia, loss of libido and impotence. Their long-continued administration is associated with a higher mortality from cardiac and cerebrovascular disease, and benefit in survival in early-stage prostatic carcinoma is outweighed by such complications (VACURG 1967). Cyproterone acetate has fewer side-effects than oestrogens and is associated with a lower incidence of cardiovascular complications. Flutamide seems to cause less sexual dysfunction than other antiandrogens, but like cyproterone may cause hepatic damage and is expensive (Drug and Therapeutics Bulletin 1986).

Orchidectomy causes similar side-effects to oestrogens, with the exception of the excess cardiovascular mortality, but carries its own psychological morbidity. Adrenalectomy and hypophysectomy are both major operative procedures and carry a small but significant mortality. Hormone replacement is subsequently required for life.

CONCLUSIONS

Radiotherapy, chemotherapy and hormone therapy are all valuable techniques for the relief of cancer pain, and those concerned with the care of cancer patients must have some knowledge of the potential of all these therapies. Side-effects caused by the inappropriate use of anticancer treatments can be very distressing, and in all cases the disadvantages of a treatment must be balanced against the palliative benefit.

In many patients the best approach to pain relief will be through interdisciplinary cooperation. Well-planned clinical trials are required because there is still much to be learned about the indications, dose, frequency and optimal administration of anticancer therapies for the relief of pain.

REFERENCES

Adamietz I A, Schöber C, Schulte R W M, Peest D, Renner Kh 1991 Palliative radiotherapy in plasma cell myeloma. Radiotherapy and Oncology 20: 111–116

Aitken-Swan J 1959 Nursing the late cancer patient at home. Practitioner 183: 64–69

Allen K L, Johnson T W, Hibbs G C 1976 Effective bone palliation as related to various treatment regimens. Cancer 37: 984–987

Arnold A M 1979 Podophyllotoxin derivative VP 16–213. Cancer Chemotherapy and Pharmacology 3: 71–80

Arnold A M, Williams C J 1979 Small-cell lung cancer: a curable disease? British Journal of Diseases of the Chest 73: 327–348

Ashby M 1991 The role of radiotherapy in palliative care. Journal of Pain and Symptom Management 6: 380–388

Ashley D J B 1978 Evans' histological appearances of tumours, 3rd edn. Churchill Livingstone, Edinburgh, p 124

Bates T D 1984 Radiotherapy in terminal care. In: Saunders C M (ed) The management of terminal malignant disease, 2nd edn. Edward Arnold, London, p 133–138

Bates T D 1987 The management of bone metastases: radiotherapy. Palliative Medicine 1: 117–120

Bates T D 1989 Radiotherapy, chemotherapy and hormone therapy in the relief of cancer pain. In: Swerdlow M, Charlton J E (eds) Relief of intractable pain. Elsevier, Amsterdam, p 329–347

Beatson G T 1896 On the treatment of inoperable cases of carcinoma of the mamma: suggestions for a new method of treatment with illustrative cases. Lancet ii: 104–107

Beierwaltes W H 1986 Carcinoma of the thyroid – radionuclide diagnosis, therapy and follow-up. In: Ackery D, Batty V (eds) Nuclear medicine in oncology. Clinics in oncology, vol 5. Baillière Tindall, London, p 23–37

Benson W J, Scarffe J H, Todd I D H, Palmer M, Crowther D 1979 Spinal cord compression in myeloma. British Medical Journal i: 1541–1544

Bissett D, Macbeth F R, Cram I 1991 The role of palliative radiotherapy in malignant mesothelioma. Clinical Oncology 3: 315–317

Bleehan N M 1986 Radiotherapy for small cell lung cancer. Chest 89 (suppl): 268–276

Bloom H J G 1971 Medroxyprogesterone acetate (Provera) in the treatment of metastatic renal cancer. British Journal of Cancer 25: 250–265

Bodley Scott R 1970 Cancer chemotherapy – the first 25 years. British Medical Journal iv: 259–265

Bonadonna G, Molinari R 1979 Role and limits of anticancer drugs in the treatment of advanced cancer pain. In: Bonica J J, Ventafridda V (eds) Advances in pain research and therapy 2. Raven Press, New York, p 131–138

Bonadonna G, Monfardini S, De Lena M, Fossati-Bellani F 1969 Clinical evolution of Adriamycin, a new anti-tumour antibiotic. British Medical Journal iii: 503–506

Bonica J J 1980 Cancer pain. In: Bonica J J (ed) Pain. Raven Press, New York, p 335–362

Borgelt B, Gelber R, Kramer S et al 1980 The palliation of brain metastases: final results of the first two studies by the Radiation Therapy Oncology Group. International Journal of Radiation Oncology, Biology, Physics 6: 1–9

Borgelt B B, Gelber R, Brady L W, Griffin T, Hendrickson F R 1981 The palliation of hepatic metastases: results of the Radiation Therapy Oncology Group pilot study. International Journal of Radiation Oncology, Biology, Physics 7: 587–591

Bradshaw J D 1964 The value of X-ray therapy in the management of oesteoclastoma. Clinical Radiology 15: 70–74

Brewin T B 1986 Quality of survival – can we measure it? In: Stoll B A (ed) Coping with cancer stress. Martinus Nijhoff, Dordrecht, p 83–93

Bridgman J F, Bruckner F, Elsen V, Tucker A, Bleehan N M 1973 Irradiation of the synovium in the treatment of rheumatoid arthritis. Quarterly Journal of Medicine 42: 357–367

British Medical Journal Editorial 1981 Pathological fracture due to bone metastasis. British Medical Journal 283: 748

Brodie A M, Dowsett M, Coombes R C 1988 Aromatase inhibitors as new endocrine therapy for breast cancer. Cancer Treatment Reviews 39: 51–65

Bruckman J E, Bloomer W D 1978 Management of spinal cord compression. Seminars in Oncology 5: 135–140

Burnet N G, Williams G, Howard N 1990 Phosphorus-32 for intractable bony pain from carcinoma of the prostate. Clinical Oncology 2: 220–223

Cady B, Oberfield R A 1974 Arterial infusion chemotherapy of hepatoma. Surgery, Gynecology and Obstetrics 138: 381–384

Calin A 1985 X-radiation in the management of rheumatoid disease. British Journal of Hospital Medicine 33: 261–265

Cancer Topics 1992 Cisplatin-cyclophosphamide versus carboplatin-cyclophosphamide. Cancer Topics 9: 31–32

Canney P A, Griffiths T, Latief T N, Priestman T J 1987 The clinical significance of tamoxifen withdrawal response. Lancet i: 36

Cappelaere P, Adenis L 1977 Intérêt de l'administration de fortes doses de succinate de 6 méthylprednisolone chez les cancéreux algiques en phase terminale. Lille Médical Actualités 22: 269–271

Closs S, Bates T D 1987 Spinal cord compression. In: Bates T D (ed) Contemporary palliation of difficult symptoms. Baillière's Clinical Oncology vol 1 no. 2. Baillière Tindall, London

Coates A 1986 Coping with cytotoxic therapy. In: Stoll B A (ed) Coping with cancer stress. Martinus Nijhoff, Dordrecht, p 33–44

Cole D J 1989 A randomised trial of a single treatment versus conventional fractionation in palliative radiotherapy of painful bone metastases. Clinical Oncology 1: 59–62

Coombes R C 1982 Metabolic manifestations of cancer. British Journal of Hospital Medicine 27: 21–27

Court-Brown W M, Doll R 1965 Mortality from cancer and other causes after radiotherapy for ankylosing spondylitis. British Medical Journal ii: 1327–1332

Crile G 1981 Endocrine therapy in thyroid cancer. In: Stoll B A (ed) Hormonal management of endocrine-related cancer. Lloyd-Luke, London, p 166–171

Curie P, Curie M, Bemont M G 1898 Sur une nouvelle substance fortement radioactive, contenue dans la pechblende. Comptes Rendus Hebdomadaires des Séances de l'Académie des Sciences 127: 1215–1217

Dahlin D C, Cupps R E, Johnson E W 1970 Giant-cell tumour: a study of 195 cases. Cancer 23: 1061–1070

Danjoux C E, Rider W D, Fitzpatrick P J 1979 The acute radiation syndrome. Clinical Radiology 30: 581–584

Dearnaley D P, Bayly R J, A'Hern R P et al 1992 Palliation of bone metastases in prostate cancer. Hemibody irradiation or Strontium-89. Clinical Oncology 4: 101–107

del Regato J A, Spjut H J, Cox J D 1985 Ackerman and del Regato's cancer diagnosis, treatment and prognosis, 6th edn. C V Mosby, St Louis, p 220, 932

DeVita V T, Hellman S, Rosenberg S A (eds) 1985 Cancer, principles and practice of oncology, 2nd edn. J B Lippincott, Philadelphia

Drug and Therapeutics Bulletin 1981 What can radiotherapy achieve now? Drug and Therapeutics Bulletin 19: 1–4

Drug and Therapeutics Bulletin 1986 Management of metastatic prostatic carcinoma. Drug and Therapeutics Bulletin 24: 85–88

Duncan W, Nias A H W 1977 Late genetic and somatic effects. In: Clinical radiobiology. Churchill Livingstone, Edinburgh, p 143–163

Ehrlich C E, Young P C M 1981 Endometrial cancer: rationale for hormone therapy. In: Stoll B A (ed) Hormone management of endocrine-related cancer. Lloyd-Luke, London, p 111–121

Einhorn L H, Donohue J 1977 Cis-diamminedichloroplatinum, vinblastine and bleomycin combination chemotherapy in disseminated testicular cancer. Annals of Internal Medicine 87: 293–298

Fallowfield L 1990 The quality of life. The missing measurement in health care. Souvenir Press, London

Farber S, Diamond L K, Mercer R D, Sylvester R F, Wolff J A 1948 Temporary remissions in acute leukaemia in children produced by folic acid antagonist 4-aminopteroyl glutamic acid. New England Journal of Medicine 238: 787–793

Fischer D S 1984 Hormonal and chemical therapy. In: Twycross R G (ed) Pain relief in cancer. Clinics in Oncology vol 3 no. 1. Baillière Tindall, London, p 55–74

Foley K M 1979 Pain syndromes in patients with cancer. In: Bonica J J, Ventafridda V (eds) Advances in pain research and therapy 2. Raven Press, New York, p 59–75

Ford H T, Yarnold J R 1983 Radiation therapy – pain relief and recalcification. In: Stoll B A, Parbhoo S (eds) Bone metastasis: monitoring and treatment. Raven Press, New York, p 343–354

Fryer C J H, Fitzpatrick P J, Rider W D, Poon P 1978 Radiation pneumonitis: experience following a large single dose of radiation. International Journal of Radiation Oncology, Biology, Physics 4: 931–936

Galasko C S B 1980 The management of skeletal metastases. Journal of the Royal College of Surgeons of Edinburgh 3: 148–151

Gallagher C J, Cairnduff F, Smith I E 1987 High-dose versus low-dose medroxyprogesterone acetate: a randomised trial in advanced breast cancer. European Journal of Clinical Oncology 23: 1890–1895

Gilbert H A, Kagan A R, Nussbaum H et al 1977 Evaluation of radiation therapy for bone metastases: pain relief and quality of life. American Journal of Roentgenology 129: 1095–1096

Gilbert R W, Kim J H, Posner J B 1978 Epidural spinal cord

compression from metastatic tumour: diagnosis and treatment. Annals of Neurology 3: 40–51
Goldenberg R R, Campbell C J, Bonfiglio M 1970 Giant-cell tumour of bone. An analysis of 218 cases. Journal of Bone and Joint Surgery 52A: 619–664
Goodman L S, Wintrobe M M, Dameshek W et al 1946 Nitrogen mustard therapy. Journal of the American Medical Association 132: 126–132
Gore M E, Selby P J, Viner C et al 1989 Intensive treatment of multiple myeloma and criteria for complete remission. Lancet ii: 879–881
Greenberger J S, Cassady J R, Jaffe N, Vawter G, Crocker A C 1979 Radiation therapy in patients with histiocytosis: management of diabetes insipidus and bone lesions. International Journal of Radiation Oncology, Biology, Physics 5: 1749–1755
Grubbé E 1933 Priority in therapeutic use of X-rays. Radiology 21: 156–162
Haram B J 1984 Facts and figures. In: Saunders C M (ed) The management of terminal malignant disease, 2nd edn. Edward Arnold, London, p 13–16
Henderson I C, Canellos G P 1980 Cancer of the breast: the past decade. New England Journal of Medicine 302: 78–90
Hertz S 1950 Modifying effect of steroid hormone therapy on human neoplastic disease as judged by radioactive phosphorus. Journal of Clinical Investigation 29: 821
Hickling P, Wright V 1981 Seronegative arthritis. Medicine International 1: 436–441
Hoskin P J 1988 Scientific and clinical aspects of radiotherapy in the relief of bone pain. Cancer Surveys 7: 69–85
Hoskin P J, Ford H T, Harmer C L 1989 Hemibody irradiation for metastatic bone pain in two histologically distinct groups of patients. Clinical Oncology 1: 67–69
Hoskin P J, Price P, Easton D et al 1992 A prospective randomised trial of 4 Gy or 8 Gy single doses in the treatment of metastatic bone pain. Radiotherapy and Oncology 23: 74–78
Hoogstraten B 1975 Adriamycin (NSC-123127) in the treatment of advanced breast cancer: studies by the southwest oncology group. Cancer Chemotherapy Report 6: 329–334
Huggins C, Hodges V C 1941 Studies on prostatic cancer. Cancer Research 1: 293–297
Jensen N H, Roesdahl K 1976 Single-dose irradiation of bone metastases. Acta Radiologica: Therapy, Physics, Biology 15: 337–339
Johnson I S, Armstrong J G, Groman M, Burnett J P 1963 The vinca alkaloids: a new class of oncolytic agents. Cancer Research 23: 1390–1427
Karnofsky D A, Burchenal J H 1949 The clinical evaluation of chemotherapeutic agents in cancer. In: Macleod C M (ed) Evaluation of chemotherapeutic agents. Columbia University Press, New York, p 191–205
Kiang D T 1981 Breast cancer: methods and results of endocrine therapy. In: Stoll B A (ed) Hormonal management of endocrine-related cancer. Lloyd-Luke, London, p 64–76
Kohorn E I 1981 Endometrial and ovarian cancer: methods and results of endocrine therapy. In: Stoll B A (ed) Hormonal management of endocrine-related cancer. Lloyd-Luke, London, p 122–127
Kornblith P L, Cassady J R 1985 Central nervous system emergencies. In: DeVita V T, Helman S, Rosenberg S A (eds) Cancer, principles and practice of oncology, 2nd edn. J B Lippincott, Philadelphia, p 1860–1866
Kramer J A 1992 Spinal cord compression in malignancy. Palliative Medicine 6: 202–211
Kramer S, Hendrickson F, Zelen M, Schotz W 1977 Therapeutic trials in the management of metastatic brain tumours by different time/dose fraction schemes of radiation therapy. In: Modern concepts in brain tumour therapy: laboratory and clinical investigations. National Cancer Institute Monograph 46: 213–221
Laing A H, Ackery D M, Bayly R J et al 1991 Strontium-89 chloride for pain palliation in prostatic skeletal malignancy. British Journal of Radiology 64: 816–822
Leake R 1981 Steroid receptors in normal and cancer tissue. In: Stoll B A (ed) Hormonal management of endocrine-related cancer. Lloyd-Luke, London, p 3–12
Lederman M 1981 The early history of radiotherapy. International Journal of Radiation Oncology, Biology, Physics 7: 639–648
Lister T A, Malpas J S 1981 Steroid therapy in leukaemia and lymphoma. In: Stoll B A (ed) Hormonal management of endocrine-related cancer. Lloyd-Luke, London, p 177–184
Maxon H R, Schroder L E, Hertzberg V S, et al 1991 Rhenium-186 (Sn) HEDP for treatment of painful osseous metastases: results of a double-blind crossover comparison with placebo. Journal of Nuclear Medicine 32: 1877–1881
Medical Research Council Committee on Leukaemia and the Working Party on Leukaemia in Childhood 1973 Treatment of acute lymphoblastic leukaemia. Effect of 'prophylactic' therapy against central nervous system leukaemia. British Medical Journal ii: 381–384
Medinger F G, Craver L F 1942 Total body irradiation with review of cases. American Journal of Roentgenology 48: 651–671
Minton M J, Knight R K, Rubens R D, Hayward J L 1981 Corticosteroids for elderly patients with breast cancer. Cancer 48: 883
Molinari R 1979 Problems of cancer pain in the head and neck. In: Bonica J J, Ventafridda V (eds) Advances in pain research and therapy 2. Raven Press, New York, p 519–522
Muss H B, White D R, Richards F et al 1978 Adriamycin versus methotrexate in five-drug combination chemotherapy for advanced breast cancer: a randomized trial. Cancer 42: 2141–2148
Nemoto T, Dao T L 1971 5-Fluorouracil and cyclophosphamide in disseminated breast cancer. New York State Journal of Medicine 71: 554–558
Nesbit M E 1986 Current concepts and treatment of histiocytosis X. In: Voûte P A, Barrett A, Bloom H J G, Lemerle J, Neidhardt M K (eds) Cancer in children. Clinical management, 2nd edn. Springer-Verlag, Berlin, p 176–184
Nobler M P, Higinbotham N L, Philips R F 1968 The cure of aneurysmal bone cysts; irradiation superior to surgery in an analysis of 33 cases. Radiology 90: 1185–1192
Paine C H 1980 Principles of radiotherapy. British Journal of Hospital Medicine 23: 544–551
Pannuti F, Martoni A, Rossi A P, Piana E 1979 The role of endocrine therapy for relief of pain due to advanced cancer. In: Bonica J J, Ventafridda V (eds) Advances in pain research and therapy 2. Raven Press, New York, p 145–165
Parmar H, Phillips R H, Rustin G, Lightman S L, Schally A V 1988 Therapy of advanced ovarian cancer with Decapeptyl. Biomedicine and Pharmacotherapy 42: 531–538
Parmar H, Phillips R H, Charlton C, Lightman S L 1990 The role of GnRH analogues in advanced breast cancer. In: Bouchard P, Haour F, Franchimont P, Schatz B (eds) Recent progress on GnRH and gonadal peptides, Elsevier, Amsterdam, p 309–317
Penn C R H 1976 Single dose and fractionated palliative irradiation for osseous metastases. Clinical Radiology 27: 405–408
Pinkel D 1959 Actinomycin D in childhood cancer. Pediatrics 23: 342–347
Portenoy R M 1992 Cancer pain: pathophysiology and syndromes. Lancet 339: 1026–1031
Posner J B 1987 Back pain and epidural spinal cord compression. Medical Clinics of North America 71: 185–205
Powles T J, Coombes R C, Smith I E et al 1980 Failure of chemotherapy to prolong survival in a group of patients with metastatic breast cancer. Lancet ii: 580–582
Powles T J, Smith I E, Coombes R C 1982 Endocrine therapy. In: Halnan K E (ed) Treatment of cancer. Chapman & Hall, London, p 103–117
Price P, Hoskin P J, Easton D et al 1986 Prospective randomised controlled trial of single and multifraction radiotherapy schedules in the treatment of painful bony metastases. Radiotherapy and Oncology 6: 247–255
Priestman T J 1989. Cancer chemotherapy–an introduction, 3rd edn. Springer-Verlag, Berlin
Priestman T J, Baum M 1976 Evaluation of quality of life in patients receiving treatment for advanced breast cancer. Lancet i: 899–901
Qasim M M 1981 Half body irradiation (HBI) in metastatic carcinomas. Clinical Radiology 32: 215–219
Rhoads C P 1946 Nitrogen mustards in the treatment of neoplastic disease. Journal of the American Medical Association 131: 656–658
Robinson R G 1986 Radionuclides for the alleviation of bone pain in

advanced malignancy. In: Ackery D, Batty V (eds) Nuclear medicine in oncology. Clinics in Oncology vol 5 no. 1. Baillière Tindall, London, p 39–49

Roentgen W C 1895 Über eine neue Art von Strahlen. Sitzungsberichte der Physikalisch-Medizinischen Gesellschaft zu Würzburg, p 132–141

Rowland C G 1979 Single fraction half body radiation therapy. Clinical Radiology 30: 1–3

Rubens R D, Knight R K, Hayward J L 1975 Chemotherapy of advanced breast cancer: a controlled randomized trial of cyclophosphamide versus a four-drug combination. British Journal of Cancer 32: 730–736

Ruiter D J, van Rijssel T G, van der Velde E A 1977. Aneurysmal bone cysts. A clinico-pathological study of 105 cases. Cancer 39: 2231–2239

Russell J A 1983 Cytotoxic therapy – pain relief and recalcification. In: Stoll B A, Parbhoo S (eds) Bone metastasis: monitoring and treatment. Raven Press, New York, p 355–368

Saenger E L, Silberstein E B, Aron B et al 1973 Whole body and partial body radiotherapy of advanced cancer. American Journal of Roentgenology 117: 670–685

Salazar O M, Rubin P, Hendrickson F R et al 1981 Single-dose half-body irradiation for the palliation of multiple bone metastases from solid tumours: a preliminary report. International Journal of Radiation Oncology, Biology, Physics 7: 773–781

Salmon S E, Jones S E 1979 Studies of the combination of Adriamycin and cyclophosphamide (alone or with other agents) for the treatment of breast cancer. Oncology 36: 40–47

Saunders C M 1984 Appropriate treatment, appropriate death. In: Saunders C M (ed) The management of terminal malignant disease, 2nd edn. Edward Arnold, London, p 1

Scarffe H 1982 Multiple myeloma. In: Halnan K E (ed) Treatment of cancer. Chapman & Hall, London, p 677–690

Sikora K, Halnan K E (eds) 1990 Treatment of cancer, 2nd edn. Chapman & Hall, London

Shay H, Zarafonetis C, Smith N, Woldow I, Sun D C H 1953 Treatment of leukaemia with triethylene thiophosphoramide (Thiotepa). Archives of Internal Medicine 92: 628–645

Smalley R V, Carpenter J, Bartolucci A, Vogel C, Krauss S 1977 A comparison of cyclophosphamide, Adriamycin, 5-fluorouracil (CAF) and cyclophosphamide, methotrexate, 5-fluorouracil, vincristine, prednisone (CMFVP) in patients with metastatic breast cancer. Cancer 40: 625–632

Smith D G, Nesbit M E, D'Angio G J, Levitt S H 1973 Histiocytosis X. Role of radiation therapy in management with special reference to dose levels employed. Radiology 106: 419–422

Souhami R L, Tobias J S 1986 Cancer and its management. Blackwell, Oxford, p 202–224

Stewart J R 1985 Hyperthermia. In: DeVita V T, Hellman S, Rosenberg S A (eds) Cancer, principles and practice of oncology, 2nd edn. J B Lippincott, Philadelphia, p 2246–2256

Stewart M J 1918 Chemical warfare. Medical Committee Report no. 12. HMSO, London

Stoll B A 1964 Rapid palliative irradiation of inoperable breast cancer. Clinical Radiology 15: 175–178

Stoll B A 1969 Hormonal management in breast cancer. Pitman Medical, London, p 38–67

Stoll B A 1981 Breast and prostatic cancer: methods and results of endocrine therapy. In: Stoll B A (ed) Hormonal management of endocrine-related cancer. Lloyd-Luke, London, p 77–91, 148–157

Stoll B A 1983 Hormonal therapy–pain relief and recalcification. In: Stoll B A, Parbhoo S (eds) Bone metastasis: monitoring and treatment. Raven Press, New York, p 321–342

Stoll B A, Andrews J T 1966 Radiation-induced peripheral neuropathy. British Medical Journal i: 834–837

Strickland P 1980 Complications of radiotherapy. British Journal of Hospital Medicine 23: 552–565

Stuart-Harris R, Dowsett M, Bozek T 1984 Low-dose aminoglutethimide in the treatment of advanced breast cancer. Lancet ii: 604–606

Szur L, Lewis S M, Goolden A W G 1959 Polycythaemia vera and its treatment with radioactive phosphorus. Quarterly Journal of Medicine 52: 397–424

Tomita T, Galicich J H, Sundaresan N 1983 Radiation therapy for spinal epidural metastases with complete block. Acta Radiologica Oncology 22: 135–143

Twycross R G, Lack S A 1983 Symptom control in far advanced cancer: pain relief. Pitman, London, p 6

van der Werf-Messing B, van Gilse H A 1971 Hormonal treatment of metastases of renal carcinoma. British Journal of Cancer 25: 423–427

Vargha Z A, Glicksman A S, Boland J 1969 Single-dose radiation therapy in the palliation of metastatic disease. Radiology 93: 1181–1184

Veterans Administration Cooperative Urological Research Group (VACURG) 1967 Carcinoma of the prostate: treatment comparisons. Journal of Urology 98: 516–522

Wang C C 1975 Radiation therapy for head and neck cancers. Cancer 36: 748–751

Wilkins M F, Keen C W 1987 Hemi-body radiotherapy in the management of metastatic carcinoma. Clinical Radiology 38: 267–268

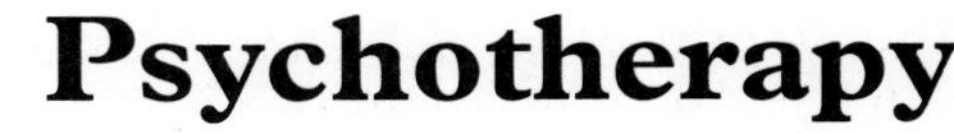

Psychotherapy

71. The placebo and the placebo response

Patrick D. Wall

INTRODUCTION

The word 'placebo' has been used since the 18th century as a term for mock medicine. Its origin and meaning is usually given as a simple translation from the Latin as 'I will please'. I find that a highly improbable use of Latin by educated men of the time who would actually have said *'Placebit'*, 'It will please'. It seems to me much more likely that the word alludes to Psalm 116:9 'Placebo Domino in regione vivorum', which appears in the King James Bible as 'I will walk before the Lord in the land of the living'. This line beginning with Placebo is the first line of the vespers for the dead. Priests and friars badgered the populace for money to sing vespers for the dead. Placebo could have been the derisory word for these unpopular and expensive prayers just as the words 'hocus pocus' comes from the first line of the Communion, *'Hoc est corpus'*, 'This is the body (of Christ)'. This is surely the way in which Geoffrey Chaucer (1340) uses the word placebo when he writes, 'Flatterers are the devil's chatterlaines for ever singing placebo' as does Frances Bacon (1625) 'Instead of giving Free Counsell sing him song of placebo'. This adds a more subtle meaning to the word where the sycophant tells the listener what he expects and wants to hear rather than the truth. That remains a placebo. The topic needs no excuse because it is full of surprise, power and paradox.

I will not attempt a precise definition of the placebo or of its effect. For those who require that, they can wade their way through the first 163 turgid pages of an otherwise lively book edited by White, Tursky & Schwarz (1985). The reason for this agonised search for an acceptable definition is that most definitions threaten to breach the general obsession with clearly separating mental from bodily sites of action. This search goes beyond the pleasures of academic, pedantic, talmudic need for acceptable precision. Legal regulations governing the introduction of a new pharmaceutical compound require that the company demonstrates that the novel molecule has a specific therapeutic action which is more powerful than the company's and doctor's and patient's belief that the novel molecule has a specific therapeutic action. A satisfactory answer is worth millions. It takes the question out of the philosopher's conundrum-riddled tutorial on to the floor of the stock market. It demands a precise dissection of the 'true' truth from the generally, even universally, accepted 'believed' truth. Whatever the definition, the placebo operates through the patient's beliefs. In this sense, placebo therapy merges with psychotherapy from one direction just as psychotherapy and pharmacology merge from another direction (Shepherd 1989). For what follows, I need go no further than Burton in 1628 in *The Anatomy of Melancholy*: 'There is no virtue in some (folk remedies) but a strong conceit and opinion alone which forceth a motion of the humours, spirits and blood which takes away the cause of the malady from the parts affected' and 'An empiric oftentimes, or a silly chirugeon, doth more strange cures than a rational physician because the patient puts more confidence in him.'

TWO EXAMPLES OF THE PLACEBO EFFECT

I wish here to give only two contemporary examples of the effect of strong conceits and opinions as samples of what is covered by the legion of placebo effects. Surgery is rarely the subject of a placebo test in spite of an admonition by Finneson (1969) in his book on surgery for pain: 'Surgery has the most potent placebo effect that can be exercised in medicine.' In the 1950s it became a common practice to ligate the internal mammary arteries as a treatment for angina pectoris. Angina is a painful condition attributed to an inadequate blood supply of muscle in the heart wall. The rationale for the operation was that if the internal mammary arteries were ligated, the blood in these arteries, being dammed up, would find alternative routes by sprouting new channels through nearby heart muscle thereby improving the circulation in the heart. This relatively simple operation was carried out in large numbers of patients to the satisfaction of many. However the rationale came under suspicion when pathologists were unable to detect any of the supposed new blood vessels in the heart. Therefore two groups of surgeons and cardiologists (Cobb et al 1959; Dimond et al 1958) decided to test the rationale by carrying out sham operations to incise the skin and expose the arteries in some patients while proceeding with the full ligation in others. The patients and their physicians did not know who had the 'true' operation and who had the 'sham'. The majority of both groups of patients greatly improved in the amount of reported pain, in their walking distance, in their consumption of vasodilating drugs and some in the shape of their electrocardiogram (ECG). The improvement in both groups was maintained over a 6-month period of observation. As an aside, it is obvious that no such trial would be permitted today for ethical reasons in spite of the fact that these tests were carried out for contemporary ethical reasons at Harvard and the University of Pennsylvania. The interest here is not only the evident power of the belief that therapeutic surgery had been completed, but that improvement was sustained over at least a 6-month period in spite of the general belief that placebos have a brief and fading action.

While this is a particularly dramatic example, Roberts et al (1993) have surveyed the reported results on five other 'treatments', which were subsequently withdrawn. They were glomectomy for asthma, evamisole for herpes simplex, photodynamic inactivation for herpes simplex, organic solvents for herpes simplex and gastric freezing for duodenal ulcers. Each of these therapies was eventually halted because they were found to lack a specific action. In spite of this, the combined literature on 7000 patients shows that they reported 30% good and 40% excellent results. It is evident that nonspecific but beneficial effects are very common during the early stages of the introduction of a new therapy even though it is later withdrawn because the therapy lacks a specific effect. It is rather extraordinary that in our obsessional search for rational and specific action, we lack respect for the powerful nonspecific effects and work hard to reject them.

The second example I wish to quote is the work of Hashish et al (1988), who examined the effect of ultrasound therapy, which others had found to be the equal of steroids in reducing pain and jaw tightness (trismus) and swelling following wisdom-tooth extraction. Wishing to determine the effective level of ultrasound, the intensity was set at different levels, including zero, in a manner which was unknown to the patient and the therapist. When the machine was set to produce no ultrasound, there was a marked beneficial effect even superior to the results of the normally used intensities. Naturally disturbed by the apparently bizarre finding, the experimenters wondered if the therapeutic effect was produced by the massage of the injured area coincident with the application of the ultrasound. They therefore trained patients to massage themselves with the inactive ultrasound head with the same movements used by professionals. This was completely ineffective. Evidently the therapeutic phenomenon required an impressive machine and someone in a white coat to transmit the effect even though the emission of ultrasound was not required. I introduce this particular example chosen from many because the placebo therapy reduced not only the pain report but also improved the ability to open the mouth and reduced the swelling.

The reduction of pain will surprise those who consider pain as a reliable and inevitable sensation associated with tissue damage. However, there are others who would categorise pain as a mental perception and therefore subject to error and manipulation. These two attitudes are practical examples of the Cartesian dualistic divide where sensation is the consequence of the working of a body mechanism while perception is a mental process. There are others who will argue that this division between body and mind is a historical artefact produced by a muddle of academic, religious, introspective argument. Whichever attitude is taken, surprise should remain that the placebo also affected the contraction of jaw muscles normally attributed to a reflex action in the flexion-reflex category which loops through the medulla. Furthermore, the placebo affected the swelling, which is a classical component of the local inflammation triggered by local damage.

FOUR REASONS FOR THE DISCOMFORT PROVOKED BY THE TOPIC.

QUACKERY

From the 18th century the word placebo became attached to quackery. As rational medicine developed, placebo could be used as a word to hammer Burton's 'empirics and silly chirugeons'. Beyond this, even the rational physicians were not above the use of a placebo as a form of deception either for diagnostic purposes or to get rid of unwanted or unprofitable patients. This, in turn, provoked the ethical and practical discussion of whether the doctor–patient relationship would survive the discovery by patients that doctors used deception on occasions. This debate on the role of truth-telling and paternalism in the clinic continues (Rawlinson 1985) with discussion of such phrases as 'the benevolent lie'. The ethical problem extends to clinical trials. If it is the doctors' duty to do their therapeutic best, how can they suggest that the patient should submit to a comparison of one therapy which the physicians believe powerful versus another they believe less effective? 'Informed consent' by the patient does not solve this ethical question since it merely recruits the patient to join in the doctors' dilemma. As awe and trust by the patient for the paternal doctor fades so does the frequency of informed consent and of the placebo response. In 1807 Thomas Jefferson wrote 'One of the most successful physicians I have ever known has assured me that he used more bread pills, drops of coloured water and powders of hickory ashes than of all other medicines put together.... 'I consider this a pious fraud.'

A TIRESOME AND EXPENSIVE ARTEFACT

A considerable fraction of the huge cost of clinical trials for a new drug resides in the legal requirement for a placebo trial. When a new idea has been developed by a clever research team, one has sympathy when their enthusiasm has to be put on hold while trials are in progress which have an apparently obvious outcome to the ethusiasts. Not only is the expensive delay assigned to the fault of a meddling bureaucracy but also the existence of a fraction of patients who show placebo responses is considered to be of no intellectual interest but simply an intrusion in the search for true mechanisms.

One attractive short cut is to compare the new therapy with an established one without a placebo stage in a cross-over trial. This, of course, does not face up to the possibility that both therapies might be placebos. The cross-over option is particularly favoured in those therapies such as surgery or psychotherapy where there is no legal requirement for placebo trials. Often an alternative therapy is not available or is so well known to the patients that it would be impossible to recruit volunteers who could openly assess differences between the two. An example is a massive study of long-term consequences of headache and backache after epidural anaesthesia during labour (MacArthur et al 1992), where the authors call for a randomised study to confirm their results. It is obvious that there is no alternative therapy which would be comparable in the mind of a patient with epidural anaesthesia. Furthermore there is a myriad of cultural, educational, social and medical reasons for a mother accepting or rejecting the offer to be assigned at random to one or another therapy, one of which was epidural anaesthesia. If there are very large ethical and practical problems in assessing the apparently straightforward question of long-term consequences of an epidural anaesthetic, it is not surprising that the majority of nonpharmaceutical therapies have never been tested or have been tested in very inadequate ways (Koes et al 1991, 1992). For example, in a large scale survey of thousands of amputees with pain, Sherman et al (1980) identified 40 different forms of therapy but only 15% of the patients reported pain relief. In a search of the literature, no rigorous trials are reported to justify any of these 40 therapies for this condition. In two surveys of tests for the effectiveness of manipulation, osteopathy and chiropracty for pain, the great majority were shown inadequate while the acceptable trials produced contradictory answers (Koes et al 1991, 1992).

A QUESTION OF LOGIC

The very mention of a placebo trial is likely to be taken as a hostile questioning of the logic on which a therapy is based. To request an investigation of the placebo component, an inevitable part of any therapy, is to invite anger. Anger confuses the question of whether something should work with the question of whether it does work.

THE REALITY OF THE SENSES

Everyone measures their own sanity by cross-checking their sensation with objective reality. On the rare occasions where there is a mismatch, special names are applied: hallucination, illusion, delusion, madness, drunkenness, etc. For anyone, there is a simple intuitive sense apparent on reading Descartes (1644): 'If for example fire comes near the foot, the minute particles of this fire, which you know move at great velocity have the power to set in motion the spot of skin of the foot which they touch, and by this means pulling on the delicate thread which is attached to the spot of the skin, they open up at the same instant the pore (in the brain) against which the delicate ends just as by pulling on one end of a rope one makes to strike at the same instant a bell which hangs at the other end.' It seems so reasonable that we should possess sensory mechanisms which represent the state of the world as reliably as the tolling of the bell represents action at the end of its rope. Furthermore it seems equally obvious and reasonable that we should possess a separate entity, the mind, which can decide whether to ignore the bell or to write a poem about it. Even a philosopher like Bertrand Russell, who questioned Cartesian dualism, still required a reliable sensory apparatus which generated sensation as the closest representation of events which the machinery would permit. Sensation for him was generated by a continous uncensored flow of information. If this flow was faulty, variable and haphazard, then even a great cognitive brain would necessarily be faulty. If the sensory apparatus was censored or corruptible, then sense could become nonsense and reality an individual construct of a particular mind. We have many reasons and facts which lead us to reject that conclusion. We trust our senses, the five senses of Aristotle. Pain appears to us as the sensation provoked by injury. A broken leg provokes an appropiate sensation and location of pain. This chapter discussess manoeuvres called placebos which in no way affect the leg and its fracture but modify the sensation of pain and its perception. No wonder the topic provokes a sense of discomfort like a cold hand in the dark.

DIVERSIONS GENERATED TO AVOID A CONSIDERATION OF THE NATURE OF PLACEBO RESPONSES

When doctors who are not involved in a therapy under trial learn that it turns out to be a placebo, they howl with laughter. It is the best example of Schadenfreude, pleasure in the discomfort of others. When you are the subject in a trial and discover that you have reacted to a placebo, as I have, you feel a fool. When you are the proponent or inventor of a therapy, whether based on contemporary rationale or old-fashioned faith, you are resentful of the need for placebo testing. If the test reveals a substantial placebo component in the response, diversions are created to eliminate consideration of the placebo effect. These add to the four general reasons for discomfort with the effect. Here I wish to examine a series of these diversions, some of which approach myths, which have in common a neglect of the placebo phenomenon.

THE PLACEBO DIFFERENTIATES BETWEEN ORGANIC AND MENTAL DISEASE

This is the most dangerous and cruel attitude which has been used by physicians and surgeons when they detect placebo responses. An example is shown in the reaction of the profession to the true or sham operation on the internal mammary artery which has been described above (Cobb et al 1959; Dimond et al 1958). Amsterdam et al (1969) describe patients with angina in whom there appears to be an adequate circulation in the coronary arteries. It is then immediately assumed, without evidence, that these are the patients who would respond to a placebo while those with true cardiac ischaemia could not. This idea had already been suggested by psychiatrists using the phrase 'somatic hallucination' (Farrer 1964). Clearly this approaches the diagnosis of hysteria (Merskey 1989) although in hysteria, the somatisation fails to initiate any known organic disease so that the alert diagnostician can differentiate hysteria from the condition it mimics. Here we have the proposal that some patients mimic an organic disease so precisely that a diagnostic test, the placebo, is needed to separate the two classes. It will be seen that the proposal is very attractive to those who seek an absolute separation of organic from mental disease and who believe that every true pain is precisely causally related to an observable organic lesion. The proposal is dangerous nonsense if one considers the hundreds of papers, of which 986 are reviewed in Turner et al (1980), where placebo responses are described in patients in pain appropriate to a diagnosed overt organic lesion as in postoperative pain, cancer, etc. Rather than a rereview of this massive literature I will simply relate two illustrative anecdotes.

A patient with classical causalgia following a near miss on his sciatic nerve by a bullet had responded to a saline injection interspersed in a regular series of morphine injections. A very senior orthopaedic surgeon concluded that there was therefore nothing wrong with the man by which he meant there could be no causative lesion in this surgeon's territory of interest (i.e. peripheral nerves and bones) and therefore this was a mental condition as proven by the placebo response. The patient's pain was abolished by a sympathectomy, an operation of which the patient had no knowledge or expectation. This patient's pain was caused by a peripheral nerve lesion and cured by a peripheral lesion.

The second anecdote is related by Professor Collins who became Head of Neurosurgery at Yale. In a forward hospital in Korea while operating on a series of casualty admissions, he began to suffer severe abdominal pain which was obviously acute appendicitis. Faced with extreme emergency casualties, he ordered the theatre sister to give him an injection of morphine. His pain subsided and he completed the surgery, after which he himself became a patient and his inflamed appendix was removed. Returning to duty after his recovery, he was leafing through the operating room report book when he came across the sister's entry, 'Major Collins ordered a 15 mg morphine injection so that he could continue operating but since he appeared distressed, I thought it best to give him an intramuscular injection of saline.'

THE PLACEBO IS THE EQUIVALENT OF NO THERAPY

This is clearly not true. The placebo has a positive effect. If cancer patients receive narcotics at regular intervals, the secret substitution of a single saline injection in the series of morphine injections results in the relief of pain and other signs and symptoms in the majority of patients. Furthermore the time course of relief imitates that produced by the administration of the narcotic. Clearly the saline injection is not the same as missing an injection since the placebo produced a decrease of pain, while missing an injection would be followed by an increase of pain.

The positive effect of the patient's belief that some therapy is in progress makes it extremely difficult to investigate the natural history of a disease which is not influenced by some form of medical intervention. On rare and special occasions, it is practically and ethically possible to disguise therapy so that the patient does not know that anything is happening. For example, it may be possible to secrete a drug in orange juice which is routinely provided or a drug may be clandestinely injected into a long intravenous drip line out of sight of the patient. Such elaborate plots have been used but are obviously limited in most practical trials and raise difficult ethical problems. One scheme to discover the natural history of a disease is simply to leave a group of patients on the waiting list while treating other groups with true or placebo therapies. There are obvious limits, depending on the society and culture, which determine how long a patient will patiently remain waiting. The richer and/or more agressive patients, or those who are in particular misery, remove themselves from the waiting list and go to another doctor, thereby tilting the nature of the remaining waiting list.

A common tactic to obtain the natural history is to study the course of other patients with the disease retrospectively before the new therapy under study appeared on the scene. This method is so full of problems that many journals now refuse to publish such studies. We can observe an accumulation of the problems of drug testing if we consider how to test a new therapy for AIDS. It is generally believed in the States that the demographic focus of AIDS has shifted from gay whites to poor blacks. We can see the precise figures for such a move in the careful figures from a very wary South African government department (DNHPD 1992). Until 1988, the great majority of the total of all cases of AIDS occurred in gay white men. From 1989–92, the number of new cases of AIDS in white men declined. During that period there was a steady, large increase among equal numbers of black men and women. Over the entire period from 1982 to the present, only eight cases of AIDS have been diagnosed in white women, four of whom had received infected transfusions. Clearly the distribution is changing so rapidly that a retrospective control would be useless. Therefore let us consider the very real problem of how to test a new AIDS therapy. We must remember that before a trial started, the media hype would have been firing on all cylinders to assure the public that a remedy had been discovered. Who in these circumstances would volunteer to take part in a placebo-controlled trial? The answer is that a small number of honest and poor people would take the 50:50 chance that they would get the new drug at no cost. The rest would buy, beg, borrow or steal for the drug. This would leave the control group as an odd minority. Even they may not be reliable since some members of just such a control group in New York have been found by blood testing to be buying the active drug under trial on the black market. It is clear that we need new and subtle methods to measure the three quite separate factors – natural history, placebo response and specific response (Finkel 1985).

A FIXED FRACTION OF PATIENTS RESPOND TO PLACEBOS

This myth is widely stated in papers and textbooks with the figure of 33% being commonly quoted. Clearly the idea is to label a fraction of the population as mentally peculiar. Where these sources quote the origin of the myth, they refer to Beecher (1955) who indeed gives the figure of 35.2%. However, had they bothered to read the paper, they would have found that this figure is an average of Beecher's own 11 studies, each of which varied widely from the average. Scanning a large number of double-blind studies shows the fraction of placebo responders varying from close to 0% (Tyler 1946) to near 100% (Liberman 1964), depending on the circumstance of the trial. Clinical pains are associated with a large number of placebo responders than experimental pains (Beecher 1959). The subtlety of the conditions has commercial as well as theoretical interest. Capsules containing coloured beads are more effective than coloured tablets which are superior to white tablets with corners which are better than round white tablets (Buchlew & Coffield, 1982). Beyond this, intramuscular saline injections are superior to any tablet but inferior to intravenous injections. Tablets taken from a bottle labelled with a well-known brand name are superior to the same tablets taken from a bottle with a typed label. My favourite is a doctor who always handled placebo tablets with forceps assuring the patient that they were too powerful to be touched by hand. On a much more serious level, we will be discussing the conversion of experimental subjects to placebo responders (Voudouris et al 1989, 1990). There is no fixed fraction of the population who respond to placebos.

PLACEBO RESPONDERS HAVE A SPECIAL MENTALITY

This proposal is an extension of the fixed-fraction myth. It proposes that there are groups in the population with distorted mental processes leading them to confuse true therapies with placebos. For those who cannot imagine that a normal person would ever make such a mistake, the idea is attractive. It was first proposed by Beecher (1968) and promptly dropped. With the rise of personality psychology, there were any number of perjorative mental tendencies which could be detected in the population by the analysis of the answers to questionnaires. Some of these seemed attractive labels to hang on those who responded to placebos to differentiate them from the normal who would never make such a silly mistake. These labels include suggestibility, hypnotisability, neurotic, extrovert, introvert, acquiescent, desire to please, lack of sophistication, acceptance of authority and so on. For anyone who rates high on masochism in a personality questionnaire, I suggest they wade their way through the 36 papers on the topic in Turner et al 1980 and the many more in White et al 1985. Most papers report no correlations with personality type and the rest are contradictory.

PAIN IS A MULTIDIMENSIONAL EXPERIENCE AND THE PLACEBO AFFECTS ONLY A FRACTION OF THE PAIN

The previous four diversions are crude myths designed to defend the indefensible. We now enter a more subtle arena. In the modern era, Beecher (1959) makes an intuitive introspective commonsense division of one's personal reaction to pain as having two separable dimensions: one deals with intensity and the other with reaction. Needless to say, there is more than a whiff here of Cartesian dualism where a mechanical sensation is followed by a mental perception. Melzack & Casey (1968) even assigned different parts of the brain to create these two dimensions which gave a new respectability to this ancient introspective idea. Melzack & Torgerson (1971) then analysed the way in which people used words about pain and derived three dimensions: sensory, affective and evaluative. From this, the widely used McGill Pain Questionnaire evolved. By now, four dimensions have been isolated (Holroyd et al 1992). It would seem entirely reasonable to examine the placebo response to discover if all dimensions of pain were equally involved. This was done by Gracely et al (1978) and Gracely (1979). They used volunteer experimental normal subjects who received gradually random shocks to the teeth or skin. The subjects were asked to rate separately the intensity of the pain and the unpleasantness of the pain (i.e. Cartesian sensation and perception or Beecher's intensity and reaction or Melzack's sensation and affect). The subjects were then given a saline injection with the assurance that they were receiving a powerful analgesic. The results are absolutely clear. The intensity of the pain was completely unaffected but at low-shock levels the unpleasantness was markedly reduced but at higher intensities was unaffected. This important experiment would seem to bring us back to the most classical position. Sensation as a body mechanism is unaffected by a placebo at any stimulus level. Minor unpleasantness as a mental perception is affected by the mental suggestion implicit in the presence of a placebo. Then the stimulus intensity rises, the appropriate unpleasant perception regains its proper place in spite of implied suggestion from the placebo. These clear experiments would seem to remove the mystery from the placebo and to return the entire subject to classical dualism. Gracely et al (1978) went on to show that diazepam, a tranquilliser, could produce exactly the same effect (i.e. intensity was unaffected but low levels of unpleasantness were reduced). Up to this point one could say that the experiments support a particular version of Cartesian dualism in which there is a reliable sensory apparatus unaffected by these manipulations and that sensation is observed by a mental apparatus which assigns unpleasantness to the pure sensation and which is subject to suggestion and to tranquillisers.

However, Gracely et al (1979) went on to investigate the effect of fentanyl, a narcotic, on the same type of pain and the result is summarised in the title 'Fentanyl reduces the intensity but not the unpleasantness of painful tooth sensations'. It will be seen that this result abolishes the idea that a reliable sensory apparatus feeds a dependent mental apparatus assigning unpleasantness. The three experiments taken together suggest with some power that there are two separate dimensions, intensity and unpleasantness, which can be manipulated independently. However, we must now return and ask if the placebo result (i.e. intensity is unaffected but low-level unpleasantness is affected) can be taken as a general statement about analgesic placebos. The first prediction would be that placebos would work on minor pains but not on severe pain but that is precisely the opposite of Beecher's (1955) observations and those of Lasagna et al (1954). The second prediction is that patients responding to a placebo would report the pain intensity unchanged while the unpleasantness is relieved but the fact is that patients with migraine or postoperative pain or cancer report relief of both aspects. Furthermore even in experimental situations (e.g. Voudouris et al 1989, 1990) both threshold and intensity are affected by placebos. My conclusion is that the identification of separate categories of pain experience is a valid and useful aspect of pain study but that the placebo effect can change these dimensions separately or together depending on the circumstances of suggestion, expectation and instruction.

THE PLACEBO RESPONSE IS PRODUCED BY ENDOGENOUS NARCOTICS

The publication of this statement by Levine et al in 1978 had an enormous and lasting impact. It gave the placebo instant respectability in 20th-century terms and partially liberated it from those doubts and denials listed above, which made people wish that the phenomenon would just go away. The logic of this reasoning for the admission of the placebo to polite society is zero. If a newspaper headline read 'Scientists discover the origin of music and poetry' followed by an article showing that music could not be performed when curare prevented the effect of acetylcholine released from motor axons, one would not be overwhelmed by the insight into the nature of music and poetry. Similarly it is not clear what insight into the overall placebo phenomenon is provided by showing that some link in the machinery involves endorphins.

In addition there are several problems with the original experiment, which reported that high doses of naloxone, an opiate antagonist, abolished the placebo reduction of pain following wisdom-tooth extraction. There are three reasons why the experiment is complex and difficult. First it is obvious that the pain did not have a steady baseline but was naturally rising and then falling during the period of observation. Second, while naloxone by itself has no effect when there is no pain (El Sobky et al 1979), in the presence of pain, naloxone by itself exaggerates the pain or reduces pain depending on the dose (Levine et al 1979). Third, some subjects were excluded from the analysis for reasons which are questionable. Mihic & Binkert (1978) were unable to show a naloxone effect on the placebo effect on cold pain. Examining naloxone and placebos on the pain of tooth extraction, Levine et al (1978) and Gracely et al (1983) concluded that the naloxone effect was independent of the placebo effect. The careful studies of Grevert et al (1983) have been quoted as supporting

Levine et al but that is not justified. They studied the effect of naloxone on a placebo reduction of experimental ischaemic pain. Each subject was tested on three occasions at 1-week intervals. On the first two tests, naloxone had no effect on the placebo response but by the 3rd week, the high dose of naloxone produced a partial decrease of the placebo response. Fields & Levine (1981, 1984) reviewed the relation between these experiments in a highly intelligent way. However, Levine & Gordon (1984) introduced a new surprising factor which they conclude demonstrates the naloxone dependence of the placebo effect, leaving me in admiration of the subtlety of the placebo but in even more doubt about the role of endorphins. Their paper, which is crucial reading for anyone working on the subject, shows that infusions delivered secretly in a long line undoubtedly included some hidden cues to the subject which were eliminated when a programmed machine without human operation delivered the various solutions. Their results show that naloxone increased pain no matter how it was given but never to the extent of the pain increase when a blank infusion was given by machine. I believe that the most generous reading of these experiments is that the question remains open.

THE PLACEBO EFFECT MAY BE DISSECTED AWAY TO REVEAL THE PURE THERAPEUTIC ACTION

For this to be true, the therapeutic effect of an active compound would have to be free of its own additional placebo component. Strong evidence shows that the two responses are not separable in practical tests. In an extensive series of tests on postoperative pain, Lasagna et al (1954) had identified placebo reactors and nonreactors. They then gave a fixed dose of morphine to the two groups and found an adequate analgesic response in 95% of the placebo reactors and only 55% of the nonreactors. A much more subtle problem was revealed by Beecher (1968) on examination of the matrix of results from double-blind cross-over studies of morphine versus saline. If, by chance, the first administration contained morphine, the patient learned that this trial involved powerful medicine and tended to give a strong response to the second administration, which was saline. The reverse was also true if, for example, the first test dose was saline, the response to the second, which contained morphine, was weak. It is obvious that this problem will also affect the results of trials where the relative effects of two active compounds are being compared. There will be a carry-over effect of the first trial on the results of the second.

It is apparent that the patient or subject is searching for subtle hints of what to expect and that these expectations affect responses. This raises the question of the comparable nature of the active test and the placebo test. It does not take a great connoisseur to differentiate between intravenous morphine and saline since the morphine produces such obvious immediate side-effects. This problem has led to the use of placebos producing some obvious effects such as vasodilatation, which are assumed to have no direct therapeutic effect but give the subject an impression of receiving powerful medicine. Clearly the introduction of active placebos produces a series of problems: the placebo and active compound rarely precisely mimic each other; the specific inactivity of the placebo is questionable; the patient may find the placebo' s side-effects distasteful. If there are serious problems in drug-testing, they obviously escalate with other forms of therapy. What is a comparable manoeuvre against which to test acupuncture?

Since, as we shall see, it is the expectation of the subject which is crucial, the obverse is the question of secrecy. It is assumed in therapeutic trials that the subject is not aware of the expectation of the enthusiastic proponent. Can that be achieved in practice? Sometimes the secrecy is shattered in obtaining consent: 'We would like you to help us in a trial of a new safer form of aspirin.' Almost always, the person who administers the therapy, and may not know which pill is blank and which is 'true', will be aware of the general nature of what is being tested (Gracely et al 1985). This person's expectations can be covertly infectious. Patients talk to each other and reach a consensus, especially when something new is brewing. The strong effects of this covert expectation are shown by Evans (1974). He examined the relation between the relative effect of analgesics versus placebos in 22 published double-blind trials. The drugs being tested varied from a strong analgesic, morphine through codeine, Darvon, Zomax, to aspirin rated as a weak analgesic. If the placebo effect was independent of the therapeutic effect, the placebo fraction of responders would have been the same in all trials, while the drugs ranged in a series of therapeutic potency. However, the results all show that the stronger the drug, the stronger the placebo response. He divided the pain reduction produced by the placebo by the pain reduction produced by the drug. The answer is a fixed 55–60% over the entire range from weak to strong analgesics. So much for the blindness of these double-blind trials. So much for the clear separation of placebo and therapeutic effects.

We have described seven reasons why we need to avoid diversions which are seven reasons why we need to consider the placebo effect with respect as a powerful phenomenon.

CLASSES OF EXPLANATION

AFFECTIVE

Gracely et al (1978) propose that the placebo affects the unpleasantness of pain while leaving the intensity dimension unaffected. We have given reasons above to support the belief that their experiments represent a special case which does not apply across the board, especially in clinical cases. Evans (1977) in another version of this approach proposes that the placebo operates by decreasing anxiety. However the results show that there is a weak and variable interaction with various types of anxiety and it is not clear that anxiety reduction is not a component of the placebo effect rather than the cause of it.

COGNITIVE

By far the commonest proposal is that the placebo effect depends on the expectation of the subject. There is nothing subtle about this. Placebo reactors can be identified before the trial by simply asking the subject what they expect to be the outcome of the therapy. Those who doubt don't respond to the placebo while those with high expectations do. The very extensive literature on this is reviewed by Bootzin (1985). Lasagna et al (1954) investigated many aspects of postoperative patients who responded to placebos and to analgesic drugs and conclude 'a positive placebo response indicated a psychological set predisposing to anticipation of pain relief'. They add: 'It is important to appreciate that this same anticipation of pain relief also predisposes to better response to morphine and other pharmacologically active drugs.' In a trial of two drugs versus placebos on 100 patients, Nash & Zimring (1969) tested specifically for the role of expectation. The two drugs had no effect which would differentiate them from the placebo, but there was a strong correlation between the measured expectation and the placebo effect. Expectation is given a number of related names – belief, faith, confidence, enthusiasm, bias, meaning, credibility, transference, anticipation, etc. – in 30 of the papers in the bibliography of Turner et al (1980).

Expectation is a learned state and therefore young children do not respond to placebos as adults do, since they have had neither the time nor the experience to learn. Similarly in adults, the learning of expected effects will depend on culture, background, experience and personality. A desire to believe, please and obey the doctor will increase the effect while hostility decreases it. Obviously, part of the expectation of the patient will depend on the expectation, enthusiasm and charisma of the therapist, and therefore there are many reports on this doctor–patient interaction. Expectation in a laboratory experiment may be more limited than in a clinical setting; this may explain why rates and intensities of placebo effects tend to be less in the laboratory than in the clinic (Beecher 1959).

CONDITIONING

There are many reports of drug anticipatory responses in animals (Hernstein 1965; Siegel 1985). These come in two forms. In the first the animal has been given one or more trials on an active drug and is then subject to a saline injection and proceeds to mimic the behavioural or physiological response which was observed after the active drug. In the second type, the animal mimics the counteractions which it mobilises to neutralise the effect of the active compound. For example, if animals have experienced a series of injections of insulin which lower the blood sugar, a saline injection in the same setting as the insulin injection results in a rise of blood sugar, which would be one of the animal's reactions to counteract the insulin-induced decrease (Siegel 1975). In cultures not raised on *Winnie the Pooh*, *Wind in the Willows* and *Watership Down*, it is customary to deny animals the luxury of cognitive processing and to ascribe such phenomena to classical Pavlovian conditioning.

This led to the proposal that the human placebo response had the characteristics of a conditioned response (Wickramasekera 1980; Reiss 1980). The idea is that active powerful drugs produce a powerful objective physiological response in the same manner that food produces salivation, the unconditioned stimuli and responses. However, giving the drug is inevitably inadvertantly associated with a pattern of other stimuli such as a hypodermic injection by a man in a white coat. It is proposed that these are the equivalent of unconditioned stimuli coupled with the conditioned stimulus. It is then proposed that if these incidentally coupled stimuli are given alone, they will provoke the same response as the original drug – just as in the dog, coupling a bell with food eventually leads to the ability of the bell by itself to provoke salivation. The similarity goes beyond the proposed production of a conditioned response. If a placebo is given repeatedly in some, but not all trials, the effect declines. This is a characteristic of Pavlovian responses where simple repeated ringing of the bells leads to a steady decline of the salivation, unless the conditioning is reinforced by occasional coupling of the bell with food.

All such comparisons between widely differing processes lead to argument about similarities and differences, identities and analogies (Wall & Safran 1986). However, the idea led to a series of clever experiments by Voudouris et al (1989, 1990). The first stage of this work was a repeat of a type of trial which had been reported many times before. Volunteer subjects were given rising electric shocks and the current was established in full view of the subject at which the shock became painful and the level at which it become intolerable. Then a bland cream was rubbed on the area, the subjects were assured that it was a powerful anaesthetic, and the shock trial was run a second time. A small fraction of the subjects demonstrated a placebo response by reporting pain and intolerable pain at a higher shock level than they had on the first trial. This part of the experiment is of no general interest, but it established the placebo response rate in these particular circumstances. They then started again with a new group of subjects and determined their threshold and tolerance shock levels. The cream was applied and now came the clever and novel part of the experiment: the strength of the electric shocks was secretly reduced unknown to the subject and observer. When the trial was now run, the subject observed that much higher numbers on the shock machine were achieved before pain was felt and before the pain reached the tolerance limit. These subjects believed that they had tested on themselves the truth of the remarkable anaesthetic properties of the cream. Next, after one such apparent demonstration of the efficacy of the cream, a trial was run in the original conditions, i.e. the strength of current was returned to its original level. The cream was put on and the shock level raised. On this trial large numbers of the subjects became placebo reactors. The only difference in these newly produced placebo responders was that they had 'experienced' in some fashion the apparently 'true' anaestheic properties of the cream. Clearly this result can have important practical implications. Whether the change in the subjects was cognitive or conditioned must remain a subject for debate and further experiment. Brewer (1974) concludes that 'there is no convincing evidence for operant or classical conditioning in adult humans' which is free of cognitive awareness of the situation. It may be that the passionately maintained differences between cognitive and conditioned responses may collapse on each other.

RESPONSE APPROPRIATE SENSATION

I wish to introduce an additional proposal which is that certain classes of sensation are locked to the response which is appropiate to the situation in contrast to the classical view that sensation is always locked to a stimulus which provokes it. I wish to stress that I refer only to certain types of body sensation and not to those sensations related to the outer world such as sight and sound, where the entire body of psychophysics shows a precise lawful relation between stimulus and sensation. However, the psychophysics of pain differs wildly from other senses (Sternbach & Tursky 1964). This special class includes pain, hunger, thirst, vertigo, fatigue, sleepiness, feeling too hot and too cold. One reason to separate this class from other sensations is that each member is associated with diseases where the sensation is not coupled with the appropriate stimulus. For pain, this is a major clinical problem to be discussed below. For hunger, the diseases include anorexia and obesity; for thirst, polydypsia; for vertigo, Menière's disease; for fatigue, postencephalitic myalgia; for sleepiness, Pickwick syndrome and narcolepsy; for extreme temperature, rigors in malaria. This proposal for a separate class of sensations has been approached in a series of steps (Wall 1974, 1979).

With pain in diseases where overt pathology is an integral part of the diagnosis, such as osteoarthritis and carpal tunnel syndrome, the amount of pain is poorly related to the amount of pathology. In other diseases such as angina pectoris and low-back pain, an appropriate evocative pathology, such as occluded coronary arteries or herniated intervertebral discs, is obvious in some cases but not all. In another series of painful conditions, no appropriate peripheral pathology has been identified. These include trigeminal neuralgia, migraine, atypical facial neuralgia, temporomandibular joint syndrome, postencephalitic myalgia syndrome and fibromyalgia. The most extreme example of an uncoupling of pain from injury occurs in emergency analgesia following abrupt injury. Beecher (1959) reported that 70% of soldiers admitted to a forward hospital with severe battle injuries did not complain of pain. In the less dramatic setting of a big city hospital 40% of patients admitted after the common accidents of civilian life reported no pain at the time of the accident (Melzack et al 1982). It is important to note that another 40% reported high levels of pain. There was no obvious relation between the location, severity or nature of the injury and the amount of pain reported at the time of the injury. Three characteristics of this analgesia are crucial to its understanding:

1. The patient is usually fully aware of the injury and its consequences but describes the initial sensation in neutral words 'bangs' 'blows' 'thumps'
2. In hospital, the analgesia is precisely located only to the original injury and does not apply to subsequent stimuli such as the introduction of an intravenous line
3. By the next day all are in the expected pain. Similar behaviour is observed in animals after injury (Wall 1979).

While the body sensations under discussion appear poorly related to a provocative stimulus, each is inevitably linked with attention and with a predictable response. For hunger, eating; for thirst, drinking; for nausea, vomiting; for fatigue, inactivity; for sleepiness, sleep; for coldness, shivering; etc. For pain, three phases of response are observed: first, to attempt to avoid further injury; second, to seek aid and safety and third, recovery from injury (Wall1979). The third phase includes immobilisation of the painful part, avoidance of contact on the painful area, withdrawal, sleep, etc. All three response patterns are observed in animals as well as in humans.

If then pain and the other sensations discussed are variably linked to the provocative stimulus but reliably locked to the response, would it not be reasonable to propose a brain mechanism by which the brain analyses some internal body states in terms of the biological relevant behaviour and that certain sensations signal the outcome of that analysis rather than the input on which the analysis was based? Just such a brain mechanism has been explored by the ethologists who followed Hess,

Tinbergen and Lorenz. In these animal schemata, the brain continuously monitors the flow of information from the internal and external sensory apparatus. Next a biological priority is assigned to a fraction of the input and the appropriate motor pattern is released. Let us propose that humans too incorporate such an apparatus in their brains and that the initial stages do not necessarily intrude on consciousness. Let us further propose that conscious pain only appears after the priority assignment stage, and that pain is sensed consciously at the same time as the release of the motor pattern. It is important to stress that the ethological motor patterns of vertebrates are not fixed-action patterns or reflex discharges. On the contrary, they too require reference to the sensory system in order to shape the correct response. The combination of an empty stomach and the sight of a nearby bill release the herring gull pecking motor pattern. However, the herring gull chick still needs to use its sensory apparatus in order to locate the red spot on the mother's bill in order to peck at it. In other words, there are two sequential uses of the sensory input. The first is used to assign priority and the second to guide the motor behaviour. It is proposed here that pain only appears as a conscious phenomenon in the second epoch of sensory analysis after the first period during which priority was established and during which consciousness is not alerted.

Turning back to pain and the placebo response, it is proposed that, before the placebo, the unconscious priority decision mechanism had assigned priority to the motor pattern and sensation of pain; after the placebo, which is a stimulus with its learned powerful association with pain relief, the unconscious priority decision mechanism reverts to selecting a nonpain state. This new situation assigns a lower priority to pain and allows the release of the next most biologically appropriate pattern. This two-stage analysis process could also provide a rational basis for the other apparently paradoxical absence of pain in emergency analgesia. Pain may be the obvious reaction to overt injury, but there may be other actions and sensations which take precedence. For the soldier in action, impending death has the well-known property of 'concentrating the mind', and much more elaborate life-preserving actions and reactions take precedence over the relative trivia of reaction to localised injury. For the footballer whose fibula is fractured in a clumsy tackle on a goal approach, precedence has been set on goal-scoring, which continues with use of a sensory input tuned to the fulfilment of that task. The horse Henbit, that won the 1980 Derby, having fractured a cannon bone 300 m from the finish, could be presumed to be operating on a nervous system similarly preset for a particular goal. All of this begs the obvious question of why should only one sensation take precedence over another. Why could they not both be felt simultaneously or at least rapidly alternating? The probable answer reinforces the linking of this type of sensation to motor pattern. It is not biologically permissable to release two motor patterns simultaneously. It would be disastrous to attempt to advance and retreat at the same time. Animals in ambiguous situations exhibit what Tinbergen called displacement activity. A herring gull in a stand-off threat posture suddenly switches on a nest-building motor pattern and rips up tufts of grass. Obviously sensation should not be considered to result from an all-or-none switch. Priorities would have a strength and a duration which would be mirrored in the strength and persistence of attention and of sensation.

For a hypothesis to be useful it has to be more than an analogy (Wall & Safran 1986) or a convenient rearrangement of old myths and vagaries. It has to be both testable and deniable. To achieve that requires probing inside the brain, but that itself requires a definition of what would be the object of the search; this leads me to the final section.

CONCLUSION

The placebo effect, as we have presented it, is clearly powerful and infiltrates all aspects of therapy. It represents a practical, ethical and scientific challenge. If a patient seeks relief from a self-proclaimed faith healer, so be it. However, if a patient approaches a physician of the traditional classical established school, the patient assumes that the recommended therapy is based on a rational, tested, scientific scheme which has been validated and which is part of the hugely successful progress of modern medicine. If the physician prescribes a placebo, he is utilising the patient's expectation which is created by the reputation and overt success of the best of modern medicine. This act of the physician goes beyond the physician's personal charisma and authority. It is a lie. If patients discover, as will inevitably sometimes occur, that they have been fooled, their expectations will be shattered, which is a disastrous side-effect of the placebo revealed and unmasked. I am not against the 'benevolent lie' provided that it is a tactial emergency solution. 'Mummy will kiss it better' is a wonderful, beautiful and effective treatment. What we need is an understanding of the nature of sensation, which is so profound that we can rationally elicit our own and our patients' expectations. The placebo reaction teaches us that pain is only felt when pain is appropriate to the situation. We must find how to manipulate this assessment of the appropriate.

REFERENCES

Amsterdam E A, Wolfson S, Garlin R 1969 New aspects of the placebo response in angina pectoris. American Journal of Cardiology 24: 305–306

Beecher H K 1955 The powerful placebo. Journal of the American Medical Association 159: 1602–1606

Beecher H K 1959 Measurement of subjective responses. Oxford University Press, New York

Beecher H K 1968 Placebo effects: a quantitative study of suggestibility. In: Non-specific factors in drug therapy. C C Thomas, Springfield, Illinois, 27–39

Bootzin R R 1985 The role of expectancy in behaviour change. In: White L P, Tursky B, Schwarz G E (eds) Placebo: theory research and mechanisms. Guilford Press, New York, Ch.10

Brewer WF 1974 There is no convincing evidence for operant or classical conditioning in adult humans. In: Weimer W B, Palermo D S (eds) Cognition and the symbolic processes. Wiley, New York, 1–42

Buchaleq L W, Coffield K E 1982 An investigation of drug expectancy as a function of colour, size and preparation. Journal of Clinical Pharmacology 2: 245–248

Cobb L A, Thomas G I, Dillard D H, Merendino K A, Bruce R A 1959 An evaluation of internal mammary artery ligation by a double blind technique. New England Journal of Medicine 20: 1115–1118

Department of National Health and Population Development, RSA, 1992 Epidemiological Comments 193

Descartes R 1641 Meditation on a first philosophy, Paris

Descartes R 1644 L'Homme, Paris

Dimond E G, Kittle C F, Crockett J E 1958 Evaluation of internal mammary ligation and sham procedure in angina pectoris. Circulation 18: 712–713

El-Sobky A, Dostrovsky J A, Wall P D 1979 Lack of effect of naloxone on pain perception in humans. Nature 263: 783–784

Evans F J 1974 The placebo response in pain reduction. In: Bonica J J (ed) Advances in neurology, vol 4. Raven Press, New York, p 289–296

Evans F J 1977 The placebo control of pain. In: Brady J P, Mendels J, Reiger W R, Orne M T (eds) Psychiatry: areas of promise and advancement. Plenum Press, New York

Farrer G R 1964 Psychoanalytic theory of placebo. Disease of the Nervous System 35: 655–662

Fields H L, Levine J D 1981 Biology of placebo analgesia. American Journal of Medicine 70: 745–746

Fields H L, Levine J D 1984 Placebo analgesia–a role for endorphins? Trends in neurosciences 7: 271–273

Finkel M J 1985 Placebo controls are not always necessary. In: White L P, Tursky B Schwarz G E (eds) Placebo: theory research and mechanisms. Guilford Press, New York, 419–422

Finneson B E 1969 Diagnosis and management of pain syndromes. W B Saunders, Philadelphia

Gracely R H 1979 Psychophysical assessment of human pain. In: Bonica J J et al (eds) Advances in pain research and therapy, vol 12. Raven Press, New York, p 211–229

Gracely R H, McGrath P, Dubner R 1978 Validity and sensitivity of ratio scales of sensory and affective verbal pain descriptors. Pain 5: 19–29

Gracely R H, McGrath P, Dubner R 1979 Fentanyl reduces the intensity but not the unpleasantness of painful tooth sensations. Science 203: 1261–1263

Gracely R H, Dubner R, Deeter W R, Wolskee P J 1983 Naloxone and placebo after postsurgical pain by separate mechanisms. Nature 306: 264–265

Gracely R H, Dubner R, Deeter W R, Wolskee P J 1985 Clinicians expectations influence placebo analgesia. Lancet 1: 8419–8423

Grevert P, Albert L H, Goldstein A 1983 Partial antagonism of placebo analgesia by naloxone. Pain 16: 126–143

Hashish I Feinman C, Harvey W 1988 Reduction of postoperative pain and swelling by ultrasound: a placebo effect. Pain 83: 303–311

Herrnstein R J 1965 Placebo effect on the rat. Science 138: 677–678

Holroyd K A, Holm J E, Keefe F J et al 1992 A multi-center evaluation of the McGill Pain Questionnaire: results from more than 1700 chronic pain patients. Pain 48: 301–312

Kantor T G, Sunshine A, Laska E, Meisner M, Hopper M 1966 Oral analgesic studies. Clinical Pharmacology and Therapeutics 7: 447–454

Koes B W, Bouter L M, Beckerman H, van der Heijden G, Knipschild P G 1991 Exercises and back pain, blinded review. British Medical Journal 302: 1572–1576

Koes B W, Bouter L M, Beckerman H 1992 Randomised clinical trials of manipulative therapy and physiotherapy. British Medical Journal 304: 601–606

Lasagna L, Mosteller F, von Felsinger J M Beecher H K 1954 A study of the placebo response. American Journal of Medicine 16: 770–779

Levine J D, Gordon N C 1984 Influence of the method of drug administration on analgesic response. Nature 312: 755–756

Levine J D, Gordon N C, Fields H L 1978 The mechanisms of placebo analgesia. Lancet 2: 654–657

Levine J D, Gordon N C, Fields H L 1979 Naloxone dose dependently produces analgesia and hyperalgesia in postoperative pain. Nature 278: 740–741

Liberman R 1964 An experimental study of the placebo response under three different situations of pain. Journal of Psychiatric Research 2: 233–246

MacArthur C, Lewis M, Knox E G 1992 Investigation of long term problems after obstetric epidural anaesthesia. British Medical Journal 304: 1279–1282

Melzack E, Casey K L 1968 Sensory, motivational and central control determinants of pain. In: Kenshalo D (ed) The skin senses. C C Thomas, Springfield, Illinois

Melzack R, Torgeson W S 1971 On the language of pain. Anesthesiology 34: 50-59

Melzack R, Wall P D, Ty T C 1982 Acute pain in an emergency clinic, latency of onset and descriptive patterns. Pain 14: 33–43

Merskey J 1989 Pain and psychological medicine. In: Wall P D, Melzack R (eds) Textbook of Pain, 2nd edn. Churchill Livingstone, Edinburgh, Ch. 46

Mikic D, Binkert E 1978 Is placebo analgesia mediated by endorphin? Paper presented at Second World Congress of Pain. Montreal, August, 1978

Nash M M, Zimring F M 1969 Prediction of reaction to placebo. Journal of Abnormal Psychology 74: 569–573

Rawlinson M C 1985 Philisophical reflections on the use of placebos in medical practice. In: White L P, Tursky B, Schwarz G E (eds) Placebo: theory research and mechanisms. Guilford Press, New York, p 403–419

Reiss S 1980 Pavlovian conditioning and human fear. An expectancy model. Behaviour Therapy 11:380–396

Roberts A H, Kewman D G, Mercier L, Hovell M 1993 The power of nonspecific effects in healing: implications for psychosocial and biological treatments. Clinical Psychology Review 1993 (in press)

Sherman R A, Sherman C J, Gall N G 1980 A survey of current phantom limb pain treatment in the United States. Pain 8: 85–99

Siegel S 1975 Conditioning insulin effects. Journal of Comparative and Physiological Psychology 89: 189–199

Siegel S 1985 Drug anticipatory responses in animals. In: White L P, Tursky B, Schwarz G E (eds) Placebo: theory, research and mechanisms. Guilford Press, New York, Ch. 16

Shepherd M 1989 Psychotherapy versus pharmacotherapy in psychiatry. Biological Psychiatry in Clinical Practice 1: 4–7

Sternbach R A, Tursky B 1964 On the psychophysical power functions in electric shock. Psychosomatic Science 1: 217–218

Turner J L, Gallimore R, Fox-Henning C 1980 An annotated bibliography of placebo research. Journal Supplement Abstract Service of the American Psychological Association 10(2): 22

Tyler D B 1946 The influence of a placebo and medication on motion sickness. American Journal of Physiology 146: 458–466

Voudouris N J, Peck C J, Coleman G 1989 Conditioned response models of placebo phenomena. Pain 38: 109–116

Voudoris N J, Peck C J, Coleman G 1990 The role of conditioning and verbal expectancy in the placebo response. Pain 43: 121–128

Wall P D 1974 'My foot hurts me', an analysis of a sentence. In: Bellairs R, Gray E G (eds) Essays on the nervous system. Clarendon, Oxford

Wall P D 1979 On the relation of injury to pain. Pain 6: 253–264

Wall P D, Jones M, 1992 Defeating pain. Plenum Press, New York

Wall P D, Safran J W 1986 Artefactual intelligence. In: Rose S Appignanesi L (eds) Science and beyond. Blackwell, Oxford

White L Tursky B, Schwarz G E (eds) 1985 Placebo: theory, research and mechanisms. Guilford Press, New York

Wickramasekera I 1980 A conditioned response model of the placebo effect. Biofeedback and Self-Regulation 5: 5–18

72. Pain and illness behaviour: assessment and management

I. Pilowsky

INTRODUCTION

Illness behaviour (Mechanic 1962) refers to the ways in which individuals think, feel and act in relation to their health status, and although illness behaviour can occur without pain, the reverse must be extremely rare. From a clinical point of view, it is reasonable to consider pain experiences and illness behaviours as essentially inseparable and to regard a statement about pain to the clinician as constituting only one facet of a patient's total illness behaviour. To understand and explain a pain experience, therefore, it is necessary to undertake an appraisal which encompasses the biological, psychological and sociocultural influences which bear on the shaping of illness behaviour.

The illness behaviours which accompany pain may be grouped into those which are adaptive and those which are pathological. The latter group comprises the various forms of abnormal illness behaviour, or dysnosognosia (Pilowsky 1969, 1978), which become particularly significant in the assessment of chronic pain whenever there appears to be a substantial discrepancy between the patient's behaviour and the degree of objective pathology.

THE DETERMINANTS OF ILLNESS BEHAVIOUR

As indicated, 'illness behaviour' refers to thoughts, feelings and behaviours. Thus in assessing patients, we have to consider their cognitive style and level of functioning, their affective status and their overt behaviours.

COGNITIVE ASPECTS

Clearly, what a person thinks about his pain will influence his feelings and actions. The ideas he forms will depend on the information he has at his disposal, which may be derived from previous experience (his own and that of others), as well as what he has read and what he has been told. The way he gathers, processes and responds to this information will depend on his cognitive style and also on the way in which his developmental history and personality structure determine the meaning of the pain experience for him. For example, it has been noted that some patients avoid exposure to information, others seek it assiduously, while still others oscillate between these extremes. These observations have led to the categorisation of patients into those who show avoidant behaviour and those who are vigilant, a dichotomy which in some ways parallels the 'augmentor-reducer' continuum studied by Petrie (1960).

Apart from the basic issue of the patient's degree of openness to information, it is also important to consider his style of gathering and processing data. Some patients who show obsessional personality traits seek to understand as many details of their illness as possible while overlooking the broader perspective. On the other hand, there are those who prefer to take a broad view and pay less attention to detail. Clearly, both styles are relevant to the clinician since he has to make allowance for them in his effort to help the patient not lose sight of the broad issues, or the details on which specific actions may depend. Thus a clinician who requires a patient to keep a record of the exercise he takes does not expect him to do so with such assiduous attention to detail that most of the day is spent in keeping a diary and very little on physical activity.

Illness behaviour may be ineffective because it is based on inaccurate information. All patients form opinions about the aetiology, pathology, treatment and prognosis of their condition. In any of these areas their understanding may be incorrect and, as a consequence, they may not be able to comprehend or accept their doctor's communications or actions, and may, therefore, produce excessive, inadequate or inappropriate responses to the demands of the situation.

Obstacles to the patient's development of an accurate appraisal of his condition may arise in a number of ways. At the most basic level, the doctor may simply not provide the patient with sufficient information or the language used to communicate with the patient may not be appropriate in the sense that it is either too technical or too abstruse. The difficulties which arise when doctor and patient do not share a common language are obvious, as are the consequences of not using a properly trained interpreter.

Apart from the fact that the doctor may not be communicating adequately, there may also be situational variables which mitigate against a desirable level of information exchange within the clinical relationship. These include inadequate time, an unsuitable interviewing area, and other extraneous intrusions on the doctor–patient relationship. Of course, ideal circumstances are rarely achieved, but it is important that the doctor should be sensitive to deficiencies and acknowledge them both to himself and the patient.

AFFECTIVE ASPECTS

It is not possible to understand an individual's feelings about his illness fully unless one has some idea of the symbolic significance of his pain and disability for him. This is not to say that it is feasible to attempt a total comprehension of the patient's symbolic life, but it is possible to know at least some of the salient implications of the pain experience, which are unique to the patient. This point may be illustrated by the case of a patient who complained of longstanding pain in her left hip, which she said bothered her when she exercised but did not prevent her from doing what she wanted (including skiing), provided she took analgesics. She said that she had learned to live with the pain, but emphasised that if it could be removed she would be grateful. It helped to understand her attitudes, when it emerged that her only child was born (when she was middle-aged) with a severe congenital cardiac malformation, and that she regularly carried him straddled on her left hip until he was 9 years old. At that age he died following cardiac surgery. She recalled postponing her own grief to support her husband, who was considerably older than she and who was devastated by the loss. She believed that constantly carrying the child had caused physical trauma to her hip and she was unaware of any emotional consequences of her experience. She had been given many treatments without success. One of the major impediments to her management was her concern not to upset her husband who had recently had a coronary artery graft and disapproved of her taking analgesics or any other form of medication. She said that there had been severe problems in her marriage, but she had learned to live with her husband.

This history also demonstrates the necessity of understanding something of the nature of a patient's body image, a term which refers to the patient's internalised concept of his own body (which as Schilder (1950) emphasised is quite a different phenomenon from the actual body). The emotional investment in the body as a whole and its various parts depends on the individual's development experiences and current life situation. For instance, it is obvious that a fashion model may have a special emotional investment in facial appearance, while a pianist will treasure the hands and a labourer, physical strength.

George Engel's (1959) classic paper on psychogenic pain is particularly helpful in the understanding of the range of meanings which pain may have for an individual. In particular, he refers to the fact that pain may be associated with ideas of punishment, guilt, loss, threat and sexual gratification, and therefore with the emotions that may be expected to accompany such ideas.

The main affects encountered with pain are depression, anxiety and anger, the latter frequently generating guilt and shame. In patients who are predisposed by earlier experiences, the affect may be particularly intense and lead to disruption of their capacity to use their customary coping strategies.

Implications for management

Depression may, on occasion, require specific treatment with an antidepressant of the tricyclic or related groups. These drugs are more likely to be helpful if there are features of an 'endogenous' or 'biological' depression such as early-morning wakening, loss of libido, loss of appetite, psychomotor retardation and constipation, but they may also have a direct ameliorating effect on pain as suggested by a number of writers (Pilowsky et al 1982a; Feinmann 1985). Psychotherapeutic support and counselling will also be necessary to deal with the sense of loss which the patient currently feels and which may be reviving memories of earlier unresolved losses.

Anxiety is often associated with pain, especially if it is acute and when experienced as a threat to personal integrity, both physical and mental. Anxiety is also provoked by fears of separation from loved ones. When severe, it may be necessary to use minor tranquillisers such as chlordiazepoxide or diazepam, but this should only be regarded as a short-term measure to render the patient accessible to a psychotherapeutic approach.

Psychotherapy includes ensuring that the patient has a realistic understanding of his illness. Where somatic factors are prominent in the genesis of the pain, and particularly where a carcinoma is involved, the patient should be allowed to ventilate his fears so that they can be discussed and placed in perspective. While it may not always be possible or appropriate to convince a patient that his ideas about his pathology are grossly distorted, it should be possible to provide reassurance that he will not be abandoned to his fate and that adequate medication will be provided at all times. The issues involved in the management of cancer-related pain have been well discussed by Saunders (1981).

Anger and resentment are affects which cannot be ignored because they may completely block effective communication with a patient if their existence is not acknowledged and accepted. This may be particularly difficult when a substantial part of the anger is displaced on to the doctor and other care-givers. In this case the patient may be guilty, anxious and ashamed as having such feelings towards those on whom he relies and from whom he expects so much. In many ways, it is safest for clinicians always to assume that such feelings may be present and to facilitate their ventilation. Above all, it is crucial not to regard feelings of anger purely as a consequence of the patient's unique perception of the situation, but to make every effort to establish any basis in reality for such feelings of hostility and resentment. There are patients who are so inhibited in their interpersonal relationships that they hesitate to convey their inner thoughts and emotions at the best of times. When ill, they may simply not inform others of the degree of pain they are suffering for fear that this will make them a focus of concern and perhaps invite physical examinations, which they find difficult to tolerate because of the sense of shame and humiliation they provoke.

BEHAVIOURAL ASPECTS

The relationship between what patients think and feel and the way they behave is not always straightforward. There are a number of reasons for this, but at the simplest level it may result from not having the doctor's (or family's) permission to take certain actions. Patients in pain sometimes want the doctor to tell them, at least once, what they must do, when they ought to do it, how often and how to tell when to stop. In other words, a patient in pain may be required to cooperate in treatment by developing skills and behaviours which he has not previously possessed or utilised. It should perhaps be emphasised that here one is not discussing the need to reshape the maladaptive behaviours shown by some patients but rather the need to faciliate the use of behavioural strategies which the patient may be only too ready to adopt. It is not uncommon for clinical staff to take for granted the patient's readiness and ability to assimilate and carry out the procedures which are a simple and routine part of their own daily work, such as changing dressings or dispensing tablets. However, when confidence is uncertain, fingers untrained or arthritic, and visual acuity less than perfect, even taking a tablet can be a problem. None of this is to say that patients should be flooded with information about everything they should or should not do every moment of the day, but that, apart from the initial presentation of facts, opportunities should be made available for patients to ask questions about their behaviours as they arise throughout the illness cycle. Some of this information may be more usefully and efficiently acquired in patient education groups or mutual-support associations such as exist in a number of centres. It is noteworthy that 'chronic pain associations' have been initiated in some communities, and it is important that clinicians maintain contact with them.

It should also be stressed that those in the patient's social setting may also need to be informed as to what the patient can and ought to do and, perhaps as importantly, what they can do to ensure that the convalescent phase of the illness does not evolve into unnecessary or excessive invalidism. In discussing these matters with the relatives, it is helpful to learn about their own views of the illness and their previous experiences of pain. A clinical episode which illustrated this point involved a factory worker who had badly injured his back but had come to terms with his residual impairment and discomfort. He was, nonetheless, referred to a pain clinic for further investigation, mainly at the urging of his wife who was extremely dependent on him as a companion. It emerged that her own father had sustained a back injury in the course of his work as a miner and had subsequently died of cancer. She believed the cancer to have been a consequence of the accident and was deeply concerned that the same outcome would befall her husband. In this case, it was she who needed explanation and reassurance so that she could accept her husband's attitude to his disability.

Overt behaviours on the patient's part can have an impact on his relationships which can, in turn, impede his ability to cope. For example, it is well known to patients that if their pain leads them to display irritability and to withdraw from others, they will find that they are increasingly isolated by their family and friends at a time when they particularly need support. Most patients are well aware of this and are able to communicate that nice mixture of displeasure at one's own illness and pleasure at the company and concern of others, so that there is no suggestion that the benefits of the sick role are being unfairly exploited. Some patients may not be aware of the fact that they are alienating others and need to be counselled. When their behaviours are not overly determined by unconscious motivations, they are usually able to modify their attitudes to others and avoid unnecessary alienation from social contacts and supports. They soon learn that, when friends ask after their health, they are generally seeking only a brief summary of the situation.

ABNORMAL ILLNESS BEHAVIOUR

In certain patients, the pain complaint represents a manifestation of illness behaviour which is part of an abnormal psychopathological state. It is helpful to place the 'abnormal illness behaviours' (AIB) or 'dysnosognosias' within the sociocultural framework provided by the 'sick role' concept of Parsons (1964). The sick role is conditionally granted to individuals who show evidence of a disordered state of body or mind over which they have no control and which brings them little benefit compared with the suffering and loss of customary pleasures they are experiencing. Those accorded the sick role are exempted from the discharge of their usual duties to an extent appropriate to the nature of their disease. For a period of time, therefore, the individual is granted special privileges, but these are graded and withdrawn by degrees as the disease resolves.

The patient is also expected to accept certain obligations and to display certain attitudes. In particular, the sick person is expected to show that he regards the sick role as undesirable and to confirm this by his efforts to divest himself of it. This requires him to seek the help of an appointed agent of society in diagnosing and treating his condition. In most industrialised societies this means that a doctor must be consulted; his task is to diagnose, treat and legitimise the sick role and to ensure in every way possible that its cost to the micro-and macrosociety is kept to a minimum.

With the sick-role concept in mind, we may regard illness as a property or attribute of a person which entitles him to 'sick-role units'. 'Illness' can, therefore, be operationally defined as 'an organismic state which fulfils the requirements of a relevant reference group for admission to the sick role' (Pilowsky 1978). In this sense, 'illness' is regarded as a currency, which is generally accepted in exchange for goods and services required to achieve health. This distinguishes illness from 'disease', which refers to the agreed objective pattern of features which form the basis of an illness. Quite often it is some time before what is considered a 'disease' by medical science is accepted as 'illness' by society.

In the case of AIB, there is a disagreement between patient and doctor as to the nature of the sick role to which the patient is entitled. In the case of chronic pain, the situation is generally one in which the patient demands or uses more sick-role units than the doctor thinks he should. AIB is defined as:

> the persistence of an inappropriate or maladaptive mode of perceiving, evaluating and acting in relation to one's own state of health, despite the fact that a doctor (or other appropriate social agent) has offered a reasonably lucid and accurate explanation of the nature of the illness and the appropriate course of management to be followed, with opportunities of discussion, negotiation and clarification, based on a thorough examination and assessment of all parameters of functioning (including the use of special investigations where necessary), and taking into account the individual's age, educational and sociocultural background (Pilowsky 1969, 1978, 1990).

AIB itself is only considered an illness when the motivation appears predominantly unconscious. When conscious, it is labelled 'malingering'. There are forms of AIB in which the patient denies the presence of illness and refuses treatment despite advice to the contrary, but these syndromes will not be discussed here since they are rarely problems associated with pain, although some patients do ignore pain and thus delay early diagnosis and treatment. (Pilowsky 1978, 1990; Strauss et al 1990).

It is also extremely important to distinguish between illness behaviours which are abnormal and those which are anomalous, atypical or unusual, but are not necessarily maladaptive and are not associated with an inability to negotiate with doctors.

Unconsciously motivated AIB in which illness is affirmed can be grouped into psychotic and neurotic forms. In the psychotic forms, the patient's belief in the presence of physical pathology is delusional. Such hypochondriacal delusions may be part of a depressive or a schizophrenic psychosis.

Hypochondriacal delusions that occur with a *depressive psychosis* often take the form of a fixed, unshakeable belief in the presence of cancer. The patient may believe that his bowels are blocked and that they are rotting within. However, the patient may not volunteer these beliefs spontaneously, and simply appear withdrawn and depressed, or complain only of pain. Indeed, in some patients with hypochondriacal delusions, the depression may not be particularly obvious. On the other hand, some patients are extremely agitated and constantly seek reassurance about their health.

Hypochondriacal or somatic delusions associated with *schizophrenia* may be bizarre and part of a wider delusional system. Thus a patient may believe that his liver is being damaged by radar waves beamed on it from a distance. Occasionally, a hypochondriacal delusion may be the patient's only obvious symptom (monosymptomatic hypochondriasis).

The treatment of psychotic hypochondriacal ideas depends on the nature of the syndrome of which they are a symptom, and this cannot be discussed in detail here. In general terms, one may say that, in the case of psychotic depression, the antidepressant drugs and electroconvulsive therapy are key treatments, while in schizophrenia, major tranquillisers are generally effective. In the case of monosymptomatic hypochondriasis, Pimozide has been found to be particularly useful.

NEUROTIC ABNORMAL ILLNESS BEHAVIOUR

There are two major forms of neurotic AIB which commonly present with pain as a leading symptom. These are hypochondriacal disorders and conversion disorders.

Hypochondriacal disorders

Hypochondriacal reactions are characterised by an overconcern with health which is out of proportion to the degree of objective pathology present. A factor-analytic study of hypochondriasis showed that three dimensions may be discerned as contributing in various combinations to the clinical form of a hypochondriacal illness (Pilowsky 1967). These emerged from a principal components analysis of the responses of 200 patients to a questionnaire, and were described as:

1. a phobic attitude to illness
2. a conviction as to the presence of disease associated with a nonresponsiveness to reassurance
3. a preoccupation with bodily symptoms.

These findings accord well with clinical anecdotal evidence as to the hypochondriacal patterns which patients may present. The phobic form of hypochondriasis is associated with feelings of anxiety and the patient's concerns may be focused on the physiological concomitants of anxiety. Thus, they are fearful that chest pains and palpitations are indicative of cardiac disease or that headaches mean a brain tumour. Usually, such patients have insight into the irrational nature of their fears, but in periods of extreme arousal their insight may be less apparent.

The other major form of hypochondriasis presents itself as an abnormal preoccupation with health and disease. Here the patients are not concerned about diseases that might befall them in the future, but rather with the symptoms they are presently aware of. The affect is one of the overconcern rather than anxiety. It is a feature of the presentation that these patients appear far more comfortable discussing their symptoms than any other problems in their lives.

The aetiology of hypochondriacal disorders is multifactorial in nature with a number of predisposing and precipitating variables involved. Patients may report a childhood in which they were regarded as frail and unwell, with frequent absences from school (Pilowsky et al 1982a) There may also have been an invalid parent who served as a model for illness behaviour.

Any stress may precipitate hypochondriasis, especially where a loss is involved. Hypochondriasis has the effect of allowing withdrawal from responsibilities, dependence on others, punishment of the self (and thus the assuagement of guilt), and the direction of hostility at others, including doctors, by the use of complaints and nonresponsiveness. The response to treatment in hypochondriasis is better when depression or anxiety are prominent, and when the history is short. In patients who have been ill for some time, who have seen many doctors and received many treatments, the prognosis is less good. Older men with a long history have a poor outcome; younger women described as having hysterical personalities also do badly (Pilowsky 1968).

On the other hand, it should be borne in mind that although they hypochondriacal fears and concerns may not disappear completely, patients may be able to cope reasonably well in their social and work settings supported by a psychotherapeutic relationship at times combined with a behavioural approach aimed at discouraging invalidism (Fordyce 1976).

Conversion disorders

These differ from hypochondriacal reactions in that the patient denies preoccupations or fears about illness, but rather complains of pain and its consequences. Classical conversion symptoms, such as motor paralysis, are apparently less common now than they once were, and pain seems to be the most frequent form of conversion disorder (Ziegler et al 1960; Ziegler & Imboden 1962). Indeed, the third edition of the Diagnostic and Statistical Manual (DSM-III) of the American Psychiatric Association (1980) included a new diagnosis of 'psychogenic pain disorder' for which the criteria are virtually the same as for conversion disorder. In the revised DSM-IIIR it is referred to as 'somatoform pain disorder'.

Although it is useful to consider hypochondriasis and conversion reactions as separate AIB syndromes, it must be acknowledged that many patients with chronic pain show a mixture of features, such that a diagnosis of 'abnormal illness behaviour' seems a useful diagnostic term in its own right. Furthermore, it is useful in these circumstances to evaluate the various components of the illness behaviour separately so as to arrive at an illness behaviour profile of the patient. This can be done clinically by assessing the patient's condition under the following headings which form the Illness Behaviour Assessment Schedule (IBAS) (Pilowsky et al 1983). Such a structured interview can also serve as a method for screening patients for research or epidemiological purposes. The IBAS is a method for establishing the congruence between the patient's and the doctor's views of the patient's health status. It can serve as an interviewing guide or checklist to ensure that areas relevant to the diagnosis of abnormal illness behaviour are covered, while also providing information concerning ideation and affect. Thus the IBAS evaluates the patient's perception of the information he has received and his acceptance of it (Items 1–6), his conceptualisation of the type of illness he has (Items 7–8), his awareness of symptoms and associated preoccupations or phobic attitudes (Items 9–11), his ideas about aetiology (Item 12), his affect state and the extent to which somatic illness is being used defensively (Items 13–19). While the IBAS uses the patient's recall of the explanation received as the yardstick against which to match his own ideas about health, it may often be the case in practice that the explanation was provided by the doctor who is actually assessing the patient's illness behaviour.

It may be seen that these items offer a basis on which to

establish whether a patient is showing clearcut AIB and what the phenomenology associated with it is.

The IBAS also allows affects to be assessed (Items 14 and 15) as well as the causes to which they are attributed. This is an important aspect of the evaluation because a distinction should be made between depression and anxiety which are part of depressive or anxiety syndromes, and affects which are part of a conversion or hypochondriacal reaction. Patients with the latter conditions, i.e. AIB, will often make complaints of depression and other psychological distress which may lead the clinician to conclude that the patient has a depressive illness. However, the patient is usually not consistently depressed and attributes the dysphoria chiefly to physical problems. The relationship between chronic pain and depression has not been entirely clarified, but recent studies suggest that it should not be regarded simply as a form of depressive illness (Pilowsky & Bassett 1982a; Roy et al 1984, Pilowsky 1988).

THE ILLNESS BEHAVIOUR QUESTIONNAIRE (IBQ)

Another approach to the assessment of patients' illness behaviour is by use of the Illness Behaviour Questionnaire (IBQ). This is a 62-item self-report questionnaire which has the advantage of not requiring an interview for its administration.

The IBQ (Pilowsky & Spence 1975, 1981) was developed from the Whiteley Index (WI) of hypochondriasis (Pilowsky 1967). In its first form of 52 items it was administered to 100 pain clinic patients and a principal component analysis was performed (Pilowsky & Spence 1975). Seven scales were constructed based on the interpretable factors which emerged. Ten items were later added to expand some of the shorter scales to a minimum of five items. The IBQ and the WI have been widely used for clinical and research purposes. Examples include studies by Metcalf et al (1988) on neurological inpatients; Jensen (1988) on pain in nonpsychotic psychiatric patients; Colgan et al (1988) on the effects of personality on pain and illness behaviour; Gourlay et al (1989) on the treatment of postoperative pain; Smith et al (1990) on the irritable bowel syndrome; Waddell et al (1989) on the assessment of low back pain and its response to treatment; and Miller & Hafner (1991) on medical visits and psychological disturbance in chronic low-back pain. Others have found the IBQ a useful item pool for new scales. For instance, Robbins et al (1990) have used 10 items as an 'Illness Worry Scale' in a study of the fibromyalgia syndrome.

Interestingly Barsky et al (1991) have demonstrated the usefulness of the Whiteley Index in a general medical setting, as an acceptable and economical screening instrument for psychiatric illness, i.e. anxiety and depression.

The names and descriptions of the IBQ scales are as follows:

1. **General hypochondriasis** (GH)

High scorers on this scale have a fearful or phobic attitude to illness, with some insight into the inappropriateness of these attitudes and a high level of arousal or anxiety.

2. **Disease conviction** (DC)

High scores indicate a strong affirmation as to the presence of physical illness and a resistance to reassurance by doctors.

3. **Psychological versus somatic focusing** (P/S)

High scores indicate a tendency to blame oneself for the illness and to be accepting of the need for psychiatric help. A low score indicates a rejection of the possibility that psychological factors are important and a tendency to focus on somatic problems.

4. **Affective inhibition** (AI)

High scores indicate difficulty in expressing personal feelings (especially negative ones) to others.

5. **Affective disturbance** (AD)

A high score indicates the presence of feelings or anxiety and depression.

6. **Denial** (D)

High scores on this scale indicate that the subject denies current life problems and, in addition, attributes the current situation entirely to physical illness.

7. **Irritability** (I)

High scores on this scale indicate feelings of anger and an awareness of interpersonal friction.

In addition to scores on the seven scales, the IBQ also provides scores on two second-order factors (AS and DA) and a discriminant function. The second-order factors have been named affective state (GH + AD +I) and disease affirmation (DC +(S-P/S)).

The discriminant function (DF) provides an index of the extent to which a conversion illness is present. It is derived from a comparison of a population of pain clinic patients (mostly with psychogenic pain disorders) and a population of unselected general practice patients. The function is a weighted combination of the scores on DC, P/S, AI, D and a constant, such that a high score indicates the likelihood that the patient shows abnormal illness behaviour of the conversion type.

The original WI items embedded in the IBQ provide a score indicating the degree to which hypochondriacal concerns and fears are present. The IBQ has been used extensively in the study of chronic pain syndromes and other conditions (Byrne & Whyte 1975; Pilowsky & Spence 1975; Chapman et al 1979; Gross et al 1980; Wise & Rosenthal 1982). The clinical utility of the instrument has been demonstrated by Keefe et al (1986), Feuerstein et al (1985) and Waddell et al (1989). In a study of more than 1000 subjects, Zonderman et al (1985) have essentially confirmed the factor structure of the IBQ and demonstrated the importance of the disease conviction scale in identifying pain clinic patients.

In order to illustrate its use in the evaluation of chronic pain, it may be helpful to examine the profiles of three representative patients.

THE ILLNESS BEHAVIOUR ASSESSMENT SCHEDULE

1. *Recall of explanations received concerning illness*
   (a) Patient says he has never received any explanation
   (b) Patient is not sure whether he has received any explanation
   (c) Patient recalls having received an explanation
2. *Interviewer's assessment of whether explanation was given*
   (a) Given (b) Uncertain (c) Not given
3. *Person who is believed or known to have given explanation*
   (a) Interviewer (b) Other
4. *Type of explanation recalled by patient*
   (a) Recalls being told there is nothing wrong at all
   (b) Recalls being told he has a minor illness, i.e. not likely to be threatening or disabling
   (c) Recalls being told he has a major illness, i.e. likely to be life-threatening or seriously disabling
   (d) Recalls more than one (different) explanation of his illness
   Not applicable (no causal explanation recalled)
5. *Type of causal explanation recalled by patient*
   (a) Patient recalls being told the illness is entirely due to somatic causes
   (b) Patient recalls being told the illness is due to a combination of somatic and psychological causes
   (c) Patient recalls being told the problems are entirely due to psychological (nonphysical) causes
   Not applicable (no causal explanation recalled)
6. *Patient's response to explanation recalled*
   (a) Accepts it completely
   (b) Accepts it partially
   (c) Rejects explanation completely
   Not applicable (no explanation recalled)
7. *Disease conviction (affirmation) – somatic*
   (a) Patient expresses certainty as to presence of specific somatic disease or pathology
   (b) Patient expresses some uncertainty as to presence of somatic disease or pathology
   (c) Patient expresses certainty as to absence of any specific somatic disease or pathology
8. *Disease conviction (affirmation) – psychological*
   (a) Patient expresses certainty as to presence of a psychological disorder
   (b) Patient expresses some uncertainty as to presence of a psychological disorder
   (c) Patient expresses certainty as to absence of a psychological disorder
9. *Symptom awareness*
   (a) Absent
   (b) Patient is aware of symptoms 50% of the time or less
   (c) Awareness of symptoms present more than 50% of the time but not constantly
   (d) Patient is constantly aware of symptoms
10. *Disease phobia – the patient reports anxious thoughts about specific disease(s) (e.g. cancer, heart attack) but feels they are unreasonable or unwarranted*
   (a) Absent
   (b) Present 50% or less of the time
   (c) Present 50% or more of the time but not constantly
11. Preoccupation with disease – patient is preoccupied with thoughts of specific disease(s) and does not regard them as irrational or unwarranted
   (a) Absent
   (b) Present 50% or less of the time
   (c) Present 50% or more of the time (but not constantly)
   (d) Present constantly
12. *Illness – causal beliefs*
   (a) Psychological: patient believes illness is a consequence of environmental and/or interpersonal stress
   (b) Mixed: patient regards illness as caused by a combination or psychological and physical factors
   (c) Somatic: patient regards illness as purely somatic and unrelated to non-physical stresses
   Not applicable
13. *Communication of affects and feelings*
   (a) Communicates affect readily
   (b) Mild inhibition: patient is inhibited about communicating feelings to others but can do so with some effort
   (c) Moderate inhibition: patient is only slightly inhibited about communicating feelings to others

(d) Marked inhibition: patient is virtually unable to express feelings to others

14. *Anxiety*
   (a) Absent
   (b) Mild: patient is aware of some feelings of vague apprehension but no physical discomforts
   (c) Moderate: feelings of apprehension are present about 50% of the time and associated with physical symptoms such as palpitations, dyspnoea, tremor and dry mouth
   (d) Marked: feelings of apprehension with physical symptoms present constantly
15. *Depression*
   (a) Absent
   (b) Mild: some occasional feelings of despondency
   (c) Moderate: patient feels sad and low-spirited more than 50% of the time but not constantly
   (d) Marked: constant feelings of despondency and sadness
16. *Attribution of affective disturbance*
   (a) Disturbance of affect attributed to environmental or interpersonal stresses
   (b) Disturbance of affect attributed to both environmental and somatic stresses
   (c) Disturbance of affect attributed entirely to somatic problems

   Not applicable (no affective disturbance reported)
17. *Denial (of current life problems)*
   (a) Absent: current life problems and difficulties are freely acknowledged
   (b) Partial: some tendency to deny life problems at first but these are acknowledged when complete absence is questioned in a neutral tone
   (c) Complete: absence of life problems maintained, even when challenged
18. *Displacement (attribution of current life problems to somatic problems)*
   (a) Absent: current life problems acknowledged and regarded as independent of somatic problems
   (b) Partial: current life problems acknowledged and partially attributed to somatic problems
   (c) Complete: current life problems acknowledged and totally attributed to physical problems

   Not applicable
19. *Irritability*
   (a) Absent
   (b) Mild: some tendency to respond excessively to mildly noxious inputs
   (c) Moderate: responds excessively to mildly noxious inputs, but can still tolerate others. Experiences substantial interpersonal friction due to the nature of own reaction to others.
   (d) Marked: reacts aversively and excessively to even the mildest of inputs.

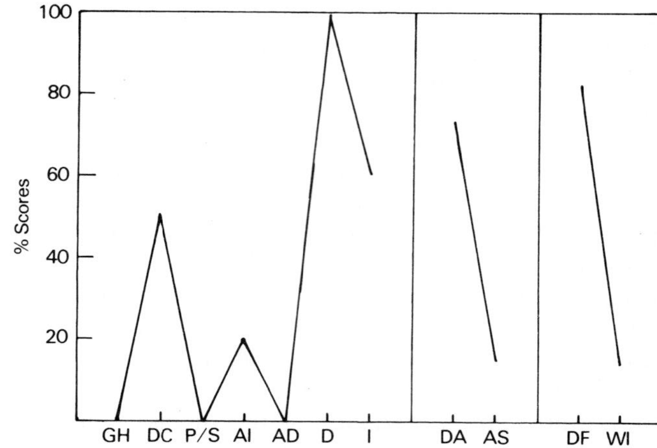

Fig. 72.1 Illness Behaviour Questionnaire profile: Patient One.

Key
GH General hypochondriasis
DC Disease conviction
P/S Psychological (high score) vs somatic focusing
AI Affective inhibition
AD Affective disturbance
D Denial
I Irritability
DA Disease affirmation
AS Affective state
DF Discriminant function (likelihood of a conversion reaction)
WI Whiteley Index (likelihood of a hypochondriacal syndrome)

Patient one

Figure 72.1 shows the IBQ profile of a 51-year-old woman who had been involved in a car accident 8 years before presentation to a pain clinic. She complained of continuous neck pain radiating down her left arm following a cervical laminectomy performed 1 year after the accident.

The IBQ profile reveals high scores on DC and D, indicating that physical illness is being strongly affirmed, while other problems are denied and all difficulties attributed to the physical disorder. The low P/S score indicates the rejection of a psychological perspective and the low AD score indicates that anxiety and depression are being completely denied. The low WI score indicates that hypochondriacal attitudes are not prominent. The second-order factor scores provide support for the profile interpretation and the discriminant score suggests a high probability of a conversion disorder.

Patient two

Figure 72.2 shows the IBQ profile of a 29-year-old woman who presented with a number of somatic complaints, including difficulties with swallowing and breathing. She was depressed and reported tension in her home between herself and her family.

The IBQ profile indicates the presence of hypochondriacal fears and concerns (high GH and WI), but with some insight into their inappropriateness. Physical disease is

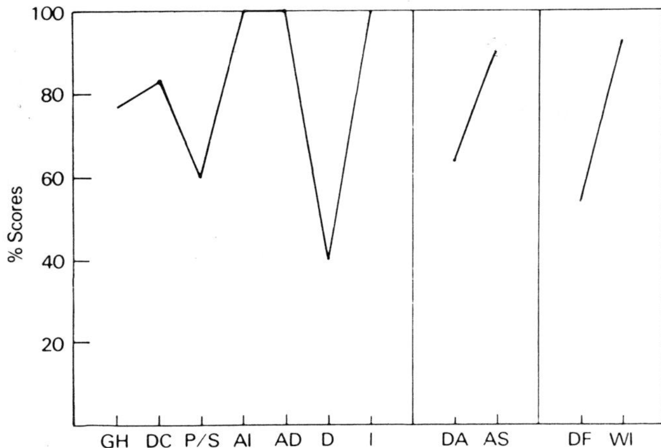

Fig. 72.2 Illness Behaviour Questionnaire profile: Patient Two. Key as in Fig. 72.1

being affirmed (high DC), but to some extent a psychological perspective is being accepted (high P/S). Marked anxiety, depression and irritability, with interpersonal friction, are being acknowledged (high AD and high I). Current life problems are being reported (low D score). The discriminant score indicates a low probability of a conversion reaction. Overall, the profile suggests a dysphoric illness with hypochondriacal features. The possibility of an endogenous component to the depression must be considered. (It is significant that this patient reported that her mother and sister had both been treated for depression in the past.)

Patient three

Figures 72.3 presents the IBQ profile of a 40-year-old male truck driver who become depressed and complained of pain following treatment for a fractured ankle. He reported longstanding psychosocial problems and he was

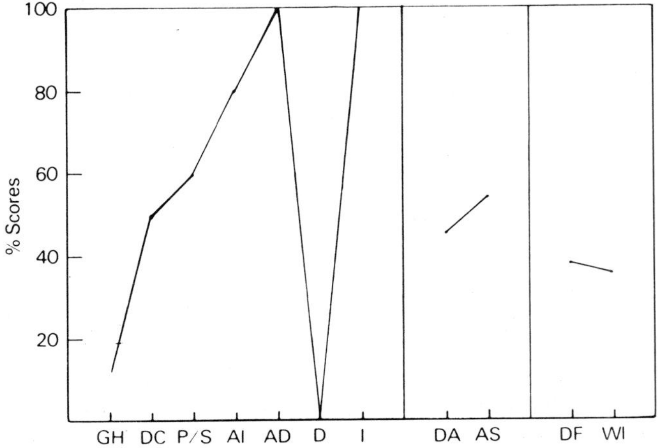

Fig. 72.3 Illness Behaviour Questionnaire profile: Patient Three. Key as in Fig.72.1

extremely dependent on his work to allay feelings of sexual and more general inadequacy.

The IBQ profile indicates marked affective disturbance (high AD) which is attributed to current life stress (low D). The discriminant score suggests a very low probability of a conversion reaction. Overall, the picture is consistent with a reactive depression in which pain is not serving a conversion function.

THE TREATMENT OF NEUROTIC ABNORMAL ILLNESS BEHAVIOUR

The major forms of treatment available for the neurotic forms of AIB are psychotherapeutic, psychopharmacological and behavioural, and they are commonly used in combination.

PSYCHOTHERAPEUTIC APPROACHES

The effectiveness of psychotherapy in the management of chronic pain syndromes is not entirely clear since relatively little research has been conducted in the area (Pilowsky & Bassett 1982b). Psychotherapy with such patients inevitably differs from conventional psychotherapy in that there must be a preparedness of move comfortably between a somatic and psychological universe of discourse. Psychotherapy is probably easier if carried out with the support of a multidisciplinary pain clinic which has thoroughly assessed the patient's needs and recommended treatment priorities. The clinic should also be available for reviewing problems as they arise during the course of psychotherapy (Bellissimo & Tunks 1984).

It would seem wisest to discuss the length of psychotherapy with the patient before embarking on a course of treatment, and it seems a reasonable approach to plan about 12 weekly sessions, each of 45 minutes' duration, as the average period of brief psychotherapy. At the completion of the series, progress can be reviewed and further treatment decided on. It is not possible in the space available to describe the treatment in any detail. However, it may be said that patients seem to find a cognitive–dynamic approach acceptable in that it includes clarification, explanation, support, and interpretation of the transference when appropriate (Pilowsky & Bassett 1982b). Furthermore, this approach has been shown in a comparative trial on a small group of pain clinic patients to be more effective in producing improved coping than brief supportive contacts (Bassett & Pilowsky 1985).

PSYCHOPHARMACOLOGICAL

Patients may be helped by the use of antidepressants. It has been suggested that the tricyclics, especially those blocking serotonin reuptake, may enhance the effectiveness of the endogenous pain-suppressing pathways. This may be so, but clinical experience suggests that dramatic responses to tricyclics occur only when there is reasonably strong evidence that the patient has symptoms of a depressive illness with endogenous features such as sleeplessness, loss of weight and psychomotor retardation (Hameroff et al 1985). Nonetheless, it may be reasonable to give patients a trial of tricyclics for up to 6 weeks, possibly in lower doses than one would ordinarily use (Pilowsky et al 1982b). This can be done by increasing the dose very gradually in an attempt to avoid side-effects and consequent noncompliance (Sternbach 1974).

COMBINED PSYCHOTHERAPY AND PSYCHOPHARMACOLOGY

Many patients are treated in outpatient clinics with combinations of psychotherapy and a tricyclic depressant such as amitriptyline. The effectiveness of this combination was investigated by Pilowsky & Barrow (1990). The main findings were that amitriptyline (AMI) was effective in improving activity levels and reducing pain intensity. Psychotherapy (consisting of 12 weekly sessions of psychodynamically oriented psychotherapy) increased pain intensity but also improved productivity. There was a complex interaction between psychotherapy and AMI in that those on supportive 'psychotherapy' (six fortnightly 15 minute sessions over 12 weeks) did better with regard to activity levels if on AMI rather than placebo. Those on AMI did worse if also receiving the higher contact psychotherapy.

COGNITIVE BEHAVIOURAL THERAPY

This approach has been well described by Fordyce (1976). Although one may not always apply it intensively to patients, for one reason or another, the insights provided by Fordyce can be applied in advising patients how to increase their activities gradually and how to prevent the relatives from reinforcing their invalidism. In patients with AIB it is particularly important not to apply behavioural methods in a mechanical way, or without fully involving the patient in planning the treatment programme. Simply ignoring the patient's pain complaints and encouraging his family to do the same can lead to severe depression and possibly suicidal behaviour. However, used in the context of a multidisciplinary approach cognitive behavioural therapy appears to have an important part to play, although we need to know a great deal more about patient–treatment interactions (Keefe 1984).

An interesting recent development has been the renewed interest in treating hypochondriacal disorders in outpatient groups using a combination of educational and cognitive methods (Barsky et al 1988; House 1989). The need to allow for a careful transitional phase of therapy, during which a new way of thinking about the illness (i.e. from both physical and psychosocial viewpoints) is introduced to the patient, is now recognised as a particularly important aspect of the therapeutic process.

CONCLUSION

It is important to assess a patient's illness behaviour as early as possible, and in particular to diagnose AIB. The sooner this is done, the less likely the doctor–patient relationship is to be placed under strain, with all the problems that inevitably follow. Quite often, the only effective way to manage AIB is in the context of a multidisciplinary pain clinic, since these patients may require care from more than one professional. Each of these will function far more effectively if all other aspects of the illness have been delineated and shared between pain clinic personnel. This would seem to be the only way to prevent what results when such patients are referred from one specialist to another without adequate collation of findings and coordination of therapies. Indeed, the patient with AIB presents one of the best arguments for the existence of pain clinics. However, once fully assessed, patients judged to have a long-term problem can be managed by a physician who is prepared to see them regularly, take symptoms seriously and not succumb to an irrational fear or malingering (Pilowsky 1985).

REFERENCES

American Psychiatric Association 1980 Diagnostic and statistical manual of mental disorders, 3rd edn. American Psychiatric Institution, Washington (revised 1987)

Barsky A J, Geringer E, Wood C A 1988 A cognitive–educational treatment programme for hypochondriasis. General Hospital Psychiatry 10: 322–327

Barsky A, Wyshak G, Klerman G L 1991 Comparison of psychiatric screening tests in a general medical setting using ROC analysis. Medical Care 29: 775–785

Bassett D L, Pilowsky I 1985 A study of brief psychotherapy for chronic pain. Journal of Psychosomatic Research 29: 259–264

Bellissimo A, Tunks E 1982 Individual psychotherapy for chronic pain. In: Roy R, Tunks E (eds) Chronic pain. Psychosocial factors in rehabilitation. Williams & Wilkins, Baltimore

Bellissimo A, Tunks E 1984 Chronic pain. The psychotherapeutic spectrum. Praeger, New York

Byrne D, Whyte H 1975 Dimensions of illness behaviour in survivors of myocardial infarction. Journal of Psychosomatic Research 26: 317–321

Chapman C R, Sola A E, Bonica J J 1979 Illness behaviour and depression compared in pain center and private practice patients. Pain 6: 1–7

Colgan S, Creed F, Klass H 1988 Symptom complaints, psychiatric disorder and abnormal illness behaviour in patients with upper abdominal pain. Psychological Medicine 18: 887–892

Engel G L 1959 Psychogenic pain and pain-prone patient. American Journal of Medicine 26: 899–918

Feinmann C 1985 Pain relief by antidepressants: possible modes of action. Pain 32: 1–8

Feuerstein M, Greenwald M, Gamache M P, Papciak A S Cook E W

1985 The pain behaviour scale: modification and validation for outpatient use. Journal of Psychopathology and Behavioural Assessment 7: 301–315
Fordyce W E 1976 Behavioural methods for chronic pain and illness. C V Mosby, St Louis.
Gourlay G K, Kowalski S R, Plummer J L et al 1989 The transdermal administration of fentanyl in the treatment of post-operative pain: pharmacokinetics and pharmacodynamic effects. Pain 37: 193–202
Gross R I, Doerr H, Caldirola D, Guzinski G Ripley H S 1980 Borderline personality syndrome and incest in chronic pelvic pain patients. International Journal of Psychiatry in Medicine 10: 79–96
Hameroff S R, Cork R C, Weiss J L, Crago B R, Davis T P 1985 Doxepin effects on chronic pain and depression: a controlled study. In: Fields H L, Dubner R, Cervero F (eds) Advances in pain research and therapy, vol 9. Raven Press, New York
Harkins S W, Price D D, Briath J 1989 Effects of extraversion and neuroticism on experimental pain, clinical pain, and illness behaviour. Pain 36: 209–218
House A 1989 Hypochondriasis and related disorders: assessment and management of patients referred for a psychiatric opinion. General Hospital Psychiatry 11; 156–165
Jensen J 1988 Pain in non-psychotic psychiatric patients: life events, symptomatology and personality traits. Acta Psychiatrica Scandinavica 78: 201–207
Keefe F J 1984 Research methods in behavioural medicine. In: Bellack A S, Hersen M (eds) Research methods in clinical psychology. Pergamon Press, New York
Keefe F J, Crisson J E, Maltbie A, Bradley L, Gil M 1986 Illness behaviour as a predictor or pain and overt behaviour patterns in chronic low back pain patients. Journal of Psychosomatic Research 30: 543–552
Mechanic D 1962 The concept of illness behaviour. Journal of Chronic Disease 156: 189–194.
Metcalf R, Firth D, Creed F 1988 Psychiatric morbidity and illness behaviour in female neurological inpatients. Journal of Neurology, Neurosurgery and Psychiatry 51: 1387–1390
Miller R J, Hafner R J 1991 Medical visits and psychological disturbance in chronic low back pain. A study of a back education class. Psychosomatics 32: 309–316
Parsons T 1964 Social structure and personality. Collier Macmillan, London.
Petrie A 1960 Some psychological aspects of pain and the relief of suffering. Annals of the New York Academy of Sciences 86: 13–27
Pilowsky I 1967 Dimensions of hypochondriasis. British Journal of Psychiatry 113: 89–93
Pilowsky I 1968 The response to treatment in hypochondriacal disorders. Australian and New Zealand Journal of Psychiatry 2: 88–94
Pilowsky I 1969 Abnormal illness behaviour. British Journal of Medical Psychology 42: 347–351
Pilowsky I 1978 A general classification of abnormal illness behaviours. British Journal of Medical Psychology 51:131–137
Pilowsky I 1985 Malingerophobia. Medical Journal of Australia 143: 571–572
Pilowsky I 1990 The concept of abnormal illness behaviour. Psychosomatics 31: 207–213
Pilowsky I, Barrow C G 1990 A controlled study of psychotherapy used individually and in combination in the treatment of chronic intractable, 'psychogenic' pain. Pain 40: 3–19
Pilowsky I, Bassett D L 1982 Pain and depression. British Journal of Psychiatry 141: 30–36
Pilowsky I, Bassett D L 1982b The place of individual psychotherapy in the treatment of chronic pain patients. In: Roy R, Tunks E (eds) Chronic pain. Psychosocial factors in rehabilitation. Williams & Wilkins, Baltimore
Pilowsky I, Spence N D 1975 Patterns of illness behaviour in patients with intractable pain. Journal of Psychosomatic Research 19: 279–287
Pilowsky I, Spence N D 1981 Manual for the illness behaviour questionnaire (IBQ). University of Adelaide, Adelaide.
Pilowsky I, Bassett D L, Begg M W, Thomas P G 1982a Childhood hospitalisation and chronic intractable pain in adults: a controlled retrospective study. International Journal of Psychiatry in Medicine 12: 75–84
Pilowsky I, Hallett E C, Bassett D L, Thomas P G, Penhall R K 1982b A controlled study of amitriptyline in the treatment of chronic pain. Pain 14: 169–179
Pilowsky I, Bassett D, Barrett R, Petrovic L, Minniti R 1983 The illness behaviour assessment schedule: reliability and validity. International Journal of Psychiatry in Medicine 13: 11–28
Robbins J M, Kirmayer L J, Kapusta M A 1990 Illness worry and disability in Fibromyalgia Syndrome. International Journal of Psychiatry in Medicine 20: 49–63
Roy R, Thomas M, Matas S 1984 Chronic pain and depression: a review. Comprehensive Psychiatry 25: 96–105
Saunders C 1981 Current views on pain relief and terminal care. In: Swerdlow M (ed) The therapy of pain. MTP Press, Lancester
Schilder P 1950 The image and appearance of the human body. International Universities Press, New York
Smith R C, Greenbaum D S, Vancouver J B et al 1990 Psychosocial factors are associated with health care seeking rather than diagnosis in irritable bowel syndrome. Gastroenterology 98: 293–301
Sternbach R A 1974 Pain patients. Traits and treatment. Academic Press, New York
Strauss D H, Spitzer R L, Muskin P R 1990 Maladaptive denial of physical illness: a proposal for DSM-IV. American Journal of Psychiatry 147: 1168–1172
Waddell G, Pilowsky I, Bond M R 1984 Clinical assessment and interpretation of abnormal illness behaviour in low back pain. Pain 32: 309–316
Wise T N, Rosenthal J B 1982 Depression, illness beliefs and severity of illness. Journal of Psychosomatic Research 26: 247–253
Ziegler F J, Imboden J B 1962 Contemporary conversion reactions. II. A conceptual model. Archives of General Psychiatry 6: 279–287
Ziegler F J, Imboden J B, Myer E 1960 Contemporay conversion reactions: a clinical study. American Journal of Psychiatry 116: 901–909
Zonderman A B, Heft M W, Costa P T Jr 1985 Does the Illness Behavior Questionnaire measure abnormal illness behavior? Health Psychology 4: 425–436

73. Relaxation and biofeedback

Barton A. Jessup and Xochitl Gallegos

INTRODUCTION

Both relaxation and biofeedback are used to treat various types of pain. Relaxation is an integrated physiological response which is characterised by generalised decreases in the sympathetic nervous system and metabolic activity (Benson 1975; Benson et al 1984). Standardised instructions (Jacobson 1938; Luthe 1969) or meditative techniques (Benson 1975; Kabat-Zinn 1982) are typically used to elicit the 'relaxation response'. Relaxation is a characteristic part of most psychological interventions for pain (Turner & Chapman 1982a).

Biofeedback is the presentation to an invidual of a sensory signal (usually visual or auditory) that changes in proportion to a biological process. The biological measures 'fed back' have included the electromyogram (EMG) of various muscles in different parts of the body, skin temperature, skin resistance, pulse volume and waveforms of the electroencephalogram (EEG). Feedback has been presented under varying conditions of amplification and electronic modification. Subjects have received differing concurrent instruction, including forms of counselling and psychotherapy, have or have not utilised relaxation training and home practice and have had the biofeedback sessions conducted in a deliberately neutral or encouraging manner. In addition, the activity level (passive versus active) or position of the body (sitting versus standing, etc.) has varied. Thus the term 'biofeedback' has come to refer to a constellation of procedures, having as their only common element the use of biofeedback itself.

This chapter examines relaxation and biofeedback effects for the most frequently treated pain syndromes. Issues in aetiology, measurement, theory and research are also considered.

CURRENT STATUS OF RELAXATION AND BIOFEEDBACK

Relaxation and biofeedback as treatments for pain have been studied extensively and have been examined in many review articles (e.g. Blanchard & Ahles 1990).

Biofeedback has been used to treat a wide variety of pain syndromes. By far the most frequent application has been EMG feedback for muscle-contraction headaches. Next in frequency has been the use of vascular feedback (skin temperature or other measures of vascular activity) for migraine. It has also been applied less frequently to other pain problems such as back pain, paediatric pain, temporomandibular joint pain, Raynaud's disease, torticollis, neck problems, gynaecological problems, arthritis, phantom-limb pain, reflex sympathetic dystrophy and other miscellaneous conditions.

In addition to variation in the syndrome treated, research subjects have varied substantially in their pain-problem histories, and pretreatment base rates of pain episodes. In different studies, subjects have consisted of college students or public research volunteers, self-referrals or medical referrals and, recently, elderly subjects.

Various physiological and self-report measures have been used to assess the outcome of the biofeedback interventions. Headaches have been measured in terms of their frequency, intensity, duration and density; intensity × duration has been used as a 'headache index' (Blanchard et al 1980).

Variability in pain syndromes, types of subject and the measures recorded should be kept in mind when considering treatment outcome. Despite the preponderance of noncontrolled studies, enough systematic data have accumulated to permit some firm conclusions about treatment efficacy.

SCALP-MUSCLE-CONTRACTION HEADACHE

This pain syndrome is the most widely studied for its responsiveness to relaxation and biofeedback. The *Classification of Chronic Pain* (International Association for the Study of Pain, IASP, 1986) defines scalp-muscle-contraction headache as 'virtually continuous head pain, usually symmetrical, associated with muscle tension, anxiety and "depression"' (IASP 1986).

BIOFEEDBACK AND RELAXATION FOR SCALP-MUSCLE-CONTRACTION HEADACHE

The literatures on biofeedback and relaxation treatments for scalp-muscle-contraction headache are intertwined to an extent that they are best considered together.

Table 73.1 presents the studies that have been published between 1986 and 1992 on muscle-contraction headache using biofeedback or relaxation or both.

In eight of the controlled studies of scalp-muscle-contraction headache, biofeedback or relaxation training in any of their varieties was compared to a no-treatment control group involving symptom monitoring, waiting list, or placebo. One study compared a self-hypnotic method of relaxation to a control group (Melis et al 1991), finding it effective. Another compared therapist-assisted relaxation to self-help relaxation (Larsson et al 1987), finding no differences between groups.

Four studies (Wisniewski et al 1988; Larson et al 1990; Passchier et al 1990; Blanchard et al 1991a) found relaxation training superior to any of the control or placebo conditions. One study (Lacroix et al 1986a, 1986b) found combined treatments better than control and waiting-list conditions in a sample of workers on compensation benefits. One study (Blanchard et al 1986) found relaxation training and biofeedback equally effective in reducing anxiety. Wallbaum et al (1991) found sensory deprivation equal to relaxation training and improvements in follow-up when both treatments were combined.

The studies reviewed in Table 73.1 support relaxation training as the treatment of choice in muscle-contraction headache. Most of the controlled studies used this technique. Only Lacroix et al (1986a, 1986b) compared biofeedback, relaxation and a combination of the two; overall they found the three equally effective when compared to a no-treatment control group. With the exception of one study (Wallbaum et al 1991), when relaxation alone was compared to conditions other than biofeedback (e.g. waiting-list, self-monitoring, medication), relaxation is clearly superior.

Three group outcome studies revealed that EMG biofeedback is equal or superior to relaxation training and other techniques (Arena et al 1988, 1991; Borgeat et al 1991). In other studies, a combination of the two was tried and found effective (Blanchard et al 1987a, 1987b; Kabela et al 1989). In two other instances, cognitive therapy was compared to relaxation training and to medication (Attanasio et al 1987; Holroyd et al 1991). Four studies found no relationship between EMG levels and improvement in headache symptomatology.

In a meta-analysis carried out in 1980, Blanchard et al determined that, 'the apparent effectiveness of EMG biofeedback for muscle-contraction-headache varies moderately across the headache measures used. With some exceptions, headache frequency tends to decrease slightly more than duration or intensity'. They found the following percentage improvements in a 'headache index' (intensity × duration) at the end of treatment and at follow-up respectively: EMG biofeedback alone 61, 58; relaxation training alone 59, 70; EMG biofeedback and relaxation combined 59, 57; headache monitoring alone 5, 21. By comparison, the corresponding figures for medication placebo were 35, 38; and for psychological placebo 35, 51.

Blanchard et al (1980) found that relaxation training or biofeedback reduced reported muscle-contraction-headache pain by about 60%. Other early reviews reached a similar figure, or occasionally slightly less, of about 50%. This improvement was almost always maintained during the following months. In contrast, the control comparison subjects, who received uninstructed self-relaxation, placebo medication or no treatment for their muscle contraction headaches consistently did not improve as much.

In considering the results for control group subjects *in the same studies* analysed by Blanchard et al (1980), other early reviewers found variable effects. Taking an average of subjects, measures and studies, reported pain tends to increase by about 8–10% in the control groups and is occasionally reported to increase much more (Haynes et al 1975; Jessup et al 1979). However, the use of a false signal as a control procedure for EMG biofeedback leads more often to a decrease in headache symptoms of about 15%.

Given an average improvement of at least 50% with EMG biofeedback, and variable outcome without treatment, EMG biofeedback is clearly an effective treatment for muscle-contraction headaches. Relaxation training on the whole is equally effective. Benefit is not due to spontaneous remission, regression to the mean, the passage of time or subject maturation.

A later meta-analysis by Malone & Strube (1988) (see also Malone & Strube 1989) reviewed 109 studies, of which 48 were used to calculate effect sizes. This sample of studies was called the effect-size sample while the remaining 61 studies were labelled the percentage-improved group. In the effect-size sample, the average sample size was 53 (range = 4–676). The average age was 35 and the average duration of pain was 9.4 years. In this group, 'All treatments were reported as extremely successful when compared with the estimated outcome effects of no-treatment control groups'. When type of outcome measure was examined, the outcome findings varied considerably, except number of symptoms, EMG recordings and mood. When these variables were taken into account, improvement was observed consistently. In contrast to Blanchard et al (1980), pill placebo was found to be more effective than biofeedback or relaxation

Table 73.1 Biofeedback and relaxation treatments for muscle-contraction headache

Authors	Treatments	No. of patients	No. of sessions	Results
Arena et al 1988	RT	10	7	Decrease in overall headache activity
Arena et al 1991	EMG	8	12	Decrease in overall headache activity
Attanasio et al 1987	RT + CT RT + CT (H)	25	3–11	Decrease in use of medical strategies
Blanchard et al 1986	RT FB	206	10–12	Reductions in anxiety and depression not attributable to specific treatments
Blanchard et al 1987a	RT FB	86	10	Muscle-contraction-headache patients improved and showed good maintenance of gains. Vascular, non-significant
Blanchard et al 1987b	FB RT	21	10–12	78% tension, 91% vascular significantly improved
Blanchard et al 1991a	RT	39	10	Treatment groups improved over control group.
Borgeat et al 1991	EMG	32	6	Patients showing a decrease of at least 10% in muscle tension in response to presence of future therapist improved more
Collet et al 1986	GSR RT	31	10	GSR significant improvement over RT in frequency, intensity and anxiety
Grazzi et al 1988	EMG	20	15	Reduction in headache attacks Reduction in anxiety and depression
Holroyd et al 1991	CT D	41	3 8	Improvements with both treatments
Juprelle & Schoenen 1990	RT EMG Trapezius	31	10	20 Ss improved 80–100% after 10 weeks of treatment
Kabela et al 1989	RT EMG EMG-N	16	10–12 7 6	10 patients improved more than 50%
Lacroix et al 1986a, 1986b	EMG-L EMG-N RT Combined	55	16	All treatment conditions equally effective. Biofeedback alone: few reports of improvement
Larsson et al 1987	RT RT (H) SM	46	9	Self-help treatment as effective as therapist-assisted treatment
Larsson et al 1990	RT (H) WL Placebo	48	'Minimal contact"	Self-help RT decrease in headache activity and other somatic complaints. Overall modest improvement
Melis et al 1991	HYPN	26	4	Reductions in headache activity
Michultka et al 1988	RT	1	19	Headache complaints reduced 48% Medication reduced 51%
Murphy et al 1989	TFB CT	1	13	Pain was not reported at follow-up
Passchier et al 1990	RT Placebo	202	10	No significant differences
Schoenen et al 1991a	EMG	32	10	No significant differences between high and low EMG level groups
Schoenen et al 1991b	EMG+RT Different positions	52	10	EMG elevated in patients not in controls
Schoenen et al 1991c	EMG RT	62	10	Pain thresholds increased after biofeedback therapy
Smith 1987	EMG TFB RT	15	7–25+	The more contact with treatment, the more improvement. Decrease of headache experience and symptoms with TFB-RT
Szekely et al 1986	RT + EMG and TFB PCT	16	12	Treatments lesser impact on menstrual associated headache than on headache not associated with menstruation

Table 73.1 *(contd)*

Authors	Treatments	No. of patients	No. of sessions	Results
Wallbaum et al 1991	REST RT	20	8	Treatment groups better than control
Wisniewski et al 1988	RT WL	10	8	Headache index scores lower in RT group than in control

CT = cognitive therapy; D = drug; EMG = frontal EMG biofeedback; EMG-L = EMG longissimus biofeedback; EMG-N = EMG neck muscle biofeedback; FB = thermal or EMG biofeedback; GSR = galvanic skin response; H = home-based; HYPN = hypnotherapy; PCT = person-centred therapy; REST = chamber-restricted environment; RT = relaxation training; SM = stress management; TFB = thermal biofeedback; Trapezius = trapezius biofeedback; WL = waiting-list condition.

training. Autogenic training was found to be superior to pill placebo, confirming the finding of Blanchard et al (1980).

In the percentage-improved sample (Malone & Strube 1988), the subjects were slightly older, had had pain for a longer period of time and the sample sizes were larger than in the effect-size sample. Based on the 'percentage-improved' method, the authors concluded that 'only relaxation training is truly effective, biofeedback training is minimally effective and the other treatments are actually less effective than no treatment at all'. The criterion for considering improvement was a 25% or greater reduction in the outcome measures (activity level, duration, EMG or temperature recordings, frequency, etc.). The percentage of improvement reported was 84% for biofeedback, 95% for relaxation, 70% for pill placebo, 72% for treatment package and 77% for no treatment.

However, Malone & Strube's meta-analysis (1988) was criticised by Holroyd & Penzien (1989). They argued that the quantitative analysis that characterises meta-analytic methodology was not used and, further, that 'type of treatment, type of pain disorder, and type of outcome measure were completely confounded'. In a rejoinder to these criticisms, Malone et al (1989) affirmed: 'In fact, the only clear conclusion that can be reached is that the research in this area is not particularly well conducted and additional work will be necessary before sound inferences are warranted.' Nevertheless, Blanchard & Ahles (1990), in a recent review of the studies of tension headache, conclude that frontal EMG biofeedback alone or with adjunctive relaxation training is more effective than placebo and at least as effective as other active psychologic treatments and drug treatments.

Relaxation training is as effective as biofeedback, is simpler to administer and is more cost-effective. The equivalent benefits of relaxation training have been repeatedly noted by researchers and reviewers, such as Turner & Chapman (1982a). Viewed even more broadly, if EMG biofeedback is effective not as a specific muscle-training technique, but as a way of training relaxation, then the key question becomes the relative effectiveness of biofeedback and relaxation training for generating relaxation. Relaxation-training studies are subject to the same sources of variability as noted earlier for EMG biofeedback, leading to some conflicting findings. Nonetheless, in a thorough review of studies comparing EMG biofeedback with relaxation training, Tarler-Benlolo (1978) concluded: 'Results of most of these [studies] indicated that either method was equally effective in producing positive results'.

MUSCLE-CONTRACTION-PAIN: TREATMENT PROCESS

The findings and conclusions from biofeedback and relaxation outcome studies have directed researchers' attention to the question of treatment process: i.e. what happens during treatment to cause improvement? One of the most incisive studies of this question was carried out by Andrasik & Holroyd (1980). They compared EMG biofeedback training for decreasing, increasing, or stabilising frontalis muscle tension with a no-treatment group. The three treatment groups showed equivalent substantial improvement in tension headaches at a 3-month follow-up. All three treatments were equally superior to the no-treatment group. Built-in checks showed that biofeedback subjects had acquired frontalis control as trained and that the treatments were equally credible. Andrasik & Holroyd (1980) concluded: 'These results suggest that the learned reduction of EMG activity may play only a minor role in outcomes obtained with biofeedback'.

The duration of treatment is not a particularly potent variable in determining treatment outcome. A minimum of 3 hours of EMG biofeedback training is usually adequate, although most clinicians use about 6–8 hours.

The source of subjects has not noticeably affected research results. Research volunteers, medical referrals and elderly subjects improve about the same amount. Subjects with lengthy headache histories, who have been refractory to other treatments, have improved with biofeedback.

Borgeat et al (1991) have suggested that a decrease of muscular tension during the first contact with the therapist can be used as predictor of success of therapy.

Schoenen et al in a series of studies (Schoenen et al 1991a, 1991b, 1991c; Juprelle & Schoenen 1990) found that EMG levels are not related to headache severity. They suggested that classification of headache populations in higher and lower EMG levels is artificial. They concluded that EMG activity of the pericranial muscles is not the cause of headaches, but rather one of the changes associated with headaches. Their data supported the hypothesis that 'diffuse disruption of central pain-modulating systems, possibly due to a modified limbic input to the brain stem, is pivotal in the pathophysiology of muscle contraction headache.' (Schoenen et al 1991c).

MIGRAINE

The Subcommittee on Taxonomy of the IASP (IASP 1986) has defined classical migraine as: 'Unilateral throbbing head pain often with a prodromal state and usually preceded by an aura which is usually visual; nausea, vomiting and photophobia often accompany the pain'. Health practitioners have turned to nonpharmacological treatments for migraine due to the harmful side effects of medication (Wilkinson 1988).

Migraine headache has been treated with finger-temperature biofeedback. Sargent et al 1973 suggested that hand-warming biofeedback could alleviate migraine by reducing sympathetic arousal. However, the outcome findings for hand-warming biofeedback are not particularly encouraging. Overall outcome effectiveness of finger-warming feedback for migraine, when objectively evaluated, has been somewhat weaker than that for EMG biofeedback applied to muscle-contraction headaches. A typical figure for migraine-symptom reduction during controlled studies of finger-warming biofeedback is about 30–35%, although occasionally no improvement has been reported. Virtually the same improvement is found in no-treatment groups, in which subjects simply keep records of their migraines, and in what should be countertherapeutic groups, in which the subjects attempt to decrease their finger temperature (Kewman & Roberts 1980).

The review of Blanchard et al (1980) was somewhat more optimistic than the present one, although their summary improvement data also overlap with the 30–35% range. Blanchard et al (1980) concluded that thermal biofeedback alone leads to a 52% improvement in migraine headache index (intensity × duration); thermal feedback with autogenic training, a 65% improvement; relaxation training, 53%; and medication placebo, 17%.

Exhaustive reviews (Holmes & Burish 1983; Chapman 1986; Litt 1986; Blanchard & Ahles 1990) all draw similar conclusions about treatment outcome when relaxation or biofeedback are used for migraine:

1. Thermal biofeedback and relaxation training are equally effective.
2. Frontalis EMG biofeedback and thermal biofeedback are equally effective in the treatment of migraine (Chapman 1986).
3. Improvement that occurs during relaxation or biofeedback continues at follow-up periods of at least up to 1 year.
4. Changes in headache parameters are not reliably associated with physiological changes postulated to mediate migraine. 'Many reports of successful headache reduction with thermal biofeedback are not paired with clear evidence that subjects learned, much less maintained or generalised, the target thermal response' (Chapman 1986).'Specific control of peripheral or cerebral vasculature through biofeedback is not deemed to be either necessary or sufficient for successful outcome in migraine treatment, either in the long term or the short term' (Litt 1986).
5. To account best for the complex and seemingly contradictory findings in *clinical* practice, an interactional model that considers 'biochemical, specific vascular, general autonomic, cognitive/affective/behavioural, dyadic and social' processes is apt to be most useful (Litt 1986). In more controlled research studies, 'the equivalent findings with biofeedback and relaxation therapies may be related to their commonality; both have involved very repetitive quiet concentration and mental and physical passivity' (Chapman 1986).

From 1986 to mid-1992, 15 studies were published involving populations of migraineurs who had been treated with biofeedback or relaxation training or both. These studies are presented in Table 73.2.

Four were controlled studies (Ellersten et al 1987; Gallegos & Espinoza 1989; Blanchard et al 1990; Gauthier & Carrier 1991) and the rest were group outcome studies. What seems clear is that biofeedback in combination with relaxation or alone is more effective in the treatment of migraine headache than placebo treatment or no treatment. However, none of the controlled studies clarified if temperature biofeedback was a better treatment per se than other more cost-effective treatments.

Holroyd & Penzien (1990) in a recent meta-analytic review reported that relaxation/biofeedback training and propranolol medication are equally effective in the prophylactic treatment of migraine. Both treatments greatly reduced headache activity in patients with migraine and differed significantly from patients in nontreatment or placebo conditions. Their study involved 2445 patients in 25 studies evaluating the effectiveness of propranolol treatment and 35 studies evaluating the effectiveness of relaxation/biofeedback treatment.

The results of this meta-analytic review differ considerably from the results of the meta-analytic study by Malone & Strube (1988) discussed earlier and those of

Table 73.2 Biofeedback and relaxation treatments for migraine

Authors	Treatments	No. of patients	No. of sessions	Results
Blanchard et al 1990	TFB+RT TFB+CT PSEUD	116	16	Treatment conditions better than no treatment. TFB better than pseudomeditation
Ellersten et al 1987	TFB	24	8	No difference between migraineurs and controls in habituation pattern. Migraineurs lower hand temperature and higher EMG
Gallegos & Espinoza 1989	TFB AT	9	16	TFB and AT raised temperature. Only TFB reduced migraine activity
Gauthier et al 1988	BVP TFB	39	12–16	Reduction in migraine activity. TFB more beneficial to classical migraine patients than to common migraine patients.
Gauthier & Carrier 1991	BVP TFB	96	12–16	Overall headache activity less at follow-up than at pretreatment
Gauthier et al 1991	TFB BVP	39	12–16	TFB effective in reducing menstrual and nonmenstrual migraine.
Guarnieri & Blanchard 1990	TFB (H & C)	16	10	Reduction in headaches. No difference between home-based and clinic-based regimen
Johansson & Ost 1987	TFB-GT TFB (H & C)	24	8	Patients who achieved temperature control showed a greater decrease in headache than those who did not
Kim & Blanchard 1992	TBF+RT (H) TBF+RT+CT (H) TBF+RT (C) TBF+RT+CT (C)	99 15	16	Reduction in headache activity after treatment
Lisspers & Ost 1990a	BVP (HM) BVP (SM)	26	9	BVP-HM group 58% headache reduction and 68% at follow-up.
Lisspers & Ost 1990b	TFB BVP RT	50	8–9	Headache reductions achieved after treatment persisted at 6 years and were enhanced
Mizener et al 1988	TFB RT	25	6	Patients became more internal about beliefs to control their health. Ignored pain sensations more after treatment
Sorbi & Tellegen 1986	RT SCT	29	9	RT patients more socially withdrawn. Stress-coping training increased their social assertiveness
Sorbi et al 1989	RT SCT	24	9	RT and SCT equally effective. Little medication in both groups since end of training. SCT improved assertiveness and active problem-solving and decreased depression
Steffek & Blanchard 1991	TFB AT	32	12	Acquisition of handwarming directly related to increase in capacity for absorption. Absorption capacity inversely related to reduction in headache activity.

AT = autogenic training; BVP = blood-volume pulse biofeedback; C = clinic-based; CT = cognitive therapy; GT = generalisation training; H = home-based; HM = headache management; PSEUD = pseudomeditation; RT = relaxation training; SCT = stress-coping training; SM = stress management; TFB = thermal biofeedback.

Mathew (1981) who reported more improvement in migraine headache activity with propranolol than with relaxation/biofeedback treatment.

Reductions in migraine activity are smaller when measured by patients' daily recordings than when measured by patients' or physicians' global reports (Holroyd & Penzien 1990). There was no evidence in this study to support either treatment, propranolol or relaxation/biofeedback, as more effective.

The findings by Holroyd & Penzien (1990) in their meta-analytic review seem to challenge the psychological interventions. If propranolol and psychological treatment are equally effective, it would seem that many patients would prefer propranolol than a lengthy and more demanding treatment such as biofeedback or relaxation training. These last treatments then would be left only for people who present with serious side-effects after the pharmacologic treatment.

A word of caution is in order regarding meta-analytic reviews. Meta-analytic reviews have been popular for some time (Devine & Cook 1986; Holroyd & Penzien 1986; Broome et al 1989; Fernandez & Turk 1989; Hyman et al 1989) and although the meta-analytic review by Holroyd & Penzien (1990) involved thousands of subjects in a considerable number of studies and followed sophisticated meta-analytic methodology, one wonders if the state of the biofeedback/relaxation literature so far is ready to conduct meta-analytic reviews and find sound conclusions. This is not to say that other types of review are better, but just to question the maturity of the research to date. If the literature is not ready yet, due to limitations in the data, such as the number of subjects in the studies, lack of adequate controls or inadequate classification of pain patients, then the conclusions of any meta-analytic review should be taken cautiously.

MIXED HEADACHE

In contrast to the extensive literature on muscle-contraction headache and migraine headache, studies involving patients with combined headache (migraine and muscle contraction) or cluster headache are rather scarce. In some clinics, patients with muscle-contraction headache, migraine or both are treated with a combined package of treatments, apparently with good results (Schwartz 1987). However, research studies of patients with combined headache and cluster headache are needed.

In a study involving a mixed population (Blanchard et al 1991b), patients with migraine or mixed headaches were assigned to one of three groups: thermal biofeedback with home practice, thermal biofeedback without home practice and a monitoring group. The groups with biofeedback treatment improved more than the monitoring group. However, there were no significant differences between the two feedback groups. The authors concluded that there was no advantage in practising at home. When the groups of patients were analysed with regard to clinically significant improvement, migraineurs responded better (64%) than patients with mixed headaches (28%). Blanchard et al (1991b) suggested that this may be due to the lack of relaxation treatment which is probably crucial for patients with mixed headache.

Evidence of the effectiveness of a combined treatment of relaxation training and biofeedback was reported by Smith (1987) with a population of mixed headache patients. Smith contacted by telephone 318 patients (muscle contraction, migraine or mixed) and analysed them in three groups according to the time since they had the last contact with biofeedback. All patients had received earlier EMG and thermal biofeedback, relaxation training, psychotherapy and physical therapy. She found that patients who had had some previous biofeedback treatment reported reduction in headache frequency and associated symptoms. The reduction was maintained in the majority of the patients for 25 months or more.

BACK PAIN

Several studies involving chronic back pain have been reviewed by Jessup (1989), although 'good research in this area has been slow to emerge compared with the profusion of studies on tension headache' (Large & Lamb 1983).

Table 73.3 presents studies on biofeedback and relaxation for back pain published between 1986 and mid-1992. The syndromes that were studied have varied. Most research subjects have had, as a minimum, recurring or nearly continuous medium to severe pain for at least 6 months. Pain histories in excess of 10 years have been typical in both clinical and research volunteer populations. Degenerative, dysfunctional, structural, inflammatory, traumatic, postsurgical and unknown aetiologies are evident. The most frequently studied classifications are fibrositis or diffuse myofascial pain syndrome, rheumatoid arthritis, chronic mechanical low-back pain, and muscle-tension pain of psychological origin (IASP 1986).

Between 20% and 85% of back-pain patients do not have differentially diagnostic physical findings. The wide range in physical findings depends on what consideration one gives to degenerative changes that do not reliably produce pain (White & Gordon 1982). Consequently, outcome findings for relaxation and biofeedback treatments of back pain have varied widely.

Relaxation training has produced some evidence of being an effective treatment for low-back pain. It also appears to be an effective component of multidimensional treatment packages (Keefe et al 1981) It produced positive results in five of the seven studies cited in Table 73.3.

The rationale for relaxation training is straightforward: sustained muscle contraction has been considered both a cause and an effect of chronic back pain, sustaining a cycle of pain–spasm–pain (Dolce & Raczynski 1985). Hence reduction of muscle contraction should be beneficial. However, muscle-tension levels in back-pain patients have been found to be lower than, equal to, or higher than those in painfree populations under various diagnostic, postural and movement conditions (Dolce & Raczynski 1985). It is also important to consider reports pointing to the fact that relaxation training may not be effective for all patients. Degner & Barkwell (1991) found that some patients consider the training too effortful or do not like it. Others report distress or withdrawal, hallucinations or psychotic manifestations if they have a history of psychosis or depression.

In two studies cited in Table 73.3, relaxation training was found to be ineffective (Shea et al 1990; Nicholas et al 1991). However in the study by Shea et al only one lecture on relaxation skills was given.

The problem of back pain is probably too complex and variable between patients to permit a simple, single-modality solution. Nonetheless, relaxation techniques are non-invasive, inexpensive, portable procedures that enjoy easy patient acceptance. They deserve further systematic study.

EMG biofeedback, usually from the paraspinal muscles, as a treatment for low-back pain has produced mixed results (Dolce & Raczynski 1985). In the studies cited in

Table 73.3 Biofeedback and relaxation treatments for back pain

Authors	Treatments	No. of patients	No. of sessions	Results
Asfour et al 1990	EMG & EXC	30	8	Gains in strength of lumbar paraspinal muscles
Biedermann et al 1989	EMG	24	10	Treatment gains in pain intensity and physical mobility for 'organic group'
Flor et al 1986	EMG PSEUD D	22	12	At 2.5 years' follow-up, EMG patients still improved and differed from control group on behavioural and cognitive responses to pain
Newshan & Balamuth 1990	RT CT IM	3	10	Treatment changed the pain experience and enabled patients to participate more fully in their lives
Nicholas et al 1991	CT BT RT	58	10	Progressive relaxation little contribution to either cognitive therapy or behavioural treatment
Nicholas et al 1992	CT RT	20	10	Combined psychological treatment improved significantly more than control. Improvement maintained at 6 months
Petrie & Azariah 1990	RT ED SM	107	2 days	RT and other techniques taught in course associated with positive affect and well-being
Shea et al 1990	RT SD	60	1	Not effective results with one lecture on relaxation skills
Spinhoven & Linssen 1991	RT IM ED	42	10	Patients reported a higher sense of perceived pain control at end of treatment. This was no longer significant at follow-up
Stuckey et al 1986	EMG RT Placebo	24	8	RT significantly superior to EMG and placebo on four measures of chronic low-back pain

BT = behavioural therapy; CT = cognitive therapy; D = drug; ED = pain education; EMG = EMG biofeedback; EXC = exercise; IM = imagery; PSEUD = pseudomeditation; RT = relaxation training; SD = sensory deprivation; SM = stress management.

Table 73.3, in general, when EMG has been used alone or in combination with other treatments, the results have been positive in terms of gains in muscular strength and physical mobility or reports in pain intensity (Flor et al 1986; Biedermann 1989; Asfour et al 1990).

BACK PAIN PROCESS ISSUES

The main aetiological issues relevant to relaxation and biofeedback training for back pain are the lack of reliable covariation between reported pain and EMG readings and evidence that for some painful back conditions training for increased rather than decreased EMG may be indicated. Diagnosis, EMG technique and patient gender are also proving to be significant factors affecting muscular activity in normal and painful backs.

Paraspinal EMG and pain report do not reliably covary in EMG biofeedback studies. Bush et al (1985) found that paraspinal EMG correlated 0.36 with subjective pain report during pretreatment assessment, but this relationship disappeared during and after treatment.

Bodily position and isometric or movement tasks during EMG affect the results (Kravitz et al 1981). Many interactions of posture, movement and site of EMG electrode placement remain to be studied more systematically. Middaugh & Kee (1987) and Middaugh (1990) propose that the traditional study and treatment of EMG biofeedback in musculoskeletal pain populations is inadequate. These authors noticed that target muscles of patients only relaxed while in the quiet sitting position but were not relaxed when other activities were performed. Their aim has been to train the target muscles to maintain good muscle control during activities. Once this training was achieved, pain relief was reported. They emphasise an individualised, dynamic, muscle-by-muscle training method (Middaugh & Kee 1987; Middaugh 1990).

Another variable that may be affecting the results obtained with EMG recordings is the location and depth of placement of electrodes. Wolf et al (1989) evaluated 10 normal women and found evidence that surface EMG recording, the type used in EMG biofeedback studies, does not reflect the activity of deeply situated muscles. They point to the importance of these findings for biofeedback treatment. Although these findings and those of Middaugh & Kee (1987) and Middaugh (1990) are important and point to a new direction in biofeedback monitoring and treatment of low-back pain, the small number of studies does not warrant definitive conclusions. Consequently, the relationship between EMG measures and back pain remains an open question.

PAEDIATRIC PAIN

Pain in children is not a separate diagnostic group in the *Classification of Chronic Pain* (IASP 1986). Schechter (1985) notes that paediatric pain is a significant and psychophysiologically complex problem, involving the interaction of a neurophysiological response with age, cognitive set, personality, ethnic background and emotional state.

Since caution has been advised regarding long-term drug therapy with children (Duckro & Cantwell-Simmons 1989), behavioural treatment seems to be a promising alternative and several researchers have studied the use of relaxation and biofeedback techniques for pain in children.

Migraine affects 2.5% of children between ages 5 and 9 years (Blanchard & Andrasik 1987). Considering that beta-blockers, which are reported to be effective in the treatment of adult migraine (Wilkinson 1988), seem to be less effective with children (Forsythe et al 1984), efforts have been made to emphasise treatment of this disorder with behavioural methods (Lascelles et al 1989).

Duckro & Cantwell-Simmons (1989), in a review article, reported on 12 studies which used behavioural treatments for headache in paediatric populations. In general, these studies supported the assumption that relaxation training with or without biofeedback is an effective treatment in the management of chronic headache in children and adolescents.

Following Duckro & Cantwell-Simmons' review, other articles have appeared in the literature that point to the effectiveness of relaxation treatment (Engel et al 1992), EMG biofeedback with mental imagery (Labbe & Ward 1990), the importance of home practice and parental support (Allen & McKeen 1991) and the difference in effectiveness of treatment when emphasis is on clinic-based or home-based treatment (Burke & Andrasik 1989; Guarnieri & Blanchard 1990).

The children's response to biofeedback and relaxation treatments is consistent with that of adults. Biofeedback and relaxation have been successfully applied to obscure or difficult pain problems, such as abdominal pain (Bodenhamer et al 1986; Sokel et al 1991). As with adult patients, clinicians working with children utilise biofeedback and relaxation in the context of more comprehensive behavioural programmes. Reviews which focused on assessment (Gascon 1984), pain treatment (Masek et al 1984) and broader psychosomatic problems (Linkenhoker 1983) have elaborated on biofeedback and relaxation applications with children. Smith & Womack (1987) described stress-management techniques such as relaxation, meditation, hypnosis and biofeedback in symptoms such as recurrent headache, chest pain, abdominal pain, syncope and dizziness. In general, in paediatric populations, biofeedback and relaxation have been primarily conceptualised as techniques for enhancing self-regulation.

OTHER PAIN SYNDROMES

Research on biofeedback treatment of a variety of pain syndromes other than functional headache shows outcomes similar to the headache research. Uncontrolled studies greatly outnumber systematic studies. Controlled research suggests that, as with headache, generalised relaxation is as effective as biofeedback and may mediate improvement in a number of syndromes.

Biofeedback treatments have been reported for the following syndromes: temporomandibular joint pain, Raynaud's disease, spasmodic torticollis, neck injury, menstrual stress, writer's cramp, duodenal ulcer, pyelonephritis, rheumatoid arthritis, phantom-limb pain, anginal pain and posttraumatic headache. They have also been applied during childbirth.

TEMPOROMANDIBULAR JOINT PAIN

Anecdotal case reports and group studies (Jessup et al 1979) suggest that masseter or temporalis muscle EMG biofeedback alone or in conjuction with cognitive–behavioural treatment is beneficial for temporomandibular joint pain and bruxism (Crocket et al 1986; Dalen et al 1986; Amen & Mostofosky 1988; Burdette & Gale 1988; Erlandson & Poppen 1989; Feehan & Marsh 1989).

RAYNAUD'S DISEASE

Three reviews of the literature on the treatment of Raynaud's disease reported contradictory findings. Sappington et al (1979) found that the most systematic studies showed that hand-warming biofeedback was no more effective than relaxation training (Keefe et al 1980). Rose & Carlson (1987) also reported inconsistent findings among major treatment studies. Several methodological and cost-effectiveness issues are raised that make it difficult to generalise across studies, settings and subject groups. In contrast, Freedman (1985) reported in a review article that temperature biofeedback is an effective treatment for idiopathic Raynaud's disease. He points to the importance of differentiating patients with Raynaud's disease, which refers to the primary form of the disorder, and 'Raynaud's phenomenon' which may be present with other tissue disorders such as scleroderma, rheumatoid arthritis, etc. Treatment with thermal biofeedback when scleroderma is present has not been as effective. The authors suggested that different aetiologies may be involved.

Freedman (1991) reported replications of controlled investigations which demonstrated that temperature biofeedback was effective in the treatment of patients suffering Raynaud's disease. Findings at the Freedman laboratory supported the hypothesis that feedback-induced vasodilatation and vasoconstriction are mediated by different physiological mechanisms, namely, vasodilatation through a β-adrenergic mechanism and vasoconstriction through the sympathetic nervous pathway. This may explain the inconsistencies between heart rate, skin conductance and other parameters during temperature biofeedback in many studies reported so far.

TORTICOLLIS

Spasmodic torticollis is a painful twisting of the head to one side due to abnormal activity of the sternocleidomastoid muscles. Nine cases reported by Cleeland (1973) and two single-case studies (Counts et al 1978; Jankel 1978) suggest that EMG biofeedback is effective for at least 90% of cases during treatment, including cases with long histories. Benefit continues for up to 3 years for about two-thirds of cases (Cleeland 1973). Extended treatment seems necessary – 40 minutes of training per day for about 20 days. Biofeedback from the sternocleidomastoid muscles bilaterally has been recommended (Jankel 1978). Not all cases show marked improvement and, even with biofeedback, sternocleidomastoid muscle tension may not decline to that of comparable controls (Martin 1981).

NECK

EMG biofeedback for trapezius muscle relaxation has benefited patients with neck injuries (Jacobs & Felton 1969).

GYNAECOLOGICAL

Time in first-stage labour and medication use during childbirth were reduced with EMG biofeedback training (Gregg 1978). EMG biofeedback augmented the benefits of Lamaze childbirth preparation (Abbott et al 1978). Recently, one controlled study (Duchene 1989) reported that primigravidae women who had been given several training sessions in biofeedback and used biofeedback equipment during labour, reported significantly lower pain from admission to delivery, at delivery and 24 hours postpartum.

Menstrual stress (dysmenorrhoea) did not improve with hand-temperature biofeedback (Russ 1977) but improved with individual or group relaxation training or a combination of relaxation training and vaginal-temperature feedback (Heczey 1978). In a multiple baseline study (Vargas et al 1987), 12 women suffering dysmenorrhoea reported less pain after relaxation training.

ARTHRITIS

Arthritis has been treated with frontalis muscle EMG biofeedback or relaxation training (Wickramasekera et al 1976; Bradley et al 1987; Rice 1989) with positive results, but negative inconclusive results have also been obtained (Noda 1979).

PHANTOM-LIMB PAIN

Phantom-limb pain was virtually eliminated in 10 of 16 cases and reduced to the point of no longer needing treatment in an additional four in a single-group study using relaxation training, EMG biofeedback and provision of information (Sherman et al 1979). These findings are particularly encouraging because 14 of the cases had suffered chronic pain for an average duration of 12 years.

REFLEX SYMPATHETIC DYSTROPHY

Reflex Sympathetic Dystrophy (RSD) has been treated with thermal biofeedback, relaxation training, psychotherapy and hypnotherapy, reducing subjective pain levels (Grunert et al 1990; Gainer 1992).

OTHER PAIN SYNDROMES

Other types of pain syndrome have been treated with biofeedback or relaxation or both and have improved various degrees. Olson (1988) reported improvement in a sample of 563 psychiatric patients suffering from different pain syndromes after treatment with biofeedback and relaxation training. Biofeedback proved to be an effective technique in one study of chronic idiopathic anal pain (Grimaud et al 1991). Relaxation was effective in the relief of oncologic pain (Graffam & Johnson 1987), postoperative pain (Flaherty & Fitzpatrick 1978; Miller 1987) and in preparation for surgery (Field 1974).

Writer's cramp has improved during EMG biofeedback in combination with desensitisation (Uchiyama et al 1977) or relaxation training (Akagi et al 1977). Preliminary work suggests that biofeedback of electrogastric activity may provide a technique for the treatment of duodenal ulcer (Walker et al 1978). Clinical relief of pain was apparent in a case of pyelonephritis treated with alpha-EEG biofeedback (Coger & Werbach 1975). The possibility of reducing angina by hand-warming biofeedback was raised in an anecdotal report of three cases (Hartman 1979).

Posttraumatic headache sufferers appear to benefit only slightly from biofeedback training (Tsushima & Hawk 1978). (See also a case report using alpha-EEG biofeedback by Gannon & Sternbach 1971.) The results with posttraumatic head pain are relatively unpromising.

In summary, the studies of biofeedback treatment of a variety of pain syndromes other than functional headache suggest that further inquiry is merited. However, as with biofeedback treatment of headache, relaxation training and other cognitive–behavioural interventions may prove to be at least as effective.

TREATMENT PROCESS CONSIDERATIONS

PAIN TAXONOMY

The *Classification of Chronic Pain* (IASP 1986), by creating a coherent pain taxonomy, could significantly aid clarification of the processes operating in biofeedback and relaxation treatment for pain. Conversely, biofeedback and relaxation research are apt to aid further clarification of pain syndromes and subtypes (Carrobles et al 1981). Qualls & Sheehan (1981) argue for more detailed analysis of subject–treatment interactions, and fear that 'the wake of biofeedback appears imminent and that EMG biofeedback will be disregarded as a relaxation procedure before it has had the chance to mature.'

Pain taxonomy is a particularly pressing problem in headache research. Although generally accepted, the belief that tension of the frontalis muscle reliably causes muscle-contraction headache is not entirely supportable (Bakal 1975) and numerous exceptions to the general opinion have been documented. Similarly, the symptoms most frequently diagnostic of migraine (prodrome, unilateral onset, nausea) occur together only slightly more frequently than by chance (Waters 1973). Factor analysis of headache syndromes yields factors that are not congruent with current diagnostic practices (Ziegler et al 1972). Subtypes of headache for which biofeedback and relaxation are specifically effective may yet be identified.

PAIN–PHYSIOLOGY DESYNCHRONY

Reduction in frontalis EMG is not necessary for improvement in muscle-contraction headaches. Evidence supporting this surprising conclusion comes from studies of the frontalis EMG–pain relationship. Muscle tension tends to be higher during muscle-contraction headaches, but many case-by-case exceptions have been observed (Haynes et al 1975; Phillips 1977). Frontalis EMG does not reliably covary with self-reported headache pain, even when a headache is occuring during EMG monitoring in the laboratory (Epstein et al 1978; Gray et al 1980).

Nuechterlein & Holroyd (1980) reviewed some of the complexities behind frontalis EMG–pain desynchrony, and emphasised the need for very discrete diagnosis (i.e. pain taxonomy) to clarify the considerable diversity within the tension headache population in the extent to which EMG alteration can be expected to change headache activity. Also noteworthy is the fact that Andrasik & Holroyd (1980) closely monitored biofeedback training that increased frontalis EMG to ensure that it would not exacerbate headache symptoms.

Although opinion is not unanimous (Basmajian 1976), reductions in frontalis EMG during biofeedback do not generalise to other, even adjacent muscles (Glaus & Kotses 1979; Thompson et al 1981). Frontalis EMG level may not be reliably related to subjective reports of relaxation (Shedivy & Kleinman 1977). However, a generalised reduction in autonomic and cortical arousal, involving changes in heart rate, skin resistance and EEG activity, has been found during extensive frontalis EMG training (Hoffman 1979). Whether the EMG biofeedback caused the generalised decrease in arousal could not be determined by Hoffman's study. However, the pattern is congruent with the state of low arousal that Benson (1975) termed the 'relaxation response'. Conceivably, EMG biofeedback treatment, like relaxation training, does lead to a generalised reduction in arousal which is nonetheless not synchronous across muscle systems, nor with self-report of experienced relaxation.

Flor & Turk (1989) carried out an exhaustive research review of the relationship between specific symptoms and psychophysiological responses in chronic-pain patients. Detailed evaluation of 60 studies against 12 theoretical and methodological criteria showed that 'baseline levels, regardless of type of physiological measure, are not generally elevated in chronic-pain patients. The presence of symptom-specific, stress-related psychophysiological responses is more commonly observed and the evidence on return to baseline is at this time inconclusive.' These findings should direct reseachers towards a more precise evaluation of biofeedback and relaxation training as methods to reduce stress-related responses.

PSYCHOSOCIAL PROCESSES

Other processes that are not necessary for improvement during biofeedback can also be clarified. Socioeconomic status probably does not have an effect on improvement during biofeedback (Acosta & Yamamoto 1978; Wachtmann 1978). Hypnotisability, usually measured by psychometric scales, is almost certainly not related to improvement during biofeedback (Crosson 1980; Frischolz & Tryon 1980; see Barabasz & McGeorge (1978) for an exception to the general findings; also Schlutter et al (1980) reported finding biofeedback equivalent in effect to hypnotic analgesia). Home practice during biofeedback training is not necessary (Wickramasekera 1973; Haynes et al 1975; Lake et al 1979). Continued practice after training may be related to continued benefit (Reinking & Hutchings 1976).

A number of processes have been proposed as mediators for improvement during biofeedback and relaxation treatment, including personality × treatment interactions, anxiety reduction, enhanced sense of self-control, cognitive changes, behavioural changes, therapist contact, instructions to relax, somatic manoeuvres and subtle changes in biological processes.

Two features of the list of possible mediators should be noted. First, the length and variety of the list suggest that no conclusive mediator has yet been found. As Turner & Chapman (1982b) note, this may reflect 'the difficulty of carrying out outcome evaluation research in the chronic-pain area, The problems are extremely complex, and many treatment packages involve a collage of interventions rather than single therapy.'

Second, a common theme of many of the mediators is increased perceived control over bodily processes and social life. Increased self-efficacy (Bandura 1977) or 'learned resourcefulness' (Meichenbaum 1976) may prove to be a potent common element explaining the similar effectiveness of diverse biofeedback, relaxation, cognitive and behavioural pain treatments.

Personality variables may also be involved in mediating improvement in biofeedback treatments of pain (Jessup et al 1979). Qualls & Sheehan (1981) argued that different relaxation procedures, including feedback, interact with certain trait dimensions in different populations to produce reliably different effects. The dimensions put forward include trait anxiety, locus of control, capacity for absorption in mental imagery and type of clinical disorder. Another personality factor put forward in headaches is the 'neuroticism', as measured by the Eysenck Personality Inventory (Eysenck 1967; Henryk-Gutt & Rees 1973; Carrobles et al 1981). The recently emerging construct of a 'disease-prone personality' which involves 'depression, anger/hostility and anxiety' may also prove to be a relevent process variable in biofeedback and relaxation treatments of pain (Friedman & Booth-Kewley 1987).

CONCLUSIONS

Three main conclusions follow from the past quarter century of biofeedback and relaxation research.

1. Biofeedback and relaxation training have been established as useful treatment interventions. In addition, biofeedback specifically can be helpful in some refractory cases. Now, however, research must focus on more specific relationships of environmental stimuli, specific physical reactivities, and clarity of aetiology.
2. Biofeedback is coming full circle to its roots in psychophysiology. This is exemplified by the work of Flor & Turk (1989) and Freedman's (1991) research on biofeedback to elucidate the different physiological mechanisms of finger warming and cooling.
3. Regrettably, the research underscores the limited utility of poorly designed research. Aetiologies and syndromes have been confounded. Research hypotheses have been too simple, and the measurement strategies too crude. The addition of further confounding treatments to already equivocal findings has added to confusion. Biofeedback and relaxation research has now reached a stage where it must be more precise and sophisticated to be of value.

REFERENCES

Abbott D W, Rollin J B, Jones J 1978 The effects of electromyographic biofeedback-assisted relaxation on Lamaze childbirth. American Journal of Clinical Biofeedback 1: 23

Acosta F X, Yamamoto J 1978 Application of electromyographic biofeedback to the relaxation training of schizophrenic, neurotic, and tension headache patients. Journal of Consulting and Clinical Psychology 46: 383–384

Akagi M, Yoshimura M, Ikemi Y 1977 A clinical study of the treatment of writer's cramp by biofeedback training. Behavioural Engineering 4: 45–50

Allen K D, McKeen L R 1991 Home-based multicomponent treatment of pediatric migraine. Headache 31: 467–472

Amen D V, Mostofofsky D I 1988 Behavioral management of myofascial pain dysfunction syndrome. Journal of the Royal Society of Health 108: 81–82, 80

Andrasik F, Holroyd K A 1980 A test of specific and nonspecific effects in the biofeedback treatment of tension headache. Journal of Consulting and Clinical Psychology 48: 575–586

Arena J G, Hightower N E, Chong G C 1988 Relaxation therapy for tension headache in the elderly: a prospective study. Psychology and Aging 3: 96–98

Arena J G, Hanah S L, Bruno G M, Meador K J 1991 Electromyographic biofeedback training for tension headache in the elderly: a prospective study. Biofeedback and Self-Regulation 16: 379–390

Asfour S S, Khalil T M, Waly S M, Goldberg M L, Rosomoff R, Rosomoff H L 1990 Biofeedback in back muscle strengthening. Spine 15: 510–513

Attanasio V, Andrasik F, Blanchard E B 1987 Cognitive therapy and relaxation training in muscle contraction headache: efficacy and cost-effectiveness. Headache 27: 254–260

Bakal D A 1975 Headache : a biophysical perspective. Psychological Bulletin 82: 369–382

Bandura A 1977 Self efficacy: toward a unifying theory of behavioral change. Psychological Review 84: 191–215

Barabasz A F, McGeorge C M 1978 Biofeedback, medicated biofeedback and hypnosis in peripheral vasodilation training. American Journal of Clinical Hypnosis 21: 28–37

Basmajian J V 1976 Facts vs. myths in EMG biofeedback. Biofeedback and Self-Regulation 1: 369–372

Benson H 1975 The relaxation response. Morrow, New York

Benson H, Pomeranz B, Kutz I 1984 The relaxation response and pain. In: Wall P, Melzack R (eds) Textbook of Pain, 1st edn. Churchill Livingstone, Edinburgh, p 817–822

Biedermann H J, Inglis J, Monga T N, Shanks G L 1989 Differential treatment responses on somatic pain indicators after EMG biofeedback training in back pain patients. International Journal of Psychosomatics 36: 53–57

Blanchard E B, Ahles T A 1990 Biofeedback therapy. In: Bonica J J, Loeser J D, Chapman C R, Fordyce W E (eds) The management of pain, 2nd edn. Lea & Febiger, Philadelphia, p 1722–1732

Blanchard E B, Andrasik F 1987 Biofeedback treatment of vascular headache. In: Hatch J P, Rugh J D, Fisher J G (eds) Biofeedback studies in clinical efficacy. Plenum Press, New York, p 1–79

Blanchard E, Andrasik F, Ahles T, Teders S, O'Keefe D 1980 Migraine and tension headache: a meta-analytic review. Behavior Therapy 11: 613–631

Blanchard E B, Andrasik F, Appelbaum K A, Evans D D, Myers P,

Barron D 1986 Three studies of the psychological changes in chronic headache patients associated with biofeedback relaxation techniques. Psychosomatic Medicine 48: 73–83
Blanchard E B, Andrasik F, Guarnieri P, Neff D F, Rodichok D 1987a Two-, three-, and four-year follow-up on the self-regulatory treatment of chronic headache. Journal of Consulting and Clinical Psychology 55: 257–259
Blanchard E B, Appelbaum K A, Guarnieri P, Morrill B, Dentinger M P 1987b Five year prospective follow-up on the treatment of chronic headache with biofeedback and/or relaxation. Headache 27: 580–583
Blanchard E B, Appelbaum K A, Radnitz C L et al 1990 A controlled evaluation of thermal biofeedback and thermal biofeedback combined with cognitive therapy in the treatment of vascular headache. Journal of Consulting and Clinical Psychology 58: 216–224
Blanchard E B, Nicholson N L, Taylor A E, Steffek B D, Radnitz C L, Appelbaum K A 1991a The role of regular home practice in the relaxation treatment of tension headache. Journal of Consulting and Clinical Psychology 59: 467–470
Blanchard E B, Nicholson N L, Radnitz C L, Steffek B D, Appelbaum K A, Dentinger M P 1991b The role of home practice in thermal biofeedback. Journal of Consulting and Clinical Psychology 59: 507–512
Bodenhamer E, Coleman C, Achterberg J 1986 Self-directed EMG training for the control of pain and spasticity and paraplegia: a case study. Biofeedback and Self-Regulation 11: 199–205
Borgeat F, Elie R, Castonguay L G 1991 Muscular response to the therapist and symptomatic improvement during biofeedback for tension headache. Biofeedback and Self-Regulation 16: 147–155
Bradley L A, Young L D, Anderson K O et al 1987 Effects of psychological therapy on pain behavior of rheumatoid arthritis patients. Arthritis and Rheumatism 30: 1105–1114
Broome M E, Lillis P P, Smith M C 1989 Pain interventions with children: a meta-analysis of research. Nursing Research 38: 154–158
Burdette B H, Gale E N 1988 The effects of treatment on masticatory muscle activity and mandibular posture in myofascial pain-dysfunction patients. Journal of Dental Research 67: 1126–1130
Burke E J, Andrasik F 1989 Home- vs. clinic-based biofeedback treatment for pediatric migraine: results of treatment through one-year follow-up. Headache 29: 434–440
Bush C, Ditto B, Feuerstein M 1985 A controlled evaluation of paraspinal EMG biofeedback in the treatment of chronic low back pain. Health Psychology 4: 307–321
Carrobles J A, Cardona A, Santacreu J 1981 Shaping and generalization procedures in the EMG–biofeedback treatment of tension headaches. British Journal of Clinical Psychology 20: 49–56
Chapman S L 1986 A review and clinical perspective on the use of EMG and thermal biofeedback for chronic headaches. Pain 27: 1–43
Cleeland C S 1973 Behavior techniques in the modification of spasmodic torticollis. Neurology 23: 1241–1247
Coger R, Werbach M 1975 Attention, anxiety and the effects of learned enhancement of EEG alpha in chronic pain: a pilot study in biofeedback. In: Crue B L (ed) Pain research and treatment. Academic Press, New York, p 297–303
Collet L, Cottraux J, Juenet C 1986 GSR feedback and Schultz relaxation in tension headaches: a comparative study. Pain 25: 205–213
Counts D K, Gutsch K U, Hutton B O 1978 Spasmodic torticollis treatment through biofeedback training. Psychotherapy: Theory, Research and Practice 15: 13–15
Crockett D J, Foreman M E, Alden L, Blasberg B 1986 A comparison of treatment modes in the management of myofascial pain dysfunction syndrome. Biofeedback and Self-Regulation 11: 279–291
Crosson B 1980 Control of skin temperature through biofeedback and suggestion with hypnotized college women. International Journal of Clinical and Experimental Hypnosis 28: 75–78
Dalen K, Ellertsen B, Espelid I, Gronningsaeter A G 1986 EMG feedback in the treatment of myofascial pain dysfunction syndrome. Acta Odontologica Scandinavica 44: 279–284
Degner L, Barkwell D 1991 Nonanalgesic approaches to pain control. Cancer Nursing 14: 105–111
Devine E C, Cook T D 1986 Clinical and cost-savings effects of psychoeducational interventions with surgical patients: a meta-analysis. Research in Nursing Health 9: 89–105
Dolce J, Raczynski J 1985 Neuromuscular activity and electromyography in painful backs: psychological and biomechanical models in assessment and treatment. Psychological Bulletin 97: 502–520
Duchene P 1989 Effects of biofeedback on childbirth pain. Journal of Pain and Symptom Management 4: 117–123
Duckro P N, Cantwell-Simmons E 1989 A review of studies evaluating biofeedback and relaxation training in the management of pediatric headache. Headache 29: 428–433
Ellersten B, Nordy H, Hammerorg D, Sigurdur Thorlacious 1987 Psychophysiologic response patterns in migraine before and after temperature feedback. Cephalalgia 7: 109–124
Engel J M, Rapoff M A, Pressman A R 1992 Long-term follow-up of relaxation training for pediatric headache disorders. Headache 32: 152–156
Epstein L H, Abel G G, Collins F, Parker L, Cinciripini P M 1978 The relationship between frontalis muscle activity and self-reports of headache pain. Behaviour Research and Therapy 16: 153–160
Erlandson P M, Poppen R 1989 Electromyographic biofeedback and rest position training of masticatory muscles in myofascial pain-dysfunction patients. Journal of Prosthetic Dentistry 62: 335–338
Eysenck H 1967 The biological basis of personality. C C Thomas, Springfield, Illinois
Feehan M, Marsh N 1989 The reduction of bruxism using contingent EMG audible biofeedback: a case study. Journal of Behavior Therapy and Experimental Psychiatry 20: 179–183
Fernandez E, Turk D C 1989 The utility of cognitive coping strategies for altering pain perception: a meta-analysis. Pain 38: 123–135
Field P B 1974 Effects of tape recorded hypnotic preparation for surgery. International Journal of Clinical and Experimental Hypnosis 22: 54–61
Flaherty G G, Fitzpatrick J J 1978 Relaxation technique to increase comfort level of postoperative patients: a preliminary study. Nursing Research 27: 352–355
Flor H, Turk D C 1989 Psychophysiology of chronic pain: do chronic pain patients exhibit symptom-specific psychophysiological responses? Psychological Bulletin 105: 215–259
Flor H, Haag G, Turk D 1986 Long-term efficacy of EMG biofeedback for chronic rheumatic back pain. Pain 27: 195–202
Forsythe W I, Gilles D, Sills M A 1984 Propranolol ("Inderal") in the treatment of childhood migraine. Development Medicine and Child Neurology 26: 737–741
Freedman R R 1985 Behavioral treatment of Raynaud's disease and phenomenon. Advances in Microcirculation 12: 138–156
Freedman R R 1991 Physiological mechanisms of temperature biofeedback. Biofeedback and Self-Regulation 16: 95–114
Friedman H, Booth-Kewley S 1987 The 'disease-prone personality': a meta-analytic view of the construct. American Psychologist 42: 539–555
Frischolz E J, Tryon W W 1980 Hypnotizability in relation to the ability to learn thermal biofeedback. American Journal of Clinical Hypnosis 23: 53–56
Gainer M J 1992 Hypnotherapy for reflex sympathetic dystrophy. American Journal of Clinical Hypnosis 34: 227–232
Gallegos X, Espinoza E 1989 Retroalimentacion biologica termal versus entrenamiento autogenico en el tratamiento de la migrana. Revista Mexicana de Psicologia 6: 55–63
Gannon L, Sternbach R 1971 Alpha enhancement as a treatment for pain: a case study. Journal of Behavior Therapy And Experimental Psychiatry 2: 209–213
Gascon G 1984 Chronic and recurrent headaches in children and adolescents. Pediatric Clinics of North America 31: 1027–1051
Gauthier J G, Carrier S 1991 Long-term effects of biofeedback on migraine headache: A prospective follow-up study. Headache 31: 605–612
Gauthier J, Fradet C, Roberge C 1988 The differential effects of biofeedback in the treatment of classical and common migraine. Headache 28: 39–46
Gauthier J G, Fournier A, Roberge C 1991 The differential effects of biofeedback in the treatment of menstrual and nonmenstrual migraine . Headache 31: 82–90
Glaus D, Kotses H 1979 Generalization of conditioned muscle tension: a closer look. Psychophysiology 16: 513–519

Graffam S, Johnson A 1987 A comparison of two relaxation strategies for the relief of pain and its distress. Journal of Pain and Symptom Management 2: 229–231

Gray L, Lyle R C, McGuire R J, Peck D F 1980 Electrode placement, EMG feedback, and relaxation for tension headaches. Behaviour Research and Therapy 18: 19–23

Grazzi L, Frediani F, Zappacosta B, Boiardi A, Bussone G 1988 Psychological assessment in tension headache before and after biofeedback treatment. Headache 28: 337–338

Gregg R H 1978 Biofeedback relaxation training effects in childbirth. Behavioral Engineering 4: 57–66

Grimaud J C, Bouvier M, Naudy B, Guien C, Salducci J 1991 Manometric and radiologic investigations and biofeedback treatment of chronic idiopathic anal pain. Diseases of the Colon and Rectum 34: 690–695

Grunert B K, Devine C A, Sanger J R, Matloub H S, Green D 1990 Thermal self-regulation for pain control in reflex sympathetic dystrophy syndrome. Journal of Hand Surgery 15: 615–618

Guarnieri P, Blanchard E B 1990 Evaluation of home-based thermal biofeedback treatment of pediatric migraine headache. Biofeedback and Self-Regulation 15: 179–184

Hartman C H 1979 Response of inguinal pain to hand warming: a clinical note. Biofeedback and Self-Regulation 4: 355–357

Haynes S N, Griffin P, Mooney D, Parise M 1975 Electromyographic biofeedback and relaxation instructions for the treatment of muscle contraction headaches. Behavior Therapy 6: 672–678

Heczey M D 1978 Effects of biofeedback and autogenic training on menstrual experiences, relationships among anxiety, locus of control, and dysmenorrhea. Dissertation Abstracts International 38(B): 5571

Henryk-Gutt R, Rees W 1973 Psychological aspects of migraine. Journal of Psychosomatic Research 17: 141–153

Hoffman E 1979 Antonomic, EEG and clinical changes in neurotic patients during EMG biofeedback training. Research Communications in Psychology, Psychiatry and Behavior 4: 209–240

Holmes D S, Burish T G 1983 Effectiveness of biofeedback for treating migraine and tension headaches: a review of the evidence. Journal of Psychosomatic Research 27: 515–532

Holroyd K A, Penzien D B 1986 Client variables and the behavioral treatment of recurrent tension headache: a meta-analytic review. Journal of Behavioral Medicine 9: 515–536

Holroyd K A, Penzien D B 1989 Meta-analysis minus the analysis: a prescription for confusion. Pain 39: 359–361

Holroyd K A, Penzien D B 1990 Pharmacological versus non-pharmacological prophylaxis of recurrent migraine headache: a meta-analytic review of clinical trials. Pain 42: 1–13

Holroyd K A, Nash J M, Pingel J D, Cordingley G E, Jerome A 1991 A comparison of pharmacological (amitriptyline HCL) and nonpharmacological (cognitive–behavioral) therapies for chronic tension headaches. Journal of Consulting and Clinical Psychology 59: 387–393

Hyman R B, Feldman H R, Harris R B, Levin R F, Malloy G B 1989 The effects of relaxation training on clinical symptoms: a meta-analysis. Nursing Research 38: 216–220

IASP 1986 International Association for the Study of Pain Subcommittee on Taxonomy Classification of chronic pain. Pain (suppl) 3

Jacobs A, Felton G S 1969 Visual feedback of myoelectric output to facilitate muscle relaxation in normal persons and patients with neck injuries. Archives of Physical and Medical Rehabilitation 50: 34–39

Jacobson E 1938 Progressive relaxation. University of Chicago Press, Chicago

Jankel W R 1978 Electromyographic feedback in spasmodic torticollis. American Journal of Clinical Biofeedback 1: 29–39

Jessup B A 1989 Relaxation and biofeedback. In: Wall P, Melzack R (eds) Textbook of Pain, 2nd edn. Churchill Livingstone, Edinburgh, p 989–1000

Jessup B A, Neufeld R W J, Merskey H 1979 Biofeedback therapy for headache and other pain: an evaluative review. Pain 7: 225–270

Johansson J, Ost L 1987 Temperature-biofeedback treatment of migraine headache. Behavior Modification 11: 182–199

Juprelle M, Schoenen J 1990 Relaxation avec biofeedback musculaire dans les cephalées de type tension: analyse multifactorielle d'un groupe de 31 patients. Revue Medicale de Liège 45: 630–637

Kabat-Zinn J 1982 An outpatient program in behavioral medicine for chronic pain based on the practice of mindfulness meditation: theoretical considerations and preliminary results. General Hospital Psychiatry 4: 33–48

Kabela E, Blanchard E B, Appelbaum K A, Nicholson N 1989 Self-regulatory treatment of headache in the elderly. Biofeedback and Self-Regulation 14: 219–228

Keefe F J, Surwit R S, Pilon R N 1980 Biofeedback, autogenic training, and progressive relaxation in the treatment of Raynaud's disease: a comparative study. Journal of Applied Behavior Analysis 13: 3–11

Keefe F, Black A, Williams R, Surwit R 1981 Behavioral treatment of chronic low back pain: clinical outcome and individual differences in pain relief. Pain 11: 221–231

Kewman D G, Roberts A H 1980 Skin temperature biofeedback and migraine headaches, a double blind study. Biofeedback and Self-Regulation 5: 327–345

Kim M, Blanchard E B 1992 Two studies of the non-pharmacological treatment of menstrually-related migraine headaches. Headache 32: 197–202

Kravitz E A, Moore M E, Glaros A 1981 Paralumbar muscle activity in chronic low back pain. Archives of Physical Medicine and Rehabilitation 62: 172–176

Labbe E E, Ward C H 1990 Electromyographic biofeedback with mental imagery and home practice in the treatment of children with muscle-contraction headache. Journal of Developmental and Behavioral Pediatrics 11: 65–68

Lacroix J M, Clarke M A, Bock J C, Doxey N C S 1986a Physiological changes after biofeedback and relaxation training for multiple-pain tension-headache patients. Perceptual and Motor Skills 63: 139–153

Lacroix J M, Clarke M A, Bock J C, Doxey N C S 1986b Muscle-contraction headache in multiple-pain patients: treatment under worsening baseline conditions. Archives of Physical Medicine and Rehabilitation 67: 14–18

Lake A E, Ramey J, Papsdolf J D 1979 Biofeedback and rational-emotive therapy in the management of migraine headache. Journal of Applied Behavior Analysis 12: 127–140

Large R, Lamb A 1983 Electromyographic (EMG) feedback in chronic musculoskeletal pain: a controlled trial. Pain 17: 167–177

Larsson B, Daleflod B, Hakansson L, Melin 1987 Therapist-assisted versus self-help relaxation treatment of chronic headaches in adolescents: a school-based intervention. Journal of Child Psychology and Psychiatry and Allied Disciplines 28: 127–136

Larsson B, Melin L, Doberl A 1990 Recurrent tension headache in adolescents treated with self-help relaxation training and a muscle relaxant drug. Headache 30: 665–671

Lascelles M A, Cunningham J, McGrath P, Sullivan M J L 1989 Teaching coping strategies to adolescents with migraine. Journal of Pain and Symptom Management 4: 135–145

Linkenhoker D 1983 Tools of behavioral medicine: applications of biofeedback treatment for children and adolescents. Journal of Developmental and Behavioral Pediatrics 4: 16–20

Lisspers J, Ost L 1990a BVP-Biofeedback in the treatment of migraine. The effects of constriction and dilatation during different phases of the migraine attack. Behavior Modification 14: 200–221

Lisspers J, Ost L 1990b Long-term follow-up of migraine treatment: do the effects remain up to six years? Behaviour Research and Therapy 28: 313–322

Litt M 1986 Mediating factors in non-medical treatment for migraine headache: toward an interactional model. Journal of Psychosomatic Research 30: 505–519

Luthe W (ed) 1969 Autogenic therapy. Grune & Stratton, New York

Malone M D, Strube M J 1988 Meta-analysis of non-medical treatments for chronic pain. Pain 34: 231–244

Malone M D, Strube M J 1989 Meta-analysis of non-medical treatments for chronic pain: corrigendum. Pain 37: 128 (Reports an error in the original article by Malone & Strube 1988, Pain 34: 231–244, the name of the 3rd author was left out. The correct version should read: Malone M D, Strube M J, Scogin F R.)

Malone M D, Strube M J, Scogin F R 1989 Reply to Holroyd and Penzien. Pain 39: 362–363

Martin P R 1981 Spasmodic torticollis: investigation and treatment using EMG feedback training. Behavior Therapy 12: 247–262

Masek B, Russo D, Varni J 1984 Behavioral approaches to the

management of chronic pain in children. Pediatric Clinics of North America 31: 1113–1131

Mathew N T 1981 Prophylaxis of migraine and mixed headache: a randomized controlled study. Headache 21: 105–109

Meichenbaum D 1976 Cognitive factors in biofeedback therapy. Biofeedback and Self-Regulation 1: 201–216

Melis P M L, Rooimans W, Spierings E L H, Hoogduin C A L 1991 Treatment of chronic tension-type headache with hypnotherapy: a single-blind time controlled study. Headache 31: 686–689

Michultka D M, Poppen R L, Blanchard E B 1988 Relaxation training as a treatment for chronic headaches in an individual having severe developmental disabilities. Biofeedback and Self-Regulation 13: 257–266

Middaugh S J 1990 On clinical efficacy: why biofeedback does and does not work. Biofeedback and Self-Regulation 15: 191–208

Middaugh S, Kee W G 1987 Advances in electromyographic monitoring and biofeedback in the treatment of chronic cervical and low back pain. Advances in Rehabilitation Technology 1: 137–172

Miller K M 1987 Deep breathing relaxation. AORN Journal 45: 484–488

Mizener D, Thomas M, Billings R 1988 Cognitive changes of migraineurs receiving biofeedback training. Headache 28: 339–343

Murphy M A, Tosi D J, Parisier R F 1989 Psychological coping and the management of pain with cognitive restructuring and biofeedback: a case study and variation of cognitive experiential therapy. Psychological Reports 64: 1343–1350

Newshan G, Balamuth R 1990 Use of imagery in a chronic pain outpatient group. Imagination, Cognition and Personality 10: 25–38

Nicholas M K, Wilson P H, Goyen J 1991 Operant-behavioural and cognitive–behavioural treatment for chronic low back pain. Behaviour Research and Therapy 29: 225–238

Nicholas M K, Wilson P H, Goyen J 1992 Comparison of cognitive–behavioral group treatment and an alternative non-psychological treatment for chronic low back pain. Pain 48: 339–347

Noda H H 1979 An exploratory study of the effects of EMG and temperature biofeedback on rheumatoid arthritis. Dissertation Abstracts International 39(B): 3532–3533

Nuechterlein K, Holroyd J 1980 Biofeedback in the treatment of tension headache. Archives of General Psychiatry 37: 866–873

Olson P 1988 A long-term, single-group follow-up study of biofeedback therapy with chronic medical and psychiatric patients. Biofeedback and Self-Regulation 13: 331–346

Passchier J, Van den Bree M B M, Emmen H H, Osterhaus S O L, Orlebeke J F, Verhage F 1990 Relaxation training in school classes does not reduce headache complaints. Headache 30: 660–664

Petrie K, Azariah R 1990 Health promoting variables as predictors of response of a brief pain management program. Clinical Journal of Pain 6: 43–46

Philips C 1977 The modification of tension headache pain using EMG biofeedback. Behaviour Research and Therapy 15: 119–129

Qualls P J, Sheehan P W 1981 Electromyograph biofeedback as a relaxation technique: a critical appraisal and reassessment. Psychological Bulletin 90: 21–42

Reinking R, Hutchings D 1976 Follow-up extension of 'Tension headaches – what method is most effective?' Proceedings of the Biofeedback Research Society Seventh Annual Meeting. Colorado Springs, p 60

Rice J M 1989 Decreasing osteoarthritis pain. (A psychological case report with follow-up data.) Clinical Journal of Pain 5: 183–188

Rose G D, Carlson J G 1987 The behavioral treatment of Raynaud's disease: a review. Biofeedback and Self-Regulation 12: 257–273

Russ C A 1977 Thermal biofeedback and menstrual distress. Dissertation Abstracts International 37: 4702B–4703B

Sappington J, Fiorito E, Brehony K 1979 Biofeedback as therapy in Raynaud's disease. Biofeedback and Self-Regulation 4: 155–169

Sargent J, Walters E, Green E 1973 Psychosomatic self-regulation of migraine headache. Seminars in Psychiatry 5: 415–428

Schechter N 1985 Pain and pain control in children. Current Problems in Pediatrics 15: 1–67

Schlutter L C, Golden C J, Blume H G 1980 A comparison of treatments for prefrontal muscle contraction headache. British Journal of Medical Psychology 53: 47–52

Schoenen J, Gerard P, De Pasqua V, Sianard-Gainko J 1991a Multiple clinical and paraclinical analyses of chronic tension-type headache associated or unassociated with disorder of pericranial muscles. Cephalalgia 11: 135–139

Schoenen J, Gerard P, De Pasqua V, Juprelle M 1991b EMG activity in pericranial muscles during postural variation and mental activity in healthy volunteers and patients with chronic tension type headache. Headache 31: 321–324

Schoenen J, Bottin D, Hardy F, Gerard P 1991c Cephalic and extracephalic pressure pain thresholds in chronic tension-type headache. Pain 47: 145–149

Schwartz M 1987 Biofeedback and stress management in the treatment of headache. Journal of Craniomandibular Disorders 1: 41–45

Shea D S, Ohnmeiss D O, Stith W J et al 1990 The effect of sensory deprivation in the reduction of pain in patients with chronic low-back pain. Spine 16: 560–561

Shedivy D I, Kleinman K M 1977 Lack of correlation between frontalis EMG and either neck EMG or verbal ratings of tension. Psychophysiology 14: 182–186

Sherman R A, Gail N, Gormly J 1979 Treatment of phantom limb pain with muscular relaxation training to disrupt the pain-anxiety-tension cycle. Pain 6: 47–55

Smith M S, Womack W M 1987 Stress management techniques in childhood and adolescence. Clinical Pediatrics 26: 581–585

Smith W B 1987 Biofeedback and relaxation training: the effect on headache and associated symptoms. Headache 27: 511–514

Sokel B, Devane S, Bentovim A 1991 Getting better with honor: individualized relaxation/self-hypnosis techniques for control of recalcitrant abdominal pain in children. Family Systems Medicine 9: 83–91

Sorbi M, Tellegen B 1986 Differential effects of training in relaxation and stress-coping in patients with migraine. Headache 26: 473–481

Sorbi M, Tellegen B, Du Long A 1989 Long-term effects of training in relaxation and stress-coping in patients with migraine: a 3-year follow-up. Headache 29: 111–121

Spinhoven P, Linssen A C G 1991 Behavioral treatment of chronic low back pain. I Relation of coping strategy use to outcome. Pain 45: 29–34

Steffek B D, Blanchard E B 1991 The role of absorption capacity in thermal biofeedback treatment of vascular headache. Biofeedback and Self-Regulation 16: 267–275

Stuckey S J, Jacobs A, Goldfarb J 1986 EMG biofeedback training, relaxation training, and placebo for the relief of chronic back pain. Perceptual and Motor Skills 63 1023–1036

Szekely B, Botwin D, Eidelmen B H, Becker M, Elman N, Schemm R 1986 Nonpharmacological treatment of menstrual headache: relaxation–biofeedback behaviour therapy and person-centred insight therapy. Headache 26: 86–92

Tarler-Benlolo L 1978 The role of relaxation in biofeedback training: a critical review of the literature. Psychological Bulletin 85: 727–755

Thompson J K, Haber J D, Tearman B H 1981 Generalization of frontalis electromyographic feedback to adjacent muscle groups: a critical review. Psychosomatic Medicine 1978 43: 19–24

Tsushima W T, Hawk A B 1978 EMG biofeedback treatment of traumatic headaches: a preliminary outcome study. American Journal of Clinical Biofeedback 1: 65–67

Turner J A, Chapman C R 1982a Psychological interventions for chronic pain: a critical review. I. Relaxation training and biofeedback. Pain 12: 1–21

Turner J A, Chapman C R 1982b Psychological interventions for chronic pain: a critical review. II. Operant conditioning, hypnosis, and cognitive–behavioral therapy. Pain 12: 23–46

Uchiyama K, Lutterjohann M, Shah M D 1977 Biofeedback-assisted desensitization treatment of writer's cramps. Journal of Behavior Therapy and Experimental Psychiatry 8: 169–171

Vargas J J, Ibanez J, Colotla V A 1987 Efecto de la relajacion en el reporte del dolor por dismenorrea. Revista Mexicana de Psicologia 4: 36–40

Wachtmann K R 1978 Effects of two modalities of treatment for tension headaches on personality within a lower socioeconomic population. Dissertation Abstracts International 38: 3918

Walker B B, Lawton C A, Sandman C A 1978 Voluntary control of electrogastric activity. Psychosomatic Medicine 40: 610–619

Wallbaum A B C, Pzewnicki R, Steele H, Svedfeld P 1991 Progressive muscle relaxation and restructured environmental stimulation therapy for chronic tension headache: a pilot study. International Journal of Psychosomatics 38: 33–39
Waters W 1973 The epidemiological enigma of migraine. International Journal of Epidemiology 2: 189–194
White A, Gordon S 1982 Synopsis: workshop on idiopathic low-back pain. Spine 7: 141–149
Wickramasekera I E 1973 Temperature feedback for the control of migraine. Journal of Behavior Therapy and Experimental Psychiatry 4: 343–345
Wickramasekera I, Truong X T, Bush M, Orr C 1976 The management of rheumatoid arthritic pain: preliminary observations. In: Wickramasekera I (ed) Biofeedback, behavior therapy and hypnosis. Nelson-Hall, Chicago, p 47–55
Wilkinson M 1988 Treatment of migraine. Headache 28: 659–661
Wisniewski J J, Genshaft J L, Mulick J A, Coury D L, Hammer D 1988 Relaxation therapy and compliance in the treatment of adolescent headache. Headache 28: 612–617
Wolf S L, Wolf L B, Segal R L 1989 The relationship of extraneous movements to lumbar paraspinal muscle activity: implications for EMG biofeedback training applications to low back pain patients. Biofeedback and Self-Regulation 14: 63–73
Ziegler D, Hassanein R, Hassanein K 1972 Headache syndromes suggested by factor analysis of symptom variables on a headache prone population. Journal of Chronic Diseases 25: 353–363

74. A cognitive–behavioural approach to pain management

Dennis C. Turk and Donald Meichenbaum

INTRODUCTION

In recent years there has been a proliferation of multidisciplinary pain clinics, so that it is estimated that there are currently over 2000 such clinics in the United States alone. These pain clinics have employed a broad range of psychological as well as somatic treatments (Turk et al 1983; Flor et al 1992). Their multifaceted treatment approach is consistent with the increasing evidence that pain extends beyond the sole contribution of sensory phenomena to include cognitive, affective and behavioural factors (Melzack & Wall 1983; Turk et al 1993).

Despite the proliferation of pain clinics and treatment modalities, relatively few comprehensive programmes have received systematic empirical evaluation (Flor et al 1992). Turner & Chapman (1982) have suggested that most research on the efficacy of pain management programmes has focused on two approaches:

1. the operant-conditioning approach developed by Fordyce and his colleagues (Fordyce et al 1973)
2. the cognitive–behavioural approach outlined by Turk et al (1983; see also Holzman et al 1986; Turk et al 1986; Turk & Rudy 1993).

In the present chapter we shall describe the central features of a cognitive–behavioural approach to pain management. For a detailed examination of the operant-conditioning approach, see Fordyce (1976) and Chapter 76 of this volume.

RATIONALE FOR THE COGNITIVE–BEHAVIOURAL APPROACH

The cognitive–behavioural perspective on pain management evolved from research on a number of psychologically-based problems (e.g. anxiety, depression and phobias). Following the initial empirical research on cognitive–behavioural techniques in the early 1970s, there have been a large number of research and clinical applications (Meichenbaum 1977, 1985; Beck et al 1979; Kendall & Hollon 1979). The common denominators across different cognitive–behavioural approaches include:

1. interest in the nature and modification of a patient's thoughts, feelings and beliefs, as well as behaviours
2. some commitment to behaviour therapy procedures in promoting change (such as graded practice, homework assignments, relaxation, relapse prevention training).

In general, the cognitive–behavioural therapist is concerned with using environmental manipulations, as are behaviour (operant-conditioning) therapists; but for the cognitive–behavioural therapist such manipulations represent informational feedback trials that provide an opportunity for the patient to question, reappraise and acquire self-control over maladaptive thoughts, feelings, behaviours and physiological responses. Thus, contrary to the suggestion of some authors (Ciccone & Grzesiak 1984; Rachlin 1985) there is no reason why the cognitive perspective and operant approaches should be viewed as incompatible or why they cannot or should not be integrated to create a cognitive–behavioural approach to treatment.

Although the cognitive–behavioural approach was developed originally for the treatment of psychologically-based disorders, the perspective has much in common with the multidimensional conceptualisations of pain that emphasise the contributions of cognitive and affective as well as sensory phenomena (Melzack & Wall 1965). Both the cognitive–behavioural perspective and the Gate Control Model of pain emphasise the important contribution of psychological variables such as the perception of control, the meaning of pain to the patient and dysphoric affect. According to Melzack & Casey (1968):

> The surgical and pharmacological attacks on pain might well profit by redirecting thinking toward the neglected and almost forgotten contribution of motivational and cognitive processes. Pain can be treated not only by trying to cut down sensory input by anesthetic blocks, surgical interventions and the like but also by influencing the motivational-affective and cognitive factors as well.

Melzack (1980) has also suggested that 'cognitive processes are at the forefront of the most exciting new psychological approaches to pain, fear and anxiety'. The cognitive–behavioural approach focuses directly on cognitive processes as well as on affect, environmental and sensory phenomena. Each of the components of pain conceptualised in the Gate Control Model is incorporated within the cognitive–behavioural treatment programme.

OVERVIEW OF THE COGNITIVE–BEHAVIOURAL PERSPECTIVE

It is important to differentiate the cognitive–behavioural perspective from cognitive–behavioural treatments. The cognitive–behavioural perspective is based on five central assumptions (Table 74.1) and can be superimposed upon any treatment approach employed with chronic-pain patients. In many cases the perspective is as important as the content of the therapeutic modalities employed, somatic as well as psychological (Turk & Holzman 1986; Turk & Rudy 1993).

The application of the cognitive–behavioural perspective to the treatment of chronic pain involves a complex clinical interaction and makes use of a wide range of tactics and techniques. Despite the specific techniques used, all cognitive–behavioural treatment approaches are characterised by being active, time-limited, and structured. Collaboration is central to the cognitive–behavioural approach. Therapists are not simply conveyers of information but serve as educators, coaches and trainers. They work in concert with the patient (and sometimes family members) to achieve mutually agreed-upon goals.

A growing body of research has demonstrated the important roles that cognitive factors (appraisals, beliefs, expectancies) play in exacerbating pain and suffering, contributing to disability and in influencing response to treatment (Turk & Rudy 1992). Thus, cognitive–behavioural interventions are designed to help patients identify maladaptive patterns and acquire, develop and practise more adaptive coping techniques. Patients are encouraged to become aware of, and monitor, the impact that negative pain-engendering thoughts and feelings play in the maintenance of maladaptive 'pain behaviours'. Additionally, patients are taught to recognise the connections linking cognition, affect and behaviour, together with their joint consequences. Finally, patients are encouraged to undertake 'personal experiments' and to test the effects of their cognitions and beliefs by means of selected homework assignments. The cognitive–behavioural therapist is concerned not only with the role that patients' cognitions play in contributing to their disorders, but, equally important, the therapist is concerned about the nature and adequacy of the patients' behavioural repertoire, since this affects resultant intrapersonal and interpersonal situations.

Table 74.1 Assumptions of the cognitive–behavioural perspective

- Individuals are active processors of information and not passive reactors
- Thoughts (e.g. appraisals, expectancies, beliefs) can elicit and influence mood, affect physiological processes, have social consequences and can also serve as an impetus for behaviour; conversely, mood, physiology, environmental factors and behaviour can influence the nature and content of thought processes
- Behaviour is reciprocally determined by *both* the individual and environmental factors
- Individuals can learn more adaptive ways of thinking, feeling, and behaving
- Individuals should be active collaborative agents in changing their maladaptive thoughts, feelings and behaviours

A cognitive–behavioural treatment programme for pain patients involves a multifaceted treatment programme for individuals or groups and may be conducted on an inpatient or outpatient basis. A detailed presentation of the comprehensive treatment programme is offered in Turk et al (1983). In this chapter we will focus only on the psychological components of the cognitive–behavioural treatment; however, it is important to acknowledge that the psychological treatment modalities described need to be considered within a broader rehabilitation model that also includes physical components, vocational components and to a greater or lesser extent involvement of significant others.

The cognitive–behavioural perspective outlined above should be considered not merely as a set of methods designed to address the psychological components of pain and disability, but as an organising strategy for more comprehensive rehabilitation (Turk & Stieg 1987). For example, patients' difficulties arising during physical therapy may be associated not only with physical limitations, but with the fear associated with anticipation of increased pain or concern about injury. Therefore, from a cognitive–behavioural perspective, physical therapists need not only to address the patient's performance of physical-therapy exercises and the accompanying attention to body mechanics, but also to address the patient's expectancies and fears. These cognitive and affective processes, including self-management concerns, need to be considered, together with traditional instructions regarding the proper performance of exercise. The same attention to the individual's thoughts and expectancies should be adopted by all members of the interdisciplinary treatment team.

The cognitive–behavioural treatment consists of five overlapping phases that are listed in Table 74.2. Although the five treatment phases are listed separately, it is important to appreciate that they overlap. The distinction between phases is designed to highlight the different components of the multidimensional treatment.

Table 74.2 Phases in cognitive–behavioural treatment

1. Initial assessment
2. Collaborative reconceptualisation of the patient's views of pain
3. Skills acquisition and skills consolidation, including cognitive and behavioural rehearsal
4. Generalisation, maintenance and relapse prevention
5. Booster sessions and follow-up

Moreover, although the treatment, as presented, follows a logical sequence, it should be implemented in a flexible, individually-tailored fashion. Patients proceed at varying paces and the therapist must be sensitive to these individual differences. At times, the therapist may decide not to move on to the next phase of the treatment as would be expected, but instead will address some pressing problems or concerns of the patient that may be interfering with progress. In short, therapists must realise that flexibility and clinical skills have to be brought into play throughout the cognitive–behavioural treatment programme.

The cognitive–behavioural treatment that we will describe is *not* designed to eliminate patients' pain per se, although the intensity and frequency of their pain may be reduced as a result of increased activity, physical reconditioning achieved during physical therapy and by means of the acquisition of various cognitive and behavioural coping skills. The treatment is designed to help patients learn to live more effective and satisfying lives, despite the presence of varying levels of discomfort. Other goals include the reduction of excessive reliance on the health-care system, reduced dependence on analgesic medications, increased functional capacity, and, whenever feasible, return to employment or usual household activities. Table 74.3 outlines the primary objectives of cognitive–behavioural treatment. The treatment programme can readily supplement other forms of somatic, pharmacological and psychological treatment.

The overriding message of the cognitive–behavioural approach, one that begins with the initial contact and is woven throughout the fabric of treatment, is that patients are not helpless in dealing with their pain nor need they view pain as an all-encompassing determinant of their lives. Rather, a variety of resources are available for confronting pain, a pain that will come to be viewed by patients in a more differentiated manner. The treatment encourages patients to maintain a problem-solving orientation and to develop a sense of resourcefulness, instead of the sense of helplessness and withdrawal that revolves around bed, physicians and pharmacists.

PHASE 1: ASSESSMENT

The assessment and reconceptualisation phases are highly interdependent. The assessment phase serves several distinct functions as outlined in Table 74.4. Assessment information is obtained by interviewing patients and significant others, as well as by using standardised self-report measures and observational procedures (see Turk & Melzack 1992 for a detailed review of assessment methods). During the assessment phase, psychosocial and behavioural factors are evaluated and the integration of this information with biomedical information is used in treatment planning. There should be a close relationship between the data acquired during the assessment phase and the nature, focus and goals of the therapeutic regimen.

PHASE 2: RECONCEPTUALISATION

A central feature of cognitive–behavioural treatment is to facilitate the emergence of a new conceptualisation of pain

Table 74.3 Primary objectives of cognitive–behavioural treatment programmes

- To combat demoralisation by assisting patients to change their view of their pain and suffering from overwhelming to manageable
- To teach patients that there are coping techniques and skills that can be used to help them to adapt and respond to pain and the resultant problems
- To assist patients to reconceptualise their view of themselves from being passive, reactive and helpless to being active, resourceful and competent
- To help patients learn the associations between thoughts, feelings and their behaviour, and subsequently to identify and alter automatic, maladaptive patterns
- To teach patients specific coping skills and, moreover, when and how to utilise these more adaptive responses
- To bolster self-confidence and to encourage patients to attribute successful outcomes to their own efforts
- To help patients anticipate problems proactively and generate solutions, thereby facilitating maintenance and generalisation

Table 74.4 Functions of assessment

- To establish the extent of physical impairment
- To identify levels and areas of psychological distress
- To establish, collaboratively, behavioural goals covering such areas as activity level, use of the health-care system, patterns of medication use and response of significant others
- To provide baseline measures against which the progress and success of treatment can be compared
- To provide detailed information about the patient's perceptions of his or her medical condition, previous treatments and expectations about current treatment
- To detail the patient's occupational history, goals vis-à-vis work
- To examine the important role of significant others in the maintenance and exacerbation of maladaptive behaviours and to determine how they can be positive resources in the change process
- To begin the reconceptualisation process by assisting patients and significant others to become aware of the situational variability of the pain and the psychological, behavioural and social factors that influence the nature and degree of pain

during the course of treatment, thereby permitting the patient's symptoms to be viewed as circumscribed and addressable problems, rather than as a vague, undifferentiated, overwhelming experience. The reconceptualisation process is designed to prepare the patient for future therapeutic interventions in a way designed to anticipate and minimise patient-resistance and treatment non-adherence (see Meichenbaum & Turk 1987 and Turk & Rudy 1991 for discussions of methods available to increase treatment adherence).

From both the assessment materials and information provided by the patient, the therapist attempts to alter the patient's conceptualisation of his or her problem from one based on a sensory view of pain to a more multifaceted view with cognitive, affective and socioenvironmental factors considered as contributors to the experience of pain. Through this process, patients are educated to think in terms of a treatment that will be effective in enhancing and providing them with greater control over their lives, even if the pain cannot be completely eliminated (Turk et al 1986).

First contact with the patient

The reconceptualisation process begins with the patient's initial contact with the therapist. The therapist is concerned with establishing the source of the referral, general details of the pain complaint, the patient's general state of health, ongoing treatment (if any), the date of the last complete physical examination and the patient's understanding of the reasons for which he or she has been referred to a nonmedical pain specialist. From the beginning, potential patients are directed toward viewing this opportunity as being unlike others they have experienced with health-care providers – they can be helped, but only if they are prepared to participate by making a serious commitment to take an active role in the intervention and in reshaping their lives. Patients are provided with information about the multiple effects of chronic pain on people's lives, general demands and specific components of the treatment programme.

As part of this initial contact, pain questionnaires are administered that are designed to elicit information regarding patients' thoughts and feelings about their capacity to exert control over pain and many other aspects of their lives (see The West Haven–Yale Multidimensional Pain Inventory (MPI), Kerns et al 1985). In addition, by means of a structured interview, questions are asked that are designed to help patients view their severest pain episodes as having a definite beginning, middle and ending; to see pain episodes as variable, but not being life-threatening; to interpret them as responses that can be controlled, and to view them as responsive to the passage of time, situational factors, and life circumstances. As part of this assessment, the therapist encourages the patient's spouse or significant other to identify the impact of the patient's pain on them, the effect of their behaviour on the patient, as well as to provide the family members with an understanding of the cognitive–behavioural treatment approach. There is increasing evidence that significant others play an important role in the maintenance and exacerbation of pain, and, moreover, are themselves affected by living with a person with chronic pain (Kerns & Turk 1984; Flor et al 1987a, 1987b).

At this point the therapist introduces the concept of 'pain behaviours' and 'operant pain' (following Fordyce) and discusses the important role that significant others may play in unwittingly, inadvertently and perhaps unknowingly reinforcing the patient's overt expression of pain and suffering. Such behaviours as grimacing, lying down, avoiding certain activities and moaning are offered as examples of 'pain behaviours'. The patient's significant other is encouraged to recall examples of the patient's specific pain behaviours. The spouse or significant other is also asked to complete a diary of the patient's pain behaviours and his or her responses. This homework assignment serves to highlight the role pain has come to have in their lives and the importance of significant others in the treatment. The question put to the spouse or significant other is: 'How do you know when your spouse is experiencing severe pain?'

The patient may be asked to complete a self-report diary for 1–2 weeks. Patients are asked to record episodes each day when they view their pain as moderate to severe and also when they are feeling particularly upset or distressed. They are also asked to record the circumstances surrounding the episode, who was present, what they thought, how they felt, what they did and whether what they did had any effect on the level of their pain. Diaries are designed so that the therapist will use them to assist patients to identify the links among thoughts, feelings, behaviours, pain intensity and distress.

Finally, patients may be provided with pain intensity rating cards to record a 2-week baseline of pain intensity. The pain-rating cards each contain a list of the hours of the day and a six-point scale of intensity with 0 = no pain to 5 = incapacitating, severe pain. Patients are instructed to rate the intensity of the pain they experience at various times during each waking day. Space is also provided on these cards for patients to indicate the time when medication is ingested and the specific incidents or thoughts and feelings that accompany intense pain (Turk et al 1983).

The pain intensity rating cards are designed to demonstrate to the patients and spouse that, contrary to their expectations, the patient rarely experiences the most intense pain over extended periods and that the intensity of the pain tends to rise and fall. Patients often find this variability surprising in view of their earlier descriptions of their pain. The identification of the pain pattern functions to encourage a sense of control-through-predictability (i.e.

pain peaks and troughs, once recognised are amenable to self-management strategies). As therapists, we can ask questions, help patients juxtapose data and provide examples that facilitate a reconceptualisation of the pain experience.

A note regarding homework assignments is in order. Since the conduct of homework assignments (such as keeping pain diaries, self-monitoring of pain levels, and so forth) are critical to cognitive–behavioural treatment, the therapist must insure that the patient and significant other understand the rationale, goals and actual procedures included with each homework assignment. A useful way to assess such understanding is to use a role-reversal procedure where the patient or significant other is required, in their own words, to explain the nature and rationale of the homework assignments to the therapist. The patient and significant other may be asked how they feel about the assignment, whether they believe they will be able to carry it out or whether they can foresee any problems or obstacles that would interfere with satisfactory completion of the assignments. If they can imagine problems developing, they are asked how they might deal with these should they occur. If no problems can be identified by the patients, the therapist may suggest some possibilities (e.g. they may forget to record a day, they may feel embarrassed to self-monitor). In order to reduce feelings of defensiveness on the part of patients, the therapist might preface specifying problems by suggesting that 'although you do not foresee any problems, some patients have told us that a problem for them was ...' and 'How would you suggest that you would deal with such a problem if it was to arise?' The therapist should anticipate and subsume any possible patient problems in conducting homework assignments within the therapeutic context.

Finally, it should be noted that the assessment should also focus on the patient's strengths and resources (e.g. coping abilities, competencies, social supports). These can be incorporated into subsequent treatment phases and contribute to the cognitive restructuring process.

Preliminary formulation of treatment goals

At this point the patient, spouse and therapist *collaborate* in establishing treatment goals that will return the patient to optimal functioning in light of any physical restriction and that are consistent with the patient's wishes. From the cognitive–behavioural perspective, collaboration is essential because it helps patients to feel that they are responsible for what occurs in treatment and for the outcomes. It is often useful to use the information obtained from the structured interview, such as 'How would your life be different if your pain could be relieved?', to generate specific goals. The goals for the patient must be specific and measurable. For example, a patient's goal 'to feel better' is inadequate. The patient needs to specify what he or she will be doing that will indicate such improvement. We have found it useful to establish collaboratively short-term, intermediate and long-term goals in order that reinforcement by goal achievement can occur early in treatment, thus enhancing patients' self-confidence. The treatment goals agreed upon – guided rather than dictated by the therapist – typically include medication reduction, increased activity (recreational, exercise), specific tasks to accomplish at home and on the job, reduction in the inappropriate use of the health-care system and other patient goals.

Towards the end of the reconceptualisation phase it is appropriate to provide a brief description of what will occur in subsequent sessions such as education and practice of specific cognitive and behavioural coping skills. It is important that patients and significant others understand the kinds of demands and expectancies of the programme and the likely impact their efforts will have on all phases of their lives. Clarification of the treatment demands at the earliest phases of the programme helps to circumvent problems that often arise later during therapy.

Graded exercise and activities

Many chronic-pain patients have developed a sedentary lifestyle that can exacerbate pain by reducing endurance, strength and flexibility. Thus, the therapist, in collaboration with a physiotherapist and the patient's physician, should develop a graded exercise–activity programme appropriate to the patient's physical status, age and gender. As is the case in operant-conditioning treatments, patients maintain activity-level charts of achievable, incremental goals from which progress can be gauged by the patient, as well as by the specific therapist and other family and treatment team members. Initial goals are set at a level that the patient should have little trouble achieving, with the requirements increasing at a gradual rate.

The exercise–activity programme has four major objectives. First, that of ameliorating physiological consequences that may exacerbate pain. Moreover, for chronic-pain patients and their families, pain is a major focus of attention. Each physical sensation, each environmental demand is viewed in terms of its significance for experiencing pain. Thus, the second objective of the exercise–activity programme is to increase the likelihood that the pain patient and his or her family develop interests other than pain. In this way 'pain' becomes more peripheral and competes for attention with other activities, rather than being the focal point of the patient's life. Thirdly, the graded exercise programme provides for success experiences and thereby will help to reduce fear of activity. Finally, the graded exercise programme reinforces the patient's perception of his or her own control and encourages self-attribution of successes.

Medication reduction

Another important issue to discuss with the patient is the usage of analgesic medication. There is sufficient evidence to indicate that many patients are overmedicated and often are dependent on analgesics. It is advantageous to help patients reduce and eventually eliminate all unnecessary medication. Since reduction of some drugs is known to be accompanied by serious side-effects, consultation with the physician is imperative.

There are two schools of thought concerning the procedure to employ during drug withdrawal. Operant-oriented treatment programmes like that of Fordyce and his colleagues (Fordyce 1976) require the patient to take medication at specific times rather than PRN (as required) and they mask the medication in a liquid medium (a 'pain cocktail') with systematic reduction of the percentage of active ingredient by the treatment manager. The patient is informed of the process of reduction prior to the initiation of the programme, but does not influence the schedule of the weaning process.

A second view regarding reduction of medication, one more congruent with the cognitive–behavioural perspective, also encourages the use of medication at specific intervals since self-control and responsibility are major factors in this approach. However, the therapist encourages the patient to systematically reduce his or her medication, helps the patient design procedures by which this can be accomplished and shares major responsibility for medication control with the patient. The patient is required to record the quantity and time of medication intake. The importance of medication reduction is stressed and the patient's medication records are carefully monitored. If the patient does not follow the guidelines in reducing the dosage, then this becomes a focus of discussion. The attempt to control medication intake is looked upon as a personal responsibility and the reasons for failure are considered in depth.

Translation process

At this time the translation or reconceptualisation process begins in a more formal manner. A simplified conceptualisation of pain based on the Gate Control Model of Melzack & Wall (1965) is presented and contrasted with the unidimensional sensory–physiological model held by many patients. The interaction of cognitions, affect and sensory aspects of a situation is presented in a clear, understandable fashion using the patient's self-monitored experiences as illustrations (Turk et al 1983). For example, the impact of anxiety is briefly considered and related to the exacerbation of pain. Data from patient diaries are extremely useful to make this point more concrete. Patients can review recent stressful episodes and examine the course his or her pain followed at that time. One coronary patient, who had been aware of a connection between periods of tension and the intensity of his pain, attributed the pain to changes in the state of his heart. As the details of his situation were examined, an alternative explanation emerged, namely, that the nature of his pain was stress-related. Muscle tension in the chest and shoulders increased when he was feeling stressed, but the heart rate and pulse remained unchanged. The patient's misattribution prevented appropriate action from being taken to reduce the muscle contraction that aggravated the chest-wall pain. The reappraisal of the pain stimulus both improved his ability to control the pain through timely and target-appropriate interventions, which in turn improved his sense of self-efficacy (Bandura 1977; Dolce et al 1986).

One item included in our pain questionnaire that we have found to be particularly suited to providing examples of how cognitive and affective factors, such as appraisal of the situation and coping resources, contribute to the pain experience asks the patient to close his or her eyes and to imagine the last time he or she had experienced intense pain ('5' on the pain-rating cards) and to record as many thoughts and feelings as possible that he or she had experienced before, during and after the episode. One patient who suffered with migraine headaches provided the following response to the item:

> For hours and hours. God, will it ever end, how much longer do I have to live this way? I have outlived my usefulness ... the hours are endless and I am alone. I wish someone could take a sharp knife and cut that artery ... How long will it be until I am sent to a mental institution? Migraines are not fatal; doctors don't care. You live through one, only to be striken with another in a few days. I am incapable of everything I used to do. How am I going to fill the rest of my life? Unemployed, can't do anything, and all alone!

This patient feels helpless, views her situation as hopeless and appraises her situation as one of continued deterioration. In such situations, patients are asked to consider the impact of such thoughts and feelings on the experience of pain and what they can do in such circumstances. In this manner, the therapist engages the patient in a Socratic dialogue in order to illustrate how such thinking may maintain and exacerbate pain and to consider alternative coping responses.

The example of Beecher's (1959) observation on the pain experienced by Second World War soldiers wounded at Anzio in Italy can be used as an example of how appraisal and meaning systems affect the perception of pain. Beecher noted that many soldiers did not report experiencing intense pain, despite having incurred life-endangering battle wounds. Beecher attributed these responses to the meaning of an experience and suggested that the individual's appraisal influences how much pain he or she perceives. The therapist uses examples from the patient's experience that illustrate similar processes.

Biofeedback equipment may be used to illustrate the relationship between stress and muscle tension. Patients can be attached to biofeedback equipment and asked to tense relevant muscles and to attend to the changes in the information fed back (visual or auditory). The therapist may then ask the patients to relax the muscles (may give some guidance in how to do this) and to observe the changes in the tones or lights. The therapist can call to patients' attention their ability to change physiological functions, thus relating muscle tension to the exacerbation of pain. This can often have a dramatic effect in helping patients to realise the relationship between thoughts, feelings, and muscle tension. Moreover, it can demonstrate to patients that they can, at least to some extent, control their own bodies. Consistent with the cognitive–behavioural perspective, biofeedback training has been found to increase pain patients' locus of control and self-efficacy, even if physiological changes have not occurred (Turk & Rudy 1992).

To facilitate this reappraisal process, the therapist introduces the notion that the patient's experience of pain can be viewed as consisting of several manageable phases, rather than one overwhelming undifferentiated assault. In this way the patient comes to view his or her pain as composed of several components that go through different phases which are, in part, influenced by his or her reactions. The patient is not the 'helpless victim' of pain. The therapist and patient have collected data to support this more differentiated view of pain, thus providing the basis for the intervention programme that will follow.

Examples are offered to show how pain can be subdivided into several steps, each of which is manageable by the patient. For example, when the patient rates his or her pain as 0 or 1 on a six-point scale (i.e. no pain or fairly low-level intensity) this is an opportunity for the patient to engage in productive coping activities. This period of low-intensity pain can function as a time when the patient can plan how he or she will deal with more intense levels of pain by means of employing cognitive and behavioural coping strategies that the patient will learn by the end of the treatment programme. Similarly, the patient can develop coping skills to employ at the higher levels of pain intensity. The patient is encouraged to view pain as a problem to be prepared for and solved. A useful analogy is the way athletic teams develop game plans. Preplanning lowers the risk of the patient becoming overwhelmed at times of more severe pain, while implicitly fostering an expectation that episodes of severe pain will pass. Patients are also encouraged to self-reinforce their efforts throughout by taking credit for their coping efforts.

Negative thoughts, pain-engendering appraisals and attributions are reviewed in treatment in order that the patient will not be surprised when and if they do arise. Rather, the patient is encouraged to use the negatively-valenced cognitions and feelings as reminders or as cues to initiate more adaptive coping strategies. The pain diaries described earlier can provide information that becomes the focus of discussion. For example, patients who recorded thoughts that they felt 'incompetent' and 'helpless' in controlling their pain during a specific episode can be encouraged to become aware of when they engage in such thinking and to appreciate how such thoughts may exacerbate their pain and become a self-fulfilling prophecy. Alternative thoughts such as a realistic appraisal of the situation and of their coping resources are encouraged and patients reinforced for using one or more of the coping strategies covered during the skills training. The patient is encouraged to divide the situation into stages as described earlier and to acknowledge that the most severe pain is usually relatively transitory. Such 'cognitive restructuring' is incorporated throughout the treatment regimen. The therapist also incorporates examples of when the patient has been resourceful in his or her life and considers how these skills can be applied in the pain situation.

PHASE 3: SKILLS-ACQUISITION AND SKILLS-CONSOLIDATION

The skills-acquisition and skills-consolidation phase begins once the basic initial goals of the treatment programme have been agreed upon. During this third phase the therapist provides practice in the use of a variety of cognitive- and behavioural-coping skills that are geared toward the alteration of the patient's response to environmental contributors to pain, to bolstering coping skills (e.g. attention diversion, relaxation skills for dealing with specific symptoms), to changing maladaptive interpretations and to changing factors that might contribute to stress (e.g. maladaptive communication patterns).

The order in which the various cognitive and behavioural strategies are covered can be varied depending upon the patient's needs. In addition to helping the patient develop specific coping skills, this phase is also designed to help patients use skills they already possess and to enhance the patient's belief in his or her ability to exercise control, further enhancing a sense of self-efficacy. The point to be underscored is that the cognitive–behavioural approach does not deal exclusively with the pain symptoms per se, but with those self-statements and environmental factors that may instigate or maintain less than optimal functioning and subsequent pain exacerbations. Alterations in lifestyle, problem-solving, communication-skills training, relaxation skills and homework assignments are woven into the fabric of the treatment.

Problem-solving

A useful way to think about pain is as a set of sequential problems, rather than simply as the presence of pain being a single overwhelming problem. That is, many patients view pain as their overriding problem and their only problem. An alternative that is encouraged by cognitive–behavioural therapists is that chronic pain presents the sufferer with an array of small and large problems – familial, occupational, social, recreational and financial, as well as physical. The therapist assists patients in identifying their problems in these areas and suggests that a method for dealing with these problems is to generate a set of alternatives and to weigh the relative advantages and disadvantages of each of these alternatives. The therapist also suggests that patients can select what they believe is the best solution and to try it out to see if it resolves or reduces the problem. It is also suggested that patients can recycle through the problem-solving process.

There are several critical features of problem-solving skills training. The important first step in problem-solving is to have patients 'operationalise' their problems in behaviourally prescriptive language (e.g. when X occurs in situation Y, I feel Z). The second step is to help patients identify what particular situations are associated with pain. The use of self-monitoring in patient diaries can help to identify such problematic situations. Patients need to think of the difficulties that they encounter as 'problems to be solved'. Next they must try out the alternative to achieve the desired outcome. Patients need to learn that there is usually not a single solution or alternative to solve problems and they need to weigh alternatives. In this way lack of success with any one attempt will not be taken as a complete failure, but rather such setbacks and lapses are viewed as learning trials and occasions to consider alternatives.

It is all too easy to conduct problem-solving during treatment but much harder to do so in the patient's natural environment. Patients may be given the homework task of formally identifying problems, generating alternative solutions, rating the solutions for likely effectiveness, trying them out and then reporting on the outcome. Throughout treatment, the therapist can use the language of problems and solutions to illustrate the value of using the problem-solving approach. The therapist uses terms and phrases like 'notice', 'catch', 'interrupt', 'plan', 'game plan', 'being in charge', 'having choices', 'performing experiments', 'setting goals' and the like.

Relaxation and controlled breathing

Relaxation and controlled-breathing exercises are especially useful in the skills-acquisition phase because they can be readily learned by almost all patients and they have a good deal of face validity. The relaxation and controlled breathing involve systematically tensing and relaxing of various muscle groups, both general and specific to the particular area of pain reported by patients. Emphasis on controlled breathing is included, due to research demonstrating that the amplitude and frequency of respiration has an effect upon heart rate and the accompanying experience of anxiety (Turk et al 1983). Instruction in the use of relaxation and controlled breathing is designed not only to teach an incompatible response, but also as a way of helping the patients develop a behavioural-coping skill that they can use in any situation in which adaptive coping is required. The practice of relaxation and controlled breathing strengthens the patients' belief that they can exert control during periods of stress and pain and that they are not helpless. Patients are encouraged to employ the relaxation skills in situations where they perceive themselves becoming tense, anxious or experiencing pain.

Relaxation is not achieved by only one method; in fact, there are a large number of relaxation techniques in the literature. At this point, there is no evidence that one relaxation approach is any more effective than any other. What is most important is to state these findings with these patients and to help them determine what relaxation technique, or set of techniques, is most effective for them. Thus, in a collaborative mode, the therapist will assist patients to learn coping strategies that they find acceptable. If the coping effort proves ineffective, this is not to be viewed as a failure of relaxation, nor a reflection of the incompetence of the patient, but rather an opportunity to seek another alternative. As in the case of problem-solving described above, it is suggested that there may not be any one best coping alternative, but rather different ones for different people, or for different situations.

Attentional training

The role of attention is a major factor in perceptual activity and therefore of primary concern in examining and changing behaviour. The act of attending has been described as having both selective and amplifying functions. Attention-diverting coping strategies (e.g. thinking about something pleasant) have been employed probably since man first experienced pain. Again it is important to underscore that the patient is viewed as a collaborator in the selection of the specific coping strategies he or she will employ. Several types of strategies are considered and the patient is encouraged to choose those that are most likely to evolve into personally-relevant resources. Patients are also assisted in generating strategies and techniques that they believe might be useful. Again, attempts are made to actively involve patients in their own treatment.

Prior to the description of the specific coping strategies, the therapist always prepares the patient for the intervention. In this instance the therapist describes to the patient how attention influences perception. The therapist notes that people can focus their attention on only one thing at a time and that people control, to some extent, what they attend to, although at times this may require active effort.

Examples are used to make this point concrete (often coming from the patient's experience). For example, the therapist uses the analogy of the stimultaneous availability of all channels on a TV, but only one channel can be fully attended to at any one time. Attention is like a TV channel-tuner: we can control what we attend to, what we avoid and the channel to which we tune. With instruction and practice the patient can gain similar control over his or her attention. This discussion prepares the way for presentation of different cognitive-coping strategies.

Both nonimagery- and imagery-based strategies are employed. Although imagery-based strategies (refocusing attention on pleasant pain-incompatible scenes and so forth) have received much attention, the results have *not* consistently demonstrated that imagery strategies are uniformly effective for all patients (Rosensteil & Keefe 1983; Turner & Clancy 1986; Fernandez & Turk 1989). The important component seems to be the patient's imaginative ability and depth or degree of absorption in using specific images. Guided imagery training is given to patients in order to enhance their abilities to employ all sensory modalities (e.g. imagine such scenes as a lemon being cut on a plate, a tennis match or a pleasant scene that incorporates all five senses). The specifics of the images seem less important than the details of sensory modalities incorporated and the patient's involvement in these images.

Following this preparation, the therapist proceeds to describe different imagery categories (e.g. pleasant, fanciful, dissociative) and once again asks the patient to generate examples that are personally relevant. The therapist asks the patient to imagine circumstances along a continuum of pain and encourages the patient to see him- or herself employing the various images to cope with the pain more effectively. The purpose of the imagery rehearsal is to foster a sense of 'learned resourcefulness' as compared to 'learned helplessness' that characterises many pain patients.

Some patients will have difficulty learning relaxation or making use of imagery techniques. In such circumstances it is often helpful to have patients use audiotapes or posters to help them focus their attention and to guide them with relaxation or imagery. The emphasis is not on one imagery method or technique, but rather on nurturing flexibility. The therapist models this by his or her own creativity in assisting patients to achieve their desired outcomes.

PHASE 4: REHEARSAL AND APPLICATION TRAINING

Next is the rehearsal phase of the treatment programme. After learning different skills, patients are asked to use them in imaginal situations in the therapist's office. For example, after learning different relaxation methods, patients can be asked to imagine themselves in various stressful situations and to see themselves employing the relaxation and coping skills in those situations. For example, patients imagine the last time their pain intensity was rated between 3 and 5 on the pain intensity rating card and to see themselves using the relaxation and other coping techniques at those times. The intent is to have the patients learn that relaxation can be employed as a general coping skill in various situations of stress and discomfort and to prepare themselves for aversive sensations as they arise.

In order to review and consolidate the training procedures, the patient may be asked to role-play a situation in which the therapist and the patient reverse roles. The patient is instructed that it will be his or her job to assume the role of the therapist and the therapist will assume the role of a new patient who has not received any cognitive–behavioural training. The role-reversal exercise is employed because research on attitude change indicates that when people have to improvise, as in a role-playing situation, they generate exactly the kinds of arguments, illustrations and motivating appeals that are most convincing. In this way the patient tailors the content of his or her roles to accommodate idiosyncratic motives, predispositions and preferences (Turk et al 1983). Such role-playing also provides the therapist with a means of assessing any conflicting thoughts, feelings or doubts that the patient may harbour.

With success, the therapist can follow up with specific homework assignments that will consolidate the skills in the patient's natural environment. For example, patients are asked to practise relaxation techniques at home at least twice a day for 15 minutes with one of the practice sessions occurring prior to the times of the most intense pain, if such times have been identified on the pain intensity rating cards. Patients are also asked to anticipate potential problems in performing the homework assignment that might arise (e.g. they forget, they fall asleep) and to generate ways that these obstacles might be addressed should they arise. In this way, attempts are made to anticipate potential difficulties before they arise and to convey the message to patients that they are capable of generating alternative solutions to problems.

As was the case with exercise, skills training follows a graded sequence. First, the therapist discusses the rationale for using a specific method. This is followed by assessing whether the skills are in the patients' repertoires and teaching the patients needed skills and having them practise them in the therapeutic setting. As patients develop proficiency, they are encouraged and challenged to use them in their homes, first in the least difficult circumstance and then building up to more stressful or difficult situations (when their pain is greater, when they are engaged in an interpersonal conflict).

PHASE 5: GENERALISATION AND MAINTENANCE

Generalisation and maintenance are fostered throughout treatment by means of the provision of guided exercise, imaginal and behavioural rehearsal and homework assignments, each of which is designed to increase the patient's sense of self-efficacy. Following the skills acquisition and rehearsal phases, patients are encouraged to 'try out' the various skills that have been covered during the treatment in a broad range of situations and to identify any difficulties that arise. During these sessions, the patient is encouraged to consider potentially problematic situations and is assisted in generating plans or scripts as to how he or she could handle these difficulties, should they arise. Plans are formulated for what the patient might do if he or she begins to lapse. The therapist attempts to anticipate problems and generate solutions, in a sense to 'inoculate' the patient against difficulties that may occur (see Marlatt & Gordon 1980 for a discussion of such relapse prevention procedures). Finally, the patient is encouraged to evaluate progress, review homework assignments and, most importantly, to attribute progress and success to his or her own coping efforts.

It is not enough to have patients change; they must learn to 'take credit' for such changes that they have been able to bring about. The therapist asks the patient a series of questions to consolidate such self-attributions. For example, 'It worked? What did you do? How did you handle the situation this time differently from how you handled it last time? When else did you do this? How did that make you feel?'

PHASE 6: TREATMENT FOLLOW-UP

During the final therapy session all aspects of the training are reviewed. Patients are provided with another set of pain intensity rating cards and a pain questionnaire (Kerns et al 1985). At 2 weeks following termination, the patient is asked to return with these materials to review progress and the maintenance of skills. At 3–6 months and 1 year, follow-up appointments are made to consider any difficulties that have arisen. Patients are also encouraged to call for appointments between specific follow-up dates if they are having difficulty with any aspect of the training. Checking in with the therapist is not viewed as a sign of failure, but rather as an occasion to reevaluate coping options.

EFFECTIVENESS OF THE COGNITIVE–BEHAVIOURAL APPROACH

Cognitive–behavioural approaches have been evaluated in a number of laboratory analogue and clinical pain studies. Laboratory studies have demonstrated the effectiveness of the cognitive–behavioural approach in the enhancement of tolerance to a variety of nociceptive procedures (Klepac et al 1981). The clinical effectiveness of the approach has been demonstrated in well over 100 studies with a wide range of pain syndromes, including headaches (Newton & Barbaree 1987; Holroyd et al 1991), arthritis (Bradley et al 1987; O'Leary et al 1988), temporomandibular pain disorders (Olson & Malow 1987), debridement of burns (Wernick et al 1981), low-back pain (Linssen & Zitman 1984; Hazard et al 1989), atypical chest pain (Klimes et al 1990), cumulative trauma injury (Spence 1989) and heterogeneous samples of chronic pain syndromes (Moore & Chaney 1985; Kerns et al 1986; Thorn et al 1986; Nicholas et al 1992). Cognitive–behavioural approaches have been used with patients across the age-span from adolescents (Lascelles et al 1989) to geriatric patients (Puder 1988). Additionally, cognitive–behavioural approaches have been employed in combination with other therapeutic modalities (Brena et al 1981; Guck et al 1985; Mayer et al 1985). A number of these studies have reported follow-up data ranging from 6 months to 2 years, indicating that the improvements have been maintained.

In summary, the cognitive–behavioural approach offers promise for use with a variety of chronic-pain syndromes. The fact that the approach has been employed in an outpatient and in a group format appears to be a particular asset, both in terms of the cost-effectiveness and the potential for generalisation and maintenance of the skills covered in the treatment programme.

An important research question is whether certain individual differences or situational constraints limit the relative efficacy of the different components of the comprehensive, multifaceted cognitive–behavioural treatment package. We know almost nothing about which treatment combinations would be most effective for what type of patient. Moreover, there is little research to determine how best to combine such psychologically-based interventions with somatically-based interventions (medications, transcutaneous nerve stimulation and so forth). Research programmes are now underway to:

- replicate the preliminary results with the inclusion of appropriate control groups (e.g. credible attention placebo and waiting-list groups)
- identify the relative effectiveness of the cognitive–behavioural treatment for different syndromes and patient populations
- assess the efficacy of treatment over a long-term follow-up period
- identify active ingredients of the treatment
- match treatment components to patient psychosocial and behavioural characteristics.

Taken as an aggregate, the available evidence suggests that the cognitive–behavioural approach has a good deal of potential as a treatment modality by itself and in conjunction with other treatment approaches. The cognitive–behavioural perspective is a reasonable way for health-care providers to think about and to deal with their patients regardless of the therapeutic modalities utilised.

SIDE-EFFECTS

Unlike more invasive medical and surgical treatments, the cognitive–behavioural approach has no known negative side-effects. However, prior to considering this approach, careful evaluation of the patient's physical condition must be conducted in order to eliminate any treatable physical causes of pain.

Finally, little is known about the limitations of the cognitive–behavioural approach. One study, conducted by Tan et al (1981), suggests that the cognitive–behavioural approach may have limited value for high-intensity pain with rapid onset (e.g. pain produced during knee arthrogram) and a follow-up study published by Sturgis et al (1984) reported no long-term benefits of a cognitive–behavioural intervention for a heterogeneous group of pain patients. It is important to identify such limitations in order that decisions about their use in more general clinical contexts can be based on data. The central question that remains to be answered is which treatment modalities are most appropriate for patients with what particular characteristics (Turk 1990)?

Although many of the elements included in the present treatment have been used for many years and many are represented in other chapters in this volume, the cognitive–behavioural treatment approach attempts to integrate these diverse features into an organised clinically-sensitive and effective intervention.

REFERENCES

Bandura A 1977 Self-efficacy: toward a unifying theory of behaviour change. Psychological Review 84: 191–215

Beck A T, Rush A J, Shaw B F, Emery G 1979 Cognitive therapy of depression. Guilford Press, New York

Beecher H K 1959 Measurement of subjective responses: quantitative effects of drugs. Oxford University Press, New York

Bradley L A, Young L D, Anderson K O et al 1987 Effects of psychological therapy on pain behaviour of rheumatoid arthritis patients. Treatment outcome and six-month follow-up. Arthritis and Rheumatism 30: 105–114

Brena S F, Chapman S L, Decker R 1981 Chronic pain as a learned experience: Emory University Pain Control Center. In: Ng L N Y (ed) New approaches to treatment of chronic pain: a review of multidisciplinary pain clinics and pain centers. DHHS publication no. (DM) 81–1089. United States Government Printing Office, Washington, DC

Ciccone D S, Grzesiak R C 1984 Cognitive dimensions of chronic pain. Social Science and Medicine 19: 1339–1346

Dolce J J, Doleys D M, Raczynski J M, Loessie J, Poole L, Smith M 1986 The role of self-efficacy expectancies in the prediction of pain tolerance. Pain 27: 261–272

Fernandez E, Turk D C 1989 The utility of cognitive coping strategies for altering pain perception: a meta-analysis. Pain 38: 123–135

Fordyce W E 1976 Behavioural methods for chronic pain and illness. C V Mosby, St Louis

Fordyce W E, Fowler R, Lehmann J, DeLateur B, Sand P, Trieschmann R 1973 Operant conditioning in the treatment of chronic pain. Archives of Physical Medicine and Rehabilitation 54: 399–408

Flor H, Kerns R D, Turk D C 1987a The role of the spouse in the maintenance of chronic pain. Journal of Psychosomatic Research 31: 251–260

Flor H, Turk D C, Scholz O B 1987b Impact of chronic pain on the spouse: marital, emotional, and physical consequences. Journal of Psychosomatic Research 31: 63–71

Flor H, Fydrich T, Turk D C 1992 Efficacy of multidisciplinary pain treatment centers: a meta-analytic review. Pain 49: 221–230

Guck T P, Skultety F M, Meilman P W, Dowd E T 1985 Multidisciplinary pain center follow-up study and evaluation with a no-treatment control group. Pain 21: 295–306

Hazard R G, Benedix A, Genwich J W 1991 Disability exaggeration as a predictor of functional restoration outcome for patients with chronic low-back pain. Spine 16: 1062–1067

Holroyd K A, Nash J M, Pingel J D, Cordingley G E, Jerome A 1991 A comparison of pharmacological (Amitriptyline HCL) and nonpharmacological (cognitive–behavioural) therapies for chronic tension headaches. Journal of Consulting and Clinical Psychology 59: 121–133

Holzman A D, Turk D C, Kerns R D 1986 The cognitive–behavioural approach in treating chronic pain. In: Holzman A D, Turk D C (eds) Pain management: a handbook of psychological treatment approaches. Pergamon Press, Elmsford, New York

Kendall P C, Hollon S D 1979 Cognitive–behavioural interventions: theory, research, and procedures. Academic Press, New York

Kerns R D, Turk D C 1984 Depression, marital satisfaction, and perceived support among chronic pain patients and their spouses. Journal of Marriage and the Family 46: 845–852

Kerns R D, Turk D C, Rudy T E 1985 The West Haven–Yale Multidimensional Pain Inventory (WHYMPI). Pain 23: 345–356

Kerns R D, Turk D C, Holzman A D, Rudy T E 1986 Efficacy of a cognitive–behavioural group approach for the treatment of chronic pain. Clinical Journal of Pain 2: 195–203

Klepac R K, Klauge G, Dowling J, McDonald M 1981 Direct and generalized effects of three components of stress inoculation for increased pain tolerance. Behaviour Therapy 12: 417–424

Klimes I, Mayou R A, Pearce M J, Fagg J R 1990 Psychological treatment for atypical non-cardiac chest pain: a controlled evaluation. Psychological Medicine 20: 605–611

Lascelles M A, Cunnigham S J, McGrath P, Sullivan M J L 1989 Teaching coping strategies to adolescents with migraine. Journal of Pain and Symptom Management 4: 135–144

Linssen A C G, Zitman F G 1984 Patient evaluation of a cognitive behavioural group program for patients with low back pain. Social Science and Medicine 19: 1361–1367

Marlatt G A, Gordon J R 1980 Determinants of relapse: implications for the maintenance of behavioural change. In: Davidson P O, Davidson S M (eds) Behavioural medicine: changing health lifestyles. Brunner/Mazel, New York

Mayer T G, Gatchel R J, Kishino N et al 1985 Objective assessment of spine function following industrial injury. A prospective study with comparison group and one-year follow-up. Spine 10: 482–493

Meichenbaum D 1977 Cognitive-behaviour modification: an integrative approach. Plenum Press, New York

Meichenbaum D 1985 Stress inoculation training. Pergamon Press, New York

Meichenbaum D, Jaremko M 1983 Stress reduction and prevention. Plenum Press, New York

Meichenbaum D, Turk D C 1987 Facilitating treatment adherence: a practitioner's guidebook. Plenum Press, New York

Melzack R 1980 Pain theory: exceptions to the rule. Behavioural and Brain Science 3: 313

Melzack R, Casey K L 1968 Sensory, motivational and central control determinants of pain: a new conceptual model. In: Kenshalo D (ed) The skin senses. C C Thomas, Springfield, Illinois

Melzack R, Wall P D 1965 Pain mechanisms: a new theory. Science 150: 971–979

Melzack R, Wall P D 1983 The challenge of pain. Basic Books , New York

Moore J E, Chaney E F 1985 Outpatient group treatment of chronic pain: effects of spouse involvement. Journal of Consulting and Clinical Psychology 53: 326–334

Newton C R, Barbaree H E 1987 Cognitive changes accompanying headache treatment: the use of a thought-sampling procedure. Cognitive Therapy and Research 11: 635–652

Nicholas M K, Wilson P H, Goyen J 1992 Comparison of cognitive-behavioural group treatment and an alternative non-psychological treatment for chronic low back pain. Pain 48: 339–347

O'Leary A, Shoor S, Lorig K, Holman H R 1988 A cognitive–behavioural treatment for rheumatoid arthritis. Health Psychology 7: 527–544

Olson R E, Malow R M 1987 Effects of biofeedback and psychotherapy on patients with myofascial pain dysfunction who are nonresponsive to conventional treatments. Rehabilitation Psychology 32: 195–205

Puder R S 1988 Age analysis of cognitive–behavioural group therapy for chronic pain outpatients. Psychology and Aging 3: 204–207

Rachlin H 1985 Pain and behaviour. Behavioural and Brain Sciences 8: 43–53

Rosenstiel A K, Keefe F J 1983 The use of coping strategies in chronic low back pain patients: relationship to patient characteristics and adjustment. Pain 17: 33–44

Spence S H 1989 Cognitive behaviour therapy in the management of chronic occupational pain of the upper limbs. Behaviour Research and Therapy 27: 435–446

Sturgis E, Schaefer C A, Sikora T L 1984 Pain center follow-up study of treated and untreated patients. Archives of Physical Medicine and Rehabilitation 65: 301–303

Thorn B E, Williams D A, Johnson P R 1986 Individualized cognitive behavioural treatment of chronic pain. Behavioural Psychotherapy 14: 210–225

Turk D C 1990 Customizing treatment for chronic patients: who, what and why. Clinical Journal of Pain 6: 255–270

Turk D C, Holzman A D 1986 Commonalities among psychological approaches in the treatment of chronic pain: specifying the meta-constructs. In: Holzman A D, Turk D C (eds) Pain management: a handbook of psychological treatment approaches, Pergamon Press, New York

Turk D C, Rudy T E 1991 Neglected factors in chronic pain treatment outcome studies – relapse, noncompliance, and adherence enhancement. Pain 44: 24–43

Turk D C, Melzack R (eds) 1992 Handbook of pain assessment. Guilford Press, New York

Turk D C, Rudy T E 1992 Cognitive factors and persistent pain: a glimpse into Pandora's box. Cognitive Therapy and Research 16: 99–122

Turk D C, Rudy T E 1993 An integrated approach to pain treatment: beyond the scalpel and syringe. In: Tollison C D (ed) Handbook of chronic pain management, 2nd edn. Williams & Wilkins, Baltimore (in press)

Turk D C, Stieg R L 1987 Chronic pain: the necessity of interdisciplinary communication. Clinical Journal of Pain 3: 163–167

Turk D C, Meichenbaum D, Genest M 1983 Pain and behavioural medicine: a cognitive–behavioural perspective. Guilford Press, New York

Turk D C, Holzman A D, Kerns R D 1986 Chronic pain. In: Holroyd K A, Creer T L (eds) Self-management of chronic disease. Academic Press, New York

Turk D C, Rudy T E, Boucek D C 1993 Psychological factors in chronic pain. In: Warfield C A (ed) Pain management techniques. Martinus Nijhoff, Boston

Turner J A, Clancy S 1986 Strategies for coping with chronic low back pain: relationship to pain and disability. Pain 24: 355–364

Wernick R, Jaremko M E, Taylor P W 1981 Pain management in severely burned patients: a test of stress-inoculation training. Journal of Behavioural Medicine 4: 103–109

75. Hypnotic analgesia

Nicholas P. Spanos, Sharon J. Carmanico and Jacqueline A. Ellis

INTRODUCTION

Procedures labelled as 'hypnotic' have been employed for well over a century to reduce the pain associated with a variety of medical disorders and medical interventions. In addition, in the last 35 years a large number of experimental studies have examined the effects of hypnotic procedures in reducing laboratory-induced pain (for reviews see Chaves 1989; Spanos 1989a, 1989b). Laboratory (as opposed to clinical) research in the area of hypnosis has been organised around two competing paradigms labelled as the special process and sociocognitive perspectives (Spanos 1986b). Special process accounts revolve around the traditional notion that hypnotic behaviour differs fundamentally from ordinary social behaviour, and reflects the operation of nonordinary states of consciousness (e.g. trance) or unusual psychological mechanisms (e.g. dissociation, trance logic). Alternatively, sociocognitive accounts emphasise the continuity between hypnotic and non-hypnotic responding, reject the positing of unusual psychological processes, and attempt to account for hypnotic behaviour by using constructs regularly employed by social and cognitive psychologists to explain other forms of social behaviour (e.g. attitudes, expectations, interpretations, role-playing, self-efficacy).

Theoretical controversies concerning hypnosis have been much less prominent in the clinical than in the experimental literature. Typically, clinical studies and reviews of the clinical literature (Frankel 1987) simply assume that the term 'hypnosis' refers to a denotable psychological state or condition, that the presence of this 'state' can be readily recognised, that it can be reliably induced through the use of rituals labelled as hypnotic induction procedures, and that once induced the 'hypnotic state' in some (often unspecified) way facilitates a therapeutic outcome.

Despite the fact that the above assumptions are routinely made in the clinical literature, all of them are open to serious question. For instance, after more than a century of research the term hypnosis remains vague and continues to be used in contradictory ways by different investigators (Barber 1969; Fellows 1986). Furthermore, physiological, behavioural and verbal report indicators that unambiguously reflect an hypnotic state (as opposed to relaxation, expectancy-induced attributions, etc.) have not been identified (Barber et al 1974; Edmonston 1980; Perlini & Spanos 1991; Radtke & Spanos 1981; Kirsch 1992). On the other hand, explanatory concepts drawn from the contemporary literature in cognitive and social psychology have proven successful at conceptualising a wide array of laboratory findings concerning hypnotic behaviour (Wagstaff 1981, 1991; Sarbin 1989; Spanos 1991; Spanos & Chaves 1989; Spanos & Coe 1992). This chapter reviews experimental and clinical findings concerning hypnotic pain reduction without adopting the assumptions of special process theories.

HYPNOTISABILITY AND ITS ASSESSMENT

People vary greatly in the extent to which they respond to hypnotic suggestions and a number of standardised scales (labelled hypnotisability scales) are available for assessing hypnotic responsiveness (see Bertrand 1989 for a review of scales). All of these scales consist of an hypnotic induction procedure followed by a standardised series of test suggestions. Hypnotisability is assessed as the number of suggestions to which subjects gave the appropriate behavioural response (i.e. the number of suggestions passed). In addition, some scales assess subjective as well as behavioural responsiveness to suggestions. At least among adults, hypnotisability is a relatively stable characteristic. All of the commonly used scales correlate with one another to at least a moderate degree, and test–retest correlations for hypnotisability are in the moderate to high range even when retest intervals are measured in decades (Gwynn et al 1988; Piccione et al 1989). On the other hand, recent evidence indicates that the cross-test and cross-temporal consistency of these scales may be strongly related to the consistency of subjects' attitudes and interpretations concerning hypnosis and hypnotic suggestions and that hypnotisability can be substantially decreased or increased by changing the way subjects think about and interpret hypnotic suggestions (Bertrand 1989; Spanos 1989b; Spanos et al 1989a). As will be seen, hypnotisability has figured prominently in debates concerning the nature of hypnotic analgesia.

LABORATORY STUDIES ON HYPNOTIC ANALGESIA

Laboratory studies on hypnotic analgesia usually employ the same basic methodology. Typically, subjects in these experiments are exposed during several trials to some harmless but painful noxious stimulus. The most commonly employed stimuli include limb immersion in circulating ice water or pressure from a heavy tapered wedge lowered on to a finger (Brown et al 1970). Ischaemia (McGlashin et al 1967) and punctate electric shock (Laurence & Perry 1981) have also been employed occasionally. The first trial of noxious stimulation is usually employed to obtain pretreatment (baseline) estimates of painfulness. A variety of procedures are available for measuring pain (Jones & Flynn 1989), but the most common in this area are pain tolerance (usually measured as the duration that the subject is willing to undergo the stimulation) and category ratings of pain intensity. Following the baseline trial, subjects are usually exposed to one of several treatment procedures (e.g. hypnotic induction plus analgesia suggestion, analgesia suggestion without preceding hypnotic induction) or to a no-treatment control condition. Finally, subjects are re-exposed to the noxious stimulation and painfulness is again assessed.

In this literature, the term 'hypnotic procedure' usually refers to repeated suggestions for eye-closure followed by further interrelated suggestions for relaxation, drowsiness and entering hypnosis. Hypnotic induction procedures vary in duration from study to study but are usually 5–15 minutes in length. In several studies, length of induction failed to influence degree of responsiveness to suggestions (Barber et al 1974). Analgesia suggestions usually consist of repeated suggestions that the area to which the noxious stimulus will be applied is becoming numb, dull and insensitive. In addition, these suggestions often instruct subjects to imagine a variety of situations that are incompatible with feeling high levels of pain (e.g. imagine lying on the beach feeling warm, comfortable and relaxed).

A large number of studies from different laboratories have now established that hypnotic procedures followed by analgesia suggestions reliably reduce reported pain and increase pain tolerance relative to no-treatment control conditions (Spanos 1989a). In the last 30 or so years, however, it has become increasingly clear that short nonhypnotic instructions designed to enhance subjects' expectations and motivations (i.e. task-motivating instructions) are as effective as hypnotic-induction procedures at enhancing responsiveness to a wide range of suggestions, including suggestions for analgesia (Barber 1969; Barber et al 1974; Spanos 1991a). In other words, analgesia suggestions without hypnotic preliminaries have been shown to reduce reported pain to the same extent as hypnotic analgesia suggestions and to a greater extent than no treatment (Barber & Hahn 1962; Evans & Paul 1970; Houle et al 1988; Spanos et al 1969; Spanos et al 1984b; Spanos & Katsanis 1989). Relatedly, two studies (Miller & Bowers 1986; Spanos et al 1986) found that hypnotic analgesia suggestions were as effective, but no more effective than nonhypnotic stress inoculation procedures.

DISSOCIATION AND HYPNOTIC ANALGESIA

Despite the consistency of the above findings, Hilgard (1977, 1986, 1987, 1991) has argued that hypnotic analgesia suggestions are more effective than nonhypnotic analgesia suggestions at least for highly hypnotisable subjects. Moreover, Hilgard has developed a two-component theory of hypnotic analgesia which holds that all subjects can reduce pain to some small degree by using such 'waking' strategies as relaxation and distraction, but that large pain reductions are produced by a psychological process of dissociation. Supposedly, only high hypnotisables can dissociate, and, therefore, only high hypnotisables who have been 'hypnotised' (i.e. placed in a condition of dissociation) can achieve large pain reductions following suggestions. Hilgard has employed three sets of experimental findings to support his hypothesis. The first set of findings purportedly shows that highly hypnotisable hypnotic subjects can reduce pain to a greater extent when 'hypnotised' than awake; the second set purportedly shows that high hypnotisables can reduce pain to a much greater extent than low hypnotisables, and the third set purportedly provides direct evidence for the dissociated 'part' of the person that 'holds' unconsciously felt pain behind an 'amnesic barrier'. Each set of findings will be briefly reviewed.

Hypnotic and nonhypnotic analgesia in high hypnotisables

In a number of experiments, highly hypnotisable subjects were administered both hypnotic and nonhypnotic suggestions for analgesia and reported greater pain reduction or larger increases in tolerance in the hypnotic than in the nonhypnotic condition (Stacher et al 1975; Hilgard et al 1978; Spanos et al 1987; Malone et al 1989). At first glance, these findings appear to support Hilgard's hypothesis that, at least for high hypnotisables, hypnotic analgesia is intrinsically more effective than nonhypnotic analgesia. Two considerations create major problems for this interpretation. First, a large number of studies that assigned different highly hypnotisable subjects to hypnotic and nonhypnotic conditions found that subjects in the two groups reported equivalent reductions in pain (Barber & Hahn 1962; Spanos et al 1979; Spanos et al 1984b; Spanos et al 1985; Jones et al 1987; Spanos & Katsanis 1989; Tenenbaum et al 1990). If hypnotic analgesia were intrinsically more effective than nonhypnotic analgesia in high hypnotisables, then its superiority should be demonstrable regardless of whether within-subject or between-subject experimental designs are employed.

These findings suggest that within-subject experiments that make use of high hypnotisables are likely to generate important context effects (Stam & Spanos 1980). According to this hypothesis, highly hypnotisable subjects are attuned to experimental demands that call for heightened performance in hypnotic conditions and are motivated to present themselves as responsive hypnotic subjects. Consequently, these subjects may perform less than optimally in nonhypnotic conditions when they are aware that they will also be tested in an hypnotic condition. To test these ideas, Stam & Spanos (1980) exposed high hypnotisables to three pain stimulation trials. Following the baseline trial, subjects were told to expect two further trials, but were given different information concerning what to expect on the third trial. Subjects who were administered nonhypnotic analgesia on the second trial when they expected (and received) hypnotic analgesia on the third trial, reported significantly less pain reduction on trial two than on trial three. Alternatively, subjects who received nonhypnotic analgesia on trial two when they expected (and received) nonhypnotic analgesia on trial three, reported as much pain reduction on trial two as on trial three. Importantly, subjects who expected hypnosis reported less pain reduction during trial two nonhypnotic analgesia than did subjects who did not expect later hypnosis. Moreover, the trial three pain reductions of subjects who received hypnotic analgesia failed to differ from the reported reductions of those given nonhypnotic analgesia on trial three. These findings very clearly fail to support the notion that hypnotic analgesia is intrinsically more effective than nonhypnotic analgesia. Instead they indicate that whether subjects rated hypnotic analgesia as less effective than waking analgesia or as equally effective as hypnotic analgesia depended upon the expectations conveyed by their treatment instructions. Thus, these findings demonstrate that the expectations and self-presentational concerns of high hypnotisables are important determinants of their pain-reporting behaviour.

Suggested analgesia in high and low hypnotisables

A large number of laboratory studies (for reviews see Hilgard 1979; Spanos 1989a) indicate that hypnotisability correlates to a moderate degree with hypnotic analgesia. Hilgard has used this finding to argue that low hypnotisables lack the 'dissociative capacity' required to experience large suggestion-induced reductions in pain (Hilgard 1977, 1987). Contrary to this hypothesis, a number of studies (Spanos et al 1984b; Spanos et al 1987; Spanos et al 1988) now indicate that the relationship between suggested analgesia and hypnotisability is context-dependent and mediated by subjects' expectations concerning their ability to reduce pain.

In studies of hypnotic analgesia, subjects are usually assessed for hypnotisability in an initial session and then tested for hypnotic or nonhypnotic analgesia in a later session. Hypnotisability scales are face obvious, and subjects who have been tested for hypnotisability are, of course, aware of how they scored. In addition, subjects who return for analgesia testing are often informed that they have been selected because of their hypnotisability. Even if not so informed, the analgesia suggestions employed in these studies are almost always imagery-based and worded in the passive voice (e.g. your hand will become numb), in the same way as the suggestions on hypnotisability scales. On the basis of these considerations, Spanos et al (1984b) hypothesised that subjects who are tested for suggested analgesia following hynotisability testing are likely to carry over expectations from their hypnotisability test session that influence their analgesia responding. More specifically, low hypnotisables are likely to believe that they will be unresponsive to analgesia suggestions and high hypnotisables are likely to be relatively confident that they will respond well to these suggestions.

Several studies (Spanos et al 1984b, 1987, 1988) tested these ideas by manipulating the expectations held by high and low hypnotisables concerning their response to analgesia situations. The findings of these studies indicated consistently that low hypnotisables who did not connect their analgesia performance with their prior hypnotisability testing, or who expected to do well at analgesia testing despite their earlier hynotisability scores, reported reduced pain following suggested analgesia suggestions to the same extent as highly hypnotisable hypnotic subjects. These findings contradict Hilgard's hypothesis that low hypnotisables lack the cognitive capacity to attain pain reductions that are as large as those of highly hypnotisable hypnotic subjects.

The hidden observer

The findings cited most commonly in support of Hilgard's dissociation hypothesis are derived from a series of 'hidden observer' experiments (Hilgard 1991). In these experiments, highly hypnotisable subjects reported pain intensity at set intervals during a baseline pain stimulation trial. Next, subjects were given an hypnotic procedure and informed that they possessed a hidden part to their mind that remained aware of their experiences even during hypnotic analgesia. Later, during hypnotic analgesia testing, subjects were instructed to give overt (verbal) reports that indexed the intensity of the pain felt by the 'conscious, hypnotised part' of their mind, and hidden reports (numerical ratings tapped out in a pretaught code) that supposedly reflected the degree of pain felt by their 'hidden part'. The high hypnotisables exposed to these procedures exhibited hypnotic analgesia by reporting relatively low levels of overt pain. In addition, many of these subjects also reported (via the pretaught code) high levels of hidden pain.

Hilgard (1977, 1979, 1991) hypothesised that hypnotically analgesic subjects simultaneously experience low levels of conscious (overt) pain and high levels of hidden pain regardless of whether or not they have been administered hidden-observer instructions. Supposedly, 'hidden pain' in hypnotically analgesic subjects normally remains dissociated from consciousness by an 'amnesic barrier' unless and until the experimenter obtains hidden reports.

A sociocognitive alternative suggests, instead, that reports of experiencing a hidden part and ratings of hidden pain reflect the obvious instructional demands of hidden observer experiments. In other words, it is these instructions, rather than an intrinsic tendency to dissociate during hypnotic analgesia, that provide subjects with the idea that they have a hidden part and with the idea that hidden pain reports should be higher than overt pain reports.

Two experiments (Spanos & Hewitt 1980; Spanos et al 1983a) obtained support for the sociocognitive hypothesis by varying the contents of hidden-observer instructions and demonstrating that hidden-observer reports were closely tied to the expectations conveyed by these instructions. Spanos et al (1983a) found that high hypnotisables rated overt and hidden pain as being of equal magnitude unless they were given explicit instructions which indicated that one type of pain was supposed to be more intense than the other. These findings clearly contradict Hilgard's (1979) hypothesis that hidden-observer instruction simply access a preexisting hidden mental system that 'holds' high levels of hidden pain. In addition, Spanos & Hewitt (1980) and Spanos et al (1983a) found that instructions which implied that hidden pain was *less* intense than overt pain (the opposite of the pain-reporting pattern predicted by Hilgard) led subjects to report lower hidden than overt pain. In other words, the high hypnotisables in these studies reported hidden pain as being equally intense, more intense or less intense than overt pain depending upon the implications of the instructions they were given. These findings indicate that the hidden-observer phenomenon is a social construction shaped by the demands to which subjects are exposed rather than an intrinsic and unsuggested aspect of hypnotic analgesia.

COGNITIVE ACTIVITY DURING HYPNOTIC ANALGESIA

The failure of the dissociation theory to provide an adequate account of hypnotic analgesia focuses attention on determining the variables that are important in this regard. People differ greatly in how they construe and respond to noxious situations and a number of studies indicate that the kind of ongoing cognitive activity carried out during noxious stimulation strongly influences perceptions and ratings of pain in both clinical and laboratory contexts (Genest et al 1977; Genest 1978; Spanos et al 1979; Spanos et al 1981; Turk et al 1983; Chaves & Brown 1987; Keefe et al 1989; Sullivan & Bishop 1992). For instance, one individual-difference variable that influences pain ratings and level of emotional responding during painful activity or painful stimulation is labelled as 'catastrophising' (Spanos et al 1979; Chaves & Brown 1983).

Catastrophising refers to the tendency of subjects to focus on and exaggerate the negative aspects of the noxious situation and the tendency to feel overwhelmed and unable to cope with or control the situation (Spanos et al 1979; Sullivan & Bishop 1992). In chronic-pain patients, catastrophising is associated with increased emotional distress and often with increased levels of reported pain (Roesenthal & Keefe 1983; Keefe et al 1989; Sullivan & D'Eon 1990). Relatedly, a number of laboratory studies found that, even before exposure to any treatment, subjects who coped with noxious stimulation by 'spontaneously' using such strategies as self-distraction and the generation of pleasant imagery reported lower levels of pain than those who catastrophised (Spanos et al 1979; Spanos et al 1981).

A large number of studies carried out within the cognitive–behavioural tradition, and unrelated to hypnosis, have found that treatment procedures designed to encourage the use of such coping strategies as self-distraction, positive imagery, and reinterpretation or transformation of noxious input, produced significant reductions in reported pain and/or significant increases in pain tolerance (Chaves & Barber 1974; Grimm & Kafner 1976; Jaremko 1978; Scott & Leonard 1978; Beers & Karoly 1979; Thelan & Fry 1981; Dubreuil et al 1987). These studies often differed in terms of the specific strategy or combination of strategies employed. Nevertheless, the underlying assumption in these studies was that subjects can gain at least partial control over their level of discomfort by controlling and directing their cognitive activities.

Subjects show wide variability in both cognitive activity and levels of reported pain even after the administration of cognitive-coping suggestions. Nevertheless, coping suggestions do lead to decreases in both catastrophising activity and reported pain and to increases in the use of coping cognitions (Spanos et al 1981, 1984a, 1989b). In addition, decrements in reported pain following coping suggestions are related to increments in coping strategy use (Spanos et al 1986).

The analgesia suggestions used in hypnosis studies, like

the coping instructions used in cognitive–behavioural studies, instruct subjects to carry out cognitive-coping activity in order to reduce pain. This suggests that the reported pain reductions associated with hypnotic analgesia and with nonhypnotic-coping instructions are mediated by the same underlying cognitive activities. Several studies (Spanos et al 1984b, 1986, 1989a; Spanos & Katsanis 1989) have examined this hypothesis by assessing catastrophising and cognitive–coping activity in both hypnotic and nonhypnotic subjects exposed to noxious stimulation. These studies consistently found that hypnotic and nonhypnotic suggestions led to equivalent reductions in catastrophising activity and reported pain and equivalent increments in cognitive–coping activity. In short, the available data indicate that the same underlying cognitive activities are associated with pain reduction in both hypnotic and nonhypnotic treatments for pain.

WHAT IS REDUCED IN HYPNOTIC ANALGESIA?

The available data clearly indicate that hypnotic and nonhypnotic treatments produce significant reductions in reported pain, and that such reporting decrements are related to subjects' ongoing cognitive activity. Nevertheless, substantial controversy remains concerning how best to conceptualise these reductions in reported pain. One hypothesis holds that suggested analgesia involves a reduction in perceptual sensitivity. Perhaps, for example, subjects divert attention away from noxious stimulation by making use of the imaginal and other strategies contained in suggestions. Such attention diversion may leave less attention available for processing the noxious stimulation and, thereby, lead to a reduction in perceptual sensitivity (McCaul & Mallot 1984). Despite the inherent plausibility of this formulation, there is little evidence to support it. The category-rating and pain-tolerance procedures used in most hypnotic analgesia experiments are subject to a number of systematic biases that preclude their use as accurate indices of pain sensitivity (Poulton, 1979; Scott 1980; Mikael et al 1986). Moreover, the use of scaling procedures that were designed to separate perceptual sensitivity from decisional biases provides little support for the reduced sensitivity hypothesis of hypnotic analgesia. For instance, neither hypnotic nor nonhypnotic analgesia appears to be consistently related to reduced perceptual sensitivity when sensitivity is measured with signal detection procedures (Clark 1974; Clark & Goodman 1974), functional measurement procedures (Jones et al 1986) or magnitude estimation/magnitude production procedures (Clum et al 1982; Spanos et al 1983b; Stam et al 1981).

The problem with the reduced-sensitivity hypothesis is highlighted in several experiments that assessed reporting bias directly and independently of any change in perceptual experience (Spanos et al 1991, 1992a, 1992b). In all of these studies subjects received three trials of noxious stimulation, and rated pain intensity 15 seconds *after* termination of each pain stimulus. The first trial was a baseline and the second was preceded by hypnotic analgesia suggestions. Following their trial-two pain rating, the hypnotic and suggestion procedures were cancelled and subjects were administered the third trial. Following termination of the trial-three pain stimulation, but before the rating of trial-three pain, subjects in a *demand* condition were administered instructions aimed at leading them to report lower levels of pain than they had actually felt on trial three. These subjects were told that hypnotic suggestions sometimes continue to operate after their cancellation. Subjects in the nondemand condition were issued no instructions following the termination of the trial-three pain stimulus. Instead, these subjects simply waited 15 seconds and again rated their pain. It is important to emphasise that, until after the termination of the trial-three pain stimulus, subjects in the demand and nondemand conditions were treated identically. Consequently, any difference in reports of trial-three pain between the demand and nondemand subjects cannot reflect a difference in the way these subjects actually experienced pain on trial three, or a difference in cognitive strategy use on trial three. Instead, any such difference must reflect a demand-induced reporting bias.

In all of these experiments, subjects in the demand condition reported less trial-three pain than nondemand subjects. In fact, nondemand subjects reported almost as much pain reduction on trial three as they had reported for hypnotic analgesia on trial two. Nondemand subjects reported approximately the same amount of pain on trial three as they had on the baseline trial. Therefore, in the demand group, the extent to which subjects reported reduced pain on trial three relative to trial one was used as an index of the extent to which they biased their trial-three pain reports.

In all of these experiments, reported pain reduction on trial two (hypnotic analgesia) was strongly correlated with reporting bias scores on trial three, for subjects in the demand condition. In addition, pretested hypnotisability correlated as highly with trial-three bias scores as it correlated with trial-two hypnotic analgesia scores. When bias scores were statistically controlled, the correlation between hypnotisability and hypnotic analgesia was substantially reduced and frequently fell to nonsignificance.

In short, all of these studies indicated that the people who reported the highest levels of hypnotic analgesia tended to be the same people who biased their trial-three reports in terms of instructional demands even though they had not experienced any reduction of pain on that trial. In addition, those with the highest hypnotic analgesia scores and the highest bias scores also tended to have the highest scores on hypnotisability.

The results of these demand-instruction experiments are open to two interpretations. The first suggests that hypnotic analgesia involves substantial levels of behavioural compliance. According to this hypothesis, hypnotic subjects given analgesia suggestions are pressured by implicit and explicit situational demands to knowingly report less pain than they actually experienced. It is clear from numerous psychological experiments that people frequently respond to social pressure from authority figures by doing and saying things that are at variance with their private beliefs and attitudes (Crutchfield 1955; Asch 1958; Milgram 1974; Wagstaff 1981; Miller 1986). Hypnosis experiments contain strong social pressures, and, consequently, it should come as no surprise that subjects may frequently misrepresent and exaggerate the extent to which they were able to generate the experiences called for by suggestions.

A second hypothesis to explain the results of these demand experiments suggests that subjects may be retrospectively reinterpreting their experiences in terms of demand instructions. Unlike the compliance hypothesis, the notion of reinterpretation does not imply that subjects are purposely deceptive. Instead, it suggests that subjects may honestly reevaluate and reclassify their experiences in terms of the demand (e.g. 'Maybe it didn't hurt as much as I first thought').

Reinterpretation can, of course, occur during painful stimulation as well as after its termination. With respect to the typical hypnotic analgesia experiment, the reinterpretation hypothesis suggests that the experiences of subjects during noxious stimulation are complex and ambiguous as well as intense. Such experiences involve a complex of diverse and changing sensations, thoughts and emotions (e.g. throbbing, prickliness, heaviness, apprehension) that subjects must periodically categorise along a painfulness dimension with a restricted range of numbers. Suggestion-induced changes in rated painfulness may reflect attentional shifts to different facets of the complex. These ratings involve the integration of multidimensional and shifting sensory–emotional–cognitive experiences and the expression of that integration as a single number (or successive set of numbers). This integration may involve weighing different aspects of the sensory–emotional–cognitive complex differently under suggestion and no-suggestion conditions. For instance, the relative weight given to 'ache', 'fear' and self-attributions of effective coping (e.g. 'This isn't so bad, as long as I keep imagining I'm OK') before and after analgesia suggestions may be particularly important in leading subjects to rate their experiences as less painful than before, even though the intensity of the sensory events has not changed (Spanos 1989a). In fact, the knowledge that they have been given purportedly effective coping strategies may be more effective than the actual strategies themselves at leading subjects to recategorise their experiences as less painful and distressing than previously.

It is worth noting that both the compliance and reinterpretation hypotheses of hypnotic analgesia are based on the notion that responsive subjects are invested in the role of being 'good subjects' and are motivated to guide their behaviour in terms of the demands associated with that role. Moreover, these two hypotheses are not mutually exclusive. Both compliance and reinterpretation may occur in the same subject. For instance, subjects in an hypnotic analgesia treatment may initially lie and report their pain as less intense than they believe it to be. However, as they reflect on their situation, on the fact that they felt less frightened and more in control than before, etc., at least some of these subjects may come to convince themselves that 'Maybe it didn't hurt as much as I thought.'

CLINICAL STUDIES OF HYPNOTIC ANALGESIA

Despite its long history as a clinical tool for the relief of pain, relatively little systematically collected information is available concerning the efficacy of hypnotic analgesia in clinical settings. Most of the studies in this area are anecdotal reports that contain no control conditions or quantitative assessment of outcome. The most dramatic of these anecdotes purport to show that hypnotic analgesia greatly reduces and sometimes eliminates the pain of major surgery (Gauld 1988; Perry et al 1988). In fact, these anecdotes contain so many methodological shortcomings (e.g. the use of local anaesthetics along with hypnotic suggestion, the confounding of hypnotic procedures with much nonhypnotic preparation, little or no information concerning subject selection, no quantitative assessment of pain) that no firm conclusions concerning this topic are possible (Chaves 1989; Spanos & Chaves 1989). In addition, there are also anecdotal reports to indicate that nonhypnotic suggestions can be employed to reduce surgical pain (Chaves 1989).

Fortunately, the last decade has seen an increase in controlled studies in this area. Frequently, however, even these more recent studies contain methodological shortcomings that make interpretations difficult. For instance, in the laboratory-pain literature the term 'hypnotic condition' usually refers to a standardised induction procedure coupled with standardised, imagery-based analgesia suggestions and nonhypnotic analgesia refers to the same analgesia suggestion without the initial hypnotic-induction procedure. In these studies, any differences between these treatments can be unambiguously attributed to the one variable that differs between them: the presence or absence of the hypnotic procedure.

In the clinical literature, however, it is often unclear to what the term 'hypnotic analgesia' actually refers. Different investigators use the term in different ways and, in some studies (e.g. Zeltzer & LeBaron 1982), procedures are considered hypnotic even when not defined as such to patients and in the absence of a formal hypnotic induction procedure. In addition, in many clinical studies that compared hypnotic and nonhypnotic analgesia treatments the two treatments differed from one another on numerous variables other than the presence of an hypnotic-induction procedure. Consequently, even if differences between treatments are obtained, it is often impossible to determine whether hypnotic procedures influenced the outcome.

In many clinical studies it is also difficult to determine the relationship between hypnotisability and outcome. Many clinical studies provide no assessment of hypnotisability. Moreover, in many studies that do assess it, the assessment does not involve the use of standardised scales. Instead, the clinician uses unknown criteria of unknown reliability and validity to make the judgement. In fact, when unstandardised procedures are employed to assess hypnotisability, it is sometimes not clear whether hypnotisability was estimated at least in part on the basis of therapeutic outcome. Obviously such a practice makes correlations between hypnotisability and outcome meaningless.

The remainder of this chapter will review clinical studies of hypnotic analgesia. Given the inherent limitations of anecdotal reports, this review will focus on controlled studies. Nevertheless, the limitations of these studies should be kept in mind. One major issue addressed by this review is whether there is evidence to support the contention that hypnotic treatments are more effective than nonhypnotic ones at alleviating clinical pain. A second major issue concerns the relationship between clinical outcome and hypnotisability for patients treated by hypnotic and nonhypnotic treatments. A number of investigators (Bowers & Kelly 1979; Wadden & Anderton 1982; Spinhoven 1988) have hypothesised that highly hypnotisable subjects are more responsive to treatments for pain that involve a suggestive component than are low hypnotisables. Others (Barber 1980), however, have suggested that, if properly prepared, low hypnotisables are as responsive to hypnotic treatments as high hypnotisables. Along these lines it is worth recalling that the literature on laboratory pain suggests that the relationship between hypnotisability and reported pain reduction is context-dependent and that depending upon such factors as subjects' expectations, hynotisability will either correlate or not correlate significantly with treatment outcome. Studies will be reviewed in terms of the syndromes the hypnotic procedures were used to treat.

HEADACHE

Recurrent headache is the clinical syndrome most commonly treated in the hypnotic analgesia literature. Case studies have reported moderate to complete success in the relief of migraine headache using hypnotic imagery techniques (Harding 1967; Friedman & Taub 1982; Milne 1982; Davidson 1987), rational stage directed hypnotherapy (Howard et al 1982) and hypnotherapy plus autogenic hand-warming suggestions (Graham 1975; Ansel 1977; Milne 1983). Hypnotherapy has also been reported to be successful in treating muscle-contraction headache (Milne 1982) and unspecified refractory headache (Singh 1989). The lack of control conditions in all of these studies makes any interpretation of their findings highly tentative.

Comparative studies

Hypnotic interventions and various nonhypnotic psychological interventions for the treatment of migraine, chronic tension, or mixed migraine/tension headache have been compared in 11 controlled outcome studies (Andreychuk & Skriver 1975; Schlutter et al 1980; Friedman & Taub 1984, 1985; Spinhoven et al 1985, 1988; Olness et al 1987; Nolan et al 1989, experiments 1 and 2; Mellis et al 1991; Zitman et al 1992; Spanos et al 1993). One study (Mellis et al 1991) compared chronic-tension headache patients administered an hypnotic treatment to those in a waiting-list control condition. Hypnotic subjects reported significant reductions in frequency and intensity of headache activity.

Five studies compared hypnotic and nonhypnotic treatments but failed to include no-treatment control groups. Four of these studies (Andreychuk & Skriver 1975; Schlutter et al 1980; Spinhoven et al 1985, 1988) found decreases in headache activity following treatment and none found differences in this regard between the hypnotic and nonhypnotic treatments. The failure to include no-treatment control conditions in these studies means that spontaneous remission cannot be ruled out as the reason for the decreases in headache activity found in both the hypnotic and nonhypnotic treatments. On the other hand, the equivalent reductions in headache activity found for hypnotic and nonhypnotic treatments in all four of these studies indicate clearly that the hypnotic treatments were never more effective than the nonhypnotic ones.

A fifth study (Zitman et al 1992) compared autogenic training against a treatment labelled as 'future-oriented imagery'. Neither of these treatments was defined as hypnosis. Chronic-tension headache patients were randomly assigned to these two treatment groups. Later, a third group of patients was added. Those in the third group were administered the 'future-oriented imagery' treatment defined as hypnosis. As part of this procedure, patients were administered a hand-levitation routine designed to induce positive expectations about hypnosis. Patients in the other two treatments did not receive a comparable expectancy-enhancing procedure. Patients in the three conditions reported equivalent headache reductions after the test. However, at a 6-month follow-up, only patients in the hypnotic treatment group reported a significant drop in headache activity. Interpretation of these findings is complicated by several methodological problems:

1. Patients assigned to the hypnotic and nonhypnotic conditions were drawn from different populations
2. Only hypnotic patients were administered an extra expectancy-enhancing procedure
3. It appears that none of the hypnotic subjects, but 24% of the nonhypnotic subjects dropped out of the study before the end of the 6-month follow-up
4. Statistical differences between treatments at follow-up were not examined.

An examination of the means suggests that there were no significant differences between the three treatments at follow-up. In fact, the largest mean baseline difference between the three treatments is larger than the largest mean follow-up difference between the treatments. In short, the limitations in this study preclude any interpretation of the findings.

Five studies that compared hypnotic and nonhypnotic treatments for headache also included a no-treatment control condition (Freidman & Taub 1984, 1985; Olness et al 1987; Nolan et al 1989; Spanos et al 1993). Friedman & Taub (1984, 1985) found that thermal biofeedback, relaxation alone, hypnotic relaxation plus thermal imagery and hypnotic relaxation alone were equally effective and more effective than no treatment at reducing the self-reported frequency and intensity of migraine headaches. However, treatment-induced decrements in headache activity were no longer evident at a 3-year follow-up (Friedman & Taub 1985).

Nolan et al (1989, experiment 1) found that imagery instructions, with and without a prior hypnotic-induction procedure, were equally effective and were more effective than no treatment at reducing self-reports of chronic tension or mixed migraine/tension headache. In a second experiment, Nolan et al (1989, experiment 2) employed the same treatments for chronic-tension headache and, in addition, compared a psychological placebo as well as no treatment. Both the hypnotic and nonhypnotic imagery treatments produced significant but equivalent decrements in self-reported headache activity. By the 4-month follow-up interval, however, headache activity in both of these treatment groups had returned to pretreatment baseline levels. Subjects in the placebo treatment group reported no significant changes in headache activity across intervals, and no-treatment control subjects reported significant increments in headache activity across intervals.

Spanos et al (1993) compared an hypnotic imagery treatment, a psychological placebo and no treatment. Subjects in the hypnotic and placebo treatments were administered either one or four sessions of their respective treatment. The number of treatments had no effect. Hypnotic and placebo subjects reported significant and equivalent decrements in headache activity over the 8-week follow-up period, whereas no-treatment control subjects reported no change.

Olness et al (1987) compared hypnotic, placebo and propranolol treatments in a double-blind, single-crossover study for the treatment of juvenile classic migraine. Patients were 6–12 years of age, and the hypnotic treatment consisted of progressive relaxation, pleasant imagery, suggestions for hand-warming and hand anaesthesia. It appears that the treatment was not defined to subjects as hypnosis and, aside from the interests of the authors, it is unclear why this is considered an experiment on hypnosis as opposed to progressive relaxation combined with suggested imagery. Children in the hypnotic treatment group reported significantly fewer headaches than those in the placebo or drug treatment groups. The severity and duration of headaches did not differ between conditions.

In summary, the available data suggest that hypnotic interventions may be of at least short-term benefit in the treatment of recurrent headache activity, but are no more effective in this regard than the same treatments without prior hypnotic induction. At least in adults, hypnotic treatments have not been shown to be consistently more effective than placebo in the treatment of headache.

Hypnotisability and outcome

Andreychuk & Skriver (1975) combined headache patients who had been treated with an hypnotic procedure, alpha biofeedback or temperature biofeedback into a single group. For the group as a whole, a significant relationship was found between hypnotisability and headache reduction. Nevertheless, the data presented make it clear that, despite the overall significant effect, the relationship between hypnotisability and outcome differed markedly between treatments. Moreover, this relationship was weakest in the hypnotic treatment. Hypnotic high hypnotisables reduced headache activity by 38% while the reduction for low hypnotisables was almost as large at 33.4%.

Friedman & Taub (1985) compared high hypnotisables given hypnotic imagery treatments with low hypnotisables instructed to simulate hypnotic imagery. Highs and lows failed to differ in headache activity following treatment or at the 6-month follow-up. However, highs reported greater headache reduction than lows at the 12-month follow-up. Unfortunately, interpretation of these findings is complicated by the fact that high hypnotisables were given hypnotic instructions without any unusual preliminaries while low hypnotisables were instructed to simulate their way through the hypnotic treatment. A good deal of experimentation indicates that the effects of hypnotic treatments are often dramatically altered when subjects are instructed to simulate (DeGroot & Gwynn 1989). In short, the confounding of hypnotisability level with instructions to simulate makes the high/low difference obtained by Friedman & Taub (1985) impossible to interpret.

Cedercreutz et al (1976) found that headache relief correlated moderately with hypnotist's ratings of 'hypnotic depth'. However, this correlation was due entirely to the fact that patients classified as showing zero depth (12% of the sample) reported no relief at all. Subjects classified as exhibiting 'light', 'medium' or 'deep' levels of hypnotic responsiveness failed to differ in treatment efficacy.

Unlike the studies reviewed thus far, Nolan et al (1989) and Spanos et al (1993) assessed hypnotisability at the end of their studies rather than before treatment administration. Neither study found a significant correlation between hypnotisability and treatment outcome in either hypnotic or nonhypnotic treatments. Relatedly, Smith et al (1989) found that hypnotisability failed to correlate with outcome of a behavioural treatment for paediatric headache.

OBSTETRICAL PAIN

Although hypnotic procedures have been used to ameliorate the pain of labour since the 19th century, most reports in this area are anecdotal case studies. The few controlled studies are now reviewed.

Comparative studies

Six published studies have investigated the comparative efficacy of hypnotic and nonhypnotic treatments in the management of obstetrical pain. In the earliest of these, Perchard (1960) assigned parturients to three sessions of either antenatal information alone, information plus relaxation techniques or information plus hypnotic suggestions for relaxation and analgesia. Subjects rated their pain retrospectively, 1 week after delivery. Perchard claimed that hypnotic subjects recalled less pain than did subjects in the other two groups. However, no statistical analysis of the findings was presented, and the 1-week delay between delivery and pain ratings raises questions about the validity of the ratings. Moreover, the fact that analgesia suggestions were given only to the hypnotic subjects would make any superiority for the hypnotic treatment uninterpretable even if it were supported statistically.

Davidson (1962) reported that six sessions of group self-hypnosis reduced reported pain more effectively than either six sessions of Reid's prepared childbirth training or 'mothercraft'. Unfortunately, subjects were not randomly assigned to treatments, but chose their preferred treatment. Importantly, only the hypnotic treatment included suggestions for analgesia. The confounding of the hypnotic procedure and analgesia suggestions, coupled with subject self-selection of treatments, makes it impossible to determine if hypnotic procedures played any important role in the results obtained.

Three studies (Rock et al 1969; Davidson et al 1985; Harmon et al 1990) assigned parturients randomly to either an hypnotic treatment or antenatal preparation. In all three studies the hypnotic treatment included suggestions for relaxation, comfort and analgesia during labour that were absent from the antenatal treatment. Rock et al (1969) found that hypnotic subjects rated their labour as less painful than did antenatal treatment subjects. Davidson et al (1985) reported that hypnotic subjects rated the first stage of labour as less painful than did those in the antenatal treatment, but subjects in these two groups failed to differ in their pain ratings of the second stage of labour. Finally, Harmon et al (1990) found that the hypnotic treatment was more effective than antenatal preparation in leading to reductions in reported pain, shorter first stage of labour and fewer requests for medication. In summary, all three of these studies found that hypnotic procedures, coupled with suggestions for relaxation and analgesia, were more effective than antenatal treatment that did not include these components in reducing pain during at least some phase of labour. Unfortunately, the confounding of hypnotic procedures with analgesia suggestions precludes the possibility of determining whether the administration of the hypnotic procedures played any role in the results obtained.

Venn (1987) compared parturients who self-selected Lamaze childbirth training, hypnotic treatment or hypnotic treatment plus Lamaze training. The hypnotic treatment consisted of an induction procedure and guided imagery suggestions for analgesia. The three groups did not differ significantly in self-reports or nurses' reports of labour pain or in medication usage.

Taken together the available data indicate that hypnotic induction procedures coupled with suggestions for relaxation and analgesia reduce the pain of labour more effectively than does antenatal treatment. Unfortunately, none of these studies compared suggestions for analgesia/relaxation with and without hypnotic procedures. As the studies on headache made clear, suggestions for analgesia in the absence of hypnotic induction can be just as effective as the same suggestions preceded by an hypnotic induction. Consequently, a facilitative role for hypnotic procedures in the reduction of labour pain has yet to be established.

Hypnotisability and outcome

Five studies assessed the relationship between hypnotisability and psychologically induced reductions in labour pain (Perchard 1960; Rock et al 1969; Samko & Schoenfeld 1975; Ven 1987; Harmon et al 1990). In all five studies hypnotisability was assessed prior to treatment, and three studies assessed hypnotisability using nonstandardised instruments. Perchard (1960) reported substantial differences between the pain reports of high and low hypnotisable parturients. Of the high hypnotisables 29% versus 54% of the low hypnotisables reported experiencing severe pain during labour. As noted earlier, however, no statistical tests were performed on the data, pain was assessed retrospectively 1 week after delivery and the criteria for determining hypnotisability are unknown.

Harmon et al (1990) reported that high hypnotisables achieved greater pain reductions than low hypnotisables in nonhypnotic as well as hypnotic treatments. On the other hand, Rock et al (1969) found no significant correlation between hypnotisability and pain reduction for hypnotic subjects and two studies (Samko & Schoenfeld 1975; Venn 1987) found that hypnotisability failed to correlate significantly with pain reduction in subjects given Lamaze, hypnosis or hypnosis plus Lamaze treatments.

ACUTE IATROGENIC PAIN

Hypnotic procedures are frequently employed to reduce the acute pain associated with such medical interventions as dental work, burn debridement and postoperative pain.

Comparison studies

McAmmond et al (1971) compared the efficacy of hypnotic induction, nonhypnotic relaxation and no treatment in the reduction of distress in a dental situation. The dependent variable was skin conductance response to pain. Reductions in skin conductance of equivalent magnitude were obtained in the hypnotic and nonhypnotic subjects.

In an uncontrolled clinical study, Barber (1976) reported a dramatic 99% success rate in performing routine dental work without the use of chemical anaesthetic, following an hypnotic procedure labelled rapid induction analgesia (RIA). Gillet & Coe (1984) failed to replicate Barber's (1976) dramatic results when comparing the relative efficacy of the original RIA procedure against an abbreviated RIA procedure. They found an overall success rate of 51.7% as indexed by reduced requests for medication and enhanced patient comfort. There were no differences between the groups. The lack of a no-treatment control group makes interpretation difficult.

Six studies have compared an hypnotic intervention to some nonhypnotic treatment or to no-treatment in the reduction of postsurgical pain. Three of these studies (Doberneck et al 1959; Werbel 1960; Bonilla et al 1961) compared hypnotic intervention to no-treatment, but failed to randomly assign subjects to conditions. All three found that hypnotic subjects required less narcotic medication postoperatively than did controls. On the other hand, Surman et al (1974) did randomly assign surgical patients to either an hypnotic treatment or no-treatment control condition and found no differences between these groups in either postoperative pain reports or pain medication. Bartlett (1966) compared an hypnotic intervention, suggestions without prior hypnotic induction and no treatment in patients undergoing a variety of surgical procedures. Subjects were not randomly assigned to conditions. Patients in the hypnotic and nonhypnotic suggestion treatment groups failed to differ. Patients in both of these conditions reported less pain and used less narcotic medication than did controls. Finally, Crowley (1980) administered either RIA or a local anaesthetic for the relief of acute pain to patients who had undergone podiatric surgery. Subjects administered the chemical analgesic reported significantly less pain than those treated with RIA.

Three controlled studies (Wakeman & Kaplan 1978; Patterson et al 1989, 1992) have assessed the effects of hypnotic intervention in reducing the pain of burn patients during debridement and dressing change. Wakeman & Kaplan (1978) compared a control condition given emotional support and medication upon request with a treatment group given the same support plus hypnotic suggestions for analgesia. Hypnotic subjects requested significantly less analgesic medication than controls. Patterson et al (1989) found significant reductions in pain during debridement for subjects given hypnotic treatment but not for control subjects given medication alone. Unfortunately, several methodological limitations complicate interpretation of these findings. Patterson et al (1989) did not randomly assign subjects to conditions and, in addition, subjects in the two conditions were not equated on total burn area. Control subjects presented with an average of 14.5% burn surface while hypnotic subjects averaged only 8.5% burn surface. Patterson et al (1992) randomly assigned subjects to an hypnotic treatment, an attention-control treatment or no-treatment. The hypnotic treatment was a modification of RIA. Pain was assessed before and after treatment. Only the hypnotic subjects reported a significant reduction in pain. Unfortunately, none of these three studies (Wakeman & Kaplan 1978; Patterson et al 1989, 1992) included a condition that received nonhypnotic suggestions for analgesia.

In summary, studies on acute iatrogenic pain have generally found that hypnotic interventions are more effective than no-treatment at producing reductions of various indices of pain. Unfortunately, very few of these studies compared hypnotic interventions to corresponding nonhypnotic interventions. The two studies that did compare hypnotic and nonhypnotic suggestions found that these procedures were equally effective at producing reductions on pain indicators.

Hypnotisability and outcome

The relationship between hypnotisability and treatment-induced relief of acute clinical pain has been assessed for dental pain (Gottfredson 1973; Barber 1976; Gillet & Coe 1984), pain associated with burn treatments (Schafer 1975) and postsurgical pain (Crowley 1980). Gottfredson (1973) found that 75% of high hypnotisables as opposed to 38.5% of low hypnotisables tolerated routine dental work without chemical analgesia and a significant negative correlation ($r = -.39$) was obtained between pain ratings and hypnotisability. On the other hand, neither Barber (1976) nor Gillet & Coe (1984) found significant correlations between pain ratings and hypnotisability in dental patients administered RIA. Relatedly, Crowley (1980) found no relationship between hypnotisability and degree of RIA-induced analgesia in patients who underwent podiatric surgery.

Schafer (1975) reported a strong relationship between hypnotically induced reductions in pain and hypnotisability in 20 burn patients. Hypnotisability was assessed by response to a series of nonstandardised suggestions. Six of Schafer's patients reported no pain relief following the hypnotic intervention, and five of these six nonresponders scored low in hypnotisability. Importantly, however, most of these nonresponders were described as too heavily drugged or in too high a state of panic to attend to the hypnotic analgesia intervention. However, if these patients were too drugged or too panic-ridden to attend to the hypnotic analgesia suggestions, then it is likely that these same factors prevented them from attending to the test suggestions used to assess hypnotisability. Thus, the strong correlation between hypnotisability and pain relief obtained by Schafer (1975) may have been produced artifactually by high levels of panic and drugs that eliminated responsiveness to both the hypnotisability test suggestions and the analgesia suggestions in a subsample of his patients.

CANCER-RELATED PAIN IN ADULTS

A number of case reports and uncontrolled clinical studies suggest that hypnotherapeutic procedures may be useful in reducing cancer-related pain in adults (Lea et al 1960; Cangello 1961, 1962). However, methodological limitations such as poorly specified treatment and assessment procedures seriously compromise the usefulness of these reports.

Comparative studies

Three comparative studies have examined hypnotic interventions for cancer-related pain in adults (Reeves et al 1983; Spiegel & Bloom 1983; Syrjala et al 1987). Spiegel & Bloom compared group therapy, group therapy plus a self-hypnosis exercise and no-treatment in women with breast cancer. The two group treatments combined produced lower reported pain on two of the four self-report pain measures. Hypnotic treatment was superior to group therapy alone on only one of the four pain measures. There are a number of problems with Spiegel & Bloom's data analyses that complicate interpretation of these results. These problems have been detailed by Stam (1989). In addition, Spiegel & Bloom confounded number of treatments (group therapy plus hypnotic treatment) with type of treatment, making it impossible to determine if the hypnotic procedures played any role in the results obtained.

Syrjala et al (1987) compared hypnotic, cognitive–behavioural, therapist contact and no-treatment control conditions for the relief of oral pain secondary to chemotherapy and radiation treatments for cancer. These investigators reported that hypnotherapy was more effective than the cognitive–behavioural treatment at reducing reported pain. However, these results were obtained only after the two control groups were dropped from the analyses. As pointed out by Stam (1989): 'It seems likely that, if the no-treatment control group were included, it would have washed out *any* treatment effects'.

To date the most methodologically-sound study of pain in adult cancer patients has been carried out by Reeves et al (1983). These investigators compared a group given two sessions of hypnotic training and a no-treatment control group in the reduction of pain induced by hyperthermia. Pain was assessed on both pretreatment and posttreatment trials. Hypnotic subjects exhibited significantly greater pain reductions than controls. Unfortunately, the role of hypnotic procedures in these results is unclear because nonhypnotic procedures for pain reduction were not included in the study.

Hypnotisability and outcome

The only adult cancer-pain study to assess the relationship between hypnotisability and pain reduction was that of Reeves et al (1983). Hypnotisability was assessed prior to treatment using a standardised scale and subjects were then assigned randomly to hypnotic or no-treatment control conditions. In the hypnotic condition, treatment-induced reductions in pain were observed for the high hypnotisables but not for the lows. There was no relationship between hypnotisability and pain reduction in the control condition.

CANCER-RELATED PAIN IN CHILDREN

A number of uncontrolled studies (Olness 1981; Hilgard & LeBaron 1982; Kellerman et al 1983) have suggested that hypnotic procedures may be useful in reducing the pain and distress of child cancer victims undergoing bone-marrow aspirations (BMA) and lumbar punctures (LP). The assessment of pain and distress in children can be problematic. Children under 5 years of age cannot apply numbers to intensities and have difficulty using visual analogue scales (McGrath et al 1985) and those under 7 years have difficulty separating pain from anxiety (Hilgard & LeBaron 1984). Consequently, investigations of pain in children typically involve the assessment of objective indices of pain instead of or as well as verbal report indices. For instance, the procedure behaviour rating scale (PBRS) was developed by Katz et al (1980) to assess objectively the distress associated with BMA and LP. The PBRS requires a trained observer who records the occurrence of such behaviours as crying, screaming, verbal resistance, verbal expression of pain and muscular rigidity. The final score reflects some combination of fear, pain and anxiety that is labelled procedural distress.

Comparative studies

Four studies compared the effects of hypnotic and nonhypnotic interventions in reducing procedural distress and other indicators of pain in children undergoing BMA/LP (Zeltzer & LeBaron 1982; Katz et al 1987a; Kuttner et al 1988; Wall & Womack 1989). Zeltzer & LeBaron (1982) compared a combination of deep-breathing exercises and nonimaginal distraction (e.g. counting, talking, hand squeezing) with an hypnotic treatment that included therapist-assisted deep breathing and pleasant imagery. The imagery-based strategy was not defined as hypnosis to either the patients or families and did not include an hypnotic-induction procedure. Thus, it is more accurately described as a guided imagery treatment than an hypnotic treatment. Both interventions were effective at reducing the pain of BMA and the anxiety associated with LP. The 'hypnotic procedure' was more effective than nonimaginal distraction at reducing the anxiety associated with BMA and the pain associated with LP. Although Zeltzer & LeBaron (1982) argued that hypnosis was more effective than a nonhypnotic technique for reducing pain and anxiety, it is more accurate to conclude that, in their study, guided imagery was more effective than distraction for reducing pain and anxiety.

Wall & Womack (1989) compared an hypnotic treatment that consisted of an induction procedure, relaxation and visual imagery to a nonhypnotic distraction procedure, for the treatment of pain and anxiety associated with BMA and LP. Patients varied in age from 5–18 years. Both interventions were equally effective for reducing self-reported pain, but neither intervention had an effect on anxiety.

Kuttner et al (1988) compared distraction, a procedure labelled as hypnosis/imaginative involvement and a standard practice control group in the reduction of procedural pain and distress during BMA in children of 3–10 years of age. Following treatment each child was assessed during two BMAs. In the distraction intervention, a therapist engaged children in blowing bubbles, counting, puppet play and looking at pop-up books during the procedure. The hypnotic group received a combination of hypnotic suggestion, guided imagery and support from the therapist. The only significant finding to emerge indicated that, among younger children (3–6 years 11 months), the hypnotic treatment produced lower distress scores than the distraction on control treatments in the first BMA only. By the second BMA the younger children in the three groups showed equivalent reductions in distress scores. There were no significant differences in self-reported pain and anxiety among the three groups. For the older children (7–10 years) there were no significant differences between the three groups in distress, self-reported pain or anxiety.

Katz et al (1987a) administered either an hypnotic procedure that included eye fixation, relaxation, imagery and coping suggestions or an attention control treatment that involved unstructured play, prior to BMA. Subjects were children 6–11 years of age preselected for high anxiety, pain and fear. Both groups showed equivalent reductions from baseline on self-reported pain and fear. Behavioural distress scores also failed to differ between the groups. Interestingly, however, these scores increased rather than decreased over the three posttest BMAs.

Hypnotisability and outcome

Hilgard & LeBaron (1982) assessed children for hypnotisability either prior to or following an hypnotic intervention for pain relief during BMA. Children classified as high hypnotisables showed larger reductions on self-reported and observer-rated pain than low hypnotisables. On the other hand, Wall & Womack (1989) found no relationship between hypnotisability and pain or anxiety-reduction scores either in BMA patients who received an hypnotic intervention or in those who received distraction. Katz et al (1987a) assessed hypnotisability using an unstandardised index and also assessed patient/therapist rapport. Although rapport correlated significantly with treatment-induced reductions in reported pain during BMA, hypnotisability failed to correlate significantly with pain reductions in either hypnotic or nonhypnotic conditions.

OTHER CHRONIC-PAIN SYNDROMES

Although hypnotic interventions have been used to treat a wide variety of chronic-pain syndromes, research in this area has been largely uncontrolled. Case series suggest that interventions involving hypnotic procedures may be useful in the treatment of arthritis (Nolan 1983; Domangue et al 1985), recurrent aphthous stomatitis (Andrews & Hall 1990) and head, facial and low-back pain (Toomey & Sanders 1983). Hypnotic procedures in combination with biofeedback and cognitive–behavioural interventions have also been employed to ease the pain associated with sickle-cell disease (Thomas et al 1984).

Comparative studies

Only three comparative studies have assessed the effects of hypnotic treatments on chronic-pain syndromes (Snow, 1979; Stam et al 1984; Edelson & Fitzpatrick 1989). Snow (1979) obtained baseline pain ratings from male paraplegics with chronic pain and then administered a single session of hypnotic analgesia suggestions followed by a single session of oral placebo. The hypnotic treatment and the placebo were found to be equally effective in reducing reported pain. The fixed order of treatment presentation and the absence of a no-treatment control group weaken the internal validity of this study.

In a well-designed study on the treatment of temporomandibular facial pain, Stam et al (1984) randomly assigned pain sufferers to either multiple sessions of progressive relaxation, multiple sessions of hypnotic induction plus relaxation or to a waiting-list control condition. Relaxation alone was as effective as hypnosis plus relaxation in reducing physician-rated pain and both treatments surpassed the control condition in this respect. Significant reductions in subjective reports of pain were observed only for subjects in the relaxation condition.

Edelson & Fitzpatrick (1989) compared the relative efficacy of cognitive–behavioural therapy, cognitive–behavioural therapy plus hypnotic induction and an attention control condition in the reduction of nonspecific chronic pain. Each treatment was administered over four sessions. Cognitive–behavioural therapy focused on the reinterpretation of the pain experience while the attention control procedure involved nondirective therapist contact. Cognitive–behaviour therapy alone was more effective than the control or the hypnosis plus cognitive–behaviour therapy treatments in increasing activity and limiting pain behaviour. Subjects in the three conditions failed to differ in subjective pain reports.

Stam et al (1984) and Edelson & Fitzpatrick (1989) are among the very few studies that unconfounded therapeutic suggestions and procedures from the presence or absence of an hypnotic induction. Neither study found that hypnotic treatments were more effective than corresponding nonhypnotic treatments and both found that, on some response dimensions, the nonhypnotic treatments were superior to the hypnotic treatments.

Hypnotisability and outcome

Three studies have assessed the relationship between hypnotisability and treatment-induced reductions in chronic pain (Snow 1979; Stam et al 1984; Andrews & Hall 1990). All three employed standardised scales to assess hypnotisability, and two of these studies (Snow 1979; Stam et al 1984) assessed hypnotisability before treatment administration. Stam et al (1984) found a significant correlation between treatment-induced reductions in temporomandibular joint pain and hypnotisability whereas Snow (1979) found no significant relationship between these variables among male paraplegics. Andrews & Hall (1990) conducted a posttreatment assessment of hypnotisability and found no relationship between hypnotisability and success in the hypnotic treatment of aphthous stomatitis.

OVERVIEW AND CONCLUSIONS

Laboratory studies have demonstrated consistently that hypnotic suggestions for analgesia are more effective than no-treatment at reducing reported pain and that analgesia suggestions without a prior hypnotic induction are as effective as hypnotic analgesia suggestions in this regard. The relevance of these laboratory findings to clinical situations has been questioned by a number of investigators (Graham 1986; Gauld 1989). Typically, these investigators argue on the basis of clinical anecdotes that hypnotic procedures are particularly powerful in reducing or even eliminating clinical pain, and that the equivalence of hypnotic and nonhypnotic procedures found in the laboratory stems from the artificiality of the laboratory situation. This review suggests, instead, that the major findings of laboratory studies generalise quite successfully to clinical situations. As with the laboratory studies, the clinical studies indicate consistently that hypnotic analgesia treatments are more effective than no-treatment in reducing reported pain. Importantly, however, clinical studies that compared hypnotic and nonhypnotic treatments usually found no differences in therapeutic efficacy. The fact that equivalent outcomes for hypnotic and nonhypnotic interventions occurred across a wide variety of pain syndromes and clinical populations supports the robustness of this finding.

A few comparison studies did find that hypnotic procedures were more effective than nonhypnotic ones at producing reductions in pain indices. Invariably, however, these studies confounded the administration of hypnotic procedures with the administration of suggestions for analgesia so that the effects of the hypnotic procedures could not be properly evaluated. The studies that avoided such confounding indicated consistently that psychological treatments in the absence of hypnotic induction were always at least as effective as the same psychological treatments preceded by hypnotic induction. In fact, two such studies (Stam et al 1984; Edelson & Fitzpatrick 1989) found that hypnotic treatments were, in some regards, less effective than corresponding nonhypnotic treatments. Future studies that assess hypnotic analgesia should include a nonhypnotic treatment that involves the same therapeutic suggestions as those given to the hypnotic subjects, as well as a no-treatment control condition.

The clinical studies reviewed here differed greatly in quality. Some, however, were well designed, clearly described the clinical interventions employed, used reliable and multidimensional indices of pain and analysed results with appropriate statistical procedures. To an even greater extent than the poorer quality studies, these well-executed clinical experiments provided results consistent with those obtained in laboratory experimentation. In short, the available clinical data provide no support whatsoever for the oft-heard but unsupported contention that hypnotic procedures are intrinsically more effective than other psychological procedures at reducing clinical pain.

Even the best of the clinical studies in this area have focused almost exclusively on outcome. Unlike the laboratory work, practically none of the clinical studies in this area has focused on the variables that mediate reductions on pain indices. Future work could profitably focus on assessing the role of hypnotic and nonhypnotic analgesia suggestions on indices of catastrophising and cognitive coping in clinical samples. Attempts to evaluate compliance-induced reporting biases in clinical samples might also prove enlightening. For example, patients in a wide range of medical settings frequently misdescribe the extent to which they adhere to prescribed regimens (Haynes 1976). Two studies (Hoelscher & Lichstein 1984; Hoelscher et al 1986) indicate that the same is true with respect to psychological interventions. In these studies, the extent to which anxious patients actually practised relaxation exercises at home was assessed unobtrusively and compared to self-reports of practice. Many patients grossly exaggerated the extent to which they practised. Clinical pain treatment settings, like laboratory pain settings, contain strong implicit demands for the reporting of lessened pain (e.g. fear of disappointing the therapist who has worked so hard to help). The extent to which patients respond to such demands has yet to be determined. It would be naive, however, to assume that subjects are always truthful in reporting their levels of pain following psychological interventions.

Of the clinical studies reviewed here, 23 examined the relationship between some index of hypnotisability and treatment outcome. Hypnotisability correlated significantly with treatment outcome in 10 of these studies, but failed to correlate significantly with treatment outcome in the remaining 13. The finding that hypnotisability failed to predict the outcome of suggestive treatments in more than half of the studies is inconsistent both with the hypothesis that high levels of hypnotisability are a requirement for achieving large psychologically-induced decrements on indices of pain and with the corresponding hypothesis that low hypnotisables are unable to attain large psychologically-induced pain reductions. What remains to be delineated are the conditions under which hypnotisability does or does not correlate with treatment outcome.

The findings from laboratory studies suggest that the relationship between hypnotisability and suggestion-induced reductions in reported pain is context-dependent and mediated by subjects' expectations. Contextual factors may also influence the relationship between these variables in clinical contexts. Along these lines it is useful to recall Katz et al's (1987a) finding that therapist/patient rapport, but not hypnotisability, predicted treatment outcome. Patient/therapist relationship variables are likely to be of particular importance in influencing patients' responses to both hypnotic and nonhypnotic treatments and such variables are likely to be much more important at influencing response in clinical contexts than in laboratory settings. However, the extent to which relationship variables also influence performance on hypnotisability tests may be related to how subjects view the connection between such tests and their own response to treatment.

Spanos (1991b) suggested that, in clinical contexts, hypnotisability and treatment outcome are likely to be related to the extent that patients see their hypnotisability test performance as being relevant to their response to treatment. If patients see hypnotisability testing as related to their response to treatment, they are likely to bring the same attitudes and motivations to the two situations and also likely to allow their hypnotisability test performance to influence their expectations of treatment success. Under these circumstances a relationship between hypnotisability and treatment outcome would likely emerge. On the other hand, if patients see their hypnotisability test performance as part of an experiment, and as unrelated to their own personal treatment goals, then the motivations and attitudes called up by the two situations may well be markedly different. Under these circumstances a significant correlation between hypnotisability and treatment outcome would not be anticipated. Unfortunately, the available clinical studies do not provide the information about subjects' perceptions of their hypnotisability testing that is required to assess these ideas. It might be useful, in future studies, to systematically vary the extent to which hynotisability performance is defined as relevant to treatment success and examine the effects of this manipulation on the relationship between hypnotisability and outcome.

REFERENCES

Andrews V H, Hall H R 1990 The effects of relaxation/imagery training on recurrent aphthous stomatis: a preliminary study. Psychosomatic Medicine 52: 526–535

Andreychuk T, Skriver C 1975 Hypnosis and biofeedback in the treatment of migraine headaches. International Journal of Clinical and Experimental Hypnosis 23:172–183

Asch S E 1958 Effects of group pressure upon modification and distortion of judgements. In: Maccoby E E, Newcomb T M, Hartley E L (eds) Readings in social psychology 3rd edn. Holt, New York, p 174–183

Barber J 1976 The efficacy of hypnotic analgesia for dental pain in individuals of both high and low hypnotic susceptibility. Unpublished doctoral dissertation, University of Southern California

Barber J 1980 Hypnosis and the unhypnotizable. American Journal of Clinical Hypnosis 23: 4–9
Barber T X 1969 Hypnosis: A scientific approach. Van Nostrand Reinhold, New York
Barber T X, Hahn K W Jr 1964 Physiological and subjective responses to pain-producing stimulation under hypnotically-suggested and waking-imagined 'analgesia'. Journal of Abnormal and Social Psychology 65: 411–418
Barber T X, Spanos N P, Chaves J F 1974 Hypnosis, imagination and human potentialities. Pergamon Press, Elmsford, New York
Bartlett E E 1966 Polypharmacy versus hypnosis in surgical patients. Pacific Medicine and Surgery 74: 109–112
Beers T M, Karoly P 1979 Cognitive strategies, expectancy and coping in the control of pain. Journal of Consulting and Clinical Psychology 47: 179–180
Bertrand L D 1989 The assessment and modification of hypnotic susceptibility. In: Spanos N P, Chaves J F (eds) Hypnosis: the cognitive–behavioral perspective. Prometheus, Buffalo, New York, p 18–31
Bonilla K B, Quigley W F, Bowers W F 1961 Experiences with hypnosis on a surgical service. Military Medicine 126: 364–370
Bowers K S, Kelly P 1979 Stress, disease, psychotherapy and hypnosis. Journal of Abnormal Psychology 88: 490–505
Brown R A, Fader K, Barber T X 1973 Responsiveness to pain: stimulus specificity versus generality. Psychological Record 23: 1–7
Cangello V W 1961 The use of hypnotic suggestion for pain relief in malignant disease. International Journal of Clinical and Experimental Hypnosis 9: 17–22
Cangello V W 1962 Hypnosis for the patient with cancer. American Journal of Clinical Hypnosis 4: 215–226
Cedercreutz C, Lahteenmaki R, Tulikoura J 1976 Hypnotic treatment of headache and vertigo in skull injured patients. International Journal of Clinical and Experimental Hypnosis 24: 195–201
Chaves J F 1989 The hypnotic control of clinical pain. In: Spanos N P, Chaves J F (eds) Hypnosis: the cognitive–behavioral perspective. Prometheus, Buffalo, New York, p 242–272
Chaves J F, Barber T X 1974 Cognitive strategies, experimenter modeling, and expectation in the attenuation of pain. Journal of Abnormal Psychology 83: 356–363
Chaves J F, Brown J 1987 Spontaneous coping strategies for pain. Journal of Behavioral Medicine 10: 263–276
Clark W C 1974 Pain sensitivity and the report of pain: an introduction to sensory decision theory. Anesthesiology 40: 272–287
Clark W C, Goodman J C 1974 Effects of suggestion on d' and Cx for pain detection and pain tolerance. Journal of Abnormal Psychology 83: 364–372
Clum G A, Luscomb R L, Scott L 1982 Relaxation training and cognitive redirection strategies in the treatment of acute pain. Pain 12: 175–183
Crowley R 1980 Effects of indirect hypnosis (rapid induction analgesia) for relief of acute pain associated with minor podiatric surgery. Dissertation Abstracts International 40: 45–49
Crutchfield R S 1955 Conformity and character. American Psychologist, 10: 191–198
Davidson G P, Garbett N D, Tozer S G 1985 An investigation into audiotaped self-hypnosis training in pregnancy and labor. In: Waxman D, Misra P C, Gibson M, Basker M A (eds) Modern trends in hypnosis. Plenum, New York, p 223–233
Davidson J A 1962 An assessment of the value of hypnosis in pregnancy and labour. British Medical Journal 2: 951–953
Davidson P 1987 Hypnosis and migraine headache: reporting a clinical series. Australian Journal of Clinical and Experimental Hypnosis 15: 111–118
deGroot H P, Gwynn M I 1989 Trance logic, duality and hidden observer responding. In: Spanos N P, Chaves J F (eds) Hypnosis: the cognitive–behavioral perspective. Prometheus, Buffalo, New York, p 187–205
D'Eon J L 1989 Hypnosis and obstetrics. In: Spanos N P, Chaves J F (eds) Hypnosis: the cognitive–behavioral perspective. Prometheus, Buffalo, New York, p 273–296
Doberneck R C, Griffen W O, Papermaster A A, Bonello F, Wangensteen O H 1959 Hypnosis as an adjunct to surgical therapy. Surgery 46: 299–304
Domangue B B, Margolis C G, Lieberman D, Kaji H 1985 Biochemical correlates of hypnoanalgesia in arthritic pain patients. Journal of Clinical Psychiatry 46: 235–238
Dubreuil D, Endler N S, Spanos N P 1988 Distraction and redefinition in the reduction of low and high intensity experimentally-induced pain. Imagination, Cognition and Personality 7: 155–164
Edelson J, Fitzpatrick J L 1989 A comparison of cognitive–behavioral and hypnotic treatments on chronic pain. Journal of Clinical Psychology 45: 316–323
Edmonston W E, Jr 1980 Hypnosis and relaxation: modern verification of an old equation. Wiley, New York
Evans M, Paul G L 1970 Effects of hypnotically suggested analgesia and subjective responses to cold pressor pain. Journal of Consulting and Clinical Psychology 35: 362–371
Fellows B J 1986 The concept of trance. In: Naish P L N (ed) What is hypnosis? Open University Press, Philadelphia
Frankel F H 1987 Significant developments in medical hypnosis during the past 25 years. The International Journal of Clinical and Experimental Hypnosis 35: 231–247
Freidman H, Taub H A 1984 Brief psychological training procedures in migraine treatment. American Journal of Clinical Hypnosis 26: 187–200
Freidman H, Taub H A 1985 Extended followup study of the effects of brief psychological procedures migraine therapy. American Journal of Clinical Hypnosis 28: 27–33
Gauld A 1988 Reflections on mesmeric analgesia. British Journal of Experimental and Clinical Hypnosis 5: 17–24
Genest M 1978 A cognitive–behavioral bibliotherapy to ameliorate pain. Paper presented at the annual meeting of the American Psychological Association, Toronto
Genest M, Meichenbaum D, Turk D C 1977 A cognitive–behavioral approach to the management of pain. Paper presented at the 11th annual convention of the Association for the Advancement of Behavior Therapy
Gillett P L, Coe W C 1984 The effects of rapid induction analgesia (RIA), hypnotic susceptibility, and the severity of discomfort on reducing dental pain. American Journal of Clinical Hypnosis 27: 81–90
Gottfredson D K 1973 Hypnosis as an anesthetic in dentistry. Unpublished doctoral dissertation, Brigham Young University, Provo, Utah
Graham K R 1986 Explaining 'virtuoso' hypnotic performance: social psychology or experiential skill? Behavioral and Brain Sciences 9: 473–474
Grimm L, Kafner F H 1976 Tolerance of aversive stimulation. Behavior Therapy 7: 593–601
Gwynn M I, Spanos N P, Gabora N J, Jarrett L E 1988 Long term and short term follow-up on the Harvard Group Scale of Hypnotic Susceptibility, Form A. British Journal of Experimental and Clinical Hypnosis 5: 117–124
Harding C H 1967 Hypnosis in the treatment of migraine. In: Lassner J (ed), Hypnosis and psychosomatic medicine. Springer-Verlag, New York
Harmon T M, Hyman M T, Tyre T E 1990 Improved obstetrical outcomes using hypnotic analgesia and skill mastery combined with childbirth education. Journal of Consulting and Clinical Psychology 58: 525–530
Haynes R B 1976 A critical review of the 'determinants' of patient compliance with therapeutic regimens. In: Sackett D L, Haynes R B (eds) Compliance with therapeutic regimens. John Hopkins University Press, Baltimore
Hilgard E R 1977 The problem of divided consciousness: a neodissociation interpretation. Annals of the New York Academy of Sciences 296: 48–59
Hilgard E R 1979 Divided consciousness in hypnosis: the implications of the hidden observer. In: Fromm E, Shor R E (eds) Hypnosis: recent developments and new perspectives Chicago, Aldine, p 45–79
Hilgard E R 1986 Divided consciousness. Wiley, New York
Hilgard E R 1987 Research advances in hypnosis: issues and methods. International Journal of Clinical and Experimental Hypnosis 35: 248–264
Hilgard E R 1991 A neodissociation interpretation of hypnosis. In: Lynn S J, Rhue J W (eds), Theories of hypnosis: current models and perspectives. Guilford, New York, p 83–104

Hilgard E R, LeBaron S 1982 Relief of anxiety and pain in children and adolescents with cancer: quantitative measures and clinical observations. International Journal of Clinical and Experimental Hypnosis 30: 417–442
Hilgard E R, LeBaron S 1984 Hypnotherapy of pain in children with Cancer. Kaufman, Los Altos, California
Hilgard E R, MacDonald H, Morgan A H, Johnson L S 1978 The reality of hypnotic analgesia: a comparison of highly hypnotizables with simulators. Journal of Abnormal Psychology 87: 239–246
Hoelscher T L, Lichstein K L 1984 Objective versus subjective assessment of relaxation compliance among anxious individuals. Behavior Research and Therapy 22: 187–193
Hoelscher T L, Rosenthal T L, Lichstein K L 1986 Home relaxation practice in hypertension treatment. Objective assessment and compliance induction. Journal of Consulting and Clinical Psychology 54: 1039–1052
Houle M, McGrath P A, Moran G, Garrett O J 1988 The efficacy of hypnosis- and relaxation-induced analgesia on two dimensions of pain for cold pressor and electrical tooth pulp stimulation. Pain 33: 241–251
Howard L, Reardon J P, Tosi D 1982 Modifying migraine headache through stage directed hypnotherapy: a cognitive experiential perspective. International Journal of Clinical and Experimental Hypnosis 30: 257–269
Jaremko M E 1978 Cognitive strategies in the control of pain tolerance. Behaviour Therapy and Experimental Psychiatry 9: 239–244
Jones B, Spanos N P, Anuza T 1987 Functional measurement analysis of suggestions for analgesia. Unpublished manuscript, Carleton University
Katz E R, Kelerman J, Ellenberg L 1987a Hypnosis in the reduction of acute pain and distress in children with cancer. Journal of Pediatric Psychology 12: 379–394
Katz E R, Kellerman J, Siegel S E 1987b Behavioral distress in children with cancer undergoing medical procedures: developmental considerations. Journal of Consulting and Clinical Psychology 48: 356–365
Keefe F J, Brown G K, Wallston K A, Caldwell D S 1989 Coping with rheumatiod arthritis: catastrophizing as a maladaptive strategy. Pain 37: 51–56
Kellerman J, Zeltzer L, Ellenberg L, Dash J 1983 Adolescents with cancer: hypnosis for the reduction of the acute pain and anxiety associated with medical procedures. Journal of Adolescent Health Care 4: 85–90
Kuttner L, Bowman M, Teasdale M 1988 Psychological treatment of distress, pain and anxiety for young children with cancer. Journal of Developmental and Behavioral Pediatrics 9: 374–382
Laurance J-R, Perry C 1981 The 'hidden observer' phenomenon in hypnosis: some additional findings. Journal of Abnormal Psychology 90: 334–344
Lea P A, Ware P D, Monroe R R 1960 The hypnotic control of intractable pain. American Journal of Clinical Hypnosis 3: 3–8
McAmmond D M, Davidson P O, Kovitz D M A 1971 Comparison of the effects of hypnosis and relaxation training on stress reactions in a dental situation. American Journal of Clinical Hypnosis 13: 233–242
McCaul K D, Malott J M 1984 Distraction and coping with pain. Psychological Bulletin 95: 516–533
McGlashin T H, Evans F J, Orne M T 1969. The nature of hypnotic analgesia and placebo response to experimental pain. Psychosomatic Medicine 31: 227–246
McGrath P A, deVeber L L, Hearn M T 1985 Multidimensional pain assessment in children. In: Fields H L, Dubner R, Cervero F (eds), Advances in Pain Research and Therapy, vol 9. Raven Press, New York, p 387–393
Malone M D, Kurtz R M, Strube M J 1989 The effects of hypnotic suggestion on pain report. American Journal of Clinical Hypnosis 31: 221–229
Mellis P M, Rooimans W, Spierings E L, Hoogdiun C A 1991 Treatment of chronic tension-type headache with hypnotherapy: a single-blind control study. Headache 31: 686–689
Mikail S F, Vandeursen J B P, von Baeyer C 1986 Rating pain or rating serenity: effects on cold pressor pain tolerance. Canadian Journal of Behavioral Science 18: 126–132
Milgram S 1974 Obedience to authority. Harper & Row, New York
Miller J A 1986 The obedience experiments. Praeger, New York
Miller M E, Bowers K W 1986 Hypnotic analgesia and stress inoculation in the reduction of pain. Journal of Abnormal Psychology 95: 6–14
Milne G 1983 Hypnotherapy with migraine. Australian Journal of Experimental and Clinical Hypnosis 11: 23–32
Nolan M 1983 A combination of hypnotherapy, megavitamins, and 'folk' medicine in the treatment of arthritis. Australian Journal of Clinical Hypnotherapy and Hypnosis 4: 21–25
Nolan R, Spanos N P, Hayward A, Scott H 1989 Hypnotic and nonhypnotic imagery based strategies in the treatment of tension and mixed tension/migraine headache. Unpublished manuscript, Carleton University
Olness K 1981 Imagery (self-hypnosis) as adjunct therapy in childhood cancer: clinical experience with 25 patients. American Journal of Pediatric Hematology/Oncology 3: 313–321
Olness K, MacDonald J T, Uden D L 1987 Comparison of self-hypnosis and propranolol in the treatment of juvenile classic migraine. Pediatrics 79: 593–597
Patterson D R, Questad K A, deLateur B J 1989 Hypnotherapy as an adjunct to narcotic analgesia for the treatment of pain for burn debridment. American Journal of Clinical Hypnosis 31: 156–163
Patterson D R, Everett J J, Burns G L, Marvin J A 1992 Hypnosis for the treatment of burn pain. Journal of Consulting and Clinical Psychology 60: 713–717
Perchard S D 1960 Hypnosis in obstetrics. Proceedings of the Royal Society of Medicine 53: 458–460
Perlini A H, Spanos N P 1991 EEG methodologies and hypnotizability: a critical review. Psychophysiology 28: 511–530
Perry C, Laurance J -R, Nadon R 1988 Hypnosis, surgery and the social-psychological position. British Journal of Experimental and Clinical Hypnosis 5: 143–149
Piccione C, Hilgard E R, Zimbardo P G 1989 On the degree of stability of measured hypnotizability over a 25 year period. Journal of Personality and Social Psychology 56: 289–295
Poulton E C 1979 Models for biases in judging sensory magnitude. Psychological Bulletin 86: 777–803
Radtke H L, Spanos N P 1981 Was I hypnotized? A social psychological analysis of hypnotic depth reports. Psychiatry 44: 359–376
Reeves J L, Redd W H, Storm F K, Minagawa R Y 1983 Hypnosis in the control of pain during hyperthermia treatment of cancer. In: Bonica J J, Lindblom U, Iggo A (eds) Advances in pain research and therapy, vol 4. Raven Press, New York, p 857–861
Rock N L, Shipley T E, Campbell C 1969 Hypnosis with untrained volunteer patients in labour. International Journal of Clinical and Experimental Hypnosis 17: 25–36
Rosenstiel A K, Keefe F J 1983 The use of coping strategies in chronic low back pain patients: relationship to patient characteristics and current adjustment. Pain 17: 33–44
Samko M A, Schoenfeld L S 1975 Hypnotic susceptibility and Lamaze childbirth experience. American Journal of Obstetrics and Gynecology 121: 631–636
Sarbin T R 1989 The construction and reconstruction of hypnosis. In: Spanos N P, Chaves J R (eds) Hypnosis: the cognitive–behavioral perspective. Prometheus, Buffalo, New York, p 400–416
Schafer D W 1975 Hypnosis use on a burn unit. International Journal of Clinical and Experimental Hypnosis 23: 1–14
Schlutter I C, Golden C, Blume H G 1980 A comparison of treatments for prefrontal muscle contraction headache. British Journal of Medical Psychology 53: 47–52
Scott D S 1980 Pain endurance induced by a subtle social variable (demand) and the 'reverse Milgram effect'. British Journal of Social and Clinical Psychology 19: 137–139
Scott D S, Leonard C E Jr 1978 Modification of pain threshold by the covert reinforcement procedure and a cognitive strategy. Psychological Record 28: 49–57
Singh R 1989 Single session treatment of refractory headache: Evaluation with three patients. Australian Journal of Clinical and Experimental Hypnosis 17: 99–105
Smith M S, Womack W M, Chen A C N 1989 Hypnotizability does not predict outcome of behavioral treatment of pediatric headache. American Journal of Clinical Hypnosis 31: 237–241
Snow L 1979 The relationship between 'Rapid Induction' and placebo

analgesia, hypnotic susceptibility and pain intensity. Dissertation Abstracts International 40: 937
Spanos N P 1986a Hypnosis and the modification of hypnotic susceptibility: a social psychological perspective. In: Naish P L N (ed) What is hypnosis? Open University Press, Philadelphia, p 85–120
Spanos N P 1986b Hypnotic behavior: a social psychological interpretation of amnesia, analgesia and trance logic. Behavioral and Brain Sciences 9: 449–502
Spanos N P 1989a Experimental research on hypnotic analgesia. In: Spanos N P, Chaves J F (eds) Hypnosis: the cognitive–behavioral perspective. Prometheus, Buffalo, New York, p 206–240
Spanos N P 1989b Interpretational sets, hypnotic responding and the modification of hypnotizability. In: Gheorghiu V A, Netter P, Eysenck H J, Rosenthal R (eds) Suggestion and suggestibility: theory and research. Springer-Verlag, New York, p 169–176
Spanos N P 1991a A sociocognitive approach to hypnosis. In: Lynn S J, Rhue J W (eds) Theories of hypnosis: current models and perspectives. Guilford, New York, p 324–361
Spanos N P 1991b Hypnosis, hypnotizability and hypnotherapy. In: Snyder C R, Forsyth D R (eds) Handbook of social and clinical psychology. Pergamon, New York, p 644–663
Spanos N P, Chaves J F 1989 Hypnosis, analgesia and surgery: in defence of the social psychological-position. British Journal of Experimental and Clinical Hypnosis 6: 131–140
Spanos N P, Coe W C 1992 Social psychological approaches to hypnosis. In: Fromm E, Nash M (eds) Contemporary hypnosis research. Plenum, New York, p 102–130
Spanos N P, Hewitt E C 1980 The hidden observer in hypnotic analgesia: discovery or experimental creation? Journal of Personality and Social Psychology 39: 1201–1214
Spanos N P, Katsanis J 1989 Effects of instructional set and attributions of nonvolition during hypnotic and nonhypnotic analgesia. Journal of Personality and Social Psychology 56: 182–188
Spanos N P, Barber T X, Lang G 1974 Cognition and self-control: cognitive control of painful sensory input. In: London H, Nisbit R E (eds) Thought and feeling: cognitive alteration of feeling states. Aldine, Chicago, p 144–158
Spanos N P, Radtke-Bodorik H L, Ferguson J, Jones B 1979 The effects of hypnotic susceptibility, suggestions for analgesia and the utilization of cognitive strategies on the reduction of pain. Journal of Abnormal Psychology 88: 282–292
Spanos N P, Brown J, Jones B, Horner D 1981 The effects of cognitive activity and suggestions for analgesia in the reduction of reported pain. Journal of Abnormal Psychology 90: 554–561
Spanos N P, Gwynn M I, Stam H J 1983a Instructional demands and ratings of overt and hidden pain during hypnotic analgesia. Journal of Abnormal Psychology 92: 479–488
Spanos N P, Jones B, Brown J, Horner D 1983b Magnitude estimates of cold pressor pain: effects of suggestions, cognitive strategy and tolerance. Perception 12: 355–362
Spanos N P, Hodgins D C, Stam H J, Gwynn M I 1984a Suffering for science: the effects of implicit social demands on response to experimentally induced pain. Journal of Personality and Social Psychology 46: 1162–1172
Spanos N P, Kennedy S K, Gwynn M I 1984b The moderating effect of contextual variables on the relationship between hypnotic susceptibility and suggested analgesia. Journal of Abnormal Psychology 93: 285–294
Spanos N P, deGroot H P, Tiller D K, Weekes J R, Bertrand L D 1985 'Trance logic' duality and hidden observer responding in hypnotic, imagination control and simulating subjects. Journal of Abnormal Psychology 94: 611–623
Spanos N P, Ollerhead V G, Gwynn M I 1986 The effects of three instructional treatments on pain magnitude and pain tolerance. Imagination, Cognition and Personality 5: 321–337
Spanos N P, Voorneveld P W, Gwynn M I 1987 The mediating effects of expectation on hypnotic and nonhypnotic pain reduction. Imagination, Cognition and Personality 6: 231–246
Spanos N P, MacDonald D K, Gwynn M I 1988 Instructional set and the relative efficacy of hypnotic and waking analgesia. Canadian Journal of Behavioural Science 26: 64–72
Spanos N P, Gabora N J, Jarrett L E, Gwynn M I 1989a Contextual determinants of hypnotizability and of the relationship between hypnotizability scales. Journal of Personality and Social Psychology 57: 271–278
Spanos N P, Perlini A H, Robertson L A 1989b Hypnosis, suggestion and placebo in the reduction of experimental pain. Journal of Abnormal Psychology 98: 285–293
Spanos N P, Perlini A H, Patrick L, Bell S, Gwynn M I 1990 The role of compliance in hypnotic and nonhypnotic analgesia. Journal of Research in Personality 24: 433–453
Spanos N P, Burgess C A, Perlini A H 1992a Compliance and suggested deafness in hypnotic and nonhypnotic subjects. Imagination, Cognition and Personality 11: 211–223
Spanos N P, Gardin A, Burgess C A 1992b Reporting bias, dissociation and expectancy in hypnotic analgesia. Unpublished manuscript, Carleton University
Spanos N P, Liddy S J, Scott H A et al 1993 Hypnotic suggestion and placebo in the treatment of chronic headache in a university volunteer sample. Cognitive Therapy and Research (in press)
Spiegel D, Bloom J R 1983 Group therapy and hypnosis reduce metastatic breast cancer pain. Psychosomatic Medicine 52: 109–114
Spinhoven P 1988 Similarities and dissimilarities in hypnotic and nonhypnotic procedures for headache control: a review. American Journal of Clinical Hypnosis 30: 183–194
Spinhoven P, Van Dyck R, Zitman F G, Linssen A C G 1985 Treating tension headache: autogenic training and hypnotic imagery. Paper presented at the 10th International Congress of Hypnosis and Psychosomatic Medicine, Toronto, Canada
Spinhoven P, Linssen A C G, Van Dyck R, Zitman F G 1988 Locus of control, cognitive strategies and hypnotizability in pain management: a preliminary report. Paper presented at the 11th International Congress of Hypnosis and Psychosomatic Medicine, The Hague, The Netherlands
Stacher G, Schuster P, Bauer P, Lahoda R, Schulze D 1975 Effects of relaxation or analgesia on pain threshold and pain tolerance in the waking and in the hypnotic state. Journal of Psychosomatic Research 19: 259–265
Stam H J 1989 From symptom relief to cure: hypnotic interventions in cancer. In: Spanos N P, Chaves J F (eds) Hypnosis: the cognitive–behavioral perspective. Prometheus, Buffalo, New York, p 313–339
Stam H J, Spanos N P 1980 Experimental designs, expectancy effects and hypnotic analgesia. Journal of Abnormal Psychology 89: 551–559
Stam H J, Petrusic W M, Spanos N P 1981 Magnitude scales for cold pressor pain. Perception and Psychophysics 29: 612–617
Stam H J, McGrath P A, Brooke R I 1984 The effects of a cognitive–behavioral treatment program on temporo-mandibular pain and dysfunction syndrome. Psychosomatic Medicine 46: 534–545
Sullivan M J L, Bishop S 1992 Catastrophizing and pain 1: scale: development validation and affective correlates. Unpublished manuscript, Dalhouse University
Sullivan M J L, D'Eon J 1990 Relation between catastrophizing and depression in chronic pain patients. Journal of Abnormal Psychology 99: 260–263
Surman O S, Hackett T P, Silverberg E L, Behrendt D M 1974 Usefulness of psychiatric intervention in patients undergoing cardiac surgery. Archives of General Psychiatry 30: 830–835
Syrjala K L, Cummings C, Donaldson G, Chapman C R 1987 Hypnosis for oral pain following chemotherapy and irradiation. Paper presented at the 5th World Conference on Pain, Hamburg, West Germany
Tenenbaum S J, Kurtz R M, Bienias J L 1990 Hypnotic susceptibility and experimental pain reduction. American Journal of Clinical Hypnosis 33: 40–49
Thomas J E, Koshy M, Patterson L, Dorn L, Thomas K 1984 Management of pain in sickle cell disease using biofeedback therapy: a preliminary study. Biofeedback and Self-Regulation 9: 413–420
Thelen M H, Fry R A 1981 The effects of modeling and selective attention on pain tolerance. Journal of Behavior Therapy and Experimental Psychiatry 12: 225–229
Toomey T C, Sanders S 1983 Group hypnotherapy as an active control strategy in chronic pain. American Journal of Clinical Hypnosis 26: 20–25
Turk D C, Meichenbaum D, Genest M 1983 Pain and behavioral medicine: a cognitive–behavioral perspective. Guilford, New York
Venn J 1987 Hypnosis and the Lamaze method: an exploratory study.

International Journal of Clinical and Experimental Hypnosis 35: 79–82
Wadden T, Anderton C H 1982 The clinical use of hypnosis. Psychological Bulletin 91: 215–243
Wagstaff G F 1981 Hypnosis compliance and belief. St Martin's Press, New York
Wagstaff G F 1991 Compliance belief and semantics in hypnosis: a nonstate sociocognitive perspective. In: Lynn S J, Rhue J W (eds), Theories of hypnosis: current models and perspectives. Guilford, New York, p 362–396
Wakeman R J, Kaplan J Z 1978 An experimental study of hypnosis in painful burns. American Journal of Clinical Hypnosis 21: 3–12
Wall V J, Womack W 1989 Hypnotic versus active cognitive strategies for alleviation of procedural distress in pediatric oncology patients. American Journal of Clinical Hypnosis 31: 181–191
Werbel E W 1963 Use of posthypnotic suggestions to reduce pain following hemorrhoidectomies. American Journal of Clinical Hypnosis 6: 132–136
Zeltzer L, LeBaron S 1982 Hypnotic and nonhypnotic techniques for the reduction of pain and anxiety during painful procedures in children and adolescents with cancer. Journal of Pediatrics 101: 1032–1035
Zitman F G, Van Dyck R, Spinhoven P, Linssen A C G 1992 Hypnosis and autogenic training in the treatment of tension headache: a two phase constructive design study with follow-up. Journal of Psychosomatic Research 36: 219–228

76. Behaviour therapy

Francis J. Keefe and John C. Lefebvre

INTRODUCTION

In the 25 years since the initial pioneering contributions of Wilbert Fordyce, behaviour therapy has had a major impact on the management of patients suffering from chronic pain. Behaviour therapy has helped many chronic-pain patients increase their activity level, reduce their dependence on medications and return to a much more effective lifestyle. Behaviour-therapy principles currently provide the conceptual foundations for many specialised inpatient and outpatient treatment programmes (Sternbach 1989). Even in pain-treatment programmes that do not strictly adhere to a behavioural viewpoint, treatment specialists frequently use behavioural-therapy techniques such as self-monitoring of activity, social reinforcement, and time-contingent pain medications.

Over the past decade, behaviour-therapy researchers have developed and refined a number of methods for assessing and treating chronic pain. Thus, to understand better the current role of behavioural therapy in pain management, one must not only be aware of the basic principles and methods of behaviour therapy, but also have an appreciation of recent developments in behavioural theory and application. This chapter seeks to provide the reader with an overview of the current status of behavioural-therapy methods used in pain management.

This chapter is divided into four sections. The first section outlines theoretical principles used to guide behavioural assessment and treatment efforts. The second section reviews a variety of established and newly-developed behavioural-assessment methods. In the third section, behavioural treatment techniques are described and critically evaluated. The concluding section highlights important conceptual and clinical issues involved in applying behaviour-therapy methods to chronic-pain patients.

THEORETICAL PRINCIPLES

Patients who have pain engage in a wide variety of pain-related behaviours such as complaining of pain, taking pain medication or moving in a slow and guarded fashion. These behaviours, which Fordyce (1976) called pain behaviours, serve to communicate to those around the patient the fact that pain is being experienced. Patients having persistent pain often exhibit a very high level of maladaptive pain behaviours (e.g. excessive reliance on narcotic medications, bed rest and an overly sedentary and restricted lifestyle), while engaging in few adaptive well behaviours (e.g. exercising, socialising or fulfilling work or home responsibilities).

Behavioural theories of persistent pain attempt to explain how pain and well behaviours are acquired and maintained. The earliest applications of behaviour therapy to the management of chronic pain were based on operant- and respondent-conditioning principles. More recently, behavioural pain management efforts have been grounded in comprehensive theoretical models that integrate conditioning and learning perspectives with an emphasis on self-regulation.

OPERANT CONDITIONING

Many of the behaviours of a patient having pain can be classified as operant behaviours because they are strongly influenced by the consequences that follow their occurrence. A low-back pain patient, for example, may rest in bed because reclining reduces pain or may avoid exercising because this activity increases pain. Operant conditioning (also known as instrumental or Skinnerian conditioning) is concerned with the relationship between such behaviours and their consequences.

A central tenet of operant conditioning is that the consequences of engaging in behaviour are an important determinant of whether those behaviours are likely to occur again in the future. The theoretical principle that outlines how consequences of behaviour can alter future behaviour was described by Thorndike (1913) in the Law of Effect. This law states that the probability of a behaviour can be increased or decreased depending on its immediate consequences. Behaviours that produce positive outcomes will be more likely to occur in the future, while behaviours that produce negative or aversive outcomes will be less likely to occur in the future.

In a series of classic studies, Skinner developed and refined many of the basic principles of operant conditioning (Skinner 1938, 1953, 1958, 1959). These principles were later extended to an analysis of abnormal behaviour in patients suffering from various psychological problems (Ullman & Krasner 1969). Fordyce (1976) was the first to argue persuasively that operant principles could be useful in understanding the behaviour of patients having chronic pain.

Fordyce (1976) described four major types of behaviour-consequence relationship that may be important in the acquisition and maintenance of pain and well behaviours. As can be seen in Figure 76.1, these relationships can be categorised along two dimensions:

1. whether the environmental stimuli involved are positive or aversive
2. whether the stimulus is delivered or withdrawn following emission of the behaviour.

The first type of behaviour–consequence relationship occurs when a behaviour leads to a positive outcome (*positive reinforcement*). Behaviours that are positively reinforced have a higher probability of being repeated. Thus, patients whose complaints about chronic pain lead to added attention and sympathy from others may be more likely to complain of pain in the future. The second type of behaviour–consequence relationship is one in which behaviour leads to an aversive outcome (*punishment*). A back-pain patient who finds that she is criticised by her husband for trying to do any household chores is less likely to attempt to do them in the future. The third relationship is one in which behaviour leads to withdrawal of a positive stimulus (*extinction*). An overly dependent chronic-pain patient who has been praised frequently by his physician for exercising may stop exercising when the physician fails to ask about, attend to or otherwise reinforce the patient for exercising. The fourth type of relationship involves the withdrawal of a negative or aversive stimulus (*negative reinforcement*). Negative reinforcement increases the likelihood of a behaviour. A patient who has constant pain while sitting or walking is likely to find reclining in bed quite reinforcing. In this case, reclining in bed is negatively reinforced by its pain-relieving effects.

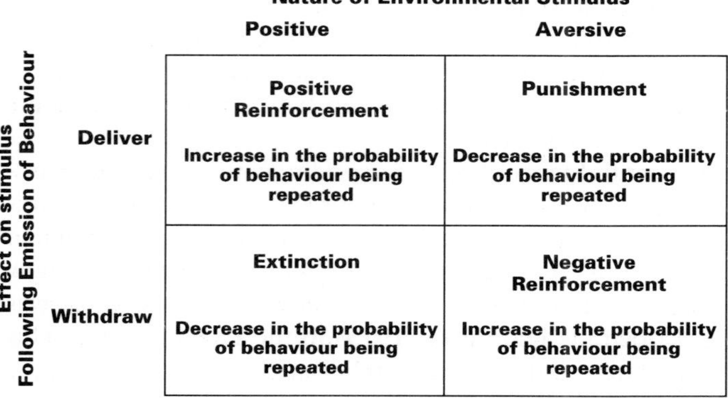

Fig. 76.1 Behaviour–consequence relations in operant conditioning.

A major tenet of operant conditioning is that one needs to carefully observe behaviour to determine whether a particular consequence is reinforcing (Catania 1984). Reinforcement is the product of experience, and different people who have different backgrounds and experiences will have different reinforcers. For some patients in pain, praise is a very effective reinforcer, while for others the opportunity to rest or read may be much more reinforcing. The best way to identify effective reinforcers is to carefully evaluate the effects that potentially reinforcing events (e.g. praise for exercising) have on future behaviour (e.g. the duration of daily exercise).

Schedules of reinforcement are very important in the acquisition and maintenance of operant behaviours. Skinner (1953, 1969) found that the most effective method for increasing the probability of behaviour is to provide immediate and constant reinforcement (*continuous reinforcement*). A patient in a hospital pain unit, for example, is likely to become much more active if he or she receives praise and attention every time he or she gets out of bed. Although one can arrange the social environment of a pain unit to provide continuous reinforcement, the behaviours acquired may rapidly extinguish once the patient leaves this specialised environment. In fact, Skinner (1953) found that behaviours that were acquired by means of continuous reinforcement were not very resistant to extinction.

Intermittent reinforcement is more effective in maintaining behaviour. For this reason, operant programmes for pain management typically employ continuous reinforcement in the early stages of treatment (e.g. praise the patient after each exercise session) and then switch to intermittent (e.g. praise the patient on a variable schedule – after a variable number of exercise sessions) later in treatment.

Fordyce (1976) has been the major proponent of operant models of chronic pain. He has maintained that, in some patients, pain behaviours that initially occur in response to acute pain can persist long after the normal healing time because these behaviours are reinforced. Given the persistent nature of certain pain conditions, there are ample opportunities for pain behaviours to be reinforced and for patients to learn to avoid well behaviours that could increase their pain. As Fordyce (1976) notes, the operant perspective not only helps one understand the persistence of such pain behaviours, it also serves to direct behavioural treatment efforts. By changing the consequences of behaviour, the frequency of maladaptive pain behaviours can be reduced and the frequency of well behaviours increased.

RESPONDENT CONDITIONING

Patients having persistent disease-related pain (e.g. patients having cancer or rheumatoid arthritis) often have evidence of underlying tissue damage that is responsible for their pain. Although the pain behaviour of these patients has an organic basis, this behaviour can be influenced by conditioning and learning factors. In these patients, stimuli associated with pain can acquire, over the course of time, the ability to elicit maladaptive pain behaviours. A burn patient who has undergone repeated wound debridements, for example, may exhibit increased tension, physiological arousal and pain as soon as he enters the room where the debridements are carried out.

Respondent conditioning focuses on the role that environmental stimuli play in eliciting pain behaviour. The pioneering work in responding conditioning (also known as classical or Pavlovian conditioning) was conducted by Ivan P. Pavlov (1849–1936). Pavlov proposed that an organism possessed a wide variety of innate reflexes. Since these reflexes were not conditional on experience, Pavlov referred to them as unconditional responses or URs. Pavlov labelled certain environmental stimuli (e.g. an intense nociceptive stimulus or very loud noise) as unconditional stimuli (US) because they produce unconditional responses. Pavlov discovered that repeated pairings of a US with a previously neutral stimulus ultimately led to a situation in which the neutral stimulus itself could elicit a response similar to UR. The previously neutral stimulus, through experience, had become a conditioned stimulus or CS, and the response it elicits is now referred to as the conditioned response (CR).

From what has been described so far, respondent conditioning may seem as merely the replacement of one stimulus by another. However, if the CS is continually presented in the absence of the US, the CR will no longer be elicited, or will extinguish. The crucial factor of respondent learning is the pairing of the US and the CS to produce behaviour. Theoretically, anything in the environment can serve as a CS, as long as it is repeatedly paired with the US. The more salient the stimulus, the faster the association develops. Stimuli that signal the onset of increased pain are particularly salient to patients having persistent pain and thus can readily acquire the ability to elicit a conditioned pain-behaviour response.

The classic example of respondent conditioning is the original experiment conducted by Pavlov. In this experiment, meat powder (the US) was placed in the mouth of a dog and the amount of salivation (the UR) was measured. Immediately prior to the presentation of the US, a neutral stimulus (a tone) was presented. After a number of pairings, Pavlov discovered that the tone (the CS) presented without the US elicited a salivary response similar to the UR, which Pavlov now referred to as the conditioned response or CR. The important factor to note is that the animal is performing the CR in anticipation of the US being delivered.

Respondent conditioning is especially useful in understanding pain behaviour in patients whose pain is related to ongoing tissue damage or disease processes. Because of underlying tissue pathology, daily activities such as walking down a few stairs or moving from one position to another can activate nociceptive input which in turn can produce pain behaviour. With repeated pairings of such activities with increased pain, previously neutral stimuli (e.g. the sight of the stairs) can acquire the ability to elicit pain behaviours.

Patients whose pain behaviour is influenced by respondent conditioning respond well to behavioural treatment (Fordyce 1976). Exposure-based therapies are often quite useful. In these therapies the patient is gradually exposed to activities that have caused increased pain in the past. With graded exposure, the association between environmental stimuli and severe pain is broken. As a result, patients can often increase their tolerance for activity and reduce the frequency of maladaptive, anticipatory pain behaviours. Patients whose pain behaviour is under respondent control are reinforced effectively by signs of their own improvement (Fordyce 1976). In these patients, progress in treatment may be rapid because operant factors (e.g. in the form of social reinforcement) play a much less important role in maintaining their pain behaviour.

SELF-REGULATION MODELS

Operant- and respondent-conditioning models emphasise the influence that the environment can have in controlling pain behaviour. These models, however, do not fully take into account the role that an individual can play in regulating his or her own behaviour. Recent behavioural theories have attempted to integrate a self-regulation perspective with earlier conditioning and learning theories.

Self-regulation theories have several basic characteristics (Hollandsworth 1986; Kanfer & Schefft 1988). First, each theory emphasises that the individual is an active agent in changing behaviour. A patient having pain, for example, can observe his or her own pain and well behaviours, set goals for changing these behaviours, and be an active participant in the entire process of behaviour change. Second, the theories are comprehensive and view behaviour as determined by multiple factors. According to self-regulation theory, the pain behaviour of a migraine headache may be influenced by respondent factors (e.g., exposure to allergens), operant factors (e.g. an opportunity to avoid a stressful examination), a breakdown in self-control efforts or a combination of these factors. Finally, self-regulation theory emphasises the interactive and dynamic nature of pain-behaviour influences. The factors affecting pain behaviour can interact with each other and also change over time.

Kanfer (1970) was one of the first to present a self-regulation model of behaviour. The model depicted in Figure 76.2 includes:

1. stimulus variables (S) – environmental stimuli that may elicit behaviour
2. organismic variables (O) – which include self-regulatory processes that may affect behaviour
3. response variables (R) – behaviour
4. contingency relationships (K) – which describe the schedule of reinforcement between response and consequence
5. consequences (C) – which include the positive and aversive contingencies of responding.

The S, R, K, and C components of Kanfer's self-regulation model had all been part of earlier conditioning and learning theories that viewed learning and reinforcement as occurring in a linear fashion. Thus, the stimulus triggers a response that prompts consequences from the environment which in turn determines the probability of the behaviour being repeated. What was new in Kanfer's model was the self-regulatory component. According to this model, self-regulation processes are activated when ongoing activities are disrupted or the individual fails to reach a desired goal. Self-regulation involves three stages. The first stage, self-monitoring, is one in which the individual attends to his or her behaviour and becomes much more aware of variations in behaviour patterns. The second stage of self-regulation, self-evaluation, is one in which current actions are compared to criteria developed from past experience or desired performance. The final stage, self-reinforcement, is a motivational stage in which the individual assigns either positive or negative consequences to his or her own behaviour. The valence of these consequences determines whether the behaviour will be continued, improved upon, replaced by different behaviours to reach the same goal or whether new goals will be set. In summary, Kanfer's original self-regulation model (1970) viewed the individual as important in monitoring, evaluating and reinforcing his or her own behaviour.

More recent versions of self-regulation theory are even more comprehensive in that they attempt to account for the interrelationships between biological factors and self-regulation (Kanfer & Schefft 1988). Schefft & Lehr (1985), for example, have presented a general systems model that is depicted in schematic fashion in Figure 76.3. This model addresses several different types of variables:

1. Alpha variables, which represent inputs from the external environment
2. Beta variables, which represent internal, psychological factors initiated and maintained by the individual
3. Gamma variables, which are the genetic and biological factors that are involved in human behaviour.

Each of the variables in the model can contribute to an individual's behaviour. However, the importance of any given variable may alter depending on the individual and the moment. In addition, each of these variables interacts with the others to determine behaviour.

The general systems model described by Schefft & Lehr (1985) includes feedback and feedforward systems that allow for interaction both among and within levels. In addition, in order to address a full range of self-regulatory processes, the model makes a distinction between corrective and anticipatory self-regulation. Corrective self-regulation involves direct contact with the environment and feedback is obtained directly from environment–action consequences. Anticipatory self-regulation, on the other hand, involves the individual imagining or thinking about the actions. The individual relies on past experience and observed results from others to determine the possible results of actions.

Given that self-regulation theory acknowledges that behaviour can be controlled by environmental influences,

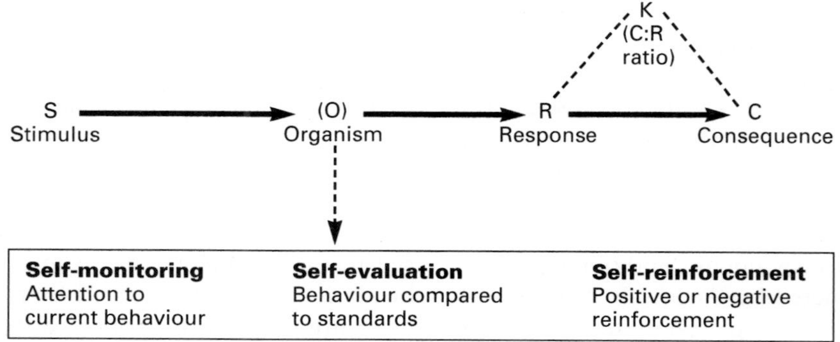

Fig. 76.2 Linear self-regulation model. (From *Guiding the Process of Therapeutic Change* (p. 48) by F. H. Kanfer and B. K. Schefft, 1988, Champaign, IL: Research Press. Copyright 1988 by the authors. Reprinted by permission.)

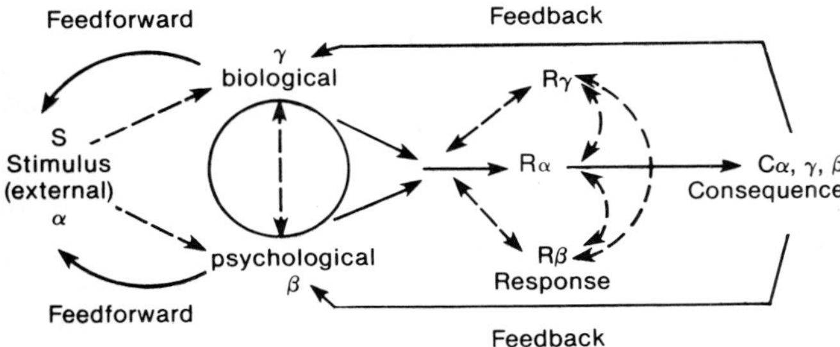

Fig. 76.3 General systems model. (From *Guiding the Process of Therapeutic Change* (p. 53) by F. H. Kanfer and B. K. Schefft, 1988, Champaign, IL: Research Press. Copyright 1988 by the authors. Reprinted by permission.)

the question arises: when are self-regulation processes activated? Kanfer (1970) maintains that self-regulation may become important when ongoing routines or activities are disrupted or the individual fails to reach a desired goal. Systems theories, such as Schefft & Lehr's (1985), maintain that since components of the system are interconnected, changes in any one component will affect others through feedback and feedforward loops. Thus, patients who receive social reinforcement for spending time up and out of the reclining position may become more aware of their own behaviour and take a more active role in trying to regulate their own activity level. Patients whose pain behaviour is clearly maintained by environmental contingencies (e.g. a patient who is addicted to narcotic medications), may be incapable of self-regulation early in the course of treatment. However, as their behaviour changes during treatment, their capacity for self-control may increase greatly.

Self-regulation theories have had several effects on behaviour-therapy approaches to chronic pain. First, these theories have underscored the need to involve patients fully in behavioural-treatment efforts. Many chronic-pain patients are capable of self-regulation and, thus, can benefit substantially from training in self-control techniques such as self-reinforcement and relaxation training. Second, self-regulation theory has directed behaviour therapists towards a more comprehensive assessment of factors that control pain behaviour. These theories suggest that patients' own coping strategies, beliefs about pain, and ability to accurately monitor their own behaviour may all be important determinants of pain behaviour. Finally, these theories have led to increased interest in outpatient behaviour-therapy treatment. If chronic-pain patients can learn to control their own behaviour, they are less likely to need to be treated in highly structured inpatient units where the reinforcement contingencies are programmed to reinforce well behaviours. Training in self-control techniques can also play an important role in enhancing the maintenance of treatment gains (Turk & Rudy 1991).

BEHAVIOURAL ASSESSMENT METHODS

Behaviour therapists have developed a wide variety of methods to assess the behaviour of chronic-pain patients. These methods include structured interviews, daily diaries, electromechanical devices, and behavioural observation.

BEHAVIOURAL INTERVIEW TECHNIQUES

Fordyce (1976) pioneered the use of structured interviewing for pain behaviour assessment. The aims of behavioural interviewing are:

1. to obtain a description of current patterns of pain and well behaviours
2. to identify factors that may control behaviour patterns
3. to select target behaviours for behavioural intervention.

Several authors have described structured interview formats for the behavioural assessment of chronic pain (Fordyce 1976; Turk et al 1983; Keefe 1988). Table 76.1 includes a topical outline of a structured interview we use in behavioural assessment. As can be seen, the interview addresses variables that are viewed important in both conditioning and self-regulation perspectives on pain behaviour.

The interview is not only a rich source of information; it also provides an opportunity to assess the patient's openness to behaviour-therapy interventions. Some chronic-pain patients seek a permanent cure for their pain and are unwilling to commit themselves to the goals of behavioural pain management. For other patients, the interview itself can be therapeutic in highlighting behavioural strategies that are effective and in pinpointing important goals for future treatment.

Interviews with the patient's spouse and family members are an important part of the behavioural assessment process (Fordyce 1976). By interviewing a spouse, one may be able to validate the patient's descriptions of daily pain and well-behaviour patterns. Areas of discrepancy between patient and spouse can be identified and then clarified through discussions with the patient. An interview with a spouse or family member also provides an opportunity to involve them in the treatment process.

DAILY DIARIES

Daily diaries are often used in the behavioural assessment of chronic pain. In contrast to interview methods that rely on retrospective reports of behaviour, diaries provide direct, immediate, and repeated measurements of important target behaviours.

The Fordyce activity diary (1976) is one of the earliest

Table 76.1 A structured behavioural interview outline*

1. Characteristics of pain
   a. Location, severity, duration
   b. Factors that increase pain
   c. Factors that decrease pain
2. Patterns of pain and well behaviour
   a. General activity level and medication intake
      (i) Estimates of daily sitting, standing and walking time
      (ii) Estimates of intake of pain medications
      (iii) Consequences of increased pain for activity and medication intake: are these consequence pain-contingent?
   b. Behaviour patterns in the home
      (i) Ability to do self-care, household and social activities
      (ii) Ability to fulfil responsibilities in the family
      (iii) Response of spouse and family members to pain and well behaviours
   c. Behaviour patterns at work
      (i) Current work status – pattern of activity over the day
      (ii) Future vocational options – for patients who are not working, explore educational level and interest in possible retraining or work options
      (iii) Incentives and disincentives for work – financial consequences of continued pain, disability support payments and financial compensation for work injury, pending litigation
   d. Pain behaviour observations
      (i) Observations of nonverbal and verbal pain behaviours during the interview and during simple activities (e.g. walking into the interview, getting up and down out of the chair)
      (ii) Observable indicators of pain status (e.g. use of a cane, wheelchair, brace, transcutaneous neural stimulator)
3. Cognitive and affective responses to pain
   a. Cognitive distortions and deficits
      (i) Negative cognitions regarding self, future, and others
      (ii) Misconceptions about the nature of pain and likely future trajectory of pain
      (iii) Problems with memory and concentration
   b. Affective disturbance
      (i) Symptoms of anxiety
      (ii) Symptoms of depression
      (iii) Relation of affective responses to pain behaviours
4. Psychophysiologic responses to pain
   a. Muscular tension responses
      (i) Effects of increased tension
      (ii) Effects of relaxation
      (iii) Muscle weakness secondary to deactivation
   b. Autonomic responses
      (i) Changes in heart rate, blood pressure, gastrointestinal symptoms
5. Self-control efforts
   a. Behavioural-coping methods
   b. Cognitive-coping methods
   c. Perceived self-control over pain
6. Basic information about behavioural treatment
   a. Treatment goals
   b. Involvement of patient and family in assessment and treatment efforts

* Based on Keefe (1988)

and most widely used daily-diary methods. This diary consists of a standard data sheet with columns for making hourly entries of the amount of time spent in three categories:

1. reclining
2. standing or walking
3. sitting

The patient is asked to fill in the diary on a daily basis for several weeks prior to treatment and then throughout the course of behavioural treatment. The data gathered are summarised on simple graphs. Activity diaries are useful in:

1. establishing baseline levels of the amount of time spent up and out of the reclining position
2. identifying problematic behaviour patterns such as the tendency to persist with activities for long periods of time followed by prolonged periods of reclining
3. documenting improvements in activity level that occur during treatment.

Fordyce (1976) recommends having the patient's spouse keep a daily diary to record the patient's activity level. Periodic recordings are especially helpful in increasing the spouse's awareness of improvements in activity level that occur with treatment. These recordings also can be used to verify the patient's own record.

Behaviour therapists often modify the Fordyce diary by including columns for recording medication intake and pain level (on a 0–10 scale). The additional information can be quite useful in determining whether increased pain leads to potentially reinforcing consequences such as rest and pain medications.

Follick et al (1984) developed and refined a comprehensive daily diary for the behavioural assessment of chronic pain. Their diary gathered information on position (e.g. sitting, reclining), time spent alone or with others, medication intake, pain, mood, tension and use of various pain-control methods (e.g. hot pack or a heating pad). Patients were systematically trained in the use of the diary and then asked to make diary entries three times daily. These diary records appeared to yield highly reliable data. Follick et al for example, found that diary measures of activity and pain tended to be consistent across days. They also reported a high level of agreement between patients' and spouses' records of activity level and medication intake. The validity of the diary was supported by the finding that patient records of time spent up and out of the reclining position correlated highly with data gathered using an automated activity monitor.

In the past five years, there have been a number of advances in daily-diary methodologies (Stone et al 1991). Behavioural researchers have begun to use sophisticated and powerful data analytic techniques that enable one to study individual differences in day-to-day reports. Affleck et al (1991) recently applied these newly developed methods to the analysis of daily-diary records of pain ratings. They asked 47 rheumatoid arthritis patients to provide daily reports of their level of joint pain over the course of 75 days. To ensure that the diary data were accurate and timely, all patients were trained in a common approach to daily recording and called by phone periodically to address any questions or difficulties they might be having. Patients complied well with the requirement that they complete and mail in the records daily. Full data were available for over 90% of the recording days. To characterise each patient's pattern of pain, sophisticated time-series regression analyses were carried out. The data analyses revealed that patients with high levels of arthritis disease rated their daily pain as more intense and more predictable from day to day. These patients also had fewer episodes of atypically severe pain than patients with less active disease. Patients who were more depressed also reported more intense daily pain over the duration of the study period.

Diary methods have long been used in the clinical assessment of pain behaviour. These methods are inexpensive and can provide high-quality data. With the development of new methods for analysing data from such diary records, new insights into how pain behaviours relate to important environmental and organismic variables may be obtained.

ELECTROMECHANICAL RECORDING DEVICES

Electromechanical recording devices can automate the process of behavioural recording and reduce demands on the patient, spouse or therapist. In the assessment of chronic-pain patients, these devices have mainly been used to assess activity level. Cairns et al (1976), for example, devised an 'uptime clock' that automatically measures the amount of time chronic-pain patients spend out of bed. Pedometers have also been used to gather data from patients involved in walking programmes (Saunders et al 1978). Both Follick et al (1985) and Sanders (1983a) have described how one can use a modified calculator timer and mercury-activated microswitch to record standing and walking time in back-pain patients.

Although electromechanical devices can provide objective data, their applicability to chronic-pain patients is sometimes questionable. For example, we evaluated an actometer, a self-winding watch modified to record movement (Morrell & Keefe 1988). The actometer has been shown to provide reliable measures of activity level in patients with depression. However, we found that its utility with chronic-pain patients was limited. Variations in movement patterns, such as greater limping while walking one day versus another, significantly reduced the reliability of the device.

Electromechanical devices are somewhat expensive and not always readily available. In general, the use of these devices has been limited to research applications.

BEHAVIOURAL OBSERVATION

Direct observation is one of the most basic and objective methods for assessing pain behaviour (Keefe 1989). Observations of pain and well behaviours can be carried out in naturalistic treatment settings. For example, Cinciripini & Floreen (1982) used a time-sampling method to record behaviours exhibited by inpatients treated on a behavioural pain-management unit. A trained staff member watched each patient on the unit for 5 minutes every half hour and recorded both pain behaviours (verbal and nonverbal pain behaviours) and well behaviours (talking about healthy topics, engaging in assertive behaviour). Over the course of treatment, patients showed a highly significant increase in the percentage of time they spent engaging in well behaviours, and a decrease in the percentage of time spent engaging in pain behaviours.

Behavioural observations can also be conducted in standardised situations designed to elicit pain behaviour. In the early 1980s we developed a behaviour-sampling approach for recording pain behaviours in chronic low-back pain patients (Keefe & Block 1982). This method involves having patients sit, stand, walk, and recline for 1–2 minute periods. The patient is videotaped as he or she completes the activities and the videotaped record is subsequently scored by a trained observer. The observer notes the occurrence of five pain behaviour coding categories:

1. guarding – stiff and interrupted movement patterns
2. bracing – pain avoidant static posturing
3. rubbing – touching or holding of the painful area
4. sighing – a pronounced exhalation of air
5. grimacing – a facial expression of pain.

A series of studies (Keefe & Block 1982) was conducted to evaluate the reliability and validity of this observation method. These studies revealed that behaviours could be coded reliably; interobserver agreement ranged from 93–99%. The observation method was also sensitive enough to detect reductions in pain behaviour occurring over the course of treatment. The construct validity of the observation method was supported by the finding that the level of recorded pain behaviours correlated highly with the patients' own ratings of pain. The method also appeared to possess discriminant validity; pain behaviour levels were substantially higher in low-back-pain patients than in painfree normal and depressed control subjects.

The observation method we developed for recording pain behaviour in low-back-pain patients has now been extended to a variety of other chronic-pain conditions. The validity of this method has been supported by research studies of patients having pain due to rheumatoid arthritis (Anderson et al 1987), cancer (Ahles et al 1990) and osteoarthritis (Keefe et al 1987).

Observational methods provide objective and useful data on pain behaviour. The major limitation of these methods is the expense entailed in training observers to gather and code behavioural data. Simplified observation methods that rely on brief behaviour samples and more practical coding methods such as rating scales are being developed and evaluated (Keefe 1989). Until these more practical methods are validated, standardised observation methods are likely to be confined primarily to research studies.

BEHAVIOURAL THERAPY TECHNIQUES

Although a wide variety of behavioural therapy techniques are used in the management of chronic pain, there are four techniques that make up the core elements of most treatment programmes: graded activation programmes, social reinforcement, time-contingent medications and training in self-control techniques. The rationale, treatment methods, and empirical findings supporting the application of each of these techniques will be presented.

GRADED ACTIVATION AND EXERCISE PROGRAMMES

Rationale

Inactivity is one of the major behavioural problems exhibited by patients having chronic pain. Many chronic patients develop an overly sedentary lifestyle in which they may spend all but 4–6 hours of their day reclining. Such inactivity has many negative consequences. The behavioural consequences of inactivity include an increased dependence on family members, a reduction in the level of pleasant events and decreased tolerance for exercise or simple daily activities. The physiological consequences of inactivity include deconditioning, increased tension and sleep difficulties. The cognitive–affective consequences of an inactive lifestyle include a narrowing of distractions from pain, fear of activity and depression.

Pain patients' efforts to increase their activity often end in increased pain and pain behaviour. One of the major reasons for this is that patients tend to work on activities or exercise until they reach the point that they have so much pain or are so tired that they have to stop and rest. Activation programmes are designed to break this tendency by having patients work to a set activity or exercise quota and then rest.

Treatment methods

Behavioural programmes for graded activation or exercise include several basic elements. First, diary records or physical evaluation data are used to establish a pretreatment baseline level of activity and exercise tolerance. Second, a rationale for graded activation is provided to the patient and agreement reached on the methods and goals of the programme. Third, the activation and exercise programme is begun with the initial goals for activity set well below the patient's activity or exercise tolerance. Finally, the goals for activity or exercise are gradually increased over a period of days and weeks.

To illustrate a typical activation programme, consider the behavioural treatment programme we instituted with Mr B, a 50-year-old chronic low-back-pain patient admitted to our inpatient pain unit. This male patient reported that he usually got out of bed each day for only short periods of time. To establish an initial baseline record of activity, he was instructed to keep a daily activity diary (Fordyce 1976) in which he made hourly entries of his 'uptime' (e.g. time up and out of the reclining position). A review of the diary records gathered during the first 3 days of admission revealed that he spent only 30–40 minutes out of bed at a time and then would rest for 1–2 hours. His total uptime over the entire day was low–varying from 4–6 hours. When asked about his activity the patient reported that his strategy was to let pain be his guide in determining when he should recline. If the pain was mild or moderate, he would persist with his activity, when the pain became extreme he would recline.

To provide a rationale for graded activation, the concept of a pain cycle was discussed with Mr B. The cycle, evident in Mr B's baseline records, consisted of continuing with activity to the point of extreme pain followed by prolonged rest. Mr B admitted that this cyclic pattern was habitual. The negative consequences of the cycle were reviewed and contrasted with the benefits that would occur if Mr B learned to pace and then increase his activities. A systematic approach to activation, labelled the activity–rest cycle was then introduced. The basic notion of the activity–rest cycle was that Mr B would engage in a moderate level of activity and then take a limited rest break. The level of activity and rest would be specified with the goal of gradually increasing the amount of activity and decreasing the amount of rest.

Mr B agreed to the activation programme and initial goals for activity were established. The activity goal, based on his baseline record of 4–6 hours of uptime, was to spend 20 minutes each hour up and out of the reclining position. Mr B was quite successful in meeting the initial activity goal and reported, after 2 days of the programme, that he had less pain than he had anticipated. He felt he could be even much more active and wanted to set a goal of 45 minutes per hour. Given his baseline records and long history of bed rest, it was felt that a goal of 30 minutes of uptime per hour was more realistic. He met this goal for the next 3 days and the activity goal was then increased to 40 minutes. The programme continued with incremental increases in daily activity goals. Mr B gradually progressed with activation so that by the end of his 3-week admission he was spending 60 minutes up and out the reclining position and resting for 10 minutes. When he returned for follow-up as an outpatient 2 months after discharge, Mr B was on a schedule of 90 minutes of activity followed by a 5-minute rest.

Empirical findings

Some of the earliest case reports of behaviour therapy for chronic pain described the effects of treatment on activity level and exercise tolerance. Progress in many cases was dramatic. Fordyce et al (1968) used a graded activation programme to increase walking tolerance in a 37-year-old woman having an 18-year history of chronic back pain and four major back operations. Over the course of inpatient treatment, the patient showed a 150% increase in walking from her initial baseline. She was able to maintain her gains in activity over a 23-week outpatient follow-up period.

The positive results of early case reports on graded activation and exercise are generally consistent with findings of later studies of groups of chronic-pain patients. For example, Fordyce et al (1973) presented outcome data gathered from a group of 36 chronic-pain patients who had participated in a behavioural treatment programme (Fordyce et al 1973). Major, statistically significant increases in activity level and exercise tolerance were reported. As a group, the patients increased their tolerance for walking, situps and time spent weaving by over 100%. Their daily uptime increased from 8.4 hours per 24 hours pretreatment to 12.7 hours per 24 hours posttreatment.

One limitation of the early research on graded activation is that this treatment technique was combined with other behavioural-treatment interventions in such a way that the relative contribution of activation to treatment outcome could not be examined. Lindstrom et al (1992) recently conducted one of the first controlled evaluations of a behavioural activation programme. A sample of 103 patients having low-back pain were randomly assigned to a graded activity programme or a routine medical care control condition. The activation programme, conducted by a physical therapist, was based on an operant model in which patients were given exercise goals that were initially set at submaximal levels and then gradually increased. Results indicated that the activation programme returned patients to work much more quickly than the routine medical care. The activation programme also resulted in significant increases in mobility, strength, and fitness.

Turner et al (1990) recently compared behavioural therapy without exercise to a graded aerobic exercise programme alone. Ninety-six chronic low-back-pain patients were randomly assigned to one of four conditions:

1. graded aerobic exercise only in which patients engaged in a walking or jogging programme based on a behavioural activation plan
2. behavioural therapy without exercise in which patients and spouses were trained in methods for socially reinforcing well behaviours and reducing reinforcement for pain behaviours
3. behavioural therapy plus graded exercise in which patients received both the behavioural intervention and graded exercise
4. a waiting-list control group.

A comprehensive set of self-report, direct observation measures and spouse's ratings was administered pretreatment, posttreatment and at 6 – and 12–month follow-ups. At the posttreatment evaluation, patients in the combined behaviour therapy and graded exercise condition showed significantly greater improvement in pain and pain behaviour than patients in the other conditions. At the follow-up evaluations, however, all three treatment groups showed similar significant improvements from their pretreatment baseline levels of pain and pain behaviour. Taken together, these findings indicate that graded exercise makes a significant contribution to the short-term positive effects of behavioural therapy for chronic pain.

SOCIAL REINFORCEMENT

Rationale

One hallmark of the behavioural approach to pain is its emphasis on the importance of the social consequences of overt pain behaviour patterns. The ways that people respond to pain behaviour can play an important role in the development and maintenance of maladaptive behaviour patterns. Positive social reinforcement in the form of attention from a solicitous spouse or family members is particularly important in reinforcing pain behaviour. At the same time that pain behaviours are being positively reinforced, the patient's efforts to engage in healthier, well behaviours may result in negative consequences. A patient may be criticised by his or her boss for trying to take on new work responsibilities despite persistent pain. This punishing consequence is likely to decrease the likelihood that he or she will take on such responsibilities in the future. Alternatively, the patient's efforts to spend more time out of bed may be ignored by family or coworkers. In some patients, the lack of meaningful social consequences may lead to extinction of important well behaviours.

Treatment methods

The major goal of social reinforcement techniques is to alter systematically the social environment so as to reward well behaviours and minimise reinforcement for pain behaviours. This goal is most easily achieved when the patient is removed from a home environment that may be reinforcing pain behaviour and admitted to an inpatient hospital setting where the social environment can be controlled and monitored. On behaviourally oriented inpatient pain units, staff members are trained to praise well behaviours and ignore or minimise the amount of attention given to pain behaviours. Immediate and dramatic reductions in pain behaviour sometimes occur when patients are admitted to behavioural pain units. This rapid change in behaviour underscores the powerful influence the home environment can have in maintaining excessively high levels of maladaptive pain behaviour. In most cases, however, changes in pain behaviour are less dramatic and staff members must use shaping principles to reward successive approximations of a full range of well behaviours.

To effectively utilise social reinforcement in the outpatient setting, one must involve the spouse and family members who have the most contact with the patient. These individuals must be educated about the rationale for social reinforcement, trained to recognise pain and well behaviour, and instructed in basic principles of reinforcement. Their perfomance also needs to be monitored and reinforced closely over time. In the absence of ongoing involvement in treatment, the tendency for spouse and family is to revert to old, maladaptive patterns of responding to pain and well behaviour.

Empirical findings

A number of research studies have examined the effects of social reinforcement on pain and pain behaviour. One of the most interesting studies (White & Sanders 1986) compared the effects of social reinforcement of discussions of pain versus well topics on subsequent ratings of pain. Each patient in this study was visited for two 5-minute periods daily and encouraged to talk about their status. During one 5-minute period, the patient was reinforced with head nods and verbal statements for talking about pain-related topics. During the other 5-minute period, reinforcement was given for talking about well topics. After each 5-minute conversation, patients rated their pain on a 0–5 scale. Figure 76.4 displays data obtained from the four chronic-pain patients who participated in this study. As can be seen, patients consistently rated their pain as more severe after being reinforced for talking about pain topics than after being reinforced for talking about well topics. What makes these findings noteworthy is the fact that they were evident after only 5 minutes of discussion. Lengthy discussions of pain-related topics presumably could have even more pronounced effects on pain report.

Patients involved in pain treatment are often provided with encouragement to exercise and to be more active. Does the way that encouragement is provided make a difference? Behavioural theory would suggest that providing patients with social encouragement and support contingent on their exercise performance is likely to be much more effective than providing social reinforcement in a noncontingent fashion. Cairns & Pasino (1977) tested the effects of contingent and noncontingent social reinforcement on walking, bicycling and uptime in chronic low-back patients. They found that noncontingent social reinforcement and the public posting of exercise/activity graphs had no effect on performance. However, when social reinforcement was given to patients during and after they engaged in exercise or activity, significant increases in performance were obtained.

When social reinforcement is used in pain management, it is typically combined with other treatment components,

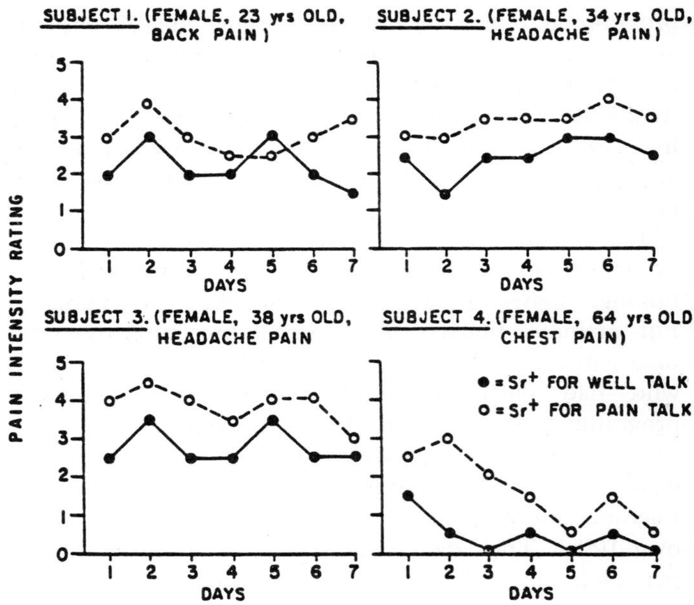

Fig. 76.4 Pain ratings under conditions of reinforcement for well talk versus reinforcement for pain talk. (Reprinted from Journal of Behavior Therapy and Experimental Psychiatry, Volume 17, p 155–159, 1985, with permission from Pergamon Press Ltd, Headington Hill Hall, Oxford OX3 0BW, UK.)

making it difficult to identify the unique effects of social reinforcement. Sanders (1983b) addressed this problem in a study in which social reinforcement was systematically compared to relaxation training, cognitive–behaviour analysis and assertiveness training. Subjects in this study were four patients suffering from chronic low-back pain. A multiple baseline design was used in which each intervention was introduced sequentially to each patient and the concomitant effects on pain and activity noted. The results revealed that social reinforcement consistently led to reductions in pain and increase in activity. The effects of social reinforcement were similar to those obtained with relaxation training and both of these interventions were more effective than cognitive–behaviour analysis and assertiveness training.

TIME-CONTINGENT MEDICATIONS

Rationale

Chronic-pain patients often take their pain medications on an as needed or PRN (pro re nata) basis. For patients having persistent pain, analgesic and narcotic medications can be potent reinforcers because they reduce pain and associated emotional distress. The delivery of medication at a time of severe pain can positively reinforce high levels of pain behaviour (Fordyce 1976). One result of this reinforcement is a vicious cycle in which increased drug use leads to increased pain behaviour, which in turn leads to increased medication intake (Berntzen & Gotestam 1987).

To break the association between pain behaviour and

medication intake, most behavioural treatment programmes use a time-contingent medication scheduling. In time-contingent medication scheduling, all pain medications are given on a fixed-interval rather than PRN basis. Thus, patients are required to take their medications at specific time periods in the day (e.g. every 6 hours). Over the course of treatment, the amount of active medication taken is gradually reduced to a zero level.

Time-contingent medication schedules effectively break the relationship between pain complaints and medication delivery. Patients on these schedules are required to take their medication at fixed times of the day regardless of whether their pain level is high or low. One pharmacologic advantage of this type of medication scheduling is that it provides an excellent means for keeping the blood level of a pain medication at a steady level. As a result, patients often report that their medications are more effective and thus they often are more compliant with efforts to taper their medication intake.

Treatment methods

The first step in implementing time-contingent medication scheduling is to obtain an estimate of the patient's pretreatment pain medication intake. In inpatient treatment settings, a baseline level of medication can be obtained by placing patients on a PRN medication schedule for the first 3–5 days. The timing and amount of medication taken can be recorded and the patient can then be carefully observed for any signs of withdrawal. Another way to establish baseline medication intake is to have patients keep diary records of their medication usage. The need for accurate reporting of medication use should be stressed (Berntzen & Gotestam 1987) since patients taking high levels of narcotics may minimise their intake.

Before implementing a time-contingent medication programme, patients need to be provided with a rationale. Most patients are reluctant to be placed on time-contingent medications, fearing that these medications will be ineffective. However, when presented with the concept of a vicious cycle with increased pain leading to increased pain-medication intake and then back to increased pain, most patients agree to a trial of time-contingent scheduling. Once time-contingent scheduling is implemented and patients notice the improvements in the levels of pain that occur, resistance to this treatment typically subsides.

To start a time-contingent medication programme, the average daily baseline intake of pain medication is typically divided into equal amounts to be delivered at regular intervals (e.g. every 6 hours) per 24 hours. In some behavioural treatment programmes, all oral pain medications are administered in tablet form at regular time intervals over a 24 hour period. In other programmes, the pain medications are converted to a miligram equivalent dose of methadone, which is then taken at fixed intervals. Often a liquid vehicle (e.g. cherry syrup or orange juice) is used to deliver the medication. This 'pain cocktail' is designed to mask the precise amount of medication so that day-to-day reductions in the dose level can be achieved without patient awareness.

The ultimate goal of time-contingent medications is to reduce the intake of medications to a zero level. To achieve this goal, the amount of pain medication is gradually reduced over a period of days or weeks. At the end of treatment, patients may simply be taking a liquid 'pain cocktail' that contains no analgesic or narcotic medications. Interestingly, we have found that at the time of discharge from the programme some patients ask for prescriptions of the cherry-syrup vehicle used to deliver the 'cocktail' even though they realise it contains no active medication.

Empirical findings

Two studies have provided support for the effectiveness of time-contingent medications in the management of pain. The first study by White & Sanders (1985) was carried out in the context of a behaviourally oriented inpatient treatment programme. In this study, eight chronic-pain patients were randomly assigned to either: (1) time-contingent medication in which they received equal doses of methadone every 6 hours with the amount per dosage gradually decreased over 5 days or (2) PRN medication in which they received four equal doses of daily methadone on an as-needed basis with the level of methadone gradually decreased over 5 days. Throughout the study, all other medications and treatments were held constant. Data analysis revealed that patients in the time-contingent condition reported significantly lower levels of pain both during and after the detoxification programme than patients in the PRN group. The patients on time-contingent medications also reported better mood that patients in the PRN group.

Berntzen & Gotestam (1987) tested the effects of time-contingent medications in a sample comprised mainly of outpatients (8 of 10 patients) having chronic pain. This study used a within-subject design in which each subject received 1 week of medications on a time-contingent basis and 1 week of medications on a PRN basis. The sequence of treatment conditions was randomised across subjects. Throughout the study, patients provided daily ratings of pain and mood level. The results indicated that pain ratings decreased significantly during time-contingent scheduling and increased during the PRN medication scheduling. Mood level also was significantly higher during the time-contingent medication regime than during the PRN medication scheduling.

SELF-CONTROL SKILLS

Rationale

When behaviour therapy is carried out in an institutional setting, the environment is carefully structured to provide opportunities for activation, reinforce well behaviours and minimise the association between pain complaints and medication delivery. However, the home and work environments that patients will return to are not so structured or regulated. If chronic-pain patients are to maintain the gains achieved in structured settings, they need to learn skills for managing their own behaviour. For this reason, training in self-control skills is viewed as essential to the generalisation of treatment effects.

Treatment techniques

Although behaviour-therapy programmes provide training in a wide variety of self-control skills, virtually all programmes emphasise three basic skills: self-monitoring, self-reinforcement and relaxation training.

Self-monitoring

In self-monitoring, patients are taught how to record important target behaviours (e.g. uptime, exercise, medication intake). Self-monitoring not only provides important information about pain and well behaviours, it can also serve to break up patterns of maladaptive pain behaviour (Kanfer & Schefft 1988). For example, a patient who keeps a record of his or her pain medication intake may become more aware of early signals of over-reliance on sedative-hypnotic drugs and decide to avoid or limit use of this medication.

Self-monitoring involves several steps. First, the behaviour to be observed is defined. The definition must specify what behaviour needs to occur (e.g. uptime consists of spending time up and out of the reclining position) and what will be recorded (e.g. the duration of uptime). Second, the method for recording needs to be specified. This might consist of a standardised data sheet (e.g. the Fordyce activity diary), an individually tailored data form or a device such as a wrist counter or tape recorder. The method chosen must be simple enough that it does not burden the patient. It should also permit the patient to record behaviour soon after it occurs. Finally, the data obtained through self-monitoring need to be periodically reviewed by the patient. In many behavioural programmes, patients graph their own data on uptime and exercise. Many patients report that a daily review of the graph helps them see their own progress and recognise early warning signs of setbacks.

Self-reinforcement

Self-reinforcement is designed to teach chronic-pain patients to reward themselves for engaging in well behaviours (e.g. exercise, socialising, returning to work). To identify rewards for use in self-reinforcement, patients are often asked to complete an inventory of pleasurable events or activities such as the pleasant events schedule (MacPhillamy & Lewinsohn 1971). They are then given basic information about reinforcement: for example, the need to deliver rewards in a contingent fashion, importance of schedules of reinforcement and the need to avoid reinforcement for maladaptive pain behaviours. Training in self-reinforcement emphasises the use of naturally occurring rewards. A patient who has increased his tolerance for walking, for example, might reward himself by walking through his favourite park.

Relaxation training

Relaxation training teaches patients to recognise and reduce excessive muscle tension that may be contributing to pain behaviour. Numerous methods can be used to teach patients to relax. Behaviour therapists typically use a modified version of Jacobson's progressive relaxation training. Progressive relaxation training involves a series of exercises in which the patient tenses and then slowly relaxes major muscle groups. The sequence of exercises progresses from the muscles of the legs and arms to muscles of the trunk and finally to muscles of the face, scalp and neck. Patients may be given a 20–30-minute audiotape that guides them through each of the exercises. To help patients generalise their skills to daily situations, they are instructed in methods for practising relaxation for brief periods (e.g. 20 seconds to 1 minute). The advantage of these brief relaxation procedures is that they can be used to keep tension at a low level during daily activities that tend to increase pain.

Empirical findings

Two recent studies have evaluated the effectiveness of training in behavioural self-control techniques for outpatients having persistent pain. In a study of chronic low-back pain patients, Kerns et al (1986) compared a behavioural programme that featured training in self-control skills with a cognitive intervention that emphasised cognitive pain-coping skills. Both treatments significantly reduced health-care use when compared with a waiting-list control condition. Nicholas et al (1991) conducted a similar study and found that training in behavioural self-control techniques produced greater initial improvements in functional impairment than cognitive treatment. Although patients in both groups were unable to maintain initial treatment gains, the very small number of patients available at follow-up may have precluded an adequate test of the long-term effects of these interventions.

ISSUES IN THE BEHAVIOURAL TREATMENT OF CHRONIC PAIN

There are a number of issues that need to be addressed in applying behavioural treatment methods with chronic-pain patients. One key issue is that changes in behaviour may not result in changes in the report of pain. Reviews of the research literature indicate that behavioural therapy is generally quite effective in increasing activity level and exercise tolerance and decreasing pain medication intake (Keefe et al 1986). The effects of behavioural therapy on pain, however, are usually more modest. Patients may report substantial initial reductions in pain, but may maintain only about 20–30% reductions in pain over long-term periods.

The inability of behaviour therapy to produce large, sustained reductions in pain report raises several interesting points. First, the magnitude of the changes in pain need to be considered in context. Patients referred for behavioural therapy usually have a long history of failure to respond to treatment. Their modest improvements in pain, therefore, need to be balanced against the typically large and significant improvements they are able to achieve in activity and medication intake. Second, chronic-pain patients entering behavioural therapy should be given an accurate description of what they might expect to gain from treatment. Specifically, they should be informed that the treatment may have its strongest impact on behaviour rather than on pain perception. Patients can then make a more informed decision about starting treatment. Many behavioural programmes formalise the process of obtaining informed consent by using a behavioural contract (Sternbach, 1974). The contract specifies patient and therapist responsibilities, the treatment techniques to be used and the likely outcomes.

A second important issue is the selection of patients for behavioural treatment. In his writings, Fordyce (1976) underscored the utility of behavioural methods for patients having an operantly based pain problem. The question arises: should behavioural treatment be restricted to operant pain? One can certainly think of situations in which behavioural methods can be used inappropriately to treat non-operantly based pain problems. For example, socially reinforcing a rheumatoid arthritis patient for progressively higher levels of activity during a period of high-disease activity is not likely to be very helpful. Nevertheless, behavioural factors appear to influence the behaviour of many chronic-pain patients, even those who have a clear organic basis for their pain complaints. The fact that a cancer patient, for example, has multiple influences affecting his or her pain, does not mean that behavioural interventions may not help reduce pain and improve functional status.

A third important issue relates to the involvement of spouses in behavioural treatment. Continuing and integral involvement of the spouse is considered to be important for the maintenance of behavioural treatment effects (Moore & Chaney 1985). Behavioural spouse training can teach the spouse how to prompt and reinforce well behaviours. It can also help prevent the spouse from unwittingly interfering with treatment goals by taking over tasks, enforcing inactivity or rest or limiting social activities. Spouse training can lead to a greater understanding of the role that behavioural methods can play in reducing pain behaviour and disability and give patient and spouse some appropriate, common activity goals to work on. Involving the spouse in treatment can also increase the spouse's confidence in the patient's capabilities.

Spouse involvement is accepted as essential in many behavioural treatment programmes. In fact, some programmes refuse to accept patients if their spouses are unwilling to participate in treatment. The literature on spouse training in behavioural pain management, however is quite limited. Only one behavioural study has directly tested the effects of involving spouses in pain management interventions (Moore & Chaney 1985). This study found no added benefits from involving spouses in behavioural treatment, but lacked sufficient power to detect differences because of small sample size (n= 11–12 patients per condition). Thus, although spouse involvement is potentially quite useful in enhancing patients response to behavioural therapy, more research is needed to evaluate the effects of spouse training.

Another key issue in the behavioural management of pain is the timing of treatment. Behavioural techniques are often used as a last resort in the management of persistent pain. Behavioural theorists, however, would predict that early intervention may be more effective. Recent studies have examined the utility of behavioural intervention in preventing pain-related disability. Fordyce et al (1986), for example, compared the efficacy of behavioural treatment and traditional medical treatment for acute back pain. Subjects were randomly assigned to one of two treatments: (1) traditional medical management in which medications, exercise, activation and return visits were all scheduled on an as needed basis or (2) behavioural treatment in which the same treatments were administered on a time-contingent basis. No differences in outcome were apparent after 6 weeks of treatment. However, at a 1-year follow-up the patients who had been treated on the behavioural protocol had returned to preinjury levels of functioning, whereas patients receiving the traditional medical treatment had significant increases in pain-related impairment. These results suggest that early, behaviourally-based intervention may be an effective in preventing the development of pain behaviour patterns.

CONCLUSION

Behaviour therapy approaches to chronic pain have advanced considerably over the past 20 years. Practitioners now have a wide variety of behavioural assessment and treatment procedures to choose from. The foundations of the behavioural approach are now more thoroughly grounded in empirical research. With the recent increase in research on behavioural methods of pain management, further advances in our ability to assess and treat the behavioural problems experienced by patients having persistent pain are likely to occur.

REFERENCES

Affleck G, Tennen H, Urrows S, Higgins P 1991 Individual differences in the day-to-day experience of chronic pain: a prospective daily study of rheumatoid arthritis patients. Health Psychology 10: 419–426

Ahles T A, Coombs D W, Jensen L, Stukel T, Maurer L H, Keefe F J 1990 Development of a behavior observation technique for the assessment of pain behaviors in cancer patients. Behavior Therapy 21: 449–460

Anderson K O, Bradley L A, McDaniel L K et al 1987 The assessment of pain in rheumatoid arthritis: validity of a behavioral observation method. Arthritis and Rheumatism 30: 36–43

Berntzen D, Gotestam K G 1987 Effects of on-demand versus fixed interval schedules in the treatment of chronic pain with analgesic compounds. Journal of Consulting and Clinical Psychology 55: 213–217

Cairns D, Pasino J 1977 Comparison of verbal reinforcement and feedback in the operant treatment of disability due to chronic low back pain. Behavior Therapy 8: 621–630

Cairns D, Thomas L, Mooney V, Pace J B 1976 A comprehensive treatment approach to chronic low back pain. Pain 2: 301–308

Catania C A 1984 Learning, 2nd edn. Prentice-Hall, New Jersey

Cinciripini P M, Floreen A 1982 An evaluation of a behavioral program for chronic pain. Journal of Behavioral Medicine 5: 375–389

Follick M J, Ahern D K, Laser-Wolston N 1984 Evaluation of a daily activity diary for chronic pain patients. Pain 19: 373–382

Follick M J, Ahern D K, Laser-Wolston N, Adams A E, Molloy A J 1985 An electromechanical recording device for the measurement of 'uptime' or 'downtime' in chronic pain patients. Archives of Physical Medicine and Rehabilitation 66: 75–79

Fordyce W E 1976 Behavioral methods for chronic pain and illness. C V Mosby, Saint Louis

Fordyce W E, Fowler R S, Lehmann J F, DeLateur B J 1968 Some implications of learning in problems of chronic pain. Journal of Chronic Diseases 21: 179–190

Fordyce W E, Fowler R S, Lehmann J R, DeLateur B J, Sand P L, Trieschmann R B 1973 Operant conditioning in the treatment of chronic pain. Archives of Physical Medicine and Rehabilitation 54: 399–408

Fordyce W E, Brockway J A, Bergman J A, Spengler D 1986 Acute back pain: a control-group comparison of behavioral versus traditional methods. Journal of Behavioral Medicine 9: 127–140

Hollandsworth J 1986 Physiology and behavior therapy. Plenum, New York

Kanfer F H 1970 Self-regulation: research, issues and speculations. In: Neuringer C, Michael L (eds) Behavior modification in clinical psychology. Appleton-Century-Crofts, New York

Kanfer F H, Schefft B K 1988 Guiding the process of therapeutic change. Research Press, Champaign, Illinois

Keefe F J 1988 Behavioral assessment methods for chronic pain. In: France R D, Krishnan K R R (eds) Chronic pain. American Psychiatric Association Press, Washington, DC. p 298–321

Keefe F J 1989 Behavioral measurement of pain. In: Chapman C R, Loeser J D (eds) Advances in pain measurement. Publishing House, p 405–424

Keefe F J, Block A R 1982 Development of an observation method for assessing pain behaviors in chronic low back pain patients. Behavior Therapy 13: 363–375

Keefe F J, Gil K M, Rose S C 1986 Behavioral approaches in the multidisciplinary management of chronic pain: programs and issues. Clinical Psychology Review 6: 87–113

Keefe F J, Caldwell D S, Queen K T et al 1987 Osteoarthritic knee pain: a behavioral analysis. Pain 28: 309–321

Kerns R D, Turk D C, Holzman A D, Rudy T E 1986 Comparison of cognitive–behavioral and behavioral approaches to the outpatient treatment of chronic pain. Clinical Journal of Pain 1: 195–203

Lindstrom I, Ohlund C, Eek C, Wallin L, Peterson L, Nachemson A 1992 Mobility, strength, and fitness after a graded activity program for patients with subacute low back pain: a randomized prospective clinical study with a behavioral therapy approach. Spine 17: 641–652

MacPhillamy D, Lewinsohn P M 1971 The pleasant events schedule. Unpublished manuscript. Eugene, Oregon, University of Oregon

Moore J E, Chaney E F 1985 Outpatient group treatment of chronic pain: effects of spouse involvement. Journal of Consulting and Clinical Psychology 53: 326–334

Morrell E M, Keefe F J 1988 The actometer: an evaluation of instrument applicability for chronic pain patients. Pain 32: 265–270

Nicholas M K, Wilson P H, Goyen J 1991 Comparison of operant-behavioral and cognitive–behavioral group treatment with and without relaxation training. Behavior Research and Therapy 29: 225–238

Sanders S H 1983a Toward a practical instrument system for automatic measurement of 'up-time' in chronic pain patients. Pain 15: 399–406

Sanders S H 1983b Component analysis of a behavioral treatment program for chronic low back pain. Behavior Therapy 14: 697–705

Saunders K J, Goldstein M K, Stein G H 1978 Automated measurement of patient activity on a hospital rehabilitation ward. Archives of Physical Medicine and Rehabilitation 59: 255–257

Schefft B K, Lehr B K 1985 A self-regulatory model of adjunctive behavior change. Behavior Modification 9: 458–476

Skinner B F 1938 The behavior of organisms. Appleton, New York

Skinner B F 1953 Science and human behavior. Macmillan, New York

Skinner B F 1958 Verbal behavior. Appleton, New York

Skinner B F 1959 Cumulative record. Appleton, New York

Skinner B F 1969 Contingencies of reinforcement: a theoretical analysis. Appleton-Century-Crofts, New York

Sternbach R A 1974 Pain patients: traits and treatment. Academic Press, New York

Sternbach R A 1989 Behavior therapy. In: Wall P D, Melzack R (eds) The textbook of pain, 2nd edn. Churchill Livingstone, Edinburgh, p 1015–1020

Stone A, Kessler R, Haythornthwaite J 1991 Measuring daily events and experiences: decisions for the researcher. Journal of Personality 59: 575–608

Thorndike E L 1913 The psychology of learning. Teachers College, New York

Turk D C, Rudy T E 1991 Neglected topics in the treatment of chronic pain – relapse compliance, and adherence enforcement. Pain 44: 5–28

Turk D C, Meichenbaum D, Genest M 1983 Pain and behavioral medicine. Guilford, New York

Turner J A, Clancy S 1988 A comparison of operant behavioral and cognitive behavioral group treatment for chronic low back pain. Journal of Consulting and Clinical Psychology 56: 261–266

Turner J A, Clancy S, McQuade K J, Cardenas D D 1990 Effectiveness of behavioral therapy for chronic low back pain: a component analysis. Journal of Consulting and Clinical Psychology 58: 573–579

Ullman L P, Krasner L 1969 A psychological approach to abnormal behavior. Prentice-Hall, Englewood Cliffs, New Jersey

White B, Sanders S H 1985 Differential effects on pain and mood in chronic pain patients with time versus pain-contingent medication delivery. Behavior Therapy 16: 28–38

White B, Sanders S H 1986 The influence of patients' pain intensity ratings of antecedent reinforcement of pain talk or well talk. Journal of Behavior Therapy and Experimental Psychiatry 17: 155–159

77. A collaborative model of care: patient, family and health professionals

K. M. Rowat, M. E. Jeans and S. M. LeFort

INTRODUCTION

The problem of chronic pain as a complex health and social concern has been well documented (Bonica 1978, 1980, 1984; Yelen et al 1980; Brena 1984; Institute of Medicine 1987). In response to this problem, diverse therapeutic approaches to specific aspects of chronic pain have emerged (Melzack & Wall 1988). Psychological approaches such as behaviour therapy, cognitive coping, group therapy and biofeedback have been utilised to deal with particular facets of the pain (Roberts & Reinhardt 1980; Kerns et al 1986; Miller 1990; Tunks et al 1990; Spinhoven & Linssen 1991; Nicholas et al 1992).

It is becoming increasingly evident, however, that many of these approaches address only part of the problem (Roy 1984). Chronic pain, like other chronic illnesses, must be viewed as a family problem (Rowat 1985a; Rowat & Knafl 1985; Turk & Kerns 1985; Turk et al 1987). Therefore the family, and not only the individual, becomes the unit of care for the health professional. A further feature of any chronic illness is that the patient and family need a general, long-term, supportive relationship within the health-care system (Turk & Kerns 1985). One of the characteristics of our current system of health care is that it is geared to short, intensive patient encounters. However, chronically ill patients, including those individuals with chronic pain, require longer encounters in which an effective dialogue can exist between the health professional and the patient (Aiken 1976).

Whether the chronic-pain patient is involved in various specialised treatments in separate facilities or is participating in a pain centre programme, one member of the health-care team (family physician, nurse or social worker) is likely to find him- or herself in the role of caregiver. Ideally this person should be the patient's case manager or coordinator who sees the patient and family on a frequent, regular basis in long-term care and follow-up.

The purpose of this chapter is to describe an approach to working with the chronic-pain patient and family within the context of a collaborative relationship. Its goals include the promotion of adaptation and improved quality of life, enhancement of pain control and facilitation of coping. This perspective is based on current research and several years of practice by the authors within a multidisciplinary pain centre. The chapter is organised so that the patient's needs are addressed first, followed by those of the family. It should be noted that there is frequent overlap between the patient and family in terms of their needs and problems. However, there also exist unique and individual issues which require distinct understanding as well as individualised interventions.

THE CHRONIC-PAIN PATIENT

One of the striking features of patients with chronic pain compared with people suffering other chronic-health problems such as diabetes or hypertension is that persons with chronic pain seldom know their diagnosis, let alone understand the nature of the problem. In most cases these patients have seen numerous different specialists throughout the course of their pain and undoubtedly have been offered a variety of possible explanatory or descriptive notions regarding their complaint. When asked what they have heard or what they believe they have been told, patients report a host of misconceptions. The majority report that at some time they have been told that nothing can be done for them and they must learn to live with the pain (Rowat 1983). Without adequate explanation of why 'nothing can be done', these patients continue their search for underlying mechanisms of explanation and a definitive treatment (Jeans et al 1979; Hilbert 1984).

The first encounter with the person suffering chronic pain reveals an individual who frequently mistrusts health professionals due to these past experiences, whose understanding of the pain may be limited, incorrect or confused and whose goal for the encounter may be at odds with the goal of the caregiver. It is at this point that the nonspecific, supportive process of working with the patient begins. The basic ingredients of this approach include support, knowledge and skills.

SUPPORT

Within the context of collaborating with the chronic-pain patient, support refers to the characteristics of the client–therapist relationship. Such a relationship provides a climate for working towards pain control, rehabilitation (which includes self-responsibilty) and an improved quality of life.

Establishing trust in the health team is a major goal. The patient's past experience has generally consisted of short-term involvement with health professionals with frequent disappointment, failure and a sense of abandonment (Rowat 1983). The patient has learned to be wary in case he or she and his or her problems are once again considered suspect and therefore rejected (Hilbert 1984).

At the outset, the role of the case manager should be explained to the patient and family with emphasis placed on the ongoing process of involvement. As Aiken (1976) has noted, one of the significant deterrents to responsive care for the chronically ill patient is lack of continuity. At the beginning of therapy, a contract can be established outlining the roles, responsibilities, accessibility and limitations of those involved in the relationship. An understanding of this assists the patient to develop trust and confidence, removing ambiguities that have existed previously with health professionals and thereby diminishing the person's somewhat desperate need to seek out new consultations. One of the important variables here appears to be the countinuing and regular visits scheduled with the patient. It provides the sense of continuity and security necessary for the work of rehabilition.

Another critical variable is that of the collaborative nature of the relationship. The patient becomes an active participant, taking responsibility for decisions and plans for intervention and change (Gottlieb & Rowat 1987; Davis 1992). This collaboration is much more than passive compliance and the cooperative provision of data from which plans are made. Rather, the patient participates in evaluating the data and making decisions about the treatment programme. The caregiver as well as the rest of the team support the patient in this role by providing honest, objective feedback, encouragement and positive reinforcement of independent and thoughtful behaviour. Chronic-pain patients, generally, are unfamiliar with this style of relationship, as they characteristically have assumed a dependent position, looking to the health professional to provide answers and solutions to the pain problem. Time and repeated help may be required for the client to assume this type of role.

Establishing goals is the first task of the collaborative work with the patient and may often be a part of the initial contract. Frequently the patient's goal is complete or permanent abolition of pain. Unfortunately this is not always possible and the alternative goal of pain control must be offered and examined in depth. Pain control is a broad concept and suggests numerous alternatives for achievement. Broadly speaking, it may mean reduced frequency and intensity of the pain with an increase in activity and an improved quality of life. The patient decides on his or her own goals in relation to pain control and an acceptable level of functioning. Once the overall goals are specified it is often useful to break these down into smaller units or subgoals. It is critical that these smaller subgoals be fairly easily achievable so that the patient does not experience failure once more.

Throughout the development and maintenance of the relationship with the patient, the caregiver acts as coordinator of the assessment and treatment programme designed for the individual. In this role an important aspect of the support is the provision of a forum for the examination of results and progress, emphasising positive gains and reinforcing the learning and changes in behaviour or symptoms achieved as a result of specific treatments. This feedback and assessment of change is conducted within the context of the goals established by the patient, family and team.

These goals, which from time to time may be evaluated and adjusted, serve as a focus for feedback and continued assessment of progress. In addition they serve as guideposts for the development of the knowledge and skills needed by the patient to engage in a meaningful way in the ongoing work of rehabilitation.

KNOWLEDGE

As stated earlier, chronic-pain patients often lack a diagnostic label and an explanation for their pain. This unknown or uncertain state usually leads to increased anxiety which in turn augments the perception of pain. It also motivates the patient to continue searching for answers and treatment.

The conceptual model of chronic pain used here is that chronic pain is a disease entity in itself and is not necessarily a symptom of some hypothetical pathology (Bonica 1973). Clarifying this understanding with the patient by providing him or her with information concerning the characteristics of chronic-pain syndromes and possible underlying mechanisms is basic to the development of a working relationship with the client.

Since people have different learning styles, this type of knowledge may need to be presented in diverse ways. Group programmes frequently incorporate knowledge of chronic pain as an important part of the overall agenda (Herman 1990; Pearce & Tunks 1990). The advantages of the group approach include the opportunity for discussion, questions and clarification as well as sharing of knowledge. Didactic lectures may also be used.

Reinforcement of this information and providing an opportunity for clarification of it may be a feature of the regular meetings that the patient has with the case manager or counsellor. Films and literature on chronic pain can also be made available to patients through a pain-centre library system. It should be noted here that there is a serious need for written material geared toward assisting patients in their understanding of chronic pain.

In addition to relevant knowledge about the mechanisms of chronic pain, patients also need a broad understanding of the numerous factors which may contribute to the modulation of pain. Identifying and understanding the complex interrelationships between these factors and the pain provides the patient with a rationale for participating in various physical and psychological treatment approaches to pain control. Such knowledge allows the patient to be a more effective collaborator and enables him or her to make intelligent choices and decisions about goals and treatment and to evaluate progress. Finally, the patient who understands the rationale for treatment is likely to be a more conscientious participant in the programme and to be more motivated to develop those skills necessary for adaptation and rehabilitation.

SKILLS

A number of treatment programmes for patients with chronic pain are directed toward the development of specific skills. These generally include skills in relaxation, cognitive coping, use of analgesics and so forth (Roberts & Reinhardt 1980; Herman & Baptiste 1990; Maruta et al 1990; Peters & Large 1990; Deardorff et al 1991). In working with chronic-pain patients over a number of years, three other skills have been identified as contributing to a higher level of functioning. These include communication skills and skills in self-observation and documentation. The identification of these skills and their development can begin from the first encounter with the patient and can continue throughout the client–therapist relationship.

Patients communicate about pain in diverse ways and to numerous people, including employers, families and health professionals. Frequently the style of the patient's communication stems from fear, misconceptions and feelings of desperation. Increasing the individual's knowledge about chronic pain may have a beneficial impact on his ability to communicate. However, additional work in this area may also be required. Knowing how, when and where to describe their pain to others is an important aspect of this learning. The more that the communication about the pain is relevant, productive and appropriate, the more likely it is that it will lead to positive outcomes for the patient. When communication skills are poor and the message is not clear or is irrelevant, decisions may be made by the receivers of this communication which may have devastating effects on the patient.

Helping the patient to develop skills in communicating about the pain can be aided by the use of such tools as the McGill Pain Questionnaire (Melzack 1975). Not only does this questionnaire help the patient to express his or her pain at the time of the interview but if used repeatedly it can influence the patient's style of describing pain.

Within the regular meetings with the patient, rehearsal techniques can also be utilised. That is, if the patient is scheduled to meet another health professional or an employer, for example, time can be devoted to practising what the patient wishes to communicate. This practice may also help the patient to feel more confident and influential in important decision-making situations. It can be useful to address the issue of communicating about pain on a regular basis. Patients often benefit from examininng their patterns of communication within the context of family and friends and as a result may gain important insight into the responses of significant others towards them and their pain.

Chronic-pain patients often appear unable observe their own behaviour and to link it to their pain (Taenzer 1981; Rowat 1983). It may be that the marked feelings of helplessness frequently noted in chronic-pain patients inhibit any attempt to search systematically for factors which may influence the pain. However, it is likely that knowledge of these relationships will increase the patient's sense of control over the pain and will subsequently diminish such feelings of helplessness.

Assisting the patient to develop self-observation skills may be achieved through the use of self-recording tools. The daily act of assessing and recording levels of physical and social activity, emotions and the pain itself serves to increase the patient's ability to observe and to derive meaning from what appeared previously to be random or unrelated events. Documentation can be of critical value for people with a chronic illness when, over time, facts and significant relationships tend to becomes less clearly remembered. This is an area where the patient's family can play an important role. They can also be assisted to observe and provide another perspective from which the patient may explore and verify his or her own observations.

THE FAMILY OF THE CHRONIC-PAIN PATIENT

Within the past decade, increased recognition has been given to the fact that a chronic illness may impinge not only on the life of the ill individual but also on the life of the whole family (Strauss 1984; Turk & Kerns 1985). It has been acknowledged that the major responsibility for the management of such chronic conditions rests with the individual and his family rather than with the health professional (Pratt 1973; Gerson & Strauss 1975; Strauss 1984). As noted above, chronic pain must be recognised as a disease state in its own right, sharing with other chronic illnesses many of the associated characteristics.

Only relatively recently has the family of the chronic-pain patient begun to receive some attention in the literature (Roy 1982, 1985). Nevertheless, the work to date has been limited and knowledge relating to the effects of the social and interpersonal context within which chronic pain occurs is at an early stage of development (Payne & Norfleet 1986; Flor et al 1987b; Turk et al 1987; Kerns et al 1991).

A popular framework within which the family of the chronic-pain patient has been considered is the operant-conditioning approach to chronic pain (Fordyce 1976). This perspective has generally implicated the family in terms of its role in predisposing, precipitating or perpetuating variables within the chronic-pain patient's experience (Fordyce 1978; Khatami & Rush 1978; Mohamed et al 1978; Hudgens 1979; Block et al 1980; Mohamed 1982; Romano et al 1991). Operating from this philosophy, the health professional's approach may be one of teaching family members to reinforce the client's healthy behaviours and to ignore behaviours associated with the sick role. Additional research based on the cognitive–behavioural and social-modelling perspective appears to support findings regarding reinforcement of pain behaviour by family members (Flor et al 1987a; 1989; Kerns et al 1990; Ehde et al 1991).

Although there is a heightened awareness of the importance of the family in the chronic-pain experience, the family is still considered primarily in terms of its influence on the individual in pain (Flor et al 1989). There is increasing support for an alternate perspective on the family of the chronic-pain patient as proposed in this chapter. This orientation is predicated on the belief that the entire family, not merely the individual designated as patient, faces the struggle of learning to live with the pain. While we do not dispute the likelihoood that family members may contribute to the pain experience in ways conceived as detrimental to the patient, the perspective taken here suggests that family members may also be attempting to deal with the pain and its effects on their lives. With this as the orientation, the family (not merely the individual in pain) becomes the unit of concern for the health professional.

Evidence is now accumulating which demonstrates the necessity of incorporating the spouse, if not all family members, into a programme of learning to live with the pain. Indeed, the health of spouses and children within chronic-pain families has been shown to be adversely affected by the experience (Block & Boyer 1984; Flor & Turk 1985; Rowat 1985b; Rowat & Knafl 1985; Turk et al 1985; Flor et al 1987c; Dura & Beck 1988; Romano et al 1989; Roy & Thomas 1989; Thomas & Roy 1989; Mikail & von Baeyer 1990; Schwartz et al 1991; Subramanian 1991; Benjamin et al 1992). The issue of control is as central to the family's experience with chronic pain as it is to the individual. Not only does the family feel impelled to control the pain, but it also faces the challenge of how best to minimise its effects on family life as a whole. When the family perceives its actions or approach as ineffectual and the pain is seen as the dominating force within family life, a sense of helplessness and distress emerges (Waring 1982; Rowat & Knafl 1985; Schwartz et al 1991). Consequently, the family also needs to have the opportunity:

1. to gain an understanding of the nature and treatment of chronic pain
2. to develop coping skills relative to pain and its effects on family life
3. to collaborate with the health professional.

UNDERSTANDING CHRONIC PAIN

One of the most critical aspects of a chronic illness is the defining process through which the individual and family must go (Stewart & Sullivan 1982). Schwenk & Hughes (1983) concluded that 'the way in which the family perceived the illness . . . was directly related to the eventual level of family stability and coping'.

For the chronic-pain family, this likewise appears to be crucial, both in terms of family adjustment (Block & Boyer 1984; Rowat & Knafl 1985; Flor et al 1987c) and treatment outcomes for the pain sufferer (Swanson & Maruta 1980; Waring 1982; Funch & Gale 1986). Chronic pain, however, presents some unique features which make the task of ascribing meaning much more difficult (Hilbert 1984). As was pointed out earlier, unlike many chronic illnesses in which a defined aetiology or pathology may be observed and confirmed, chronic pain frequently presents no such clear picture and the patient and family are left to deal with an amorphous, vague situation. The unique characteristics of chronic pain are found to be puzzling and distressing to family members. 'I've never heard of people having pain for which there's no apparent cure – people with pains that can't be explained', stated one spouse.

In the face of such uncertainty, family members also engage in the struggle to establish some meaning for the pain. They often use other experiences such as their own as a basis for comparison. Frequently these pain episodes have been of an acute nature, bearing little resemblance to the present picture of chronic pain. The inability to find standards in prior experiences generally serves to heighten the family's sense of uncertainty and distress.

In order to fill the existing void, family members then develop their own explanations of the pain which may be inappropriate (Benjamin et al 1992). For some the pain may mean nothing more than a sign of impending 'old age', while still others may question whether or not it signifies a dread disease such as cancer. In addition, sequelae that often accompany chronic pain such as depression and social withdrawal on the part of the patient may be misunderstood and interpreted as rejection of family members.

The distress engendered by these uncertainties arises out of a lack of understanding of the phenomenon of chronic pain. The extent to which such uncertainty can be reduced and meanings clarified through total family involvement in the learning process may be one approach to assisting families to cope more effectively with living with pain.

DEVELOPMENT OF COPING SKILLS

The feeling of helplessness experienced by the spouses of chronic-pain patients in terms of being unable to effect any change in their mate's pain appears to be a major contributor to the distress experienced by these spouses (Vachon et al 1977; Rowat & Knafl 1985). Such feelings of impotence and subsequent distress emphasise the importance of incorporating family members into the teaching aspect of the programme in order that appropriate coping strategies may be developed.

Factors that augment or reduce pain often go unrecognised by family members and attempts at pain management are generally haphazard and ill-conceived. Engaging the family in a deliberative and conscious process of assessment and planning may not only facilitate their development of pain-management skills but may also work towards altering their perceptions of helplessness.

One means of assisting family members with learning coping skills is through the use of spouse or family groups, or combined patient/family groups (Langelier & Gallagher 1989). The provision of such a forum for the sharing of experiences and the identification of successful coping strategies is seen as an important facet of the overall programme of assisting families to deal and live with chronic pain. To know that one is not alone and that one's situation is not unique may have a major therapeutic effect in itself.

For the majority of families this may be their first encounter with a chronic health problem. Coping skills which were found to be effective in the past in dealing with acute crises may now be found to be inappropriate. As one spouse stated, 'He's had other illnesses which we've coped with as crises, but this is not a crisis, this is a chronic situation and I have to learn to live with it.' Assisting families to recognise that control over the pain and pain-related stressors may lie in their hands can be an important feature of the caregiver's work with chronic-pain families.

COLLABORATION WITH THE HEALTH PROFESSIONAL

Communication and collaboration with the health professional within a positive and trusting atmosphere (Waring 1982) is an essential aspect of the family's learning to live chronic pain (Rowat 1983). Families readily identify that a chronic-pain problem is a family affair. However, family members report that they have been offered little information about possible causes and treatment of chronic pain and have been told nothing regarding how they could help (Benjamin et al 1992). In their search for assistance, families frequently confront a health-care system which is geared to the individual: 'The rest of the family – I don't think the doctors know they exist; there's nobody we can see, which leaves me feeling there's no one to help.' This statement illustrates that the sense of abandonment experienced by the patient is shared by the family.

When family members are incorporated into the team which deals with the chronic pain and when they perceive that health professionals are accessible to them, not only is family distress as a whole reduced, but energies become channelled in a constructive way to deal with the problem. Often merely knowing that help is available to them is sufficient.

CONCLUSION

Learning to live with chronic pain is a family affair. It is proposed that this learning is best accomplished within the context of a supportive relationship, one characterised by continuity and collaboration. Patient, family and health professional join forces as together they strive for the ultimate goal, that of a positive quality of life for the family which includes a person with chronic pain.

REFERENCES

Aiken L 1976 Chronic illness and responsive ambulatory care. In: Mechanic D (ed) The growth of bureaucratic medicine. John Wiley, New York, p 239–251

Benjamin S, Mawer J, Lennon S 1992 The knowledge and beliefs of family care givers about chronic pain patients. Journal of Psychosomatic Medicine 36: 211–217

Block A, Boyer S 1984 The spouse's adjustment to chronic pain: cognitive and emotional factors. Social Science in Medicine 19: 1313–1317

Block A, Kremer E, Gaylor M 1980 Behavioral treatment of chronic pain: the spouse as a discriminative cue for pain behavior. Pain 9: 243–252

Bonica J 1973 Management of pain. Postgraduate Medicine 53: 56–57

Bonica J 1978 Introduction. In: Brena S (ed) Chronic pain: America's hidden epidemic. Atheneum/SMI, New York, p v–ix

Bonica J 1980 Conclusion. In: Bonica J (ed) Pain research publication. Association for research on nervous and mental disease. Raven Press, New York, p 381–384

Bonica J 1984 Pain research and therapy: recent advances and future needs. In: Kruger L, Liebeskind J (eds) Advances in pain research and therapy. Raven Press, New York, p 1–22

Brena S F 1984 Pain and litigation. In: Wall P D, Melzack R (eds)Textbook of pain, 1st edn. Churchill Livingstone, New York, p 832–839

Davis G 1992 The meaning of pain management: a concept analysis. Advances in Nursing Science 15: 77–86

Deardroff W, Rubin H, Scott D 1991 Comprehensive multidisciplinary treatment of chronic pain: a follow-up study of treated and non-treated groups. Pain 45: 35–43

Dura J, Beck S 1988 A comparison of family functioning when mothers have chronic pain. Pain 35: 79–89

Ehde D, Holm J, Metzger D 1991 The role of family structure, functioning and pain modeling in headache. Headache 31: 35–40

Flor H, Kerns R, Turk D 1987a The role of spouse reinforcement, perceived pain, and activity levels of chronic pain patients. Journal of Psychosomatic Research 31: 251–259

Flor H, Turk D, Rudy T 1987b Pain and families. II. Assessment and treatment. Pain 30: 29–45

Flor H, Turk D, Scholz B 1987c Impact of chronic pain on the spouse: marital, emotional and physical consequences. Journal of Psychosomatic Research 31: 63–71

Flor H, Turk D, Rudy T 1989 Relationship of pain impact and significant other reinforcement of pain behaviors: the mediating role of gender, marital status and marital satisfaction. Pain 38: 45–50

Fordyce W 1976 Behavioral methods for chronic pain and illness. C V Mosby, St Louis

Fordyce W 1978 Learning processes in pain. In: Sternbach R (ed) The psychology of pain. Raven Press, New York

Funch D, Gale E 1986 Predicting treatment completion in a behavioral therapy program for chronic temporomandibular pain. Journal of Psychosomatic Research 30: 57–62

Gerson E, Strauss A 1975 Time for living: problems in chronic illness care. Social Policy 6: 12–18

Gottlieb L, Rowat K 1987 The McGill model of nursing: a practice derived model. Advances in Nursing Science 9: 51–61

Herman E 1990 Group experience as healing process. In: Miller T (ed) Chronic pain, vol 2. International Universities Press, Madison, Connecticut, p 459–497

Herman E, Baptiste S 1990 Group therapy: a cognitive behavioral model. In: Tunks E, Bellissimo A, Roy R (eds) Chronic pain: psychological factors in rehabilitation. Robert E Publishing, Malabar, Florida, p 212–228

Hilbert R 1984 The acultural dimensions of chronic pain: flawed reality construction and the problem of meaning. Social Problems 31: 365–378

Hudgens A 1979 Family oriented treatment of chronic pain. Journal of Marital and Family Therapy 5: 67–78

Institute of Medicine 1987 Committee on Pain, Disability and Chronic Illness Behavior. Pain and disability: clinical, behavioral and public policy perspectives. National Academy Press, Washington, DC

Jeans M E, Stratford J, Melzack R, Monks R 1979 Assessment of pain. Canadian Family Physician 25: 159–162

Kerns R, Turk D, Holzman A, Rudy T 1986 Comparison of cognitive–behavioral group approach for the treatment of chronic pain. Clinical Journal of Pain 2: 195–203

Kerns R, Haythornwaite S, Southwick S, Giller E 1990 The role of marital interaction in chronic pain and depressive symptom severity. Journal of Psychosomatic Research 34: 401–408

Kerns R, Southwick S, Giller E, Haythornwaite J, Jacob M, Rosenberg R 1991 The relationship between reports of pain-related social interactions and expressions of pain and affective distress, Behavior Therapy 22: 101–111

Khatami M, Rush J 1978 A pilot study of the treatment of outpatients with chronic pain: symptom control, stimulus control and social system intervention. Pain 5: 163–172

Langelier R, Gallagher R, 1989 Outpatient treatment of chronic pain groups for couples. Clinical Journal of Pain 5: 227–231

Maruta T, Swanson D, McHardy M J 1990 Three year follow-up of patients with chronic pain who were treated in a multidisciplinary pain management center. Pain 41: 47–53

Melzack R 1975 The McGill pain questionnaire: major properties and scoring methods. Pain 1: 227–299

Melzack R, Wall P D 1988 The challenge of pain. Penguin Books, Harmondsworth, Middlesex

Mikail S, von Baeyer C 1990 Pain, somatic focus and emotional adjusment in children of chronic headache sufferers and controls. Social Science in Medicine 31: 51–59

Miller T (ed) 1990 Chronic pain, vol 2. International Universities Press, Madison, Connecticut

Mohamed S 1982 The patient and his family. In: Roy R, Turks E (eds) Chronic pain. Psychosocial factors in rehabilitation Williams & Wilkins, Baltimore, p 145–150

Mohamed S, Weisz G, Waring E 1978 The relationship of chronic pain to depression, marital adjustment and family dynamics. Pain 5: 285–292

Nicholas M, Wilson P, Goyen J 1992 Comparison of cognitive–behavioral group treatment and an alternative non-psychological treatment for chronic low back pain. Pain 48: 339–343

Payne B, Norfleet M 1986 Chronic pain and the family: a review. Pain 26: 1–22

Pearce T, Tunks E 1990 Multimodal treatment for chronic pain. In: Tunks E, Bellissimo A, Roy R (eds) Chronic pain: psychological factors in rehabilitation. Robert E Publishing, Malabar, Florida, p 255–270

Peters J, Large R 1990 A randomised control trial evaluating in- and outpatient programmes. Pain 41: 283–293

Pratt L 1973 The significance of the family in medication. Journal of Comparative Family Studies IV: 13–35

Roberts A H, Reinhardt L 1980 The behavioral management of chronic pain: long-term follow-up with comparison groups. Pain 8: 151–163

Romano J, Turner J, Clancy S 1989 Sex differences in the relationship of pain patient dysfunction to spouse adjustment. Pain 39: 289–295

Romano J, Turner J, Freidman L, Bulcroft R, Jensen M, Hops H 1991 Observational assessment of chronic pain patients – spouse behavioral interactions. Behavior Therapy 22: 549–567

Rowat K M 1983 The meaning and management of chronic pain: the family's perspective. Doctoral dissertation. University of Illinois at Chicago Health Sciences Center, Chicago

Rowat K 1985a Chronic pain: a family affair. In: King K (ed) Recent advances in nursing: long term care, vol 13. Churchill Livingstone, London, p 137–149

Rowat K 1985b Assessing the 'chronic pain family'. International Journal of Family Therapy 7: 284–296

Rowat K, Knafl K 1985 Living with chronic pain: the spouse's perspective. Pain 23: 259–271

Roy R 1982 Marital and family issues in patients with chronic pain: a review. Psychotherapy Psychosomatic 37: 1–12

Roy R 1985 Family treatment for chronic pain: state of the art. International Journal of Family Therapy 7: 297–309

Roy R, Thomas M 1989 Nature of marital relations among chronic pain patients. Contemporary Family Therapy 11: 277–285

Schwartz L, Slater M, Birchler G, Atkinson J 1991 Depression in spouses of chronic pain patients: the role of patient pain and anger, and marital satisfaction. Pain 44: 61–67

Schwenk T, Hughes C 1983 The family as patient in family medicine. Social Science in Medicine 17: 1–16

Spinhoven P, Linssen A 1991 Behavioral treatment of chronic low back pain. I. Relation of coping strategy use to outcome. Pain 45: 29–34

Stewart D, Sullivan T 1982 Illness behavior and the sick role in chronic disease: the case of multiple sclerosis. Social Science in Medicine 16: 1397–1404

Strauss A 1984 Chronic illness and the quality of life, 2nd edn. C V Mosby, St Louis

Subramanian K 1991 The multidimensional impact of chronic pain on the spouse: a pilot study. Social Work in Health Care 15: 47–62

Swanson D, Maruta T 1980 The family's viewpoint of chronic pain. Pain 8: 163–166

Taenzer P 1981 Personal communication

Thomas M, Roy R 1989 Pain patients and marital relations. The Clinical Journal of Pain 5: 255–259

Tunks E, Bellissimo A, Roy R 1990 Chronic pain: psychosocial factors in rehabilitation. Robert E Publishing, Malabar, Florida

Turk D, Kerns R (eds) 1985 Health, illness and families. Wiley, New York

Turk D, Rudy T, Flor H 1985 Why a family perspective for pain? International Journal of Family Therapy 7: 223–233

Turk D, Flor H, Rudy T 1987 Pain and families. I. Etiology, maintenance, and psychosocial impact. Pain 30: 3–27

Vachon M L, Freedman K, Formo A, Rogers J, Lyall W, Freeman S 1977 The final illness in cancer: the widow's perspective. Canadian Medical Association Journal 117: 1151–1154

Waring E 1982 Conjoint marital aid and family therapy. In: Roy R, Turks E (eds) Chronic pain: psychosocial factors in rehabilitation. Williams & Wilkins, Baltimore, p 151–165

Yelen E, Nevitt M, Epstein W 1980 Toward an epidemiology of work disability. Health and Society 58: 386

78. Chronic pain and compensation issues

George Mendelson

INTRODUCTION

The first reported case of an employee seeking compensation from an employer for a work injury reached the High Court in England during 1837. The plaintiff employee had been travelling in his employer's van which 'broke down, and the plaintiff was thrown with violence to the ground, and his thigh was thereby fractured'. The lower court entered a verdict of £100 in favour of the plaintiff. On appeal, it was noted that 'It is admitted that there is no precedent for the present action by a servant against a master.' The Court of Appeal reversed the judgement which had been made in favour of the plaintiff, Lord Abinger C.B. noting that 'if the master be liable to the servant in this action, the principle of that liability will be found to carry us to an alarming extent' (Priestley v. Fowler 1837). Subsequent actions for damages brought by employees against employers, seeking compensation at common law for work injuries, under headings of damages including 'pain and suffering', met with mixed success in what was termed by some a 'forensic lottery'.

This unsatisfactory situation continued in Great Britain until 1897, when the Workmen's Compensation Act introduced a statutory scheme which provided income support for injured workers on a *no fault* basis (Bartrip & Burman 1983), based on similar legislation introduced earlier by Bismarck in Germany. Laws providing for statutory benefits for injured workers were subsequently also adopted in other countries and similar legislation was passed during the early part of this century in the United States (Larson 1952).

Although such statutory provisions were hailed by many as an important and progressive social-welfare measure, the new legislation also encountered criticism from those who regarded the financial benefits to which injured workers were entitled as conducive to false claims.

Parry, writing in 1911, stated '[T]he strain, sprain, or rupture of a muscle is one of the easiest things to allege and one of the hardest things to disprove. Pain in the back has become a byword among workmen, who are fully aware that "if you say you have got a pain in your back, nobody can't say you haven't got it".' According to Parry '[T]he duration of cure in a sprained muscle should not exceed fourteen to twenty-eight days. An extra week for complete recovery is all the further period of rest that need be allowed. If four or five weeks after a sprain a man still complains of pain in his back you should be very suspicious of malingering.'

Concern about prolonged complaints of back pain was also expressed by Morley (1914), who described his technique for the detection of malingering in the following terms 'I often quietly knock some article of the man's clothing, such as his cap, tie-clip, or belt, off the chair or table where it has been placed, and I have been amused to watch the man afterwards stoop freely and pick it up, though his chief complaint throughout the previous examination had been that it was impossible to stoop.'

In a discussion of the effects of the introduction of workers' compensation laws, Collie summed up the views of many authors when he stated that 'fraud is a product of the age, of the Workmen's Compensation Act, of Trade Unions and allied Clubs. There are no malingerers in countries where there is no Workmen's Compensation Act' (Collie 1932). With reference to pain, Collie wrote:

> [I]n dealing with a back injury, it is necessary to make up one's mind on two points. First, is the pain real, psychic or assumed; second, is it due to disease or accident? In the vast majority of cases, alleged pain in the back is mental and not physical. The idea of a tender spot or of pain takes possession of the patient, and has the same effect and requires the same tratment as obsessions in regard to other parts of the body. (Collie 1932).

Another author who dealt with the subject of pain and compensation during the early part of this century was Slot (1927). Among the issues discussed by Slot were the problem of the definition of pain as well as 'the causes of pain'. With reference to the medicolegal aspects of pain, Slot wrote '[P]ain itself is however the more frequent complaint; here of course it is of cardinal importance, from the medicolegal aspect, to decide whether the pain is real or not, and whether it was caused by the accident or other cause claimed, and how great is the extent of the incapacity.' These concerns are echoed in the questions which continue to be posed in present-day medicolegal practice in letters from solicitors seeking reports about plaintiffs.

Until 1970 the predominant theme in the professional literature dealing with the medicolegal aspects of compensation was concern about the putative clinical entities of 'accident neurosis' (Miller 1961) or 'compensation neurosis'. In an oft-quoted aphorism, Foster Kennedy (1946) defined 'compensation neurosis' as 'a state of mind, born out of fear, kept alive by avarice, stimulated by lawyers, and cured by a verdict'. The continuing difficulties faced by the legal system and by statutory schemes in providing appropriate compensation for pain have been comprehensively discussed in an important review by Pryor (1991).

This chapter will review the current status of the concept of 'compensation neurosis', the relationship between chronic pain complaints and compensation, approaches to the rating of pain-related impairment and the problems of psychiatric diagnosis in cases of chronic pain among recipients of compensation where the subjective complaint of pain and the alleged resultant disability appear disproportionate to the extent of objectively demonstrable organic pathology or evidence of continuing physical injury.

Although the term 'compensation' will be employed throughout this chapter, it will be taken as referring not only to those individuals who are in receipt of workers' compensation benefits under the relevant statutory schemes, but also to those who are seeking damages through litigation following injuries which have led to persistent pain and those who are in receipt of pensions or disability benefits under the terms of social security legislation.

COMPENSATION NEUROSIS

'Compensation neurosis' has been one of numerous terms which have been used to describe the occurrence of subjective symptoms in circumstances which led to litigation or entitlement to compensation payments where such symptoms cannot be attributed to a demonstrable physical lesion. The essential component of the concept of compensation neurosis is that of complaints which are motivated by the prospect of pecuniary gain, albeit at an 'unconscious' level (and thus distinguished from malingering) and which cannot be attributed to any recognised or diagnosable physical disorder. A large number of terms have been used as the equivalents of compensation neurosis to describe the sequelae of compensable accidents; these have been listed elsewhere (Mendelson 1988).

Foster Kennedy's 'definition' of compensation neurosis has been cited above. Another description of this putative condition can be derived from the writings of Henry Miller, also a neurologist, whose Milroy Lectures in 1961 were on the subject he termed 'accident neurosis'. Miller put forward the following five propositions which, in his view, defined this condition:

1. an absolute failure to respond to therapy until the compensation issue was settled
2. the accident . . . must have occurred in circumstances where payment of financial compensation is potentially involved
3. it is comparatively uncommon where injury has been severe . . . the inverse relationship to the severity of injury . . . is crucial to its understanding
4. such a development is favoured by a low social and occupational status
5. after [the compensation issue was settled] nearly all the cases described recovered completely without treatment.

Terms such as 'compensation neurosis', 'accident neurosis', 'functional overlay' and 'litigation neurosis' are still encountered fairly frequently in medicolegal reports and, although their use presupposes that they have a degree of diagnostic validity, these terms tend to be used loosely and usually in an idiosyncratic way, the authors frequently failing to define the way in which the particular 'label' is to be understood. According to Sindell & Perr (1963) the term 'compensation neurosis' has acquired 'an unfavourable connotation: it is a dirty word implying an admixture of lying or malingering and/or unconscious exaggeration of symptoms in order to obtain something positive for the patient involved. For purposes of medical testimony it is not an accurate expression . . . ' A critical examination of terms such as compensation neurosis and what they imply shows that these in fact do not meet the usual validity criteria which have been developed as part of the modern system of nomenclature in medicine. While it is easy to demonstrate that patients labelled as having a compensation neurosis are homogeneous in respect of one specific variable, namely receipt of compensation or involvement in litigation following a compensable injury, and to that extent are different from other patient groups, studies have failed to detect any other difference between litigants and comparable groups of nonlitigants. Such studies which have specifically compared pain patients are reviewed below.

Research findings indicate that, using standard criteria of diagnostic validity, and in particular those of content validity, compensation claimants cannot be distinguished from nonlitigants with similar symptoms and that the assumed 'predictive' value of the label compensation neurosis, namely that litigants improve after the case is finalised, is similarly not supported (Mendelson 1988).

Specifically in relation to patients with chronic back pain, Guest & Drummond (1992) have found that following settlement patients continued to show evidence of emotional distress and that reports of pain intensity did not differ between compensation recipients and those who had settled their claim.

THE EFFECT OF COMPENSATION STATUS ON CHRONIC PAIN

Studies which have explored the interaction between compensation and chronic pain complaints can be categorised as having utilised one of the following three approaches:

1. Comparison of the described pain experience of compensation recipients (or litigants) with that of pain patients with similar complaints not involved in litigation and not receiving pain-contingent benefits
2. Comparison of treatment response between comparable pain patient groups where members of one group are involved in litigation or receive compensation, and the others do not
3. Examination of the presentation and duration of chronic pain complaints under different systems of compensation.

COMPENSATION STATUS AND PAIN DESCRIPTION

Peck et al (1978) compared two groups of injured workers: one group consisted of 105 persons who had made a third-party tort claim and the other group included 103 subjects who did not make a third-party claim. Comparison of the two groups failed to show any significant difference in pain behaviour; thus, the presence of a third-party claim did not increase pain behaviour. However, this study is open to criticism on the grounds that both patient groups were in receipt of compensation, the only difference between them being the presence of an additional tort claim.

Another method of comparison between patients with chronic low-back pain receiving compensation and those who had no such claims was utilised by Leavitt et al (1982), who compared the two groups on pain measures such as duration, intensity, locus of pain, pain description and the quality of pain. The results of the comparison indicated that patients who had objective evidence of injury but showed no significant psychological disturbance, and were receiving compensation, reported more intense sensory discomfort. However, no other differences between the compensation and noncompensation groups were found.

Pain ratings, using the McGill Pain Questionnaire (Melzack 1975) and the visual analogue scale, were recorded by 80 patients with chronic low-back pain who had been referred for assessment and/or treatment at a pain clinic (Mendelson 1984). The patients were divided into two groups according to whether or not they were claiming compensation, and the groups compared with respect to psychological and pain variables. In the group of 47 patients receiving compensation there were almost equal numbers of males and females, whereas among the 33 patients in the noncompensation group females outnumbered males by a ratio slightly greater than 2.5:1. Comparison of the various measures of pain severity, the visual analogue scale scores, and the mean scores on the categories of the McGill Pain Questionnaire checklist failed to demonstrate any significant difference in either the severity or the characteristics of low-back pain described by the compensation group and the noncompensation group.

The role of compensation in chronic pain was also examined by Melzack et al (1985). These authors reported on a group of 145 patients with chronic pain of at least 6 months' duration, who had been referred to the Pain Clinic at Montreal General Hospital. There were 81 patients with chronic low-back pain (of these, 27 were receiving compensation and 54 were not). Among these, 64 patients had musculoskeletal pain, mainly affecting the upper back, shoulders, or lower limbs (of these 15 were on compensation and 49 were not). The patients in this study were an unselected consecutive sample of Pain Clinic referrals. Analysis of results for the low-back pain group showed that there was a 'remarkable consistency with which low-back pain patients describe their pain regardless of whether or not they receive financial compensation for their illness'.

Analysis of results for the musculoskeletal pain group showed that compensation patients subjectively evaluated the overall pain intensity as lower than the noncompensation group; the conpensation group had also sought the opinion of fewer consultants. Thus, contrary to the common notion of pain exaggeration by litigants, in this group of patients those involved in litigation described their pain as less severe when compared with a group not involved in litigation.

Chronic-pain patients in receipt of compensation or involved in personal injury litigation have also been compared with similar patients not involved in litigation nor receiving pain-related compensation on measures of illness behaviour, using the illness behaviour questionnaire (IBQ) developed by Pilowsky & Spence (1975). No differences between these two groups were found in the mean group scores on the scales of the IBQ (Mendelson 1987a) or on the conscious exaggeration scale of the IBQ which, it had been asserted, can detect deception with the object of financial gain among chronic-pain patients involved in litigation (Mendelson 1987b).

THE EFFECT OF COMPENSATION ON TREATMENT OUTCOME AND DISABILITY

It has been generally considered that recipients of compensation benefits have more marked disability and show reduced motivation for effective treatment. Fowler & Mayfield (1969), in a study comparing 327 patients receiving disability compensation with 613 patients not in receipt of compensation, commented that compensation beneficiaries (although manifesting less symptoms) had a significantly poorer occupational adjustment than the noncompensation group.

Studies of the effect of compensation on treatment outcome of chronic pain, published prior to 1983 and reviewed elsewhere by this author (Mendelson 1983), were in general agreement that patients in receipt of compensation and/or involved in litigation had a worse prognosis than those with similar complaints who were not in receipt of such payments nor involved in litigation. A representative study from that period was that by Hammonds et al (1978), who found that among 26 patients with chronic pain not receiving pain-contingent financial benefits, 18 (69%) showed significant benefit from a rehabilitation programme, whereas only 15 out of 35 patients (43%) of a group in receipt of compensation payments showed comparable improvement.

The presence or absence of litigation was one of several factors considered by Gore & Sepic (1984) in an evaluation of the results of cervical disc fusion. Among the 146 patients in this study there were 45 who attributed their neck problems to a specific injury and of these 22 were involved in litigation; the litigation had been finalised in 17 cases at the time of evaluation. Of all patients, 97% were considered to have benefited from surgery and 78% were painfree. There was no significant correlation between presence or absence of litigation and improvement following surgery. Patients with pain in the upper limbs had better results than those with neck and head pains and there was a significant negative correlation between pain duration and postoperative improvement.

Cairns et al (1984) compared the results of inpatient and outpatient treatment of patients with chronic spinal pain; there were 100 subjects in each group. Among the inpatients, 58% were receiving Workers' Compensation payments, social security disability pensions or both; the corresponding figure for the outpatient group was 68%. Analysis of results showed that 42% of those outpatients who had been receiving Workers' Compensation payments returned to work, whereas only two out of the 20 inpatients who had been receiving such payments returned to work. The authors commented that although the presence of litigation generally lowered the expectation that patients with low-back pain will return to work, the finding that 42% of outpatients receiving compensation payments returned to work 'suggests that litigation may not limit return to work as much as expected'.

Catchlove & Cohen (1983) compared the return to work rates of a group of 20 pain patients claiming compensation (who were treated without any specific instruction concerning resumption of work) with that of a group of 27 patients who received similar treatment at a pain clinic but who also had been given a specific 'return to work as part of the therapy' instruction. The two groups were compared on variables such as age, sex, pain duration, site of pain and treatment duration and no significant difference between the two groups was found. However, among the 'instruction' group, 16 out of the 27 patients (59%) returned to work during treatment at the Pain Management Unit, whereas among the 'no-instruction' group five out of 20 patients had resumed work (25%). Follow-up data were obtained for 15 patients in each of the two groups. Of 10 patients in the 'instruction' group who had returned to work and were available for follow-up (a mean of 9.6 months after termination of treatment), nine were continuing to work; among patients from the 'no-instruction' group, three out of four were working a mean of 19.9 months after treatment ceased. It was concluded that a directive approach of this type was an important part of the 'holistic' treatment of patients with chronic pain receiving Workers' Compensation.

Dworkin et al (1985) noted that outcome studies which have evaluated the treatment response of pain patients in receipt of compensation had shown inconsistent results. Their study involved a total of 454 chronic pain patients and the influence of employment and compensation on treatment outcome was examined by a multiple regression analysis. The results showed that only employment was a statistically significant predictor of long-term outcome. The authors of this study concluded that it was important to direct attention 'toward the roles of activity and employment in the treatment and rehabilitation of chronic pain patients', within the individual's limitations. They also specifically noted the 'deleterious effects' of terms such as compensation neurosis which are used to label patients and which may divert attention away from the need to involve the patient in an active treatment programme.

Sander & Meyers (1986) compared the period of work disability following a low-back sprain/strain injury among two groups of patients drawn from railway employees covered by a Federal disability scheme in the United States. One group consisted of those injured while at work and the other comprised those who had been injured off duty. The two groups were matched for type of injury and for gender. The authors found that the 35 subjects who had been injured at work, and who were therefore in receipt of pain-contingent compensation benefits, were away from work for a mean of 14.2 months, as compared with 4.9 months for the 30 subjects injured off duty. This difference was statistically significant and the authors concluded that 'the financial rewards of compensation' were responsible for the prolonged recovery of those injured at work. In a similar study of the duration of time off work due to low-back pain, Leavitt (1990) found that, among a group of 1373 patients with pain following a work injury, 23.7% were disabled for longer than 12 months, whereas among 417 patients with similar pain not receiving compensation benefits 13.2% were off work for longer than 12 months.

Although the studies reviewed above have indicated that the receipt of compensation has a negative effect on treatment outcome and tends to prolong work disability, it has been demonstrated that specific treatment programmes can reduce the likelihood of progression to pain chronicity following work injuries (Wiesel et al 1984). Similarly, Fordyce et al (1986) have shown that a treatment programme for low-back pain which incorporates behavioural methods is more effective than traditional management. Thus, the adverse effect of compensation on the outcome of treatment for acute pain following work injuries can be modified by specific programmes which stress early mobilisation and return to the workplace, appropriate activity and exercises and avoidance of other factors which may promote 'learned pain behaviour' (Tyrer 1986; see below). Peters et al (1992) have also demonstrated that a cognitive–behavioural treatment programme for chronic pain patients can be effective in helping the patients who come off compensation or sickness benefits and resume work, with a consequent saving to the state by returning people to work.

THE COMPENSATION SYSTEM AND CHRONIC PAIN

In examining the influence of compensation on chronic pain, it is also useful to compare populations which have different systems of compensation and litigation. It is therefore fortuitous that in 1974 New Zealand instituted an universal system of compensation for injuries. Under this system:

1. the traditional Workers' Compensation Scheme was abolished
2. the right to sue in civil courts at common law for personal injuries was abolished
3. a new scheme was established to provide benefits to all who suffer an injury, irrespective of fault or circumstances
4. the new scheme was universal in that it covered all persons in New Zealand.

There have been two reports which have compared chronic pain patients in New Zealand with those in countries which continued to have the traditional common law systems and Workers' Compensation schemes. These systems allow for personal-injury claims to be litigated in court, with the plaintiff seeking damages from the wrongdoer, and similarly allow an injured worker to sue the employer if negligence can be established as having caused or contributed to the injury.

Carron et al (1985) examined the pain and disability ratings of patients referred for treatment and related the treatment outcome to the type of compensation or disability benefits received by the patients in New Zealand and the United States. The Accident Compensation Commission in New Zealand meets the full cost of medical care, and provides income security, for all accident victims irrespective of fault, thus avoiding litigation with its concomitant 'adversary' system within which many personal injury cases are played out. The authors found that 49% of the sample from the United States and 17% of the New Zealand sample were receiving pain-related compensation at the time of referral to the pain clinic. A significantly greater proportion of US patients reported sleep disturbance, reduced social and recreational activities and impaired libido. At follow-up, although the US compensation patients reported a higher degree of subjective improvement, they reported a higher degree of pain intensity and frequency, a greater limitation of activities and a lower return to full activity and ability to work. It was noted by the authors of this study that 'the differential effects linked to compensation status are quite small, and almost nonexistent in the New Zealand sample'. Carron et al concluded that the difference between the patient groups in the two countries was related to the no-fault system in New Zealand which automatically provided income compensation for accidental injury, without the need to prove injury at work, and the consequent absence of an adversarial relationship between the claimant, employer and insurer.

Mills & Horne (1986) compared data for motor-vehicle accidents in New Zealand and Victoria, Australia, for the 12-month period to 30 June 1983. They analysed the number of motor-vehicle accidents, rear-end collisions, claims for 'whiplash' injuries and the mean compensation paid to each claimant. They found that in New Zealand there had been 422 'whiplash' claims during that 12-month period, arising from 547 rear-end collisions. The comparable figures in Victoria were 4231 claims arising from 2181 rear-end collisions. Thus, in New Zealand there were 77 claims per 100 rear-end collisions, whereas in Victoria there were 194 claims per 100 rear-end collisions, a rate of claims almost three times greater. It was also found that in New Zealand the mean compensation paid per claim was NZ $1038, as compared with a mean of Aust. $3265 in Victoria.

In commenting on these findings, the authors noted that 'the striking difference in the incidence of whiplash injury in the two groups suggests that litigation and the expectation of financial compensation may have an influence on development of whiplash symptoms'. Mills & Horne also suggested that 'because patients in Victoria would seek compensation for an injury through the common law system... they are more conversant with and more attuned to receiving compensation for injury, which may in itself be stimulus for claiming for an injury that they would not normally have claimed for' whereas that stimulus 'does not exist in New Zealand'. Mills & Horne also analysed the statistics for 'time off work' of the two patient groups. Data were available for 227 cases in New Zealand and for 1558 cases in Victoria. Of the New Zealand group, 212 (93.4%) returned to work within 6 months; the comparable figure for Victoria was 1126 (72.3%). This difference was statistically significant.

The relationship between societal expectations concerning illness and illness behaviour was explored by Balla (1982) in an analysis of the 'late whiplash syndrome' as manifested in Australia and in Singapore. The 'late whiplash syndrome' was defined as a condition which follows a motor-vehicle accident, usually after a rear-end collision. The injured person complains of persistent pain and other symptoms, long after the acute pain resulting from the soft-tissue injury would have been expected to subside. Typically, the patient complains of neck pain and stiffness, headache, pain in the arms, problems in carrying out usual daily activities, sleep disturbance and loss of libido. Other symptoms which may be present include irritability, anxiousness, poor memory and concentration and feelings of depression. Balla found that this condition, which is well known in Australia, 'was unheard of' in Singapore except 'for the odd case seen in those with European backgrounds'. A prospective study of 20 patients with an acute whiplash injury, whose 'original acute complaints of pain in the head and neck region were the same as seen in Australia', showed that the symptoms resolved and that the patients did not go on to develop the 'late whiplash syndrome'.

On the basis of these findings, Balla postulated that the 'late whiplash syndrome' is a 'culturally constructed illness behavior based on indigenous categories and social structural determinants'. He also noted that in Australia such a condition had been accepted as compensable by the courts, and that this provided a positive reinforcement for 'illness behaviour' following the acute phase of 'whiplash'. Balla commented that because there were 'no clear and frequent precedents' in Singapore following an acute whiplash injury, this was 'likely to be one explanation for significant differences in behavior in association with an illness which may have taken place'.

It is also instructive to examine the effects that a change in the laws concerning compensation and common-law rights has on the rate of claims. In Victoria, Australia, over a period of 7 years prior to 30 June 1985 there had been a dramatic increase in claims for 'sprain or strain of the neck' (that is, the so-called 'whiplash' injury) following a motor-vehicle accident. Claims for this type of injury (which is usually a 'nondemonstrable injury' with minimal or absent objective abnormal findings or signs) had increased during that 7-year period at an average annual growth rate of 25.9%; the comparable figure was 2% for major-injury claims and 5.7% for minor-injury claims (Motor Accidents Board 1986).

That pattern of a continuing increase in the number of 'whiplash' claims has been dramatically reversed since 1984/85. The annual report of the Transport Accident Commission for the year to 30 June 1989 (Transport Accident Commission 1989) indicated that a total of 2004 new 'whiplash' claims were lodged during that period, as compared with a 'high' of 6364 such claims in 1986. There has thus been a reduction of almost 70% in the number of new 'whiplash' claims.

It has been suggested that reasons for the dramatic reduction in the rate of claims were related to legislative changes in the new Transport Accident Act which was proclaimed in January 1987. These changes included making eligibility for benefits dependent upon the accident being reported to the police, discouraging minor claims by the introduction of a medical services excess fee and limiting the entitlement to sue at common law to those seriously injured and impaired. In addition, wide media publicity given to antifraud activities may have had an effect in discouraging claims for a nondemonstrable injury such as 'whiplash'.

Legislative changes can also have the opposite effect. Among the objectives of the WorkCare scheme, which was introduced in Victoria, Australia, on 1 September 1985, were (1) to provide suitable and just compensation to injured workers and (2) to speedily and efficiently decide claims for compensation and deliver compensation to injured workers. The scheme provided for compensation benefits of 80–85% of preinjury earnings; such benefits were, on average, some 20% higher than the benefits provided under the previous scheme. However, as had been made clear in an annual report of the Accident Compensation Commission which administers the WorkCare scheme, in some instances workers 'actually received more in benefits than they would have if they returned to their preinjury employment' (Accident Compensation Commission 1988). This anomaly was subsequently corrected by legislation.

It has been estimated that following the introduction of the WorkCare scheme up to 98.4% of all claims were accepted. This figure was significantly higher than the estimated initial acceptance rate of 60–80% of claims under the previous system. Whereas under the previous Workers' Compensation scheme only about 2.5% of claims continued beyond 12 months, the comparable figure reported by the Accident Compensation Commission for the 1986–87 period was 18% and for the 1987–88 period it was 12.5% (Accident Compensation

Commission 1988). The 1986–87 report showed that the percentage of claimants receiving more than 80% of their former earnings was much higher among those on payments for longer than 12 months than those in the 'short-term claims' group.

One of the features of the WorkCare system introduced in 1985 was its 'open-ended' nature; that is, entitlement to compensation benefits continues until the statutory age of retirement. The effects of such 'unlimited' availability of compensation payments on pain behaviour and treatment outcome among patients with chronic pain have been studied by Jamison et al (1988). They reported on three groups of male patients with chronic low-back pain treated at a multidisciplinary pain clinic: one group was not in receipt of compensation payments, the second group received time-limited Workers' Compensation benefits and the final group received 'unlimited' social security disability benefits. The three patient groups did not differ on variables such as age, pain duration or baseline pain severity levels. Follow-up was undertaken some 12 months after completion of treatment. The study found that, at follow-up, significantly more of the noncompensation and 'time-limited' compensation group who were initially not employed due to pain had returned to work compared with the 'unlimited time' compensation group. The authors interpreted these findings as suggesting that time-limited compensation may not affect treatment outcome or reduce the likelihood of return to work to a significant extent, whereas 'unlimited time' compensation may have an adverse effect on the likelihood that the recipients will return to work. It is interesting to compare the figures concerning WorkCare recipients, cited above, with data presented at Congressional hearings in the United States during 1976, quoted by Nachemson (1983), which showed that 'the threshold of increased disability claims lies at about 55% of net income; if the income received during sickness is greater than this percentage, the number of claims increases drastically'.

An Australian study of work injury and absence from work has found 'a very important role for compensation benefits and the unemployment rate in influencing accident frequency', with each 1% rise in compensation benefits leading to a 3.3% rise in the frequency of claims (Woden et al 1987). This estimated 'elasticity' of 3.3% for accident claims with respect to compensation payments was contrasted by the authors with the comparable figure of −0.3 for the rate of accident claims with respect to the unemployment rate.

The influence of the compensation system and public perception of what constitutes a legitimately 'compensable' condition has been well illustrated in Australia in relation to regional pain syndrome of the upper limb (the preferred term for 'repetitive strain injury' or 'RSI'). The rise and fall of that 'epidemic' in Australia has been documented by Ferguson (1984, 1987) and will not be detailed here. The 1987/88 annual report of the Accident Compensation Commission in Victoria (which administers WorkCare) had indicated that the proportion of such claims decreased by half among female workers over the previous 3 years (from 10.59% to 5.01% of all claims), while it had shown very little change among male workers during that period (from 1.73% to 1.4% of all claims). It is instructive to consider the changes in the public perception in Australia of the 'RSI' phenomenon over a period of several years. Whereas initially the lay media and some medical publications gave rather alarmist publicity to this putative 'crippling' condition, more responsible medical observers (Brooks 1986) and trade unions drew attention to the deleterious effects of such publicity and cautioned against the impact that this was having in promoting complaints and disability. It is a matter for speculation as to whether or not the widely publicised compensation claim in March 1987, which was lost by the plaintiff who had sued the Australian Taxation Office in the Supreme Court of Victoria, had been a factor in the reduction of new compensation claims for 'RSI'. In that case, the jury found that the plaintiff 'had not contracted repetitive strain injury while working at the Taxation Office'.

In a subsequent case decided on appeal in the Federal Court of Australia, the bench (by a 2:1 majority) found against a plaintiff who had sued her employers (a Canberra legal firm) in respect of 'RSI'. The majority held that the employers were not obliged to 'act upon the alarmist views about R.S.I. presented in some publications', and that the evidence of the two doctors called on behalf of the plaintiff 'was to be rejected' as ' these doctors could not agree as to what caused R.S.I'. (Phipson Nominees Pty Limited v. French 1988).

The Australian experience of the 'RSI epidemic' was compared with that in the states of Colorado and Arizona among employees of a large US telecommunications company (Hadler 1992). Many of the Denver, Colorado workers who presented with upper-limb pain were subjected to inappropriate surgery which left them 'permanently disabled'. Hadler noted that it was the individual worker's perception of the implications of 'regional musculoskeletal symptoms of the upper extremity' that, to a large extent, determined the person's response. According to Hadler, 'the worker's perceptions of the implications of the discomfort, personal resources on and off the job, job flexibility and alternatives, and personal satisfactions on and off the job are potential confounders of the experience of any illness. The arm discomfort is real, but the quality of the experience is perturbable by these and other confounders.' Reviewing the Australian and US experiences of such 'epidemics' of upper-limb pain, an advisory committee of the British Orthopaedic Association concluded that 'no condition should be prescribed as an industrial disease unless it can be unambiguously defined both clinically and pathologically' (Barton et al 1992).

Two such conditions are currently recognised in Great Britain: 'cramp of the hand or forearm, in people with an occupation entailing prolonged periods of handwriting, typing, or other repetitive movements of the fingers, hand, or arm' and 'traumatic inflammation of the tendons of the hand or forearm or the associated tendon sheaths in any occupation entailing manual labour or frequent or repeated movements of the hand or wrist' (Barton et al 1992). These authors stated that '[A]t present there is insufficient conclusive evidence of occupational causation to prescribe any further types of "repetitive strain injuries".'

RATING PAIN-RELATED IMPAIRMENT

In the context of the medicolegal evaluation of a compensation recipient or litigant with chronic pain, it is important to distinguish between the concepts of impairment and disability, as defined by the World Health Organisation (1980). Impairment is defined as the 'loss or abnormality of psychological, physiological, or anatomical structure or function', whereas disability is defined as the 'restriction or lack (resulting from an impairment) of ability to perform an activity in the manner or within the range considered normal for a human being'. It is generally accepted that the evaluation and rating of impairment is the task of the clinician, whereas the determination of disability is an administrative and legal issue which depends upon the specific circumstances of the claimant and the relevant statutory provisions.

These considerations have been summed up in the following terms by Curran et al (1990):

> [I]t is desirable that 'impairment' and 'disability' not be used interchangeably. The evaluation of impairment is alone a medical responsibility, while the evaluation of disability is essentially an administrative responsibility. While the uniquely medical character of the former is self-evident, the determination of disability involves review, not only of medical factors but of legal, psychological, social, and vocational considerations as well.

Guidelines for the evaluation and rating of permanent impairment due to pain have been set out in an appendix to the third edition of the Guides published by the American Medical Association (1988) and have been reprinted without change in its revision (AMA 1990). These offer little assistance for impairment rating, but caution that '[S]ince chronic pain by definition is primarily a perceptual, maladaptive behavioral problem; since pain per se cannot be validated objectively or quantitated, and since the underlying substrate of somatic pathology is minimal or nonexistent, it follows that little, if any, impairment exists in most instances of the chronic-pain syndrome.'

The Guides also consider pain-related disability in the following terms:

> [S]ince the chronic pain syndrome is a bio-psycho-social problem with major social, economic, and environmental ramifications, it would seem that disability may become a major issue. Chronic pain patients may, indeed, have major limitations of functional capacity over and above any possible impairment. Such disability must be defined by the individual's limitations of functional capacity in the sphere of activities of daily living, social interaction, recreational pursuits, and work endeavors. This will require nonmedical assessment, particularly when countervailing nonmedical influences, such as legal or occupational problems, motivate the patient to maximise the chronic pain syndrome.'

Thus, the American Medical Association Guides lack specific criteria for the rating of impairment due to chronic pain in the absence of a demonstrable organic abnormality.

Turk et al (1988) have suggested a set of multiaxial criteria for the determination of 'impairment due primarily to pain'. The criteria they have proposed combine both physical findings *or* behavioural manifestations *and* functional loss. Thus, whether or not abnormal physical findings were present, there would need also to be significant functional loss in the areas of 'daily living, social functioning, time efficiency in completing routine tasks of living, and the performance of basic work behaviours'. These authors also discussed the various procedures used in the evaluation of pain patients and recommended that additional measures such as observation of pain behaviours, assessment of coping skills, cognitive style and vocational factors be utilised in the determination of impairment due primarily to chronic pain.

In a subsequent article, Turk & Rudy (1991) further discussed the problems in assessment due to the 'minimal association between the extent of impairment and degree of disability, and between the magnitude of physical pathology and severity of the pain report'. They have commented that '[T]he most prominent behavioural component of persistent pain and disability is associated with the principles of operant conditioning.' In relation to pain complaints which are attributed to work injuries, Turk & Rudy observed that:

> [A]nother operant-conditioning principle that is relevant to persistent pain is that of response costs that can operate to decrease 'well behaviors', for example, when injured workers are told by attorneys, employers, or union representatives that they will lose their pending litigation cases or compensation benefits if they are observed engaging in normal activities. Because of established reinforcement contigencies, pain behaviors persist long after the initial tissue pathology is resolved or greatly reduced. These behaviors, then, become an important set of factors in understanding reports of pain and disability and thus are among the targets of assessment and elimination.

Other factors which act to reinforce 'pain behaviours' are

discussed below in the section dealing with 'psychiatric diagnosis' in relation to learned pain behaviour.

Turk & Rudy have suggested that the focus of impairment and disability evaluation be on the injured worker rather than on biomedical diagnosis, and that psychological, behavioural and job-related factors also need to be considered. The benefits of such an approach for the vocational rehabilitation of injured workers have been demonstrated by the success of funtional restoration (Mayer et al 1987; Moreno et al 1991) and work hardening (Matheson et al 1985) programmes. In relation to such programmes, it is relevant to note that 'disability exaggeration' is a poor predictor of the success of functional restoration programmes for patients with chronic low-back pain (Hazard et al 1991). These authors have commented that, in fact, when disability exaggeration did correlate significantly with a positive treatment outcome, the correlation was negative.

It is clear that any proposed system of rating of impairment due to chronic pain will need to take into consideration relevant occupational factors in translating impairment into disability. McBride (1963), in an important yet relatively neglected work on the evaluation of disability, provided an extensive listing of various occupations, indicating those parts of the body which may be functionally impaired and the individual 'still work at the designated job'. Nachemson (1983) has emphasised that, with respect to chronic low-back pain, return to work is possible and indeed 'well justified from a medical, psychologic, and economic point of view' for the approximate 80% of patients who do not have an objectively demonstrable organic cause for the pain complaint or significant physical impairment. There is an urgent need for the type of classification of suitable occupations initially devised by McBride to be updated. Robinson (1990) has presented a list of 89 occupations which he termed 'potentially appropriate' for individuals who are unable to return to their usual work because of low-back pain. The approach which he used to identify these occupations, based on the Worker Rehabilitation Questionnaire, is a promising one and deserves further evaluation.

In discussing the concepts of impairment and disability due to chronic pain it also must be noted that the Committee on Pain, Disability, and Chronic Illness Behavior of the Institute of Medicine, in an important report, recommended that '... "chronic pain" alone should not be added to the SSA [Social Security Administration, USA] regulatory listing of impairments that allow a presumption of disability, nor should 'chronic-pain syndrome' be added to the listings. Likewise, "illness behavior" should be neither a diagnosis nor a listing.' (Osterweis et al 1987). Thus, the Committee recommended that the complaint of chronic pain per se, in the absence of a specific diagnosable physical disease or mental disorder, should not be accepted as a cause of work incapacity leading to entitlement to disability benefits.

CHRONIC PAIN, COMPENSATION AND PSYCHIATRIC DIAGNOSIS

Psychiatrists are very frequently asked to assess patients with chronic pain complaints whose subjective description of pain severity, and the extent of alleged disability, cannot be explained on the basis of objectively demonstrable organic abnormality. Such is often the case when litigants or compensation recipients with chronic pain are referred for psychiatric examination and the question is posed as to whether the individual is suffering from a mental disorder which could 'explain' the complaint of persistent pain.

The 'classification of chronic pain' published by the International Association for the Study of Pain (IASP) (Merskey 1986) recognises 'pain of psychological origin' (Code I-16) resulting from three different mechanisms: through chronic muscle tension; delusional or hallucinatory pain, and hysterical or hypochondriacal pain. Muscle-tension pain of psychological origin is defined as 'virtually continuous pain in any part of the body due to sustained muscle contraction and provoked by emotional causes or by persistent overuse of particular muscles'. Delusional or hallucinatory pain of psychological origin is defined as 'pain of psychological origin and attributed by the patient to a specific delusional cause'. Finally, the IASP classification defines hysterical or hypochondriacal pain as being 'specifically attributable to the thought processes, emotional state or personality of the patient in the absence of an organic or delusional cause or tension mechanism'.

It may be that the patient has pain associated with a clinically significant psychiatric disorder such as major depression; if such is the case, with appropriate treatment, the depression and pain resolve. More commonly the patient may have some symptoms which overlap those found in mental disorders, such as sleep disturbance or dysphoria, but the nature of the psychiatric symptoms elicited and the findings on mental state examination do not warrant the formal diagnosis of a specific mental disorder such as a depressive illness, a generalised anxiety disorder or a psychotic condition.

In the absence of a specific mental disorder which could explain the presence of pain which cannot be attributed to a demonstrable organic lesion, or which is disproportionate to the extent of any objectively demonstrable pathology or evidence of continuing physical injury, clinicians may use a variety of terms such as 'psychogenic pain disorder' (American Psychiatric Association 1980), 'somatoform pain disorder' (American Psychiatric Association 1987), or 'learned pain behaviour' (Tyrer 1986). Although there had been considerable disagreement in the psychiatric literature as to whether pain can be legitimately considered to be a conversion symptom, the work of Engel (1959), Walters (1961) and Merskey (1965) has led to the general acceptance of that view.

The clinical entity of psychogenic pain disorder was introduced in the Diagnostic and Statistical Manual of Mental Disorders, third edition published in 1980 (DSM-III, American Psychiatric Association 1980), with the following diagnostic criteria:

1. Severe and prolonged pain is the predominant disturbance.
2. The pain presented as a symptom is inconsistent with the anatomical distribution of the nervous system; after extensive evaluation, no organic pathology or pathophysiological mechanism can be found to account for the pain; or, when there is some related organic pathology, the complaint of pain is grossly in excess of what would be expected from the physical findings.
3. Psychological factors are judged to be aetiologically involved in the pain, as evidenced by at least one of the following:
   a. a temporal relationship between an environmental stimulus that is apparently related to a psychological conflict or need and the initiation or exacerbation of the pain
   b. the pain's enabling the individual to avoid some activity that is noxious to him or her
   c. the pain's enabling the individual to get support from the environment that otherwise might not be forthcoming.
4. Not due to another mental disorder.

In the revised edition of DSM-III published in 1987 (DSM-III-R, American Psychiatric Association 1987), the term psychogenic pain disorder was omitted, and instead the 'new' clinical entity of somatoform pain disorder was introduced with the following diagnostic criteria:

1. Preoccupation with pain for at least 6 months.
2. Either (a) or (b):
   a. appropriate evaluation uncovers no organic pathology or pathophysiological mechanism (e.g. a physical disorder or the effects of injury) to account for the pain
   b. when there is related organic pathology, the complaint of pain or resulting social or occupational impairment is grossly in excess of what would be expected from the physical findings.

The specified diagnostic criteria for somatoform pain disorder are unsatisfactory, as they do not require the presence of any specific psychiatric findings and are merely based on the absence of an adequate organic basis for the 'preoccupation' with pain. It has been one of the tenets of clinical psychiatry that a conversion disorder (or hysteria, to use the older term) cannot be diagnosed simply because the symptoms and signs manifested by the patient cannot be explained by an organic cause at the time the diagnosis is made. In the absence of some specific psychiatric findings which can explain the individual's complaints, the diagnosis of hysteria frequently has been demonstrated to be incorrect on follow-up (Slater 1961). The term 'preoccupation' itself is vague and not defined in this context; the diagnostic criteria do not require the individual specifically to experience pain, as had been the case with psychogenic pain disorder.

Although the more detailed diagnostic criteria for psychogenic pain disorder appear more satisfactory than those for somatoform pain disorder, in the assessment of compensation claimants with chronic pain, the use of the former diagnosis is of limited, if any, utility in explaining the persistence of pain complaints and pain behaviour. It is very infrequent for such a patient to acknowledge the presence of any preinjury emotional problems or psychological conflict which could 'explain' the persistence of disproportionate pain and resultant disability following the injury. In the absence of any understandable intrapsychic basis for the 'psychogenesis' of chronic pain, it is usually postulated that the pain persists beyond the usual duration of healing because of environmental factors which reinforce the pain complaints and pain behaviour, that is, criteria 3b and 3c of those listed above.

For that reason, in the context of the psychiatric evaluation of a patient with chronic pain – where the pain cannot be attributed to a physical lesion – in a medicolegal setting, it is inaccurate to make the diagnosis of psychogenic pain disorder, which is a mental disorder, unless there is some specific evidence of preexisting intrapsychic conflict or psychological disturbance. In such a situation the presentation of a somatic complaint (i.e. pain) allows the individual to avoid acknowledging and dealing with the conflict and thus also avoid the experience of anxiety which that would provoke (primary gain). For that reason, in my view, the term 'learned pain behaviour' (Tyrer 1986) provides a more accurate description of the psychological mechanisms which lead to the persistence of pain following an injury in compensable circumstances. Tyrer has described factors which promote pain complaints and pain behaviour, such as sympathetic attention from those of importance to the individual or permission to avoid unpleasant activities. Block et al (1980) have demonstrated empirically that patients with 'sympathetic spouses' showed more marked pain behaviour when they were told that the spouse was observing the interview through a one-way mirror. In general, other such environmental factors which may reinforce pain behaviour include the availability of medications prescribed on a 'pain contingent' basis as well as, in some cases, availability or entitlement to 'pain contingent' compensation benefits. Such factors which tend to promote pain complaints and pain behaviour have been termed 'secondary gains'.

Finally, 'tertiary gain' which may also perpetuate pain

complaints is that which is obtained by others in the patient's environment who obtain some form of benefit from the patient's continuing sick role (Dansak 1973). Tertiary gain may accrue to spouses, children and relatives of the patient, as well as to that individual's medical and paramedical attendants and lawyers (Bokan et al 1981). Westin & Reiss (1979) have commented that a family which is 'fearful, suspicious or highly competitive' may undermine a rehabilitation programme, and have emphasised the need to identify such families and design intervention strategies which will minimise the risk that such a family may adversely affect the patient's progress towards recovery.

Bayer (1985) has provided an illuminating discussion of the mechanisms of self-deception in patients with pain of nonorganic origin, discussing patterns of abnormal illness behaviour shown by such patients in relation to cognitive dissonance theory. This approach also helps to explain the mental processes which lead to disproportionate disability among individuals who have no or minimal discernible physical basis for the complaint of pain. It is also noteworthy that dissatisfaction with the concept of psychogenic pain disorder led Stoudemire & Sandhu (1987) to recommend that the term 'idiopathic pain syndrome' be introduced, as this made no aetiological assumption concerning the origin of pain complaints which could not be explained on the basis of a demonstrable physical lesion.

The term somatoform pain disorder which was introduced in DSM-III-R has also been considered unsatisfactory, and this led to the suggestion that the next edition of DSM introduce a new diagnostic category of 'pain disorder' with four subtypes (King & Strain 1992). The proposed criteria for 'pain disorder' are 'first, that pain in one (or more) anatomical site(s) is a major part of the clinical presentation, and, second, that the pain causes significant impairment in occupational or social functioning or causes marked distress'. The four suggested subtypes are 'psychological type, secondary type due to nonpsychiatric medical condition, combined type and unspecified type'. The introduction of these proposed subtypes, as indicated by the authors, is likely to perpetuate the problem of deciding whether the pain disorder is properly classified as 'psychological' or 'combined' and the inclusion of the subtype 'secondary due to nonpsychiatric medical condition' in what is a diagnostic manual of mental disorders is also likely to cause some difficulty.

In the area of psychiatric diagnosis of chronic pain patients in receipt of, or seeking, compensation, lies also the question frequently asked of the psychiatrist by solicitors or insurance agents, namely 'Does this person have real pain or is he or she malingering?' The recent introduction of technological equipment in an attempt to assess impairment 'objectively' has given rise to claims that such equipment can be used to 'catch malingerers'. It needs to be emphasised that malingering is not a medical or psychiatric diagnosis, but an act which is properly assessed by a tribunal or a court of law. Jayson (1992) has shown that, in relation to low-back pain, dynamometric techniques which may indicate that a submaximal effort has been made cannot be used as 'the final arbiter' of malingering. Poor motor performance due to submaximal effort on dynamometry among patients with low-back pain may be due to a failure to understand instructions about the nature of the examination, nociception provoked by movement (and as such distinguished from the patient's experience of low-back pain), anxiety due to the test situation, depression, fear of pain and what can be termed 'unconscious symptom magnification' (Hirsch et al 1991). These authors have also shown that patients with a high Waddell score, indicating the presence of nonorganic signs on physical examination, tend to have a lower performance on lumbar dynamometry.

DISCUSSION

The studies concerning the relationship between chronic pain and compensation, reviewed above, indicate that:

1. There is no support for the view that compensation recipients, including those with chronic pain, have a specific 'condition' frequently labelled compensation neurosis.
2. The prevalence of chronic pain complaints is positively correlated with compensation systems which provide pain-contingent benefits and allow litigation at common law, and the rate and duration of claims is influenced by the level of compensation payments.
3. Compensation and litigation often have an adverse effect on treatment response in chronic pain, but this effect is modified by work and by the provision of specific treatment programmes.
4. There is no evidence to support the view that chronic pain patients – as a group – involved in litigation or receiving compensation describe their pain as more severe or more distressing than similar patients with pain which is not compensable.

The studies by Balla (1982), Carron et al (1985) and Mills & Horne (1986) have demonstrated that the assessment of chronic pain patients needs to take into consideration societal expectations, and that attitudes to illness and illness behaviour must also be considered. The impact of the compensation system and of litigation on the process of becoming a chronic-pain patient has important social policy implications which thus far have been generally neglected by governments and by policy-makers.

The studies comparing the pain description by litigants with that by nonlitigants do not support the frequent assertion that – as a group – patients claiming compensation describe their pain as more severe than a comparable group of pain patients not seeking compensation payments. The only study to find a significant difference between the two groups was that by Leavitt et al (1982), who found that litigants with objective evidence of injury, and free of significant psychological disturbance, reported more intense sensory discomfort. The authors suggested this may have been the result of overemphasis on the symptoms of the actual initial injury among patients who may have considered that the injury was 'not regarded with sufficient seriousness by the employer'.

There is also no support for the view that litigants with chronic pain are significantly more psychologically disturbed than similar patients not claiming compensation (Mendelson 1984). This finding contradicts the view that patients involved in litigation develop the putative psychiatric condition termed 'accident neurosis' or 'compensation neurosis', as these patients could not be distinguished on psychometric testing from those not seeking compensation. Dworkin et al (1985) have specifically commented on the deleterious effect of using such labels, which have no clinical validity.

The above findings suggest that the effect of compensation on chronic pain complaints and disability can best be conceptualised as occurring at an unconscious rather than a conscious level, as do other secondary gains which tend to perpetuate psychogenic symptoms. These factors have been well reviewed by Merskey (1979). For that reason the simplistic notion of 'compensation neurosis' as a 'state' which is totally reversible once the claim is finalised is invalid. Emotional factors which perpetuate psychogenic symptoms also lead to other changes in the individual's level of functioning and, once established, can perpetuate the symptoms after litigation has been finalised. This emphasises the need to carefully evaluate each litigant with chronic pain to assess the relative importance of compensation and other factors and to avoid stereotyping or labelling litigants as universally motivated by potential financial gains.

Weijel (1974) has examined the relationship between social security systems in affluent countries and illness behaviour. He noted that among the many factors which might determine an individual's presentation of somatic complaints to a doctor are 'decreasing vitality, early ageing, inability to keep up the pace of work, shift-work or piece work, insufficient vocational training, character disturbances, problems originating in the working environment or at home' as well as disease. If the social matrix and the shared belief system of the patient and doctor promote the attribution of somatic complaints to the adverse effects of work, then the stage is set for a compensation claim or litigation.

In considering the social policy implications of the interaction between chronic pain complaints, compensation payments and litigation, it is relevant to note that the studies reviewed above indicate that where litigation and/or continued receipt of compensation payments are pain-contingent, the complaint of chronic pain may become the 'badge' of alleged continuing work incapacity and, as such, resistant to treatment. Most compensation systems are adversarial in nature, and the resultant combination of anger, resentment, bureaucracy, entitlement attitudes and peer-group expectations creates a climate in which the complaint of chronic pain may persist long after any possible initial physical cause has resolved.

In the evaluation of pain-related impairment for medicolegal purposes, there is still no generally accepted rating scheme which would provide a reproducible and valid score based on physical and psychiatric examination. The multiaxial approach described by Turk et al (1988) does not as yet provide for a rating system of impairment which could be used to meet legal and administrative requirements in situations where rating of permanent impairment is necessary to establish entitlements to benefits.

As noted above, the Committee on Pain, Disability, and Chronic Illness Behaviour of the Institute of Medicine has stated that '. . . "chronic pain" alone should not be added to the SSA [Social Security Administration, USA] regulatory listing of impairments that allow a presumption of disability, nor should "chronic pain syndrome" be added to the listings' (Osterweis et al 1987). Thus, if this principle is to be followed in the medicolegal evaluation of impairment due to chronic pain, one of the essential 'axes' in the assessment process would be the rating of any specific diagnosable underlying physical or mental disorder, without which pain-related impairment would not entitle the individual to compensation or other benefits.

In the diagnostic evaluation of patients with chronic pain seeking compensation, in the absence of an objectively demonstrable organic lesion or evidence of continuing physical injury which could explain the persistence of pain, diagnoses such as psychogenic pain disorder are problematic.

Dworkin (1991) has cogently discussed the limited current understanding of factors responsible for the 'psycho-genesis of chronic pain'. His article highlighted the difficulties inherent in retrospectively attributing a causative role to factors which, although present in association with chronic pain complaints, may in fact be consequences of the experience of persistent pain. Dworkin's review is a useful reminder that we need to exercise caution in using a diagnostic term such as psychogenic pain disorder, which has certain specific aetiological implications.

This issue also has caused difficulty for courts which have to make decisions concerning entitlement to benefits, and contradictory judgments have been reported. In Carr v. Sullivan (1991), the applicant for social security benefits was successful on the basis of complaints of back pain where a diagnosis of 'somatoform disorder' had been made. However, in Miller v. Sullivan (1991) the court held that a claimant 'with back problems and degenerative disc disease' was not disabled 'despite his complaints of pain ... even though the treating physician declared the claimant to be totally disabled'.

A legal solution to this dilemma has been adopted by the Workers' Compensation Appeals Tribunal of Ontario (1987). In a lengthy decision on a pension application by a worker who had sustained some injuries when a wall collapsed, but whose subsequent chronic-pain complaints were described as predominantly psychogenic, the Tribunal held, in effect, that if pain which is considered to be psychogenic persists after a physical injury has resolved, the claimant would be entitled to benefits. It was noted that in the Tribunal's view 'a non-organic element in the chronic condition is compensable', and that '[T]he Tribunal determined that the injuries resulting from the fall were a significant contributing factor in the development of both the organic and the non-organic components of the worker's chronic pain condition'.

It might well be that rather than concentrate on the question of deciding whether or not work-related pain is 'organic' or 'psychogenic', more attention should be paid to factors which determine the reporting of pain in the workplace. Bigos et al (1991) have reported that, in a prospective study of 3020 subjects, those who had indicated lack of job satisfaction were 2.5 times more likely to report a back injury than those who had indicated that they 'almost always enjoyed' their job tasks. The results of this study potentially also have important implications for the understanding of factors which promote pain chronicity after the initial report of work-related low-back pain.

The finding that there has been a significant decrease in the rate of compensation claims for 'whiplash' and 'repetitive strain injury', as has occurred in Australia over the past few years, indicates that when societal validation of specific types of chronic pain complaints is withdrawn, the frequency of those clinical entities diminishes. These observations have important implications not just for pain clinicians and lawyers, but also for policy-makers, legislators and sociologists, and hopefully will in time lead to the development of innovative approaches to the management of work-related pain which minimises the likelihood of progression to disability and involvement within the compensation system.

REFERENCES

Accident Compensation Commission 1988 Annual Report 1987–88. ACC, Melbourne, p 23

American Medical Association 1988 Guides to the evaluation of permanent impairment, 3rd edn. AMA, Chicago

American Medical Association 1990 Guides to the evaluation of permanent impairment, 3rd edn revised. AMA, Chicago

American Psychiatric Association 1980 Diagnostic and statistical manual of mental disorders, 3rd edn. APA,Washington, DC

American Psychiatric Association 1987 Diagnostic and statistical manual of mental disorders, 3rd edn revised. APA, Washington, DC

Balla J I 1982 The late whiplash syndrome: a study of an illness in Australia and Singapore. Culture, Medicine and Psychiatry 6: 191–210

Barton N U, Hooper G, Noble J, Steel W M 1992 Occupational causes of disorders in the upper limbs. British Medical Journal 304: 309–311

Bartrip P W J, Burman S B 1983 The wounded soldiers of industry: industrial compensation policy 1833–1897. Clarendon Press, Oxford

Bayer T L 1985 Weaving a tangled web: the psychology of deception and self deception in psychogenic pain. Social Science and Medicine 20: 517–527

Bigos S J, Battie M C, Spengler D M et al 1991 A prospective study of work perceptions and psychosocial factors affecting the reporting of back injury. Spine 16: 1–6

Block A R, Kremer E F, Gaylor M 1980 Behavioral treatment of chronic pain: the spouse as a discriminative cue for pain behavior. Pain 9: 243–252

Bokan J A, Ries R K, Katon W U 1981 Tertiary gain and chronic pain. Pain 10: 331–335

Brooks P M 1986 Occupational pain syndromes. Medical Journal of Australia 144: 170–171

Cairns D, Mooney V, Crane P 1984 Spinal pain rehabilitation: inpatient and outpatient treatment results and development of predictors for outcome. Spine 9: 91–95

Carr v. Sullivan, 772 F. Supp. 522 (E.D. Wash. 1991)

Carron H, DeGood D E, Tait R 1985 A comparison of low back pain patients in the United States and New Zealand: psychosocial and economic factors affecting severity of disability. Pain 21: 77–89

Catchlove R, Cohen K 1983 Directive approach with workmen's compensation patients. Advances in Pain Research and Therapy 5: 913–918

Collie J 1913 Malingering and feigned sickness. Edward Arnold, London

Collie J 1932 Fraud in medico-legal practice, 2nd edn. Edward Arnold, London

Curran W J, Hall M A, Kaye D H 1990 Health care law, forensic science, and public policy, 4th edn. Little, Brown, Boston, p 16–17

Dansak D A 1973 On the tertiary gain of illness. Comprehensive Psychiatry 14: 523–534

Dworkin R H 1991 What do we really know about the psychological origins of chronic pain? American Pain Society Bulletin 1: 7–11

Dworkin R H, Handlin D S, Richlin D M, Brand L, Vannucci C 1985 Unravelling the effects of compensation, litigation, and employment on treatment response in chronic pain. Pain 23: 49–59

Engel G L 1959 'Psychogenic' pain and the pain prone patient. American Journal of Medicine 26: 899–918

Ferguson D 1984 The 'new' industrial epidemic. Medical Journal of Australia 140: 318–319

Ferguson D 1987 RSI: putting the epidemic to rest. Medical Journal of Australia 147: 213–214

Feuerstein M, Thebarge R W 1991 Perceptions of disability and occupational stress as discriminators of work disability in patients with chronic pain. Journal of Occupational Rehabilitation 1: 185–195

Fordyce W E, Brockway J A, Bergman J A, Spengler D 1986 Acute back pain: a control group comparison of behavioral vs. traditional management methods. Journal of Behavioral Medicine 9: 127–140

Fowler D R, Mayfield D G 1969 Effect of disability compensation: disability symptoms and motivation for treatment. Archives of Environmental Health 19: 719–725

Gore D R, Sepic S B 1984 Anterior cervical fusion for degenerated or protruded discs: a review of one hundred and forty-six patients. Spine 9: 667–671

Guest G H, Drummond P D 1992 Effect of compensation on emotional state and disability in chronic back pain. Pain 48: 125–130
Hadler N M 1992 Arm pain in the workplace: a small area analysis. Journal of Occupational Medicine 34: 113–119
Hammonds W, Brena S F, Unikel I P 1978 Compensation for work-related injuries and rehabilitation of patients with chronic pain. Southern Medical Journal 71: 664–666
Hazard R G, Bendix A, Fenwick J W 1991 Disability exaggeration as a predictor of functional restoration outcomes for patients with chronic low-back pain. Spine 16: 1062–1067
Hirsch G, Beach G, Cooke C, Menard M, Locke S 1991 Relationship between performance on lumbar dynamometry and Waddell score in a population with low-back pain. Spine 16: 1039–1043
Jamison R N, Matt D A, Parris W C V 1988 Effects of time-limited vs. unlimited compensation on pain behavior and treatment outcome in low back pain patients. Journal of Psychosomatic Research 32: 277–283
Jayson M I V 1992 Trauma, back pain, malingering, and compensation. British Medical Journal 305: 7–8
Kennedy F 1946 The mind of the injured worker: its effect on disability periods. Compensation Medicine 1: 19–24
King S A, Strain J J 1992 Revising the category of somatoform pain disorder. Hospital and Community Psychiatry 43: 217–219
Leavitt F 1990 The role of psychological disturbance in extending disability time among compensable back injured industrial workers. Journal of Psychosomatic Research 34: 447–453
Leavitt F, Garron D C, McNeill T W, Whisler W W 1982 Organic status, psychological disturbance, and pain report characteristics in low-back-pain patients on compensation. Spine 7: 398–402
McBride E D 1963 Disability evaluation and principles of treatment of compensable injuries, 6th edn. J B Lippincott, Philadelphia
Matheson L N, Ogden L D, Violette K 1985 Work hardening: occupational therapy in vocational rehabilitation. American Journal of Occupational Therapy 39: 314–321
Mayer T, Gatchel R, Mayer H, Kishino N, Keeley J, Mooney V 1987 A prospective two-year study of functional restoration in industrial low back injury: an objective assessment procedure. Journal of the American Medical Association 258: 1763–1767
Melzack R 1975 The McGill Pain Questionnaire: major properties and scoring methods. Pain 1: 277–299
Melzack R, Katz J, Jeans M E 1985 The role of compensation in chronic pain: analysis using a new method of scoring the McGill Pain Questionnaire. Pain 23: 101–112
Mendelson G 1983 The effect of compensation and litigation on disability following compensable injuries. American Journal of Forensic Psychiatry 4: 97–112
Mendelson G 1984 Compensation, pain complaints, and psychological disturbance. Pain 20: 169–177
Mendelson G 1987a Illness behaviour, pain and personal injury litigation. Psychiatric Medicine 5: 39–48
Mendelson G 1987b Measurement of conscious symptom exaggeration by questionnaire: a clinical study. Journal of Psychosomatic Research 31: 703–711
Mendelson G 1988 Psychiatric aspects of personal injury claims. C C Thomas, Springfield, Illinois
Merskey H 1965 Psychiatric patients with persistent pain. Journal of Psychosomatic Research 9: 299–309
Merskey H 1979 The analysis of hysteria. Bailliere Tindall, London
Merskey H (ed) 1986 Classification of chronic pain: descriptions of chronic pain syndromes and definitions of pain terms. Pain (suppl 3)
Miller H 1961 Accident neurosis. British Medical Journal 1: 919–925, 992–998
Miller v. Sullivan, 769 F. Supp. 1073 (E.D. Mo. 1991)
Mills H, Horne G 1986 Whiplash – manmade disease? New Zealand Medical Journal 99: 373–374
Moreno R, Cunningham A C, Gatchel R J, Mayer T G 1991 Functional restoration for chronic low back pain: changes in depression, cognitive distortion, and disability. Journal of Occupational Rehabilitation 1: 207–216
Morley A S 1914 Injuries of the back, considered from their medico-legal aspect. Transactions of the Medico-Legal Society 11: 1–19
Motor Accidents Board 1986 Statistics of persons killed or injured in road accidents occurring year ended 30th June 1985 for which claims were registered with the board. MAB, Melbourne
Nachemson A 1983 Work for all – for those with low back pain as well. Clinical Orthopaedics 179: 77–85
Ontario Workers' Compensation Appeals Tribunal 1987 Decision no. 915. Research Publications Department, WCAT, Toronto
Osterweis M, Kleinman A, Mechanic D (eds) 1987 Pain and disability: clinical, behavioral, and public policy perspectives. National Academy Press, Washington, D C, p 267
Parry L A 1911 Some cases under the Workmen's Compensation Act, and others of medico-legal interest. British Medical Journal 1: 989–992
Peck C J, Fordyce W E, Black R G 1978 The effect of pendency of claims for compensation upon behavior indicative of pain. Washington Law Review 53: 251–278
Peters J, Large R G, Elkind G 1992 Follow-up results from a randomized controlled trial evaluating in- and outpatient pain management programmes. Pain 50: 41–50
Phipson Nominees Pty. Limited v. French, 1988 Australian Torts Reports, 80–196
Pilowsky I, Spence N D 1975 Patterns of illness behaviour in patients with intractable pain. Journal of Psychosomatic Research 19: 279–287
Priestley v. Fowler 1837 3 M. & W. 1030–1033
Pryor E S 1991 Compensation and the ineradicable problems of pain. George Washington Law Review 59: 239–306
Robinson D D 1990 Occupations potentially appropriate for persons with low back pain (abstract). Pain (suppl 5): S394
Sander R A, Meyers J E 1986 The relationship of disability to compensation status in railroad workers. Spine 11: 141–143
Sindell D I, Perr I N 1963 Subjective complaints v. objective signs. Cleveland-Marshall Law Review 12: 42–58
Slater E 1961 Hysteria 311. Journal of Mental Science 107: 359–381
Slot G 1927 Pain in its medico-legal aspect. Transactions of the Medico-Legal Society 22: 74–91
Stoudemire A, Sandhu J 1987 Psychogenic/idiopathic pain syndromes. General Hospital Psychiatry 9: 79–86
Tait R C, Chibnall J T, Richardson W D 1990 Litigation and employment status: effects on patients with chronic pain. Pain 43: 37–46
Transport Accident Commission 1989 Third annual report, 1989. TAC, Melbourne
Turk D C, Rudy T E 1991 Pain and the injured worker: integrating biomedical, psychosocial and behavioral factors in assessment. Journal of Occupational Rehabilitation 1: 159–179
Turk D C, Rudy T E, Stieg R L 1988 The disability determination dilemma: toward a multiaxial solution. Pain 34: 217–229
Tyrer S P 1986 Learned pain behaviour. British Medical Journal 292: 1–2
Walters A 1961 Psychogenic regional pain alias hysterical pain. Brain 84: 1–18
Weijel J A 1974 The influence of social security in an affluent society on illness behaviour. Psychotherapy and Psychosomatics 23: 272–282
Westin M T, Reiss D 1979 The family's role in rehabilitation. Journal of Rehabilitation 45: 26–29
Wiesel S W, Feffer H L, Rothman R H 1984 Industrial low back pain: a prospective evaluation of a standardized diagnostic and treatment protocol. Spine 9: 199–203
Woden M, Dawkins P, Kenyon P 1987 Illness, injury and absence from work: an analysis of the health survey and other ABS data sources. National Institute of Labour Studies Inc., Adelaide, p 187
World Health Organization 1980 International classification of impairments, disabilities, and handicaps. WHO, Geneva

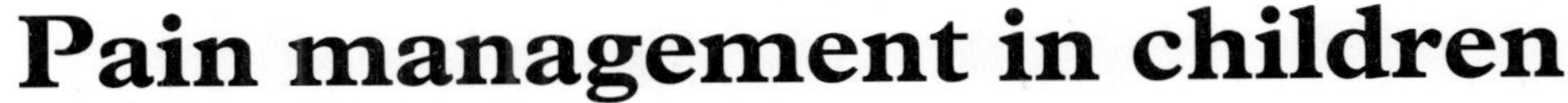

Pain management in children

79. Alleviating children's pain: a cognitive–behavioural approach

Patricia A. McGrath

INTRODUCTION

During the past decade, unprecedented scientific and clinical attention has focused on the special pain problems of infants, children and adolescents, so that there have been enormous advances in our understanding of children's pain perception and in our ability to alleviate their pain (for review see Ch. 41; McGrath & Unruh 1987; Ross & Ross 1988; Schechter 1989; McGrath 1990b; Tyler & Krane 1990; Bush & Harkins 1991; Schechter et al 1993). The myths underlying our treatment of children's pain have been refuted. We now know that children, like adults, can experience many different types of acute, recurrent, and chronic pain throughout their lives. We recognise that infants perceive pain at birth and that the failure to alleviate their pain has adverse physiological effects, in addition to the suffering that they experience. We know that children with severe pain require potent analgesics for pain relief, and that the fear of addiction associated with opioid analgesia in children has been unduly exaggerated. We know that children can describe their pain qualitatively, using language that reflects their own experiences and that they can rate their pain quantitatively using a variety of standardised scales. Yet the most remarkable advance (due to its important implications for pain management) has been our gradual realisation that the system that mediates children's pain perceptions is a marvel of subtlety and complexity.

Children's nociceptive systems function as active integrative mechanisms, not as fixed and rigid systems that passively relay pain information. The neural responses initiated by tissue damage can be modified by a diverse array of physical and psychological factors, so that children can experience very different pains from the same type of tissue damage. Therefore, the concept that guided much of the past management of children's pain – namely, that a child's pain is simply and directly proportional to the nature and extent of tissue damage – is no longer credible. Instead, a child's age, sex, developmental level, prior pain experience and relevant contextual and psychological factors will affect how his or her nociceptive system responds to tissue damage. We now know that we cannot completely control a child's pain by gearing our interventions solely to the source of tissue damage. Instead, we must also control the primary physical and psychological factors that affect a child's nociceptive processing.

Optimal pain control for children requires a dual focus on appropriate analgesic selection and administration, in relation to the intensity and source of tissue damage and on selective modification of all factors that exacerbate their pain, regardless of the primary pain source. Adequate analgesics should be administered at regular dosing intervals and should be complemented by a consistent cognitive–behavioural approach (see Ch. 81). This chapter delineates the relevant factors that exacerbate children's acute, recurrent and chronic pain, describes some practical physical, cognitive and behavioural interventions to modify these factors and thereby lessen children's pain and presents information on how to routinely integrate these interventions into a cognitive–behavioural approach for clinical practice. The emphasis is on a practical approach for optimally controlling children's pain from a multidimensional perspective, consistent with the neural and psychological mechanisms that mediate their pain.

THE COMPLEXITY AND PLASTICITY OF CHILDREN'S PAIN PERCEPTION

Like adults, children's nociceptive systems have the capacity to respond differently to the same amount of tissue damage. Children's pain perception depends upon complex gating mechanisms, where impulses generated by tissue damage are modulated by both ascending systems activated by innocuous stimuli and descending pain-inhibitory systems activated by varied environmental and psychological factors (Basbaum & Fields 1984; Wall 1984; Willis 1985; McGrath 1990b; Price 1988; Fitzgerald & Anand 1993). Much research has been conducted to identify the critical factors that activate this system (Lewis 1942; Beecher 1956, 1959; Zborowski 1962; Collins

1965; Hilgard 1969; Johnson et al 1970, 1971; Melzack 1973; Barrell & Price 1975; Weisenberg & Tursky 1976; Weisenberg 1977, 1984; von Graffenried et al 1978; Craig 1980; Dubner et al 1981; Hayes et al 1981; McGrath et al 1981; Thompson 1981; Watkins & Mayer 1982; Craig et al 1984; Price 1984, 1988; Dworkin et al 1986; Duncan et al 1987; McGrath 1993). Comparable results from physiological studies on nociceptive mechanisms in monkeys and from parallel psychological studies on pain perception in adults confirm that several situational, behavioural and emotional factors modify both the neuronal responses as well as the pain evoked by a constant noxious stimulus. Furthermore, subsequent research studies and clinical reports indicate that children's pains are modified by these same factors (Johnson et al 1975; Peterson & Shigetomi 1981; Siegel & Peterson 1981; Beales 1983; Beales et al 1983; Jay et al 1985; McGrath & deVeber 1986; Katz et al 1987; Ross & Ross 1988; Kavanagh et al 1991; Routh & Sanfilippo 1991; McGrath 1993). Moreover, a child's pain may be even more plastic that that of an adult and, therefore, easier to modulate by altering relevant context-specific factors (McGrath 1990b).

A model depicting the diverse array of factors that affect children's pain perception is shown in Fig. 79.1. A noxious stimulus initiates a sequence of neural events that may lead to pain, but many factors can intervene to alter the sequence of nociceptive transmission and thereby modify a child's pain perception. Children vary in sex, age, cognitive level, previous pain experience, family and cultural background (shown in the closed box). These child characteristics represent relatively stable influencing factors and shape how children generally interpret the various sensations evoked by tissue damage. In contrast, the situational, behavioural and emotional factors (listed at the top of the figure) vary dynamically depending on the context in which a child experiences pain. These context-specific factors exert a profound impact on children's pain. What children understand about the tissue damage, how they and their parents behave and how they feel all affect their pain. These factors mutually influence one another to modify a child's pain through complex interactions that occur at spinal and supraspinal levels in the nociceptive system. Context-specific factors can account for why the same tissue damage can evoke different pains and can partially explain why the effectiveness of proven analgesic interventions (pharmacological and nonpharmacological) may vary among children and vary for the same child at different times.

Situational factors refer to the particular combination of psychological and contextual factors that exist in a specific pain situation (McGrath 1983, 1990b; Ross & Ross 1988). They represent a unique interaction between the child experiencing pain and the context in which the pain is experienced. These include children's understanding about the pain source, their expectations regarding the quality and intensity of pain sensations, their ability to control what will happen, their primary focus of attention, their ability to use a pain-reducing strategy and the relevance or meaning of the pain to them. Situational factors vary extensively not only for different children experiencing the same tissue damage, but also for the same child experiencing the same tissue damage at different times.

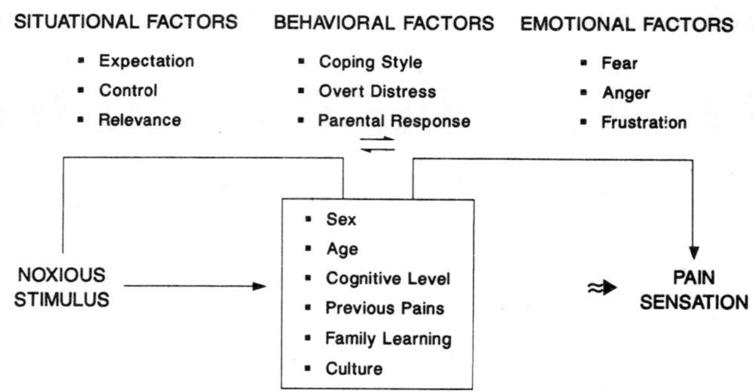

Fig. 79.1 A model of the situational, behavioural, and emotional factors that modify a child's pain perception. (From McGrath 1990a with permission.)

Multiple aspects of a child's behaviours are encompassed by the term 'behavioural factors'. These include children's overt behaviours when they experience pain (e.g. crying, grimacing, modifying their posture) and their parents' or health staff's behaviours in response to children (e.g. providing comfort and reassurance, administering medication, encouraging children to maintain normal activities). The term also refers to the effects of prolonged or recurrent pain on children's lives, including their ability to attend school, participate in sports and social activities with peers and assume typical family and household responsibilities. Like situational factors, behavioural factors share a powerful modulating role in children's pain. Some behaviours promote a healthy recovery, while other behaviours may initiate, exacerbate or maintain children's pain.

Children's emotions affect their ability to understand what is happening, their ability to cope in a particular situation, their behavioural responses and subsequently, their pain experience. Children's emotional reactions to pain may vary extensively from a relatively calm acceptance to fear, anger, anxiety, depression, or frustration. In general, the more fearful and anxious a child is, the stronger and more unpleasant the pain. Moreover, children's emotions are influenced by the myriad situational factors described previously. When children lack understanding, control and positive coping behaviours, their emotional distress increases and their pain intensifies.

Since its inception in 1983, the dual focus of the pain clinic at the Children's Hospital of Western Ontario

(CHWO) has been to evaluate and treat children's pain from the theoretical perspective depicted in Fig. 79.1. The sources of nociceptive activity are determined, relevant contributing factors are identified and then the most appropriate pharmacological and nonpharmacological interventions are administered. Some common contributing factors for acute treatment-induced pain, recurrent pain syndromes, and chronic pain have been identified from the many pain assessments conducted throughout the past decade. Although each child with pain experiences a unique set of physical, psychological, social, and emotional changes, Table 79.1 lists the typical factors that must be addressed to fully control their pain (McGrath 1993). This list provides a convenient reference for controlling pain in relation to the child experiencing it, rather than as an entity apart from the child.

COMMON FACTORS THAT EXACERBATE CHILDREN'S PAIN

SITUATIONAL FACTORS

Acute pain signals a warning about physical injury, so that the pain generally has an adaptive biological significance. Children do not usually experience any prolonged emotional distress because the pain diminishes progressively as the injury heals. They perceive their pain more as the occasionally inevitable result of daily activities than as something to fear. They quickly learn that the cause of their pain is physical damage, often easily visible, that their pain is relatively brief, and that many interventions can alleviate their discomfort. Children usually have accurate age-appropriate information about acute pain and positive expectations for pain relief. They believe that they have some control because they have developed some pain-reducing strategies, such as seeking a parent for a special hug, cleansing and bandaging an injured area, or swallowing medication. The aversive significance is determined more by the actual pain intensity and by any disruption in children's normal activities than by concerns of continued pain and disability.

However, the situational factors present for acute treatment-induced pain are quite different (McGrath 1990b; Anderson et al 1993; Carr et al 1993). Children often believe that they have no control in a medical situation. They may be uncertain about what to expect, they may not understand the need for a treatment that will hurt, particularly if they do not feel sick, and they may not know any simple tools to use to help them cope with their anxiety and pain. In fact, children may be told how to cope during a painful treatment in a manner that makes the procedure easier for the adult administering the treatment, but that does not necessarily make it better for the children receiving the treatment. Children's lack of understanding about pain, their expectations of continued pain, their uncertainty about obtaining eventual pain relief, and their lack control over the pain are common situational factors for children experiencing acute treatment-induced pain (e.g. blood sampling, intramuscular injections, lumbar punctures), recurrent pain syndromes (e.g. headaches, abdominal pain, limb pain) and chronic pain (e.g. cancer, reflex sympathetic dystrophy, arthritis) (Beales 1983; Beales et al 1983; Ross & Ross 1988; McGrath 1990b, 1992). Few children and adolescents

Table 79.1 Common factors that increase children's pain perception

	Acute treatment-induced pain	Recurrent pain syndrome	Chronic pain
Situational			
Inaccurate information regarding:			
cause/sensations/treatment efficacy	S	A	U
Little perceived control	U	U	S
Few independent pain-reducing strategies	U	U	S
Aversive significance	U	S	A
Learned pain triggers	S	A	R
Behavioural			
Overt distress behaviours	U	S	S
Inconsistent parental responses	S	U	S
Prolonged physical distress	R	S	U
Limited physical activity	S	S	U
Limited peer and social activities	S	S	U
Emotional			
Specific anxiety and fear regarding:			
diagnosis/treatment	S	A	U
future implications	S	U	U
General anxiety/stress	S	U	S
Inability to identify and express emotions	R	U	R
High expectations for achievement	R	U	R

Note: A, always present; U, usually present; S, sometimes present; R, rarely present
(From McGrath 1993a with permission.)

Table 79.2 Objectives for a cognitive–behavioural programme

Pain assessment – evaluate factors that contribute to pain
Situational
Behavioural
Emotional
Familial
Education – child, parent
Nociceptive system
Pain control strategies
Treatment – equipment and rationale
Need for children's control
Behaviour – child, parent
Increase coping behaviours
Decrease anxiety increasing behaviours
Reduce overt distress behaviours
Clinic – staff awareness
Adequate analgesic medications
Improve predictability
Minimise waiting period
Encourage child to use pain strategies
Use consistent approach
Encourage active play preprocedures

(From McGrath 1990b with permission).

have an age-appropriate understanding of the source of their pain, probable contributing factors, and the rationale for the treatments they receive. Most children do not know any practical physical, behavioural or cognitive pain-reducing methods that they can use conveniently. Consequently, children often lack any independent control over the pain, intensifying their emotional distress.

Recurrent pain syndromes are chronic-like conditions in which otherwise healthy and painfree children experience frequent episodes of headaches, abdominal pains or limb pains (Apley et al 1978; Chutorian 1978; Barr 1981, 1983; Shinnar & D'Souza 1981; McGrath 1987; Rappaport & Leichtner 1993; Rothner 1993). Their pains are not symptoms of an underlying condition that requires medical treatment; instead, their pains are the disorder. However, parents and children often receive inconsistent information about pain diagnosis and prognosis from various specialists, with the result that their anxiety progressively increases as their expectations for a clear-cut aetiology and a favourable outcome decrease (McGrath 1990b). The absence of clearly defined external causes for the apparently unpredictable headaches causes parents to search for some environmental triggers; they tentatively identify certain foods, weather conditions and some of their children's normal activities as probable causes. Parents then become so anxious that these neutral events might cause a headache, that they focus undue attention on the children's activities in an attempt to isolate the children from these supposed pain triggers. Children's increasing anxiety about these triggers eventually evokes a painful episode, thus confirming their suspicions (Joffe et al 1983; Andrasik et al 1986). The longer children endure recurrent headaches, the greater the number of 'learned' or 'conditioned' pain triggers – stimuli that they believe cause their pains (McGrath 1990b). Children who experience recurrent headaches usually have extremely low expectations that any treatment will alleviate their pain and suffering; they lack practical independent strategies for reducing the painfulness of individual headaches and for coping with the syndrome. Instead, children assume an increasingly passive role, depending primarily on parents and rest, rather than learning how to actively modify the circumstances that evoke headaches. The unpredictable headaches, the uncertainty of eventual pain relief, a progressive tendency to assume a passive patient role and an increasing number of conditioned pain triggers create ideal circumstances for initiating new pain episodes and for exacerbating pain intensity (McGrath 1990b).

Children can experience various types of chronic pain caused by disease, injury and emotional distress (McGrath & Unruh 1987; Ross & Ross, 1988; McGrath 1990b; Walco & Ilowite 1991; Miser 1993; Olsson & Berde 1993; Shapiro 1993; Walco & Oberlander 1993). Although many of the situational factors described previously can exacerbate children's chronic pain, the most salient situational factor is probably the relevance or aversive significance of the prolonged pain and any accompanying disability. The impact of chronic pain is profound for children and their families; all aspects of a child's life are immediately and adversely affected. Parents are distressed by the condition and its implications for their child's future – the life-threatening potential (if any), continuing pain and progressive disability. Parents tend to emphasise the future consequences of the child's physical condition and the pain, whereas children are more preoccupied by the immediate consequences. The dynamics within the family inevitably change as chronic pain prevents children from pursuing their normal activities and as each family member adjusts to the altered circumstances. Children endure a prolonged period of physical disability, continuous pain and varied medical treatments.

Although most children receive accurate information about their disease and required treatments, few receive concrete information about their pain, the external and internal factors that can attenuate or exacerbate it, and effective nonpharmacological pain-reducing strategies. Thus, most children do not know simple interventions that they can incorporate into their daily activities to complement the medical management of their disease. Also, they do not know that prescribed pain-control treatments may vary in efficacy at different periods throughout their treatment due to variations in disease activity or in situational factors. Without this knowledge, children's (and parents') confidence in certain therapies can decrease, even though these therapies would effectively alleviate pain at another time period. Children's expectations that they will experience persistent pain, that they must rely exclusively on potent analgesic medication for partial pain relief, and that they will always live their lives differently from other children, create enormous emotional distress – distress that can exacerbate their pain and disability (Beales et al 1983a, 1983b; McGrath 1992, 1993). Similar to chronic pain in adults, children's chronic pain is complicated by decreased independence, reduced control and an uncertain prognosis.

BEHAVIOURAL FACTORS

Children learn about pain from their own experiences and from the responses of their parents and families. They learn how to communicate their distress to others through their words and their behaviours and they learn techniques to alleviate their suffering. Yet, some behaviours can intensify rather than alleviate children's pain. Generally, the more overtly distressed a child is, the greater his or her pain (Katz et al 1980; Jay et al 1983, 1985; Schechter 1985; McGrath & deVeber 1986; Kuttner et al 1988). Children with diseases or injuries requiring long-term medical management are at risk for developing progressively more pain-exacerbating behaviours throughout the course of their treatment, including overt distress behaviours during procedures (e.g. crying, tensing muscles) and more subtle changes in their daily activities (e.g. acting more aggressively toward siblings, withdrawing socially). Some distress behaviours during invasive procedures may reflect a child's underlying emotional distress, while other behaviours, particularly stalling, may represent a simple conditioned response. If parents or staff inadvertently reinforce children by delaying treatment or by inconsistent coaching, reassuring or coercing, then children will exhibit increasing distress so that they can delay aversive procedures.

Parents' behaviours are important determinants of children's behaviours when they experience pain, particularly when children experience repeated or prolonged pain – multiple invasive treatments, recurrent pain syndromes or chronic pain (Ross & Ross 1988). In particular, children with recurrent pains are at risk to develop heightened pain complaints and pain behaviours due to their parents' responses. Because parents do not receive any information about how to manage recurrent pain syndromes, they often respond inconsistently to children's pain complaints – providing excessive emotional and physical support during some pain episodes and suggesting that children should manage on their own during other pain episodes. The implicit message that children receive is that their pain or pain complaints need to be stronger to convince their parents that they need the maximum level of support. Some children gradually learn to exaggerate their complaints or to develop new symptoms so that they can gain their parents' attention (McGrath 1990b). Parents may inadvertently increase children's recurrent pains when they allow children to remain at home instead of attending school, encourage them to withdraw from potentially stressful sports or social situations and relieve them from their usual family responsibilities. These secondary gains may prolong the length of a pain episode or provoke new episodes when children are stressed. In addition, children's specific physical behaviours may exacerbate their pain intensity. Some children may tense specific muscle groups for extended periods, alter their usual sitting or standing posture or progressively restrict their physical activities because they are concerned that their normal physical movements or sports could trigger additional pain. Yet, the abnormal sensory input from these altered behaviours might actually increase their pain (McGrath 1990b, 1992).

Although chronic pain resulting from disease or injury causes prolonged physical and emotional distress for children, the nature of their distress has not been well documented. We do know that children's normal motions are restricted, with the degree of disability related to the extent of tissue damage. Their prolonged physical restrictions are probably the most relevant behavioural factors for these children. They may gradually withdraw from many activities with peers and from most physical sports. Since the major focus of children's social activities is school and play, children may then become isolated, frustrated, and anxious. As children's general physical activity and normal exercise decrease, abnormal sensory input may increase, producing concomitant increases in pain. This problem can be confounded by the responses of children's parents and siblings. Parents who encourage children to adopt passive patient roles, to behave differently than other children and to depend primarily on others for pain control, will undoubtedly create a situation wherein children's chronic pain is maximised. Parents who encourage children to resume as many of their normal activities as possible create a situation wherein children's pain should be minimised.

EMOTIONAL FACTORS

The aversive, unpleasant aspect of most childhood pain (i.e. acute pain caused by minor injuries during normal play) provides children with an unequivocal warning signal to teach them about potentially harmful activities. There are no prolonged emotional consequences from these 'protective' acute pains. However, acute pain evoked by serious injury, acute treatment-induced pain, recurrent pain syndrome and chronic pain share a distinctively aversive nature in that they all cause prolonged emotional distress to children and their families. Children can become anxious, frightened, frustrated, angry, sad and depressed – emotions that can exacerbate pain. And, as the pain continues, children's emotional distress intensifies, creating a steadily increasing pain–emotional distress–pain cycle (McGrath 1993b).

All children experience some anxiety, fear, and sadness incidental to their pain. Yet, children requiring repeated medical procedures are at risk to develop excessive fear and anxiety towards their diagnosed medical condition, invasive procedures, and the future implications of their condition (Katz et al 1980; Jay et al 1985; McGrath & deVeber 1986; Kuttner 1989; Zeltzer et al 1989; McGrath 1990b; Peterson et al 1990). Usually young children are affected more adversely by the immediate effects of the diagnosis – medical tests, treatments, hospitalisation, and separation from family – than by the future consequences of the disease. Older children are distressed by both the immediate effects and by the future implications for a normal healthy childhood and life. Parents may be overwhelmed with fear about the disease or injury, particularly the possibility of more severe complications or death. Parents' emotional distress as they adjust to their children's diagnosis can exacerbate children's own anxiety, and subsequently their pain.

Children with recurrent pain syndrome usually are extremely anxious about the true aetiology of their pain, the effectiveness of different drugs for alleviating painful episodes, and the future implications. For example, many children with recurrent headaches develop painful episodes in response to stressful situations – stress that they fail to recognise and are unable to resolve effectively (Leviton et al 1984; Apley 1975). Their pains remove them temporarily from the source of stress and may lead to some positive benefits through increased parental attention and decreased expectations of achievement. As a result, their bodies' pain responses to stress are gradually reinforced so that their headaches become involuntary protective reactions that recur in potentially stressful or aversive situations. As shown in Table 79.1, the inability to identify or express emotions is rarely present as a pain-exacerbating factor in children with acute treatment-induced pain or children with chronic pain, but is usually present in children with recurrent pain syndrome. These children are generally unable to identify typical stress-inducing situations and unable to recognise their bodies' reaction to stress. For example, children with recurring headaches did not differ in stress levels from children without headaches (Andrasik et al 1988), but they seem to respond differently to typical everyday stressors (Andrasik et al 1986). Many children with recurrent pains have not learned effective and practical responses that truly alleviate the source of anxiety. Instead, their emotions are suppressed and eventually released in pain episodes. As children learn to recognise and express their feelings, the frequency and intensity of their recurrent pain episodes decrease (McGrath 1987, 1990b).

Many children with recurrent pains have extremely high expectations for personal achievement in all aspects of their lives (e.g. scholastic, familial, sports), unlike children with other types of pain. They repeatedly set such high standards for themselves that they are not fully satisfied, despite consistently positive performance. They place excessive demands on themselves to achieve at progressively higher levels and frequently monitor their own performance, perceiving that they are not fulfilling their expectations. As a consequence, they are frustrated more readily by routine school and play activities than other children and subsequently are at risk to develop more stress-related somatic complaints.

Children with chronic pain feel anxious and distressed by their prolonged suffering. Medications may cause various adverse effects, including hair loss, nausea, limb aches, bloating, and some disfigurement. Children can become overly self-conscious about their physical appearance and their inability to participate in daily activities, so that they become ill at ease with their peers. They may withdraw socially because they anticipate negative reactions from their friends. Increased withdrawal and social isolation can exacerbate their pain. Children may eventually depend exclusively on their parents to support and entertain them, even though they continue to miss their friends and become increasingly sad. When their prognosis is uncertain, they may feel extremely anxious and frightened. Some children may become increasingly irritable and may act out by provoking arguments, disobeying parents and not completing assigned school work. Other children may outwardly cope with the pain and accept required treatments, but may actually suppress their true emotional reactions – anger, anxiety, or depression. These children then develop progressively more somatic complaints, as other outlets for their emotional expression diminish.

In summary, the gradual recognition that a child's pain is not simply and directly related to the nature and extent of tissue damage has profound implications for the management of children's pain. Clinical emphasis broadens from an exclusive focus on the source of tissue damage to a more comprehensive focus on the source of tissue damage and the relevant factors that modulate nociceptive processing. Inaccurate understanding, limited control, negative expectations of treatment efficacy, behavioural restrictions, prolonged physical distress, heightened fear and anxiety, can all increase children's acute pain, trigger or intensify episodes of recurrent pain and exacerbate chronic pain. Therefore, it is essential to mitigate their pain-increasing effects as part of any child's pain-management programme. Our current knowledge about the critical pain-modulating role of situational, behavioural, and emotional factors guides us to adopt a consistent cognitive–behaviour focus to control the factors that can exacerbate children's pain, regardless of the specific pharmacological and nonpharmacological interventions they receive.

CHILDREN'S PAIN CONTROL: EMERGING INSIGHTS FOR CLINICAL PRACTICE

Optimal pain control begins with a thorough medical examination and comprehensive pain assessment. They provide the foundation of an accurate differential diagnosis of a child's pain complaint, in relation to both the underlying physical trauma/condition which initiates activity in nociceptive afferents and the relevant factors that modulate nociceptive activity. When all initiating and contributing sources of nociceptive activity are identified, an effective treatment plan can be designed to manage adequately the child's condition and alleviate his or her suffering. For most moderate-to-severe pains caused by tissue damage, a treatment plan should include a primary pharmacological intervention, either analgesics or anaesthetics, plus a cognitive, physical, or behavioural intervention as outlined in Fig. 79.2 (McGrath 1992). Analgesics or anaesthetics attenuate nociceptive activity and often constitute the foundation for a child's pain

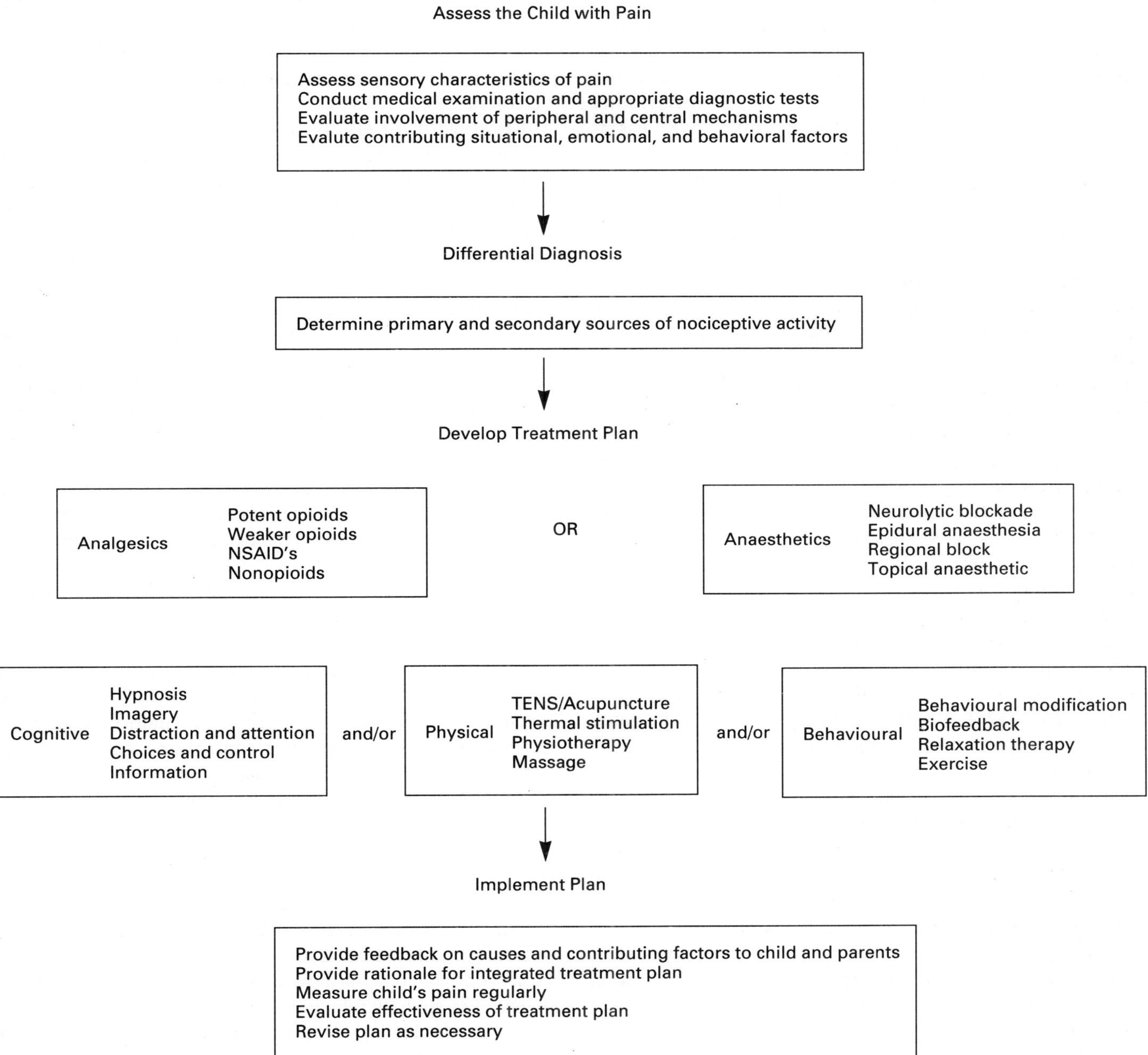

Fig. 79.2 A model of an integrated pharmacological and nonpharmacological approach for controlling a child's pain. (From McGrath 1992 with permission.)

management, but nonpharmacological interventions are required to mitigate the pain-exacerbating impact of situational, behavioural and emotional factors so as to fully alleviate a child's pain. The cognitive, physical, and behavioural interventions are listed in a manner similar to the analgesic ladder, in which the methods required to manage increasingly intense or more prolonged pains are listed in an ascending rank.

Nonpharmacological interventions are categorised according to whether they are focused primarily on modifying a child's thoughts and coping abilities, sensory systems, or behaviours. Although each of the interventions in Fig. 79.2 is listed within a principal category, the three categories are not mutually exclusive. Instead, most nonpharmacological methods vary in the particular combination of cognitive, physical and behavioural modulation that is involved. For example, hypnosis is considered primarily a cognitive intervention because children learn to reduce pain through their mental concentration, even though an hypnotic induction process often includes a behavioural component (muscle relaxation).

Cognitive interventions are probably the most important and versatile nonpharmacological pain therapies for children. Their understanding and expectations exert a powerful influence on their pain perceptions. Even though the provision of age-appropriate information about a pain source or instruction about a simple coping strategy has not been regarded as a specific cognitive intervention, each constitutes a practical, effective method for alleviating a child's pain and distress. In particular, accurate information about a pain source should be considered as an essential component of any child's pain management. Information enables health staff to increase children's understanding, their control, and the predictability of aversive events – whether they are specific treatments, seemingly unpredictable headaches or the natural pain fluctuations caused by chronic-pain disease. Thus, appropriate information reduces children's pain and emotional distress. Moreover, simple information about pain gates and about some pain-reducing strategies for children will further reduce their pain.

Distraction and attention, as well as guided imagery, provide practical tools for use in hospitals, clinics and homes. Unfortunately, distraction is often not used appropriately because health professionals have perceived it incorrectly as a simple diversionary tactic, in which a child passively focuses away from pain. The implication is that the pain is still there, but that the child is momentarily focused elsewhere. However, distraction and attention from pain – when the child's attention is fully involved in an activity or topic other than pain – is a very active process that can actually reduce the neuronal responses to a noxious stimulus. Children are not simply ignoring their pain, but are actually reducing it. Parents and staff can assist children to concentrate fully on something else besides their pain. Music, lights, coloured objects, toys and other children are effective 'attention-grabbing' stimuli for infants and young children; conversation, games, computers and interesting movies are effective diversions for older children and adolescents (Fowler-Kerry & Lander 1987; Ross & Ross 1988; Field 1990; McGrath 1990b). Imagery is a specific method to distract attention; children are guided to recall or vividly describe some previous positive experience, a story or a sensation, such as a numb sensation induced by a topical anaesthetic. The more vividly children imagine this positive experience, the less pain they experience. Hypnosis has successfully relieved anxiety, pain and distress in children with cancer, burns, migraine headaches, and haemophilia (LaBaw, 1973; Olness & MacDonald 1981; Varni et al 1981; Hilgard & LeBaron 1984; Kuttner, 1993).

Physical therapies include a variety of techniques to reduce pain by selectively stimulating non-nociceptive afferents or by generally stimulating different body regions. Children seem to naturally rub painful areas when they experience stubbed toes, muscle pain, stomachaches or acute pain after injections. They know that this physical stimulation relieves pain. Their knowledge enables staff to use simple physical interventions, such as deep rubbing and cold compresses, more routinely in clinical practice. Deep rubbing stimulates nonnociceptive afferents and is particularly beneficial before and after painful injections and to relieve sore muscles during headaches or stomachaches. Physiotherapy, simple stretching and conditioning exercises are valuable interventions for children with cancer, arthritis or any disease that prevents them from participating in normal activities (McGrath 1990b; Allen et al 1993). Their bodies may gradually lose flexibility as they withdraw from their accustomed physical activities. Other sources of pain may develop from the abnormal sensory input. Simple stretching exercises for 15 minutes prescribed four times per week can help children maintain their flexibility. Another benefit is that children are actively participating in their own pain-management programmes, improving their control and becoming less reliant on medications or parents for assistance.

Behavioural therapies for reducing children's pain typically consist of methods that are targeted at the children themselves or the adults that respond to them. Simple exercise and relaxation therapy provide convenient tools for most children experiencing acute pain during invasive treatments. At these times, children seem to naturally tense their muscles and hold their breath. However, when children consistently perform certain behaviours such as relaxing and loosening a fist, rhythmically moving a leg or deep breathing, they can sometimes naturally relax other body areas and then experience dramatic pain relief during invasive treatments. The benefits of physical exercise for promoting general health and alleviating stress have been well documented. Exercise is an important therapy for children with acute treatment-related, recurrent or chronic pain. An exercise programme is based on the sports and activities that are enjoyable and physically possible for children. The objective is to restore as many of the children's normal physical activities as possible in order to provide them with enjoyment, increase their participation in other events beyond their pain and help them to reduce stress. Generally children with recurrent and chronic pain improve both their physical health and mental outlook through an exercise programme. They become more involved in the world and less preoccupied with their pain. Exercise also helps to normalise any abnormal sensory input caused when children restrict body movements or physical activities. Although biofeedback, modelling, desensitisation, and operant conditioning are more specialised therapies, which are not routinely provided by health staff (McGrath 1992), their underlying principles can be adopted by all staff in their interactions with children. These are to increase children's physical activity, decrease their fear and anxiety, decrease their reliance on medication or parents for pain relief, reduce maladaptive pain behaviours, and thereby reduce their pain.

The majority of cognitive, physical, and behavioural methods for alleviating children's pain are used in conjunction with one another rather than independently. The term 'cognitive–behavioural' has evolved as the most appropriate description for a comprehensive approach to pain management, in which the primary objectives are:

1. to provide children with accurate information and realistic expectations about their pain
2. to improve their control by teaching them specific pain-reducing strategies
3. to modify any behaviours (child or staff) that intensify pain
4. to reduce a child's emotional distress by reducing the aversive significance or meaning of the pain to the child and family.

A COGNITIVE–BEHAVIOURAL APPROACH TO CLINICAL PRACTICE

Although some of the interventions described in the previous section are ideally suited for use with certain types of acute, recurrent or chronic pain, many interventions should be integrated into all clinical programmes for children, regardless of the specific source of noxious stimulation. Children's pain control should be enhanced when a consistent cognitive–behavioural approach is adopted throughout a hospital. Medical and health staff can modify the relevant environmental factors that exacerbate children's pain and can teach children several simple, effective pain-control strategies. The starting point for a consistent cognitive–behavioural approach should be a uniform attitude towards preparing children for aversive procedures. In most children's hospitals, it is common to observe many different approaches to inserting an intravenous line, administering an intramuscular injection or accessing a portacatheter site. The approaches vary in the extent to which children receive information about the specific sensations they might experience, hear the words 'pain' or 'hurt', are active, have choices, use pain-coping strategies or are physically restrained. Although some variation in approach may be due to differences among children, most of it is due to differences in the attitudes of the adults who conduct these procedures. Their approaches are based on their personal assumptions about what is best for children rather than on objective facts. Some adults believe that they should surprise a child with an invasive procedure, so that he or she cannot become overly distressed ahead of time, or that they should reassure a child that he or she will not hurt, even though the procedure will probably cause some pain. Some adults assume that it is best for all children to be distracted, while others may advocate that children should participate in any procedure when possible. Yet, regardless of discrepant personal beliefs, we already know that inaccurate expectations about what will happen during a treatment (lack of perceived control during noxious procedures, heightened fear and anxiety, lack of a simple pain-coping strategy, expressed parental fears and anxiety and physical restraints) can increase children's pain and distress. This knowledge alone should not only guide the way health professionals conduct painful procedures but also provide the foundation for a cognitive–behavioural approach in paediatrics to control the primary factors that exacerbate children's pain.

PAIN-CONTROL PROGRAMMES

After adequate pain control in all children is recognised as a primary objective for a children's hospital, an integrated pharmacological and nonpharmacological approach can then be developed to meet the specific requirements of different acute, recurrent, and chronic childhood pains (McGrath 1990b). Because all disciplines have a unique role in pain management, a cohesive programme requires an interdisciplinary approach. Each discipline (e.g. medicine, nursing, psychology, social work) should share in developing a comprehensive hospital-based, rather than a discipline-based, pain-control programme whose sole mandate is to provide adequate pain control in infants, children, and adolescents. Programme members would share the responsibility for identifying and resolving pain problems in the hospital environment (e.g. the place of analgesia during invasive procedures in neonates or in older children on certain cancer protocols). Interventions should be designed to integrate the skills and expertise of each relevant discipline, including subspecialists (e.g. neonatology, oncology). General hospital guidelines for analgesic and anaesthetic administration (described in Ch. 81) and guidelines for a cognitive–behavioural approach (as listed in Table 79.2) can be adopted. The educational and clinical components of a pain control programme must be practical so they can be easily implemented without disrupting staff.

Individual pain-control programmes begin with an objective evaluation of a child's specific pain complaint or the general pain problem within a particular medical setting. A thorough assessment is conducted to identify the specific factors that intensify pain from the perspective of all those involved – the child, parents, physicians, nurses and other relevant health professionals – because each person has a unique perspective on a child's pain problem. When the primary source of noxious stimulation is known (e.g. postsurgical trauma, chemotherapy effects), situational factors may be assessed during brief interviews or observations. When the source of noxious stimulation is not known (e.g. pain complaints in the absence of clear-cut tissue damage), systematic diagnostic investigations should be conducted concurrently with pain interviews. In order to illustrate how a consistent pain management approach may be adapted to meet the needs of children in all clinical areas, two programmes are presented that were developed in our pain clinic to address different pain problems from a cohesive framework – one for infants in the critical care unit and one for children receiving cancer treatments in the ambulatory clinic.

Much attention has focused recently on the special problems of assessing and controlling pain in infants, particularly newborns. Yet, few specific guidelines existed until relatively recently. In 1986 several concerns were raised about staff's ability to manage pain adequately in critically ill infants. In order to design an effective pain-management programme for those infants, it was essential first to survey the professional staff (medical and nursing) to identify the specific pain problems they confronted while treating infants. Staff were interviewed independently by a member of the pain programme to ensure that they could freely express all their concerns so that all pain problems would be identified.

The major concern was that infants' pain might not be adequately controlled during invasive procedures. There was a general lack of knowledge about infants' nociceptive systems, opioid pharmacokinetics and pharmacodynamics in newborns and infants and feasible methods of assessing pain in critically ill children. In order to address these issues, an education and research plan was implemented. Staff rounds focused on our improved understanding of the nociceptive system in infants, appropriate analgesic and physical interventions and the need to use available physiological data as distress measures for infants. Several specific questions, such as which intravenous site (scalp or arm) produces less stress for an infant, or does the infiltration prior to conducting a lumbar puncture in newborns cause more pain than the procedure alone, could not be answered without conducting randomised controlled trials. Thus, it was essential to collect baseline data on infants' normal distress responses, since most published information had been obtained from healthy infants. The Critical Care Unit has recently obtained this information (manuscript in preparation).

The second major focus of our pain-control programme is the management of acute pain produced during repeated medical procedures, particularly in children with cancer. Despite seemingly adequate sedation, appropriate analgesic administration and the increasing use of porta-catheters to reduce the number of intravenous insertions, many children with cancer continue to experience intense pain during invasive procedures, seemingly out of proportion to the tissue damage produced. Initial observational studies of our clinical population revealed that several situational, behavioural and emotional factors were responsible for the heightened pain, fear and anxiety experienced by the children (McGrath & deVeber 1986). These results led to the development of a structured congnitive – behavioural pain management programme to improve understanding and pain control in children by providing accurate age-appropriate information, by teaching them how to relax using guided imagery and progressive relaxation exercises and by restructuring negative sensations so that they could be more positive and therapeutic. Although the specific goals for each child depended on age, sex, previous experience and the major source of fear and anxiety, desensitisation procedures, guided imagery, hypnotic-like suggestions for analgesia, relaxation training and cognitive information on the purpose of each procedure were essential components of all children's pain control programmes.

The oncology programme is evaluated and updated every 2–3 years. At present, the programme focuses on structured behavioural management programmes for very young children (because staff and parents inadvertently reward their distress behaviours by delaying procedures), formal hypnosis (because it has proven more effective for adolescents) and a physical-exercise component for children suffering from treatment-induced bone or muscle pain. Specific pain-management tools have been refined on the basis of our improved understanding of children's pain perceptions, their ability to use different coping strategies and the emerging literature on the effectiveness of specific cognitive–behavioural interventions for children with cancer.

An effective cognitive–behavioural approach can be adapted within a hospital for the management of all pains in infants and children when there is an integrated emphasis on a comprehensive pain assessment, on the consistent application of available pain control methodology, and on an objective evaluation of treatment efficacy. The model in Figure 79.1 provides the framework for evaluating the primary factors that determine children's pain. After the relative contributions of these factors to a pain problem are assessed, a consistent management programme with the most appropriate pharmacological and nonpharmacological interventions can be developed to minimise a child's pain, regardless of the nature of the pain or the age of the child. The efficacy of the interventions must then be objectively evaluated and refined if necessary.

PRACTICAL METHODS FOR REDUCING CHILDREN'S PAIN

When possible, children should learn some simple methods to reduce their pain and distress. Even very young children can easily learn to use a variety of practical pain-control strategies. In fact, children seem more adept than adults at using nonpharmacological interventions, perhaps because they are usually less biased than adults about the potential efficacy of nondrug therapies. However, since adults teach children how to use these interventions, adult biases (either parents or staff) can weaken treatment efficacy. Therefore, staff must understand the rationale for a general cognitive–behavioural approach, as well as the rationale for the specific pain-reducing methods children will use. Pain-control strategies should be selected according to the type of pain, the child's age or cognitive level and the situational, behavioural, emotional and familial factors relevant for that child (as shown in Table 79.1). As children mature, they generally gain a better understanding of their pain, acquire more coping strategies and exhibit less overt behavioural distress. However, they may have learned some exaggerated or maladaptive pain behaviours. Their emotions vary from situation-specific fear and anxiety related to the immediate effects of pain and treatment to deep fear, anxiety or depression related to the future consequences of pain or their disease. Thus, children under 7 years old often require a behavioural-management component to reduce the number of overt distress behaviours and any learned pain behaviours, while many adolescents with recurrent or persistent pain require a counselling component to address the emotional effects of the disease, trauma or syndrome causing their pain. All parents should learn how their behaviours affect their children's pain, their expressions of pain and their abilities to cope with pain.

Pain-control strategies are based on the principal factors that contribute to children's pain problems rather than on the specific diseases responsible for their pain. These strategies are used in conjunction with the medical treatment of any underlying disease and with any prescribed pharmacological therapies. The emphasis of the pain-control programme shifts depending on whether the pain is acute, recurrent or chronic and the application of the programme shifts according to a child's age, cognitive level and family support. Individual differences among children, their families, and relevant situational factors require that all pain programmes should be flexible so that they can be adapted to the special needs of each child, family, and pain problem. However, the factors listed in Table 79.1 provide a framework for a consistent cognitive–behavioural programme with four major objectives:

1. to provide children and parents with accurate information about the pain problem in relation to nociceptive systems and the factors that modify pain perception
2. to alter the situational factors that usually increase pain – for example to reduce waiting time for invasive procedures (acute pain), to decrease excessive reliance on parents or medication for pain relief (all types of pain), to increase regular physical activities (recurrent and chronic pain) and to reduce anxiety-related or conditioned pain behaviours (all types of pain)
3. to improve children's control by teaching them simple ways to cope with or reduce pain
4. to encourage children to be actively involved in pain management, using a positive and consistent approach from staff and parents, with appropriate support for parents (McGrath 1990b).

TEACHING CHILDREN HOW TO REDUCE THEIR PAIN

Several general methods should be taught to each child so that he or she can develop a flexible repertoire of pain-coping strategies. The same strategy is often not effective for all occurrences of a child's pain, since the strength, quality, extent and unpleasantness of the pain undoubtedly vary. Emphasis should be placed on the children's attitudes towards reducing the pain rather than on the magical benefits of any one method. In essence, children should learn some principles of pain management so that they can naturally evolve their own techniques for reducing pain. They should not be encouraged to develop a false reliance on a particular pain-coping strategy. Children must acquire a rationale for controlling their pain based on the plasticity and complexity of their nociceptive systems.

Children with persistent pain or who require prolonged medical care should receive more in-depth, age-appropriate information about pain. Their parents should learn that the study of pain in children represents a relatively new area. Children and parents should learn that the nociceptive system is plastic and complex, that pain is not simply and directly related to the intensity of a noxious stimulus and that many environmental and internal factors can modify their pain perception. This information can be presented in a straightforward manner, with the emphasis on the concept of the plasticity and modifiability of neuronal coding rather than on the specific terminology or mechanisms. Figures 79.1 and 79.2 can be used to illustrate information in a concrete and tangible manner. Thus, parents learn that the spinal cord is a major site (or pain gate) for modifying nociceptive input, that internal opioid and nonopioid systems can be activated to inhibit pain and that several environmental and internal factors can activate these systems.

Two simple examples of pain modulation can be provided at a child's pain assessment. Children should learn that rubbing their fingers after a finger prick can help to lessen pain, because they are activating nerves that can partially close the pain gate. Even very young children understand that messages (voices on telephones, films on television, sounds on radios) are transmitted along wires and that the transmission can be blocked by other signals. Parents and children are then reminded that they may not feel pain from an injury (e.g., cut, scrape or headache) when their attention is focused on something other than the injury (e.g., an interesting show, a conversation, a sports activity). They are asked to describe situations from their own experience in which this has happened; they often cite injuries sustained during play.

The term 'situational factors' is introduced to teach families about the tremendous potential impact of contextual and situational cues for modifying children's pain. A figure depicting a wide-dynamic-range neuron's differential response to the same noxious stimulus presented in two different contexts, (signalled and nonsignalled) is used to demonstrate how situational factors alter neuronal responses and may reduce pain (Hayes et al 1981). Another figure is shown to illustrate the pain reduction produced when noxious stimuli are signalled to adult volunteers (Price et al 1980). Parents and children are asked to describe the implications of this research for children's pain, to help them understand that they can apply techniques of pain management. Figure 79.2 helps families to understand that nondrug therapies complement drug therapies and are selected and prescribed in a complementary manner. Using this format and these figures, information about the plasticity and complexity of the nociceptive system can be introduced in about 15 minutes so that families understand that their children's pain can be reduced by various methods in addition to directly attenuating the source of noxious stimulation.

Children can easily learn several methods for reducing their pain. The approach that has proven most beneficial in our clinic has been to teach children a few basic cognitive, physical and behavioural methods and then to encourage them to personalise these methods or to design new methods with their parents and families. Although some information about pain-reducing strategies is provided in the initial interview, children learn various pain-control interventions in relatively brief pain-management programmes, usually 4–12 sessions depending on the nature of their pain. The sessions are structured to enable children to achieve definite objectives throughout the course of the programme, beginning with the acquisition of standard pain-coping strategies and culminating in the design of a versatile repertoire of skills. The sessions are scheduled weekly for children referred for acute pain management, such as children who are receiving medical or dental treatments that evoke pain, while sessions are usually scheduled biweekly or monthly for chidren referred for recurrent or chronic pain management (depending on the frequency and intensity of their pain). Outpatients, who receive invasive procedures on a daily or weekly basis, require a pain-management programme that enables them to learn, practise, and refine their pain control strategies in the normal course of their treatment. Inpatients may require daily sessions depending on the factors affecting their pain or the number of invasive procedures they receive. Children with recurrent or chronic pain seem to respond to the programme better when sessions are scheduled monthly, which allows them sufficient time to practise management techniques.

Logical, age-appropriate rationales are presented to explain why these strategies should lessen their pain. Strategies which are easiest for all children to understand and use are taught in the first few sessions. Then, more abstract methods are gradually introduced as children master the concrete methods. In general, the younger the child, the more concrete the methods selected. Children first learn to rub their fingertips deeply and continuously after a finger prick to shorten and reduce any pain, because all children have already experienced acute pain from a finger prick. Most children remember that they have instinctively rubbed a painful body area to lessen the pain or that their mothers have massaged a painful site to reduce their discomfort. Pain reduction produced by physically rubbing the finger makes sense to them. They understand that the pain reduction is due to the physiological mechanisms that were described to them. Adolescents benefit when the relatively simple mechanism of rubbing is compared to the more complex mechanisms of acupuncture, to illustrate that some physiological mechanisms are common to both.

Another physical intervention provides the second pain strategy for children. The pain-reducing potential of a relaxed body state is taught to children through discussion, progressive muscle relaxation and biofeedback. Children easily distinguish between a tight tense fist and a relaxed open hand. They can visualise that it is harder to insert a needle (a concrete image for producing pain) into a tensed arm than a relaxed arm, with the probable result that the needle produces more pain in the tensed state. In fact, any type of pain could be intensified if the muscles are always tightened. Since fear or anxiety creates some body tension, children need to recognise when they are tense and learn to relax. Again, the need for altering a physical state that can exacerbate their pain makes sense to children so that they are motivated to learn how to control their bodies. Biofeedback is an excellent tool for teaching children how their bodies react to pain-inducing stimuli or stressful situations. Children watch or listen to their body responses and use deep breathing, progressive muscle relaxation, guided imagery or hypnosis to lower the amplified signals. Children select the methods that produce the most relaxation for them. They then attempt to use the same method when they are in pain or when they expect pain (medical procedures or the onset of a headache).

Some cognitive interventions are introduced as children learn these concrete physical interventions. Since children already understand the model in Figure 79.1, they then substitute the concepts of 'thinking, doing and feeling' in the model as positive factors that can reduce their pain. They help to select the thoughts, actions and emotions that they should have in order to manage their pain. Special attention is focused on children's ability to reduce pain by controlling their minds in a similar manner to how they learned to control their bodies. The most important feature is that they must concentrate fully on 'something else' such as a distracting situation (a story, a conversation, a cartoon) or an activity (singing a song, playing a game, assisting with the procedure).

The optimal use of cognitive pain interventions necessitates that children understand the importance of their full concentration. A practical auditory analogy has been useful in our programme. Children are reminded that they often do not hear when parents call them because they are concentrating on television or actively playing a game. In a sense, they selectively tuned out noises that weren't interesting or relevant to what they were doing. At this point in the session, we usually remind them to listen to the hum of the ventilation system. They are aware that the sound was present throughout the session, but that they really did not hear it throughout most of our discussion. They can learn to do a similar 'tuning out' with pain. The same distracting situation or activity will not be consistently effective for all children. Instead, children choose those techniques that facilitate their complete mental absorption. Their full concentration is the critical component for pain reduction, not the particular method they use to achieve it. Young children choose counting aloud, singing songs, squeezing a hand in proportion to the strength of any pain and describing parties, cartoons, trips and books as methods to absorb their attention during invasive procedures. Older children generally prefer conversations and hypnosis. Children with recurrent or chronic pain use primarily relaxation, induced by progressive muscle relaxation, guided imagery, music and exercise, to lessen their pain.

The analogy of tuning out sound is also useful in teaching children how to use cognitive intervention. The therapist tells a child, 'Imagine that you and I are watching a movie in a downtown theatre. Two people come in and sit in front of us. They are eating a jumbo box of popcorn and candies in crinkly plastic wrappers. They are making a lot of noise with their crunching and unwrapping. What if I told you not to pay attention to the noise that they are making, but to only concentrate on the movie?' Most children respond that if they tried too hard to block out the noise of the people eating, they would probably pay more attention to them than if they simply forgot them and watched the movie. We use this example to teach children that they should not constantly monitor how well their pain-reduction technique is working; they should simply use it when they are feeling pain and they can evaluate its efficacy with the therapist later.

The last cognitive interventions children learn are the more abstract methods of hypnosis or hypnotic-like suggestions for analgesia. As yet, there are no clear criteria to determine which children will benefit from these interventions. Instead, these techniques are introduced to most children. The common approach is to explain that their mind can move pain to different body areas, similar to the way they can attend to sensations in their arm, leg or head while ignoring sensations in other body areas. Children learn that this method is called hypnosis; adolescents receive more information about the hypnotic process and may participate in a standard induction procedure.

In our clinic, most of the pain-reduction children achieve from cognitive interventions derives from hypnotic-like suggestions for analgesia, rather than from a standard hypnotic-induction procedure. The term, hypnotic-like, refers to the fact that the suggestions are similar to those used to induce analgesia under hypnosis. Two familiar sensations provide a framework for explaining to children how these suggestions can lessen their pain. They have usually experienced tingling sensations followed by numbness due to a lack of circulation while sitting or sleeping or due to local anaesthetic at the dentist. So children can readily accept that they will not feel pain as strongly when different parts of their bodies fall asleep. Similarly, children with cancer, who have used EMLA (topical anaesthetic cream, eutectic mixture of local anaesthetics) benefit from imagining the same tingling and numb sensations produced by EMLA. Many children can learn to induce similar anaesthesia in different body regions. The loss of sensation associated with posture, novocaine or EMLA is a concrete experience that children remember. Their memories enable them to accept that physical pain reduction can be accomplished in a somewhat indirect, intangible manner, as well as by direct, tangible techniques. They learn that they can imagine a magic gas with properties similar to nitrous oxide sedation or a magic cream like EMLA so that they can numb a body region by imagining that it is going to sleep or is saturated with the cream. The usual sequence for introducing these suggestions is described below with typical instructions and coaching for a 5-year-old boy referred for acute-pain management.

'We know that your brain can shut off pain so that the injection won't hurt as much. But we don't know, yet, which method is best for you and the easiest for you to use. So, let's practise some today and we'll try them together during your next treatment. Okay?

First, you already said that you remember when the doctor froze your leg so that you wouldn't feel anything when he stitched your cut. Sometimes, you can produce that same freezing or numbing feeling by yourself, just by thinking very hard about how if felt. In fact, you can make your hand go to sleep as if the doctor made it numb. Would you like to try it? It might feel as if you had played in the snow too long without mittens or as if you put your hands in very cold water. There's a funny sensation that feels different to different people. What does it feel like to you?' (McGraw 1945; McGrath 1990b).

The specific examples depend on the child's past experience about what types of numbness they remember. If they do not have any memories of how pain may be blocked, even when their skin looks the same and they are alert, the therapist may use a local anaesthetic spray or cream to demonstrate a slight loss of pain sensation when it is applied. The cream is placed on the therapist's hand so that the child can observe and touch the skin. The therapist reports that the child's touch feels different (usually less strong and distinct) on that hand and encourages the child to try it on him- or herself. This demonstration provides children with a more concrete image of pain reduction produced by a quick and noninvasive method. Children can easily imagine altered sensations, which they generally describe as slightly more fuzzy, blurred or weak in comparison to the other hand. When a sharp object is gently placed on the skin, they might say that it feels blunt, while the same object placed on the other hand might cause a startle response. The therapist coaches children who are responsive to these suggestions to try to numb another body part in the same way or to move the numb area to a different site. The major goal is to enable children to numb the painful region. Another goal for young children is to encourage them to move the pain from the painful region to a neutral place, such as the therapist's hand, where the pain can then be shaken off when enough has accumulated. Children tell the therapist when to shake it off and sometimes, to stamp on it after it has been shaken onto the floor. Some children, including very young children and adolescents, respond almost immediately to these simple suggestions, while others are not able to adopt any of these suggestions for reducing their pain. Adolescents may benefit from a more adult approach with a standard hypnotic-induction technique, with encouragement to activate their own natural, endogenous opiate pain-inhibitory systems (Hilgard & LeBaron 1984; Olness & Gardner 1988).

These pain-control strategies may be used by children above 5 years of age to modify their acute, recurrent or chronic pain. The principles of pain management are consistent regardless of the children's age or type of pain. However, the particular methods for applying these principles depend on the type of pain, children's ages and parental support. Children from 3–5 years old benefit from a structured behavioural programme in which their use of a concrete pain-control tool (squeezing a hand, singing a song, conversing about a trip, breathing special calming air called 'magic sparklies') is rewarded to encourage them to use it, even if they do not understand the principle, and to encourage parents to assist children to cope more independently. Older children and adolescents usually adopt and refine these strategies with minimal encouragement from parents and staff.

CONCLUSION

A comprehensive pain-management programme evolves from a theoretical perspective in which a child's pain is regarded as a complex perception, usually initiated by tissue damage, but always modified by situational and emotional factors. A thorough assessment is conducted to identify the factors that intensify pain from the unique perspective of the child, parents, and relevant health professionals. A consistent management programme can then be developed to minimise children's pain by selecting the most appropriate analgesic or anaesthetic treatments to modify nociceptive input and selecting the most appropriate cognitive, physical, and behavioural interventions to modify the environmental and internal factors that modulate their pain perception.

The benefits of allowing children more choice, improved control, increased participation, and a better understanding of invasive treatments are revealed dramatically by reductions in children's overt distress, anxiety and pain. Most children can easily understand about 'closing their pain gates' and eagerly learn new methods to shut the gate to lessen pain. Although some children require special programmes from an experienced pain therapist, all children benefit from a general cognitive–behavioural approach in which the primary focus is to modify the contextual factors that exacerbate the neuronal activity initiated by a noxious stimulus. Unfortunately, few nonpharmacological interventions are used consistently for children, even though many represent practical, versatile, inexpensive and effective pain-reducing techniques that can be adopted within a short time.

In summary, children's pain control must be viewed from a multidimensional perspective because many factors contribute to a child's pain, no matter how seemingly clear-cut the aetiology. Since pain is not determined solely by the nature of the noxious stimulus, adequate analgesic prescriptions administered at regular dosing intervals must be complemented by a practical cognitive–behavioural approach to ensure optimal pain relief. The challenge of alleviating children's pain requires a dual emphasis on appropriate analgesic selection and administration in relation to the intensity and source of the pain, and on selective modification of the primary situational, behavioural, emotional, and familial factors that can exacerbate pain, regardless of the pain source.

REFERENCES

Allen J, Jedlinsky B P, Wilson T L, McCarthy C F 1993 Physical therapy management of pain in children. In: Schechter N L, Berde C B, Yaster M (eds) Pain in infants, children, and adolescents. Williams & Wilkins, Baltimore p 317–330

Anderson C T M, Zeltzer L K, Fanurik D 1993 Procedural pain. In: Schechter N L, Berde C B, Yaster M (eds) Pain in infants, children and adolescents. Williams & Wilkins, Baltimore, p 435–457

Andrasik F, Blake D D, McCarran M S 1986 A biobehavioral analysis of pediatric headache. In: Krasnegor N A, Arasteh J D, Cataldo M F (eds) Child health behavior: a behavioral pediatrics perspective. Wiley Interscience, New York, p 394–434

Andrasik F, Kabela E, Quinn S, Attanasio V, Blanchard E B, Rosenblum E L 1988 Psychological functioning of children who have recurrent migraine. Pain 34: 43–52

Apley J 1975 The child with abdominal pains. Blackwell, Oxford

Apley J, MacKeith R, Meadow R 1978 The child and his symptoms: a comprehensive approach. Blackwell, Oxford

Barr R G 1981 Recurrent abdominal pain. In: Gabel S (ed) Behavioural problems in childhood: a primary care approach. Grune & Stratton, New York, p 229–241

Barr R G 1983 Recurrent abdominal pain. In: Levine M D, Carey W B, Crocker A C, Gross R T (eds) Developmental–behavioral pediatrics. W B Saunders, Philadelphia, p 521–528

Barr R G 1989 Pain in children. In: Wall P D, Melzack R (eds) Textbook of pain, 2nd edn. Churchill Livingstone, Edinburgh, p 568–588

Barrell J J, Price D D 1975 The perception of first and second pain as a function of psychological set. Perception and Psychophysics 17: 163–166

Barrell J J, Price D D 1977 Two experiential orientations toward a stressful situation and their related somatic and visceral responses. Psychophysiology 14: 517–521

Basbaum A I, Fields H L 1984 Endogenous pain control systems: brainstem spinal pathways and endorphin circuitry. Annual Review of Neuroscience 7: 309–338

Beales J G 1983 Factors influencing the expectation of pain among patients in a children's burn unit. Burns 9: 187–192

Beales J G, Holt P J L, Keen J H, Mellor V P 1983a Children with juvenile chronic arthritis: their beliefs about their illness and therapy. Annals of the Rheumatic Diseases 42: 481–486

Beales J G, Keen J H, Holt P J L 1983b The child's perception of the disease and the experience of pain in juvenile chronic arthritis. Journal of Rheumatology 10: 61–65

Beecher H K 1956 Relationship of significance of wound to pain experienced. Journal of the American Medical Association 161: 1609–1613

Beecher H K 1959 The measurement of subjective responses: quantitative effects of drugs. Oxford University Press, New York

Bush J P, Harkins S W (eds) 1991 Children in pain: clinical and research issues from a developmental perspective. Springer-Verlag, New York

Carr D B, Osgood P F, Szyfelbein S K 1993 Treatment of pain in acutely burned children. In: Schechter N L, Berde C B, Yaster M (eds) Pain in infants, children and adolescents. Williams & Wilkins, Baltimore, p 495–504

Chutorian A M 1978 Migrainous syndromes in children. In: Thompson R A, Green J R (eds) Pediatric neurology and neurosurgery. Spectrum, Jamaica, p 183–204

Collins G L 1965 Pain sensitivity and ratings of childhood experience. Perceptual and Motor Skills 21: 349–350

Craig K D 1980 Ontogenetic and cultural influences on the expression of pain in man. In: Kosterlitz H W, Terenius L Y (eds) Pain and society. Verlag Chemie, Weinheim, Germany, p 37–52

Craig K D, McMahon R J, Morison J D, Zaskow C 1984 Developmental changes in infant pain expression during immunization injections. Social Science and Medicine 19: 1331–1337

Dubner R, Hoffman D S, Hayes R L 1981 Neuronal activity in medullary dorsal horn of awake monkeys trained in a thermal discrimination task. III. Task-related responses and their functional role. Journal of Neurophysiology 46: 444–464

Duncan G H, Bushnell M C, Bates R, Dubner R 1987 Task-related responses of monkey medullary dorsal horn neurons. Journal of Neurophysiology 57: 289–310

Dworkin S F, Schubert M M, Chen A C N, Clark D W 1986 Psychological preparation influences nitrous oxide analgesia: replication of laboratory findings in a clinical setting. Oral Surgery, Oral Medicine, Oral Pathology 61: 108–112

Field T 1990 Alleviating stress in newborn infants in the intensive care unit. Clinical Perinatology 17: 1–10

Fitzgerald M Anand K J S 1993 Developmental neuroanatomy and neurophysiology of pain. In: Schechter N L, Berde C B, Yaster M (eds) Pain in infants, children and adolescents. Williams & Wilkins, Baltimore, p 11–31

Fowler-Kerry S, Lander J R 1987 Management of injection pain in children. Pain 30: 169–175

Hayes R L, Dubner R, Hoffman D S 1981 Neuronal activity in medullary dorsal horn of awake monkeys trained in a thermal discrimination task; II. Behavioral modulation of responses to thermal and mechanical stimuli. Journal of Neurophysiology 46: 428–443

Hilgard E R 1969 Pain as a puzzle for psychology and physiology. American Psychologist 24: 103–113

Hilgard J R, LeBaron S 1984 Hypnotherapy of pain in children with cancer. William Kaufman, Los Altos, California

Jay S M, Ozolins M, Elliott C H, Caldwell S 1983 Assessment of children's distress during painful medical procedures. Health Psychology 2: 133–147

Jay S M, Elliott C H, Ozolins M, Olson R A, Pruitt S D 1985 Behavioural management of children's distress during painful medical procedures. Behaviour Research and Therapy 23: 513–552

Joffe R, Bakal D A, Kaganov J 1983 A self-observation study of headache symptoms in children. Headache 23: 20–25

Johnson J E, Dabbs J M Jr, Leventhal H 1970 Psychosocial factors in the welfare of surgical patients. Nursing Research 19: 18–29

Johnson J E, Leventhal H, Dabbs J M Jr 1971 Contributions of emotional and instrumental response processes in adaptation to surgery. Journal of Personality and Social Psychology 20: 55–64

Johnson J E, Kirchhoff K T, Endress M P 1975 Altering children's distress behavior during orthopedic cast removal. Nursing Research 24: 404–410

Katz E R, Kellerman J, Siegel S E 1980 Behavioral distress in children with cancer undergoing medical procedures: developmental considerations. Journal of Consulting Clinical Psychology 48: 356–365

Katz E R, Kellerman J, Ellenberg L 1987 Hypnosis in the reduction of acute pain and distress in children with cancer. Journal of Pediatric Psychology 12: 379–394

Kavanagh C K, Lasoff E, Eide Y et al 1991 Learned helplessness and the pediatric burn patient: dressing change behavior and serum cortisol and beta-endorphin. In: Barness L (ed) Advances in pediatrics, vol 38. Mosby-Year Book, St Louis, p 335–363

Kuttner L 1989 Management of young children's acute pain and anxiety during invasive medical procedures. Pediatrician 16: 39–44

Kuttner L 1993 Hypnotic interventions for children in pain. In: Schechter N L, Berde C B, Yaster M (eds) Pain in infants, children, and adolescents. Williams & Wilkins, Baltimore, p 229–236

Kuttner L, Bowman M, Teasdale M 1988 Psychological treatment of distress, pain and anxiety for young children with cancer. Journal of Developmental and Behavioral Pediatrics 9: 374–381

LaBaw W L 1973 Adjunctive trance therapy with severely burned children. International Journal of Child Psychotherapy 2: 80–92

Leviton A, Slack W V, Masek B, Bana D Graham J R 1984 A computerized behavioral assessment for children with headaches. Headache 24: 182–185

Lewis T 1942 Pain. MacMillan, London

McGrath P A 1983 Biologic basis of pain and analgesia: the role of situational variables in pain control. Anesthesia Progress 30: 137–146

McGrath P A 1987 The management of chronic pain in children. In: Burrows G D, Elton D Stanley G V (eds) Handbook of chronic pain management. Elsevier, Amsterdam, p 205–216

McGrath P A 1990a Pain assessment in children – a practical approach. In: Tyler D C, Krane E J (eds) Advances in pain research and therapy, vol 15. Raven Press, New York

McGrath P A 1990b Pain in children: nature, assessment and treatment. Guilford Publications, New York

McGrath P A 1992 Pain control in children. In: Weiner R S (ed) Innovations in pain management: a practical guide for clinicians. Paul M Deutsch Press, Orlando, Florida, p 32-1–32-79

McGrath P A 1993 Psychological aspects of pain perception. In: Schechter N L, Berde C B, Yaster M (eds) Pain in infants, children and adolescents. Williams & Wilkins, Baltimore, pp 39–63

McGrath P A, deVeber L L 1986 The management of acute pain evoked by medical procedures in children with cancer. Journal of Pain and Symptom Management 1: 145–150

McGrath P A, Brooke R I, Varkey M 1981 Analgesic efficacy and subject expectation for clinical and experimental pain. Pain (suppl 1): S13

McGrath P J, Unruh A 1987 Pain in children and adolescents. Elsevier, Amsterdam

McGraw M B 1945 The neuromuscular maturation of the human infant. Hafner, New York

Melzack R 1973 The puzzle of pain. Basic Books, New York

Miser A M 1993 Management of pain associated with childhood cancer. In: Schechter N L, Berde C B, Yaster M (eds) Pain in infants, children and adolescents. Williams & Wilkins, Baltimore, p 411–423

Olness K, Gardner G G 1988 Hypnosis and hypnotherapy with children. Grune & Stratton, Philadelphia

Olness K, MacDonald J 1981 Self-hypnosis and biofeedback in the management of juvenile migraine. Journal of Developmental and Behavioral Pediatrics 2: 168–170

Olsson G, Berde C 1993 Neuropathic pain in children and adolescents. In: Schechter N L, Berde C B, Yaster M (eds) Pain in infants, children and adolescents. Williams & Wilkins, Baltimore, p 473–493

Peterson L, Shigetomi C 1981 The use of coping techniques to minimize anxiety in hospitalized children. Behavior Therapy 12: 1–14

Peterson L, Harbeck C, Chaney J, Farmer J, Muir Thomas A 1990 Children's coping with medical procedures: a conceptual overview and integration. Behavioral Assessment 12: 197–212

Price D D 1984 Dorsal horn mechanisms of pain. In: Davidoff R A (ed) The handbook of the spinal cord. Marcel Dekker, New York, p 751–777

Price D D 1988 Psychological and neural mechanisms of pain. Raven Press, New York

Price D D, Barrell J J, Gracely R H 1980 A psychophysical analysis of experiential factors that selectively influence the affective dimension of pain. Pain 8: 137–149

Rappaport L A, Leichtner A M 1993 Recurrent abdominal pain. In: Schechter N L, Berde C B, Yaster M (eds) Pain in infants, children and adolescents. Williams & Wilkins, Baltimore, p 561–569

Ross D M, Ross S A 1988 Childhood pain: current issues, research, and management. Urban & Schwarzenberg, Baltimore

Rothner A D 1993 Diagnosis and management of headaches in children and adolescents. In: Schechter N L, Berde C B, Yaster M (eds) Pain in infants, children and adolescents. Williams & Wilkins, Baltimore, pp 547–554

Routh D K, Sanfilippo M D 1991 Helping children cope with painful medical procedures. In: Bush J P, Harkins S W (eds) Children in pain: clinical and research issues from a developmental perspective. Springer-Verlag, New York

Schechter N L 1985 Pain and pain control in children. Current Problems in Pediatrics 15: 1–67

Schechter N L 1989 Acute pain in children. Pediatric Clinics of North America 36: 781–1052

Schechter N L, Berde C, Yaster M (eds) 1993 Pain management in children and adolescents. Williams & Wilkins, Baltimore

Shapiro B S 1993 Management of painful episodes in sickle cell disease. In: Schechter N L, Berde C B, Yaster M (eds) Pain in infants, children and adolescents. Williams & Wilkins, Baltimore, p 385–410

Shinnar S, D'Souza B J 1981 The diagnosis and management of headaches in childhood. Pediatric Clinics of North America 29: 79–94

Siegel L J, Peterson L 1981 Maintenance effects of coping skills and sensory information on young children's response to repeated dental procedures. Behavior Therapy 12: 530–535

Thompson S C 1981 Will it hurt less if I can control it? A complex answer to a simple question. Psychological Bulletin 90: 89–101

Tyler D C, Krane E J (eds) 1990 Advances in pain research and therapy. Raven Press, New York

Varni J W, Gilbert A, Dietrich S L 1981 Behavioral medicine in pain and analgesia management for the hemophilic child with Factor VIII inhibitor. Pain 11: 121–126

von Graffenried B, Adler R, Abt K, Nuesch E, Spiegel R 1978 The influence of anxiety and pain sensitivity on experimental pain in man. Pain 4: 253–263

Walco G A, Ilowite N T 1991 Vertical versus horizontal visual analogue scales of pain intensity in children. Journal of Pain and Symptom Management 6: 200

Walco G A, Oberlander T F 1993 Musculoskeletal pain syndromes in children. In: Schechter N L, Berde C B, Yaster M (eds) Pain in infants, children and adolescents. Williams & Wilkins, Baltimore, p 459–471

Wall P D 1984 Mechanisms of acute and chronic pain. In: Kruger L, Liebeskind J C (eds) Advances in pain research and therapy, vol 6. Raven Press, New York, p 95–104

Watkins L R, Mayer D J 1982 Organization of endogenous opiate and nonopiate pain control systems. Science 216: 1185–1192

Weisenberg M 1977 Pain and pain control. Psychological Bulletin 84: 1008–1041

Weisenberg M 1984 Cognitive aspects of pain. In: Wall P D Melzack R (eds) Textbook of pain. Churchill Livingstone, Edinburgh, p 162–172

Weisenberg M, Tursky B 1976 Pain: new perspectives in therapy and research. Plenum Press, New York

Willis W D 1985 The pain system: the neural basis of nociceptive transmission in the mammalian nervous system. Karger, Basel

Zborowski M 1962 Cultural components in responses to pain. Journal of Social Issues 8: 16–30

Zeltzer L K, Jay S M, Fisher D M 1989 The management of pain associated with pediatric procedures. Pediatric Clinics of North America 36: 941–964

80. Treatment of pain in children

Constance S. Houck Todd Troshynski and Charles B. Berde

INTRODUCTION

Undertreatment of actue pain in children has been widespread in the past. This was due to:

1. lack of information regarding the safety and efficacy of analgesics in young children
2. difficulty in distinguishing pain from anxiety, hunger or fear
3. concerns regarding the increased risk of respiratory depression with opioids in infants
4. societal fears of opioid addiction
5. lack of advocacy.

During the past 10 years, there has been considerable progress in studies of paediatric analgesic pharmacology. In addition, multidisciplinary paediatric pain-management teams have done much to improve the treatment of pain in children and adolescents and have applied pain-treatment modalities such as patient-controlled analgesia, epidural analgesia and regional blockade (nonneuraxial) for postoperative analgesia.

This chapter provides an overview of the medical management of acute and chronic pain in children.

DEVELOPMENTAL ISSUES IN ANALGESIC PHARMACOLOGY

Although most of the major organ systems are anatomically well developed at birth, their functional maturity is often delayed. In the first months of life in both preterm and fullterm newborns, these systems mature rapidly, most approaching a functional level similar to adults before 3 months of age. General principles of newborn physiology and its effects on the pharmacology of opioids and local anaesthetics are summarised below:

1. Most analgesics are conjugated in the liver. Newborns, and especially prematures, have delayed maturation of enzyme systems involved in drug conjugation, including sulphation, glucuronidation, and oxidation. The cytochrome P450 system which, along with the mixed-function oxidases, catalyses these reactions in the liver is quite immature at birth and does not reach adult levels until the first month of life.

2. Glomerular filtration rates are diminished in the first week of life, but generally are sufficiently mature to clear medications and metabolites by 2 weeks of age.

3. Newborns have a higher percentage of body weight as water and less as fat than older patients. Water-soluble drugs, therefore, often have larger volumes of distribution.

4. Newborns have reduced plasma concentrations of albumin and alpha-1 acid glycoprotein than older children and adults. In some circumstances, this results in a greater availability of active drug at receptors and increased risk of acute toxicity.

5. Brain and viscera account for a greater proportion of body mass and muscle and fat account for smaller proportions of body mass than in adults. In term neonates, and especially in prematures, there is increased passage into the brain of naturally occurring toxins, such as bilirubin, as well as drugs, such as morphine.

6. Newborns, and especially prematures, have diminished ventilatory responses to hypoxaemia and hypercarbia.

NONOPIOID ANALGESICS

Except in the newborn period, the pharmacodynamics and pharmacokinetics of acetaminophen, salicylates and the nonsteroidal antiinflammatory agents (NSAIDs) in children are not much different than in adults. The choice of agent is dependent on a variety of factors, including cost, duration of action, requirements for antiinflammatory effect, whether the oral or intravenous route is to be used and which side-effects are to be avoided.

Acetaminophen (paracetamol) remains the most popular analgesic in infants and children and has been found to be safe and effective in newborns as well. In fact, the immaturity of hepatic metabolic systems in the newborn may be protective and lead to diminished production of the toxic metabolites of this drug. The elimination rate of unchanged acetaminophen is similar in neonates, children and adults (Miller et al 1976). Doses of 10–15 mg/kg every 4 hours given orally and 20–25 mg/kg every 4 hours given rectally produce relatively low plasma levels (Gaudreault et al 1988) and provide analgesia similar to the NSAIDs.

Acetylsalicylic acid (ASA), with its antiinflammatory qualities, continues to be widely used for the treatment of mild to moderate pain in children, especially when the pain is of inflammatory origin. Oral dosages are similar to those for acetaminophen. Neonates eliminate ASA much more slowly than adults but the elimination half-life of this drug reaches adult levels within the first year of life (Levy & Garretson 1974). The association between the use of this agent to treat febrile illness and the development of Reye's syndrome, combined with the higher incidence of gastrointestinal side-effects and platelet dysfunction, has resulted in a marked decrease in the use of ASA in children in recent years (Hurwitz et al 1985). Therefore, other NSAIDs have become much more popular for the treatment of acute pain in children and adolescents. These include ibuprofen, naprosyn, indomethacin, choline magnesium trisalicylate and ketorolac. Dosage guidelines for their use in children can be found in Table 80.1.

Ibuprofen is frequently chosen for mild to moderate pain because it is available in a liquid form, allowing easy administration to younger children. A recent study of this drug compared to ASA for the treatment of juvenile rheumatoid arthritis indicated that it is of equal efficacy and tends to be better tolerated for long-term administration (Giannini et al 1990). Since it is also available as a rectal preparation in Canada, it has been used as a 'prophylactic' analgesic for postoperative pain, reducing the need for additional narcotic analgesics by approximately 30% (Maunuksela et al 1992).

Indomethacin is available intravenously and, because of its use in premature infants to promote closure of the patent ductus arteriosus, there has been considerable clinical experience with its use in young children (Brash et al 1982). Though elimination of this drug is delayed in premature infants, volume of distribution and elimination half-life approach that of adults by 1 year of age (Olkkola et al 1989). Oliguria, weight gain and hyponatraemia have been noted in premature infants after administration of indomethacin, but no such effects have been noted in children over the age of 1 year (Maunuksela et al 1987). In a recent study of the use of indomethacin by continuous intravenous infusion for postoperative pain, it was found to provide excellent adjunctive pain relief and provide greater patient satisfaction than 'prn' narcotics alone (Maunuksela et al 1988).

Choline magnesium trisalicylate (Trilisate) is a long-acting nonacetylated salicylate that generally leads to less gastrointestinal upset and platelet dysfunction than ASA (Stuart & Pisko 1981). It is also available in a liquid form and has been investigated for the treatment of juvenile rheumatoid arthritis in children as young as 6 years of age. It is most often used when once- or twice-daily dosing is preferred or when other nonsteroidal antiinflammatory agents are not well tolerated. Though no reports of Reye's syndrome have been associated with this compound, it is recommended that its use should also be avoided during febrile illness in children.

The nonsteroidal antiinflammatory drug ketorolac tromethamine has become widely available for use by the intravenous, intramuscular and oral routes. This drug, given intravenously, has proven to be valuable as both an adjuvant to supplement opioid agents and as a single agent for the treatment of postoperative pain in children and adolescents (Maunuksela et al 1993). In doses of 1 mg/kg/dose as an initial loading dose followed by 0.5 mg/kg/dose every 6 hours for a total of 48 hours, pain relief has been suggested to equal that obtained with morphine in the dose of 0.1 mg/kg for less painful surgical procedures. It has also been associated with less postoperative nausea and vomiting (Watcha et al 1992). Side-effects of ketorolac are similar to those found with oral NSAIDs. Therefore, nausea, gastrointestinal bleeding, platelet dysfunction and interstitial nephritis may occur with this drug, though the incidence of renal impairment when used

Table 80.1 Pediatric dosage of nonsteroidal antiinflammatory drugs used as analgesics

	Single dose mg/kg	Number of daily doses	Maximum dose mg/kg/day
Acetaminophen	10–15	4–6	60
Acetylsalicylic acid	10–15	4–6	60
Ibuprofen	5–10	3–4	40
Indomethacin	1	3	3
Choline magnesium trisalicylate	25	2	50
Naprosyn	7	2	15
Ketorolac (po) – adolescents	10 mg/dose	3–4	40 mg/day
Ketorolac (IV or IM)	0.5	4	2
initial loading	1.0		

on a short-term basis appears very low. Ketorolac does not produce tolerance, physical or psychological dependence and is not associated with sedation or respiratory depression. It is therefore particularly useful for patients whose opioid use is limited by respiratory depressant effects. We have used IV ketorolac along with either patient-controlled analgesia or nurse-administered prn morphine in over 400 patients at Children's Hospital, Boston. Many patients, especially those who have undergone orthopaedic procedures, report excellent postoperative analgesia and little requirement for additional opioids.

OPIOID ANALGESICS

Opioids are useful for the treatment of pain in patients of all ages. They are the most commonly used analgesic agents in postoperative patients and the most commonly used analgesic agents in patients with other forms of moderate to severe acute pain. For the vast majority of children, opioids produce excellent analgesia with a wide margin of safety. There is, however, marked individual variation in opioid dose requirements and doses must be adjusted to effect. For the treatment of acute pain, the correct dose of opioid is that which treats the pain, yet does not result in excessive somnolence or respiratory depression.

The use of opioids for the treatment of pain in infants mandates an understanding of the unique pharmacokinetics of opioids in these patients. Though less is known about the newer synthetic opioids, the pharmacokinetics of morphine have been extensively studied in newborns and children. The elimination half-life of morphine is more than twice as long in newborns in the first week of life than older children or adults and even longer in premature infants (Lynn & Slattery 1987; Bhat et al 1990). This appears to be due to several factors, most important of which is the immaturity of the newborn infant's hepatic enzyme systems. Clearance of morphine is dependent on conjugation of the drug to the inactive metabolite morphine-3-glucuronide and the active metabolite morphine-6-glucuronide. This reaction is catalysed by mixed function oxidases (cytochrome P450); concentrations of which are very low in newborns. Glomerular filtration rate is also reduced in the first week of life leading to a further decrease in elimination. In addition, many of the infants who require postoperative opioids have undergone abdominal procedures such as gastroschisis, omphalocele or malrotation repair and will have delayed opioid clearance secondary to decreased hepatic blood flow.

Studies in newborn rats suggest that newborns are less sensitive to the analgesic effects of morphine but more sensitive to the respiratory depressant effects of this drug than older rats (Pasternak et al 1980). This is speculated to be a result of age-related changes in the number and subtypes of mu receptors. In addition, morphine is approximately 20% bound to serum protein in preterm and fullterm infants younger than 5 days of age, as compared to 35% in adults, allowing a greater proportion of active drug to penetrate the blood–brain barrier. These physiological differences, combined with the known delay in clearance, appear to account for the greatly increased risk of respiratory depression when morphine is administered to newborn infants. This has led to a recommendation for cardiorespiratory monitoring and careful observation whenever opioids are administered to infants less than 2 months of age (Yaster & Maxwell 1993).

Less is known about the receptor properties of the other commonly used opioids in infants and children but elimination appears to be delayed in a fashion similar to morphine. Fentanyl, sufentanil, meperidine and methadone all undergo biotransformation in the liver and therefore will have prolonged elimination until hepatic enzyme systems mature.

Opioids can be administered by a number of routes – orally, intravenously, intramuscularly, subcutaneously, rectally, transdermally or transmucosally. Oral administration is generally the easiest and can lead to relatively constant drug levels with regular administration. After minor, less painful surgery, oral opioids are usually well tolerated and provide excellent postoperative pain relief. This route, however, is often not appropriate for severe acute pain. Delayed onset of effect, inconsistent gastric absorption and the inability to tolerate oral medications make it a poor choice for patients immediately after major surgery.

Codeine is available in an elixir form and is therefore the most commonly administered oral opioid in young children. It is often given in combination with acetaminophen. In fact, this combined form is not only more effective than the single drug alone, but also may, unlike most opioids in the United States, be prescribed over the phone. Dosage guidelines for this and other opioid analgesics can be found in Table 80.2.

Oxycodone is usually administered to older children because it is available only as a tablet. To increase its analgesic efficacy, it is frequently combined with acetaminophen or aspirin. Many practitioners prefer this agent to codeine because it appears to cause less gastrointestinal upset at equianalgesic doses.

Methadone when administered orally is well absorbed in the gastrointestinal tract, leading to predictable serum drug levels and clinical effect. Its long duration of action provides excellent pain relief when administered every 6–12 hours. With its 70–90% biovailability after absorption from the gastrointestinal tract, it can provide good analgesia without the need for intravenous or intramuscular injections.

Intramuscular (IM) administration of opioids has been popular for the treatment of postoperative pain in adults

Table 80.2 Opioid analgesics for pediatric pain

	Equipotent IV dose (mg/kg)	Comments
Morphine	0.1	Histamine release, vasodilation. Use caution with asthmatics or patients with haemodynamic compromise
Meperidine	1.0	Metabolite produces seizures – not recommended for chronic use. Catastrophic interaction with monoamine oxidase inhibitors
Methadone	0.1	Very effective by the intravenous, intramuscular or oral route
Fentanyl	0.001	Chest-wall rigidity. Decreases heart rate but causes minimal haemodynamic change
Codeine	1.2	Oral use only
Hydromorphone (Dilaudid)	0.015 – 0.02	Associated with less itching and nausea than morphine May be used by either IV or epidural route
Oxycodone	0.15	Better oral bioavailability than morphine Often used when weaning from IV to oral pain meds

because it provides more constant serum opioid levels than intravenous administration and can be administered every 3–4 hours. Children in pain, however, often prefer to remain in pain rather than receive a 'shot'. Many will deny that they are having pain despite clear evidence that they are uncomfortable. Because this fear of injections often leads to undertreatment of pain, IM injections of opioids are discouraged in most instances.

Opioids, therefore, are often administered to children postoperatively via the intravenous (IV) route. Intermittent boluses of morphine, meperidine, fentanyl or sufentanil can provide rapid pain relief but their duration of action is short, resulting in marked fluctuations in serum opioid levels during the dosage period. Children, after receiving an IV bolus, are predictably sedated; then as the blood level declines, can become quite uncomfortable before the next scheduled dose. Therefore, patient-controlled analgesia and continuous infusions of opioids have become much more popular in recent years to provide a more steady level of analgesia.

PATIENT-CONTROLLED ANALGESIA

Patient-controlled analgesia (PCA) is now a widely used method of providing postoperative pain relief to adults. In recent years, it has also emerged as an important method of providing analgesia to children and adolescents (Dodd et al 1988; Means et al 1988; Broadman et al 1989; Gaukroger et al 1989; Lawrie et al 1990; Berde et al 1991a). PCA was initiated first in adolescents but soon was found to be a safe and effective method of pain control in younger children. It not only eliminates the need for 'shots' but also gives the child a greater sense of control. Berde et al (1991a) compared PCA in a randomised prospective study to IM injection of morphine in postoperative paediatric patients and demonstrated both lower pain scores and greater overall satisfaction with PCA.

The most important factors in the successful use of this technique appear to be the child's ability to understand the concept of patient-controlled pain relief and the ability to push the button. With appropriate preoperative teaching and encouragement, children as young as 7 years of age can independently use the PCA pump to provide good postoperative pain relief. Children between the ages of 4 and 6, however, often require encouragement from their parents and nursing staff to push the button before anticipated painful movements or procedures. Even with encouragement, the failure rate among 4- and 5-year-olds with PCA appears quite high.

An early report suggested that parents may be relied upon to administer PCA to younger children and those otherwise unable to use the apparatus (Rodgers et al 1988). This has generally not been recommended because it removes the safeguards inherent in patient-administered dosing. In addition, parents are usually too emotionally involved with their children to assume sole management of their child's pain. Broadman (1990) at the Children's National Medical Center has suggested a modified method which he calls 'parent-assisted analgesia'. This method involves communication between the parent and child who then jointly decide whether the pain is intense enough to press the button. This 'assistance' is generally not required beyond the first 24 hours postoperatively. We discourage parent-controlled analgesia in the postoperative setting, but use it freely in children with chronic pain due to cancer or AIDS.

PCA may be administered either alone or in conjunction with a low-dose continuous infusion. Initial parameters for postoperative patients include: morphine bolus doses of 0.02–0.03 mg/kg/dose and a lockout interval of 7 minutes. If a basal infusion is used, a rate of 0.01–0.02 mg/kg/h is usually chosen. If the pump is capable of maintaining a 4-hour limit, this is set at approximately 0.3 mg/kg.

Meperidine may also be used for PCA, but continuous infusions of this drug are generally avoided. A metabolite of meperidine, normeperidine, which may cause seizures if allowed to accumulate, precludes the use of continuous, long-term infusions. Meperidine bolus doses are 10 times the morphine dose (i.e. 0.2–0.3 mg/dose) and a 4-hour limit may be set at 3 mg/kg. Fentanyl, dilaudid and sufentanil may also be administered through a PCA pump and may be effective for children who cannot otherwise tolerate morphine or meperidine.

The issue of whether to use a background infusion of opioids along with PCA to provide better analgesia during periods of sleep has been a controversial one, especially for elderly adults who may be slow at eliminating drugs.This had not clinically posed much of a problem in children (Berde et al 1991a). Recently, however, McNeely et al found more episodes of hypoxaemia during sleep among children receiving a basal infusion than those receiving bolus doses only (McNeely et al 1992). To lessen the risks inherent in continuous infusions, we have begun combining bolus-dose PCA with round-the-clock intravenous ketorolac in opioid-naive postoperative patients. This regimen provides excellent pain relief in all but the most painful surgeries. In contrast, it is our experience that most oncology patients using PCA are significantly more comfortable when provided with a basal infusion. For disease-related pain, we try to provide at least 60% of the overall opioid requirement in the basal infusion.

Opioid-induced nausea and vomiting and urinary retention appear to be no more frequent with PCA than with intramuscular opioids (Gaukroger et al 1989). Respiratory depression has been extremely rare except with the concomitant use of drugs with sedative effects. A study of 1589 patients at the Children's Hospital, Boston, receiving PCA during a 3-year period demonstrated only two episodes of significant respiratory depression (Wilder et al 1992). Both of these occurred during concurrent administration of perphenazine and diphenhydramine for the treatment of nausea, neither patient was apnoeic and although naloxone was administered in each case, no further treatment was needed and no sequelae resulted.

CONTINUOUS OPIOID INFUSIONS

Continuous IV infusions of opioids (most commonly morphine) can provide very effective analgesia for postoperative patients who, because of young age or cognitive or physical handicaps, are unable to use a PCA pump. The infusion maintains a constant level of opioid but requires initial loading with 0.05–0.10 mg/kg of morphine or its equivalent. This initial loading is often achieved while the patient is in the operating room. The continuous infusion is begun in the postanaesthesia care unit once the child is deemed sufficiently recovered from anaesthesia. Since neonates and young infants metabolise and excrete morphine and its metabolites more slowly than older children, the initial infusion rate is usually about one-half to one-third that of their more mature counterparts. Generally, the infusion for neonates and infants less than 3 months of age is begun at 0.01–0.015 mg/kg/h and for older children, 0.025–0.03 mg/kg/h.

A technologically simple regimen involving loading doses (usually 0.1–0.2 mg/kg) and small bolus doses of methadone has been shown to be very effective for postoperative analgesia (Gourlay et al 1984, 1986; Berde et al 1988). The elimination half-life of methadone in children averages 19 hours. A practical and simple method of administration of methadone is sometimes referred to as the 'reverse prn' method (Berde et al 1991b). Patients are assessed by the nursing staff at regular intervals (usually every 3–4 hours). A 'sliding scale' regimen is ordered so that the nurse may administer additional doses every 4 hours based on her assessment of the child's pain as either severe (0.08 mg/kg), moderate (0.05 mg/kg) or mild (0.03 mg/kg). In this way, methadone is 'titrated' to a level that keeps the child comfortable.

Continuous infusions of fentanyl and sufentanil are frequently used to sedate neonates and older children who require prolonged endotracheal intubation. Infusions of high doses (the fentanyl equivalent of 10–20 mcg/kg/hr) not only block the haemodynamic and pulmonary responses to pain but also appear to blunt the endocrine stress response as well (Anand et al 1990; Anand & Hickey 1992). Older children and those who have not undergone surgery can often be rendered comfortable with infusions of 1–3 mcg/kg/h. Newborns who receive fentanyl infusions to help maintain haemodynamic stability during extracorporeal membrane oxygenation (ECMO) or prolonged mechanical ventilation often require daily increases in their infusion rate to achieve similar levels of sedation. This implies an unusually rapid development of opioid tolerance in these young patients (Arnold et al 1990, 1991).

For patients with cancer or AIDS who are unable to take oral opioids and have no intravenous access, the subcutaneous administration of opioids has proven to be very effective (Urquhart 1988; Taylor et al 1989). Morphine and hydromorphone (Dilaudid™) are well suited to this method of administration and are available in more concentrated solutions. Though usually well tolerated, itching and redness often occur at the insertion site and may be bothersome to some children. Needle insertion sites need only be changed as needed (usually every 2–3 days).

Transdermal fentanyl has been used on a limited basis in children for treatment of cancer pain. Since there is a considerable lag before therapeutic blood concentrations are reached and elimination is slow, it is useful only for chronic ongoing pain. Nevertheless, supplemental opioids are often needed for acute exacerbations of pain in these patients.

Transmucosal fentanyl, the 'fentanyl lollipop', has been investigated as an analgesic and sedative agent prior to painful procedures in children (Schechter et al 1991; Weisman et al 1991). The onset of effect is usually noted in 10–30 minutes, so 'titration' of this agent is possible. Though readily accepted by children, there is a relatively high incidence of nausea and vomiting and facial pruritus with this drug (Nelson et al 1989).

REGIONAL ANAESTHESIA AND ANALGESIA

Recently there has been increased interest in the use of regional anaesthetic techniques to decrease general anaesthetic requirements and aid in postoperative pain management in children and adolescents. These techniques range from local infiltration to the deposition of local anaesthetics or opioids along the neuraxis (epidural or subarachnoid). Peripheral nerve blocks can also provide long-lasting pain relief after many common paediatric operations.

The most frequently used local anaesthetics for postoperative pain relief are lidocaine and bupivacaine, both amide local anaesthetics. Bupivacaine has the advantage of a prolonged duration of action and, perhaps, in dilute concentrations, a relative preference for sensory blockade over motor blockade. The pharmacokinetic parameters and recommended maximum doses of these two agents are found in Table 80.3.

Caution must be exercised when local anaesthetics are administered to neonates and young children. Neonates have low concentrations of albumin and alpha-1 acid glycoprotein which can lead to decreased protein binding of local anaesthetics and increases in the plasma concentrations of the unbound drug. As well, amide local anaesthetics are metabolised by the microsomal P450 enzyme system in the liver which does not exhibit full activity for weeks after birth. This, combined with a decrease in liver blood flow found with respiratory diseases and cardiac insufficiency, can lead to a significantly prolonged terminal half-life of these agents in sick newborns.

Ester local anaesthetics (procaine, chloroprocaine and tetracaine) are broken down by plasma cholinesterases. Since the activity of these enzymes is diminished in the first 6 months of life, clearance of the ester local anaesthetics may theoretically be prolonged. However, a recent study of the use of 2-chloroprocaine for continuous caudal anaesthesia revealed that neonates have the ability to clear this drug effectively even at high infusion rates (Hendersen et al 1992).

LOCAL INFILTRATION AND TOPICAL ANAESTHESIA

Infiltration of the wound edges with bupivacaine is an effective adjunct providing postoperative analgesia for common paediatric surgeries such as inguinal herniorrhaphy. The pain relief with this method was indistinguishable from that provided by ilioinguinal nerve block for inguinal herniorrhaphy in one series (Casey et al 1990). One must take care to avoid toxic doses of local anaesthetics when performing wound infiltration, especially in newborns and younger infants and and no more than 2.0–2.5 mg/kg of bupivacaine should be administered. This is equivalent to approximately 0.5 ml/kg of 0.5% bupivacaine or 1.0 mg/kg of 0.25% bupivacaine. More dilute solutions are generally used in younger children to provide adequate spread of the anaesthetic without exceeding the recommended limits. Solutions containing epinephrine are desirable in highly vascular areas to slow vascular uptake of local anaesthetics and to prolong the duration of effect. However, they should be avoided when procedures are performed on the distal extremities or penis to avoid ischaemic injury to these areas (e.g. when performing digital and penile blocks).

Transdermal administration of local anaesthetics has become much more popular in recent years with the development of a eutectic mixture of local anaesthetics (EMLA). EMLA is a mixture of lidocaine and prilocaine base in a weight ratio of 1:1. The crystalline powders of the two anaesthetics melt at a lower temperature than they do separately and, as a result, constitute a liquid at room temperature. This physical feature permits a higher effective concentration at the stratum corneum and increases the rate of uptake (Bodin et al 1984). The usefulness of EMLA cream for the placement of intravenous lines in the paediatric population has been demonstrated in several

Table 80.3 Pharmacology of the most commonly used local anaesthetics for nerve blocks

Agent	Potency	Onset (min)	Duration after infiltration (min)	Maximum dose in children (mg/ml)	Protein binding (%)	Lipid solubility	Clearance (L/min)	Elimination half-time (min)
Lidocaine	1	rapid	60–120	5 (10 W/EPI)	70	2.9	0.95	96
Bupivacaine	4	slow	240–280	3	95	28	0.47	210

Data from Stoelting 1987.

recent studies (Maunuksela et al 1986; Soliman et al 1988; Halperin et al 1989). Its use is limited by the fact that the cream must be placed on the intended puncture site and covered with an occlusive dressing for a minimum of 40–60 minutes prior to the procedure. In addition, the duration of effect is usually less than 1 hour. It has value, however, for anticipated venous cannulation, lumbar punctures and other elective procedures. Caution must be observed in the use of EMLA in infants less than 3 months of age because the metabolism of prilocaine results in the production of oxidants that can lead to the development of methaemoglobinaemia. Neonates are especially at risk, not only because they have decreased levels of methaemoglobin reductase, but also because fetal haemoglobin is more easily oxidised to methaemoglobin (Yaster & Maxwell 1989). Newer and more lipophilic preparations of topical local anaesthetics such as amethocaine have been studied in Europe and provide excellent anaesthesia in approximately 30 minutes with a duration of effect of more than 3 hours (McCafferty et al 1989).

PERIPHERAL NERVE BLOCKS

Regional anaesthetic techniques that are simple to perform in children and provide excellent postoperative analgesia include:

1. penile nerve block (dorsal or ring) for circumcision or hypospadias repair
2. ilioinguinal/iliohypogastric nerve blocks for inguinal hernia repair
3. fascia iliaca compartment block for surgical procedures involving the femur and thigh.

The fascia iliaca block deserves particular mention because it is not only simple to perform, but an excellent method to provide postoperative pain relief for femur fractures (Dalens et al 1989a). Since the femoral, lateral cutaneous, genitofemoral and obturator nerves all pass over the iliacus muscle, it follows that injection of sufficient quantities of local anaesthetic beneath the fascia iliaca will result in blockade of all four nerves.

Using the anterior superior iliac spine and the spine of the pubic tubercle as landmarks, a line is drawn between the two. At a point where the medial two-thirds meets the lateral one-third, a needle is inserted at right angles to the skin while gentle pressure is applied to the barrel of a syringe filled with local anaesthetic. A loss of resistance is first felt when the needle passes through the fascia lata and a second loss of resistance is felt when the needle passes through the fascia iliaca into the compartment below. After negative aspiration, approximately 1cc/kg (maximum of 40 cc) of bupivacaine 0.25% with epinephrine is then deposited into the compartment. Recommended volumes of 0.25% bupivacaine with epinephrine for the most commonly performed peripheral nerve blocks are given in Table 80.4.

Intercostal nerve blocks have been used to treat the pain associated with rib fractures, thoracotomy and upper abdominal incisions. When used to treat the pain of rib fractures, the results can be quite remarkable with the patient able to cough, deep breathe and ambulate almost immediately after the needle is removed. However, intercostal nerve blocks produce the highest peak plasma concentrations of local anaesthetics of any regional anaesthetic technique (Moore et al 1976; Rothstein et al 1986). Because of the increased risk of local anaesthetic toxicity, the requirement for repeated needle injections and the limited duration of these blocks, we generally prefer thoracic epidural analgesia for these patients.

Brachial plexus anaesthesia can be an important adjunct after revascularisation procedures to improve blood flow and reduce vascular spasm. In addition, patients who are at increased risk for respiratory depression with opioid analgesics may obtain prolonged analgesia for 6–18 hours after the performance of a brachial plexus block. Since children are rarely able to cooperate for performance of these blocks, they are usually performed under conscious sedation or a general anaesthetic. This requires care in avoiding intravascular or subarachnoid injection and the use of a nerve stimulator to help confirm proper placement of the block needle. Epinephrine-containing solutions are generally used to aid in the detection of intravascular injection and the dose is given slowly over at least 90–120 seconds, intermittently stopping and aspirating for blood throughout injection.

The two most common approaches to the brachial plexus in the anaesthetised child include the interscalene approach and the axillary approach. The axillary block has proven to be virtually free of complications and is usually the first choice (Dalens 1990). When the axillary route is

Table 80.4 Recommended volumes of anaesthetic solution for common peripheral block procedures

Procedure	Under 20 kg	20 – 29 kg	30 – 45 kg	Over 45 kg
Supraclavicular block	0.5 –1 ml/kg	15 – 20 ml	20 – 22.5 ml	22.5 – 25 ml
Axillary block	0.3 – 0.6 ml/kg	10 –15 ml	13 –18 ml	18 – 20 ml
Fascia iliaca block	1 ml/kg	20 – 25 ml	25 – 30 ml	30 – 35 ml
Lumbar plexus block	0.7 ml/kg	10 –12.5 ml	12.5 –15 ml	15 –17.5 ml
Penile block	0.1 ml/kg	2 – 2.5 ml	3 – 4 ml	5 ml

Adapted from Dalens 1993.

unsuitable because of axillary lymphadenopathy, unstable fractures, or decreased mobility of the limb, the interscalene route may be used. Since there is always a small risk of pneumothorax whenever a supraclavicular route is used, the block should be attempted only on one side (Dalens 1987).

Penile nerve blocks for the performance of neonatal circumcision have gained popularity in recent years with the advent of studies suggesting there are adverse behavioural and physiological effects of circumcision performed without the benefit of anaesthesia (Anders & Chalemian 1974; Marshall et al 1980). Two methods have generally been advocated for use in the neonatal population.

The dorsal nerve block of the penis is performed by injecting local anaesthetic immediately below the symphysis pubis, 0.5–1.0 cm lateral to the midline (Dalens et al 1989b). A small needle is inserted through the two layers of the fascia superficialis and approximately 0.05 cc/kg of bupivacaine is injected on each side. Care must be taken to avoid accidental puncture of either the paired dorsal arteries or dorsal vein, which lie below Buck's fascia. Two cases of gangrene of the skin of the glans were reported after circumcisions performed with dorsal nerve blocks (Sara & Lowry 1984).

This complication has led investigators to advocate the use of a simple ring block of the penis (Broadman et al 1987a; Broadman & Rice 1988). This is performed by injecting local anaesthetic around the shaft of the penis near the base with a small (23 gauge) needle. Superficial vascular structures are avoided and frequent aspirations are performed during infiltration to minimise intravascular injection. Though one institution has had excellent results with this technique, a higher volume of local anaesthetic is generally required and increased swelling at the base of the penis has been noted.

The ilioinguinal and iliohypogastric nerve blocks are commonly performed to provide adjunctive anaesthesia and postoperative analgesia for inguinal herniorrhaphy and orchidopexy. One technique consists of injecting local anaesthetics in a fan shape both subcutaneously and immediately below the aponeurosis of the external oblique muscle (Dalens 1993). A second technique involves infiltration of the abdominal wall muscles through the lateral edge of the skin incision in the area just medial to the anterior superior iliac spine (Broadman & Rice 1988).

EPIDURAL ANALGESIA

Epidural analgesia can provide excellent postoperative analgesia in children undergoing thoracic, abdominal, perineal and lower extremity surgery. In our view, it is the most versatile analgesic technique for children undergoing major surgery.

The epidural space may be approached at any level, but is most frequently approached via the lumbar or caudal route in children. For upper abdominal or thoracic procedures, a thoracic epidural approach may be used, but this is commonly reserved for older children who can cooperate with the procedure under light sedation. Performance of thoracic puncture under general anaesthesia should be performed only by personnel experienced with this approach in younger children. Alternatively, a lumbar or caudal catheter may be placed and threaded cephalad. Several studies have shown that a catheter can be reliably threaded to the thoracic region from a caudal approach in neonates (Bosenberg et al 1988). In addition, our experience has demonstrated that lumbar epidural catheters can be advanced to the thoracic region in many cases. Placement can be verified by the injection of radio-opaque dye through the catheter followed by radiography.

Single-shot caudal blockade is frequently performed in a paediatric outpatients undergoing perineal, lower abdominal or orthopaedic procedures and has a relatively low incidence of side-effects or toxicity. Broadman et al (1987b) demonstrated the safety and efficacy of this method in over 1100 outpatient procedures at the Children's National Medical Center in Washington, DC. 'Kiddie caudals' have become extremely popular because they are easy to perform and can reduce general anaesthetic requirements for perineal and lower extremity procedures. In some instances, this may reduce the need for endotracheal intubation and increase operating-room efficiency. Despite the low-morbidity and high-success rate with this block, care must be taken to maintain strict asepsis and avoid intravascular or intrathecal injection. Frequent aspiration looking for evidence of blood or cerebrospinal fluid must be scruptiously adhered to throughout the injection of the local anaesthetic and care must be taken not to inject the solution too quickly. It is speculated that some cases of local-anaesthetic toxicity associated with this technique may be due to rapid uptake from sacral intraosseous injection.

Patients undergoing more complex thoracic, abdominal or lower extremity procedures requiring several days of postoperative pain relief may have catheters placed and continuous infusions of opioids, local anaesthetics or local anaesthetic/opioid combinations continued postoperatively. The safety and efficacy of these infusions in children have been demonstrated in several recent studies (Ecoffey et al 1986; Desparmet et al 1987; Berde et al 1990a). In 1983 Meignier first showed that children with severe pulmonary disease recover rapidly following thoracic epidural anaesthesia combined with light general anaesthesia (Meignier et al 1983). Two recent retrospective studies (Bosenberg et al 1991; McNeely 1991) suggest that intensive care unit and hospital stays can be shortened when regional anaesthesia is combined with general anaesthesia and continued in the postoperative period for thoracic and upper abdominal surgical procedures. McNeely and his colleagues (1991, 1992) found significantly lower oxygen requirements and days of hospitalisation after Nissen fundoplication when epidural anaesthesia was used. In addition, Bosenberg et al (1991) found a significant difference in the requirement of postoperative mechanical ventilation when a caudal epidural catheter was placed and threaded cephalad to the thoracic area during repair of tracheoesophageal fistula. Prospective studies are needed to confirm these reports.

Epidural morphine in the range of 30–50 mcg/kg has been shown to be both efficacious and safe in children (Attia et al 1986; Krane et al 1987). The risks of respiratory depression can be reduced by avoidance of systemic opioids and sedatives, and by restricting doses to no more than 50 mcg/kg every 6–12 hours as needed (Krane 1988). Hydromorphone is roughly 3–5 times as potent as morphine via the epidural route and may also be used when cephalad spread of the epidural opioid is required. Studies in adult patients suggest that the analgesic efficacy is similar but the incidence of moderate to severe pruritus is much less with hydromorphone than with morphine (Chaplan et al 1992). Hydrophilic opioids are useful via the caudal or lumbar routes even for thoracic surgery. Further studies are needed to determine the dose response and safety of epidural hydromorphone in children.

At the Children's Hospital, Boston, we commonly use a solution of 0.1% bupivacaine combined with 2 mcg/cc of fentanyl for postoperative epidural infusions. After lower abdominal and lower extremity procedures, between 0.2 and 0.3 cc/kg/h of this solution is generally required in the first postoperative day. If local anaesthetics and/or hydrophobic opioids such as fentanyl are to be used, it is crucial that the catheter be placed at spinal levels innervating the operative site.

Continuous epidural anaesthesia/analgesia can be safely administered on the surgical and medical wards if there is proper observation and a management protocol. The nursing staff must be educated about the potential complications that may arise with these infusions and the appropriate measures to take if such complications arise. Details of the protocol used at the Children's Hospital, Boston, are found in Table 80.5. We have applied these protocols to over 2000 children in Boston over the past 6 years.

Two recent case reports and an analysis of retrospective data from 13 pediatric institutions have identified risk factors for systemic toxicity (primarily seizures) with the use of continuous epidural infusions of local anaesthetics (Agarwal et al 1992; McCloskey et al 1992). Based on the available data, it has been recommended that the initial epidural bolus of bupivacaine (caudal or lumbar) not exceed 2–2.5 mg/kg and that subsequent infusions of bupivacaine be maintained in doses no greater than 0.4 mg/kg/h. For infants less than 3 months of age the infusion should probably not exceed 0.25–0.3 mg/kg/h.

Table 80.5 Pain service guidelines for epidural infusions

1. A representative of the paediatric pain service or the anaesthesia department is available in the hospital 24 hours a day to rapidly deal with any complication that may arise
2. Respiratory rates and quality along with level of sedation are monitored and recorded every hour for at least the first 24 hours postoperatively.
3. Heart rate, blood pressure and pain scales are recorded at least every 4 hours.
4. The patient is evaluated by a member of the pain service at least once a day.
5. Any changes in respiratory rate, quality or level of sedation must be promptly reported to a member of the pain service.
6. Any patient under the age of 6 months, having severe neurologic deficits, receiving hydrophilic opioids or at an otherwise increased risk for respiratory depression should be placed on a cardiorespiratory monitor.
7. Heels should be padded to prevent pressure necrosis.
8. No systemic opioids are given concurrent with epidural opioids.

Adapted from: Protocols for Pain Management – Report of an Ad Hoc Committee, Children's Hospital, Boston, Massachusetts.

CHRONIC PAIN IN CHILDREN

Barr, PJ McGrath, and others have noted that recurrent pains (painful episodes interspersed with painfree intervals) occur commonly in children who are otherwise medically and psychologically well (Barr 1983; McGrath & Unruh 1987). As described in Chapter 25, recurrent headaches, abdominal pains, chest pains and limb pains occur in 5–10% of school children. Chronic persistent pain in children is less common and is more often associated either with neuropathic pain syndromes or with chronic medical conditions, such as cancer, sickle cell anaemia or arthritis.

NEUROPATHIC PAIN

Neuropathic pain is seen commonly among children and adolescents referred to our clinic. Peripheral nerve injuries may occur from a variety of causes ranging from motor-vehicle accidents to sciatic nerve injuries resulting from improper injection techniques during immunisation.

Animal research suggests that there may be marked age-related differences in both healing and plasticity following nerve injury and in the expression of chronic pain following injury (Fitzgerald 1991). While adults who suffer a plexus injury very commonly experience severe pain, it has been traditionally stated that infants with birth injury to the brachial plexus do not show signs of pain. Despite this general impression, Rossitch et al (1992) reported on an infant with self-mutilation following plexus injury and we have recently cared for an infant with apparent neuropathic pain of the arm and shoulder and sympathetic dysfunction following birth trauma to the brachial plexus.

Reflex sympathetic dystrophy (RSD) is being recognised with increasing frequency among children and adolescents. In the past 6 years, over 200 patients under age 18 have been referred to our clinic. Recently, we completed a long-term follow-up study of the first 70 patients (Wilder et al 1992a). The population was overwhelmingly female and lower extremity cases predominated. A high percentage participated in sports, ballet and gymnastics. Many had coexisting problems, including eating disorders, posttraumatic stress syndrome and family dysfunction.

In the adult anaesthesia/pain literature, there is a strong belief that early and aggressive sympathetic blockade is the cornerstone of treatment for RSD. The available literature in paediatrics in this regard is somewhat mixed. Bernstein et al (1978) first reported a high rate of success with treatment of children with an aggressive programme of physical therapy and biobehavioural treatments in an inpatient rehabilitation milieu. Others have suggested that transcutaneous electrical nerve stimulation (TENS) and sympathetic blocks are helpful. We chose a hybrid approach with an initial trial of physical therapy and cognitive and behavioural therapies for all patients. Sympathetic blockade was reserved for those who did not progress with an extended trial of physical therapy, or whose circulatory dysfunction and profound allodynia made prolonged aggressive attempts at physical therapy impossible. In long-term follow-up, it appeared that over half of children could have excellent improvement in both pain scores and function scores with conservative treatment. In those who did not respond to physical therapy and biobehavioural treatment, sympathetic blockade had a high success rate.

Physical therapy has proven to be an essential element in the treatment of overuse syndromes, RSD, myofascial pain and other forms of chronic pain in childhood. The child's emotional maturity, behavioural development and level of independence influence the goals and interventions chosen. The short attention span of a child, combined with a limited pain tolerance, may necessitate dividing the treatments into more frequent, shorter sessions.

The therapist must be flexible and focus on the most appropriate portion of the evaluation as the patient's tolerance permits. Procedures performed with the patient in the upright position are less threatening than those done supine. Starting with the child in the standing or sitting position will maximise his feeling of self-control during the therapy session.

Psychosocial elements need consideration and can heavily influence the patient's compliance. Activities must be found which are motivating to do. Socialisation may be incorporated into an activity such as walking to the shops, playing ball or swimming.

Ultrasound, though quite effective in older children and adults by delivering deep heating effects to tissues and promoting healing, is contraindicated in younger children in whom growth plates have not closed.

Biobehavioural treatment of chronic headache has gained wide acceptance recently and these techniques also show promise for the treatment of neuropathic pain. Children 7 years of age and older can be taught to control their pain by a combination of techniques. Biobehavioural treatment refers to a collection of techniques that fall into two different categories. These include:

1. self-control skills such as biofeedback and relaxation training.
2. procedures to modify the behaviour that increases the pain such as pain-behaviour management and cogntive–behavioural techniques.

As a part of the treatment, attempts are made to identify the antecedent stressors and consequences of the pain. A diary is often helpful to keep an accurate record of the activities and thoughts that surround the pain. Treatment then focuses on the teaching of relaxation techniques utilising meditation, imagery and progressive muscle relaxation. Biofeedback is useful to motivate the child to monitor and attenuate arousal in stressful circumstances and at the first signs of pain. Parents can then implement pain-behaviour management techniques by eliminating sources of reinforcement maintaining pain behaviour and promote active coping and normal activity. The child is then taught cognitive–behavioural strategies to deal with the negative thoughts which interfere with coping. In addition, children are taught problem-solving skills to help them deal with the stresses in their lives.

Opinions regarding optimal timing of the various treatment modalities in neuropathic pain remain mixed. In the view of Olsson et al (1990), early sympathetic blockade is indicated to shorten the overall course of the condition. Prospective study of this issue is warranted.

The use of regional and sympathetic blocks for the treatment of chronic pain has become routine in adult patients but their use in children is far less common. Utilising these blocks in children can be much more difficult due to the frequent need for heavy intravenous sedation or even general anaesthesia during performance of the block.

Prior to the performance of a regional nerve block in children, it is important that meticulous attention is paid to the psychological preparation of the child and his or her parents. Most children will cooperate much more if they know exactly how the block is performed and the extent of numbness or extremity weakness after the procedure. It is also imperative that an additonal anaesthesiologist is available during the block to monitor the patient and provide general anaesthesia or conscious sedation during performance of the block. Fasting guidelines must be carefully explained to the parent and child and immediate availability of emergency resuscitative drugs and equipment must be a priority. A nerve stimulator is frequently required as an aid for successful location of the nerves to be blocked. In addition, fluoroscopy may be used in a variety of circumstances, most notably when the nerves are not easily accessible (such as a lumber sympathetic or coeliac plexus block) or when the anatomy is distorted by disease or previous surgery.

Older children can usually cooperate with a regional block with incremental doses of sedative agents that allow assessment of

1. paraesthesias
2. the effect of a local anaesthetic test dose
3. evidence of inadvertent intravascular or subarachnoid needle placement.

If patient cooperation cannot be assured, general anaesthesia with endotracheal intubation is often the safest option to allow performance of the block.

Continuous catheter techniques rather than repeated injections are generally preferred in children due to the frequent need for heavy sedation or general anaesthesia for placement. Children tend to be much more cooperative for their subsequent physical therapy if nerve blocks have been done in a nontraumatic manner.

Medical management of neuropathic pain in children requires further study. Most prescribing is based on extrapolation from adult studies. Although we frequently prescribe tricyclic antidepressants, there are no prospective studies of their efficacy in neuropathic pain in childhood. Use of tricyclics requires assessment of the small but real risk of sudden cardiac events in children. Similarly, long term use of anticonvulsants in children with neuropathic pain requires weighing of risks associated with allergic and autoimmune reactions, hepatic and haematological toxicities, and behavioural alterations.

Antidepressant medications have been used as adjuvants for the treatment of chronic-pain syndromes in adults such as chronic headaches, denervation syndromes, postherpetic pain, rheumatic pain and facial pain (Getto et al 1987). Their effectiveness is thought to be related to increases in serotonin, a critical neurotransmitter in pain modulation (Snyder & Peroutha 1984). When using these agents in children, several guidelines have been developed to aid in choosing the most appropriate agent. First, it is reasonable to prescribe an antidepressant for pain in conditions where antidepressants have been shown to be effective in adults. The choice of a particular agent is usually made on the basis of side-effect profiles. Doxepin is available in an elixir and nortriptyline in a solution so they may be prescribed when ingestion of tablets is not possible. Trazadone has been associated with priapism and is therefore not recommended for younger males.

Children metabolise and eliminate tricyclic antidepressants more efficiently than adults do and may therefore require twice-daily dosing of these agents, particularly when antidepressant effects are sought (Geller et al 1987). The dose may be determined on a mg/kg basis but the optimal dose must still be based on effect within these guidelines. These drugs are usually started at low doses and gradually increased until some improvement is noted. More specific guidelines for the use of these drugs can be found in Table 80.6.

The use of opioids in chronic pain management in adults has been controversial. Similar considerations apply for children and adolescents. Among our clinic population of 500 patients annually, there are typically 6–12 who chronically receive opioids for noncancer/nonterminal painful conditions. As with adults, prescribing of opioids in this setting requires careful consideration of the patient's social functioning and optimisation of nonopioid alternatives. The developmental consequences of long-term opioid treatment in childhood are poorly understood.

PHANTOM-LIMB PAIN

Until recently, it was widely accepted that children do not experience phantom pain after limb amputation. Though there had been several case reports describing phantom pain in children prior to this, it was not until 1991 when Krane et al reported on their experience in the Seattle area, that it was shown that not only did phantom limb pain occur in paediatric amputees but the incidence was quite high. This pain was largely ignored or disregarded by health-care providers despite the fact that the pain was described as severe in many cases. Little is known about the best treatments for this type of pain in children. A treatment plan including epidural analgesia prior to and for several days after amputation, followed by physical therapy, TENS, low-dose tricyclic antidepressant agents and biobehavioural therapy has been recommended (McGrath & Hillier 1992).

Table 80.6 Psychotropic adjuvant analgesics

Drug	Starting dose mg	Maximum daily dose mg/kg/day
Tricyclic antidepressants		
Amitriptyline	10	3 – 5
Imipramine	10	3 – 5
Clomipramine	25	3 – 5
Nortriptyline	10	1– 3
Doxepin	12.5	12.5 –100 mg/day
Novel antidepressants		
Fluoxetine	10	10 – 20 mg/day
Antihistamines		
Hydroxyzine	25	25 –100 mg/day
Psychostimulants		
Methylphenidate	2.5	5 – 20 mg/dose
Dextroamphetamine	2.5	2.5 –10 mg/dose

Adapted from Heiligenstein & Gerrity 1993.

MEDICAL ILLNESSES ASSOCIATED WITH CHRONIC PAIN

Cancer

Children with cancer experience pain due to tumour infiltration or impingement and as a result of the various medical procedures they must undergo as a part of their treatment. Childhood cancer has several epidemiological differences compared to adult cancer that have important therapeutic implications. Childhood cancers have a considerably higher cure rate with chemotherapy and radiation than adult cancers. Chemotherapy is a major pain-relieving modality in many cases. Although moderate and severe pain are common in children with advanced disease, there are fewer patients with long-term pain and slowly fatal metastases, as occur with adult tumours such as breast or prostate cancer.

There has not been a detailed description of cancer-pain syndromes in children analogous to that pioneered by Foley et al (1976) in adults. However, several authors have studied the incidence of pain in this population and found that procedure-related pain is much more common than tumour-related pain once treatment is established (Cornaglia et al 1984; Miser et al 1987). Leukaemias, lymphomas, and visceral solid tumours frequently produce pain associated with infiltration of viscera. Sarcomas, including osteosarcoma, Ewing's sarcoma and primitive neuroectodermal tumours are associated with a relatively high incidence of severe pain in bone and soft tissues, as well as involvement of roots, plexuses and the epidural space. Brain tumours of posterior fossa origin are quite common and are often associated with headache.

Neuropathic pain is not rare in childhood cancer. It may be related to tumour involvement of peripheral nerves, plexuses and the epidural space. Deafferentation pain is often produced by surgical resection of limb sarcomas, particularly with limb-sparing procedures.

The World Health Organization's 'analgesic ladder' has been successfully applied to children in several series (Cancer Pain Relief 1986). Because of particular concerns with platelet dysfunction, acetaminophen, not aspirin, is the preferred first step of the ladder. In addition, codeine and oxycodone are acceptable second-step agents, but the mixed agonist-antagonists are not recommended. Oral morphine is widely regarded as the drug of first choice in children with cancer requiring a strong opioid. While most school-aged children and adolescents can swallow timed-release morphine tablets whole, the use of these agents in infants and toddlers is limited somewhat by the fact that crushing the tablets accelerates drug release. Methadone and levorphanol are both slowly eliminated in children and methadone elixir in our practice has become a convenient method to provide prolonged analgesia in infants unable to swallow tablets.

In a series of children studied by Pichard-Leandri et al (1990) and by Richter et al (1990), constipation was the most frequent side-effect of morphine treatment, though it was readily treated with cathartics. Nausea and pruritus were also common and could be adequately treated with phenothiazines and antihistamines. In a group of children undergoing bone-marrow transplantation with refractory pruritus from morphine, infusion of fentanyl was associated with good efficacy and a diminished incidence of pruritus (Miser et al 1987).

In a significant percentage of children, use of oral opioids is made difficult by ileus, bowel obstruction, refractory nausea, painful swallowing due mucositis or delirium associated with terminal illness. The choice of intravenous versus subcutaneous routes for parenteral infusions is determined by venous access and local custom. In the United States, a high percentage of children with cancer have long-term tunnelled silastic central venous catheters. In those who do not, subcutaneous infusions can be used according to the principles described elsewhere (Miser et al 1983; Bruera et al 1988, 1990).

Opioid requirements in children are extraordinarily variable. While a median morphine infusion rate of 0.04 mg/kg/h was described by Miser et al (1980), it is not rare in our experience for children to require 20–100 mg/kg/h in the setting of terminal disease. In many cases, these infusion rates provide comfort while preserving a clear sensorium. In some cases, there remains no margin between inadequate analgesia and persistent somnolence. As with adults, there appears to be some benefit from the use of amphetamines in children to antagonise somnolence (Bruera et al 1989). In our experience, tricyclic antidepressants also appear quite useful in the management of sleep disturbance, as well as the treatment of vincristine neuropathy or tumour involvement of peripheral nerves. The choice of agents parallels that for adults. In children unable to tolerate oral tricyclics, slow intravenous infusion of amitriptyline may be considered.

PCA appears quite useful for children with cancer. Although a basal infusion for postoperative pain is discouraged by some, it appears uniformly necessary when PCA is used for disease-related cancer pain (Kerr et al 1988). While parent-controlled or nurse-controlled analgesia is discouraged for postoperative patients, it appears extremely useful for the management of breakthrough pain in infants and toddlers with AIDS and cancer.

There remains a small subgroup of children with intolerable somnolence or delirium with very high opioid infusion rates. For selected patients, use of epidural and subarachnoid opioids and local anaesthetics can widen the therapeutic ratio. Each of these cases requires individual consideration of a variety of issues, including:

1. the patient's and parent's wishes for alertness versus sedation

2. the site of tumour spread, especially related to spinal involvement
3. the nature of the limiting side-effects
4. the contribution of nonnociceptive forms of suffering, including air hunger, fear of dying, anxiety, depression and isolation.

It has been our common experience that epidural or preferably subarachnoid local anaesthetic infusions may be required in addition to neuraxial opioids in order to adequately widen the therapeutic ratio. In these cases, systemic requirements are unpredictable and either acute somnolence or withdrawal can occur. Neurolytic blockade is used only extremely rarely for children (Berde et al 1990b).

A major feature of childhood cancer is the frequent requirement of brief noxious diagnostic and therapeutic procedures, including bone-marrow biopsy and aspiration and lumbar puncture. These procedures produce great fear and anxiety among children, and many survivors of childhood cancer regard these as the worst aspect of their cancer treatment. The distress of these procedures can be diminished by a variety of behavioural treatments (Jay et al 1987; Zeltzer et al 1989). In addition, there is a definite role for conscious sedation or brief general anaesthesia in many cases. Conscious sedation has been made more convenient by the recent development of short-acting opioids of the fentanyl series, short-acting benzodiazepines such as midazolam, and ultra-short-acting intravenous anaesthetics, such as propofol. We recently examined the issue of whether conscious sedation using midazolam with or without opioids can be applied safely in a paediatric oncology clinic without anaesthetists in attendance (Sievers et al 1991). With application of a standardised protocol (Table 80.7), all patients tolerated the procedure without mishap. Brief episodes of hypoxaemia occurred, but all resolved with encouragement to breathe deeply or with application of oxygen by face mask. Our findings support the routine use of pulse oximetry and constant observation throughout the procedure.

Cystic fibrosis

Children with cystic fibrosis have multiple medical problems which can cause them significant pain throughout their lives. Specific pain syndromes have been identified with this disease and strategies have been developed to deal with them. The major problem for these children is chest pain. This may arise from muscle overuse, chest wall disease or rib fracture (not an uncommon finding in these children). In addition, pneumothorax and chest tube insertion can cause considerable pain and make cooperation with chest physiotherapy quite difficult. Chest pain from overuse may respond to low-dose tricyclic antidepressants, TENS and antiinflammatory medications.

Table 80.7 Conscious sedation for oncology procedures: suggested guidelines

Full-time observer
Pulse oximetry
Oxygen
Bag and mask
Airway equipment
Resuscitative drugs
Reversal drugs (naloxone, flumazenil)

In addition, cautious use of opioids often combined with the parenteral nonsteroidal antiinflammatory agent, ketorolac, can be helpful. Caution must be used not to depress respiratory drive with these agents.

Headache is not uncommon in these children as a result of hypercarbia, muscle tension, sinusitis or migraine and may respond favourably to physical therapy, TENS units or acupuncture in addition to the routine treatments. These patients have an increased incidence of other types of pain as well, including abdominal, oesophageal, maxillofacial and orthopaedic pain.

AIDS

The pain associated with AIDS can be of peripheral or central origin. Peripheral neuropathies are relatively common along with headaches associated with the disease-related encephalopathy. Strafford et al (1993) investigated the sources of pain in patients with AIDS and found that abdominal pain, oesophagitis and pancreatitis were extremely common, occurring in most patients at some point in the disease progression. Respiratory distress and air hunger in the terminal stages of the illness were also a source of significant discomfort. Pain could usually be adequately treated with judicious use of opioids and comfort measures surrounding the performance of medical procedures.

Sickle-cell crisis

Vaso-occlusive crises in sickle-cell disease can produce severe episodic bouts of pain. Pharmacologic therapies are usually the mainstay of treatment and almost always involve some type of opioid. Nonsteroidal antiinflammatory agents such as ketorolac provide good adjunctive pain relief but are usually insufficient as single agents to control the pain. Oral opioids are used whenever possible but intravenous administration is often required. Continuous opioid infusions in younger patients and PCA in older children have proven to be effective in maintaining the pain at a manageable level (Batenhorst et al 1987; Schechter et al 1988; Holbrook 1990). Though tolerance and addiction are always a concern when long-term opioids are used, treatment with these agents should not be withheld during periods of intense pain. For those patients whose pain relief is limited by respiratory depression or extreme somnolence, epidural local anaesthetics and opioids have been used. However, they are generally reserved for pain crises that are considered much worse than usual (Finer et al 1988). Heating pads and hot baths may be helpful for many patients as well. Biobehavioural techniques can be taught during relatively painfree periods and enhance coping skills during the intermittent periods of intense pain.

Haemophilia

Haemophilia A is an X-linked disorders that can cause considerable pain throughout childhood due to recurrent bleeding into the joints. Treatment includes titrated use of opioid analgesics during these episodes. Nonsteroidal antiinflammatory agents are contraindicated.

Rheumatologic disease

Children with arthritis, lupus, scleroderma or mixed connective tissue disease may have chronic pain associated with either joint inflammation or a variety of associated vascular problems, including ischaemia of fingers and toes, and entrapment neuropathies. Nonsteroidals form the mainstay of analgesic therapy for children with milder forms of arthritis. Selected adolescents with severe Raynaud's disease associated with vasculopathy have benefited from sympathetic blockade.

CONCLUSIONS

In conclusion, the development of comprehensive paediatric pain-treatment teams has done much to improve the lives of children experiencing acute or chronic pain. Progress in the understanding of the pharmacology of opioids and the use of regional anaesthetics in children has made the treatment of pain easier and the prevention of pain a reality for certain patients. Undertreatment of pain in infants and children can no longer be justified by claims of an insufficient basis in pharmacologic studies.

REFERENCES

Agarwal R, Gutlove D P, Lockhart C H 1992 Seizures occurring in pediatric patients receiving continuous infusion of bupivacaine. Anesthesia and Analgesia 75: 284–286

Anand K J S, Hickey P R 1992 Halothane–morphine compared with high-dose sufentanil for anesthesia and postoperative analgesia in neonatal cardiac surgery. New England Journal of Medicine 326: 1–9

Anand K J S, Hansen D D, Hickey P R 1990 Hormonal–metabolic stress responses in neonates undergoing cardiac surgery. Anesthesiology 73: 661–670

Anders T F, Chalemian R J 1974 The effects of circumcision on sleep–wake states in human neonates. Psychosomatic Medicine 36: 174–179

Arnold J H, Truog R D, Orav E J, Scavone J M, Hershenson M B 1990 Tolerance and dependence in neonates sedated with fentanyl during extracorporeal membrane oxygenation. Anesthesiology 73: 1136–1140

Arnold J H, Truog R D, Scavone J M, Fenton T 1991 Changes in the pharmacodynamic response to fentanyl in neonates during continuous infusion. Journal of Pediatrics 119: 639–643

Attia J, Ecoffey C, Sandouk P et al 1986 Epidural morphine in children: pharmacokinetics and CO_2 sensitivity. Anesthesiology 65: 590–594.

Barr R G 1983 Recurrent abdominal pain. In: Levine M D, Carey W B, Crocker A C, Gross R T (eds) Developmental–behavioral pediatrics. W B Saunders, Philadelphia, p 521–528

Batenhorst R L, Maurer H S, Bertch K A et al 1987 Patient controlled analgesia in uncomplicated sickle cell pain crisis. Blood 70: S58a

Berde C B, Holzman R S, Sethna N F, Dickerson R B, Brustowicz R M 1988 A comparison of methadone and morphine for postoperative analgesia in children and adolescents. Anesthesiology 69: (suppl): A768

Berde C B, Sethna N F, Yemen T A 1990a Continuous epidural bupivacaine–fentanyl infusions in children following ureteral reimplantation. Anesthesia and Analgesia 73: A1128

Berde C B, Sethna N F, Fisher D E et al 1990b Celiac plexus blockade for a 3-year-old boy with hepatoblastoma and refractory pain. Pediatrics 85: 779–781

Berde C B, Lehn B M, Yee J D et al 1991a Patient-controlled analgesia in children and adolescents: a randomized, prospective comparison with intramuscular morphine for postoperative analgesia. Journal of Pediatrics 118: 460–466

Berde C B, Beyer J E, Bournaki M C et al 1991b Comparison of morphine and methadone for prevention of postoperative pain in 3- to 7-year-old children. Journal of Pediatrics 119: 136–141

Bernstein B H, Singsen B H, Kent J T et al 1978 Reflex neurovascular dystrophy in childhood. Journal of Pediatrics 93: 211–215

Bhat R, Chori G, Gulati A et al 1990 Pharmacokinetics of a single dose of morphine in preterm infants during the first week of life. Journal of Pediatrics 117: 477–481

Bodin A, Nyqvist-Mayer A, Wadsten T et al 1984 Phase diagram and aqueous solubility of the lidocaine-prilocaine binary system. Journal of Pharmaceutical Sciences 73: 481

Bosenberg A T, Bland B A, Schulte–Steinberg O 1988 Thoracic epidural anesthesia via caudal route in infants. Anesthesiology 69: 265–269

Bosenberg A T, Hadley G P, Murray W B 1991 Postoperative ventilation requirements following esophageal atresia repair. Journal of Pain and Symptom Management 6: 209

Brash A R, Hickey D E, Graham T P et al 1982 Pharmacokinetics of indomethacin in the neonate: relation of plasma indomethacin levels to response of the ductus arteriosus. New England Journal of Medicine 305: 67–72

Broadman L M 1990 Patient-controlled analgesia in children and adolescents. In: Ferrante F M, Ostheimer G W, Covino B G, (eds) Patient–controlled analgesia. Blackwell, Oxford, p 129–138

Broadman L M, Rice L J 1988 Pediatric regional anesthesia and perioperative analgesia. Problems in Anesthesia 2: 386–407

Broadman L M, Hannallah R S, Belman A B et al 1987a Postcircumcision pain – a prospective evaluation of subcutaneous ring block of the penis. Anesthesiology 67: 399–402

Broadman L M, Hannallah R S, Norden J M et al 1987b 'Kiddie caudals' experience with 1154 consecutive cases without complications. Anesthesia and Analgesia 66: S18

Broadman L M, Brown R E, Rice L J, Higgins T, Vaughan M 1989 Patient-controlled analgesia in children and adolescents: a report of postoperative pain management in 150 patients. Anesthesiology 71: A1171

Bruera E, Brenneis C, Michaud M et al 1988 Use of the subcutaneous route for the administration of narcotics in patients with cancer pain. Cancer 62: 407–411

Bruera E, Brenneis C, Paterson A H et al 1989 Use of methylphenidate as an adjuvant to narcotic analgesics in patients with advanced cancer. Journal of Pain and Symptom Management 4: 3–6

Bruera E, Legris M A, Kuehn N et al 1990 Hypodermoclysis for the administration of fluids and narcotic analgesics in patients with advanced cancer. Journal of Pain and Symptom Management 5: 78–82

Cancer Pain Relief 1986 World Health Organization, Geneva

Casey W F, Rice L J, Hannallah R S et al 1990 A comparison between bupivacaine instillation versus ilioinguinal/iliohypogastric nerve block for postoperative analgesia following inguinal herniorrhaphy in children. Anesthesiology 72: 637–639

Chaplan S R, Duncan S R, Brodsky J B et al 1992 Morphine and hydromorphone epidural analgesia. A prospective, randomized comparison. Anesthesiology 77: 1090–1094

Cornaglia C, Massimo L, Haupt R et al 1984 Incidence of pain in children with neoplastic disease. Pain 2 (Suppl): S28

Dalens B J 1990 Infraclavicular brachial plexus blocks. In: Dalens B J (ed) Pediatric Regional Anesthesia. CRC Press Boca Raton, p 241–255

Dalens B 1993 Peripheral nerve blockade in the management of postoperative pain in children. In: Schecter N L, Berde C B, Yaster M (eds) Pain in infants, children and adolescents. Williams & Wilkins, Baltimore, p 261–280

Dalens B, Vanneuville G, Tanguy A 1987 A new parascalene approach to the brachial plexus in children: comparison with the supraclavicular approach. Anesthesia and Analgesia 66: 1264–1271

Dalens B, Vanneuville G, Tanguy A 1989a Comparison of the fascia iliaca compartment block with the 3-in-1 block in children. Anesthesia and Analgesia 69: 705–713

Dalens B, Vanneuville G, Dechelotte P 1989b Penile block via the subpubic space in 100 children. Anesthesia and Analgesia 69: 41–45

Desparmet J, Meistelman C, Barre J, Saint-Maurice C 1987 Continuous epidural infusion of bupivacaine for postoperative pain relief in children. Anesthesiology 67: 108–110

Dodd E, Wang J M, Rauck R L 1988 Patient controlled analgesia for post-surgical pediatric patients aged 6–16 years. Anesthesiology 69: A372

Ecoffey C, Debousset A M, Samii K 1986 Lumbar and thoracic epidural anesthesia for urologic and upper abdominal surgery in infants and children. Anesthesiology 65: 87–90.

Finer P, Blair J, Rowe P 1988 Epidural analgesia in the management of labor pain and sickle cell crisis – a case report. Anesthesiology 68: 799–800

Fitzgerald M 1991 The developmental neurobiology of pain. In: Bond M R, Charlton J E, Woolf C J, (eds) Proceedings of the VIth World Congress on Pain, Pain Research and Clinical Management, vol. 4. Elsevier, Amsterdam, p 253–262

Foley K M 1976 Pain syndromes in patients with cancer. In: Bonica J J, Ventafridda V (eds) Advances in pain research and therapy. Raven Press, New York, p 59–75

Gaudreault P, Guay J, Nicol O et al 1988 Pharmacokinetics and clinical efficacy of intrarectal solution of acetaminophen. Canadian Journal of Anaesthesia 35: 149–152

Gaukroger P B, Tomkins D P, Van der Walt J H 1989 Patient-controlled analgesia in children. Anaesthesia and Intensive Care 17: 264–268

Geller B, Cooper T B, Schluchter M D et al 1987 Child and adolescent nortriptyline single dose pharmacokinetic parameters: final report. Journal of Clinical Psychopharmacology 7: 321–323

Getto C J, Sorkness C A, Howell T 1987 Antidepressants and chronic nonmalignant pain: a review. Journal of Pain Symptom and Management 2: 9–18

Giannini E H, Brewer E J, Miller M L et al 1990 Ibuprofen suspension in the treatment of juvenile rheumatoid arthritis. Pediatric Rheumatology Collaborative Study Group. Journal of Pediatrics 117: 645–652

Gourlay G K, Willis R J, Wilson P R 1984 Postoperative pain control with methadone: influence of supplementary methadone doses and blood-concentration-response relationships. Anesthesiology 61: 19–26

Gourlay G K, Willis R J, Lamberty J 1986 A double-blind comparison of the efficacy of methadone and morphine in postoperative pain control. Anesthesiology 64: 322–327

Halperin D L, Koren G, Attias D et al 1989 Topical skin anesthesia for venous, subcutaneous drug reservoir and lumbar punctures in children. Pediatrics 84: 281–284

Heiligenstein E, Gerrity S 1993 Psychotropics as adjuvant analgestics. In: Schechter N L, Berde C B, Yaster M (eds) Pain in infants, children and adolescents. Williams & Wilkins, Baltimore

Hendersen K, Sethna N F, Berde C B 1993 Continuous caudal anesthesia for inguinal hernia repair in former preterm infants. Journal of Clinical Anesthesia 5: 129–133

Holbrook C T 1990 Patient-controlled analgesia pain management for children with sickle cell disease. Journal of the Association of the Academy of Minority Physicians 1: 93–96

Hurwitz E S, Barret M J, Bregman D et al 1985 Public Health Service Study on Reye's syndrome and medications. Report of the pilot phase. New England Journal of Medicine 313: 849–857

Jay S M, Elliott C H, Katz E R et al 1987 Cognitive behavioral and pharmacologic interventions for children undergoing painful medical procedures. Journal of Consulting and Clinical Psychology 55: 860–865

Kerr I G, Sone M, DeAngelis C et al 1988 Continuous narcotic infusion with patient controlled analgesia for chronic cancer pain in outpatients. Annals of Internal Medicine 108: 554–557

Krane E J 1988 Delayed respiratory depression in a child after caudal epidural morphine. Anesthesia and Analgesia 67: 79–82

Krane E J, Jacobson L E, Lynn A M et al 1987 Caudal morphine for postoperative analgesia in children: a comparison with caudal bupivacaine and intravenous morphine. Anesthesia and Analgesia 66: 647–653

Krane E J, Heller E B, Pomietto M L 1991 Incidence of phantom sensation and pain in pediatric amputees. Anesthesiology 75: A69

Lawrie S C, Forbes D W, Akhtar T M, Morton N S 1990 Patient-controlled analgesia in children. Anaesthesia 46: 1074–1076

Levy G, Garretson L K 1974 Kinetics of salicylate elimination by newborn infants of mothers who ingested aspirin before delivery. Pediatrics 53: 201–210

Lynn A M, Slattery J T 1987 Morphine pharmacokinetics in early infancy. Anesthesiology 66: 136–139

McCafferty D F, Woolfson A D, Boston V 1989 In vivo assessment of percutaneous local anaesthetic preparations. British Journal of Anaesthesia 62: 17–21

McCloskey J J, Haun S E, Deshpande J K 1992 Bupivacaine toxicity secondary to continuous caudal epidural infusion in children. Anesthesia and Analgesia 75: 287–290

McGrath P A, Hillier J A 1992 Phantom limb sensations in adolescents: a case study to illustrate the utility of sensation and pain logs in pediatric clinical practice. Journal of Pain and Symptom Management 7: 46–52

McGrath P J, Unruh A 1987 Pain in children and adolescents. Elsevier Amsterdam

McNeely J M 1991 Comparison of epidural opioids and intravenous opioids in the postoperative management of pediatric antireflux surgery. Anesthesiology 75: A689

McNeely J M, Pontus S P, Trentadue N C 1992 Comparison of patient controlled analgesia with and without basal morphine infusion for postoperative pain control in children. Anesthesiology 77: A814

Marshall R E, Stratton W C, Moore J A et al 1980 Circumcision 1. Effects upon newborn behavior. Infant Behavior and Development 3: 1–14

Maunuksela E L, Korpela R 1986 Double-blind evaluation of a lignocaine-prilocaine cream (EMLA) in children: effect on the pain associated with venous cannulation. British Journal of Anaesthesia 58: 1242

Maunuksela E-L, Olkkola K T, Korpela R 1987 Intravenous indomethacin as postoperative analgesic in children: acute effects on blood pressure, heart rate, body temperature and bleeding. Annals of Clinical Research 19: 359–363

Maunuksela E-L, Olkkola K T, Korpela R 1988 Does prophylactic intravenous infusion of indomethacin improve the management of postoperative pain in children? Canadian Journal of Anesthesia 35: 123–127

Maunuksela E-L, Ryhanen P, Janhunen L 1992 Efficacy of rectal ibuprofen in controlling postoperative pain in children. Canadian Journal of Anaesthesia 39: 226–230

Maunuksela E-L, Kokki H, Bullingham R E S 1993 Comparison of IV ketorolac with morphine for postoperative pain in children. Clinical Pharmacology and Therapeutics
Means L J, Allen H M, Lookabill S J, Krishna G 1988 Recovery room initiation of patient-controlled analgesia in pediatric patients. Anesthesiology 69: A772
Meignier M, Souron R, Le Neel J C 1983 Postoperative dorsal epidural analgesia in the child with respiratory disabilities. Anesthesiology 59: 473–475
Miller R P, Roberts R J, Fischer L J 1976 Acetaminophen elimination kinetics in neonates, children and adults. Clinical Pharmacology and Therapeutics 19: 284–294
Miser A W, Miser J S, Clark B S 1980 Continuous intravenous infusion of morphine sulfate for control of severe pain in children with terminal malignancy. Journal of Pediatrics 96: 930–932
Miser A W, Davis D M, Hughes C S, et al 1983 Continuous subcutaneous infusion of morphine in children with cancer. American Journal of Diseases of Children 137: 383–385
Miser A W, Dothage J A, Wesley R A, Miser J S 1987 The prevalence of pain in a pediatric and young adult cancer population. Pain 29: 73–83
Miser A W, Dothage J A, Miser J S 1987b Continuous intravenous fentanyl for pain control in children and young adults with cancer. Clinical Journal of Pain 3: 152–157
Moore D C, Mather L E, Bridenbaugh P O et al 1976 Arterial and venous plasma levels of bupivacaine following epidural and bilateral intercostal nerve blocks. Anesthesiology 45: 39–45
Nelson P S, Streisand J B, Mulder S M et al 1989 Comparison of oral transmucosal fentanyl citrate and an oral solution of meperidine, diazepam, and atropine for premedication in children. Anesthesiology 70: 616–621
Olkkola K T, Maunuksela E-L, Korpela R 1989 Pharmacokinetics of postoperative intravenous indomethacin in children. Pharmacology and Toxicology 64: 157–160
Olsson G I, Arner S, Hirsch G 1990 Reflex sympathetic dystrophy in children. Advances in Pain Research and Therapy 15: 323–331
Pasternak G W, Zhang A Z, Tecott L 1980 Developmental differences between high and low affinity opiate binding sites: their relationship to analgesia and respiratory depression. Life Sciences 27: 1185–1190
Pichard-Leandri E, Poulain P H, Gauvain A 1990 Evaluation of the side effects related to long term opioid treatment in cancer pain children. Pain (suppl 5): S8
Richards M P M, Bernal J F, Brackbill Y 1976 Early behavioural differences: gender or circumcision? Developmental Psychobiology 9: 89–95
Richter R C, Sittl R J C Sorge J 1990 Results of a multicenter study of the German Society of Pediatric Oncology concerning pain management in children. Pain (suppl 5): S26
Rodgers B M, Webb C J, Stergios D et al 1988 Patient-controlled analgesia in pediatric surgery. Journal of Pediatric Surgery 23: 259–262
Rossitch E Jr, Oakes W J, Ovelman-Levitt J et al 1992 Self-mutilation following brachial plexus injury sustained at birth. Pain 50: 209–211
Rothstein P, Arthur G R, Feldman H S et al 1986 Bupivacaine for intercostal nerve blocks in children: blood concentrations and pharmacokinetics. Anesthesia and Analgesia 65: 625–632
Sara C A, Lowry C J 1984 A complication of circumcision and dorsal nerve block of the penis. Anaesthesia and Intensive Care 13: 79 – 85
Schechter N L, Berrian F B, Katz S M, 1988 The use of patient-controlled analgesia in adolescents with sickle cell pain crisis: a preliminary report. Journal of Pain and Symptom Management 3: 109–113
Schechter N L, Weisman S J, Rosenblum M et al 1991 Oral transmucosal fentanyl citrate for pediatric procedures. Journal of Pain and Symptom Management 6: 178
Sievers T D, Yee J D, Foley M E et al 1991 Midazolam for conscious sedation during pediatric oncology procedures: safety and recovery parameters. Pediatrics 88: 1172–1179
Snyder S H, Peroutha S J 1984 Antidepressants and neurotransmitter receptors. In: Post R M, Ballenger J C (eds) Neurobiology of mood disorders. Williams & Wilkins, Baltimore p 686–697
Soliman I E, Broadman L M, Hannallah R S et al 1988 Comparison of the analgesic effects of EMLA (eutectic mixture of local anesthetics) to intradermal lidocaine infiltration prior to venous cannulation in unpremedicated children. Anesthesiology 68: 804–806
Stang H J, Gunnar M R, Snellman L et al 1988 Local anesthesia for neonatal circumcision-effects on distress and cortisol response. Journal of the American Medical Association 259: 1507–1511
Stoelting R K 1987 Pharmacology and physiology in anesthetic practice. J B Lippincott, Philadelphia
Strafford M A, Cahill C A, Schwartz T, Berde C B 1993 Pain in children with AIDS. (submitted)
Stuart J J, Pisko E J 1981 Choline magnesium trisalicylate does not impair platelet aggregation. Pharmatherapeutica 2: 547
Talbert L M, Kraybill E N, Potter H D 1976 Adrenal cortical response to circumcision in the neonate. Obstetrics and Gynecology 48: 208–210
Taylor E, White P F, Urquhart M L 1989 Postoperative analgesia: SQ–PCA vs IV–PCA. Anesthesiology 71: A685
Urquhart M L, Klapp K, White P F 1988 Patient-controlled analgesia: a comparison of intravenous versus subcutaneous hydromorphone. Anesthesiology 69: 428–432
Watcha M F, Jones M B, Lagueruela R G et al 1992 Comparison of ketorolac and morphine as adjuvants during pediatric surgery. Anesthesiology 76: 368–372
Weisman S J, Schechter N L, Rosenblum M 1991 Safety and efficacy of oral transmucosal fentanyl for procedures in children. Journal of Pain and Symptom Management 6: 142
Wilder R T, Berde C B, Wolohan M et al 1992a Reflex sympathetic dystrophy in children: clinical characteristics and follow-up in seventy patients. Journal of Bone and Joint Surgery 74A: 910–919
Wilder R T, Berde C B, Troshynski T J et al 1992b Patient-controlled analgesia in children and adolescents: safety and outcome among 1589 patients. Anesthesiology 77: A1187
Yaster M, Maxwell L G 1989 Pediatric regional anesthesia. Anesthesiology 70: 323–338
Yaster M, Maxwell L G 1993 Opioid agonists and antagonists. In: Schechter N L, Berde C B, Yaster M (eds) Pain in infants, children and adolescents. Williams & Wilkins, Baltimore p 145–171
Zeltzer L K, Jay S M, Fisher D M 1989 The management of pain associated with pediatric procedures. Pediatric Clinics of North America 36: 941– 964

Management of cancer pain

81. Practical issues in the management of cancer pain

Nathan I. Cherny and Russell K. Portenoy

INTRODUCTION

Pain is among the most prevalent symptoms experienced by patients with cancer (Bonica et al 1990b; Coyle et al 1990; Ventafridda et al 1990; Henteleff 1991; Johanson 1991). Although established analgesic strategies could benefit most patients (Takeda 1986; Ventafridda et al 1987b; Walker et al 1988; Jorgensen et al 1990; Schug et al 1990; Grond et al 1991), undertreatment is common (Bonica 1985; Stjernsward & Teoh 1990). Inadequate understanding of the principles of cancer pain therapy contributes greatly to undertreatment (Cleeland et al 1986; Schauer et al 1988; Cleeland 1989; Musto 1989; Von Roenn et al 1993) and efforts to redress this situation are both a therapeutic and an ethical imperative (Edwards 1989; Martin 1989; Wanzer et al 1989).

The success of cancer pain therapy depends on the ability of the clinician to assess the presenting problems, identify and evaluate pain syndromes and formulate a plan for comprehensive continuing care (Foley & Inturrisi 1987; Belgrade 1989; Ferrell et al 1989). This requires familiarity with a range of therapeutic options (Table 81.1) and an approach to long-term care that is responsive to the changing needs of the patient (Coyle 1987; Ventafridda 1989; Shegda & McCorkle 1990). This approach emphasises the need to incorporate pain treatment within a broader therapeutic agenda, in which tumour control, symptom palliation (physical and psychological) and functional rehabilitation are concurrently addressed (Ventafridda 1989; World Health Organization 1990).

Table 81.1 Analgesic therapies for cancer pain

Therapy	Examples
Primary therapy	Chemotherapy Radiotherapy Hormone therapy Immunotherapy Surgery Antibiotics
Systemic analgesic pharmacotherapy	Nonopioid analgesics Opioids Adjuvant analgesics
Anaesthetic techniques	Intraspinal opioids ± local anaesthetic Chemical rhizotomy Somatic neurolysis Sympathetic blockade
Neurosurgical techniques	Rhizotomy Cordotomy Cingulotomy Pituitary ablation Dorsal root entry zone lesions
Physiatric techniques	Orthoses Physical therapy
Psychological techniques	Relaxation training Distraction techniques
Neurostimulatory techniques	Transcutaneous electrical nerve stimulation Dorsal column stimulation Deep brain stimulation Acupuncture

COMPREHENSIVE ASSESSMENT

The formulation of an effective therapeutic strategy for the management of pain and other symptoms is predicated on a comprehensive assessment of the patient (described in Ch. 43). The assessment should clarify the characteristics of the pain, including its impact on function and psychological well-being, the pain syndrome and the putative mechanisms that may underlie the pain. In addition, the assessment defines and evaluates both the nature and extent of the underlying disease and identifies concurrent problems (physical, psychological and social) that are contributing, or may soon contribute, to patient distress.

The particular therapeutic strategy that evolves from this information depends on the goals of care. These goals are diverse, but can generally be grouped into three broad categories:

1. prolonging survival
2. optimising comfort
3. optimising function.

The relative priority of these goals provides an essential context for therapeutic decision-making. The therapeutic strategy should address a prioritised problem list that best serves both the current goals of the patient and the anticipated problems that would benefit from advanced planning.

Most cancer patients can attain satisfactory relief of pain through an approach that incorporates primary treatments, systemic analgesic therapy and at times, other noninvasive techniques (such as psychological or rehabilitative interventions). Some patients whose pain is refractory to this approach benefit from invasive anaesthetic or neurosurgical treatments. Such patients should have access to specialists in pain management or palliative medicine, who can provide additional expertise in addressing these complex problems.

PRIMARY THERAPY

The assessment process may reveal a cause for the pain that is amenable to primary therapy (i.e. therapy that is directed at the aetiology of the pain). This therapy may improve comfort, function or duration of survival. For example, pain that is produced by tumour infiltration may respond to antineoplastic treatment with surgery, radiotherapy or chemotherapy and pain caused by infections may be relieved with antibiotic therapy or drainage procedures. Specific analgesic treatments are usually required as an adjunct to the primary therapy.

RADIOTHERAPY

Radiotherapy has a pivotal role in the treatment of cancer pain and other oncological conditions (Bates 1992; Bates et al 1992; Coia 1992). Before this approach is selected for symptom palliation, however, the clinician should ensure that there is a high likelihood of efficacy and a low risk of adverse effects. The duration of treatment should be short and it should offer a more favourable risk: benefit ratio than other available therapeutic modalities (Bosch 1984). In some situations, such as the treatment of bone metastases (Bates 1992; Bates et al 1992), epidural neoplasm (Bates 1992) and cerebral metastases (Coia 1992), the value of radiotherapy is documented by abundant data and a favourable clinical experience. In other settings, however, there is a paucity of data, and the use of radiotherapy is empirical. For example, the results with perineal pain due to low sacral plexopathy appear to be encouraging (Bosch 1984; Dobrowsky & Schmidt 1985) and hepatic radiotherapy (e.g. 2000–3000 cGy) can be well tolerated and effective for the pain of hepatic capsular distension in 50–90% of patients (Prassad et al 1977; Sherman et al 1978; Borgelt et al 1981; Minsky & Leibel 1989).

CHEMOTHERAPY

Despite a paucity of data concerning the specific analgesic benefits of chemotherapy (MacDonald 1990), there is a strong clinical impression that tumour shrinkage is generally associated with relief of pain. Although there are some reports of analgesic value even in the absence of significant tumour shrinkage (Patt et al 1985), the likelihood of a successful effect on pain is generally related to the likelihood of tumour response. Hence, benefit can be anticipated in chemotherapy-responsive tumours, such as lymphoma, small-cell lung cancer, germ-cell tumours and previously untreated breast cancer. In all situations, the decision to administer chemotherapy solely for the treatment of symptoms should be promptly reconsidered unless the patient demonstrates a clearly favourable balance between relief and adverse effects.

SURGERY

Surgery may have a role in the relief of symptoms caused by specific problems, such as obstruction of a hollow viscus, unstable bony structures and compression of neural tissues (Williams 1984; Boraas 1985; Petrelli et al 1985; Sundaresan & DiGiacinto 1987; MacDonald 1990). The potential benefits must be weighed against the risks of surgery, the anticipated length of hospitalisation and convalescence, and the predicted duration of benefit (Boraas 1985). Clinical experience has generally been most effective when surgery has been used to stabilise pathological fractures, relieve bowel obstructions or drain symptomatic ascites. Large volume (up to 5–10 litres) paracentesis, for example, may provide prompt and prolonged relief from the pain and discomfort of tense ascites (Boraas 1985; Ross et al 1989), with a small risk of hypotension (Cruikshank & Buchsbaum 1973; Ross et al 1989) or hypoproteinaemia (Lifshitz & Buchsbaum 1976). Radical surgery to excise locally advanced disease in patients with no evidence of metastatic spread may be palliative, and potentially increase the survival of some patients (Takagi et al 1985; Williams et al 1988; Montesani et al 1991; Temple & Ketcham 1992).

ANTIBIOTIC THERAPY

Antibiotics may be analgesic when the source of the pain involves infection. Illustrative examples include chronic sinus infections, pelvic abscess, pyonephrosis and osteitis pubis (Butch et al 1985; Burney & Faulkner 1988). In some cases, infection may be occult and confirmed only by the symptomatic relief provided by empiric treatment with these drugs (Bruera & McDonald 1986; Coyle & Portenoy 1991).

SYSTEMIC ANALGESIC PHARMACOTHERAPY

THE 'ANALGESIC LADDER'

Analgesic pharmacotherapy is the mainstay of cancer pain management (Foley 1985; World Health Organization 1986, 1990). Although concurrent use of other interventions is valuable in many patients, and essential in some, analgesic drugs are needed in almost every case. Based on clinical convention, analgesic drugs can be separated into three groups:

1. the nonopioid analgesics
2. the opioid analgesics
3. adjuvant analgesics, which are drugs with other primary indications that can be effective analgesics in specific circumstances.

The guiding principle of care is the individualisation of therapy. Through a process of repeated evaluations, drug selection and administration is individualised so that a favorable balance between pain relief and adverse pharmacological effects is achieved and maintained (Foley & Inturrisi 1987; Belgrade 1989; Ferrell et al 1989).

An expert committee convened by the Cancer Unit of the World Health Organization (WHO) has proposed a useful approach to drug selection for cancer pain, which has become known as the 'analgesic ladder' (World Health Organization 1986). When combined with appropriate dosing guidelines, this approach is capable of providing adequate relief to 70–90% of patients (Takeda 1986; Ventafridda et al 1987b; Walker et al 1988; Schug et al 1990; Grond et al 1991). Emphasising that pain intensity should be the prime consideration in analgesic selection, the approach advocates three basic steps (Fig. 81.1).

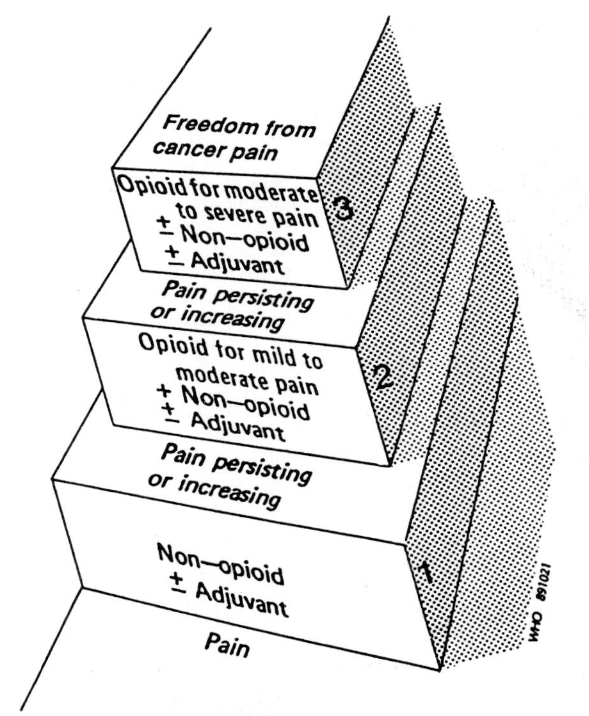

Fig. 81.1 WHO analgesic ladder. (From World Health Organization 1990 with permission.)

Step 1

Patients with mild to moderate cancer-related pain should be treated with a nonopioid analgesic, which should be combined with an adjuvant analgesic if a specific indication for one exists. For example, a patient with mild to moderate arm pain caused by radiation-induced brachial plexopathy may benefit when a tricyclic antidepressant is added to acetaminophen.

Step 2

Patients who are relatively nontolerant and present with moderate to severe pain, or who fail to achieve adequate relief after a trial of a nonopioid analgesic, should be treated with an opioid conventionally used to treat pain of this intensity. This treatment is typically accomplished using a combination product containing a nonopioid (e.g. aspirin or acetaminophen) and an opioid (such as codeine, oxycodone or propoxyphene). This drug can also be coadministered with an adjuvant analgesic.

Step 3

Patients who present with severe pain, or fail to achieve adequate relief following appropriate administration of drugs on the second rung of the 'analgesic ladder', should receive an opioid agonist conventionally used for pain of this intensity. This drug may also be combined with a nonopioid analgesic or an adjuvant drug.

NONOPIOID ANALGESICS

The nonopioid analgesics (aspirin, acetaminophen and the nonsteroidal antiinflammatory drugs (NSAIDs)) are useful alone for mild to moderate pain (Step 1 of the analgesic ladder) and provide additive analgesia when combined with opioid drugs in the treatment of more severe pain. Unlike opioid analgesics, the nonopioid analgesics have a 'ceiling' effect for analgesia and produce neither tolerance nor physical dependence.

The nonopioid analgesics constitute a heterogeneous group of compounds that differ in chemical structure but share many pharmacological actions (see Ch. 48) (Table 81.2). Some of these agents, like aspirin and the NSAIDs, inhibit the enzyme cyclo-oxygenase and consequently block the biosynthesis of prostaglandins, inflammatory

Table 81.2 Nonopioid analgesics

Chemical class	Generic name
Nonacidic	Acetaminophen
	Nabumetone
Acidic	
Salicylates	Aspirin
	Diflunisal
	Choline magnesium trisalicylate
	Salsalate
Proprionic acids	Ibuprofen
	Naproxen
	Fenoprofen
	Ketoprofen
	Flurbiprofen
	Suprofen
Acetic acids	Indomethacin
	Tolmentin
	Sulindac
	Diclofenac
	Ketorolac
Oxicams	Piroxicam
Fenemates	Mefenamic acid
	Meclofenamic acid

mediators known to sensitise peripheral nociceptors (Vane 1971). A central mechanism is also likely (Willer et al 1989; Malmberg & Yaksh 1992) and appears to predominate in acetaminophen analgesia (Piletta et al 1991).

The safe administration of nonopioid analgesics requires familiarity with their potential adverse effects (Brooks & Wood 1991). Aspirin and the other NSAIDs have a broad spectrum of potential toxicity; bleeding diathesis due to inhibition of platelet aggregation, gastroduodenopahy (including peptic ulcer disease) and renal impairment are the most common. The less common adverse effects include confusion, precipitation of cardiac failure and exacerbation of hypertension. Particular caution is required in the administration of these agents to patients at increased risk of adverse effects, including the elderly and those with blood-clotting disorders, predilection to peptic ulceration, impaired renal function and concurrent corticosteroid therapy. Of the NSAIDs, the nonacetylated salicylates (choline magnesium trisalicylate and salsalate) are preferred in patients who have a predilection to bleeding; these drugs have less effect on platelet aggregation and no effect on bleeding time at the usual clinical doses (Insel 1990). Acetaminophen also rarely produces gastrointestinal toxicity and there are no adverse effects on platelet function; hepatic toxicity is possible, however and patients with chronic alcoholism and liver disease can develop severe hepatotoxicity at the usual therapeutic doses (Seeff et al 1986).

The optimal administration of nonopioid analgesics requires an understanding of their clinical pharmacology (Brooks & Wood 1991). There is no certain knowledge of the minimal effective analgesic dose, ceiling dose or toxic dose for any individual patient with cancer pain. These doses may be higher or lower than the usual dose ranges recommended for the drug involved. Recommended doses are usually derived from studies performed in relatively healthy patients who have an inflammatory disease, a population clearly dissimilar from those with cancer pain, who often have coexistent organ failure and may be receiving multiple other drugs. Given that the effects of these drugs are (at least partially) dose-dependent, in the cancer population the minimal effective analgesic dose is unknown. These observations support an approach to the administration of NSAIDs that incorporates both low initial doses and dose titration. Through a process of gradual dose escalation, it may be possible to identify the ceiling dose and reduce the risk of significant toxicity. Several weeks are needed to evaluate the efficacy of a dose when NSAIDs are used in the treatment of grossly inflammatory lesions, such as arthritis. Clinical experience suggests that a shorter period, usually a week, is adequate for the same purpose in the patient with cancer pain. Based on clinical experience, an upper limit for dose titration is usually set at 1.5–2 times the standard recommended dose of the drug in question. Since failure with one NSAID can be followed by success with another, sequential trials of several NSAIDs may be useful to identify a drug with a favourable balance between analgesia and side-effects.

OPIOID ANALGESICS

Cancer pain of moderate or greater intensity should generally be treated with a systemically administered opioid analgesic. Optimal use of opioid analgesics requires a sound understanding of the general principles of opioid pharmacology (see Ch. 49), the pharmacological characteristics of each of the commonly used drugs and principles of administration, include:

1. drug selection
2. routes of administration
3. dosing and dose titration
4. adverse effects and their management.

General principles of opioid pharmacology

The clinical implications of opioid classification

Based on their interactions with the various receptor subtypes, opioid compounds can be divided into agonist, agonist-antagonist and antagonist classes (Table 81.3) (Jaffe & Martin 1990). The pure agonist drugs (Table 81.4) are most commonly used in clinical pain management. The mixed agonist-antagonist opioids (pentazocine, nalbuphine and butorphanol) and the partial agonist opioids (buprenorphine and probably dezocine) play a minor role in the management of cancer pain (Foley 1985; Foley & Inturrisi 1987) because of the existence of a

Table 81.3 Analgesic opioid classification based on receptor interactions

Agonists	Partial agonists	Agonist/antagonists
Morphine	Buprenorphine	Pentazocine
Codeine	Dezocine	Butorphanol
Oxycodone		Nalbuphine
Hydrocodone		
Dihydrocodeine		
Heroin		
Oxymorphone		
Meperidine		
Levorphanol		
Hydromorphone		
Methadone		
Fentanyl		
Sufentanil		
Alfentanil		
Propoxyphene		

ceiling effect for analgesia, the potential for precipitation of withdrawal in patients physically dependent to opioid agonists, and in the case of mixed agonist-antagonists, the problem of dose-dependent psychotomimetic side-effects that exceed those of pure agonist drugs.

The pure agonist opioid drugs appear to have no ceiling effect for analgesia. As the dose is raised, analgesic effects increase until either analgesia is achieved or the patient loses consciousness. This increase in effect occurs as a log-linear function: dose increments on a logarithmic scale yield linear increases in analgesia. In practice, it is the appearance of adverse effects, including confusion, sedation, nausea, vomiting or respiratory depression, that imposes a limit on the useful dose. The overall efficacy of any drug in a specific patient will be determined by the balance between analgesia and side-effects that occurs during dose escalation (Portenoy et al 1990).

Relative potency and equianalgesic doses

Relative analgesic potency is the ratio of the dose of two analgesics required to produce the same analgesic effect. By convention, the relative potency of each of the commonly used opioids is based upon a comparison to 10 mg of parenteral morphine (Houde et al 1966). Equianalgesic dose information (Table 81.4) provides guidelines for dose selection when the drug or route of administration is changed. Equianalgesic doses provide a useful reference point but should not be considered as standard starting doses or a firm guideline when switching between opioids. Numerous variables may influence the appropriate dose for the individual patient, including pain severity, prior opioid exposure (and the degree of cross-tolerance this confers), age, route of administration, level of consciousness and metabolic abnormalities (see below).

'Weak' versus 'strong' opioids

The division of opioid agonists into 'weak' versus 'strong' opioids was incorporated into the original 'analgesic ladder' proposed by the World Health Organization

Table 81.4 Opioid agonist drugs

Drug	Dose (mg) equianalgesic to 10 mg I M Morphine I M	P O	Half-life (hrs)	Duration of action (hrs)	Comments
Codeine	130	200	2–3	2–4	Usually combined with a nonopioid
Oxycodone	15	30	2–3	2–4	Usually combined with a nonopioid
Propoxyphene	50	100	2–3	2–4	Usually combined with nonopioid. Norpropoxyphene toxicity may cause seizures
Morphine	10	30 (repeated dose) 60 (single dose)	2–3	3–4	Multiple routes of administration available. Controlled release available. M6G accumulation in renal failure
Hydromorphone	1.5	7.5	2–3	2–4	No known active metabolites. Multiple routes available
Methadone	10	20	15–190	4–8	Plasma accumulation may lead to delayed toxicity. Dosing should be initiated on a PRN basis
Meperidine	75	300	2–3	2–4	Low oral bioavailability. Normeperidine toxicity limits utility. Contraindicated in patients with renal failure and those receiving MAO inhibitors
Oxymorphone	1	10 (PR)	2–3	3–4	No oral formulation available. Less histamine release
Heroin	5	60	0.5	3–4	High solubility. Morphine prodrug
Levorphanol	2	4	12–15	4–8	Plasma accumulation may lead to delayed toxicity
Fentanyl transdermal system	NA	NA		48–72	Patches available to deliver 25, 50, 75 and 100 μg/h

(1986). This distinction was not based on a fundamental difference in the pharmacology of the pure agonist opioids, but rather reflected the customary manner in which these drugs were used. The opioids customarily used for moderate pain (Step 2 of the analgesic ladder) in the United States include codeine, dihydrocodeine, hydrocodone, oxycodone and propoxyhene.

Selecting patients for opioid therapy

A trial of systemic opioid therapy should be administered to all cancer patients with pain of moderate or greater severity. This is true regardless of the pain mechanism (Portenoy et al 1990; Cherny et al 1992; Jadad et al 1992; McQuay et al 1992). Although somatic and visceral pain appear to be relatively more responsive to opioid analgesics than neuropathic pain, a neuropathic mechanism does not confer ‘opioid resistance’ or ‘opioid unresponsiveness’ (Twycross & Lack 1984; Arner & Meyerson 1988; Reidenberg et al 1988). Opioid responsiveness is a continuum that may vary with any of a large number of pain-related factors (Portenoy et al 1990; Cherny et al 1992), and appropriate dose escalation will identify many patients with neuropathic pain who can achieve adequate relief (Portenoy et al 1990; McQuay et al 1992).

Patients who present with severe pain should be treated with a ‘strong’ opioid from the start. Patients with moderate pain are commonly treated with a combination drug containing acetaminophen or aspirin plus codeine, oxycodone or propoxyphene. The dose of these combination products can be increased until the maximum dose of the nonopioid coanalgesic is attained (e.g. 4000–6000 mg acetaminophen). If pain relief is inadequate at this dose, the opioid contained in the combination product can be increased as a single agent (e.g. oxycodone tablets or syrup can be used to supplement an oxycodone–aspirin combination product) or the patient can be switched to an opioid customarily used to treat severe pain.

Important factors in opioid selection

Besides pain intensity, there are numerous other factors that must be considered in the selection of an appropriate opioid. Among the most important are patient age, prior opioid therapy, the influence of underlying illness and characteristics of the opioid and concurrent medications.

Patient age

For the younger patient without major organ failure, any of the available agonist opioids could be selected. Convenience of administration should be a major determinant; morphine sulphate may be preferred since it is available as a controlled release preparation that allows an 8–12 hour dosing interval. For the elderly and those with major organ failure, short half-life drugs (e.g. morphine, hydromorphone or oxycodone), which are simpler to titrate due to the relatively short period required to approach steady-state plasma concentrations, are preferred. The clearance of morphine is decreased in individuals older than 50 years, and this age-related difference in pharmacokinetics may explain, in part, the greater tendency of older patients to adverse effects of morphine (Kaiko 1980).

Pharmacological considerations

As discussed previously, the mixed agonist-antagonist opioids (pentazocine, nalbuphine and butorphanol) and the partial agonist opioids (buprenorphine and probably dezocine) are not preferred in the management of cancer pain (Foley 1985; Foley & Inturrisi 1987). Similarly the pharmacological characteristics of meperidine limit its role in the cancer population. Meperidine is N-demethylated to normeperidine, which is an active metabolite that is twice as potent as a convulsant and one-half as potent as an analgesic than its parent compound. The half-life of normeperidine is 12–16 hours, approximately 4–5 times the half-life of meperidine. Accumulation of normeperidine after repetitive dosing of meperidine is initiated can result in central nervous system toxicity characterised by subtle adverse mood effects, tremulousness, multifocal myoclonus and, occasionally, seizures (Szeto et al 1977; Eisendrath et al 1987). Although accumulation of normeperidine is most likely to affect the elderly and patients with overt renal disease, toxicity is sometimes observed in younger patients with normal renal function (Szeto et al 1977; Kaiko et al 1983).

The most serious toxicity associated with meperidine is normeperidine-induced seizures. Naloxone does not reverse this effect and indeed, could theoretically precipitate seizures in patients receiving meperidine by blocking the depressant action of meperidine and allowing the convulsant activity of normeperidine to become manifest (Umans & Inturrisi 1982). If naloxone must be administered to a patient receiving meperidine, it should be diluted and slowly titrated while appropriate seizure precautions are taken. Selective toxicity of meperidine can also occur following administration to patients receiving monoamine oxidase inhibitors. This combination may produce a syndrome characterised by hyperpyrexia, muscle rigidity and seizures (Inturrisi & Umans 1986). The pathophysiology of this syndrome is unknown.

Coexisting disease

Pharmacokinetic studies of meperidine, pentazocine and propoxyphene have revealed that liver disease may decrease the clearance and increase the bioavailability and half-lives of these drugs (Neal et al 1979; Giacomini et al 1980). These changes may eventuate in plasma concentrations higher than normal. Mild or moderate hepatic impairment has only minor impact on morphine clearance (Patwardhan et al 1981; Crotty et al 1989); however, advanced disease may be associated with reduced elimination (Hasselstrom et al 1990).

Patients with renal impairment may accumulate the active metabolites of propoxyphene (norpropoxyphene), meperidine (normeperidine) and morphine (morphine-6-glucuronide) (Sawe et al 1985; Osborne et al 1986; Chan & Matzke 1987; McQuay et al 1990; Hagen et al 1991; Portenoy et al 1991). In the setting of renal failure or unstable renal function, titration of these drugs requires caution and close monitoring; alternative opioids are often recommended.

Response to previous trials of opioid therapy

The report of inadequate analgesia with previous trials of opioid analgesics due to dose-limiting drug toxicity may influence subsequent drug selection. Clinical experience supports sequential trials of different opioid drugs, which may identify an agent with a more acceptable balance between analgesia and side-effects. Interindividual differences in opioid responses, and the existence of incomplete cross-tolerance to the analgesic effects and adverse effects of different opioid drugs may explain the potential utility of this approach (Galer et al 1992).

Selecting the appropriate route of systemic opioid administration

Routes of systemic administration may be classified on the basis of invasiveness (Table 81.5). Opioids should be administered by the least invasive and safest route capable of providing adequate analgesia. In a survey of patients with advanced cancer, more than half required two or more routes of administration prior to death and almost a quarter required three or more (Coyle et al 1990).

Noninvasive routes

The oral route of opioid administration is the preferred approach in routine practice. Alternative routes are necessary for patients who have impaired swallowing or gastrointestinal dysfunction, those who require a very rapid onset of analgesia and those who are unable to manage either the logistics or side-effects associated with the oral route. For highly tolerant patients, the inability to prescribe a manageable oral opioid programme due to excessive number of tablets or volume of oral solution may be an indication for the use of a nonoral route.

Table 81.5 Routes of systemic opioid administration

Noninvasive	Invasive
Oral	Intramuscular
Rectal	Intravenous
Transdermal	Subcutaneous
Intranasal	
Sublingual	
Transmucosal	

Noninvasive alternatives to the oral route of opioid administration for relatively nontolerant patients include the rectal, transdermal and sublingual routes. Rectal suppositories containing oxycodone, hydromorphone, oxymorphone and morphine have been formulated and controlled-release morphine tablets can also be administered per rectum (Kaiko et al 1989). The potency of opioids administered rectally is believed to approximate oral dosing (Beaver & Feise 1977; Hanning 1990).

Fentanyl is the only opioid available as a transdermal preparation. The fentanyl transdermal system consists of a drug reservoir that is separated from the skin by a copolymer membrane that controls the rate of drug delivery to the skin surface such that the drug is released into the skin at a nearly constant amount per unit time. The system has been demonstrated to be effective in postoperative pain and cancer pain (Miser et al 1989; Gourlay et al 1990; Calis et al 1992). The dosing interval for each system is usually 72 hours (Varvel et al 1989), but some patients require a 48-hour schedule. There is some interindividual variability in fentanyl bioavailability by this route, and this phenomenon, combined with large differences in elimination pharmacokinetics, necessitates dose titration in most cases (Holley & Van-Steennis 1988; Gourlay et al 1990; Portenoy et al 1993). Transdermal patches capable of delivering 25, 50, 75 and 100 μg/h are available. Multiple patches may be used simultaneously for patients who require higher doses. At the present time, the limitations of the transdermal delivery system include its cost and the requirement for an alternative short-acting opioid for breakthrough pain.

Sublingual absorption of any opioid could potentially yield clinical benefit, but bioavailability is very poor with drugs that are not highly lipophilic and the likelihood of an adequate response is consequently low (Weinberg et al 1988). Sublingual buprenorphine, a relatively lipophilic partial agonist, can provide adequate relief of mild to moderate cancer pain (Bullingham et al 1982). Anecdotally, sublingual morphine has also been reported to be effective; but this drug has poor sublingual absorption (Weinberg et al 1988) and efficacy may be related, in part, to swallowing of the dose (Hirsch 1984). Both fentanyl and methadone are relatively well absorbed through the buccal mucosa (Weinberg et al 1988) and sublingual administration of an injectable formulation is occasionally performed in the relatively nontolerant patient who transiently loses the option of oral dosing.

Overall, however, the sublingual route has limited value due to the lack of formulations, poor absorption of most drugs and the inability to deliver high doses or prevent swallowing of the dose.

An oral transmucosal formulation of fentanyl, which incorporates the drug into a candy base, is under evaluation (Stanley et al 1989). A pilot study in cancer patients suggested that it may be useful to provide rapid relief of breakthrough pain (Fine et al 1991).

Invasive routes

For patients undergoing a trial of systemic drug administration, a parenteral route must be considered when the oral route is precluded or there is need for rapid onset of analgesia or a more convenient regimen. Repeated parenteral bolus injections, which may be administered by the intravenous (IV), intramuscular (IM) or subcutaneous (SC) routes, may be useful in some patients, but are often compromised by the occurrence of prominent 'bolus' effects (toxicity at peak concentration and/or pain breakthrough at the trough). Repetitive IM injections are a common practice, but they are painful and offer no pharmacokinetic advantage; their use is not recommended (American Pain Society 1992). Repeated bolus doses without frequent skin punctures can be accomplished through the use of an indwelling IV or SC infusion device. To deliver repeated SC injections, a 27-gauge infusion device (a 'butterfly') can be left under the skin for up to a week.

Intravenous bolus administration provides the most rapid onset and shortest duration of action. Time to peak effect correlates with the lipid solubility of the opioid and ranges from 2–5 minutes for methadone to 10–15 minutes for morphine (Sawe et al 1981; Chapman et al 1990; Inturrisi et al 1990). This approach is appropriate in two settings:

1. to provide parenteral opioids, usually transiently, to patients who already have venous access and are unable to tolerate oral opioids
2. to treat very severe pain, for which IV doses can be repeated at an interval as brief as that determined by the time to peak effect, if necessary, until adequate relief is achieved.

Continuous parenteral infusions are useful for many patients who cannot be maintained on oral opioids. Long-term infusions may be administered IV or SC. In practice, the major indication for continuous infusion occurs in patients who are unable to swallow or absorb opioids. Continuous infusion is also used in some patients whose high opioid requirement renders oral treatment impractical (Twycross & Lack 1984; Coyle et al 1986; Portenoy 1987; Bruera et al 1988a, 1988b; Swanson et al 1989; Storey et al 1990).

Continuous SC infusion can be easily used by ambulatory patients. A recent study demonstrated that the bioavailability of hydromorphone is 78% by this route (Moulin et al 1991) and clinical experience suggests that dosing may proceed in a manner identical to continuous IV infusion. A range of pumps is available, which vary in complexity, cost and ability to provide patient-controlled 'rescue doses' as an adjunct to a continuous basal infusion (Swanson et al 1989). Opioids suitable for continuous SC infusion must be soluble, well absorbed and nonirritant. Extensive experience has been reported with heroin, hydromorphone, oxymorphone and morphine (Twycross & Lack 1984; Coyle et al 1986; Bruera et al 1988b, 1990; Swanson et al 1989; Storey et al 1990; Moulin et al 1991, 1992). Methadone appears to be relatively irritating and is not preferred (Bruera et al 1991). To maintain the comfort of an infusion site, the SC infusion rate should not exceed 5 cc/h. Patients who require high doses may benefit from the use of concentrated solutions. A high concentration hydromorphone (10 mg/cc) is available commercially and the organic salt of morphine, morphine tartrate, is available in some countries as an 80 mg/cc solution. In selected cases, concentrated opioid solutions can be compounded specifically for continuous SC infusion.

Subcutaneous infusion, like repeated SC bolus injections, can usually be administered using a 27-gauge 'butterfly' needle. The infraclavicular and anterior chest sites provide the greatest freedom of movement for patients, but other sites may be used. A single infusion site can usually be maintained for 5–7 days (Coyle et al 1986; Bruera et al 1988a). Occasional patients develop focal erythematous swelling at the site of injection (Bruera et al 1991); this appears to be a common complication with methadone and has also been described with morphine and hydromorphone.

Continuous SC delivery of drug combinations may be indicated when pain is accompanied by nausea, anxiety or agitation. An antiemetic, neuroleptic or anxiolytic may be combined with an opioid, provided that it is nonirritant, miscible and stable in combined solution. Experience has been reported with metoclopromide, haloperidol, scopolamine, cyclizine, methotrimeprazine, chlorpromazine and midazolam (Dover 1987; Oliver 1988; Amesbury 1989).

In some circumstances, continuous IV infusion may be the most appropriate way of delivering an opioid. The need for very large doses, or treatment with methadone, may suggest the utility of this approach. If continuous IV infusion is to be continued on a long-term basis, a permanent central venous port is recommended.

Changing routes of administration

The switch between oral and parenteral routes should be guided by a knowledge of relative potency (Table 81.4) to avoid subsequent overdosing or underdosing. In calculating the equianalgesic dose, the potencies of the IV, SC and IM routes are considered equivalent. In recognition of the imprecision in the accepted equianalgesic doses and the risk of toxicity from potential overdose, a modest reduction in the equianalgesic dose is prudent. The problems associated with switching the route of administration can be minimised by accomplishing the change in steps (e.g. slowly reducing the parenteral dose and increasing the oral dose over a 2–3 day period).

Scheduling of opioid administration

The schedule of opioid administration should be individualised to optimise the balance between patient comfort and convenience. 'Around-the-clock' dosing and 'as needed' dosing both have a place in clinical practice.

'Around-the-clock' (ATC) dosing

Patients with continuous or frequent pain generally benefit from scheduled 'around-the-clock' dosing, which can provide the patient with continuous relief by preventing the pain from recurring. Clinical vigilance is required, however, when this approach is used in patients with no previous opioid exposure and when administering drugs that have long half-lives (methadone or levorphanol) or produce metabolites with long half-lives (e.g. morphine-6-glucuronide and norpropoxyphene). In the latter situations, delayed toxicity may develop as plasma drug (or metabolite) concentrations rise towards steady state levels.

Most patients who receive an 'around-the-clock' opioid regimen should also be provided a so-called 'rescue dose', which is a supplemental dose offered on an 'as needed' basis to treat pain that breaks through the regular schedule. The frequency with which the rescue dose can be offered depends on the route of administration and the time to peak effect for the particular drug. Oral rescue doses are usually offered up to every 1–2 hours and parenteral doses can be offered as frequently as every 15–30 minutes. Clinical experience suggests that the size of the rescue dose should be equivalent to approximately 50–100% of the dose administered every 4 hours for oral or parenteral bolus medications or 50–100% of the hourly infusion rate for patients receiving continuous infusions. Alternatively, this may be calculated as 5–15% of the 24–hour baseline dose. The drug used for the rescue dose is usually identical to that administered on a scheduled basis, with the exception of transdermal fentanyl and methadone; the use of an alternative short half-life opioid for the rescue dose is recommended in the latter cases.

The integration of 'around-the-clock' dosing with 'rescue doses' provides a method for safe and rational stepwise dose escalation, which is applicable to all routes of opioid administration. Patients who require more than 4–6 rescue doses per 24 hours should generally undergo escalation of the baseline dose. The quantity of the rescue medication consumed can be used to guide the dose increment. Alternatively, each dose increment can be set at 33–50% of the preexisting dose. In all cases, escalation of the baseline dose should be accompanied by a proportionate increase in the rescue dose, so that the size of the supplemental dose remains a constant percentage of the fixed dose (Table 81.6).

Controlled release drug formulations

Controlled release preparations of oral opioids can lessen the inconvenience associated with the use of 'around-the-clock' administration of drugs with a short duration of action (Arkinstall et al 1989). Numerous studies have demonstrated the safety and efficacy of these preparations in cancer patients with pain (Kaiko 1990, 1991; Shepherd 1990; Kim & Chung 1991; Walsh et al 1992). In the United States, controlled release morphine sulphate is available in 15, 30, 60 and 100 mg tablets and formula-

Table 81.6 Examples of stepwise dose escalation of morphine sulphate administered as (A) oral immediate release preparation, (B) oral controlled release and (C) continuous infusion

A Oral immediate release morphine sulphate

Step*	mg q4h ATC	Rescue dose mg
1	15	7.5 PRN q1h
2	30	15.0 PRN q1h
3	45	22.5 PRN q1h
4	60	30.0 PRN q1h
5	90	45.0 PRN q1h

B Oral controlled release morphine sulphate (immediate release rescue dose)

Step*	mg ATC	Immediate release rescue dose mg
1	30 q12	7.5 PRN q1h
2	30 q8	15.0 PRN q1h
3	60 q12	15.0 PRN q1h
4	100 q12	30.0 PRN q1h
5	100 q8	45.0 PRN q1h

C Continuous morphine infusion

Step*	mg/h	Rescue dose mg
1	3	2.0 PRN q30min
2	5	2.5 PRN q30min
3	7	3.5 PRN q30min
4	10	5.0 PRN q30min
5	15	7.5 PRN q30min

* Suggested indications for progression from one step to the next include:
1. requirement of > 2 rescue dose in any 4-hour interval or
2. requirement of > 6 rescue doses in 24 hours.

ATC = around-the clock; PRN = as needed; q = every.

tions of controlled release oxycodone and hydromorphone are under development. Controlled release preparations of morphine sulphate typically achieve peak levels 3–5 hours after administration and have a duration of effect of 8–12 hours (Shepherd 1990). Most patients who are administered controlled release morphine should also be provided a 'rescue dose' of immediate release opioid to treat pain that breaks through the regular controlled release schedule (Warfield 1991) (Table 81.6).

Clinical experience suggests that controlled release morphine should not be used to rapidly titrate the dose in patients with severe pain (Warfield 1991). The time required to approach steady-state plasma concentration after dosing is initiated or changed (at least 24 hours) may complicate efforts to identify rapidly the appropriate dose. Repeat-dose adjustments in patients with severe pain are performed more efficiently with a short-acting morphine preparation, which may be changed to a controlled release preparation when the effective 'around-the-clock' dose is identified. This change from short-acting morphine to controlled release morphine should be a milligram to milligram conversion which results in the same total 'around-the-clock' dose of the opioid.

'As Needed' (PRN) dosing

In some situations, opioid administration on an 'as needed' basis, without an 'around-the-clock' dosing regimen, may be beneficial. In the opioid-naive patient, 'as needed' dosing may provide additional safety during the initiation of opioid therapy, particularly when rapid dose escalation is needed or therapy with a long half-life opioid such as methadone or levorphanol is begun. 'As needed' dosing may also be appropriate for patients who have rapidly decreasing analgesic requirement or intermittent pains separated by painfree intervals.

Patient-controlled analgesia

Patient-controlled analgesia (PCA) generally refers to a technique of parenteral drug administration in which the patient controls an infusion device that delivers a bolus of analgesic drug 'on demand' according to parameters set by the physician. Use of a PCA device allows the patient to overcome variations in both pharmacokinetic and pharmacodynamic factors by carefully titrating the rate of opioid administration to meet individual analgesic needs (Citron et al 1986; Kerr et al 1988; Lange et al 1988; Chapman 1989; Egbert et al 1990; Hill et al 1991). Although it should be recognised that the use of oral 'rescue doses' is, in fact, a form of PCA, the term is not commonly applied to this situation.

Long-term PCA in cancer patients is most commonly accomplished via the subcutaneous route using an ambulatory infusion device (Coyle et al 1986; Bruera et al 1988b; Swanson et al 1989). In most cases, PCA is added to a basal infusion rate and acts essentially as a rescue dose. Rare patients have benefited from PCA alone to manage episodic pains characterised by an onset so rapid that an oral dose could not provide sufficiently prompt relief (Portenoy & Hagen 1990). Long-term intravenous PCA (Citron et al 1986; Urquhart et al 1988) can be used for patients who require doses that cannot be comfortably tolerated via the subcutaneous route or in those who develop local reactions to subcutaneous infusion.

Dose selection and titration

Selecting a starting dose

A patient who is relatively nontolerant, having had only some exposure to an opioid typically used on the second rung of the 'analgesic ladder' for moderate pain, should generally begin one of the opioids typically used for severe pain at a dose equivalent to 5–10 morphine IM every 4 hours. If morphine is used, a PO:IM relative potency ratio of 3:1 is conventional, based on survey data and clinical experience in the cancer population (Sawe et al 1981; Twycross & Lack 1984). When patients on higher doses of opioids are switched to an alternative opioid drug, the starting dose of the new drug should be reduced to 50–75% of the equianalgesic dose to account for incomplete cross-tolerance. Based on clinical experience, the switch to methadone should be considered the exception to this guideline. The change to methadone is accomplished more safely with a reduction of 50–70% in the equianalgesic dose.

Dose adjustment

Adjustment of the opioid dose is essential at the start of therapy and is usually necessary repeatedly during the patient's course. At all times, inadequate relief should be addressed through gradual escalation of dose until adequate analgesia is reported or intolerable and unmanageable side-effects supervene. Because opioid response increases linearly with the log of the dose, a dose increment of less than 30–50% is not likely to significantly improve analgesia. Doses can become extremely large during this process of titration. The absolute dose is immaterial as long as administration is not compromised by cost, inconvenience or discomfort.

Rate of dose titration

The rate of dose titration depends on the severity of the pain, the medical condition of the patient and the goals of care. Patients who present with very severe pain are sometimes best managed by repeated parenteral administration of a dose every 15–30 minutes until pain is partially relieved. Empiric guidelines have been proposed for the calculation of hourly maintenance, dosing after this parenteral loading has been accomplished with a short half-life opioid such as morphine, hydromorphone or fentanyl (Edwards & Breed 1990); these guidelines, which can be reasonably extrapolated to the cancer population, recommend that the starting hourly maintenance dose of the short half-life opioid can be approximated by dividing the total loading dose by twice the elimination half-life of the drug. For example, the starting maintenance dose for a patient who has required a total intravenous loading dose of 60 mg of morphine sulphate (half-life approximately 3 hours) to achieve adequate relief, would be 10 mg per hour.

Patients with moderate pain may not require a loading dose of the opioid. In this situation, dose increments of 30–50% can be administered at intervals greater than that required to reach steady state following each change (Table 81.6). The dose of morphine (tablets or elixir), hydromorphone or oxycodone can be increased on a twice-daily basis, and the dose of controlled release oral morphine or transdermal fentanyl can be increased every 24–48 hours.

The problem of tolerance

Patients vary greatly in the opioid dose required to manage pain. A survey of patients with advanced cancer observed that the average daily opioid requirement was equivalent to 400–600 mg of intramuscular morphine; approximately 10% of patients in the survey required greater than 2000 mg and one patient required over 35 000 mg per 24 hours (Coyle et al 1990).

The need for escalating doses is a complex phenomena. Most patients reach a dose that remains constant for prolonged periods (Kanner & Foley 1981; Brescia et al 1992). When the need for dose escalation arises, any of a variety of distinct processes may be involved. Clinical experience suggest that true analgesic tolerance is a much less common reason than disease progression or increasing psychological distress. Changes in the pharmacokinetics of an analgesic drug could potentially be involved as well.

In true pharmacologic tolerance, which presumably involves changes at the receptor level (Foley 1991; Lutfy & Yoburn 1991), continued drug administration itself induces an attenuation of effect. Clinically, tolerance to the nonanalgesic effects of opioids appears to occur commonly (Foley 1991), albeit at varying rates for different effects. For example, tolerance to respiratory depression, somnolence and nausea generally develops rapidly, whereas tolerance to opioid-induced constipation develops very slowly, if at all (Foley 1991). Tolerance to these opioid side-effects is not a clinical problem and, indeed, is a desirable outcome that allows effective dose titration to proceed.

The induction of true analgesic tolerance, which could compromise the utility of treatment, can only be said to occur if a patient manifests the need for increasing opioid doses in the absence of other factors (e.g. progressive disease) that would be capable of explaining the increase in pain. Extensive clinical experience suggests that most patients who require an escalation in dose to manage increasing pain have demonstrable progression of disease (Kanner & Foley 1981; Coyle et al 1988; Foley 1989a, 1991). These observations suggest that true pharmacological tolerance to the analgesic effects of opioids is not a common clinical problem. This conclusion has two important implications:

1. concern about tolerance should not impede the use of opioids early in the course of the disease
2. worsening pain in a patient receiving a stable dose of opioids should not be attributed to tolerance, but should be assessed as presumptive evidence of disease progression or, less commonly, increasing psychological distress.

Management of opioid adverse effects

Successful opioid therapy requires that the benefits of analgesia and other desired effects clearly outweigh treatment-related adverse effects. This implies that a detailed understanding of adverse opioid effects and the strategies used to prevent and manage them are essential skills for everyone involved in cancer-pain management.

The pathophysiological mechanisms that contribute to adverse opioid effects are incompletely understood. The appearance of these effects depends on a number of factors, including patient age, extent of disease, concurrent organ dysfunction, other drugs, prior opioid exposure and the route of drug administration (Payne & Inturrisi 1985; Foley & Inturrisi 1987). There is a paucity of data from controlled studies that compare the adverse effects of one opioid analgesic to another or that compare the adverse effects produced by the same opioid given by various routes of administration.

Adverse drug interactions

The potential for additive side-effects and serious toxicity from drug combinations must be recognised. The sedative effect of an opioid may add to that produced by numerous other centrally-acting drugs, such as anxiolytics, neuroleptics and antidepressants. Likewise, the constipatory effects of opioids are probably worsened by drugs with anticholinergic effects. As noted previously, a severe adverse reaction, including excitation, hyperpyrexia, convulsions and death, has been reported after the administration of meperidine to patients treated with a monoamine oxidase inhibitor (Inturrisi & Umans 1986).

Respiratory depression

Respiratory depression is potentially the most serious adverse effect of opioid therapy. All phases of respiratory activity (rate, minute volume and tidal exchange) may be impaired by these drugs. It is important to recognise that a compensatory increase in respiratory rate may obscure the degree of respiratory insufficiency initially produced by an opioid. Consequently, patients who appear to have normal respiration during opioid therapy may be predisposed to respiratory compromise if any pulmonary insult occurs. Clinically significant respiratory depression is always accompanied by other signs of central nervous system depression, including sedation and mental clouding. Respiratory compromise accompanied by tachypnoea and anxiety is never a primary opioid event.

With repeated opioid administration, tolerance appears to develop rapidly to the respiratory depressant effects of the opioid drugs (Foley 1991). As a result, opioid analgesics can be used in the management of chronic cancer pain without significant risk of respiratory depression. Indeed, clinically important respiratory depression is a very rare event in the cancer patient whose opioid dose has been titrated against pain. When respiratory depression occurs in such patients, alternative explanations (e.g. pneumonia or pulmonary embolism) should be sought. Opioid-induced respiratory depression can occur, however, if pain is suddenly eliminated (such as may occur following neurolytic procedures) and the opioid dose is not reduced. This latter observation suggests that patients whose respiratory function is well compensated following repeated opioid administration do not entirely lack opioid effect on respiration, but rather have respiratory function that reflects a balance between ongoing opioid effects and factors that increase the respiratory drive, including pain, anxiety and alertness.

When respiratory depression occurs in patients on chronic opioid therapy, administration of the specific opioid antagonist, naloxone, usually improves ventilation. This is true even if the primary cause of the respiratory event was not the opioid itself, but rather an intercurrent cardiac or pulmonary process. A response to naloxone, therefore, should not be taken as proof that the event was due to the opioid alone and an evaluation for these other processes should ensue.

Naloxone can precipitate a severe abstinence syndrome and should be administered only if strongly indicated. If the patient is bradypnoeic but readily arousable, and the peak plasma level of the last opioid dose has already been reached, the opioid should be withheld and the patient monitored until improved. If severe hypoventilation occurs (regardless of the associated factors that may be contributing to respiratory compromise) or the patient is bradypnoeic and unarousable, naloxone should be administered. To reduce the risk of severe withdrawal following a period of opioid administration, dilute naloxone (1:10) should be used in doses titrated to respiratory rate and level of consciousness (Bradberry & Reabel 1981; Goldfrank et al 1986). It is neither necessary nor desirable to reverse analgesia during the treatment of analgesic-induced respiratory depression. In the comatose patient, it may be prudent to insert an endotracheal tube to prevent aspiration following administration of naloxone. As mentioned previously, naloxone should be used cautiously in patients who have received chronic meperidine therapy, since it may precipitate seizures (Umans & Inturrisi 1982).

Sedation

Initiation of opioid therapy or significant dose escalation commonly induces sedation that usually persists until tolerance to this effect develops, usually in days to weeks. It is useful to forewarn patients of this potential, and thereby reduce anxiety and encourage avoidance of activities, such as driving, that may be dangerous if sedation occurs. Some patients have a persistent problem with sedation, particularly if other confounding factors exist. These factors include the use of other sedating drugs or coexistent diseases such as dementia, metabolic encephalopathy or brain metastases. Management of persistent sedation is best accomplished with a stepwise approach (Table 81.7).

Both dextroamphetamine (Forrest et al 1977) and methylphenidate (Bruera et al 1987, 1989a) have been widely used in the treatment of opioid-induced sedation. There has also been some anecdotal experience with the related compound, pemoline, which has relatively minor sympathomimetic effects and is available in a chewable tablet. A controlled study of oral methylphenidate in patients with advanced cancer demonstrated that this drug can improve analgesia and reverse opioid-induced sedation in the majority of patients (Bruera et al 1987). A survey of 50 similar patients observed early toxicity in two patients (hallucinations and a paranoid reaction, respectively), beneficial effects in more than 90% of the remaining group, no late toxicity and the need for escalating doses to maintain effects in some patients (Bruera et al 1989b). Treatment with methylphenidate or dextroamphetamine is typically begun at 2.5–5 mg in the

Table 81.7 Management of opioid-induced sedation

1. Discontinue nonessential central nervous system depressant medications.
2. If analgesia is satisfactory, reduce opioid dose by 25%.
3. If analgesia is unsatisfactory, try addition of a psychostimulant: (methylphenidate, dextroamphetamine or pemoline).
4. If somnolence persists, consider:
    a. addition of coanalgesic that will allow reduction in opioid dose
    b. change to an alternative opioid drug
    c. a change in opioid route to the intraspinal route (± local anaesthetic)
    d. a trial of other anaesthetic or neurosurgical options.

morning, which is repeated at midday if necessary to maintain effects until evening. Doses are then increased gradually if needed. Few patients require more than 40 mg per 24 hours in divided doses. At the doses used clinically, the risks associated with this treatment appear to be very small. Relative contraindications are generally considered to be cardiac arrhythmias, agitated delirium, paranoid personality and past amphetamine abuse.

Confusion and delirium

For patients and their families, confusion is a greatly feared effect of the opioid drugs (Cleeland 1989). Mild cognitive impairment is common following the initiation of opioid therapy or dose escalation (Bruera et al 1989b). Similar to sedation, however, pure opioid-induced encephalopathy appears to be transient in most patients, persisting from days to 1–2 weeks. Although persistent confusion attributable to opioid alone occurs, the aetiology of persistent delirium is usually related to the combined effect of the opioid and other contributing factors, including electrolyte disorders, neoplastic involvement of central nervous system, sepsis, vital organ failure and hypoxemia (Breitbart & Holland 1988). A stepwise approach to management (Table 81.8) often culminates in a trial of a neuroleptic drug. Haloperidol in low doses (0.5–1.0 mg PO or 0.25–0.5 mg IV or IM) is most commonly recommended because of its efficacy and low incidence of cardiovascular and anticholinergic effects.

Constipation

Constipation is the most common adverse effect of chronic opioid therapy in patients with advanced cancer (Twycross & Lack 1984; Foley 1985; Foley & Inturrisi 1987; Hill & Fields 1989; Inturrisi 1989; McQuay et al 1990; Walsh 1990b; Sykes 1991). The likelihood of opioid-induced constipation is so great that laxative medications should be prescribed prophylactically to most cancer patients (Twycross & Lack 1984; Foley 1985; Foley & Inturrisi 1987; Hill & Fields 1989; Inturrisi 1989; McQuay et al 1990; Walsh 1990b; Sykes 1991). This is particularly true for patients who are otherwise predisposed to constipation by advanced age, immobility, abdominal disease or concurrent medications. There are no controlled comparisons of the various laxatives for opioid-induced constipation and published recommendations are based entirely on anecdotal experience (Table 81.9). Combination therapy is frequently used, particularly coadministration of a softening agent (docusate) and a cathartic (e.g. senna, bisocodyl or phenophthalein). The doses of these drugs should be increased as necessary, and an osmotic laxative (e.g. milk of magnesia) should be added if needed. Chronic lactulose therapy is an alternative that some patients prefer and occasional patients are managed with intermittent colonic lavage using an oral bowel preparation such as 'Golytely'.

Table 81.8 Management of opioid-induced delirium

1. Discontinue nonessential centrally acting medications.
2. If analgesia is satisfactory, reduce opioid dose by 25%.
3. Exclude sepsis or metabolic derangement.
4. Exclude CNS involvement by tumour.
5. If delirium persists, consider:
   a. trial of a neuroleptic (e.g. haloperidol)
   b. change to an alternative opioid drug
   c. a change in opioid route to the intraspinal route (± local anaesthetic)
   d. a trial of other anaesthetic or neurosurgical options.

Rare patients with refractory constipation can undergo a trial of oral naloxone, which has a bioavailability less than 3% and presumably acts selectively on opioid receptors in the gut. A small series of patients has been reported in whom an oral dose of 3–12 mg reversed constipation without compromising analgesia or precipitating systemic withdrawal (Sykes 1991). Systemic withdrawal can be produced, however, if doses are escalated (Culpepper-Morgan et al 1992). Hence, the initial dose should be small (0.8–1.2 mg once or twice per 24 hours) and the dose should be escalated slowly until either favourable effects occur or the patient develops abdominal cramps, diarrhoea or any other adverse effect.

Nausea and vomiting

Opioids may produce nausea and vomiting through both central and peripheral mechanisms. These drugs stimulate the medullary chemoreceptor trigger zone, increase vestibular sensitivity and have effects on the gastrointestinal tract (including increased gastric antral tone, diminished motility and delayed gastric emptying) (Rogers & Cerda 1989). In ambulatory patients, the incidence of nausea and vomiting has been estimated to be 10–40% and 15–40%, respectively (Jaffe & Martin 1990; Campora et al 1991). The likelihood of these effects is greatest at the start of opioid therapy (Walsh 1990b). With the initiation of opioid therapy, patients should be informed that nausea can occur and that it is usually transitory and controllable. Tolerance typically develops within weeks. Routine prophylactic administration of an antiemetic is not necessary, except in patients with a history of severe opioid-induced nausea and vomiting (Walsh 1990b), but patients should have access to an antiemetic at the start of therapy if the need for one arises. Anecdotally, the use of prochlorperazine and metoclopramide has usually been sufficient.

In patients with more severe or persistent symptoms, the most appropriate antiemetic treatment may be suggested by the clinical features. For nausea associated with early satiety, bloating or postprandial vomiting, all of which are features of delayed gastric emptying, metoclopramide is the most reasonable initial treatment. Patients

Table 81.9 Laxative medications

Class	Drug	Usual starting dose	Comments
Stool softeners	Docusate sodium	200 mg/day	
Osmotic agents	Lactulose	15–30 cc	May cause abdominal cramps or flatulence
	Milk of magnesia	30–60 cc	
Stimulants	Senna	2 tab at bedtime	Delayed onset of action
	Bisacodyl	10–15 mg	Delayed onset of action
	Phenolphthalein	60–120 mg	Allergic rash 5%
Bulk agents	Psyllium	4–6 g	May constipate if oral fluid intake is low
Oral lavage	'Golytely'	100 cc tid	
Opioid antagonist	Oral naloxone	0.8–1.2 mg bid	Escalate dose by small steps until either favourable effect or the development of abdominal cramps, diarrhoea or signs of systemic withdrawal

with vertigo, or prominent movement-induced nausea, may benefit from the use of an antivertigenous drug such as prochlorperazine, scopolamine or meclizine. If neither signs of gastroparesis nor vestibular dysfunction are prominent, treatment is usually begun with a neuroleptic, such as prochlorperazine or metoclopramide. Drug combinations are sometimes used and, in all cases, doses are escalated if initial treatment is unsuccessful. If these drugs are ineffective at relatively high doses, other options include trials of alternative opioids or treatment with antihistamines (e.g. diphenhydramine or hydroxyzine), other neuroleptics (e.g. haloperidol, chlorpromazine or droperidol), benzodiazepines (e.g. lorazepam) or steroids (e.g. dexamethasone). The new serotonin antagonists (e.g. ondansetron) are not likely to be effective with opioid-induced symptoms since they do not eliminate apomorphine-induced vomiting and motion sickness (Stott et al 1989), which appear to be appropriate models for opioid effects. Clinical trials of the latter agents are needed to confirm this conclusion.

Multifocal myoclonus

All opioid analgesics can produce myoclonus. The mechanism of this effect is not known and patients with advanced cancer often have multiple potential contributing factors. The opioid effect is dose-related and is most prominent with meperidine, presumably as a result of metabolite accumulation. Mild and infrequent myoclonus is common and may resolve spontaneously with the development of tolerance to this effect. In occasional patients, myoclonus can be distressing or contribute to breakthrough pain that occurs with the involuntary movement. In this situation, a benzodiazepine (particularly clonazepam) (Eisele et al 1992), barbiturate or an anticonvulsant may be of value in the management of this symptom.

Urinary retention

Opioid analgesics increase smooth muscle tone and can occasionally cause bladder spasm or urinary retention (due to an increase in sphincter tone) (Jaffe & Martin 1990). This is an infrequent problem that is usually observed in elderly male patients. Tolerance can develop rapidly but catheterisation may be necessary to manage transient problems.

Pulmonary oedema

Noncardiogenic pulmonary oedema has been observed in patients treated with high, escalating opioid doses (Bruera & Miller 1989). A clear cause-and-effect relationship with the opioid has not been established, but is suspected. The mechanism, if opioid-related, is obscure.

Dependence and addiction

Confusion about physical dependence and addiction augment the fear of opioid drugs and contribute substantially to the undertreatment of pain (Cleeland 1989; Foley 1989b; Hill & Fields 1989; Jaffe 1989; Morgan 1989; Schuster 1989). To understand these phenomena as they relate to opioid pharmacotherapy for cancer pain, it is useful first to present a concept that might be called 'therapeutic dependence'. Patients who require a specific pharmacotherapy to control a symptom or disease process are clearly dependent on the therapeutic efficacy of the drugs in question. Examples of this 'therapeutic dependence' include the requirements of patients with congestive cardiac failure for cardiotonic and diuretic medications or the reliance of insulin-dependent diabetics on insulin therapy. In these patients, undermedication or withdrawal of treatment results in serious untoward consequences for the patient, the fear of which could conceivably induce aberrant psychological responses and drug-seeking behaviours. Patients with chronic cancer pain have an analogous relationship to their analgesic pharmacotherapy. This relationship may or may not be associated with the development of physical dependence, but is virtually never associated with addiction.

Physical dependence

Physical dependence is a pharmacological property of opioid drugs defined by the development of an abstinence (withdrawal) syndrome following either abrupt dose reduction or administration of an antagonist. Despite the observation that physical dependence is most commonly observed in patients taking large doses for a prolonged period of time, withdrawal has also been observed in patients after low doses or short duration of treatment. Physical dependence never becomes a clinical problem if:

1. patients are warned to avoid abrupt discontinuation of the drug
2. a tapering schedule is used if treatment cessation is indicated
3. opioid antagonist drugs (including agonist-antagonist analgesics) are avoided.

Addiction

The term addiction refers to a psychological and behavioural syndrome characterised by a continued craving for an opioid drug to achieve a psychic effect (psychological dependence) and associated aberrant drug-related behaviours, such as compulsive drug-seeking, unsanctioned use or dose escalation and use despite harm to self or others. Addiction should be suspected if patients demonstrate compulsive use, loss of control over drug use and continuing use despite harm.

The medical use of opioids is very rarely associated with the development of addiction (Chapman & Hill 1989; Foley 1989a; Schuster 1989). In the largest prospective study, only four cases could be identified among 11 882 patients with no history of addiction who received at least one opioid preparation in the hospital setting (Porter & Jick 1980). Although there are no prospective studies in patients with chronic cancer pain, there is an extensive clinical experience that affirms the extremely low risk of addiction in this population (American College of Physicians Health and Public Policy Committee 1983; Twycross & Lack 1984; Foley 1985, 1989a, 1989b; World Health Organization 1986, 1990; Chapman & Hill 1989; Hill & Fields 1989; Inturrisi 1989; Walsh 1990b; American Pain Society 1992). Health-care providers, patients and families often require vigorous and repeated reassurance that the risk of addiction is extremely small.

'Pseudoaddiction'

The distress engendered in patients who have a therapeutic dependence on analgesic pharmacotherapy but who continue to experience unrelieved pain is occasionally expressed in behaviours that are reminiscent of addiction, such as intense concern about opioid availability and unsanctioned dose escalation. Pain relief, usually produced by dose escalation, eliminates these aberrant behaviours and distinguishes the patient from the true addict. This syndrome has been termed 'pseudoaddiction' (Weissman & Haddox 1989). Misunderstanding of these phenomena may lead the clinician to inappropriately stigmatise the patient with the label 'addict', which may compromise care and erode the doctor–patient relationship. In the setting of unrelieved pain, aberrant drug-related behaviours require careful assessment, renewed efforts to manage pain and avoidance of stigmatising labels.

THE PATIENT REFRACTORY TO SYSTEMIC OPIOID THERAPY

All patients who are candidates for opioid therapy should undergo a trial of systemic opioid administration guided by the foregoing principles. Some patients, however, fail to attain adequate relief despite escalation of the dose to levels associated with intolerable and unmanageable side-effects. A stepwise strategy (Table 81.10) can be considered when dose escalation of a systemically administered opioid fails to yield a satisfactory result.

The first step in this strategy includes interventions that may improve the balance between the analgesic and adverse effects of systemic opioid therapy. If dose-limiting side-effects cannot be ameliorated, it may be possible to reduce the requirement for opioid therapy by the concurrent use of an appropriate primary therapy or other non-invasive analgesic approach. The latter comprise

Table 81.10 A stepwise strategy for the management of the patient with dose-limiting toxicity from systemic opioid therapy

Step	Intervention
1.	Noninvasive interventions to improve the therapeutic index of systemic opioid therapy: a. treat dose-limiting opioid side-effect b. reduce opioid requirement by: appropriate primary therapy addition of nonopioid analgesic addition of an adjuvant analgesic use of cognitive or behavioural techniques use of an orthotic device or other physical medicine approach use of transcutaneous electrical nerve stimulation c. switch to another opioid
2.	Consider invasive interventions to lower systemic opioid requirement and preserve cognitive function: a. regional analgesic techniques (spinal or intraventricular opioids) b. neural blockade c. neuroablative techniques d. invasive neurostimulatory approach
3.	Consider increased sedation

pharmacological treatments (a nonopioid or an adjuvant analgesic) and a diverse group of psychological, rehabilitative and neurostimulatory techniques (e.g. transcutaneous electrical nerve stimulation). A switch to another opioid, as described previously, may also improve the therapeutic outcome (Galer et al 1992).

Patients unable to achieve a satisfactory analgesic outcome despite these interventions are candidates for the use of invasive analgesic techniques. The use of these approaches should be based on a careful evaluation of the likelihood and duration of analgesic benefit, the immediate risks and morbidity of the procedure (including the anticipated length of hospitalisation), and the risks of long-term neurological sequelae. Anaesthetic approaches using opioids or local anaesthetics, such as epidural infusion, are usually considered first because they can reduce the requirement for systemically administered opioids without compromising function. Neurodestructive procedures that involve chemical or surgical neurolysis are very valuable in a small subset of patients; some of these procedures, such as coeliac plexus blockade in patients with pancreatic cancer, may have a sufficiently favourable risk: benefit ratio that early treatment is warranted. Finally, some patients with advanced cancer who have comfort as the overriding goal of care can elect to be deeply sedated rather than endure further trials of invasive analgesic therapy.

ADJUVANT ANALGESICS

The term 'adjuvant analgesic' describes a drug that has a primary indication other than pain but is analgesic in some conditions. A large group of such drugs, which are derived from diverse pharmacological classes, is now used to manage nonmalignant pain (see Ch. 50). In the cancer population, these drugs may be combined with primary analgesics in any of the three steps of the 'analgesic ladder' to improve the outcome for patients who cannot otherwise attain an acceptable balance between relief and side-effects. The potential utility of an adjuvant analgesic is usually suggested by the characteristics of the pain or by the existence of another symptom that may be amenable to a nonanalgesic effect of the drug.

Whenever an adjuvant analgesic is selected, differences between the use of the drug for its primary indication and its use as an analgesic must be appreciated. Since the nature of dose-dependent analgesic effects has not been characterised for most of these drugs, dose titration is reasonable with virtually all. Low initial doses are appropriate given the desire to avoid early side-effects. The use of low initial doses and dose titration may delay the onset of analgesia, however, and patients must be forewarned of this possibility to improve compliance with the therapy.

There is great interindividual variability in the response to all adjuvant analgesics. Although patient characteristics, such as advanced age or coexistent major organ failure, may increase the likelihood of some (usually adverse) responses, neither favourable effects nor specific side-effects can be reliably predicted in the individual patient. Furthermore, there is remarkable intraindividual variability in the response to different drugs, including those within the same class. These observations suggest the potential utility of sequential trials of adjuvant analgesics. The process of sequential drug trials, like the use of low initial doses and dose titration, should be explained to the patient at the start of therapy to enhance compliance and reduce the distress that may occur if treatments fail.

In the management of cancer pain, adjuvant analgesics can be broadly classified based on conventional use. Three groups are distinguished:

1. multipurpose adjuvant analgesics
2. adjuvant analgesics used for neuropathic pain
3. adjuvant analgesics used for bone pain.

Multipurpose adjuvant analgesics

Corticosteroids

Corticosteroids are among the most widely used adjuvant analgesics (Ettinger & Portenoy 1988; Walsh 1990a). They have been demonstrated to have analgesic effects (Bruera et al 1985), to improve significantly quality of life (Della Cuna et al 1989; Popiela et al 1989; Tannock et al 1989); and to have beneficial effects on appetite, nausea, mood and malaise in the cancer population (Moertel et al 1974; Wilcox et al 1984; Bruera et al 1985). Painful conditions that commonly respond to corticosteroids are listed in Table 81.11. The mechanism of analgesia produced by these drugs may involve antioedema effects (Yamada et al 1983), antiinflammatory effects and a direct influence on the electrical activity in damaged nerves (Devor et al 1985).

The relative risks and benefits of the various corticosteroids are unknown and dosing is largely empirical. In the United States, the most commonly used drug is dexamethasone, a choice that gains theoretical support from the relatively low mineralocorticoid effect of this agent. Dexamethasone also has been conventionally used for

Table 81.11 Painful conditions commonly responding to corticosteroid therapy

Raised intracranial pressure
Acute spinal cord compression
Superior vena cava syndrome
Metastatic bone pain
Neuropathic pain due to infiltration or compression by tumour
Symptomatic lymphoedema
Hepatic capsular distension

raised intracranial pressure and spinal cord compression. Prednisone (Tannock et al 1989), methylprednisolone (Hanks et al 1983; Bruera et al 1985) and prednisolone have also been used for other indications.

Patients with advanced cancer who experience pain and other symptoms may respond favourably to a relatively small dose of corticosteroid (e.g. dexamethasone 1–2 mg twice daily). In some settings, however, a high dose regimen may be appropriate. For example, patients with an acute episode of very severe bone pain or neuropathic pain that cannot be promptly reduced with opioids may respond dramatically to a short course of relatively high doses (e.g. dexamethasone 100 mg, followed initially by 96 mg per 24 hours in divided doses) (Greenberg et al 1980). This dose can be tapered over weeks, concurrent with initiation of other analgesic approaches, such as radiotherapy. Although high steroid doses are more likely to lead to adverse effects (Walsh 1990b), clinical experience with this approach has been successful.

Although the effects produced by corticosteroids in patients with advanced cancer are often very gratifying, side-effects are potentially serious and increase with prolonged usage. The varying constellations of adverse effects associated with brief or prolonged administration, or with the withdrawal of these drugs following long-term use, are generally appreciated by the medical community (Haynes 1990). In a study of advanced cancer patients chronically administered prednisolone or dexamethasone at varying doses, oropharyngeal candidiasis occurred in approximately one-third, oedema or cushingoid habitus developed in almost one-fifth, dyspepsia, weight gain, neuropsychological changes or ecchymoses were observed in 5–10%, and the incidence of other adverse effects, such as hyperglycemia, myopathy and osteoporosis was extremely low (Hanks et al 1983). The risk of peptic ulcer is approximately doubled in patients chronically treated with corticosteroids (Messer et al 1983) and coadministration of corticosteroid with aspirin or a NSAID further increases the risk of gastroduodenopathy and is not recommended. Active peptic ulcer disease and systemic infection are relative contraindications to the use of corticosteroids as adjuvant analgesics.

Neuroleptics

The role of neuroleptic drugs in the management of cancer pain is limited. Methotrimeprazine is a proven analgesic (Beaver et al 1966; Lasagna & DeKornfeld 1961; Montilla et al 1963) that has been very useful in bedridden patients with advanced cancer who experience pain associated with anxiety, restlessness or nausea. In this setting, the sedative, anxiolytic and antiemetic effects of this drug can be highly favourable, and side-effects, such as orthostatic hypotension, are less an issue. In the United States, methotrimeprazine is approved for intramuscular administration , but extensive experience has affirmed that it may also be given by continuous SC administration (Storey et al 1990), SC bolus injection or brief IV infusion (administration over 20–30 minutes). A prudent dosing schedule begins with 5–10 mg every 6 hours, or a comparable dose delivered by infusion, which is gradually increased as needed. Most patients will not require more than 20–50 mg every 6 hours to gain the desired effects.

Given their potential for serious toxicity and the limited evidence in support of analgesic efficacy, other neuroleptics, such as fluphenazine and haloperidol, should only be considered for therapeutic trials as analgesics in patients with refractory neuropathic pains who have failed trials with other agents. The primary use of these drugs is for the treatment of delirium and nausea.

Antihistamines

Despite evidence of analgesic effects in single dose studies of various antihistamines (Batterman 1965; Beaver & Feise 1976; Gold 1978; Campos & Solis 1980; Hupert et al 1980; McColl & Durkin 1982; Stambaugh & Lance 1983; Sunshine et al 1989), clinical experience has failed to confirm significant analgesic utility from this class of drugs. The use of these agents must also be tempered by the potential for additive side-effects, including sedation and dry mouth. These drugs should only be considered in patients who have a primary indication other than pain. A trial of hydroxyzine, for example, is sometimes selected in cancer patients where pain is complicated by anxiety, nausea or itch.

Benzodiazepines

Benzodiazepines have analgesic effects (Caccia 1975; Singh et al 1981; Swerdlow & Cundill 1981; Miller et al 1986; Fernandez et al 1987), but this must be balanced by the potential for side-effects, including sedation and confusion. With the important exception of clonazepam, which is widely accepted for the management of neuropathic pain (Caccia 1975; Swerdlow & Cundill 1981), these drugs are generally used only if another indication exists, such as anxiety or insomnia. The evidence that diazepam reduces muscle spasm, however, suggests that this drug may be appropriate for an analgesic indication alone if pain is believed to have such an aetiology.

Adjuvants used for neuropathic pain

Neuropathic pains are generally less responsive to opioid therapy than nociceptive pains (Portenoy et al 1990; Cherny et al 1992; McQuay et al 1992). The therapeutic outcome of pharmacotherapy may be improved by the addition of an adjuvant medication selected for the particular clinical characteristics of the prevailing neuropathic pain problem. The distinction between continuous, lancinating and sympathetically maintained neuropathic pain has important implications for the selection of an appropriate drug (Table 81.12).

Antidepressants

In the cancer population, antidepressant drugs are commonly used to manage continuous neuropathic pains that have not responded adequately to an opioid and lancinating neuropathic pains that are refractory to opioids and other specific adjuvant agents (see below) (Walsh 1983, 1986; Magni et al 1987; Ventafridda et al 1987a; Panerai et al 1991; Portenoy 1993). The evidence for analgesic efficacy is greatest for the tertiary amine tricyclic drugs, such as amitriptyline, doxepin and imipramine (Hugues et al 1963; Breivik & Rennemo 1982; Walsh 1986; Magni et al 1987; Panerai et al 1991). The secondary amine tricyclic antidepressants (such as desipramine and nortriptyline) have fewer side-effects and are preferred when concern about sedation, anticholinergic effects or cardiovascular toxicity is high (Portenoy 1993). The evidence of analgesic effect for most of the 'newer' antidepressants, such as maprotiline (Watson et al 1992), trazodone (Davidoff et al 1987; Magni et al 1987; Ventafridda et al 1987a), zimelidine (Johansson & Von Knorring 1979; Watson & Evans 1985), paroxetine (Sindrup et al 1990) and fluoxetine (Max et al 1992) is less abundant. Monoamine oxidase inhibitors may have analgesic effects in selected disorders (Anthony & Lance 1969), but the meager supporting data and the potential for serious toxicity suggest that there is a very limited role for these agents in the patient with pain due to progressive medical illness.

The starting dose of a tricyclic antidepressant should be low (e.g. amitriptyline 10 mg in the elderly and 25 mg in younger patients). Doses can be increased every few days and the initial dosing increments are usually the same size as the starting dose. When doses have reached the usual effective range (e.g. amitriptyline 50–150 mg), it is prudent to observe effects for a week before continuing upward dose titration. Analgesia usually occurs within a week after achieving an effective dosing level. Although most patients can be treated with a single nighttime dose, some patients have less morning 'hangover', and some report less late afternoon pain, if doses are divided. It is reasonable to continue upward dose titration beyond the usual analgesic doses in patients who fail to achieve benefit and have no limiting side-effects. Plasma drug concentration, if available, may provide useful information and should be followed during the course of therapy. Very low levels in nonresponders suggest either poor compliance or an unusually rapid metabolism. In the latter case, doses can be increased while repeatedly monitoring the plasma drug level. Likewise, nonresponders whose plasma concentration is not very low, but is lower than the antidepressant range, should be considered for a trial of higher doses if side-effects are not a problem.

Table 81.12 A guide to the selection of adjuvant analgesics for neuropathic pain based on clinical characteristics

Continuous pain	Lancinating pain	Sympathetically-maintained pain
Antidepressants	Anticonvulsant drugs	Phenoxybenzamine
Amitriptyline	Carbamazepine	Prazosin
Doxepin	Phenytoin	Corticosteroid
Imipramine	Clonazepam	Nifedipine
Desipramine	Valproate	Propranolol
Nortriptyline	Baclofen	Calcitonin
Trazodone	Oral local anaesthetics	
Maprotiline		
Oral local anaestheics		
Mexiletine		
Clonidine		
Capsaicin		

Oral local anaesthetics

Local anaesthetic drugs may be useful in the management of neuropathic pains characterised by either continuous or lancinating dysaesthesias. Controlled trials have demonstrated the efficacy of tocainide (Lindstrom & Lindblom 1987) and mexiletine (Dejgard et al 1988; Chabal et al 1992), and there is clinical evidence that suggests similar effects from flecainide (Dunlop et al 1989) and subcutaneous lidocaine (Brose & Cousins 1991). Experience with oral local anaesthetics in the cancer population is still limited and recommendations are largely empirical. It is reasonable to undertake a trial with an oral local anaesthetic in patients with continuous dysaesthesias who fail to respond adequately, or who cannot tolerate the tricyclic antidepressants, and in patients with lancinating pains refractory to trials of anticonvulsant drugs and baclofen (see p. 1455). Mexiletine is the safest of the oral local anaesthetics (Horn et al 1980; CAST (Cardiac Arrhythmia Suppression Trial) Investigators 1989; Portenoy 1993) and is preferred. Dosing with mexiletine should usually be started at 100–150 mg per 24 hours. If intolerable side-effects do not occur, the dose can be increased by a like amount every few days, until the usual maximum dose of 300 mg three times per 24 hours is reached. Plasma drug concentrations, if available, can provide information similar to that described previously for the tricyclic antidepressants.

Clonidine

Clonidine is an alpha-2 adrenergic agonist that has established analgesic effects (Shafar et al 1972; Tan & Croese 1986; Boico et al 1988; Bonnet et al 1988; Max et al 1988; Mok et al 1988; Portenoy 1993). In the cancer population, a trial of oral or transdermal clonidine can be considered in the management of continuous neuropathic pain refractory to opioids and other adjuvants.

Capsaicin

Topical administration of capsaicin depletes peptides in small primary afferent neurons, including those that are putative mediators of nociceptive transmission (e.g. substance P) (Jessel & Dodd 1989; Dubner 1991). This effect suggests that long-term use of the drug could reduce the central transmission of information about a noxious stimulus. Analgesic effects have been suggested in postherpetic neuralgia, painful peripheral neuropathies and postmastectomy pain (Watson et al 1988, 1989; Scheffler et al 1991; The Capsaicin Study Group 1991; Tandan et al 1992). Although the dose-response relationship has not been evaluated in controlled studies, data from phase II studies of 0.075% and 0.025% preparations are suggestive of the phenomenon and it is reasonable to use the higher concentration for either the initial trial or a subsequent trial following failure of the lower concentration product. A burning sensation can follow the topical application of capsaicin. This wanes spontaneously in some patients and others can reduce it through the prior use of an oral analgesic or cutaneous application of lidocaine 5% ointment. A proportion of patients report intolerable burning and cannot use the drug. In those who tolerate the drug, an adequate trial should be considered of at least four applications per 24 hours for 4 weeks.

Anticonvulsant drugs

Selected anticonvulsant drugs appear to be analgesic for the lancinating dysaesthesias that characterise diverse types of neuropathic pain (Swerdlow 1984; Portenoy 1993). Clinical experience also supports the use of these agents in patients with paroxysmal neuropathic pains that may not be lancinating and, to a far lesser extent, in those with neuropathic pains characterised solely by continuous dysaesthesias. Although most practitioners prefer to begin with carbamazepine because of the extraordinarily good response rate observed in trigeminal neuralgia (Rockliff & Davis 1966; Lloyd-Smith & Sachdev 1969; Taylor et al 1980a, 1980b; Tomson & Bertilsson 1984), this drug must be used cautiously in cancer patients with thrombocytopenia, those at risk for marrow failure (e.g. following chemotherapy) and those whose blood counts must be monitored to determine disease status. If carbamazepine is used, a complete blood count should be obtained prior to the start of therapy, after 2 and 4 weeks, and then every 3–4 months thereafter. A leucocyte count below 4000 is usually considered to be a contraindication to treatment and a decline to less than 3000, or an absolute neutrophil count of less than 1500 during therapy, should prompt discontinuation of the drug.

Other anticonvulsant drugs may also be useful for patients with lancinating dysaesthesias following nerve injury. Published reports and clinical experience support trials with phenytoin (Ianmore et al 1958; Braham & Saia 1960; Green 1961; Ellenberg 1968; Hallag & Harris 1968; Cantor 1972; Ekbom 1972; Lockman et al 1973; Mladinich 1974; Raskin et al 1974; Hatangdi et al 1976; Taylor et al 1977; Swerdlow 1984; Chadda & Mathur 1978), clonazepam (Caccia 1975; Martin 1981; Swerdlow & Cundill 1981) and valproate (Raftery 1979; Peiris et al 1980).

The use of all these drugs as adjuvant analgesics customarily follows the dosing guidelines employed in the treatment of seizures. Low initial doses are appropriate for carbamazepine, valproate and clonazepam and the administration of phenytoin often begins with the presumed therapeutic dose (e.g. 300 mg per 24 hours) or a prudent oral loading regimen (e.g. 500 mg twice, separated by hours). When low initial doses are used, dose escalation should ensue until a favourable effect occurs, intolerable side-effects supervene or the plasma drug concentration has reached a predetermined level, which is customarily at the upper end of the therapeutic range for seizure management. This approach is empirical, since there are no data-relating plasma concentration to analgesic effects. The variability in the response to these drugs is great and sequential trials in patients with refractory pain is amply justified by clinical experience.

Baclofen

Baclofen is a GABA-agonist that has proven efficacy in the treatment of trigeminal neuralgia (Fromm et al 1984; Fromm 1989). On this basis, a trial of this drug is commonly employed in the management of paroxysmal neuropathic pains of any type. Dosing is generally undertaken in a manner similar to the use of the drug for its primary indication, spasticity. A starting dose of 5 mg 2–3 times per 24 hours is gradually escalated to 30–90 mg per 24 hours, and sometimes higher if side-effects do not occur. The most common adverse effects are sedation and confusion.

Calcitonin

In a placebo-controlled trial, calcitonin (200 IU per 24 hours) has been shown to be an active analgesic in the management of continuous neuropathic phantom limb pain (Jaeger & Maier 1992). Experience with this drug in the treatment of neuropathic pain is very limited and it should be considered only after trials of other drugs have failed.

Pimozide

Pimozide, a phenothiazine neuroleptic with activity against lancinating neuropathic pain, is rarely used in the cancer population. Given its high incidence of adverse effects, including physical and mental slowing, tremour and slight parkinsonian symptoms (Lechin et al 1989), it also should be considered following failed trials with other drugs.

Adjuvant drugs for sympathetically-maintained pain

Sympathetically-maintained pain that occurs in the cancer patient can often be ameliorated with sympathetic nerve blocks. Occasionally, sympathetically-maintained pain is strongly suspected (pain associated with local signs of autonomic dysregulation, such as oedema, vasomotor instability or sweating abnormalities), but nerve blocks are contraindicated or fail. In this situation, adjuvant analgesics that have been employed specifically for this type of neuropathic pain may be considered.

Phenoxybenzamine, 60–120 mg per 24 hours, has been reported to be effective in a survey of patients with causalgia (Ghostine et al 1984). The risk of orthostatic hypotension limits this treatment to younger patients with intact cardiovascular reflexes. There is limited evidence for the efficacy of prazosin (Abram & Lightfoot 1981), propranolol (Simson 1974; Scadding 1982), and nifedipine (Prough et al 1985). A recent controlled trial suggests that calcitonin may also be useful in some patients with sympathetically-maintained pain (Gobelet et al 1992).

Adjuvant analgesics used for bone pain

Antiinflammatory drugs

Anecdotally, nonsteroidal antiinflammatory drugs appear to be particularly efficacious for malignant bone pain. Corticosteroids are often advocated in difficult cases (Nielsen et al 1991; Portenoy 1993).

Bisphosphonates

Bisphosphonates (previously known as diphosphonates) are analogues of inorganic pyrophosphate that inhibit osteoclast activity and consequently reduce bone resorption in a variety of illnesses. This effect presumably underlines the putative analgesic efficacy of these compounds in bone pain. Controlled and uncontrolled trials of pamidronate in patients with advanced cancer have demonstrated significant reduction of bone pain (Clarke et al 1991; Coleman et al 1988; Morton et al 1988; Thiebaud et al 1991; Van Holten-Verzantvoort et al 1991). A controlled trial of clodronate (Ernst et al 1992) was similarly successful, but a study that evaluated sodium etidronate demonstrated no beneficial effects (Smith 1989). On balance, the data are sufficient to recommend a trial of one of these agents in patients with refractory bone pain; currently the evidence for analgesic effects is best for pamidronate. Potential differences in the analgesia produced by various drugs in this class require additional study and neither dose-dependent effects nor long-term risks or benefits in cancer patients are known. The use of any bisphosphonate requires monitoring of serum calcium, phosphate, magnesium and potassium.

Radiopharmaceuticals

Radiolabelled agents that are absorbed into areas of high bone turnover have been evaluated as potential therapies for metastatic bone disease. Systemically administered phosphorus-32 has long been known to be an effective agent in the management of metastatic bone pain, but its utility is limited by significant bone-marrow depression (Silberstein et al 1992). More recently, bone-seeking radiopharmaceuticals that link a radioisotope with a bisphosphonate compound have been synthesised. Significant clinical response with acceptable haematological toxicity has been observed with strontium-89 (Silberstein & Williams 1985; Robinson et al 1992), samarium-153-ethylenediaminetetramethylene phosphonic acid (Turner et al 1989; Turner & Claringbold 1991; Holmes 1992), and rhenium-186-hydroxyethylidene diphosphonate (Maxon et al 1988, 1992; Holmes 1992). Further studies are needed to identify the risks and benefits of each agent and the durability of the effects produced. If is likely that such agents will become available in the future and represent an important means of treating refractory bone pain from metastatic disease.

Calcitonin

There is limited evidence that repeated doses of subcutaneous calcitonin can reduce bone pain (Hindley et al 1982; Blomquist et al 1988). Nonetheless, it is reasonable to consider a trial with this drug (e.g. salmon calcitonin 100–200 IU twice daily subcutaneously for several weeks) in refractory cases.

OTHER NONINVASIVE ANALGESIC TECHNIQUES

PSYCHOLOGICAL THERAPIES IN CANCER PAIN

Psychological approaches are an integral part of the care of the cancer patient with pain. All patients can benefit from psychological assessment and support and some are good candidates for specific psychological interventions including those commonly used in the management of pain. Cognitive–behavioural interventions can help some patients decrease the perception of distress engendered by the pain through the development of new coping skills and the modification of thoughts, feeling and behaviours (Fordyce 1976; Fishman 1990). Relaxation methods may be able to reduce muscular tension and emotional arousal or enhance pain tolerance (Linton & Melin 1983). Other approaches reduce anticipatory anxiety that may lead to avoidant behaviours or lessen the distress associated with the pain (Turk et al 1983). Successful implementation of these approaches in the cancer population requires a cognitively intact patient and a dedicated, well-trained clinician (Fishman 1990).

PHYSIATRIC TECHNIQUES

Physiatric techniques can be used to optimise the function of the patient with chronic cancer pain (Gamble et al 1990) or enhance analgesia through application of modalities such as electrical stimulation, heat or cryotherapy. The treatment of lymphoedema by use of wraps, pressure stockings or pneumatic pump devices can both improve function and relieve pain and heaviness (Brennan 1992). The use of orthotic devices can immobilise and support painful or weakened structures and assistive devices can be of great value to patients with pain precipitated by weight bearing or ambulation.

TRANSCUTANEOUS ELECTRICAL NERVE STIMULATION (TENS)

The mechanisms by which transcutaneous electrical stimulation reduce pain are not well defined; local neural blockade and activation of a central inhibitory systems have been proposed as explanations (Bushnell et al 1991; Long 1991). Clinical experience suggests that this modality can be a useful adjunct in the management of mild to moderate musculoskeletal or neuropathic pain.

INVASIVE ANALGESIC TECHNIQUES

ANAESTHETIC AND NEUROSURGICAL TECHNIQUES

The results of the WHO 'analgesic ladder' validation studies suggest that 10–30% or patients with cancer pain do not achieve a satisfactory balance between relief and side-effects using systemic pharmacotherapy alone without unacceptable drug toxicity (Takeda 1986; Ventafridda et al 1987b; Walker et al 1988; Schug et al 1990; Grond et al 1991). Anaesthetic and neurosurgical techniques (Tables 81.13 and 81.14) may reduce or eliminate the requirement for systemically administered opioids to achieve adequate analgesia.

Regional opioid analgesia

Epidural and intrathecal opioids

The delivery of low opioid doses near the sites of action in the spinal cord may decrease supraspinally-mediated adverse effects. Compared to neuroablative therapies, spinal opioids have the advantage of preserving sensation, strength and sympathetic function. Contraindications include bleeding diathesis, profound leucopenia and sepsis. A temporary trial of spinal opioid therapy should be performed to assess the potential benefits of this approach

Table 81.13 Commonly performed anaesthetic and neurosurgical analgesic techniques for pain refractory to systemic pharmacotherapy

Class	Technique	Clinical situation
Regional analgesia	Spinal opioids and/or local anaesthetics	Systemic opioid analgesia complicated by unmanageable supraspinally-mediated adverse effects
Sympathetic blockade and neurolysis	Coeliac plexus block	Refractory malignant pain involving the upper abdominal viscera including the upper retroperitoneum, liver, small bowel and proximal colon
	Lumbar sympathetic blockade	Sympathetically-maintained pain involving the legs
	Stellate ganglion blockade	Sympathetically-maintained pain involving the head, neck or arms
Somatic neurolysis or pathway ablation	Chemical rhizotomy	Refractory brachial plexopathy or arm pain Intercostal nerve pain, chest-wall pain Refractory bilateral pelvic or lumbosacral plexus pain in patient with urinary diversion and who is confined to bed.
	Trigeminal neurolysis	Refractory unilateral facial pain
	Transacral neurolysis	Refractory pain limited to the perineum
	Cordotomy	Refractory unilateral pain arising in the torso or lower extremity
High centre ablation	Cingulotomy	Refractory multifocal pain
	Pituitary ablation	Refractory multifocal pain

Table 81.14 A guide to the selection of invasive analgesic techniques according to the site of pain

Site	Procedure
Face: unilateral	Gasserian gangliolysis
	Trigeminal neurolysis
	Intraventricular opioid
Pharyngeal	Glossopharyngeal neurolysis
	Intraventricular opioid
Arm/brachial plexus	Spinal opioid ± local anaesthetic
	Chemical rhizotomy
	Surgical rhizotomy
Chest wall	Spinal opioid ± local anaesthetic
	Intercostal neurolysis
	Paravertebral neurolysis
	Chemical rhizotomy
	Surgical rhizotomy
Abdominal: somatic	Spinal opioid ± local anaesthetic
	Chemical rhizotomy
	Surgical rhizotomy
	Cordotomy (unilateral pain)
Upper abdomen: visceral	Coeliac plexus neurolysis
Lower abdomen: visceral	Hypogastric neurolysis
Perineum	Spinal opioid ± local anaesthetic
	Chemical rhizotomy
	Surgical rhizotomy
	Transsacral S4 neurolysis
Pelvis + lower limb	Spinal opioid ± local anaesthetic
	Chemical rhizotomy
	Surgical rhizotomy
Unilateral lower quadrant	Cordotomy
Multifocal or generalized pain	Pituitary ablation
	Cingulotomy

before implantation of a permanent catheter. Opioid selection for intraspinal delivery is influenced by several factors. Hydrophilic drugs, such as morphine and hydromorphone, have a prolonged half-life in cerebrospinal fluid and significant rostral redistribution (Max et al 1985; Moulin et al 1986; Brose et al 1991). Lipophilic opioids, such as fentanyl and sufentanil, have less rostral redistribution (Chrubasik et al 1988) and may be preferable for segmental analgesia at the level of spinal infusion. In some patients, the addition of a low concentration of a local anaesthetic, such as 0.125–0.25% bupivacaine, to an epidural opioid has been demonstrated to increase analgesic effect without increasing toxicity (Du Pen & Ramsey 1988; Nitescu et al 1990; Hogan et al 1991; Sjoberg et al 1991). The potential morbidity for these procedures indicates the need for a well-trained clinician and long-term monitoring.

Intraventricular opioids

Administration of an opioid into the cerebral ventricles has been used to treat selected patients with severe chronic pain (Lobato et al 1987; Obbens et al 1987). This technique is usually considered for patients with upper body or head pain, or severe diffuse pain (De Castro et al 1991). In relatively nontolerant patients, the analgesia produced by a dose of morphine has a rapid onset and a long duration (Sandouk et al 1991).

Anaesthetic techniques for sympathetically-maintained pain and visceral pain

Coeliac plexus block

Neurolytic coeliac plexus blockade can be considered in the management of pain caused by neoplastic infiltration of the upper abdominal viscera, including the pancreas, upper retroperitoneum, liver, gall bladder and proximal small bowel (Brown et al 1987; Cousins et al 1988; Bonica et al 1990a). Reported analgesic response rates in patients with pancreatic cancer are 50–90%, with the duration of effect lasting from 1–12 months (Brown et al 1987; Cousins et al 1988; Bonica et al 1990a). Common transient complications include postural hypotension and diarrhoea (Brown et al 1987; Cousins et al 1988; Bonica et al 1990a). Posterior spread of neurolytic solution can lead to involvement of lower thoracic and lumbar somatic nerves and potentially result in neuropathic pain in the region of the lower rib cage or upper thigh. Uncommon complications include pneumothorax, retroperitoneal haematoma and paraparesis.

Sympathetic blockade of somatic structures

Sympathetically-maintained pain syndromes may be relieved by interruption of sympathetic outflow to the affected region of the body. Lumbar sympathetic blockade should be considered for sympathetically-maintained pain involving the legs and stellate ganglion blockade may be useful for sympathetically-maintained pain involving the face or arms.

Neuroablative techniques for somatic and neuropathic pain

Chemical rhizotomy

Chemical rhizotomy, which may be produced by the instillation of a neurolytic solution into either the epidural or intrathecal space, can be an effective method of pain control for patients with otherwise refractory localised pain syndromes (Ischia et al 1984; Hellendoorn & Overweg van Kints 1988). The technique is most commonly used in the management of chest-wall pain due to tumour invasion of somatic and neural structures. Other indications include refractory upper limb, lower limb, pelvic or perineal pain. Because of the significant risk of increased disability through weakness, sphincter incompetence and loss of positional sense, chemical rhizotomy of lumbosacral nerve roots is best reserved for patients with limited function and preexistent urinary diversion.

Satisfactory analgesia is achieved in about 50% of patients who undergo epidural or intrathecal neurolysis (Cousins et al 1988). Adverse effects can be related to the injection technique (spinal headache, mechanical neural damage, infection and arachnoiditis) or to the destruction of nonnociceptive nerve fibres. Specific complications of the procedure depend on the site of neurolysis. Complications of lumbosacral neurolysis include paresis (5–20%) sphincter dysfunction (5–60%), impairment of touch and proprioception and dysaesthesias. Fortunately, neurological deficits are usually transient, although fatal meningitis, paraplegia, and permanent impairment of sphincter function have been recorded (Cousins et al 1988). Patient counselling regarding the risks involved in these techniques is essential.

Other chemical neurolyses

Neurolysis of primary afferent nerves may provide significant relief for selected patients with localised pain. Refractory unilateral facial or pharyngeal pain may be amenable to trigeminal neurolysis, Gasserian gangliolysis or glossopharyngeal neurolysis. Intercostal or paravertebral neurolysis is an alternative to rhizotomy for patients with chest-wall pain. Severe pain limited to the perineum may be treated by neurolysis of the S4 nerve root via the ipsilateral posterior sacral foramen, a procedure that carries a minimal risk of motor or sphincter impairment (Robertson 1983).

Cordotomy

During cordotomy, the anterolateral spinothalamic tract is sectioned to produce contralateral loss of pain and temperature sensibility (Rosomoff et al 1965; Arbit 1990). The patient with severe unilateral pain arising in the torso or lower extremity is most likely to benefit from this procedure (Ischia et al 1984). The percutaneous technique is generally preferred (Arbit 1990); open cordotomy is usually reserved for patients who are unable to lie in the supine position or are not cooperative enough to undergo a percutaneous procedure (Arbit 1990).

Significant pain relief is achieved in more than 90% of patients during the period immediately following cordotomy (Rosomoff et al 1965; Ischia et al 1984; Tasker et al 1988; Arbit 1990). Of surviving patients 50% have recurrent pain after 1 year. Repeat cordotomy can sometimes be effective. The neurological complications of cordotomy include paresis, ataxia and bladder dysfunction (Tasker et al 1988). The complications are usually transient, but are protracted and disabling in approximately 5% of cases. Rarely, patients with a long duration of survival (>12 months) develop a delayed-onset dysaesthetic pain. The most serious potential complication is respiratory dysfunction, which may occur in the form of phrenic nerve paralysis or as sleep-induced apnoea (Polatty & Cooper 1986). Because of the latter concern, bilateral high cervical cordotomies or a unilateral cervical cordotomy ipsilateral to the site of the only functioning lung are not recommended.

Dorsal root entry zone lesions

The dorsal root entry zone (DREZ) procedure is performed under general anaesthesia and requires a multilevel laminectomy. With the exception of pain associated with nerve-root avulsion, for which this technique appears to be very successful, the overall analgesic efficacy is only 30–50% (Ishijima et al 1988). There is very little experience in the application of this technique to cancer pain. Complications of DREZ procedures include increasing neurological dysfunction, loss of proprioception and dysaesthesias.

Pituitary ablation

Pituitary ablation by chemical or surgical hypophysectomy has been reported to relieve diffuse and multifocal pain syndromes that have been refractory to opioid therapy and are unsuitable for any regional neuroablative procedure (see Ch. 61 and Levin & Ramirez 1984; Bonica et al 1990a). Pain relief has been observed from pain due to both hormone-dependent and hormone-independent tumours (Levin & Ramirez 1984; Bonica et al 1990a).

Cingulotomy

Anecdotal reports also support the efficacy of cingulotomy (Hassenbusch et al 1990) in the management of diffuse pain syndromes that have been refractory to opioid therapy. The mode of action is unknown and the procedure is considered rarely.

SEDATION AS PAIN THERAPY

Some patients with advanced disease develop severe pain that is poorly controlled despite maximally tolerated systemic pharmacotherapy, with or without the use of concurrent anaesthetic or neurosurgical techniques. The incidence of this phenomenon has been variably estimated at 5–25%. In one study 52% of terminally ill patients developed otherwise unendurable symptoms requiring deep sedation for adequate relief; in just under half of these patients, pain was the predominant symptom (Ventafridda et al 1990).

Thus, the patient with advanced cancer with uncontrolled symptoms has an option other than continued efforts to identify an effective pharmacologic or nonpharmacological therapy. The patient may choose an approach designed to provide adequate sedation until death or may choose to continue trials of analgesic therapies, with or without the transitory use of sedating therapies. The ethical basis of this approach is predicated upon informed consent and an acknowledgement of the 'principle of double effect', which distinguishes between the compelling primary therapeutic intent (to relieve suffering) and unavoidable untoward consequences (the possible foreshortening of the process of dying) (Latimer 1991). This approach recognises the rights of dying patients to adequate relief of pain, and to chose between appropriate therapeutic options. In the advanced stages of disease, the relief from discomfort is an ethical imperative; no patient should have to ask to be killed because of persistently unrelieved pain (Edwards 1989; Martin 1989; Wanzer et al 1989).

Choosing among these options requires sensitive and supportive communication between the clinician and the patient. Informed decision-making is predicated on a candid discussion that clarifies the difficulties in the prevailing clinical situation, the limitations of alternative analgesic options (including sedation) and the reality of the patient's suffering. The potentially conflicting goals of comfort versus function may need to be made explicit to the patient. Other relevant considerations include existential, ethical, religious and familial concerns that may benefit from the participation of a religious counsellor, social worker or clinical ethics specialist.

Sedation can potentially be accomplished through the use of systemic opioids, with either a benzodiazepine (e.g. lorazepam or midazolam), a neuroleptic (e.g. chlorpromazine or methotrimeprazine) or a barbiturate (e.g. thiopental). Experience has been reported in the use of opioids in conjunction with continuous infusions of midazolam (Burke et al 1991) or thiopental (Greene & Davis 1991). It is the responsibility of the physician to ensure that the patient and family, and staff as well, have a comprehensive understanding of this intervention.

CONCLUSION

The goal of analgesic therapy in the cancer population is to optimise analgesia with the minimum of side-effects and inconvenience. Currently available techniques can provide adequate relief to a vast majority of patients. Most will require ongoing pain treatment and analgesic requirements often change as the disease progresses. Patients with refractory pain, or unremitting suffering related to other losses or distressing symptoms, should have access to specialists in pain management or palliative medicine who can provide an approach capable of addressing these complex problems.

REFERENCES

Abram S E, Lightfoot R W 1981 Treatment of longstanding causalgia with prazosin. Regional Anesthesia 6: 79–81

American College of Physicians Health and Public Policy Committee 1983 Drug therapy for severe chronic pain in terminal illness. Annals Internal Medicine 99: 870–880

American Pain Society 1992 Principles of analgesic use in the treatment of acute pain and chronic cancer pain. A concise guide to medical practice, 3rd edn. American Pain Society, Skokie, Illinois

Amesbury B D W 1989 Use of SC Midazolam in the home care setting. Palliative Medicine 3: 299–301

Anthony M, Lance J W 1969 Monoamine oxidase inhibitors in the treatment of migraine. Archives of Neurology 21: 263–268

Arbit E 1990 Neurosurgical management of cancer pain. In: Foley K M, Bonica J J, Ventafrida V (eds) Second international congress on cancer pain. Advances in pain research and therapy, vol 16. Raven Press, New York, p 289–300

Arkinstall W W, Goughnour B R, White J A, Stewart J H 1989 Control of severe pain with sustained-release morphine tablets v. oral morphine solution. Canadian Medical Association Journal 140: 653–657

Arner S, Meyerson B A 1988 Lack of analgesic effect of opioids on neuropathic and idiopathic forms of pain. Pain 33: 11–23

Bates T 1992 A review of local radiotherapy in the treatment of bone metastases and cord compression. International Journal of Radiation Oncology, Biology, Physics 23: 217–222

Bates T, Yarnold J R, Blitzer P, Nelson O S, Rubin P, Maher J 1992 Bone metastasis consensus statement. International Journal of Radiation Oncology, Biology, Physics 23: 215–216

Batterman R C 1965 Methodology of analgesic evaluation: experience with orphenadrine citrate compound. Current Therapeutic Research 7: 639–647

Beaver W T, Feise G 1976 Comparison of the analgesic effect of morphine, hydroxyzine and their combination in patients with postoperative pain. In: Bonica J J, Albe-Fessard D (eds) First International Congress on Pain. Advances in pain research and therapy. Raven Press, New York, p 553–557

Beaver W T, Feise G 1977 Comparison of the analgesic effect of oxymorphone by rectal suppository and intramuscular injection in patients with postoperative pain. Journal of Clinical Pharmacology 17: 276

Beaver W T, Wallenstein S, Houde R W, Rogers A 1966 A comparison of the analgesic effects of methotrimeprazine and morphine in patients with cancer. Clinical Pharmacology and Therapeutics 7: 436–446

Belgrade M J 1989 Control of pain in cancer patients. Postgraduate Medicine 85: 319–323

Blomquist C, Elomaa I, Porkka L, Karonen S L, Lamberg-Allardt C 1988 Evaluation of salmon calcitonin treatment in bone metastases from breast cancer – a controlled trial. Bone 9: 45–51

Boico O, Bonnet F, Rostaing S, Loriferne J F, Quintin L, Ghignone M 1988 Epidural clonidine produces postoperative analgesia. Anesthesiology 69: A388

Bonica J J 1985 Treatment of cancer pain: current status and future needs. In: Fields H L, Dubner R, Cervero F (eds) Advances in pain research and therapy, vol 9. Raven Press, New York, p 589–616

Bonica J J, Buckley F P, Moricca G, Murphey T M 1990a Neurolytic blockade and hypohysectomy. In: Bonica J J (ed) The management of pain, 2nd edn. Lea & Febiger, Philadelphia, vol 2, p 1980–2039

Bonica J J, Ventafridda V, Twycross R G 1990b Cancer pain. In: Bonica J J (ed) The management of pain. 2nd edn. Lea & Febiger, Philadelphia, p 400–460

Bonnet F, Boico O, Rostaing S, Loriferne J F, Quintin L, Ghignone M 1988 Clonidine for postoperative analgesia: epidural vs. IM study. Anesthesiology 69: A395

Boraas M 1985 Palliative surgery. Seminars in Oncology 12: 368–374

Borgelt B B, Gelber R, Brady L W et al 1981 The palliation of hepatic metastases. Results of a Radiation Therapy Oncology Group pilot study. International Journal of Radiation Oncology, Biology, Physics 7: 587–591

Bosch A 1984 Radiotherapy. Clinics in Oncology 3: 47–53

Bradberry J C, Reabel M A 1981 Continuous infusion of naloxone in the treatment of narcotic overdose. Drug Intelligence and Clinical Pharmacy 15: 85–90

Braham J, Saia A 1960 Treatment of diabetic neuropathy with diphenylhydantoin. New York State Journal of Medicine 68: 2633–2655

Breitbart W, Holland J C 1988 Psychiatric complications of cancer. Current Therapeutics in Hematologic Oncology 3: 268–275

Breivik H, Rennemo F 1982 Clinical evaluation of combined treatment with methadone and psychotropic drugs in cancer patients. Acta Anaesthetica Scandinavica 74: 135–140

Brennan M J 1992 Management of lymphedema: review of pathophysiology and treatment. Journal of Pain and Symptom Management 7: 110–116

Brescia F J, Portenoy R K, Ryan M, Krasnoff L, Gray G 1992 Pain, opioid use, and survival in hospitalized patients with advanced cancer. Journal of Clinical Oncology 10: 149–155

Brooks P M, Wood A J J 1991 Nonsteroidal antiinflammatory drugs – differences and similarities. New England Journal Of Medicine 324: 1716–1725

Brose W G, Cousins M J 1991 Subcutaneous lidocaine for treatment of neuropathic cancer pain. Pain 45: 145–148

Brose W G, Tanalian D L, Brodsky J B, Mark J B D, Cousins M J 1991 CSF and blood pharmacokinetics of hydromorphone and morphine following lumbar epidural administration. Pain 45: 11–17

Brown D L, Bulley C K, Quiel E C 1987 Neurolytic celiac plexus blockade for pancreatic cancer pain. Anesthesia and Analgesia 66: 869–873

Bruera E, McDonald N 1986 Intractable pain in patients with advanced head and neck tumors: a possible role of local infection. Cancer Treatment Report 70: 691–692

Bruera E, Miller M J 1989 Non-cardiogenic pulmonary edema after narcotic treatment for cancer pain. Pain 39: 297–300

Bruera E, Roca E, Cedaro L, Carraro S, Chacon R 1985 Action of oral methylprednisolone in terminal cancer patients: a prospective randomized double-blind study. Cancer Treatment Report 69: 751–754

Bruera E, Chadwich S, Brenneis C, Hanson J, MacDonald R N 1987 Methylphenidate associated with narcotics for the treatment of cancer pain. Cancer Treatment Report 71: 67–70

Bruera E, Brenneis C, Michaud M et al 1988a Use of the subcutaneous route for the administration of narcotics in patients with cancer pain. Cancer 62: 407–411

Bruera E, Brenneis C, Michaud M, Macmillan K, Hanson J, MacDonald R N 1988b Patient-controlled subcutaneous hydromorphone versus continuous subcutaneous infusion for the treatment of cancer pain. Journal of the National Cancer Institute 80(14): 1152–1154

Bruera E, Brenneis C, Paterson A H, MacDonald R N 1989a Use of methylphenedate as an adjuvant to narcotic analgesics in patients with advanced cancer. Journal of Pain and Symptom Management 4: 3–6

Bruera E, Macmillan K, Hanson J, MacDonald R N 1989b The cognitive effects of the administration of narcotic analgesics in patients with cancer pain. Pain 39: 13–6

Bruera E, Macmillan K, Selmser P, MacDonald R N 1990 Decreased local toxicity with subcutaneous diamorphine (heroin): a preliminary report. Pain 43: 91–94

Bruera E, Fainsinger R, Moore M, Thibault R, Spoldi E, Ventafridda V 1991 Local toxicity with subcutaneous methadone. Experience of two centers. Pain 45: 141–145

Bullingham R, McQuay H, Porter E, Allen M, Moore R 1982 Sublingual buprenorphine used postoperatively: ten hour plasma drug concentration analysis. British Journal of Clinical Pharmacology 13: 665–673

Burke A L, Diamond P L, Hulbert J, Yeatman J, Farr E A 1991 Terminal restlessness – its management and the role of midazolam. Medical Journal of Australia 155: 485–487

Burney R E, Faulkner D J 1988 Recurrent abdominal abscess caused by retained colorectum after proctocolectomy. Surgery 104: 580–582

Bushnell M C, Marchand S, Tremblay N, Duncan G H 1991 Electrical stimulation of peripheral and central pathways for the relief of musculoskeletal pain. Canadian Journal of Physiology and Pharmacology 69: 697–703

Butch R J, Wittenberg J, Mueller P R, Simeone J F, Meyer J E, Ferrucci J J 1985 Presacral masses after abdominoperineal resection for colorectal carcinoma: the need for needle biopsy. American Journal of Roentgenology 144: 309–12

Caccia M R 1975 Clonazepam in facial neuralgia and cluster headache: clinical and electrophysiological study. European Neurology 13: 560–563

Calis K A, Kohler D R, Corso D M 1992 Transdermally administered fentanyl for pain management. Clinical Pharmacology 11: 22–36

Campora E, Merlini L, Pace M et al 1991 The incidence of narcotic induced emesis. Journal of Pain and Symptom Management 6: 428–430

Campos V M, Solis E L 1980 The analgesic and hypothermic effects of nefopam, morphine, aspirin, diphenhydramine and placebo. Journal of Clinical Pharmacology 20: 42–49

Cantor F K 1972 Phenytoin treatment of thalamic pain. British Medical Journal 2: 590

CAST (Cardiac Arrhythmia Suppression Trial) Investigators 1989 Preliminary report: effect of encainide and flecainide on mortality in a randomized trial of arrhythmia suppression after acute myocardial infarction. New England Journal of Medicine 321: 406–412

Chabal C, Jacobson L, Mariano A, Chaney E, Britell C W 1992 The use of oral mexiletine for the treatment of pain after peripheral nerve injury. Anesthesiology 76: 513–517

Chadda V S, Mathur M S 1978 Double-blind study of the effects of diphenylhydantoin sodium in diabetic neuropathy. Journal of the Association of Physicians of India 26: 403–406

Chan G L, Matzke G R 1987 Effects of renal insufficiency on the pharmacokinetics and pharmacodynamics of opioid analgesics. Drug Intelligence and Clinical Pharmacy 21: 773–783

Chapman C R 1989 Giving the patient control of opioid analgesic administration. In: Hill C S, Fielda W S (eds) Drug treatment of cancer pain in a drug oriented society. Advances in pain research and therapy, vol 11. Raven Press, New York, p 339–351

Chapman C R, Hill H F 1989 Prolonged morphine self-administration and addiction liability. Cancer 63: 1636–1644

Chapman C R, Hill H F, Saeger L, Gavrin J 1990 Profiles of opioid analgesia in humans after intravenous bolus administration: alfentanil, fentanyl and morphine compared on experimental pain. Pain 43: 47–55

Cherny N I, Thaler H T, Friedlander-Klar H, Lapin J, Portenoy R K 1992 Opioid responsiveness of neuropathic cancer pain: combined analysis of single-dose analgesic trials. Proceedings of the American Society of Clinical Oncology 11: abstract 1330

Chrubasik J, Wust H, Schulte M J, Thon K, Zindler M 1988 Relative analgesic potency of epidural fentanyl, alfentanil, and morphine in treatment of postoperative pain. Anesthesiology 68: 929–933

Citron M, Johnston-Early A Boyer M, Brasnow S, Hood M, Cohen M 1986 Patient-controlled analgesia for severe cancer pain. Archives of Internal Medicine 146: 734–736

Clarke N W, Holbrook I B, McClure J, George N J 1991 Osteoclast inhibition by pamidronate in metastatic prostate cancer: a preliminary study. British Journal of Cancer 63: 420–423

Cleeland C S 1989 Pain control: public and physician's attitudes. In: Hill C S, Fields W S (eds) Drug treatment of cancer pain in a drug-oriented society. Advances in pain research and therapy, vol 11. Raven Press, New York, p 81–89

Cleeland C S, Cleeland L M, Dar R, Rinehardt L C 1986 Factors influencing physician management of cancer pain. Cancer 58: 796–800

Coia L R 1992 The role of radiotherapy in the treatment of brain metastases. International Journal Of Radiation Oncology, Biology, Physics 23: 239–244

Coleman R E, Woll P J, Miles M, Scrivener W, Rubens R D 1988 Treatment of bone metastases with (3 amino-1-hydroxyprpylidene)-1, 1-bisphosphonate (APD). British Journal of Cancer 58: 621–625

Cousins M J, Dwyer B, Gibb D 1988 Chronic pain and neurolytic blockade. In: Cousins M J, Bridenbaugh P O (eds) Neural blockade in clinical anesthesia and management of pain, 2nd edn. J B Lippincott, Philadelphia, p 1053–1084

Coyle N 1987 A model of continuity of care for cancer patients with chronic pain. Medical Clinics of North America 71: 259–270

Coyle N, Portenoy R K 1991 Infection as a cause of rapidly increasing pain in cancer patients. Journal of Pain and Symptom Management 6: 266–269

Coyle N, Mauskop A, Maggard J 1986 Continuous subcutaneous infusions of opiates in cancer patients with pain. Oncology Nursing Forum 13: 53–57

Coyle N, Adelhardt J, Foley K M 1988 Disease progression and tolerance in the cancer pain patient. 2nd International Congress on Cancer Pain. Journal of Pain and Symptom Management 3: S25

Coyle N, Adelhardt J, Foley K M, Portenoy R K 1990 Character of terminal illness in the advanced cancer patient: pain and other symptoms during last four weeks of life. Journal of Pain and Symptom Management 5: 83–89

Crotty B, Watson K J R, Desmond P V et al 1989 Hepatic extraction of morphine is impaired in cirrhosis. European Journal of Clinical Pharmacology 36: 501–506

Cruikshank D P Buchsbaum H J 1973 Effects of rapid paracentesis. Cardiovascular dynamics and body fluid composition. JAMA 225: 1361–1365

Culpepper-Morgan J A, Inturrisi C E, Portenoy R K et al 1992 Treatment of opioid induced constipation with oral naloxone: a pilot study. Clinical Pharmacology and Therapeutics 52: 90–95

Davidoff G, Guarracini M, Roth E, Sliwa J, Yarkony G 1987 Trazodone hydrochloride in the treatment of dysesthetic pain in traumatic myelopathy: a randomized, double-blind, placebo-controlled study. Pain 29: 151–161

De Castro M D, Meynadier M D, Zenz M D 1991 Regional opioid analgesia. Developments in critical care medicine and anesthesiology, vol 20. Kluwer Academic Publishers, Dordrecht

Dejgard A, Petersen P Kastrup J 1988 Mexiletine for treatment of chronic painful diabetic neuropathy. Lancet 1: 9–11

Della Cuna G R, et al 1989 Effect of methylprednisolone sodium succinate on quality of life in preterminal cancer patients. A placebo-control multicenter study. European Journal of Clinical Oncology 29: 1817–1821

Devor M, Govrin-Lippman R, Raber P 1985 Corticosteroids reduce neuroma hyperexcitability. In: Fields H L, Dubner R, Cervero F (eds) Proceedings of the Fourth World Congress on Pain. Advances in Pain Research and Therapy, vol 9. Raven Press, New York, p 451–455

Dobrowsky W, Schmidt A P 1985 Radiotherapy for presacral recurrence following radical surgery for rectal carcinoma. Diseases of the Colon and Rectum 28: 917–919

Dover S B 1987 Syringe driver in terminal care. British Medical Journal 294: 553–555

Du Pen S L, Ramsey D H 1988 Compounding local anaesthetics and narcotics for epidural analgesia in cancer outpatients. Anesthesiology 69: A404

Dubner R 1991 Topical capsaicin therapy for neuropathic pain. Pain 47: 247–248

Dunlop R, Davies R J, Hockley J, Turner P 1989 Letter to the Editor. Lancet 1: 420–421

Edwards R B 1989 Pain management and the values of health care providers. In: Hill C S, Fields W S (eds) Drug treatment of cancer pain in a drug-oriented society. Advances in pain research and therapy, vol 11. Raven Press, New York, p 101–112

Edwards W T, Breed R J 1990 Treatment of postoperative pain in the post anesthesia care unit. Anesthesiology Clinics of North America 8: 235–265

Egbert A M, Parks L H, Short L M, Burnett M L 1990 Randomized trial of postoperative patient-controlled analgesia vs intramuscular narcotics in frail elderly men. Archives of Internal Medicine 150: 1897–1903

Eisele J H, Grigsby E J, Dea G 1992 Clonazepam treatment of myoclonic contractions associated with high dose opioids: a case report. Pain 49: 231–232

Eisendrath S J, Goldman B, Douglas J, Dimatteo L, Van D C 1987 Meperidine-induced delirium. American Journal of Psychiatry 144: 1062–1065

Ekbom K 1972 Carbamazepine in the treatment of tabetic lightning pains. Archives of Neurology 26: 374–378

Ellenberg M 1968 Treatment of diabetic neuropathy with diphenylhydantoin. New York State Journal of Medicine 68: 2633–2655

Ernst D S, MacDonald R N, Paterson A H G, Jensen J, Brasher P, Bruera E 1992 A double blind, crossover trial of IV clodronate in metastatic bone pain. Journal of Pain and Symptom Management 7: 4–11

Ettinger A B, Portenoy R K 1988 The use of corticosteroids in the treatment of symptoms associated with cancer. Journal of Pain and Symptom Management 3: 99–103

Fernandez F, Adams F, Holmes V F 1987 Analgesic effect of alprazolam in patients with chronic, organic pain of malignant origin. Journal of Clinical Psychopharmacology 3: 167–169

Ferrell B R, Wisdom C, Wenzl C 1989 Quality of life as an outcome variable in the management of cancer pain. Cancer 11: 2321–2327

Fine P G, Marcus M, DeBoer A J, Van der Oord B 1991 An open label study of oral transmucosal fentanyl citrate (OTFC) for the treatment of breakthrough cancer pain. Pain 45: 149–155

Fishman B 1990 The treatment of suffering in patients with cancer pain: cognitive behavioral approaches. In: Foley K M, Bonica J J, Ventafridda V (eds) Second International Congress on Cancer Pain. Advances in pain research and therapy, vol 16. Raven Press, New York, p 301–316

Foley K M 1985 The treatment of cancer pain. New England Journal of Medicine 313: 84–95

Foley K M 1989a Controversies in cancer pain: medical perspective. Cancer 63: 2257–2265

Foley K M 1989b The decriminalization of cancer pain. In: Hill C S, Field H, (ed) Drug treatment of cancer pain in a drug-oriented society. Advances in pain research and therapy, vol 11. Raven Press, New York, p 5–18

Foley K M 1991 Clinical tolerance to opioids. In: Basbaum A I, Bessom J M (eds) Towards a new pharmacotherapy of pain, Dahlem Konfrenzen. John Wiley, Chichester, p 181–204

Foley K M, Inturrisi C E 1987 Analgesic drug therapy in cancer pain: principles and practice. Medical Clinics of North America 71: 207–232

Fordyce W E 1976 Behavioral methods for chronic pain and illness C V Mosby, St Louis

Forrest W H, Brown B W, Brown C R et al 1977 Dextroamphetamine with morphine for the treatment of postoperative pain. New England Journal of Medicine 296: 712–715

Fromm G H 1989 Trigeminal neuralgia and related disorders. In: Portenoy R K (ed) Pain: mechanisms and syndromes. Neurologic clinics, vol 7. W B Saunders, Philadelphia, p 305–319

Fromm G H, Terrence C F, Chattha A S 1984 Baclofen in the treatment of trigeminal neuralgia: double-blind study and long-term follow-up. Annals of Neurology 15: 240–244

Galer B S, Coyle N, Pasternak G W, Portenoy R K 1992 Individual variability in the response to different opioids: report of five cases. Pain 49: 87–91

Gamble G L, Kinney C L, Brown P S, Maloney F P 1990 Cardiovascular, pulmonary, and cancer rehabilitation. 5. Cancer rehabilitation: management of pain, neurologic and other clinical problems. Archives of Physical Medicine and Rehabilitation 71: S248–S251

Ghostine S Y, Comair Y G, Turner D M, Kassell N F, Azar C G 1984 Phenoxybenzamine in the treatment of causalgia. Journal of Neurosurgery 60: 1263–1268

Giacomini K M, Giacomini J C, Gibson T P, Levy G 1980 Propoxyphene and norpropoxyphene plasma concentrations after oral propoxyphene in cirrhotic patients with and without surgically constructed portacaval shunt. Clinical Pharmacology and Therapeutics 28: 417–424

Gobelet C, Waldburger M, Meier J L 1992 The effect of adding calcitonin to physical treatment on reflex sympathetic dystrophy. Pain 48: 171–5

Gold R H 1978 Treatment of low back pain syndrome with oral orphenadrine citrate. Current Therapeutic Research 23: 271–276

Goldfrank L, Weisman R S, Errick J K, Lo M W 1986 A dosing nomogram for continuous infusion of intravenous naloxone. Annals of Emergency Medicine 15: 91–95

Gourlay G K, Kowalski S R, Plummer J L et al 1990 The efficacy of transdermal fentanyl in the treatment of postoperative pain: a double blind comparison of fentanyl and placebo systems. Pain 40: 21–28

Green J B 1961 Dilantin in the treatment of lightning pains. Neurology 11: 257–258
Greenberg H S, Kim J, Posner J B 1980 Epidural spinal cord compression from metastatic tumor: results with a new treatment protocol. Annals of Neurology 8: 361–366
Greene W R, Davis W H 1991 Titrated intravenous barbiturates in the control of symptoms in patients with terminal cancer. Southern Medical Journal 84: 332–7
Grond S, Zech D, Schug S A, Lynch J, Lehman K A 1991 Validation of the World Health Organization guidelines for cancer pain relief during the last days and hours of life. Journal of Pain and Symptom Management 6: 411–422
Hagen N, Foley K M, Cerbones D J, Portenoy R K, Inturrisi C E 1991 Chronic nausea and morphine-6-glucuronide. Journal of Pain and Symptom Management 6: 125–128
Hallag I Y, Harris J D 1968 The syndrome of postherpetic neuralgia: complications and an approach to therapy. Journal of the American Osteopathic Association 681: 1256–1258
Hanks G W, Trueman T, Twycross R G 1983 Corticosteroids in terminal cancer. Postgraduate Medical Journal 59: 702–706
Hanning C D 1990 The rectal absorption of opioids. In: Benedetti C, Chapman C R, Giron G (eds) Opioid analgesia. Advances in pain research and therapy, vol 14. Raven Press, New York, p 259–269
Hasselstrom J, Eriksson L S, Persson A, Rane A, Svensson J, Sawe J 1990 The metabolism and bioavailability of morphine in patients with severe liver cirrhosic patients. British Journal of Clinical Pharmacology 29: 289–297
Hassenbusch S J, Pillay P K, Barnett G M 1990 Radiofrequency cingulotomy for intractable cancer pain using stereotaxis guided by magnetic resonance imaging. Neurosurgery 27: 220–223
Hatangdi V S, Boas R A, Richards E G 1976 Postherpetic neuralgia: management with antiepileptic and tricyclic drugs. In: Bonica J J, Albe-Fessard D (eds) Advances in pain research and therapy, vol 1. Raven Press, New York, p 583–587
Haynes R C 1990 Adrenocorticotrophic hormone: adrenocortical steroids and their synthetic analogs: inhibitors of the synthesis and actions of adrenocortical hormones. In: Gilman A G, Rall T W, Nies A S, Taylor P (eds) The pharmacological basis of therapeutics, 8th edn. Pergamon Press, New York, p 1431–1462
Hellendoorn S M, Overweg van Kints J 1988 Perineal pain: a case report. European Journal of Surgical Oncology 14: 197–8
Henteleff P D 1991 Symptom prevalence and control during cancer patients' last days of life (letter). Journal of Palliative Care 7: 50–1
Hill C S, Fields W S (eds) 1989 Drug treatment of cancer pain in a drug-oriented society. Advances in pain research and therapy, vol 11. Raven Press, New York
Hill H F, Mackie A M, Coda B A, Iverson K, Chapman C R 1991 Patient-controlled analgesic administration. A comparison of steady-state morphine infusions with bolus doses. Cancer 67: 873–882
Hindley A C, Hill A B, Leyland M J, Wiles A E 1982 A double-blind controlled trial of salmon calcitonin in pain due to malignancy. Cancer Chemotherapy and Pharmacology 9: 71–74
Hirsch J D 1984 Sublingual morphine sulphate in chronic pain management. Clinical Pharmacy 3: 585
Hogan Q, Haddox J D, Abram S, Weissman D, Taylor M L, Janjan N 1991 Epidural opiates and local anesthetics for the management of cancer pain. Pain 46: 271–279
Holley F O, Van-Steennis C 1988 Postoperative analgesia with fentanyl: pharmacokinetics and pharmacodynamics of constant-rate IV and transdermal delivery. Br Journal of Anaesthesia 60: 608–613
Holmes R A 1992 [153Sm]EDTMP: a potential therapy for bone cancer pain. Seminars in Nuclear Medicine 22: 41–45
Horn H R, Hadidian Z, Johnson J L, Vasallo H G, Williams J H, Young M D 1980 Safety evaluation of tocainide in an American emergency use program. American Heart Journal 100: 1037–1040
Houde R W, Wallenstein S L, Beaver W T 1966 Evaluation of analgesics in patients with cancer pain. In: Lasagna L (ed) International encyclopedia of pharmacology and therapeutics, vol 1. Pergamon Press, New York, p 59–67
Hugues A, Chauvergne J, Lissilour T, Lagarde C 1963 L'imipramine utilisée comme antalgique majeur en carcinologie: étude de 118 cas. Presse Medicale 71: 1073–1074
Hupert C, Yacoub M, Turgeon L R 1980 Effect of hydroxyzine on morphine analgesia for the treatment of postoperative pain. Anesthesia and Analgesia 59: 690–696
Ianmore A, Baker A R, Morrell F 1958 Dilantin in the treatment of trigeminal neuralgia. Neurology 8: 126–128
Insel P A 1990 Analgesic-antipyretics and antiinflammatory agents: drugs employed in the treatment of rheumatoid arthritis and gout. In: Gilman A G, Rall T W, Nies A S, Teylor P (eds) The pharmacological basis of therapeutics, 8th edn. Permagon Press, New York, p 638–681
Inturrisi C E 1989 Management of cancer pain. Cancer 63: 2308–2320
Inturrisi C E, Umans J G 1986 Meperidine biotransformation and central nervous system toxicity in animals and humans. In: Foley K M, Inturrisi C E (eds) Opioid analgesics in the management of clinical pain. Advances in pain research and therapy, vol 8. Raven Press, New York, p 143–154
Inturrisi C E, Portenoy R K, Max M B, Colburn W A, Foley K M 1990 Pharmacokinetic-pharmacodynamic (PK-PD) relationships of methadone infusions in patients with cancer pain. Clinical Pharmacology and Therapeutics 47: 565–570
Ischia S, Luzzani A, Ischia A, Magon F, Toscano D 1984 Subarachnoid neurolytic block (L5-S1) and unilateral percutaneous cervical cordotomy in the treatment of pain secondary to pelvic malignant disease. Pain 20: 139–49
Ishijima B, Shimoji K, Shimizu H, Takahashi H, Suzuki I 1988 Lesions of spinal and trigeminal dorsal root entry zone for deafferentation pain. Experience of 35 cases. Applied Neurophysiology 51: 175–187
Jadad A R, Carroll D, Glynn C J, Moore R A, McQuay H J 1992 Morphine responsiveness of chronic pain: double blind randomised crossover study with patient controlled analgesia. Lancet 339: 1367–1371
Jaeger H, Maier C 1992 Calcitonin in phantom limb pain: a double-blind study. Pain 48: 21–27
Jaffe J H 1989 Misinformation: euphoria and addiction. In: Hill C S, Fields W S (eds) Drug treatment of cancer pain in a drug oriented society. Advances in pain research and therapy, vol 11. Raven Press, New York, p 163–174
Jaffe J H, Martin W R 1990 Opioid analgesics and antagonists. In: Gilman AG, Rall T W, Nies A S, Teylor P (eds) The pharmacological basis of therapeutics, 8th edn. Permagon Press, New York, p 485–521
Jessel T M, Dodd J 1989 Functional chemistry of primary afferent neurons. In: Wall P D, Melzack R (eds) Textbook of pain, 2nd edn. Churchill Livingstone, Edinburgh, p 82–99
Johanson G A 1991 Symptom character and prevalence during cancer patients' last days of life. American Journal of Hospital Palliative Care 8: 6–8
Johansson F, Von Knorring L 1979 A double-blind controlled study of a serotonin uptake inhibitor (zimelidine) versus placebo in chronic pain patients. Pain 7: 69–78
Jorgensen L, Mortensen M B, Jensen N H, Eriksen J 1990 Treatment of cancer pain patients in a multidisciplinary pain clinic. Pain Clinic 3: 83–89
Kaiko R F 1980 Age and morphine analgesia in cancer patients with postoperative pain. Clinical Pharmacology and Therapeutics 28: 823–826
Kaiko R F 1990 Controlled-release oral morphine for cancer-related pain: European and North American experiences. In: Foley K M, Bonica J J, Ventafridda (eds) Second International Congress on Cancer Pain. Advances in pain research and therapy, vol 16. Raven Press, New York, p 171–189
Kaiko R F 1991 Clinical protocol and role of controlled release morphine the surgical patient. In: Stanley T H, Ashburn M A, Fine P G (eds) Anesthesiology in pain management. Kluwer Academic, Dordrecht, p 193–212
Kaiko R F, Foley K M, Grabinski P V et al 1983 Central nervous system excitatory effects of meperidine in cancer patients. Annals of Neurology 13: 180–185
Kaiko R F, Cronin C, Healy N, Pav J, Thomas G, Goldenheim P D 1989 Bioavailibility of rectal and oral MS-Contin. Proceedings of the American Society of Clinical Oncology 8: abstract 1307
Kanner R M, Foley K M 1981 Patterns of narcotic drug use in a cancer pain clinic. Annals of the New York Academy of Sciences 362: 161–172

Kerr I G, Sone M, Deangelis C, Iscoe N, MacKenzie R, Schueller T 1988 Continuous narcotic infusion with patient-controlled analgesia for chronic cancer pain in outpatients. Annals of Internal Medicine 108: 554–557

Kim B S, Chung H C 1991 Experience with a controlled-release oral morphine for cancer pain management. Postgraduate Medical Journal 67: 6–10

Lange M P, Dahn M S, Jacobs L A 1988 Patient-controlled analgesia versus intermittent analgesia dosing. Heart and Lung 17: 495–498

Lasagna L, DeKornfeld T J 1961 Methotrimeprazine, a new phenothiazine derivative with analgesic properties. Journal of the American Medical Association 178: 887–890

Latimer E J 1991 Ethical decision-making in the care of the dying and its applications to clinical practice. Journal of Pain and Symptom Management 6: 329–336

Lechin F, van der Dijs B, Lechin M E et al 1989 Pimozide therapy for trigeminal neuralgia. Archives of Neurology 9: 960–962

Levin A B, Ramirez L L 1984 Treatment of cancer pain with hypophysectomy: surgical and chemical. In: Benedetti C, Chapman C R, Moricca G (eds) Recent advances in the management of pain. Advances in pain research and therapy, vol 7. Raven Press, New York, p 631–645

Lifshitz S, Buchsbaum H J 1976 The effect of paracentesis on serum proteins. Gynecological Oncology 4: 347–351

Lindstrom P, Lindblom U 1987 The analgesic effect of tocainide in trigeminal neuralgia. Pain 28: 45–50

Linton S L, Melin L 1983 Applied relaxation in the management of cancer pain. Behavioral Psychotherapy 11: 337–350

Llyod-Smith D L, Sachdev K K 1969 A long-term, low dosage study of carbamazepine in trigeminal neuralgia. Headache 9: 64–72

Lobato R D, Madrid J L, Fatela L V, Sarabia R, Rivas J J, Gozalo A 1987 Intraventicular morphine for intractable cancer pain: rationale, methods, clinical results. Acta Anaesthesiologica Scandinavica (suppl 31): 68–74

Lockman L A, Hunninghake D B, Drivit W, Desnick R J 1973 Relief of pain of Fabry's disease by diphenylhydantoin. Neurology 23: 871–875

Long D M 1991 Fifteen years of transcutaneous electrical stimulation for pain control. Stereotactic and Functional Neurosurgery 56: 2–19

Lutfy K, Yoburn B C 1991 The role of opioid receptor density in morphine tolerance. Journal of Pharmacology and Experimental Therapeutics 256: 575–80

McColl J D, Durkin W 1982 The effect of pyrilamine on relief of symtoms of the premenstrual syndrome (PMS) and primary dysmenorrhea. Federation Proceedings 41: 5572

MacDonald N 1990 The role of medical and surgical oncology in the management of cancer pain. In: Foley K M, Bonica J J, Ventafridda V (eds) Second International Congress on Cancer Pain. Advances in pain research and therapy, vol 16. Raven Press, New York, p 27–39

McQuay H J, Carroll D, Faura C C, Gavaghan D J, Hand C W, Moore R A 1990 Oral morphine in cancer pain: influences on morphine and metabolite concentration. Clinical Pharmacology and Therapeutics 48: 236–244

McQuay H J, Jadad A R, Carnoll D et al 1992 Opioid sensitivity of chronic pain: a patient controlled analgesia method. Anaesthesia 47: 757–767

Magni G, Arsie D, DeLeo D 1987 Antidepressants in the treatment of cancer pain. A survey in Italy. Pain 29: 347–353

Malmberg A B, Yaksh T L 1992 Hyperalagesia mediated by spinal glutamate and substance P receptors blocked by spinal cyclooxygenase inhibition. Science 92: 1276–1279

Martin G 1981 The management of pain following laminectomy for lumbar disc lesions. Annals of the Royal College of Surgeons of England 63: 244–252

Martin R S 1989 Mortal values: healing, pain and suffering. In: Hill C S, Fields W S (eds) Drug treatment of cancer pain in a drug-oriented society. Advances in pain research and therapy, vol 11. Raven Press, New York, p 19–26

Max M B, Inturrisi C E, Kaiko R F, Grabinski P Y, Li C H, Foley K M 1985 Epidural and intrathecal opiates: cerebrospinal fluid and plasma profiles in patients with chronic cancer pain. Clinical Pharmacology and Therapeutics 38: 631–641

Max M B, Schafer S C, Culnane M, Dubner R, Gracely R H 1988 Association of pain relief with drug side effects in postherpetic neuralgia: a single dose study of clonidine, codeine, ibuprofen and placebo. Clinical Pharmacology and Therapeutics 43: 363–371

Max M B, Lynch S A, Muir J, Shoaf S E, Smoller B, Dubner R 1992 Effects of desipramine, amitriptyline, and fluoxetine on pain in diabetic neuropathy. New England Journal of Medicine 326: 1250–1256

Maxon H R, Deutsch E A, Thomas S R et al 1988 Initial experience with 186-Re(Sn)-HEDP in the treatment of painful skeletal metastases. Journal of Nuclear Medicine 29: 776

Maxon H, Thomas S R, Hertzberg V S et al 1992 Rhenium-186 hydroxyethylidene diphosphonate for the treatment of painful osseous metastases. Seminars in Nuclear Medicine 22: 33–40

Messer J, Reitman D, Sacks H S, Smith H, Chalmers T 1983 Association of adrenocorticorticosteroid therapy and peptic ulcer disease. New England Journal of Medicine 309: 21–24

Miller R, Eisenkraft J B, Cohen M, Toth C, Mora C T, Bernstein J L 1986 Midazolam as an adjunct to meperidine analgesia for postoperative pain. Clinical Journal of Pain 2; 37–43

Minsky B D, Leibel S 1989 The treatment of hepatic metastases from colorectal cancer with radiation therapy alone or combined with cemotherapy or misonidazole. Cancer Treatment Reviews 16: 213–219

Miser A W, Narang P K, Dothage J A, Young R C, Sindelar W, Miser J S 1989 Transdermal fentanyl for pain control in patients with cancer. Pain 37: 15–21

Mladinich E K 1974 Diphenylhydantoin in the Wallenberg syndrome. Journal of the American Medical Association 230: 372–373

Moertel C G, Shutte A, Reitemeier R et al 1974 Corticosteroid therapy of preterminal gastrointestinal cancer. Cancer 33: 1607–1609

Mok M S, Wang J J, Chan J H, Liu S E, Lippmann M 1988 Analgesic effect of epidural clonidine and nalbuphine in combined use. Anesthesiology 69: A398

Montesani C, Ribotta G, De M R et al 1991 Extended resection in the treatment of colorectal cancer. International Journal of Colorectal Disease 6: 161–164

Montilla E, Frederick W S, Cass L J 1963 Analgesic effects of methotrimeprazine and morphine. Archives of Internal Medicine 111: 725–728

Morgan J P 1989 American opiophobia: customary underutilization of opioid analgesics. In: Hill C S, Fields W S (eds) Drug treatment of cancer pain in a drug-oriented society, vol 11. Raven Press, New York, p 181–189

Morton A R, Cantrill J A, Pillai G V, McMahon A, Anderson D C, Howell A 1988 Sclerosis of lytic bony metastases after aminohydroxypropylidene bisphosphonate (APD) in patients with breast cancer. British Medical Journal 297: 772–773

Moulin D E, Inturrisi C E, Foley K M 1986 Epidural and intrathecal opioids: cerebrospinal fluid and plasma pharmacokinetics in cancer pain patients. In: Foley K M, Inturrisi C E (eds) Opioid analgesics in the management of clinical pain. Advances in pain research and therapy, vol 8. Raven Press, New York, p 369–384

Moulin D E, Kreeft J H, Murray P N, Bouquillon A I 1991 Comparison of continuous subcutaneous and intravenous hydromorphone infusions for management of cancer pain. Lancet 337: 465–468

Moulin D E, Johnson N G, Murray P N, Geoghegan M F, Goodwin V A, Chester M A 1992 Subcutaneous narcotic infusions for cancer pain: treatment outcome and guidelines for use. Canadian Medical Association Journal 146: 891–7

Musto D F 1989 Physicians' attitudes towards narcotics. In: Hill C S, Fields W S (eds) Drug treatment of cancer pain in a drug oriented society. Advances in pain research and therapy, vol 11. Raven Press, New York, p 51–60

Neal E A, Meffin P J, Gregory P B, Blaschke T F 1979 Enhanced bioavailability and decreased clearance of analgesics in patients with cirrhosis. Gastroenterology 77: 96–102

Nielsen O S, Munro A J, Tannock I F 1991 Bone metastases: pathophysiology and management policy. Journal of Clinical Oncology 9: 509–524

Nitescu P, Appelgren L, Linder L E et al 1990 Epidural versus intrathecal morphine-bupivacaine: assessment of consecutive treatment in advanced cancer pain. Journal of Pain and Symptom Management 5: 18–26

Obbens E A M T, Hill C S, Leavens M E, Ruthenbeck S S, Otis F 1987 Intraventricular morphine administration for control of chronic cancer pain. Pain 28: 61–68

Oliver D J 1988 Syringe drivers in palliative care: a review. Palliative Medicine 2: 21–26

Osborne R J, Joel S P, Slevin M L 1986 Morphine intoxication in renal failure: the role of morphine-6-glucuronide. British Medical Journal 292: 1548–1549

Panerai A E, Bianchi M, Sacerdote P, Ripamonti C, Ventafridda V, De Conno F 1991 Antidepressants in cancer pain. Journal of Palliative Care 7: 42–44

Patt Y Z, Peters R E, Chuang V P, Wallace S, Claghorn L, Mavligit G 1985 Palliation of pelvic recurrence of colorectal cancer with intra-arterial 5-fluorouracil and mitomycin. Cancer 56: 2175–2180

Patwardhan R, Johnson R F, Hoyumpa A et al 1981 Normal metabolism of morphine in cirrhosis. Gastroenterology 77: 96–102

Payne R, Inturrisi C E 1985 CSF distribution of morphine, methadone and sucrose after intrathecal injection. Life Sciences 37: 1137–1144

Peiris J B, Perera G L S, Davendra S V, Lionel N D W 1980 Sodium valproate in trigeminal neuralgia. Medical Journal of Australia 2: 278

Petrelli N J, Velez A, Herrera L, Walsh D, Mittelman A 1985 Ileal conduits for recurrent unresectable colorectal adenocarcinoma. American Journal of Surgery 150: 239–242

Piletta P, Porchet H C, Dayer P 1991 Central analgesic effect of acetaminophen but not of aspirin. Clinical Pharmacology and Therapeutics 49: 350–354

Polatty R C, Cooper K R 1986 Respiratory failure after percutaneous cordotomy. Southern Medical Journal 79: 367–379

Popiela T, Lucchi R, Giongo F 1989 Methylprednisolone as palliative therapy for female terminal cancer patients. The Methylprednisolone Female Preterminal Cancer Study Group. European Journal of Cancer and Clinical Oncology 25: 1823–1829

Portenoy R K 1987 Continuous intravenous infusions of opioid drugs. Medical Clinics of North America 71: 233–241

Portenoy R K 1993 Adjuvant analgesics. In: Doyle D, Hanks G W, MacDonald N (eds) Oxford textbook of palliative medicine. Oxford University Press, Oxford, p 187–203

Portenoy R K, Hagen N A 1990 Breakthrough pain: definition, prevalence and characteristics. Pain 41: 273–281

Portenoy R K, Foley K M, Inturrisi C E 1990 The nature of opioid responsiveness and its implications for neuropathic pain: new hypotheses derived from studies of opioid infusions. Pain 43: 273–286

Portenoy R K, Foley K M, Stulman J et al 1991 Plasma morphine and morphine-6-glucuronide during chronic morphine therapy for cancer pain: plasma profiles, steady state concentrations and the consequences of renal failure. Pain 47: 13–19

Portenoy R K, Southam M, Gupta S K et al 1993 Transdermal fentanyl for cancer pain repeated dose pharmacokinetics. Anesthesiology 28: 36–43

Porter J, Jick H 1980 Addiction rate in patients treated with narcotics (letter). New England Journal of Medicine 302: 123

Prassad B, Lee M, Hendrickson F R 1977 Irradiation of hepatic metastases. International Journal of Radiation Oncology, Biology, Physics 2: 129–132

Prough D S, McLeskey C H, Poehling G G, et al 1985 Efficacy of oral nifedipine in the treatment of reflex sympathetic dystrophy. Anesthesiology 62: 796–799

Raftery H 1979 The management of postherpetic pain using sodium valproate and amitriptyline. Journal of the Irish Medical Association 72: 399–401

Raskin N H, Levinson S A, Hoffman P M, Pickett J B E, Fields H L 1974 Postsympathectomy neuralgia: amelioration with diphenylhydantoin and carbamazepine. American Journal of Surgery 128: 75–78

Reidenberg M M, Goodman H, Erle H et al 1988 Hydromorphone levels and pain control in patients with severe chronic pain. Clinical Pharmacology and Therapeutics 44: 376–382

Robertson D H 1983 Transsacral neurolytic nerve block. An alternative approach to intractable perineal pain. British Journal of Anaesthesia 55: 873–875

Robinson R G, Preston D F, Spicer J A, Baxter K G 1992 Radionuclide therapy of intractable bone pain: emphasis on strontium-89. Seminars in Nuclear Medicine 22: 28–32

Rockliff B W, Davis E H 1966 Controlled sequential trials of carbamazepine in trigeminal neuralgia. Archives of Neurology 15: 129–136

Rogers M, Cerda J J 1989 The narcotic bowel syndrome. Journal of Clinical Gastroenterology 11: 132–135

Rosomoff H L, Carroll F, Brown J 1965 Percutaneous radiofrequency cervical cordotomy: technique. Journal of Neurosurgery 23: 639–644

Ross G J, Kessler H B, Clair M R, Gatenby R A, Hartz W H, Ross L V 1989 Sonographically guided paracentesis for palliation of symptomatic malignant ascites. American Journal of Roentgenology 153: 1309–1311

Sandouk P, Serrie A, Urtizberea M, Debray M, Got P, Scherrmann M J 1991 Morphine pharmacokinetics and pain assessment after intracerebroventricular administration in patients with terminal cancer. Clinical Pharmacology and Therapeutics 49: 422–448

Sawe J, Dahlstrom B, Paazlow L, Rane A 1981 Morphine kinetics in cancer patients. Clinical Pharmacology and Therapeutics 30: 629–634

Sawe J, Svensson J O, Odar-Cederlof I 1985 Kinetics of morphine in patients with renal failure (letter). Lancet 2: 211

Scadding J W 1982 Clinical trial of propranolol in post-traumatic neuralgia. Pain 14: 283–292

Schauer P K, Wettermann T L, Schauer A R 1988 Physicians' attitudes and knowledge about the management of cancer-related pain. Connecticut Medicine 52: 705–7

Scheffler N M, Sheitel P L, Lipton M N 1991 Treatment of painful diabetic neuropathy with capsaicin 0.075%. Journal of the American Podiatric Medical Association 81; 288–293

Schug S A, Zech D, Dorr U 1990 Cancer pain management according to WHO analgesic guidelines. Journal of Pain and Symptom Management 5: 27–32

Schuster C R 1989 Does treatment of cancer pain with narcotics produce junkies? In: Hill C S, Fields W S (ed) Drug treatment of cancer pain in a drug oriented society. Advances in pain research and therapy, vol 11. Raven Press, New York, p 1–3

Seeff L B, Cuccherini B A, Zimmerman H I, Adler E, Benjamin S 1986 Acetaminophen hepatotoxicity in alcoholics. Annals of Internal Medicine 104: 399–404

Shafar J, Tallett E R, Knowlson P A 1972 Evaluation of clonidine in prophylaxis of migraine. Lancet 1: 403–407

Shegda L M, McCorkle R 1990 Continuing care in the community. Journal of Pain and Symptom Management 5: 279–286

Shepherd K 1990 Review of a controlled-release morphine preparation. In: Foley K M, Bonica J J, Ventafridda V (eds) Second International Congress on Cancer Pain. Advances in pain research and therapy, vol 16. Raven Press, New York, p 191–202

Sherman D M, Weichselbaum R, Order S E et al 1978 Palliation of hepatic metastases. Cancer 41: 2013–2017

Silberstein E B, Williams C 1985 Strontium-89 therapy for the pain of osseous metastases. Journal of Nuclear Medicine 26: 345–348

Silberstein E B, Elgazzar A H, Kapilivsky A 1992 Phosphorus-32 radiopharmaceuticals for the treatment of painful osseous metastases. Seminars in Nuclear Medicine 22: 17–27

Simson G 1974 Propranolol for causalgia and Sudek's atrophy. Journal of the American Medical Association 227: 327

Sindrup S H, Gram L F, Brosen K, Eshoj O, Mogensen E F 1990 The selective serotonin reuptake inhibitor paroxetine is effective in the treatment of diabetic neuropathy symptoms. Pain 42: 135–144

Singh P N, Sharma P, Gupta P K, Pandey K 1981 Clinical evaluation of diazepam for relief of postoperative pain. British Journal of Anaesthesia 53: 831–836

Sjoberg M, Appelgren L, Einarsson S et al 1991 Long-term intrathecal morphine and bupivacaine in 'refractory' cancer pain. Results from the first series of 52 patients. Acta Anaesthesiologica Scandinavica 35: 30–43

Smith J A 1989 Palliation of painful bone metastases from prostate cancer using sodium etidronate: results of a randomized, prospective, double-blind, placebo-controlled study. Journal of Urology 141: 85–87

Stambaugh J E, Lance C 1983 Analgesic efficacy and pharmacokinetic evaluation of meperidine and hydroxyzine, alone and in combination. Cancer Investigation 1: 111–117

Stanley T H, Hague B, Mock D L et al 1989 Oral transmucosal fentanyl citrate (lollipop) premedications in human volunteers. Anesthesia and Analgesia 69: 21–27

Stjernsward J, Teoh N 1990 The scope of the cancer pain problem. In: Foley K M, Bonica J J, Ventafridda V (eds) Second International Congress on Cancer Pain. Advances in pain research and therapy, vol 16. Raven Press, New York, p 7–12

Storey P, Hill H H, St Louis R, Tarver E E 1990 Subcutaneous infusions for control of cancer symptoms. Journal of Pain and Symptom Management 5: 33–41

Stott J R R, Barnes G R, Wright R J, Ruddock C J S 1989 The effect on motion sickness and occulomotor function of GR38032F: a 5-HT3 receptor antagonist with anti-emetic properties. Journal of Clinical Pharmacology 27: 147–157

Sundaresan N, DiGiacinto G V 1987 Antitumor and antinociceptive approaches to control cancer pain. Medical Clinics of North America 71: 329–348

Sunshine A, Zighelboim I, De Castro A et al 1989 Augmentation of acetaminophen analgesia by the antihistamine phenyltoloxamine. Journal of Clinical Pharmacology 29: 660–664

Swanson G, Smith J, Bulich R, New P, Shiffman R 1989 Patient-controlled analgesia for chronic cancer pain in the ambulatory setting: a report of 117 patients. Journal of Clinical Oncology 7: 1903–1908

Swerdlow M 1984 Anticonvulsant drugs and chronic pain. Clinical Neuropharmacology 7: 51–82

Swerdlow M, Cundill J G 1981 Anticonvulsant drugs used in the treatment of lancinating pains. A comparison. Anesthesia 36: 1129–1132

Sykes N P 1991 Oral naloxone in opioid associated constipation. Lancet 337: 1475

Szeto H H, Inturrisi C E, Houde R et al 1977 Accumulation of normeperidine an active metabolite of meperidine, in patients with renal failure or cancer. Annals of Internal Medicine 85: 738–741

Takagi H, Morimoto T, Yasue M, Kato K, Yamada E, Suzuki R 1985 Total pelvic exenteration for advanced carcinoma of the lower colon. Journal of Surgical Oncology 28: 59–62

Takeda F 1986 Results of field-testing in Japan of WHO draft interim guidelines on relief of cancer pain. The Pain Clinic 1: 83–89

Tan Y-M, Croese J 1986 Clonidine and diabetic patients with leg pains. Annals of Internal Medicine 105: 633

Tandan R, Lewis G A, Krusinski P B, Badger G B, Fries T J 1992 Topical capsaicin in painful diabetic neuropathy. Controlled study with long-term follow-up. Diabetes Care 15: 8–14

Tannock I, Gospodarowicz M, Meakin W, Panzarella T, Stewart L, Rider W 1989 Treatment of metastatic prostatic cancer with low-dose prednisone: evaluation of pain and quality of life as pragmatic indices of response. Journal of Clinical Oncology 7: 590–597

Tasker R R, Tsuda T, Howrylyshn P 1988 Percutaneous cordotomy – the lateral high cervical technique. In: Schmidek H H, Sweet W H (eds) Operative neurosurgical technique indications, methods and results. Grune & Stratton, New York, p 1191–1205

Taylor J C, Brauer S, Espir M L E 1980 Long-term treatment of trigeminal neuralgia with carbamazepine. Postgraduate Medical Journal 57: 16–18

Taylor P H, Gray K, Bicknell R G, Rees J R 1977 Glossopharyngeal neuralgia with syncope. Journal of Laryngology and Otology 91: 859–868

Temple W J, Ketcham A S 1992 Sacral resection for control of pelvic tumours. American Journal of Surgery 163: 370–374

The Capsaicin Study Group 1991 Treatment of painful diabetic neuropathy with topical capsaicin. A multicenter, double-blind, vehicle-controlled study. Archives of Internal Medicine 151: 2225–2229

Thiebaud D, Leyvraz S, von Fliedner V et al 1991 Treatment of bone metastases from breast cancer and myeloma with pamidronate. European Journal of Cancer 27: 37–41

Tomson T, Bertilsson L 1984 Potent therapeutic effects of carbamazepine 10, 11-epoxide in trigeminal neuralgia. Archives of Neurology 41: 598–601

Turk D, Meichenbaum D, Genest M 1983 Pain and behavioral medicine. Guilford Press, New York

Turner J H, Claringbold B G 1991 A phase II study of treatment of painful multifocal skeletal metastases with single and repeated dose samarium-153 ethylenediaminetetramethylene phosphonate. European Journal of Cancer 27(9): 1084–1086

Turner J H, Claringbold B G, Heatherington E L, Sorby P, Martindal A A 1989 A phase 1 study of samarium-153 ethylenediaminetetramethylene phosphonate therapy for disseminated skeletal metastases. Journal of Clinical Oncology 7: 1926–1931

Twycross R G, Lack S A 1984 Symptom control in far-advanced cancer: pain relief. Pitman, London

Umans J G, Inturrisi C E 1982 Antinociceptive activity and toxicity of meperidine and normeperidine in mice. Journal of Pharmacology and Experimental Therapeutics 223: 203–206

Urquhart M L, Klapp K, White P F 1988 Patient-controlled analgesia: a comparison of intravenous versus subcutaneous hydromorphone. Anesthesiology 69: 428–32

Vane J R 1971 Inhibition of prostaglandin synthesis as a mechanism of action for aspirin-like drugs. Nature: New Biology 234: 231–238

Van Holten-Verzantvoort A T M, Zwinderman A H, Aaronson N K et al 1991 The effect of supportive pamidronate treatment on aspects of quality of life of patients with advanced breast cancer. European Journal of Cancer 27: 544–549

Varvel J R, Shafer S L, Hwang S S, Coen P A, Stanski D R 1989 Absorption characteristics of transdermally administered fentanyl. Anesthesiology 70: 928–934

Ventafridda V 1989 Continuing care: a major issue in cancer pain management. Pain 36: 137–143

Ventafridda V, Ripamonti C, DeConno F, Bianchi M, Pazzuconi F, Panerai A E 1987a Antidepressants for cancer pain and other painful syndromes with deafferentation component: comparison of amitriptyline and trazodone. Italian Journal of Neurological Science 8: 579–587

Ventafridda V, Tamburini M, Caraceni A, DeConno F, Naldi F 1987b A validation study of the WHO method for cancer pain relief. Cancer 59: 851–856

Ventafridda V, Ripamonti C, De Conno F, Tamburini M, Cassileth B R 1990 Symptom prevalence and control during cancer patients' last days of life. Journal of Palliative Care 6: 7–11

Von Roenn J H, Cleeland C S, Gonin R, Hatfield A, Pandya K J 1993 Physicians' attitudes and practice in cancer pain management. A survey from the Eastern Cooperative Oncology Group. Annals of Internal Medicine 119: 121–126

Walker V A, Hoskin P J, Hanks G W et al 1988 Evaluation of WHO analgesic guidelines for cancer pain in a hospital-based palliative care unit. Journal of Pain and Symptom Management 3: 145–150

Walsh T D 1983 Antidepressants in chronic pain. Clinical Neuropharmacology 6: 271–295

Walsh T D 1986 Controlled study of imipramine and morphine in chronic pain due to cancer (abstract). In: American Society of Clinical Oncology, vol 5, p 237

Walsh T D 1990a Adjuvant analgesic therapy in cancer pain. In: Foley K M, Bonica J J, Ventafridda V (eds) The Second International Conference on Cancer Pain. Advances in pain research and therapy, vol 16. New York, New York, p 155–168

Walsh T D 1990b Prevention of opioid side effects. Journal of Pain and Symptom Management 5: 363–367

Walsh T D, MacDonald N, Bruera E, Shepard K V, Michaud M, Zanes R 1992 A controlled study of sustained-release morphine sulfate tablets in chronic pain from advanced cancer. American Journal of Clinical Oncology 15: 268–272

Wanzer S H, Federman D D, Adelstein S J et al 1989 The physician's responsibility toward hopelessly ill patients–a second look. New England Journal of Medicine 120: 844–849

Warfield C A 1991 Guidelines for the use of MS Contin tablets in the management of cancer pain. Postgraduate Medical Journal 67 (suppl 2): 9–13

Watson C P N, Evans R J 1985 A comparative trial of amitriptyline and zimelidine in postherpetic neuralgia. Pain 23: 387–394

Watson C P N, Evans R J, Watt V R 1988 Postherpetic neuralgia and topical capsaicin. Pain 33: 333–340

Watson C P N, Evans R J, Watt V R 1989 The post-mastectomy pain syndrome and the effect of topical capsaicin. Pain 38: 177–186

Watson C P, Chipman M, Reed K, Evans R J, Birkett N 1992 Amitriptyline versus maprotiline in postherpetic neuralgia: a randomized, double-blind, crossover trial. Pain 48: 29–36
Weinberg D S, Inturrisi C E, Reidenberg B et al 1988 Sublingual absorption of selected opioid analgesics. Clinical Pharmacology and Therapeutics 44: 335–342
Weissman D E, Haddox J D 1989 Opioid pseudoaddiction – an iatrogenic syndrome. Pain 36: 363–366
Wilcox J C, Corr J, Shaw J, Richardson M, Calman K C 1984 Prednisolone as appetite stimulant in patients with cancer. British Medical Journal 288: 27
Willer J C, DeBrouckert T, Bussel B et al 1989 Central analgesic effect of ketoprofen in humans: electrophysiologic evidence for a supraspinal mechanism in a double-blind and cross-over study. Pain 38: 1–8
Williams L J, Huddleston C B, Sawyers J L, Potts J, Sharp K W, McDougal S W 1988 Is total pelvic exenteration reasonable primary treatment for rectal carcinoma? Annals of Surgery 207: 670–678
Williams M R 1984 The place of surgery in terminal care. In: Saunders C (ed) The management of terminal disease. Edward Arnold, London, p 148–153
World Health Organization 1986 Cancer pain relief. World Health Organization, Geneva
World Health Organization 1990 Cancer pain relief and palliative care. World Health Organization, Geneva
Yamada K, Ushio Y, Hayakawa T, Arita N, Yamada N, Mogami H 1983 Effects of methylprednisolone on peritumoral brain edema. A quantitative autoradiographic study. Journal of Neurosurgery 59: 612–619

Index